FOR INSTRUCTORS

INSTRUCTOR'S ELECTRONIC RESOURCE

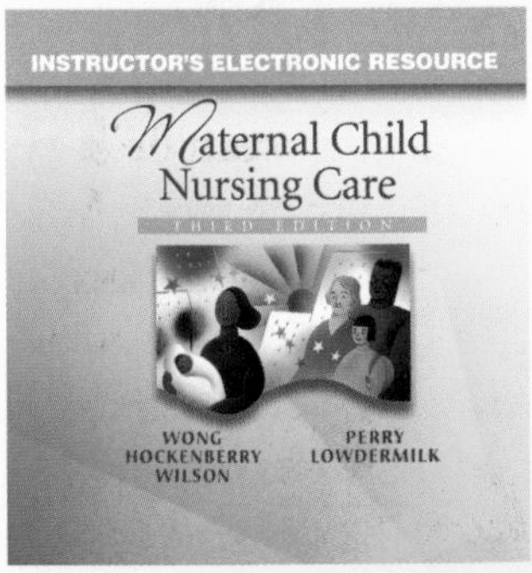

0-323-03702-X

Available in CD and online formats, this helpful instructor's package provides all of the tools needed to quickly and consistently develop lectures and student assignments and evaluate student comprehension. The *Instructor's Manual* includes chapter outlines and teaching strategies, activities for students, case studies, curriculum guides for courses of various lengths, and open-book quizzes. The ExamView *Test Bank* contains questions in NCLEX® format, including new alternate format questions, and an answer key with page references to the text, rationales, and NCLEX® coding. Also included are a full-color *Image Collection* and *PowerPoint Lecture Slides* for building presentations and developing lectures.

EVOLVE COURSE MANAGEMENT SYSTEM

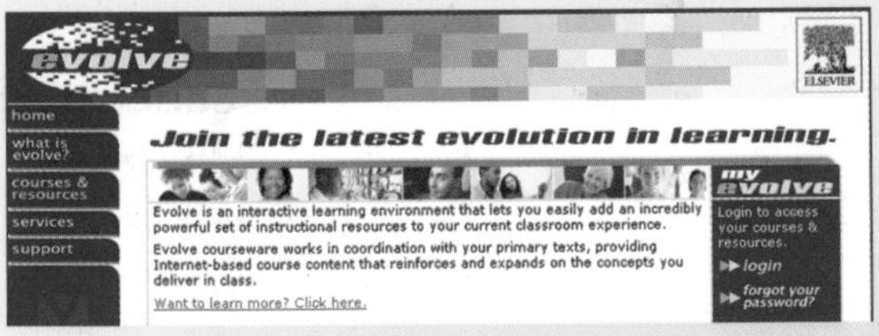

http://evolve.elsevier.com/Wong/maternal/

Evolve is an interactive teaching and learning environment that works in coordination with *Maternal Child Nursing Care, Third Edition,* providing Internet-based course content that reinforces and expands on the concepts that instructors deliver in class. In addition to the resources available to students, instructors are able to access all of the components of the *Instructor's Electronic Resource,* including the computerized test bank and PowerPoint slides. Instructors can also use Evolve to do the following: publish class syllabi, outline, and lecture notes; set up "virtual office hours" and e-mail communication; share important dates and information through the online class *Calendar;* and encourage student participation through *Chat Rooms* and *Discussion Boards.* Instructors are encouraged to contact their sales representative for more information about integrating Evolve into their curriculum.

Contents

Companion CD

DONNA L. WONG,
PhD, RN, PNP, CPN, FAAN
Nursing Consultant,
The Children's Hospital at Saint Francis;
Adjunct Associate Professor, Department of Pediatrics
University of Oklahoma College of Medicine – Tulsa;
Adjunct Professor
University of Oklahoma College of Nursing;
Adjunct Professor and Consultant
Oral Roberts University Anna Vaughn School of Nursing
Tulsa, Oklahoma

SHANNON E. PERY,
RN, CNS, PhD, FAAN
Instructional Faculty, Summer Session
Professor Emerita, School of Nursing
San Francisco State University
San Francisco, California;
Nurse Consultant
International Education Research Foundation
Culver City, California

MARILYN J. HOCKENBERRY,
PhD, RN-CS, PNP, FAAN
Director, Center for Research and Evidence-Based Practice
Nurse Scientist, Texas Children's Hospital;
Director of Nurse Practitioners
Texas Children's Cancer Center;
Professor, Department of Pediatrics
Baylor College of Medicine
Houston, Texas

DEITRA LEONARD LOWDERMILK,
RNC, PhD, FAAN
Clinical Professor, School of Nursing
Nursing Education and Curriculum Consultant
University of North Carolina at Chapel Hill
Chapel Hill, North Carolina

DAVID WILSON,
MS, RNC
Adjunct Faculty
Langston University School of Nursing;
Adjunct Faculty
Southern Nazarene University;
Staff Nurse
Children's Hospital Urgent Care Center
Saint Francis Hospital
Tulsa, Oklahoma

Maternal Child Nursing Care

THIRD EDITION

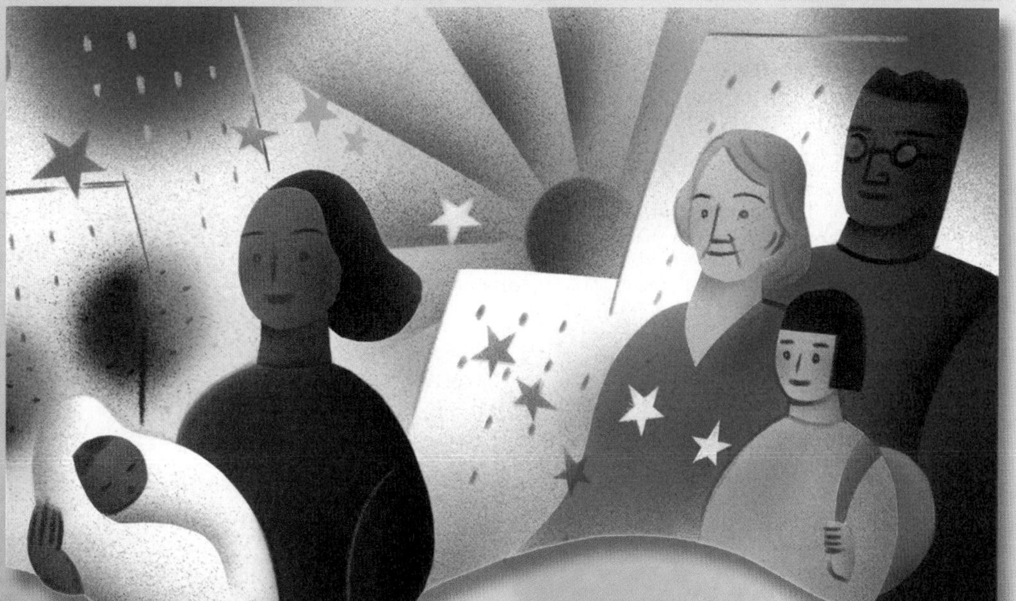

MOSBY
ELSEVIER

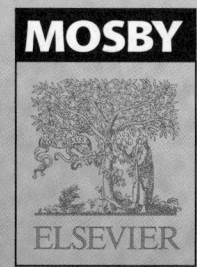

MOSBY
ELSEVIER

11830 Westline Industrial Drive
St. Louis, Missouri 63146

MATERNAL CHILD NURSING CARE, THIRD EDITION
ISBN-13: 978–0–323–02865–3
ISBN-10: 0–323–02865–9

Notice

Knowledge and best practice in this field are constantly changing. As new research and experience broaden our knowledge, changes in practice, treatment and drug therapy may become necessary or appropriate. Readers are advised to check the most current information provided (i) on procedures featured or (ii) by the manufacturer of each product to be administered, to verify the recommended dose or formula, the method and duration of administration, and contraindications. It is the responsibility of the practitioner, relying on their own experience and knowledge of the patient, to make diagnoses, to determine dosages and the best treatment for each individual patient, and to take all appropriate safety precautions. To the fullest extent of the law, neither the Publisher nor the Authors assume any liability for any injury and/or damage to persons or property arising out of or related to any use of the material contained in this book.

Library of Congress Cataloging-in-Publication Data

Maternal child nursing care / Shannon E. Perry ... [et al.]. —3re ed.
p. ; cm.
Rev. ed. of: Maternal child nursing care / Donna L. Wong. 2nd ed. 2002.
Includes bibliographical references and index.
ISBN-13: 978–0–323–02865–3 ISBN-10: 0–323–02865–9
1. Maternity nursing. 2. Pediatric nursing. I. Perry, Shannon E. II. Wong, Donna L., 1948-. Maternal child nursing care.
[DNLM: 1. Maternal-Child Nursing—methods. 2. Pediatric Nursing—methods. WY 157.3 M4254 2006]
RG951.W87 2006
618.92′00231—dc22

2005051380

Acquisitions Editor: Catherine Jackson
Managing Editor: Michele D. Hayden
Senior Developmental Editor: Laurie K. Gower
Publishing Services Manager: Jeff Patterson
Senior Project Manager: Anne Konopka
Design Manager: Julia Dummitt

ISBN-13: 978–0–323–02865–3
ISBN-10: 0–323–02865–9

Printed in China

Last digit is the print number: 9 8 7 6 5 4 3

Contributing Editor

PATRICK F. BARRERA, BS
Assistant Director
Center for Research and Evidence-Based Practice
Texas Children's Hospital
Houston, Texas

Reviewers

DEBBIE FRASER ASKIN, MN, RNC
Assistant Professor, Faculty of Nursing
University of Manitoba;
Neonatal Nurse Practitioner
St. Boniface General Hospital
Winnipeg, Manitoba, Canada

LOUISE AURILIO, PhD, RNC, CNA
Assistant Professor, Nursing Department
Youngstown State University
Youngstown, Ohio

JOHNETT BENSON-SOROS, RN, MSN, CNP
Assistant Professor, College of Nursing
Kent State University—Ashtabula
Ashtabula, Ohio

PATRICIA COYLE-ROGERS, PhD, MSN, RN, BC
Assistant Professor, Director of Continuing Education
Purdue University School of Nursing
West Lafayette, Indiana

LISA M. KRITZ, RNC, MA
Associate Professor
Clarke College
Dubuque, Iowa

TERRIE SNOW, MSN, RN, CPNP
Nursing Instructor
Shasta College
Redding, California

BARBARA L.W. ST. JOHN, RN, DNSc
Nursing Instructor
Blue Ridge Community College
Flat Rock, North Carolina

IVY S. RAZMUS, MSN, RN
Clinical Manager
Children's Hospital of Saint Francis
Tulsa, Oklahoma

SUE G. THACKER, PHD, RNC, AS, BSN, MS
Professor, Nursing Department
Wytheville Community College
Wytheville, Virginia

LORETTA WACK, MSN, RN, PNP, FNP
Associate Professor, Nursing Program Coordinator
Blue Ridge Community College
Weyers Cave, Virginia

Preface

This third edition of *Maternal Child Nursing Care* combines essential information on maternity and pediatric nursing into one text. The text focuses on the care of women during their reproductive years and on children from newborn through adolescence. Issues and concerns of childbearing women and the health care of children are the primary concentrations. The promotion of wellness and the management of common women's health problems and child development are also addressed. As we move further into the twenty-first century, this third edition of *Maternal Child Nursing Care* is designed to address the changing needs of women during their childbearing years and children during their developing years.

Maternal Child Nursing Care was developed to provide students with the knowledge and skills they need to become competent, critical thinkers, and to attain the sensitivity needed to become caring nurses. This third edition has been revised and refined in response to comments and suggestions from educators, clinicians, and students. It includes the most accurate, current, and clinically relevant information available.

APPROACH

Professional nursing practice continues to evolve and adapt to society's changing health priorities. The rapidly changing health care delivery system offers new opportunities for nurses to alter the practice of maternity and pediatric nursing and to improve the way care is given. Increasingly, nursing practice must be evidence based. It is incumbent on nurses to use the most up-to-date and scientifically supported information on which to base their care. To assist nurses in providing this type of care, *Evidence-Based Practice* boxes with implications for practice and research are included throughout the text.

Consumers of maternity and pediatric care vary in age, ethnicity, culture, language, social status, marital status, and sexual orientation. They seek care from obstetricians, gynecologists, pediatricians, family practice physicians, nurse-midwives, nurse practitioners, and other health care providers in a variety of health care settings, including the home. To meet the needs of these consumers, clinical education must offer students a variety of health care experiences in settings that include hospitals and birth centers, homes, clinics, private physicians' offices, shelters for the homeless or for women and children in need of protection, and other community-based settings.

Care Management has been used as an organizing framework for discussion in the nursing care chapters. This approach demonstrates how nursing must collaborate with other health care disciplines to provide the most comprehensive care possible to women and children. Assessments, nursing diagnoses, expected outcomes, nursing implementation, and evaluation of care are highlighted throughout the chapters. Nursing care plans reinforce the problem-solving approach to patient care. In chapters that focus on complications of childbearing, reproductive conditions, and childhood illnesses, medical interventions are presented first and are followed by nursing care management. Throughout the discussion of assessment and care, we alert the nurse to signs of potential problems and provide information boxes that highlight warning signs and emergency situations.

Patient education is an essential component of nursing care of women and children. The chapter on women's health promotion and screening emphasizes teaching for self-care to promote wellness and to encourage preventive care. The chapter on transition to parenthood focuses on teaching for new mothers and infants at home. Special boxes highlight community care throughout the text. *Family Focus* boxes incorporate family considerations important to care of women and children. Issues concerning grandparents, siblings, and different family constellations are addressed. In the pediatric chapters, these boxes focus on the special learning needs of families caring for their child. Legal tips are integrated throughout the maternity section to emphasize these issues as they relate to the care of women and infants.

FEATURES

This third edition features a contemporary design with logical, easy-to-follow headings and attractive four-color design that highlights important content and increases visual appeal. Hundreds of color photographs and drawings throughout the text, many of them new, illustrate important concepts and techniques to further enhance comprehension.

To help students learn essential information quickly and efficiently, we have included numerous features that prioritize, condense, simplify, and emphasize important aspects of nursing care. In addition, the text encourages students to *think critically.* The organizing framework, *Care Management,* is used consistently to discuss nursing care. The five steps of the *Nursing Process* are incorporated into this framework. *Nursing Care Plans* are included to help students apply the nursing process in the clinical setting. The *Nursing Care Plans* use NANDA-approved nursing diagnoses, describe expected outcomes, and provide rationales for interventions. *Care Paths, Protocols,* and *Procedures* are included to provide students with examples of various approaches to the implementation of care.

SPECIAL FEATURES

- **Electronic Resources** providing additional information related to chapter content are placed at the beginning of each chapter and highlighted throughout the text.
- **Learning Objectives** focus students' attention on the important content to be mastered.
- **Critical Thinking Exercises** present students with real-life situations and encourage them to make appropriate clinical judgments. Answer guidelines are provided at the end of the chapter.
- **Evidence-Based Practice** boxes are incorporated throughout the book. In Part One these boxes summarize findings from the **Cochrane Pregnancy and Childbirth Database**. Findings that confirm effective practices or that identify practices with unknown, ineffective, or harmful effects are identified by the icon in the margin.
- **Home Care** boxes emphasize patient and family self-care and provide information to help students transfer learning from the hospital to the home setting.
- **Cultural Awareness** boxes describe beliefs and practices about pregnancy, childbirth, parenting, and women's health concerns.
- **Guidelines/Guías** boxes in Part One provide common English-to-Spanish phrases for patient assessment and teaching.
- **Family Focus** boxes highlight the needs or concerns of families that should be addressed when family-centered care is provided.
- **Community Focus** boxes emphasize community issues, provide resources and guidance, and illustrate nursing care in a variety of settings.
- **Nursing Care Plans** are provided for all commonly encountered situations and disorders. NANDA-accepted nursing diagnoses are included as well as rationales for nursing interventions that might not be immediately evident to students.
- **Patient Teaching** boxes assist students to help patients and families become involved in their own care with optimal outcomes.
- **Alternative and Complementary Therapies** are discussed for many pregnancy-related problems and are identified in the text by a **new** icon in the margin.
- **Atraumatic Care** boxes emphasize the importance of providing competent care while minimizing undue physical and psychologic distress for the child and family.
- **Emergency** boxes alert students to the signs and symptoms of various emergency situations and provide interventions for immediate implementation.
- **Nurse Alerts** call the reader's attention to critical information that could lead to deteriorating or emergency situations.
- During assessment, the nurse must be alert for **Signs of Potential Complications;** these are included in chapters that cover uncomplicated pregnancy and childbirth.
- **Care Paths, Protocols, and Procedures** provide students with examples of various approaches to implementation of care.
- **Medication Guide** boxes include key information about medications used in maternity and newborn care, including their indications, adverse effects, and nursing considerations.
- **Legal Tips** are integrated throughout Part One to provide students with relevant information to deal with important legal areas in the context of maternity nursing.
- **Key Points,** located at the end of each chapter, help the reader summarize major points, make connections, and synthesize information.
- **Resources,** including Web sites and contact information for organizations and educational resources available for the topics discussed, are listed throughout.
- A highly detailed, cross-referenced **index** allows readers to quickly access needed information.

ACKNOWLEDGMENTS

Thanks to Pat Gingrich for preparing the Evidence-Based Practice boxes in Part One; to Jo Garner for her assistance with the Spanish translations; to Julie Perry Nelson, Gilbert, AZ, for many new photographs; and to those parents who permitted us to use photos of their infants and families. Special words of gratitude are extended to Michael Ledbetter for his encouragement and assistance. Very special thanks to Catherine Jackson and Laurie Gower, whose support was crucial for the completion of this project, and to Anne Konopka for her exceptional attention to detail.

Shannon E. Perry
Deitra Leonard Lowdermilk

Special thanks to Patrick Barrera for his continued support of the Wong legacy textbooks. We are so thankful for the supportive staff at Elsevier, Shelly Hayden, Heather Bays, and Anne Konopka, for their continued devotion to excellence in pediatric nursing education.

Marilyn J. Hockenberry
David Wilson

The authors would like to acknowledge the following individuals for contributions to the seventh edition of *Wong's Essentials of Pediatric Nursing*:

Chris L. Algren, EdD, MSN, RN; Debra Arnow, MSN, RN, CNA, BC; Debbie Fraser Askin, MN, RNC; Rose A. Urdiales Baker, MSN, RN, CS; Patrick Barrera, BS; Carol C. Bowman, MS, RD, LD; Christine A. Brosnan, DrPH, RN; Rosalind Bryant, MN, RN-CS, PNP; Kimberly Childers, MS, RN, CEN, CPNP; Christine Chordas, MSN, RN, CPNP; Helen Currier, BSN, RN, CNN; Martha R. Curry, MS, RN, CPNP; Carolyn V. Daigneau, MS, RN-CS, PNP; Susan O. Fernbach, BSN, RN; Melody Brown Hellsten, MSN, RN, APRN-BC, PNP; Mary C. Hooke, MSN, RN, CPON, CNS; Linda M. Kollar, MSN, RN; Kerri Lemance, RN; Shannon Stone McCord, MS, RN, CPNP, CNS, WOCN, CCRN; Mary A. Mondozzi, MSN, RN, CPNP; Barbara Montagnino, MS, RN, CNS; Patricia A. Murray, MN, CPNP, HNC; Patricia O'Brien, MSN, RN-CS, PNP; Amy Nadel Romanczuk, MSN, RN; Rebecca J. Schultz, MSN, RN, CPNP; Sandra Upchurch, PhD, RN, CDE

Special Features

Nursing Process is used to format major diseases, disorders, and conditions.

Critical Thinking Exercises depict real-life situations that challenge students to choose the best interventions and make good clinical judgments.

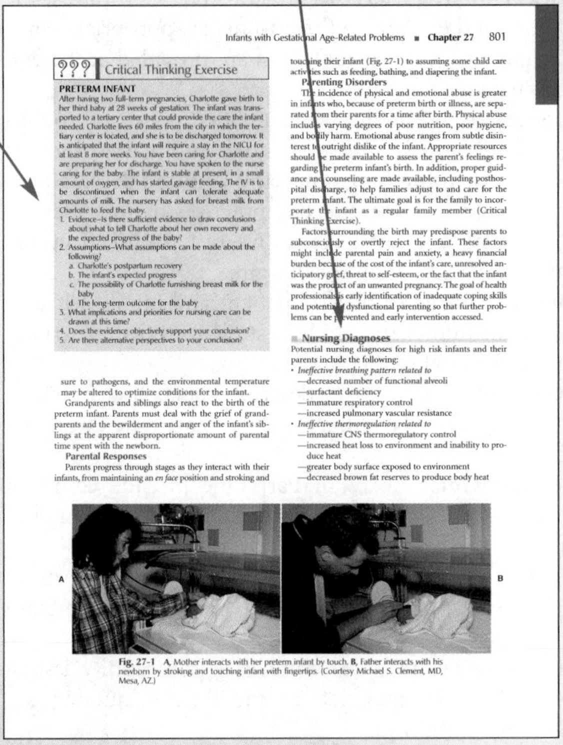
Infants with Gestational Age-Related Problems ■ Chapter 27 801

Critical Thinking Exercise

PRETERM INFANT

After having two full-term pregnancies, Charlotte gave birth to her third baby at 28 weeks of gestation. The infant was transported to a tertiary center that could provide the care the infant needed. Charlotte lives 60 miles from the city in which the tertiary center is located, and she is to be discharged tomorrow. It is anticipated that the infant will require a stay in the NICU for at least 8 more weeks. You have been caring for Charlotte and are preparing her for discharge. You have spoken to the nurse caring for the baby. The infant is stable at present, in a small amount of oxygen, and has started gavage feeding. The IV is to be discontinued when the infant can tolerate adequate amounts of milk. The nursery has asked for breast milk from Charlotte to feed the baby.

1. Evidence—Is there sufficient evidence to draw conclusions about what to tell Charlotte about her own recovery and the expected progress of the baby?
2. Assumptions—What assumptions can be made about the following?
   a. Charlotte's postpartum recovery
   b. The infant's expected progress
   c. The possibility of Charlotte furnishing breast milk for the baby
   d. The long-term outcome for the baby
3. What implications and priorities for nursing care can be drawn at this time?
4. Does the evidence objectively support your conclusion?
5. Are there alternative perspectives to your conclusion?

sure to pathogens, and the environmental temperature may be altered to optimize conditions for the infant.

Grandparents and siblings also react to the birth of the preterm infant. Parents must deal with the grief of grandparents and the bewilderment and anger of the infant's siblings at the apparent disproportionate amount of parental time spent with the newborn.

Parental Responses

Parents progress through stages as they interact with their infants, from maintaining an *en face* position and stroking and touching their infant (Fig. 27-1) to assuming some child care activities such as feeding, bathing, and diapering the infant.

Parenting Disorders

The incidence of physical and emotional abuse is greater in infants who, because of preterm birth or illness, are separated from their parents for a time after birth. Physical abuse includes varying degrees of poor nutrition, poor hygiene, and bodily harm. Emotional abuse ranges from subtle disinterest to outright dislike of the infant. Appropriate resources should be made available to assess the parent's feelings regarding the preterm infant's birth. In addition, proper guidance and counseling are made available, including posthospital discharge, to help families adjust to and care for the preterm infant. The ultimate goal is for the family to incorporate the infant as a regular family member (Critical Thinking Exercise).

Factors surrounding the birth may predispose parents to subconsciously or overtly reject the infant. These factors might include parental pain and anxiety, a heavy financial burden because of the cost of the infant's care, unresolved anticipatory grief, threat to self-esteem, or the fact that the infant was the product of an unwanted pregnancy. The goal of health professionals is early identification of inadequate coping skills and potential dysfunctional parenting so that further problems can be prevented and early intervention accessed.

Nursing Diagnoses

Potential nursing diagnoses for high risk infants and their parents include the following:

- *Ineffective breathing pattern related to*
  - —decreased number of functional alveoli
  - —surfactant deficiency
  - —immature respiratory control
  - —increased pulmonary vascular resistance
- *Ineffective thermoregulation related to*
  - —immature CNS thermoregulatory control
  - —increased heat loss to environment and inability to produce heat
  - —greater body surface exposed to environment
  - —decreased brown fat reserves to produce body heat

A B

Fig. 27-1 A, Mother interacts with her preterm infant by touch. B, Father interacts with his newborn by stroking and touching infant with fingertips. (Courtesy Michael S. Clement, MD, Mesa, AZ.)

Evidence-Based Practice boxes highlight both research and critical thought processes that support and guide the outcomes of nursing care.

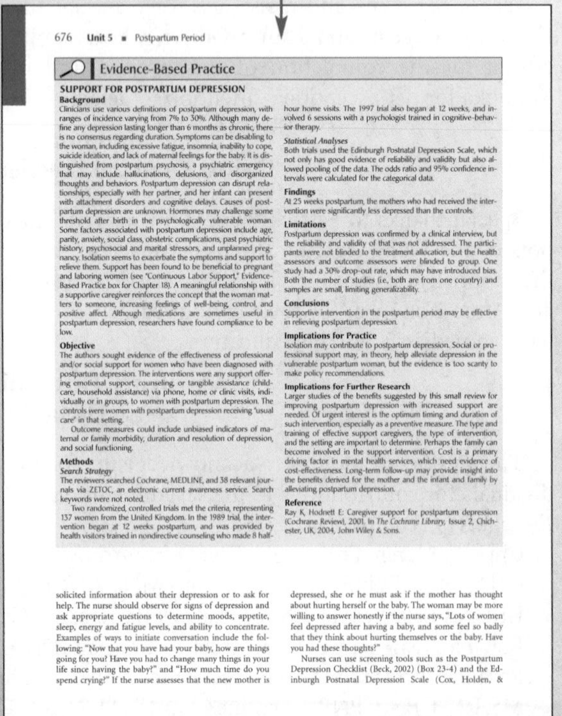
676 Unit 5 ■ Postpartum Period

Evidence-Based Practice

SUPPORT FOR POSTPARTUM DEPRESSION

Background

Clinicians use various definitions of postpartum depression, with ranges of incidence varying from 7% to 30%. Although many define any depression lasting longer than 6 months as chronic, there is no consensus regarding duration. Symptoms can be disabling to the woman, including excessive fatigue, insomnia, inability to cope, suicide ideation, and lack of maternal feelings for the baby. It is distinguished from postpartum psychosis, a psychiatric emergency that may include hallucinations, delusions, and disorganized thoughts and behaviors. Postpartum depression can disrupt relationships, especially with her partner, and her infant can present with attachment disorders and cognitive delays. Causes of postpartum depression are unknown. Hormones may challenge some threshold after birth in the psychologically vulnerable woman. Some factors associated with postpartum depression include age, parity, anxiety, social class, obstetric complications, past psychiatric history, psychosocial and marital stressors, and unplanned pregnancy. Isolation seems to exacerbate the symptoms and support to relieve them. Support has been found to be beneficial to pregnant and laboring women (see "Continuous Labor Support," Evidence-Based Practice box for Chapter 18). A meaningful relationship with a supportive caregiver reinforces the concept that the woman matters to someone, increasing feelings of well-being, control, and positive affect. Although medications are sometimes useful in postpartum depression, researchers have found compliance to be low.

Objective

The authors sought evidence of the effectiveness of professional and/or social support for women who have been diagnosed with postpartum depression. The interventions were any support offering emotional support, counseling, or tangible assistance (child-care, household assistance) via phone, home or clinic visits, individually or in groups, to women with postpartum depression. The controls were women with postpartum depression receiving "usual care" in that setting.

Outcome measures could include unbiased indicators of maternal or family morbidity, duration and resolution of depression, and social functioning.

Methods

Search Strategy

The reviewers searched Cochrane, MEDLINE, and 38 relevant journals via ZETOC, an electronic current awareness service. Search keywords were not noted.

Two randomized, controlled trials met the criteria, representing 137 women from the United Kingdom. In the 1989 trial, the intervention began at 12 weeks postpartum, and was provided by health visitors trained in nondirective counseling who made 8 half-hour home visits. The 1997 trial also began at 12 weeks, and involved 6 sessions with a psychologist trained in cognitive-behavior therapy.

Statistical Analyses

Both trials used the Edinburgh Postnatal Depression Scale, which not only has good evidence of reliability and validity but also allowed pooling of the data. The odds ratio and 95% confidence intervals were calculated for the categorical data.

Findings

At 25 weeks postpartum, the mothers who had received the intervention were significantly less depressed than the controls.

Limitations

Postpartum depression was confirmed by a clinical interview, but the reliability and validity of that was not addressed. The participants were not blinded to the treatment allocation, but the health assessors and outcome assessors were blinded to group. One study had a 30% drop-out rate, which may have introduced bias. Both the number of studies (i.e., both are from one country) and samples are small, limiting generalizability.

Conclusions

Supportive intervention in the postpartum period may be effective in relieving postpartum depression.

Implications for Practice

Isolation may contribute to postpartum depression. Social or professional support may, in theory, help alleviate depression in the vulnerable postpartum woman, but the evidence is too scanty to make policy recommendations.

Implications for Further Research

Larger studies of the benefits suggested by this small review for improving postpartum depression with increased support are needed. Of urgent interest is the optimum timing and duration of such intervention, especially as a preventive measure. The type and training of effective support caregivers, the type of intervention, and the setting are important to determine. Perhaps the family can become involved in the support intervention. Cost is a primary driving factor in mental health services, which need evidence of cost-effectiveness. Long-term follow-up may provide insight into the benefits derived for the mother and the infant and family by alleviating postpartum depression.

Reference

Ray K, Hodnett E: Caregiver support for postpartum depression (Cochrane Review), 2001. In *The Cochrane Library*, Issue 2, Chichester, UK, 2004, John Wiley & Sons.

solicited information about their depression or to ask for help. The nurse should observe for signs of depression and ask appropriate questions to determine moods, appetite, sleep, energy and fatigue levels, and ability to concentrate. Examples of ways to initiate conversation include the following: "Now that you have had your baby, how are things going for you? Have you had to change many things in your life since having the baby?" and "How much time do you spend crying?" If the nurse assesses that the new mother is depressed, she or he must ask if the mother has thought about hurting herself or the baby. The woman may be more willing to answer honestly if the nurse says, "Lots of women feel depressed after having a baby, and some feel so badly that they think about hurting themselves or the baby. Have you had these thoughts?"

Nurses can use screening tools such as the Postpartum Depression Checklist (Beck, 2002) (Box 23-4) and the Edinburgh Postnatal Depression Scale (Cox, Holden, &

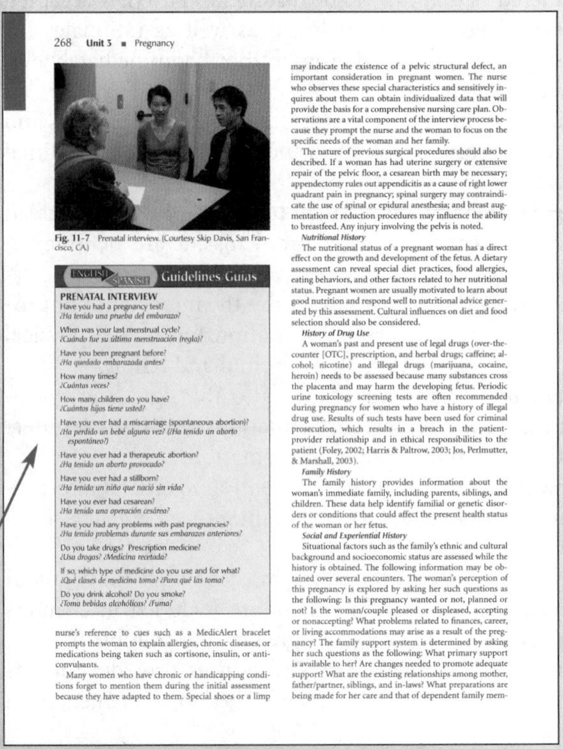
268 Unit 3 ■ Pregnancy

Fig. 11-7 Prenatal interview. (Courtesy Skip Davis, San Francisco, CA)

ENGLISH SPANISH Guidelines/Guías

PRENATAL INTERVIEW

Have you had a pregnancy test?
¿Ha tenido una prueba del embarazo?

When was your last menstrual cycle?
¿Cuándo fue su última menstruación (regla)?

Have you been pregnant before?
¿Ha quedado embarazada antes?

How many times?
¿Cuántas veces?

How many children do you have?
¿Cuántos hijos tiene usted?

Have you ever had a miscarriage (spontaneous abortion)?
¿Ha perdido un bebé alguna vez? ¿Ha tenido un aborto espontáneo?

Have you ever had a therapeutic abortion?
¿Ha tenido un aborto provocado?

Have you ever had a stillborn?
¿Ha tenido un niño que nació sin vida?

Have you ever had cesarean?
¿Ha tenido una operación cesárea?

Have you had any problems with past pregnancies?
¿Ha tenido problemas durante sus embarazos anteriores?

Do you take drugs? Prescription medicine?
¿Usa drogas? ¿Medicina recetada?

If so, which type of medicine do you use and for what?
¿Qué clases de medicina toma? ¿Para qué las toma?

Do you drink alcohol? Do you smoke?
¿Toma bebidas alcohólicas? ¿Fuma?

nurse's reference to cues such as a MedicAlert bracelet prompts the woman to explain allergies, chronic diseases, or medications being taken such as cortisone, insulin, or anticonvulsants.

Many women who have chronic or handicapping conditions forget to mention them during the initial assessment because they have adapted to them. Special shoes or a limp may indicate the existence of a pelvic structural defect, an important consideration in pregnant women. The nurse who observes these special characteristics and sensitively inquires about them can obtain individualized data that will provide the basis for a comprehensive nursing care plan. Observations are a vital component of the interview process because they prompt the nurse and the woman to focus on the specific needs of the woman and her family.

The nature of previous surgical procedures should also be described. If a woman has had uterine surgery or extensive repair of the pelvic floor, a cesarean birth may be necessary; appendectomy rules out appendicitis as a cause of right lower quadrant pain in pregnancy; spinal surgery may contraindicate the use of spinal or epidural anesthesia; and breast augmentation or reduction procedures may influence the ability to breastfeed. Any injury involving the pelvis is noted.

Nutritional History

The nutritional status of a pregnant woman has a direct effect on the growth and development of the fetus. A dietary assessment can reveal special diet practices, food allergies, eating behaviors, and other factors related to her nutritional status. Pregnant women are usually motivated to learn about good nutrition and respond well to nutritional advice generated by this assessment. Cultural influences on diet and food selection should also be considered.

History of Drug Use

A woman's past and present use of legal drugs (over-the-counter [OTC], prescription, and herbal drugs; caffeine; alcohol; nicotine) and illegal drugs (marijuana, cocaine, heroin) needs to be assessed because many substances cross the placenta and may harm the developing fetus. Periodic urine toxicology screening tests are often recommended during pregnancy for women who have a history of illegal drug use. Results of such tests have been used for criminal prosecution, which results in a breach in the patient-provider relationship and in ethical responsibilities to the patient (Foley, 2002; Harris & Paltrow, 2003; Jos, Perlmutter, & Marshall, 2003).

Family History

The family history provides information about the woman's immediate family, including parents, siblings, and children. These data help identify familial or genetic disorders or conditions that could affect the present health status of the woman or her fetus.

Social and Experiential History

Situational factors such as the family's ethnic and cultural background and socioeconomic status are assessed while the history is obtained. The following information may be obtained over several encounters. The woman's perception of this pregnancy is explored by asking her such questions as the following: Is this pregnancy wanted or not, planned or not? Is the woman/couple pleased or displeased, accepting or nonaccepting? What problems related to finances, career, or living accommodations may arise as a result of the pregnancy? The family support system is determined by asking her such questions as the following: What primary support is available to her? Are changes needed to promote adequate support? What are the existing relationships among mother, father/partner, siblings, and in-laws? What preparations are being made for her care and that of dependent family mem-

English-Spanish Guidelines boxes assist students in translating key words and phrases to better serve Spanish-speaking patients.

Nurse Alerts point out critical information students should not overlook when treating patients.

Community Focus boxes provide thoughtful consideration of issues that expand to the community.

1212 **Unit 9** ■ Health Promotion and Special Health Problems

Suicide

Suicide is defined as the deliberate act of self-injury with the intent that the injury results in death. Most experts distinguish between suicidal ideation, suicide attempt (or parasuicide), and suicide.

Suicidal ideation involves a preoccupation with thoughts about committing suicide and may be a precursor to suicide. Although it is not uncommon for adolescents to experience occasional suicidal thoughts, expressions of preoccupation with suicide should be taken seriously, and an assessment should be conducted for appropriate referral. A *suicide attempt* is intended to cause injury or death. The term *parasuicide* is used to refer to behaviors ranging from gestures to serious attempts to kill oneself. Parasuicide is a preferred term because it makes no reference to intent and because a person's motive may be too difficult or complex to determine. However, all parasuicidal activity should be taken seriously.

NURSE ALERT A history of a previous suicide attempt is a serious indicator for possible suicide completion in the future. Studies of adolescent suicides have found that as many as half of the adolescents had made previous attempts. ■

Recent results from the Youth Risk Behavior Survey, 2001, indicated that 8.8% of students nationwide had attempted suicide at least once during the 12 months preceding the survey (Grunbaum et al, 2002). This number represented a significant increase from 7.8% who reported attempts in 1999 (Division of Adolescent and School Health, 2000). Approximately 15% of the students in this survey reported that they had made a specific plan to attempt suicide in the 12 months preceding the survey. In the United States, the suicide rate for adolescents has increased dramatically in the last few decades. Suicide is currently the third leading cause of death during the teenage years, surpassed only by death from injury and homicide (see Chapter 29).

Etiology

Individual, family, and social-environmental factors have all been implicated in suicide. The single most important individual factor is the presence of an active psychiatric disorder (depression, bipolar disorder, psychosis, substance abuse, or conduct disorder). Comorbidity of an affective disorder and substance abuse also increases the risk for suicide. Alcohol use has been associated with more than 50% of suicides (AAP, Committee on Adolescence, 2000). Gay and lesbian adolescents are at particularly high risk for suicide completion, especially if raised in an environment in which they are denied support systems (Community Focus box). Family factors influencing suicide include parental loss; family disruption; a family history of suicide, depression, substance abuse, or emotional disturbance; child abuse or neglect; unavailable parents; poor communication and isolation within the family; family conflict; and unrealistically high parental expectations or parental indifference with low expectations. Social/environmental factors include incarceration, isolation, acute loss of a boyfriend or girlfriend, lack of future options, and availability of firearms in the home.

Community Focus

SUICIDE, SEXUAL IDENTITY, AND SEXUAL ORIENTATION

A significant number of teenage suicides occur among homosexual youths. Gay or lesbian adolescents who live in families or communities that do not accept homosexuality are likely to suffer low self-esteem, self-loathing, depression, and hopelessness as a result of lack of acceptance from their family or community. Such internalization, without treatment and support, can lead to substance abuse and, eventually, suicide. Youths most at risk are those who struggle with gender identity issues such as gay identity formation at a young age, intrapersonal conflict regarding sexuality, and nondisclosure of orientation to others.

Supportive parents, friends, or relationships serve as protective factors against suicide. However, many gay, lesbian, and bisexual adolescents do not feel supported, understood, or accepted by their friends, parents, and families. Nurses who interact with adolescents must be aware of the association between suicide and adolescent homosexuality and gender nonconformity. School nurses may be the first individuals to discuss issues of sexual identity and orientation with adolescents and/or their families. In their professional capacity, nurses can also serve as support persons for these adolescents. Nurses can also provide guidance and resources to families so that they know and understand how best to nurture and support their child.

Nurses must also capitalize on opportunities or experiences that promote the healthy development of self-esteem in youths who choose nontraditional sexual orientation. Educational programs to raise the level of consciousness about the risk factors for and warning signs of suicide are one example. Another possibility could be programs conducted in or outside of school that are designed to foster peer relationships and competency in social skills among high-risk adolescents and young adults, such as support groups and social organizations for these young people.

Methods

Firearms are by far the most commonly used instruments in completed suicides among males and females (AAP, Committee on Adolescence, 2000). For adolescent males, the second and third most common means of suicide are hanging and overdose, respectively; for females, the second and third most common means are overdose and strangulation.

The most common method of suicide attempt is overdose or ingestion of a potentially toxic substance, such as drugs. The second most common method of suicide attempt is self-inflicted laceration.

NURSE ALERT Given what is known about youth suicide, nurses should ask parents, especially those with at-risk teenagers, if firearms are available in the house and, if so, recommend their removal. Parents must ensure that their children, especially those who are depressed, have poor problem-solving skills, or use drugs or alcohol, do not have access to firearms. Parents must also be educated on the warning signs of suicide (Box 40-8). ■

Learning Objectives begin each chapter to focus attention on the important content to be mastered.

Electronic Resources related to chapter content are included at the beginning of each chapter and highlighted throughout the text.

Unit 9

38 The Preschooler and Family

LEARNING OBJECTIVES

On completion of this chapter the reader will be able to:

- Identify the major biologic, psychosocial, cognitive, moral, spiritual, and social developments that occur during the preschool years.
- List the benefits of imaginary playmates.
- Prepare preschoolers for preschool or day care experience.
- Provide parents with guidelines for sex education.
- Provide parents with guidelines for dealing with a child's fears, stresses, aggression, and sleep problems.
- Recognize the causes of stuttering during the preschool years.
- Offer parents suggestions for preventing speech problems.
- Recognize feeding patterns of preschoolers.
- Provide anticipatory guidance to parents regarding injury prevention based on the preschooler's developmental achievements.
- State three factors thought to be associated with child abuse.
- State four areas of the history that should arouse suspicion of abuse.
- Describe the nursing care of the abused child.

ELECTRONIC RESOURCES

Additional information related to the content in Chapter 38 can be found on

the companion website at evolve
http://evolve.elsevier.com/Wong/maternal/

- NCLEX Review Questions
- Case Study–Sleep Problems
- Case Study–Varicella in Spite of Vaccine
- WebLinks

or the interactive student CD-ROM
Activities for Chapter 38 include the following:

- NCLEX Review Questions
- Case Study–Chickenpox (Varicella)
- Critical Thinking Exercise–Imitative Play
- Nursing Care Plan–The Child with a Communicable Disease
- Nursing Care Plan–The Child Who Is Maltreated

PROMOTING OPTIMUM GROWTH AND DEVELOPMENT

The combined biologic, psychosocial, cognitive, spiritual, and social achievements during the *preschool period* (3 to 5 years of age) prepare preschoolers for their most significant change in lifestyle—entrance into school. Their control of bodily functions, experience of brief and prolonged periods of separation, ability to interact cooperatively with other children and adults, use of language for mental symbolization, and increased attention span and memory ready them for the next major period—the school years. Successful achievement of previous levels of growth and development is essential for preschoolers to refine many of the tasks that were mastered during the toddler years.

Biologic Development

The rate of physical growth slows and stabilizes during the preschool years. The average *weight* is 14.6 kg (32 pounds) at 3 years, 16.7 kg (36.75 pounds) at 4 years, and 18.7 kg (41.25 pounds) at 5 years. The average weight gain per year remains approximately 2.3 kg (5 pounds).

Growth in *height* also remains steady at a yearly increase of 6.75 to 7.5 cm (2.5 to 3 inches) and generally occurs in elongation of the legs rather than of the trunk. The average height is 95 cm (37.25 inches) at 3 years, 103 cm (40.5 inches) at 4 years, and 110 cm (43.25 inches) at 5 years.

Physical proportions no longer resemble those of the squat, potbellied toddler. The preschooler is slender but sturdy, graceful, agile, and posturally erect. There is little difference in physical characteristics according to gender, except as dictated by such factors as dress and hairstyle.

1114

1006 **Unit 8** ■ Assessment of the Child and Family

them for the procedure by allowing them to play with the instrument, demonstrating how it works, and stressing the importance of remaining still. A helpful suggestion is to let them observe you examining the parent's ear. Restraint is needed for younger children because the ear examination upsets them (Atraumatic Care box).

As you insert the speculum into the meatus, move it around the outer rim to accustom the child to the feel of something entering the ear. If examining a painful ear, touch a nonpainful part of the affected ear, then examine the unaffected ear, and finally return to the painful ear. By this time the child is usually less fearful of anything causing discomfort to the ear and will cooperate more.

For their protection and safety, infants and toddlers must be restrained for the otoscopic examination. There are two general positions of restraint. In one the child is seated sideways in the parent's lap with one arm "hugging" the parent and the other arm at the side. The ear to be examined is toward the nurse. With one arm the parent holds the child's head firmly against his or her chest, and with the other arm "hugs" the child, thereby securing the child's free arm. The ear is examined using the same procedure for holding the otoscope as described later (Fig. 35-17, *A*).

The other position involves placing the child on the side, back, or abdomen with the arms at the side and the head turned so that the ear to be examined points toward the ceiling. Lean over the child and use the upper part of the body to restrain the arms and upper trunk movements, and the examining hand to stabilize the head. This position is practical for young infants or for older children who need minimal restraining, but it may not be feasible for other children who protest vigorously. For safety enlist the parent's or an assistant's help in immobilizing the head by firmly placing one hand above the ear and the other on the child's side, abdomen, or back (Fig. 35-17, *B*).

With cooperative children examine the ear with the child in a side-lying, sitting, or standing position. One disadvantage to standing is that the child may "walk away" as the otoscope enters the canal. If the child is standing or sitting, tilt the head slightly toward the child's opposite shoulder to achieve a better view of the drum (Fig. 35-18).

With the thumb and forefinger of the free (usually nondominant) hand, grasp the auricle. For the two positions of restraint, hold the otoscope upside down at the junction of its head and handle with the thumb and index finger. Place the other fingers against the skull to allow the otoscope to

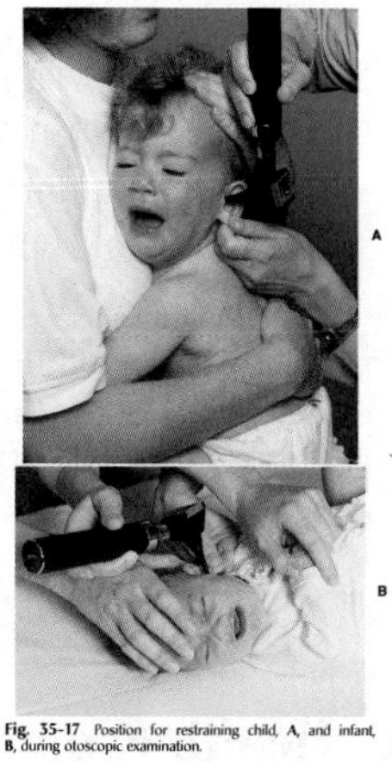

A

B

Fig. 35-17 Position for restraining child, **A**, and infant, **B**, during otoscopic examination.

move with the child in case of sudden movement. In examining a cooperative child, hold the handle with the otic head upright or upside down. Use the dominant hand to examine both ears or reverse hands for each ear, whichever is more comfortable.

Before using the otoscope, visualize the external ear and the tympanic membrane as being superimposed on a clock (Fig. 35-19). The numbers become important geographic landmarks. Introduce the speculum into the meatus between the 3 and 9 o'clock positions in a *downward* and *forward* position. Because the canal is curved, the speculum does not permit a panoramic view of the tympanic membrane unless the canal is straightened. In infants the canal curves upward. Therefore pull the pinna *down* and *back* to the 6 to 9 o'clock range to straighten the canal (Fig. 35-20, *A*).

With older children, usually those older than 3 years of age, the canal curves downward and forward. Therefore pull the pinna *up* and *back* toward a 10 o'clock position (Fig.

Atraumatic Care

REDUCING DISTRESS FROM OTOSCOPY IN YOUNG CHILDREN

Make examining the ear a game by explaining that you are looking for a "big elephant" in the ear. This kind of make-believe is an absorbing distraction and usually elicits cooperation. After the ear has been examined, clarify that "looking for elephants" was only pretend and thank the child for letting you look in his or her ear. You can also ask the child to put a finger on the opposite ear to keep the light from getting out, which is a great distraction technique.

Full-color photographs and illustrations help clarify information.

Atraumatic Care boxes teach the importance of minimizing undue physical and psychologic distress for the child and family.

Contents

PART I
Maternity Nursing

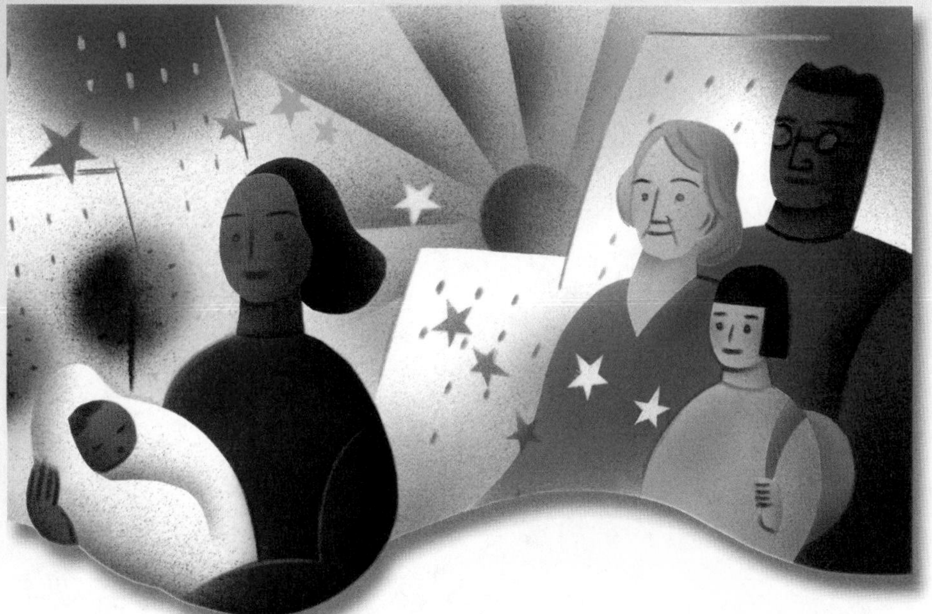

Contemporary Maternity Nursing 1

LEARNING OBJECTIVES

On completion of this chapter the reader will be able to:

- Describe the scope of maternity nursing.
- Evaluate contemporary issues and trends in maternity nursing.
- Describe sociopolitical issues affecting the care of women and infants.
- Compare selected biostatistical data among races and countries.
- Examine social concerns in maternity nursing.
- Explain quality management and standards of practice in the delivery of nursing care.
- Debate ethical issues in perinatal nursing.
- Examine the *Healthy People 2010* goals related to maternal and infant care.

ELECTRONIC RESOURCES

Additional information related to the content in Chapter 1 can be found on

the companion website at evolve
http://evolve.elsevier.com/Wong/maternal/
- NCLEX Review Questions
- WebLinks

or the interactive student CD-ROM
Activities for Chapter 1 include the following:
- NCLEX Review Questions

Maternity nursing focuses on the care of childbearing women and their families through all stages of pregnancy and childbirth, as well as the first 4 weeks after birth. Throughout the prenatal period, nurses, nurse practitioners, and nurse-midwives provide care for women in clinics and physicians' offices and teach classes to help families prepare for childbirth. Nurses care for childbearing families during labor and birth in hospitals, in birthing centers, and in the home. Nurses with special training may provide intensive care for high risk neonates in special care units and for high risk mothers in antepartum units, in critical care obstetric units, or in the home. Maternity nurses teach about pregnancy; the process of labor, birth, and recovery; and parenting skills. They provide continuity of care throughout the childbearing cycle. The Vision for Women and Their Health of the International Confederation of Midwives provides an excellent model for nurses who care for women and children (Box 1-1).

Tremendous advances in the care of mothers and their infants have taken place during the past 150 years (Box 1-2). However, in the United States, serious problems exist related to the health and health care of mothers and infants. Lack of access to prepregnancy and pregnancy-related care for all women and lack of reproductive health services for adolescents are major concerns. Sexually transmitted infections, including acquired immunodeficiency syndrome (AIDS), continue to adversely affect reproduction. One fifth of all Americans, 58 million people, lack health insurance for a year or more (Marwick, 2002).

Racial and ethnic diversity are increasing within North America. It is estimated that by the year 2050, 50% of the population will be European-American, 15% will be African-American, 24% will be Hispanic, and 8% will be Asian-American (U.S. Census Bureau, 2004). This provides a challenge for health care providers to provide culturally sensitive health care (Box 1-3).

Although the United States has made great strides in public health, significant disparity exists in health outcomes among people of various racial and ethnic groups. In addition, people may have lifestyles, health needs, and health care preferences related to their ethnic or cultural backgrounds. They may have dietary preferences and health practices that are not understood by caregivers. To meet the health care needs of a culturally diverse society, the nursing workforce must reflect the diversity of its patient population.

The focus of the first part of this book is maternity nursing. Chapter 1 presents a general overview of issues and trends related to the health and health care of women and infants during the maternity cycle. The second part, which begins with Chapter 29, addresses the issues and trends related to the health care of children.

BOX 1-1

The Vision for Women and Their Health

The International Confederation of Midwives envisions a world where

- Women are respected and treated as persons in their own right in all societies.
- Women stand as equal partners with men in the world order.
- Women are recognized as crucial to the health of any nation.
- Women and their families are part of a health care system with high-quality care and easy access when needed.
- Women have the right to choose from among safe options for care throughout their lives, including high-quality, state-of-the-art care from competent providers who truly care about the woman and her health.
- Women are educated and empowered to delight in a strong sense of self, to trust their bodies, to plan their pregnancies, and to make wise choices in their health care.
- Women experience a reasonable standard of living, including a clean and safe environment, healthy food, and a reasonable place to live.
- Women need have no fear for their lives or the lives of their babies when they are pregnant.
- Women believe that birth is normal and prefer to avoid unnecessary intervention.

From The International Confederation of Midwives: Internet document available at www.internationalmidwives.org/vision.htm (accessed June 15, 2002).

CONTEMPORARY ISSUES AND TRENDS

Structure of Health Care Delivery

The changing health care delivery system offers opportunities for nurses to alter nursing practice and improve the way care is delivered through managed care, integrated delivery systems (IDSs), and redefined roles. Nurses have been critically important in developing strategies to improve the well-being of women and their infants and have led the efforts to implement clinical practice guidelines and to practice using an evidence-based approach. Through professional associations, nurses can have a voice in setting standards and in influencing health policy by actively participating in the education of the public and of state and federal legislators.

Changes in the health care market are influencing the way health care providers can care for their patients. Health spending varies considerably among nations (Table 1-1). In the United States during 2001 health spending accounted for 13.9% of the gross domestic product (GDP); in Canada 9.7% of the GDP was spent on health care (Reinhart, Hussey, & Anderson, 2004). A national nursing shortage exists; the number of professional nurses in hospitals has declined, and unlicensed assistive personnel and multiskilled workers have been substituted. A minimum nurse-patient ratio has been legislated.

The role of the nurse is evolving from primary caregiver to the leader of an interdisciplinary care team. Documenta-

BOX 1-2

Historic Milestones in the Care of Mothers and Infants

1847—James Young Simpson in Edinburgh, Scotland, used ether for an internal podalic version and birth; the first reported use of obstetric anesthesia
1861—Ignaz Semmelwies wrote *The Cause, Concept, and Prophylaxis of Childbed Fever*
1906—First program for prenatal nursing care established
1908—Childbirth classes started by the American Red Cross
1909—First White House Conference on Children convened
1911—First milk bank in the United States established in Boston
1912—U.S. Children's Bureau established
1916—Margaret Sanger established first American birth control clinic in Brooklyn, NY
1923—First U.S. hospital center for premature infant care established at Sarah Morris Hospital in Chicago
1933—*Natural Childbirth* published by Grantly Dick-Read
1941—Penicillin used as a treatment for infection
1953—Virginia Apgar, an anesthesiologist, published Apgar scoring system of neonatal assessment
1956—Oxygen determined to cause retrolental fibroplasia (RLF) (now known as retinopathy of prematurity [ROP])
1958—Edward Hon reported on the recording of the fetal electrocardiogram (ECG) from the maternal abdomen (first commercial electronic fetal monitor produced in the late 1960s)
1958—Ian Donald, a Glasgow physician, was the first to report clinical use of ultrasound to examine the fetus
1959—*Thank You, Dr. Lamaze* published by Marjorie Karmel
1959—Cytologic studies demonstrate that Down syndrome is associated with a particular form of nondisjunction now known as trisomy 21.
1960—American Society for Psychoprophylaxis in Obstetrics (ASPO/Lamaze) formed
1960—International Childbirth Education Association formed
1960—Birth control pill introduced in the United States
1962—Thalidomide found to cause birth defects
1963—Title V of the Social Security Act amended to include comprehensive maternity and infant care for women who were low income and high risk
1965—Supreme Court ruled married people have the right to use birth control
1967—Rh_o(D) immune globulin produced
1967—Reva Rubin published article on Maternal Role Attainment
1968—Rubella vaccine available
1969—Nurses Association of the American College of Obstetricians and Gynecologists (NAACOG) founded; renamed Association of Women's Health, Obstetric, and Neonatal Nurses (AWHONN) and incorporated as a 501(c)3 organization in 1993
1972—Special Supplemental Food Program for Women, Infants, and Children (WIC) started
1973—Abortion legalized
1974—First standards for obstetric, gynecologic, and neonatal nursing published by NAACOG
1975—The Pregnant Patient's Bill of Rights published by the International Childbirth Education Association
1978—Louise Brown, first test-tube baby, born
1991—Society for Advancement of Women's Health Research founded
1992—Office of Research on Women's Health authorized by U.S. Congress
1993—Human embryos cloned at George Washington University
1993—Family and Medical Leave Act enacted
1998—Newborns' and Mothers' Health Act put into effect
2000—Working draft of sequence and analysis of human genome completed

BOX 1-3

Terms Describing Cross-Cultural Capacity

Cultural Knowledge
Familiarization with selected cultural characteristics, history, values, belief systems, and behaviors of the members of another ethnic group

Cultural Awareness
Developing sensitivity and understanding of another ethnic group

Cultural Sensitivity
Knowing that cultural differences and similarities exist, without assigning values (i.e., better or worse, right or wrong) to those cultural differences

Cultural Competence
A set of congruent behaviors, attitudes, and policies that enable persons to work together in cross-cultural situations; emphasizes the idea of effectively operating in different cultural contexts.

Source: Internet document available at www.geocities.com/artmasp/CulSens.html (accessed April 12, 2004).

tion of patient outcomes has become essential (see later discussion). Advanced practice roles will increase as nurses assume more responsibility for patient care.

Integrative Health Care

Integrative health care encompasses complementary and alternative therapies in combination with conventional Western modalities of treatment. Many popular alternative healing modalities offer human-centered care based on philosophies that recognize the value of the patient's input and honor the individual's beliefs, values, and desires (Fig. 1-1). The focus of these modalities is on the whole person, not just on a disease complex. Patients often find that alternative modalities are more consistent with their own belief systems and also allow for more patient autonomy in health care decisions (Fig. 1-2). Complementary and alternative therapies are identified throughout the text with an icon. ( )

Increasing numbers of American adults are seeking alternative and complementary health care, which exceeds visits paid to U.S. primary care physicians. Use of complementary and alternative therapies is increasing rapidly in Canada (Verhoef & Findlay, 2003). Approximately 40% of the general population uses complementary and alternative therapies (Barrett, 2003), and most of these users do not tell their physicians. Annual expenditures related to alternative therapies are estimated at $27 billion, over half of which is out-of-pocket expense not covered by medical insurance (Eisenberg et al, 1998). Throughout the world, the use of traditional medicine presents unique challenges in terms of policy, efficacy, accessibility, and utilization (World Health Organization, 2002).

In 1992 the National Institutes of Health (NIH) developed the Office of Alternative Medicine (OAM). Mandated by Congress, the OAM was designed to support research and evaluation of various alternative and complementary modalities and to provide information to health care con-

Table 1-1

International Comparison of Percentage of Gross Domestic Product (GDP) Spent on Health Care in 2001

COUNTRY	PERCENTAGE
United States	13.9
Switzerland	11.1
Germany	10.7
Canada	9.7
France	9.5
Australia	9.2
New Zealand	8.1
Japan	8.0
United Kingdom	7.6

Source: Reinhardt UE, Hussey PS, Anderson GF: U.S. Health care spending in an international context, *Health Affairs* 23(3):10-25, 2004.

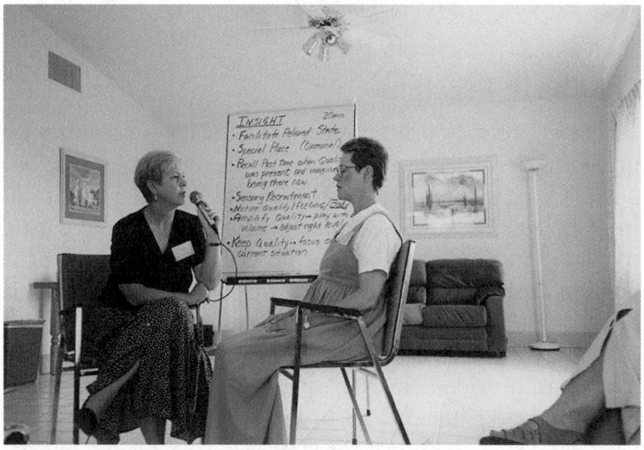

Fig. 1-1 Nurse and patient during guided imagery session. (Courtesy Nurses Certificate Program in Interactive Imagery, Foster City, CA.)

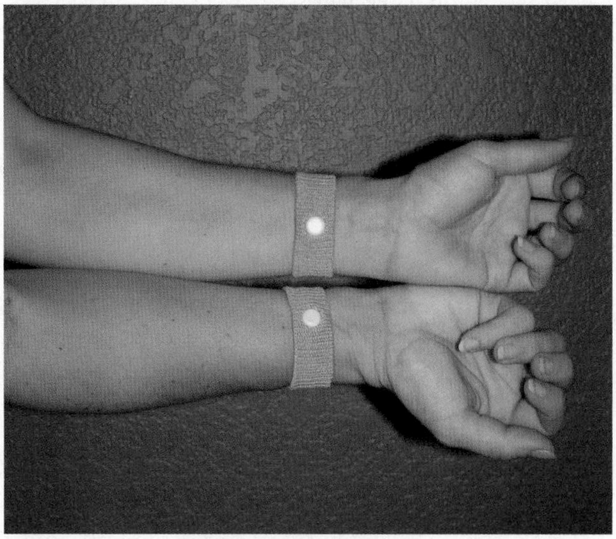

Fig. 1-2 Sea Bands used for stimulation of acupressure point P6. (Courtesy Julie Perry Nelson, Gilbert, AZ.)

BOX 1-4

Five Types or Classifications of Complementary or Alternative Therapies

Alternative medical systems (e.g., homeopathic and naturopathic medicine; traditional Chinese medicine)
Mind-body interventions (e.g., patient support groups, cognitive-behavioral therapy; meditation, prayer, art, music, dance)
Biologically based therapies (e.g., herbs, foods, vitamins)
Manipulative and body-based methods (e.g., chiropractic or osteopathic manipulation, massage)
Energy therapies (e.g., qi gong, Reiki, therapeutic touch, use of electromagnetic fields)

Source: Hawks JH, Moyad MA: CAM: definition and classification overview, *Urol Nurs* 23(3):221-223, 2003.

sumers about such modalities (Box 1-4). In 1998 Congress instituted the National Center for Complementary and Alternative Medicine (NCCAM), which incorporates the work of the OAM in its mission and function. With additional funding, NCCAM will expand its research focus (Dossey, 1998; NCCAM, 2002) (Table 1-2).

Table 1-2

National Institutes of Health Categories of Alternative Healing Modalities

CATEGORY	EXAMPLES
Alternative systems of medical practice	Acupuncture Ayurveda Environmental medicine Homeopathy Native American healing Naturopathic medicine Shamanism Traditional Chinese medicine
Bioelectromagnetic applications	Electroacupuncture Neuromagnetic stimulation devices
Diet, nutrition, lifestyle changes	Changes in lifestyle Diet Macrobiotics Megavitamins and other nutritional supplements
Herbal medicine	Herbal approaches from a variety of cultures including the Americas, Europe, and the Far East
Manual healing	Acupressure Chiropractic Massage therapy Osteopathy Reflexology Therapeutic touch/healing touch Trager method
Mind/body control	Art therapy Biofeedback Counseling Dance therapy Guided imagery and hypnosis Humor therapy Meditation Music therapy Prayer Psychotherapy Relaxation Support and self-help groups Yoga
Pharmacologic and biologic treatments	Antioxidizing agents Chelation therapy Oxidizing agents Vaccines (not currently accepted by mainstream medicine)

Sources: Dossey BM: Holistic modalities and healing moments, *Am J Nurs* 98(6):44-47, 1998; National Center for Complementary and Alternative Medicine (NCCAM). Internet document available at http://nccam.nih.gov (accessed November 27, 2004).

Childbirth Practices

Prenatal care may promote better pregnancy outcomes by providing early risk assessment and promoting healthy behaviors such as improved nutrition and smoking cessation. In 2002, 83.7% of all women received care in the first trimester and 3.6% had late or no prenatal care. This proportion rose to more than 5% for black, Hispanic, and American Indian mothers (Martin et al, 2003).

Women can choose physicians or nurse-midwives as primary care providers. In 2002, physicians attended 91% and nurse-midwives attended 8% of all births (Martin et al, 2003). Hospital births accounted for 99% of births. Of the out-of-hospital births, 65% were in the home, 27% in free-standing birth centers, and 2% in clinics or doctor's offices (Martin et al, 2003). Cesarean births increased to 26.1% of live births in the United States in 2002, the highest rate ever in the United States, whereas the rate of vaginal births after cesarean (VBACs) declined to 12.6% (Martin et al, 2003). Women who choose nurse-midwives as their primary providers actively participate in childbirth decisions and receive fewer interventions such as epidural analgesia for labor (Jackson et al, 2003) (Table 1-3).

Changes are occurring in the conduct of the second stage of labor (from 10 cm dilation to birth of the baby); positions are varied, with more emphasis on upright posture. The arbitrary limit of 2 hours for the second stage is less rigid as delayed pushing (waiting until the forces of labor propel the fetus down in the birth canal instead of encouraging pushing as soon as the cervix is 10 cm dilated) is instituted. Delayed pushing conserves the energy of the mother, results in fewer instrumental deliveries, and is less costly. The rates of episiotomy are declining, resulting in fewer severe perineal lacerations. Midwives perform fewer episiotomies than do physicians.

The method of analgesia varies, depending on the condition and choice of the mother and the preferences of the providers. Mothers typically are awake and aware during labor and birth. Contrasting philosophies exist regarding analgesia during labor. Some women prefer to experience the sensations of birth with little or no analgesia; others opt for epidural analgesia to provide comfort and control over their behavior during the experience.

Table 1-3

Percent of Women Receiving Six Obstetric Procedures

PROCEDURE	%
Electronic fetal monitoring	85.2
Ultrasound	68.0
Induction of labor	20.6
Stimulation of labor	17.3
Tocolysis	2.1
Amniocentesis	2.0

Data from Martin JA et al: Births: final data for 2002, *Natl Vital Stat Rep* 52(10):1-114, 2003.

With family-centered care, fathers, partners, grandparents, siblings, and friends may be present for labor and birth. Fathers or partners may be present for cesarean births. Fathers may participate by cutting the umbilical cord (Fig. 1-3). Doulas—trained and experienced female labor attendants—provide a continuous, one-on-one, caring presence throughout the labor and birth. Newborn infants remain with the mother and are encouraged to breastfeed immediately after birth. Parents participate in the care of their infants in nurseries and neonatal intensive care units.

Childbirth education and parenting classes encourage the participation of a support person, teach breathing and relaxation techniques, and give general information about birth, infant development, and parenting. Other classes or parent support groups may be organized for the weeks and months after birth.

In some cases, a woman labors, gives birth, and recovers in the same room (labor-delivery-recovery); she may stay in the same room for the entire birth experience (labor-delivery-recovery-postpartum). Instead of having one nurse care for the baby and another nurse care for the mother, some hospitals have one nurse care for both the mother and baby (couplet or mother-baby care). In some hospitals, central nurseries have been eliminated, and babies "room-in" with their mothers. Many hospitals use lactation consultants to assist mothers with breastfeeding.

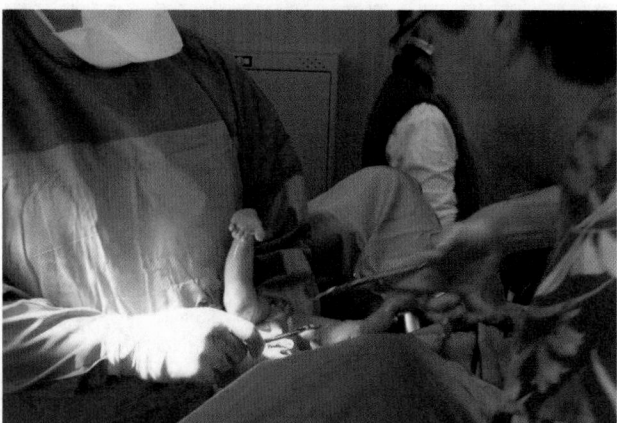

Fig. 1-3 Father cutting cord of his newborn daughter. (Courtesy Tricia Olson, North Ogden, UT.)

Discharge of a mother and baby within 24 hours of birth has created a growing need for follow-up or home care. In some settings, discharge may occur as early as 6 hours after birth. Legislation has been enacted to ensure that mothers and babies are permitted to stay in the hospital at least 48 hours after vaginal birth and 96 hours after cesarean birth. Focused and efficient teaching is necessary to enable the parents and infant to make a safe transition from hospital to home. Nurses may use follow-up telephone calls or home visits to assist families needing information and reassurance.

Neonatal security in the hospital setting is of concern. A number of cases of "baby-napping" and of sending parents home with the wrong baby have been reported. Security systems are being placed in nurseries, and nurses are required to wear photo identification or some other security badge.

Certified Nurse-Midwives

Certified nurse-midwives (CNMs) are registered nurses with education in the two disciplines of nursing and midwifery. Certified midwives (direct-entry midwives) are educated only in the discipline of midwifery. In the United States, certification of midwives is through the American College of Nurse-Midwives, the professional association for midwives in the United States. The Royal College of Midwives is the professional association for midwives in the United Kingdom. In Canada, the Association of Ontario Midwives is the professional association, and the College of Midwives of Ontario is the regulatory body for midwives in Ontario; the other provinces of Canada have similar regulatory bodies. Many national associations belong to the International Confederation of Midwives, which comprises 83 member associations from 70 countries in the Americas and Europe, Africa, and the Asia-Pacific region.

Views of Women

Women must be viewed holistically and in the context in which they live. Their physical, mental, and social factors must be considered because these interdependent components influence health and illness. Even the language health care professionals use to describe women and their problems needs to be examined (Freda, 1995). For example, practitioners describe women who have an "incompetent cervix," who "fail to progress," or who have an "arrest" of labor. They may describe a fetus as having intrauterine growth "retardation." They also "allow" women a "trial" of labor. Freda suggests that practitioners use phrases such as "women who have recurrent premature dilation of the cervix" or "fetuses whose intrauterine growth has been restricted." There is a movement to refer to spontaneous pregnancy loss as a "miscarriage" instead of the more politically charged "abortion," especially when talking to patients (Freda, 1999).

Breastfeeding in the Workplace

Women are a significant proportion of the workforce. Companies are recognizing that it is good business to retain good employees and are making provisions for women returning to work after childbirth. Lactation rooms that provide space and privacy for pumping are available at many work sites and on college campuses (Fig. 1-4). In some instances, breastfeeding women bring their babies to work. Since 1999, by law, women may breastfeed in federal buildings and on federal property. Some states have enacted legislation to ensure that mothers can breastfeed their babies in public places. These efforts may help mothers breastfeed longer and meet the recommendation of the American Academy of Pediatrics that breastfeeding continue for at least 1 year.

Family Leave

The Family and Medical Leave Act of 1993 provides for up to 12 weeks' unpaid leave to eligible employees for birth, adoption, or foster placement; for care of a child, spouse, or parent who is seriously ill; or for the employee's own illness. This is of great benefit to women because they are usually the primary caretakers of family members.

Violence

Violence is a major factor affecting pregnant women. This includes battering (which may increase during pregnancy), rape or other sexual assaults, and attacks with various weapons. Approximately 8% of pregnant women are battered. Violence is associated with complications of pregnancy such as bleeding.

HIV/AIDS in Pregnancy and the Newborn

Cases of perinatally acquired human immunodeficiency virus (HIV) infection and AIDS peaked in 1992; since then the rate of AIDS among infants has continued to decline. Treatment of mothers who tested positive for HIV before giving birth with zidovudine has resulted in a dramatic decrease in the number of infants infected with the virus (Cohan, 2003). Universal HIV testing and access to quality prenatal care will contribute to reducing the transmission of HIV and prolonging survival. For women in labor who have had no prenatal care, rapid HIV testing is available (Cohan, 2003).

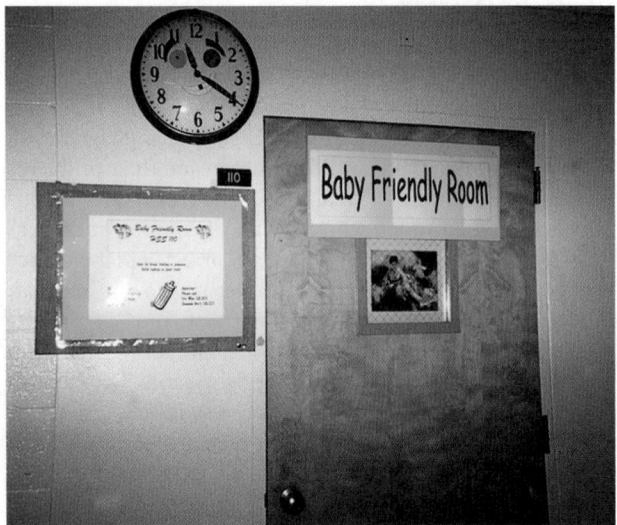

Fig. 1-4 Room on a university campus dedicated to parents and infants. The room contains comfortable furniture, a breast pump, a refrigerator, a baby changing table, and a television and VCR for instructional purposes. The room is available to students, faculty, and staff. (Courtesy Shannon Perry, Phoenix, AZ.)

International Concerns

Female genital mutilation, infibulation, and *circumcision* are terms used to describe procedures in which part or all of the female external genitalia are removed for cultural reasons (Parkin, 2001). Worldwide, many women undergo such procedures. With the growing number of immigrants from Africa and other countries where female genital mutilation is practiced, nurses will increasingly encounter women who have undergone the procedure. The International Council of Nurses and other health professionals have spoken out against the procedures as harmful to women's health.

Healthy People 2010 Goals

Healthy People 2010 is the nation's agenda for improving health. It has two overarching goals: to increase the quality and years of healthy life and to eliminate health disparities. Within *Healthy People 2010,* there are 467 objectives to improve health that are organized into 28 specific focus areas including one related to maternal, infant, and child health (Box 1-5). Current information about the goals of *Healthy People 2010* is available on the Internet at www.health.gov/healthypeople.

Trends in Fertility and Birthrate

Fertility trends and birthrates reflect women's needs for health care. Box 1-6 defines biostatistical terminology useful in analyzing maternity health care. In 2002 the fertility rate, the number of births per 1000 women from 15 to 44 years of age, was 64.8 (Arias et al, 2003). This is a slight decline from the 65.3 live births per 1000 women reported in 2001. The highest birthrates (number of births per 1000 women) were for women between ages 25 and 29 (113.4 per 1000), but the

BOX 1-5

***Healthy People 2010,* Focus Area 16, Maternal, Infant, and Child Health**

Goal: Improve the health and well-being of women, infants, children, and families

Fetal, infant, and child deaths
Maternal death and illness
Prenatal care
Obstetric care
Risk factors
Developmental disabilities and neural tube defects
Prenatal substance exposure
Breastfeeding, newborn screening, and service systems

From US Department of Health and Human Services: *Healthy People 2010* (conference edition, two volumes), Washington, DC, 2000, USDHHS.

BOX 1-6

Maternal-Infant Biostatistical Terminology

Abortus: An embryo or fetus that is removed or expelled from the uterus at 20 weeks of gestation or less, weighs 500 g or less, or measures 25 cm or less
Birthrate: Number of live births in 1 year per 1000 population
Fertility rate: Number of births per 1000 women between the ages of 15 and 44 years (inclusive), calculated on a yearly basis
Infant mortality rate: Number of deaths of infants under 1 year of age per 1000 live births
Maternal mortality rate: Number of maternal deaths from births and complications of pregnancy, childbirth, and puerperium (the first 42 days after termination of the pregnancy) per 100,000 live births
Neonatal mortality rate: Number of deaths of infants under 28 days of age per 1000 live births
Perinatal mortality rate: Number of stillbirths and the number of neonatal deaths per 1000 live births
Stillbirth: An infant who, at birth, demonstrates no signs of life, such as breathing, heartbeat, or voluntary muscle movements

birthrate for women in their forties (8.1 per 1000) continues to increase (Arias et al, 2003). One third (33.8%) of all births in the United States in 2002 were to unmarried women, with much variation in proportion among racial groups (African-American 68%, Hispanic 43.4%, Caucasian 28.4%, non-Hispanic white 22.9%) (Arias et al, 2003). Births to unmarried women are often related to less favorable outcomes, such as low birth weight or preterm birth, because there are typically a large number of teenagers in the unmarried group.

The rates of pregnancy and abortion among adolescents have declined (Martin et al, 2003) but are still higher in the United States than in any other industrialized country (Fig. 1-5).

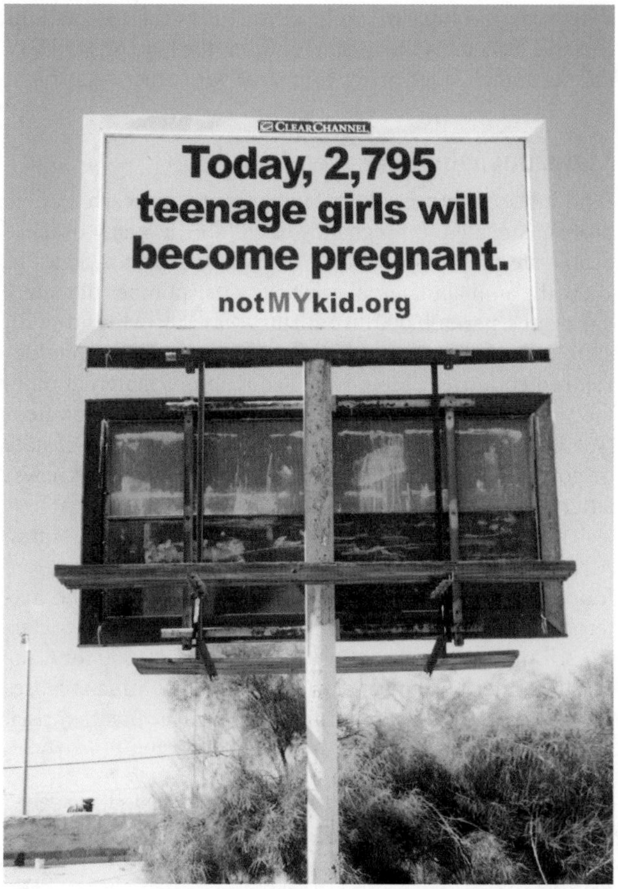
CLEARCHANNEL
Today, 2,795
teenage girls will
become pregnant.
notMYkid.org

Fig. 1-5 Billboard calling attention to problem of teenage pregnancy. (Courtesy Shannon Perry, Phoenix, AZ.)

Incidence of Low Birth Weight

Babies born weighing less than 2500 g are classified as low birth weight (LBW), and their risks for morbidity and mortality increase. In 2002 the incidence of LBW was 7.8%, and the incidence of very low birth weight (VLBW; less than 1500 g) was 1.4% (Arias et al, 2003). There is racial disparity in the incidence of LBW. African-American babies are twice as likely as Caucasian babies to be LBW and to die within the first year of life. By race, the incidence of LBW for African-American births was 13.3%; for Hispanic births, 6.5%; and for Caucasian births, 6.8%. Cigarette smoking is associated with LBW, prematurity, and intrauterine growth restriction. In 2001, 12.0% of pregnant women smoked, a proportion that has declined by 38% since 1989 (Arias et al, 2003).

The proportion of preterm infants (i.e., those born before 38 weeks of gestation) was 17.5% for African-American births, 11.6% for Hispanic births, and 11.1% for Caucasian births (Arias et al, 2003). Multiple births accounted for 3.2% of births in 2001, with most of the increase associated with increased use of fertility drugs and older age at childbearing (Arias et al, 2003).

Infant Mortality in the United States

A common indicator of the adequacy of prenatal care and the health of a nation as a whole is the infant mortality rate, the number of deaths of infants younger than 1 year of age per 1000 live births. The neonatal mortality rate is the number of deaths of infants younger than 28 days of age per 1000 live births. The perinatal mortality rate is the number of stillbirths plus the number of neonatal deaths per 1000 live births. The provisional infant mortality rate for 2002 was 6.9, up slightly from the 2001 rate of 6.8 (Arias et al, 2003). The infant mortality rate continues to be higher for African-American babies (14.0 per 1000) than for Caucasian (5.7 per 1000) and Hispanic (5.5 per 1000) babies (Arias et al, 2003). Limited maternal education, young maternal age, unmarried status, poverty, and lack of prenatal care appear to be associated with higher infant mortality rates. Poor nutrition, smoking and alcohol use, and maternal conditions such as poor health or hypertension are also important contributors to infant mortality. A shift from the current emphasis on high-technology medical interventions to a focus on improving access to preventive care for low-income families is necessary to reduce the disparity.

International Trends in Infant Mortality

The infant mortality rate of Canada (5.3 per 1000 in 1999) ranks sixteenth and that of the United States ranks twenty-sixth when compared with other industrialized nations (Arias et al, 2003). One reason for this is the high rate of LBW infants in the United States compared with other countries.

Maternal Mortality Trends

Worldwide, approximately 1600 women die each day of problems related to pregnancy or childbirth; many of these deaths are preventable (Table 1-4). In the United States in 2000, the annual maternal mortality rate (number of maternal deaths per 100,000 live births) was 9.8 (Minino et al, 2002). The United States is tied for seventeenth among developed countries (Table 1-5). Reduction of maternal mortality rates is a key goal of the Millennium Development Goals endorsed by 189 member states and 149 heads of state or government in December 2000 (*Safe Motherhood* newsletter is back, 2002).

There are significant racial differences in the rates: African-American women have a maternal mortality rate four times higher than that of Caucasian women. The maternal mortality rate was 30 per 100,000 for African-American women, in contrast with 8.1 per 100,000 for Caucasian women (Chang et al, 2003). The predominant causes of these deaths are embolism, hemorrhage, preeclampsia, and infection (Chang et al, 2003). The *Healthy People 2010* goal of 3.3 maternal deaths per 100,000 poses a significant challenge. To achieve this goal, early diagnosis and appropriate intervention must occur. Worldwide strategies to reduce maternal mortality rates include improving access to skilled attendants at birth, providing postabortion care, improving family planning services, and providing adolescents with better reproductive health services (Liljestrand, 2000).

Involving Consumers and Promoting Self-Care

Self-care is appealing to both patients and the health care system because of its potential to reduce health care costs. Maternity care is especially suited to self-care because childbearing is essentially health focused, women are usually well when they enter the system, and visits to health care providers can present the opportunity for health and illness interventions. Measures to improve health and reduce risks associated with poor pregnancy outcomes and illness can be addressed. Topics such as nutrition education, stress management, smoking cessation, alcohol and drug treatment, improvement of social supports, and parenting education are appropriate for such encounters.

Table 1-4

Maternal Mortality per 100,000 Births 1985–1999 in 20 Countries with Highest Rates

COUNTRY	RATE
Mozambique	1100
Malawi	1100
Central African Republic	1100
Eritrea	1000
Guinea-Bissau	910
Chad	830
Zimbabwe	700
Zambia	650
Laos	650
Cote d'Ivoire	600
Niger	590
Kenya	590
Mali	580
Senegal	580
Solomon Islands	550 (approx)
Sudan	550
Mauritania	550 (approx)
Nepal	540
India	540
Guinea	540

Source: Health: maternal mortality. Internet document available at www.nationmaster.com/graph-T/hea_mat_mor (accessed June 22, 2004).

Table 1-5

Maternal Mortality per 100,000 Births 1985–1999 in 20 Countries with Lowest Rates

COUNTRY	RATE
Greece	1
Grenada	1
United Arab Emirates	3
Israel	5
Kuwait	5
Sweden	5
Switzerland	5
Spain	6
Norway	6
Finland	6
Singapore	6
Ireland	6
Croatia	6
Italy	7
United Kingdom	7
Netherlands	7
United States	8
Portugal	8
Germany	8
Poland	8

Source: Health: maternal mortality. Internet document available at www.nationmaster.com/graph-T/hea_mat_mor (accessed June 22, 2004).

Efforts to Reduce Health Disparities

Significant disparities in morbidity and mortality rates are experienced by African-Americans, Native Americans, Hispanics, Alaska Natives, and Asians/Pacific Islanders. Shorter life expectancy, higher infant and maternal mortality rates, more birth defects, and more sexually transmitted infections are found among these groups. The cause-specific mortality ratio was three to four times higher for black women when compared with white women for each cause of death (Chang et al, 2003). The disparities are thought to result from a complex interaction among biologic factors, environment, and health behaviors. Disparities in education and income are associated with differences in occurrence of morbidity and mortality. The National Institutes of Health has a commitment to improve the health of minorities and provides funding for research and training of minority researchers. The National Institute of Nursing Research has included the goal of reducing disparities in its strategic plan and supports research for that purpose. The nation must make a concerted effort to eliminate health disparities.

Health Literacy

Almost half of all American adults have difficulty in understanding and using health information (Nielsen-Bohlman, Panzer, & Kindig, 2004). Health literacy is "the degree to which individuals have the capacity to obtain, process, and understand basic health information and services needed to make appropriate health decisions" (Ratzan & Parker, 2000). Literacy encompasses a set of skills including reading, writing, mathematics, and speech and speech comprehension. Health literacy involves a spectrum of abilities, ranging from reading an appointment slip to interpreting medication instructions. These skills must be assessed routinely to recognize a problem and accommodate patients with limited literacy skills. An excellent resource is *Teaching Patients with Low Literacy Skills,* second edition (Doak, Doak, & Root, 1996).

Individuals and groups for whom English is a second language often lack the skills necessary to seek medical care and function adequately in the health care setting. Lack of English fluency is a barrier, and communication difficulties continue to affect access to care, particularly in such areas as making appointments, applying for services, and obtaining transportation. As a result of the increasingly multicultural U.S. population, there is a more urgent need to address health literacy as a component of culturally and linguistically competent care. Health care providers contribute to health literacy by using simple common words, avoiding jargon, and assessing whether the patient is understanding the discussion. Speaking slowly and clearly and focusing on what is important will increase understanding (Roberts, 2004).

??? Critical Thinking Exercise

HEALTH LITERACY

Maria speaks English as her second language; she speaks Spanish at home. She has been diagnosed with a urinary tract infection. While giving Maria instructions about perineal hygiene and medication administration, the nurse noted that Maria listened intently to her instructions, nodded affirmatively, and looked at the patient information handout.

1. Evidence—Is there sufficient evidence to draw conclusions about Maria's comprehension of the oral and written instructions?
2. Assumptions—What assumptions can be made about patient understanding of information and instructions?
   a. Mode of patient education
   b. Reading and comprehension
   c. Processing of information
   d. Nonverbal language
   e. Clarity and use of words
   f. Use of interpreters
3. What implications and priorities for nursing care can be drawn at this time?
4. Does the evidence objectively support your conclusion?
5. Are there alternative perspectives to your conclusion?

High-Technology Care

Advances in scientific knowledge and the large number of high risk pregnancies have contributed to a health care system that emphasizes high-technology care. Maternity care has extended to preconception counseling, more and better scientific techniques to monitor the mother and fetus, more definitive tests for hypoxia and acidosis, and neonatal intensive care units. Point-of-care testing is available. Personal data assistants are used to enhance comprehensive care (Lewis & Sommers, 2003). Virtually all women are monitored electronically during labor despite the lack of evidence of efficacy of such monitoring.

Telemedicine is an umbrella term for the use of communication technologies and electronic information to provide or support health care when the participants are separated by distance. Telemedicine permits specialists, including nurses, to provide health care and consultation when distance separates them from those needing care. For example, Baby CareLink (Gray et al, 2000) is an Internet-based program that incorporates teleconferencing and the World Wide Web to enhance interactions among health care providers, families, and community providers. It includes distance learning, virtual home visits, and remote monitoring of the infant after discharge. This technology has the potential to save billions of dollars annually for health care.

Strides are being made in identifying genetic codes, and genetic engineering is taking place. In general, high-technology care has flourished while "health" care has been relatively neglected. These technologic advances have also contributed to higher health care costs. Nurses must use caution and prospective planning and assess the effect of the emerging technology.

Community-Based Care

A shift in settings, from acute care institutions to the home, has been occurring. Even childbearing women at high risk are cared for in the home. Technology previously available only in the hospital is now found in the home. This has affected the organizational structure of care, the skills required to provide such care, and the cost to consumers.

Home health care also has a community focus. Nurses are involved in caring for women and infants in homeless shelters, in caring for adolescents in school-based clinics, and in promoting health at community sites, churches, and shopping malls. Nursing education curricula are increasingly community based.

Increase in High Risk Pregnancies

The number of high risk pregnancies has increased, which means that a greater number of women are at risk for poor pregnancy outcomes. Escalating drug use (ranging from 11% to 27% of pregnant women, depending on geographic location) has contributed to higher incidences of prematurity, LBW, congenital defects, learning disabilities, and withdrawal symptoms in infants. Alcohol use in pregnancy has been associated with miscarriages, mental retardation, LBW, and fetal alcohol syndrome.

The two most frequently reported maternal medical risk factors are hypertension associated with pregnancy and diabetes. The birthrate of higher-order multiples (triplet, quadruplet, and greater) rose 2% from 2000 to 2001 (Arias et al, 2003). Multiple births now account for 3.2% of all births (Arias et al, 2003). The cesarean birthrate increased to 26.1% in 2002, with primary cesareans rising to 18.0% and vaginal births after cesarean dropping 23% from 2001 to 12.7% per 100 in 2002 (Arias et al, 2003). This cesarean rate is significantly higher than the *Healthy People 2010* goal of 15%. Births of babies born vaginally assisted with forceps or with vacuum extraction decreased to 5.9%.

High Cost of Health Care

Health care is one of the fastest-growing sectors of the U.S. economy. Even though the United States spends proportionately more on health care than any of the other 190 countries that make up the World Health Organization, it ranks thirty-seventh in quality (Rubin, 2000). A shift in demographics, an increased emphasis on high-cost technology, and the liability costs of a litigious society contribute to the high cost of care. Most researchers agree that the cost of caring for the increased number of LBW infants in neonatal intensive care units contributes significantly to the overall health care costs.

Midwifery care has helped contain some health care costs. However, not all insurance carriers reimburse nurse practitioners and clinical nurse specialists as direct care providers. Nor do they reimburse for all services provided by nurse-midwives, a situation that continues to be a problem. Nurses must become involved in the politics of cost containment because they, as knowledgeable experts, can provide solutions to many of the health care problems at a relatively low cost.

Early postpartum discharge programs also are used to reduce costs. The American Academy of Pediatrics has published minimal criteria for early discharge of a newborn (American Academy of Pediatrics Committee on Fetus and Newborn, 1995) (see Box 21-3).

Limited Access to Care

Barriers to access must be removed so pregnancy outcomes can be improved. The most significant barrier to access is the inability to pay. Lack of transportation and dependent child care are other barriers. In addition to a lack of insurance and high costs, a lack of providers for low-income women exists. Many physicians either refuse to take Medicaid patients or take only a few such patients. This presents a serious problem because a significant proportion of births are to mothers who receive Medicaid.

TRENDS IN NURSING PRACTICE

The increasing complexity of care for maternity and women's health patients has contributed to specialization of nurses working with these patients. This specialized knowledge is gained through experience, advanced degrees, and certification programs. Nurses in advanced practice (e.g., nurse practitioners and nurse-midwives) may provide primary care throughout a woman's life, including during the pregnancy cycle. In some settings, the clinical nurse specialist and nurse practitioner roles are blended, and nurses deliver high-quality, comprehensive, and cost-effective care in a variety of settings. Lactation consultants provide services in the postpartum unit or on an outpatient basis, including home visits.

Nursing Interventions Classification

When the National Institute of Medicine proposed that all patient records be computerized by the year 2000, a need for a common language to describe the contributions of nurses to patient care became evident. Nurses from the University of Iowa developed a comprehensive standardized language that describes interventions that are performed by generalist or specialist nurses. This language is included in the Nursing Interventions Classification (NIC) (Dochterman & Bulechek, 2004). Interventions commonly used by maternal-child nurses include those in Box 1-7.

Evidence-Based Practice

Evidence-based practice—providing care based on evidence gained through research and clinical trials—is being increasingly emphasized. Although not all practice can be evidence based, practitioners must use the best available information on which to base their interventions. The Association of Women's Health, Obstetric, and Neonatal Nurses (AWHONN) *Standards and Guidelines for Professional Nursing Practice in the Care of Women and Newborns* (1998) and the *Standards for Professional Perinatal Nursing Practice and Certification in Canada* (2002) include an evidence-based approach to practice. Discussion of nursing care and evidence-based nursing boxes throughout this text provide examples of evidence-based practice in perinatal nursing.

AWHONN has conducted six research-based practice projects (Box 1-8). These projects were conducted in several

BOX 1-7

Childbearing Care Interventions

Level 1 Domain: Family
Care that supports the family

Level 2 Class: Childbearing Care
Interventions to assist in the preparation for childbirth and management of the psychologic and physiologic changes before, during, and immediately following childbirth

Level 3: Interventions
Amnioinfusion
Birthing
Bleeding reduction: antepartum uterus
Bleeding reduction: postpartum uterus
Breastfeeding assistance
Cesarean section care
Childbirth preparation
Circumcision care
Electronic fetal monitoring: antepartum
Electronic fetal monitoring: intrapartum
Environmental management: attachment process
Family integrity promotion: childbearing family
Family planning: contraception
Family planning: infertility
Family planning: unplanned pregnancy
Fertility preservation
Genetic counseling
Grief work facilitation: perinatal death
High risk pregnancy care
Intrapartal care
Intrapartal care: high risk delivery
Kangaroo care
Labor induction
Labor suppression
Lactation suppression
Newborn care
Newborn monitoring
Nonnutritive sucking
Phototherapy: neonate
Postpartal care
Preconception counseling
Pregnancy termination care
Prenatal care
Reproductive technology management
Resuscitation: fetus
Resuscitation: neonate
Risk identification: childbearing family
Surveillance: late pregnancy
Tube care: umbilical line
Ultrasonography: limited obstetric

From Dochterman JM, Bulechek GM: *Nursing interventions classification (NIC),* ed 4, St Louis, 2004, Mosby.

BOX 1-8

Association of Women's Health, Obstetric, and Neonatal Nurses (AWHONN) Research-Based Practice Programs

Transition of the Preterm Infant to an Open Crib
Management of Women in Second-Stage Labor
Continence for Women
Neonatal Skin Care
Cyclic Pelvic Pain and Discomfort Management
Setting Universal Cessation Counseling, Education, and Screening Standards: Nursing Care for Pregnant Women Who Smoke (SUCCESS)

states, and staff nurses were involved in their implementation and in data collection. The AWHONN practice guidelines incorporate evidence-based practices for second-stage labor management, continence for women, breastfeeding support, midlife well-being, perianesthesia care, neonatal skin care, and cardiac health. By using such guidelines and published reports, nurses can develop protocols and procedures based on published research and incorporate an evidence base into their practice. AWHONN research priorities include the aforementioned topics, as well as family violence, fetal surveillance, genetics, infertility, and early parenting (Box 1-9). The incorporation of research findings into practice is essential in developing a science-based practice.

Introduction to Evidence-Based Practice Reviews

Identifying the Need for a Review. Suppose you are asked to be on a multidisciplinary committee to write a discharge protocol for your maternity unit. As a professional nurse, you read journal articles and individual studies. Some studies say that "early discharge" after birth is beneficial for mother and baby, whereas others say it may be riskier. How do you make sense of all these conflicting findings?

Evidence-based practice review groups systematically examine all relevant research studies on a certain topic and efficiently communicate it to the professionals who make clinical decisions and write protocols for clinical practice. Many studies are too small to be generalizable to the general population. By combining the studies, several smaller studies together achieve more "power," or predictive value. The review by Brown and colleagues (2002), for example, combined eight smaller trials with a total of 3600 women.

To perform a review, the review group starts with a brief *background statement* defining the problem. This is followed by the *objective,* or purpose for the review. The group members ask a list of ideal questions that they would like to see answered by research.

Before they begin the review process, they define their *methods,* or criteria by which they will select and analyze studies. This includes the *search strategy,* usually which *keywords* they used to search databases for relevant articles. They may choose to review only randomized trials, because these are the most generalizable to the larger population. In addition, they may choose only controlled trials (one group gets the intervention and one group, the control, does not), which makes a stronger case that any difference between the groups is actually due to the intervention, and not due to some other influence. *Data (statistical) analysis* describes how the trials will be compared and combined. This would

BOX 1-9

Association of Women's Health, Obstetric, and Neonatal Nurses (AWHONN) Research Priorities for Women's and Neonatal Health

Strategies to Promote Healthy Behaviors in Women Across the Lifespan
- Prevention of unintended pregnancy
- Cardiovascular health, including smoking cessation
- Weight management and nutrition
- Menstrual and menopausal adjustment and symptom management
- Cancer screening and risk reduction
- Chronic illness self-care (e.g., diabetes)
- Social risks (poverty, addiction, sexual risks, violence)
- Promotion of women's mental health and stress management

Reducing Health Disparities
- Delivering culturally competent care
- Enhancing access to and utilization of health care
- Reducing disparities in rates of low birth weight
- Improving breastfeeding rates among low-income and minority women
- Reducing genetically determined risk through appropriate screening

Models of Nursing Care Delivery
- Strategies to increase diversity of the nursing workforce
- Effect of workforce diversity on patient outcomes
- Comparative studies of quality, patient outcomes, and cost across the following:
  - Providers (physicians, nurses, advanced practice nurses)
  - Delivery settings (medical centers, birth centers, primary care, home care)
  - Practice decisions and decision making (levels and types of clinical decision making and interventions)
  - Staff development and support models
  - Models of care delivery in prenatal and antepartum care

Approved by AWHONN Research Committee, July 2001.

be easy if all the studies used the same definitions and measured the same outcomes, but this is rare. Reviewers rely on creativity and common sense to compare and contrast the studies. Sometimes, they just have to report that it is comparing apples to oranges. In the Evidence-Based Practice box, the studies ranged from 1962 to 2000 and were from North America, Sweden, the United Kingdom, and Australia. The standard length of stay after normal birth ranged from 2 to 5 days, and early discharge ranged from 6 hours to 4 days, so considerable overlap prevented some calculations from all the studies together. In this case, the reviewers combined studies with similar definitions.

Findings are determined by whether the difference between the control and intervention group is significant. This means that the difference between two groups was large enough that it cannot be accounted for by chance alone. The difference between groups may be due to the intervention, or to some third factor, but the chance of it occurring randomly is very small. For example, in the cited review, the studies were pooled to find the overall readmission rate for new mothers who were discharged early, compared to mothers who had standard length of stay. The difference between groups fell within the same range as 95% of any other two groups in the population, and therefore may be due to chance alone. Therefore the readmission rates for early versus standard discharge mothers were not significantly different.

Limitations identify the weaknesses of the studies and of the overall review. There are *always* limitations in the research process. In the case of this review, the varied definitions of "early discharge" from study to study made comparison a challenge. There were also differences between studies in what prenatal education and postpartum follow-up visits were offered. Randomization was compromised, because some women decided not to stick with their assigned length of stay, or they developed problems, necessitating longer stays. This may have introduced some bias, or uncontrolled influence, on the results.

Conclusions are sometimes surprising. This is the review committee's best recommendations for clinical practice, based on the best available evidence. Reviewers may find that some of our long-standing assumptions about clinical care are not beneficial, or may even be harmful for mother or baby. In this review, the trend was toward improvement in most outcome measures with early discharge, but there were no statistically significant differences. Therefore the conclusion is that early discharge appears to do no harm, but adverse outcomes cannot be ruled out, due to limitations in the studies. *Implications for practice* includes some of the ways that these conclusions can be integrated into clinical nursing practice. *Implications for further research* provides guidance for future research questions and methods.

Cochrane Pregnancy and Childbirth Database

The Cochrane Pregnancy and Childbirth Database was first planned in 1976 with a small grant from the World Health Organization to Dr. Iain Chalmers and colleagues at Oxford. In 1993, the Cochrane Collaboration was formed, and the Oxford Database of Perinatal Trials became known as the Cochrane Pregnancy and Childbirth Database. The Cochrane Collaboration oversees up-to-date, systematic reviews of randomized controlled trials of health care and disseminates these reviews. The premise of the project is that these types of studies provide the most reliable evidence about the effects of care.

The evidence from these studies should encourage practitioners to implement useful measures and to abandon those that are useless or harmful. Studies are ranked in six categories:

1. Beneficial forms of care
2. Forms of care that are likely to be beneficial
3. Forms of care with a trade-off between beneficial and adverse effects
4. Forms of care with unknown effectiveness

Evidence-Based Practice

EARLY POSTNATAL DISCHARGE OF HEALTHY MOTHERS AND BABIES

Background

Since the 1970s the trend has been toward shorter postpartum length of stay. Current average stays in the United States are typically 12 to 24 hours for uncomplicated vaginal births and 48 to 72 hours for uncomplicated cesarean births. Many have debated the consequences to mothers and babies of this change in practice. Risks include delay in detecting maternal and infant morbidity, readmission of mothers and babies, breastfeeding problems, decreased maternal satisfaction in care, and decreased confidence in infant care. Advantages include family-centered bonding, better sleep for the mother in her own home, decreased exposure to nosocomial infections for mother and baby, increased maternal satisfaction in care, and decreased cost.

Objectives

Specific research questions include identifying whether early postnatal discharge leads to any of the following:

1. Increased maternal or infant readmissions or physical problems
2. Increased maternal fatigue, depression, or anxiety
3. Breastfeeding problems
4. Change in maternal satisfaction levels with health care
5. Increased paternal anxiety
6. Increased costs, including any prenatal teaching and support following discharge

Methods

Search Strategy

The search strategy included searching in the Cochrane, Medline, CINAHL, and EMBASE databases. Search keywords were *postnatal care, postpartum, puerpera, childbirth, length of stay, discharge, hospitalization,* and *readmission.*

The reviewers selected eight randomized, controlled studies, involving a total of 3600 women and their babies. The studies were published from 1962 to 2000 and involved Australia, Canada, the United States, the United Kingdom, and Sweden. All studies had some cointervention to accompany early discharge, such as antenatal education and postdischarge midwife or nurse visits or calls.

Statistical Analysis

Reviewers independently analyzed the studies and then met to resolve disagreements. "Early" and "standard" time frames overlapped, so the reviewers agreed to accept the "standard" of the setting of each study. Statistical analysis enabled comparison of outcomes, such as readmissions or breastfeeding problems, of early versus standard discharge patients (using the standards of that particular study).

Findings

The reviewers found no significant differences between early versus standard discharge groups in numbers of readmissions of infants or mothers. One study found significantly increased depression scores (indicating more depression) in the standard discharge group at 1 month. There was no significant difference in maternal fatigue. Both groups were the most exhausted the day after discharge.

Early discharge mothers were more confident at 1 week, but there was no difference between the groups by 1 month.

Trends were mixed for breastfeeding, which may reflect the cultural differences of the time frame (1950s to present) and countries. The reviewers identified no significant differences.

There was a trend toward higher maternal satisfaction with care in the early discharge group that was not statistically significant.

Fathers spent significantly more time with the baby who was discharged early. No data about paternal anxiety were found.

One study showed that early discharge cost was considerably less than standard care, even with the costs of multiple home visits and acute care visits factored in.

Limitations

Many studies had low recruitment rates (only 24% to 44%) and high exclusion rates after randomization and withdrawals for reasons such as not following the assigned protocol. Some women changed their minds about their length of stay or developed problems and stayed longer. Cointerventions included some combination of prenatal education and from one to seven postnatal visits by midwives or nurses. Available postnatal primary and specialist medical support varied. Definitions of "standard" versus "early" discharge overlapped. The three studies that measured depression scores did not use validated depression screening tools. The studies were too heterogeneous to assess breastfeeding success or maternal satisfaction with care. Few studies reported costs.

Conclusions

The review committee found no evidence of adverse outcomes from early discharge. However, methodologic limitations may obscure adverse outcomes.

Implications for Practice

Health care providers can include in their prenatal education the information that all women feel the most exhausted on the first day after discharge. Maternal confidence seems to increase with time after discharge. Early discharge may allow more time for paternal bonding before the father must return to work.

Implications for Further Research

The authors call for large, well-designed trials, using standardized approaches, factoring in the likely attrition rates. Much remains to be clarified in further research regarding the importance of postdischarge nursing and midwifery care.

Reference

Brown S et al: Early postnatal discharge from hospital for healthy mothers and term infants (Cochrane Review), 2002. In *The Cochrane Library,* Issue 2, Chichester, UK, 2004, John Wiley & Sons.

5. Forms of care that are unlikely to be beneficial
6. Forms of care that are likely to be ineffective or harmful

Practices that have been reviewed by the Collaboration are identified with a symbol (⊞) throughout this text.

Outcomes-Oriented Practice

Outcomes of care (that is, the effectiveness of interventions and quality of care) are receiving increased emphasis. Outcomes-oriented care measures effectiveness of care against benchmarks or standards. It is a measure of the value of nursing using quality indicators and answers the question, "Did the patient benefit or not benefit from the care provided?" (Moorhead, Johnson, & Maas, 2004). The Outcome Assessment Information Set (OASIS) is an example of an outcome system important for nursing. Its use is required by the Centers for Medicare and Medicaid Services, formerly the Health Care Financing Administration (HCFA), in all home health organizations that are Medicare accredited. The Nursing Outcomes Classification (NOC) is

Table 1-6

Nursing Outcomes Classification (NOC)

TAXONOMY

Level 1: Domain IV—Health Knowledge and Behavior

Outcomes that describe attitudes, comprehension, and actions with respect to health and illness

Level 2: Q—Health Behavior

Outcomes that describe an individual's actions to promote, maintain, or restore health

Level 3: 1607—Prenatal Health Behavior

Care Recipient: Data Source:

Scale(s)—*Never demonstrated* to *Consistently demonstrated* (m)

Definition: Personal actions to promote a healthy pregnancy and a healthy newborn

OUTCOME TARGET RATING: Maintain at ________ Increase to ________

Prenatal Health Behavior Overall Rating		**Never demonstrated 1**	**Rarely demonstrated 2**	**Sometimes demonstrated 3**	**Often demonstrated 4**	**Consistently demonstrated 5**	**NA**
Indicators:							
160701	Maintains healthy preconceptual state	1	2	3	4	5	NA
160702	Uses proper body mechanics	1	2	3	4	5	NA
160703	Keeps appointments for prenatal care	1	2	3	4	5	NA
160704	Maintains healthy weight gain pattern	1	2	3	4	5	NA
160705	Receives proper dental care	1	2	3	4	5	NA
160706	Uses seat belt appropriately	1	2	3	4	5	NA
160707	Attends childbirth education classes	1	2	3	4	5	NA
160709	Participates in regular exercise	1	2	3	4	5	NA
160710	Maintains adequate nutrient intake for pregnancy	1	2	3	4	5	NA
160711	Practices safe sex	1	2	3	4	5	NA
160721	Uses medications as prescribed	1	2	3	4	5	NA
160712	Consults health care professional concerning use of non-prescription drugs	1	2	3	4	5	NA
160713	Avoids environmental hazards	1	2	3	4	5	NA
160714	Avoids exposure to infectious diseases	1	2	3	4	5	NA
160715	Avoids recreational drugs	1	2	3	4	5	NA
160716	Abstains from alcohol	1	2	3	4	5	NA
160717	Abstains from tobacco use	1	2	3	4	5	NA
160718	Avoids teratogenic agents	1	2	3	4	5	NA
160719	Avoids abusive situations	1	2	3	4	5	NA

Outcome Content References: Bell R, O'Neill M: Exercise and pregnancy: a review, *Birth* 21(2):85-95, 1994; Crowell DT: Weight change in the postpartum period: a review of the literature, *J Nurs Midwifery* 40(5):418-423, 1995; Freda MC et al: What pregnant women want to know: a comparison of client and provider perceptions, *J Obstet Gynecol Neonatal Nurs* 22(3):237, 1993; Kearney MH et al: Salvaging self: a grounded theory of pregnancy on crack cocaine, *Nurs Res* 44(4):208-213, 1995; McFarlane J et al: Abuse during pregnancy: associations with maternal health and infant birth weight, *Nurs Res* 45(1):37-42, 1996; Olds S et al: *Maternal-newborn nursing: a family-centered approach*, ed 5, Menlo Park, CA, 1996, Addison-Wesley; Shapiro HR: Prenatal education in the work place, *AWHONN's Clin Issues Perinat Women's Health Nurs* 4(1):113-121, 1993; Summers L: Preconception care: an opportunity to maximize health in pregnancy, *J Nurs Midwifery* 38(4):188-198, 1993.

Source: Moorhead S, Johnson M, Maas M: *Nursing Outcomes Classification (NOC)*, ed 3, St Louis, 2004, Mosby.

BOX 1-10

Strategic Directions for Nursing and Midwifery Services

Health and human resource planning
Management of health personnel
Evidence-based practice
Education
Stewardship and regulation

Source: Al-Gasseer N, Persaud V: Measuring progress in nursing and midwifery globally, *J Nurs Sch* 35(4):309-315, 2003.

an effort to identify outcomes and related measures that can be used for evaluation of care of individuals, families, and communities across the care continuum (Moorhead et al, 2004). An example of outcomes classification is provided in Table 1-6.

Best Practices as Goal of Care

A program or service that has been recognized for excellence is considered to be a best practice. A best practice must provide a better or a new way to achieve goals and be sound from operational, clinical, and financial perspectives. To determine best practices, information is collected from similar institutions. Staff members then identify solutions that have been successful in addressing specific needs and select one that incorporates the best resolutions of the problem that fit the agency's unique population and mission characteristics. The agency continually compares its performance against the best in the industry and the best of a specific function.

Clinical Benchmarking

Clinical benchmarking is a process used to compare one's own performance against the performance of the best in an area of service. Benchmarking supports and promotes continual quality improvement and helps the organization remain competitive in the health care market.

The Best Practices Network uses collaborative benchmarking, which involves sharing strategies and outcomes and leads to the development of new best practices (Reclaiming benchmarking, 1999/2000). Areas of practice routinely monitored in perinatal nursing include hospital length of stay, maternal mortality rate, infant mortality rate, cesarean birthrate, epidural rate, and episiotomy rate.

A Global Perspective

Advances in medicine and nursing have resulted in increased knowledge and understanding in the care of mothers and infants and reduced perinatal morbidity and mortality rates. However, these advances have affected predominantly the industrialized nations. For example, the majority of the 3.2 million children living with HIV or AIDS acquired the infection through perinatal transmission and live in sub-Saharan Africa. This illustrates the inequities that exist between industrialized and resource-poor parts of the world

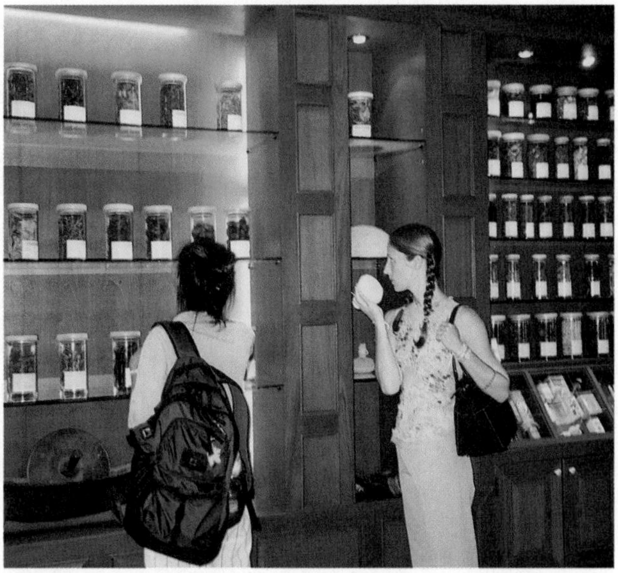

Fig. 1-6 U.S. nursing students examining herbal remedies in a traditional medicine museum in Thailand as part of an international perspectives in nursing course. (Courtesy Shannon Perry, Phoenix, AZ.)

(Cohan, 2003). The World Health Organization and partners in nursing developed Strategic Directions for Nursing and Midwifery Services (Box 1-10). Action in the key areas identified will promote health and reduce disability, morbidity, and mortality (Al-Gasseer & Persaud, 2003).

As the world becomes smaller because of travel and communication technologies, nurses and other health care providers are gaining a global perspective and participating in activities to improve the health and health care of people worldwide (Katz & Hirsch, 2003). Nurses participate in medical outreach, providing obstetric, surgical, ophthalmologic, orthopedic, or other services; attend international meetings; conduct research; and provide international consultation. International student and faculty exchanges occur (Fig. 1-6). More articles about health and health care in various countries are appearing in nursing journals. Several schools of nursing in the United States are World Health Organization Collaborating Centers.

STANDARDS OF PRACTICE AND LEGAL ISSUES IN DELIVERY OF CARE

Nursing standards of practice in perinatal nursing have been described by several organizations, including the American Nurses Association (ANA), which publishes standards for maternal-child health nursing; AWHONN, which publishes standards of practice and education for perinatal nurses (Box 1-11); the American College of Nurse Midwives (ACNM), which publishes standards of practice for midwives; and the National Association of Neonatal Nurses (NANN), which publishes standards of practice for neonatal nurses. These standards reflect current knowledge, represent levels of practice agreed on by leaders in the specialty, and can be used for clinical benchmarking.

BOX 1-11

Standards of Care for Women and Newborns

Standards That Define the Nurse's Responsibility to the Patient

Assessment
Collection of health data of the woman or newborn

Diagnosis
Analysis of data to determine nursing diagnosis

Outcome Identification
Identification of expected outcomes that are individualized

Planning
Development of a plan of care

Implementation
Performance of interventions for the plan of care

Evaluation
Evaluation of the effectiveness of interventions in relation to expected outcomes

Standards of Professional Performance That Delineate Roles and Behaviors for Which the Professional Nurse Is Accountable

Quality of Care
Systemic evaluation of nursing practice

Peformance Appraisal
Self-evaluation in relation to professional practice standards and other regulations

Education
Participation in ongoing educational activities to maintain knowledge for practice

Collegiality
Contribution to the development of peers, students, and others

Ethics
Use of Code for Nurses to guide practice

Collaboration
Involvement of patient, significant others, and other health care providers in the provision of patient care

Research
Use of research findings in practice

Resource Utilization
Consideration of factors related to safety, effectiveness, and costs in planning and delivering patient care

Practice Environment
Contribution to the environment of care delivery

Accountability
Legal and professional responsibility for practice

Source: Association of Women's Health, Obstetric, and Neonatal Nurses (AWHONN): *Standards and guidelines for professional nursing practice in the care of women and newborns,* ed 5, Washington, DC, 1998, AWHONN.

In addition to these more formalized standards, agencies have their own policy and procedure books that outline standards to be followed in that setting. In legal terms, the standard of care is that level of practice that a reasonably prudent nurse would provide. In determining legal negligence, the care given is compared with the standard of care. If the standard was not met and harm resulted, negligence occurred. The number of legal suits in the perinatal area has typically been high. As a consequence, malpractice insurance costs are high for physicians, nurse-midwives, and nurses who work in labor and delivery.

LEGAL TIP **Standard of Care** When you are uncertain about how to perform a procedure, consult the agency procedure book and follow the guidelines printed therein. These guidelines are the standard of care for that agency. ■

Risk Management

Risk management is an evolving process that identifies risks, establishes preventive practices, develops reporting mechanisms, and delineates procedures for managing lawsuits. Nurses should be familiar with concepts of risk management and their implications for nursing practice. These concepts can be viewed as systems of checks and balances that ensure high-quality patient care from preconception until after birth. Effective risk management minimizes the risk of injury to patients and the number of lawsuits against nurses. Each facility or site develops site-specific risk management procedures based on accepted standards and guidelines. The procedures and guidelines must be reviewed periodically (Brott, 2000).

To decrease risk of errors in the administration of medications, the Joint Commission on Accreditation of Healthcare Organizations has developed a list of abbreviations, acronyms, and symbols *not* to use (Table 1-7).

ETHICAL ISSUES IN PERINATAL NURSING

Ethical concerns and debates have multiplied with the increased use of technology and with scientific advances. For example, with reproductive technology, pregnancy is now possible in women who thought they would never bear children, including some who are menopausal or postmenopausal. Should scarce resources be devoted to achieving pregnancies in older women? Is giving birth to a child at an older age worth the risks involved? Should older parents be encouraged to conceive a baby when they may not live to see the child reach adulthood? Should a woman who is HIV-positive have access to assisted reproduction services? Should third-party payers assume the costs of reproductive technology? With induced ovulation and in vitro fertilization, multiple pregnancies occur, and multifetal pregnancy reduction (selectively terminating one or more fetuses) may be considered. Innovations such as intrauterine fetal surgery, fetoscopy, therapeutic insemination, genetic engineering, stem cell research, surrogate childbearing, surgery for infer-

Table 1-7

JCAHO "Do Not Use" List

ABBREVIATION	POTENTIAL PROBLEM	PREFERRED TERM
U (for unit)	Mistaken as zero, four, or cc.	Write "unit."
IU (for international unit)	Mistaken as IV (intravenous) or 10 (ten).	Write "international unit."
Q.D., Q.O.D. (Latin abbreviations for once daily and every other day)	Mistaken for each other. The period after the Q can be mistaken for an "I." The "O" can be mistaken for "I."	Write "daily" and "every other day."
Trailing zero (X.0 mg); lack of leading zero (.X mg)	Decimal point is missed.	Never write a zero by itself after a decimal point (X mg), and always use a zero before a decimal point (0.X mg).
MS MSO_4 $MgSO_4$	Confused for one another. Can mean morphine sulfate or magnesium sulfate.	Write "morphine sulfate" or "magnesium sulfate."

Source: "Do not use" list required in 2004, *LTC Update,* Issue 3, 2003.

tility, "test-tube" babies, fetal research, and treatment of VLBW babies have resulted in questions about informed consent and allocation of resources. The introduction of long-acting contraceptives has created moral choices and policy dilemmas for health care providers and legislators; that is, should some women (substance abusers, women with low incomes, or women who are HIV positive) be required to take the contraceptives? With the potential for great good that can come from fetal tissue transplantation, what research is ethical? What are the rights of the embryo? Should cloning of humans be permitted? Discussion and debate about these issues will continue for many years. Nurses and patients, as well as scientists, physicians, attorneys, lawmakers, ethicists, and clergy, must be involved in the discussions.

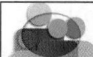

Community Focus

REPRODUCTIVE HEALTH

Examine a daily newspaper for 7 days. Identify articles reporting topics related to maternity or reproductive health.

- How many articles did you identify? What are the topics? Are they local or national issues?
- Is the reporter a health reporter, local or national columnist, male or female?
- What is the "slant" of the articles? Are the reports favorable to women and reproductive health? Does the tenor of the articles limit reproductive freedom or infringe on women's rights?
- What conclusions can you draw related to the treatment of women's issues and reproductive health in your community?

RESEARCH IN PERINATAL NURSING

Research plays a vital role in the establishment of a maternity nursing science. Nurses should promote research funding and conduct research on maternity and women's health, especially concerning the effectiveness of nursing strategies for these patients. Research can validate that nursing care makes a difference. For example, although prenatal care is clearly associated with healthier infants, no one knows exactly which nursing interventions produce this outcome. Many possible areas of research exist in maternity and women's health care. The clinician can identify problems in the health and health care of women and infants. Through research, nurses can make a difference for these patients.

Ethical Guidelines for Nursing Research

Nurses must protect the rights of human subjects (that is, patients) in all of their research. For example, nurses may collect data on or care for patients who are participating in clinical trials. The nurse ensures that the particpants are fully informed and aware of their rights as subjects. Research with perinatal patients may create ethical dilemmas for the nurse. For example, participating in research may cause additional stress to a woman concerned about outcomes of genetic testing or one who is waiting for an invasive procedure. Obtaining amniotic fluid samples or performing cordocentesis poses risks to the fetus. The nurse may be involved in determining whether the benefits of research outweigh the risks to the mother and the fetus. Following the ANA ethical guidelines in the conduct, dissemination, and implementation of nursing research helps nurses ensure that research is conducted ethically (Silva, 1995).

Key Points

- Maternity nursing focuses on women and their infants and families during the childbearing cycle.
- Nurses caring for women can play an active role in shaping health care systems to be responsive to the needs of contemporary women.
- Childbirth practices have changed to become more family-focused and to allow alternatives in care.
- Canada ranks sixteenth and the United States ranks twenty-sixth among industrialized nations in infant mortality.

- Integrative medicine combines modern technology with ancient healing practices and encompasses the whole of body, mind, and spirit.
- Evidence-based practice, outcomes orientation, best practices, and clinical benchmarking are emphasized in current practice.
- *Healthy People 2010* provides goals for maternal and infant health.
- Ethical concerns have multiplied with increasing use of technology and scientific advances.

Answer Guidelines to Critical Thinking Exercise

Health Literacy

1. No. The nurse should assess Maria's understanding of the instructions.
2. (a) Patients must be able to read and understand written information if the nurse is relying on that mode of patient education. (b) Reading—looking at the written instructions does not indicate that Maria can read or understand English or can comprehend the information that is in the material. (c) Patients of different cultures may process information differently. (d) Patients' nonverbal language may vary based on their culture. (e) Patients are more likely to understand information if it is given clearly and slowly, while using simple and common words. (f) Interpreters (unless professional) may not interpret completely and accurately.
3. Maria must receive information about perineal hygiene and taking her prescribed medications. She must have information about contraindications and side effects of the medication. She needs to know when to call her health care provider.
4. Yes. Standards of practice guide patient education and administration of medication.
5. Sensitivity to diversity and culture is necessary in a setting where patients are from a variety of cultures and speak other languages. Interpreters who are not family members should be available; patients have the right to an interpreter. Nurses in this type of setting should increase their language capabilities and work with other staff to prepare patient education materials in a variety of languages to meet the needs of the patients they see.

Resources

Alternative Health News Online
www.altmedicine.com

Alternative Medicine Foundation
www.amfoundation.org

Alternative Medicine: Health Care Information Resources
www-hsl.mcmaster.ca/tomflem/altmed.hyml

American College of Nurse Midwives
www.acnm.org

American Massage Therapy Association
www.amtamassage.org/health_pract.html

Ask NOAH: Complementary and Alternative Medicine
www.noah-health.org/english/alternative/alternative.html

Association of Nurse Advocates for Childbirth Solutions
www.anacs.org/html/index/php

Birthing from Within
www.birthpower.com

CAM on PubMEd
www.nlm.nih.gov/nccam/camonpubmed.html

Childbirth.Org
www.childbirth.org

Doulas of North America
www.dona.org

Emerging Infectious Diseases (Centers for Disease Control and Prevention)
www.cdc.gov/ncidod/eid/index.htm

Global Health Council
www.globalhealthcouncil.org

HerbMed
www.herbmed.org

Homebirth Information
www.changesurfer.com/hlth/homebirth.html

International Council of Nurses (ICN)
www.icn.ch

Internet Health Library
www.internethealthlibrary.com

MEDLINEplus: Alternative Medicine
www.nlm.nih.gov/medlineplus/alternative medicine.html

Midwives Alliance of North America
www.mana.org

National Association of Childbearing Centers
www.birthcenters.org

National Center for Complementary and Alternative Medicine
P.O. Box 8218
Silver Spring, MD 20907-8218
888-644-6226
nccam.nih.gov/nccam

Ounce of Prevention Fund
122 S. Michigan Avenue, Suite 2050
Chicago, IL 60603-6107
312-922-3863
www.ounceofprevention.org

The Alternative Medicine Homepage
www.pitt.edu/~cbw/altm.html

The Natural Pharmacist
www.tnp.com

The Office of Dietary Supplements
Dietary-supplements.info.nih.gov/

Touch Research Institutes (University of Miami, School of Medicine)
www.miami.edu/touch-research/

Virtual Library on International Development
www.acdi-cida.gc.ca/virtual.nsf

UNICEF
www.unicef.org

Waterbirth International
Waterbirth.org/spa/index.php

WholeHealthMD
www.wholehealthmd.com

Wholenurse Alternative and Holistic Webcenters
www.wholenurse.com

World Health Organization (WHO)
www.who.org

References

Al-Gasseer N, Persaud V: Measuring progress in nursing and midwifery globally, *J Nurs Sch* 35(4):309-315, 2003.

American Academy of Pediatrics Committee on Fetus and Newborn: hospital stay for healthy term newborns, *Pediatrics* 96(4 pt 1):788-790, 1995.

Arias E et al: Annual summary of vital statistics—2002, *Pediatrics* 112(6 pt 1):1215-1230, 2003.

Association of Women's Health, Obstetric, and Neonatal Nurses (AWHONN): *Standards and guidelines for professional nursing practice in the care of women and newborns,* ed 5, Washington, DC, 1998, AWHONN.

Association of Women's Health, Obstetric, and Neonatal Nurses (AWHONN): *Standards for professional perinatal nursing practice and certification in Canada,* Washington, DC, 2002, AWHONN.

Barrett B: Alternative, complementary, and conventional medicine: is integration upon us? *J Altern Complement Med* 9(3):417-427, 2003.

Brott L: Risk management and obstetrics, *Community Health Forum* 1(1):54-57, 2000.

Brown S et al: Early postnatal discharge from hospital for healthy mothers and term infants (Cochrane Review), 2002. In *The Cochrane Library,* Issue 2, Chichester, UK, 2004, John Wiley & Sons.

Chang J et al: Pregnancy-related mortality surveillance—United States, 1991-1999, *Morb Mortal Wkly Rep Surveill Summ* 52(SS02):1-8, 2003.

Cohan D: Perinatal HIV: special considerations, *Top HIV Med* 11(6):200-213, 2003.

"Do not use" list required in 2004: LTC Update, Issue 3. Internet document available at www.jcaho.org/accredited+organizations/long+term+care/ltc+update/2003 issue3/npsg_04.htm (accessed April 4, 2004.)

Doak CC, Doak LG, Root JH: *Teaching patients with low literacy skills,* ed 2, Philadelphia, 1996, JB Lippincott.

Dochterman JM, Bulechek GM: *Nursing interventions classification (NIC),* ed 4, St Louis, 2004, Mosby.

Dossey BM: Holistic modalities and healing moments, *Am J Nurs* 98(6):44-47, 1998.

Eisenberg DM et al: Trends in alternative medicine use in the United States, 1990-1997: results of a follow-up national survey, *JAMA* 280(18):1569-1575, 1998.

Freda MC: Arrest, trial, and failure, *J Obstet Gynecol Neonatal Nurs* 24(5):393-394, 1995.

Freda MC: MCN editorial: the power of words, *MCN Am J Matern Child Nurs* 24(1):63, 1999.

Gray JE et al: Baby CareLink: using the Internet and telemedicine to improve care for high-risk infants, *Pediatrics* 106(6):1318-1324, 2000.

Hawks JH, Moyad MA: CAM: Definition and classification overview, *Urol Nurs* 23(3):221-223, 2003.

Jackson DJ et al: Outcomes, safety and resource utilization in a collaborative care birth center program compared with traditional physician-based perinatal care, *Am J Public Health* 93(6):999-1006, 2003.

Katz JR, Hirsch AM: When global health is local health, *Am J Nurs* 103(1):75-79, 2003.

Lewis JA, Sommers CO: Personal data assistants: using new technology to enhance nursing practice, *MCN Am J Matern Child Nurs* 28(2):66-73, 2003.

Liljestrand J: Strategies to reduce maternal mortality worldwide, *Curr Opin Obstet Gynecol* 12(6):513-517, 2000.

Martin JA et al: Births: final data for 2002, *Natl Vital Stat Rep* 52(10):1-114, 2003.

Marwick C: A total of 58 million Americans lack health insurance, *BMJ* 325(7366):678, 2002.

Minino A et al: Deaths: final data for 2000, *Natl Vital Stat Rep* 50(15):1-119, 2002.

Moorhead S, Johnson M, Maas ML: *Nursing outcomes classification (NOC),* ed 3, St Louis, 2004, Mosby.

National Center for Complementary and Alternative Medicine (NCCAM): 2002. Internet document available at nccam.nih.gov (accessed November 25, 2004).

Nielsen-Bohlman L, Panzer AM, Kindig DA, eds: *Health literacy: a prescription to end confusion* (pp. 31-58), Washington, DC, 2004, Institute of Medicine.

Parkin J: Female genital mutilation: a midwife's perspective, *Br J Midwifery* 9(7):421-424, 2001.

Ratzan SC, Parker RM: Introduction. In Selden CR et al, eds: *National Library of Medicine current bibliographies in medicine: health literacy,* vol NLM, pub no CBM 2000-1, Bethesda, MD, 2000, National Institutes of Health, US Department of Health and Human Services.

Reclaiming benchmarking for clinicians, *AWHONN Lifelines* 3(6):41, 1999/2000.

Reinhardt UE, Hussey PS, Anderson GF: U.S. Health care spending in an international context, *Health Affairs* (Millwood) 23(3):10-25, 2004.

Roberts K: Simplify, simplify: tackling health literacy by addressing reading literacy, *Am J Nurs* 104(3):118-119, 2004.

Rubin R: U.S. ranks 37th in health care, *USA Today,* June 21, 2000, p 1.

Safe Motherhood newsletter is back, *Safe Mother* 29(1):1, 2002.

Silva M: *Ethical guidelines in the conduct, dissemination, and implementation of nursing research,* Washington, DC, 1995, American Nurses Association.

US Census Bureau: U.S. interim projections by age, sex, race, and Hispanic origin. Internet document available at www.census.gov/ipc/www/usinterimproj/ (accessed April 13, 2004).

US Department of Health and Human Services (USDHHS): *Healthy People 2010* (conference edition in two volumes), Washington, DC, 2000, USDHHS.

Verhoef M, Findlay B: Maturation of complementary and alternative healthcare in Canada, *Healthc Pap* 3(5):56-61, 2003.

World Health Organization: *Traditional medicine: growing needs and potential, WHO Policy Perspectives on Medicine,* Geneva, No. 2, May 2002, WHO. Internet document available at www.who.int/medicines/organization/trm/orgtrmmain.htm (accessed November 25, 2004).

Unit 1

2 The Family and Culture

LEARNING OBJECTIVES

On completion of this chapter the reader will be able to:

- Describe the main characteristics of contemporary family forms.
- Identify key factors influencing family health.
- Explain family functions that contribute to the well-being of its members and society.
- Explain family dynamics and how family dynamics contribute to accomplishing family functions.
- Compare theoretic approaches for working with childbearing families.
- Relate the impact of culture on childbearing families.
- Discuss cultural competence in relation to one's own nursing practice.

ELECTRONIC RESOURCES

Additional information related to the content in Chapter 2 can be found on

the companion website at evolve
http://evolve.elsevier.com/Wong/maternal/
- NCLEX Review Questions
- WebLinks

or the interactive student CD-ROM
Activities for Chapter 2 include the following:
- NCLEX Review Questions
- Critical Thinking Exercise–Cultural Health and the Family
- Nursing Care Plan–Incorporating the Infant into the Family
- Nursing Care Plan–The Family Newly Immigrated

THE FAMILY IN CULTURAL AND COMMUNITY CONTEXT

The family and its cultural context play an important role in defining the work of maternity nurses. Family structure and function, care-seeking behavior, and relationships with providers are all influenced by culturally related health beliefs and values. Ultimately all of these factors have the power to affect maternal and child health outcomes. It is therefore important to recognize these influences, discuss current trends in families, and explore nursing implications.

DEFINING FAMILY

The family has traditionally been viewed as the primary unit of socialization, the basic structural unit within a community. Family is "the primary institution in society that preserves and transmits culture" (Chen & Rankin, 2002). Family also plays a pivotal role in health care, representing the primary target of health care delivery for maternal and newborn nurses. Most models of health behavior view family as a "system" within the larger social framework of a community. These definitions and understandings affect our approaches to health and health care of individuals within the family unit.

The family assumes major responsibility for the introduction and socialization of children. It transmits its fundamental cultural background to its members. Despite modern stresses and strains, the family, through its structure and function, forms a social network that acts as a potent support system for its members. The current emphasis in working with families is on wellness and empowerment for families to achieve control over their lives.

Family Organization and Structure

Census data indicate significant alterations in the definition and social configuration of families over the past several decades. The Urban Institute recognizes four categories of families: the two-parent family, the single-parent family, blended families, and no-parent families (Staveteig & Wigton, 2000). A broader view of the contemporary family is as "a group of two or more persons related by blood, marriage, adoption, or emotional commitment who have a permanent relationship and who work together to meet life goals and needs" (Brooks, 2002).

When members are gained or lost through events (e.g., marriage, divorce, birth, death, abandonment, or incarceration), the family composition is altered and roles must be redefined or redistributed. Children may belong to several different family groups during their lifetimes.

Evidence-Based Practice

PROMOTING CERVICAL SCREENING

Background

Cervical cancer is the third most common cancer worldwide, with 400,000 cases and 200,000 deaths every year. Most, if not all, cervical cancers are due to human papillomavirus (HPV). Risk factors for cervical cancer include smoking, early sexual activity, multiple lifetime sexual partners, sexually transmitted infection, and impaired immunologic status. Primary prevention of cervical cancer involves avoiding the risk factors (see "Primary Prevention of Human Papillomavirus in Women," Evidence-Based Practice box in Chapter 4). Secondary prevention includes achieving regular cervical screening. The Papanicolaou test can increase survival rates, depending on the skill of the clinician collecting the endocervical and ectocervical cells from the transformation zone, and the skill of the cytologist evaluating the smear. Typing for HPV can also screen for the aggressive types, of which types 16 and 18 cause 80% of all cervical cancers. Cervical screening is generally recommended every 1 to 3 years for women age 20 to 65 years. Compliance ranges from 84% in England, which has a well-established national screening program, to about 5% in developing countries, where 80% of all cervical cancer cases occur. In most countries, being older, less well educated, lower socioeconomic, and rural is associated with the poorest screening rate. Barriers to screening include feelings of embarrassment and vulnerability; cost; lack of perceived benefit; fear of cancer; and, in the case of HPV typing, connotation of sexual promiscuity.

Critics of cervical screening point out the false negatives (averaging 20% to 60% of all Papanicolaou tests), and the possible harm they may cause: anxiety, false alarm, unnecessary colposcopy or biopsy, overtesting, and overtreatment. Some lower-grade cervical lesions resolve spontaneously. Treatment can injure cervical structure and function. Women need to be informed of these risks before testing.

Objective

The reviewers' goal was to examine the interventions that promote both compliance with cervical screening recommendations and informed consent. The following types of interventions were sought: invitations, reminders, educational materials, positive or negative message framing, counseling, risk factor assessment, procedures to ease the screening procedure, and economic incentives. Primary outcomes included receiving a cervical screen, and informed consent about the details of the procedure and its risks and benefits. Reviewers hoped for intermediate outcomes of booking appointments, intentions to attend screening, knowledge of screening, and satisfaction with screening, as well as costs.

Methods

Search Strategy

Reviewers searched Cochrane, MEDLINE, BIDS, Cancer lit, DHSS date, Dissertation Abstracts, HealthStat, ASSIA, Pascal, SIGLE, CINAHL, Sociofile, Psycinfo, SHARE, NHS CRD DARE, and National Research Register, as well as bibliographies, specialists, and the *Journal of American Screening.* Keywords included *vaginal smears, Pap tests, Papanicolaou, cytology, pap smear, with attitude, accept, encourage, improve, promote, uptake,* and *utilization.* The reviewers found 35 controlled studies, representing over 57,000 women from the United States, Australia, the United Kingdom, Canada, Italy, and Belgium. Of these trials, 27 were randomized and 8 were quasi-randomized.

Statistical Analysis

Similar data were pooled. Reviewers calculated relative risks for dichotomous (categorical) data, and weighted mean differences for continuous data. Results outside the 95% confidence interval were accepted as significantly different.

Findings

Women were significantly more likely to use cervical screening when they received an invitation, especially when the letter was from the woman's general practitioner health care provider and when they were provided with a fixed appointment in the letter. There was a trend toward greater participation when the letter revealed the gender of the clinician who would be taking the smear, and when using a health promotion nurse, but none of these reached the level of statistical significance. Response to telephone calls was equivocal. There was a greater response from women who received educational materials than controls. There was limited evidence of a beneficial effect of having a lay community member involved in promoting the screening.

Limitations

None of the studies were in developing countries. Invitations may not work in an area of frequent migration, illiteracy, or transportation from remote areas. Many address lists were outdated, and thus many subjects were lost to follow-up. None of the trials examined informed consent related to risks and benefits. The assumption throughout the trials was that screening was always beneficial. The reviewers noted methodologic problems with the trial sizes, randomization, blinding of assessors, concealment of treatment allocation, and numbers lost to follow-up, as well as the way the statistical analysis of some of the data was handled.

Conclusions

Invitations and educational material appear to be effective at increasing participation in cervical screening in developed countries. Modifications of these methods may increase use of cervical screening in developing countries. Revealing the gender of the clinician and making a fixed appointment seem to be promising.

Implications for Practice

To increase rates of cervical screening, health care providers can institute a program of written invitations with fixed appointments. The letter should include the gender of the health care provider. Educational materials should be distributed widely.

Implications for Further Research

Trials that account for the methodologic problems of randomization, concealment, blinding the assessor, and follow-up would strengthen the data pool. Research is still needed on informed consent. Much more information is needed about promotional interventions in developing countries, which stand to benefit greatly from cervical screening.

Reference

Forbes C, Jepson R, Martin-Hirsch P: Interventions targeted at women to encourage the uptake of cervical screening (Cochrane Review), 2001. In *The Cochrane Library,* Issue 2, Chichester, UK, 2004, John Wiley & Sons.

The nuclear family has long represented the traditional American family in which male and female partners and their children live as an independent unit, sharing roles, responsibilities, and economic resources (Fig. 2-1). In contemporary society, this idealized family structure actually represents only a relatively small number of families. Two-parent families (biologic or adoptive parents) account for approximately 64% of American families, representing 72% of Cau-

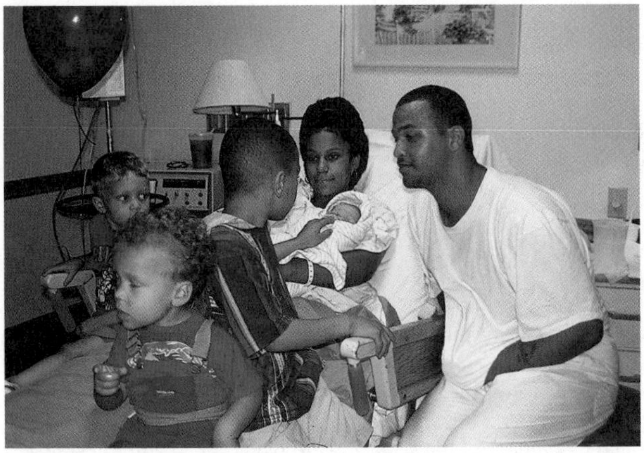

Fig. 2-1 Nuclear family. (Courtesy Marjorie Pyle, RNC, Lifecircle, Costa Mesa, CA.)

casian, 60% of Latino, and 29% of African-American families (Staveteig & Wigton, 2000). The binuclear family is an alternate form of the traditional nuclear family arrangement that results from divorce. Children of remarried parents then become members of both the maternal and paternal nuclear households. In joint custody, the court assigns divorcing parents equal rights to and responsibilities for the minor child or children.

Many nuclear families have other relatives living in the same household. These extended family members, called *kin,* are grandparents, aunts or uncles, or other people related by blood (Fig. 2-2). For some groups, such as African-American and Latin-American women, the family kin network is an important resource in terms of preventive health behavior (Clarke L, 2001; Williams et al, 2001). The extended family is becoming more common as American society ages. The need to care for elderly parents within the same household often creates a "sandwich generation" in which parents of the nuclear family provide care for their children as well as for elderly grandparents or other relatives.

Single-parent families comprise an unmarried biologic or adoptive parent who may or may not be living with other adults. The single-parent family may result from the loss of spouse by death, divorce, separation, or desertion; from either an unplanned or a planned pregnancy; or from the adoption of a child by an unmarried woman or man. This family structure is becoming more prevalent, with current estimates at one fifth of Caucasian families, one third of Hispanic families, and more than half of African-American families in the United States. Although the number of single-parent households has decreased for most groups, the number of single-parent families among African-American households has remained fairly steady at approximately 55% (Staveteig & Wigton, 2000).

Current research takes opposing perspectives on the merits and challenges of single-parent households. In many cases, the single-parent family tends to be vulnerable economically and socially, creating an unstable and deprived environment for the growth potential of children. Research demonstrates the impact of single-parenthood not only in economic instability but also in relation to health status, school achievement, and high risk behaviors for these children. Single mothers are more likely to live in poverty and have poor perinatal outcomes (U.S. Department of Health and Human Services [USDHHS], 2000).

In recent years, single parenting has become a common and acceptable choice in society. Individuals for whom the single-parent family is a chosen lifestyle often enjoy a free and open system for the development of parents and children. In these families, decision making and communication are seen as joint commitments between parent and child. The parent-child relationship is considered a major source of life fulfillment. The most frequently identified strength in these families was emotional closeness (Ford-Gilboe, 2000).

Reconstituted or blended families, those formed as the result of divorce and remarriage, consist of unrelated family members (stepparents, stepchildren, and stepsiblings) who join together to create a new household. These family groups

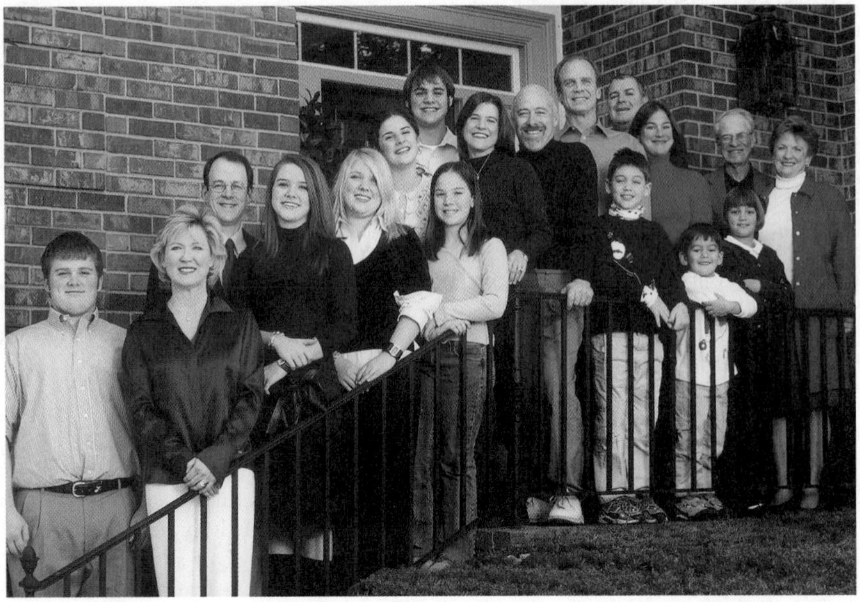

Fig. 2-2 Extended family. (Courtesy Frances M. Edwards, Nashville, TN.)

frequently involve a biologic or adoptive parent whose spouse has not adopted the child.

Other family configurations, which are less well documented, include children in families whose parents are cohabiting and an increasing number of homosexual (lesbian and gay) families, who may live together with or without children (Federal Interagency Forum on Children and Family Statistics, 2004). Children in homosexual (lesbian and gay) families may be the offspring of previous heterosexual unions, conceived by one member of a lesbian couple through therapeutic insemination, or adopted. These trends reflect the increased opportunities for alternate forms of parenthood within our society, owing both to more liberal social mores and to technologic and medical advances that offer the possibility of parenthood to single men and women. Despite increasing recognition of the biologic and psychologic needs of homosexual families, social acceptance and attitudes of health care providers often present significant barriers to quality health care (Clarke V, 2001).

Family Functions

Although family functions have evolved and adapted over time in response to social and economic changes (Friedman, 2002), the family progresses through its life cycle (Table 2-1) and continues to carry out certain functions for the well-being of family members and the wider society.

Friedman (2003) described the family functions as affective, socialization, reproductive, economic, and health care functions. The affective function is one of the most vital and focuses on meeting family members' needs for affection and understanding. The socialization function refers to the learning experiences provided within the family to teach children their culture and how to function and assume adult social roles. This is a lifelong process. The reproductive function ensures family continuity over the generations and the survival of society (Fig. 2-3). Economic functions involve the family's provision and allocation of sufficient resources. Health care functions are met by the provision of

Table 2-1

Stages of the Family Life Cycle

STAGE OF FAMILY LIFE CYCLE	EMOTIONAL PROCESS OF TRANSITION: KEY PRINCIPLES	SECOND-ORDER CHANGES IN FAMILY STATUS REQUIRED TO PROCEED DEVELOPMENTALLY
Leaving home: single young adults	Accepting emotional and financial responsibility for self	Differentiation of self in relation to family of origin Development of intimate peer relationships Establishment of self through work and financial independence
Joining of families through marriage: new couple	Commitment to new system	Formation of marital system Realignment of relationships with extended families and friends to include spouse
Families with young children	Accepting new members into system	Adjusting marital system to make space for child(ren) Joining in childrearing, financial, and household tasks Realignment of relationships with extended family to include parenting and grandparenting roles
Families with adolescents	Increasing flexibility of family boundaries to include children's independence and grandparents' frailties	Shifting of parent-child relationships to permit adolescent to move in and out of system Refocus on midlife marital and career issues Beginning shift toward joint caring for older generation
Launching children and moving on	Accepting multitude of exits from and entries into the family system	Renegotiation of marital system as a dyad Development of adult-to-adult relationships between grown children and their parents Realignment of relationships to include in-laws and grandchildren
Families in later life	Accepting shifting of generational roles	Dealing with disabilities and death of parents (grandparents) Maintaining own and/or couple functioning and interests in face of physiologic decline; exploration of new familial and social role options Support for a more central role of middle generation Making room in the system for wisdom and experience of elderly members; supporting older generation without overfunctioning for them Dealing with loss of spouse, siblings, and other peers and preparation for own death; life review and integration

From Carter B, McGoldrick M: *The expanded family life cycle: individual, family, and social perspectives*, ed 3, Boston, 1999, Allyn & Bacon.

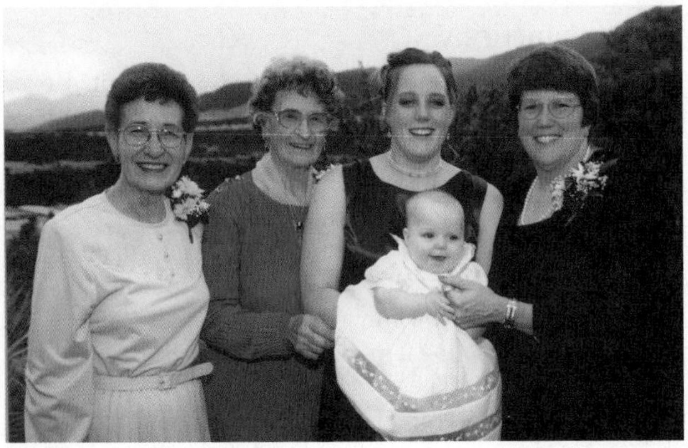

Fig. 2-3 Five generations of a family. (Courtesy Kathleen Sawin, Milwaukee, WI.)

such physical necessities as food, clothing, shelter, and health care.

Some functions are emphasized more in one phase of a family's life cycle; others are continuous for the family's survival and progress. Many functions previously performed almost exclusively by one gender (e.g., child care and financial support) are today shared between genders. Although goals for socialization and childrearing practices differ from culture to culture, in most societies the family appears to have three major objectives in relation to children: caregiving, nurturing, and training.

Family Dynamics

Families work cooperatively to accomplish family functions. Through family dynamics (interactions and communication), family members assume appropriate social roles. Social roles in the family are learned in pairs (e.g., mother-father, parent-child, and brother-sister). Role pairing enables social interactions to take place in an orderly, predictable manner; the roles are said to be complementary. Some families maintain a traditional pairing of roles, whereas other families change behavior patterns to suit a change in family lifestyle. Rather than mother-father, brother-sister, the roles may be mother-daughter, mother-son. Negotiation brings these pair roles into a new alignment. Negotiation is essential to maintain family equilibrium.

Ideally, the family uses its resources to provide a safe, intimate environment for the biopsychosocial development of the family members. The family provides for the nurturing of the newborn and the gradual socialization of the growing child. Children form their earliest and closest relationships with their parents or parenting persons; these affiliations continue throughout a lifetime. For better or worse, parent-child relationships influence self-worth and the ability to form later relationships. The family also influences the child's perceptions of the outside world. The family provides the growing child with an identity that possesses both a past and a sense of the future. Cultural values and rituals are passed from one generation to the next through the family (Friedman, 2003).

Through everyday interactions, the family develops and uses its own patterns of verbal and nonverbal communication. These patterns give insight into the emotional exchange within a family and act as reliable indicators of interpersonal functioning. Family members not only react to the communication or actions of other family members, but also interpret and define them.

Over time the family develops protocols for problem solving, particularly regarding important decisions such as having a baby, buying a house, or sending children to college. The criteria used in making decisions are based on family values and attitudes about the appropriateness of the behavior and the moral, social, political, and economic events of society. The power to make critical decisions is given to a family member through tradition or negotiation. This power is not always stated. Power reflects the family's concepts of male or female dominance and cultural practices, social customs, and community norms. As a result, family members attain certain statuses or hierarchies. They play out these statuses by assuming various roles. Most families have a member who "takes charge" or "is supportive" or "can't be expected to do anything."

Critical Thinking Exercise

FAMILY ROLES AND FUNCTIONS

Angelina is a 25-year-old married woman. She is having a protracted labor with fetal distress, and the obstetrician has recommended a cesarean birth. Her husband is at home with their two other children. The obstetrician talked with Angelina and, coming out of her room, asked the nurse to get the operative permit signed. When the nurse approached Angelina for her signature, she said that her husband has to sign the permit. The nurse responded that, "Oh, no. You have to sign it. Just sign right here." Was the nurse's response appropriate?

1. Evidence—Is there sufficient evidence to draw conclusions about the appropriateness of the nurse's response?
2. Assumptions—What assumptions can be made about the appropriateness of the response in relation to:
   a. Legal requirements for informed consent.
   b. Who is the decision-maker in the family.
   c. The patient's preferences.
   d. Culture of the patient and family.
   e. Values of the patient.
3. What implications and priorities for nursing care can be drawn at this time?
4. Does the evidence objectively support your conclusion?
5. Are there alternative perspectives to your conclusion?

The Family in Society

The social context for the family can be viewed in relation to social and demographic trends that define the population as a whole. Current U.S. census data indicate that the racial and ethnic diversity of the population has grown dramatically in the last three decades. This increased diversity—first manifested among children, and soon to be evident in the older population—is projected to increase in the future (Federal Interagency Forum on Children and Family Statistics, 2004).

Each family sets up boundaries between itself and society. People are conscious of the difference between "family members" and "outsiders," or people without kinship status. Some families isolate themselves from the outside community; others have a wide community network to help in times of stress. Although boundaries exist for every family, family members set up channels through which they interact with society. These channels also ensure that the family receives its share of social resources.

THEORETIC APPROACHES TO UNDERSTANDING FAMILIES

A family theory can be used to describe families and how the family unit responds to events both within and outside the family. Each family theory makes certain assumptions about the family and has inherent strengths and limitations. Most nurses use a combination of theories in their work with families. A brief discussion of a theory commonly used with families, systems theory, and the implications of this theory for maternal-child nursing is presented. A brief synopsis of several other theories useful in working with families is included in Table 2-2.

Family Systems Theory

Among the caring disciplines, a systems approach to understanding the family is almost universally applied. Many systems concepts are central to the delivery of holistic nursing care. These include recognition that changes occurring in one member affect the entire family, and an appreciation that nurses who work with families also enter into a systemic relationship with them. This is especially true for nurses who provide perinatal nursing care through community- or home-based agencies. Understanding how family members influence and interact with each other can help the nurse develop empathy with and respect for different ways of functioning.

When applied to families, the systems theory allows nurses to "view the family as a unit and thus focus on observing the interaction among family members rather than studying family members individually" (Wright & Leahey, 2000). Within a systems framework, the individual takes on several roles as a unique and important person in his or her own system and as part of one or more subsystems within the larger family. For example, an individual may belong to one of several subsystems, such as a child subsystem or a parental subsystem. When considering more than one generation of a family, a married woman may belong to a parental subsystem in her own home and to a subsystem of children when considered in relationship to her own parents.

Wright and Leahy (2000) outlined the key characteristics of family systems theory:

- A family system is part of a larger suprasystem and comprises many subsystems.

Table 2-2

Theories and Models Relevant to Family Nursing Practice

THEORY	SYNOPSIS OF THEORY
Family Life Cycle (Developmental) Theory (Carter & McGoldrick, 1999)	Families move through stages. The family life cycle is the context in which to examine the identity and development of the individual. Relationships among family members go through transitions. Although families have roles and functions, a family's main value is in relationships that are irreplaceable. The family involves different structures and cultures organized in various ways. Developmental stresses may disrupt the life cycle process.
Family Stress Theory (Boss, 2002)	Concerned with ways families react to stressful events. Family stress can be studied within the internal and external contexts in which the family is living. The internal context involves elements that a family can change or control, such as family structure, psychologic defenses, and philosophic values and beliefs. The external context consists of the time and place in which a particular family finds itself and over which the family has no control, such as the culture of the larger society, the time in history, the economic state of society, maturity of the individuals involved, success of the family in coping with stressors, and genetic inheritance.
McGill Model of Nursing (Allen, 1997)	Strength-based focus in clinical practice with families rather than a deficit approach. Identification of family strengths and resources; provision of feedback about strengths; assist family to develop and elicit strengths and use resources.
Health Belief Model (Becker, 1974; Janz & Becker, 1984)	The goal of the model is to reduce cultural and environmental barriers that interfere with access to health care. Key elements of the Health Belief Model include the following: perceived susceptibility, perceived severity, perceived benefits, perceived barriers, cues to action, and confidence.
Human Developmental Ecology (Bronfenbrenner, 1979, 1989)	Behavior is a function of interaction of traits and abilities with the environment. Major concepts include ecosystem, niches (social roles), adaptive range, and ontogenetic development. Individuals are "embedded in a microsystem (role and relations), a mesosystem (interrelations between two or more settings), an exosystem (external settings that do not include the person), and a macrosystem (culture)" (Klein & White, 1996). Change over time is incorporated in the chronosystem.

- The family as a whole is greater than the sum of its individual members.
- A change in one family member affects all family members.
- The family is able to create a balance between change and stability.
- Family members' behaviors are best understood from a view of circular rather than linear causality; that is, an individual's behavior affects and is affected by the behavior of others.

The family systems theory encourages nurses to view individual family members as part of a larger family system influenced by and influencing others. Application of these concepts can guide assessment and interventions for the family. For example, the childbearing family interacts as a system with many elements in the environmental suprasystem, including the health care community. The extent to which this suprasystem influences the family in matters such as prenatal care, childbirth education, and infant care depends on the family's boundary permeability. A relatively closed family may want instructions only from others within the family, whereas a relatively open family may be more receptive to instructions from health care providers.

Using Theories to Guide Practice

People interact effectively with each other in many ways. The nurse must understand that countless factors influence ways in which family members relate among themselves and with the health care community. Some of these factors include the natural history of the family, culture, roles, values, beliefs, and traditional customs. Because so many variables affect ways of relating, the nurse must be aware that most family members will interact and communicate with each other in ways that are very different from those of the nurse's own family of origin. Most families will hold at least some beliefs about health that are very different from those of the nurse. In some instances, their beliefs will conflict with principles of health care management predominant in the Western health care system. Therefore, to be effective in working with families, the nurse must possess a degree of personal openness and acceptance and be willing to work with families in a way that is respectful and adapts to their ways of learning and communicating.

Because family relationships are always complex, viewing the interaction of the whole family helps nurses to understand more fully the functioning of individual family members. A family that has recently immigrated to this country may want to receive health information only from others within the family or the immediate cultural community, whereas a family that has more experience in dealing with the American health care system may be more receptive to nurses who are culturally different. When interacting with family members, the nurse becomes part of a system with them. The behaviors and interaction style of the nurse affect not just the individual who is identified as the "patient" but also contribute to family members' responses to each other. Finally, the quality of the nurse-family system strongly influences how the family will interact with the greater health care community in the future.

Knowing about the phases of the life cycle can assist nurses in providing anticipatory guidance for families. For example, helping childbearing families prepare for the birth of a newborn may minimize the development of crises (Nursing Care Plan). By using developmental theory, a nurse can anticipate that a family who delivers a child with a serious anomaly might experience a crisis or state of disequilibrium because the birth of an ill child is not a normative event. Because such a family may revert to a state of dependence, the nurse will realize that their need for extra support and nurturing from the nurse is a natural response to stress.

Because today's families experience a great deal of pressure, they must develop effective stress-management strategies. Maternity nurses working in community settings may care for a full range of family situations including healthy but highly stressed families and families coping with the extraordinary stress of ill infants or mothers who have recently had major surgical procedures such as cesarean births. Nurses can assist families in changing their stress levels by helping families control internal and external context factors. The nurse can intervene through educational strategies to correct misconceptions and reduce stress. Explaining normal infant growth and development (maturation) may reduce the stress of parenting.

In planning the care of a family or an individual family member, the nurse may find it useful to view the family at a developmental phase in the life cycle, facing stressful life events, and operating as a system. A family assessment tool such as the one outlined by Friedman (2002) (Fig. 2-4) can be used as a guide for assessing aspects of the family discussed in this chapter. A family genogram (family tree format depicting relationships of family members over at least three generations) (Fig. 2-5) provides valuable information about a family and can be placed in the nursing care plan for easy access by care providers.

By using the Health Belief Model as a guide to assessment, nurses can better address concerns specific to an individual from a different cultural group, motivating the individual to take action on his or her own behalf. Understanding a woman's concerns from her own point of view can help the nurse to provide interventions that will place women at ease in the health care setting. For example, the nurse can modify or adjust her care in assessing uterine involution as part of postpartum care for a woman who holds traditional Mexican beliefs and fears of having cold enter her uterus during a normal examination. The culturally competent nurse can close the door to the room, pull curtains to minimize air flow around the woman, position the woman so that the perineum is facing away from the door or air vents, and keep the perineum draped so that the examination takes place with a minimum of exposure.

Within the larger society, individuals and families have a variety of stressors that affect their ability to function and to engage consistently in behaviors that will promote health and wellness. These individuals and families fall into high risk or vulnerable populations. Their stresses relate to many aspects of life: ethnic and cultural minority status, immigration status, poverty, challenges with English language fluency and literacy, malnutrition, and limited access to housing.

Nursing Care Plan

INCORPORATING THE INFANT INTO THE FAMILY

NURSING DIAGNOSIS: Readiness for enhanced family coping related to adaptation of family to new infant

EXPECTED OUTCOME

Family members will verbalize that individual and family goals are met during a smooth transition of new family member into the home.

NURSING INTERVENTIONS/*RATIONALES*

Assess type and amount of support available to family on a daily basis during the postpartal period *to facilitate adaptation of the family to situation of a new member.*

Encourage family to use past successful coping mechanisms *to enhance ability to cope with new situation and promote self-esteem.*

Encourage mother to use family and other support or services to carry out daily household tasks *to permit her to focus on herself and infant.*

Suggest that woman take time to rest when infant sleeps *to conserve energy for healing and limit responsibility to herself and infant.*

Give suggestions regarding potential roles of siblings and grandparents, taking into account developmental stages and availability of grandparents *to include all family members in creative ways and facilitate goals of all family members.*

Assess family structure and relationships, including culture, *to evaluate if longer period of adjustment may be expected.*

Teach family about sensory needs and capabilities of infant *to motivate family to meet infant's needs and set realistic expectations for infant's capabilities.*

Refer to parent support group or community agencies, as needed, *to facilitate and validate ongoing positive adjustment of family to new family member.*

NURSING DIAGNOSIS: Ineffective role performance related to developmental challenge of addition of new family member

EXPECTED OUTCOME

Each family member will verbalize realistic expectations regarding his or her role in the family and formulate a plan to incorporate role into overall family goals.

NURSING INTERVENTIONS/*RATIONALES*

Assess family structure, roles, and each member's perception of his or her role in the family *to evaluate the impact of the new member on the structure and roles of the family as perceived by the members.*

Evaluate individual's perception of goals and new roles during this transition *to promote early intervention and correct any misinterpretation.*

Encourage discussion of family members' thoughts and feelings regarding this transition *to promote open communication and trust.*

Demonstrate positive interactions and behaviors *to provide a role model for transition to new roles.*

Provide positive reinforcement for family members' actions that promote a positive environment for the infant *to increase self-esteem and provide encouragement.*

Refer to community support groups *to provide group reinforcement and further assistance.*

Give information about sibling and grandparent classes and support groups as available *to promote empowerment and self-esteem for significant others in the family.*

Some families have multiple stressors, placing them at especially high risk for poor health outcomes. It should be noted, however, that not only low-income or minority groups are at high risk for morbidity and mortality. Some stressors affect families at all strata of society. Even those who are well educated and in a higher socioeconomic class can have life stressors that make them highly vulnerable to health problems. These antecedents to vulnerability include mental illness; substance use; domestic violence; and reduced access to medical care due to unemployment, loss of medical insurance, or inadequate insurance coverage. Nurses cannot make the assumption that a family is immune to vulnerability because its members live in an exclusive neighborhood, are well educated, and are fully employed. The concepts of high risk and vulnerability potentially apply to everyone.

CULTURAL FACTORS RELATED TO FAMILY HEALTH

Cultural Context of the Family

Culture has many definitions. Thomas (2001) defined culture as "a unified set of values, ideas, beliefs, and standards of behavior shared by a group of people; it is the way a person accepts, orders, interprets, and understands experiences throughout the life course." Willis (1999) added to that explanation, stating, "Culture is an integrated dynamic system of values, beliefs and practices shaped by close ties, teachings, and common interactions from conception and throughout the lifespan." Williams and colleagues (2001) described culture as a "set of interlocking cognitive schemata that construct and give meaning to what people do in their everyday lives." The political, social, and economic context of people's lives also is part of the cultural experience. All of these definitions include the recognition that culture helps shape a person's interpretation of every life experience.

Culture is influenced by religion, environment, and historic events, and plays a powerful role in the individual's behavior and patterns of human interaction (Doyle & Ward, 2001). Culture is not static; it is an ongoing process that influences people throughout their entire lives, from birth to death. Culture is an essential element of what defines us as people.

Cultural knowledge includes beliefs and values about each facet of life and is passed from one generation to the next. Cultural beliefs and traditions relate to food, language, religion, art, health and healing practices, kinship relationships, and all other aspects of community, family, and individual life. Culture also has been shown to have a direct effect on health behaviors. Values, attitudes, and beliefs that are culturally acquired may influence perceptions of illness,

The Friedman Family Assessment Model (Short Form)

Identifying Data

1. Family name
2. Address and phone
3. Family composition
4. Type of family form
5. Cultural (ethnic) background
6. Religious identification
7. Social class status
8. Family's recreational or leisure-time activities

Developmental Stage and History of Family

9. Family's present developmental stage
10. Extent of family developmental tasks fulfillment
11. Nuclear family history
12. History of family of origin of both parents

Environmental Data

13. Characteristics of home
14. Characteristics of neighborhood and larger community
15. Family's geographic mobility
16. Family's associations and transactions with community
17. Family's social support system or network

Family Structure

18. Communication patterns
    - Extent of functional and dysfunctional communication (types of recurring patterns)
    - Extent of emotional (affective) messages and how expressed
    - Characteristics of communication within family subsystems
    - Extent of congruent and incongruent messages
    - Types of dysfunctional communication processes seen in family
    - Areas of open and closed communication
    - Familial and contextual variables affecting communication
19. Power structure
    - Power outcomes
    - Decision-making process
    - Power bases
    - Variables affecting family power
    - Overall family system and subsystem power (Family power continuum placement)
20. Role structure
    - Formal role structure
    - Informal role structure
    - Analysis of role models (optional)
    - Variables affecting role structure
21. Family values
    Compare the family to American or family's reference group values and/or identify important family values and their importance (priority) in family.
    - Congruence between the family's values and the family's reference group or wider community
    - Congruence between the family's values and family member's values
    - Variables influencing family values
    - Values consciously or unconsciously held
    - Presence of value conflicts in family
    - Effect of the above values and value conflicts on health status of family

Family Functions

22. Affective function
    - Family's need–response patterns
    - Mutual nurturance, closeness, and identification
    - Separateness and connectedness
23. Socialization function
    - Family child-rearing practices
    - Adaptability of child-rearing practices for family form and family's situation
    - Who is (are) socializing agent(s) for child(ren)?
    - Value of children in family
    - Cultural beliefs that influence family's child-rearing patterns
    - Social class influence on child-rearing patterns
    - Estimation about whether family is at risk for child-rearing problems and if so, indication of high risk factors
    - Adequacy of home environment for children's need to play
24. Health care function
    - Family's health beliefs, values, and behavior
    - Family's definitions of health–illness and their level of knowledge
    - Family's perceived health status and illness susceptibility
    - Family's dietary practices
    - Adequacy of family diet (recommended 3-day food history record)
    - Function of mealtimes and attitudes toward food and mealtimes
    - Shopping (and its planning) practices
    - Person(s) responsible for planning, shopping, and preparation of meals
    - Sleep and rest habits
    - Physical activity and recreation practices (not covered earlier)
    - Family's drug habits
    - Family's role in self-care practices
    - Medically based preventive measures (physicals, eye and hearing tests, and immunizations)
    - Dental health practices
    - Family health history (both general and specific diseases—environmentally and genetically related)
    - Health care services received
    - Feelings and perceptions regarding health services
    - Emergency health services
    - Source of payments for health and other services
    - Logistics of receiving care

Family Stress and Coping

25. Short- and long-term familial stressors and strengths
26. Extent of family's ability to respond, based on objective appraisal of stress-producing situations
27. Coping strategies utilized (present/past)
    - Differences in family members' ways of coping
    - Family's inner coping strategies
    - Family's external coping strategies
28. Dysfunctional adaptive strategies utilized (present/past; extent of usage)

Family Composition Form

Name (last, first)	Gender	Relationship	Date/place of birth	Occupation	Education
1. (Father)					
2. (Mother)					
3. (Oldest child)					
4.					
5.					
6.					
7.					
8.					

Fig. 2-4 The Friedman Family Assessment Model (Short Form). (From Friedman M: *Family nursing theory and assessment,* ed 4, New York, 1998, Appleton & Lange.)

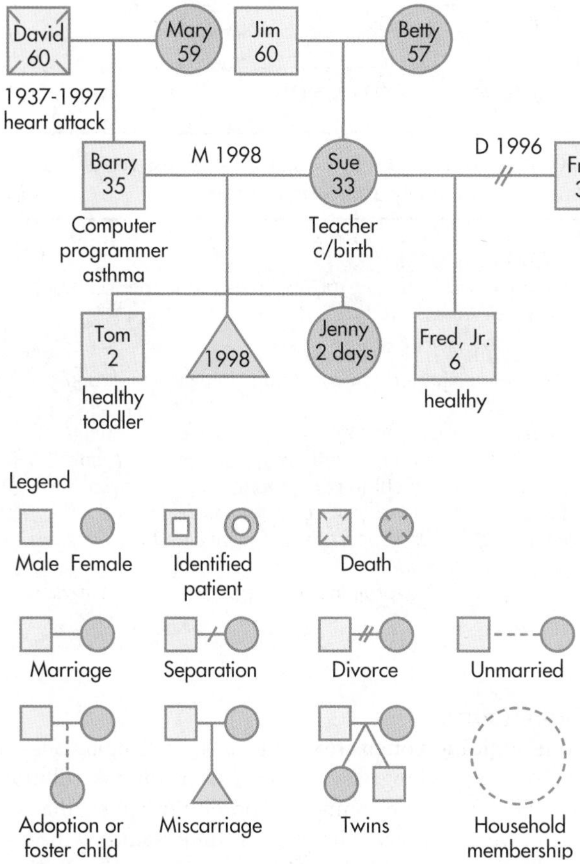

Fig. 2-5 Example of a family genogram.

as well as health care–seeking behavior and response to treatment (National Academy Press, 2002). The impact of these influences must be assessed by health professionals in providing health care and developing effective intervention strategies (Williams et al, 2001).

Many subcultures may be found within each culture. Subculture refers to a group existing within a larger cultural system that retains its own characteristics. A subculture may be an ethnic group or a group organized in other ways. In the United States, there are many ethnic subcultures (e.g., African-Americans, Asian-Americans, Hispanics), as well as subcultures within these groups. In addition, the Caucasian population in America has diverse and multiple subcultures (e.g., Italian-Americans, Polish-Americans, German-Americans). Because every identified cultural group has subcultures, and because it is impossible to study every subculture in depth, greater differences may exist among and between groups than is generally acknowledged.

Each subculture holds rich and complex traditions, including health practices, that have proved effective over time. These traditions vary from group to group. In a multicultural society, many groups can influence traditions and practices. As cultural groups come in contact with each other, acculturation and assimilation may occur.

Acculturation refers to changes that occur within one group or among several groups when people from different cultures come in contact with one another. People may retain some of their own culture while adopting some of the cultural practices of the dominant society. This familiarization among cultural groups results in some overt behavioral similarity, especially in mannerisms, styles, and practices. Dress, language patterns, food choices, and health practices especially show differences among cultural groups. In the United States, acculturation is generally thought to take three generations. An adult grandchild of an immigrant is usually fully Americanized. An example of acculturation is the adoption of ethnic food practices in the United States.

During times of family transitions such as childbearing, or during crisis or illness, a woman may rely on old cultural patterns even after she has become acculturated in many ways. This is consistent with family developmental theory that states that during times of stress, people revert to practices and behaviors that are most comfortable and familiar.

Assimilation, on the other hand, occurs when a cultural group loses its identity and becomes part of the dominant culture. According to Friedman (1998), "assimilation denotes the more complete and one-way process of one culture being absorbed into the other." Assimilation is the process by which groups "melt" into the mainstream, thus accounting for the notion of a "melting pot," a phenomenon that has been said to occur in the United States. This is illustrated by individuals who identify themselves as being of "Irish" or "German" descent, without having any remaining cultural practices or values linked specifically to that culture, such as food preparation techniques, style of dress, or proficiency in the language associated with their reported cultural heritage. Spector (2004) asserts that in the United States, the melting pot, with its dream of a common culture, "has proved to be a myth and has faded; it is now time to identify the mosaic phenomenon and both accept and appreciate the differences among people."

The family process within its cultural context is a central concern in nursing, especially when the nurse is providing care to the childbearing family. A critical life experience, such as childbearing, is often bound by traditional beliefs and practices. A culture's beliefs and practices regarding childbearing are embedded in its economic, religious, kinship, and political structures. All cultures have behavioral norms and expectations for each stage of the perinatal cycle. These norms and expectations relate to each culture's view of how people stay healthy and prevent illness. Patients have the right to expect that their physiologic and psychologic health care needs will be met and that their cultural beliefs will be respected. Cultural sensitivity, compassion, and a critical awareness of family dynamics and social stressors that will affect health-related decision making are critical components in developing an effective plan of care (see Nursing Care Plan).

Understanding the concepts of ethnocentrism and cultural relativism may be helpful to nurses caring for families in a multicultural society.

Ethnocentrism is a belief in the rightness of one's culture's way of doing things. Essentially, ethnocentrism supports the notion that "my group is the best." Although the United States is a culturally diverse nation, the prevailing practice of health care is based on beliefs and practices held by members of the dominant culture, primarily Caucasians of European descent. This practice is based on the biomedical model that

Nursing Care Plan

THE FAMILY NEWLY IMMIGRATED FROM A NON–ENGLISH-SPEAKING COUNTRY

NURSING DIAGNOSIS: Impaired verbal communication related to inability to speak or understand English

EXPECTED OUTCOME

Family and health care providers will communicate using bilingual health care providers or interpreters.

NURSING INTERVENTIONS/*RATIONALES*

Determine language of patient *to provide a basis for facilitating communication.*

Enlist assistance of bilingual health care provider or interpreter *to complete assessment and health teaching.*

Prepare health education materials in languages of patients commonly seen in the agency *to facilitate patient education.*

Listen actively *to indicate concern for family and reduce anxiety.*

Identify patient education materials that use pictures or symbols *to enhance understanding.*

NURSING DIAGNOSIS: Risk for loneliness related to separation from family and country of origin

EXPECTED OUTCOME

Family members will form new relationships within the community and reduce their loneliness.

NURSING INTERVENTIONS/*RATIONALES*

Provide emotional support *to assist family in developing coping skills.*

Introduce family to a support group of people from a similar culture *to enhance developing relationships and provide comfort.*

Promote family involvement in new parent groups or neighborhood activities *to enhance participation in activities that enhance parenting skills, support the development of relationships, and help reduce loneliness.*

Refer to clergy of choice for spiritual support *to enhance coping skills.*

focuses on curing disease states. From this biomedical perspective, pregnancy and childbirth are viewed as processes with inherent risks that are most appropriately managed by using scientific knowledge and advanced technology. The medical perspective stands in direct contrast with the belief systems of many cultures. Among many women, birth is traditionally viewed as a completely normal process that can be managed with a minimum of involvement from health practitioners. When encountering behavior in women unfamiliar with the biomedical model, the nurse may become frustrated and impatient. The nurse may label the woman's behavior inappropriate and believe that it conflicts with "good" health practices. If the Western health care system provides the nurse's only standard for judgment, the behavior of the nurse is called ethnocentric.

Cultural relativism is the opposite of ethnocentrism. It refers to learning about and applying the standards of another person's culture to activities within that culture. To be culturally relativistic, the nurse recognizes that people from different cultural backgrounds comprehend the same objects and situations differently. In other words, culture determines a person's viewpoint.

Cultural relativism does not require nurses to accept the beliefs and values of another culture. Instead, nurses recognize that the behavior of others may be based on a system of logic different from their own. Cultural relativism affirms the uniqueness and value of every culture.

Childbearing Beliefs and Practices

Nurses working with childbearing families care for families from many different cultures and ethnic groups. To provide culturally competent care, the nurse must assess the beliefs and practices of patients. A nurse should consider all aspects of culture, including communication, space, time orientation, and family roles, when working with childbearing families.

Communication

Communication often creates the most challenging obstacle for nurses working with patients from diverse cultural groups. This is because communication is not merely the exchange of words. Instead it involves (1) understanding the individual's language, including subtle variations in meaning and distinctive dialects; (2) appreciation of individual differences in interpersonal style; and (3) accurate interpretation of the volume of speech, as well as the meanings of touch and gestures. For example, members of some cultural groups tend to speak more loudly, with great emotion, and with vigorous and animated gestures when they are excited; this is true whether their excitement is related to positive or negative events or emotions. It is important, therefore, for the nurse to avoid rushing to judgment regarding a patient's intent when the patient is speaking, especially in a language not understood by the nurse. In these situations, it is critical that the nurse avoid instantaneous responses that may well be based on an incorrect interpretation of the patient's gestures and meaning. Instead, the nurse should withhold an interpretation of what has been communicated until it is possible to clarify the patient's intent. The nurse needs to enlist the assistance of a person who can help and verify with the patient the true intent and meaning of the communication.

Use of Interpreters

Inconsistencies between the language of patients and the language of providers present a significant barrier to effective health care. Because of the diversity of cultures and languages within the U.S. and Canadian populations, health care agencies are increasingly seeking the services of interpreters (of oral communication from one language to another) or translators (of written words from one language to another) to bridge these gaps and fulfill their obligation for culturally and linguistically appropriate health care (Box 2-1). Finding the best possible interpreter in the circumstance also is critically important. A number of personal at-

BOX 2-1

Working with an Interpreter

Step 1: Before the Interview

A. Outline your statements and questions. List the key pieces of information you want/need to know.
B. Learn something about the culture so that you can converse informally with the interpreter.

Step 2: Meeting with the Interpreter

A. Introduce yourself to the interpreter and converse informally. This is the time to find out how well he or she speaks English. No matter how proficient or what age the interpreter is, be respectful. Some ways to show respect are to ask a cultural question to acknowledge that you can learn from the interpreter, or you could learn one word or phrase from the interpreter.
B. Emphasize that you do want the patient to ask questions because some cultures consider this inappropriate behavior.
C. Make sure the interpreter is comfortable with the technical terms you need to use. If not, take some time to explain them.

Step 3: During the Interview

A. Ask your questions and explain your statements (see Step 1).
B. Make sure that the interpreter understands which parts of the interview are most important. You usually have limited time with the interpreter, and you want to have adequate time at the end for patient questions.
C. Try to get a "feel" for how much is "getting through." No matter what the language is, if in relating information to the patient the interpreter uses far fewer or far more words than you do, "something else" is going on.
D. Stop every now and then and ask the interpreter, "How is it going?" You may not get a totally accurate answer, but you will have emphasized to the interpreter your strong desire to focus on the task at hand. If there are language problems: (1) speak *slowly;* (2) use gestures (e.g., fingers to count or point to body parts); and (3) use pictures.
E. Ask the interpreter to elicit questions. This may be difficult, but it is worth the effort.
F. Identify cultural issues that may conflict with your requests or instructions.
G. Use the interpreter to help problem solve or at least give insight into possibilities for solutions.

Step 4: After the Interview

A. Speak to the interpreter and try to get an idea of what went well and what could be improved. This will help you to be more effective with this or another interpreter.
B. Make notes on what you learned for your future reference or to help a colleague.

Remember:

Your interview is a *collaboration* between you and the interpreter. *Listen* as well as speak.

Notes:

1. The interpreter may be a child, grandchild, or sibling of the patient. Be sensitive to the fact that the child is playing an adult role.
2. Be sensitive to cultural and situational differences (e.g., an interview with someone from urban Germany will likely be different from an interview with someone from a transitional refugee camp).
3. Younger females telling older males what to do may be a problem for both a female nurse and a female interpreter. This is not the time to pioneer new gender relations. Be aware that in some cultures it is difficult for a woman to talk about some topics with a husband or a father present.

Courtesy Elizabeth Whalley, PhD, San Francisco State University.

tributes and qualifications contribute to an interpreter's potential to be effective. Ideally, interpreters should have the same native language and be of the same religion or have the same country of origin as the patient (Murray et al, 2001). Interpreters should have specific health-related language skills and experience and help bridge the language and cultural barriers between the patient and the health care provider (Howard et al, 2001). The person interpreting also should be mature enough to be trusted with private information. However, because the nature of nursing care is not always predictable and because nursing care that is provided in a home or community setting does not always allow expert, experienced, or mature adult interpreters, ideal interpretive services sometimes are impossible to find when they are needed. In crisis or emergency situations, or when family members are having extreme stress or emotional upset, it may be necessary to use relatives, neighbors, or children as interpreters. If this situation occurs, the nurse must ensure that the patient is in agreement and comfortable with using the available interpreter to assist.

When using an interpreter, the nurse respects the family by creating an atmosphere of respect and privacy. Questions should be addressed to the woman and not to the interpreter. Even though an interpreter will of necessity be exposed to sensitive and privileged information about the family, the nurse should take care to ensure that confidentiality is maintained. A quiet location free from interruptions is the ideal place for interpretive services to take place. In addition, culturally and linguistically appropriate educational materials that are easy to read, with appropriate text and graphics, should be available to assist the woman and her family in understanding health care information (Simmons et al, 2002). When using interpretive services, the nurse demonstrates respect for the woman and helps her maintain a sense of dignity by taking care to do all of the following:

- Respect the woman's wishes
- Involve her in the decision about who will be the most appropriate person to interpret under the circumstances
- Provide as much privacy as possible
- Use culturally appropriate learning aids

Personal Space

Cultural traditions define the appropriate personal space for various social interactions. Although the need for personal space varies from person to person and with the situation, the actual physical dimensions of comfort zones differ from culture to culture. Actions such as touching, placing the woman in proximity to others, taking away personal possessions, and making decisions for the woman can decrease

Cultural Awareness

QUESTIONS TO OBTAIN CULTURAL EXPECTATIONS ABOUT CHILDBEARING

1. What do you and your family think you should do to remain healthy during pregnancy?
2. What are the things you can do or cannot do to improve your health and the health of your baby?
3. Who do you want with you during your labor?
4. What actions are important for you and your family to do after the baby's birth?
5. What do you and your family expect from the nurse(s) caring for you?
6. How will family members participate in your pregnancy, childbirth, and parenting?

personal security and heighten anxiety. Conversely, if nurses respect the need for distance, they allow the woman to maintain control over personal space and support personal autonomy, thereby increasing her sense of security. For example, many Asian groups have reserved attitudes about physical contact, and touching a woman may at times create anxiety when health care is delivered. Nurses must touch patients. However, they frequently do so without any awareness of the emotional distress they may be causing their patients.

Time Orientation

Time orientation also is a fundamental way in which culture affects health behaviors. People in cultural groups may be relatively more oriented to past, present, or future. Those who focus on the past strive to maintain tradition or the status quo and have little motivation for formulating future goals. In contrast, individuals who focus primarily on the present neither plan for the future nor consider the experiences of the past. These individuals do not necessarily adhere to strict schedules and are often described as "living for the moment" or "marching to the beat of their own drummer." Individuals oriented to the future maintain a focus on achieving long-term goals.

The time orientation of the childbearing family may affect nursing care. For example, talking to a family about bringing the infant to the clinic for follow-up examinations (events in the future) may be difficult for the family that is focused on the present concerns of day-to-day survival. Because a family with a future-oriented sense of time plans far in advance, thinking about the long-term consequences of present actions, they may be more likely to return as scheduled for follow-up visits. Despite the differences in time orientation, each family may be equally concerned for the well-being of its newborn.

Family Roles

Family roles involve the expectations and behaviors associated with a member's position in the family (e.g., mother, father, grandparent). Social class and cultural norms also affect these roles, with distinct expectations for men and women clearly determined by social norms. For example, culture may influence whether a man actively participates in pregnancy and childbirth, yet maternity care practitioners working in the Western health care system expect fathers to be involved. This can create a significant conflict between the nurse and the role expectations of very traditional Mexican or Arab families, who usually view the birthing experience as a female affair (see Cultural Awareness box). The way that health care practitioners manage such a family's care molds its experience and perception of the Western health care system.

In maternity nursing, the nurse supports and nurtures the beliefs that promote physical or emotional adaptation to childbearing. However, if certain beliefs might be harmful, the nurse should carefully explore them with the woman and use them in the reeducation and modification process. Strategies for care delivery and providing appropriate care are presented in Box 2-2.

BOX 2-2

Strategies for Care Delivery and Providing Appropriate Care

Strategies for Care Delivery
- Break down the language barriers
- Explain your rationale and reasons for suggestions
- Integrate folk and Western treatments
- Enlist the family caretaker and others
- Get consent from the right person
- Provide language-appropriate materials

Providing Appropriate Care
- Ask about traditional beliefs, such as the role of hot and cold
- Be sensitive regarding interpreters and language barriers
- Ask about important dietary practices, particularly related to events such as childbirth
- Ask about group practices and beliefs
- Ask about a woman's fears, and those of her family, regarding an unfamiliar care setting

From Mattson S: Providing culturally competent care: strategies and approaches for perinatal clients, *AWHONN Lifelines* 4(5):37-39, 2000.

Table 2-3 provides examples of some cultural beliefs and practices surrounding childbearing. The cultural beliefs and customs in this table are categorized based on distinct cultural traditions and are not practiced by all members of the cultural group in every part of the country. Women from these cultural and ethnic groups may adhere to some, all, or none of the practices listed.

In using Table 2-3 as a guide, the nurse should use caution to avoid making stereotypic assumptions about any person based on sociocultural-spiritual affiliations. Nurses should exercise sensitivity in working with every family, being careful to assess the ways in which they apply their own mixture of cultural traditions.

DEVELOPING CULTURAL COMPETENCE

Cultural competence has many names and definitions, all of which have subtle shades of difference, but which are essentially the same: multiculturalism, cultural sensitivity, and intercultural effectiveness. It involves the "ability to think, feel, and act in ways that acknowledge, respect and build upon ethnic, [socio]cultural, and linguistic diversity" (Lynch & Hanson, 1998). Willis (1999) noted that culturally competent professionals are able to act in ways that meet the needs

Table 2-3

Traditional* Cultural Beliefs and Practices: Childbearing and Parenting

PREGNANCY	CHILDBIRTH	PARENTING
HISPANIC (Based primarily on knowledge of Mexican-Americans; members of the Hispanic community have their origins in Spain, Cuba, Central and South America, Mexico, Puerto Rico, and other Spanish-speaking countries.)		
Pregnancy Pregnancy desired soon after marriage Late prenatal care Expectant mother influenced strongly by mother or mother-in-law Cool air in motion considered dangerous during pregnancy Unsatisfied food cravings thought to cause a birthmark Some pica observed in the eating of ashes or dirt (not common) Milk avoided because it causes large babies and difficult births Many predictions about sex of baby May be unacceptable and frightening to have pelvic examination by male health care provider Use of herbs to treat common complaints of pregnancy Drinking chamomile tea thought to ensure effective labor	**Labor** Use of "partera" or lay midwife preferred in some places; may prefer presence of mother rather than husband After birth of baby, mother's legs brought together to prevent air from entering uterus Loud behavior in labor **Postpartum** Diet may be restricted after birth; for first 2 days only boiled milk and toasted tortillas permitted (special foods to restore warmth to body) Bed rest for 3 days after birth Keep warm Delay bathing Mother's head and feet protected from cold air; bathing permitted after 14 days Mother often cared for by her own mother 40-day restriction on sexual intercourse	**Newborn** Breastfeeding begun after third day; colostrum may be considered "filthy" or "spoiled" Olive oil or castor oil given to stimulate passage of meconium Male infant not circumcised Female infant's ears pierced Belly band used to prevent umbilical hernia Religious medal worn by mother during pregnancy; placed around infant's neck Infant protected from "evil eye" Various remedies used to treat "mal ojo" (evil eye) and fallen fontanel (depressed fontanel)
AFRICAN-AMERICAN (Members of the African-American community, many of whom are descendants of slaves, have different origins. Today a number of black Americans have emigrated from Africa, the West Indian Islands, the Dominican Republic, Haiti, and Jamaica.)		
Pregnancy Acceptance of pregnancy depends on economic status Pregnancy thought to be state of "wellness," which is often the reason for delay in seeking prenatal care, especially by lower-income African-Americans "Old wives' tales" include having a picture taken during pregnancy will cause stillbirth and reaching up will cause cord to strangle baby Craving for certain foods, including chicken, greens, clay, starch, and dirt Pregnancy may be viewed by African-American men as a sign of their virility Self-treatment for various discomforts of pregnancy, including constipation, nausea, vomiting, headache, and heartburn	**Labor** Use of "Granny midwife" in certain parts of United States Varied emotional responses: some cry out, some display stoic behavior to avoid calling attention to selves Patient may arrive at hospital in far-advanced labor Emotional support often provided by other women, especially own mother **Postpartum** Vaginal bleeding seen as sign of sickness; tub baths and shampooing of hair prohibited Sassafras tea thought to have healing power Eating liver thought to cause heavier vaginal bleeding because of its high "blood" content	**Newborn** Feeding very important: "Good" baby thought to eat well Early introduction of solid foods May breastfeed or bottle-feed; breastfeeding may be considered embarrassing Parents fearful of spoiling baby Commonly call baby by nicknames May use excessive clothing to keep baby warm Belly band used to prevent umbilical hernia Abundant use of oil on baby's scalp and skin Strong feeling of family, community, and religion

Data from Amaro H: Women in the Mexican-American community: religion, culture, and reproductive attitudes and experiences, *J Comp Psych* 16(1):6-19, 1994; Bar-yam NB: Learning about culture: a guide for birth practitioners, *Int J Childbirth Educ* 9(2):8-10, 1994; Galanti G: *Caring for patients from different cultures: case studies from American hospitals,* ed 2, Philadelphia, 1997, University of Pennsylvania Press; D'Avanzo CE, Geissler EM: *Pocket guide to cultural assessment,* ed 3, St Louis, 2003, Mosby; Mattson S: Culturally sensitive prenatal care for Southeastern Asians, *J Obstet Gynecol Neonatal Nurs* 24(4):335-341, 1995; Spector RE: *Cultural diversity in health and illness,* ed 6, Upper Saddle River, NJ, 2004, Prentice Hall Health; and Williams R: Issues in women's health care. In Johnson B (ed): *Psychiatric mental health nursing: adaptation and growth,* Philadelphia, 1989, JB Lippincott.

NOTE: Most of these cultural beliefs and customs reflect the traditional culture and are not universally practiced. These lists are not intended to stereotype patients but rather to serve as guidelines while discussing meaningful cultural beliefs with a patient and her family. Examples of other cultural beliefs and practices are found throughout this text.

*Variations in some beliefs and practices exist within subcultures of each group.

Continued

Table 2-3

Traditional Cultural Beliefs and Practices: Childbearing and Parenting—cont'd

PREGNANCY	CHILDBIRTH	PARENTING
ASIAN-AMERICAN (Typically refers to groups from China, Korea, the Philippines, Japan, Southeast Asia [particularly Thailand], Indochina, and Vietnam).		
Pregnancy Pregnancy considered time when mother "has happiness in her body" Pregnancy seen as natural process Strong preference for female health care provider Belief in theory of hot and cold May omit soy sauce in diet to prevent dark-skinned baby Prefer soup made with ginseng root as general strength tonic Milk usually excluded from diet because it causes stomach distress Inactivity or sleeping late may cause difficult delivery	**Labor** Mother admitted by other women, especially her own mother Father does not actively participate Labor in silence Cesarean birth not welcome **Postpartum** Must protect self from yin (cold forces) for 30 days Ambulation limited Shower and bathing prohibited Warm room Chinese mother avoids fruits and vegetables Diet: Warm fluids Some patients are vegetarians Korean mother served seaweed soup with rice Chinese diet high in hot foods	**Newborn** Concept of family important and valued Father is head of household; wife plays a subordinate role Birth of boy preferred May delay naming child Some groups (e.g., Vietnamese) believe colostrum is dirty; therefore they may delay breastfeeding until milk comes in
EUROPEAN-AMERICAN (Members of the European-American [Caucasian] community have their origins in countries such as Ireland, Great Britain, Germany, Italy, and France.)		
Pregnancy Pregnancy viewed as a condition that requires medical attention to ensure health Emphasis on early prenatal care Variety of childbirth education programs available and participation encouraged Technology driven Emphasis on nutritional science Involvement of the father valued Written source of information valued	**Labor** Birth is a public concern Technology dominated Birthing process in institutional setting valued Involvement of father expected Physician seen as head of team **Postpartum** Emphasis or focus on early bonding Medical interventions for dealing with discomfort Early ambulation and activity emphasized Self-care valued	**Newborn** Increased popularity of breastfeeding Breastfeeding begins as soon as possible after childbirth **Parenting** Motherhood and transition to parenting seen as stressful time Nuclear family valued, although single parenting and other forms of parenting more acceptable than in the past Women often deal with multiple roles Early return to prenatal activities
NATIVE AMERICAN (Many different tribes exist within the Native American culture; viewpoints vary according to tribal customs and beliefs.)		
Pregnancy Pregnancy considered as a normal, natural process Late prenatal care Avoid heavy lifting Herb teas encouraged	**Labor** Prefers female attendant, although husband, mother, or father may assist with birth Birth may be attended by whole family Herbs may be used to promote uterine activity Birth may occur in squatting position **Postpartum** Herb teas to stop bleeding	**Newborn** Infant not fed colostrum Use of herbs to increase flow of milk Use of cradle boards for infant Babies not handled often

of the patient and are respectful of ways and traditions that may be very different from their own. In today's society, it is of critical importance that nurses develop more than technical skill. Nurses at every level of preparation, and throughout their professional lives, must engage in a continual process of developing and refining attitudes and behaviors that will promote culturally competent care (Ryan, Carlton, & Ali, 2000).

In addition to issues of preserving and promoting human dignity, the development of cultural competence is of equal importance in terms of health outcomes. Nurses who relate effectively with patients are able to motivate them in the direction of health-promoting behaviors. In that way, cultural competence becomes an issue of cost-effectiveness as well (USDHHS, 2001).

Pathways to the Development of Cultural Competence

Cultural competence proceeds along a continuum. Out of her research into nursing cultural competence, Willis (1999) devised a framework for developing competence. Her framework comprises seven steps that can move a professional from a lower level of development to higher levels of culturally competent professionalism (Box 2-3).

Programs that promote values important to the cultural identity of the community build on the values of mutual support, cohesiveness, and self-sufficiency and therefore result in better health outcomes for community members. The use of community advocates most effectively reaches underserved populations through a network of existing social relationships (Williams et al, 2001). This can be especially true in isolated communities such as those that exist in remote or rural areas. Using local health workers builds on preexisting trust relationships. Moreover, local health workers are in a position to reinforce health teaching and best practices in health maintenance even when nurses or other heath professionals are absent.

BOX 2-3

Willis's Seven-Step Framework for Cultural Competence

Step 1
Knowledge of one's own cultural affiliation (beliefs, values, lifeways)

Step 2
Knowledge of others' cultural beliefs, values, lifeways

Step 3
Nonthreatening, non–fear-provoking interactions with others

Step 4
Tolerance

Step 5
Inclusion

Step 6
Appreciation for and acceptance of difference

Step 7
Competence

From Willis WO: Culturally competent care during the perinatal period, *J Perinat Neonatal Nurs* 13(3):45-49, 1999.

Integrating Cultural Competence with the Nursing Care Plan

In many cultures, family members make most of the decisions for the patient, and therefore the central relationship between the nurse and patient is mediated directly by the family. The nurse must recognize the cultural importance of family in supporting the patient, guiding decision making, and preserving cultural integrity in the health care interaction.

Engebretson and Littleton (2001) noted that all nursing care is delivered in multiple cultural contexts. These include the cultures of the patient, of the nurse, and of the health care system, as well as the larger culture of the society in which health care is delivered. If any of these cultural groups is excluded from the nurse's assessment and consideration, nursing care may fail to achieve its goals and may be culturally insensitive.

Implications for Nursing

According to Huff and Kline (1999), there are four areas of focus for culturally competent care: (1) developing cultural awareness or sensitivity to differences; (2) gaining cultural knowledge of values, beliefs, and lifeways of other groups; (3) developing skills in cultural assessment as a basis for intervention; and (4) engaging in direct cultural encounters or immersion in cultural experiences. These approaches build a basis for effective care strategies, enabling the nurse to promote self-care and effective lifestyle changes (Pender, Murdaugh, & Parsons, 2002). Cross-cultural experiences also present an opportunity for the health care professional to expand cultural sensitivity, awareness, and skills.

All cultures maintain behavioral norms and expectations for each stage of the perinatal cycle. These norms and expectations evolve from a culture's view of how people stay healthy and prevent illness. A culture's economic, religious, kinship, and political structures pervade its beliefs and practices regarding childbearing. To practice with cultural competence, nurses must understand the ways in which people of different cultures perceive life events and the health care system. Patients have a right to expect that their physiologic and psychologic health care needs will be met and that their cultural and spiritual beliefs will be respected.

CARE MANAGEMENT

Assessment

When nurses develop plans of care for patients who are culturally different from themselves or from the dominant culture of the community, they should be certain to include an assessment that addresses psychosocial issues related to that diversity. No nursing care plan is complete without attention to nursing diagnoses that address cultural diversity issues.

Community Focus

CULTURE AND VIEWS OF HEALTH

In a prenatal clinic, interview families from at least two different cultural backgrounds.

- What do they believe will keep them healthy in pregnancy?
- What are the roles of men and women in childbirth? Who should be present at birth?
- What is the role of technology in the childbirth process?
- Are there restrictions on activity and diet in the postpartum period?
- What is the preferred method of infant feeding? How soon after birth should breastfeeding begin?
- Are there special foods that should be eaten during pregnancy or after childbirth?
- What will keep the infant healthy after birth?

Did the responses to these questions differ significantly between the two families? Did the responses differ from what you have learned as the "correct way" to keep healthy? How can you use this information?

Nursing Diagnoses

- *Impaired verbal communication related to*
  —inability to speak or understand English
- *Risk for loneliness related to*
  —separation from family and country of origin
- *Social isolation related to*
  —separation from family and friends due to immigration status
- *Chronic sorrow related to*
  —refugee status, separation from family, and death of family members

Expected Outcomes

Examples of expected outcomes for perinatal patients include that the woman/family will do the following:

- Verbalize understanding of treatments.
- Report decreased anxiety about performing procedures (e.g., blood glucose monitoring).
- Use support systems to cope effectively with problems (e.g., pregnancy complications, newborn complications or treatments).
- Perform procedures accurately, as evidenced by return demonstration.
- Verbalize decreased role strain.

Plan of Care and Implementation

The nursing plan of care is developed in collaboration with the patient, based on the health care needs of the individual.

Evaluation

Evaluation is based on the expected outcomes of care. The plan is revised as necessary.

Key Points

- Contemporary American society recognizes and accepts a variety of family forms.
- The family is a social network that acts as an important support system for its members.
- Ideally, the family provides a safe, intimate environment for the biopsychosocial development of its children and adult members.
- Family theories provide nurses with useful guidelines for understanding family function.
- Family socioeconomics, response to stress, and culture are key factors influencing family health.
- The reproductive beliefs and practices of a culture are embedded in its economic, religious, kinship, and political structures.
- To provide quality care to women in their childbearing years and beyond, nurses should be aware of the cultural beliefs and practices important to individual families.

Answer Guidelines to Critical Thinking Exercise

Family Roles and Functions

1. Yes. The nurse's response is not appropriate. Legally, the patient must sign the consent for her surgery. However, in some cultures and some families, the decision maker may be another person such as the husband or parent. The patient, the obstetrician, or the nurse should contact the husband, explain the situation to him, and obtain his consent, and then the patient will sign the consent form.
2. (a) Legal requirements for obtaining informed consent must be met. (b) The patient may not always be the decision maker. (c) The wishes of the patient must be ascertained. (d) To provide culturally competent care, the family's culture, roles, and responsibilities must be respected. (e) Patients may have values that do not fit with the Western biomedical model of care.
3. To protect the mother and the fetus, the fetus must be delivered. This requires informed consent for the procedure. The priority for the nurse is to ensure that the woman and her husband have a clear understanding of the need for the procedure and that a written consent is obtained. (A physician is responsible for obtaining informed consent; a nurse can obtain a signature on a consent form.)
4. Yes, the evidence supports this conclusion.
5. The values of patients and their families may differ from those of health care providers. Ultimately, the patient has the right to consent to or refuse treatment even if health care providers believe that the decision is wrong or may result in harm.

Resources

Child and Family Policy Center
www.cfpciowa.org

Federal Interagency Forum on Children and Family Statistics
www.childstats.gov

"From Generation to Generation: The Health and Well-being of Children in Immigrant Families"
search.nap.edu/html/generation/summary.html

The Harriet and Robert Heilbrunn Department of Population and Family Health
cpmcnet.columbia.edu/dept/sph/popfam/

Health Literacy Toolbox 2000
www.prenataled.com/healthlit/hlt2k/script/index.asp

Indian Health Services
www.ihs.gov

Institute for the Support of Latino Families and Communities
www.uiowa.edu/nrcfcp/new/Latinos/1st%20latino%20page.htm

Institute for Urban Family Health
www.institute2000.org/

Kaiser Family Foundation
www.kff.org/

Maternal and Child Health Bureau
mchb.hrsa.gov/

Maternal and Neonatal Health Resources
www.jhuccp.org/mmc/mnh/index.stm

National Alliance for Hispanic Health
www.hispanichealth.org

National Center for the Study of Adult Learning and Literacy
www.hsph.harvard.edu/healthliteracy/

The National Multicultural Institute
www.nmci.org

National Resource Center on Family Centered Practice (NRC/FCP)
www.uiowa.edu/nrcfcp/new/index.html

Survey on Women's Health in the United States
www.kff.org/content/2002/20020507a/

Urban Institute: National Survey of America's Families
newfederalism.urban.org/nsaf/

References

Allen M: Comparative theories of the expanded role in nursing and implications for nursing practice: a working paper, *Nurs Pap* 9(2):38-45, 1997.

Amaro H: Women in the Mexican-American community: religion, culture, and reproductive attitudes and experiences, *J Comp Psychol* 16(1):6-19, 1994.

Bar-yam NB: Learning about culture: a guide for birth practitioners, *Int J Childbirth Educ* 9(2):8-10, 1994.

Becker M: The Health Belief Model and sick role behavior, *Health Educ Monogr* 2:409-419, 1974.

Boss P: *Family stress management,* ed 2, Thousand Oaks, CA, 2002, Sage.

Bronfenbrenner U: *The ecology of human development: experiments by nature and design,* Cambridge, MA, 1979, Harvard University Press.

Bronfenbrenner U: Ecological systems theory. In R.Vasta (ed): *Annals of child development* (vol 6, pp 187-249), Greenwich, CT, 1989, JAI.

Brooks E: Family assessment and cultural diversity. In Clemen-Stone S, McGuire SL, Eigsti DG (eds): *Comprehensive community health nursing: family, aggregate, and community practice,* ed 6, St Louis, 2002, Mosby.

Carter B, McGoldrick M: *The expanded family life cycle: individual, family, and social perspectives,* ed 3, Boston, 1999, Allyn & Bacon.

Chen JL, Rankin SH: Using the resiliency model to deliver culturally sensitive care to Chinese families, *J Pediatr Nurs* 17(3):157-166, 2002.

Clarke L: La familia: methodological issues in the assessment of perinatal social support for Mexicanas living in the United States, *Soc Sci Med* 53(10):1303-1320, 2001.

Clarke V: What about the children? Arguments against lesbian and gay parenting, *Womens Stud Int Forum* 24(5):555-570, 2001.

D'Avanzo CE, Geissler EM: *Pocket guide to cultural assessment,* ed 3, St Louis, 2003, Mosby.

Doyle EI, Ward SE: *The process of community health education and health promotion,* Mountain View, CA, 2001, Mayfield.

Engebretson J, Littleton LY: Cultural negotiation: a constructivist-based model for nursing practice, *Nurs Outlook* 49(5):223-230, 2001.

Federal Interagency Forum on Children and Family Statistics: Population and family characteristics, 2004. Internet document available at www.childstats.gov (accessed November 28, 2004).

Forbes C, Jepson R, Martin-Hirsch P: Interventions targeted at women to encourage the uptake of cervical screening (Cochrane Review), 2001. In *The Cochrane Library,* Issue 2, Chichester, UK, 2004, John Wiley & Sons.

Ford-Gilboe M: Dispelling myths and creating opportunity: a comparison of the strengths of single-parent and two-parent families, *ANS Adv Nurs Sci* 23(1):41-58, 2000.

Friedman MM: *Family nursing theory and assessment,* ed 4, New York, 1998, Appleton & Lange.

Friedman MM, Bowden VR, Jones EG: *Family nursing: research, theory, and practice,* ed 5, Upper Saddle River, NJ, 2003, Prentice Hall.

Galanti G: *Caring for patients from different cultures: case studies from American hospitals,* Philadelphia, 1997, University of Pennsylvania.

Howard CA, Andrade SJ, Byrd T: The ethical dimensions of cultural competence in border health care settings, *Fam Community Health* 23(4):36-49, 2001.

Huff RM, Kline MV: *Promoting health in multicultural populations,* Thousand Oaks, CA, 1999, Sage.

Janz NK, Becker MH: The Health Belief Model: a decade later, *Health Educ Q* 11(1):1-47, 1984.

Klein D, White J: *Family theories: an introduction,* Newberry Park, CA, 1996, Sage.

Lee R, Cubbin C: Neighborhood context and youth cardiovascular health behaviors, *Am J Public Health* 92(3):428-436, 2002.

Lynch EW, Hanson MJ: *Developing cross-cultural competence: a guide for working with children and their families,* Baltimore, 1998, Paul H Brookes.

Mattson S: Culturally sensitive prenatal care for Southeastern Asians, *J Obstet Gynecol Neonatal Nurs* 24(4):335-341, 1995.

Mattson S: Providing culturally competent care: strategies and approaches for perinatal clients, *AWHONN Lifelines* 4(5):37-39, 2000.

Murray RB, Zentner JP, Samiezade-Yazd C: Sociocultural influences on the person and family. In Murray RB, Zentner JP (eds): *Health promotion strategies through the life span,* ed 7, Upper Saddle River, NJ, 2001, Prentice-Hall.

National Academy Press: *From generation to generation: the health and well-being of children in immigrant families,* 2002. Internet document available at search.nap.edu/html/generation/summary.html (accessed November 28, 2004).

Pender NJ, Murdaugh CL, Parsons MA: *Health promotion in nursing practice,* Upper Saddle River, NJ, 2002, Prentice-Hall.

Ryan M, Carlton KH, Ali N: Transcultural nursing concepts and experiences in nursing curricula, *J Transcult Nurs* 11(4):300-307, 2000.

Simmons R et al: Health education and cultural diversity in the health care setting: tips for the practitioner, *Health Promot Pract* 3(1):8-11, 2002.

Spector RE: *Cultural diversity in health and illness,* ed 6, Upper Saddle River, NJ, 2004, Prentice Hall Health.

Staveteig S, Wigton A: *Key findings by race and ethnicity: findings from the National Survey of America's Families,* Washington, DC, 2000, Urban Institute. Internet document available at www.urban.org (accessed November 28, 2004).

Thomas ND: The importance of culture throughout all of life and beyond, *Holist Nurs Pract* 15(2):40-46, 2001.

US Department of Health and Human Services: *Healthy People 2010,* Chapter 16: Maternal, infant, and child health, 2000. Internet document available at www.health.gov/healthypeople/Document/HTML/Volume2/16MICH.htm (accessed November 28, 2004).

US Department of Health and Human Services, Office on Women's Health: Women's health issues: an overview, 2001. Internet document available at www.4woman.gov (accessed November 28, 2004).

Williams M et al: Promoting early breast cancer screening: strategies with rural African American women, *Am J Health Stud* 17(2):65-73, 2001.

Williams R: Issues in women's health care. In Johnson B (ed): *Psychiatric mental health nursing: adaptation and growth,* Philadelphia, 1989, Lippincott.

Willis WO: Culturally competent nursing care during the perinatal period, *J Perinat Neonatal Nurs* 13(3):45-59, 1999.

Wright LM, Leahey M: *Nurses and families: a guide to family assessment and intervention,* ed 3, Philadelphia, 2000, FA Davis.

Unit 1

3 Community and Home Care

LEARNING OBJECTIVES

On completion of this chapter the reader will be able to:

- Compare community-based health care and community health (population- or aggregate-focused) care.
- Identify key components of the community assessment process.
- List indicators of community health status and their relevance to perinatal health.
- Describe data sources and methods for obtaining information about community health status.
- Identify predisposing factors and characteristics of vulnerable populations.
- List the potential advantages and disadvantages of home visits.
- Explore telephonic nursing care options in perinatal nursing.
- Describe how home care fits into the maternity continuum of care.
- Identify and define common perinatal conditions amenable to home care.
- Discuss safety and infection control principles as they apply to the care of patients in their homes.
- Describe the nurse's role in perinatal home care.

ELECTRONIC RESOURCES

Additional information related to the content in Chapter 3 can be found on

the companion website at evolve
http://evolve.elsevier.com/Wong/maternal/
- NCLEX Review Questions
- WebLinks

or the interactive student CD-ROM
Activities for Chapter 3 include the following:
- NCLEX Review Questions
- Critical Thinking Exercise–Community Resources for Families
- Nursing Care Plan–Community and Home Care

Health care in the United States has evolved rapidly in recent years, with notable shifts in both the nature of health priorities and the ways that health care is delivered to populations, families, and individuals. Greater emphasis is placed on the prevention of disease and disability, rather than the curative focus of past decades.

One major shift in health care delivery is an increased emphasis on brief hospital stays that serve to reduce the financial burden for individuals, agencies, and insurance carriers. Hospital stays after childbirth may be abbreviated. By minimizing inpatient length of stay, much of acute care nursing has been transferred to home-based nursing services in local communities.

The U.S. national health objectives in *Healthy People 2010* focus attention on the unequal distribution of disease and disability and the need to reach out to vulnerable populations not being adequately served by the current health system (U.S. Department of Health and Human Services [USDHHS], 2000a). Hospital-based nurses are increasingly involved in follow-up of patients and families after discharge.

Trends in maternal and infant health in the United States reveal that progress has been made in relation to reduced infant and fetal deaths, use of prenatal care, and rates of cesarean births (see Chapter 1), but notable gaps remain in many other target areas. Some critical measures, such as low birth weight (LBW) and very low birth weight (VLBW), have increased, with significant disparities in infant mortality rates between Caucasians and other racial and ethnic groups in the United States. Despite favorable trends in early prenatal care and cesarean births, maternal mortality has not decreased significantly since 1982, with disproportionate rates among African-American and Hispanic women (USDHHS, 2000b). That many of these outcomes are preventable through access to prenatal care and use of preventive health practices clearly demonstrates the need for comprehensive, community-based care for mothers, infants, and families.

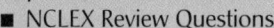

Changing demands on the community-based nurse evolve out of these societal, economic, and health-related trends. Acuity of illness of home care patients may be far greater than in the past, requiring the community nurse to become more adept in maternal assessment, direct care, and teaching. Assessment of the neonate requires knowledge of parameters for measuring the health of a newborn within the first days of life. Skill in assisting with breastfeeding is essential. Knowledge of an ever-widening array of diverse family traditions, beliefs, and expectations related to childbearing becomes even more critical for the nurse to facilitate effectively the transition required when a family moves through the stages of incorporating a new family member.

Community and family cannot be considered apart. Furthermore, as population demographics change, nurses are assuming greater roles in assessing community health status and providing health promotion and disease prevention interventions across the perinatal health continuum. Chapter 2 contains an overview of family and cultural theory and assessment. The integration of community and home care is discussed within the context of family-focused nursing in relation to *Healthy People 2010* and perinatal health outcomes. Methods of community assessment and the special perinatal health needs of vulnerable aggregates in the population are discussed.

HEALTH AND WELLNESS IN THE COMMUNITY

In the context of community-based health care, both the aggregate (group of people who have shared characteristics) and the population become the focus of intervention. Health professionals are required not only to determine health priorities but also to develop successful plans of care to be delivered in the health clinic, the community health center, or the patient's home.

Community Health Status Indicators

The data collected about communities can be compared with state or national standards to assess the well-being of the population as a whole and answer questions such as the following: Do most women begin prenatal care in the first trimester? What are the fetal and infant mortality rates?

Box 3-1 displays a set of community health status indicators developed by a committee of experts from many community health-related organizations. Infant mortality, because it is affected by the preconceptional health and prenatal and intrapartal care of the mother, as well as living conditions for the infant after birth, is a statistic widely used to compare the health status of different populations. Three of the five indicators of risk (i.e., incidence of low birth weight, adolescent pregnancy, and early prenatal care) refer to maternal-infant health. Poverty and a high percentage of young children in a community are strongly associated with significant community health needs (Zyzanski, Williams, & Flocke, 1996).

BOX 3-1

Consensus Set of Indicators* for Assessing Community Health Status

Indicators of Health Status Outcome

1. Race/ethnicity-specific infant mortality, as measured by the rate (per 1000 live births) of deaths among infants younger than 1 year of age

Death rates (per 100,000 population)† for

2. Motor vehicle crashes
3. Work-related injury
4. Suicide
5. Lung cancer
6. Breast cancer
7. Cardiovascular disease
8. Homicide
9. All causes

Reported incidence (per 100,000 population) of

10. Acquired immunodeficiency syndrome
11. Measles
12. Tuberculosis
13. Primary and secondary syphilis

Indicators of Risk Factors

14. Incidence of LBW, as measured by percentage of total number of live-born infants weighing less than 2500 g at birth
15. Births to adolescents (females age 10 to 17 years) as a percentage of total live births
16. Prenatal care, as measured by percentage of mothers delivering live infants who did not receive prenatal care during first trimester
17. Childhood poverty, as measured by the proportion of children younger than 15 years of age living in families at or below the poverty level
18. Proportion of persons living in counties exceeding U.S. Environmental Protection Agency standards for air quality during previous year

From US Department of Health and Human Services: Consensus set of indicators for assessing community health status, *MMWR* 40(27):449, 1991.
*Position or number of the indicator does not imply priority.
†Age-adjusted to the 1940 standard population.

VULNERABLE POPULATIONS

Several broad categories of high risk or vulnerable populations are of special interest to perinatal nurses working in the community. These include the following categories.

Women

One of the primary factors compromising women's health is lack of access to acceptable-quality health care, which may take many forms: lack of health insurance, living in a medically underserved area, or an inability to obtain needed services, particularly basic services such as prenatal care. For example, some rural areas have few obstetricians, pediatricians, and nurse-midwives; women may have to travel hundreds of miles for this kind of care (Bushy, 1998, 2001). Women often have lower incomes and less education and are therefore considered at high risk. Infant mortality is nearly two times higher for mothers without a high school education (USDHHS, 2000b).

Within the larger group of vulnerable women, a number of subgroups present challenges to the community-based perinatal nurse.

Adolescent Girls

Youth and adults younger than 24 years are the least medically served of all age groups in the United States (USDHHS, 2001). Lifestyle choices related to substance use, sexually transmitted infections, and human immunodeficiency virus (HIV) represent high risk behaviors with both immediate and long-term health consequences. Many engage in "survival sex," exchanging sexual favors for food, clothing, and shelter, making them vulnerable to sexually transmitted infections and unintended pregnancies. Young women, particularly African-Americans and Hispanics, are less likely to have access to routine care and often fail to seek care because of inability to pay, lack of transportation, or confidentiality issues (USDHHS, 2000c).

Minority Women

In the United States, disparities continue to exist in health and health care. Higher infant and maternal mortality rates are evident in African-American and Hispanic women and among some Native American and Alaskan Native communities. Women with underlying health conditions are at especially high risk for poor obstetric outcomes for both themselves and their infants. They have high rates of preterm labor and preeclampsia, and often have intrauterine growth restriction resulting in the birth of infants who are small for gestational age. These are the patients for whom the community-based perinatal nurse will be providing care, and their needs are complex, demanding expertise and high levels of skill.

Migrant Women

An estimated 3 to 5 million people, 16% of whom are women, are classified as migrant farm workers in the United States (Maternal Child Health Bureau, 1997). Migrant laborers establish temporary residence in various areas on a seasonal basis to obtain employment. Although many acquire temporary housing for at least 6 months, others move continuously throughout the year. Diverse ethnic groups are represented among migrants: African-Americans, European-Americans, Hispanics, Haitians, and Southeast Asians.

Migrant laborers and their families face many problems, including financial instability, child labor, poor housing, lack of education, language and cultural barriers, and limited access to health and social services (McGuire, 2002). Poor dental health, diabetes, hypertension, malnutrition, tuberculosis, and parasitic infections are common health issues among migrant populations. The average life expectancy for migrant laborers is 49 years (as compared with 79 years for the population as a whole). Substance abuse and domestic violence are significant problems.

Numerous reproductive health issues exist for migrant women, including less consistent use of contraception and increased rates of sexually transmitted infections. Migrants are less likely to receive early prenatal care and have a greater incidence of inadequate weight gain during pregnancy than do other poor women. The infant mortality rate among migrant workers is estimated to be 25 times higher than the national average (Murray, Zentner, & Samiezade-Yazd, 2001).

Federally funded migrant health centers have been established in many regions of the United States, but they are unable to meet the demands of the 3 to 5 million migrants. Many seek care at local hospitals and clinics in the areas in which they work, but access is limited by lack of time and financial constraints. Even if services are free, the loss of wages incurred in leaving the field is a deterrent to preventive care. Lack of trust or fear of being reported to the Immigration and Naturalization Services prevents many undocumented workers from seeking care.

??? Critical Thinking Exercise

HEALTH NEEDS OF A MIGRANT WORKER

The home care agency receives a referral for a home visit to a 16-year-old Vietnamese-speaking mother, Linh, who is a migrant worker. She has a 2-week-old infant and is expected to return to the fields to work. Before visiting Linh, the nurse establishes as priorities to promote breastfeeding, encourage use of birth control, and involve the father of the baby in child care.

1. Evidence—Is there sufficient evidence to draw conclusions about the appropriateness of the nurse's plan of care?
2. Assumptions—What assumptions can be made about the needs of this mother and baby in regard to the following issues?
   a. The priorities for care
   b. Conditions for effective breastfeeding
   c. Feasibility of maintaining breastfeeding while working in the field
   d. Cultural relevancy of involving the father
3. What implications and priorities for nursing care can be drawn at this time?
4. Does the evidence objectively support your conclusion?
5. Are there alternative perspectives to your conclusion?

Rural versus Urban Community Settings

Rural refers to a town or community area that has a population of less than 2500 or to a county with fewer than 50,000 people. A number of common characteristics define rural groups: They lack anonymity, are isolated, and tend to be content to live independently (Bushy, 2000; Murray et al, 2001). Geographic and socioeconomic factors present barriers to accessing prenatal care associated with transportation and provider inaccessibility.

Homeless Women

An estimated 2.5 to 3.5 million people are homeless nationally, with 6.5% of adults reporting homelessness each year. This includes increasing numbers of women, children, and adolescents who are disenfranchised from their homes, families, and services for various reasons, resulting in a 17% increase in the demand for family assistance (Bureau of Primary Health Care, 2001). Depending on the cause of homelessness and the availability of services, a person may be homeless for weeks or months, intermittently, or on a prolonged basis.

The most significant causes of homelessness in the United States relate to mental illness (approximately 50%) and substance use (nearly 75% among homeless men). Violent relationships and a history of abuse are significant contributing factors to homelessness for women.

Although the homeless population is generally higher in urban areas, a growing number of the homeless are found in rural agricultural, mining, and fishing regions, where they seek temporary employment. Often these families remain hidden within the community. Sometimes the family stays in a local hotel (paying on a daily basis while they work), lives out of their car, resides in an unoccupied building, or may camp in a national park. Couples with children form the largest group among rural homeless. Lack of visibility and community resources in rural areas frequently results in longer periods of poverty and homelessness for these families (Bushy, 2000).

Health issues among the homeless are numerous, resulting primarily from a lack of preventive care and a lack of resources in general. Because very few are able to access primary care, most of the homeless population are forced to use the emergency room for routine health problems. Mental health and substance abuse services for the homeless are extremely limited in many communities, in particular in medically underserved rural regions of the United States (Bureau of Primary Health Care, 2001).

For women, the emotional and psychologic trauma of the homeless experience is often exacerbated by physical or sexual assault; 36% of homeless women report being a victim of a crime while living on the streets. Approximately 24% of women become pregnant while they are homeless. Although many women are eligible for Medicaid and public health services, few receive prenatal care.

Refugees and Immigrants

Refugees are defined as those who are displaced suddenly or forced to leave their country of origin because of persecution, civil unrest, or war. Families are thus forced from their own homes to seek residence and employment elsewhere (Murray et al, 2001). Often these groups are extremely impoverished and face extreme physical and emotional stress when they arrive in the United States. Some refugees have a history of arrival in a new country by precarious means, such as crossing wide oceans in fragile boats. Many survivors of such journeys have memories of relatives and friends who died at sea. Many have been raped by modern pirates who prey on those who are desperate for a better life. The traumatic stress of having witnessed the murders of their families as a result of war haunts many refugees. Many have profound grief over the loss of loved ones, their homelands, and all they owned. Both refugees and immigrants are saddened by the knowledge that it will be difficult or impossible to go "home" to the people, traditions, and customs that were familiar and comforting.

Along with their profound resilience and determination, refugees and immigrants have brought rich diversity to the United States in several important dimensions, including cultural heritage and customs, economic productivity, and enhanced national vitality. At the same time, multiple challenges accompany the dramatic influx of individuals and families from other countries.

In general, refugees are more likely to live in poverty than are immigrants (Murray et al, 2001). Over time, measures of health and well-being actually decline for the immigrant population as they become part of American society (National Academy Press [NAP], 2002). Many of the conditions or illnesses that they acquire contribute to the persistence of disparities in maternal and neonatal health outcomes for both immigrants and refugees.

Implications for Nursing

Working in the community or in the home with the full spectrum of family organizational styles, vulnerable populations, and cultural groups presents challenges for the nurse. Whether it involves perinatal care focused on women and their newborns, or women's health care directed toward treatment and prevention of other health conditions such as communicable diseases and sexually transmitted infections, nursing must exhibit a high degree of professionalism. Cultural sensitivity, compassion, and a critical awareness of family dynamics and social stressors that will affect health-related decision making are critical components in developing an effective plan of care.

Although the long-term consequences of contemporary immigration for American society are unclear, the successful incorporation of immigrant families depends on the resources, benefits, and policies that ensure their healthy development and successful social adjustment. Culturally competent health care and involvement of the immigrant community in health care programs are recommended strategies for improving the access to and effectiveness of health care for this population (NAP, 2002).

The use of camp volunteers, known as "romatoras," has been effective in assisting families living in migrant worker camps to obtain prenatal, postpartum, and infant care (see Resources at the end of the chapter). Working in partnership with health professionals such as nurses, lay camp aides have been used effectively for outreach and health education; however, more strategies are needed to link traditional practices with the formal health care system. Guidance and information about other health resources are available to health care providers through the National Migrant Resource Program and the Migrant Clinicians Network.

Nurses working with homeless women and families are challenged to treat them with dignity and respect to establish a therapeutic relationship. Case management is recommended to coordinate the services and disciplines that may be involved in meeting the complex needs of these families. Whenever possible, health services must be provided when the woman seeks treatment, as this may be the only opportunity to provide health information and intervention. Building on existing coping strategies and strengths, the health care provider helps the woman and her family to reconnect with a social support system. Nurses also have an important role in advocating for funding to support homeless health services and to improve access to preventive care for all homeless populations.

ASSESSING THE COMMUNITIES IN WHICH FAMILIES LIVE

Mothers assume much of the health-related decision making for their families (USDHHS, 2001), with up to 83% of them having sole or shared responsibility for financial decisions affecting family health. A significant link exists between the maternal roles of health care provider and decision maker and family health behavior. The health and well-being of women and children will be in jeopardy as long as the communities in which they live are ill prepared to provide the quantity and quality of services they need.

Important measures of community health include access to care, level of provider services available, and other social and economic factors. For women and infants, access to a consistent source of care is critical. Those with a regular source of care are more likely to use preventive services and receive timely treatment for illness and injury (USDHHS, 2000c), but current statistics indicate that more than 16% of Medicaid-covered women as compared with 13.4% of privately insured women lack access to a usual source of care or rely primarily on emergency services. Consequently, many of these women report unmet health or dental needs (Almeida, Dubay, & Ko, 2001).

Methods of Community Assessment

Community, in its broadest definition, refers to a geographically defined area; its residents; their cultural, religious, and ethnic characteristics; and the activities or functions through which the needs of the residents are met. The health of individuals or groups is inextricably linked to the health status of each community.

With the community as the focus of perinatal health care, the nurse must become familiar with the neighborhoods and resources that influence patients. Community assessment is a complex although well-defined process through which the unique characteristics of the populations and their special needs are identified to plan and evaluate health services for the community as a whole. The desired outcome of this process is identification of direct service, as well as advocacy needs of the targeted aggregate or group and improved health for the community as a whole (Kuehnert, 2002).

Data Collection and Sources of Community Health Data

A community assessment framework or model provides criteria for conducting a community assessment, identifies types and methods of data collection, and organizes the data of a community assessment (Ervin, 2002) (Fig. 3-1).

Data collection is often the most time-consuming phase of the community assessment process, but it provides an important definition and description of the community (Ervin, 2002). A broad range of health information is available for

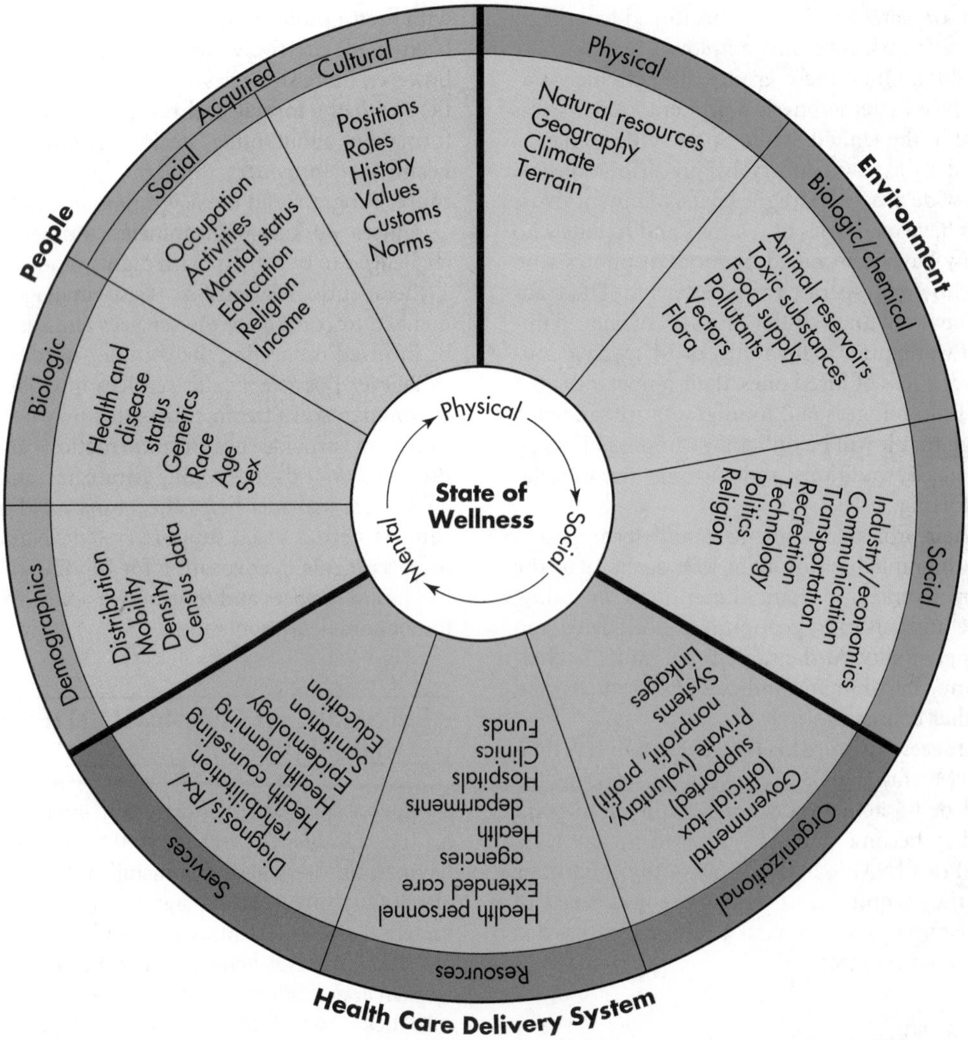

Fig. 3-1 Community health assessment wheel. (From Clemen-Stone S: Community assessment and diagnosis. In Clemen-Stone S, McGuire S, Eigsti D (eds): *Comprehensive community health nursing: family, aggregate, and community practice,* ed 6, St Louis, 2002, Mosby.)

nurses in conducting a community assessment. The most critical indicators of perinatal health in a community are related to access to health care; maternal mortality; infant mortality; low birth weight; first trimester prenatal care; and rates for mammography, Pap smears, and other similar screening tests (USDHHS, 2000c). Nurses may use these indicators as a reflection of access, quality, and continuity of health care in a community.

The U.S. government census provides data on population size, age ranges, sex, racial and ethnic distribution, socioeconomic status, educational level, employment, and housing characteristics. Summary data are available for most large metropolitan areas, arranged by zip code and census tract, which usually corresponds to a neighborhood (approximately 3000 to 6000 people). Looking at individual census tracts within a community helps to identify subpopulations or aggregates whose needs may differ from those of the larger community. For example, women at high risk for inadequate prenatal care according to age, race, and ethnic or cultural group may be readily identified, and outreach activities may be appropriately targeted.

City, county, and state health departments provide annual reports of births and deaths. Maternal and infant death rates are particularly important, as they reflect health outcomes that may be preventable (McDevitt & Wilbur, 2002). Local health departments also compile extensive statistics about the birth complications, causes of death, and leading causes of morbidity and mortality for each age group. The National Health Survey, which describes national health trends, is published annually by the National Center for Health Statistics.

Other sources of useful information are hospitals and voluntary health agencies. The March of Dimes Birth Defects Foundation, for example, has supported perinatal needs assessments in many communities across the United States. Other community health resources include health care providers or administrators, government officials, religious leaders, and representatives of voluntary health agencies. Community or county health councils exist in many areas, with oversight of specific health initiatives or programs for that region. These key informants often provide a unique perspective that may be inaccessible through other sources.

The perinatal health nurse also may explore community health program reports, records of preventive health screenings, and other informal data. Established programs often provide good indicators of the health promotion and disease prevention characteristics of the population.

Professional publications are a rich and readily accessible source of information for all nurses. In addition to nursing and public health journals, behavioral and social science literature offers diverse perspectives on community health status for specific populations and subgroups. The Internet has increased the availability and accessibility of national, state, and local health data as well. Use of Web-based resources for health information requires some caution, however, as the reliability and the validity of the data are difficult to verify. Some guidelines for evaluation of Internet health resources can be found at the Health on the Net Web site at www.hon.org. Additional health Web sites are identified at the end of the chapter.

Data collection methods may be either qualitative or quantitative, including visual surveys that can be completed by walking through a community, participant observation, interviews, focus groups, and analysis of existing data. Potential patients and health care consumers may be asked to participate in focus groups or community forums to present their views on needed community services and programs. Formal surveys, either by mail, by telephone, or by face-to-face interviews, can be a valuable source of information not available from national databases or other secondary sources. Several drawbacks exist with this method: surveys are generally expensive to develop and time consuming to administer. In addition to the cost of such surveys, poor response rates often preclude a sufficiently representative response on which to base nursing interventions.

A walking survey is generally conducted by a walk-through observation of the community (Box 3-2), taking note of specific characteristics of the population, economic and social environment, transportation, health care services, and other resources This method allows the nurse to collect subjective data and may facilitate other aspects of the assessment (Ervin, 2002). Figure 3-2 is an example of an accommodation for expectant and new mothers that might be noticed during such a survey.

Participant observation is another useful assessment method in which the nurse actively participates in the community to understand the community more fully and to validate observations.

Finally, as part of the assessment process, nurses working in multiethnic and multicultural groups need an in-depth assessment of culturally driven behaviors (Williams et al, 2001). Needs assessment for these groups should focus on epidemiologic data and population needs and interests.

Analysis and synthesis of data obtained during the assessment process helps to generate a comprehensive picture of the community's health status, needs, and problem areas, as well as its strengths and resources for addressing these concerns. The goal of this process is to assign priorities to community health needs and to develop a plan of action for correcting them. A comparison of community health data with state and national statistics may be useful in identification of appropriate target populations, as well as interventions to improve health outcomes.

Successful community-based health initiatives involve understanding of community relationships and resources, as well as participation of community leaders (Lauderdale, 2001). Failure to recognize and involve individuals, families, and communities in the process often results in failed or short-lived health interventions (Bruhn, 2001).

Comprehensive community assessment and the use of timely, high-quality data sources can help prevent poor birth outcomes and promote maternal health by identifying aggregates at risk and giving direction to preventive interventions. Often the outcomes of local and state assessments are used to determine policy and resource allocation, which directly or indirectly affect health for the most needy and vulnerable populations. Decisions related to funding of community health promotion initiatives also are linked to these data sources (Doyle & Ward, 2001).

BOX 3-2

Learning about the Community on Foot

I. Community Core

1. **History**—What can you glean by looking (e.g., old, established neighborhoods; new subdivision)? Ask people willing to talk: How long have you lived here? Has the area changed? As you talk, ask if there is an "old-timer" who knows the history of the area.
2. **Demographics**—What sorts of people do you see? Young? Old? Homeless? Alone? Families? What races do you see? Is the population homogeneous?
3. **Ethnicity**—Do you note indicators of different ethnic groups (e.g., restaurants, festivals)? What signs do you see of different cultural groups?
4. **Values and beliefs**—Are there churches, mosques, temples? Does it appear homogeneous? Are the lawns cared for? With flowers? Gardens? Signs of art? Culture? Heritage? Historical markers?

II. Subsystems

1. **Physical environment**—How does the community look? What do you note about air quality, flora, housing, zoning, space, green areas, animals, people, human-made structures, natural beauty, water, climate? Can you find or develop a map of the area? What is the size (e.g., square miles, blocks)?
2. **Health and social services**—Evidence of acute or chronic conditions? Shelters? "Traditional" healers (e.g., curanderos, herbalists)? Are there clinics, hospitals, practitioners' offices, public health services, home health agencies, emergency centers, nursing homes, social service facilities, mental health services? Are there resources outside the community but accessible to them?
3. **Economy**—Is it a "thriving" community or does it feel "seedy?" Are there industries, stores, places for employment? Where do people shop? Are there signs that food stamps are used/accepted? What is the unemployment rate?
4. **Transportation and safety**—How do people get around? What types of private and public transportation are available? Do you see buses, bicycles, taxis? Are there sidewalks, bike trails? Is getting around in the community possible for persons with disabilities? What types of protective services are there (e.g., fire, police, sanitation)? Is air quality monitored? What are the types of crimes committed? Do people feel safe?
5. **Politics and government**—Are there signs of political activity (e.g., posters, meetings)? What party affiliation predominates? What is the governmental jurisdiction of the community (e.g., elected mayor, city council with single-member districts)? Are people involved in decision making in their local governmental unit?
6. **Communication**—Are there "common areas" where people gather? What newspapers do you see in the stands? Do people have TVs and radios? What do they watch/listen to? What are the formal and informal means of communication?
7. **Education**—Are there schools in the area? How do they look? Are there libraries? Is there a local board of education? How does it function? What is the reputation of the school(s)? What are major educational issues? What are the dropout rates? Are there extracurricular activities available? Are they used? Is there a school health service? A school nurse?
8. **Recreation**—Where do children play? What are the major forms of recreation? Who participates? What facilities for recreation do you see?

III. Perceptions

1. **The residents**—How do people feel about the community? What do they identify as its strengths? Problems? Ask several people from different groups (e.g., old, young, field worker, factory worker, professional, minister, housewife) and keep track of who gives what answer.
2. **Your perceptions**—General statements about the "health" of this community. What are its strengths? What problems or potential problems can you identify?

From Anderson ET, McFarlane J: *Community as partner: theory and practice in nursing,* ed 4, Philadelphia, 2004, Lippincott Williams & Wilkins.
NOTE: Supplement your impressions with information from the census, police records, school statistics, chamber of commerce data, health department reports, etc., to confirm or refute your conclusions. Tables, graphs, and maps are helpful and will aid in your analysis.

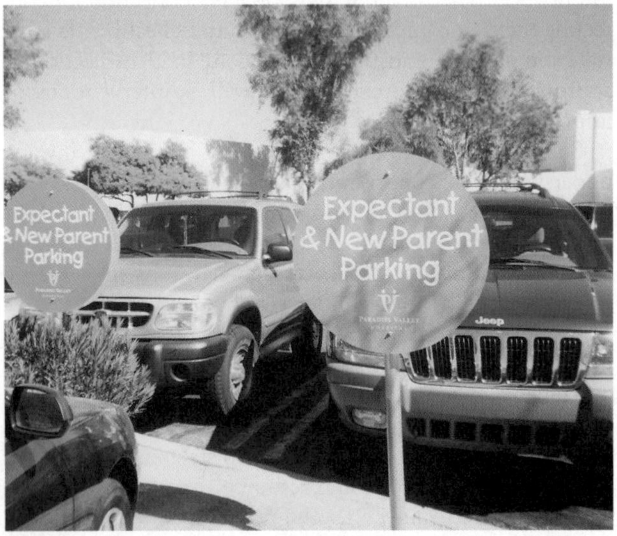

Fig. 3-2 Community accommodation for expectant and new parents. (Courtesy Shannon Perry, Phoenix, AZ.)

LEVELS OF PREVENTIVE CARE

Population-based care involves prevention activities focused on target needs identified in the community assessment process. These levels of prevention provide a framework for nursing interventions. Primary prevention involves health promotion and disease prevention activities to decrease the occurrence of illness and enhance general health and quality of life. Sometimes referred to as "true prevention," primary prevention precedes disease or dysfunction and encourages individuals to achieve the optimal level of health possible. This includes the use of specific health protections such as recommended immunizations, infant car seats, and school health education to prevent tobacco use.

Early detection of health problems is the focus of secondary prevention. Persons who are asymptomatic or who have nonspecific disease symptoms are targeted to receive curative treatment and reduce disease prevalence (Marks & Wilcox, 1999). At this level, various methods of health screening and testing facilitate early treatment of the pathologic process. The goal is to shorten disease duration and severity, thus enabling an individual to return to normal function as quickly as possible (Murray et al, 2001).

Tertiary prevention follows the occurrence of a defect or disability that is permanent and irreversible (Murray et al, 2001). Persons who have developed disease are provided with treatment and rehabilitation to prevent complications and further deterioration and to maintain their optimal level of function.

Because most women are healthy during pregnancy, maternal-newborn nursing emphasizes primary and secondary prevention activities regardless of where care is provided. Tertiary prevention is frequently the focus for the ill patient at home or in the hospital.

Primordial prevention, which refers to genetic modifications that prevent susceptibility to some conditions, is an emerging concept made possible through recent genetic research and the advances of the Human Genome Project (Marks & Wilcox, 1999).

COMMUNITY HEALTH PROMOTION

The emphasis on community-based health promotion has grown in recent years, with recognition that many health issues require the collaborative efforts of a diverse community network to achieve public health goals (Marks & Wilcox, 1999). Pender and colleagues (2002) also noted the benefits of community-based, coordinated health promotion programs with the potential for widespread change in community health status. These efforts are particularly relevant in relation to maternal-newborn health, which encompasses multiple public health issues: lack of health insurance, teen pregnancy, substance abuse, and the consequences of inadequate prenatal care.

Health promotion efforts for childbearing families are primarily focused on early intervention through prenatal care and prevention of complications during the perinatal period. Often this early exposure to health information sets the stage for a successful birth and positive outcomes for mother and baby. Involving expectant mothers and fathers in identification of their learning needs is an essential first step to securing their participation in the health promotion process.

A wide variety of strategies have been used to disseminate heath information to women in the community. Prenatal classes are a well-established mechanism for increasing awareness of healthy behaviors during pregnancy and preparing parents for the care of themselves and their newborn during the postpartum period. Mass media efforts such as those presented by the March of Dimes "Baby Your Baby" advertisements are clear, consumer-friendly messages designed to reach a large target audience. Other venues include public health education in newspapers and magazines, and health department programs such as the Special Supplemental Program for Women, Infants, and Children (WIC), which offers a variety of health education and written information to mothers. The Association of Women's Health, Obstetric, and Neonatal Nurses' (AWHONN's) education guide, *Every Woman: The Essential Guide for Healthy Living,* is an evidence-based practice guide distributed to women by their nurses.

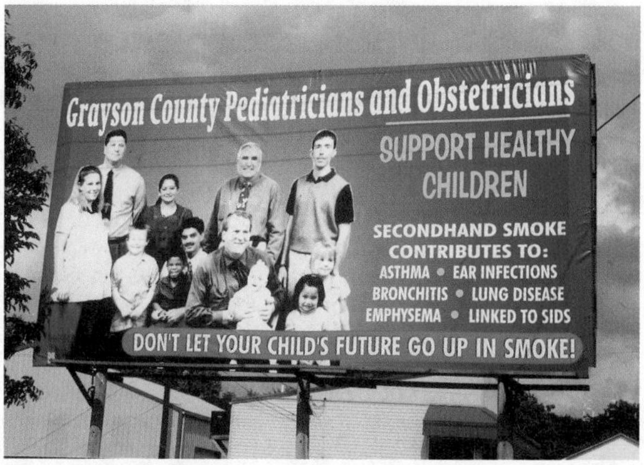
Grayson County Pediatricians and Obstetricians
SUPPORT HEALTHY CHILDREN
SECONDHAND SMOKE CONTRIBUTES TO:
ASTHMA • EAR INFECTIONS
BRONCHITIS • LUNG DISEASE
EMPHYSEMA • LINKED TO SIDS
DON'T LET YOUR CHILD'S FUTURE GO UP IN SMOKE!

Fig. 3-3 Billboard illustrating the hazards of smoking. (Courtesy Joan R. Vogel, Boca Raton, FL.)

Many communities have organized coalitions to address specific health promotion agendas related to sharing information, educating community members, or advocating for health policies around maternal and child health issues. An example of this is Healthy Start, a community-based initiative to reduce infant mortality and improve the health and well-being of women, children, and families (Goldman & DeLaCruz, 1999). Smoking presents major health risks for women, fetuses, and infants. There are major smoking cessation efforts directed toward pregnant women (Fig. 3-3). Adolescent health is another broad target area for community health promotion efforts, including both health education and policy initiatives. Issues related to adolescent sexuality, teen pregnancy, and substance abuse are particularly problematic, requiring aggressive prevention programs and community outreach (Maehr & Felice, 1999).

Community-based health promotion for childbearing families is often a challenge, because those who are most in need are less able to access such services. For example, low-income, uneducated, or homeless women, who frequently delay seeking prenatal care, also are disenfranchised in relation to other health promotion activities. Failure to address these social and environmental barriers and inability to engage the target audience often limits the benefits and sustainability of health promotion initiatives (Bruhn, 2001). Efforts should thus be focused on increasing awareness of health promotion activities, as well as ensuring access for all community groups.

PERINATAL CONTINUUM OF CARE

Within the community, perinatal care is provided on a continuum. A *continuum of care* is defined as a range of clinical services provided for an individual or group that reflects care given during a single hospitalization or care for multiple conditions over a lifetime. Home care is one delivery

Evidence-Based Practice

PARENTING GROUPS FOR TEENAGE PARENTS

Background

In the developed world, teen pregnancy is highest in the United States (55/1000 women age 15 to 19 years), followed by New Zealand (33/1000) and Canada (25/1000). The United Kingdom (23/1000) has the highest rate in Europe. Where deprivation and poverty are high, so is teen pregnancy. There is evidence that teen mothers have lower aspirations for themselves and come from family backgrounds of low educational expectations. Early parenthood brings the needs of the still-developing teen in direct competition with the needs of the fetus and baby, and usually truncates the mother's opportunities. Younger parents may lack realistic expectations of child development and parenting and disciplinary skills. They may experience stress, depression, low self-esteem, and socioeconomic deprivation. Infants of teen mothers may have developmental delays, behavioral problems, intellectual deficits, and lower educational achievement. Child abuse may be present for all these reasons, rather than young parental age alone. The prevention of teen pregnancy remains the primary intervention to prevent these vulnerabilities. After birth, however, early interventions such as parenting programs show promise as a way to compensate the immature and inexperienced parent for a lack of life exposure and perspective.

Objectives

The reviewers' goal was to assess the impact of parenting skills education on the health and well-being of teen parents and their babies. The ideal interventions would be individually or group formatted, offered during pregnancy or after birth to teen parents, and structured to improve parenting attitudes, skills, or knowledge. Outcomes sought were maternal anxiety, stress, depression, self-esteem, sense of parenting competence, and parenting and child development knowledge, and infant cognitive, social, and mental development.

Methods

Search Strategy

The authors searched Cochrane, MEDLINE, EMBASE, CINAHL, Psyclit, Sociofile, Social Science Citation Index, ASSIA, National Research Registry, ERIC, and reference lists. Search keywords included *parent, program, train, education, promotion, health, adolescent, mother, teen, father, pregnancy,* and combinations of these words.

Four randomized, controlled trials were selected, for a subject pool of 247 teen mothers who volunteered for a parenting program. The studies were published between 1977 and 1999 and were all from the United States. The trials used a variety of settings, including a school, a health setting, a residential maternity home, community health clinics, and family support centers.

Statistical Analyses

The reviewer calculated a treatment effect for each available and reliable outcome. This enabled assessment of how strongly the intervention was associated with the outcomes.

Findings

When compared with the controls, the parenting intervention group showed a significant increase in maternal sensitivity, identity as a mother, parenting knowledge, maternal-child interaction, mealtime attitudes and communication, and cognitive growth fostering capacities. There were trends of improvement in maternal self-confidence and motivation, but not to the level of statistical significance. Infants whose mothers were receiving the parenting intervention had nonsignificant trends toward responsiveness to parent, clearer interaction, and language scores, up to 2 years of age.

Limitations

The small number of studies, and the fact that they were all from the same country, limits generalizability of the results. Some of the data were collected with tools that had no reported reliability or validity. The treatment effects may have seemed stronger than they actually were, due to the statistical handling of cluster randomization (groups in a school who were divided into groups by classroom), dropouts, and subjects lost to follow-up. Dropout rates were marked in one study (33%), but remarkably low in the other three studies, considering that dropout rates are usually increased with teenagers, low socioeconomic status, and ethnic minorities.

There were no data on fathers. All the subjects were volunteers, and so may have self-selected for motivation, the maturity to identify their own deficits, self-esteem, or some other confounding influence. A strength of the review was the variety of settings where pregnant teens were seen.

Conclusions

Interventions facilitating parenting skills for vulnerable teen parents foster improved outcomes for both the mother and (probably) the child.

Implications for Practice

Interventions to foster parenting skills should be provided for teen parents. Health care providers need to give some thought to which setting might maximize the effects of which interventions. There needs to be some coordination among various providers. Teen fathers, often absent due to lack of commitment, mistrust in the services, illiteracy, and personality, need interventions tailored to their special needs as teens and parents.

Implications for Further Research

More trials are needed, with attention to large numbers, minimizing dropouts, and statistical rigor for confounding effects. Some methods to recruit and randomize nonvolunteers would improve the generalizability of the results. Of particular interest are the influences of peers in the group. The skill of the facilitator is critical to the process and tone of the group, but none of the studies discussed this variable. Data on the long-term outcomes of the children are needed.

Reference

Coren E, Barlow J: Individual and group-based parenting programmes for improving psychosocial outcomes for teenage parents and their children (Cochrane Review), 2001. In *The Cochrane Library,* Issue 2, Chichester, UK, 2004, John Wiley & Sons.

component available along the perinatal continuum of care (Fig. 3-4). This continuum begins with family planning and continues with preconception care, prenatal care, intrapartum care, postpartum care, newborn care, interconception care, and infant care until the infant is 1 year old. Independent self-care, ambulatory care, home care, low risk hospitalization, or specialized intensive care may be appropriate at different points along this continuum.

Clinical integration of services can improve services. The goals of clinical integration are improved coordination of

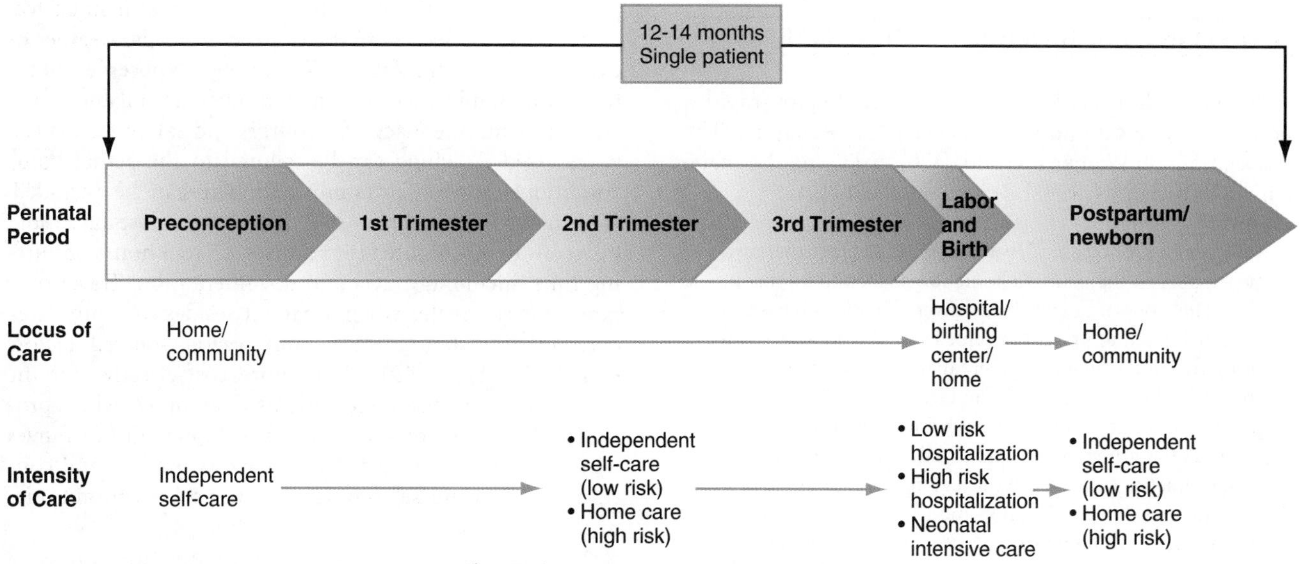

Fig. 3-4 Perinatal continuum of care.

care and care outcomes; better communication among health care providers; increased patient, payer, and provider satisfaction; and reduced cost. With clinical integration, the focus changes from illness to health, from the individual to the population, and from care provided in one setting to care across the continuum. The following factors make home care an important area in perinatal services:

- Interest in family birthing alternatives
- Shortened hospital stays
- New technologies that allow sophisticated assessments and treatments to be performed in the home
- Reimbursement by third-party payers

Modern home care nursing has its foundation in public health nursing, which provided comprehensive care to sick and well patients in their own homes. Specialized maternity home care nursing services began in the 1980s when public health maternity nursing services were limited and services had not kept pace with the changing practices of high risk obstetrics and emerging technology. Lengthy antepartal hospitalizations for such conditions as preterm labor and preeclampsia created nursing care challenges for staff members of inpatient units. Many women expressed their concern for the negative effect of antepartal hospitalizations on the family. Although clinical indications showed that a new nursing care approach was needed, home health care did not become a viable alternative until third-party payers (i.e., public or private organizations or employer groups that pay for health care) pushed for cost containment in maternity services.

COMMUNICATION TO BRIDGE THE CONTINUUM

As maternity care continues to consist of frequent and brief contacts with health care providers throughout the prenatal and postpartum periods, services that link maternity patients throughout the perinatal continuum of care have assumed increasing importance. These services include critical pathways, telephonic nursing assessments, discharge planning, specialized education programs, parent support groups, home visiting programs, nurse advice lines, and perinatal home care. Some hospitals provide cross-training for hospital-based nurses to make postpartum home visits or to staff outpatient centers for postpartum follow-up.

Telephonic Nursing Care

Telephonic nursing care through services such as "warm lines," nurse advice lines, and telephonic nursing assessments is a valuable means of managing health care problems and bridging the gaps among acute, outpatient, and home care services. Some providers are using the Internet to communicate with patients who have an Internet service provider (ISP). Nursing care that occurs by telephone is interactive and responsive to immediate health care questions about particular health care needs. Warm lines are telephone lines that are offered as a community service to provide new parents with support, encouragement, and basic parenting education. Nurse advice lines, or toll-free nurse consultation services, often are supported by third-party payers or health maintenance organization/managed care organization (HMO/MCO) nurse case managers and are designed to provide answers to medical questions. These nurses are prepared to guide callers through urgent health care situations, suggest treatment options, and provide health education (Bleich, 1998). Telephonic nursing assessments, or nurse consultation, assessment, and health education that take place during a telephone conversation, can be added to the plan of care in conjunction with skilled nursing visits or may be a separate nursing contact for the woman. Telephonic nursing assessments are commonly used after a postpartum home care visit to reassess a woman's knowledge about the signs and symptoms of adequate hydration in breastfeeding, or, after initiating home phototherapy, to assess the caregiver's knowledge regarding problems with equipment.

GUIDELINES FOR NURSING PRACTICE

Although the home care industry continues to grow rapidly, perinatal home care nursing practice is still emerging. The Association of Women's Health, Obstetric, and Neonatal Nurses (AWHONN, 1998) defined *home care* as

> the provision of technical, psychologic, and other therapeutic support in the patient's home rather than in an institution. The scope of nursing care delivered in the home is necessarily limited to practices deemed safe and appropriate to be carried out in an environment that is physically separated from a health care institution and its resources. . . . Nursing practice at home is consistent with federal and state regulations . . . that direct home care practice. The nurse demonstrates practice competence through formalized orientation and ongoing clinical education and performance evaluation in the respective home care agency. Standards for practice from key specialty organizations such as AWHONN, the American College of Obstetricians and Gynecologists (ACOG), the American Academy of Pediatrics (AAP), and the Intravenous Nursing Society (INS) provide the basis for clinical protocols and pathways and organizational programs in home care practice. The Joint Commission on Accreditation of Health Care Organizations (JCAHO) provides criteria for home care operations based on Centers for Medicare and Medicaid Services regulations.

AWHONN (1994) developed standards of practice and identified essential knowledge and skills to provide safe perinatal home care. Health care agencies and individuals can use these to assess the nurse's skills and learning needs.

A wide range of professional health care services and health products can be delivered or used in the home with technology and telecommunication. For example, telehealth and telemedicine make it possible for patients in the home to be interviewed and assessed by a specialist located hundreds of miles away. Some view home health care as an extension of in-hospital care. Essentially, the primary difference between health care in a hospital and home care is the absence of the continuous presence of professional health care providers in a patient's home. Generally, but not always, home health care entails intermittent care by a professional who visits the patient's home for a particular reason and/or provides care on site for fewer than 4 hours at a time. The home health care agency maintains on-call professional staff to assist home care patients who have questions about their care and for emergencies, such as equipment failure.

HOME CARE PERINATAL SERVICES

Home care perinatal services may be provided by hospital-based programs, independent proprietary (for-profit) agencies or nonprofit home care agencies, and official or tax-supported agencies. Innovative programs may be supported by research grants for a period of years, but ultimately they must be sponsored by an agency with long-term funding. Home visits have both advantages and disadvantages. The pregnant woman is able to maintain bed rest if indicated, and vulnerable neonates are not exposed to the weather or external sources of infection. The nurse can observe and interact with family members in their most natural and secure environment. Adequacy of resources and safety factors can be assessed. Teaching can be tailored to the actual home conditions, and other family members can be included. A home visit is less expensive than a day's hospitalization, but a 60- to 90-minute visit requires 2.5 to 3 hours of nursing time, including travel and documentation. Travel time may be even greater when a patient resides in a rural area because of distance, travel, and weather-related factors (Bosch & Bushy, 1997). It is more cost-effective for the health care provider to see patients in an office, where professional time is not spent in travel. Availability of nurses with expertise in maternity care may be limited, and concerns about the nurse's physical safety in some communities may limit visits.

Visits for outreach and health promotion are an integral part of community (or public) health nursing. In countries with national health systems, a nurse or midwife may see all women during pregnancy and after birth. In the United States, visits of this sort have been provided mainly to low-income families without health insurance and Medicaid recipients who use the clinics provided by local health departments (Koniak-Griffin et al, 1999; Olds et al, 1997). Until recently, private insurers did not reimburse for health promotion visits. MCOs now recognize that anticipatory guidance can be cost-effective, but home visitation programs for the most part still target specific high risk populations, such as adolescents and women at risk for preterm labor.

Home care agencies are subject to regulation by governmental and professional organizations. They provide interdisciplinary services including social work, nutrition, and occupational and physical therapy. Increasingly their case loads are made up of patients who require high-technology care, such as infusions or home monitoring. Although the home health nurse develops the care plan, all care must be ordered by a physician. Additionally, interventions must meet the insurer's criteria for reimbursement, and services are limited to registered patients. Preconception care and low risk antepartum care can usually be provided more efficiently in offices and are not currently reimbursable. High risk antepartum care is often provided by home care agencies. For example, women with hyperemesis gravidarum who require parenteral nutrition may be treated at home. Conditions requiring bed rest, such as preterm labor and hypertension, are other common indications for home care. Other conditions may include cardiac disease, substance abuse, and diabetes in pregnancy.

Some insurers reimburse for at least one postpartum visit to families after early discharge or in the presence of high risk factors. Home phototherapy is used for treatment of neonatal hyperbilirubinemia and to avoid separation of mother and infant. Many other neonates who require long-term high-technology care also are managed with home care. The American Academy of Pediatrics (1998) recommends home visits as an effective early intervention strategy to improve child health in families at risk.

Patient Selection and Referral

The office- or hospital-based nurse is often the key person in making effective referrals to home care. When considering a referral to home care, the following factors are evaluated:

- Health status of mother and fetus or infant: Is the condition serious enough to warrant home care? Is it stable enough for intermittent observation to be sufficient?
- Availability of professionals to provide the needed services within the patient's community
- Family resources, including psychosocial, social, and economic resources: Will the family be able to provide care between nursing visits? Are relationships supportive? Is third-party reimbursement available, or can it be negotiated with the insurer? Could a voluntary or tax-supported community agency provide needed care without payment?
- Cost-effectiveness: Is it more reasonable for the patient to receive these services at home or to go to a local outpatient facility to receive them?

Community referrals should not be limited to women with physiologic complications of pregnancy that require medical treatment. Patients at risk (e.g., young adolescents, families with a history of abuse, members of vulnerable population groups, developmentally disabled individuals) may need follow-up care at home. In consultation with the social worker, the hospital-based nurse should become familiar with agencies in the community that accept such referrals. When the patient lives in a rural area, hospital-based nurses should familiarize themselves with available formal and informal resources in that community, as these may be different from those in a more populated setting (Bushy, 2000).

Standardized referral forms simplify the referral process and ensure that all needed information will be forwarded to the home health agency. The nursing assessment should include the woman's physical and psychologic status, her level of knowledge about self-care activities, her willingness to learn, the availability of caregivers and social support in the home, and her level of comfort with home care. If the referral is for a mother and infant home care visit, the nursing assessment should include newborn data.

High-technology home care requires additional information to be collected from the medical record and consultation with the referring physician and other members of the health care team before making a home care referral. These additional data include the medical diagnosis, medical prognosis, prescribed therapies, medication history, drug-dosing information, potential ancillary supplies, type of infusion access device, and the available systems of social support for the patient and family. The nursing assessment and therapies data provide baseline information for the home care nurse and other types of health care providers involved in the care plan.

Whenever a referral is called in to a home health care agency, a member of the nursing or admission staff determines the agency's ability to accept the patient for service. The use of telecommunication such as fax machines, cellular phones, and the Internet to transmit information has eliminated delays in initiating home care services, even in more remote rural areas.

Preparing for the Home Visit

The home care nurse reviews the available clinical data, demographic information, and completed plan of care form and consults with the home care pharmacist or other health care team members who have previously contacted the woman to determine the goals of the visit. At this point, the nurse uses the medical diagnosis and place on the perinatal continuum as a starting point to organize the woman's care. The nurse reviews agency policies and procedures, professional literature about diagnosis, and community resources as part of the previsit preparation work (Box 3-3).

Before going on a home visit, the nurse contacts the woman to make necessary arrangements and obtain detailed instructions on the location of the home. Contact by telephone has several goals besides establishing a convenient time to visit and exact directions; it also sets the stage for the first home care visit.

The nurse identifies himself or herself by name, title, and agency. He or she then explains who referred the woman to the agency for home care and the purpose of the home care visits. The nurse briefly explains what will occur during the visit and approximately how long the visit will last. The woman should be asked to restrain any pets during the visit. Last, the nurse asks about health supplies that may be needed for the woman's care.

Before the first visit, the home care nurse collects the woman's clinical record, patient education materials, medical supplies, and equipment necessary for the visit. Medications and specialized equipment should be ordered before the visit and delivered at the time of the scheduled visit.

CARE MANAGEMENT

First Home Care Visit

Making the first home care visit can be stressful for the nurse and the woman. The home care nurse is faced with an unknown environment controlled by the woman and her family. The woman and her family also experience feelings about the unknown, such as anxiety about the way the nurse will treat them or what the nurse will do during the visit. The challenge for the home care nurse is to establish a nurse-patient relationship and provide the prescribed home care services within the time provided for the initial home visit. One of the most important roles of the home care nurse is modeling health-related behaviors for the patient and others who are in the home during the visit.

Introductions generally begin the visit; the nurse identifies himself or herself and the home care agency. The woman introduces herself and the other family members who are present. Sometimes the woman may feel uncertain of her role or be uncomfortable in taking the lead in introductions, so other people in the home may not be introduced to the nurse. In these situations, the nurse can politely ask about other people in the home and their relationship to the woman.

In the first visit to the home, the home care nurse completes extensive documentation with the patient (Fig. 3-5).

BOX 3-3

Protocol for Perinatal Home Visits

Previsit Interventions

1. Contact family to arrange details for home visit.
   a. Identify self, credentials, and agency role.
   b. Review purpose of home visit follow-up.
   c. Schedule convenient time for visit.
   d. Confirm address and route to family home.
2. Review and clarify appropriate data.
   a. All available assessment data for mother and fetus or infant (i.e., referral forms, hospital discharge summaries, family-identified learning needs).
   b. Review records of any previous nursing contacts.
   c. Contact other professional caregivers as necessary to clarify data (i.e., obstetrician, nurse-midwife, pediatrician, referring nurse).
3. Identify community resources and teaching materials appropriate to meet needs already identified.
4. Plan the visit, and prepare bag with equipment, supplies, and materials necessary for assessments of mother and fetus or infant, actual care anticipated, and teaching.

In-Home Interventions: Establishing a Relationship

1. Reintroduce self and establish purpose of visit for mother, infant, and family; offer family opportunity to clarify their expectations of contact.
2. Spend brief time socially interacting with family to become acquainted and establish trusting relationship.

In-Home Interventions: Working with Family

1. Conduct systematic assessment of mother and fetus or newborn to determine physiologic adjustment and any existing complications.
2. Throughout visit, collect data to assess the emotional adjustment of individual family members to pregnancy or birth and lifestyle changes. Note evidence of family-newborn bonding and sibling rivalry; note relationships among mother, father, children, and grandparents.
3. Determine adequacy of support system.
   a. To what extent does someone help with cooking, cleaning, and other home management tasks?
   b. To what extent is help being provided in caring for the newborn and any other children?
   c. Are support persons encouraging the new mother to care for herself and get adequate rest?
   d. Who is providing helpful information? Emotional support?
4. Throughout the visit, observe home environment for adequacy of resources:
   a. Space: privacy, safe play of children, sleeping.
   b. Overall cleanliness and state of repair.
   c. Number of steps pregnant woman/new mother must climb.
   d. Adequacy of cooking arrangements.
   e. Adequacy of refrigeration and other food storage areas.
   f. Adequacy of bathing, toilet, and laundry facilities.
   g. Arrangements in home for newborn: sleeping, bathing, formula preparation (if needed), layette items, and diapers.
5. Throughout the visit, observe home environment for overall state of repair and existence of safety hazards:
   a. Storage of medications, household cleaners, and other substances hazardous to children.
   b. Presence of peeling paint on furniture, walls, or pipes.
   c. Factors that contribute to falls, such as dim lighting, broken steps, scatter rugs.
   d. Presence of vermin.
   e. Use of crib or playpen that fails to meet safety guidelines.
   f. Existence of emergency plan in case of fire; fire alarm or extinguisher.
6. Provide care to mother, newborn, or both as prescribed by their respective primary care provider or in accord with agency protocol.
7 Provide teaching on basis of previously identified needs.
8. Refer family to appropriate community agencies or resources, such as warm lines and support groups.
9. Ascertain that woman knows potential problems to watch for and whom to call if they occur.
10. Ensure that used disposable items have been handled appropriately and that reusable items are cleaned and repacked appropriately in the nurse's bag.

In-Home Interventions: Ending the Visit

1. Summarize the activities and main points of the visit.
2. Clarify future expectations, including schedule of next visit.
3. Review teaching plan and provide major points in writing.
4. Provide information about reaching the nurse or agency if needed before the next scheduled visit.

Postvisit Interventions

1. Document the visit thoroughly, using the necessary agency forms to serve as a legal record of the visit and to allow third-party reimbursement, as possible.
2. Initiate the plan of care on which the next encounter with the woman/family will be based.
3. Communicate appropriately (by telephone, letter, progress notes, or referral form) with primary care provider, other health professionals, or referral agencies on behalf of woman/family.

Before performing any services, the nurse must obtain written agreement and consent for the home health care services. This consent-for-care serves two major purposes: agreement for care and authorization to release medical information. Many third-party payers require written documentation of the services provided; therefore the agency obtains authorization from the woman to give information to her physician and any individual or company involved in payment for the services. Agencies that bill third-party payers for the rendered services will include agreement language for assignment of benefits and financial remuneration. By agreeing to assign insurance benefits to the agency, the woman allows her insurance company to pay the home health care agency directly.

All patients have the right to participate actively in their plan of care. These patient rights and responsibilities should begin the discussion about the nurse and patient roles during this initial visit.

Assessment

The primary goals of the assessment phase are to develop a trusting relationship and collect data by various methods to obtain a comprehensive patient profile. It may not be feasible or appropriate to collect in-depth information about all areas of assessment during the first visit. In many instances, however, the nurse may be limited to one visit and must ob-

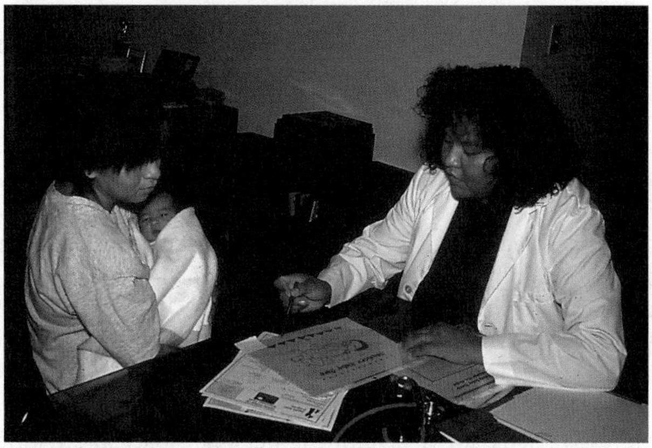

Fig. 3-5 Home care nurse visiting with woman and her infant. (Courtesy Michael S. Clement, MD, Mesa, AZ.)

tain information pertinent to the current situation in that hour.

The establishment of a trusting relationship begins with the previsit telephone call. An interview style that reflects sensitivity; a nonjudgmental, accepting attitude; and respect for the woman's rights facilitates the development of that trusting relationship. A skillful interviewer avoids barriers to communication such as false reassurance, advice giving, excessive talking, and the showing of approval or disapproval. This nurse-patient relationship continues to develop over the course of home visits.

The nurse is a guest in the woman's home and should show respect for her and her belongings. Some adaptation of the home visit schedule may be made if numerous distractions interrupt a visit, such as caring for the needs of small children. The nurse may ask to have the volume of the television reduced or suggest moving to another room where it is more quiet and private.

The major areas of the assessment are demographics, medical history, general health history, medication history, sociocultural assessment, home and community environment, and physical assessment. Some of this information can be obtained from patient records sent to the home care agency at the time of referral or from the previsit interview. These data will be used to develop the nursing care plan and complete the plan of care, which is required for many licensed home health care agencies. Two areas requiring further discussion are the social assessment and the home environment assessment.

Social assessment includes information regarding the number in the family and the roles of each household member, which family members or individuals have taken on the roles of caregivers, and the woman's social support network (Box 3-4). Identifying the roles of each member is helpful for developing the plan of care.

Physical assessment of the home environment is an essential element of the home care assessment. The major areas of the home environment assessment include physical features of the home, access to the home, sanitary conditions, the presence of utilities (e.g., indoor plumbing, telephone, electricity), safety features, and access to transportation and emergency support. Although some of this information can be collected during an interview, physically

BOX 3-4

Psychosocial Assessment

Language

Identify the primary language spoken in the home.
Assess whether there are any language barriers to receiving support.

Community Resources/Access to Care

Identify primary and secondary means of transportation.
Identify community agencies family currently uses for health care and support.
Assess cultural and psychosocial barriers to receiving care.

Social Support

Determine the people living with the pregnant woman.
Identify who assists with household chores.
Identify who assists with child care/parenting activities.
Identify who the pregnant woman turns to for problems or during a crisis.

Interpersonal Relationship

Identify the way decisions are made in the family.
Identify the family's perception of the need for home care.
Identify roles of adults in caring for family members.

Caregiver

Identify the primary caregiver for home care treatments.
Identify other caregivers and their roles.
Assess the caregiver's knowledge of treatments and care process.
Identify potential strain from the caregiver role.
Identify the level of satisfaction with the caregiver role.

Stress and Coping

Identify what the woman perceives as lifestyle changes and their impact on her and her family.
Identify the changes she and her family have made to adjust to her health condition and home health care treatments.

inspecting many areas of the home essential to care is a critical part of developing an accurate nursing plan of care. Before any physical inspection, the home care nurse should ask the woman or the caregiver for permission and assistance in identifying areas in the home that will be involved in the caregiving activities. During the physical inspection, careful consideration should be taken to avoid moving personal belongings that are not affected by the care.

Each plan of care has a different emphasis in the home environment. For example, women receiving infusion therapy for hyperemesis gravidarum need a safe place to store medications and infusion supplies that is out of reach of small children living in the home. The home care nurse should incorporate the agency policies and procedures for the storage and handling of infusion supplies into her walk-through inspection. During the walk through, the home care nurse looks at the potential storage areas that are dry, that are clean, and where the temperature can be maintained. The home care nurse should include an inspection of work areas, such as countertops, tabletops, sinks, and trash areas, that the woman or caregiver may use for mixing medications, changing infusion tubing, handling supplies, or disposing of used equipment and supplies.

The homes of patients using electronic home health care equipment, such as phototherapy equipment or infusion pumps, require physical inspection of electrical outlets, electrical cords, and extension cords that will be used. Homes with faulty electrical wiring may place the patient at risk for being involved in an electrical fire. Faulty wiring may require inspection and repair by a professional electrician before electronic devices are used. Findings from the assessment are incorporated into the plan of care.

Nursing Diagnoses

Nursing diagnoses are derived from the data collected at the first home visit. Nursing diagnoses for perinatal home health care patients include the following:

- *Deficient knowledge related to*
  —management of therapeutic regimen (e.g., nausea and vomiting, preterm labor, gestational diabetes)
  —newborn care and feeding
- *Compromised family coping related to*
  —lack of child care while mother is on bed rest
  —care of newborn receiving oxygen therapy
- *Impaired parenting related to*
  —maternal immaturity and lack of family support
- *Deficient diversional activity related to*
  —prolonged bed rest

Expected Outcomes

Examples of expected outcomes for perinatal patients include that the woman/family will do the following:

- Verbalize understanding of treatments
- Report decreased anxiety about performing procedures (e.g., blood glucose monitoring)
- Use support systems to cope effectively with problems (e.g., pregnancy complications, newborn complications or treatments)
- Perform procedures accurately, as evidenced by return demonstration
- Verbalize decreased role strain

Plan of Care and Implementation

The nursing plan of care is developed in collaboration with the patient, based on the health care needs of the individual. Home care nurses working in home health care agencies regulated by the Centers for Medicare and Medicaid Services use a plan of care that includes patient demographics, the health care provider's orders, home care goals, and the level of functioning. This document is initiated at the time of referral to the home care agency and must be updated every 60 days or as specified by state regulations.

The frequency of the skilled nursing visit may vary with the individual plan of care and reimbursement criteria established by the third-party payers.

Nurse safety and infection control are two important aspects specific to home care.

Safety Issues for the Home Care Nurse

The nurse should be fully aware of the home environment and neighborhood in which the home care is being provided. Unlike hospitals, in which the environment is more predictable and controlled, the patient's neighborhood and home have the potential for uncertainty. Home care nurses should take necessary safety precautions and avoid dangerous areas.

Agencies that serve patients in high crime areas may conduct a violence potential assessment by telephone before the visit and enlist the patient's cooperation in minimizing risk. Others have hired full-time security personnel to accompany nurses on their visits. Personal strategies recommended for nurses visiting families with a history of violence or substance abuse include (1) self-awareness; (2) environmental assessment; (3) using listening and observation skills with patients to be aware of behavioral changes indicating aggression or lack of impulse control; (4) planning for dealing with aggressive behavior (i.e., allowing personal space and taking a nonaggressive stance); (5) making visits in pairs; and (6) having access to a cellular phone at all times.

Personal Safety

The home care nurse must be aware of personal safety behaviors before going on a home visit. Dress should be casual but professional in appearance, with a name identification tag. Limited jewelry should be worn. Valuable personal items, such as an expensive purse or coat, should not be worn on a visit. Carrying an extra set of car keys in the nursing home care bag saves time and frustration if the nurse becomes locked out of the automobile. Automobile keys spread between the fingers with sharp ends outward can be used as a weapon if necessary. The same commonsense behaviors and precautions that guide a person's behavior when alone in any setting should be followed by home care nurses.

The agency should have a copy of the nurse's home care itinerary, including contact telephone numbers if a patient does not have a telephone and information on the nurse's car (make, model, color, and license plate number). Many home care nurses carry agency-provided pagers or cellular telephones that allow the agency to contact the nurse throughout the day to give information about patient updates, changes in orders or services, schedule changes, and new patients who require an initial visit. The telephone also is useful to notify patients when the nurse is delayed.

The automobile used for the home care visits, whether a personal or an agency-owned vehicle, should have regular preventive maintenance checks, an adequate fuel level, and road safety items stored in the trunk. Items to carry in the vehicle include change for telephone calls and tolls, maps, emergency telephone numbers, a flashlight, a first aid kit, flares, a blanket, and equipment for inclement weather conditions. When making a visit to a patient in a more remote rural setting, other travel considerations may be needed, as well as taking additional supplies or medication to the patient (Bosch & Bushy, 1997).

Home care nurses should park and lock their cars in a safe place that is visible from the street and the patient's home and away from hidden alleys. While driving to the patient's home, the nurse should assess the neighborhood for safety, especially if the neighborhood is unfamiliar. All valuable items should be stored out of sight before leaving the office. While walking to the patient's home, nurses should not walk near groups of strangers hanging out in doorways or alleys, enter into vacant buildings, or enter a yard that has an unrestrained dog. The home or building should not be en-

Nursing Care Plan

COMMUNITY AND HOME CARE

NURSING DIAGNOSIS: Readiness for enhanced family coping, related to family growth and development in new community as evidenced by family report

EXPECTED OUTCOME

Family will identify at least three community groups that can serve as appropriate resources for an expectant family with small children.

NURSING INTERVENTIONS/*RATIONALES*

Assess family structure and availability of significant others, friends, or family members to assist family with new baby and siblings *to provide database for further interventions.*

Encourage family to enlist assistance of individuals who are available to help family at birth of new baby *to provide physical and emotional support.*

Using therapeutic communication, assist the family to assess coping strategies used in the past for new situations *to provide clarification and promote empowerment of family in new situations.*

Suggest strategies to find resources available in the community *to assist family during pregnancy, with new baby, and small siblings.*

Give information regarding community workshops, classes, or support groups *to promote networking, community bonding, and support.*

NURSING DIAGNOSIS: Ineffective community management of therapeutic regimen related to meeting the needs of new members in the community as evidenced by inadequate community programs to meet needs of newcomers

EXPECTED OUTCOME

The community will develop programs to meet the needs of new members of the community.

NURSING INTERVENTIONS/*RATIONALES*

Conduct a needs assessment of the community *to identify priority needs for new members of the community.*

Initiate health education programs based on topics identified in the needs assessment *to meet the needs of members of the community.*

Identify risks in the community (e.g., environmental hazards, drug sales) *to provide a target for community improvement.*

With community leaders, develop a plan to cope with and reduce environmental hazards *to improve public health and safety.*

Develop a monitoring/surveillance system *to ensure that progress made will continue and new problems are identified.*

NURSING DIAGNOSIS: Ineffective community coping related to providing a safe and healthy environment as evidenced by presence of hazards in the environment

EXPECTED OUTCOME

Health status of the community will improve.

NURSING INTERVENTIONS/*RATIONALES*

Initiate health screening programs for community members *to identify effects of environmental hazards in the community.*

Work with politicians and policy makers to develop the community *to provide a safe environment with means of economic survival for community members.*

Initiate programs such as Block Watch, Safe Houses, and Neighborhood Watch *to enhance the safety of the environment.*

Work with community leaders to develop or clean up playgrounds *to provide a safe place for children to play.*

With community leaders, develop community grass roots initiatives *to enable community members to take ownership in the community.*

Identify sites of lead exposure *to decrease the potential for lead poisoning in children.*

Participate in immunization/vaccination clinics *to reduce the risk in the community of infectious diseases.*

tered if the nurse has any safety concerns. Responsibility for safety of home care staff is the responsibility of the agency (McPhaul, 2004). All home care agencies should have policies to follow for such situations.

Unsafe Situations in the Patient's Home

Once inside the woman's home, the nurse may encounter unsafe situations such as the presence of weapons, abusive behavior, or health hazards. Each potentially hazardous situation must be dealt with according to agency policies and procedures. If abuse or neglect is reasonably suspected, the home care nurse should follow home care agency and state and federal regulations for reporting and documenting the situation. Nurses should maintain their own safety first and act accordingly throughout the visit.

Infection Control

The nurse carries the necessary supplies and equipment to provide nursing care to the woman. Home care bags should contain infection control supplies, such as personal protection equipment; disposable nonsterile, sterile, and utility gloves; disinfectants; disposable cardiopulmonary resuscitation (CPR) masks; gowns; shoe covers; caps; leak-proof and puncture-resistant specimen containers; sharps container; dry hand disinfectants; and leak-proof barriers. Proper infection control techniques should be used in stocking, storing, handling, and transporting this bag. When a procedure is to be performed, the nurse should set up a clean area for necessary supplies. A "dirty" area is designated with a trash bag for the collection of soiled equipment and supplies. Hands are washed before all supplies and equipment for the visit are removed from the bag and placed in a clean area.

The importance of infection control does not diminish because nursing care is provided in the patient's home rather than in a hospital. Patients are not likely to become infected because of their home environment, but the nurse may become exposed to an infectious disease.

Standard Precautions should be used whenever a treatment is performed because it is difficult to determine which patients have a communicable disease (see Box 6-5).

Handwashing remains the single most important infection-control procedure, and the caregiver is in a position to educate about the importance of this practice in preventing disease. Hands should be washed before and after each patient contact. Wearing gloves does not eliminate the necessity for handwashing. If running water or clean facilities are unavailable, the hands can be cleaned with a self-drying antiseptic solution.

Using gloves reduces the incidence of exposure to bloodborne pathogens. Gloves should be selected according to the nursing activity to be performed. Nonsterile latex or vinyl gloves should be worn with each procedure that has the potential for contact with bodily substances (e.g., performing venipunctures, heel sticks on the newborn, perineal care). Sterile gloves should be worn with clinical procedures requiring sterile technique, such as insertion of peripherally inserted central lines and certain dressing changes. General purpose utility gloves should be used for housekeeping activities, such as cleaning equipment or spills. Nonsterile and sterile gloves should be discarded after each use in a leak-resistant waste receptacle. Utility gloves may be disinfected and reused.

Disposable personal protection equipment should be removed after each use and discarded in a plastic trash container. Safety glasses or goggles can be cleaned with soap and water after each use.

Whenever specimens are collected, Standard Precautions should be used. Any specimen of bodily fluids should be placed in a leak-proof bag and secured in a puncture-proof container. The outside of the container is washed off, if it was soiled, before transporting it. Specimens should be labeled with the woman's or infant's name and additional identifying information according to the home health care agency or laboratory policies. If specimens are being transported, they should be placed in a container on a flat surface in the vehicle. An insulated container may be used to keep specimens cool in transit. The nurse should be aware of the time-sensitive laboratory procedures for certain types of specimens.

Sharps containers are puncture-proof and leak-proof containers labeled with a biohazard sign on the outside and should be used to collect needles and sharp objects. Patients are instructed to fill containers between two-thirds and three-fourths full to prevent spillage of their contents. As part of the patient teaching process, information about storage and handling is covered by the home care nurse. When the container reaches its maximal capacity, it should be returned to the home health care agency and replaced. Medical waste, such as urine and secretions, can be discarded through the sewer or septic system.

Contaminated dressings and disposable supplies should be placed in a leak-proof plastic bag and securely fastened for disposal at the patient's home. The patient should be instructed regarding the proper disposal of medical waste in the home. Agency policies and procedures and local waste management ordinances should be consulted before the patient is instructed.

Nursing Considerations

In home care, the woman or family members are responsible for administration of medications in the absence of the nurse. A careful medication history should be obtained to see if the woman is taking her medications correctly and understands the desired action and potential side effects. Sometimes when orders are changed, women continue to take both the old and new prescriptions, which can lead to dangerous overdoses or medication interactions. The nurse ensures that there is an adequate supply and a safe place for proper storage of medications to prevent deterioration or accidental ingestion by children or pets. The nurse inquires about any other medications that the woman might be taking concurrently. Over-the-counter drugs or herbal supplements may not be considered medications by the women and not mentioned unless such information is specifically asked for. Even more important is ensuring that the patient and her caregivers fully understand the information that they are exposed to by health care providers.

High-technology home care involves many diagnostic and therapeutic procedures. A focused physical assessment is always part of the visit. Nurses involved in perinatal home care must be skilled in prenatal, postpartal, and newborn assessment. Many women require additional diagnostic tests. The nurse may need to collect blood or other specimens. Portable fetal monitoring equipment or even ultrasound can be used in the home for fetal assessment. Home infusion for women with hyperemesis gravidarum often replaces hospitalization. Women with preterm labor may receive parenteral tocolytic therapy. Phototherapy or apnea monitors can be provided in the home for newborns. The power supply and wiring must be reliable. Family members may need to be taught to monitor equipment between nurse visits and to prevent accidental damage.

Medical emergencies may occur during or between the nurse's visits to the home. Prior planning and education can reduce the risk of problems. All parents of newborns should know infant CPR. There should be immediate telephone access to call for emergency medical assistance. Women and their families should be taught to recognize danger signs related to their condition. For example, women at risk for preterm labor should learn to palpate the uterus and recognize contractions in the absence of pain; women with diabetes must learn the signs of hypoglycemia and what to do if it occurs; women with preeclampsia must know the danger signs that indicate worsening of their condition and notify the health care provider immediately. In a more remote rural community that does not have an obstetrician in the region, the nurse may need to assist the patient's family to arrange for "boarding" somewhere that is closer to a medical specialist.

Patient and family education in home care includes information about the specific high risk condition(s) involved, implications for pregnancy outcome, and measures for self-monitoring. Verbal explanations should be supplemented with clearly written instructions. General information to promote well-being, such as about nutrition and common discomforts of pregnancy, also should be included. The need for preparation for childbirth can be addressed by using books or videos and supplemented by individual teaching at home. Coping with bed rest or other limitation of activity is a problem for many women with high risk pregnancies. The nurse may share strategies that others have used, help with time management, and provide information about support

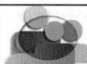

Community Focus

HEALTH NEEDS OF VULNERABLE POPULATIONS

Read your local newspaper and identify articles describing health needs of vulnerable populations in your community. Consult the yellow pages of the telephone book. Are there agencies in your area that specifically deal with meeting those needs? If you encountered a patient with one of the needs, to whom would you refer her?

services. Teaching about infant care or the special needs of the preterm infant may be appropriate during the prenatal period.

Clear documentation of assessments, problems identified, treatments and interventions performed, and the patient's responses is essential. Third-party payers base reimbursement on the nurse's written record of providing skilled nursing care and assessments that support the woman's continuing need for those services. The nurse must promptly inform the health care provider by telephone or facsimile of any significant changes. When new orders are transmitted by telephone, a written copy must be sent for the physician's signature.

The home care nurse continually reassesses the patient's condition and response to the interventions during every home visit and revises the nursing diagnoses and plan of care. Nursing documentation should reflect an objective description of the nursing assessment data collected at each visit. Statements such as "no change" or "same as last visit" do not accurately reflect the monitoring of the patient condition that occurred during the skilled nursing visit. Once the home care outcomes are achieved and the patient is discharged from the home care agency, documentation should include information about the patient's status at the time of discharge, progress toward attaining health care goals, and plans for follow-up care.

The role of the clinical record in home care has been affected by social, economic, and legal health care changes. Appropriate care should be taken to complete the necessary home health care records accurately and in a timely manner. Documentation guidelines include writing or dictating notes or using a laptop computer at the patient's home or shortly after the visit.

Evaluation

Evaluation is based on the expected outcomes of care. The plan is revised as necessary.

Key Points

- A community is defined as a locality-based entity composed of systems of societal institutions, informal groups, and aggregates that are interdependent and whose function is to meet a wide variety of collective needs.
- Of necessity, most changes aimed at improving community health involve partnerships among community residents and health workers.
- Methods of collecting data useful to the nurse working in the community include walking surveys, analysis of existing data, informant interviews, and participant observation.
- Vulnerable populations are groups who are at higher risk for developing physical, mental, or social health problems.
- Perinatal home care is a unique nursing practice that incorporates knowledge from community health nursing, acute care nursing, family therapy, health promotion, and patient education.
- Social and economic factors affect the scope of perinatal nursing practice.
- Perinatal home care can be provided for women and infants throughout the perinatal period, beginning before conception and ending in the postpartum period.
- Perinatal home care nurses should incorporate personal safety and infection control practices in the nursing plan of care.
- Telephonic nurse advice lines, telephonic nursing assessments, and warm lines are low-cost health care services that facilitate continuous patient education, support, and health care decision making, even though health care is delivered in multiple sites.
- Communication protocols among members of the home health care team are critical to diminish fragmentation and duplication of health care services.

Answer Guidelines to Critical Thinking Exercise

Health Needs of a Migrant Worker

1. No, there is not sufficient evidence. The nurse needs to establish baseline data and understanding of the mother within her culture and perform an assessment before mutual goal setting.
2. (a) The goals must be realistic, not just idealistic. (b) Both mother and infant need adequate nutrition and rest. (c) Maintaining breastfeeding while working long hours in the field is difficult if not impossible. (d) Including other family members in the care of the infant will assist the mother. Including the father may not be culturally appropriate or possible given work hours.
3. Priority for care is to ensure that the infant and mother obtain adequate nutrition. If the mother cannot breastfeed, a safe source of nutrition must be provided. Refrigeration must be available, as well as a source of safe water. WIC may be a source of formula for the infant and food for the mother. In this setting, powdered formula may be the safest form of milk because each feeding can be prepared at the time of feeding.
4. Yes. Standards of care dictate that the mother and infant need adequate nutrition, as well as sleep and rest.
5. There are no data to indicate whether or not the father of the baby is involved or that his involvement is culturally appropriate. Because the mother is Vietnamese speaking, a nurse who speaks Vietnamese or an interpreter must be involved. There also may be need for a bed and clothing and other supplies for the infant. Sources of family support should be ascertained. Whether there are other community agencies or groups that can provide assistance should be ascertained.

Resources

Association of Women's Health, Obstetric, and Neonatal Nurses (AWHONN): *Every woman: the essential guide for healthy living,* ed 5, Washington, DC, 2004, AWHONN.

Bushy A: *Resource manual: rural minorities, their health issues and resources,* Kansas City, MO, 2002, National Rural Health Association.

Centers for Medicare and Medicaid Services
cms.hhs.gov

Community Health Status Indicators
www.phf.org

National Association of County and City Health Officials
www.naccho.org/

Online Content for Low-Income and Underserved Americans: The Digital Divide's New Frontier
www.childrenspartnership.org/pub/low_income/index.html

Population and Family Health Sciences (Johns Hopkins)
www.jhsph.edu/pfhs/

Provider's Guide to Quality and Care
erc.msh.org/quality&culture

U.S. Department of Health and Human Services, Health Resources and Services Administration (HRSA)
www.hrsa.gov/

U.S. Department of Health and Human Services, Centers for Disease Control and Prevention: *CDC Fact Book 2000/2001*
www.cdc.gov

U.S. Department of Health and Human Services, Health Resources and Services Administration: Community health status report: Data sources, definitions, and notes
www.communityhealth.hrsa.gov

References

Almeida R, Dubay L, Ko G: Access to care and use of health services by low-income women, *Health Care Financing Rev* 22(4):27-47, 2001.

American Academy of Pediatrics Council on Child and Adolescent Health: The role of home-visitation programs in improving health outcomes for children and families, *Pediatrics* 101:486-489, 1998.

Anderson ET, McFarlane J: *Community-as-partner: theory and practice in nursing,* ed 4, Philadelphia, 2004, Lippincott Williams & Wilkins.

Association of Women's Health, Obstetric, and Neonatal Nurses (AWHONN): *Didactic content and clinical skills verification for professional nurse providers of perinatal home care,* Washington, DC, 1994, AWHONN.

Association of Women's Health, Obstetric, and Neonatal Nurses (AWHONN): *Standards and guidelines for professional nursing practice in the care of women and newborns,* ed 5, Washington, DC, 1998, AWHONN.

Bleich M: Growth strategies to optimize the functions of telephonic nursing call centers, *Nurs Econ* 4(6):215-218, 1998.

Bosch D, Bushy A: Case management: implementing home care in rural areas, *Home Health Cons* 4(7):19-42, 1997.

Bruhn J: Ethical issues in intervention outcomes, *Fam Comm Health* 23(4):24-35, 2001.

Bureau of Primary Health Care: *Homeless population statistics,* Washington, DC, 2001, Bureau of Primary Health Care. Internet document available at www.hrsa.bphc.gov (accessed November 29, 2004).

Bushy A: Health issues of women in rural environments: an overview, *J Am Med Womens Assoc* 53(2):53-56, 1998.

Bushy A: *Orientation to nursing in the rural community,* Thousand Oaks, CA, 2000, Sage.

Bushy A: Panel 1: Framing issues in rural women's health issues—Speaker 3. *Women's Health Issues* 11(1):26-9. 2001.

Clemen-Stone S: Community assessment and diagnosis. In Clemen-Stone S, McGuire S, Eigsti D (eds): *Comprehensive community health nursing: family, aggregate, and community practice,* ed 6, St Louis, 2002, Mosby.

Coren E, Barlow J: Individual and group-based parenting programmes for improving psychosocial outcomes for teenage parents and their children (Cochrane Review), 2001. In *The Cochrane Library,* Issue 2, Chichester, UK, 2004, John Wiley & Sons.

Doyle E, Ward S: *The process of community health education and health promotion,* Mountain View, CA, 2001, Mayfield.

Ervin N: *Advanced community health nursing practice: population-focused care,* Upper Saddle River, NJ, 2002, Prentice Hall.

Goldman T, DeLaCruz D: The Healthy Start Initiative. In Wallace H et al (eds): *Health and welfare for families in the 21st century,* Sudbury, MA, 1999, Jones & Bartlett.

Koniak-Griffin D et al: An early intervention program for adolescent mothers: a nursing demonstration project, *J Obstet Gynecol Neonatal Nurs* 28:51-59, 1999.

Kuehnert P: Overview of program planning. In Ervin N (ed): *Advanced community health nursing practice,* Upper Saddle River, NJ, 2002, Prentice Hall.

Lauderdale M: Issues in securing the community's sanction before making an intervention, *Fam Comm Health* 23(4):1-8, 2001.

Maehr J, Felice M: Adolescent health and welfare reform. In Wallace H et al (eds): *Health and welfare for families in the 21st century,* Sudbury, MA, 1999, Jones & Bartlett.

Marks J, Wilcox L: The future of prevention. In Wallace H et al (eds): *Health and welfare for families in the 21st century,* Sudbury, MA, 1999, Jones & Bartlett.

Maternal Child Health Bureau: Pregnancy-related behaviors among migrant farm workers: four states, 1989-1993, *MMWR* 46(13):283, 1997.

McDevitt J, Wilbur J: Locating sources of data. In Ervin N (ed): *Advanced community health nursing practice: population-focused care,* Upper Saddle River, NJ, 2002, Prentice Hall.

McGuire SL: Occupational health nursing. In Clemen-Stone S, McGuire S, Eigsti D (eds): *Comprehensive community health nursing: family, aggregate, and community practice,* ed 6, St Louis, 2002, Mosby.

McPhaul K: Health & Safety. Home care security, *Am J Nurs* 104(9):96, 2004.

Murray R, Zentner J, Samiezade-Yazd C: Sociocultural influences on the person and family. In Murray R, Zentner J (eds): *Health promotion strategies through the lifespan,* ed 7, Upper Saddle River, NJ, 2001, Prentice Hall.

National Academy Press: *From generation to generation: the health and well-being of children in immigrant families, 2002.* Internet document available at search.nap.edu/html/generation/summary.html (accessed November 29, 2004).

Olds D et al: Long term effects of home visitation on maternal life-course and child abuse and neglect, *JAMA* 278(8):637-643, 1997.

Pender N, Murdaugh C, Parsons M: *Health promotion in nursing practice,* Upper Saddle River, NJ, 2002, Prentice-Hall.

US Department of Health and Human Services: *Healthy people 2010: understanding and improving health,* Washington, DC, 2000a, US Department of Health and Human Services, US Government Printing Office.

US Department of Health and Human Services: *Healthy People 2010,* Chapter 16: Maternal, infant, and child health, 2000b. Internet document available at www.health.gov/healthypeople/Document/HTML/Volume2/16MICH.htm (accessed November 28, 2004).

US Department of Health and Human Services: *CDC fact book, 2000/2001,* Atlanta, GA, 2000c, Centers for Disease Control and Prevention.

US Department of Health and Human Services, Office on Women's Health: *Women's health issues: an overview, 2001.* Internet document available at www.4woman.gov (accessed November 28, 2004).

Williams M et al: Promoting early breast cancer screening: strategies with rural African American women, *Am J Health Stud* 17(2):65-73, 2001.

Zyzanski S, Williams R, Flocke S: Selection of key community descriptors for community-oriented primary care, *Fam Prac* 13(3):280-288, 1996.

Health Promotion and Prevention 4

LEARNING OBJECTIVES

On completion of this chapter the reader will be able to:

- Identify reasons women enter the health care delivery system.
- Analyze financial, cultural, and communication barriers that may affect a woman's decision to seek and follow through with health care.
- Analyze conditions and characteristics that increase health risks for women during their childbearing years.
- Evaluate programs of anticipatory guidance that promote health and prevention of disease.
- Suggest community resources to combat violence against women.
- Explain the cycle of violence and its use in assessment and intervention for battered women.
- Discuss the incidence of battering in pregnant women.
- Outline health-screening schedules for women in the childbearing years.

ELECTRONIC RESOURCES

Additional information related to the content in Chapter 4 can be found on

the companion website at evolve
http://evolve.elsevier.com/Wong/maternal/
- NCLEX Review Questions
- WebLinks

or the interactive student CD-ROM
Activities for Chapter 4 include the following:
- NCLEX Review Questions

REASONS FOR ENTERING THE HEALTH CARE SYSTEM

Many women initially enter the health care system because of some reproductive system–related situation such as pregnancy, irregular menses, a desire for contraception, or an episodic illness such as a vaginal infection. It is important that health care providers recognize the importance of health promotion and preventive health maintenance and to offer these services across the life span of women. This chapter addresses barriers to seeking health care and contains an overview of conditions and circumstances that increase health risks across the life span. Anticipatory guidance suggestions, including nutrition and stress management, are also included. Intimate partner violence and battering of women is discussed.

Preconception Counseling

Preconception health promotion provides women and their partners with information that is needed to make decisions about their reproductive future. Preconception counseling guides couples on how to avoid unintended pregnancies, how to identify and manage risk factors in their lives and their environment, and how to identify healthy behaviors that promote the well-being of the woman and her potential fetus.

Activities that promote healthy mothers and babies must be initiated before the period of critical fetal organ development, which is between 17 and 56 days after fertilization. By the end of the eighth week after conception and certainly by the end of the first trimester, any major structural anomalies in the fetus are already present. Because many women do not realize that they are pregnant, and do not seek prenatal care until well into the first trimester, the rapidly growing fetus may be exposed to many types of intrauterine environmental hazards during this most vulnerable developmental phase. Thus preconception health care should occur well in advance of an actual pregnancy.

Preconception care is important for women who have had a problem with a previous pregnancy (e.g., miscarriage or preterm birth). Although causes are not always identifiable, in many cases problems can be identified and treated and do not recur in subsequent pregnancies. Preconception care is also important to minimize fetal malformations. For example, the offspring of women who have type 1 diabetes mellitus have significantly more congenital anomalies than do children of mothers without diabetes. The rate of malformation is greatly reduced when the insulin-dependent diabetic woman has excellent blood glucose control when she becomes pregnant and maintains euglycemia (normal blood sugar) throughout the period of organ development in the fetus. The incidence of neural tube defects such as spina bifida and anencephaly is significantly decreased with the intake of 400 mcg of supplemental folic acid.

Many examples illustrate effects of maternal age or illnesses; conditions that produce anomalies in the fetus (teratogenic agents), such as drugs, viruses, and chemicals; genetically inherited diseases; or other conditions that might be harmful to the woman should a pregnancy occur. In many instances, counseling can allow for behavior modification before damage is done, or the woman can make an informed decision about her willingness to accept potential hazards. The components of preconception care, such as health promotion, risk assessment, and interventions, are outlined in Box 4-1.

Pregnancy

A woman's entry into health care is often associated with pregnancy, either for diagnosis or for actual care. Early entry into prenatal care, within the first 12 weeks, allows for identification of the woman at risk for complications and initiation of measures to prevent problems or treat them if they arise. Major goals of prenatal care are listed in Box 4-2 and should be addressed in the first visit. Extensive discussion of pregnancy is found in Unit 3.

Well-Woman Care

Many women first enter the health care delivery system for a Papanicolaou (Pap) smear or for contraception. Visits to the nurse may be their only contact with the system unless they become ill. Some women postpone examination until a specific need arises, such as pregnancy, infertility, pain, abnormal bleeding, or vaginal discharge.

Fertility Control and Infertility

More than half of the pregnancies in the United States each year are unintended, and the majority of these occur in the 7% of women who do not use birth control (Alan Guttmacher Institute, 2002). Education is the key to encouraging women to make family planning choices based on preference and actual benefit-to-risk ratios. Providers can influence the user's motivation and ability to use the method correctly (see Chapter 7 for further discussion of contraception).

The concept of health promotion applies to contraception, as can be seen in Box 4-3. The nurse can provide information regarding the need for child spacing, methods of family planning that are consistent with religious and per-

BOX 4-1

Components of Preconception Care

Health Promotion: General Teaching

- Nutrition
  - Healthy diet, including folic acid
  - Optimum weight
- Exercise and rest
- Avoidance of substance abuse (tobacco, alcohol, "recreational" drugs)
- Use of safer sex practices
- Attending to family and social needs

Risk Factor Assessment

- Medical history
  - Immune status (e.g., rubella, hepatitis B)
  - Family history (e.g., genetic disorders)
  - Illnesses (e.g., infections)
  - Current use of medications (prescription, nonprescription)
- Reproductive history
  - Contraceptive
  - Obstetric
- Psychosocial history
  - Spouse/partner and family situation, including domestic violence
  - Availability of family or other support systems
  - Readiness for pregnancy (e.g., age, life goals, stress)
- Financial resources
- Environmental (home, workplace) conditions
  - Safety hazards
  - Toxic chemicals
  - Radiation

Interventions

- Anticipatory guidance/teaching
- Treatment of medical conditions and results
  - Medications
  - Cessation/reduction in substance use/abuse
  - Immunizations (e.g., rubella, tuberculosis, hepatitis)
- Nutrition, diet, and weight management
- Exercise
- Referral for genetic counseling
- Referral to and use of
  - Family planning services
  - Family and social needs management

BOX 4-2

Major Goals of Prenatal Care

- Define health status of mother and fetus.
- Determine the gestational age of the fetus, and monitor fetal development.
- Identify the woman at risk for complications, and minimize the risk whenever possible.
- Provide appropriate education and counseling.

BOX 4-3

Contraceptive Health Promotion

- Child spacing and quality maternity care improve perinatal outcomes and health in general of mother and children.
- Achieving desired family size enables a better sharing of all resources with attendant increases in education, health care, and other positive societal parameters.
- Contraceptives themselves may positively affect future health. For example, use of condoms may prevent acquisition of HIV infection; combined oral contraceptives (OCs) may provide some protection against later development of cancer of ovary and endometrium; barrier methods decrease transmission of STIs, which can develop into pelvic inflammatory disease with resultant infertility or sterility and thus affect future childbearing capacity.

sonal preferences, noncontraceptive benefits of certain methods, the appropriate use of methods selected, and the protection of future fertility when so desired.

Women also enter the health care system because of their desire to achieve a pregnancy. Approximately 15% of couples in the United States have some degree of infertility. Infertility can cause emotional pain for many couples, and the inability to produce an offspring sometimes results in feelings of failure and inordinate stress on the couple relationship. Significant amounts of time, money, and emotional investment can be used for testing and treatment in efforts to build a family.

Infertility appears to be an ever-increasing problem. There are more couples trying to have babies in their thirties or forties, exposing them to situations negatively affecting fertility such as age-related infertility. Sexually transmitted infections (STIs), which can predispose to decreased fertility, are becoming more common, and many women and men are in workplaces and home settings where they may be exposed to reproductive hazards in the environment.

Steps toward prevention of infertility should be undertaken as part of ongoing routine health care, and such information is especially appropriate in preconception counseling. Primary care providers can undertake initial evaluation and counseling before couples are referred to specialists. For additional information about infertility, see Chapter 7.

BARRIERS TO SEEKING HEALTH CARE

Financial Issues

The United States spends almost 15% of its gross domestic product on health, far more than any other industrialized nation in the world, yet major problems still exist. Employment-based financing of health insurance has resulted in a system in which one's health insurance is linked to a job. This system is working well for fewer and fewer people, especially women. Fourteen percent of young women have no health insurance, and 5 million more have coverage so inadequate that it does not even include maternity care (National Women's Law Center, 2000).

In the United States, disparity among races and socioeconomic classes affects many facets of life, including health. With limited money and awareness, there is a lack of access to care, delay in seeking care, few prevention activities, and little accurate information about health and the health care system. Women use health services more often than do men but are more likely than men to have difficulty in financing the services. They are twice as often underinsured (i.e., have limited coverage with high-cost copayments or deductibles). Women make up the majority of Medicaid recipients; however, only 42% of poor women are eligible. Medicaid includes special benefits for pregnant women, but the benefits are limited to treatment of pregnancy-related conditions and terminate 60 days after birth. More and more states are requiring their Medicaid recipients to enroll in managed care programs; whether this improves access and outcomes is yet to be determined.

Insurance coverage varies significantly by age, marital status, race, and ethnicity. Caucasians of all ages are more likely than African-Americans and other racial or ethnic groups to have private insurance. Caucasians possess insurance 2.5 times more often than Hispanics and 1.8 times more often than African-Americans. Single, separated, or divorced individuals are less likely to have insurance. Often unmarried teenagers, who are usually covered by their parents' medical insurance, do not have maternity coverage because policies have exclusion statements and cover only the employee or spouse. Midwifery care has helped contain some health care costs, but reimbursement issues still exist in some areas. The existing health care system continues to be oriented to treatment of acute or episodic conditions rather than the promotion of health and comprehensive care.

Cultural Issues

As our nation becomes more racially, ethnically, and culturally diverse, the health of minority groups becomes a major issue. A variety of reasons are given to explain some of the differences in accessing care when financial barriers are adjusted. Some women experience racial discrimination, or disrespectful, disillusioning, or discouraging encounters with community service providers such as social services and health care providers. A lack of cross-cultural communication also presents problems. Desired health outcomes are best achieved when the health care provider has knowledge of and understanding about the culture, language, values, priorities, and health beliefs of those in minority groups. Conversely, members of the group should understand the health goals to be achieved and the methods proposed to do so. Language differences can produce profound barriers between patients and providers. Even with an interpreter, misinformation can occur on both sides of the communication.

Providers must consider culturally based differences that could affect the treatment of diverse groups of women, and the women themselves must share practices and beliefs that could influence their management responses or willingness to comply (Mattson, 2000). For example, women in some cultures value privacy to such an extent that they are reluctant to disrobe and as a result avoid physical examination unless absolutely necessary. Other women rely on their husbands to make major decisions, including those affecting the woman's health. Religious beliefs may dictate a plan of care, as with birth control measures or blood transfusions. Some cultural groups prefer folk medicine, homeopathy, or prayer to traditional Western medicine, and others attempt combinations of some or all practices. In any event, it is incumbent on health care providers to value and appreciate their own and their patients' various sources of information and beliefs about sickness and health. Although there is an increasing amount of health information on the World Wide Web, information in languages other than English is limited.

Gender Issues

Gender influences provider-patient communication and may influence access to health care in general. The most obvious gender consideration is that between men and women.

Researchers have reported significant male-female differences in receipt of major diagnostic and therapeutic interventions, especially with cardiac and kidney problems. Women tend to use primary care services more often than do men and, some believe, more effectively. The gender of the provider plays a role; studies have shown that female patients have Pap smears and mammograms more consistently if they are seen by female providers.

Sexual orientation may produce another barrier. Some lesbians may not disclose their sexual orientation to health care providers because they feel they may be at risk for hostility, inadequate health care, or breach of confidentiality. In many health care settings, heterosexuality is assumed, and the setting may be one in which the woman does not feel welcome (magazines, brochures, and environment reflect heterosexual couples, or the health care provider shows discomfort interacting with the woman). Another problem is that lesbians themselves may hold beliefs that are incorrect, such as that they have immunity to human immunodeficiency virus (HIV), STIs, and certain cancers (e.g., cervical). The perceived lack of risk can result in lesbians avoiding medical care, as well as in health care providers giving incorrect advice or not doing appropriate cancer screening for these women. Not all gynecologic cancers are related to sexual activity; lesbians who have never had children may be more at risk for breast, ovarian, and endometrial cancer. Their risk for heart disease, cancer of the lung, and colon cancer is not different from that of the heterosexual woman. To offset stereotypes, it is necessary for providers to develop an approach that does not assume that all patients are heterosexual (Stevens & Hall, 2001).

HEALTH RISKS IN THE CHILDBEARING YEARS

Maintaining optimal health is a goal for all women. Essential components of health maintenance are the identification of unrecognized problems and potential risks and the education and health promotion needed to reduce them. This is especially important for a woman in her childbearing years, because conditions that increase a woman's health risks not only are of concern for her well-being but also may be associated with negative outcomes for both mother and baby in the event of a pregnancy. Prenatal care is an example of prevention that is practiced after conception. However, prevention and health maintenance are needed before conception because many of the mother's risks can be identified and then eliminated, or at least modified. An overview of conditions and circumstances that increase health risks in the childbearing years follows.

Age

Adolescents

As a female progresses through developmental ages and stages, she is faced with conditions that are age related. All teens undergo progressive growth of sexual characteristics. They also undertake the developmental tasks of adolescence such as establishing identity, developing sexual preference, emancipating from family, and establishing career goals. Some of these situations can produce great stress for the adolescent, and the health care provider should treat her very carefully. Female teenagers who enter the health care system usually do so for screening (Pap smears start at age 18 or when sexually active) or because of a problem such as episodic illness or accidents. Gynecologic problems are often associated with menses (either bleeding irregularities or dysmenorrhea), vaginitis or leukorrhea, STI, contraception, or pregnancy.

Most young women begin having sex in the mid to late teens; for those who do not, the likelihood of having intercourse increases steadily with age. A sexually active teen who does not use contraception has a 90% chance of pregnancy within 1 year (Alan Guttmacher Institute, 2002).

Teenage Pregnancy

Pregnancy in the teenager who is 16 years of age or younger often introduces additional stress on an already stressful developmental period. The emotional level of such teens is commonly characterized by impulsiveness and self-centered behavior, and they often place primary importance on the beliefs and actions of their peers. In attempts to establish a personal and independent identity, many teens do not realize the consequences of their behavior; their thinking processes do not include planning for the future.

Unless very young, teens are sufficiently mature for physical support of the pregnancy, but they may not adhere to healthy prenatal behaviors, especially appropriate nutrition and continuing care. Children of teen mothers may be at risk for abuse or neglect because of the teen's inadequate knowledge of growth, development, and parenting. Implementation of specialized adolescent programs in schools, communities, and health care systems is demonstrating continued success in lowering the birth rate in teens as evidenced by a 31% decline in teenage pregnancy since 1991 (Arias et al, 2003).

Young and Middle Adulthood

Because women age 20 to 40 years have a need for contraception, pelvic and breast screening, and pregnancy care, they may prefer to use their gynecologic or obstetric provider as their primary care provider. During these years the woman may be "juggling" family, home, and career responsibilities with resulting increases in stress-related conditions. Health maintenance includes not only pelvic and breast screening but also promotion of a healthy lifestyle: that is, good nutrition, regular exercise, no smoking, moderate or no alcohol consumption, sufficient rest, stress reduction, and referral for medical conditions and other specific problems. Common conditions in well-woman care include vaginitis, urinary tract infections, menstrual variations, obesity, sexual and relationship issues, and pregnancy.

Parenthood after Age 35

The woman older than 35 years does not have a different physical response to a pregnancy per se, but rather has had health status changes as a result of time and the aging process. These changes may be responsible for age-related pregnancy conditions. For example, a woman with type 2 diabetes may not have had expression of her diabetes at age 22

Evidence-Based Practice

PRIMARY AND SECONDARY PREVENTION OF CERVICAL CANCER

Background

Cervical cancer has been primarily a disease of aging. Younger women, ages 20 to 40 years, test positive for premalignant conditions, which may progress to invasive cervical carcinoma after age 50. Risk factors include the following:

- Contact with human papillomavirus (HPV), especially the more aggressive types 16 and 18. Nearly all cervical cancer is caused by HPV.
- Early exposure to HPV may damage the developing cervix, especially soon after menarche.
- Smoking impairs the immune system and concentrates carcinogens in the cervix.
- Low socioeconomic women have higher rates of smoking and earlier intercourse than middle class women. These factors may have a synergistic effect on risk for cervical cancer.
- History of more lifetime partners means a greater possible exposure to HPV.
- Use of oral contraceptive pills may decrease condom use. Unknown hormonal changes of the cervix may leave it more vulnerable to HPV uptake.
- Sexually transmitted infections (STIs) are associated with greater incidences of HPV.
- Poor hygiene may indicate lack of basic knowledge about healthy body norms, and consequently delay treatment for abnormal conditions.

There has been a recent trend, however, to more invasive disease in younger women. This effect may be due to increased screening, increased risky behavior, or the more aggressive types of HPV.

In public health, primary prevention is the promotion of healthy lifestyles and behaviors in order to minimize risk factors and prevent the disease entirely. An intervention to teach teens to use condoms and delay intercourse is an example of primary prevention. Secondary prevention is concerned with the early detection and treatment of disease. The intervention to promote regular Papanicolaou (Pap) smears for women who have been sexually active is an example of secondary prevention (see "Promoting Cervical Screening," evidence-based research box in Chapter 2). An integrated approach of primary and secondary prevention would provide the most comprehensive approach to preventing cervical cancer.

Interventions for promoting behaviors that decrease risk for cervical cancer would need to teach at least three concepts: delaying onset of intercourse, using condoms, and negotiating a safer sex approach, such as sex with an uninfected partner and a commitment to use condoms with any outside relationship. Interventions aimed at prevention of STIs and smoking may also decrease cervical cancer. There have been promising results with interventions using peer educators. Positive outcomes tend to fade with time, so the intervention would be most effective if some long-term refreshers were built in.

To evaluate such a program, the best long-term outcome would be a decrease in abnormal Pap smears. Pragmatically, the best short-term outcomes would be reported condom use, delayed intercourse, and a drop in STI rate.

Objective

The reviewers sought to assess the effectiveness of health education interventions on reducing behaviors that increase risk for transmission of HPV. Any educational interventions in any setting, delivered by any provider, were acceptable. Behavioral outcomes would ideally be condom use for vaginal intercourse, reduction in the numbers of sexual partners, development of sexual negotiation skills, delayed first intercourse, and abstinence. Clinical outcomes could be evidence of STI or cervical cancer.

Methods

Search Strategy

The reviewers searched EMBASE, ERIC, MEDLINE, Psyclit, Social Science Citation Index, Cochrane Library, and 11 journals. Search keywords were not noted. Ten controlled studies were selected, representing 5089 women, ages 11 to 54 years. The countries mentioned included Canada, India, and the United States, but countries were not listed with the trials. Eight trials were randomized. All trials aimed to decrease exposure to STIs, including human immunodeficiency virus (HIV), but not specifically HPV. The trials took place in a wide variety of settings.

Statistical Analysis

Statistical analyses involved process evaluation, which evaluates the factors together that may influence the outcome of an intervention. Meta-analysis was not possible, due to the heterogeneity of the trials.

Findings

All studies showed a short-term reduction in sexual risk reduction outcomes in the intervention group. A combination of factual information and negotiation skills development, often through role-playing, significantly increased reported condom use more effectively than either intervention alone or control. Duration of this effect is unknown. The evidence suggested that peer educators leading small group discussion sessions with a variety of media can be effective.

Limitations

Generalizability was compromised when all trials were not randomized, and when the trial subjects were all lower socioeconomic women. Groups within trials were not always equivalent. Rigorous criteria may have kept several insightful studies from inclusion. Some ethical problems may exist about use of prisoners or sex workers as to whether they were genuinely free to decline consent. Short-term behavior change may not mean long-term gains.

Conclusions

Sexual risk behaviors were reduced in the intervention group. Factual information and negotiation skills development were effective in increasing reported use of condoms.

Implications for Practice

Negotiation skills development, along with factual information, can be adapted to many situations. Peer educators running small discussion groups and using a variety of media, such as videos, brochures, and posters, can be effective at bringing about behavior changes that decrease exposure to HPV. Long-term reinforcement should be built into the intervention.

Implications for Further Research

Long-term data are needed on behavior change after short-term and long-term interventions, with information from women and men from all socioeconomic levels. Further measures of attitude, motivation, and self-efficacy (the belief that one has control over the outcome) need to be refined.

Reference

Shepherd J et al: Interventions for encouraging sexual lifestyles and behaviours intended to prevent cervical cancer (Cochrane Review), 2001. In *The Cochrane Library,* Issue 2, Chichester, UK, 2004, John Wiley & Sons.

Critical Thinking Exercise

PRECONCEPTION COUNSELING

Marcia and Robert are in their late thirties and have been married for 2 years. They have been successfully using natural family planning. Marcia has a family history of diabetes (mother and sister have type 2 diabetes). Robert has a sister who has Down syndrome. Marcia has a body mass index (BMI) of 28. Marcia and Robert are now ready to start a family. They have come to see a nurse-midwife for preconception care. The nurse-midwife identified several risk factors for the couple, including age over 35, being overweight, a family history of diabetes, and a family history of Down syndrome.

1. Evidence—Is there sufficient evidence to draw conclusions about risk factors for Marcia and Robert?
2. Assumptions—What assumptions can be made about the following risks of pregnancy for Marcia and Robert?
   a. Marcia's age
   b. Planning conception
   c. Economics
   d. Environment.
3. What implications and priorities for nursing care can be drawn at this time?
4. Does the evidence objectively support your conclusion?
5. Are there alternative perspectives to your conclusion?

years but may have full-blown disease when she is 38 years old. Other chronic or debilitating diseases or conditions increase in severity with time and these, in turn, may predispose to increased risks during pregnancy. Of significance to women in this age group is the risk for certain genetic anomalies (e.g., Down syndrome). The opportunity for genetic counseling should be available to all (see Chapter 8).

Late Reproductive Age

Women of later reproductive age are often experiencing change and reordering personal priorities. In general, the goals of education, career, marriage, and family have been achieved, and now the woman has increased time and opportunity for new interests and activities. Divorce rates are high at this age, and children leaving home may produce an "empty nest syndrome" that results in increased levels of depression. Chronic diseases also become more apparent. Most problems for the well woman are associated with perimenopause (e.g., bleeding irregularities and vasomotor symptoms). Health maintenance screening continues to be of importance because some conditions such as breast disease or ovarian cancer occur more often during this stage.

Social/Cultural

Differences exist among people from different socioeconomic levels and ethnic groups with respect to risk for illness and distribution of disease and death. Some diseases are more common among people of selected ethnicity; for example, sickle cell anemia in African-Americans, Tay-Sachs disease in Ashkenazi Jews, adult lactase deficiency in Chinese, β-thalassemia in Mediterranean peoples, and cystic fibrosis in northern Europeans. Cultural and religious influences also increase health risks because the woman and her family may have life and societal values and a view of health and illness that dictate practices different from those expected in the Judeo-Christian Western model. These may include food taboos or frequencies, methods of hygiene, effects of climate, care-seeking behaviors, willingness to undergo screening and diagnostic procedures, and value conflicts.

Socioeconomic status affects birth outcomes. The rates of perinatal and maternal deaths, preterm births, and low-birth-weight babies are considerably higher in disadvantaged populations (Arias et al, 2003). Social consequences for poor women as single parents are great because many mothers with few skills are caught in the bind of insufficient income to afford child care. These families generate fewer and fewer resources and increase their risks for health problems. Multiple roles for women in general produce overload, conflict, and stress, resulting in higher risks for psychologic illness.

Substance Use and Abuse

Use of illicit drugs and the inappropriate use of prescription drugs continue to increase; the problem is found in all ages, races, ethnic groups, and socioeconomic strata. When abused, psychoactive (mind-altering) drugs can disturb relationships, cause psychologic and physical dependency, and create serious health problems. Such substances interfere with the brain's neurotransmitters and normal chemistry; this in turn affects an individual's moods. They particularly affect the part of the brain that produces euphoria, pleasure, or pain release and, as a result, lead easily to abuse. Risk increases with the strength, amount, frequency, and route of administration.

Smoking

Tobacco use is the leading cause of preventable death and illness. Smoking is linked to cardiovascular heart disease, various types of cancers (especially lung and cervical), chronic lung disease, and negative pregnancy outcomes. Tobacco contains nicotine, which is an addictive substance that creates physical and psychologic dependence. Tobacco smoke contains known carcinogens. The average cigarette smoker shortens his or her life by 6 to 8 years.

Smoking rates vary among women in different U.S. ethnic groups. Of women smokers in the United States, Native American and non-Hispanic white women have the highest rates of all ethnic groups. African-American and Puerto Rican women have the next highest rates, whereas Asian-American and other Hispanic women have the lowest prevalence. Teen smoking rate decreased slightly to 17.5% from 2000 to 2001, reversing the upward trend since 1994 (Arias et al, 2003).

Cigarette smoking impairs fertility in both women and men, may reduce the age for menopause, and increases the risk for osteoporosis after menopause. Passive, or secondhand, smoke (environmental tobacco smoke [ETS]) contains similar hazards and presents additional problems for the smoker, as well as harm for the nonsmoker. Smoking in pregnancy is known to cause a decrease in placental perfusion and is one cause of low birth weight in infants.

Alcohol

Women ages 35 to 49 years have the highest rates of chronic alcoholism, but women ages 21 to 34 years have the highest rates of specific alcohol-related problems. About one third of alcoholics are women, and many relate the onset of their drinking problem to stressful events. Women who are problem drinkers are often depressed, have more motor vehicle injuries, and have a higher incidence of attempted suicide than do women in the general population. They are also at risk for alcohol-related liver damage. Early case finding and early treatment are important in alcoholism for both the ill individual and for family members.

Alcohol abuse during pregnancy is the leading cause of mental retardation in the United States. In addition, alcohol abuse during pregnancy has been associated with fetal growth restriction, altered facies, and developmental problems. For this reason, abstinence from alcohol consumption during pregnancy is recommended.

Prescription Medications

Psychotherapeutic medications such as stimulants, sleeping pills, tranquilizers, and pain relievers are used by an estimated 2% of American women. Such medications can bring relief from undesirable conditions such as insomnia, anxiety, and pain. Because the medications have mind-altering capacity, misuse can produce psychologic and physical dependency in the same manner as illicit drugs. Risk-to-benefit ratios should be considered when such medications are used for more than a very short period of time.

Depression is the most common mental health problem in women. Many kinds of medications are used to treat depression. All of these psychotherapeutic drugs can have some effect on the fetus and must be very carefully monitored.

Illicit Drugs

Cocaine

Cocaine is a powerful central nervous system stimulant that is addictive because of the tremendous sense of pleasure that it creates. It can be snorted, smoked, or injected. Crack or rock cocaine is a form of the drug that is exceedingly potent and even more highly addictive. (Some say that an individual is "hooked" after the first use or, at the least, after two or three "hits.") After ingestion of cocaine, an intensely pleasurable high results that is followed by an uncomfortable low; this increases the urge to repeat the drug.

Cocaine affects all of the major body systems. Among other complications, it produces cardiovascular stress that can lead to heart attack or stroke, liver disease, central nervous system stimulation that can cause seizures, and even perforation of the nasal septum. Users are often poorly nourished and commonly have STIs. If the user is pregnant, there is an increased incidence of miscarriage, preterm labor, small-for-gestational-age babies, abruption of placenta, and stillbirth. Anomalies have been reported.

Heroin

Heroin is an opiate that is usually injected but can also be smoked or snorted. It produces euphoria, relaxation, relief from pain, and "nodding out" (i.e., apathy, detachment from reality, impaired judgment, and drowsiness). Signs and symptoms are constricted pupils, nausea, constipation, slurred speech, and respiratory depression. Users are at increased risk for HIV and hepatitis B, C, and D virus infection, primarily because of sharing needles that contain contaminated blood. Perinatal effects include interference with fetal growth, premature rupture of membranes, preterm labor, and prematurity. Newborns can be born addicted to heroin and may need to undergo a withdrawal process.

Marijuana

Marijuana is a substance derived from the cannabis plant. It is usually rolled into cigarettes and smoked. It may also be mixed into food and eaten. It produces an intoxicating and sensory-distorting high. Marijuana smoke has the same characteristics as tobacco smoke and, for this reason, has similar dangers. It also readily crosses the placenta and has the effect of increasing carbon monoxide levels in the mother's blood, reducing the oxygen supply to the fetus.

Other Illicit Drugs

A number of other street drugs pose risk to users. A few are derived from organic materials, but more and more are synthetically produced in laboratories. Variations of stimulants (e.g., "speed," "meth," and "ice") produce signs and symptoms similar to cocaine, although fewer maternal and fetal complications have been attributed to them. Sedatives such as "downers," "yellow jackets," or "red devils" are used to come off of "highs." Hallucinogens alter perception and body function. PCP ("angel dust") and LSD produce vivid changes in sensation, often with agitation, euphoria, paranoia, and a tendency toward antisocial behavior. Their use may lead to flashbacks, chronic psychosis, and violent behavior. Hallucinogens taken during pregnancy may have negative neurobehavioral effects on the newborn.

Caffeine

Caffeine is found in society's most popular drinks: coffee, tea, and soft drinks. It is a stimulant that can affect mood and interrupt body functions by producing anxiety and sleep interruptions. Heart arrhythmias may be made worse by caffeine, and there can be interactions with certain medications such as lithium. Birth defects have not been related to caffeine consumption; however, high intake has been related to a slight decrease in birth weight. The U.S. Food and Drug Administration recommends that pregnant women eliminate or limit their consumption of caffeine to less than 300 mg per day (three cups of coffee or cola).

Nutrition

Good nutrition is essential to good health. A well-balanced diet helps prevent illness and also is used to treat certain health problems. Conversely, poor eating habits, eating disorders, and obesity are linked to disease and discomfort.

Nutritional Deficiencies

Overt disease caused by a lack of certain nutrients is rarely seen in the United States. However, insufficient amounts or imbalances of nutrients do pose problems for individuals and families. Overweight or underweight status, malabsorption, listlessness, fatigue, frequent colds and other minor infections, constipation, dull hair and nails, and dental caries are examples of problems that could be nutritionally related and indicate the need for further nutritional assessment. Poor nutrition, especially related to obesity and high fat and cholesterol intake, may lead to more serious conditions and is said to contribute to 4 of the 10 leading causes of death in the United States: diseases of the heart, malignant neoplasms, cerebrovascular diseases, and diabetes (Minino & Smith, 2001).

Obesity

During the past 20 years, there has been a dramatic increase in obesity in the United States. It is estimated that 25% of the women older than 20 years are obese (body mass index [BMI], 30 or higher), and 51% of the women older than 20 years are overweight (BMI, 25 to 25.9) (National Center for Chronic Disease Prevention and Health Promotion, 2000). The BMI is defined as a measure of an adult's weight in relation to his or her height, specifically the adult's weight in kilograms divided by the square of his or her height in meters (Box 4-4)

Overweight and obesity are known risk factors for diabetes, heart disease, stroke, hypertension, gallbladder disease, osteoarthritis, sleep apnea, and some types of cancer (uterine, breast, colorectal, kidney, and gallbladder) (American Cancer Society, 2004). In addition, obesity is associated with high cholesterol, menstrual irregularities, hirsutism (excess body/facial hair), stress incontinence, depression, complications of pregnancy, increased surgical risk, and shortened life span. Pregnant women who are morbidly obese are at increased risk for hypertension, diabetes, gallbladder disease, postterm pregnancy, and musculoskeletal problems.

Other Considerations

Other dietary extremes also can produce risk. For example, insufficient amounts of calcium can lead to osteoporosis, too much sodium can aggravate hypertension, and megadoses of vitamins can cause adverse effects in several body systems. Fad weight-loss programs and yo-yo dieting (repeated weight gain and weight loss) result in nutritional imbalances and, in some instances, medical problems. Such diets and programs are not appropriate for weight maintenance. Adolescent pregnancy produces special nutritional requirements because the metabolic needs of pregnancy are superimposed on the teen's own needs for growth and maturation at a time when eating habits are less than ideal. Neural tube defects are more common in infants born of women with a diet poor in folate. In their childbearing years, women should ingest at least 0.4 mg (400 mcg) of folic acid daily in addition to consuming a diet rich in folate-containing foods.

Anorexia Nervosa

Some women have a distorted view of their bodies and, no matter what their weight, perceive themselves to be much too heavy. As a result, they undertake strict and severe diets and rigorous extreme exercise. This chronic eating disorder is known as anorexia nervosa. A coexisting depression usually accompanies anorexia. Women can carry this condition to the point of starvation, with resulting endocrine and metabolic abnormalities. If not corrected, significant complications of arrhythmias, amenorrhea, cardiomyopathy, and congestive heart failure occur and, in the extreme, can lead to death. The condition commonly begins during adolescence in young women who have some degree of personality disorder. They gradually lose weight over several months, have amenorrhea, and are abnormally concerned with body image. The condition requires both psychiatric and medical intervention.

Bulimia Nervosa

Bulimia refers to secret, uncontrolled binge eating alternating with methods to prevent weight gain: self-induced vomiting, laxatives or diuretics, strict diets, fasting, and rigorous exercise. During a binge episode, large numbers of calories are consumed, usually consisting of sweets and "junk foods." Binges occur at least twice per week. Bulimia usually begins in early adulthood (ages 18 to 25 years) and is found primarily in females. Complications can include dehydration and electrolyte imbalance, gastrointestinal abnormalities, and cardiac arrhythmias. Bulimia is somewhat similar to anorexia in that it is an eating disorder and usually involves some degree of depression. Unlike those with anorexia, individuals with bulimia may feel shame or disgust about their disorder and tend to seek help earlier.

BOX 4-4

Ideal Body Weight with Body Mass Index (BMI)

BMI ≤ 18.5: underweight
BMI 18.5 to 24.9: normal weight
BMI 25.0 to 29.9: overweight
BMI 30.0 to 34.5: obese
BMI 35.0 to 40: very obese

Source: Weiss J, Scott L: Stalking the no. 1 killer of women: detecting diabetes and heart diseases, *AWHONN Lifelines* 5(5):26-34, 2001.

Physical Fitness and Exercise

Exercise contributes to good health by lowering risks for a variety of conditions that are influenced by obesity and a sedentary lifestyle. It is effective in the prevention of cardiovascular disease and in the management of chronic conditions such as hypertension, arthritis, diabetes, respiratory disorders, and osteoporosis (Fig. 4-1). Exercise also contributes to stress reduction and weight maintenance. Women report that engaging in regular exercise improves their body image and self-esteem and acts as a mood enhancer. Aerobic exercise produces cardiovascular involvement because increasing amounts of oxygen are delivered to working muscles. Anaerobic exercise, such as weight training, improves individual muscle mass without stress on the cardiovascular system (Fig. 4-2). Because women are concerned about both cardiovascular and bone health, weight-bearing aerobic exercises such as walking, running, racket sports, and dancing are preferred. However, excessive or strenuous exercise can

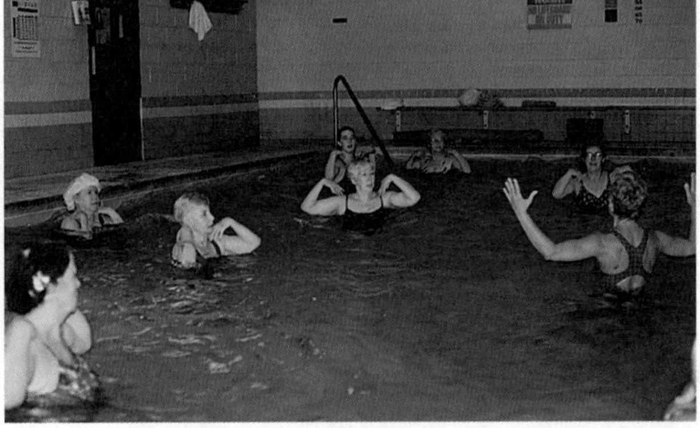

Fig. 4-1 Water aerobics improves cardiovascular function. (Courtesy Jonas McCoy, Raleigh, NC.)

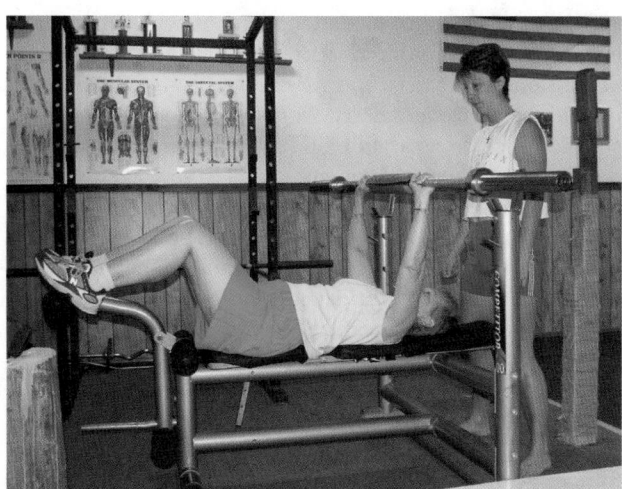

Fig. 4-2 Weight training improves muscle mass without stress on the cardiovascular system. (Courtesy Julie Perry Nelson, Gilbert, AZ.)

lead to hormonal imbalances, resulting in amenorrhea and its consequences. Physical injury is also a potential risk.

Physical activity and exercise counseling for persons of all ages should be undertaken at schools, work sites, and primary care settings. Specific recommendations include 20 to 30 minutes of moderate activity at least three times per week. Few Americans exercise this often, and physical inactivity increases with age, especially during adolescence and early adulthood. Even small increases in activity can be beneficial. During pregnancy, an ongoing exercise regimen can be continued but should be decreased in intensity and duration. Sedentary women should obtain medical clearance to initiate exercise during pregnancy, and should begin with low-intensity and low-impact workouts.

Kegel Exercises

Kegel exercises, or pelvic muscle exercises, were developed to strengthen the supportive pelvic floor muscles to control or reduce involuntary urine loss (Patient Teaching box). These exercises are also beneficial during pregnancy and postpartum. They strengthen the muscles of the pelvic floor, providing support for the pelvic organs and control of the muscles surrounding the vagina and urethra.

Stress

The modern woman faces increasing levels of stress and, as a result, is prone to a variety of stress-induced complaints and illnesses. Stress often occurs because of multiple roles in which coping with job and financial responsibilities conflicts with parenting and duties at home. To add to this burden, women are socialized to be caretakers, which is emotionally draining in itself. They also may find themselves in positions of minimal power that do not allow them control over their everyday environments. Some stress is normal and contributes to positive outcomes. Many women thrive in busy surroundings. However, excessive or high levels of ongoing stress trigger physical reactions such as rapid heart rate, elevated blood pressure, slowed digestion, release of additional

Patient Teaching

KEGEL EXERCISES

Description and Rationale

Kegel exercise, or pelvic muscle exercise, is a technique used to strengthen the muscles that support the pelvic floor. This exercise involves regularly tightening (contracting) and relaxing the muscles that support the bladder and urethra. By strengthening these pelvic muscles, a woman can prevent or reduce accidental urine loss.

Technique

The woman needs to learn how to target the muscles for training and how to contract them correctly. One suggestion for teaching is to have the woman pretend she is trying to prevent the passage of intestinal gas. Have her use this tightening motion on the muscles around her vagina and the upper pelvis. She should feel these muscles drawing inward and upward. Other suggested techniques are to have the woman pretend she is trying to stop the flow of urine in midstream or to have her think about how her vagina is able to contract around and move up the length of the penis during intercourse.

The woman should avoid straining or bearing-down motions while performing the exercise. She should be taught how bearing down feels by having her take a breath, hold it, and push down with her abdominal muscles as though she were trying to have a bowel movement. Then the woman can be taught how to avoid straining down by exhaling gently and keeping her mouth open each time she contracts her pelvic muscles.

Specific Instructions

1. Each contraction should be as intense as possible without contracting the abdomen, thighs, or buttocks.
2. Contractions should be held for at least 10 seconds. The woman may have to start with as little as 2 seconds per contraction until her muscles get stronger.
3. The woman should rest for 10 seconds or more between contractions so that the muscles have time to recover and each contraction can be as strong as the woman can make it.
4. The woman should feel the pulling up and over the three muscle layers so that the contraction reaches the highest level of her pelvis.

Other Suggestions for Implementation

1. At first the woman should set aside about 15 minutes a day to do the Kegel exercises.
2. The woman may want to put up reminders, such as notes on her bathroom mirror, her refrigerator, her TV, or a calendar, to do the exercises.
3. Guidelines for practicing Kegel exercises suggest performing between 30 and 80 contractions a day; however, positive results can be achieved with only 30 a day.
4. The best position for learning how to do Kegel exercises is to lie supine with the knees bent. Another position to use is on the hands and knees. Once the woman learns the proper technique, she can perform the exercises in other positions such as standing or sitting.

Sources: Sampselle CM: Behavioral interventions for urinary incontinence in women: evidence for practice, *J Midwifery Womens Health* 45(2):94-103, 2000; Sampselle CM et al: Continence for women: evidence-based practice, *J Obstet Gynecol Neonatal Nurs* 26(4):375-385, 1997.

neurotransmitters and hormones, muscle tenseness, and a weakened immune system. Consequently, constant stress can contribute to clinical illnesses such as flare-ups of arthritis or asthma, frequent colds or infections, gastrointestinal upsets, cardiovascular problems, and infertility. Box 4-5 lists symptoms that may be related to chronic or extreme stress. Psychologic symptoms such as anxiety, irritability, eating disorders, depression, insomnia, and substance abuse have also been associated with stress.

Stress Management

Because it is neither possible nor desirable to avoid all stress, women must learn how to manage stress. The nurse should assess each woman for signs of stress, using therapeutic communication skills to determine risk factors and the woman's ability to function.

Some women must be referred for counseling or other mental health therapy. Women are twice as likely as men to suffer from depression, anxiety, or panic attacks. Nurses must be alert to the symptoms of serious mental disorders, such as depression and anxiety, and make referrals to mental health practitioners when necessary. Women experiencing major life changes, such as separation and divorce, bereavement, serious illness, and unemployment, also need special attention.

Many centers offer support groups to help women prevent or manage stress. Social support and good coping skills can improve a woman's self-esteem and give her a sense of mastery. Anticipatory guidance for developmental or expected situational crises can help her plan strategies for dealing with potentially stressful events. Role-playing, relaxation techniques, biofeedback, meditation, desensitization, imagery, assertiveness training, yoga, diet, exercise, and weight control are all techniques nurses can include in their repertoire of helping skills.

BOX 4-5

Stress Symptoms

Physical

Perspiration/sweaty hands
Increased heart rate
Trembling
Nervous tics
Dryness of throat and mouth
Tiring easily
Urinating frequently
Sleeping problems
Diarrhea, indigestion, vomiting
Butterflies in stomach
Headaches
Premenstrual tension
Pain in the neck and lower back
Loss of appetite or overeating
Susceptibility to illness
Behavior
- Stuttering and other speech difficulties
- Crying for no apparent reason
- Acting impulsively
- Startling easily
- Laughing in a high-pitched and nervous tone of voice
- Grinding teeth
- Increasing smoking
- Increasing use of drugs and alcohol
- Being accident prone
- Losing appetite or overeating

Psychologic

Feeling anxious
Feeling scared
Feeling irritable
Feeling moody
Low self-esteem
Fear of failure
Inability to concentrate
Embarrassing easily
Worrying about the future
Preoccupation with thoughts or tasks
Forgetfulness

Modified from State University of New York Counseling Center: *Stress management*, Buffalo, NY, 2002, University of Buffalo, State University of New York.

Sexual Practices

Potential risks related to sexual activity include undesired pregnancy and STIs. The risks are particularly high for adolescents and young adults who engage in sexual intercourse at earlier and earlier ages. Adolescents report many reasons for wanting to be sexually active: peer pressure, desire to love and be loved, experimentation, to enhance self-esteem, and to have fun. However, many teens do not have the decision-making or values-clarification skills needed to take this important step. They may also lack knowledge about contraception and STIs. Many do not believe that becoming pregnant or acquiring an STI will happen to them.

Although some STIs can be cured with antibiotics, many cause significant problems. Possible sequelae include infertility, ectopic pregnancy, neonatal morbidity and mortality, genital cancers, acquired immunodeficiency syndrome, and even death. STIs are increasing rapidly and are in epidemic proportion. Choice of contraception has an impact on the risk of contracting an STI. No method of contraception offers complete protection. (See Chapter 6 for a discussion of STIs and Chapter 7 for a discussion of contraception.)

Safer Sexual Practices

Prevention of STIs is predicated on the reduction of high risk behaviors by educating toward a behavioral change. Behaviors of concern include multiple and casual sexual partners and unsafe sexual practices. Specific self-care measures for safer sex are listed in Box 4-6. The abuse of alcohol and drugs is also a high risk behavior resulting in impaired judgment and thoughtless acts. Behavioral changes must come from within, and therefore the nurse must provide sufficient information for the individual or group to "buy into" the need for change. Education is a powerful tool in health promotion and prevention of STIs and pregnancy. However, it works best when delivered in a way that takes into account the language, culture, and lifestyle of the intended listener.

Medical Conditions

Most women of reproductive age are relatively healthy. Heart disease; lung, breast, colon, and other nongynecologic cancers; chronic lung disease; and diabetes are all concerns for adult women, as they are among the leading causes of death

BOX 4-6

Safer Sex

- Safer sex is possible only if there is no oral, genital, or rectal exchange of body fluids or if a person is in a long-term, mutually monogamous relationship with an uninfected partner.
- Correct use of latex condoms, although greatly reducing risk, is not exclusively protective.
- Sexual partners should be selected with great care.
- Partners should be asked about history of STIs.
- A new condom should be used for each act of sexual intercourse when a partner's infection status is unknown or if the partner is infected with HIV or another STI.
- Abstinence from sexual intercourse is encouraged for persons who are being treated for an STI or whose partners are being treated.

Source: Centers for Disease Control and Prevention: Sexually transmitted diseases treatment guidelines 2002, *MMWR* 51(RR-6):1-80, 2002.

in women. Certain medical conditions present during pregnancy can have deleterious effects on both the woman and the fetus. Of particular concern are risks from all forms of diabetes, urinary tract disorders, thyroid disease, hypertensive disorders of pregnancy, cardiac disease, and seizure disorders. Effects on the fetus vary and include intrauterine growth restriction, macrosomia, anemia, prematurity, immaturity, and stillbirth. Effects on the woman also can be severe. These conditions are discussed in later chapters.

Gynecologic Conditions

Women are at risk for pelvic inflammatory disease, endometriosis, STIs and other vaginal infections, uterine fibroids, uterine deformities such as bicornuate uterus, ovarian cysts, and urinary incontinence related to pelvic relaxation throughout their reproductive years. These gynecologic conditions may contribute negatively to pregnancy by causing infertility, miscarriage, preterm labor, and fetal and neonatal problems. Gynecologic cancers also affect women's health, although the risk for most cancers is low in pregnancy. Risk factors depend on the type of cancer. The impact of developing a gynecologic problem or cancer on women and their families is shaped by a number of factors, including the specific type of problem or cancer, the implications of the diagnosis for the woman and her family, and the timing of the occurrence in the woman's and the family's lives.

Female Genital Mutilation

Female genital mutilation is practiced in more than 45 countries, with the majority of these countries being in Africa. These procedures involve the intentional removal of all or part of the external female genitalia (Affara, 2000). As emigrants from those countries arrive in North America, nurses in the United States and Canada will see patients who have had such procedures performed. Complications of female genital mutilation include infection, hemorrhage, and urinary complications, as well as higher maternal and infant morbidity and mortality rates during labor (Affara, 2000).

Environmental and Workplace Hazards

Environmental hazards in the home, workplace, and community can contribute to poor health at all ages. Categories and examples of health-damaging hazards include the following: (1) pathogenic agents (viruses, bacteria, fungi, parasites); (2) natural and synthetic chemicals (natural toxins from animals, insects, and plants; consumer and industrial products such as pesticides and hydrocarbon gases; medical and diagnostic devices; tobacco; fuels; and drug and alcohol abuse); (3) radiation (radon, heat waves, sound waves); (4) food substances (added components that are not necessary for nutrition); and (5) physical objects (moving vehicles, machinery, weapons, water, and building materials).

Environmental hazards can affect fertility, fetal development, live birth, and the child's future mental and physical development. Children are at special risk for poisoning from lead found in paint and soil. Everyone is at risk from air pollutants such as tobacco smoke, carbon monoxide, smog, suspended particles (dust, ash, and asbestos), and cleaning solvents; noise pollution; pesticides; chemical additives; and poor preparation of food. Workers also face safety and health risks caused by ergonomically poor workstations and stress. The lists could go on and on. It is important that risk assessments continue to be in effect to identify and understand environmental public health problems.

ANTICIPATORY GUIDANCE FOR HEALTH PROMOTION AND PREVENTION

Over the last several decades, women have made tremendous strides in education, careers, policy making, and overall participation in today's complex society. There have been costs for these advances, and although women are living longer, they may not be living better. As a result, the health care system needs to pay greater attention to the health consequences for women. Women must be active participants in their own health promotion and illness prevention.

Community Focus

ANTICIPATORY GUIDANCE FOR HEALTH PROMOTION

Prepare a consultation plan that uses community resources for a 35-year-old, divorced, nulliparous woman needing general anticipatory guidance for health promotion and prevention.

- Ascertain her opinion regarding her health status.
- Identify need for counseling regarding nutrition, exercise, stress management, and safer sexual practices.
- Suggest recommendations for screening based on information obtained.
- Are there nurse practitioners available in the community?
- What health education programs are available in the community?
- In consultation with the woman, develop an exercise program for her.
- What resources in the community are available to her?
- What resources in the community are available for low-income women?

Nurses have a major opportunity and responsibility to help women understand risk factors and to motivate them to adopt healthy lifestyles that prevent disease. Lifestyle factors that affect health—and that the woman has some control over—include diet; tobacco, alcohol, and substance use; exercise; sunlight exposure; stress management; and sexual practices. Other influences, such as genetic and environmental factors, may be beyond the woman's control, although some opportunities for prevention exist (e.g., through environmental legislative activism or genetic counseling services).

Knowledge alone is not enough to bring about healthy behaviors. The woman must be convinced that she has some control over her life and that healthy life habits, including periodic health examinations, are a sound investment. She must believe in the efficacy of prevention, early detection, and therapy, and in her ability to perform self-care practices such as breast self-examination. Many people believe that they have little control over their health, or they become so immobilized by fear and anxiety in the face of life-threatening illnesses, such as cancer, that they delay seeking treatment. The nurse must explore the reality of each woman's perceptions about health behaviors and individualize teaching if it is to be effective.

Substance Use Cessation

All women at all ages will receive substantial and immediate benefits from smoking cessation. This is not easy, however, and most people will attempt to stop several times before they accomplish their goal. Many are never able to do so.

New approaches are needed to increase cessation among smokers and to discourage smoking among young women, especially in adolescence and during pregnancy. Health care providers can have an impact on smoking behavior and should attempt to motivate smokers to stop (Box 4-7). Raising questions about social consequences (e.g., stained teeth and foul-smelling breath and clothes) is sometimes effective with young people.

Those who wish to stop smoking can be referred to a smoking cessation program in which individualized methods can be implemented. At the very least, individuals should be guided to self-help materials available from the March of Dimes Birth Defects Foundation, the American Lung Association, and the American Cancer Society. During pregnancy, women seem to be highly motivated to stop or at least to limit smoking to 10 or fewer cigarettes a day. Insult to the fetus can be reduced or even avoided if this is done by the end of the first trimester.

Alcohol and other drugs exact a staggering toll on society, not only in terms of personal health, but also in their association with poverty and homelessness, family disorganization, violence, crime, motor vehicle injuries, reduced productivity, and economic costs. The abuse of alcohol and other drugs increases the risk of victimization and date rape and of acquiring HIV through shared needles or sexual contact. Alcohol use and drug use are the leading preventable causes of birth defects.

A national awareness of the seriousness of problems associated with substance abuse has led to raising the legal drinking age to 21 in all states and to tighter controls on advertising. Stronger regulation of advertising and tougher laws and law enforcement for alcohol- and drug-related offenses are being implemented. There is still much that must be done to increase the accessibility to care for low-income people, minorities, and young people. Women—especially pregnant women and the mothers of young children—have special needs that must be addressed.

All primary care providers should screen for alcohol and other drug use problems, with an understanding of the obvious problems in relying on self-reporting of these behaviors. The use of over-the-counter drugs by women should also be explored. Counseling women who appear to be drinking excessively or using drugs may include strategies to increase self-esteem and teaching new coping skills to resist and maintain resistance to alcohol abuse and drug use. Appropriate referrals should be made, with the health care provider arranging the contact and then following up to ensure that appointments are kept. General referral to sources of support should also be provided. National groups that provide information and support for those who are chemically dependent are listed in Resources at the end of the chapter. Many of these organizations have local branches or contacts that are listed in the telephone book.

Anticipatory guidance includes teaching about the health and safety risks of alcohol and mind-altering substances and discouraging drug experimentation among preteen and high school students, because the use of drugs at an early age tends to predict greater involvement later.

BOX 4-7

Interventions for Smoking Cessation: The Four *A's*

Ask
What was her age when she started smoking? How many cigarettes does she smoke a day? When was her last cigarette? Has she tried to quit? Does she want to quit?

Assess
What are her reasons for not being able to quit before, or what made her start again? Does she have anyone who can help her? Does anyone else smoke at home? Does she have friends or family who have quit successfully?

Advise
Give her information about the effects of smoking on pregnancy and her fetus, on her own future health, and on the members of her household.

Assist
Provide support; give self-help materials. Encourage her to set a quit date. Refer to a smoking cessation program or provide information about nicotine replacement products (not recommended during pregnancy) if she is interested. Teach and encourage use of stress reduction activities. Provide for follow-up with a phone call, letter, or clinic visit.

Source: American College of Obstetricians and Gynecologists (ACOG): *Smoking and women's health,* ACOG Tech Bull no 240, Washington, DC, 1997, ACOG.

Health Screening Schedule

Periodic health screening includes history, physical examination, education, counseling, and selected diagnostic and laboratory tests. This regimen provides the basis for overall health promotion, prevention of illness, early diagnosis of problems, and referral for appropriate management. Such screening should be customized according to a woman's age and risk factors. In most instances it is completed in health care offices, clinics, or hospitals; however, portions of the screening are now being carried out at events such as community health fairs. An overview of health screening recommendations for women over 18 years of age is provided in Table 4-1. Consistent with information provided earlier in this chapter, it is important for the nurse to continually educate and counsel on diet, exercise, cessation of smoking, alcohol moderation, help for drug abuse, and stress management.

Health Risk Prevention

Often, simple safety factors are forgotten or perceived not to be important; yet injuries continue to have a major impact on the health status of all age groups. Awareness of hazards and implementation of safety guidelines will reduce risks. The nurse should regularly reinforce the following commonsense concepts that will protect the individual:

- Wear seat belts at all times in a moving vehicle.
- Wear safety helmets when riding a motorcycle or bicycle.
- Follow driving rules of the road.
- Have working smoke alarms in place throughout the home and workplace.
- Avoid secondhand smoke.
- Reduce noise pollution or safeguard against hearing loss.
- Protect skin from ultraviolet light via sunscreen and clothing.
- Handle and store firearms appropriately.
- Practice water safety.

Taking necessary precautions and avoiding dangerous situations are imperative.

Health Protection

Nurses can make a difference in stopping violence against women and in preventing further injury. Educating women that abuse is a violation of their rights and facilitating their access to protective and legal services constitutes a first step. Encouraging health care institutions to implement appropriate domestic violence screening programs is also of great value. Other measures that may help women avoid falling into abusive relationships are promoting assertiveness and self-defense courses; suggesting support and self-help groups that encourage positive self-regard, confidence, and empowerment; and recommending educational and skills development classes that will enhance independence (or at least the ability to take care of oneself).

Many national and local organizations provide information and assistance for women in abusive situations. Nurses and victims may find these resources helpful (see Resources at end of chapter). All nurses who work in women's health care should become familiar with local services and legal options.

Violence Against Women

Violence against women is a significant social problem and a major health care problem in the United States. It is estimated that 25% of women worldwide have been victims of intimate partner violence (IPV) (Tjaden & Thoennes, 2000). An average of three women a day are murdered by their intimate partners (Walton-Moss & Campbell, 2002). Pregnancy is often a time when violence begins or escalates. Women who are abused during pregnancy have a threefold increase in risk of being murdered (McFarlane et al, 2002). A *Healthy People 2010* objective is to decrease the rate of IPV to 4 per 1000 women older than 12 years (U.S. Department of Health and Human Services [USDHHS], 2000).

Although IPV is the preferred term, *wife battering, spouse abuse,* and *domestic* or *family violence* are all terms that may be applied to a pattern of assaultive and coercive behaviors inflicted by a male partner in a marriage or other heterosexual, significant, intimate relationships. Relationship violence rarely consists of a single episode but is a pattern that may start with intimidation or threats (Fig. 4-3) and progress to more aggressive physical and sexual acts resulting in injury to the woman. Common elements of battering are economic deprivation, sexual abuse, intimidation, isolation, and stalking and terrorizing victims and their children (National Women's Health Information Center [NWHIC], 2002).

Maternity and women's health nurses, by the very nature of their practice, are in a unique position to identify and assist in the treatment of women experiencing any type of violence or sexual assault; to help prevent further harm through identification, treatment and education; and to influence public policy in decreasing violence.

Characteristics of Women in Abusive Relationships

Women of all races and of all ethnic, educational, religious, and socioeconomic backgrounds are affected. In the United States, Caucasian women report less IPV than do non-Caucasians. Native American/Alaskan Native women report significantly more instances of IPV than do women of any other racial background; Asian women report significantly less IPV than do other racial groups (Tjaden & Thoennes, 2000). Reporting rates may not reflect the magnitude of the problem, as many women do not disclose violence because of fear, embarrassment, or not having been asked by those from whom they seek help. Poor and uneducated women tend to be disproportionately represented because they are seen in emergency departments (EDs), they are financially more dependent, they have fewer resources and support systems, and they may have fewer problem-solving skills.

Battered women may believe they are to blame for their situations because they are "not good enough, not efficient enough, not pretty enough." The woman may blame herself for bringing on the violent behavior in her relationship because she believes she must "try harder" to please the abuser. In many cases, a traumatic bonding with the man hinges on loyalty, fear, terror, and learned helplessness. Some women

Table 4-1

Health Screening Recommendations for Women Age 18 Years and Older

INTERVENTION	RECOMMENDATION*
PHYSICAL EXAMINATION	
Blood pressure	Every visit, but at least every 2 years
Height and weight	Every visit, but at least every 2 years
Pelvic examination	Annually until age 70; recommended for any woman who has ever been sexually active
Breast examination	
Self-examination	Initiated/taught at time of first pelvic examination; done monthly at end of menses
Clinical examination†	Every 3 years, ages 20 to 39; annually after age 40
High risk	Annually after age 18 with history of premenopausal breast cancer in first-degree relative
Risk groups	At least annually
Skin examination	Family history of skin cancer or increased exposure to sunlight after age 40; every 3 years between ages 20 and 40; monthly self-examinations also recommended
Oral cavity examination	Mouth lesion or exposure to tobacco or excessive alcohol
LABORATORY/DIAGNOSTIC TESTS	
Blood cholesterol (fasting lipoprotein analysis)	Every 5 years
High risk	More often per clinical judgment with potential for cardiac or lipid abnormalities
Papanicolaou (Pap) smear†	Initially, 3 years after becoming sexually active but no later than age 21; yearly with conventional Pap test or every 2 years with liquid-based Pap tests; after age 30 and after three normal test results in a row, every 2 to 3 years; after age 70 and no abnormal test results in 10 years, screening may be stopped
Mammography‡	Annually over age 50 Annually over age 40 Every 1 to 2 years between ages 40 and 49 and annually thereafter
Colon cancer screening	Fecal occult blood test annually and flexible sigmoidoscopy every 5 years after age 50; more often if family history of colon cancer or polyps
RISK GROUPS	
Fasting blood sugar	Annually with family history of diabetes, gestational diabetes, or significantly obese; every 3 to 5 years for all women older than 45 years of age
Hearing screen	Annually with exposure to excessive noise or when loss is suspected
Sexually transmitted infection screen	As needed with multiple sexual partners
Tuberculin skin test	Annually with exposure to persons with tuberculosis or in risk categories for close contact with the disease
Endometrial biopsy	At menopause for women at risk for endometrial cancer
Vision	Every 2 years between ages 40 and 64; annually after age 65
Bone mineral density testing	All women age 65 and older; younger women with risk for osteoporosis may need periodic screenings
IMMUNIZATIONS	
Tetanus-diphtheria	Booster is given every 10 years after primary series
Measles, mumps, rubella	Once if born after 1956 and no evidence of immunity
Hepatitis B	Primary series of three for all who are in risk categories
Influenza	Annually after age 65 or in risk categories, such as chronic diseases, immunosuppression, renal dysfunction

*Unless otherwise noted, the recommended intervention should be performed routinely every 1 to 3 years.

†Sources: American Cancer Society: *Cancer facts and figures 2003,* New York, 2003, American Cancer Society; Centers for Disease Control and Prevention: Sexually transmitted diseases treatment guidelines 2002, *MMWR* 51(RR-6):1-80, 2002; Expert Panel on Detection, Evaluation, and Treatment of High Blood Cholesterol in Adults: executive summary of the third report of the National Education Program (NCEP) expert panel on detection, evaluation, and treatment of high blood cholesterol in adults (adult treatment panel III), *JAMA* 285(19):2486-2497, 2001; National Women's Health Resource Center: Screening tests and women's health, *National Women's Health Report* 23(6):1-7, 2001; US Preventive Services Task Force: *Guide to clinical preventive services,* ed 2, Baltimore, 1996, Williams & Wilkins; US Preventive Services Task Force: *Screening for cervical cancers,* AHRQ pub 03-535, Rockville, MD, 2003, Agency for Healthcare Research and Quality.

‡NOTE: There is no consensus regarding mammograms for women between 40 and 49 years of age; thus various recommendations are listed. Women are urged to discuss circumstances with their health care provider.

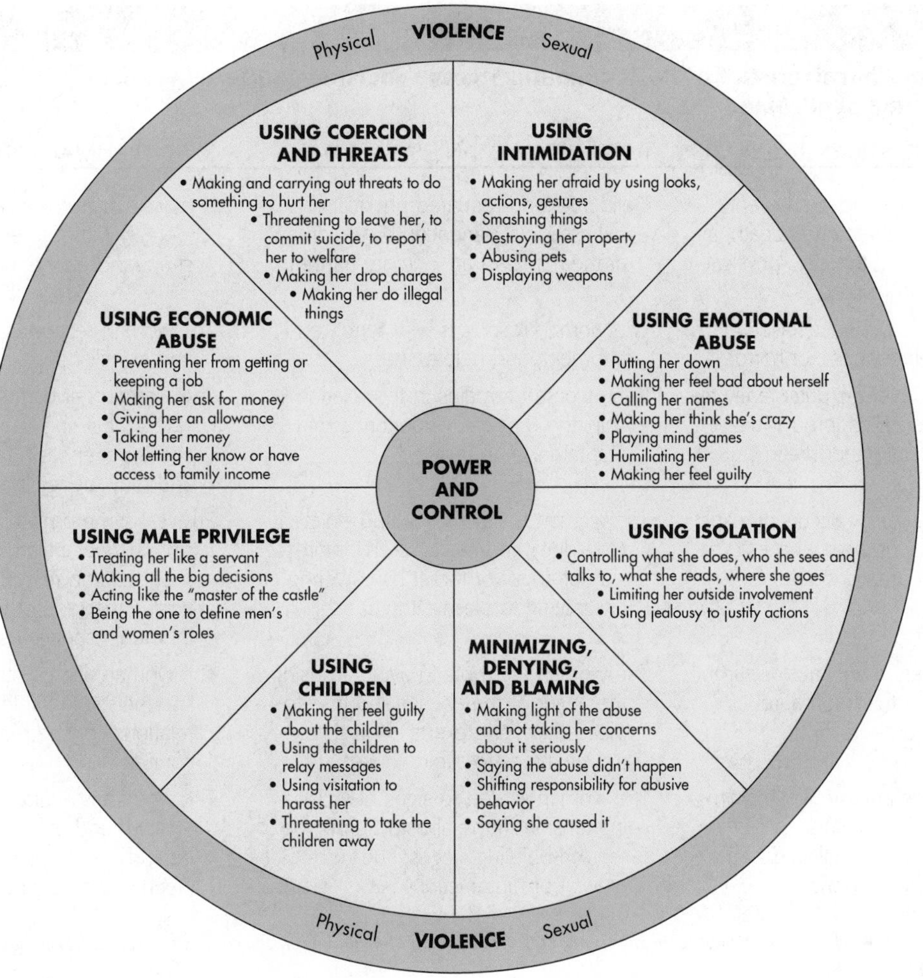

Fig. 4-3 Model of how power and control issues perpetuate battering. (From Duluth Domestic Abuse Intervention Project: *Power and control: tactics of men who batter,* Duluth, MN, 1986, Author.)

have low self-esteem and may have histories of domestic violence in their families of origin. They fear societal rejection if they discuss their problem openly.

The battered woman's syndrome may be formally diagnosed in the fourth edition of the *Diagnostic and Statistical Manual of Mental Disorders* (DSM-IV) (American Psychiatric Association, 2000) as *posttraumatic stress disorder (PTSD),* provided that the symptoms meet the criteria. Table 4-2 compares the characteristics of PTSD with battered woman's syndrome. Professionals making the diagnosis must guard against implying that the woman's problems are her issues alone (Box 4-8). Table 4-3 lists some myths and facts about abuse and battering.

Cycle of Violence: The Dynamics of Battering

Battering is neither random nor constant; rather, it occurs in repeated cycles. A three-phase cyclic pattern to the battering behavior includes a period of *increasing tension* leading to the *battery,* which is then followed by a period of *calm and remorse* in which the male partner displays kind, loving behavior and pleas for forgiveness. This "honeymoon" phase lasts until stress or other factors cause conflict and tension to mount again toward another episode of battering. Over time, the tension and battering phases last longer and the calm phase becomes shorter until there is no honeymoon phase.

Battering during Pregnancy

Estimates of prevalence of battering in pregnancy vary, ranging from 4% to 8% (Martin et al, 2001). Most women abused before pregnancy will be abused during the pregnancy; the incidence may escalate. Abuse also may happen for the first time during pregnancy. Pregnant adolescents are abused at higher rates than are adult women, so they should be considered at high risk.

Physical abuse is harmful not only to the mother; the risk of fetal injury is very high. Studies have demonstrated that battery during pregnancy also results in a higher rate of low-birth-weight newborns and maternal complications of depression, suicide, low weight gain, infections, bleeding, and anemia (McFarlane et al, 2002). In addition, the woman may smoke or use alcohol or other drugs as means of coping with IPV. These activities are significantly related to low-birth-weight infants (Humphreys, Parker, & Campbell, 2001).

During pregnancy, the nurse should assess for abuse at each prenatal visit and on admission to labor. Battering episodes initiate or increase in pregnancy for a variety of reasons: (1) the biopsychosocial stresses of pregnancy may strain the relationship beyond the couple's ability to cope, and frustration is followed by violence; (2) the man may be jealous of the fetus, resenting the intrusion into the couple's

Table 4-2

Comparison of Characteristics of Posttraumatic Stress Syndrome, Battered Woman's Syndrome, and Rape-Trauma Syndrome

POSTTRAUMATIC STRESS SYNDROME*	BATTERED WOMAN'S SYNDROME	RAPE-TRAUMA SYNDROME
1. The person experienced an event that involved or threatened death, a serious injury, or a threat to physical integrity of self or other.	Deliberate and repeated physical or sexual assault experienced by a woman at the hands of an intimate partner.	A violent, aggressive sexual assault on a woman without her consent from a stranger or someone she knows.
2. The person's response involved intense fear, helplessness, or horror.	The woman responds with terror, entrapment, and helplessness.	The woman responds with shock, terror, and humiliation.
3. The traumatic event is persistently reexperienced, such as through distressing recollections or dreams.	If the woman remains in the relationship, the repeated experience may be real rather than recalled.	The woman relives the scene and considers what she "should have done"; she experiences a range of emotions and may feel guilty.
4. Psychologic reactivity occurs on exposure to internal or external cues symbolic of the traumatic event.	The woman feels anxious and isolated (or alone) and reacts to any expression of anger or threat by cowering or attempting to placate the abuser.	Physical symptoms such as muscle tension, hyperventilation, and flushing may occur in response to reexperiencing the rape or when approached by men, especially strangers.
5. The person persistently avoids stimuli associated with the trauma; responses are numbed.	The woman attempts to avoid arousing the anger of the abuser and tries to please him; she exerts effort to control situations to avoid abuse.	The woman avoids situations in which she feels vulnerable; if in an intimate relationship, she may avoid intercourse.
6. The person has persistent symptoms of increased arousal, such as difficulty sleeping, hypervigilance, and exaggerated startle response.	The woman is alert to signs of increasing tension in the abuser during the tension-building stages; she withdraws from interaction.	The woman is afraid of being alone or in a crowd and of being attacked from behind; she takes extra precautions when going out and is suspicious.

*Modified from American Psychiatric Association: *Diagnostic and statistical manual of mental disorders,* ed 4, text revision, Washington, DC, 2000, American Psychiatric Association.

BOX 4-8

What Not to Say to a Battered Woman and What You Can Say and Do

What *Not* to Say
1. Do not ask "why." This question "revictimizes" and blames the victim.
2. Do not talk negatively about the abuser to the victim. She may become defensive and stop talking.
3. Do not talk directly to the abuser about your suspicions of abuse. The abuser will assume the victim told you, and the victim risks retaliation.

What to Do
1. Empower the victim.
2. Sit down with her.
3. Assure her of total privacy and confidentiality (but only if you can).
4. Use your best listening skills.
5. Call 911 and report any incident of imminent danger.
6. Give the woman the telephone number of the nearest battered women's shelter.

What to Say
1. "I'm afraid for your safety (and the safety of your children)."
2. "I believe you."
3. "It is progressive and will only get worse."
4. "You deserve better than this. You deserve to be treated with respect."
5. "You are not alone."
6. "It is a crime."
7. "I am here for you."

Adapted from *A few dangerous myths.* Internet document available at www.batteredwomen.com (accessed November 30, 2004).

relationship and the woman's displacement of attention; (3) the man may be angry at the unborn child or the woman; and (4) the beating may be the man's conscious or subconscious attempt to end the pregnancy. After birth, the mother may be so physically and emotionally drained that she may have difficulty bonding with her infant (Lindgren, 2001). She may be at risk of becoming an abusive mother whether or not she remains in the abusive relationship.

During pregnancy, the target body parts change during abusive episodes. Women report physical blows directed to the head, breasts, abdomen, and genitalia. Sexual assault is common. Physical and sexual assaults also increase the rate of miscarriages and preterm and stillborn infants. The battered woman should be treated as an obstetric patient at high risk.

If the pregnant woman remains with her partner, she is at additional risk for repeated physical and psychologic trauma

Table 4-3

Myths and Facts about Intimate Partner Violence

MYTHS	FACTS
Battering occurs in a small percentage of the population.	One fourth of all women experience battering by an intimate partner.
Being pregnant protects the woman from battering.	From 4% to 8% of all women who are battered are battered during pregnancy. Battering frequently begins or escalates in frequency and intensity during pregnancy. Pregnancy may be the result of forced sex or of the man's control of contraception.
Battering occurs only in "problem" or lower-class families.	Intimate partner violence can occur in any family. Although lower-income families have a higher reported incidence of battering, it also occurs in middle- and upper-income families. Incidence is not accurately known because of the tendency of middle- and upper-income families to hide their battering.
Battered women like to be beaten and deliberately provoke the attack. They are masochistic.	Women are terrified of their assailants and go to great lengths to avoid a confrontation. In some cases, the woman may provoke her partner to release tension that, if left unchecked, might lead to a more severe beating and possible death.
Only men with psychologic problems abuse women.	Many batterers are successful professionals, including politicians, ministers, physicians, and lawyers. Research indicates that only a small number of abusers have psychologic problems.
Only people who come from abusive families end up in abusive relationships.	Most battered women report that their partners were the first person to beat them.
Alcohol and drug abuse cause battering.	Although alcohol may be involved in abusive incidents, it is not the cause. Many batterers use alcohol as an excuse to batter and shift the blame to the alcohol.
Women would leave the relationship if the abuse were really that bad.	Those women who stay in the relationship do so out of fear and financial dependence. Shelters have long waiting lists.
Batterers and battered women cannot change.	Counseling may effectively help both batterers and battered women.

From Gelles R: *Intimate violence in families,* ed 3, Thousand Oaks, CA, 1997, Sage; National Institute on Alcohol and Alcoholism: Alcohol violence and aggression, *Alcohol Alert* 38:1-6, 1997; National Women's Health Information Center: *Violence against women,* 2002. Internet document available at www.4woman.gov/violence/index.cfm (accessed August 14, 2002).

and even death (McFarlane et al, 2002). If battering begins in pregnancy, it is likely to continue after the birth. This information is vital to share with the woman and other nurses involved in her care.

Assessment and Nursing Diagnoses

All women entering the health care system should be assessed for potential abuse (McFarlane et al, 2002). At least the following questions should be asked (American College of Obstetricians and Gynecologists [ACOG], 2002): (1) Are you with a spouse or partner who threatens or physically hurts you? (2) Within the past year or in this pregnancy has anyone hit, slapped, kicked, or otherwise hurt you? and (3) Has anyone forced you to have sexual activities that made you uncomfortable? These questions give a woman permission to disclose sensitive information.

In the United States, a pregnant woman is often accompanied by her husband to the antepartum appointment if the woman does not speak English and the husband does. Unless an interpreter is available, it is difficult to interview the woman alone; in addition, asking questions about abuse through an interpreter is more difficult unless the interpreter is a woman and can communicate the nurse's sensitivity and concern accurately. See the Guidelines/Guías box for descriptions of abusive relationships and how a woman can recognize whether she is in one.

Plan of Care and Interventions

A therapeutic relationship and skillful interviewing help women disclose and describe their abuse. Language is important when talking with women. For example, using the term *victim* connotes powerlessness and hopelessness; a more empowering term is *survivor*. Women who have identified their abuse may appear passive, hostile, anxious, depressed, or hysterical because they may think they are at the mercy of the man's temper or may feel that he is "out of control." In addition, they may be embarrassed, afraid, angry, sad, and shocked.

The most significant part of the intervention is to ensure that the woman has knowledge of the resources available to her and a plan of action should she stay with the battering partner. First, services and telephone numbers of a hotline and the battered women's shelter or other safe haven should be provided by the nurse (see Resources at end of chapter). The woman can be offered a telephone to call the shelter if

ENGLISH SPANISH **Guidelines/Guías**

RECOGNIZING VIOLENCE IN A RELATIONSHIP

ARE YOU IN A RELATIONSHIP IN WHICH YOU ARE . . .
¿TIENE UNA RELACIÓN CON SU PAREJA EN LA QUE . . .

afraid of your partner's temper?
tiene miedo de que él pierda los estribos?

afraid to break up because your partner has threatened to hurt someone?
tiene miedo de dejarlo porque él ha amenazado con pegar o lastimar a alguien?

constantly apologizing for or defending your partner's behavior?
constantemente tiene que disculparse por o defender el comportamiento de su pareja?

afraid to disagree with your partner?
tiene miedo de discutir con su pareja?

isolated from your family or friends?
está aislada de su familia o sus amigos?

embarrassed in front of others because of your partner's words or actions?
las palabras o acciones de su pareja delante de otra gente le dan vergüenza?

intimidated by your partner and forced into having sex?
su pareja le intimida a usted y le obliga a tener relaciones sexuales con él?

depressed and jumpy?
está deprimida y/o nerviosa?

A PERSON WHO IS VIOLENT IN A RELATIONSHIP OFTEN . . .
UNA PERSONA QUE TIENE UN CARÁCTER VIOLENTO EN UNA RELACIÓN A MENUDO . . .

has an explosive temper.
pierde los estribos.

is possessive or jealous of his partner's time, friends, or family.
es posesivo o tiene celos de que su pareja pase tiempo con la familia o los amigos.

constantly criticizes his partner's thoughts, feelings or appearance.
critica constantemente los sentimientos, ideas o apariencia física de su pareja.

pinches, slaps, grabs, shoves, or throws things at his partner.
pellizca, pega, agarra, empuja, o lanza objetos que pueden lastimar a su pareja.

forces his partner into having sex.
obliga a su pareja a tener relaciones sexuales.

causes his partner to be afraid.
causa que su pareja tenga miedo.

this is an option she chooses. If she chooses to go back to the abuser, a safety plan includes necessities for a quick escape: a bag packed with personal items for an overnight stay (can be hidden or left with a neighbor), money or a checkbook, an extra set of car keys, and any legal documents for identification. Legal options, such as those for restraining orders or arrest of the perpetrator, also are important aspects of the safety plan. A restraining order can be obtained 24 hours a day from the county court or police department. Shelters also can be helpful with assistance in obtaining orders of protection. If the woman chooses not to act in the middle of a violent episode, she may use the hotline or shelter for some counseling when the threat of harm is no longer present.

LEGAL TIP Mandatory Reporting of Domestic Violence
Domestic violence is considered a crime in all states, but it varies between misdemeanor and felony offenses, the majority being misdemeanors. Forty states and the District of Columbia have laws that mandate reporting by health care providers in situations in which the woman has an injury that may be caused by a deadly weapon. Some states also require reports when there is a reason to believe that the woman's injury may have resulted from an illegal act or act of violence.

Because of the wide variation from state to state in mandatory reporting, nurses *must* be knowledgeable about the reporting requirements of the state in which they practice. Nurses can check the Family Violence Prevention Fund (2002) for a current listing and evaluation of reporting laws listed in the Resources section of this chapter, or they can call the local shelter for assistance. ■

Prevention

Nurses can make a difference in stopping the violence and preventing further injury. Educating women that abuse is a violation of their rights and facilitating their access to protective and legal services is a first step. Other helpful measures for women to discourage the risk of abusive relationships are promoting assertiveness and self-defense courses; suggesting support and self-help groups that encourage positive self-regard, confidence, and empowerment; and recommending educational and skills-development classes that will enhance independence or at least the ability to take care of oneself. Classes for English language learning may be particularly helpful to immigrant women. Nurses can offer information on local classes.

SEXUAL ABUSE

It is estimated that 3% to 27% of women and 2% to 16% of men have experienced childhood sexual abuse (Molnar, Buka, & Kessler, 2001) (see Chapter 28). If a stranger commits sexual abuse, it is considered sexual assault. Childhood sexual abuse continues over time and gradually escalates. This continuing victimization and accompanying feeling of helplessness, together with lack of confiding, lead to the long-term behavioral and relationship consequences seen in adult survivors of sexual assault (Molnar et al, 2001). Common psychopathologic consequences are dissociative identity disorder, borderline personality disorder, substance abuse, and generalized anxiety disorder. Women who experience symptoms of PTSD, sexual dysfunction, depression, anxiety, or substance abuse problems may be seen in obstetric and gynecologic practice. Female sexual abuse and assault victims appear to be the largest single group to experience PTSD.

Collaborative Care

Patients usually do not resent or object to being asked about their sexual abuse; they feel some relief because of the possibility of being relieved of the psychologic burden. The history obtained from an interview and review of medical records may reveal clues suggestive of sexual abuse. A history of dreams, flashbacks, or terror attacks may indicate PTSD (Silva et al, 1997). Patients may exhibit feelings of self-blame, shame, body rejection, anxiety, fear, mistrust, and hatred. They may dislike physical examinations more than do other women.

Overall planning for the adult survivor of childhood sexual abuse must acknowledge that the survivor is able to recognize that the abuse occurred, to share her story, and to begin a healing process. Heritage (1998) stated that disclosing must be done whenever and however the survivor chooses, that it be done with someone she trusts, and that the survivor believes she can disclose without experiencing further alienation. Either verbal or nonverbal shock and horror reactions from the nurse are particularly devastating. Professional demeanor and professional empathy are essential.

Nursing Care

The survivor needs support on many different levels, and a nurse may be the first person to whom she relates her story. Therapeutic communication skills and listening are initial interventions. Interventions may focus on empowering the victim to develop a sense of self-worth, mastery, competence, and control toward a resolution of the incest trauma.

Psychologic support is a necessary intervention when the survivor experiences flashbacks, learns to express feelings of anger without fear of losing control, and expresses needs without guilt. Consistently reinforcing that the adult was the responsible party is important.

Referral of incest survivors to appropriate support and recovery groups who assist each other in decreasing depression, anger, and guilt; reducing isolation; improving self-esteem; and developing effective coping mechanisms are effective interventions.

Nurses must be aware that women who have been sexually abused may be very anxious and uncomfortable about being examined and being touched. Sensitivity, gentleness, patience, and tact are essential.

SEXUAL ASSAULT

Sexual assault is a broad term that encompasses a wide range of sexual victimization, including rape, and includes unwanted or uncomfortable touches, kisses, hugs, petting, intercourse, or other sexual acts (Kaplan et al, 2001). It consists of sexual contact with or without penetration but with force or physical coercion. Rape is an act of violence and is a legal and not a medical term. In its strictest sense, rape is forced sexual intercourse or the penile penetration of the female sex organ or labia without consent; it may or may not include the use of a weapon. Molestation consists of noncoital sexual activity between a child and an adolescent or adult. Statutory rape involves penetration by a person who is 18 years or older of a person under the age of consent, which varies from state to state.

The key feature to establish rape is the absence of consent: threat or coercion implies the lack of consent. The victim who is mentally retarded, who is unconscious or otherwise physically unable to move, who has been drugged without her knowledge, or who is a minor (statutory rape) is not capable of giving consent. The court must prove absence of consent; thus the term *alleged rape* or *alleged sexual assault* is used in medical records.

More than 300,000 women are raped each year in the United States (NWHIC, 2002). Adolescents have the highest rates of rape and sexual assault. More than half of all rape victims are females younger than 25, and most perpetrators are acquaintances or a relative (Kaplan et al, 2001). Drugs often are involved in date rapes, and alcohol potentiates the effects. Date rape drugs (flunitrazepam and gamma-hydroxybutyrate) are often available at bars and clubs (Poirier, 2002). Signs indicating that a woman may have been drugged include no recall after taking a drink, feeling as if sex has occurred but not having any memory of the incident, feeling more intoxicated than a usual response to the amount of alcohol consumed, or feeling fuzzy on awakening (American College of Emergency Physicians [ACEP], 1999).

Elderly women also are victims. Gerophiles often seek employment in nursing homes and may be aggressive male residents or strangers who rape older women. Postassault examinations in this population may be traumatic, difficult, and uncomfortable, and more so if the victim is cognitively impaired or has dementia. This group may be neglected and not identified but are vulnerable (Burgess, Dowdell, & Brown, 2000).

Many factors deter a woman from reporting the crime, so accurate statistics concerning psychosocial and demographic variables relating to rape are not available. It is estimated that one in every six women will be raped during her lifetime. Women do not report rape because of the associated stigma; embarrassment; guilt that in some way they provoked the assault; fear of retribution from the rapist or his friends; dread of being humiliated and figuratively "raped" again by the criminal justice system publicity; and discouragement generated by the dismally small number of convictions. Fewer than one third of all rapes are reported (McConkey, Sole, & Holcomb, 2001). Victims often fear the reactions of husbands, lovers, friends, family, and children and prefer to suffer alone.

The types of rape are reported as date or acquaintance rape, marital rape, gang rape, stranger rape, and psychic rape. *Acquaintance rape* involves persons who know one another, such as a classmate, neighbor, family member, or date; it is sexual assault that occurs when the trust of a relationship is violated, and one person is forced by another into sexual activity (Stuart & Laraia, 2001). Victims of date and acquaintance rape are most often between the ages of 15 and 19 years.

Marital rape occurs partly because some men believe it is their right to engage in sex whenever they desire, regardless of the partner's desire or condition. It frequently occurs when there is physical abuse of the woman. Marital rape is particularly devastating to the woman because she is in a committed relationship and living with the partner (Stuart & Laraia, 2001). Most states now recognize marital rape as a legitimate, reportable crime.

Gang rape occurs when one woman is raped by two or more men. *Stranger rape* describes an unknown attacker actively seeking a woman who is vulnerable. This is the type of rape most feared by women.

Psychic rape occurs when one's personal dignity and self-respect are assaulted (Stuart & Laraia, 2001). *Sexual harassment*, although not classified as rape, is another form of using power and control tactics to victimize women sexually, particularly in workplaces.

Dynamics of Rape

Rape is not an act of lust or overzealous passion. Rape is a violent, aggressive assault on the victim's body and integrity. As one victim said, "No matter how terrible people think rape is, it's worse than they know. It's like a bomb going off at the center of your soul." Sexual assault is the use of power and control tactics and is often motivated by a desire to humiliate, defile, and dominate the victim (Stuart & Laraia, 2001).

The rapist has no regard for his victim's age, race, sexual attraction, or physical condition: 10-day-old infants as well as handicapped elderly women confined to wheelchairs have been sexually assaulted. Most rapes occur intraracially rather than interracially.

Collaborative Care

Nurses in women's health care and EDs are most likely to see rape victims in the acute phase. However, all women who manifest any of the signs of other phases should be assessed for posttraumatic experiences.

Facilities that treat rape victims vary in protocols and resources (see Community Focus Box—Resources for Rape Survivors). The Joint Commission on Accreditation of Healthcare Organizations (JCAHO) requires EDs and ambulatory care departments to have protocols on physical assault; rape or sexual assault; and domestic abuse of elders, spouses, partners, and children. These protocols must address patient consent, examination, and treatment guidelines and the health care facility's responsibility for collecting evidence, photographing injuries, and releasing evidence to law enforcement officials. In addition, the EDs and ambulatory care departments must provide to victims a referral list of community-based and private service agencies dealing with family violence. The nurse interacting with the sexual assault patient should be guided by the particular treatment center's protocol (Box 4-9).

Many treatment centers have initiated the use of sexual assault nurse examiners (SANEs). A SANE is educated in the specialty of forensic nursing and is prepared to examine patients; recognize, collect, and preserve evidence; counsel the patient; link the patient with vital community resources; follow up cases; and, if necessary, testify in court (Stermac & Stirpe, 2002). If SANEs are not available in a particular facility, JCAHO member organizations must implement a plan for educating an appropriate staff member about identifying, treating, and referring abuse victims. Additional resources may include a social worker who is called when a woman who has been raped is admitted. A local rape crisis center may have volunteers on call who may help by providing emotional support; providing transportation; helping the woman interact with her family, friends, and various authorities; informing her of rape-trauma syndrome (see Table 4-2); and finding other resources for her as needed. Male volunteers may counsel male members of the victim's family and her male friends.

History taking is an important first step in care, and the patient should be informed of all the steps involved in the rape examination and follow-up examination. Because rape is a crime, the first nurse to see the sexually assaulted patient must consider the need to preserve evidence (see Legal Tip). However, the preservation of evidence should not overshadow a victim's rights: to be treated as a human being with respect, courtesy, and dignity.

LEGAL TIP Collector of Evidence Consent forms must be signed before evidence can be collected and released to the police and before photographs can be taken. If the victim is under 16 years of age, a pediatrician is notified. A parent or guardian is required to sign the consent forms. A children's protective service may need to be called to facilitate consent. ■

History includes a statement of the traumatic event. Box 4-10 lists information to be collected. The woman needs privacy but should not be left alone. She also needs assurance of confidentiality and may need a great deal of support and assistance in verbalizing the offender's acts. For example, giving the woman permission to describe the situation however she chooses and restating what the patient has said (without minimizing) will show empathy. It is important to tell the woman that she is safe, that the incident is not her fault, and that she is not alone in what she has experienced. It also is important to obtain sexual, gynecologic, and obstetric histories. Because determination of rape is made in court, the wording of the history should reflect the woman's report, and her exact words should be used as often as possible (Poirier, 2002).

The nurse may assist with or, if trained, may perform the physical examination, which is conducted after the procedure is explained to the woman and consent is obtained

Community Focus

RESOURCES FOR RAPE SURVIVORS

Investigate resources in your community for victims of rape. Do local hospitals have rape counselors? Are there SANE nurses in your community? What educational efforts have the police made? Are there telephone hotlines for advice and referral? How would a victim of rape learn of these resources? Prepare a list of community resources appropriate for distribution in the community.

BOX 4-9

Adult Sexual Assault Protocol: Emergency Department

Purpose

To outline nursing care of sexual assault (rape or other sexual offense) patients, which includes participation in the collection of forensic evidence and in the referral of patients for follow-up treatment.

Whenever possible, the sexual assault patient will be cared for by a sexual assault nurse examiner (SANE) registered nurse (RN). These nurses have successfully completed a continuing education course in forensic and sexual assault evidence collection. This course provides those nurses with the information and skills to care properly for patients after sexual assault by recognizing, collecting, and preserving evidence; interviewing the patient; and linking the patient to vital community resources for follow-up.

Assessment

1. Assess the patient for any life-threatening injuries.
2. Assess the patient's level of coping, coherence, and ability to control behavior.
3. Assess the patient's priorities:
   - Is patient seeking care for prevention of pregnancy or disease only?
   - Is patient seeking forensic evidence collection?
   - Does the patient want both?

   NOTE: Notify a SANE nurse to perform the examination if the patient is seeking evidence collection for filing of police charges either at this time or in the future.
4. Assess the patient's entire body for bruises, lacerations, and/or other skeletal or soft-tissue injuries.
5. Initiate the collection of evidence using the sexual assault collection kit if patient consents:
   - If SANE nurse is available:
     - SANE: Complete collection.
     - SANE: Examine the vagina and rectum to include the speculum examination.

       (NOTE: A toluidine blue dye and colposcope may be used to collect evidence.)
   - Physician performs the bimanual examination.
   - If SANE nurse is not available:
     - Primary nurse initiates collection with the exception of vaginal, rectal, and bimanual examinations.
     - Physician performs vaginal, rectal, and bimanual examinations.
6. Ask patient whether or not those who are with the patient know that the patient has been sexually assaulted.

   NOTE: This information cannot be given to secondary victims without the patient's permission.

Safety

7. Notify hospital police when a sexual assault patient enters the emergency department.

   NOTE: Hospital police will complete a risk assessment of patient safety.

Care

8. Provide care for any physical injuries.
9. Provide for patient privacy and nonjudgmental support.
10. Protect patient confidentiality by identifying the patient as "7273" rather than by name or chief complaint.
11. Assign one nurse to the patient for the duration of his or her stay and disposition of evidence collection.
12. Notify the sexual assault advocate office.

    NOTE: The patient has the right to refuse an advocate. It is the policy of the emergency department to allow the advocate to offer services directly to the patient unless the patient expressly forbids it. Notify the advocate of any secondary victims who may have accompanied the patient if the secondary victim is aware that the patient has been sexually assaulted.
13. Reassure the patient that he or she is safe.
14. Reassure the patient that the incident is not his or her fault.
15. Prepare the patient for the possibility that some questions asked may be embarrassing.
16. Obtain informed consent for the physical examination, to include photographs of injuries.

    NOTE: If the patient permits the release of information to law enforcement agencies, explain to the victim that the evidence will be turned over to the appropriate jurisdiction for processing. If the patient is unwilling to have law enforcement notified at this time, the patient should mark "do not" on the release form. The patient may later change this if he or she chooses to file charges or have law enforcement involved.
17. Collect the evidence as directed and in accordance with patient consent.

    NOTE: All evidence should be marked with the patient's identification. Any photographs taken should be labeled with the patient's information and described in the nursing notes. These photographs should then be sealed in an envelope and secured per Department of Emergency Medicine policy. The evidence *must* remain in the possession of *one nurse* throughout the entire assessment procedure and treatment period, until it is released to a police agency.
18. Perform a urine test for pregnancy; the urine can also be tested for drugs if the patient suspects that he or she was drugged.
19. Provide the opportunity for bathing and clean clothing after the examination.
20. Discuss and provide emergency contraception and prophylaxis against STIs, including HIV if desired.
21. Arrange for follow-up care per patient preference for any medical or psychologic problems or injury.

Patient/Significant Other (SO) Teaching

22. Explain to the patient/SO:
    - All procedures and rationale
    - That feelings of anger, anxiety, and fear are normal
    - That options for medical, legal, and emotional counseling are available to both primary and secondary victims

    NOTE: Do not assume that a friend or SO is aware of the assault (see no. 6).
23. Inform patient/SO of resources available:
    - Judicial system options (e.g., official police report, "blind" report)
    - Financial assistance
    - *Other available resources:*
      - Local rape crisis center
      - Mental health agency
      - Sites and phone numbers for HIV counseling and testing
      - Resource list of phone numbers (e.g., law enforcement)

Documentation

24. Complete the forms for sexual assault evidence collection.
25. Attach forms to appropriate documents.
26. Seal the evidence kit as directed, and deliver it to a sworn law enforcement officer.
27. Seal all photographs in an envelope marked with patient identification, and secure per Department of Emergency Medicine policy.
28. Document care rendered, teaching done, and patient response and level of understanding on emergency department nursing record.

BOX 4-10

Sexual Assault History Taking and Assessment

- Assess the patient for life-threatening injuries.
- Assess the patient's level of coping, coherency, and ability to control behavior.
- Assess the patient's priorities:
  Is the patient seeking care for prevention of disease or pregnancy only?
  Is the patient seeking forensic evidence collection?
  Does the patient want both?
- Ask patient to describe the event:
  Time and place of the event
  Relationship to the assailant, if any
  Nature of suspected physical and sexual acts
  Time lapse between assault and current examination
- Did the woman bathe, douche, or shower? Did she urinate or defecate?
- Ask patient whether those who are with the patient know that the patient has been sexually assaulted.
- Ask the patient if she can think of any other information that would help in her care, and inform her that it is safe and confidential to say whatever she needs to.
- Inspect the entire body for bruises, lacerations, and other injuries.
- Initiate collection of evidence using the sexual assault collection kit (or notify the sexual assault nurse examiner).

(Box 4-11). Preservation of the woman's dignity is of utmost importance during the examination. A female attendant, rape counselor, or other person of her choice may remain with her during the examination. The physician or nurse practitioner informs her of every step of the procedure.

Necessary equipment for the examination is usually packaged in standard rape kits, which should be available in most EDs. Sexual assault kits that are intended to facilitate collection of specimens, particularly if they are to be used as evidence should the woman decide to report the rape, give specific instructions on what specimens to collect from what body parts or articles of clothing and ways to preserve the evidence.

During the examination, the woman's emotional status is assessed, and findings are recorded: what reactions she exhibits to the assault; her orientation to time and place; and her attention span, affect, and verbal description and feelings about the assault. The availability of family or peer-support systems is assessed. She is asked about her plans to report or not to report the crime to the police.

After the physical examination, the woman should be allowed to shower and offered fresh clothes or a gown. She may be offered time to rest and to talk with the nurse, rape crisis counselor, family, or friends.

Nursing diagnoses for the rape victim during the immediate posttrauma period include the following:

- *Anxiety/fear related to*
  —rape-trauma experience
  —interactions with police and caregivers
  —physical examination to assess injury and collect evidence
- *Acute pain related to*
  —physical injury from rape
  —examination

BOX 4-11

Physical Examination of Rape Victim

- Inspect clothing for stains, tears, and foreign material. Clothing is handled only by the woman and may be collected and sealed in a bag to be checked for evidence.
- Inspect body for bruises, swelling, scratches, lacerations, stab wounds, and body lice. A head-to-toe examination is performed. Many victims have injuries to other parts of their body, mostly involving head, face, and neck (Poirier, 2002). Special attention is given to the area assaulted, that is, pelvic structures and genitalia. External genitals, thighs, buttocks, and lower abdomen are assessed. If there are injuries, photographs may be taken or drawings made.
- Pubic and scalp hair is combed for collection of evidence.
- Perianal, oral, and vaginal swabs are collected.
- If the victim scratched her attacker, her nails are scraped to obtain material that may aid in identification.
- A speculum examination is performed gently to detect tears or bruises and to collect appropriate specimens. Most victims have some type of genital injury, even if it is asymptomatic. The cervix is cultured for *Neisseria gonorrhoeae*, *Chlamydia* organisms, and herpes simplex virus, and vaginal fluid is aspirated for analysis. One slide is fixed and dried to be stained and examined for sperm. Fluid is evaluated for seminal contents, including acid phosphatase (an enzyme found in high concentrations in seminal fluid), p30 protein (specific to the prostate and indicates ejaculation), and seminal vesicle specific antigen and ABO antigens (McGregor, Mont, & Myhr, 2002).
- Cultures for gonorrhea and chlamydia may be obtained from any other sites of penetration or contact such as vagina, anus, and pharynx. Standard wet-mount slides and cultures also may be obtained to test for trichomoniasis.
- Colposcopy may be used to visualize small abrasions. Some care providers use a handheld magnifying glass.
- A bimanual pelvic examination is performed carefully to determine the size and position of the uterus and adnexa. If a pelvic mass is palpated, it may be caused by bleeding into the broad ligament. Internal pelvic assessment ends with a rectovaginal examination if the woman has given consent and it is deemed necessary.
- Laboratory tests may include a urine or serum pregnancy test and serum tests for syphilis, hepatitis B virus, and human immunodeficiency virus (Centers for Disease Control and Prevention, 2002).

- *Disturbed body image related to*
  —the rape
- *Rape-trauma syndrome related to*
  —aftermath of being sexually assaulted
  —feelings of being unclean and humiliation
  —silent reaction of being unable to discuss the rape
- *Decisional conflict related to*
  —discussing rape with family
  —possible pregnancy

Nursing diagnoses for the rape victim during the later posttrauma period include the following:

- *Risk for infection with sexually transmitted infections related to*
  —sexual assault by an assailant of unknown sexual history
- *Impaired social interaction related to*
  —the rape

Immediate Care

Medical management includes (1) treating the physical injuries, including tetanus toxoid booster if indicated; (2) providing prophylactic antibiotic therapy for STIs (e.g., gonorrhea, syphilis); and (3) providing prophylaxis for pregnancy if the woman is not pregnant. If physical trauma is life threatening, appropriate intervention takes precedence over collecting evidence.

If the victim is at risk for pregnancy, emergency contraception should be discussed with her. Approximately 5% of women who are raped become pregnant. Emergency contraception with progestin only or combined estrogen and progestin pills must be used within 72 hours of the sexual assault (American College of Obstetricians and Gynecologists, 2001) (see Table 7-3). The woman is told that the therapy might cause nausea and that she should expect withdrawal bleeding shortly after finishing the therapy. Antinausea therapy, such as prochlorperazine preparation (Compazine) or dimenhydrinate (Dramamine), may be prescribed to counter the side effects of estrogens. She is advised, before she takes the drug, about the possible teratogenic effects of estrogen in emergency contraception doses, if a pregnancy occurs. She should be advised that emergency contraception does not guarantee pregnancy prevention, and that she should repeat the pregnancy test if she has not had a menstrual period within 3 to 4 weeks. The woman is apprised of the availability of abortion or menstrual extraction as a backup measure. If the woman is pregnant at the time of the assault, she should be observed for several hours for uterine contractility.

The woman may be provided with prophylactic antibiotic therapy to prevent STIs, hepatitis B immunization if needed, and HIV prophylaxis (Centers for Disease Control and Prevention, 2002).

Discharge

The woman is discharged with medications and printed instructions about their use, printed instructions for self-care, and names and telephone numbers of resource people if she requires assistance. Money as needed and transportation to wherever she is staying (an alternative place may be found for her) add to the woman's comfort and perception of being in control. A medical follow-up examination in the gynecology or pediatric clinic is scheduled in 1 to 2 weeks for repeated cultures for gonorrhea and other STIs; at 6 weeks for assessment of healing injuries; and at 6, 12, and 24 weeks for repeated serology tests for syphilis and HIV infection if initial test results were negative. The woman and her counselor determine whether there is a need for an additional medical or psychologic follow-up examination between the scheduled visits. The woman has a choice of site for follow-up testing. Some women choose to continue with the health care provider who first performed the examination; others prefer their primary health care provider; and still others need referral to a clinic in the area (city, state) in which they live.

Nurses must be aware that responses to rape are variable. Self-blame and humiliation may alternate with anger and fear. The patient needs to be reassured again before she leaves that her feelings are normal and that she is not alone. The initial care of a woman will affect her recovery and her decision to return for follow-up care. Nurses can assist patients through an examination that is as nontraumatic as possible, with kindness, skill, and empathy.

After Discharge

Because of the phases of recovery, telephone contact by the health care provider to whom the woman is referred is continued until the woman has no further need for such help. Education in prevention strategies is often offered by community agencies or rape-awareness groups (see Resources at end of chapter). The focus of the classes is usually on increasing women's awareness of situations that put them at high risk for rape or sexual assault. Other courses may teach self-defense methods or how to change personal behaviors to reduce the risk of being victimized, such as avoiding being alone in isolated places and being alert to unusual activities or persons in one's environment. Still other courses may focus on changing societal attitudes about rape. Nurses can play a role in preventive education by offering courses or participating in courses offered by community or health care groups. Nurses must be knowledgeable about the epidemiology of sexual assault, reporting requirements, and services available in their community for victims, and nurses should screen all women for a history of assault and any sequelae.

Key Points

- Culture, religion, socioeconomic status, personal circumstances, the uniqueness of the individual, and the stage of development influence a person's recognition of need for care and the response to the health care system and therapy.
- Preconception counseling allows identification and possible remediation of potentially harmful personal and social conditions, medical and psychologic conditions, environmental conditions, and barriers to care before pregnancy occurs.
- Conditions that increase a woman's health risks also increase risks for her offspring.
- Periodic health screening provides the basis for overall health promotion, prevention of illness, early diagnosis of problems, and referral for management.
- Health promotion and prevention of illness assists women to actualize health potential by increasing motivation, providing information, and suggesting how to access specific resources.
- Intimate partner violence against women is a major social and health care problem in the United States and includes physical, sexual, emotional, psychologic, and economic abuse.
- Battering affects all races; all socioeconomic, educational, and religious groups; and many pregnant women.

Answer Guidelines to Critical Thinking Exercise

Preconception Counseling

1. Yes. The nurse-midwife identified several risk factors. Based on these identified factors, the nurse-midwife,

Marcia, and Robert can make plans to decrease risks in pregnancy (such as participating in a weight loss program before pregnancy), performing assessment tests (e.g., assessing Marcia's blood sugar level), and counseling about nutrition (e.g., adequate calcium intake; at least 400 mcg supplemental folic acid daily).
2. (a) Age over 35 is a theoretic risk factor. If Marcia is in good health, maintains proper nutrition, exercises, and loses weight, her risks for problems in pregnancy are low. (b) Having successfully practiced natural family planning, Marcia and Robert are cognizant of how to determine fertile periods. (c) They have resources to support an infant. (d) Marcia and Robert are interested in creating an optimum environment for an embryo and fetus.
3. Priorities for care include assessing Marcia's blood sugar levels; obtaining a more complete family history for Robert; gathering further information about Robert's sibling with Down syndrome; counseling about nutrition, weight loss, and exercise; determining need for counseling regarding sexuality, including fertile times; and answering questions about pregnancy testing.
4. Yes. Marcia and Robert appropriately sought preconception counseling and care. The nurse-midwife provided assessment, counseling, and testing that meets the standard of care.
5. Referral to a geneticist may be appropriate. Ascertaining family and community supports would provide further data to help meet the needs of Marcia and Robert. Introducing the topic of breastfeeding and sources for educational materials would benefit the couple and their hoped-for child.

Resources

Al-Anon World Service Office
1600 Corporate Landing Parkway
Virginia Beach, VA 23454-5617
757-563-1600
757-563-1655 (fax)
wso@al-anon.org
www.al-anon-alateen.org

Alcoholics Anonymous World Services, Inc.
Grand Central Station
PO Box 459
New York, NY 10163
212-870-3400 (for local numbers, look for Alcoholics Anonymous in your telephone directory)
www.alcoholics-anonymous.org

American Cancer Society
1599 Clifton Rd., NE
Atlanta, GA 30329
800-ACS-2345
www.cancer.org

American Lung Association
61 Broadway, 6th Floor
New York, NY 10006
212-315-8700
www.lungusa.org

Association of Women's Health, Obstetric, and Neonatal Nurses
2000 L St. NW
Washington, DC 20024
800-673-8499
www.awhonn.org

Center for Women Policy Studies
2000 P St. NW, Suite 508
Washington, DC 20036
202-872-1770

COCAINE Hotline
1-800-COCAINE

Family Violence Prevention Fund
383 Rhode Island St., Suite 304
San Francisco, CA 94103-5133
415-252-8900
www.fvpf.org
www.endabuse.org

March of Dimes Birth Defects Foundation
1275 Mamaroneck Avenue
White Plains, NY 10605
914-428-7100
888-663-4637 (888-MODIMES)
800-537-2238 (information line)
www.modimes.org

Narcotics Anonymous (for drug abusers)
1-888-336-4066

National Alcohol and Drug Abuse Hotline
1-800-252-6465

National Center on Women and Family Law
799 Broadway, Room 402
New York, NY 10003
212-674-8200

National Child Abuse Hotline
800-422-4453

National Coalition Against Domestic Violence
PO Box 34103
Washington, DC 20043-4301
202-638-8638
www.ncadv.org

National Coalition Against Sexual Assault
912 North 2nd St.
Harrisburg, PA 17102
717-232-6771

National Domestic Violence/Abuse Hotline
800-799-SAFE (7233)
(Many states have local coalitions against domestic violence.)

National Electronic Network on Violence Against Women (VAWnet)
6400 Flank Drive, Suite 1300
Harrisburg, PA 17112-2778
800-537-2238
800-553-2508 (TTY)
717-545-9456 (fax)
www.vawnet.org

National Organization for Women (NOW) Legal Defense and Education Fund
99 Hudson St.
New York, NY 10013-2871
212-925-6635

National Resource Center for Domestic Violence
800-537-2238

National Women's Health Information Center
Office on Women's Health
Department of Health and Human Resources
800-994-9662
www.4woman.gov

No Safe Place
www.pbs.org/kued/nosafeplace

Rape, Abuse and Incest National Network (RAINN)
www.rainn.org
800-656-HOPE (4673)

Violence Against Women Office at the Department of Justice
810 Seventh St. NW
Washington, DC 20531
www.ojp.usdoj.gov/vawo

References

A few dangerous myths. Internet document available at www.batteredwomen.com (accessed November 30, 2004).

Affara FA: Correspondence from abroad. When tradition maims, *Am J Nurs* 100(8):52-60, 2000.

Alan Guttmacher Institute: Sexuality education, *Facts in Brief,* 2002. Internet document available at www.agi-usa.org/pubs/fb_sex_ed02 (accessed November 30, 2004).

American Cancer Society (ACS): *Cancer facts and figures 2004,* New York, 2004, ACS.

American College of Emergency Physicians (ACEP): *Evaluation and management of the sexually assaulted or sexually abused patient,* Dallas, 1999, ACEP.

American College of Obstetricians and Gynecologists (ACOG): *Smoking and women's health,* ACOG Tech Bull no 240, Washington, DC, 1997, ACOG.

American College of Obstetricians and Gynecologists (ACOG): *Emergency contraception,* ACOG Pract Bull no 25, Washington, DC, 2001, ACOG.

American College of Obstetricians and Gynecologists: *Screening tools for domestic violence.* ACOG violence against women home page, 2002. Internet document available at www.acog.org (accessed August 16, 2002).

American Psychiatric Association: *Diagnostic and statistical manual of mental disorders,* ed 4 rev, Washington, DC, 2000, American Psychiatric Association.

Arias E et al: Annual summary of vital statistics—2002, *Pediatrics* 112(6):1215-1230, 2003.

Burgess AW, Dowdell EB, Brown K: The elderly rape victim: stereotypes, perpetrators and implications for practice, *J Emerg Nurs* 26(5):516-518, 2000.

Centers for Disease Control and Prevention: Sexually transmitted diseases treatment guidelines 2002, *MMWR* 51(RR-6):1-80, 2002.

Expert Panel on Detection, Evaluation, and Treatment of High Blood Cholesterol in Adults: Executive summary of the third report of the National Education Program (NCEP) expert panel on detection, evaluation, and treatment of high blood cholesterol in adults (adult treatment panel III), *JAMA* 285(19):2486-2497, 2001.

Family Violence Prevention Fund (FVPF): *Preventing domestic violence: clinical guidelines on routine screening,* San Francisco, 2002, FVPF. Internet document available at http://action.endabuse.org/fvpf/home/ (accessed June 1, 2002).

Gelles R: *Intimate violence in families,* ed 3, Thousand Oaks, CA, Sage, 1997.

Heritage C: Working with childhood sexual abuse survivors during pregnancy, labor, and birth, *J Obstet Gynecol Neonatal Nurs* 27(6):671-676, 1998.

Humphreys J, Parker B, Campbell JC: Intimate partner violence against women, *Ann Rev Nurs Res* 19:275-306, 2001.

Kaplan D et al: Care of the adolescent sexual assault victim, *Pediatrics* 107(6):1476-1479, 2001.

Lindgren K: Relationships among maternal fetal attachment, prenatal depression, and health practices in pregnancy, *Res Nurs Health* 24(3):203-217, 2001.

Martin SL et al: Physical abuse of women before, during, and after pregnancy, *JAMA* 285(12):1581-1584, 2001.

Mattson S: Providing culturally competent care: strategies and approaches for perinatal clients, *AWHONN Lifelines* 4(5):37-39, 2000.

McConkey T, Sole M, Holcomb L: Assessing the female sexual assault survivor, *Nurse Pract* 26(7):8-39, 2001.

McFarlane J et al: Abuse during pregnancy and femicide: urgent implications for women's health, *Obstet Gynecol* 100(1):27-36, 2002.

McGregor M, Mont J, & Myhr T: Sexual assault forensic medical examination: is evidence related to successful prosecution? *Ann Emerg Med* 39(6):639-647, 2002.

Minino A, Smith B: Deaths: preliminary data for 2000, *Nat Vital Stat Rep* (vol 49, no 12), Hyattsville, MD, 2001, National Center for Health Statistics.

Molnar BE, Buka SL, Kessler RC: Child sexual abuse and subsequent psychopathology: results from the national comorbidity survey, *Am J Public Health* 91(5):753-760, 2001.

National Center for Chronic Disease Prevention and Health Promotion: *U.S. obesity trends 1985 to 2000,* Atlanta, 2000, Centers for Disease Control and Prevention.

National Institute on Alcohol and Alcoholism: Alcohol violence and aggression, *Alcohol Alert* 38:1-6, 1997.

National Women's Health Information Center: *Violence against women, 2002.* Internet document available at www.4woman.gov/violence/index.cfm (accessed August 14, 2002).

National Women's Health Resource Center: Screening tests and women's health, *National Women's Health Report* 23(6):1-7, 2001.

National Women's Law Center: *Making the grade on women's health: a national and state-by-state report card,* Washington, DC, 2000, National Women's Law Center.

Poirier MP: Care of the female adolescent rape victim, *Pediatr Emerg Care* 18(1):53-59, 2002.

Sampselle CM: Behavioral interventions for urinary incontinence in women: evidence for practice, *J Midwifery Womens' Health* 45(2):94-103, 2000.

Sampselle CM et al: Continence for women: evidence-based practice, *J Obstet Gynecol Neonatal Nurs* 26(4):375-385, 1997.

Shepherd J et al: Interventions for encouraging sexual lifestyles and behaviours intended to prevent cervical cancer (Cochrane Review), 2001. In *The Cochrane Library,* Issue 2, Chichester, UK, 2004, John Wiley & Sons.

Silva C et al: Symptoms of posttraumatic stress disorder in abused women in a primary care setting, *J Women's Health* 6(5):543-552, 1997.

State University of New York Counseling Center: *Stress management,* Buffalo, NY, 2002, University of Buffalo, State University of New York.

Stermac LE, Stirpe TS: Efficacy of a 2-year-old sexual assault nurse examiner program in a Canadian hospital, *J Emerg Nurs* 28(1):18-23, 2002.

Stevens PE, Hall JM: Sexuality and safer sex: the issue of lesbians and bisexual women, *J Obstet Gynecol Neonatal Nurs* 39(4):439-447, 2001.

Stuart GW, Laraia MT: *Principles and practice of psychiatric nursing,* ed 7, St Louis, 2001, Mosby.

Tjaden P, Thoennes N: *Extent, nature and consequences of intimate partner violence: findings from the national violence against women survey,* Washington, DC, 2000, US Department of Justice.

US Department of Health and Human Services: *Healthy people 2010: national health promotion and disease prevention objectives,* Washington, DC, 2000, US Department of Health and Human Services.

US Preventive Services Task Force: *Guide to clinical preventive services,* ed 2, Baltimore, 1996, Williams & Wilkins.

US Preventive Services Task Force: *Screening for cervical cancers,* AHRQ pub 03-535, Rockville, MD, 2003, Agency for Healthcare Research and Quality.

Walton-Moss BJ, Campbell J: Intimate partner violence: implications for nursing, *Online J Issues Nurs* 7(1):6, 2002.

Weiss J, Scott L: Stalking the no. 1 killer of women: detecting diabetes and heart diseases, *AWHONN Lifelines* 5(5):26-34, 2001.

Unit 2

5 Health Assessment

LEARNING OBJECTIVES

On completion of this chapter the reader will be able to:

- Identify the structures and functions of the female reproductive system.
- Differentiate the menstrual cycle in relation to hormonal, ovarian, and endometrial responses.
- Identify the four phases of the sexual response cycle.
- Investigate how the history and physical examination can be adapted for women with special needs.
- Identify indications of abuse, appropriate screening, and referral to community agencies.
- Describe components of taking a woman's history and performing a physical examination.
- Identify the correct procedure for assisting with and collecting Papanicolaou smear specimens.
- Review patient teaching of breast self-examination.

ELECTRONIC RESOURCES

Additional information related to the content in Chapter 5 can be found on

the companion website at evolve
http://evolve.elsevier.com/Wong/maternal/
- NCLEX Review Questions
- Case Study—Health Assessment
- WebLinks

or the interactive student CD-ROM
Activities for Chapter 5 include the following:
- NCLEX Review Questions
- Case Study—Health Assessment
- Critical Thinking Exercise—Women's Health and Safety
- Skill—Breast Self-Examination

The purpose of this chapter is to review female anatomy and physiology, the menstrual cycle, and gynecologic health assessment.

FEMALE REPRODUCTIVE SYSTEM

The female reproductive system consists of external structures visible from the pubis to the perineum and internal structures located in the pelvic cavity. The external and internal female reproductive structures develop and mature in response to estrogen and progesterone. This process starts in fetal life and continues through puberty and the childbearing years. Reproductive structures atrophy with age or in response to a decrease in ovarian hormone production. A complex nerve and blood supply supports the functions of these structures. The appearance of the external genitalia varies greatly among women. Heredity, age, race, and the number of children a woman has borne influence the size, shape, and color of her external organs.

External Structures

The external genital organs, or vulva, include all structures visible externally from the pubis to the perineum. These include the mons pubis, labia majora, labia minora, clitoris, vestibular glands, vaginal vestibule, vaginal orifice, and urethral opening. The external genital organs are illustrated in Fig. 5-1.

The mons pubis is a fatty pad that lies over the anterior surface of the symphysis pubis. In the postpubertal female, the mons is covered with coarse, curly hair. The labia majora are two rounded folds of fatty tissue covered with skin that extend downward and backward from the mons pubis. The labia are highly vascular structures that develop hair on the outer surfaces after puberty. They protect the inner vulvar structures. The labia minora are two flat, reddish folds of tissue visible when the labia majora are separated. There are no hair follicles on the labia minora, but many sebaceous follicles and a few sweat glands are present. The interior of the labia minora is composed of connective tissue and smooth muscle, and is supplied with extremely sensitive nerve endings. Anteriorly, the labia minora fuse to form the prepuce (the hoodlike covering of the clitoris) and the frenulum (the fold of tissue under the clitoris). The labia minora join to form a thin, flat tissue called the fourchette underneath the vaginal opening at midline. The clitoris is located underneath the prepuce. It is a small structure composed of erectile tissue with numerous sensory nerve endings. During sexual arousal the clitoris increases in size.

The vaginal vestibule is an almond-shaped area enclosed by the labia minora that contains openings to the urethra, Skene's glands, vagina, and Bartholin's glands. The urethra is

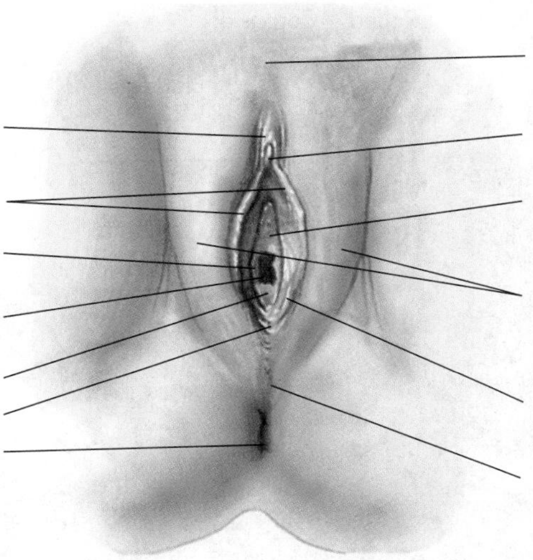

Fig. 5-1 External female genitalia.

not a reproductive organ but is discussed here because of its location. It usually is found about 2.5 cm below the clitoris. Skene's glands are located on each side of the urethra and produce mucus, which aids in lubrication of the vagina. The vaginal opening is in the lower portion of the vestibule and varies in shape and size. The hymen, a connective tissue membrane that surrounds the vaginal opening, can be perforated during strenuous exercise, insertion of tampons, masturbation, and vaginal intercourse. Bartholin's glands lie under the constrictor muscles of the vagina and are located posteriorly on the sides of the vaginal opening, although the ductal openings are usually not visible. During sexual arousal the glands secrete clear mucus to lubricate the vaginal introitus.

The area between the fourchette and the anus is the perineum, a skin-covered muscular area that covers the pelvic structures. The perineum forms the base of the perineal body, a wedge-shaped mass that serves as an anchor for the muscles, fascia, and ligaments of the pelvis. The muscles and ligaments form a sling that supports the pelvic organs.

Internal Structures

The internal structures include the vagina, uterus, uterine tubes, and ovaries.

The vagina is a fibromuscular, collapsible, tubular structure that lies between the bladder and rectum and extends from the vulva to the uterus. During the reproductive years the mucosal lining is arranged in transverse folds called rugae. These rugae allow the vagina to expand during childbirth. Estrogen deprivation that occurs after childbirth, during lactation, and at menopause causes dryness and thinning of the vaginal walls and smoothing of the rugae. The vagina, particularly the lower segment, has few sensory nerve endings. Vaginal secretions are slightly acidic (pH 4 to 5) so that vaginal susceptibility to infections is limited. The vagina serves as a passageway for menstrual flow, as a female organ of copulation, and as a part of the birth canal for vaginal childbirth. The uterine cervix projects into a blind vault at the upper end of the vagina. There are anterior, posterior, and lateral pockets called fornices (singular: fornix) that surround the cervix. The internal pelvic organs can be palpated through the thin walls of these fornices.

The uterus is a muscular organ shaped like an upside-down pear that sits midline in the pelvic cavity between the bladder and rectum and above the vagina. Four pairs of ligaments support the uterus: the cardinal, uterosacral, round, and broad. Single anterior and posterior ligaments also support the uterus. The cul-de-sac of Douglas is a deep pouch, or recess, posterior to the cervix formed by the posterior ligament.

The uterus is divided into two major parts, an upper triangular portion called the corpus and a lower cylindrical portion called the cervix (Fig. 5-2). The fundus is the dome-shaped top of the uterus and is the site at which the uterine tubes enter the uterus. The isthmus, or lower uterine segment, is a short, constricted portion that separates the corpus from the cervix.

The uterus serves for reception, implantation, retention, and nutrition of the fertilized ovum and later of the fetus during pregnancy and for expulsion of the fetus during childbirth. It also is responsible for cyclic menstruation.

The uterine wall comprises three layers: the endometrium, the myometrium, and part of the peritoneum. The endometrium is a highly vascular lining made up of three layers, the outer two of which are shed during menstruation. The myometrium is made up of layers of smooth muscles that extend in three different directions (longitudinal, transverse, and oblique) (Fig. 5-3). Longitudinal fibers of the outer myometrial layer are found mostly in the fundus, and this arrangement assists in expelling the fetus during the birth process. The middle layer contains fibers from all three directions, which form a figure-eight pattern encircling large blood vessels. These fibers assist in ligating blood vessels after childbirth and control blood loss. Most of the circular fibers of the inner myometrial layer are around the site where the uterine tubes enter the uterus and around the internal cervical os (opening). These fibers help keep the cervix closed during pregnancy and prevent menstrual blood from flowing back into the uterine tubes during menstruation.

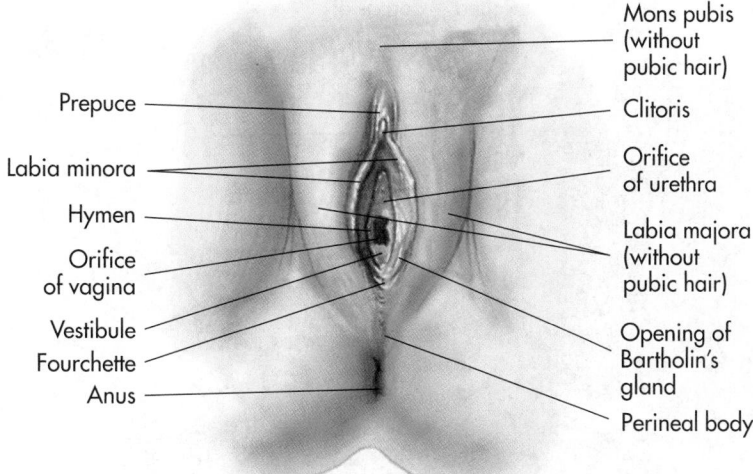

The cervix is made up of mostly fibrous connective tissues and elastic tissue, making it possible for the cervix to

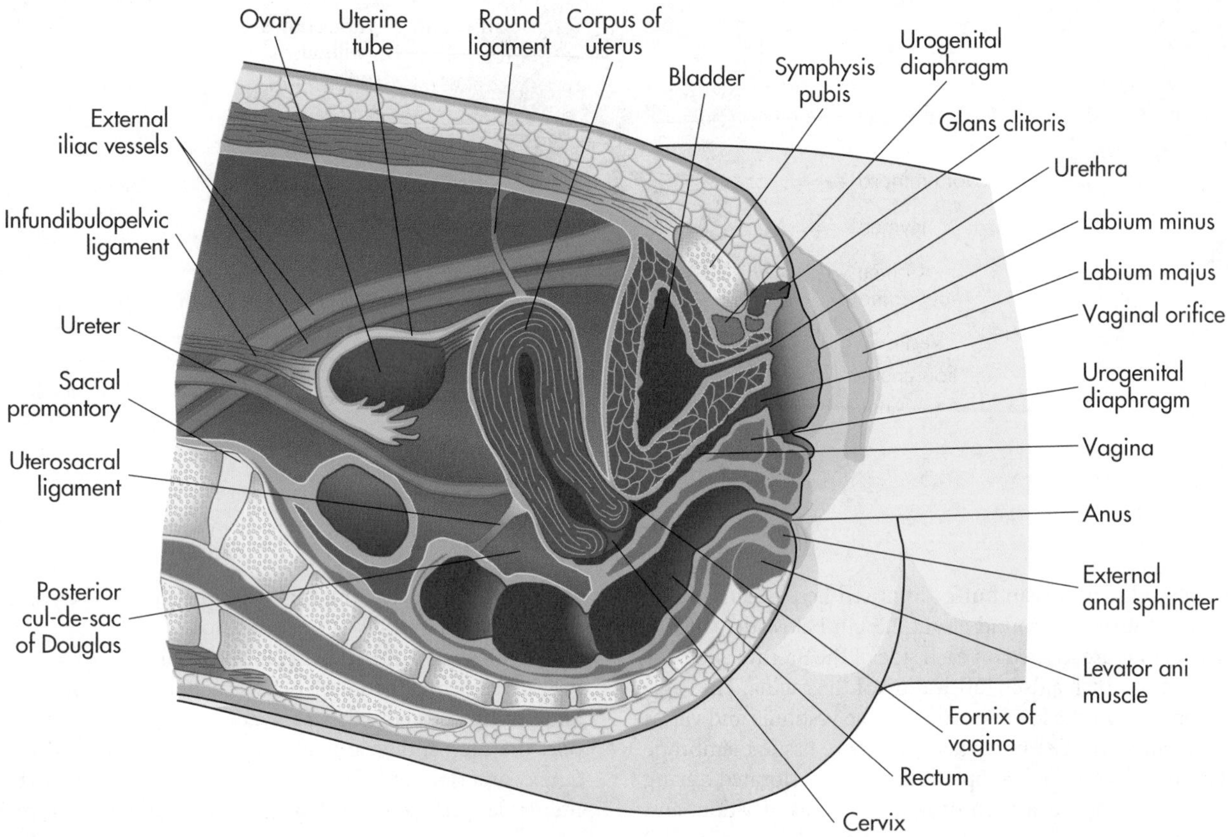

Fig. 5-2 Midsagittal view of female pelvic organs with woman lying supine.

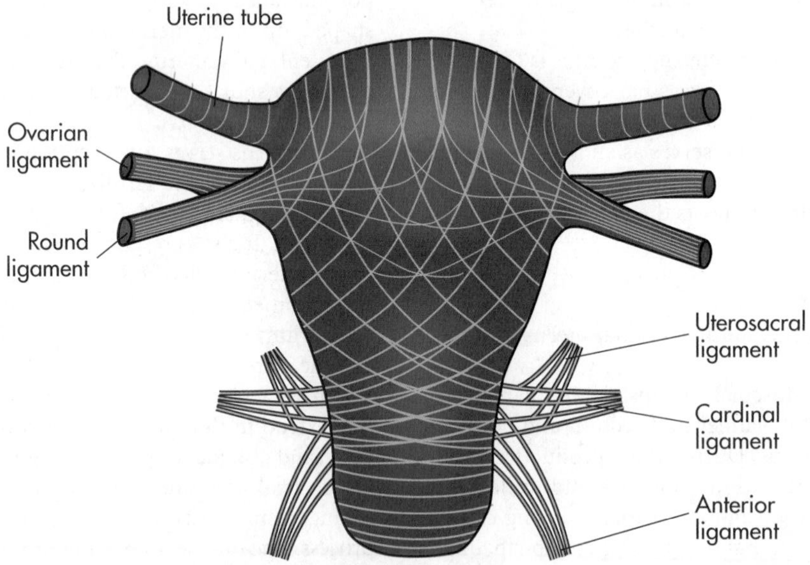

Fig. 5-3 Schematic arrangement of directions of muscle fibers. Note that uterine muscle fibers are continuous with supportive ligaments of uterus.

stretch during vaginal childbirth. The opening between the uterine cavity and the canal that connects the uterine cavity to the vagina (endocervical canal) is the internal os. The narrowed opening between the endocervix and the vagina is the external os, a small circular opening in women who have never been pregnant. The cervix feels firm (like the end of a nose) with a dimple in the center that marks the external os.

The outer cervix is covered with a layer of squamous epithelium. The mucosa of the cervical canal is covered with columnar epithelium and contains numerous glands that secrete mucus in response to ovarian hormones. The squamocolumnar junction, where the two types of cells meet, is usually located just inside the cervical os. This junction also is called the transformation zone and is the most common site for neoplastic changes. Cells from this site are scraped for the Papanicolaou (Pap) test.

The uterine tubes (fallopian tubes) attach to the uterine fundus. The tubes are supported by the broad ligaments and range from 8 to 14 cm in length. The tubes are divided into four sections: the interstitial portion is closest to the uterus; the isthmus and the ampulla are the middle portions; and the infundibulum is closest to the ovary (Fig. 5-4). The uterine tubes provide a passage between the ovaries and the uterus for the movement of the ovum. The infundibulum has fimbriated (fringed) ends, which pull the ovum into the tube. The ovum is pushed along the tubes to the uterus by rhythmic contractions of muscles of the tubes and by the current produced by the movement of the cilia that line the tubes. The ovum is usually fertilized by the sperm in the ampulla portion of one of the tubes.

The ovaries are almond-shaped organs located on each side of the uterus below and behind the uterine tubes. During the reproductive years, they are approximately 3 cm long, 2 cm wide, and 1 cm thick; they diminish in size after menopause. Before menarche, each ovary has a smooth surface; after menarche they become nodular because of repeated ruptures of follicles at ovulation. The two functions of the ovaries are ovulation and hormone production. Ovulation is the release of a mature ovum from the ovary at intervals (usually monthly). Estrogen, progesterone, and androgen are the hormones produced by the ovaries.

The Bony Pelvis

The bony pelvis serves three primary purposes: protection of the pelvic structures, accommodation of the growing fetus during pregnancy, and anchorage of the pelvic support structures. The pelvis comprises four bones: the two innominate (hip) bones (consisting of ilium, ischium, and pubis); the sacrum; and the coccyx (Fig. 5-5). Cartilage and ligaments form the symphysis pubis, sacrococcygeal joint, and two sacroiliac joints that separate the pelvic bones.

The pelvis is divided into two parts: the false pelvis and the true pelvis (Fig. 5-6). The false pelvis is the upper portion above the pelvic brim or inlet. The true pelvis is the lower curved bony canal, which includes the inlet, the cavity, and the outlet through which the fetus passes during vaginal birth. The upper portion of the outlet is at the level of the ischial spines, and the lower portion is at the level of the ischial tuberosities and the pubic arch (see Fig. 5-5). Variations that occur in the size and shape of the pelvis are usually due to age, race, and sex. Pelvic ossification is complete at about 20 years of age.

Breasts

The breasts are paired mammary glands located between the second and sixth ribs (Fig. 5-7). About two thirds of the breast overlies the pectoralis major muscle, between the sternum and midaxillary line, with an extension to the axilla referred to as the tail of Spence. The lower one third of the breast overlies the serratus anterior muscle. The breasts are attached to the muscles by connective tissue or fascia.

The breasts of the healthy, mature woman are approximately equal in size and shape, but often are not absolutely symmetric. The size and shape vary with the woman's age, heredity, and nutrition. However, the contour should be smooth with no retractions, dimpling, or masses. Estrogen stimulates growth of the breast by inducing fat deposition in the breasts, increase in the amount and elasticity of stromal tissue, and growth of the extensive ductile system. Estrogen also increases the vascularity of breast tissue.

Once ovulation begins in puberty, progesterone levels increase. The increase in progesterone causes maturation of mammary gland tissue, specifically the lobules and acinar

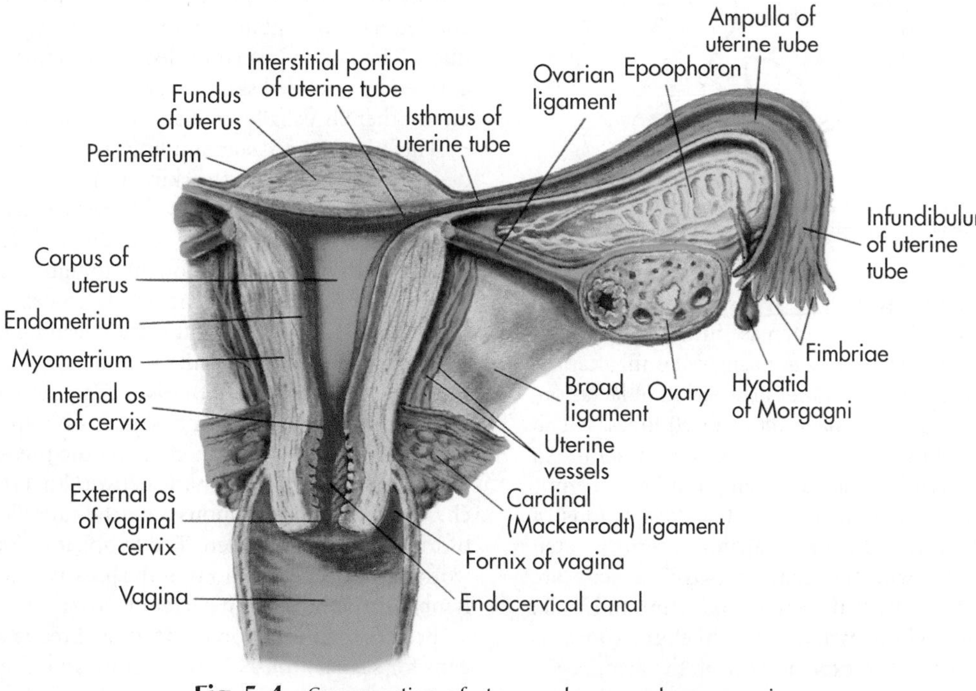

Fig. 5-4 Cross section of uterus, adnexa, and upper vagina.

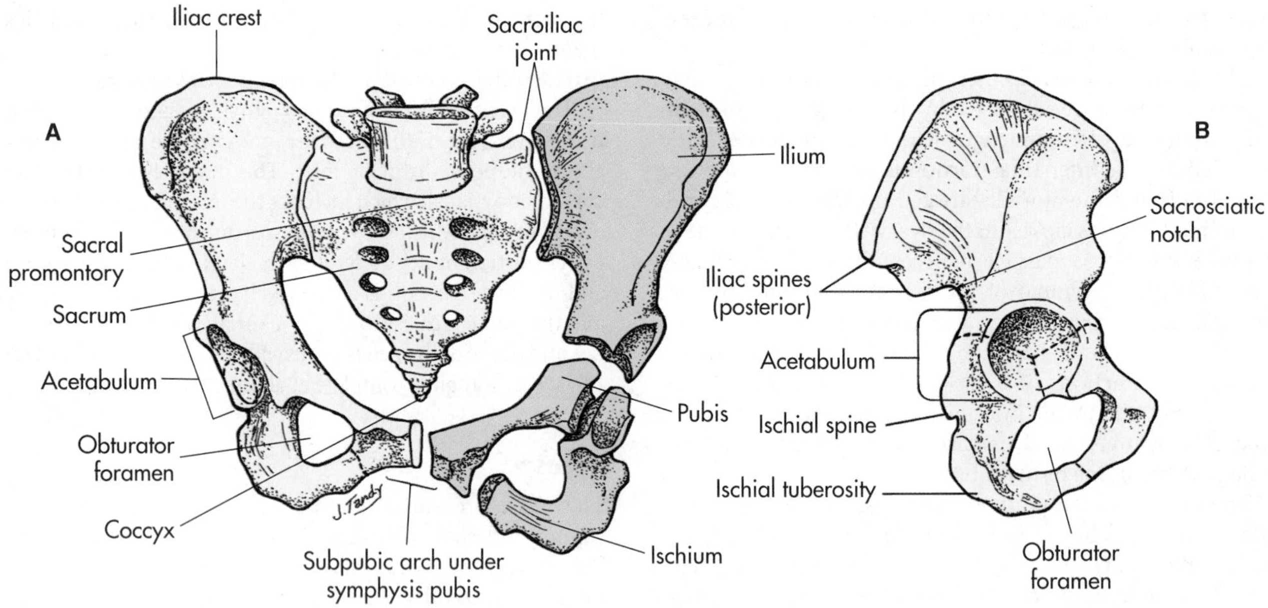

Fig. 5-5 Adult female pelvis. **A,** Anterior view. **B,** External view of innominate bone (fused).

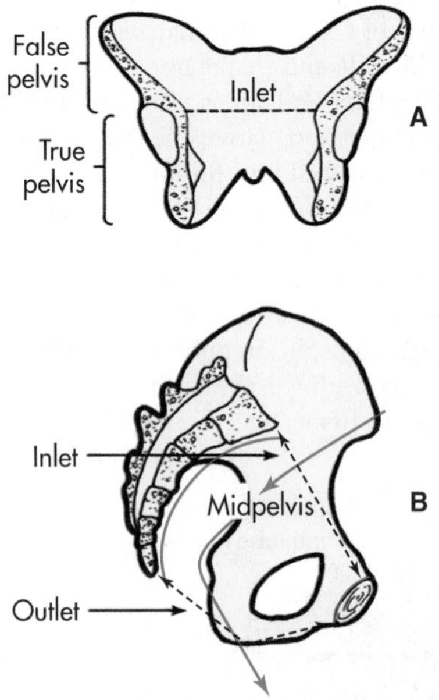

Fig. 5-6 Female pelvis. **A,** Cavity of false pelvis is shallow. **B,** Cavity of true pelvis is an irregularly curved canal *(arrows).*

structures. During adolescence, fat deposition and growth of fibrous tissue contribute to the increase in the glands' size. Full development of the breasts is not achieved until after the end of the first pregnancy or in the early period of lactation.

Each mammary gland is made of 15 to 20 lobes, which are divided into lobules. Lobules are clusters of acini. An acinus is a saclike terminal part of a compound gland emptying through a narrow lumen or duct. In discussions of mammary glands, *acinus,* the correct anatomic term, is often used interchangeably with the term *alveolus.* The acini are lined with epithelial cells that secrete colostrum and milk. Just below the epithelium is the myoepithelium (*myo,* or muscle), which contracts to expel milk from the acini.

The ducts from the clusters of acini that form the lobules merge to form larger ducts draining the lobes. Ducts from the lobes converge in a single nipple (mammary papilla) surrounded by an areola. Just as the ducts converge, they dilate to form common lactiferous sinuses, which are also called ampullae. The lactiferous sinuses serve as milk reservoirs. Many tiny lactiferous ducts drain the ampullae and exit in the nipple.

The glandular structures and ducts are surrounded by protective fatty tissue and are separated and supported by fibrous suspensory Cooper's ligaments. Cooper's ligaments provide support to the mammary glands while permitting their mobility on the chest wall (see Fig. 5-7). The nipple is usually round, slightly elevated, and projects slightly upward and laterally. It contains 15 to 20 openings from lactiferous ducts. The nipple is surrounded by fibromuscular tissue and covered by wrinkled skin. Except during pregnancy and lactation, there is usually no discharge from the nipple.

The nipple and surrounding areola are usually more deeply pigmented than the skin of the breast. The rough appearance of the areola is caused by sebaceous glands, Montgomery tubercles, directly beneath the skin. These glands secrete a fatty substance thought to lubricate the nipple. Smooth muscle fibers in the areola contract to stiffen the nipple to make it easier for the breastfeeding infant to grasp.

The vascular supply to the mammary gland is abundant. In the nonpregnant state the skin does not have an obvious vascular pattern. The normal skin is smooth without tightness or shininess. The skin covering the breasts contains an extensive superficial lymphatic network that serves the entire chest wall and is continuous with the superficial lymphatics of the neck and abdomen. The lymphatics form a rich network in the deeper portions of the breasts. The primary deep lymphatic pathway drains laterally toward the axillae.

Besides their function of lactation, breasts function as organs for sexual arousal in the mature adult.

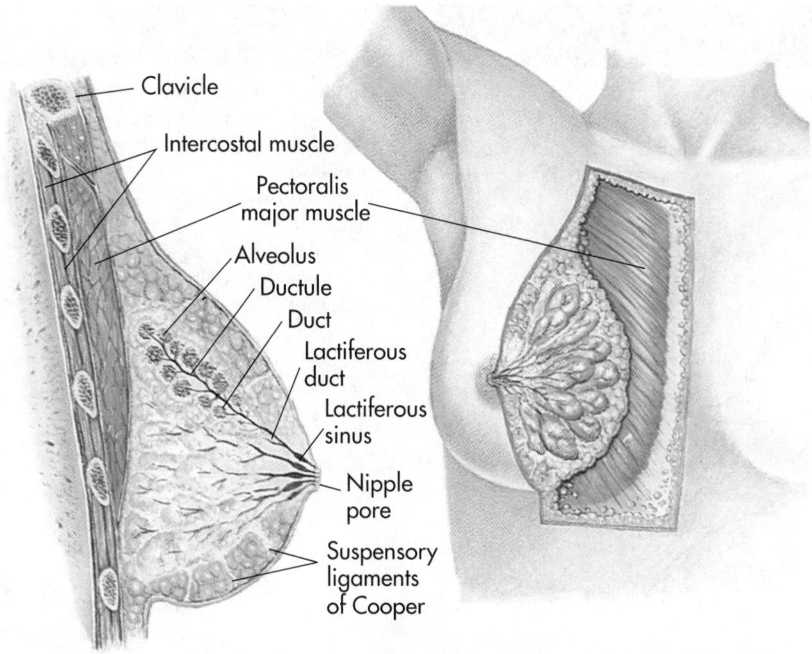

Fig. 5-7 Anatomy of the breast, showing position and major structures. (From Seidel HM et al: *Mosby's guide to physical examination,* ed 5, St Louis, 2003, Mosby.)

The breasts change in size and nodularity in response to cyclic ovarian changes throughout reproductive life. Increasing levels of both estrogen and progesterone in the 3 to 4 days before menstruation increase vascularity of the breasts, induce growth of the ducts and acini, and promote water retention. The epithelial cells lining the ducts proliferate in number, the ducts dilate, and the lobules distend. The acini become enlarged and secretory, and lipid (fat) is deposited within their epithelial cell lining. As a result, breast swelling, tenderness, and discomfort are common symptoms just before the onset of menstruation. After menstruation, cellular proliferation begins to regress, acini begin to decrease in size, and retained water is lost. After breasts have undergone changes numerous times in response to the ovarian cycle, the proliferation and involution (regression) are not uniform throughout the breast. In time, after repeated hormonal stimulation, small persistent areas of nodulations may develop. This normal physiologic change must be remembered when breast tissue is examined. Nodules may develop just before and during menstruation, when the breast is most active. The physiologic alterations in breast size and activity reach their minimum level about 5 to 7 days after menstruation stops. Therefore breast self-examination (BSE), which is the systematic palpation of breasts to detect signs of breast cancer or other changes, is best carried out during this phase of the menstrual cycle (Guidelines box).

MENSTRUATION

Menarche and Puberty

Although young girls secrete small, rather constant amounts of estrogen, a marked increase occurs between 8 and 11 years of age. The term *menarche* denotes first menstruation. *Puberty* is a broader term that denotes the entire transitional stage between childhood and sexual maturity. Increasing amounts and variations in gonadotropin and estrogen secretion develop into a cyclic pattern at least a year before menarche. In North America this occurs in most girls at about 13 years of age.

Initially menstrual periods are irregular, unpredictable, painless, and anovulatory (no ovum is released from the ovary). After 1 or more years, a hypothalamic-pituitary rhythm develops, and the ovary produces adequate cyclic estrogen to make a mature ovum. Ovulatory (ovum released from the ovary) periods tend to be regular, monitored by progesterone.

Although pregnancy can occur in exceptional cases of true precocious puberty, most pregnancies in young girls occur after the normally timed menarche. All young adolescents of both sexes would benefit from knowing that pregnancy can occur at any time after the onset of menses.

Menstrual Cycle

Menstruation is the periodic uterine bleeding that begins approximately 14 days after ovulation. It is controlled by a feedback system of three cycles: endometrial, hypothalamic-pituitary, and ovarian. The average length of a menstrual cycle is 28 days, but variations are normal. The first day of bleeding is designated as day 1 of the menstrual cycle, or menses (Fig. 5-8). The average duration of menstrual flow is 5 days (with a range of 3 to 6 days) and the average blood loss is 50 ml (with a range of 20 to 80 ml), but these vary greatly.

For about 50% of women, menstrual blood does not appear to clot. The menstrual blood clots within the uterus, but the clot usually liquefies before being discharged. Uterine

Guidelines

BREAST SELF-EXAMINATION

1. The best time to do breast self-examination is after your period, when breasts are not tender or swollen. If you do not have regular periods or sometimes skip a month, do it on the same day every month.
2. Lie down and put a pillow under your right shoulder. Place your right arm behind your head (Fig. 1).

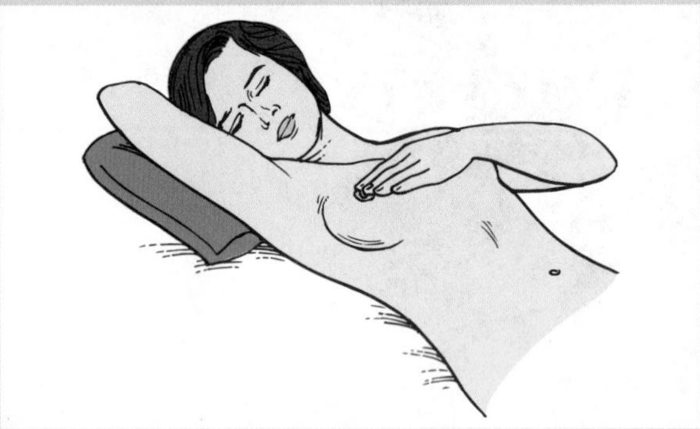

3. Use the finger pads of your three middle fingers on your left hand to feel for lumps or thickening. Your finger pads are the top third of each finger.
4. Press firmly enough to know how your breast feels. If you're not sure how hard to press, ask your health care provider, or try to copy the way your health care provider uses the finger pads during a breast examination. Learn what your breast feels like most of the time. A firm ridge in the lower curve of each breast is normal.
5. Move around the breast in a set way. You can choose either circles (Fig. 2, *A*), vertical lines (Fig. 2, *B*), or wedges (Fig. 2, *C*). Do it the same way every time. It will help you to make sure that you've gone over the entire breast area and to remember how your breast feels.

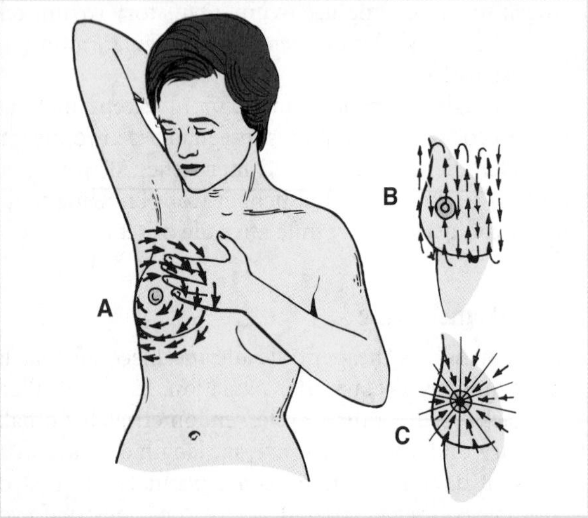

6. Gently compress the nipple between your thumb and forefinger and look for discharge.
7. Now examine your left breast using the finger pads of your right hand.
8. If you find any changes, see your health care provider right away.
9. You may want to check your breasts while standing in front of a mirror right after you do your breast self-examination each month. See if there are any changes in the way your breasts look: dimpling of the skin, changes in the nipple, or redness or swelling.
10. You may also want to do an extra breast self-examination while you're in the shower (Fig. 3). Your soapy hands will glide over the wet skin, making it easy to check how your breasts feel.

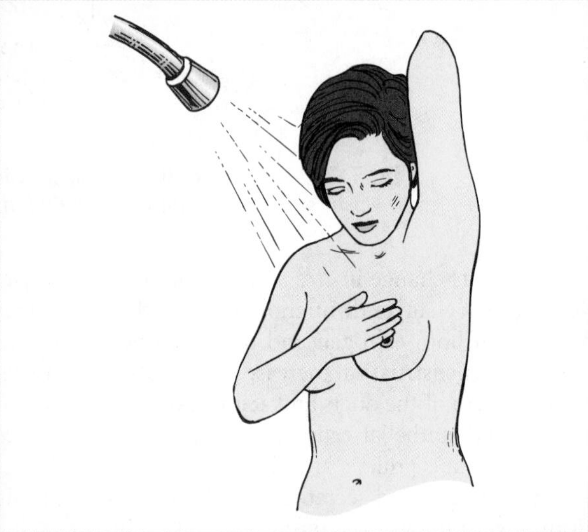

11. It is important to check the area between the breast and the underarm and the underarm itself. Also examine the area above the breast to the collarbone and to the shoulder.

discharge includes mucus and epithelial cells in addition to blood.

The menstrual cycle is a complex interplay of events that occur simultaneously in the endometrium, hypothalamus and pituitary glands, and ovaries. The menstrual cycle prepares the uterus for pregnancy. When pregnancy does not occur, menstruation follows. A woman's age, physical and emotional status, and environment influence the regularity of her menstrual cycles.

Endometrial Cycle

The four phases of the endometrial cycle are (1) the menstrual phase, (2) the proliferative phase, (3) the secretory phase,

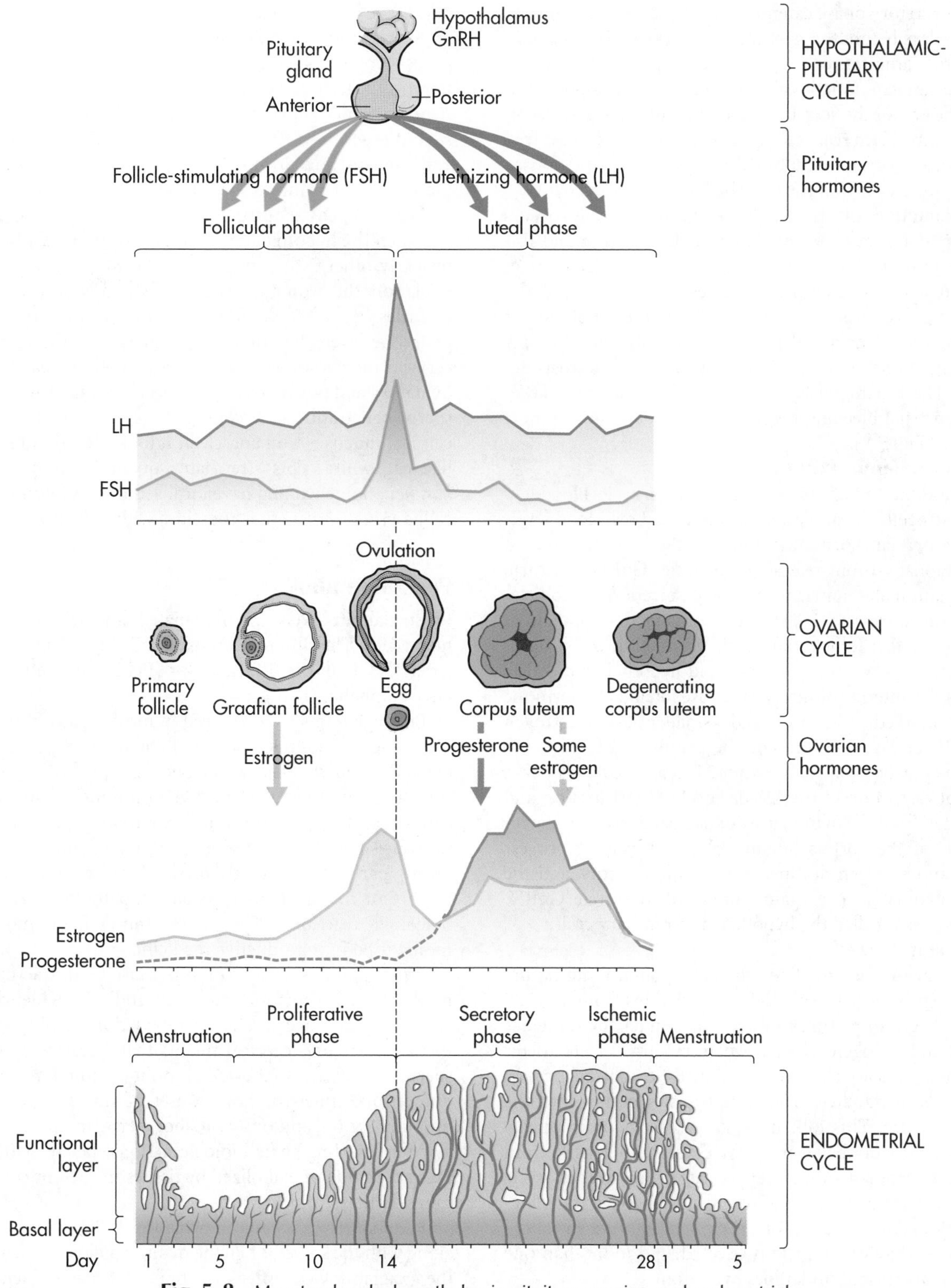

Fig. 5-8 Menstrual cycle: hypothalamic-pituitary, ovarian, and endometrial.

and (4) the ischemic phase (see Fig. 5-8). During the menstrual phase, shedding of the functional two thirds of the endometrium (the compact and spongy layers) is initiated by periodic vasoconstriction in the upper layers of the endometrium. The basal layer is always retained, and regeneration begins near the end of the cycle from cells derived from the remaining glandular remnants or stromal cells in this layer.

The proliferative phase is a period of rapid growth lasting from about the fifth day to the time of ovulation. The endometrial surface is completely restored in approximately 4 days, or slightly before bleeding ceases. From this point on an eightfold to tenfold thickening occurs, with a leveling off of growth at ovulation. The proliferative phase depends on estrogen stimulation derived from ovarian follicles.

The secretory phase extends from the day of ovulation to about 3 days before the next menstrual period. After ovulation, larger amounts of progesterone are produced. An edematous, vascular, functional endometrium is now apparent.

At the end of the secretory phase the fully matured secretory endometrium reaches the thickness of heavy, soft velvet. It becomes luxuriant with blood and glandular secretions, a suitable protective and nutritive bed for a fertilized ovum.

Implantation of the fertilized ovum generally occurs about 7 to 10 days after ovulation. If fertilization and implantation do not occur, the corpus luteum, which secretes estrogen and progesterone, regresses. With the rapid decrease in progesterone and estrogen levels, the spiral arteries go into spasm. During the ischemic phase, the blood supply to the functional endometrium is blocked and necrosis develops. The functional layer separates from the basal layer, and menstrual bleeding begins, marking day 1 of the next cycle (see Fig. 5-8).

Hypothalamic-Pituitary Cycle

Toward the end of the normal menstrual cycle, blood levels of estrogen and progesterone decrease. Low blood levels of these ovarian hormones stimulate the hypothalamus to secrete gonadotropin-releasing hormone (GnRH). In turn, GnRH stimulates anterior pituitary secretion of follicle-stimulating hormone (FSH). FSH stimulates development of ovarian graafian follicles and their production of estrogen. Estrogen levels begin to decrease, and hypothalamic GnRH triggers the anterior pituitary to release luteinizing hormone (LH). A marked surge of LH and a smaller peak of estrogen (day 12; see Fig. 5-8) precede the expulsion of the ovum from the graafian follicle by about 24 to 36 hours. LH peaks at about day 13 or 14 of a 28-day cycle. If fertilization and implantation of the ovum have not occurred by this time, regression of the corpus luteum follows. Levels of progesterone and estrogen decline, menstruation occurs, and the hypothalamus is once again stimulated to secrete GnRH. This process is called the hypothalamic-pituitary cycle.

Ovarian Cycle

The primitive graafian follicles contain immature oocytes (primordial ova). Before ovulation, from 1 to 30 follicles begin to mature in each ovary under the influence of FSH and estrogen. The preovulatory surge of LH affects a selected follicle. The oocyte matures, ovulation occurs, and the empty follicle begins its transformation into the corpus luteum. This follicular phase (preovulatory phase) (see Fig. 5-8) of the ovarian cycle varies in length from woman to woman. Almost all variations in ovarian cycle length are the result of variations in the length of the follicular phase. On rare occasions (i.e., 1 in 100 menstrual cycles) more than one follicle is selected, and more than one oocyte matures and undergoes ovulation.

After ovulation, estrogen levels drop. For 90% of women, only a small amount of withdrawal bleeding occurs and it goes unnoticed. In 10% of women, there is sufficient bleeding for it to be visible, resulting in what is termed *midcycle bleeding.*

The luteal phase begins immediately after ovulation and ends with the start of menstruation. This postovulatory phase of the ovarian cycle usually requires 14 days (range, 13 to 15 days). The corpus luteum reaches its peak of functional activity 8 days after ovulation, secreting the steroids estrogen and progesterone. Coincident with this time of peak luteal functioning, the fertilized ovum is implanted in the endometrium. If no implantation occurs, the corpus luteum regresses and steroid levels drop. Two weeks after ovulation, if fertilization and implantation do not occur, the functional layer of the uterine endometrium is shed through menstruation.

Other Cyclic Changes

When the hypothalamic-pituitary-ovarian axis functions properly, other tissues undergo predictable responses. Before ovulation the woman's basal body temperature (BBT) is often less than 37° C; after ovulation, with increasing progesterone levels, her BBT rises. Changes in the cervix and cervical mucus follow a generally predictable pattern. Preovulatory and postovulatory mucus is viscous (thick) so that sperm penetration is discouraged. At the time of ovulation, cervical mucus is thin and clear. It looks, feels, and stretches like egg white. This stretchable quality is termed *spinnbarkheit.* Some women have localized lower abdominal pain called *mittelschmerz* that coincides with ovulation.

Prostaglandins

Prostaglandins (PGs) are oxygenated fatty acids classified as hormones. The different kinds of PGs are distinguished by letters (PGE and PGF), numbers (PGE_2), and letters of the Greek alphabet ($PGF_{2\alpha}$).

Prostaglandins are produced in most organs of the body, including the uterus. Menstrual blood is a potent prostaglandin source. PGs are metabolized quickly by most tissues. They are biologically active in minute amounts in the cardiovascular, gastrointestinal, respiratory, urogenital, and nervous systems. They also exert a marked effect on metabolism, particularly on glycolysis. Prostaglandins play an important role in many physiologic, pathologic, and pharmacologic reactions. $PGF_{2\alpha}$, PGE_4, and PGE_2 are most commonly used in reproductive medicine.

Prostaglandins affect smooth muscle contractility and modulation of hormonal activity. Indirect evidence indicates that PGs have an effect on ovulation, fertility, changes in the cervix and cervical mucus that affect receptivity to sperm, tubal and uterine motility, sloughing of endometrium (menstruation), onset of miscarriage and induced abortion, and onset of labor (term and preterm).

After exerting their biologic actions, newly synthesized PGs are rapidly metabolized by tissues in such organs as the lungs, kidneys, and liver.

PGs may play a key role in ovulation. If PG levels do not rise along with the surge of LH, the ovum remains trapped within the graafian follicle. After ovulation, PGs may influence production of estrogen and progesterone by the corpus luteum.

The introduction of PGs into the vagina or into the uterine cavity (from ejaculated semen) increases the motility of uterine musculature, which may assist the transport of sperm through the uterus and into the oviduct.

Prostaglandins produced by the woman cause regression of the corpus luteum; regression of the endometrium; and sloughing of the endometrium, resulting in menstruation.

PGs increase myometrial response to oxytocic stimulation, enhance uterine contractions, and cause cervical dilation. They may be a factor in the initiation of labor, the maintenance of labor, or both. They may also be involved in dysmenorrhea (see Chapter 6) and preeclampsia-eclampsia (see Chapter 14).

Climacteric and Menopause

The climacteric is a transitional phase during which ovarian function and hormone production decline. This phase spans the years from the onset of premenopausal ovarian decline to the postmenopausal time when symptoms stop. Menopause (from the Latin *mensis,* month, and Greek *pauses,* to cease) refers only to the last menstrual period. Unlike menarche, however, menopause can be dated with certainty only 1 year after menstruation ceases. The average age at natural menopause is 51.4 years, with an age range of 35 to 60 years. Perimenopause is a period between 2 and 8 years before menopause, with an onset between the age of 39 and 51 years.

SEXUAL RESPONSE

The hypothalamus and anterior pituitary glands in females regulate the production of FSH and LH. The target tissue for these hormones is the ovary, which produces ova and secretes estrogen and progesterone. A feedback mechanism between hormone secretion from the ovaries, the hypothalamus, and the anterior pituitary aids in the control of the production of sex cells and steroid sex hormone secretion.

Although the first outward appearance of maturing sexual development occurs at an earlier age in females, both females and males achieve physical maturity at approximately 17 years of age; however, individual development varies greatly. Anatomic and reproductive differences notwithstanding, women and men are more alike than different in their physiologic response to sexual excitement and orgasm. For example, the glans clitoris and the glans penis are embryonic homologues. Little difference exists between female and male sexual response; the physical response is essentially the same whether stimulated by coitus, fantasy, or masturbation. Physiologic sexual response can be analyzed in terms of two processes: vasocongestion and myotonia.

Sexual stimulation results in increase in circulation to circumvaginal blood vessels (lubrication in the female), causing engorgement and distention of the genitalia. Venous congestion is localized primarily in the genitalia, but it also occurs to a lesser degree in the breasts and in other parts of the body. Arousal is characterized by myotonia (increased muscular tension), resulting in voluntary and involuntary rhythmic contractions. Examples of sexually stimulated myotonia are pelvic thrusting, facial grimacing, and spasms of the hands and feet (carpopedal spasms).

The sexual response cycle is divided into four phases: excitement phase, plateau phase, orgasmic phase, and resolution phase. The four phases occur progressively, with no sharp dividing line between any two phases. Specific body changes take place in sequence. The time, intensity, and duration for cyclic completion also vary for individuals and situations. Table 5-1 compares male and female body changes during each of the four phases of the sexual response cycle.

HEALTH ASSESSMENT

Current women's health trends have expanded beyond a reproductive focus to include a holistic approach to health care across the life span. Women's health assessment and screening focus on a systems evaluation that begins with a careful history and physical examination. During the assessment and evaluation, the responsibility for self-care, health promotion, and enhancement of wellness is emphasized. Nursing is an interactive process that begins with establishing trust and a caring relationship, with the broader goal of enhancing and maintaining wellness. The nurse provides care that includes assessment, planning, education, counseling, and referral as needed, as well as commendations for good self-care that the woman has practiced. This enables women to make informed decisions about their own health care.

A nurse often takes the history, orders diagnostic tests, interprets test results, makes referrals, coordinates care, and directs attention to problems requiring medical intervention. Advanced practice nurses who have specialized in women's health, such as nurse practitioners, clinical nurse specialists, and nurse-midwives, perform complete physical examinations including gynecologic examinations.

Culturally competent nursing care should be delivered with an awareness of cultural diversity while respecting the unique qualities of each woman. Such care cannot be provided in the absence of self-awareness. Nurses must acknowledge their own values, beliefs, and communication styles to understand what they contribute to cross-cultural communication (Mattson, 2000b).

Interview

Contact with the woman usually begins with an interview. This interview should be conducted in a private, comfortable, and relaxed setting (Fig. 5-9). The nurse is seated and makes sure the woman is comfortable. The woman is addressed by her title and name (e.g., Mrs. Martinez) and the nurse introduces herself or himself using name and title. It is important to phrase questions in a sensitive and nonjudgmental manner. Body language should match oral communication. The nurse is aware of a woman's vulnerability and assures her of strict confidentiality. For many women, fear, anxiety, and modesty make the examination a dreaded and stressful experience. Many women are uninformed, misguided by myths, or afraid they will appear ignorant by asking questions about sexual or reproductive functioning. The woman is assured that no question is irrelevant.

The history begins with an open-ended question such as, "What brings you into the office/clinic/ hospital today?" and is furthered by other questions such as "Anything else?" and

Table 5-1

Four Phases of Sexual Response

REACTIONS COMMON TO BOTH SEXES	FEMALE REACTIONS	MALE REACTIONS
EXCITEMENT PHASE		
Heart rate and blood pressure increase. Nipples become erect. Myotonia begins.	Clitoris increases in diameter and swells. External genitals become congested and darken. Vaginal lubrication occurs; upper two thirds of vagina lengthen and extend. Cervix and uterus pull upward. Breast size increases.	Erection of the penis begins; penis increases in length and diameter. Scrotal skin becomes congested and thickens. Testes begin to increase in size and elevate toward the body.
PLATEAU PHASE		
Heart rate and blood pressure continue to increase. Respirations increase. Myotonia becomes pronounced; grimacing occurs.	Clitoral head retracts under the clitoral hood. Lower one third of vagina becomes engorged. Skin color changes occur—red flush may be observed across breasts, abdomen, or other surfaces.	Head of penis may enlarge slightly. Scrotum continues to grow tense and thicken. Testes continue to elevate and enlarge. Preorgasmic emission of two or three drops of fluid appears on the head of the penis.
ORGASMIC PHASE		
Heart rate, blood pressure, and respirations increase to maximum levels. Involuntary muscle spasms occur. External rectal sphincter contracts.	Strong rhythmic contractions are felt in the clitoris, vagina, and uterus. Sensations of warmth spread through the pelvic area.	Testes elevate to maximum level. Point of "inevitability" occurs just before ejaculation and an awareness of fluid in the urethra. Rhythmic contractions occur in the penis. Ejaculation of semen occurs.
RESOLUTION PHASE		
Heart rate, blood pressure, and respirations return to normal. Nipple erection subsides. Myotonia subsides.	Engorgement in external genitalia and vagina resolves. Uterus descends to normal position. Cervix dips into seminal pool. Breast size decreases. Skin flush disappears.	Fifty percent of erection is lost immediately with ejaculation; penis gradually returns to normal size. Testes and scrotum return to normal size. Refractory period (time needed for erection to occur again) varies according to age and general physical condition.

"Tell me about it." Additional ways to encourage women to share information include the following:

- *Facilitation*—Using a word or posture that communicates interest, such as leaning forward, making eye contact, or saying "Mm-hmmm" or "Go on."
- *Reflection*—Repeating a word or phrase that a woman has used.
- *Clarification*—Asking the woman what is meant by a stated word or phrase.
- *Empathic responses*—Acknowledging the feelings of a woman by statements such as "That must have been frightening."
- *Confrontation*—Identifying something about the woman's behavior or feelings not expressed verbally or apparently inconsistent with her history.
- *Interpretation*—Putting into words what you infer about the woman's feelings or about the meaning of her symptoms, events, or other matters.

Direct questions may be necessary to elicit specific details. These should be worded in language that is understandable to the woman and expressed neutrally so that the woman will not be led into a specific response. The nurse asks about one item at a time and proceeds from the general to the specific (Seidel et al, 2003).

Cultural Considerations and Communication Variations

Recognizing signs and symptoms of disease and deciding to seek treatment are influenced by cultural perceptions. Culture evolves over time and is a system of symbols that are learned, shared, and passed on through generations of a social group. Cultural competence in nursing is a complex combination of knowledge, attitudes, and skills mixed with personal attributes of flexibility, empathy, and language facility. It is more than simply acquiring knowledge about another ethnic group. It is essential that a nurse have respect for the rich and unique qualities that cultural diversity brings to individuals. In recognizing the value of these differences, the nurse can modify the plan of care to meet the needs of each woman. Trust that the woman is the expert on her life, culture, and experiences. If the nurse asks with respect and a genuine desire to learn, the woman will tell the nurse how to care for her (Mattson, 2000a). The nurse communicates in an even-toned and nonjudgmental manner, keeps a calm facial expression, and recognizes that modifica-

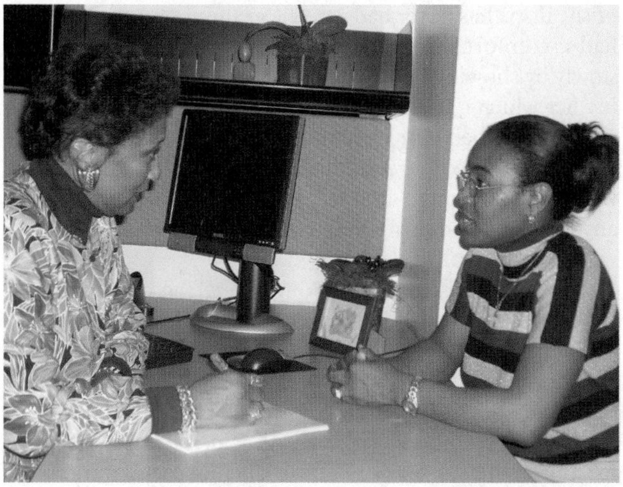

Fig. 5-9 Nurse interviews patient as part of annual physical examination. (Courtesy Julie Perry Nelson, Gilbert, AZ.)

tions may be necessary for the physical examination. In some cultures, it may be considered inappropriate for the woman to disrobe completely for the physical examination. In many cultures, a woman examiner is preferred.

Women with Special Needs

Women with Disabilities

Women with emotional or physical disorders have special needs. Women who have vision, hearing, emotional, or physical disabilities should be respected and involved in the assessment and physical examination to the full extent of their capabilities. The nurse should communicate openly and directly and with sensitivity. It is often helpful to learn about the disability directly from the woman while maintaining eye contact. Family and significant others should be relied on only when absolutely necessary. The assessment and physical examination can be adapted to each woman's individual needs.

Communication with a woman who is hearing impaired can be accomplished without difficulty. Many of these women read lips, write, or both. The interviewer who speaks and enunciates each word slowly and in full view may be easily understood. If a woman is not comfortable with lip reading, she may use an interpreter. In this case, it is important to continue to address the woman directly, avoiding the temptation to speak directly with the interpreter. The visually impaired woman needs to be oriented to the examination room and may have her guide dog with her. As with all patients, the visually impaired woman needs a full explanation of what the examination entails before proceeding. Before touching her, the nurse explains, "Now I am going to take your blood pressure. I am going to place the cuff on your right arm." The woman can be asked if she would like to touch each of the items that will be used in the examination to reduce her anxiety.

Many women with physical disabilities cannot comfortably lie in the lithotomy position for the pelvic examination. Several alternative positions may be used, including a lateral (side-lying) position, a V-shaped position, a diamond-shaped position, and an M-shaped position (Fig. 5-10). The woman can be asked what has worked best for her previ-

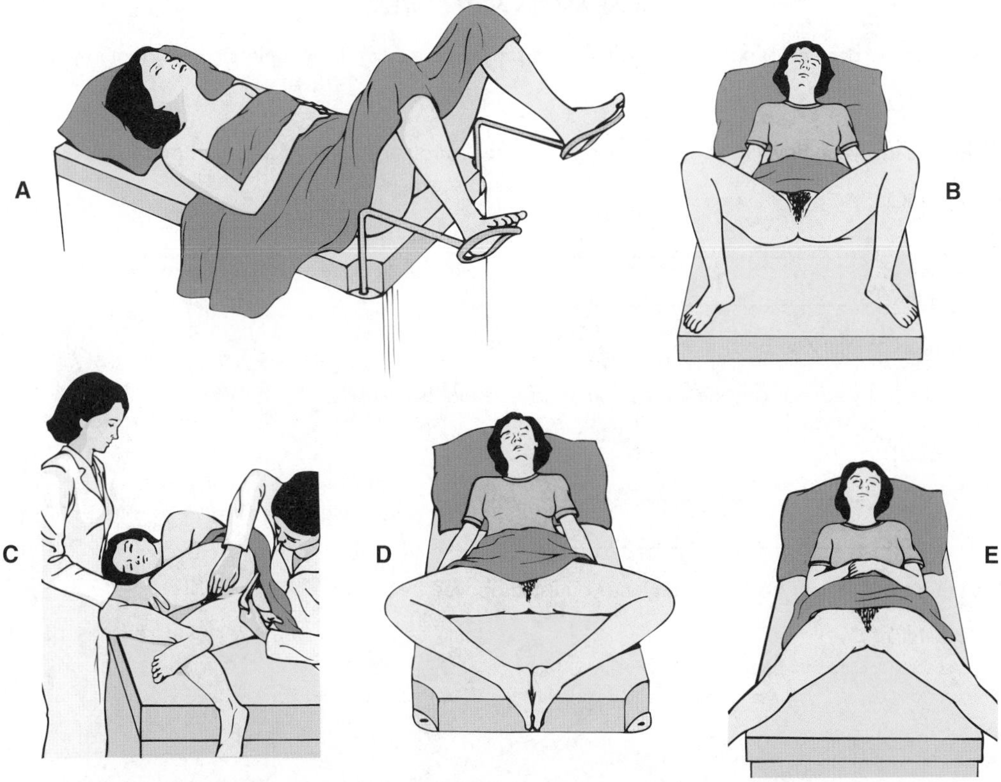

Fig. 5-10 Lithotomy and variable positions for women who have a disability. **A**, Lithotomy position. **B**, M-shaped position. **C**, Side-lying position. **D**, Diamond-shaped position. **E**, V-shaped position.

Critical Thinking Exercise

CARING FOR A WOMAN WITH A PHYSICAL DISABILITY

Giana, a 36-year-old woman with severe scoliosis who uses a wheelchair, arrives at the clinic for a physical examination and Pap smear. She states that she needs a physical examination to qualify for insurance through her place of employment. She informs the nurse practitioner that she has only had one pelvic examination in her life because the first one was such an awful experience. "They wouldn't listen to me when I told them the best way to check me."

1. Evidence—Is there sufficient evidence to draw conclusions about the possibility of performing a pain-free physical examination on Giana including a pelvic examination and Pap smear?
2. Assumptions—What assumptions about the following factors can be made about performing a physical examination on a woman with a disability?
   a. Accessibility of the clinic.
   b. The nurse's usual assessment procedure.
   c. Alternative positions for performing a pelvic examination.
   d. Necessary accommodations.
3. What implications and priorities for nursing care can be drawn at this time?
4. Does the evidence objectively support your conclusion?
5. Are there alternative perspectives to your conclusion?

ously. If she has never had a pelvic examination, or has never had a comfortable pelvic examination, the nurse proceeds slowly by showing her a picture of various positions and asking her which one she prefers. The nurse's support and reassurance can help the woman to relax, which will make the examination go more smoothly. The woman is informed that she is in charge, and if the examination must stop for any reason, it can be rescheduled at a later date.

Abused Women

Nurses should screen all women entering the health care system for abuse. Abuse is a life-threatening public health problem that affects millions of women and their children. The risk for intimate partner violence increases during pregnancy and after separation or divorce. Help for the woman may depend on the sensitivity with which the nurse screens for abuse, the discovery of abuse, and subsequent intervention. The nurse must be familiar with the laws governing abuse in the state in which she or he practices.

Pocket cards listing emergency numbers (abuse counseling, legal protection, and emergency shelter) may be obtained from local police departments, women's shelters, or emergency departments. It is helpful to have these on hand in the setting where screening is done. An abuse assessment screen (Fig. 5-11) can be used as part of the interview or written history. If a male partner is present, he should be asked to leave the room because the woman may not disclose experiences of abuse in his presence, or he may try to answer questions for her to protect himself. The same procedure

ABUSE ASSESSMENT SCREEN

1. Have you ever been emotionally or physically abused by your partner or someone important to you?

YES ☐ NO ☐

2. Within the last year, have you been hit, slapped, kicked, or otherwise physically hurt by someone?

YES ☐ NO ☐

If YES, by whom ____________________

Number of times ____________________

Mark the area of injury on body map.

3. Within the last year, has anyone forced you to have sexual activities?

YES ☐ NO ☐

If YES, by whom ____________________

Number of times ____________________

4. Are you afraid of your partner or anyone you listed above?

YES ☐ NO ☐

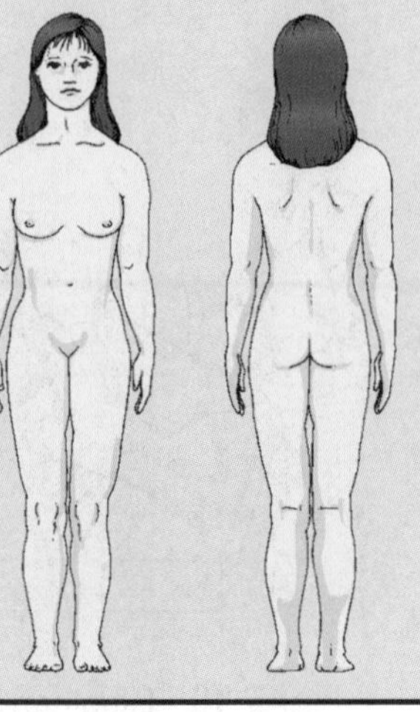

Fig. 5-11 Abuse assessment screen. (Modified from the Nursing Research Consortium on Violence and Abuse, 1991.)

would apply for partners of lesbians or the adult children of older women.

Fear, guilt, and embarrassment may keep many women from giving information about family violence. Clues in the history and evidence of injuries on physical examination should give a high index of suspicion. The areas most commonly injured in women are the head, neck, chest, abdomen, breasts, and upper extremities. Burns and bruises in patterns resembling hands, belts, cords, or other weapons may be seen, as well as multiple traumatic injuries. Attention should be given to women who repeatedly seek treatment for somatic complaints such as headaches, insomnia, choking sensations, hyperventilation, gastrointestinal symptoms, and pain in the chest, back, or pelvis. During pregnancy, the nurse should assess for injuries to the breasts, abdomen, and genitalia. See Chapter 4 for further discussion of violence.

Adolescents (Ages 13 to 19 Years)

A maturing young woman should be asked the same questions that are included in any history. Particular attention should be paid to hints about risky behaviors, eating disorders, and depression. Sexual activity is addressed after rapport has been established. It is best to talk to a teen with the parent (or partner or friend) out of the room. Questions should be asked with sensitivity and in a gentle and nonjudgmental manner (Seidel et al, 2003).

Injury prevention should be a part of the counseling at routine health examinations, with special attention to seat belts, helmets, firearms, recreational hazards, and sports involvement. The use of drugs and alcohol and the nonuse of seat belts contribute to motor vehicle injuries, accounting for the greatest proportion of accidental deaths in women (Arias et al, 2003). Contraceptive options, including the use of condoms, should be addressed during visits.

To provide developmentally appropriate care, it is important to review the major tasks for women in this stage of life. Major tasks for teens include values assessment; education and work goal setting; formation of peer relationships that focus on love, commitment, and becoming comfortable with sexuality; and separation from parents. The teen is egocentric as she progresses rapidly through emotional and physical change. Her feelings of invulnerability may lead to misconceptions such as the belief that unprotected sexual intercourse will not lead to pregnancy.

History

At a woman's first visit, she is often expected to fill out a form with biographic and historic data before meeting with the examiner. This form aids the health care provider in completing the history. This medical history usually includes the following:

1. Identifying data: Name, age, race, living household preference, occupation, religion, culture, and ethnicity are obtained.
2. Chief complaint(s): A verbatim response to the question, "What problem or symptom brought you here today?" is recorded. If a lengthy list is recited, it may be necessary to tell the woman that her two complaints with the highest priority will be addressed today. To give all of her problems the full attention they deserve, a follow-up appointment can be scheduled.
3. History of present illness: A chronologic narrative that includes onset of the problem, the setting in which it developed, its manifestations, and any treatments received are noted. The woman's state of health before the onset of the present problem is determined. If the problem is of long standing, the reason for seeking attention at this time is elicited. The principal symptoms should be described as to the following:
   - Location
   - Quality
   - Quantity or severity
   - Timing (onset, duration, frequency)
   - Setting
   - Factors that aggravate or relieve
   - Associated manifestations
4. Medical history: Determine general state of health and strength:
   - Infectious diseases: measles, mumps, rubella, whooping cough, chickenpox, rheumatic fever, scarlet fever, diphtheria, polio, tuberculosis (TB), hepatitis
   - Chronic disease and system disorders: arthritis, cancer, diabetes, heart, lung, kidney, seizures, thyroid, stroke, ulcers
   - Adult injuries, accidents, illnesses, disabilities, hospitalizations, blood transfusions; note if the injury occurred on the job (workers' compensation) or if potential litigation is being considered
5. Present health status:
   - Allergies: medications, previous transfusion reactions, environmental allergies
   - Immunizations: diphtheria; pertussis; tetanus; polio; measles, mumps, rubella (MMR); hepatitis B; varicella; influenza; pneumococcal vaccine; last TB skin test
   - Screening tests: Pap smear, mammogram, stool for occult blood, sigmoidoscopy/colonoscopy, chest radiograph, hematocrit, hemoglobin, rubella titer, urinalysis, cholesterol test; blood type/Rh; last eye examination; last dental examination
   - Environmental/chemical hazards: home, school, work, and leisure setting; exposure to extreme heat or cold, noise, industrial toxins such as asbestos or lead, pesticides, diethylstilbestrol (DES), radiation exposure, cat feces, cigarette smoke
   - Use of safety measures: seat belts, bicycle helmets, athletic protective devices, designated driver
   - Exercise and leisure activities; stress-relieving activities
   - Sleep patterns: length and quality
   - Sexuality: Is she sexually active? With men, women, or both? Does she use condoms?
   - Diet, including beverages: 24-hour dietary recall; brushes teeth three times daily; flosses daily
   - Medications: name, dose, frequency, duration, reason for taking, and compliance with prescription medications; home remedies, over-the-counter drugs, vitamin and mineral or herbal supplements used over a 24-hour period
   - Nicotine, alcohol, or recreational drugs: type, amount, frequency, duration, and reactions

- Caffeine: coffee, tea, cola, or chocolate intake

6. Surgical history: Type, date, reason, outcome, and any complications should be noted.
7. Family history: Information about age and health of family members may be presented in narrative or genogram: age, health/death of parents, siblings, spouse, children. Check for history of diabetes, heart disease, hypertension, stroke, respiratory diseases, renal conditions, thyroid problems, cancer, bleeding disorders, hepatitis, allergies, asthma, arthritis, TB, epilepsy, mental illness, human immunodeficiency virus (HIV), or other disorders.
8. Social history: Note birthplace, education, employment, marital status, living accommodations, children, persons at home, and hobbies. Does she enjoy what she is doing?
   - Screen for abuse: Has she ever been hit, kicked, slapped, or forced to have sex against her wishes? Verbally or emotionally abused? History of childhood sexual abuse? If yes, has she received counseling or does she need referral?
9. Review of systems: It is probable that all questions in each system will not be included every time a history is taken. Some questions regarding each system should be included in every history. The essential areas to be explored are listed in the following head-to-toe sequence. If a woman gives a positive response to a question about an essential area, more detailed questions should be asked.
   - General: weight change, fatigue, weakness, fever, chills, or night sweats
   - Skin: skin, hair, and nail changes; itching, bruising, bleeding, rashes, sores, lumps, or moles
   - Lymph nodes: enlargement, inflammation, pain, suppuration (pus), or drainage
   - Head, eyes, ears, nose, and throat:
     Head: trauma, vertigo (dizziness), convulsive disorder, syncope (fainting), headache location, frequency, pain type, nausea/vomiting, or visual symptoms
     Eyes: glasses, contact lenses, blurriness, tearing, itching, photophobia, diplopia, inflammation, trauma, cataracts, glaucoma, or acute visual loss
     Ears: hearing loss, tinnitus (ringing), vertigo, discharge, pain, fullness, recurrent infections, or mastoiditis
     Nose/sinuses: trauma, rhinitis, nasal discharge, epistaxis, obstruction, sneezing, itching, allergy, or smelling impairment
     Mouth/throat/neck: hoarseness, voice changes, soreness, ulcers, bleeding gums, goiter, swelling, or enlarged nodes
   - Breasts: masses, pain, lumps, dimpling, nipple discharge, fibrocystic changes, or implants; BSE practice
   - Respiratory: shortness of breath, wheezing, cough, sputum, hemoptysis, pneumonia, pleurisy, asthma, bronchitis, emphysema, or TB; last chest radiograph
   - Cardiac: hypertension, rheumatic fever, murmurs, angina, palpitations, dyspnea, tachycardia, orthopnea, edema, chest pain, cough, cyanosis, cold extremities, ascites, intermittent claudication (leg pain caused by poor circulation to the leg muscles), phlebitis, or skin-color changes
   - Gastrointestinal: appetite, nausea, vomiting, indigestion, dysphagia, abdominal pain, ulcers, hematochezia (bleeding with stools), melena (black, tarry stools), bowel-habit changes, diarrhea, constipation, bowel-movement frequency, food intolerance, hemorrhoids, jaundice, or hepatitis; sigmoidoscopy, colonoscopy, barium enema, ultrasound
   - Genitourinary: frequency, hesitancy, urgency, polyuria, dysuria, hematuria, nocturia, incontinence, stones, infection, or urethral discharge; dysmenorrhea, intermenstrual bleeding, dyspareunia, discharge, sores, itching, sexually transmitted infections, gravidity (G), parity (P), problems in pregnancy, contraception, menopause, hot flashes, or sweats (may be included here or as part of endocrine)
   - Vascular: leg edema, claudication, varicose veins, thromboses, or emboli
   - Endocrine: heat/cold intolerance, dry skin, excessive sweating, polyuria, polydipsia, polyphagia, thyroid problems, diabetes, or secondary sex characteristic changes; age at menarche, length/flow of menses, last menstrual period (LMP), age at menopause, libido, or sexual concerns
   - Hematologic: anemia, easy bruising, bleeding, petechiae, purpura, or transfusions
   - Musculoskeletal: muscle weakness, pain, joint stiffness, scoliosis, lordosis, kyphosis, range-of-motion instability, redness, swelling, arthritis, or gout
   - Neurologic: loss of sensation, numbness, tingling, tremors, weakness, vertigo, paralysis, fainting, twitching, blackouts, seizures, convulsions, loss of consciousness or memory
   - Psychiatric: moodiness, depression, anxiety, obsessions, delusions, illusions, or hallucinations
   - Functional assessment: should be done on women with disabilities and women 70 years of age and older (see previous discussion)

Physical Examination

In preparation for the physical examination, the woman is instructed on undressing and given a gown to wear during the examination. She is usually given the opportunity to undress privately. Some guidelines for assisting the Spanish-speaking woman during a physical examination are listed in the Guidelines/Guías box.

Objective data are recorded by system or location. A general statement of overall health status is a good way to start. Findings are described in detail.

- General appearance: age, race, sex, state of health, posture, height, weight, development, dress, hygiene, affect, alertness, orientation, cooperativeness, and communication skills
- Vital signs: temperature, pulse, respiration, blood pressure
- Skin: color; integrity; texture; hydration; temperature; edema; excessive perspiration; unusual odor; presence and description of lesions; hair texture and distribution; nail configuration, color, texture, condition, or presence of nail clubbing
- Head: size, shape, trauma, masses, scars, rashes, or scaling; facial symmetry; presence of edema or puffiness
- Eyes: pupil size, shape, reactivity, conjunctival injection, scleral icterus, fundal papilledema, hemorrhage, lids, extraocular movements, visual fields and acuity

evolve CASE STUDY–HEALTH ASSESSMENT

- Ears: shape and symmetry, tenderness, discharge, external canal, and tympanic membranes; hearing—Weber should be midline (loudness of sound equal in both ears) and Rinne negative (no conductive or sensorineural hearing loss); should be able to hear whisper at 3 feet
- Nose: symmetry, tenderness, discharge, mucosa, turbinate inflammation, frontal or maxillary sinus tenderness; discrimination of odors
- Mouth and throat: hygiene, condition of teeth, dentures, appearance of lips, tongue, buccal and oral mucosa, erythema, edema, exudate, tonsillar enlargement, palate, uvula, gag reflex, ulcers
- Neck: mobility, masses, range of motion, trachea deviation, thyroid size, carotid bruits
- Lymphatic: cervical, intraclavicular, axillary, trochlear, or inguinal adenopathy; size, shape, tenderness, and consistency
- Breasts: skin changes, dimpling, symmetry, scars, tenderness, discharge, or masses; characteristics of nipples and areolae
- Heart: rate, rhythm, murmurs, rubs, gallops, clicks, heaves, or precordial movements
- Peripheral vascular: jugular vein distention, bruits, edema, swelling, vein distention, Homans' sign, or tenderness of extremities
- Lungs: chest symmetry with respirations, wheezes, crackles, rhonchi, vocal fremitus, whispered pectoriloquy, percussion, and diaphragmatic excursion; breath sounds equal and clear bilaterally
- Abdomen: shape, scars, bowel sounds, consistency, tenderness, rebound, masses, guarding, organomegaly, liver span, percussion (tympany, shifting, dullness), costovertebral angle tenderness
- Extremities: edema, ulceration, tenderness, varicosities, erythema, tremor, or deformity
- Genitourinary: external genitalia, perineum, vaginal mucosa, cervix, inflammation, tenderness, discharge, bleeding, ulcers, nodules, masses, internal vaginal support, bimanual, and rectovaginal; palpation of cervix, uterus, and adnexae
- Rectal: sphincter tone, masses, hemorrhoids, rectal wall contour, tenderness, and stool for occult blood
- Musculoskeletal: posture, symmetry of muscle mass, muscle atrophy, weakness, appearance of joints, tenderness or crepitus, joint range of motion, instability, redness, swelling, or spine deviation
- Neurologic: mental status, orientation, memory, mood, speech clarity and comprehension, cranial nerves II to XII, sensation, strength, deep tendon and superficial reflexes, gait, balance, and coordination with rapid alternating motions

Pelvic Examination

Many women fear the gynecologic portion of the physical examination. The nurse can be instrumental in allaying these fears by providing information and assisting the woman to express her feelings to the examiner (Box 5-1).

The woman is assisted into the lithotomy position (see Fig. 5-10, *A*) for the pelvic examination. When she is in the

---

ENGLISH SPANISH Guidelines/Guías

PHYSICAL EXAMINATION

Take off all your clothes, please.
Quítese toda la ropa, por favor.

Put on the gown, please.
Póngase la bata, por favor.

I am going to examine you.
Le voy a examinar.

You will feel less discomfort if you relax.
Se sentirá más cómoda si se relaja el cuerpo.

Lie down, please.
Acuéstese, por favor.

Put your feet in the stirrups.
Póngase los pies en los estribos.

Open your legs, please.
Sepárese las piernas, por favor.

I am going to take a sample from the lining of the cervix (Pap smear).
Le voy a tomar una muestra del cuello uterino (el examen de Papanicolao).

We will test this sample for cancer.
Haremos un análisis de esta muestra para determinar si hay cáncer.

It won't hurt.
No le va a doler.

Everything looks fine.
Todo está bien.

You may get dressed.
Puede vestirse.

BOX 5-1

Procedure: Assisting with Pelvic Examination (see Fig. 5-13)

Wash hands. Assemble equipment.
Ask woman to empty her bladder before the examination (obtain clean-catch urine specimen as needed).
Assist with relaxation techniques. Have the woman place her hands on her chest at about the level of the diaphragm, breathe deeply and slowly (in through her nose and out through her O-shaped mouth), concentrate on the rhythm of breathing, and relax all body muscles with each exhalation (Barkauskas, Baumann, & Darling-Fisher, 2002).
Encourage the woman to become involved with the examination if she shows interest. For example, a mirror can be placed so that she can see the area being examined.
Assess for and treat signs of problems such as supine hypotension.
Warm the speculum in warm water if a prewarmed one is not available.
Instruct the woman to bear down when the speculum is being inserted.
Apply gloves and assist the examiner with collection of specimens for cytologic examination, such as a Pap test. After handling specimens, remove gloves and wash hands.
Lubricate the examiner's fingers with water or water-soluble lubricant before bimanual examination.
Assist the woman to a sitting position at completion of the examination.
Provide tissues to wipe lubricant from perineum.
Provide privacy for the woman while she is dressing.

lithotomy position, the woman's hips and knees are flexed, with buttocks at the edge of the table, and her feet are supported by heel or knee stirrups.

Some women prefer to keep their shoes or socks on, especially if the stirrups are not padded. Many women express feelings of vulnerability and strangeness when in the lithotomy position. During the procedure, the nurse assists the woman with relaxation techniques.

One method of helping the woman relax is to have her place her hands on her chest at about the level of the diaphragm, breathe deeply and slowly (in through her nose and out through her O-shaped mouth), concentrate on the rhythm of breathing, and relax all body muscles with each exhalation. This breathing technique is particularly helpful for the adolescent and for the woman whose introitus may be especially tight or for whom the experience is new or may provoke tension. Some women relax when they are encouraged to become involved with the examination with a mirror placed so that they can view the area being examined. This type of participation helps with health teaching as well. Distraction is another technique that can be used effectively (e.g., placing interesting pictures on the ceiling over the head of the table).

Many women find it distressing to attempt to converse in the lithotomy position. Most women appreciate an explanation of the procedure as it unfolds, as well as coaching for the type of sensations they may expect. Generally, however, women prefer not to have to respond to questions until they are again upright and at eye level with the examiner. Questioning during the procedure, especially if they cannot see their questioner's eyes, may make women tense.

A teen's first speculum examination is the most important because she will develop perceptions that will remain with her for future examinations. What the examination entails should be discussed with the teen while she is dressed. Models or illustrations can be used to show exactly what will happen. All of the necessary equipment should be assembled so that there are no interruptions (Fig. 5-12). Pediatric specula that are 1 to 1.5 cm wide can be inserted with minimal discomfort. If the teen is sexually active, a small adult speculum may be used.

External Inspection and Palpation

The examiner proceeds with the examination using inspection and palpation. The examiner wears gloves and sits at the foot of the table for the inspection of the external genitalia and for the speculum examination. To facilitate open communication, and to help the woman relax, the woman's head is raised on a pillow and the drape is arranged so that eye-to-eye contact can be maintained. In good lighting, external genitalia are inspected for sexual maturity, clitoris, labia, and perineum. After childbirth or other trauma there may be healed scars.

Before touching the woman, the examiner explains what is going to be done and what the woman should expect to feel (e.g., pressure). The examiner may touch the woman in a less sensitive area such as the inner thigh to alert her that the genital examination is beginning. This gesture may put the woman more at ease. The labia are spread apart to expose the structures in the vestibule: urinary meatus, Skene's glands, vaginal orifice, and Bartholin's glands (Fig. 5-13). To assess the Skene's glands, the examiner inserts one finger into the vagina and "milks" the area of the urethra. Any exudate from the urethra or the Skene's glands is cultured. Masses and erythema of either structure are assessed further. Ordinarily the openings to the Skene's glands are not visible; prominent openings may be seen if the glands are infected (e.g., with gonorrhea). During the examination, the examiner keeps in mind the data from the review of systems, such as history of burning on urination.

The vaginal orifice is examined. Hymenal tags are normal findings. With one finger still in the vagina, the examiner repositions the index finger near the posterior part of the orifice. With the thumb outside the posterior part of the labia majora, the examiner compresses the area of Bartholin's glands located at the 8 o'clock and 4 o'clock positions and looks for swelling, discharge, and pain.

The support of the anterior and posterior vaginal wall is assessed. The examiner spreads the labia with the index and middle finger and asks the woman to strain down. Any bulge from the anterior wall (urethrocele or cystocele) or posterior wall (rectocele) is noted and compared with the history, such as constipation or difficulty starting the stream of urine.

The perineum (area between the vagina and anus) is assessed for scars from old lacerations or episiotomies, thinning, fistulas, masses, lesions, and inflammation. The anus is assessed for hemorrhoids, hemorrhoidal tags, and in-

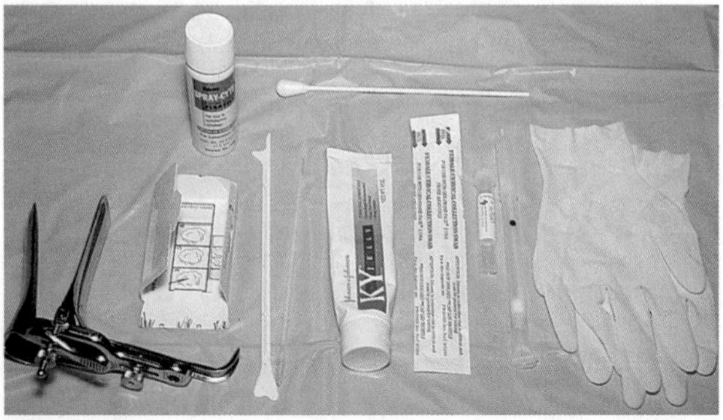

Fig. 5-12 Equipment used for pelvic examination. (Courtesy Michael S. Clement, MD, Mesa, AZ.)

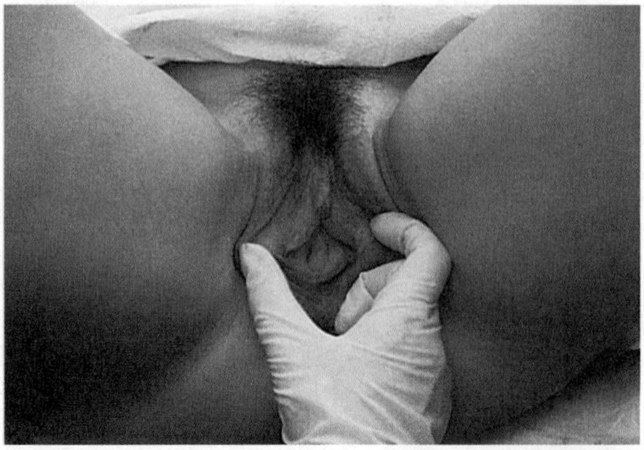

Fig. 5-13 External examination. Separation of the labia. (From Edge V, Miller M: *Women's health care,* St Louis, 1994, Mosby.)

tegrity of the anal sphincter. The anal area is also assessed for lesions, masses, abscesses, and tumors. If there is a history of sexually transmitted infection, the examiner may want to obtain a culture specimen from the anal canal at this time. Throughout the genital examination, the examiner notes any odor, which may indicate infection or poor hygiene.

Vulvar Self-Examination

The pelvic examination provides a good opportunity for the practitioner to emphasize the need for regular vulvar self-examination (VSE) and to teach this procedure. Because there has been a dramatic increase in cancerous and precancerous conditions of the vulva in recent years, a VSE should be an integral part of preventive health care for all women who are sexually active or 18 years of age or older. VSE should be performed monthly between menses or more often if there are symptoms or a history of serious vulvar disease. Most lesions, including malignancy, condyloma acuminatum (wartlike growth), and Bartholin cysts, can be seen or palpated and are easily treated if diagnosed early.

The VSE can be performed by the practitioner and woman together, by using a mirror. A simple diagram of the anatomy of the vulva can be given to the woman, with instructions to perform the examination herself that evening to reinforce what she has learned. She does the examination in a sitting position with adequate lighting, holding a mirror in one hand and using the other hand to expose the tissues surrounding the vaginal introitus. She then systematically examines the mons pubis, clitoris, urethra, labia majora, perineum, and perianal area and palpates the vulva, noting any changes in appearance or abnormalities, such as ulcers, lumps, warts, and changes in pigmentation.

Internal Examination

A vaginal speculum consists of two blades and a handle. Specula come in a variety of types and styles. A vaginal speculum is used to view the vaginal vault and cervix. The speculum is gently introduced into the vagina and inserted to the back of the vaginal vault. The blades are opened to reveal the cervix and are locked into the open position. The cervix is inspected for position and appearance of the os: color, lesions, bleeding, and discharge (Fig. 5-14). Cervical findings not within normal limits include ulcerations, masses, inflammation, and excessive protrusion into the vaginal vault. Anomalies, such as a cockscomb (a protrusion over the cervix that looks like a rooster's comb), a hooded or collared cervix (seen in DES daughters [Box 5-2]), or polyps, are noted.

Collection of Specimens

The collection of specimens for cytologic examination is an important part of the gynecologic examination. Infection can be diagnosed by examination of specimens collected during the pelvic examination. These infections include candidiasis, trichomoniasis, bacterial vaginosis, group B streptococcus, gonorrhea, chlamydia, and herpes simplex virus. Once the diagnoses have been made, treatment can be instituted.

Papanicolaou (Pap) Smear

Carcinogenic conditions, whether potential or actual, can be determined by examination of cells from the cervix collected during the pelvic examination (Box 5-3, Fig. 5-15). This examination is a Pap smear.

Vaginal Examination

After the specimens are obtained, the vagina is viewed when the speculum is rotated. The speculum blades are unlocked and partially closed. As the speculum is withdrawn, it is rotated and the vaginal walls are inspected for color, lesions, rugae, fistulas, and bulging.

Bimanual Palpation

The examiner stands for this part of the examination. A small amount of lubricant is placed on the first and second fingers of the gloved hand for the internal examination. To avoid tissue trauma and contamination, the thumb is abducted and the ring and little fingers are flexed into the palm (Fig. 5-16).

The vagina is palpated for distensibility, lesions, and tenderness. The cervix is examined for position, shape, consistency, motility, and lesions. The fornix around the cervix is palpated.

The other hand is placed on the abdomen halfway between the umbilicus and symphysis pubis and exerts pressure downward toward the pelvic hand. Upward pressure from the pelvic hand traps reproductive structures for assessment by palpation. The uterus is assessed for position, size, shape, consistency, regularity, motility, masses, and tenderness.

With the abdominal hand moving to the right lower quadrant and the fingers of the pelvic hand in the right lateral fornix, the adnexa is assessed for position, size, tenderness, and masses. The examination is repeated on the woman's left side.

Just before the intravaginal fingers are withdrawn, the woman is asked to tighten her vagina around the fingers as much as she can. If the muscle response is weak, the woman is assessed for her knowledge about Kegel exercises.

Rectovaginal Palpation

To prevent contamination of the rectum from organisms in the vagina (such as *Neisseria gonorrhoeae*), it is necessary to change gloves, add fresh lubricant, and then reinsert the index finger into the vagina and the middle finger into the rectum (Fig. 5-17). Insertion is facilitated if the woman strains down. The maneuvers of the abdominovaginal examination are repeated. The rectovaginal examination permits assessment of the rectovaginal septum, the posterior surface of the uterus, and the region behind the cervix and the adnexa. The vaginal finger is removed and folded into the palm, leaving the middle finger free to rotate 360 degrees. The rectum is palpated for rectal tenderness and masses.

After the rectal examination, the woman is assisted into a sitting position, given tissues or wipes to cleanse herself, and afforded privacy to dress. The examiner returns after the woman is dressed to discuss findings and the plan of care.

Pelvic Examination During Pregnancy

The pelvic examination is done in the same way as it is during a routine examination on a nonpregnant woman. Pelvic measurements are completed, and uterine size is estimated. A Pap smear may be done initially, as well as collection of cytologic specimens to test for gonorrhea, chlamy-

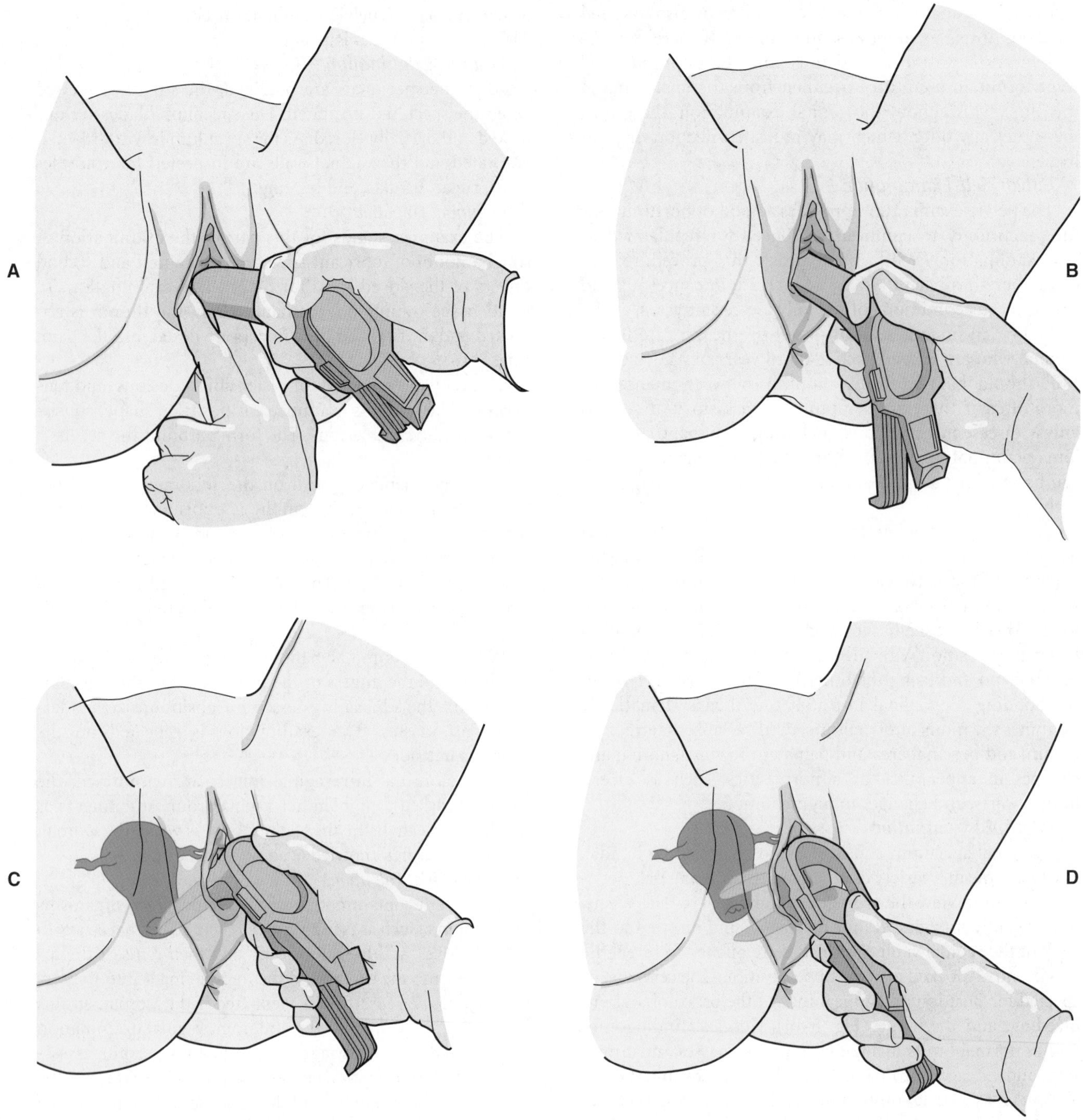

Fig. 5-14 Insertion of speculum for vaginal examination. **A,** Opening of the introitus. **B,** Oblique insertion of the speculum. **C,** Final insertion of the speculum. **D,** Opening of the speculum blades. (From Barkauskas VH, Baumann LC, Darling-Fisher CS: *Health and physical assessment,* ed 3, St Louis, 2002, Mosby.)

dia, human papillomavirus, herpes simplex virus, and group B streptococci. As the pregnancy progresses, the nurse will inspect the woman's abdomen, palpate fetal size and position, auscultate fetal heart tones, and measure fundal height at each visit.

While the pregnant woman is in lithotomy position, the nurse must watch for supine hypotension (decrease in BP), caused by the weight of the uterus pressing on the vena cava and aorta. Symptoms of supine hypotension include pallor, dizziness, faintness, breathlessness, tachycardia, nausea, clammy skin, and sweating. The woman should be positioned on her side until symptoms resolve and vital signs stabilize. The vaginal examination can be done with the woman in lateral position.

BOX 5-2

Diethylstilbestrol—Yesterday and Today

Between 1938 and 1971, 5 to 10 million pregnant women who had previously experienced a miscarriage or premature birth received diethylstilbestrol (DES) to improve their chances of having a successful pregnancy. In 1971, researchers discovered that prenatal exposure to DES increases the risk of clear cell adenocarcinoma (CCA) of the cervix and vagina. At that time, the Food and Drug Administration (FDA) issued a warning and advised physicians to stop prescribing DES. Today researchers are discovering more adverse effects of exposure to DES. The women who received DES while pregnant have a moderate increase in the risk of breast cancer. DES daughters have an increased risk of pregnancy complications and infertility and structural differences of the reproductive tract such as a T-shaped uterus. DES sons have an increased risk of noncancerous epididymal cysts. There are no known effects on granddaughters of women who received DES, but grandsons are 20 times more likely than those in the general population to have hypospadias.

Source: A drug of the past still haunts some, *Am J Nurs* 103[8]: 20, 2003.

Laboratory and Diagnostic Procedures

The following laboratory and diagnostic procedures are ordered at the discretion of the clinician, considering the patient and family history: hemoglobin, fasting blood glucose, total blood cholesterol, lipid profile, urinalysis, syphilis serology (VDRL or RPR) and other screening tests for sexu-

A

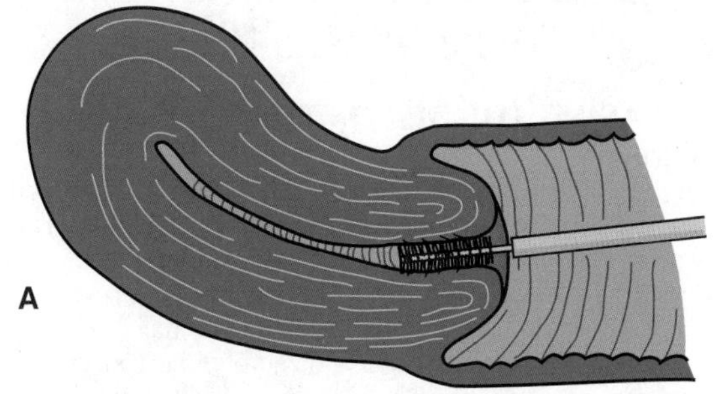

B

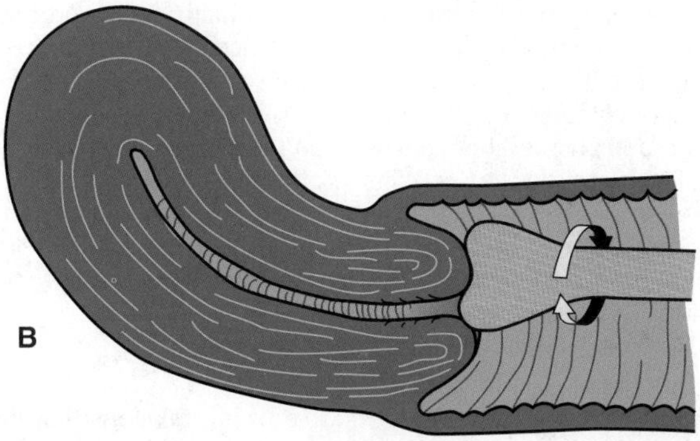

Fig. 5-15 Pap smear. **A,** Collecting cells from the endocervix using a cytobrush. **B,** Obtaining cells from the transformation zone using a wooden spatula. (From Stenchever M et al: *Comprehensive gynecology,* ed 4, St Louis, 2001, Mosby.)

BOX 5-3

Procedure: Papanicolaou (Pap) Smear

In preparation, make sure the woman has not douched, used vaginal medications, or had sexual intercourse for at least 24 hours before the procedure. Reschedule the test if the woman is menstruating. Midcycle is the best time to test.

The woman is assisted into a lithotomy position. A speculum is inserted into the vagina.

Explain to the woman the purpose of the test and what sensations she will feel as the specimen is obtained (e.g., pressure but not pain).

The cytologic specimen is obtained before any digital examination of the vagina is made or endocervical bacteriologic specimens are taken with cotton swabbing of the cervix.

The Pap smear is obtained by using an endocervical sampling device (Cytobrush, Cervex-Brush, papette, or broom) (see Fig. 5-15). If the two-sample method of obtaining cells is used, the cytobrush is inserted into the canal and rotated 90 to 180 degrees, followed by a gentle smear of the entire transformation zone using a spatula. Broom devices are inserted and rotated 360 degrees five times. They obtain endocervical and ectocervical samples at the same time. If the patient has had a hysterectomy, the vaginal cuff is sampled. Areas that appear abnormal on visualization will require colposcopy and biopsy. If using a one-slide technique, the spatula sample is smeared first. This is followed by applying the cytobrush sample (rolling the brush in the opposite direction from which it was obtained), which is less subject to drying artifact, and then the slide is sprayed with preservative within 5 seconds.

The ThinPrep Pap Test is an improved method of preserving cells that reduces blood, mucus, and inflammation. The Pap specimen is obtained in the manner described previously, and the collection device (brush, spatula, or broom) is simply rinsed in a vial of preserving solution that is provided by the laboratory. The sealed vial with solution is sent off to the appropriate laboratory. A special processing device filters the contents, and a thin layer of cervical cells is deposited on a slide, which is then examined microscopically. Initial reports state that specimen adequacy is improved by 50% and detection of low-grade and more severe lesions is improved by 65%. The Autopap and Papnet tests are similar to the ThinPrep test.

Label the slides with the woman's name and site. Include on the form to accompany the slides the woman's name, age, LMP, parity, and chief complaint or reason for taking the cytologic specimens.

Send specimens to the pathology laboratory promptly for staining, evaluation, and a written report, with special reference to abnormal elements, including cancer cells.

Advise the woman that repeat smears may be necessary if the specimen is not adequate.

Instruct the woman concerning routine checkups for cervical and vaginal cancer. The American Cancer Society advises that women over 18 years of age and those under 18 who are sexually active have the test at least every 3 years, but only after they have had three negative Pap tests a year apart. A pelvic examination is recommended every 3 years from age 20 to 40 and every 1 to 3 years thereafter.

Record the examination date on the woman's record.

Evidence-Based Practice

DECREASING THE DISCOMFORT AND PAIN OF MAMMOGRAPHY

Background

Mammography, the radiographic screening test for breast cancer, has been shown by randomized, controlled trials to decrease mortality rates. Each breast is pressed between two plates horizontally, then vertically, and a low-level x-ray is taken of each view. Mammography can find breast lumps that are too small to be palpable, thus enabling life-saving surgery to remove the cancer before it metastasizes. In spite of all these advantages, studies show that some women never return after their first mammogram. From 32% to 53% of women reported discomfort or pain with the procedure. It is important to make mammograms acceptable to the women who need them as a screening tool. Causes of pain may include the level of compression of the breast, a woman's expectations of the procedure, her level of confidence in the procedure and the technician, breast density, and timing of the mammogram during the woman's menstrual cycle. It is important to measure the pain accurately, with a standardized scale that has demonstrable reliability and validity (meaning, a tool that measures exactly what it claims to measure and nothing else).

Objectives

The reviewers were seeking evidence of interventions that might relieve the discomfort and pain of mammography. Interventions might include technique and manner of staff and facility, the woman's preparation for the procedure (including analgesia and alternative therapy), the procedure itself, and her participation in the procedure. Outcomes would be the pain and discomfort, and some way to standardize these measures. Quality of mammogram is also an important outcome, because false positives and recalls decrease the woman's confidence in the process.

Methods

Search Strategy

The search was extensive, and used Cochrane, EBM Reviews, AMED, CANCERLIT, CINAHL, Current Contents, EMBASE, HealthSTAR, PREMEDLINE, MEDLINE, PsycINFO, dissertation and theses databases, and five journals, as well as relevant organizations and specialists. Search keywords were *pain, mammogram,* and *screen,* and the search was limited to humans and females. Three randomized, controlled trials were included in the review, dated 1993 to 1998, representing 574 women.

Statistical Analyses

Meta-analysis was not possible, due to the heterogeneity of the trials. Discomfort scales were not standardized, ranging from "comfortable–not comfortable" to a six-point visual analog scale from comfortable to very uncomfortable.

Findings

Trial findings are presented separately.

Study 1 compared the comfort level of technician compression of one breast and patient-controlled compression of the other. This design enabled the woman to serve as her own control for comparison. Women reported significantly less pain in self-controlled compression than when the technician compressed the other breast, regardless of which went first. The qualities of the mammogram images were equal when the technician went first, but were of significantly poorer quality when the patient controlled the first compression. This suggests that there was some modeling during the first compression, so that the women knew approximately how much compression was desirable.

Study 2 was a master's thesis, and compared the discomfort level in women who were given acetaminophen before the procedure with the control group with no pretreatment. There were no differences in discomfort levels between groups.

Study 3 measured the discomfort levels of a standard mammogram compression on one breast with a standard compression that was loosened for one second on the other breast. No significant differences were found. More than half (57%) noted no difference, 23% felt the firmer compression to be the more uncomfortable side, and 20% felt the loosened compression to be the more uncomfortable side.

Limitations

The small number of trials, and their small numbers of subjects, limits the power of the findings. Pain and discomfort could lend themselves well to standardized scales, which could then be meta-analyzed across trials, increasing their generalizability. Even though pain is discussed, the measures are all of discomfort, and they are not standardized. The quality of mammogram interpretation across trials was also not addressed.

Conclusions

There are not enough data to draw conclusions about how to reduce the discomfort of mammograms. Increasing the woman's control of the procedure seemed to decrease her discomfort, but mild analgesics did not.

Implications for Practice

Some women may find the experience less unpleasant if they are given the option to control their own mammograms. The role of perception of control in alleviating pain is well documented in patient-controlled analgesia. Preparing a woman for a mammogram should include an honest description of the procedure and the sensations.

Implications for Further Research

More replication and further research into creative intervention to alleviate mammogram discomfort is needed. Measures of women's attitudes and confidence in the procedure still need research. This seems an ideal area in which to explore alternative interventions, such as hypnosis, guided imagery, aromatherapy, massage, temperature, acupressure, music, and distraction. Research into pretreatment with other analgesics, such as nonsteroidal antiinflammatory drugs (NSAIDs), may show more promise than acetaminophen.

Reference

Miller D, Martin I, Herbison P: Interventions for relieving the pain and discomfort of screening mammography (Cochrane Review), 2003. In *The Cochrane Library,* Issue 2, Chichester, UK, 2004, John Wiley & Sons.

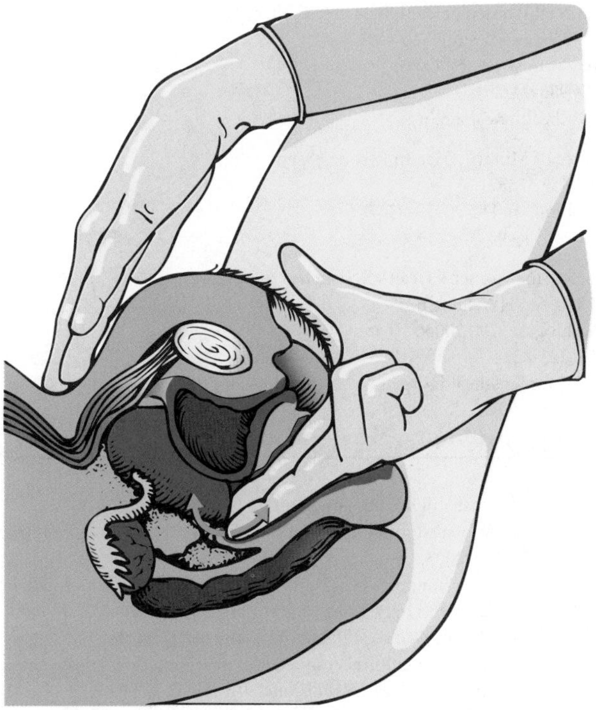

Fig. 5-16 Bimanual palpation of the uterus.

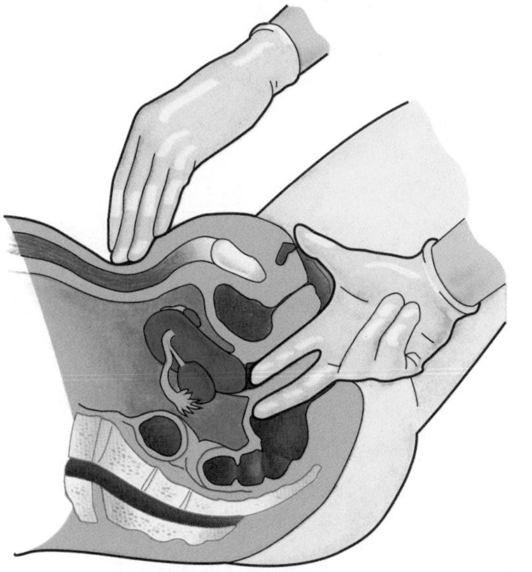

Fig. 5-17 Rectovaginal examination. (From Seidel HM et al: *Mosby's guide to physical examination,* ed 5, St Louis, 2003, Mosby.)

ally transmitted infections, mammogram, tuberculosis skin testing, hearing, visual acuity, electrocardiogram, chest x-ray, pulmonary function, fecal occult blood, flexible sigmoidoscopy, and bone mineral density (DEXA scan). Tests for HIV, hepatitis B, and drug screening may be offered with informed consent in high risk populations.

Community Focus

REFERRAL RESOURCES

Analyze resources in your community for referring the following women: a woman desiring tattoo removal; a lesbian who has just lost her partner to acquired immunodeficiency syndrome (AIDS) and is in need of counseling; a teenager with a body mass index (BMI) greater than 30 desiring a fitness program. Evaluate the resources in terms of access, confidentiality, cost, and follow-up services. Develop a resource file for each.

Key Points

- Normal feedback regulation of the menstrual cycle depends on an intact hypothalamic-pituitary-gonadal mechanism.
- The female's reproductive tract structures and breasts respond predictably to changing levels of sex steroids across her life span.
- The myometrium of the uterus is uniquely designed to expel the fetus and promote hemostasis after birth.
- Health promotion and prevention assist women to actualize health potential by increasing motivation, providing information, and suggesting how to access specific resources.
- Periodic health screening, including history, physical examination, and diagnostic and laboratory tests, provides the basis for overall health promotion, prevention of illness, early diagnosis of problems, and referral for management.
- Monthly breast self-examination, routine screening mammography, and yearly breast examinations by practitioners are recommended for early detection of breast cancer.

Answer Guidelines to Critical Thinking Exercise

Caring for a Woman with a Physical Disability

1. Although the nurse practitioner (NP) will need to do an assessment of Giana's capabilities, it is probable that the physical examination and pelvic examination can be performed with a minimum of discomfort by progressing slowly and checking with Giana about the easiest way for her to move and position herself.
2. (a) Any obstacles in the clinic setting that would prevent patients with disabilities from receiving appropriate care must be removed. (b) The nurse's usual assessment procedure will need to be modified to accommodate Giana's disability; that is, Giana cannot assume the lithotomy position for the pelvic examination and an alternative position will need to be used. (c) The NP needs to be cognizant of a variety of positions for performing a pelvic examination. (d) Giana is the best person to inform the nurse what accommodations must be made to enable the NP to provide appropriate care.
3. Giana needs to have the examination; she has expressed her willingness to have the examination by coming to the clinic. Reduction of anxiety and fear will be necessary to

enable Giana to relax for the examination. Informing her of what is to happen each step of the way will assist in reducing anxiety.

4. Yes. Women with disabilities need physical examinations for the same reasons as other women. Giana has a right to accessible health care. It is incumbent on health care providers to provide such care in the least restrictive environment.
5. It is possible that during Giana's first examination, her fear and anxiety interfered to such an extent that the health care provider was unable to perform a pelvic examination with a minimum of discomfort. In that case, it would have been better to reschedule the appointment and offer some patient education regarding the examination and anxiety reduction. Having a support person to accompany her might also be useful.

Resources

Integration of Prevention Services into Reproductive Health Services
Centers for Disease Control and Prevention
770-488-5227
www.cdc.gov/nccdphp/drh

Mental Health Education Campaigns
Depression awareness: 800-421-4211
Anxiety disorders: 888-8-ANXIETY
Panic disorders: 800-64-PANIC

National Council of Women's Organizations
Women's Health
1126 16th St., NW, Suite 411
Washington, DC 20036
202-331-7343
womensorganizations.org

National Women's Health Information Center
Office on Women's Health
Department of Health and Human Services
800-994-9662
www.4woman.gov

National Women's Health Resource Center
120 Albany St., Suite 820
New Brunswick, NJ 08901
877-986-9472
www.healthywomen.org

Office of Minority Health Resource Center
PO Box 37337
Washington, DC 20013-7337
301-587-1938

Society for Women's Health Research
1828 L St., NW, Suite 625
Washington, DC 20036
202-223-8224
www.womens-health.org

References

A drug of the past still haunts some, *Am J Nurs* 103[8]: 20, 2003.

Arias E et al: Annual summary of vital statistics—2002, *Pediatrics* 112(6 pt 1):1215-1230, 2003.

Barkauskas VH, Baumann LC, Darling-Fisher CS: *Health and physical assessment,* ed 3, St Louis, 2002, Mosby.

Edge V, Miller M: *Women's health care,* St Louis, 1994, Mosby.

Mattson S: Striving for cultural competence: providing care for the changing face of the U.S., *AWHONN Lifelines* 4(3):48-52, 2000a.

Mattson S: Providing culturally competent care: strategies and approaches for perinatal clients, *AWHONN Lifelines* 4(5):37-39, 2000b.

Miller D, Martin I, Herbison P: Interventions for relieving the pain and discomfort of screening mammography (Cochrane Review), 2003. In *The Cochrane Library,* Issue 2, Chichester, UK, 2004, John Wiley & Sons.

Seidel HM et al: *Mosby's guide to physical examination,* ed 5, St Louis, 2003, Mosby.

Stenchever MA et al: *Comprehensive gynecology,* ed 4, St Louis, 2001, Mosby.

Common Health Problems 6

LEARNING OBJECTIVES

On completion of this chapter the reader will be able to:

- Develop a nursing care plan for the woman with primary dysmenorrhea.
- Outline patient teaching about premenstrual syndrome.
- Relate the pathophysiology of endometriosis to associated symptoms.
- Evaluate the use of alternative therapies for menstrual disorders.
- Describe prevention and treatment of sexually transmitted infections in women.
- Summarize the care of women with selected viral infections (i.e., human immunodeficiency virus and hepatitis B virus).
- Differentiate signs, symptoms, and management of selected vaginal infections.
- Review principles of infection control for human immunodeficiency virus and blood-borne pathogens.
- Discuss the pathophysiology and emotional effects of selected benign breast conditions and malignant neoplasms of the breasts found in women.

ELECTRONIC RESOURCES

Additional information related to the content in Chapter 6 can be found on

the companion website at evolve
http://evolve.elsevier.com/Wong/maternal/
- NCLEX Review Questions
- Case Study–Breast Cancer
- WebLinks

or the interactive student CD-ROM
Activities for Chapter 6 include the following:
- NCLEX Review Questions
- Case Study–Breast Cancer
- Nursing Care Plan–Premenstrual Syndrome
- Nursing Care Plan–Breast Cancer

At some point in her lifetime the average woman is likely to have some concerns related to her menstrual and gynecologic health and will experience bleeding, pain, or discharge or infections associated with her reproductive organs or functions. This chapter provides information on common menstrual problems, sexually transmitted infections, and selected other infections that can affect reproductive functions. Benign breast conditions are also discussed. Breast cancer is also included as the most common reproductive cancer occurring in women.

MENSTRUAL DISORDERS

Normal menstrual patterns are averages based on observations and reports from large groups of healthy women. Generally a woman's menstrual frequency stabilizes at 28 days within 1 to 2 years after puberty, with a range of 26 to 34 days (Blackburn, 2003). Although no woman's cycle is exactly the same length every month, the typical month-to-month variation in an individual's cycle is usually plus or minus 2 days. However, greater but still normal variations are commonly noted.

Women typically have menstrual cycles for about 40 years. Once a cyclic, predictable pattern of monthly bleeding is established, women may worry about any deviation from that pattern or from what they have been told is normal for all menstruating women. A woman may be concerned about her ability to conceive and bear children or believe that she is not really a woman without monthly evidence. A sign such as amenorrhea or excess menstrual bleeding can be a source of severe distress and concern for a woman.

Amenorrhea

Amenorrhea, the absence of menstrual flow, is a clinical symptom of a variety of disorders. Generally, the following circumstances should be evaluated: (1) the absence of both menarche and secondary sexual characteristics by age 14 years; (2) the absence of menses by age 16, regardless of normal growth and development (primary amenorrhea); or (3) a 3- to 6-month cessation of menses after a period of menstruation (secondary amenorrhea) (Harlow, 2000).

Amenorrhea is most commonly the result of pregnancy. Although amenorrhea is not a disease, it is often a sign of disease. It may occur from any defect or interruption in the hypothalamic-pituitary-ovarian-uterine axis. It may also result from anatomic abnormalities; other endocrine disorders, such as hypothyroidism or hyperthyroidism; chronic diseases such as type 1 diabetes; medications, such as phenytoin (Dilantin); eating disorders; strenuous exercise; emotional stress; and oral contraceptive use.

Assessment of amenorrhea begins with a thorough history and physical examination. An important initial step is to be sure that the woman is not pregnant. Specific components of the assessment process depend on a patient's age—adolescent, young adult, or perimenopausal—and whether she has previously menstruated.

Hypogonadotropic Amenorrhea

Hypogonadotropic amenorrhea reflects a problem in the central hypothalamic-pituitary axis. In rare instances, a pituitary lesion or genetic inability to produce follicle-stimulating hormone (FSH) and luteinizing hormone (LH) is at fault. Once pregnancy has been ruled out by a β-human chorionic gonadotropin (hCG) pregnancy test, diagnostic tests may include FSH level, thyroid-stimulating hormone (TSH) and prolactin levels, radiographic or computed tomography scan of the sella turcica, and a progestational challenge (Hall, 2002).

Hypogonadotropic amenorrhea often results from hypothalamic suppression as a result of stress (in the home, school, or workplace) or a sudden and severe weight loss, eating disorders, strenuous exercise, or mental illness (Parent-Stevens & Burns, 2000). Research on the interaction between nervous system or neurotransmitter functions and hormonal regulation throughout the body has demonstated a biologic basis for the relation of stress to physiologic processes. Women who are more than 20% underweight for height or who have had rapid weight loss may report amenorrhea, as may women with eating disorders such as anorexia nervosa (Alexander, Shrimp, & Smith, 2000; Parent-Stevens & Burns, 2000). Amenorrhea is one of the classic signs of anorexia nervosa, and the interrelation of disordered eating, amenorrhea, and premature osteoporosis has been described as the female athlete triad (Kleposki, 2002; Sabatini, 2001). A loss of calcium from the bone, comparable to that seen in postmenopausal women, may occur with this type of amenorrhea.

Exercise-associated amenorrhea can occur in women undergoing vigorous physical and athletic training (Sanborn et al, 2000) and is thought to be associated with many factors, including body composition (height, weight, and percentage of body fat); type, intensity, and frequency of exercise; nutritional status; and presence of emotional or physical stressors (Kleposki, 2002). Women who participate in sports emphasizing low body weight are at greatest risk, including dance, gymnastics, and figure skating (sports in which scoring is subjective and prepubertal body shape favors success); distance running and cycling (endurance sports that favor low body weight); swimming, diving, and volleyball (in which body contour–revealing clothing is worn); and rowing and martial arts (which have weight categories) (Sabatini, 2001).

Management

When amenorrhea is due to hypothalamic disturbances, the nurse is an ideal health professional to assist women because many of the causes are potentially reversible (e.g., stress, weight loss for nonorganic reasons). Counseling and education are interventions and appropriate nursing roles. When a stressor known to predispose a woman to hypothalamic amenorrhea is identified, initial management involves addressing the stressor. Together the woman and nurse plan how the woman can decrease or discontinue medications known to affect menstruation, correct weight loss, deal more effectively with psychologic stress, address emotional distress, and alter exercise routine.

The nurse works with the woman to help her identify, cope with, and eliminate sources of stress in her life. Deep-breathing exercises and relaxation techniques are simple yet effective stress-reduction measures. Referral for biofeedback or massage therapy also may be useful. In some instances, referrals for psychotherapy may be indicated.

If a woman's exercise program is thought to contribute to her amenorrhea, several options exist for management. She may decide to decrease the intensity or duration of her training or to gain 2% to 3% in body weight. Accepting this alternative may be difficult for one who is committed to a strenuous exercise regimen. The woman and nurse may have several sessions before the woman elects to try exercise reduction. Many young female athletes may not understand the consequences of low bone density or osteoporosis; nurses can point out the connection between low bone density and stress fractures. The nurse and woman should also investigate other factors that may be contributing to the amenorrhea and develop plans for altering lifestyle and decreasing stress.

A daily calcium intake of 1200 to 1500 mg, accomplished by drinking three glasses of skim milk or by taking a calcium supplement, is recommended for women experiencing amenorrhea associated with the female athlete triad (West, 1998).

Dysmenorrhea

Dysmenorrhea, pain during or shortly before menstruation, is one of the most common gynecologic problems in women of all ages. Most adolescents have dysmenorrhea in the first 3 years after menarche. Young adult women ages 17 to 24 years are most likely to report painful menses. Dysmenorrhea improves in most women after a full-term pregnancy. Between 30% and 40% of women report some level of discomfort associated with menses, and 7% to 15% report severe dysmenorrhea (Parent-Stevens & Burns, 2000). The amount of disruption caused in women's lives, however, is difficult to determine. It has been estimated that up to 10% of women with dysmenorrhea have pain severe enough to interfere with their functioning for 1 to 3 days a month. Menstrual problems, including dysmenorrhea, are more common in women who smoke and who are obese. Traditionally dysmenorrhea is differentiated as primary or secondary. Symptoms usually begin with menstruation, although some women have discomfort several hours before onset of flow. The range and severity of symptoms differ from woman to woman and from cycle to cycle in the same woman. Symptoms of dysmenorrhea may last several hours or several days.

Primary Dysmenorrhea

Primary dysmenorrhea, a condition associated with abnormally increased uterine activity, is due to myometrium contractions induced by prostaglandins in the second half of the menstrual cycle. During the luteal phase and subsequent menstrual flow, prostaglandin $F_{2\alpha}$ ($PGF_{2\alpha}$) is secreted. The uterine muscle of both normal and dysmenorrheic women is sensitive to prostaglandins; however, the amount of prostaglandin produced is the major differentiating factor (Stenchever et al, 2001). Excessive release of $PGF_{2\alpha}$ increases the amplitude and frequency of uterine contractions and causes vasospasm of the uterine arterioles, resulting in ischemia and cyclic lower abdominal cramps. Systemic responses to $PGF_{2\alpha}$ include backache, weakness, sweating, gastrointestinal symptoms (anorexia, nausea, vomiting, and diarrhea), and central nervous system symptoms (dizziness, syncope, headache, and poor concentration). Pain begins at the onset of menstrual flow and lasts from 8 to 48 hours. The release of most prostaglandins during menstruation occurs in the first 48 hours, which coincides with the greatest intensity of symptoms (Stenchever et al, 2001).

Primary dysmenorrhea is not caused by underlying pathology. Rather, it is the occurrence of a physiologic alteration in some women. Primary dysmenorrhea usually appears within 6 to 12 months after menarche when ovulation is established. Anovulatory bleeding, common in the first few months or years after menarche, is painless. Because both estrogen and progesterone are necessary for primary dysmenorrhea to occur, it is experienced only with ovulatory cycles. This problem is most common in women in their late teens and early twenties; the incidence declines with age.

Management

Management of primary dysmenorrhea depends on the severity of the problem and an individual woman's response to various treatments. Information and support are important components of nursing care. Because menstruation is so closely linked to reproduction and sexuality, menstrual problems can have a negative influence on sexuality and self-worth. Nurses can correct myths and misinformation about menstruation and dysmenorrhea by providing facts about what is normal.

Often more than one alternative for alleviating menstrual discomfort and dysmenorrhea can be offered. Women can then try options and decide which ones work best for them. Heat (heating pad or hot bath) minimizes cramping by increasing vasodilation and muscle relaxation and minimizing uterine ischemia. Massaging the lower back can reduce pain by relaxing paravertebral muscles and increasing pelvic blood supply. Soft rhythmic rubbing of the abdomen (effleurage) may be useful because it provides distraction and an alternative focal point. Guided imagery, progressive relaxation, hatha yoga, and meditation also have been used successfully to decrease menstrual discomfort (Fig. 6-1).

Exercise helps relieve menstrual discomfort through increased vasodilation and subsequent decreased ischemia; release of endogenous opiates, specifically β-endorphins; suppression of prostaglandins; and shunting of blood flow away from the viscera, resulting in less pelvic congestion. Specific exercises that nurses can suggest to their patients include pelvic rock and the heels-over-the-head yoga position.

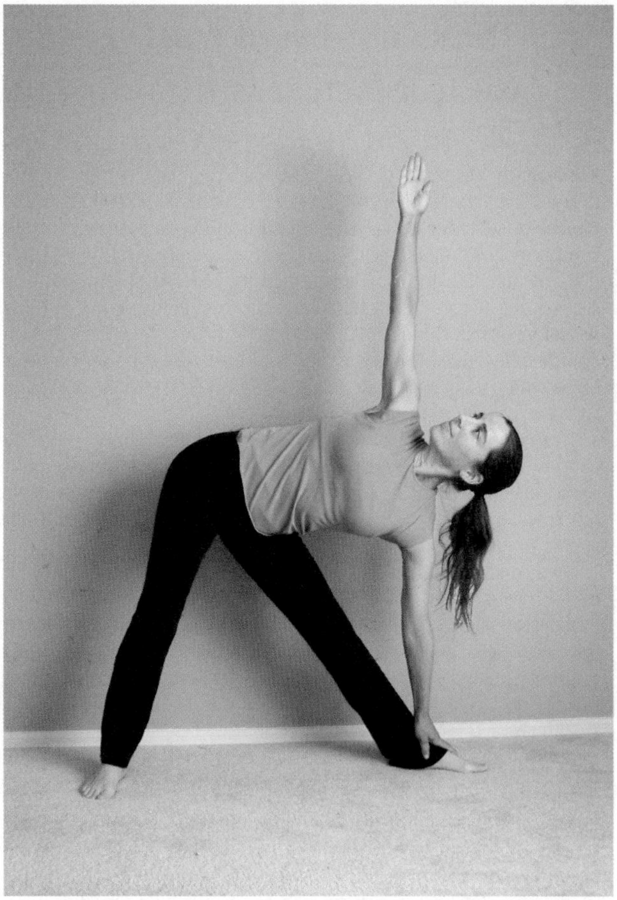

Fig. 6-1 Yoga asana: triangle pose. Helpful for assisting digestion and for stretching and strengthening the spine; also used for dysmenorrhea and pelvic congestion. (Courtesy Julie Perry Nelson, Gilbert, AZ.)

In addition to maintaining good nutrition at all times, specific dietary changes may be helpful in decreasing some of the systemic symptoms associated with dysmenorrhea. Decreased salt and refined sugar intake in the 7 to 10 days before expected menses may reduce fluid retention. Increasing water intake may serve as a natural diuretic. Natural diuretics such as asparagus, cranberry juice, peaches, parsley, and watermelon may help reduce edema and related discomforts. Decreasing red meat intake and switching to a low-fat diet may also help minimize dysmenorrheal symptoms.

Medications used to treat primary dysmenorrhea in women not desiring contraception include prostaglandin synthesis inhibitors, primarily nonsteroidal antiinflammatory drugs (NSAIDs) (Parent-Stevens & Burns, 2000) (Table 6-1). NSAIDs are effective if begun 2 to 3 days before menses or with the first sign of bleeding. This regimen decreases the possibility of a woman taking these drugs early in pregnancy (Stenchever et al, 2001). Often if one NSAID is ineffective, a different one will be effective. All NSAIDs have potential gastrointestinal side effects, including nausea, vomiting, and indigestion. All women taking NSAIDs should be warned to report dark-colored stools, which may be an indication of gastrointestinal bleeding. Women with a history of aspirin sensitivity or allergy should avoid all NSAIDs. Approximately 80% of dysmenorrheic women obtain relief with prostaglandin inhibitors.

Evidence-Based Practice

TENS AND ACUPUNCTURE AS ALTERNATIVE THERAPY FOR DYSMENORRHEA

Background

Dysmenorrhea affects up to half of all childbearing-aged women, significantly decreasing productivity and quality of life. Primary dysmenorrhea occurs in the absence of organic pathology, with a typical onset coinciding with establishment of ovulatory cycles. Symptoms, often incapacitating, occur during the first two to three days of menstrual flow. Medical treatment for dysmenorrhea decreases the uterine muscle spasms and resulting painful ischemia by using nonsteroidal antiinflammatory drugs (NSAIDs) and oral contraceptive pills. Additional alternative therapies provide options for women who experience side effects with medical therapy, or who prefer nonpharmacologic treatment.

Transcutaneous electrical nerve stimulation (TENS) has been used to provide noninvasive pain relief for certain types of chronic pain. Low-frequency stimulation (1-4 HZ) of the skin causes rhythmic muscle contractions. High-frequency stimulation (50-120 HZ) seems to alter the sensation of pain.

Acupuncture is the 2500-year-old traditional Chinese practice of balancing Qi (life force energy) by inserting needles into skin and tissues at exact points. Western explanations of its mechanism have included neurologic, neurohormonal, and/or psychologic hypotheses. Like TENS, acupuncture also seems to block pain impulses, and is now recommended by the National Institutes of Health as a treatment for dysmenorrhea. Few adverse reactions (pneumothorax, infection, cardiac injury) have been reported.

Objective

The reviewers sought to compare the efficacy of TENS and acupuncture as alternatives to medical therapy for relief of the pain of primary dysmenorrhea. They wished to compare high- and low-frequency TENS, acupuncture, placebo, control, and medical treatment. Participants would have severe primary dysmenorrhea in greater than half their cycles. Outcome measures included pain levels, adverse effects, additional medication requirements, daily activity restrictions, and absences from school or work.

Methods

Search Strategy

Reviewers searched the Menstrual Disorders and Subfertility Group's Specialized Register, MEDLINE, EMBASE, CINAHL, Bio Abstracts, Psyclit, SPORTDiscus, the National Research Register, the Clinical Trials Register, and the Cochrane Complementary Medicine Field's register, and several TENS and acupuncture investigators. Keywords included *dysmenorrhea, pelvic pain, TENS, nerve stimulation,* and *acupuncture.*

The reviewers accepted nine randomized, controlled trials, representing 217 women from the United States and Sweden. Four were of a crossover design, where the intervention was switched in the same subject at some point, enabling the woman to become her own control.

For TENS placebos, investigators placed electrodes and told the subjects that they were getting ultra-high frequencies, and may not feel them. Placebo acupuncture groups received needles in noncritical areas. Controls received no intervention. The outcome was pain, measured by subjective scales.

Statistical Analyses

Similar data were pooled. Reviewers calculated relative risks for dichotomous (categorical) data, and weighted mean differences for continuous data. Results outside the 95% confidence interval were accepted as significantly different.

Findings

High-frequency TENS (HF-TENS) was significantly more effective at relieving pain and decreasing analgesia use when compared to low-frequency TENS, placebo, and control. Ibuprofen provided significantly better pain relief than HF-TENS. There was no difference in pain between the group given naproxen and HF-TENS.

Pain relief was significantly greater with the acupuncture than placebo or control groups.

No study compared TENS to acupuncture.

One trial reported adverse effects of TENS in 4 out of 32 women: muscle vibrations and tightness, headaches, and slight skin redness or burning. No adverse effects were noted with placebo TENS.

Limitations

These trials included a very small number of subjects and wide confidence intervals, which greatly limits their generalizability. Primary dysmenorrhea is a diagnosis of exclusion, and some of the studies did not rule out organic causes by examination. Concealment of treatment allocation was nearly impossible, although some deception was possible with naïve subjects within groups. The studies that used sham (placebo) TENS and acupuncture may actually have caused some unintended stimulation that confounds the results. TENS administration was not standardized. Acupuncture results may vary by the skill of the practitioner.

Conclusions

HF-TENS relieves pain and decreases analgesia use; however, Ibuprofen provided significantly better pain relief than HF-TENS. Acupuncture relieved more pain than a placebo. There were few adverse effects.

Implications for Practice

Alternative therapy is particularly important for women who have side effects with medical therapy, and may be beneficial as complementary treatment. This review establishes measurable benefits of TENS and acupuncture for the relief of primary dysmenorrhea, with few adverse reactions.

Implications for Further Research

Larger randomized, controlled trials can give more information about dose and frequency of TENS and acupuncture. Comparison of the two methods and other complementary and alternative medicine therapies may demonstrate some potentiation of pain relief with certain combinations. Pain relief measures for dysmenorrhea may generalize to other forms of ischemic pain.

Reference

Proctor ML et al: Transcutaneous electrical nerve stimulation and acupuncture for primary dysmenorrhea (Cochrane Review). In *The Cochrane Database of Systematic Reviews,* Issue 1, 2002, Chichester, UK, John Wiley & Sons.

Oral contraceptive pills (OCPs) are a reasonable choice for women who do not want to become pregnant. The benefits of OCP use are attributed to decreased prostaglandin synthesis associated with an atrophic decidualized endometrium (Stenchever et al, 2001). No single OCP has been shown to be superior to another for the relief of primary dysmenorrhea. Although generally prescribed on a 21-day cycle of hormones, followed by 7 hormone-free days, OCPs can be used continuously in an attempt to produce amenorrhea if women have severe dysmenorrhea during withdrawal bleeding. Since OCPs have side effects, women may not wish to use them for dysmenorrhea. OCPs may be contraindicated for some women. (See Chapter 7 for a complete discussion of OCPs.)

Table 6-1

Medications Used to Treat Dysmenorrhea

DRUG	COMMON SIDE EFFECTS*	COMMENTS
Diclofenac (Cataflam Rx)	Nausea, diarrhea, constipation, abdominal distress, dyspepsia, flatulence.	Enteric coated: immediate release.
Fenoprofen† (Nalfon Rx)	Nausea, diarrhea, constipation, abdominal distress, dyspepsia, flatulence.	Use for mild to moderate pain only if other NSAIDs are not effective; take with meals; avoid alcohol.
Ibuprofen (Motrin Rx) (Advil OTC, Nuprin OTC, Motrin IB OTC)	Nausea, dyspepsia, rash, pruritus.	If GI upset occurs, take with food, milk, or antacids; avoid alcoholic beverages; do not take with aspirin.
Ketoprofen (Orudis Rx) (Orudis KT OTC) (Actron OTC)	Nausea, diarrhea, constipation, abdominal distress, dyspepsia, flatulence.	See ibuprofen.
Meclofenamate (Meclomen Rx)	Dizziness, headache, severe diarrhea, nausea, abnormal liver function tests.	See ibuprofen.
Mefenamic acid (Ponstel Rx)	Severe diarrhea, nausea, and vomiting.	Very potent and effective prostaglandin-synthesis inhibitor. Antagonizes already formed prostaglandins. Increased incidence of adverse GI side effects.
Naproxen (Naprosyn Rx)	See ibuprofen.	See ibuprofen.
Naproxen sodium (Anaprox Rx) (Aleve OTC)	See ibuprofen.	See ibuprofen.

Sources: Facts and Comparisons: *Loose-leaf drug information service*, St Louis, 2002, Facts and Comparisons; Parent-Stevens L, Burns E: Menstrual disorders. In Smith M, Shimp L (eds): *20 common problems in women's health care*, New York, 2000, McGraw-Hill.

NOTE: For all NSAIDs: Do not give if patient has hemophilia or bleeding ulcers; do not give if patient has had an allergic or anaphylactic reaction to aspirin or another NSAID; do not give if patient is taking anticoagulant medication.

*Risk with all NSAIDs is gastrointestinal ulceration, possible bleeding, and prolonged bleeding time. Incidence of side effects is dose related. Reported incidence, 3% to 9%.

†Unlabeled indications for use in treating dysmenorrhea.

Rx, prescription; *OTC*, over-the-counter; *GI*, gastrointestinal.

Community Focus

ALTERNATIVE THERAPIES FOR MENSTRUAL PROBLEMS

Review the literature for studies determining effectiveness of alternative therapies for menstrual problems. Identify therapies that have been shown to be beneficial, are likely to be beneficial, have unknown effects, or have effects that are likely not to be beneficial or may be harmful. Visit a pharmacy, health food store, and a nutritional supplement outlet. Are the therapies available in these locations? Are there patient warnings clearly identified on labels? Observe customers. Are there more men or women? Did any of the women purchase any of the therapies you identified?

Over-the-counter (OTC) preparations that are indicated for primary dysmenorrhea contain the same active ingredients (e.g., ibuprofen or naproxen sodium) as prescription preparations. However, the labeled recommended dose may be subtherapeutic. Preparations containing acetaminophen are even less effective because acetaminophen does not have the antiprostaglandin properties of NSAIDs.

Herbal preparations have long been used for management of menstrual problems, including dysmenorrhea (Table 6-2). Herbal medicines may be valuable in treating dysmenorrhea. However, it is essential that women understand that these therapies are not without potential toxicity and may cause drug interactions.

NURSE ALERT Nurses must routinely ask women about use of herbal and other alternative therapies and document their use. ■

Secondary Dysmenorrhea

Secondary dysmenorrhea is menstrual pain that develops later in life than primary dysmenorrhea, typically after age 25. It is associated with pelvic pathology such as adenomyosis, endometriosis, pelvic inflammatory disease, endometrial polyps, or submucous or interstitial myomas (fibroids). Women with secondary dysmenorrhea often have other symptoms that may suggest the underlying cause. For example, heavy menstrual flow with dysmenorrhea suggests a diagnosis of leiomyomata, adenomyosis, or

Table 6-2

Herbal Medicinals Taken Orally for Menstrual Disorders

SYMPTOMS/ INDICATIONS	HERBAL	ACTION	CONTRAINDICATIONS	ADVERSE REACTIONS	DRUG INTERACTIONS
Menstrual cramping	Black haw	Uterine anti-spasmodic; β_2-agonist activity	None known	None known	None known
Premenstrual discomfort (anxiety, tension, depression), dysmenorrhea	Black cohosh root	Estrogen-like LH suppressant, binds to estrogen receptors	Pregnancy	Gastric irritation, CNS side effects at high doses	None known
Tension, breast pain	Bugleweed	Antigonadotropic, antithyrotropic, decreased prolactin levels	Thyroid disease	Thyroid enlargement with prolonged high dose	Interferes with diagnostic radioactive isotopes
Mastodynia, premenstrual discomfort, menstrual cycle irregularities	Chaste tree fruit	Decreased prolactin levels	None known	Itching, urticaria	Possible antagonism of dopaminergic antagonists
Menstrual cramping	Ginger	Antiinflammatory			
Dysmenorrhea	Potentilla	Increased tonus and contraction frequency in uterus	Pregnancy and lactation	Gastric irritation	None known
Menorrhea and metrorrhagia	Shepard's purse	Increased uterine contractions	None known	None known	None known
Dysmenorrhea	Dong quai	Stimulate/relax uterus; antiinflammatory; possibly analgesic activity	Phototoxicity Liver and renal damage in animal studies Abortifacient	Pregnancy	Coumarin components may increase risk of bleeding

Sources: Bascom A: *Incorporating herbal medicine into clinical practice,* Philadelphia, 2002, FA Davis; Fugh-Berman A, Awang D: Black cohosh, *Altern Ther Womens Health* 39(11):81-85, 2001; Dog L: *An integrative approach to dysmenorrhea,* Corrales, NM, 2000, Integrative Medicine Education Association; Dog L: *Endocrinology and women's issues,* Third Annual Conference on Clinical Relevance of Medicinal Herbs and Nutritional Supplements in the Management of Major Medical Problems, September 21-23, 2001; Schellenberg R: Treatment for the premenstrual syndrome with *Agnus castus* fruit extract: prospective, randomized, placebo controlled study, *BMJ* 322(7279):134-137, 2001; Stevinson C, Ernst E: Complementary/alternative therapies for premenstrual syndrome: a systemic review of random controlled trials, *Am J Obstet Gynecol* 185(1):227-235, 2001.
CNS, central nervous system; *LH,* luteinizing hormone.

endometrial polyps. Pain associated with endometriosis often begins a few days before menses, but can be present at ovulation and continue through the first days of menses or start after menstrual flow has begun. In contrast to primary dysmenorrhea, the pain of secondary dysmenorrhea is often characterized by dull, lower abdominal aching that radiates to the back or thighs. Often women experience feelings of bloating or pelvic fullness. In addition to a physical examination with a careful pelvic examination, diagnosis may be assisted by ultrasound examination, dilation and curettage (D&C), endometrial biopsy, or laparoscopy. Treatment is directed toward removal of the underlying pathology. Many of the measures described for pain relief of primary dysmenorrhea are also helpful for women with secondary dysmenorrhea.

Premenstrual Syndrome

Premenstrual sundrome (PMS) is a complex, poorly understood condition that includes a number of cyclic symptoms occurring in the luteal phase of the menstrual cycle. Estimates of the number of women with some degree of problems related to their menstrual cycle range from 5% to 95%, with 40% of women reporting some degree of disruption of their daily activities (Cronje & Studd, 2002; Lin & Thompson, 2001; Stenchever et al, 2001). All age groups are affected, with women in their twenties and thirties most often reporting symptoms. Ovarian function is necessary for the condition to occur. PMS does not occur before puberty, after menopause, or during pregnancy. The condition is not dependent on the presence of monthly menses, because women who have had a hysterectomy

Critical Thinking Exercise

UTERINE FIBROIDS AND PREGNANCY

Tracy, a 30-year-old married woman, has been diagnosed with large uterine fibroids. She had experienced dysmenorrhea until she started using Depo-Provera as a contraceptive. She and her husband are now considering starting a family. Her physician informed her that she might have trouble getting pregnant and maintaining the pregnancy with her fibroids and recommended that she have the fibroids removed before trying to get pregnant. She has come to her nurse practitioner (NP) for information and advice. What information and advice should the nurse practitioner provide?

1. Evidence—Is there sufficient evidence to draw conclusions about what advice the NP should provide?
2. Assumptions—Describe underlying assumptions about each of the following topics:
   a. The relationship between uterine fibroids and pregnancy
   b. The risks of surgery to remove uterine fibroids
   c. The effects of Depo-Provera on ovulation and dysmenorrhea
3. What implications and priorities for nursing care can be drawn at this time?
4. Does the evidence objectively support your conclusion?
5. Are there alternative perspectives to your conclusion?

without bilateral salpingo-oophorectomy still can have cyclic symptoms.

It is difficult to establish a universal definition of PMS because so many symptoms have been associated with the condition. At least two different syndromes have been recognized: PMS and premenstrual dysphoric disorder (PDD). PMS is a cluster of physical, psychologic, and behavioral symptoms (more than 100) beginning in the luteal phase of the menstrual cycle, occurring to such a degree that lifestyle or work is affected, and followed by a symptom-free period. Symptoms include fluid retention (abdominal bloating, pelvic fullness, edema of the lower extremities, breast tenderness, and weight gain); behavioral or emotional changes (depression, crying spells, irritability, panic attacks, and impaired ability to concentrate); premenstrual cravings (sweets, salt, increased appetite, and food binges); and headache, fatigue, and backache. PDD is a more severe variant of PMS in which women have marked irritability, dysphoria, mood lability, anxiety, fatigue, appetite changes, and a sense of feeling overwhelmed (Elliot, 2002).

A diagnosis of PMS is made only if the following criteria are met:

- Symptoms occur in the luteal phase and resolve within a few days of onset of menses.
- A symptom-free period occurs in the follicular phase.
- Symptoms are recurrent.

Readers are encouraged to explore current feminist, medical, and social science literature for more information on PMS.

Management

There is little agreement on management. A careful, detailed history and daily log of symptoms and mood fluctuations spanning several cycles may give direction to a plan of management. Any changes that assist a woman with PMS to exert control over her life have a positive impact.

Education is an important component of the management of PMS. Nurses can advise women that self-help modalities often result in significant symptom improvement. Women have found a number of complementary and alternative therapies to be useful in managing the symptoms of PMS. Diet and exercise changes are a useful way to begin and provide symptom relief for some women. Nurses can suggest that patients not smoke and limit their consumption of refined sugar (less than 5 tbsp/day), salt (less than 3 g/day), red meat (less than 3 oz/day), alcohol (less than 1 oz/day), and caffeinated beverages.

Patients can be encouraged to include whole grains, legumes, seeds, nuts, vegetables, fruits, and vegetable oils in their diet. Use of natural diuretics (see the section on dysmenorrhea management earlier in this chapter) may help reduce fluid retention. Nutritional supplements may assist in symptom relief. Calcium (1000 to 1200 mg/day), magnesium (300 to 400 mg/day), and vitamin E (100 to 150 mg/day) have been shown to be moderately effective in relieving symptoms, to have few side effects, and to be safe. Daily supplements of evening primrose oil are thought to relieve breast symptoms with minimal side effects.

Regular exercise (aerobic exercise three to four times a week), especially in the luteal phase, is widely recommended for relief of PMS symptoms. A monthly program that varies in intensity and type of exercise according to PMS symptoms is best. Women who exercise regularly seem to have less premenstrual anxiety than nonathletic women. It is thought that aerobic exercise increases β-endorphin levels to offset symptoms of depression and to elevate mood.

Yoga, acupuncture, hypnosis, chiropractic therapy, and massage therapy have all been reported to have a beneficial effect on the woman with PMS. Herbal therapies have long been used to treat PMS; specific suggestions are found in Table 6-2.

Counseling, in the form of support groups or individual or couple counseling, may be helpful. Stress-reduction techniques may also assist with symptom management.

Community Focus

PREMENSTRUAL SYNDROME IN ADOLESCENTS

Premenstrual syndrome (PMS) is characterized by physical, psychologic, and behavioral changes that are severe enough to interfere with daily activities and interpersonal relationships. Almost 30% of women have PMS, and 14% to 88% of adolescent girls have symptoms that are moderate to severe. Older adolescents have more severe symptoms than do younger adolescents. Nurses in schools and clinics will encounter adolescents with symptoms of PMS. They can assist the adolescent to keep a symptom diary and counsel her to decrease salt, caffeine, alcohol, and simple carbohydrate intake. They can advise incorporation of aerobic exercise into the adolescent's daily routine and recommend alternative therapies for symptom relief. Counseling and stress management may also assist in reducing symptoms. Creating a special support group for adolescents with symptoms of PMS would be beneficial.

Data from Clark LR: Premenstrual syndrome, *eMedicine Specialties,* February 18, 2004. Internet document available at www.emedicine.com (accessed July 14, 2004).

Nursing Care Plan

PREMENSTRUAL SYNDROME

NURSING DIAGNOSIS: Pain related to cyclic breast changes as evidenced by patient report

EXPECTED OUTCOME
Patient will report a decrease in the intensity of pain or discomfort following interventions.

NURSING INTERVENTIONS/*RATIONALES*
Assess timing and intensity of pain or discomfort *to validate relationship to cyclic changes.*
Administer hormonal medications or diuretics if prescribed *to minimize breast tenderness.*
Suggest that patient wear a supportive bra *to minimize breast tenderness.*

NURSING DIAGNOSIS: Situational low self-esteem related to cyclic hormonal changes as evidenced by patient verbal report

EXPECTED OUTCOME
Patient will report increased number of feelings of self-worth.

NURSING INTERVENTIONS/*RATIONALES*
Provide therapeutic communication *to validate patient feelings of depression and mood swings.*
Encourage patient to limit caffeine intake and eat small, frequent meals *to lessen irritability aggravated by caffeine and hypoglycemia.*
Refer patient to support groups *to encourage the sharing of experiences, feelings, and self-help tips.*

NURSING DIAGNOSIS: Excess fluid volume related to cyclic hormonal influences as evidenced by weight gain before start of menstrual period

EXPECTED OUTCOME
Patient will report no significant changes in body weight before start of menstrual period.

NURSING INTERVENTIONS/*RATIONALES*
Encourage patient to limit intake of salt- and sodium-containing foods *to decrease fluid retention.*
Administer diuretics as prescribed *to facilitate fluid excretion.*

If these strategies do not provide significant symptom relief in 1 to 2 months, medication is often begun. Many medications have been used in treatment of PMS, but no single medication alleviates all PMS symptoms. Medications often used in the treatment of PMS include diuretics, prostaglandin inhibitors (NSAIDs), progesterone, and OCPs. Fluoxetine (Sarafem or Prozac), a selective serotonin reuptake inhibitor (SSRI), is the only Food and Drug Administration (FDA)–approved agent for PMS. Use of this medication results in a decrease in emotional symptoms, especially depression (Jones, 2001; Lin & Thompson, 2001) (Nursing Care Plan).

Endometriosis

Endometriosis is characterized by the presence and growth of endometrial tissue outside of the uterus. The tissue may be implanted on the ovaries, cul-de-sac, uterine ligaments, rectovaginal septum, sigmoid colon, pelvic peritoneum, cervix, and inguinal area (Fig. 6-2). Endometrial lesions have been found in the vagina and surgical scars, as well as on the vulva, perineum, and bladder. Lesions have also been found on sites far from the pelvic area such as the thoracic cavity, gallbladder, and heart. A cystic lesion of endometriosis found in the ovary is sometimes described as a chocolate cyst because of the dark coloring of the contents of the cyst caused by the presence of old blood.

Endometrial tissue contains glands and stoma and responds to cyclic hormonal stimulation in the same way that the uterine endometrium does but often out of phase with it. The endometrial tissue grows during the proliferative and secretory phases of the cycle. During or immediately after menstruation, the tissue bleeds, resulting in an inflammatory response with subsequent fibrosis and adhesions to adjacent organs.

The overall incidence of endometriosis is 5% to 15% in reproductive-age women, 30% to 45% in infertile women, and 33% in women with chronic pelvic pain (Stenchever et al, 2001). Although the condition usually develops in the

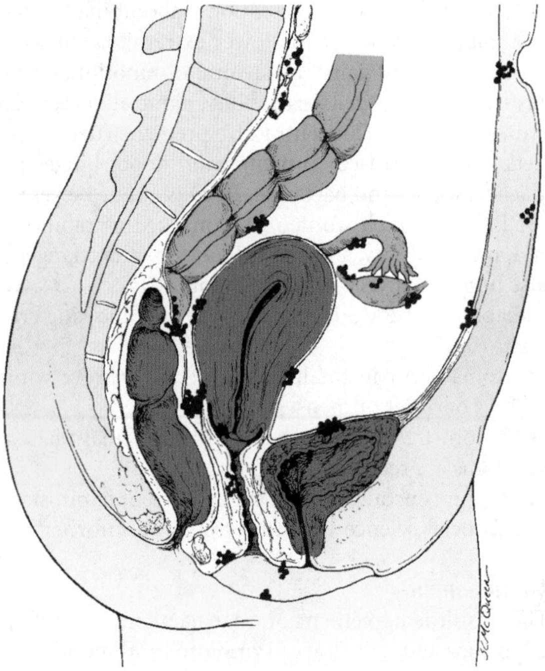

Fig. 6-2 Common sites of endometriosis. (From Stenchever M et al: *Comprehensive gynecology,* ed 4, St Louis, 2001, Mosby.)

third or fourth decade of life, endometriosis has been found in adolescents with disabling pelvic pain or abnormal vaginal bleeding. Endometriosis may worsen with repeated cycles, or it may remain asymptomatic and undiagnosed, eventually disappearing after menopause. The condition appears equally in Caucasian, African-American, and Asian women (Nakad & Isaacson, 2002). It occurs across all socioeconomic levels. There appears to be a familial tendency to develop endometriosis.

Several theories of the cause of endometriosis have been suggested. However, the etiology and pathology of this condition continue to be poorly understood. One of the most widely accepted theories is transplantation or retrograde menstruation. According to this theory, endometrial tissue is refluxed through the uterine tubes during menstruation into the peritoneal cavity, where it implants on the ovaries and other organs. Retrograde menstruation has been documented in a number of surgical studies and is estimated to occur in 96% of menstruating women. For most women, endometrial tissue outside the uterus is destroyed before it can implant or seed in the peritoneal cavity or elsewhere.

Symptoms, from nonexistent to incapacitating, vary among women. Severity of symptoms can change over time and may not reflect the extent of the disease. The major symptoms of endometriosis are dysmenorrhea and deep pelvic dyspareunia (painful intercourse). Women also have chronic noncyclic pelvic pain, pelvic heaviness, or pain radiating into the thighs. Many women report bowel symptoms such as diarrhea, pain with defecation, and constipation caused by avoiding defecation because of the pain. Less common symptoms include abnormal bleeding (hypermenorrhea, menorrhagia, or premenstrual staining) and pain during exercise as a result of adhesions.

Impaired fertility may result from adhesions around the uterus that pull the uterus into a fixed, retroverted position. Adhesions around the uterine tubes may block the fimbriated ends or prevent the spontaneous movement that carries the ovum to the uterus or blocks the fimbriated ends.

Management

Treatment is based on the severity of symptoms and the goals of the woman or couple. Women without pain who do not want to become pregnant need no treatment. In women with mild pain who may desire a future pregnancy, treatment may be limited to use of NSAIDs during menstruation (see earlier discussion of these medications).

Suppression of endogenous estrogen production and subsequent endometrial lesion growth is the cornerstone of management of the disease. Two main classes of medications are currently used to suppress endogenous estrogen levels: gonadotropin-releasing hormone (GnRH) agonists and androgen derivatives. GnRH agonist therapy (leuprolide [Lupron] or nafarelin [Synarel]) acts by suppressing pituitary gonadotropin secretion. FSH and LH stimulation of the ovary declines markedly, and ovarian function decreases significantly. A medically induced menopause develops, resulting in anovulation and amenorrhea. Shrinkage of already established endometrial tissue, significant pain relief, and an interruption in further lesion development follow. The hypoestrogenism results in hot flashes in almost all women. Trabecular bone loss is common, although most loss is reversible within 12 to 18 months after the medication is stopped. Both leuprolide (3.75 mg intramuscular injection given once a month) and nafarelin (200 mg administered twice daily by nasal spray) are effective and well tolerated. Both medications reduce endometrial lesions and pelvic pain associated with endometriosis and have posttreatment pregnancy rates similar to that of danazol therapy (Stenchever et al, 2001). Common side effects of these drugs are those of natural menopause—hot flashes and vaginal dryness. Occasionally women report headaches and muscle aches. Treatment is usually limited to 6 months to minimize bone loss. Although unlikely, it is possible for a woman to become pregnant while taking a GnRH agonist. Because the potential teratogenicity of this drug is unclear, women should use a barrier contraceptive during treatment.

Danazol (Danocrine), a mildly androgenic synthetic steroid, suppresses FSH and LH secretion, thus producing anovulation and hypogonadotropism. This results in decreased secretion of estrogen and progesterone and regression of endometrial tissue. Danazol can produce side effects severe enough to cause a woman to discontinue the drug. Side effects include masculinizing traits in the woman (weight gain, edema, decreased breast size, oily skin, hirsutism, and deepening of the voice), all of which often disappear when treatment is discontinued (Selak et al, 2004). Other side effects are amenorrhea, hot flashes, vaginal dryness, insomnia, and decreased libido. Migraine headaches, dizziness, fatigue, and depression are also reported. Danazol treatment has been reported to adversely affect lipids, with a decrease in high-density lipoprotein (HDL) levels and an increase in low-density lipoprotein (LDL) levels. Danazol should never be prescribed when pregnancy is suspected, and contraception should be used with it because ovulation may not be suppressed. Danazol can produce pseudohermaphroditism in female fetuses. The medication is contraindicated in women with liver disease and should be used with caution in women with cardiac and renal disease.

Women who have early symptomatic disease and who can postpone pregnancy may be treated with continuous oral contraceptives that have a low estrogen-to-progestin ratio to shrink endometrial tissue. Any low-dose OCPs can be used if taken for 15 weeks followed by 1 week of withdrawal. This

Community Focus

RESPONSES OF A WOMAN TO ENDOMETRIOSIS

While in the clinic, interview a woman with endometriosis to determine her responses to the condition.

- What are her perceptions about how others view her condition?
- Examine how her responses compare with theoretic responses, as well as your own perceptions.
- Does she know other women with this condition?
- What therapies has she used to treat her condition? How effective were the therapies?
- Develop patient teaching guidelines for women with endometriosis. Have the guidelines translated into Spanish and other languages of women using that clinic.

therapy is associated with minimal side effects and can be taken for extended periods (Nakad & Isaacson, 2002).

Surgical intervention is often needed for severe, acute, or incapacitating symptoms. Decisions regarding the extent and type of surgery are influenced by a woman's age, desire for children, and location of the disease. For women who do not want to preserve their ability to have children, the only definite cure is total abdominal hysterectomy with bilateral salpingo-oophorectomy (TAH with BSO). In women who are in their childbearing years and who want children, and in whom the disease does not prevent it, reproductive capacity should be retained through careful removal by surgery or laser therapy of all endometrial tissue possible with retention of ovarian function (Nakad & Isaacson, 2002).

Regardless of the type of treatment (short of TAH with BSO), endometriosis recurs in approximately 40% of women. Thus for many women endometriosis is a chronic disease with conditions such as chronic pain or infertility. Counseling and education are critical components of nursing care for women with endometriosis. Women need an honest discussion of treatment options, with potential risks and benefits of each option reviewed. Because pelvic pain is a subjective, personal experience that can be frightening, support is important. Sexual dysfunction resulting from dyspareunia is common and may necessitate referral for counseling. Support groups for women with endometriosis may be found in some locations. Resolve, an organization for infertile couples, may also be helpful. The nursing care discussed in the section on dysmenorrhea and premenstrual syndrome is appropriate for managing chronic pelvic pain and dysmenorrhea experienced by women with endometriosis or premenstrual syndrome (see Resources and Nursing Care Plan on p. 114).

Abnormal Uterine Bleeding

Abnormal uterine bleeding (AUB) is any form of uterine bleeding that is irregular in amount, duration, or timing and not related to regular menstrual bleeding. Box 6-1 lists possible causes of AUB. Although often used interchangeably, the terms *AUB* and *dysfunctional uterine bleeding (DUB)* are not synonymous. Dysfunctional uterine bleeding is a subset of AUB defined as "excessive uterine bleeding with no demonstrable organic cause, genital or extragenital" (Stenchever et al, 2001). DUB is most frequently caused by anovulation at the extremes of a woman's reproductive years—when the menstrual cycle is just becoming established at menarche or when it draws to a close at menopause. A diagnosis of DUB is made only after all other causes of abnormal menstrual bleeding have been ruled out (ACNM Clinical Bulletin, 2002).

Oligomenorrhea/Hypomenorrhea

The term *oligomenorrhea* often is used to describe decreased menstruation, either in amount, time, or both. However, oligomenorrhea more correctly refers to infrequent menstrual periods characterized by intervals of 40 to 45 days or longer, and hypomenorrhea, to scanty bleeding at normal intervals. The causes of oligomenorrhea are often abnormalities of hypothalamic, pituitary, or ovarian function. Oligomenorrhea also can be physiologic, or part of a woman's normal pattern for the first few years after menarche or for several years before menopause.

Treatment is aimed at reversing the underlying cause, if possible. Hormonal therapy using progestins, with or without estrogens, also may be used to prevent complications of unopposed estrogen production (endometrial hyperplasia or carcinoma) or of absent estrogen (vaginal dryness, hot flashes or flushes, osteoporosis).

Women with menstruation characterized by prolonged intervals between cycles need education and counseling. The cause of the condition and the rationale for a specific treatment should be discussed, as should advantages and disadvantages of hormonal therapy. If a woman chooses medical intervention, she should be provided with written instructions, taught how to take the medications, and made aware of side effects of any medications. Teaching and counseling should emphasize the importance of the woman keeping careful records of her vaginal bleeding.

Metrorrhagia

Metrorrhagia, or intermenstrual bleeding, refers to any episode of bleeding, whether spotting, menses, or hemorrhage, that occurs at a time other than the normal menses.

BOX 6-1

Possible Causes of Abnormal Uterine Bleeding

Anovulation
- Hypothalamic dysfunction
- Polycystic ovary syndrome

Pregnancy-Related Conditions
- Threatened or spontaneous abortion
- Retained products of conception after elective abortion
- Ectopic pregnancy

Lower Reproductive Tract Infections
- Chlamydial cervicitis
- Pelvic inflammatory disease

Neoplasms
- Endometrial hyperplasia
- Cancer of cervix and endometrium
- Endometrial polyps
- Hormonally active tumors (rare)
- Leiomyomata
- Vaginal tumors (rare)

Trauma
- Genital injury (accidental, coital trauma, sexual abuse)
- Foreign body
- Primary coagulation disorders

Systemic Diseases
- Diabetes mellitus
- Thyroid dysfunction (hypothyroidism, hyperthyroidism)
- Severe organ disease (renal or liver failure)

Iatrogenic Causes
- Exogenous hormone use (oral contraceptives, menopausal hormone therapy)
- Medications with estrogenic activity
- Herbal preparation (ginseng)

Sources: Hillard P: Diagnosing and controlling abnormal uterine bleeding, *Contemp Adolescent Gynecol* 4(1):4-11, 1999; Stenchever M et al: *Comprehensive gynecology,* ed 4, St Louis, 2001, Mosby.

Mittlestaining, a small amount of bleeding or spotting that occurs at the time of ovulation (14 days before onset of the next menses), is considered normal.

Women taking OCPs may have midcycle bleeding or spotting. (See Chapter 7 for a discussion of the side effects of OCPs.) If the OCP does not sufficiently maintain a hypoplastic endometrium, the endometrium will begin to shed, usually in small amounts at a time, a process termed *breakthrough bleeding.* Suggesting that women take their pill at exactly the same time each day may alleviate the problem. If the spotting continues, a different formulation of OCP that increases either the estrogen or progestin component of the pill can be tried.

Women with an intrauterine device (IUD) may have spotting between their periods and a heavier menstrual flow.

The causes of intermenstrual bleeding are varied (Table 6-3). It is important that the nurse always consider the possibility that any woman who has not undergone menopause and who seeks care for intermenstrual bleeding is or recently has been pregnant.

Treatment depends on the cause and may include reassurance and education concerning mittlestaining, observation of three menstrual cycles for presumed functional ovarian cyst, adjustment of an OCP, removal of foreign bodies, and treatment for vaginal infections. More complex treatment may consist of removal of polyps; evaluation and treatment of an abnormal Papanicolaou (Pap) smear, including colposcopy, biopsy, cautery, cryosurgery, or conization; and surgery, chemotherapy, or radiation treatment for malignancy. Important nursing roles include reassurance, counseling, education, and support.

Menorrhagia

Menorrhagia (hypermenorrhea) is defined as excessive menstrual bleeding, in either duration or amount. A single episode of heavy bleeding may occur, or a woman may have regular flooding as a pattern in which she changes tampons or pads every few hours for several days. The causes of heavy menstrual bleeding are many, including an early pregnancy loss, hormonal disturbances, systemic disease, blood dyscrasias, benign and malignant neoplasms, infection, and contraception (IUDs). Medications, including chemotherapy, anticoagulants, neuroleptics, and steroid hormone therapy, may cause abnormal bleeding.

Table 6-3

Causes of Intermenstrual Bleeding

REPRODUCTIVE DISORDER
Functional ovarian cyst
Cervical erosion infection
Leiomyoma
Polyps, uterine or endocervix
Trauma
Foreign body
Malignancy of reproductive tract
PREGNANCY PROBLEMS
Pregnancy: implantation
Miscarriage
Ectopic pregnancy
Molar pregnancy
Retained placenta: miscarriage or induced abortion
Retained placenta: birth
INFECTIONS
Endometritis
Sexually transmitted infections

NURSE ALERT If the woman herself considers the amount or duration of bleeding to be excessive, the problem should be investigated. ■

Hemoglobin and hematocrit provide objective indicators to actual blood loss and should always be assessed. If pregnancy is suspected, a serum β-hCG pregnancy test should be done.

Uterine leiomyomata (fibroids or myomas) are a common cause of menorrhagia. Fibroids are benign tumors of the smooth muscle of the uterus, the etiology of which is unknown. Fibroids occur in one fourth of women of reproductive age; the incidence of fibroids is two to three times higher in African-American women than in Caucasian or Hispanic women (Friedman & Carlson, 2002).

Treatment for menorrhagia depends on the cause of the bleeding. Treatment options include medical and surgical management. Most fibroids can be monitored by frequent examinations to judge growth, if any, and correction of anemia, if present. Women with menorrhagia should be warned not to use aspirin because of its tendency to increase bleeding. Medical treatment is directed toward temporarily reducing symptoms, shrinking the myoma, and reducing its blood supply. This reduction is often accomplished with the use of a GnRH agonist. If the woman wishes to retain childbearing potential, a myomectomy, or removal of the tumors only, may be done. For more severe cases, hysterectomy or endometrial ablation (laser surgery or electrocoagulation) may be done (Stenchever et al, 2001).

Management

When uterine bleeding is severe and a woman's hemoglobin level is less than 8 g/100 ml (hematocrit of 23% or 24%), the woman may be hospitalized and given conjugated estrogens (Premarin) intravenously (Stenchever et al, 2001) until bleeding stops or slows significantly. If the bleeding has not stopped in 12 to 24 hours, dilation and curettage (D&C) may be done to control severe bleeding and hemorrhage. An endometrial biopsy may be done at the same time to evaluate endometrial tissue or to rule out endometrial cancer. After this treatment, oral conjugated estrogen is given for 21 days. During the last 7 to 10 days of this estrogen regimen, progesterone (e.g., medroxyprogesterone [Provera]) is added. Alternatively, a combined OCP is given for 21 days after intravenous therapy. Once the acute phase has passed, the woman is maintained on cyclic, low-dose oral contraceptives for 3 to 6 months. Such long-term treatment will help prevent recurrence of the pattern of dysfunctional uterine bleeding and hemorrhage. If she wants contraception, she should continue to take OCPs. If the woman has no need for contraception, the treatment may be stopped to assess her bleeding pattern.

If her menses does not resume, a progestin regimen may be prescribed after ruling out pregnancy. This is done to prevent persistent anovulation with chronic unopposed endogenous estrogen hyperstimulation of the endometrium, which can result in eventual atypical tissue changes.

If the recurrent, heavy bleeding is not controlled by hormonal therapy or D&C, ablation of the endometrium through laser treatment may be performed. Nursing roles include informing patients of their options, counseling and education as indicated, and referring to the appropriate specialists and health care services.

Care Management

Assessment

In addition to taking a careful menstrual, obstetric, sexual, and contraceptive history, the nurse should explore the woman's perceptions of her condition, cultural or ethnic influences, experiences with other caregivers, lifestyle, and patterns of coping. The amount of pain or bleeding experienced and its effect on daily activities should be evaluated (see Guidelines/Guías). Home remedies and prescriptions to relieve discomfort are noted. A symptom diary, in which the woman records emotions, behaviors, physical symptoms, diet, and exercise and rest patterns, is a useful diagnostic tool.

Nursing Diagnoses

Nursing diagnoses for women with menstrual disorders include the following:

- *Ineffective individual or family coping related to*
  —insufficient knowledge of the cause of the disorder
  —emotional and physiologic effects of the disorder
- *Deficient knowledge related to*
  —self-care
  —available therapy for the disorder
- *Risk for disturbed body image related to*
  —menstrual disorder
  —sexual dysfunction
- *Acute pain related to*
  —menstrual disorder

ENGLISH SPANISH Guidelines/Guías

MENSTRUATION

At what age did you begin to menstruate?
¿A qué edad empezó a menstruar?

When was your last menstrual cycle?
¿Cuándo fue su última menstruación (regla)?

Was it normal?
¿Fue normal?

Do you have pains with your period?
¿Tiene algún dolor con la menstruación (regla)?

How many days does your period last?
¿Por cuántos días dura su menstruación (regla)?

Is the flow light or heavy?
¿Tiene mucha o poquita hemorragia durante su menstruación (regla)?

Expected Outcomes

The expected outcomes for the woman with a menstrual disorder are that she will do the following:

- Verbalize understanding of reproductive anatomy, etiology of her disorder, medication regimen, and diary use.
- Develop personal goals that benefit her emotionally and physically.
- Choose appropriate therapeutic measures for her menstrual problems.
- Adapt successfully to the condition if cure is not possible.

Plan of Care and Implementation

During the history and diagnostic workup, the clinician's concern for and acceptance of the woman's symptoms as valid are in themselves therapeutic. Data from the daily diary about emotional status, subjective feelings, and physical state are correlated with physiologic changes. If the woman has a partner, the woman and her partner should keep separate diaries that include how each perceives the other's responses day by day. Through the diaries, feelings are vented, problems are identified and clarified, insights occur, and possible solutions begin to develop. The clinician facilitates insights and suggests therapeutic options. The woman (or couple) makes choices considered best for her (or them).

Nurses should discuss the options available to women with menstrual disorders. Women must understand basic information about anatomy and physiology, pathophysiology, psychologic impact, and treatment for the condition, including alternative therapies. Support groups are an important resource. Nurses can use a local women's center or clinic to bring together women who want to learn more about their condition and support each other.

Evaluation

The nurse can be assured that care has been effective when the woman reports improvement in the quality of her life, skill in self-care, and a positive self-concept and body image.

INFECTIONS

Sexually Transmitted Infections

Sexually transmitted infections (STIs), or sexually transmitted diseases (STDs), are infections or infectious disease syndromes primarily transmitted by close, intimate contact (Box 6-2). These terms, used interchangeably in this text, have replaced the older designation, venereal disease, which primarily described gonorrhea and syphilis. Caused by a wide spectrum of bacteria, viruses, protozoa, and ectoparasites (organisms that live on the outside of the body, such as a louse), STIs are a direct cause of tremendous human suffering, place heavy demands on health care services, and cost hundreds of millions of dollars to treat. The phrase *sexually transmitted disease* is not specific for any one disease; rather the term includes more than 25 infectious organisms that are transmitted through sexual activity and the dozens of clinical syndromes that they cause (Institute of Medicine, Committee on Prevention and Control of Sexually Transmitted Diseases, 1997). The U.S. Surgeon General has targeted STIs as a priority for prevention and control efforts. Still, STIs are among

BOX 6-2

Sexually Transmitted Infections

Bacteria
Chlamydia
Gonorrhea
Syphilis
Chancroid
Lymphogranuloma venereum
Genital mycoplasmas
Group B streptococci

Viruses
Human immunodeficiency virus
Herpes simplex virus, types 1 and 2
Cytomegalovirus
Viral hepatitis A and B
Human papillomavirus

Protozoa
Trichomoniasis

Parasites
Pediculosis (may or may not be sexually transmitted)
Scabies (may or may not be sexually transmitted)

the most common health problems in the United States (Institute of Medicine, 1997). The Centers for Disease Control and Prevention (CDC) estimates that more than 15 million Americans are infected with STIs every year (Workowski, Levine, & Wasserheit, 2002). The most common STIs in women are chlamydia, human papillomavirus, gonorrhea, herpes simplex virus type 2, syphilis, and human immunodeficiency virus (HIV) infection. These are discussed in this chapter. Neonatal effects of STIs are discussed in Chapter 28.

Prevention

Preventing infection (primary prevention) is the most effective way of reducing the adverse consequences of STIs for women and for society. With the advent of serious and potentially lethal STIs that are either not readily cured or incurable, primary prevention becomes critical. Prompt diagnosis and treatment of current infections (secondary prevention) can prevent personal complications and transmission to others.

Preventing the spread of STIs requires that women at risk for transmitting or acquiring infections change their behavior. A critical first step is for the nurse to include questions about a woman's sexual history, sexual risk behaviors, and drug-related risky behaviors as a part of her assessment (Box 6-3). When risk factors or risky behaviors are identified, the nurse has an opportunity to provide prevention counseling. Effective techniques in providing prevention counseling include using open-ended questions, using understandable language, and reassuring the woman that treatment will be provided regardless of consideration such as ability to pay, language spoken, or lifestyle (CDC, 2002). Prevention messages should include descriptions of specific actions to be taken to avoid acquiring or transmitting STIs (e.g., refrain from sexual activity if you have STI-related symptoms) and should be tailored to the individual woman with attention given to her specific risk factors (Guidelines box).

To be motivated to take preventive actions, a woman must believe that catching a disease will be serious for her

BOX 6-3

Assessing STI/HIV Risk Behaviors

Answer these questions for all the times in your life from 1977* to now.

Sexual Risk
Are you sexually active now?
If no, have you had sex in the past?
Ever had an oral, vaginal, or anal sexual experience with another person?
With how many different people? 1? 2 or 3? 4 to 10? More than 10?
Have your partners been men, women, both?
Ever thought that a sex partner put you at risk for AIDS/STI (IV drug user, bisexual)?
Ever had an STI (herpes, gonorrhea, genital warts, chlamydia)?
Ever had sex against your will?
What do you do to protect yourself from AIDS/STIs?
Do you use male condoms? Female condoms? Other barriers?

Drug Use–Related Risk
Ever injected drugs using shared equipment, including street drugs, steroids?
Ever had sex with a person who uses and shares?
Ever had sex while stoned, high, or drunk, so that you can't remember the details?
Ever exchanged sex for drugs, money, shelter?

Blood-Related Risks
Ever had a blood transfusion?
Ever had sex with a person who had a blood transfusion?
Ever had sex with a person with hemophilia?
Ever received donor semen, egg, transplanted organ or tissue?
Ever shared equipment for tattoo, body piercing?

Other
Ever had a test for HIV?
Ever worried about AIDS and would like to talk with someone about it?

Adapted from Hatcher R et al: *Contraceptive technology,* ed 17, New York, 1998, Ardent Media.
*Relates to risk of HIV—infection not known to exist in humans until this time.

Guidelines

PREVENTION OF GENITAL TRACT INFECTIONS IN WOMEN

- Practice genital hygiene.
- Choose underwear or hosiery with a cotton crotch.
- Avoid tight-fitting clothing (especially tight jeans).
- Select cloth car seat covers instead of vinyl.
- Limit the time spent in damp exercise clothes (especially swimsuits, leotards, and tights).
- Limit exposure to bath salts or bubble bath.
- Avoid colored or scented toilet tissue.
- If sensitive, discontinue use of feminine hygiene deodorant sprays.
- Use condoms.
- Void before and after intercourse.
- Decrease dietary sugar.
- Drink yeast-active milk and eat yogurt (with lactobacilli).
- Do not douche.

Table 6-4

Safer Sex Guidelines

SAFEST	LOW RISK	POSSIBLY RISKY (POSSIBLE EXPOSURE)	HIGH RISK (UNSAFE)
BEHAVIOR			
Abstinence Self-masturbation Monogamous (both partners and no high risk activities) Hugging,* massage,* touching* Dry kissing Mutual masturbation§ Drug abstinence Sexual fantasy Erotic conversation, books, movies, videos Erotic bathing, showering Eroticizing feet, fingers, buttocks, abdomen, ears	Wet kissing* Vaginal intercourse with condom Anal intercourse with condom Urine contact with intact skin	Cunnilingus† Fellatio‡ Mutual masturbation with skin breaks Vaginal intercourse after anal contact without new condom	Unprotected anal intercourse Unprotected vaginal intercourse Oral-anal contact Any sex (fisting, rough vaginal or anal intercourse, rape) that causes tissue damage or bleeding Multiple sexual partners Sharing sex toys, douche equipment Sharing needles Blood contact, including menstrual blood
PREVENTION			
Avoid high risk behaviors	Avoid exposure to potentially infected body fluids Consistent use of condom and spermicide Avoid anal intercourse	Use dental dam or female condom with cunnilingus Use condom with fellatio Use latex gloves	Avoid exposure to potentially infected body fluids Use condom and spermicide consistently Avoid anal penetration If anal penetration occurs, use condom with intercourse, latex glove with hand penetration Avoid oral-anal contact Do not share sex toys, needles, douching equipment If sharing needles, clean with bleach before and after use

Adapted from Centers for Disease Control and Prevention: Sexually transmitted diseases treatment guidelines, 2002, *MMWR* 51(RR-6):1-82, 2002; Fogel CI: Female sexuality. In Breslin E, Lucas V (eds): *AWHONN women's health nursing: toward evidence-based practice*, Philadelphia, 2003, WB Saunders.
*Assumes no breaks in skin.
†Cunnilingus: oral stimulation of the female genitalia.
‡Fellatio: oral stimulation of the male genitalia.
§Assumes no contact with semen or vaginal secretions.

and that she is at risk for infection. Most individuals tend to underestimate their personal risk of infection in a given situation. Thus many women may not perceive themselves as being at risk for contracting an STI, and telling them that they need to carry condoms may not be well received. Although levels of awareness of STIs are generally high, widespread misconceptions or specific gaps in knowledge also exist. Therefore nurses have a responsibility to ensure that their patients have accurate, complete knowledge about transmission and symptoms of STIs and the behaviors that place them at risk for contracting an infection.

Primary preventive measures are individual activities aimed at avoiding infection. Risk-free options include complete abstinence from sexual activities that transmit semen, blood, or other body fluids or that allow for skin-to-skin contact (CDC, 2002). Involvement in a mutually monogamous relationship with an uninfected partner also eliminates risk of contracting STIs. When neither of these options is realistic for a woman, the nurse must focus on other, more feasible measures.

Safer Sex Practices

An essential component of primary prevention is counseling women regarding safer sex practices, including knowledge of her partner, reduction of number of partners, low risk sex, and avoiding the exchange of body fluids.

No aspect of prevention is more important than knowing one's partner. Reducing the number of partners and avoiding partners who have had many previous sexual partners decreases a woman's chances of contracting an STI. Deciding not to have sexual contact with casual acquaintances also may be helpful. Discussing each new partner's previous sexual history and exposure to STIs will augment other efforts to reduce risk; however, sexual partners are not always truthful about their sexual history.

Sexually active persons also may benefit from carefully examining a partner for lesions, sores, ulcerations, rashes, redness, discharge, swelling, and odor before initiating sexual activity.

Women should be taught low risk sexual practices, as well as which sexual practices to avoid (Table 6-4). Sexual fantasizing is safe, as are caressing, hugging, body rubbing, and massage. Mutual masturbation is low risk as long as there is no contact with a partner's semen or vaginal secretions. All sexual activities are safe when both partners are monogamous, trustworthy, and known (by testing) to be free of disease.

The physical barrier promoted for the prevention of sexual transmission of HIV and other STIs is the condom (male and female). Discussing the use of condoms gives women permission to discuss any concerns, misconceptions, or hesitations they may have about using condoms. The discussion can include the following:

- How and where to purchase and use a condom, price range, and sizes
- The importance of using latex or plastic male condoms rather than natural skin condoms for STI protection
- The importance of using a condom with every sexual encounter and using each condom only once
- The importance of checking the expiration date
- The importance of handling the condom carefully to avoid damaging it with fingernails, teeth, or other sharp objects

Condoms should be stored away from high heat. Although it is not ideal, women may safely carry condoms in wallets, shoes, or inside a bra. Explicit instructions for how to apply a male condom are included in Box 7-8.

The female condom—a lubricated polyurethane sheath with a ring on each end that is inserted into the vagina—has been shown in laboratory studies to be an effective mechanical barrier to viruses, including HIV. Although no clinical studies have been completed to evaluate the efficacy of female condoms in protecting against STIs, the CDC (2002) states that, when used correctly and consistently, the female condom may substantially reduce STI risk and recommends its use when a male condom cannot be used properly. What is important and should be stressed by nurses is the consistent use of condoms for every act of sexual intimacy where there is the possibility of transmission of disease (Box 6-4).

Recent evidence has shown that vaginal spermicides do not protect against certain STIs (e.g., chlamydia, cervical gonorrhea). Frequent use of spermicides containing nonoxynol-9 has been associated with genital lesions and may increase HIV transmission (Wilkinson et al, 2002). Condoms lubricated with nonoxynol-9 are not recommended (CDC, 2002).

Women should be counseled to watch out for situations that make it hard to talk about and practice safer sex. These include romantic times when condoms are not available and when alcohol or drugs make it impossible to make wise decisions about safer sex.

Certain sexual practices should be avoided to reduce one's risk of infection. Abstinence from any sexual activities that could result in exchange of infective body fluids will help decrease risk. Anal-genital intercourse, anal-oral contact, and anal-digital activity are high risk sexual behaviors and should be avoided. Sexual transmission occurs through direct skin or mucous membrane contact with infectious lesions or body fluids. Because mucosal linings are delicate and subject to considerable mechanical trauma during intercourse, small abrasions often may occur, facilitating entry of infectious agents into the bloodstream. The rectal epithelium is especially easy to traumatize with penetration. Sexual practices that increase the likelihood of tissue damage or bleeding, such as fisting (inserting a fist into the rectum), should be avoided. Deep kissing when lips, gums, or other tissues are raw or broken also should be avoided (Fogel, 2003). Because enteric infections are transmitted by oral-fecal contact, avoiding oral-anal activities, "rimming" (licking the anal area), and digital-anal activities should reduce the likelihood of infection. Vaginal intercourse should never follow anal contact unless a condom has been used and then removed and replaced with a new condom.

BOX 6-4

Strategies to Enhance a Woman's Negotiation and Communication Skills Regarding Condom Use

Suggest that the woman talk with her partner about condom use at a time removed from sexual activity.
Role play possible partner reactions with a woman and her alternative responses.
Ask a woman who appears particularly uncomfortable to rehearse how she might approach the topic of condom use.
Women may feel more comfortable and in control of the situation if they sort out their feelings and fears before talking with their partners. Women can be reassured that it is natural to be uncomfortable and that the hardest part is getting started.
Clarify for herself what she will and will not do sexually.
Suggest that the woman begin by saying, "I need to talk with you about something that is important to both of us. It's hard for me, and I feel embarrassed, but I think we need to talk about safer sex."
The partner may need time to think about what he has heard.
If the partner resists safer sex, the woman may wish to reconsider the relationship.

Sexually Transmitted Bacterial Infections

Chlamydia

Chlamydia trachomatis is the most common and fastest-spreading STI in American women, with an estimated 3 million new cases each year (Walsh & Irwin, 2002). These infections are often silent and highly destructive. Their sequelae and complications can be very serious. In women, chlamydial infections are difficult to diagnose; the symptoms, if present, are nonspecific, and culturing the organism is expensive.

Early identification of *C. trachomatis* is important because untreated infection often leads to acute salpingitis or pelvic inflammatory disease. Pelvic inflammatory disease is the most serious complication of chlamydial infections, and past chlamydial infections are associated with an increased risk of ectopic pregnancy and tubal factor infertility. Chlamydial infection of the cervix causes inflammation that results in microscopic cervical ulcerations. These ulcerations may increase the risk of acquiring HIV infection.

Sexually active women younger than age 20 years are two to three times as likely to become infected with chlamydia as women between age 20 and 29 years. Women over age 30 years have the lowest rate of infection. Risky behaviors, including multiple partners and nonuse of barrier methods of birth control, increase a woman's risk of chlamydial infection. Lower socioeconomic status may be a risk factor, especially with respect to treatment-seeking behaviors.

Screening and Diagnosis

In addition to obtaining information about the presence of risk factors, the nurse should inquire about the presence of any symptoms. The CDC (2002) and the U.S. Preventive Services Task Force (USPSTF, 2001a) strongly urge screening of asymptomatic, high risk women in whom infection would otherwise go undetected. CDC guidelines recommend screening of sexually active adolescents, women between ages 20 and 34 years, women who do not use barrier contraceptives, and women with new or multiple partners. In addition, whenever possible, all women with two or more of the risk factors for chlamydia should be cultured.

All pregnant women should have cervical cultures for chlamydia at the first prenatal visit. Repeat culturing late in the third trimester (36 weeks) should be carried out if the woman was previously positive or if she is younger than age 25 years or has a new sex partner or multiple sex partners.

Although chlamydia infections are usually asymptomatic, some women may experience spotting or postcoital bleeding, mucoid or purulent cervical discharge, or dysuria. Bleeding results from inflammation and erosion of the cervical columnar epithelium. Women taking oral contraceptives may have breakthrough bleeding.

Diagnosis of chlamydia is by culture (expensive and labor intensive), DNA probe (less expensive but less sensitivity), enzyme immunoassay (less expensive but less sensitivity), and nucleic acid amplification (expensive but about 90% sensitivity) (Rawlins, 2001). Special culture media and proper handling of specimens are important, so the nurse should always know what is required in the individual practice site.

Management

CDC recommendations for the treatment of urethral, cervical, and rectal chlamydial infections are doxycycline or azithromycin (CDC, 2002). Azithromycin is often prescribed when compliance may be a problem because only one dose is needed; however, expense is a concern with this medication. If the woman is pregnant, erythromycin or amoxicillin is used. Women who have a chlamydial infection and are also infected with HIV should be treated with the same regimen as those who are not infected with HIV.

Because chlamydia is often asymptomatic, the woman should be cautioned to take all medication prescribed. All exposed sexual partners should be treated. Women treated with doxycycline or azithromycin do not need to be retested unless symptoms continue. Women treated with erythromycin may be retested 3 weeks after completing the medication, although the validity of this practice has not been established (CDC, 2002).

Gonorrhea

Gonorrhea is probably the oldest communicable disease in the United States. An estimated 600,000 American men and women contract gonorrhea each year (CDC, 2002). The incidence of drug-resistant cases of gonorrhea, in particular penicillinase-producing *Neisseria gonorrhoeae* (PPNG), is increasing dramatically in the United States.

Gonorrhea is caused by the aerobic, gram-negative diplococci *Neisseria gonorrhoeae.* The principal means of transmission is genital-to-genital contact during sexual activity; however, it is also spread by oral-genital and anal-genital contact. There is also evidence that infection may spread in females from vagina to rectum. Although the organism has been recovered from inanimate objects artificially inoculated with the bacteria, there is no evidence that natural transmission occurs this way.

Age is probably the most important risk factor associated with gonorrhea. The majority of those contracting gonorrhea are younger than 20 years of age. The reported incidence of gonococcal disease is higher in minority groups. Many of the apparent differences in infection rates can be explained by the disproportionate representation of African-Americans among the nation's poor and among inner city dwellers. Rates of gonorrhea are higher in urban areas than in rural areas, with even higher rates in the inner city. Sex workers and their partners, intravenous drug users, and crack cocaine users are considered groups at high risk. Other risk factors include early onset of sexual activity and multiple sexual partners.

Women are often asymptomatic, with one third of infections in adolescent women going unnoticed. When symptoms are present, they are often less specific than the symptoms in men. Women may have a purulent endocervical discharge, but discharge is usually minimal or absent. Menstrual irregularities may be the initial symptom, or women may complain of pain: chronic or acute severe pelvic or lower abdominal pain or longer, more painful menses. Infrequently, dysuria, vague abdominal pain, or low backache prompts a woman to seek care. Gonococcal rectal infection may occur in women following anal intercourse. Ten percent to 30% of urogenital infections are accompanied by rectal infection. Rectal gonorrhea may be completely asymptomatic or, conversely, cause severe symptoms with profuse purulent anal discharge, rectal pain, and blood in the stool. Rectal itching, fullness, pressure, and pain are also common symptoms, as is diarrhea. A diffuse vaginitis with vulvitis is the most common form of gonococcal infection in prepubertal girls. There may be few signs of infection; or vaginal discharge, dysuria, and swollen, reddened labia may be present.

Gonococcal infections in pregnancy potentially affect both mother and infant. Women with cervical gonorrhea may develop salpingitis in the first trimester. Perinatal complications of gonococcal infection include premature rupture of membranes, preterm birth, chorioamnionitis, neonatal sepsis, intrauterine growth restriction, and maternal postpartum sepsis. Amniotic infection syndrome—manifested by placental, fetal, and umbilical cord inflammation following premature rupture of the membranes—may result from gonorrheal infection during pregnancy.

Screening and Diagnosis

Because gonococcal infections in women often are asymptomatic, the CDC (2002) recommends screening all women at risk for gonorrhea. All pregnant women should be screened at the first prenatal visit, and infected women and those identified with risky behaviors rescreened at 36 weeks of gestation. Gonococcal infection cannot be diagnosed reliably by clinical signs and symptoms alone. Cultures should be obtained from the endocervix, the rectum, and, when indicated, the pharynx. Because coinfection is common, any woman suspected of having gonorrhea should have a chlamydial culture and serologic test for syphilis unless one has been done within the past 2 months.

Management

Management of gonorrhea is straightforward, and with appropriate antibiotic therapy, the cure is usually rapid. Single-dose efficacy is a major consideration in selecting an antibiotic regimen for women with gonorrhea. Another important consideration is the high proportion (45%) of women with coexisting chlamydial infections. The treatment of choice for uncomplicated urethral, endocervical, and rectal infections in pregnant and nonpregnant women is cefixime (400 mg orally once) or ceftriaxone (125 mg IM once). The CDC (2002) recommends concomitant treatment for chlamydia because coinfection is common. All women with both gonorrhea and syphilis should also be treated for syphilis according to CDC guidelines (see discussion of syphilis later in this chapter).

Gonorrhea is highly communicable. Recent (past 30 days) sexual partners should be examined, cultured, and treated with appropriate regimens. Most treatment failures result from reinfection. The patient needs to be informed of this, as well as of the consequences of reinfection in terms of chronicity, complications, and potential infertility. Women are counseled to use condoms. All patients with gonorrhea should be offered confidential counseling and testing for HIV infection.

LEGAL TIP Gonorrhea Gonorrhea is a reportable communicable disease. Health care providers are legally responsible for reporting all cases of gonorrhea to health authorities, usually the local health department in the patient's county of residence. Women should be informed that the case will be reported, told why, and informed of the possibility of being contacted by a health department epidemiologist. ■

Treatment failure following combined ceftriaxone/doxycycline therapy is rare; therefore follow-up culture (test of cure) is not essential. A more cost-effective approach is reexamination with a culture 1 to 2 months after treatment. This approach will detect both treatment failures and reinfections. Patients should be counseled to return if symptoms persist after treatment.

Syphilis

Syphilis, one of the earliest described STIs, is caused by *Treponema pallidum,* a motile spirochete. Transmission is thought to be by entry in the subcutaneous tissue through microscopic abrasions that can occur during sexual intercourse. The disease can also be transmitted through kissing, biting, or oral-genital sex. Transplacental transmission may occur at any time during pregnancy; the degree of risk is related to the quantity of spirochetes in the maternal bloodstream.

The rate of primary and secondary syphilis in the United States in 2002 was 2.4 per 100,000, a rate slightly up from 2001(Primary and secondary syphilis, 2003). Rates are highest among adolescents and women of color, and in southern states (Primary and secondary syphilis, 2003). Much of the increase in cases seen since 1990 is directly attributable to illicit drug use, particularly crack cocaine, and the exchange of sex for drugs and money.

Syphilis is a complex disease that can lead to serious systemic disease and even death when untreated. Infection manifests itself in distinct stages with different symptoms and clinical manifestations. Primary syphilis is characterized by a primary lesion, the chancre, that appears 5 to 90 days after infection. This lesion often begins as a painless papule at the site of inoculation and then erodes to form a nontender, shallow, indurated, clean ulcer several millimeters to centimeters in size (Fig. 6-3). Secondary syphilis occurs 6 weeks to 6 months after the appearance of the chancre. It is characterized by a widespread, symmetric, maculopapular rash on the palms and soles and generalized lymphadenopathy. The infected individual also may experience fever, headache, and malaise.

Condylomata lata (broad, painless, pink-gray, wartlike infectious lesions) may develop on the vulva, perineum, or anus. If the woman is untreated, she enters a latent phase that

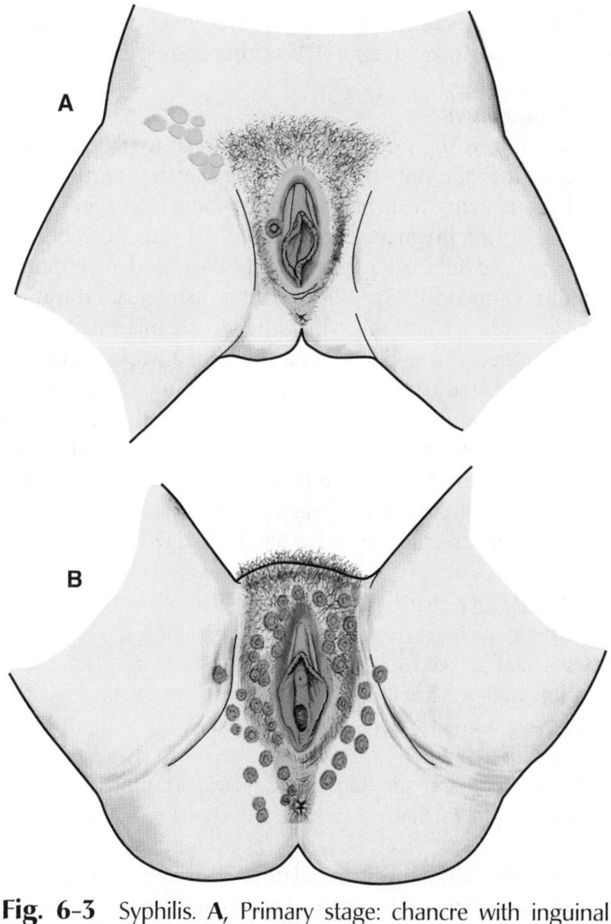

Fig. 6-3 Syphilis. **A,** Primary stage: chancre with inguinal adenopathy. **B,** Secondary stage: condylomata lata.

is asymptomatic for the majority of individuals. Left untreated, about one third of these women will develop tertiary syphilis. Neurologic, cardiovascular, musculoskeletal, or multiorgan system complications can develop in the third stage.

Screening and Diagnosis

All women who are diagnosed with another STI or with HIV should be screened for syphilis. All pregnant women should be screened for syphilis at the first prenatal visit and again in the late third trimester. Diagnosis is dependent on microscopic examination of primary and secondary lesion tissue and serology during latency and late infection. A test for antibodies may not be reactive in the presence of active infection because it takes time for the body's immune system to develop antibodies to any antigens. Up to one third of people in early primary syphilis may have nonreactive serologic tests. Two types of serologic tests are used: nontreponemal and treponemal. Nontreponemal antibody tests such as the Venereal Disease Research Laboratories (VDRL) and rapid plasma reagin (RPR) are used as screening tests. False-positive results are not unusual, particularly when conditions such as acute infection, autoimmune disorders, malignancy, pregnancy, and drug addiction exist and after immunization or vaccination. The treponemal tests, fluorescent treponemal antibody absorbed (FTA-ABS) and microhemagglutination assays for antibody to *T. pallidum* (MHA-TP), are used to confirm positive results. Test results in patients with early primary or incubating syphilis may be negative. Seroconversion usually takes place 6 to 8 weeks after exposure, so testing should be repeated in 1 to 2 months when a suspicious genital lesion exists.

Tests for concomitant STIs (e.g., wet preps and cultures) should be performed, and HIV testing should be offered if indicated.

Management

Penicillin is the preferred drug for treating patients with syphilis. It is the only proven therapy that has been widely used for patients with neurosyphilis, congenital syphilis, or syphilis during pregnancy. Intramuscular penicillin G benzathine is used to treat primary, secondary, and early latent syphilis. Women with syphilis of greater than 1 year's duration (late latent or tertiary stages) require weekly treatment of 2.4 million units of penicillin G benzathine for 3 weeks. Although doxycycline, tetracycline, and erythromycin are alternative treatments for penicillin-allergic patients, both tetracycline and doxycycline are contraindicated in pregnancy, and erythromycin is unlikely to cure a fetal infection. Therefore pregnant women should, if necessary, receive skin testing and be treated with penicillin, or be desensitized (CDC, 2002).

NURSE ALERT Patients treated for syphilis may experience a Jarisch-Herxheimer reaction. This is an acute febrile reaction often accompanied by headache, myalgias, and arthralgias that develop within the first 24 hours of treatment. Women treated in the second half of pregnancy are at risk for preterm labor and birth if treatment precipitates this reaction. They should be advised to contact their health care provider if they notice any change in fetal movement or have any contractions. ■

Monthly follow-up is mandatory so that repeated treatment may be given if needed. The nurse should emphasize the necessity of long-term serologic testing even in the absence of symptoms. The woman should be advised to practice sexual abstinence until treatment is completed, all evidence of primary and secondary syphilis is gone, and serologic evidence of a cure is demonstrated. Women should be told to notify all partners who may have been exposed. They should be informed that the disease is reportable. Preventive measures should be discussed.

Pelvic Inflammatory Disease

Pelvic inflammatory disease (PID) is an infectious process that most commonly involves the uterine tubes, causing salpingitis; the uterus, causing endometritis; and, more rarely, the ovaries and peritoneal surfaces. Multiple organisms have been found to cause PID; most cases are associated with more than one organism. In the past the most common causative agent was thought to be *N. gonorrhoeae;* however, *C. trachomatis* is now estimated to cause one half of all cases of PID. In addition to gonorrhea and chlamydia, a wide variety of anaerobic and aerobic bacteria cause PID. PID encompasses a wide variety of pathologic processes; the infection can either be acute, subacute, or chronic and can have a wide range of symptoms.

Most PID results from the ascending spread of microorganisms from the vagina and endocervix to the upper genital tract. This spread most commonly happens at the end of or just after menses following reception of an infectious agent. During the menstrual period, several factors facilitate the development of an infection: the cervical os is slightly open, the cervical mucus barrier is absent, and menstrual blood is an excellent medium for growth. PID also may develop after an abortion, pelvic surgery, or childbirth.

PID is the single most frequent serious infection encountered by women. Each year more than 1 million women in the United States have an episode of symptomatic PID (Institute of Medicine, 1997). Risk factors for acquiring PID are those associated with the risk of contracting an STI, including young age, multiple partners, high rate of new partners, and a history of STIs. Women who use IUDs may be at increased risk for PID if they have more than one sexual partner or if the partner has other sexual partners because they are at higher risk for acquiring an STI (World Health Organization, 2000). Most of this risk occurs in the first months after IUD insertion. PID tends to recur, with nearly one in five patients experiencing recurrent PID.

Women who have had PID are at increased risk for ectopic pregnancy, infertility, and chronic pelvic pain. Other problems associated with PID include dyspareunia, pyosalpinx (pus in the uterine tubes), tuboovarian abscess, and pelvic adhesions.

The symptoms of PID vary depending on whether the infection is acute, subacute, or chronic. However, pain is common to all clinical presentations. It may be dull, cramping, and intermittent (subacute); or severe, persistent, and incapacitating (acute). The woman with acute PID also may complain of intermenstrual bleeding. Physical examination reveals adnexal tenderness, with or without rebound, and exquisite tenderness with cervical movement (Chandelier sign). Pelvic tenderness is usually bilateral. There may or may not be a palpable adnexal swelling or thickening. A urethral or cervical discharge, often purulent in nature, may be present. A fever of 39° C or above is characteristic. Significant laboratory data include an elevated white blood cell count and markedly elevated erythrocyte sedimentation rate. Fever and peritonitis are more characteristic of gonococcal PID than of PID caused by other organisms that are more likely to be "silent." Because PID caused by chlamydia is more commonly asymptomatic, it more often results in tubal obstruction from delayed diagnosis or inadequate treatment.

Screening and Diagnosis

A careful history is necessary to distinguish between PID and other conditions that cause abdominal pain, such as an ectopic pregnancy or appendicitis. A menstrual history is useful in establishing the relationship of onset of pain to menses and in identifying any variations from normal in the cycle. Other relevant history includes recent pelvic surgery, birth, induced abortion, or dilation of the cervix; purulent vaginal discharge; irregular bleeding; and a longer, heavier menstrual period. A sexual history will assist in identifying possible increased risk for STI exposure. Symptoms of an STI in a woman's partner(s) also should be noted.

Vital signs are obtained and a complete physical examination is performed. CDC routine criteria for diagnosing PID include oral temperature greater than 38.3° C, abnormal cervical or vaginal discharge, elevated erythrocyte sedimentation rate, and laboratory documentation of cervical infection with *N. gonorrhoeae* or *C. trachomatis.* Physical findings of lower abdominal tenderness, bilateral adnexal tenderness, and cervical motion tenderness are important in making a clinical diagnosis of PID. Essential laboratory data are a complete blood count with differential and cervical cultures for gonorrhea and chlamydia.

Management

Perhaps the most important nursing intervention is prevention. Primary prevention is education to avoid acquisition of STIs, whereas secondary prevention involves preventing a lower genital tract infection from ascending to the upper genital tract. Instructing women in self-protective behaviors such as practicing safer sex and using barrier methods is critical. Women using hormonal contraception or an IUD and those who have chosen tubal ligation must be reminded to use a condom with intercourse when indicated. Also important is the detection of asymptomatic gonorrheal and chlamydial infections through routine screening of women who practice risky behaviors or have specific risk factors such as age. Partner notification when an STI is diagnosed is essential to prevent reinfection.

When and if women with PID are hospitalized varies. The CDC recommends hospitalization in the following situations (CDC, 2002):

- Surgical emergencies such as appendicitis cannot be excluded.
- The woman has a tuboovarian abscess.
- The woman is pregnant.
- Severe illness precludes outpatient management.
- The woman is unable to tolerate or follow an outpatient oral regimen.
- The woman has failed to respond to oral outpatient therapy.

Although treatment regimens vary with the infecting organism, generally a broad-spectrum antibiotic is used. Several antimicrobial regimens have proved to be effective, and no single therapeutic regimen of choice exists. The woman with acute PID should be on bed rest in a semi-Fowler's position. Comfort measures include analgesics for pain and all other nursing measures applicable to a patient confined to bed. Few pelvic examinations should be done during the acute phase of the disease. During the recovery phase, the woman should restrict her activity and make every effort to get adequate rest and a nutritionally sound diet. Follow-up laboratory work after treatment should include endocervical cultures for a test of cure.

Health education is central to effective management of PID. Nurses should explain the nature of the disease to women and should encourage them to comply with all therapy and prevention recommendations, emphasizing the need to take all medication, even if symptoms disappear. Any problems that could prevent a woman from completing a course of treatment (such as a lack of money for prescriptions or a lack of transportation to return for follow-up appointments) should be identified. The importance of follow-up visits should be stressed. Women should be counseled to refrain from sexual intercourse until their treatment is completed. Contraceptive counseling, including information on barrier methods such as condoms, the contraceptive sponge, and the diaphragm, should be provided. A woman with a history of PID should not use an IUD as her contraceptive method.

Because PID is so closely tied to sexuality, body image, and self-concept, the woman diagnosed with it will need supportive care. Her feelings should be discussed and her partner(s) included when appropriate.

Sexually Transmitted Viral Infections

Human Papillomavirus

Human papillomavirus (HPV) infection, previously named genital or venereal warts, is a sexually transmitted infection that was first described in 25 AD and is now the most common viral STI seen in ambulatory health care settings. HPV, a double-stranded DNA virus, has over 40 known serotypes; more than 20 types can infect the genital tract. Most HPV infections are asymptomatic, subclinical, or unrecognized. The visible genital lesions are usually caused by HPV types 6 and 11. Other types (e.g., 16, 18, 31, 33, and 35) have the highest oncogenic potential, with types 16 and 18 associated with the highest mortality rate from cervical cancer (Thomas, 2001; Workowski et al, 2002). HPV types 31, 33, and 35 have an intermediate oncogenic potential and are commonly associated with squamous cell carcinoma in situ (Canavan & Doshi, 2000).

Because health care providers are not required to report HPV infections, the true incidence of these infections is not known. An estimated 24 million Americans are infected with HPV, and as many as 1 million new infections occur yearly (CDC, 2002). In addition to the general risk factors for STIs noted earlier, cigarette smoking and use of oral contraceptives for more than 5 years have been found to be risk factors for HPV.

In women, HPV lesions (also called condylomata acuminata) are most commonly seen in the posterior part of the introitus. Lesions also are found on the buttocks, vulva, vagina, anus, and cervix (Fig. 6-4). Typically the lesions are

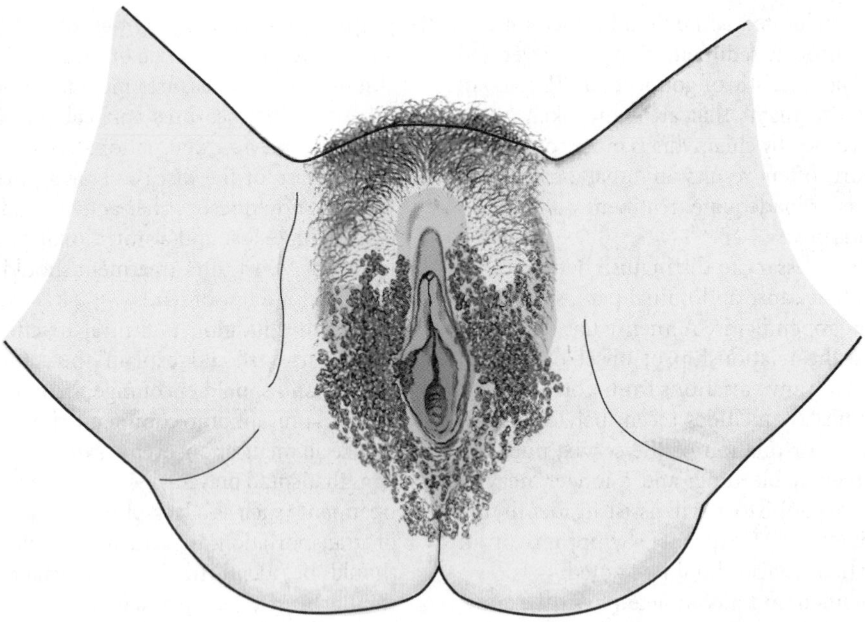

Fig. 6-4 HPV infection. Genital warts or condylomata acuminata.

small, 2 to 3 mm in diameter and 10 to 15 mm in height, soft, papillary swellings occurring singly or in clusters on the genital and anal-rectal region. Infections of long duration may appear as a cauliflower-like mass. In moist areas such as the vaginal introitus, the lesions may appear to have multiple, fine, fingerlike projections. Vaginal lesions are often multiple. Flat-topped papules, 1 to 4 mm in diameter, are seen most often on the cervix. Often these lesions are visualized only under magnification. Warts are usually flesh colored or slightly darker on Caucasian women, black on African-American women, and brownish on Asian women. Usually painless, the lesions may also be uncomfortable, particularly when very large, inflamed, or ulcerated. Chronic vaginal discharge, pruritus, or dyspareunia can occur.

HPV infections are thought to be more common in pregnant than in nonpregnant women, with an increase in incidence from the first trimester to the third. Furthermore, a significant proportion of preexisting HPV lesions enlarge greatly during pregnancy, a proliferation presumably resulting from the relative state of immunosuppression present during pregnancy. Lesions may become so large during pregnancy that they affect urination, defecation, mobility, and fetal descent, although birth by cesarean is rarely necessary (Thomas, 2001). Cesarean birth may be performed when extensive growths are present. Initial observation of large growths can be misleading, suggesting that the entire vagina is involved. However, all of the growth may derive from one stalk, and in such cases it may be possible to push the large mass to the side, allowing the baby to pass through.

Screening and Diagnosis

A woman with HPV lesions may complain of symptoms such as a profuse, irritating vaginal discharge, itching, dyspareunia, or postcoital bleeding. She also may report "bumps" on her vulva or labia. History of a known exposure is important; however, because of the potentially long latency period and the possibility of subclinical infections in men, the lack of a history of known exposure cannot be used to exclude a diagnosis of HPV infection.

Physical inspection of the vulva, perineum, anus, vagina, and cervix is essential whenever HPV lesions are suspected or seen in one area. Because speculum examination of the vagina may block some lesions, it is important to rotate the speculum blades until all areas are visualized. When lesions are visible, the characteristic appearance previously described is considered diagnostic. However, in many instances, cervical lesions are not visible, and some vaginal or vulvar lesions also may be unobservable to the naked eye. Because of the potential spread of vulvar or vaginal lesions to the anus, gloves should be changed between vaginal and rectal examinations.

Diagnosis is made by colposcopy and direct visualization of the growths or by biopsy. Cervical examination with a Papanicolaou (Pap) smear is imperative for women who either have vulvar HPV or who have partners with HPV. Pap smears of the cervical transformation zone are used as a screening technique; however, because of false-negative results, a negative Pap smear does not indicate absence of disease. The severity of any cervical lesion reported on a Pap smear is best determined by colposcopy and biopsy. Vinegar solution may be used to highlight early or flat cervical lesions; however, it is important to note that a positive reaction may also be obtained with any inflammatory reaction, after sexual intercourse, and with vaginal trauma. DNA testing for high risk types of HPV also is recommended for Pap smears showing cervical abnormalities (Wright et al, 2002).

HPV lesions must be differentiated from molluscum contagiosum and condylomata lata. Molluscum contagiosum lesions are half-domed, smooth, flesh-colored to pearly white papules with depressed centers. Condylomata lata are a form of secondary syphilis and generally are flatter and wider than genital warts. A serologic test for syphilis would confirm the diagnosis of secondary syphilis.

Management

Treatment of genital warts is often difficult. No therapy has been shown to eradicate HPV. The goal of treatment therefore is removal of warts and relief of signs and symptoms, not the eradication of HPV (CDC, 2002). Often the patient must make multiple office visits; commonly, many different treatment modalities will be used. Eradication of the virus is not considered conclusive even after there is no visible evidence of wart tissue because of the high incidence of recurrence.

Treatment of genital warts should be guided by preference of the woman, available resources, and experience of the health care provider. None of the treatments is superior to all other treatments, and no one treatment is ideal for all warts (CDC, 2002). Imiquimod, podophyllin, and podofilox are common treatments, but should not be used during pregnancy. Because the lesions can proliferate and become friable during pregnancy, many experts recommend their removal using cryotherapy or various surgical techniques (CDC, 2002).

Women who have discomfort associated with genital warts may find that bathing with an oatmeal solution and drying the area with cool air from a hair dryer will provide some relief. Keeping the area clean and dry will also decrease the growth of the warts. Cotton underwear and loose-fitting clothes that decrease friction and irritation also may lessen discomfort. Women should be advised to maintain a healthy lifestyle to aid the immune system and be counseled regarding diet, rest, stress reduction, and exercise.

Patient counseling should address how the virus is transmitted and stress that no immunity is conferred with infection and that reacquisition of the infection is likely with repeated contact. Women need to know that partners should be checked even if they are asymptomatic. Because HPV is highly contagious, the majority of women's partners will be infected and should be treated. All sexually active women with multiple partners or a history of HPV should be encouraged to use latex condoms and a vaginal spermicide for intercourse to decrease acquisition or transmission of condylomata.

Instructions for all medications and treatments must be detailed. Women should be informed before treatment of the possibility of posttreatment pain associated with specific therapies. The importance of thorough treatment of concurrent vaginitis or STI should be emphasized. The link between cervical cancer and HPV infections and the need for close follow-up should be discussed.

Women should be counseled to have regular Pap screening, as recommended for women without genital warts. The presence of genital warts is not an indication for a change in Pap smear test frequency or for cervical colposcopy (CDC, 2002).

Women with HPV infection may radically alter their sexual practices both from fear of transmission to and from a partner and from genital discomfort associated with treatment, which may have a negative impact on their sexual relationships. Unless the partner accepts and understands the necessary precautions, it may be difficult for the woman to follow the treatment regimen. The nurse can offer to discuss feelings that the woman may have. When indicated, joint counseling can be suggested.

Herpes Simplex Virus

Unknown until the middle of the twentieth century, herpes simplex virus (HSV) infection is now widespread in the United States, especially in women. HSV infection results in painful, recurrent genital ulcers. It is caused by two different antigen subtypes of herpes simplex virus: herpes simplex virus type 1 (HSV-1) and herpes simplex virus type 2 (HSV-2). HSV-2 is usually transmitted sexually and HSV-1 nonsexually. Although HSV-1 is more commonly associated with gingivostomatitis and oral labial ulcers (fever blisters) and HSV-2 with genital lesions, neither type is exclusively associated with the respective sites.

Although HSV infection is not a reportable disease, it is estimated that about one in five people in the United States are infected with genital herpes and that up to one million new infections occur each year (CDC, 2002). Recurrent HSV infections are much more common. Most persons infected with HSV-2 have not been diagnosed, and most infections are transmitted by persons unaware that they are infected.

An initial HSV genital infection is characterized by multiple painful lesions, fever, chills, malaise, and severe dysuria, and may last 2 to 3 weeks. Women generally have a more severe clinical course than do men. Women with primary genital herpes have many lesions that progress from macules to papules; they then progress to form vesicles, pustules, and ulcers that crust and heal without scarring (Fig. 6-5). These ulcers are extremely tender, and primary infections may be bilateral. Women also may have itching, inguinal tenderness, and lymphadenopathy. Severe vulvar edema may develop, and women may have difficulty sitting. HSV cervicitis also is common with initial HSV-2 infections. The cervix may appear normal or be friable, reddened, ulcerated, or necrotic. A heavy, watery to purulent vaginal discharge is common. Extragenital lesions may be present because of autoinoculation. Urinary retention and dysuria may occur secondary to autonomic involvement of the sacral nerve root.

Women with recurrent episodes of HSV infections commonly have only local symptoms that are usually less severe than those associated with the initial infection. Systemic symptoms are usually absent, although the characteristic prodromal genital tingling is common. Recurrent lesions are unilateral, are less severe, and usually last 5 to 7 days. Lesions begin as vesicles and progress rapidly to ulcers. Few women with recurrent disease have cervicitis.

During pregnancy, maternal infection with HSV-2 can have adverse effects on both the mother and fetus. Viremia occurs during the primary infection, and congenital infection is possible, though rare. Primary infections during the first trimester have been associated with increased miscarriage rates. The most severe complication of HSV infection is neonatal herpes, a potentially fatal or severely disabling disease occurring at a rate of 1 in 2000 to 1 in 10,000 live births. Most mothers of infants who contract neonatal herpes lack a history of clinically evident genital herpes. Risk of neonatal infection is highest among women with primary herpes infection who are near term; risk is low among women with recurrent herpes (CDC, 2002).

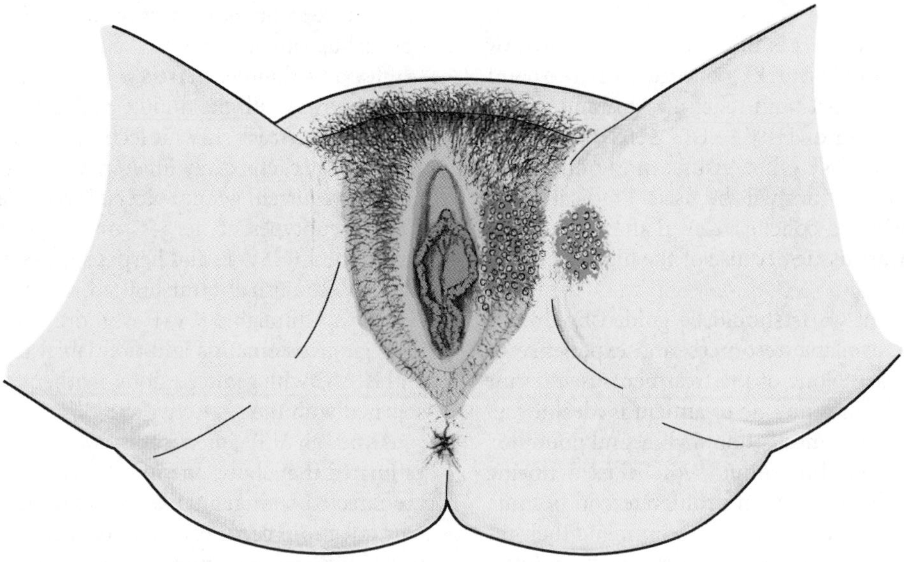

Fig. 6-5 Herpes genitalis.

An association between cervical cancer and HSV-2 has been observed. It is theorized that genital herpes is a marker for high risk sexual behaviors that could transmit other STIs, including HPV (DiSaia & Creasman, 2002).

Screening and Diagnosis

A diagnosis of herpes is facilitated by a careful history. A history of exposure to an infected person is important, although infection from an asymptomatic individual is possible. A history of viral symptoms such as malaise, headache, fever, or myalgia is suggestive. Local symptoms such as vulvar pain, dysuria, itching, or burning at the site of infection, and painful genital lesions that heal spontaneously are also highly suggestive of HSV infections. The nurse should ask about history of a primary infection, prodromal symptoms, vaginal discharge, and dyspareunia. Pregnant women should be asked whether they or their partner(s) have had genital lesions.

During the physical examination, the nurse should assess for inguinal and generalized lymphadenopathy and elevated temperature. The entire vulvar, perineal, vaginal, and cervical areas should be carefully inspected for vesicles or ulcerated or crusted areas. A speculum examination may be very difficult for the woman because of the extreme tenderness often associated with herpes infections. Any suspicious or recurrent lesions found during pregnancy should be cultured to document HSV. Although a diagnosis of herpes infection may be suspected from the history and physical, it is confirmed by laboratory studies. A viral culture is obtained by swabbing exudate during the vesicular stage of the disease. In primary HSV infection, viral shedding is prolonged and HSV is more easily isolated.

Management

Genital herpes is a chronic and recurring disease for which there is no known cure. Management is directed toward specific treatment during primary and recurrent infections, prevention, self-help measures, and psychologic support.

Systemic antiviral medications partially control the symptoms and signs of HSV infections when used for the primary or recurrent episodes or when used as daily suppressive therapy. However, these medications do not eradicate the infection, nor do they alter subsequent risk, frequency, or recurrences after the medication is stopped. Three antiviral medications provide clinical benefit: acyclovir, valacyclovir, and famciclovir. Safety and efficacy have been clearly shown in persons taking acyclovir daily for up to 3 years. The safety of acyclovir, valacyclovir, and famciclovir therapy during pregnancy has not been established; however, the first clinical episode of genital herpes during pregnancy may be treated with oral acyclovir. In the presence of life-threatening maternal HSV infection, intravenous (IV) acyclovir is indicated (CDC, 2002). Continued investigation of HSV therapy with these medications during pregnancy is needed.

Cleaning lesions twice a day with saline will help prevent secondary infection. Bacterial infection must be treated with appropriate antibiotics. Measures that may increase comfort for women when lesions are active include warm sitz baths with baking soda; keeping lesions dry by using cool air from a hair dryer or by patting dry with a soft towel; wearing cotton underwear and loose clothing; using drying aids such as hydrogen peroxide, Burow's solution, or oatmeal baths; applying cool, wet, black tea bags to lesions; and applying compresses with an infusion of cloves or peppermint oil and clove oil to lesions.

Oral analgesics such as aspirin or ibuprofen may be used to relieve pain and systemic symptoms associated with initial infections. Because the mucous membranes affected by herpes are extremely sensitive, any topical agents should be used with caution. Nonantiviral ointments, especially those containing cortisone, should be avoided. A thin layer of lidocaine ointment or an antiseptic spray may be applied to decrease discomfort, especially if walking is difficult.

A diet rich in vitamin C, B-complex vitamins, zinc, and calcium is thought to help prevent recurrences. The amino acid L-lysine has been used in doses of 750 to 1000 mg daily while lesions are active and doses of 500 mg during asymptomatic periods. It is thought that L-lysine has an inhibitory effect on the multiplication of the herpes simplex virus.

Counseling and education are critical components of the nursing care of women with herpes infections. Information regarding the etiology, signs and symptoms, transmission, and treatment should be provided. The nurse should explain that each woman is unique in her response to herpes and emphasize the variability of symptoms. Women should be helped to understand when viral shedding and thus transmission to a partner is most likely. They should be counseled to refrain from sexual contact from the onset of prodrome until complete healing of lesions.

Some authorities recommend consistent use of condoms for all persons with genital herpes. Condoms may not prevent transmission, particularly male-to-female transmission; however, this does not mean that the partners should avoid all intimacy. Women can be encouraged to maintain close contact with their partners while avoiding contact with lesions. Women should be taught how to look for herpetic lesions using a mirror and good light source and a wet cloth or finger covered with a finger cot to rub lightly over the labia. The nurse should ensure that women understand that when lesions are active, sharing intimate articles (e.g., washcloths or wet towels) that come into contact with the lesions should be avoided. Plain soap and water is all that is needed to clean hands that have come in contact with herpetic lesions; isolation is neither necessary nor appropriate.

The role of precipitating factors in the reactivation of the latent virus and recurrent episodes should be discussed. Stress, menstruation, trauma, febrile illnesses, chronic illness, and ultraviolet light have all been found to trigger genital herpes. Women may wish to keep a diary to identify stressors that seem to be associated with recurrent herpes attacks so that they can then avoid these stressors when possible. The role of exercise in reducing stress can be discussed. Referral for stress-reduction therapy, yoga, or meditation classes may be indicated. Avoiding excessive heat and sun and hot baths and using a lubricant during sexual intercourse to reduce friction may also be helpful. Women in their childbearing years should be counseled regarding the risk of herpes infection during pregnancy. They should be instructed to use condoms if there is any risk of contracting an STI from a sexual partner. If they are using acyclovir therapy, they should be counseled to use contraception because of the potential teratogenicity of acyclovir. Women who are breastfeeding should use acyclovir with caution because it concentrates in the milk.

Because neonatal HSV infection is such a devastating disease, prevention is critical. Current recommendations include carefully examining and questioning all women about symptoms at onset of labor (CDC, 2002). If visible lesions are not present at onset of labor, vaginal birth is acceptable. Cesarean birth within 4 hours after labor begins or membranes rupture is recommended if visible lesions are present. Infants who are delivered through an infected vagina should be carefully observed and cultured. Some experts recommend presumptive treatment of infants who were exposed to HSV during birth. Because HSV infection may be associated with cervical dysplasia, women must be encouraged to have yearly Pap smears and gynecologic examinations.

The emotional impact of contracting herpes is considerable. No cure is available, and most women experience recurrences. At diagnosis many emotions may surface—helplessness, anger, denial, guilt, anxiety, shame, or inadequacy. Women need the opportunity to discuss their feelings and help in learning to live with the disease. A woman can be encouraged to think of herself as someone who is healthy and merely inconvenienced from time to time. Herpes can affect a woman's sexuality, her sexual practices, and her current and future relationships. She may need help in discussing her HSV status with her partner or with future partners.

Viral Hepatitis

Five different viruses (hepatitis viruses A, B, C, D, and E) account for almost all cases of viral hepatitis in humans. Hepatitis viruses A, B, and C are discussed. Hepatitis D and E viruses, common among users of intravenous drugs and recipients of multiple blood transfusions, are not included in this discussion.

Hepatitis A

Hepatitis A virus (HAV) infection is acquired primarily through a fecal-oral route by ingestion of contaminated food, particularly milk, shellfish, or polluted water, or person-to-person contact. Hepatitis A, like other enteric infections, can be transmitted during sexual activity. Women living in the western United States, Native Americans, Alaskan Natives, and children and employees in day care centers are at high risk.

HAV infection is characterized by flu-like symptoms with malaise, fatigue, anorexia, nausea, pruritus, fever, and upper right quadrant pain. Serologic testing to detect the immunoglobulin M (IgM) antibody is done to confirm acute infections. The IgM antibody is detectable 5 to 10 days after exposure and can remain positive for up to 6 months. Because HAV infection is self-limited and does not result in chronic infection or chronic liver disease, treatment is usually supportive. Women who become dehydrated from nausea and vomiting or who have fulminating hepatitis A may need to be hospitalized. Medications that might cause liver damage or that are metabolized in the liver should be used with caution. No specific diet or activity restrictions are necessary. Immune globulin (gamma globulin) or immune-specific globulin is indicated for any pregnant woman exposed to HAV to provide passive immunity through injected antibodies. All household contacts of the woman should also receive gamma globulin. Vaccination is the most effective means of preventing HAV transmission; maintenance of "good personal hygiene" has not been successful in preventing HAV outbreaks.

Hepatitis B

Hepatitis B virus (HBV) infection is a sexually transmitted disease and is the virus most threatening to the fetus and neonate. It is caused by a large DNA virus and is associated with three antigens and their antibodies: hepatitis B surface antigen (HBsAg), HBV antigen (HBeAg), HBV core antigen (HBcAg), antibody to HBsAg (anti-HBs), antibody to HBeAg (anti-HBe), and antibody to HBcAg (anti-HBc). Screening for active or chronic disease or disease immunity is based on testing for these antigens and their antibodies.

Factors considered to place a woman at risk for HBV are those associated with STI risk in general: history of multiple sexual partners, multiple STIs, and intravenous drug use; and behaviors that are associated with blood contact (e.g., work or treatment in a dialysis unit, history of multiple blood transfusions, public safety workers exposed to blood in the workplace, and health care workers). Although HBV can be transmitted through blood transfusion, the incidence of such infections has decreased significantly since testing of blood for HBsAg became a routine procedure. Drug abusers who share needles are at risk, as are health care workers exposed to blood and needle sticks. In addition, women of Asian, Pacific Island (e.g., Polynesian, Micronesian, and Melanesian), or Alaskan Eskimo descent and of Haitian or sub-Saharan Africa birth are considered to be at risk.

HBV infection can be transmitted parenterally, perinatally, and, rarely, orally, as well as through intimate contact. It is 50 to 100 times more contagious than HIV. The hepatitis B carrier state affects 5% of the world's population, with higher percentages found in tropical areas and Southeast Asia. HBsAg has been found in blood, saliva, sweat, tears, vaginal secretions, and semen. Perinatal transmission does occur; however, the fetus is not at risk until it comes in contact with contaminated blood during birth. Infants born to mothers who are highly infectious (positive for both HBsAg and HBeAg) have a 10% to 90% chance of acquiring perinatal hepatitis B infection (Thomas, 2001). Approximately 85% to 90% of infected infants will become chronic carriers. HBV has also been transmitted by artificial insemination.

HBV infection is a disease of the liver and is often a silent infection. In the adult, the course of the infection can be fulminating and the outcome fatal. Symptoms of HBV infection are similar to those of hepatitis A: arthralgias, arthritis, lassitude, anorexia, nausea, vomiting, headache, fever, and mild abdominal pain. Later the woman may have clay-colored stools, dark urine, increased abdominal pain, and jaundice. Between 5% and 10% of individuals with HBV have persistence of HBsAg and become chronic hepatitis B carriers. Twenty-five percent of chronic carriers die of primary hepatocellular carcinoma or cirrhosis of the liver.

Screening and Diagnosis

All women at high risk for contracting HBV should be screened on a regular basis. Since screening only individuals at high risk may not identify up to 50% of HBsAg-positive women, current CDC guidelines recommend screening for the presence of HBsAg on all women at the first prenatal visit, regardless of whether they have been tested previously. Testing should be repeated later in pregnancy for women with high risk behaviors (CDC, 2002).

Testing for HBV is complex. Patients with acute hepatitis B generally have detectable serum HBsAg levels in the late incubation phase of the disease, 2 to 5 weeks before symptoms appear. Anti-HBs with a negative HBsAg test signals immunity. Anti-HBs with a positive antigen denotes a chronic carrier state. During this time, the disease can be transmitted. During the recovery phase, the patient may continue to be infectious even though HBsAg cannot be detected. This is called the "window phase" and is identified by anti-HBc in the absence of anti-HBs. Women should be prepared for repeat testing because HBV screening tests may also be used to monitor the progression of the disease.

Components of the history to be obtained when hepatitis B is suspected include inquiry about the symptoms of the disease and risk factors outlined earlier. Physical examination includes inspection of the skin for rashes, inspection of the skin and conjunctiva for jaundice, and palpation of the liver for enlargement and tenderness. Weight loss, fever, and general debilitation should be noted. If the HBsAg is positive, further laboratory studies may be ordered (anti-HBe, anti-HBc, serum glutamic-oxaloacetic transaminase [SGOT], alkaline phosphatase, and liver panel). If the HBsAg is negative in early pregnancy and the woman could be in the window phase, or if high risk behaviors continue during pregnancy, a repeat HBsAg should be ordered in the third trimester.

Management

There is no specific treatment for hepatitis B. Recovery is usually spontaneous in 3 to 16 weeks. Pregnancies complicated by acute viral hepatitis are managed on an outpatient basis. Women should be advised to increase bed rest; eat a high-protein, low-fat diet; and increase their fluid intake. They should avoid medications metabolized in the liver, drugs, and alcohol. Pregnant women with a definite exposure to HBV should be given hepatitis B immune globulin and should begin the hepatitis B vaccine series within 14 days of the most recent contact to prevent infection (CDC, 2002). Vaccination during pregnancy is not thought to pose risks to the fetus.

All nonimmune women at high or moderate risk of hepatitis should be informed of the existence of hepatitis B vaccine. Vaccination is recommended for all individuals who have had multiple sex partners within the past 6 months (CDC, 2002). In addition, intravenous drug users, residents of correctional or long-term care facilities, persons seeking care for an STI, prostitutes, women whose partners are intravenous drug users or bisexual, and women whose occupation exposes them to high risk should be vaccinated. The vaccine is given in a series of three (four if rapid protection is needed) doses over a 6-month period with the first two doses given at least 1 month apart. The vaccine is given in the deltoid muscle (CDC, 2002).

Patient education includes explaining the meaning of hepatitis B infection, including transmission, state of infectivity, and sequelae. The nurse should also explain the need for immunoprophylaxis for household members and sexual contacts. To decrease transmission of the virus, women with hepatitis B or who test positive for HBV should be advised to maintain a high level of personal hygiene (e.g., wash hands after using the toilet; carefully dispose of tampons, pads, and bandages in plastic bags; do not share razor blades, toothbrushes, needles, or manicure implements; have male partner use a condom if unvaccinated and without hepatitis; avoid sharing saliva through kissing, or through sharing of silverware or dishes; and wipe up blood spills immediately with soap and water). They should inform all health care providers of their carrier state. Breastfeeding is not contraindicated if the infant receives prophylaxis at birth and is currently on the immunization schedule.

Hepatitis C

Hepatitis C virus (HCV) infection is the most common blood-borne infection in the United States; 1.8% of Americans are infected with HCV (National Center for Infectious Diseases, 2004). Because 75% to 85% of patients with HCV infection progress to chronic hepatitis, hepatitis C represents nearly 50% of chronic viral hepatitis. The most common risk factor for pregnant women is a history of intravenous drug use. Other risk factors include STIs such as hepatitis B and HIV, multiple sexual partners, and a history of blood transfusions. Hepatitis C is readily transmitted through exposure to blood. It is transmitted much less efficiently through semen, saliva, and urine.

Most patients with hepatitis C are asymptomatic or have general flu-like symptoms similar to hepatitis A. HCV infection is confirmed by the presence of anti-C antibody during laboratory testing. Routine HCV testing is recommended for women who have ever injected drugs; women who received a blood transfusion before July 1992; children of HCV-positive women; health care, emergency, medical, and public safety workers; and women with chronic liver disease (CDC, 2002).

Interferon alfa-2b and ribavirin are the main treatment for HCV infection. Currently there is no vaccine to prevent hepatitis C. Transmission of HCV through breastfeeding has not been reported.

Human Immunodeficiency Virus

Although HIV has been thought of as a disease primarily related to homosexual behavior, heterosexual transmission is now the most common means of transmission in women. Furthermore, women are now the fastest-growing population of individuals with HIV infection and acquired immunodeficiency syndrome (AIDS). Between 1985 and 1997, the proportion of women with AIDS tripled. HIV/AIDS infections are seen disproportionately in women of color (African-American and Hispanic).

Transmission of HIV, a retrovirus, occurs primarily through exchange of body fluids (semen, blood, or vaginal secretions). Severe depression of the cellular immune system associated with HIV infection characterizes AIDS. For both men and women, the most commonly reported opportunistic diseases are *Pneumocystis carinii* pneumonia (PCP), candida esophagitis, and wasting syndrome. Other viral infections such as HSV and cytomegalovirus infections seem to be more prevalent in women than men. PID may be more severe in HIV-infected women, and rates of HPV and cervical dysplasia may be higher. The clinical course of HPV infection in women with HIV infection is accelerated, and recurrence is more frequent.

Once HIV enters the body, seroconversion to HIV positivity usually occurs within 6 to 12 weeks. Although HIV seroconversion may be totally asymptomatic, it usually is accompanied by a viremic, influenza-like response. Symptoms include fever, headache, night sweats, malaise, generalized lymphadenopathy, myalgias, nausea, diarrhea, weight loss, sore throat, and rash.

Laboratory studies may reveal leukopenia, thrombocytopenia, anemia, and an elevated erythrocyte sedimentation rate. HIV has a strong affinity for surface-marker proteins on T lymphocytes. This affinity leads to significant T-cell destruction. Both clinical and epidemiologic studies have shown that declining CD4 levels are strongly associated with increased incidence of AIDS-related diseases and death in many different groups of HIV-infected persons.

Screening and Diagnosis

Screening, teaching, and counseling regarding HIV risk factors, indications for being tested, and testing are major roles for nurses caring for women today. A number of behaviors place women at risk for HIV infection. These include intravenous drug use, high risk sex partners, multiple sex partners, and a previous history of multiple STIs. HIV infection is usually diagnosed by using HIV-1 and HIV-2 antibody tests. Antibody testing is done first with a sensitive screening test such as the enzyme immunoassay (EIA). Reactive screening tests must be confirmed by an additional test, such as the Western blot or an immunofluorescence assay. If a positive antibody test is confirmed by a supplemental test, it means that a woman is infected with HIV and is capable of infecting others. HIV antibodies are detectable in at least 95% of patients within 3 months after infection. Although a negative antibody test usually indicates that a person is not infected, antibody tests cannot exclude recent infection. Because HIV antibody crosses the placenta, definite diagnosis of HIV in children younger than 18 months is based on laboratory evidence of HIV in blood or tissues by culture, nucleic acid, or antigen detection (CDC, 2002).

CDC guidelines recommend offering HIV testing to all women whose behavior places them at risk for HIV infection (CDC, 2002). It may be useful to allow women to self-select for HIV testing. On entry to the health care system a woman can be handed written information about the risk factors for the AIDS virus and asked to inform the nurse if she believes she is at risk. She should be told that she does not have to say why she may be at risk, only that she thinks she might be.

Counseling for HIV Testing

Counseling before and after HIV testing is standard nursing practice. It is a nursing responsibility to assess a woman's understanding of the information such a test would provide and ensure that the patient thoroughly understands the emotional, legal, and medical implications of a positive or negative test before she is ready to take an HIV test. One's life is profoundly altered by knowledge of HIV seropositivity. A unique stigma associated with HIV infection can have a profound impact on the quality of life of those infected. This stigma extends to those who are asymptomatic but seropositive.

Pregnancy is not encouraged for women who are HIV positive. Preconception counseling is recommended; contraceptive counseling should be offered to HIV-positive women who do not desire pregnancy. HIV-infected women should be informed specifically about the risks for perinatal infection. Current evidence indicates that 15% to 25% of infants born to untreated HIV-infected women are infected with HIV; an additional 12% to 14% are infected when breastfeeding continues after age 1 year (CDC, 2002).

All pregnant women should be offered counseling and HIV testing as early in pregnancy as possible (Allen et al, 2001; CDC, 2002). This recommendation is essential because of the available treatments that can reduce the likelihood of perinatal transmission and maintain the health of the woman.

Perinatal transmission of HIV has decreased significantly in the past decade because of the administration of antiretroviral prophylaxis (zidovudine [ZDV, AZT, Retrovir]) to pregnant women in the prenatal and perinatal period. Oral ZDV is initiated between 14 and 34 weeks of pregnancy and continued until labor. During labor, intravenous ZDV is administered. The newborn infant then receives oral ZDV for 6 weeks after birth. The transmission rate of HIV to the newborn with this protocol demonstrated a 66% decrease in the Pediatric AIDS Clinical Trials Group (PACTG protocol 076) in the early 1990s (Allen et al, 2001). The suspected means of protection for the fetus is preexposure prophylaxis. With this standard of care, rates of perinatal transmission to the fetus have been reported as low as 4%.

Other factors identified as potentially influencing perinatal transmission of HIV to the fetus include length of time membranes are ruptured before birth; mode of birth; duration of labor, especially prolonged second stage expulsion efforts; increased maternal viral load levels; and multiple births. Exposure to cervical and vaginal secretions is the likely mechanism of transmission to the newborn, rather than in utero exposure. Cesarean birth has been shown to be of benefit for preventing vertical transmission of HIV. However, complications after cesarean birth are more common in HIV-positive women than in uninfected women.

Given the strong social stigma attached to HIV infection, nurses must consider confidentiality and documentation before providing counseling and offering HIV testing to patients.

LEGAL TIP **HIV Testing** If test results are placed in the woman's chart—the appropriate place for all health information—they are available to all who have access to the chart. The woman must be informed of this before testing. Informed consent must be obtained before an HIV test is performed. In some states written consent is mandated. All pretest and posttest counseling should be documented. ■

There is generally a 1- to 3-week waiting period after testing for HIV, and this can be a very anxious time for the woman. It is helpful if the nurse informs her that this time period between blood drawing and test results is routine. Test results, whatever they are, must always be communicated in person, and women should be informed in advance that this is the procedure. Whenever possible, the person who provided the pretest counseling should also tell the woman her test results.

Some women, when informed of negative results, may escalate risk behaviors because they equate negativity with immunity. Others may believe that negative means "bad" and positive means "good." The woman's reaction to a negative test should be explored by asking, "How do you feel?" Counseling sessions for women with an HIV-negative result are another opportunity to provide education. Emphasis can be placed on ways in which a woman can remain HIV free. She should be reminded that if she has been exposed to HIV in the past 6 months she should be retested, and that she should have ongoing testing if she continues high risk behaviors.

As the number of HIV-infected women escalates, prevention, education, and counseling activities must be directed toward all women. It is very difficult to keep abreast of the ever-changing picture of AIDS. Sources of information are listed in the Resources at the end of the chapter.

Management

During the initial contact with an HIV-infected woman, the nurse should establish what the woman knows about HIV infection. The nurse should ensure that the woman is being cared for by a medical practitioner or a facility with expertise in caring for persons with HIV infections, including AIDS. Psychologic referral also may be indicated. Resources such as counseling for financial assistance, suicide prevention, death and dying, and legal advocacy may be appropriate. All women who are drug users should be referred to a substance abuse program. A major focus of counseling is prevention of transmission of HIV to partners.

Nurses counseling seropositive women who wish to receive contraceptive information may recommend (1) oral contraceptives and latex condoms, or (2) tubal sterilization or vasectomy and latex condoms. The IUD is not an ideal choice for the HIV-infected woman because of increased risk of infection. Insertion in a woman who is immunocompromised should be avoided (World Health Organization, 2000). Female condoms or abstinence can be offered to women whose partners refuse to use condoms.

No cure is available for HIV infection. Rare and unusual diseases are characteristic of HIV infection. Opportunistic infections and concurrent diseases should be managed vigorously with treatment specific to the infection or disease. HIV-positive women should be screened for syphilis, gonorrhea, chlamydia, and other vaginal infections.

Discussion of the medical care of HIV-positive women and women with AIDS is beyond the scope of this chapter. The reader is referred to the Centers for Disease Control and Prevention, AIDS hotlines, and Internet Web sites for current information and recommendations (see Resources at end of chapter).

Vaginal Infections

Vaginal discharge and itching of the vulva and vagina are among the most common reasons a woman seeks help from a health care provider. More women complain of vaginal discharge than of any other gynecologic symptom. Women who have adequate endogenous or exogenous estrogen will have vaginal secretions. Vaginal discharge resulting from infection must be distinguished from normal secretions. Normal vaginal secretions (or leukorrhea) are clear to cloudy in appearance. The discharge may turn yellow after drying; is slightly slimy; is nonirritating; and has a mild, inoffensive odor. Normal vaginal secretions are acidic, with a pH range of 4 to 5. The amount of leukorrhea differs with phases of the menstrual cycle, with greater amounts occurring at ovulation and just before menses. Leukorrhea is also increased during pregnancy. Normal vaginal secretions contain lactobacilli and epithelial cells.

Abnormal vaginal discharge (or vaginitis) is an infection caused by a microorganism. The most common vaginal infections are bacterial vaginosis, candidiasis, and trichomoniasis. Inflammation of the vulva and vagina (or vulvovaginitis) may be caused by vaginal infection; copious leukorrhea, which can cause maceration of tissues; and chemical irritants, allergens, and foreign bodies, which may produce inflammatory reactions.

Bacterial Vaginosis

Bacterial vaginosis (BV), formerly called nonspecific vaginitis, *Haemophilus* vaginitis, or *Gardnerella*, is the most common type of vaginitis. BV is associated with preterm labor and birth; treatment with antibiotics does not prevent preterm birth in the general obstetric population (Carey et al, 2000) but does reduce the rate of preterm birth in women with a history of previous preterm birth (Brocklehurst, Hannah, & McDonald, 2000). The exact etiology of BV is unknown. It is a syndrome in which normal H_2O_2–producing lactobacilli are replaced with high concentrations of anaerobic bacteria (*Gardnerella* and *Mobiluncus*). With the proliferation of anaerobes, the level of vaginal amines is raised and the normal acidic pH of the vagina is altered. Epithelial cells slough and numerous bacteria attach to their surfaces (clue cells). When the amines are volatilized, the characteristic odor of BV occurs.

Screening and Diagnosis

A careful history may help distinguish BV from other vaginal infections if the woman is symptomatic. Women with previous occurrence of similar symptoms, diagnosis, and treatment should be queried, because women with BV often have been treated incorrectly because of misdiagnosis.

Most women with BV complain of a characteristic "fishy odor." The odor may be noticed by the woman or her partner after heterosexual intercourse because semen releases the vaginal amines. When present, the BV discharge is usually profuse; thin; and white, gray, or milky in appearance. Some women also may experience mild irritation or pruritus.

Microscopic examination of vaginal secretions is always done (Table 6-5). Both normal saline and 10% potassium hydroxide (KOH) smears should be made. The presence of clue cells (vaginal epithelial cells coated with bacteria) confirmed by wet smear is highly diagnostic because the phenomenon is specific to BV (USPSTF, 2001b). Vaginal secretions should be tested for pH and amine odor. Nitrazine paper is sensitive enough to detect a pH of 4.5 or greater. The fishy odor of BV will be released when KOH is added to vaginal secretions on the lip of the withdrawn speculum.

Management

Treatment of bacterial vaginosis with oral metronidazole (Flagyl) is most effective (CDC, 2002). Metronidazole is an antiprotozoal and antibacterial agent. In the past metronidazole was contraindicated in the first trimester of pregnancy; however, because of the increased risk of preterm birth, current CDC guidelines recommend treatment of all high risk asymptomatic pregnant women, as well as all symptomatic pregnant women (CDC, 2002). The medication is contraindicated if the woman is breastfeeding because high concentrations have been found in infants. If it is necessary to prescribe metronidazole for the lactating woman, she can suspend breastfeeding temporarily (pump and discard milk to maintain supply), and resume it 48 to 72 hours after taking the last dose. Metronidazole is contraindicated in patients with blood dyscrasia or central nervous system disease because in rare cases it may affect the hematopoietic or central nervous system.

Side effects of metronidazole include a sharp, unpleasant metallic taste in the mouth; furry tongue; central nervous system reactions; and urinary tract disturbances. When oral metronidazole is taken, the patient is advised not to drink alcoholic beverages because they produce severe side effects of abdominal distress, nausea, vomiting, and headache. Gastrointestinal symptoms are common whether alcohol is consumed or not. Treatment of sexual partners is not recommended because sexual transmission of BV has not been proven (CDC, 2002).

Candidiasis

Vulvovaginal candidiasis, or yeast infection, is the second most common type of vaginal infection in the United States. Although vaginal candidiasis infections are common in healthy women, those seen in women with HIV infection are often more severe and persistent. Genital candidiasis lesions may be painful, coalescing ulcerations necessitating continuous, prophylactic therapy.

The most common organism is *Candida albicans.* It is estimated that 80% to 95% of yeast infections in women are caused by this organism. However, in the past 10 years, the incidence of non–*C. albicans* infections has increased steadily. Women with chronic or recurrent infections often are infected with a higher percentage of non–*C. albicans* species than are women with their first infection or who have few recurrences.

Numerous factors have been identified as predisposing a woman to yeast infections. These include antibiotic therapy, particularly broad-spectrum antibiotics such as ampicillin, tetracycline, cephalosporins, and metronidazole; diabetes, especially when uncontrolled; pregnancy; obesity; diets high in refined sugars or artificial sweeteners; use of corticosteroids and exogenous hormones; and immunosuppressed states. Clinical observations and research have suggested that tight-fitting clothing and underwear or pantyhose made of nonabsorbent materials create an environment in which a vaginal fungus can grow.

The most common symptom of yeast infection is vulvar and possibly vaginal pruritus. The itching may be mild or intense, may interfere with rest and activities, and may occur during or after intercourse. Some women report a feeling of dryness. Others may have painful urination as the urine flows over the vulva. The latter usually occurs in women who have excoriations resulting from scratching. Most often the discharge is thick, white, lumpy, and cottage cheese–like. The discharge may be found in patches on the vaginal walls,

Table 6-5

Wet Smear Tests for Vaginal Infections

INFECTION	TEST	POSITIVE FINDINGS
Trichomoniasis	Saline wet smear (vaginal secretions mixed with normal saline on a glass slide)	Presence of many white blood cell protozoa
Candidiasis	Potassium hydroxide (KOH) prep (vaginal secretions mixed with KOH on a glass slide)	Presence of hyphae and pseudohyphae (buds and branches of yeast cells)
Bacterial vaginosis	Normal saline smear	Presence of clue cells (vaginal epithelial cells coated with bacteria)
	Whiff test (vaginal secretions mixed with KOH)	Release of fishy odor

cervix, and labia. Commonly the vulva is red and swollen, as are the labial folds, vagina, and cervix. Although there is no odor characteristic of yeast infections, sometimes a yeasty or musty smell is noted.

Screening and Diagnosis

In addition to noting the woman's symptoms, their onset, and their course, the history is a valuable screening tool for identifying predisposing risk factors. Physical examination should include a thorough inspection of the vulva and vagina. A speculum examination is always done. Commonly saline and KOH wet smear and vaginal pH are obtained. Vaginal pH is normal with a yeast infection; if the pH is greater than 4.5, trichomoniasis or BV should be suspected. The characteristic pseudohyphae (bud or branching of a fungus) may be seen on a wet smear done with normal saline; however, they may be confused with other cells and artifacts.

Management

A number of antifungal preparations are available for the treatment of *C. albicans.* In 1990 many of these medications (Monistat and Gyne-Lotrimin) were made available as over-the-counter agents. The first time a woman suspects that she may have a yeast infection, she should see a health care provider for confirmation of the diagnosis and treatment recommendation. If she experiences another infection, she may wish to purchase an OTC preparation and self-treat. If she elects to do this, she should always be counseled to seek care for numerous recurrent or chronic yeast infections. If vaginal discharge is extremely thick and copious, vaginal debridement with a cotton swab followed by application of vaginal medication may be effective.

Women who have extensive irritation, swelling, and discomfort of the labia and vulva may find sitz baths helpful in decreasing inflammation and increasing comfort. Adding Aveeno powder to the bath may also increase the woman's comfort. Not wearing underpants to bed may help decrease symptoms and prevent recurrences. Completing the full course of treatment prescribed is essential to removing the pathogen. Medication should be continued even during menstruation. Women should be counseled not to use tampons during menses because the medication will be absorbed by the tampon. If possible, intercourse is avoided during treatment; if this is not feasible, the woman's partner should use a condom to prevent introduction of more organisms.

Trichomoniasis

Trichomoniasis is a cause of up to 25% of all vaginal infections and is almost always a sexually transmitted infection. Trichomoniasis is caused by *Trichomonas vaginalis,* an anaerobic, one-celled protozoan with characteristic flagella. Although trichomoniasis may be asymptomatic, commonly women have yellowish to greenish, frothy, mucopurulent, copious, and malodorous discharge. Inflammation of the vulva, vagina, or both may be present, and the woman may complain of irritation and pruritus. Dysuria and dyspareunia are often present. Typically, the discharge worsens during and after menstruation. Often the cervix and vaginal walls demonstrate the characteristic "strawberry spots" or tiny petechiae, and the cervix may bleed on contact. In severe infections, the vaginal walls, cervix, and occasionally the vulva may be acutely inflamed.

Screening and Diagnosis

In addition to obtaining a history of current symptoms, a careful sexual history should be obtained. Any history of similar symptoms in the past and any treatments used should be noted. The nurse should determine whether the patient's partner(s) were treated, and if she has had subsequent sexual relations with new partners.

A speculum examination is always done, even though it may be very uncomfortable for the woman; relaxation techniques and breathing exercises may help the woman with the procedure. Any of the classic signs may or may not be present on physical examination. The typical one-celled flagellate trichomonads are easily distinguished on a normal saline wet prep. Trichomoniasis also may be identified on Pap smears. Because trichomoniasis is an STI, once diagnosis is confirmed, appropriate laboratory studies for other STIs should be carried out.

Management

The recommended treatment is metronidazole, 2 g orally in a single dose (CDC, 2002). Although the male partner is usually asymptomatic, it is recommended that he receive treatment also, because he often harbors the trichomonads in the urethra or prostate. It is important that nurses discuss the importance of partner treatment with patients because it

Patient Teaching

YEAST INFECTION–INADEQUATE PATIENT EDUCATION

Marcella, an 82 year old widow, had a precancerous lesion excised from her forehead and was placed on a broad-spectrum antibiotic for one week. She later presented to the clinic with profuse, white vaginal discharge, severe itching, and excoriation on her labia, in her groin, and extending onto her buttocks and lower abdomen. When she expressed hesitance in talking to the physician, the nurse assured her that she would be with her during the examination. Marcella said that wasn't the problem. When the nurse examined Marcella, she said that her problem looked like a yeast infection and asked Marcella if she had been taking antibiotics. The nurse explained that yeast infections are common when taking antibiotics. The physician verified the diagnosis and prescribed Monistat. On further discussion, the nurse determined that Marcella had thought that she picked up an STI when she used a public restroom and was ashamed and embarrassed to discuss her problem so had not told anyone or sought treatment earlier. When Marcella returned home and told her daughter that she had seen a physician, her daughter stated "You have a yeast infection." When Marcella asked how she knew that, the daughter said that her friend and her daughter both had yeast infections when on antibiotics.

This situation could have been avoided if the physician who prescribed the antibiotic or the nurse had told Marcella that yeast infections are common when antibiotics are taken or if Marcella had discussed the condition with her daughter. Marcella can be counseled to discuss problems and seek care in early stages of a problem, even when discussing the condition may be embarrassing. Had she discussed this with her daughter, treatment could have been started much sooner and Marcella would have avoided the distress she experienced. Marcella also needs some teaching about the transmission of STIs.

is likely that the infection will recur if partners are not treated.

Women with trichomoniasis need to understand the sexual transmission of this disease. The patient must know that the organism may be present without symptoms being present, perhaps for several months, and that it is not possible to determine when she became infected. Women should be informed of the necessity for treating all sexual partners and helped with ways to raise the issue with their partner(s).

Group B Streptococcus

Group B streptococcus (GBS) may be considered a normal vaginal flora in a woman who is not pregnant. It is present in 9% to 23% of healthy pregnant women. However, GBS infection is associated with poor pregnancy outcomes (Guise et al, 2001). GBS infections are an important factor in perinatal and neonatal morbidity and mortality, usually resulting from vertical transmission from the birth canal of the infected mother to the infant during birth.

Risk factors for neonatal GBS infection include positive prenatal culture for GBS in the current pregnancy; preterm birth of less than 37 weeks of gestation; premature rupture of membranes for longer than 18 hours; intrapartum maternal fever higher than 38° C; and a positive history for early-onset neonatal GBS.

To decrease the risk of neonatal GBS infection, it is recommended that all women be screened at 35 to 37 weeks of gestation for GBS using a rectovaginal culture and that intravenous antibiotic prophylaxis (IAP) be offered to all who test positive. If a culture is not available at onset of labor or if risk factors are present, IAP is also offered. IAP is not recommended before a cesarean birth if labor or rupture of membranes has not occurred. The recommended treatment is penicillin G, 5 million units IV loading dose, and then 2.5 million units IV every 4 hours during labor. Ampicillin, 2 g loading dose IV, followed by 1 g IV every 4 hours, is an alternative therapy (Home Care box).

Home Care

SEXUALLY TRANSMITTED INFECTIONS

Take your medication as directed.
Use comfort measures for symptom relief as suggested by your health care provider.
Keep your appointment for repeat cultures or checkups after your treatment to make sure your infection is cured.
Inform your sexual partner(s) to be tested and treated, if necessary.
Abstain from sexual intercourse until your treatment is completed or for as long as you are advised by your health care provider.
Use safer sex practices when sexual intercourse is resumed.
Call your health care provider immediately if you notice bumps, sores, rashes, or discharges.
Keep all future appointments with your health care provider, even if things appear normal.

INFECTION CONTROL

Infection control measures are essential to protect care providers and to prevent nosocomial infection of patients, regardless of the infectious agent. The risk for occupational transmission varies with the disease. Even when the risk is low, as with HIV, the existence of any risk warrants reasonable precautions. Precautions against airborne disease transmission are available in all health care agencies. Standard Precautions (precautions to use in care of all persons for infection control) and additional precautions for labor and birth settings are listed in Box 6-5.

PROBLEMS OF THE BREAST

Fibrocystic Changes

The most common benign breast problem is fibrocystic change. Fibrocystic change is not a disease but a condition found in varying degrees in healthy women's breasts. Fibrocystic changes are palpable thickenings in the breast usually associated with pain and tenderness. The pain and tenderness fluctuate with the menstrual cycle and can become progressively worse until menopause (American Cancer Society, 2003). Only about 5% of fibrocystic conditions have changes that indicate a risk factor for breast cancer.

Etiology

No known etiologic agent is responsible for benign breast disease, although an imbalance of estrogen and progesterone may be responsible. One theory is that estrogen excess and progesterone deficiency in the luteal phase of the menstrual cycle may cause changes in breast tissue. Risk factors are associated with benign breast disease, including nulliparity, low parity, late menopause, and estrogen therapy. Researchers have found no substantial association between smoking, alcohol or caffeine consumption, and risk of benign breast disease (Friedenreich et al, 2000).

Clinical Manifestations and Diagnosis

The usual clinical presentation of fibrocystic change is lumpiness in both breasts. However, single simple cysts may also occur. Symptoms usually develop about a week before menstruation begins and subside about a week after menstruation ends. They include dull, heavy pain and a sense of fullness and tenderness that increases premenstrually. The woman with fibrocystic change may form cysts that manifest as painful enlarging lumps in her breasts. Cysts are common in premenopausal women who are not receiving estrogen therapy. The cysts are soft on palpation, well differentiated, and movable. Deeper cysts, especially aggregations of cysts, are indistinguishable by palpation from carcinomas, which are malignant growths that infiltrate surrounding tissue.

A first step in the workup of a breast lump is ultrasonography to determine if it is fluid filled or solid. Fluid-filled cysts are aspirated, and the woman is monitored on a routine basis for development of other cysts. If the lump is solid, mammography is obtained if the woman is older than 35 years. A fine-needle aspiration (FNA) is then performed, regardless of the woman's age, to determine the nature of the lump. In some cases, a core biopsy may be needed after FNA to harvest adequate amounts of tissue for pathologic examination (Stenchever et al, 2001). The "triple test" (not an ac-

BOX 6-5

Standard Precautions

Medical history and examination cannot reliably identify all persons infected with HIV or other blood-borne pathogens. Standard Precautions should therefore be used consistently in the care of all persons. These precautions apply to blood, body fluids, and all secretions and excretions, except sweat, nonintact skin, and mucous membranes. Standard Precautions are recommended to reduce the risk of transmission of microorganisms from known and unknown sources of infection (CDC, 2004).

1. Handwashing is recommended promptly and thoroughly between patient contacts. Hands and other skin surfaces should be washed immediately and thoroughly if contaminated with blood or other body fluids. Hands should be washed immediately after gloves are removed.
2. In addition to handwashing, all health care workers should routinely use appropriate barrier precautions to prevent skin and mucous membrane exposure when contact with blood or other body fluids of any person is anticipated. *Latex gloves* should be worn for touching blood and body fluids, mucous membranes, or nonintact skin of all persons; for handling items or surfaces soiled with blood or body fluids; and for performing venipuncture and other vascular access procedures. Gloves should be changed after contact with each patient. *Masks and protective eyewear* or face shields should be worn during procedures that are likely to generate droplets of blood or other body fluids to prevent exposure of mucous membranes of the mouth, nose, and eyes. *Gown or aprons* should be worn during procedures that are likely to generate splashes of blood or other body fluids. Leg coverings, boots, or shoe covers also can be worn to provide protection against splashes and may be recommended for certain procedures such as surgery.
3. All health care workers should take precautions to prevent injuries caused by needles, scalpels, and other sharp instruments or devices during procedures; when cleaning used instruments; during disposal of used needles; and when handling sharp instruments after procedures. *To prevent needle-stick injuries,* needles should not be recapped, purposely bent or broken by hand, removed from disposable syringes, or otherwise manipulated by hand. After they are used, disposable syringes and needles, scalpel blades, and other sharp items should be immediately placed in a puncture-resistant container for disposal; puncture-resistant containers should be located as close as is practical to the use area.
4. Although saliva has not been implicated in HIV transmission, to minimize the need for emergency mouth-to-mouth resuscitation, mouthpieces, resuscitation bags, or other ventilation devices should be available for use in areas in which the need for resuscitation is predictable.
5. Health care workers who have exudative lesions or weeping dermatitis should refrain from all direct patient care and from handling patient care equipment until the condition resolves.

Precautions for Invasive Procedures

An invasive procedure is surgical entry into tissues, cavities, or organs or repair of major traumatic injuries (1) in an operating or birthing room, emergency department, or out-of-hospital setting, including both physicians' and dentists' offices; and (2) a vaginal or cesarean birth or other invasive obstetric procedure during which bleeding may occur. Standard Precautions, combined with the following precautions, should serve as minimum precautions for all such invasive procedures:

1. All health care workers who participate in invasive procedures must routinely use appropriate barrier precautions to prevent skin and mucous membrane contact with blood and other body fluids of all patients. Gloves and surgical masks must be worn for all invasive procedures. Protective eyewear or face shields should be worn for procedures that commonly result in the generation of droplets, splashing of blood or other body fluids, or the generation of bone chips. Gowns or aprons made of materials that provide an effective barrier should be worn during invasive procedures that are likely to result in the splashing of blood or other body fluids. All health care workers who perform or assist in vaginal or cesarean births should wear gloves and gowns when handling the placenta or the infant until blood and amniotic fluid have been removed from the infant's skin. Gloves should be worn during infant eye prophylaxis, care of the umbilical cord and circumcision site, parenteral procedures, diaper changes, contact with colostrum, and postpartum assessments.
2. If a glove is torn or a needle stick or other injury occurs, the glove should be removed and a new glove used as promptly as patient safety permits; the needle or instrument involved in the incident also should be removed from the sterile field.
3. Any needle stick or other injury should be reported and appropriate treatment obtained as specified by the health care facility.

tual test) correlates the findings from the breast physical examination, mammography, and FNA. If findings from all three indicate that the condition is benign, the condition can be considered benign with 98% accuracy (American Cancer Society, 2003).

Management

Treatment for fibrocystic change is usually conservative with diuretics and restriction of salt and fluid. Vitamin E supplements also have been recommended, although megadose therapy should be avoided. Even though no research support has been found, some advocate eliminating dimethylxanthines, such as caffeine. Some women report relief of symptoms by avoiding smoking and the consumption of alcohol. Recommended pain-relief measures include taking analgesics or nonsteroidal antiinflammatory drugs (NSAIDs) such as ibuprofen, wearing a supportive bra, and applying heat to the breasts. Some women report relief while taking oral contraceptives, but others report worsening of symptoms. Women may need to try several approaches for a number of months before improvement is noted. The recommended therapies are based on mostly anecdotal evidence; scientific validation of treatment strategies is lacking.

Surgical removal of nodules is attempted only in selected cases. In the presence of multiple nodules, the surgical approach involves multiple incisions and tissue manipulation and may not prevent the development of more nodules.

Fibroadenomas

The next most common benign condition of the breast is fibroadenoma. Fibroadenomas occur in women from puberty through menopause. Masses are solid, encapsulated, nontender, and most often found in the upper outer quadrant of the breast.

The cause of fibroadenomas is unknown. Fibroadenomas are characterized by discrete, usually solitary lumps less than 3 cm in diameter. Occasionally the woman with a fibroadenoma will experience tenderness in the tumor during the menstrual cycle. Fibroadenomas increase in size during pregnancy and shrink as the woman ages. Fibroadenomas do not increase in size in response to the menstrual cycle (in contrast to fibrocystic cysts). The mass tends to remain the same size or increase in size slowly over time (American Cancer Society, 2003).

Diagnosis is made by a review of the history and physical examination. Mammography, ultrasonography, or magnetic resonance imaging (MRI) may be used to determine the type of lesion. FNA may be used to determine the underlying disorder. Surgical excision may be necessary if the lump is suspicious or if the symptoms are severe. Fibroadenomas do not respond to either dietary changes or hormonal therapy. Periodic observation of masses by professional physical examination or mammography may be all that is necessary for those masses not needing surgical intervention.

Lipomas

A lipoma is a tumor, composed of fat, that is soft and has discrete borders. The cause of lipoma is unknown. Lipomas are often found in women over 45 years of age, usually on the chest wall and breast. They are characterized as palpable soft masses that are mobile and nontender. Mammography can be used to make a diagnosis; biopsy usually is not needed. Lipomas can be surgically excised if removal is desired.

Nipple Discharge

Nipple discharge is a common occurrence that concerns many women. Although most nipple discharge is physiologic, each woman who has this problem must be evaluated carefully. A small percentage will be found to have a serious endocrine disorder or malignancy. Bilateral, serous discharge expressed during nipple stimulation can be considered a normal finding. Patient education and reassurance are indicated (American Cancer Society, 2003).

Another form of breast discharge not related to malignancy is galactorrhea. Galactorrhea manifests as a bilaterally spontaneous, milky, sticky discharge. It is a normal finding in pregnancy. It can also occur as the result of elevated prolactin levels. Increased prolactin levels may occur as a result of a thyroid disorder, pituitary tumor, or chest wall surgery or trauma. A complete medication history is essential. Oral contraceptives and neuroleptic drugs are known to precipitate galactorrhea in some women. The optimal time to draw blood to determine a prolactin level is between 8 and 10 AM. Ideally, prolactin levels should not be determined directly after a breast examination, sexual activity, or exercise session. Diagnostic tests that may be indicated include prolactin levels, microscopic analysis of the discharge, a thyroid profile, a pregnancy test, and a mammogram (Shenenberger & Knee, 2004).

Mammary Duct Ectasia

Mammary duct ectasia is an inflammation of the ducts behind the nipple. The cause of mammary duct ectasia is unknown, although chronic inflammation and dilation of the lactiferous ducts has been suggested. It occurs most often in perimenopausal women and is characterized by a nipple discharge that is thick; sticky; and white, brown, green, or purple. Often the patient will experience a burning pain, itching, or a palpable mass behind the nipple.

The workup includes a mammogram, and aspiration and culture of fluid. Duct ectasia is usually self-limiting, requiring only reassurance of the woman (American Cancer Society, 2003). Development of an infection in the inflamed area requires antibiotic therapy. Incision and drainage is necessary if an abscess develops. Treatment also may include a local excision of the affected duct(s) if the woman has no future plans to breastfeed.

Intraductal Papilloma

Intraductal papilloma is a rare, benign condition that develops in the terminal nipple ducts. The cause is unknown. It usually occurs in women between ages 30 and 50 years. Usually too small to be palpated (less than 0.5 cm), this papilloma causes serous, serosanguineous, or bloody nipple discharge. The discharge is unilateral and spontaneous. After the possibility of malignancy is eliminated, the affected segments of the ducts and breasts are surgically excised (American Cancer Society, 2003).

Table 6-6 compares common manifestations of benign breast masses.

Care Management

Assessment should include a careful history and physical examination. The history should focus on risk factors for breast diseases, events related to the breast mass, and health maintenance practices. Risk factors for breast cancer are discussed later in this chapter. Information related to the breast mass should include how, when, and by whom the mass was discovered. The interval between discovery and seeking care is crucial. The answers to these questions can give clues about breast self-examination (BSE) practice and access to care. The nurse should document the following patient information: pain, whether symptoms increase with menses, dietary habits, smoking habits, use of oral contraceptives, regular BSE, and the examination technique used. The woman's emotional status, including her stress level, fears, and concerns, and her ability to cope should also be assessed.

Physical examination may include assessment of the breasts for symmetry, masses (size, number, consistency, and mobility), and nipple discharge.

Nursing actions might include the following:

- Demonstrate correct BSE technique.
- Discuss the intervals for and facets of breast screening, including professional examination and mammography. Women with breast implants may need special views of the breast and precautions taken not to rupture the implant during mammography.
- Provide written educational materials in the woman's primary language.

Table 6-6

Comparison of Common Manifestations of Benign Breast Masses

FIBROCYSTIC CHANGES	FIBROADENOMA	LIPOMA	INTRADUCTAL PAPILLOMA	MAMMARY DUCT ECTASIA
Multiple lumps	Single lump	Single lump	Single or multiple	Mass behind nipple
Nodular	Well delineated	Well delineated	Not well delineated	Not well delineated
Palpable	Palpable	Palpable	Nonpalpable	Palpable
Movable	Movable	Movable	Nonmobile	Nonmobile
Round, smooth	Round, lobular	Round, lobular	Small, ball-like	Irregular
Firm or soft	Firm	Soft	Firm or soft	Firm
Tenderness influenced by menstrual cycle	Usually asymptomatic	Nontender	Usually nontender	Painful, burning, itching
Bilateral	Unilateral	Unilateral	Unilateral	Unilateral
May or may not have nipple discharge	No nipple discharge	No nipple discharge	Serous or bloody nipple discharge	Thick, sticky nipple discharge

- Encourage the verbalization of fears and concerns about treatment and prognosis.
- Provide specific information regarding the woman's condition and treatment, including dietary changes, drug therapy, comfort measures, stress management, and surgery.
- Describe pain-relieving strategies in detail, and collaborate with the primary health care provider to ensure effective pain control.
- Encourage discussion of feelings about body image.
- Refer to a support group or stress management resource if needed to cope with long-term consequences of benign breast conditions.

CASE STUDY—BREAST CANCER

Malignant Conditions of the Breast

The United States has one of the highest rates of breast carcinoma in the world. One in eight American women will develop breast cancer in her lifetime. The incidence of breast cancer rose about 4% per year beginning in 1980 and leveled off in the 1990s to about 110 cases per 100,000 women (American Cancer Society, 2004). Increasing incidence may be related to better detection of early-stage breast cancer. The incidence of breast cancer is higher in Caucasian women than in African-American women, but the mortality rate for African-American women with breast cancer is higher (Fig. 6-6). Even though African-American women practice BSE and obtain clinical breast examinations and mammograms by a professional with a frequency the same as or greater than that of Caucasian women, more African-American women are initially diagnosed with a later stage of breast cancer (American Cancer Society, 2004).

Etiology

Although the exact cause of breast cancer continues to elude investigators, certain factors that increase a women's risk for developing a malignancy have been identified. The factors are listed in Box 6-6.

The most important predictor of risk for breast cancer is age. A woman's risk of breast cancer increases as her age increases. Most of the other risk factors involve the effects of the menstrual-reproductive cycle (probably the effect of estrogen or progesterone) on the development of breast cancer. Fewer menstrual cycles and early childbearing appear to have a protective effect.

Although most breast cancers are not related to genetic factors, the identification of the BRCA1 and BRCA2 genes demonstrated the role of heredity and genetic mutations in this disease. Only about 5% of all breast cancers are attributed to heredity, but it is believed that mutations in the BRCA1 and BRCA2 genes are involved in 30% to 70% of all inherited cases of breast cancer (Nogueira & Appling, 2000).

Some known and suspected environmental risk factors include exposure to organochlorine pesticides and other synthetic chemicals, hormonal factors (both exogenous and endogenous), diet, tobacco and alcohol use, radiation, and magnetic fields (Johnson-Thompson & Guthrie, 2000). Exposure to radiation has been observed to double breast cancer risk, particularly when exposure occurs during rapid breast formation, as in teenage years (McPherson, Steel, & Dixon, 2000). Risk factors help to identify fewer than 30% of women who will eventually develop breast cancer. Women at increased risk should be screened more frequently.

Maintaining normal weight, eating a diet rich in fruits and vegetables and low in fat, and regular exercise seem to exert a protective effect against the development of breast cancer (McPherson et al, 2000).

Information about breast cancer risks can be confusing, and women can overestimate or underestimate their risks. The Breast Cancer Risk Assessment Tool can be used by women and health professionals to calculate risk. This tool was developed and verified by the National Cancer Institute (NCI) to predict the risk of breast cancer in 5 years and over the lifetime (to age 90 years) of a woman. The risk factors used are listed in Box 6-7. The tool is available on the Internet at the NCI Web site (see Resources at the end of chapter).

A comprehensive review of the research discussion about possible links between breast cancer and hormonal therapy revealed such a confounding range of variables that it has

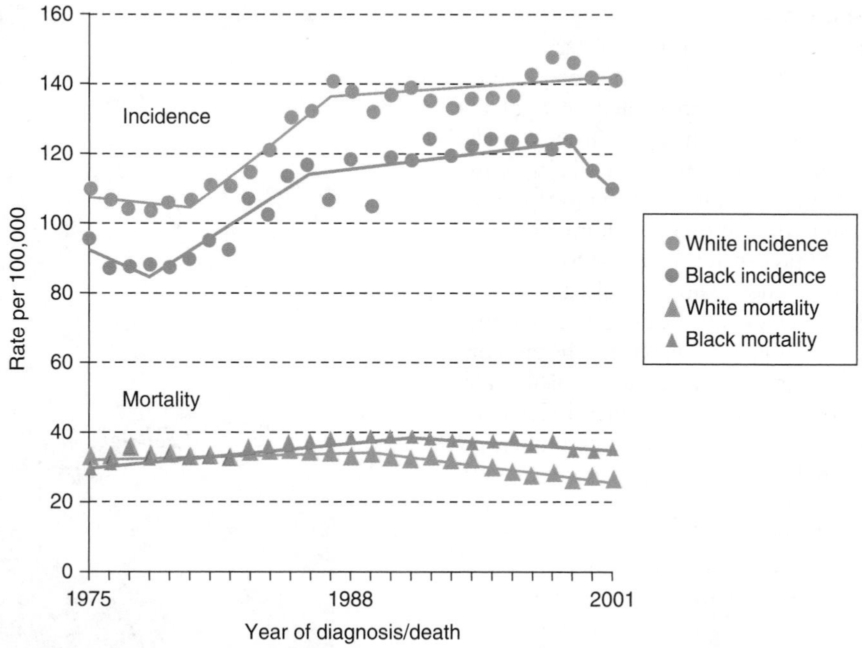

Fig. 6-6 Breast cancer incidence and mortality rates–Caucasian females vs. African-American females. (Courtesy National Cancer Institute, Washington, DC.)

BOX 6-6

Risk Factors for Breast Cancer*

Age
Previous history of breast cancer
Family history of breast cancer, especially a mother or sister (particularly significant if premenopausally)
Previous history of ovarian, endometrial, colon, or thyroid cancer
Early menarche (before age 12 years)
Late menopause (after age 55 years)
Nulliparity or first pregnancy after age 30 years
Use of estrogen replacement therapy
Daily alcohol use
Obesity after menopause
Previous history of benign breast disease with epithelial hyperplasia
Race (Caucasian women have highest incidence)
High socioeconomic status
Sedentary lifestyle

*Risk factors are cumulative—the more risk factors present, the greater the likelihood of breast cancer occurring.

BOX 6-7

Risk Factors Included in the Breast Cancer Risk Assessment Tool

Woman's age
Number of first-degree relatives affected
Age of woman at menarche
Age of woman at first live birth
Number of breast biopsies
History of abnormal hyperplasia in biopsy specimens

been impossible to draw definitive conclusions about hormonal replacement therapy and the risk of breast cancer. Observational data suggest that long-term use of estrogen replacement therapy (longer than 10 years) may slightly increase the risk, but the risk decreases after discontinuing use (Marsden, 2002).

Chemoprevention

Ongoing studies by the NCI and other groups are investigating the role of tamoxifen and raloxifene in the prevention of breast cancer (National Cancer Institute, 2002; Vogel et al, 2002). Raloxifene prevents osteoporosis without the possible increased cancer risks of estrogen replacement. This medication may be an ideal choice for the woman at high risk for both osteoporosis and breast cancer. Tamoxifen reduces the recurrence of breast cancer in women with prior breast malignancies. The risk of occasional serious side effects demands careful consideration before prescribing tamoxifen (Kinsinger et al, 2002) (see later discussion).

Pathophysiology

Breast cancer occurs when there are genetic alterations in the deoxyribonucleic acid (DNA) of breast epithelial cells. Many types of breast cancer exist. Genetic alterations are found in the epithelial cells, compromising ductal or lobular tissue. These genetic abnormalities may have been inherited or may have developed spontaneously (Rosenzweig, Rust, & Hoss, 2000). These cancers can be either invasive (infiltrating) or noninvasive (in situ). The most frequently occurring cancer of the breast is invasive ductal carcinoma. Ductal carcinoma originates in the lactiferous ducts and invades surrounding breast structures. The tumor is usually unilateral, not well delineated, solid, nonmobile, and nontender.

Metastasis results from seeding of the breast cancer cells into the blood and lymph systems, leading to tumor development in the bones, lungs, brain, and liver.

Clinical Manifestations and Diagnosis

Breast cancer in its earliest form can be detected on a mammogram before it can be felt by the woman or her health care provider. However, approximately 90% of all breast lumps are detected by the woman. Of this 90%, only 20% to 25% are malignant. More than half of all lumps are discovered in the upper outer quadrant of the breast (Fig. 6-7). The most common initial symptom is a lump or thickening of the breast. The lump may feel hard and fixed or soft and spongy. It may have well-defined or irregular borders. It may be fixed to the skin, thereby causing dimpling to occur. A bloody or clear unilateral nipple discharge may be present.

Early detection and diagnosis reduce the mortality rate because the cancer is found when it is smaller, lesions are more localized, and there tends to be a lower percentage of positive nodes. Regular BSE, the use of clinical examination by a qualified health care provider, and screening mammography (x-ray filming of the breast) (Fig. 6-8) may aid in the early detection of breast cancers. Table 6-7 lists the current recommendations of the American Cancer Society for breast cancer screening.

When a suspicious finding on mammogram is noted, or when a lump is detected, diagnosis is confirmed by FNA, core needle biopsy, or needle localization biopsy. The latter procedure requires the collaborative efforts of both the radiologist and the surgeon. This often requires that the procedure take place in two different environments (radiology and surgery). Patients need specific information regarding procedures, duration, and outcomes.

Major barriers to screening behaviors are cost, lack of access to health care, and lack of availability of mammography services. Cultural factors may influence a woman's decision to participate in breast cancer screening. Knowledge of these factors and use of culturally sensitive tailored messages and materials that appeal to the unique concerns, beliefs, and reading abilities of target groups of underutilizers may assist the nurse in helping women overcome barriers to seeking care (Cultural Awareness box).

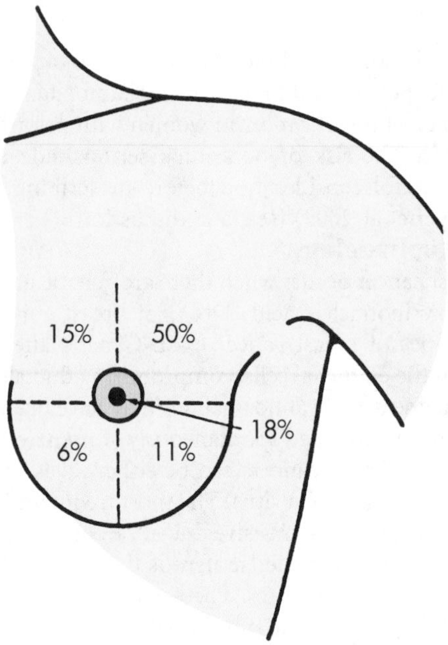

Fig. 6-7 Relative location of malignant lesions of the breast (Modified from DiSaia PJ, Creasman WT: *Clinical gynecologic oncology,* ed 6, St Louis, 2002, Mosby.)

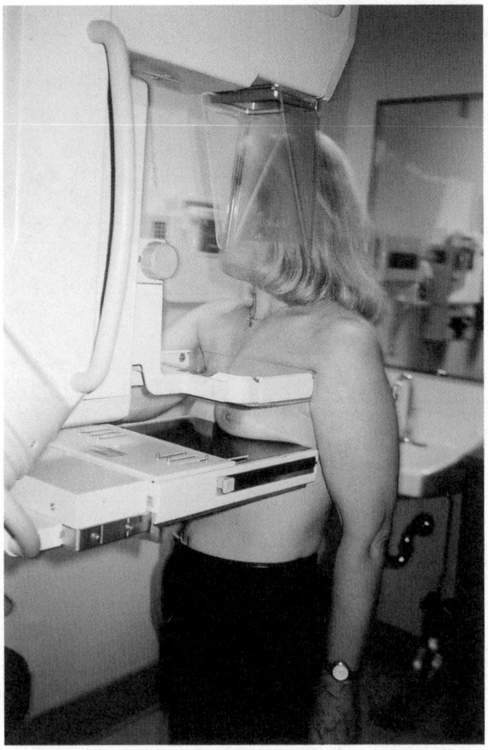

Fig. 6-8 Mammography. (Courtesy Shannon Perry, Phoenix, AZ.)

Laboratory diagnosis of breast cancer and possible cancer metastasis includes complete blood count, liver enzyme levels, serum calcium level, and alkaline phosphatase level. Elevated liver enzyme levels indicate possible liver metastasis, and increased serum calcium and alkaline phosphatase levels may indicate bone metastasis.

Prognosis

Major advances in understanding the biology of cancer have occurred in the past 10 years. Many studies support the theory that breast cancer is a systemic disease; micrometastasis could be present at the initial presentation with or without nodal involvement. However, nodal involvement and tumor

Table 6-7

Screening Guidelines for Breast Cancer: Detection in Asymptomatic Women Recommended by the American Cancer Society

AGE (YR)	EXAMINATION	FREQUENCY
20-39	Breast self-examination (BSE)	Monthly
	Clinical breast examination	Every 3 yr
40 and older	BSE	Monthly
	Clinical breast examination	Yearly
	Mammography	Yearly

Source: American Cancer Society: *Cancer facts and figures, 2004,* New York, 2004, American Cancer Society.

Cultural Awareness

BREAST SCREENING PRACTICES

Lower-income Hispanic women with less than a high school education were found to be more likely not to have participated in screening mammography. Reasons given by the women included fear of the test, misconceptions about cancer, embarrassment, and lack of knowledge (Fernandez, Tortolero-Luna, Gold, 1998). African-American women reported not participating in early breast cancer screening because breast cancer comes from chance, because getting it is determined by a higher being, because of fear of gynecologic examinations, because of doubting the value of early diagnosis and treatment, and because of not believing in vulnerability to cancer because no one in their family has had cancer (Barroso et al, 2000; Lawson, 1998). Both Hispanic and African-American women reported lack of available money to spend on health care, lack of insurance, and perceptions of being treated with prejudice by health care providers because of their race, age, income, or sexual orientation as reasons that they did not participate in breast cancer screening (Facione, 1999).

Chinese-American women were found to believe that they are not likely to get breast cancer and that getting cancer is related to bad luck. If they have symptoms of breast cancer, they are more likely to try Chinese medicine before Western medical treatments (Facione N et al: Perceived risk and help-seeking behavior for breast cancer: a Chinese-American perspective. *Cancer Nurs* 23(4):258-267, 2000).

size are the most significant prognostic criteria for long-term survival (Fig. 6-9). Women with estrogen receptor (ER) tumors respond better to therapy and have higher survival rates.

Management

Medical management of breast cancer includes surgery, breast reconstruction, radiation therapy, adjuvant hormone therapy, and chemotherapy.

Surgery

The most commonly recommended surgical approaches are lumpectomy and modified radical mastectomy (Fig. 6-10). Lumpectomy involves the removal of the breast tumor, a small amount of surrounding tissue, and a sampling of axillary lymph nodes, leaving the pectoralis major muscle intact. Partial mastectomy includes tylectomy, wide excision, and quadrantectomy or segmental mastectomy and involves removal of different amounts of tissue along with the tumor. Sampling of axillary lymph nodes is usually done through a separate incision at the time of these procedures, and surgery is usually followed by radiation therapy to the remaining breast tissue (Crane-Okada, 2001; DiSaia & Creasman, 2002). Total mastectomy (also called simple mastectomy) is the removal of all breast tissue, nipple, and areola; the axillary nodes and pectoral muscles are not removed. Lumpectomy offers survival equivalent to that with modified radical mastectomy (DiSaia & Creasman, 2002).

Modified radical mastectomy is the removal of the entire breast and a sample of axillary lymph nodes, sparing the pectoral muscles. A radical mastectomy, although rarely performed, removes the entire breast, axillary nodes, and the pectoral muscles. Mastectomy is used for the treatment of early-stage breast cancer when the woman fits the criteria listed in Box 6-8. Women who are found to have metastatic

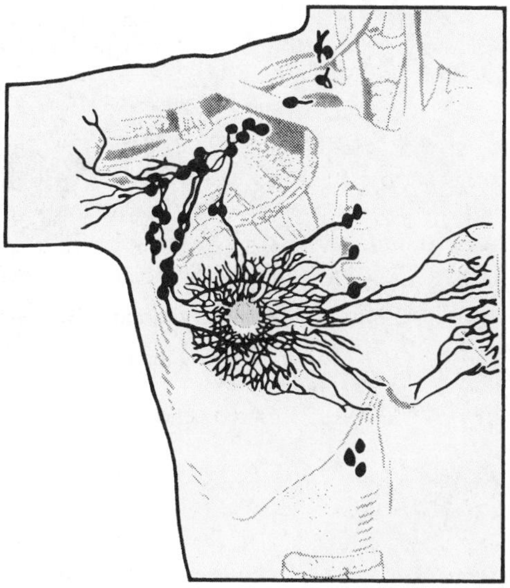

Fig. 6-9 Lymphatic spread of breast cancer.

breast cancer at the time of diagnosis usually do not have a mastectomy because it does not offer increased chances of survival.

Women who have these surgeries experience cosmetic changes. Change in shape (because of lumpectomy) or loss of a breast results in a change in body image, which can cause significant alterations in perceptions of femininity and sexual image and interest.

Breast Reconstruction

The goals of surgical breast reconstruction are achievement of symmetry and preservation of body image (Fig. 6-11). Surgical reconstruction can be done immediately or at a later date. Immediate reconstruction at the time of mastectomy does not change survival rates or interfere with therapy or the treatment of recurrent disease.

Autologous flap reconstruction involves the use of the woman's own tissue to create a breast. The three types of autologous flaps are the latissimus dorsi flap, the transverse rectus abdominis myocutaneous (TRAM) flap, and the inferior gluteus free flap. The latissimus dorsi and TRAM flaps are the most common (Fig. 6-12). After the reconstruction is done, postoperative care specific to the procedure focuses on monitoring the skin flap for signs of decreased capillary refill, hematoma, infection, and necrosis. Standard mastectomy activity restrictions and patient education points are followed.

The breast may also be reconstructed using saline-filled tissue expanders. A tissue expander is placed under the chest tissue to stretch the surrounding tissue to create adequate space for the permanent implant. The tissue expander is slowly filled with saline, through an injection port, over a period of months, to stretch the skin gradually until the desired symmetry is attained (Resnick & Belcher, 2002). As with all implantation procedures, risks of surgical complications such as hematoma, infection, and delayed wound healing are possible, as well as the possibility of capsular contractions from, or leakage of, the implant (Resnick & Belcher, 2002).

The safety of silicone breast implants continues to be controversial. Since 1992, the U.S. Food and Drug Adminis-

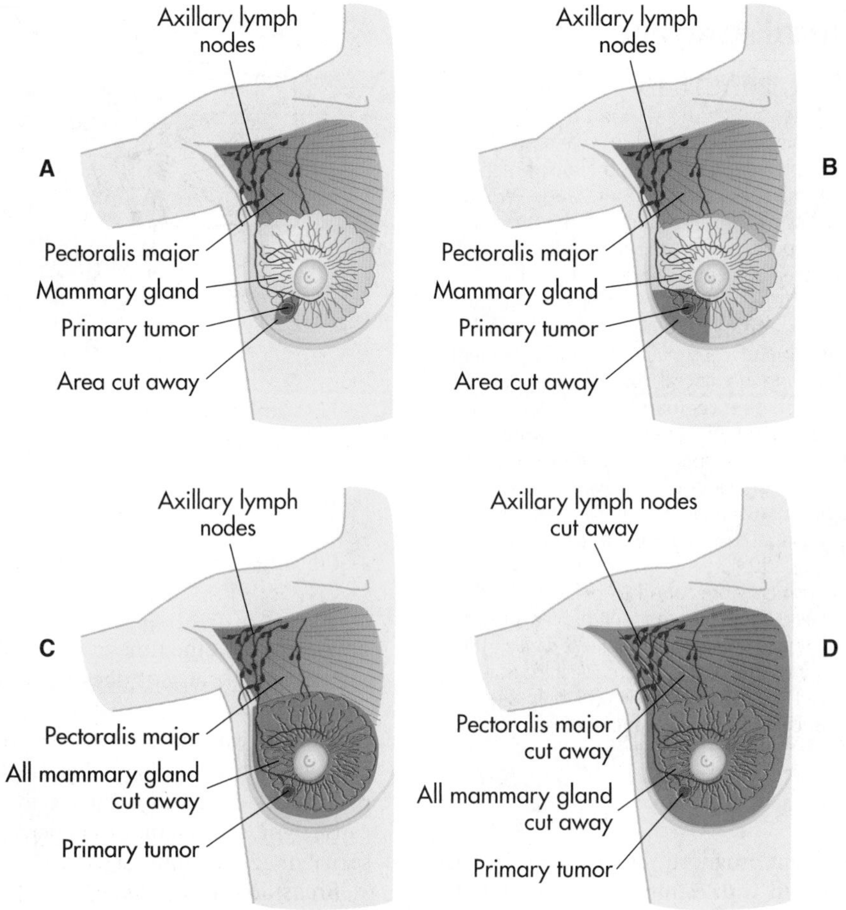

Fig. 6-10 Surgical alternatives for breast cancer. **A**, Lumpectomy (tylectomy). **B**, Quadrantectomy (segmental resection). **C**, Total (simple) mastectomy. **D**, Radical mastectomy.

BOX 6-8

Contraindications for Breast Conservation Treatment

- Presence of multiple tumors, especially in different parts of the breast
- Tumor removal alone would produce a cosmetically unacceptable result
- Previous breast radiation
- Pregnancy in the first or second trimester
- Persistent positive margins after reasonable surgery
- Possible history of collagen-vascular disease

Sources: DiSaia PJ, Creasman WT: *Clinical gynecologic oncology,* ed 6, St Louis, 2002, Mosby; Shuster TD et al: Multidisciplinary care for patients with breast cancer, *Surg Clin North Am* 80(2):505-533, 2000.

tration (FDA) has restricted use of silicone breast implants to women who are undergoing reconstruction after mastectomy, who have had severe breast injuries, who have birth defects that affect the breasts, who have a medical condition causing a severe breast abnormality, or who need to replace an existing implant (Zuckerman, 2002). Women interested in these implants should be informed of all the risks before making a decision (Resnick & Belcher, 2002).

Radiation

The conservative approach to treatment involves lumpectomy followed by radiation therapy as standard therapy for early stage breast cancer. Radiation to the breast destroys tumor cells remaining after manipulation and handling of the tumor during surgery. Side effects of radiation therapy include swelling and heaviness in the breast, sunburnlike skin changes in the treated area, and fatigue. Changes to the breast tissue and skin usually resolve in 6 to 12 months. Radiation therapy in the area of the axilla can cause lymphedema of the ipsilateral arm. Close medical follow-up is important after conservative surgery and radiation. Recommended guidelines include a breast physical examination every 4 to 6 months for 2 years, twice a year for 3 years, and then yearly. A mammogram is recommended 6 months after radiation and then annually (National Comprehensive Cancer Network, 2002).

Adjuvant Therapy

Chemotherapy administered soon after initial diagnosis and surgical removal of the tumor is referred to as adjuvant chemotherapy. Adjuvant chemotherapy (chemotherapy and endocrine therapy) is used to either eradicate or impede the growth of micrometastatic (microscopic cell metastasis) disease. Adjuvant chemotherapy significantly reduces the risks for recurrence and mortality in patients with node-positive disease (Shuster et al, 2000).

Hormonal Therapy

To determine whether a woman is a candidate for hormonal therapy, a receptor assay is done. The presence of a receptor on the cell wall indicates that the woman is positive for that type of hormone receptor. If these receptors are present, the growth of the woman's breast cancer may be influenced by estrogen, progesterone, or both. It is unknown exactly how these hormones affect breast cancer growth. Some premenopausal women may undergo bilateral oophorectomy to decrease the supply of hormones available for tumor growth (Shuster et al, 2000).

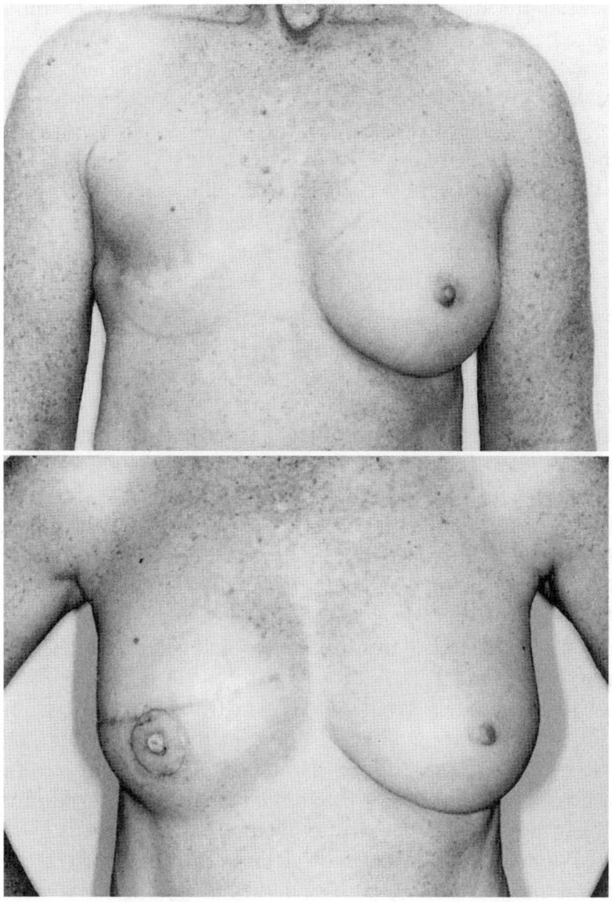

Fig. 6-11 Latissimus dorsi reconstruction after radical mastectomy.

Tamoxifen is an oral antiestrogen medication that mimics progesterone and estrogen. Tamoxifen attaches to the hormone receptors on cancer cells and prevents natural hormones from attaching to the receptors. When tamoxifen fits into the receptors, the cell is unable to grow. Adjuvant hormonal therapy using tamoxifen, recommended for all women over 50 years of age, improves disease-free survival and in some cases length of survival. The side effects of hormonal therapy include hot flashes, nausea, vomiting, fluid retention, weight gain, and thrombocytopenia. Tamoxifen therapy also increases the risk of endometrial cancer and deep vein thrombosis (Medication Guide box).

Chemotherapy

Chemotherapy drugs are most effective when used in combination. Chemotherapy drugs include methotrexate, 5-fluorouracil, cyclophosphamide, doxorubicin, and a taxane (DiSaia & Creasman, 2002; Shuster et al, 2000). Because chemotherapy drugs are designed to kill rapidly reproducing cells, normal body cells that rapidly reproduce (red and white blood cells, gastric mucosa, and hair) also can be affected during treatment. Thus chemotherapy can cause leukopenia, neutropenia, thrombocytopenia, anemia, gastrointestinal side effects (nausea, vomiting, anorexia, mucositis), and partial or full hair loss.

Chemotherapy treatments are usually given to ambulatory patients, once or twice per month. Depending on the medications used, the treatments may include intravenous, subcutaneous, and oral medications. Often a long-term central venous catheter is inserted when the women will be receiving chemotherapy for an extended period or when she will receive medications that may damage the vein.

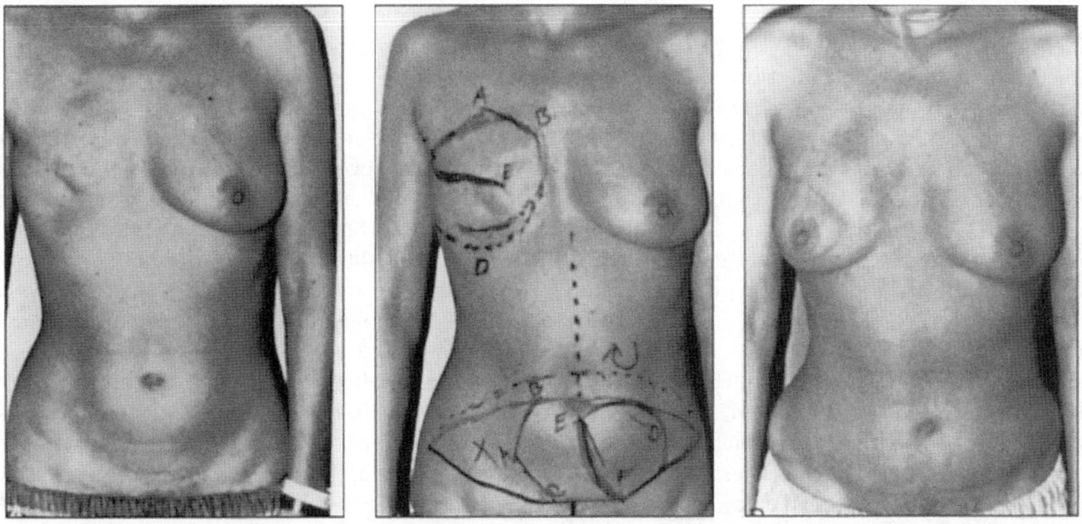

Fig. 6-12 Transverse rectus abdominis myocutaneous (TRAM) flap reconstruction. (From Harden JT, Girard N: Breast reconstruction using an innovative flap procedure, *AORN J* 60[2]:184-192, 1994.)

Medication Guide

TAMOXIFEN (NOLVADEX)

Action

Antiestrogenic effects; attaches to hormone receptors on cancer cells and prevents natural hormones from attaching to the receptors.

Indication

For treatment of metastatic breast cancer; treatment of breast cancer in postmenopausal women after breast cancer surgery and radiation therapy; to reduce the incidence of breast cancer in women at high risk.

Dosage

20 to 40 mg orally, daily. Dosages greater than 20 mg should be given in divided doses (AM and PM).

Adverse Reactions

Common side effects include hot flashes, nausea, vomiting, vaginal bleeding or discharge, menstrual irregularities, and rash. Hair loss is an uncommon effect. Serious side effects include deep vein thrombosis, increased risk of endometrial cancer, and stroke.

Nursing Considerations

The medication may be taken on an empty stomach or with food. Missed doses should be taken as soon as possible, but taking two doses at once is not recommended. A barrier or nonhormonal form of contraception is recommended in premenopausal women because tamoxifen may be harmful to the fetus.

Breast cancer treatment often causes changes in reproductive function. The postmenopausal woman may have to cope with hair loss and other unpleasant side effects from chemotherapy and loss of part or all of her breast. The premenopausal woman may experience these changes along with symptoms of menopause and possible infertility. The young woman with breast cancer may become devastated by an early and abrupt menopause and the possibility of jeopardized reproductive function. These factors can seriously affect the quality of life of the young woman (Sammarco, 2001) (Evidence-Based Practice box).

Chemotherapy is a mutagen and a teratogen. Any woman who is of childbearing age and receiving chemotherapy, even though no longer menstruating, must use birth control.

With the advance in monoclonal antibody technology, it is now possible to test for residual disease with a serum tumor marker, CA 15-3, if it is secreted by the patient's tumor. This technology is used to determine effectiveness of therapy for cancer without the need for second-look diagnostic surgery.

Care Management

Preoperatively, women need to be assessed for psychologic preparation and specific teaching needs. General preoperative teaching and care are given, including expectations regarding physical appearance, pain management, equipment to be used (e.g., intravenous therapy, drains), and emotional support. The emotional reaction to the diagnosis of cancer is always intense, and the many disruptions caused by the disease challenge the woman's and family's ability to cope. A visit from a woman who has had a similar experience may be beneficial preoperatively, as well as postoperatively. The woman is reminded that when she awakens after surgery, her arm on the affected side will feel tight.

Postoperative nursing care focuses on recovery. After recovery from anesthesia, the woman is returned to her room. Special precautions must be observed to prevent or to minimize lymphedema of the affected arm.

NURSE ALERT When vital signs are taken, never apply the blood pressure cuff on the affected arm. ■

The affected arm is elevated with pillows above the level of the right atrium. Blood is not drawn from this arm, and this arm is not used for intravenous therapy. Early arm movement is encouraged. Any increase in the circumference of that arm is reported immediately.

Nursing care of the wound involves observation for signs of hemorrhage (dressing, drainage tubes, and Hemovac or Jackson-Pratt drainage reservoirs are emptied at least every 8 hours and more frequently as needed), shock, and infection. Dressings are reinforced as necessary. The woman is asked to turn (alternating between unaffected side and back), cough (while the nurse or the woman applies support to the chest), and deep breathe every 2 hours. Breath sounds are auscultated every 4 hours. Active range-of-motion (ROM) exercise of legs is encouraged. Parenteral fluids are given until adequate oral intake is possible. Emotional support is continued.

The woman is given self-care instructions and usually discharged to home after 24 hours or more, depending on the type of procedure done (Home Care box). Lumpectomy is an outpatient procedure, and the patient will return home a few hours after surgery. A women is discharged 24 to 48 hours after modified radical mastectomy. A referral for home nursing care may be made if the woman needs assistance caring for her incision. A referral to the American Cancer Society's Reach to Recovery program will result in a visit by a breast cancer survivor who has been trained in how to offer information. The resources offered may include such things as a list of sources for prostheses and lingerie. Arm exercises are encouraged at least four times daily (Box 6-9).

Exercise is increased as tolerated and is stopped at the point of pain. Initially the woman alternately clenches and extends her fingers and then progresses to wrist and elbow exercises, gradually abducting her arm and raising it to and over her head. She is encouraged to exercise by assisting with her care—washing her face, brushing her teeth, and eating with her hand and arm on the affected side. Physical therapy may be prescribed to improve strength and mobility of the affected arm.

Concerns about appearance after breast surgery may affect the woman's self-concept. Before surgery, the woman and her partner need information about what the woman's postoperative appearance will be like. Both the woman and her partner need to be able to discuss feelings and concerns about accepting the changes. Information about community resources and support groups such as Reach to Recovery may be beneficial. Invaluable resources are the National

Home Care

AFTER A MASTECTOMY

Wash hands well before and after touching incision area or drains.

Empty surgical drains twice a day and as needed, recording the date, time, drain site (if more than one drain is present), and amount of drainage in milliliters in a diary you will take to each surgical checkup until your drains are removed. (Before discharge, you may receive a graduated container for emptying drains and measuring drainage.)

Avoid driving, lifting more than 10 pounds, or reaching above your head until given permission by surgeon.

Take medications for pain as soon as pain begins.

Perform arm exercises as directed.

Call physician if inflammation of incision or swelling of the incision or the arm occurs.

Avoid tight clothing, tight jewelry, and other causes of decreased circulation in the affected arm.

Until drains are removed, wear loose-fitting underwear (camisole or half-slip) and clothes, pinning surgical drains inside of clothing. (You will be taught how to do this safely.)

After drains are removed and surgical sites are healing and still tender, wear a mastectomy bra or camisole with a cotton-filled, muslin temporary prosthesis. Temporary prostheses of this type are often available from Reach to Recovery.

Avoid depilatory creams, strong deodorants, and shaving of affected chest area, axilla, and arm.

Sponge bathe until drains are removed.

Return to the surgeon's office for incision check, drain inspection, and possible drain removal as directed.

Contact Reach to Recovery for assistance obtaining external prosthesis and lingerie when dressings, drains, and staples are removed and wound is healing and nontender.

Contact insurance company for information about coverage of prosthesis and wig if needed. Obtain prescriptions for prosthesis and wig to submit with receipts of purchase for these items to the insurance company. If insurance does not pay for these items, contact hospital or agency social worker or local American Cancer Society for assistance.

Continue with monthly BSE of unaffected side and affected surgical site and axilla.

Encourage mother, sisters, and daughters (if applicable) to learn and practice monthly BSE and to have annual professional breast examinations and mammography (if appropriate).

Keep follow-up visits for professional examination, mammography, and testing to detect recurrent breast cancer.

Expect decreased sensation and tingling at incision sites and in the affected arm for weeks to months after surgery.

Resume sexual activities as desired.

BOX 6-9

Arm Exercises After Lymph Node Dissection

Check with your health care provider before performing these exercises. Perform exercises slowly to stretch the muscle gently. Repeat exercises several times a day with time to rest in between.

Exercise: Climbing the Wall

1. Stand facing wall with toes close to wall.
2. Bend elbows and place palms of hands against wall at shoulder level.
3. Move both hands parallel to each other up the wall as far as possible until incisional pull or pain occurs.
4. Move both hands down to starting position either by sliding them back down or walking them back down.
5. Goal is to reach all the way up with arm in complete extension with elbow straight. Repeat several times.
6. Perform activities that use the same action: reaching top shelves, washing windows, blow-drying hair.

Exercise: Rope Pull

1. Attach a 6-foot rope over a shower rod or a hook at the top of a door.
2. Grasp one end of the rope in each hand, and extend your arms to your sides. Pull down on one end while raising the other arm, raising arm as high as you can (on affected side to a point of incisional pull or pain). Reverse the exercise, with the raised arm being lowered and raising the lower arm.
3. Shorten rope over time until arm on affected side is raised almost directly overhead.

Exercise: Elbow Spread

1. Clasp hands behind neck.
2. Raise elbows to chin level, holding head erect; move slowly and rest when incisional pull or pain occurs.
3. Gradually spread elbows apart; rest when pull or pain occurs. Repeat several times.

Exercise: Arm Over Head

1. Lie down with your arms by your side.
2. Raise the arm on the surgery side straight up and reach over your head. Repeat several times.

Community Focus

CHOICES REGARDING RECONSTRUCTIVE SURGERY AFTER MASTECTOMY

Interview a woman who selected reconstructive surgery after mastectomy to treat breast cancer and one who did not select such surgery.

- What were their reasons for their decisions?
- What influence did their partners have on their decisions?
- Did their age affect their treatment decision?
- What social and community support did they receive to deal with their diagnoses and treatment?
- What additional social and community support would they recommend be available for women with breast cancer?
- How will this information assist you in caring for patients having mastectomy, with or without reconstructive surgery?

Nursing Care Plan

THE WOMAN WITH BREAST CANCER

NURSING DIAGNOSIS: Pain related to surgical incision and surgical drains as evidenced by patient verbalizations

EXPECTED OUTCOME

Patient will report minimal intensity and decreased number of painful episodes.

NURSING INTERVENTIONS/*RATIONALES*

Use pain scale to assess for type and intensity of pain *to provide accurate database.*

Administer analgesics as ordered *to decrease perception of pain.*

Reposition patient with affected arm elevated *to promote comfort and lymphatic channel return.*

NURSING DIAGNOSIS: Risk for infection related to disruption of skin integrity and removal of lymph nodes as evidenced by clinical manifestations

EXPECTED OUTCOME

Patient will experience no clinical manifestations of infection.

NURSING INTERVENTIONS/*RATIONALES*

Assess for clinical manifestations of infection at the incision and drain sites that may include redness, swelling, localized heat, fever, increasing pain, and foul-smelling drainage *to facilitate prompt treatment.*

Demonstrate the procedure for emptying and recording the amount of drainage from the Jackson-Pratt drain(s) *to provide information to the surgeon as to the appropriate removal time of drains. Drains are usually removed when 24 hours of drainage does not exceed 30 ml of fluid.*

Explain the need to avoid trauma or irritation to the affected arm *to reinforce to the patient that alterations in sensation and removal of some lymph nodes may affect ability to sense irritation and prevent infection.*

Reinforce to patient the need to protect arm from injury and to avoid venipunctures or blood pressures to be taken on the affected arm *to avoid trauma and infection, since decreased sensation may be present as well as decreased lymphatic return.*

Explain the importance of reporting any clinical manifestations of infection to the caregiver as soon as possible *to provide identification and treatment of problem.*

NURSING DIAGNOSIS: Disturbed body image related to loss of all or part of a breast as evidenced by patient statements

EXPECTED OUTCOME

Patient will maintain a positive body image.

NURSING INTERVENTIONS/*RATIONALES*

Provide opportunity through therapeutic communication to express feelings about body image changes *to clarify and validate feelings.*

Provide information about breast prostheses and other cosmetic devices *to assist in maintaining an intact body image.*

Encourage woman to speak to physician about the possibility of breast reconstructive surgery *to provide additional resources for body image enhancement.*

Refer to support groups *to facilitate verbalization of feelings with women who have similar concerns.*

Comprehensive Cancer Network (NCCN) and the American Cancer Society, which provide specific, up-to-date recommendations on breast cancer treatments on the Internet.

Before discharge, considerable time should be spent counseling the woman and her family about the aspects of self-care. Printed instructions should be given to the woman and her family.

Care of the woman with breast cancer is effective if the woman verbalizes satisfaction with the decision-making process about treatment options and if she gets appropriate support from significant others through all stages of treatment and recovery (Nursing Care Plan).

Key Points

- Menstrual disorders diminish the quality of life for affected women and their families.
- Premenstrual syndrome (PMS) is a disorder that begins in the luteal phase of the menstrual cycle and ends with the onset of menses.
- Endometriosis is characterized by secondary amenorrhea, dyspareunia, abnormal uterine bleeding, and infertility.
- Alternative therapies are beneficial in relieving some discomforts associated with menstrual disorders.
- Safer sex practices are key STI prevention strategies.
- STIs are responsible for substantial mortality and morbidity, great personal suffering, and heavy economic burden in the United States.
- Pregnancy confers no immunity against infection; both mother and fetus must be considered when a pregnant woman contracts an infection.
- Blood and body fluid precautions should be used consistently for everyone all the time.
- Approximately 50% of women experience a breast problem at some point in their adult life; the risk of an American woman developing breast cancer is 1 in 8.
- Monthly BSE, yearly clinical breast examinations by a health care provider, and routine screening mammograms are recommended for early detection of breast cancer.

- Treatment for breast cancer includes surgery, radiation, and chemotherapy.

Answer Guidelines to Critical Thinking Exercise

Uterine Fibroids and Pregnancy

1. Yes, there is sufficient evidence to draw conclusions about what information and advice to provide Tracy.
2. (a) Depending on size and location, fibroids may interfere with implantation of a fertilized ovum, the enlarging embryo/fetus, and expulsion of the fetus during labor. Based on physical examination, ultrasound, and other diagnostic tests, the physician can provide Tracy with information about the probabilities of problems. (b) The risks of surgery are well documented. Tracy can be advised about criteria to use to select a surgeon, an anesthesiologist, and a hospital if she chooses to have surgery. Her options may be limited by her insurance. (c) If Tracy chooses to try to achieve pregnancy, she will need to allow time for the effects of her last injection of Depo-Provera to wear off and to be prepared for a return of dysmenorrhea. If she chooses to have surgery, the dysmenorrhea may lessen after the fibroids are removed.
3. Tracy is seeking information and advice. The NP can refer her to written information, provide her with statistics and criteria for making health care decisions. The NP needs to collaborate with the physician so that Tracy is provided the best information and choices available. The NP can assist Tracy with her decision-making process, but should refrain from making the decision for Tracy. The decision must be made by Tracy and her husband.
4. Yes, the statistics on fibroids, pregnancy, surgery, and dysmenorrhea are available.
5. Tracy can also choose to try to become pregnant without the surgery to remove the fibroids. If she is able to achieve and maintain a pregnancy, a cesarean birth is an option if the fibroids are at the cervical os and would interfere with a vaginal birth. Tracy and her husband could also choose not to become pregnant but to have a child through adoption or to remain childless.

Resources

American Cancer Society
1599 Clifton Rd., NE
Atlanta, GA 30329
800-ACS-2345
www.cancer.org

American College of Obstetricians and Gynecologists
409 12th St.
Washington, DC 20024
800-762-2264
www.acog.org

Association of Women's Health, Obstetric, and Neonatal Nurses (AWHONN)
2000 L St., NW, Suite 740
Washington, DC 20036
800-673-8499 (United States)
800-245-0231 (Canada)
www.awhonn.org

Endometriosis Association
8585 North 76th Place
Milwaukee, WI 53223
414-355-2200
800-992-3636
www.ivf.com/endohtml.html

Food and Drug Administration (FDA)
Office of Consumer Affairs
Public Inquiries
5600 Fishers Lane (HFE-88)
Rockville, MD 20857
301-443-3170
www.fda.gov

Jacob's Institute for Women's Health
409 12th St., SW
Washington, DC 20024
National AIDS Hotline
1-800-342-2437 (English)
1-800-344-7432 (Spanish)
1-800-243-7889 (hearing-impaired)

National AIDS Information Clearing House
PO Box 6003
Rockville, MD 20850
1-800-458-5231

National Women's Health Resource Center
120 Albany St., Suite 820
New Brunswick, NJ 08901
877-986-9472
www.healthywomen.org

Premenstrual Syndrome Action
PO Box 16292
Irvine, CA 92713
714-854-4407

References

ACNM Clinical Bulletin: Clinical Bulletin no. 6: abnormal and dysfunctional uterine bleeding, *J Midwifery Womens Health* 47(3):207-213, 2002.

Alexander E, Shimp L, Smith M: Obesity and eating disorders. In Smith M, Shimp L (eds): *20 common problems in women's health care,* New York, 2000, McGraw-Hill.

Allen D et al: Revised recommendations for HIV screening of pregnant women, *MMWR* 50(RR-19):59-86, 2001.

American Cancer Society: *Cancer facts and figures 2004,* New York, 2004, American Cancer Society.

American Cancer Society: Benign breast conditions. Updated May 15, 2003. Internet document available at www.cancer.org/docroot/CRI/content/CRI_2_6X_benign_breast_conditions_59.asp (accessed July 14, 2004).

Barroso J et al: Comparison between African-American and white women in their beliefs about breast cancer and their health locus of control, *Cancer Nurs* 23(4): 268-276, 2000.

Bascom A: *Incorporating herbal medicine into clinical practice,* Philadelphia, 2002, FA Davis.

Blackburn ST: *Maternal, fetal, and neonatal physiology: a clinical perspective,* ed 2, St Louis, 2003, WB Saunders.

Bolyard EA et al: Guidelines for infection control in health care personnel, 1998, *Am J Infect Control* 26:289-354, 1998.

Brocklehurst P, Hannah M, McDonald H: Interventions for treating bacterial vaginosis in pregnancy, *Cochrane Database Syst Rev* (2):CD000262, 2000.

Canavan TP, Doshi NR: Cervical cancer, *Am Fam Physician* 61(5): 1369-1376, 2000.

Carey JC et al: Metronidazole to prevent preterm delivery in pregnant women with asymptomatic bacterial vaginosis. National Institute of Child Health and Human Development Network of Maternal-Fetal Medicine Units, *N Engl J Med* 342(8):534-540, 2000.

Centers for Disease Control and Prevention: Sexually transmitted diseases treatment guidelines 2002, *MMWR* 51(RR-6):1-82, 2002.

Centers for Disease Control and Prevention: Standard precautions: excerpted from Guideline for isolation precautions in hospitals, January 1996. Updated November 3, 2004. Web document available from www.cdc.gov/ncidod/hip/ISOLAT/std_prec_excerpt.htm (accessed December 4, 2004).

Clark LR: Premenstrual syndrome, *eMedicine Specialties,* February 18, 2004. Internet document available at www.emedicine.com (accessed July 14, 2004).

Crane-Okada R: Breast cancers. In Otto S (ed): *Oncology nursing,* ed 4, St Louis, 2001, Mosby.

Cronje WH, Studd JW: Premenstrual syndrome and premenstrual dysphoric disorder, *Prim Care* 29(1):1-12, 2002.

DiSaia PJ, Creasman WT: *Clinical gynecologic oncology,* ed 6, St Louis, 2002, Mosby.

Dog L: *An integrative approach to dysmenorrhea,* Corrales, NM, 2000, Integrative Medicine Education Association.

Dog L: *Endocrinology and women's issues,* Third Annual Conference on Clinical Relevance of Medicinal Herbs and Nutritional Supplements in the Management of Major Medical Problems, September 21-23, 2001.

Elliot H: Premenstrual dysphoric disorder, *North Carolina Med J* 63(2): 72-75, 2002.

Facione N: Breast cancer screening in relation to access to health services, *Onc Nurs Forum* 26(4): 689-696, 1999.

Facts and Comparisons: *Loose-leaf drug information service,* St Louis, 2002, Facts and Comparisons.

Fernandez M, Tortolero-Luna G, Gold R: Mammography and Pap test screening among low-income foreign-born Hispanic women in USA, *Cadernos de Saude Publica* 14(suppl 3):133-147, 1998.

Fogel CI: Female sexuality. In Breslin E, Lucas V (eds): *AWHONN women's health nursing: toward evidence-based practice*, Philadelphia, 2003, WB Saunders.

Friedenreich CM et al: Risk factors for benign proliferative breast disease, *Int J Epidemiol* 29(4):637-644, 2000.

Friedman A, Carlson K: Uterine fibroids. In Carlson K et al (eds): *Primary care of women,* ed 2, St Louis, 2002, Mosby.

Fugh-Berman A, Awang D: Black cohosh, *Altern Ther Womens Health* 39(11):81-85, 2001.

Guise JM et al: Screening for bacterial vaginosis in pregnancy, *Am J Prev Med* 20(3 suppl):62-72, 2001.

Hall J: Amenorrhea. In Carlson K et al (eds): *Primary care of women,* ed 2, St Louis, 2002, Mosby.

Harden JT, Girard N: Breast reconstruction using an innovative flap procedure, *AORN J* 60(2):184-192, 1994.

Harlow S: Menstruation and menstrual disorders. In Goldman M, Hatch M (eds): *Women and health,* San Diego, 2000, Academic Press.

Hillard P: Diagnosing and controlling abnormal uterine bleeding, *Contemp Adolescent Gynecol* 4(1):4-11, 1999.

Institute of Medicine, Committee on Prevention and Control of Sexually Transmitted Diseases: *The hidden epidemic: confronting sexually transmitted diseases,* Washington, DC, 1997, National Academy of Sciences.

Johnson-Thompson M, Guthrie J: Ongoing research to identify environmental risk factors in breast carcinoma, *Cancer* 88(5):1224-1229, 2000.

Jones C: Premenstrual dysphoric disorder: a protocol for management, *Adv Nurse Pract* 9(3):87-90, 2001.

Kinsinger LS et al: Chemoprevention of breast cancer: a summary of the evidence for the US Preventive Services Task Force, *Ann Intern Med* 137(1):59-69, 2002.

Kleposki RW: The female athlete triad: a terrible trio, implications for primary care, *J Am Acad Nurse Pract* 14(1):26-31, 2002.

Lawson E: A narrative analysis: a black woman's perception of breast cancer risks and early breast cancer detection, *Cancer Nurs* 21(6): 421-429, 1998.

Lin J, Thompson DS: Treating premenstrual dysphoric disorder using serotonin agents, *J Womens Health Gen Based Med* 10(8):745-750, 2001.

Marsden J: Hormone-replacement therapy and breast cancer, *Lancet Oncol* 3(5):303-311, 2002.

McPherson K, Steel CM, Dixon JM: ABC of breast diseases: breast cancer epidemiology, risk factors, and genetics, *BMJ* 321(7261):624-628, 2000.

Nakad T, Isaacson K: Endometriosis. In Carlson K et al (eds): *Primary care of women,* ed 2, St Louis, 2002, Mosby.

National Cancer Institute: Cancer trials information. Internet document available at www.nci.nih.gov/clinicaltrials/ (accessed May 22, 2002).

National Center for Infectious Diseases: Viral hepatitis C. Fact sheet. Internet document available at www.cdc/ncidod/diseases/hepatitis/c/fact.htm (accessed July 14, 2004).

National Comprehensive Cancer Network: Breast cancer treatment guidelines for patients, 2002. Internet document available at www.nccn.org (accessed June 4, 2002).

Nogueira SM, Appling SE: Breast cancer: genetics, risks, and strategies, *Nurs Clin North Am* 35(3):663-669, 2000.

Parent-Stevens L, Burns E: Menstrual disorders. In Smith M, Shimp L (eds): *20 common problems in women's health care,* New York, 2000, McGraw-Hill.

Primary and secondary syphilis—United States, 2002, *MMWR* 52(46): 1117-1120, 2003.

Rawlins S: Nonviral sexually transmitted infections, *J Obstet Gynecol Neonatal Nurs* 30(3):324-331, 2001.

Resnick B, Belcher AE: Breast reconstruction: options, answers, and support for patients making a difficult personal decision, *Am J Nurs* 102(4):26-33, 2002.

Rosenzweig MQ, Rust D, Hoss J: Prognostic information in breast cancer care: helping patients utilize important information, *Clin J Oncol Nurs* 4(6):271-278, 2000.

Sabatini S: The female athlete triad, *Am J Med Sci* 322(4):193-195, 2001.

Sammarco A: Perceived social support, uncertainty, and quality of life of younger breast cancer survivors, *Cancer Nurs* 24(3):212-218, 2001.

Sanborn CF et al: Disordered eating and the female athlete triad, *Clin Sports Med* 19(2):199-213, 2000.

Schellenberg R: Treatment for the premenstrual syndrome with *Agnus castus* fruit extract: prospective, randomized, placebo controlled study, *BMJ* 322(7279):134-137, 2001.

Selak V et al: Danazol for pelvic pain associated with endometriosis (Cochrane Review), 2004. In *The Cochrane Library*, Issue 4, Chichester, UK, 2004, John Wiley & Sons.

Shenenberger D, Knee T: Hyperprolactinemia, *eMedicine Specialties,* June 4, 2004. Internet document available at emedicine.com/med/topic1098.htm (accessed July 14, 2004).

Shuster TD et al: Multidisciplinary care for patients with breast cancer, *Surg Clin North Am* 80(2):505-533, 2000.

Stenchever M et al: *Comprehensive gynecology,* ed 4, St Louis, 2001, Mosby.

Stevinson C, Ernst E: Complementary/alternative therapies for premenstrual syndrome: a systemic review of random controlled trials, *Am J Obstet Gynecol* 185(1):227-235, 2001.

Thomas DJ: Sexually transmitted viral infections: epidemiology and treatment, *J Obstet Gynecol Neonatal Nurs* 30(3):316-323, 2001.

US Preventive Services Task Force: Screening for chlamydial infection: recommendations and rationale, *Am J Prev Med* 20(3S):90-94, 2001a.

US Preventive Services Task Force: Screening for bacterial vaginosis in pregnancy: recommendations and rationale, *Am J Nurs* 102(8):91-93, 2001b.

Vogel VG et al: The study of tamoxifen and raloxifene: preliminary enrollment data from a randomized breast cancer risk reduction trial, *Clin Breast Cancer* 3(2):153-159, 2002.

Walsh C, Irwin K: Combating the silent *Chlamydia* epidemic, *Contemp OB/GYN* 47(4):90-100, 103-104, 2002.

West RV: The female athlete. The triad of disordered eating, amenorrhoea, and osteoporosis, *Sports Med* 26(2):63-71, 1998.

Wilkinson D et al: Nonoxynol-9 spermicide for prevention of vaginally acquired HIV and other sexually transmitted infections: systematic review and meta-analysis of randomized controlled trials including more than 5000 women, *Lancet Infect Dis* 2(10):613-617, 2002.

Workowski KA, Levine WC, Wasserheit JN: US Centers for Disease Control and Prevention guidelines for the treatment of sexually transmitted diseases: an opportunity to unify clinical and public health practice, *Ann Intern Med* 137(4):255-262, 2002.

World Health Organization (WHO), Department of Reproductive Health and Research: *Improving access to quality care in family planning: medical eligibility criteria for contraceptive use,* ed 2, Geneva, 2000, WHO.

Wright TC Jr et al: 2001 consensus guidelines for the management of women with cervical cytology abnormalities, *JAMA* 287(16):2120-2129, 2002.

Zuckerman D: The breast cancer information gap, *RN* 65(2):39-41, 2002.

Unit 2

7 Infertility, Contraception, and Abortion

LEARNING OBJECTIVES

On completion of this chapter the reader will be able to:

- List common causes of infertility.
- Discuss the psychologic impact of infertility.
- List common diagnoses and treatments for infertility.
- Compare reproductive alternatives for couples experiencing infertility.
- State the advantages and disadvantages of methods of contraception.
- Explain common nursing interventions that facilitate contraceptive use.
- Describe the techniques used for medical and surgical interruption of pregnancy.
- Recognize ethical, legal, cultural, and religious considerations of infertility, contraception, and elective abortion.

ELECTRONIC RESOURCES

Additional information related to the content in Chapter 7 can be found on

the companion website at evolve
http://evolve.elsevier.com/Wong/maternal/
- NCLEX Review Questions
- WebLinks

or the interactive student CD-ROM
Activities for Chapter 7 include the following:
- NCLEX Review Questions
- Critical Thinking Exercise—Patient Teaching: Contraception
- Nursing Care Plan—Sexual Activity/Contraception
- Nursing Care Plan—Infertility

This chapter addresses infertility, associated tests, and common therapies; contraception; and abortion. Available alternatives and psychosocial implications are discussed.

INFERTILITY

Incidence

Infertility is a serious medical concern that affects quality of life and is a problem for approximately 10% of reproductive-age couples (American Society for Reproductive Medicine [ASRM], 2004). Infertility implies subfertility, a prolonged time to conceive, as opposed to sterility, or the inability to conceive. A fertile couple has approximately a 25% chance of conception in each ovulatory cycle. Primary infertility applies to a woman who has never been pregnant. Secondary infertility applies to a woman who has been pregnant in the past.

The prevalence of infertility is relatively stable among the overall population; in the individual, it increases with the age of the woman. Probable causes of infertility include the trend toward delaying pregnancy until later in life, when fertility decreases naturally and the prevalence of diseases such as endometriosis and ovulatory dysfunction increases.

The diagnosis and treatment of infertility have considerable physical, emotional, psychologic, and social effects (King, 2003; Sherrod, 2004) and require financial investment over an extended period. Men and women often perceive infertility differently, with women having more stress from tests and treatments, placing greater importance on having children, being more accepting of indicated treatments, and wanting children more than men. Feelings connected with infertility are many and complex. The attitude, sensitivity, and caring nature of those who are involved in the assessment and treatment of infertility lay the foundation for the patients' ability to cope with the many tests and treatments they must undergo. Team members must respect individuals' and couples' desires in choosing to stop treatment and to select other alternatives such as remaining childless or adoption.

Factors Associated with Infertility

Many factors, in both the male and female, contribute to normal fertility. A normally developed reproductive tract in both the male and female partner is essential. Normal functioning of an intact hypothalamic-pituitary-gonadal axis supports gametogenesis (the formation of sperm and ova). Timing of intercourse is critical: infertility may be caused by something as simple as poor timing or inadequate frequency of intercourse. Although sperm remain viable in the female's reproductive tract for 48 hours or more, probably only a few retain fertilization potential for more than 24 hours. Ova remain viable for about 24 hours, but the optimum time for fertilization may be no more than 1 to 2 hours (Cunningham et al, 2001). Implantation of the blastocyst must occur within 7 to 10 days in a hormone-prepared endometrium. The conceptus must develop normally, reach viability, and be born in good condition for extrauterine life.

An alteration in one or more of these structures, functions, or processes results in some degree of impaired fertility. In general, a female factor such as ovulatory dysfunction or pelvic factors is responsible for infertility in one third of infertile couples and a male factor (sperm and semen abnormalities) is responsible for infertility in about one third of couples. In the remaining couples, a combination of female and male factors or unexplained factors and unusual problems account for infertility (ASRM, 2004). Box 7-1 lists factors affecting female fertility; Box 7-2 lists factors affecting male fertility.

Care Management

Assessment

The nurse assists in the assessment by obtaining data relevant to fertility through interview and physical examination. The database must include information to identify whether infertility is primary or secondary. Religious, cultural, and ethnic data are noted because these may place restrictions on tests and treatments (Box 7-3 and Cultural Awareness box).

Some of the data needed to investigate impaired fertility are of a sensitive, personal nature. Obtaining these data may be viewed as an invasion of privacy. The tests and examinations are occasionally painful and intrusive and can take the romance out of lovemaking. A high level of motivation is needed to endure the investigation.

Because multiple factors involving both partners are common, the investigation of impaired fertility is conducted systematically and simultaneously for both male and female partners. Both partners must be interested in the solution to the problem. The medical investigation requires time (3 to 4 months) and considerable financial expense (Box 7-4). It also causes emotional distress and strain on the couple's interpersonal relationship (King, 2003). Couples should be cautioned that everything can be normal and conception may still not occur; and conversely, that poor test results do not mean a pregnancy will not occur.

Assessment of Female Infertility

Investigation of impaired fertility begins for the woman with a complete history and physical examination. The history explores the duration of infertility and past obstetric events and contains a detailed sexual history. Medical and surgical conditions are evaluated. Exposure to reproductive hazards in the home (e.g., mutagens such as vinyl chlorides, teratogens such as alcohol, and emotional stresses) and workplace are explored.

BOX 7-1

Factors Affecting Female Fertility

Congenital or Developmental Factors
Abnormal external genitals
Absence of internal reproductive structures

Ovarian Factors
Anovulation—primary
Pituitary or hypothalamic hormone disorder
Adrenal gland disorder
Congenital adrenal hyperplasia
Anovulation—secondary
Disruption of hypothalamic-pituitary-ovarian axis
Amenorrhea after discontinuing oral contraceptive pills
Early menopause
Increased prolactin levels

Tubal/Peritoneal Factors
Tubal motility reduced
Absence of fimbriated end of tube
Absence of a tube
Inflammation within the tube
Tubal adhesions

Uterine Factors
Developmental anomalies
Endometrial and myometrial tumors
Asherman syndrome (uterine adhesions or scar tissue)

BOX 7-2

Factors Affecting Male Fertility

Structural or Hormonal Disorders
Undescended testes
Hypospadias
Varicocele
Low testosterone levels
Testicular damage caused by mumps

Other Factors
Endocrine disorders
Genetic disorders
Psychologic disorders
Sexually transmitted infections
Exposure to workplace hazards such as radiation or toxic substances
Exposure of scrotum to high temperatures

Substance Abuse
Changes in sperm
- Smoking, heroin, marijuana, amyl nitrate, butyl nitrate, ethyl chloride, methaqualone
- Monoamine oxidase

Decrease in sperm
- Hypopituitarism
- Debilitating or chronic disease
- Trauma
- Gonadotropic inadequacy

Decrease in libido
- Heroin, methadone, selective serotonin reuptake inhibitors, and barbiturates

Impotence
- Alcohol
- Antihypertensive medications

Obstructive Lesions of the Epididymis and Vas Deferens

Nutritional Deficiencies

BOX 7-3

Religious Considerations of Infertility

Civil laws and religious proscriptions about sex must always be kept in mind by the health care provider.

Conservative and reform Jewish couples are accepting of most infertility treatment; however, the Orthodox Jewish husband and wife may face infertility investigation and management problems because of religious laws that govern marital relations. For example, according to Jewish law, the Orthodox couple may not engage in marital relations during menstruation and through the following 7 "preparatory days." The wife then is immersed in a ritual bath *(Mikvah)* before relations can resume. Fertility problems can arise when the woman has a short cycle (i.e., a cycle of 24 days or fewer, when ovulation would occur on day 10 or earlier).

The Roman Catholic Church regards the embryo as a human being from the first moment of existence and regards as unacceptable technical procedures such as in vitro fertilization, therapeutic donor insemination, and freezing embryos.

Other religious groups may have ethical concerns about infertility tests and treatments. For example, most Protestant denominations and Muslims usually support infertility management as long as in vitro fertilization (IVF) is done with the husband's sperm, there is no reduction of fetuses, and insemination is done with the husband's sperm. These groups are less supportive of surrogacy and use of donor sperm and eggs. Christian Scientists do not permit surgical procedures or IVF but do permit insemination with husband and donor sperm.

Care providers should seek to understand the woman's spirituality and how it affects her perception of health care, especially in relation to infertility. Women may wish to seek infertility treatment but have questions about proposed diagnostic and therapeutic procedures because of religious proscriptions. These women are encouraged to consult their minister, rabbi, priest, or other spiritual leader for advice.

A complete general physical examination is followed by a specific assessment of the reproductive tract. The endocrine system is evaluated for abnormalities. Inadequate development of secondary sex characteristics (e.g., inappropriate distribution of body fat and hair) may point to problems with the hypothalamic-pituitary-ovarian axis or genetic aberrations (e.g., polycystic ovarian syndrome, Turner's syndrome).

A woman may have an abnormal uterus and tubes (Fig. 7-1) as a result of in utero exposure to diethylstilbestrol (DES) (See Box 5-2). A history of infection of the genitourinary system is noted. Bimanual examination of internal organs may reveal lack of mobility of the uterus or abnormal contours of the uterus and adnexa. Laboratory data, including routine urine and blood tests, are collected.

Cultural Awareness

FERTILITY/INFERTILITY

Worldwide cultures continue to use symbols and rites that celebrate fertility. One fertility rite that persists today is the custom of throwing rice at the bride and groom. Other fertility symbols and rites include passing out congratulatory cigars, candy, or pencils by a new father and baby showers held in anticipation of a child's birth.

In many cultures, the responsibility for infertility is usually attributed to the woman. A woman's inability to conceive may be due to her sins, to evil spirits, or to the fact that she is an inadequate person. The virility of a man in some cultures remains in question until he demonstrates his ability to reproduce by having at least one child (D'Avanzo & Geissler, 2003).

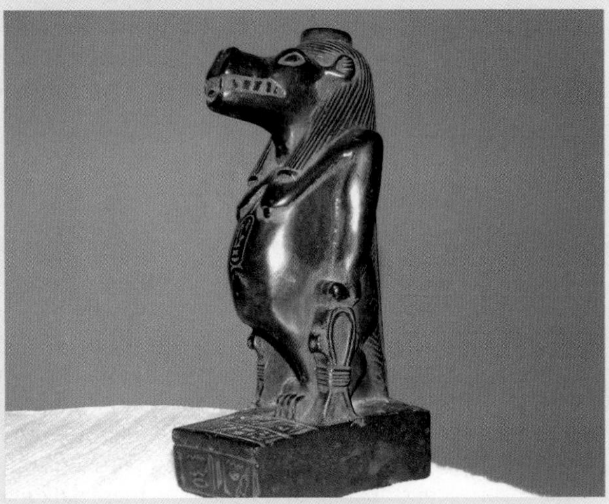

Taweret, goddess of fertility, Egypt (Courtesy Julie Perry Nelson, Phoenix, AZ).

BOX 7-4

Insurance Coverage for Infertility

In 2004 only 15 states had mandated some form of insurance coverage for infertility (Jones & Cohen, 2004). These mandates included in vitro fertilization in some states, whereas others only covered some diagnostic tests. Some states require health maintenance organizations (HMOs) to cover some costs, whereas in others, HMOs are exempt. Patients need information about what they can expect from their insurers. The Web site for the American Society for Reproductive Medicine (www.asrm.org) has more complete information.

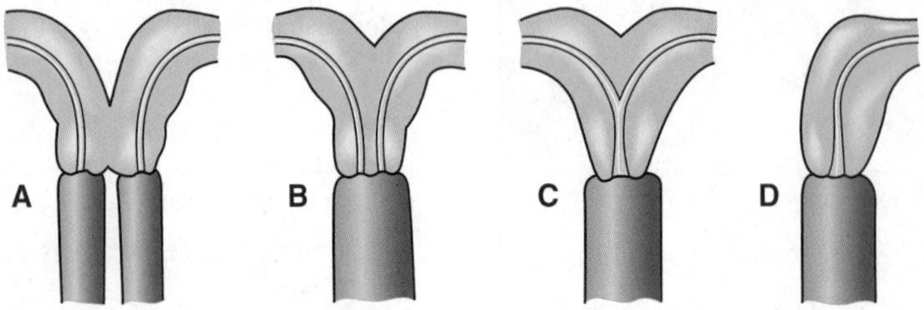

Fig. 7-1 Abnormal uterus. **A**, Complete bicornuate uterus with vagina divided by a septum. **B**, Complete bicornuate uterus with normal vagina. **C**, Partial bicornuate uterus with normal vagina. **D**, Unicornuate uterus.

Diagnosis

The basic infertility survey of the female involves evaluation of the cervix, uterus, tubes, and peritoneum; detection of ovulation; hormone analysis; assessment of immunologic compatibility; and evaluation of psychogenic factors (Table 7-1). Ultrasonography, timed (during the luteal phase) endometrial biopsy, hysterosalpingography (x-ray of the uterine cavity and tubes after instillation of radiopaque contrast material through the cervix), and laparoscopy (to detect and possibly treat problems such as endometriosis or adhesions in the peritoneal cavity) may be performed. The nurse can alleviate some of the anxiety associated with testing by explaining the timing and rationale for each test. Test findings that are favorable to fertility are summarized in Box 7-5.

Table 7-1

Tests for Impaired Fertility

TEST/EXAMINATION	TIMING (MENSTRUAL CYCLE DAYS)	RATIONALE
Hysterosalpingogram	7-10	Late follicular, early proliferative phase; will not disrupt a fertilized ovum; may open uterine tubes before time of ovulation
Postcoital test	1-2 days before ovulation	Ovulatory late proliferative phase; look for normal motile sperm in cervical mucus
Sperm immobilization antigen-antibody reaction	Variable, ovulation	Immunologic test to determine sperm and cervical mucus interaction
Assessment of cervical mucus	Variable, ovulation	Cervical mucus should have low viscosity, high spinnbarkeit
Ultrasound diagnosis of follicular collapse	Ovulation	Collapsed follicle is seen after ovulation
Serum assay of plasma progesterone	20-25	Midluteal midsecretory phase; check adequacy of corpus luteal production of progesterone
Basal body temperature (BBT)	Chart entire cycle	Elevation occurs in response to progesterone, documents ovulation
Endometrial biopsy	21-27	Late luteal, late secretory phase; check endometrial response to progesterone and adequacy of luteal phase
Sperm penetration assay	After 2 days but ≤1 wk of abstinence	Evaluation of ability of sperm to penetrate an egg

BOX 7-5

Summary of Findings Favorable to Fertility

1. Follicular development, ovulation, and luteal development are supportive of pregnancy:
   a. BBT (presumptive evidence of ovulatory cycles) is biphasic, with temperature elevation that persists for 12 to 14 days before menstruation.
   b. Cervical mucus characteristics change appropriately during phases of the menstrual cycle.
   c. Laparoscopic visualization of pelvic organs verifies follicular and luteal development.
2. The luteal phase is supportive of pregnancy:
   a. Levels of plasma progesterone are adequate.
   b. Findings from endometrial biopsy samples are consistent with day of cycle.
3. Cervical factors are receptive to sperm during expected time of ovulation:
   a. Cervical os is open.
   b. Cervical mucus is clear, watery, abundant, and slippery and demonstrates good spinnbarkeit and arborization (fern pattern).
   c. Cervical examination does not reveal lesions or infections.
   d. Postcoital test findings are satisfactory (adequate number of live, motile, normal sperm present in cervical mucus).
   e. No immunity to sperm is demonstrated.
4. The uterus and uterine tubes are supportive of pregnancy:
   a. Uterine and tubal patency are documented by
      (1) Spillage of dye into the peritoneal cavity.
      (2) Outlines of uterine and tubal cavities of adequate size and shape, with no abnormalities.
   b. Laparoscopic examination verifies normal development of internal genitals and absence of adhesions, infections, endometriosis, and other lesions.
5. The male partner's reproductive structures are normal:
   a. No evidence of developmental anomalies of penis, testicular atrophy, or varicocele (varicose veins on the spermatic vein in the groin).
   b. No evidence of infection in prostate, seminal vesicles, and urethra.
   c. Testes are >4 cm in largest diameter.
6. Semen is supportive of pregnancy:
   a. Sperm (number per milliliter) are adequate in ejaculate.
   b. Most sperm show normal morphology.
   c. Most sperm are motile, forward moving.
   d. No autoimmunity exists.
   e. Seminal fluid is normal.

Assessment of Male Infertility

The systematic investigation of infertility in the male patient begins with a thorough history and physical examination. Assessment of the male patient starts with noninvasive tests.

Semen Analysis

The basic test for male infertility is the semen analysis. A complete semen analysis, study of the effects of cervical mucus on sperm forward motility and survival, and evaluation of the sperm's ability to penetrate an ovum provide basic information. Sperm counts vary from day to day and are dependent on emotional and physical status and sexual activity. Therefore a single analysis may be inconclusive. A minimum of two analyses must be performed several weeks apart to assess male fertility (Keye, 2000).

Semen is collected by ejaculation into a clean container or a plastic sheath that does not contain a spermicidal agent. The specimen is usually collected by masturbation following 2 to 3 days of abstinence from ejaculation (Stenchever et al, 2001). The semen is examined at the collection site or taken to the laboratory in a sealed container within 2 hours of ejaculation. Exposure to excessive heat or cold is avoided. Commonly accepted values for semen characteristics are given in Box 7-6.

Hormone analyses are done for testosterone, gonadotropin, follicle-stimulating hormone (FSH), and luteinizing hormone (LH). The sperm penetration assay may be used to evaluate the ability of sperm to penetrate an egg. Because human oocytes are not readily available, hamster eggs are used as a substitute to evaluate sperm penetration abilities (no actual fertilization occurs). Testicular biopsy may be warranted.

Assessment of the Couple

Postcoital Test

The postcoital test (PCT), also called the Sims-Huhner test, is one method used to test for adequacy of coital technique, cervical mucus, sperm, and degree of sperm penetration through cervical mucus. The test is performed within several hours after ejaculation of semen into the vagina. A specimen of cervical mucus is obtained from the cervical os and examined under a microscope. The quality of mucus and the number of forward-moving sperm are noted. A PCT with good mucus and motile sperm is associated with fertility.

Intercourse is synchronized with the expected time of ovulation (as determined from evaluation of basal body temperature [BBT], cervical mucus changes, and usual length of menstrual cycle or use of LH detection kit to determine LH surge). Intercourse is performed only in the absence of vaginal infection. Couples may experience some difficulty abstaining from intercourse for 2 to 4 days before expected ovulation, and then having intercourse with ejaculation on schedule. Sex on demand may strain the couple's interpersonal relationship. A problem may arise if the expected day of ovulation occurs when facilities or the physician is unavailable (such as over a weekend or holiday).

BOX 7-6

Semen Analysis

- Liquefaction usually complete within 10 to 20 minutes
- Semen volume 2 to 5 ml (range 1 to 7 ml)
- Semen pH 7.2 to 7.8
- Sperm density 20 to 200 million cells/ml
- Normal morphology, ≥60% normal oval
- Motility (important consideration in sperm evaluation), percentage of forward-moving sperm estimated with respect to abnormally motile and nonmotile sperm ≥50%
- Ovum penetration test (may be done if further evaluation necessary)

NOTE: These values are not absolute, only relative to final evaluation of the couple as a single reproductive unit.

Nursing Diagnoses

Examples of nursing diagnoses related to impaired fertility include the following:

- *Disturbed body image* or *risk for situational low self-esteem related to*
  —impaired fertility
- *Decisional conflict* related to
  —therapies for impaired fertility
  —alternatives to therapy (e.g., childfree living or adoption)
- *Sexual dysfunction* related to
  —loss of libido secondary to medically imposed restrictions
- *Social isolation* related to
  —impaired fertility, its investigation, and its management

Expected Outcomes

The expected outcomes are phrased in patient-centered terms and may include that the couple will do the following:

- Verbalize understanding of the anatomy and physiology of the reproductive system.
- Verbalize understanding of treatment for any abnormalities identified through various tests and examinations and be able to make an informed decision about treatment.
- Resolve guilt feelings and not need to focus blame.
- Conceive or, failing to conceive, decide on an alternative acceptable to both of them (childfree living or adoption).

Plan of Care and Implementation

Psychosocial

In the United States, feelings connected to impaired fertility are numerous and complex. Infertility is recognized as a major life stressor that can affect self-esteem; relations with the spouse, family, and friends; and careers. Couples often need assistance in separating their concepts of success and failure related to treatment for infertility from personal success and failure. The woman or couple facing infertility may exhibit grieving behaviors usually associated with other types of loss. Recognizing the significance of infertility as a loss, and resolving these feelings, is crucial to putting infertility into perspective, even if treatment is successful. Nurses can help couples express and discuss their feelings as honestly as possible. Ventilation may help couples to unburden themselves of negative feelings. Referral for mental health counseling may be beneficial.

Psychologic responses to the diagnosis of infertility may tax a couple's capacity for giving and receiving physical and sexual closeness. The prescriptions and proscriptions for achieving conception may add tension to a couple's sexual functioning. Couples may report decreased desire for intercourse, orgasmic dysfunction, or midcycle erectile disorders.

To be able to deal comfortably with a couple's sexuality, nurses must be comfortable with their own sexuality so that they can better help couples understand why the private act of lovemaking needs to be shared with health care professionals. Nurses need up-to-date factual knowledge about human sexual practices, and must be accepting of the preferences and activities of others without being judgmental. They must be skilled in interviewing and in therapeutic use of self, sensitive to the nonverbal cues of others, and knowledgeable regarding each couple's sociocultural and religious tenets.

The support systems of the couple with impaired fertility need to be explored. This exploration should include data about persons available to assist, their relationship to the couple, their ages, their availability, and the cultural or religious support that is available.

If the couple conceives, the concerns and problems of the previously infertile couple may not be over. Many couples are overjoyed with the pregnancy; however, some are not. Some couples rearrange their lives, sense of self, and personal goals within their acceptance of their infertile state. The couple may feel that those who worked with them to identify and treat impaired fertility expect them to be happy with the pregnancy. The couple may be shocked to find that they feel resentment because the pregnancy, once a cherished dream, now necessitates another change in goals, aspirations, and identities. The normal ambivalence toward pregnancy may be perceived as reneging on the original choice to become parents. The couple might choose to abort the pregnancy at this time. Other couples worry about miscarriage. If the couple wishes to continue with the pregnancy, they will need the care other expectant couples need.

If the couple does not conceive, they are assessed regarding their desire to be referred for help with adoption, therapeutic intrauterine insemination, other reproductive alternatives, or choosing a childfree state. The couple may find helpful a list of agencies, support groups, and other resources in their community (see Resources at end of chapter).

??? Critical Thinking Exercise

INFERTILITY WORKUP

Jane and Andrew are in their early thirties. They have been trying to achieve pregnancy for the 10 years of their marriage. They have come for an infertility workup. The nurse will do the initial intake interview and some counseling. Jane and Andrew express discouragement, disillusionment, and anxiety. They have many questions about the probability of achieving pregnancy after this length of time.

1. Evidence—Is there sufficient evidence to draw conclusions about the probability of achieving pregnancy?
2. Assumptions—What assumptions can be made about a couple experiencing infertility?
3. What implications and priorities for nursing care can be drawn at this time?
4. Does the evidence objectively support your conclusion?
5. Are there alternative perspectives to your conclusion?

Nonmedical

Simple changes in lifestyle may be effective in the treatment of subfertile men. Only water-soluble lubricants should be used during intercourse because many commonly used lubricants contain spermicides or have spermicidal properties. High scrotal temperatures may be caused by daily hot tub baths or saunas that keep the testes at temperatures too high for efficient spermatogenesis.

Treatment is available for women who have immunologic reactions to sperm. The use of condoms during genital intercourse for 6 to 12 months will reduce female antibody production in most women who have elevated antisperm antibody titers. After the serum reaction subsides, condoms are used at all times except at the expected time of ovulation. Approximately one third of couples with this problem conceive by following this course of action.

Change in nutrition and habits may increase fertility for both men and women. For example, a well-balanced diet, exercise, decreased alcohol intake, not smoking or abusing drugs, and stress management may be effective.

Herbal Alternative Measures

Most herbal remedies have not been proven clinically to promote fertility or to be safe in early pregnancy and should be taken by the woman only as prescribed by a physician or nurse-midwife who has expertise in herbology. Relaxation, stress management, and nutritional and exercise counseling have been reported to increase pregnancy rates in some women. Herbal remedies that promote fertility in general include red clover flowers, nettle leaves, *dong quai,* and false unicorn root (Weed, 1986). Vitamin E, calcium, and magnesium may promote fertility and conception (Tiran & Mack, 2000). Herbs to avoid while trying to conceive include licorice root, yarrow, wormwood, ephedra, fennel, goldenseal, lavender, juniper, flaxseed, pennyroyal, passionflower, wild cherry, cascara, sage, thyme, and periwinkle (Kennedy, Griffin, & Frishman, 1998).

Medical

Pharmacologic therapy for female infertility is often directed at treating ovulatory dysfunction either by stimulating ovulation or by enhancing ovulation so that more oocytes mature. These medications include clomiphene citrate, human menopausal gonadotropin (HMG), FSH, recombinant FSH (rFSH), and human chorionic gonadotropin (hCG). Gonadotropin-releasing hormone (GnRH) agonists, progesterone, and bromocriptine (Parlodel) also are used.

These medications are extremely potent and require daily monitoring with ovarian ultrasonography and monitoring of estradiol levels to prevent hyperstimulation. The incidence of multiple pregnancy with the use of these medications is greater than 25%. When failure to ovulate is caused either by hypothalamic-pituitary dysfunction or failure, or failure to respond to clomiphene, GnRH may be used. Thyroid-stimulating hormone (Synthroid) is indicated if the woman has hypothyroidism.

The woman who has low estrogen levels may be a candidate for conjugated estrogens and medroxyprogesterone. A hypoestrogenic condition may result from a high stress level or from a decreased percentage of body fat as a result of an eating disorder (e.g., anorexia nervosa) or excessive exercise. Hydroxyprogesterone supplementation with vaginal suppositories or intramuscular injection is used to treat luteal phase defects. In the presence of adrenal hyperplasia, prednisone, a glucocorticoid, is taken orally. Treatment of endometriosis may include danazol, progesterones, combined oral contraceptives, or GnRH agonists (Stenchever et al, 2001). Infections are treated with appropriate antimicrobial formulations.

Drug therapy may be indicated for male infertility. Problems with the thyroid or adrenal glands are corrected with appropriate medications. Infections are identified and treated with antimicrobials. FSH, HMG, and clomiphene may be used to stimulate spermatogenesis in men with hypogonadism (Leibowitz & Hoffman, 2000).

Surgical

A number of surgical procedures can be used for problems causing female infertility. Ovarian tumors must be excised. Whenever possible, functional ovarian tissue is left intact. Scar tissue adhesions caused by chronic infections may cover much or all of the ovary. These adhesions usually necessitate surgery to free and expose the ovary so that ovulation can occur.

Hysterosalpingography is useful for identification of tubal obstruction and also for the release of blockage (Fig. 7-2). During laparoscopy, delicate adhesions may be divided and removed and endometrial implants may be destroyed by electrocoagulation or laser (Fig. 7-3). Laparotomy and even microsurgery may be required to do extensive repair of the damaged tube. Prognosis is dependent on the degree to which tubal patency and function can be restored.

A woman with a relatively small uterus may become pregnant, but the uterus may be incapable of accommodating the enlarging fetus, and a miscarriage may result. In such cases recurrent or habitual (three or more) miscarriages often occur. No medical therapy has been effective for the enlargement of an abnormally small uterus. Observation suggests that women who do become pregnant, but who miscarry, often abort at a later time with each successive pregnancy. After two or three pregnancy losses, they may finally give birth to a viable infant. Apparently, actual growth of the uterus occurs with each pregnancy. Reconstructive surgery (e.g., the unification operation for bicornuate uterus) often improves a woman's ability to conceive and carry the fetus to term.

Surgical removal of tumors or fibroids involving the endometrium or uterus often improves the woman's chance of conceiving and maintaining the pregnancy to viability. Surgical treatment of uterine tumors or maldevelopment that results in successful pregnancy usually requires birth by cesarean surgery near term gestation. The uterus may rupture as a result of weakness in the area of surgical healing.

Chronic inflammation and infection can be eliminated by radial chemocautery (destruction of tissue with chemicals) or thermocautery (destruction of tissue with heat, usually electrical) of the cervix; cryosurgery (destruction of tissue by application of extreme cold, usually liquid nitrogen); or conization (excision of a cone-shaped piece of tissue from the endocervix). When the cervix has been deeply cauterized or frozen, or when extensive conization has been performed, extreme limitation of mucous production by the cervix may result. The absence of a mucous bridge from the vagina to the uterus may therefore make sperm migration difficult or impossible. Therapeutic intrauterine insemination may be necessary to carry the sperm directly through the internal os of the cervix.

Surgical procedures may also be used for problems causing male infertility. Surgical repair of varicocele has been relatively successful in increasing sperm count but not fertility rates. A varicocele on the left side is found in a substantial number of subfertile men.

Microsurgery to reanastomose (restore tubal continuity) the sperm ducts can result in pregnancy rates greater than 50%. The rate of success decreases as the time since the procedure increases.

Reproductive Alternatives

Although there have been remarkable developments in reproductive medicine, assisted reproductive therapies (ARTs) account for less than 1% of all U.S. births (Centers for Disease Control and Prevention [CDC], 2001). ARTs are creating ethical and legal dilemmas. The lack of information, or misleading information about success rates and the risks and benefits of treatment alternatives, prevents couples from making in-

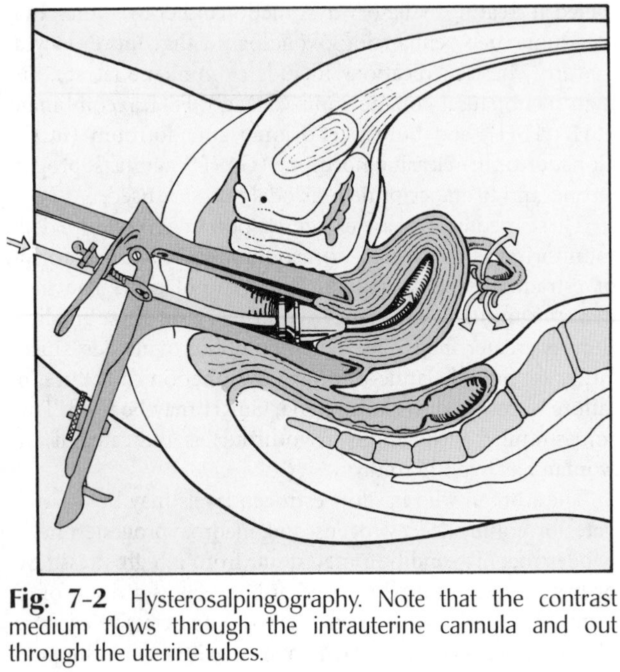

Fig. 7-2 Hysterosalpingography. Note that the contrast medium flows through the intrauterine cannula and out through the uterine tubes.

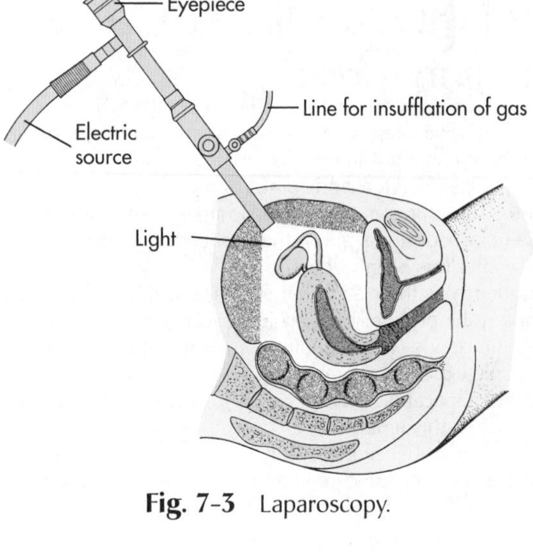

Fig. 7-3 Laparoscopy.

formed decisions. Some of the ARTs for treatment of infertility include in vitro fertilization–embryo transfer (IVF-ET), gamete intrafallopian transfer (GIFT) (Fig. 7-4), zygote intrafallopian transfer (ZIFT), ovum transfer (oocyte donation), embryo adoption, embryo hosting and surrogate parenting, and therapeutic donor insemination (TDI). Table 7-2 describes these procedures and the possible indications for ARTs. Other options include intracytoplasmic sperm injection, assisted hatching, and adoption.

LEGAL TIP **Cryopreservation of Human Embryos** Couples who have excess embryos frozen for later transfer must be fully informed before consenting to the procedure, to make decisions regarding the disposal of embryos in the event of death, divorce, or the decision that the couple no longer wants the embryos at a later time. ■

Complications

Other than the established risks associated with laparoscopy and general anesthesia, few risks are associated with IVF-ET, GIFT, and ZIFT. The more common transvaginal needle aspiration requires only local or intravenous analgesia. Congenital anomalies occur no more frequently than among naturally conceived embryos. Ectopic pregnancies do occur more often, however, and these carry a significant maternal risk. There is no increase in maternal or perinatal complications with TDI; the same incidences of anomalies (about 5%) and obstetric complications (between 5% and 10%) that accompany natural insemination (through sexual intercourse) also apply to TDI.

Preimplantation Genetic Diagnosis

Preimplantation genetic diagnosis (PGD) is a form of early genetic testing designed to eliminate embryos with serious genetic diseases before implantation through one of the ARTs and to avoid future termination of pregnancy for genetic reasons. There are over 20 centers around the world where PGD is used clinically. Couples must be counseled about their options and choices, as well as the implications of their choices, when genetic analysis is considered (Jones, 2000).

Adoption

Couples may choose to build their family by adopting children who are not their own biologically. With increased availability of birth control and abortion, and an increase in single mothers who choose to keep their babies, the availability of Caucasian infants for adoption is extremely limited. Minority infants, infants with special needs, older children, and foreign adoptions are other options (Fig. 7-5).

Couples who seek to adopt a child have decided that being a parent and having a child is more important than the actual process of birthing the child. The birth process is a very small aspect of having a baby and becoming a parent. The question to be answered by couples who want to adopt is, "Do you want to have a baby, or do you want to become parents?" Nurses should have information on options for adoption available for couples or refer to community resources for further assistance (see Resources at end of chapter).

Surrogate Mothers

Surrogate motherhood can be achieved by two methods. The first is to have the surrogate mother inseminated with semen from the infertile woman's partner and carry the baby until the birth. The baby is then formally adopted by the infertile couple. The second, less common method is to retrieve an ovum from the infertile woman, fertilize it with her partner's sperm, and place it into the uterus of a surrogate, who becomes a gestational carrier. These newer interventions raise considerable legal and ethical issues that require extensive counseling of couples and the women who choose to become pregnant.

Evaluation

Evaluation of the effectiveness of care of the couple experiencing impaired fertility is based on the previously stated outcomes (Nursing Care Plan).

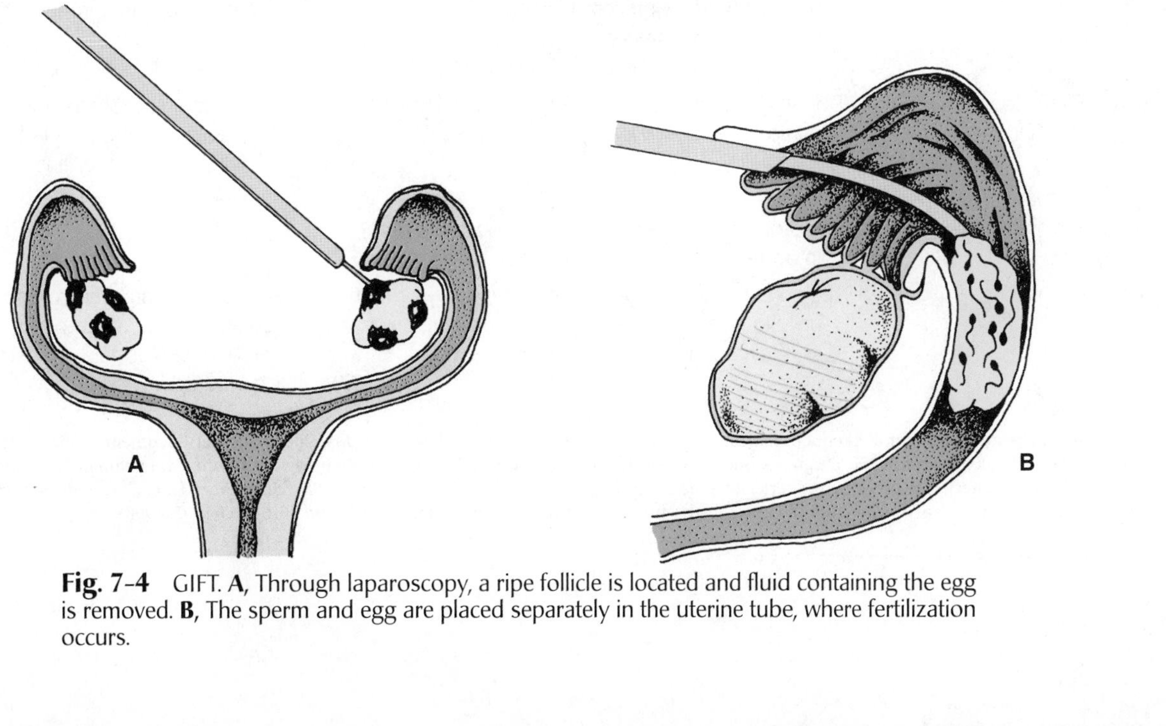

Fig. 7-4 GIFT. **A,** Through laparoscopy, a ripe follicle is located and fluid containing the egg is removed. **B,** The sperm and egg are placed separately in the uterine tube, where fertilization occurs.

Table 7-2

Assisted Reproductive Therapies (ARTs)

PROCEDURE	DEFINITION	INDICATIONS
In vitro fertilization–embryo transfer (IVF-ET)	A woman's eggs are collected from her ovaries, fertilized in the laboratory with sperm, and transferred to her uterus after normal embryo development has occurred.	Tubal disease or blockage; severe male infertility; endometriosis; unexplained infertility; cervical factor; immunologic infertility
Gamete intrafallopian transfer (GIFT)	Oocytes are retrieved from the ovary, placed in a catheter with washed motile sperm, and immediately transferred into the fimbriated end of the uterine tube. Fertilization occurs in the uterine tube.	Same as for IVF-ET, except there must be normal tubal anatomy, patency, and absence of previous tubal disease in at least one uterine tube
IVF-ET and GIFT with donor sperm	This process is the same as described above except in cases where the husband's fertility is severely compromised and donor sperm can be used; if donor sperm are used, the wife must have indications for IVF and GIFT.	Severe male infertility; azoospermia; indications for IVF-ET or GIFT
Zygote intrafallopian transfer (ZIFT)	This process is similar to IVF-ET; after in vitro fertilization the ova are placed in one uterine tube during the zygote stage.	Same as for GIFT
Donor oocyte	Eggs are donated by an IVF procedure, and the donated eggs are inseminated. The embryos are transferred into the recipient's uterus, which is hormonally prepared with estrogen/progesterone therapy.	Early menopause; surgical removal of ovaries; congenitally absent ovaries; autosomal or sex-linked disorders; lack of fertilization in repeated IVF attempts because of subtle oocyte abnormalities or defects in oocyte/spermatozoa interaction
Donor embryo (embryo adoption)	A donated embryo is transferred to the uterus of an infertile woman at the appropriate time (normal or induced) of the menstrual cycle.	Infertility not resolved by less aggressive forms of therapy; absence of ovaries; male partner is azoospermic or is severely compromised
Gestational carrier (embryo host); surrogate mother	A couple undertakes an IVF cycle and the embryo(s) is transferred to another woman's uterus (the carrier) who has contracted with the couple to carry the baby to term. The carrier has no genetic investment in the child. Surrogate motherhood is a process by which a woman is inseminated with semen from the infertile woman's partner and then carries the baby until birth.	Congenital absence or surgical removal of uterus; a reproductively impaired uterus, myomas, uterine adhesions, or other congenital abnormalities; a medical condition that might be life-threatening during pregnancy, such as diabetes, immunologic problems, or severe heart, kidney, or liver disease
Therapeutic donor insemination (TDI)	Donor sperm are used to inseminate the female partner.	Male partner is azoospermic or has a very low sperm count; couple has a genetic defect; male partner has antisperm antibodies
Intracytoplasmic sperm injection	Selection of one sperm cell that is injected directly into the egg to achieve fertilization. Used with IVF.	Same as TDI
Assisted hatching	The zona pellucida is penetrated chemically or manually to create an opening for the dividing embryo to hatch and implant into the uterine wall.	Recurrent miscarriages; to improve implantation rate in women with previously unsuccessful IVF attempts; advanced age

Data from American Society for Reproductive Medicine: *Frequently asked questions about infertility,* 2002. Internet document available at www.asrm.org (accessed March 5, 2005); Angard NT: Diagnosis infertility, *AWHONN Lifelines* 3(3):22-29, 1999; Kennedy HP, Griffin M, Frishman G: Enabling conception and pregnancy: midwifery care of women experiencing infertility, *J Nurse Midwifery* 43(3):190-207, 1998; Stenchever MA et al: *Comprehensive gynecology,* ed 4, St Louis, 2001, Mosby; Van Voorhis BJ et al: Cost-effective treatment of the infertile couple, *Fertil Steril* 70(6):995-1005, 1998.

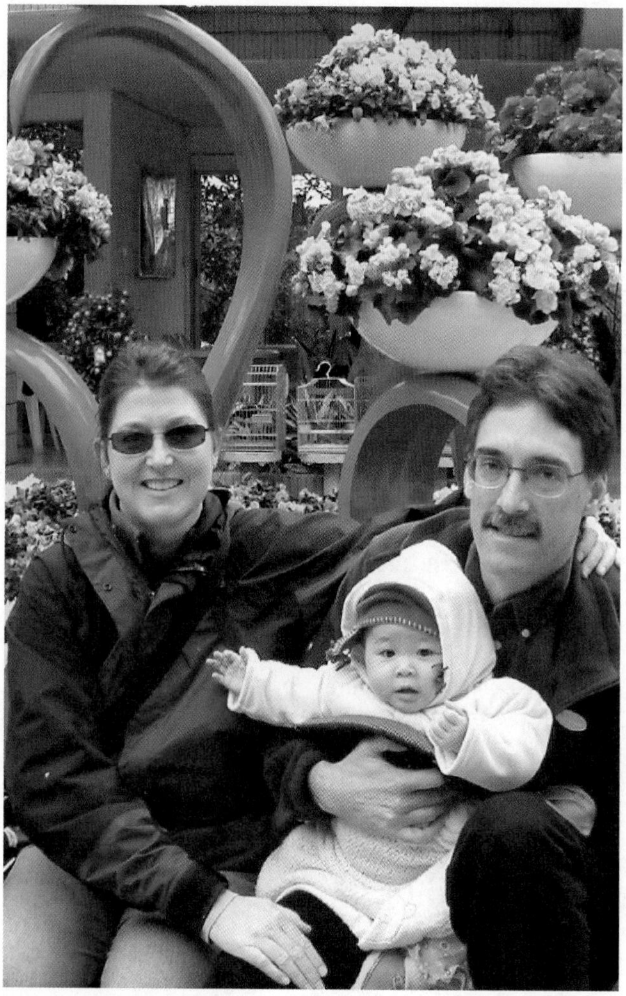

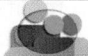

Fig. 7-5 After 2 miscarriages, this couple chose foreign adoption. (Courtesy Shannon Perry, Phoenix, AZ.)

CONTRACEPTION

Contraception is the voluntary prevention of pregnancy. Despite the large numbers of men and women who use contraception, more than half of pregnancies in the United States every year in women 20 years and younger are unintended (U.S. Department of Health and Human Services, 2002). Those who use contraception may still be at risk for pregnancy if their choice of contraceptive method is not perfect or is used incorrectly. Providing adequate instruction about how to use a contraceptive method, when to use a backup method, and when to use emergency contraception could decrease the risk of unintended pregnancy (Hatcher et al, 2004) (Community Focus).

Community Focus

EDUCATION FOR CONTRACEPTIVE USE

Education on contraceptive use in the postpartum period is a common component of discharge planning in many countries, with wide variation among health care delivery systems. Education at this time assumes women's receptiveness to information about contraception, and that education or receptiveness to such information will be less at a later period. Clinical trials have not demonstrated the effectiveness of education in the immediate postpartum period. When assessing effectiveness of contraceptive education, attendance at family planning clinics, cessation of breastfeeding, knowledge about contraception, unplanned pregnancies, and satisfaction with care should be included as factors affecting or measuring effectiveness. The content, timing, and organization of contraceptive education offered in the postpartum period needs to be addressed. Nurses provide discharge planning after childbirth; they commonly staff family planning clinics and provide contraceptive information. Evaluation of the effectiveness of their efforts must be implemented and results used to make appropriate changes.

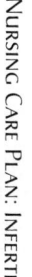

Critical Thinking Exercise—Patient Teaching: Contraception

Nursing Care Plan

THE COUPLE EXPERIENCING INFERTILITY

NURSING DIAGNOSIS: Deficient knowledge related to lack of understanding of the reproductive process with regard to conception as evidenced by patient questions

EXPECTED OUTCOME

Patient and partner will verbalize understanding of the components of the reproductive process, common problems leading to infertility, usual infertility testing, and the importance of completing testing in a timely manner.

NURSING INTERVENTIONS/*RATIONALES*

Assess woman's current level of understanding of the factors promoting conception *to identify gaps or misconceptions in knowledge base.*

Provide information in a supportive manner regarding factors promoting conception, including common factors leading to infertility of either partner, *to raise couples' awareness and promote trust in caregiver.*

Identify and describe the basic infertility tests and the rationale for precise scheduling *to enhance completion of the diagnostic phase of the infertility workup.*

NURSING DIAGNOSIS: Risk for ineffective individual/family coping related to inability to conceive as evidenced by patient and partner statements

EXPECTED OUTCOME

Patient and partner will identify situational stressors and positive coping methods to deal with testing and unknown outcomes.

NURSING INTERVENTIONS/*RATIONALES*

Provide opportunities through therapeutic communication to discuss feelings and concerns *to identify common feelings and perceived stressors.*

Evaluate couple's support system, including support of each other during this process, *to identify any barriers to effective coping.*

Identify support groups and refer as needed *to enhance coping by sharing experiences with other couples experiencing similar problems.*

Nursing Care Plan: Infertility

CARE MANAGEMENT

A multidisciplinary approach may assist a woman in choosing and correctly using an appropriate contraceptive method. Nurses, nurse-midwives, nurse practitioners, and other advanced practice nurses and physicians have the knowledge and expertise to assist a woman in making decisions about contraception that will satisfy the woman's personal, social, cultural, and interpersonal needs.

Assessment

A history (including menstrual, contraceptive, and obstetric), physical examination (including pelvic examination), and laboratory tests are usually completed. The woman's knowledge about contraception and her sexual partner's commitment to any particular method are determined (Fig. 7-6). Data are required about the frequency of coitus, number of sexual partners, level of contraceptive involvement, and her or her partner's objections to any specific method(s). The woman's level of comfort and willingness to touch her genitals and cervical mucus are assessed. Myths are identified, and religious and cultural factors are determined (Guidelines/Guías). The woman's verbal and nonverbal responses to hearing about the various available methods are carefully noted. An individual's reproductive life plan must be considered.

Informed consent is a vital component in the education of the woman concerning contraception or sterilization. The nurse has the responsibility of documenting information provided and the understanding of that information by the woman.

Nursing Diagnoses

Examples of nursing diagnoses regarding contraception include the following:

- *Decisional conflict related to*
  —contraceptive alternatives
  —partner's willingness to agree on a contraceptive method
- *Risk for infection related to*
  —unprotected sexual intercourse
  —use of contraceptive method
  —broken skin or mucous membrane secondary to surgery, intrauterine device (IUD) insertion, or hormonal implant
- *Spiritual distress related to*
  —discrepancy between religious or cultural beliefs and choice of contraception

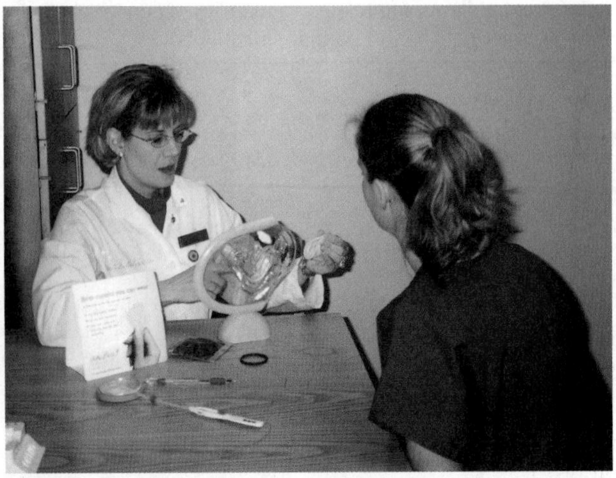

Fig. 7-6 Nurse counseling woman about contraceptive methods. (Courtesy Dee Lowdermilk, Chapel Hill, NC.)

Expected Outcomes

The expected outcomes are stated in patient-centered terms and may include that the woman or couple will do the following:

- Verbalize understanding about contraceptive methods.
- State comfort and satisfaction with the method chosen.
- Use the contraceptive method correctly and consistently.
- Experience no adverse sequelae as a result of the chosen method of contraception.
- Prevent unplanned pregnancy or plan a pregnancy.

Plan of Care and Implementation

Unbiased patient teaching is fundamental to initiating and maintaining any form of contraception. The nurse counters myths with facts, clarifies misinformation, and fills in gaps of knowledge. The ideal contraceptive should be safe, easily available, economical, acceptable, simple to use, and

ENGLISH SPANISH **Guidelines/Guías**

CONTRACEPTION

Do you plan to have more children?
¿Piensa tener más hijos?

Are you sexually active?
¿Tiene relaciones sexuales?

Do you have many partners?
¿Tiene muchas parejas sexuales?

Have you had many partners in the past?
¿Ha tenido muchas parejas sexuales en el pasado?

Do you presently use contraception/birth control?
¿Usa anticonceptivos/control de natalidad actualmente?

The Pill? Condoms? The diaphragm? The IUD?
¿La píldora anticonceptiva? ¿Los condones (preservativos)? ¿El diafragma? ¿El dispositivo intrauterino (DIU)?

Spermicides? The rhythm method? Injection (Depo-Provera)?
¿Los espermaticidas? ¿El método del ritmo? ¿La inyección (Depo-Provera)?

How long have you used this method?
¿Por cuánto tiempo ha usado este método?

Do you like this method?
¿Le gusta este método?

Why did you stop using it?
¿Por qué dejó de usarlo?

Do you want to change to a different method?
¿Quiere cambiar a otro método?

Have you had a tubal ligation?
¿Ha tenido una ligadura de trompas?

Has he had a vasectomy?
¿Tuvo él una vasectomía?

BOX 7-7

Factors Affecting Method Effectiveness

Frequency of intercourse
Motivation to prevent pregnancy
Understanding of how to use the method
Adherence to method
Provision of short-term or long-term protection
Likelihood of pregnancy for the individual woman
Consistent use of method

promptly reversible. Although no method may ever achieve all these objectives, impressive progress has been made.

Contraceptive failure rate refers to the percentage of contraceptive users expected to have an accidental pregnancy during the first year even when they use a method consistently and correctly. Contraceptive effectiveness varies from couple to couple and depends on both the properties of the method and the characteristics of the user (Hatcher et al, 2004) (Box 7-7). Failure rates decrease over time, either because a user gains experience with and uses a method more appropriately or because the less effective users stop using the method.

Safety of a method depends on the woman's medical history. Barrier methods offer some protection from sexually transmitted infections (STIs), and oral contraceptives may lower the incidence of ovarian and endometrial cancer but increase the risk of thromboembolic problems.

Methods of Contraception

The following discussion of contraceptive methods provides the nurse with information needed for patient teaching. After implementing the appropriate teaching for contraceptive use, the nurse supervises return demonstrations and practice to assess patient understanding. The woman is given written instructions and phone numbers for questions. If the woman has difficulty understanding written instructions, she (and her partner, if available) is offered graphic material and a phone number to call as necessary or is offered an opportunity to return for further instruction.

Coitus Interruptus

Coitus interruptus (withdrawal) involves the man withdrawing his penis from the woman's vagina before he ejaculates. Although coitus interruptus has been criticized as being an ineffective method of contraception, it is a good choice for couples who do not have another contraceptive available (Hatcher et al, 2004). Effectiveness is similar to barrier methods and depends on the man's ability to withdraw his penis before ejaculation. The percentage of women who will experience an unintended pregnancy within the first year of typical use (failure rate) of withdrawal is about 27% (Trussell, 2004). Coitus interruptus does not protect against STIs or human immunodeficiency virus (HIV) infection.

Natural Family Planning and Fertility Awareness Methods

Natural Family Planning

Natural family planning (NFP) provides contraception by using methods that rely on avoidance of intercourse during fertile days. It is the only method of contraception acceptable to the Roman Catholic Church. Fertility awareness methods combine the charting of signs and symptoms of the menstrual cycle with the use of abstinence or other contraceptive methods during fertile periods. Techniques used to determine fertility include the calendar method, the cervical mucus ovulation-detection method, the basal body temperature (BBT) method, the postovulation method, and the symptothermal method (Hatcher et al, 2004).

Critical Thinking Exercise

CONTRACEPTION FOR ADOLESCENTS

Alicia is a 15-year-old second-generation Chinese-American female who comes to the family planning clinic seeking contraception. She has recently become sexually active and tells the nurse she is concerned that her mother will find out. She also has many questions about the type of contraception to use. She seeks the nurse's advice to help in her decision making.

1. Evidence—Is there sufficient evidence to draw conclusions about what advice to give Alicia?
2. Assumptions—What assumptions can be made about contraception for adolescents (types, legal issues, and implications of culture on choice)?
3. What implications and priorities for nursing care can be drawn at this time?
4. Does the evidence objectively support your conclusion?
5. Are there alternative perspectives to your conclusion?

The human ovum can be fertilized no later than 16 to 24 hours after ovulation. Motile sperm have been recovered from the uterus and the oviducts as long as 7 days after coitus. However, their ability to fertilize the ovum probably lasts no longer than 24 to 48 hours. Pregnancy is unlikely to occur if a couple abstains from intercourse for 4 days before and for 3 or 4 days after ovulation (fertile period). Unprotected intercourse on the other days of the cycle (safe period) should not result in pregnancy. However, the exact time of ovulation cannot be predicted accurately, and couples may find it difficult to abstain from sexual intercourse for several days before and after ovulation. Women with irregular menstrual periods have the greatest risk of failure with this form of contraception. The typical failure rate for all fertility awareness methods is 25% during the first year of use (Trussell, 2004).

Calendar Method

Practice of the calendar method (also called the rhythm method) is based on the number of days in each cycle counting from the first day of menses (Hatcher et al, 2004). The fertile period is determined after accurately recording the lengths of menstrual cycles for 6 months. The beginning of the fertile period is estimated by subtracting 18 days from the length of the shortest cycle. The end of the fertile period is determined by subtracting 11 days from the length of the longest cycle. If the shortest cycle is 24 days and the longest is 30 days, application of the formula is as follows:

Shortest cycle, $24 - 18 =$ day 6
Longest cycle, $30 - 11 =$ day 19

To avoid conception the couple would abstain during the fertile period, days 6 through 19.

If the woman has very regular cycles of 28 days each, the formula indicates the fertile days to be as follows:

$$\text{Shortest cycle, } 28 - 18 = \text{day } 10$$
$$\text{Longest cycle, } 28 - 11 = \text{day } 17$$

To avoid conception, the couple would abstain from day 10 through 17 because ovulation occurs on day 14 ± 2 days. A major drawback of the calendar method is that one is trying to predict future events with past data. The unpredictability of the menstrual cycle is also not taken into consideration. The calendar rhythm method is most useful as an adjunct to the BBT or cervical mucus method.

Basal Body Temperature Method

The BBT is the lowest body temperature of a healthy person, taken immediately after waking and before getting out of bed. The BBT usually varies from 36.2° to 36.3° C during menses and for approximately 5 to 7 days afterward (Fig. 7-7).

About the time of ovulation, a slight drop in temperature (approximately 0.05° C) may occur in some women, but others may have no decrease at all. After ovulation, in concert with the increasing progesterone levels of the early luteal phase of the cycle, the BBT increases slightly (approximately 0.4° to 0.8° C) (Hatcher et al, 2004). The temperature remains on an elevated plateau until 2 to 4 days before menstruation. Then it decreases to the low levels recorded during the previous cycle unless pregnancy has occurred. In that event, the temperature remains elevated.

If ovulation fails to occur, the pattern of lower body temperature continues throughout the cycle. Infection, fatigue, less than 3 hours of sleep per night, awakening late, and anxiety may cause temperature fluctuations and alter the expected pattern. If a new BBT thermometer is purchased, this fact is noted on the chart because the readings may vary slightly. Jet lag, alcohol taken the evening before, or sleeping in a heated waterbed must also be noted on the chart because these affect the BBT.

The decrease and subsequent increase in temperature are referred to as the thermal shift. When the entire month's temperatures are recorded on a graph, the pattern described is more apparent. It is more difficult to perceive day-to-day variations without the entire picture (Guidelines box). Therefore, the BBT alone is not a reliable method of predicting ovulation (Hatcher et al, 2004). To determine if an increase in temperature is indeed the thermal shift, the woman must be aware of other signs of approaching ovulation while she continues to assess the BBT (see later discussion of the symptothermal method for other indicators of ovulation).

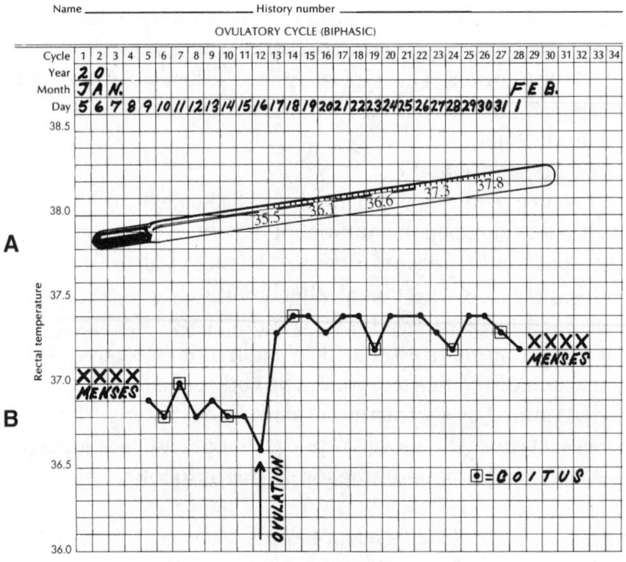

Fig. 7-7 **A,** Special thermometer for recording BBT, marked in tenths to enable person to read more easily. **B,** Basal temperature record shows decrease and sharp increase at time of ovulation. Biphasic curve indicates ovulatory cycle.

Cervical Mucus Ovulation-Detection Method

The cervical mucus ovulation-detection method requires that the woman recognize and interpret the characteristic cyclic changes in amount and consistency that characterize her own unique pattern of cervical mucus changes. The cervical mucus that accompanies ovulation is necessary for viability and motility of sperm. To ensure an accurate assessment of changes, the cervical mucus should be free from semen, contraceptive gels or foams, and blood or discharge from vaginal infections for at least one full cycle. Other factors that create difficulty in identifying mucus changes include douches and vaginal deodorants, being in the sexually aroused state (which thins the mucus), and taking medications such as antihistamines, which dry the mucus.

Some women may find this method unacceptable if they are uncomfortable touching their genitals. Whether or not a woman wants to use this method for contraception, it is to her advantage to learn to recognize mucus characteristics at ovulation (Guidelines box).

Symptothermal Method

The symptothermal method combines the BBT and cervical mucus methods with awareness of secondary, cycle phase–related symptoms. The woman gains fertility awareness as she learns the psychologic and physiologic symptoms that mark the phases of her cycle. Secondary symptoms include increased libido, midcycle spotting, mittelschmerz, pelvic fullness or tenderness, and vulvar fullness.

Guidelines

BASAL BODY TEMPERATURE

Discuss BBT with the woman.

Show the woman a diagram depicting the phases of the menstrual cycle.

Discuss the hormones in the woman's body that are responsible for her menstrual cycle and ovulation. Leave time for questions.

Show the woman a sample BBT graph (see Fig. 7-7) and the biphasic line seen in ovulatory cycles.

Show the woman the BBT thermometer and how it is calibrated.

Provide a demonstration.

Encourage the woman to demonstrate taking and reading the thermometer and graphing the temperature while the nurse watches.

Encourage the woman to start a log to keep track of any other activity that might interfere with her true BBT.

Guidelines

CERVICAL MUCUS CHARACTERISTICS

Setting the Stage

- Show charts of menstrual cycle along with changes in the cervical mucus.
- Have the woman practice with raw egg white.
- Supply her with a BBT log and graph if she does not already have one.
- Explain that the assessment of cervical mucus characteristics is best when mucus is not mixed with semen, contraceptive jellies or foams, or discharge from infections.

Content Related to Cervical Mucus

- Explain to the woman (or couple) how cervical mucus changes throughout the menstrual cycle.
- Right before ovulation, the watery, thin, clear mucus becomes more abundant and thick. It feels like a lubricant and can be stretched approximately 5 cm between the thumb and forefinger; this is called *spinnbarkeit.* This characteristic indicates the period of maximum fertility. Sperm deposited in this type of mucus can survive until ovulation occurs.

Assessment Technique

- Stress that good handwashing is imperative to begin and end all self-assessment.
- Start observation from last day of menstrual flow.
- Assess cervical mucus several times a day for several cycles. Mucus can be obtained from vaginal introitus; no need to reach into vagina to cervix.
- Record findings on the same record on which her BBT is entered.

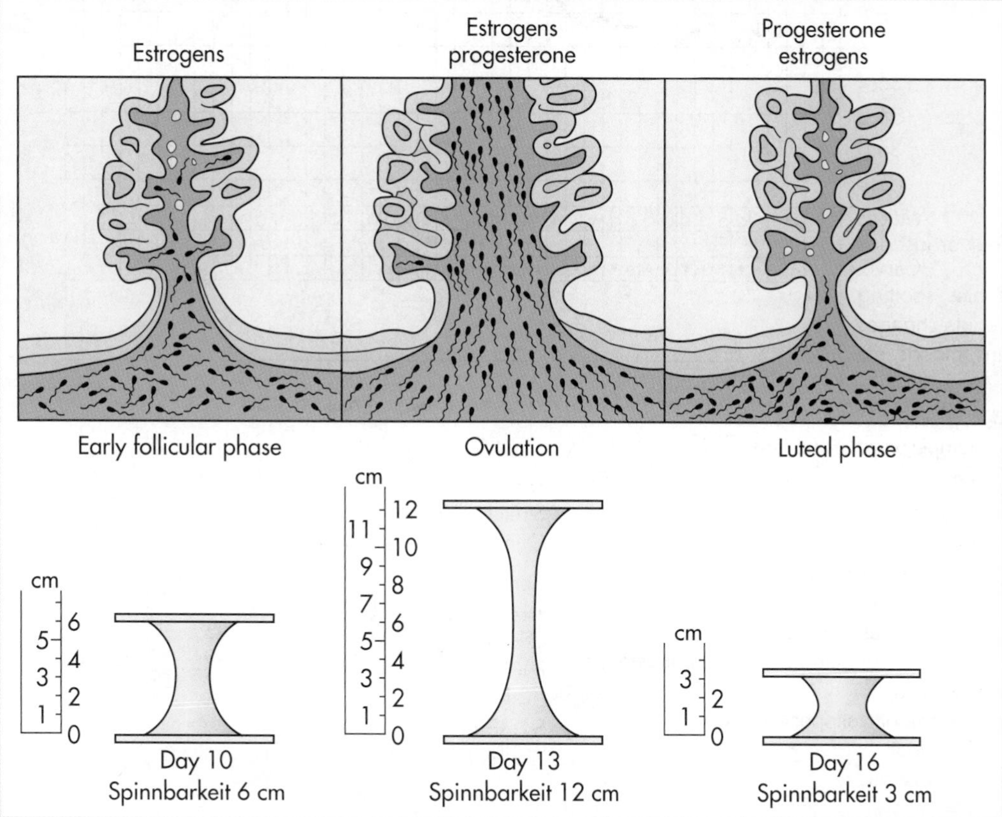

The woman is taught to palpate the cervix to assess for changes indicating ovulation: the cervical os dilates slightly, the cervix softens and rises in the vagina, and cervical mucus is copious and slippery. The woman notes days on which coitus, changes in routine, illness, and so on have occurred (Fig. 7-8). Calendar calculations and cervical mucus changes are used to estimate the onset of the fertile period; changes in cervical mucus or the BBT are used to estimate its end.

Predictor Test for Ovulation

All the methods previously discussed are indicative of ovulation but do not prove its occurrence or exact timing. The predictor test for ovulation is a major addition to the NFP and fertility-awareness methods to help women who want to plan the time of their pregnancies and for women who are trying to conceive. The predictor test for ovulation detects the sudden surge of LH that occurs approximately 12 to 24 hours before ovulation. Unlike BBT, the test is not affected by illness, emotional upset, or physical activity. A test kit is available for home use. The test kit contains sufficient material for several days' testing during each cycle. A positive response indicating an LH surge is noted by a color change that is easy to read. Directions for use of this home test kit vary with the manufacturer.

Barrier Methods

Barrier contraceptives have gained in popularity not only as a contraceptive method but also as protection against the

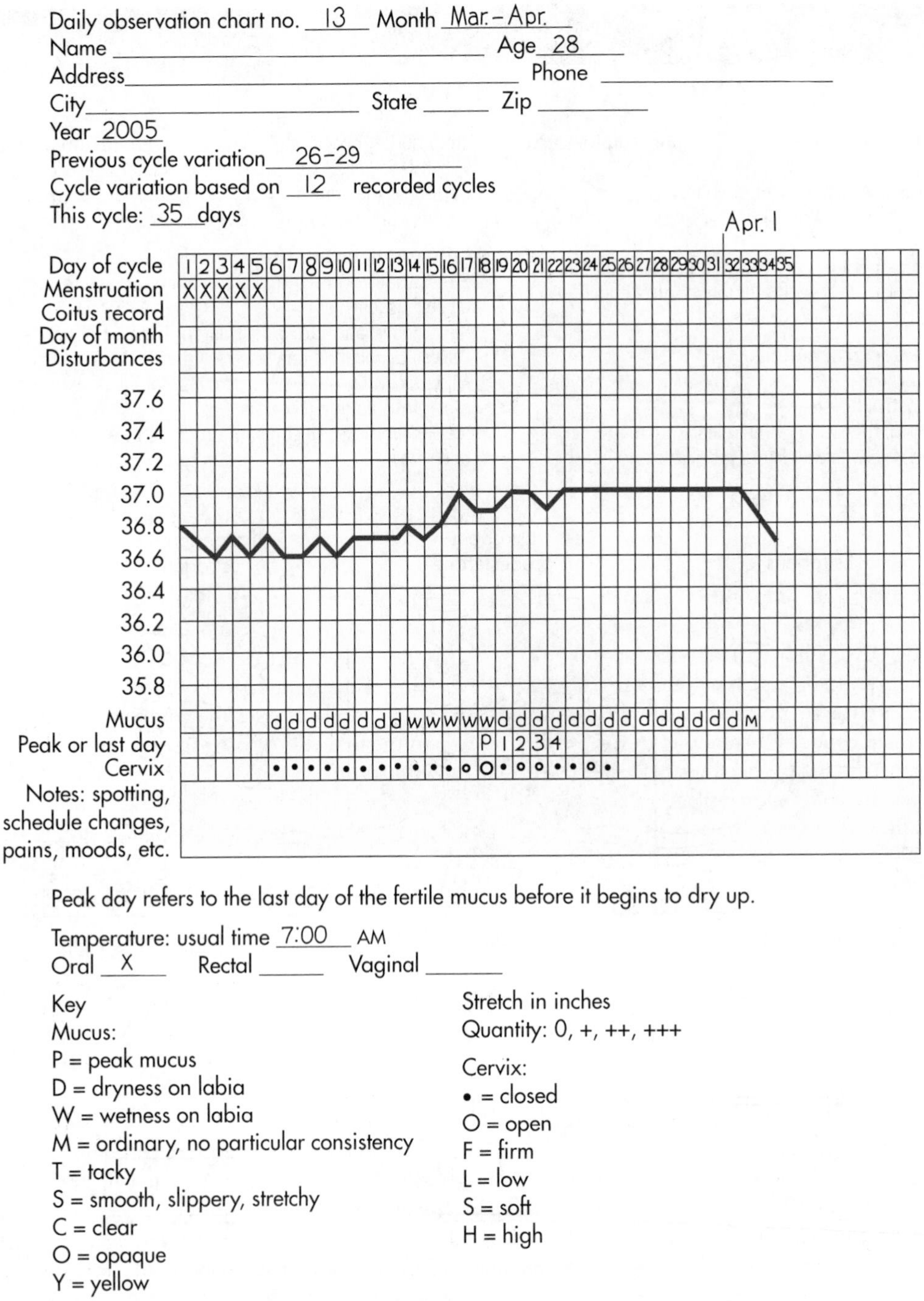

Fig. 7-8 Example of completed symptothermal chart.

spread of STIs. Chemical barriers (spermicides) such as nonoxynol-9 may reduce the risk of some STIs (e.g., human papillomavirus) but are not effective against chlamydia and gonorrhea or HIV infection (CDC, 2002). Male and female condoms provide a mechanical barrier to STIs, including HIV (Hatcher et al, 2004).

Spermicides

A vaginal spermicide is a physical barrier to sperm penetration that also has a chemical action on sperm. Nonoxynol-9 is the most commonly used spermicidal chemical in the United States. However, frequent use of nonoxynol-9 may increase the transmission of HIV and can cause genital lesions (CDC, 2002). Intravaginal spermicides are marketed and sold without prescriptions as aerosol foams, suppositories, creams, films, and gels (Fig. 7-9). Preloaded, single-dose applicators small enough to be carried in a small purse are available. Effectiveness of spermicides depends on consistent and accurate use. Not more than 1 hour before sexual intercourse, the spermicide should be inserted into the vagina so that it makes contact with the cervix. Typical failure rate in the first year of spermicidal use alone is 29% (Trussell, 2004).

Condoms

The male condom is a thin, stretchable sheath that covers the penis (Fig. 7-10). Condoms are made of latex rubber, which provides a barrier to sperm, as well as STIs (including HIV); polyurethane; or natural membranes. Latex condoms

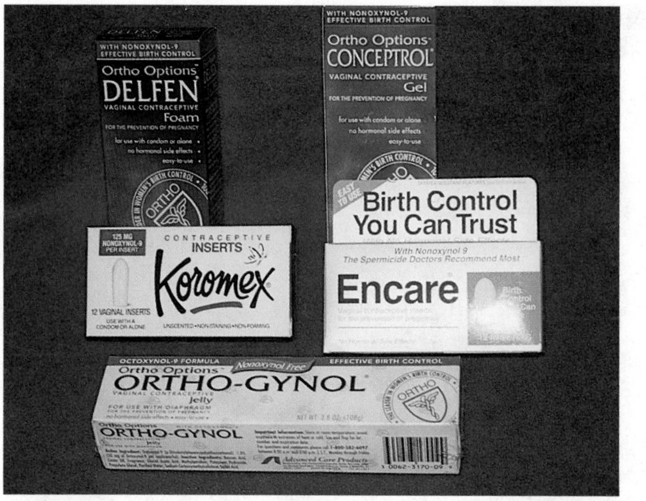

Fig. 7-9 Spermicides. (Courtesy Marjorie Pyle, RNC. Life Circle, Costa Mesa, CA.)

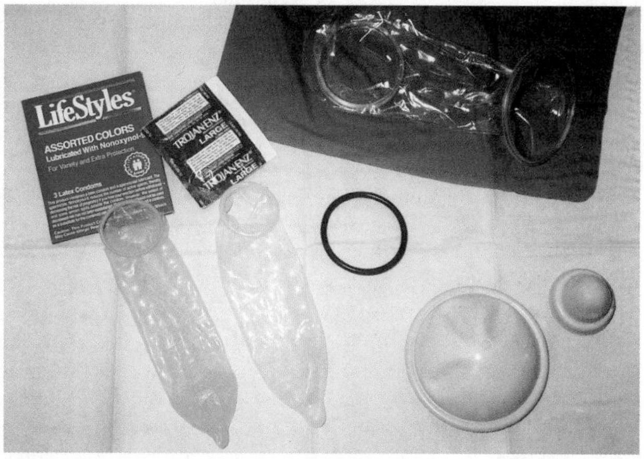

Fig. 7-10 Mechanical barriers. *Clockwise from top:* female condom, cervical cap, diaphragm, types of male condoms, vaginal ring (hormonal) *(center).* (Courtesy Donna Rowe, University of North Carolina Student Health, Chapel Hill, NC.)

will break down with oil-based lubricants (e.g., petroleum jelly and suntan oil) and should be used only with water-based lubricants (e.g., K-Y jelly). A small percentage of condoms are made from the intestinal cecum of lambs (natural skin). These condoms do not provide the same protection against STIs and HIV infection. Natural skin condoms contain small pores that could allow passage of viruses such as hepatitis B, herpes simplex, and HIV. More recently, condom manufacturers have begun using polyurethane, a material that is thinner and stronger than latex. Polyurethane condoms can be used with oil-based lubricants (Hatcher et al, 2004). Research is being conducted to determine the effectiveness of polyurethane condoms in protecting against STIs and HIV.

NURSE ALERT All patients should be questioned about the potential for latex allergy. Latex condom use is contraindicated for patients with latex sensitivity. ■

A functional difference in condom shape is the presence or absence of a sperm reservoir tip. To enhance vaginal stimulation, some condoms are contoured and rippled or have ribbed or roughened surfaces. Thinner construction increases heat transmission and sensitivity; a variety of colors increases their acceptability and attractiveness (Hatcher et al., 2004). A wet jelly or dry powder lubricates some condoms. Spermicide is added to the interior or exterior surfaces of some condoms. Typical failure rate for the first year of use of the male condom is 15% (Trussell, 2004).

NURSE ALERT It is a false assumption that everyone knows how to use condoms. To prevent unintended pregnancy and the spread of STIs, it is essential that condoms be used correctly. Proper instructions in use must be provided. The sheath is applied over the erect penis before insertion and before the loss of preejaculatory drops of semen (Box 7-8). ■

The vaginal sheath (female condom) is made of polyurethane and has flexible rings at both ends (Fig. 7-10). The closed end of the pouch is inserted into the vagina and is anchored around the cervix; the open ring covers the labia. The female condom can be inserted up to 8 hours before intercourse and is intended for one-time use. Both women and men report that intercourse with the sheath is generally as satisfying as intercourse without the sheath. It comes in one size and is available over the counter. Typical failure rate is 21% in the first year of use (Trussell, 2004).

Diaphragm

The vaginal diaphragm is a shallow, dome-shaped, rubber device with a flexible rim that covers the cervix (Fig. 7-10). The diaphragm is a mechanical barrier to the meeting of sperm with the ovum. By holding spermicide in place against the cervix for the 6 hours it takes to destroy the sperm, the diaphragm also provides a chemical barrier to pregnancy. Diaphragms are available in a wide range of diameters (50 to 95 mm) and differ in the inner construction of the circular rim. The types of rims are flat spring, coil spring, arcing spring, and wide-seal rim. The diaphragm should feel comfortable. It should be the largest size the woman can wear without being aware of its presence. Typical failure rate of the diaphragm combined with spermicide is 16% in the first year of use (Trussell, 2004).

Nursing Considerations

The woman using a diaphragm needs an annual gynecologic examination to assess the fit of the diaphragm. The device should be replaced every 2 years and may need to be refitted after a weight loss or gain, term birth, or a second-trimester miscarriage (Hatcher et al, 2004). Because there are various types of diaphragms on the market, the package insert is used for teaching the woman how to use and care for the diaphragm (Home Care box).

Except for occasional allergic responses to the diaphragm or spermicide, there are no side effects from a well-fitted device. The diaphragm can be inserted as long as 6 hours before intercourse, but spermicide must be inserted into the vagina each time intercourse is repeated (Hatcher et al, 2004). The diaphragm must be left in place for at least 6 hours after the last intercourse. The woman who engages in intercourse infrequently may choose this barrier method. The spermicide offers additional lubrication if it is needed. A decreased incidence of vaginitis, cervicitis (including cer-

BOX 7-8

Male Condoms

Mechanism of Action

Sheath is applied over the erect penis before insertion or loss of preejaculatory drops of semen. Used correctly, condoms prevent sperm from entering the cervix. Spermicide-coated condoms cause ejaculated sperm to be immobilized rapidly, thus increasing contraceptive effectiveness.

Failure Rate

Typical users, 15%

Correct and consistent users, 2%

Advantages

- Safe.
- No side effects.
- Readily available.
- Premalignant changes in cervix can be prevented or ameliorated in women whose partners use condoms.
- Method of male nonsurgical contraception.

Disadvantages

- Must interrupt lovemaking to apply sheath.
- Sensation may be altered.
- If used improperly, spillage of sperm can result in pregnancy.
- Condoms occasionally may tear during intercourse.

STI Protection

If a condom is used throughout the act of intercourse and there is no unprotected contact with female genitals, a latex rubber condom, which is impermeable to viruses, can act as a protective measure against STIs.

Nursing Considerations

Teach man to do the following:

- Use a new condom (check expiration date) for each act of sexual intercourse or other acts between partners that involve contact with the penis.
- Place condom after penis is erect and before intimate contact.
- Place condom on head of penis (Fig. A) and unroll it all the way to the base (Fig. B).
- Leave an empty space at the tip (Fig. A); remove any air remaining in the tip by gently pressing air out toward the base of the penis.

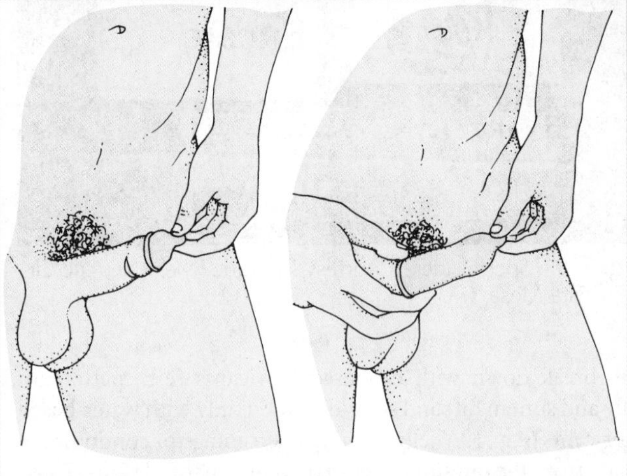

Fig. A Fig. B

- If a lubricant is desired, use water-based products such as K-Y lubricating jelly. Do not use petroleum-based products because they can cause the condom to break.
- After ejaculation, carefully withdraw the still-erect penis from the vagina, holding onto condom rim; remove and discard the condom.
- Store unused condoms in cool, dry place.
- Do not use condoms that are sticky, brittle, or obviously damaged.

vicitis caused by *Chlamydia trachomatis* and *Neisseria gonorrhoeae*), and pelvic inflammatory disease (PID) has been reported among women who use contraceptive creams, foams, and gels with the diaphragm. A reduced risk of cervical dysplasia has been reported among women who use a diaphragm (Hatcher et al, 2004).

Disadvantages of using a diaphragm include the reluctance of some women to insert and remove the device. A cold diaphragm and a cold gel temporarily reduce vaginal response to sexual stimulation if insertion of the diaphragm occurs immediately before intercourse. Some women or couples object to the messiness of the spermicide. These annoyances of diaphragm use, along with failure to insert the device once foreplay has begun, are the most common reasons for failures of this method. Side effects may include irritation of tissues from contact with spermicides. Urethritis and recurrent cystitis caused by upward pressure of the diaphragm rim against the urethra may be increased by use of the contraceptive diaphragm. Diaphragms are contraindicated for women with pelvic relaxation (uterine prolapse) or a large cystocele. Women with a latex allergy should not use latex diaphragms.

Toxic shock syndrome (TSS), although reported in very small numbers, can occur in association with the use of the contraceptive diaphragm (Hatcher et al, 2004). Measures to reduce the risk for TSS include handwashing before insertion and removal, prompt removal 6 to 8 hours after intercourse, not using the diaphragm during menses, and learning and watching for danger signs of TSS.

NURSE ALERT The nurse should be alert for signs of TSS in women who use a diaphragm or cervical cap as a contraceptive method. The most common signs include sudden onset of a fever greater than 38.4° C, hypotension (systolic blood pressure less than 90 mm Hg or orthostatic dizziness), and a rash. ■

Cervical Cap

The cervical cap has a soft, natural rubber dome with a firm but pliable rim (Fig. 7-10). It fits snugly around the base of the cervix close to the junction of the cervix and vaginal fornices. The device is available in four sizes (22, 25, 28, and 31 mm). It is recommended that the cap remain in place no less than 8 hours and not more than 48 hours at a time. It is left in place at least 6 hours after the last act of intercourse. The seal provides a physical barrier to sperm; spermicide inside the cap adds a chemical barrier.

Home Care

USE AND CARE OF THE DIAPHRAGM

Positions for Insertion of Diaphragm

Squatting

- Squatting is the most commonly used position, and most women find it satisfactory.

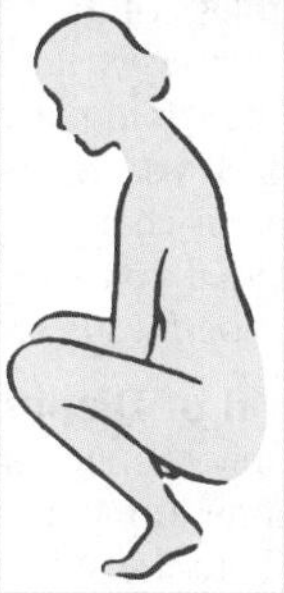

Leg-up Method

- Another position is to raise the left foot (if right hand is used for insertion) on a low stool and, while in a bending position, insert the diaphragm.

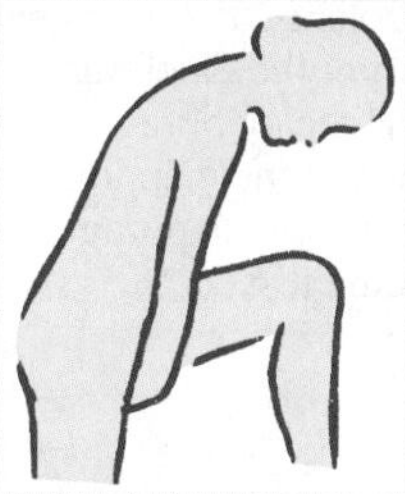

Chair Method

- Another practical method for diaphragm insertion is to sit far forward on the edge of a chair.

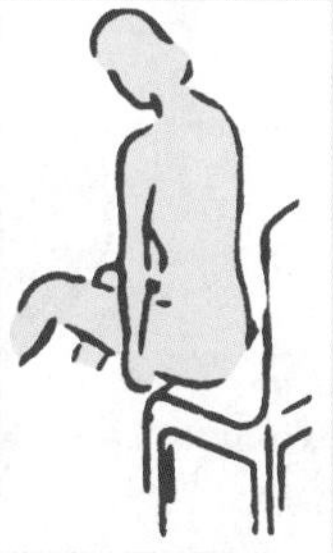

Reclining

- You may prefer to insert the diaphragm while in a semireclining position in bed.

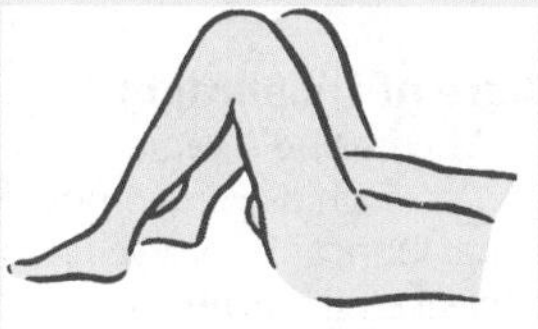

Inspection of Diaphragm

Your diaphragm must be inspected carefully before each use. The best way to do this is as follows:

- Hold the diaphragm up to a light source. Carefully stretch the diaphragm at the area of the rim, on all sides, to make sure there are no holes. Remember, it is possible to puncture the diaphragm with sharp fingernails.
- Another way to check for pinholes is to carefully fill the diaphragm with water. If there is any problem, it will be seen immediately.
- If your diaphragm is puckered, especially near the rim, this could mean thin spots.
- The diaphragm should not be used if you see any of these; consult your health care provider.

Preparation of Diaphragm

- Rinse off cornstarch. Your diaphragm must always be used with a spermicidal lubricant to be effective. Pregnancy cannot be prevented effectively by the diaphragm alone.
- Always empty your bladder before inserting the diaphragm. Place about 2 teaspoonfuls of contraceptive jelly or contraceptive cream on the side of the diaphragm that will rest against the cervix (or whichever way you have been instructed). Spread it around to coat the surface and the rim. This aids in insertion and offers a more complete seal. Many women also spread some jelly or cream on the other side of the diaphragm (Fig. A).

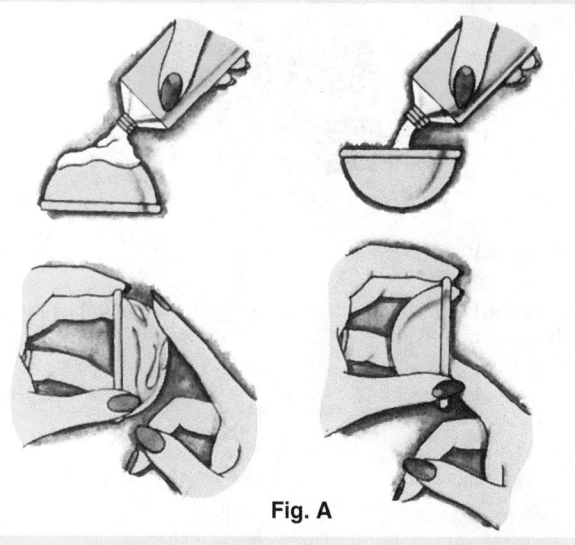

Fig. A

Insertion of Diaphragm

- The diaphragm can be inserted as long as 6 hours before intercourse. Hold the diaphragm between your thumb and fingers. The dome can either be up or down, as directed by your health care provider. Place your index finger on the outer rim of the compressed diaphragm (Fig. B).
- Use the fingers of the other hand to spread the labia (lips of the vagina). This will assist in guiding the diaphragm into place.

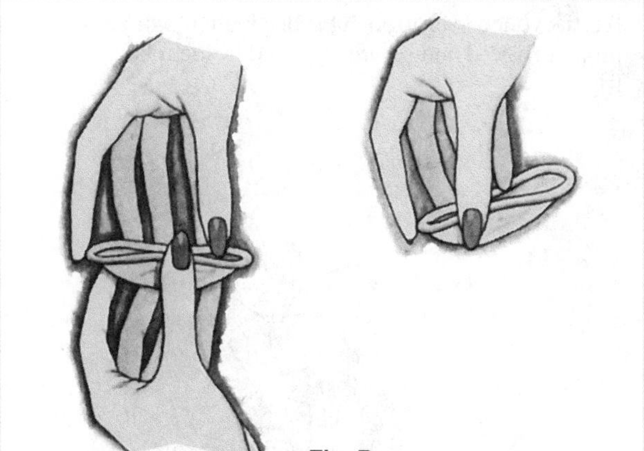

Fig. B

Continued

Home Care

USE AND CARE OF THE DIAPHRAGM—CONT'D

Insertion of Diaphragm—cont'd

- Insert the diaphragm into the vagina. Direct it inward and downward as far as it will go to the space behind and below the cervix (Fig. C).

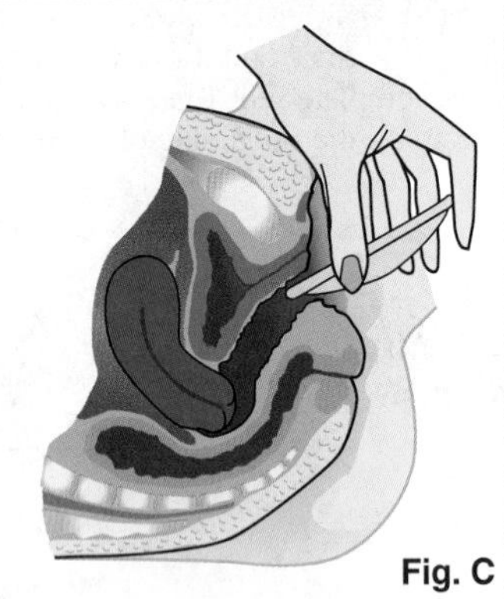

Fig. C

- Tuck the front of the rim of the diaphragm behind the pubic bone so that the rubber hugs the front wall of the vagina (Fig. D).

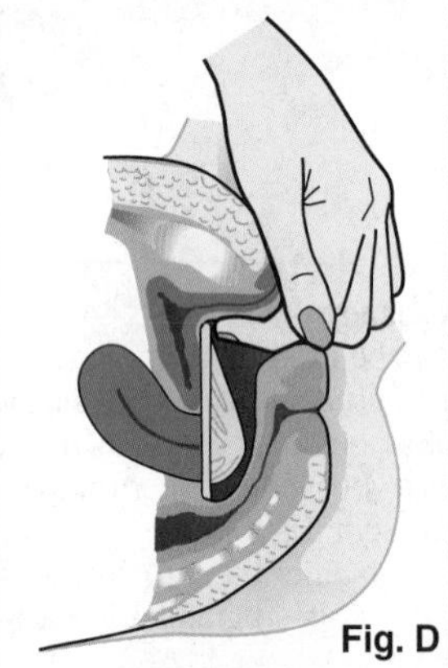

Fig. D

- Feel for your cervix through the diaphragm to be certain it is properly placed and securely covered by the rubber dome (Fig. E).

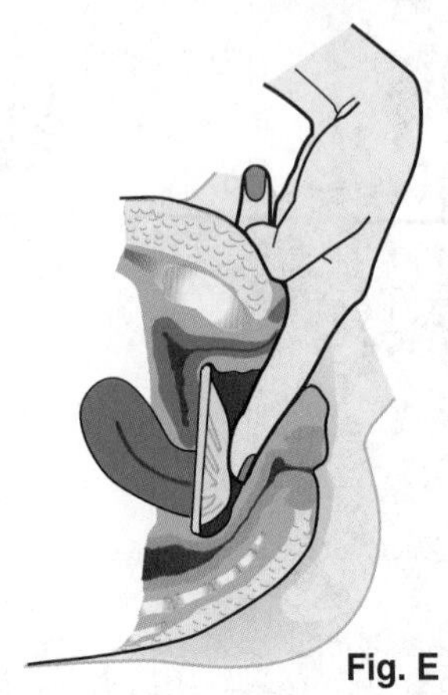

Fig. E

General Information

- Regardless of the time of the month, you must use your diaphragm every time intercourse takes place. Your diaphragm must be left in place for at least 6 hours after the last intercourse. If you remove your diaphragm before the 6-hour period, your chance of becoming pregnant could be greatly increased. If you have repeated acts of intercourse, you must add more spermicide for each act of intercourse.

Removal of Diaphragm

- The only proper way to remove the diaphragm is to insert your forefinger up and over the top side of the diaphragm and slightly to the side.
- Next, turn the palm of your hand downward and backward, hooking the forefinger firmly on top of the inside of the upper rim of the diaphragm, breaking the suction.
- Pull the diaphragm down and out. This avoids the possibility of tearing the diaphragm with the fingernails. You should not remove the diaphragm by trying to catch the rim from below the dome (Fig. F).

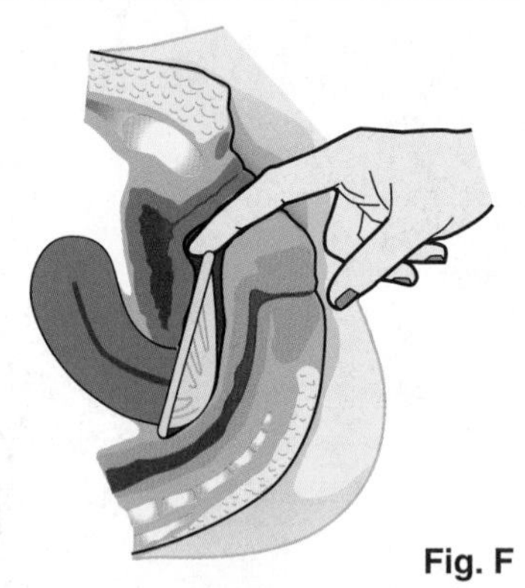

Fig. F

Care of Diaphragm

- When using a vaginal diaphragm, avoid using oil-based products, such as certain body lubricants, mineral oil, baby oil, vaginal lubricants, or vaginitis preparations. These products can weaken the rubber.
- A little care means longer wear for your diaphragm. After each use, wash the diaphragm in warm water and mild soap. Do not use detergent soaps, cold-cream soaps, deodorant soaps, and soaps containing oil products, because they can weaken the rubber.
- After washing, dry the diaphragm thoroughly. All water and moisture should be removed with a towel. Then dust the diaphragm with cornstarch. Scented talc, body powder, baby powder, and the like should not be used because they can weaken the rubber.
- To clean the introducer (if one is used), wash with mild soap and warm water, rinse, and dry thoroughly.
- Place the diaphragm back in the plastic case for storage. Do not store it near a radiator or heat source or exposed to light for an extended period.

The extended period of wear is an added convenience for women who previously used the diaphragm. Instructions for the actual insertion and use of the cervical cap closely resemble the instructions for use of the contraceptive diaphragm. Some of the differences are that the cervical cap can be inserted hours before sexual intercourse without a later need for additional spermicide, the cervical cap requires less spermicide than the diaphragm when initially inserted, and no additional spermicide is required for repeated acts of intercourse.

Women who are not good candidates for wearing the cervical cap include those with abnormal Papanicolaou (Pap) test results, those who cannot be fitted properly with the existing cap sizes or who find the insertion and removal of the device too difficult, those with a history of TSS or with vaginal or cervical infections, and those who experience allergic responses to the cap or to spermicide.

Nursing Considerations

The angle of the uterus, the vaginal muscle tone, and the shape of the cervix may interfere with the ease of fitting and use of the cervical cap. Correct fitting requires time, effort, and skill of both the woman and the clinician. The woman must check the position of the cap before and after each act of intercourse. A Pap smear should be done after 3 months of use because of increased risk of cervical dysplasia at 3 months. No increased risk of dysplasia is found at 1 year (Hatcher et al, 2004).

Although no link has been discovered between TSS and the use of the cervical cap, such an association is possible. The package insert recommends that another form of birth control be used during menstrual bleeding and for at least 6 weeks postpartum. The cap should be checked for proper fit after any gynecologic surgery or birth and after major weight loss or gain. Otherwise, the size should be checked at least once a year.

Strong patient motivation is the most important criterion for successful cap use. Failure rate with typical use for parous women is 32% and for nulliparous women is 16% (Trussell, 2004). The nurse should assess the woman's understanding and skill in the use of the cervical cap (Home Care box).

Contraceptive Sponge

The vaginal sponge was taken off the market in the United States in 1995 because of production problems of the manufacturer, and as of this writing (2005), the contraceptive sponge (Today sponge) is still unavailable in the United States. The manufacturer is awaiting full marketing approval in the United States. For updates on the status, send e-mail to questions@todaysponge.com. It is available in other countries, including Canada. The vaginal sponge is a small, round, polyurethane sponge that contains a spermicide. It is designed to fit over the cervix (one size fits all). The side that is placed next to the cervix is concave for better fit. The opposite side has a woven polyester loop to be used in removing the sponge.

The sponge should be moistened with water before it is inserted into the vagina to cover the cervix. It provides protection for up to 24 hours and for numerous instances of sexual intercourse. The sponge should be left in place for at least 6 hours after the last act of sexual intercourse. Longer wearing time (greater than 24 to 30 hours) is not recommended because the woman may be at risk for TSS (Hatcher et al, 2004).

Home Care

USE OF THE CERVICAL CAP

- Push cap up into vagina until it covers cervix.

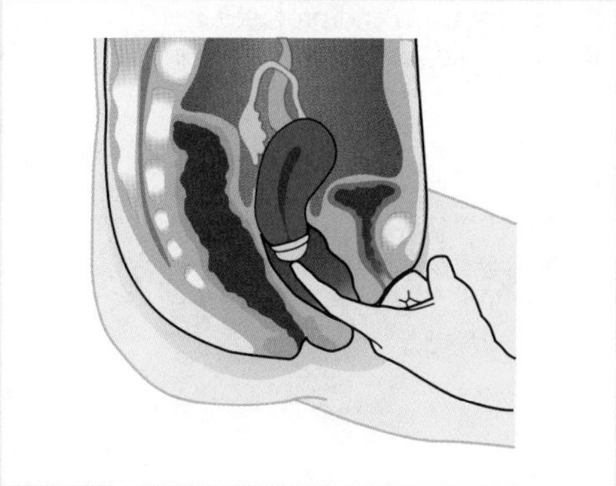

- Press rim against cervix to create a seal.

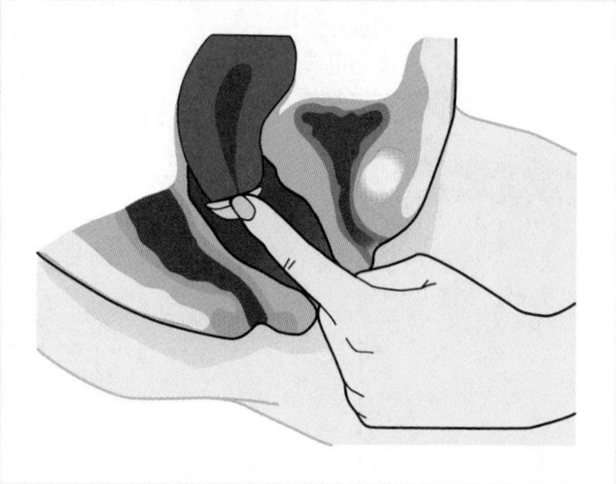

- To remove, push rim toward right or left hip to loosen from cervix, and then withdraw.

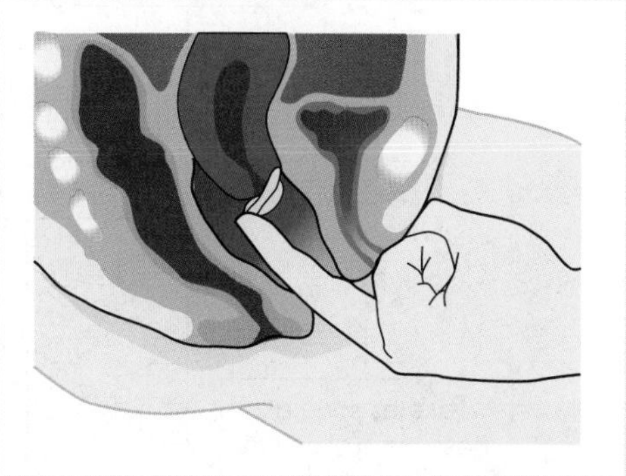

- The woman can assume several positions to insert the cervical cap. See the four positions shown for inserting the diaphragm.

Hormonal Methods

More than 30 different hormonal contraceptive formulations are available in the United States today. General classes are described in Table 7-3. Because of the wide variety of preparations available, the woman and nurse must read the

Table 7-3

Hormonal Contraception

COMPOSITION	ROUTE OF ADMINISTRATION	DURATION OF EFFECT
Combination estrogen and progestin (synthetic estrogens and progestins in varying doses and formulations)	Oral	24 hours
	Transdermal patch	7 days
	Intramuscular injection	28 ± 5 days
	Vaginal ring insertion	3 weeks
Progestin only	Oral	24 hours
Norethindrone, norgestrel	Intramuscular injection	3 months
Medroxyprogesterone acetate	Subdermal implant	Up to 5 years
Levonorgestrel	Intrauterine device	1 year

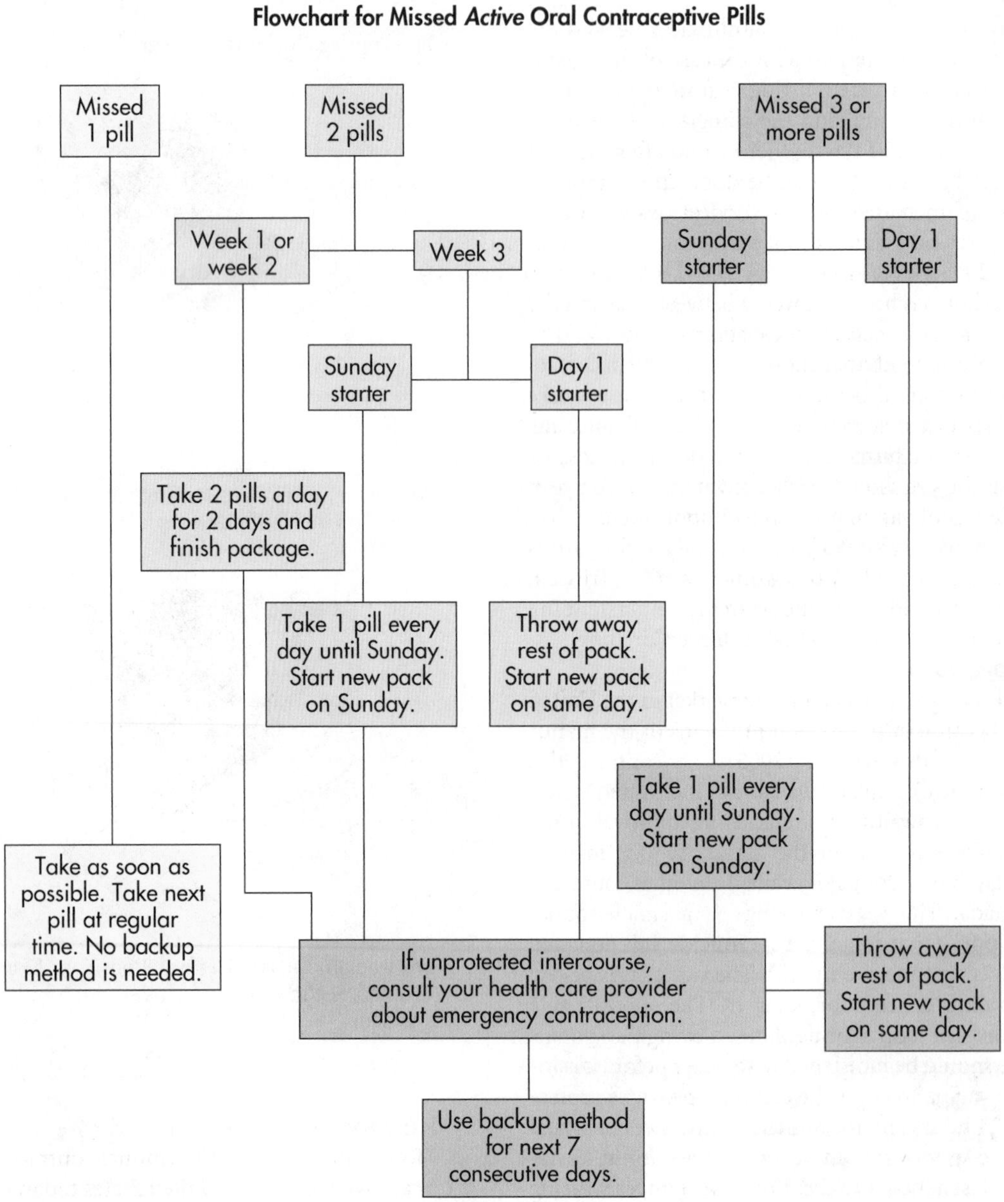

Fig. 7-11 Flowchart for missed contraceptive pills. (Courtesy Patsy Huff, PharmD, Chapel Hill, NC.)

package insert for information about specific products prescribed. Formulations include combined estrogen-progestin steroidal medications or progestational agents. The formulations are administered orally, transdermally, vaginally, by implantation, or by injection.

Combined Estrogen-Progestin Contraceptives

Oral Contraceptives

Regular ingestion of combined oral contraceptive (COC) pills suppresses the action of the hypothalamus and anterior pituitary, leading to inappropriate secretion of FSH and LH; therefore follicles do not mature and ovulation is inhibited. COCs also affect the endometrium so that from 1 to 4 days after the COC is taken, the endometrium sloughs and bleeds (withdrawal bleeding) as a result of hormone withdrawal. The withdrawal bleeding usually is less profuse than that of normal menstruation and may last only 2 to 3 days. Some women have no bleeding at all.

Monophasic pills provide fixed dosages of estrogen and progestin. Multiphasic pills alter the amount of progestin and sometimes the amount of estrogen within each cycle. These preparations reduce the total dosage of hormones in a single cycle without sacrificing contraceptive efficacy (Wallach & Grimes, 2000). To maintain adequate hormonal levels for contraception and enhance compliance, COCs should be taken at the same time each day. Taken exactly as directed, oral contraceptives prevent ovulation, and pregnancy cannot occur. The overall effectiveness rate is almost 100%.

Contraindications for COC use include a history of thromboembolic disorders, cerebrovascular or coronary artery disease, breast cancer, estrogen-dependent tumors, pregnancy, impaired liver function, liver tumor, lactation less than 6 weeks postpartum, smoking if older than 35 years (more than 15 cigarettes a day), headaches with focal neurologic symptoms, surgery with prolonged immobilization or any surgery on the legs, hypertension (160/100), and diabetes mellitus (of more than 20 years' duration) with vascular disease (World Health Organization, 2000).

The effectiveness of oral contraceptives is decreased when the following medications are taken simultaneously:

- Anticonvulsants (phenytoin, sodium, carbamazepine, primidone, topiramate)
- Griseofulvin
- Rifampin

After discontinuing oral contraception, return of fertility usually happens quickly, but fertility rates are slightly lower the first 3 to 12 months after discontinuation (Wallach & Grimes, 2000).

Nursing Considerations

Many different preparations of oral hormonal contraceptives are available. Because of the wide variations, each woman must be clear about the unique dosage regimen for the preparation prescribed for her and follow directions on the package insert. Directions for care after missing one or two tablets also vary (Fig. 7-11). Signs of potential complications associated with the use of oral contraceptives must be reviewed with the woman (Box 7-9). Oral contraceptives do not protect a woman against STIs. A barrier method such as condoms and spermicide should be used for protection.

BOX 7-9

Signs of Potential Complications with Oral Contraceptives

Before oral contraceptives are prescribed and periodically throughout hormone therapy, the woman is alerted to stop taking the pill and to report immediately any of the following symptoms to the health care provider. The word *aches* helps in remembering this list:

A—Abdominal pain: may indicate a problem with the liver or gallbladder
C—Chest pain or shortness of breath: may indicate possible clot problem within lungs or heart
H—Headaches (sudden or persistent): may be caused by cardiovascular accident or hypertension
E—Eye problems: may indicate vascular accident or hypertension
S—Severe leg pain: may indicate a thromboembolic process

Data from Hiller J, Griffith E: Education for contraceptive use by women after childbirth (Cochrane Review), *The Cochrane Library,* Issue 3, Oxford, 2000, Update Software.

Combined Estrogen and Progestin Injection

The combined injectable contraceptive (e.g., Lunelle) is injected intramuscularly in the deltoid or gluteus maximus muscle every 28 ± 5 days. Typical failure rate in the first year of use is 3% (Trussell, 2004). Mechanisms of action, contraindications, and side effects are similar to those of COCs.

Transdermal Contraceptive System

The contraceptive patch delivers continuous levels of progesterone and ethynyl estradiol. The patch can be applied to the lower abdomen, upper outer arm, buttock, or upper torso (except the breast). Application is on the same day once a week for 3 weeks, followed by a week without the patch. Withdrawal bleeding occurs during the "no patch" week. Mechanisms of action, contraindications, and side effects are similar to those of COCs.

Vaginal Ring

The vaginal ring (made of ethylene vinyl acetate copolymer) delivers continuous levels of progesterone and ethynyl estradiol. One vaginal ring is worn for 3 weeks, followed by a week without the ring. Withdrawal bleeding occurs during the "no ring" week. The ring can be inserted by the woman and does not have to be fitted. Mechanisms of action, contraindications, and side effects are similar to those of COCs.

Progestin-Only Contraception

Progestin-only methods impair fertility by inhibiting ovulation, thickening and decreasing the amount of cervical mucus, thinning the endometrium, and altering cilia in the uterine tubes (Hatcher et al, 2004).

Oral Progestins (Minipill)

Progestin-only pills are less effective than COCs. Failure rate for typical users is 8% in the first year of use (Trussell, 2004). Effectiveness is increased if minipills are taken correctly. Because minipills contain such a low dose of progestin, the minipill must be taken at the same time every day. Users often complain of irregular vaginal bleeding.

Injectable Progestins

Depot medroxyprogesterone acetate (DMPA; Depo-Provera) is given intramuscularly in the deltoid or gluteus maximus muscle. Injections should be administered every 12 weeks. Typical failure rate is 3% in the first year of use (Trussell, 2004).

NURSE ALERT When administering an intramuscular injection of progestin (e.g., Depo-Provera), the site should not be massaged after the injection because this action can hasten the absorption and shorten the period of effectiveness. ■

Advantages of Depo-Provera include a contraceptive effectiveness comparable to combined oral contraceptives, long-lasting effects, the requirement of injections only four times a year, and lactation not likely to be impaired (Cunningham et al, 2001; Hatcher et al, 2004). Disadvantages are prolonged amenorrhea or uterine bleeding, increased risk of venous thrombosis and thromboembolism, and no protection against STIs (including HIV).

Implantable Progestins (Norplant)

The Norplant system consists of six flexible, nonbiodegradable polymeric silicone (Silastic) capsules. The Silastic capsules contain progestin and provide up to 5 years of contraception. Insertion and removal of the capsules are minor surgical procedures involving a local anesthetic, a small incision, and no sutures. The capsules are placed subdermally in the inner aspect of the upper arm. The progestin prevents some, but not all, ovulatory cycles and thickens cervical mucus. Other advantages include reversibility and long-term continuous contraception that is not coitus related. The effectiveness is greater than 99% over 5 years.

Irregular menstrual bleeding is the most common side effect. Less common side effects include headaches, nervousness, nausea, skin changes, and vertigo. No STI protection is provided with the Norplant method; condoms should be used for protection. The drug was withdrawn from the U.S. market in 2002.

Emergency Contraception

Emergency contraception is used within 72 hours of unprotected intercourse to prevent pregnancy. The three methods available in the United States include high doses of oral progestins or COCs and insertion of the copper IUD (Hatcher et al, 2004).

The Food and Drug Administration (FDA) has approved an emergency contraception kit (Preven) with the exact dosage and instructions for use. There is no medical contraindication for emergency contraception except pregnancy and undiagnosed abnormal vaginal bleeding. Emergency contraception is ineffective if the woman is pregnant. Pregnancy rates are reduced by at least 75% (Trussell, 2004).

To minimize the side effect of nausea that occurs with high doses of estrogen and progestin, the woman can be advised to take an over-the-counter antiemetic 1 hour before each dose. If the woman does not begin menstruation within 21 days after taking the pills, she should be evaluated for pregnancy.

Intrauterine devices containing copper (see later discussion) provide another emergency contraception option. The intrauterine device should be inserted within 7 days of unprotected intercourse (Hatcher et al, 2004). This method is suggested only for women who wish to have the benefit of long-term contraception.

Contraceptive counseling, including a discussion of modification of risky sexual behaviors to prevent STIs and unwanted pregnancy, should be provided to all women requesting emergency contraception.

Intrauterine Devices

An intrauterine device (IUD) is a small T-shaped device inserted into the uterine cavity. Medicated IUDs are loaded with either copper or a progestational agent (Fig. 7-12). These chemically active substances are released continuously (copper-bearing devices for up to 10 years and progesterone devices for up to 5 years) (Hatcher et al, 2004). IUDs are impregnated with barium sulfate for radiopacity. The copper-bearing IUD damages sperm in transit to the uterine tubes and few sperm reach the ovum, thus preventing fertilization.

The progesterone-bearing IUD causes progestin-related effects on cervical mucus and endometrial maturation. The effect is primarily local, but there are some systemic effects, such as irregular menstrual bleeding. After 1 year of use, women usually experience amenorrhea or regular menses. The typical failure rate of the IUD ranges from 0.8% to 2.0% (Trussell, 2004).

The IUD offers constant contraception without the need to remember to take pills each day or engage in other manipulation before or between coital acts. If pregnancy can be excluded, an IUD can be placed at any time during the menstrual cycle. An IUD may be inserted immediately after childbirth or first trimester abortion. Contraceptive effects are reversible. When pregnancy is desired, the IUD may be removed by the health care provider.

The progesterone IUD offers two important noncontraceptive progesterone-related advantages: less blood loss during menstruation and decreased primary dysmenorrhea. The average blood loss is increased for the copper IUD. The IUD is contraindicated for women with a history of PID, known or suspected pregnancy, undiagnosed genital bleeding, suspected genital malignancy, or a distorted intrauterine cavity.

Disadvantages of IUD use include increased risk of PID in the first 20 days after insertion, and risk of bacterial vaginosis and uterine perforation. The IUD offers no protection

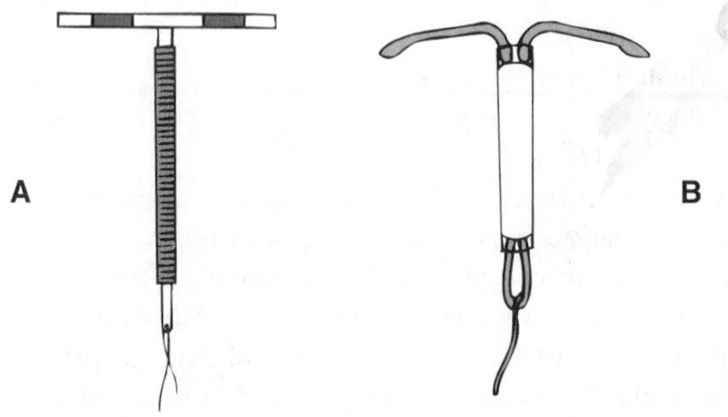

Fig. 7-12 Intrauterine devices. **A**, Copper T380A. **B**, Levonorgestrel-releasing IUD.

against STIs or HIV. The IUD is recommended primarily for women who want long-term contraception, who have had at least one child, and who are involved in stable monogamous relationships (Hatcher et al, 2004).

Nursing Considerations

The woman should be taught to check for the presence of the IUD thread after menstruation to rule out expulsion of the device. If pregnancy occurs with the IUD in place, the IUD should be removed immediately in the first trimester if the strings are visible. Later in pregnancy, ultrasound examination should be used to localize the IUD and to rule out placenta previa. Retention of the IUD during pregnancy increases the risk of septic miscarriage and ectopic pregnancy (Hatcher et al, 2004). Some women allergic to copper develop a rash, necessitating removal of the copper-bearing IUD. Signs of potential complications are listed in Box 7-10.

Sterilization

Sterilization refers to surgical procedures intended to render the person infertile. Most procedures involve the occlusion of the passageways for the ova and sperm (Fig. 7-13, A). For the female, the oviducts (uterine tubes) are occluded; for the male, the sperm ducts (vas deferens) are occluded. Only surgical removal of the ovaries (oophorectomy) or uterus (hysterectomy) or both will result in absolute sterility for the woman. All other sterilization procedures have a small but definite failure rate; that is, pregnancy may result.

Female Sterilization

Female sterilization (bilateral tubal ligation) may be done immediately after giving birth (within 24 to 48 hours), concomitantly with abortion, or as an interval procedure (during any phase of the menstrual cycle). Half of all sterilization procedures are performed immediately after a pregnancy. Sterilization procedures can be done safely on an outpatient basis. Failure rate for methods of female sterilization vary by the method and the woman's age, but the average is 0.5% (Trussell, 2004).

Tubal Occlusion

A laparoscopic approach or a minilaparotomy may be used for tubal ligation (Fig. 7-14), tubal electrocoagulation, or for the application of bands or clips. Electrocoagulation and ligation are considered to be permanent methods. Use of the bands or clips has the theoretic advantage of possible removal and return of tubal patency (Guidelines box).

BOX 7-10

Signs of Potential Complications with Intrauterine Devices (IUDs)

Signs of potential complications related to IUDs can be remembered using the *pains* mnemonic:

P–Period late, abnormal spotting or bleeding
A–Abdominal pain, pain with intercourse
I–Infection exposure, abnormal vaginal discharge
N–Not feeling well, fever, or chills
S–String missing; shorter or longer

Data from Hatcher R et al: *A pocket guide to managing contraception 2004-2005 edition*, Tiger, GA, 2004, Bridging the Gap Foundation.

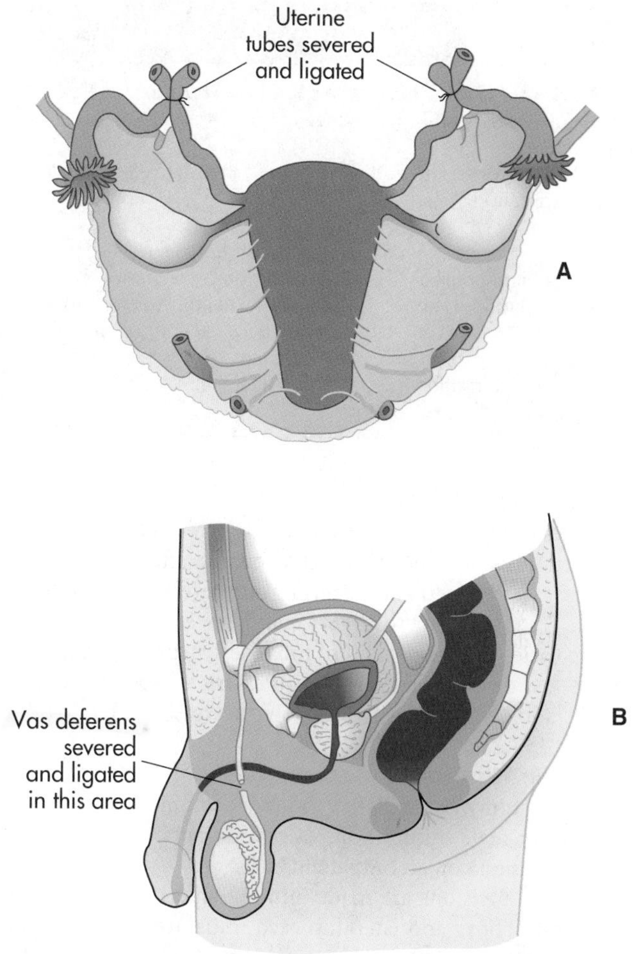

Fig. 7-13 Sterilization. **A**, Uterine tubes ligated and severed (tubal ligation). **B**, Sperm duct ligated and severed (vasectomy).

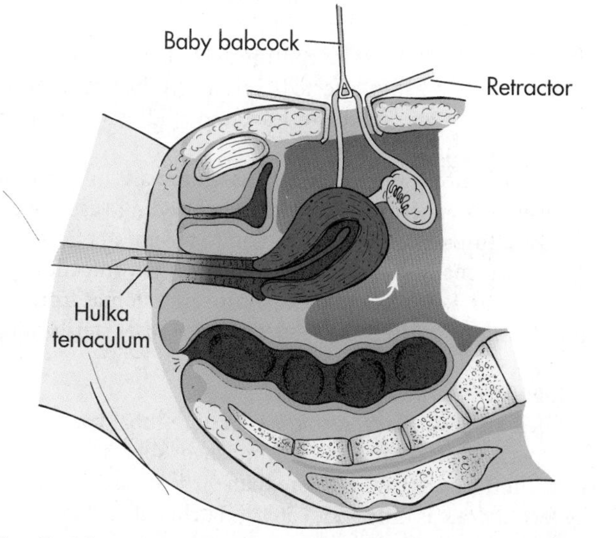

Fig. 7-14 Use of minilaparotomy to gain access to uterine tubes for occlusion procedures. Tenaculum is used to lift uterus upward *(arrow)* toward incision.

Guidelines

WHAT TO EXPECT AFTER TUBAL LIGATION

- You should expect no change in hormones and their influence.
- Your menstrual period will be about the same as before the sterilization.
- You may feel pain at ovulation.
- The ovum disintegrates within the abdominal cavity.
- It is highly unlikely that you will become pregnant.
- You should not have a change in sexual functioning; you may enjoy sexual relations more because you will not be concerned about becoming pregnant.
- Sterilization offers no protection against STIs. Therefore you may need to use condoms.

Tubal Reconstruction

Restoration of tubal continuity (reanastomosis) and function is technically feasible except after laparoscopic tubal electrocoagulation. Sterilization reversal is costly, difficult (requiring microsurgery), and uncertain. The success rate varies with the extent of tubal destruction and removal. The loss of a segment of tube necessary for sperm capacitation and fertilization is probably the reason for low pregnancy rates.

Male Sterilization

Vasectomy is the easiest and most commonly used operation for male sterilization. Vasectomy can be done with local anesthesia on an outpatient basis.

Small incisions are made into the anterior aspect of the scrotum above and lateral to each testis over the spermatic cord (Fig. 7-13, *B*). Each vas deferens is identified, doubly ligated, and then severed between the ligatures. Occasionally the surgeon cauterizes the cut stumps of the sperm ducts. Many surgeons bury the cut ends in scrotal fascia to lessen the chance of reunion. Then the skin incisions are closed. Usually one suture is used for closure of each skin incision and a dressing is applied.

Vasectomy has no effect on potency (ability to achieve and maintain erection) or volume of ejaculate. Endocrine production of testosterone continues so that secondary sex characteristics are not affected. Sperm production continues, but sperm are unable to leave the epididymis and are lysed by the immune system.

Complications after bilateral vasectomy are uncommon and usually not serious. They include bleeding (usually external), suture reaction, and reaction to the anesthetic agent. Men occasionally may develop a hematoma, infection, or epididymitis. Less common are painful granulomas from accumulation of sperm. The failure rate for male sterilization is 0.15% (Trussell, 2004).

Tubal Reconstruction

Microsurgery to reanastomose (restore tubal continuity) the sperm ducts can be accomplished successfully (i.e., sperm in the ejaculate) in more than 90% of cases; however, the fertility rate is only about 50% (Hatcher et al, 2004). The vasectomy may result in permanent changes in the testes that leave men unable to father children. The changes are those ordinarily seen only in the elderly (e.g., interstitial fibrosis [scar tissue between the seminiferous tubules]). Some men develop antibodies against their own sperm (autoimmunization).

Laws and Regulations

All states have strict regulations for informed consent. Many states permit voluntary sterilization of any mature, rational woman without reference to her marital or pregnancy status. Although the partner's consent is not required by law, the woman is encouraged to discuss the situation with her partner, and health care providers may request the partner's consent. Sterilization of minors or mentally incompetent individuals is restricted by most states and often requires the approval of a board of eugenicists or other court-appointed individuals.

LEGAL TIP Sterilization If federal funds are used for sterilization, the person must be at least 21 years old.

Informed consent must include an explanation of the risks, benefits, and alternatives; a statement that describes sterilization as a permanent, irreversible method of birth control; and a statement that mandates a 30-day waiting period between giving consent and the sterilization.

Informed consent must be in the person's native language, or an interpreter must be provided to read the consent form to the person. ■

Nursing Considerations

The nurse plays an important role in assisting people with decision making so that all requirements for informed consent are met. The nurse also provides information about alternatives to sterilization, such as contraception.

Information must be given about what is entailed in the various procedures, how much discomfort or pain can be expected, and what type of care is needed. Many individuals fear sterilization procedures because of the imagined effect on their sexual life. They need reassurance concerning the hormonal and psychologic basis for sexual function, and that uterine tube occlusion or vasectomy has no biologic sequelae in terms of sexual adequacy.

Preoperative care includes health assessment, which includes a psychologic assessment, physical examination, and laboratory tests. The nurse confirms the woman's understanding of printed instructions. Ambivalence and extreme fear of the procedure are reported to the physician.

Postoperative care depends on the procedure performed (e.g., laparoscopy, laparotomy for tubal occlusion, or vasectomy). General care includes recovery after anesthesia, vital signs, fluid-electrolyte balance (intake and output, laboratory values), prevention of or early identification and treatment of infection or hemorrhage, control of discomfort, and assessment of emotional response to the procedure and recovery.

Discharge planning depends on the type of procedure performed. In general, the patient is given written instructions about observing for and reporting symptoms and signs of complications, the type of recovery to be expected, and the date and time for a follow-up appointment.

Evaluation

The nurse can be reasonably assured that care was effective when the patient-centered expected outcomes have been achieved (Nursing Care Plan).

Nursing Care Plan

SEXUAL ACTIVITY AND CONTRACEPTION

NURSING DIAGNOSIS: Decisional conflict related to contraceptive alternatives as evidenced by patients' comments

EXPECTED OUTCOME
Patient and partner will verbalize understanding of different methods of contraception and will choose the method best suited for their needs.

NURSING INTERVENTIONS/*RATIONALES*
Provide information regarding reliability, use, indications, contraindications, and side effects of different methods of contraception *to facilitate the decision-making process.*
Use privacy and therapeutic communication during discussion of sexual activity and methods of contraception *to provide clarification of information and patient trust of caregiver.*

NURSING DIAGNOSIS: Risk for infection related to ongoing sexual activity as evidenced by patient history

EXPECTED OUTCOME
Patient and her partner will remain free of sexually transmitted infections (STIs).

NURSING INTERVENTIONS/*RATIONALES*
Provide information regarding safer sex practices, use of spermicides, and use of barrier methods *to raise patient awareness of methods to prevent infection.*
Educate patient (and partner if available) about signs and symptoms of STIs *to encourage diagnosis and treatment of STIs if they occur.*

ABORTION

Induced abortion is the purposeful interruption of a pregnancy before 20 weeks of gestation. (Miscarriage is discussed in Chapter 14.) If the abortion is performed at the woman's request, the term *elective abortion* is usually used; if performed for reasons of maternal or fetal health or disease, the term *therapeutic abortion* applies. Many factors contribute to a woman's decision to have an abortion. Indications include (1) preservation of the life or health of the mother, (2) genetic disorders of the fetus, (3) rape or incest, and (4) the pregnant woman's request. The control of birth, dealing as it does with human sexuality and the question of life and death, is one of the most emotional components of health care. It has been the most controversial social issue in the last half of the twentieth century and the beginning of the twenty-first century. Regulations exist to protect the mother from the complications of abortion.

The U.S. Supreme Court set aside previous antiabortion laws in January 1973, holding that first trimester abortion is permissible inasmuch as the mortality rate from interruption of early gestation is less than the mortality rate after normal term birth; 90% of abortions are performed at this point in pregnancy. Second trimester abortion was left to the discretion of the individual states (Hatcher et al, 2004). Hospitals maintained by Roman Catholics, and some of those maintained by strict fundamentalists, forbid abortion (and often sterilization) despite legal challenges.

LEGAL TIP **Induced Abortion** It is important for nurses to know the laws regarding abortion in their state of practice before they offer abortion counseling or nursing care to a woman choosing an abortion. Many states enforce a mandatory delay or state-directed counseling before a woman may legally obtain an abortion. ■

Rates of biologic complications after abortions such as ectopic pregnancy, infection, or hemorrhage tend to be low if the woman aborts during the first trimester. Psychologic sequelae of induced abortion are uncommon and may be related to circumstances and support systems surrounding the pregnant woman such as the attitudes reflected by friends, family, and health care workers. The woman facing an abortion is pregnant and will exhibit the emotional responses shared by all pregnant women, including the possibility of postbirth depression.

Nurses often struggle with the same values and moral convictions as those of the pregnant woman. The conflicts and doubts of the nurse can be readily communicated to women who are already anxious and overly sensitive. Health care professionals need assistance to identify and come to terms with their own feelings. It is not uncommon for confusion to arise when beliefs are challenged by the reality of care.

NURSE ALERT Nurses whose religious or moral beliefs do not support abortion have the right to refuse such an assignment. Reassignment is usually an option so that the abortion patient receives needed care. ■

First Trimester Abortion

Methods for performing early elective abortion include vacuum aspiration and medical methods (mifepristone with prostaglandin; methotrexate with misoprostol).

Vacuum Aspiration

Vacuum aspiration abortion is the most common procedure, with about 97% of all procedures being performed by suction curettage. Very early abortions (menstrual extraction, endometrial aspiration) can be done with a small, flexible, plastic cannula without cervical dilation or anesthesia. The insertion of a small laminaria tent (cone of dried seaweed that swells as it absorbs moisture and dilates the cervix) retained by a vaginal tampon for 4 to 24 hours will atraumatically dilate the cervix two or three times its original diameter. This usually facilitates the purposeful interruption of a first trimester pregnancy greater than 8 weeks of gestation (Hatcher et al, 2004). On removal of the laminaria tent, the insertion of an adequate-sized aspiration cannula (8.5 to 10.5

mm) is almost always possible. Prostaglandin gel may also be used to soften the cervix (Cunningham et al, 2001).

Aspiration abortion may be performed in a physician's office, clinic, or hospital. The ideal time for performing this procedure is 8 to 12 weeks after the last menstrual period. The suction procedure for performing an early elective abortion usually requires less than 5 minutes. During the procedure, the woman is kept informed about what to expect next (e.g., menstrual-like cramping and sounds of the suction machine). The nurse assesses her vital signs. The aspirated uterine contents must be carefully inspected to ascertain whether all fetal parts and adequate placental tissue have been evacuated. After the abortion the woman rests on the table until she is ready to stand. She then remains in the recovery area or waiting room for 1 to 3 hours for detection of excessive cramping or bleeding. She may be discharged alone or in the company of a relative or friend, depending on the anesthetic used. If the procedure is done in the physician's office, preoperative sedation is usually not given, and local anesthesia is usually used.

Bleeding after the operation is normally about the equivalent of a heavy menstrual period, and cramps are rarely severe. Excessive vaginal bleeding and infection, such as endometritis or salpingitis, are the most common complications of induced abortion. Retained products of conception are the primary cause of vaginal bleeding. Evacuation of the uterus, uterine massage, and administration of oxytocin or methylergonovine (Methergine) may be necessary. Prophylactic antibiotics have been shown to decrease the risk of infection and should be considered (Hatcher et al, 2004).

Nursing Considerations

Postabortal instructions differ among health care providers (e.g., tampons should not be used for at least 3 days or should be avoided for up to 3 weeks, and resumption of sexual intercourse may be permitted within 1 week or discouraged for 3 weeks). The woman may shower daily. Instruction is given to watch for excessive bleeding (i.e., more than one large pad per hour for 4 hours), cramps, or fever, and to avoid douches of any type. The woman may expect her menstrual period to resume 4 to 6 weeks after the day of the procedure. The nurse offers information about the birth control method the woman prefers, if this has not been done during the counseling interview that usually precedes the decision to have an abortion. The woman must be strongly encouraged to return for her follow-up visit so that complications can be detected and an acceptable contraceptive method prescribed. A pregnancy test may also be performed to determine if the pregnancy has been successfully terminated.

Methotrexate

Methotrexate is a cytotoxic drug that causes early abortion by blocking folic acid in fetal cells so they cannot divide. Methotrexate can be given intramuscularly or orally, followed by vaginal placement of misoprostol (prostaglandin analog). Women commonly have nausea, vomiting, and cramping after the misoprostol insertion. If abortion does not occur, misoprostol is repeated or vacuum aspiration is performed (Hatcher et al, 2004).

Critical Thinking Exercise

TERMINATION OF PREGNANCY

Tricia is a 24-year-old single woman, engaged to be married, whose contraceptive failed. She is 6 weeks pregnant and is seeking termination of the pregnancy. She has many questions for the nurse in the family planning clinic: What procedure is most likely to be chosen at this gestation? What are the risks associated with the procedure? Should her fiancé be involved in the decision to terminate the pregnancy?

1. Evidence—Is there sufficient evidence to draw conclusions about what information the nurse should provide Tricia?
2. Assumptions—What assumptions can be made about Tricia's reaction to termination of the pregnancy?
   a. Psychologic/emotional reaction and sequelae
   b. Physical response
   c. Future childbearing
   d. Relationship with her fiancé
3. What implications and priorities for nursing care can be drawn at this time?
4. Does the evidence objectively support your conclusion?
5. Are there alternative perspectives to your conclusion?

Mifepristone

Mifepristone (RU 486) can be used up to 9 weeks after conception. The effectiveness of mifepristone is inversely related to gestational age as determined by β-human chorionic gonadotropin levels and the duration of amenorrhea (Hatcher et al, 2004). However, it is considered to be an effective and safe method for termination of early pregnancy.

Uterine bleeding begins within 4 days of administration of the first dose. Usually a period of painless heavy bleeding is reported. Termination of pregnancy occurs for most women. When mifepristone is combined with administration of a prostaglandin agent (misoprostol) 36 to 48 hours later, the rate of abortion increases.

Supporters of this method believe that even with known disadvantages, mifepristone offers a reasonable alternative to surgical abortion, which carries the risk of anesthesia, surgical complications, and infertility (Hatcher et al, 2004). Others have taken a strong stand against the use of mifepristone. Mifepristone was approved by the FDA for use in the United States in October 2000 but is not available for use. It is popular in France and other European countries and in China (Hatcher et al, 2004).

Second Trimester Abortion

Second trimester abortion is associated with an increase in complications and costs. Dilation and evacuation, induction of uterine contractions, and major operations are the methods used.

Dilation and Evacuation

Dilation and evacuation (D&E) can be performed at up to 20 weeks of gestation but is more appropriate between 13 and 16 weeks. The cervix requires more dilation because the products of conception are larger. Often laminaria are inserted several hours or several days before the procedure. Nursing care includes monitoring vital signs, providing emotional support, administering analgesics, and postoper-

Evidence-Based Practice

COMPARING MEDICAL AND SURGICAL ABORTIONS

Background

Abortion has been with us for millennia. Historically, it has included both medical and instrumental methods, sometimes inflicting grave injury and death. Approximately 53 million abortions are performed each year. An estimated one third of these are performed in unsafe circumstances, mostly in developing countries, and account for one out of eight maternal deaths worldwide. Surgical abortion in safe settings has the lowest complication rates at 7 to 8 weeks from last menses. Complications are 2.3 times higher for dilation and curettage (D&C), where the contents of the uterus are gently scraped out, as compared with vacuum aspiration, which uses a suction pump connected to a tube with a curette on the end. Complications of surgical abortion include infection, incomplete evacuation, cervical trauma, uterine perforation, hemorrhage, complications with anesthesia, and possible associations with infertility, miscarriages, and low birth weight in subsequent pregnancies. Medical abortions use pharmaceuticals to terminate pregnancy growth or stimulate expulsion of uterine contents. Four protocols are commonly used: misoprostol (prostaglandin E_1), mifepristone, mifepristone with misoprostol, and methotrexate with misoprostol. Mifepristone is still widely unavailable in some countries, including the United States. Methotrexate is used in chemotherapy to treat cancer by stopping rapid cell replication. It was used successfully to stop cell replication in ectopic pregnancies, and now is used successfully to terminate intrauterine pregnancies. Misoprostol causes uterine contractions. Both methotrexate and misoprostol are teratogenic, should the pregnancy fail to abort. Side effects of medical abortion are moderate to heavy bleeding, pain, nausea, vomiting, diarrhea, and more observed blood loss and passage of tissue. Women have reported that they chose medical abortion to avoid anesthesia and because it was more simple and natural. Women report that they chose surgical abortion to avoid awareness, because of worries about pain and bleeding, and to "get it over with."

Objectives

The reviewers desired to compare medical versus surgical methods of abortion. Intervention included any type of first trimester abortion, up to 98 days (14 weeks) from last menses.

Outcomes were efficacy, side effects, and acceptability of the procedure. Specific primary outcomes may include incomplete abortion, pelvic infection, blood transfusion, blood loss or hemoglobin drop, uterine perforation, cervical injury, and readmission. Secondary outcomes may include hospital stay exceeding 24 hours, duration of bleeding, use of uterotonic or antibiotic drugs not routinely given, pain or analgesia use, vomiting, diarrhea, and dissatisfaction.

Methods

Search Strategy

The authors searched Cochrane, MEDLINE, and Popline, and contacted experts at the World Health Organization (WHO). Search keywords included *abortion, pregnancy termination, first trimester, vacuum aspiration, suction, dilatation and curettage, D&C, mifepristone, misoprostol, prostaglandin, methotrexate,* and *RU 486.*

Five randomized trials comparing medical versus surgical abortion were chosen. The trials represented a total of 989 women from Sweden, Denmark, the United Kingdom, the United States, and a WHO multicenter trial from India, Vietnam, Slovenia, Zambia, China, Sweden, and Hungary. The trials were published from 1984 to 2000.

Statistical Analyses

Outcomes of each medical abortion protocol were compared with outcomes of vacuum aspiration, the surgical treatment of choice for first trimester abortion. Differences were analyzed as to whether they were significant or could have been caused by chance alone.

Findings

- *Misoprostol alone, versus vacuum aspiration:* The misoprostol group resulted in significantly more incomplete abortions and increased bleeding and pain, compared with vacuum aspiration. No significant differences were found between groups in infection rates.
- *Mifepristone alone, versus vacuum aspiration:* No significant differences were found between groups in infection rates, incomplete abortions, or perforations.
- *Mifepristone plus misoprostol, versus vacuum aspiration:* No difference in blood loss, but the medical group had significantly longer duration of bleeding.
- *Methotrexate plus misoprostol, versus vacuum aspiration:* Duration of bleeding and use of analgesia for pain were both significantly greater in the medical abortion group. No differences between groups were found in incomplete abortion rates.

Overall efficacy rate for medical abortions was 76% to 97%, and for surgical abortions, it was 94% to 100%. Mifepristone alone had the lowest efficacy, at 76%. One perforation occurred in the surgical groups. Medical intervention groups experienced more days of bleeding than surgical patients, which may reflect the surgical capture of more blood during the suction procedure, leaving less lining in the uterus to bleed later. The medical group also experienced more pain, which may also reflect the use of analgesia during the surgical procedure. The longer the gestation, the less acceptable the medical procedure was to the women. In one study, 63% of the medical group would choose that method again, whereas 92% of the surgical group would opt to repeat the surgical procedure, should the need arise. Overall, vacuum aspiration may be more effective than misoprostol alone, and seems to be associated with less pain and bleeding.

Limitations

Small number of trials and small sample sizes limit the generalizability of the results to the larger population. One trial allowed some participants to choose their methods and combined the data of both the randomized and nonrandomized subjects, thus decreasing generalizability. Many were lost to follow-up.

Conclusions

Both medical and surgical abortion are effective and safe; vacuum extraction was more effective than medical abortion and was associated with less pain and bleeding.

Implications for Practice

The decision between medical versus surgical abortions carries trade-offs. Careful counseling is necessary to prepare the woman for realistic expectations of each protocol, with careful attention to the attitude toward pregnancy and abortion. The decision to have an abortion and what type of abortion to undergo may be within the context of high emotions, and it needs to be made with guidance and sensitivity. The setting may dictate one procedure over another, depending on whether a safe surgical procedure is available, or the proximity of a woman to a health facility for the duration of the medical abortion. All women who are ending a pregnancy deserve contraceptive counseling. Abortion provides a golden "teachable moment" for contraceptive education.

Implications for Further Research

Much more information is needed regarding women's attitudes regarding unintended and unwanted pregnancies, abortions, and contraception. Larger studies about women's preferences for methods of abortions, and the efficacy of the methods, are needed. More information about the pain experienced in abortion would be illuminating, much as the pain in childbirth has been investigated, such as preparation techniques, precounseling, alternative therapies, and support person present.

Reference

Say L et al: Medical versus surgical methods for first trimester termination of pregnancy (Cochrane Review), 2002. In *The Cochrane Library,* Issue 2, Chichester, UK, 2004, John Wiley & Sons.

ative monitoring. Disadvantages of D&E may be long-term harmful effects on the cervix.

Prostaglandins

The most common technique for medical termination in the second trimester is the administration of prostaglandins. Prostaglandins can be administered in suppository form, as a gel, or by intrauterine injection. Unpleasant side effects (e.g., nausea, vomiting, diarrhea) usually occur. Repeated doses may be needed for expulsion of the products of conception.

Hypertonic and Uterotonic Agents

Hypertonic solutions (saline, urea) injected directly into the uterus and uterotonic agents (misoprostol and dinoprostone) account for fewer than 1% of all abortions because other methods are safer and easier to use.

Nursing Considerations

The woman considering an abortion will need help to explore the meaning of the various alternatives and consequences to herself and her significant others. It is often difficult for a woman to express her true feelings (e.g., what abortion means to her now and in the future and what support or regret her friends and peers may demonstrate). A calm, matter-of-fact approach on the part of the nurse can be helpful. Clarifying, restating, and reflecting statements; open-ended questions; and feedback are communication techniques that can be used to maintain a realistic focus on the situation and bring the woman's problems into the open. Once a decision has been made to have an abortion, the woman must be assured of continued support. Information must be given about what various procedures entail, how much discomfort or pain can be expected, and what type of care is needed. If family or friends cannot be involved, scheduling time for nursing personnel to give the necessary support is an essential component of the care plan.

After the abortion, nurses must assess women for grief reactions and facilitate the grieving process through active listening and nonjudgmental support and care.

Key Points

- Infertility is the inability to conceive and to carry a fetus to term gestation at a time the couple has chosen to do so.
- Infertility affects about 10% of otherwise healthy adults. Infertility increases in women older than 35 years.
- In the United States, about one third of infertility is related to female causes; one third is related to male causes; and 20% of the causes are unexplained.
- Common etiologic factors of infertility include decreased sperm production, ovulation disorders, tubal occlusion, and endometriosis.
- Reproductive alternatives for family building include IVF-ET, GIFT, ZIFT, oocyte donation, embryo donation, TDI, surrogate motherhood, and adoption.
- A variety of contraceptive methods with various effectiveness rates, advantages, and disadvantages are available.
- Women and their partners should choose the contraceptive method(s) best suited to them.
- Effective contraceptives are available through both prescription and nonprescription sources.
- Proper concurrent use of spermicides and latex condoms provides protection against STIs.
- Tubal ligations and vasectomies are permanent sterilization methods used by increasing numbers of women and men.
- Induced abortion performed in the first trimester is safer and less complex than an abortion performed in the second trimester.
- The most common complications of induced abortion include infection, retained products of conception, and excessive vaginal bleeding.

Answer Guidelines to Critical Thinking Exercises

Infertility Workup

1. Yes. There are general statistics available, as well as the success rates of treatment at this particular clinic. However, a guarantee of success is not possible.
2. (a) There are a number of psychosocial issues and pressures that such a couple face. (b) Jane may be more interested than Andrew in undergoing fertility treatment. (c) An infertility workup and in vitro or other assisted reproductive technologies may not be covered by the couple's insurance. (d) There are many myths about how to achieve pregnancy.
3. The priorities for nursing care are to take a thorough medical and sexual history, offer support, and provide information about infertility treatment.
4. Yes, the evidence objectively supports this conclusion.
5. After hearing the choices available and the cost of treatment, Jane and Andrew may decide to remain childless or to adopt. Health care providers must give reasonable and realistic information to assist in a couple's decision making.

Contraception for Adolescents

1. There is sufficient theoretic knowledge for a basis for advice. However, Alicia will have to be interviewed to determine her preferences and issues of concern based on her age and culture.
2. (a) There are many issues facing sexually active adolescents. (b) The legality of prescribing contraception may vary from state to state; nurses must be knowledgeable about the law in their state of practice. (c) Culture may affect use of contraception. (d) There are advantages and disadvantages to a 15-year-old female of various types of contraceptives.
3. Priorities for nursing care are to determine Alicia's knowledge of sexuality, provide information as needed, ascertain Alicia's preferences regarding type of contraception, provide education about sexually transmitted infections and how to prevent them, and encourage communication with her mother.
4. Yes, there is evidence to support this conclusion.
5. Abstinence can be encouraged. Monogamy can be encouraged.

Termination of Pregnancy

1. Yes. At this stage of pregnancy, vacuum suction is the procedure of choice. There are risks of uterine perforation, infection, excessive bleeding, and cervical damage. However, abortion at this gestation is safer than carrying a fetus to term. Legally, the fiancé is not required to be involved. However, for the sake of their relationship, he should be involved in the decision.
2. (a) Tricia is likely to experience some fear and anxiety during the procedure. With good support from the nurse and Tricia's family, she will be able to cope with these. There are few or no psychologic sequelae to an early abortion. (b) The procedure takes about 5 minutes. Tricia will have to remain in the clinic/office for 2 to 3 hours to be sure there is no excessive bleeding or other complication. She will experience some bleeding and minimal cramping. Menses will resume in 4 to 6 weeks. (c) The abortion is not likely to affect future childbearing. She needs counseling about contraception. Since she had a contraceptive failure, she may need to change methods. If she retains the same method, the nurse should ensure that she knows the proper way to use the method. (d) Tricia and her fiancé need to maintain good communication. Ideally, the decision to have an abortion would be agreed on by both parties. A difference of opinion could introduce friction between the couple at a very stressful time.
3. Priorities for care are to ensure that Tricia knows the options available and then to support her in her decision. Patient teaching regarding the procedure and contraception are necessary.
4. Yes. There are excellent data about the safety of the procedure and sequelae and a woman's response to the procedure.
5. Abortion is a very emotion-laden topic. A nurse may believe that terminating a pregnancy in a healthy young woman because the pregnancy is inconvenient is not a good enough reason for the procedure. A nurse may feel differently if a woman is pregnant as a result of rape or incest or if the fetus has congenital anomalies incompatible with life. Nurses need to examine their own values and beliefs regarding abortion.

Resources

American College of Obstetricians and Gynecologists
409 12th St. SW
Washington, DC 20024
800-762-2264
www.acog.com

American Fertility Foundation
2131 Magnolia Ave., Suite 201
Birmingham, AL 35256
205-251-9764

American Society for Reproductive Medicine
1209 Montgomery Hwy.
Birmingham, AL 35316
205-978-5000
www.asrm.org

Association of Reproductive Health Professionals
2401 Pennsylvania Ave. NW, Suite 350
Washington, DC 20037
202-466-3825
www.arhp.org

Center for the Evaluation of Risks to Human Reproduction (CERHR)
National Toxicology Program
U.S. Department of Health and Human Services
cerhr.niehs.nih.gov

Emergency Contraception Hotline
PO Box 33344
Washington, DC 20033
888-668-2528
www.not-2-late.com

Infertility Resources
www.ihr.com/infertility/index.html

International Council on Infertility Information Dissemination
PO Box 6836
Arlington, VA 22206
703-379-9178
www.inciid.org

Internet Health Resources
www.ihr.com

National Abortion Federation Consumer Hotline
1156 15th St. NW, Suite 700
Washington, DC 20005
800-772-9100

National Adoption Information Clearing House
330 C St. SW
Washington, DC 20447
888-251-0075
www.calib.com/naic

National Clearinghouse for Family Planning Information
PO Box 10716
Rockville, MD 20850
703-558-4990

National Women's Health Resource Center
120 Albany St., Suite 820
New Brunswick, NJ 08901
877-986-9472
www.healthywomen.org

Planned Parenthood Federation of America, Inc.
810 Seventh Ave.
New York, NY 10019
800-669-0156
www.plannedparenthood.org

Resolve, Inc.
1310 Broadway, Dept
Somerville, MA 02144
617-623-1156
888-623-0744
info@resolve.org
www.resolve.org

References

American Society for Reproductive Medicine: *Frequently asked questions about infertility,* 2002. Internet document available at www.asrm.org (accessed July 15, 2004).

Angard NT: Diagnosis infertility, *AWHONN Lifelines* 3(3):22-29, 1999.

Centers for Disease Control and Prevention: 1999 assisted reproduction technology success rates. Results generated from SART/ASRM, CDC, and Resolve. Internet document available www.cdc.bov/nccdphp/drh (accessed October 1, 2002).

Centers for Disease Control and Prevention: Sexually transmitted disease treatment guidelines, *MMWR* 51(RR6):1-80, 2002.

Cunningham FG et al: *Williams obstetrics,* ed 21, New York, 2001, McGraw-Hill.

D'Avanzo CE, Geissler EM: *Pocket guide to cultural health assessment,* ed 3, St Louis, 2003, Mosby.

Hatcher R et al: *A pocket guide to managing contraception 2004-2005 edition,* Tiger, GA, 2004, Bridging the Gap Foundation.

Hiller J, Griffith E: Education for contraceptive use by women after childbirth (Cochrane Review), *The Cochrane Library,* Issue 3, Oxford, 2000, Update Software.

Jones HW, Cohen J: IFFS Surveillance 04. *Fertil Steril* 81(5) (Suppl 4): S1-S54, 2004.

Jones SL: Reproductive genetic technologies: exploring ethical and policy implication, *AWHONN Lifelines* 4(5):33-36, 2000.

Kennedy HP, Griffin M, Frishman G: Enabling conception and pregnancy: midwifery care of women experiencing infertility, *J Nurse Midwifery* 43(3):190-207, 1998.

Keye W: Medical aspects of infertility for the counselor. In Burns H, Covington S (eds): *Infertility counseling: a comprehensive handbook for clinicians,* New York, 2000, Parthenon Publishing Group.

King RB: Subfecundity and anxiety in a nationally representative sample, *Soc Sci Med* 56(4):739-751, 2003.

Leibowitz D, Hoffman J: Fertility drug therapies: past present, and future, *J Obstet Gynecol Neonatal Nurs* 29(2):201-210, 2000.

Say L et al: Medical versus surgical methods for first trimester termination of pregnancy (Cochrane Review), 2002. In *The Cochrane Library,* Issue 2, Chichester, UK, 2004, John Wiley & Sons.

Sherrod RA: Understanding the emotional aspects of infertility: implications for nursing practice, *J Psychosoc Nurs Ment Health Serv* 42(3):40-49, 2004.

Stenchever MA et al: *Comprehensive gynecology,* ed 4, St Louis, 2001, Mosby.

Tiran D, Mack S: *Complementary therapies for pregnancy and childbirth,* Edinburgh, 2000, Bailliere Tindall.

Trussell J: The essentials of contraception: efficacy, safety, and personal considerations. In Hatcher R et al (eds): *Contraceptive technology,* ed 18, New York, 2004, Ardent Media.

US Department of Health and Human Services, Health Resources and Service Administration, Maternal and Child Health Bureau: *Women's health USA 2002,* Rockville, MD, 2002, US Department of Health and Human Services.

Van Voorhis BJ et al: Cost-effective treatment of the infertile couple, *Fertil Steril* 70(6):995-1005, 1998.

Wallach M, Grimes D: *Modern oral contraception: updates from The Contraceptive Report,* Totowa, NJ, 2000, Emron.

Weed S: *Wise woman herbal for the childbearing year,* Woodstock, NY, 1986, Ash Tree Publishing.

World Health Organization: *Improving access to quality care in family planning: medical eligibility criteria for contraceptive use,* ed 2, Geneva, 2000, World Health Organization.

Genetics, Conception, and Fetal Development

8

LEARNING OBJECTIVES

On completion of this chapter the reader will be able to:

- Explain the key concepts of basic human genetics.
- Discuss the purpose, key findings, and potential outcomes of the Human Genome Project.
- Describe expanded roles for nurses in genetics and genetic counseling.
- Examine ethical dimensions of genetic screening.
- Discuss the current status of gene therapy (gene transfer).
- Summarize the process of fertilization.
- Describe the development, structure, and functions of the placenta.
- Describe the composition and functions of the amniotic fluid.
- Identify three organs or tissues arising from each of the three primary germ layers.
- Summarize the significant changes in growth and development of the embryo and fetus.
- Identify the potential effects of teratogens during vulnerable periods of embryonic and fetal development.

ELECTRONIC RESOURCES

Additional information related to the content in Chapter 8 can be found on

the companion website at evolve
http://evolve.elsevier.com/Wong/maternal/
- NCLEX Review Questions
- WebLinks

or the interactive student CD-ROM
Activities for Chapter 8 include the following:
- NCLEX Review Questions
- Critical Thinking Exercise–Genetic Counseling
- Nursing Care Plan–Down Syndrome

This chapter presents a brief discussion of genetics and the role of the nurse in genetics. It also provides an overview of the process of fertilization and of the development of the normal embryo and fetus.

GENETICS

Genetics is currently recognized as a contributing factor in virtually all human illnesses (Hamilton & Wynshaw-Boris, 2004). In maternity care, genetics issues occur before, during, and after pregnancy (Hamilton & Wynshaw-Boris, 2004). With growing public interest in genetics, increasing commercial pressures, and Web-based opportunities for individuals, families, and communities to participate in the direction and design of their genetic health care, genetic services are rapidly becoming an integral part of routine health care (Collins & Guttmacher, 2001; Collins & McKusick, 2001).

For most genetic conditions, therapeutic or preventive measures do not exist or are very limited. Consequently, the most useful means of reducing the incidence of these disorders is by preventing their transmission. It is standard practice to assess all pregnant women for heritable disorders to identify potential problems. The incidence of chromosomal aberrations is estimated to be 0.5% to 0.6% in newborns. Approximately 62% of miscarriages and 5% to 7% of stillbirths and perinatal deaths are caused by chromosomal abnormalities (Hamilton & Wynshaw-Boris, 2004; Lashley, 1998).

Genetic disease affects people of all ages, from all socioeconomic levels, and from all racial and ethnic backgrounds. Genetic disease affects not only individuals, but also families, communities, and society. Advances in genetic testing and genetically based treatments have altered the care provided to affected individuals. Improvements in diagnostic capability have resulted in earlier diagnosis and enabled individuals who previously would have died in childhood to survive into adulthood (Lashley, 1998). The genetic aberrations that lead to disease are present at birth but may not be manifested for many years, or possibly never manifested.

Some disorders appear more often in ethnic groups. Examples include Tay-Sachs disease in Ashkenazi Jews, French Canadians of the Eastern St. Laurence River valley area of Quebec, Cajuns from Louisiana, and the Amish in Pennsylvania; β-thalassemia in Mediterranean, Middle Eastern, Transcaucasus, Central Asian, Indian, and Far Eastern groups, as well as those of African heritage; sickle cell anemia in African-Americans; α-thalassemia in those from Southeast Asia, South China, the Philippine Islands, Thailand, Greece, and Cyprus; lactase deficiency in adult Chinese and Thailanders; neural tube defects in Irish, Scots, and Welsh; phenylketonuria in Irish, Scots, Scandinavians, Icelanders, and Polish; cystic fibrosis in Caucasians, Ashkenazi Jews, and Hispanics; and Niemann-Pick disease, type A, in Ashkenazi Jews (Hamilton & Wynshaw-Boris, 2004; Jenkins & Wapner, 2004).

Relevance of Genetics to Nursing

Genetic disorders span every clinical practice specialty and site, including school, clinic, office, hospital, mental health agency, and community health settings. Because the potential impact on families and the community is significant (Box 8-1), genetics must be integrated into nursing education and practice. A genetic paradigm must be embraced; that is, genetic information, technology, and testing must be incorporated in health care services (Anderson et al., 2000).

Although many of the roles for nurses in genetics are being expanded or developed, all nurses should be prepared to collaborate in interdisciplinary clinical partnerships and provide five main genetics-related nursing activities (International Society of Nurses in Genetics [ISONG], 1998; Lea, Feetham, & Monsen, 2002; Lea, Jenkins, & Francomano, 1998). The five main activities are as follows:

- Collecting, reporting, and recording genetics information
- Offering genetics information and resources to patients and families
- Participating in the informed consent process and facilitating informed decision making
- Participating in management of patients and families affected by genetic conditions
- Evaluating and monitoring the impact of genetics information, testing, and treatment on patients and their families

These activities are not limited to particular practice settings, nor are they limited to specific specialty areas.

Genetics-related activities that all nurses should be able to provide are further delineated in the *Statement on the Scope and Standards of Genetics Clinical Nursing Practice* (ISONG, 1998). This document includes standards and levels of practice for genetics nursing that were established cooperatively by ISONG and the American Nurses Association (ANA).

Although diagnosis and treatment of genetic disorders requires medical skills, nurses with advanced preparation are assuming important roles in counseling people about genetically transmitted or genetically influenced conditions. Nurses are usually the ones who provide follow-up care and maintain contact with the patients. Community health nurses can identify groups within populations that are high risk for illness, as well as provide care to individuals, families, and groups. They are a vital link in follow-up for newborns who may need newborn screening.

Referral to appropriate agencies is an essential part of the follow-up management. Many organizations and foundations (e.g., the Cystic Fibrosis Foundation and the Muscular Dystrophy Association) help provide services and equipment for affected children. There are also numerous parent groups in which the family can share experiences and derive mutual support from other families with similar problems.

Probably the most important of all nursing functions is providing emotional support to the family during all aspects of the counseling process. Feelings that are generated under the real or imagined threat posed by a genetic disorder are as varied as the people being counseled (McGowan, 1999). Responses may include a variety of stress reactions such as apathy, denial, anger, hostility, fear, embarrassment, grief, and loss of self-esteem.

BOX 8-1

Potential Impact of Genetic Disease on Family and Community

- Financial cost to family
- Decrease in planned family size
- Loss of geographic mobility
- Decreased opportunities for siblings
- Loss of family integrity
- Loss of career opportunities and job flexibility
- Social isolation
- Lifestyle alterations
- Reduction in contributions to their community by families
- Disruption of husband-wife or partner relationship
- Threatened family self-concept
- Coping with intolerant public attitudes
- Psychologic effects
- Stresses and uncertainty of treatment
- Physical health problems
- Loss of dreams and aspirations
- Cost to society of institutionalization or home or community care
- Cost to society because of additional problems and needs of other family members
- Cost of long-term care
- Housing and living arrangement changes

From Lashley F: *Clinical genetics in nursing practice,* ed 2, New York, 1998, Springer.

CRITICAL THINKING EXERCISE—GENETIC COUNSELING

Genetic History-Taking and Genetic Counseling Services

It is standard practice in obstetrics to determine whether a heritable disorder exists in a couple or in anyone in either of their families. The goal of screening is to detect or define risk for disease in low risk populations and identify those for whom diagnostic testing may be appropriate. A nurse can obtain a genetics history using a questionnaire or checklist such as the one in Fig. 8-1.

Genetic counseling that follows may occur in the office, or referral to a geneticist may be necessary. The most efficient counseling services are associated with the larger universities and major medical centers. This is also where support services are available (e.g., biochemistry and cytology laboratories), usually from a group of specialists under the leadership of a physician trained in medical genetics. Health professionals should become familiar with people who provide genetic counseling and the places that offer counseling

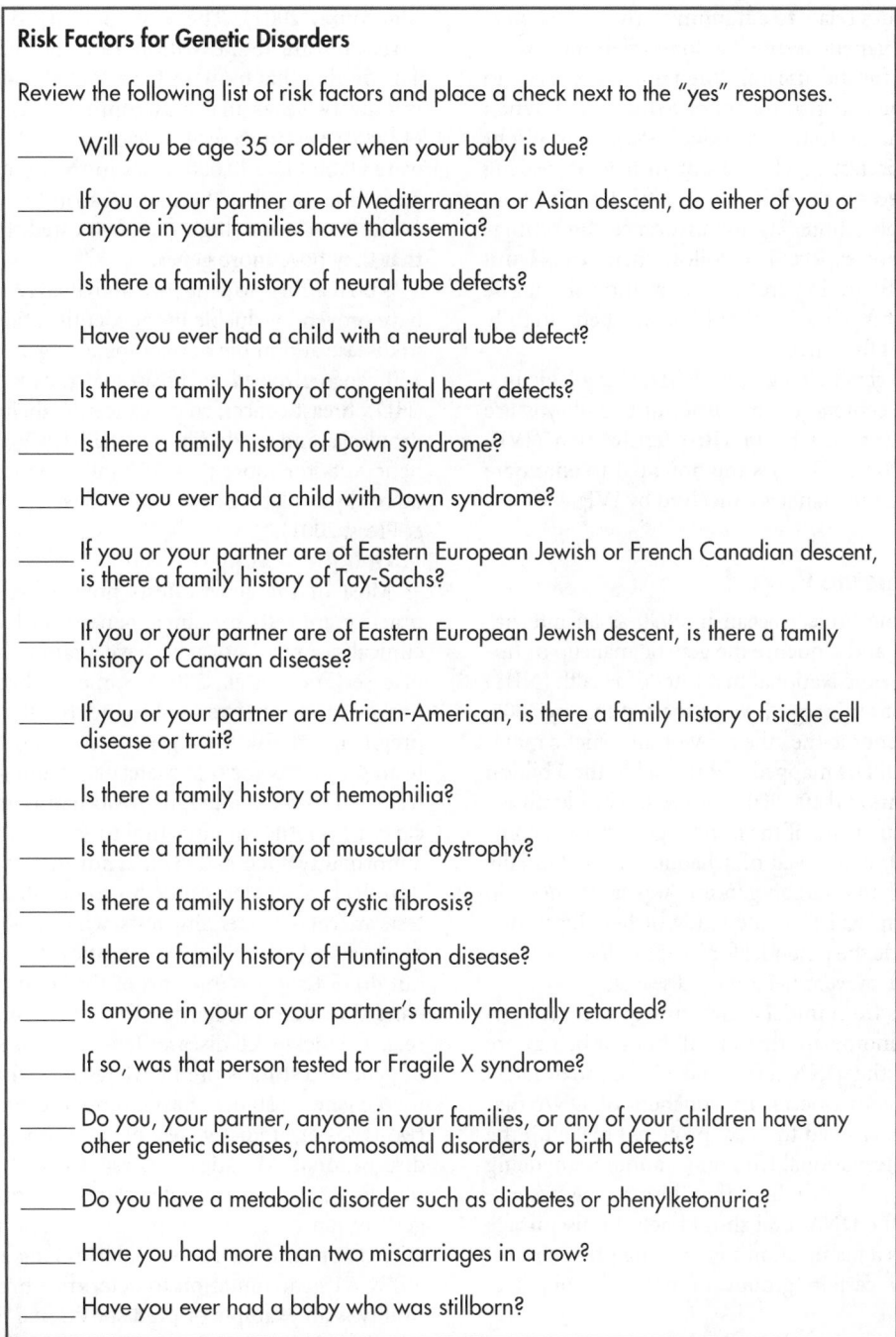

Risk Factors for Genetic Disorders

Review the following list of risk factors and place a check next to the "yes" responses.

_____ Will you be age 35 or older when your baby is due?

_____ If you or your partner are of Mediterranean or Asian descent, do either of you or anyone in your families have thalassemia?

_____ Is there a family history of neural tube defects?

_____ Have you ever had a child with a neural tube defect?

_____ Is there a family history of congenital heart defects?

_____ Is there a family history of Down syndrome?

_____ Have you ever had a child with Down syndrome?

_____ If you or your partner are of Eastern European Jewish or French Canadian descent, is there a family history of Tay-Sachs?

_____ If you or your partner are of Eastern European Jewish descent, is there a family history of Canavan disease?

_____ If you or your partner are African-American, is there a family history of sickle cell disease or trait?

_____ Is there a family history of hemophilia?

_____ Is there a family history of muscular dystrophy?

_____ Is there a family history of cystic fibrosis?

_____ Is there a family history of Huntington disease?

_____ Is anyone in your or your partner's family mentally retarded?

_____ If so, was that person tested for Fragile X syndrome?

_____ Do you, your partner, anyone in your families, or any of your children have any other genetic diseases, chromosomal disorders, or birth defects?

_____ Do you have a metabolic disorder such as diabetes or phenylketonuria?

_____ Have you had more than two miscarriages in a row?

_____ Have you ever had a baby who was stillborn?

Fig. 8-1 Questionnaire for identifying couples having increased risk for offspring with genetic disorders. (Courtesy American College of Obstetricians and Gynecologists: *Planning your pregnancy and birth,* ed 4, Washington, DC, 2005, ACOG.)

services in their area of practice. See Resources at the end of this chapter for information on genetics resources.

Ethical Considerations

Researchers have proposed using fetal neurologic, liver, and pancreatic tissues to treat adults with Parkinson disease, metabolic disorders, or head and spinal cord injury. The use of fetal tissue in research was banned in the United States for several years, but the ban was lifted in 1993.

Most genetic testing is offered prenatally in order to identify genetic disorders in fetuses (Jenkins & Wapner, 2004). When an affected fetus is identified, termination of the pregnancy is an option. Other requests for genetic testing occur for sex selection or for late-onset disorders. An ethic of social responsibility should guide genetic counselors in their interactions with patients (White, 1999) while recognizing that people make their choices by integrating personal values and beliefs with their new knowledge of genetic risk and medical treatments (Anderson, 1998).

Other ethical issues relate to autonomy, privacy, and confidentiality. Should genetic testing be done when there is no treatment available for the disease? When is it appropriate to warn family members at risk for inherited diseases? When should presymptomatic testing be done? Some who might benefit from genetic testing choose not to have it, fearing discrimination based on the risk of a genetic disorder. Several states have prohibitions against insurance discrimination; other states are expected to follow their lead. Until guidelines for genetic testing are created, caution should be exercised. The benefits of testing should be weighed carefully against the potential for harm.

Preimplantation genetic diagnosis (PGD) is available in a limited number of centers. In this procedure, embryos are tested before implantation by in vitro fertilization (IVF) (Jones & Fallon, 2002). PGD has the potential to eliminate specific disorders in pregnancies conceived by IVF.

The Human Genome Project

The Human Genome Project began in 1990 as an international effort to map and sequence the genetic makeup of humans; it is funded by the National Institutes of Health (NIH) and the Department of Energy. It was expected that by 2005, the entire human genome (i.e., the copy of the genetic material in humans) would be mapped and that all of the 5 billion nucleic acid base pairs and 100,000 genes would be identified. However, initial sequencing of the human genome was completed in June 2000, well ahead of schedule. A substantially complete version of the human genome was announced in April 2002. The map will facilitate study of hereditary diseases and will provide the potential for making changes at the gene level to treat or prevent hereditary diseases.

Two key findings from initial efforts to sequence and analyze the human genome are that (1) all human beings are 99.9% identical at the DNA level, and (2) approximately 30,000 to 40,000 genes (pieces or sequences of DNA that contain information needed to make proteins) make up the human genome (International Human Genome Sequencing Consortium, 2001). The finding that human beings are 99.9% identical at the DNA level should help to discourage the use of science as a justification for drawing precise racial boundaries around certain groups of people (Collins & Mansoura, 2001). The vast majority of the 0.1% genetic variations are found within and not between populations. The finding that humans have 30,000 to 40,000 genes, which is only twice as many as roundworms (18,000) and flies (13,000), was unexpected. Scientists had estimated that there were 80,000 to 150,000 genes in the human genome. It had been assumed that the main reason that humans are more evolved and more highly sophisticated than other species is that they have more genes.

> **Community Focus**
>
> **USE OF GENETIC MATERIALS AND INFORMATION**
>
> Rapid technologic advances have created complex questions for which there are no easy answers. Mapping of the human genome and other advances occurred before adequate debate on legal, ethical, social, and clinical issues by professionals and the public had taken place. Currently there are inadequate laws to protect the interests of stakeholders: donors, researchers, and insurers. There is no agreement on what encompasses "proper use" of such information. Continued discussion and debate must occur among ethicists, health professionals, representatives of the legal profession, and the public.
>
> Data from Giarelli E, Jacobs L: Issues related to the use of genetic material and information, *Oncol Nurs Forum* 27(3):459-467, 2000.

Initial efforts to sequence and analyze the human genome have proven invaluable in the identification of genes involved in disease and in the development of genetic tests. More than 100 genes involved in diseases such as Huntington's Disease (HD), breast cancer, colon cancer, Alzheimer disease, achondroplasia, and cystic fibrosis (CF) have been identified. Genetic tests for more than 700 inherited conditions are commercially available or in research development (Burke, Pinsky, & Press, 2001).

Genetic Testing

Most of the genetic tests now being offered in clinical practice are tests for single-gene disorders in patients with clinical symptoms or who have a family history of a genetic disease (Yoon et al., 2001). Some of these genetic tests are prenatal tests or tests used to identify the genetic status of a pregnancy at risk for a genetic condition. Current prenatal testing options include maternal serum screening (a blood test used to see if a pregnant woman is at increased risk for carrying a fetus with a neural tube defect or a chromosomal abnormality such as Down syndrome) and invasive procedures (amniocentesis and chorionic villus sampling). Other tests are carrier screening tests, which are used to identify individuals who have a gene mutation for a genetic condition but do not show symptoms of the condition, because it is a condition that is inherited in an autosomal recessive form (e.g., CF, sickle cell disease, Tay-Sachs disease). Another type of genetic testing is predictive testing, which is used to clarify the genetic status of asymptomatic family members. The two types of predictive testing are presymptomatic and predispositional. Mutation analysis for HD, a neurodegenerative disorder, is an example of presymptomatic testing. If the gene mutation for HD is present, symptoms of HD are certain to appear if the individual lives long enough. Testing for a BRCA1 gene mutation to determine breast cancer susceptibility is an example of predispositional testing. Predispositional testing differs from presymptomatic testing in that a positive result (indicating that a BRCA1 mutation is present) does not indicate a 100% risk of developing the condition (breast cancer).

Pharmacogenomics

One of the most immediate clinical applications of the Human Genome Project may be pharmacogenomics, or the use of genetic information to individualize drug therapy (Phillips et al, 2001). There has been speculation that pharmacogenomics may become part of standard practice for a large number of disorders and drugs by 2020 (Collins & McKusick, 2001). The expectation is that by identifying common variants in genes that are associated with the likelihood of a good or bad response to a specific drug, drug prescriptions can be individualized, based on the individual's unique genetic makeup (Roses, 2000). A primary benefit of pharmacogenomics is the potential to reduce adverse drug reactions.

Gene Therapy (Gene Transfer)

In the early 1990s, a great deal of optimism was felt about the possibility of using genetic information to provide quick solutions to a long list of health problems (Collins & McKusick, 2001). However, the field of gene therapy, also known as gene transfer, has sustained a number of major disappointments during the past few years. Although the early optimism about gene therapy was probably never fully justified, it is likely that the development of safer and more effective methods for gene delivery will ensure a significant role for gene therapy in the treatment of some diseases (Collins & McKusick, 2001). Major challenges include targeting the right gene to the right location in the right cells, expressing the transferred gene at the right time, and minimizing adverse reactions (Brower, 2001). Some reports detail exciting possibilities regarding the application of gene therapy for hemophilia B (Kay et al, 2000) and severe combined immunodeficiency (Anderson, 2000; Cavazzana-Calvo et al, 2000). According to a scientist who is very active in the field of gene therapy, "Gene therapy will succeed with time. And it is important that it does, because no other area of medicine holds as much promise for providing cures for the many devastating diseases that ravage humankind" (Anderson, 2000).

Ethical, Legal, and Social Implications

An integral part of the Human Genome Project is the Ethical, Legal, and Social Implications (ELSI) program; 5% of the Human Genome Project budget was designated for the study of the ELSI of human genome research. This program addresses the potential that genetic information may be used to discriminate against individuals or for eugenic purposes. Continued awareness of and vigilance against such misuse of information is the collective responsibility of health care providers, ethicists, and society.

BOX 8-2

Stem Cells

Stem cells are able to divide for indefinite periods and can differentiate into the many different types of cells that make up an organism. Embryonic stem cells are derived from the blastocyst before it implants in the uterine wall. A zygote is described as *totipotent* because it has the potential to produce all the cells and tissues that compose an embryo and to support its in utero development. The term *pluripotent* is used to describe stem cells that generate cells derived from the three embryonic germ layers (endoderm, mesoderm, and ectoderm). The embryonic stem cell is pluripotent. Human stem cells were derived and maintained for the first time in 1998 by Thomson and colleagues by using blastocysts donated by couples undergoing in vitro fertilization. Potential uses of human embryonic stem cells include transplant therapy, in which tissues damaged by disease or injury are replaced or restored, as for example, in diabetes, Parkinson disease, heart disease, and multiple sclerosis. Stem cell research engenders ethical concerns related to the source of human embryonic stem cells (embryos left over from in vitro fertilization and aborted fetuses). Currently federal support for research is restricted to existing cell lines.

From National Institutes of Health: Stem cells: scientific progress and future research directions, 2001. Internet document available at www.nih.gov/news/stemcell/scireport.htm (accessed June 9, 2002).

Management of Genetic Disorders

At this time, no cures exist for genetic disorders, although remedies can be implemented to prevent or reduce the harmful effects of a few disorders. Structural defects can sometimes be modified to produce normal or near-normal function. Surgical therapy is employed for congenital heart defects and cosmetic defects such as cleft lip. Advances in fetal surgery are occurring. Other conditions are treated with product replacement (e.g., thyroid for hereditary cretinism), diet modification (e.g., low-phenylalanine diet for phenylketonuria), and corrective devices for missing limbs. Research is being conducted on methods to influence or change genes directly by placing substitute DNA in the cells of those with a genetic mutation, thereby preventing or curing the disease process or relieving symptoms.

The possibility exists that understanding embryonic stem cells (primitive cells that can develop into all types of body tissue, including muscles, nerves, and bones) will lead to new medical discoveries (Box 8-2). The successful cloning of sheep, cattle, mice, and pigs; the production of rhesus monkeys through nuclear transfer of embryonic cells; and the isolation of stem cells constitute breakthroughs in technology. They also raise other ethical questions. On August 25, 2000, the NIH published guidelines for research using human stem cells (National Institutes of Health, 2000). The nurse involved in genetics must keep abreast of new developments and be prepared to discuss ethical implications with patients and other health care providers.

Estimation of Risk

The risks of recurrence of a genetic disorder are determined by the mode of inheritance. The risk of recurrence for disorders caused by a factor that segregates during cell division (i.e., genes and chromosomes) can be estimated with a high degree of accuracy by application of mendelian principles. In a dominant disorder the risk is 50%, or one in two, that a subsequent offspring will be affected; an autosomal recessive disease carries a one-in-four risk of recurrence; and an X-linked disorder is related to the child's sex, as described in the section related to X-linked inheritance. Translocation chromosomes have a high risk of recurrence.

Disorders in which a subsequent pregnancy would carry no more risk than there is for pregnancy alone (estimated at 1 in 30) include those resulting from isolated incidences not likely

Community Focus

WEB RESOURCES ON GENETICS

Select two Web addresses for resources on genetics for parents from the Resource list provided in this chapter. Access the sites.

- Compare and contrast the appearance, the readability, and the information contained in the sites.
- To whom would you recommend these sites?
- Is the information contained culturally relevant?
- What information would parents need?
- How could you as a nurse use this information?

to be present in another pregnancy. These disorders include maternal infections (e.g., rubella and toxoplasmosis), maternal ingestion of drugs, most chromosomal abnormalities, and a disorder determined to be the result of a fresh mutation.

Interpretation of Risk

Counselors explain the risk estimates to patients without making recommendations or decisions and without allowing their own biases to interfere. The counselor provides appropriate information about the nature of the disorder, the extent of the risks in the specific case, the probable consequences, and (if appropriate) alternative options available; however, the final decision to become pregnant or to continue a pregnancy must be left to the family. An important nursing role is reinforcing the information the families are given and continuing to interpret this information on their level of understanding.

The most important concept that must be emphasized to families is that *each pregnancy is an independent event.* For example, in monogenic disorders, in which the risk factor is one in four that the child will be affected, the risk remains the same no matter how many affected children are already in the family. Families may make the erroneous assumption that the presence of one affected child ensures that the next three will be free of the disorder. However, "chance has no memory." The risk is one in four for each pregnancy. On the other hand, in a family with a child who has a disorder with multifactorial causes, the risk increases with each subsequent child born with the disorder.

GENES AND CHROMOSOMES

The hereditary material carried in the nucleus of each somatic (body) cell determines an individual's physical characteristics. This material, called deoxyribonucleic acid (DNA), forms threadlike strands known as chromosomes. Each chromosome is composed of many smaller segments of DNA referred to as genes. Genes or combinations of genes contain coded information that determines an individual's unique characteristics. The code consists of the specific linear order of the molecules that combine to form the strands of DNA. Genes never act in isolation; they always interact with other genes and the environment.

All normal human somatic cells contain 46 chromosomes arranged as 23 pairs of homologous (matched) chromosomes; one chromosome of each pair is inherited from each parent. There are 22 pairs of autosomes, which control most traits in the body, and one pair of sex chromosomes, which determines sex and some other traits. The large female chromosome is called the X; the tiny male chromosome is the Y. When one X chromosome and one Y chromosome are present, the embryo develops as a male. When two X chromosomes are present, the embryo develops as a female.

Because each gene occupies a specific chromosome location, and because chromosomes are inherited as homologous pairs, each person has two genes for every trait. In other words, if an autosome has a gene for hair color, its partner also has a gene for hair color—in the same location on the chromosome. Although both genes code for hair color, they may not code for the same hair color. Different genes coding for different variations of the same trait are called alleles. An individual with two copies of the same allele for a given trait is said to be homozygous for that trait. With two different alleles, the person is heterozygous for the trait.

The term *genotype* typically is used to refer to the genetic makeup of an individual when discussing a specific gene pair, but at times, genotype is used to refer to an individual's entire genetic makeup or all the genes that the individual can pass on to future generations. Phenotype refers to the observable expression of an individual's genotype, such as physical features, a biochemical or molecular trait, and even a psychologic trait. A trait or disorder is considered dominant if it is expressed or phenotypically apparent when only one copy of the gene is present. It is considered recessive if it is expressed only when two copies of the gene are present.

The pictorial analysis of the number, form, and size of an individual's chromosomes is known as a karyotype. Cells from any nucleated, replicating body tissue (not red blood cells, nerves, or muscles) can be used (Scheuerle, 2001). The most commonly used tissues are white blood cells and fetal cells in amniotic fluid. The cells are grown in a culture and arrested when they are in metaphase, and then the cells are dropped onto a slide. This breaks the cell membranes and spreads the chromosomes, making them easier to visualize. The cells are stained with special stains (e.g., Giemsa stain) that create striping or "banding" patterns. Once the chromosome spreads are photographed or scanned by a computer, they are cut out and arranged in a specific numeric order according to their length and shape. The chromosomes are numbered from largest to smallest, 1 to 22, and the sex chromosomes are designated by the letter X or Y. Each chromosome is divided into two "arms" designated by p (short arm) and q (long arm). A female karyotype is designated as 46, XX and a male karyotype is designated as 46, XY. Figure 8-2 illustrates the chromosomes in a body cell and a karyotype. Karyotypes can be used to determine the sex of a child and the presence of any gross chromosomal abnormalities.

Chromosomal Abnormalities

Chromosomal abnormalities account for approximately 4% to 7% of perinatal deaths and 0.5% to 1% of infants born with multiple anomalies (Gelehrter, Collins, & Ginsberg, 1998; Jones, 1997). Errors resulting in chromosomal abnormalities can occur in mitosis or meiosis. These occur in either the autosomes or the sex chromosomes. Even without the presence of obvious structural malformations, small deviations in chromosomes can cause problems in fetal development.

Autosomal Abnormalities

Autosomal abnormalities involve differences in the number or structure of chromosomes resulting from unequal distribution of the genetic material during gamete formation.

Abnormalities of Chromosome Number

Euploidy denotes the correct number of chromosomes. Deviations from the correct number of chromosomes can be one of two types: (1) polyploidy, in which the deviation is an exact multiple of the haploid number of chromosomes or one chromosome set (23 chromosomes); or (2) aneuploidy, in which the numerical deviation is not an exact multiple of the haploid set (Lashley, 1998).

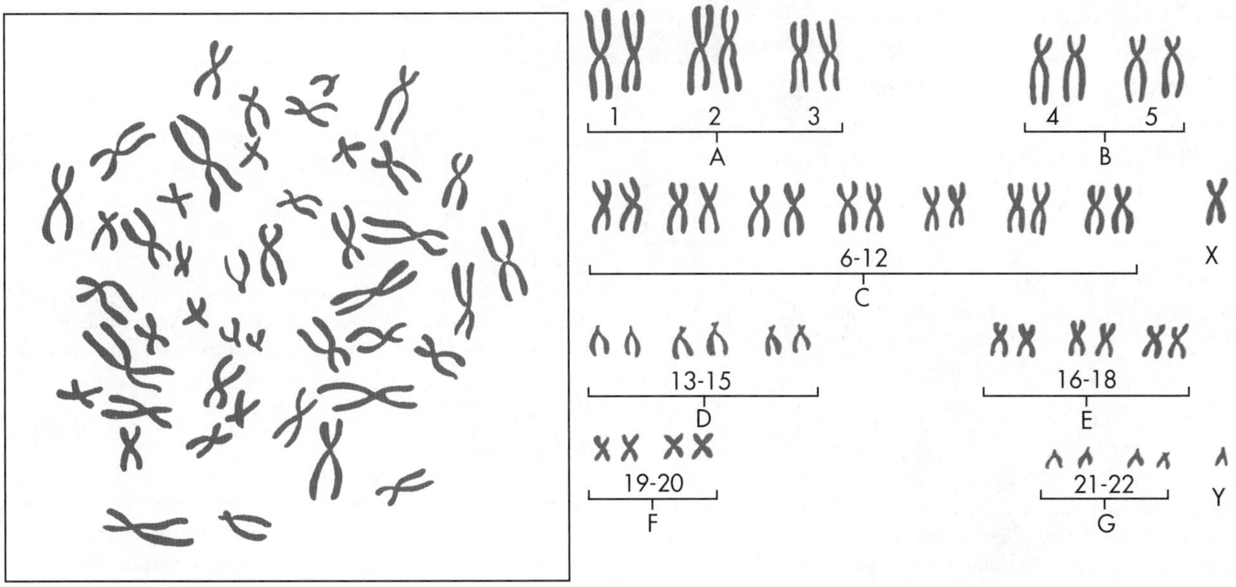

Fig. 8-2 Chromosomes during cell division. **A,** Example of photomicrograph. **B,** Chromosomes arranged in karyotype; female and male sex-determining chromosomes.

Aneuploidy is the most commonly identified chromosome abnormality in humans. Aneuploidy occurs in at least 5% of all clinically recognized pregnancies, and it is the leading known cause of pregnancy loss (Hassold & Hunt, 2001). Aneuploidy also is the leading genetic cause of mental retardation. The two most common aneuploid conditions are monosomies and trisomies. A monosomy is the product of the union between a normal gamete and a gamete that is missing a chromosome. Monosomic individuals only have 45 chromosomes in each of their cells. The product of the union of a normal gamete with a gamete containing an extra chromosome is a trisomy. Trisomies are more common than monosomies. Trisomic individuals have 47 chromosomes in each of their cells.

Limited data are available concerning the origin of monosomies because when an embryo is missing an autosomal chromosome, the embryo never survives. Most trisomies are caused by nondisjunction during the first meiotic division. That is, one pair of chromosomes fails to separate. One of the resulting cells contains two chromosomes, and the other contains none.

The most common trisomal abnormality is Down syndrome, or trisomy 21 (Nursing Care Plan) (see Fig. 42-5 and discussion in Chapter 42). Other autosomal trisomies that have been identified are trisomy 18 (Edwards syndrome) and trisomy 13 (Patau syndrome). Both conditions have a very poor prognosis, and most affected children die from cardiac or respiratory complications within 6 months of birth.

The product of the union of a normal gamete (ovum or sperm) with a gamete that is missing a chromosome is a monosomy. This individual would have only 45 chromosomes in each cell. The lack of an autosomal chromosome always results in death of the embryo.

Nondisjunction can also occur during mitosis. If this occurs early in development, when cell lines are forming, the individual has a mixture of cells, some with a normal number of chromosomes and others either missing a chromosome or containing an extra chromosome. This condition is known as mosaicism.

Abnormalities of Chromosome Structure

Abnormalities of chromosome structure involve chromosome breakage, usually resulting from one of two events: (1) translocation and (2) additions or deletions (or both). Translocation occurs when genetic material is transferred from one chromosome to another, different chromosome. Thus instead of two normal pairs of chromosomes, the individual has one normal chromosome of each pair and a third chromosome that is a fusion of the other two chromosomes. As long as all genetic material is retained in the cell, the individual is unaffected but is a carrier of a balanced translocation.

If a gamete receives the two normal chromosomes or the fused chromosome, the resulting offspring will be clinically normal. If the gamete receives one of the two normal chromosomes and the fused version, the resulting offspring will have an extra copy of one of the chromosomes. This condition is called an unbalanced translocation and often has serious clinical effects.

Whenever a portion of a chromosome is deleted from one chromosome and added to another, the gamete produced may have either extra copies of genes or too few copies. The clinical effects produced may be mild or severe depending on the amount of genetic material involved.

Sex Chromosome Abnormalities

Several sex chromosome abnormalities are caused by nondisjunction during gametogenesis in either parent. The most common deviation in females is Turner's syndrome, or monosomy X (having only one X chromosome); the affected female exhibits juvenile external genitalia with undeveloped ovaries. She is usually short in stature with webbing of the neck. Intelligence may be impaired. Most affected embryos miscarry spontaneously.

The most common deviation in males is Klinefelter's syndrome, or trisomy XXY. The affected male has poorly developed secondary sexual characteristics and small testes. He is

Nursing Care Plan

THE FAMILY WITH DOWN SYNDROME

NURSING DIAGNOSIS: Risk for interrupted family processes related to birth of a neonate with an inherited disorder

EXPECTED OUTCOME

The couple will verbalize accurate information about Down syndrome, including implications for future pregnancies.

NURSING INTERVENTIONS/*RATIONALES*

Assess knowledge base of couple regarding the clinical signs and symptoms of Down syndrome and inheritance patterns *to correct any misconceptions and establish basis for teaching plan.*

Provide information throughout the genetics evaluation regarding risk status and clinical signs and symptoms of Down syndrome *to give couple a realistic picture of neonate's defects and assist with decision making for future pregnancies.*

Use therapeutic communication during discussions with the couple *to provide opportunity for expression of concern.*

Refer to support groups, social services, or counseling *to assist with family cohesive actions and decision making.*

Refer to child development specialist *to provide family with realistic expectations regarding cognitive and behavioral differences of child with Down syndrome.*

NURSING DIAGNOSIS: Situational low self-esteem related to diagnosis of inherited disorder as evidenced by parents' statements of guilt and shame

EXPECTED OUTCOME

The parents will express an increased number of positive statements regarding the birth of a neonate with Down syndrome.

NURSING INTERVENTIONS/*RATIONALES*

Assist parents to list strengths and coping strategies that have been helpful in past situations *to use appropriate strategies during this situational crisis.*

Encourage expression of feelings using therapeutic communication *to provide clarification and emotional support.*

Clarify and provide information regarding Down syndrome *to decrease feelings of guilt and gradually increase feelings of positive self-esteem.*

Refer for further counseling as needed *to provide more in-depth and ongoing support.*

NURSING DIAGNOSIS: Risk for impaired parenting related to birth of neonate with Down syndrome

EXPECTED OUTCOME

Parents demonstrate competent skills in parenting a child with Down syndrome and willingness to care for neonate.

NURSING INTERVENTIONS/*RATIONALES*

Assist parents to see and describe normal aspects of infant *to promote bonding.*

Encourage and assist with breastfeeding if that is parents' choice of feeding method *to facilitate closeness with infant and provide benefits of breast milk.*

Assure parents that information regarding the neonate will remain confidential *to assist the parents to maintain some situational control and allow for time to work through their feelings.*

Discuss and role play with parents ways of informing family and friends of infant's diagnosis and prognosis *to promote positive aspects of infant and decrease potential isolation from social interactions.*

Provide anticipatory guidance about what to expect as infant develops *to assist family to be prepared for behavior problems or mental deficits.*

NURSING DIAGNOSIS: Spiritual distress related to situational crisis of child born with Down syndrome

EXPECTED OUTCOME

Parents seek appropriate support persons (family members, priest, minister, rabbi) for assistance.

NURSING INTERVENTIONS/*RATIONALES*

Listen for cues indicative of parents' feelings ("Why did God do this to us?") *to identify messages indicating spiritual distress.*

Acknowledge parents' spiritual concerns and encourage expression of feelings *to help build a therapeutic relationship.*

Facilitate visits from clergy and provide privacy during visits *to demonstrate respect for parents' relationship with clergy.*

Encourage parents to discuss concerns with clergy *to use expert spiritual care resources to help the parents.*

Facilitate interaction with family members and other support persons *to encourage expressions of concern and seek comfort.*

NURSING DIAGNOSIS: Risk for social isolation related to full-time caretaking responsibilities for a neonate with Down syndrome

EXPECTED OUTCOME

Parents will describe a plan to utilize resources to prevent social isolation.

NURSING INTERVENTIONS/*RATIONALES*

Provide opportunity for parents to express feelings about caring for a neonate with Down syndrome *to facilitate effective communication and trust.*

Discuss with parents their expectations about caring for the neonate *to identify potential areas of concern.*

Assist parents to identify potential caregiving resources *to permit parents to return to a routine at home.*

Identify appropriate referrals for home care *to provide continuity of care.*

Refer to support groups of parents of children with Down Syndrome *to enlist support, understanding, and strategies for coping.*

infertile, usually tall, and effeminate. Males who are mosaic for Klinefelter's syndrome may be fertile. Subnormal intelligence is usually present.

Patterns of Genetic Transmission

Heritable characteristics are those that can be passed on to offspring. The patterns by which genetic material is transmitted to the next generation are affected by the number of genes involved in the expression of the trait. Many phenotypic characteristics result from two or more genes on different chromosomes acting together (referred to as multifactorial inheritance); others are controlled by a single gene (unifactorial inheritance).

Defects at the gene level cannot be determined by conventional laboratory methods such as karyotyping. Instead, genetic specialists predict the probability of the presence of an abnormal gene from the known occurrence of the trait in the individual's family and the known patterns by which the trait is inherited.

Multifactorial Inheritance

Most common congenital malformations, such as cleft lip and palate and neural tube defects, result from multifactorial inheritance, a combination of genetic and environmental factors. Each malformation may range from mild to severe, depending on the number of genes for the defect present or the amount of environmental influence. Multifactorial disorders tend to occur in families. Some malformations occur more often in one sex than the other. For example, pyloric stenosis and cleft lip are more common in males, and cleft palate is more common in females.

Unifactorial Inheritance

If a single gene controls a particular trait, disorder, or defect, its pattern of inheritance is referred to as unifactorial mendelian or single-gene inheritance. The number of unifactorial abnormalities far exceeds the number of chromosomal abnormalities. This is understandable, considering that 30,000 to 40,000 genes in the haploid number (23) of chromosomes are passed on to an offspring from each parent.

Unifactorial or single-gene disorders follow the inheritance patterns of dominance, segregation, and independent assortment described by Mendel and include autosomal dominant, autosomal recessive, and X-linked dominant and recessive modes of inheritance (Fig. 8-3).

Autosomal Dominant Inheritance

Autosomal dominant inheritance disorders are those in which the abnormal gene for the trait is expressed even when the other member of the pair is normal. The abnormal gene may appear as a result of a mutation, a spontaneous and permanent change in the normal gene structure. In this case the disorder occurs for the first time in the family. Usually an affected individual comes from multiple generations having the disorder (Fig. 8-3, *B* and *C*). Males and females are equally affected.

Examples of common autosomal dominantly inherited disorders are Marfan syndrome (a disorder of connective tissue resulting in skeletal, ocular, and cardiovascular abnormalities), achondroplasia (dwarfism), polydactyly (extra digits), Huntington disease, and polycystic kidney disease.

Neurofibromatosis (NF) is a progressive disorder of the nervous system that causes tumors to form on nerves anywhere in the body. NF affects all races, all ethnic groups, and both sexes equally. Half of the cases of NF result from spontaneous genetic mutation, whereas the other half are inherited in an autosomal dominant manner. Two genetically distinct forms of NF are NF1, the most common type, with an incidence of 1 in 3000 (Mueller & Young, 2001), and NF2, with an incidence of 1 in 35,000. The most notable features of NF1 are the small pigmented skin lesions known as café-au-lait spots and the neurofibromata (small, soft, fleshy growths). Other clinical features of NF1 are axillary freckling, mild developmental delay, large head, and Lisch nodules (small, harmless, raised pigmented areas in the iris). Individuals with NF1 generally are able to live a normal, healthy life. Café-au-lait spots and neurofibromata can occur with NF2, but they are far less common than with NF1.

NF1 is inherited in an autosomal dominant manner with almost complete penetrance by age 5 years (Mueller & Young, 2001). The NF1 gene, located on chromosome 17, functions as a tumor suppressor. When it is missing or mutated, tumors grow. More than 100 mutations have been identified in the NF1 gene. The NF2 gene has been mapped to chromosome 22. No treatment for NF is available, other than the surgical removal of the tumors. Once removed, the tumors may grow back.

Autosomal Recessive Inheritance

Autosomal recessive inheritance disorders are those in which both genes of a pair must be abnormal for the disorder to be expressed. Heterozygous individuals have only one abnormal gene and are unaffected clinically because their normal gene overshadows the abnormal gene. They are known as carriers of the recessive trait. For the trait to be expressed, two carriers must each contribute the abnormal gene to the offspring (Fig. 8-3, *C*). Males and females are equally affected. Most inborn errors of metabolism, such as phenylketonuria, galactosemia, maple syrup urine disease, Tay-Sachs disease, sickle cell anemia, and cystic fibrosis, are autosomal recessive inherited disorders.

X-Linked Dominant Inheritance

X-linked dominant inheritance disorders occur in males and heterozygous females. Because the females also have a normal gene, the effects are less severe than in affected males. Affected males transmit the abnormal gene only to their daughters on the X chromosome. Fragile X syndrome and vitamin D–resistant rickets are examples of X-linked dominant inherited disorders. (See discussion in Chapter 42.)

X-Linked Recessive Inheritance

Abnormal genes for X-linked recessive inheritance disorders are carried on the X chromosome. Females may be heterozygous or homozygous for traits carried on the X chromosome because they have two X chromosomes. Males are hemizygous because they have only one X chromosome carrying genes, with no alleles on the Y chromosome. Therefore X-linked recessive disorders are most often manifested in the male with the abnormal gene on his single X chromosome. Hemophilia, color blindness, and Duchenne muscular dystrophy are all X-linked recessive disorders.

Evidence-Based Practice

FOLATE SUPPLEMENTS TO PREVENT NEURAL TUBE DEFECTS

Background

Within 3 weeks of implantation, the embryonic neural groove is formed on the dorsum, and will give rise to the brain and spinal cord. The groove folds into a tube by 1 month postfertilization (6 weeks from last menstrual period). Defects in this closure can lead to anencephaly (absence of brain, cranial vault, and covering skin), which is incompatible with survival, and spina bifida (herniation of the spinal cord and/or meninges), which has a high mortality rate and mild to extreme neural damage. Neural tube defects (NTDs) may be attributed to both genetic and environmental causes. Screening during the second trimester, using maternal serum alpha-fetoprotein estimation or fetal ultrasound, can identify NTDs, while the pregnancy can still be terminated. This has led to a decrease in birth rates of infants with NTDs, but it does not address primary prevention.

Higher dietary folate, taken periconceptionally (before conception and during the first 2 months of pregnancy), seems to greatly decrease the incidence of NTDs.

Objectives

The reviewers' primary objective was to inquire as to whether periconceptional folate or multivitamins can decrease the prevalence of neural tube defects.

Interventions were the folate supplements or multivitamins. Outcomes, aside from neural tube defects, might include other defects, spontaneous abortion, multiple pregnancy, preterm birth, perinatal and infant mortality, length of supplementation before conception, blood and tissue levels of folate, and attitudes toward and knowledge of NTDs in the population and among practitioners.

Methods

Search Strategy

The reviewers searched Cochrane, MEDLINE, and ZETOC, using the search keywords neural tube defects.

Four randomized or quasi-randomized, controlled trials, representing 6425 women, were selected. One dissemination trial looked at the impact of printed materials on six communities. The trials took place in Hungary, Republic of Ireland, the United Kingdom, Israel, Australia, Canada, the former USSR, and France, from 1981 to1994.

Statistical Analyses

Statistical analyses of homogeneous data were performed, using relative risks with 95% confidence intervals.

Findings

Neural tube defects were significantly decreased by periconceptional folate supplementation. There was a consistent increase in multiple pregnancies across three trials, though it did not reach statistical significance. There were no associations of folate supplementation with other birth defects, ectopic pregnancies, stillbirths, miscarriages, or increase in conception. The doses of folate ranged from 0.36 to 4 mg/day. In one trial, the folate group experienced less nausea and vomiting of pregnancy in the first trimester than the controls.

Multivitamins alone did not decrease the rate of NTDs.

In the literature dissemination trial, there was a significant increase in knowledge and intervention in the sample studied. Many women were not aware that folate was required periconceptionally for effective prevention.

Limitations

Randomization was not clear, nor was the dropout rate discussed in the review. These studies did not reach those whose pregnancy was unplanned, which can number half of all pregnancies in some areas. There was little information about the effects of folate on other drugs. None of the trials looked at dietary folate, which may be more practical in certain developing countries than supplementation.

Conclusions

There is evidence that folate supplementation reduces the incidence of neural tube defects.

Implications for Practice

Most national policy statements call for 0.4 mg/day for all women of childbearing age, especially if they are contemplating pregnancy. For women with a history of an affected prior pregnancy, the recommended dose is 4 mg/day. Printed materials are a cost-effective way to educate and reinforce the message about folate supplementation. Most prenatal multivitamins now include the recommended dose of folate. Certain drugs may alter folate metabolism, such as antiseizure medication, which causes higher risk of NTD.

Implications for Further Research

New trials on cost-effective information dissemination can identify the most effective methods to educate childbearing-age women, so that they can take folate before pregnancy. Large randomized, controlled trials can determine any side effects of folate, such as multiple births, which could change the relative risks and benefits of folate supplementation substantially. Trials involving food products that contain added folate would be informative. Folate deficiency recently has been tied to cardiovascular disease. Some trials in the future may establish the need for increased folate throughout life.

Reference

Lumley J et al: Periconceptional supplementation with folate and/or multivitamins for preventing neural tube defects (Cochrane Review), 2001. In *The Cochrane Library,* Issue 2, Chichester, UK, 2004, John Wiley & Sons.

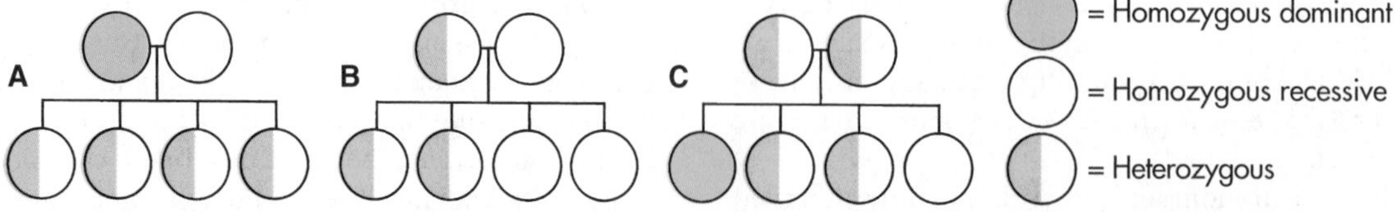

Fig. 8-3 Possible offspring in three types of matings. **A,** Homozygous-dominant parent and homozygous-recessive parent. Children: all heterozygous, displaying dominant trait. **B,** Heterozygous parent and homozygous-recessive parent. Children: 50% heterozygous, displaying dominant trait; 50% homozygous, displaying recessive trait. **C,** Both parents heterozygous. Children: 25% homozygous, displaying dominant trait; 25% homozygous, displaying recessive trait; 50% heterozygous, displaying dominant trait.

Inborn Errors of Metabolism

Disorders of protein, fat, or carbohydrate metabolism that reflect absent or defective enzymes generally follow a recessive pattern of inheritance. Enzymes, the actions of which are genetically determined, are essential for all the physical and chemical processes that sustain body systems. Defective enzyme action interrupts the normal series of chemical reactions from the affected point onward. The result may be an accumulation of a damaging product such as phenylalanine or the absence of a necessary product such as thyroxin or melanin. (See Table 25-3 for screening tests for inborn errors of metabolism.)

Phenylketonuria (PKU) is an uncommon disorder caused by autosomal recessive genes. A deficiency in the liver enzyme phenylalanine hydroxylase results in failure to metabolize the amino acid phenylalanine, allowing its metabolites to accumulate in the blood. The incidence of this disorder is 1 in every 10,000 to 20,000 births. The highest incidence is found in Caucasians (from northern Europe and the United States). It is rarely seen in Jewish, African, or Japanese populations. Screening for PKU is routinely performed on all infants through a blood test.

Tay-Sachs disease, inherited as an autosomal recessive trait, results from a deficiency in hexosaminidase. It occurs more commonly in Ashkenazi Jews and French-Canadians from Quebec. Infants appear normal until 4 to 6 months of age, then the clinical symptoms appear: apathy and regression in motor and social development, and decreased vision. Death occurs between ages 3 and 4 years. No treatment exists.

Cystic fibrosis (mucoviscidosis or fibrocystic disease of the pancreas) is inherited as an autosomal recessive trait and is characterized by generalized involvement of exocrine glands. Clinical features are related to the altered viscosity of mucus-secreting glands throughout the body. Overall incidence is 1 per every 2000 births. Advances in diagnosis and treatment have improved the prognosis; many affected individuals live to adulthood. Some affected women have borne children, but men generally are sterile.

Meconium ileus occurs in about 10% of newborns with cystic fibrosis. Although an initial stool may be passed from the rectum with none thereafter, usually no meconium is passed during the first 24 to 48 hours. The abdomen becomes increasingly distended, and eventually the newborn requires a laparotomy for diagnosis and treatment of the condition. (See discussion in Chapter 46.)

Nongenetic Factors Influencing Development

Not all congenital disorders are inherited. Congenital means that the condition was present at birth. Some congenital malformations may be the result of teratogens, that is, environmental substances or exposures that result in functional or structural disability. In contrast to other forms of developmental disabilities, disabilities caused by teratogens are, in theory, totally preventable. Known human teratogens are drugs and chemicals, infections, exposure to radiation (Scialli, 1997), and certain maternal conditions such as diabetes and PKU (Box 8-3). A teratogen has the greatest effect on the organs and parts of an embryo during its periods of rapid differentiation. This occurs during the embryonic period, specifically from days 15 to 60. During the first 2 weeks of development, teratogens either have no effect on the embryo or have effects so severe that they cause miscarriage. Brain growth and development continue during the fetal period, and teratogens can severely affect mental development throughout gestation (Fig. 8-4).

In addition to genetic makeup and the influence of teratogens, the adequacy of maternal nutrition influences development. The embryo and fetus must obtain the nutrients they need from the mother's diet; they cannot tap the maternal reserves. Malnutrition during pregnancy produces low-birth-weight newborns who are susceptible to infection. Malnutrition also affects brain development during the latter half of gestation and may result in learning disabilities in the child. Inadequate folic acid is associated with neural tube defects.

The field of human behavioral genetics seeks to understand genetic and environmental influences on variations in human behavior (McInerney, 2004). Behavior involves multiple genes. Study of behavior and genes requires analysis of families and populations to compare those who have the trait with those who do not. The result is an estimate of the amount of variation in the population attributable to genetic factors. The findings of this research have significant political and social implications. For example, what are the social consequences of determining a genetic diagnosis of traits such as intelligence, criminality, or homosexuality? Caution must be exercised in accepting discoveries in behavioral genetics until there is substantial scientific corroboration (McInerney & Rothstein, 2004).

BOX 8-3

Etiology of Human Malformations

Environmental

Maternal conditions
- Alcoholism, diabetes, endocrinopathies, phenylketonuria, smoking, nutritional problems

Infectious agents
- Rubella, toxoplasmosis, syphilis, herpes simplex, cytomegalic inclusion disease, varicella, Venezuelan equine encephalitis

Mechanical problems (deformations)
- Amniotic band constrictions, umbilical cord constraint, disparity in uterine size and uterine contents

Chemicals, drugs, radiation, hyperthermia

Genetic

Single-gene disorders
Chromosomal abnormalities

Unknown

Polygenic/multifactorial (gene-environment interactions)
"Spontaneous" errors of development
Other unknowns

Modified from Hudgins L, Cassidy SB: Congenital anomalies. In Fanaroff AA, Martin RJ (eds): *Neonatal-perinatal medicine: diseases of the fetus and infant,* ed 7, St Louis, 2002, Mosby.

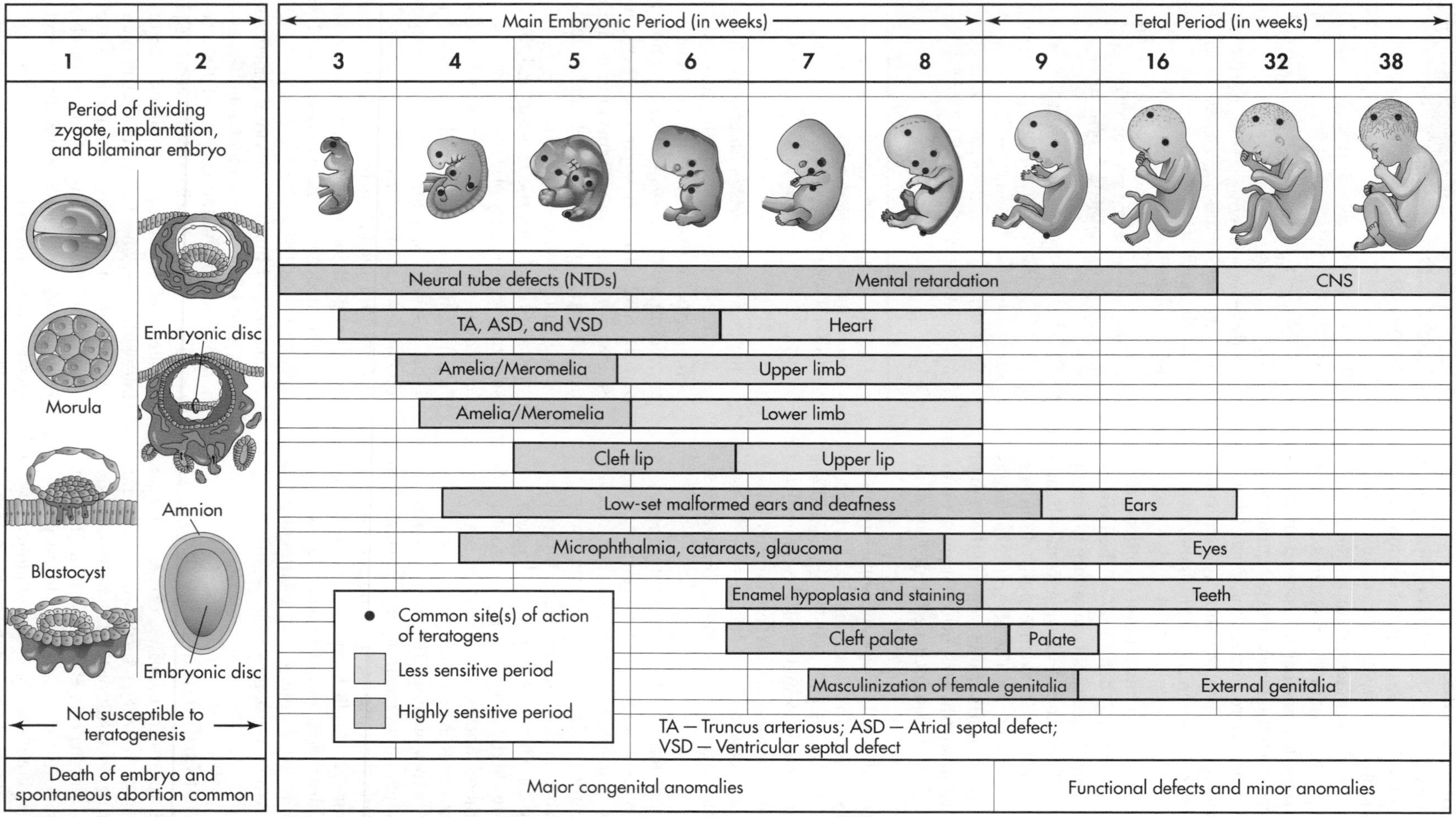

Fig. 8-4 Sensitive, or critical, periods in human development. *Dark color* denotes highly sensitive periods; *light color* indicates stages that are less sensitive to teratogens. (From Moore KL, Persaud TVN: *Before we are born: essentials of embryology and birth defects,* ed 6, Philadelphia, 2003, WB Saunders.)

CONCEPTION

Cell Division

Cells are reproduced by two different methods: mitosis and meiosis. In mitosis, the body cells replicate to yield two cells with the same genetic makeup as the parent cell. First the cell makes a copy of its DNA; then it divides, with each daughter cell receiving one copy of the genetic material. Mitotic division facilitates growth and development or cell replacement.

Meiosis, the process by which germ cells divide and decrease their chromosomal number by half, produces gametes (eggs and sperm). Each homologous pair of chromosomes contains one chromosome received from the mother and one from the father; thus meiosis results in cells that contain one of each of the 23 pairs of chromosomes. Because these germ cells contain 23 single chromosomes, half of the genetic material of a normal somatic cell, they are called haploid. When the female gamete (egg or ovum) and the male gamete (spermatozoon) unite to form the zygote, the diploid number of human chromosomes (46, or 23 pairs) is restored.

The process of DNA replication and cell division in meiosis allows different alleles for genes to be distributed at random by each parent and then rearranged on the paired chromosomes. The chromosomes then separate and proceed to different gametes. Because the two parents have genotypes derived from four different grandparents, many combinations of genes on each chromosome are possible. This random mixing of alleles accounts for the variation of traits seen in the offspring of the same two parents.

Gametogenesis

When a male reaches puberty, his testes begin the process of spermatogenesis. The cells that undergo meiosis in the male are called spermatocytes. The primary spermatocyte, which undergoes the first meiotic division, contains the diploid number of chromosomes. The cell has already copied its DNA before division, so four alleles for each gene are present. Because the copies are bound together (i.e., one allele plus its copy on each chromosome), the cell is still considered diploid.

During the first meiotic division, two haploid secondary spermatocytes are formed. Each secondary spermatocyte contains 22 autosomes and one sex chromosome; one contains the X chromosome (plus its copy) and the other the Y chromosome (plus its copy). During the second meiotic division the male produces two gametes with an X chromosome and two gametes with a Y chromosome, all of which will develop into viable sperm (Fig. 8-5, *A*).

Oogenesis, the process of egg (ovum) formation, begins during fetal life of the female. All the cells that may undergo meiosis in a woman's lifetime are contained in her ovaries at birth. The majority of the estimated 2 million primary oocytes (the cells that undergo the first meiotic division) degenerate spontaneously. Only 400 to 500 ova will mature during the approximately 35 years of a woman's reproductive life. The primary oocytes begin the first meiotic division (i.e., they replicate their DNA) during fetal life, but remain suspended at this stage until puberty (Fig. 8-5, *B*). Then, usually monthly, one primary oocyte matures and completes the first meiotic division, yielding two unequal cells: the secondary oocyte and a small polar body. Both contain 22 autosomes and one X sex chromosome.

At ovulation the second meiotic division begins. However, the ovum does not complete the second meiotic division unless fertilization occurs. At fertilization, a second polar body and the zygote (the united egg and sperm) are produced (Fig. 8-5, *C*). The three polar bodies degenerate. If fertilization does not occur, the ovum also degenerates.

Conception

Conception, defined as the union of a single egg and sperm, marks the beginning of a pregnancy. Conception occurs not as an isolated event but as part of a sequential process. This sequential process includes gamete (egg and sperm) formation, ovulation (release of the egg), union of the gametes (which results in an embryo), and implantation in the uterus.

Ovum

Meiosis is the process by which germ cells divide and decrease their chromosomal number by half. In the female this meiotic process occurs in the ovarian follicles and produces an egg, or ovum. Each month, one ovum matures with a host of surrounding supportive cells.

At ovulation the ovum is released from the ruptured ovarian follicle. High estrogen levels increase the motility of the uterine tubes so that their cilia are able to capture the ovum and propel it through the tube toward the uterine cavity. An ovum cannot move by itself.

Two protective layers surround the ovum (Fig. 8-6). The inner layer is a thick, acellular layer called the zona pellucida. The outer layer, called the corona radiata, is composed of elongated cells.

Ova are considered fertile for about 24 hours after ovulation. If unfertilized by a sperm, the ovum degenerates and is reabsorbed.

Sperm

Ejaculation during sexual intercourse normally propels almost a teaspoon of semen containing as many as 200 to 500 million sperm into the vagina. The sperm swim by means of the flagellar movement of their tails. Some sperm can reach the site of fertilization within 5 minutes, but average transit time is 4 to 6 hours. Sperm remain viable within the woman's reproductive system for an average of 2 to 3 days. Most sperm are lost in the vagina, within the cervical mucus, or in the endometrium; or they enter the tube that contains no ovum.

As sperm travel through the female reproductive tract, enzymes are produced to aid in their capacitation. Capacitation is a physiologic change that removes the protective coating from the heads of the sperm. Small perforations then form in the acrosome (a cap on the sperm) and allow enzymes (e.g., hyaluronidase) to escape. These enzymes are necessary for the sperm to penetrate the protective layers of the ovum before fertilization.

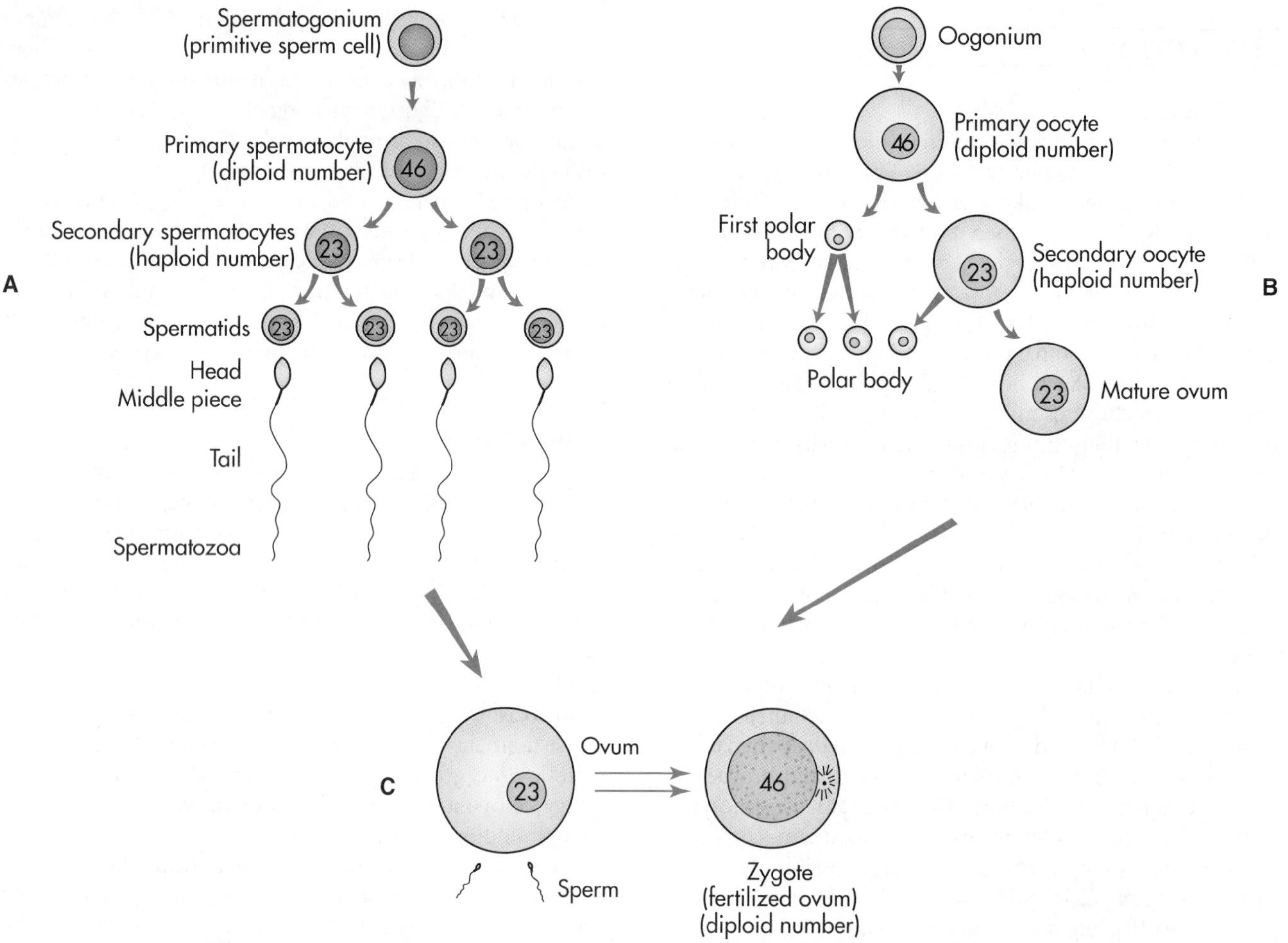

Fig. 8-5 Spermatogenesis. **A**, Gametogenesis in the male produces four mature gametes, the sperm. **B**, Oogenesis. Gametogenesis in the female produces one mature ovum and three polar bodies. Note relative difference in overall size between ovum and sperm. **C**, Fertilization results in the single-cell zygote and restoration of the diploid number of chromosomes.

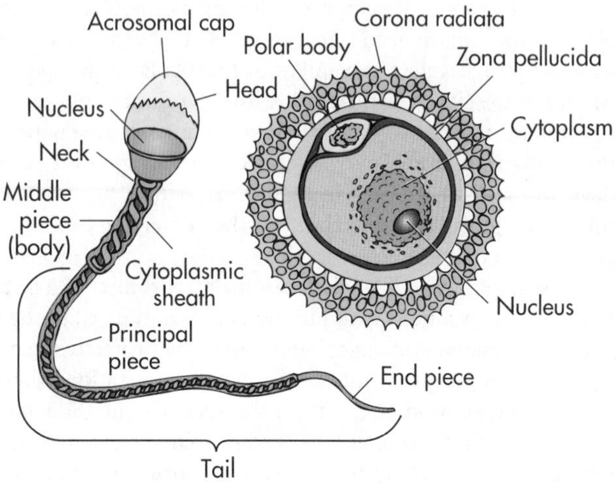

Fig. 8-6 Sperm and ovum.

Fertilization

Fertilization takes place in the ampulla (the outer third) of the uterine tube. When a sperm successfully penetrates the membrane surrounding the ovum, both sperm and ovum are enclosed within the membrane, and the membrane becomes impenetrable to other sperm; this process is termed the *zona reaction.* The second meiotic division of the oocyte is then completed, and the ovum nucleus becomes the female pronucleus. The head of the sperm enlarges to become the male pronucleus, and the tail degenerates. The nuclei fuse and the chromosomes combine, restoring the diploid number (46) (Fig. 8-7). Conception, the formation of the zygote (the first cell of the new individual), has been achieved.

Mitotic cellular replication, called cleavage, begins as the zygote travels the length of the uterine tube into the uterus. This voyage takes 3 to 4 days. Because the fertilized egg divides rapidly with no increase in size, successively smaller cells, called blastomeres, are formed with each division. A 16-cell morula, a solid ball of cells, is produced within 3 days, and is still surrounded by the protective zona pellucida

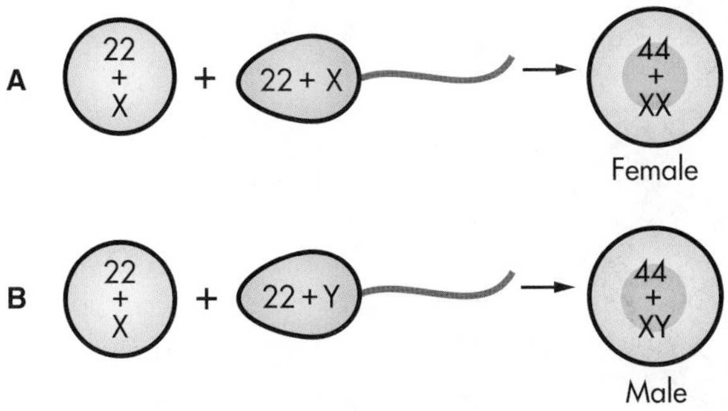

Fig. 8-7 Fertilization. **A**, Ovum fertilized by X-bearing sperm to form female zygote. **B**, Ovum fertilized by Y-bearing sperm to form male zygote.

(Fig. 8-8, *A*). Further development occurs as the morula floats freely within the uterus. Fluid passes through the zona pellucida into the intercellular spaces between the blastomeres, separating them into two parts: the trophoblast (which gives rise to the placenta) and the embryoblast (which gives rise to the embryo). A cavity forms within the cell mass as the spaces come together, forming a structure called the blastocyst cavity. When the cavity becomes recognizable, the whole structure of the developing embryo is known as the blastocyst. Stem cells are derived from the inner cell mass of the blastocyst. The outer layer of cells surrounding the cavity is the trophoblast.

Implantation

The zona pellucida degenerates, and the trophoblast attaches itself to the uterine endometrium, usually in the anterior or posterior fundal region. Between 6 and 10 days after conception, the trophoblast secretes enzymes that enable it to burrow into the endometrium until the entire blastocyst is covered. This is known as implantation. Endometrial blood vessels erode, and some women experience slight implantation bleeding (slight spotting and bleeding during the time of the first missed menstrual period). Chorionic villi, or fingerlike projections, develop out of the trophoblast and extend into the blood-filled spaces of the endometrium. These villi are vascular processes that obtain oxygen and nutrients from the maternal bloodstream and dispose of carbon dioxide and waste products into the maternal blood.

After implantation, the endometrium is called the decidua. The portion directly under the blastocyst, where the chorionic villi tap into the maternal blood vessels, is the decidua basalis. The portion covering the blastocyst is the decidua capsularis, and the portion lining the rest of the uterus is the decidua vera (Fig. 8-9).

THE EMBRYO AND FETUS

Pregnancy lasts approximately 10 lunar months, 9 calendar months, 40 weeks, or 280 days. Length of pregnancy is computed from the first day of the last menstrual period (LMP)

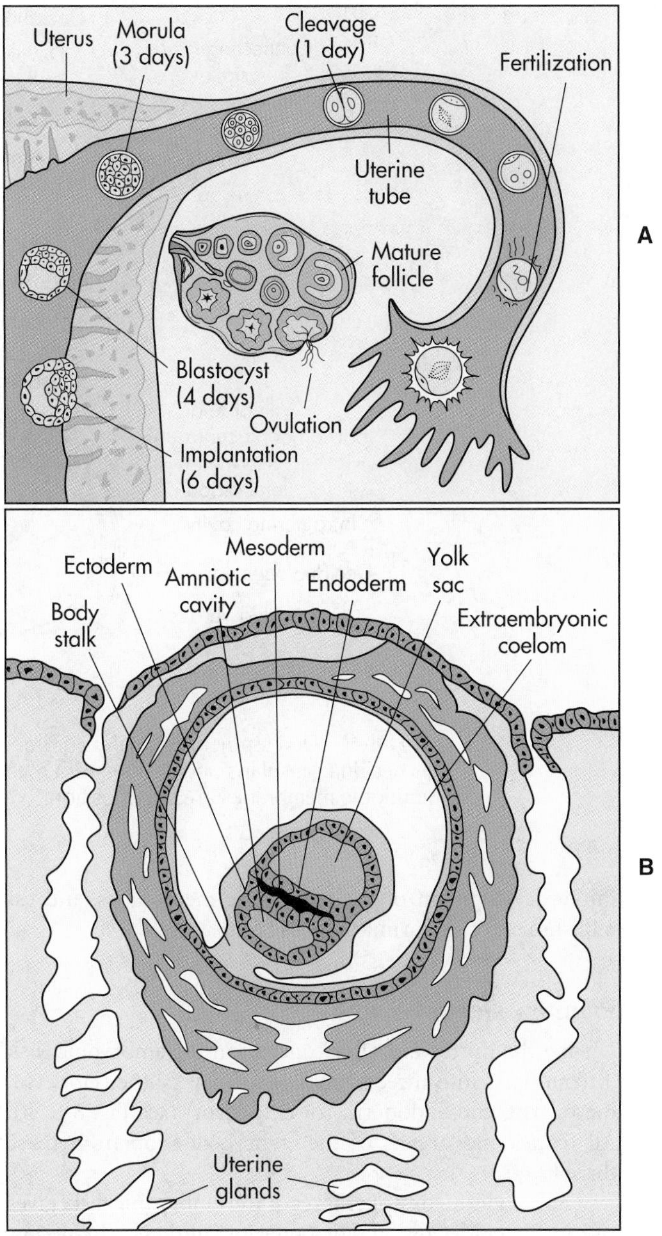

Fig. 8-8 **A**, First weeks of human development. Follicular development in ovary, ovulation, fertilization, and transport of early embryo down uterine tube and into uterus, where implantation occurs. **B**, Blastocyst embedded in endometrium. Germ layers forming. (*A*, From Carlson B: *Human embryology and developmental biology*, ed 3, St Louis, 2004, Mosby. *B*, Adapted from Langley L et al: *Dynamic human anatomy and physiology*, ed 5, New York, 1980, McGraw-Hill.)

until the day of birth. However, conception occurs approximately 2 weeks after the first day of the LMP. Thus the postconception age of the fetus is 2 weeks less, for a total of 266 days or 38 weeks. Postconception age is used in the discussion of fetal development.

Intrauterine development is divided into three stages: ovum or preembryonic, embryo, and fetus (see Fig. 8-4). The stage of the ovum lasts from conception until day 14. This period covers cellular replication, blastocyst formation,

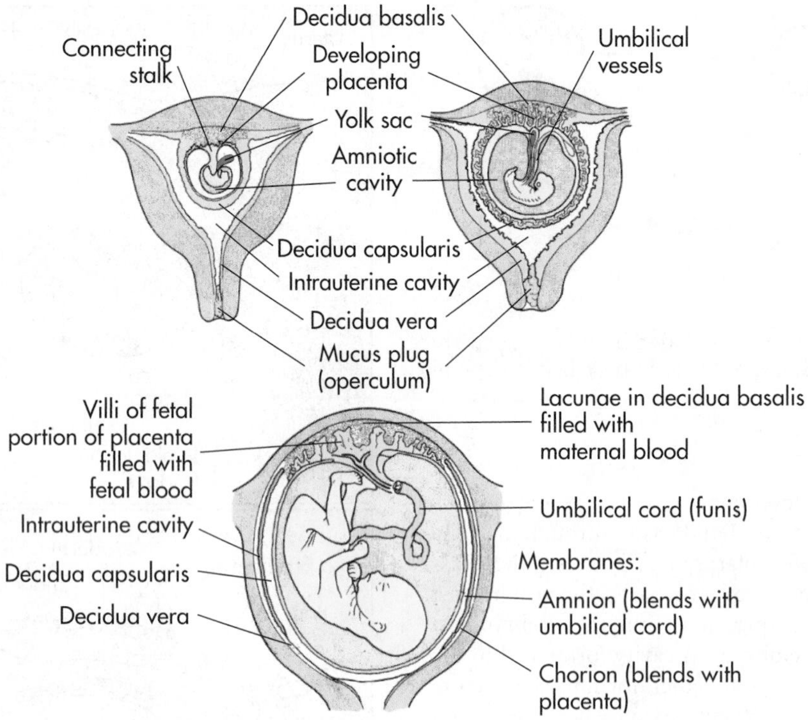

Fig. 8-9 Development of fetal membranes. Note gradual obliteration of intrauterine cavity as decidua capsularis and decidua vera meet. Also note thinning of uterine wall. Chorionic and amnionic membranes are in apposition to each other but may be peeled apart.

initial development of the embryonic membranes, and establishment of the primary germ layers.

Primary Germ Layers

During the third week after conception the embryonic disk differentiates into three primary germ layers: the ectoderm, mesoderm, and endoderm (or entoderm) (see Fig. 8-8, *B*). All tissues and organs of the embryo develop from these three layers.

The ectoderm, or upper layer of the embryonic disk, gives rise to the epidermis, glands (anterior pituitary, cutaneous, and mammary), nails and hair, central and peripheral nervous systems, lens of the eye, tooth enamel, and floor of the amniotic cavity.

The mesoderm, or middle layer, develops into the bones and teeth, muscles (skeletal, smooth, and cardiac), dermis and connective tissue, cardiovascular system and spleen, and urogenital system.

The endoderm, or lower layer, gives rise to the epithelium lining the respiratory tract and digestive tract, including the oropharynx, liver and pancreas, urethra, bladder, and vagina. The endoderm forms the roof of the yolk sac.

Development of the Embryo

The stage of the embryo lasts from day 15 until approximately 8 weeks after conception, when the embryo measures approximately 3 cm from crown to rump. The embryonic stage is the most critical time in the development of the organ systems and the main external features. Developing areas with rapid cell division are the most vulnerable to malformation by environmental teratogens. At the end of the eighth week, all organ systems and external structures are present, and the embryo is unmistakably human (Fig. 8-4).

Membranes

At the time of implantation, two fetal membranes that will surround the developing embryo begin to form. The chorion develops from the trophoblast and contains the chorionic villi on its surface. The villi burrow into the decidua basalis and increase in size and complexity as the vascular processes develop into the placenta. The chorion becomes the covering of the fetal side of the placenta. It contains the major umbilical blood vessels that branch out over the surface of the placenta. As the embryo grows, the decidua capsularis stretches. The chorionic villi on this side atrophy and degenerate, leaving a smooth chorionic membrane.

The inner cell membrane, the amnion, develops from the interior cells of the blastocyst. The cavity that develops between this inner cell mass and the outer layer of cells (trophoblast) is the amniotic cavity (see Fig. 8-8, *B*). As it grows larger, the amnion forms on the side opposite the developing blastocyst (see Fig. 8-8, *B*, and Fig. 8-9). The developing embryo draws the amnion around itself to form a fluid-filled sac. The amnion becomes the covering of the umbilical cord and covers the chorion on the fetal surface of the placenta. As the embryo grows larger, the amnion enlarges to accommodate the embryo/fetus and the surrounding amniotic

Critical Thinking Exercise

ULTRASOUND DATING OF PREGNANCY

Sandra believes she is 8 weeks pregnant, but her obstetrician believes she is closer to 12 weeks of gestation. Sandra has come to the clinic for an ultrasound examination for dating. She has many questions for the nurse: How can they tell what gestation she is? What would the fetus look like at this time if she is 8 weeks of gestation? If she is 12 weeks of gestation? What fetal structures would be apparent on ultrasound if she is 8 weeks pregnant? If she is 12 weeks pregnant? Would any structural anomalies be apparent at 8 weeks? At 12 weeks? Why is it important to date a pregnancy accurately?

What information should the nurse provide Sandra?

1. Evidence—Is there sufficient evidence to draw conclusions about what information the nurse should provide Sandra?
2. Assumptions—What assumptions can be made about the following factors?
   a. Sandra's motivation to learn about fetal development
   b. Sandra's understanding of fetal development
   c. Sandra's knowledge about ultrasound examinations
   d. Why dating the pregnancy is important
3. What implications and priorities for nursing care can be drawn at this time?
4. Does the evidence objectively support your conclusion?
5. Are there alternative perspectives to your conclusion?

fluid. The amnion eventually comes in contact with the chorion surrounding the fetus.

Amniotic Fluid

At first the amniotic cavity derives its fluid by diffusion from the maternal blood. The amount of fluid increases weekly, and 800 to 1200 ml of transparent liquid are normally present at term. The volume of amniotic fluid changes constantly. The fetus swallows fluid, and fluid flows into and out of the fetal lungs. The fetus urinates into the fluid, greatly increasing its volume.

The amniotic fluid serves many functions for the embryo/fetus. Amniotic fluid helps maintain a constant body temperature. It serves as a source of oral fluid and as a repository for waste. It cushions the fetus from trauma by blunting and dispersing outside forces. It allows freedom of movement for musculoskeletal development. The fluid keeps the embryo from tangling with the membranes, facilitating symmetric growth of the fetus. If the embryo does become tangled with the membranes, amputations of extremities or other deformities can occur from constricting amniotic bands.

The volume of amniotic fluid is an important factor in assessing fetal well-being. Having less than 300 ml of amniotic fluid (oligohydramnios) is associated with fetal renal abnormalities. Having more than 2 L of amniotic fluid (hydramnios) is associated with gastrointestinal and other malformations.

Amniotic fluid contains albumin, urea, uric acid, creatinine, lecithin, sphingomyelin, bilirubin, fructose, fat, leukocytes, proteins, epithelial cells, enzymes, and lanugo hair. Study of fetal cells in amniotic fluid through amniocentesis yields much information about the fetus. Genetic studies (karyotyping) provide knowledge about the sex and the number and structure of chromosomes. Other studies such as the lecithin/sphingomyelin (L/S) ratio determine the health or maturity of the fetus.

Yolk Sac

At the same time the amniotic cavity and amnion are forming, another blastocyst cavity forms on the other side of the developing embryonic disk (see Fig. 8-8, *B*). This cavity becomes surrounded by a membrane, forming the yolk sac. The yolk sac aids in transferring maternal nutrients and oxygen, which have diffused through the chorion, to the embryo. Blood vessels form to aid transport. Blood cells and plasma are manufactured in the yolk sac during the second and third weeks. At the end of the third week, the primitive heart begins to beat and circulate the blood through the embryo, connecting stalk, chorion, and yolk sac.

The folding in of the embryo during the fourth week results in incorporation of part of the yolk sac into the embryo's body as the primitive digestive system. Primordial germ cells arise in the yolk sac and move into the embryo. The shrinking remains of the yolk sac degenerate (see Fig. 8-8, *B*), and by the fifth or sixth week, the remnant has separated from the embryo.

Umbilical Cord

By day 14 after conception the embryonic disk, amniotic sac, and yolk sac are attached to the chorionic villi by the connecting stalk. During the third week the blood vessels develop to supply the embryo with maternal nutrients and oxygen. During the fifth week, the embryo has curved inward on itself from both ends (bringing the connecting stalk to the ventral side of the embryo) and the connecting stalk becomes compressed from both sides by the amnion and forms the narrower umbilical cord (see Fig. 8-9). Two arteries carry blood to the chorionic villi from the embryo, and one vein returns blood to the embryo. Approximately 1% of umbilical cords contain only two vessels: one artery and one vein. This occurrence is sometimes associated with congenital malformations.

The cord rapidly increases in length. At term the cord is 2 cm in diameter and ranges from 30 to 90 cm in length (with an average of 55 cm). It twists spirally on itself and loops around the embryo/fetus. A true knot is rare, but false knots occur as folds or kinks in the cord and may jeopardize circulation to the fetus. Connective tissue called Wharton's jelly prevents compression of the blood vessels and ensures continued nourishment of the embryo/fetus. Compression can occur if the cord lies between the fetal head and the pelvis or is twisted around the fetal body. When the cord is wrapped around the fetal neck, it is called a nuchal cord.

Because the placenta develops from the chorionic villi, the umbilical cord is usually located centrally. A peripheral location is less common and is known as a battledore placenta. The blood vessels are arrayed out from the center to all parts of the placenta.

A

B

C

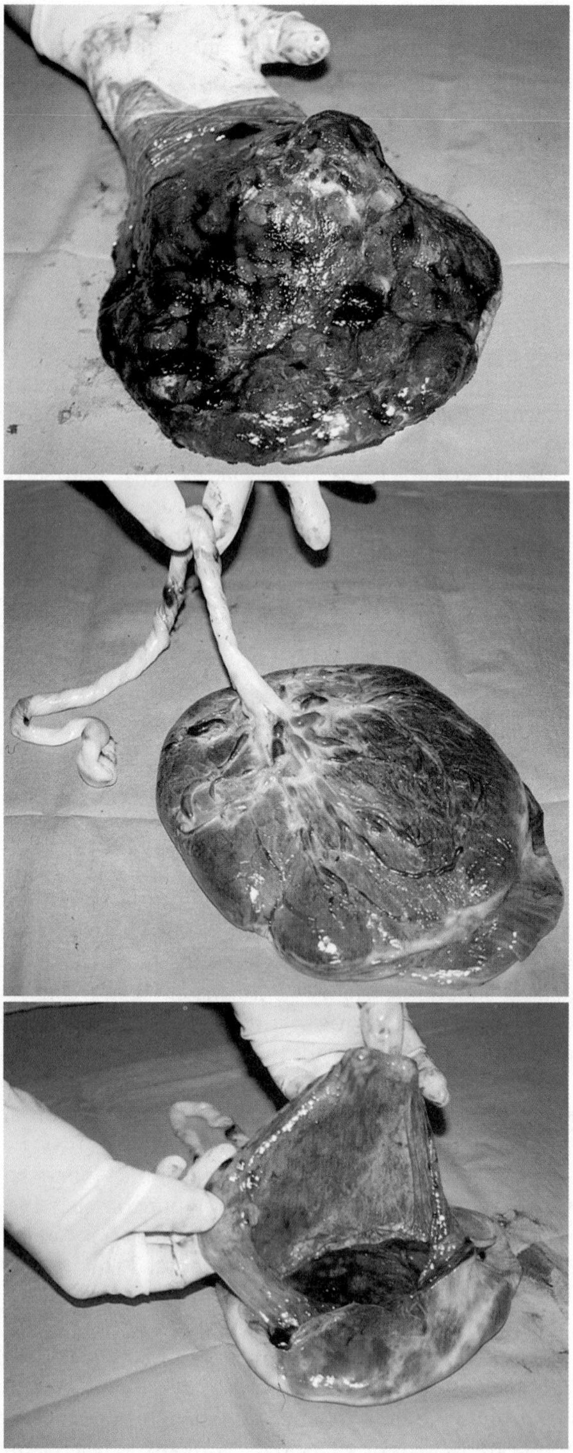

Fig. 8-10 Full-term placenta. **A**, Maternal (or uterine) surface, showing cotyledons and grooves. **B**, Fetal (or amniotic) surface, showing blood vessels running under amnion and converging to form umbilical vessels at attachment of umbilical cord. **C**, Amnion and smooth chorion are arranged to show that they are (1) fused and (2) continuous with margins of placenta. (Courtesy Marjorie Pyle, RNC, Lifecircle, Costa Mesa, CA.)

Placenta

Structure

The placenta begins to form at implantation. During the third week after conception the trophoblast cells of the chorionic villi continue to invade the decidua basalis. As the uterine capillaries are tapped, the endometrial spiral arteries fill with maternal blood. The chorionic villi grow into the spaces with two layers of cells: the outer syncytium and the inner cytotrophoblast. A third layer develops into anchoring septa, dividing the projecting decidua into separate areas called cotyledons. In each of the 15 to 20 cotyledons, the chorionic villi branch out, and a complex system of fetal blood vessels forms. Each cotyledon is a functional unit. The whole structure is the placenta (Fig. 8-10).

The maternal-placental-embryonic circulation is in place by day 17, when the embryonic heart starts beating. By the end of the third week, embryonic blood is circulating between the embryo and the chorionic villi. In the intervillous spaces, maternal blood supplies oxygen and nutrients to the embryonic capillaries in the villi (Fig. 8-11). Waste products and carbon dioxide diffuse into the maternal blood.

The placenta functions as a means of metabolic exchange. Exchange is minimal at this time because the two cell layers of the villous membrane are too thick. Permeability increases as the cytotrophoblast thins and disappears; by the fifth month, only the single layer of syncytium is left between the maternal blood and the fetal capillaries. The syncytium is the functional layer of the placenta. By the eighth week, genetic testing may be done on a sample of chorionic villi obtained by aspiration biopsy; however, limb defects have been associated with chorionic villi sampling done before 10 weeks. The structure of the placenta is complete by the twelfth week. The placenta continues to grow wider until 20 weeks, when it covers about half of the uterine surface. It then continues to grow thicker. The branching villi continue to develop within the body of the placenta, increasing the functional surface area.

Functions

One of the early functions of the placenta is as an endocrine gland that produces four hormones necessary to maintain the pregnancy and support the embryo/fetus. The hormones are produced in the syncytium.

The protein hormone human chorionic gonadotropin (hCG) can be detected in the maternal serum by 8 to 10 days after conception, shortly after implantation. This hormone is the basis for pregnancy tests. The hCG preserves the function of the ovarian corpus luteum, ensuring a continued supply of estrogen and progesterone needed to maintain the pregnancy. Miscarriage occurs if the corpus luteum stops functioning before the placenta can produce sufficient estrogen and progesterone. The hCG reaches its maximum level at 50 to 70 days, then begins to decrease.

The other protein hormone produced by the placenta is human chorionic somatomammotropin (hCS) or human placental lactogen (hPL). This substance is similar to a growth hormone and stimulates maternal metabolism to supply needed nutrients for fetal growth. This hormone increases the resistance to insulin, facilitates glucose transport

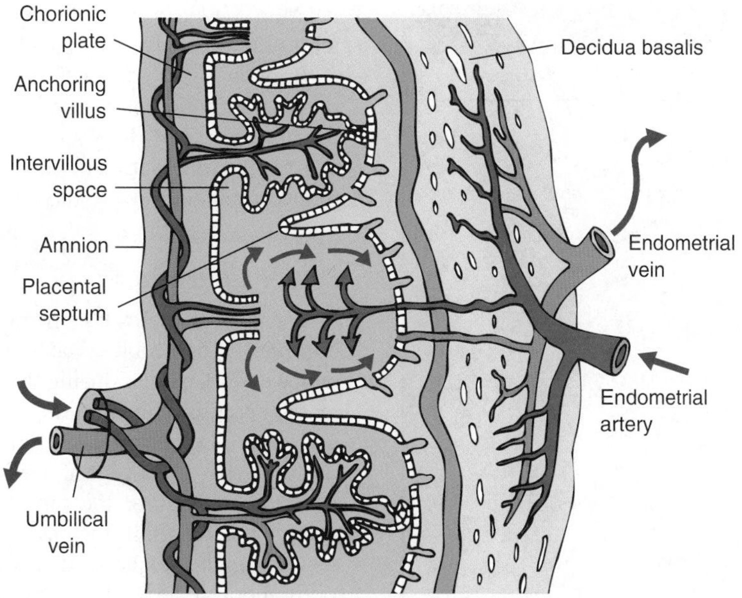

Fig. 8-11 Schematic drawing of placenta illustrating how it supplies oxygen and nutrition to embryo and removes its waste products. Deoxygenated blood leaves fetus through the umbilical arteries and enters placenta, where it is oxygenated. Oxygenated blood leaves placenta through the umbilical vein, which enters the fetus via the umbilical cord.

across the placental membrane, and stimulates breast development to prepare for lactation.

The placenta eventually produces more of the steroid hormone progesterone than the corpus luteum does during the first few months of pregnancy. Progesterone maintains the endometrium, decreases the contractility of the uterus, and stimulates development of breast alveoli and maternal metabolism.

By 7 weeks after fertilization, the placenta is producing most of the maternal estrogens, which are steroid hormones. The major estrogen secreted by the placenta is estriol, whereas the ovaries produce mostly estradiol. Measuring estriol levels is a clinical assay for placental functioning. Estrogen stimulates uterine growth and uteroplacental blood flow. It causes a proliferation of the breast glandular tissue and stimulates myometrial contractility. Placental estrogen production increases greatly toward the end of pregnancy. One theory for the cause of the onset of labor is the decrease in circulating levels of progesterone and the increased levels of estrogen.

The metabolic functions of the placenta are respiration, nutrition, excretion, and storage. Oxygen diffuses from the maternal blood across the placental membrane into the fetal blood, and carbon dioxide diffuses in the opposite direction. In this way the placenta functions as a lung for the fetus.

Carbohydrates, proteins, calcium, and iron are stored in the placenta for ready access to meet fetal needs. Water, inorganic salts, carbohydrates, proteins, fats, and vitamins pass from the maternal blood supply across the placental membrane into the fetal blood, supplying nutrition. Water and most electrolytes with a molecular weight less than 500 readily diffuse through the membrane. Hydrostatic and osmotic pressures aid in the flow of water and some solutions. Facilitated and active transport assists in the transfer of glucose, amino acids, calcium, iron, and substances with higher molecular weights. Amino acids and calcium are transported against the concentration gradient between the maternal blood and fetal blood.

The fetal concentration of glucose is lower than the glucose level in the maternal blood because of its rapid metabolism by the fetus. This fetal requirement demands larger concentrations of glucose than simple diffusion can provide. Therefore maternal glucose moves into the fetal circulation by active transport.

Pinocytosis is a mechanism used for transferring large molecules such as albumin and gamma globulins across the placental membrane. This mechanism conveys the maternal immunoglobulins that provide early passive immunity to the fetus.

Metabolic waste products of the fetus cross the placental membrane from the fetal blood into the maternal blood. The maternal kidneys then excrete them. Many viruses can cross the placental membrane and infect the fetus. Some bacteria and protozoa first infect the placenta and then infect the fetus. Drugs can also cross the placental membrane and may harm the fetus. Caffeine, alcohol, nicotine, carbon monoxide and other toxic substances in cigarette smoke, and prescription and recreational drugs (such as marijuana and cocaine) readily cross the placenta (Box 8-4).

Although no direct link exists between the fetal blood in the vessels of the chorionic villi and the maternal blood in the intervillous spaces, only one cell layer separates them. Breaks occasionally occur in the placental membrane. Fetal erythrocytes then leak into the maternal circulation, and the mother may develop antibodies to the fetal red blood cells. This is often the way the Rh-negative mother becomes sensitized to the erythrocytes of her Rh-positive fetus (see the discussion of isoimmunization in Chapter 28).

BOX 8-4

Developmentally Toxic Exposures in Humans

Aminopterin
Androgens
Angiotensin-converting enzyme inhibitors
Carbamazepine
Cigarette smoking
Cocaine
Coumarin anticoagulants
Cytomegalovirus
Diethylstilbestrol
Ethanol (>1 drink/day)
Etretinate
Hyperthermia
Iodides
Ionizing radiation (>10 rads)
Isotretinoin
Lead
Lithium
Methimazole
Methyl mercury
Parvovirus B19
Penicillamine
Phenytoin
Radioiodine
Rubella
Syphilis
Tetracycline
Thalidomide
Toxoplasmosis
Trimethadione
Valproic acid
Varicella

Though the placenta and fetus are living tissue transplants, they are not destroyed by the host mother (Silver Peltier, & Branch, 2004). Either the placental hormones suppress the immunologic response, or the tissue evokes no response.

Placental function depends on the maternal blood pressure supplying the circulation. Maternal arterial blood, under pressure in the small uterine spiral arteries, spurts into the intervillous spaces (see Fig. 8-11). As long as rich arterial blood continues to be supplied, pressure is exerted on the blood already in the intervillous spaces, pushing it toward drainage by the low-pressure uterine veins. At term gestation, 10% of the maternal cardiac output goes to the uterus.

If there is interference with the circulation to the placenta, the placenta cannot supply the embryo or fetus. Vasoconstriction, such as that caused by hypertension or cocaine use, diminishes uterine blood flow. Decreased maternal blood pressure or decreased cardiac output also diminishes uterine blood flow.

When a woman lies on her back with the pressure of the uterus compressing the vena cava, blood return to the right atrium is diminished (see the discussion of supine hypotension in Chapter 11). Excessive maternal exercise that diverts blood to the muscles away from the uterus compromises placental circulation. Optimum circulation is achieved when the woman is lying at rest on her side. Decreased uterine circulation may lead to intrauterine growth restriction of the fetus and infants who are small for gestational age.

Braxton Hicks contractions seem to enhance the movement of blood through the intervillous spaces, aiding placental circulation. However, prolonged contractions or too-short intervals between contractions during labor can reduce the blood flow to the placenta.

Fetal Maturation

The stage of the fetus lasts from 9 weeks (when the embryo becomes recognizable as a human being) until the pregnancy ends. Changes during the fetal period are not as dramatic, because refinement of structure and function is taking place. The fetus is less vulnerable to teratogens, except for those that affect central nervous system functioning.

Viability refers to the capability of the fetus to survive outside the uterus. In the past the earliest age at which fetal survival could be expected was 28 weeks after conception. With modern technology and advances in maternal and neonatal care, viability is now possible at 20 weeks after conception (22 weeks since LMP; fetal weight of 500 g or more). The limitations on survival outside the uterus are based on central nervous system function and oxygenation capability of the lungs.

Respiratory System

The respiratory system begins development during embryonic life and continues through fetal life and into childhood. The development of the respiratory tract begins in week 4 and continues through week 17 with formation of the trachea, bronchi, and lung buds. Between 16 and 24 weeks the bronchi and terminal bronchioles enlarge, and vascular structures and primitive alveoli are formed. Between 24 weeks and term birth, more alveoli form. Specialized alveolar cells, type I and type II cells, secrete pulmonary surfactants to line the interior of the alveoli. After 32 weeks, sufficient surfactant is present in developed alveoli to provide infants with a good chance of survival.

Pulmonary Surfactants

The detection of the presence of pulmonary surfactants (surface-active phospholipids) in amniotic fluid has been used to determine the degree of fetal lung maturity, or the ability of the lungs to function after birth. Lecithin (L) is the most critical alveolar surfactant required for postnatal lung expansion. It is detectable at approximately 21 weeks and increases in amount after week 24. Another pulmonary phospholipid, sphingomyelin (S), remains constant in amount. Thus the measure of lecithin in relation to sphingomyelin, or the L/S ratio, is used to determine fetal lung maturity. When the L/S ratio reaches 2:1, the infant's lungs are considered to be mature. This occurs at approximately 35 weeks of gestation (Mercer, 2004).

Certain maternal conditions that cause decreased maternal placental blood flow, such as maternal hypertension, placental dysfunction, infection, or corticosteroid use, accelerate lung maturity. This apparently is caused by the resulting fetal hypoxia, which stresses the fetus and increases the blood levels of corticosteroids that accelerate alveolar and surfactant development.

Conditions such as gestational diabetes and chronic glomerulonephritis can retard fetal lung maturity. The use of intrabronchial synthetic surfactant in the treatment of respiratory distress syndrome in the newborn has greatly improved the chances of survival for preterm infants.

Fetal respiratory movements have been seen on ultrasound as early as the eleventh week. These fetal respiratory movements may aid in development of the chest wall muscles and regulate lung fluid volume. The fetal lungs produce fluid that expands the air spaces in the lungs. The fluid drains into the amniotic fluid or is swallowed by the fetus.

Before birth, secretion of lung fluid decreases. The normal birth process squeezes out approximately one third of the fluid. Infants of cesarean births do not benefit from this squeezing process; thus they may have more respiratory difficulty at birth. The fluid remaining in the lungs at birth is usually reabsorbed into the infant's bloodstream within 2 hours of birth.

Fetal Circulatory System

The cardiovascular system is the first organ system to function in the developing human. Blood vessel and blood cell formation begins in the third week and supplies the embryo with oxygen and nutrients from the mother. By the end of the third week the tubular heart begins to beat, and the primitive cardiovascular system links the embryo, connecting stalk, chorion, and yolk sac. During the fourth and fifth weeks the heart develops into a four-chambered organ. By the end of the embryonic stage, the heart is developmentally complete.

The fetal lungs do not function for respiratory gas exchange, so a special circulatory pathway, the ductus arteriosus, bypasses the lungs. Oxygen-rich blood from the placenta flows rapidly through the umbilical vein into the fetal abdomen (Fig. 8-12). When the umbilical vein reaches the liver, it divides into two branches. One branch circulates some oxygenated blood through the liver. Most of the blood

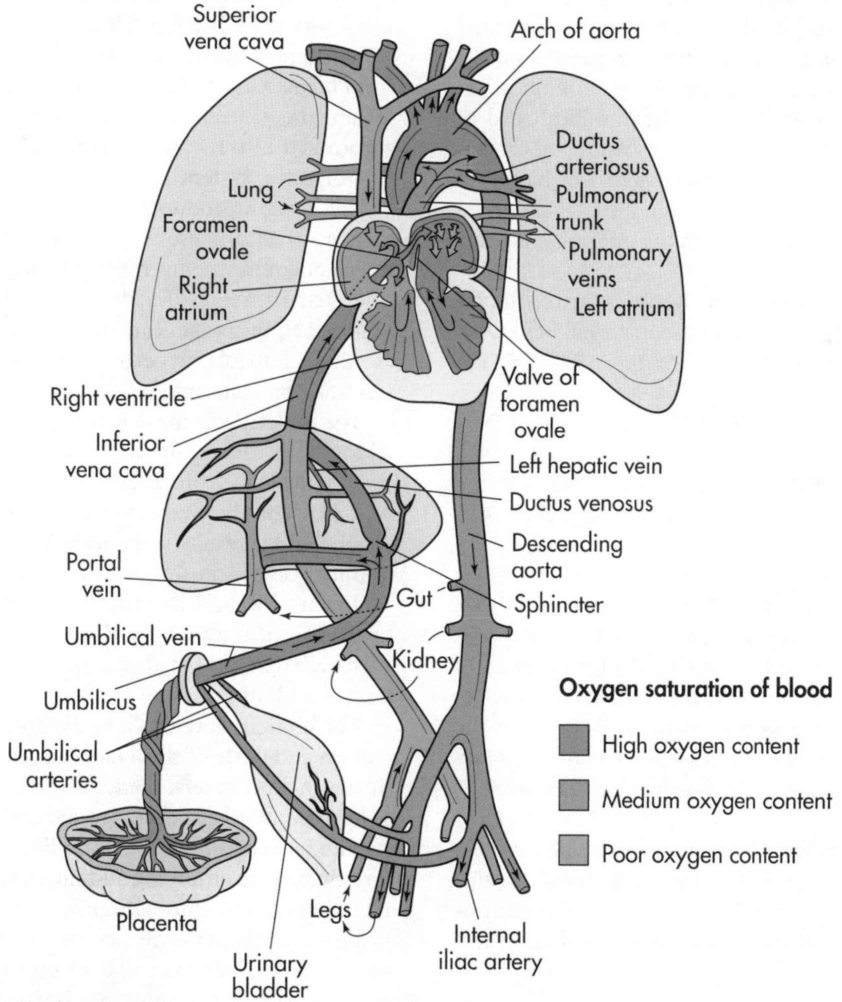

Fig. 8-12 Schematic illustration of the fetal circulation. The colors indicate the oxygen saturation of the blood, and the arrows show the course of the blood from the placenta to the heart. The organs are not drawn to scale. Observe that three shunts permit most of the blood to bypass the liver and lungs: (1) ductus venosus, (2) foramen ovale, and (3) ductus arteriosus. The poorly oxygenated blood returns to the placenta for oxygen and nutrients through the umbilical arteries. (From Moore KL, Persaud TVN: *Before we are born: essentials of embryology and birth defects,* ed 6, Philadelphia, 2003, WB Saunders.)

passes through the ductus venosus into the inferior vena cava. There it mixes with the deoxygenated blood from the fetal legs and abdomen on its way to the right atrium. Most of this blood passes straight through the right atrium and through the foramen ovale, an opening into the left atrium. There it mixes with the small amount of deoxygenated blood returning from the fetal lungs through the pulmonary veins.

The blood flows into the left ventricle and is squeezed out into the aorta, where the arteries supplying the heart, head, neck, and arms receive most of the oxygen-rich blood. This pattern of supplying the highest levels of oxygen and nutrients to the head, neck, and arms enhances the cephalocaudal (head-to-rump) development of the embryo/fetus.

Deoxygenated blood returning from the head and arms enters the right atrium through the superior vena cava. This blood is directed downward into the right ventricle, where it is squeezed into the pulmonary artery. A small amount of blood circulates through the resistant lung tissue, but the majority follows the path with less resistance through the ductus arteriosus into the aorta, distal to the point of exit of the arteries supplying the head and arms with oxygenated blood. The oxygen-poor blood flows through the abdominal aorta into the internal iliac arteries, where the umbilical arteries direct most of it back through the umbilical cord to the placenta. There the blood gives up its wastes and carbon dioxide in exchange for nutrients and oxygen. The blood remaining in the iliac arteries flows through the fetal abdomen and legs, ultimately returning through the inferior vena cava to the heart.

The following three special characteristics enable the fetus to obtain sufficient oxygen from the maternal blood:

- Fetal hemoglobin carries 20% to 30% more oxygen than maternal hemoglobin.
- The hemoglobin concentration of the fetus is about 50% greater than that of the mother.
- The fetal heart rate (FHR) is 110 to 160 beats/min, making the cardiac output per unit of body weight higher than that of an adult.

Hematopoietic System

Hematopoiesis, the formation of blood, occurs in the yolk sac (see Fig. 8-8, *B*) beginning in the third week. Hematopoietic stem cells seed the fetal liver during the fifth week, and hematopoiesis begins there during the sixth week. This accounts for the relatively large size of the liver between the seventh and ninth weeks. Stem cells seed the fetal bone marrow, spleen and thymus, and lymph nodes between weeks 8 and 11.

The antigenic factors that determine blood type are present in the erythrocytes soon after the sixth week. For this reason the Rh-negative woman is at risk for isoimmunization in any pregnancy that lasts longer than 6 weeks after fertilization.

Hepatic System

The liver and biliary tract develop from the foregut during the fourth week of gestation. Hematopoiesis begins during the sixth week and requires that the liver be large. The embryonic liver is prominent, occupying most of the abdominal cavity. Bile, a constituent of meconium, begins to form in the twelfth week.

Glycogen is stored in the fetal liver beginning at week 9 or 10. At term, glycogen stores are twice those of the adult. Glycogen is the major source of energy for the fetus and for the neonate stressed by in utero hypoxia, extrauterine loss of the maternal glucose supply, the work of breathing, or cold stress. Iron is also stored in the fetal liver. If maternal intake is sufficient, the fetus can store enough iron to last for 5 months after birth.

During fetal life the liver does not have to conjugate bilirubin for excretion because the unconjugated bilirubin is cleared by the placenta. Therefore the glucuronyl transferase enzyme needed for conjugation is present in the fetal liver in amounts less than those required after birth. This predisposes the neonate, especially the preterm infant, to hyperbilirubinemia.

Coagulation factors II, VII, IX, and X cannot be synthesized in the fetal liver because of the lack of vitamin K synthesis in the sterile fetal gut. This coagulation deficiency persists after birth for several days and is the rationale for the prophylactic administration of vitamin K to the newborn.

Gastrointestinal System

During the fourth week the shape of the embryo changes from being almost straight to a C shape as both ends fold in toward the ventral surface. A portion of the yolk sac is incorporated into the body from head to tail as the primitive gut (digestive system).

The foregut produces the pharynx, part of the lower respiratory tract, the esophagus, the stomach, the first half of the duodenum, the liver, the pancreas, and the gallbladder. These structures evolve during the fifth and sixth weeks. Malformations that can occur in these areas include esophageal atresia, hypertrophic pyloric stenosis, duodenal stenosis or atresia, and biliary atresia.

The midgut becomes the distal half of the duodenum, the jejunum and ileum, the cecum and appendix, and the proximal half of the colon. The midgut loop projects into the umbilical cord between weeks 5 and 10. A malformation (or omphalocele) results if the midgut fails to return to the abdominal cavity, causing the intestines to protrude from the umbilicus. Meckel's diverticulum is the most common malformation of the midgut. It occurs when a remnant of the yolk stalk that has failed to degenerate attaches to the ileum, leaving a blind sac.

The hindgut develops into the distal half of the colon, the rectum and parts of the anal canal, the urinary bladder, and the urethra. Anorectal malformations are the most common abnormalities of the digestive system.

The fetus swallows amniotic fluid beginning in the fifth month. Gastric emptying and intestinal peristalsis occur. Fetal nutrition and elimination needs are taken care of by the placenta. As the fetus nears term, fetal waste products accumulate in the intestines as dark green to black, tarry meconium. Normally this substance is passed through the rectum within 24 hours of birth. Sometimes with a breech presentation or fetal hypoxia, meconium is passed in utero into the amniotic fluid. The failure to pass meconium after birth may indicate atresia somewhere in the digestive tract; an imperforate anus; or meconium ileus, in which a firm meconium plug blocks passage (seen in infants with cystic fibrosis).

The metabolic rate of the fetus is relatively low, but the infant has great growth and development needs. Beginning in week 9 the fetus synthesizes glycogen for storage in the liver. Between 26 and 30 weeks the fetus begins to lay down stores of brown fat in preparation for extrauterine cold stress. Thermoregulation in the neonate requires increased metabolism and adequate oxygenation.

The gastrointestinal system is mature by 36 weeks. Digestive enzymes (except pancreatic amylase and lipase) are present in sufficient quantity to facilitate digestion. The neonate cannot digest starches or fats efficiently. Little saliva is produced.

Renal System

The kidneys form during the fifth week and begin to function approximately 4 weeks later. Urine is excreted into the amniotic fluid and forms a major part of the amniotic fluid volume. Oligohydramnios is indicative of renal dysfunction. Because the placenta acts as the organ of excretion and maintains fetal water and electrolyte balance, the fetus does not need functioning kidneys while in utero. At birth, however, the kidneys are required immediately for excretory and acid-base regulatory functions.

A fetal renal malformation can be diagnosed in utero. Corrective or palliative fetal surgery may treat the malformation successfully, or plans can be made for treatment immediately after birth.

At term the fetus has fully developed kidneys. However, the glomerular filtration rate (GFR) is low, and the kidneys lack the ability to concentrate urine. This makes the newborn more susceptible to both overhydration and dehydration.

Most newborns void within 24 hours of birth. With the loss of the swallowed amniotic fluid and the metabolism of nutrients provided by the placenta, voidings for the first days of life are scant until fluid intake increases.

Neurologic System

The nervous system originates from the ectoderm during the third week after fertilization. The open neural tube forms during the fourth week. It initially closes at what will be the junction of the brain and spinal cord, leaving both ends open. The embryo folds in on itself lengthwise at this time, forming a head fold in the neural tube at this junction. The cranial end of the neural tube closes, then the caudal end closes. During week 5, different growth rates cause more flexures in the neural tube, delineating three brain areas: the forebrain, midbrain, and hindbrain.

The forebrain develops into the eyes (cranial nerve II) and cerebral hemispheres. The development of all areas of the cerebral cortex continues throughout fetal life and into childhood. The olfactory system (cranial nerve I) and thalamus also develop from the forebrain. Cranial nerves III and IV (oculomotor and trochlear) form from the midbrain. The hindbrain forms the medulla, the pons, the cerebellum, and the remainder of the cranial nerves. Brain waves can be recorded on an electroencephalogram by week 8.

The spinal cord develops from the long end of the neural tube. Another ectodermal structure, the neural crest, develops into the peripheral nervous system. By the eighth week, nerve fibers traverse throughout the body. By week 11 or 12 the fetus makes respiratory movements, moves all extremities, and changes position in utero. The fetus can suck his or her thumb, swim in the amniotic fluid pool, and turn somersaults, and sometimes ties a knot in the umbilical cord. Box 8-5 describes the major types of fetal movements. Sometime between 16 and 20 weeks, when the movements are strong enough to be perceived by the mother as "the baby moving," quickening has occurred. The perception of movement occurs earlier in the multipara than in the primipara. The mother also becomes aware of the sleep and wake cycles of the fetus.

Sensory Awareness

Purposeful movements of the fetus have been demonstrated in response to a firm touch transmitted through the mother's abdomen. Because it can feel, the fetus requires anesthesia when invasive procedures are done.

Fetuses respond to sound by 24 weeks. Different types of music evoke different movements. The fetus can be soothed by the sound of the mother's voice. Acoustic stimulation can be used to evoke a fetal heart rate response. The fetus becomes accustomed (habituates) to noises heard repeatedly. Hearing is fully developed at birth.

The fetus is able to distinguish taste. By the fifth month, when the fetus is swallowing amniotic fluid, a sweetener

BOX 8-5

Major Types of Fetal Movements

General movements. These slow, gross movements involve the whole body. Their duration is from several seconds to a minute.

Startle movements. These quick (less than 1 second), generalized movements always start in the limbs and may spread to the trunk and neck.

Hiccups. These are repetitive phasic contractions of the diaphragm. A bout may last several minutes.

Fetal breathing movements. These are paradoxic movements in which the thorax moves inward and the abdomen outward with each contraction of the diaphragm.

Isolated arm or leg movements. These movements of extremities occur without movement of the trunk.

Hand-face contact. This occurs any time the moving hand makes contact with the face or mouth.

Retroflexion of the head. This is a slow to jerky backward bending of the head.

Lateral rotation of the head. This involves isolated turning of the head from side to side.

Anteflexion of the head. This is a normally slow forward bending of the head.

Opening of the mouth. This isolated movement may be accompanied by protrusion of the tongue.

Yawn. The mouth is slowly opened and rapidly closed after a few seconds.

Sucking. This burst of rhythmic jaw movements is sometimes followed by swallowing. With this movement the fetus may be drinking amniotic fluid.

Stretch. This complex movement involves overextension of the spine, retroflexion of the head, and elevation of the arms.

From Carlson B: *Human embryology and developmental biology,* ed 3, St Louis, 2004, Mosby.

added to the fluid causes the fetus to swallow faster. The fetus also reacts to temperature changes. A cold solution placed into the amniotic fluid can cause fetal hiccups.

The fetus can see. Eyes have both rods and cones in the retina by the seventh month. A bright light shone on the mother's abdomen in late pregnancy causes abrupt fetal movements. During sleep time, rapid eye movements (REMs) have been observed similar to those occurring in children and adults while dreaming.

At term the fetal brain is approximately one fourth the size of an adult brain. Neurologic development continues. Stressors on the fetus and neonate (e.g., chronic poor nutrition or hypoxia, drugs, environmental toxins, trauma, or disease) cause damage to the central nervous system long after the vulnerable embryonic time for malformations in other organ systems. Neurologic insult can result in cerebral palsy, neuromuscular impairment, mental retardation, and learning disabilities.

Endocrine System

The thyroid gland develops along with structures in the head and neck during the third and fourth weeks. The secretion of thyroxine begins during the eighth week. Maternal thyroxine does not readily cross the placenta; therefore the fetus that does not produce thyroid hormones will be born with congenital hypothyroidism. If untreated, hypothyroidism can result in severe mental retardation. Screening for hypothyroidism is typically included in the testing when screening for PKU after birth.

The adrenal cortex is formed during the sixth week and produces hormones by the eighth or ninth week. As term approaches, the fetus produces more cortisol. This is believed to aid in initiation of labor by decreasing the maternal progesterone and stimulating production of prostaglandins.

The pancreas forms from the foregut during the fifth through eighth weeks. The islets of Langerhans develop during the twelfth week. Insulin is produced by the twentieth week. In infants of mothers with uncontrolled diabetes, maternal hyperglycemia produces fetal hyperglycemia, stimulating hyperinsulinemia and islet cell hyperplasia. This results in a macrosomatic (large-sized) fetus. The hyperinsulinemia also blocks lung maturation, placing the neonate at risk for respiratory distress and hypoglycemia when the maternal glucose source is lost at birth. Control of the maternal glucose level before and during pregnancy minimizes problems for the fetus and infant.

Reproductive System

Sex differentiation begins in the embryo during the seventh week. Distinguishing characteristics appear around the ninth week and are fully differentiated by the twelfth week. When a Y chromosome is present, testes are formed. By the end of the embryonic period, testosterone is being secreted and causes formation of the male genitalia. By week 28 the testes begin descending into the scrotum. After birth, low levels of testosterone continue to be secreted until the pubertal surge.

The female, with two X chromosomes, forms ovaries and female external genitalia. By the sixteenth week, oogenesis has been established. At birth the ovaries contain the female's lifetime supply of ova. Most female hormone production is delayed until puberty. However, the fetal endometrium responds to maternal hormones, and withdrawal bleeding or vaginal discharge (pseudomenstruation) may occur at birth when these hormones are lost. The high level of maternal estrogen also stimulates mammary engorgement and secretion of fluid ("witch's milk") in newborn infants of both sexes.

Musculoskeletal System

Bones and muscles develop from the mesoderm by the fourth week of embryonic development. At that time the cardiac muscle is already beating. The mesoderm next to the neural tube forms the vertebral column and ribs. The parts of the vertebral column grow toward each other to enclose the developing spinal cord. Ossification, or bone formation, begins. If there is a defect in the bony fusion, various forms of spina bifida may occur. A large defect affecting several vertebrae may allow the membranes and spinal cord to pouch out from the back, producing neurologic deficits and skeletal deformity.

The flat bones of the skull develop during the embryonic period, and ossification continues throughout childhood. At birth, connective tissue sutures exist where the bones of the skull meet. The areas where more than two bones meet (called fontanels) are especially prominent. The sutures and fontanels allow the bones of the skull to mold, or move during birth, enabling the head to pass through the birth canal.

The bones of the shoulders, arms, hips, and legs appear in the sixth week as a continuous skeleton with no joints. Differentiation occurs, producing separate bones and joints. Ossification will continue through childhood to allow growth. Beginning in the seventh week, muscles contract spontaneously. Arm and leg movements are visible on ultrasound, although the mother does not perceive them until sometime between 16 and 20 weeks.

Integumentary System

The epidermis begins as a single layer of cells derived from the ectoderm at 4 weeks. By the seventh week, there are two layers of cells. The cells of the superficial layer are sloughed and become mixed with the sebaceous gland secretions to form the white, cheesy vernix caseosa, the material that protects the skin of the fetus. The vernix is thick at 24 weeks but becomes scant by term.

The basal layer of the epidermis is the germinal layer, which replaces lost cells. Until 17 weeks the skin is thin and wrinkled, with blood vessels visible underneath. The skin thickens, and all layers are present at term. After 32 weeks, as subcutaneous fat is deposited under the dermis, the skin becomes less wrinkled and red in appearance.

By 16 weeks the epidermal ridges are present on the palms of the hands, the fingers, the bottom of the feet, and the toes. These handprints and footprints are unique to that infant.

Hairs form from hair bulbs in the epidermis that project into the dermis. Cells in the hair bulb keratinize to form the hair shaft. As the cells at the base of the hair shaft proliferate, the hair grows to the surface of the epithelium. Very fine hairs, called lanugo, appear first at 12 weeks on the eyebrows and upper lip. By 20 weeks they cover the entire body. At this time the eyelashes, eyebrows, and scalp hair are beginning to grow. By 28 weeks the scalp hair is longer than the lanugo, which thins and may disappear by term gestation.

Fingernails and toenails develop from thickened epidermis at the tips of the digits beginning during the tenth week. They grow slowly. Fingernails usually reach the fingertips by 32 weeks, and toenails reach toetips by 36 weeks.

Immunologic System

During the third trimester, albumin and globulin are present in the fetus. The only immunoglobulin (Ig) that crosses the placenta, IgG, provides passive acquired immunity to specific bacterial toxins. The fetus produces IgM immunoglobulins by the end of the first trimester. These are produced in response to blood group antigens, gram-negative enteric organisms, and some viruses. IgA immunoglobulins are not produced by the fetus; however, colostrum, the precursor to breast milk, contains large amounts of IgA and can provide passive immunity to the neonate who is breastfed (Table 8-1).

The normal term neonate can fight infection, but not as effectively as an older child. The preterm infant is at much greater risk for infection.

Table 8-2 summarizes embryonic and fetal development.

Multifetal Pregnancy

Twins

The incidence of twinning is 1 in 43 pregnancies (Benirschke, 2004). There has been a steady rise in multiple births since 1973. This is partly attributed to delayed childbearing. The use of ovulation-enhancing drugs is also a factor.

Dizygotic Twins

When two mature ova are produced in one ovarian cycle, both have the potential to be fertilized by separate sperm. This results in two zygotes, or dizygotic twins (Fig. 8-13). There are always two amnions, two chorions, and two placentas that may be fused together. These dizygotic or fraternal twins may be the same sex or different sexes and are genetically no more alike than siblings born at different times. Dizygotic twinning occurs in families, is more common among African-American women than Caucasian women, and is least common among Asian-American women. Dizygotic twinning increases in frequency with maternal age up to 35 years, with parity, and with the use of fertility drugs.

Monozygotic Twins

Identical or monozygotic twins develop from one fertilized ovum, which then divides (Fig. 8-14). They are the same sex and have the same genotype. If division occurs soon after fertilization, two embryos, two amnions, two chorions, and two placentas that may be fused will develop. Most often, division occurs between 4 and 8 days after fertilization, and there are two embryos, two amnions, one chorion, and one placenta. Rarely, division occurs after the eighth day following fertilization. In this case there are two embryos within a common amnion and a common chorion with one placenta. This often causes circulatory problems because the umbilical cords may tangle together, and one or both fetuses may die. If division occurs very late, cleavage may not be complete, and conjoined or "Siamese" twins could result. Monozygotic twinning occurs in approximately 1 of 250 births (Benirschke, 2004). There is no association with race, heredity, maternal age, or parity. Fertility drugs increase the incidence of monozygotic twinning.

Other Multifetal Pregnancies

The occurrence of multifetal pregnancies with three or more fetuses has increased with the use of fertility drugs and in vitro fertilization. Triplets occur in about 1 of 1341 pregnancies (Benirschke, 2004). They can occur from the division of one zygote into two, with one of the two dividing again, producing identical triplets. Triplets can also be produced from two zygotes, one dividing into a set of identical twins and the second zygote a single fraternal sibling, or from three zygotes. Quadruplets, quintuplets, sextuplets, and so on have similar possible derivations.

Table 8-1

Characteristics of Immunoglobulins

CLASS	LOCATION	CHARACTERISTICS
IgG	Plasma, interstitial fluid	Only immunoglobulin that crosses placenta Responsible for secondary immune response
IgA	Body secretions, including tears, saliva, breast milk, colostrum	Lines mucous membranes and protects body surfaces
IgM	Plasma	Responsible for primary immune response Forms antibodies to ABO blood antigens
IgD	Plasma	Present on lymphocyte surface Assists in the differentiation of B lymphocytes
IgE	Plasma, interstitial fluids	Causes symptoms of allergic reactions Fixes to mast cells and basophils Assists in defense against parasitic infections

Modified from Lewis SM, Heitkemper MM, Dirksen SR: *Medical-surgical nursing: assessment and management of clinical problems,* ed 6, St Louis, 2004, Mosby.

Table 8-2

Milestones in Human Development before Birth since Last Menstrual Period (LMP)

4 WEEKS	8 WEEKS	12 WEEKS
EXTERNAL APPEARANCE		
Body flexed, C shaped; arm and leg buds present; head at right angles to body	Body fairly well formed; nose flat, eyes far apart; digits well formed; head elevating; tail almost disappeared; eyes, ears, nose, and mouth recognizable	Nails appearing; resembles a human; head erect but disproportionately large; skin pink, delicate
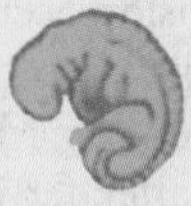	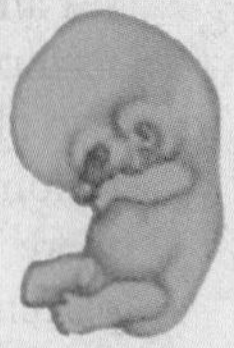	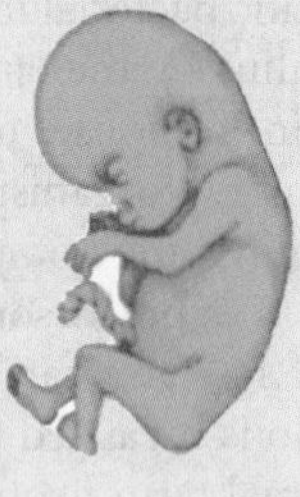
CROWN-TO-RUMP MEASUREMENT; WEIGHT		
0.4 to 0.5 cm; 0.4 g	2.5 to 3 cm; 2 g	6 to 9 cm; 19 g
GASTROINTESTINAL SYSTEM		
Stomach at midline and fusiform; conspicuous liver; esophagus short; intestine a short tube	Intestinal villi developing; small intestines coil within umbilical cord; palatal folds present; liver very large	Bile secreted; palatal fushion complete; intestines have withdrawn from cord and assume characteristic positions
MUSCULOSKELETAL SYSTEM		
All somites present	First indication of ossification—occiput, mandible, and humerus; fetus capable of some movement; definitive muscles of trunk, limbs, and head well represented	Some bones well outlined, ossification spreading; upper cervical to lower sacral arches and bodies ossify; smooth muscle layers indicated in hollow viscera
CIRCULATORY SYSTEM		
Heart develops, double chambers visible, begins to beat; aortic arch and major veins completed	Main blood vessels assume final plan; enucleated red cells predominate in blood	Blood forming in marrow
RESPIRATORY SYSTEM		
Primary lung buds appear	Pleural and pericardial cavities forming; branching bronchioles; nostrils closed by epithelial plugs	Lungs acquire definite shape; vocal cords appear
RENAL SYSTEM		
Rudimentary ureteral buds appear	Earliest secretory tubules differentiating; bladder-urethra separates from rectum	Kidney able to secrete urine; bladder expands as a sac
NERVOUS SYSTEM		
Well-marked midbrain flexure; no hindbrain or cervical flexures; neural groove closed	Cerebral cortex begins to acquire typical cells; differentiation of cerebral cortex, meninges, ventricular foramina, cerebrospinal fluid circulation; spinal cord extends entire length of spine	Brain structural configuration almost complete; cord shows cervical and lumbar enlargements; fourth ventricle foramina are developed; sucking present
SENSORY ORGANS		
Eye and ear appearing as optic vessel and otocyst	Primordial choroid plexuses develop; ventricles large relative to cortex; development progressing; eyes converging rapidly; internal ear developing	Earliest taste buds indicated; characteristic organization of eye attained
GENITAL SYSTEM		
Genital ridge appears (fifth week)	Testes and ovaries distinguishable; external genitalia sexless but begin to differentiate	Sex recognizable; internal and external sex organs specific

16 WEEKS	20 WEEKS	24 WEEKS
EXTERNAL APPEARANCE		
Head still dominant; face looks human; eyes, ears, and nose approach typical appearance on gross examination; arm/leg ratio proportionate; scalp hair appears	Vernix caseosa appears; lanugo appears; legs lengthen considerably; sebaceous glands appear	Body lean but fairly well proportioned; skin red and wrinkled; vernix caseosa present; sweat glands forming
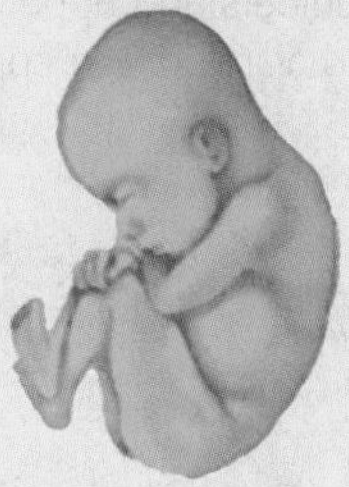	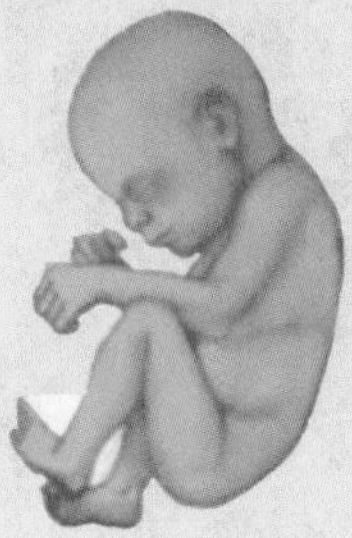	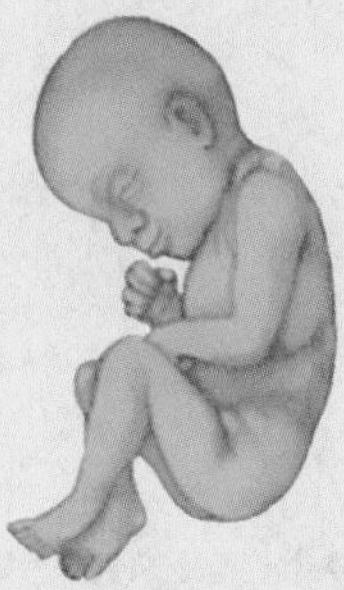
CROWN-TO-RUMP MEASUREMENT; WEIGHT		
11.5 to 13.5 cm; 100 g	16 to 18.5 cm; 300 g	23 cm; 600 g
GASTROINTESTINAL SYSTEM		
Meconium in bowel; some enzyme secretion; anus open	Enamel and dentine depositing; ascending colon recognizable	
MUSCULOSKELETAL SYSTEM		
Most bones distinctly indicated throughout body; joint cavities appear; muscular movements can be detected	Sternum ossifies; fetal movements strong enough for mother to feel	
CIRCULATORY SYSTEM		
Heart muscle well developed; blood formation active in spleen		Blood formation increases in bone marrow and decreases in liver
RESPIRATORY SYSTEM		
Elastic fibers appear in lungs; terminal and respiratory bronchioles appear	Nostrils reopen; primitive respiratory-like movements begin	Alveolar ducts and sacs present; lecithin begins to appear in amniotic fluid (weeks 26 to 27)
RENAL SYSTEM		
Kidney in position; attains typical shape and plan		
NERVOUS SYSTEM		
Cerebral lobes delineated; cerebellum assumes some prominence	Brain grossly formed; cord myelination begins; spinal cord ends at level of first sacral vertebra (S-1)	Cerebral cortex layered typically; neuronal proliferation in cerebral cortex ends
SENSORY ORGANS		
General sense organs differentiated	Nose and ears ossify	Can hear
GENITAL SYSTEM		
Testes in position for descent into scrotum: vagina open		Testes at inguinal ring in descent to scrotum

Continued

Table 8-2

Milestones in Human Development before Birth since Last Menstrual Period (LMP)—cont'd

28 WEEKS	30-31 WEEKS	36 AND 40 WEEKS
EXTERNAL APPEARANCE		
Lean body, less wrinkled and red; nails appear	Subcutaneous fat beginning to collect; more rounded appearance; skin pink and smooth; has assumed birth position 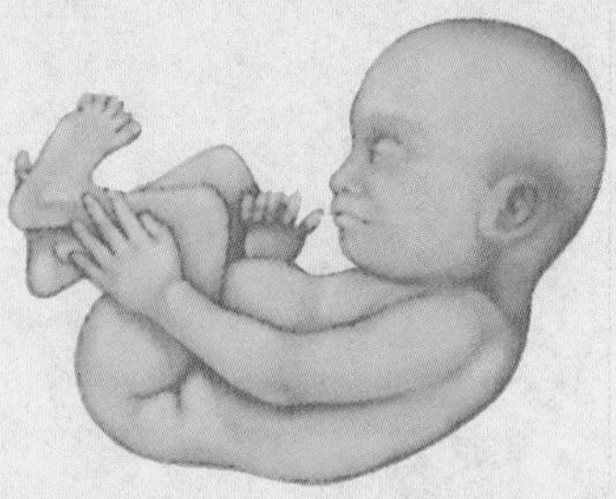	**36 Weeks** Skin pink, body rounded; general lanugo disappearing; body usually plump **40 Weeks** Skin smooth and pink; scant vernix caseosa; moderate to profuse hair; lanugo on shoulders and upper body only; nasal and alar cartilage apparent
CROWN-TO-RUMP MEASUREMENT; WEIGHT		
27 cm; 1100 g	31 cm; 1800 to 2100 g	**36 Weeks** 35 cm; 2200 to 2900 g **40 Weeks** 40 cm: 3200+ g
MUSCULOSKELETAL SYSTEM		
Astragalus (talus, ankle bone) ossifies; weak, fleeting movements, minimum tone	Middle fourth phalanxes ossify; permanent teeth primordia seen; can turn head to side	**36 Weeks** Distal femoral ossification centers present; sustained, definite movements; fair tone; can turn and elevate head **40 Weeks** Active, sustained movement; good tone; may lift head
RESPIRATORY SYSTEM		
Lecithin forming on alveolar surfaces	L/S ratio = 1.2:1	**36 Weeks** L/S ratio ≥2:1 **40 Weeks** Pulmonary branching only two-thirds complete
RENAL SYSTEM		**36 Weeks** Formation of new nephrons ceases
NERVOUS SYSTEM		
Appearance of cerebral fissures, convolutions rapidly appearing; indefinite sleep-wake cycle; cry weak or absent; weak suck reflex		**36 Weeks** End of spinal cord at level of third lumbar vertebra (L-3); definite sleep-wake cycle **40 Weeks** Myelination of brain begins; patterned sleep-wake cycle with alert periods; cries when hungry or uncomfortable; strong suck reflex
SENSORY ORGANS		
Eyelids reopen; retinal layers completed, light receptive; pupils capable of reacting to light	Sense of taste present; aware of sounds outside mother's body	
GENITAL SYSTEM		
	Testes descending to scrotum	**40 Weeks** Testes in scrotum; labia majora well developed

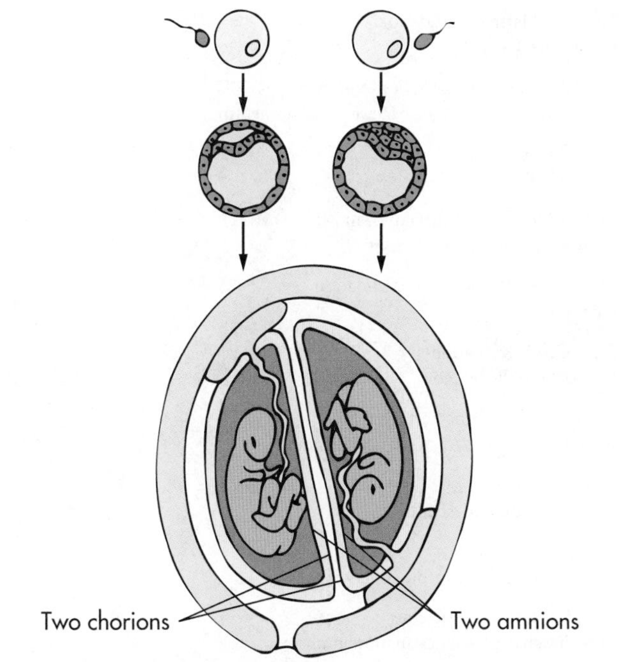

Fig. 8-13 Formation of dizygotic twins. There is fertilization of two ova, two implantations, two placentas, two chorions, and two amnions.

Key Points

- Genetic disease affects people of all ages, from all socioeconomic levels, and from all racial and ethnic backgrounds.
- Genetic disorders span every clinical practice specialty.
- Nurses with advanced preparation are assuming important roles in genetic counseling.
- Genes are the basic units of heredity responsible for all human characteristics. They comprise 23 pairs of chromosomes: 22 pairs of autosomes and one pair of sex chromosomes.
- Genetic disorders follow mendelian inheritance patterns of dominance, segregation, and independent assortment of normal genetic transmission.
- Multifactorial inheritance includes both genetic and environmental contributions.
- Human gestation is approximately 280 days after the LMP or 266 days after conception.
- Fertilization occurs in the uterine tube within 24 hours of ovulation. The zygote undergoes mitotic divisions, creating a 16-cell morula.

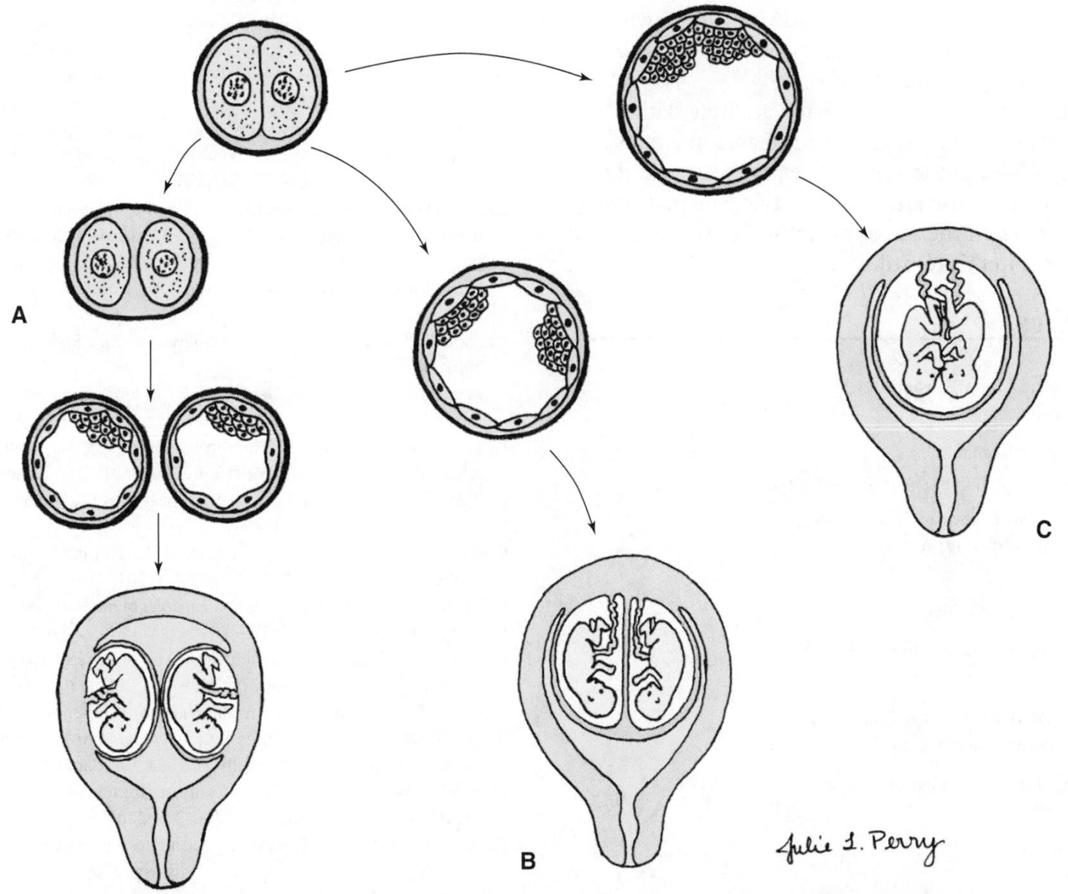

Fig. 8-14 Formation of monozygotic twins. **A**, One fertilization: blastomeres separate, resulting in two implantations, two placentas, and two sets of membranes. **B**, One blastomere with two inner cell masses, one fused placenta, one chorion, and separate amnions. **C**, One blastomere with incomplete separation of cell mass resulting in conjoined twins.

- Critical periods occur in human development during which the embryo/fetus is vulnerable to environmental teratogens.

Answer Guidelines to Critical Thinking Exercise

Ultrasound Dating of Pregnancy

1. Yes. Ultrasound dating of pregnancies is well established. The nurse can use photographs or drawings of a fetus to educate Sandra about the appearance of a fetus at different gestational ages. In addition, charts of embryonic development including critical periods of development can be used.
2. The nurse can assume the following: (a) Sandra wants to learn about fetal development. (b) Depending on prior education, Sandra may know little about embryonic and fetal development. (c) Sandra has the right to know the risks and benefits of ultrasound examination and to give informed consent for the procedure. (d) Dating the pregnancy is important to identify and prepare for variations from normal.
3. Priorities for nursing care include educating Sandra about fetal development, ensuring that she is aware of the risks and benefits of ultrasound testing, obtaining a signature for the procedure on a consent form (if her physician has not already done so), informing Sandra what ultrasound testing entails, and providing support as necessary during the procedure.
4. Yes. Ultrasound testing can provide accurate dating of a pregnancy and detect structural anomalies in a fetus.
5. Sandra has the right to refuse to learn about fetal development and to refuse ultrasound testing. She may or may not want to learn the sex of the fetus; her wishes should be respected in this regard.

Resources

Alliance of Genetic Support Groups
www.geneticalliance.org

Ask NOAH About: Pregnancy
www.noah.cuny.edu/pregnancy/pregnancy.html

Family Guide to Cystic Fibrosis Genetic Testing
www.phd.msu.edu/cf/fam.html

Gene Tests
www.hslib.washington.edu/helix

International Society of Nurses in Genetics (ISONG)
www.nursing.creighton.edu/isong

MEDLINE: PubMed and Internet Grateful Med
www.nlm.nih.gov/databases/freemedl.html

National Center for Human Genome Research
www.nhgri.nih.gov

National Down Syndrome Society
www.ndss.org

National Fragile X Foundation
www.nfxf.org

National Marfan Foundation
www.marfan.org

National Society of Genetic Counselors
http://members.aol.com/nsgcweb/nsgchome.htm

Neurofibromatosis
www.nf.org/

Online Mendelian Inheritance in Man (OMIM)
www.ncbi.nlm.nih.gov/Omim

Osteogenesis Imperfecta Foundation
www.oif.org

Stem Cell Information
http://stemcells.nih.gov

Understanding Gene Testing
www.gene.com/ae/AE/AEPC/NIH/index.html

Visible Embryo
http://visembryo.ucsf.edu

Webget
http://med.upenn.edu/bioethic/webget

World of Genetics Societies
http://faseb.org/genetics/mainmenu.htm

References

Anderson G: Storytelling: a holistic foundation for genetic nursing, *Holist Nurs Pract* 12(3):64-76, 1998.

Anderson G et al: Preparing the nursing profession for participation in a genetic paradigm in health care, *Nurs Outlook* 48(1):23-27, 2000.

Anderson WF: Gene therapy: the best of times, the worst of times, *Science* 288(5466):627-628, 2000.

Benirschke K: Multiple gestation. The biology of twinning. In Creasy RK, Resnik R, Iams JD (eds): *Maternal-fetal medicine: principles and practice,* ed 5, Philadelphia, 2004, WB Saunders.

Brower V: Gene therapy revisited: in spite of problems and drawbacks, gene therapy moves forward, *EMBO Rep* 2(12):1064-1065, 2001.

Burke W, Pinsky LE, Press NA: Categorizing genetic tests to identify their ethical, legal, and social implications, *Am J Med Genet* 106(3):233-240, 2001.

Carlson B: *Human embryology and developmental biology,* ed 3, St Louis, 2004, Mosby.

Cavazzana-Calvo M et al: Gene therapy of human severe combined immunodeficiency (SCID)-X1 disease, *Science* 288(5466):669-672, 2000.

Collins F, Mansoura M: The Human Genome Project: revealing the shared inheritance of all humankind, *Cancer Suppl* 91:221-225, 2001.

Collins FS, Guttmacher AE: Genetics moves into the medical mainstream, *JAMA* 286(18):2322-2324, 2001.

Collins FS, McKusick VA: Implications of the Human Genome Project for medical science, *JAMA* 285(5):540-544, 2001.

Gelehrter T, Collins F, Ginsberg D: *Principles of medical genetics,* ed 2, Baltimore, 1998, Williams & Wilkins.

Giarelli E, Jacobs L: Issues related to the use of genetic material and information, *Oncol Nurs Forum* 27(3):459-467, 2000.

Hamilton BA, Wynshaw-Boris A: Basic genetics and patterns of inheritance. In Creasy RK, Resnik R, Iams JD (eds): *Maternal-fetal medicine: principles and practice,* ed 5, Philadelphia, 2004, WB Saunders.

Hassold T, Hunt P: To err (meiotically) is human: the genesis of human aneuploidy, *Nat Rev Genet* 2(4):280-291, 2001.

Hudgins L, Cassidy SB: Congenital anomalies. In Fanaroff AA, Martin RJ (eds): *Neonatal-perinatal medicine: diseases of the fetus and infant,* ed 7, St Louis, 2002, Mosby.

International Human Genome Sequencing Consortium: Initial sequencing and analysis of the human genome, *Nature* 409(6822):860-921, 2001.

International Society of Nurses in Genetics (ISONG): *Statement on the scope and standards of genetics clinical nursing practice,* Washington, DC, 1998, American Nurses Association.

Jenkins TM, Wapner RJ: Prenatal diagnosis of congenital disorders. In Creasy RK, Resnik R, Iams JD (eds): *Maternal-fetal medicine: principles and practice,* ed 5, Philadelphia, 2004, WB Saunders.

Jones K: *Smith's recognizable patterns of human malformation,* ed 5, Philadelphia, 1997, WB Saunders.

Jones SL, Fallon LA: Reproductive options for individuals at risk for transmission of a genetic disorder, *J Obstet Gynecol Neonat Nurs* 31(2):193-199, 2002.

Kay M et al: Evidence for gene transfer and expression of factor IX in haemophilia B patients treated with an AAV vector, *Nat Genet* 24(3):257-261, 2000.

Langley L et al: *Dynamic human anatomy and physiology,* ed 5, New York, 1980, McGraw-Hill.

Lashley F: *Clinical genetics in nursing practice,* ed 2, New York, 1998, Springer.

Lea D, Jenkins J, Francomano C: *Genetics in clinical practice: new directions for nursing and health care,* Sudbury, MA, 1998, Jones & Bartlett.

Lea DH, Feetham SL, Monsen RB: Genomic-based health care in nursing: a bi-directional approach to bringing genetics into nursing's body of knowledge, *J Prof Nurs* 18(3):120-129, 2002.

Lewis SM, Heitkemper MM, Dirksen SR: *Medical-surgical nursing: assessment and management of clinical problems,* ed 6, St Louis, 2004, Mosby.

Lumley J et al: Periconceptional supplementation with folate and/or multivitamins for preventing neural tube defects (Cochrane Review), 2001. In *The Cochrane Library,* Issue 2, Chichester, UK, 2004, John Wiley & Sons.

McGowan R: Beyond the disorder: one parent's reflection on genetic counseling, *J Med Ethics* 25(2):195-199, 1999.

McInerney J: What is behavioral genetics? Human Genome Project Information. Internet document available at www.ornl.bov/sci/techresources/Human_Genome/elsi/behavior.shtml (accessed August 12, 2004).

McInerney J, Rothstein M: *What implications does behavioral genetics research have for society?* Human Genome Project Information. Internet document available at www.ornl.bov/sci/techresources/Human_Genome/elsi/behavior.shtml (accessed August 12, 2004).

Mercer BM: Assessment and induction of fetal pulmonary maturity. In Creasy RK, Resnik R, Iams JD (eds): *Maternal-fetal medicine: principles and practice,* ed 5, Philadelphia, 2004, WB Saunders.

Moore KL, Persaud TVN: *Before we are born: essentials of embryology and birth defects,* ed 6, Philadelphia, 2003, WB Saunders.

Mueller R, Young I: *Emery's elements of medical genetics,* ed 11, New York, 2001, Churchill Livingstone.

National Institutes of Health: *NIH publishes final guidelines for stem cell research.* News release. Internet document available at www.nih.gov/news/pr/aug2000 (accessed December 13, 2004).

National Institutes of Health: *Stem cells: scientific progress and future research directions,* 2001. Internet document available at www.nih.gov/news/stemcell/scireport.htm (accessed June 9, 2002).

Phillips KA et al: Potential role of pharmacogenomics in reducing adverse drug reactions, *JAMA* 286(18):2270-2279, 2001.

Roses A: Pharmacogenetics and the practice of medicine, *Nature* 405:857-865, 2000.

Scheuerle A: Diagnosis of genetic disease. In Mahowald M et al (eds): *Genetics in the clinic: clinical, ethical, and social implications for primary care,* St Louis, 2001, Mosby.

Scialli A: Toxicology, *Contemp Ob Gyn* 42(5):15, 1997.

Silver RM, Peltier MR, Branch EW: The immunology of pregnancy. In Creasy RK, Resnik R, Iams JD (eds): *Maternal-fetal medicine: principles and practice,* ed 5, Philadelphia, 2004, WB Saunders.

Simpson JL, Elias S: *Genetics in obstetrics and gynecology,* Philadelphia, 2003, WB Saunders.

Thomson JA et al: Embryonic stem cell lines derived from human blastocysts, *Science* 282, 1145-1147, 1998.

White M: Making responsible decisions: an interpretive ethic for genetic decision-making, *Hastings Cent Rep* 29(1):14-21, 1999.

Yoon PW et al: Public health impact of genetic tests at the end of the 20th century, *Genet Med* 3(6):405-410, 2001.

Unit 3

9 Assessment for Risk Factors

LEARNING OBJECTIVES

On completion of this chapter the reader will be able to:

- Explore the scope of high risk pregnancy.
- Discuss regionalization of health care services.
- Examine risk factors identified through history, physical examination, and diagnostic techniques.
- Describe diagnostic techniques and implications of findings.
- Describe the nursing role in antepartal risk assessment.

ELECTRONIC RESOURCES

Additional information related to the content in Chapter 9 can be found on

the companion website at evolve
http://evolve.elsevier.com/Wong/maternal/
- NCLEX Review Questions
- WebLinks

or the interactive student CD-ROM
Activities for Chapter 9 include the following:
- NCLEX Review Questions

Approximately 500,000 of the 4 million births that occur in the United States each year are categorized as high risk because of maternal or fetal complications. Perinatal outcome depends on the early recognition and management of problems. Identification of the risks, together with appropriate and timely intervention during the perinatal period, can prevent morbidity and mortality among mothers and infants.

With the changing demographics in the United States, more women and families can be identified as at risk because of factors other than biophysical criteria. Among those at risk are homeless, single, and uninsured pregnant women, who are unlikely to be able to access prenatal care early or at all. Psychosocial factors that involve maternal behaviors and adverse lifestyles have a negative effect on the health of the mother and fetus.

Care of these high risk patients requires the unified efforts of medical and nursing personnel. The high risk patient and the factors associated with a diagnosis of high risk are discussed in this chapter. Diagnostic techniques used to monitor the maternal-fetal unit are also described.

DEFINITION AND SCOPE OF THE PROBLEM

A high risk pregnancy is one in which the life or health of the mother or infant is jeopardized by a disorder coincidental with or unique to pregnancy. For the mother, the high risk status arbitrarily extends through the puerperium (30 days after childbirth). Postbirth maternal complications usually are resolved within 1 month of birth, but perinatal morbidity may continue for months or years.

High risk pregnancy is a critical problem for modern medical and nursing care. The new social emphasis on the quality of life and the wanted child has resulted in a reduction of family size and the number of unwanted pregnancies. At the same time, technologic advances have facilitated pregnancies in previously infertile couples. As a consequence, emphasis is on the safe birth of normal infants who can develop to their potential. Scientific and technologic advances have allowed perinatal health care to reach a level far beyond that previously available.

The diagnosis of high risk imposes a situational crisis on the family (e.g., loss of pregnancy before the anticipated date, development of gestational diabetes mellitus with its potential complications, or birth of a neonate who does not meet cultural, societal, or familial norms and expectations).

Maternal Health Problems

The leading causes of maternal death attributable to pregnancy differ throughout the world. In general, three major causes have persisted for the last 50 years: hypertensive disorders, infection, and hemorrhage.

The maternal death rate in the United States in 2000 was 9.8 per 100,000 live births. Factors that are strongly related to maternal death include age (younger than 20 years and 35 years or older), lack of prenatal care, low educational attainment, unmarried status, and nonwhite race. African-American maternal mortality rates are more than three times higher than those for Caucasian women (Minino et al, 2002).

Although the overall number of maternal deaths is small, maternal mortality remains a significant problem because a high proportion of these deaths are preventable, primarily through improving access to and use of prenatal care services. Nurses can be instrumental in educating the public about the importance of obtaining early and regular care during pregnancy. Reaching the *Healthy People 2010* goal of 3.3 maternal deaths per 100,000 poses a significant challenge.

Fetal and Neonatal Health Problems

The leading causes of death in the neonatal period are congenital anomalies, disorders relating to short gestation and low birth weight (LBW), respiratory distress syndrome, and the effects of maternal complications. Racial differences in the infant mortality rates continue to challenge public health experts. Increased rates of survival during the neonatal period have resulted largely from high-quality prenatal care and the improvement in perinatal services, including technologic advances in neonatal intensive care and obstetrics.

To achieve significant decline of the infant mortality rate and to eliminate racial and ethnic differences in pregnancy outcomes, a national, state, and local commitment to these goals is necessary. Reducing infant mortality rates requires the removal of financial, educational, sociocultural, and logistic barriers to care so that pregnant women can seek and receive health services. Perinatal services must be modified to meet contemporary health care needs (American College of Obstetricians and Gynecologists [ACOG], 2004b). Mortality rate decreases when high risk status is identified and when intensive care is applied. Follow-up studies have shown that serious residual handicaps (both physical and mental) of surviving infants have been dramatically reduced when such identification and intervention exist.

It is neither feasible nor reasonable for each hospital to develop and maintain the full spectrum of services required for high risk perinatal patients. As a consequence, regionalization of health care emerged (i.e., facilities within a geographic region organized to provide different levels of care).

However, regionalization alone has not consistently improved perinatal outcomes. Furthermore, managed care markets and other financial pressures have forced some providers to be more competitive. To meet this challenge, facilities began to extend the kind of perinatal services offered. Perinatal services in some areas were duplicated, creating an imbalance in the provision of services within a geographic area.

Clearer guidelines were established regarding the level of care that could be expected at any given facility. In ambulatory settings, providers must distinguish themselves by the level of care they provide. *Basic care* is provided by obstetricians, family physicians, certified nurse-midwives, and other advanced practice clinicians approved by local governance. Routine risk-oriented prenatal care, education, and support are included. Providers offering *specialty* care are obstetricians who must provide fetal diagnostic testing and management of obstetric and medical complications in addition to basic care. *Subspecialty care* is provided by maternal-fetal medicine specialists and includes the aforementioned, as well as genetic testing, advanced fetal therapies, and management of severe maternal and fetal complications (American Academy of Pediatrics/American College of Obstetricians and Gynecologists [AAP/ACOG], 1997).

In hospital settings, perinatal services are also designated as basic, specialty, or subspecialty. Criteria for basic perinatal services include care of all patients admitted to the service, with an established triage system for high risk patients who should be transferred to a higher level of care; ability to perform a cesarean birth within 30 minutes of a decision to do so; availability of blood and blood products; availability of radiology, anesthesia, and laboratory services on a 24-hour basis; presence of nursery and postpartum care; resuscitation and stabilization of all neonates born in the hospital; availability of transport for all sick neonates; family visitation; and data collection and retrieval (AAP/ACOG, 1997).

Specialty hospital care includes the aforementioned requirements in addition to care of high risk mothers and fetuses, stabilization of ill neonates before transfer, and care of preterm infants with a birth weight of 1500 g or more. Preterm labor or impending births of 32 weeks of gestation or less should be transferred for subspecialty care. Other criteria for subspecialty care include comprehensive prenatal services, research and educational support, and use of high risk technologies. Collaboration among providers to meet the patient's needs is key in reducing perinatal morbidity and mortality (AAP/ACOG, 1997).

Assessment for Risk Factors

Pregnancies can be designated as high risk for any of several undesirable outcomes. Those considered to be at risk for uteroplacental insufficiency carry a serious threat for fetal growth restriction, intrauterine fetal death, intrapartum death, intrapartum fetal distress, and various types of neonatal morbidity.

When using a medical model perspective, a patient is at risk only from medical, obstetric, or physiologic factors. Today a more comprehensive approach to high risk pregnancy is used, and the factors associated with high risk childbearing are grouped into broad categories based on threats to health and pregnancy outcome (Guidelines/Guías box). Categories of risk include biophysical, psychosocial, sociodemographic, and environmental (Gilbert & Harmon, 2003) (Box 9-1).

Biophysical risks include factors that originate within the mother or fetus and affect the development or functioning of either or both. Examples include genetic disorders, nutritional and general health status, and medical or obstetric-related illnesses.

Psychosocial risks comprise maternal behaviors and adverse lifestyles that have a negative effect on the health of the mother or fetus (or both). These risks may include emotional distress and disturbed interpersonal relationships, inadequate social support, and unsafe cultural practices (Box 9-2).

Sociodemographic risks arise from the mother and her family and place the mother and fetus at risk. Examples include lack of prenatal care, low income, marital status, and ethnicity (see Box 9-1).

Environmental risks include hazards of the workplace and the woman's general environment. These risks may include

ENGLISH SPANISH **Guidelines/Guías**

HIGH RISK FACTORS

High Risk Assessment	Potential Problem
Have you had any problems with this pregnancy? *¿Ha tenido problemas con este embarazo?*	General assessment
Have you had blurred vision? *¿Ha tenido visión borrosa?*	Preeclampsia
Have you had severe headaches? *¿Ha tenido dolores fuertes de cabeza?*	Preeclampsia
Have you had difficulty breathing? *¿Ha tenido dificultad para respirar?*	Cardiac disease
Have you had heart palpitations? *¿Ha tenido palpitaciones del corazón?*	Cardiac disease
Have you been vomiting? *¿Ha tenido vómitos?*	Hyperemesis gravidarum
Have you had any infections? *¿Ha tenido alguna infección?*	Sexually transmitted infections/vaginal infections
Have you had swelling? *¿Ha tenido hinchazón?*	Preeclampsia
Were all your pregnancies term? *¿Llegaron a las cuarenta semanas todos sus embarazos?*	Preterm labor
Have you ever had diabetes? *¿Ha tenido diabetes?*	Diabetes
Have you ever had high blood pressure? *¿Ha tenido alta presión sanguínea?*	Preeclampsia
Have you ever had anemia? *¿Ha estado anémica?*	Anemia
Do you take drugs? Prescription medicine? *¿Usa drogas? ¿Medicina recetada?*	Substance abuse
Do you drink alcohol? Smoke? *¿Toma bebidas alcohólicas? ¿Fuma?*	Substance abuse

noxious chemicals, radiation, infections, and pollutants (Boxes 8-3 and 8-4).

Risk factors are interrelated and cumulative in their effects. Specific pregnancy problems and risk factors are listed in Box 9-3. Risk factors of the postpartum woman and the neonate are outlined in Box 9-4. The development of a comprehensive database for pregnancy risk assessment will help generate appropriate nursing diagnoses (Box 9-5).

ANTEPARTUM TESTING/BIOPHYSICAL ASSESSMENT

The major expected outcome of antepartum testing is the detection of potential fetal compromise. Ideally the technique used will identify fetal compromise before intrauterine asphyxia of the fetus occurs so that the health care provider can take measures to prevent or minimize adverse perinatal outcomes. No single test can provide this information. Assessment tests should be selected based on their effectiveness, and the results must be interpreted in light of the complete clinical picture. The most reliable evidence for effectiveness is provided by randomized controlled trials. Nurses can be informed about the most recent research on fetal assessment by using an up-to-date systematic review such as the Cochrane Database of Systematic Reviews (Enkin et al, 2000). Table 9-1 lists evidence for recommending care for fetal assessment screening based on this database.

Daily Fetal Movement Count

Assessment of fetal activity by the mother is a simple yet valuable method for monitoring the condition of the fetus. The daily fetal movement count (DFMC) (also called "kick counts") can be done at home, is simple to understand, is noninvasive, and does not interfere with a daily routine. The DFMC is frequently used to monitor the fetus in pregnancies complicated by conditions that may affect fetal oxygenation. These conditions include but are not limited to gestational hypertension or chronic hypertension and diabetes. The presence of fetal movements is generally a reassuring sign of fetal health.

Several protocols are used for counting. Generally it is recommended that mothers count fetal activity two or three times daily for 60 minutes each time. Except for noting a very

Critical Thinking Exercise

FETAL ACTIVITY MONITORING

Barbra is an elementary school teacher. She is at 30 weeks of gestation with her first baby. This is a planned pregnancy, and Barbra and her husband are excited about becoming parents. They have read extensively about pregnancy and selected midwifery care after a careful review of the literature on childbirth and interviewing other patients of the midwife they selected to provide care. Barbra has kept all of her recommended appointments with the nurse-midwife. On the last two visits to her nurse-midwife, Barbra's blood pressure has been elevated. She has been advised to monitor fetal activity at home. As her nurse, you are responsible for developing a teaching plan that includes the following: the purpose of monitoring fetal activity; the significance of fetal activity; the times when monitoring is to take place; and instructing Barbra on the way to count movements, the best time of the day to complete the counts, how to record the counts, and when to notify you or her nurse-midwife with findings.

1. Evidence—Is there sufficient evidence to draw conclusions about the benefits of monitoring fetal activity?
2. Assumptions—Describe an underlying assumption about each of the following topics:
   a. Barbra's motivation for learning about fetal activity monitoring
   b. Barbra's motivation to perform fetal activity monitoring
   c. The best time of the day for Barbra to complete the counts
   d. Barbra's ability to comply with instructions
3. What implications and priorities for nursing care can be drawn at this time?
4. Does the evidence objectively support your conclusion?
5. Are there alternative perspectives to your conclusion?

BOX 9-1

Categories of High Risk Factors

Biophysical

1. Genetic—may interfere with normal fetal/neonatal development, result in congenital anomalies, or create difficulties for the mother. Includes defective genes, transmittable inherited disorders, chromosome anomalies, multiple pregnancy, large fetal size, and ABO incompatibility.
2. Nutritional status—one of the most important determinants of pregnancy outcome. Fetal growth and development cannot progress normally without adequate nutrition. Includes very young age; three pregnancies in the past 2 years; tobacco, alcohol, or drug use; inadequate intake because of chronic illness or food fads; inadequate or excessive weight gain; and hematocrit less than 33%.
3. Medical and obstetric—medical complications of current and past pregnancies, obstetric-related illnesses, and pregnancy losses. See Box 9-3.

Psychosocial

1. Smoking—strong, consistent, causal relationship between maternal smoking and reduced birth weight has been established. Risks include LBW infants, especially with increased age; higher neonatal mortality rates; increased miscarriages; and increased incidence of premature rupture of membranes. Risks aggravated by low socioeconomic status, poor nutritional status, and concurrent use of alcohol.
2. Caffeine—not been shown to cause birth defects in humans. High intake (three or more cups of coffee per day) has been related to a slight decrease in birth weight.
3. Alcohol—although exact effects of use in pregnancy have not been quantified and mode of action is largely unexplained, alcohol exerts adverse effects on the fetus, resulting in fetal alcohol syndrome (FAS) and fetal alcohol effects (FAEs), learning disabilities, and hyperactivity.
4. Drugs—may adversely affect a developing fetus through several mechanisms: they can be teratogenic, cause metabolic disturbances, produce chemical effects, or cause depression or alteration of central nervous system function. Includes medications prescribed by health care provider or bought over the counter, as well as commonly abused drugs such as heroin, cocaine, and marijuana.
5. Psychologic status—childbearing triggers profound and complex physiologic, psychologic, and social changes, with evidence to suggest a relationship between emotional distress and birth complications. Includes specific intrapsychic disturbances and addictive lifestyles; history of child or spouse abuse; inadequate support systems; family disruption or dissolution; maternal role changes/conflicts; noncompliance with cultural norms; unsafe cultural, ethnic, or religious practices; and situational crises.

Sociodemographic

1. Low income—poverty underlies many other risk factors and leads to inadequate financial resources for food and prenatal care, poor general health, and increased risk of medical complications of pregnancy; adverse environmental influences more prevalent.
2. Lack of prenatal care—major factor in placing woman at risk because opportunity is lost for early diagnosis and treatment of complications. May be caused by financial barriers or lack of access to care; depersonalization of the system resulting in long waits, routine visits, variability in health care personnel, and unpleasant physical surroundings; lack of understanding of need for early and continued care or cultural beliefs that do not support the need; and fear of health care providers and the system.
3. Age—women at both ends of the childbearing years have a higher incidence of poor outcomes; age may not be a risk factor in all patients. Both physiologic and psychologic risks should be evaluated.
   Adolescents: More complications are seen in the very young (younger than 15 years old), who have a 60% higher mortality rate than those over age 20. Complications include anemia, preeclampsia, prolonged labor, contracted pelvis, and cephalopelvic disproportion. Long-term social implications of early motherhood are lower educational attainment, lower income, increased dependence on government support programs, higher divorce rates, and higher parity.
   Mature mothers: Risks do not arise from age alone, but are affected by other factors, such as number and spacing of previous pregnancies; genetic disposition of the parents; and medical history, lifestyle, nutrition, and prenatal care. Increased likelihood of chronic diseases that adversely affect pregnancy outcomes; more invasive medical management of older women's pregnancies and labors, with resulting complications; and demographic characteristics put an older woman at risk. Medical conditions more likely to be experienced by mature women include hypertension and preeclampsia, diabetes, extended labor, cesarean birth, placenta previa, abruptio placentae, and death. Their fetuses are at greater risk for both LBW and macrosomia, chromosomal abnormalities, congenital malformations, and neonatal death.
4. Parity—number of previous pregnancies is a risk factor associated with age. Includes all first pregnancies and first pregnancy at either end of the childbearing age continuum; incidence of preeclampsia and dystocia is higher with a first birth.
5. Marital status—mortality and morbidity rates are higher for nonmarried women. Includes greater risk for preeclampsia and inadequate prenatal care; occurs more often in lower age groups.
6. Residence—availability and quality of prenatal care vary greatly with geographic region. Women in metropolitan areas have more prenatal visits than those in rural areas; those in rural areas have higher incidence of maternal mortality and have fewer opportunities for specialized care. Health care in an inner city may be of poorer quality than in a more affluent section, and those women are usually poorer and begin childbearing earlier and continue longer.
7. Ethnicity—although ethnicity alone is not a major risk, race is an indicator of other sociodemographic factors. Non-Caucasian women are more than three times as likely as Caucasian women to die of pregnancy-related causes; infant mortality rates among African-Americans are more than twice as high as those among Caucasians; and African-American babies have the highest rates of prematurity and LBW.

Environmental

Various environmental substances can affect fertility and fetal development, the chance of a live birth, and the child's subsequent mental and physical development. Environmental influences include infections, radiation, chemicals such as pesticides, therapeutic drugs, illicit drugs, industrial pollutants, cigarette smoke, stress, and diet. Paternal exposure to mutagenic agents in the workplace has been associated with increased risk of miscarriage.

BOX 9-2

Antepartum Cultural Assessment

All cultures recognize pregnancy as a special transitional period and have particular customs and beliefs that dictate behavior during this time. In the antepartum period the nurse should assess the following:
- Beliefs of whether pregnancy is a state of illness or health
- Behavioral expectations of the mother and of the health care provider
- Dietary prescriptions or restrictions (e.g., hot/cold balance theory, pica)
- Activity restrictions or prescriptions (e.g., use of massage)
- Availability of advice (e.g., from whom and at what time advice will be sought and when prenatal care will begin [if at all])
- Considerations of modesty

low number of daily fetal movements (FMs) or a trend toward decreased motion, the clinical value of the absolute number of FMs has not been established. The only exception is if FMs cease entirely for 12 hours (the fetal alarm signal). A count of fewer than three FMs within 1 hour warrants further evaluation by nonstress or contraction stress testing, biophysical profile (BPP), or a combination of these. Women should be taught the significance of both the presence and the absence of fetal movements, the procedure to use for counting, how to record findings on a daily fetal movement record, and when to notify their health care provider (Fig. 9-1).

NURSE ALERT In assessing fetal movements, it is important to remember that they are usually not present during the fetal sleep cycle; they may be temporarily reduced if the woman is taking depressant medication, drinking alcohol, or smoking a cigarette. They do not usually decrease as the woman nears term. Obesity decreases the ability of the mother to assess fetal movement. ■

Ultrasonography

Sound is a form of wave energy that causes small particles in a medium to oscillate. The frequency of sound, which refers to the number of peaks or waves that move over a given point per unit of time, is expressed in hertz (Hz). Sound with a frequency of 1 cycle, or one peak per second, has a frequency of 1 Hz. When directional beams of sound strike an object, an echo is returned. The time delay between the emission of the sound and the return of the echo and the direction of the echo are noted. From these data, the distance and location of an object can be calculated. Ultrasound is sound frequency higher than that detectable by humans (greater than 20,000 Hz). Diagnostic ultrasound instruments operate within a frequency range of 2 to 10 million Hz (or 2 to 10 MHz), which is below the range used by sonar and radar equipment.

BOX 9-3

Specific Pregnancy Problems and Related Risk Factors

Preterm Labor
Age below 16 or over 35 years
Low socioeconomic status
Maternal weight below 50 kg (110 lb)
Poor nutrition
Previous preterm birth
Incompetent cervix
Uterine anomalies
Smoking
Drug addiction and alcohol abuse
Pyelonephritis, pneumonia
Multiple gestation
Anemia
Abnormal fetal presentation
Preterm rupture of membranes
Placental abnormalities
Infection

Polyhydramnios
Diabetes mellitus
Multiple gestation
Fetal congenital abnormalities
Isoimmunization (Rh or ABO)
Nonimmune hydrops
Abnormal fetal presentation

Intrauterine Growth Restriction (IUGR)
Multiple gestation
Poor nutrition

Intrauterine Growth Restriction (IUGR)—cont'd
Maternal cyanotic heart disease
Chronic hypertension
Gestational hypertension
Recurrent antepartum hemorrhage
Smoking
Maternal diabetes with vasculopathy
Fetal infections
Fetal cardiovascular anomalies
Drug addiction and alcohol abuse
Fetal congenital anomalies
Hemoglobinopathies

Oligohydramnios
Renal agenesis (Potter's syndrome)
Prolonged rupture of membranes
Intrauterine growth restriction
Intrauterine fetal demise

Postterm Pregnancy
Anencephaly
Placental sulfatase deficiency
Perinatal hypoxia, acidosis
Placental insufficiency

Chromosomal Abnormalities
Maternal age 35 years or more at delivery
Balanced translocation (maternal and paternal)

From Gillen-Goldstein J et al: Methods of assessment for pregnancy at risk. In DeCherney AH, Nathan L (eds): *Current obstetric and gynecologic diagnosis and treatment,* ed 9, New York, 2003, Lange Medical Books/McGraw-Hill.

BOX 9-4

Factors that Place the Postpartum Woman and Neonate at High Risk

Mother
Hemorrhage
Infection
Abnormal vital signs
Traumatic labor of birth
Psychosocial factors

Infant (for Admission to NICU)
High Risk Category
Infants continuing or developing signs of RDS or other respiratory distress
Asphyxiated infants (Apgar scores less than 6 at 5 minutes); resuscitation required at birth
Preterm infants; dysmature infants
Infants with cyanosis or suspected cardiovascular disease; persistent cyanosis
Infants with major congenital malformations requiring surgery; chromosomal anomalies
Infants with convulsions, sepsis, hemorrhagic diathesis, or shock
Meconium aspiration syndrome
CNS depression for longer than 24 hours
Hypoglycemia
Hypocalcemia
Hyperbilirubinemia

Moderate Risk Category
Dysmaturity
Prematurity (weight between 2000 and 2500 g)
Apgar score less than 5 at 1 minute
Feeding problems
Multifetal birth
Transient tachypnea
Hypomagnesemia or hypermagnesemia
Hypoparathyroidism
Failure to gain weight
Jitteriness or hyperactivity
Cardiac anomalies not requiring immediate catheterization
Heart murmur
Anemia
CNS depression for less than 24 hours

CNS, central nervous system; *NICU*, neonatal intensive care unit; *RDS*, respiratory distress syndrome.

BOX 9-5

PRAMS, the Pregnancy Risk Assessment Monitoring System

PRAMS is a surveillance project of the Centers for Disease Control and Prevention and state health departments. It was started in 1987 to improve the health of mothers and infants by reducing adverse outcomes. The sample in PRAMS is chosen from all women who recently had a live birth. Currently, 31 states and New York City participate in PRAMS. The PRAMS questionnaire contains questions asked by all states and some state-specific questions. Data are used to plan maternal and infant health programs and develop partnerships between agencies that have important contributions to make in developing programs.

Information from www.cdc.gov/reproductivehealth/srv_prams.htm (accessed August 17, 2004).

Diagnostic ultrasonography is an important technique in antepartum fetal surveillance (Fig. 9-2). Ultrasound examination can be done abdominally or transvaginally during pregnancy. Both methods produce a three-dimensional view from which a pictorial image is obtained. Abdominal ultrasonography is more useful after the first trimester when the pregnant uterus becomes an abdominal organ. For the procedure the woman is usually required to have a full bladder (to push the uterus up) to get a better image of the fetus. Transmission gel or paste is applied to the abdomen before a transducer is moved over the skin to enhance transmission and reception of the sound waves.

Transvaginal ultrasonography, in which the probe is inserted into the vagina, allows pelvic anatomy to be evaluated in greater detail and allows intrauterine pregnancy to be diagnosed earlier (Manning, 2004). A transvaginal ultrasound examination is well tolerated by most patients because it alleviates the need for a full bladder. It is especially useful in obese patients whose thick abdominal layers cannot be penetrated adequately by an abdominal approach. Transvaginal ultrasonography is used in the first trimester to detect ectopic pregnancies, monitor the developing embryo, help identify abnormalities, and help establish gestational age. In some instances it may be used as an adjunct to abdominal scanning to evaluate preterm labor in second- and third-trimester pregnancies.

For an abdominal ultrasound the woman is positioned comfortably with small pillows under her head and knees. The display panel should be positioned so that the woman and her partner can observe the images on the screen if they desire.

A transvaginal ultrasound may be performed either with the woman in a lithotomy position or with her pelvis elevated by towels, cushions, or a folded pillow. This pelvic tilt is optimal to image the pelvic structures. A protective cover such as a condom, the finger of a clean rubber surgical glove, or a special cover provided by the manufacturer is used to cover the probe. The probe is lubricated with a water-soluble gel and placed in the vagina either by the examiner or by the woman herself. During the examination the position of the probe or the tilt of the examining table may be changed to view the complete pelvis. The procedure is not physically painful, although the woman will feel pressure as the probe is moved.

Levels of Ultrasonography

Perinatal care providers and ultrasonographers have come to a tentative agreement on terminology describing two different levels of ultrasonography. The basic screening or limited examination is used most frequently and can be performed by ultrasonographers or other health care professionals, including nurses, who have had special training. Targeted or comprehensive examinations are performed if a woman is suspected of carrying an anatomically or a physiologically abnormal fetus. Indications for a comprehensive

Table 9-1

Fetal Assessment Screening: Recommendations for Care

FETAL ASSESSMENT TEST	RECOMMENDATION/CONCLUSION
• Doppler ultrasound use in pregnancy at high risk for fetal compromise • Ultrasound use to estimate gestational age in first and early second trimesters • Ultrasound use to confirm suspected multiple pregnancy • Ultrasound use for placental location in suspected placenta previa • Ultrasound use to assess amniotic fluid volume • Early second-trimester amniocentesis for identification of chromosomal abnormalities • Transabdominal instead of transvaginal chorionic villus sampling (CVS)	Beneficial effects Effects likely to be beneficial
• Formal systems of risk scoring • Routine use of early ultrasound • CVS versus amniocentesis for diagnosing chromosomal abnormalities • Serum alpha-fetoprotein screening for neural tube defects • Triple screen test for Down syndrome and neural tube defects	Trade-off between beneficial and adverse effects
• Placental grading by ultrasound to improve perinatal outcome • Biophysical profile for fetal surveillance • Routine fetal movement counts to improve perinatal outcome	Unknown effectiveness
• Routine use of ultrasound for fetal anthropometry (body measurements) in late pregnancy • Use of Doppler ultrasound screening in all pregnancies • Measurement of placental hormones (estriol and human placental lactogen)	Unlikely to be beneficial
• Nipple stimulation test to improve perinatal outcome • Nonselective nonstress test to improve perinatal outcome • Contraction stress test to improve perinatal outcome	Likely to be ineffective or harmful

Source: Enkin M et al: Effective care in pregnancy and childbirth: a synopsis, *Birth* 28(1):41-51, 2001.

examination include abnormal findings on clinical examination, especially with polyhydramnios or oligohydramnios, elevated alpha-fetoprotein (AFP) levels, and a history of offspring with anomalies that can be detected by ultrasound examination. Comprehensive ultrasonography is performed by highly trained and experienced personnel.

Indications for Use

Major indications for the use of obstetric sonography vary by trimester (Table 9-2). During the first trimester, ultrasound examination is performed to obtain information on the following: (1) number, size, and location of gestational sacs; (2) presence or absence of fetal cardiac and body movements; (3) presence or absence of uterine abnormalities (e.g., bicornuate uterus or fibroids) or adnexal masses (e.g., ovarian cysts or an ectopic pregnancy); (4) pregnancy dating (i.e., by measuring crown-rump length); and (5) presence and location of an intrauterine contraceptive device.

During the second and third trimesters, information on the following is sought: (1) fetal viability, number, position, gestational age, growth pattern, and anomalies; (2) amniotic fluid volume; (3) placental location and maturity; (4) uterine fibroids and anomalies; (5) adnexal masses; and (6) cervical length.

Ultrasonography can lead to earlier diagnosis, allowing therapy to be instituted early in pregnancy. This decreases the severity and duration of morbidity, both physical and emotional, for the family.

Fetal Heart Activity

Fetal heart activity can be demonstrated as early as 6 to 7 weeks by real-time echo scanners and at 10 to 12 weeks by Doppler mode. By 9 to 10 weeks, gestational trophoblastic disease can be diagnosed. Fetal death can be confirmed by lack of heart motion, the presence of fetal scalp edema, and maceration and overlap of the cranial bones.

Gestational Age

Gestational dating by ultrasonography is indicated for conditions such as the following: (1) uncertain dates for the last normal menstrual period, (2) recent discontinuation of oral contraceptives, (3) bleeding episode during the first trimester, (4) uterine size that does not agree with dates, and (5) other high risk conditions.

During the first 20 weeks of gestation, ultrasonography provides an accurate assessment of gestational age because most normal fetuses grow at the same rate. With increased fetal age, the accuracy of gestational age estimates using ultrasound also increases because more variables are measured. Four methods of fetal age estimation are used: (1) determination of gestational sac dimensions (at about 8 weeks), (2) measurement of crown-rump length (between 7 and 12 weeks), (3) measurement of the biparietal diameter (BPD) (after 12 weeks), and (4) measurement of femur length (after 12 weeks). Fetal BPD at 36 weeks should be approximately 8.7 cm. Term pregnancy and fetal maturity can be diagnosed with some confidence if the biparietal

FORMULARIO PARA LOS MOVIMIENTOS DEL FETO

1. Este formulario servirá para ver como progresa el niño.
2. Con cuidado cuente el número de movimientos del niño durante la misma hora cada noche. (El niño se mueve mas durante la noche.) Ejemplo: 8-9 PM cada noche.
3. Si el niño no sea movido por 12 horas, es importante que usted notifique la clínica (555-1234). Si la clínica está cerrada, un mensaje se le dara con instrucciones para que llamé al doctor.
4. Triaga este formulario con usted cuando venga a la clínica o hospital.

FORMULARIO DIARIO DE MOVIMIENTOS DEL FETO

DÍAS DE LA SEMANA	LUN	MAR	MIER	JUEV	VIER	SAB	DOM
FECHA							
MOVIMIENTOS							
FECHA							
MOVIMIENTOS							
FECHA							
MOVIMIENTOS							
FECHA							
MOVIMIENTOS							
FECHA							
MOVIMIENTOS							
FECHA							
MOVIMIENTOS							
FECHA							
MOVIMIENTOS							
FECHA							
MOVIMIENTOS							
FECHA							
MOVIMIENTOS							

X-IMR-2211 (03/C1) OTHER

FETAL MOVEMENT CHART

1. This chart will help us find out how your baby is doing.
2. Carefully count the number of baby movements during the same hour every evening. (Baby moves more during the evening hours.) Example: 8-9 PM every evening.
3. If the baby has not moved for 12 hours, it is important that you notify the clinic (555-1234). If the clinic is closed, a recorded message will further instruct you for contacting a doctor who is on-call.
4. Bring this chart with you whenever you come to the clinic or hospital.

DAILY CHART OF BABY KICKS

DAYS OF WEEK	MON	TUES	WED	THURS	FRI	SAT	SUN
DATE							
KICKS							
DATE							
KICKS							
DATE							
KICKS							
DATE							
KICKS							
DATE							
KICKS							
DATE							
KICKS							
DATE							
KICKS							
DATE							
KICKS							
DATE							
KICKS							

X-IMR-2211 (03/C1) OTHER

Fig. 9-1 Fetal movement (kick count) chart. (Courtesy St. Joseph Hospital and Medical Center, Phoenix, AZ.)

A

B

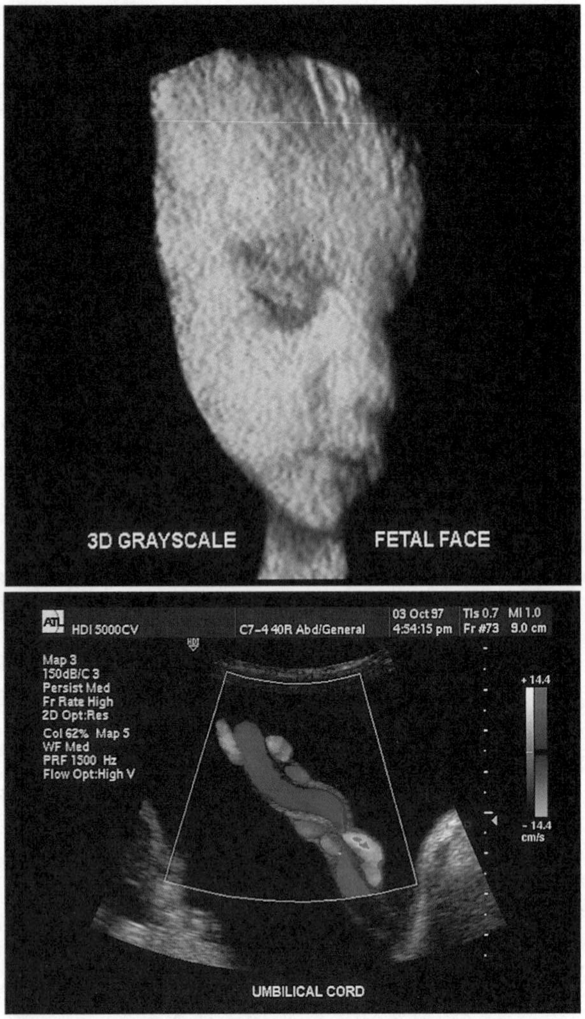

Fig. 9-2 Two views of the fetus during ultrasonography. **A**, Fetal face (20 weeks). **B**, Umbilical cord (26 weeks). (Courtesy Advanced Technology Laboratories, Bothell, WA.)

measurement by ultrasound is greater than 9.8 cm (Figs. 9-3 and 9-4, Table 9-3), especially when this is combined with appropriate femur length measurement.

In later gestational periods, the accuracy of fetal age determination is enhanced by serial measurements. Two and preferably three composite measurements are recommended, at least 2 weeks apart, and these are plotted against standard fetal growth curves. When applied between 24 and 32 weeks of gestation, this method yields an estimation error of 10 days more or less than the actual age (Manning, 2004).

Fetal Growth

Fetal growth is a result of interaction between intrinsic growth potential and the environmental factors that may enhance or inhibit that growth. Conditions that indicate the need for ultrasound assessment of fetal growth include the following: (1) poor maternal weight gain or pattern of weight gain, (2) previous intrauterine growth restriction (IUGR), (3) chronic infections, (4) ingestion of drugs (e.g., tobacco, alcohol, over-the-counter drugs, and street drugs), (5) maternal diabetes mellitus, (6) hypertension, (7) multifetal pregnancy, and (8) other medical or surgical complications.

Serial evaluations of BPD and limb length can differentiate between size discrepancy resulting from inaccurate dates and true IUGR. IUGR may be symmetric (i.e., the fetus is small in all parameters) or asymmetric (i.e., head and body growth vary). Symmetric IUGR implies a chronic or long-standing insult and may be caused by low genetic growth potential, intrauterine infection, maternal undernutrition, heavy smoking, or chromosomal aberration. Asymmetric growth reflects an acute or late-occurring deprivation such as placental insufficiency resulting from hypertension, renal disease, or cardiovascular disease. Reduced fetal growth is still one of the most frequent conditions associated with stillbirth.

Macrosomic infants (those weighing 4000 g or more) are at increased risk for dystocia, traumatic injury, and asphyxia during birth. Fetal macrosomia associated with maternal glucose intolerance carries an increased risk of intrauterine death. Macrosomia in the infant of a diabetic mother is

Table 9-2

Major Uses of Ultrasonography during Pregnancy

FIRST TRIMESTER	SECOND TRIMESTER	THIRD TRIMESTER
Confirm pregnancy	Establish or confirm dates	Confirm gestational age
Confirm viability	Confirm viability	Confirm viability
Determine gestational age	Detect polyhydramnios, oligohydramnios	Detect macrosomia
Rule out ectopic pregnancy	Detect congenital anomalies	Detect congenital anomalies
Detect multiple gestation	Detect intrauterine growth restriction (IUGR)	Detect IUGR
Visualization during chorionic villus sampling	Confirm placenta placement	Determine fetal position
Detect maternal abnormalities such as bicornuate uterus, ovarian cysts, fibroids	Visualization during amniocentesis	Detect placenta previa or abruptio placentae
		Visualization during amniocentesis, external version
		Biophysical profile
		Amniotic fluid volume assessment
		Doppler flow studies
		Detect placental maturity

asymmetric and characterized by increases in fat and muscle in the abdomen and shoulders, while head circumference remains normal. Macrosomia in an infant whose mother is obese without glucose intolerance results in symmetric changes—excessive growth of abdominal and head circumferences (Chervenak & Gabbe, 2002).

Fetal Anatomy

Depending on the gestational age, the following structures may be identified: head (including ventricles and blood vessels), neck, spine, heart, stomach, small bowel, liver, kidneys, bladder, limbs, and umbilical cord. Ultrasonography permits the confirmation of normal anatomy (Fig. 9-5) as well as the detection of major fetal malformations. The presence of an anomaly may influence the birth location (e.g., delivery room instead of a labor-delivery-recovery room or a subspecialty center versus a basic care center) and the method of birth to optimize neonatal outcomes.

The number of fetuses and their presentation also may be assessed by ultrasonography, allowing plans for therapy and mode of birth to be made in advance.

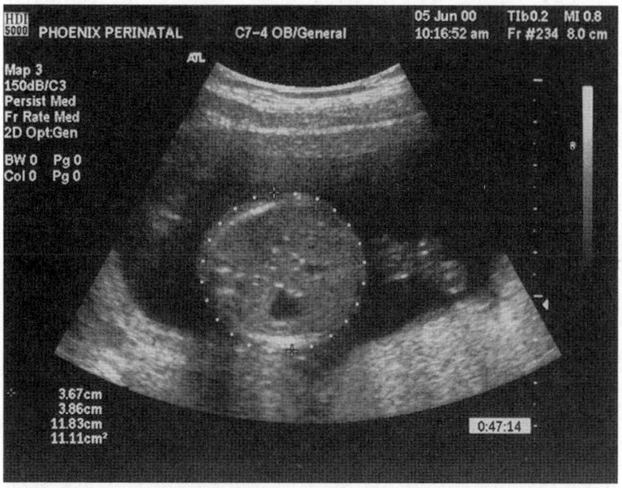

Fig. 9-3 Biparietal cephalometry by ultrasound. (Courtesy Michael S. Clement, MD, Mesa, AZ.)

Fetal Genetic Disorders and Physical Anomalies

A prenatal screening technique called fetal nuchal translucency (FNT) screening uses ultrasound measurement of fluid in the nape of the fetal neck between 10 and 14 weeks of gestation to identify possible fetal abnormalities. A finding of abnormal fluid collection that is greater than 2.5 mm is considered abnormal, whereas a measurement of 3 mm or greater is highly indicative of genetic disorders or physical anomalies. If the FNT is abnormal, diagnostic genetic testing is recommended (ACOG, 2004a).

Placental Position and Function

The pattern of uterine and placental growth and the fullness of the maternal bladder influence the apparent location of the placenta as viewed by ultrasonography. By 14 to 16 weeks the placenta can be clearly defined, but its relationship to the internal cervical os can sometimes be altered dramatically by changing the degree of fullness of the maternal bladder. In approximately 15% to 20% of all pregnancies in which ultrasound scanning is performed in the second trimester, the placenta seems to be overlying the os, but at term the incidence of placenta previa is only 0.5%. Thus the diagnosis of placenta previa can seldom be confirmed before 27 weeks, primarily because of the elongation of the lower uterine segment as pregnancy advances.

Another use of ultrasound is the grading of placental maturation (Box 9-6). Calcium deposits are of significance

Table 9-3

Correlation of Fetal Weight and BPD

BPD (cm)	ESTIMATED FETAL WEIGHT
8.2	2290 g
8.5	2500 g
8.8	2730 g
9.4	3180 g
10.0	3630 g
10.6	4070 g

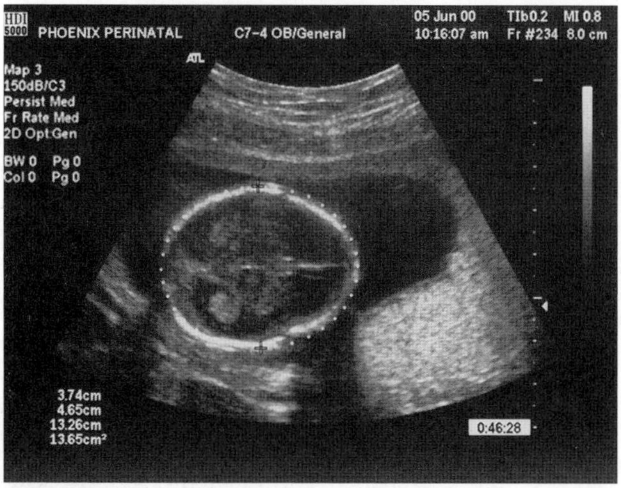

Fig. 9-4 Head circumference. (Courtesy Michael S. Clement, MD, Mesa, AZ.)

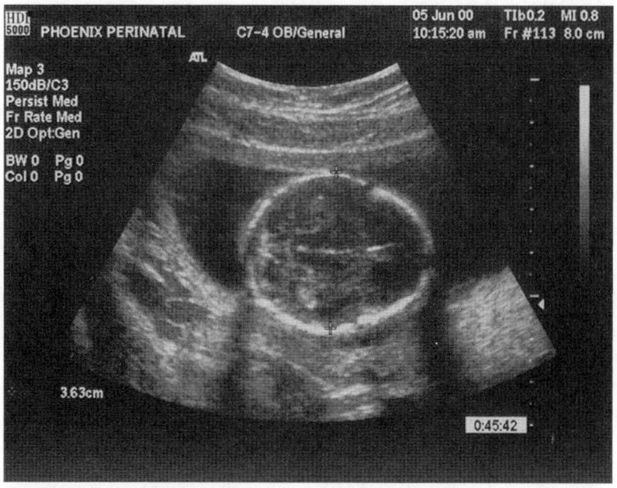

Fig. 9-5 Abdominal circumference. (Courtesy Michael S. Clement, MD, Mesa, AZ.)

BOX 9-6

Placental Grading

Third-trimester grading of placental maturation can be accomplished by ultrasound scanning. The placenta undergoes detectable maturational changes throughout gestation; a relation has been noted between advancing placental grade and fetal pulmonary maturity. Placentas are graded 0, I, II, and III (with grade III placentas being the most mature) on the basis of the identification and distribution of calcium deposits within the fetal portion (Manning, 2004). Ultrasound examination can identify changes in the chorionic plate, placental substance, and basal layer of the placenta that correspond to the various grades: (1) grade 0 placentas are seen in the first and second trimesters, (2) grade I placentas appear between 30 and 32 weeks and may even persist until term, (3) grade II placentas are observed at around 36 weeks and persist until term in 45% of pregnancies, and (4) grade III placentas are seen at 38 weeks and reflect the greatest maturation. However, only a small number of placentas are grade III.

in postterm pregnancies because as they increase, the available surface area that can be adequately bathed by maternal blood decreases. At exactly what point this results in fetal wastage and hypoxia cannot be determined precisely; however, effects usually are observable by 42 weeks and are progressive (Gilbert & Harmon, 2003).

Adjunct to Amniocentesis, Percutaneous Umbilical Blood Sampling, and Chorionic Villus Sampling

The safety of amniocentesis is increased when the physician knows the exact position of the fetus, placenta, and pockets of amniotic fluid. Ultrasound scanning has reduced the risks previously associated with amniocentesis, such as fetomaternal hemorrhage from a pierced placenta. Percutaneous umbilical blood sampling (PUBS) and chorionic villus sampling (CVS) are also guided by ultrasound to identify accurately the cord and chorion frondosum (Fig. 9-2, *B*).

Fetal Well-Being

Physiologic measurements that can be performed with ultrasound scanning include amniotic fluid volume, vascular waveforms from the fetal circulation, heart motion, fetal breathing movements, fetal urine production, and fetal limb and head movements. Assessment of these parameters, singly or in combination, yields a fairly reliable picture of fetal well-being. The significance of these findings is discussed in the following sections.

Amniotic Fluid Volume

Abnormalities of amniotic fluid volume (AFV), whether excessive or diminished, are often associated with fetal disorders. Subjective criteria for the assessment of oligohydramnios (decreased fluid) include the absence of fluid pockets in the uterine cavity and the impression of crowding of fetal small parts (arms and legs). An objective criterion of decreased AFV is met when the largest pocket of fluid measured in two perpendicular planes is less than 2 cm. In the case of hydramnios (increased fluid), the criteria include multiple large pockets of fluid greater than 12 cm in the vertical axis, the impression of a floating fetus, and free movement of fetal limbs (Manning, 2004). The total AFV can be evaluated by a method in which the depths (in centimeters) of amniotic fluid in all four quadrants surrounding the maternal umbilicus are totaled, resulting in an amniotic fluid index (AFI). An AFI is normal if the summed value is more than 80 mm and less than 180 mm (Manning, 2004).

Oligohydramnios is associated with rupture of the membranes and congenital anomalies (such as renal agenesis), IUGR, and fetal distress in labor. Hydramnios is associated with neural tube defects, obstruction of the fetal gastrointestinal tract, multiple fetuses, and fetal hydrops.

Doppler Blood Flow Analysis

One of the major advances in perinatal medicine is the ability to study blood flow noninvasively in the fetus and placenta. Doppler ultrasound is a useful adjunct in the management of pregnancies at risk because of hypertension, IUGR, diabetes mellitus, multiple fetuses, or preterm labor.

When a sound wave is reflected from a moving target, there is a change in frequency of the reflected wave relative to the transmitted wave. This is called the *Doppler effect.* An ultrasound beam scattered by a group of red blood cells (RBCs) is an example of this effect. The velocity of the RBCs can be determined by measuring the change in the frequency in the sound wave reflected off them.

The shifted frequencies can be displayed as a plot of velocity versus time, and the shape of these waveforms can be analyzed to give information about blood flow and resistance in a given circulation. Velocity waveforms from umbilical and uterine arteries, reported in systolic/diastolic (S/D) ratios, can be first detected at 15 weeks of pregnancy. Because of progressive decline in resistance in both the umbilical and the uterine arteries, this ratio decreases as pregnancy advances. Most fetuses achieve an S/D ratio of 3 or less by 30 weeks (Fig. 9-6). Persistent elevation of S/D ratios after 30 weeks is associated with IUGR, usually resulting from uteroplacental insufficiency (UPI) (Druzin, Gabbe, & Reed, 2002). In postterm pregnancies evaluated by Doppler umbilical flow studies, an elevated S/D ratio indicates a poorly perfused placenta. Abnormal velocity study results are also seen with certain chromosomal abnormalities (i.e., trisomy 13 and 18) and with lupus erythematosus in the mother. Exposure to nicotine from maternal smoking also increases the S/D ratio.

Biophysical Profile

Real-time ultrasound permits detailed assessment of the physical and physiologic characteristics of the developing fe-

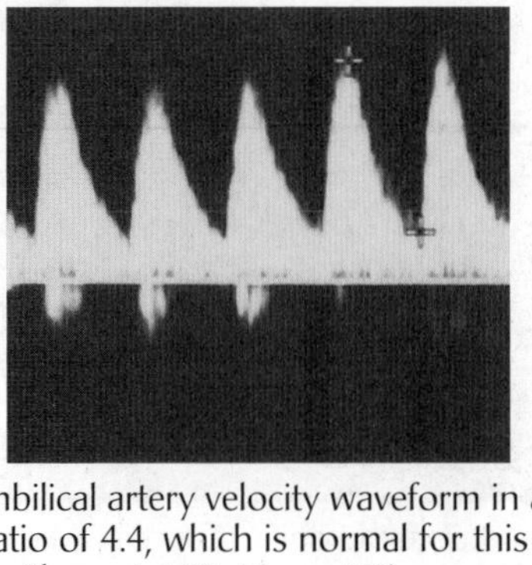

Fig. 9-6 Umbilical artery velocity waveform in a 17-week fetus with S/D ratio of 4.4, which is normal for this stage. (Courtesy Michael S. Clement, MD, Mesa, AZ.)

tus to such an extent that it is possible to examine the fetus in detail and to catalog normal and abnormal biophysical responses to stimuli. The biophysical profile (BPP) is a noninvasive dynamic assessment of a fetus that is based on the assessment of acute and chronic markers of fetal disease.

The BPP includes fetal breathing movements, fetal movements, fetal tone, fetal heart rate (FHR) patterns by means of a nonstress test (NST), and AFV.

The BPP may be considered as a physical examination of the fetus, including determination of vital signs. The fetus responds to central hypoxia by alteration in movement, muscle tone, breathing, and heart rate patterns. The presence of normal fetal biophysical activities shows that the central nervous system is fully functional and that therefore the fetus is not hypoxemic (Harman, 2004). BPP variables and scoring are detailed in Table 9-4.

The BPP is an accurate indicator of impending fetal death. Fetal acidosis can be diagnosed early with a nonreactive NST and absent fetal breathing movements. When an abnormal score and oligohydramnios are encountered, labor induction is warranted (Harman, 2004). Fetal infection in women whose membranes rupture prematurely (at less than 37 weeks of gestation) can be diagnosed early by changes in biophysical activities that precede the clinical signs of infection and indicate the necessity for immediate birth. When the BPP score is normal and the risk of fetal death low, intervention is indicated only for obstetric or maternal factors.

Nursing Role

Although a growing number of nurses perform ultrasound scans and BPPs in certain centers, the main role of nurses is in counseling and educating women about the procedure. Providing accurate information regarding the procedure is imperative to allay the mother's anxiety. Women should be provided ample opportunity to ask questions and be reassured that the procedure is safe. In the 30 years that diagnostic ultrasonography has been used, no conclusive evidence of any harmful effects on humans has emerged. Although the possibility of unidentified biologic effects exists, the benefits to the woman of prudent use of diagnostic ultrasonography appear to outweigh any possible risk (Chervenak & Gabbe, 2002).

LEGAL TIP Performance of Limited Ultrasound Examinations Nurses who have the training and competence may perform limited ultrasound examinations if it is within the scope of practice in their state or area and consistent with regulations of the agencies in which they practice. Limited ultrasound examinations include identification of fetal number, fetal presentation, fetal cardiac activity, location of the placenta, and BPP, including AFV assessment. Women should be informed about the limited information provided by these examinations. They are not meant to evaluate or identify fetal anomalies, assess fetal age, or estimate fetal weight. The obstetric health care

Table 9-4

Interpretation of Biophysical Profile Score Variables

FETAL VARIABLE	NORMAL BEHAVIOR (SCORE = 2)	ABNORMAL BEHAVIOR (SCORE = 0)
Fetal breathing movements	Intermittent multiple episodes of more than 30-sec duration, within 30-min BPS time frame. Hiccups count. Continuous FBM for 30 min = exclude fetal acidosis.	Continuous breathing without cessation. Completely absent breathing or no sustained episodes.
Body or limb movements	At least four discrete body movements in 30 min. Continuous active movement episodes = single movement. Includes fine motor movements, rolling movements, and so on, but not REM or mouthing movements.	Three or fewer body/limb movements in a 30-min observation period.
Fetal tone/posture	Demonstration of active extension with rapid return to flexion of fetal limbs and brisk repositioning/trunk rotation. Opening and closing of hand, mouth, kicking, and so on.	Low-velocity movement only. Incomplete flexion, flaccid extremity positions, abnormal fetal posture. Must score = 0 when FM completely absent.
Cardiotocogram	Normal mean variation (computerized FHR interpretation), accelerations associated with maternal palpation of FM (accelerations graded for gestation), 20-min CTG.	Fetal movement and accelerations not coupled. Insufficient accelerations, absent accelerations, or decelerative trace. Mean variation <20 on numerical analysis of CTG.
Amniotic fluid evaluation	At least one pocket >3 cm with no umbilical cord. See text regarding subjectively decreased fluid.	No cord-free pocket >2 cm or elements of subjectively reduced amniotic fluid volume definite.

From Harman CR: Assessment of fetal health. In Creasy RK, Resnik R, Iams JD (eds): *Maternal-fetal medicine: principles and practice,* ed 5, Philadelphia, 2004, WB Saunders, p 363.
BPS, biophysical profile score; *CTG,* cardiotocogram; *FBM,* fetal breathing movements; *FHR,* fetal heart rate; *FM,* fetal movement; *REM,* rapid eye movement.

provider is responsible for obtaining a more comprehensive ultrasound examination when complete patient assessment is necessary (Association of Women's Health, Obstetric and Neonatal Nurses, 1998). ■

Magnetic Resonance Imaging

Magnetic resonance imaging (MRI) is a noninvasive tool that can be used for obstetric and gynecologic diagnosis. Like computed tomography (CT), MRI provides excellent pictures of soft tissue. Unlike CT, ionizing radiation is not used; thus vascular structures within the body can be visualized and evaluated without injection of an iodinated contrast medium, thus eliminating any known biologic risk. Like sonography, MRI is noninvasive and can provide images in multiple planes, but there is no interference from skeletal, fatty, or gas-filled structures, and imaging of deep pelvic structures does not require a full bladder.

With MRI, the examiner can evaluate (1) fetal structure (central nervous system, thorax, abdomen, genitourinary tract, and musculoskeletal system) and overall growth; (2) placenta (position, density, and presence of gestational trophoblastic disease); (3) amniotic fluid quantity; (4) maternal structures (uterus, cervix, adnexa, and pelvis); (5) biochemical status (pH and adenosine triphosphate content) of tissues and organs; and (6) soft tissue, metabolic, or functional malformations.

The woman is placed on a table in a supine position and slid into the bore of the main magnet, which is similar in appearance to a CT scanner. Depending on the reason for the study, the entire procedure may take from 20 to 60 minutes, during which time the woman must be perfectly still except for short respites. Because of the long time needed to produce magnetic resonance images, it is likely that the fetus will move and obscure anatomic details. The only way to ensure that this does not occur is to administer a sedative to the mother, but this approach should be reserved for selected cases in which visualization of fetal detail is critical.

MRI has little effect on the fetus; concerns that the FHR or fetal movement would decrease have not been supported.

BIOCHEMICAL ASSESSMENT

Biochemical assessment involves the study of biologic components such as genes or exfoliated cells and chemical components such as the lecithin/sphingomyelin (L/S) ratio and bilirubin levels (Table 9-5). Procedures used to obtain the specimens for study include amniocentesis, percutaneous umbilical blood sampling, chorionic villus sampling, and maternal assays (see Box 9-10).

Amniocentesis

Amniocentesis is performed to obtain amniotic fluid, which contains fetal cells. Under direct ultrasonographic visualization, a needle is inserted transabdominally into the uterus, amniotic fluid is withdrawn into a syringe, and various assessments are performed. Amniocentesis is possible after week 14 of pregnancy, when the uterus becomes an abdominal organ and sufficient amniotic fluid is available for testing (see Table 9-5, Fig. 9-7). Indications for the procedure include prenatal diagnosis of genetic disorders or congenital anomalies (neural tube defects in particular),

Table 9-5

Summary of Biochemical Monitoring Techniques

TEST	POSSIBLE FINDINGS	CLINICAL SIGNIFICANCE
MATERNAL BLOOD		
Coombs' test	Titer of 1:8 and rising	Significant Rh incompatibility
AFP	See below	See below
AMNIOTIC FLUID ANALYSIS		
Color	Meconium	Possible hypoxia or asphyxia
Lung profile		
• L/S ratio	>2	Fetal lung maturity
• Phosphatidylglycerol	Present	Fetal lung maturity
Creatinine	>2 mg/dl	Gestational age >36 weeks
Bilirubin (ΔOD 450/nm)	<0.015 High levels	Gestational age >36 weeks, normal pregnancy Fetal hemolytic disease in Rh-isoimmunized pregnancies
Lipid cells	>10%	Gestational age >35 weeks
AFP	High levels after 15-week gestation	Open neural tube or other defect
Osmolality	Decline after 20-week gestation	Advancing nonspecific gestational age
Genetic disorders • Sex-linked • Chromosomal • Metabolic	Dependent on cultured cells for karyotype and enzymatic activity	Counseling possibly required

assessment of pulmonary maturity, and diagnosis of fetal hemolytic disease.

Complications in the mother and fetus occur in less than 1% of cases and include the following:

Maternal—Hemorrhage, fetomaternal hemorrhage with possible maternal Rh isoimmunization, infection, labor, abruptio placentae, inadvertent damage to the intestines or bladder, and amniotic fluid embolism. Because of the possibility of fetomaternal hemorrhage, it is standard practice to administer immune globulin D (RhoGAM) to the woman who is Rh negative after an amniocentesis.

Fetal—Death, hemorrhage, infection (amnionitis), direct injury from the needle, miscarriage or preterm labor, and leakage of amniotic fluid.

Many of the complications have been minimized or eliminated by performing the procedure under ultrasound guidance.

Indications for Use

Genetic Concerns

Prenatal assessment of genetic disorders is indicated for women over age 35 years (Box 9-7), for those with a previous child with a chromosomal abnormality, and those with a family history of chromosomal anomalies. Inherited errors of metabolism and other disorders for which marker genes are known may also be detected.

Cells are cultured for karyotyping of chromosomes (see Chapter 8). The incidence of fetal chromosomal aberrations increases with age of the mother. Fetal cells can be assessed for sex chromatin; sex determination is important if a sex-linked disorder is suspected.

Alpha-fetoprotein (AFP) levels are assessed as a follow-up for elevated levels of maternal serum AFP. High AFP levels in the amniotic fluid occur in the presence of an open neural tube

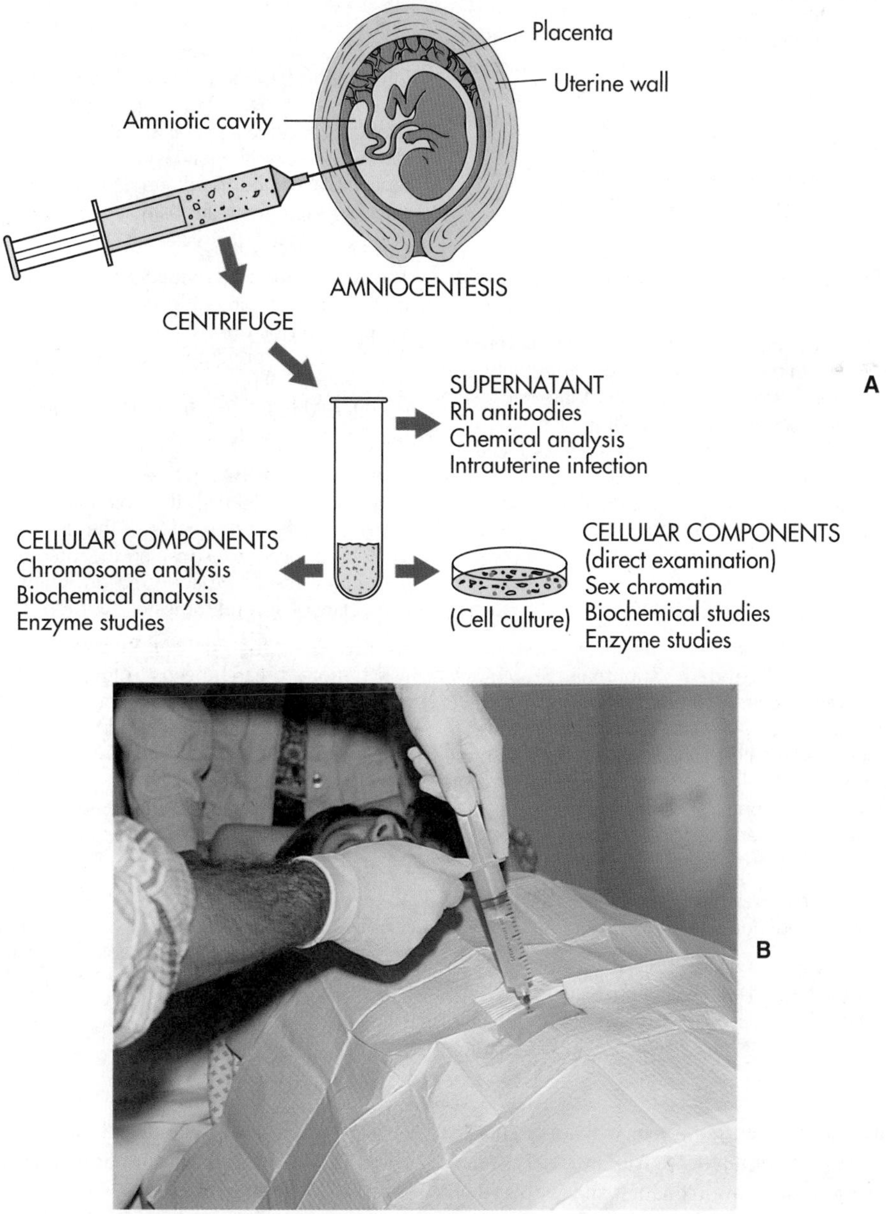

Fig. 9-7 **A**, Amniocentesis and laboratory use of amniotic fluid aspirant. **B**, Transabdominal amniocentesis. (*B*, Courtesy Marjorie Pyle, RNC, Lifecircle, Costa Mesa, CA.)

Evidence-Based Practice

PRENATAL DIAGNOSTICS: AMNIOCENTESIS AND CHORIONIC VILLI SAMPLING

Background

Women requesting prenatal diagnostic testing may have anxiety while waiting, receive false-positive results (abnormal results but a normal fetus), and have a lack of options if the test is abnormal. Many women want the testing done early enough that they may consider pregnancy termination if the results are abnormal. The method of choice for diagnosing anatomic problems is ultrasonography. Maternal serum screening can show markers for certain abnormalities, such as Down syndrome. Diagnostic testing for genetic abnormality, however, must be done on fetal cells. Techniques to obtain those cells are all invasive, and carry risks for fetal injury and loss.

Amniocentesis is conventionally done at approximately 16 weeks of gestation. The amount of amniotic fluid is sufficient by then to permit the withdrawal of the 10 to 20 ml that is required to yield an adequate number of fetal cells. Removal of that much amniotic fluid earlier may lead to increased orthopedic problems and respiratory distress syndrome. Genetic results are returned after 18 weeks, in time for the woman to choose a second trimester termination. The wait is agonizing for parents, and second trimester abortion is not always a personal option, nor is it always available.

There is pressure for earlier diagnostic procedures, such as chorionic villi sampling (CVS) of the placenta, accessed either transabdominally or transcervically. Most clinicians delay this procedure until after 9 weeks of gestation, due to some early clusters of limb reduction (missing or hypoplastic limbs) seen after early CVS. Early amniocentesis is another option, requiring skillful removal of amniotic fluid from the inner amniotic sac only, filtering for fetal cells, and replacing the fluid. Both early procedures may cause pregnancy loss.

Objective

The reviewers' goal was to compare early and late amniocentesis and CVS (both transabdominal and transcervical) for safety and accuracy. The interventions were these four tests. Outcomes were the technical difficulties encountered in sampling, problems with the genetic analysis, pregnancy complications such as bleeding, leaking fluid, preterm labor, any pregnancy losses and stillbirths, and neonatal abnormalities, such as talipes (clubfoot), hemangiomas, limb reduction, respiratory distress syndrome, low birth weight, and admission to special care nursery.

Methods

Search Strategy

The reviewers searched Cochrane, MEDLINE, 30 journals, and a weekly awareness search that covered 37 journals. Search keywords included *amniocentesis* and *chorionic villi sampling*.

There were 14 randomized studies that were accepted into this review, ranging in publication dates from 1986 to 1999. The number of women was not reported for every study, but totaled more than 15,000. The countries of origin included Denmark, Sweden, Finland, Italy, the United States, and Canada.

Statistical Analyses

Statistical analyses allowed a weighted estimate of risk for each outcome, and the results were pooled from the studies.

Findings

Pregnancy loss following second-trimester amniocentesis was 3%, which was not significantly increased over the general population risk of 2%. However, amniocentesis was associated with an increased risk of spontaneous miscarriage and amniotic fluid leakage. Second-trimester amniocentesis was safer and easier than early amniocentesis, with fewer fetal anomalies, fewer needle inserts, fewer laboratory failures (due to inadequate fetal cells), and fewer false-negative results. Transcervical CVS was associated with significantly more pregnancy loss, more laboratory failures, and more vaginal bleeding than second-trimester amniocentesis. Transabdominal CVS appears to be safer than the transcervical procedure. Early amniocentesis appeared to cause more spontaneous miscarriage than transabdominal CVS. The incidence of anomalies was not increased significantly.

Limitations

The expertise of the operators varied, because CVS was fairly new in 1991. This, however, may not necessarily be a limitation, because it reflects the reality that there are always practitioners of varying skill levels practicing. Some studies "randomized" by giving women the choice of procedures. During the course of some of the trials, information became publicized about CVS leading to limb reduction (never replicated in later, larger studies), so recruitment and dropouts became a problem. None of the trials assessed the laboratory accuracy adequately. One large trial excluded 70% of potential CVS-randomized women because of placental position, thus reducing generalizability.

Conclusions

The second-trimester amniocentesis appears to be the safest and most accurate prenatal diagnostic procedure. Amniocentesis should never be done before 15 weeks of gestation. The transabdominal CVS is preferable if an early procedure is warranted. If the transabdominal procedure is contraindicated, the transcervical CVS is preferred in the first trimester and amniocentesis is preferred in the second trimester.

Implications for Practice

Women presented with the possibility of fetal anomalies need to know the risks and benefits of the diagnostic procedures offered. They also need to consider the therapeutic options available, should the results be abnormal, including the availability and acceptability of second trimester abortion.

Implications for Further Research

Much more research needs to focus on the acceptability and satisfaction of women with the procedures, and their decision making. The unavailability of second trimester abortion in some areas creates hardships that deserve research. All new prenatal procedures should be rigorously tested before general use. Outcomes should include antenatal and neonatal loss, details about anomalies, and diagnostic accuracy. Neonatal assessors should be blinded as to procedure used.

Reference

Alfirevic Z, Sunberg K, Brigham S: Amniocentesis and chorionic villi sampling for prenatal diagnosis (Cochrane Review). In *The Cochrane Library*, Issue 2, Chichester, UK, 2004, John Wiley & Sons.

defect such as spina bifida or anencephaly, or with an open abdominal wall defect such as omphalocele. AFP levels also may be elevated in a normal multifetal pregnancy and with intestinal atresia, presumably caused by lack of fetal swallowing. The presence of acetylcholinesterase in amniotic fluid almost always indicates a fetal defect (Jenkins & Wapner, 2004). Follow-up ultrasound examination is recommended.

Fetal Maturity

Accurate assessment of fetal maturity is possible through examination of amniotic fluid or its exfoliated cellular con-

BOX 9-7

Elimination of Maternal Age as an Indication for Invasive Prenatal Diagnosis

Maternal age of 35 years and older has been a standard indication for invasive prenatal testing since 1979 despite a sensitivity of only 30%. The importance of age as a single indication for testing is being reevaluated as serum screening has evolved. The most effective use of resources involves screening the whole population of pregnant women. Presently many centers offer the option of screening before invasive testing for women over 35 years of age (Jenkins & Wapner, 2004).

BOX 9-8

Shake Test for the Presence of Phospholipids

A quick means of determining an approximate L/S ratio is the shake test, foam test, or bubble stability test. Serial dilutions of fresh amniotic fluid are mixed with ethanol and shaken. After 15 minutes, the amount of bubbles present at different dilutions indicates the presence of surfactant.

tents (Box 9-8). Table 9-5 includes laboratory studies that are used to demonstrate term pregnancy and fetal maturity.

Fetal Hemolytic Disease

Amniocentesis is used to identify and follow up fetal hemolytic disease in cases of isoimmunization. The procedure is usually not done until the mother's serum antibody titer reaches 1:8 and is rising. Currently, PUBS is the procedure of choice to evaluate and treat fetal hemolytic disease.

Meconium

The presence of meconium in the amniotic fluid is usually determined by visual inspection of the sample. The significance of meconium in the amniotic fluid varies depending on when it is found.

Antepartal Period

Meconium in the amniotic fluid before early labor begins is not usually associated with an adverse fetal outcome. The finding may be the result of an acute and subsequently corrected fetal stress, chronic ongoing stress, or simply the physiologic passage of meconium. Because there is some association between meconium in amniotic fluid in the third trimester and hypertensive conditions and postmaturity, the fetus should undergo further antepartum evaluation if the birth is not imminent (Glantz & Woods, 2004).

Intrapartal Period

Intrapartal meconium-stained amniotic fluid is an indication for more careful evaluation by electronic fetal monitoring (EFM) and perhaps fetal scalp blood sampling. The presence of meconium, however, should not be the sole indicator for intervention.

Three possible reasons exist for the passage of meconium during the intrapartal period: (1) it is a normal physiologic function that occurs with maturity (meconium passage is uncommon before weeks 23 to 24, but there is an increased incidence after 38 weeks); (2) it is the result of hypoxia-induced peristalsis and sphincter relaxation; and (3) it may be a sequel to umbilical cord compression–induced vagal stimulation in mature fetuses. Thick, fresh meconium passed for the first time in late labor, associated with nonremediable severe variable or late FHR decelerations, is an ominous sign.

Suctioning the nasopharynx of the neonate at time of the birth before the first breath is taken is common practice. Suctioning at this time is thought to be effective in reducing the incidence and severity of meconium aspiration in the neonate. However, Vain and colleagues (2004) studied 2514 patients with meconium-stained amniotic fluid randomly assigned to suction or no suction groups. They found no significant difference between groups in the incidence of meconium aspiration syndrome.

Use of amniocentesis and CVS is declining because of advances in noninvasive screening techniques. These techniques include measurement of nuchal translucency, maternal serum screening tests in the first and second trimesters, and ultrasonography in the second trimester (ACOG, 2004b).

Percutaneous Umbilical Blood Sampling

Direct access to the fetal circulation during the second and third trimesters is possible through percutaneous umbilical blood sampling (PUBS), or cordocentesis. PUBS is the most widely used method for fetal blood sampling and transfusion. PUBS involves the insertion of a needle directly into the fetal umbilical vessel under ultrasound guidance. Ideally, the umbilical cord is punctured 1 to 2 cm from its placental insertion (Fig. 9-8). At this point the cord is well anchored and will not move, and the risk of maternal blood contamination (from the placenta) is slight. Generally, 1 to 4 ml of blood is removed during the puncture and tested immediately by the Kleihauer-Betke procedure to ensure that it is fetal blood. Indications for use of PUBS include prenatal diagnosis of inherited blood disorders, karyotyping of malformed fetuses, detection of fetal infection, determination of the acid-base status of fetuses with IUGR, and assessment and treatment of isoimmunization and thrombocytopenia (Jenkins & Wapner, 2004). Complications that can occur include leaking of blood from the puncture site, cord laceration, thromboembolism, preterm labor, premature rupture of membranes, and infection.

In fetuses at risk for isoimmune hemolytic anemia, PUBS permits precise identification of fetal blood type and RBC count and may eliminate the need for further intervention. If the fetus is positive for the presence of maternal antibodies, a direct blood test can confirm the degree of anemia resulting from hemolysis. Intrauterine transfusion of severely anemic fetuses can be done 4 to 5 weeks earlier than through the intraperitoneal route.

Follow-up includes continuous FHR monitoring for several minutes to 1 hour and a repeat ultrasound examination 1 hour later to ensure that no bleeding or hematoma formation has occurred.

Chorionic Villus Sampling

The combined advantages of earlier diagnosis and rapid results have made chorionic villus sampling a popular technique for genetic studies, although some risks to the fetus exist. Indications for CVS are similar to those for amniocen-

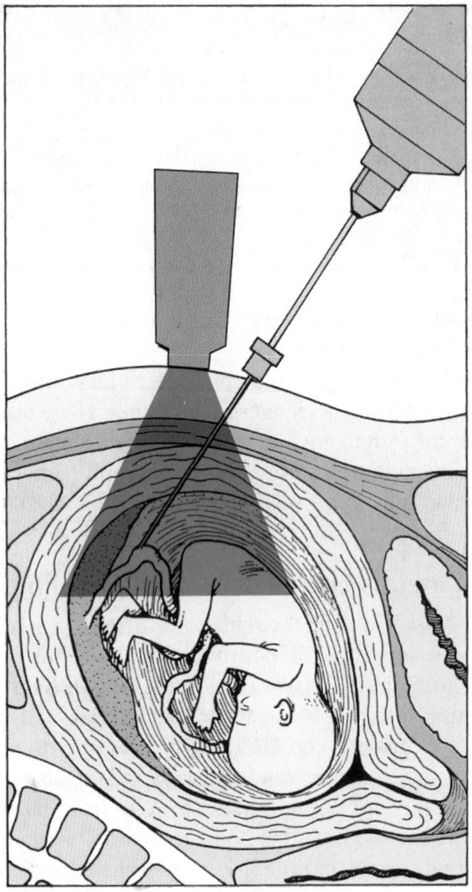

Fig. 9-8 Technique for PUBS guided by ultrasound.

tesis, however, second trimester amniocentesis appears to be safer than CVS (Alfirevic, Sunberg, & Brigham, 2004). The benefits of earlier diagnosis must be weighed against the increased risk of pregnancy loss and risk of anomalies.

The procedure is performed between 10 and 12 weeks of gestation and involves the removal of a small tissue specimen from the fetal portion of the placenta. Because chorionic villi originate in the zygote, that tissue reflects the genetic makeup of the fetus.

CVS can be accomplished either transcervically or transabdominally. In transcervical sampling, a sterile catheter is introduced into the cervix under continuous ultrasonographic guidance and a small portion of the chorionic villi is aspirated with a syringe. The aspiration cannula and obturator must be placed at a suitable site, and rupture of the amniotic sac must be avoided.

If the abdominal approach is used, an 18-gauge spinal needle with stylet is inserted under sterile conditions through the abdominal wall into the chorion frondosum under ultrasound guidance. The stylet is then withdrawn, and the chorionic tissue is aspirated into a syringe (Fig. 9-9).

Complications of the procedure include vaginal spotting or bleeding immediately afterward (Box 9-9), miscarriage (0.3%), rupture of membranes (0.1%), and chorioamnionitis (0.5%). Because of the possibility of fetomaternal hemorrhage, women who are Rh negative should receive RhoGAM to avoid isoimmunization (Gilbert & Harmon, 2003). An increased risk of limb anomalies has been noted when CVS is done before 10 weeks of gestation (Box 9-10).

BOX 9-9

Apt Test for Differentiation of Maternal and Fetal Blood

The Apt test is used to differentiate maternal and fetal blood when vaginal bleeding occurs during pregnancy or labor. It may be performed quickly by the following method: Add 0.5 ml of bloody fluid to 4.5 ml of distilled water and shake. Add 1 ml of 0.25 N sodium hydroxide. Fetal and cord blood remains pink for 1 to 2 minutes. Maternal blood turns brown in 30 seconds. A Kleihauer-Betke procedure can be done in the laboratory to confirm the presence of fetal blood.

Maternal Assays

Alpha-Fetoprotein

AFP is produced by the fetal liver and is detectable in increasing quantities in the serum of pregnant women from 14 to 34 weeks. Maternal serum AFP (MSAFP) is used in pregnancy as a screening tool for neural tube defects (NTDs) and is usually done between 15 and 22 weeks of gestation (ideally between 16 and 18 weeks) (Jenkins & Wapner, 2004). Screening is recommended for all pregnant women. Once the maternal level of AFP is determined, it is compared with normal values for each week of gestation. Values also should be correlated with maternal age, weight, race, and whether the woman has insulin-dependent diabetes. If findings are abnormal, follow-up procedures include genetic counseling for families with a history of NTD, repeat AFP, ultrasound examination, and possibly amniocentesis.

Through MSAFP, approximately 80% to 85% of all open NTDs and open abdominal defects, can be detected early in pregnancy. The cause of NTDs is not well understood, but 95% of all affected infants are born to women with no family history of similar anomalies. The defect occurs in 7 per 10,000 births in the United States (U.S., Irish Researchers Identify Important Clue to Genetic Basis for Neural Tube Defects, 2004). The birth of one affected child increases the risk of NTD recurrence in future pregnancies to 1% to 5%.

Down syndrome—and probably other autosomal trisomies—is associated with lower-than-normal levels of MSAFP and amniotic fluid AFP. The triple-marker test is also performed at 16 to 18 weeks of gestation and uses the levels of three markers, MSAFP, unconjugated estriol, and human chorionic gonadotropin (hCG), in combination with maternal age to calculate a new risk. If a fetus has Down syndrome, the MSAFP and unconjugated estriol levels are low and the hCG level is elevated. With these two additional screening tests, approximately 60% of fetuses with Down syndrome can be identified. Other maternal markers are being investigated as predictors of fetal abnormalities as well. Serum pregnancy-associated placental protein A (PAPP-A) is low in Down syndrome, whereas another substance, inhibin-A, is elevated in Down syndrome and other trisomies (Simpson, 2002).

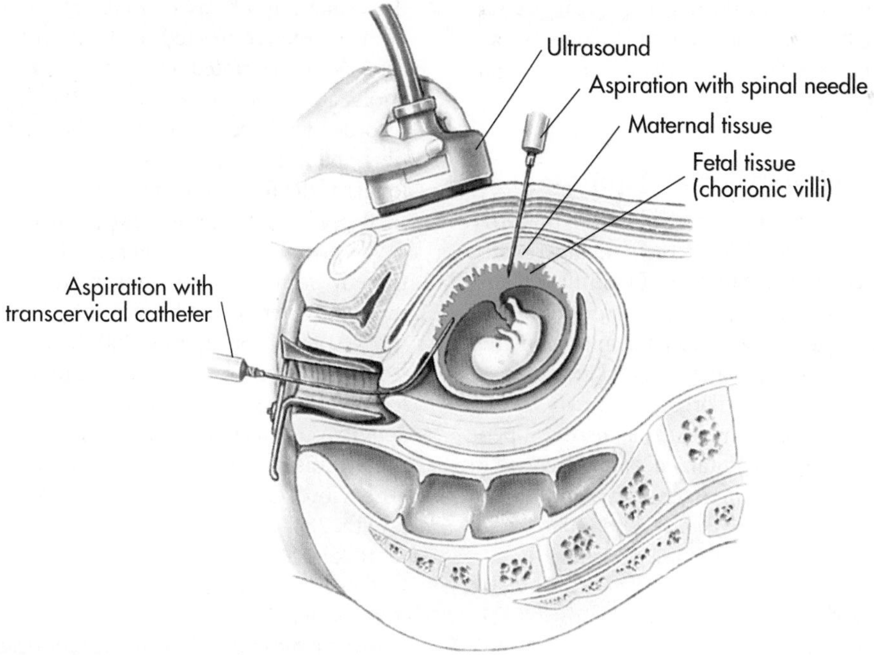

Fig. 9-9 Chorionic villi sampling (abdominal and transcervical methods). (Courtesy Medical and Scientific Illustration, Crozet, VA.)

BOX 9-10

Fetal Rights

Amniocentesis, PUBS, and CVS are prenatal tests used for diagnosing fetal defects in pregnancy. They are invasive and carry risks to the mother and fetus. A consideration of abortion is linked to the performance of these tests because there is no treatment for genetically affected fetuses. Thus the issue of fetal rights is a key ethical concern in prenatal testing for fetal defects.

As with MSAFP, these tests are screening procedures only and are not diagnostic. A definitive examination of amniotic fluid for AFP and chromosomal analysis, combined with ultrasound visualization of the fetus, is necessary for diagnosis.

Coombs' Test

The Coombs' test for Rh incompatibility is discussed in Chapter 28. If the maternal titer for Rh antibodies is greater than 1:8, amniocentesis for bilirubin in amniotic fluid or PUBS is indicated to determine the severity of fetal anemia from hemolysis. The Coombs' test can also detect other antibodies that may place the fetus at risk for incompatibility with maternal antigens.

ASSESSMENT USING ELECTRONIC FETAL MONITORING

Indications

Assessment during the first and second trimesters is directed primarily at the diagnosis of fetal anomalies. The goal of third-trimester testing is to determine whether the intrauterine environment continues to be supportive to the fetus. The testing is often used to determine the timing of childbirth for patients at risk for uteroplacental insufficiency (i.e., the gradual decline in the delivery of needed substances to the fetus). Gradual loss of placental function results in inadequate nutrient delivery to the fetus leading to IUGR. Subsequently, respiratory function is compromised, resulting in fetal hypoxia. Indications for the nonstress test (NST) (or fetal activity determination [FAD]) and the contraction stress test (CST) are listed in Box 9-11.

BOX 9-11

Indications for the Nonstress Test and the Contraction Stress Test

Maternal diabetes mellitus
Chronic hypertension
Hypertensive disorders in pregnancy
IUGR
Sickle cell disease
Maternal cyanotic heart disease
Postmaturity
History of previous stillbirth
Decreased fetal movement
Isoimmunization
Meconium-stained amniotic fluid at third-trimester amniocentesis
Hyperthyroidism
Collagen disease
Older pregnant woman
Chronic renal disease

No clinical contraindications exist for the NST, but results may be inconclusive if gestation is 26 weeks or less. Absolute contraindications for the CST are rupture of membranes, previous classic incision for cesarean birth, preterm labor, placenta previa, and abruptio placentae. Multifetal pregnancy, previous preterm labor, hydramnios, more than

36 weeks of gestation, and incompetent cervix are relative contraindications for CST. As a rule, reactive patterns with the NST or negative results with the CST are associated with favorable outcomes.

Fetal Responses to Hypoxia and Asphyxia

Hypoxia or asphyxia elicit a number of responses in the fetus. There is a redistribution of blood flow to certain vital organs. This series of responses (redistribution of blood flow favoring vital organs, decreased total oxygen consumption, and anaerobic glycolysis) is a temporary mechanism that enables the fetus to survive up to 30 minutes of limited oxygen supply without decompensation of vital organs. However, during more severe asphyxia or sustained hypoxemia, these compensatory responses are no longer maintained, and a decrease in the cardiac output, arterial blood pressure, and blood flow to the brain and heart occurs (Parer & Nageotte, 2004), with characteristic FHR patterns reflecting these changes.

Variability

Considerable evidence supports the clinical belief that FHR variability indicates an intact nervous pathway through the cerebral cortex, midbrain, vagus nerve, and cardiac conduction system. With 98% accuracy in predicting fetal well-being, the presence of normal FHR variability is a reassuring indicator. Input from various areas of the brain decreases after cerebral asphyxia, leading to a decrease in variability after failure of the fetal hemodynamic compensatory mechanisms to maintain cerebral oxygenation (Parer & Nageotte, 2004).

Nonstress Test (Fetal Activity Determination)

The NST is the most widely applied technique for antepartum evaluation of the fetus. The basis for the NST, or FAD, is that the normal fetus produces characteristic FHR patterns in response to fetal movements (FMs). In the healthy fetus with an intact central nervous system, 90% of gross fetal body movements are associated with FHR accelerations. An absence of acceleration is most commonly associated with the fetal sleep cycle but may result from depression of the central nervous system (e.g., from hypoxemia, anomalies, or drugs) (Tucker, 2004).

NST can be performed easily in an outpatient setting because it is noninvasive. It also is relatively inexpensive and has no known contraindications. Disadvantages center around the high rate of false-positive results for nonreactivity as a result of fetal sleep cycles, medications, and fetal immaturity. The test is slightly less sensitive in detecting fetal compromise than are the CST or BPP.

Procedure

The woman is seated in a reclining chair (or in a semi-Fowler position) with a slight left tilt to optimize uterine perfusion and avoid supine hypotension. The FHR is recorded with a Doppler transducer, and a tocodynamometer is applied to detect uterine contractions or fetal movements. The tracing is observed for signs of fetal activity and a concurrent acceleration of FHR. If evidence of FM is not apparent on the strip, the woman may be asked to depress a button on a hand-held event marker connected to the monitor when she feels FM. The FM is then noted on the strip. Because almost all accelerations are accompanied by FM, the movements need not be recorded with accelerations for the test to be considered reactive. The test usually takes 20 to 30 minutes, but it may take longer if the fetus needs to be awakened from a sleep state.

It has been suggested that the woman drink orange juice or be given glucose to increase her blood sugar level and thereby stimulate fetal movements. This practice is common; however, research has not proven this practice to be effective (Tan & Sabapathy, 2004). Some sources suggest that fetal movements increase when maternal glucose levels are low. Other methods that have been used to stimulate fetal activity, such as manipulating the woman's abdomen or using a transvaginal light, have not been very effective either. Only vibroacoustic stimulation has had some impact (Tan & Smyth, 2004).

Interpretation

Generally accepted criteria for a reactive tracing are as follows (Fig. 9-10):

- Two or more accelerations of 15 beats/min lasting for 15 seconds over a 20-minute period
- Normal baseline rate
- Long-term variability amplitude of 10 or more beats/min

If the test does not meet the criteria after 40 minutes, it is considered nonreactive (Fig. 9-11, Table 9-6), in which case further assessments are needed with a CST or BPP. The current recommendation is that NST be performed twice weekly (after 28 weeks of gestation) with patients who have diabetes or are at risk for fetal death (Druzin et al, 2002).

Vibroacoustic Stimulation

Vibroacoustic stimulation (also called fetal acoustic stimulation test) is another method of testing antepartum FHR response. The test takes approximately 15 minutes to complete, with the fetus monitored for 5 to 10 minutes before stimulation to obtain a baseline FHR. If the fetal baseline pattern is nonreactive, the sound source (usually a laryngeal stimulator) is then activated for 3 seconds on the maternal abdomen over the fetal head. Monitoring continues for another 5 minutes, after which the monitor tracing is assessed. A test is considered reactive if there is an immediate and sustained increase in long-term variability and heart rate accel-

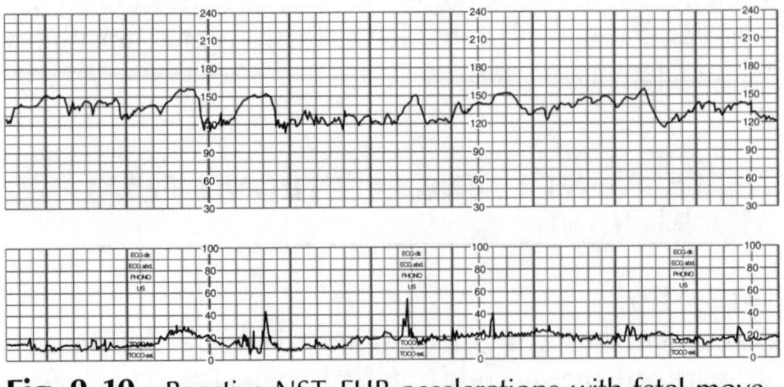

Fig. 9-10 Reactive NST. FHR accelerations with fetal movement. (From Tucker SM: *Pocket guide to fetal monitoring and assessment,* ed 5, St Louis, 2004, Mosby.)

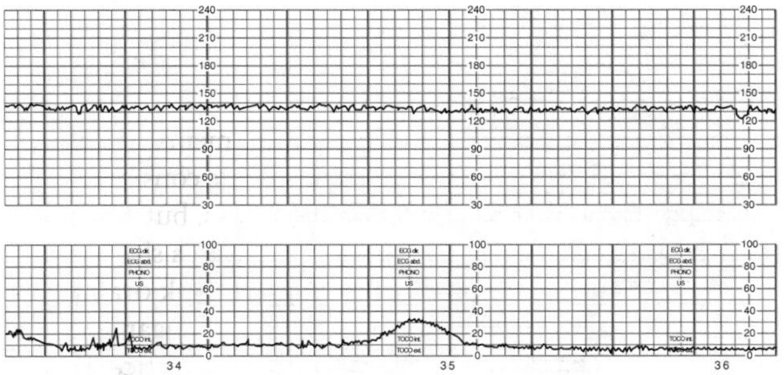

Fig. 9-11 Nonreactive nonstress test (no fetal heart rate accelerations). (From Tucker SM: *Pocket guide to fetal monitoring and assessment,* ed 5, St Louis, 2004, Mosby.)

erations. The test may be repeated at 1-minute intervals up to three times when there is no response. Further evaluation is needed with BPP or CST if the pattern is still nonreactive (Druzin et al, 2002)

Contraction Stress Test

The CST was one of the first electronic methods to be developed for assessment of fetal well-being. It was devised as a graded stress test of the fetus. Its purpose was to identify the fetus in jeopardy who was stable at rest but showed evidence of compromise with stress. Uterine contractions decrease uterine blood flow and placental perfusion. If this decrease is sufficient to produce hypoxia in the fetus, a deceleration in FHR results, beginning at the peak of the contraction and persisting after its conclusion (late deceleration).

NURSE ALERT In a healthy fetoplacental unit, uterine contractions usually do not produce late decelerations; when there is underlying uteroplacental insufficiency, contractions will produce late decelerations. ■

The CST provides a warning of fetal compromise earlier than the NST and with fewer false-positive tests. In addition to the contraindications described earlier, CST is more time-consuming and expensive than an NST. It also is an invasive procedure if exogenous oxytocin stimulation is required.

Procedure

The woman is placed in semi-Fowler position or sits in a reclining chair with a slight lateral tilt to optimize uterine perfusion and avoid supine hypotension. She is monitored electronically with the fetal ultrasound transducer and uterine tocodynamometer. The tracing is observed for 10 to 20 minutes for baseline rate, long-term variability, and the possible occurrence of spontaneous contractions. Two methods of CST are the nipple-stimulated contraction test and the oxytocin-stimulated contraction test.

Nipple-Stimulated Contraction Test

Several methods of nipple stimulation have been described. In one approach, the woman applies warm, moist washcloths to both breasts for several minutes. The woman is then asked to massage one nipple for 10 minutes. Massaging the nipples causes a release of oxytocin from the posterior pituitary. An alternative approach is for her to massage the nipple for 2 minutes, rest for 5 minutes, and repeat the cycles of massage and rest as necessary to achieve adequate uterine activity. When adequate contractions or hyperstimulation (defined as uterine contractions lasting more than 90 seconds or five or more contractions in 10 minutes) occurs, stimulation should be stopped (Druzin et al, 2002).

Oxytocin-Stimulated Contraction Test

Exogenous oxytocin can also be used to stimulate uterine contractions. An intravenous (IV) infusion is begun with a scalp needle. The oxytocin is diluted in an IV solution (usually 10 units in 1000 ml of fluid) and infused through a piggyback port into the tubing of the main IV device. An infusion pump is used to ensure accurate dosage. The oxytocin infusion usually is begun at 0.5 milliunits/min and increased by 0.5 milliunits/min at 15- to 30-minute intervals until three uterine contractions of good quality are observed within a 10-minute period. A rate of 10 milliunits/min is usually adequate to elicit uterine contractions (Druzin et al, 2002).

Interpretation

If no late decelerations are observed with the contractions, the findings are considered to be negative (Fig. 9-12). Repet-

Table 9-6

Interpretation of the Nonstress Test

RESULT	INTERPRETATION	CLINICAL SIGNIFICANCE
Reactive	Two or more accelerations of FHR of 15 beats/min lasting 15 sec or more, associated with each FM in a 20-min period	As long as twice-weekly NSTs remain reactive, most high risk pregnancies are allowed to continue.
Nonreactive	Any tracing with either no FHR accelerations or accelerations <15 beats/min or lasting <15 sec throughout any FM during testing period	Further indirect monitoring may be attempted with abdominal fetal electrocardiography (ECG) in an effort to clarify FHR pattern and quantitative variability; external monitoring should continue, and a CST or BPP should be done.
Unsatisfactory	Quality of FHR recording not adequate for interpretation	Test is repeated in 24 hr or a CST is done, depending on the clinical situation.

BPP, biophysical profile; *CST,* contraction stress test; *FHR,* fetal heart rate; *FM,* fetal movements; *NST,* nonstress test.

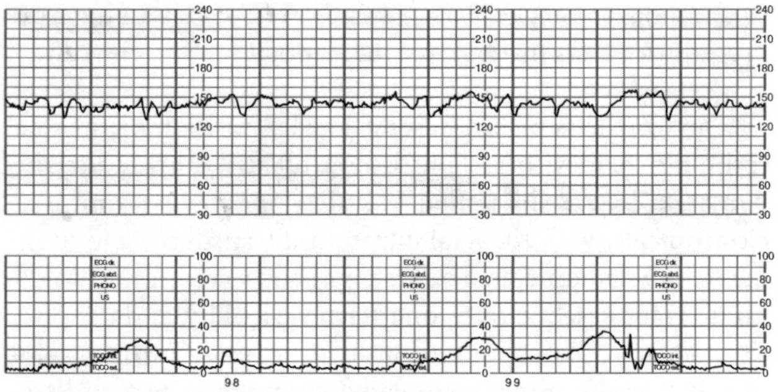

Fig. 9-12 Negative contraction stress test (reassuring external fetal heart rate tracing). (From Tucker SM: *Pocket guide to fetal monitoring and assessment,* ed 5, St Louis, 2004, Mosby.)

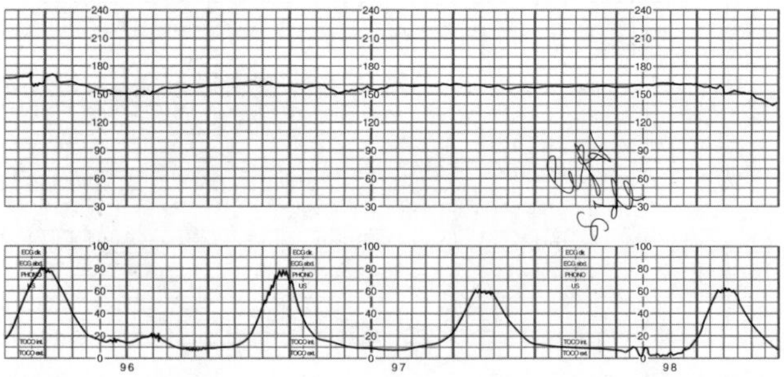

Fig. 9-13 Positive contraction stress test (nonreassuring late decelerations with uterine contractions). (From Tucker SM: *Pocket guide to fetal monitoring and assessment,* ed 5, St Louis, 2004, Mosby.)

itive late decelerations render the test results positive (Fig. 9-13, Table 9-7).

After interpretation of the FHR pattern, the oxytocin infusion is discontinued, and the maintenance IV solution is infused until the uterine activity has returned to the prestimulation level. If the CST is negative, the IV device is removed and the fetal monitor disconnected. If the CST is positive, continued monitoring and further evaluation of fetal well-being are indicated.

NURSING ROLE IN ANTENATAL ASSESSMENT FOR RISK

The nurse's role is that of educator and support person when the woman is undergoing examinations such as ultrasonography, MRI, CVS, PUBS, and amniocentesis. In some instances the nurse may assist the physician with the procedure. In many antenatal settings, nurses perform NSTs, CSTs, BPPs, and basic ultrasonography; conduct an initial assessment;

Table 9-7

Interpretation of the Contraction Stress Test

INTERPRETATION	CLINICAL SIGNIFICANCE
NEGATIVE	
No late decelerations, with minimum of three uterine contractions lasting 40 to 60 sec within 10-min period (see Fig. 9-12)	Reassurance that the fetus is likely to survive labor should it occur within 1 wk; more frequent testing may be indicated by clinical situation
POSITIVE	
Persistent and consistent late decelerations occurring with more than half of contractions (see Fig. 9-13)	Management lies between use of other tools of fetal assessment such as BPP and termination of pregnancy; a positive test result indicates that fetus is at increased risk for perinatal morbidity and mortality; physician may perform expeditious vaginal birth after successful induction or may proceed directly to cesarean birth; decision to intervene is determined by fetal monitoring and presence of FHR reactivity
SUSPICIOUS	
Late decelerations occurring in less than half of uterine contractions once adequate contraction pattern established	NST and CST should be repeated within 24 hr; if interpretable data cannot be achieved, other methods of fetal assessment must be used*
HYPERSTIMULATION	
Late decelerations occurring with excessive uterine activity (contractions more often than every 2 min or lasting longer than 90 sec) or persistent increase in uterine tone	
UNSATISFACTORY	
Inadequate uterine contraction pattern or tracing too poor to interpret	

*Applies to results noted as suspicious, hyperstimulation, or unsatisfactory.
BPP, biophysical profile; *FHR,* fetal heart rate; *NST,* nonstress test; *CST,* contraction stress test.

Community Focus

SUPPORT FOR AT-RISK PREGNANT WOMEN

Researchers have consistently found a relationship between social disadvantage and low-birth-weight babies. Multiple trials of providing social support to women believed to be at risk for giving birth to low-birth-weight babies have been conducted. Nurses, social workers, and midwives—as well as trained lay persons—have provided support. The assistance provided was emotional support such as counseling, sympathetic listening, reassurance, and education or advice at home or in the clinic. In addition, transportation to the clinic or assistance with care of children in the home has been provided. Although such programs have demonstrated improved short-term psychosocial outcomes, medical outcomes have not improved. Preterm births still pose a significant problem in the care of pregnant women and their families. Efforts to reduce the incidence of preterm births must continue.

Reference: Hodnett E: Support during pregnancy for women at increased risk of low birthweight babies (Cochrane Review). In *The Cochrane Library*, Issue 3, Oxford, 2000, Update Software.

and begin necessary interventions for nonreassuring patterns. These nursing procedures are accomplished after additional education and training, under guidance of established protocols, and in collaboration with physicians. Patient teaching, which is an integral component of this role, involves preparing the patient for the procedure, interpreting the findings, and providing psychosocial support when needed.

All women who undergo antenatal assessments are at risk for real and potential problems and may be anxious. With rare exceptions, the tests are ordered because of suspected fetal compromise or deterioration of a maternal condition, or both. In the third trimester, pregnant women are most concerned about protecting themselves and their fetuses and consider themselves most vulnerable to outside influences. The label of high risk will increase this sense of vulnerability.

If the woman is fearful for her own well-being, she may continue to feel ambivalence about the pregnancy or not accept the reality of the pregnancy. She may not be able to complete preparations for the baby or go to childbirth classes if she is on bed rest or hospitalized. The family may become frustrated because they cannot engage in these activities that prepare them for parenthood.

Most patients have incomplete knowledge related to the procedures, the implications of findings, or the need for further evaluation or counseling. Perinatal nurses can provide the required education, and by keeping the patients well informed, can also promote a positive parental self-image in these high risk individuals.

Key Points

- A high risk pregnancy is one in which the life or well-being of the mother or infant is jeopardized by a biophysical or psychosocial disorder coincidental with or unique to pregnancy.
- The pregnancy, fetus, or neonate can be placed at risk by biophysical, sociodemographic, psychosocial, and environmental factors.
- Psychosocial perinatal warning indicators include characteristics of the parents, the child, their support systems, and family circumstances.
- There are racial and ethnic disparities in maternal and perinatal mortality rates in the United States.
- Mortality rate decreases when risks are identified early and intensive care is applied.
- Biophysical assessment techniques include fetal movement counts, ultrasonography, and MRI.
- Biochemical monitoring techniques include amniocentesis, PUBS, CVS, and MSAFP.
- Reactive NSTs and negative CSTs suggest fetal well-being.
- Most assessment tests have some degree of risk for the mother and fetus, and usually cause some anxiety for the woman and her family.

Answer Guidelines to Critical Thinking Exercise

Fetal Activity Monitoring

1. Yes, there is sufficient evidence. Fetal movement may decrease or cease before fetal death. Theoretically, this change in movement could be noted by fetal activity monitoring and appropriate actions can be taken to reduce jeopardy or deliver the infant early. In two large studies, there was no evidence that fetal movement counting improved pregnancy outcome. Reduction in fetal movement resulted in an increase in other techniques of fetal testing, more frequent antepartum hospitalization, and an increased use of elective delivery. This resulted in an increased use of resources without compensatory benefits (Enkin et al, 2000). However, fetal movement counting is commonly recommended by obstetric health care providers.
2. (a) Barbra selected a nurse-midwife as a care provider after careful study. She and her husband have read extensively. You can safely assume that Barbra and her husband are motivated to learn about fetal activity monitoring. (b) Barbra is motivated to provide a safe environment for her fetus; she has been actively seeking prenatal care. There is every expectation that she will follow the recommendations of her nurse-midwife. (c) Fetal activity monitoring can occur any time of the day that is convenient for the woman. Thus the best time of the day for Barbra to monitor fetal activity is a time that fits in with her schedule and that she can plan to count at the same time each day. (d) Barbra is a teacher; you can assume that she can read and understand written instruction and follow oral instruction. However, her anxiety may interfere with learning. Following your teaching session, you need to obtain feedback from Barbra and verify that she has indeed understood the instructions.
3. Priorities for nursing care include determining Barbra's knowledge of fetal movement counting, its purpose, the method of counting and recording the counts, and information about when to notify you or the nurse-midwife. Allaying her anxiety about the reason for the need for counting is also important.
4. While the evidence from the two studies does not verify the value of fetal activity monitoring in preventing fetal

death in late pregnancy, health care providers commonly recommend kick counts. Monitoring may give information about pending fetal asphyxia; decreases in fetal oxygenation have been linked to decreases in gross fetal body movements (Druzin et al, 2002). Monitoring fetal activity can give the woman some sense of control in a situation where the fetus may be at risk. It also ensures that she will be in contact with her health care provider, who may decide there is need for further testing.

5. Yes. Since there is no documented value to fetal activity counting and it leads to additional testing, hospitalization, and early birth, an educated consumer may refuse to do the counts but continue the recommended pattern of prenatal visits.

Resources

Healthy Mothers, Healthy Babies Coalition
409 12th St. SW
Washington, DC 20024
202-863-2458

March of Dimes Birth Defects Foundation
National Foundation/March of Dimes
1275 Mamaroneck Ave.
White Plains, NY 10605
914-428-7100
888-663-4637 (MODIMES)
www.modimes.org

National Center for Education in Maternal and Child Health
Georgetown University
Box 571272
Washington, DC 20057-1272
202-784-9770
202-784-9777 (fax)
email: mchlibrary@ncemch.org

National Institute of Child Health and Human Development (NICHD)
National Institutes of Health
9000 Rockville Pike
Bldg. 31, Room 2A32
Bethesda, MD 20892
301-496-4000
www.nih.gov

Parenthood after Thirty
451 Vermont
Berkeley, CA 94707
415-524-6635

Spina Bifida Association of America
4590 McArthur Blvd. NW, Suite 250
Washington, DC 20007-4226
800-621-3141

References

Alfirevic Z, Sunberg K, Brigham S: Amniocentesis and chorionic villi sampling for prenatal diagnosis (Cochrane Review). In *The Cochrane Library*, Issue 2, Chichester, UK, 2004, John Wiley & Sons.

American Academy of Pediatrics/American College of Obstetricians and Gynecologists (AAP/ACOG): *Guidelines for perinatal care,* ed 4, Elk Grove, IL, 1997, AAP/ACOG.

American College of Obstetricians and Gynecologists: News release. *ACOG issues position on first-trimester screening methods, 2004a.* Internet document available at www.acog.org/from_home/publications/press_releases/nr06-30-04.cfm (accessed August 17, 2004).

American College of Obstetricians and Gynecologists: News release. *Amniocentesis and CVS tests decline despite increase in number of older mothers,* 2004b. Internet document available at www.acog.org/from_home/publications/press_releases/nr05-31-04-1.cfm (accessed August 17, 2004).

Association of Women's Health, Obstetric and Neonatal Nurses (AWHONN): *Nursing practice competencies and educational guidelines for limited ultrasound examination in obstetric and gynecology/infertility settings,* ed 2, Washington, DC, 1998, AWHONN.

Chervenak F, Gabbe S: Obstetric ultrasound: assessment of fetal growth and anatomy. In Gabbe SG, Niebyl JR, Simpson JL (eds): *Obstetrics: normal and problem pregnancies,* ed 4, New York, 2002, Churchill Livingstone.

Druzin M, Gabbe S, Reed K: Antepartum fetal evaluation. In Gabbe SG, Niebyl JR, Simpson JL (eds): *Obstetrics: normal and problem pregnancies,* ed 4, New York, 2002, Churchill Livingstone.

Enkin M et al: *A guide to effective care in pregnancy and childbirth,* ed 3, Oxford, 2000, Oxford University Press.

Enkin M et al: Effective care in pregnancy and childbirth: a synopsis, *Birth* 28(1):41-51, 2001.

Gilbert ES, Harmon JS: *Manual of high risk pregnancy and delivery,* ed 3, St Louis, 2003, Mosby.

Gillen-Goldstein J et al: Methods of assessment for pregnancy at risk. In DeCherney AH, Nathan L (eds): *Current obstetric and gynecologic diagnosis and treatment,* ed 9, New York, 2003, Lange Medical Books/McGraw-Hill.

Glantz J, Woods J: Significance of amniotic fluid meconium. In Creasy RK, Resnik R, Iams JD (eds): *Maternal-fetal medicine: principles and practice,* ed 5, Philadelphia, 2004, WB Saunders.

Harman CR: Assessment of fetal health. In Creasy RK, Resnik R, Iams JD (eds): *Maternal-fetal medicine: principles and practice,* ed 5, Philadelphia, 2004, WB Saunders.

Hodnett E: Support during pregnancy for women at increased risk of low birthweight babies (Cochrane Review). In *The Cochrane Library,* Issue 3, Oxford, 2000, Update Software.

Jenkins TM, Wapner RJ: Prenatal diagnosis of congenital disorders. In Creasy RK, Resnik R, Iams JD (eds): *Maternal-fetal medicine: principles and practice,* ed 5, Philadelphia, 2004, WB Saunders.

Manning F: General principles and applications of ultrasonography. In Creasy RK, Resnik R, Iams JD (eds): *Maternal-fetal medicine: principles and practice,* ed 5, Philadelphia, 2004, WB Saunders.

Minino A et al: Deaths: final data for 2000, *Natl Vital Stat Rep* 50(15):1-119, 2002.

Parer J, Nageotte MP: Intrapartum fetal surveillance. In Creasy RK, Resnik R, Iams JD (eds): *Maternal-fetal medicine: principles and practice,* ed 5, Philadelphia, 2004, WB Saunders.

PRAMS: Internet document available from www.cdc.gov/reproductivehealth/srv_prams.htm (accessed August 17, 2004).

Simpson J: Genetic counseling and prenatal diagnosis. In Gabbe SG, Niebyl JR, Simpson JL (eds): *Obstetrics: normal and problem pregnancies,* ed 4, New York, 2002, Churchill Livingstone.

Tan KH, Sabapathy A: Maternal glucose administration for facilitating tests of fetal wellbeing (Cochrane Review). In *The Cochrane Library,* Issue 3, Chichester, UK, 2004, John Wiley & Sons.

Tan KH, Smyth R: Fetal vibroacoustic stimulation for facilitation of tests of fetal wellbeing (Cochrane Review). In *The Cochrane Library,* Issue 3, Chichester, UK, 2004, John Wiley & Sons.

Tucker SM: *Pocket guide to fetal monitoring and assessment,* ed 5, St Louis, 2004, Mosby.

U.S., *Irish researchers identify important clue to genetic basis for neural tube defects,* USDHHS NICHD, *NIH News,* March 21, 2004. Internet document available at www.nichd.nih.gov/new/releases/genetic_basis.cfm (accessed August 16, 2004).

Vain NE et al: Oropharyngeal and nasopharyngeal suctioning of meconium-stained neonates before delivery of their shoulders: multicentre, randomized controlled trial, *Lancet* 364(9434): 597-602, 2004.

Anatomy and Physiology of Pregnancy

10

LEARNING OBJECTIVES

On completion of this chapter the reader will be able to:

- Determine gravidity and parity using the five- and four-digit systems.
- Explain the expected maternal anatomic and physiologic adaptations to pregnancy.
- Differentiate among presumptive, probable, and positive signs of pregnancy.
- Identify maternal hormones produced during pregnancy, their target organs, and their major effects on pregnancy.
- Compare the characteristics of the abdomen, vulva, and cervix of the nullipara and multipara.
- Describe the various types of pregnancy tests, including timing of tests and interpretation of results.

ELECTRONIC RESOURCES

Additional information related to the content in Chapter 10 can be found on

the companion website at evolve
http://evolve.elsevier.com/Wong/maternal/
- NCLEX Review Questions
- WebLinks

or the interactive student CD-ROM
Activities for Chapter 10 include the following:
- NCLEX Review Questions

The goal of maternity care is a healthy pregnancy with a physically safe and emotionally satisfying outcome for mother, infant, and family. Consistent health supervision and surveillance are of utmost importance. Many maternal adaptations are unfamiliar to pregnant women and their families. Helping the pregnant woman recognize the relationship between her physical status and the plan for her care assists her in making decisions and encourages her to participate in her own care.

GRAVIDITY AND PARITY

An understanding of the following terms used to describe pregnancy and the pregnant woman is essential to the study of maternity care:

- **Gravida**—A woman who is pregnant
- **Gravidity**—Pregnancy
- **Multigravida**—A woman who has had two or more pregnancies
- **Multipara**—A woman who has completed two or more pregnancies to the stage of fetal viability
- **Nulligravida**—A woman who has never been pregnant
- **Nullipara**—A woman who has not completed a pregnancy with a fetus or fetuses who have reached the stage of viability
- **Parity**—The number of pregnancies in which the fetus or fetuses have reached viability, not the number of fetuses (e.g., twins) born; not affected by whether the fetus is born alive or is stillborn (i.e., showing no signs of life at birth) after viability is reached
- **Postdate or postterm**—Pregnancy that goes beyond 42 weeks of gestation
- **Preterm**—Born after 20 weeks of gestation but before completion of 37 weeks of gestation
- **Primigravida**—A woman who is pregnant for the first time
- **Primipara**—A woman who has completed one pregnancy with a fetus or fetuses who have reached the stage of fetal viability
- **Term**—Born between the beginning of week 38 of gestation and the end of week 42 of gestation
- **Viability**—Capacity to live outside the uterus, occurring about 22 to 24 weeks since last menstrual period or when weight of fetus is greater than 500 g

Gravidity and parity information is obtained during history-taking interviews and may be recorded in several ways in patient records. A two-digit system uses abbreviations that stand for gravity and parity. For example, the abbreviation "I/0" means that a woman is pregnant for the first time (primigravida) and has not carried a pregnancy to viability (nullipara).

Table 10-1

Gravidity and Parity Using Five-Digit (GTPAL) and Two-Digit Systems

	Five-Digit System					Two-Digit System
CONDITION	PREGNANCIES (GRAVIDITY, G)	TERM BIRTH (T)	PRETERM BIRTH (P)	ABORTIONS (A)	LIVING CHILDREN (L)	GRAVIDITY/PARITY
Kathy is pregnant for the first time.	1	0	0	0	0	I/O
She carries the pregnancy to term, and the neonate survives.	1	1	0	0	1	I/I
She is pregnant again.	2	1	0	0	1	II/I
Her second pregnancy ends in abortion (miscarriage).	2	1	0	1	1	II/I
During her third pregnancy, she gives birth to preterm twins.	3	1	1	1	3	III/II

BOX 10-1

Using TPAL to Define Parity

T, term birth(s)
P, preterm birth(s)
A, abortion(s), miscarriage(s)
L, living children

Another abbreviation commonly employed in maternity centers is more detailed. It consists of five digits with hyphens for separation. The first digit represents the total number of pregnancies, including the present one (gravidity); the second digit represents the total number of full-term births; the third indicates the number of preterm births; the fourth identifies the number of abortions (miscarriage or elective termination of pregnancy before viability); and the fifth is the number of children currently living. The acronym GTPAL may be helpful in remembering this numeric abbreviation. For example, if a woman pregnant only once with twins gives birth at the thirty-fifth week and the babies survive, the abbreviation that represents this information is "1-0-1-0-2." During her next pregnancy the abbreviation is "2-0-1-0-2." Table 10-1 provides additional examples.

Others prefer a four-digit system. The first digit of the five-digit system, which signifies gravidity, is dropped. The acronym TPAL may be useful in remembering what the four digits stand for (Box 10-1).

PREGNANCY TESTS

Early detection of pregnancy allows for early initiation of care. Human chorionic gonadotropin (hCG) is the biologic marker on which pregnancy tests are based. Production of hCG begins as early as the day of implantation and can be detected in the blood as early as 6 to 11 days after conception if very sensitive tests are used (Buster & Carson, 2002), or about 20 days since the last menstrual period (LMP), and in urine about 26 days after conception (Cunningham et al, 2001). The level of hCG rises until it peaks at about 60 to 70 days of pregnancy and then begins to decline. The lowest level is reached at about 140 days of pregnancy. Higher than normal levels of hCG may indicate ectopic pregnancy, abnormal gestation (e.g., fetus with Down syndrome), or multiple gestation; abnormally slow increase or a decrease in hCG levels may indicate impending miscarriage (Buster & Carson, 2002).

Serum and urine pregnancy tests are performed in clinics, offices, women's health centers, and laboratory settings. Urine pregnancy tests may be performed at home (Community Focus box). Both serum tests and urine tests provide accurate results. A 7- to 10-ml sample of venous blood is collected for serum testing. Most urine tests require a first-voided morning urine specimen because it contains levels of hCG approximately the same as those in serum. Random urine samples usually have lower levels. Urine tests are less expensive and provide more immediate results than serum tests (Hatcher et al, 2004).

Many different pregnancy tests are available, but they all depend on recognition of hCG or a beta subunit of hCG. The wide variety of tests precludes discussion of each; however, the nurse should read the manufacturer's directions for the test to be used.

Immunoassay or agglutination inhibition tests (AITs) depend on an antigen-antibody reaction between hCG and an

Community Focus

OTC PREGNANCY HOME TEST KITS

In a pharmacy in your neighborhood, how many different types of OTC pregnancy home test kits are available? Read the labels on three different types of OTC pregnancy home test kits. Do the kits provide for more than one test? Are the directions printed in more than one language? After reading the directions, do you have questions about how to perform the test or how to interpret the results? If so, what does that say about the likelihood that the tests will be used correctly?

antiserum. Usually the antiserum is mixed with urine, and hCG-coated particles (e.g., latex or blood cells) are added. If hCG is present in the urine, agglutination does not occur because the hCG neutralizes the hCG antibody, and the test is considered positive (Cunningham et al, 2001). Although immunologic tests are accurate from 4 to 10 days after a missed period, they are most appropriate for confirming a pregnancy at or after the sixth week of gestation (Hatcher et al, 2004).

Radioimmunoassay (RIA) pregnancy tests for the beta subunit of hCG in serum or urine samples use radioactively labeled markers and are usually performed in a laboratory. These tests are accurate with low hCG levels and can confirm pregnancy 1 week after conception (Hatcher et al, 2004).

Radioreceptor assay (RRA) is a serum test that measures the ability of a blood sample to inhibit the binding of radiolabeled hCG to receptors. The test is 90% to 95% accurate from 6 to 8 days after conception (Pagana & Pagana, 2003).

Enzyme-linked immunosorbent assay (ELISA) testing is the most popular testing procedure for pregnancy. It uses a specific monoclonal antibody (anti-hCG) with enzymes that bond with hCG in urine. Depending on the specific test, levels of hCG as low as 5 to 50 milli international units/ml can be detected as early as 7 to 10 days after conception (Hatcher et al, 2004). As an office or home procedure, it requires minimal time and offers results in 1 to 3 minutes. A positive test is indicated by a simple color change reaction.

ELISA technology is the basis for most over-the-counter (OTC) home pregnancy tests. With these one-step tests, the woman usually applies urine to a strip and reads the results. The test kit comes with directions for collection of the specimen, the testing procedure, and reading of results. Most manufacturers of the kits provide a toll-free telephone number to call if users have concerns and questions about test procedures or results. The most common error in performing home pregnancy tests is doing the test too early in pregnancy (Hatcher et al, 2004).

Interpreting the results of pregnancy tests requires some judgment. The type of pregnancy test and its degree of sensitivity (the ability to detect low levels of a substance) and specificity (the ability to discern the absence of a substance) must be considered in conjunction with the woman's history. This includes the date of the last normal menstrual period (LNMP), her usual cycle length, and results of previous pregnancy tests. It is important to know if the woman abuses substances, and what medications she is taking. Medications such as anticonvulsants and tranquilizers can cause false-positive results, whereas diuretics and promethazine can cause false-negative results (Pagana & Pagana, 2003). Improper collection of the specimen, hormone-producing tumors, and laboratory errors may also be responsible for inaccurate results. When there is any question, further evaluation or retesting may be appropriate.

Critical Thinking Exercise

AWARENESS OF PHYSIOLOGIC CHANGES OF PREGNANCY

Marlys is pregnant with her first child and Janice is pregnant with her third child. They are both at approximately 18 weeks of gestation and have come to a prenatal appointment. While they are in the waiting room, you overhear Marlys asking Janice about some "old wives' tales" that she has heard:

- If she raises her arms above her head, the cord will wrap around the baby's neck.
- Putting a knife under the bed while she is laboring will "cut" the pain.
- If she dangles a needle in front of her abdomen, she will be able to tell if the baby is a boy or a girl.
- A rapid fetal heartbeat means the baby will be a boy.

Marlys says that she has not felt her baby move yet, whereas Janice says that she has been feeling fetal movement for over 2 weeks. Marlys also has questions about some of the changes in her body that she has experienced or expects to experience. Janice bases her responses on her own experience. Based on the conversation you have overheard, you identify a need to spend some time with Marlys and Janice discussing physiologic changes of pregnancy.

1. Evidence—Is there sufficient evidence to draw conclusions about the normal physiologic changes in pregnancy in primiparas and multiparas that the nurse should discuss with Marlys and Janice?
2. Assumptions—Describe an underlying assumption about each of the following topics:
   a. Differences in the normal physiologic changes in pregnancy between primiparas and multiparas
   b. Reversibility of these physiologic changes in pregnancy
   c. Information provided by the health care provider
   d. Deviations from normal in the physiologic changes of pregnancy
3. What implications and priorities for nursing care can be drawn at this time?
4. Does the evidence objectively support your conclusion?
5. Are there alternative perspectives to your conclusion?

ADAPTATIONS TO PREGNANCY

Maternal physiologic adaptations are attributed to the hormones of pregnancy and to mechanical pressures arising from the enlarging uterus and other tissues. These adaptations protect the woman's normal physiologic functioning, meet the metabolic demands that pregnancy imposes on her body, and provide a nurturing environment for fetal development and growth. Although pregnancy is a normal phenomenon, problems can occur. The nurse needs a foundation in normal maternal physiology to provide optimal nursing care.

Signs of Pregnancy

Some physiologic adaptations are recognized as the signs and symptoms of pregnancy. Three commonly used categories of these signs and symptoms are (1) presumptive, those changes felt by the woman (e.g., amenorrhea, fatigue, and breast changes); (2) probable, those changes observed by an examiner (e.g., Hegar's sign, ballottement, and pregnancy tests); and (3) positive, those signs attributed only to the presence of the fetus (e.g., hearing fetal heart tones, visualizing the fetus, and palpating fetal movements). Table 10-2 summarizes these signs of pregnancy in relation to when they might occur and gives other possible causes for their occurrence.

Table 10-2

Signs of Pregnancy

TIME OF OCCURRENCE (GESTATIONAL AGE)	SIGN	OTHER POSSIBLE CAUSES
	PRESUMPTIVE	
3-4 weeks	Breast changes	Premenstrual changes, oral contraceptives
4 weeks	Amenorrhea	Stress, vigorous exercise, early menopause, endocrine problems, malnutrition
4-14 weeks	Nausea, vomiting	Gastrointestinal virus, food poisoning
6-12 weeks	Urinary frequency	Infection, pelvic tumors
12 weeks	Fatigue	Stress, illness
16-20 weeks	Quickening	Gas, peristalsis
	PROBABLE	
5 weeks	Goodell's sign	Pelvic congestion
6-8 weeks	Chadwick's sign	Pelvic congestion
6-12 weeks	Hegar's sign	Pelvic congestion
4-12 weeks	Positive pregnancy test (serum)	Hydatidiform mole, choriocarcinoma
6-12 weeks	Positive pregnancy test (urine)	Pelvic infection, tumors
16 weeks	Braxton Hicks contractions	Myomas, other tumors
16-28 weeks	Ballottement	Tumors, cervical polyps
	POSITIVE	
5-6 weeks	Visualization of fetus by ultrasound, x-ray films	No other causes
6 weeks	Fetal heart tones (FHTs) by ultrasound	
10-17 weeks	FHTs by Doppler	
17-19 weeks	FHTs by stethoscope	
19-22 weeks	Fetal movements palpated	
Late pregnancy	Visible	

Reproductive System and Breasts

Uterus

Changes in Size, Shape, and Position

High levels of estrogen and progesterone stimulate phenomenal uterine growth in the first trimester. Early uterine enlargement results from increased vascularity and dilation of blood vessels, hyperplasia (production of new muscle fibers and fibroelastic tissue) and hypertrophy (enlargement of preexisting muscle fibers and fibroelastic tissue), and development of the decidua. By 7 weeks of gestation the uterus is the size of a large hen's egg; by 10 weeks it is the size of an orange (twice its nonpregnant size); and by 12 weeks it is the size of a grapefruit. After the third month, uterine enlargement is primarily the result of mechanical pressure of the growing fetus.

As the uterus enlarges, it also changes in shape and position. At conception the uterus is shaped like an upside-down pear. During the second trimester, as the muscular walls strengthen and become more elastic, the uterus becomes spherical or globular. Later, as the fetus lengthens, the uterus becomes larger and more ovoid and rises out of the pelvis into the abdominal cavity.

The pregnancy may "show" after the fourteenth week, although this depends to some degree on the woman's height and weight. Abdominal enlargement may be less apparent in the nullipara with good abdominal muscle tone (Fig. 10-1). Posture also influences the type and degree of abdominal enlargement that occurs. In normal pregnancies the uterus enlarges at a predictable rate.

As the uterus grows and fills the pelvic cavity, it is elevated out of the pelvic area. It may be palpated above the symphysis pubis sometime between the twelfth and fourteenth weeks of pregnancy (Fig. 10-2). The uterus rises gradually to the level of the umbilicus at 22 to 24 weeks of gestation, and nearly reaches the xiphoid process at term. Between weeks 38 and 40, fundal height decreases as the fetus begins to descend and engage in the pelvis (lightening). Generally, lightening occurs in the nullipara about 2 weeks before the onset of labor and at the start of labor in the multipara.

Uterine enlargement is determined by measuring fundal height (see Fig. 11-8). This measurement is commonly used to estimate the duration of pregnancy. However, variation in the position of the fundus or the fetus, variations in the amount of amniotic fluid present, the presence of more than one fetus, maternal obesity, and variation in examiner tech-

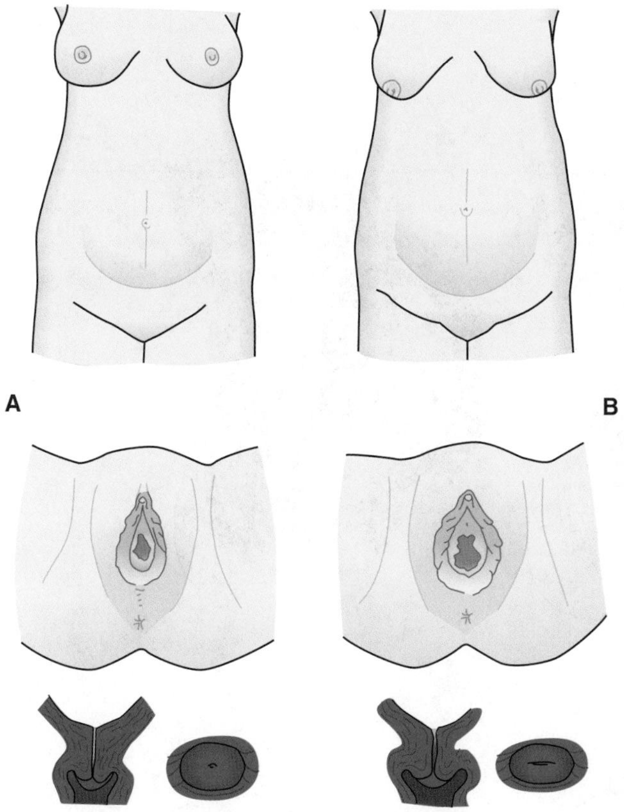

Fig. 10-1 Comparison of abdomen, vulva, and cervix in **A**, nullipara, and **B**, multipara, at the same stage of pregnancy.

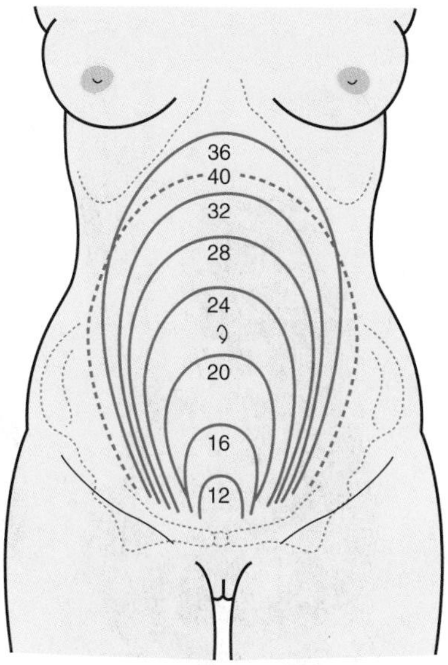

Fig. 10-2 Height of fundus by weeks of normal gestation with a single fetus. *Dashed line,* height after lightening.

nique can reduce the accuracy of this estimation of the duration of pregnancy.

Generally the uterus rotates to the right as it elevates, probably because of the presence of the rectosigmoid colon on the left side. However, the extensive hypertrophy (enlargement) of the round ligaments keeps the uterus in the midline. Eventually the growing uterus touches the anterior abdominal wall and displaces the intestines to either side of the abdomen (Fig. 10-3). When a pregnant woman stands, most of her uterus rests against the anterior abdominal wall and contributes to altering her center of gravity.

During the early weeks of pregnancy an increase in uterine blood flow and lymph causes pelvic congestion and edema. As a result, the uterus, cervix, and isthmus soften perceptibly and progressively, and the cervix takes on a bluish color (Chadwick's sign, a probable sign of pregnancy).

At approximately 6 weeks of gestation, softening and compressibility of the lower uterine segment (uterine isthmus) occurs (Hegar's sign). This results in exaggerated uterine anteflexion during the first 3 months of pregnancy (Fig. 10-4). In this position the uterine fundus presses on the urinary bladder, causing the woman to experience urinary frequency.

Changes in Contractility

Soon after the fourth month of pregnancy, uterine contractions can be felt through the abdominal wall. These contractions are referred to as Braxton Hicks contractions, a probable sign of pregnancy. Braxton Hicks contractions are irregular, painless contractions that occur intermittently throughout pregnancy. These contractions facilitate uterine blood flow through the intervillous spaces of the placenta and promote oxygen delivery to the fetus. Although Braxton Hicks contractions are not painful, some women do complain that they are annoying. After the twenty-eighth week, these contractions become more definite, but they usually cease with walking or exercise. Braxton Hicks contractions can be mistaken for true labor; however, they do not increase in intensity or duration or cause cervical dilation. Conversely, premature labor contractions can be mistaken for Braxton Hicks contractions and lead to a delay in seeking treatment.

Uteroplacental Blood Flow

Placental perfusion depends on the maternal blood flow to the uterus. Blood flow increases rapidly as the uterus increases in size. Although uterine blood flow increases twentyfold, the fetoplacental unit grows even more rapidly. Consequently, more oxygen is extracted from the uterine blood during the latter part of pregnancy. In a normal term pregnancy, one sixth of the total maternal blood volume is within the uterine vascular system. The rate of blood flow through the uterus averages 500 ml/min, and oxygen consumption of the gravid uterus increases to meet fetal needs. Three factors known to decrease uterine blood flow are low mean maternal arterial pressure, contractions of the uterus, and maternal position. Estrogen stimulation may increase uterine blood flow. Doppler ultrasound examination can be used to measure uterine blood flow velocity, especially in pregnancies at risk because of conditions associated with decreased placental perfusion such as hypertension, intrauterine growth restriction, diabetes mellitus, and multiple gestation.

Using an ultrasound device or a fetal stethoscope, the examiner may hear the uterine souffle or bruit, a rushing or blowing sound of maternal blood flowing through uterine arteries to the placenta that is synchronous with the maternal pulse. The funic souffle, which is synchronous with the fetal heart rate and is caused by fetal blood coursing through the umbilical cord, may also be heard, as well as the actual heartbeat of the fetus.

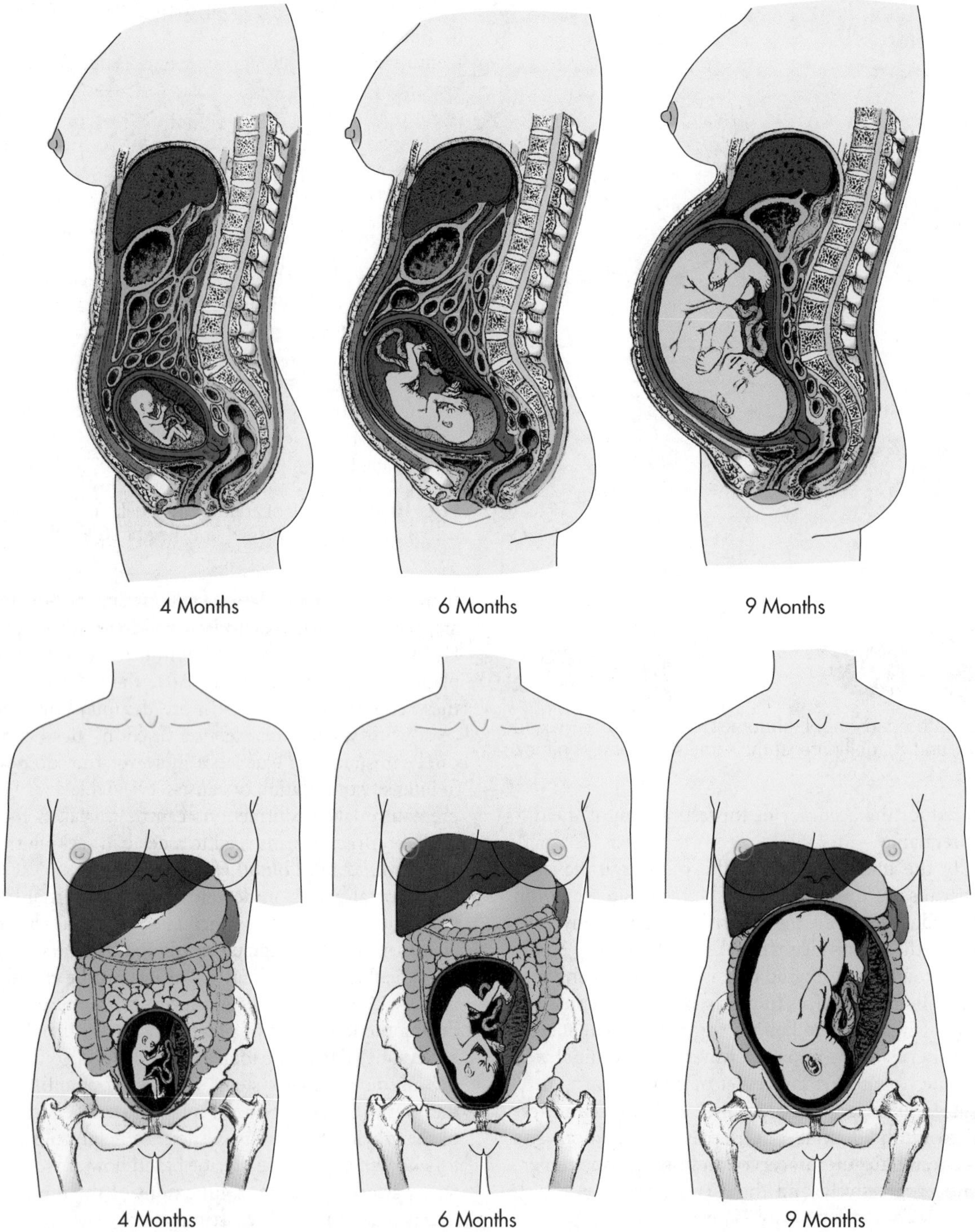

Fig. 10-3 Displacement of internal abdominal structures and diaphragm by the enlarging uterus at 4, 6, and 9 months of gestation.

Cervical Changes

In a normal, unscarred cervix, a softening of the cervical tip may be observed about the beginning of the sixth week. This probable sign of pregnancy, Goodell's sign, is brought about by increased vascularity, slight hypertrophy, and hyperplasia (increase in number of cells). The muscle and its collagen-rich connective tissue become loose, edematous, highly elastic, and increased in volume. The glands near the external os proliferate beneath the stratified squamous epithelium, giving the cervix the velvety consistency characteristic of pregnancy. Friability is increased; that is, the cervix bleeds easily when scraped or touched. Increased friability is the cause of the few drops of blood seen after coitus with deep penetration or after vaginal examination. These few drops are usually within normal limits.

Pregnancy can also cause the squamocolumnar junction (the site for obtaining cells for cervical cancer screening) to be located away from the cervix. Because of these changes, evaluation of abnormal Papanicolaou tests during pregnancy can be complicated. However, a careful assessment of

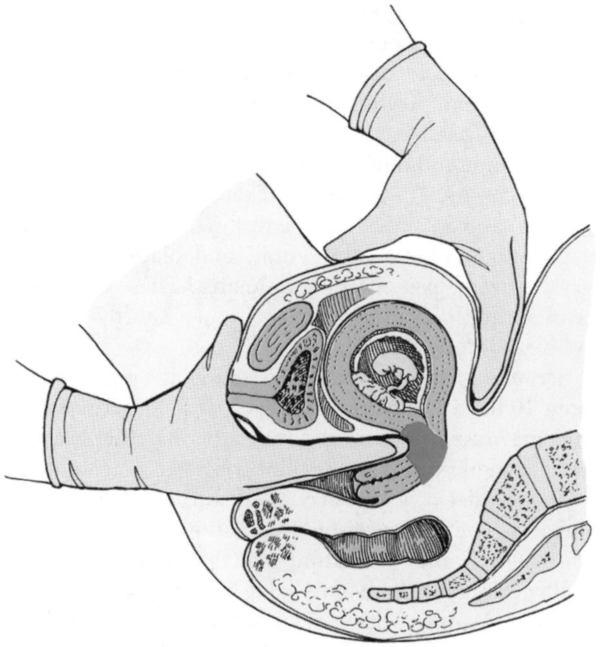

Fig. 10-4 Hegar's sign. Bimanual examination for assessing compressibility and softening of isthmus (lower uterine segment) while the cervix is still firm.

all pregnant women is important because about 3% of all cervical cancers are diagnosed during pregnancy (Berman, Di Saia, & Tewari, 2004).

The cervix of the nullipara is rounded. Lacerations of the cervix almost always occur during the birth process. With or without lacerations, after childbirth the cervix becomes more oval in the horizontal plane, and the external os appears as a transverse slit (see Fig. 10-1).

Changes Related to the Presence of the Fetus

Passive movement of the unengaged fetus is called ballottement and can be identified generally between the sixteenth and eighteenth week. Ballottement is a technique of palpating a floating structure by bouncing it gently and feeling it rebound. To palpate the fetus, the examiner places a finger within the vagina and taps gently upward, causing the fetus to rise. The fetus then sinks, and a gentle tap is felt on the finger (Fig. 10-5). Internal ballottement of a fetus within a uterus is a probable objective sign of pregnancy.

The first recognition of fetal movements, or "feeling life," by the multiparous woman may occur as early as the sixteenth week. The nulliparous woman may not notice these sensations until the eighteenth week or later. Quickening, a presumptive sign of pregnancy, is commonly described as a flutter and is difficult to distinguish from peristalsis. Fetal movements gradually increase in intensity and frequency. The week in which quickening occurs provides a tentative clue in dating the duration of gestation.

Vagina and Vulva

Pregnancy hormones prepare the vagina for stretching during labor and birth by causing the vaginal mucosa to thicken, connective tissue to loosen, smooth muscle to hypertrophy, and the vaginal vault to lengthen. Increased vascularity results in a violet-blue color of the vaginal mucosa and cervix. The deepened color, termed *Chadwick's sign,* may be evident as early as the sixth week but is easily noted by the eighth week of pregnancy.

Leukorrhea is a white or slightly gray mucoid discharge with a faint musty odor. This copious mucoid fluid occurs in response to cervical stimulation by estrogen and progesterone. The fluid is whitish because of the presence of many exfoliated vaginal epithelial cells caused by normal pregnancy hyperplasia. This vaginal discharge is never pruritic or blood stained. Because of the progesterone effect, ferning usually does not occur in the dried cervical mucus smear, as it would in a smear of amniotic fluid. Instead, a beaded or cellular crystallizing pattern formed in the dried mucus is seen. The mucus fills the endocervical canal, resulting in the formation of the mucous plug (operculum) (Monga & Sanborn, 2004). The operculum acts as a barrier against bacterial invasion during pregnancy.

The pH of vaginal secretions is more acidic during pregnancy, ranging from about 3.5 to about 6.0. This is the result of increased production of lactic acid caused by *Lactobacillus acidophilus* acting on glycogen in the vaginal epithelium The pregnant woman is more vulnerable to vaginal infections, especially yeast infections, because the glycogen-rich environment of the vagina is more susceptible to *Candida albicans* (Murray, 2003).

The increased vascularity of the vagina and other pelvic viscera results in a marked increase in sensitivity. The increased sensitivity may lead to a high degree of sexual interest and arousal, especially during the second trimester of pregnancy. The increased congestion, plus the relaxed walls

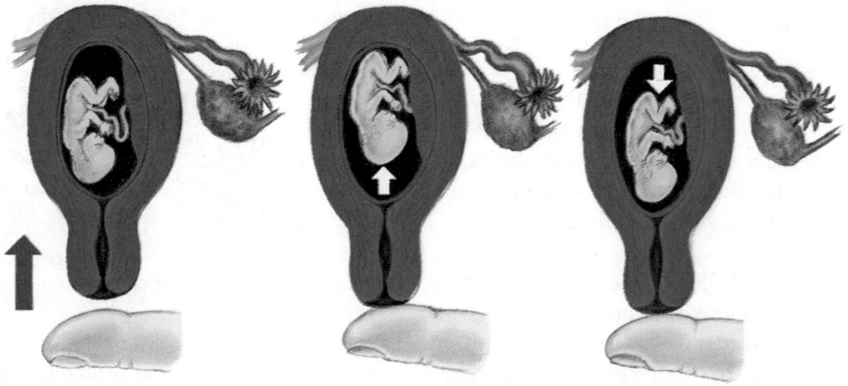

Fig. 10-5 Internal ballottement (18 weeks).

of the blood vessels and the heavy uterus, may result in edema and varicosities of the vulva. The edema and varicosities usually resolve during the postpartum period.

External structures of the perineum are enlarged during pregnancy because of an increase in vasculature, hypertrophy of the perineal body, and deposition of fat. The labia majora of nullipara approximate and obscure the vaginal introitus; those of the parous woman separate and gape after childbirth and perineal or vaginal injury (see Fig. 10-1).

Breasts

Fullness, heightened sensitivity, tingling, and heaviness of the breasts begin as early as the sixth week of gestation in response to increased levels of estrogen and progesterone. These changes are considered presumptive signs of pregnancy because other factors can cause them to occur. Breast sensitivity varies from mild tingling to sharp pain. Nipples and areolae become more pigmented; secondary pinkish areolae develop, extending beyond the primary areolae; and nipples become more erectile. Hypertrophy of the sebaceous (oil) glands embedded in the primary areolae, called Montgomery tubercles, may be seen around the nipples. These sebaceous glands may have a protective role in that they keep the nipples lubricated for breastfeeding.

The richer blood supply causes the vessels beneath the skin to dilate. Once barely noticeable, the blood vessels become visible, often appearing in an intertwining blue network beneath the surface of the skin. Venous congestion in the breasts is more obvious in the primigravida. Striae gravidarum may appear at the outer aspects of the breasts.

During the second and third trimesters, growth of the mammary glands accounts for the progressive breast enlargement (see Fig 10-8). The high levels of luteal and placental hormones in pregnancy promote proliferation of the lactiferous ducts and lobule-alveolar tissue; thus palpation of the breasts reveals a generalized, coarse nodularity. Glandular tissue displaces connective tissue, and as a result the tissue becomes softer and looser.

Although development of the mammary glands is functionally complete by midpregnancy, lactation is inhibited until a drop in estrogen level occurs after birth. A thin, clear, viscous secretory material (precolostrum) can be found in the acini cells by the third month of gestation. Colostrum, the creamy, white-to-yellowish-to-orange premilk fluid, may be expressed from the nipples as early as 16 weeks of gestation. See Chapter 26 for discussion of lactation.

General Body Systems

Cardiovascular System

Maternal adjustments to pregnancy involve extensive anatomic and physiologic changes in the cardiovascular system. Cardiovascular adaptations protect the woman's normal physiologic functioning, meet the metabolic demands pregnancy imposes on her body, and provide for fetal developmental and growth needs.

Slight cardiac hypertrophy (enlargement) is probably secondary to increased blood volume and cardiac output. The heart returns to its normal size after childbirth. As the diaphragm is displaced upward by the enlarging uterus, the heart is elevated upward and rotated forward to the left (Fig. 10-6). The apical impulse, a point of maximum intensity (PMI), is shifted upward and laterally about 1 to 1.5 cm. The degree of shift depends on the duration of pregnancy and the size and position of the uterus.

The changes in heart size and position, and increases in blood volume and cardiac output, contribute to auscultatory changes common in pregnancy. There is more audible splitting of S_1 and S_2, and S_3 may be readily heard after 20 weeks of gestation. Additionally, systolic and diastolic murmurs may be heard over the pulmonic area. These changes are transient and disappear in most women shortly after they give birth (Monga, 2004).

Between 14 and 20 weeks of gestation, the pulse increases about 10 to 15 beats/min and this persists to term. Palpitations may occur. In twin gestations the maternal heart rate increases significantly in the third trimester.

The cardiac rhythm may be disturbed. The pregnant woman may experience sinus arrhythmia, premature atrial contractions, and premature ventricular systole. In the healthy woman with no underlying heart disease, no therapy is needed. Women with preexisting heart disease will need close medical and obstetric supervision during pregnancy (see Chapter 13).

Blood Pressure

Arterial blood pressure (brachial artery) varies with age, activity level, presence of health problems, and circadian rhythm (Hermida et al, 2001). Additional factors must be considered during pregnancy. These factors include maternal anxiety, maternal position, and type of blood pressure apparatus.

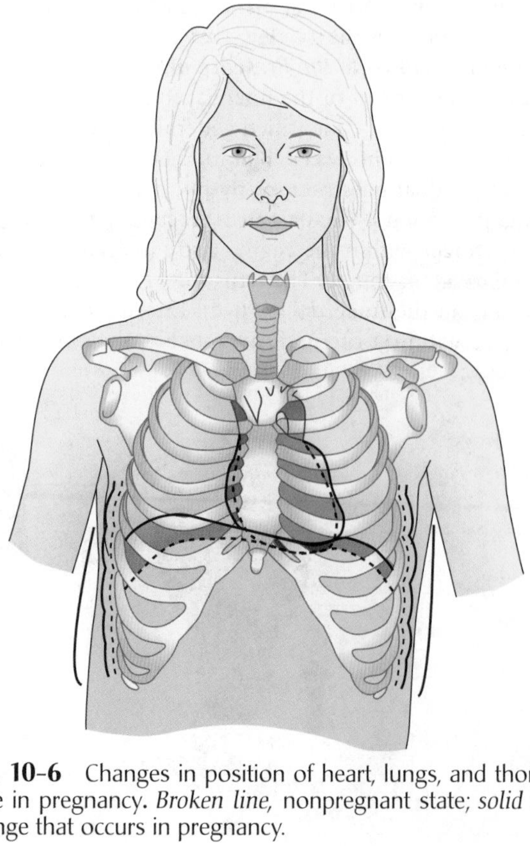

Fig. 10-6 Changes in position of heart, lungs, and thoracic cage in pregnancy. *Broken line,* nonpregnant state; *solid line,* change that occurs in pregnancy.

Maternal anxiety can elevate readings. If an elevated reading is found, the woman is given time to rest, and the reading is repeated.

Maternal position affects readings. Brachial blood pressure is highest when the woman is sitting; lowest when she is lying in the lateral recumbent position; and intermediate when she is supine, except for some women who experience hypotensive syndrome (see discussion later). Therefore at each prenatal visit the reading should be obtained in the same arm and with the woman in the same position. The position and arm used should be recorded along with the reading.

The proper size of cuff is essential for accurate readings. The cuff should be 20% wider than the diameter of the patient's arm (i.e., about 12 to 14 cm for average-sized individuals and 18 to 20 cm for obese persons). A cuff that is too small yields a falsely high reading; a cuff that is too large yields a falsely low reading. Caution should be used when comparing auscultatory and oscillatory blood pressure readings because discrepancies can occur.

In the first trimester, blood pressure usually remains at the prepregnancy level. During the second trimester of pregnancy, both systolic pressure and diastolic pressure decrease about 5 to 10 mm Hg. This decrease is probably the result of peripheral vasodilation caused by hormonal changes during pregnancy. During the third trimester, maternal blood pressure should return to first trimester levels.

Calculating the mean arterial pressure (MAP) (mean of the blood pressure in the arterial circulation) increases the diagnostic value of the findings. Normal MAP readings in the nonpregnant woman are 86.4 ± 7.5 mm Hg. MAP readings for a pregnant woman are slightly higher (Gonik & Foley, 2004). Box 10-2 illustrates one way to calculate MAP.

Some degree of compression of the vena cava occurs in all women who lie on their backs during the second half of pregnancy. Some women experience a fall of more than 30 mm Hg in their systolic pressure. After 4 to 5 minutes a reflex bradycardia is noted, cardiac output is reduced by half, and the woman feels faint. This condition is called supine hypotensive syndrome (Monga, 2004).

Compression of the iliac veins and inferior vena cava by the uterus causes increased venous pressure and reduced blood flow in the legs, except when the woman is in the lateral position. These alterations contribute to the dependent edema, varicose veins in the legs and vulva, and hemorrhoids experienced by women in the latter part of term pregnancy (Fig. 10-7).

BOX 10-2

Calculation of Mean Arterial Pressure

Blood pressure: 106/70

Formula: $\dfrac{\text{Systolic} + 2(\text{Diastolic})}{3}$

$\dfrac{106 + 2(70)}{3}$

$\dfrac{106 + 140}{3}$

246/3 = 82 mm Hg

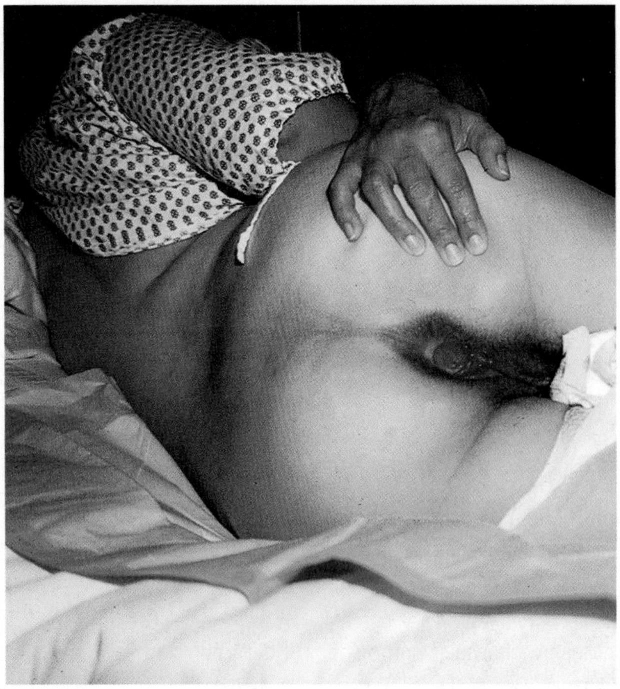

Fig. 10-7 Hemorrhoids. (Courtesy Marjorie Pyle, RNC, Lifecircle, Costa Mesa, CA.)

Blood Volume and Composition

The degree of blood volume expansion varies considerably. Blood volume increases by approximately 1500 ml, or 40% to 50% above nonpregnancy levels. This increase consists of 1000 ml of plasma plus 450 ml of red blood cells (RBCs). The increase in volume starts at weeks 10 to 12, peaks at weeks 32 to 34, and decreases slightly at week 40. The volume in a multiple gestation increases above that for a single pregnancy. Increased blood volume is a protective mechanism. It is essential for meeting the blood needs of the hypertrophied vascular system of the enlarged uterus, for adequately hydrating fetal and maternal tissues when the woman assumes an erect or supine position, and for providing a fluid reserve to compensate for blood loss during birth and the puerperium. Peripheral vasodilation maintains a normal blood pressure despite the increased blood volume in pregnancy.

During pregnancy there is an accelerated production of RBCs (normal, 4.2 to 5.4 million/mm^3). The RBC mass increases by about 20% to 30%. The percentage of increase depends on the amount of iron available (Monga, 2004).

Because the plasma increase is greater than the increase in RBC production, there is a decrease in normal hemoglobin values (12 to 16 g/dl blood) and hematocrit values (37% to 47%). This state of hemodilution is referred to as physiologic anemia. The decrease is more noticeable during the second trimester, when rapid expansion of blood volume occurs faster than RBC production. If the hemoglobin value drops to 10 g/dl or less, or if the hematocrit decreases to 35% or less, the woman is considered anemic.

The total white blood cell count increases during the second trimester and peaks during the third trimester. This increase is primarily in the granulocytes; the lymphocyte count stays about the same throughout pregnancy. See Table 10-3 for laboratory values during pregnancy.

Table 10-3

Laboratory Values for Pregnant and Nonpregnant Women

VALUES	NONPREGNANT	PREGNANT
HEMATOLOGIC		
Complete Blood Count (CBC)		
Hemoglobin, g/dl	12-16*	>11*
Hematocrit, PCV, %	37-47	>33*
Red blood cell (RBC) volume, per ml	1600	1500-1900
Plasma volume, per ml	2400	3700
RBC count, million/mm^3	4.2-5.4	5-6.25
White blood cells, total per mm^3	5000-10,000	5000-15,000
Neutophils, %	55-70	60-85
Lymphocytes, %	20-40	15-40
Erythrocyte sedimentation rate, mm/hr	20	Elevated in second and third trimesters
Mean corpuscular hemoglobin concentration (MCHC), g/dl packed RBCs	32-36	No change in hemoglobin concentration
Mean corpuscular hemoglobin (MCH), pg	27-31	No change per pg (less than 1 ng)
Mean corpuscular volume (MCV), mcm^3	80-95	No change per mcm^3
Blood Coagulation and Fibrinolytic Activity†		
Factor VII	65-140	Increase in pregnancy, return to normal in early puerperium; factor VIII increases during and immediately after birth
Factor VIII	55-145	
Factor IX	60-140	
Factor X	45-155	
Factor XI	65-135	Decrease in pregnancy
Factor XII	50-150	
Prothrombin time (PT), sec	11-12.5	Slight decrease in pregnancy
Partial thromboplastin time (PTT), sec	60-70	Slight decrease in pregnancy and decrease during second and third stage of labor (indicates clotting at placental site)
Bleeding time, min	1-9 (Ivy)	No appreciable change
Coagulation time, min	6-10 (Lee/White)	No appreciable change
Platelets, per mm^3	150,000-400,000	No significant change until 3-5 days after birth and then a rapid increase (may predispose woman to thrombosis) and gradual return to normal

Data from Gordon M: Maternal physiology in pregnancy. In Gabbe SG, Niebyl JR, Simpson JL (eds): *Obstetrics: normal and problem pregnancies,* ed 4, New York, 2002, Churchill Livingstone; Pagana KD, Pagana TJ: *Mosby's diagnostic and laboratory test reference,* ed 6, St Louis, 2003, Mosby.
*At sea level. Permanent residents of higher levels (e.g., Denver) require higher levels of hemoglobin.
†Pregnancy represents a hypercoagulable state.
Pg, picogram; *mm/hr,* millimeters/hours; *ng,* nanogram; *mcm³,* cubic micrometer; *mm³,* cubic millimeter; *PCV,* packed cell volume.

Cardiac Output

Cardiac output increases from 30% to 50% by week 32 of pregnancy; this declines to about a 20% increase at 40 weeks of gestation. This elevated cardiac output is largely a result of increased stroke volume and heart rate and occurs in response to increased tissue demands for oxygen (Monga, 2004).

Cardiac output in late pregnancy is appreciably higher when the woman is in the lateral recumbent position than when she is supine. In the supine position the large, heavy uterus often impedes venous return to the heart and affects blood pressure. Cardiac output increases with any exertion, such as labor and birth. Box 10-3 summarizes cardiovascular changes in pregnancy.

Circulation and Coagulation Times

The circulation time decreases slightly by week 32. It returns to near normal at term. There is a greater tendency for blood to coagulate (clot) during pregnancy because of increases in various clotting factors (i.e., factors VII, VIII, IX, X, and fibrinogen). This, combined with the fact that fibrinolytic activity (the splitting up or dissolving of a clot) is de-

Table 10-3

Laboratory Values for Pregnant and Nonpregnant Women—cont'd

VALUES	NONPREGNANT	PREGNANT
Blood Coagulation and Fibrinolytic Activity—*cont'd*		
Fibrinolytic activity		Decreases in pregnancy and then abrupt return to normal (protection against thromboembolism)
Fibrinogen, mg/dl	200-400	Increased levels late in pregnancy
Mineral/Vitamin Concentrations		
Vitamin B_{12}, folic acid, ascorbic acid	Normal	Moderate decrease
Serum Proteins		
Total, g/dl	6.4-8.3	5.5-7.5
Albumin, g/dl	3.5-5	Slight increase
Globulin, total, g/dl	2.3-3.4	3.0-4.0
Blood Glucose		
Fasting, mg/dl	70-105	Decreases
2-hr postprandial, mg/dl	<140	<140 after a 100 g-carbohydrate meal is considered normal
Acid-Base Values in Arterial Blood		
Po_2, mm Hg	80-100	104-108 (increased)
Pco_2, mm Hg	35-45	27-32 (decreased)
Sodium bicarbonate (HCO_3), mEq/L	21-28	18-31 (decreased)
Blood pH	7.35-7.45	7.40-7.45 (slightly increased, more alkaline)
HEPATIC		
Bilirubin, total, mg/dl	≤1	Unchanged
Serum cholesterol, mg/dl	120-200	Increases from 16 to 32 weeks of pregnancy; remains at this level until after birth
Serum alkaline phosphatase, U/L	30-120	Increases from week 12 of pregnancy to 6 weeks after birth
Serum albumin, g/dl	3.5-5	Slight increase
RENAL		
Bladder capacity, ml	1300	1500
Renal plasma flow (RPF), ml/min	490-700	Increase by 25%-30%
Glomerular filtration rate (GFR), ml/min	88-128	Increase by 30%-50%
Nonprotein nitrogen (NPN), mg/dl	25-40	Decreases
Blood urea nitrogen (BUN), mg/dl	10-20	Decreases
Serum creatinine, mg/dl	0.5-1.1	Decreases
Serum uric acid, mg/dl	2.7-7.3	Decreases
Urine glucose	Negative	Present in 20% of pregnant women
Intravenous pyelogram (IVP)	Normal	Slight-to-moderate hydroureter and hydronephrosis; right kidney larger than left kidney

Note: Abbreviations should not be used in practice.
Mg/dl, milligrams/deciliter; *g/dl,* grams/deciliter; *mm Hg,* millimeters of mercury; *mEg/l,* milliequivalents/liter; *ml,* milliliter; *ml/min,* milliliter/minute; *U/L,* units/liter.

pressed during pregnancy and the postpartum period, provides a protective function to decrease the chance of bleeding but also makes the woman more vulnerable to thrombosis, especially after cesarean birth.

Respiratory System

Structural and ventilatory adaptations occur during pregnancy to provide for both maternal and fetal needs. Maternal oxygen requirements increase in response to the acceleration in metabolic rate and the need to add to the tissue mass in the uterus and breasts. In addition, the fetus requires oxygen and a way to eliminate carbon dioxide.

Elevated levels of estrogen cause the ligaments of the rib cage to relax, permitting increased chest expansion (see Fig. 10-6). The transverse diameter of the thoracic cage increases by about 2 cm and the circumference by 6 cm. The costal angle increases and the lower rib cage appears to flare out

BOX 10-3

Cardiovascular Changes in Pregnancy

Heart rate	Increases 10-15 beats/min
Blood pressure	Remains at prepregnancy levels in first trimester Slight decrease in second trimester Returns to prepregnancy levels in third trimester
Blood volume	Increased by 1500 ml or 40%-50% above prepregnancy level
Red blood cell mass	Increases 17%
Hemoglobin	Decreases
Hematocrit	Decreases
White blood cell count	Increases in second and third trimesters
Cardiac output	Increases 30%-50%

BOX 10-4

Respiratory Changes in Pregnancy

Respiratory rate	Unchanged or slightly increased
Tidal volume	Increased 30%-40%
Vital capacity	Unchanged
Inspiratory capacity	Increased
Expiratory volume	Decreased
Total lung capacity	Unchanged to slightly decreased
Oxygen consumption	Increased 15%-20%

(Whitty & Dombrowski, 2004). The chest may not return to its prepregnant state after birth.

The diaphragm is displaced by as much as 4 cm during pregnancy. With advancing pregnancy, chest breathing replaces abdominal breathing, and descent of the diaphragm with inspiration becomes less possible. Thoracic breathing is primarily accomplished by the diaphragm rather than by the costal muscles.

The upper respiratory tract becomes more vascular in response to elevated levels of estrogen. As the capillaries become engorged, edema and hyperemia develop within the nose, pharynx, larynx, trachea, and bronchi. This congestion within the tissues of the respiratory tract gives rise to several conditions commonly seen during pregnancy, including nasal and sinus stuffiness, epistaxis (nosebleed), changes in the voice, and marked inflammatory response to even a mild upper respiratory infection.

Increased vascularity of the upper respiratory tract also can cause the tympanic membranes and eustachian tubes to swell, giving rise to symptoms of impaired hearing, earaches, or a sense of fullness in the ears.

Pulmonary Function

The pregnant woman breathes deeper, increasing her tidal volume (i.e., the volume of gas moved into or out of the respiratory tract with each breath). The respiratory rate remains unchanged or is only slightly increased (by about two breaths per minute). The expiratory reserve volume and residual volume decrease progressively during pregnancy. The inspiratory capacity increases slightly, whereas the vital capacity remains unchanged. The total lung capacity decreases slightly. These changes are related to the elevation of the diaphragm and chest wall changes. Box 10-4 lists respiratory changes in pregnancy.

During pregnancy, changes in the respiratory center result in a lowered threshold for carbon dioxide. Progesterone and estrogen are presumed to be responsible for the increased sensitivity of the respiratory center to carbon dioxide. In addition, pregnant women experience increased awareness of the need to breathe; some may complain of dyspnea at rest.

Although pulmonary function is not impaired by pregnancy, diseases of the respiratory tract may be more serious during this time. One important factor responsible for this may be the increase in oxygen requirements.

Basal Metabolic Rate

The basal metabolic rate (BMR) varies considerably in women at the beginning and during pregnancy; it usually increases 15% to 20% by term. The BMR returns to nonpregnant levels by 5 to 6 days postpartum. The elevation in BMR reflects increased oxygen demands of the uterine-placental-fetal unit and greater oxygen consumption because of increased maternal cardiac work. Peripheral vasodilation and acceleration of sweat gland activity help dissipate the excess heat resulting from the increased BMR during pregnancy. Pregnant women may experience heat intolerance. Lassitude and fatigability after only slight exertion are experienced by many women in early pregnancy. These feelings, along with a greater need for sleep, may persist and may be caused in part by the increased metabolic activity.

Acid-Base Balance

Progesterone may be responsible for increasing the sensitivity of the respiratory center receptors, so that tidal volume is increased and P_{CO_2} falls, the base excess (HCO_3, or bicarbonate) falls, and pH rises slightly. These alterations in acid-base balance indicate that pregnancy is a state of respiratory alkalosis compensated by mild metabolic acidosis (Monga, 2004). These changes also facilitate the transport of CO_2 from the fetus and O_2 release from the mother to the fetus. Table 10-3 lists laboratory values for pregnant and nonpregnant women.

Renal System

The kidneys are responsible for maintaining electrolyte and acid-base balance, regulating extracellular fluid volume, excreting waste products, and conserving essential nutrients.

Anatomic Changes

Changes in renal structure result from hormonal activity (estrogen and progesterone), pressure from an enlarging uterus, and an increase in blood volume. As early as the tenth week of pregnancy, the renal pelves and the ureters dilate. Dilation of the ureters is more pronounced above the pelvic brim, in part because they are compressed between the uterus and the pelvic brim. In most women the ureters below the pelvic brim are of normal size. The smooth-muscle walls of the ureters undergo hyperplasia and hypertrophy and muscle tone relaxation. The ureters elongate, become tortuous, and form single or double curves. In the latter part of pregnancy the renal pelvis and ureter dilate more on the right side than on the left because the heavy uterus is displaced to the right by the sigmoid colon.

Because of these changes, a larger volume of urine is held in the pelves and ureters, and urine flow rate is slowed. Urinary stasis or stagnation has several consequences:

- There is a lag between the time urine is formed and when it reaches the bladder. Therefore clearance test results may reflect substances contained in glomerular filtrate several hours before.
- Stagnated urine is an excellent medium for the growth of microorganisms. In addition, the urine of pregnant women contains more nutrients, including glucose, that increase the pH (make the urine more alkaline). Pregnant women are therefore more susceptible to urinary tract infection.

Bladder irritability, nocturia, and urinary frequency and urgency (without dysuria) are commonly reported in early pregnancy. These bladder symptoms may return near term, especially after lightening occurs.

Urinary frequency results initially from increased bladder sensitivity and later from compression of the bladder. In the second trimester the bladder is pulled up out of the true pelvis into the abdomen. The urethra lengthens to 7.5 cm as the bladder is displaced upward. The pelvic congestion that occurs in pregnancy is reflected in hyperemia of the bladder and urethra. This increased vascularity causes the bladder mucosa to be traumatized and bleed easily. Bladder tone may decrease, which increases the bladder capacity to 1500 ml. At the same time, the bladder is compressed by the enlarging uterus, resulting in the urge to void even if the bladder contains only a small amount of urine.

Functional Changes

In normal pregnancy, renal function is altered considerably. Glomerular filtration rate (GFR) and renal plasma flow (RPF) increase early in pregnancy (Monga, 2004). These changes are caused by pregnancy hormones; an increase in blood volume; and the woman's posture, physical activity, and nutritional intake. The woman's kidneys must manage the increased metabolic and circulatory demands of the maternal body and also the excretion of fetal waste products.

Renal function is most efficient when the woman lies in the lateral recumbent position and least efficient when the woman assumes a supine position. A side-lying position increases renal perfusion, which increases urine output and decreases edema. When the pregnant woman is lying supine, the heavy uterus compresses the vena cava and the aorta, and cardiac output decreases. As a result, blood flow to the brain and heart is continued at the expense of other organs, including the kidneys and uterus.

Fluid and Electrolyte Balance

Selective renal tubular reabsorption maintains sodium and water balance regardless of changes in dietary intake and losses through sweat, vomitus, or diarrhea. From 500 to 900 mEq of sodium is normally retained during pregnancy to meet fetal needs. To prevent excessive sodium depletion, the maternal kidneys undergo a significant adaptation by increasing tubular reabsorption. Because of the need for increased maternal intravascular and extracellular fluid volume, additional sodium is needed to expand fluid volume and to maintain an isotonic state. As efficient as the renal system is, it can be overstressed by excessive dietary sodium intake or restriction, or by use of diuretics. Severe hypovolemia and reduced placental perfusion are two consequences of using diuretics during pregnancy.

The capacity of the kidneys to excrete water is more efficient during the early weeks than later in pregnancy. As a result, some women feel thirsty in early pregnancy because of the greater amount of water loss. The pooling of fluid in the legs in the latter part of pregnancy decreases renal blood flow and GFR. This pooling is sometimes referred to as physiologic or dependent edema, and requires no treatment. The normal diuretic response to the water load is triggered when the woman lies down, preferably on her side, and the pooled fluid reenters general circulation.

Normally the kidney reabsorbs almost all the glucose and other nutrients from the plasma filtrate. In pregnant women, however, tubular reabsorption of glucose is impaired so that glucosuria occurs at varying times and to varying degrees. Normal values range from 0 to 20 mg/dl, meaning that during any day, the urine is sometimes positive and sometimes negative for glucose. In nonpregnant women, blood glucose levels must be at 160 to 180 mg/dl before glucose is "spilled" into the urine (not reabsorbed). During pregnancy, glucosuria occurs when maternal glucose levels are lower than 160 mg/dl. Why glucose, as well as other nutrients such as amino acids, is wasted during pregnancy is not understood, nor has the exact mechanism been discovered. Although glucosuria may be found in normal pregnancies (1+ levels may be seen with increased anxiety states), the possibility of diabetes mellitus and gestational diabetes must be kept in mind.

Proteinuria does not usually occur in normal pregnancy except during labor or after birth. However, the increased amounts of amino acids that need to be filtered may exceed the capacity of the renal tubules to absorb them, and small amounts of protein may be lost in the urine. Values of trace to 1+ protein (by dipstick assessment), or less than 300 mg/24 hr, are acceptable during pregnancy. However, a pregnant woman with hypertension and proteinuria must be carefully evaluated because she may be at greater risk for an adverse pregnancy outcome. Box 10-5 lists renal changes during pregnancy.

Integumentary System

Alterations in hormonal balance and mechanical stretching are responsible for several changes in the integumentary system during pregnancy. General changes include increases in skin thickness and subdermal fat, hyperpigmentation, increased hair and nail growth, accelerated sweat and sebaceous gland activity, and increased circulation and vasomotor activity. Cutaneous elastic tissues are more fragile,

BOX 10-5

Renal Changes in Pregnancy

Bladder capacity	Increased
Glomerular filtration rate (GFR)	Increased 30%-50%
Renal plasma flow (RPF)	Increased 30%
Blood urea nitrogen (BUN)	Decreased
Creatinine	Decreased
Glucose (in urine)	Present in 20% of pregnant women

resulting in striae gravidarum (or "stretch marks"). Cutaneous allergic responses are enhanced.

Hyperpigmentation is stimulated by the anterior pituitary hormone melanotropin, which is increased during pregnancy. Darkening of the nipples, areolae, axillae, and vulva occurs at about the sixteenth week of gestation (Fig. 10-8). Facial melasma (also called chloasma or mask of pregnancy) is a blotchy, brownish hyperpigmentation of the skin over the cheeks, nose, and forehead, especially in pregnant women with dark complexions. Chloasma appears in 50% to 70% of pregnant women, beginning after the sixteenth week and increasing gradually until term. The sun intensifies this pigmentation in susceptible women. Chloasma caused by normal pregnancy usually fades after birth.

The linea nigra (Fig. 10-9) is a pigmented line extending from the symphysis pubis to the top of the fundus in the midline. This line is known as the linea alba before hormone-induced pigmentation. In primigravidas the extension of the linea nigra, beginning in the third month, keeps pace with the rising height of the fundus; in multigravidas the entire line often appears earlier than the third month. Not all pregnant women develop lineae nigra, and some women notice hair growth along the line with or without the change in pigmentation.

Striae gravidarum (see Fig. 10-8) appear over the lower abdomen in 50% to 90% of pregnant women during the second half of pregnancy. These may be caused by the action of adrenocorticosteroids. Striae reflect separation within the underlying connective (collagen) tissue of the skin. These slightly depressed streaks tend to occur over areas of maximum stretch (the abdomen, thighs, and breasts). The stretching sometimes causes a sensation that resembles itching. The tendency to develop striae may be familial. After birth they usually fade, although they never disappear completely. Color of striae varies depending on the pregnant woman's skin color. The striae appear pinkish on a woman with light skin and are lighter than the surrounding skin in dark-skinned women. In the multipara, in addition to the striae of the present pregnancy, glistening silvery lines (in light-skinned women) or purplish lines (in dark-skinned women) are commonly seen. These represent the scars of striae from previous pregnancies.

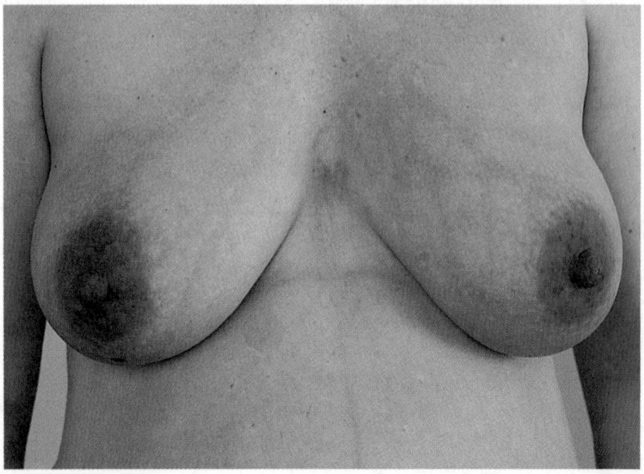

Fig. 10-8 Enlarged breasts in pregnancy with venous network and darkened areolae and nipples. (From Seidel HM et al: *Mosby's guide to physical examination,* ed 5, St. Louis, 2003, Mosby.)

Angiomas are commonly referred to as vascular spiders. These tiny, star-shaped or branched, slightly raised, and pulsating end-arterioles are usually found on the neck, thorax, face, and arms. They occur as a result of elevated levels of circulating estrogens. The spiders are bluish in color and do not blanch with pressure. Vascular spiders appear during the second to fifth month of pregnancy in 65% of Caucasian women and 10% of African-American women. The spiders usually disappear after birth.

Pinkish red, diffusely mottled or well-defined blotches are seen over the palmar surfaces of the hands in about 60% of Caucasian women and 35% of African-American women during pregnancy. These color changes, called palmar erythema, are related primarily to increased estrogen levels. Box 10-6 lists ethnic considerations for skin assessment during pregnancy.

Some dermatologic conditions have been identified as unique to pregnancy or as having an increased incidence during pregnancy. Pruritus is a relatively common dermatologic symptom in pregnancy. The goal of management is to relieve the itching. Topical steroids are the usual treatment, although systemic steroids may be needed. The problem usually resolves in the postpartum period (Stambuk & Colven, 2002).

BOX 10-6

Ethnic Considerations for Skin Assessment during Pregnancy

Integumentary system changes vary greatly among women of different racial backgrounds. For example, vascular spiders and palmar erythema are seen more often in Caucasian women than in African-American women. Areolar pigmentation varies by race: African-American women have the darkest areolae, Caucasian women have the lightest, and Asian women and Native American women have intermediate pigmentation. When performing physical assessments, the color of the woman's skin should be noted along with any changes that may be attributed to pregnancy.

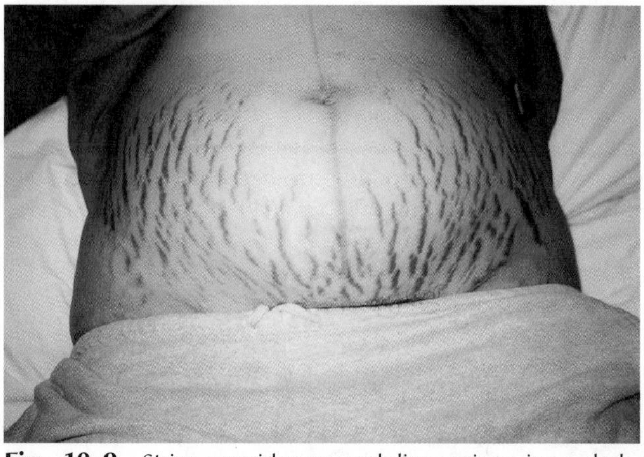

Fig. 10-9 Striae gravidarum and linea nigra in a dark-skinned person. (Courtesy Shannon Perry, Phoenix, AZ.)

Gum hypertrophy may occur. An epulis (gingival granuloma gravidarum) is a red, raised nodule on the gums that bleeds easily. This lesion may develop around the third month and usually continues to enlarge as pregnancy progresses. It is usually managed by avoiding trauma to the gums (e.g., using a soft toothbrush). An epulis usually regresses spontaneously after birth.

Nail growth may be accelerated. Some women may notice thinning and softening of the nails. Oily skin and acne vulgaris may occur during pregnancy.

NURSE ALERT Women with severe acne taking isotretinoin (Accutane) should avoid pregnancy while receiving the treatment because it is teratogenic and is associated with major fetal malformations. ■

For other women the skin clears and looks radiant. Hirsutism, the excessive growth of hair or growth of hair in unusual places, is commonly reported. An increase in fine hair growth may occur but tends to disappear after pregnancy. However, growth of coarse or bristly hair does not usually disappear after pregnancy.

Increased blood supply to the skin leads to increased perspiration. Women feel hotter during pregnancy, possibly related to a progesterone-induced increase in body temperature and the increased BMR.

Musculoskeletal System

The gradually changing body and increasing weight of the pregnant woman usually cause noticeable changes in her posture (Fig. 10-10) and in the way she walks. The great abdominal distention gives the pelvis a forward tilt, decreased abdominal muscle tone, and increased weight bearing. The woman's center of gravity shifts forward, requiring a realignment of the spinal curvatures. An increase in the normal lumbosacral curve (lordosis) develops, and a compensatory curvature in the cervicodorsal region (exaggerated anterior flexion of the head) develops to help her maintain balance. Aching, numbness, and weakness of the upper extremities may result. Large breasts and a stoop-shouldered stance will further accentuate the lumbar and dorsal curves. Walking is more difficult, and the waddling gait of the pregnant woman, called "the proud walk of pregnancy" by Shakespeare, is well known. The ligamentous and muscular structures of the middle and lower spine may be severely stressed. These and related changes often cause musculoskeletal discomfort.

The young, well-muscled woman may tolerate these changes without complaint. However, older women or those with a back disorder or a faulty sense of balance may have a considerable amount of back pain during and just after pregnancy.

Slight relaxation and increased mobility of the pelvic joints is normal during pregnancy. This is secondary to the exaggerated elasticity and softening of connective and collagen tissue caused by increased circulating steroid sex hormones, especially estrogen. Relaxin, an ovarian hormone, assists in this relaxation and softening. These adaptations permit enlargement of pelvic dimensions to facilitate labor and birth. The degree of relaxation varies, but considerable separation of the symphysis pubis and the instability of the sacroiliac joints may cause pain and difficulty in walking. Obesity or multifetal pregnancy tend to increase the pelvic instability. Peripheral joint laxity also increases as pregnancy progresses, but the cause is not known.

The muscles of the abdominal wall stretch and ultimately lose some tone. During the third trimester the rectus abdominis muscles may separate (Fig. 10-11), allowing abdominal contents to protrude at the midline. The umbilicus flattens or protrudes. After birth the muscles gradually regain

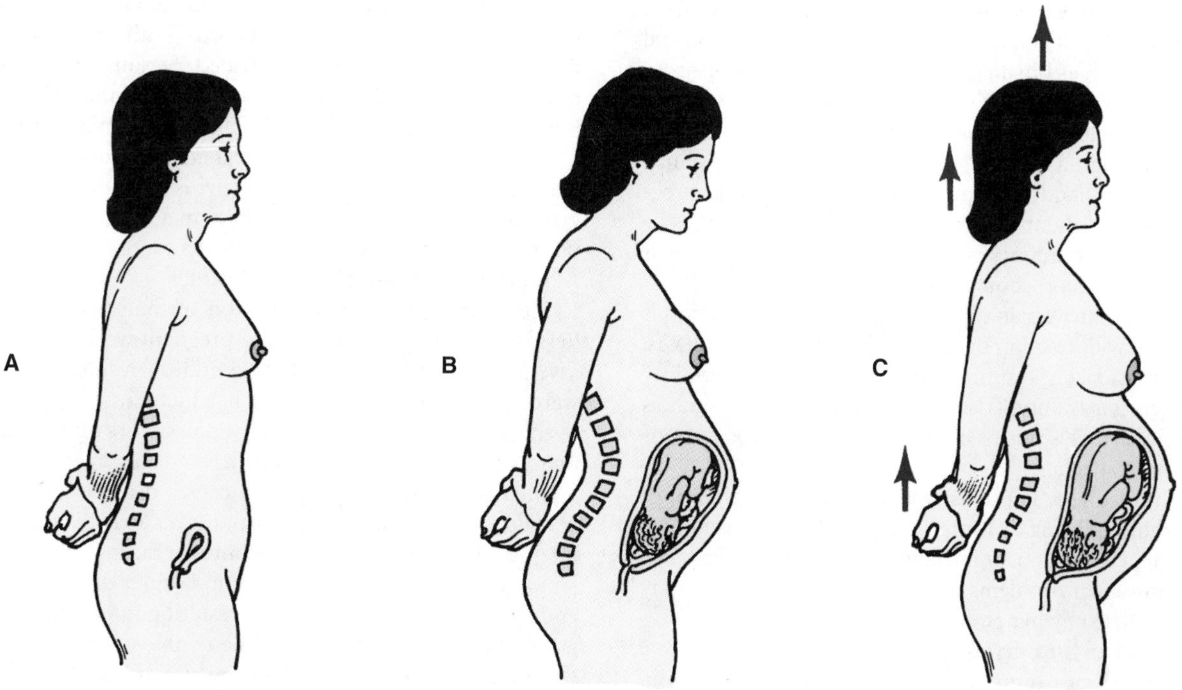

Fig. 10-10 Postural changes during pregnancy. **A**, Nonpregnant. **B**, Incorrect posture during pregnancy. **C**, Correct posture during pregnancy.

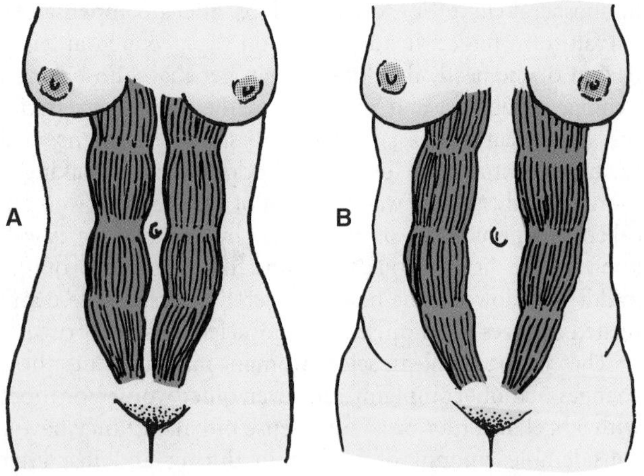

Fig. 10-11 Possible change in rectus abdominis muscles during pregnancy. **A**, Normal position in nonpregnant woman. **B**, Diastasis recti abdominis in pregnant women.

tone. However, separation of the muscles (diastasis recti abdominis) may persist.

Neurologic System

Little is known regarding specific alterations in function of the neurologic system during pregnancy, aside from hypothalamic-pituitary neurohormonal changes. Specific physiologic alterations resulting from pregnancy may cause the following neurologic or neuromuscular symptoms:

- Sensory changes in the legs as a result of compression of pelvic nerves or vascular stasis caused by enlargement of the uterus.
- Pain from dorsolumbar lordosis because of traction on nerves or compression of nerve roots.
- Carpal tunnel syndrome from edema of the peripheral nerves during the third trimester. The edema compresses the median nerve beneath the carpal ligament of the wrist. The syndrome is characterized by paresthesia (abnormal sensation such as burning or tingling caused by a disorder of the sensory nervous system) and pain in the hand, radiating to the elbow. The dominant hand is usually affected most, although as many as 80% of women report symptoms in both hands. Symptoms usually regress after pregnancy. Some patients may require surgical treatment.
- Acroesthesia (numbness and tingling of the hands) is caused by the stoop-shouldered stance (see Fig. 10-10, *B*) assumed by some women during pregnancy. The condition is associated with traction on segments of the brachial plexus.
- Tension headache is common when anxiety or uncertainty complicates gestation. However, vision problems such as refractive errors, sinusitis, or migraine may also be responsible for headaches.
- Light-headedness, faintness, and even syncope (fainting) are common during early pregnancy. Vasomotor instability, postural hypotension, or hypoglycemia may be responsible.
- Neuromuscular problems such as muscle cramps or tetany may be caused by hypocalcemia.

Gastrointestinal System

A variety of gastrointestinal system changes occur during pregnancy. The appetite fluctuates, intestinal secretion is reduced, liver function is altered, and absorption of nutrients is enhanced. Early in pregnancy, some women have nausea with or without vomiting (morning sickness), possibly in response to increasing levels of hCG and altered carbohydrate metabolism (Gordon, 2002). Whenever the vomiting is severe or persists beyond the first trimester, or when it is accompanied by fever, pain, or weight loss, further evaluation is necessary, and medical intervention is likely. The colon is displaced laterally upward and posteriorly. Peristaltic activity (motility) decreases. As a result, bowel sounds are diminished and constipation, nausea, and vomiting are common. Blood flow to the pelvis increases, as does venous pressure, contributing to hemorrhoid formation in later pregnancy. (For further discussion of nutrition in pregnancy, see Chapter 12.)

Women may have changes in their sense of taste, leading to cravings and changes in dietary intake. Some women have nonfood cravings (pica), such as for ice, clay, and laundry starch. Usually the subjects of these cravings, if consumed in moderation, are not harmful to the pregnancy if the woman has adequate nutrition with appropriate weight gain (Gordon, 2002).

Mouth

The gums are hyperemic, spongy, and swollen during pregnancy. They tend to bleed easily because the increasing levels of estrogen cause selective increased vascularity and connective tissue proliferation (a nonspecific gingivitis). Epulis (discussed in the section on the integumentary system) may develop at the gumline. Some pregnant women complain of ptyalism (excessive salivation), which may be caused by the decrease in unconscious swallowing by the woman when nauseated or from stimulation of salivary glands by eating starch.

Teeth

The pregnant woman requires about 1.2 g of calcium and approximately the same amount of phosphorus every day during pregnancy. This is an increase of about 0.4 g of each of these elements over nonpregnant needs. With a well-balanced diet, these requirements are satisfied. Serious dietary deficiency may deplete the mother's bony stores of these elements, but does not draw on calcium in her teeth. Demineralization of teeth does not occur during pregnancy; the old adage, "for every child a tooth" is untrue. Gingivitis and poor dental hygiene during pregnancy (or anytime) may contribute to dental caries, which can lead to the loss of a tooth.

Esophagus, Stomach, and Intestines

Herniation of the upper portion of the stomach (hiatal hernia) occurs in 15% to 20% of pregnant women after the seventh or eighth month. This condition results from upward displacement of the stomach, which causes a widening of the hiatus of the diaphragm. It occurs more often in multiparas and older or obese women.

Increased estrogen production causes decreased secretion of hydrochloric acid. Therefore peptic ulcer formation or flare-up of existing peptic ulcers is uncommon during pregnancy.

Increased progesterone production causes decreased tone and motility of smooth muscles resulting in esophageal regurgitation, slower emptying time of the stomach, and reverse peristalsis. As a result, the woman may experience "acid indigestion" or heartburn (pyrosis).

Evidence-Based Practice

RELIEF FOR FIRST-TRIMESTER NAUSEA AND VOMITING

Background

In the first trimester of pregnancy, nausea affects 70% to 85% of all women, and vomiting affects 50%. The discomfort can last all day, and, for 13% of affected women, can persist beyond the twentieth week. About one pregnant woman in three loses some time from work or home duties. In its most severe form, hyperemesis gravidarum can cause dehydration and starvation, and even death. Before the current era of easy replacement with intravenous fluids, hyperemesis was a major reason for pregnancy termination. It has been speculated that nausea and vomiting of pregnancy is due to the level of human chorionic gonadatropin. Nausea and vomiting is low in women who eventually have a miscarriage and high in women with multiple pregnancies.

Objectives

The authors of this review wished to discover any effective interventions for relief of nausea and vomiting of early pregnancy.

Intervention for nausea and vomiting of pregnancy could include antihistamine or antiemetic medications, pyridoxine (vitamin B_6), acupuncture, or acupressure at the P6 point, which is the inner aspect of the wrist, between the two tendons, about three fingerbreadths proximal from the wrist. For hyperemesis gravidarum, interventions could include ginger, corticosteroid or adrenocorticotropic hormone (ACTH) injections, intravenous diazepam, oral ondansetron, and acupuncture. Outcome measures included nausea, vomiting, retching, side effects of medications, and fetal outcomes.

Methods

Search Strategy

Search strategy included Cochrane, MEDLINE, hand searches of 30 journals, and weekly awareness service of 37 journals. Search keywords included *nausea and vomiting* and *pregnancy.*

Twenty-eight trials met the inclusion criteria, representing 3577 women. Publication dates ranged from 1958 to 2000. Countries were not noted in the review.

Statistical Analyses

Statistical analyses of homogeneous data enabled pooling. All data were assigned an odds ratio with a 95% confidence interval. Analysis revealed if the differences between groups were possibly from chance alone (insignificant).

Findings

Antiemetic drugs (12 trials): Nausea is significantly reduced by use of antiemetic drugs, but the medications may cause sleepiness. Bendectin was withdrawn from the market in 1983, due to fears of causing birth defects, but subsequent large, randomized, controlled trials showed no evidence of teratogenicity.

Pyridoxine (vitamin B_6): Two trials found significantly reduced nausea, but no effect on vomiting in the pyridoxine groups, compared with controls. There may be greater effect of 75 mg/day than with 30 mg/day.

Ginger: One trial reported that ginger is significantly helpful with nausea and vomiting.

Acupuncture or P6 acupressure: Six trials found that P6 or acupuncture was significantly more effective at relieving nausea and vomiting than sham acupuncture or sham acupressure at incorrect sites.

No intervention helped hyperemesis gravidarum, but oral methylprednisone or intravenous diazepam were associated with lower readmission rates. Ginger showed some promise, but not significantly.

There was no evidence of birth defects caused by the interventions in these trials.

Limitations

The challenges in reviewing such a large pool of studies are the diverse protocols, variable periods of observation, and diverse sample criteria. Several trials did not report how they randomized, or what happened to their dropouts, thus limiting generalizability. Most of the trials were small. The long time span (42 years) in which the trials occurred makes comparisons problematic, where technology has solved some problems (such as ease of intravenous hydration) and created others (such as side effects of antiemetic drugs).

Conclusions

Several therapies are effective in reducing nausea and vomiting of early pregnancy. These therapies include pyridoxine, fresh ginger root, Sea Bands, and antiemetic drugs.

Implications for Practice

Women may benefit from taking 10 to 25 mg of pyridoxine three times a day for nausea and vomiting of early pregnancy. Fresh ginger root may be beneficial. Women can try Sea Bands, which are elastic wristbands with a plastic knob, to be applied to the P6 acupressure site. Remedies may not work consistently. Antiemetic drugs are available, if necessary.

Implications for Further Research

More information about hyperemesis gravidarum is necessary to identify interventions for this intractable disease. More information about the fetal outcomes of antiemetic medications is essential.

Reference

Jewell D, Young G: Interventions for nausea and vomiting in early pregnancy (Cochrane Review), 2003. In *The Cochrane Library,* Issue 2, Chichester, UK, 2004, John Wiley & Sons.

In response to increased needs during pregnancy, iron is absorbed more readily in the small intestine. Even if the woman is deficient in iron, it will continue to be absorbed in sufficient amounts for the fetus to have a normal hemoglobin level.

Increased progesterone (which causes loss of smooth muscle tone and decreased peristalsis) results in an increase in water absorption from the colon and may cause constipation. Constipation can also result from hypoperistalsis (sluggishness of the bowel), food choices, lack of fluids, iron supplementation, decreased activity level, abdominal distention by the pregnant uterus, and displacement and compression of the intestines. If the pregnant woman has hemorrhoids (see Fig. 10-7) and is constipated, the hemorrhoids can evert or bleed during straining at stool.

Gallbladder and Liver

The gallbladder is often distended because of its decreased muscle tone during pregnancy. Increased emptying time and thickening of bile caused by prolonged retention are typical changes. These features, together with slight hypercholesterolemia from increased progesterone levels, may account for the development of gallstones during pregnancy.

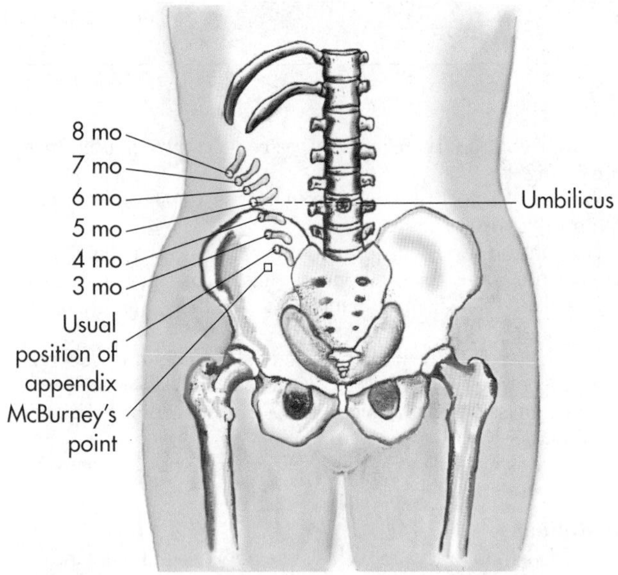

Fig. 10-12 Change in position of appendix in pregnancy. Note McBurney's point.

Hepatic function is difficult to appraise during pregnancy. However, only minor changes in liver function develop. Occasionally, intrahepatic cholestasis (retention and accumulation of bile in the liver caused by factors within the liver) occurs late in pregnancy in response to placental steroids. It may result in pruritus gravidarum (severe itching) with or without jaundice. These distressing symptoms subside soon after birth.

Abdominal Discomfort

Intraabdominal alterations that can cause discomfort include pelvic heaviness or pressure, round ligament tension, flatulence, distention and bowel cramping, and uterine contractions. In addition to displacement of intestines, pressure from the expanding uterus causes an increase in venous pressure in the pelvic organs. Although most abdominal discomfort is a consequence of normal maternal alterations, the health care provider must be constantly alert to the possibility of disorders such as bowel obstruction or an inflammatory process.

Appendicitis may be difficult to diagnose in pregnancy because the appendix is displaced upward and laterally, high and to the right, away from McBurney's point (Fig. 10-12).

Table 10-4

Hormones and Effects of Changes during Pregnancy

HORMONE	SOURCE	EFFECTS OF CHANGES DURING PREGNANCY
Human chorionic gonadotropin (hCG)	Fertilized ovum and chorionic villi	Maintains corpus luteum's production of estrogen and progesterone until placenta takes over the function
Progesterone	Corpus luteum until 14 weeks of gestation, then the placenta	Suppresses secretion of FSH and LH by the anterior pituitary; maintains pregnancy by relaxing smooth muscles, decreasing uterine contractility; causes fat to deposit in subcutaneous tissues over the maternal abdomen, back, and upper thighs; decreases mother's ability to use insulin
Estrogen	Corpus luteum until 14 weeks of gestation, then the placenta	Suppresses secretion of FSH and LH by the anterior pituitary; causes fat to deposit in subcutaneous tissues over the maternal abdomen, back, and upper thighs; promotes enlargement of genitals, uterus, and breasts; increases vascularity; relaxes pelvic ligaments and joints, interferes with folic acid metabolism, increases the level of total body proteins, promotes retention of sodium and water; decreases secretion of hydrochloric acid and pepsin; decreases mother's ability to use insulin
Serum prolactin	Anterior pituitary	Responsible for initial lactation
Oxytocin	Posterior pituitary	Stimulates uterine contractions; stimulates the let-down or milk-ejection reflex
Human chorionic somatomammotropin (previously called human placental lactogen)	Placenta	Acts as a growth hormone; contributes to breast development; decreases maternal metabolism of glucose; increases the amount of fatty acids for metabolic needs
Thyroxine-binding globulin, thyroxine, triiodothyronine	Thyroid	Causes moderate enlargement of the thyroid gland but woman remains euthyroid; possibly plays role in early neural development of the fetus
Parathyroid	Parathyroid	Controls calcium and magnesium metabolism
Insulin	Pancreas	Decreases production of insulin to protect fetus and its need for glucose
Cortisol	Adrenal glands	Stimulates production of insulin; increases peripheral resistance to insulin
Aldosterone	Adrenal glands	Stimulates reabsorption of excess sodium from the renal tubules

FSH, follicle-stimulating hormone; *LH*, luteinizing hormone.

Endocrine System

Profound endocrine changes are essential for pregnancy maintenance, normal fetal growth, and postpartum recovery. Hormones, their sources, and their effects on the pregnancy are presented in Table 10-4.

Key Points

- Adaptations to pregnancy protect the woman's normal physiologic functioning, meet the metabolic demands that pregnancy imposes, and provide for fetal developmental and growth needs.
- Maternal adaptations are attributed to the hormones of pregnancy and to mechanical pressures arising from the enlarging uterus and other tissues.
- The ability to recognize the beta subunit of hCG through monoclonal antibody technology has revolutionized endocrine tests for pregnancy.
- Presumptive, probable, and positive signs of pregnancy aid in the diagnosis of pregnancy; only positive signs (identification of a fetal heart tone, verification of fetal movements, and visualization of the fetus) can establish the diagnosis of pregnancy.
- Although the pH of the pregnant woman's vaginal secretions is more acidic, she is more vulnerable to some vaginal infections, especially yeast infections.
- Increased vascularity and sensitivity of the vagina and other pelvic viscera may lead to a high degree of sexual interest and arousal.
- Some adaptations to pregnancy result in discomforts such as fatigue, urinary frequency, nausea, constipation, and breast sensitivity.
- Balance and coordination are affected by changes in joints and in the woman's center of gravity as pregnancy progresses.

Answer Guidelines to Critical Thinking Exercise

Awareness of Physiologic Changes of Pregnancy

1. Yes. The physiologic changes of pregnancy and the differences in those changes between primiparas and multiparas are well documented. In addition, each pregnancy is unique; thus what happens in one pregnancy may not happen in the next pregnancy.
2. (a) Differences in the normal physiologic changes in pregnancy between primiparas and multiparas usually relate to the gestational age at which the changes occur. For example, multiparas are usually able to perceive fetal movement earlier than do primiparas. (b) Most of the differences in the normal physiologic changes in pregnancy are reversible; however, some changes are permanent. For example, chloasma fades, the areolae return to the former appearance, the linea nigra disappears, but the appearance of the vulva and cervix changes and scars of striae gravidarum remain. (c) The health care provider usually has a routine for providing information about the changes of pregnancy; that is, at the first visit, some information is given. At subsequent visits, the woman is prepared for what will happen in the next month or two. In addition, childbirth classes include information on physiologic changes in pregnancy. It is important to listen to women to be sure that their questions are answered. (d) Deviations from normal in the physiologic changes of pregnancy may signal problems in the pregnancy and warrant further investigation.
3. Priorities for nursing care are to ascertain what questions Marlys and Janice have about their pregnancies, provide education on the physiologic changes of pregnancy and the differences in those changes between primiparas and multiparas, and answer any other questions the two women might have; perform the assessments appropriate for their gestations; and schedule their next prenatal appointments. Childbirth education classes can be recommended and written material provided.
4. Yes, the evidence objectively supports the conclusion. There has been a great deal of research on the physiologic changes of pregnancy, what causes them, meaning and treatment of deviations from normal, and the efficacy of childbirth education in answering questions and allaying anxiety of women in pregnancy.
5. Yes. There is still a great deal that is unknown about physiologic changes of pregnancy and their meaning, as well as the cause of deviations from normal and the advisibility and appropriateness of treating the deviations. Different women react differently to pregnancy, and each pregnancy is unique. What happens in one pregnancy may not happen in the next. Not all women want information about physiology or possibility of deviations from normal. Not all women seek care from Western medical practitioners. Some women use traditional practitioners and traditional medicine to meet their needs. Women learn in various ways and obtain answers to their questions from a variety of sources. A great deal of information is available on the World Wide Web. Education about how to judge the trustworthiness of the information is important.

Resources

Alexian Brothers Medical Center (information on physiologic and emotional aspects of pregnancy)
Elk Grove, IL
www.alexian.org/progserv/babies/babytoo.html

Babyonline.com (source of information on pregnancy and baby care)
www.babyonline.com

Childbirth.org (source of links to other sites related to pregnancy and birth)
www.childbirth.org

New York Online Access to Health (consumer-level information site; includes information on tests, fetal development, postnatal topics, etc., in English and Spanish)
www.noah-health.org/english/pregnancy

Official site of the Perinatal Education Associates, Inc.
www.birthsource.com

References

Berman ML, Di Saia PJ, Tewari KS: Pelvic malignancies, gestational trophoblastic neoplasia, and nonpelvic malignancies. In Creasy RK, Resnik R, Iams JD (eds): *Maternal-fetal medicine: principles and practice,* ed 5, Philadelphia, 2004, WB Saunders.

Buster J, Carson S: Endocrinology and diagnosis of pregnancy. In Gabbe SG, Niebyl JR, Simpson JL (eds): *Obstetrics: normal and problem pregnancies,* ed 4, New York, 2002, Churchill Livingstone.

Cunningham F et al: *Williams obstetrics,* ed 21, New York, 2001, McGraw-Hill.

Gonik B, Foley MR: Intensive care monitoring of the critically ill pregnant patient. In Creasy RK, Resnik R, Iams JD (eds): *Maternal-fetal medicine: principles and practice,* ed 5, Philadelphia, 2004, WB Saunders.

Gordon M: Maternal physiology in pregnancy. In Gabbe SG, Niebyl JR, Simpson JL (eds): *Obstetrics: normal and problem pregnancies,* ed 4, New York, 2002, Churchill Livingstone.

Hatcher R et al: *A pocket guide to managing contraception,* Tiger, GA, 2004, Bridging the Gap Foundation.

Hermida R et al: Time-qualified reference values for ambulatory blood pressure monitoring in pregnancy, *Hypertension* 38(3 Pt 2):746-752, 2001.

Jewell D, Young G: Interventions for nausea and vomiting in early pregnancy (Cochrane Review), 2003. In *The Cochrane Library,* Issue 2, Chichester, UK, 2004, John Wiley & Sons.

Monga M: Maternal cardiovascular and renal adaptation to pregnancy. In Creasy RK, Resnik R, Iams JD (eds): *Maternal-fetal medicine: principles and practice,* ed 5, Philadelphia, 2004, WB Saunders.

Monga M, Sanborn BM: Biology and physiology of the reproductive tract and control of myometrial contraction. In Creasy RK, Resnik R, Iams JD (eds): *Maternal-fetal medicine: principles and practice,* ed 5, Philadelphia, 2004, WB Saunders.

Murray I: Change and adaptation in pregnancy. In Fraser DM, Cooper MA: *Myles textbook for midwives,* ed 14, Edinburgh, 2003, Churchill Livingstone.

Pagana KD, Pagana TJ: Mosby's *diagnostic and laboratory test reference,* ed 6, St Louis, 2003, Mosby.

Stambuk R, Colven R: Dermatologic disorders. In Gabbe SG, Niebyl JR, Simpson JL (eds): *Obstetrics: normal and problem pregnancies,* ed 4, New York, 2002, Churchill Livingstone.

Whitty JE, Dombrowski MP: Respiratory diseases in pregnancy. In Creasy RK, Resnik R, Iams JD (eds): *Maternal-fetal medicine: principles and practice,* ed 5, Philadelphia, 2004, WB Saunders.

Nursing Care during Pregnancy 11

LEARNING OBJECTIVES

On completion of this chapter the reader will be able to:

- Describe the processes of confirming pregnancy and estimating the date of birth.
- Summarize the physical, psychosocial, and behavioral changes that usually occur as the mother and other family members adapt to pregnancy.
- Discuss the benefits of prenatal care and problems of accessibility for some women.
- Outline the patterns of health care provided to assess maternal and fetal health status at the initial visit and at follow-up visits during pregnancy.
- Identify the typical nursing assessments, diagnoses, interventions, and methods of evaluation in providing care for the pregnant woman.
- Discuss education needed by pregnant women to understand physical discomforts related to pregnancy and to recognize the signs and symptoms of potential complications.
- Explain the impact of culture, age, parity, and number of fetuses on the response of the family to the pregnancy and on the prenatal care provided.
- Identify the purposes of childbirth education.
- Compare the advantages and disadvantages of choosing different care providers.

ELECTRONIC RESOURCES

Additional information related to the content in Chapter 11 can be found on

the companion website at evolve
http://evolve.elsevier.com/Wong/maternal/
- NCLEX Review Questions
- Case Study–First Trimester
- Case Study–Second Trimester
- Case Study–Third Trimester
- WebLinks

or the interactive student CD-ROM
Activities for Chapter 11 include the following:
- NCLEX Review Questions
- Case Study–First Trimester
- Case Study–Second Trimester
- Case Study–Third Trimester
- Nursing Care Plan–Discomforts of Pregnancy
- Nursing Care Plan–Adolescent Pregnancy

The prenatal period is a time of physical and psychologic preparation for birth and parenthood. Becoming a parent represents one of the maturational milestones of adult life, and as such, it is a time of intense learning for parents and those close to them. The prenatal period provides a unique opportunity for nurses and other members of the health care team to influence family health. During this period, essentially healthy women seek regular care and guidance. The nurse's health promotion interventions can affect the well-being of the woman, her unborn child, and the rest of her family for many years.

Regular prenatal visits, ideally beginning soon after the first missed menstrual period, offer opportunities to ensure the health of the expectant mother and her infant. Prenatal health care permits diagnosis and treatment of preexisting maternal disorders and those that may develop during the pregnancy. Care is designed to monitor the growth and development of the fetus and to identify abnormalities that may interfere with the course of normal labor. The woman and her family can seek support to reduce stress and to learn parenting skills.

Pregnancy lasts 9 calendar months. However, health care providers use the concept of lunar months, which last 28 days (or 4 weeks) to describe the duration of pregnancy or gestational age. Thus normal pregnancy lasts about 10 lunar months, that is, 40 weeks, or 280 days. Pregnancy is divided into three 3-month periods, or trimesters. The first trimester covers weeks 1 through 13; the second, weeks 14 through 26; and the third, weeks 27 through term gestation (38 to 40 weeks). Prenatal care during each trimester focuses on different priorities of care. The focus of this chapter is on meeting the health needs of the expectant family over the course of pregnancy, which is known as the prenatal period.

DIAGNOSIS OF PREGNANCY

Women may suspect pregnancy when they miss a menstrual period. Many women come to the first visit after a positive home pregnancy test. However, the clinical diagnosis of pregnancy before the second missed period may be difficult in some women. Factors such as physical variations, lack of relaxation, obesity, or tumors may confound even the experienced examiner. Accuracy is important, however, because emotional, social, medical, or legal consequences related to an inaccurate diagnosis, either positive or negative, can be extremely serious. A correct date for the first day of the last (normal) menstrual period (LMP), the date of intercourse, or the basal body temperature (BBT) record may be of great value in the accurate diagnosis of pregnancy (see Chapter 7).

Signs and Symptoms

Great variability is possible in the subjective and objective symptoms of pregnancy. Therefore the diagnosis of pregnancy may be uncertain for a time. The diagnosis of pregnancy is based on signs and symptoms that are reported during history taking or found during physical examination. These signs and symptoms are classified as presumptive, probable, and positive (see Table 10-2).

Estimating Date of Birth

When pregnancy is confirmed, the woman's first question usually concerns when she will give birth. This date has traditionally been called the estimated date of confinement (EDC) or estimated date of delivery (EDD). However, to promote a more positive perception of both pregnancy and birth, the term *estimated date of birth* (EDB) is now used. Because the exact date of conception is usually unknown, several formulas have been suggested for calculating the EDB. None of these guides is infallible, but Nägele's rule is reasonably accurate and is the method usually used.

Nägele's rule is as follows: After determining the first day of the LMP, subtract 3 months, add 7 days and 1 year; or alternatively, add 7 days to the LMP and count forward 9 months. For example, if the first day of the LMP was July 10, 2004, the EDB is April 17, 2005.

Nägele's rule assumes that the woman has a 28-day menstrual cycle and that the pregnancy occurred on the fourteenth day of the cycle. An adjustment is in order if the cycle is longer or shorter than 28 days. Only about 5% of pregnant women give birth spontaneously on the EDB as determined by Nägele's rule. Most women give birth during the period extending from 7 days before to 7 days after the EDB.

ADAPTATION TO PREGNANCY

Pregnancy affects all family members, and each family member must adapt to the pregnancy and interpret its meaning in light of his or her own needs. This process of family adaptation to pregnancy takes place within a cultural environment influenced by societal trends. Dramatic changes have occurred in Western society in recent years, and the nurse must be prepared to support single-parent families, reconstituted families, dual-career families, and alternative families, as well as traditional families, in the childbirth experience.

Much of the investigation of family dynamics in pregnancy by scholars in the United States and Canada has been done with Caucasian, middle-class nuclear families, and findings may not apply to families who do not fit the traditional North American model. Terms such as *spouse, husband,* and *wife,* for example, are used consistently in family literature but may not fit the configuration of a given family in the nurse's care.

Maternal Adaptation

Women of all ages use the months of pregnancy to adapt to the maternal role. Early in pregnancy nothing seems to be happening, and much time is spent sleeping. With the perception of fetal movement in the second trimester, the woman turns her attention inward to her pregnancy (Family Focus box).

Pregnancy is a maturational milestone and requires mastery of certain developmental tasks: accepting the pregnancy, identifying with the role of mother, reordering the relationships between herself and her mother and between herself and her partner, establishing a relationship with the unborn child, and preparing for the birth experience (Lederman, 1996). The partner's emotional support is an important factor in the successful accomplishment of these developmental tasks. Single women with limited support may have difficulty making this adaptation.

Accepting the Pregnancy

The first step in adapting to the maternal role is accepting the idea of pregnancy and assimilating the pregnant state into the woman's way of life. Mercer (1995) described this process as cognitive restructuring and credited Reva Rubin (1984) as the nurse theorist who pioneered our understanding of maternal role attainment.

The degree of acceptance is reflected in the woman's emotional responses. Initially, many women are dismayed at finding themselves pregnant. Eventual acceptance of pregnancy parallels the growing acceptance of the reality of a child. Nonacceptance of the pregnancy should not be equated with rejection of the child. A woman may dislike being pregnant but feel love for the child to be born. Women who are happy and pleased about their pregnancy have high self-esteem and tend to be confident about outcomes for themselves, their babies, and other family members.

Despite a general feeling of well-being, many pregnant women are surprised to experience emotional lability, that is, rapid and unpredictable changes in mood. These swings in emotions and increased sensitivity to others are disconcerting to the expectant mother and those around her. Increased irritability, explosions of tears and anger, and feelings of great joy and cheerfulness alternate, apparently with little or no provocation. Profound hormonal changes that are part of the maternal response to pregnancy may be responsible for mood changes.

Most women experience ambivalent feelings during pregnancy. Ambivalence, or having conflicting feelings at the

Family Focus

MATERNAL ADAPTATION

Adaptation to the maternal role involves a complex social and cognitive learning process. Pregnancy functions as a rite of passage and indicates that maturity has been reached. Reva Rubin began studying maternal role adaptation in the 1960s. She described the *developmental tasks* of pregnancy as accepting the pregnancy, identifying the role of mother, reordering the relationships between her mother and herself and between herself and her partner, establishing a relationship with the unborn child, and preparing for the birth experience.

The partner's emotional support is an important factor in the successful accomplishment of these developmental tasks. Women who are prepared to accept a pregnancy seek medical validation early. When pregnancy is confirmed, a woman's emotional responses may range from delight to shock, disbelief, and despair. A general state of well-being predominates, but emotional lability is common. These rapid mood changes include increased irritability, explosions of tears and anger, and feelings of great joy and cheerfulness. Such changes are often attributed to hormonal changes.

Rubin described changes in pregnancy as follows. The subjective experience of time and space changes during pregnancy; early in pregnancy, nothing seems to be happening, and the woman spends much time sleeping. With quickening (feelings of fetal movement) in the second trimester, there is a reduction of time and space, both geographic and social, as the woman turns her attention inward to her pregnancy. She examines or fosters relationships with her mother and other women who have been or are pregnant. With the third trimester, there is a slower pace and a sense that time is running out as the woman's activities are curtailed. A mother's reaction to her daughter's pregnancy signifies her acceptance of the grandchild and of her daughter. If the mother is supportive, the daughter has an opportunity to discuss pregnancy and labor and her feelings of joy or ambivalence with a knowledgeable and accepting woman.

Women express two major needs within the partner relationship during pregnancy: feeling loved and valued, and having the child accepted by the partner. The addition of a child changes forever the nature of the bond between partners. The partner can be a stabilizing influence, a good listener to expressions of doubts and fears, and a source of physical and emotional reassurance. The partner can also feel jealous of the unborn baby. Lesbian and unpartnered women have received little attention in the literature. Some suggest that a woman partner may be better able to understand and meet more effectively the needs of her partner for nurturing. An unpartnered woman may seek out her mother or other women friends to meet her dependence needs.

Data from Mercer R: *Becoming a mother,* New York, 1995, Springer.

same time, is considered a normal response in people preparing for a new role. Even women who are pleased to be pregnant may experience feelings of hostility toward the pregnancy or the unborn child from time to time. Intense feelings of ambivalence that persist through the third trimester may indicate an unresolved conflict with the motherhood role (Mercer, 1995). After the birth of a healthy child, memories of these ambivalent feelings usually are dismissed. If the child is born with a defect, a woman may look back at the times when she did not want the pregnancy and feel intense guilt; she may believe that her ambivalence caused the birth defect. She will need reassurance that her feelings were not responsible for the problem.

Identifying with the Mother Role

The process of identifying with the mother role begins early in each woman's life when she is being mothered as a child. Practice roles, such as playing with dolls, baby-sitting, and taking care of siblings, may increase her understanding of what being a mother entails.

Many women have always wanted a baby; they like children, and look forward to motherhood. Their high motivation to become a parent promotes acceptance of pregnancy and eventual prenatal and parental adaptation. Other women apparently have not considered in any detail what motherhood means to them. During pregnancy, conflicts such as not wanting the pregnancy and career-related decisions need to be resolved.

Reordering Personal Relationships

Close relationships held by the pregnant woman undergo change as she prepares emotionally for the new role of mother. As family members learn their new roles, periods of tension and conflict may occur. Promoting effective communication patterns between the expectant mother and her own mother and between the expectant mother and her partner are common nursing interventions provided during the prenatal visits.

The woman's relationship with her mother is significant in adapting to pregnancy and motherhood. Important components in the pregnant woman's relationship with her mother are the mother's availability (past and present), her reactions to the daughter's pregnancy, respect for her daughter's autonomy, and the willingness to reminisce (Mercer, 1995).

The mother's reaction to the daughter's pregnancy signifies her acceptance of the grandchild and of her daughter. If the mother is supportive, the daughter has an opportunity to discuss pregnancy and labor and her feelings of joy or ambivalence with a knowledgeable and accepting woman (Fig. 11-1). Reminiscing about the pregnant woman's early childhood and sharing the grandmother-to-be's account of her childbirth experience help the daughter anticipate and prepare for labor and birth.

Although the woman's relationship with her mother is significant in considering her adaptation in pregnancy, the most important person to the pregnant woman is usually the father of her child. A woman who is nurtured by her partner during pregnancy has fewer emotional and physical symptoms, fewer labor and childbirth complications, and an easier postpartum adjustment.

The marital or committed relationship is not static but evolves over time. The addition of a child changes forever the nature of the bond between partners. Partners who trust and support each other are able to share mutual-dependency needs (Mercer, 1995).

Myths about body functions and fantasies about the influence of the fetus as a third party in lovemaking are commonly expressed. An individual may also inaccurately attribute anomalies, mental retardation, and other injuries to the fetus and mother to sexual relations during pregnancy. Some couples fear that the woman's genitals will be drastically changed by the birth process.

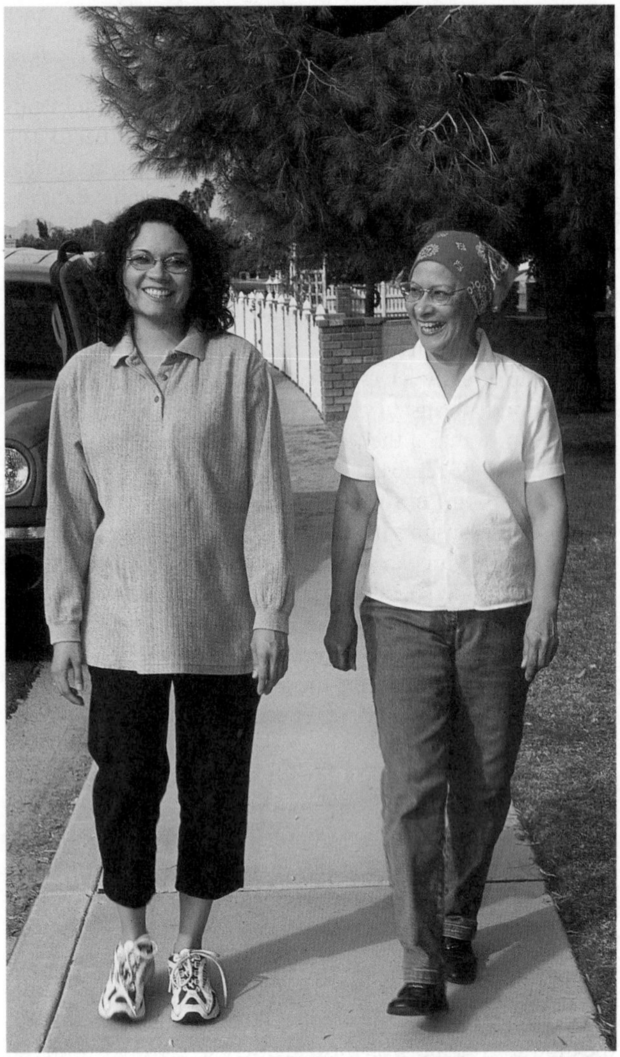

Fig. 11-1 A pregnant woman and her mother enjoy a walk together. (Courtesy Michael S. Clement, MD, Mesa, AZ.)

As pregnancy progresses, changes in body shape, body image, and levels of discomfort influence both partners' desire for sexual expression. During the first trimester the woman's sexual desire may decrease, especially if she experiences breast tenderness, nausea, fatigue, or sleepiness. As she progresses into the second trimester, her sense of well-being, combined with the increased pelvic congestion that occurs at this time, may increase her desire for sexual release. In the third trimester, somatic complaints and physical bulkiness may increase her physical discomfort and diminish her interest in sex.

Establishing a Relationship with the Fetus

Parental concern for the health of the child seems to vary during the course of pregnancy. The first concern appears in the first trimester and relates to the possibility of miscarriage. Many women delay telling others about the pregnancy until this time passes. As the child becomes more of a reality, with movement and an audible heartbeat and through ultrasound examination, parental anxiety focuses on possible defects in the child.

Emotional attachment to the child begins during the prenatal period as women use fantasizing and daydreaming to prepare themselves for motherhood (Rubin, 1975). They think of themselves as mothers and imagine maternal qualities they would like to possess. Expectant parents desire to be warm, loving, and close to their child. The mother-child relationship progresses through pregnancy as a developmental process. Three phases in the developmental pattern become apparent.

In phase 1 the woman accepts the biologic fact of pregnancy. She needs to be able to state, "I am pregnant." In phase 2 the woman accepts the growing fetus as distinct from herself and as a person to nurture. She can now say, "I am going to have a baby." Attachment by a mother to her child is enhanced by experiencing a planned pregnancy, and it increases when ultrasound examination and quickening confirm the reality of the fetus. During phase 3, the woman prepares realistically for the birth and parenting of the child. She expresses the thought, "I am going to be a mother," and defines the nature and characteristics of the child. She may, for example, speculate about the child's sex and personality traits based on patterns of fetal activity. Although the mother alone experiences the child within, both parents and siblings believe the unborn child responds in a very individualized, personal manner. Family members may interact with the unborn child by talking to the fetus and stroking the mother's abdomen, especially when the fetus shifts position.

Preparing for Childbirth

Many women actively prepare for birth. They read books, view films, attend parenting classes, and talk to other women. They seek the best caregiver possible for advice, monitoring, and caring. The multipara has her own history of labor and birth, which influences her approach to preparation for this childbirth experience.

Anxiety can arise from concern about safe passage for herself and her child during the birth process (Mercer, 1995; Rubin, 1975). This concern may not be expressed overtly, but cues are given as the nurse listens to plans women make for care of the new baby and other children in case "anything should happen." These feelings persist despite statistical evidence about the safe outcome of pregnancy for mothers and their infants. Many women fear the pain of childbirth or mutilation because they do not understand anatomy and the birth process. Education by the nurse can alleviate many of these fears.

Toward the end of the third trimester breathing is difficult and fetal movements become vigorous enough to disturb the mother's sleep. Backaches, frequency and urgency of urination, constipation, and varicose veins can become troublesome. The bulkiness and awkwardness of her body interfere with the woman's ability to care for other children, perform routine work-related duties, and assume a comfortable position for sleep and rest. A strong desire to see the end of pregnancy, to be over and done with it, makes women at this stage ready to move on to childbirth.

Paternal Adaptation

The father's beliefs and feelings about the ideal mother and father and his cultural expectation of appropriate behavior during pregnancy affect his response to his partner's need for him. For most men, pregnancy can be a time of preparation for the parental role with intense learning (Family Focus box).

Family Focus

PATERNAL ADAPTATION

A man's emotional responses to becoming a father, his concerns, and his informational needs change during the course of pregnancy. Three styles of involvement provide examples of different ways men can experience pregnancy (May, 1980, 1982). Men may be involved in pregnancy as an observer, that is, avoiding direct involvement in activities such as parent education classes and decisions about breastfeeding. Others are more expressive and display a strong emotional response to pregnancy and a desire to be a full partner in the project. Some expectant fathers experience the couvade syndrome and have pregnancy-like symptoms such as nausea and other gastrointestinal complaints, fatigue, and other physical discomforts. Other fathers adopt the instrumental style, seeing tasks they can perform in their role as manager of the pregnancy. They feel responsible for the outcome of pregnancy and are protective and supportive of their wives.

The father's beliefs and feelings about the ideal mother and father and his cultural expectation of appropriate behavior during pregnancy affect his response to his partner's need for him. One man may engage in nurturing behavior; another may feel lonely and alienated as the woman becomes physically and emotionally engrossed in the unborn child. The man may seek comfort and understanding outside the home, or become interested in a new hobby or involved with his work. Some men view pregnancy as a proof of their masculinity and their dominant role. To others, pregnancy has no meaning in terms of responsibility to either mother or child. For most men, however, pregnancy is a time of preparation for the parental role, of fantasy, of great pleasure, and of intense learning.

Accepting the Pregnancy

In older societies, the man enacted the ritual couvades; that is, he behaved in specific ways and respected taboos associated with pregnancy and giving birth. In this way the man's new status was recognized and endorsed. His behavior acknowledged his psychosocial and biologic relationship to the mother and child. During the past 30 years, changing cultural and professional attitudes have encouraged fathers' participation in the birth experience (Fig. 11-2).

Identifying with the Father Role

Each father brings to pregnancy attitudes that affect the way in which he adjusts to the pregnancy and parental role. His memories of the fathering he received from his own father, the experiences he has had with child care, and the perceptions of the male and father roles within his social group will guide his selection of the tasks and responsibilities he will assume. Some men are highly motivated to nurture and love a child. They may be excited and pleased about the anticipated role of father. Others may be more detached or even hostile to the idea of fatherhood.

Reordering Personal Relationships

The partner's main role in pregnancy is to nurture and respond to the pregnant woman's feelings of vulnerability. The partner also must deal with the reality of the pregnancy. The partner's support indicates involvement in the pregnancy and preparation for attachment to the child.

Some aspects of a partner's behavior indicate rivalry. Direct rivalry with the fetus may be evident, especially during sexual activity. Men may protest that fetal movements prevent sexual gratification, or that the fetus is watching them during sexual activity. Feelings of rivalry may be unconscious and not verbalized, but expressed in subtle behaviors.

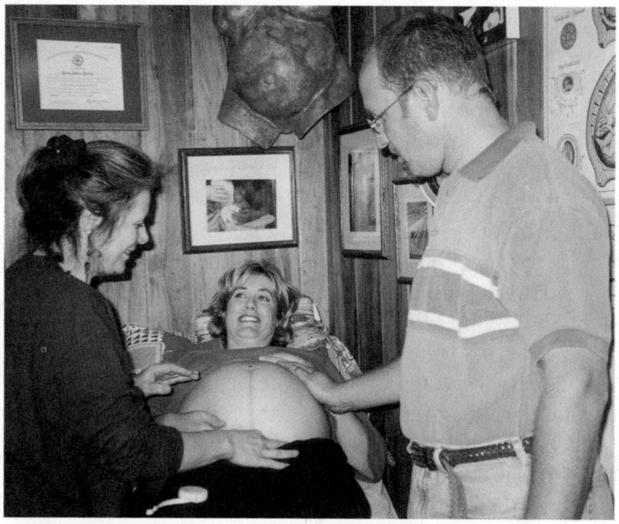

Fig. 11-2 Father participating in prenatal visit. Nurse-midwife instructs him in palpating fundus. (Courtesy Shannon Perry, Phoenix, AZ.)

The woman's increased introspection may cause her partner to feel uneasy as she becomes preoccupied with thoughts of the child and of motherhood, with her growing dependence on her physician or midwife, and with her reevaluation of the couple's relationship. Couples who are told early in the pregnancy that ambivalence, anxiety, and increased tensions are common experiences for expectant couples then can devote energy to managing the changes.

Establishing a Relationship with the Fetus

The father-child attachment can be as strong as the mother-child relationship, and fathers can be as competent as mothers in nurturing their infants. The father-child attachment begins in pregnancy. A father may rub or kiss the maternal abdomen; try to listen, talk, or sing to the fetus; or play with the fetus as he notes fetal movement.

Men prepare for fatherhood in many of the same ways that women prepare for motherhood—by reading and fantasizing. Daydreaming about their role as father is common in the last weeks before the birth; men rarely describe their thoughts unless they are reassured that such daydreams are normal. They may adjust work commitments or plan vacations so that they can spend time with their new family.

As the birth day approaches, fathers have more questions about fetal and newborn behaviors. Some fathers are shocked or amazed at the small size of the clothes and furniture for the baby. The nurse can tell the father about the unborn child's ability to respond to light, sound, and touch and encourage him to feel and talk to the fetus. A tour of a newborn nursery may be welcomed.

Some men become involved by picking the child's name and anticipating the child's sex, if it is not already known. Some couples select the name of the child as early as the first month of pregnancy. Family tradition, religious customs, and the continuation of the parent's name or names of relatives or friends are important in the selection process. Calling the unborn child by name helps to confirm the reality of pregnancy and promote attachment.

Parents may occasionally show or voice disappointment over the sex of the child. The parents may experience grief and a sense of loss at birth as they release their fantasized image of the child and begin to accept the real child. These negative responses toward a normal, healthy baby may be difficult for nurses to understand; however, most such responses are temporary. Providing an accepting environment for parental reactions facilitates the parent's ability to move beyond disappointment to acceptance.

evolve CASE STUDY—SECOND TRIMESTER

Preparing for Childbirth

The father's major concerns are getting the mother to a medical facility in time for the birth and not appearing ignorant. He may fantasize about different situations and plan what he will do in response to them; he may rehearse taking various routes to the hospital, timing each route at different times of the day. Some prospective fathers have questions about the labor suite's furniture, nursing staff, and location, as well as the availability of the physician and anesthesiologist. Others want to know what is expected of them when their partners are in labor. The father may have fears concerning safe passage of his partner and the mutilation or death of his partner or child. With the exception of childbirth preparation classes, a father has few opportunities to learn ways to be an involved and active partner in this rite of passage into parenthood (Family Focus box).

CASE STUDY—SECOND TRIMESTER

The same fears, questions, and concerns may affect birth partners who are not the biologic fathers. Birth partners need to be kept informed, supported, and included in all activities in which the mother desires their participation. The nurse can do much to promote pregnancy and birth as a family experience.

Family Focus

MATERNAL-PATERNAL-FETAL RELATIONSHIP

Emotional attachment to the child begins during the prenatal period. Parents fantasize and daydream to prepare for parenthood. Early in pregnancy the woman accepts the biologic fact of pregnancy and incorporates the idea of a child into her body and self-image. When the fetus is viewed on ultrasound, it becomes more real. During the second trimester there is growing awareness of the child as a separate being. When she accepts the reality of the child, the woman becomes more introspective. She seems to withdraw and to concentrate her interest on the unborn child. Her partner may feel left out, and other children in the family become more demanding in efforts to redirect the mother's attention to themselves.

The *fantasy child* may have familial characteristics and superior abilities; its appearance may be that of a 3- or 4-month-old infant. Both parents and siblings believe the unborn child responds in an individualized, personal manner. Some families become involved by picking the child's name and anticipating the child's sex if it is not already known. Some families select the child's name as early as the first month of pregnancy. Family tradition, religious customs, and continuation of one's own name or names of relatives and friends are important in the selection process. Family members may interact a great deal with the unborn child by trying to listen to, talk to, and play with the fetus and stroking or kissing the mother's abdomen, especially when the fetus moves.

Nurses must continue to seek to understand and foster attitudes and behaviors that promote early attachment and reduce the risk of negative long-term effects such as child neglect and abuse. More research relating psychologic variables to prenatal attachment and maternal-paternal-fetal interaction with maternal-paternal-child interaction is needed, including research with lesbian couples and unpartnered women. Tools to measure maternal-fetal attachment are the Maternal-Fetal Attachment Scale (MFAS)* and the Prenatal Attachment Inventory (PAI).†

*Cranley MS: Development of a tool for the measurement of maternal attachment during pregnancy, *Nurs Res* 30(5):281-284, 1981.

†Müller ME: Development of the prenatal attachment inventory, *West J Nurs Res* 15(2):199-211, 1993.

Sibling Adaptation

Sharing the spotlight with a new brother or sister may be the first major crisis for a child. The older child often experiences a sense of loss or feels jealous at being "replaced" by the new baby. Some of the factors that influence the child's response are age, the parents' attitudes, the father's role, the length of separation from the mother, the hospital's visitation policy, and how the child has been prepared for the change.

By age 3 or 4 years, children like to be told the story of their own beginning and accept its being compared to the present pregnancy. They like to listen to heartbeats and feel the baby moving in utero (Fig. 11-3). Sometimes they worry about how the baby is being fed and what it wears.

The mother with other children must devote time and energy to reorganizing her relationships with these children. She needs to prepare siblings for the birth of the baby (Box 11-1). She can begin the process of role transition in the

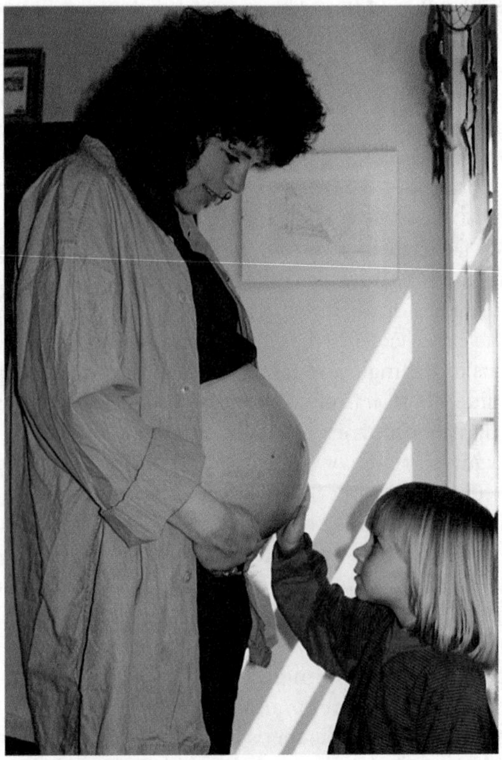

Fig. 11-3 A sibling feels the movement of a fetus. (Courtesy Kim Molloy, Knoxville, IA.)

BOX 11-1

Tips for Sibling Preparation

Prenatal

1. Adjust the timing and content of information about an anticipated infant to the age and understanding of the older child.
2. Take your child on a prenatal visit. Let the child listen to the fetal heartbeat and feel the baby move.
3. Involve the child in preparations for the baby, such as helping decorate the baby's room.
4. Move the child to a bed (if still sleeping in a crib) at least 2 months before the baby is due.
5. Read books, show videos, or take child to sibling preparation classes, including a hospital tour.
6. Answer your child's questions about the coming birth, what babies are like, and any other questions.
7. Take your child to the homes of friends who have babies so that the child has realistic expectations of what babies are like.

During the Hospital Stay

1. Have someone bring the child to the hospital to visit you and the baby (unless you plan to have the child attend the birth).
2. Don't force interactions between the child and the baby. Often the child will be more interested in seeing you and being reassured of your love.
3. Help the child explore the infant by showing how and where to touch the baby.
4. Give the child a gift (from you or from you, the father, and the baby).

Going Home

1. Leave the child at home with a relative or baby-sitter.
2. Have someone else carry the baby from the car so that you can hug the child first.

Adjustment after the Baby Is Home

1. Arrange for a special time with the child alone with each parent.
2. Don't exclude the child during infant feeding times. The child can sit with you and the baby and feed a doll or drink juice or milk with you or sit quietly with a game.
3. Prepare small gifts for the child so that when the baby gets gifts, the sibling won't feel left out. The child can also help open the baby gifts.
4. Praise the child for acting age appropriately (so that being a baby does not seem better than being older).

family by including the children in the pregnancy and being sympathetic to older children's concerns about losing their places in the family hierarchy. No child willingly gives up a familiar position.

Classes to prepare children for the birth of a new brother or sister are available in many communities (Fig. 11-4) (Family Focus box).

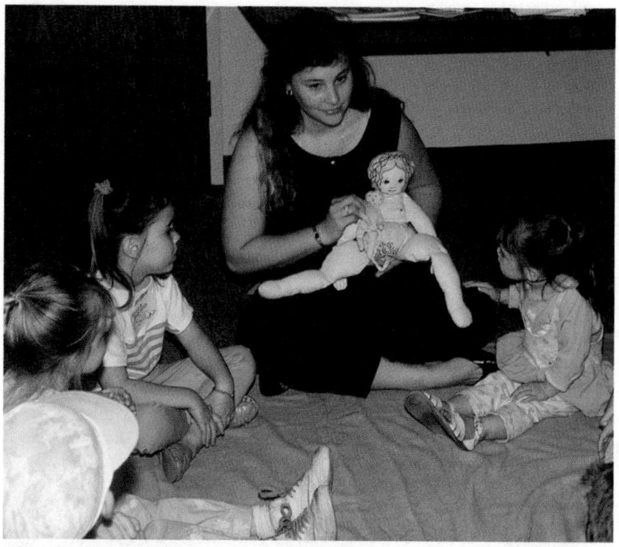

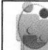

Fig. 11-4 A sibling class of preschoolers learns about childbirth and infant care using dolls. (Courtesy Marjorie Pyle, RNC, Lifecircle, Costa Mesa, CA.)

Family Focus

SIBLING ADAPTATION TO PREGNANCY AND BIRTH

Sibling responses to pregnancy vary with age and dependency needs. The 1-year-old infant seems largely unaware of the process, but the 2-year-old child notices the change in the mother's appearance and may comment, "Mommy's fat." The 2-year-old child's need for sameness in the environment makes the child aware of any change. Toddlers may exhibit more clinging behavior and revert to dependent behaviors in toilet training or eating.

By age 3 or 4 years, children like to be told the story of their own beginning and accept its being compared to the present pregnancy. They like to listen to heartbeats and feel the baby moving in utero (see Fig. 11-3). Sometimes they worry about how the baby is being fed and what it wears.

School-age children take a more clinical interest in their mother's pregnancy. They may want to know in more detail, "How did the baby get in there?" and "How will it get out?" Children in this age group notice pregnant women in stores, churches, and schools and sometimes seem shy if they need to approach a pregnant woman directly. On the whole they look forward to the new baby, see themselves as "mothers" or "fathers," and enjoy buying baby supplies and readying a place for the baby. Because they still think in concrete terms and base judgments on the here and now, they respond positively to their mother's current good health.

Early and middle adolescents, preoccupied with the establishment of their own sexual identity, may have difficulty accepting the overwhelming evidence of the sexual activity of their parents. They reason that if they are too young for such activity, certainly their parents are too old. They seem to take on a critical parental role and may ask, "What will people think?" or "How can you let yourself get so fat?" Many pregnant women with teenage children confess that their teenagers are the most difficult factor in their current pregnancy.

Late adolescents do not appear to be unduly disturbed. They realize that they soon will be gone from home. Parents usually report that they are comforting and act more like other adults than children.

Grandparent Adaptation

Expectant grandparenthood can represent a maturational milestone for the parent of an expectant parent. Some grandparents describe having a grandchild as the best thing that ever happened to them; they can enjoy the child without assuming responsibility for its care. For other grandpar-

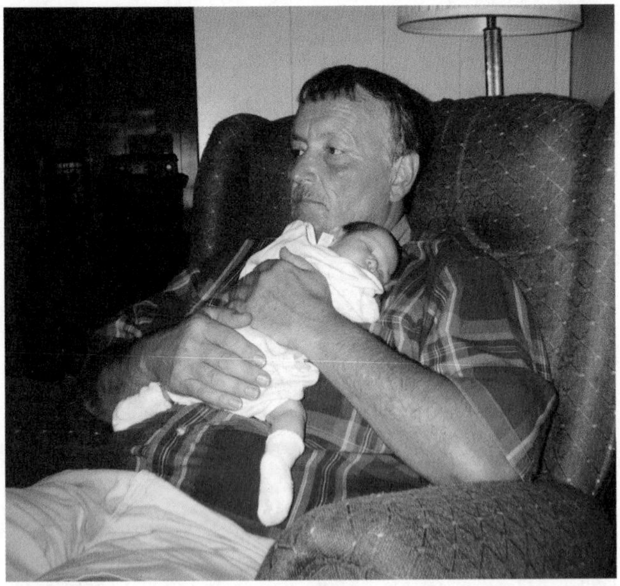

Fig. 11-5 A grandfather relaxes with his granddaughter. (Courtesy Gregory Vogel, Bloomington, IL.)

ents, when the mother is a young adolescent or for other reasons such as a substance-abusing mother, the grandchild may mean assuming care and raising another child when they thought childrearing was over.

The grandparent is the historian who transmits the family history, a resource person who shares knowledge based on experience, a role model, and a support person. The grandparent's presence and support can strengthen family systems by widening the circle of support and nurturance (Fig. 11-5).

To be truly family oriented, maternity care must include the grandparent in the implementation of the nursing process with the whole childbearing family. A class for grandparents is one method of incorporating the grandparents into the family system and encouraging communication between the generations (Family Focus box).

CARE MANAGEMENT

The purpose of prenatal care is to identify existing risk factors and other deviations from normal so that pregnancy outcomes may be enhanced. Major emphasis is placed on preventive aspects of care, primarily to motivate the pregnant woman to practice optimal self-care and to report unusual changes early so that problems can be minimized or prevented. In providing holistic care, nurses also provide information and guidance about the psychosocial impact of pregnancy on the woman and members of her family. The goals of prenatal nursing care, therefore, are not only to foster a safe birth for the infant and mother but also to promote satisfaction of the mother and family with the pregnancy and birth experience (Box 11-2).

Advances have been made in the number of women in the United States who receive adequate prenatal care, currently at 84% (Martin et al, 2003). Prenatal care is sought routinely by women of middle or high socioeconomic status. However, women living in poverty or who lack health insurance may not be able to use public medical services or gain access to private care. Lack of culturally sensitive care providers and barriers in communication caused by differences in language also interfere with access to care (Shaffer, 2002). Immigrant women from cultures in which prenatal care is not emphasized may not know to seek routine prenatal care. Birth outcomes in these populations are thus less positive, with higher rates of maternal and fetal or newborn complications. In particular, problems with low birth weight (less than 2500 g) and infant mortality have been associated with inadequate prenatal care.

Barriers to obtaining health care during pregnancy include inadequate numbers of health care providers, unpleasant clinic facilities or procedures, inconvenient clinic hours, distance from health care facilities, lack of transportation, fragmentation of services, inadequate finances, and personal attitudes (Boyle et al, 2003; Handler et al, 2003; Sword, 2003). The availability and accessibility of prenatal care may be improved by sharing care among health care providers, including increasing the use of advanced practice nurses in

Family Focus

GRANDPARENT ADAPTATION TO PREGNANCY AND BIRTH

Every pregnancy affects all family relationships. For expectant grandparents, a first pregnancy in a child is undeniable evidence that they are growing older. Many think of a grandparent as old, white haired, and becoming feeble of mind and body; however, some people face grandparenthood while still in their thirties or forties. A mother-to-be announcing her pregnancy to her mother may be greeted by a negative response that indicates she is not ready to be a grandmother. Both daughter and mother may be startled and hurt by the response.

Some expectant grandparents not only are nonsupportive but also use subtle means to decrease the self-esteem of the young parents-to-be. Mothers may talk about their terrible pregnancies; fathers may discuss the endless cost of rearing children; and mothers-in-law may complain that their sons are neglecting them because their concern is now directed toward the pregnant daughters-in-law.

However, most grandparents are delighted with the prospect of a new baby in the family. It reawakens their feelings of their own youth, the excitement of giving birth, and their delight in the behavior of the parents-to-be when they were infants. They set up a memory store of their child's first smiles, first words, and first steps that can be used later for "claiming" the newborn as a member of the family. Their and the parents' satisfaction comes with the realization that continuity between past and present is guaranteed.

The grandparent is the historian who transmits the family history, a resource person who shares knowledge based on experience, a role model, and a support person. The grandparent's presence and support can strengthen family systems by widening the circle of support and nurturance (see Fig. 11-5). Other sources of information cannot replace the unique contribution that grandparents make.

Many women report that their pregnancies bridged the final gap between them and their own mothers. The estrangement that began in adolescence disappears as the now-pregnant daughter experiences joys, concerns, and anxieties similar to those her mother felt before her.

evolve CASE STUDY–FIRST TRIMESTER

CASE STUDY–FIRST TRIMESTER

BOX 11-2

Lamaze Philosophy of Birth

Birth is normal, natural, and healthy.
The experience of birth profoundly affects women and their families.
Women's inner wisdom guides them through birth.
Women's confidence and ability to give birth is either enhanced or diminished by the care provider and place of birth.
Women have the right to give birth free from routine medical interventions.
Birth can safely take place in birth centers and homes.
Childbirth education empowers women to make informed choices in health care, to assume responsibility for their health, and to trust their inner wisdom.

Source: http://normalbirth.lamaze.org/About/PhilosophyofBirth.asp (accessed December 16, 2004)

collaborative practice with physicians or midwives (Boyle et al, 2003) (Box 11-3). The effectiveness of a regular schedule of home visiting by nurses during pregnancy also has been validated (Fetrick, Christensen, & Mitchell, 2003).

The current model for provision of prenatal care has been used for more than a century. The initial visit usually occurs in the first trimester, with monthly visits through week 28 of pregnancy. Thereafter, visits are scheduled every 2 weeks until week 36, and then every week until birth. This model is currently being questioned, and in some practices, there is a growing tendency to have fewer visits with women who are at low risk for complications (Villar et al, 2002).

Prenatal care is ideally a multidisciplinary activity in which nurses work with physicians or midwives, nutritionists, social workers, and others. Collaboration among these individuals is necessary to provide holistic care.

Assessment

Once the presence of pregnancy has been confirmed and the woman's desire to continue the pregnancy has been validated, prenatal care is begun. The assessment process begins at the initial prenatal visit and is continued throughout the pregnancy. Assessment techniques include the interview, physical examination, and laboratory tests. Because the initial visit and follow-up visits are distinctly different in content and process, they are described separately.

BOX 11-3

Sharing Care—Planning Safe Passage

Pamela, a 38-year-old professional, pregnant with her second child, planned a home birth. After successfully giving birth to her first child at home, she contracted with a home birth lay midwife for pregnancy care and birth for the second child. During pregnancy, she scheduled three visits with an obstetrician to ensure that, in the case of problems, a skilled practitioner with access to high risk hospital care was familiar with her. She was able to give birth at home with family and friends in attendance. She was able to fulfill her desire for a home birth while at the same time assuring expert care in the event of problems.

Initial Visit

The initial evaluation includes a comprehensive health history that emphasizes the current pregnancy, previous pregnancies, the family, a psychosocial profile, a physical assessment, diagnostic testing, and an overall risk assessment. A prenatal history form (Fig. 11-6) is the best way to document information obtained.

Interview

The therapeutic relationship between the nurse and the woman is established during the initial assessment interview (Fig. 11-7). It is a time for planned, purposeful communication that focuses on specific content. The data collected are of two types: the woman's subjective appraisal of her health status and the nurse's objective observations. The nurse observes the woman's affect, posture, body language, skin color, and other physical and emotional signs.

Often the pregnant woman is accompanied by one or more family members. The nurse needs to build a relationship with these people as part of the social context of the patient. With her permission, those accompanying the woman can be included in the initial prenatal interview, and the observations and information about the woman's family form part of the database. For example, if the woman is accompanied by small children, the nurse can ask about her plans for child care during the time of labor and birth. Special needs are noted at this time (e.g., wheelchair access, assistance in getting on and off the examining table, and cognitive deficits).

Reason for Seeking Care

Although pregnant women are scheduled for "routine" prenatal visits, they often come to the health care provider seeking information or reassurance about a particular concern. When the woman is asked a broad, open-ended question such as "How have you been feeling?" she may reveal problems that could otherwise be overlooked. The woman's chief concerns should be recorded in her own words to alert other personnel to the priority of needs identified by her. A typical desire at the initial visit is for information about what is normal in the course of pregnancy (Guidelines/Guías box).

Current Pregnancy

The presumptive signs of pregnancy may be of great concern to the woman. A review of symptoms she is experiencing and how she is coping with them helps establish a database to develop a plan of care. Some early teaching may be provided at this time.

Obstetric/Gynecologic History

Data are gathered on the woman's age at menarche, menstrual history, contraceptive history, the nature of any infertility or gynecologic conditions, history of any sexually transmitted infections (STIs), her sexual history, and a detailed history of all her pregnancies, including the present one, and their outcomes. The date of the last Papanicolaou (Pap) test and the result are noted. The date of her LMP is obtained to establish the EDB.

Medical History

The medical history includes those medical or surgical conditions that may affect the pregnancy or that may be affected by the pregnancy. For example, a pregnant woman who has diabetes or epilepsy requires special care. Because most women are anxious during the initial interview, the

Text continued on page 268.

Patient Addressograph

DATE ____________________

NAME ____
LAST FIRST MIDDLE

ID # ______________ HOSPITAL OF DELIVERY ______________

NEWBORN'S PHYSICIAN ______________ REFERRED BY ______________

FINAL EDD ______________ PRIMARY PROVIDER/GROUP ______________

BIRTH DATE MONTH DAY YEAR	AGE	RACE	MARITAL STATUS S M W D SEP	ADDRESS
OCCUPATION		EDUCATION (LAST GRADE COMPLETED)		ZIP PHONE (H) (O)
LANGUAGE				INSURANCE CARRIER/MEDICAID #
HUSBAND/DOMESTIC PARTNER		PHONE		POLICY #
FATHER OF BABY		PHONE		EMERGENCY CONTACT PHONE

TOTAL PREG	FULL TERM	PREMATURE	AB. INDUCED	AB. SPONTANEOUS	ECTOPICS	MULTIPLE BIRTHS	LIVING

MENSTRUAL HISTORY

LMP ☐ DEFINITE ☐ APPROXIMATE (MONTH KNOWN) MENSES MONTHLY ☐ YES ☐ NO FREQUENCY: Q ____ DAYS MENARCHE ____ (AGE ONSET)
☐ UNKNOWN ☐ NORMAL AMOUNT/DURATION PRIOR MENSES ____ DATE ON BCP AT CONCEPT ☐ YES ☐ NO hCG + __/__/__
☐ FINAL ____

PAST PREGNANCIES (LAST SIX)

DATE MONTH/ YEAR	GA WEEKS	LENGTH OF LABOR	BIRTH WEIGHT	SEX M/F	TYPE DELIVERY	ANES.	PLACE OF DELIVERY	PRETERM LABOR YES/NO	COMMENTS/ COMPLICATIONS

MEDICAL HISTORY

	O Neg. + Pos.	DETAIL POSITIVE REMARKS INCLUDE DATE & TREATMENT		O Neg. + Pos.	DETAIL POSITIVE REMARKS INCLUDE DATE & TREATMENT
1. DIABETES			17. D (Rh) SENSITIZED		
2. HYPERTENSION			18. PULMONARY (TB, ASTHMA)		
3. HEART DISEASE			19. SEASONAL ALLERGIES		
4. AUTOIMMUNE DISORDER			20. DRUG/LATEX ALLERGIES/ REACTIONS		
5. KIDNEY DISEASE/UTI					
6. NEUROLOGIC/EPILEPSY			21. BREAST		
7. PSYCHIATRIC			22. GYN SURGERY		
8. DEPRESSION/POSTPARTUM DEPRESSION					
9. HEPATITIS/LIVER DISEASE			23. OPERATIONS/ HOSPITALIZATIONS (YEAR & REASON)		
10. VARICOSITIES/PHLEBITIS					
11. THYROID DYSFUNCTION			24. ANESTHETIC COMPLICATIONS		
12. TRAUMA/VIOLENCE			25. HISTORY OF ABNORMAL PAP		
13. HISTORY OF BLOOD TRANSFUS.			26. UTERINE ANOMALY/DES		

	AMT/DAY PREPREG	AMT/DAY PREG	# YEARS USE			
				27. INFERTILITY		
14. TOBACCO				28. RELEVANT FAMILY HISTORY		
15. ALCOHOL						
16. ILLICIT/RECREATIONAL DRUGS				29. OTHER		

COMMENTS ____

 AA129 12345/76543

ACOG ANTEPARTUM RECORD (FORM A)

Fig. 11-6 A sample prenatal history form. (Copyright © 2003 The American College of Obstetricians and Gynecologists, 409 12th Street, SW, PO Box 96920, Washington, DC 20090-6920.)

Patient Addressograph

SYMPTOMS SINCE LMP

GENETIC SCREENING/TERATOLOGY COUNSELING INCLUDES PATIENT, BABY'S FATHER, OR ANYONE IN EITHER FAMILY WITH:	YES	NO		YES	NO
1. PATIENT'S AGE ≥35 YEARS AS OF ESTIMATED DATE OF DELIVERY			12. HUNTINGTON'S CHOREA		
2. THALASSEMIA (ITALIAN, GREEK, MEDITERRANEAN, OR ASIAN BACKGROUND): MCV <80			13. MENTAL RETARDATION/AUTISM		
			IF YES, WAS PERSON TESTED FOR FRAGILE X?		
3. NEURAL TUBE DEFECT (MENINGOMYELOCELE, SPINA BIFIDA, OR ANENCEPHALY)			14. OTHER INHERITED GENETIC OR CHROMOSOMAL DISORDER		
4. CONGENITAL HEART DEFECT			15. MATERNAL METABOLIC DISORDER (EG, TYPE 1 DIABETES, PKU)		
5. DOWN SYNDROME			16. PATIENT OR BABY'S FATHER HAD A CHILD WITH BIRTH DEFECTS NOT LISTED ABOVE		
6. TAY-SACHS (EG, JEWISH, CAJUN, FRENCH CANADIAN)					
7. CANAVAN DISEASE			17. RECURRENT PREGNANCY LOSS, OR A STILLBIRTH		
8. SICKLE CELL DISEASE OR TRAIT (AFRICAN)			18. MEDICATIONS (INCLUDING SUPPLEMENTS, VITAMINS, HERBS OR OTC DRUGS)/ILLICIT/RECREATIONAL DRUGS/ALCOHOL SINCE LAST MENSTRUAL PERIOD		
9. HEMOPHILIA OR OTHER BLOOD DISORDERS					
10. MUSCULAR DYSTROPHY			IF YES, AGENT(S) AND STRENGTH/DOSAGE		
11. CYSTIC FIBROSIS			19. ANY OTHER		

COMMENTS/COUNSELING ______________________________

INFECTION HISTORY	YES	NO		YES	NO
1. LIVE WITH SOMEONE WITH TB OR EXPOSED TO TB			4. HISTORY OF STD, GONORRHEA, CHLAMYDIA, HPV, SYPHILIS		
2. PATIENT OR PARTNER HAS HISTORY OF GENITAL HERPES					
3. RASH OR VIRAL ILLNESS SINCE LAST MENSTRUAL PERIOD			5. OTHER (See Comments)		

COMMENTS ______________________________

______________________________ **INTERVIEWER'S SIGNATURE** ______________________________

INITIAL PHYSICAL EXAMINATION						
DATE ____/____/____	HEIGHT ______	BP ______				
1. HEENT	☐ NORMAL	☐ ABNORMAL	12. VULVA	☐ NORMAL	☐ CONDYLOMA	☐ LESIONS
2. FUNDI	☐ NORMAL	☐ ABNORMAL	13. VAGINA	☐ NORMAL	☐ INFLAMMATION	☐ DISCHARGE
3. TEETH	☐ NORMAL	☐ ABNORMAL	14. CERVIX	☐ NORMAL	☐ INFLAMMATION	☐ LESIONS
4. THYROID	☐ NORMAL	☐ ABNORMAL	15. UTERUS SIZE	______ WEEKS		☐ FIBROIDS
5. BREASTS	☐ NORMAL	☐ ABNORMAL	16. ADNEXA	☐ NORMAL	☐ MASS	
6. LUNGS	☐ NORMAL	☐ ABNORMAL	17. RECTUM	☐ NORMAL	☐ ABNORMAL	
7. HEART	☐ NORMAL	☐ ABNORMAL	18. DIAGONAL CONJUGATE	☐ REACHED	☐ NO	______ CM
8. ABDOMEN	☐ NORMAL	☐ ABNORMAL	19. SPINES	☐ AVERAGE	☐ PROMINENT	☐ BLUNT
9. EXTREMITIES	☐ NORMAL	☐ ABNORMAL	20. SACRUM	☐ CONCAVE	☐ STRAIGHT	☐ ANTERIOR
10. SKIN	☐ NORMAL	☐ ABNORMAL	21. SUBPUBIC ARCH	☐ NORMAL	☐ WIDE	☐ NARROW
11. LYMPH NODES	☐ NORMAL	☐ ABNORMAL	22. GYNECOID PELVIC TYPE	☐ YES	☐ NO	

COMMENTS (Number and explain abnormals) ______________________________

______________________________ **EXAM BY** ______________________________

ACOG ANTEPARTUM RECORD (FORM B)

Fig. 11-6, cont'd
For legend see opposite page.

Continued

Patient Addressograph

NAME ____
LAST FIRST MIDDLE

DRUG ALLERGY	LATEX ALLERGY	
IS BLOOD TRANSFUSION ACCEPTABLE IN AN EMERGENCY? ☐ YES ☐ NO		ANESTHESIA CONSULT PLANNED ☐ YES ☐ NO

PROBLEMS/PLANS	MEDICATION LIST	Start date	Stop date
1.	1.	__/__/__	__/__/__
2.	2.	__/__/__	__/__/__
3.	3.	__/__/__	__/__/__
4.	4.	__/__/__	__/__/__
5.	5.	__/__/__	__/__/__
6.	6.	/ /	/ /

EDD CONFIRMATION

INITIAL EDD

LMP	__/__/__	= EDD __/__/__
INITIAL EXAM	__/__/__	= __ WKS = EDD __/__/__
ULTRASOUND	__/__/__	= __ WKS = EDD __/__/__
INITIAL EDD	__/__/__	INITIALED BY ______

18–20-WEEK EDD UPDATE

QUICKENING	__/__/__	+22 WKS = __/__/__
FUNDAL HT. AT UMBIL.	__/__/__	+20 WKS = __/__/__
ULTRASOUND	__/__/__	= __ WKS = __/__/__
FINAL EDD	__/__/__	INITIALED BY ______

PREPREGNANCY WEIGHT ________

	WEEKS GEST. (BEST EST.)	FUNDAL HEIGHT (CM)	PRESENTATION	FHR	FETAL MOVEMENT	PRETERM LABOR SIGNS/SYMPTOMS + = PRESENT o = ABSENT	CERVIX EXAM (DIL/EFF/STA.) ULTRASOUND LENGTH	BLOOD PRESSURE	WEIGHT	URINE (ALBUMIN/GLUCOSE)	NEXT APPOINTMENT	PROVIDER (INITIALS)

COMMENTS

PROBLEMS ____________________

COMMENTS ____________________

ACOG ANTEPARTUM RECORD (FORM C)

Fig. 11-6, cont'd A sample prenatal history form. (Copyright © 2003 The American College of Obstetricians and Gynecologists, 409 12th Street, SW, PO Box 96920, Washington, DC 20090-6920.)

Patient Addressograph

LABORATORY AND EDUCATION

INITIAL LABS	DATE	RESULT	REVIEWED
BLOOD TYPE	/ /	A B AB O	
D (Rh) TYPE	/ /		
ANTIBODY SCREEN	/ /		
HCT/HGB	/ /	_______ % _______ g/dL	
PAP TEST	/ /	NORMAL/ABNORMAL _______	
RUBELLA	/ /		
VDRL	/ /		
URINE CULTURE/SCREEN	/ /		
HBsAg	/ /		
HIV COUNSELING/TESTING*	/ /	POS. NEG. DECLINED	
OPTIONAL LABS	**DATE**	**RESULT**	**REVIEWED**
HGB ELECTROPHORESIS	/ /	AA AS SS AC SC AF ↑A_2	
PPD	/ /		
CHLAMYDIA	/ /		
GONORRHEA	/ /		
GENETIC SCREENING TESTS (SEE FORM B)	/ /		
OTHER			
8–18-WEEK LABS (WHEN INDICATED/ ELECTED)	**DATE**	**RESULT**	
ULTRASOUND	/ /		
MSAFP/MULTIPLE MARKERS	/ /		
AMNIO/CVS	/ /		
KARYOTYPE	/ /	46,XX OR 46,XY/OTHER _____	
AMNIOTIC FLUID (AFP)	/ /	NORMAL _____ ABNORMAL _____	
24–28-WEEK LABS (WHEN INDICATED)	**DATE**	**RESULT**	
HCT/HGB	/ /	_______ % _______ g/dL	
DIABETES SCREEN	/ /	1 HOUR _______________	
GTT (IF SCREEN ABNORMAL)	/ /	_____ FBS _____ 1 HOUR _____ 2 HOUR _____ 3 HOUR	
D (Rh) ANTIBODY SCREEN	/ /		
ANTI-D IMMUNE GLOBULIN (RhIG) GIVEN (28 WKS)	/ /	SIGNATURE _______________	
32–36-WEEK LABS	**DATE**	**RESULT**	
HCT/HGB	/ /	_______ % _______ g/dL	
ULTRASOUND (WHEN INDICATED)	/ /		
VDRL (WHEN INDICATED)	/ /		
GONORRHEA (WHEN INDICATED)	/ /		
CHLAMYDIA (WHEN INDICATED)	/ /		
GROUP B STREP	/ /		

COMMENTS/ADDITIONAL LABS

*Check state requirements before recording results.

PROVIDER SIGNATURE (AS REQUIRED) ____

ACOG ANTEPARTUM RECORD (FORM D)

Fig. 11-6, cont'd
For legend see opposite page.

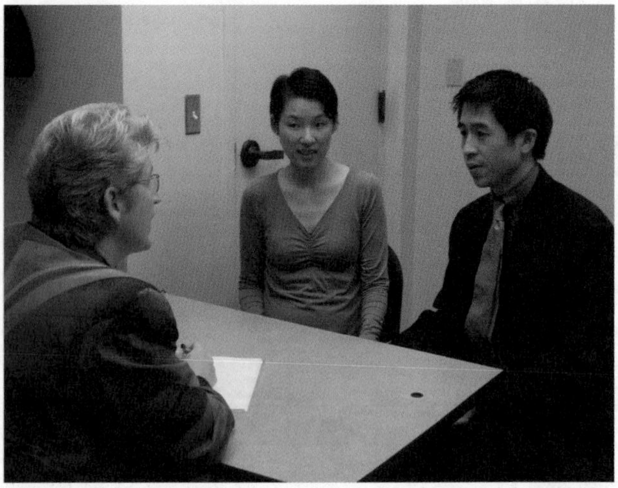

Fig. 11-7 Prenatal interview. (Courtesy Skip Davis, San Francisco, CA.)

ENGLISH SPANISH **Guidelines/Guías**

PRENATAL INTERVIEW

Have you had a pregnancy test?
¿Ha tenido una prueba del embarazo?

When was your last menstrual cycle?
¿Cuándo fue su última menstruación (regla)?

Have you been pregnant before?
¿Ha quedado embarazada antes?

How many times?
¿Cuántas veces?

How many children do you have?
¿Cuántos hijos tiene usted?

Have you ever had a miscarriage (spontaneous abortion)?
¿Ha perdido un bebé alguna vez? (¿Ha tenido un aborto espontáneo?)

Have you ever had a therapeutic abortion?
¿Ha tenido un aborto provocado?

Have you ever had a stillborn?
¿Ha tenido un niño que nació sin vida?

Have you ever had cesarean?
¿Ha tenido una operación cesárea?

Have you had any problems with past pregnancies?
¿Ha tenido problemas durante sus embarazos anteriores?

Do you take drugs? Prescription medicine?
¿Usa drogas? ¿Medicina recetada?

If so, which type of medicine do you use and for what?
¿Qué clases de medicina toma? ¿Para qué las toma?

Do you drink alcohol? Do you smoke?
¿Toma bebidas alcohólicas? ¿Fuma?

nurse's reference to cues such as a MedicAlert bracelet prompts the woman to explain allergies, chronic diseases, or medications being taken such as cortisone, insulin, or anticonvulsants.

Many women who have chronic or handicapping conditions forget to mention them during the initial assessment because they have adapted to them. Special shoes or a limp may indicate the existence of a pelvic structural defect, an important consideration in pregnant women. The nurse who observes these special characteristics and sensitively inquires about them can obtain individualized data that will provide the basis for a comprehensive nursing care plan. Observations are a vital component of the interview process because they prompt the nurse and the woman to focus on the specific needs of the woman and her family.

The nature of previous surgical procedures should also be described. If a woman has had uterine surgery or extensive repair of the pelvic floor, a cesarean birth may be necessary; appendectomy rules out appendicitis as a cause of right lower quadrant pain in pregnancy; spinal surgery may contraindicate the use of spinal or epidural anesthesia; and breast augmentation or reduction procedures may influence the ability to breastfeed. Any injury involving the pelvis is noted.

Nutritional History

The nutritional status of a pregnant woman has a direct effect on the growth and development of the fetus. A dietary assessment can reveal special diet practices, food allergies, eating behaviors, and other factors related to her nutritional status. Pregnant women are usually motivated to learn about good nutrition and respond well to nutritional advice generated by this assessment. Cultural influences on diet and food selection should also be considered.

History of Drug Use

A woman's past and present use of legal drugs (over-the-counter [OTC], prescription, and herbal drugs; caffeine; alcohol; nicotine) and illegal drugs (marijuana, cocaine, heroin) needs to be assessed because many substances cross the placenta and may harm the developing fetus. Periodic urine toxicology screening tests are often recommended during pregnancy for women who have a history of illegal drug use. Results of such tests have been used for criminal prosecution, which results in a breach in the patient-provider relationship and in ethical responsibilities to the patient (Foley, 2002; Harris & Paltrow, 2003; Jos, Perlmutter, & Marshall, 2003).

Family History

The family history provides information about the woman's immediate family, including parents, siblings, and children. These data help identify familial or genetic disorders or conditions that could affect the present health status of the woman or her fetus.

Social and Experiential History

Situational factors such as the family's ethnic and cultural background and socioeconomic status are assessed while the history is obtained. The following information may be obtained over several encounters. The woman's perception of this pregnancy is explored by asking her such questions as the following: Is this pregnancy wanted or not, planned or not? Is the woman/couple pleased or displeased, accepting or nonaccepting? What problems related to finances, career, or living accommodations may arise as a result of the pregnancy? The family support system is determined by asking her such questions as the following: What primary support is available to her? Are changes needed to promote adequate support? What are the existing relationships among mother, father/partner, siblings, and in-laws? What preparations are being made for her care and that of dependent family members during labor and for the care of the infant after birth? Is financial, educational, or other support needed from the community? What are the woman's ideas about childbearing, her expectations of the infant's behavior, and her outlook on life and the female role?

Other such questions that should be asked include the following: What does the woman think it will be like to have a baby in the home? How is her life going to change by having a baby? What plans will having a baby interrupt? In interviews throughout the pregnancy, the nurse should remain alert for the appearance of potential parenting problems such as depression, lack of family support, and inadequate living conditions. The nurse needs to assess the woman's attitude toward health care, particularly during childbearing; her expectations of health care providers; and her view of the relationship between herself and the nurse.

Coping mechanisms and patterns of interacting are identified. Early in the pregnancy the nurse should determine the woman's knowledge of pregnancy, maternal changes, fetal growth, self-care, and care of the newborn, including feeding. It is important to ask about attitudes toward unmedicated or medicated childbirth and about her knowledge of the availability of parenting skills classes. Before planning for nursing care, the nurse needs information about the woman's decision-making abilities and living habits (e.g., exercise, sleep, diet, diversional interests, personal hygiene, clothing). Common stressors during childbearing include the baby's welfare, the labor and birth process, the behaviors of the newborn, the relationship with the baby's father, changes in body image, and physical symptoms.

Attitudes concerning the range of acceptable sexual behaviors during pregnancy are explored. Questions such as the following could be asked: What has your family (partner, friends) told you about sex during pregnancy? The woman's sexual self-concept is given emphasis by asking questions such as the following: How do you feel about the changes in your appearance? How does your partner feel about your body now? How do you feel about wearing maternity clothes?

History of Physical Abuse

All women should be assessed for a history or risk of physical abuse, particularly since the likelihood of abuse increases during pregnancy. Although visual cues from the woman's appearance or behavior may suggest the possibility of abuse, no one profile of the battered woman exists. Identification of abuse and immediate clinical intervention that includes information about safety can result in behavior that may prevent future abuse and increase the safety and well-being of the woman and her infant.

Review of Systems

During this portion of the interview, the woman is asked to identify and describe preexisting or concurrent problems with any of the body systems, and her mental status is assessed. The woman is questioned about physical symptoms she has experienced, such as shortness of breath or pain. Pregnancy affects and is affected by all body systems; therefore information on the present status of body systems is important in planning care. For each sign or symptom described, the following additional data should be obtained: body location, quality, quantity, chronology, aggravating or alleviating factors, and associated manifestations (onset, character, and course) (Seidel et al, 2003).

Physical Examination

The initial physical examination provides the baseline for assessing subsequent changes. The examiner should determine the woman's needs for basic information regarding reproductive anatomy and provide this information, along with a demonstration of the equipment that may be used during the examination and an explanation of the procedure itself. The interaction requires an unhurried, sensitive, and gentle approach with a matter-of-fact attitude.

The physical examination begins with assessment of vital signs, including blood pressure, height, and weight. The bladder should be empty before pelvic examination. This may provide the opportunity to collect a urine specimen to test for protein, glucose, or leukocytes, or for other tests.

Each examiner develops a routine for proceeding with the physical examination; most choose the head-to-toe progression. Heart and breath sounds are evaluated and extremities examined. The skin is assessed for changes in pigmentation, rashes, and edema. Distribution, amount, and quality of body hair is of particular importance because the findings reflect nutritional status, endocrine function, and attention to hygiene. The thyroid gland is assessed carefully, as are the breasts and abdomen. The height of the fundus is noted if the first examination occurs after the first trimester of pregnancy. The typical basic examination is usually completed without much discomfort for the healthy woman. During the examination, the examiner needs to remain alert to the woman's cues that give direction to the remainder of the assessment and that indicate imminent untoward response such as supine hypotension (low blood pressure that occurs while the woman is lying on her back, causing feelings of faintness). See Chapter 5 for a detailed description of the physical examination.

Whenever a pelvic examination is performed, the tone of the pelvic musculature and the woman's knowledge of Kegel exercises are assessed. Particular attention is paid to the size of the uterus because this is an indication of the duration of gestation. The nurse present during the examination can coach the woman at this time in breathing and relaxation techniques as needed. One vaginal examination during pregnancy is recommended, but another is usually not done unless medically indicated.

Laboratory Tests

The data yielded by laboratory examination of specimens obtained during the examination add important information concerning the symptoms of pregnancy and the woman's health status. Both nursing and medical diagnoses stem from such information.

Specimens are collected at the initial visit so that any abnormal findings can be treated. Blood is drawn for a variety of tests (Table 11-1). A sickle cell screen is recommended for women of African, Asian, or Middle Eastern descent. The folacin level is measured when indicated. Testing for antibody to the human immunodeficiency virus (HIV) is strongly recommended for all pregnant women (Box 11-4). Culture and sensitivity tests are ordered as necessary. During the pelvic examination, cervical and vaginal smears may be obtained for cytologic studies and for diagnosis of infection (e.g., *Chlamydia*, gonorrhea).

Table 11-1

Laboratory Tests in Prenatal Period

LABORATORY TEST	PURPOSE
Hemoglobin, hematocrit/WBC, differential	Detects anemia/detects infection
Hemoglobin electrophoresis	Identifies women with hemoglobinopathies (e.g., sickle cell anemia, thalassemia)
Blood type, Rh, and irregular antibody	Identifies those fetuses at risk for developing erythroblastosis fetalis or hyperbilirubinemia in neonatal period
Rubella titer	Determines immunity to rubella
Tuberculin skin testing; chest film after 20 weeks of gestation in women with reactive tuberculin tests	Screens for exposure to tuberculosis
Urinalysis, including microscopic examination of urinary sediment; pH, specific gravity, color, glucose, albumin, protein, RBCs, WBCs, casts, acetone; hCG	Identifies women with unsuspected diabetes mellitus, renal disease, hypertensive disease of pregnancy; infection; occult hematuria
Urine culture	Identifies women with asymptomatic bacteriuria
Renal function tests: BUN, creatinine, electrolytes, creatinine clearance, total protein excretion	Evaluates level of possible renal compromise in women with a history of diabetes, hypertension, or renal disease
Papanicolaou (Pap) test	Screens for cervical intraepithelial neoplasia, herpes simplex type 2, and HPV
Vaginal or rectal smear for *Neisseria gonorrhoeae, Chlamydia,* HPV, GBS	Screens high risk population for asymptomatic infection; GBS done at 35-37 weeks
RPR/VDRL/FTA-ABS	Identifies women with untreated syphilis
HIV antibody,* hepatitis B surface antigen, toxoplasmosis	Screens for infection
1-hr glucose tolerance	Screens for gestational diabetes; done at initial visit for women with risk factors; done at 28 weeks for all pregnant women
3-hr glucose tolerance	Screens for diabetes in women with elevated glucose level after 1-hr test; must have two elevated readings for diagnosis
Cardiac evaluation: ECG, chest x-ray film, and echocardiogram	Evaluates cardiac function in women with a history of hypertension or cardiac disease

BUN, blood urea nitrogen; *ECG,* electrocardiogram; *FTA-ABS,* fluorescent treponemal antibody absorption test; *GBS,* group B streptococcus; *hCG,* human chorionic gonadotropin; *HIV,* human immunodeficiency virus; *HPV,* human papillomavirus; *RBC,* red blood cell; *RPR,* rapid plasma reagin; *VDRL,* Venereal Disease Research Laboratories; *WBC,* white blood cell.
*With patient permission.

The finding of risk factors during pregnancy may indicate the need to repeat some tests at other times. For example, exposure to tuberculosis or an STI would necessitate repeat testing. STIs are common in pregnancy and may have negative effects on mother and fetus. Careful assessment and thorough screening are essential.

Follow-up Visits

Monthly visits are scheduled routinely during the first and second trimesters, although additional appointments may be made as the need arises. During the third trimester, however, the possibility for complications increases, and closer monitoring is warranted. Starting with week 28, visits are scheduled every 2 weeks until week 36, and then every week until birth, unless the health care provider individualizes the schedule. Individual needs and risks of the pregnant woman may warrant visits more or less often. The pattern of interviewing the woman first and then assessing physical changes and performing laboratory tests is maintained.

Interview

Follow-up visits are less intensive than the initial prenatal visit. At each of these follow-up visits, the woman is asked to summarize relevant events that have occurred since the previous visit. She is asked about her general emotional and physiologic well-being, any complaints or problems, and any questions she may have. Personal and family needs are identified and explored.

Emotional changes are common during pregnancy. A woman's emotional state can affect her and her family's general well-being. Therefore it is logical that the nurse ask whether the woman has experienced any mood swings, reactions to changes in her body image, bad dreams, or worries. The reactions of family members to the pregnancy and the woman's progression through the developmental tasks of pregnancy also are assessed and recorded.

During the third trimester, current family situations and their effect on the woman are assessed (e.g., the response of

BOX 11-4

HIV Screening

Pregnant women are ethically obligated to seek reasonable care during pregnancy and to avoid causing harm to the fetus. Maternity nurses should be advocates for the fetus but not at the expense of the pregnant woman.

The incidence of perinatal transmission from an HIV-positive mother to her fetus ranges from 25% to 35%. Zidovudine decreases perinatal transmission and the risk of infant death (Brocklehurst & Volmink, 2002). Elective cesarean birth significantly reduces the risk of transmission from the mother to child (Brocklehurst, 2002). Thus testing has the potential to identify HIV-positive women who can then be treated. Health care providers have an obligation to ensure that pregnant women are well informed about HIV symptoms, testing, and methods of decreasing maternal-fetal transmission. However, mandatory HIV screening involves ethical issues related to privacy invasion, discrimination, social stigma, and reproductive risks to the pregnant woman. Although some professional groups advocate mandatory testing, the Association of Women's Health, Obstetric, and Neonatal Nurses (AWHONN) does not support either mandatory or universal HIV testing of pregnant women because these models do not have the same standards of confidentiality and counseling that are present with voluntary, confidential testing with counseling (AWHONN, 1999).

siblings and grandparents to the pregnancy and the coming child). The nurse needs to assess the parents' understanding of the following: the warning signs of emergencies, such as bleeding and abdominal pain; the signs of preterm and term labor; the labor process and anxieties about labor; fetal development; and methods to assess fetal well-being. The nurse should ascertain whether the woman is planning to attend childbirth preparation classes, and what she knows about the control of discomfort during labor. If she is having a home birth, she should be queried as to whether all the necessary supplies have been obtained.

A review of the woman's physical systems is appropriate at each visit, and any suggestive signs or symptoms are assessed in depth. Discomforts reflecting adaptations to pregnancy are identified. Special inquiries are made about possible infections (e.g., genitourinary tract, respiratory tract). The woman's knowledge of and success with self-care measures are assessed, as well as outcomes of prescribed therapy.

Physical Examination

Reevaluation is a constant aspect of a pregnant woman's care. (See Guidelines/Guías box for phrases in Spanish for prenatal physical assessment.) Each woman reacts differently to pregnancy. As a result, careful monitoring of the pregnancy and her reactions to care is vital. Physiologic changes are documented as the pregnancy progresses and reviewed for possible deviations from normal progress.

At each visit, physical parameters are measured. Blood pressure (BP) is taken at every visit using the same arm and with the woman seated. Her weight is measured and the appropriateness of the weight gain is evaluated. Urine may be checked by dipstick. The presence and degree of edema are noted. For examination of the abdomen, the woman lies on her back with her arms by her side and head supported by a pillow. The bladder should be empty. Abdominal inspection is followed by measurement of the height of the fundus (Fig. 11-8). While the woman lies on her back, the nurse should be alert for the occurrence of supine hypotension (Emergency box). When a woman is lying in this position, the weight of the abdominal contents may compress the vena cava and aorta, causing a drop in BP and a feeling of faintness.

The findings revealed during the interview and physical examination reflect the status of maternal adaptations. When any of the findings is suspicious, an in-depth examination is performed. For example, careful interpretation of BP is important in the risk factor analysis of all pregnant women. BP is evaluated on the basis of absolute values and the length of gestation and is interpreted in the light of modifying factors.

ENGLISH SPANISH Guidelines/Guías

PRENATAL PHYSICAL ASSESSMENT

Get up on the scale, please.
Súbase a la balanza, por favor.

I need a urine sample.
Necesito una muestra de orina.

Go to the bathroom, please.
Vaya al baño, por favor.

I need to take your blood pressure.
Necesito verificar su presión sanguínea.

I am going to listen to the baby's heartbeat.
Voy a escuchar el latido del corazón del bebé.

The doctor is going to examine you.
El doctor le va a examinar.

Don't be afraid.
No tenga miedo.

Lie down, please.
Acuéstese, por favor.

Open your legs, please.
Sepárese las piernas, por favor.

Relax.
Afloje los músculos.

Go to the laboratory for a blood test, please.
Vaya al laboratorio para un análisis de sangre, por favor.

Go to this office for your ultrasound, please.
Vaya a esta oficina para que le haga el ultrasonido, por favor.

NURSE ALERT Individuals whose systolic blood pressure is 120 to 139 mm Hg or whose diastolic blood pressure is 80 to 89 mm Hg should be viewed as prehypertensive. To prevent cardiovascular disease, they require health-promoting lifestyle modifications (National High Blood Pressure Education Program, 2003). ■

An absolute systolic BP (SBP) of 140 mm Hg or more and a diastolic BP (DBP) of 90 mm Hg or more suggests the presence of hypertension. An SBP $\geq$125 mm Hg or a DBP $\geq$75 mm Hg in midpregnancy or an SBP $\geq$130 mm Hg or a DBP $\geq$85 mm Hg in later pregnancy are indicative of

A

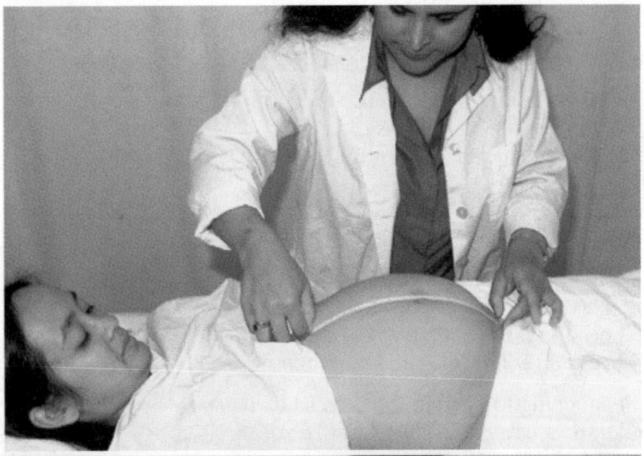

B

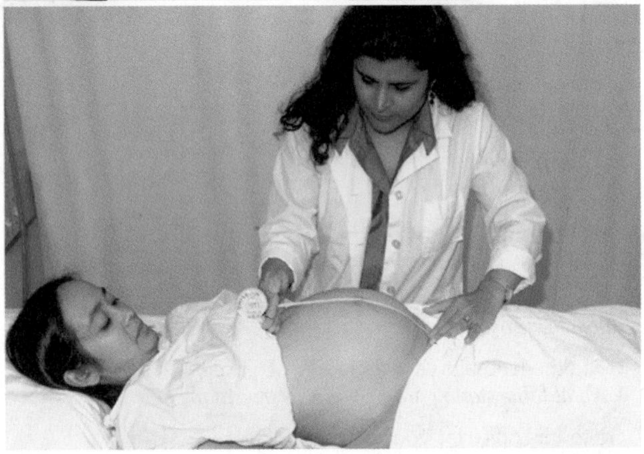

Fig. 11-8 Measurement of fundal height from symphysis that **A**, includes the upper curve of the fundus and **B**, does not include the upper curve of the fundus. Note position of hands and measuring tape. (Courtesy Chris Rozales, San Francisco, CA.)

Emergency

SUPINE HYPOTENSION

Signs/Symptoms

Pallor
Dizziness, faintness, breathlessness
Tachycardia
Nausea
Clammy (damp, cool) skin; sweating

Interventions

Position woman on her side until her signs/symptoms subside and vital signs stabilize within normal limits.

problems and should be reported to the primary health care provider immediately (Peters & Flack, 2004).

A rise in SBP of 30 mm Hg more than the baseline pressure, or a rise in the DBP of 15 mm Hg more than the baseline pressure, is also a significant finding regardless of the absolute values. An increase of 20 mm Hg or more in the mean arterial pressure (MAP) is also an indicator of hypertension (Gilbert & Harmon, 2003). See Chapter 14 for an in-depth discussion of problems associated with hypertension.

The pregnant woman is monitored continuously for a range of signs and symptoms that indicate potential complications in addition to hypertension. For example, persistent and excessive vomiting and ketonuria may indicate the development of hyperemesis gravidarum. Uterine cramping and vaginal bleeding are signs of threatened miscarriage. Chills and fever are symptoms of infection. Discharge from the vagina may be amniotic fluid or associated with infection (Box 11-5).

BOX 11-5

Signs of Potential Complications during the First, Second, and Third Trimesters

First Trimester

Signs/Symptoms	*Possible Causes*
Severe vomiting	Hyperemesis gravidarum
Chills, fever	Infection
Burning on urination	Infection
Diarrhea	Infection
Abdominal cramping; vaginal bleeding	Miscarriage, ectopic pregnancy

Second and Third Trimesters

Signs/Symptoms	*Possible Causes*
Persistent, severe vomiting	Hyperemesis gravidarum, hypertension, preeclampsia
Sudden discharge of fluid from vagina before 37 weeks	Premature rupture of membranes (PROM)
Vaginal bleeding, severe abdominal pain	Miscarriage, placenta previa, abruptio placentae
Chills, fever, burning on urination, diarrhea	Infection
Severe backache or flank pain	Kidney infection or stones; preterm labor
Change in fetal movements: absence of fetal movements after quickening, any unusual change in pattern or amount	Fetal jeopardy or intrauterine fetal death
Uterine contractions; pressure; cramping before 37 weeks	Preterm labor
Visual disturbances: blurring, double vision, or spots	Hypertensive conditions, preeclampsia
Swelling of face or fingers and over sacrum	Hypertensive conditions, preeclampsia
Headaches: severe, frequent, or continuous	Hypertensive conditions, preeclampsia
Muscular irritability or convulsions	Hypertensive conditions, preeclampsia
Epigastric or abdominal pain (perceived as severe stomachache)	Hypertensive conditions, preeclampsia, abruptio placentae
Glycosuria, positive glucose tolerance test reaction	Gestational diabetes mellitus

Fetal Assessment

Toward the end of the first trimester, before the uterus is an abdominal organ, the fetal heart tones (FHTs) can be heard with an ultrasound fetoscope or an ultrasound stethoscope. To hear the FHTs the instrument is placed in the midline, just above the symphysis pubis, and firm pressure is applied. The woman and her family should be offered the opportunity to listen to the FHTs. The health status of the fetus is assessed at each visit for the remainder of the pregnancy.

Fundal Height

During the second trimester, the uterus becomes an abdominal organ. The fundal height, or measurement of the height of the uterus above the symphysis pubis, is used as one indicator of fetal growth. The measurement also provides a gross estimate of the duration of pregnancy. During the second and third trimesters (weeks 18 to 30), the height of the fundus in centimeters is approximately the same as the number of weeks of gestation, if the woman's bladder is empty at the time of measurement. Measurement of fundal height may aid in the identification of high risk factors. A stable or decreased fundal height may indicate the presence of intrauterine growth restriction (IUGR); an excessive increase could indicate the presence of multifetal gestation (more than one fetus) or hydramnios.

A paper tape measure or a pelvimeter may be used to measure fundal height. To increase the reliability of the measurement, the same person could examine the pregnant woman at each of her prenatal visits; often this is not possible. All clinicians who examine a particular pregnant woman should be consistent in their measurement technique. Ideally a protocol should be established for the setting in which the measurement technique is explicitly set forth, and the woman's position on the examining table, the measuring device, and method of measurement used are specified. Figure 11-8 presents two methods of measuring fundal height.

Gestational Age

In an uncomplicated pregnancy, fetal gestational age is estimated after the duration of pregnancy and the EDB are determined. Fetal gestational age is determined from the menstrual history, contraceptive history, and pregnancy test results, and the following findings obtained from the clinical evaluation:

- First uterine size estimate: date, size
- Fetal heart rate first heard: date, method (Doppler stethoscope, fetoscope)
- Date of quickening
- Current fundal height, estimated fetal weight (EFW)
- Current week of gestation by history of LMP or ultrasound examination (or both)
- Ultrasound examination: date, week of gestation, biparietal diameter (BPD)
- Reliability of dates

Quickening ("feeling life") refers to the mother's first perception of fetal movement. It usually occurs between weeks 16 and 20 of gestation and is initially experienced as a fluttering sensation. The mother's report should be recorded.

Routine use of ultrasound examination (also called a sonogram) in early pregnancy has been recommended, and many health care providers have this equipment available in the office. This procedure may be used to establish the duration of pregnancy if the woman cannot give a precise date for her LMP or if the size of the uterus does not conform to the EDB as calculated by Nägele's rule. Ultrasound also provides information about the well-being of the fetus. However, the routine use of ultrasound has not been found to substantively improve fetal outcome (Bricker & Neilson, 2004).

Health Status

The assessment of fetal health status includes consideration of fetal movement. The mother is instructed to note the extent and timing of fetal movements and to report immediately if the pattern changes or if movement ceases. Regular movement has been found to be a reliable indicator of fetal health.

The fetal heart rate (FHR) is checked on routine visits once it has been heard (Fig. 11-9). Early in the second trimester the heartbeat may be heard with the Doppler stethoscope (Fig. 11-9, *B*). Before the fetus can be palpated by Leopold's maneuvers (see Fig. 18-6), the scope is moved around the abdomen until the heartbeat is heard. Each nurse develops a set pattern for searching the abdomen for the heartbeat: for example, starting in the midline about 2 to 3 cm above the symphysis, followed by the left lower quadrant, and so on. The FHR is counted, and the quality and rhythm are noted. Later in the second trimester the FHR can be determined with the fetoscope or Pinard's stethoscope (Fig. 11-9, *A* and *C*). A normal rate and rhythm are other good indicators of fetal health. Once the heartbeat is noted, its absence is cause for immediate investigation.

Intensive investigation of fetal health status is initiated if any maternal or fetal complications arise (e.g., maternal hypertension, IUGR, premature rupture of membranes [PROM], irregular or absent FHR, absence of fetal movements after quickening). Careful, precise, and concise recording of patient responses and laboratory results contributes to the continuous supervision vital to ensuring the well-being of the mother and fetus.

Laboratory Tests

The number of routine laboratory tests done during pregnancy is limited.

A clean-catch urine specimen is used to test for levels of glucose, protein, and nitrites and leukocytes at each follow-up visit. Urine specimens for culture and sensitivity, as well as blood samples, are obtained only if signs and symptoms warrant. A hematocrit determination is done at each visit in some offices.

The multiple marker test, or triple screen test, is used to detect Down syndrome and other chromosomal abnormalities. Done between 16 and 18 weeks of gestation, it measures maternal serum alpha-fetoprotein (MSAFP), human chorionic gonadotropin (hCG), and unconjugated estriol. Combining these three markers with maternal age allows a high detection rate for Down syndrome. High levels are associated with neural tube defects, and abnormally low levels may be associated with Down syndrome or other trisomies (Gilbert & Harmon, 2003).

Other blood tests are repeated as necessary: RPR/VDRL (rapid plasma reagin/Venereal Disease Research Laboratories) test for syphilis; complete blood count (CBC) with hematocrit, hemoglobin, and differential values; antibody screen (Kell, Duffy, rubella, toxoplasmosis, anti-Rh, HIV); sickle cell; and level of folacin when indicated. Cervical and vaginal smears are repeated as necessary to examine for

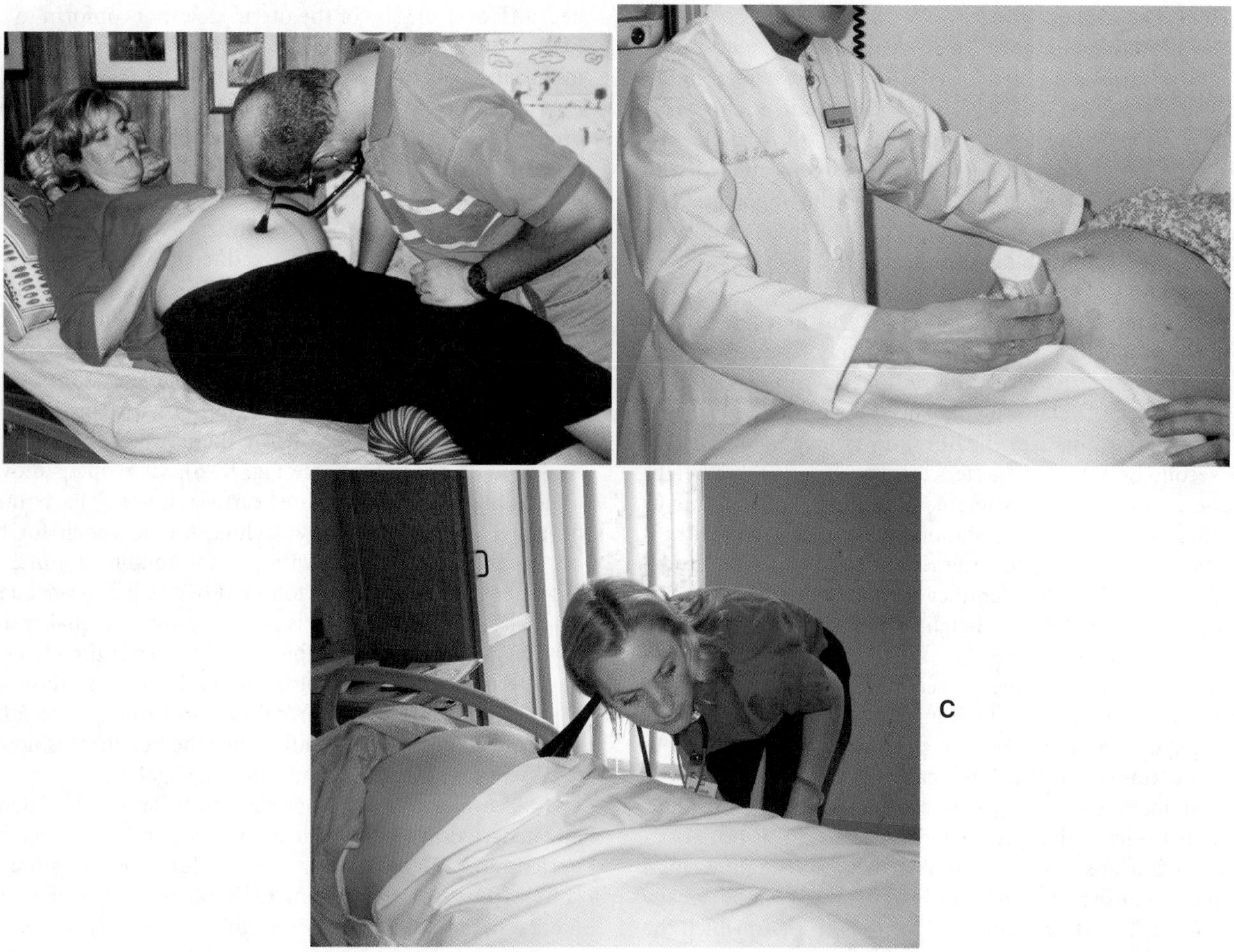

Fig. 11-9 Detecting fetal heartbeat. **A**, Father can listen to the fetal heart with a fetoscope (first detectable at 18 to 20 weeks with a fetoscope). **B**, Doppler ultrasound stethoscope (fetal heartbeat detectable at 12 weeks). **C**, Pinard's stethoscope. NOTE: Hands should not touch stethoscope while nurse is listening. (*A*, Courtesy Shannon Perry, Phoenix, AZ. *B*, Courtesy Dee Lowdermilk, Chapel Hill, NC. *C*, Courtesy Julie Perry Nelson, Gilbert, AZ.)

chlamydia organisms, gonorrhea, and herpes simplex virus (HSV) types 1 and 2. Group B streptococcus (GBS) testing is done between 35 and 37 weeks of gestation; cultures collected earlier will not accurately predict GBS status at time of birth.

If not done earlier in pregnancy, a glucose screen in women over age 25 is performed. A glucose challenge is usually done between 24 and 28 weeks of gestation.

Other Tests

Other diagnostic tests are available to assess the health status of both the pregnant woman and the fetus. Ultrasonography, for example, may be performed to determine the status of the pregnancy and to confirm gestational age of the fetus. Amniocentesis, a procedure used to obtain amniotic fluid for analysis, may be needed to evaluate the fetus for genetic disorders or gestational maturity. These and other tests used to determine health risks for the mother and infant are described in Chapters 9 and 17.

Nursing Diagnoses

The diagnoses that follow are examples of the nursing diagnoses that may be appropriate in the prenatal period:

- *Anxiety related to*
  - —physical discomforts of pregnancy
  - —ambivalent and labile emotions
  - —changes in family dynamics
  - —fetal well-being
  - —ability to manage anticipated labor
- *Interrupted family processes related to*
  - —changing roles and responsibilities
  - —inadequate understanding of physical and emotional changes in pregnancy
  - —increased concern about labor
- *Deficient knowledge regarding self-care measures for*
  - —posture and body mechanics
  - —rest and relaxation
  - —personal hygiene
  - —activity and exercise
  - —safety
- *Disturbed sleep pattern related to*
  - —discomforts of late pregnancy
  - —anxiety about approaching labor

Expected Outcomes

Individualized plans that are developed mutually with the pregnant woman are more likely to result in desirable outcomes than are those developed by the nurse for the woman.

Measured outcomes of prenatal care include not only physical outcomes but also developmental and psychosocial outcomes. The following are examples of outcomes that may be expected. The pregnant woman will achieve the following:

- Indicate decreased anxiety about the health of her fetus and herself.
- Describe improved family dynamics.
- Show appropriate weight gain patterns.
- Report signs and symptoms of complications.
- Describe appropriate measures taken to relieve physical discomforts.
- Develop a realistic birth plan.

Plan of Care and Implementation

The nurse-patient relationship is critical in setting the tone for further interaction. The techniques of listening with an attentive expression, touching, and using eye contact have their place, as does recognizing the woman's feelings and her right to express these feelings. The clinic, home visits, and telephone conversations all provide opportunities for contact and can be used effectively.

Sometimes women repeatedly seek information about a particular problem. At other times the woman may be reluctant to bring up another underlying problem. The nurse must be perceptive in identifying such unvoiced needs and can help the woman by asking for a patient-generated solution and a subsequent report of its effectiveness. Supportive care involves developing, augmenting, or changing the mechanisms used by women and their families in coping with stress. The woman must be a willing partner in a purely voluntary relationship. As such, the relationship can be refused or terminated at any time by the pregnant woman or her family.

Care Paths

Because of the large number of health care professionals involved in care of the expectant mother, unintentional gaps or overlaps in care may occur. To better coordinate prenatal care services for childbearing families, care paths are used to improve consistency of care and reduce costs. Although the Care Path (p. 276) focuses only on prenatal education, it is an example of the type of form that might be developed to guide health care providers in carrying out the appropriate assessments and interventions in a timely way. Use of care paths also may contribute to improved satisfaction of families with the prenatal care provided, and members of the health care team may function more efficiently and effectively.

Education about Maternal and Fetal Changes

Expectant parents are typically curious about the growth and development of the fetus and the consequent changes that occur in the mother's body. Mothers may be more tolerant of the discomforts related to the continuing pregnancy if they understand the underlying causes. Commercial literature that describes the fetal and maternal changes is often available and can be used in explaining changes as they occur.

Education for Self-Care

The expectant mother needs information on many topics. The nurse who is observant, listens, and knows typical concerns of expectant parents can anticipate what questions will be asked and prompt mothers and their partners to discuss what is on their minds. Printed literature can be given to supplement the individualized teaching the nurse provides, and women often avidly read books and pamphlets related to their own experience. When nurses read the literature before they distribute it, they have an opportunity to point out areas that may not correspond with local health care practices. Increasingly, information about pregnancy is available on the World Wide Web. The nurse should review material on Web sites before recommending them to patients. Patients who receive conflicting advice or instruction are likely to grow increasingly frustrated with members of the health care team and the care provided. Several topics that may cause concern in pregnant women are discussed in the following sections.

Nutrition

Good nutrition is important in the maintenance of maternal health during pregnancy and in the provision of adequate nutrients for embryonic and fetal development. The nourishment the fetus receives from its mother influences health in later life. Assessing a woman's nutritional status and providing information on nutrition are part of the nurse's responsibilities in providing prenatal care. In some settings, a registered dietitian conducts classes for pregnant women on the topics of nutritional status and nutrition during pregnancy or interviews them to assess their knowledge of these topics. Nurses can refer women to a registered dietitian if a need is revealed during the nursing assessment. (For detailed information concerning maternal and fetal nutritional needs and related nursing care, see Chapter 12.)

Personal Hygiene

During pregnancy, the sebaceous (sweat) glands are highly active because of hormonal influences, and women often perspire freely. They may be reassured that the increase is normal and that their previous patterns of perspiration will return after the postpartum period. Washing the body regularly is basic to good personal hygiene. Baths and warm showers can be therapeutic because they relax tense, tired muscles; help counter insomnia; and make the pregnant woman feel fresh. Tub bathing is permitted even in late pregnancy because little water enters the vagina unless under pressure. However, later in pregnancy, when the woman's center of gravity lowers, she is at risk for falling. Tub bathing is contraindicated after rupture of the membranes.

Prevention of Urinary Tract Infection

Because of dramatic changes that occur in the renal system during pregnancy (see Chapter 10), urinary tract infections are common, but they may be asymptomatic. Over-the-counter tests for urinary tract infection are available (Fig. 11-10). Women should be instructed to inform their health care provider if blood or pain occurs with urination. These infections pose a risk to the mother and fetus; thus the prevention or early treatment of these infections is essential.

The nurse can assess the woman's understanding and use of good handwashing techniques before and after urinating and whether she knows to wipe from front to back. Soft, absorbent toilet tissue, preferably white and unscented, should be used; harsh, scented, or printed toilet paper may cause irritation. Bubble bath or other bath oils should be avoided because these may be irritating to the urethra. Women should wear underpants and panty hose with a cotton crotch and avoid wearing tight-fitting slacks or jeans for long peri-

Care Path

PRENATAL CARE

PRENATAL EDUCATION CLINICAL PATHWAY

INITIAL VISIT AND ORIENTATION: ______ SOCIAL SERVICE: ______ DIETITIAN: ______

I. EARLY PREGNANCY (WEEKS 1-20) (initial and date after education given)

Fetal growth and development	______	Testing: Labs	Ultrasound ______
Maternal changes	______	Possible complications:	
		a. Threatened miscarriage	______
Lifestyle: exercise/stress/nutrition	______	b. Diabetes	______
Drugs, OTC, tobacco, alcohol	______	c. ______	______
STIs	______		
		Introduction to breastfeeding	______
Psycho/social adjustments:			
FOB involved/accepts	______	Acceptance	______
Baby for adoption	______	and childbirth preparation	______
		Dietary follow-up	______

II. MIDPREGNANCY (WEEKS 21-27) (initial and date after education given)

Fetal growth and development	______	Breastfeeding or bottle-feeding	______
Maternal changes	______	Birth plan initiated	______
Daily fetal movement	______	Childbirth preparation	______
Possible complications:			
a. Preterm labor prevention	______	Dietary follow-up	______
b. GH symptoms	______		
c. ______	______		

III. LATE PREGNANCY (WEEKS 28-40) (initial and date after education given)

Fetal growth and development	______	Childbirth preparation:	
		S/S of labor; labor process	______
Fetal evaluation:		Pain management: natural childbirth, meds, epidural	______
Daily movement ______	NSTs ______	Cesarean; VBAC	______
		Birth plan complete	______
Kick counts ______	BPPs ______	Review hospital policies	______
Maternal changes	______	Parenting preparation:	
		Pediatrician ______	Child care ______
Possible complications:		Siblings ______	Immunizations ______
a. Preterm labor prevention	______	Car seat/safety ______	
b. GH symptoms	______		
c. ______	______	Postpartum:	
		PP care/checkup	______
Breastfeeding preparation:		Emotional changes	______
Nipple assessment	______	BC options	______
		Safer sex/STIs	______
Dietary follow-up	______		

Signature: ______ ______ ______ ______

BC, birth control; *BPP,* biophysical profile; *FOB,* father of baby; *GH,* gestational hypertension; *NST,* nonstress test; *OTC,* over the counter; *PP,* postpartum; *S/S,* signs and symptoms; *STI,* sexually transmitted infection; *VBAC,* vaginal birth after cesarean.

ods. Anything that allows a buildup of heat and moisture in the genital area may foster the growth of bacteria.

Some women do not consume enough fluid and food. After ascertaining the woman's food preferences, the nurse should advise the woman to drink at least 2 L (eight glasses) of liquid a day to maintain an adequate fluid intake that ensures frequent urination. Pregnant women should not limit fluids in an effort to reduce the frequency of urination. Women need to know that if urine looks dark (concentrated), they need to increase their fluid intake. Vitamin C

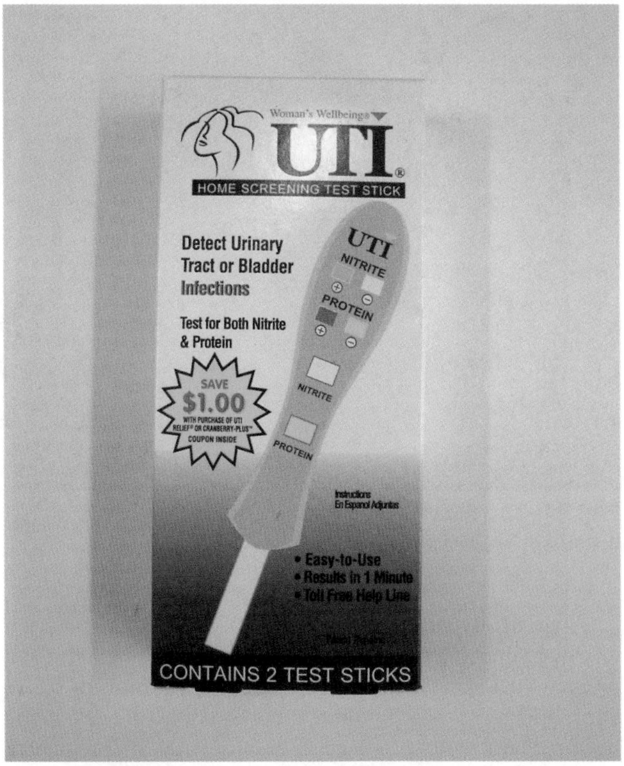

Fig. 11-10 Over-the-counter urinary tract infection detection kit. (Courtesy Julie Perry Nelson, Gilbert, AZ.)

makes the urinary tract less hospitable to bacteria by lowering the pH. The consumption of yogurt and acidophilus milk may also help prevent urinary tract and vaginal infections. Although drinking cranberry juice is often recommended, that sold to consumers is too dilute to lower the pH of urine.

The nurse should review healthy urination practices with the woman. Women should be told not to ignore the urge to urinate because holding urine lengthens the time bacteria are in the bladder and allows them to multiply. Women should plan ahead when faced with situations that may normally require them to delay urination (e.g., a long car ride). They should always urinate before going to bed at night. Bacteria also can be introduced during intercourse. Women are therefore advised to urinate before and after intercourse and then drink a large glass of water to promote additional urination.

Kegel Exercises

Kegel exercises, deliberate contraction and relaxation of the pubococcygeus muscle, strengthen the muscles around the reproductive organs and improve muscle tone. Many women are not aware of the muscles of the pelvic floor until it is pointed out that these are the muscles used during urination and sexual intercourse and they can be consciously controlled. The pelvic floor muscles encircle the vaginal outlet, and they need to be exercised. An exercised muscle can stretch and contract readily at birth. Practice of pelvic muscle exercise during pregnancy also results in fewer complaints of urinary incontinence in late pregnancy and postpartum (see Patient Teaching box, p. 67).

Preparation for Breastfeeding the Newborn

Pregnant women are usually eager to discuss their plans for feeding the newborn. Breast milk is the food of choice, in part because breastfeeding is associated with a decreased incidence in perinatal morbidity and mortality. The American Academy of Pediatrics recommends breastfeeding for at least 1 year. However, a deep-seated aversion to breastfeeding by the mother or partner; the mother's need for certain medications; and certain medical complications, such as active tuberculosis and newly diagnosed breast cancer, are contraindications to breastfeeding. Although hepatitis B antigen has not been shown to be transmitted through breast milk, it is recommended, as an added precaution, that infants born to hepatitis B antigen–positive women receive hepatitis B vaccine and hepatitis B immune globulin (HBIG) immediately after birth. Nursing is discouraged in women who are HIV positive because of the risk of HIV transmission (Lawrence & Lawrence, 2005).

A woman's decision about the method of infant feeding is made before pregnancy; thus it is essential to educate women of childbearing age about the benefits of breastfeeding. The woman and her partner are encouraged to decide what method of feeding is suitable for them; however, the benefits of breastfeeding should be emphasized. Once the couple has been given information about the advantages and disadvantages of breastfeeding and bottle-feeding, they can make an informed choice. Health care providers support these decisions and provide any needed assistance.

Women with inverted nipples need special consideration if they are planning to breastfeed. The pinch test is done to determine whether the nipple is everted or inverted (Fig. 11-11). To perform the pinch test, the woman places her thumb and forefinger on her areola and presses inward gently. This action will cause her nipple either to stand erect or to invert. Most nipples will stand erect.

Exercises to break the adhesions that cause the nipple to invert do not work and may in fact cause uterine contractions (Lawrence & Lawrence, 2005). The use of breast shells, small plastic devices that fit over the nipple, by women with flat or inverted nipples is sometimes recommended (Fig. 11-12). However, in a large multicenter trial of shells, Hoffman exercises, and no prenatal treatment, "no treatment" was most effective (cited in Lawrence & Lawrence, 2005). Breast shells exert a continuous, gentle pressure around the areola that pushes the nipple through a central opening in the inner shield. If breast shells are recommended, they should be worn for 1 to 2 hours daily during the last trimester of pregnancy. Breast stimulation is contraindicated in women at risk for preterm labor; therefore the decision to suggest the use of breast shells to women with flat or inverted nipples must be made judiciously.

The woman is taught to cleanse the nipples with warm water to prevent blocking of the ducts with dried colostrum. Soap, ointments, alcohol, and tinctures should not be applied because they remove protective oils that keep nipples supple. The use of these substances may cause the nipple to crack during early lactation (Lawrence & Lawrence, 2005).

The woman who plans to breastfeed should purchase a nursing bra that will accommodate her increased breast size during the last few months of pregnancy and during lacta-

A

B

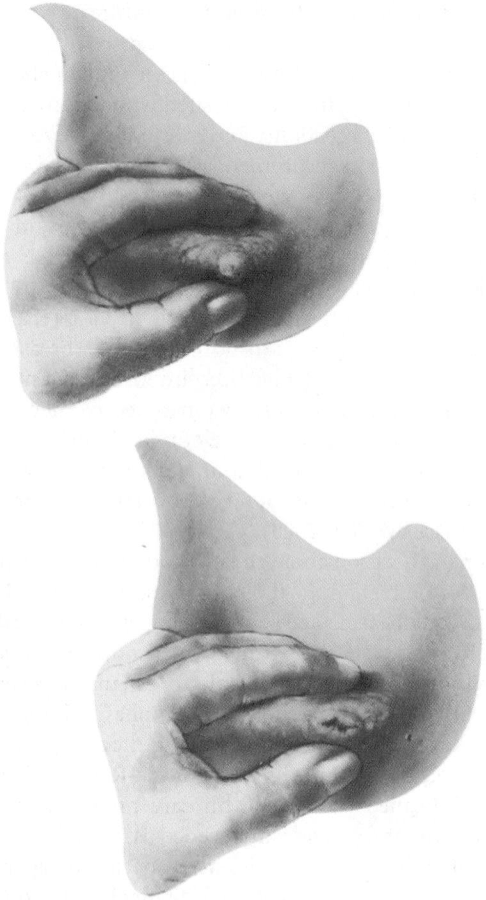

Fig. 11-11 Pinch test. **A,** Normal nipple everts with gentle pressure. **B,** Inverted nipple inverts with gentle pressure. (Modified from Lawrence RA, Lawrence RM: *Breastfeeding: a guide for the medical profession,* ed 5, St Louis, 1999, Mosby.)

tion. If her breasts are very heavy, or if the woman feels uncomfortable with the weight unsupported, the bra can be worn day and night.

Dental Health

Dental care during pregnancy is especially important because nausea during pregnancy may lead to poor oral hygiene and allow dental caries to develop. However, no physiologic alteration during gestation can cause dental caries. A fluoride toothpaste should be used daily. Inflammation and infection of the gingival and periodontal tissues may occur (Carl, Roux, & Matacale, 2000). There is some evidence linking periodontal infections and preterm birth and low birth weight (Jared et al, 1999).

Because calcium and phosphorus in the teeth are fixed in enamel, the old adage "for every child a tooth" is not true. There is no scientific evidence indicating that filling teeth or even dental extraction using local or nitrous oxide–oxygen anesthesia causes miscarriage or premature labor. Antibacterial therapy should be considered for sepsis, however, especially in pregnant women who have had rheumatic heart disease or nephritis. Emergency dental surgery is not contraindicated during pregnancy; however, the risks and benefits of surgery need to be explained to the mother. If dental treatment is necessary, the woman will be most comfortable during the second trimester (Carl, Roux, & Matacale, 2000).

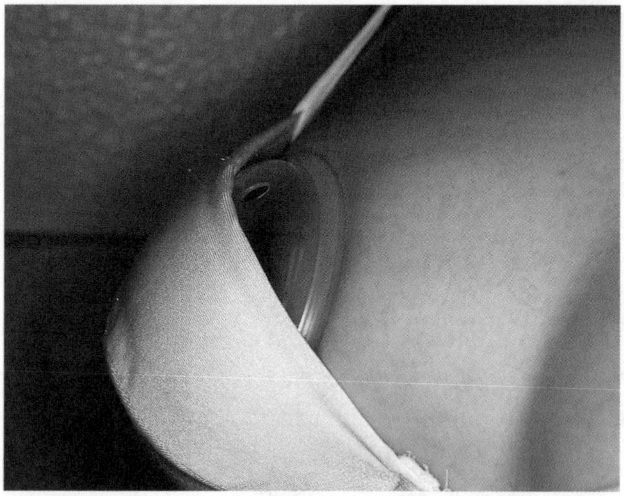

Fig. 11-12 Breast shell in place inside bra to evert nipple. (Courtesy Michael S. Clement, MD, Mesa, AZ.)

Physical Activity

Physical activity promotes a feeling of well-being in the pregnant woman. It improves circulation, promotes relaxation and rest, and counteracts boredom, as it does in the nonpregnant woman. Detailed exercise tips for pregnancy are presented in the Home Care box.

Exercises that help relieve the low back pain that often arises during the second trimester because of the increased weight of the fetus are demonstrated in Fig. 11-13.

Posture and Body Mechanics

Many maternal adaptations predispose the woman to backache and incurring possible injury. The pregnant woman's center of gravity changes, pelvic joints soften and relax, and stress is placed on abdominal musculature as pregnancy progresses. Poor posture and body mechanics contribute to the discomfort and potential for injury. To minimize these problems, women can acquire a kinesthetic sense for good body posture (Fig. 11-14; see also Fig. 10-10). The activities described in the Home Care box can also promote greater physical comfort. (See also Patient Teaching box, p. 283.)

Rest and Relaxation

The pregnant woman is encouraged to plan regular rest periods, particularly as pregnancy advances. The side-lying position is recommended to promote uterine perfusion and fetoplacental oxygenation by eliminating pressure on the ascending vena cava and descending aorta, which can lead to supine hypotension (Fig. 11-15). The mother should also be shown the way to rise slowly from a side-lying position to prevent strain on the back and to minimize the orthostatic hypotension caused by changes in position common in the latter part of pregnancy. To stretch and rest back muscles at home or at work, the nurse can suggest the woman do the following exercises:

- Stand behind a chair. Support and balance yourself using the back of the chair (Fig. 11-16). Squat for 30 seconds; stand for 15 seconds. Repeat six times, in several sets per day, as needed.
- While sitting in a chair, lower your head to your knees for 30 seconds. Raise your head up. Repeat six times, several times per day, as needed.

Home Care

EXERCISE TIPS FOR PREGNANT WOMEN

Consult your health care provider when you know or suspect you are pregnant. Discuss your medical and obstetric history, your current exercise regimen, and the exercises you would like to continue throughout pregnancy.

Seek help in determining an exercise routine that is well within your limit of tolerance, especially if you have not been exercising regularly.

Consider decreasing weight-bearing exercises (jogging, running) and concentrating on non–weight-bearing activities such as swimming, cycling, or stretching. If you are a runner, starting in your seventh month, you may wish to walk instead.

Avoid risky activities such as surfing, mountain climbing, skydiving, and racquetball because such activities that require precise balance and coordination may be dangerous. Avoid activities that require holding your breath and bearing down (Valsalva's maneuver). Jerky, bouncy motions also should be avoided.

Exercise regularly at least three times a week, as long as you are healthy, to improve muscle tone and increase or maintain your stamina. If you do exercises sporadically, this may put undue strain on your muscles. Limit activity to shorter intervals. Exercise for 10 to 15 minutes, rest for 2 to 3 minutes, then exercise for another 10 to 15 minutes.

Decrease your exercise level as your pregnancy progresses. The normal alterations of advancing pregnancy, such as decreased cardiac reserve and increased respiratory effort, may produce physiologic stress if you exercise strenuously for a long time.

Take your pulse every 10 to 15 minutes while you are exercising. If it is more than 140 beats/min, slow down until it returns to a maximum of 90 beats/min. You should be able to converse easily while exercising. If you cannot, you need to slow down.

Avoid becoming overheated for extended periods of time. It is best not to exercise for more than 35 minutes, especially in hot, humid weather. As your body temperature rises, the heat is transmitted to your fetus. Prolonged or repeated elevation of fetal temperature may result in birth defects, especially during the first 3 months. Your temperature should not exceed 38° C.

Do not use hot tubs and saunas.

Warm-up and stretching exercises prepare your joints for more strenuous exercise and lessen the likelihood of strain or injury to your joints. After the fourth month of gestation you should not perform exercises flat on your back.

A cool-down period of mild activity involving your legs after an exercise period will help bring your respiration, heart, and metabolic rates back to normal and prevent the pooling of blood in the exercised muscles.

Rest for 10 minutes after exercising, lying on your side. As the uterus grows, it puts pressure on a major vein in your abdomen, which carries blood to your heart. Lying on your side removes the pressure and promotes return circulation from your extremities and muscles to your heart, thereby increasing blood flow to your placenta and fetus. You should rise gradually from the floor to prevent dizziness or fainting (orthostatic hypotension).

Drink two or three 8-oz glasses of water after you exercise to replace the body fluids lost through perspiration. While exercising, drink water whenever you feel the need.

Increase your caloric intake to replace the calories burned during exercise and provide the extra energy needs of pregnancy. (Pregnancy alone requires an additional 300 kcal/day.) Choose such high-protein foods as fish, milk, cheese, eggs, or meat.

Take your time. This is not the time to be competitive or train for activities requiring speed or long endurance.

Wear a supportive bra. Your increased breast weight may cause changes in posture and put pressure on the ulnar nerve.

Wear supportive shoes. As your uterus grows, your center of gravity shifts and you compensate for this by arching your back. These natural changes may make you feel off balance and more likely to fall.

Stop exercising immediately if you experience shortness of breath, dizziness, numbness, tingling, pain of any kind, more than four uterine contractions per hour, decreased fetal activity, or vaginal bleeding, and consult your health care provider.

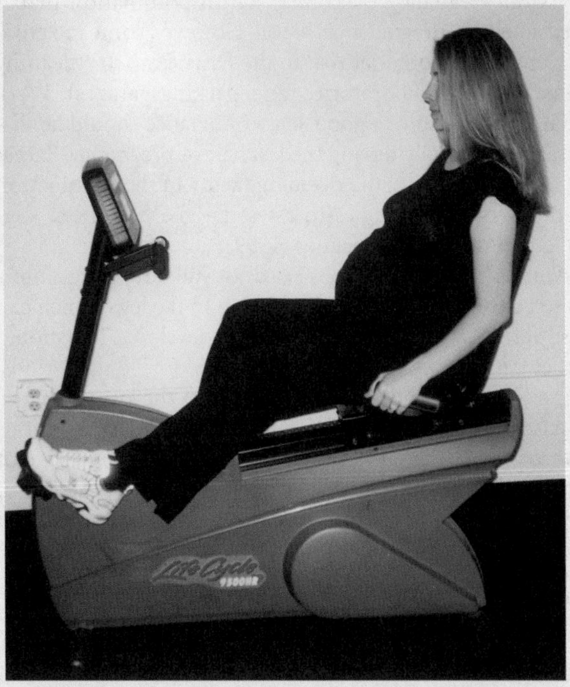

Riding a recumbent bicycle provides exercise while supplying back support. (Courtesy Shannon Perry, Phoenix, AZ.)

Modified from Artal R, Subak-Sharpe G: *Pregnancy and exercise,* New York, 1992, Delacorte Press; Fishbein EG, Phillips M: How safe is exercise during pregnancy? *J Obstet Gynecol Neonatal Nurs* 19(1):45-49, 1990; ACOG: Exercise during pregnancy and the postpartum period, *Technical Bulletin*189, 1994; Pivarnik JM: Maternal exercise in pregnancy, *Sports Med* 18(4):215-217, 1994.

Conscious relaxation is the process of releasing tension from the mind and body through deliberate effort and practice. The ability to relax consciously and intentionally can be beneficial for the following reasons:

- Relief of the normal discomforts related to pregnancy.
- Reduction of stress and to diminish pain perception during the childbearing cycle.
- Heighten self-awareness and trust in one's own ability to control responses and functions.
- Help cope with stress in everyday life situations, whether pregnant or not.

The techniques for conscious relaxation are numerous and varied. The guidelines given in Box 11-6 can be used by anyone.

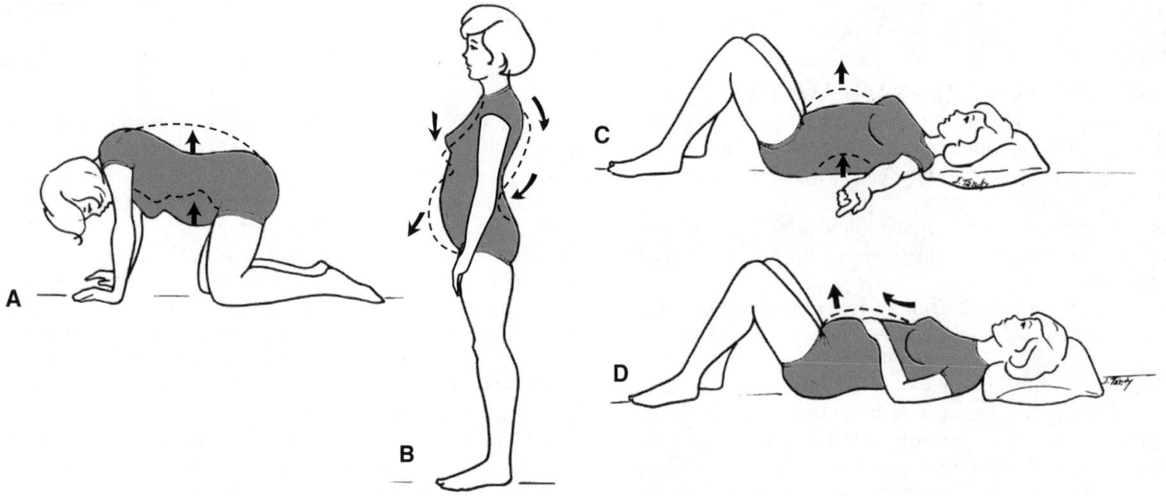

Fig. 11-13 Exercises. **A, B, C,** Pelvic rocking relieves low backache (excellent for relief of menstrual cramps as well). **D,** Abdominal breathing aids relaxation and lifts abdominal wall off uterus.

Employment

Employment of pregnant women usually has no adverse effects on pregnancy outcomes. Job discrimination that is based solely on pregnancy is illegal. However, some job environments pose potential risk to the fetus (e.g., dry cleaning plants, chemical laboratories, and parking garages). Work activities that require a good sense of balance should be discouraged, especially during the last half of pregnancy. Excessive fatigue is usually the deciding factor in the termination of employment; strategies to assess fatigue have been suggested by Pugh and colleagues (1999).

Women in sedentary jobs need to walk around at intervals to counter the sluggish circulation in the legs, which can cause varices and thrombophlebitis to develop. They should neither sit nor stand in one position for long periods. Women should avoid crossing their legs at the knees because this also fosters such conditions. Standing for long periods also increases the risk of preterm labor. The pregnant woman's chair should provide adequate back support. Use of a footstool can prevent pressure on veins, relieve strain on varicosities, and minimize swelling of feet.

Clothing

Comfortable, loose clothing is best. Washable fabrics (e.g., absorbent cottons) are often preferred. Maternity clothes may be purchased new or found in good condition at thrift shops or garage sales because they rarely wear out. Tight bras and belts, stretch pants, garters, tight-top knee socks, panty girdles, and other constrictive clothing should be avoided because tight clothing over the perineum encourages vaginitis and miliaria (heat rash), and impaired circulation in the legs can cause varicosities.

Maternity bras are constructed to accommodate the increased breast weight, chest circumference, and size of breast tail tissue (under the arm). These bras have drop-flaps over the nipples to facilitate breastfeeding. A good bra can help prevent neckache and backache.

Elastic hose give considerable comfort and promote greater venous emptying in women with large varicose veins. Ideally, support stockings should be put on before the woman gets out of bed in the morning. Figure 11-17 demonstrates a position to rest the legs and reduce swelling.

Comfortable shoes that provide firm support and promote good posture and balance are advisable. Very high heels and platform shoes are not recommended because of the woman's changed center of gravity, which can cause her to lose her balance. In addition, the woman's pelvis tilts for-

Home Care

POSTURE AND BODY MECHANICS

To Prevent or Relieve Backache

Do pelvic tilt:

- Pelvic tilt (rock) on hands and knees (see Fig. 11-13, *A*) and while sitting in straight-back chair.
- Pelvic tilt (rock) in standing position against a wall, or lying on floor (see Fig. 11-13, *B* and *C*).
- Perform abdominal muscle contractions during pelvic tilt while standing, lying, or sitting to help strengthen rectus abdominis muscle (see Fig. 11-13, *D*).
- Use good body mechanics.
- Use leg muscles to reach objects on or near floor. Bend at the knees, not the back. Knees are bent to lower body to squatting position. Feet are kept 12 to 18 inches apart to provide a solid base to maintain balance (Fig. 11-14, *A*).
- Lift with the legs. To lift a heavy object (e.g., young child), one foot is placed slightly in front of the other and kept flat as the woman lowers herself onto one knee. She lifts the weight holding it close to her body and never higher than the chest. To stand up or sit down, one leg is placed slightly behind the other as she raises or lowers herself (Fig. 11-14, *B*).

To Restrict the Lumbar Curve

For prolonged standing (e.g., ironing or because of employment), place one foot on low footstool or box; change positions often.

Move car seat forward so that knees are bent and higher than hips. If needed, use a small pillow to support low back area.

Sit in chairs low enough to allow both feet to be placed on floor, preferably with knees higher than hips.

A

B

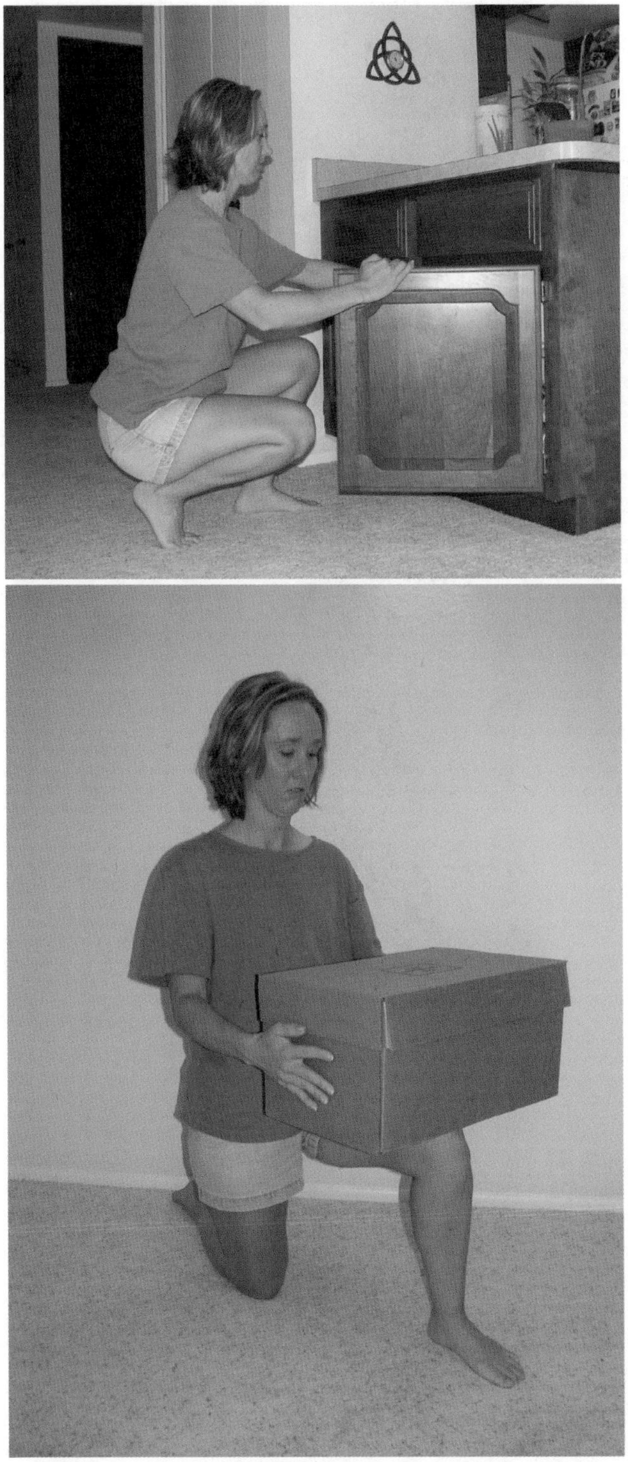

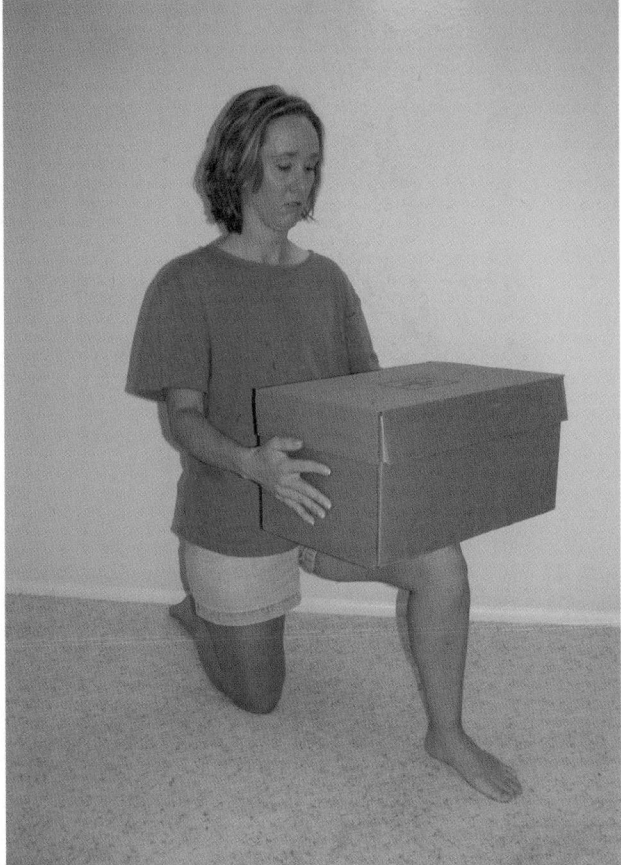

Fig. 11-14 Correct body mechanics. **A,** Squatting. **B,** Lifting. (Courtesy Julie Perry Nelson, Gilbert, AZ.)

ward in the third trimester, increasing her lumbar curve. The resulting leg aches and cramps will be aggravated by shoes that do not provide good support. Figure 11-18 shows exercises to relieve leg cramps.

Travel

Travel is not contraindicated for low risk pregnant women, but those with high risk pregnancies are advised to avoid long-distance travel after fetal viability has been

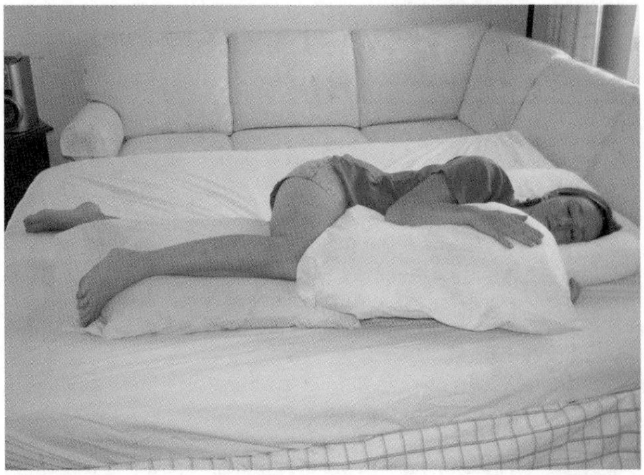

Fig. 11-15 Side-lying position for rest and relaxation. (Courtesy Julie Perry Nelson, Gilbert, AZ.)

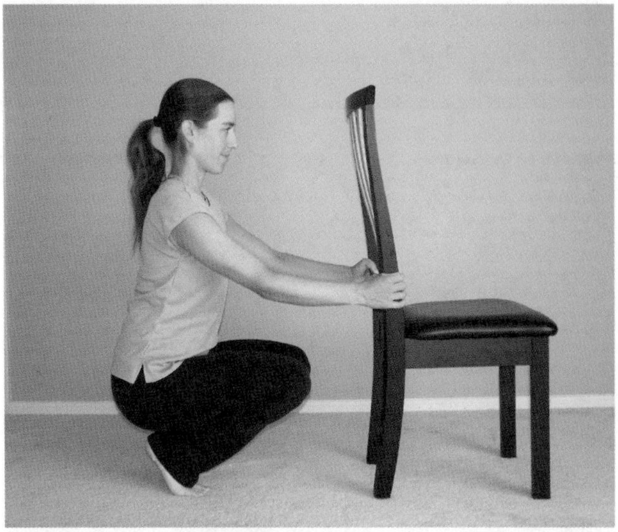

Fig. 11-16 Squatting for muscle relaxation and strengthening and for keeping leg and hip joints flexible. (Courtesy Julie Perry Nelson, Gilbert, AZ.)

reached to avert the economic and psychologic consequences of giving birth to a preterm infant far from home. Travel to areas where medical care is poor, water is untreated, and malaria is prevalent should be avoided if possible. Women who contemplate foreign travel should be aware that many health insurance carriers do not cover birth in a foreign setting or even hospitalization for preterm labor.

Pregnant women who travel for long distances should schedule periods of activity and rest. While sitting the woman can practice deep breathing, foot circling, and alternately contracting and relaxing different muscle groups. She should avoid becoming fatigued. Although travel in itself is not a cause of adverse outcomes such as miscarriage or preterm labor, certain precautions are recommended while traveling in a car. The woman should always use automobile restraints; a combination lap belt and shoulder harness is the most effective automobile restraint. Both shoulder and lap belts should be used. The lap belt should be worn low across the hip bones and as snug as is comfortable (Fig. 11-19). The shoulder belt should be worn above the pregnant uterus and below the

BOX 11-6

Conscious Relaxation Tips

Preparation: Loosen clothing, assume a comfortable sitting or side-lying position with all parts of body well supported with pillows. The use of soothing music is optional.

Beginning: Allow self to feel warm and comfortable. Inhale and exhale slowly, and imagine peaceful relaxation coming over each part of the body, starting with the neck and working down to the toes. People who learn conscious relaxation often speak of feeling relaxed even if some discomfort is present.

Maintenance: Use imagery (fantasy or daydream) to maintain the state of relaxation. Using *active imagery,* imagine yourself moving or doing some activity and experiencing its sensations. Using *passive imagery,* imagine yourself watching a scene, such as a lovely sunset.

Awakening: Return to the wakeful state gradually. Slowly begin to take in stimuli from the surrounding environment.

Further retention and development of the skill: Practice regularly for some periods each day, for example, at the same hour for 10 to 15 minutes each day, to feel refreshed, revitalized, and invigorated.

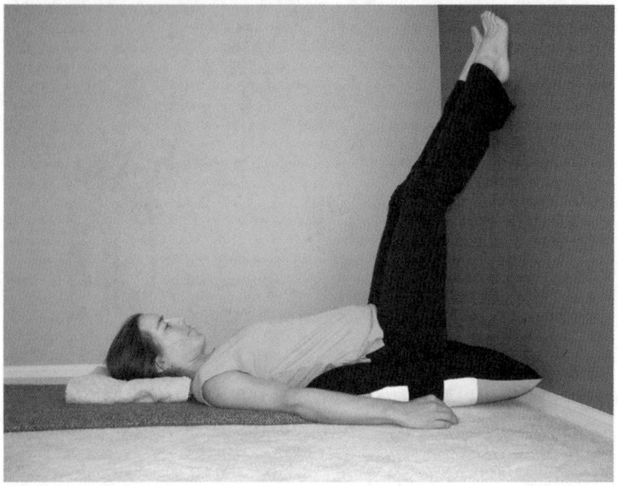

Fig. 11-17 Position for resting legs and for reducing edema and varicosities. Encourage the woman with vulvar varicosities to include a pillow under her hips. (Courtesy Julie Perry Nelson, Gilbert, AZ.)

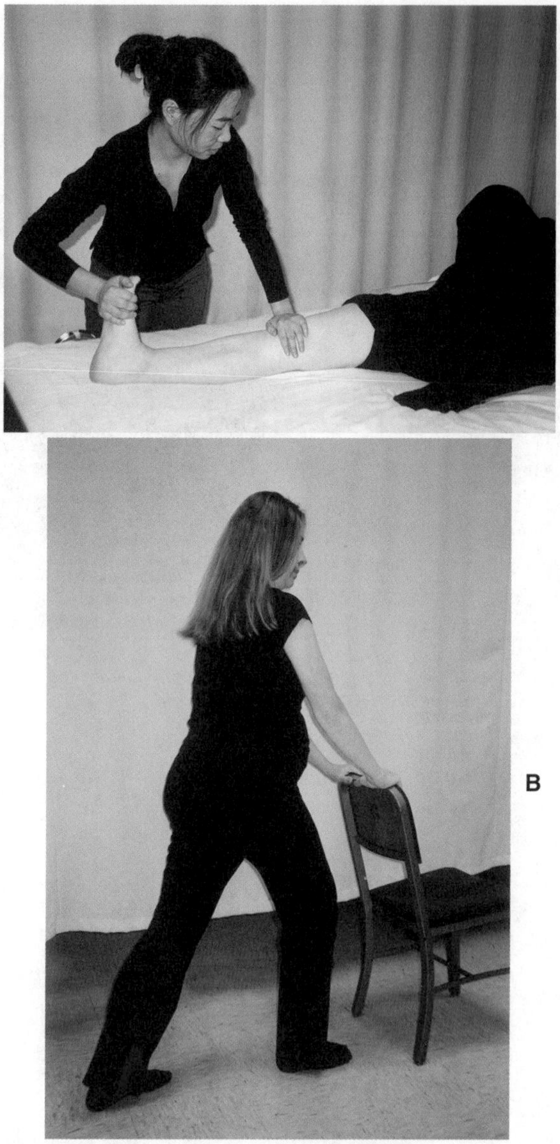

Fig. 11-18 Relief of muscle spasm (leg cramps). **A,** Another person dorsiflexes foot with knee extended. **B,** Woman stands and leans forward, thereby dorsiflexing foot of affected leg. (Courtesy Shannon Perry, Phoenix, AZ.)

neck to avoid chafing. The pregnant woman should sit upright. The headrest should be used to avoid a whiplash injury.

Maternal death as a result of injury is the most common cause of fetal death. The next most common cause is placental separation that occurs because body contours change in reaction to the force of a collision. The uterus as a muscular organ can adapt its shape to that of the body, but the placenta is not resilient. At the impact of collision, placental separation can occur.

Air travel in large commercial jets usually poses little risk to the pregnant woman, but policies vary from airline to airline. The pregnant woman is advised to inquire about restrictions or recommendations from her carrier. Magnetometers (metal detectors) used at airport security checkpoints are not harmful to the fetus. The 8% humidity at which cabins are maintained in commercial airlines may result in some water loss; hydration (with water) should be maintained under these conditions. Sitting in the cramped seat of an airliner for prolonged periods may increase the risk of superficial and deep thrombophlebitis. A pregnant woman is encouraged to take a 15-minute walk around the aircraft during each hour of travel to minimize this risk (see the Patient Teaching box earlier in this chapter).

Medications

Although much has been learned in recent years about fetal drug toxicity, the possible teratogenicity of many drugs, both prescription and OTC, is still unknown. This is especially true for new medications and combinations of medications. Moreover, certain subclinical errors or deficiencies in intermediate metabolism in the fetus may cause an otherwise harmless drug to be converted into a hazardous one. The greatest danger of drug-caused developmental defects in the fetus extends from the time of fertilization through the first trimester, a time when the woman may not realize she is pregnant. Self-treatment

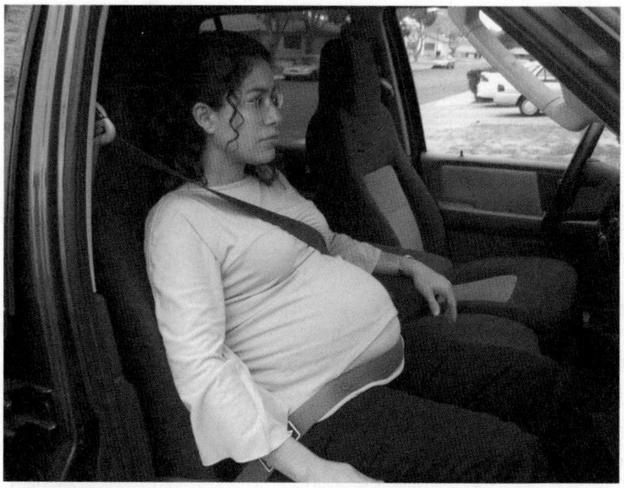

Fig. 11-19 Proper use of seat belt and headrest. (Courtesy Brian Sallee, Las Vegas, NV.)

must be discouraged. The use of all drugs, including OTC medications and vitamins, should be limited and a careful record kept of all therapeutic agents used.

Immunization

Some concern has been raised over the safety of various immunization practices during pregnancy. Immunization with live or attenuated live viruses is contraindicated during pregnancy because of potential teratogenicity. Live virus vaccines include measles (rubeola and rubella), chickenpox, mumps, and the Sabin (oral) poliomyelitis vaccine (no longer used in the United States). Vaccines with killed viruses that may be administered in pregnancy include tetanus, diphtheria, recombinant hepatitis B, rabies, and flu vaccines.

Alcohol, Cigarette Smoke and Other Substances

A safe level of alcohol consumption during pregnancy has not yet been established. Although the consumption of occasional alcoholic beverages may not be harmful to the mother or her developing embryo or fetus, complete abstinence is strongly advised. Maternal alcoholism is associated with high rates of miscarriage and fetal alcohol syndrome; the risk for miscarriage is dose related (three or more drinks per day) in the first trimester. Although nonpregnant women report more alcohol use than do those who are pregnant, the use of at least some alcohol among pregnant women is still too high. This finding underscores the need for more systematic public health efforts to educate women about the hazards of alcohol consumption in pregnancy.

Cigarette smoking or continued exposure to secondhand smoke (even if the mother does not smoke) is associated with fetal growth restriction (IUGR) and an increase in perinatal and infant morbidity and mortality. Smoking is associated with an increased frequency of preterm labor, PROM, abruptio placentae, placenta previa, and fetal death, possibly resulting from decreased placental perfusion.

All women who smoke should be strongly encouraged to quit or at least reduce the number of cigarettes they smoke. Pregnant women need to be told about the negative effects of secondhand smoke on the fetus and encouraged to avoid such environments (Andres, 2004). Efforts focused on preventing girls and women from beginning to smoke should be intensified.

Patient Teaching

SAFETY DURING PREGNANCY

Changes in the body caused by pregnancy include relaxation of joints, alteration to center of gravity, faintness, and discomforts. Problems with coordination and balance are common. Therefore the woman should follow these guidelines:

- Use good body mechanics.
- Use safety features on tools/vehicles (safety seat belts, shoulder harnesses, headrests, goggles, helmets) as specified.
- Avoid activities requiring coordination, balance, and concentration.
- Take rest periods; reschedule daily activities to meet rest and relaxation needs.

Embryonic and fetal development are vulnerable to environmental teratogens. Many potentially dangerous chemicals are present in the home, yard, and workplace: cleaning agents, paints, sprays, herbicides, and pesticides. The soil and water supply may be unsafe. Therefore the woman should follow these guidelines:

- Read all labels for ingredients and proper use of product.
- Ensure adequate ventilation with clean air.
- Dispose of wastes appropriately.
- Wear gloves when handling chemicals.
- Change job assignments or workplace as necessary.
- Avoid high altitudes (not in pressurized aircraft), which could jeopardize oxygen intake.

Most studies of human pregnancy have revealed no association between caffeine consumption and birth defects or low birth weight (LBW) (Andres, 2004). Because other effects are unknown, however, pregnant women are advised to limit their caffeine intake.

Any drug or environmental agent that enters the pregnant woman's bloodstream has the potential to cross the placenta and harm the fetus. Marijuana, heroin, and cocaine are common examples of such substances. Although substance abuse in pregnancy is a major public health concern, comprehensive care of drug-addicted women improves maternal and neonatal outcomes (see Chapter 13).

Normal Discomforts

Pregnant women are confronted with symptoms that would be considered abnormal in the nonpregnant state. Much of prenatal care requested by women pregnant for the first time is prompted by the need for explanations of the causes of the discomforts and for advice on ways to relieve the discomforts. The discomforts are fairly specific to each trimester of pregnancy. Table 11-2 provides information about the physiology, prevention, and self-care of discomforts experienced during the three trimesters. Nurses can do much to allay a first-time mother's anxiety about such symptoms by telling her about them in advance, using terminology that the woman (or couple) can understand. Women who understand the physical discomforts of pregnancy are less apt to become overly anxious about their health. In addition, understanding the rationale for treatment promotes their participation in their care. Interventions should be individualized, with attention given to the woman's lifestyle and culture.

Evidence-Based Practice

PROMOTING SMOKING CESSATION DURING PREGNANCY

Background

Smoking during pregnancy is linked with low birth weight (less than 2500 g), very preterm birth (less than 32 weeks), perinatal death, low rates of breastfeeding, and shorter duration of breastfeeding. Characteristics of women likely to smoke during pregnancy include being of significantly higher parity and lower socioeconomic status, experiencing depression and job strain, and being more likely to be without a partner or practical support system. Even when they have these characteristics, however, certain groups still have lower smoking prevalence rates in pregnancy than the general population, as a result of cultural influences. For example, Mexican-American and African-American women have lower smoking rates in pregnancy, although the rate is rising. Widespread campaigns to discourage smoking during pregnancy may have decreased the incidence, but the women who continue to smoke experience guilt, anxiety, and stress on their relationships with families and health care providers. Smokers are notoriously unreliable in self-reporting how much they smoke, and this is exacerbated in pregnancy, leading to measurement errors in research. Some women erroneously believe that low birth weight is desirable for an easy delivery.

Objectives

The reviewers searched for studies comparing the efficacy of smoking cessation interventions in pregnancy. Interventions included information on the risks of smoking, advice to quit, individual counseling, group counseling, feedback of the pathophysiologic effects of smoking on mother or fetus, pictures of the fetus, nicotine replacement therapy, self-help manuals on strategies for quitting, and rewards and incentives. Outcomes included birth weight, gestation at birth, perinatal mortality, method of delivery, breastfeeding initiation and duration, maternal anxiety, depression, family functioning, duration of smoking cessation, and knowledge, attitudes, and behavior of health professionals regarding smoking in pregnancy.

Methods

Search Strategy

The authors searched the Cochrane database and the Cochrane Tobacco Addiction Group trials register. Search keywords were not reported. Thirty-seven trials, representing 16,916 women, were selected, dated 1976 to 1999. Most of the trials (27) took place in the United States, but other countries represented included the United Kingdom, Argentina, Brazil, Cuba, Mexico, New Zealand, Sweden, Australia, Canada, and Norway.

Statistical Analyses

The trials were grouped by type and intensity of the intervention. Similar data were pooled. Secondary analyses looked at some outcomes separately.

Findings

There was a significant decrease in smoking during late pregnancy in the intervention groups. The absolute difference between groups was 6.4%: of 100 women smokers, 10 will stop smoking as a result of "usual care," and a further 6 to 7 will stop as a result of intervention. Smoking cessation interventions were associated with significantly fewer low-birth-weight babies and preterm births, and increased mean birth weight. No differences were detected in very-low-birth-weight (less than 1500 g) and perinatal mortality rates.

Five trials had a smoking relapse prevention intervention, with even fewer women in late pregnancy smoking. About 25% of women who quit smoking during pregnancy relapse while still pregnant. Some data suggested that the stages of change (precontemplation, contemplation, preparation, and action) may be different in pregnancy, and that changes made in early pregnancy may not be sustained.

Limitations

A number of trials did not offer informed consent. Many trials did not discuss the method of randomization, and many were quasi-randomized. Since the interventions were not concealed, outside influence may have skewed the results. Intervention protocols varied quite a bit, as did duration of intervention and follow-up. Interventions may not have been culturally appropriate for every setting. The amount of smoking cessation intervention that occurs in the "usual care" control group more recently may exceed the intervention groups of decades ago. Health providers may find it difficult to treat women differently according to their randomized group allocation. Many withdrawals and dropouts in the trials leave gaps in the data. Women who had a fetal death or a preterm infant may not have been counted as late-pregnancy smokers, because they never reached 36 weeks. Self-report inaccuracies may be replaced with biochemical results.

Conclusions

Intervention is effective in assisting women to decrease smoking during late pregnancy. The women who quit smoking had fewer low-birth-weight babies and preterm births, but the interventions made no difference in incidence of very-low-birth-weight (less than 1500 g) babies or perinatal mortality rate.

Implications for Practice

All maternity settings need smoking cessation programs. This review makes it clear that smoking cessation groups perform poorly. Further education can be fostered with programs that take into account the concerns of women who smoke, the staff who counsel them, and cognitive-behavioral strategies and relapse prevention. Health care providers need to team with other community educators to prevent smoking onset in young people and address socioeconomic inequities and stresses.

Implications for Further Research

Standardization of intervention and outcome measures would strengthen the ability to determine which smoking cessation interventions are successful in pregnancy. Biochemical markers are better indicators of smoking behavior than self-report. Targeting teens would benefit a subset of the population already at risk for low-birth-weight babies. These trials did not measure methods of delivery, breastfeeding, or maternal or family psychologic well-being.

Reference

Lumley J, Oliver S, Waters E: Interventions for promoting smoking cessation during pregnancy (Cochrane Review), 1999. In *The Cochrane Library,* Issue 2, Chichester, UK, 2004, John Wiley & Sons.

NURSE ALERT Although complementary and alternative therapies may benefit the woman during pregnancy, some practices should be avoided because they may cause miscarriage or preterm labor (Beal, 1998). It is important to ask the woman what therapies she may be using (Box 11-7). ■

Recognizing Potential Complications

One of the most important responsibilities of care providers is to alert the pregnant woman to signs and symptoms that indicate a potential complication of pregnancy. The woman needs to know how and to whom such warning

Text continued on p. 288.

Table 11-2

Discomforts Related to Pregnancy

First Trimester		
DISCOMFORT	PHYSIOLOGY	EDUCATION FOR SELF-CARE
Breast changes, new sensation; pain, tingling, tenderness	Hypertrophy of mammary glandular tissue and increased vascularization, pigmentation, and size and prominence of nipples and areolae caused by hormonal stimulation	Wear supportive maternity bras with pads to absorb discharge, may be worn at night; wash with warm water and keep dry; breast tenderness may interfere with sexual expression/foreplay but is temporary
Urgency and frequency of urination	Vascular engorgement and altered bladder function caused by hormones; bladder capacity reduced by enlarging uterus and fetal presenting part	Empty bladder regularly; perform Kegel exercises; limit fluid intake before bedtime; wear perineal pad; report pain or burning sensation to primary health care provider
Languor and malaise; fatigue (early pregnancy, most commonly)	Unexplained; may be caused by increasing levels of estrogen, progesterone, and hCG or by elevated BBT; psychologic response to pregnancy and its required physical/psychologic adaptations	Rest as needed; eat well-balanced diet to prevent anemia
Nausea and vomiting, morning sickness—occurs in 50%-75% of pregnant women; starts between first and second missed periods and lasts until about fourth missed period; may occur any time during day; fathers also may have symptoms	Cause unknown; may result from hormonal changes, possibly hCG; may be partly emotional, reflecting pride in, ambivalence about, or rejection of pregnant state	Avoid empty or overloaded stomach; maintain good posture—give stomach ample room; stop smoking; eat dry carbohydrate on awakening; remain in bed until feeling subsides, or alternate dry carbohydrate 1 hr with fluids such as hot herbal decaffeinated tea, milk, or clear coffee the next hour until feeling subsides; eat five to six small meals per day; avoid fried, odorous, spicy, greasy, or gas-forming foods; consult primary health care provider if intractable vomiting occurs
Ptyalism (excessive salivation) may occur starting 2 to 3 weeks after first missed period	Possibly caused by elevated estrogen levels; may be related to reluctance to swallow because of nausea	Use astringent mouthwash, chew gum, eat hard candy as comfort measures
Gingivitis and epulis (hyperemia, hypertrophy, bleeding, tenderness); condition will disappear spontaneously 1 to 2 months after birth	Increased vascularity and proliferation of connective tissue from estrogen stimulation	Eat well-balanced diet, with adequate protein and fresh fruits and vegetables; brush teeth gently and observe good dental hygiene; avoid infection; see dentist
Nasal stuffiness; epistaxis (nosebleed)	Hyperemia of mucous membranes related to high estrogen levels	Use humidifier; avoid trauma; normal saline nose drops or spray may be used
Leukorrhea: often noted throughout pregnancy	Hormonally stimulated cervix becomes hypertrophic and hyperactive, producing abundant amount of mucus	Not preventable; do not douche; wear perineal pads; perform hygienic practices such as wiping front to back; report to primary health care provider if accompanied by pruritus, foul odor, or change in character or color
Psychosocial dynamics, mood swings, mixed feelings	Hormonal and metabolic adaptations; feelings about female role, sexuality, timing of pregnancy, and resultant changes in life and lifestyle	Participate in pregnancy support group; communicate concerns to partner, family, and others; request referral for supportive services if needed (financial assistance)

BBT, basal body temperature; *hCG*, human chorionic gonadotropin.

Continued

Table 11-2

Discomforts Related to Pregnancy—cont'd

Second Trimester		
DISCOMFORT	PHYSIOLOGY	EDUCATION FOR SELF-CARE
Pigmentation deepens, acne, oily skin	Melanocyte-stimulating hormone (from anterior pituitary)	Not preventable; usually resolves during puerperium
Spider nevi (angiomas) appear over neck, thorax, face, and arms during second or third trimester	Focal networks of dilated arterioles (end-arteries) from increased concentration of estrogens	Not preventable; they fade slowly during late puerperium; rarely disappear completely
Palmar erythema occurs in 50% of pregnant women; may accompany spider nevi	Diffuse reddish mottling over palms and suffused skin over thenar eminences and fingertips; may be caused by genetic predisposition or hyperestrogenism	Not preventable; condition will fade within 1 week after giving birth
Pruritus (noninflammatory)	Unknown cause; various types as follows: nonpapular; closely aggregated pruritic papules	Keep fingernails short and clean; contact primary health care provider for diagnosis of cause
	Increased excretory function of skin and stretching of skin possible factors	Not preventable; symptomatic; Keri baths; mild sedation
		Distraction; tepid baths with sodium bicarbonate or oatmeal added to water; lotions and oils; change of soaps or reduction in use of soap; loose clothing
Palpitations	Unknown; should not be accompanied by persistent cardiac irregularity	Not preventable; contact primary health care provider if accompanied by symptoms of cardiac decompensation
Supine hypotension (vena cava syndrome) and bradycardia	Induced by pressure of gravid uterus on ascending vena cava when woman is supine; reduces uteroplacental and renal perfusion	Side-lying position or semisitting posture, with knees slightly flexed (see also Emergency box, p. 272.)
Faintness and, rarely, syncope (orthostatic hypotension) may persist throughout pregnancy	Vasomotor lability or postural hypotension from hormones; in late pregnancy may be caused by venous stasis in lower extremities	Moderate exercise, deep breathing, vigorous leg movement; avoid sudden changes in position* and warm crowded areas; move slowly and deliberately; keep environment cool; avoid hypoglycemia by eating five to six small meals per day; wear elastic hose; sit as necessary; if symptoms are serious, contact primary health care provider
Food cravings	Cause unknown; craving determined by culture or geographic area	Not preventable; satisfy craving unless it interferes with well-balanced diet; report unusual cravings to primary health care provider
Heartburn (pyrosis or acid indigestion): burning sensation, occasionally with burping and regurgitation of a little sour-tasting fluid	Progesterone slows gastrointestinal (GI) tract motility and digestion, reverses peristalsis, relaxes cardiac sphincter, and delays emptying time of stomach; stomach displaced upward and compressed by enlarging uterus	Limit or avoid gas-producing or fatty foods and large meals; maintain good posture; sip milk for temporary relief; hot herbal tea; primary health care provider may prescribe antacid between meals; contact primary health care provider for persistent symptoms

*Caution woman to rise slowly and sit on edge of bed or to assume hands-and-knees posture before rising, and to get up slowly after sitting or squatting.

Table 11-2

Discomforts Related to Pregnancy—cont'd

Second Trimester—cont'd		
DISCOMFORT	PHYSIOLOGY	EDUCATION FOR SELF-CARE
Constipation	GI tract motility slowed because of progesterone, resulting in increased resorption of water and drying of stool; intestines compressed by enlarging uterus; predisposition to constipation because of oral iron supplementation	Drink six glasses of water per day; include roughage in diet; moderate exercise; maintain regular schedule for bowel movements; use relaxation techniques and deep breathing; do not take stool softener, laxatives, mineral oil, other drugs, or enemas without first consulting primary health care provider
Flatulence with bloating and belching	Reduced GI motility because of hormones, allowing time for bacterial action that produces gas; swallowing air	Chew foods slowly and thoroughly; avoid gas-producing foods, fatty foods, large meals; exercise, maintain regular bowel habits
Varicose veins (varicosities): may be associated with aching legs and tenderness; may be present in legs and vulva; hemorrhoids are varicosities in perianal area	Hereditary predisposition; relaxation of smooth muscle walls of veins because of hormones causing tortuous dilated veins in legs and pelvic vasocongestion; condition aggravated by enlarging uterus, gravity, and bearing down for bowel movements; thrombi from leg varices rare but may be produced by hemorrhoids	Avoid obesity, lengthy standing or sitting, constrictive clothing, and constipation and bearing down with bowel movements; moderate exercises; rest with legs and hips elevated (see Fig. 11-17); wear support stockings; thrombosed hemorrhoid may be evacuated; relieve swelling and pain with warm sitz baths, local application of astringent compresses
Leukorrhea: often noted throughout pregnancy	Hormonally stimulated cervix becomes hypertrophic and hyperactive, producing abundant amount of mucus	Not preventable; do not douche; maintain good hygiene; wear perineal pads; report to primary health care provider if accompanied by pruritus, foul odor, or change in character or color
Headaches (through week 26)	Emotional tension (more common than vascular migraine headache); eye strain (refractory errors); vascular engorgement and congestion of sinuses resulting from hormone stimulation	Conscious relaxation; contact primary health care provider for constant "splitting" headache to assess for preeclampsia
Carpal tunnel syndrome (involves thumb, second and third fingers, lateral side of little finger)	Compression of median nerve resulting from changes in surrounding tissues; pain, numbness, tingling, burning; loss of skilled movements (typing); dropping of objects	Not preventable; elevate affected arms; splinting of affected hand may help; regressive after pregnancy; surgery is curative
Periodic numbness, tingling of fingers (acrodysesthesia) occurs in 5% of pregnant women	Brachial plexus traction syndrome resulting from drooping of shoulders during pregnancy (occurs especially at night and early morning)	Maintain good posture; wear supportive maternity bra; condition will disappear if lifting and carrying baby does not aggravate it
Round ligament pain (tenderness)	Stretching of ligament caused by enlarging uterus	Not preventable; rest, maintain good body mechanics to avoid overstretching ligament; relieve cramping by squatting or bringing knees to chest, sometimes heat helps
Joint pain, backache, and pelvic pressure; hypermobility of joints	Relaxation of symphyseal and sacroiliac joints because of hormones, resulting in unstable pelvis; exaggerated lumbar and cervicothoracic curves caused by change in center of gravity resulting from enlarging abdomen	Maintain good posture and body mechanics; avoid fatigue; wear low-heeled shoes; abdominal supports may be useful; conscious relaxation; sleep on firm mattress; apply local heat or ice; get back rubs; do pelvic rock exercise; rest; condition will disappear 6 to 8 weeks after birth

Continued

Table 11-2

Discomforts Related to Pregnancy—cont'd

Third Trimester		
DISCOMFORT	PHYSIOLOGY	EDUCATION FOR SELF-CARE
Shortness of breath and dyspnea occur in 60% of pregnant women	Expansion of diaphragm limited by enlarging uterus; diaphragm is elevated about 4 cm; some relief after lightening	Good posture; sleep with extra pillows; avoid overloading stomach; stop smoking; contact health care provider if symptoms worsen to rule out anemia, emphysema, and asthma
Insomnia (later weeks of pregnancy)	Fetal movements, muscle cramping, urinary frequency, shortness of breath, or other discomforts	Reassurance; conscious relaxation; back massage or effleurage; support of body parts with pillows; warm milk or warm shower before retiring
Psychosocial responses: mood swings, mixed feelings, increased anxiety	Hormonal and metabolic adaptations; feelings about impending labor, birth, and parenthood	Reassurance and support from significant other and nurse; improved communication with partner, family, and others
Gingivitis and epulis (hyperemia, hypertrophy, bleeding, tenderness): condition will disappear spontaneously 1 to 2 months after birth	Increased vascularity and proliferation of connective tissue from estrogen stimulation	Well-balanced diet with adequate protein and fresh fruits and vegetables; gentle brushing and good dental hygiene; avoid infection; see dentist for teeth cleaning
Urinary frequency and urgency return	Vascular engorgement and altered bladder function caused by hormones; bladder capacity reduced by enlarging uterus and fetal presenting part	Empty bladder regularly, Kegel exercises; limit fluid intake before bedtime; reassurance; wear perineal pad; contact health care provider for pain or burning sensation
Perineal discomfort and pressure	Pressure from enlarging uterus, especially when standing or walking; multifetal gestation	Rest, conscious relaxation, and good posture; contact health care provider for assessment and treatment if pain is present
Leg cramps (gastrocnemius spasm), especially when reclining	Compression of nerves supplying lower extremities because of enlarging uterus; reduced level of diffusible serum calcium or elevation of serum phosphorus; aggravating factors: fatigue, poor peripheral circulation, pointing toes when stretching legs or when walking, drinking more than 1 L (1 qt) of milk per day	Check for Homans' sign; if negative, use massage and heat over affected muscle; dorsiflex foot until spasm relaxes (see Fig. 11-18); stand on cold surface; oral supplementation with calcium carbonate or calcium lactate tablets; aluminum hydroxide gel, 30 ml, with each meal removes phosphorus by absorbing it
Ankle edema (nonpitting) to lower extremities	Edema aggravated by prolonged standing, sitting, poor posture, lack of exercise, constrictive clothing (e.g., garters), or by hot weather	Ample fluid intake for natural diuretic effect; put on support stockings before arising; rest periodically with legs and hips elevated (see Fig. 11-17); exercise moderately; contact health care provider if generalized edema develops; *diuretics are contraindicated*

signs should be reported (see Box 11-5). It is difficult to remember specifics when stressed by a disturbing symptom. Therefore the woman and her family can be reassured if they receive and use a printed form listing the signs and symptoms that warrant an investigation and the phone numbers to call with questions or in an emergency.

The nurse must answer questions honestly as they arise during pregnancy. Pregnant women often have difficulty deciding when to report signs and symptoms. The mother is encouraged to refer to the printed list of potential complications and to listen to her body. If she senses that something is wrong, she should call her care provider immediately. Several signs and symptoms must be discussed more extensively. These include vaginal bleeding, alteration in fetal movements, symptoms of preeclampsia, rupture of membranes, and preterm labor.

BOX 11-7

Complementary and Alternative Therapies Used in Pregnancy

Morning Sickness and Hyperemesis
Acupuncture
Acupressure (see Figs. 1-2 and 16-6)
Shiatzu
Herbal remedies*
- Peppermint
- Spearmint
- Ginger root
- Raspberry leaf
- Fennel
- Chamomile
- Hops
- Meadowsweet
- Wild yam root

Relaxation and Muscle-Ache Relief
Yoga
Biofeedback
Reflexology
Therapeutic touch

From Beal MW: Women's use of complementary and alternative therapies in reproductive health, *J Nurse Midwifery* 43(3):224-233, 1998; and Schirmer G: *Herbal medicine*, Bedford, TX, 1998, MED2000 Inc.
*Some herbs can cause miscarriage, preterm labor, or fetal or maternal injury. Pregnant women should discuss use with pregnancy health care provider, as well as an expert qualified in the use of the herb.

Recognizing Preterm Labor

Teaching each expectant mother to recognize preterm labor is necessary. Preterm labor occurs after the twentieth week but before the thirty-seventh week of pregnancy. It consists of uterine contractions that, if untreated, cause the cervix to open earlier than normal, resulting in preterm birth.

Although certain factors, such as multifetal pregnancy, may increase a woman's chances of going into preterm labor, the specific cause (or causes) is usually not known. An increased incidence of preterm birth is associated with sociodemographic factors such as poverty, low educational level, lack of social support, smoking, domestic violence, and stress (Challis & Lye, 2004). The rate of prematurity is almost twice as high in the African-American population as in Caucasians.

If a woman knows the warning signs and symptoms of preterm labor and seeks care early enough, prevention of preterm birth may be possible. Warning signs and symptoms of preterm labor are given in the Home Care box. Fig. 11-20 shows where in the body the signs and symptoms of preterm labor may be located.

Moore and colleagues (1998) demonstrated that nursing telephone support to at-risk women can result in a significant decrease in LBW and preterm births in African-American women. This study and others demonstrate the power of nursing care, nursing support, and patient education in the care of women at highest risk for preterm birth.

Sexual Counseling

Sexual counseling of expectant couples includes countering misinformation, providing reassurance of normality, and suggesting alternative behaviors. The uniqueness of each couple is considered within a biopsychosocial framework (Guidelines box).

Many women merely need "permission" to be sexually active during pregnancy. Many other women, however, need information about the physiologic changes that occur during pregnancy and to dispel myths associated with sex during pregnancy. Such tasks are within the purview of the

Home Care

HOW TO RECOGNIZE PRETERM LABOR

Because the onset of preterm labor is subtle and often hard to recognize, it is important to know how to feel your abdomen for uterine contractions. You can feel for contractions in the following way. While lying down, place your fingertips on the top of your uterus. A contraction is the periodic tightening or hardening of your uterus. If your uterus is contracting, you will actually feel your abdomen get tight or hard and then feel it relax or soften when the contraction is over.

If you think you are having any of the other signs and symptoms of preterm labor, empty your bladder, drink three to four glasses of water for hydration, lie down tilted toward your side, and place a pillow at your back for support.

Check for contractions for 1 hour. To tell how often contractions are occurring, check the minutes that elapse from the beginning of one contraction to the beginning of the next.

It is *not normal* to have frequent uterine contractions (every 10 minutes or more often for 1 hour).

Contractions of labor are regular, frequent, and hard. They also may be felt as a tightening of the abdomen or a backache. This type of contraction causes the cervix to efface and dilate.

Call your doctor, nurse-midwife, clinic, or labor and birth unit, or go to the hospital, if any of the following signs occur:
- You have uterine contractions every 10 minutes or more often for 1 hour or
- You have any of the other signs and symptoms for 1 hour or
- You have any bloody spotting or leaking of fluid from your vagina

It is often difficult to identify preterm labor. Accurate diagnosis requires assessment by the health care provider, usually in the hospital or clinic.

Post these instructions where they can be seen by everyone in the family.

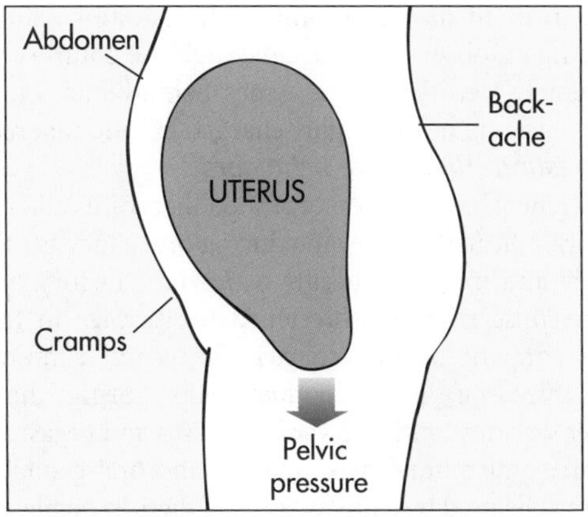

Fig. 11-20 Symptoms of preterm labor.

Guidelines

SEXUALITY IN PREGNANCY

- Be aware that maternal physiologic changes, such as breast enlargement, nausea, fatigue, abdominal changes, perineal enlargement, leukorrhea, pelvic vasocongestion, and orgasmic responses, may affect sexuality and sexual expression.
- Discuss responses to pregnancy with your partner.
- Keep in mind that cultural prescriptions (do's) and proscriptions (don'ts) may affect your responses.
- Although your libido may be depressed during the first trimester, it often increases during the second and third trimesters.
- Discuss and explore with your partner:
  Alternative behaviors (e.g., mutual masturbation, foot massage, cuddling)
  Alternative positions (e.g., female superior, side lying) for sexual intercourse
- Intercourse is safe as long as it is not uncomfortable. There is no correlation between intercourse and miscarriage, but observe the following precautions:
  Abstain from intercourse if you experience uterine cramping or vaginal bleeding; report event to your caregiver as soon as possible.
  Abstain from intercourse (or any activity that results in orgasm) if you have a history of premature dilation of the cervix until the problem is corrected.
- Continue to use "safer sex" behaviors. Women at risk for acquiring or conveying STIs are encouraged to use condoms during sexual intercourse throughout pregnancy.

maternity nurse and should be an integral component of the health care provided. However, not all maternity nurses are comfortable dealing with the sexual concerns of their patients.

Some couples need to be referred for sex therapy or family therapy. Couples whose long-standing sexual dysfunction is intensified by pregnancy are good candidates for sex therapy. When a sexual problem is a symptom of a more serious relationship problem, the couple would benefit from family therapy.

Countering Misinformation

Many myths and much of the misinformation related to sex and pregnancy are masked by seemingly unrelated issues. For example, a discussion about the baby's ability to hear and see in utero may be prompted by questions about the baby being an observer of lovemaking. The counselor must be extremely sensitive to the issues behind such questions when counseling in this highly charged emotional area.

Suggesting Alternative Behaviors

Researchers have not demonstrated that coitus and orgasm are contraindicated at any time during pregnancy for the obstetrically and medically healthy woman. A history of more than one miscarriage; a threatened miscarriage in the first trimester; impending miscarriage in the second trimester; and PROM, bleeding, or abdominal pain during the third trimester warrant caution regarding coitus and orgasm.

Solitary and mutual masturbation and oral-genital intercourse may be used by couples as alternatives to penile-vaginal intercourse. Partners who enjoy cunnilingus (oral stimulation of the clitoris or vagina) may feel "turned off" by the normal increase in amount and odor of vaginal discharge during pregnancy. Couples who practice cunnilingus should be cautioned against the blowing of air into the vagina, particularly during the last few weeks of pregnancy, when the cervix may be slightly open. An air embolism can occur if air is forced between the uterine wall and fetal membranes and enters the maternal vascular system through the placenta.

Showing the woman or couple illustrations of the possible variations of coital position is helpful (Fig. 11-21). The female-superior, side-by-side, rear-entry, and facing-each-other positions are alternatives to the traditional male-superior position. The woman astride (superior position) allows her to control the angle and depth of penile penetration, as well as protect her breasts and abdomen. During the third trimester, the side-by-side position or any position that places less pressure on the pregnant abdomen and requires less energy may be preferred.

Multiparous women sometimes experience significant breast tenderness in the first trimester. A coital position that avoids direct pressure on the woman's breasts, and decreased breast fondling during love play, can be recommended to such couples. The woman should also be reassured that this condition is normal and temporary.

Some women complain of lower abdominal cramping and backache after orgasm during the first and third trimesters. A back rub can often relieve some of the discomfort and provide a pleasant experience. A tonic uterine contraction, often lasting up to a minute, replaces the rhythmic contractions of orgasm during the third trimester. Changes in FHR without fetal distress have also been reported.

The objective of "safer sex" is to provide prophylaxis against the acquisition and transmission of STIs (e.g., HSV, human papillomavirus, and HIV). Because these diseases may be transmitted to the woman and her fetus, the use of condoms is recommended throughout pregnancy if the woman is at risk for an STI.

Well-informed nurses who are comfortable with their own sexuality and the sexual counseling needs of expectant couples can offer information and advice in this valuable but often neglected area. They can establish an open environment in which couples can feel free to introduce their concerns about sexual adjustment and seek support and guidance. This intervention is as important for lesbian women and their partners as it is for women partnered with men.

Psychosocial Support

Esteem, affection, trust, concern, consideration of cultural and religious responses, and listening are all components of the emotional support given to the pregnant woman and her family. The woman's satisfaction with her relationships and support, her feeling of competence, and her sense of being in control are important issues to be addressed in the third trimester. A discussion of fetal responses to stimuli such as sound, light, maternal posture, and tension, as well as patterns of sleeping and waking, can be helpful. Also discussed are emotional tensions that can arise in relation to the childbirth experience, such as those stemming from fear of pain, loss of control, and possible birth of the infant before reaching the hospital. Parental concerns about the responsibilities and tasks of parenthood; about the safety of the mother and unborn child; about siblings and their ac-

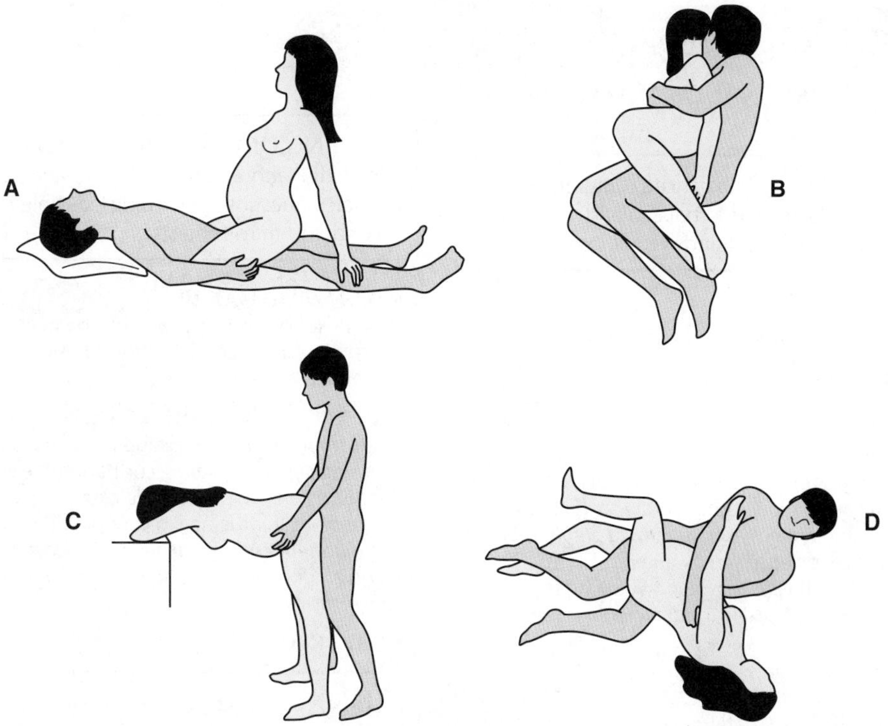

Fig. 11-21 Positions for sexual intercourse during pregnancy. **A**, Female superior. **B**, Side by side. **C**, Rear entry. **D**, Facing each other.

ceptance of the new baby; about social and economic responsibilities; and about possible conflicts in cultural, religious, or personal value systems are addressed.

The father's or partner's commitment to the pregnancy, the couple's relationship, and their concerns about sexuality and sexual expression can emerge as issues for many expectant parents. Validation, feedback, and social comparison characterize the support given.

Providing the prospective mother and father with opportunities to discuss their concerns and validating the normality of their responses can meet their needs to some degree. Nurses must also recognize that men feel more vulnerable during their partner's pregnancy. Female partners may also have these feelings. Anticipatory guidance and health promotion strategies can help partners cope with their concerns. Nursing intervention may help them to deal with such concerns either directly through counseling or indirectly through the education of the mothers. Health care providers can stimulate and encourage open dialogue between the couple.

Evaluation

Evaluation of the effectiveness of care of the woman during pregnancy is based on the previously stated outcomes. More effort is needed in evaluating outcomes of nursing care during the prenatal period. A formal systematic follow-up on quality of care is not common but needs to be developed and incorporated in all settings (Nursing Care Plan).

Variations in Prenatal Care

The course of prenatal care described thus far may seem to suggest that the experiences of childbearing women are similar and that nursing interventions are uniform across all populations. Although typical patterns of response to pregnancy are easily recognized, and many aspects of prenatal care indeed are consistent, pregnant women enter the health care system with individual concerns and needs. The nurse's ability to assess unique needs and to tailor interventions to the individual is the hallmark of expertise in providing care. Variations that influence prenatal care include culture, age, and number of fetuses.

Cultural Influences

Prenatal care as North Americans know it is a phenomenon of Western medicine. In the Western biomedical model of care, women are encouraged to seek prenatal care as early as possible in their pregnancy by visiting a physician, nurse-midwife, office, or clinic. Such visits are routine and follow a systematic sequence, with the initial visit followed by monthly, then semimonthly, then weekly visits. Monitoring weight and blood pressure; testing blood and urine; teaching specific information about diet, rest, and activity; and preparing for childbirth are common components of prenatal care. This model is not only unfamiliar but may seem strange to many groups. Different models for providing prenatal care for women in other parts of the world are being explored (Chalmers, Mangiaterra, & Porter, 2001).

Many cultural variations in prenatal care exist. Even if the prenatal care described is familiar to a woman, some practices may conflict with the beliefs and practices of a subculture group to which she belongs. Because of these and other factors, such as lack of money, lack of transportation, and poor communication on the part of health care providers, women from many such groups do not participate in the prenatal care system. The nurse may misinterpret their behavior as uncaring, lazy, or ignorant.

Nursing Care Plan

DISCOMFORTS OF PREGNANCY AND WARNING SIGNS

FIRST TRIMESTER

NURSING DIAGNOSIS: Imbalanced nutrition: less than body requirements, related to nausea and vomiting as evidenced by woman's report and weight loss

EXPECTED OUTCOME

Woman will gain 1 to 2.5 kg during the first trimester.

NURSING INTERVENTIONS/*RATIONALES*

Obtain diet history *to identify current meal patterns and foods that may be implicated in nausea.*

Advise woman to consume small frequent meals and avoid having empty stomach *to avoid further nausea episodes.*

Suggest that woman eat a simple carbohydrate such as dry crackers before arising in the morning *to avoid empty stomach and decrease incidence of nausea and vomiting.*

Advise woman to call health care provider if vomiting is persistent and severe *to identify possible incidence of hyperemesis gravidarum.*

NURSING DIAGNOSIS: Fatigue related to hormonal changes in the first trimester as evidenced by woman's complaints

EXPECTED OUTCOME

Woman will report a decreased number of episodes of fatigue.

NURSING INTERVENTIONS/*RATIONALES*

Rest as needed *to avoid increasing feeling of fatigue.*

Eat a well-balanced diet *to meet increased metabolic demands and avoid anemia.*

Discuss the use of support systems to help with household responsibilities *to decrease workload at home and decrease fatigue.*

Reinforce to woman the transitory nature of first trimester fatigue *to provide emotional support.*

SECOND TRIMESTER

NURSING DIAGNOSIS: Constipation related to progesterone influence on GI tract as evidenced by woman's report of altered patterns of elimination

EXPECTED OUTCOME

Woman will report a return to normal bowel elimination pattern following implementation of interventions.

NURSING INTERVENTIONS/*RATIONALES*

Provide information to woman regarding pregnancy-related causes: progesterone slowing gastrointestinal motility, growing uterus compressing intestines, and influence of iron supplementation *to provide basic information for self-care during pregnancy.*

Assist woman to plan a diet that will promote regular bowel movements, such as increasing amount of oral fluid intake to at least six glasses of water a day and increasing the amount of fiber in daily diet, and to maintain moderate exercise *to promote self-care.*

NURSING DIAGNOSIS: Anxiety related to deficient knowledge about course of pregnancy as evidenced by woman's questions regarding possible complications of second and third trimesters

EXPECTED OUTCOME

Woman will correctly list signs of potential complications that can occur during the second and third trimesters and exhibit no overt signs of stress.

NURSING INTERVENTIONS/*RATIONALES*

Provide information concerning the potential complications or warning signs that can occur during the second and third trimesters, including possible causes of signs and the importance of calling the health care provider immediately, *to ensure identification and treatment of problems in a timely manner.*

Provide a written list of complications *to have a reference list for emergencies.*

THIRD TRIMESTER

NURSING DIAGNOSIS: Disturbed sleep pattern related to discomforts/insomnia of third trimester as evidenced by woman's report of inadequate rest

EXPECTED OUTCOME

Woman will report an improvement of quality and quantity of rest and sleep.

NURSING INTERVENTIONS/*RATIONALES*

Assess current sleep pattern and review need for increased requirement during pregnancy *to identify need for change in sleep patterns.*

Suggest change of position to side-lying position with pillows between legs or to sleep in semi-Fowler position *to increase support and decrease any problems with dyspnea or heartburn.*

Reinforce the possibility of the use of various sleep aids such as relaxation techniques, reading, and decreased activity before bedtime *to decrease the possibility of anxiety or physical discomforts before bedtime.*

NURSING DIAGNOSIS: Ineffective sexuality patterns related to changes in comfort level and fatigue

EXPECTED OUTCOME

Woman will verbalize feelings regarding changes in sexual desire.

NURSING INTERVENTIONS/*RATIONALES*

Assess couple's usual sexual patterns *to determine how patterns have been altered by pregnancy.*

Provide information regarding expected changes in sexual patterns during pregnancy *to correct any misconceptions.*

Allow the couple to express feelings in a nonjudgmental atmosphere *to promote trust.*

Suggest alternative sexual positions *to decrease pressure on enlarging abdomen of woman and increase sexual comfort and satisfaction of couple.*

Refer couple for counseling as appropriate *to assist the couple to cope with sexuality pattern changes.*

For many women, concern for modesty is a deterrent for seeking prenatal care. Some women consider exposing body parts, especially to a man, a major violation of their modesty. For many women, invasive procedures such as vaginal examination may be so threatening that they cannot be discussed even with their own husbands. Thus many women prefer a female over a male health care provider. Most women value and appreciate efforts to maintain their modesty.

In many cultural groups a physician is deemed appropriate only in times of illness. Because pregnancy is considered a normal process and the woman is in a state of health, the services of a physician are considered inappropriate. Even if what are considered problems with pregnancy by standards of Western medicine do develop, they may not be perceived as problems by members of other cultural groups.

Although pregnancy is considered normal by many, certain practices are expected of women of all cultures to ensure a good outcome. Cultural prescriptions tell women what to do, whereas cultural proscriptions establish taboos. The purposes of these practices are to prevent maternal illness caused by a pregnancy-induced imbalanced state and to protect the vulnerable fetus. Prescriptions and proscriptions regulate the woman's emotional response, clothing, physical activity and rest, sexual activity, and dietary practices. Exploration of the woman's beliefs, perceptions of the meaning of childbearing, and health care practices may help health care providers foster her self-actualization, promote attainment of the maternal role, and positively influence her relationship with her spouse.

To provide culturally sensitive care, the nurse must be knowledgeable about practices and customs, although it is not possible to know all there is to know about every culture and subculture or the many lifestyles that exist (Fig. 11-22). When exploring cultural beliefs and practices related to childbearing, the nurse can support and nurture those beliefs that promote physical or emotional adaptation. However, if potentially harmful beliefs or activities are identified, the nurse should sensitively provide education and propose modifications.

Emotional Response

Virtually all cultures emphasize the importance of maintaining a socially harmonious and agreeable environment for the pregnant woman. An absence of stress is important in ensuring a successful outcome for mother and baby. Harmony with other people must be fostered, and visits from extended family members may be required to demonstrate pleasant and noncontroversial relationships. If discord exists in a relationship, it is usually dealt with in culturally prescribed ways.

Besides proscriptions regarding food, other proscriptions involve imitative magic. For example, some Mexicans believe pregnant women should not be allowed to witness an eclipse of the moon because it may cause a cleft palate in the infant. They also believe that exposure to an earthquake may precipitate preterm birth, miscarriage, or a breech presentation. In some cultures, a pregnant woman must not ridicule someone with an affliction for fear her child might be born with the

Community Focus

CULTURE AND CHILDBIRTH BELIEFS AND PRACTICES

Select an immigrant or other minority group in your community and identify childbirth-related beliefs and practices that are unique to that group. Are there stores in the area that sell items that meet the needs of that group? Does the community center have activities or classes that are directed toward that group? Are there childbirth education programs available that provide essential information while incorporating cultural patterns? What could you, as a nurse, contribute to the community that would help meet the needs of that group?

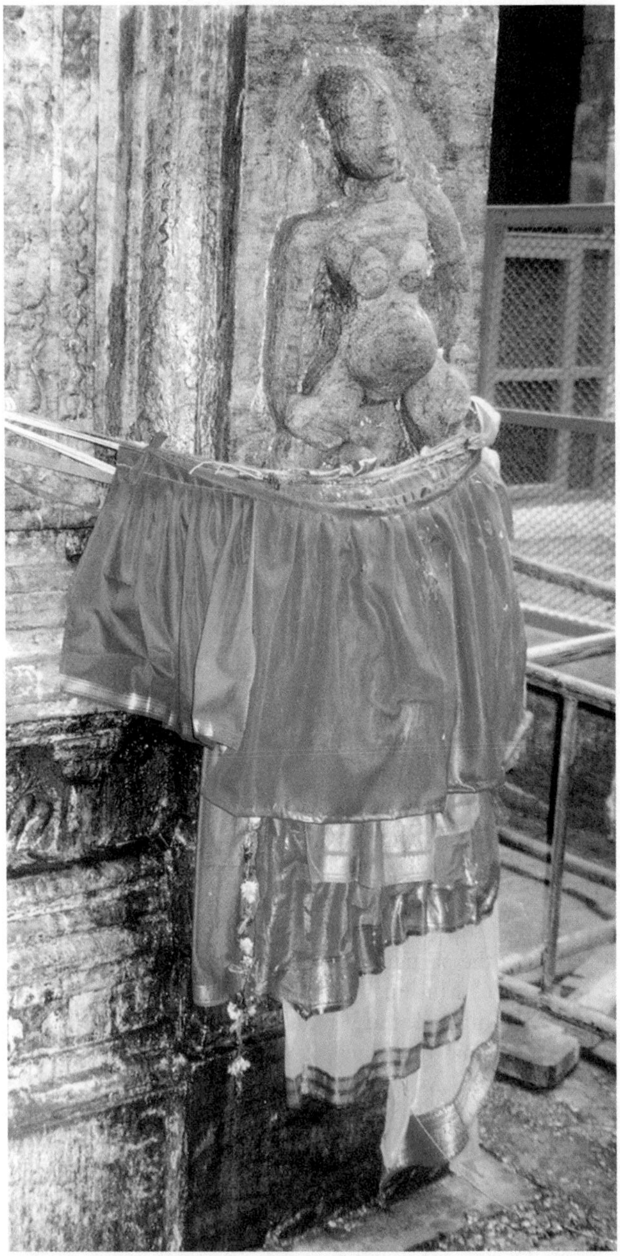

Fig. 11-22 Pregnant Hindu goddess in a temple in India. Women leave offerings and pray for a healthy baby and pregnancy and a safe delivery. (Courtesy Joan Vogel, Boca Raton, FL.)

same handicap. A mother should not hate a person lest her child resemble that person, and dental work should not be done during pregnancy because it may cause a baby to have a "harelip." A folk belief widely held in many cultures is that the pregnant woman should refrain from raising her arms above her head and from tying knots because such movements tie knots in the umbilical cord and may cause it to wrap around the baby's neck. Another belief is that placing a knife under the bed of a laboring woman will "cut" her pain.

Clothing

Although most cultural groups do not prescribe specific clothing for pregnancy, modesty is an expectation for many. Some Mexican women of the Southwest wear a cord beneath the breasts and knotted over the umbilicus. This cord, called a muñeco, is thought to prevent morning sickness and ensure a safe birth. Amulets, medals, and beads also may be worn to ward off evil spirits.

Physical Activity and Rest

Norms that regulate physical activity of mothers during pregnancy vary tremendously. Many groups, including Native Americans and some Asian groups, encourage women to be active, to walk, and to engage in normal although not strenuous activities to ensure that the baby is healthy and not too large. Other groups, such as Filipinos, believe that any activity is dangerous, and others willingly take over the work of the pregnant woman. Some Filipinos believe that this inactivity protects the mother and child. The mother is encouraged simply to produce the succeeding generation. If health care providers do not know of this belief, they could misinterpret this behavior as laziness or noncompliance with the desired prenatal health care regimen. It is important for the nurse to find out the way each pregnant woman views activity and rest.

Sexual Activity

In most cultures, sexual activity is not prohibited until the end of pregnancy. Some Latinos view sexual activity as necessary to keep the birth canal lubricated. Conversely, some Vietnamese may have definite proscriptions about sexual intercourse, requiring abstinence throughout the pregnancy because it is thought that sexual intercourse may harm the mother and the fetus.

Diet

Nutritional information given by Western health care providers may be a source of conflict for many cultural groups. Such a conflict commonly is not known by health care providers unless they understand the dietary beliefs and practices of the particular people for whom they are caring. For example, Muslims have strict regulations regarding preparation of food, and if meat cannot be prepared as prescribed, they may omit meat from their diets. Many cultures permit pregnant women to eat only warm foods.

Age

The age of the childbearing couple may have a significant influence on their physical and psychosocial adaptation to pregnancy. Normal developmental processes that occur in both very young and older mothers are interrupted by pregnancy and require a different type of adaptation to pregnancy than that of the woman of typical childbearing age. Although the individuality of each pregnant woman is recognized, special needs of expectant mothers age 15 years or younger or those age 35 years or older are summarized here.

Adolescents

About 1 million adolescent females in the United States, or 4 out of every 10 girls, become pregnant each year. Most of the pregnancies are unintended; 56% end in live birth; 29% end in induced abortion; and 15% end in miscarriage (Arias et al, 2003). Adolescents are responsible for almost 500,000 births in the United States annually. Hispanic adolescents currently have the highest birth rate, although the rate for African-American adolescents also is high. Of girls who become pregnant, 21% are repeat pregnancies (Arias et al, 2003). Most of these young women are unmarried, and many are not ready for the emotional, psychosocial, and financial responsibilities of parenthood.

Despite these alarming statistics, and the fact that the United States has the highest adolescent birth rate in the industrialized world, the birth rate for adolescents has steadily declined since 1991 (Arias et al, 2003). Concentrated national efforts have spawned a host of adolescent pregnancy prevention programs that have had varying degrees of success (Ford et al, 2002). Characteristics of programs that make a difference are those that have sustained commitment to adolescents over a long period, involve the parents and other adults in the community, promote abstinence and personal responsibility, and assist adolescents to develop a clear strategy for reaching future goals such as a college education or a career.

When adolescents become pregnant and decide to give birth, they are much less likely than older women to receive adequate prenatal care, with many receiving no care at all (Ford et al, 2002). These young women also are more likely to smoke and less likely to gain adequate weight during pregnancy. As a result of these and other factors, babies born to adolescents are at greatly increased risk of LBW, of serious and long-term disability, and of dying during the first year of life.

Delayed entry into prenatal care may be the result of late recognition of pregnancy, denial of pregnancy, or confusion about the services that are available. Such a delay in care may leave an inadequate time before birth to attend to correctable problems. The very young pregnant adolescent is at higher risk for each of the confounding variables associated with poor pregnancy outcomes (e.g., socioeconomic factors) and for those conditions associated with a first pregnancy regardless of age (e.g., preeclampsia). However, when prenatal care is initiated early and consistently, and confounding variables are controlled, very young pregnant adolescents are at no greater risk (nor are their infants) for an adverse outcome than older pregnant women. Thus the role of the nurse in reducing the risks and consequences of adolescent pregnancy is twofold: first, to encourage early and continued prenatal care; and second, to refer the adolescent, if necessary, for appropriate social support services, which can help reverse the effects of a negative socioeconomic environment (Fig. 11-23; Nursing Care Plan).

Women Older Than 35 Years of Age

Two groups have emerged in the population of women having a child late in their childbearing years. One group consists of women who have many children or who have an

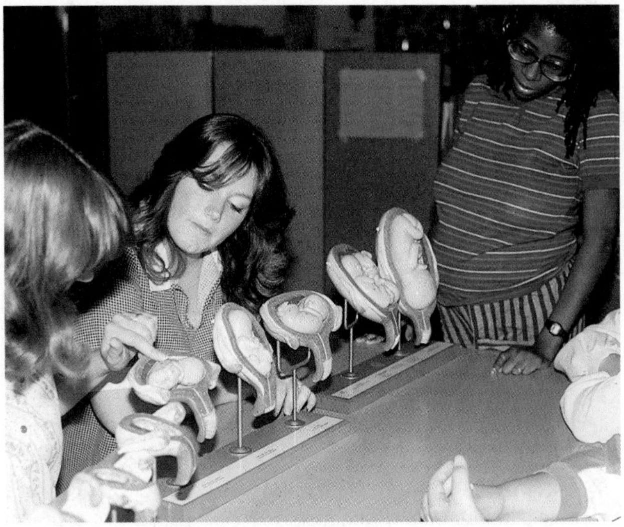

Fig. 11-23 Pregnant adolescents review fetal development. (Courtesy Marjorie Pyle, RNC, Lifecircle, Costa Mesa, CA).

additional child during the menopausal period. The other group consists of relative newcomers to maternity care. These are women who have deliberately delayed childbearing until their late thirties or early forties.

Multiparous Women

Multiparous women may have never used contraceptives because of personal choice or because of a lack of knowledge concerning contraceptives. They also may be women who have used contraceptives successfully during the childbearing years but, as menopause approaches, cease menstruating regularly, stop using contraception, and subsequently become pregnant. The older multiparous woman may feel that pregnancy separates her from her peer group and that her age is a hindrance to close associations with young mothers. Other parents welcome the unexpected infant as evidence of continuing maternal and paternal roles.

Nulliparous Women

The number of first-time pregnancies in women between ages 35 and 40 years has increased significantly over the last three decades (Tough et al, 2002). It is common now to see women in their late thirties or early forties pregnant for the first time. Reasons for delaying pregnancy include advanced education, career priorities, better contraceptive measures, and infertility.

These women choose parenthood over a childfree lifestyle. They often are established in a career and a lifestyle with a partner that includes time for self-attention, the establishment of a home with accumulated possessions, and freedom to travel. Questioned as to why they chose pregnancy later in life, many reply, "Because time is running out."

The dilemma of choice includes recognition that being a parent will have both positive and negative consequences. Couples need to discuss the consequences of childbearing and childrearing before committing themselves to this lifelong venture. Partners in this group seem to share the preparation for parenthood, the planning for a family-centered birth, and the desire to be loving and competent parents. However, the reality of child care may prove difficult for such parents.

As with mothers of all ages, the mother over 35 who is accustomed to the stimulation of and contact with other adults may find isolation with her infant difficult to accept. Anger and resentment toward the father (or infant) can result, even with anticipatory guidance for these aspects of parenting.

First-time mothers older than 35 years select the "right time" for pregnancy; this time is influenced by their awareness of the increasing possibility of infertility or of genetic defects in the infants of older women. Such women seek information about pregnancy from books and friends. They actively try to prevent fetal disorders and are careful in searching for the best possible maternity care. They identify sources of stress in their lives. They have concerns about having enough energy and stamina to meet the demands of parenting and their new roles and relationships.

If they become pregnant after treatment for infertility, they may suddenly have negative or ambivalent feelings about the pregnancy. They may experience a multifetal pregnancy that may create emotional and physical problems. Adjusting to parenting two or more infants requires adaptability and additional resources.

During pregnancy, parents explore the possibilities and responsibilities of changing identities and new roles. They must prepare a safe and nurturing environment during pregnancy and after birth. They must integrate the child into an established family system and negotiate new roles (e.g., parent roles, sibling roles, and grandparent roles) for family members.

Adverse perinatal outcomes are more common in older primiparas than in younger women, even when they receive good prenatal care. Women 35 years of age and older are more likely than younger primiparas to have LBW infants, premature birth, IUGR, and abruptio placentae (Tough et al, 2002). The incidence of malpresentation also is more common in older primiparas, and they are more likely to have a cesarean birth. In uncomplicated pregnancies, older mothers have significantly less fear of helplessness and loss of control in labor than younger women. Age and education are thought to balance the concerns of the older mothers related to age.

Multifetal Pregnancy

A multifetal pregnancy, or pregnancy with more than one fetus, places the mother and fetuses at risk. The maternal blood volume is increased, resulting in an increased strain on the maternal cardiovascular system. Anemia often develops because of a greater demand for iron by the fetuses. Marked uterine distention and increased pressure on the adjacent viscera and pelvic vasculature and diastasis of the two rectus abdominis muscles may occur (see Fig. 10-11). Placenta previa develops more commonly in multifetal pregnancies because of the large size or placement of the placentas (Clark, 2004). Premature separation of the placenta may occur before the second and any subsequent fetuses are born.

Twin pregnancies often end prematurely. Spontaneous rupture of membranes before term is common. Congenital malformations are twice as common in monozygotic twins as in singletons. No increase is seen in the incidence of congenital anomalies in dizygotic twins. Two-vessel cords (i.e.,

Nursing Care Plan

ADOLESCENT PREGNANCY

NURSING DIAGNOSIS: Imbalanced nutrition: less than body requirements related to intake insufficient to meet metabolic needs of fetus and adolescent patient

EXPECTED OUTCOMES

Patient will gain weight as prescribed by age, take prenatal vitamins/iron as prescribed, and maintain normal hematocrit and hemoglobin.

NURSING INTERVENTIONS/*RATIONALES*

Assess current diet history/intake *to determine prescriptions for additions or changes in present dietary pattern.*

Compare prepregnancy weight with current weight *to determine if pattern is consistent with appropriate fetal growth and development.*

Provide information concerning food prescriptions for appropriate weight gain, considering preferences for "fast food" and peer influences, *to correct any misconceptions and increase chances for compliance with diet.*

Include patient's immediate family or support system during instruction *to ensure that person preparing family meals receives information.*

NURSING DIAGNOSIS: Risk for injury, maternal or fetal, related to inadequate prenatal care and screening

EXPECTED OUTCOMES

Patient will experience uncomplicated pregnancy and give birth to a healthy fetus at term.

NURSING INTERVENTIONS/*RATIONALES*

Provide information, using therapeutic communication and confidentiality, *to establish relationship and build trust.*

Discuss importance of ongoing prenatal care and possible risks to adolescent patient and fetus *to reinforce that ongoing assessment is crucial to health and well-being of patient and fetus, even if patient feels well. The adolescent patient is more at risk for certain complications that may be avoided or managed early if prenatal visits are maintained.*

Discuss risks of alcohol, tobacco, and recreational drug use during pregnancy *to minimize risks to patient and fetus, because adolescent patients have a higher abuse rate than the rest of the pregnant population.*

Assess for evidence of sexually transmitted infection (STI) and provide information regarding safer sexual practices *to minimize risk to patient and fetus, because adolescent is more at risk for STIs.*

Screen for preeclampsia on an ongoing basis *to minimize risk, because adolescent population is more at risk for preeclampsia.*

NURSING DIAGNOSIS: Social isolation related to body image changes of pregnant adolescent as evidenced by patient statements and concerns

EXPECTED OUTCOMES

Patient will identify support systems and report decreased feelings of social isolation.

NURSING INTERVENTIONS/*RATIONALES*

Establish a therapeutic relationship *to listen objectively and establish trust.*

Discuss with patient changes in relationships that have occurred as a result of the pregnancy *to determine extent of isolation from family, peers, and father of the baby.*

Provide referrals and resources appropriate for developmental stage of patient *to give information for patient support.*

Provide information regarding parenting classes, breastfeeding classes, and childbirth-preparation classes *to give further information and group support, which lessens social isolation.*

NURSING DIAGNOSIS: Interrupted family processes related to adolescent pregnancy

EXPECTED OUTCOME

Patient will reestablish relationship with her mother and father of baby.

NURSING INTERVENTIONS/*RATIONALES*

Encourage communication with mother *to clarify roles and relationships related to birth of infant.*

Encourage communication with father of baby (if she desires continued contact) *to ascertain level of support to be expected of father of baby.*

Refer to support group *to learn more effective problem-solving methods and reduce conflict within the family.*

NURSING DIAGNOSIS: Disturbed body image related to situational crisis of pregnancy

EXPECTED OUTCOME

Pregnant adolescent will verbalize positive comments regarding her body image during the pregnancy.

NURSING INTERVENTIONS/*RATIONALES*

Assess pregnant adolescent's perception of self related to pregnancy *to provide basis for further interventions.*

Give information regarding expected body changes occurring during pregnancy *to provide a realistic view of these temporary changes.*

Provide opportunity to discuss personal feelings and concerns *to promote trust and support.*

NURSING DIAGNOSIS: Risk for impaired parenting related to immaturity and lack of experience in new role of adolescent mother

EXPECTED OUTCOME

Parents will demonstrate parenting roles with confidence.

NURSING INTERVENTIONS/*RATIONALES*

Provide information on growth and development *to enhance knowledge so that adolescent mother can have basis for caring for her infant.*

Refer to parenting classes *to enhance knowledge and obtain support for providing appropriate care to newborn and infant.*

Initiate discussion of child care *to assist adolescent in problem solving for future needs.*

Assess parenting abilities of adolescent mother and father *to provide baseline for education.*

Provide information on parenting classes that are appropriate for parents' developmental stage *to give opportunity to share common feelings and concerns.*

Assist parents to identify pertinent support systems *to give assistance with parenting as needed.*

cords with a single umbilical artery) occur more often in twins than in singletons; this abnormality is most common in monozygotic twins. The most serious problem for the fetus is the local shunting of blood between placentas (twin-to-twin transfusion); this causes the recipient twin to be larger and the donor twin to be small, pallid, dehydrated, malnourished, and hypovolemic. However, the larger twin may develop congenital heart failure during the first 24 hours after birth.

The clinical diagnosis of multifetal pregnancy is accurate in about 90% of cases. The likelihood of a multifetal pregnancy is increased if any one or a combination of the following factors is noted during a careful assessment:

- History of dizygotic twins in the female lineage
- Use of fertility drugs
- More rapid uterine growth for the number of weeks of gestation
- Hydramnios
- Palpation of more than the expected number of small or large parts
- Asynchronous fetal heartbeats or more than one fetal electrocardiographic tracing
- Ultrasonographic evidence of more than one fetus

The diagnosis of multifetal pregnancy can come as a shock to many expectant parents, and they may need additional support and education to help them cope with the changes they face. The mother needs nutrition counseling so that she gains more weight than that needed for a singleton birth. She should also be counseled that maternal adaptations will probably be more uncomfortable, and provided with information about the possibility of a preterm birth.

If the presence of more than three fetuses is diagnosed, the parents may receive counseling regarding selective reduction of the fetuses to reduce the incidence of premature birth and improve the opportunities for the remaining fetuses to grow to term gestation (Malone & D'Alton, 2004). This situation poses an ethical dilemma for many couples, especially those who have worked hard to overcome problems with infertility and those who harbor strong values regarding the right to life. The nurse able to engage the couple in discussion to identify what resources could help the couple (e.g., a minister, priest, rabbi, or mental health counselor) can make the decision-making process somewhat less traumatic.

Prenatal care given to women with multifetal pregnancies includes changes in the pattern of care and modifications in other aspects such as the amount of weight gained and the nutritional intake observed. The prenatal visits of these mothers are scheduled at least every 2 weeks in the second trimester and weekly thereafter. The recommended weight gain in twin gestations is 16 to 20 kg. No specific recommendation for weight gain for women with higher-order multifetal pregnancies has been made, but it is likely to be more than with twin gestation (Malone & D'Alton, 2004). Iron and vitamin supplements are desirable. Attempts are made to prevent preeclampsia and eclampsia, which occur more commonly during multifetal pregnancies, and vaginitis; if these conditions cannot be prevented, they are treated.

The considerable uterine distention involved can cause the backache commonly experienced by pregnant women to be even worse. Elastic stockings or maternity tights may be worn to control leg varicosities. If risk factors for preterm birth such as premature dilation of the cervix or bleeding are present, abstinence from orgasm and nipple stimulation during the last trimester is recommended to help prevent preterm labor. Frequent ultrasound examinations and heart rate monitoring will occur. Some practitioners recommend bed rest beginning at 20 weeks to prevent preterm labor in women carrying multiple fetuses. Other practitioners question the value of prolonged bed rest. If bed rest is recommended, the mother needs to assume the lateral position to promote increased placental perfusion. If birth is delayed until after the thirty-sixth week, the risk of morbidity and mortality decreases for the neonates.

Multiple newborns will likely place a strain on finances, space, workload, and the mother's and family's coping abilities. Lifestyle changes may be necessary. Parents will need assistance in making realistic plans for the care of the babies, for example, whether to breastfeed and whether to raise them as "alike" or as separate individuals. Parents should be referred to national organizations such as Parents of Twins, Mothers of Multiples, and the La Leche League for further support.

Childbirth and Perinatal Education

The goal of childbirth and perinatal education is to assist individuals and their family members to make informed, safe decisions about pregnancy, birth, and early parenthood. It also is to assist them to comprehend the long-lasting potential that empowering birth experiences have in the lives of women and that early experiences have on the development of children and the family. The perinatal education program is an expansion of the earlier childbirth education movement that originally offered a set of classes in the third trimester of pregnancy to prepare parents for birth. Today perinatal education programs consist of a menu of class series and activities from preconception through the early months of parenting.

Preconception education and care are designed to foster conscious conception and health maintenance, to promote healthy behaviors for the health of the woman and her potential fetus, and to foster risk management as needed. Preconception and early pregnancy education, therefore, fosters behaviors in potential parents to do the following:

- Establish lifestyle behaviors to maintain optimal health (e.g., eating a healthy diet, including sources of folic acid; getting enough rest and exercise; and avoiding alcohol use, smoking, and other drugs).
- Prepare psychologically for pregnancy and the responsibilities that come with parenthood and build a support system to sustain the new family throughout the perinatal year.
- Identify, minimize, or treat risk factors before conception (e.g., medical conditions such as diabetes mellitus, substance abuse, use of medications for chronic illness, or infections, including STIs).
- Screen for health hazards in the workplace or home.
- Obtain, when warranted, genetic counseling to identify carriers of inherited diseases (i.e., Tay-Sachs disease, sickle cell disease, or thalassemia).

- Compare the quality and philosophic bases of the perinatal care options available.

The components of general preconception education, such as health promotion, risk assessment, and interventions, are outlined in Box 11-8.

All health-promoting education should be provided in a context that emphasizes how well designed a healthy body is to adapt to the changes that accompany pregnancy. Without this context of health, routine care and testing for risks may contribute to a mindset of families that pregnancy is a pathologic as opposed to a healthy mind-body-spirit event (Strong, 2002).

Some of the decisions the childbearing family must consider are the decision to have a baby, followed by choices of a care provider and type of care (a midwifery [natural-oriented] model versus a medical [intervention-oriented] model), the place for birth (hospital, birthing center, home), and the type of infant feeding (breast or bottle) and care. If a woman has had a previous cesarean birth, she may consider having a vaginal birth. This section discusses these choices and the nurse's role in educating childbearing families to make informed decisions about them.

Previous pregnancy and childbirth experiences are important elements that influence current learning needs. The patient's (and support person's) age, cultural background, personal philosophy in regard to childbirth, socioeconomic status, spiritual beliefs, and learning styles all need to be assessed to develop the best plan to help the woman meet her needs.

Most childbirth education classes are attended by the pregnant woman and her partner, although a friend, teenage daughter, or parent may be the designated support person. Classes may also be held for grandparents and siblings to prepare them for their attendance at birth or the arrival of the baby (see Fig. 11-4). Siblings often see a film about birth and learn ways they can help welcome the baby. They also learn to cope with changes that include a reduction in parental time and attention. Grandparents learn about current child care practices and how to help their adult children adapt to parenting in a supportive way.

BOX 11-8

Components of Preconception Care

Health Promotion: General Teaching

Nutrition
- Healthy diet, including folic acid
- Optimal weight

Exercise and rest

Avoidance of substance abuse (tobacco, alcohol, "recreational" drugs)

Use of safer sex practices

Attending to family and social needs

Risk Factor Assessment

Medical history
- Immune status (e.g., rubella)
- Family history (e.g., genetic disorders)
- Illnesses (e.g., infections)
- Current use of medication (prescription, nonprescription, herbal)

Reproductive history
- Contraceptive
- Obstetric

Psychosocial history
- Spouse/partner and family situation, including domestic violence
- Availability of family or other support systems
- Readiness for pregnancy (e.g., age, life goals, stress)

Financial resources

Environmental (home, workplace) conditions
- Safety hazards
- Toxic chemicals
- Radiation

Interventions as Indicated

Anticipatory guidance/teaching

Treatment of medical conditions and results
- Medications
- Cessation/reduction in substance use/abuse
- Immunizations (e.g., rubella, hepatitis)

Nutrition, diet, and weight management

Exercise

Referral for genetic counseling

Referral to and use of
- Family planning services
- Family and social needs management

Perinatal Care Choices

The Coalition to Improve Maternity Services (CIMS), a group of more than 50 nursing and maternity care–oriented organizations, produced a document to assist women in selecting their perinatal care. After some explanation of choices, women are encouraged to ask potential care providers the following questions:

- Who can be with me during labor and birth?
- What happens during a normal labor and birth in your setting?
- How do you allow for differences in culture and beliefs?
- Can I walk and move around during labor? What position do you suggest for birth?
- How do you make sure everything goes smoothly when my nurse, doctor, midwife, or agency work with each other?
- What things do you normally do to a woman in labor?
- How do you help mothers stay as comfortable as they can be? Besides drugs, how do you help mothers relieve the pain of labor?
- What if my baby is born early or has special problems?
- Do you circumcise babies?
- How do you help mothers who want to breastfeed?

The entire document can be downloaded from www.motherfriendly.org. By using a related CIMS questionnaire provided by Hotelling (2004), hospitals and birthing centers can apply to CIMS to be designated Mother Friendly, and such ratings can be passed on to expectant parents.

Childbirth Education

Childbirth, when one is prepared and well supported, presents to women a unique and powerful opportunity to find their core strength in a manner that forever changes their self-perception. Expectant parents and their families have different interests and information needs as the pregnancy progresses.

Early pregnancy ("early bird") classes provide fundamental information. Classes are developed around the following areas: (1) early fetal development, (2) physiologic and emotional changes of pregnancy, (3) human sexuality, and (4) the nutritional needs of the mother and fetus. Environmental and workplace hazards may be addressed. Exercises, nutrition, warning signs, drugs, and self-medication are topics of interest and concern.

Midpregnancy classes emphasize the woman's participation in self-care. Classes provide information on preparation for breastfeeding and formula feeding; infant care; basic hygiene; common complaints and simple, safe remedies; infant health; parenting; and updating and refining the birth plans.

Late pregnancy classes emphasize labor and birth. Different methods of coping with labor and birth have been developed and are often the basis for various prenatal classes. These include Lamaze, Bradley, and Dick-Read. A hospital tour is usually included.

Throughout the series of classes there is discussion of support systems that people can use during pregnancy and after birth. Such support systems help parents function independently and effectively. During all the classes the open expression of feelings and concerns about any aspect of pregnancy, birth, and parenting is welcomed.

Fathers or partners often worry about their role during childbirth classes and labor and birth, as well as the safety of their partner and baby during the birth. Many fathers elect to participate actively during labor and the birth of their child. As noted earlier, however, some men, through personal or cultural conception of the father role, neither want nor intend to participate. It is important that the partners agree on each other's roles.

Current Practices in Childbirth Education

A variety of approaches to childbirth education have evolved as childbirth educators attempt to meet learning needs. In addition to classes designed specifically for pregnant adolescents, their partners, or parents, classes exist for other groups with special learning needs. These include classes for first-time mothers over 35, single women, adoptive parents, and parents of twins. Refresher classes for parents with children not only review coping techniques for labor and birth but also help couples prepare for sibling reactions and adjustments to a new baby. Cesarean birth classes are offered for couples who have this kind of birth scheduled because of breech position or other risk factors. Other classes focus on vaginal birth after cesarean (VBAC), because many women successfully give birth vaginally after previous cesarean birth.

Strategies for Childbirth Education

Because of the multicultural composition of the population in North America, there is great diversity in attitudes, expectations, and behaviors judged appropriate during pregnancy and early parenthood. No one approach can meet all needs. For example, classes for new immigrants are particularly effective when taught in a native language (e.g., Spanish, Tagalog, Cantonese). For classes to be meaningful, parent educators must understand the value systems in other cultures and their influence on issues such as nutrition, exercise, valuing of early prenatal care, maternal weight gain, and infant feeding practices. Parent educators must establish rapport, be understood, and build on cultural practices, reinforcing the positive and promoting change only if a practice, such as pica, is directly harmful.

Options for Care Providers

Often the first decision the woman makes is who will be her primary health care provider for the pregnancy and birth. This decision is doubly important because it usually affects where the birth will take place. The nurse can provide information about the different types of health care providers and what kind of care to expect from each type.

Physicians

Physicians (obstetricians, family practice physicians) attend about 91% of births in the United States and Canada (Martin et al, 2003). They see low risk and high risk patients. Care often includes pharmacologic and medical management of problems, as well as use of technologic procedures. Family practice physicians may need backup by obstetricians if a specialist is needed for a problem (e.g., a cesarean birth). Most physicians manage births in a hospital setting.

Nurse-Midwives

Nurse-midwives are registered nurses with advanced training in care of obstetric patients. They provide care for about 8% of the births in the United States and Canada (Martin et al, 2003). Nurse-midwives may practice with physicians or independently with an arrangement for physician backup. They usually see low risk obstetric patients. Care is often noninterventionist, and the woman and her family are encouraged to be active participants in the care. Nurse-midwives must refer patients to physicians for complications. Most births are managed in hospital settings or alternative birth centers; a few may be managed in a home setting.

Direct-Entry Midwives

Direct-entry midwives are trained in midwifery schools or universities as a profession distinct from nursing. Increasing numbers of midwives in the United Kingdom and Ireland are in this category.

Independent Midwives

Independent midwives, who also may be called lay midwives, are nonprofessional caregivers. Their training varies greatly, from formal training to self-teaching. They manage about 1% of births in the United States and Canada. Patients who develop problems need to be seen by a physician. A majority (61%) of births are managed in the home setting.

Doula

A doula is professionally trained to provide labor support, including physical, emotional, and informational support to women and their partners during labor and birth. The doula does not become involved with clinical tasks (Doulas of North America, 1999a, 1999b, 1999c). A doula typically meets with the mother and her partner before labor to ascertain their expectations and desires for the birth experience. Working collaboratively with other health care providers and the woman's supportive individuals, the doula focuses efforts on assisting the woman to achieve her goals. Box 11-9 provides questions to ask when interviewing a prospective doula. See Resources at the end of this chapter for organizations that offer information or referral services.

Although the doula role originally developed as an assistant during labor, some women need assistance during the postpartum period. There are small but growing numbers of

evolve CASE STUDY: THIRD TRIMESTER

CASE STUDY: THIRD TRIMESTER

BOX 11-9

Questions to Ask When Choosing a Doula

To discover the specific training, experience, and services offered by anyone who provides labor support, potential patients, nursing supervisors, physicians, midwives, and others should ask the following questions of that person:

- What training have you had?
- Tell me about your experience with birth, personally and as a doula.
- What is your philosophy about childbirth and supporting women and their partners through labor?
- May we meet to discuss our birth plans and the role you will play in supporting me through childbirth?
- May we call you with questions or concerns before and after the birth?
- When do you try to join women in labor? Do you come to our home or meet us at the hospital?
- Do you meet with us after the birth to review the labor and answer questions?
- Do you work with one or more backup doulas for times when you are not available? May we meet them?
- What is your fee?

From Simkin P, Way K: *DONA position paper: the doula's contributions to modern maternity care,* Seattle, WA, 1998, Doulas of North America.

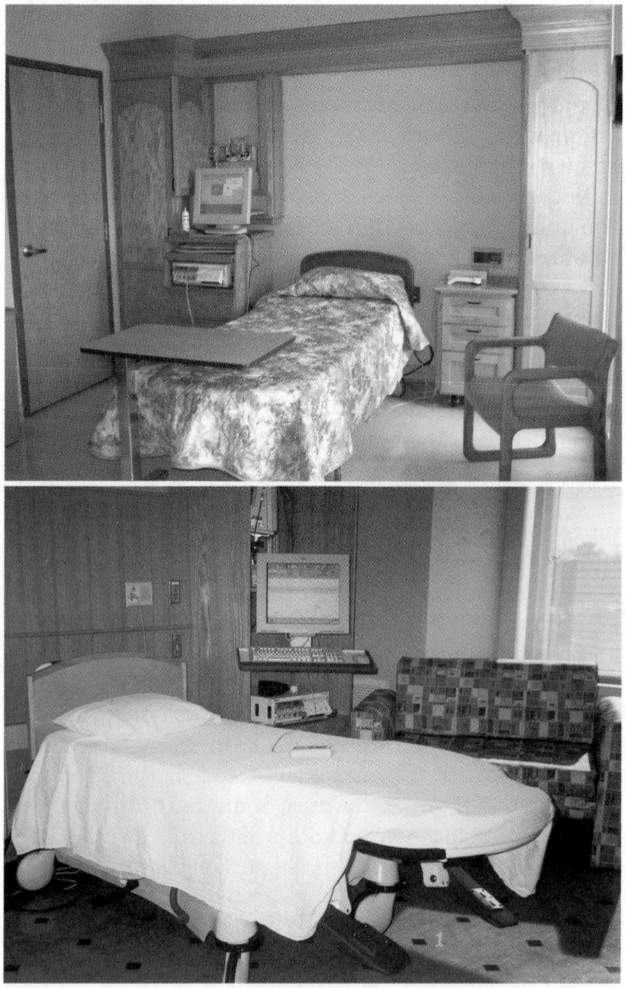

A

B

Fig. 11-24 **A,** LDR unit. **B,** LDRP unit. (*A,* Courtesy Julie Perry Nelson, Gilbert, AZ. *B,* Courtesy Dee Lowdermilk, Chapel Hill, NC.)

postnatal doulas, who provide assistance to the new mother as she develops competence with infant care, feeding, and other maternal tasks.

Birth Setting Choices

With careful thought, the concept of natural, family, or woman-centered maternity care can be implemented in any setting. The three primary options for birth settings today are the hospital, birth center, and home. Women consider several factors in choosing a setting for childbirth, including the preference of their health care provider, characteristics of the birthing unit, and preference of their third-party payer. Approximately 99% of all births in the United States take place in a hospital setting (Martin et al, 2003). However, the types of labor and birth services vary greatly, from the traditional labor and delivery rooms with separate postpartum and newborn units, to in-hospital birthing centers where all or almost all care takes place in a single unit.

Labor, Delivery, Recovery, Postpartum (Birthing) Rooms

Labor, delivery, and recovery (LDR) and labor, delivery, recovery, and postpartum (LDRP) rooms offer families a comfortable, private space for childbirth (Fig. 11-24). Women are admitted to LDR units, labor and give birth, and spend the first 1 to 2 hours postpartum there for immediate recovery and to have time with their families to bond with their newborns. After this period of recovery, the mothers and newborns are transferred to a postpartum unit and nursery or mother-baby unit for the duration of their stay.

In LDRP units, total care is provided from admission for labor through postpartum discharge in the same room and usually by the same nursing staff. The woman and her family may stay in this unit for 6 to 48 hours after giving birth. The units are furnished in a homelike atmosphere, similar to LDR units, but have accommodations for family members to stay overnight (see Fig. 11-24, *B*).

Both units are equipped with fetal monitors, emergency resuscitation equipment for both mother and newborn, and heated cribs or warming units for the newborn. Often this equipment is out of sight in cabinets or closets when it is not being used (see Fig. 11-24, *A*).

Birth Centers

Free-standing birth centers are usually built in locations separate from the hospital but may be located nearby in case transfer of the woman or newborn is needed. These birth centers are intended to offer families a safe and cost-effective alternative to hospital or home birth. The centers are usually staffed by nurse-midwives or physicians who also have privileges at the local hospital. Only women at low risk for complications are included for care. Attendance at childbirth and parenting classes is required of all patients. The family is admitted to the birth center for labor and birth and will remain there until discharge, which often takes place within 6 hours of the birth.

Birth centers typically have homelike accommodations, including a double bed for the couple and a crib for the newborn (Fig. 11-25, *A*). Emergency equipment and drugs are

A

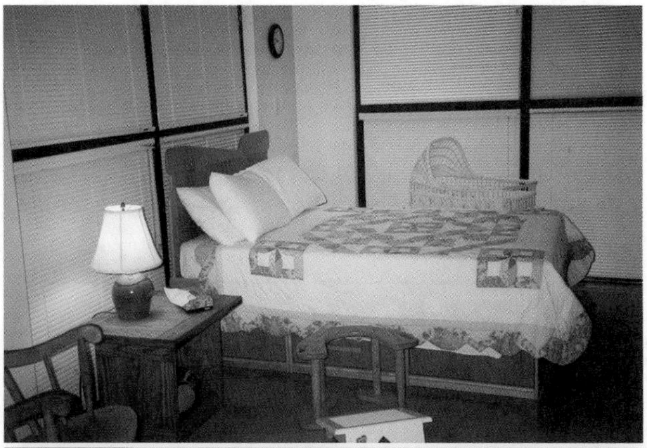

B

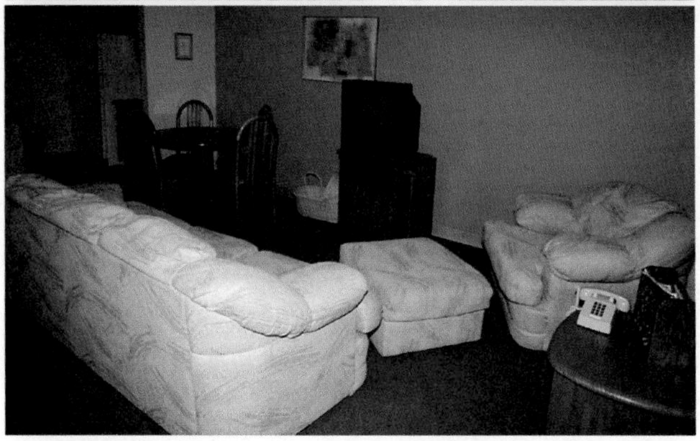

Fig. 11-25 Birth center. **A,** Note double bed, baby crib, and birthing stool. **B,** Lounge and kitchen. (*A,* Courtesy Dee Lowdermilk, Chapel Hill, NC. *B,* Courtesy Michael S. Clement, MD, Mesa, AZ. Photo location: Bethany Birth Center, Phoenix, AZ.)

stored discreetly within cupboards, out of view but easily accessible. Private bathroom facilities are incorporated into each birth unit. There may be an early labor lounge or a living room and small kitchen (Fig. 11-25, *B*).

Services provided by the free-standing birth centers include those necessary for safe management during the childbearing cycle. Patients must understand that some situations require transfer to a hospital, and they must agree to abide by those guidelines. Expectant families develop birth plans, that is, the practices and procedures they would like to either include or exclude from their childbirth experience.

Birth centers, as well as a hospital with a comprehensive birthing program, may have resources for parents, such as a lending library that includes books and videotapes; reference files on related topics; recycled maternity clothes, baby clothes, and equipment; and supplies and reference materials for childbirth educators. The centers may also have referral files for community resources that offer services relating to childbirth and early parenting, including support groups (e.g., for single parents, for postbirth support, and for parents of twins), genetic counseling, women's issues, and consumer action.

When births occur in a birth center or a home setting, they should be located close to a major hospital so that quick transfer to that institution is possible when necessary. Ambulance service and emergency procedures must be readily available. Fees vary with the services provided but typically are less than or equal to those charged by local hospitals. Some base fees on the ability of the family to pay (a reduced-fee sliding scale). Several third-party payers, as well as Medicaid and the Civilian Health and Medical Programs of the Uniformed Services (TRICARE/CHAMPUS), recognize and reimburse these centers.

Home Birth

Home birth has always been popular in certain countries, such as Sweden and The Netherlands. In developing countries, hospitals or adequate lying-in facilities often are unavailable to most pregnant women, and home birth is a necessity. In North America, home births account for less than 1% of births (Martin et al, 2003).

National groups supporting home birth are the Home Oriented Maternity Experience (HOME) and the National Association of Parents for Safe Alternatives in Childbirth (NAPSAC). These groups work to foster more humane childbearing practices at all levels, integrating the alternatives for childbirth to meet the needs of the total population.

With a home birth the family is in control of the experience, and the birth may be more physiologically natural in familiar surroundings. The mother may be more relaxed than she would be in the hospital environment. The family can assist in and be a part of the birth, and the mother-father/partner-infant (and sibling-infant) contact is immediate and sustained. Home birth may be less expensive than a hospital confinement. Serious infection may be less likely (assuming strict aseptic principles are followed) because it is usual for people to be relatively immune to the bacteria in their own home.

Although some physicians and nurses support home births that use good medical and emergency backup systems, many regard this practice as exposing the mother and the fetus to unnecessary danger. Thus home births are not widely accepted by the North American medical community. This makes it difficult for a family to find a qualified health care provider willing to give prenatal care and to attend the birth. Backup emergency care by a physician in a hospital may be difficult to arrange in advance. If an emergency birth is necessary, no effective way exists to do this rapidly in the home setting.

Factors Increasing the Safety of Birth at Home

Most health care providers agree that if home birth is the woman's choice, certain criteria promote a safe home birth experience. The woman must be comfortable with her decision to have her baby at home. She should be in good health. Home birth is not indicated for women with a high risk pregnancy. A drive to the hospital (if needed) should take no more than 10 to 15 minutes. The woman should be attended by a well-trained physician or midwife with adequate medical supplies and resuscitation equipment, including oxygen.

Pain Management

Fear of pain in labor is a key issue for pregnant women and the reason many give for attending childbirth education classes. Numerous studies show that women who have received childbirth preparation later report no less pain but do report greater ability to cope with the pain during labor and birth and increased birth satisfaction than unprepared

Critical Thinking Exercise

DECIDING ABOUT A HOME BIRTH

Millie, 28 years old and gravida 1, para 0, is interested in having a home birth. She is currently 14 weeks pregnant and her pregnancy is progressing normally. According to an ultrasound examination, she has one fetus, which is appropriate size for gestational age with no detectable anomalies. She asks a nurse on the obstetric clinic about how to find a midwife who will attend a home birth.

1. Evidence–Is there sufficient evidence to draw conclusions about the safety of a home birth for Millie?
2. Assumptions–Describe an underlying assumption about each of the following issues:
   a. Assessments that are necessary to identify whether it is feasible and safe for Millie to have a home birth
   b. Supports necessary for a home birth
   c. How to identify providers who are willing to attend a home birth
   d. Ethics of the nurse assisting Millie to find a midwife who will attend a home birth
3. What implications and priorities for nursing care can be drawn at this time?
4. Does the evidence objectively support your conclusion?
5. Are there alternative perspectives to your conclusion?

women. Thus although pain management strategies are an essential component of childbirth education, pain eradication is not the primary source of birth satisfaction. Control in childbirth, meaning participation in decision making, has been repeatedly found to be the primary source of birth satisfaction (Nichols & Gennaro, 2000).

Pain management strategies are an essential component of childbirth education. Couples need information about the advantages and disadvantages of pain medication and about other techniques for coping with labor. An emphasis on nonpharmacologic pain management strategies helps couples manage the labor and birth with dignity and increased comfort. Most instructors teach a flexible approach, which helps couples learn and master many techniques that can be used during labor. Couples are taught techniques such as massage, pressure on the palms or soles of the feet, hot compresses to the perineum, perineal massage, applications of heat or cold, breathing patterns, and focusing of attention on visual or other stimuli as ways to increase coping and decrease the distress from labor pain.

Other valuable tools are vocalization, or "sounding," to relieve tension during pregnancy and labor; subdued lighting; warm water for showers or bathing during labor; and aromatherapy. Some hospitals have Jacuzzi bathtubs for use during labor (see Fig. 16-4, *C*). Childbearing couples are taught to recognize labor's start and to practice coping skills such as relaxation, slow breathing, and other nonpharmacologic strategies (see Chapter 16).

Relaxation counters the effects of sympathetic nervous system arousal. It produces a balance between the sympathetic and parasympathetic systems, slows heart and breathing rates, increases uterine contractility, and produces a sense of security and tranquility. To be effective, varied relaxation techniques must be incorporated into every class session. Paced breathing, biofeedback, therapeutic touch, acupressure, imagery and visualization, and music are relaxation techniques that can be used (see Chapter 16). A variety of skills taught in childbirth classes augment relaxation during the pregnancy, as well as in labor. All can be taught as lifetime skills that are useful to the couple and that can be used to teach their children to cope with the stresses of life.

Key Points

- The prenatal period is a preparatory one, both physically and psychologically.
- Psychosocial aspects of care may affect pregnancy, childbirth, and the adjustment of the new family.
- The pregnant woman's readiness to learn is at a high level, making this an excellent time to help her expand her self-care skills.
- Maternal physical and familial adaptations to pregnancy generate needs that the nurse can anticipate and meet.
- Even with a normal pregnancy the nurse must remain alert to hazards such as supine hypotension, warning signs and symptoms, and signs of family maladaptations.
- Each pregnant woman needs to know how to recognize and report preterm labor.
- Parent-child, sibling-child, and grandparent-child relationships are affected by pregnancy.
- Cultural prescriptions and proscriptions influence responses to pregnancy and to the health care delivery system.
- Childbirth education is a process designed to help parents make the transition from the role of expectant parents to the role and responsibilities of parents of a new baby.

Answer Guidelines to Critical Thinking Exercise

Deciding about a Home Birth

1. Yes, there is sufficient evidence to draw conclusions about the safety of a home birth for Millie.
2. (a) Millie needs to have a low risk pregnancy, have education about requirements of a home birth, have supports available, be able to secure the equipment necessary, and have made plans for hospital or emergency care as needed. (b) Millie needs to have a partner or family or friends who will support her; there needs to be a backup plan for emergencies. (c) Midwives are listed in telephone directories. Names of home birth midwives can be obtained from midwifery associations, from boards of registered nursing, from telephone directories, and by word of mouth. (d) Women have the right to select their care provider. Part of the role of a nurse is appropriate referral; thus referral to a home birth midwife is ethical.
3. Priorities for care include ensuring that Millie has access to prenatal care, providing information about home birth and other options for care such as a birth center, and making appropriate referrals.
4. Yes, information about the importance of prenatal care and the safety of home birth is available and supports the conclusion.

5. The nurse might explore with Millie her reasons for seeking a home birth, her tolerance of pain and willingness to forego use of analgesic medications during labor, and her previous experiences with physicians, nurses, and midwives.

Resources

Association of Labor Assistants and Childbirth Educators (ALACE)
PO Box 382724
Cambridge, MA 02238
617-441-2500

Babyonline.com (source of articles on pregnancy and baby care)
www.babyonline.com

Childbirth.org (source of links to other sites related to pregnancy and birth)
www.childbirth.org

COPE—Coping with the Overall Pregnancy/Parenting Experience
37 Clarendon St.
Boston, MA 02116
617-357-5588

Doulas of North America (DONA)
1100 23rd Ave. East
Seattle, WA 98112
206-324-5440

Healthy Mothers, Healthy Babies Coalition
409 12th St., SW
Washington, DC 20024
202-863-2458

International Childbirth Education Association (ICEA)
PO Box 20048
Minneapolis, MN 55420
800-624-4934

La Leche League International
1400 North Meacham Road
PO Box 4097
Schaumburg, IL 60168
800-525-3243
www.lalecheleague.org

Lamaze International
1200 19th St. NW, Suite 300
Washington, DC 20036
202-857-1100 800-368-4404
202-223-4579 (fax)
www.lamaze-childbirth.com

Lesbian Mother's Support Society
www.lesbian.org/lesbian-moms

Midwife Alliance of North America (MANA)
309 Main Street
Concord, NH 03301
316-283-4543

National Center for Complementary and Alternative Medicine (NCCAM) Clearinghouse
PO Box 7923
Gaithersburg, MD 20898
www.nccam.nih.gov

National Organization of Mothers of Twins Clubs, Inc.
PO Box 23188
Albuquerque, NM 87192
505-275-0955
www.nomotc.org

National Organization on Adolescent Pregnancy, Parenting, and Prevention
2401 Pennsylvania Ave., Suite 350
Washington, DC 20037
202-293-8370

Parenthood After Thirty
451 Vermont
Berkeley, CA 94707
415-524-6635

Sex Information and Education Council of the United States (provides publications [e.g., "Sexual Relations in Pregnancy and Postpartum"] and teaching aids)
130 W. 42nd St., Suite 350
New York, NY 10036
www.siecus.org

Stepping Up: Prevention Strategies for Pregnancy, Parenting and Infancy
www.steppingup.washington.edu

References

American College of Obstetricians and Gynecologists: Exercise during pregnancy and the postpartum period, *Technical Bulletin* 189, 1994.

Andres RL: Effects of therapeutic, diagnostic, and environmental agents and exposure to social and illicit drugs. In Creasy RK, Resnik R, Iams JD (eds): *Maternal-fetal medicine: principles and practice,* ed 5, Philadelphia, 2004, WB Saunders.

Arias E et al: Annual summary of vital statistics—2002. *Pediatrics* 112 (6), 1215-1230, 2003.

Artal R, Subak-Sharpe G: *Pregnancy and exercise,* New York, 1992, Delacorte Press.

Association of Women's Health, Obstetric, and Neonatal Nurses: *HIV testing and disclosure for pregnant women and newborns.* Policy Position Statement, 1999. Available online from www.awhonn.org. (Accessed December 16, 2004).

Beal MW: Women's use of complementary and alternative therapies in reproductive health, *J Nurse Midwifery* 43(3):224-233, 1998.

Boyle GB et al: Sharing maternity care, *Fam Pract Manag* 10(3):37-40, 2003.

Bricker L, Neilson JP: Routine Doppler ultrasound in pregnancy (Cochrane Review). In *The Cochrane Library,* Issue 3, Chichester, UK, 2004, John Wiley & Sons.

Brocklehurst P: Interventions for reducing the risk of mother-to-child transmission of HIV infection (Cochrane Review). In *The Cochrane Library*, Issue 3, Oxford, 2002, Update software.

Brocklehurst P, Volmink J: Antiretrovirals for reducing the risk of mother-to-chld transmission of HIV infection (Cochrane Review). In *The Cochrane Library*, Issue 3, Oxford, 2002, Update Software.

Carl DL, Roux G, Matacale R: Exploring dental hygiene and perinatal outcomes: oral health implications for pregnancy and early childhood, *AWHONN Lifelines* 4(1):22-27, 2000.

Challis JRG, Lye SJ: Characteristics of parturition. In Creasy RK, Resnik R, Iams JD (eds): *Maternal-fetal medicine: principles and practice,* ed 5, Philadelphia, 2004, WB Saunders.

Chalmers B, Mangiaterra V, Porter R: WHO principles of prenatal care: the essential antenatal, perinatal, and postpartum care course, *Birth* 28(3): 202-207, 2001.

Clark SL: Placenta previa and abruption placentae. In Creasy RK, Resnik R, Iams JD (eds): *Maternal-fetal medicine: principles and practice,* ed 5, Philadelphia, 2004, WB Saunders.

Cranley MS: Development of a tool for the measurement of maternal attachment during pregnancy, *Nurs Res* 30(5):281-284, 1981.

Doulas of North America: *Do I need a doula?* 1999a. Internet document available at www.dona.com.faq.html (accessed December 16, 2004).

Doulas of North America: *Doulas of North America position paper: the doula's contribution to modern maternity care,* 1999b. Internet document available at www.dona.com/positionpapers.html (accessed December 16, 2004).

Doulas of North America: *Mission statement,* 1999c. Internet document available at www.dona.com/mission.html (accessed December 16, 2004).

Fetrick A, Christensen M, Mitchell C: Does public health nurse home visitation make a difference in the health outcomes of pregnant clients and their offspring? *Public Health Nurs* 20(3):184-189, 2003.

Fishbein EG, Phillips M: How safe is exercise during pregnancy? *J Obstet Gynecol Neonatal Nurs* 19(1):45-49, 1990.

Foley EM: Drug screening and criminal prosecution of pregnant women, *J Obstet Gynecol Neonat Nurs* 33(2):133-137, 2002.

Ford K et al: Effects of a prenatal care intervention for adolescent mothers on birth weight, repeat pregnancy, and educational outcomes at one year postpartum, *J Perinat Educ* 11(1):35-38, 2002.

Gilbert ES, Harmon JS: *Manual of high risk pregnancy and delivery,* ed 3, St Louis, 2003, Mosby.

Handler A et al: Prenatal care characteristics and African-American women's satisfaction with care in a managed care organization, *Womens Health Issues* 13(3):93-103, 2003.

Harris LH, Paltrow L: The status of pregnant women and fetuses in US criminal law, *JAMA* 289(13):1697-1699, 2003.

Hotelling BA: Is your perinatal practice mother-friendly? A strategy for improving maternity care, *Birth* 31(2):143-147, 2004.

Jared JH et al: Perioperative periodontal disease and low birth weight: a critical link? *Access* 13(3):32, 34-37, 1999.

Jos PH, Perlmutter M, Marshall MF: Substance abuse during pregnancy: clinical and public health approaches, *J Law Med Ethics* 31(3):340-350, 2003.

Lawrence RA, Lawrence RM: *Breastfeeding: a guide for the medical profession,* ed 5, St Louis, 2005, Mosby.

Lederman R: *Psychosocial adaptation in pregnancy,* ed 2, New York, 1996, Springer.

Lumley J, Oliver S, Waters E: Interventions for promoting smoking cessation during pregnancy (Cochrane Review), 1999. In *The Cochrane Library,* Issue 2, Chichester, UK, 2004, John Wiley & Sons.

Malone FD, D'Alton ME: Multiple gestation. Clinical characteristics and management. In Creasy RK, Resnik R, Iams JD (eds): *Maternal-fetal medicine: principles and practice,* ed 5, Philadelphia, 2004, WB Saunders.

Martin et al: Births: final data for 2002, *Natl Vit Stat Rep* 52(10):1-114, 2003.

May K: A typology of detachment and involvement styles adopted during pregnancy by first-time expectant fathers, *West J Nurs Res* 2(2):444-461, 1980.

May KA: Three phases of father involvement in pregnancy, *Nurs Res* 31(6):337-342, 1982.

Mercer R: *Becoming a mother,* New York, 1995, Springer.

Moore M et al: A randomized trial of nurse intervention to reduce preterm and low birthweight births, *Obstet Gynecol* 91: 656-661,1998.

Müller ME: Development of the prenatal attachment inventory, *West J Nurs Res* 15(2):199-211, 1993.

National High Blood Pressure Education Program: *Seventh report of the Joint National Committee on Prevention, Detection, Evaluation, and Treatment of High Blood Pressure,* Bethesda, MD, 2003, USDHHS, NIH, NHLBI.

Nichols F, Gennaro S: The childbirth experience. In Nichols F, Humenick S (eds): *Childbirth education: practice, research and theory,* ed 2, Philadelphia, 2000, WB Saunders.

Philosophy of birth. Internet document available at normalbirth.lamaze.org/About/PhilosophyofBirth.asp (accessed December 16, 2004).

Peters RM, Flack JM: Hypertensive disorders of pregnancy, *J Obstet Gynecol Neonatal Nurs* 33(2):209-220, 2004.

Pivarnik JM: Maternal exercise in pregnancy, *Sports Med* 18(4):215-217, 1994.

Pugh L et al: Clinical approaches in the assessment of childbearing fatigue, *J Obstet Gynecol Neonat Nurs* 28(1):74-80, 1999.

Rubin R: Maternal tasks in pregnancy, *Matern Child Nurs J* 4(3):143-153, 1975.

Rubin R: *Maternity identity and the maternal experience,* New York, 1984, Springer.

Schirmer G: *Herbal medicine,* Bedford, TX, 1998, MED2000 Inc.

Seidel HM et al: *Mosby's guide to physical examination,* ed 5, St Louis, 2003, Mosby.

Shaffer CF: Factors influencing the access to prenatal care by Hispanic pregnant women, *J Am Acad Nurse Pract* 14(2):93-98, 2002.

Simkin P, Way K: *DONA position paper: the doula's contributions to modern maternity care,* Seattle, WA, 1998, Doulas of North America.

Strong T: *Expecting trouble: the myth of prenatal care in America,* New York, 2002, New York University Press.

Sword W: Prenatal care use among women of low income: a matter of "taking care of self," *Qual Health Res* 13(3):319-332, 2003.

Tough SC et al: Delayed childbearing and its impact on population rate changes in lower birth weight, multiple birth, and preterm delivery, *Pediatrics* 109(3):399-403, 2002.

Villar J et al: Patterns of routine antenatal care for low-risk pregnancy. In *The Cochrane Library,* Issue 4, Oxford, 2002, Update Software.

Unit 3

Maternal and Fetal Nutrition 12

LEARNING OBJECTIVES

On completion of this chapter the reader will be able to:

- Explain recommended maternal weight gain during pregnancy.
- Compare the recommended level of intake of energy sources, protein, and key vitamins and minerals during pregnancy and lactation.
- Give examples of the food sources that provide the nutrients required for optimal maternal nutrition during pregnancy and lactation.
- Examine the role of nutrition supplements during pregnancy.
- List five nutritional risk factors during pregnancy.
- Compare the dietary needs of adolescent and mature pregnant women.
- Give examples of cultural food patterns and possible dietary problems for two ethnic groups or for two alternative eating patterns.
- Assess nutritional status during pregnancy.

ELECTRONIC RESOURCES

Additional information related to the content in Chapter 12 can be found on

the companion website at evolve
http://evolve.elsevier.com/Wong/maternal/
- NCLEX Review Questions
- WebLinks

or the interactive student CD-ROM
Activities for Chapter 12 include the following:
- NCLEX Review Questions
- Critical Thinking Exercise–Nutrition Education
- Nursing Care Plan–Nutrition during Pregnancy

Nutrition is one of the many factors that influence the outcome of pregnancy (Fig. 12-1). However, maternal nutritional status is an especially significant factor, both because it is potentially alterable and because good nutrition before and during pregnancy is an important preventive measure for a variety of problems. These problems include birth of low-birth-weight and preterm infants. It is essential that the importance of good nutrition be emphasized to all women of childbearing potential. Nutrition assessment, intervention, and evaluation must be an integral part of the nursing care provided to all pregnant women.

The Pregnancy Nutrition Surveillance System (PNSS) was developed to help health professionals identify and reduce pregnancy-related health risks (Centers for Disease Control and Prevention [CDC], 2004). The data collected from programs such as the Special Supplemental Program for Women, Infants, and Children (WIC) and prenatal clinics funded by Maternal and Child Health Program Block Grants are submitted to the CDC. Annual data summaries allow states to monitor trends in prevalence of prenatal risk factors that predict low birth weight and infant mortality, as well as monitor infant feeding practices.

NUTRIENT NEEDS BEFORE CONCEPTION

The first trimester of pregnancy is a crucial one for embryonic and fetal organ development. A healthful diet before conception is the best way to ensure that adequate nutrients are available for the developing fetus. Folate or folic acid intake is of particular concern in the periconceptual period. *Folate* is the form in which this vitamin is found naturally in foods, and *folic acid* is the form used in fortification of grain products and other foods and in vitamin supplements. Neural tube defects, or failure in closure of the neural tube, are more common in infants of women with poor folic acid intake. It is estimated that the incidence of neural tube defects could be halved if all women had an adequate folic acid intake during the periconceptual period (Kilpatrick & Laros, 2004). All women capable of becoming pregnant are advised to consume 400 mcg of folic acid daily in fortified foods (e.g., ready-to-eat cereals and enriched grain products) or supplements in addition to a diet rich in folate-containing foods such as green leafy vegetables, whole grains, and fruits.

Both maternal and fetal risks in pregnancy are increased when the mother is significantly underweight or overweight

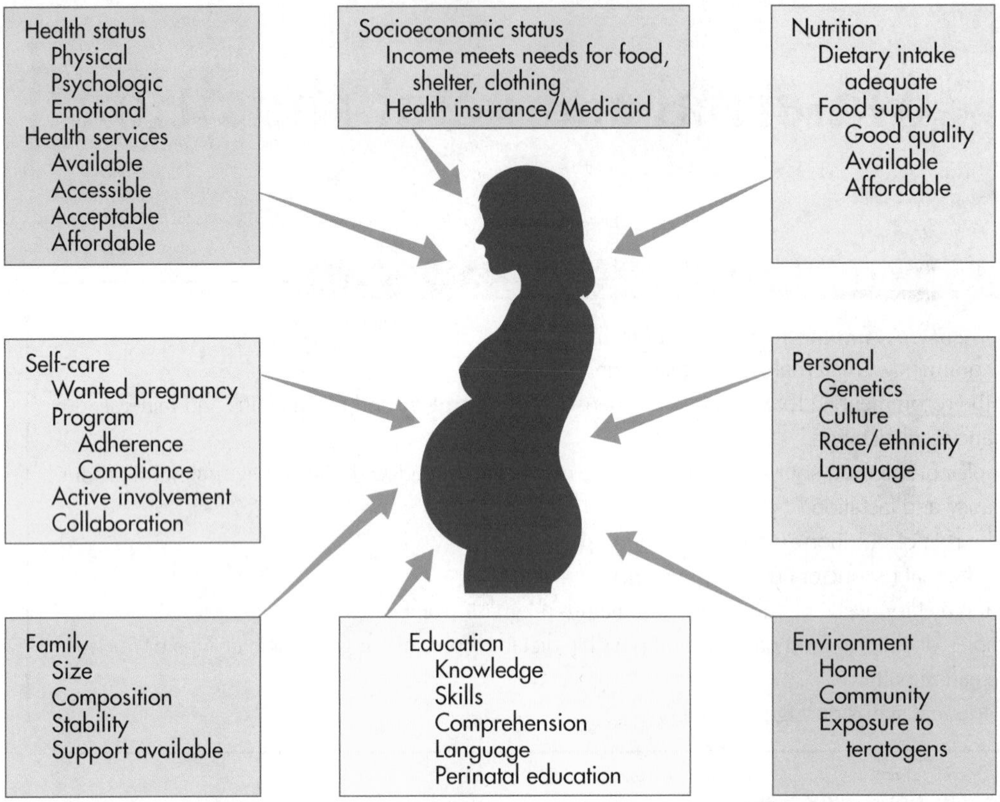

Fig. 12-1 Factors that influence the outcome of pregnancy.

when pregnancy begins. Ideally, all women would achieve their desirable body weights before conception.

NUTRIENT NEEDS DURING PREGNANCY

Nutrient needs are determined, at least in part, by the stage of gestation. The amount of fetal growth varies during the different stages of pregnancy. During the first trimester, the synthesis of fetal tissues places relatively few demands on maternal nutrition. Therefore the first trimester needs, when the embryo or fetus is very small, are only slightly increased over those before pregnancy. In contrast, the last trimester is a period of noticeable fetal growth when most of the fetal stores of energy sources and minerals are deposited. Basal metabolic rates (BMRs), when expressed as kilocalories (kcal) per minute, are approximately 20% higher in pregnant women than in nonpregnant women. This increase includes the energy cost for tissue synthesis.

The Food and Nutrition Board of the National Academy of Sciences publishes recommendations for the people of the United States, the Dietary Reference Intakes (DRIs). The DRIs consist of Recommended Dietary Allowances (RDAs) and Adequate Intakes (AIs), as well as Upper Limits (ULs), guidelines for avoiding excessive intakes of nutrients that may be toxic if consumed in excess. RDAs for some nutrients have been available for many years, and they have been revised periodically. RDAs are recommendations for daily nutritional intakes that meet the needs of almost all (97% to 98%) of the healthy members of the population. AIs are similar to the RDAs and are believed to cover the needs for virtually all healthy individuals in a group, except that they deal with nutrients for which there are not enough data to be certain of their requirements. The RDAs and AIs include a wide variety of nutrients and food components, and they are divided into age, sex, and life-stage categories (e.g., infancy, pregnancy, and lactation). They can be used as goals in planning the diets of individuals (Table 12-1).

Energy Needs

Energy (kilocalories or kcal) needs are met by carbohydrate, fat, and protein in the diet. No specific recommendations exist for the amount of carbohydrate and fat in the diet of the pregnant woman. However, intake of these nutrients should be adequate to support the recommended weight gain. Although protein can be used to supply energy, its primary role is to provide amino acids for the synthesis of new tissues (see the discussion later in this chapter). The RDA during the second and third trimesters of pregnancy is 300 kcal greater than prepregnancy needs. Very underweight or active women or those with multifetal gestations will require more than 300 additional kcal to sustain the desired rate of weight gain.

Weight Gain

The optimal weight gain during pregnancy is not known precisely. It is known, however, that the amount of weight gained by the mother during pregnancy has an important bearing on the course and outcome of pregnancy. Adequate weight gain does not necessarily indicate that the diet is nutritionally adequate, but it is associated with a reduced risk of giving birth to a small-for-gestational-age (SGA) or preterm infant.

Table 12-1

Recommendations for Daily Intakes of Selected Nutrients during Pregnancy and Lactation

NUTRIENT (UNIT)	RECOMMENDATION FOR NONPREGNANT WOMAN	RECOMMENDATION FOR PREGNANCY*	RECOMMENDATION FOR LACTATION*	ROLE IN RELATION TO PREGNANCY AND LACTATION	FOOD SOURCES
Energy (kilocalories [kcal] or kilojoules [kJ]†)	Variable	First trimester, same as nonpregnant; second and third trimesters, nonpregnant + 300 kcal or 72 kJ	Nonpregnant + 500 kcal or 120 kJ	Growth of fetal and maternal tissues; milk production	Carbohydrate, fat, and protein
Protein (g)	50	60	65	Synthesis of the products of conception; growth of maternal tissue and expansion of blood volume; secretion of milk protein during lactation	Meats, eggs, cheese, yogurt, legumes (dry beans and peas, peanuts), nuts, grains
MINERALS					
Calcium (mg)	1300/1000	1300/1000	1300/1000	Fetal and infant skeleton and tooth formation; maintenance of maternal bone and tooth mineralization	Milk, cheese, yogurt, sardines or other fish eaten with bones left in, deep green leafy vegetables except spinach or Swiss chard, calcium-set tofu, baked beans, tortillas
Iron (mg)	15/18	27	10/9	Maternal hemoglobin formation, fetal liver iron storage	Liver, meats, whole grain or enriched breads and cereals, deep green leafy vegetables, legumes, dried fruits
Zinc (mg)	9/8	12/11	13/12	Component of numerous enzyme systems, possibly important in preventing congenital malformations	Liver, shellfish, meats, whole grains, milk
Iodine (mcg)	150	220	290	Increased maternal metabolic rate	Iodized salt, seafood, milk and milk products, commercial yeast breads, rolls, and donuts
Magnesium (mg)	360/320	400/360	350/320	Involved in energy and protein metabolism, tissue growth, muscle action	Nuts, legumes, cocoa, meats, whole grains

Recommendations are the Dietary Reference Intakes (RDA or AI, see text), where available.

Sources: Food and Nutrition Board, National Academy of Sciences, Institute of Medicine, 1997; *Dietary Reference Intakes for calcium, phosphorus, magnesium, vitamin D, and fluoride*, 1998; *Dietary Reference Intakes for thiamin, riboflavin, niacin, vitamin* B_6, *folate, vitamin* B_{12}, *pantothenic acid, biotin, and choline*, 2000; *Dietary Reference Intakes for vitamin C, vitamin E, selenium, and carotenoids*, 2001; *Dietary Reference Intakes for vitamin A, vitamin K, arsenic, boron, chromium, copper, iodine, iron, manganese, molybdenum, nickel, silicon, vanadium, and zinc*, Washington, DC, 2001, National Academy Press. Where DRIs are not available, the values are taken from Food and Nutrition Board, National Academy of Sciences, National Research Council: *Recommended dietary allowances*, ed 10, Washington, DC, 1989, National Academy Press.

*When two values appear, separated by a diagonal slash, the first is for females younger than 19 years, and the second is for those 19 to 50 years of age.

†The international metric unit of energy measurement is the joule (J).

1 kcal = 4.184 kJ.

Continued

Table 12-1

Recommendations for Daily Intakes of Selected Nutrients during Pregnancy and Lactation—cont'd

NUTRIENT (UNIT)	RECOMMENDATION FOR NONPREGNANT WOMAN	RECOMMENDATION FOR PREGNANCY*	RECOMMENDATION FOR LACTATION*	ROLE IN RELATION TO PREGNANCY AND LACTATION	FOOD SOURCES
FAT-SOLUBLE VITAMINS					
A (mcg)	700	750/770	1200/1300	Essential for cell development, tooth bud formation, bone growth	Deep green leafy vegetables; dark yellow vegetables; and fruits, chili peppers, liver, fortified margarine and butter
D (mcg)	5	5	5	Involved in absorption of calcium and phosphorus, improves mineralization	Fortified milk and margarine, egg yolk, butter, liver, seafood
E (mg)	15	15	19	Antioxidant (protects cell membranes from damage), especially important for preventing breakdown of RBCs	Vegetable oils, green leafy vegetables, whole grains, liver, nuts and seeds, cheese, fish
WATER-SOLUBLE VITAMINS					
C (mg)	65/75	80/85	115/120	Tissue formation and integrity, formation of connective tissue, enhancement of iron absorption	Citrus fruits, strawberries, melons, broccoli, tomatoes, peppers, raw deep green leafy vegetables
Folate (mcg)	400	600	500	Prevention of neural tube defects, support for increased maternal RBC formation	Fortified ready-to-eat cereals and other grain products, green leafy vegetables, oranges, broccoli, asparagus, artichokes, liver
B_6 or pyridoxine (mg)	1.2/1.3	1.9	2.0	Involved in protein metabolism	Meat, liver, deep green vegetables, whole grains
B_{12} (mcg)	2.4	2.6	2.8	Production of nucleic acids and proteins, especially important in formation of RBCs and neural functioning	Milk and milk products, egg, meat, liver, fortified soy milk

RBCs, red blood cells.

The desirable weight gain during pregnancy varies among women. The primary factor to consider in making a weight gain recommendation is the appropriateness of the prepregnancy weight for the woman's height. Maternal and fetal risks in pregnancy are increased when the mother is either significantly underweight or overweight before pregnancy, and when weight gain during pregnancy is either too low or too high. Severely underweight women are more likely to have preterm labor and to give birth to low-birth-weight (LBW) infants. Women with inadequate weight gain have an increased risk of delivering an infant with intrauterine growth restriction (IUGR). Greater-than-expected weight gain during pregnancy may occur for many reasons, including multiple gestation, edema, preeclampsia, and overeating. When obesity is present (either preexisting or developed during pregnancy), there is an increased likelihood of macrosomia and fetopelvic disproportion; operative birth; emergency cesarean birth; postpartum hemorrhage; wound, genital tract, or urinary tract infection; birth trauma; and late fetal death. Obese women are more likely than normal-weight women to have preeclampsia and gestational diabetes; their risk of giving birth to a child with a major congenital defect is double that of normal-weight women.

A commonly used method of evaluating the appropriateness of weight for height is the body mass index (BMI), which is calculated by the following formula:

$$BMI = weight/height^2$$

where the weight is in kilograms and height is in meters. Thus for a woman who weighed 51 kg before pregnancy and is 1.57 m tall:

$$BMI = 51/(1.57)^2, \text{ or } 20.7$$

Prepregnant BMI can be classified into the following categories: less than 19.8, underweight or low; 19.8 to 26.0, normal; 26.0 to 29.0, overweight or high; and greater than 29.0, obese (Institute of Medicine, 1992).

For women with single fetuses, current recommendations are that women with a normal BMI should gain 11.5 to 16 kg during pregnancy, underweight women should gain 12.5 to 18 kg, overweight women should gain 7 to 11.5 kg, and obese women should gain at least 7 kg (Institute of Medicine, 1992). Adolescents are encouraged to strive for weight gains at the upper end of the recommended range for their BMI because it appears that the fetus and the still-growing mother compete for nutrients. The risk of mechanical complications at birth is reduced if the weight gain of short adult women (shorter than 157 cm) is near the lower end of their recommended range. In twin gestations, gains of approximately 16 to 20 kg appear to be associated with the best outcomes (Malone & D'Alton, 2004).

Pattern of Weight Gain

Weight gain should take place throughout pregnancy. The risk of delivering an SGA infant is greater when the weight gain early in pregnancy has been poor. The likelihood of preterm birth is greater when the gains during the last half of pregnancy have been inadequate. These risks exist even when the total gain for the pregnancy is in the recommended range.

The optimal rate of weight gain depends on the stage of pregnancy. During the first and second trimesters, growth takes place primarily in maternal tissue; during the third trimester, growth occurs primarily in fetal tissues. During the first trimester there is an average total weight gain of only 1 to 2.5 kg. Thereafter the recommended weight gain increases to approximately 0.4 kg per week for a woman of normal weight (Fig. 12-2). The recommended weekly weight gain for overweight women during the second and third trimesters is 0.3 kg, and for underweight women it is 0.5 kg. The recommended caloric intake corresponds to this pattern of gain. For the first trimester there is no increment; during the second and third trimesters an additional 300 kcal/day over the prepregnant intake is recommended. The amount of food providing 300 kcal is not great. It can be provided by one additional serving from any one of the following groups: milk, yogurt, or cheese (all skim milk products); fruits; vegetables; and bread, cereal, rice, or pasta.

The reasons for an inadequate weight gain (less than 1 kg per month for normal-weight women or less than 0.5 kg per month for obese women during the last two trimesters) or excessive weight gain (more than 3 kg per month) should be thoroughly evaluated. Possible reasons for deviations from the expected rate of weight gain, besides inadequate or excessive dietary intake, include measurement or recording errors, differences in weight of clothing, time of day, and accumulation of fluids. An exceptionally high gain is likely to be caused by an accumulation of fluids, and a gain of more than 3 kg in a month, especially after the twentieth week of gestation, often heralds the development of preeclampsia.

Hazards of Restricting Adequate Weight Gain

Figure-conscious women may find it difficult to make the transition from guarding against weight gain before pregnancy to valuing weight gain during pregnancy. In counseling these women, the nurse can emphasize the positive effects of good nutrition, as well as the adverse effects of maternal malnutrition (manifested by poor weight gain) on infant growth and development. This counseling includes information on the components of weight gain during pregnancy (Table 12-2) and the amount of this weight that will be lost at birth. Early in a woman's pregnancy, explaining ways to lose weight in the postpartum period helps relieve her concerns. Because lactation can help to reduce maternal energy stores gradually, this provides an opportunity to promote breastfeeding.

Pregnancy is not a time for a weight-reduction diet. Even overweight or obese pregnant women need to gain at least enough weight to equal the weight of the products of conception (fetus, placenta, and amniotic fluid). If they limit their caloric intake to prevent weight gain, they may also excessively limit their intake of important nutrients. Moreover, dietary restriction results in catabolism of fat stores, which in turn augments the production of ketones. The long-term effects of mild ketonemia during pregnancy are not known, but ketonuria has been found to be correlated with the occurrence of preterm labor. It should be stressed to obese women (and to all pregnant women) that the quality of the weight gain is

??? Critical Thinking Exercise

NUTRITION AND THE OVERWEIGHT PREGNANT WOMAN

Tamara, of African-American and Asian heritage, is 3 months pregnant and comes to her initial appointment for diagnosis and care. She appears to be overweight for her height. To provide optimum care for her, you plan to calculate her prepregnancy BMI. When her pregnancy is confirmed, you are asked to plan a diet with Tamara that meets the minimum daily requirements and allows for growth of the pregnancy. You know that it is important to include consideration of personal preferences and cultural factors in your plan. With Tamara, identify barriers to implementing the plan.

1. Evidence—Is there sufficient evidence to draw conclusions about an appropriate nutrition plan, taking into consideration personal preferences and cultural factors?
2. Assumptions—Describe underlying assumptions about each of the following issues:
   a. Dietary Reference Intakes for pregnancy and lactation
   b. Indicators of nutritional risk in pregnancy
   c. Daily food guide for pregnancy and lactation
   d. Sources of calcium for women who do not drink milk
3. What implications and priorities for nursing care can be drawn at this time?
4. Does the evidence objectively support your conclusion?
5. Are there alternative perspectives to your conclusion?

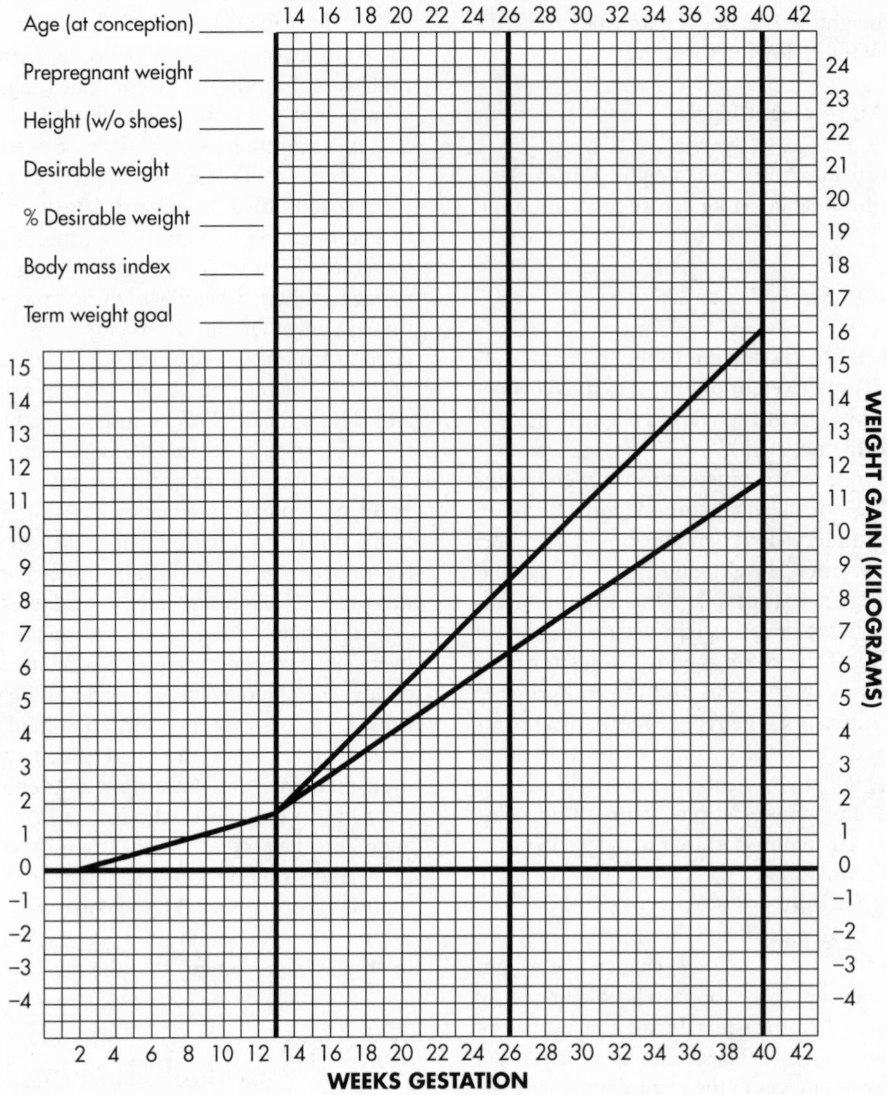

Fig. 12-2 Prenatal weight gain chart for plotting weight gain of normal-weight women. NOTE: Young adolescents, African-American women, and smokers should aim for the upper end of the recommended range; short women (<157 cm) should strive for gains at the lower end of the range.

Table 12-2

Tissues Contributing to Maternal Weight Gain at 40 Weeks of Gestation

TISSUE	POUNDS
Fetus	7-8.5
Placenta	2-2.5
Amniotic fluid	2
Increase in uterine tissue	2
Breast tissue	1-4
Increased blood volume	4-5
Increased tissue fluid	3-5
Increased stores (fat)	4-6

important, with emphasis placed on the consumption of nutrient-dense foods and the avoidance of empty-calorie foods.

Weight gain is important, but pregnancy is not an excuse for uncontrolled dietary indulgence. Excessive weight gained during pregnancy may be difficult to lose after pregnancy, thus contributing to chronic overweight or obesity, an etiologic factor in a host of chronic diseases including hypertension, diabetes mellitus, and arteriosclerotic heart disease. The woman who gains 18 kg or more during pregnancy is especially at risk.

Protein

Protein, with its essential constituent nitrogen, is the nutritional element basic to growth. Adequate protein intake is essential to meet increasing demands in pregnancy. These demands arise from the rapid growth of the fetus; the enlargement of the uterus and its supporting structures, mammary glands, and placenta; an increase in maternal circulating blood volume and subsequent demand for increased amounts of plasma protein to maintain colloidal osmotic pressure; and the formation of amniotic fluid.

Milk, meat, eggs, and cheese are complete-protein foods with a high biologic value. Legumes (dried beans and peas), whole grains, and nuts are also valuable sources of protein. In addition, these protein-rich foods are a source of other nutrients such as calcium, iron, and B vitamins; plant sources of protein often provide needed dietary fiber. The recommended daily food plan (Table 12-3) is a guide to the amounts of these foods that would supply the quantities of protein needed. The recommendations provide for only a modest increase in protein intake over the prepregnant levels in adult women. Protein intake in many people in the United States is relatively high, so many women may not need to increase their protein intake at all during pregnancy. Three servings of milk, yogurt, or cheese (four for adolescents) and 5 to 6 ounces (140 to 168 g) (two servings) of meat, poultry, or fish supply the recommended protein for the pregnant woman. Additional protein is provided by vegetables and breads, cereals, rice, and pasta. Pregnant adolescents, women from impoverished backgrounds, and women adhering to unusual diets, such as a macrobiotic (highly restricted vegetarian) diet, are those most likely to have inadequate protein intake. The use of high-protein supplements is not recommended, because these have been associated with an increased incidence of preterm births.

Fluids

Essential during the exchange of nutrients and waste products across cell membranes, water is the main substance of cells, blood, lymph, amniotic fluid, and other vital body fluids. It also aids in maintaining body temperature. A good fluid intake promotes good bowel function, which is sometimes a problem during pregnancy. The recommended daily intake is about six to eight glasses (1500 to 2000 ml) of fluid. Water, milk, and juices are good fluid sources. Dehydration may increase the risk of cramping, contractions, and preterm labor.

Women who consume more than 300 mg of caffeine daily (equivalent to about 500 to 750 ml of coffee) may be at increased risk of miscarriage and of giving birth to infants with IUGR. The ill effects of caffeine have been proposed to result from vasoconstriction of the blood vessels supplying the uterus or from interference with cell division in the developing fetus. Consequently, caffeine-containing products such as caffeinated coffee, tea, soft drinks, and cocoa beverages should be avoided or consumed only in limited quantities.

Aspartame (Nutrasweet, Equal) and acesulfame potassium (Sunett), and sucralose (Splenda), artificial sweeteners

Table 12-3

Daily Food Guide for Pregnancy and Lactation

FOOD GROUP	SERVING SIZE	Suggested Number of Servings: NONPREGNANT, NONLACTATING WOMAN	PREGNANT WOMAN	LACTATING WOMAN
GRAIN PRODUCTS				
Include whole-grain and enriched breads, cereals, pasta, and rice.	1 slice bread; ½ bun, bagel, or English muffin; 1 oz ready-to-eat cereal; ½ c cooked grains	6-11	6-11	6-11
VEGETABLES				
Eat dark green leafy and deep yellow often. Eat dried beans and peas often; count ½ c cooked dried beans or peas as a serving of vegetables or 1 oz from meat group.	1 c raw leafy greens; ½ c of others	3-5	3-5	3-5
FRUITS				
Include citrus fruits, strawberries, or melons frequently.	1 medium apple, orange, banana, peach, etc; ½ c small or diced fruit; ¾ c juice	2-4	2-4	2-4
MILK AND MILK PRODUCTS	1 c milk or yogurt; 1½ oz cheese	2-3	3 or more	4 or more
MEAT, POULTRY, FISH, DRY BEANS, NUTS, AND EGGS				
Eat peanut butter or nuts rarely to avoid excessive fat intake. Limit egg intake to reduce cholesterol intake; trim fat from meat, and remove skin from poultry.	½ c cooked dried beans, 1 egg, or 1½ T peanut butter is equivalent to 1 oz of meat	Up to 6 oz total	Up to 6 oz total	Up to 6 oz total

c, cup; *T*, tablespoon.

commonly used in low- or no-calorie beverages and low-calorie food products, have not been found to have adverse effects on the normal mother or fetus. Aspartame, which contains phenylalanine, should be avoided by the mother with phenylketonuria (PKU) (Box 12-1).

Minerals and Vitamins

In general, the nutrient needs of pregnant women, except perhaps the need for folate and iron, can be met through dietary sources. Counseling about the need for a varied diet rich in vitamins and minerals should be a part of every pregnant woman's early prenatal care and should be reinforced throughout pregnancy. Supplements of certain nutrients (listed in the following discussion) are recommended whenever the woman's diet is very poor or whenever significant nutritional risk factors are present. Nutritional risk factors in pregnancy are listed in Box 12-2.

Iron

Iron is needed both to allow transfer of adequate iron to the fetus and to permit expansion of the maternal red blood cell (RBC) mass. Beginning in the latter part of the first trimester, the blood volume of the mother increases steadily, peaking at about 1500 ml more than that in the nonpregnant state. In twin gestations, the increase is at least 500 ml greater than that in pregnancies with single fetuses. Plasma volume increases more than RBC mass, with the difference between plasma and RBCs being greatest during the second trimester. The relative excess of plasma causes a modest decrease in the hemoglobin concentration and hematocrit, termed *physiologic anemia of pregnancy.* This is a normal adaptation during pregnancy.

BOX 12-1

Use of Artificial Sweeteners during Pregnancy

All of the following sweeteners are approved for use in all age groups, including pregnant women, in the United States:

Acesulfame K
- Brand names: Sunett, Sweet One
- Primary uses: baked goods, frozen desserts, candies, beverages
- Sweetness: 200 times sweeter than sugar
- Shelf life: long
- Suitability for cooking: good, does not break down when heated
- Health concerns: none known

Aspartame
- Brand names: Equal, NutraSweet, NatraTaste
- Primary uses: beverages, frozen desserts, dairy products, chewing gum, breakfast cereals, table-top sweetener
- Sweetness: 180 times sweeter than sugar
- Shelf life: relatively short (about 5 months in a soft drink)
- Suitability for cooking: breaks down and loses sweetness if cooked at high temperatures or for long periods
- Health concerns: contains phenylalanine, a consideration in the diets of people with phenylketonuria

Neotame
- Brand names: none (not currently available)
- Primary uses: approved in the United States but not currently marketed; proposed use in beverages, frozen desserts, yogurt, chewing gum, toppings, fillings, fruit spreads, table-top sweetener
- Sweetness: 8000 times sweeter than sugar
- Shelf life: similar to aspartame (about 5 months in a soft drink)
- Suitability for cooking: good, but loses sweetness if cooked at high temperatures or for prolonged periods
- Health concerns: none known; contains phenylalanine but not in a form that can be metabolized

Saccharin
- Brand name: Sweet'n Low
- Primary uses: fountain drinks, chewable vitamins and medications, table-top sweetener
- Sweetness: 300 times sweeter than sugar
- Shelf life: long
- Suitable for cooking: good, does not lose sweetness during cooking
- Health concerns: linked to bladder cancer in rats

Sucralose
- Brand name: Splenda
- Primary uses: baked goods, beverages, frozen desserts, gelatins, table-top sweetener
- Sweetness: 600 times sweeter than sugar
- Shelf life: long
- Suitability for cooking: very good, does not break down during cooking (maltodextrin is added to give products better bulk and texture)
- Health concerns: none known

Sugar alcohols (not technically artificial sweeteners; contain almost as many calories as sugar)
- Types: sorbitol, xylitol, lactitol, mannitol, and maltitol
- Primary uses: sugar-free candy, cookies, and chewing gum
- Sweetness: most are about 70% as sweet as sugar; xylitol equals sugar in sweetness
- Shelf life: long
- Suitability for cooking: good
- Advantages over sugar: do not promote tooth decay, more slowly metabolized so that they do not create a rapid peak in blood glucose
- Health concerns: diarrhea can occur with large intakes

NOTE: Sugar is important for the volume and moisture of baked goods. Artificial sweeteners may produce a good-tasting product, but some sugar is necessary in many recipes to yield normal volume and texture.

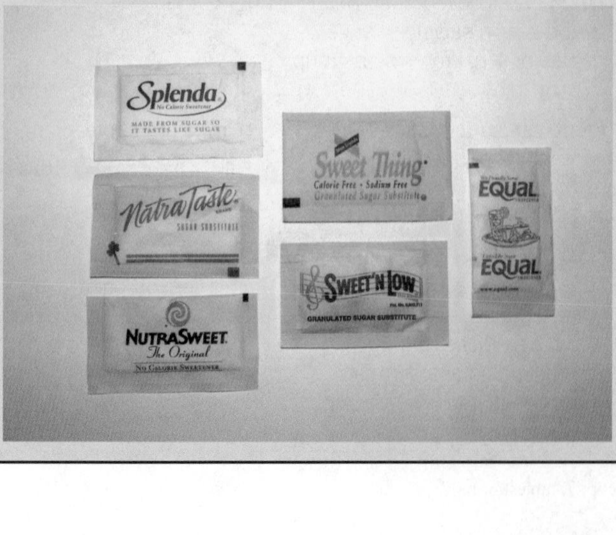

BOX 12-2

Indicators of Nutritional Risk in Pregnancy

Adolescence
Frequent pregnancies: three within 2 years
Poor fetal outcome in a previous pregnancy
Poverty
Poor diet habits with resistance to change
Use of tobacco, alcohol, or drugs
Weight at conception under or over normal weight
Problems with weight gain
Any weight loss
Weight gain of less than 1 kg/mo after the first trimester
Weight gain of more than 1 kg/wk after the first trimester
Multifetal pregnancy
Low hemoglobin or hematocrit values (or both)

However, poor iron intake and absorption, which can result in iron deficiency anemia, is relatively common among women in the childbearing years. It affects nearly one fifth of the pregnant women in industrialized countries. The maternal mortality rate is increased among anemic women, who are poorly prepared to tolerate hemorrhage at the time of birth. In addition, anemic women may have a greater likelihood of cardiac failure during labor, postpartum infections, and poor wound healing. The fetus is also affected by maternal anemia. The risk of preterm birth is about threefold greater in anemic women, and fetal iron stores may also be reduced by maternal anemia. Anemia is more common among adolescents and African-American women than among adult Caucasian women.

The Institute of Medicine (1992) recommended that all pregnant women receive a supplement of 30 mg of ferrous iron daily, starting by 12 weeks of gestation. (Iron supplements may be poorly tolerated during the nausea that is prevalent in the first trimester.) If maternal iron deficiency anemia is present (preferably diagnosed by measurement of serum ferritin, a storage form of iron), increased dosages (60 to 100 mg daily) are recommended. Certain foods taken with an iron supplement can promote or inhibit absorption of iron from the supplement. Even when a woman is taking an iron supplement, she should include good food sources of iron in her daily diet (see Table 12-1).

Calcium

There is no increase in the DRI of calcium during pregnancy and lactation, in comparison with the recommendation for the nonpregnant woman (see Table 12-1). The DRI (1000 mg daily for women 19 and older and 1300 mg for those younger than 19) appears to provide sufficient calcium for fetal bone and tooth development to proceed while maintaining maternal bone mass.

Milk and yogurt are especially rich sources of calcium, providing approximately 300 mg per cup (240 ml). Nevertheless, many women do not consume these foods or do not consume adequate amounts to provide the recommended intakes of calcium. One problem that can interfere with milk consumption is lactose intolerance, which is the inability to digest milk sugar (lactose) caused by the absence of the lactase enzyme in the small intestine. Lactose intolerance is relatively common in adults, particularly African-Americans, Asians, Native Americans, and Inuits. Milk consumption may cause abdominal cramping, bloating, and diarrhea in such people. Yogurt, sweet acidophilus milk, buttermilk, cheese, chocolate milk, and cocoa may be tolerated even when fresh fluid milk is not. Commercial products that contain lactase (e.g., Lactaid) are widely available. Many supermarkets stock lactase-treated milk. The lactase in these products hydrolyzes, or digests, the lactose in milk, making it possible for lactose-intolerant people to drink milk.

In some cultures, adults rarely drink milk. For example, Puerto Ricans and other Hispanic people may use milk only as an additive in coffee. Pregnant women from these cultures may need to consume nondairy sources of calcium. Vegetarian diets may also be deficient in calcium (Box 12-3). If calcium intake appears low, and the woman does not change her dietary habits despite counseling, a daily supplement containing 600 mg of elemental calcium may be needed. Calcium supplements may also be recommended when a pregnant woman experiences leg cramps caused by an imbalance in the calcium/phosphorus ratio.

Sodium

During pregnancy the need for sodium increases slightly, primarily because the body water is expanding (e.g., the expanding blood volume). Sodium is essential for maintaining body water balance. In the past, dietary sodium was routinely restricted in an effort to control the peripheral edema that commonly occurs during pregnancy. It is now recognized that moderate peripheral edema is normal in pregnancy, occurring as a response to the fluid-retaining effects of elevated

BOX 12-3

Calcium Sources for Women Who Do Not Drink Milk

Each of the following provides approximately the same amount of calcium as 1 cup of milk:

Fish
3 oz can of sardines
4½ oz can of salmon (if bones are eaten)

Beans and Legumes
3 cups of cooked dried beans
2½ cups of refried beans
2 cups of baked beans with molasses
1 cup of tofu (calcium is added in processing)

Greens
1 cup of collards
1½ cups of kale or turnip greens

Baked Products
3 pieces of cornbread
3 English muffins
4 slices of French toast
2 waffles (7 inches in diameter)

Fruits
11 dried figs
1⅛ cups of orange juice with calcium added

Sauces
3 oz of pesto sauce
5 oz of cheese sauce

Evidence-Based Practice

CALCIUM SUPPLEMENTATION FOR PREVENTING PREECLAMPSIA

Background

Hypertensive disorders of pregnancy are associated with maternal and fetal death and morbidity. Hypertension leads to poor uterine perfusion, preterm birth, fetal distress, low birth weight, and perinatal fetal mortality. In the mother, preeclampsia can lead to edema; seizures; renal failure; the syndrome of hemolysis, elevated liver enzymes, and low platelets (HELLP); admission to intensive care; cesarean birth; and maternal death. *Gestational hypertension* (GH) is usually defined as new-onset diastolic blood pressure over 90 mm Hg, or a rise over baseline for systolic blood pressure of 30 mm Hg or diastolic rise of 15 mm Hg. Preeclampsia is diagnosed when GH is accompanied by proteinuria of 2+, or 300 mg in 24 hours. Blood pressure climbs when the endothelial walls become inflamed from unknown causes. Low calcium intake may stimulate either parathyroid hormone or renin release, which increases cellular uptake of calcium, leading to vasospasm. Calcium supplementation reduces parathyroid hormone, thus reducing intravascular inflammation, and may be a treatment for GH. Calcium may also relax the smooth muscles in the uterus, reducing the risk of preterm labor. Calcium is cost-effective, familiar, and available. No risk of renal stones has been noted.

Objectives

The goal of the review was to determine whether calcium supplementation during pregnancy affected preeclampsia, and related adverse maternal and fetal outcomes. Of interest were comparisons of women at low risk for preeclampsia with high risk mothers (teens, women with history of preeclampsia or prepregnancy hypertension, increased sensitivity to angiotensin II) and comparisons of women with low dietary calcium baselines (under 900 mg/day) with women with adequate dietary calcium. The intervention was oral calcium, at least 1 g/day. The controls took a placebo. Maternal outcome measures included hypertension, proteinuria, placental abruption, cesarean birth, mother's length of stay, eclampsia, renal failure, HELLP, intensive care unit admission, and maternal death. Fetal/neonatal outcomes included preterm labor (before 37 weeks), low birth weight, small for gestational age, admission to neonatal intensive care unit (NICU), length of stay longer than seven days, perinatal death, long-term disability, and childhood hypertension (greater than 95th percentile).

Methods

Search Strategy

The reviewers searched the Cochrane database, MEDLINE, 30 journals and conferences, and a weekly current awareness service of 37 journals. Search keywords were *calcium, hypertension, pregnancy, blood pressure,* and combinations of these terms.

Eleven randomized, placebo-controlled trials were selected, representing 6894 women from Argentina, the United States, Australia, Ecuador, and India. The trials were published from 1989 to 2001.

Statistical Analyses

Similar data were pooled, and effect size (the difference between intervention and control groups in each trial) was calculated. The calculations comparing high risk and low risk women, and baseline low and adequate dietary calcium, were analyzed post hoc (after the main calculations).

Findings

Calcium supplementation was associated with significantly less high blood pressure than placebo. The difference was more marked in the group of women at high risk for GH and in the group of women with low baseline dietary calcium. Preeclampsia was likewise significantly reduced with calcium in low risk women and markedly reduced in high risk women and women with low baseline dietary calcium, but the effect was not significant with women who had adequate baseline dietary calcium. The risk of preterm birth and low birth weight was significantly decreased among high risk women taking calcium. There was no difference in cesarean births, admission to NICU, or perinatal death. Data were inadequate to make determinations about maternal death or serious morbidity, placental abruptions, mother's length of stay, small-for-gestational-age babies, or childhood disabilities. One follow-up study of children at 7 years of age found fewer elevated blood pressures in the calcium group than placebo, suggesting a lingering benefit for the offspring. No side effects of calcium were recorded in these trials.

Limitations

The doses and types of calcium differed, as did the definitions of high risk and the baseline dietary calcium intake, causing heterogeneity in the trials and limiting generalizability. Some randomization was not well described. In general, however, these were strong trials in that they were large, double-blinded, and placebo-controlled trials.

Conclusions

Supplemental calcium is associated with less hypertension and less preeclampsia, as well as less preterm birth and low birth weight, especially in those women at high risk.

Implications for Practice

Health care providers should support calcium supplementation for women at high risk for GH, as well as in communities with low baseline calcium intake.

Implications for Further Research

Research should focus on women at high risk for GH and communities with low baseline dietary calcium, and on ideal dosages of calcium. The one study of long-term benefits for offspring was promising. Researchers should distinguish between small-for-gestational-age babies and preterm babies, because they are different processes and have different prognoses.

Reference

Atallah A, Hofmeyr G, Duley L: Calcium supplementation during pregnancy for preventing hypertensive disorders and related problems (Cochrane Review), 2003. In *The Cochrane Library,* Issue 2, Chichester, UK, 2004, John Wiley & Sons.

levels of estrogen. An excessive emphasis on sodium restriction may make it difficult for pregnant women to achieve an adequate diet. Grain, milk, and meat products, which are good sources of other nutrients needed during pregnancy, are significant sources of sodium. In addition, sodium restriction may stress the adrenal glands and the kidney as they attempt to retain adequate sodium. In general, sodium restriction is necessary only if the woman has a medical condition such as renal or liver failure or hypertension.

Excessive intake of sodium is discouraged during pregnancy just as it is in nonpregnant women, because it may contribute to abnormal fluid retention and edema. Table salt (sodium chloride) is the richest source of sodium. Most canned foods contain added salt unless the label specifically states otherwise. Large amounts of sodium are also found in many processed foods, including meats (e.g., smoked or cured meats, cold cuts, and corned beef), baked goods, mixes for casseroles or grain products, soups, and condiments.

Products low in nutritive value and excessively high in sodium include pretzels, potato and other chips, pickles, catsup, prepared mustard, steak and Worcestershire sauces, some soft drinks, and bouillon. A moderate sodium intake can usually be achieved by salting food lightly in cooking; adding no additional salt at the table; and avoiding low-nutrient, high-sodium foods.

Zinc

Zinc is a constituent of numerous enzymes involved in major metabolic pathways. Zinc deficiency is associated with malformations of the central nervous system in infants. When large amounts of iron and folic acid are consumed, the absorption of zinc is inhibited and serum zinc levels are reduced as a result. Because iron and folic acid supplements are commonly prescribed during pregnancy, pregnant women should be encouraged to consume good sources of zinc daily (see Table 12-1). Women with anemia who receive high-dose iron supplements also need supplements of zinc and copper (King, 2000).

Fluoride

There is no evidence that prenatal fluoride supplementation reduces the child's likelihood of tooth decay during the preschool years (Fluoride Recommendations Working Group, 2001). No increase in fluoride intake over the nonpregnant DRI is currently recommended during pregnancy.

Fat-Soluble Vitamins

Fat-soluble vitamins—A, D, E, and K—are stored in the body tissues. With chronic overdoses, these vitamins can reach toxic levels. Because of the high potential for toxicity, pregnant women are advised to take fat-soluble vitamin supplements only as prescribed. Vitamins A and D deserve special mention.

Adequate intake of vitamin A is needed so that sufficient amounts can be stored in the fetus. Dietary sources can readily supply sufficient amounts. Congenital malformations have occurred in infants of mothers who took excessive amounts of vitamin A during pregnancy, and thus supplements are not recommended for pregnant women. Vitamin A analogs such as isotretinoin (Accutane), which are prescribed for the treatment of cystic acne, are a special concern. Isotretinoin use during early pregnancy has been associated with an increased incidence of heart malformations, facial abnormalities, cleft palate, hydrocephalus, and deafness and blindness in the infant, as well as an increased risk of miscarriage. Topical agents such as tretinoin (Retin-A) do not appear to enter the circulation in any substantial amounts, but their safety in pregnancy has not been confirmed.

Vitamin D plays an important role in absorption and metabolism of calcium. The main food sources of this vitamin are enriched or fortified foods such as milk and ready-to-eat cereals. Vitamin D is also produced in the skin by the action of ultraviolet light (in sunlight). Severe deficiency may lead to neonatal hypocalcemia and tetany, as well as hypoplasia of the tooth enamel. Women with lactose intolerance and those who do not include milk in their diet for any reason are at risk for vitamin D deficiency. Other risk factors are dark skin; habitual use of clothing that covers most of the skin (e.g., Arab women with extensive body covering); and living in northern latitudes where sunlight exposure is limited, especially during the winter. Use of recommended amounts of sunscreen with a sun protection factor (SPF) rating of 15 reduces skin vitamin D production by as much as 99% (Scanlon, 2001), reinforcing the need for regular intake of fortified foods or a supplement.

Water-Soluble Vitamins

Body stores of water-soluble vitamins are much smaller than those of fat-soluble vitamins. Water-soluble vitamins, in contrast to fat-soluble vitamins, are readily excreted in the urine. Therefore good sources of these vitamins must be consumed frequently. Toxicity with overdose is less likely than with fat-soluble vitamins.

Because of the increase in RBC production during pregnancy, as well as the nutritional requirements of the rapidly growing cells in the fetus and placenta, pregnant women should consume about 50% more folic acid than nonpregnant women, or about 0.6 mg (600 mcg) daily. In the United States, all enriched grain products (this includes most white breads, flour, and pasta) must contain folic acid at a level of 1.4 mg/kg of flour. This level of fortification is designed to supply approximately 0.1 mg of folic acid daily in the average American diet and has significantly increased folic acid consumption in the population as a whole (Boushey, Edmonds, & Welshimer, 2001). All women of childbearing potential need careful counseling about including good sources of folic acid in their diet (Box 12-4; see Table 12-1). Supplemental folic acid is usually prescribed to ensure that intake is adequate. Women who have borne a child with a neural tube defect are advised to consume 4 mg of folic acid daily, and a supplement is required for them to achieve this level of intake.

Pyridoxine, or vitamin B_6, is involved in protein metabolism. Although levels of a pyridoxine-containing enzyme have been reported to be low in women with preeclampsia, there is no evidence that supplementation prevents or corrects the condition. No supplement is recommended routinely, but women with poor diets and those at nutritional risk (see Box 12-2) may need a supplement providing 2 mg/day.

Vitamin C, or ascorbic acid, plays an important role in tissue formation and enhances the absorption of iron. The vitamin C needs of most women are readily met by a diet that includes at least one daily serving of citrus fruit or juice or another good source of the vitamin (see Table 12-1), but women who smoke need more. For women at nutritional risk, a supplement of 50 mg/day is recommended. However, if the mother takes excessive doses of this vitamin during pregnancy, a vitamin C deficiency may develop in the infant after birth.

Multivitamin-Multimineral Supplements during Pregnancy

The consensus of the 1992 Institute of Medicine committee is that food can and should be the normal vehicle to meet the additional needs imposed by pregnancy, except for iron. Recall that a supplemental dose of 30 mg per day is recommended. In addition, the recommended folate intake may be difficult for some women to achieve. Some women habitually consume diets that are deficient in necessary nutrients and, for whatever reason, may be unable to change this intake. For these women, a multivitamin-multimineral supplement should be considered to ensure that they consume the RDA for most known vitamins and minerals. It is important that the pregnant woman understand that the use of a vitamin-mineral supplement does not lessen the need to consume a nutritious, well-balanced diet.

BOX 12-4

Food Sources of Folate

Foods Providing 500 mcg or More per Serving
Liver: chicken, turkey, goose (3.5 oz)

Foods Providing 200 mcg or More per Serving
Liver: lamb, beef, veal (3.5 oz)

Foods Providing 100 mcg or More per Serving
Legumes, cooked (½ cup)
Peas: black-eye, chickpea (garbanzo)
Beans: black, kidney, pinto, red, navy
Lentils
Vegetables (½ cup)
Asparagus
Spinach, cooked
Papaya (1 medium)
Breakfast cereal, ready-to-eat (½ to 1 cup)
Wheat germ (¼ cup)

Foods Providing 50 mcg or More per Serving
Vegetables (½ cup)
Broccoli
Beans: lima beans, baked beans, or pork and beans
Greens: collards or mustard, cooked
Spinach, raw
Fruits (½ cup)
Avocado
Orange or orange juice
Pasta, cooked (1 cup)
Rice, cooked (1 cup)

Foods Providing 20 mcg or More per Serving
Bread (1 slice)
Egg (1 large)
Corn (½ cup)

Other Nutritional Issues during Pregnancy

Pica and Food Cravings

Pica, the practice of consuming nonfood substances (e.g., clay, dirt, and laundry starch) or excessive amounts of foodstuffs low in nutritional value (e.g., cornstarch, ice, baking powder, and baking soda), is often influenced by the woman's cultural background (Fig. 12-3). In the United States it appears to be most common among African-American women, women from rural areas, and women with a family history of pica. Regular and heavy consumption of low-nutrient products may cause more nutritious foods to be displaced from the diet, and the items consumed may interfere with the absorption of nutrients, especially minerals. Women with pica have lower hemoglobin levels than those without pica. The possibility of pica must be considered when pregnant women are found to be anemic. The nurse should provide counseling about the health risks associated with pica.

The existence of pica, as well as details of the type and amounts of products ingested, is likely to be discovered only by the sensitive interviewer who has developed a relationship of trust with the woman. It has been proposed that pica and food cravings (e.g., the urge to consume ice cream, pickles, or pizza) during pregnancy are caused by an innate drive to consume nutrients missing from the diet. However, research has not supported this hypothesis.

Adolescent Pregnancy Needs

Many adolescent females have diets that provide less than the recommended intakes of key nutrients, including energy, calcium, and iron. Pregnant adolescents and their infants are at increased risk of complications during pregnancy and parturition. Growth of the pelvis is delayed in comparison with growth in stature, and this helps to explain why cephalopelvic disproportion and other mechanical problems associated with labor are common among young adolescents. Competition for nutrients between the growing adolescent and the fetus may also contribute to some of the poor outcomes apparent in teen pregnancies. Pregnant adolescents are encouraged to choose a weight gain goal at the upper end of the range for their BMI.

Efforts to improve the nutritional health of pregnant adolescents focus on improving the nutrition knowledge, meal planning, and food preparation and selection skills of young women; promoting access to prenatal care; developing nutrition interventions and educational programs that are effective with adolescents; and striving to understand the factors that create barriers to change in the adolescent population.

Preeclampsia

The cause of preeclampsia is not known. There has been speculation that the poor intake of several nutrients, including calcium, magnesium, vitamin B_6, and protein, might foster its development. There is no definite evidence that nutritional deficiencies are causes or that nutrition supplements can help prevent it. At present, a diet adequate in the recommended nutrients (see Table 12-1) appears to be the best means of reducing the risk of preeclampsia.

Exercise during Pregnancy

Moderate exercise during pregnancy yields numerous benefits, including improving muscle tone, potentially shortening the course of labor, and promoting a sense of well-being. If no medical or obstetric problems contraindicate physical activity, pregnant women should obtain 30 minutes of moderate physical exercise on most, if not all, days of the week (American College of Obstetricians and Gynecologists, 2002). Two nutritional concepts are especially important for women who choose to exercise during pregnancy. First, a liberal amount of fluid should be consumed before, during, and after exercise because dehydration can trigger premature labor. Second, the calorie intake should be sufficient to meet the increased needs of pregnancy and the demands of exercise.

NUTRIENT NEEDS DURING LACTATION

Nutritional needs during lactation are similar in many ways to those during pregnancy (see Table 12-1). Needs for energy (calories), protein, calcium, iodine, zinc, the B vitamins (thiamine, riboflavin, niacin, pyridoxine, and vitamin B_{12}), and vitamin C remain greater than nonpregnant needs. The recommendations for some of these (e.g., vitamin C, zinc, and protein) are slightly to moderately higher than during pregnancy (see Table 12-1). This allowance covers the amount of the nutrients released in the milk, as well as the needs of the mother for tissue maintenance. In the case of iron and folic acid, the recommendation during lactation is lower than during pregnancy. Both of these nutrients are essential for RBC

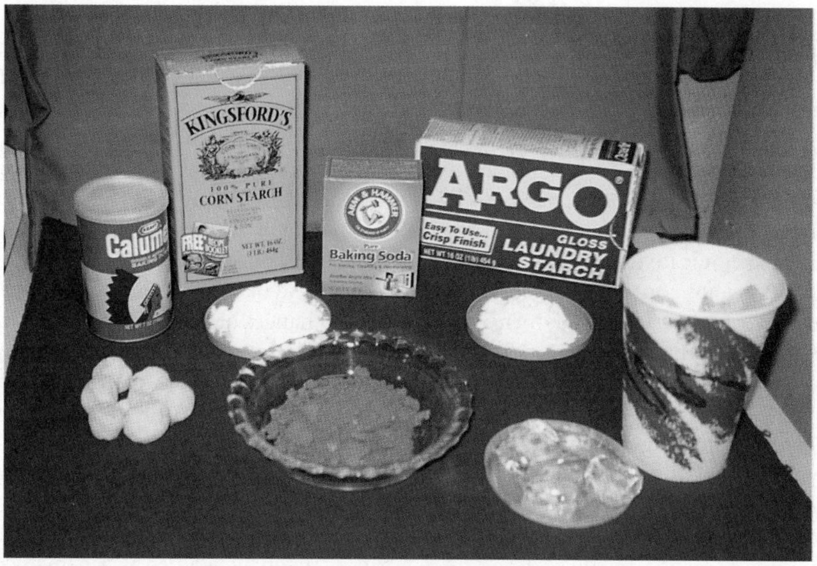

Fig. 12-3 Nonfood substances consumed in pica: red clay from Georgia, Nzu from Eastern Nigeria, baking powder, corn starch, baking soda, laundry starch, and ice. Some individuals practice poly-pica (consuming more than one of these substances). (Courtesy Shannon Perry, Phoenix, AZ.)

formation, and thus for maintaining the increase in the blood volume that occurs during pregnancy. With the decrease in maternal blood volume to nonpregnant levels after birth, maternal iron and folic acid needs also decrease. Many lactating women have a delay in the return of menses; this conserves blood cells and reduces iron and folic acid needs. It is especially important that the calcium intake be adequate; if it is not and the women does not respond to diet counseling, a supplement of 600 mg of calcium per day may be needed.

The recommended energy intake is an increase of 500 kcal more than the woman's nonpregnant intake. The Institute of Medicine (1992) recommends that lactating women consume at least 1800 kcal per day; it is difficult to obtain adequate nutrients for maintenance of lactation at levels below that. Because of the deposition of energy stores, the woman who has gained the optimal amount of weight during pregnancy is heavier after birth than at the beginning of pregnancy. As a result of the caloric demands of lactation, however, the lactating mother usually experiences a gradual but steady weight loss. Most women rapidly lose several pounds during the first month after birth whether or not they breastfeed. After the first month the average loss during lactation is 0.5 to 1.0 kg a month. Fluid intake must be adequate to maintain milk production, but the mother's level of thirst is the best guide to the right amount. There is no need to consume more fluids than those needed to satisfy thirst.

Smoking, alcohol intake, and excessive caffeine intake should be avoided during lactation. Smoking may not only impair milk production, but also expose the infant to the risk of passive smoking. It is speculated that the infant's psychomotor development may be affected by maternal alcohol use, and alcoholic beverages (two drinks per day) may impair the milk ejection reflex. Coffee intake may lead to a reduced iron concentration in milk and consequently contribute to the development of anemia in the infant. The caffeine concentration in milk is only approximately 1% of the mother's plasma level, but caffeine seems to accumulate in the infant. Breastfed infants of mothers who drink large amounts of coffee or caffeine-containing soft drinks may be unusually active and wakeful.

Community Focus

NUTRITION EDUCATION IN THE PRENATAL CLINIC

Visit a prenatal clinic. Identify sources of nutrition education that are evident in the waiting room. Does the clinic employ a nutritionist/dietitian? Who provides nutrition counseling in the clinic? Are print materials available in multiple languages? Are interpreters available? Are there sources of free materials on nutrition that could be placed in the clinic? Identify strengths and weaknesses of nutrition education in that setting. Develop a feasible plan for improving nutrition education in the clinic.

Care Management

During pregnancy, nutrition plays a key role in achieving an optimum outcome for the mother and her unborn baby. Motivation to learn about nutrition is usually higher during pregnancy as parents strive to "do what's right for the baby." Optimum nutrition cannot eliminate all problems that may arise during pregnancy, but it does establish a good foundation for supporting the needs of the mother and her unborn baby (Community Focus).

Assessment

Assessment is based on a diet history (a description of the woman's usual food and beverage intake and factors affecting her nutritional status, such as medications being taken and adequacy of income to allow her to purchase the necessary foods) obtained from an interview and review of the woman's health records, physical examination, and laboratory results. Ideally, a nutritional assessment is performed before conception so that any recommended changes in diet, lifestyle, and weight can be undertaken before the woman becomes pregnant.

Diet History

Obstetric and Gynecologic Effects on Nutrition

Nutritional reserves may be depleted in the multiparous woman or one who has had frequent pregnancies (especially three pregnancies within 2 years). A history of preterm birth or the birth of an LBW or SGA infant may indicate inadequate dietary intake. Preeclampsia may also be a factor in poor maternal nutrition. Birth of a large-for-gestational-age (LGA) infant may indicate the existence of maternal diabetes mellitus. Previous contraceptive methods also may affect reproductive health. Increased menstrual blood loss often occurs during the first 3 to 6 months after placement of an intrauterine contraceptive device. Consequently the user may have low iron stores or even iron deficiency anemia. Oral contraceptive agents, on the other hand, are associated with decreased menstrual losses and increased iron stores. Oral contraceptives, however, may interfere with folic acid metabolism.

Medical History

Chronic maternal illnesses such as diabetes mellitus, renal disease, liver disease, cystic fibrosis or other malabsorptive disorders, seizure disorders and the use of anticonvulsant agents, hypertension, and PKU may affect a woman's nutritional status and dietary needs. In women with illnesses that have resulted in nutritional deficits or that require dietary treatment (e.g., diabetes mellitus, PKU), it is extremely important for nutritional care to be started and for the condition to be optimally controlled before conception. A registered dietitian can provide in-depth counseling for the woman who requires a therapeutic diet during pregnancy and lactation.

Usual Maternal Diet

The woman's usual food and beverage intake, adequacy of income and other resources to meet her nutritional needs, any dietary modifications, food allergies and intolerances, and all medications and nutrition supplements being taken, as well as pica and cultural dietary requirements, should be ascertained. In addition, the presence and severity of nutrition-related discomforts of pregnancy, such as morning sickness, constipation, and pyrosis (heartburn), should be determined. The nurse should be alert to any evidence of eating disorders such as anorexia nervosa, bulimia, or frequent and rigorous dieting before or during pregnancy.

The impact of food allergies and intolerances on nutritional status ranges from very important to almost nil. Lactose intolerance is of special concern in pregnant and lactating women because no other food group equals milk and milk products in terms of calcium content. If a woman has lactose intolerance, the interviewer should explore her intake of other calcium sources (see Box 12-3).

The assessment must include an evaluation of the woman's financial status and her knowledge of sound dietary practices. The quality of the diet improves with increasing socioeconomic status and educational level. Poor women may not have access to adequate refrigeration and cooking facilities and may find it difficult to obtain adequate nutritious food. The pregnancy rates are high among homeless women, and many such women cannot or do not take advantage of services such as food stamps.

Box 12-5 provides a simple tool for obtaining diet history information. When potential problems are identified, they should be followed up with a careful interview.

Physical Examination

Anthropometric (body) measurements provide short- and long-term information on a woman's nutritional status and are thus essential to the assessment. At a minimum, the woman's height and weight must be determined at the time of her first prenatal visit, and her weight should be measured at each subsequent visit (see earlier discussion of BMI).

A careful physical examination can reveal objective signs of malnutrition (Table 12-4). It is important to note, however, that some of these signs are nonspecific and that the physiologic changes of pregnancy may complicate the interpretation of physical findings. For example, lower extremity edema often occurs in calorie and protein deficiency, but it may also be a normal finding in the third trimester of pregnancy. Interpretation of physical findings is made easier by a thorough health history and by laboratory testing, if indicated.

Laboratory Testing

The only nutrition-related laboratory testing needed by most pregnant women is a hematocrit or hemoglobin measurement to screen for the presence of anemia. Because of the physiologic anemia of pregnancy, the reference values for hemoglobin and hematocrit must be adjusted during pregnancy. The lower limit of the normal range for hemoglobin during pregnancy is 11 g/dl in the first and third trimesters and 10.5 g/dl in the second trimester (compared with 12 g/dl in the nonpregnant state). The lower limit of the normal range for hematocrit is 33% during the first and third trimesters and 32% in the second trimester (compared with 36% in the nonpregnant state). Cutoff values for anemia are higher in women who smoke or who live at high altitudes, because the decreased oxygen-carrying capacity of their RBCs causes them to produce more RBCs than other women (Institute of Medicine, 1992).

A woman's history or physical findings may indicate the need for additional testing, such as a complete blood cell count with a differential to identify megaloblastic or macrocytic anemia and measurement of levels of specific vitamins or minerals believed to be lacking in the diet.

The assessment gives a basis for making appropriate nursing diagnoses.

Nursing Diagnoses

- *Imbalanced nutrition: less than body requirements related to*
  —inadequate information about nutritional needs and weight gain during pregnancy
  —misperceptions regarding normal body changes during pregnancy and inappropriate fear of becoming fat
  —inadequate income or skills in meal planning and preparation
- *Imbalanced nutrition: more than body requirements related to*
  —excessive intake of energy (calories) or decrease in activity during pregnancy
  —use of unnecessary dietary supplements
- *Constipation related to*
  —decrease in gastrointestinal motility because of elevated progesterone levels
  —compression of intestines by the enlarging uterus
  —oral iron supplementation

Expected Outcomes

An individualized plan of care based on the nursing diagnoses should be developed in collaboration with the woman.

BOX 12-5

Food Intake Questionnaire

Which of the following did you eat or drink yesterday? If the way you ate yesterday wasn't the way you usually eat, choose a recent day that was typical for you.

Food or Drink	Number of Servings	Food or Drink	Number of Servings
Beer, wine, other alcoholic drinks		Orange or grapefruit juice	
Tea		Fruit juice other than orange or grapefruit	
Coffee		Soft drinks	
Fruit drink		Milk	
Water		Cereal with milk	
Cheese		Yogurt	
Macaroni and cheese		Pizza	
Other foods with cheese (such as lasagna, enchiladas, cheeseburgers)		Melon (such as watermelon, cantaloupe, honeydew)	
Orange or grapefruit		Berries (kind) ________________	
Bananas		Apples	
Peaches or apricots		Other fruit	
Green salad		Broccoli	
Spinach or greens		Green beans	
Green peas		Potatoes (other than fried)	
Sweet potatoes		Corn	
Carrots		Other vegetables	
Meat		Chicken or turkey	
Fish		Egg	
Peanut butter		Nuts	
Dried beans or peas		Hot dog	
Bacon or sausage		Cold cuts	
Bread		Roll	
Rice		Cereal	
Spaghetti or other pasta		Noodles	
Tortillas		Chips	
French fries		Cake	
Cookie		Donut or pastry	
Pie			

Are you often bothered by any of the following? (Circle all that apply)
Nausea   Vomiting   Heartburn   Constipation
Are you on a special diet? No ______ Yes ______ If yes, what kind? ____________
Do you try to limit the amount or kind of food you eat to control your weight? No ______ Yes ______
Do you avoid any foods for health or religious reasons? No ______ Yes ______ If yes, what foods? ____________
Do you take any prescribed drugs or medications? No ______ Yes ______ If yes, what are they? ____________
Do you take any over-the-counter medications (such as aspirin, cold medicines, Tylenol)? No ______ Yes ______
If yes, what are they? ______________________________
Do you ever have trouble affording the food you need? No ______ Yes ______
Do you have any help getting the food you need? No ______ Yes ______ (Circle all that apply)
Food stamps   WIC   School lunch or breakfast
Food from a food pantry, soup kitchen, or food bank

For many women with uncomplicated pregnancies, the nurse can serve as the primary source of nutrition education during pregnancy. The registered dietitian, who has specialized training in diet evaluation and planning, nutritional needs during illness, and ethnic and cultural food patterns, as well as translating nutrient needs into food patterns, often serves as a consultant. Pregnant women with serious nutritional problems, those with intervening illnesses such as diabetes (either preexisting or gestational), and any others requiring in-depth dietary counseling should be referred to the dietitian. The nurse, dietitian, physician, and nurse-midwife collaborate in helping the woman achieve nutrition-related expected outcomes. Some common nutrition-related outcomes are that the woman will take the following actions:

- Achieve an appropriate weight gain during pregnancy. An appropriate goal for weight gain takes into account such factors as prepregnancy weight, whether she is overweight/obese or underweight, and whether the pregnancy is single or multifetal.
- Consume adequate nutrients from the diet and supplements to meet estimated needs.
- Cope successfully with nutrition-related discomforts associated with pregnancy, such as morning sickness, pyrosis (heartburn), and constipation.
- Avoid or reduce potentially harmful practices such as smoking, alcohol consumption, and caffeine intake.
- Return to prepregnancy weight (or an appropriate weight for height) within 6 months of giving birth.

Plan of Care and Implementation

Nutritional care and teaching generally involves the following: (1) acquainting the woman with nutritional needs dur-

Table 12-4

Physical Assessment of Nutritional Status

SIGNS OF GOOD NUTRITION	SIGNS OF POOR NUTRITION
GENERAL APPEARANCE	
Alert, responsive, energetic, good endurance	Listless, apathetic, cachectic, easily fatigued, looks tired
MUSCLES	
Well developed, firm, good tone, some fat under skin	Flaccid, poor tone, undeveloped, tender, "wasted" appearance
NERVOUS CONTROL	
Good attention span, not irritable or restless, normal reflexes, psychologic stability	Inattentive, irritable, confused, burning and tingling of hands and feet, loss of position and vibratory sense, weakness and tenderness of muscles, decrease or loss of ankle and knee reflexes
GASTROINTESTINAL FUNCTION	
Good appetite and digestion, normal regular elimination, no palpable organs or masses	Anorexia, indigestion, constipation or diarrhea, liver or spleen enlargement
CARDIOVASCULAR FUNCTION	
Normal heart rate and rhythm, no murmurs, normal blood pressure for age	Rapid heart rate, enlarged heart, abnormal rhythm, elevated blood pressure
HAIR	
Shiny, lustrous, firm, not easily plucked, healthy scalp	Stringy, dull, brittle, dry, thin and sparse, depigmented, can be easily plucked
SKIN (GENERAL)	
Smooth, slightly moist, good color	Rough, dry, scaly, pale, pigmented, irritated, easily bruised, petechiae
FACE AND NECK	
Skin color uniform, smooth, pink, healthy appearance; no enlargement of thyroid gland; lips not chapped or swollen	Scaly, swollen, skin dark over cheeks and under eyes, lumpiness or flakiness of skin around nose and mouth; thyroid enlarged; lips swollen, angular lesions or fissures at corners of mouth
ORAL CAVITY	
Reddish pink mucous membranes and gums; no swelling or bleeding of gums; tongue healthy pink or deep reddish in appearance, not swollen or smooth, surface papillae present; teeth bright and clean, no cavities, no pain, no discoloration	Gums spongy, bleed easily, inflamed or receding; tongue swollen, scarlet and raw, magenta color, beefy, hyperemic and hypertrophic papillae, atrophic papillae; teeth with unfilled caries, absent teeth, worn surfaces, mottled
EYES	
Bright, clear, shiny, no sores at corners of eyelids, membranes moist and healthy pink color, no prominent blood vessels or mound of tissue (Bitot's spots) on sclera, no fatigue circles beneath	Eye membranes pale, redness of membrane, dryness, signs of infection, Bitot's spots, redness and fissuring of eyelid corners, dryness of eye membrane, dull appearance of cornea, soft cornea, blue sclerae
EXTREMITIES	
No tenderness, weakness, or swelling; nails firm and pink	Edema, tender calves, tingling, weakness; nails spoon-shaped, brittle
SKELETON	
No malformations	Bowlegs, knock-knees, chest deformity at diaphragm, beaded ribs, prominent scapulas

ing pregnancy and, if necessary, the characteristics of an adequate diet; (2) helping her individualize her diet so that she achieves an adequate intake while conforming to her personal, cultural, financial, and health circumstances; (3) acquainting her with strategies for coping with the nutrition-related discomforts of pregnancy; (4) helping her use nutrition supplements appropriately; and (5) consulting with and making referrals to other professionals or services as indicated. Two programs that provide nutrition services are the food stamp program and the Special Supplemental Program for Women, Infants, and Children (WIC). These programs provide vouchers for selected foods to pregnant and lactating women, as well as infants and children at nutritional risk. WIC foods include items such as eggs, cheese, milk, juice, and fortified cereals—foods chosen because they provide iron, protein, vitamin C, and other vitamins.

Adequate Dietary Intake

Diet teaching can take place in a one-on-one interview or in a group setting. In either case, teaching should emphasize the importance of choosing a varied diet composed of readily available foods, rather than specialized diet supplements. Good nutrition practices (and avoidance of poor practices such as smoking and alcohol or drug use) are essential content for prenatal classes designed for women in early pregnancy (see Guidelines/Guías box).

The USDA Food Guide is an eating pattern integrating dietary recommendations designed to provide a healthy way to eat for most people. The eating pattern includes a range of calorie levels that meet the needs of different age and gender groups. For a healthful diet, a variety of nutrient-dense foods and beverages from basic food groups should be consumed. Pregnant women or those who may become pregnant need to ingest foods high in heme-iron and iron-rich plant foods as well as synthetic folic acid and good forms of folate. For a 2,000 calorie diet, 2 cups of fruit and 2½ cups of vegetables per day are recommended (Fig. 12-4). Vegetables should be selected from all five vegetable subgroups. Three or more ounces of whole-grain products should be consumed each day as well as 3 cups per day of fat-free or low-fat milk or their equivalents. Pregnant women should not eat or drink unpasteurized milk or products made from unpasteurized milk, or raw or undercooked eggs, meat, poultry, fish or shellfish, juices, or raw sprouts.

Pregnancy

The pregnant woman must understand what adequate weight gain during pregnancy means, recognize the reasons for its importance, and be able to evaluate her own gain in terms of the desirable pattern. Many women, particularly those who have worked hard to control their weight before pregnancy, may find it difficult to understand why the weight gain goal is so high when a newborn infant is so

ENGLISH SPANISH **Guidelines/Guías**

DIET AND NUTRITION

You need to gain weight.
Usted necesita aumentar de peso.

You need to control your weight gain.
Usted necesita controlar su aumento de peso.

Eat nutritious foods.
Coma alimentos nutritivos.

Eat foods high in protein, calcium, vitamins, and iron.
Coma alimentos altos en proteínas, calcio, vitaminas, y hierro.

Eat a lot of fruits and vegetables.
Coma muchas frutas y vegetales.

Drink four glasses of milk a day.
Tome cuatro vasos de leche diariamente.

Drink low-fat instead of whole milk.
Tome la leche baja en grasa en lugar de la leche entera.

Avoid salty foods like sausage, hot dogs, and french fries.
Evite alimentos muy salados como, calchichas, perros calientes y papitas fritas.

Avoid fried foods.
Evite las frituras.

Avoid caffeine.
Evite la cafeína.

There is caffeine in Coca-Cola, tea, and chocolate.
Hay cafeína en la Coca-Cola, el té, y el chocolate.

Take prenatal vitamins.
Tome vitaminas prenatales.

Suggested amounts of food to consume from the basic food groups, subgroups, and oils to meet recommended nutrient intakes at the 2,000 calorie level are as follows. Nutrient and energy contributions from each group are calculated according to the nutrient-dense forms of foods in each group (e.g., lean meats and fat-free milk). The table also shows the discretionary calorie allowance that can be accommodated in addition to the suggested amounts of nutrient-dense forms of foods in each group.

DAILY AMOUNT OF FOOD FROM EACH GROUP (vegetable subgroup amounts are per week) FOR A 2,000 CALORIE LEVEL

Food Group	Food Items Included in Each Group and Subgroup	Amount and Number of Servings
Fruits	All fresh, frozen, canned, and dried fruits and fruit juices	2 cups (4 servings)
Vegetables		2.5 cups (5 servings)
Dark green	All fresh, frozen, and canned dark green vegetables, cooked or raw (e.g., broccoli, spinach, collard)	3 cups/wk
Orange	All fresh, frozen, and canned orange and deep yellow vegetables, cooked or raw (e.g., carrots, sweet potatoes, winter squash)	2 cups/wk
Legumes	All cooked dry beans and peas and soybean products (e.g., pinto beans lentils, tofu)	3 cups/wk
Starchy	All fresh, frozen, and canned starchy vegetables (e.g., white potatoes, corn, green peas)	3 cups/wk
Other	All fresh, frozen, and canned other vegetables, cooked or raw (e.g., tomatoes, lettuce, green beans, onions)	6.5 cups/wk
Grains		6 oz equivalent
Whole grains	All whole-grain products and whole grains used as ingredients (e.g., whole-wheat or rye bread, whole-grain cereals and crackers, oatmeal, brown rice)	3
Other grains	All refined grain produces and refined grains used as ingredients (e.g., white bread, enriched grain cereals and crackers, enriched pasta, white rice)	3
Lean meat and beans	All meat, poultry, fish, dry beans and peas, eggs, nuts, seeds (most choices should be lean or low-fat). Dry beans and peas and soybean products are considered part of this group as well as the vegetable groups, but should be counted on one group only.	5.5 oz equivalent
Milk	All milks, yogurts, frozen yogurts, dairy desserts, cheeses (low-fat or fat-free)	3 cups
Oils	Oils and soft margarine added to foods during processing, cooking, or at the table	27 g
Discretionary calorie allowance	Remaining amount of calories after selecting the specified number of nutrient-dense forms of foods in each group. Solid fat and sugar calories always need to be counted as discretionary calories	267

Fig. 12-4 USDA Food Guide. From Dietary Guidelines for Americans, 2005. Available online at www.healthierus.gov/dietaryguidelines (accessed March 1, 2005). Consult the website for additional explanations and recommended nutrient intakes at 11 more calorie levels.

small. The nurse can explain that maternal weight gain consists of increments in the weight of many tissues, not just the growing fetus (see Table 12-2).

Dietary overindulgence, which may result in excessive fat stores that persist after giving birth, should be discouraged. Nevertheless, it is best not to focus unduly on weight gain because this could result in feelings of stress and guilt in the woman who does not follow the preferred pattern of gain. Teaching regarding weight gain during pregnancy is summarized in Box 12-6.

Postpartum

The need for a varied diet with portions of food from all food groups continues throughout lactation. As mentioned previously, the lactating woman should be advised to consume at least 1800 kcal daily, and she should receive counseling if her diet appears to be inadequate in any nutrients. Special attention should be given to her zinc, vitamin B_6, and folic acid intake because the recommendations for these remain higher than for nonpregnant women (see Table 12-1). Sufficient calcium is needed to allow for both milk formation and for maintenance of maternal bone mass. It may be difficult for lactating women to consume enough of these nutrients without careful diet planning.

The woman who does not breastfeed loses weight gradually if she consumes a balanced diet that provides slightly less than her daily energy expenditure. Lactating and nonlactating women should know that fat is the most concentrated source of calories in the diet (9 kcal/g vs. 4 kcal/g in carbohydrates and proteins). Therefore the first step in weight reduction (or preventing excessive weight gain) is to evaluate sources of fat in the diet and explore with the woman ways of reducing them. Even foods such as vegetables that are naturally low in fat can become high in fat when fried or sautéed, served with excessive amounts of salad dressing, consumed with high-fat dips or sauces, or seasoned with butter or bacon drippings. A reasonable weight loss goal for nonlactating women is 0.5 to 1 kg per week; a loss of 1 kg per month is recommended for most lactating women who need to lose weight. A woman who is overweight may be able to lose up to 2 kg per month without decreasing her milk supply.

BOX 12-6

Weight Gain during Pregnancy

- Progressive weight gain during pregnancy is essential to ensure normal fetal growth and development and the deposition of maternal stores that promote successful lactation.
- Recommended weight gain during pregnancy is determined largely by prepregnancy weight for height: normal-weight women, 11.5-16 kg; underweight women, 12.5-18 kg; overweight women, 7-11.5 kg.
- Weight gain should be achieved through a balanced diet of regular foods chosen from all the different food groups (see Table 12-4).
- The pattern of weight gain is important: approximately 0.4 kg per week during the second and third trimesters for normal-weight women; 0.5 kg per week for underweight women; and 0.3 kg per week for overweight women.

Daily Food Guide and Menu Planning

The daily food plan (see Table 12-2 and Fig. 12-4) can be used as a guide for educating women about nutritional needs during pregnancy and lactation. This food plan is general enough to be used by women from a variety of cultures, including those following a vegetarian diet. One of the more helpful teaching strategies is to assist the woman to plan daily menus that follow the food plan and are affordable, have realistic preparation times, and are compatible with personal preferences and cultural practices. Information regarding cultural food patterns is provided later in this chapter.

Medical Nutrition Therapy

During pregnancy and lactation, the food plan for women with special medical nutrition therapy (therapeutic diets) may have to be modified. The registered dietitian can instruct these women about their diets and assist them in meal planning. However, the nurse should understand the basic principles of the diet and be able to reinforce the diet teaching.

The nurse should be especially aware of the dietary modifications necessary for women with diabetes mellitus (either gestational or preexisting). This is necessary because this disease is relatively common and because fetal deformity and death occur more often in pregnancies complicated by hyperglycemia or hypoglycemia (see discussion of diabetes in Chapter 13).

Counseling about Iron Supplementation

As mentioned earlier, the nutrition supplement most commonly needed during pregnancy is iron. However, a variety of dietary factors can affect the completeness of absorption of an iron supplement. The following points should be addressed in patient education:

- Bran, milk, egg yolks, coffee, tea, or oxalate-containing vegetables such as spinach and Swiss chard will inhibit iron absorption if consumed at the same time as iron.
- Iron absorption is promoted by a diet rich in vitamin C (e.g., citrus fruits and melons) or "heme iron" (found in red meats, fish, and poultry).
- Iron supplements are best absorbed on an empty stomach; thus they can be taken between meals with beverages other than milk, tea, or coffee.
- Some women have gastrointestinal discomfort when they take the supplement on an empty stomach; therefore a good time for them to take the supplement is just before bedtime.
- Constipation is common with iron supplementation.
- Iron supplements should be kept away from any children in the household because their ingestion could result in acute iron poisoning and even death.

Coping with Nutrition-Related Discomforts of Pregnancy

The most common nutrition-related discomforts of pregnancy are nausea and vomiting (or "morning sickness"), constipation, and pyrosis.

Nausea and Vomiting

Nausea and vomiting are most common during the first trimester. Usually, nausea and vomiting cause only mild to moderate problems nutritionally, although they may cause substantial discomfort. Antiemetic medications, vitamin B_6, and P6 acupressure (Fig. 12-5) may be effective in reducing

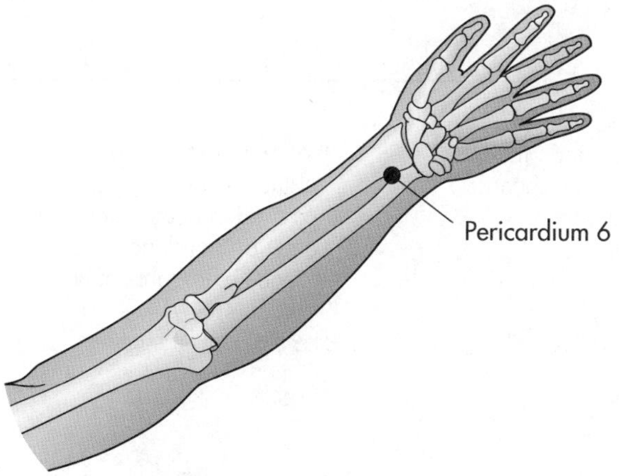

Fig. 12-5 Pericardium 6 (P6) acupressure/acupuncture point for nausea.

the severity of nausea (Jewell & Young, 2004). The pregnant woman may find the following suggestions helpful in alleviating the problems:

- Eat dry, starchy foods such as dry toast, Melba toast, or crackers on awakening in the morning and at other times when nausea occurs.
- Avoid consuming excessive amounts of fluids early in the day or when nauseated (but compensate by drinking fluids at other times).
- Eat small amounts frequently (every 2 to 3 hours) and avoid large meals that distend the stomach.
- Avoid skipping meals and thus becoming extremely hungry, which may worsen nausea. Have a snack such as cereal with milk, a small sandwich, or yogurt before bedtime.
- Avoid sudden movements. Get out of bed slowly.
- Decrease intake of fried and other fatty foods. Starches such as pastas, rice, and breads and low-fat, high-protein foods such as skinless broiled or baked poultry, cooked dry beans or peas, lean meats, and broiled or canned fish are good choices.
- Some women find that tart foods or drinks (e.g., lemonade) or salty foods (e.g., potato chips) are tolerated during periods of nausea.
- Fresh air may help relieve nausea. Keep the environment well ventilated (e.g., open a window), go for a walk outside, or decrease cooking odors by using an exhaust fan.
- During periods of nausea, eat foods served at cool temperatures and foods that give off little aroma.
- Try herbal teas such as those made with raspberry leaf or peppermint to decrease nausea.
- Ginger root may be effective in reducing nausea.
- Avoid brushing teeth immediately after eating.

Hyperemesis gravidarum (severe and persistent vomiting causing weight loss, dehydration, and electrolyte abnormalities) occurs in up to 1% of pregnant women. Intravenous fluid and electrolyte replacement is usually necessary for women who lose 5% of their body weight. Often this is followed by improved tolerance of oral intake; therapy then consists of frequently consuming small amounts of low-fat foods. Enteral tube feeding using small-bore nasogastric tubes has been successful for some women. Because pulmonary aspiration of the feeding is a potential complication if vomiting occurs, antiemetic medications are sometimes used in conjunction with tube feedings. Tube feedings may be used to supplement oral intake, with the volume of the tube feeding gradually being decreased as oral intake improves. In some instances, total parenteral nutrition (balanced intravenous feedings of amino acids, carbohydrate, lipid, vitamins, and minerals) is used to nourish women with hyperemesis gravidarum when their nutritional status has been severely impaired.

Constipation

Improved bowel function generally results from increasing the intake of fiber (e.g., wheat bran and whole-wheat products, popcorn, and raw or lightly steamed vegetables) in the diet. Fiber helps retain water within the stool, creating a bulky stool that stimulates intestinal peristalsis. The recommendation for adults for fiber is 25 to 35 g per day. An increase of approximately 15% would be optimal. An adequate fluid intake (at least 50 ml/kg/day) helps hydrate the fiber and increase the bulk of the stool. Making a habit of regular exercise that uses large muscle groups (walking, swimming, cycling) also helps stimulate bowel motility.

Pyrosis

Pyrosis, or heartburn, is usually caused by reflux of gastric contents into the esophagus. This condition can be minimized by eating small, frequent meals rather than two or three larger meals daily. Because fluids increase the distention of the stomach, they should not be consumed with foods. The woman needs to be sure to drink adequate amounts between meals. Avoiding spicy foods may help alleviate the problem. Lying down immediately after eating and wearing clothing that is tight across the abdomen can contribute to the problem of reflux.

Cultural Influences

Consideration of a woman's cultural food preferences enhances communication and provides a greater opportunity for following the agreed-on pattern of intake. Women in most cultures are encouraged to eat a diet typical for them. The nurse needs to be aware of what constitutes a typical diet for each cultural or ethnic group. However, several variations may occur within one cultural group. Thus a careful exploration of individual preferences is needed. Although ethnic and cultural food beliefs may seem, at first glance, to conflict with the dietary instruction provided by physicians, nurses, and dietitians, it is often possible for the empathic health care provider to identify cultural beliefs that are congruent with the modern understanding of pregnancy and fetal development. Many cultural food practices have some merit or the culture would not have survived. Food cravings during pregnancy are considered normal by many cultures, but the kinds of cravings often are culturally specific. In most cultures women crave acceptable foods, such as chicken, fish, and greens among African-Americans. Cultural influences on food intake usually lessen if the woman and her family become more integrated into the dominant culture. Nutrition beliefs and the practices of selected cultural groups are summarized in Table 12-5.

Vegetarian Diets

Vegetarian diets represent another cultural effect on nutritional status. Foods basic to almost all vegetarian diets are vegetables, fruits, legumes, nuts, seeds, and grains. However,

Text continued on p. 326.

Table 12-5

Characteristic Food Patterns of Selected Cultures

MILK GROUP	PROTEIN GROUP	FRUITS AND VEGETABLES	BREADS AND CEREALS	POSSIBLE DIETARY PROBLEMS
NATIVE AMERICAN (MANY TRIBAL VARIATIONS; MANY "AMERICANIZED")				
Fresh milk Evaporated milk for cooking Ice cream Cream pie	Pork, beef, lamb, rabbit Fowl, fish, eggs Legumes Sunflower seeds Nuts: walnuts, acorn, pine, peanut butter Game meat	Green peas, beans Beets, turnips Leafy green and other vegetables Grapes, bananas, peaches, other fresh fruits Roots	Refined bread Whole wheat Cornmeal Rice Dry cereals "Fry" bread Tortillas	Obesity, diabetes, alcoholism, nutritional deficiencies expressed in dental problems and iron deficiency anemia Inadequate amounts of all nutrients Excessive use of sugar
MIDDLE EASTERN* (ARMENIAN, GREEK, SYRIAN, TURKISH)				
Yogurt Little butter	Lamb Nuts Dried peas, beans, lentils Sesame seeds	Peppers, tomatoes, cabbage, grape leaves, cucumbers, squash Dried apricots, raisins, dates	Cracked wheat and dark bread	Fry many meats and vegetables Lack of fresh fruits Insufficient foods from milk group High consumption of sweetenings, lamb fat, and olive oil
AFRICAN-AMERICAN (PARTICULARLY SOUTHERN AND RURAL)				
Milk† Ice cream Cheese: longhorn, American	Pork: all cuts, plus organs, chitterlings Beef, lamb Chicken, giblets Eggs Nuts Legumes Fish, game	Leafy vegetables Green and yellow vegetables Potato: white, sweet Stewed fruit Bananas and other fresh fruit	Cornmeal and hominy grits Rice Biscuits, pancakes, white breads Puddings: bread, rice	Extensive use of frying, smothering in gravy, or simmering Fats: salt pork, bacon drippings, lard, and gravies High consumption of sweets Insufficient citrus Vegetables often boiled for long periods with pork fat and much salt Limited amounts from milk group†
CHINESE (CANTONESE MOST PREVALENT)				
Milk: water buffalo	Pork sausage‡ Eggs and pigeon eggs Fish Lamb, beef, goat Fowl: chicken, duck Nuts Legumes Soybean curd (tofu)	Many vegetables Radish leaves Bean, bamboo sprouts	Rice/rice flour products Cereals, noodles Wheat, corn, millet seed	Tendency of some immigrants to use large amounts of grease in cooking Limited use of milk and milk products Often low in protein, calories, or both Soy sauce (high sodium)
FILIPINO (SPANISH-CHINESE INFLUENCE)				
Flavored milk Milk in coffee Cheese: gouda, cheddar	Pork, beef, goat, rabbit Chicken Fish Eggs, nuts, legumes	Many vegetables and fruits	Rice, cooked cereals Noodles: rice, wheat	Limited use of milk and milk products Tendency to prewash rice Tendency to have only small portions of protein foods
ITALIAN				
Cheese Some ice cream	Meat Eggs Dried beans	Leafy vegetables Potatoes Eggplant, tomatoes, peppers Fruits	Pasta White breads, some whole wheat Farina Cereals	Prefer expensive imported cheeses; reluctant to substitute less expensive domestic varieties Tendency to overcook vegetables Limited use of whole grains High consumption of sweets Extensive use of olive oil Insufficient servings from milk group

MSG, monosodium L-glutamate.
*Religious holidays may involve fasting, which is believed to increase the likelihood of preterm labor. Fasting requirement may be waived during pregnancy.
†Lactose intolerance relatively common in adults.
‡Lower in fat content than Western sausage.

Table 12-5

Characteristic Food Patterns of Selected Cultures—cont'd

MILK GROUP	PROTEIN GROUP	FRUITS AND VEGETABLES	BREADS AND CEREALS	POSSIBLE DIETARY PROBLEMS
JAPANESE (ISEI, MORE JAPANESE INFLUENCE; NISEI, MORE WESTERNIZED)				
Increasing amounts being used by younger generations	Pork, beef, chicken Fish Eggs Legumes: soys, red, lima beans Tofu Nuts	Many vegetables and fruits Seaweed	Rice, rice cakes Wheat noodles Refined bread, noodles	Excessive sodium: pickles, salty crisp seaweed, MSG, and soy sauce Insufficient servings from milk group May use prewashed rice
HISPANIC, MEXICAN-AMERICAN				
Milk Cheese Flan, ice cream	Beef, pork, lamb, chicken, tripe, hot sausage, beef intestines Fish Eggs Nuts Dry beans: pinto, chickpeas (often eaten more than once daily)	Spinach, wild greens, tomatoes, chilies, corn, cactus leaves, cabbage, avocado, potatoes Pumpkin, zapote, peaches, guava, papaya, citrus	Rice, cornmeal Sweet bread, pastries Tortilla: corn, flour Vermicelli *(fideo)*	Limited meats primarily due to cost Limited use of milk and milk products Large amounts of lard Abundant use of sugar Tendency to boil vegetables for long periods
PUERTO RICAN				
Limited use of milk products Coffee with milk *(café con leche)*	Pork Poultry Eggs (Fridays) Dried codfish Beans *(habichuelas)*	Avocado, okra Eggplant Sweet yams Starchy vegetables and fruits *(viandas)*	Rice Cornmeal	Small amounts of pork and poultry Extensive use of fat, lard, salt pork, and olive oil Lack of milk products
SCANDINAVIAN (DANISH, FINNISH, NORWEGIAN, SWEDISH)				
Cream Butter Cheeses	Wild game Reindeer Fish (fresh or dried) Eggs	Berries Dried fruit Vegetables: cole slaw, roots	Whole wheat, rye, barley, sweets (cookies and sweet breads)	Insufficient fresh fruits and vegetables High consumption of sweets, pickled or salted meats, and fish
SOUTHEAST ASIAN (VIETNAMESE, CAMBODIAN)				
Generally not taken Coffee with condensed cow's milk Plain yogurt Ice cream (rare) Soybean milk	Fish (daily): fresh, dried, salted Poultry/eggs: duck, chicken Pork Beef (seldom) Dry beans Tofu	Seasonal variety: fresh or preserved Green, leafy vegetables Yams Corn	Rice: grains, flour, noodles French bread "Cellophane" (bean starch) noodles	Fresh milk products generally not consumed Poultry/eggs may be limited Meat considered "unclean" is avoided Preference for a diet high in salt and pepper, as well as rice and pork High intake of MSG and soy sauce
JEWISH: ORTHODOX*				
Milk† Cheese†	Meat (bloodless; Kosher prepared): beef, lamb, goat, deer, poultry (all types), no pork Fish with fins and scales only No crustaceans	Wide variety	Wide variety	High intake of sodium in meat products

there are many variations in vegetarian diets. Semivegetarians, who are not truly vegetarians, include fish, poultry, eggs, and dairy products in their diets but do not eat beef or pork. Such a diet can be completely adequate for pregnant women. Besides plant products, lacto-ovo vegetarians also eat dairy products and eggs. Iron and zinc intake may not be adequate in these women, but such diets can be otherwise nutritionally sound. Strict vegetarians, or vegans, consume only plant products. Because vitamin B_{12} is found only in foods of animal origin, this diet is therefore deficient in vitamin B_{12}. As a result, strict vegetarians should take a supplement or regularly consume vitamin B_{12}–fortified foods (e.g., soy milk). Vitamin B_{12} deficiency can result in megaloblastic anemia, glossitis (inflamed red tongue), and neurologic deficits in

Nursing Care Plan

NUTRITION DURING PREGNANCY

NURSING DIAGNOSIS: Deficient knowledge related to nutritional requirements during pregnancy

EXPECTED OUTCOMES

The patient will delineate nutritional requirements and exhibit evidence of incorporating requirements into diet.

NURSING INTERVENTIONS/*RATIONALES*

Review basic nutritional requirements for a healthy diet using recommended dietary guidelines and the USDA Food Guide *to provide knowledge baseline for discussion.*

Discuss increased nutrient needs (calories, protein, minerals, vitamins) that occur as a result of being pregnant *to increase knowledge needed for altered dietary requirements.*

Discuss the relationship between weight gain and fetal growth *to reinforce interdependence of fetus and mother.*

Calculate the appropriate total weight gain range during pregnancy using the woman's body mass index as a guide and discuss recommended rates of weight gain during the various trimesters of pregnancy *to provide concrete measures of dietary success.*

Review food preferences, cultural eating patterns or beliefs, and prepregnancy eating patterns *to enhance integration of new dietary needs.*

Discuss how to fit nutritional needs into usual dietary patterns and how to alter any identified nutritional deficits or excesses *to increase chances of success with dietary alterations.*

Discuss food aversions or cravings that may occur during pregnancy and strategies to deal with these if they are detrimental to fetus (e.g., pica) *to ensure well-being of fetus.*

Have woman keep a food diary delineating eating habits, dietary alterations, aversions, and cravings *to track eating habits and potential problem areas.*

NURSING DIAGNOSIS: Imbalanced nutrition: more than body requirements related to excessive intake or inadequate activity levels (or both)

EXPECTED OUTCOME

The patient's weekly weight gain will be reduced to the appropriate rate using her body mass index (BMI) and recommended weight gain ranges as guidelines.

NURSING INTERVENTIONS/*RATIONALES*

Review recent diet history (including food cravings) using a food diary, 24-hour recall, or food frequency approach *to ascertain food excesses contributing to excess weight gain.*

Review normal activity and exercise routines *to determine level of energy expenditure;* discuss eating patterns and reasons that lead to increased food intake (e.g., cultural beliefs or myths, increased stress, boredom) *to identify habits that contribute to excess weight gain.*

Review optimal weight gain guidelines and their rationale *to ensure that woman is knowledgeable about healthful weight gain rates.*

Set target weight gains for the remaining weeks of the pregnancy *to establish set goals.*

Discuss with the woman what changes can be made in diet, activity, and lifestyle *to enhance chances of meeting weight gain goals and dietary needs.* Weight-reduction diets should be avoided, *because they may deprive the mother and fetus of needed nutrients and lead to ketonemia.*

NURSING DIAGNOSIS: Imbalanced nutrition: less than body requirements related to inadequate intake of needed nutrients

EXPECTED OUTCOME

The woman's weekly weight gain will be increased to the appropriate rate using her BMI and recommended weight gain ranges as guidelines.

NURSING INTERVENTIONS/*RATIONALES*

Review recent diet history (including food aversions) using a food diary, 24-hour recall, or food frequency approach *to ascertain dietary inadequacies contributing to lack of sufficient weight gain.*

Review normal activity and exercise routines *to determine level of energy expenditure;* discuss eating patterns and reasons that lead to decreased food intake (e.g., morning sickness, pica, fear of becoming fat, stress, boredom) *to identify habits that contribute to inadequate weight gain.*

Review optimal weight gain guidelines and their rationale *to ensure that woman is knowledgeable about healthful weight gain rates.*

Set target weight gains for the remaining weeks of the pregnancy *to establish set goals.*

Review increased nutrient needs (calories, protein, minerals, vitamins) that occur as a result of being pregnant *to ensure woman is knowledgeable about altered dietary requirements.*

Review relationship between weight gain and fetal growth *to reinforce that adequate weight gain is needed to promote fetal well-being.*

Discuss with woman what changes can be made in diet, activity, and lifestyle *to enhance chances of meeting set weight gain goals and nutrient needs of mother and fetus.*

If woman has fear of being fat, if symptoms of an eating disorder are evident, or if problems in adjusting to a changing body image surface, refer woman to the appropriate mental health professional for evaluation, because intensive treatment and follow-up may be required *to ensure fetal health.*

the mother. Infants born to affected mothers are likely to have megaloblastic anemia and exhibit neurodevelopmental delays. Iron, calcium, zinc, and vitamin B_6 intake may also be low in women on this diet, and some strict vegetarians have excessively low caloric intakes. The protein intake should be assessed especially carefully because plant proteins tend to be incomplete in that they lack one or more amino acids required for growth and maintenance of body tissues. The daily consumption of a variety of different plant proteins (grains, dried beans and peas, nuts, and seeds) helps provide all of the essential amino acids.

Evaluation

In evaluating the adequacy of nutritional intake during pregnancy, the woman's weight gain can be compared with standardized grids showing recommended patterns (see Fig. 12-2). These grids are based on mean data and do not always account for factors such as ethnic or racial variations. To evaluate the adequacy of the woman's diet, it can be compared with the plan in Table 12-2. It is essential that individual factors affecting nutritional needs and dietary intake be considered.

Physical examination and laboratory testing can be used to confirm that nutritional status is adequate (see the section on assessment). When weight gain is inadequate or when nutritional deficits appear, the nurse must reassess the woman and her understanding of her nutritional needs, reinforce teaching as needed, and continue to reevaluate her nutritional status regularly (Nursing Care Plan).

Key Points

- A woman's nutritional status before, during, and after pregnancy contributes significantly to her well-being and that of her infant.
- Many physiologic changes occurring during pregnancy influence the need for additional nutrients and the efficiency with which the body uses them.
- Both the total maternal weight gain and the pattern of weight gain are important determinants of the outcome of pregnancy.
- The appropriateness of the mother's prepregnancy weight for height (BMI) is a major determinant of her recommended weight gain during pregnancy.
- Nutritional risk factors include adolescent pregnancy, nicotine use, alcohol or drug use, bizarre or faddish food habits, a low weight for height, and frequent pregnancies.
- Iron supplementation is usually routinely recommended during pregnancy. Other supplements may be warranted when nutritional risk factors are present.
- The nurse and the woman are influenced by cultural and personal values and beliefs during nutrition counseling.
- Pregnancy complications that may be nutrition related include anemia, preeclampsia, gestational diabetes, and intrauterine growth restriction.
- Dietary adaptation can be an effective intervention for some of the common discomforts of pregnancy, including nausea and vomiting, constipation, and heartburn.

Answer Guidelines to Critical Thinking Exercise

Nutrition and the Overweight Pregnant Woman

1. Yes. A dietary assessment using a food intake questionnaire should be conducted and a physical assessment of nutritional status performed. Based on these data, the desired pattern of weight gain during pregnancy, and a knowledge of characteristic food patterns of African-American and Asian people, planning can begin.
2. (a) A list of Dietary Reference Intakes for pregnancy and lactation can be shared with Tamara. Through discussion, you can determine whether Tamara is ingesting adequate amounts of these important elements and whether supplementation of vitamins and minerals is necessary. (b) While reviewing indicators of nutritional risk in pregnancy with Tamara, problem areas can be identified, and recommendations for change provided as needed. (c) The daily food guide for pregnancy and lactation can be shared with Tamara. It can provide a basis for planning appropriate menus to provide the necessary nutrients and avoid consuming more energy (calories) than is desired. (d) As someone with Asian heritage, Tamara may be lactose intolerant and need sources of calcium other than milk. Through careful questioning, her lactose status can be determined and counseling provided about nonmilk sources of calcium.
3. As part of her prenatal care, Tamara (and all pregnant women) should receive nutrition counseling. Tamara is currently overweight. Although reduction diets are contraindicated in pregnancy, Tamara can be assisted to plan menus that allow a slow but adequate weight gain to support growth of the pregnancy and the fetus and avoid excess weight gain.
4. Yes, there is ample evidence about DRIs in pregnancy and lactation. Nutrition counseling should be part of the plan of care for Tamara.
5. Tamara could have metabolic problems, including diabetes mellitus, that contribute to her weight. Ethnic and cultural patterns of eating could also be a factor. Enlisting the support of her family would likely be helpful in planning appropriate meals.

Resources

American Botanical Council
PO Box 144345
Austin, TX 78714-4345
512-926-4900
www.herbalgram.org

American Diabetes Association
Diabetes Information Service Center
1660 Duke St.
Alexandria, VA 22314
800-342-2383
www.diabetes.org

American Dietetic Association
216 West Jackson Blvd., Suite 800
Chicago, IL 60606-6995
www.eatright.org

American Medical Association
Department of Foods and Nutrition
515 North State St.
Chicago, IL 60610
www.ama-assn.org

Anorexia Nervosa and Related Eating Disorders, Inc.
www.anred.com

Body Mass Index Calculator
National Heart, Lung, and Blood Institute Information Center
PO Box 30105
Bethesda, MD 20824-0105
301-592-8573
www.nhlbisupport.com/bmi

Center for Food Safety and Applied Nutrition
Food and Drug Administration
200 C St., SW
Washington, DC 20250
202-720-2791
www.usda.gov/usda.htm

Food and Nutrition Board
Institute of Medicine
2101 Constitution Ave., NW
Washington, DC 20418
202-334-1732
www.iom.edu
E-mail: fnb@nas.edu

National Dairy Council
6300 N. River Rd.
Rosemont, IL 60018
www.nutritionexplorations.org

Nutritional content of foods
www.nal.usda.gov/fnic/foodcomp

Office of Dietary Supplements
National Institutes of Health
31 Center Dr., Room 1829
Bethesda, MD 20892-2086
301-435-2920
www.odp.od.nih.gov/ods

RDAs according to age and sex
www.nal.usda.gov/fnic/dga/rda/htm

Society of Nutrition Education
1001 Connecticut Ave., NW, Suite 529
Washington, DC 20036-5528
202-452-8534
www.sne.org
E-mail: info@sne.org

Special Supplemental Nutrition Program for Women, Infants, and Children (WIC)
Food and Consumer Service
3101 Park Center Dr., Room 819
Alexandria, VA 22302
703-305-2286
www.usda.gov/fns/wic.html

U.S. Department of Agriculture
Food and Nutrition Information Center
14th and Independence Ave., SW
Washington, DC 20250
202-720-2791
www.usda.gov/usda.htm
www.health.gov/dietaryguidelines/dga2005/report/

References

American College of Obstetricians and Gynecologists: ACOG committee opinion: exercise during pregnancy and the postpartum period, number 267, *Obstet Gynecol* 99(1):171-173, 2002.

Atallah A, Hofmeyr G, Duley L: Calcium supplementation during pregnancy for preventing hypertensive disorders and related problems (Cochrane Review), 2003. In *The Cochrane Library,* Issue 2, Chichester, UK, 2004, John Wiley & Sons.

Boushey CJ, Edmonds JW, Welshimer KJ: Estimates of the effects of folic-acid fortification and folic-acid bioavailability for women, *Nutrition* 17(10):873-879, 2001.

Centers for Disease Control and Prevention: PNSS pregnancy nutrition surveillance system. Internet document available at www.ced.gov/nccdphp/dnpa/PNSS.htm (accessed August 22, 2004).

Fluoride Recommendations Work Group: Recommendations for using fluoride to prevent and control dental caries in the United States, *MMWR* 50(RR-14):1-42, 2001.

Food and Nutrition Board, Institute of Medicine: *Dietary reference intakes for calcium, phosphorus, magnesium, vitamin D, and fluoride.* Washington, DC, 1997, National Academy Press.

Food and Nutrition Board, Institute of Medicine: *Dietary reference intakes for thiamine, riboflavin, niacin, vitamin B_6, folate, vitamin B_{12}, pantothenic acid, biotin, and choline.* Washington, DC, 1998, National Academy Press.

Food and Nutrition Board, Institute of Medicine: *Dietary reference intakes for vitamin C, vitamin E, selenium, and carotenoids.* Washington, DC, 2000, National Academy Press.

Food and Nutrition Board, Institute of Medicine: *Dietary reference intakes for vitamin A, vitamin K, arsenic, boron, chromium, copper, iodine, iron, manganese, molybdenum, nickel, silicon, vanadium, and zinc.* Washington, DC, 2001, National Academy Press.

Food and Nutrition Board, National Academy of Science, National Research Council: *Recommended dietary allowances,* ed 10, Washington, DC, 1989, National Academy Press.

Institute of Medicine: *Nutrition during pregnancy and lactation: an implementation guide,* Washington, DC, 1992, National Academy Press.

Jewell D, Young G: Interventions for nausea and vomiting in early pregnancy (Cochrane Review), 2004. In *The Cochrane Library,* Issue 4, Chichester, UK, 2004, John Wiley & Sons.

Kilpatrick SJ, Laros RK: Maternal hematologic disorders. In Creasy RK, Resnik R, Iams JD (eds): *Maternal-fetal medicine: principles and practice,* ed 5, Philadelphia, 2004, WB Saunders.

King JC: Determinants of maternal zinc status during pregnancy, *Am J Clin Nutr* 71(5 suppl):1334S-1343S, 2000.

Malone FD, D'Alton ME: Multiple gestation: clinical characteristics and management. In Creasy RK, Resnik R, Iams JD (eds): *Maternal-fetal medicine: principles and practice,* ed 5, Philadelphia, 2004, WB Saunders.

Scanlon K (ed): *Final report of the vitamin D expert panel,* Atlanta, 2001, Centers for Disease Control and Prevention.

Pregnancy at Risk: Preexisting Conditions

13

LEARNING OBJECTIVES

On completion of this chapter the reader will be able to:

- Differentiate the types of diabetes mellitus and their respective risk factors in pregnancy.
- Compare insulin requirements during pregnancy, the postpartum period, and lactation.
- Identify maternal and fetal risks or complications associated with diabetes in pregnancy.
- Develop a plan of care for the pregnant woman with pregestational or gestational diabetes.
- Compare the management of a pregnant woman with hyperthyroidism with one who has hypothyroidism.
- Differentiate the management of various cardiovascular disorders in pregnant women.
- Discuss the different types of anemia and their effects during pregnancy.
- Explain the care of pregnant women with pulmonary disorders.
- Describe the effect of gastrointestinal disorders on pregnancy.
- Review the effects of neurologic disorders on pregnancy.
- Describe the care of women whose pregnancies are complicated by autoimmune disorders.
- Explain the effects on and the management of pregnant women with human immunodeficiency virus (HIV).
- Discuss the care of pregnant women who use, abuse, or are dependent on alcohol or illicit or prescription drugs.

ELECTRONIC RESOURCES

Additional information related to the content in Chapter 13 can be found on

the companion website at evolve
http://evolve.elsevier.com/Wong/maternal/
- NCLEX Review Questions
- Case Study–Pregestational Diabetes
- Case Study–Class III Cardiac Disorder
- WebLinks

or the interactive student CD-ROM
Activities for Chapter 13 include the following:
- NCLEX Review Questions
- Case Study–Pregestational Diabetes
- Case Study–Class III Cardiac Disorder
- Nursing Care Plan–Pregestational Diabetes
- Nursing Care Plan–Heart Disease

For most women, pregnancy represents a normal part of life. However, for some women, pregnancy represents a significant risk because it is superimposed on a chronic illness. With well-motivated patients who actively participate in the treatment plan, and with careful management from a multidisciplinary health care team, positive pregnancy outcomes are often possible today.

Providing safe and effective care for women experiencing high risk pregnancy and their fetuses is a challenge. While unique maternal and fetal needs prompted by these conditions exist, these women also experience many of the same pregnancy-related feelings, needs, and concerns as their "normal" counterparts. The primary objective of nursing care must be to guide and support the woman and her family in achieving optimal outcome for both the pregnant woman and the fetus.

This chapter focuses on metabolic disorders, including diabetes mellitus and thyroid disorders; cardiovascular disorders; selected disorders of the respiratory, gastrointestinal, integumentary, and central nervous systems; and autoimmune disorders. Substance abuse and human immunodeficiency virus (HIV) infection are also discussed.

METABOLIC DISORDERS

Diabetes Mellitus

Despite advances in care, pregnancy complicated by diabetes is still considered high risk. It is most successfully managed with a multidisciplinary approach involving the obstetrician, internist or diabetologist, neonatologist, nurse, nutritionist, and social worker. Favorable outcome of pregnancy complicated by diabetes requires commitment and active participation by the woman and her family. The woman must comply with a schedule of frequent prenatal visits, strict adherence to the dietary regimen, regular self-monitoring of blood glucose level, frequent laboratory evaluation, intensive fetal surveillance, and possible hospitalization.

The perinatal mortality rate for well-managed diabetic pregnancies, excluding major congenital malformations, is about the same as that for any other pregnancy (Moore, 2004). The incidence of major congenital malformations in infants born to women with diabetes has not changed significantly over time. Experts have concluded that the key to optimal pregnancy outcome is strict maternal glucose control before conception, as well as throughout the pregnancy. Consequently, much emphasis is placed on preconception counseling for women with diabetes.

Care of the pregnant woman who has diabetes requires that the nurse fully understand the normal physiologic responses to pregnancy, as well as the altered metabolism of diabetes. Furthermore, the nurse must understand the relationship between pregnancy and diabetes, including psychosocial implications, to assess the woman accurately, plan for her care, and intervene appropriately.

Pathogenesis

Diabetes mellitus is a group of metabolic diseases characterized by hyperglycemia resulting from defects in insulin secretion, insulin action, or both (Expert Committee on the Diagnosis and Classification of Diabetes Mellitus, 2003). Insulin, produced by beta cells in the islets of Langerhans in the pancreas, regulates blood glucose levels by enabling glucose to enter adipose and muscle cells where it is used for energy. Insulin also stimulates protein synthesis and storage of free fatty acids. When insulin is insufficient or ineffective in promoting glucose uptake by the muscle and adipose cells, glucose accumulates in the bloodstream and hyperglycemia results. Hyperglycemia causes hyperosmolarity of the blood, which attracts intracellular fluid into the vascular system, resulting in cellular dehydration and expanded blood volume. Consequently the kidneys function to excrete large volumes of urine (polyuria) in an attempt to regulate excess vascular volume and to excrete the unusable glucose (glycosuria). Polyuria and cellular dehydration cause excessive thirst (polydipsia).

The body compensates for its inability to convert carbohydrate (glucose) into energy by burning proteins (muscle) and fats. The end products of this metabolism are ketones and fatty acids, which in excess quantity produce ketoacidosis and acetonuria. Weight loss occurs because of the breakdown of fat and muscle tissue. This tissue breakdown causes a state of starvation that compels the individual to eat excessive amounts of food (polyphagia).

Over time, diabetes causes significant changes in both the microvascular and macrovascular circulations. These structural changes affect a variety of organ systems, primarily the heart, eyes, kidneys, and nerves. Complications resulting from diabetes include premature atherosclerosis, retinopathy, nephropathy, and neuropathy.

Diabetes may be caused by either impaired insulin secretion, when beta cells of the pancreas are destroyed by an autoimmune process; or by inadequate insulin action in target tissues at one or more points along the metabolic pathway. Both of these conditions are commonly present in the same person, and it is unclear which abnormality, if either, is the primary cause of the disease (Expert Committee on the Diagnosis and Classification of Diabetes Mellitus, 2003).

Classification

The classification and diagnosis of diabetes were revised in 1997 by an international Expert Committee working under the sponsorship of the American Diabetes Association (ADA). The current classification system includes four groups: type 1 diabetes, type 2 diabetes, other specific types (e.g., diabetes caused by infection or drug-induced diabetes), and gestational diabetes mellitus. A major change proposed by the Expert Committee was a move away from a system that classified the disease by its pharmacologic management to one based on disease etiology (Expert Committee on the Diagnosis and Classification of Diabetes Mellitus, 2003).

Type 1 diabetes includes those cases that are primarily due to pancreatic islet beta cell destruction and that are prone to ketoacidosis. People with type 1 diabetes usually have an absolute insulin deficiency. Type 1 diabetes includes cases currently thought to be caused by an autoimmune process, as well as those for which the cause is unknown (Expert Committee on the Diagnosis and Classification of Diabetes Mellitus, 2003).

Type 2 diabetes is the most prevalent form of the disease and includes individuals who have insulin resistance and usually relative (rather than absolute) insulin deficiency. Specific etiologies for type 2 diabetes are unknown at this time. Type 2 diabetes often goes undiagnosed for years because hyperglycemia develops gradually and often is not severe enough for the person to recognize the classic signs of polyuria, polydipsia, and polyphagia. Many people who develop type 2 diabetes are obese or have an increased amount of body fat distributed primarily in the abdominal area. Other risk factors include aging, a sedentary lifestyle, hypertension, and prior gestational diabetes. Type 2 diabetes often has a strong genetic predisposition (Expert Committee on the Diagnosis and Classification of Diabetes Mellitus, 2003).

Pregestational diabetes is the label sometimes given to type 1 or type 2 diabetes that existed before pregnancy.

Gestational diabetes mellitus (GDM) is any degree of glucose intolerance with its onset or first recognition during pregnancy. This definition is appropriate whether or not insulin is used for treatment or whether the diabetes persists after pregnancy. It does not exclude the possibility that the glucose intolerance preceded the pregnancy. Women experiencing gestational diabetes should be reclassified 6 weeks or more after the pregnancy ends (Expert Committee on the Diagnosis and Classification of Diabetes Mellitus, 2003).

Prediabetes

Hyperglycemia that is not sufficient to meet the criteria for a diagnosis of diabetes is categorized as impaired fasting glucose (IFG). IFG is identified through fasting plasma glucose or impaired glucose tolerance (IGT) if identified through an oral glucose tolerance test. Recently, IFG (fasting plasma glucose of 100 to 125 mg/dl) and IGT (2-hour plasma glucose of 140 to 199 mg/dl) have been classified as prediabetes. Both categories are risk factors for diabetes and cardiovascular disease. The rate of progression to type 2 diabetes can be reduced by weight loss and regular physical activity (ADA, 2004b).

Metabolic Changes Associated with Pregnancy

Normal pregnancy is characterized by complex alterations in maternal glucose metabolism, insulin production, and metabolic homeostasis. During normal pregnancy, adjustments in maternal metabolism allow for adequate nutrition for both the mother and the developing fetus. Glucose, the primary fuel used by the fetus, is transported across the placenta through the process of carrier-mediated facilitated diffusion. This means that the glucose levels in the fetus are directly proportional to maternal levels. Although glucose crosses the placenta, insulin does not. By the tenth week of gestation the embryo or fetus secretes its own insulin at levels adequate to use the glucose obtained from the mother. Thus as maternal glucose levels rise, fetal glucose levels are increased, resulting in increased fetal insulin secretion.

During the first trimester of pregnancy, the pregnant woman's metabolic status is significantly influenced by the rising levels of estrogen and progesterone. These hormones stimulate the beta cells in the pancreas to increase insulin production, which promotes increased peripheral utilization of glucose and decreased blood glucose with fasting levels being reduced by approximately 10% (Fig. 13-1, *A*). There is a concomitant increase in tissue glycogen stores and a decrease in hepatic glucose production, which further encourage lower fasting glucose levels. As a result of these normal metabolic changes of pregnancy, women with insulin-dependent diabetes are prone to hypoglycemia (low blood glucose) during the first trimester.

During the second and third trimesters, pregnancy exerts a diabetogenic effect on the maternal metabolic status. Because of the major hormonal changes, there is decreased tolerance to glucose, increased insulin resistance, decreased hepatic glycogen stores, and increased hepatic production of glucose. Increasing levels of human chorionic somatomammotropin (hCS), estrogen, progesterone, prolactin, cortisol, and insulinase increase insulin resistance through their actions as insulin antagonists. Insulin resistance is a glucose-sparing mechanism that ensures an abundant supply of glucose for the fetus. Maternal insulin requirements gradually increase from about 18 to 24 weeks of gestation to about 36 weeks of gestation. At this time, insulin requirements usually level off until labor begins (Fig. 13-1, *B* and *C*).

At birth, expulsion of the placenta prompts an abrupt decrease in levels of circulating placental hormones, cortisol, and insulinase (Fig. 13-1, *D*). Maternal tissues quickly regain their prepregnancy sensitivity to insulin. For the nonbreastfeeding mother, the prepregnancy insulin-carbohydrate balance usually returns in about 7 to 10 days (Fig. 13-1, *E*). Lactation uses maternal glucose; thus the breastfeeding mother's insulin requirements will remain low as long as she is nursing (Fig. 13-1, *E*). On completion of weaning, the mother's prepregnancy insulin requirement is reestablished (Fig. 13-1, *F*).

Pregestational Diabetes Mellitus

Approximately 2 per 1000 pregnancies are complicated by preexisting diabetes. Women with pregestational diabetes may have either type 1 or type 2 diabetes, with type 1 now the more common diagnosis. As the incidence of type 2 diabetes increases in the general population, it may become the more prevalent form of the disease in childbearing-age women. Fetal risks for women with type 1 and type 2 diabetes are about the same. Maternal risks, however, tend to be greater in women with type 1 diabetes. Their blood sugar control is usually more erratic because of their absolute lack of insulin production. They also are more likely to have the vascular, retinal, or renal complications that often accompany the disease, because their duration of illness is usually

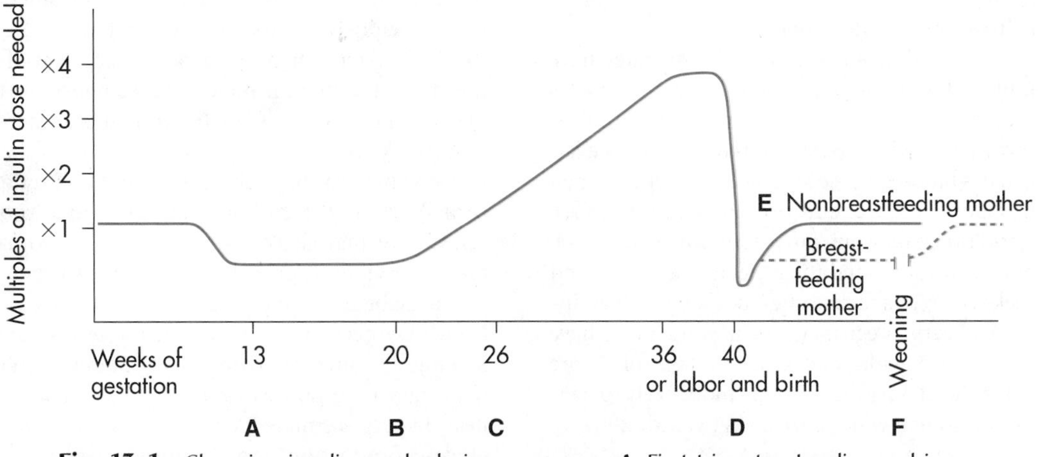

Fig. 13-1 Changing insulin needs during pregnancy. **A**, First trimester: Insulin need is reduced because of increased insulin production by the pancreas and increased peripheral sensitivity to insulin; nausea, vomiting, and decreased food intake by mother and glucose transfer to embryo/fetus contribute to hypoglycemia. **B**, Second trimester: Insulin need increases as placental hormones, cortisol, and insulinase act as insulin antagonists, decreasing insulin's effectiveness. **C**, Third trimester: Insulin requirements gradually increase until about 36 weeks of gestation. **D**, Day of delivery: Maternal insulin requirements drop drastically to approach prepregnancy levels. **E**, Breastfeeding mother maintains lower insulin requirements, as much as 25% less than prepregnancy; insulin need of nonbreastfeeding mother returns to prepregnancy levels in 7 to 10 days. **F**, At weaning of breastfeeding infant, mother's insulin need returns to prepregnancy levels.

longer than that of women with type 2 diabetes. Almost all women with pregestational diabetes are insulin dependent during pregnancy.

Preconception Counseling

Preconception counseling, which is recommended for all women of reproductive age with diabetes, is associated with an improved pregnancy outcome (Moore, 2004). Under ideal circumstances, the pregestational diabetic woman is counseled before the time of conception to plan the optimal time for pregnancy, establish glycemic control before conception, and diagnose any vascular complications of diabetes. However, it has been estimated that in the United States, fewer than 20% of women with diabetes participate in preconception counseling (Landon, Catalano, & Gabbe, 2002).

CASE STUDY—PREGESTATIONAL DIABETES

Preconception counseling is particularly important because strict metabolic control before conception and in the early weeks of gestation is instrumental in decreasing the risk of congenital anomalies (Landon et al, 2002; Moore, 2004) (Box 13-1).

Oral hypoglycemic agents are discontinued in the preconception period in women with type 2 diabetes. These women are started on insulin before pregnancy when the pregnancy is planned, or as soon as the pregnancy is diagnosed when it is unplanned.

The woman's partner should be included in the counseling to assess the couple's level of understanding related to the effects of pregnancy on the diabetic condition and of the potential complications of pregnancy as a result of diabetes. The couple also should be informed of the anticipated alterations in management of diabetes during pregnancy and the need for a multidisciplinary team approach to health care. Financial implications of diabetic pregnancy and other demands related to frequent maternal and fetal surveillance should be discussed. Contraception is an important aspect of preconception counseling to assist the couple in planning effectively for pregnancy.

Maternal Risks and Complications

Although maternal morbidity and mortality rates have improved significantly, the pregnant woman with diabetes remains at risk for the development of significant complications during pregnancy. Risk assessment is best done by evaluating the woman's blood glucose and blood vessels. Women with excellent glucose control and no blood vessel disease should have good pregnancy outcomes (Landon et al, 2002).

Poor glycemic control around the time of conception and in the early weeks of pregnancy may be associated with an increased incidence of early pregnancy loss in women who have diabetes. Those women with good glycemic control before conception and in the first trimester are no more likely to have a miscarriage than women without diabetes (Moore, 2004).

BOX 13-1

Goals for Self-Monitored Glucose Levels in Preconceptional Period

Before meals:
Capillary plasma glucose: 80-110 mg/dl
2 hr after meals:
Capillary plasma glucose: <155 mg/dl

Poor glycemic control later in pregnancy, particularly in women without vascular disease, increases the rate of fetal macrosomia, or excessive growth. Macrosomia occurs in 25% to 45% of diabetic pregnancies (Lindsay, 2002). These large infants tend to have a disproportionate increase in shoulder and trunk size; consequently, the risk of shoulder dystocia is greater in these babies than in other macrosomic infants. Thus women with diabetes face an increased likelihood of cesarean birth (because of failure to progress or failure of descent) or operative vaginal birth (birth using episiotomy, forceps, or vacuum extraction) (Moore, 2004).

Hypertensive disorders, such as preeclampsia or eclampsia, occur much more frequently in women with pregestational diabetes, particularly in those who already have renal dysfunction (Moore, 2004). Preterm labor/birth also is more likely to occur, especially with more severe diabetes, elevated glucose levels, and genital or urinary tract infections. The risk for induced preterm birth also is greater in women with pregestational diabetes.

Hydramnios (polyhydramnios), or amniotic fluid in excess of 2000 ml, occurs about 10 times more often in diabetic pregnancies than in nondiabetic pregnancies. Overdistention of the uterus caused by hydramnios increases the possibility of compression of maternal abdominal blood vessels (vena cava and aorta), causing supine hypotension. Premature rupture of the membranes, preterm labor, and postpartum hemorrhage are associated with hydramnios.

Infections are more common and more serious in pregnant women with diabetes. Disorders of carbohydrate metabolism alter the body's normal resistance to infection. The inflammatory response, leukocyte function, and vaginal pH are all affected. Vaginal infections, particularly monilial vaginitis, are more common. Urinary tract infections also are more prevalent. Infection is serious because it causes increased insulin resistance and may result in ketoacidosis. Postpartum infection is more common among women who are insulin dependent.

Ketoacidosis occurs most often during the second and third trimesters when the diabetogenic effect of pregnancy is the greatest. When the maternal metabolism is stressed by illness or infection, the diabetic woman is at increased risk for diabetic ketoacidosis (DKA). The use of betasympathomimetic medications such as terbutaline (Brethine) may also contribute to the risk for hyperglycemia and subsequent DKA. DKA may also occur because of the woman's failure to take insulin appropriately. The onset of previously undiagnosed diabetes during pregnancy is another cause of DKA. DKA may occur with blood glucose levels barely exceeding 200 mg/dl, compared with 300 to 350 mg/dl in the nonpregnant state. In response to stress factors such as infection or illness, hyperglycemia occurs as a result of increased hepatic glucose production and decreased peripheral glucose use. Stress hormones, which act to impair insulin action and further contribute to insulin deficiency, are released. Fatty acids are mobilized from fat stores into the circulation. As they are oxidized, ketone bodies are released into the peripheral circulation. The woman's buffering system is unable to compensate, and metabolic acidosis develops. The excessive blood glucose and ketone bodies result in osmotic diuresis with subsequent loss of fluid and electrolytes, volume depletion, and cellular dehydration. Prompt treatment of DKA is necessary to avoid maternal coma or death. Ketoacidosis at any time during pregnancy can lead to intrauterine fetal death; it is also a cause of preterm labor. The perinatal mortality rate is about 10% with maternal ketoacidosis (Moore, 2004).

The risk of hypoglycemia is also increased. Early in pregnancy, when hepatic production of glucose is diminished and peripheral use of glucose is enhanced, hypoglycemia occurs frequently, often during sleep. Later in pregnancy, hypoglycemia may also result as insulin doses are adjusted to maintain normoglycemia. Women with a prepregnancy history of severe hypoglycemia are at increased risk for severe hypoglycemia during gestation. Mild to moderate hypoglycemic episodes do not appear to have significant deleterious effects on fetal well-being. The long-term fetal effects of severe maternal hypoglycemia are as yet uncertain.

Fetal and Neonatal Risks and Complications

Despite the improvements in care of pregnant women with diabetes, sudden and unexplained stillbirth is still a significant risk (Moore, 2004). The other major cause of perinatal deaths in pregnancies complicated by diabetes is congenital anomalies. The incidence of congenital anomalies in infants born to women with diabetes is 6% to 10%, a twofold to fourfold increase over that of the general population (Landon et al, 2002). Cardiac defects are the most common anomalies seen, followed by central nervous system and skeletal defects (Moore, 2004).

Other problems that cause significant neonatal morbidity include macrosomia, hypoglycemia, respiratory distress syndrome, polycythemia, and hyperbilirubinemia (Landon et al, 2002; Moore, 2004). See Chapter 27 for further discussion of neonatal risks associated with maternal diabetes.

Care Management

Assessment

Interview

When a pregnant woman with diabetes initiates prenatal care, a thorough evaluation of her health status is completed. In addition to routine prenatal assessment, a detailed history regarding the onset and course of the diabetes and the degree of glycemic control before pregnancy is obtained. Effective management of diabetic pregnancy depends on the woman's adherence to a plan of care. For the woman to care for her diabetes on a daily basis, she must have an adequate understanding of her disease and the prescribed regimen. Thus with the initial prenatal visit, the woman's knowledge regarding diabetes and pregnancy, potential maternal and fetal complications, and the plan of care are assessed. With subsequent visits, follow-up assessments are completed. Data from these assessments are used to identify the woman's specific learning needs. The support person's knowledge of diabetes is also assessed, and teaching needs are identified.

The woman's emotional status is assessed to determine how she is coping with pregnancy superimposed on preexisting diabetes. Although normal pregnancy typically evokes some degree of stress and anxiety, pregnancy designated "high risk" will compound anxiety and stress levels. Fear of maternal and fetal complications is a major concern. Strict adherence to the plan of care necessitates alterations in patterns of daily living and may be an additional source of stress.

The woman's support system is assessed to identify those people significant to her and their roles in her life. It is important to assess the reactions of family members and the partner to the pregnancy and to the strict management plan, and their involvement in the treatment regimen. Socioeconomic factors are reviewed. Areas of emotional stress are identified because such stress can precipitate complications.

Physical Examination

At the initial visit, a thorough physical examination is performed to assess the woman's current health status. In addition to the routine prenatal examination, specific efforts are made to assess the effects of diabetes. A baseline electrocardiogram may be done to assess cardiovascular status. Evaluation for retinopathy is done, with follow-up as needed by an ophthalmologist each trimester and more often if retinopathy is diagnosed. Blood pressure is monitored carefully throughout pregnancy because of the increased risk for preeclampsia. The woman's weight gain is also monitored at each visit. Fundal height is measured, noting any abnormal increase in size for dates, which may indicate hydramnios or fetal macrosomia.

Laboratory Tests

Routine prenatal laboratory examinations include assessment of baseline renal function with a 24-hour urine collection for total protein excretion and creatinine clearance. Urinalysis and culture are performed on the initial prenatal visit and throughout the pregnancy to assess for the presence of urinary tract infection, which is common in diabetic pregnancy. At each visit, urine is tested for the presence of ketones. Because of the risk of coexisting thyroid disease, thyroid function tests may also be performed (see later discussion of thyroid disorders).

For the woman with pregestational type 1 or type 2 diabetes, laboratory tests may be done to assess past glycemic control. At the initial prenatal visit, the glycosylated hemoglobin A_{1c} level may be measured. With prolonged hyperglycemia, some of the hemoglobin remains saturated with glucose for the life of the red blood cell. Therefore a test for glycosylated hemoglobin provides a measurement of glycemic control over time, specifically over the previous 4 to 6 weeks. Regular measurements of glycosylated hemoglobin provide data for altering the treatment plan and lead to improvement of glycemic control. Values for the measurement of hemoglobin A_{1c}, the most commonly used index of glycosylated hemoglobin, are as follows (Pagana & Pagana, 2003):

- Adult/elderly (nondiabetic): 2.2% to 4.8%
- Good diabetic control: 2.5% to 5.9%
- Fair diabetic control: 6% to 8%
- Poor diabetic control: greater than 8%

Fasting blood glucose and random (1 to 2 hours after eating) glucose levels may be assessed during antepartum visits (Fig. 13-2). Blood glucose self-monitoring records may also be reviewed.

Nursing Diagnoses

Nursing diagnoses for the woman with pregestational diabetes include the following:

- *Deficient knowledge related to*
  —diabetic pregnancy, management, and potential effects on pregnant woman and fetus

A

B

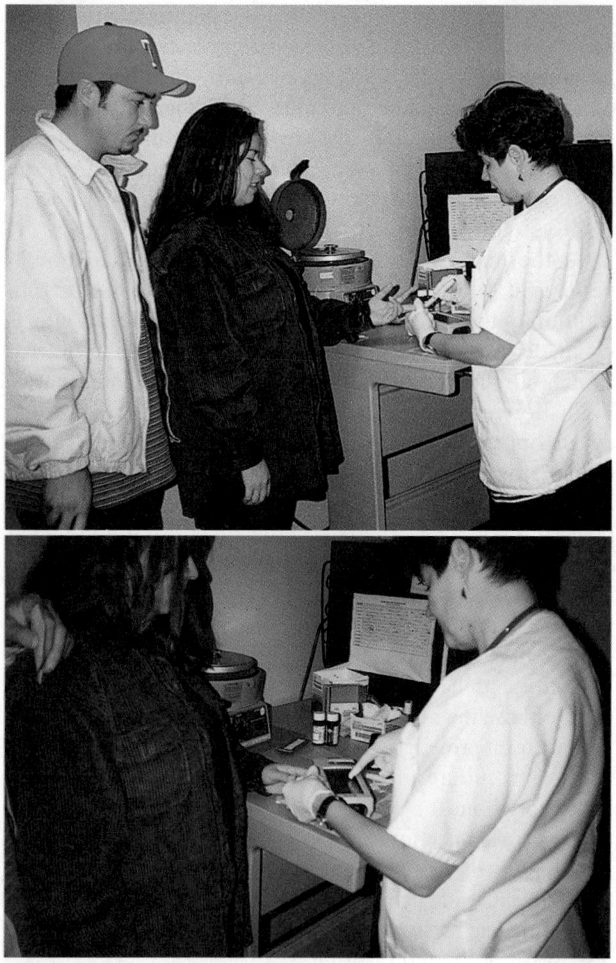

Fig. 13-2 **A,** Clinic nurse collects blood to determine glucose level. **B,** Nurse interprets glucose value displayed by monitor. (Courtesy Dee Lowdermilk, UNC Ambulatory Care Clinics, Chapel Hill, NC.)

- *Anxiety, fear, dysfunctional grieving, powerlessness, disturbed body-image, situational low self-esteem, spiritual distress, ineffective role performance, interrupted family processes related to*
  —stigma of being labeled diabetic
  —effects of diabetes and its potential sequelae on the pregnant woman and the fetus
- *Risk for injury to fetus related to*
  —uteroplacental insufficiency
  —birth trauma
- *Risk for injury to mother related to*
  —improper insulin administration
  —hypoglycemia and hyperglycemia
  —cesarean or operative vaginal birth
  —postpartum infection

Expected Outcomes

Expected outcomes of care for the pregnant woman with pregestational diabetes include that she will do the following:

- Demonstrate or verbalize understanding of diabetic pregnancy, the plan of care, and the importance of glycemic control.
- Achieve and maintain glycemic control.
- Demonstrate effective coping.
- Experience no complications (maternal morbidity or mortality).
- Give birth to a healthy infant at term.

Plan of Care and Implementation

Antepartum

Because of her high risk status, the woman with diabetes is monitored much more frequently and thoroughly than are other pregnant women. During the first and second trimesters of pregnancy, her routine prenatal care visits may be scheduled every 1 to 2 weeks. In the last trimester, she will probably be seen one or two times each week. In the past, routine hospitalization for management of the diabetes, such as insulin dose changes, was common. With the availability of better home glucose monitoring, and the growing reluctance of third-party payers to reimburse for hospitalization, pregnant women with diabetes are now generally managed as outpatients. Some patient and family education and maternal and fetal assessment may be done in the home, depending on the woman's insurance coverage and care provider preference.

Achieving and maintaining *euglycemia* (normal blood glucose level; also called *normogylcemia*), with blood glucose levels in the range of 60 to 120 mg/dl (Table 13-1), is the primary goal of medical therapy for the pregnant woman with diabetes. Euglycemia is achieved through a combination of diet, insulin, exercise, and blood glucose determinations. Providing the woman with the knowledge, skill, and motivation she needs to achieve and maintain excellent blood glucose control is the primary nursing goal.

Achieving euglycemia requires commitment of the woman and her family to make the necessary lifestyle changes, which can sometimes seem overwhelming. Maintaining tight blood glucose control necessitates that the woman follow a consistent daily schedule. She must go to bed and get up, eat, exercise, and take insulin at the same time every day. Blood glucose measurements are done frequently to determine how well the major components of therapy (diet, insulin, and exercise) are working together to control blood glucose levels.

Table 13-1

Target Blood Glucose Levels during Pregnancy

TIME OF MEASUREMENT	TARGET GLUCOSE LEVEL (mg/dl)*
Fasting	60 to 90
Premeal (lunch, dinner)	60 to 105
Bedtime	90 to 120
Postmeal	
1 hr	100 to 120
2 hr	90 to 120
2 AM to 4 AM	60 to 120

Source: American Diabetes Association: *Medical management of pregnancy complicated by diabetes,* ed 3, Alexandria, VA, 2000, The Association.
*Add 15% if plasma values are used.

The woman should wear an identification bracelet at all times and carry insulin, syringes, and "glucose boosters" with her whenever she is away from home. She should be given written instructions for reporting the development of problems such as nausea, vomiting, and infections; and directions for reaching her health care provider by phone at night and on weekends and holidays (Guidelines box).

Because the diabetic woman is at risk for infections, eye problems, and neurologic changes, foot care and general skin care are important. A daily bath that includes good perineal care and foot care is important. Lotions, creams, or oils can be applied to dry skin. Tight clothing should be avoided. Shoes or slippers that fit properly should be worn at all times and are best worn with socks or stockings. Feet should be inspected regularly; toenails should be cut straight across; and professional help should be sought for any foot problems. Extremes of temperature should be avoided.

Diet

The woman with pregestational diabetes has usually had nutritional counseling regarding the management of diabetes. Because pregnancy precipitates special nutritional concerns and needs, the woman must be educated to incorporate these changes into dietary planning. Nutritional counseling is usually provided by a registered dietitian.

Dietary management during diabetic pregnancy must be based on blood (not urine) glucose levels. The diet is individualized to allow for increased fetal and metabolic requirements, with consideration of such factors as prepregnancy weight and dietary habits, overall health, ethnic background, lifestyle, stage of pregnancy, knowledge of nutrition, and insulin therapy. The dietary goals are to provide weight gain consistent with a normal pregnancy, prevent ketoacidosis, and minimize wide fluctuation of blood glucose levels.

Guidelines

TREATMENT FOR HYPOGLYCEMIA

- Be familiar with signs and symptoms of hypoglycemia (nervousness, headache, shaking, irritability, personality change, hunger, blurred vision, sweaty skin, tingling of mouth or extremities).
- Check blood glucose level immediately when hypoglycemic symptoms occur.
- If blood glucose is <60 mg/dl, immediately eat or drink something that contains 10 to 15 g of simple carbohydrate. Examples:
  - ½ cup (4 ounces) unsweetened fruit juice
  - ½ cup (4 ounces) regular (not diet) soda
  - 5 to 6 Life Savers candies
  - 1 tablespoon honey or corn (Karo) syrup
  - 1 cup (8 ounces) milk
  - 2 to 3 glucose tablets
- Rest for 15 min, then recheck blood glucose.
- If glucose level is still <60 mg/dl, eat or drink another serving of one of the "glucose boosters" listed above.
- Wait 15 min, then recheck blood glucose. If it is still <60 mg/dl, notify health care provider immediately.

Source: American Diabetes Association: *Medical management of pregnancy complicated by diabetes,* ed 3, Alexandria, VA, 2000, The Association; Becton Dickinson & Co: *Controlling low blood sugar reactions,* Franklin Lakes, NJ, 1997, Becton Dickinson.

Energy needs are usually calculated on the basis of 30 to 35 calories per kilogram of ideal body weight, with the average diet including 2200 calories (first trimester) to 2500 calories (second and third trimesters). Total calories may be distributed among three meals and one evening snack, or, more commonly, three meals and at least two snacks. Meals should be eaten on time and never skipped. Snacks must be carefully planned in accordance with insulin therapy to avoid fluctuations in blood glucose levels. A large bedtime snack of at least 25 g of carbohydrate with some protein is recommended to help prevent hypoglycemia and starvation ketosis during the night.

The ratio of carbohydrates, protein, and fat is important to meet the metabolic needs of the woman and the fetus. Approximately 50% to 60% of the total calories should be carbohydrates, with a minimum of 250 g per day. Simple carbohydrates are limited; complex carbohydrates that are high in fiber content are recommended because the starch and protein in such foods help regulate the blood glucose level by more sustained glucose release. Protein intake should constitute 12% to 20% of the total kilocalories; 20% to 30% of the daily caloric intake should come from fat, with no more than 10% saturated fats (Home Care box). Weight gain for most women should be about 12 kg during the pregnancy (Gilbert & Harmon, 2003).

Exercise

Although exercise enhances the utilization of glucose and decreases insulin need in nonpregnant women with diabetes, there are limited data regarding exercise during pregnancy. Any prescription of exercise during pregnancy for a woman with diabetes should be done by the primary health care provider and should be monitored closely to prevent complications. For those women with vasculopathy, only mild exercise is recommended because exercise causes a redistribution of blood flow, which increases the potential for ischemic injury to the placenta and already compromised organs. Women with vasculopathy typically depend completely on exogenous insulin and are at greater risk for wide fluctuations in blood glucose levels and ketoacidosis, which can be worsened by exercise.

Home Care

DIETARY MANAGEMENT OF DIABETIC PREGNANCY

- Follow the prescribed diet plan.
- Eat a well-balanced diet, including daily food requirements for a normal pregnancy.
- Divide daily food intake between three meals and two to four snacks, depending on individual needs.
- Eat a substantial bedtime snack to prevent a severe drop in blood glucose level during the night.
- Limit the intake of fats if weight gain occurs too rapidly.
- Take daily vitamins and iron as prescribed by the health care provider.
- Avoid foods high in refined sugar.
- Eat consistently each day; never skip meals or snacks.
- Reduce the intake of saturated fat and cholesterol.
- Eat foods high in dietary fiber.
- Avoid alcohol and caffeine.

When exercise is prescribed by the health care provider as part of the treatment plan, careful instructions are given. The exercise need not be vigorous to be beneficial: 15 to 30 minutes of walking four to six times a week is satisfactory for most pregnant women. Other exercises that may be recommended include non–weight-bearing activities such as arm ergometry or use of a recumbent bicycle. The best time for exercise is after meals when the blood glucose level is rising. To monitor the effect of insulin on blood glucose levels, the woman can measure blood glucose before, during, and after exercise (see also Exercise Tips for Pregnant Women in Chapter 11).

Insulin Therapy

Adequate insulinization is the primary factor in the maintenance of normoglycemia during pregnancy, thus ensuring proper glucose metabolism of the mother and fetus. Insulin requirements during pregnancy change dramatically as the pregnancy progresses, necessitating frequent adjustments in insulin dosage. In the first trimester, little or no change occurs in prepregnancy insulin requirements; however, insulin dosage may need to be decreased because of hypoglycemia. During the second and third trimesters, because of insulin resistance, the dosage must be increased to maintain target glucose levels.

The goal of administration of exogenous insulin during pregnancy is to achieve diurnal glucose levels that are similar to those of a nondiabetic pregnant woman. The insulin regimen for a pregnant woman differs from that which is effective in the nonpregnant state in combinations and timing of insulin injections (Moore, 2004). Thus, for the woman with type 1 pregestational diabetes who has typically been accustomed to one injection per day of intermediate-acting insulin, multiple daily injections of mixed insulin are a new experience. The woman with type 2 diabetes previously treated with oral hypoglycemics is faced with the task of learning to self-administer injections of insulin. The nurse is instrumental in education and support with regard to insulin administration and the adjustment of insulin dosage to maintain normoglycemia (Patient Teaching box).

Many types of insulin are available today. Beef and pork insulin have largely been replaced by biosynthetic human insulin preparations (Humulin or Novolin), which are less likely to cause antibody formation. Patients with new onset of diabetes are almost always started on this type of insulin. Lispro (Humalog) is a rapid-acting insulin preparation that has an onset of action within 15 minutes of injection and peaks in 2 to 3 hours. Advantages of lispro include convenience, because it is injected immediately before mealtime; less hyperglycemia after meals; and fewer hypoglycemic episodes. Lispro insulin has a total duration of action of 3 to 4 hours (Landon et al, 2002) (Table 13-2).

Insulin-dependent diabetes is managed in most women with two to three injections per day. Usually two thirds of the daily insulin dose, with longer-acting (NPH) and short-acting (regular or Lispro) insulin combined in a 2:1 ratio, is given before breakfast. The remaining one third, again a combination of longer- and short-acting insulin, is administered in the evening before dinner. To reduce the risk of hypoglycemia during the night, separate injections often are administered, with short-acting insulin given before dinner, followed by longer-acting insulin at bedtime. An alternative insulin regimen that works well for some women is to administer short-acting insulin before each meal and longer-acting insulin at bedtime (Moore, 2004).

Although subcutaneous insulin injections are most commonly used, increasing numbers of pregnant women are using continuous insulin infusion systems. The insulin pump is designed to mimic more closely the function of the pancreas in secreting insulin (Fig. 13-3). This portable, battery-powered device is worn, like a pager, during most daily activities.

Patient Teaching

ADMINISTRATION OF INSULIN

Procedure for Mixing NPH (Intermediate-Acting) and Regular (Short-Acting) Insulin

- Wash hands thoroughly and gather supplies. Be sure the insulin syringe corresponds to the concentration of insulin you are using.
- Check insulin bottle to be certain it is the appropriate type and check the expiration date.
- Gently rotate (do not shake) the insulin vial to mix the insulin.
- Wipe off rubber stopper of each vial with alcohol.
- Draw into syringe the amount of air equal to total dose.
- Inject air equal to NPH (intermediate-acting) dose into NPH vial. Remove syringe from vial.
- Inject air equal to regular insulin dose into regular insulin vial.
- Invert regular insulin bottle and withdraw regular insulin dose.
- Without adding more air to NPH vial, carefully withdraw NPH dose.

Procedure for Self-Injection of Insulin

- Select proper injection site (remember to rotate sites).
- Injection site should be clean. Use of alcohol is not necessary. If alcohol is used, let it dry before injecting.
- Pinch the skin up to form a subcutaneous pocket and, holding the syringe like a pencil, puncture the skin at a 45- to 90-degree angle. If there is a great deal of fatty tissue at the site, spread the skin taut and inject the syringe at a 90-degree angle.
- Slowly inject the insulin.
- As you withdraw the needle, cover the injection site with sterile gauze and apply gentle pressure to prevent bleeding.
- Record insulin dosage and time of injection.

Table 13-2

Insulin Administration during Pregnancy: Expected Time of Action

TYPE OF INSULIN	ONSET	PEAK	DURATION
Lispro (rapid acting)	Within 15 min	2-3 hr	3-4 hr
Regular (short acting)	30 min	3-4 hr	6-8 hr
Intermediate acting	2-4 hr	4-12 hr	12-24 hr
Long acting	3-4 hr	14-24 hr	24-36 hr

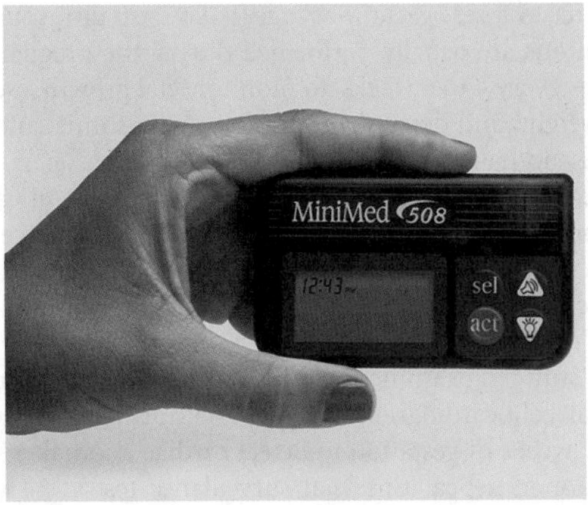

Fig. 13-3 Insulin pump shows basal rate for pregnant women with diabetes. (Courtesy MiniMed, Inc., Sylmar, CA.)

The pump infuses regular insulin at a set basal rate and has the capacity to deliver up to four different basal rates in 24 hours. It also delivers bolus doses of insulin before meals to control postprandial blood glucose levels. A fine-gauge plastic catheter is inserted into subcutaneous tissue, usually in the abdomen, and attached to the pump syringe by connecting tubing. The subcutaneous catheter and connecting tubing are changed every 2 to 3 days. Although the insulin pump is convenient and generally provides good glycemic control, complications such as DKA, infection, or hypoglycemic coma can still develop. Use of the insulin pump requires a knowledgeable, motivated patient; skilled health care providers; and 24-hour availability of emergency assistance (Moore, 2004).

Monitoring Blood Glucose Levels

Blood glucose testing at home is the commonly accepted method for monitoring blood glucose levels. It is the most important tool available to the woman to assess her degree of glycemic control. In addition, this monitoring provides motivation to continue the prescribed treatment plan. The data obtained facilitate interaction with the health care team in maintaining glycemic control and minimizing fetal risk (Home Care box).

Women with pregestational diabetes are often familiar with self-monitoring of blood glucose levels because it is typically included in the management plan for type 1 and some cases of type 2 diabetes. However, a thorough assessment of the woman's knowledge and skill related to blood glucose testing is essential to ensure accurate monitoring of glucose levels during pregnancy. The nurse observes the woman performing blood glucose monitoring to determine her accuracy and comfort with the system. The family also is included in the assessment and in subsequent instruction.

Meters incorporate memory to store a large number of readings; however, the woman is still encouraged to keep written records of glucose levels. She should bring her written records, her meter containing stored test results, or both with her to each appointment. It is important that the monitoring equipment be checked for accuracy at intervals by comparing the woman's results on her machine with the results of a laboratory test done at the same time on a capillary whole blood sample.

Home Care

TESTING BLOOD GLUCOSE LEVEL

- Gather supplies, check expiration date, and read instructions on testing materials. Prepare glucose reflectance meter for use according to manufacturer's directions.
- Wash hands in warm water (warmth increases circulation).
- Select site on side of any finger (all fingers should be used in rotation).
- Pierce site with lancet (may use automatic, spring-loaded, puncturing device). Cleaning the site with alcohol is not necessary.
- Drop hand down to side; with other hand gently squeeze finger from hand to fingertip.
- Allow blood to drop onto testing strip. Be sure to cover entire reagent area.
- Determine blood glucose value using the glucose reflectance meter, following manufacturer's instructions.
- Record results.
- Repeat daily as instructed by health care provider and as needed for signs of hypoglycemia or hyperglycemia.

Source: American Diabetes Association: *Medical management of pregnancy complicated by diabetes*, ed 3, Alexandria, VA, 2000, The Association.

Blood glucose levels are routinely measured at various times throughout the day such as before breakfast, lunch, and dinner; 2 hours after meals; at bedtime; and in the middle of the night. The primary health care provider will determine for each individual woman the number and timing of routine blood glucose determinations. Because hyperglycemia is to be avoided, postprandial measurements are often performed.

NURSE ALERT Hyperglycemia will most likely be identified in the 2-hour postprandial values because blood glucose levels peak about 2 hours after a meal. ■

Special circumstances may necessitate more frequent testing. Women are instructed to check glucose levels at any sign of hypoglycemia or hyperglycemia. When there is any readjustment in insulin dosage or diet, more frequent measurement of blood glucose is warranted. If nausea, vomiting, or diarrhea occurs, or if any infection is present, the woman will probably be asked to monitor her blood glucose levels more closely.

Target levels of blood glucose during pregnancy are lower than nonpregnant values. Acceptable fasting levels are generally between 60 and 90 mg/dl, and 2-hour postprandial levels should be less than 120 mg/dl (see Table 13-1) (ADA, 2000). The woman should be told to report episodes of hypoglycemia (less than 60 mg/dl) and hyperglycemia (greater than 200 mg/dl) to her health care provider immediately so that adjustments in diet or insulin therapy can be made.

Pregnant women with diabetes are much more likely to develop hypoglycemia than hyperglycemia, because the goal of therapy is to maintain the blood glucose in a narrow, low-normal range of 60 to 120 mg/dl. Although a blood glucose level greater than 120 mg/dl is considered too high for a pregnant woman, it will not produce the classic signs and symptoms of hyperglycemia. However, many women will have signs and symptoms of hypoglycemia with blood glucose levels below 60 mg/dl.

Most episodes of mild or moderate hypoglycemia can be treated with oral intake of 10 to 15 g of simple carbohydrates (see Guidelines box on p. 335). If severe hypoglycemia occurs in which the woman experiences a decrease in or loss of consciousness or an inability to swallow, she will require a parenteral injection of glucagon or intravenous (IV) glucose. Because hypoglycemia can develop rapidly, and because impaired judgment can be associated with even moderate episodes, it is vital that family members, friends, and work colleagues be able to recognize signs and symptoms quickly and initiate proper treatment if necessary.

Although hyperglycemia is less likely to occur, it is still a dangerous complication. Hyperglycemia can rapidly progress to diabetic ketoacidosis. Women and family members should be alert for signs and symptoms of hyperglycemia, especially when infections or other illnesses occur (Home Care box).

Complications Requiring Hospitalization

Occasionally hospitalization may be required to regulate insulin dosage and stabilize glucose levels. Hospitalization offers a controlled situation to initiate and regulate insulin therapy while providing opportunity for intensive education in self-administration of insulin and regulation of blood glucose. Infection, which can lead to hyperglycemia and diabetic ketoacidosis, is an indication for hospitalization, regardless of gestational age. Hospitalization during the third trimester for closer maternal and fetal observation may be indicated for women whose diabetes is poorly controlled or who also have hypertension.

Fetal Surveillance

Diagnostic techniques for fetal surveillance are often performed during a pregnancy complicated by diabetes to assess fetal growth and well-being. The goals of fetal surveillance are to detect fetal compromise as early as possible and to prevent intrauterine fetal death or unnecessary preterm birth. The majority of fetal surveillance measures are concentrated in the third trimester, when the risk of fetal compromise is greatest.

Early in pregnancy, the estimated date of birth (EDB) is determined. A baseline sonogram is done during the first trimester to assess gestational age. Follow-up ultrasound examinations are usually performed during the pregnancy, as often as every 4 to 6 weeks, to monitor fetal growth, estimate fetal weight, and detect hydramnios, macrosomia, and congenital anomalies.

Because a fetus in a diabetic pregnancy is at greater risk for neural tube defects (e.g., spina bifida, anencephaly, microcephaly), measurement of maternal serum alphafetoprotein is performed between 16 and 18 weeks of gestation. This is often done in conjunction with a detailed ultrasound study to examine the fetus for neural tube defects.

Fetal echocardiography may be performed between 18 and 22 weeks of gestation to detect cardiac anomalies. Some practitioners repeat this fetal surveillance test at 34 weeks. Doppler studies of the umbilical artery may be performed to detect placental compromise in women with vascular disease.

Maternal evaluation of fetal movements (kick counts) is used primarily as a screening technique in fetal surveillance. Nonstress tests (NSTs) to evaluate fetal well-being may be used weekly or more often, typically beginning around 28 to 32 weeks of gestation (see Chapter 9). After 32 weeks, testing may be done twice weekly. For the woman with vascular disease, testing may begin earlier and continue more frequently. In the presence of a nonreactive NST, a contraction stress test or fetal biophysical profile may be used to evaluate fetal well-being (Moore, 2004).

Determination of Birth Date and Mode of Delivery

Today the majority of diabetic pregnancies are allowed to progress to term (38 to 40 weeks of gestation), as long as good metabolic control is maintained and all parameters of antepartum fetal surveillance remain within normal limits. Reasons to proceed with delivery before term include poor metabolic control, worsening hypertensive disorders, fetal macrosomia, or fetal growth restriction (Moore, 2004).

Many practitioners plan elective labor induction between 38 and 40 weeks provided maternal glucose levels are well controlled. To confirm fetal lung maturity before birth, an amniocentesis may be performed in pregnancies of less than 39 weeks. For the pregnancy complicated by diabetes, fetal lung maturation is better predicted by the amniotic fluid phosphatidylglycerol (PG) than by the lecithin/sphingomyelin (L/S) ratio. If the fetal lungs are still immature, birth should be postponed as long as the results of fetal assessment remain reassuring. Induced labor and birth despite poor fetal lung maturity may be essential when testing suggests fetal compromise or if preeclampsia, deteriorating vision due to proliferative retinopathy, or worsening renal function develops (Landon et al, 2002).

The mode of birth for women with pregestational diabetes is a subject of controversy among practitioners. The rate of cesarean births for these women is high, around 45%. Cesarean birth is often performed when antepartum testing suggests fetal distress or the estimated fetal weight is 4000 to 4500 g. When induction of labor is desired and the cervix fails to respond, cesarean birth often is necessary (Landon et al, 2002; Moore, 2004).

Intrapartum

During the intrapartum period the woman with pregestational diabetes must be monitored closely to prevent complications related to dehydration, hypoglycemia, and hyper-

Home Care

WHAT TO DO WHEN ILLNESS OCCURS

- Be sure to take insulin even though appetite and food intake may be less than normal. (Insulin needs are increased with illness or infection.)
- Call the health care provider and relay the following information:
  Symptoms of illness (e.g., nausea, vomiting, diarrhea)
  Fever
  Most recent blood glucose level
  Urine ketones
  Time and amount of last insulin dose
- Increase oral intake of fluids to prevent dehydration.
- Rest as much as possible.
- If unable to reach health care provider and blood glucose exceeds 200 mg/dl with urine ketones present, seek emergency treatment at the nearest health care facility. Do not attempt to self-treat for this.

glycemia. Most women use large amounts of energy (calories) to accomplish the work and manage the stress of labor and birth; however, this calorie expenditure varies with the individual. Blood glucose levels and hydration must be carefully controlled during labor. An IV line is inserted for infusion of a maintenance fluid such as lactated Ringer's solution or 5% dextrose in lactated Ringer's solution. Insulin may be administered by continuous infusion or by intermittent subcutaneous injection.

Determinations of blood glucose are made every hour, and fluids and insulin are adjusted to maintain blood glucose levels between 70 and 90 mg/dl or capillary whole blood glucose levels at 60 to 80 mg/dl. It is essential that these target glucose levels be maintained because hyperglycemia during labor can precipitate metabolic problems in the neonate, particularly hypoglycemia.

During labor, continuous fetal heart monitoring is necessary. The mother should assume an upright or side-lying position during bed rest in labor to prevent supine hypotension because of a large fetus or polyhydramnios. Labor is allowed to progress without intervention, provided normal rates of cervical dilation, fetal descent, and fetal well-being are maintained. Failure to progress may indicate a macrosomic infant and cephalopelvic disproportion, necessitating cesarean birth. The woman is observed and treated during labor for diabetic complications such as hyperglycemia, ketosis, ketoacidosis, and glycosuria. During second-stage labor, the nurse should be alert for the possibility of shoulder dystocia if delivery of a macrosomic infant is attempted and be prepared to assist with maneuvers to free the fetal shoulder that is lodged behind the symphysis pubis (see Chapter 19). A neonatologist, pediatrician, or neonatal nurse practitioner may be present at the birth to initiate assessment and neonatal care.

If a cesarean birth is planned, it should be scheduled in the early morning to facilitate glycemic control. The morning dose of insulin is withheld and the woman given nothing by mouth. Epidural anesthesia is recommended because hypoglycemia can be detected earlier if the woman is awake.

Postpartum

In the immediate postpartum period, insulin requirements decrease substantially because the major source of insulin resistance, the placenta, has been removed. Women with type 1 diabetes may require only one half the prenatal insulin dose on the first postpartum day, provided that they are eating a full diet. It takes several days after delivery to reestablish carbohydrate homeostasis. Blood glucose levels are monitored in the postpartum period, and insulin dosage is adjusted accordingly. Blood glucose levels do not require as tight control after birth. Usually insulin is not given until the blood glucose level is greater than 200 mg/dl. The woman who is insulin dependent must realize the importance of eating on time even if the baby needs feeding or other pressing demands exist. Women with type 2 diabetes often require no insulin in the postpartum period and are able to maintain normoglycemia through diet alone or with oral hypoglycemics.

Possible postpartum complications include preeclampsia-eclampsia, hemorrhage, and infection. Hemorrhage is a possibility if the mother's uterus was overdistended (by hydramnios or a macrosomic fetus) or overstimulated (by oxytocin induction). Postpartum infections such as endometritis are more likely to occur in a woman with diabetes.

Mothers are encouraged to breastfeed. In addition to the advantages of maternal satisfaction and pleasure, breastfeeding has an antidiabetogenic effect. Insulin requirements may be half of prepregnancy levels because of the carbohydrate used in human milk production. Because glucose levels are lower, breastfeeding women are at increased risk for hypoglycemia, especially in the early postpartum period and after breastfeeding sessions.

The mother may have early breastfeeding difficulties. Poor metabolic control may delay lactogenesis and contribute to decreased milk production. Because many women give birth by cesarean, the effects of anesthesia and postoperative discomfort may delay maternal attachment and make breastfeeding more difficult. Initial contact and opportunity to breastfeed the infant are often delayed because many institutions place infants of mothers with diabetes in neonatal intensive care units or special care nurseries for observation during the first few hours after birth. Support and assistance from nursing staff and lactation specialists can facilitate the mother's early experience with breastfeeding and encourage her to continue.

Infants who are exclusively breastfed are less likely to develop diabetes; exposure to cow's milk products before 8 days of age is an important risk factor for the disease.

Breastfeeding mothers with diabetes may be at increased risk for mastitis and yeast infections of the breast. Insulin dosage, which is decreased during lactation, must be recalculated at the time of weaning.

Family Planning and Contraception

The new mother needs information about family planning and contraception. While family planning is important for all women, it is essential for the woman with diabetes to safeguard her own health and to promote optimal outcomes in future pregnancies. Because excellent glucose control at conception is crucial for all diabetics, the importance of conscientiously using a reliable contraceptive method until another pregnancy is desired should be stressed. No one best form of contraception exists for diabetic women. Instead, emphasis should be placed on consistent use of a reliable and effective birth control method. The risks and benefits of contraceptive methods should be discussed with the mother and her partner before discharge from the hospital.

The barrier methods are often recommended as safe, inexpensive options that have no inherent risks for women with diabetes (Landon et al, 2002). However, barrier methods are not as effective as some other forms of contraception.

Use of oral contraceptives is controversial because of the risk of thromboembolic and vascular complications and the effect on carbohydrate metabolism. In women without vascular disease or other risk factors, combination low-dose oral contraceptives may be prescribed. Close monitoring of blood pressure and lipid levels is necessary to detect complications (Landon et al, 2002). Progestin-only oral contraceptives also may be used, because they minimally affect carbohydrate metabolism (Cunningham et al, 2001; Landon et al, 2002).

Some health care providers are reluctant to use intrauterine contraceptive devices (IUDs) in women with diabetes because of concerns about infection. However, this method has been used successfully by these women (Landon et al, 2002).

Opinion is divided about the use of long-acting parenteral or implantable progestins, such as Depo-Provera. Some authorities recommend their use, especially in women who may not be compliant with daily dosing for oral contraceptives or appropriate follow-up care. Others believe that these methods may adversely affect diabetic control (Landon et al, 2002).

The woman and her partner should be informed that the risks associated with pregnancy increase with the duration and severity of the diabetic condition, and that pregnancy may contribute to vascular changes associated with diabetes. Therefore sterilization should be discussed with the woman who has completed her family or who has significant vasculopathy.

Evidence-Based Practice

SOCIAL SUPPORT FOR PREVENTION OF LOW-BIRTH-WEIGHT BABIES

Background

Low-birth-weight (LBW) babies includes small-for-gestational-age (SGA) babies, who have not grown adequately during gestation, and preterm babies, who are normal size for gestation but are born too soon (less than 37 weeks). These two conditions have different prognoses and treatments. The SGA baby may be at a greater long-term deficit, particularly if brain growth has been compromised. Prematurity is a more acute problem of survival until the lungs mature. One of the major risk factors for LBW babies (less than 2500 g) is chronic poverty, which can lead to malnutrition, unhealthy living conditions, infections, and increased stress. Psychologic stress increases the likelihood of pregnancy and labor complications, fetal growth restriction, preterm birth, and poor health in mother and child. Social support may mitigate this stress somewhat. Accordingly, many countries have attempted to decrease their LBW rates by offering social support programs to women in distress. The programs usually include advice and counseling, tangible assistance, and emotional support. Support is offered by multidisciplinary teams, which may include lay peer counselors. Health care workers have the knowledge and training, but may not have experienced social disadvantage, as the lay peer counselor would.

Objectives

Reviewers sought to determine the effects of social support for women at high risk for LBW babies, compared with routine care. The authors also planned to compare the effectiveness of health care workers with that of peer counselors. Interventions included some form of emotional support, such as counseling, reassurance, and sympathetic listening, with or without advice about nutrition, rest, stress management, and substance abuse. Tangible assistance included transportation to clinic appointment and household help. Support could start during the first or second trimester, and continue at least until birth. Settings could be clinics or home visits, with telephone follow-up. Outcome could include preterm birth, LBW, miscarriage, pregnancy termination, complications of pregnancy or labor, hospitalization, distress, operative birth, perinatal death, length of stay, and postnatal physical or mental health.

Methods

Search Strategy

The reviewers searched Cochrane, MEDLINE, 30 journals and conference proceedings, and a current awareness service of 37 journals. Search keywords were not noted.

Sixteen randomized, controlled trials were selected, representing 13,651 women from Australia, the United Kingdom, France, Latin America, the Netherlands, South Africa, and the United States. The trials were dated 1986–2001.

Statistical Analyses

Similar data were pooled. Categorical data were reported by effect size. Continuous data were assigned a weighted mean difference (between intervention and control group).

Findings

Additional social support did not significantly lower the rate of LBW or preterm births. It did significantly decrease the cesarean birthrate. Women who received additional support were three times more likely to terminate their pregnancy than controls. There was equivocal evidence that the support group required less analgesia than controls. Supported women had improved psychosocial outcomes of significantly less worry and increased satisfaction. No comparison was possible of lay versus professional support.

Limitations

The definitions of "high risk for low birth weight" and "social disadvantage" were murky. There was no way to blind the subjects or evaluators to the presence or absence of additional support. Some subjects were lost to follow-up, so long-term data were not available. Various support teams included nurses, doctors, midwives, social workers, psychologists, and trained lay women. Randomization was not consistent.

Conclusions

Social support was not able to mitigate the effects on birth weight or prematurity of chronic poverty and the stresses caused by that poverty, or psychologic stress. However, other positive outcomes were seen: a reduction in cesarean birthrate and less worry and increased satisfaction.

Implications for Practice

The decrease in cesarean birthrate and the improved psychosocial outcomes are reasons to offer support to high risk pregnant women. The additional support may not be powerful enough to overcome the social disadvantage associated with LBW and preterm birth. The marked increase in number of pregnancy terminations in the supported group may have been a result of their increased awareness of their fragile situation, and feelings of empowerment to change it.

Implications for Further Research

Researchers have not identified how social disadvantage causes preterm birth and low birth weight. Clear definitions of high risk women may better show any benefits of additional support. The value of lay peer counselors is yet undecided. Lay peer counselors have insight into the lives of the women that professionals may lack, and may offer a cost-effective support system that benefits the community.

Reference

Hodnett ED, Fredericks S: Support during pregnancy for women at increased risk of low birthweight babies (Cochrane Review), 2003. In *The Cochrane Library,* Issue 2, Chichester, UK, 2004, John Wiley & Sons.

Evaluation

Evaluation of the care of the pregnant woman with pregestational diabetes is based on the previously stated expected outcomes, which are closely associated with the degree of maternal metabolic control during pregnancy (Nursing Care Plan).

Gestational Diabetes Mellitus

Gestational diabetes mellitus (GDM) complicates approximately 7% of all pregnancies in the United States and accounts for 90% of all cases of diabetic pregnancy (ADA, 2004a). Prevalence varies by race and ethnicity (Cultural Awareness box). GDM is more likely to occur among Hispanic, Native American, Asian, and African-American populations than in Caucasians (Centers for Disease Control and Prevention, 2004; Landon et al, 2002). Women with GDM are at significant risk of developing glucose intolerance later in life; about 50% will be diagnosed as diabetic within 5 years. This is especially true of women whose GDM is diagnosed early in pregnancy and who also are obese (Landon

Nursing Care Plan

PREGNANCY COMPLICATED BY PREGESTATIONAL DIABETES

NURSING DIAGNOSIS: Deficient knowledge related to lack of recall of information as evidenced by patient questions and concerns

EXPECTED OUTCOMES

Patient will be able to verbalize important information regarding diabetes, its management, and potential effects on the pregnant woman and fetus.

NURSING INTERVENTIONS/*RATIONALES*

Assess patient's current knowledge base regarding disease process, management, effects on pregnancy and fetus, and potential complications *to provide database for further teaching.*

Review the pathophysiology of diabetes, effects on pregnancy and fetus, and potential complications *to promote patient recall of information and compliance with treatment plan.*

Review procedure for insulin administration, demonstrate procedure for blood glucose monitoring and insulin measurement and administration, and obtain return demonstration *to establish patient comfort and competence with procedures.*

Discuss diet and exercise as prescribed by diabetologist *to promote self-care.*

Review signs and symptoms of complications of hypoglycemia and hyperglycemia and appropriate interventions *to promote prompt recognition of complications and self-care.*

Provide contact numbers for health care team for prompt interventions and answers to questions on an ongoing basis *to promote patient and health team collaboration.*

NURSING DIAGNOSIS: Risk for fetal injury related to elevated maternal glucose levels

EXPECTED OUTCOMES

Fetus will remain free of injury and be born at term in a healthy state.

NURSING INTERVENTIONS/*RATIONALES*

Assess patient's current diabetic control *to identify risk for fetal death and congenital anomalies.*

Monitor fundal height during each prenatal visit *to identify appropriate fetal growth.*

Monitor for signs and symptoms of pregnancy-induced hypertension *to identify early manifestations because pregnant women with diabetes are more at risk.*

Assess fetal movement and heart rate during each prenatal visit, and perform weekly nonstress tests during the last 4 weeks of pregnancy, *to assess fetal well-being.*

Review procedure for blood glucose testing and insulin administration *to promote self-care.*

NURSING DIAGNOSIS: Anxiety related to threat to maternal and fetal well-being as evidenced by patient verbal expressions of concern

EXPECTED OUTCOMES

Patient will identify sources of anxiety and report feeling less anxious.

NURSING INTERVENTIONS/*RATIONALES*

Through therapeutic communication, promote an open relationship with patient *to promote patient trust.*

Listen to patient's feelings and concerns *to assess for any misconception or misinformation that may be contributing to anxiety.*

Review potential dangers by providing factual information *to correct any misconceptions or misinformation.*

Encourage patient to share concerns with her health care team *to promote patient and team collaboration in her care.*

NURSING DIAGNOSIS: Risk for imbalanced nutrition: less than body requirements related to inability to ingest nutrients that are needed for pregnancy complicated by diabetes

EXPECTED OUTCOMES

Patient will verbalize understanding of dietary needs during pregnancy, gain weight that is consistent with a normal pregnancy, and maintain blood sugar levels between 65 and 130 mg/dl.

NURSING INTERVENTIONS/*RATIONALES*

Assess caloric intake and dietary pattern using 24-hour recall *to evaluate patient understanding and adherence to dietary regimen.*

Review importance of regularity of meals and snacks *to promote compliance with treatment plan.*

Review blood glucose monitoring *to determine if patient is competent with procedure.*

Weigh patient at each prenatal visit *to assess appropriate weight gain.*

Refer to dietitian for individualized counseling if needed *to plan diet that assists the woman to maintain normoglycemia and to gain the appropriate amount of weight.*

Cultural Awareness

PREVALENCE OF DIABETES IN PERSONS AGED 20 AND OVER IN THE UNITED STATES (2002) BY RACE/ETHNICITY

Non-Hispanic whites	8.4%
Non-Hispanic blacks	11.4%
Hispanic/Latino Americans	8.2%
American Indians/Alaska Natives who receive care from the Indian Health Service	14.9%
Regional Level	
Alaska Natives	8.2%
American Indians in southeastern United States and southern Arizona	27.8%
Asian Americans and Native Hawaiian or other Pacific Islanders	Data are limited, but Native Hawaiians, Japanese, Hawaiians/other Pacific Islanders, and Filipino residents of Hawaii are approximately twice as likely to have diabetes as white residents of Hawaii.

Data from Centers for Disease Control and Prevention: National diabetes fact sheet. Internet document available at www.cdc.gov/diabetes/pubs/estimates.htm (accessed September 5, 2004).

et al, 2002). Classic risk factors for GDM include maternal age older than 30 years; obesity; family history of type 2 diabetes; and an obstetric history of an infant weighing more than 9 pounds, hydramnios, unexplained stillbirth, miscarriage, or an infant with congenital anomalies. Other factors include hypertensive disorders, recurrent monilial vaginitis, and glucosuria on two consecutive visits to the clinic or office (ADA, 2004a).

The diagnosis of gestational diabetes is usually made during the second half of pregnancy. As fetal nutrient demands rise during the late second and third trimesters, maternal nutrient ingestion induces greater and more sustained levels of blood glucose. At the same time, maternal insulin resistance is also increasing as a result of the insulin antagonistic effects of the placental hormones, cortisol and insulinase. Consequently, maternal insulin demands rise as much as threefold. The majority of pregnant women are capable of increasing insulin production to compensate for the insulin resistance and to maintain normoglycemia. When the pancreas is unable to produce sufficient insulin or the insulin is not used effectively, gestational diabetes can result.

Maternal and Fetal Risks

Women with GDM have twice the risk of developing hypertensive disorders compared with normal pregnant women. They also have increased risk for fetal macrosomia, which can lead to increased rates of perineal lacerations, episiotomy, and cesarean birth. In addition, fetal macrosomia may be associated with shoulder dystocia and birth trauma. GDM also places the neonate at increased risk for hypoglycemia, hypocalcemia, hyperbilirubinemia, thrombocytopenia, polycythemia, and respiratory distress syndrome.

The overall incidence of congenital anomalies among infants of women with gestational diabetes approaches that of the general population because gestational diabetes usually develops after week 20 of pregnancy—after the critical period of organogenesis (first trimester) has passed.

Screening for Gestational Diabetes Mellitus

Nurses involved in prenatal care delivery can be instrumental in the identification of women with GDM. Although protocols regarding which women will undergo screening and exactly how the screening will be done vary among care providers, nurses are often responsible for ensuring that the screen is performed on the identified group of women at the proper gestational age. Careful adherence to screening protocols is crucial to identify women with GDM correctly.

The American College of Obstetricians and Gynecologists (ACOG) recommends that all pregnant women be screened for GDM, either by history, clinical risk factors, or laboratory screening of blood glucose levels (ACOG, 2001). Based on history and clinical risk factors, some women are at such low risk for the development of GDM that glucose testing is neither necessary nor cost-effective (Expert Committee on the Diagnosis and Classification of Diabetes Mellitus, 2003). This group at low risk includes normal-weight women younger than 25 years who have no family history of diabetes, are not members of an ethnic or a racial group known to have a high prevalence of the disease, and have no previous history of abnormal glucose tolerance or adverse obstetric outcomes usually associated with GDM (ACOG, 2001; Expert Committee on the Diagnosis and Classification of Diabetes Mellitus, 2003). Women at high risk for developing GDM should be screened at the first prenatal visit and again at 24 to 28 weeks of gestation (ADA, 2004a).

The screening test used most often in North America (Glucola screening) consists of a 50 g oral glucose load, followed 1 hour later by a plasma glucose determination. Screening should be performed at 24 to 28 weeks of gestation. It is not necessary that the woman be fasting. A glucose value of 140 mg/dl is usually considered a positive screen. A positive Glucola screen requires follow-up with a 3-hour oral glucose tolerance test (OGTT). The 3-hour OGTT is administered after an overnight fast and at least 3 days of unrestricted diet (at least 150 g carbohydrate) and physical activity. The woman is instructed to avoid caffeine because it tends to increase glucose levels, and to abstain from smoking for 12 hours before and during the test. A fasting blood glucose level is drawn before giving a 100 g glucose load. Blood glucose levels are then drawn 1, 2, and 3 hours later. The woman is diagnosed with gestational diabetes if two or more values are met or exceeded (Fig. 13-4).

Nursing diagnoses and expected outcomes of care for the woman with GDM are basically the same as those for women with pregestational diabetes; however, the time frame for planning may be shortened with GDM because the diagnosis is usually made later in pregnancy.

Interventions

Antepartum

When the diagnosis of gestational diabetes is made, treatment begins immediately, allowing little or no time for the woman and her family to adjust to the diagnosis before they are expected to participate in the treatment plan. This is in contrast to the woman with pregestational diabetes who may have had years to learn about the disease and adapt to dietary modifications, self-monitoring of glucose, and insulin

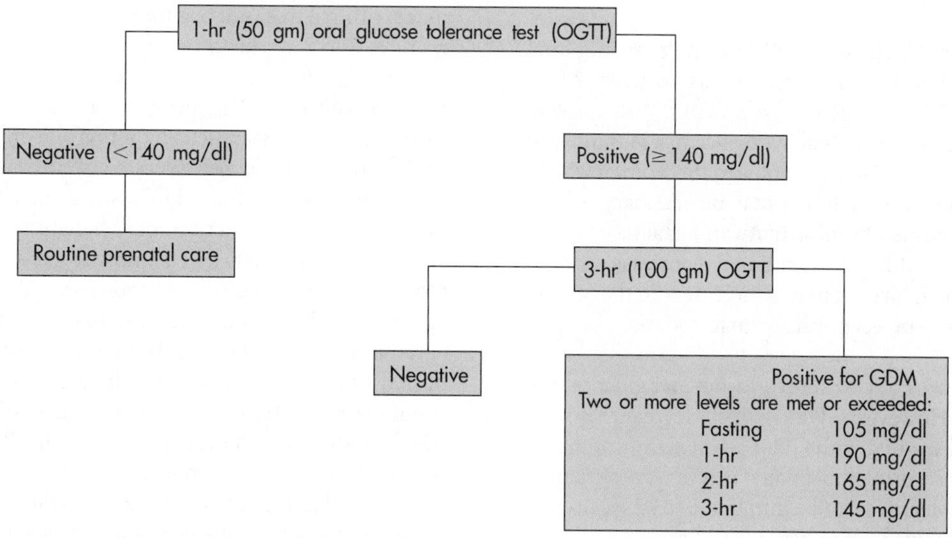

Fig. 13-4 Screening and diagnosis for gestational diabetes. (From American Diabetes Association: Position statement: gestational diabetes mellitus, *Diabetes Care* 27[suppl 1]:S88-S90, 2004.)

administration. With each step of the treatment plan, the nurse and other health care providers should educate the woman and her family, providing detailed and comprehensive explanations to ensure understanding, participation, and adherence to the necessary interventions. Potential complications should be discussed, and the need for maintenance of normoglycemia throughout the remainder of the pregnancy is reinforced. It may be reassuring for the woman and her family to know that gestational diabetes typically disappears when the pregnancy is over.

As with pregestational diabetes, the aim of therapy in women with GDM is meticulous blood glucose control. Fasting blood glucose levels should be between 60 and 90 mg/dl, and 2-hour postprandial blood levels should be between 90 and 120 mg/dl (ADA, 2000).

Diet

Dietary modification is the mainstay of treatment for GDM. The woman with GDM is placed on a standard diabetic diet immediately on diagnosis. Some authorities recommend fewer calories for overweight or morbidly obese women, believing that such a diet will cause less hyperglycemia and reduce the need for insulin (Landon et al, 2002). Dietary counseling by a nutritionist is recommended.

Exercise

Exercise in women with GDM appears to be safe. It helps lower blood glucose levels and may be instrumental in eliminating the need for insulin.

Monitoring Blood Glucose Levels

Regular blood glucose monitoring is necessary to determine if euglycemia can be maintained by diet and exercise. However, the optimal frequency and timing of blood glucose monitoring has not been established (ACOG, 2001). Some women with GDM are provided with reflectance meters and encouraged to perform frequent self-monitoring at home, or monitoring may be done only at the clinic or office visit.

Insulin Therapy

Up to 20% of women with GDM will require insulin during the pregnancy to maintain adequate blood glucose levels, despite compliance with the prescribed diet. The nurse should never assume that increased blood glucose levels in the woman with GDM have been caused by dietary indiscretion alone without first taking a thorough history.

Women who repeatedly exceed glucose thresholds for fasting and 2-hour postprandial values are usually started on insulin therapy. Again, there is no consensus regarding the exact glucose values that warrant insulin use (ACOG, 2001; Landon et al, 2002). The woman and her family should be taught the necessary skills to manage insulin administration. Langer and colleagues (2000) compared the use of glyburide, a second-generation oral hypoglycemic agent, and insulin in women with GDM. They found similar improvement in maternal glucose levels in both groups. Furthermore, the incidence of fetal macrosomia and neonatal hypoglycemia in the two study groups also was similar. More studies must be done, however, before oral hypoglycemic agents become widely used in GDM.

Fetal Surveillance

There is no standard recommendation for fetal surveillance in pregnancies complicated by GDM. Women whose blood glucose levels are well controlled by diet are at low risk for fetal death. Many practitioners do not routinely perform antepartum fetal testing on them so long as their fasting and 2-hour postprandial blood glucose levels remain within normal limits and they have no other risk factors. Usually these women are allowed to progress to term and spontaneous labor without intervention. Once the woman reaches 40 weeks of gestation, fetal surveillance once or twice weekly is usually instituted (ACOG, 2001; Landon et al, 2002).

Women with GDM whose blood glucose levels are not well controlled or who require insulin therapy, have hypertension, or have a history of previous stillbirth generally receive more intensive fetal biophysical monitoring. There is no standard recommendation regarding initiation of testing. Nonstress tests and biophysical profiles are often performed weekly, beginning from 32 to 36 weeks of gestation (ACOG, 2001; Landon et al, 2002).

Intrapartum

During labor and birth, blood glucose levels are monitored at least every 2 hours to maintain levels between 70 and 90 mg/dl (ADA, 2000). Glucose levels within this range will decrease the severity of neonatal hypoglycemia. IV fluids containing glucose are not given as a bolus to the woman who has gestational diabetes, although they may be necessary as maintenance fluids. Routine uterine activity and fetal heart rate assessments are done. Although gestational diabetes is not an indication for cesarean birth, it may be necessary in the presence of problems such as preeclampsia or macrosomia.

Postpartum

Most women with GDM return to normal glucose levels after childbirth. However, GDM is likely to recur in future pregnancies, and women with GDM are at significant risk of developing glucose intolerance later in life. Assessment for carbohydrate intolerance can be initiated 6 to 12 weeks postpartum or after breastfeeding has stopped and should be repeated at regular intervals throughout the woman's life. Obesity is a major risk factor for the later development of diabetes. Thus women with a history of GDM, particularly those who are overweight, should be encouraged to make lifestyle changes that include weight loss and exercise to reduce this risk. Because offspring of women with GDM are at risk to develop obesity and diabetes in childhood or adolescence, regular health care for these children is essential.

Thyroid Disorders

Hyperthyroidism

Hyperthyroidism occurs in approximately 2 of every 1000 pregnancies (Nader, 2004). In 90% to 95% of pregnant women, it is caused by Graves' disease. Other rare but possible causes include toxic nodular goiter and thyroiditis (Nader, 2004). Clinical manifestations of hyperthyroidism are associated with an increased basal metabolic rate and increased sympathetic nervous system activity. Typical symptoms include fatigue, heat intolerance, warm skin, diaphoresis, emotional lability, tremulousness, and a wide pulse pressure. Many of these symptoms also occur with pregnancy, so the disorder can be difficult to diagnose. Signs that may help differentiate hyperthyroidism from normal pregnancy include unplanned weight loss, onycholysis (loose nails), and a pulse rate greater than 100 beats per minute that does not decrease with the Valsalva maneuver. Laboratory findings include an elevated free thyroxine (T_4) level and a suppressed serum thyroid-stimulating hormone (TSH) level. Mild hyperthyroidism is not thought to impair fertility, although it is rare to find severe disease in early pregnancy. Hyperthyroidism is best treated before pregnancy. Moderate and severe hyperthyroidism must be treated during pregnancy; untreated or inadequately treated women give birth to infants with low birth weight and more minor fetal anomalies (Nader, 2004). Women with hyperthyroidism are also at increased risk to develop severe preeclampsia. Hyperemesis gravidarum is often associated with elevated thyroid hormone levels (Mestman, 2002).

The primary treatment of hyperthyroidism during pregnancy is drug therapy; the medication of choice is propylthiouracil (PTU). Patients generally show clinical improvement within 2 weeks of beginning therapy, but the medication requires 6 to 8 weeks to reach full effectiveness. During therapy the woman's free T_4 levels are measured monthly and the results used to taper the drug to the smallest effective dosage to prevent unnecessary fetal hypothyroidism (Mestman, 2002; Nader, 2004). PTU is well tolerated by most patients. Rare side effects include pruritus, skin rash, a metallic taste, nausea, bronchospasm, oral ulcerations, hepatitis, and a lupus-like syndrome (Nader, 2004). The most severe side effect is agranulocytosis, which is more common in women over 40 years of age and in those taking high doses of PTU. Symptoms of agranulocytosis are fever and sore throat, which should be reported immediately to the health care provider; the woman should stop taking the PTU. Leukopenia of a transient and benign nature may occur as a result of PTU therapy. PTU readily crosses the placenta and may induce fetal hypothyroidism and goiter (Mestman, 2002; Nader, 2004).

Beta-adrenergic blockers such as propranolol may be used in severe hyperthyroidism. Long-term use is not recommended because of the potential for intrauterine growth restriction (IUGR) and altered response to anoxic stress, postnatal bradycardia, and hypoglycemia.

Radioactive iodine must not be used in diagnosis or treatment of hyperthyroidism because it may compromise the fetal thyroid. If a mother taking hyperthyroid medication chooses to breastfeed, she needs to be aware that physiologically significant doses of the drug are passed to the infant through the breast milk. The infant's thyroid status should be monitored periodically so hypothyroidism can be prevented.

In severe cases, surgical treatment of hyperthyroidism (subtotal thyroidectomy) may be performed during the second or third trimester. Because of the increased risk of miscarriage and preterm labor associated with major surgery, this treatment is usually reserved for women with severe disease, those for whom drug therapy proves toxic, and those who are unable to adhere to the prescribed medical regimen. Postoperative hypothyroidism is common, occurring in at least 20% of women with hyperthyroidism.

NURSE ALERT A serious but uncommon complication of undiagnosed or partially treated hyperthyroidism is thyroid storm, which may occur in response to stresses such as infection, birth, or surgery. A woman experiencing this emergent condition may have fever, restlessness, tachycardia, vomiting, hypotension, or stupor. Congestive heart failure frequently occurs. Prompt treatment is essential; IV fluids and oxygen are administered along with high doses of PTU. Potassium iodide, antipyretics, glucocorticoids, and beta-adrenergic blockers may also be given; sedation may be necessary for extreme restlessness (Nader, 2004). ■

Hypothyroidism

Hypothyroidism during pregnancy is rare because women with this condition are often infertile. Hypothyroidism is usually the result of Hashimoto's disease, thyroid gland ablation by radiation, previous surgery, or antithyroid medications. Reduced thyroid function because of hypothalamic or pituitary failure is rare, with only a few reported cases. Iodine deficiency in the United States is also rare (Nader, 2004).

Characteristic symptoms of hypothyroidism include fatigue, weight gain, cold intolerance, constipation, cool and dry skin, coarsened hair, and muscle weakness. Laboratory findings during pregnancy include low or low-normal T_3 and T_4 levels and elevated levels of TSH.

Pregnant women with untreated hypothyroidism are at risk for preeclampsia, placental abruption, and stillbirth. Infants born to mothers with hypothyroidism may be of low birth weight, but for the most part are healthy, without evidence of thyroid dysfunction.

Thyroid hormone supplements are used to treat hypothyroidism. Levothyroxine (L-thyroxine [Synthroid]) is most often prescribed during pregnancy. As pregnancy progresses, the woman usually requires increased amounts of L-thyroxine. The aim of drug therapy is to maintain the woman's TSH level within the normal range for pregnant women. Dosage adjustments are made as necessary by measuring TSH levels periodically. Each dosage change should be followed 4 to 6 weeks later by determining the TSH level.

NURSE ALERT Pregnant women should be told to take L-thyroxine 2 hours before or after iron tablets, because ferrous sulfate lowers the effectiveness of the medication (Diehl, 1998). ■

The fetus depends on maternal thyroid hormones until 12 weeks of gestation, when fetal production begins. Thus maternal hypothyroidism does not cause fetal hypothyroidism. However, maternal treatment of hypothyroidism may result in increased fetal levels of thyroid hormones. Careful monitoring of the neonate's thyroid status is important to detect any abnormalities.

Nursing Care

Education of the pregnant woman with thyroid dysfunction is essential to promote compliance with the plan of treatment. The woman is instructed regarding the disorder and its potential impact on herself and her fetus, the medication regimen and possible side effects, the need for continuing medical supervision, and the importance of compliance. The family is incorporated into the plan of care to foster mutuality and support among the members.

NURSE ALERT Thyroid medication should be stored in a dark bottle to prevent deterioration. The woman should be counseled not to change brands of thyroid medication without physician approval because hormone content varies between brands. ■

The woman often needs assistance from the nurse in coping with the discomforts and frustrations associated with symptoms of the disorder. For example, the woman with hyperthyroidism who has nervousness and hyperactivity concomitant with weakness and fatigue may benefit from suggestions to channel excess energies into quiet diversional activities such as reading or crafts. Discomfort associated with hypersensitivity to heat (hyperthyroidism) or cold intolerance (hypothyroidism) can be minimized by appropriate clothing and regulation of environmental temperatures, when possible, and by avoidance of temperature extremes.

Nutrition counseling with a registered dietitian may provide guidance in selecting a well-balanced diet. The woman with hyperthyroidism who has increased appetite and poor weight gain and the hypothyroid woman who has anorexia and lethargy need counseling to ensure adequate intake of nutritionally sound foods to meet both maternal and fetal needs.

Maternal Phenylketonuria

Phenylketonuria (PKU), a recognized cause of mental retardation, is an inborn error of metabolism caused by an autosomal recessive trait that creates a deficiency in the enzyme phenylalanine hydrolase. Absence of this enzyme impairs the body's ability to metabolize the amino acid phenylalanine, found in all protein foods. Consequently, there is toxic accumulation of phenylalanine in the blood, which interferes with brain development and function. PKU affects approximately 1 of every 15,000 infants in the United States (Mayo Clinic Staff, 2004).

All newborns are tested for this disorder soon after birth; prompt diagnosis and therapy with a phenylalanine-restricted diet significantly decreases the incidence of mental retardation. Dietary therapy for PKU is recommended to continue throughout life (Rouse & Azen, 2004). Subtle but detrimental effects of elevated levels of phenylalanine on neurologic, behavioral, and intellectual function have been found in women who discontinued treatment in childhood.

The key to prevention of fetal anomalies caused by PKU is the identification of women in their reproductive years who have the disorder. Screening programs during the school years and in the premarital period may help identify those individuals with PKU so that dietary therapy can be instituted before conception occurs. Before conception, these women and their families should be educated about the potential risks to the fetus if phenylalanine levels are not controlled.

Screening for undiagnosed maternal PKU at the first prenatal visit may be warranted, especially in individuals with a family history of the disorder, with low intelligence of uncertain etiology, or who have given birth to microcephalic infants. Although it may be too late to improve the current pregnancy outcome through diet therapy, the woman and her family will be aware of the problem and the necessary treatment should future pregnancies occur.

Normal pregnancy weight gain reduces the incidence of microcephaly and should be encouraged. Adequate protein and vitamin intake early in pregnancy may prevent congenital heart disease even when the blood phenylalanine level is elevated (Matalon, Acosta, & Azen, 2003).

Women with PKU have been discouraged from breastfeeding because their milk contains a high concentration of phenylalanine. Infants diagnosed with PKU can be safely breastfed if the amount of breast milk ingested is monitored so that phenylalanine levels do not get too high. Mothers who choose to breastfeed must supplement the infant's diet with a special milk preparation that contains little or no phenylalanine.

CARDIOVASCULAR DISORDERS

During a normal pregnancy the maternal cardiovascular system undergoes many changes that put a physiologic strain on the heart. The major cardiovascular changes that occur during a normal pregnancy and that affect the patient with cardiac disease are increased intravascular volume, decreased systemic vascular resistance, cardiac output changes occurring during labor and birth, and the intravascular volume changes that occur just after childbirth. The strain is present during pregnancy and continues for a few weeks after birth. The normal heart can compensate for the increased workload, and pregnancy, labor, and birth are generally well tolerated; but the diseased heart is hemodynamically challenged.

If the cardiovascular changes are not well tolerated, cardiac failure can develop during pregnancy, labor, or the postpartum period. In addition, if myocardial disease develops, valvular disease exists, or a congenital heart defect is present, cardiac decompensation (inability of the heart to maintain a sufficient cardiac output) may occur.

From 0.4% to 4% of pregnancies are complicated by heart disease (Grewal, Biswas, & Perloff, 2003), the leading cause of nonobstetric maternal death. Rheumatic fever is responsible for about 50% of cardiac complications; congenital diseases and mitral valve disease are the next most common causes. Other cardiac diseases are uncommon (Gilbert & Harmon, 2003). Cardiac disease ranks fourth overall as a cause of maternal death. A maternal mortality rate of up to 50% is anticipated in women with persistent cardiac decompensation. Box 13-2 lists maternal cardiac disease risk groups.

The degree of disability experienced by the woman with cardiac disease is often more important in the treatment and prognosis of cardiac disease complicating pregnancy than is the diagnosis of cardiovascular disease. The New York Heart Association's (NYHA's) classification of functional capacity of patients with heart disease, a widely accepted standard, is as follows (Criteria Committee of the New York Heart Association, 1994):

Class I—Asymptomatic at normal levels of activity
Class II—Symptomatic with ordinary activity
Class III—Symptomatic with less than ordinary activity
Class IV—Symptomatic at rest

No classification of heart disease can be considered rigid or absolute, but the NYHA classification offers a basic practical guide for treatment, assuming that frequent prenatal visits, good patient cooperation, and appropriate obstetric care occur. Medical therapy is conducted by a team approach that includes the cardiologist, obstetrician, and nurses. The functional classification may change over the course of the pregnancy because of the hemodynamic changes that occur in the cardiovascular system. There is a 30% to 45% increase in cardiac output compared with nonpregnancy resting values, with the majority of the increase in the first trimester and the peak at 20 to 24 weeks of gestation (Blanchard & Shabetai, 2004). The functional classification of the disease is determined at 3 months and again at 7 or 8 months of gestation. Pregnant women may progress from class I or II to III or IV during pregnancy. Women with cyanotic congenital heart disease do not fit into the NYHA classification because their exercise-induced symptoms have causes not related to heart failure. An Ability Index was developed for assessment of these patients (Gei & Hankins, 2001).

Contraindications to pregnancy in women with heart disease are listed in Box 13-3. The incidence of miscarriage is increased, and preterm labor and birth are more prevalent in the pregnant woman with cardiac problems. In addition,

evolve CASE STUDY—CLASS III CARDIAC DISORDER

BOX 13-2

Maternal Cardiac Disease Risk Groups

Group I (Mortality Rate 1%)
Corrected tetralogy of Fallot
Pulmonic/tricuspid disease
Mitral stenosis (classes I, II)
Patent ductus arteriosus
Ventricular septal defect
Atrial septal defect
Porcine valve

Group II (Mortality Rate 5%-15%)
Mitral stenosis with atrial fibrillation
Artificial heart valves
Mitral stenosis (classes III, IV)
Uncorrected tetralogy of Fallot
Aortic coarctation (uncomplicated)
Aortic stenosis
Marfan syndrome with normal aorta

Group III (Mortality Rate 25%-50%)
Aortic coarctation (complicated)
Myocardial infarction (previous)
Marfan syndrome with aortic involvement
Pulmonary hypertension

From Gilbert ES, Harmon JS: *Manual of high risk pregnancy and delivery,* ed 3, St Louis, 2003, Mosby.

BOX 13-3

Contraindications to Pregnancy in a Woman with Heart Disease

Dilated cardiomyopathy
Primary pulmonary hypertension
Eisenmenger's syndrome
Marfan syndrome with aortic root dilation

Source: Blanchard DG, Shabetai R: Cardiac diseases. In Creasy RK, Resnik R, Iams JD (eds): *Maternal-fetal medicine: principles and practice,* ed 5, Philadelphia, 2004, WB Saunders.

IUGR is common, probably because of low oxygen pressure (Po_2) in the mother. The incidence of congenital heart lesions is increased in children of mothers with congenital heart disease; thus preconception counseling is important.

A diagnosis of cardiac disease depends on the history, physical examination, x-ray findings, and, if indicated, sonogram results. The differential diagnosis of heart disease also involves ruling out respiratory problems and other potential causes of chest pain.

Maternal mortality rate of more than 50% during pregnancy has been associated with pulmonary hypertension; it is vital that the woman with cardiac disease be assessed and the diagnosis established as soon as possible (Blanchard & Shabetai, 2004).

CASE STUDY—CLASS III CARDIAC DISORDER

Peripartum Cardiomyopathy

The criteria for the diagnosis of peripartum cardiomyopathy (PPCM) include development of congestive heart failure in the last month of pregnancy or within the first 5 postpartum months, lack of another cause for heart failure, and absence of heart disease before the last month of pregnancy (Blanchard & Shabetai, 2004). Some data suggest that this definition be expanded, because the diagnosis of PPCM has been made at other times during gestation. The etiology of the disease is unknown; theories suggest genetic predisposition, autoimmunity, and viral infections.

Peripartum cardiomyopathy is more common in African-American women, in twin pregnancies, and in women with preeclampsia (Grewal et al, 2003). In the United States, the incidence is 1 in 3000 to 4000 live births. Maternal mortality rate has been estimated in the range of 25% to 50%, whereas infant mortality rate is approximately 10% (Ramsey, Ramin, & Ramin, 2001). Symptoms include breathlessness, tachydysrhythmias, and edema, with radiologic findings of cardiomegaly. The prognosis is good if cardiomegaly does not persist after 6 months postpartum. Women whose hearts remain enlarged after 6 months postpartum will have PPCM in future pregnancies (Blanchard & Shabetai, 2004). Pregnancy is contraindicated for women with persistent cardiomegaly or cardiac dysfunction.

Medical management of cardiomyopathy during pregnancy includes a regimen used for congestive heart failure and the potential for thromboembolism: diuretics, sodium restriction, afterload-reducing agents, anticoagulants, and digoxin. Angiotensin-converting enzyme inhibitors can be used only in the postpartum period, because they are teratogenic agents. The nursing care of women with PPCM is essentially the same as that for women with other types of cardiac problems.

Rheumatic Heart Disease

Rheumatic fever is increasingly uncommon in the United States. When it occurs, it usually develops suddenly, often several symptom-free weeks after an inadequately treated group A beta-hemolytic streptococcal throat infection. Episodes of rheumatic fever create an autoimmune reaction in the heart tissue that leads to permanent damage of heart valves (usually the mitral valve) and the chorda tendineae cordis. This damage is referred to as *rheumatic heart disease* (RHD). RHD may be evident during acute rheumatic fever or discovered years later. Recurrences of rheumatic fever are common; each has the potential to increase the severity of heart damage. If a woman has had rheumatic fever in the past, it can recur during pregnancy. The American Heart Association recommends lifelong prophylaxis with penicillin G benzathine, even during pregnancy. For those with penicillin allergies, erythromycin is an acceptable alternative during pregnancy. Heart murmurs, resulting from stenosis, valvular insufficiency, or thickening of the walls of the heart, characterize RHD. Abnormal pulse rate and rhythm, as well as congestive heart failure, are common.

Mitral Valve Stenosis

Mitral valve stenosis (narrowing of the opening of the mitral valve caused by stiffening of valve leaflets, thereby obstructing blood flow from the atrium to the ventricles) is the characteristic lesion resulting from RHD (Blanchard & Shabetai, 2004). Even though a history of rheumatic fever may be absent, it remains the most likely cause of mitral stenosis. As the mitral valve narrows, dyspnea worsens, occurring first on exertion and eventually at rest. A tight stenosis, plus the increase in blood volume and cardiac output of normal pregnancy, may cause ventricular failure and pulmonary edema; hemoptysis may occur. About 25% of women with mitral valve stenosis may become symptomatic for the first time during pregnancy (Ramsey et al, 2001).

The care of the woman with mitral stenosis typically is managed by reducing her activity, restricting dietary sodium, and increasing bed rest. The pregnant woman with mitral stenosis should be monitored clinically for symptoms and with echocardiograms to monitor the atrial and ventricular size, as well as heart valve function. Prophylaxis for intrapartum endocarditis and pulmonary infections may be provided for women at high risk (Easterling & Otto, 2002) (Box 13-4).

For patients with NYHA class III or IV cardiac disease, mitral balloon valvuloplasty can be considered. This procedure should be considered only when symptoms cannot be controlled by standard means. Mitral balloon valvuloplasty is optimally performed after 20 weeks of gestation to decrease radiation risks to the fetus.

Mitral Valve Prolapse

Mitral valve prolapse (MVP) is a common, usually benign, condition occurring in 5% to 8% of women of reproductive age (Grewal et al, 2003). The mitral valve leaflets prolapse into the left atrium during ventricular systole, allowing some backflow of blood. Midsystolic click and late systolic murmur are hallmarks of this syndrome. Most cases are asymptomatic. A few women have atypical chest pain (sharp and located in the left side of the chest) that occurs at rest, is unrelated to exercise, and does not respond to nitrates. They may have anxiety, palpitations, dyspnea on exertion, and syncope. Specific treatment is usually not necessary except

BOX 13-4

Prophylaxis for Bacterial Endocarditis

High Risk Patients

In active labor: ampicillin 2 g IV or IM plus gentamicin 1.5 mg/kg (not to exceed 120 mg)

6 hr later: ampicillin 1 g IV or IM or amoxicillin 1 g PO

Penicillin-Allergic Patients

In active labor: vancomycin 1 g IV over 1-2 hr plus gentamicin as above

Moderate Risk Patients

In active labor: amoxicillin 2 g PO or ampicillin 2 g IV or IM

Penicillin-Allergic Patients

In active labor: vancomycin 1 g IV over 1-2 hr

Sources: Dajani AS et al: Prevention of bacterial endocarditis: recommendations by the American Heart Association, *JAMA* 277(22):1794-1801, 1997; Easterling TR, Otto C: Heart disease. In Gabbe SG, Niebyl JR, Simpson JL (eds): *Obstetrics: normal and problem pregnancies,* ed 4, New York, 2002, Churchill Livingstone.

IM, intramuscular administration; *IV,* intravenous administration; *PO,* by mouth (from Latin, *per os*).

for symptomatic tachyarrhythmias. Pregnancy and its associated hemodynamic changes may change or alleviate the murmur and click of MVP, as well as its symptoms. As with RHD, antibiotic prophylaxis may be given before invasive procedures for at-risk patients and for complicated vaginal deliveries in patients with MVP.

Infective Endocarditis

Infective endocarditis, or inflammation of the innermost lining (endocardium) of the heart caused by invasion of microorganisms, is an uncommon disorder during pregnancy. It may be seen in women taking street drugs intravenously. Bacterial endocarditis, leading to incompetence of heart valves and thus congestive heart failure and cerebral emboli, can result in death. Treatment is with antibiotics (see Box 13-4).

Eisenmenger's Syndrome

Eisenmenger's syndrome is a right-to-left or bidirectional shunting that can be at the atrial or ventricular level and is combined with elevated pulmonary vascular resistance (Blanchard & Shabetai, 2004). The syndrome is associated with a mortality rate of approximately 50%; thus pregnancy is contraindicated. If pregnancy occurs, termination may be recommended if the woman has significant pulmonary hypertension.

In women who continue pregnancy despite the risks, physical activity is strictly limited; prophylactic anticoagulation is considered (Blanchard & Shabetai, 2004). Intensive care monitoring during labor and birth, including a Swan-Ganz catheter, and skilled obstetric anesthesia care are essential.

Atrial Septal Defect

Atrial septal defect (ASD; abnormal opening between the atria), one of the causes of a left-to-right shunt, is the most common congenital defect seen during pregnancy. This defect may go undetected because the woman usually is asymptomatic. The pregnant woman with an ASD will most likely have an uncomplicated pregnancy. Some women may have right-sided heart failure or arrhythmias as the pregnancy progresses, as a result of increased plasma volume.

Tetralogy of Fallot

Tetralogy of Fallot is the most common cyanotic heart disease present during pregnancy. Other cyanotic congenital heart diseases are rarely seen during pregnancy because women with these conditions rarely survive to adulthood. Components of tetralogy of Fallot include a ventricular septal defect (VSD), pulmonary stenosis, overriding aorta, and right ventricular hypertrophy, leading to a right-to-left shunt. Women with corrected tetralogy of Fallot have a mortality rate of less than 1%; however, women with uncorrected tetralogy of Fallot have a 5% to 15% mortality rate (Gei & Hankins, 2001). Medical management for women with uncorrected tetralogy of Fallot includes anticoagulant therapy, high-concentration oxygen administration, and hemodynamic monitoring during labor and birth.

Marfan Syndrome

Marfan syndrome is an autosomal dominant genetic disorder characterized by generalized weakness of the connective tissue, resulting in joint deformities, ocular lens dislocation, and weakness of the aortic wall and root (Blanchard & Shabetai, 2004). About 90% of individuals with this syndrome have MVP, and 25% have aortic insufficiency, with an increased risk of aortic dissection and rupture during pregnancy. Excruciating chest pain is the most common symptom of aortic dissection. Aortic dissection most often occurs in the third trimester or postpartally. Therapy includes limiting physical activity, preventing hypertensive complications, and administering beta-blockers. Preconception genetic counseling is recommended to make women aware of the risks of pregnancy with this condition, with a 50% risk of inheritance of the syndrome (Blanchard & Shabetai, 2004).

Heart Transplantation

Increasing numbers of heart recipients are successfully completing pregnancies. Before conception, the woman should be assessed for quality of ventricular function and potential rejection of the transplant. The woman should be stabilized on the immunosuppressant regimen. Conception should be postponed for at least 1 year after transplantation to avoid acute rejection episodes (Ramsey et al, 2001). Risks to the woman include hypertension, preeclampsia, preterm labor, renal insufficiency, small-for-gestational-age neonate, and infections. During labor, beta-blocking agents may be needed to prevent tachycardia due to vagal denervation from the transplant surgery. Vaginal birth is desired, but transplant recipients have an increased rate of cesarean births. Management of the intrapartal period requires the coordination of care among all health care providers involved in the care of the woman and her fetus.

After birth, the neonate may exhibit immunosuppressive effects during the first week of life. Breastfeeding is not advised for infants of mothers taking cyclosporine.

Care Management

Nursing care of the woman with a cardiovascular disorder combines routine peripartum care with care specific for the cardiac diagnosis and function. Cardiac conditions vary in their impact on pregnancy because of acuteness or chronicity.

The presence of cardiac disease makes the decision to become pregnant more difficult. Planned pregnancy requires that the woman understand the peripartum risks. If the pregnancy is unplanned, the nurse needs to explore the woman's desire to continue the pregnancy. The nurse should review with the woman options for pregnancy termination if her cardiac status is tenuous and abortion is an acceptable alternative. The woman's significant other and family should be included in the discussion. Teaching sessions for the woman and her support people should be offered as indicated by their learning needs.

Care of these women at high risk requires a multidisciplinary approach. The multidisciplinary team includes a cardiologist who is familiar with expected cardiovascular changes in pregnancy; a perinatologist; an anesthesiologist; and nurses expert in labor and fetal and hemodynamic monitoring.

Assessment

The pregnant woman with cardiac disease requires detailed assessment throughout the peripartum period to determine the potential for optimal maternal health and a viable fetus. If she chooses to continue the pregnancy, the high risk pregnant woman's condition may be assessed as often as weekly.

Interview

The nurse elicits information from the woman regarding her personal medical history and that of her family. Special notation is made of diseases of cardiovascular significance, including congenital heart disease, streptococcal infections, rheumatic fever, valvular disease, endocarditis, congestive heart failure, angina, or myocardial infarction.

The nurse assesses for factors that would increase stress on the heart, such as anemia, infection, and edema, as well as how the woman is adapting to the physiologic changes of pregnancy. Special attention is given to the review of the cardiovascular and pulmonary systems. The nurse should determine whether the patient has experienced chest pain at rest or on exertion; edema of the face, hands, or feet; hypertension; heart murmurs; palpitations; paroxysmal nocturnal dyspnea; diaphoresis; and pallor or syncope. Pulmonary symptoms such as cough, hemoptysis, shortness of breath, and orthopnea also can be signs of cardiac disease. Table 13-3 lists the normal and abnormal cardiovascular signs and symptoms during pregnancy.

The nurse documents all medications taken by the woman—including over-the-counter medications such as supplemental iron—and is alert to their potential side effects and interactions. The woman is also assessed for undue emotional stress that might further compromise cardiac status. Examples of emotional stress are depression, anxiety or fear of morbidity or death for herself and the fetus, financial concerns related to extended hospitalization, anger because of impaired social interaction, and feelings of inadequacy regarding her inability to meet family and household demands.

The woman's cultural background may affect the amount of support that she is able to receive from significant others. Family size (number of children and extended family members in the home), and role expectations within the family, may be dictated by cultural norms. For the woman with cardiac impairment, family expectations may be a cause of major stress if she is unable to bear the expected number of children or if it is unacceptable to receive help with domestic chores. The nurse should be aware of the cultural customs of the pregnant woman and her family.

Physical Examination

Routine assessments continue during the prenatal period, including monitoring the amount and pattern of edema, vital signs, discomforts of pregnancy, and amount and pattern of weight gain. The woman is observed for signs of cardiac decompensation, that is, progressive generalized edema, crackles at the base of the lungs, or pulse irregularity (Box 13-5). Symptoms of cardiac decompensation may appear

Table 13-3

Cardiovascular Signs and Symptoms during Pregnancy

NORMAL	ABNORMAL
Signs	
Neck vein pulsation	Neck vein distention
Diffuse/displaced apical pulse	Cardiomegaly; heave
Split S_1, accentuated S_2	Loud P_2; wide split of S_2
Third heart sound	Summation gallop
Systolic murmur (1-2/6)	Loud systolic murmur (4-6/6)
Venous hum	Diastolic murmur
Sinus dysrhythmia	Sustained dysrhythmia
Peripheral edema	Clubbing/cyanosis
Symptoms	
Fatigue	Symptoms at rest
Chest pain	Exertional chest pain
Dyspnea	Exertional, severe dyspnea
Orthopnea	Orthopnea (progressive)
Hyperpnea	Paroxysmal nocturnal dyspnea
Palpitations	Tachycardia (>120 beats/min); dysrhythmia
Syncope (vasovagal)	Exertional syncope

Adapted from Mendelson MA: Congenital cardiac disease and pregnancy, *Clin Perinatol* 24(2):467-482, 1997.

BOX 13-5

Signs of Potential Complications

Cardiac Decompensation

Pregnant Woman: Subjective Symptoms

- Increasing fatigue or difficulty breathing, or both, with usual activities
- Feeling of smothering
- Frequent cough
- Palpitations; feeling that her heart is racing
- Swelling of face, feet, legs, fingers (e.g., rings do not fit anymore)

Nurse: Objective Signs

- Irregular weak, rapid pulse (≥100 beats/min)
- Progressive, generalized edema
- Crackles at base of lungs after two inspirations and exhalations
- Orthopnea; increasing dyspnea
- Rapid respirations (≥25 breaths/min)
- Moist, frequent cough
- Increasing fatigue
- Cyanosis of lips and nail beds

abruptly or gradually. Medical intervention must be instituted immediately to maintain optimal cardiac status. Dyspnea, palpitations, syncope, and edema commonly occur in pregnant women and can mask the symptoms of a developing or worsening cardiovascular disorder. A woman's sudden inability to perform activities she previously was comfortable doing may indicate cardiovascular decompensation.

Laboratory and Diagnostic Tests

Routine urinalysis and blood work (complete blood count and blood chemistry) are done during the initial visit. The woman with cardiac impairment requires a baseline 12-lead electrocardiogram (ECG) at the beginning of her pregnancy, if not before pregnancy, which permits vital diagnostic comparisons with subsequent ECGs. Echocardiograms and pulse oximetry studies may be performed as indicated. Chest films may be necessary during late pregnancy; the abdomen must be carefully shielded. In addition, fetal ultrasound, fetal movement studies, or fetal nonstress tests may be used to determine fetal well-being.

Nursing Diagnoses

The following examples are some nursing diagnoses that may be formulated. As always, individualizing diagnoses is vital.

Prenatal period:
- *Fear related to*
  —increased peripartum risk
- *Deficient knowledge related to*
  —cardiac condition
  —pregnancy and how it affects cardiac condition
  —requirements to alter self-care activities
- *Activity intolerance related to*
  —cardiac condition
- *Risk for self-care deficit (bathing, grooming, and dressing) related to*
  —fatigue or activity intolerance
  —need for bed rest
- *Impaired home maintenance related to*
  —woman's confinement to bed or limited activity level

Postpartum period:
- *Anxiety related to*
  —fear for infant's safety
- *Fear of dying related to*
  —perceived physiologic inability to cope with stress of labor
- *Risk for impaired gas exchange related to*
  —cardiac condition
- *Risk for excess fluid volume related to*
  —extravascular fluid shifts
- *Ineffective breastfeeding related to*
  —fatigue from cardiac condition

Expected Outcomes

The pregnant woman with cardiovascular problems faces curtailment of her activities. Bed rest during pregnancy affects all of the organ systems, but especially the cardiovascular and musculoskeletal. In addition, psychologic side effects can be debilitating, especially stress (Cunningham et al, 2001; Maloni, Brezinski-Tomasi, & Johnson, 2001). The community health nurse, social worker, and physical or occupational therapist are some of the resource people whose services may be incorporated into the plan of care. Expected outcomes might include that the pregnant woman (and family, if appropriate) will do the following:

- Verbalize understanding of the disorder, management, and probable outcome.
- Describe her role in management, including when and how to take medication, adjust diet, and prepare for and participate in treatment.
- Cope with emotional reactions to pregnancy and an infant at risk.
- Adapt to the physiologic stressors of pregnancy, labor, and birth.
- Identify and use support systems.
- Carry her fetus to viability or to term.

Plan of Care and Implementation

Therapy for the pregnant woman with heart disease is focused on minimizing stress on the heart. This stress is greatest between 28 and 32 weeks as the hemodynamic changes reach their maximum. The workload of the cardiovascular system is reduced by appropriate treatment of any coexisting emotional stress, hypertension, anemia, hyperthyroidism, or obesity.

Signs and symptoms of cardiac decompensation are reviewed with the pregnant woman and her family. The woman with class I or II heart disease requires 8 to 10 hours of sleep every day and should take 30-minute naps after meals. Her activities are restricted, with housework, shopping, and exercise limited to the amount recommended for the functional classification of her heart disease.

The woman with class II cardiac disease should avoid heavy exertion and should stop any activity that causes even minor signs and symptoms of cardiac decompensation. She should be admitted to the hospital near term (or earlier if signs of cardiac overload or dysrhythmia develop) for evaluation and treatment.

Bed rest for much of the day is necessary for pregnant women with class III cardiac disease. About 30% of these women experience cardiac decompensation during pregnancy. These women may require hospitalization for the remainder of the pregnancy.

Because decompensation occurs even at rest in persons with class IV cardiac disease, a major initial effort must be made to improve the cardiac status of the pregnant woman in this category who chooses to continue her pregnancy (Patient Teaching box).

Infections are treated promptly. Women who have valvular disorders should receive prophylactic antibiotics against bacterial endocarditis during gestation (see Box 13-4).

Nutrition counseling is necessary, and optimally takes place with the woman's family present. The woman needs a well-balanced diet with iron and folic acid supplementation, high protein, and adequate calories to gain weight. Iron supplements tend to cause constipation. The pregnant woman should increase her intake of fluids and fiber. A stool softener may be prescribed. It is important that the pregnant woman with cardiac disease avoid straining during defecation, thus causing the Valsalva maneuver (forced expiration against a closed airway, which when released causes blood to

Patient Teaching

THE PREGNANT WOMAN AT RISK FOR CARDIAC DECOMPENSATION

- Assess lifestyle patterns, emotional status, and environment of woman.
- Arrange for consultations as needed (i.e., dietitian, home care, child care, social work).
- Determine woman's and her family's understanding of her heart disease and how the disease affects her pregnancy.
- Determine stressors in the woman's life. Assist woman in identifying effective coping strategies.
- Instruct woman to report signs of cardiac decompensation or congestive heart failure: generalized edema, distention of neck veins, dyspnea, pulmonary crackles, cough, palpitations, sudden weight gain.
- Instruct woman to be watchful for signs of thromboembolism, such as redness, tenderness, pain, or swelling of the legs. Instruct woman to seek medical help immediately if such symptoms occur.
- Instruct woman to avoid constipation and thus straining with bowel movements (Valsalva maneuver) by taking in adequate fluids and fiber. A stool softener may be ordered.
- Explore with woman ways to obtain the needed rest throughout the day. Depending on the level of her cardiac disease, she may need to sleep 10 hours per night and rest for 30 minutes after meals (class I or II) or rest for most of the day (class III or IV).
- Help woman make use of community resources, including support groups, as indicated.
- Emphasize the importance of keeping her prenatal visits.

From Gilbert ES, Harmon JS: *Manual of high risk pregnancy and delivery,* ed 3, St Louis, 2003, Mosby; Health Care Resources: *Handbook of high risk perinatal home care,* St Louis, 1997, Mosby; Lowdermilk DL, Grohar J: *High risk antepartal home care,* White Plains, NY, 1998, March of Dimes.

rush to the heart and overload the cardiac system) (see Patient Teaching box). If sodium restriction is necessary, the amount should not be less than 2.5 g/day (Gilbert & Harmon, 2003). The woman's intake of potassium is monitored to prevent hypokalemia, especially if she is taking diuretics. A referral to a registered dietitian may be necessary.

Cardiac medications are prescribed as needed for the pregnant woman, with attention to fetal well-being. The hemodynamic changes that occur during pregnancy, such as increased plasma volume and increased renal clearance of drugs, can alter the amount of medication needed to establish and maintain a therapeutic drug level (Blanchard & Shabetai, 2004). Monitoring of the drug levels during the pregnancy is crucial to maintain effective therapy for the woman while minimizing risk to the fetus. Research on the effects of cardiovascular drugs on the fetus and pregnant woman has been limited. The nurse should review current pharmacologic literature, especially when administering any medication to a pregnant woman (Table 13-4).

If anticoagulant therapy is required during pregnancy for conditions such as recurrent venous thrombosis, pulmonary embolus, rheumatic heart disease, prosthetic valves, or cyanotic congenital heart defects, heparin may be used because this large-molecule drug does not cross the placenta (Blanchard & Shabetai, 2004). The nurse should closely monitor the woman's blood work, including clotting factors. The woman may need to learn to self-administer heparin. She also requires specific nutritional teaching to avoid foods high in vitamin K such as raw dark green and leafy vegetables, which counteract the effects of the heparin. In addition, she will require a folic acid supplement.

Tests for fetal maturity and well-being and placental sufficiency may be necessary. Other therapy is directly related to the functional classification of heart disease. The nurse may need to reinforce the need for close medical supervision.

LEGAL TIP **Cardiac and Metabolic Emergencies** The management of emergencies such as maternal cardiopulmonary distress or arrest or maternal metabolic crisis should be documented in policies, procedures, and protocols. Any independent nursing actions appropriate to the emergency should be clearly identified. ■

Heart Surgery during Pregnancy

Ideally, a woman would have surgical correction of the cardiac lesion before pregnancy; however, cardiac disease may be diagnosed for the first time during pregnancy. When medical therapy for a pregnant woman fails, cardiac surgery may be performed. Early in the second trimester is the best time for surgery. The woman, fetus, and uterine activity must be monitored carefully during surgery. Closed cardiac surgery, such as release of a stenotic mitral orifice, can be accomplished with little risk to mother or fetus. Open heart surgery requires extracorporeal circulation, and under these circumstances, hypoxia and fetal bradycardia may occur as a result of low blood-flow rates. Periods of hypoxemia for the fetus can lead to various kinds of neurologic insults. Increase in flow rates on cardiopulmonary bypass may correct fetal bradycardia. Uterine contractions also increase in frequency before and during cardiopulmonary bypass and can be alleviated by medication.

Intrapartum

For all pregnant women, the intrapartum period evokes the most apprehension in patients and caregivers. The woman with impaired cardiac function has additional reasons to be anxious because labor and giving birth place an additional burden on her already compromised cardiovascular system.

Assessments include the routine assessments for all laboring women, as well as assessments for cardiac decompensation. In addition, arterial blood gases (ABGs) may be needed to assess for adequate oxygenation. A Swan-Ganz catheter may be inserted to monitor hemodynamic status accurately during labor and birth. ECG monitoring and continuous monitoring of blood pressure and pulse oximetry are usually instituted for the woman, and the fetus is continuously monitored electronically.

NURSE ALERT A pulse rate of 100 beats/min or greater or a respiratory rate of 25 breaths/min or greater is a concern. Respiratory status is checked frequently for developing dyspnea, coughing, or crackles at the base of the lungs. The color and temperature of the skin are noted. Pale, cool, clammy skin may indicate cardiac shock. ■

Nursing care during labor and birth focuses on the promotion of cardiac function. Anxiety is minimized by maintaining a calm atmosphere in the labor and birth rooms. The

Table 13-4

Medications Used in Pregnancy for Cardiac Conditions

MEDICATION	SELECTED MATERNAL INDICATIONS	FDA PREGNANCY CATEGORY*	POSSIBLE ADVERSE FETAL EFFECTS
CARDIAC GLYCOSIDE			
Digoxin, digitoxin	Arrhythmia	C	Maternal overdose can cause fetal toxicity and death
ANTICOAGULANTS			
Heparin	Thrombophlebitis Pulmonary hypertension	Does not cross the placenta	Heparin considered safe in pregnancy for the fetus
Warfarin	Same as heparin	X	Fetal anomalies, congenital malformations, hemorrhage; contraindicated in first trimester and at term
DIURETICS			
Furosemide	Hypertension	C	No known teratogenic effects; possible growth restriction
Thiazides			Neonatal jaundice, thrombocytopenia, hemolytic anemia, hypoglycemia
BETA-BLOCKERS			
Propranolol Metoprolol	Angina, hypertension, mitral valve prolapse, arrhythmia	C	During labor can cause bradycardia; after birth can cause hypoglycemia, hyperbilirubinemia
VASODILATORS			
Hydralazine	Severe hypertension, pulmonary hypertension	C	Leukopenia and thrombocytopenia reported in newborns
CALCIUM CHANNEL BLOCKERS			
Nifedipine Verapamil	Angina, hypertension, arrhythmia (verapamil only)	C	Considered safe for use in pregnancy but no controlled human studies on fetal effects
ANTIARRHYTHMIAS			
Quinidine Procainamide	Arrhythmia	C	Neonatal thrombocytopenia reported; quinidine preferred over procainaminde

References: Blanchard DG, Shabetai T: Cardiac diseases. In Creasy RK, Resnik R, Iams JD (eds): *Maternal-fetal medicine: principles and practice,* ed 5, Philadelphia, 2004, WB Saunders; Gilbert ES, Harmon JS: *Manual of high risk pregnancy and delivery,* ed 3, St Louis, 2003, Mosby.

*U.S. Food and Drug Administration (FDA) pregnancy categories:

Category A: Controlled studies have not demonstrated a risk to the fetus.

Category C: Animal studies have shown no adverse effects on the fetus, but there are no adequate studies in humans; potential benefits may be acceptable despite potential risks.

Category X: Studies demonstrate fetal risk or abnormalities; risks outweigh potential benefits.

nurse provides anticipatory guidance by keeping the woman and her family informed of labor progress and events that will probably occur, as well as answering any questions they have. The woman's childbirth preparation method should be supported to the degree it is feasible for her cardiac condition. Nursing techniques that promote comfort, such as back massage, are used.

Cardiac function is supported by keeping the woman's head and shoulders elevated and body parts resting on pillows. The side-lying position usually facilitates hemodynamics during labor. Discomfort is relieved with medication and supportive care. Epidural regional analgesia provides better pain relief than narcotics and causes fewer alterations in hemodynamics. Hypotension must be avoided.

The woman may require other types of medication (e.g., anticoagulants, prophylactic antibiotics). If evidence of cardiac decompensation appears, the physician may order deslanoside (Cedilanid-D) for rapid digitalization, furosemide (Lasix) for rapid diuresis, and oxygen by intermittent positive pressure to decrease the development of pulmonary edema.

Beta-adrenergic agents (i.e., ritodrine and terbutaline) should not be used for tocolysis. These medications are associated with various cardiac side effects, including tachycardia and myocardial ischemia. A synthetic oxytocin (Syntocinon) can be used for induction of labor. This drug does not appear to cause significant coronary artery constriction in doses prescribed for labor induction or control of postpartum uterine atony. Cervical ripening agents containing prostaglandin are not contraindicated, but reports of use in pregnant women with cardiac disease are not available.

If there are no obstetric problems, vaginal birth is recommended and may be accomplished with the woman in a side-lying position to facilitate uterine perfusion. If the supine position is used, a pad is positioned under the hip to displace the uterus laterally and minimize the danger of supine hypotension. The knees are flexed, and the feet are flat on the bed. To prevent compression of popliteal veins and an increase in blood volume in the chest and trunk as a result of the effects of gravity, stirrups are not used. Open-glottis pushing is recommended, and the Valsalva maneuver must be avoided during pushing in the second stage of labor because it reduces diastolic ventricular filling and obstructs left ventricular outflow. Mask oxygen is important.

Episiotomy and vacuum extraction or outlet forceps may be used because these procedures decrease the length of the second stage of labor and decrease the workload of the heart in second-stage labor. Cesarean birth is not routinely recommended for women who have cardiovascular disease because there is risk of dramatic fluid shifts, sustained hemodynamic changes, and increased blood loss.

Penicillin prophylaxis may be ordered for nonallergic pregnant women with class II or higher cardiac disease to protect against bacterial endocarditis in labor and during early puerperium. Dilute IV oxytocin immediately after birth may be employed to prevent hemorrhage. Ergot products should not be used because they tend to increase blood pressure. Fluid balance should be maintained and blood loss replaced. If tubal sterilization is desired, surgery is delayed at least several days to ensure homeostasis.

Postpartum

Monitoring for cardiac decompensation in the postpartum period is essential. The first 24 to 48 hours postpartum are the most hemodynamically difficult for the woman. Hemorrhage or infection, or both, may worsen the cardiac condition. The woman with a cardiac disorder may continue to require a Swan-Ganz catheter and ABG monitoring.

NURSE ALERT The immediate postbirth period is hazardous for a woman whose heart function is compromised. Cardiac output increases rapidly as extravascular fluid is remobilized into the vascular compartment. At the moment of birth, intraabdominal pressure is reduced drastically; pressure on veins is removed, the splanchnic vessels engorge, and blood flow to the heart is increased. When blood flow increases to the heart, a reflex bradycardia may result. ■

Care in the postpartum period is tailored to the woman's functional capacity. Postpartum assessment of the woman with cardiac disease includes vital signs, oxygen saturation levels, lung and heart auscultation, edema, amount and character of bleeding, uterine tone and fundal height, urinary output, pain (especially chest pain), the activity-rest pattern, dietary intake, mother-infant interactions, and emotional state. The head of the bed is elevated and the woman is encouraged to lie on her side. Bed rest may be ordered, with or without bathroom privileges. Progressive ambulation may be permitted as tolerated. The nurse may help the woman meet her grooming and hygiene needs and other activities. Bowel movements without stress or strain for the woman are promoted with stool softeners, diet, and fluids.

The woman may need a family member to help in the care of the infant. Breastfeeding is not contraindicated, but not all women with heart disease will be able to nurse their infants. The woman who chooses to breastfeed will need the support of her family and the nursing staff to be successful. The woman may need assistance in positioning herself or the infant for feeding. To conserve the woman's energy, the infant may need to be brought to the mother and taken from her after the feeding. Women who breastfeed may need less medication for their cardiac condition, especially diuretics. Because diuretics can cause neonatal diuresis that can lead to dehydration, lactating women must be monitored closely to determine if medication doses can be reduced and still be effective.

If the woman is unable to breastfeed and her energies do not allow her to bottle-feed the infant, the baby can be kept at the bedside so she can look at and touch her baby to establish an emotional bond with her baby with a low expenditure of energy. The infant should be held at the mother's eye level and near her lips and brought to her fingers.

Preparation for discharge is carefully planned with the woman and family. Provision of help for the woman in the home by relatives, friends, and others must be addressed. The family is referred to community resources (e.g., homemaking services) as appropriate. Rest and sleep periods, activity, and diet must be planned. The couple may need information about reestablishing sexual relations and contraception or sterilization. Potential hazards of a subsequent pregnancy need to be examined by the woman and her partner. If sterilization is selected as a method of contraception, the risks of surgery, especially for the woman with class III or IV heart disease, need to be explained. Oral contraceptives are often contraindicated because of the risk of thromboembolism. IUDs may put the woman at risk for infection, especially if she has a valve replacement. Injectable progestins are effective and safe (Easterling & Otto, 2002). Both the woman and her partner need to be involved in the decision-making process.

Monitoring for cardiac decompensation continues through the first few weeks after birth because of hormonal shifts that affect hemodynamics. Maternal cardiac output is usually stabilized by 2 weeks postpartum (Easterling & Otto, 2002).

CARDIOPULMONARY RESUSCITATION OF THE PREGNANT WOMAN

Cardiac arrest in a pregnant woman is most often related to events at the time of birth such as amniotic fluid embolism, eclampsia, and drug toxicity. It can also be related to congestive cardiomyopathy, aortic dissection, pulmonary embolism, or hemorrhage that is due to a pregnancy-related pathologic condition. Other problems are motor vehicle accidents, falls, assault, suicide attempts, and trauma (stabbing, gunshot wounds) (American Heart Association [AHA], 2000). Preexisting disorders, such as heart or pulmonary disease, hypertension, or autoimmune collagen vascular disease, increase this risk.

Various protocols exist for cardiopulmonary resuscitation (CPR) during pregnancy. The most widely used guide is the AHA's advanced cardiac life support (ACLS) protocol (AHA, 2000). This protocol recommends standard CPR with the uterus displaced laterally, fluid volume restoration, and defibrillation if indicated. The decision for cesarean birth must be made within 4 to 5 minutes of the mother's cardiac arrest. The gestational age of the infant and the presence of skilled pediatric support personnel must be considered in the decision. No matter what protocol is used, nurses and other health care providers must be prepared if CPR is to be successful.

In the event of cardiac arrest, standard resuscitative efforts with a few modifications are implemented. To prevent supine hypotension, the woman is placed on a flat, firm surface with the uterus displaced laterally either manually or with a wedge or rolled towel under her right hip or on her side supported by angled thighs of several rescuers or angled backs of several chairs (AHA, 2000). If defibrillation is needed, the paddles need to be placed one rib interspace higher than usual because the heart is slightly displaced by the enlarged uterus. If possible, the fetus should be monitored during the cardiac arrest (Emergency box).

Complications that may be associated with CPR of a pregnant woman include laceration of the liver, rupture of the uterus, hemothorax, and hemoperitoneum. Fetal complications that may occur include cardiac dysrhythmia or asystole related to maternal defibrillation and medications, central nervous system (CNS) depression related to antidysrhythmic drugs and inadequate uteroplacental perfusion, and onset of preterm labor.

If there is successful resuscitation, the woman and her fetus must receive careful monitoring. The woman remains at increased risk for recurrent pulmonary arrest and dysrhythmias (ventricular tachycardia, supraventricular tachycardia, and bradycardia). Therefore her cardiovascular, pulmonary, and neurologic status should be assessed continuously. Uterine activity and resting tone must be monitored. Fetal status and gestational age should be determined and used in decision making regarding continuation of the pregnancy or the timing and route of birth.

Emergency

CARDIOPULMONARY RESUSCITATION OF THE PREGNANT WOMAN

Airway

Determine unresponsiveness.

Activate emergency medical system and get the automated external defibrillator (AED) if available.

Position woman on flat, firm surface with uterus displaced laterally with a wedge (e.g., a rolled towel placed under her hip) or manually, or place her in a lateral position.

Open airway with head tilt–chin lift maneuver.

Breathing

Determine breathlessness (look, listen, feel).

If the woman is not breathing, give two slow breaths.

Circulation

Determine pulselessness by feeling carotid pulse.

If there is no pulse, begin chest compressions at rate of 100 per minute. Chest compressions may be performed slightly higher on the sternum if the uterus is enlarged enough to displace the diaphragm into a higher position.

After four cycles of 15 compressions and two breaths, check her pulse. If pulse is not present, continue CPR.

Defibrillation

Use an AED according to standard protocol to analyze heart rhythm and deliver shock if indicated.

Relief of Foreign-Body Airway Obstruction

If the pregnant woman is unable to speak or cough, perform chest thrusts. Stand behind the woman and place your arms under her armpits to encircle her chest. Press backward with quick thrusts until the foreign body is expelled (see Fig. 13-5). If the woman becomes unresponsive, follow the steps for victims who become unresponsive, but use chest thrusts instead of abdominal thrusts.

Data from Stapleton E et al: *Fundamentals of BLS for healthcare providers*, Dallas, 2001, American Heart Association.

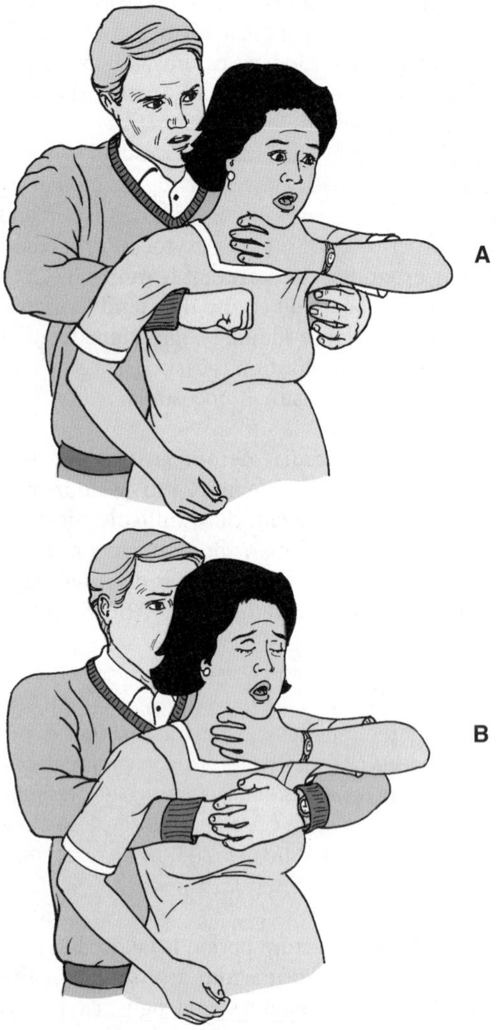

Fig. 13-5 Heimlich maneuver. Clearing airway obstruction in a woman in the late stages of pregnancy (can also be used in markedly obese person). **A,** Standing behind victim, place your arms under woman's armpits and across the chest. Place thumb side of your clenched fist against the middle of the sternum and place other hand over fist. **B,** Perform backward chest thrusts until foreign body is expelled or woman loses consciousness. If pregnant woman becomes unconscious because of foreign body airway obstruction, place her on her back and kneel close to her side. (Be sure uterus is displaced laterally by using, for example, a rolled blanket under her hip.) Open her mouth with tongue-jaw lift, perform finger sweep, and attempt rescue breathing. If unable to ventilate, position hands as for chest compression. Deliver five chest thrusts firmly to remove the obstruction. Repeat the sequence of Heimlich maneuver, finger sweep, and attempt to ventilate. Continue sequence until pregnant woman's airway is clear of obstruction or help has arrived to relieve you. If woman is unconscious, give chest compressions as for woman without a pulse.

Clearing an airway obstruction in a woman in the second or third trimester of pregnancy also requires a modification of the Heimlich maneuver (Fig. 13-5).

Evaluation

The nurse uses the previously stated expected outcomes as criteria to evaluate the care of the woman with cardiac disease (Nursing Care Plan).

ANEMIA

Anemia is the most common medical disorder of pregnancy, affecting at least 20% of pregnant women. Anemia results in reduction of the oxygen-carrying capacity of the blood, and the heart tries to compensate by increasing the cardiac output. This effort increases the workload of the heart and

Nursing Care Plan

THE PREGNANT WOMAN WITH HEART DISEASE

NURSING DIAGNOSIS: Activity intolerance related to effects of pregnancy on the patient with rheumatic heart disease with mitral valve stenosis

EXPECTED OUTCOME

Woman will verbalize a plan to change her lifestyle throughout pregnancy to avoid risk of cardiac decompensation.

NURSING INTERVENTIONS/*RATIONALES*

Assist woman to identify factors that decrease activity tolerance and explore extent of limitations *to establish a baseline for evaluation.*

Help woman to develop an individualized program of activity and rest, taking into account the living and working environment, as well as support of family and friends, *to maintain sufficient cardiac output.*

Teach woman to monitor physiologic response to activity (i.e., pulse rate, respiratory rate) and reduce activity that causes fatigue or pain *to maintain sufficient cardiac output and prevent potential injury to fetus.*

Enlist family and friends to assist woman in pacing activities and to provide support in performing role functions and self-care activities that are too strenuous *to increase chances of compliance with activity restrictions.*

Suggest that woman maintain an activity log that records activities, time, duration, intensity, and physiologic response *to evaluate effectiveness of and adherence to activity program.*

Discuss various quiet diversional activities that could be done by the woman *to decrease the potential for boredom during rest periods*

NURSING DIAGNOSIS: Risk for ineffective therapeutic regimen management related to woman's first pregnancy and perceived sense of wellness

EXPECTED OUTCOME

Woman will participate in an effective therapeutic regimen for pregnancy complicated by heart disease.

NURSING INTERVENTIONS/*RATIONALES*

Identify factors that could inhibit the woman from participating in a therapeutic regimen, such as insufficient knowledge about the effect of cardiac disease on pregnancy, *to promote early interventions, such as teaching about the importance of rest.*

Teach woman and family about factors such as lack of rest or not taking prescribed medications that could adversely affect the pregnancy *to provide information and promote empowerment over the situation.*

Encourage expression of feelings about the disease and its potential effect on the pregnancy *to promote a sense of trust.*

Identify resources in the community *to provide a shared sense of common experiences.*

Encourage woman to verbalize her plan for carrying out the regimen of care *to evaluate the effects of teaching.*

NURSING DIAGNOSIS: Decreased cardiac output related to increased circulatory volume secondary to pregnancy and cardiac disease

EXPECTED OUTCOME

The woman will exhibit signs of adequate cardiac output (i.e., normal pulse and blood pressure, normal heart and breath sounds, normal skin color, tone, and turgor, normal capillary refill, normal urine output, and no evidence of edema).

NURSING INTERVENTIONS/*RATIONALES*

Reinforce the importance of activity/rest cycles *to prevent cardiac complications.*

Plan with woman a frequent visit schedule to caregiver *to provide adequate surveillance of high risk pregnancy.*

Teach woman to lie in lateral position *to increase uteroplacental blood flow* and to elevate legs while sitting *to promote venous return.*

Monitor intake and output and check for edema *to assess for renal complications or venous return problems.*

Monitor fetal heart rate (FHR) and fetal activity, perform NST as indicated, *to assess fetal status and detect uteroplacental insufficiency.*

NURSING DIAGNOSIS: Risk for ineffective tissue perfusion related to cardiac condition secondary to increased circulatory needs during pregnancy

EXPECTED OUTCOMES

The woman will exhibit signs of hemodynamic stability (i.e., blood pressure, pulse, ABGs, and WBC counts are within normal limits). The fetus will exhibit signs of well-being (i.e., fetal activity and FHR are within normal limits).

NURSING INTERVENTIONS/*RATIONALES*

Monitor heart rate and rhythm, blood pressure, skin color and temperature, WBCs, hemoglobin and hematocrit, and ABGs *to detect early signs of cardiac failure/hypoxia.*

Monitor fetal activity and FHR, and perform NST as indicated, *to assess fetal status and detect uteroplacental insufficiency.*

Teach woman how to detect and report early signs of cardiac decompensation *to prevent maternal/fetal complications.*

stresses ventricular function. Therefore anemia that occurs with any other complication (e.g., preeclampsia) may result in congestive heart failure.

An indirect index of the oxygen-carrying capacity is the packed red blood cell volume, or hematocrit level. The normal hematocrit range in nonpregnant women is 37% to 47%. Normal values for pregnant women with adequate iron stores may be as low as 34%. This has been explained by hydremia (dilution of blood), also called the physiologic anemia of pregnancy.

At or near sea level, the pregnant woman in the first trimester is anemic when her hemoglobin level is less than 11 g/dl or the hematocrit is less than 34%. At high altitudes, much higher values indicate anemia; for example, at 1500 m (5000 ft) above sea level, a hemoglobin level less than 14 g/dl indicates anemia (Pagana & Pagana, 2003).

When a woman has anemia during pregnancy, the loss of blood at birth, even if minimal, is not well tolerated. She is at an increased risk for requiring blood transfusions. Women with anemia have a higher incidence of puerperal complications such as infection than do pregnant women with normal hematologic values (Box 13-6).

Nursing care of the pregnant woman with anemia requires that the nurse be able to distinguish between the normal physiologic anemia of pregnancy and the disease states. About 90% of cases of anemia in pregnancy are of the iron deficiency type. The remaining 10% embrace a considerable variety of acquired and hereditary anemias, including folic acid deficiency, sickle cell anemia, and thalassemia.

During prenatal visits the nurse should take a diet history and provide dietary teaching as appropriate. Pregnancy may cause increased fatigue, stress, and financial difficulties for a woman with anemia as she copes with her activities of daily living. The nurse should assess the pregnant woman's needs and provide her with appropriate resources or referral.

Iron Deficiency Anemia

Pathologic anemia of pregnancy is mainly the result of iron deficiency. Without iron therapy even pregnant women who enjoy excellent nutrition conclude pregnancy with an iron deficit. Iron is actively transported across the placenta for fetal erythropoiesis. Diet alone cannot replace gestational iron losses. Inadequate nutrition without therapy will certainly mean iron deficiency anemia during late pregnancy and the puerperium.

If iron deficiency anemia is diagnosed, increased iron dosages are recommended (elemental iron, 60 to 120 mg per day). It is important to teach the pregnant woman the significance of iron therapy (see Table 12-1). In addition, the woman should be instructed in dietary ways to decrease the gastrointestinal side effects of iron therapy. Some pregnant women cannot tolerate the prescribed oral iron because of nausea and vomiting. In such cases the woman should receive parenteral iron such as an iron-dextran complex (Imferon).

BOX 13-6

Restless Legs Syndrome

Restless legs syndrome (RLS) is a sensorimotor disorder characterized by discomfort of the legs and an urge to move the legs, usually during rest or inactivity. The discomfort is relieved by movement. RLS occurs mostly in the evening. RLS is generally idiopathic but is associated with anemia and pregnancy. Pregnant women have two to three times the risk of having RLS than the general population. Preexisting RLS worsens during pregnancy, having the highest degree of severity in the third trimester, and disappears at the time of birth.

Sources: Manconi M et al: Pregnancy as a risk factor for restless legs syndrome, *Sleep Med* 5(3):305-308, 2004; Zucconi M, Ferini-Strambi L: Epidemiology and clinical findings of restless legs syndrome, *Sleep Med* 5(3):293-299, 2004.

Folic Acid Deficiency Anemia

Folic acid deficiency during conception and early pregnancy increases the incidence of neural tube defects, cleft lip, and cleft palate. Even in well-nourished women, it is common to have a folate deficiency. Poor diet, cooking with large volumes of water, or home canning of food (especially vegetables) may lead to folate deficiency. Malabsorption may play a part in the development of anemia caused by a lack of folic acid. Folic acid deficiency is common in multiple gestations. During pregnancy the recommended daily intake is 600 mcg per day of folic acid, although women who have a deficiency may need 1 mg or more per day (see Box 12-4).

Since 1998, the U.S. Food and Drug Administration has required the addition of folic acid to cereals, pasta, breads, and other food that are labeled "enriched." However, the amount added is small and most pregnant women will need a supplement.

Sickle Cell Hemoglobinopathy

Sickle cell hemoglobinopathy is a disease caused by the presence of abnormal hemoglobin in the blood. Sickle cell trait (SA hemoglobin pattern), sickling of the red blood cells but with a normal red blood cell life span, usually causes only mild clinical symptoms. Sickle cell anemia (sickle cell disease) is a recessive, hereditary, familial hemolytic anemia that affects those of African-American or Mediterranean ancestry. These individuals usually have abnormal hemoglobin types (SS or SC). People with sickle cell anemia have recurrent attacks (crises) of fever and pain in the abdomen or extremities. These attacks are attributed to vascular occlusion (from

Community Focus

FOODS ENRICHED WITH FOLIC ACID

For foods to be labeled "enriched," they must include folic acid. Examine at least five items in a grocery store that are labeled enriched. How much folic acid does a single serving of each contain? Can a pregnant woman obtain the recommended amount of folic acid through eating these items? Plan a menu that includes foods high in folic acid. In the prenatal or women's health clinic, note information about folic acid. Is it prominently displayed? Interview one of the women in the clinic regarding her knowledge of the need for folic acid and of which foods contain folic acid. If she is agreeable, plan with her a diet rich in folic acid that takes into consideration her food preferences and cultural factors.

abnormal cells), tissue hypoxia, edema, and red blood cell destruction. Crises are associated with normochromic anemia, jaundice, reticulocytosis, a positive sickle cell test, and the demonstration of abnormal hemoglobin (usually SS or SC).

Almost 10% of African-Americans in North America have the sickle cell trait, but fewer than 1% have sickle cell anemia. The anemia often is complicated by iron and folic acid deficiency.

Women with sickle cell trait usually do well in pregnancy, although they are at increased risk for urinary tract infections and may be deficient in iron (Kilpatrick & Laros, 2004). If the woman has sickle cell anemia, the anemia that occurs in normal pregnancies may aggravate the condition and bring on more crises. Fetal complications include being small for gestational age, IUGR, and skeletal changes. Pregnant women with sickle cell anemia are prone to pyelonephritis, leg ulcers, bone abnormalities, strokes, cardiopathy, congestive heart failure, and preeclampsia. UTIs and hematuria are common. An aplastic crisis may follow serious infection. Transfusions of the woman have been the usual treatment for symptomatic patients; however, partial exchange transfusions or prophylactic transfusions are common as well and significantly reduce the number of painful crises (Kilpatrick & Laros, 2004). Cesarean birth is warranted only for obstetric indications. Oral contraceptives are contraindicated.

Table 13-5 identifies some potential problems faced by the woman with sickle cell disease and some preventive and maintenance interventions.

Table 13-5

Sickle Cell Anemia: Potential Problems, Prevention, and Maintenance

POTENTIAL PROBLEM	PREVENTION AND MAINTENANCE
1. Inadequate oxygen to meet needs of labor and prevent sickling	1. a. Monitor Hb level and HCT to maintain Hb at ≥8 g and HCT at ≥20%. b. Have typed and crossmatched blood available. c. Assist with transfusions. d. Administer oxygen continuously during labor. e. Coach for relaxation and to lessen anxiety.
2. Infection: UTI, pyelonephritis, pneumonia	2. a. Continue actions as under No. 1. b. Maintain adequate hydration. c. Administer antibiotics as ordered. d. Maintain strict asepsis. e. Encourage frequent voiding to keep bladder empty.
3. Sequestration crisis caused by need for and destruction of RBCs	3. Administer folic acid supplement (1 mg/day) to decrease erythropoietic demands and reduce probability of capillary stasis.
4. Crisis caused by hypoxia, hypotension, acidosis, dehydration, exertion, sudden cooling, low-grade fever	4. a. Continue actions as under No. 1. b. Avoid supine hypotension. c. Maintain adequate hydration. d. Maintain comfortable room temperature: use warm blankets or cool cloths as needed. e. Assist with analgesia and anesthesia.
5. Pseudotoxemia (hypertension, proteinuria, no large weight gain); often accompanying bone pain crisis	5. a. If true preeclampsia occurs, care is the same as for preeclampsia. b. Monitor blood pressure and urine.
6. Thromboembolism (from increased blood viscosity)	6. a. Monitor for positive Homans' sign. b. Initiate bed rest if Homans' sign is positive or if reddened, warm areas or lump appears in the calf. c. Maintain adequate hydration. d. Administer heparin as ordered. e. Apply warm compresses. f. Apply antiembolism stockings.
7. Congestive heart failure	7. a. Assess pulse, respiratory rate. b. Place in semirecumbent position; lateral position for labor. c. Auscultate frequently for crackles in the lungs. d. Administer oxygen and medications (e.g., digitalis, antibiotics, diuretics, analgesics). e. Regional analgesia for pain relief in labor.
8. Pulmonary infarction (hemoptysis, cough, temperature to 38.9° C, friction rub)	8. Assess for this possible complication to facilitate early diagnosis.
9. Postpartum hemorrhage (resulting from heparin therapy)	9. Administer ordered oxytocic medication.

Hb, hemoglobin; *HCT*, hematocrit; *RBCs*, red blood cells; *UTI*, urinary tract infection.

Thalassemia

Thalassemia (Mediterranean or Cooley anemia) is a relatively common anemia in which an insufficient amount of globin is produced to fill the red blood cells (RBCs). The condition eventually manifests itself in severe bone deformities caused by massive marrow tissue expansion. Thalassemia is a hereditary disorder that involves the abnormal synthesis of the alpha (α) or beta (β) chains of hemoglobin. β-Thalassemia is the more common variety in the United States and is more common in individuals of Mediterranean, Middle Eastern, and Asian descent (Kilpatrick & Laros, 2004). The unbalanced synthesis of hemoglobin leads to premature RBC death, resulting in severe anemia. Thalassemia major is the homozygous form of the disorder; thalassemia minor is the heterozygous form. Couples with the thalassemia trait should seek genetic counseling. Women with the thalassemia trait usually have an uncomplicated pregnancy.

Women with thalassemia major or minor have infertility problems, so few pregnancies will result. As many as 50% of these pregnancies have been complicated by stillbirth, IUGR, preeclampsia, and preterm birth. Medical management consists of ongoing monitoring and transfusion therapy.

Women with thalassemia minor have a mild, persistent anemia, but the RBC level may be normal or even elevated. However, no systemic problems are caused by the anemia. Thalassemia minor must be distinguished from iron deficiency anemia.

The anemia will not respond to iron therapy, and prolonged parenteral iron therapy can lead to harmful, excessive iron storage. People with thalassemia minor should have a normal life span despite a moderately reduced hemoglobin level.

ENGLISH SPANISH **Guidelines/Guías**

ASSESSMENT OF RESPIRATORY SYMPTOMS

When did you first notice the cough?
¿Cuándo se notó la tos por primera vez?

Is the cough constant or does it come and go?
¿Es la tos continua o va y viene?

What are the characteristics of your cough? Is it a dry cough?
¿Puede describir la tos? ¿Es seca la tos?

Are you coughing up sputum or phlegm?
¿Escupe esputo o flema?

What does the sputum look like?
¿Puede describir el esputo?

Do you have pain in your chest? Where is it located?
¿Siente dolor en el pecho? ¿Dónde le duele?

Do you have shortness of breath?
¿Respira con dificultad?

Is it harder to inhale or exhale or are both the same?
¿Tiene más dificultad al aspirar o exhalar, o son lo mismo?

Do the symptoms interfere with your activities?
¿Afectan los síntomas sus actividades?

Do you think the shortness of breath is getting better or worse?
¿Cree que la respiración dificultosa se está mejorando o está empeorando?

Do you use oxygen or an inhaler at home?
¿Usa oxígeno o un inhalador en casa?

PULMONARY DISORDERS

As pregnancy advances and the uterus impinges on the thoracic cavity, any pregnant woman may have increased respiratory difficulty. This difficulty will be compounded by pulmonary disease.

A pregnant woman with a pulmonary disorder requires assessment, planning, and interventions specific to the disease process, in addition to the routine peripartum care (see Guidelines/Guías box). The nurse also must be alert to pulmonary complications precipitated by the pregnancy.

Asthma

Bronchial asthma is an acute respiratory illness caused by allergens, by marked change in ambient temperature, or by emotional tension. In many cases the cause may be unknown. A family history of allergy is common in people with asthma. In response to stimuli, there is widespread but reversible narrowing of the hyperreactive airways, making it difficult to breathe. The clinical manifestations are some or all of the following: expiratory wheezing, productive cough, thick sputum, and dyspnea.

Up to 4% of pregnant women have diagnosed asthma (Whitty & Dombrowski, 2004). The effect of pregnancy on asthma is unpredictable. About one half will improve, one fourth will stay the same, and one fourth will worsen (Wendel, 2001). Asthma has been associated with IUGR and preterm birth (Whitty & Dombrowski, 2004). Physiologic alterations induced by pregnancy do not make the pregnant woman more prone to asthmatic attacks. Women often have few symptoms of asthma in the first trimester and in the last weeks of pregnancy. The severity of symptoms usually peaks between 29 and 36 weeks of gestation (Burton & Reyes, 2001).

The ultimate goal of therapy for asthma is to prevent hypoxic episodes in the mother and fetus. The therapy has three objectives: (1) relief of the acute attack, (2) prevention or limitation of later attacks, and (3) adequate maternal and fetal oxygenation. These goals can be achieved in pregnancy by eliminating environmental triggers (dust mites, animal dander, pollen), drug therapy (e.g., bronchodilators and antiinflammatory agents), and patient education. Respiratory infections should be treated, and mist or steam inhalation should be used to aid expectoration of mucus. Acute episodes may require albuterol, steroids, aminophylline, beta-adrenergic agents, and oxygen. Almost all asthma medications are considered safe in pregnancy (Burton & Reyes, 2001; Murdock, 2002) (Table 13-6). Patients should determine their peak expiratory flow rate (PEFR) before taking medications (Whitty & Dombrowski, 2004).

Asthma attacks can occur in labor; thus medications for asthma are continued in labor and postpartum. Pulse oxime-

Table 13-6

Medications Used in Pregnancy in Patients with Asthma

STAGE/CONDITION OF PREGNANCY	PREFERRED MEDICATION	MEDICATION(S) TO AVOID (RATIONALE)
Labor	Continue asthma medications	
Induction	Oxytocin	Prostaglandins (may cause bronchoconstriction or bronchospasm)
Pain relief	Fentanyl Epidural anesthesia	Morphine and meperidine (Demerol) (release histamine)
Preterm labor	Magnesium sulfate, nifedipine, β-agonist	β-Agonist if patient is already taking one for her asthma (may cause respiratory distress) NSAIDs (may exacerbate asthma)
Postpartum hemorrhage	Oxytocin	Methylergonovine and 15-methyl prostaglandin $F_2\alpha$ (may worsen asthma)

Data from Barbour L: Asthma. In Lee R et al (eds): *Medical care of the pregnant patient,* Philadelphia, 2000, American College of Physicians; Wendel PJ: Asthma in pregnancy, *Obstet Gynecol Clin North Am* 28(3):537-549, 2001.
NSAIDs, nonsteroidal antiinflammatory drugs.

try should be instituted during labor. Epidural analgesia reduces oxygen consumption and minute ventilation during labor. Meperidine is a histamine-releasing narcotic but rarely causes bronchospasm (Whitty & Dombrowski, 2004).

During the postpartum period, women who have asthma are at increased risk for hemorrhage. If excessive bleeding occurs, oxytocin is the recommended drug. Asthma medications are usually safe for administration during the postpartum period and lactation. The woman usually returns to her prepregnancy asthma status within 3 months after giving birth.

Cystic Fibrosis

Cystic fibrosis is a common autosomal recessive genetic disorder in which the exocrine glands produce excessive viscous secretions, causing problems with both respiratory and digestive functions. There is an increase in pulmonary capillary permeability, decrease of lung volume, and shunting, which results in arterial hypoxemia. Respiratory failure and early death (in the early twenties) may occur.

The gene for cystic fibrosis was identified in 1989. All infants born to mothers with cystic fibrosis will be carriers of the gene. The disease occurs in 1 in 3000 live white births (Whitty & Dombrowski, 2004). Improvements in diagnosis and treatment have allowed an increasing number of women with cystic fibrosis to survive to adulthood. The median age of survival for women with pancreatic insufficiency is 27 years (Whitty & Dombrowski, 2004). Preconception counseling is essential for women with cystic fibrosis. Infertility appears to relate to changes in cervical mucus.

In women with good nutritional status, mild obstructive lung disease, and minimal impairment of lung function, pregnancy is tolerated well. In those with severe disease, the pregnancy is often complicated by chronic hypoxia and frequent pulmonary infections. Women with cystic fibrosis show a decrease in their residual lung volume during pregnancy, as do normal pregnant women, and are unable to maintain vital capacity. Presumably, the pulmonary vasculature cannot accommodate the increased cardiac output of pregnancy. The results are decreased oxygen to the myocardium, decreased cardiac output, and increased hypoxia. A pregnant woman with less than 50% of expected vital capacity usually has a difficult pregnancy. Increased maternal and perinatal mortality rates are related to severe pulmonary infection. There is an increased incidence of preterm births, IUGR, and neonatal deaths in patients with cystic fibrosis. Predictors of adverse effects to the fetus and neonate are inadequate weight gain, dyspnea, and cyanosis.

In addition to the respiratory problems, women with cystic fibrosis may develop gestational diabetes and liver disease. Pancreatic insufficiency may put the woman at risk for malnutrition, because she cannot meet the increased nutritional requirements of pregnancy. Fat-soluble vitamins may not be used because of diminished absorption.

Weight and symptoms of malabsorption should be monitored at each prenatal visit, and pancreatic enzymes should be adjusted as necessary. Women with severe pancreatic insufficiency may require total parenteral nutrition. A glucose tolerance test should be done at 20 weeks of gestation. Routine respiratory management is continued throughout the pregnancy. Antibiotics such as cephalosporins, aminoglycosides, and antipseudomonal penicillins can be used safely in pregnancy (Pickard, 2000). Nonstress testing should be initiated at 32 weeks.

During labor, monitoring for fluid and electrolyte balance is required. The amount of sodium lost through sweat can be significant, and hypovolemia can occur. Conversely, if the woman has any degree of cor pulmonale, fluid overload is a concern. Oxygen is given freely during labor, and monitoring by pulse oximetry is recommended. Epidural or local anesthesia is the preferred analgesic for birth. Vaginal birth is preferable; cesarean birth should be reserved for the usual obstetric indications.

Breastfeeding appears to be safe as long as the sodium content of the mother's milk is not abnormal. Pumping and discarding the milk is done until the sodium content has been determined. Milk samples should be tested periodically for sodium, chloride, and total fat and the infant's growth pattern should be followed (Lawrence & Lawrence, 1999).

GASTROINTESTINAL DISORDERS

Compromise of gastrointestinal function during pregnancy is a concern. Obvious physiologic alterations, such as the greatly enlarged uterus, and less apparent changes, such as hormonal differences and hypochlorhydria (deficiency of hydrochloric acid in the stomach's gastric juice), require understanding for proper diagnosis and treatment. Gallbladder disease and inflammatory bowel disease are two gastrointestinal disorders that may occur during pregnancy.

Cholelithiasis and Cholecystitis

Women are twice as likely to have cholelithiasis (presence of gallstones in the gallbladder) than are men, and pregnancy seems to make the woman more vulnerable to gallstone formation. Decreased muscle tone allows gallbladder distention, thickening of the bile, and prolongs emptying time. Increased progesterone levels result in a slight hypercholesterolemia. Nutritional counseling is important (Home Care box).

Cholecystitis (inflammation of the gallbladder) may also occur during pregnancy, probably because pressure of the enlarged uterus interferes with the normal circulation and drainage of the gallbladder. Acute cholecystitis occurs most often in older women who have been pregnant several times and who have a history of previous attacks.

Women with acute cholecystitis usually have fatty food intolerance along with colicky abdominal pain radiating to the back or shoulder, nausea, and vomiting. Fever and an increased leukocyte count may also be present. Ultrasound is often used to detect the presence of stones or dilation of the common bile duct.

Generally, gallbladder surgery should be postponed until the puerperium. Usually the woman can be treated with medical therapy, consisting of antibiotics, analgesics, intravenous fluids, bowel rest, and nasogastric suctioning. Total parenteral nutrition (TPN) can be used in some cases as an alternative to surgery. Morphine should not be used as an analgesic because it may cause ductal spasm. The woman's condition should improve significantly within 48 hours of beginning treatment. Surgery may be necessary if the woman has repeated attacks of biliary colic, acute cholecystitis, obstructive jaundice, peritonitis, or pancreatitis. Laparoscopic cholecystectomy performed in the second trimester poses minimal risk to both mother and fetus. Other procedures performed may be endoscopic retrograde cholangiopancreatography (ERCP) or open cholecystectomy (Landon, 2004).

> **Home Care**
>
> **NUTRITIONAL COUNSELING FOR THE PREGNANT WOMAN WITH CHOLECYSTITIS OR CHOLELITHIASIS**
>
> - Assess your diet for foods that cause discomfort and flatulence, and omit foods that trigger episodes.
> - Reduce dietary fat intake to 40 to 50 g/day.
> - Limit protein to 10% to 12% of total calories.
> - Choose foods so that most of the calories come from carbohydrates.
> - Prepare food without adding fats or oils as much as possible.
> - Avoid fried foods.

Inflammatory Bowel Disease

Treatment of inflammatory bowel disease is the same for the pregnant woman as it is for the nonpregnant woman. Medications include prednisone and sulfasalazine. Vitamin and folic acid supplementation is especially important because of problems with malabsorption. Effects of inflammatory bowel disease on pregnancy are usually minimal; however, if the woman is severely debilitated, miscarriage, preterm birth, or fetal death can occur.

INTEGUMENTARY DISORDERS

The skin surface may exhibit many physiologic and pathologic conditions during pregnancy. Dermatologic disorders induced by pregnancy include melasma (chloasma), vascular "spiders," palmar erythema, and striae gravidarum. Skin problems generally aggravated by pregnancy are acne vulgaris (in the first trimester), erythema multiforme, herpetiform dermatitis (fever blisters and genital herpes), granuloma inguinale (Donovan bodies), condylomata acuminata (genital warts), neurofibromatosis (von Recklinghausen disease), and pemphigus. Dermatologic disorders usually improved by pregnancy include acne vulgaris (in the third trimester), seborrheic dermatitis (dandruff), and psoriasis. An unpredictable course during pregnancy may be expected in atopic dermatitis, lupus erythematosus, and herpes simplex. Disease processes during and soon after pregnancy may be extremely difficult to diagnose and treat.

NURSE ALERT Isotretinoin (Accutane), commonly prescribed for acne, is contraindicated in pregnancy because of its high teratogenicity. Fetuses exposed to this medication are at increased risk for craniofacial, cardiac, and CNS anomalies. ■

Pruritis is a common symptom in pregnancy-specific inflammatory skin diseases. The most common pregnancy-specific causes of pruritis are polymorphic eruption of pregnancy (also known as pruritic urticarial papules and plaques of pregnancy [PUPPP]) (Fig. 13-6), prurigo gestationis, and cholestasis of pregnancy. Symptoms usually appear in the third trimester and usually subside in the postpartum period. The abdomen is usually affected, but lesions can spread to the arms, thighs, back, and buttocks. Topical steroid therapy usually provides relief, but some women may require systemic steroid therapy for severe symptoms (Stambuk & Colven, 2002).

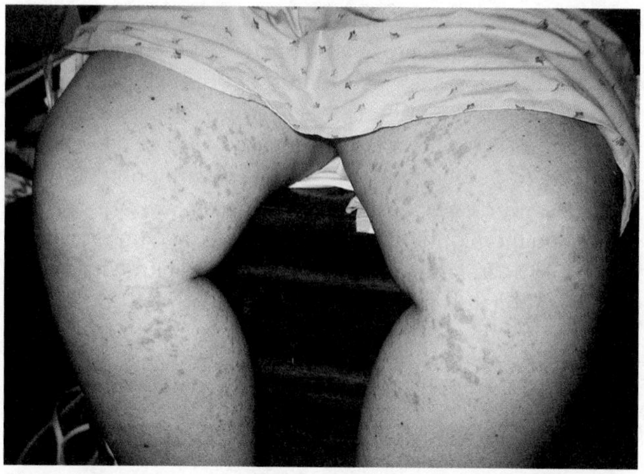

Fig. 13-6 Woman with pruritic urticarial papules and plaques of pregnancy. Lesions also are present on her arms, back, abdomen, and buttocks. (Courtesy Shannon Perry, Phoenix, AZ.)

NEUROLOGIC DISORDERS

The pregnant woman with a neurologic disorder needs to deal with the potential teratogenic effects of prescribed medications, changes of mobility during pregnancy, and impaired ability to care for the baby. The nurse should be aware of all drugs the pregnant woman is taking and the associated potential for producing congenital anomalies. As the pregnancy progresses, the woman's center of gravity shifts and causes balance and gait changes. The woman should be advised of these expected changes and suggest safety measures as appropriate. Family and community resources should be assessed to provide child care for the neurologically impaired woman.

Epilepsy

Epilepsy is a disorder of the brain causing recurrent seizures and is the most common neurologic disorder accompanying pregnancy. Epilepsy may result from developmental abnormalities or injury, or have no identified cause. Convulsive seizures may be more frequent or severe during complications of pregnancy such as edema, alkalosis, fluid-electrolyte imbalance, cerebral hypoxia, hypoglycemia, and hypocalcemia. They also may be related to hormonal changes, fatigue, or sleep deprivation.

NURSE ALERT Anticonvulsants and oral contraceptive agents may have interactions that decrease the effectiveness of the contraceptive, leading to unplanned pregnancy. ■

The effects of pregnancy on epilepsy are unpredictable. Most women have no change in seizure activity during pregnancy; some have an increase whereas others have a decrease in seizures.

The differential diagnosis between epilepsy and eclampsia may pose a problem. Epilepsy and eclampsia can coexist. However, a history of seizures and a normal plasma uric acid level, as well as the absence of hypertension, generalized edema, or proteinuria, point to epilepsy.

During pregnancy, risk of vaginal bleeding is doubled, and there is a threefold risk of abruptio placentae. Abnormal presentations are more common in labor and delivery. There is an increased possibility that the fetus will experience seizures in utero.

Metabolic changes in pregnancy usually alter pharmacokinetics. In addition, nausea and vomiting may interfere with ingestion and absorption of medication.

Failure to take medications is a common factor leading to worsening of seizure activity during pregnancy. This is largely due to the message that drugs are harmful to the fetus. Teratogenicity of antiepileptic drugs (AEDs) has been described thoroughly, but the risks to the infant have been exaggerated. Congenital anomalies associated with AEDs include cleft lip or palate, congenital heart disease, urogenital defects, and neural tube defects. AEDs should be monotherapeutic and used in the smallest therapeutic dose. Daily folic acid supplementation is important because of the depletion that occurs when taking AEDs.

A small risk of seizure activity exists during labor. If the woman cannot take oral AEDs, phenytoin can be administered intravenously. Serum levels of AEDs should be checked within 48 hours and at 1 to 2 weeks after birth, because levels can change quickly, and toxicity can develop.

During the neonatal period, infants can have a hemorrhagic disorder associated with AED-induced vitamin K deficiency. Prophylaxis consists of administering vitamin K, 20 mg orally, daily during the last month of pregnancy and administering 1 mg intramuscularly to the newborn at birth. Neonates also should be monitored for drug withdrawal. With the exception of phenobarbital, clonazepam, and ethosuxamide, all AEDs are compatible with breastfeeding (Barbour & Pickard, 2000).

Multiple Sclerosis

Multiple sclerosis (MS), a patchy demyelinization of the spinal cord and CNS, may be a viral disorder. Women are affected twice as often as men, with the most common onset occurring during the childbearing years between ages 20 and 40. MS does not affect the normal course of pregnancy or birth (Aminoff, 2004).

MS may occasionally complicate pregnancy, but exacerbations and remissions are unrelated to the pregnant state. Bed rest and steroids are commonly used to treat acute exacerbations. Nursing care of the pregnant woman with MS is similar to the care of the normal pregnant woman. Women with MS occasionally may have an almost painless labor, although the character of uterine contractions is unaffected by the disease.

Bell's Palsy

An association between Bell's palsy (idiopathic facial paralysis) and pregnancy was first cited by Bell in 1830. The incidence of Bell's palsy in pregnancy is about 57 per 100,000 per year. The clinical manifestations include the sudden development of a unilateral facial weakness, often discovered first thing in the morning. In addition, taste on the anterior two thirds of the tongue may be lost, depending on the location of the lesion. Pain may occur in and around the ear. The incidence usually peaks during the third trimester and the puerperium. There is no relationship between the appearance of Bell's palsy and any complications of pregnancy.

No effects of maternal Bell's palsy have been observed in infants. Maternal outcome is generally good unless there is a complete block in nerve conduction. Steroids sometimes are prescribed for the condition, but they do not hasten recovery. In most affected women, 90% or more of facial function can be expected to return. Supportive care includes prevention of injury to the exposed cornea, facial muscle massage, careful chewing and manual removal of food from inside the affected cheek, and reassurance that return of total neurologic function is likely.

AUTOIMMUNE DISORDERS

Autoimmune disorders make up a large group of diseases that disrupt the function of the immune system of the body. In these types of disorders, the body develops antibodies that attack its normally present antigens, causing tissue damage. Autoimmune disorders have a predilection for women in their reproductive years; therefore associations with pregnancy are not uncommon. Pregnancy may affect the disease process. Some disorders adversely affect the course of pregnancy or are detrimental to the fetus. Autoimmune disorders of concern in pregnancy include systemic lupus erythematosus, myasthenia gravis, and rheumatoid arthritis.

Systemic Lupus Erythematosus

One of the most common serious disorders in women of childbearing age, systemic lupus erythematosus (SLE), is a chronic multisystem inflammatory disease characterized by autoimmune antibody production that affects skin, joints, kidneys, lungs, CNS, liver, and other body organs. The exact cause is unknown, but viral infection and hormonal and genetic factors may be related. SLE affects approximately 1 in 2000 to 3000 births (Hankins & Suarez, 2004). It is three times more common in African-American than in Caucasian women.

Early symptoms such as fatigue, fever, skin rashes, weight loss, and arthralgias may be overlooked. Pericarditis is often the initial symptom. Eventually all organs become involved. The condition is characterized by a series of exacerbations and remissions.

If the diagnosis has been established and the woman desires a child, she is advised to wait until she has been in remission for at least 6 months before attempting to get pregnant (Gilbert & Harmon, 2003). An exacerbation of SLE during pregnancy or postpartum occurs in 21% to 60% of women (Hankins & Suarez, 2004).

SLE during pregnancy is associated with increased rates of preterm deliveries, IUGR, stillbirth, postpartum hemorrhage, and perinatal death. Complications such as preeclampsia and HELLP syndrome are common.

Medical therapy is kept to a minimum in women who are in remission or who have a mild form of SLE. Antiinflammatory medications such as prednisone and aspirin may be used. Immunosuppressive medications are not recommended during pregnancy but may be used in some situations when there is more risk in not treating SLE. Nursing care focuses on early recognition of signs of SLE exacerbation and pregnancy complications, education and support of the woman and her family, and assessment of fetal well-being.

Vaginal birth is preferred, but cesarean birth is common because of maternal and fetal complications. During labor, efforts are aimed at reducing the risk of infection, which is the leading cause of death in women with SLE.

During the postpartum period, the mother should rest as much as possible to prevent an exacerbation of SLE. Breastfeeding is encouraged unless the mother is taking immunosuppressive agents. Women with SLE should limit their number of pregnancies because of increased adverse perinatal outcomes, as well as the guarded maternal prognosis (Hankins & Suarez, 2004). Family planning is important. Oral contraceptives with synthetic estrogens should not be used in women with active lupus nephritis.

Myasthenia Gravis

Myasthenia gravis (MG), an autoimmune motor (muscle) end-plate disorder that involves acetylcholine use, affects the motor function at the myoneural junction. Muscle weakness results, particularly in the eyes, face, tongue, neck, limbs, and respiratory muscles. Symptoms include easy fatigability, intermittent double vision (diplopia), upper eyelid drooping, and difficulty speaking, swallowing, and clearing secretions. In more serious cases, upper arm weakness and breathing difficulty are seen. The response of women with MG to pregnancy is unpredictable; remission, exacerbation, or remaining stable during pregnancy may occur.

Pregnancy may complicate the disorder, although some women experience remission during gestation. If preterm labor occurs, magnesium sulfate, which interferes with neuromuscular transmission, is absolutely contraindicated (Gilbert & Harmon, 2003).

Treatment is the same as that for a nonpregnant woman. Usual medications include immunosuppressive medications and acetylcholinesterase inhibitors. Monitoring blood glucose values is important because hyperglycemia may be the result of corticosteroid therapy. Thymectomy may result in remission of the disease but is best performed before or after pregnancy, if at all possible. For severe weakness, plasmapheresis or intravenous immunoglobulin therapy may be needed.

Women with MG usually tolerate labor well, but vacuum or forceps assistance for birth may be required because of muscle weakness. Oxytocin may be given, but magnesium sulfate is contraindicated because it inhibits the release of acetylcholine. Narcotic analgesia should be avoided because it may precipitate respiratory depression. Regional analgesia is preferred. After birth, women must be carefully supervised because relapses often occur during the puerperium.

In approximately 10% to 15% of neonates, neonatal myasthenia develops, with symptoms of feeble cry, respiratory distress, and weak suck. These neonates may require ventilatory support. With proper management, complete recovery of the neonate should occur within 6 weeks (Aminoff, 2004).

HUMAN IMMUNODEFICIENCY VIRUS AND ACQUIRED IMMUNODEFICIENCY SYNDROME

Infection with the human immunodeficiency virus (HIV) and the resultant acquired immunodeficiency syndrome (AIDS) are increasingly occurring in women. Although HIV and AIDS have been traditionally associated with homosexual populations, women are now the fastest-growing population of individuals with HIV infection and AIDS. Women are more likely to have acquired the infection through heterosexual contact or IV drug use. Women of color are disproportionately affected; about 78% of HIV-infected women are African-American or Hispanic. This section addresses management of the pregnant woman who is HIV positive or who has developed full-blown AIDS. See Chapter 6 for more information about the diagnosis and management of nonpregnant women with HIV and Chapter 28 for a discussion of HIV/AIDS in infants.

Preconception Counseling

Pregnancy is not encouraged in HIV-positive women; preconception counseling is recommended. Exposure to the virus has a significant impact on the pregnancy, neonatal feeding method, and neonatal health status. HIV-positive women should be counseled extensively about the risk of perinatal transmission and possible obstetric complications. Pregnancy itself does not appear to significantly accelerate the progression of HIV infection. HIV-positive women should be encouraged to seek prenatal care immediately if they suspect pregnancy in order to maximize chances for a positive outcome.

Pregnancy Risks

Perinatal Transmission

About 90% of all pediatric AIDS cases are due to transmission of the virus from mother to child during the perinatal period. Exposure may occur to the fetus through the maternal circulation as early as the first trimester of pregnancy; to the infant during labor and birth by inoculation or ingestion of maternal blood and other infected fluids; or to the infant through breast milk. The frequency of perinatal transmission has been reported from a low of 5% to 10% to a high of 50% to 60%. Most researchers report transmission rates of 20% to 30%. Factors that increase the likelihood of perinatal viral transmission are listed in Box 13-7.

Treatment of HIV-infected women with the antiviral drug zidovudine (AZT) during pregnancy and intrapartum, and treatment of their infants for the first 6 weeks of life with zidovudine, decreases the rate of viral transmission from 25.5% to 8.3%. All women should be given the option of having a scheduled cesarean birth at 38 weeks to decrease the risk of transmission of HIV to their infant.

BOX 13-7

Factors That Increase the Risk of Perinatal HIV Transmission

Previous history of a child with HIV infection
AIDS
Preterm birth
Decreased maternal CD4 count
Firstborn twin
Chorioamnionitis
Intrapartum blood exposure
Failure to treat mother and fetus with zidovudine during the perinatal period

Source: Minkoff HL: Human immunodeficiency virus. In Creasy RK, Resnik R, Iams JD (eds): *Maternal-fetal medicine: principles and practice,* ed 5, Philadelphia, 2004, WB Saunders.

Obstetric Complications

It is difficult to determine obstetric risk in persons with HIV infection because so many confounding variables are often present. Many HIV-positive women also suffer from drug and alcohol addiction, poor nutrition, limited access to prenatal care, or concurrent sexually transmitted infections (STIs). HIV-positive women are probably at risk for preterm labor and birth, premature rupture of membranes, IUGR, perinatal death, and postpartum endometritis.

Care Management

HIV counseling and testing should be offered to all women at their initial entry into prenatal care. Most states in the United States have enacted legislation to ensure that this is offered. If only those presumed to be at high risk are screened, about half of all HIV-positive women will not be detected. Identification of HIV-positive pregnant women is especially important because antepartum and intrapartum antiviral drug therapy has been shown to greatly decrease the risk of viral transmission to the fetus.

HIV-infected women should also be tested for other STIs such as gonorrhea; syphilis; chlamydial infection; hepatitis B, C, and D; and herpes. Cytomegalovirus (CMV) and toxoplasmosis antibody testing should be done because both infections can cause significant maternal and fetal complications and can be successfully treated with antimicrobial agents. Any history of vaccination and immune status should be documented, and chickenpox (varicella) and rubella titers should be determined. A tuberculin skin test should be performed; a positive test necessitates a chest x-ray film to identify active pulmonary disease. Also, a Papanicolaou (Pap) smear should be done.

All HIV-infected women should be treated with zidovudine during pregnancy regardless of the CD4 counts. The major side effect of this drug is bone marrow suppression. Periodic hematocrit, white blood cell (WBC) count, and platelet count assessments should be performed. Women with CD4 counts of less than 200 cells/mm^3 should receive prophylactic treatment for *Pneumocystis carinii* pneumonia with daily trimethoprim-sulfamethoxazole. Any other opportunistic infections should be treated with medications

Critical Thinking Exercise

THE PREGNANT WOMAN WHO IS HIV POSITIVE

Betsy is being seen in the prenatal clinic at 34 weeks of gestation. She is HIV positive and has a past history of IV cocaine and heroin use. She has been drug free for the last 18 months. She tells you she is taking "some AIDS drug" during pregnancy but does not seem to know much about it. As part of your care, you will be providing information regarding risk factors in her lifestyle and future planning for her own care and that of her infant.

1. Evidence—Is there sufficient evidence to draw conclusions about the necessity of continued treatment for Betsy and her infant? Can risk factors in Betsy's background be identified?
2. Assumptions—What assumptions can be made about the following issues?
   a. The drug Betsy has most likely been taking and the rationale for its use
   b. Continuation of the therapy during the intrapartum and postpartum periods
   c. Therapy for the infant
   d. Risk factors for acquiring HIV infection present in Betsy's background
   e. Precautions necessary to protect yourself as you provide care for Betsy
3. What implications and priorities for nursing care can be drawn at this time?
4. Does the evidence objectively support your conclusion?
5. Are there alternative perspectives to your conclusion?

specific for the infection; often dosages must be higher for women with HIV infection or AIDS.

Women who are HIV positive should also be vaccinated against hepatitis B, pneumococcal infection, hemophilus B influenza, and viral influenza. To support any pregnant woman's immune system, appropriate counseling is provided about optimal nutrition, sleep, rest, exercise, and stress reduction. The HIV-infected woman needs a greater amount of nutritional support and counseling about diet choices, food preparation, and food handling. Weight gain or maintenance in pregnancy is a challenge with the HIV-infected patient. The infected patient is counseled regarding "safer sex" techniques. Use of condoms and a spermicide is encouraged to minimize further exposure to HIV if her partner is the source. Orogenital sex is discouraged.

The woman is referred for drug rehabilitation as necessary to discontinue substance abuse. Abuse of alcohol, methamphetamines ("speed," "ice"), marijuana, cocaine, nitrites ("poppers," "snappers"), or other drugs compromises the body's immune system and increases the risks of AIDS and associated conditions. It also interferes with many medical and alternative therapies for AIDS. In addition, alcohol and other drugs affect the judgment of abusers, who may be more likely to engage in high risk activities that increase their exposure to HIV.

IV zidovudine is administered to the HIV-positive woman during the intrapartum period. A loading dose is initiated on her admission in labor, followed by a continuous maintenance dose throughout labor.

Every effort should be made during the birthing process to decrease the neonate's exposure to infected maternal blood and secretions. If feasible, the membranes should be left intact until the birth. Women who give birth within 4 hours after membrane rupture are less likely to transmit the virus to their neonates than are women who experience a longer interval between rupture and birth (Gilbert & Harmon, 2003). Fetal scalp electrode and scalp pH sampling should be avoided because these procedures may result in inoculation of the virus into the fetus. The use of forceps and vacuum extractor should also be avoided when possible. Episiotomy does not seem to greatly influence the infection rate (Gilbert & Harmon, 2003).

Immediately after birth, infants should be wiped free of all body fluids and then bathed as soon as they are in stable condition. All staff working with the mother or infant must adhere strictly to infection control techniques and observe Standard Precautions for blood and other body fluids (Gilbert & Harmon, 2003).

The postpartum period for the woman infected with HIV may be notable for infection, hemorrhage, or both. Women without symptoms may have an unremarkable postpartum course; on the other hand, immunosuppressed women with symptoms may be at increased risk for postpartum UTIs, vaginitis, postpartum endometritis, and poor wound healing. HIV-related thrombocytopenias may also increase the risk of hemorrhage.

The cleansed neonate can be with the mother after birth, but breastfeeding is discouraged because of the risk of transmission through breast milk. After discharge, the woman and her infant are referred to physicians who are experienced in the treatment of AIDS and associated conditions.

SUBSTANCE ABUSE

The damaging effects of alcohol and illicit drugs on pregnant women and their unborn babies are well documented (Armstrong et al, 2003). Alcohol and other drugs easily pass from a mother to her baby through the placenta. Smoking during pregnancy has serious health risks, including bleeding complications, miscarriage, stillbirth, prematurity, placenta previa, placental abruption, low birth weight, and sudden infant death syndrome (Andres, 2004; Jos, Perlmutter, & Marshall, 2003). Congenital abnormalities have occurred in infants of mothers who have taken drugs (Andres, 2004). The safest pregnancy is one in which the mother is totally drug and alcohol free, with one exception: For pregnant women addicted to heroin, methadone maintenance is safer for the fetus than acute opiate detoxification.

Substance abuse refers to the continued use of substances despite related problems in physical, social, or interpersonal areas. Recurrent abuse results in failure to fulfill major role obligations, and there may be substance-related legal problems.

Barriers to Treatment

Pregnant women often do not seek help because of the fear of losing custody of the child or of criminal prosecution.

Pregnant women who abuse substances commonly have little understanding of the ways in which these substances affect them, their pregnancies, and their babies. They often delay seeking prenatal care until labor begins. Stigma, shame, and guilt lead to a high denial of drinking or drug problems both by the woman herself and by family members and friends, who conceal the abuse from outsiders to protect the abuser (Jos et al, 2003). Traditionally, substance-abuse treatment programs have not addressed issues that affect pregnant women, such as concurrent need for obstetric care and child care for other children. Long waiting lists and lack of health insurance present further barriers to treatment.

Legal Considerations

Because of the risks to the unborn children, pregnant women who abuse substances may face criminal charges under expanded interpretations of child abuse and drug-trafficking statutes. At least 35 states have prosecuted pregnant women on a variety of charges for suspected harm to the fetus (Jos et al, 2003). Some policymakers have proposed that pregnant women who abuse substances should be jailed, placed under house arrest, or committed to psychiatric hospitals for the remainder of their pregnancies. Nurses who screen for substance abuse in pregnancy and encourage prenatal care, counseling, and treatment will be of greater benefit to the mother and child than will prosecution (Foley, 2002). A public health approach to substance abuse can inspire macrolevel policy that is designed to strengthen communities, as well as specific treatment and prevention programs embedded in the communities (Jos et al, 2003).

LEGAL TIP **Drug Testing during Pregnancy** There is no state requirement for a health care provider to test either the mother or the newborn for the presence of drugs. However, nurses need to know the practices of the states in which they are working. In some states, a woman whose urine drug screen test is positive at the time of labor and birth must be referred to child protective services. If the mother is not in a drug treatment program or is judged unable to provide care, the infant may be placed in foster care. In all states, the U.S. Supreme Court has ruled that it is unlawful to test for drug use without the pregnant woman's permission (Harris & Paltrow, 2003). ■

Care Management

The care of the substance-dependent pregnant woman is based on historical data, symptoms, physical findings, and laboratory results. Screening questions for alcohol and drug abuse should be included in the overall assessment of the first prenatal visit of all women. Because women often deny or greatly underreport usage when asked directly about drug or alcohol consumption, it is crucial that the nurse display a nonjudgmental and matter-of-fact attitude while taking the history in order to gain the woman's trust and elicit a reasonably accurate estimate. Information about drug use should be obtained by first asking about the woman's intake of over-the-counter and prescribed medications. Next, her usage of "legal" drugs such as caffeine, nicotine, and alcohol should be ascertained. Finally, the woman should be questioned about her use of illicit drugs, such as cocaine, heroin, and marijuana. The approximate frequency and amount should be documented for each drug used.

Screening questionnaires generally ask about consequences of heavy drinking, alcohol intake, or both. The Michigan Alcoholism Screening Test (MAST) and the CAGE test are two well-known screens that are used. The T-ACE (Hankin & Sokol, 1995) (Box 13-8) and the TWEAK (Russell, 1994) (Box 13-9) have been developed to screen specifically for alcohol use during pregnancy. Urine screening is unreliable because alcohol is undetectable within a few hours following ingestion. Abnormal liver function studies can provide diagnostic data about the physical effects of alcohol abuse.

Urine toxicology testing is often performed to screen for illicit drug use. Drugs may be found in urine days to weeks after ingestion, depending on how quickly they are metabolized and excreted from the body. Meconium (from the

BOX 13-8

T-ACE Test

- How many drinks can you hold before getting sleepy or passing out? (TOLERANCE)
- Have people ANNOYED you by criticizing your drinking?
- Have you ever felt you ought to CUT DOWN on your drinking?
- Have you ever had a drink first thing in the morning to steady your nerves or get rid of a hangover? (EYE-OPENER)

Scoring: Two points are given for the TOLERANCE question for the ability to hold at least a six-pack of beer or a bottle of wine. A "yes" answer to any of the other questions receives one point. An overall score of ≥2 indicates a high probability that the woman is a risk drinker.

From Hankin JR, Sokol RJ: Identification and care of problems associated with alcohol ingestion in pregnancy, *Semin Perinatol* 19(4):286-292, 1995.

BOX 13-9

TWEAK Test

- How many drinks can you hold before getting sleepy or passing out? (TOLERANCE)
- Have close friends or relatives WORRIED or complained about your drinking during the past year?
- Do you sometimes take a drink in the morning when you first get up? (EYE-OPENER)
- Has a friend or family member ever told you about things you said or did while you were drinking that you could not remember? (AMNESIA)
- Do you sometimes feel the need to KUT/CUT down on your drinking?

Scoring: Two points are given for the TOLERANCE question for the ability to hold more than five drinks. A "yes" answer to the WORRY question receives two points. A "yes" answer to any of the other questions receives one point. An overall score of ≥2 indicates that the woman is likely to be a risk drinker.

From Russell M: New assessment tools for risk drinking during pregnancy: T-ACE, TWEAK, and others, *Alcohol Health Res World* 18(1):55, 1994.

neonate) and hair can also be analyzed to determine past drug use over a longer period of time (Gilbert & Harmon, 2003).

In addition to screening for alcohol and drug abuse, the nurse should also screen for physical and sexual abuse and history of psychiatric illness, because these are risk factors in women who abuse substances.

Initial and serial ultrasound studies are usually performed to determine gestational age because the woman may have had amenorrhea as a result of her drug use or may not know when her last menstrual period occurred. Because of concerns about stillbirth, an increased frequency of the birth of small-for-gestational-age (SGA) infants, and the potential for hypoxia, some experts recommend that nonstress testing be done in women who are known substance abusers.

Planning the care for a pregnant woman who is a substance abuser must take into consideration the woman's lifestyle and habits. Although the ideal long-term outcome is total abstinence, it is not likely that the woman will either desire or be able to stop alcohol and drug use suddenly. Indeed, it may be harmful to the fetus for her to do so. A realistic goal may be to decrease substance use, and short-term outcomes will be necessary.

An interdisciplinary model is essential when planning the care for women who abuse substances. Major issues that must be addressed in treatment for women that generally are not part of treatment for men are low self-esteem, stigmatization, high probability of sexual abuse and physical abuse, lack of social support, need for social services and child care, need for women's health services, and need for support and education in the mothering role. Drug-free public housing or residential communities may offer an ideal route to stabilization in a safe environment. Treatment must demonstrate cultural sensitivity and responsiveness to recognize ethnicity and culture as an important part of her identity. Other needs of many women include relationship counseling, coping skills training, and vocational and legal assistance (Jos et al, 2003).

Intervention with the pregnant substance abuser begins with education about specific effects on pregnancy, the fetus, and the newborn for each drug used. Consequences of perinatal drug use should be clearly communicated and abstinence recommended as the safest course of action. Women are often more receptive to making lifestyle changes during pregnancy than at any other time in their lives. The casual, experimental, or recreational drug user is often able to achieve and maintain sobriety when she receives education, support, and continued monitoring throughout pregnancy. Periodic screening during pregnancy of women who have admitted to drug use may help them to continue abstinence (Gilbert & Harmon, 2003). Pregnancy presents a window of opportunity for motivating women to stop their abuse of substances.

Treatment for substance abuse will be individualized for each woman depending on the type of drug used and the frequency and amount of use. Detoxification, short-term inpatient or outpatient treatment, long-term residential treatment, aftercare services, and self-help support groups are all possible options. Neonatal outcomes are improved among infants whose mothers received an integration of substance abuse treatment with prenatal care (Armstrong et al, 2003).

Women for Sobriety may be a more helpful organization for women than Alcoholics Anonymous or Narcotics Anonymous, which are based on the 12-step program. The emphasis on powerlessness over addiction and avoidance of codependency found in 12-step programs may disempower and isolate women, particularly women of color. The confrontational techniques of the 12-step program, developed to break down denial in men, may be especially threatening to women, who often feel unworthy and full of shame and guilt.

In general, long-term treatment of any sort is becoming increasingly more difficult to obtain, particularly for women who lack insurance coverage. Although some programs allow a woman to keep her child with her at the treatment facility, far too few are available to meet the demand (Gilbert & Harmon, 2003).

Methadone treatment for pregnant women dependent on heroin or other narcotics is controversial. If women withdraw from heroin during pregnancy, blood flow to the placenta is impaired. Methadone, however, can cause detrimental fetal effects, and the newborn will have to withdraw from it after birth (Gilbert & Harmon, 2003).

Cocaine use during pregnancy has increased dramatically in the last few years. A number of maternal and fetal complications accompany cocaine use, including placental abruption and stillbirth, prematurity, and SGA infants. When it is determined that a pregnant woman is using cocaine, she should be advised to stop using immediately. She will need a great deal of assistance, such as an alcohol and drug treatment program, individual or group counseling, and participation in self-help support groups, to successfully accomplish this major lifestyle change.

Because of the lifestyle often associated with drug use, substance-abusing women are at risk for STIs, including HIV. Laboratory assessments will likely include screening for STIs such as gonorrhea and chlamydial infection and antibody determinations for hepatitis B and HIV. A chest x-ray film may be taken to assess for pulmonary problems such as hilar lymphadenopathy, pulmonary edema, bacterial pneumonia, and foreign-body emboli. A skin test to screen for tuberculosis may also be ordered.

Although substance abusers may be difficult to care for at any time, they are often particularly challenging during the intrapartum and postpartum periods because of manipulative and demanding behavior. Typically, these women display poor control over their behavior and a low threshold for pain. Increased dependency needs and poor parenting skills may also be apparent.

Nurses must understand that substance abuse is an illness and that these women deserve to be treated with patience, kindness, consistency, and firmness when necessary (Box 13-10). Even women who are actively abusing drugs will experience pain during labor and after giving birth. Withholding analgesia or anesthesia in an attempt to "punish" them for prenatal substance abuse is not helpful and should be avoided. It is helpful to develop a standardized plan of care so that patients have limited opportunities to play staff members against each other. Mother-infant attachment should be promoted by identifying the woman's strengths and by reinforcing positive maternal feelings and behaviors.

BOX 13-10

Dealing with Pregnant Substance Abusers

- Realize that the decision to become and remain sober can *only* be made by the substance abuser.
- Understand that nurses do not have the power to cure anyone. We are only cheerleaders and supporters!
- Educate yourself about the effects of drug use in general and its effect on pregnancy and the newborn specifically.
- Treat substance abusers with the same respect and consideration you show other people.
- Become familiar with your local treatment centers. Learn which of them will accept pregnant women. Keep an up-to-date list of groups meeting in your community.
- Remember that there are no "hopeless cases." It is *never* too late to quit!
- Practice patience and persistence. It may take months or years to see the effects of your work.

Staffing should be sufficient to ensure strict surveillance of visitors and prevent unsupervised drug use.

Advice regarding breastfeeding must be individualized. Although all abuse substances appear in breast milk, some in greater amounts than others, breastfeeding is definitely contraindicated in women who continue to use amphetamines, alcohol, cocaine, heroin, or marijuana. The baby's nutrition and safety needs are of primary importance in this consideration. For some women, a desire to breastfeed may provide strong motivation to achieve and maintain sobriety.

Before a known substance abuser is discharged with her baby, the home situation must be assessed to determine that the environment is safe and that someone will be available to meet the infant's needs if the mother proves unable to do so. Usually the hospital's social services department will be involved in interviewing the mother before discharge to ensure that the infant's needs will be met. Sometimes family members or friends will be asked to become actively involved with the mother before discharge. A home care or public health nurse may be asked to make home visits to assess the mother's ability to care for the baby and provide guidance and support. If serious questions about the infant's well-being exist, the case will probably be referred to the state's child protective services agency for further action.

Key Points

- Careful monitoring of blood glucose levels, insulin administration when necessary, and dietary counseling are used to create a normal intrauterine environment for fetal growth and development in the pregnancy complicated by diabetes mellitus.
- Poor maternal glycemic control before conception and in the first trimester of pregnancy may be responsible for fetal congenital malformations and for maternal complications such as miscarriage, infection, preeclampsia, and dystocia (difficult labor) caused by macrosomia.
- Maternal insulin requirements increase as the pregnancy progresses and may quadruple by term as a result of insulin resistance created by placental hormones, insulinase, and cortisol.
- Thyroid dysfunction during pregnancy requires close monitoring of thyroid hormone levels to regulate therapy and prevent fetal insult.
- High levels of phenylalanine in the maternal bloodstream cross the placenta and are teratogenic to the fetus. Damage can be prevented or minimized by dietary restriction of phenylalanine.
- The stress of the normal maternal adaptations to pregnancy on a heart whose functions are already taxed may cause cardiac decompensation.
- In the case of a cardiac arrest in a pregnant woman, the standard advanced cardiac life support (ACLS) guidelines should be implemented without modification.
- Anemia, the most common medical disorder of pregnancy, affects at least 20% of pregnant women.
- Women in their reproductive years show a predilection for autoimmune disorders (e.g., systemic lupus erythematosus and myasthenia gravis); therefore they may occur during pregnancy.
- Perinatal administration of zidovudine (AZT) is recommended to decrease transmission of HIV from mother to fetus.
- Support from a variety of sources—including family and friends, health care providers, and the recovery community—is needed to help perinatal substance abusers achieve and maintain sobriety.

Answer Guidelines to Critical Thinking Exercise

The Pregnant Woman Who Is HIV Positive

1. Yes, there is sufficient evidence to support teaching the need for continued therapy for Betsy and for treatment of her infant at birth. The incidence of perinatal transmission of HIV has been reduced significantly with the use of AZT. Counseling Betsy about avoiding risky behaviors; maintaining good nutrition; getting adequate sleep, rest, and exercise; and reducing stress will support her immune system and help Betsy attain a good perinatal outcome.
2. (a) Betsy has most likely been taking AZT. It has demonstrated effectiveness in the prevention of transmission of HIV to the fetus/newborn. (b) Continuation of the therapy during the intrapartum and postpartum periods reduces perinatal transmission of HIV to the fetus. In addition, Betsy should be given the option of having a cesarean birth scheduled at 38 weeks to reduce the risk of transmission. (c) Therapy with AZT for the infant will be continued for the first 6 weeks of life. Betsy should not breastfeed because the virus can be transmitted through breast milk. (d) Betsy has a number of risk factors for acquiring HIV infection in her background; a past history of IV cocaine and heroin use has been identified. Further questions will elicit other factors such as a partner who is also an IV drug user, other STIs, poor nutrition, low socioeconomic status, and high stress in her life. (e) Standard Precautions are necessary to protect yourself as you provide care for Betsy.

3. Betsy needs some education about the medication she is taking and encouragement to continue with her prenatal care. Her home situation needs to be assessed. The option to have a scheduled cesarean birth needs to be discussed with her.
4. There are many good studies about the effectiveness of AZT to prevent transmission of HIV, as well as how to care for an infant whose mother is HIV positive.
5. Studies continue about how to care for women and infants exposed to HIV. More research is needed on how to motivate people to stay drug free and to pursue healthy lifestyles. Differences in incidence and response to treatment of different ethnic groups need to be addressed.

Resources

American Diabetes Association
Diabetes Information Service Center
1660 Duke St.
Alexandria, VA 22314
800-342-2383
www.diabetes.org

COPE (Coping with the Overall Pregnancy/Parenting Experience)
37 Clarendon St.
Boston, MA 02116
617-357-5588

March of Dimes Birth Defects Foundation
1275 Mamaroneck Ave.
White Plains, NY 10605
914-428-7100
888-663-4637
www.modimes.org

National Phenylketonuria Foundation
6301 Tejas Drive
Pasadena, TX 77503
713-487-4802

Pregnancy and Infant Loss
1421 East Wayzata Blvd., Suite 40
Wayzata, MN 55391
614-473-9372

Women for Sobriety, Inc.
PO Box 618
Quakertown, PA 18951-0618
215-536-8026
215-538-9026 (fax)
www.womenforsobriety.org

References

American College of Obstetricians and Gynecologists: *Gestational diabetes. ACOG Practice Bulletin number 30,* Washington, DC, 2001, American College of Obstetricians and Gynecologists.

American Diabetes Association: *Medical management of pregnancy complicated by diabetes,* ed 3, Alexandria, VA, 2000, The Association.

American Diabetes Association: Position statement: gestational diabetes mellitus, *Diabetes Care* 27(suppl 1):S88-S90, 2004a.

American Diabetes Association: Standards of medical care in diabetes, *Diabetes Care* 27(suppl 1): S15-S35, 2004b.

American Heart Association: Part 8: advanced challenges in resuscitation. Section 3: special challenges in ECC. 3F: cardiac arrest associated with pregnancy, *Resuscitation* 46:293-295, 2000.

Aminoff MJ: Neurologic disorders. In Creasy RK, Resnik R, Iams JD (eds): *Maternal-fetal medicine: principles and practice,* ed 5, Philadelphia, 2004, WB Saunders.

Andres RL: Effects of therapeutic, diagnostic, and environmental agents and exposure to social and illicit drugs. In Creasy RK, Resnik R, Iams JD (eds): *Maternal-fetal medicine: principles and practice,* ed 5, Philadelphia, 2004, WB Saunders.

Armstrong MA et al: Perinatal substance abuse intervention in obstetric clinics decreases adverse neonatal outcomes, *J Perinatol* 23(1):3-9, 2003.

Barbour L: Asthma. In Lee R et al (eds): *Medical care of the pregnant patient,* Philadelphia, 2000, American College of Physicians.

Barbour L, Pickard J: Epilepsy. In Lee R et al (eds): *Medical care of the pregnant patient,* Philadelphia, 2000, American College of Physicians.

Becton Dickinson & Co: *Controlling low blood sugar reactions,* Franklin Lakes, NJ, 1997, Becton Dickinson.

Blanchard DG, Shabetai R: Cardiac diseases. In Creasy RK, Resnik R, Iams JD (eds): *Maternal-fetal medicine: principles and practice,* ed 5, Philadelphia, 2004, WB Saunders.

Burton J, Reyes J: Breathe in, breathe out, controlling asthma during pregnancy, *AWHONN Lifelines* 5(1):24-30, 2001.

Centers for Disease Control and Prevention: National diabetes fact sheet. Internet document available at www.cdc.gov/diabetes/pubs/estimates.htm (accessed September 5, 2004).

Criteria Committee of the New York Heart Association: *Nomenclature and criteria for diagnosis of diseases of the heart and great vessels,* ed 9, Boston, 1994, Little, Brown.

Cunningham FG et al: *Williams obstetrics,* ed 21, New York, 2001, McGraw-Hill.

Dajani AS et al: Prevention of bacterial endocarditis: recommendations by the American Heart Association, *JAMA* 277(22):1794-1801, 1997.

Diehl K: Thyroid dysfunction in pregnancy, *J Perinat Neonatal Nurs* 11(4):1-12, 1998.

Easterling TR, Otto C: Heart disease. In Gabbe SG, Niebyl JR, Simpson JL (eds): *Obstetrics: normal and problem pregnancies,* ed 4, New York, 2002, Churchill Livingstone.

Expert Committee on the Diagnosis and Classification of Diabetes Mellitus: Report of the Expert Committee, *Diabetes Care* 26(suppl 1):S5-S20, 2003.

Foley EM: Drug screening and criminal prosecution of pregnant women, *J Obstet Gynecol Neonat Nurs* 31(2):133-137, 2002.

Gei AF, Hankins GD: Cardiac disease and pregnancy, *Obstet Gynecol Clin North Am* 28(3):465-512, 2001.

Gilbert ES, Harmon JS: *Manual of high risk pregnancy and delivery,* ed 3, St Louis, 2003, Mosby.

Grewal M, Biswas MK, Perloff D: Cardiac, hematologic, pulmonary, renal and urinary tract disorders in pregnancy. In DeCherney AH, Nathan L: *Current obstetric and gynecologic diagnosis and treatment,* ed 9, New York, 2003, Lange Medical Books/McGraw-Hill.

Hankin JR, Sokol RJ: Identification and care of problems associated with alcohol ingestion in pregnancy, *Semin Perinatol* 19(4):286-292, 1995.

Hankins GDV, Suarez VR: Rheumatologic and connective tissue disorders. In Creasy RK, Resnik R, Iams JD (eds): *Maternal-fetal medicine: principles and practice,* ed 5, Philadelphia, 2004, WB Saunders.

Harris LH, Paltrow L: The status of pregnant women and fetuses in US criminal law, *JAMA* 289(13):1697-1699, 2003.

Health Care Resources: *Handbook of high risk perinatal home care,* St Louis, 1997, Mosby.

Hodnett ED, Fredericks S: Support during pregnancy for women at increased risk of low birthweight babies (Cochrane Review), 2003. In *The Cochrane Library,* Issue 2, Chichester, UK, 2004, John Wiley & Sons.

Jos PH, Perlmutter M, Marshall MF: Substance abuse during pregnancy: clinical and public health approaches, *J Law Med Ethics* 31(3):340-350, 2003.

Kilpatrick SJ, Laros RK: Maternal hematologic disorders. In Creasy RK, Resnik R, Iams JD (eds): *Maternal-fetal medicine: principles and practice,* ed 5, Philadelphia, 2004, WB Saunders.

Landon MB: Diseases of the liver, biliary system, and pancreas. In Creasy RK, Resnik R, Iams JD (eds): *Maternal-fetal medicine: principles and practice,* ed 5, Philadelphia, 2004, WB Saunders.

Landon MB, Catalano PM, Gabbe SG: Diabetes mellitus. In Gabbe SG, Niebyl JR, Simpson JL (eds): *Obstetrics: normal and problem pregnancies,* ed 4, New York, 2002, Churchill Livingstone.

Langer O et al: A comparison of glyburide and insulin in women with gestational diabetes mellitus, *N Engl J Med* 343(16):1134-1138, 2000.

Lawrence RA, Lawrence RM: *Breastfeeding: a guide for the medical profession,* ed 5, St Louis, 1999, Mosby.

Lindsay CA: Pregnancy complicated by diabetes mellitus. In Fanaroff AA, Martin RJ (eds): *Neonatal-perinatal medicine: diseases of the fetus and infant,* ed 7, St Louis, 2002, Mosby.

Lowdermilk DL, Grohar J: *High risk antepartal home care,* White Plains, NY, 1998, March of Dimes.

Maloni JA, Brezinski-Tomasi JE, Johnson LA: Antepartum bed rest: effect upon the family, *J Obstet Gynecol Neonat Nurs* 30(2):67-77, 2001.

Manconi M et al: Pregnancy as a risk factor for restless legs syndrome, *Sleep Med* 5(3):305-308, 2004.

Matalon KM, Acosta PB, Azen C: Role of nutrition in pregnancy with phenylketonuria and birth defects, *Pediatrics* 112(6 pt 2):1534-1536, 2003.

Mayo Clinic Staff: *Phenylketonuria.* Internet document available at www.mayoclinic.com/invoke.cfm?id=DS00514&dsection=1 (accessed September 4, 2004).

Mendelson MA: Congenital cardiac disease and pregnancy, *Clin Perinatol* 24(2):467-482, 1997.

Mestman JH: Endocrine diseases in pregnancy. In Gabbe SG, Niebyl JR, Simpson JL (eds): *Obstetrics: normal and problem pregnancies,* ed 4, New York, 2002, Churchill Livingstone.

Minkoff HL: Human immunodeficiency virus. In Creasy RK, Resnik R, Iams JD (eds): *Maternal-fetal medicine: principles and practice,* ed 5, Philadelphia, 2004, WB Saunders.

Moore TR: Diabetes in pregnancy. In Creasy RK, Resnik R, Iams JD (eds): *Maternal-fetal medicine: principles and practice,* ed 5, Philadelphia, 2004, WB Saunders.

Murdock MP: Asthma in pregnancy, *J Perinat Neonatal Nurs* 15(4):27-36, 2002.

Nader S: Thyroid disease and pregnancy. In Creasy RK, Resnik R, Iams JD (eds): *Maternal-fetal medicine: principles and practice,* ed 5, Philadelphia, 2004, WB Saunders.

Pagana KD, Pagana TJ: *Mosby's diagnostic and laboratory test reference,* ed 6, St Louis, 2003, Mosby.

Pickard J: Chronic lung disease. In Lee R et al (eds): *Medical care of the pregnant patient,* Philadelphia, 2000, American College of Physicians.

Ramsey PS, Ramin KD, Ramin SM: Cardiac disease in pregnancy, *Am J Perinatol* 18(5):245-266, 2001.

Rouse B, Azen C: Effect of high maternal blood phenylalanine on offspring congenital anomalies and developmental outcome at ages 4 and 6 years: the importance of strict dietary control preconception and throughout pregnancy, *J Pediatr* 144(2):235-239, 2004.

Russell M: New assessment tools for risk drinking during pregnancy: T-ACE, TWEAK, and others, *Alcohol Health Res World* 18(1):55, 1994.

Stambuk R, Colven R: Dermatologic disorders. In Gabbe SG, Niebyl JR, Simpson JL (eds): *Obstetrics: normal and problem pregnancies,* ed 4, New York, 2002, Churchill Livingstone.

Stapleton E et al: *Fundamentals of BLS for healthcare providers,* Dallas, 2001, American Heart Association.

Wendel PJ: Asthma in pregnancy, *Obstet Gynecol Clin North Am* 28(3):537-551, 2001.

Whitty JE, Dombrowski MP: Respiratory diseases in pregnancy. In Creasy RK, Resnik R, Iams JD (eds): *Maternal-fetal medicine: principles and practice,* ed 5, Philadelphia, 2004, WB Saunders.

Zucconi M, Ferini-Strambi L: Epidemiology and clinical findings of restless legs syndrome, *Sleep Med* 5(3):293-299, 2004.

14 Pregnancy at Risk: Gestational Conditions

LEARNING OBJECTIVES

On completion of this chapter the reader will be able to:

- Differentiate among gestational hypertension, preeclampsia/eclampsia, and chronic hypertension.
- Describe the etiologic theories and pathophysiology of preeclampsia.
- Compare care management of women with mild preeclampsia versus care management of women with severe preeclampsia.
- Describe HELLP syndrome, including appropriate nursing actions.
- Explain the effects of hyperemesis gravidarum on maternal and fetal well-being.
- Differentiate among causes, signs and symptoms, possible complications, and management of miscarriage, ectopic pregnancy, incompetent cervix, and hydatidiform mole.
- Compare and contrast placenta previa and abruptio placentae in relation to signs and symptoms, complications, and management.
- Discuss the diagnosis and management of disseminated intravascular coagulation.
- Explain the basic principles of care for a pregnant woman undergoing abdominal surgery.
- Discuss implications of trauma on mother and fetus during pregnancy.
- Identify priorities in assessment and stabilization measures for the pregnant trauma victim.
- Differentiate signs and symptoms; effects on pregnancy, fetus, and newborn; and management during pregnancy of common sexually transmitted infections.
- Describe signs, symptoms, and management of pregnant women with TORCH infections.

ELECTRONIC RESOURCES

Additional information related to the content in Chapter 14 can be found on

the companion website at evolve
http://evolve.elsevier.com/Wong/maternal/
- NCLEX Review Questions
- Case Study—Preeclampsia
- WebLinks

or the interactive student CD-ROM
Activities for Chapter 14 include the following:
- NCLEX Review Questions
- Case Study—Preeclampsia
- Nursing Care Plan—Mild Preeclampsia
- Nursing Care Plan—Severe Preeclampsia
- Nursing Care Plan—Hyperemesis Gravidarum
- Nursing Care Plan—Placenta Previa

Providing safe and effective care for the high risk patient requires a joint effort from all members of the health care team, with each member contributing unique skills and talents to provide optimum outcomes for mother and infant. This chapter discusses a wide range of disorders that did not exist before pregnancy, all of which have at least one thing in common: their occurrence in pregnancy puts the woman and fetus at risk. Hypertension in pregnancy, hyperemesis gravidarum, hemorrhagic complications of early and late pregnancy, surgery during pregnancy, trauma, and sexually transmitted infections (STIs) are discussed.

HYPERTENSION IN PREGNANCY

Significance and Incidence

Hypertensive disorders are the most common medical complication of pregnancy (Martin et al, 2003). A significant contributor to maternal and perinatal morbidity and mortality, preeclampsia complicates approximately 12% to 20% of all pregnancies not terminating in first-trimester miscarriage (American College of Obstetricians and Gynecologists [ACOG], 2002b). The rate of pregnancy-related hypertension has risen steadily, by about 30% to 40%, since 1990 for all ages, races, and ethnic groups to the current rate of 37.8 per 1000 live births (Martin et al, 2003). Rates for chronic hypertension have increased moderately (8.4 per 1000), whereas the rate for eclampsia has declined (4.0 per 1000 live births) (Martin et al, 2003). Age distribution remains U shaped, with women younger than 20 years and older than 40 years having the highest rates of occurrence for hypertension. Maternal race also influences the rate of pregnancy-associated hypertension, with the highest rates seen in Native American (46.5 per 1000) and African-American (41.5 per 1000) women. The rate for white women is 38.1 per 1000. Hispanic women have an intermediate rate (26.3 per 1000), and Asian or Pacific Islander women have the lowest rate for hypertension complicating pregnancy (20.8 per 1000) (Martin et al, 2003).

Morbidity and Mortality

In the United States, preeclampsia ranks second only to embolic events as a cause of maternal mortality and accounts for almost 15% of these deaths (National High Blood Pressure Education Program: *Working Group Report on High Blood Pressure in Pregnancy* [Working Group], 2000). Preeclampsia/eclampsia predisposes the woman to potentially lethal complications such as abruptio placentae, disseminated intravascular coagulation (DIC), cerebral hemorrhage, hepatic failure, and acute renal failure (Working Group, 2000).

Hypertension (chronic and gestational) complicating pregnancy increases the woman's risk for a cesarean birth, which further increases the risk of morbidity and mortality. The final report of birth certificate data for 2002 indicated that of the total rates of cesarean birth for selected conditions, 46.4% were for women with chronic hypertension, 41.6% for women with pregnancy-associated hypertension, and 53.4% for women with eclampsia (Martin et al, 2003). When primary indications were reported, the rates of cesarean births were as follows: 35.2% for women with chronic hypertension, 35.7% for women with pregnancy-associated hypertension, and 48.4% for women with eclampsia (Martin et al, 2003).

Preeclampsia occurs primarily after the second trimester of pregnancy (earlier with hydatidiform mole and hydrops) and contributes to intrauterine fetal death and perinatal mortality (Working Group, 2000). Causes of perinatal death related to preeclampsia are uteroplacental insufficiency and abruptio placentae, which lead to intrauterine death, preterm birth, and low birth weight.

Eclampsia (characterized by seizures) from profound cerebral effects of preeclampsia is the major maternal hazard. As a rule, maternal and perinatal morbidity and mortality rates are highest when eclampsia is seen early in gestation (before 28 weeks), maternal age is greater than 25 years, the woman is a multigravida, and chronic hypertension or renal disease is present. The fetus of the eclamptic woman is at increased risk from abruptio placentae, preterm birth, intrauterine growth restriction (IUGR), and acute hypoxia.

Classification

Several groups have published classification schemes and diagnostic criteria for the hypertensive disorders of pregnancy, causing confusion for health care providers caring for women with hypertensive complications during pregnancy and childbirth. The classification system most commonly used in the United States today is based on reports from the American College of Obstetricians and Gynecologists (2002b) and the National High Blood Pressure Education Program Working Group on High Blood Pressure in Pregnancy (2000). This classification system is summarized in Table 14-1.

Gestational Hypertension

Gestational hypertension is the onset of hypertension without proteinuria after week 20 of pregnancy (ACOG, 2002b; Report of the National High Blood Pressure Education

Table 14-1

Classification of Hypertensive States of Pregnancy

TYPE	DESCRIPTION
Gestational hypertension	Blood pressure elevation detected first time after midpregnancy without proteinuria. (Previously known as pregnancy-induced hypertension [PIH].)
Transient hypertension	Gestational hypertension with no signs of preeclampsia present at the time of birth and hypertension resolves by 12 weeks postpartum. This is a retrospective diagnosis.
Preeclampsia	Pregnancy-specific syndrome that usually occurs after 20 weeks of gestation and is determined by gestational hypertension plus proteinuria.
Eclampsia	The occurrence of seizures in a woman with preeclampsia that cannot be attributed to other causes.
Chronic hypertension	Hypertension that is present and observable before pregnancy or that is diagnosed before week 20 of gestation.
Preeclampsia superimposed on chronic hypertension	Chronic hypertension with new proteinuria or an exacerbation of hypertension (previously well controlled) or proteinuria, thrombocytopenia, or increases in hepatocellular enzymes.

Adapted from American College of Obstetricians and Gynecologists: *Diagnosis and management of preeclampsia and eclampsia: ACOG Practice Bulletin number 33,* Washington, DC, 2002b, American College of Obstetricians and Gynecologists; Blackburn ST: *Maternal, fetal, and neonatal physiology: a clinical perspective,* ed 2, St Louis, 2003, WB Saunders; National High Blood Pressure Education Program: *Working Group Report on High Blood Pressure in Pregnancy:* NIH pub no 00-3029, Bethesda, MD, 2000, National Institutes of Health, National Heart, Lung, and Blood Institute.

Program Working Group on High Blood Pressure in Pregnancy [Summary Report], 2000; Working Group, 2000). *Gestational hypertension* is a nonspecific term that replaces the term *pregnancy-induced hypertension,* or PIH. Chronic hypertension and gestational hypertension may occur independently or simultaneously. Gestational hypertension is further classified according to the maternal organ systems affected.

The final diagnosis and differentiation between gestational hypertension and preeclampsia is made in the postpartum period. If the woman has not developed preeclampsia and her blood pressure (BP) returns to normal values by 12 weeks after birth, the woman is said to have *transient hypertension.* If BP values remain elevated, the diagnosis of chronic hypertension is made (ACOG, 2002b; Summary Report, 2000; Working Group, 2000).

Preeclampsia

Preeclampsia is a pregnancy-specific syndrome in which hypertension develops after 20 weeks of gestation in a previously normotensive woman. It is a multisystem, vasospastic disease process of reduced organ perfusion characterized by the presence of hypertension and proteinuria (ACOG, 2002b; Summary Report, 2000; Working Group, 2000). Preeclampsia is usually categorized as mild or severe in terms of management (Table 14-2).

Hypertension, whether gestational or chronic, is defined as a systolic BP greater than 140 mm Hg, or a diastolic BP greater than 90 mm Hg, or a mean arterial pressure (MAP) greater than 105 mm Hg (ACOG, 2002b; Summary Report, 2000; Working Group, 2000). The diagnosis of a new onset of hypertension during pregnancy is based on at least two measurements that meet the criteria for gestational BP elevation.

Elevations over prepregnancy values are no longer considered diagnostic for preeclampsia. However, women who demonstrate an increase of 30 mm Hg systolic or 15 mm Hg diastolic warrant closer observation if the BP elevation occurs with proteinuria and hyperuricemia (uric acid of 6 mg/dl or more) (ACOG, 2002b; Summary Report, 2000; Working Group, 2000).

Accurate and consistent BP assessment is important for establishing a baseline and monitoring subtle changes

Table 14-2

Differentiation between Mild and Severe Preeclampsia

	MILD PREECLAMPSIA	SEVERE PREECLAMPSIA
MATERNAL EFFECTS		
Blood pressure (BP)	BP reading of 140/90 mm Hg ×2, >4-6 hr apart, no more than 1 wk apart	Rise to ≥160/110 mm Hg on two separate occasions
Mean arterial pressure (MAP)	>105 mm Hg	>105 mm Hg
Proteinuria		
Quantitative 24-hr analysis	Proteinuria of >0.3 g in a 24-hr specimen	Proteinuria of >2 g in 24 hr
Qualitative dipstick	≥30 mg/dl on dipstick	2+ to 3+ protein on dipstick
Reflexes	May be normal	Hyperreflexia >3+, possible ankle clonus
Urine output	Output matching intake, ≥30 ml/hr or <650 ml/24 hr	20 ml/hr or <400 ml to 500 ml/24 hr
Headache	Absent/transient	Severe
Visual problems	Absent	Blurred, photophobia, blind spots on funduscopy
Irritability/changes in affect	Transient	Severe
Epigastric pain	Absent	Present
Serum creatinine	Normal	Elevated
Thrombocytopenia	Absent	Present
AST elevation	Normal or minimal	Marked
FETAL EFFECTS		
Placental perfusion	Reduced	Decreased perfusion expressing as IUGR in fetus; FHR: late decelerations
Premature placental aging	Not apparent	At birth, placenta appearing smaller than normal for duration of pregnancy, premature aging apparent with numerous areas of broken syncytia, ischemic necroses (white infarcts); numerous, intervillous fibrin deposition (red infarcts)

Sources: American College of Obstetricians and Gynecologists: *Diagnosis and management of preeclampsia and eclampsia, ACOG Practice Bulletin number 33,* Washington, DC, 2002b, American College of Obstetricians and Gynecologists; Report of the National High Blood Pressure Education Program Working Group on High Blood Pressure in Pregnancy: Summary report, *Am J Obstet Gynecol* 183(1): S1-S22, 2002.
AST, aspartate aminotransferase; *FHR,* fetal heart rate; *IUGR,* intrauterine growth restriction.

throughout the pregnancy. BP readings are affected by maternal position and measurement techniques. Consistency must be ensured in that proper equipment and cuff size are used, the woman is correctly positioned with a rest period before recording the pressure, and Korotkoff phase V (disappearance of sound) is recorded (ACOG, 2002b; Summary Report, 2000; Working Group, 2000). Korotkoff phase IV (muffling sound) is typically 5 to 10 mm Hg higher than phase V. Ideally, BP measurements should be recorded with the woman in a semi-Fowler position with the arm at heart level. If the initial measurement indicates an elevation, the woman should be allowed to relax and have a repeated measurement, again in a semi-Fowler position (ACOG, 2002b; Summary Report, 2000; Working Group, 2000). Assessment focuses on trends, not on a single reading. Box 14-1 presents recommendations for standardizing this procedure.

Proteinuria is defined as a concentration of 30 mg/dl (1+ or greater on dipstick measurement) or more in at least two random urine specimens collected at least 6 hours apart. In a 24-hour specimen, proteinuria is defined as a concentration of 0.3 g/L or greater per 24 hours (Box 14-2).

Pathologic edema is clinically evident, generalized accumulation of fluid in the face, hands, or abdomen that is not responsive to 12 hours of bed rest. It may also be manifested as a rapid weight gain of more than 2 kg in 1 week. Edema occurs in too many normal pregnancies to be used as a marker for preeclampsia; therefore the presence of edema is no longer considered diagnostic of preeclampsia (ACOG, 2002b; Summary Report, 2000; Working Group, 2000).

BOX 14-1

Protocol for Blood Pressure Measurement

- Measure blood pressure in the same arm with the woman in the same position each time (e.g., seated or in a 30-degree tilt on her left side).
- After positioning, allow the woman 5 minutes of quiet rest before blood pressure measurement, to encourage relaxation.
- If the woman is seated, her arm should be resting on a surface at the level of her heart.
- If the woman is in a lateral position, the lower arm should be positioned so the woman is not lying on the arm, and the blood pressure is then taken in the dependent arm. This more closely approximates the arterial pressure, whereas using the arm of the opposite side will falsely reduce the measurement.
- Use the proper-size cuff (cuff should cover 80% of the upper arm).
- In women who have an upper arm too large for a standard-size cuff (cuff is too short), the more accurate measure is obtained by taking the blood pressure with the cuff placed on the forearm, and Korotkoff phase V is recorded at the radial artery.
- Maintain a slow, steady deflation rate.
- Take the average of two readings 6 hours apart to minimize recorded blood pressure variations across time.
- Use Korotkoff phase V (disappearance of sound) for recording the diastolic value (some sources recommend recording both phase IV [the muffled sound] and phase V).
- Use accurate equipment.
- If interchanging manual and electronic devices, use caution in interpreting different blood pressure values.

BOX 14-2

Urine Protein Values

Protein readings are designated as follows:

0	Negative
Trace	Trace
+1	30 mg/dl (equivalent to 0.3 g/L)
+2	100 mg/dl
+3	300 mg/dl
+4	>1000 mg (1 g)/dl

Severe Preeclampsia

Severe preeclampsia is the presence of any one of the following in the woman diagnosed with preeclampsia: (1) systolic blood pressure of at least 160 mm Hg or diastolic blood pressure of at least 110 mm Hg; (2) proteinuria of greater than 2 g protein excreted in a 24-hour specimen, or greater than 2+ to 3+ on dipstick measurement; (3) oliguria, less than 400 to 500 ml of urine output over 24 hours; (4) cerebral or visual disturbances, such as altered level of consciousness, headache, or blurred vision; (5) hepatic involvement, including epigastric pain or elevated liver enzymes; (6) thrombocytopenia with a platelet count less than 100,000/mm^3; (7) pulmonary or cardiac involvement; (8) development of eclampsia; (9) development of the HELLP syndrome (defined later in this chapter); (10) increased serum creatinine (1.2 mg/dl or greater unless known to be elevated; or (11) certain cases of severe fetal growth restriction (ACOG, 2002b; Sibai, 2002b; Summary Report, 2000; Working Group, 2000).

Eclampsia

Eclampsia is the onset of seizure activity or coma in the woman diagnosed with preeclampsia, with no history of preexisting pathology that can result in seizure activity (ACOG, 2002b; Summary Report, 2000; Working Group, 2000). A seizure can be the initial sign for a pregnancy complicated by preeclampsia.

Chronic Hypertension

Chronic hypertension is defined as hypertension present before the pregnancy or diagnosed before the twentieth week of gestation. Hypertension that persists longer than 12 weeks postpartum is also classified as chronic hypertension. There is no widely accepted definition of mild hypertension. *Severe hypertension* is usually defined as a diastolic blood pressure of 110 mm Hg or higher (ACOG, 2002b; Summary Report, 2000; Working Group, 2000). Preconception counseling is recommended for women with chronic hypertension about the increased risk of superimposed preeclampsia and lifestyle adjustments that may be necessary.

Chronic Hypertension with Superimposed Preeclampsia

Women with chronic hypertension may develop preeclampsia or eclampsia. Chronic hypertension with superimposed preeclampsia is defined in the presence of the following findings (ACOG, 2002b; Summary Report, 2000; Working Group, 2000):

- In women with hypertension and no proteinuria early in pregnancy (before 20 weeks), new-onset proteinuria, defined as the urinary excretion of 0.3 g or greater in a 24-hour specimen
- In women with hypertension and proteinuria before 20 weeks of gestation
- Sudden increase in proteinuria
- A sudden increase in BP in a woman whose hypertension has previously been well controlled
- Thrombocytopenia
- An increase in hepatocellular markers for hepatic dysfunction

Preeclampsia

Etiology

Preeclampsia is a condition unique to human pregnancy; signs and symptoms develop only during pregnancy and disappear soon after birth of the fetus and placenta. No single patient profile identifies the woman who will have preeclampsia. However, certain high risk factors are associated with development of the disease: primigravidity, multifetal pregnancy, and morbid obesity (Box 14-3).

Proposed causes of hypertension in pregnancy are multiple and have been the subject of extensive research and much speculation. The ultimate cause is unknown. Several major concepts contribute to current theories regarding the etiology of preeclampsia: vasoconstrictor tone, abnormal prostaglandin action, endothelial cell dysfunction, coagulation abnormalities, abnormal trophoblast invasion, and dietary deficiencies or excesses (Sibai, 2002b). Immunologic factors and genetic disposition may play an important role.

Preeclampsia is characterized by vasospasms, changes in the coagulation system, and disturbances in systems related to volume and blood pressure control. Vasospasms result from an increased sensitivity to circulating pressors, such as angiotensin II, and possibly an imbalance between the prostaglandins prostacyclin and thromboxane A_2 (ACOG, 2002b; Summary Report, 2000; Working Group, 2000).

Endothelial cell dysfunction, believed to result from decreased placental perfusion, may account for many changes in preeclampsia, as depicted in Fig. 14-1. Arteriolar vasospasm may cause endothelial damage and contribute to an increased capillary permeability. This increases edema and further decreases intravascular volume, predisposing the woman with preeclampsia to pulmonary edema (Working Group, 2000).

Immunologic factors may play an important role in the development of preeclampsia (Sibai, 2002b). The presence of foreign protein, the placenta, or the fetus may trigger an adverse immunologic response. This theory is supported by the increased incidence of preeclampsia or eclampsia in first-time mothers (first exposure to fetal tissue) and multiparous women pregnant by a new partner (different genetic material) (Li & Wi, 2000). Preeclampsia may be an immune complex disease in which the maternal antibody system is overwhelmed from excessive fetal antigens in the maternal circulation. This theory seems compatible with the high incidence of preeclampsia among women exposed to a large mass of trophoblastic tissue as seen in twins and hydatidiform moles.

BOX 14-3

Risk Factors Associated with the Development of Preeclampsia

Chronic renal disease
Chronic hypertension
Family history of preeclampsia
Multifetal gestation
Primigravidity or new partner
Maternal age younger than 19 years or 40 years or older
Diabetes
Rh incompatibility
Obesity

Data from American College of Obstetricians and Gynecologists: *Diagnosis and management of preeclampsia and eclampsia: ACOG Practice Bulletin number 33,* Washington, DC, 2002b, American College of Obstetricians and Gynecologists; National High Blood Pressure Education Program: *Working Group Report on High Blood Pressure in Pregnancy,* NIH pub no 00-3029, Bethesda, MD, 2000, National Institutes of Health, National Heart, Lung, and Blood Institute; Roberts J: Pregnancy-related hypertension. In Creasy RK, Resnik R, Iams JD (eds): *Maternal-fetal medicine: principles and practice,* ed 5, Philadelphia, 2004, WB Saunders.

Community Focus

THE ADOLESCENT WITH PREECLAMPSIA

Marilyn, a 15-year-old, G1 P0, high school sophomore, is seen in the clinic for her routine prenatal visit at 30 weeks of gestation. On examination, you note that she has gained 7 pounds since her last clinic visit 2 weeks ago, her blood pressure is 148/92, and on a urine dipstick she has 1+ proteinuria.

- What is the likely diagnosis for Marilyn? What other signs and symptoms of this condition might you find? Develop a nursing care plan for Marilyn. What teaching about diet, rest, signs and symptoms to observe, and fetal assessment should be included in the plan?
- Contact the nurse in a high school near you. What type of sex education is available in the school? Do adolescent men as well as women receive information about parenting? Are there prenatal classes directed toward adolescents available in your community? What supports exist in your community for pregnant and parenting adolescents?

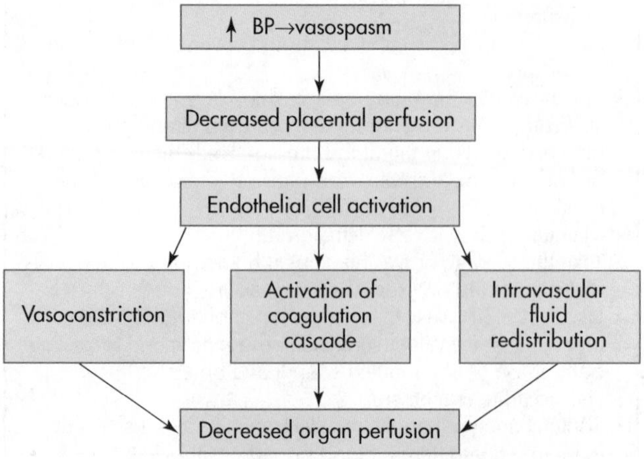

Fig. 14-1 Etiology of gestational hypertension.

Genetic predisposition may be another immunologic factor. Dekker (2001) reported a greater frequency of preeclampsia and eclampsia among daughters and granddaughters of women with a history of eclampsia, which suggests an autosomal recessive gene controlling the maternal immune response. Paternal factors also are being examined (Robillard, 2002).

Diets inadequate in nutrients, especially protein, calcium, sodium, magnesium, and vitamins E and C, may be an etiologic factor in preeclampsia. Proponents of this theory prescribe high-protein diets without caloric or sodium restriction in prevention and treatment of this disorder. However, data are inconclusive for an association between diet and the development of preeclampsia.

Pathophysiology

Preeclampsia progresses along a continuum from mild disease to severe preeclampsia, HELLP syndrome, or eclampsia. The pathophysiology of preeclampsia reflects alterations in the normal adaptations of pregnancy. Normal physiologic adaptations to pregnancy include increased blood plasma volume, vasodilation, decreased systemic vascular resistance, elevated cardiac output, and decreased colloid osmotic pressure (Box 14-4).

Pathologic changes in the endothelial cells of the glomeruli are uniquely characteristic of preeclampsia, particularly in nulliparous women. The main pathogenic factor is not an increase in blood pressure but poor perfusion as a result of vasospasm. Arteriolar vasospasm diminishes the diameter of blood vessels, which impedes blood flow to all organs and raises blood pressure (Working Group, 2000).

BOX 14-4

Normal Physiologic Adaptations to Pregnancy

Cardiovascular

↑ Blood volume; plasma volume expansion greater than red cell mass expansion, leading to physiologic anemia of pregnancy
↓ Total peripheral resistance, decreases in blood pressure readings and MAP
↑ Cardiac output resulting from increased blood volume, slight increase in heart rate to compensate for peripheral relaxation
↑ Oxygen consumption
Physiologic edema related to ↓ plasma colloid osmotic pressure and ↑ venous capillary hydrostatic pressure

Hematologic

↑ Clotting factors, predisposing to DIC and clotting
↓ Serum albumin resulting in decreases in colloid osmotic pressure, predisposing to pulmonary edema

Renal

↑ Renal plasma flow and glomerular filtration rate

Endocrine

↑ Estrogen production resulting in ↑ renin–angiotensin II–aldosterone secretion
↑ Progesterone production blocking aldosterone effect (slight ↓ Na)
↑ Vasodilator prostaglandins resulting in resistance to angiotensin II (slight ↓ blood pressure)

DIC, disseminated intravascular coagulation; *MAP*, mean arterial pressure.

Function in organs such as the placenta, kidneys, liver, and brain is depressed by as much as 40% to 60%. The pathophysiologic sequelae are shown in Fig. 14-2.

HELLP Syndrome

HELLP syndrome is a laboratory diagnosis for a variant of severe preeclampsia that involves hepatic dysfunction, characterized by hemolysis *(H)*, elevated liver enzymes *(EL)*, and low platelets *(LP)* (ACOG, 2002b). To have a diagnosis of HELLP syndrome, the platelet count must be less than 100,000/mm^3, liver enzyme levels (aspartate aminotransferase [AST] and alanine aminotransferase [ALT]) must be elevated, and there must be some evidence of intravascular hemolysis (burr cells on peripheral smear or elevated bilirubin level). A unique form of coagulopathy (not DIC) occurs with HELLP syndrome. The platelet count is low, but coagulation factor assays, prothrombin time (PT), partial thromboplastin time (PTT), and bleeding time remain normal. In some instances, hemolysis does not occur and the condition is termed ELLP (Sibai, 2004).

A diagnosis of HELLP syndrome is associated with an increased risk for adverse perinatal outcomes, including placental abruption, acute renal failure, subcapsular hepatic hematoma, hepatic rupture, recurrent preeclampsia, preterm birth, and fetal and maternal death (ACOG, 2002b; Sibai, 2004).

HELLP syndrome appears in only 2% to 12% of severely preeclamptic women, or about 1 in 1000 pregnancies. Although the exact mechanism is unknown, HELLP syndrome is thought to occur secondary to changes occurring with preeclampsia (see Fig. 14-2). Arterial vasospasm, endothelial damage, and platelet aggregation with resultant tissue hypoxia are the underlying mechanisms for the pathophysiology of HELLP syndrome. The syndrome is associated with an increased risk of maternal death. Perinatal mortality rates range from 7.4% to 20.4% (Sibai, 2004).

Most commonly, HELLP syndrome is seen in older, Caucasian, multiparous women. About 90% of women report a history of malaise for several days. Many women (65%) experience epigastric or right upper quadrant abdominal pain (possibly related to hepatic ischemia), and approximately half develop nausea and vomiting. It is extremely important to understand that many women with HELLP syndrome may not have signs and symptoms of severe preeclampsia; many are normotensive and have no proteinuria. As a result, women with HELLP syndrome are often misdiagnosed with a variety of other medical or surgical disorders (Sibai, 2004).

Recognition of the clinical and laboratory findings associated with HELLP syndrome is important if early, aggressive therapy is to be initiated to prevent maternal and neonatal death. Complications reported with HELLP syndrome include renal failure, pulmonary edema, ruptured liver hematoma, DIC, and abruptio placentae (Sibai, 2004).

Care Management

Assessment

Hypertensive disorders of pregnancy can occur without warning or with the gradual development of symptoms. A

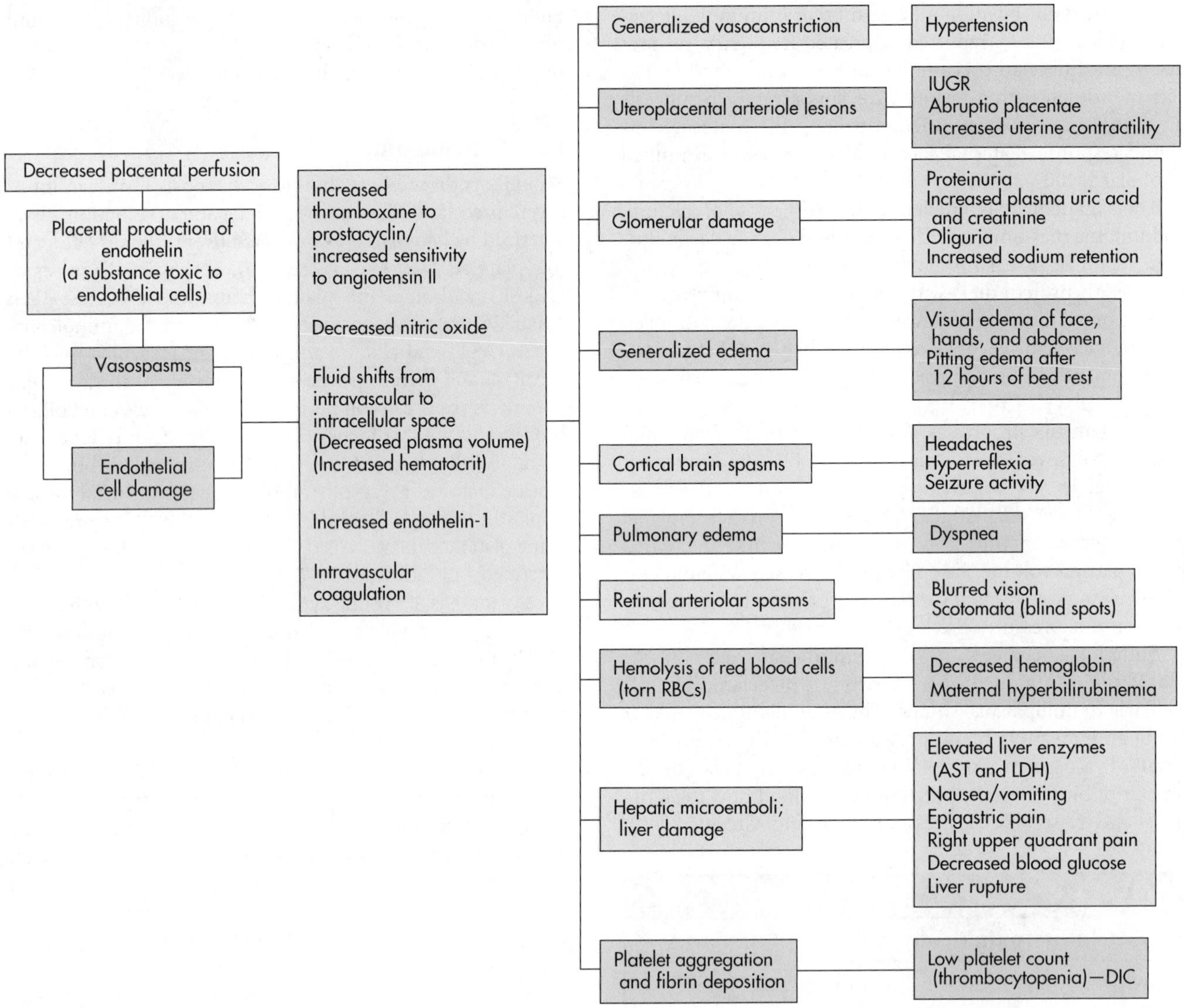

Fig. 14-2 Pathophysiology of preeclampsia. (Modified from Gilbert ES, Harmon JS: *Manual of high risk pregnancy and delivery,* ed 3, St Louis, 2003, Mosby.)

key goal is early identification of pregnant women at risk for the development of preeclampsia in order to prevent catastrophic maternal and fetal sequelae. Therefore each woman is assessed for etiologic factors during the first prenatal visit (see Box 14-3). During each subsequent visit the woman is assessed for signs and symptoms that suggest the onset or presence of preeclampsia.

Interview

The nurse reviews the woman's admission form and prenatal record. The nurse conducts the interview to clarify, expand, or complete the form. Medical history is reviewed, especially the presence of diabetes mellitus, renal disease, and hypertension. Family history is explored for occurrence of preeclamptic or hypertensive conditions, diabetes mellitus, and other chronic conditions. The social and experiential history provides information about the woman's marital status, nutritional status, cultural beliefs, activity level, and health habits such as smoking, drug use, and alcohol consumption.

A review of systems adds to the database for detecting BP changes from baseline and the presence of proteinuria. It is important to note whether the woman is having unusual, frequent, or severe headaches; visual disturbances; or epigastric pain. Abnormal amount and pattern of weight gain and increased signs of edema may be present even though they may not be specifically diagnostic signs of preeclampsia.

Physical Examination

Personnel caring for pregnant women must be consistent in taking and recording BP measurements in the standardized manner (see Box 14-1). If electronic BP devices are used, a manual reading should be taken to validate the electronic device reading. Electronic BP devices show a widening of the pulse pressure as compared with manual readings; the MAP, however, remains unchanged. Electronic BP devices are less accurate in high-flow states such as pregnancy or in hypertensive/hypotensive states.

Observation of edema in addition to hypertension warrants additional investigation. Edema is assessed for distribu-

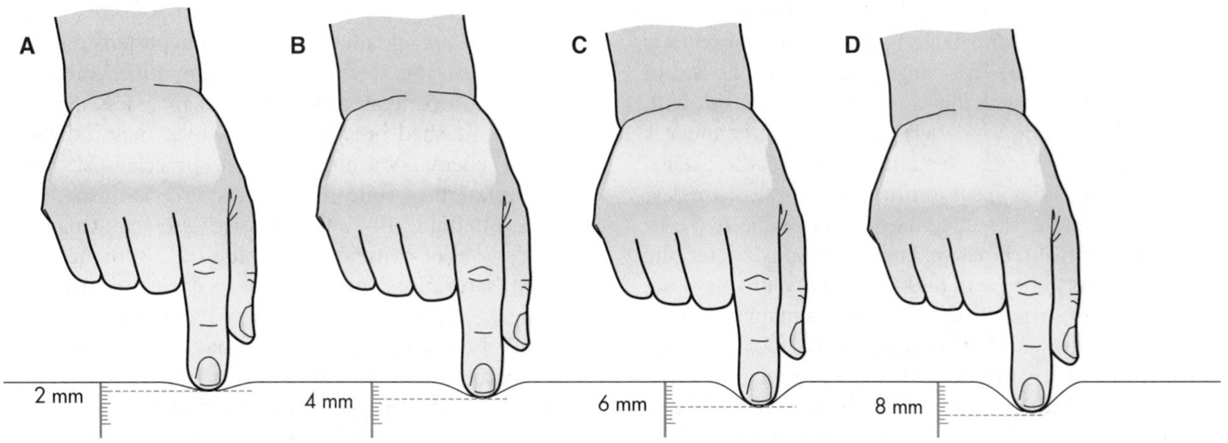

Fig. 14-3 Assessment of pitting edema. **A**, 1+; **B**, 2+; **C**, 3+; **D**, 4+.

tion, degree, and pitting. If periorbital or facial edema is not obvious, the pregnant woman is asked if it was present when she awoke. Edema may be described as dependent or pitting.

Dependent edema is edema of the lower or most dependent parts of the body, where hydrostatic pressure is greatest. If a pregnant woman is ambulatory, this edema may first be evident in the feet and ankles. If the woman is confined to bed, the edema is more likely to occur in the sacral region.

Pitting edema is edema that leaves a small depression or pit after finger pressure is applied to the swollen area. The pit, caused by movement of fluid away from the point of pressure to adjacent tissues, normally disappears within 10 to 30 seconds. Although the amount of edema is difficult to quantify, the method shown in Fig. 14-3 may be used to record relative degrees of edema formation.

Symptoms reflecting central nervous system (CNS) and visual system involvement usually accompany facial edema. Although it is not a routine assessment during the prenatal period, evaluation of the fundus of the eye yields valuable data. An initial baseline finding of normal eyegrounds assists in differentiating a preexisting from a new disease process. Other symptoms such as epigastric pain or oliguria may or may not be present. Respirations are assessed for crackles, which may indicate pulmonary edema, a sign associated with severe preeclampsia.

Deep tendon reflexes (DTRs) are evaluated if preeclampsia is suspected. The biceps and patellar reflexes and ankle clonus are assessed and the findings recorded (Fig. 14-4, Table 14-3). The evaluation of DTRs is especially important if the woman is being treated with magnesium sulfate. Absence of DTRs is an early indication of impending magnesium toxicity.

To elicit the biceps reflex a downward blow is struck over the thumb, which is placed over the biceps tendon. Normal re-

Table 14-3

Assessing Deep Tendon Reflexes

GRADE	DEEP TENDON REFLEX RESPONSE
0	No response
1+	Sluggish or diminished
2+	Active or expected response
3+	More brisk than expected, slightly hyperactive
4+	Brisk, hyperactive, with intermittent or transient clonus

From Seidel HM et al: *Mosby's guide to physical examination,* ed 5, St Louis, 2003, Mosby.

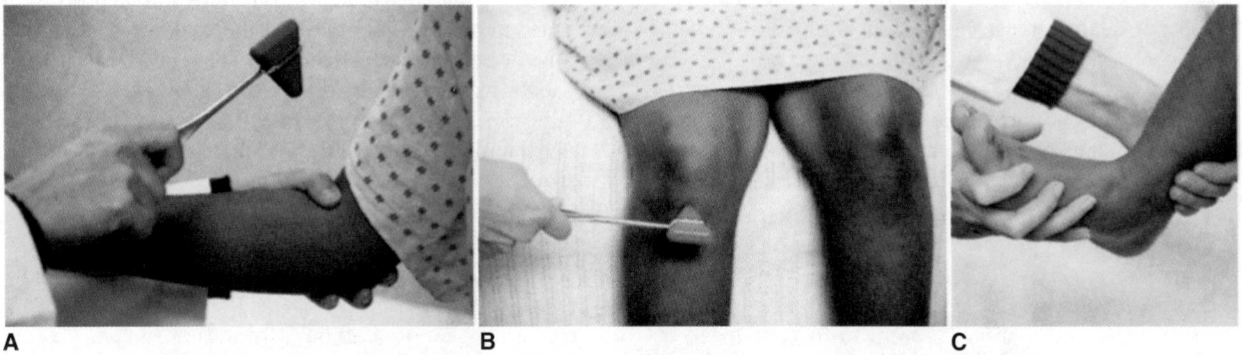

Fig. 14-4 DTRs. **A**, Biceps reflex. **B**, Patellar reflex with woman's legs hanging freely over end of examining table. **C**, Test for ankle clonus. (From Seidel HM et al: *Mosby's guide to physical examination,* ed 5, St Louis, 2003, Mosby.)

sponse is flexion of the arm at the elbow, described as a 2+ response (see Fig. 14-4, *A,* and Table 14-3). The patellar reflex is elicited with the woman's legs hanging freely over the end of the examining table, or with the woman lying on her side with the knee slightly flexed. A blow with a percussion hammer is dealt directly to the patellar tendon, inferior to the patella. Normal response is the extension or kicking out of the leg, which is recorded as 2+ (see Fig. 14-4, *B,* and Table 14-3). To assess for hyperactive reflexes (clonus) at the ankle joint, the examiner supports the leg with the knee flexed. With one hand, the examiner sharply dorsiflexes the foot, maintains the position for a moment, and then releases the foot (see Fig. 14-4, *C*). Normal (negative clonus) response is elicited when no rhythmic oscillations (jerks) are felt while the foot is held in dorsiflexion. When the foot is released, no oscillations are seen as the foot drops to the plantar-flexed position. Abnormal (positive clonus) response is recognized by rhythmic oscillations of one or more beats felt when the foot is in dorsiflexion and seen as the foot drops to the plantar-flexed position.

An important assessment is determination of fetal status. Uteroplacental perfusion is decreased in women with preeclampsia, placing the fetus in jeopardy. The fetal heart rate (FHR) is assessed for baseline rate and the presence of variability and accelerations, which indicate an intact oxygenated fetal CNS. Abnormal baseline rate, decreased or absent variability, and late or variable decelerations are indications of fetal intolerance to the intrauterine environment. Biophysical or biochemical monitoring, such as nonstress testing, contraction stress testing, biophysical profile, and serial ultrasonography, is also used to assess fetal status.

Doppler flow velocimetry studies are used for evaluating maternal and fetal well-being (see Chapter 17). Uteroplacental perfusion is assessed by measuring the velocity of blood flow through the uterine artery, umbilical arteries, or both. Abnormal uterine artery Doppler flow is associated with risk of IUGR in women with HELLP syndrome (Bush, O'Brien, & Barton, 2001). Currently this diagnostic test is not recommended as a general screening test for preeclampsia (Sibai, 2002b).

Uterine tonicity is evaluated for signs of labor and abruptio placentae. If labor is suspected, a vaginal examination for cervical changes is indicated. Women with hypertension are at increased risk for an abruption.

NURSE ALERT Uterine tenderness in the presence of increasing tone may be the earliest finding of an abruption. Idiopathic preterm contractions also may be an early sign. ■

During the physical examination, the pregnant woman is examined for signs of progression of mild preeclampsia to severe preeclampsia or eclampsia. Signs of worsening liver involvement, renal failure, worsening hypertension, cerebral involvement, and developing coagulopathies must be assessed and documented. Respirations are assessed for crackles or diminished breath sounds, which may indicate pulmonary edema. Warning signs of preeclampsia and the differentiation of mild from severe preeclampsia are summarized in Table 14-2. Noninvasive assessment parameters include level of consciousness, blood pressure, hemoglobin oxygen saturation (pulse oximetry), electrocardiographic findings, and urine output. Invasive hemodynamic monitoring may be indicated in selected patients (ACOG, 2002b). Eclampsia usually is preceded by various premonitory symptoms and signs, including headache, severe epigastric pain, hyperreflexia, and hemoconcentration. However, convulsions can appear suddenly and without warning in a seemingly stable woman with only minimum blood pressure elevations (Sibai, 2004).

The convulsions that occur in eclampsia are frightening to observe. Increased hypertension and tonic contractions of all body muscles (arms flexed, hands clenched, legs inverted) precede the tonic-clonic convulsions (Fig. 14-5). During this stage, muscles alternately relax and contract. Respirations are halted and then begin again with long, deep, stertorous inhalation. Hypotension follows, and coma ensues. Nystagmus and muscular twitching persist for a time. Disorientation and amnesia cloud the immediate recovery. Oliguria and anuria are notable. Seizures may recur within minutes of the first convulsion, or the woman may never have another. During the convulsion the mother and fetus are not receiving oxygen, so eclamptic seizures produce a marked metabolic insult to both mother and fetus.

Laboratory Tests

The nurse assists in obtaining a number of blood and urine specimens to aid in the diagnosis of preeclampsia, HELLP syndrome, and chronic hypertension. Baseline laboratory test information is useful in the early diagnosis of preeclampsia because it can be compared with later results to evaluate progression and severity of disease. An initial blood specimen is obtained for the following tests to assess the disease process and its effect on renal and hepatic functioning:

- Complete blood cell count (CBC) (including a platelet count)
- Clotting studies (including bleeding time, prothrombin time, partial thromboplastin time, and fibrinogen)
- Liver enzymes (lactic dehydrogenase [LDH], AST, ALT)
- Chemistry panel (blood urea nitrogen [BUN], creatinine, glucose, uric acid)
- Type and screen, possible crossmatch

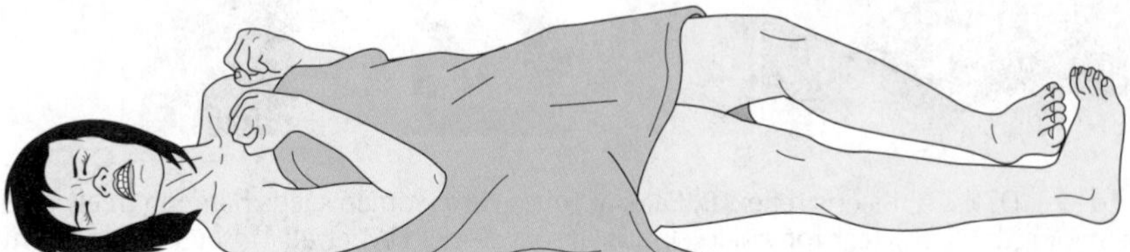

Fig. 14-5 Eclampsia (convulsion or seizure).

The hematocrit, hemoglobin, and platelet levels are monitored closely for changes indicating a worsening of patient status. Because hepatic involvement is a possible complication, serum glucose levels are monitored if liver function tests indicate elevated liver enzymes. Once the platelet count drops below 100,000/mm^3, coagulation profiles are needed to identify developing DIC (Sibai, 2002b).

Urine output is assessed for volume of at least 30 ml/hr or 120 ml in 4 hours. Proteinuria is determined from dipstick testing of a clean-catch or catheterized urine specimen. A reading of 2+ or 3+ on two or more occasions, at least 6 hours apart, should be followed by a 24-hour urine collection. A 24-hour collection for protein and creatinine clearance is more reflective of true renal status. Proteinuria usually is a late sign in the course of preeclampsia (Working Group, 2000).

Renal laboratory assessments include monitoring trends in serum creatine and BUN levels. As renal function becomes compromised, renal excretion of creatinine and other waste products, including magnesium sulfate, decreases. As renal excretion decreases, serum levels for creatinine, BUN, uric acid, and magnesium increase.

Nursing Diagnoses

Nursing diagnoses for the woman with hypertensive disorders in pregnancy include the following:

- *Anxiety related to*
  —preeclampsia and its effect on woman and infant
- *Ineffective individual/family coping related to*
  —the woman's restricted activity and concern over a complicated pregnancy
  —the woman's inability to work outside the home
  —the transfer of the woman to a tertiary center for more intensive management
- *Powerlessness related to*
  —inability to prevent or control condition and outcomes
- *Ineffective tissue perfusion related to*
  —hypertension
  —cyclic vasospasms
  —cerebral edema
  —hemorrhage
- *Risk for injury to fetus related to*
  —uteroplacental insufficiency
  —preterm birth
  —abruptio placentae

Expected Outcomes

Expected outcomes for care of patients with hypertensive disorders of pregnancy include that the woman will do the following:

- Recognize and immediately report abnormal signs and symptoms indicative of worsening condition.
- Adhere to the medical regimen to minimize risk to herself and her fetus.
- Identify and use available support systems.
- Verbalize her fears and concerns to cope with the condition and situation.
- Develop no signs of eclampsia and its complications.
- Give birth to a healthy infant.
- Develop no adverse sequelae from her condition or its management.

Plan of Care and Implementation

Nursing actions are derived from medical management, health care provider directives, and nursing diagnoses. The most effective therapy is prevention. Early prenatal care, identification of at-risk women during pregnancy, and recognition and reporting of physical warning signs are essential components for optimizing maternal and perinatal outcomes. The nurse's skills in assessing the woman for factors and symptoms of preeclampsia and educating her about reporting symptoms cannot be overestimated.

The goals of therapy are to ensure maternal safety and to deliver a healthy newborn, as close to term as possible. At or near term, the woman with preeclampsia will most likely have an induction of labor, preceded if necessary by cervical ripening.

When preeclampsia is diagnosed in a woman who is at less than 37 weeks of gestation, however, immediate delivery may not be in the best interest of the infant. In this situation, a thorough evaluation of the condition of both the mother and fetus will be done in the hospital, in a high risk clinic, or in a physician's office. A multidisciplinary plan of care is then developed, based on the assessment findings.

Emotional and psychologic support is essential to help the woman and her family cope. Their perceptions of the disease process, the reasons for it, and the care received will affect their compliance with and participation in treatment. The family will need to use coping mechanisms and support systems to help them through this crisis. A plan of care specifically designed for the woman with preeclampsia is superimposed on the nursing care all women need during pregnancy, and the labor and the birth process.

Mild Preeclampsia and Home Care

If the woman has mild preeclampsia (BP is stable, urine protein is less than 300 mg in a 24-hour collection, and no subjective complaints), she may be managed expectantly, usually at home. The maternal-fetal condition should be assessed two or three times per week. Many agencies are able to provide this assessment in the home. Arrangements for this service may be made, depending on the woman's insurance coverage. If home nursing is not possible, the woman may be asked to perform self-assessment daily, including weight, urine dipstick, protein determinations, BP measurement, and fetal movement counting. She will be instructed to report immediately any subjective symptoms (Home Care box). In this case, she will likely be seen in the high risk clinic or physician's office at least twice each week for continued fetal assessment.

The fetal condition also is closely monitored because the only reason for expectant management of preeclampsia is to allow additional time for fetal growth and maturation. An evaluation of fetal growth by ultrasound should be obtained at diagnosis and repeated every 3 weeks. Fetal movements are counted daily. Other fetal assessment tests include a nonstress test once or twice a week and a biophysical profile as needed. Fetal jeopardy as evidenced by inappropriate growth or abnormal testing necessitates immediate delivery (ACOG, 2002b; Summary Report, 2000; Working Group, 2000).

Activity Restriction

Bed rest in the lateral recumbent position is a traditional therapy for preeclampsia and may improve uteroplacental

Evidence-Based Practice

ADVISABILITY OF ROUTINE BED REST FOR MULTIPLE PREGNANCY

Background

Since the early 1950s, it has been standard practice to admit all women pregnant with twins to the hospital for bed rest to prolong pregnancy, improve fetal growth, and manage labor. Although multiple pregnancy is associated with perinatal death as a result of preterm birth and intrauterine growth restriction, no controlled trials provided evidence of benefit from hospitalization. Half a century later, it is still widely accepted. Women frequently reported that the hospitalization and bed rest was distressing and disruptive to their families. Hospitalization is costly, and staffing resources are limited.

Objectives

The reviewers' goals were to determine the effects of the intervention (routine hospitalization for bed rest of women with multiple pregnancies) on the outcomes of preterm birth, perinatal death, perinatal morbidity, and women's satisfaction with care.

Methods

Search Strategy

The reviewers searched the Cochrane database. Search keywords were *hospital, pregnancy, multiple pregnancy, twin pregnancy, triplet pregnancy,* and combinations of these words.

Six randomized, controlled trials met the selection criteria. The trials represented 600 women and 1400 babies, from Zimbabwe, Finland, and Australia and were conducted 1985-1991.

Statistical Analyses

Similar data were pooled. Reviewers calculated relative risks for dichotomous (categorical) data, and weighted mean differences for continuous data. Results outside the 95% range were accepted as significant differences.

Findings

Routine hospitalization for bed rest for women with multiple pregnancies did not result in a decrease of preterm birth. There was equivocal evidence of a trend to decreased low birth weight. There were no differences in very-low-birth-weight (less than 1500 g) infants between groups. The hospitalized group did not have a lower rate of low Apgar (less than 7), need for admission to the neonatal unit, or a stay of 7 days or more. Some equivocal evidence showed a decreased risk of hypertension in hospitalized women. One trial measured psychosocial outcomes and reported that 6% "appreciated admission," whereas 18% found it "distressing."

In twin pregnancies, significantly more hospitalized women gave birth very preterm (less than 34 weeks), and there was a nonsignificant trend to lower gestation ages at birth than controls. No difference was found in perinatal mortality rate.

In triplet pregnancies, hospitalization showed more beneficial effects and a trend to decreased very-low-birth-weight births, although the results did not reach significance.

Twin pregnancies with cervical effacement and dilation before labor showed no differences between the hospitalized group and the controls in any outcomes.

Limitations

The small number of studies and small sample sizes limit the power of the study to draw conclusions. Four of the trials took place in Zimbabwe, and all the trials are more than a decade old, further limiting their generalizability. There were some randomization problems. No information about costs was reported.

Conclusions

There is no evidence that supports recommending a policy of routine hospitalization for bed rest for women with multiple pregnancies.

Implications for Practice

A policy of routine hospitalization for bed rest for women with multiple pregnancies may, in fact, be harmful by increasing the risk of very preterm births in twins. There was some evidence of beneficial effects for triplets, but it could not be determined if the effects were due to chance alone. Some women found the hospitalization distressing. When women are hospitalized because of multiple gestation, nurses can support them and help them deal with the inactivity and boredom that occurs. Families can be included. The woman and her family need to be kept informed of the condition of the fetuses.

Implications for Further Research

Important long-term developmental outcome of the infants remains unknown. Only one trial addressed the psychosocial effects of hospitalization, yet it is very disruptive to the family, leaving other family members to not only care for the woman, but also perform the family duties she cannot perform. Hospitalization frequently puts a financial burden on the family because of medical costs and lost income. Any future research should include these burdens and costs in their outcomes.

Reference

Crowther C: Hospitalisation and bed rest for multiple pregnancy (Cochrane Review), 2000. In *The Cochrane Library,* Issue 2, Chichester, UK, 2004, John Wiley & Sons.

blood flow during pregnancy. However, recommending bed rest for all high risk pregnant women is becoming more controversial. Maloni (1998; Maloni et al, 2004) documented adverse physiologic outcomes related to complete bed rest, including cardiovascular deconditioning; diuresis with accompanying fluid, electrolyte, and weight loss; muscle atrophy; and psychologic stress. These changes begin on the first day of bed rest and continue for the duration of therapy. Sibai (2002b) recommends rest at home, rather than strict bed rest, and allows women hospitalized with mild preeclampsia to be out of bed.

Bed rest has been shown to be beneficial in decreasing blood pressure and promoting diuresis. Women with mild preeclampsia feel reasonably well; thus boredom from the restriction is common. Diversionary activities, visits from friends, telephone conversations, and creation of a comfortable and convenient environment are ways to cope with the boredom (Home Care box). Gentle exercise (e.g., range of motion, stretching, Kegel exercises, and pelvic tilts) is important in maintaining muscle tone, blood flow, regularity of bowel function, and a sense of well-being. Relaxation techniques can help reduce stress associated with the high risk condition and prepare the woman for labor and the birth.

Diet

Diet and fluid recommendations are much the same as for healthy pregnant women. Diets high in protein and low in salt have been suggested to prevent preeclampsia; however, the efficacy of this has not been proven. Sibai (2004) recommends a regular diet with no salt restriction. Because pregnant women with hypertension have a lower plasma

Home Care

ASSESSING AND REPORTING CLINICAL SIGNS OF PREECLAMPSIA

Report immediately any increase in your blood pressure, protein in urine, weight gain, decreased fetal movement.*

Take your blood pressure on the same arm in a sitting position each time for consistent and accurate readings. Support arm on a table in a horizontal position at heart level.

Use the same scale, wearing the same clothes, at the same time each day, after voiding, before breakfast, for reliable daily weights.

Dipstick test your clean-catch urine sample to assess proteinuria; report frequency or burning on urination.

Assess your baby's activity daily. Decreased activity (three or fewer movements per hour) may indicate fetal compromise.

It is important to keep your scheduled prenatal appointments so that any changes in your or your baby's condition can be detected immediately.

Keep a daily log or diary of your assessments for your home health care nurse, or bring it with you to your next prenatal visit.

*Thresholds for blood pressure, weight gain, fetal movement counts, and proteinuria are set by the physician or institutional protocol.

Home Care

COPING WITH BED REST

In bed, lie on your side. This allows more blood to get to your uterus (womb) and baby. The bed or sofa should be near a window and a bathroom.

Increase your fluid intake to eight glasses per day and add roughage (bran, fruits, leafy vegetables) to your diet to decrease constipation. Keep a bowl of fruit and a large container full of water close by.

Include diversionary activities, such as puzzles, reading, and crafts, to reduce boredom. Place a box or table within reach to store magazines, books, telephone, and other useful items.

Do gentle exercises, such as circling your hands and feet or gently tensing and relaxing arm and leg muscles. This improves muscle tone, circulation, and sense of well-being.

Encourage family participation in your care.

Have significant others assist you with care of the house, children, and so on.

Use relaxation to help cope with stress. Relax your body one muscle at a time, or imagine some pleasant scene, word, or image. Soothing music can also help you relax.

volume than do normotensive women, sodium restriction is not necessary. Women need salt for maintenance of blood volume and placental perfusion. The exception may be the woman with chronic hypertension that was successfully controlled with a low-salt diet before the pregnancy. Adequate fluid intake helps maintain optimum fluid volume and aids in renal perfusion and filtration. The nurse uses assessment data regarding the woman's diet to counsel her in areas of deficiency, if needed (Guidelines box).

Successful home care requires that the woman be well educated about preeclampsia and motivated to follow the plan of care. She must be reliable about keeping appointments. The home environment must be assessed and the woman's ability to assume responsibility determined. In addition, the effects of illness, language, age, culture, beliefs, and support systems must be considered. The woman's support systems must be mobilized and involved in planning and implementing her care. During the period of instruction for the woman and her family, time must be allowed for assimilation of information, questions, and concerns. A patient's understanding is usually directly associated with compliance with the prescribed treatment program. Methods for enhancing learning include visual aids, videotapes, handouts, and demonstrations with return demonstrations (Nursing Care Plan).

Severe Preeclampsia/HELLP Syndrome

If the woman's condition worsens, or if she already has severe preeclampsia or HELLP syndrome and is critically ill, she should receive appropriate management (usually in a tertiary care center) ranging from immediate birth to conservative management of the pregnancy (ACOG, 2002b; Sibai, 2004; Summary Report, 2000; Working Group, 2000). Recognition of the clinical and laboratory findings of severe preeclampsia or HELLP syndrome is important if early, aggressive therapy is to be initiated to prevent maternal and perinatal death. An unfavorable (uneffaced and undilated) cervix resulting from gestational age and the aggressive nature of this disorder supports cesarean birth. Prolonged induction of labor could increase maternal morbidity.

Guidelines

NUTRITION

Eat a nutritious, balanced diet (60 to 70 g protein; 1200 mg calcium; and adequate zinc, magnesium, and vitamins). Consult with registered dietitian on the diet best suited for you as an individual.

There is no sodium restriction; however, consider limiting excessively salty foods (luncheon meats, pretzels, potato chips, pickles, sauerkraut).

Eat foods with roughage (whole grains, raw fruits, and vegetables).

Drink six to eight 8 oz glasses of water per day.

Avoid alcohol, and limit caffeine intake.

The administration of magnesium sulfate as prophylaxis against seizures and the administration of an antihypertensive agent if diastolic BP is higher than 100 to 110 mm Hg are important components of management.

Hospital Care

The woman with severe preeclampsia or HELLP syndrome has multiple problems and provides a complex challenge for the health care team. Nursing care must focus on both mother and fetus.

Antepartum care focuses on stabilization and preparation for birth. The woman may be admitted to an antepartum or a labor and birth unit, depending on the hospital. If the woman's condition is severe, she may be placed in an intensive care unit for hemodynamic monitoring. Maternal and fetal surveillance, patient education regarding the disease process, and supportive measures directed toward the woman and her family are initiated. Assessments include review of the cardiovascular, pulmonary, renal, hematologic, and central nervous systems. Monitoring urinary output is

Nursing Care Plan

MILD PREECLAMPSIA: HOME CARE

NURSING DIAGNOSIS: Risk for injury related to signs of preeclampsia

EXPECTED OUTCOMES

Patient will demonstrate ability to assess self and fetus for signs of worsening preeclampsia; no adverse sequelae will occur as result of preeclamptic condition.

NURSING INTERVENTIONS/*RATIONALES*

Review warning signs/symptoms of preeclampsia *to ensure adequate knowledge base exists for decision making.*

Assess home environment, including woman's ability to assume self-care responsibilities, support systems, language, age, culture, beliefs, and effects of illness, *to determine if home care is viable option.*

Teach woman how to do a self-assessment for clinical signs of preeclampsia (take and record blood pressure, measure urine protein, maintain daily weight log, assess edema formation, assess fetal activity) *to provide immediate evidence of a worsening condition.*

Teach woman to report any increases in blood pressure, ≥2 proteinuria, weight gain, and decreased fetal activity to her health care provider immediately *to prevent worsening of preeclamptic condition.*

Teach woman about use of rest and relaxation as palliative treatment options *to decrease blood pressure and promote diuresis.*

NURSING DIAGNOSIS: Fear/anxiety related to preeclampsia and its effect on the fetus

EXPECTED OUTCOME

Patient's feelings and symptoms of fear/anxiety will decrease/ease.

NURSING INTERVENTIONS/*RATIONALES*

Provide a calm, soothing atmosphere and teach family to provide emotional support *to facilitate coping.*

Encourage verbalization of fears *to decrease intensity of emotional response.*

Involve woman and family in the management of her preeclamptic condition *to promote a greater sense of control.*

Help woman identify and use appropriate coping strategies and support systems *to reduce fear/anxiety.*

Explore use of desensitization strategies such as progressive muscle relaxation, visual imagery, or thought stopping *to reduce fear-related emotions and related physical symptoms.*

NURSING DIAGNOSIS: Deficient diversional activity related to imposed bed rest

EXPECTED OUTCOME

Patient will verbalize diminished feelings of boredom.

NURSING INTERVENTIONS/*RATIONALES*

Assist woman to creatively explore personally meaningful activities that can be pursued from the bed *to ensure activities that have meaning, purpose, and value to the individual.*

Maintain emphasis on personal choices of woman *to promote control and minimize imposition of routines by others.*

Evaluate what support and system resources are available in the environment *to assist in providing diversional activities.*

Explore ways for woman to remain an active participant in home management and decision making *to promote control.*

Engage support of family and friends in carrying out chosen activities and making necessary environmental alterations *to ensure success.*

Teach woman about stress-management and relaxation techniques *to help manage tension of confinement.*

NURSING CARE PLAN–MILD PREECLAMPSIA

critical because magnesium is excreted by the kidneys. Fetal assessments for well-being (e.g., nonstress testing, biophysical profile [BPP], fetal movement counts) are important because of the potential for hypoxia related to uteroplacental insufficiency. Baseline laboratory assessments include metabolic studies for liver enzyme (AST, ALT, LDH) determination, CBC with platelets, coagulation profile to assess for DIC, and electrolyte studies to establish renal functioning.

Weight is measured on admission and every day thereafter. An indwelling urinary catheter facilitates monitoring of renal function and effectiveness of therapy. If appropriate, vaginal examination may be done to check for cervical changes. Abdominal palpation establishes uterine tonicity and fetal size, activity, and position. Electronic monitoring to determine fetal status is initiated at least once a day. The nurse's skill in implementing the techniques described here can be reassuring to the woman and her family. The woman's room must be close to staff and to emergency drugs, supplies, and equipment. Noise and external stimuli must be minimized. Seizure precautions are taken (Box 14-5).

Bed rest or restricted activity is commonly ordered even though there is lack of scientific evidence to support the efficacy of such restriction (Enkin et al, 2001; Working Group, 2000). The nurse's ingenuity may be called on to help the woman cope physically and psychologically with the side effects of immobility and an environment limited in stimuli and support. Thromboembolic events, a risk factor during normal pregnancy, pose an even greater risk with preeclampsia (Nursing Care Plan).

BOX 14-5

Hospital Precautionary Measures

- Environment
  - Quiet
  - Nonstimulating
  - Lighting subdued
- Seizure precautions
  - Suction equipment tested and ready to use
  - Oxygen administration equipment tested and ready to use
- Call button within easy reach
- Emergency medication tray immediately accessible
  - Hydralazine or other antihypertensive medication and magnesium sulfate in or adjacent to woman's room
  - Calcium gluconate immediately available
- Emergency birth pack accessible

Nursing Care Plan

SEVERE PREECLAMPSIA: HOSPITAL CARE

NURSING DIAGNOSIS: Risk for injury to mother and fetus related to CNS irritability

EXPECTED OUTCOMES

Patient will show diminished signs of CNS irritability (e.g., DTRs 2+, absence of clonus) and have no convulsions.

NURSING INTERVENTIONS/*RATIONALES*

Establish baseline data (e.g., DTRs, clonus) *to use as basis for evaluating effectiveness of treatment.*

Administer IV magnesium sulfate per physician's orders *to decrease hyperreflexia and minimize risk of convulsions.*

Monitor maternal vital signs, FHR, urine output, DTRs, IV flow rate, and serum levels of magnesium sulfate *to assess for and prevent magnesium sulfate toxicity* (e.g., depressed respirations, oliguria, sudden drop in blood pressure, hyporeflexia, fetal distress).

Have calcium gluconate at bedside if needed *as antidote for magnesium sulfate toxicity.*

Maintain a quiet, darkened environment *to avoid stimuli that may precipitate seizure activity.*

NURSING DIAGNOSIS: Ineffective tissue perfusion related to preeclampsia secondary to arteriolar vasospasm

EXPECTED OUTCOME

Patient will exhibit signs of increased vasodilation (diuresis, decreased edema, weight loss).

NURSING INTERVENTIONS/*RATIONALES*

Establish baseline data (weight, degree of edema) *to use as basis for evaluating effectiveness of treatment.*

Administer IV magnesium sulfate per physician order, *which serves to relax vasospasms and increase renal perfusion.*

Place woman on bed rest in a side-lying position *to maximize uteroplacental blood flow, reduce blood pressure, and promote diuresis.*

Monitor intake and output, edema, and weight *to assess for evidence of vasodilation and increased tissue perfusion.*

NURSING DIAGNOSIS: Risk for

- Excess fluid volume related to increased sodium retention secondary to administration of magnesium sulfate
- Impaired gas exchange related to pulmonary edema secondary to increased vascular resistance
- Decreased cardiac output related to use of antihypertensive drugs
- Injury to fetus related to uteroplacental insufficiency secondary to use of antihypertensive medications

EXPECTED OUTCOMES

Patient will exhibit signs of normal fluid volume (balanced intake and output, normal serum creatinine levels, normal breath sounds); adequate oxygenation (normal respirations; fully oriented to person, time, and place); normal range of cardiac output (normal pulse rate and rhythm); and fetal well-being (adequate fetal movement, normal FHR).

NURSING INTERVENTIONS/*RATIONALES*

Monitor woman for signs of fluid volume excess (increased edema, decreased urine output, elevated serum creatinine level, weight gain, dyspnea, crackles) *to prevent complications.*

Monitor woman for signs of impaired gas exchange (increased respirations, dyspnea, altered blood gases, hypoxemia) *to prevent complications.*

Monitor woman for signs of decreased cardiac output (altered pulse rate and rhythm) *to prevent complications.*

Monitor fetus for signs of difficulty (decreased fetal activity, decreased FHR) *to prevent complications.*

Record findings and report signs of increasing problems to physician *to enable timely interventions.*

CNS, central nervous system; *DTRs*, deep tendon reflexes; *FHR*, fetal heart rate.

Intrapartum nursing care of the woman with severe preeclampsia or the HELLP syndrome involves continuous maternal and fetal assessments as labor progresses. The assessment for and prevention of tissue hypoxia and hemorrhage, both of which can lead to permanent compromise of vital organs, continue throughout the intrapartum and postpartum periods.

Magnesium Sulfate

One of the important goals of care for the woman with severe preeclampsia is prevention or control of convulsions. Magnesium sulfate is the drug of choice in the prevention and treatment of convulsions caused by preeclampsia or eclampsia (ACOG, 2002b; Magpie Trial Collaborative Group, 2002). The use of magnesium sulfate in the management of preeclampsia halves the risk of eclampsia and probably reduces the risk of maternal death (Magpie Trial Collaborative Group, 2002). The routine use of magnesium sulfate is indicated for severe preeclampsia, HELLP syndrome, or eclampsia; however, no data support routine use of magnesium sulfate for women diagnosed with mild preeclampsia or gestational hypertension (Summary Report, 2000; Working Group, 2000).

Magnesium sulfate is administered as a secondary infusion ("piggyback") to the main intravenous (IV) line by volumetric infusion pump. An initial loading dose of 4 to 6 g diluted in 100 ml of IV fluid per protocol or physician's order is infused over 15 to 30 minutes. This dose is followed by a maintenance dose of magnesium sulfate diluted in an IV solution per physician's order (e.g., 40 g of magnesium sulfate in 1000 ml of lactated Ringer's solution) and administered by infusion pump at 2 g per hour (Gilbert & Harmon, 2003). This dose should maintain a therapeutic serum magnesium level of 4 to 8 mg/dl. No data exist to support the routine drawing of serial serum magnesium levels, although levels are often checked daily (Gilbert & Harmon, 2003) (Box 14-6).

After the loading dose, there may be a transient lowering of the arterial blood pressure secondary to relaxation of smooth muscle.

BOX 14-6

Protocol for Care of Patient with Preeclampsia Receiving Magnesium Sulfate

Magnesium Sulfate Administration

Patient and Family Teaching

Explain technique, rationale, and reactions to expect
- Route and rate
- Purpose of "piggyback"

Reasons for use
- Tailor information to patient's readiness to learn
- Explain that it is to prevent disease progression
- Explain that it is to prevent seizures

Reactions to expect from medication
- Initially patient will feel flushed, hot, sedated, especially during the bolus
- Sedation will continue

Monitoring to anticipate
- Maternal: blood pressure, pulse, DTRs, level of consciousness, urine output (indwelling catheter likely), presence of headache, visual disturbances, epigastric pain
- Fetal: FHR and activity

Administration
- Verify physician order
- Position woman in side-lying position
- Prepare solution and administer with an infusion control device (pump)
- Piggyback a solution of 40 g of magnesium sulfate in 1000 ml of lactated Ringer's solution with an infusion control device at the ordered rates: loading dose: initial bolus of 4-6 g over 15-30 min; maintenance dose: 1-3 g/hr

Maternal and Fetal Assessments
- Monitor blood pressure, pulse, respiratory rate, FHR, and contractions every 15-30 min, depending on patient condition
- Monitor intake and output, proteinuria, DTRs, presence of headache, visual disturbances, and epigastric pain at least hourly
- Restrict hourly fluid intake to a total of 100-125 ml/hr; urinary output should be ≥30 ml/hr

Reportable Conditions
- Blood pressure: systolic, 160 mm Hg; diastolic, 110 mm Hg, or both
- Respiratory rate: 12 breaths/min
- Urinary output <30 ml/hr
- Presence of headache, visual disturbances, or epigastric pain
- Increasing severity or loss of DTRs, increasing edema, proteinuria
- Any abnormal laboratory values (magnesium levels, platelet count, creatinine clearance, levels of uric acid, AST, ALT, prothrombin time, partial thromboplastin time, fibrinogen, fibrin split products)
- Any other significant change in maternal or fetal status

Emergency Measures
- Keep emergency drug tray at bedside with calcium gluconate and intubation equipment
- Keep side rails up
- Keep lights dimmed, and maintain a quiet environment

Documentation
- All of the above

ALT, alanine aminotransferase; *AST,* aspartate aminotransferase; *DTRs,* deep tendon reflexes; *FHR,* fetal heart rate.

NURSE ALERT The woman's BP, pulse, and respiratory status should be monitored closely while the loading dose is being administered intravenously and every 15 to 30 minutes at other times, depending on the stability of the woman's condition. Administration of magnesium sulfate is continued for at least the first 12 to 24 hours postpartum to prevent seizures. ■

Intramuscular (IM) magnesium sulfate is used rarely because the absorption rate cannot be controlled, injections are painful, and tissue necrosis can occur. The IM route may be used with some women who are being transported to a tertiary care center. The IM dose is 4 to 5 g given in each buttock, for a total of 10 g (1% procaine may be ordered to be added to the solution to reduce injection pain), and can be repeated at 4-hour intervals. Z-track technique should be used for the deep IM injection, followed by gentle massage at the site.

Magnesium sulfate interferes with the release of acetylcholine at the synapses, decreasing neuromuscular irritability, depressing cardiac conduction, and decreasing CNS irritability. Because magnesium circulates free and unbound to protein and is excreted in the urine, accurate recordings of maternal urine output must be obtained.

Diuresis within 24 to 48 hours is an excellent prognostic sign. It is considered evidence that perfusion of the kidneys has improved as a result of relaxation of arteriolar spasm. With improved perfusion, fluid moves from interstitial spaces to the intravascular bed and edema is reduced. Diuresis results in weight loss. Although diuresis generally indicates improvement, diuresis in the presence of worsening clinical status may indicate impending renal failure. As renal function declines and serum creatinine levels rise, renal filtration is compromised. The woman can excrete large volumes of urine (greater than 200 ml/hr) but will not excrete magnesium sulfate.

Because magnesium sulfate is a CNS depressant, the nurse assesses for signs and symptoms of magnesium toxicity (see Box 14-6). Serum magnesium levels are obtained on the basis of the woman's response and if any signs of toxicity are present. Early symptoms of toxicity include decreased DTRs, nausea, a feeling of warmth, flushing, muscle weakness, decreased reflexes, and slurred speech.

NURSE ALERT Loss of patellar reflexes, respiratory depression, oliguria, and decreased level of consciousness are signs of magnesium toxicity. Actions are needed to prevent respiratory or cardiac arrest. If magnesium toxicity is suspected, the infusion should be discontinued immediately. Calcium gluconate, the antidote for magnesium sulfate, may also be ordered (10 ml of a 10% solution, or 1 g) and given by slow IV push (usually by the physician) over at least 3 minutes to avoid undesirable reactions such as dysrhythmias, bradycardia, and ventricular fibrillation. ■

Because magnesium sulfate is also a tocolytic agent, its use may increase the duration of labor.

NURSE ALERT The labor of a woman with preeclampsia receiving magnesium sulfate may need augmentation with oxytocin. The amount of oxytocin needed to stimulate labor may be more than that needed for a woman who is not on magnesium sulfate. ■

Magnesium sulfate does not seem to affect FHR variability in a healthy term fetus, and rarely is toxic in the healthy term newborn whose weight is within normal range for gestational age. Neonatal serum magnesium levels approximate those of the mother, and toxic levels can cause depressed respirations and hyporeflexia. The neonate with hypermagnesemia can be treated with calcium and exchange transfusion with citrated blood or may require assisted mechanical ventilation until serum levels normalize. A follow-up study is being conducted to determine whether there are long-term effects of magnesium administration on mothers and infants (Magpie Trial Follow Up Study Management Group, 2004).

If eclampsia develops after the initiation of magnesium sulfate therapy, additional magnesium sulfate or another anticonvulsant (e.g., diazepam or phenobarbital) may be administered (Roberts, 2004) (Emergency box). Rarely, the woman will continue to experience seizures despite adequate blood magnesium levels.

Diazepam has fetal and neonatal effects. The FHR loses variability, a reflection of fetal oxygenation. High levels of these medications in the newborn depress sucking ability, cause hypotonia, and may result in temperature instability. The newborn's respiratory rate may be decreased. Careful surveillance of both maternal and fetal or neonatal status is necessary.

Control of Blood Pressure

For the severely hypertensive woman with preeclampsia, antihypertensive medications are usually ordered to lower the BP. Initiation of antihypertensive therapy reduces risk of maternal morbidity and mortality associated with left ventricular failure and cerebral hemorrhage. Because a degree of maternal hypertension is necessary to maintain uteroplacental perfusion, antihypertensive therapy must not decrease the arterial pressure too much or too rapidly. The target range for the diastolic pressure is 95 to 100 mm Hg (Roberts, 2004).

Intravenous hydralazine remains the antihypertensive agent of choice for the treatment of hypertension in severe preeclampsia. Intravenous labetalol hydrochloride may also be used (ACOG, 2002b; Summary Report, 2000; Working Group, 2000). The choice of agent depends on patient response and physician preference. Table 14-4 compares antihypertensive agents used to treat hypertension in pregnancy. Nifedipine may be used as an antihypertensive agent in nonacute settings; however, the use for the control of severe hypertension or during a hypertensive crisis is contraindicated.

Emergency

MAGNESIUM SULFATE TOXICITY

Signs/Symptoms

Respirations <12/min
Hyporeflexia, absence of reflexes
Urine output <30 ml/hr
Toxic serum levels >9.6 mg/dl
Signs of fetal stress (e.g., fetal tachycardia or bradycardia)
Significant drop in maternal pulse or blood pressure

Interventions

Discontinue magnesium sulfate immediately, and change to maintenance solution.
Call for assistance and notify health care provider for immediate care.
Administer calcium gluconate as ordered (e.g., 1 g for IV injection given over 3 minutes).
Monitor return of DTRs, respiratory rate and quality, pulse rate and quality, and urine output.
Monitor magnesium sulfate level as indicated by patient response.

DTRs, deep tendon reflexes.

NURSE ALERT When administering antihypertensive therapy, the nurse must remember that the drug effects are dependent on intravascular volume. Because preeclampsia is associated with contracted intravascular volume, initial doses should be given with caution and maternal response monitored closely. ■

Eclampsia

Immediate Care

The immediate care during a convulsion is to ensure a patent airway (Emergency box). When convulsions occur, the woman is turned to her side to prevent aspiration of vomitus and supine hypotension syndrome. After the convulsion ceases, food and fluid are suctioned from the glottis or trachea, and oxygen is given by face mask. Magnesium sulfate or another anticonvulsant is given as ordered. If an IV infusion is not in place, one is begun with a large-bore needle. Time, duration, and a description of the convulsions are recorded, and any urinary or fecal incontinence is noted. The fetus is monitored for adverse effects. Transient fetal bradycardia and decreased FHR variability are common.

Aspiration is a leading cause of maternal morbidity and mortality following an eclamptic seizure. After initial stabilization and airway management, the nurse should anticipate orders for a chest x-ray film and possibly arterial blood gases to determine whether aspiration occurred.

A rapid assessment of uterine activity, cervical status, and fetal status is performed after a convulsion. During the convulsion, membranes may rupture and the cervix may dilate because the uterus becomes hypercontractile and hypertonic; birth may be imminent. If birth is not imminent, once the woman's seizure activity and BP are controlled, a decision should be made regarding whether birth should take place. The more serious the condition of the woman, the greater the need to proceed to the birth, which is the definitive cure for the disease. The means of birth—induction of labor vs. cesarean birth—depends on maternal and fetal condition. If fetal lungs are not mature, and the birth can be delayed for 48 hours, steroids such as betamethasone may be given.

The woman may have been incontinent of urine and stool or the membranes may have ruptured during the convulsion; she will need assistance with hygiene and a change of gown. Oral care with a soft toothbrush may be of comfort.

Table 14-4

Pharmacologic Control of Hypertension in Pregnancy

ACTION	TARGET TISSUE	Effects: MATERNAL	Effects: FETAL	NURSING ACTIONS
HYDRALAZINE (APRESOLINE, NEOPRESOL)				
Arteriolar vasodilator	Peripheral arterioles: to decrease muscle tone, decrease peripheral resistance; hypothalamus and medullary vasomotor center for minor decrease in sympathetic tone	Headache, flushing, palpitation, tachycardia, some decrease in uteroplacental blood flow, increase in heart rate and cardiac output, increase in oxygen consumption, nausea and vomiting	Tachycardia; late decelerations and bradycardia if maternal diastolic pressure <90 mm Hg	Assess for effects of medications, alert woman (family) to expected effects of medications, assess blood pressure frequently because precipitate decrease can lead to shock and perhaps abruptio placentae; assess urinary output; maintain bed rest in a lateral position with side rails up; use with caution in presence of maternal tachycardia
LABETALOL HYDROCHLORIDE (NORMODYNE)				
β-Blocking agent causing vasodilation without significant change in cardiac output	Peripheral arterioles (see hydralazine)	Minimal: flushing, tremulousness; minimal change in pulse rate	Minimal, if any	See hydralazine; less likely to cause excessive hypotension and tachycardia; less rebound hypertension than hydralazine
METHYLDOPA (ALDOMET)				
Maintenance therapy if needed: 250-500 mg orally every 8 hr (α_2-receptor agonist)	Postganglionic nerve endings: interferes with chemical neurotransmission to reduce peripheral vascular resistance, causes CNS sedation	Sleepiness, postural hypotension, constipation; rare: drug-induced fever in 1% of women and positive Coombs' test result in 20%	After 4 mo maternal therapy, positive Coombs' test result in infant	See hydralazine
NIFEDIPINE (PROCARDIA)				
Calcium channel blocker	Arterioles: to reduce systemic vascular resistance by relaxation of arterial smooth muscle	Headache, flushing; possible potentiation of effects on CNS if administered concurrent with magnesium sulfate, may interfere with labor	Minimal	See hydralazine; use caution if patient also getting magnesium sulfate

CNS, central nervous system.

NURSE ALERT Immediately after a seizure, the woman may be very confused and can be combative, necessitating the temporary use of restraints. It may take several hours for the woman to regain her usual level of mental functioning. The health care provider explains procedures briefly and quietly. The woman is never left alone. The family is kept informed of management, the rationale for treatment, and the woman's progress. ■

Determination of central venous pressure (CVP) or pulmonary artery wedge pressure (PAWP) (Swan-Ganz catheter) may occasionally be required for accurate fluid monitoring in the presence of pulmonary edema or acute renal failure (ACOG, 2002b). No oral intake is permitted if the woman is convulsing or has symptoms of severe preeclampsia. An indwelling catheter is required for accurate hourly measurement of urine output. For correction of hypovolemia, crystalloids (e.g., 0.9% saline or lactated Ringer's solution) are infused intravenously at a rate that maintains a urine output of at least 25 to 30 ml/hr. Maternal response to therapy is recorded.

Medications (e.g., magnesium sulfate and antihypertensive agents) are given as directed. The woman's response is monitored and recorded, and all drugs, doses, and times are recorded. Laboratory tests are ordered to assess for HELLP syndrome and to have blood typed and crossmatched for administration of packed red blood cells as needed. Blood is kept available for emergency transfusion; abruptio placentae,

Emergency

ECLAMPSIA

Tonic-Clonic Convulsion Signs

Stage of invasion: 2-3 sec, eyes are fixed, twitching of facial muscles occurs
Stage of contraction: 15-20 sec, eyes protrude and are bloodshot, all body muscles are in tonic contraction
Stage of convulsion: Muscles relax and contract alternately (clonic), respirations are halted and then begin again with long, deep, stertorous inhalation, coma ensues

Intervention

Keep airway patent: Turn head to one side, place pillow under one shoulder or back if possible
Call for assistance
Protect with side rails up
Observe and record convulsion activity

After Convulsion or Seizure

Do not leave unattended until fully alert
Observe for postconvulsion coma, incontinence
Use suction as needed
Administer oxygen via face mask at 10 L/min
Start IV fluids and monitor for potential fluid overload
Give magnesium sulfate or anticonvulsant drug as ordered
Insert indwelling urinary catheter
Monitor blood pressure
Monitor fetal and uterine status
Expedite laboratory work as ordered to monitor kidney function, liver function, coagulation system, and drug levels
Provide hygiene and a quiet environment
Support and keep woman and family informed
Be prepared to assist with birth when woman is in stable condition

with accompanying hemorrhage and shock, often occurs in women with eclampsia. Other tests include determination of electrolytes; a liver function battery; and complete hemogram and clotting profile, including platelet count and fibrin split product levels (to assess for DIC).

Postpartum Nursing Care

After birth the symptoms of preeclampsia or eclampsia resolve quickly, usually within 48 hours; however, symptoms have been reported up to several weeks after birth. The hematopoietic and hepatic complications of HELLP syndrome may persist longer. These patients often show an abrupt decrease in platelet count with a concomitant increase in LDH and AST levels after a trend toward normalization of values has begun. Generally, the laboratory abnormalities seen with HELLP syndrome resolve in 72 to 96 hours.

The nursing care of the woman with hypertensive disease differs in a number of respects from that required in a normal postpartum period. These variations in the nursing process are described in the following paragraphs.

Careful assessment of the woman with a hypertensive disorder continues throughout the postpartum period. Blood pressure is measured at least every 4 hours for 48 hours, or more often as the woman's condition warrants. Even if no convulsions occurred before the birth, they may occur within this period. Magnesium sulfate infusion is usually continued 12 to 24 hours after birth. The same assessments continue until the medication is discontinued.

NURSE ALERT The woman is at risk for a boggy uterus and a large lochial flow as a result of magnesium sulfate therapy. Uterine tone and lochial flow must be monitored closely. ■

The preeclamptic woman is hemoconcentrated and unable to tolerate excessive postpartum blood loss. Oxytocin or prostaglandin products are used to control bleeding. Ergot products (e.g., Ergotrate and Methergine) are contraindicated because they increase BP. The woman is asked to report symptoms such as headaches and blurred vision. The nurse assesses affect, level of consciousness, blood pressure, pulse, and respiratory status before an analgesic is given for headache. Magnesium sulfate potentiates the action of narcotics, CNS depressants, and calcium channel blockers; these medications must be administered with caution. The woman may need to continue antihypertensive medication if her diastolic blood pressure exceeds 100 mm Hg at discharge.

The woman's and family's responses to labor, the birth, and the newborn are monitored. Interactions and involvement in the care of the newborn are encouraged as much as the woman and her family desire. In addition, the woman and her family need opportunities to discuss their emotional response to complications. The nurse also provides information concerning the prognosis. Preeclampsia and eclampsia do not necessarily recur in subsequent pregnancies (recurrence rate is approximately 30%), but prenatal care is essential for assessment and early intervention. If the outcome for the mother or baby is unfavorable, the family is assisted in coping with loss and grief.

Prevention

The etiology of preeclampsia continues to be unknown. Numerous clinical trials of various methods to prevent preeclampsia have been conducted. Interventions used in the clinical trials include the use of low-dose aspirin, calcium, magnesium, zinc, and fish oil dietary supplementation. Continued research in prevention is needed because no strategies have proven to have beneficial effects. Nurses should be aware of strategies being studied and use the most reliable evidence about the results to counsel pregnant women about interventions that are likely to be beneficial. One resource is the Cochrane Pregnancy and Childbirth Database (www.cochrane.org).

Evaluation

Evaluation of the effectiveness of care of the woman with preeclampsia is based on the expected outcomes.

Chronic Hypertension

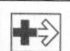

Chronic hypertension occurs in up to 5% of pregnant women, with the incidence higher in African-American women and all women older than 40 years (Livingston & Sibai, 2001). Chronic hypertension in pregnancy is associated with increased incidence of abruptio placentae and superimposed preeclampsia, and adverse pregnancy outcomes are increased in women in whom these complications develop (Sibai, 2002a). Postpartum complications include pulmonary edema, renal failure, and hypertensive encephalopathy (Sibai, 2002a). The risk of perinatal deaths is increased, as are the rates of preterm birth and small-for-gestational-age (SGA) infants in women with chronic hypertension (Livingston & Sibai, 2001).

Women with chronic hypertension ideally should be screened before conception or at the first prenatal visit. Medications that could have adverse effects on the fetus should be discussed and may be discontinued or changed to another medication. Based on the history and physical findings, women with chronic hypertension are identified as either at high or low risk for pregnancy complications (Sibai, 2002a). Women who are high risk are usually managed with antihypertensive therapy and frequent assessments of maternal and fetal well-being. Methyldopa (Aldomet) is usually the drug of choice, although beta-blockers and calcium channel blockers also are used (Working Group, 2000). Antihypertensive therapy may or may not be beneficial for women who are at low risk for complications (Sibai, 2002a).

Lifestyle changes may be necessary; for example, limiting sodium in the diet, limiting exercise during pregnancy, not smoking or using alcohol, limiting caffeine, and losing weight in the preconception period if overweight (Gilbert & Harmon, 2003). The woman should be taught how to monitor her BP.

The time of birth is individualized, but a woman at low risk can usually wait until her cervix is favorable for induction at 40 to 41 weeks of gestation. The woman at high risk should not continue her pregnancy past 40 weeks (Livingston & Sibai, 2001). In the postpartum period, women with chronic hypertension, especially if at high risk, should be monitored for signs of complications such as renal failure, pulmonary edema, heart failure, and encephalopathy. All antihypertensive drugs are found in breast milk. If the woman wishes to breastfeed and needs medication to control her BP, methyldopa is the usual choice.

HYPEREMESIS GRAVIDARUM

Nausea and vomiting complicates approximately 70% of all pregnancies, and is usually confined to the first trimester (Scott & Abu-Hamda, 2004). Although these manifestations are distressing, they are typically benign, with no significant alterations or risks to the mother or fetus. Women with nausea and vomiting in pregnancy have a lower proportion of premature births (Czeizel & Puho, 2004).

When vomiting during pregnancy becomes excessive (i.e., enough to cause weight loss of at least 5% of prepregnancy weight) and is accompanied by dehydration, electrolyte imbalance, ketosis, and acetonuria, the disorder is termed *hyperemesis gravidarum.* The estimated incidence varies from 3.3 to 10 per 1000 pregnancies (Scott & Abu-Hamda, 2004). Hyperemesis gravidarum usually begins during the first 10 weeks of pregnancy. Women with hyperemesis tend to be nulliparous, be overweight, and have a twin gestation.

Etiology

The etiology of hyperemesis gravidarum remains obscure. Several theories have been proposed as to the cause, although none of them adequately explains the disorder. Hyperemesis gravidarum may be related to high levels of estrogen or human chorionic gonadotropin and may be associated with transient hyperthyroidism during pregnancy. It may be accompanied by liver dysfunction manifested by elevated transaminase and abnormal bilirubin level and prothrombin time. Other possible causes include vitamin B deficiencies and increased sensitivity to circulating sex steroid hormones (Scott & Abu-Hamda, 2004).

Psychologic and social factors may also play a part in the development of hyperemesis gravidarum. Ambivalence toward the pregnancy and difficult relationships with mothers or partners have been identified as causative factors. High stress levels are probably also associated with this condition. Conflicting feelings regarding prospective motherhood, body changes, and lifestyle alterations—all normal reactions to pregnancy—may contribute to episodes of vomiting, particularly if these feelings are excessive or unresolved.

Clinical Manifestations

The woman with hyperemesis usually has significant weight loss and dehydration. She may have a decreased blood pressure, increased pulse rate, and poor skin turgor (Scott & Abu-Hamda, 2004). She is almost always unable to keep down even clear liquids taken by mouth. Laboratory tests may reveal electrolyte imbalances.

Collaborative Care

Whenever a pregnant woman has a complaint of nausea and vomiting, the first priority is a thorough assessment to determine the severity of the problem. In most cases, the woman should be told to come immediately to the health care provider's office or to the emergency department, because the severity of illness is often difficult to determine by phone. Assessments should be made of the frequency, severity, and duration of episodes of nausea and vomiting. Other symptoms such as diarrhea, indigestion, and abdominal pain or distention are also identified. Pharmacologic and nonpharmacologic treatments should be recorded.

The woman's weight and vital signs are measured and a complete physical examination is performed, with attention to signs of fluid and electrolyte imbalance and nutritional status. The most important initial laboratory test to be obtained is a dipstick determination of ketonuria. Other laboratory tests that may be ordered include a urinalysis, CBC, electrolytes, liver enzymes, and bilirubin levels. These tests help rule out the presence of underlying diseases such as pyelonephritis, pancreatitis, cholecystitis, and hepatitis. Because of the recognized association between hyperemesis gravidarum and hyperthyroidism, thyroid function may also be assessed (Scott & Abu-Hamda, 2004).

Psychosocial assessment includes asking the woman about anxiety, fears, and concerns related to her own health and the effects on pregnancy outcome. Family members should be assessed both for anxiety and in regard to their role in providing support for the woman.

Initial Care

Initially the woman who is unable to keep down clear liquids by mouth will require IV therapy for correction of fluid and electrolyte imbalances. She should receive nothing by mouth until dehydration has been resolved and for at least 48 hours after vomiting has stopped. In the past, women requiring IV therapy were admitted to the hospital. Today, they often are successfully managed at home. Antiemetic medications may be used if nausea and vomiting are uncontrolled; commonly used medications include pyridoxine, droperidol, diphenhydramine, and metoclopramide. Corticosteroids have also been used successfully to treat refractory hyperemesis gravidarum. Some women also benefit from psychotherapy or stress reduction techniques (Scott & Abu-Hamda, 2004). When the woman begins responding to therapy, limited amounts of oral fluids and bland foods such as crackers and toast are begun. The diet is progressed slowly as tolerated by the woman until she is able to consume a nutritionally sound diet.

In severe cases of hyperemesis gravidarum, enteral nutrition through a feeding tube or parenteral nutrition may be necessary to correct maternal nutritional deprivation. Total parenteral nutrition has also been used successfully (Scott & Abu-Hamda, 2004).

Interventions may include initiating and monitoring IV therapy, administering drugs and nutritional supplements, and monitoring the woman's response to interventions. The nurse observes the woman for any signs of complications such as metabolic acidosis, jaundice, or hemorrhage and alerts the physician should these occur. Accurate intake and output, including the amount of emesis, is an important aspect of nursing care. Oral hygiene while the woman is on nothing-by-mouth status and after episodes of vomiting helps allay associated discomforts. Assistance with positioning and providing a quiet, restful environment that is free from odors may increase the woman's comfort. Promoting adequate rest is important for the woman with hyperemesis; the nurse can assist in coordinating treatment measures and periods of visitation to provide opportunity for rest periods (Nursing Care Plan).

NURSING CARE PLAN—HYPEREMESIS GRAVIDARUM

Nursing Care Plan

HYPEREMESIS GRAVIDARUM

NURSING DIAGNOSIS: Imbalanced nutrition: less than body requirements related to nausea and persistent vomiting as evidenced by weight decrease as compared with prepregnant weight

EXPECTED OUTCOMES

Patient will exhibit no further weight losses, and weight will stabilize. Patient will tolerate regular diet with adequate nutrients for pregnancy with no further nausea and vomiting.

NURSING INTERVENTIONS/*RATIONALES*

Ascertain patient's prepregnant weight, and monitor patient's current weight and intake and output *to provide a database for care planning.*

Resume oral diet as tolerated and prescribed by caregiver *to provide oral nutrition at optimal time.*

Provide small, frequent bland meals as patient tolerates *to assess patient's response to limited oral intake.*

Administer antiemetic medications as prescribed *to decrease or eliminate episodes of vomiting.*

Provide a quiet, restful environment *to decrease associated discomforts.*

Teach patient the importance of a low-fat, high-protein diet with fluids between meals *to provide optimal nutrition for fetal growth and keep nausea to a minimum.*

Refer to dietitian to develop optimal diet plan individualized to patient's current preferences, culture, and lifestyle *to encourage ongoing compliance.*

Discuss with patient the importance of contacting health care provider if intractable nausea and vomiting recur *to provide prompt treatment and avoid complications.*

NURSING DIAGNOSIS: Deficient fluid volume related to excessive vomiting as evidenced by fluid and electrolyte imbalance

EXPECTED OUTCOME

Patient's fluid and electrolyte balance will be restored.

NURSING INTERVENTIONS/*RATIONALES*

Assess and document skin turgor, condition of mucous membranes, vital signs, and urine specific gravity *to provide database for planning care.*

Obtain daily weight *to provide ongoing evaluation of care.*

Monitor laboratory values and report deviations from normal *to prevent complications.*

Maintain accurate intake and output record *to assess for evidence of fluid deficit.*

Initiate and maintain IV therapy carefully *to maintain fluid balance.*

Administer antiemetics as prescribed *to inhibit nausea and vomiting.*

Begin oral fluids slowly and carefully *to increase tolerance and restore fluid balance.*

NURSING DIAGNOSIS: Anxiety related to effects of hyperemesis on fetal well-being as evidenced by patient statements of concern

EXPECTED OUTCOME

Patient will exhibit decreased anxiety.

NURSING INTERVENTIONS/*RATIONALES*

Use therapeutic communication to listen to patient concerns *to maintain a relationship and feeling of trust.*

Provide information regarding any potential risks to the fetus *to alleviate anxiety.*

Assist patient to identify personal strengths and previous coping mechanisms *to reinforce to patient those strengths and coping mechanisms that may be of assistance during this illness.*

Help patient identify sources of support and mobilize support person or group of her choice *to provide support as needed.*

Refer to social services as needed *for ongoing evaluation and assistance.*

Follow-up Care

Most women are able to take nourishment by mouth after several days of treatment. Women should be encouraged to eat small, frequent meals consisting of low-fat, high-protein foods; to avoid greasy and highly seasoned foods; and to increase dietary intake of potassium and magnesium. Herbal teas such as chamomile and raspberry leaf may decrease nausea. Taking fluids between meals rather than with them sometimes helps decrease nausea. Many pregnant women find exposure to cooking odors nauseating; having other family members cook may decrease nausea. The woman is counseled to contact her health care provider immediately if the nausea and vomiting recur, especially if accompanied by abdominal pain, dehydration, or weight loss greater than 2.3 kg (5 lb) in 1 week.

A few women will continue to experience intractable nausea and vomiting throughout pregnancy. Rarely it may be necessary to maintain a woman on enteral, parenteral, or total parenteral nutrition in order to provide adequate nutrition for the mother and fetus. Many home health agencies are able to provide these services, and arrangements for service may be made depending on the woman's insurance coverage.

Regardless of the site of care, the woman needs calm, compassionate, and sympathetic care. Irritability, tearfulness, and mood changes are often consistent with this disorder. Fetal well-being is a primary concern of the woman. The nurse can provide an environment conducive to discussion of those concerns and assist the woman in identifying and mobilizing sources of support. Family members should be included in the plan of care whenever possible. Their participation may help alleviate some of the emotional stress associated with this disorder. Psychologic counseling may be needed, as well as referral to a social worker. Education of the woman and her family about hyperemesis, its causes, potential complications, and a management plan is necessary at the onset because understanding enhances adherence to the treatment plan and influences maternal and fetal outcomes.

HEMORRHAGIC DISORDERS

Bleeding in pregnancy may jeopardize maternal and fetal well-being. Maternal blood loss decreases oxygen-carrying capacity; predisposes the woman to increased risk for hypovolemia, anemia, infection, preterm labor, and preterm birth; and adversely affects oxygen delivery to the fetus. Fetal risks from maternal hemorrhage include blood loss or anemia, hypoxemia, hypoxia, anoxia, and preterm birth.

Hemorrhagic disorders in pregnancy are medical emergencies. The incidence and type of bleeding vary by trimester. In the first trimester, most bleeding is a result of miscarriage and ectopic pregnancy. Approximately 50% of bleeding in the third trimester is caused by placenta previa and abruptio placentae. Antepartal hemorrhage is a leading cause of maternal death, with ectopic pregnancy rupture and abruptio placentae being responsible for most maternal deaths.

With approximately 650 ml/min (15% of maternal cardiac output) of blood flow to the uterine vasculature and placenta, disruption of vascular integrity has the potential for maternal exsanguination within 8 to 10 minutes. Prompt, expert teamwork on the part of the health care providers is essential to save the lives of the mother and infant.

Early Pregnancy Bleeding

Bleeding during early pregnancy is alarming to the woman and of concern to health care providers. The common bleeding disorders of early pregnancy include miscarriage, premature dilation of the cervix, ectopic pregnancy, and hydatidiform mole (molar pregnancy).

Miscarriage (Spontaneous Abortion)

A pregnancy that ends before 20 weeks of gestation is defined as a *miscarriage* or *spontaneous abortion*. This 20-week marker is considered to be the point of viability, when a fetus may survive in an extrauterine environment. A fetal weight less than 500 g may also be used to define a miscarriage (Garmel, 2003).

A miscarriage results from natural causes. *Miscarriage* is suggested as a more appropriate term to use with patients because *abortion* may be an insensitive term to use with families who are grieving a pregnancy loss (Freda, 1999). The term *miscarriage* is used throughout this discussion. The term *abortion* is used when discussing therapeutic or elective induced abortion (see Chapter 7).

Incidence and Etiology

Approximately 10% to 15% of all clinically recognized pregnancies end in miscarriage (Simpson, 2002). An early miscarriage is one that occurs before 12 weeks of gestation. At least 50% of all clinically recognized pregnancy losses result from chromosomal abnormalities (Simpson, 2002). More than 90% of miscarriages occur early, before 8 weeks of gestation (Simpson, 2002). The causes of early miscarriage may include endocrine imbalance (as in women who have luteal phase defects or who have insulin-dependent diabetes mellitus with high blood-glucose levels in the first trimester), immunologic factors (e.g., antiphospholipid antibodies), infections (e.g., bacteriuria and *Chlamydia trachomatis*), systemic disorders (e.g., lupus erythematosus), and genetic factors (Gilbert & Harmon, 2003).

A late miscarriage occurs between 12 and 20 weeks of gestation. It usually results from maternal causes such as advancing maternal age and parity, chronic infections, premature dilation of the cervix and other anomalies of the reproductive tract, chronic debilitating diseases, inadequate nutrition, and recreational drug use (Cunningham et al, 2001). Little can be done to avoid genetic causes of pregnancy loss, but correction of maternal disorders, immunization against infectious diseases, adequate early prenatal care, and treatment of pregnancy complications can do much to prevent miscarriage.

Types

The types of miscarriage include threatened, inevitable, incomplete, complete, and missed (Fig. 14-6). All but the threatened miscarriage can lead to infection.

Clinical Manifestations

Signs and symptoms of miscarriage depend on the duration of the pregnancy. The presence of uterine bleeding, uterine contractions, or uterine pain is an ominous sign in early pregnancy and must be considered a threatened miscarriage until proven otherwise.

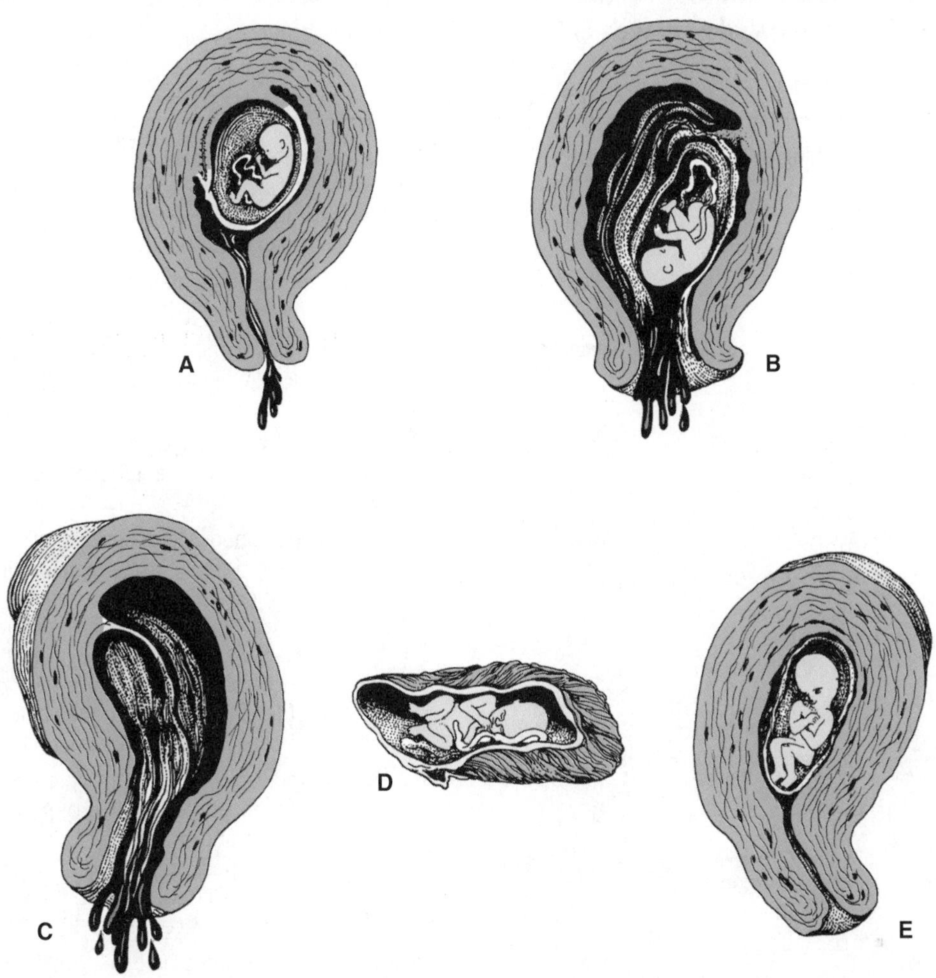

Fig. 14-6 Miscarriage. **A**, Threatened. **B**, Inevitable. **C**, Incomplete. **D**, Complete. **E**, Missed.

If miscarriage occurs before the sixth week of pregnancy, the woman may report a heavy menstrual flow. Miscarriage that occurs between the sixth and twelfth weeks of pregnancy causes moderate discomfort and blood loss. After the twelfth week, miscarriage is typified by more severe pain—similar to that of labor—because the fetus must be expelled. Diagnosis of the type of miscarriage is based on the signs and symptoms present (Table 14-5).

Symptoms of a threatened miscarriage (see Fig. 14-6, *A*) include spotting of blood with a closed cervical os. Mild uterine cramping may be present.

Inevitable (see Fig. 14-6, *B*) and incomplete (see Fig. 14-6, *C*) miscarriages involve a moderate to heavy amount of bleeding with an open cervical os. Tissue may be present with the bleeding. Mild to severe uterine cramping may be present. An inevitable miscarriage is often accompanied by rupture of membranes (ROM) and cervical dilation; passage of the products of conception will occur. An incomplete miscarriage involves the expulsion of the fetus with retention of the placenta (Cunningham et al, 2001).

In a complete miscarriage (see Fig. 14-6, *D*), all the fetal tissue is passed, the cervix is closed, and there may be slight bleeding. Mild uterine cramping may be present.

The term *missed miscarriage* (see Fig. 14-6, *E*) refers to a pregnancy in which the fetus has died but the products of conception are retained in utero for up to several weeks. It may be diagnosed by ultrasonic examination after the uterus stops increasing in size or even decreases in size. There may be no bleeding or cramping, and the cervical os remains closed. If the products of conception are retained after a missed miscarriage, they may calcify, forming a uterine lithopedion or "womb stone" (see Fig. 14-6, *E*).

Recurrent early (habitual) miscarriage is the loss of two or more previable pregnancies (historically, recurrent miscarriage was defined as three or more pregnancy losses) (Hill, 2004).

Miscarriage can become septic, although this is not a common occurrence. Symptoms of sepsis include fever and abdominal tenderness. Vaginal bleeding, which may be slight to heavy, is usually malodorous.

Care Management

Assessment

Whenever a woman has vaginal bleeding early in pregnancy, a thorough assessment should be performed (Box 14-7). The data to be collected include pain, bleeding, and last menstrual period (LMP) to determine the approximate length of gestation. The initial database includes vital signs (a temperature higher than 38° C may indicate infection), previous pregnancies, previous pregnancy losses, type and location of pain, quantity and nature of bleeding, allergies,

Table 14-5

Types of Miscarriage and Usual Management

TYPE OF MISCARRIAGE	AMOUNT OF BLEEDING	UTERINE CRAMPING	PASSAGE OF TISSUE	CERVICAL DILATION	MANAGEMENT
Threatened	Slight, spotting	Mild	No	No	Bed rest, sedation, and avoidance of stress and orgasm usually recommended. Further treatment depends on woman's response to treatment.
Inevitable	Moderate	Mild to severe	No	Yes	Prompt termination of pregnancy is accomplished, usually by dilation and curettage.
Incomplete	Heavy, profuse	Severe	Yes	Yes, with tissue in cervix	Prompt termination of pregnancy is accomplished, usually by dilation and curettage.
Complete	Slight	Mild	Yes	No	No further intervention may be needed if uterine contractions are adequate to prevent hemorrhage and there is no infection.
Missed	None, spotting	None	No	No	If spontaneous evacuation of the uterus does not occur within 1 mo, pregnancy is terminated by method appropriate to duration of pregnancy. Blood clotting factors are monitored until uterus is empty. DIC and incoagulability of blood with uncontrolled hemorrhage may develop in cases of fetal death after the twelfth week, if products of conception are retained for >5 wk.
Septic	Varies, usually malodorous	Varies	Varies	Yes, usually	Immediate termination of pregnancy by method appropriate to duration of pregnancy. Cervical culture and sensitivity studies are done, and broad-spectrum antibiotic therapy (e.g., ampicillin) is started. Treatment for septic shock is initiated if necessary.
Recurrent	Varies	Varies	Yes	Yes, usually	Varies, depends on type. Prophylactic cerclage may be done if premature cervical dilation is the cause.

Adapted from Gilbert ES, Harmon JS: *Manual of high risk pregnancy and delivery,* ed 3, St Louis, 2003, Mosby.
DIC, disseminated intravascular coagulation.

BOX 14-7

Assessment of Bleeding in Pregnancy

Initial Database
- Chief complaint
- Vital signs
- Gravidity, parity
- Last menstrual period/estimated date of birth
- Pregnancy history (previous and current)
- Allergies
- Nausea and vomiting
- Pain (onset, quality, precipitating event, location)
- Bleeding or coagulation problems
- Level of consciousness
- Emotional status

Early Pregnancy
- Confirmation of pregnancy
- Bleeding (bright or dark, intermittent or continuous)
- Pain (type, intensity, persistence)
- Vaginal discharge

Late Pregnancy
- Estimated date of birth
- Bleeding (quantity, associated pain)
- Vaginal discharge
- Amniotic membrane status
- Uterine activity
- Abdominal pain
- Fetal status/viability

ENGLISH SPANISH Guidelines/Guías

ASSESSMENT OF BLEEDING IN EARLY PREGNANCY

When was your last menstrual period?
¿Cuándo fue su última regla?

When did the bleeding start?
¿Cuándo empezó la hemorragia?

What color is the blood? Is it bright red or dark red?
¿Qué color tiene la sangre? ¿Es un rojo fuerte o un rojo oscuro?

Were there any clots or tissue in the blood?
¿Había algunos coágulos o tejido en la sangre?

Is the bleeding continuous or intermittent (starts and stops then starts again)?
¿Es la hemorragia continua o intermitente (corre y deja de correr, luego corre de nuevo)?

How much are you bleeding? How many pads or towels have you saturated since you started bleeding?
¿Cuánta sangre le sale? ¿Cuántas toallas femeninas o toallas se han empapado con sangre desde que empezara la hemorragia?

Do you have any pain with the bleeding?
¿Le duele cuando le sale la sangre?

and emotional status. It is not uncommon for the woman and her family to be anxious and fearful regarding what may happen to her and to her pregnancy.

Various laboratory findings are characteristic of miscarriage. Evaluation of the placental hormone human chorionic gonadotropin (hCG) is used in the diagnosis of pregnancy and pregnancy loss. Human chorionic gonadotropin is produced by the syncytiotrophoblast, and the beta subunit of hCG (β-hCG) can be detected in maternal plasma and urine 8 to 9 days after ovulation if the woman is pregnant. In early pregnancy, the concentration of β-hCG should double every 1.4 to 2.0 days until about 60 or 70 days of gestation (Cunningham et al, 2001). Before 8 weeks of gestation, if miscarriage is suspected, two serum quantitative β-hCG levels are measured 48 hours apart. If a normal pregnancy is present, the β-hCG level doubles within that time. Ultrasonography can then be used to determine the presence of a viable gestational sac. With considerable or persistent blood loss, anemia is likely (hemoglobin level less than 11g/dl). If infection is present, the white blood cell count is greater than 12,000/mm^3. Sedimentation rate is not helpful for differential diagnostic purposes because an increased sedimentation rate occurs with pregnancy, anemia, or infection.

Nursing Diagnoses

The following nursing diagnoses are appropriate for the woman experiencing a miscarriage:

- *Anxiety/fear related to*
  —unknown outcome and unfamiliarity with medical procedures
- *Deficient fluid volume related to*
  —excessive bleeding secondary to miscarriage
- *Anticipatory grieving related to*
  —unexpected pregnancy outcome
- *Situational low self-esteem related to*
  —inability to successfully carry a pregnancy to term gestation

Expected Outcomes

Expected outcomes for the woman experiencing miscarriage include that the woman will do the following:

- Discuss the impact of the loss on her and her family.
- Identify and use available support systems.
- Develop no signs and symptoms of complications (e.g., hemorrhage or infection).
- Verbalize relief from pain.

Plan of Care and Implementation

Medical-Surgical Management

Medical management of miscarriage (see Table 14-5) depends on the classification of the miscarriage and on signs and symptoms. Traditionally, threatened miscarriages have been managed with bed rest and supportive care. Follow-up treatment depends on whether the threatened miscarriage progresses to actual miscarriage, or symptoms subside and the pregnancy remains intact. Dilation and curettage (D&C) is a surgical procedure in which the cervix is dilated and a curette is inserted to scrape the uterine walls and remove uterine contents. A D&C is commonly used to treat inevitable and incomplete miscarriages. The nurse reinforces explanations, answers any questions or concerns, and prepares the woman for surgery.

Dilation and evacuation, performed after 16 weeks of gestation, consists of wide cervical dilation followed by instrumental removal of the uterine contents.

Before either surgical procedure is performed, a full history should be obtained, and general and pelvic examinations should be performed. General preoperative and postoperative care is appropriate for the woman requiring surgical intervention. Analgesia and anesthesia appropriate to the procedure are used.

For late incomplete, inevitable miscarriages, or missed miscarriages (16 to 20 weeks), prostaglandins may be administered into the amniotic sac or by vaginal suppository to augment or induce labor and cause the products of conception to be expelled. Intravenous oxytocin may also be used.

Nursing Care

Immediate nursing care focuses on physiologic stabilization. Typical orders to be followed are initiation of an IV line, request for blood testing of hemoglobin and hematocrit, blood type and Rh, and indirect Coombs' screen. An ultrasound examination is performed for diagnostic confirmation.

Nursing care is similar to care for any woman whose labor is being induced (see Chapter 19). Special care may be needed for management of side effects of prostaglandin such as nausea, vomiting, and diarrhea. If the products of conception are not passed in entirety, the woman may be prepared for manual or surgical evacuation of the uterus.

After evacuation of the uterus, 10 to 20 units of oxytocin in 1000 ml of fluids may be given to prevent hemorrhage. For excessive bleeding, ergot products such as ergonovine, or a prostaglandin derivative such as carboprost tromethamine, may be given to contract the uterus. Three or four doses of ergonovine (e.g., 0.2 mg orally or intramuscularly every 4 hours) may be given if the woman is normotensive. A 25 mg dose of carboprost may be given intramuscularly every 15 to 90 minutes for as many as eight doses (Cunningham et al, 2001). Antibiotics are given as necessary. Analgesics, such as antiprostaglandin agents, may decrease discomfort from cramping. Transfusion may be required for shock or anemia. The woman who is Rh negative and has not developed isoimmunization is given an IM injection of Rh_o(D) immune globulin within 72 hours of the miscarriage.

Psychosocial aspects of care focus on what the pregnancy loss means to the woman and her family. Women experience feelings of grief and loss after a miscarriage; they have more intense feelings for a longer period of time than do men (Abboud & Liamputtong, 2003; Broen et al, 2004). Explanations of expected procedures, possible complications, and future implications for childbearing are provided. Culturally sensitive education regarding recognition of grief responses and how to manage these responses effectively may prevent adverse outcomes (Van & Meleis, 2003).

As with other fetal or neonatal loss, the woman should be offered the option of seeing the products of conception. She may also want to know what the hospital does with the products of conception or whether she needs to make a decision about final disposition of fetal remains.

NURSE ALERT Procedures for disposition of the fetal remains vary from hospital to hospital and state to state. The nurse should know what the usual procedures are in his or her setting. ■

Home Care

The woman will usually be discharged home postoperatively after a D&C when vital signs are stable, vaginal bleeding remains minimal, and she has recovered from anesthesia. Discharge teaching emphasizes the need for rest. If significant blood loss occurred, iron supplementation may be ordered. Teaching includes information about normal physical findings, such as cramping and type and amount of bleeding, resumption of sexual activity, and family planning. Follow-up care is needed to assess the woman's physical and emotional recovery. Referrals to local support groups or counseling are provided as necessary (see Resources at end of chapter) (Patient Teaching box).

Follow-up phone calls after a loss are important. The woman may appreciate a phone call on what would have been her due date. These calls provide opportunities for the woman to ask questions, seek advice, and receive information to help process her grief.

Evaluation

Evaluation is based on the predetermined patient-centered outcomes.

Recurrent Premature Dilation of Cervix (Incompetent Cervix)

Passive and painless dilation of the cervical os without labor or contractions of the uterus (incompetent cervix) may occur in the second trimester or early in the third trimester of pregnancy; miscarriage or preterm birth may result. This description assumes an "all or nothing" role for the cervix; it is either "competent" or "incompetent." Current researchers contend that cervical competence is variable and exists as a continuum that is determined in part by cervical length. Other related causative factors include composition of the cervical tissue and the individual circumstances associated with the pregnancy in terms of maternal stress and lifestyle. Iams (2004) refers to this condition as *abnormal* or *reduced cervical competence,* whereas Freda (1999) prefers the term *premature dilation of the cervix.*

Etiology

Etiologic factors include a history of cervical trauma such as lacerations during childbirth, excessive cervical dilation for curettage or biopsy, and ingestion of diethylstilbestrol (DES) by the woman's mother while pregnant with the woman (see Community Focus Box). Other causes are a congenitally short cervix and cervical or uterine anomalies. Reduced cervical competence is a clinical diagnosis based on history. Short labors and recurring loss of the pregnancy at progressively earlier gestational ages are characteristics of reduced cervical competence. Diagnostic criteria for ultrasound are (1) a short cervix (i.e., less than 20 mm in length) and (2) funneling of the internal os of 30% to 40% of the length of the cervix (Iams, 2004).

Collaborative Care

Medical Management

Conservative management consists of bed rest, progesterone, antiinflammatory drugs, and antibiotics (Iams, 2004). A cervical cerclage may be performed before (rare) or during pregnancy. During pregnancy a Shirodkar or McDonald procedure may be performed. In the Shirodkar, maternal fascia lata is threaded submucosally in the cervix anteriorly and posteriorly and tied. In the McDonald cerclage, nonabsorbable ribbon (Mersilene) is placed around

Patient Teaching

DISCHARGE TEACHING FOR THE WOMAN AFTER EARLY MISCARRIAGE

- Advise the woman to report any heavy, profuse, or bright-red bleeding to health care provider.
- Reassure the woman that a scant, dark discharge may persist for 1 to 2 weeks.
- To reduce the risk of infection, remind the woman not to put anything into the vagina for 2 weeks or until bleeding has stopped (e.g., no tampons, no vaginal intercourse). She should take antibiotics as prescribed.
- Advise the woman to eat foods high in iron and protein.
- Acknowledge that the woman has experienced a loss and that time is required for recovery. She may have mood swings and depression.
- Refer the woman to support groups, clergy, or professional counseling as needed.
- Advise the woman that attempts at pregnancy should be postponed for at least 2 months to allow her body to recover.

From Gilbert ES, Harmon JS: *Manual of high risk pregnancy and delivery,* ed 3, St Louis, 2003, Mosby.

Community Focus

DES EXPOSURE

Diethylstilbesterol (DES), a synthetic nonsteroidal estrogen, was used in the United States between 1938 and 1971 to prevent miscarriage and other pregnancy complications. When a relationship was found between exposure to DES and clear cell adenocarcinoma of the vagina and cervix in young women whose mothers had taken DES while pregnant, the U.S. Food and Drug Administration (FDA) issued a warning in 1971 about the use of DES. Although DES has not been given to pregnant women for more than 30 years, effects continue to be seen. Women who took DES during pregnancy have a higher risk of breast cancer than other women. Women who were exposed to DES in utero have a higher incidence of structural reproductive tract anomalies, increased infertility, and poorer pregnancy outcomes than women who were not exposed. They also have a higher rate of miscarriage, ectopic pregnancy, and preterm birth. Male offspring of women who took DES while pregnant have more genital abnormalities and a possible increased risk of prostate and testicular cancer. Women who took DES during pregnancy should be encouraged to have regular mammography. Women exposed to DES in utero should have vaginal and cervical digital palpation to assess for clear cell adenocarcinoma. Colposcopic examination may be indicated. Men exposed to DES in utero should have routine prostate cancer screening and perform testicular self-examination.

Source: Schrager S, Potter BE: Diethylstilbestrol exposure, *Am Fam Physician* 69(10):2395-2400, 2004.

the cervix beneath the mucosa to constrict the internal os of the cervix (Fig. 14-7).

Prophylactic cerclage is placed at 11 to 15 weeks of gestation, after which the woman is told to refrain from intercourse, prolonged (i.e., more than 90 minutes) standing, and heavy lifting (Iams, 2004). She is monitored during the rest of her pregnancy with ultrasound scans to assess for cervical shortening and funneling. The cerclage is electively removed (usually an office or a clinic procedure) when the woman reaches 37 weeks of gestation, or it may be left in place and a cesarean birth performed. If removed, the cerclage must be repeated with each successive pregnancy.

The cerclage left in place permanently in the woman who anticipates future pregnancies rarely causes problems. Births are accomplished by cesarean. Recent data suggest that prophylactic cerclage may have no advantage over surveillance by ultrasound (Iams, 2004).

A woman whose reduced cervical competence is diagnosed during the current pregnancy may undergo emergency cerclage placement. Risks of the procedure include premature rupture of membranes (PROM), preterm labor, and chorioamnionitis. Because of these risks, and because bed rest and tocolytic therapy can be used to prolong the pregnancy, cerclage is rarely performed after 25 weeks of gestation (Iams, 2004).

Nursing Management

If a cervical cerclage is performed, the nurse monitors the woman postoperatively for contractions, PROM, and signs of infection. Discharge teaching focuses on continued monitoring of these aspects at home. Home uterine monitoring may be indicated with follow-up from a home health agency.

The nurse assesses the woman's feelings about her pregnancy and her understanding of reduced cervical competence. Because the diagnosis of reduced cervical competence is usually not made until the woman has lost one or two pregnancies, she may feel guilty or to blame for this impending loss. It is therefore important to assess for previous reactions to stresses and appropriateness of coping responses. It is important to evaluate the woman's support systems. She needs the support of her health care providers, as well as that of her family.

Home Care

The woman must understand the importance of activity restriction at home and the need for close observation and supervision. Instruction includes the rationale for bed rest or activity restriction and the need to report signs of preterm labor, PROM, and infection.

Tocolytics may be given to prevent uterine contractions and further dilation of the cervix. The woman must be instructed on the importance of taking oral tocolytic medication as prescribed, on the expected response, and about possible side effects. If home uterine monitoring is implemented, the women is taught how to apply a uterine contraction monitor and transmit the monitor tracing by telephone to the monitoring center. Nurses at the monitoring center assess the tracing for contractions, answer questions, provide emotional support and education, and report information to the woman's physician or midwife. The woman should know the signs that warrant immediate transfer to the hospital, including strong contractions less than 5 minutes apart, rupture of membranes, severe perineal pressure, and an urge to push. If management is unsuccessful and the fetus is born before viability, appropriate grief support should be provided. If the fetus is born prematurely, appropriate anticipatory guidance and support are necessary.

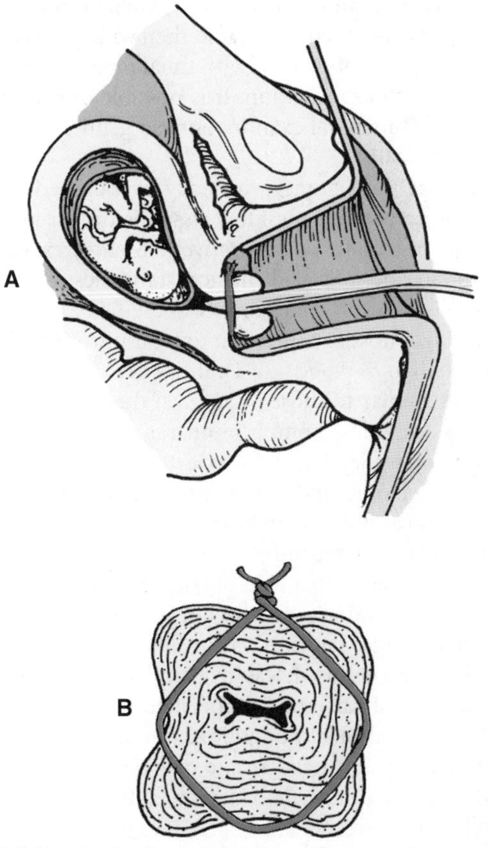

Fig. 14-7 **A**, Cerclage correction of recurrent premature dilation of cervix. **B**, Cross section of closed internal os.

Ectopic Pregnancy

Incidence and Etiology

An ectopic pregnancy is one in which the fertilized ovum is implanted outside the uterine cavity (Fig. 14-8). It accounts for 2% of all pregnancies in the United States (Sepilian & Wood, 2004).

About 95% of ectopic pregnancies occur in the uterine (fallopian) tube, with most located on the ampullar or

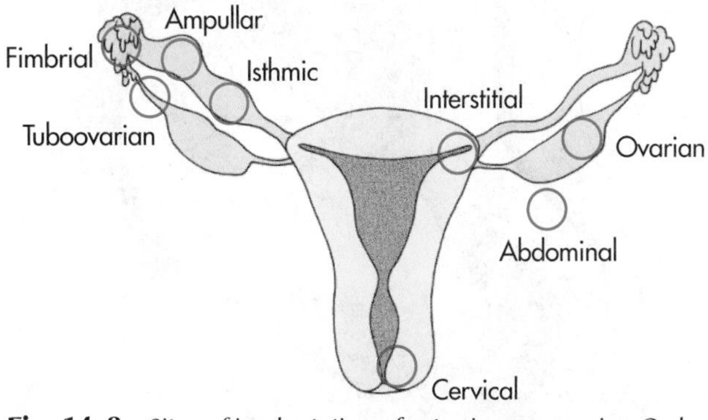

Fig. 14-8 Sites of implantation of ectopic pregnancies. Order of frequency of occurrence is ampullar, isthmic, interstitial, fimbrial, tuboovarian ligament, ovarian, abdominal cavity, and cervical (external os).

largest portion of the tube. Other sites include the ovary (0.5%), abdominal cavity (1.5%), and cervix (0.3%) (Gilbert & Harmon, 2003).

Ectopic pregnancy is the leading pregnancy-related cause of first trimester maternal death and is responsible for 9% to 13% of pregnancy-related deaths (Sepilian & Wood, 2004). Ectopic pregnancy is a leading cause of infertility. Women who have been treated surgically for ectopic pregnancy have a subsequent intrauterine pregnancy rate of 25% to 70%; recurrent ectopic pregnancy rate is up to 28%. Women treated with methotrexate have an intrauterine pregnancy rate of 64%; recurrent ectopic pregnancy rate is approximately 11% (Sepilian & Wood, 2004).

The incidence of ectopic pregnancy is rising as a result of improved diagnostic techniques and an increased incidence of STIs, better treatment of pelvic inflammatory disease (which formerly would have caused sterility), increased numbers of tubal sterilizations, and surgical reversal of tubal sterilizations (Sepilian & Wood, 2004).

Ectopic pregnancy is classified according to the site of implantation (e.g., tubal, ovarian). The uterus is the only organ capable of containing and sustaining a term pregnancy. However, 5% to 25% of abdominal pregnancies, with birth by laparotomy, may result in a living infant (Fig. 14-9). The risk of deformity in these infants is as high as 40% (Gilbert & Harmon, 2003).

Clinical Manifestations

A missed menstrual period, adnexal fullness, and tenderness may suggest an unruptured tubal pregnancy. The tenderness can progress from a dull pain to a colicky pain when the tube stretches. Pain may be unilateral, bilateral, or diffuse over the abdomen. Dark red or brown abnormal vaginal bleeding occurs in 50% to 80% of women. If the ectopic pregnancy ruptures, pain increases. This pain may be generalized, unilateral, or acute deep lower quadrant pain caused by blood irritating the peritoneum. Referred shoulder pain can occur from diaphragmatic irritation caused by blood in the peritoneal cavity. The woman may exhibit signs of shock

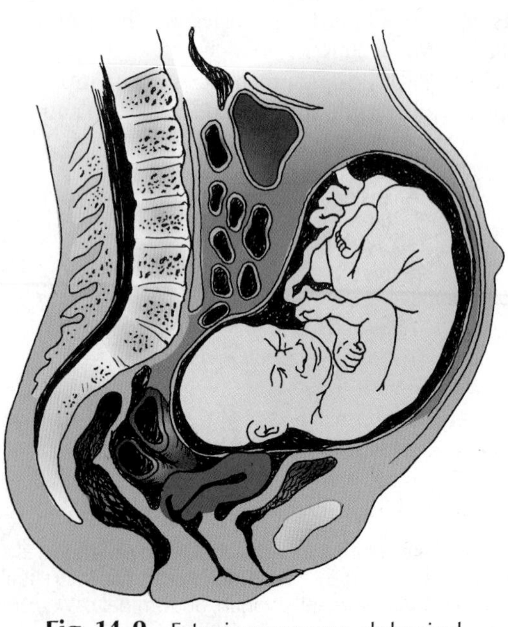

Fig. 14-9 Ectopic pregnancy, abdominal.

related to the amount of bleeding in the abdominal cavity and not necessarily related to obvious vaginal bleeding. An ecchymotic blueness around the umbilicus (Cullen's sign), indicating hematoperitoneum, may develop in an undiagnosed, ruptured intraabdominal ectopic pregnancy.

Diagnosis

The differential diagnosis of ectopic pregnancy involves consideration of numerous disorders that share many signs and symptoms. Miscarriage, ruptured corpus luteum cyst, appendicitis, salpingitis, ovarian cysts, torsion of the ovary, and urinary tract infection must be considered (Table 14-6). The key to early detection of ectopic pregnancy is having a high index of suspicion for this condition. Any woman with complaints of abdominal pain, vaginal spotting or bleeding, and a positive pregnancy test should undergo screening for ectopic pregnancy.

Laboratory screening includes determination of serum progesterone and β-hCG levels. If either of these values is lower than would be expected for a normal pregnancy, the woman is asked to return within 48 hours for serial measurements. At this time, the woman also will undergo transvaginal ultrasound to confirm intrauterine or tubal pregnancy Most ectopic pregnancies occur in the uterine tube; in the past, these were usually diagnosed at the time of rupture, when the major management problem was hemorrhage. Often laparotomy, followed by removal of the entire uterine tube, is the treatment necessary to control bleeding and save the woman's life.

The woman should be assessed for the presence of active bleeding, which is associated with tubal rupture. If internal bleeding is present, the woman may have vertigo, shoulder pain, hypotension, and tachycardia. A vaginal examination should be performed only once, and then with great caution. Approximately half of women with tubal pregnancies have a palpable mass on examination. It is possible to rupture the mass during a bimanual examination, so gentleness is critical (Simpson, 2002).

Removal of the ectopic pregnancy by salpingostomy is possible before rupture. Residual tissue is dissolved with a dose of methotrexate postoperatively. Methotrexate is an antimetabolite and folic acid antagonist that destroys rapidly dividing cells (Wilson, Shannon, & Stang, 2002). It may be used in a single-dose IM injection to treat unruptured pregnancies (Sepilian & Wood, 2004). It has been shown to produce results similar to those of surgical therapy in terms of high success rate, low complication rate, and good reproductive potential (Sepilian & Wood, 2004).

Advanced ectopic abdominal pregnancy requires laparotomy as soon as the woman has been stabilized for surgery. If the placenta of a second- or third-trimester abdominal pregnancy is attached to a vital organ, such as the liver, separation and removal are usually not attempted because of risk of hemorrhage. The cord is cut flush with the placenta and the abdomen is closed, leaving the placenta in place. Degeneration and absorption of the placenta usually occur without complication, although infection and intestinal obstruction may occur. Methotrexate may be given to dissolve the residual tissue (Gilbert & Harmon, 2003).

Hospital Care

If surgery is planned, general preoperative and postoperative care is appropriate for the woman with an ectopic preg-

Table 14-6

Differential Diagnosis of Ectopic Pregnancy

	ECTOPIC PREGNANCY	APPENDICITIS	SALPINGITIS	RUPTURED OVARIAN CYST	MISCARRIAGE
Pain	Unilateral cramps and tenderness before rupture May be colicky after rupture Sudden sharp abdominal pelvic pain Abdominal tenderness	Epigastric, periumbilical, then right lower quadrant pain, tenderness localizing at McBurney's point, rebound tenderness	Usually in both lower quadrants with or without rebound Mild to severe pelvic pressure	Unilateral, becoming general with progressive bleeding, dull cramping	Mild uterine cramps to severe uterine pain
Nausea and vomiting	Occasionally before, frequently after rupture	Usual, precedes shift of pain to right lower quadrant	Infrequent	Rare	Almost never
Menstruation	Some aberration, missed period, spotting	Unrelated to menses	Hypermenorrhea, metrorrhagia, or both	Period delayed, then bleeding, often with pain	Amenorrhea, then spotting, then brisk bleeding
Temperature, pulse, and blood pressure	37.2°-37.8° C, pulse variable, normal before and rapid after rupture, ↓BP after rupture	37.2°-37.8° C, pulse rapid	37.2°-40° C, pulse elevated in proportion to fever	Not >37.2° C, pulse normal unless blood loss marked, then rapid	To 37.2° C Signs of shock related to obvious bleeding
Pelvic examination	Unilateral tenderness, especially on movement of cervix, crepitant mass on one side or in cul-de-sac; dark red or brown vaginal discharge	No masses, rectal tenderness high on right side No vaginal discharge	Bilateral tenderness on movement of cervix Purulent discharge	Tenderness over affected ovary, no masses	Cervix open or closed, uterus slightly enlarged, irregularly softened, tender with infection, vaginal bleeding
Laboratory findings	White blood cell count (WBC) to 15,000/mm³ Pregnancy test positive Ultrasound to rule out pregnancy after 6 wk	WBC 10,000-18,000/mm³ (rarely normal) Pregnancy test negative unless also pregnant	WBC 15,000-30,000/mm³ Pregnancy test negative unless also pregnant	WBC normal to 10,000/mm³ Pregnancy test negative unless also pregnant Ultrasound will show ovarian cyst	WBC normal Pregnancy test positive

Modified from Gilbert ES, Harmon JS: *Manual of high risk pregnancy and delivery,* ed 3, St Louis, 2003, Mosby.

nancy. Vital signs (pulse, respirations, and blood pressure) are assessed every 15 minutes or as needed based on severity of the bleeding and the woman's condition. Preoperative laboratory tests include determination of blood type and Rh factor, CBC, and serum quantitative β-hCG assay. Ultrasonography is used to confirm an extrauterine pregnancy. Blood replacement may be necessary. The nurse verifies the woman's Rh and antibody status and administers Rh_o(D) immune globulin if appropriate. The woman should be encouraged to verbalize her feelings related to the loss. Referral to community resources may be appropriate.

Home Care

Hemodynamically stable women with ectopic pregnancies are eligible for methotrexate therapy if the mass is unruptured and measures less than 3.5 cm in diameter by ultrasound (Sepilian & Wood, 2004). Methotrexate therapy avoids surgery and is a safe, effective, and cost-effective way of managing many cases of tubal pregnancy. Management is almost always accomplished on an outpatient basis.

The woman is informed about how the medication works, what adverse effects are possible, who to call if she has concerns or if problems develop, and the importance of follow-up care. After receiving the single methotrexate injection, the woman must return at least weekly for follow-up laboratory studies for an average of 2 to 8 weeks (Kumtepe & Kadanali, 2004; Sepilian & Wood, 2004). A repeat dose may be necessary if hCG titers do not drop to 15% by day 7. Multiple-dose regimens may also be given (Sepilian & Wood, 2004). During that time, she is instructed to put nothing in the vagina (i.e., no tampons, douches, or intercourse) and to avoid sun exposure because the drug will make her more photosensitive.

NURSE ALERT The woman receiving methotrexate therapy who drinks alcohol and takes vitamins continuing folic acid (e.g., prenatal vitamins) increases her risk of having side effects of the drug or of exacerbating the ectopic rupture. ■

Future fertility should be discussed. Any woman who has been diagnosed with an ectopic pregnancy should be told to contact her health care provider as soon as she suspects that she might be pregnant because of the increased risk for recurrent ectopic pregnancy. These women may need referral to grief or infertility support groups. In addition to the loss of the current pregnancy, they are faced with the possibility of future pregnancy losses and infertility.

Gestational Trophoblastic Disease

Gestational trophoblastic disease (GTD) includes disorders that arise from the placental trophoblast. It includes hydatidiform mole, invasive mole, and choriocarcinoma. Gestational trophoblastic neoplasia (GTN) refers to persistent trophoblastic tissue that is presumed to be malignant (Berman, DiSaia, & Tewari, 2004; Gilbert & Harmon 2003). Once almost invariably fatal, the treatment has progessed until today GTN is the most curable gynecologic malignancy (Berman, DiSaia, & Tewari, 2004).

Hydatidiform Mole

Hydatidiform mole (molar pregnancy) is a GTD. There are two distinct types: complete (or classic) mole and partial mole.

Incidence and Etiology

Hydatidiform mole occurs in 1 in 1200 pregnancies in the United States, but a higher incidence has been reported in Asian countries (Berman, DiSaia, & Tewari, 2004). The etiology is unknown, although there may be an ovular defect or nutritional deficiency. Women at higher risk for hydatidiform mole are those in their early teens or over age 40. The risk of developing a second mole is 1% to 2%.

Types

The complete mole results from fertilization of an egg whose nucleus has been lost or inactivated. The nucleus of a sperm (23,X) duplicates itself (resulting in the diploid number, 46,XX) because the ovum has no genetic material or the material is inactive. The mole resembles a bunch of white grapes (Fig. 14-10). The hydropic (fluid-filled) vesicles grow rapidly, causing the uterus to be larger than expected for the duration of the pregnancy. Usually the complete mole contains no fetus, placenta, amniotic membranes, or fluid. Maternal blood has no placenta to receive it; therefore hemorrhage into the uterine cavity and vaginal bleeding occur. In about 20% of complete moles, progression toward choriocarcinoma occurs.

A partial mole occurs as a result of two sperm fertilizing an apparently normal ovum. Partial moles often have embryonic or fetal parts and an amniotic sac. Congenital anomalies are usually present. The potential for malignant transformation is less than 6% (Copeland & Landon, 2002).

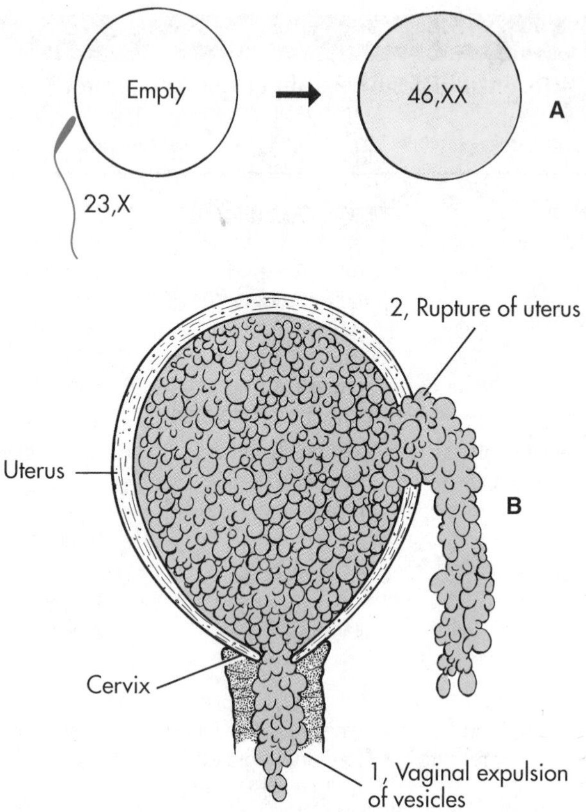

Fig. 14-10 **A,** Chromosomal origin of complete mole. Single sperm (in color) fertilizes an "empty" ovum. Reduplication of sperm's 23,X set gives completely homozygous diploid 46,XX. Similar process follows fertilization of empty ovum by two sperm with two independently drawn sets of 23,X or 23,Y; both karyotypes of 46,XX and 46,YY can therefore result. **B,** Uterine rupture with hydatidiform mole. *1,* Evacuation of mole through cervix. *2,* Rupture of uterus and spillage of mole into peritoneal cavity (rare).

Clinical Manifestations

In the early stages the clinical manifestations of a complete hydatidiform mole cannot be distinguished from normal pregnancy. Vaginal bleeding occurs in almost 95% of patients. The vaginal discharge may be dark brown (resembling prune juice) or bright red, and either scant or profuse. It may continue for only a few days or intermittently for weeks. In early pregnancy, in about half of affected women, the uterus is significantly larger than expected from menstrual dates.

Anemia from blood loss, excessive nausea and vomiting (hyperemesis gravidarum), and abdominal cramps caused by uterine distention are relatively common findings. Preeclampsia occurs in about 15% of cases (usually between 9 and 12 weeks of gestation), but any symptoms of gestational hypertension before 24 weeks of gestation may suggest hydatidiform mole. Hyperthyroidism and pulmonary embolization of trophoblastic elements occur less commonly but are serious complications of hydatidiform mole. Partial mole causes few of these symptoms and may be mistaken for an incomplete miscarriage or a missed miscarriage.

Medical-Surgical Management

Although most moles pass spontaneously, suction curettage offers a safe, rapid, and effective method of evacuation of hydatidiform mole if necessary (Gilbert & Harmon, 2003).

Induction of labor with oxytocic agents or prostaglandins is not recommended because of the increased risk of embolization of trophoblastic tissue (Copeland & Landon, 2002). Administration of $Rh_o(D)$ immune globulin to women who are Rh negative is needed to prevent isoimmunization.

Nursing Care

Nursing assessments during prenatal visits should include observation for signs of molar pregnancy during the first 24 weeks. If hydatidiform mole is suspected, ultrasonography and serial β-hCG immunoassays will be used to confirm the diagnosis. The sonographic pattern of a molar pregnancy is characterized by a diffuse snowstorm appearance. The hCG titer remains high or rises above the normal peak after the time it normally drops (i.e., 70 to 100 days).

The nurse provides the woman and her family with information about the disease process, the necessity for a long course of follow-up, and the possible consequences of the disease. The nurse helps the woman understand and cope with pregnancy loss and recognize that the pregnancy was abnormal. The woman and her family are encouraged to express their feelings, and information is provided about support groups or counseling resources if needed.

Home Care

Follow-up management includes frequent physical and pelvic examinations along with measurement of serum β-hCG until the level drops to normal and remains normal for 3 weeks. Monthly measurements are taken for 6 months, then every 2 months for a total of 1 year. A rising titer and an enlarging uterus may indicate choriocarcinoma.

NURSE ALERT To avoid confusing the signs of choriocarcinoma with the signs of pregnancy, pregnancy should be avoided for 1 year. Any contraceptive method except the intrauterine device is acceptable. Oral contraceptives are highly effective. ■

Gestational Trophoblastic Neoplasia

These types of tumors are classified as nonmetastatic, metastatic low risk, and metastatic high risk. Almost 50% of these tumors occur after a hydatidiform mole. Approximately 30% follow an ectopic pregnancy or miscarriage, and 20% occur after an apparently normal birth at term. There is almost a 100% cure rate after nonmetastatic and low risk metastatic GTN. Common sites of metastasis are the lungs, vagina, pelvis, liver, and brain (Gilbert & Harmon, 2003). There is a 10% risk of maternal death after high risk GTN.

Continued bleeding after evacuation of a hydatidiform mole is usually the most suggestive symptom of GTN. Other clinical signs include abdominal pain and uterine and ovarian enlargement. Signs of metastasis include pulmonary symptoms (e.g., dyspnea, cough). The diagnosis is usually confirmed by increasing or plateauing hCG levels after evacuation of a molar pregnancy. Once diagnosis is confirmed, other clinical studies (e.g., computed tomography scan of lungs and brain, chest x-ray, pelvic ultrasound, and liver scan) are done to determine the extent of the disease.

For women who wish to preserve their fertility, single-agent chemotherapy is chosen. Methotrexate has been the treatment of choice for years. High-dose methotrexate followed by folinic acid "rescue" within 24 hours also has shown excellent results and causes fewer toxic effects (Berman, Di Saia, & Tewari, 2004). Dactinomycin also has been used with equally good results and is used for women with liver or renal disease, both of which are contraindications for methotrexate. Hysterectomy with adjuvant chemotherapy is often the choice of treatment for nonmetastatic tumors in women who have completed their childbearing.

Therapy is continued until negative hCG levels are obtained. Follow-up after successful chemotherapy is by serum hCG levels obtained every 2 weeks for 3 months, every month for 3 months, every other month for 6 months, and then every 6 months indefinitely. Physical examinations should be done at least yearly, and chest radiographs are done if indicated. Contraception is needed until the woman has been in remission for at least 6 months (Berman, DiSaia, & Tewari, 2004). Oral contraceptives are preferred, but barrier methods are acceptable if oral contraceptives are contraindicated. During a subsequent pregnancy, pelvic ultrasonography is recommended because the woman is at higher risk to develop another molar pregnancy. Serum hCG levels should be obtained 6 weeks after the birth (Berman, DiSaia, & Tewari, 2004).

Late Pregnancy Bleeding

Late pregnancy bleeding disorders include placenta previa, premature separation of placenta (abruptio placentae), and variations in the insertion of the cord and the placenta (Fig. 14-11). Expedient assessment for and diagnosis of the cause of bleeding are essential to reduce the risk of maternal and perinatal morbidity and mortality.

Placenta Previa

In placenta previa, the placenta is implanted in the lower uterine segment near or over the internal cervical os. The degree to which the internal cervical os is covered by the placenta has traditionally been used to classify three types of placenta previa (Fig. 14-12). Placenta previa often is described as complete, total, or central if the internal os is entirely covered by the placenta when the cervix is fully dilated. Partial placenta previa implies incomplete coverage of the internal os. Marginal placenta previa indicates that only an edge of the placenta extends to the internal os, but it may extend onto the os during dilation of the cervix during labor. The term *low-lying placenta* is used when the placenta is implanted in the lower uterine segment but does not reach the os.

Recent advances in sonographic diagnosis and a better understanding of the changing relationship of the internal cervical os and the placenta as pregnancy progresses have made these traditional definitions and classifications obsolete. During the second trimester, the placenta may appear to cover the cervical os; however, at term, it does not cover the os (Clark, 2004). A more descriptive classification is placenta previa (in the third trimester, the placenta covers the internal os) and marginal placenta previa (the distance of the placenta is 2 to 3 cm from the internal os and does not cover it). When the exact relationship of the os to the placenta has not been determined or in cases of apparent placenta previa in the second trimester, the term *low-lying placenta* can be used (Clark, 2004) (see Fig. 14-12).

Incidence and Etiology

The incidence of placenta previa is approximately 0.5% of births. The most important risk factors are previous placenta

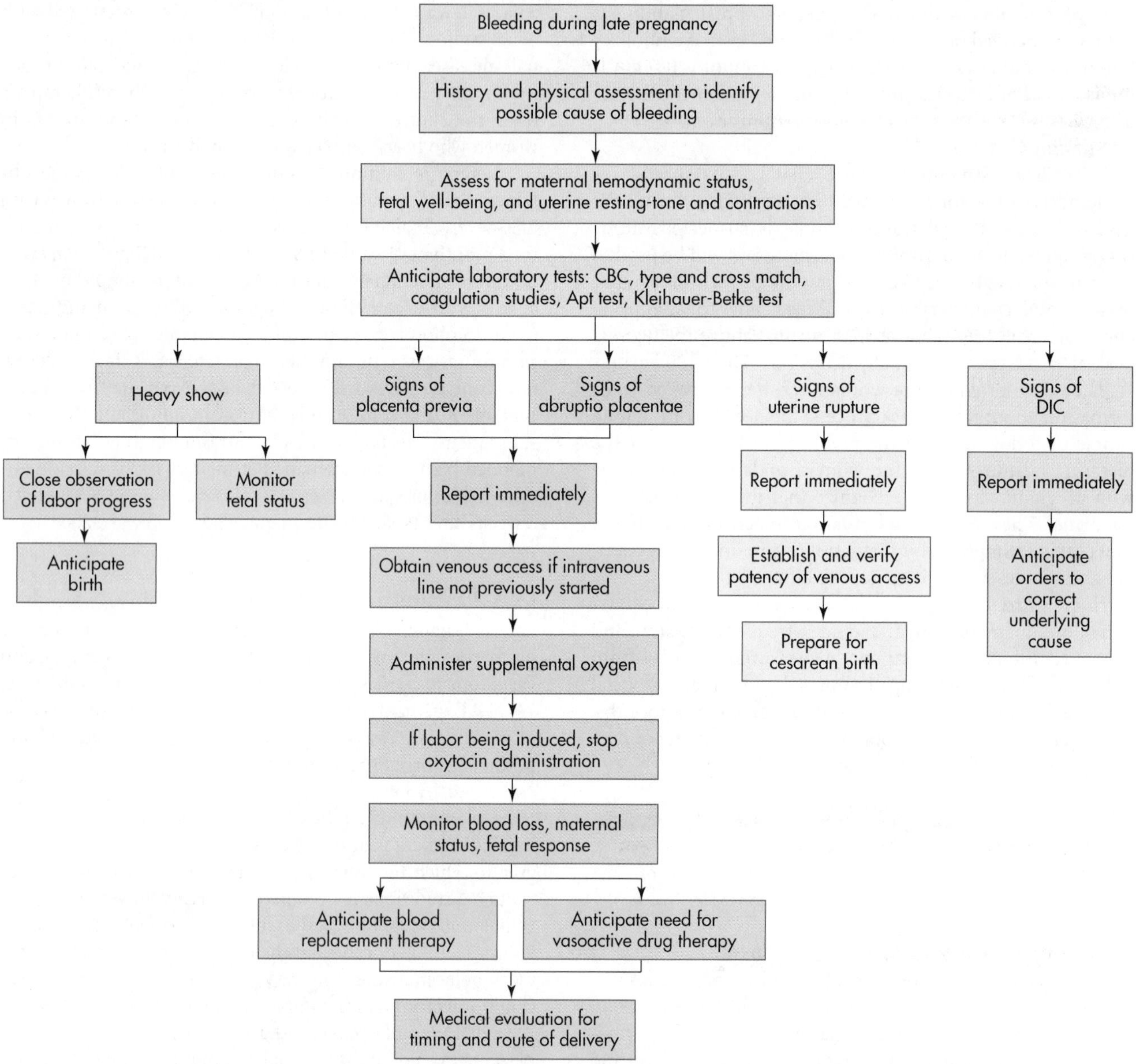

Fig. 14-11 Bleeding during late pregnancy.

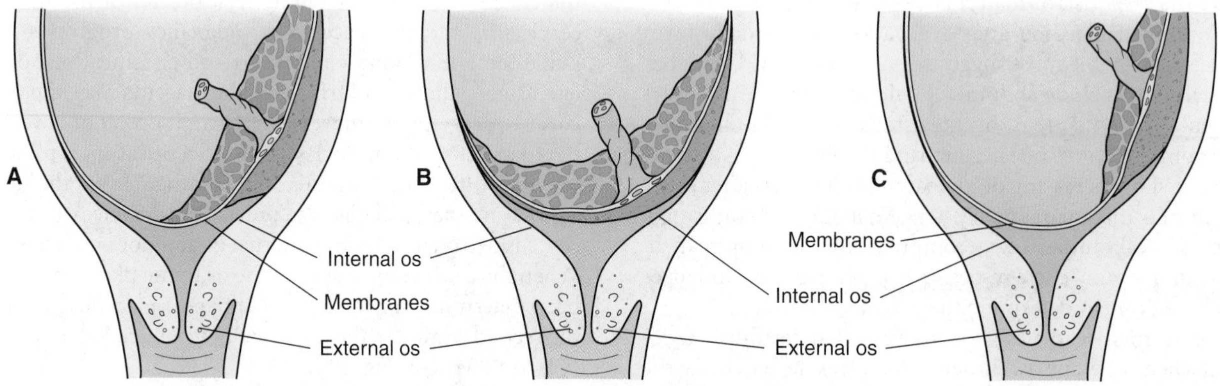

Fig. 14-12 Types of placenta previa. **A**, Low-lying placenta in second trimester. **B**, Placenta previa. **C**, Marginal placenta previa.

previa, previous cesarean birth, and suction curettage for miscarriage or induced abortion, possibly related to endometrial scarring. The risk also increases with multiple gestation (because of the larger placental area), closely spaced pregnancies, maternal age over 35 years, African or Asian ethnicity, male fetal gender, smoking, and cocaine use (Clark, 2004).

Clinical Manifestations

About 70% of women with placenta previa have painless uterine bleeding; 20% have vaginal bleeding associated with uterine activity. Previa should be suspected whenever vaginal bleeding occurs after 20 weeks of gestation. This bleeding is associated with the stretching and thinning of the lower uterine segment that occurs during the third trimester. Placental attachment is gradually disrupted, and bleeding occurs when the uterus is not able to contract adequately and stop blood flow from open vessels. The initial bleeding is usually a small amount and stops as clots form; however, it can recur at any time (Table 14-7). It is bright red.

Vital signs may be normal even with heavy blood loss, because a pregnant woman can lose up to 40% of blood volume without showing signs of shock. Clinical presentation and decreasing urinary output may be better indicators of acute blood loss than vital signs alone. The fetal heart rate is reassuring unless there is a major detachment of the placenta (Gilbert & Harmon, 2003).

Abdominal examination usually reveals a soft, relaxed, nontender uterus with normal tone. If the fetus is lying longitudinally, the fundal height is usually greater than expected for gestational age because the low placenta hinders descent of the presenting fetal part. Leopold's maneuvers may reveal a fetus in an oblique or breech position or lying transverse because of the abnormal site of placental implantation.

Table 14-7

Summary of Findings: Abruptio Placentae and Placenta Previa

	Abruptio Placentae			Placenta Previa
	GRADE 1 MILD SEPARATION (10% TO 20%)	GRADE 2 MODERATE SEPARATION (20% TO 50%)	GRADE 3 SEVERE SEPARATION (>50%)	
Bleeding, external, vaginal	Minimal	Absent or moderate	Absent to moderate	Minimal to severe and life threatening
Total amount of blood loss	<500 ml	1000-1500 ml	>1500 ml	Varies
Color of blood	Dark red	Dark red	Dark red	Bright red
Shock	Rare; none	Mild shock	Common, often sudden, profound	Uncommon
Coagulopathy	Rare; none	Occasional DIC	Frequent DIC	None
Uterine tonicity	Normal	Increased, may be localized to one region or diffuse over uterus, uterus fails to relax between contractions	Tetanic, persistent uterine contraction, boardlike uterus	Normal
Tenderness (pain)	Usually absent	Present	Agonizing, unremitting uterine pain	Absent
Ultrasonographic findings				
Location of placenta	Normal, upper uterine segment	Normal, upper uterine segment	Normal, upper uterine segment	Abnormal, lower uterine segment
Station of presenting part	Variable to engaged	Variable to engaged	Variable to engaged	High, not engaged
Fetal position	Usual distribution*	Usual distribution*	Usual distribution*	Commonly transverse, breech, or oblique
Gestational or chronic hypertension	Usual distribution*	Commonly present	Commonly present	Usual distribution*
Fetal effects	Normal fetal heart rate pattern	Nonreassuring fetal heart rate pattern	Nonreassuring fetal heart rate pattern; death can occur	Normal fetal heart rate and pattern

**Usual distribution* refers to the usual variations of incidence seen when there is no concurrent problem.
DIC, disseminated intravascular coagulation.

Maternal and Fetal Outcome

The maternal morbidity rate is about 5%, and the mortality rate is less than 1% with placenta previa (Clark, 2004). Complications associated with placenta previa include PROM, preterm labor and birth, surgery-related trauma to structures adjacent to the uterus, anesthesia complications, blood transfusion reactions, overinfusion of fluids, abnormal placental attachments, postpartum hemorrhage, anemia, thrombophlebitis, and infection (Crane et al, 2000).

The greatest risk of fetal death is caused by preterm birth. Other fetal risks include malpresentation and congenital anomalies (Clark, 2004; Gilbert & Harmon, 2003). Infants who are small for gestational age or have intrauterine growth restriction also have been associated with placenta previa; this association may be related to poor placental exchange or hypovolemia resulting from maternal blood loss and maternal anemia (Clark, 2004).

Diagnosis and Medical Management

The standard for the diagnosis of placenta previa is a transabdominal ultrasound examination. It is accurate 93% to 97% of the time. Transvaginal ultrasound also is used for placental location, particularly when the exact relation of the lower placental margin to the internal os is not clearly seen with transabdominal examination (Clark, 2004). If ultrasonographic scanning reveals a normally implanted placenta, a speculum examination is performed to rule out local causes of bleeding (e.g., cervicitis, polyps, or carcinoma of the cervix), and a coagulation profile is obtained to rule out other causes of bleeding.

Management of placenta previa depends on the gestational age and condition of the fetus and the amount of bleeding present. It includes expectant management and cesarean birth. Expectant management (observation and bed rest) usually is implemented when the fetus is not mature. Women may be placed in the hospital on complete bed rest or managed at home. If a woman is bleeding, she is usually placed in the labor and birth unit, where she and the fetus can be closely monitored.

Critical Thinking Exercise

PLACENTA PREVIA

Marta is a 26-year-old woman who is G6, P4, Ab1 at 26 weeks of gestation seen in the emergency department with bright-red vaginal bleeding. She asks you what is wrong and whether this means she will lose the baby.

1. Evidence—Is there sufficient evidence to draw conclusions about her diagnosis and preferred treatment?
2. Assumptions—What assumptions can be made about the following items?
   a. Possible diagnoses for Marta
   b. Physical assessment, laboratory tests, and diagnostic procedures that will be done to make a diagnosis
   c. The circumstances under which Marta would be transferred to the antepartum unit
   d. The circumstances under which Marta would be discharged home
3. What implications and priorities for nursing care can be drawn at this time?
4. Does the evidence objectively support your conclusion?
5. Are there alternative perspectives to your conclusion?

If expectant management is to be implemented, a vaginal speculum examination is postponed until fetal viability is reached (preferably after 34 weeks of gestation). If a pelvic examination is needed before that time, anticipate the possibility that an immediate cesarean birth may be required. The woman is taken to a delivery room or an operating room set up for cesarean birth because profound hemorrhage can occur during the examination. This type of vaginal examination, known as the double-setup procedure, is not often performed.

Care Management

Assessment

A woman with third trimester vaginal bleeding requires immediate evaluation. Necessary history data include gravidity, parity, estimated date of birth, general status, bleeding (i.e., quantity, precipitating event, and associated pain), vital signs, and fetal status. Laboratory studies include a complete blood cell count, determination of blood type and Rh factor, coagulation profile, and possible type and crossmatch.

Nursing Diagnoses

Potential nursing diagnoses for the woman with a placenta previa include the following:

- *Decreased cardiac output related to*
  —excessive blood loss secondary to placenta previa
- *Deficient fluid volume related to*
  —excessive blood loss secondary to placenta previa
- *Ineffective peripheral tissue perfusion related to*
  —hypovolemia and shunting of blood to central circulation
- *Anxiety/fear related to*
  —maternal condition and pregnancy outcome
- *Anticipatory grieving related to*
  —actual/perceived threat to self, pregnancy, or infant

Expected Outcomes

Expected outcomes for the woman experiencing placenta previa may include that the woman will do the following:

- Verbalize understanding of her condition and its management.
- Identify and use available support systems.
- Demonstrate compliance with prescribed activity limitations.
- Develop no complications related to bleeding.
- Give birth to a healthy term infant.

Plan of Care and Implementation

Hospital Care

Active Management

Once placenta previa has been diagnosed, a management plan is developed based on gestational age, amount of bleeding, and fetal condition. If the woman is at term (longer than or equal to 37 weeks of gestation) and in labor or bleeding persistently, immediate delivery by cesarean is almost always indicated. In women who have minimal bleeding, vaginal birth may be attempted. Vaginal birth also may be indicated for previable gestations or births involving intrauterine fetal demise (Benedetti, 2002).

If cesarean birth is undertaken, the nurse continuously assesses maternal and fetal status while preparing the woman for surgery. Maternal vital signs are assessed frequently for decreasing BP, increasing pulse rate, changes in level of consciousness, and oliguria. Fetal assessment is maintained by continuous electronic fetal monitoring to assess for signs of hypoxia.

Blood loss may not cease with the infant's birth. The large vascular channels in the lower uterine segment may continue to bleed because of the diminished muscle content in that region. The natural mechanism to control bleeding—the interlacing muscle bundles contracting around open vessels (the "living ligature" characteristic of the upper part of the uterus)—is absent in the lower part of the uterus. Postpartum hemorrhage may occur even if the fundus is contracted firmly.

Emotional support for the woman and her family is extremely important. The actively bleeding woman is concerned not only for her own well-being but for the well-being of her fetus. All procedures should be explained, and a support person should be present. The woman should be encouraged to express her concerns and feelings. If the woman and her support person or family desire pastoral support, the nurse can notify the hospital chaplain service or provide information about other supportive resources.

Expectant Management

If the woman is less than 36 weeks of gestation, is not in labor, and the bleeding is mild or has stopped, expectant management (i.e., rest and close observation) is generally the treatment of choice to give the fetus time to mature in utero. The woman may remain in the hospital on bed rest with bathroom privileges and limited activity (up in a wheelchair for short periods of time). Bleeding is assessed by checking the amount of bleeding on perineal pads, bed pads, and linens. Weighing pads, although not often used, is one way to more accurately assess blood loss; 1 g is equal to 1 ml of blood.

Ultrasonographic examinations may be done every 2 to 3 weeks. Fetal surveillance may include nonstress testing (NST) or BPPs once or twice weekly. Serial laboratory values are evaluated for decreasing hemoglobin and hematocrit levels and changes in coagulation values. Venous access with an IV infusion or heparin lock may be placed in case blood or blood component therapy is needed. Antepartum steroids (betamethasone) may be ordered to promote fetal lung maturity if the woman is at less than 34 weeks of gestation. No vaginal or rectal examinations are performed, and the woman is placed on pelvic rest (nothing in the vagina). Once she reaches 37 weeks of gestation, and fetal lung maturity is documented, cesarean birth can be scheduled.

The woman with placenta previa should always be considered a potential emergency because massive blood loss with resulting hypovolemic shock can occur quickly if bleeding resumes. Placenta previa in a preterm gestation may be an indication for admission to a tertiary perinatal center because many community hospitals are not equipped to perform emergency cesarean births 24 hours per day, 7 days per week, nor to provide neonatal intensive care.

Home Care

Criteria for home care management vary among primary perinatal providers and home care agencies and are usually determined on a case-by-case basis. To be considered for home care referral, the woman must be in stable condition with no evidence of active bleeding and must have resources to be able to return to the hospital immediately if active bleeding resumes.

She must have close supervision by family or friends in the home. She should be taught how to assess fetal and uterine activity and bleeding; and told to avoid intercourse, douching, and enemas. She should limit her activities according to the advice of her physician and be advised to keep all appointments for fetal testing, laboratory assessments, and prenatal care. Visits by a perinatal home care nurse may be arranged.

Evaluation

The expected outcomes of care are used to evaluate the care for the woman with placenta previa (Nursing Care Plan).

Premature Separation of Placenta

Premature separation of the placenta, or abruptio placentae, is the detachment of part or all of the placenta from its implantation site (Fig. 14-13). Separation occurs in the area of the decidua basalis after 20 weeks of pregnancy and before birth of the baby.

Incidence and Etiology

Premature separation of the placenta is a serious event that accounts for significant maternal and fetal morbidity and mor-

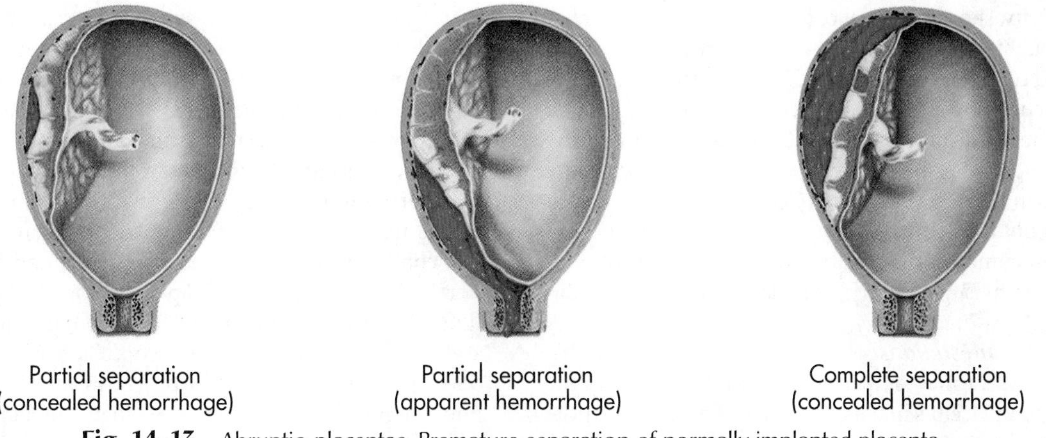

Fig. 14-13 Abruptio placentae. Premature separation of normally implanted placenta.

Nursing Care Plan

PLACENTA PREVIA

NURSING DIAGNOSIS: Decreased cardiac output related to bleeding secondary to placenta previa

EXPECTED OUTCOME

Patient will exhibit signs of increased blood volume and restoration of cardiac output (i.e., normal pulse and blood pressure; normal heart and breath sounds; normal skin color, tone, and turgor; normal capillary refill).

NURSING INTERVENTIONS/*RATIONALES*

Palpate uterus for tenderness and tone; assess bleeding rate, amount, color, degree of bleeding, CBC values, and coagulation profile *to determine severity of situation.* Do not perform vaginal examination *because it may stimulate further bleeding.*

Establish baseline data for cardiac output (vital signs; heart and breath sounds; skin color, tone, turgor; capillary refill; level of consciousness; urinary output; pulse oximetry) *to use as basis for evaluating effectiveness of treatment.*

Initiate intravenous therapy or blood transfusions and medications per physician order *to restore blood volume and prevent organ compromise to mother and fetus.*

Place woman on bed rest *to decrease oxygen demands.*

Monitor vital signs, intake and output, hemodynamic status, and laboratory values *to evaluate treatment response.*

Provide emotional support to woman and her family (e.g., explain procedures and their rationale; explain what is happening and what to expect; keep support person present) *to allay fears and provide the family with some sense of control.*

After stabilization, teach woman home management, including bed rest, watching for spotting/bleeding, close follow-up with her health care provider, and preparation for immediate return to hospital if needed *to prevent or stem further complications.*

NURSING DIAGNOSIS: Risk for injury to the fetus related to decreased uterine/placental perfusion secondary to bleeding

EXPECTED OUTCOME

Patient will exhibit ongoing signs of fetal well-being (i.e., adequate fetal movement, normal fetal heart rate, reactive NST, normal BPP).

NURSING INTERVENTIONS/*RATIONALES*

Monitor fetus daily for signs of tachycardia, decreased movement, loss of reactivity on NST *to identify and treat changes in fetal status early.*

Obtain BPP per physician order *to assess for signs of chronic asphyxia.*

Maintain maternal side-lying position *to prevent compression of aorta and vena cava.*

NURSING DIAGNOSIS: Risk for infection related to anemia and bleeding secondary to placenta previa

EXPECTED OUTCOME

Patient will show no signs of intrauterine infection.

NURSING INTERVENTIONS/*RATIONALES*

Monitor vital signs for elevated temperature, pulse, and decreased blood pressure; monitor laboratory results for elevated white blood cell count, differential shift; check for uterine tenderness and malodorous vaginal discharge *to detect early signs of infection resulting from exposure of placental tissue.*

Provide/teach perineal hygiene *to decrease the risk of ascending infection.*

BPP, biophysical profile; *CBC,* complete blood count; *NST,* nonstress test.

tality. Maternal hypertension is probably the most consistently identified risk factor for abruption (Benedetti, 2002). Cocaine use also is a risk factor, possibly because cocaine use is associated with the development of hypertension (Andres & Day, 2000). Blunt external abdominal trauma, most often the result of motor vehicle accidents or maternal battering, is an increasingly significant cause of placental abruption (Benedetti, 2002). Maternal smoking and poor nutrition may be associated with an increased risk. In the past, maternal age older than 35 years, parity, short umbilical cord, and folic acid deficiency were all thought to increase risk; however, more recent research has failed to confirm this (Benedetti, 2002). Abruption is more likely to occur in twin gestation. There is a significant (5% to 17%) recurrence risk for placental abruption. A woman who has had two previous premature separations has a recurrence risk of 25% in the next pregnancy (Clark, 2004).

Classification Systems

The most common classification of placental abruption is according to type and severity. This classification is summarized in Table 14-7.

Clinical Manifestations

The separation may be partial or complete, or only the margin of the placenta may be involved. Bleeding from the placental site may dissect (separate) the membranes from the decidua basalis and flow out through the vagina; it may remain concealed (retroplacental hemorrhage); or it may do both (see Fig. 14-13). Clinical symptoms vary with the degree of separation (see Table 14-7).

Typically, vaginal bleeding, abdominal pain, and uterine tenderness and contractions are seen with abruptio placentae. Although abdominal pain and uterine tenderness are characteristic of abruption, either finding may be absent in the presence of a silent abruption (Clark, 2004). Bleeding may result in maternal hypovolemia (i.e., shock, oliguria, and anuria) and coagulopathy. Mild to severe uterine hypertonicity is present. Pain is mild to severe and localized over one region of the uterus or diffuse over the uterus with a boardlike abdomen.

Extensive myometrial bleeding damages the uterine muscle. If blood accumulates between the separated placenta and the uterine wall, it may produce a Couvelaire uterus. The uterus appears purplish and copper colored, it is ecchymotic, and contractility is lost. Shock may occur and is out of proportion to blood loss. The Apt test (for blood in amniotic fluid) is positive, hemoglobin and hematocrit levels drop, and coagulation factor levels drop. Clotting defects (DIC) develop in 10% to 30% of women, in most cases within 8 hours of hospital admission. A Kleihauer-Betke stain may be ordered to determine the presence of fetal-to-maternal bleeding (transplacental hemorrhage), although this test appears to be of no value in the general workup of patients with placental abruption (Clark, 2004).

Maternal, Fetal, and Neonatal Outcomes

Maternal mortality rate approaches 1% in abruptio placentae; this condition remains a leading cause of maternal death. The mother's prognosis depends on the extent of placental detachment, overall blood loss, degree of DIC, and time between placental detachment and birth.

Maternal complications are associated with the abruption or its treatment. Hemorrhage, hypovolemic shock, hypofibrinogenemia, and thrombocytopenia are associated with severe abruption. Couvelaire uterus, DIC, and infection may occur. Renal failure and pituitary necrosis (Sheehan's syndrome) may result from ischemia. In rare cases, women who are Rh negative can become sensitized if fetal-to-maternal hemorrhage occurs and the fetal blood type is Rh positive.

Perinatal mortality rate ranges from 15% to 30%. Death occurs from fetal hypoxia, preterm birth, and SGA status. Risks of neurologic deficits are increased. Fetal complications include congenital anomalies (Clark, 2004).

Collaborative Care

Abruptio placentae should be strongly suspected in the woman who has a sudden onset of intense, usually localized, uterine pain, with or without vaginal bleeding. Initial assessment is much the same as for placenta previa. Physical examination usually reveals abdominal pain, uterine tenderness, and contractions. The fundal height may be measured over time, because increasing fundal height indicates concealed bleeding. Approximately 60% of live fetuses exhibit nonreassuring signs on the electronic fetal heart monitor, such as loss of variability and late decelerations; uterine hyperstimulation and increased resting tone may also be noted on the monitor tracing (Benedetti, 2002).

Many women demonstrate coagulopathy, as evidenced by abnormal clotting studies (fibrinogen, platelet count, prothrombin time, partial thromboplastin time, fibrin split products). Sonographic examination is used to rule out placenta previa; however, it is not always diagnostic for abruption. A retroplacental mass may be detected with ultrasonographic examination, but negative findings do not rule out a life-threatening abruption (Clark, 2004).

Nursing diagnoses and expected outcomes are similar to those described for placenta previa.

Hospital Care

Treatment depends on severity of blood loss and fetal maturity and status. If the abruption is mild, expectant management is implemented if the fetus is less than 36 weeks of gestation and not in distress. The woman is hospitalized and closely observed for signs of bleeding and labor. The fetal status is monitored with intermittent FHR monitoring and NST or BPP until fetal maturity is achieved or until the woman's condition deteriorates and immediate birth is indicated. Use of corticosteroids to accelerate fetal lung maturity is appropriately included in the plan of care for the woman managed expectantly (ACOG, 2002a; Antenatal Corticosteroids Revisited, 2000; Purdy & Wiley, 2004). Women who are Rh negative may be given $Rh_o(D)$ immune globulin if fetal-to-maternal hemorrhage occurs and the fetal blood is Rh positive.

If the mother is hemodynamically stable, a vaginal birth may be attempted if the fetus is alive and in no acute distress or if the fetus is dead. In the presence of fetal compromise, severe hemorrhage, coagulopathy, poor labor progress, or increasing uterine resting tone, a cesarean birth is performed. At least one large-bore (16-gauge) IV line should be started. Maternal vital signs are monitored frequently to observe for signs of declining hemodynamic status such as increasing pulse rate and decreasing BP. Serial laboratory studies include hematocrit or hemoglobin determinations and clotting studies. Continuous electronic fetal monitoring is mandatory. An indwelling Foley catheter is inserted for continuous assessment of urine output, an excellent indirect measure of maternal organ perfusion.

Blood and fluid volume replacement will most likely be ordered, with the goals of maintaining the urine output at 30 ml/hr or more and the hematocrit at 30% or more. If these goals are not reached despite vigorous attempts at replacement, hemodynamic monitoring may be necessary. Fresh frozen plasma or cryoprecipitate may be given to maintain the fibrinogen level at a minimum of 100 to 150 mg/dl.

Emotional support for the woman and her family is extremely important. If actively bleeding, the woman is concerned not only for her own well-being but also for the well-being of her fetus. All procedures should be explained, and a support person should be present.

Home Care

Women with abruptio placentae are usually not managed out of the hospital because the placenta can separate at any time and immediate intervention or birth may be necessary.

Cord Insertion and Placental Variations

Velamentous insertion of the cord (vasa previa) is a rare placental anomaly associated with placenta previa and multiple gestation. The cord vessels begin to branch at the membranes and then course onto the placenta (Fig. 14-14, *A*). ROM or traction on the cord may tear one or more of the fetal vessels. As a result, the fetus may rapidly bleed to death. Battledore (marginal) insertion of the cord (Fig. 14-14, *B*) increases the risk of fetal hemorrhage, especially after marginal separation of the placenta.

Rarely, the placenta may be divided into two or more separate lobes, resulting in succenturiate placenta (Fig. 14-14, *C*). Each lobe has a distinct circulation. The vessels collect at the periphery, and the main trunks eventually unite to form the vessels of the cord. Blood vessels joining the lobes may be supported only by the fetal membranes and are therefore in danger of tearing during labor, birth, or expulsion of the placenta. During expulsion of the placenta, one or more of the separate lobes may remain attached to the decidua basalis, preventing uterine contraction and increasing the risk of postpartum hemorrhage.

Clotting Disorders in Pregnancy

Normal Clotting

Normally a delicate balance (homeostasis) is maintained between the opposing hemostatic system and fibrinolytic systems. The hemostatic system is involved in the life-saving process by stopping the flow of blood from injured vessels, in part through the formation of insoluble fibrin, which acts as a hemostatic platelet plug. The coagulation process involves an interaction of the coagulation factors in which

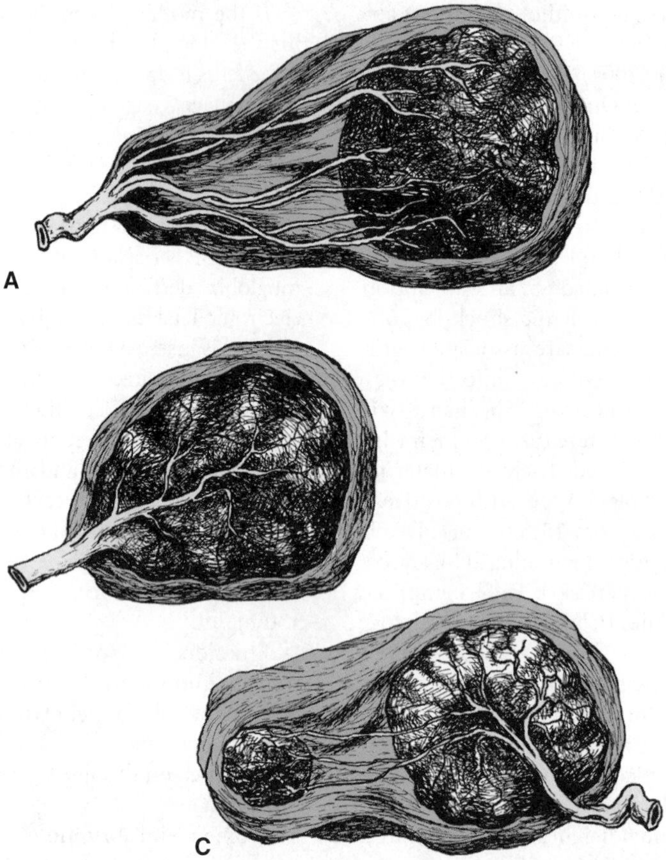

Fig. 14-14 Cord insertion and placental variations. **A,** Velamentous insertion of cord. **B,** Battledore placenta. **C,** Succenturiate placenta.

each factor sequentially activates the factor next in line, the "cascade effect" sequence. The fibrinolytic system is the process by which the fibrin is split into fibrin degradation products and circulation is restored.

Clotting Problems

A history of abnormal bleeding, inheritance of unusual bleeding tendencies, or a report of significant aberrations of laboratory findings indicates a bleeding or clotting problem. For the pregnant woman, bleeding disorders are suspected if the woman has gestational hypertension, HELLP syndrome, retained dead fetus syndrome, amniotic fluid embolism, sepsis, or hemorrhage. Determination of hemostasis is made by testing the usual mechanisms for the control of bleeding, the function of platelets, and the necessary clotting factors. Most clotting disorders are more a concern in the immediate postpartum period. Recognition in the antepartal period may decrease hemorrhagic problems.

Disseminated Intravascular Coagulation

DIC is a pathologic form of clotting that is diffuse and consumes large amounts of clotting factors, causing widespread external or internal bleeding (or both). DIC is an overactivation of the clotting cascade and the fibrinolytic system resulting in depletion of platelets and clotting factors. This results in the formation of multiple fibrin clots throughout the body's vasculature, even in the microcirculation. Blood cells are destroyed as they pass through these fibrin-choked vessels. Thus DIC results in a clinical picture of hemorrhage, anemia, and ischemia.

DIC is always a secondary diagnosis. In the obstetric population, DIC is most often triggered by the release of large amounts of tissue thromboplastin; this occurs in abruptio placentae, retained dead fetus, and amniotic fluid embolus. Severe preeclampsia, HELLP syndrome, and gram-negative sepsis are examples of conditions that can trigger DIC because of widespread damage to vascular integrity.

Medical Management

The diagnosis of DIC is based on clinical findings and laboratory markers. Physical examination reveals unusual bleeding. Spontaneous bleeding from the woman's gums or nose may be noted. Petechiae may appear around the blood pressure cuff placed on her arm. Excessive bleeding may occur from the site of a slight trauma (e.g., venipuncture sites, IM or subcutaneous injection sites, or injury from insertion of urinary catheter). Maternal symptoms may include tachycardia and diaphoresis.

Laboratory tests reveal decreased platelets, fibrinogen, proaccelerin, antihemophilic factor, and prothrombin (the factors consumed during coagulation). Other factors should be normal. Fibrinolysis is first increased but is later severely depressed. Degradation of fibrin leads to the accumulation of fibrin split products in the blood. Fibrin split products have anticoagulant properties and thus prolong the PT. Bleeding time is normal; coagulation time shows no clot; clot retraction time shows no clot; and PTT is increased. DIC must be distinguished from other clotting disorders before therapy is initiated.

The primary management of DIC involves correction of the underlying cause, which may be removal of the dead fetus, treatment of existing infection or preeclampsia or eclampsia, or removal of a placental abruption. Concomitantly, treatment is directed toward support of maternal physiologic functioning and replacing essential factors faster than the body can consume them. Intravenous fluids are given to replace volume lost through severe bleeding. Packed red blood cells are administered to maintain enough circulating red blood cells to ensure tissue oxygenation. Fresh frozen plasma or cryoprecipitate is given to replace fibrinogen and coagulation factors. Platelets may also be administered.

Nursing Care Management

The nurse caring for the woman at risk for DIC must be aware of risk factors. Careful and thorough assessment is required, with particular attention to the signs of bleeding (e.g., petechiae, oozing from injection sites, and hematuria). Because renal failure is one consequence of DIC, urinary output is carefully monitored using an indwelling Foley catheter. Urine output must be maintained at more than 30 ml/hr. Vital signs are assessed frequently.

Supportive measures include keeping the pregnant woman in a side-lying tilt to maximize blood flow to the uterus. Oxygen may be administered through a tight-fitting rebreathing mask at 8 to 10 L/min or per hospital protocol or physician order. Blood and blood products must be administered safely. Fetal assessments are done to monitor fetal well-being.

The educational and emotional needs of the woman and her family must be recognized and supported. They need information about her condition and explanations of unfamiliar equipment and procedures and will most likely be very anxious about the health of the mother and baby.

von Willebrand Disease

von Willebrand disease, a type of hemophilia, is probably the most common of all hereditary bleeding disorders. It results from a factor VIII deficiency and platelet dysfunction. It is transmitted as an incomplete autosomal dominant trait to both sexes. Although von Willebrand disease is rare, it is one of the most common congenital clotting defects in American women of childbearing age. Symptoms include a familial bleeding tendency, previous bleeding episodes, prolonged bleeding time (the most important test), factor VIII deficiency (mild to moderate), and bleeding from mucous membranes. Factor VIII increases during pregnancy, and this increase may be sufficient to offset danger from hemorrhage during childbirth. von Willebrand disease is variable in its clinical course, severity, and laboratory values, so it is possible for this condition to go undetected throughout pregnancy until bleeding problems develop after birth. If the woman is known to have von Willebrand disease before labor, factor VIII levels should be monitored and cryoprecipitate given as needed to maintain activity at 40% of normal near term gestation (Kilpatrick & Laros, 2004).

INFECTIONS IN PREGNANCY

In this section, infections that may occur in pregnancy and affect the pregnancy and the fetus are discussed. Sexually transmitted infections and TORCH infections are addressed. Other infections may also adversely affect the pregnant woman (Box 14-8).

Sexually Transmitted Infections

Sexually transmitted infections are responsible for significant morbidity and mortality in pregnancy. Some consequences of maternal infection, such as infertility and sterility, last a lifetime. Psychosocial sequelae may include altered interpersonal relationships and lowered self-esteem. Congenitally acquired infection may affect the length and quality of a child's life.

Chapter 6 discusses the diagnosis and management of STIs. Chapter 28 discusses neonatal effects and management. This discussion focuses only on the effects of several common STIs on pregnancy and the fetus. Effects on the pregnancy and the fetus vary according to whether or not the infection has been treated at the time of labor and birth.

Sexually transmitted infections (STIs) are infections or infectious disease syndromes primarily transmitted by close, intimate contact. STIs are a direct cause of tremendous human suffering, place heavy demands on health care services, and cost hundreds of millions of dollars to treat. The term *sexually transmitted infection* is not specific for any one disease; rather the term includes more than 25 infectious organisms that are transmitted through sexual activity and the dozens of clinical syndromes that they cause (Institute of Medicine, Committee on Prevention and Control of Sexually Transmitted Diseases, 1997). Despite the U.S. Surgeon General's targeting STIs as a priority for prevention and control efforts, STIs are among the most common health problems in the United States (Institute of Medicine, Committee on Prevention and Control of Sexually Transmitted Diseases, 1997). The Centers for Disease Control and Prevention (CDC) estimates that more than 15 million Americans are infected with STIs every year

BOX 14-8

West Nile Virus in Pregnancy

Humans contract West Nile virus (WNV) from infected mosquitoes. WNV has been associated with miscarriage and illness in the newborn. One woman who had WNV gave birth to an infant with congenital cerebral anomalies; no causative link was established. The Centers for Disease Control and Prevention (CDC) recommends that women who live in an area where the virus has been found and who develop unexplained high fever, meningitis, encephalitis, or acute flaccid paralysis during pregnancy have blood and, if indicated, cerebrospinal fluid testing. If WNV is diagnosed during pregnancy, ultrasonography to assess for structural abnormalities should be performed. Products of conception (if a spontaneous or an induced abortion) and the placenta should be analyzed for viral infection. Infants born to women with suspected or confirmed infection should have a comprehensive clinical examination. Pregnant women should take preventive measures: avoid mosquito-infested areas, wear long sleeves and pants, and use a Deet-containing insect repellent on skin and clothes. The CDC is gathering data on the outcome of pregnancy of approximately 70 women who had WNV during pregnancy.

Source: Centers for Disease Control and Prevention: Interim guidelines for the evaluation of infants born to mothers infected with West Nile virus during pregnancy, *MMWR Morb Mortal Wkly Rep* 53(7):154-157, 2004.

Table 14-8

Maternal, Fetal, and Neonatal Effects and Treatment of Common Sexually Transmitted Infections

INFECTION	MATERNAL EFFECTS	FETAL/NEONATAL EFFECTS	MANAGEMENT
Chlamydia trachomatis (bacteria)	Asymptomatic; may cause salpingitis, ectopic pregnancy, PID, infertility and sterility, postpartum endometritis	Preterm birth, low birth weight; stillbirth, neonatal death; conjunctivitis, pneumonia	Single dose of azithromycin or 7 days of doxycycline; amoxycillin or erythromycin may also be used. Use erythromycin in pregnancy. Test all sexual partners.
Gonorrhea (diplococci)	May cause PID and lead to ectopic pregnancy and sterility, PROM, and chorionitis; if untreated, may have postpartum gonococcal endometritis, acute salpingitis, dermatitis, and arthritis	Preterm birth, ophthalmia neonatorum and pneumonia	Spread by direct contact with lesions and indirectly by transfer by fomites. Treated with a single dose of ceftriaxone, cefixime, ciprofloxacin, or ofloxacin.
Syphilis (spirochete)	Primary: chancre Secondary: maculopopular rash on palms and soles, lymphadenopathy, fever, headache, malaise Tertiary: neurologic, cardiovascular, musculoskeletal, or multiorgan system complications	Late miscarriage and stillbirth; congenital syphilis	Acquired through sexual contact. Parenteral penicillin is preferred for treatment of all stages of syphilis.
Human immunodeficiency virus/acquired immunodeficiency syndrome (virus)	Fatigue, anorexia, weight loss, chronic diarrhea, and fever Virus present in breast milk Postpartum: increased risk for URIs, vaginitis, postpartum endometritis, and poor wound healing	Maternal-fetal transmission of virus	Transmitted through contact with body fluids. Pregnancy is not recommended; preconception counseling is advised. Primary drug for treatment is zidovudine (AZT). Elective cesarean birth reduces rate of vertical transmission. Breastfeeding is contraindicated.
Human papillomavirus (genital warts) (virus)	Proliferation and increased friability of lesions	Neonatal respiratory or laryngeal papillomatosis	Sexually transmitted. Recommend removal of large, outward-growing lesions; carbon dioxide laser treatments have been used.
Vaginal candidiasis (yeast)	Pain, itching, vaginal discharge; increased rate of infection during pregnancy	Oral candidiasis in newborns	Spread by direct contact. Mother is treated with clotrimazole, miconazole, butoconazole, or terconazole. Newborn is treated with oral nystatin.
Trichomonas vaginalis (protozoa)	May be present on nipples of breastfeeding mother	Fever and irritability	Metronidazole should be administered to pregnant women only in the second and third trimesters.
Group B streptococci (GBS) (diplococci)	Miscarriage, stillbirth, preterm birth, fever, septicemia, and puerperal infection	Sepsis and meningitis, blindness, deafness, mental retardation, learning disabilities, death	Normal flora; vertical transmission to newborn during passage through birth canal. Treated with penicillin, ampicillin, cephalothin, or erythromycin. Intrapartum treatment of women who are GBS carriers reduces the incidence of neonatal infection.
Varicella (virus)	Severe disseminated, epidemic type of varicella can be fatal to mother	Miscarriage; severe disseminated, epidemic type of varicella can be fatal to fetus. If maternal varicella occurs in the first trimester, fetus may develop varicella syndrome; chorioretinitis, hydrocephalus	Newborn may receive prophylactic treatment. Transmitted by direct contact. Give VZIG to exposed pregnant women. Treat severe infections with IV acyclovir or vidarabine.

IV, intravenous; *PID*, pelvic inflammatory disease; *PROM*, premature rupture of membranes; *URI*, upper respiratory infection; *VZIG*, varicella-zoster immune globulin.

(Workowski, Levine, & Wasserheit, 2002). The most common STIs in women are chlamydia, human papillomavirus, gonorrhea, herpes simplex virus type 2, syphilis, and human immunodeficiency virus (HIV) infection.

Factors that influence the development and management of STIs during pregnancy include previous history of STI or pelvic inflammatory disease, number of current sexual partners, frequency of intercourse, and anticipated sexual activity during pregnancy. Lifestyle choices also may affect STIs in the perinatal period. Women who use IV drugs or who have partners that use IV drugs are at risk. Other lifestyle factors that increase susceptibility to STIs (through suppressive effects on the immune system) include smoking, alcohol use, inadequate or poor nutrition, and high levels of fatigue or personal stress.

Physical examination and laboratory studies to determine the presence of STIs in the pregnant woman are the same as those done in nonpregnant women (see Chapter 6).

Treatment of specific STIs may be different for the pregnant woman and may even be different at different stages of pregnancy. Table 14-8 describes the maternal, fetal, and neonatal effects and treatment during pregnancy of common STIs (i.e., chlamydial infections, gonorrhea, syphilis, HIV, human papillomavirus, vaginal candidiasis, *Trichomonas vaginalis,* and group B streptococci). Varicella may also place a woman at risk during the childbearing cycle and is included in Table 14-8.

Infected women need instruction on how to take prescribed medications, information on whether their partner(s) also need to be evaluated and treated, and a review of preventive measures to avoid reinfection.

TORCH Infections

TORCH infections can affect a pregnant woman and her fetus. *T*oxoplasmosis, *o*ther infections (e.g., hepatitis), *r*ubella virus, *c*ytomegalovirus, and *h*erpes simplex viruses, known collectively as TORCH infections, are a group of organisms capable of crossing the placenta and adversely affecting the development of the fetus. Generally, all TORCH infections produce influenza-like symptoms in the mother, but fetal and neonatal effects are more serious. TORCH infections and their maternal and fetal effects are presented in Table 14-9.

Infection Control

Infection control measures are essential to protect care providers and to prevent nosocomial infection of patients, regardless of the infectious agent. The risk for occupational transmission varies with the disease. Even when the risk is low, as with HIV, the existence of any risk warrants reasonable precautions. Precautions against airborne disease transmission are available in all health care agencies. Standard Precautions (precautions to use in care of all persons for infection control) are listed in Box 6-5, and additional precautions for labor and birth settings are listed in Box 18-4.

SURGERY DURING PREGNANCY

The incidence of surgery requiring anesthesia during pregnancy ranges from 0.2% to 2.2%, affecting an estimated 50,000 women each year (Ludmir & Stubblefield, 2002). The need for abdominal surgery occurs as often among pregnant women as among nonpregnant women of comparable age. However, diagnosis is more difficult in the pregnant woman. An enlarged uterus and displaced internal organs may make abdominal palpation more difficult, may alter the position of an affected organ, or may change the usual signs associated with a particular disorder. The most common conditions necessitating abdominal surgery during pregnancy are appendicitis, intestinal obstruction, and gynecologic problems.

Appendicitis

Appendicitis occurs approximately once in 2000 pregnancies. Appendicitis occurs in approximately the same frequency during each trimester of pregnancy and in the postpartum period (Ludmir & Stubblefield, 2002). The diagnosis is often delayed because the usual signs and symptoms mimic some normal changes of pregnancy such as nausea and vomiting and increased white blood cell (WBC) count. As pregnancy progresses, the appendix is pushed upward and to the right from its usual anatomic location (see Fig. 10-12). Because of these changes, appendiceal rupture and peritonitis occur two to three times more often in pregnant women than in nonpregnant women.

The woman with appendicitis most commonly has right lower quadrant pain, nausea and vomiting, and loss of appetite. Approximately half of these women will have muscle guarding. Temperature may be normal or mildly increased (to 38.3° C). Because of the physiologic increase in WBCs that occurs in pregnancy, significant increases associated with appendicitis must be documented either by rising levels on serial samples or by an increasing left shift.

The diagnosis of appendicitis requires a high level of suspicion because the typical signs and symptoms are similar to those found in many other conditions, including pyelonephritis, round ligament pain, placental abruption, torsion of an ovarian cyst, cholecystitis, and preterm labor (Ludmir & Stubblefield, 2002).

Appendectomy before rupture usually does not require either antibiotic or tocolytic therapy. If surgery is delayed until after rupture, multiple antibiotics are ordered. Rupture is likely to result in preterm labor and necessitate the use of tocolytic agents.

Intestinal Obstruction

The second most common nonobstetric abdominal emergency in pregnancy is intestinal obstruction. Any woman with a laparotomy scar is more likely to have an intestinal obstruction (adynamic ileus) during gestation. Adhesions as a result of previous surgery or pelvic inflammatory disease, an enlarging uterus, and displacement of the intestines are etiologic factors.

Constipation; persistent cramplike, abdominal pain; vomiting; auscultatory rushes within the abdomen; and "laddering" of the intestinal shadows on x-ray films aid in the diagnosis of intestinal obstruction. Immediate surgical intervention is required for release of the obstruction. Pregnancy is rarely affected by the surgery, assuming the absence of complications such as peritonitis.

Table 14-9

Maternal Infection: TORCH

INFECTION	MATERNAL EFFECTS	FETAL EFFECTS	COUNSELING: PREVENTION, IDENTIFICATION, AND MANAGEMENT
Toxoplasmosis (protozoa)	Acute infection similar to influenza, lymphadenopathy Woman immune after first episode (except in immunocompromised patients)	With maternal acute infection, parasitemia Less likely to occur with maternal chronic infection Miscarriage likely with acute infection early in pregnancy	Use good handwashing technique. Avoid eating raw meat; avoid exposure to litter used by infected cats; if cats in house, have toxoplasma titer checked. If titer is rising during early pregnancy, abortion may be considered an option.
Other			
Hepatitis A (infectious hepatitis) (virus)	Miscarriage, cause of liver failure during pregnancy Fever, malaise, nausea, and abdominal discomfort	Exposure during first trimester, fetal anomalies, fetal or neonatal hepatitis, preterm birth, intrauterine fetal death	Usually spread by droplet or hand contact especially by culinary workers; gammaglobulin can be given as prophylaxis for hepatitis A; vaccine is available for populations at risk.
Hepatitis B (serum hepatitis) (virus)	Symptoms variable: fever, rash, arthralgia, depressed appetite, dyspepsia, abdominal pain, generalized aching, malaise, weakness, jaundice, tender and enlarged liver	Infection occurs during birth Maternal vaccination during pregnancy presents no risk for fetus	Generally passed by contaminated needles, syringes, or blood transfusions or sexually; also can be transmitted orally (but incubation period is longer); hepatitis B immune globulin can be given prophylactically after exposure. Hepatitis B vaccination recommendations: universal infant immunizations, universal immunizations of previously unvaccinated adolescents age 11-12 yr, adolescents and adults at increased risk. Populations at risk are women from Asia, Pacific Islands, Indochina, Haiti, South Africa, Alaska (women of Eskimo descent); other women at risk include health care providers, users of intravenous drugs, those sexually active with multiple partners or single partner with multiple risks.
Rubella (3-day German measles) (virus)	Joint pain, muscle aches, rash, fever, mild symptoms; suboccipital lymph nodes may be swollen; some photophobia Occasionally arthritis or encephalitis Miscarriage	Incidence of congenital anomalies: first trimester 50%-90% Exposure during first 2 mo: malformations of heart, eyes, ears, or brain; abnormal dermatoglyphics Exposure after fourth mo: hearing loss, psychomotor retardation, systemic infection, hepatosplenomegaly, intrauterine growth restriction, rash, heart disease, cataracts	Vaccination of pregnant women contraindicated; pregnancy should be prevented for 3 mo after vaccination; pregnant women nonreactive to hemagglutinin-inhibition antigen can be safely vaccinated after birth.
Cytomegalovirus (CMV) (a herpesvirus)	Respiratory or sexually transmitted asymptomatic illness or mononucleosis-like syndrome, may have cervical discharge No immunity develops	Fetal death or severe, generalized disease: hemolytic anemia and jaundice, hydrocephaly or microcephaly, pneumonitis, hepatosplenomegaly, deafness, mental retardation	Virus may be reactivated and cause disease in utero or during birth in subsequent pregnancies; fetal infection may occur during passage through infected birth canal; disease is commonly progressive through infancy and childhood.
Herpes genitalis (herpes simplex virus, type 2 [HSV-2])	Primary blisters, rash, fever, malaise, nausea, headache; pregnancy risks include miscarriage, preterm labor, stillbirths	Transmission occurs after rupture of membranes; congenital effects include skin lesions and scarring, IUGR, mental retardation, microcephaly Active HSV in first trimester, there is 20%-50% miscarriage/stillbirth rate	Risk of transmission is greatest during vaginal birth if woman has active lesions. Acyclovir not recommended in pregnancy; treat symptomatically.

Sources: Centers for Disease Control and Prevention: Sexually transmitted diseases treatment guidelines 2002, *MMWR Morb Mortal Wkly Rep* 51(RR-6):1-82, 2002; Cowles TA, Gonik B: Perinatal infections. In Fanaroff AA, Martin RJ (eds): *Neonatal-perinatal medicine: diseases of the fetus and infant*, ed 7, St Louis, 2002, Mosby.

Gynecologic Problems

Pregnancy predisposes a woman to ovarian problems, especially during the first trimester. Ovarian cysts and twisting of ovarian cysts or adnexal tissues may occur. Other problems include retained or enlarged cystic corpus luteum of pregnancy and bacterial invasion of reproductive or other intraperitoneal organs.

Laparotomy or laparoscopy may be required to discriminate between ovarian problems and early ectopic pregnancy, appendicitis, or an infectious process.

Care Management

Initial assessment of the pregnant woman requiring surgery focuses on her signs and symptoms. A thorough history and a physical examination are performed. Laboratory testing includes, at a minimum, a CBC with differential and a urinalysis. Fetal heart rate and activity and uterine activity should be monitored; constant vigilance is maintained for symptoms of impending obstetric complications. The extent of preoperative assessment is determined by the immediacy of surgical intervention and the specific condition that requires surgery.

Hospital Care

The woman and her family are concerned about fetal well-being; their greatest fear related to surgery is of losing the baby. An important part of preoperative nursing care is encouraging the woman to express her fears, concerns, and questions.

Preoperative care for a pregnant woman differs from that of a nonpregnant woman in one significant aspect: the presence of at least one other person—the fetus. Continuous FHR and uterine contraction monitoring should be performed if the fetus is considered viable. Procedures such as preparation of the operative site and time of insertion of IV lines and urinary retention catheters vary with the physician and the facility. However, in every instance, there is total restriction of solid food and fluids or a clear specification of the type, amount, and time at which clear liquids may be taken before surgery. Some bowel preparation such as clear liquids and laxatives may be required before surgery. Food by mouth is restricted for several hours before a scheduled procedure. If the woman experiences a prolonged NPO status, IV fluids with dextrose should be given. Even if she has had nothing by mouth—but more important, if surgery is unexpected—the woman is in danger of vomiting and aspirating, and special precautions are taken before the anesthetic is administered (e.g., administering an antacid).

Intraoperatively, perinatal nurses may collaborate with the surgical staff to provide for the special needs of pregnant women undergoing surgery. To improve fetal oxygenation, the woman should be positioned on the operating table with a lateral tilt to avoid maternal compression of the vena cava. Continuous fetal and uterine monitoring during the procedure is recommended because the risk of preterm labor is great. Monitoring can be accomplished using sterile Aquasonic gel and a sterile sleeve for the transducer. Uterine contractions may be palpated manually.

In the immediate recovery period, general observations and care pertinent to postoperative recovery are initiated. Frequent assessments are carried out for several hours after surgery. Whether the woman is cared for in the surgical postanesthesia recovery area or in a labor and delivery unit, continuous fetal and uterine monitoring will likely be initiated or resumed because of the increased risk of preterm labor. Tocolysis may be necessary if preterm labor occurs.

Home Care

Plans for the woman's return home and for convalescent care should be completed as early as possible before discharge. Depending on her insurance coverage, nursing care may be provided through a home health agency. If not, the woman and other support persons must be taught necessary skills and procedures, such as wound care. Provision should be made for supervised practice before discharge. Box 14-9 lists information that should be included in discharge teaching for the postoperative patient. The woman may also need referrals to various community agencies for evaluation of the home situation, child care, home health care, and financial or other assistance.

BOX 14-9

Discharge Teaching for Home Care

- Care of incision site
- Diet and elimination related to gastrointestinal function
- Signs and symptoms of developing complications; wound infection, thrombophlebitis, pneumonia
- Equipment needed and technique for assessing temperature
- Recommended schedule for resumption of activities of daily living
- Treatments and medications ordered
- List of resource persons and their telephone numbers
- Schedule of follow-up visits

If birth has not occurred:

- Assessment of fetal activity (kick counts)
- Signs of preterm labor

TRAUMA DURING PREGNANCY

Trauma is a common complication during pregnancy because the majority of pregnant women in the United States continue activities as usual. Thus pregnant women are at the same risk as others for vehicular crashes, falls, burns, industrial mishaps, violence, gunshot wounds, and other injuries in the home and community. Treatment of pregnant trauma victims is complicated because doctors and nurses who have expertise in the care of trauma victims rarely have similar expertise in the care of pregnant women.

Significance

Approximately 8% of pregnancies are complicated by physical trauma (Van Hook, 2002). As pregnancy progresses, the risk of trauma seems to increase because more cases of trauma are reported in the third trimester than earlier in gestation.

Special considerations for mother and fetus are necessary when trauma occurs during pregnancy because of the physiologic alterations that accompany pregnancy and because of the presence of the fetus. Fetal survival depends on maternal survival; therefore the pregnant woman must receive immediate stabilization and appropriate care for optimal fetal outcome.

Acts of violence are a significant health problem in the United States. The risk of trauma caused by battering and abuse is increased during pregnancy, and rates of recurrence are high. Women who are abused during pregnancy have a threefold risk of being murdered compared with their nonpregnant abused controls (McFarlane et al, 2002). African-American women have a threefold higher risk than Caucasion women in the same pregnancy group (McFarlane et al, 2002).

Trauma is the leading nonobstetric cause of maternal death. Maternal death caused by trauma is usually the result of head injury or hemorrhagic shock. Fetal death usually occurs as a sequela to maternal death or as a result of placental abruption.

The majority of trauma injuries during pregnancy are minor and have no impact on pregnancy outcome. However, each case of trauma during pregnancy must be evaluated carefully because pregnancy can mask signs of severe injury. Trauma increases the incidence of miscarriage, preterm labor, abruptio placentae, and stillbirth. Less serious trauma is associated with numerous complications for pregnancy, including fetomaternal hemorrhage, abruptio placentae, intrauterine fetal death, and preterm labor and birth (Gilbert & Harmon, 2003). The effect of trauma on pregnancy is influenced by the length of gestation, type and severity of the trauma, and degree of disruption of uterine and fetal physiologic features. Careful evaluation of mother and fetus after all types of trauma is imperative.

Maternal Physiologic Characteristics

Optimal care for the pregnant woman after trauma is dependent on understanding the physiologic state of pregnancy and its effects on trauma. The pregnant woman's body will exhibit responses different from those of a nonpregnant person to the same traumatic insults. Because of the different responses to injury during pregnancy, management strategies must be adapted for appropriate resuscitation, fluid therapy, positioning, assessments, and most other interventions.

The uterus and bladder are confined to the bony pelvis during the first trimester of pregnancy and are at reduced risk for injury in cases of abdominal trauma. After pregnancy progresses beyond the fourteenth week, the uterus becomes an abdominal organ, and the risk for injury increases in cases of abdominal trauma. During the second and third trimesters, the distended bladder becomes an abdominal organ and is at increased risk for injury and rupture. Bowel injuries occur less often during pregnancy because of the protection provided by the enlarged uterus.

The elevated levels of progesterone that accompany pregnancy relax smooth muscle and profoundly affect the gastrointestinal tract. Gastrointestinal motility decreases, with a resultant increased time required for gastric emptying, whereas the production of hydrochloric acid increases in the last trimester, and the gastroesophageal sphincter relaxes. Airway management of the unconscious pregnant woman is of critical importance.

NURSE ALERT The unconscious pregnant woman is at increased risk for regurgitation of gastric contents and aspiration whenever her head is positioned lower than her stomach or if abdominal pressure is applied. ■

A pregnant woman has decreased tolerance for hypoxia and apnea because of her decreased functional residual capacity and increased renal loss of bicarbonate. Acidosis develops more quickly in the pregnant than in the nonpregnant state.

Cardiac output (CO) increases 44% to 50% over prepregnancy values and is positionally dependent in the third trimester. Because of compression of the inferior vena cava and descending aorta by the pregnant uterus, CO will decrease dramatically if the woman is placed in the supine position. The supine position must be avoided, even in women with cervical spine injuries. It is a primary priority that lateral uterine displacement be accomplished without any head movement. As soon as the neck is immobilized, the stretcher should be tilted laterally.

Circulating blood volume increases 50% during gestation, and pregnant women can tolerate a 1000 ml blood loss readily without demonstrating clinical signs. Hemodynamic instability that indicates the need for transfusion may not be apparent until blood loss nears 1500 to 2000 ml. Clinical signs of hemorrhage do not appear until after a 30% loss of circulating volume occurs. Although heart rate increases with pregnancy, a maternal heart rate greater than 100 beats/min should be considered abnormal.

Fetal Physiologic Characteristics

Perfusion of the uterine arteries, which provide the primary blood supply to the uteroplacental unit, depends on adequate maternal arterial pressure because these vessels lack autoregulation. Therefore maternal hypotension decreases uterine and fetal perfusion. Maternal shock results in splanchnic and uterine artery vasoconstriction, which decreases blood flow and oxygen transport to the fetus. Electronic fetal monitoring (EFM) tracings can assist in the evaluation of maternal status after trauma. EFM tracings reflect fetal cardiac responses to hypoxia and hypoperfusion, including tachycardia or bradycardia, decreased or absent baseline variability, and late decelerations.

Careful monitoring of fetal status assists greatly in maternal assessment, because the fetal monitor tracing works as an "oximeter" of internal maternal well-being. Hypoperfusion may be present in the pregnant woman before the onset of clinical signs of shock. The EFM tracings show the first signs of maternal compromise, such as when maternal heart rate, BP, and color appear normal, yet the EFM printout shows signs of fetal hypoxia (Murray, 1997).

Mechanisms of Trauma

Blunt Abdominal Trauma

Blunt abdominal trauma is most commonly the result of motor vehicle crashes but also may be the result of battering or falls. Maternal and fetal morbidity and mortality rates associated with motor vehicle accidents are directly correlated with whether the mother remains inside the vehicle or is ejected. Maternal death is usually the result of a head injury or exsanguination from a major vessel rupture. Serious retroperitoneal hemorrhage after lower abdominal and pelvic trauma is reported more often during pregnancy. Serious maternal abdominal injuries are usually the result of splenic rupture or liver and renal injury.

When maternal survival of trauma occurs, fetal death is usually the result of abruptio placentae. Placental separation is thought to be a result of deformation of the elastic myometrium around the relatively inelastic placenta. Shearing of the placental edge from the underlying decidua basalis results and is worsened by the increased intrauterine pressure resulting from the impact. It is imperative that all pregnant victims be carefully evaluated for signs and symptoms of abruptio placentae after even minor blunt abdominal trauma.

NURSE ALERT Signs and symptoms of abruptio placentae include uterine tenderness or pain, uterine irritability, uterine contractions, vaginal bleeding, leaking of amniotic fluid, and a change in fetal heart rate characteristics. ■

Pelvic fracture may result from severe injury and may produce bladder trauma or retroperitoneal bleeding with two-point displacement of pelvic bones that usually occurs. One point of displacement is commonly at the symphysis pubis and the second point is posterior, because of the structure of the pelvis. Careful evaluation for clinical signs of internal hemorrhage is indicated.

Direct fetal injury as a complication of trauma during pregnancy most often involves the fetal skull and brain (Gilbert & Harmon, 2003). Most commonly this injury accompanies maternal pelvic fracture in late gestation, after the fetal head becomes engaged. When the force of the impact is great enough to fracture the maternal pelvis, the fetus will often sustain a skull fracture. Evaluation for fetal skull fracture or intracranial hemorrhage is indicated.

Uterine rupture as a result of trauma is rare, occurring in only 0.6% of all reported cases of trauma during pregnancy. Uterine rupture depends on numerous factors, including gestational age; the intensity of the impact; and the presence of a predisposing factor, such as a distended uterus caused by polyhydramnios or multiple gestation, or the presence of a uterine scar from previous uterine surgery. When uterine rupture occurs, the force responsible is usually a direct, high-energy blow. Fetal death is common with traumatic uterine rupture. However, maternal death occurs less than 10% of the time, and when it occurs it is usually the result of massive injuries sustained from an impact severe enough to rupture the uterus.

Penetrating Abdominal Trauma

Bullet wounds are the most frequent cause of penetrating abdominal injury, followed by stab wounds. In the majority of cases of penetrating abdominal wounds, the woman survives, but the fetus does not. The enlarged uterus may protect other maternal organs, but the fetus is more vulnerable.

Numerous factors determine the extent and severity of maternal and fetal injury from a bullet wound, including size and velocity of the bullet, anatomic region penetrated, angle of entry, path of the bullet, organs damaged, gestational age, and exit wound. Once the bullet enters the body, it may ricochet several times as it encounters organs or bone, or it may sever a large blood vessel. During the second half of pregnancy, the fetus usually sustains a direct injury from the bullet. Gunshot wounds require surgical exploration to determine the extent of injury and repair damage as needed.

Stab wounds are limited by the length and width of the penetrating object and are usually confined to the pathway of the weapon. Maternal and fetal injury are less if the stab wound is located in the upper abdomen and if the angle of penetration is downward rather than upward. Stab wounds usually require surgical exploration to clean out debris, determine extent of injury, and repair damage.

Thoracic Trauma

Thoracic trauma is reported to produce 25% of all trauma deaths. Pulmonary contusion results from nearly 75% of blunt thoracic trauma and is a potentially life-threatening condition. Pulmonary contusion can be difficult to recognize, especially if flail chest also is present or if there is no evidence of thoracic injury. Pulmonary contusion should be suspected in cases of thoracic injury, especially after blunt acceleration or deceleration trauma, such as that occurring when a rapidly moving vehicle crashes into an immovable object.

Penetrating wounds into the chest can result in pneumothorax or hemothorax. This type of injury is usually caused by a vehicular crash that results in impalement by the steering column or a loose article in the vehicle that became a projectile with the force of impact. Stab wounds into the chest also may occur as a result of violence.

Care Management

Immediate Stabilization

Immediate priorities for stabilization of the pregnant woman after trauma should be identical to those of the nonpregnant trauma patient. Pregnancy should not result in any restriction of the usual diagnostic, pharmacologic, or resuscitative procedures or maneuvers. Fetal survival depends on maternal survival, and stabilization of the mother improves fetal chance of survival. The perinatal nurse is often called on to function collaboratively with emergency department or trauma unit staff members in providing care for the pregnant trauma victim.

NURSE ALERT Priorities of care for the pregnant woman after trauma must be to resuscitate the woman and stabilize her condition *first,* and then consider fetal needs. ■

In cases of minor trauma, the woman is evaluated for vaginal bleeding, uterine irritability, abdominal tenderness, abdominal pain or cramps, and evidence of hypovolemia. A change in, or absence of, FHR or fetal activity; leakage of amniotic fluid; and presence of fetal cells in the maternal circulation are also included in the assessment.

Primary Survey

In cases of major trauma, the systematic evaluation begins with a primary survey and the initial ABCs of resuscitation:

- *Airway:* Establish and maintain an airway.
- *Breathing:* Ensure adequate breathing.
- *Circulation:* Maintain an adequate circulatory volume.

Increased oxygen needs during gestation necessitate a rapid response. The presence of a cervical spine injury is always assumed.

NURSE ALERT Hyperextension of the neck is avoided; instead jaw thrust is used to establish an airway for the trauma victim. ■

Once an airway is established, assessment should focus on adequacy of oxygenation. The chest wall is observed for movement. If breathing is absent, ventilations and endotracheal intubation are initiated. Supplemental oxygen should be administered with a tight-fitting, nonrebreathing face mask at 10 to 12 L per minute to maintain a maternal arterial oxygen tension (PaO_2) greater than 60 mm Hg and a hemoglobin saturation greater than 90% to maintain fetal status. The chest wall is assessed for penetrating chest wound or flail chest. Breathing with a flail chest will be rapid and labored; chest wall movements will be uncoordinated and asymmetric; crepitus from bony fragments may be palpated.

Rapid placement of two large-bore (14- to 16-gauge) IV lines is necessary in the majority of seriously injured patients. It is important to place the lines while veins are still distended. Infusion of crystalloids such as Ringer's solution or normal saline solution should be given as a 3:1 ratio; that is, 3 ml of crystalloid replacement to 1 ml of the estimated blood loss is given over the first 30 to 60 minutes of acute resuscitation. Because of the 50% increase in blood volume during pregnancy, published formulas for nonpregnant adults used for estimating crystalloid and blood replacement to counter blood loss must be adjusted upward for pregnancy.

Replacement of red blood cells and other blood components is anticipated, and blood is drawn for type, crossmatch, CBC, and platelet count. Vasopressor drugs to restore maternal arterial BP should be avoided, if possible, until volume replacement is administered.

After 20 weeks of gestation, venous return to the heart is best accomplished by positioning the uterus to one side to eliminate the weight of the uterus compressing the inferior vena cava or the descending aorta. This facilitates efforts to establish the forward flow of blood through resuscitation and stabilization. If a lateral position is not possible because of resuscitative efforts or cervical spine immobilization, the uterus can be manually deflected to the left, or a wedge can be inserted underneath the right side of the backboard or stretcher.

Signs of bleeding may be more difficult to recognize in the pregnant woman because a 30% to 35% loss of maternal blood volume may produce only a minimal change in maternal MAP. Hypovolemia can be detrimental for the fetus because the vascular bed of the uterus is a low-resistance system that depends on adequate maternal arterial pressure to maintain uterine and fetal perfusion. Maternal hypovolemia can be fatal for the fetus.

Establishing a baseline neurologic status (level of consciousness, pupil size and reactivity) is essential. The Glasgow Coma Scale is commonly used at the scene of the accident to help determine the extent of the head injury. The scale is simple and easy to use (Box 14-10).

Secondary Survey

After immediate resuscitation and successful stabilization measures, a more detailed secondary survey of the mother and fetus should be accomplished. A complete physical assessment including all body systems is performed.

BOX 14-10

Glasgow Coma Scale

Eyes	Open	Spontaneously	4
		To verbal command	3
		To pain	2
		No response	1
Best motor response	To verbal command	Obeys	6
	To painful stimulus	Localizes pain	5
		Flexion-withdrawal	4
		Flexion-abnormal (decorticate rigidity)	3
		Extension (decerebrate rigidity)	2
		No response	1
Best verbal response		Oriented and converses	5
		Disoriented and converses	4
		Inappropriate words	3
		Incomprehensible sounds	2
		No response	1
Total			3-15

The maternal abdomen should be evaluated carefully, because a large percentage of serious injuries involve the uterus, intraperitoneal structures, and retroperitoneum. The pregnant woman's stomach is assumed to be full. A nasogastric tube can be used to empty the stomach to help prevent acid aspiration syndrome. An empty stomach facilitates respiratory efforts. The uterus should be evaluated for evidence of gross deformity, tenderness, irritability, or contractions.

The greatest clinical concern after vehicular crashes is abruptio placentae, because up to 40% of these women will have an abruption (Van Hook, 2002). Assessments should focus on recognition of this complication, with careful evaluation of fetal monitor tracings, uterine tenderness, labor, or vaginal bleeding. Ultrasound examination may be performed to determine gestational age, viability of fetus, and placental location. However, ultrasound studies cannot exclude abruptio placentae.

If trauma is the result of a penetrating wound, the woman should be completely undressed and carefully examined for all entrance and exit wounds. A bullet may be located on x-ray films. Exploratory laparotomy is necessary after a gunshot wound to explore the abdominal cavity for organ damage and to repair any damage present, with careful examination of all organs, the entire bowel, and posterior vessels. If uterine injury is determined, a careful evaluation of the risks and benefits of cesarean birth is quickly accomplished. A cesarean birth is desirable if the fetus is alive and near term and may be necessary for the preterm fetus because of the high incidence of fetal injury in these cases. Tetanus prophylaxis guidelines are not changed by pregnancy. The fetus usually tolerates surgery and anesthesia if adequate uterine perfusion and oxygenation are maintained.

Electronic Fetal Monitoring

Continuous EFM may show early signs of abruptio placentae, including a change in baseline rate, loss of accelerations, or the presence of late decelerations. Fetal monitoring should be initiated soon after the woman is stable because abruptio placentae usually becomes apparent shortly after the injury. Fetal monitoring should be continued and further evaluation initiated if any of the aforementioned signs occur. Palpation is required to evaluate the intensity of contractions and the uterine resting tone. It is important to palpate between contractions to verify that the uterus is well relaxed. If the uterus does not relax between contractions, abruptio placentae could be present.

Abruptio placentae occurring after trauma may be delayed up to 48 hours after the incident. EFM periods of 2 to 6 hours after minor trauma are adequate if there are no uterine contractions, uterine tenderness, or bleeding.

LEGAL TIP Care of the Pregnant Woman after Minor Trauma After minor trauma, the pregnant woman may be discharged after an adequate period of EFM that demonstrates fetal reassurance and absence of uterine contractions. However, clear instructions must be given for immediate return if vaginal bleeding, leaking of amniotic fluid, decreased fetal movement, or abdominal pain occurs. ■

In addition to assisting with stabilization of the woman, the nurse provides emotional support for the injured woman and her family. If the trauma is the result of a motor vehicle accident, other family members may also have been critically injured or killed. The nurse collaborates with other staff to make sure that questions are answered and consistent information given. Grief support may be necessary.

Perimortem Cesarean Delivery

In the presence of multisystem trauma, perimortem cesarean birth may be indicated. Removal of the stressor of pregnancy early in the process of resuscitation may increase the chance for maternal survival. Fetal survival is unlikely if cesarean birth is accomplished more than 20 minutes after maternal death. Therefore, to facilitate resuscitative efforts, consideration may be given to cesarean birth for maternal benefit after 5 minutes of resuscitative efforts that produce no response in the mother.

Discharge Planning

The woman may be discharged home after several hours of evaluation following minor trauma. Her vital signs should be stable, with no evidence of bleeding at the time of discharge. The fetal tracing should be reassuring before monitoring is discontinued and the woman discharged. Education for the woman and her family is very important. She should be instructed to contact her health care provider immediately if changes in fetal movement or signs and symptoms indicative of preterm labor, premature rupture of membranes, or placental abruption develop. If the trauma occurred as a result of a motor vehicle accident, the importance of wearing a seat belt should be reinforced and she should be given directions for using it correctly during pregnancy (i.e., position the lap belt over hips and thighs rather than across the abdomen; see Fig. 11-19). If the trauma occurred as a result of domestic violence, the woman may need information about the abuse cycle; referral to a crisis center, law enforcement agency, or counseling center; and help in forming a safety plan.

Key Points

- Hypertensive disorders during pregnancy are a leading cause of maternal and perinatal morbidity and mortality worldwide.
- The cause of preeclampsia is unknown, and there are no known reliable tests for predicting women at risk for developing preeclampsia/eclampsia.
- Preeclampsia/eclampsia is a multisystem disease, and the pathologic changes are present long before clinical manifestations, such as hypertension, are evident.
- Once preeclampsia becomes clinically evident, therapeutic interventions are palliative (e.g., bed rest and diet) and may slow the progression of the disease, allowing the pregnancy to continue, but the underlying pathology continues.
- The HELLP syndrome, which usually becomes apparent during the third trimester, is considered life threatening.
- Magnesium sulfate, the anticonvulsant of choice for preventing eclampsia, requires careful monitoring of reflexes, respirations, and renal function; its antidote, calcium gluconate, should be at the bedside.
- Intent of emergency interventions for eclampsia is to prevent self-injury, ensure adequate oxygenation, reduce aspiration risk, and establish control with magnesium sulfate.
- Blood loss during pregnancy should always be regarded as a warning sign until ruled out by the woman's health care provider.
- Ectopic pregnancy is a significant cause of maternal morbidity and mortality even in developed countries.
- Abruptio placentae and placenta previa are differentiated by type of bleeding, uterine tonicity, and presence or absence of pain.
- Clotting disorders are associated with many obstetric complications.
- The physiologic adaptations of pregnancy mask warning signs and changes in vital signs during early shock states.
- The potential hazards of therapeutic interventions may further compromise the woman experiencing hemorrhagic disorders.
- Pregnancy confers no immunity against infection, and both mother and fetus must be considered when the pregnant woman contracts an infection.
- HIV is transmitted through blood, semen, and perinatal events.
- *Chlamydia trachomatis* is the most common sexually transmitted bacterial pathogen in the United States and is responsible for substantial morbidity, personal suffering, and economic burden.
- STIs often occur in groups; what appear to be resistant infections actually may be multiple infections or reinfections.
- Abuse of alcohol and drugs compromises the body's immune system and increases the risk for HIV infection and associated conditions.
- Because medical history and examination cannot reliably identify all persons with HIV or other blood-borne pathogens, blood and body fluid precautions should be used consistently for everyone.

- STIs and genital and perigenital infections are biologic events, for which all individuals have a right to expect objective, compassionate, and effective health care.
- Preoperative care for a pregnant woman differs from that for a nonpregnant woman in one significant aspect: the presence of at least one other person—the fetus.
- Trauma from accidents is the most common cause of death in women of childbearing age.
- Fetal survival depends on maternal survival. After trauma, the first priority is resuscitation and stabilization of the mother before consideration of fetal concerns.
- Minor trauma is associated with major complications for the pregnancy, including abruptio placentae, fetomaternal hemorrhage, preterm labor and birth, and fetal death.

Answer Guidelines to Critical Thinking Exercise

Placenta Previa

1. Without further assessments a diagnosis cannot be made. Many tools are available to assist in gathering data that will enable the diagnosis to be made. Of major concern is the amount of bleeding and the fetal tolerance of this insult.
2. (a) Possible diagnoses for Marta at her stage in pregnancy include placenta previa and placental abruption. Less likely diagnoses are clotting disorders of pregnancy because these are associated with other problems such as hypertension, retained dead fetus syndrome, or von Willebrand disease. (b) Marta will need a physical assessment that focuses on the cardiovascular and circulatory systems, uterine resting tone, and fetal assessment. A bimanual vaginal examination will not be done; a speculum examination may be indicated. Laboratory tests likely to be ordered include a CBC; crossmatched blood should be made available. The standard for the diagnosis of placenta previa is a transabdominal ultrasound. If the bleeding is active, an IV line should be established. (c) Marta will be transferred to the antepartum unit if her bright-red bleeding continues, the fetus is experiencing distress, she is having uterine contractions, her membranes rupture, or she has an elevated temperature. (d) Marta will be discharged home if a placenta previa is identified, the bleeding decreases or turns to a darker brown color, she has no contractions, the fetus is active and stable, and her CBC is normal.
3. Priorities for nursing care at this time include monitoring the amount and color of bleeding, uterine contractions, and fetal heart rate; providing education and reassurance to Marta and her family; decreasing her anxiety and stress; starting an IV line if ordered; ensuring that laboratory specimens are collected; and preparing her for a sonogram.
4. There is good evidence that a placenta previa will be detected by ultrasound examination in the great majority of cases. Expectant management is based on clinical trials.
5. Alternative perspectives include other problems that may be detected during a thorough history. For example, Marta has had one abortion. When was it; was it spontaneous or induced? Has she experienced any trauma that might cause the bleeding? Has she self-inflicted harm in an effort to cause a miscarriage? Does she have family support? Who is taking care of her other children?

Resources

American College of Obstetricians and Gynecologists
409 12th St. SW
Washington, DC 20024
800-762-2264
www.acog.com

COPE (Coping with the Overall Pregnancy/Parenting Experience)
37 Clarendon St.
Boston, MA 02116
617-357-5588

Family Violence Prevention Fund
383 Rhode Island St., Suite 304
San Francisco, CA 94103
415-252-8900
www.fvpf.org

Pregnancy and Infant Loss
1421 East Wayzata Blvd., Suite 40
Wayzata, MN 55391
614-473-9372

References

Abboud LN, Liamputtong P: Pregnancy loss: what it means to women who miscarry and their partners, *Soc Work Health Care* 36(3):37-62, 2003.

American College of Obstetricians and Gynecologists: *Antenatal corticosteroid therapy for fetal maturation. ACOG Committee Opinion No. 210,* Washington, DC, 2002a, American College of Obstetricians and Gynecologists.

American College of Obstetricians and Gynecologists: *Diagnosis and management of preeclampsia and eclampsia. ACOG Practice Bulletin number 33,* Washington, DC, 2002b, American College of Obstetricians and Gynecologists.

Andres R, Day M: Perinatal complications associated with maternal tobacco use, *Semin Neonatol* 5(3):231-234, 2000.

Antenatal Corticosteroids Revisited: Repeat Courses. NIH Consensus Statement Online 2000 August 17-18; 17(2):1-10. Internet document available at consensus.nih.gov (accessed January 15, 2005).

Benedetti T: Obstetric hemorrhage. In Gabbe SG, Niebyl JR, Simpson JL (eds): *Obstetrics: normal and problem pregnancies,* ed 4, New York, 2002, Churchill Livingstone.

Berman ML, DiSaia PJ, Tewari KS: Pelvic malignancies, gestational trophoblastic neoplasia, and nonpelvic malignancies. In Creasy RK, Resnik R, Iams JD (eds): *Maternal-fetal medicine: principles and practice,* ed 5, Philadelphia, 2004, WB Saunders.

Blackburn ST: *Maternal, fetal, and neonatal physiology: a clinical perspective,* ed 2, St Louis, 2003, WB Saunders.

Broen AN et al: Psychological impact on women of miscarriage versus induced abortion: a 2-year follow-up study, *Psychosom Med* 66(2):265-271, 2004.

Bush K, O'Brien J, Barton J: The utility of umbilical artery Doppler investigation in women with HELLP (hemolysis, elevated liver enzymes, and low platelets) syndrome, *Am J Obstet Gynecol* 184(6):1087-1089, 2001.

Centers for Disease Control and Prevention: Interim guidelines for the evaluation of infants born to mothers infected with West Nile virus during pregnancy, *MMWR Morb Mortal Wkly Rep* 53(7):154-157, 2004.

Centers for Disease Control and Prevention: Sexually transmitted diseases treatment guidelines 2002, *MMWR Morb Mortal Wkly Rep* 51(RR-6): 1-82, 2002.

Clark SL: Placenta previa and abruptio placentae. In Creasy RK, Resnik R, Iams JD (eds): *Maternal-fetal medicine: principles and practice,* ed 5, Philadelphia, 2004, WB Saunders.

Copeland L, Landon M: Malignant diseases and pregnancy. In Gabbe SG, Niebyl JR, Simpson JL (eds): *Obstetrics: normal and problem pregnancies,* ed 4, New York, 2002, Churchill Livingstone.

Cowles TA, Gonik B: Perinatal infections. In Fanaroff AA, Martin RJ (eds): *Neonatal-perinatal medicine: diseases of the fetus and infant,* ed 7, St Louis, 2002, Mosby.

Crane J et al: Maternal complications with placenta previa, *Am J Perinatol* 17(2):101-105, 2000.

Crowther C: Hospitalisation and bed rest for multiple pregnancy (Cochrane Review), 2000. In *The Cochrane Library,* Issue 2, Chichester, UK, 2004, John Wiley & Sons.

Cunningham F et al: *Williams obstetrics,* ed 21, New York, 2001, McGraw-Hill.

Czeizel AI, Puho E: Associaton between severe nausea and vomiting in pregnancy and lower rate of preterm births, *Paediatr Perinat Epidemiol* 18(4):253-259, 2004.

Dekker G: Prevention of preeclampsia. In Sibai B (ed): *Hypertensive disorders in women,* Philadelphia, 2001, WB Saunders.

Enkin M et al: Effective care in pregnancy and childbirth: a synopsis, *Birth* 28(1):41-51, 2001.

Freda M: The power of words, *MCN Am J Matern Child Nurs* 24(2):63, 1999.

Garmel SH: Early pregnancy risks. In DeCherney AH, Nathan L: *Current obstetric and gynecologic diagnosis and treatment,* ed 9, New York, 2003, Lange Medical Books/McGraw-Hill.

Gilbert ES, Harmon JS: *Manual of high risk pregnancy and delivery,* ed 3, St Louis, 2003, Mosby.

Hill JA: Recurrent pregnancy loss. In Creasy RK, Resnik R, Iams JD (eds): *Maternal-fetal medicine: principles and practice,* ed 5, Philadelphia, 2004, WB Saunders.

Iams JD: Abnormal cervical competence. In Creasy RK, Resnik R, Iams JD (eds): *Maternal-fetal medicine: principles and practice,* ed 5, Philadelphia, 2004, WB Saunders.

Institute of Medicine, Committee on Prevention and Control of Sexually Transmitted Diseases: *The hidden epidemic: confronting sexually transmitted diseases,* Washington, DC, 1997, National Academy of Sciences.

Kilpatrick SJ, Laros RK: Maternal hematologic disorders. In Creasy RK, Resnik R, Iams JD (eds): *Maternal-fetal medicine: principles and practice,* ed 5, Philadelphia, 2004, WB Saunders.

Kumtepe Y, Kadanali I: Medical treatment of ruptured with hemodynamically stable and unruptured ectopic pregnancy patients, *Eur J Obstet Gynecol Reprod Biol* 116(2):221-225, 2004.

Li DK, Wi S: Changing paternity and the risk of preeclampsia/eclampsia in the subsequent pregnancy, *Am J Epidemiol* 151(1):57-62, 2000.

Livingston J, Sibai B: Chronic hypertension in pregnancy, *Obstet Gynecol Clin* 28(3):1-15, 2001.

Ludmir J, Stubblefield P: Surgical procedures in pregnancy. In Gabbe SG, Niebyl JR, Simpson JL (eds): *Obstetrics: normal and problem pregnancies,* ed 4, New York, 2002, Churchill Livingstone.

Magpie Trial Collaborative Group: Do women with pre-eclampsia, and their babies, benefit from magnesium sulfate? The Magpie Trial: a randomised placebo-controlled trial, *Lancet* 359(9321):1877-1890, 2002.

Magpie Trial Follow Up Study Management Group: The Magpie Trial follow-up study: outcome after discharge from hospital for women and children recruited to a trial comparing magnesium sulphate with placebo for pre-eclampsia, *BMC Pregnancy Childbirth* 4(1):5, 2004.

Maloni J: *Antepartum bed rest: case studies, research and nursing care,* Washington, DC, 1998, Association of Women's Health, Obstetric and Neonatal Nurses.

Maloni JA et al: Antepartum bed rest: maternal weight change and infant birth weight, *Biol Res Nurs* 5(3):177-186, 2004.

Martin J et al: Births: final data for 2000, *Natl Vital Stat Rep* 50(5):1-114, 2003.

McFarlane J et al: Abuse during pregnancy and femicide: urgent implications for women's health, *Obstet Gynecol* 100(1):27-36, 2002.

Murray M: *Antepartal and intrapartal fetal monitoring,* ed 2, Albuquerque, NM,1997, Learning Resources International.

National High Blood Pressure Education Program: *Working Group Report on High Blood Pressure in Pregnancy,* NIH pub no 00-3029, Bethesda, MD, 2000, National Institutes of Health, National Heart, Lung, and Blood Institute. Available at www.nhlbi.nih.gov/health/prog/heart/hbp_preg.htm (accessed January 15, 2005).

Purdy IB, Wiley DJ: Perinatal corticosteroids: a review of research. Part I: antenatal administration, *Neonat Netw* 23(2):15-30, 2004.

Report of the National High Blood Pressure Education Program Working Group on High Blood Pressure in Pregnancy: Summary report, *Am J Obstet Gynecol* 183(1):S1-S22, 2000.

Roberts J: Pregnancy-related hypertension. In Creasy RK, Resnik R, Iams JD (eds): *Maternal-fetal medicine: principles and practice,* ed 5, Philadelphia, 2004, WB Saunders.

Robillard P: Interest in preeclampsia for researchers in reproduction, *J Reprod Immunol* 53(1-2):279-287, 2002.

Scott LD, Abu-Hamda E: Gastrointestinal disease in pregnancy. In Creasy RK, Resnik R, Iams JD (eds): *Maternal-fetal medicine: principles and practice,* ed 5, Philadelphia, 2004, WB Saunders.

Seidel HM et al: *Mosby's guide to physical examination,* ed 5, St Louis, 2003, Mosby.

Sepilian V, Wood E: Ectopic pregnancy, *Emedicine.* Internet document available at www.emedicine.com/med/topic3212.htm (accessed September 12, 2004).

Sibai B: Chronic hypertension in pregnancy, *Obstet Gynecol* 100(2):369-377, 2002a.

Sibai B: Hypertension in pregnancy. In Gabbe SG, Niebyl JR, Simpson JL (eds): *Obstetrics: normal and problem pregnancies,* ed 4, New York, 2002b, Churchill Livingstone.

Sibai B: Diagnosis, controversies, and management of the syndrome of hemolysis, elevated liver enzymes, and low platelet count, *Obstet Gynecol* 103(5 pt 1):981-991, 2004.

Simpson J: Fetal wastage. In Gabbe SG, Niebyl JR, Simpson JL (eds): *Obstetrics: normal and problem pregnancies,* ed 4, New York, 2002, Churchill Livingstone.

Van P, Meleis AI: Coping with grief after involuntary pregnancy loss: perspectives of African American women, *J Obstet Gynecol Neonatal Nurs* 32(1):28-39, 2003.

Van Hook J: Trauma in pregnancy, *Clin Obstet Gynecol* 45(2):414-424, 2002.

Wilson BA, Shannon MT, Stang CL: *Nurse's drug guide 2002,* Upper Saddle River, NJ, 2002, Prentice-Hall.

Workowski K, Levine W, Wasserheit J: US Centers for Disease Control and Prevention guidelines for the treatment of sexually transmitted diseases: an opportunity to unify clinical and public health practice, *Ann Intern Med* 137(4):255-262, 2002.

Unit 4

15 Labor and Birth Processes

LEARNING OBJECTIVES

On completion of this chapter the reader will be able to:

- Explain the five factors that affect the labor process.
- Describe the anatomic structure of the bony pelvis.
- Recognize the normal measurements of the diameters of the pelvic inlet, cavity, and outlet.
- Explain the significance of the size and position of the fetal head during labor and birth.
- Summarize the cardinal movements of the mechanism of labor for a vertex presentation.
- Assess the maternal anatomic and physiologic adaptations to labor.
- Describe fetal adaptations to labor.

ELECTRONIC RESOURCES

Additional information related to the content in Chapter 15 can be found on

the companion website at evolve
http://evolve.elsevier.com/Wong/maternal/
- NCLEX Review Questions
- WebLinks

or the interactive student CD-ROM
Activities for Chapter 15 include the following:
- NCLEX Review Questions

During late pregnancy, the woman and fetus prepare for the labor process. The fetus has grown and developed in preparation for extrauterine life. The woman has undergone various physiologic adaptations during pregnancy that prepare her for birth and motherhood. Labor and birth represent the end of pregnancy, the beginning of extrauterine life for the newborn, and a change in the lives of the family. This chapter discusses the factors affecting labor, the processes involved, the normal progression of events, and the adaptations made by both the woman and fetus.

FACTORS AFFECTING LABOR

At least five factors affect the process of labor and birth. These are easily remembered as the five *P*'s: passenger (fetus and placenta), passageway (birth canal), powers (contractions), position of the mother, and psychologic response. The first four factors are presented here as the basis of understanding the physiologic process of labor. The fifth factor is discussed in Chapter 18. Other factors that may be a part of the woman's labor experience may be important as well. VandeVusse (1999) identified external forces including place of birth, preparation, type of provider (especially nurses), and procedures. Physiology (sensations) was identified as an internal force. These factors are discussed generally in Chapter 18 as they relate to nursing care during labor. Further research investigating essential forces of labor is recommended.

Passenger

The movement of the passenger, or fetus, through the birth canal is determined by several interacting factors: the size of the fetal head, fetal presentation, fetal lie, fetal attitude, and fetal position. Because the placenta also must pass through the birth canal, it can be considered a passenger along with the fetus; however, the placenta rarely impedes the process of labor in normal vaginal birth. An exception is the case of placenta previa (see Chapter 14).

Size of the Fetal Head

Because of its size and relative rigidity, the fetal head has a major effect on the birth process. The fetal skull is composed of two parietal bones, two temporal bones, the frontal bone, and the occipital bone (Fig. 15-1, *A*). These bones are united by membranous sutures: the sagittal, lambdoidal, coronal, and frontal (Fig. 15-1, *B*). Membrane-filled spaces called fontanels are located where the sutures intersect. During labor, after rupture of membranes, palpation of fontanels and sutures during vaginal examination reveals fetal presentation, position, and attitude.

The two most important fontanels are the anterior and posterior ones (see Fig. 15-1, *B*). The larger of these, the anterior fontanel, is diamond shaped, about 3 cm by 2 cm, and

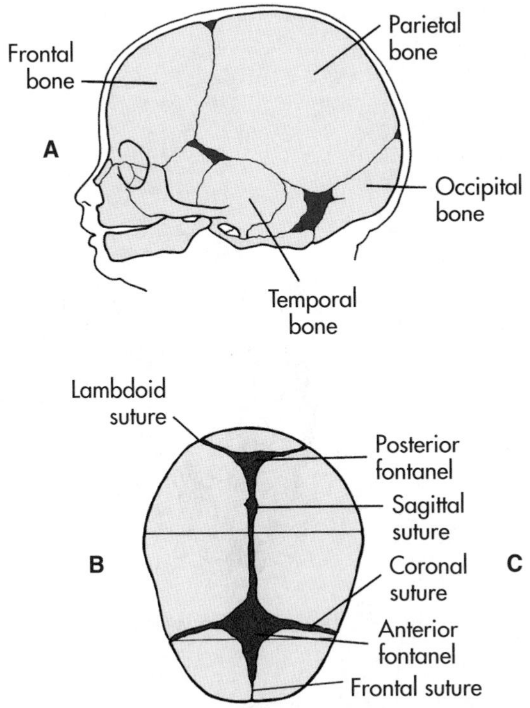

Fig. 15-1 Fetal head at term. **A**, Bones. **B**, **C**, Sutures and fontanels.

lies at the junction of the sagittal, coronal, and frontal sutures. It closes by 18 months after birth. The posterior fontanel lies at the junction of the sutures of the two parietal bones and the one occipital bone, is triangular, and is about 1 cm by 2 cm. It closes 6 to 8 weeks after birth.

Sutures and fontanels make the skull flexible to accommodate the infant brain, which continues to grow for some time after birth. Because the bones are not firmly united, however, slight overlapping of the bones, or molding of the shape of the head, occurs during labor. This capacity of the bones to slide over one another also permits adaptation to the various diameters of the maternal pelvis. Molding can be extensive, but the heads of most newborns assume their normal shape within 3 days after birth.

Although the size of the fetal shoulders may affect passage, their position can be altered relatively easily during labor, so that one shoulder may occupy a lower level than the other. This creates a shoulder diameter that is smaller than the skull, facilitating passage through the birth canal. The circumference of the fetal hips is usually small enough not to create problems.

Fetal Presentation

Presentation refers to the part of the fetus that enters the pelvic inlet first and leads through the birth canal during labor at term. The three main presentations are cephalic presentation (head first), occurring in 96% of births (Fig. 15-2); breech presentation (buttocks or feet first), occurring in 3% of births (Fig. 15-3, *A-C*); and shoulder presentation, seen in 1% of births (Fig. 15-3, *D*). *Presenting part* refers to that part of the fetal body first felt by the examining finger during a vaginal examination. In a cephalic presentation, the presenting part is usually the occiput; in a breech presentation, it is the sacrum; in the shoulder presentation, it is the scapula. When the presenting part is the occiput, the presentation is noted as vertex (see Fig. 15-2). Factors that determine the presenting part include fetal lie, fetal attitude, and extension or flexion of the fetal head.

Fetal Lie

Lie is the relation of the long axis (spine) of the fetus to the long axis (spine) of the mother. The two primary lies are *longitudinal*, or vertical, in which the long axis of the fetus is parallel with the long axis of the mother (see Fig. 15-2); and *transverse*, horizontal, or oblique, in which the long axis of the fetus is at a right angle diagonal to the long axis of the mother (see Fig. 15-3, *D*). Longitudinal lies are either cephalic or breech presentations, depending on the fetal structure that first enters the mother's pelvis. Vaginal birth cannot occur when the fetus stays in a transverse lie. An oblique lie, one in which the long axis of the fetus is lying at an angle to the long axis of the mother, is less common and usually converts to a longitudinal or transverse lie during labor (Cunningham et al, 2001).

Fetal Attitude

Attitude is the relation of the fetal body parts to each other. The fetus assumes a characteristic posture (attitude) in utero partly because of the mode of fetal growth and partly because of the way the fetus conforms to the shape of the uterine cavity. Normally the back of the fetus is rounded so that the chin is flexed on the chest, the thighs are flexed on the abdomen, and the legs are flexed at the knees. The arms are crossed over the thorax, and the umbilical cord lies between the arms and the legs. This attitude is termed *general flexion* (see Fig. 15-2).

Deviations from the normal attitude may cause difficulties in childbirth. For example, in a cephalic presentation, the fetal head may be extended or flexed in a manner that presents a head diameter that exceeds the limits of the maternal pelvis, leading to prolonged labor, forceps- or vacuum-assisted birth, or cesarean birth (see Fig. 15-5).

Certain critical diameters of the fetal head are usually measured. The biparietal diameter, which is about 9.25 cm at term, is the largest transverse diameter and an important indicator of fetal head size (Fig. 15-4, *B*). In a well-flexed cephalic presentation, the biparietal diameter will be the widest part of the head entering the pelvic inlet. Of the several anteroposterior diameters, the smallest and the most critical one is the suboccipitobregmatic diameter (about 9.5 cm at term). When the head is in complete flexion, this diameter allows the fetal head to pass through the true pelvis easily (Fig. 15-5, *A*). As the head is more extended, the anteroposterior diameter widens, and the head may not be able to enter the true pelvis (see Fig. 15-5, *B, C*).

Fetal Position

The presentation or presenting part indicates the portion of the fetus that overlies the pelvic inlet. *Position* is the relation of the presenting part (occiput, sacrum, mentum [chin], or sinciput [deflexed vertex]) to the four quadrants of the mother's pelvis (see Fig. 15-2). Position is denoted by a three-letter abbreviation. The first letter of the abbreviation denotes the location of the presenting part in the right (R) or left (L) side of the mother's pelvis. The middle letter

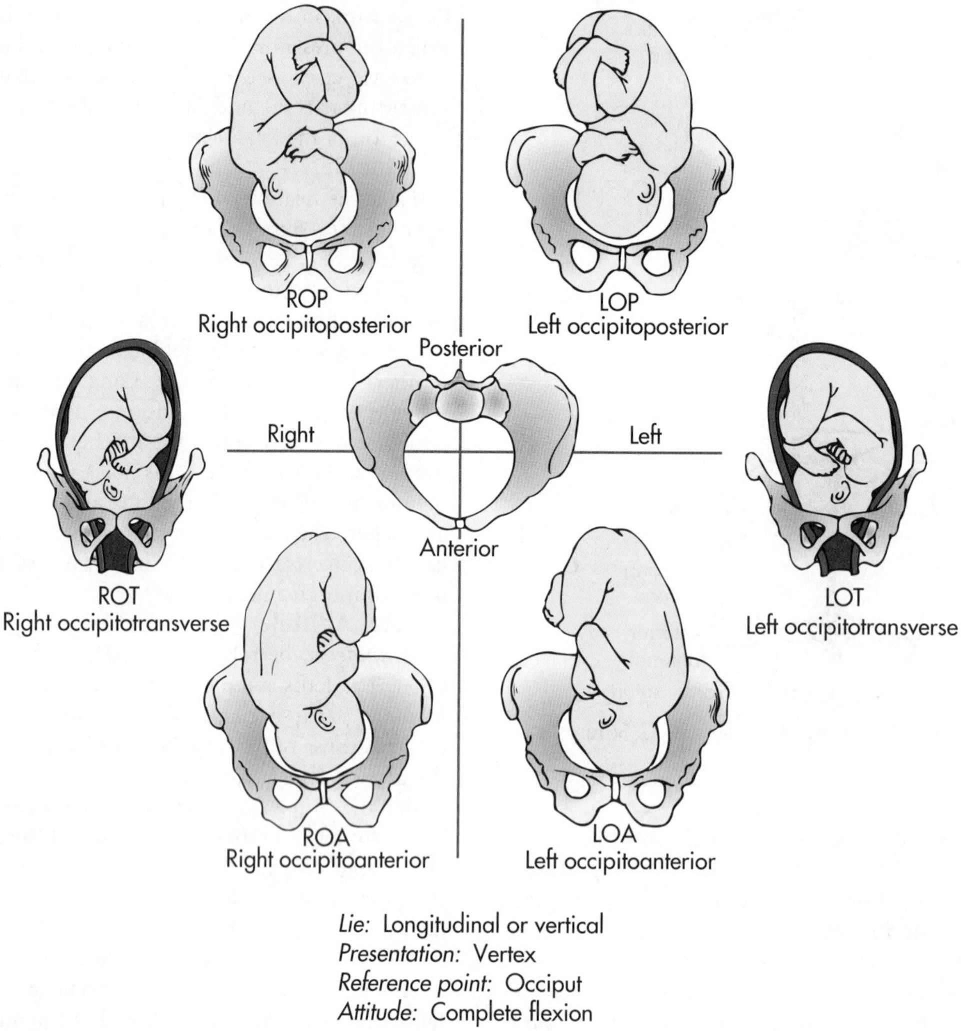

Fig. 15-2 Examples of fetal vertex (occiput) presentations in relation to front, back, or side of maternal pelvis

stands for the specific presenting part of the fetus (O for occiput, S for sacrum, M for mentum [chin], and Sc for scapula [shoulder]). The third letter stands for the location of the presenting part in relation to the anterior (A), posterior (P), or transverse (T) portion of the maternal pelvis. For example, ROA means that the occiput is the presenting part and is located in the right anterior quadrant of the maternal pelvis (see Fig. 15-2). LSP means that the sacrum is the presenting part and is located in the left posterior quadrant of the maternal pelvis (see Fig. 15-3).

Station is the relation of the presenting part of the fetus to an imaginary line drawn between the maternal ischial spines and is a measure of the degree of descent of the presenting part of the fetus through the birth canal. The placement of the presenting part is measured in centimeters above or below the ischial spines (Fig. 15-6). For example, when the lowermost portion of the presenting part is 1 cm above the spines, it is noted as being minus (–) 1. At the level of the spines, the station is referred to as 0 (zero). When the presenting part is 1 cm below the spines, the station is said to be plus (+) 1. Birth is imminent when the presenting part is at +4 to +5 cm. The station of the presenting part should be determined when labor begins so that the rate of descent of the fetus during labor can be accurately determined.

Engagement is the term used to indicate that the largest transverse diameter of the presenting part (usually the biparietal diameter) has passed through the maternal pelvic brim or inlet into the true pelvis and usually corresponds to station 0. Engagement often occurs in the weeks just before labor begins in nulliparas and may occur before or during labor in multiparas. Engagement can be determined by abdominal or vaginal examination.

Passageway

The *passageway*, or birth canal, is composed of the mother's rigid bony pelvis and the soft tissues of the cervix, pelvic floor, vagina, and introitus (the external opening to the vagina). Although the soft tissues, particularly the muscular layers of the pelvic floor, contribute to vaginal birth of the fetus, the maternal pelvis plays a far greater role in the labor process because the fetus must successfully accommodate

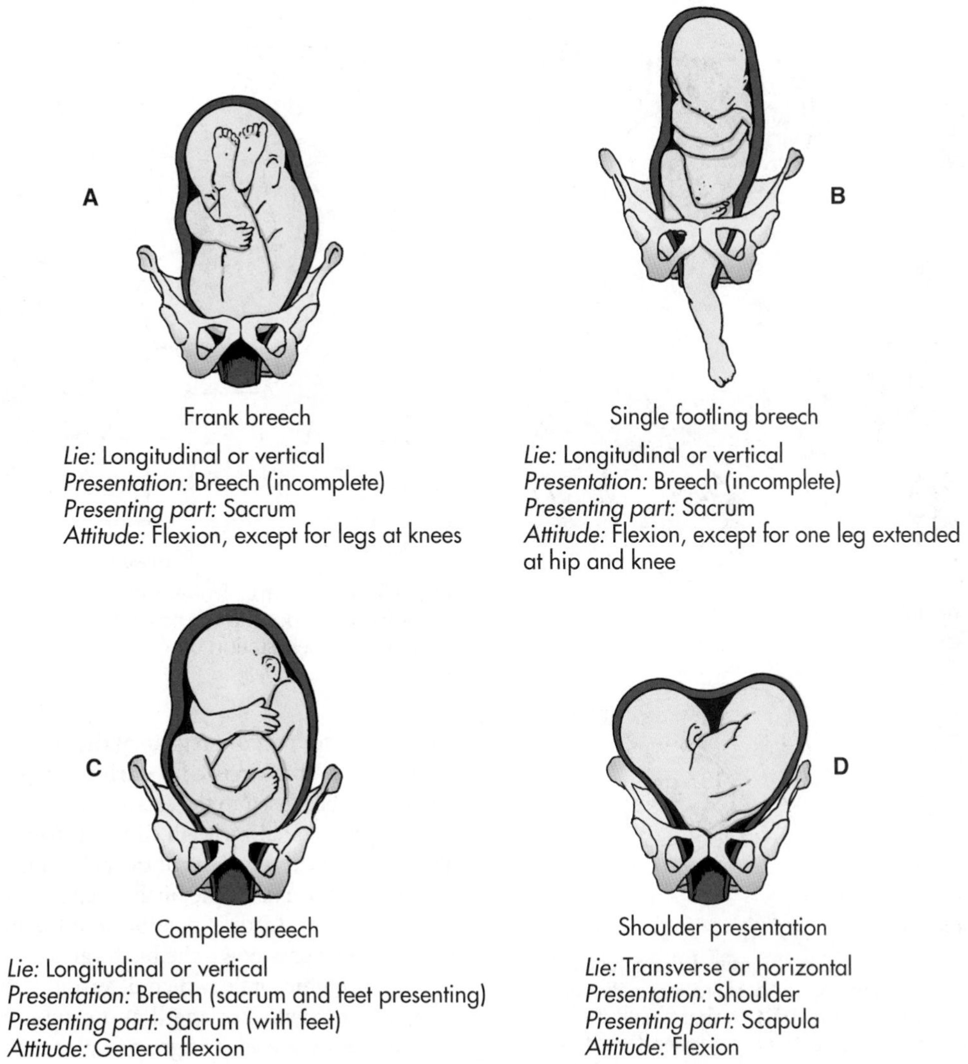
A
B
Frank breech
Lie: Longitudinal or vertical
Presentation: Breech (incomplete)
Presenting part: Sacrum
Attitude: Flexion, except for legs at knees
Single footling breech
Lie: Longitudinal or vertical
Presentation: Breech (incomplete)
Presenting part: Sacrum
Attitude: Flexion, except for one leg extended at hip and knee
C
D
Complete breech
Lie: Longitudinal or vertical
Presentation: Breech (sacrum and feet presenting)
Presenting part: Sacrum (with feet)
Attitude: General flexion
Shoulder presentation
Lie: Transverse or horizontal
Presentation: Shoulder
Presenting part: Scapula
Attitude: Flexion

Fig. 15-3 Fetal presentations. **A**, **B**, **C**, Breech (sacral) presentation. **D**, Shoulder presentation.

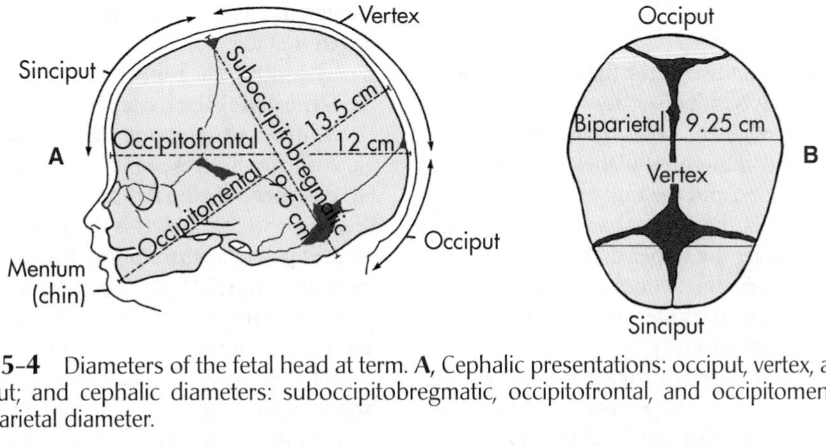

Fig. 15-4 Diameters of the fetal head at term. **A**, Cephalic presentations: occiput, vertex, and sinciput; and cephalic diameters: suboccipitobregmatic, occipitofrontal, and occipitomental. **B**, Biparietal diameter.

itself to this relatively rigid passageway. Therefore the size and shape of the pelvis must be determined before childbirth begins.

Bony Pelvis

The anatomy of the bony pelvis is described in Chapter 5. The following discussion focuses on the importance of pelvic configurations as they relate to the labor process. (It may be helpful to refer to Figs. 5-5 and 5-6.)

The bony pelvis is formed by the fusion of the ilium, ischium, pubis, and sacral bones. The four pelvic joints are the symphysis pubis, the right and left sacroiliac joints, and the sacrococcygeal joint (Fig. 15-7, *A*). The bony pelvis is sepa-

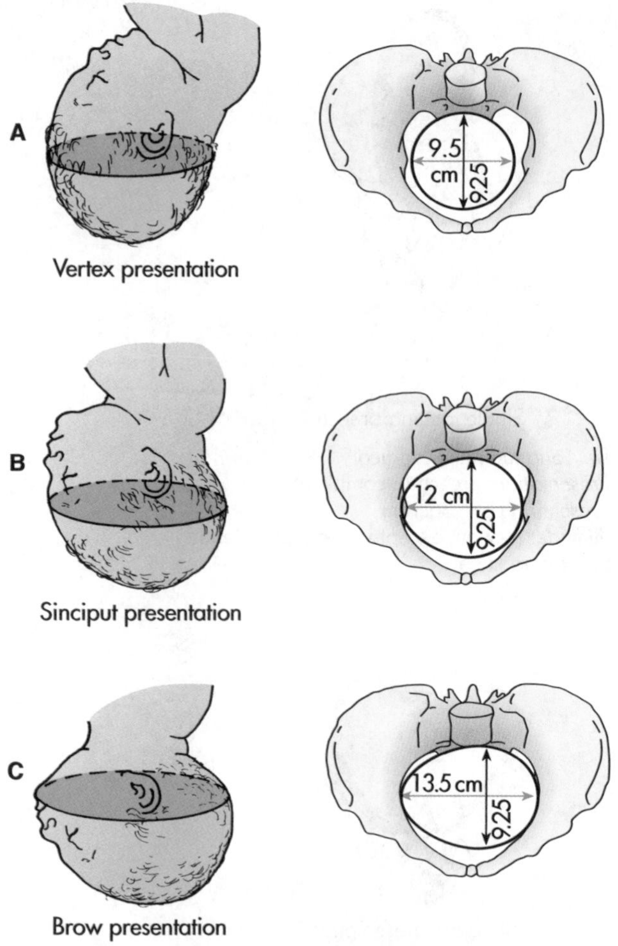

Fig. 15-5 Head entering pelvis. Biparietal diameter is indicated with shading (9.25 cm). **A**, Suboccipitobregmatic diameter: complete flexion of head on chest so that smallest diameter enters. **B**, Occipitofrontal diameter: moderate extension (military attitude) so that large diameter enters. **C**, Occipitomental diameter: marked extension (deflection) so that the largest diameter, which is too large to permit head to enter pelvis, is presenting

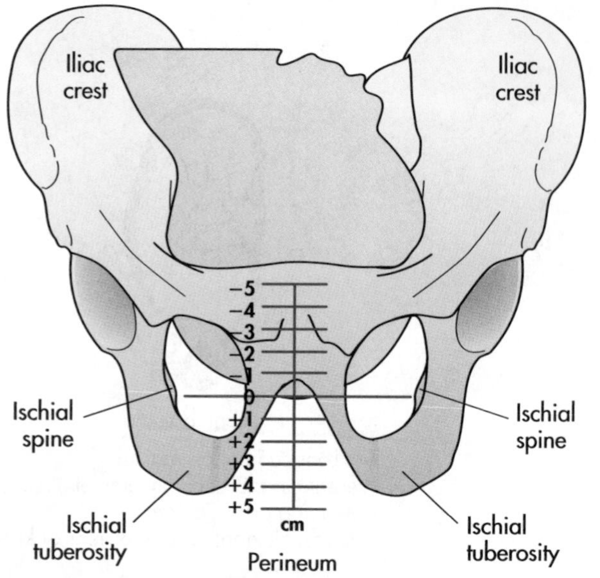

Fig. 15-6 Stations of presenting part, or degree of descent. The lowermost portion of the presenting part is at the level of the ischial spines, station 0.

rated by the brim, or inlet, into two parts: the false pelvis and the true pelvis. The false pelvis is the part above the brim and plays no part in childbearing. The true pelvis, the part involved in birth, is divided into three planes: the inlet, or brim; the midpelvis, or cavity; and the outlet.

The pelvic inlet, which is the upper border of the true pelvis, is formed anteriorly by the upper margins of the pubic bone, laterally by the iliopectineal lines along the innominate bones, and posteriorly by the anterior, upper margin of the sacrum and the sacral promontory.

The pelvic cavity, or midpelvis, is a curved passage with a short anterior wall and a much longer concave posterior wall. It is bounded by the posterior aspect of the symphysis pubis, the ischium, a portion of the ilium, the sacrum, and the coccyx.

The pelvic outlet is the lower border of the true pelvis. Viewed from below, it is ovoid; somewhat diamond shaped; and bounded by the pubic arch anteriorly, the ischial tuberosities laterally, and the tip of the coccyx posteriorly (Fig. 15-7, *B*). In the latter part of pregnancy, the coccyx is movable (unless it has been broken in a fall during skiing or skating, for example, and has fused to the sacrum during healing).

The pelvic canal varies in size and shape at various levels. The diameters at the plane of the pelvic inlet, midpelvis, and outlet, plus the axis of the birth canal (Fig. 15-8), determine whether vaginal birth is possible and the manner by which the fetus may pass down the birth canal.

The subpubic angle, which determines the type of pubic arch, together with the length of the pubic rami and the intertuberous diameter, is of great importance. Because the fetus must first pass beneath the pubic arch, a narrow subpubic angle will be less accommodating than a rounded wide arch. The method of measurement of the subpubic arch is shown in Fig. 15-9. A summary of obstetric measurements is given in Table 15-1.

The four basic types of pelvis are classified as follows:

1. Gynecoid (the classic female type)
2. Android (resembling the male pelvis)
3. Anthropoid (resembling the pelvis of anthropoid apes)
4. Platypelloid (the flat pelvis)

The gynecoid pelvis is the most common, with major gynecoid pelvic features present in 50% of all women. Anthropoid and android features are less common, and platypelloid pelvic features are the least common. Mixed types of pelves are more common than are pure types (Cunningham et al, 2001). Examples of pelvic variations and their effects on mode of birth are given in Table 15-2.

Assessment of the bony pelvis can be performed during the first prenatal evaluation and need not be repeated if the pelvis is of adequate size and suitable shape. In the third trimester of pregnancy, the examination of the bony pelvis may be more thorough and the results more accurate because there is relaxation and increased mobility of the pelvic joints and ligaments due to hormonal influences. Widening

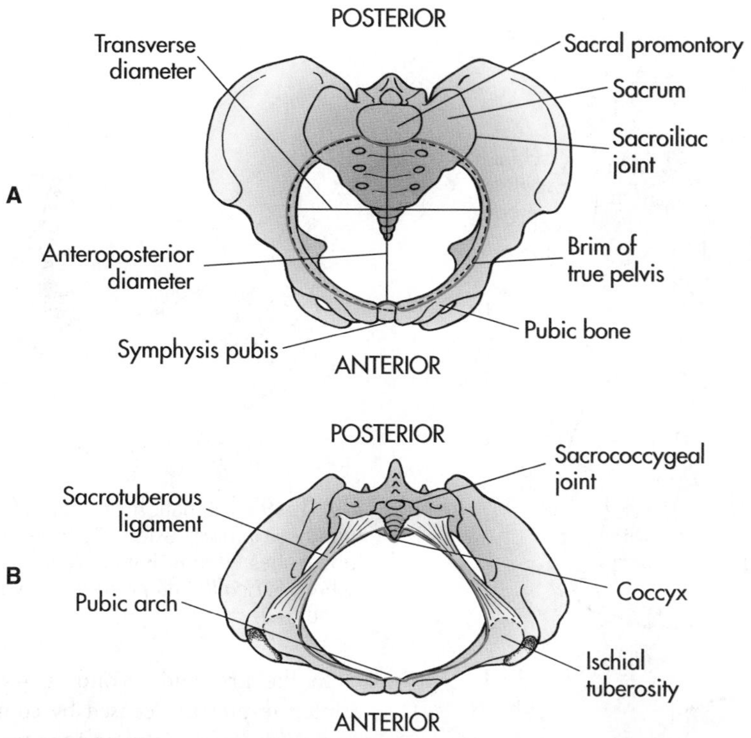

Fig. 15-7 Female pelvis. **A**, Pelvic brim above. **B**, Pelvic outlet from below.

of the joint of the symphysis pubis and the resulting instability may cause pain in any or all of the pelvic joints.

Because the examiner does not have direct access to the bony structures and because the bones are covered with varying amounts of soft tissue, estimates of size and shape are approximate. Precise bony pelvis measurements can be determined by use of computed tomography, ultrasound, or x-ray films. However, radiographic examination is rarely done during pregnancy because the x-rays may damage the developing fetus.

Soft Tissues

The soft tissues of the passageway include the distensible lower uterine segment, cervix, pelvic floor muscles, vagina, and introitus. Before labor begins, the uterus is composed of the uterine body (corpus) and cervix (neck). After labor has begun, uterine contractions cause the uterine body to have a thick and muscular upper segment and a thin-walled, passive, muscular lower segment. A physiologic retraction ring separates the two segments (Fig. 15-10). The lower uterine segment gradually distends to accommodate the intrauterine contents as the wall of the upper segment thickens and its accommodating capacity is reduced. The contractions of the uterine body thus exert downward pressure on the fetus, pushing it against the cervix.

The cervix effaces (thins) and dilates (opens) sufficiently to allow the first fetal portion to descend into the vagina. As the fetus descends, the cervix is actually drawn upward and over this first portion.

The pelvic floor is a muscular layer that separates the pelvic cavity above from the perineal space below. This structure helps the fetus rotate anteriorly as it passes through the birth canal. As noted earlier, the soft tissues of the vagina develop throughout pregnancy until at term the vagina can dilate to accommodate the fetus and permit passage of the fetus to the external world.

Powers

Involuntary and voluntary powers combine to expel the fetus and the placenta from the uterus. Involuntary uterine contractions, called the *primary powers,* signal the beginning of labor. Once the cervix has dilated, voluntary bearing-down efforts by the woman, called the *secondary powers,* augment the force of the involuntary contractions.

Primary Powers

The involuntary contractions originate at certain pacemaker points in the thickened muscle layers of the upper uterine segment. From the pacemaker points, contractions move downward over the uterus in waves, separated by short rest periods. Terms used to describe these involuntary contractions include *frequency* (the time from the beginning of one contraction to the beginning of the next), *duration* (length of contraction), and *intensity* (strength of contraction).

The primary powers are responsible for the effacement and dilation of the cervix and descent of the fetus. Effacement of the cervix means the shortening and thinning of the cervix during the first stage of labor. The cervix, normally 2 to 3 cm long and about 1 cm thick, is obliterated or "taken up" by a shortening of the uterine muscle bundles during the thinning of the lower uterine segment that occurs in advancing labor. Only a thin edge of the cervix can be palpated when effacement is complete. Effacement generally is advanced in first-time term pregnancy before more than slight

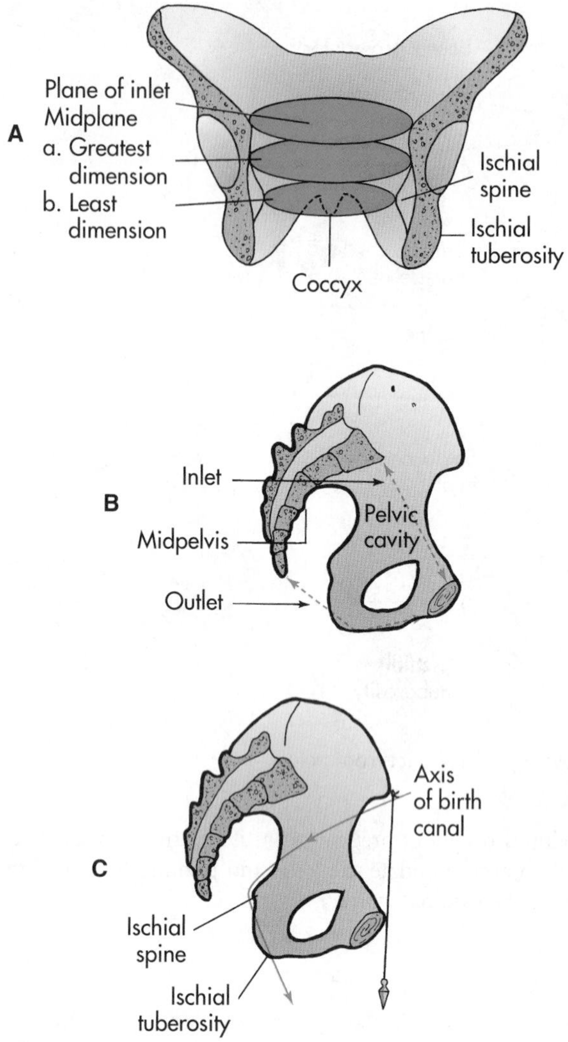

Fig. 15-8 Pelvic cavity. **A,** Inlet and midplane. Outlet not shown. **B,** Cavity of true pelvis. **C,** Note curve of sacrum and axis of birth canal.

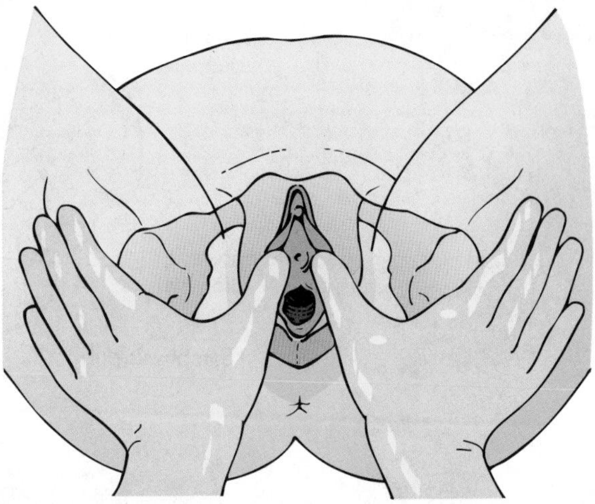

Fig. 15-9 Estimation of angle of subpubic arch. With both thumbs, examiner externally traces descending rami down to tuberosities. (From Barkauskas VH, Baumann LC, Darling-Fisher CS: *Health and physical assessment,* ed 3, St Louis, 2002, Mosby.)

dilation occurs. In subsequent pregnancies, effacement and dilation of the cervix tend to progress together. Degree of effacement is expressed in percentages, from 0% to 100% (e.g., a cervix is 50% effaced) (Fig. 15-11, *A–C*).

Dilation of the cervix is the enlargement or widening of the cervical opening and the cervical canal that occurs once labor has begun. The diameter of the cervix increases from less than 1 cm to full dilation (approximately 10 cm) to allow birth of a term fetus. When the cervix is fully dilated (and completely retracted), it can no longer be palpated (Fig. 15-11, *D*). Full cervical dilation marks the end of the first stage of labor.

Dilation of the cervix occurs by the drawing upward of the musculofibrous components of the cervix, caused by strong uterine contractions. Pressure exerted by the amniotic fluid while the membranes are intact or by the force applied by the presenting part can promote cervical dilation. Scarring of the cervix as a result of prior infection or surgery may slow cervical dilation.

In the first and second stages of labor, increased intrauterine pressure caused by contractions exerts pressure on the descending fetus and the cervix. When the presenting part of the fetus reaches the perineal floor, mechanical stretching of the cervix occurs. Stretch receptors in the posterior vagina cause release of endogenous oxytocin that triggers the maternal urge to bear down, or the Ferguson reflex.

Uterine contractions are usually independent of external forces. For example, laboring women who are paraplegic will have normal but painless uterine contractions (Aminoff, 2004). However, uterine contractions may decrease temporarily in frequency and intensity if narcotic analgesic medication is given early in labor. Studies of effects of epidural analgesia have demonstrated prolonged length of labor for nulliparas both in the active phase of first-stage labor and in second-stage labor (Alexander et al, 2002; Sharma & Leveno, 2003).

Secondary Powers

As soon as the presenting part reaches the pelvic floor, the contractions change in character and become expulsive. The laboring woman experiences an involuntary urge to push. She uses secondary powers (bearing-down efforts) to aid in expulsion of the fetus as she contracts her diaphragm and abdominal muscles and pushes. These bearing-down efforts result in increased intraabdominal pressure that compresses the uterus on all sides and adds to the power of the expulsive forces.

The secondary powers have no effect on cervical dilation, but they are of considerable importance in the expulsion of the infant from the uterus and vagina after the cervix is fully dilated. Studies have shown that pushing in the second stage is more effective and the woman is less fatigued when she begins to push only after she has the urge to do so rather than beginning to push when she is fully dilated without an urge to do so (Roberts, 2002, 2003).

When and how a woman pushes in the second stage is a much-debated topic. Studies have investigated the effects of

Text continued on p. 427.

Table 15-1

Obstetric Measurements

PLANE	DIAMETER	MEASUREMENTS
Inlet (superior strait)		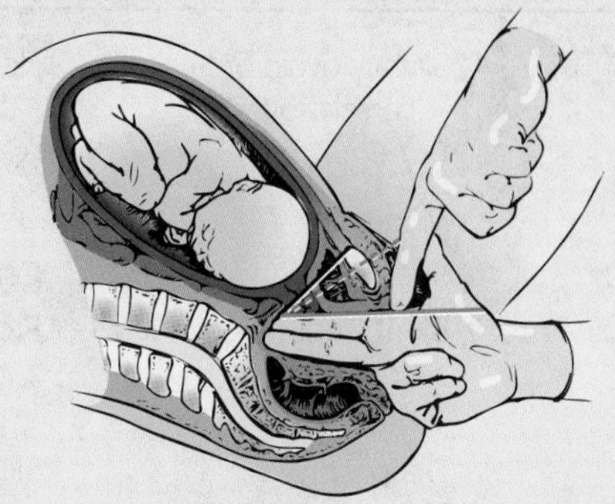 Length of diagonal conjugate (solid colored line), obstetric conjugate (broken colored line), and true conjugate (black line)*
Conjugates		
Diagonal	12.5-13 cm	
Obstetric: measurement that determines whether presenting part can engage or enter superior strait	1.5-2 cm less than diagonal (radiographic)	
True (vera) (anteroposterior)	≥11 cm (12.5) (radiographic)	
Midplane		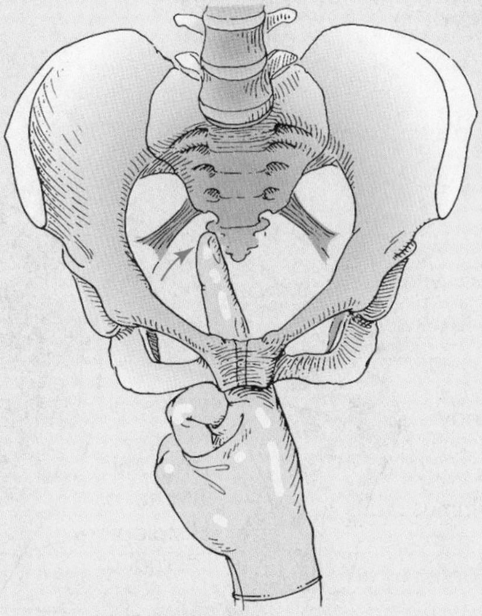 Measurement of interspinous diameter*
Transverse diameter (interspinous diameter)	10.5 cm	
The midplane of the pelvis normally is its largest plane and the one of greatest diameter.		
Outlet		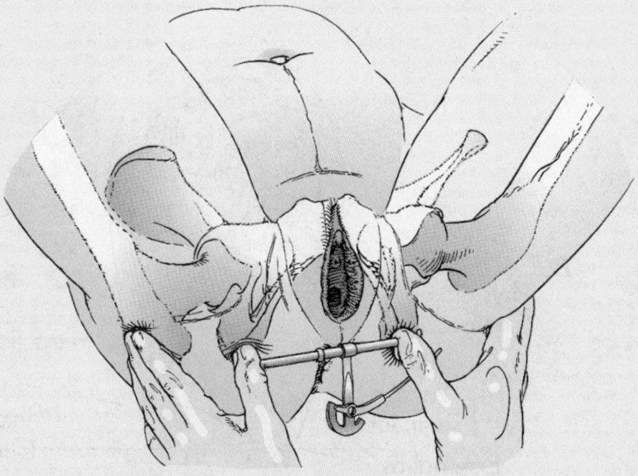 Use of Thom's pelvimeter to measure intertuberous diameter*
Transverse diameter (intertuberous diameter) (biischial)	≥8 cm	
The outlet presents the smallest plane of the pelvic canal.		

*From Seidel HM et al: *Mosby's guide to physical examination,* ed 5, St Louis, 2003, Mosby.

Table 15-2

Comparison of Pelvic Types

	GYNECOID (50% OF WOMEN)	ANDROID (23% OF WOMEN)	ANTHROPOID (24% OF WOMEN)	PLATYPELLOID (3% OF WOMEN)
Brim	Slightly ovoid or transversely rounded ○ Round	Heart shaped, angulated ♡ Heart	Oval, wider anteroposteriorly 0 Oval	Flattened anteroposteriorly, wide transversely ⊂⊃ Flat
Depth	Moderate	Deep	Deep	Shallow
Side walls	Straight	Convergent	Straight	Straight
Ischial spines	Blunt, somewhat widely separated	Prominent, narrow interspinous diameter	Prominent, often with narrow interspinous diameter	Blunt, widely separated
Sacrum	Deep, curved	Slightly curved, terminal portion often beaked	Slightly curved	Slightly curved
Subpubic arch	Wide	Narrow	Narrow	Wide
Usual mode of birth	Vaginal Spontaneous Occipitoanterior position	Cesarean Vaginal Difficult with forceps	Forceps/spontaneous Occipitoposterior or occipitoanterior position	Vaginal Spontaneous

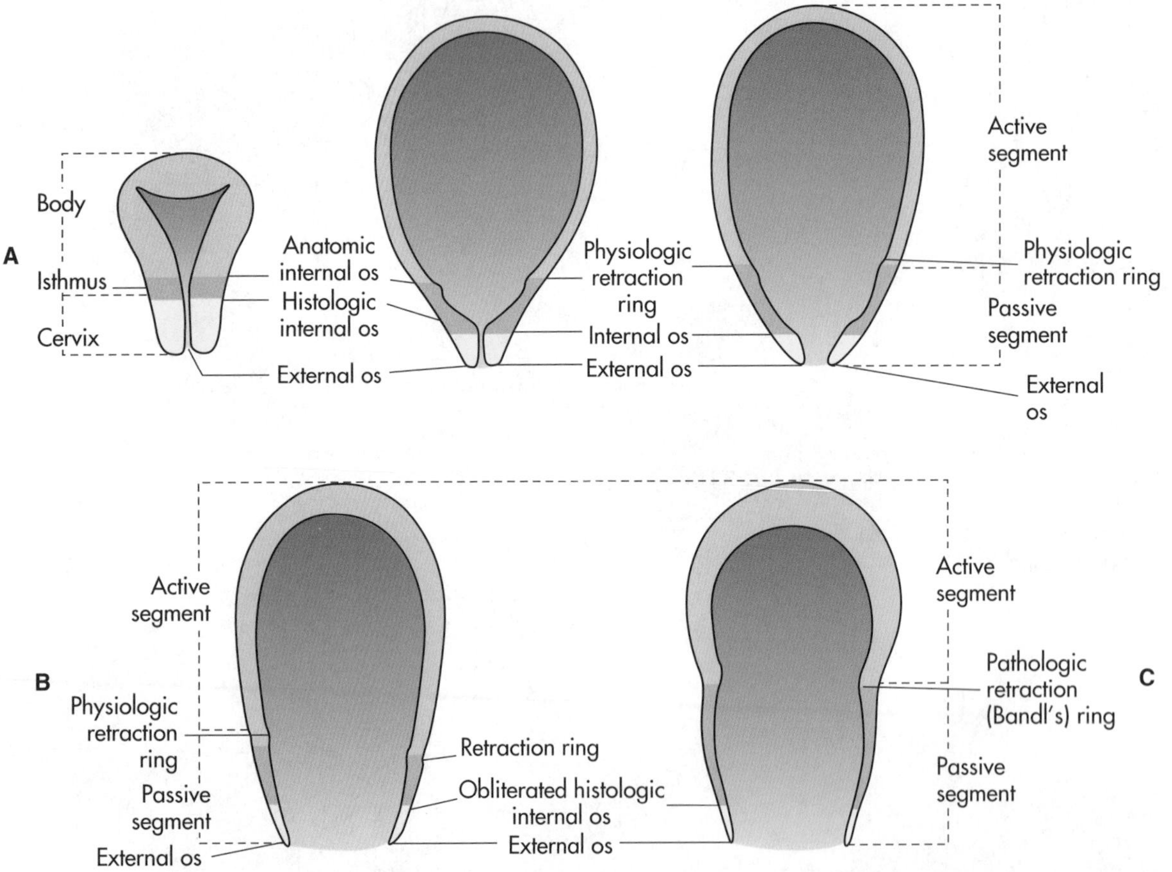

Fig. 15-10 **A,** Uterus in normal labor in early first stage, and **B,** in second stage. Passive segment is derived from lower uterine segment (isthmus) and cervix, and physiologic retraction ring is derived from anatomic internal os. **C,** Uterus in abnormal labor in second-stage dystocia. Pathologic retraction (Bandl's) ring that forms under abnormal conditions develops from the physiologic ring.

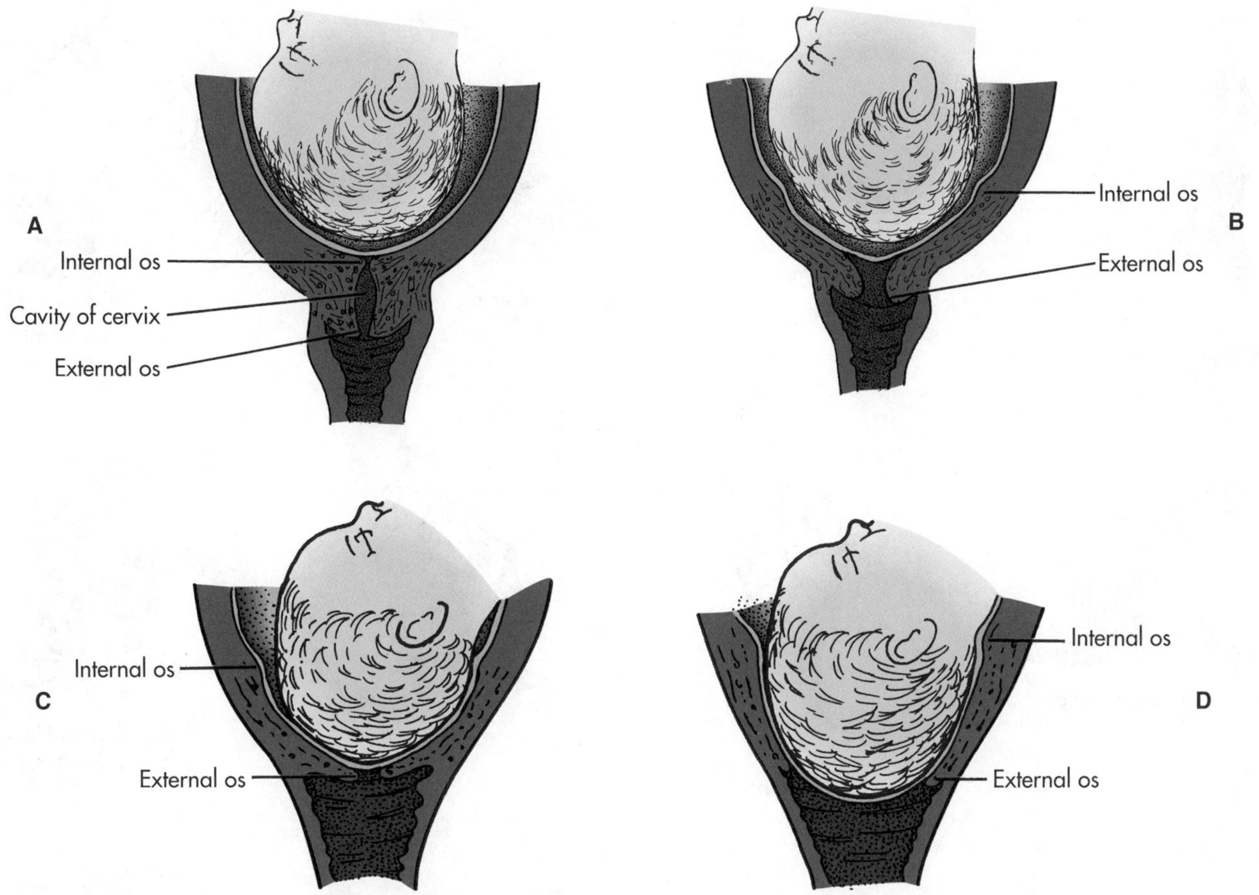

Fig. 15-11 Cervical effacement and dilation. Note how cervix is drawn up around presenting part (internal os). Membranes are intact, and head is not well applied to cervix. **A**, Before labor. **B**, Early effacement. **C**, Complete effacement (100%). Head is well applied to cervix. **D**, Complete dilation (10 cm). Cranial bones overlap somewhat, and membranes are still intact.

spontaneous bearing-down efforts, directed pushing, delayed pushing, Valsalva (closed glottis and prolonged bearing down) pushing, and open glottis pushing (Hansen, Clark, & Foster, 2002; Mayberry et al, 2000; Minato, 2000/2001; Petrou, Coyle, & Fraser, 2000). Although no significant differences have been found in the duration of second-stage labor, adverse consequences have been reported. Fetal hypoxia and subsequent acidosis have been associated with prolonged breath holding and forceful pushing efforts (Roberts, 2002). Perineal tears have been associated with directed pushing (Fraser et al, 2000). Continued study is needed to determine the effectiveness and appropriateness of strategies used by nurses to teach pushing techniques, the suitability and effectiveness of various pushing techniques related to nonreassuring fetal heart patterns, and the standards for length of pushing in terms of maternal and fetal outcomes (Roberts, 2003).

Position of the Laboring Woman

Position affects the woman's anatomic and physiologic adaptations to labor. Frequent changes in position relieve fatigue, increase comfort, and improve circulation (Gupta & Nikodem, 2001). Therefore a laboring woman should be encouraged to find positions that are most comfortable to her (Fig. 15-12, *A*).

An upright position (walking, sitting, kneeling, or squatting) offers a number of advantages. Gravity can promote the descent of the fetus. Uterine contractions are generally stronger and more efficient in effacing and dilating the cervix, resulting in shorter labor (Gupta & Nikodem, 2001; Simkin & Ancheta, 2000).

An upright position also is beneficial to the mother's cardiac output, which normally increases during labor as uterine contractions return blood to the vascular bed. The increased cardiac output improves blood flow to the uteroplacental unit and the maternal kidneys. Cardiac output is compromised if the descending aorta and ascending vena cava are compressed during labor. Compression of these major vessels may result in supine hypotension that decreases placental perfusion. With the woman in an upright position, pressure on the maternal vessels is reduced, and compression is prevented. If the woman wishes to lie down, a lateral position is suggested (Blackburn, 2003).

The "all fours" position (hands and knees) may be used to relieve backache if the fetus is in an occipitoposterior position and may assist in anterior rotation of the fetus and in

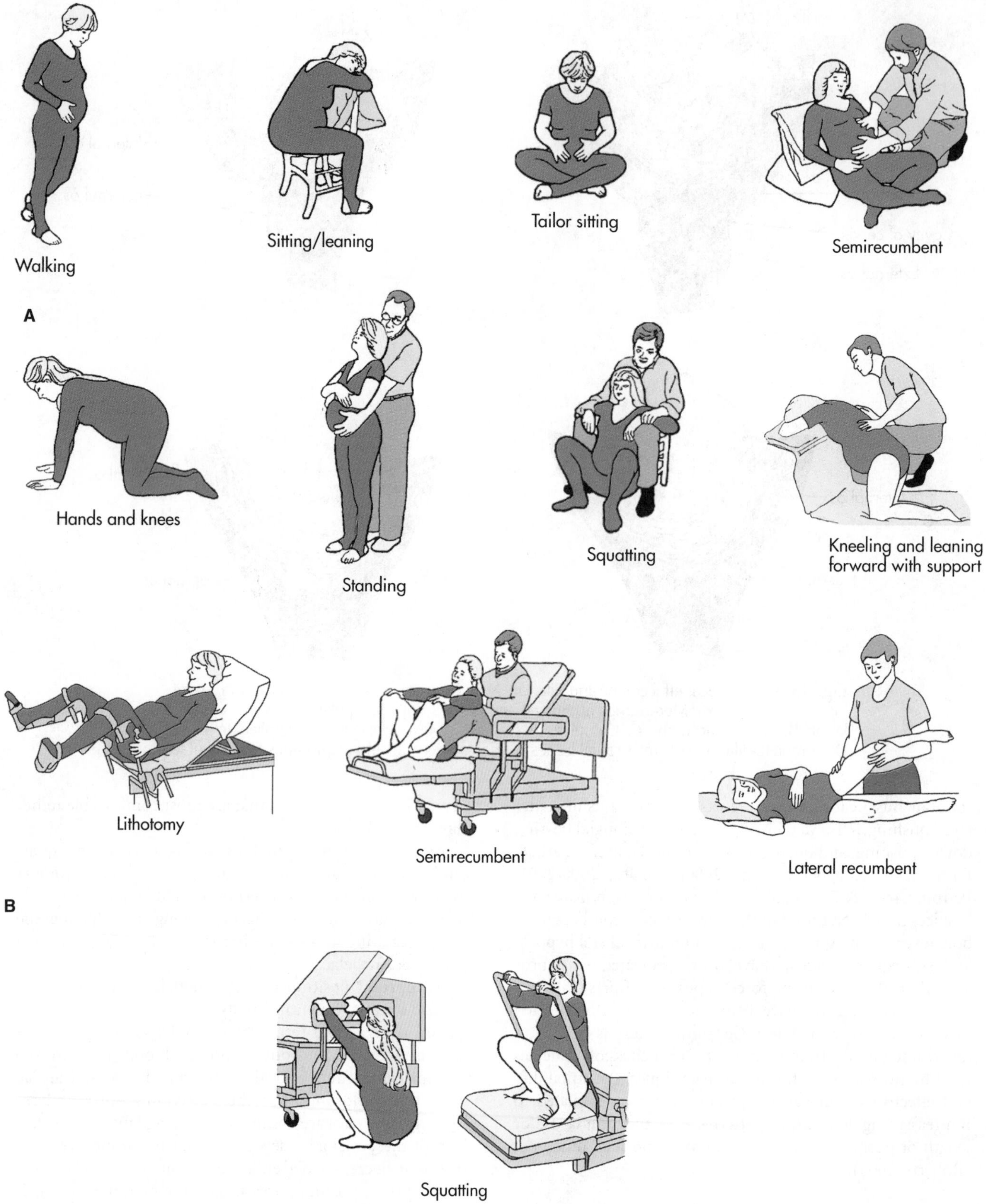

Fig. 15-12 Positions for labor and birth. **A,** Positions for labor. **B,** Positions for birth.

cases of shoulder dystocia (Hofmeyr & Kulier, 2000; Simkin & Ancheta, 2000).

Positioning for second-stage labor (Fig. 15-12, *B*) may be determined by the woman's preference, but it is constrained by the condition of the woman or fetus, the environment, and the health care provider's confidence in assisting in a birth in a specific position (Simkin & Ancheta, 2000). The predominant position in the United States in physician-attended births is the lithotomy position. Alternative positions and position changes that result in more births over an intact perineum are more commonly practiced by nurse-midwives (Shorten, Donsante, & Shorten, 2002).

A woman who pushes in a semirecumbent position needs adequate body support to push effectively because her weight will be on her sacrum, moving the coccyx forward and causing a reduction in the pelvic outlet. In a sitting or squatting position, abdominal muscles work in greater synchrony with uterine contractions during bearing-down efforts. Kneeling or squatting moves the uterus forward and aligns the fetus with the pelvic inlet and can facilitate the second stage of labor by increasing the pelvic outlet (Simkin & Ancheta, 2000).

The lateral position can be used by the woman to help rotate a fetus that is in a posterior position. It also can be used when there is a need for less force to be used during bearing down, such as when there is a need to control the speed of a precipitate birth (Simkin & Ancheta, 2000).

No evidence exists that any of these positions suggested for second-stage labor increases the need for use of operative techniques (e.g., forceps- or vacuum-assisted birth, cesarean birth, episiotomy) or causes perineal trauma. No evidence has been found that use of any of these positions adversely affects the newborn (Mayberry et al, 2000).

PROCESS OF LABOR

Labor is the process of moving the fetus, placenta, and membranes out of the uterus and through the birth canal. Various changes take place in the woman's reproductive system in the days and weeks before labor begins. Labor itself can be discussed in terms of the mechanisms involved in the process and the stages the woman moves through.

Signs Preceding Labor

In first-time pregnancies, the uterus sinks downward and forward about 2 weeks before term, when the fetus's presenting part (usually the fetal head) descends into the true pelvis. This settling is called lightening, or "dropping," and usually happens gradually. After lightening, women feel less congested and breathe more easily, but usually more bladder pressure results from this shift and consequently there is a return of urinary frequency. In a multiparous pregnancy, lightening may not take place until after uterine contractions are established and true labor is in progress.

The woman may complain of persistent low backache and sacroiliac distress as a result of relaxation of the pelvic joints. She may identify strong, frequent, but irregular uterine (Braxton Hicks) contractions.

The vaginal mucus becomes more profuse in response to the extreme congestion of the vaginal mucous membranes. Brownish or blood-tinged cervical mucus may be passed (bloody show). The cervix becomes soft (ripens), becomes partially effaced, and may begin to dilate. The membranes may rupture spontaneously.

Other phenomena are common in the days preceding labor: (1) loss of 0.5 to 1.5 kg in weight, caused by water loss resulting from electrolyte shifts that in turn are produced by changes in estrogen and progesterone levels; and (2) a surge of energy. Women speak of having a burst of energy that they often use to clean the house and put everything in order. Less commonly, some women have diarrhea, nausea, vomiting, and indigestion. Box 15-1 lists signs that may precede labor.

Onset of Labor

The onset of true labor cannot be ascribed to a single cause. Many factors, including changes in the maternal uterus, cervix, and pituitary gland, are involved. Hormones produced by the normal fetal hypothalamus, pituitary, and adrenal cortex probably contribute to the onset of labor. Progressive uterine distention, increasing intrauterine pressure, and aging of the placenta seem to be associated with in-

Community Focus

CHILDBIRTH CLASS FOR SPANISH-SPEAKING NULLIPARAS

You have been asked by the staff at the community health center to prepare a childbirth class on the signs that precede labor for a group of Spanish-speaking nulliparas.

1. Identify essential content to be covered, and describe how you would collect data about the group's knowledge and educational levels (e.g., through an interpreter).
2. Plan a 5- to 10-minute class, including audiovisuals. Discuss the plan with your faculty.
3. Give the class (through an interpreter if needed), and ask the staff at the health center to evaluate it in terms of level of content and appropriate cultural content.

BOX 15-1

Signs Preceding Labor

Lightening
Return of urinary frequency
Backache
Stronger Braxton Hicks contractions
Weight loss of 0.5 to 1.5 kg
Surge of energy
Increased vaginal discharge; bloody show
Cervical ripening
Rupture of membranes

creasing myometrial irritability. This is a result of increased concentrations of estrogen and prostaglandins, as well as decreasing progesterone levels. The mutually coordinated effects of these factors result in the occurrence of strong, regular, rhythmic uterine contractions. The outcome of these factors working together is normally the birth of the fetus and the expulsion of the placenta; however, how certain alterations trigger others and how proper checks and balances are maintained is not known.

Fetal fibronectin is a protein found in plasma and cervicovaginal secretions of pregnant women before the onset of labor. Assessment for the presence of fetal fibronectin is being used to predict the likelihood of preterm labor in women who are at increased risk for this complication (Goldenberg et al, 2003). The value of detection of fetal fibronectin in management of women with preterm labor has yet to be determined; therefore the test is not indicated for screening for preterm labor in low risk pregnant women (Bernhardt & Dorman, 2004).

Stages of Labor

Labor is considered "normal" when the woman is at or near term, no complications exist, a single fetus presents by vertex, and labor is completed within 18 hours. The course of normal labor, which is remarkably constant, consists of (1) regular progression of uterine contractions, (2) effacement and progressive dilation of the cervix, and (3) progress in descent of the presenting part. Four stages of labor are recognized. These stages are discussed in greater detail, along with nursing care for the laboring woman and family, in Chapter 18.

The first stage of labor is considered to last from the onset of regular uterine contractions to full dilation of the cervix. Commonly the onset of labor is difficult to establish because the woman may be admitted to the labor unit just before birth, and the beginning of labor may be only an estimate. The first stage is much longer than the second and third combined. Great variability is the rule, however, depending on the factors discussed previously in this chapter. Full dilation may occur in less than 1 hour in some multiparous pregnancies. In first-time pregnancy, complete dilation of the cervix can take up to 20 hours. Variations may reflect differences in the patient population (e.g., risk status, age) or in clinical management of the labor and birth.

The first stage of labor has been divided into three phases: a latent phase, an active phase, and a transition phase. During the *latent phase,* there is more progress in effacement of the cervix and little increase in descent. During the *active phase* and the *transition phase,* there is more rapid dilation of the cervix and increased rate of descent of the presenting part.

The second stage of labor lasts from the time the cervix is fully dilated to the birth of the fetus. The second stage takes an average of 20 minutes for a multiparous woman and 50 minutes for a nulliparous woman. Labor of up to 2 hours has been considered within the normal range for the second stage, but there can be significant variations. For example, a woman who has received epidural analgesia may take up to 3 hours (Zhang et al, 2001). Ethnicity may shorten the length of the second stage of labor for African-American and Puerto Rican women (Diegmann, Andrews, & Niemczura, 2000).

Simkin and Ancheta (2000) described the latent and active phases of second-stage labor. The latent phase is a period that begins about the time of complete dilation of the uterus when the contractions are weak or not noticeable and the woman is not feeling the urge to push, is resting, or is exerting only small bearing-down efforts with contractions. The active phase is a period when contractions resume, the woman is making strong bearing-down efforts, and the fetal station is advancing.

The third stage of labor lasts from the birth of the fetus until the placenta is delivered. The placenta normally separates with the third or fourth strong uterine contraction after the infant has been born. After it has separated, the placenta can be delivered with the next uterine contraction. The duration of the third stage may be as short as 3 to 5 minutes, although up to 1 hour is considered within normal limits. The risk of hemorrhage increases as the length of the third stage increases (Cunningham et al, 2001).

The fourth stage of labor arbitrarily lasts about 2 hours after delivery of the placenta. It is the period of immediate recovery, when homeostasis is reestablished. It is an important period of observation for complications, such as abnormal bleeding (see Chapter 23).

Mechanism of Labor

As already discussed, the female pelvis has varied contours and diameters at different levels, and the presenting part of the passenger is large in proportion to the passage. Therefore for vaginal birth to occur, the fetus must adapt to the birth canal during the descent. The turns and other adjustments necessary in the human birth process are termed the *mechanism of labor* (Fig. 15-13). The seven cardinal movements of the mechanism of labor that occur in a vertex presentation

Critical Thinking Exercise

PUSHING IN SECOND-STAGE LABOR

During your clinical experience in the labor and birth unit, you are assigned to a woman having her first baby. Her cervix is fully dilated and effaced and the fetus is at station 0. She has an epidural and does not feel the urge to push, but her mother is telling her that she needs to push with each contraction, holding her breath as long as she can while she is pushing. What intervention would you suggest?

1. Evidence—Is there sufficient evidence to draw conclusions about what intervention is needed?
2. Assumptions—Describe underlying assumptions about the following issues:
   a. Phases of second-stage labor
   b. Effects of epidurals on labor for nulliparas
   c. Delayed versus directed pushing
   d. Valsalva (prolonged bearing down) pushing
3. What implications and priorities for nursing care can be made at this time?
4. Does the evidence objectively support your conclusion?
5. Are there alternative perspectives to your conclusions?

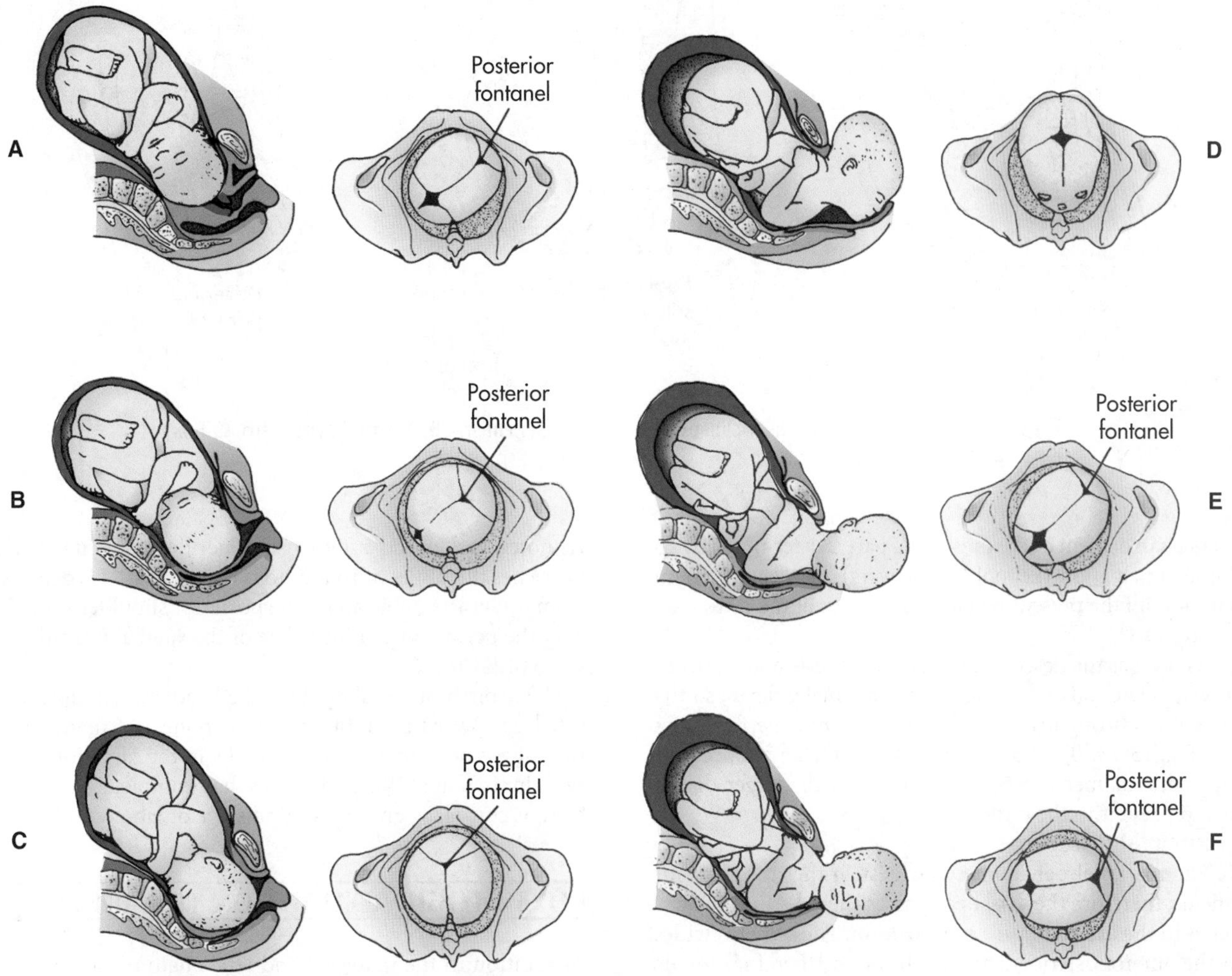

Fig. 15-13 Cardinal movements of the mechanism of labor. Left occipitoanterior (LOA) position. **A**, Engagement and descent. **B**, Flexion. **C**, Internal rotation to occipitoanterior (OA) position. **D**, Extension. **E**, External rotation beginning (restitution). **F**, External rotation.

are engagement, descent, flexion, internal rotation, extension, external rotation (restitution), and finally birth by expulsion. Although these movements are discussed separately, in actuality, a combination of movements occurs simultaneously. For example, engagement involves both descent and flexion.

Engagement

When the biparietal diameter of the head passes the pelvic inlet, the head is said to be engaged in the pelvic inlet (Fig. 15-13, *A*). In most nulliparous pregnancies, this occurs before the onset of active labor because the firmer abdominal muscles direct the presenting part into the pelvis. In multiparous pregnancies, in which the abdominal musculature is more relaxed, the head often remains freely moveable above the pelvic brim until labor is established.

Asynclitism

The head usually engages in the pelvis in a synclitic position, one that is parallel to the anteroposterior plane of the pelvis. Frequently asynclitism occurs (the head is deflected anteriorly or posteriorly in the pelvis), which can facilitate descent because the head is being positioned to accommodate to the pelvic cavity (Fig. 15-14). Extreme asynclitism can cause cephalopelvic disproportion, even in a normal-size pelvis, because the head is positioned so that it cannot descend.

Descent

Descent refers to the progress of the presenting part through the pelvis. Descent depends on at least four forces: (1) pressure exerted by the amniotic fluid, (2) direct pressure exerted by the contracting fundus on the fetus, (3) force of the contraction of the maternal diaphragm and abdominal muscles in the second stage of labor, and (4) extension and straightening of the fetal body. The effects of these forces are modified by the size and shape of the maternal pelvic planes and the size of the fetal head and its capacity to mold.

The degree of descent is measured by the station of the presenting part (see Fig. 15-6). As mentioned, little descent occurs during the latent phase of the first stage of labor. Descent accelerates in the active phase when the cervix has dilated to 5 to 7 cm. It is especially apparent when the membranes have ruptured.

In a first-time pregnancy, descent is usually slow but steady; in subsequent pregnancies descent may be rapid.

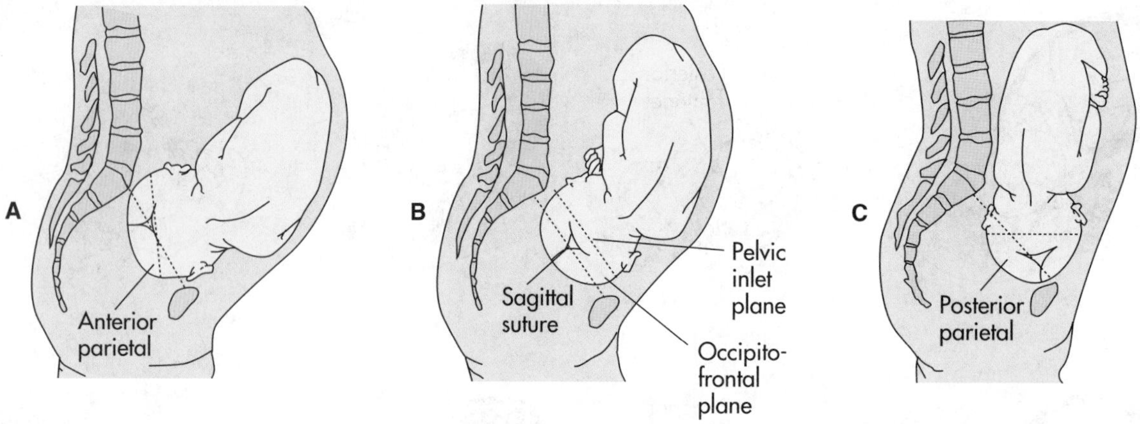

Fig. 15-14 Synclitism and asynclitism. **A,** Anterior asynclitism. **B,** Normal synclitism. **C,** Posterior asynclitism.

Progress in descent of the presenting part is determined by abdominal palpation (Leopold maneuvers) and vaginal examination until the presenting part can be seen at the introitus.

Flexion

As soon as the descending head meets resistance from the cervix, pelvic wall, or pelvic floor, it normally flexes, so that the chin is brought into closer contact with the fetal chest (see Fig. 15-13, *B*). Flexion permits the smaller suboccipitobregmatic diameter (9.5 cm) rather than the larger diameters to present to the outlet.

Internal Rotation

The maternal pelvic inlet is widest in the transverse diameter; therefore the fetal head passes the inlet into the true pelvis in the occipitotransverse position. The outlet is widest in the anteroposterior diameter, however; therefore for the fetus to exit, the head must rotate. Internal rotation begins at the level of the ischial spines but is not completed until the presenting part reaches the lower pelvis. As the occiput rotates anteriorly, the face rotates posteriorly. With each contraction, the fetal head is guided by the bony pelvis and the muscles of the pelvic floor. Eventually the occiput will be in the midline beneath the pubic arch. The head is almost always rotated by the time it reaches the pelvic floor (see Fig. 15-13, *C*). Both the levator ani muscles and the bony pelvis are important for achieving anterior rotation. A previous childbirth injury or regional anesthesia may compromise the function of the levator sling.

Extension

When the fetal head reaches the perineum for birth, it is deflected anteriorly by the perineum. The occiput passes under the lower border of the symphysis pubis first, and then the head emerges by extension: first the occiput, then the face, and finally the chin (see Fig. 15-13, *D*).

Restitution and External Rotation

After the head is born, it rotates briefly to the position it occupied when it was engaged in the inlet. This movement is referred to as restitution (see Fig. 15-13, *E*). The 45-degree turn realigns the infant's head with her or his back and shoulders. The head can then be seen to rotate further. This external rotation occurs as the shoulders engage and descend in maneuvers similar to those of the head (see Fig. 15-13, *F*). As noted earlier, the anterior shoulder descends first. When it reaches the outlet, it rotates to the midline and is delivered from under the pubic arch. The posterior shoulder is guided over the perineum until it is free of the vaginal introitus.

Expulsion

After birth of the shoulders, the head and shoulders are lifted up toward the mother's pubic bone and the trunk of the baby is born by flexing it laterally in the direction of the symphysis pubis. When the baby has completely emerged, birth is complete, and the second stage of labor ends.

PHYSIOLOGIC ADAPTATION TO LABOR

In addition to the maternal and fetal anatomic adaptations that occur during birth, physiologic adaptations must occur. Accurate assessment of the laboring woman and fetus requires knowledge of these expected adaptations.

Fetal Adaptation

Several important physiologic adaptations occur in the fetus. These changes occur in fetal heart rate (FHR), fetal circulation, respiratory movements, and other behaviors.

Fetal Heart Rate

FHR monitoring provides reliable and predictive information about the condition of the fetus related to oxygenation. The average FHR at term is 140 beats/min. The normal range is 110 to 160 beats/min. Earlier in gestation, the FHR is higher, with an average of approximately 160 beats/min at 20 weeks of gestation. The rate decreases progressively as the maturing fetus reaches term. However, temporary accelerations and slight early decelerations of the FHR can be expected in response to spontaneous fetal movement, vaginal examination, fundal pressure, uterine contractions, abdominal palpation, and fetal head compression. Stresses to the uterofetoplacental unit result in characteristic FHR patterns (see Chapter 17 for further discussion).

Fetal Circulation

Fetal circulation can be affected by many factors, including maternal position, uterine contractions, blood pressure, and umbilical cord blood flow. Uterine contractions during labor tend to decrease circulation through the spiral arterioles and subsequent perfusion through the intervillous space. Most healthy fetuses are well able to compensate for this stress and exposure to increased pressure while moving passively through the birth canal during labor. Usually umbilical cord blood flow is undisturbed by uterine contractions or fetal position (Uçkar & Townsend, 1999).

Fetal Respiration

Certain changes stimulate chemoreceptors in the aorta and carotid bodies to prepare the fetus for initiating respirations immediately after birth (Rosenberg, 2002; Uçkar & Townsend, 1999). These changes include the following:

- Fetal lung fluid is cleared from the air passages during labor and (vaginal) birth.
- Fetal oxygen pressure (PO_2) decreases.
- Arterial carbon dioxide pressure (PCO_2) increases.
- Arterial pH decreases.
- Bicarbonate level decreases.
- Fetal respiratory movements decrease during labor.

Maternal Adaptation

As the woman progresses through the stages of labor, various body system adaptations cause the woman to exhibit both objective and subjective symptoms (Box 15-2).

Cardiovascular Changes

During each contraction, an average of 400 ml of blood is emptied from the uterus into the maternal vascular system. This increases cardiac output by about 12% to 31% in the first stage and by about 50% in the second stage. The heart rate increases slightly (Monga, 2004).

Changes in the woman's blood pressure also occur. Blood flow, which is reduced in the uterine artery by contractions, is redirected to peripheral vessels. As a result, peripheral resistance increases, and blood pressure increases (Monga, 2004). During the first stage of labor, uterine contractions cause systolic readings to increase by about 10 mm Hg; assessing blood pressure between contractions therefore provides more accurate readings. During the second stage, contractions may cause systolic pressures to increase by 30 mm Hg and diastolic readings to increase by 25 mm Hg, with both systolic and diastolic pressures remaining somewhat elevated even between contractions (Monga, 2004). Therefore the woman already at risk for hypertension is at increased risk for complications such as cerebral hemorrhage.

Supine hypotension (see Fig. 18-5) occurs when the ascending vena cava and descending aorta are compressed. The laboring woman is at greater risk for supine hypotension if the uterus is particularly large because of multifetal pregnancy, hydramnios, or obesity or if the woman is dehydrated or hypovolemic. In addition, anxiety and pain, as well as some medications, can cause hypotension.

The woman should be discouraged from using the Valsalva maneuver (holding one's breath and tightening abdominal muscles) for pushing during the second stage. This activity increases intrathoracic pressure, reduces venous return, and increases venous pressure. The cardiac output and blood pressure increase and the pulse slows temporarily. During the Valsalva maneuver, fetal hypoxia may occur. The process is reversed when the woman takes a breath.

The white blood cell (WBC) count can increase (Pagana & Pagana, 2003). Although the mechanism leading to this increase in WBCs is unknown, it may be secondary to physical or emotional stress or to tissue trauma. Labor is strenuous, and physical exercise alone can increase the WBC count.

Some peripheral vascular changes occur, perhaps in response to cervical dilation or to compression of maternal vessels by the fetus passing through the birth canal. Flushed cheeks, hot or cold feet, and eversion of hemorrhoids may result.

Respiratory Changes

Increased physical activity with greater oxygen consumption is reflected in an increase in the respiratory rate. Hyperventilation may cause respiratory alkalosis (an increase in pH), hypoxia, and hypocapnia (decrease in carbon dioxide). In the unmedicated woman in the second stage, oxygen consumption almost doubles. Anxiety also increases oxygen consumption.

Renal Changes

During labor, spontaneous voiding may be difficult for various reasons: tissue edema caused by pressure from the presenting part, discomfort, analgesia, and embarrassment. Proteinuria of +1 is a normal finding because it can occur in response to the breakdown of muscle tissue from the physical work of labor.

Integumentary Changes

The integumentary system changes are evident, especially in the great distensibility (stretching) in the area of the vaginal introitus. The degree of distensibility varies with the individual. Despite this ability to stretch, even in the absence of episiotomy or lacerations, minute tears in the skin around the vaginal introitus occur.

Musculoskeletal Changes

The musculoskeletal system is stressed during labor. Diaphoresis, fatigue, proteinuria (+1), and possibly an increased temperature accompany the marked increase in muscle activity. Backache and joint ache (unrelated to fetal position) occur as a result of increased joint laxity at term.

BOX 15-2

Maternal Physiologic Changes during Labor

Cardiac output increases 10% to 15% in first stage; 30% to 50% in second stage.
Heart rate increases slightly in first and second stages.
Systolic blood pressure increases during uterine contractions in first stage; systolic and diastolic pressures increase during uterine contractions in second stage.
White blood cell count increases.
Respiratory rate increases.
Temperature may be slightly elevated.
Proteinuria (+1) may occur.
Gastric motility and absorption of solid food is decreased; nausea and vomiting may occur during transition to second-stage labor.
Blood glucose level decreases.

Evidence-Based Practice

BIRTHING CENTERS VERSUS HOSPITAL BIRTHS

Background

A frequent complaint of the hospital birthing experience is the focus on technology, what some have called the "cascade of interventions" that some women feel grows out of their control. One outcome of the consumer movement has been a demand for a more homelike birthing environment, with a focus on the natural process of birthing. In the 1970s and 1980s, many women in the United States chose to give birth at home, attended by lay midwives or nurse-midwives. Hospitals responded to this with a mid-level solution: homelike birthing centers, staffed by professionals and in close proximity to specialty emergency services. Women at low risk for complications could be seen antenatally, and labor, give birth, and recover in the same environment, accompanied by family. Some birthing centers are owned and staffed by the institution; others are affiliated with a hospital, but staffed independently. Birthing centers share a philosophy that many women can labor and deliver without medication and technology, if only they have the appropriate preparation and support. Birthing center staff feel that the pain cycle of fear-tension-pain can be broken by having the woman in a safe, supportive, familiar environment. Low risk obstetrics is lucrative for hospitals, and most have responded to the competition by offering attractive homelike birthing centers.

Objective

The reviewers planned to compare the maternal and fetal outcomes of birthing center to conventional hospital births. They hoped to compare hospital-based centers to free-standing centers. The intervention was labor and delivery at a birthing center, and the control was conventional hospital care. Outcome measures of interest were intrapartal medical interventions, complications, method of delivery, perinatal death, maternal satisfaction, neonatal health, and adjustment to parenting.

Methods

Search Strategy

The authors looked for randomized or quasi-randomized, controlled trials in Cochrane, MEDLINE, and ZETOC, a weekly awareness service of 37 relevant journals. Search keywords were not noted.

The reviewers selected six trials, involving 8677 women, from the United Kingdom, Sweden, Canada, and Australia, published 1984 to 2000.

Statistical Analyses

Similar data were pooled. Reviewers calculated relative risks for dichotomous (categorical) data, and weighted mean differences for continuous data. The reviewers accepted results outside the 95% confidence intervals as significant differences.

Findings

The birthing center group used less pain medication and less labor augmentation than the hospitalized group. The women were more mobile during labor. There were fewer fetal heart abnormalities and fewer operative deliveries (forceps, vacuum extraction, or cesarean birth). Episiotomy was less frequent, but perineal tears were more frequent. All of these differences were significant. There was no difference between groups in the number that had discontinued breastfeeding by 6 to 8 weeks postpartum. One trial noted significantly more sore nipples and mastitis in the birthing center group. There was a trend toward increased perinatal mortality rate in the birthing center group across three trials, but it did not reach the level of significance. No data were available on the type of caregivers or the continuity of care.

Limitations

Substantial numbers of women (29% to 77%) in the birthing center group transferred to the hospital during labor. Reasons included medical problems, no longer meeting the eligibility criteria for birthing center, and desire for epidural pain medication. This may introduce a selection bias.

Conclusions

Women who give birth in a birthing center have fewer interventions than women who give birth in a hospital. Their outcomes are similar to the birth outcomes of women who give birth in a hospital.

Implications for Practice

The decreased use of pain medication and labor augmentation reflects their limited access in birthing centers. Electronic fetal monitors are not commonly used at birthing centers, so there would be fewer reports of fetal heart abnormalities, and women are freer to move around without monitors or intravenous lines. Many of the results mirror other evidence of the benefits of continuous support during labor and delivery (see "Evidence-Based Practice: Continuous Labor Support," Chapter 18). Hospitals would be wise to focus more on the benefits of continuous care for women in childbirth than the décor of the environment.

The trend toward increased perinatal mortality rate, although not significant, was consistent across three trials. The focus on normality may cause caregivers to miss subtle early warnings of problems, or delay action. All staff members need to be alert to trouble and be able to expedite transfer to hospital care without delay.

Implications for Further Research

Solving the bias problem would be a significant step toward generalizable results. This includes randomization, dropouts, and addressing the inevitable transfers. Cost is a major driving force in policy and choice, yet it was not addressed in these trials. Further exploration of the perinatal mortality trend is warranted.

Reference

Hodnett E: Home-like versus conventional institutional settings for birth (Cochrane Review), 2001. In *The Cochrane Library,* Issue 2, Chichester, UK, 2004, John Wiley & Sons.

The labor process itself and the woman's pointing her toes can cause leg cramps.

Neurologic Changes

Sensorial changes occur as the woman moves through phases of the first stage of labor and as she moves from one stage to the next. Initially she may be euphoric. Euphoria gives way to increased seriousness, then to amnesia between contractions during the second stage, and finally to elation or fatigue after giving birth. Endogenous endorphins (morphine-like chemicals produced naturally by the body) raise the pain threshold and produce sedation. In addition, physiologic anesthesia of perineal tissues, caused by pressure of the presenting part, decreases perception of pain.

Gastrointestinal Changes

During labor, gastrointestinal motility and absorption of solid foods are decreased, and stomach-emptying time is slowed. Nausea and vomiting of undigested food eaten after onset of labor are common. Nausea and belching also occur as a reflex response to full cervical dilation. The woman may state that diarrhea accompanied the onset of labor, or the nurse may palpate the presence of hard or impacted stool in the rectum.

Endocrine Changes

The onset of labor may be triggered by decreasing levels of progesterone and increasing levels of estrogen, prostaglandins, and oxytocin. Metabolism increases, and blood glucose levels may decrease with the work of labor.

Accurate assessment of the mother and fetus during labor and birth depends on knowledge of these expected adaptations so that appropriate interventions can be implemented.

Key Points

- Labor and birth are affected by the five *P*'s: passenger, passageway, powers, position of the woman, and psychologic response.
- Because of its size and relative rigidity, the fetal head is a major factor in determining the course of birth.
- The diameters at the plane of the pelvic inlet, midpelvis, and outlet, plus the axis of the birth canal, determine whether vaginal birth is possible and the manner in which the fetus passes down the birth canal.
- Involuntary uterine contractions act to expel the fetus and placenta during the first stage of labor; these are augmented by voluntary bearing-down efforts during the second stage.
- The first stage of labor lasts from the time dilation begins to the time when the cervix is fully dilated. The second stage of labor lasts from the time of full dilation to the birth of the infant. The third stage of labor lasts from the infant's birth to the expulsion of the placenta. The fourth stage is the first 2 hours after birth.
- The cardinal movements of the mechanism of labor are engagement, descent, flexion, internal rotation, extension, restitution and external rotation, and expulsion of the infant.
- Although the events precipitating the onset of labor are unknown, many factors, including changes in the maternal uterus, cervix, and pituitary gland, are thought to be involved.
- A healthy fetus with an adequate uterofetoplacental circulation will be able to compensate for the stress of uterine contractions.
- As the woman progresses through labor, various body systems adapt to the birth process.

Answer Guidelines to Critical Thinking Exercise

Pushing in Second-Stage Labor

1. Yes, there is sufficient evidence to draw conclusions about what action should be implemented for this patient in second-stage labor.
2. (a) There are variations in the time when a woman feels the initial urge to push. These are related to the fetal station and position of the presenting part. Second-stage labor has an early phase when the woman may not feel an urge to push; the uterine contractions may be weak. The active or last phase is when the woman feels a strong urge to push, usually when the fetal head has advanced to the pelvic floor and the Ferguson reflex is triggered. Passive descent and rotation of the fetal head (i.e., not encouraging the woman to push with contractions) in the early phase may prevent maternal and fetal complications. Pushing may also be more effective if the woman begins to push only after she has an urge to do so. (b) Nulliparas who have an epidural are more likely to have a longer second-stage labor than nulliparas who do not have an epidural, but research has not demonstrated harmful effects on the mother or fetus. With epidurals, the woman may not feel her contractions and may not feel an urge to push. A period of "laboring down" (not pushing with contractions), which allows the fetus to descend and rotate, is one approach to managing patients with epidurals in second-stage labor. (c) Directed bearing down (pushing in a manner that the care provider thinks is effective or that is based on the appearance of contractions on the electronic monitor) may trigger the Valsalva maneuver, which can cause an increase in maternal blood pressure and nonreassuring fetal heart rate patterns. The woman with an epidural may be directed to push too soon and become tired before the contractions are strong again. Directed pushing also has been associated with perineal tears. Delayed or spontaneous pushing has been shown to have fewer effects on maternal blood pressure and fetal status. Fewer interventions are needed (e.g., episiotomies and forceps or vacuum assistance). Delayed pushing for women with epidurals (i.e., laboring down) allows fetal descent and rotation before pushing is initiated. Even though there is evidence for this practice, it is not yet widely used in labor and birth units. (d) Use of prolonged strenuous pushing during contractions can affect maternal and fetal status. Maternal cardiac output may decrease, resulting in decreased blood flow to the uterus and decreased fetal oxygenation, resulting in fetal hypoxia and acidosis. This practice has been found to be harmful or ineffective and should be discouraged.
3. The nursing priority is to help the woman in having a safe and effective second stage of labor with no maternal or fetal complications. Assessments for maternal and fetal effects of directed prolonged pushing need to be made. Explanations about the positive effects of delayed pushing are needed. The woman's mother needs to be included in the discussion about delayed pushing so that she becomes a better support for her daughter. When pushing is needed, demonstration and encouragement of taking cleansing breaths as the contraction starts, pushing with the greatest force of the contraction, and taking breaths between bearing-down efforts during the contraction are appropriate interventions. Continued nursing support, coaching, and encouragement for the patient and her mother during the second stage are needed.
4. Yes, there is evidence to support these conclusions about delayed second-stage pushing for nulliparous women

with epidurals (see AWHONN's Nursing Management of the Second Stage of Labor, 2000).

5. Some studies have not found a difference in length of second-stage labor regardless of whether the woman delays pushing. If the woman wants to keep pushing, she should be encouraged to use the open glottis method rather than the closed glottis method.

Resources

Alexian Brothers Medical Center
Elk Grove, IL
Information on stages of labor and other labor and birth topics
847-437-5500
www.alexian.org/progserv/babies/babytoo.html

Baby Center
Source for expectant parents
www.babycenter.com/pregnancy

Childbirth Graphics
PO Box 21207
Waco, TX 76702
800-229-3366
www.childbirthgraphics.com

Childbirth Organization
Source of links to other sites related to labor and birth
www.childbirth.org

References

Alexander JM et al: Epidural analgesia lengthens the Friedman active phase of labor, *Obstet Gynecol* 100(1):46-50, 2002.

Aminoff MJ: Neurologic disorders. In Creasy RK, Resnik R, Iams JD (eds): *Maternal-fetal medicine: principles and practice,* ed 5, Philadelphia, 2004, WB Saunders.

Association of Women's Health, Obstetric, and Neonatal Nurses: *Nursing management of the second stage of labor,* Washington, DC, 2000, AWHONN.

Barkauskas VH, Baumann LC, Darling-Fisher CS: *Health and physical assessment,* ed 3, St Louis, 2002, Mosby.

Bernhardt J, Dorman K: Pre-term birth risk assessment tools: exploring fetal fibronectin and cervical length for validating risk, *AWHONN Lifelines* 8(1):38-44, 2004.

Blackburn ST: *Maternal, fetal, and neonatal physiology: a clinical perspective,* ed 2, St Louis, 2003, WB Saunders.

Cunningham F et al: *Williams obstetrics,* ed 21, New York, 2001, McGraw-Hill.

Diegmann EK, Andrews CM, Niemczura CA: The length of the second stage of labor in uncomplicated, nulliparous African American and Puerto Rican women, *J Midwifery Womens Health* 45(1):67-71, 2000.

Fraser WD et al: Multicentered, randomized, controlled trial of delaying pushing for nulliparopus women in the second stage of labor with continuous epidural analgesia, *Am J Obstet Gynecol* 182(5):1165-1172, 2000.

Goldenberg RL et al: What have we learned about the predictors of preterm birth? *Semin Perinatol* 27(3):185-193, 2003.

Gupta J, Nikodem V: Woman's position during second stage of labor (Cochrane Review). In *The Cochrane Library,* Issue 2, Oxford, 2001, Update Software.

Hansen SL, Clark SL, Foster JC: Active pushing versus passive fetal descent in the second stage of labor: a randomized controlled trial, *Obstet Gynecol* 99(1):29-34, 2002.

Hodnett E: Home-like versus conventional institutional settings for birth (Cochrane Review), 2001. In *The Cochrane Library,* Issue 2, Chichester, UK, 2004, John Wiley & Sons.

Hofmeyr G, Kulier R: Hands/knees posture in later pregnancy or labour for fetal malposition (lateral or posterior) (Cochrane Review). In *The Cochrane Library,* Issue 2, Oxford, 2000, Update Software.

Mayberry L et al: *AWHONN symposium: second-stage labor management: promotion of evidence-based practice and a collaborative approach to patient care,* Washington, DC, 2000, Association of Women's Health, Obstetric, and Neonatal Nurses.

Minato JF: Is it time to push? Examining rest in second-stage labor, *AWHONN Lifelines* 4(6):20-23, 2000/2001.

Monga M: Maternal cardiovascular and renal adaptations to pregnancy. In Creasy RK, Resnik R, Iams JD (eds): *Maternal-fetal medicine: principles and practice,* ed 5, Philadelphia, 2004, WB Saunders.

Pagana KD, Pagana TJ: *Mosby's diagnostic and laboratory test reference,* ed 6, St Louis, 2003, Mosby.

Petrou S, Coyle D, Fraser WD: Cost-effectiveness of a delayed pushing policy for patients with epidural anesthesia: the PEOPLE (Pushing Early or Pushing Late with Epidural) Study Group, *Am J Obstet Gynecol* 182(5):1158-1164, 2000.

Roberts JE: The "push" for evidence: management of the second stage, *J Midwifery Womens Health* 47(1):2-15, 2002.

Roberts JE: A new understanding of the second stage of labor: implications for nursing care, *J Obstet Gynecol Neonat Nurs* 32(6):794-801, 2003.

Rosenberg A: The neonate. In Gabbe SG, Niebyl JR, Simpson JL (eds): *Obstetrics: normal and problem pregnancies,* ed 4, New York, 2002, Churchill Livingstone.

Seidel HM et al: *Mosby's guide to physical examination,* ed 5, St Louis, 2003, Mosby.

Sharma SK, Leveno KJ: Regional analgesia and progress of labor, *Clin Obstet Gynecol* 46(3):633-645, 2003.

Shorten A, Donsante J, Shorten B: Birth position, accoucheur, and perineal outcomes: informing women about choices for vaginal birth, *Birth* 29(1):18-27, 2002.

Simkin P, Ancheta R: *The labor progress handbook: early interventions to prevent and treat dystocia,* Oxford, 2000, Blackwell Science.

Uçkar E, Townsend N: Fetal adaptation. In Mandeville L, Troiano N (eds): *AWHONN's high-risk and critical care intrapartum nursing,* ed 2, Philadelphia, 1999, Lippincott.

VandeVusse L: The essential forces of labor revisited: 13 Ps reported in womens' stories, *MCN Am J Matern Child Nurs* 24(4):176-184, 1999.

Zhang J et al: Does epidural analgesia prolong labor and increase risk of cesarean delivery? A natural experiment, *Am J Obstet Gynecol* 185(1): 128-134, 2001.

Management of Discomfort 16

LEARNING OBJECTIVES

On completion of this chapter the reader will be able to:

- Compare various childbirth preparation methods.
- Describe breathing and relaxation techniques used for each stage of labor.
- Identify nonpharmacologic strategies to enhance relaxation and decrease discomfort during labor.
- Discuss types of analgesia and anesthesia used during labor.
- Compare pharmacologic methods of relief of discomfort in different stages of labor and for different methods of birth.
- Describe nursing responsibilities appropriate for a woman receiving analgesia and anesthesia during labor.

ELECTRONIC RESOURCES

Additional information related to the content in Chapter 16 can be found on

the companion website at evolve
http://evolve.elsevier.com/Wong/maternal/
- NCLEX Review Questions
- WebLinks

or the interactive student CD-ROM
Activities for Chapter 16 include the following:
- NCLEX Review Questions
- Critical Thinking Exercise–Patient Receiving Epidural Block
- Nursing Care Plan–Nonpharmacologic Management of Discomfort
- Nursing Care Plan–Epidural Block during Labor

Pain is an unpleasant, complex, highly individualized phenomenon with both sensory and emotional components. Pregnant women commonly worry about the pain they will experience during labor and birth and how they will react to and deal with that pain. Many physiologic, psychosocial, and environmental factors influence the nature and degree of pain of a woman in labor and the manner in which she will respond to and cope with the pain (Lowe, 2002). A variety of childbirth preparation methods are available to help the woman or couple cope with the discomfort of labor. The methods selected depend on the situation, availability, and the preferences of the woman and her primary health care provider.

The discomforts experienced during labor are discussed in this chapter, as are nonpharmacologic and pharmacologic interventions to relieve the discomforts during the different stages of labor. This information provides the basis for understanding the nurse's role in management of maternal discomfort during labor.

DISCOMFORT DURING LABOR AND BIRTH

Neurologic Origins

The pain and discomfort experienced during labor has two origins: visceral and somatic (Lowe, 2002). During the first stage of labor, uterine contractions cause cervical dilation and effacement. Uterine ischemia (decreased blood flow and therefore local oxygen deficit) results from compression of the arteries supplying the myometrium during uterine contractions. Pain impulses during the first stage of labor are transmitted through the T10 to T12 spinal nerve segment and accessory lower thoracic and upper lumbar sympathetic nerves. These nerves originate in the uterine body and cervix.

The pain from cervical changes, distention of the lower uterine segment, and uterine ischemia that predominates during the first stage of labor is visceral pain. It is located over the lower portion of the abdomen. Referred pain occurs when the pain that originates in the uterus radiates to the abdominal wall, lumbosacral area of the back, iliac crests, gluteal area, and down the thighs. Usually the woman experiences discomfort only during contractions and is free of pain between contractions, although some women have continuous contraction-related low back pain, even in the interval between contractions (Lowe, 2002).

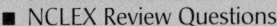

During the second stage of labor, the stage of expulsion of the baby, the woman experiences somatic pain. This pain is often described as intense, sharp, burning, and well localized. Pain results from stretching and distention of perineal tissues and the pelvic floor to allow passage of the fetus, from distention and traction on the peritoneum and uterocervical supports during contractions, and from lacerations of soft tissue (e.g., cervix, vagina, perineum). Discomfort also can be produced by expulsive forces or by pressure exerted by the presenting part on the bladder, bowel, or other sensitive pelvic structures. Pain impulses during the second stage of labor are carried from perineal tissues via the S2 to S4 spinal nerve segments and the parasympathetic system (Lowe, 2002).

Pain during the third stage of labor and the afterpains of the early postpartum period are uterine, similar to that experienced early in the first stage of labor. Areas of discomfort during labor are illustrated in Fig. 16-1.

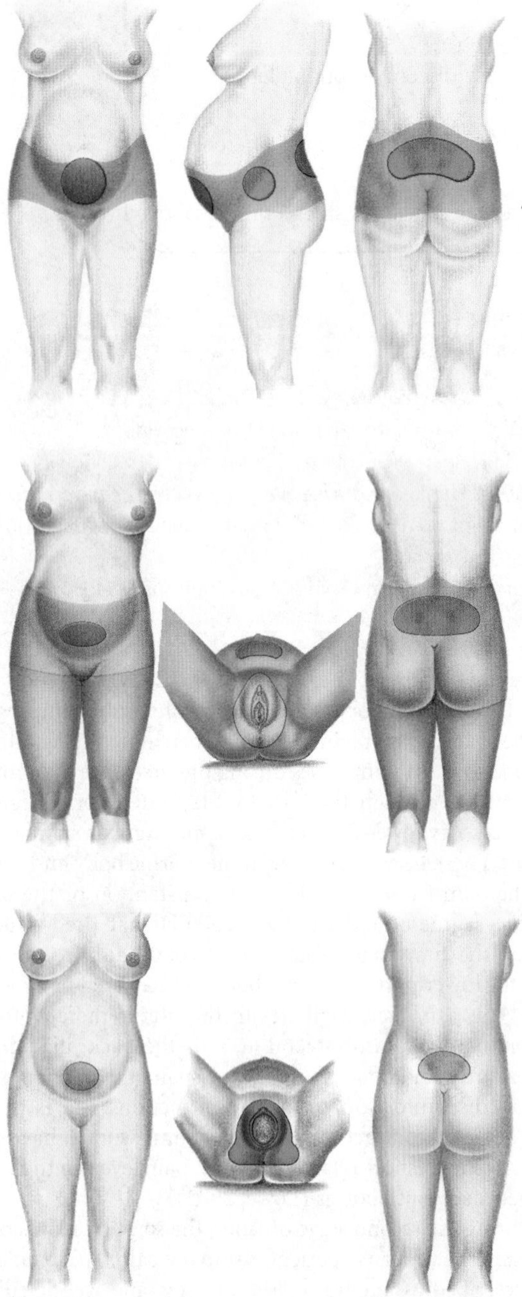

Fig. 16-1 Discomfort during labor. **A,** Distribution of labor pain during first stage. **B,** Distribution of labor pain during later phase of first stage and early phase of second stage. **C,** Distribution of labor pain during later phase of second stage and during birth. (*Gray shading* indicates areas of mild discomfort; *light-colored shading* indicates areas of moderate discomfort; *dark-colored shading* indicates areas of intense discomfort.)

Perception of Pain

Although the pain threshold is remarkably similar in all persons regardless of gender, social, ethnic, or cultural differences, these differences play a definite role in the person's perception of and behavioral responses to pain. The effects of factors such as culture, counterstimuli, and distraction in coping with pain are not fully understood. The meaning of pain and the verbal and nonverbal expressions given to pain are apparently learned from interactions within the primary social group. Cultural influences may impose unrealistic expectations. For instance, Asian women typically believe it shameful to scream or show pain, and they avoid verbal expression (Weber, 1996).

Expression of Pain

Pain results in physiologic effects and sensory and emotional (affective) responses. During childbirth, pain gives rise to identifiable physiologic effects. Sympathetic nervous system activity is stimulated in response to intensifying pain, resulting in increased catecholamine levels. Blood pressure and heart rate increase. Maternal respiratory patterns change in response to an increase in oxygen consumption. Hyperventilation, sometimes accompanied by respiratory alkalosis, can occur as pain intensifies. Pallor and diaphoresis may be seen. Gastric acidity increases, and nausea and vomiting are common in the active phase of labor. Placental perfusion may decrease, and uterine activity may diminish, potentially prolonging labor and affecting fetal well-being.

The sensory quality of visceral and somatic pain has been described as prickling, stabbing, burning, bursting, aching, heavy, pulling, throbbing, sharp, shooting, stinging, or cramping. The emotional (affective) quality of pain has been described as tiring, exhausting, annoying, sickening, and nauseating (Lowe, 2002).

Certain emotional (affective) expressions of suffering are often seen. Such changes include increasing anxiety with lessened perceptual field, writhing, crying, groaning, gesturing (hand clenching and wringing), and excessive muscular excitability throughout the body. Cultural expression of pain may vary. For example, Native American women may endure pain quietly, whereas Hispanic women may endure pain stoically, because it is expected and esteemed, but consider it acceptable to cry out (Villarruel, 1995).

Factors Influencing Pain Response

Each woman's pain during childbirth is unique and is influenced by a variety of factors.

Physiologic Factors

A variety of physiologic factors can affect the intensity of pain experienced by women during childbirth. Women with a history of dysmenorrhea may experience increased pain during childbirth as a result of higher prostaglandin levels. Back pain associated with menstruation also may increase the likelihood of contraction-related low back pain. Upright positions, when assumed during labor, seem to result in decreased pain and an overall increase in comfort when compared with the supine position. Women also report that being able to move freely to find a position of comfort is an important factor in reducing pain and muscle tension and maintaining control during labor. The relation of fetal size to the dimensions of the maternal pelvis may influence pain intensity (Lowe, 2002; Simkin & O'Hara, 2002).

Endorphins are endogenous opioids secreted by the pituitary gland that act on the central and peripheral nervous systems to reduce pain. Beta-endorphin is the most potent of the endorphins. Although the physiologic role of endorphins is not completely understood, it is thought that endorphin levels increase during pregnancy and birth in humans. Higher endorphin levels may increase the ability of women in labor to tolerate acute pain and may reduce their irritability and anxiety. Levels of beta-endorphins are higher when a woman experiences a spontaneous, natural childbirth (Righard, 2001).

Culture

The obstetric population reflects the increasingly multicultural nature of U.S. society. As nurses care for women and families from a variety of cultural backgrounds, they must have knowledge and understanding of how culture mediates pain (Lee & Essoka, 1998; Mattson, 2000). An understanding of the beliefs, values, expectations, and practices of various cultures will narrow the cultural gap and help the nurse to assess the laboring woman's pain experience more accurately and to provide culturally sensitive care by using appropriate pain relief measures (Cultural Awareness) (see Table 18-1). The nurse must take care not to have *cultural blindness,* an inability to see other courses of action, which may lead to cultural clashes, resulting in less than optimal care and less than satisfied women of a culture different from that of the nurse (Weber, 1996). It is important for the nurse to recognize that although a woman's behavior in response to pain may vary according to her cultural background, it may not accurately reflect the intensity of the pain she is experiencing. The nurse must assess the woman for the physiologic effects of pain and must listen to the words the woman uses to describe the sensory and affective qualities of her pain (Lowe, 2002).

Anxiety and Fear

Anxiety and fear are commonly associated with increased pain during labor. Mild anxiety is considered normal for a woman during labor and birth. However, excessive anxiety and fear cause catecholamine secretion, resulting in more pelvic pain stimuli reaching the brain; this in turn magnifies pain perception (Lowe, 2002). As anxiety heightens, muscle tension increases, the effectiveness of the uterine contractions decreases, and discomfort intensifies; a cycle of increased fear and anxiety begins. Ultimately this cycle will slow the progress of labor. The woman's confidence in her ability to cope with pain will be diminished, potentially resulting in reduced effectiveness of pain relief measures being used.

Previous Experience

Previous experience with pain and childbirth may affect a woman's description of her pain and her ability to cope with the pain. Childbirth, for a healthy young adult woman, may be her first experience with significant pain, and as a result, she may not have developed effective pain coping strategies. She may describe the intensity of even early labor pain as pain "as bad as it can be." Sensory pain for nulliparous women is often greater than that for multiparous women during early labor (dilation less than 5 cm) because their reproductive tract structures are less supple. During the transition phase of the first stage of labor and during the second stage of labor, multiparous women may experience greater sensory pain than nulliparous women because their more supple tissue increases the speed of fetal descent and thereby intensifies pain. The firmer tissue of nulliparous women results in a slower, more gradual descent. Affective pain is usually greater for nulliparous women throughout the first stage of labor but decreases for both nulliparous and multiparous women during the second stage of labor (Lowe, 2002).

For women who have had a difficult and painful previous birth experience, anxiety and fear from this past experience may lead to increased perception of pain. Conversely, a woman who experienced a labor and birth in which the degree of pain matched expectations and her coping skills were successful may have decreased anxiety. However, if those previously successful coping skills no longer work because of a more difficult labor, anxiety will increase.

Cultural Awareness

SOME CULTURAL BELIEFS ABOUT PAIN

The following are only examples of how women of different cultural backgrounds may react to pain. Because they are generalizations, the nurse must assess each woman experiencing pain related to childbirth.

- Chinese women may not exhibit reactions to pain, although it is acceptable to exhibit pain during childbirth. They consider it impolite to accept something when it is first offered; therefore pain interventions may need to be offered more than once. Acupuncture may be used for pain relief.
- Arab or Middle Eastern women may be vocal in response to labor pain. They may prefer medication for pain relief.
- Japanese women may be stoic in response to labor pain, but they may request medication when pain becomes severe.
- Southeast Asian women may endure severe pain before requesting relief.
- Hispanic women may be stoic until late in labor, when they may become vocal and request pain relief.
- Native American women may use medications or remedies made from indigenous plants. They are often stoic in response to labor pain.
- African-American women may express pain openly. Use of medication for pain relief varies.

Community Focus

CULTURE AND PAIN

Talk to a woman from a culture different from your own who has experienced childbirth. Ask her to describe her reactions to pain, how she sought relief of pain, the atmosphere of the childbirth setting, and the attitudes of the health care providers. How did her culture influence her response to labor and the associated pain? What expressions of pain are "acceptable" in her culture? What is the role of support persons in the labor process? Are her responses different from your responses to those same questions?

Women with a history of substance abuse have as much pain during labor as other women. Although it is usually unnecessary to withhold pain medications, close monitoring for complications associated with each substance is part of the nursing assessment. For example, opioid antagonists or opioid agonist-antagonists should be avoided for women with a history of opioid abuse because abstinence syndrome (withdrawal) may be precipitated in the woman and her newborn (Hawkins, Chestnut, & Gibbs, 2002).

Pain is a personal response in each individual. As pain is experienced, people develop various coping mechanisms to deal with it. Emotional tension from anxiety and fear may increase pain and perception of pain during labor (see the discussion of the Dick-Read method later in this chapter). Pain, or the possibility of pain, can induce fear in which anxiety borders on panic. Fatigue and sleep deprivation magnify pain. Parity may affect perception of labor pain because nulliparous women often have longer labors and thus greater fatigue, causing a vicious circle of increased pain, fatigue, reduced ability to cope, and a more likely use of pharmacologic support.

Childbirth Preparation

Even particularly intense pain can, at times, be ignored. This is possible because certain nerve cell groupings within the spinal cord, brainstem, and cerebral cortex have the ability to modulate the pain impulse through a blocking mechanism. The gate-control theory of pain helps explain the way hypnosis and the pain relief techniques taught in childbirth preparation classes work to relieve the pain of labor. According to this theory, pain sensations travel along sensory nerve pathways to the brain, but only a limited number of sensations, or messages, can travel through these nerve pathways at one time. By using distraction techniques such as massage or stroking, music, focal points, and imagery, the capacity of nerve pathways to transmit pain is reduced or completely blocked. These distractions are thought to work by closing down a hypothetic gate in the spinal cord, thus preventing pain signals from reaching the brain. Perception of pain stimuli is thereby diminished.

In addition, when the woman in labor engages in neuromuscular and motor activity, activity within the spinal cord itself further modifies the transmission of pain. Cognitive work involving concentration on breathing and relaxation requires selective and directed cortical activity that activates and closes the gating mechanism as well. As labor intensifies, more complex cognitive techniques are required to maintain effectiveness. The gate-control theory therefore underscores the need for a supportive birth setting that allows the laboring woman to relax and use various higher mental activities.

Comfort

Although the predominant medical approach to labor is that it is painful and the pain must be removed, an alternative view is that labor is a natural process and women can experience comfort and transcend the discomfort or pain to reach the joyful outcome of birth. Having needs and desires met engenders a feeling of comfort. Comfort may be viewed as strengthening; this represents a paradigm shift in the interpretation of pain in labor (Schuiling & Sampselle, 1999). The most helpful interventions in enhancing comfort are a caring nursing approach and a supportive presence.

Support

The pain occurring during childbirth, and the management of this pain, belongs to the woman experiencing the pain. The nurse must engage in a cooperative effort to provide whatever external tools the woman requires to manage her pain experience. These tools include both nonpharmacologic and pharmacologic interventions. A woman's satisfaction with her childbirth experience is primarily influenced by the attitudes and behaviors of her caregivers, including the caregivers' ability to communicate and to be helpful, supportive, accepting, and kind. In addition, satisfaction is influenced by the degree to which she was able to stay in control of her labor and to participate in decision making regarding her labor, including the pain relief measures to be used (Hodnett, 2002).

The presence of a person (e.g., doula, partner, family member, friend, nurse) who provides continuous physical, emotional, and psychologic support of the woman in labor is a beneficial form of care. Continuous support significantly relieves pain, improves outcomes, decreases interventions (e.g., use of pharmacologic pain relief measures) and complication rates (e.g., cesarean births) associated with labor, and enhances overall maternal satisfaction (Enkin et al, 2000; Hodnett et al, 2004; Righard, 2001; Simkin & O'Hara, 2002). The Hawthorne effect may in part explain the positive benefit of continuous support during labor and birth. According to this effect, the woman in labor will perform better when receiving special attention and encouragement from a support person (Jiménez, 2000).

Environment

According to Lowe (2002), environment should be viewed in terms of the persons present (e.g., how they communicate, their philosophy of care, practice policies, and quality of support) and the physical space in which the labor occurs. The quality of the environment can influence a woman's ability to cope with the pain of labor. Women prefer to be cared for by familiar caregivers in a comfortable, homelike setting (Hodnett, 2002). An environment should be safe and private, allowing a woman to feel free to be herself as she tries out different comfort measures. Stimuli such as light, noise, and temperature should be adjusted according to the woman's preferences. There should be space for movement, and equipment should be readily available for a variety of nonpharmacologic pain relief measures such as birth balls, comfortable chairs, tubs, and showers. The familiarity of the environment can be enhanced by bringing items from home such as pillows, objects for a focal point, music, and videos.

NONPHARMACOLOGIC MANAGEMENT OF DISCOMFORT

The alleviation of pain is important. Commonly it is not the amount of pain the woman experiences, but whether she meets her goals for herself in coping with the pain that influences her perception of the birth experience as "good" or "bad." The observant nurse looks for cues to identify the woman's desired level of control in the management of pain and its relief.

Nonpharmacologic measures are often simple, safe, and relatively inexpensive. They provide the woman with a sense of control over her childbirth as she makes choices about the measures that are best for her. She should be encouraged to write a birth plan that lists her preferences for pain relief measures. Using these measures requires the woman's active participation and support from her partner and caregivers.

The woman who chooses to deal with childbirth pain by using nonpharmacologic methods needs care and support from nurses and other care providers who are skilled in pain management. Nonpharmacologic methods for relief of discomfort are taught in many different types of prenatal preparation classes, or the woman or couple may have read various books and magazine articles on the subject in advance. Many of these methods require practice for best results (e.g., hypnosis, patterned breathing and controlled relaxation techniques, biofeedback), although the nurse may use some of them successfully without the woman or couple having prior knowledge (e.g., slow-paced breathing, massage and touch, effleurage, counterpressure). Women should be encouraged to try a variety of methods and to seek alternatives, including pharmacologic methods, if the measure being used is no longer effective (Box 16-1).

Childbirth Education

Childbirth, when one is prepared and well supported, presents to women a unique and powerful opportunity to find their core strength in a manner that forever changes their self-perception. Additionally, it can offer women an experience in trusting their body wisdom in a way that may alter how they respond throughout life to health challenges. Most health care providers recommend or offer childbirth preparation classes to expectant parents.

Most proponents of prepared childbirth agree that the major causes of pain in labor are fear and tension. All childbirth methods attempt to reduce these two factors and eliminate pain by increasing the woman's knowledge of the labor and birth process, enhancing her self-confidence and sense of control, preparing a support person, and training the woman in physical conditioning and relaxation breathing.

There are a few fine differences in approach. For example, in the Lamaze method, external focusing and distraction are stressed. In the Bradley method, women are discouraged from using medication and encouraged to focus inwardly and to take direction from their own body. In reality, few instructors adhere strictly to one particular method but instead incorporate a variety of strategies aimed at increasing the woman's ability to cope with labor and minimize her need for medication.

Early methods of childbirth education included the Dick-Read method, or natural childbirth; the Lamaze, or psychoprophylactic, method; and the Bradley, or husband-coached, method.

Dick-Read Method

An English physician, Grantly Dick-Read, published two books (*Natural Childbirth*, 1933; *Childbirth without Fear,* 1944) in which he theorized that pain in childbirth is socially conditioned and caused by a fear-tension-pain syndrome. The Grantly Dick-Read method, referred to as *Childbirth without Fear,* initially recommended deep abdominal breathing during early first-stage contractions, shallow breathing for later first stage, and sustained pushing with breath holding (Dick-Read, 1987). Women were taught to relax different muscle groups through the entire body, consciously and progressively, until a high degree of skill at relaxation was achieved. Consequently a woman was taught to relax completely between contractions and keep all muscles except the uterus relaxed during contractions.

Lamaze Method

During the 1960s the Lamaze method, originally known as the psychoprophylactic method (PPM), was introduced in the United States by Marjorie Karmel in her book *Thank You, Dr. Lamaze,* published in 1959. PPM offered new perspectives on preparation for childbirth by emphasizing control by using the mind. PPM combined controlled muscular relaxation and breathing techniques. Active relaxation has been an integral part of the Lamaze method. The woman was taught to contract specific muscle groups (neuromuscular control) while relaxing the remainder of her body. She thus learned to relax the uninvolved muscles in her body while her uterus contracted. Instead of tensing during uterine contractions, women were conditioned to respond with relaxation and breathing patterns.

Bradley Method

The Bradley method, also called husband-coached childbirth, was devised based on observations of animal behavior

BOX 16-1

Nonpharmacologic Strategies to Encourage Relaxation and Relieve Pain

Cutaneous Stimulation Strategies
- Counterpressure*
- Effleurage (light massage)*
- Therapeutic touch and massage*
- Walking*
- Rocking*
- Changing positions*
- Application of heat or cold*
- Transcutaneous electrical nerve stimulation
- Acupressure
- Water therapy (hydrotherapy)
- Intradermal water block

Sensory Stimulation Strategies
- Aromatherapy
- Breathing techniques*
- Music*
- Imagery*
- Use of focal points*

Cognitive Strategies
- Childbirth education*
- Hypnosis
- Biofeedback

*Forms of care likely to be beneficial (Enkin et al, 2000).

during birth. It emphasizes working in harmony with the body, using breath control and abdominal breathing, and promoting general body relaxation (Bradley, 1981). The husband or partner takes an active role in assisting the woman to relax and use correct breathing techniques. This method also stresses environmental factors such as darkness, solitude, and quiet to make childbirth a more natural experience. Women using the Bradley method often appear to be sleeping during labor because they are in such a deep state of mental relaxation. Medication is discouraged.

Today there are a variety of groups who have adopted many of the elements of these earlier methods. They have in common the belief that childbirth is a natural process and that interventions should be kept to a minimum.

The Coalition to Improve Maternity Services (CIMS) was founded in 1996. The group drafted standards for normal birth entitled the Mother Friendly Childbirth Initiative (MFCI). This document was ratified by Lamaze International; La Leche League; Birth Works; the American Academy of Husband-Coached Childbirth; the American College of Nurse Midwives (ACNM); the Association of Women's Health, Obstetric, and Neonatal Nurses (AWHONN); International Childbirth Education Association (ICEA); the Midwife Alliance of North America (MANA); and Physicians for Midwifery.

The Lamaze International Philosophy (2005) is illustrative of the philosophy of birth held by many individuals and groups today:

- Birth is normal, natural, and healthy.
- The experience of birth profoundly affects women and their families.
- Women's inner wisdom guides them through birth.
- Women's confidence and ability to give birth is either enhanced or diminished by the care provider and place of birth.
- Women have a right to give birth free from routine medical interventions.
- Birth can safely take place in birth centers and homes.
- Childbirth education empowers women to make informed choices in health care, to assume responsibility for their health, and to trust their inner wisdom.

Three organizations that function with this or a similar philosophy are HypnoBirthing, Birthing From Within, and the Childbirth and Postpartum Professional Association (CAPPA).

HypnoBirthing

HypnoBirthing, the Mongan Method, grew out of the work of Dr. Grantly Dick-Read, an English obstetrician, who taught that fear (of pain or birth) and tension (resulting from the fear) lead to pain (HypnoBirthing, 2004). In HypnoBirthing, pregnant women (couples) learn how the birthing muscles work when the woman is in a state of relaxation. The woman will be relaxed and in control. She will experience surges (contractions) while calm and relaxed, free of fear and tension. Testimonials from birthing women and their attendants attest to the effectiveness of this technique, describing births as rapid and pain free (HypnoBirthing, 2004).

Birthing From Within

Birthing From Within mentors (teachers) believe that childbirth is not a medical event but a profound rite of passage. Parents are taught the power of birthing-in-awareness. Mentors create a safe, nurturing class experience and assist parents to find their personal strength and wisdom. Birth is taught from four perspectives: mother, father, baby, and culture. Parents are assisted to develop a pain-coping mindset. Parents deserve support for whatever birth option they choose. Fathers provide most help as loving partners and birth guardians, not coaches (Birthing From Within, 2004).

Childbirth and Postpartum Professional Association

CAPPA is a nonprofit, international organization, formed in 1998, that provides professional membership and training to antepartum doulas, childbirth educators, labor doulas, postpartum doulas, and lactation educators. They are proponents of evidence-based practice in childbirth education. Their childbirth educators teach parents that childbirth is painful but there are ways to deal with the pain. They generally recommend deep, abdominal breathing in labor. Relaxation is vital to achieve their goals. Vocalization, position changes, walking, frequent urination, and hydrotherapy are useful techniques (CAPPA, 2004).

Relaxation and Breathing Techniques

Relaxation

Relaxation is a technique promoted by virtually all childbirth education organizations. Learning relaxation in childbirth education classes can help couples with the stresses of pregnancy, childbirth, and adjustment to parenting and can be a form of stress management throughout life (Fig. 16-2). The research is clear that relaxation skill is the most effective nonpharmacologic strategy for coping with the stress of labor (Humenick, Schrock, & Libresco, 2000). Relaxation is ideally combined with activity such as walking, slow dancing, rocking, and position changes that help the baby rotate through the pelvis.

Approaches to relaxation can include neuromuscular relaxation, autogenic training, meditation, imagery, hypnosis, or touch relaxation. Women vary unpredictably in their re-

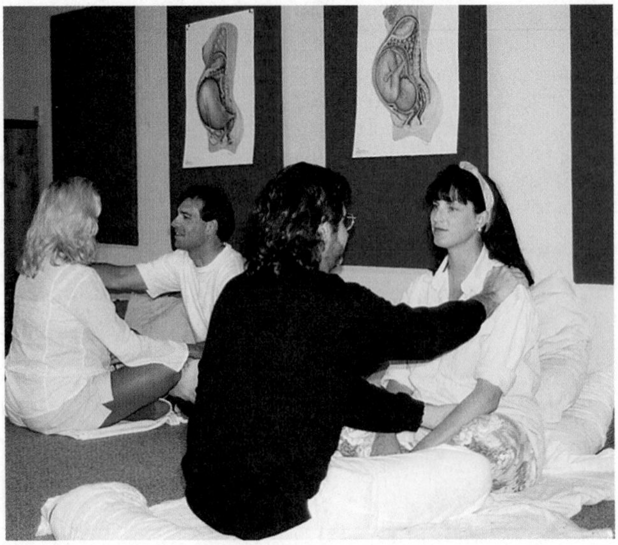

Fig. 16-2 Expectant parents learning relaxation techniques. (Courtesy Marjorie Pyle, RNC, Lifecircle, Costa Mesa, CA.)

laxation technique preferences during labor, so it is useful to teach them a variety of approaches. When couples work together in class to learn relaxation, they also increase communication skills. For example, by using massage with a light touch to encourage relaxation, they can learn to give each other positive reinforcement and enhance their sense of being a team.

Imagery and Visualization

Imagery and visualization are useful techniques in preparation for birth. Although research on their use is scant, clinical reports suggest that imagery and visualization can be used to produce a sense of well-being during pregnancy, as well as assist with cervical dilation and decrease the experience of pain and tension during labor. Imagery involves techniques such as imagining a walk through a restful garden or breathing in light, energy, and healing color and breathing out worries and tension. A variety of skills taught in childbirth classes augment relaxation during the pregnancy, as well as in labor. All can be taught as lifetime skills useful to the couple and used to teach their children to cope with the stresses of life.

Music

Music, taped or live, enhances relaxation during labor, thereby reducing stress, anxiety, and the perception of pain. It can be used to promote relaxation in early labor and to stimulate movement as labor progresses. Women can prepare their musical preferences in advance and bring their tape or compact disc player to the hospital or birthing center. Use of a headset or earphones may increase the effectiveness of the music because other sounds will be shut out. Live music provided at the bedside by a support person may also be very helpful in transmitting energy that decreases tension and elevates mood (Gentz, 2001). Ocean waves and Baroque and New Age music assist in relaxation (Wiand, 1997). Changing the tempo of the music to coincide with the rate and rhythm of each breathing technique may facilitate proper pacing (Di Franco, 2000; Gentz, 2001).

Touch and Massage

Touch and massage have been an integral part of the traditional care process for women in labor. They are likely to be beneficial in relieving labor pain (Enkin et al, 2000). Touch can be as simple as holding the woman's hand, stroking her body, and embracing her. Head, hand, back, and foot massage may be very effective in reducing tension and enhancing comfort. Hand and foot massage may be especially relaxing in advanced labor when hyperesthesia limits a woman's tolerance for touch on other parts of her body. The woman and her partner should be encouraged to experiment with different types of massage during pregnancy to determine what might feel best and be most relaxing during labor. When using touch to communicate caring, reassurance, and concern, it is important that the woman's preferences for touch (e.g., who can touch her, where they can touch her, and how they can touch her) and responses to touch be determined (Simkin & O'Hara, 2002).

Touch also can involve highly specialized techniques that require manipulation of the human energy field. Therapeutic touch (TT) uses the concept of energy fields within the body termed *prana.* Prana are thought to be deficient in some people who are in pain. Therapeutic touch uses the laying on of hands by a specially trained person to redirect energy fields associated with pain. Therapeutic touch requires a subjective, intuitive approach and may be taught by having the partners first experience their own energy field between their palms. They then learn the phases of centering, assessing differences of energy flow across the body, unruffling the field, and directing energy (usually over the uterus or back) to restore harmony (Marks, 2000).

Healing touch (HT) is another energy-based healing modality. Whereas TT emphasizes a single sequence of energy modulation, HT combines a variety of techniques from a series of disciplines. This gives the practitioner an array of "tools" to use with clients. Practitioners are taught energetic diagnosis and treatment forms and the means of documenting the patient's response and progress. These techniques are said to align and balance the human energy field, thereby enhancing the body's ability to heal itself. HT has been used in labor management, but no studies have been published about its effectiveness (Hover-Kramer et al, 2001).

Breathing Techniques

Different approaches to childbirth preparation use varying breathing techniques to help the woman maintain control through contractions (Fig. 16-3). In the first stage of labor, such breathing techniques can promote relaxation of abdominal muscles and thereby increase the size of the abdominal cavity. This lessens the friction and discomfort between the uterus and abdominal wall during contractions. Because the muscles of the genital area also become more relaxed, they do not interfere with descent. In the second stage, breathing is used to increase abdominal pressure and thereby assist in expelling the fetus. It also is used to relax the pudendal muscles to prevent precipitate expulsion of the fetal head.

Paced breathing is the technique most associated with prepared childbirth. The Lamaze method uses a slow-paced, modified, and patterned breathing technique with the understanding that each labor is different and that couples need to adapt breathing techniques to their individual birth experience.

All patterns begin with the routine cleansing breath and end with a deep breath exhaled to "blow the contraction

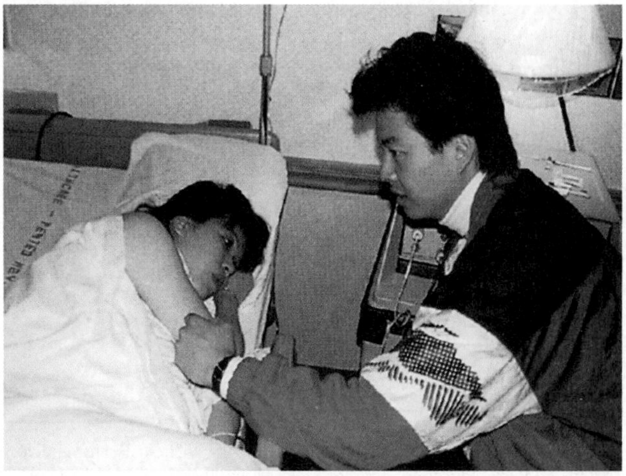

Fig. 16-3 Laboring woman using focusing and breathing techniques during contraction with coaching from her partner. (Courtesy Marjorie Pyle, RNC, Lifecircle, Costa Mesa, CA.)

away." In general, slow abdominal breathing, approximately half the woman's normal breathing rate, is initiated when the woman can no longer walk or talk through contractions (Box 16-2). As contractions increase in frequency and intensity, the woman may need to change to chest breathing, which is more shallow and approximately twice her normal rate of breathing.

The most difficult time to maintain control during contractions comes when the cervix dilates to 8 to 10 cm. This period is also called the transition period. Even for the woman who has prepared for labor, concentration on breathing techniques is difficult to maintain. The type of technique used at this stage may be the 4:1 pattern: breath, breath, breath, breath, blow (as though blowing out a candle). This ratio may be increased to 6:1 or 8:1. However, an undesirable side effect of this type of breathing may be hyperventilation. The woman and her support person must be aware of and watch for symptoms of the resultant respiratory alkalosis: light-headedness, dizziness, tingling of fingers, or circumoral numbness. Such alkalosis may be eliminated by having the woman breathe into a paper bag held tightly around the mouth and nose. This enables her to rebreathe carbon dioxide and replace the bicarbonate ion. She can also breathe into her cupped hands if no bag is available.

As the fetal head reaches the pelvic floor, the woman may experience the urge to push and may automatically begin to exert downward pressure by contracting her abdominal muscles. Nurses guide couples in the application of breathing and relaxation methods during labor, adapting methods to their particular needs, and using pushing techniques for birth that avoid a Valsalva response. Such techniques often involve moaning or other noise as the woman pushes without holding her breath.

The woman can control the urge to push by taking panting breaths or by slowly exhaling through pursed lips. This is good practice for the type of breathing to be used as the fetal head is slowly born.

BOX 16-2

Breathing Techniques

Cleansing Breath

Relaxed breath in through nose and out mouth. Used at the beginning and end of each contraction.

Slow-Paced Breathing (Approximately 6 to 8 Breaths per Minute)

Not less than half normal breathing rate (no. breaths/min divided by 2)

In-2-3-4/Out-2-3-4/In-2-3-4/Out-2-3-4 . . .

Modified-Paced Breathing (Approximately 32 to 40 Breaths per Minute)

Not more than twice normal breathing rate (no. breaths/min times 2)

In-Out/In-Out/In-Out/In-Out . . .

For more flexibility and variety, the woman may combine the slow and modified breathing by using the slow breathing for beginnings and ends of contractions and modified breathing for more intense peaks. This technique conserves energy and lessens fatigue.

Patterned-Paced Breathing (Same Rate as Modified)

Enhances concentration

a. 3:1 Patterned breathing
   In-Out/In-Out/In-Out/In-Blow
   (repeat through contraction)
b. 4:1 Patterned breathing
   In-Out/In-Out/In-Out/In-Out/In-Blow
   (repeat through contraction)
   You may do any pattern desired, although ratios of 5:1 or higher tend to be very tiring. Some people like to do patterned breathing to a tune ("Yankee Doodle," "Old McDonald"), to a repeated phrase ("I think I can, I think I can"), or in a pyramid pattern such as 1:1, 2:1, 3:1, 4:1, 5:1–5:1, 4:1, 3:1, 2:1, 1:1.
c. Coach call: May be used when the woman needs more distraction and concentration (e.g., during transition). The woman's coach signals the breathing ratio with his or her fingers or by verbal cues, changing the ratio after each "In-Blow."
   Example:
   In-Out/In-Out/In-Blow
   In-Out/In-Out/In-Out/In-Out/In-Blow
   In-Out/In-Blow

From Nichols F: Paced breathing techniques. In Nichols F, Humenick S (eds): *Childbirth education: practice, research and theory,* ed 2, Philadelphia, 2000, WB Saunders; Perinatal Education Association: *Breathing through labor and birth*, 2003. Retrieved from www.birthsource.com, December 7, 2004.

Effleurage and Counterpressure

Effleurage (light massage) and counterpressure bring relief to many women during the first stage of labor. The gate-control theory may explain the effectiveness of these measures. Effleurage is a light stroking, usually of the abdomen, in rhythm with breathing during contractions. It is used to distract the woman from contraction pain. Often the presence of monitor belts makes it difficult to perform effleurage on the abdomen; thus a thigh or the chest may be used.

Counterpressure is steady pressure in the sacral area with the fist or heel of the hand, which may help the woman cope with the sensations of internal pressure and pain in the lower back.

Water Therapy (Hydrotherapy)

Bathing, showering, or jet hydrotherapy (whirlpool baths) using warm water are nonpharmacologic measures that can be used to promote comfort and relaxation during labor (Fig. 16-4). Sitting in a tub of water up to the shoulders for 1 to 2 hours has several immediate benefits. Buoyancy in the water results in general body relaxation and temporary relief from discomfort and pain. This reduces the woman's anxiety and enhances a feeling of well-being. Catecholamine production decreases. This triggers an increase in the levels of oxytocin (to stimulate uterine contractions) and endorphins (to reduce pain perception). In addition, the bubbles and gentle lapping of the water stimulate the nipples, also triggering an increase in oxytocin production; this has not been observed to cause uterine hyperstimulation. The cervix has often been observed to dilate 2 to 3 cm in 30 minutes of whirlpool therapy. In addition, it promotes diuresis and a decrease in blood pressure (Simkin, 1995). Whirlpool baths in labor also have been found to have positive effects on analgesia requirements, instrumentation rates, condition of the perineum, and personal satisfaction with labor (Simkin & O'Hara, 2002).

If the woman is experiencing "back labor" as a result of an occiput posterior or transverse position, she is encouraged to assume the hands-and-knees or the side-lying position in the tub. Because this position decreases pain and increases relaxation and the production of oxytocin, the fetus can rotate spontaneously to the occiput anterior position.

In some settings, jet hydrotherapy may need to be approved by the woman's primary health care provider. The woman's vital signs must be within normal limits and she should be in the active phase of the first stage of labor. If she is in the latent phase, her contractions may slow down (Mackey, 2001). Fetal well-being must also be documented.

Fetal heart rate (FHR) monitoring is done by Doppler device, fetoscope, or wireless external monitor device (see Fig. 16-4, *C*). Placement of internal electrodes is contraindicated for jet hydrotherapy. The woman's membranes may be intact or ruptured. If the membranes are ruptured, the fluid must be clear or only lightly stained with meconium (Mackey, 2001).

There is no limit to the time women can stay in the bath, and often women are encouraged to stay in it as long as desired. However, most women use jet hydrotherapy for 30 to 60 minutes at a time. During the bath, if the woman's temperature and the FHR increase, if the labor slows or becomes too intense, or if relief of pain is reduced, the woman can come out of the bath and return at a later time. Repeated baths with occasional breaks may be more effective in relieving pain in long labors than unlimited amounts of time in the water. Fluids to maintain hydration and ice chips and a cool face cloth are offered during the bath (Mackey, 2001; Simkin & O'Hara, 2002).

Transcutaneous Electrical Nerve Stimulation

Transcutaneous electrical nerve stimulation (TENS) involves placing two pairs of electrodes on either side of the woman's thoracic and sacral spine (Fig. 16-5). These electrodes provide continuous mild electrical current from a battery-operated device. During a contraction, the woman increases the stimulation by turning control knobs on the device. Women describe the resulting sensation as a tingling or buzzing and pain relief as good or very good. TENS is most useful for lower back pain during the early first stage of labor. The use of TENS poses no risk to the mother or fetus, and it is credited with reducing or eliminating the need for analgesia and with increasing the woman's perception of control over the experience. It may be effective because of the placebo effect; that is, confidence in the effectiveness of TENS may stimulate the release of endogenous opiates (enkephalins) in the woman's body and thus alleviate the discomfort (Gentz, 2001; Scott et al, 1999). The nurse assists the mother in using TENS by explaining the device and its use, by carefully placing and securing the electrodes, and by closely evaluating its effectiveness. TENS is considered a form of care with insufficient quality data to recommend its use (Enkin et al, 2000) (Nursing Care Plan).

Acupressure

Acupressure techniques can be used in pregnancy, labor, and postpartum to relieve pain and other discomforts. Pressure, heat, or cold is applied to acupuncture points termed *tsubos*. These points have an increased density of neuroreceptors and increased electrical conductivity. Acupressure is best applied over the skin without using lubricants. Pressure is

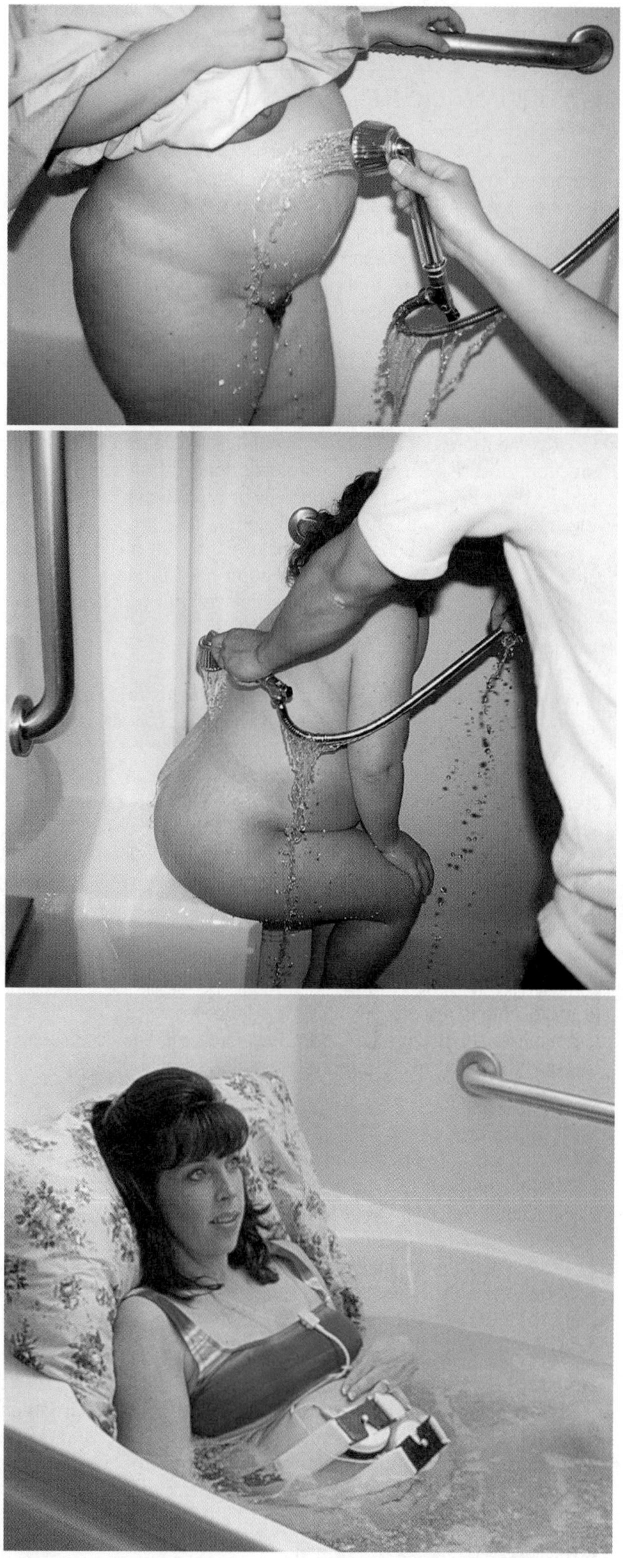
A
B
C

Fig. 16-4 Water therapy during labor. **A,** Use of shower during labor. **B,** Woman experiencing back labor relaxes as husband sprays warm water on her back. **C,** Woman relaxing in Jacuzzi. (*A, B,* Courtesy Marjorie Pyle, RNC, Lifecircle, Costa Mesa, CA. *C,* Courtesy Spacelabs Medical, Redmond, WA.)

Evidence-Based Practice

WATER IMMERSION DURING LABOR

Background

Many lay and professional caregivers and researchers have advocated warm water immersion for their obstetric patients. Immersion may help decrease edema and blood pressure during pregnancy. During labor, the buoyancy of immersion may relieve pressure and tension, decrease catecholamines and pain, and decrease maternal anxiety. Some postulate that nipple stimulation from the water may increase oxytocin and speed cervical dilation and decrease use of pitocin to augment labor. Water immersion may increase uterine perfusion. The mother may benefit from decreased blood pressure and increased satisfaction. Water births may increase elasticity of the birth canal, resulting in fewer tears and episiotomies.

Adverse maternal effects may include restricted mobility, risk of infection, and risk for water embolism. Reduced uterine tone may lead to decreased contraction effectiveness, postpartum bleeding, and need for manual removal of placenta.

Adverse neonatal effects may include inhalation of water, possibly leading to hemodilution, or pneumonitis due to additives.

Emergency interventions may be delayed during water immersion, and caregivers may risk back injuries.

Objectives

Research questions included evidence of benefits and risks of water immersion during pregnancy, early and late first-stage labor, and second-stage labor.

The reviewers also questioned if any difference in outcomes occurred in moving versus still water, or if water additives, such as essential oils or salt, were present.

Reviewers looked for the following outcomes in trials: maternal satisfaction, pain, use of analgesia/anesthesia, labor augmentation, maternal blood pressure and pulse, duration of labor and delivery, mode of delivery, perineal trauma, blood loss, postnatal infection, maternal self-esteem, postpartum depression, and breastfeeding. Fetal/infant outcomes were fetal heart rate patterns and neonatal Apgar, cord pH, neonatal intensive care unit (NICU) admission, respiratory support, temperature at birth, infection, neurologic outcome (e.g., cerebral palsy, death, and cord injuries), and caregiver satisfaction and injuries.

Methods

Search Strategy

Search strategy involved searches in Cochrane Central Registry of Controlled trials, MEDLINE, hand searches in 30 journals, and a weekly alert service for 37 other journals. Keywords were not noted.

Eight randomized, controlled trials were selected, for a total of 2939 women from Belgium, Australia, Sweden, South Africa, Canada, and the United States. The studies were published from 1993 to 2003. All studies used warm water immersion as their intervention, and standard institutional labor care for the controls.

Statistical Analyses

Statistical analyses compared similar outcome measures. Interventions varied, such as water temperature (37° to 38° C) and the intermittent or continuous presence of a one-to-one caregiver (which is known to benefit laboring women; see Evidence-Based Practice: Continuous Support during Childbirth, Chapter 18).

Findings

During first-stage labor, women using water immersion demonstrated a statistically significant decrease in perception of pain and use of epidural/spinal/cervical analgesia or anesthesia when compared with controls. Blood pressure was significantly lower for the water immersion group. No difference was noted between groups in labor or birth duration, operative or assisted birth, perineal trauma, tears, or episiotomies. Infants of mothers using water immersion during first-stage labor had no difference from the controls in number of low Apgar scores or NICU admissions. This was true even when the gestation was less than 34 weeks.

During second-stage labor, one trial reported that women in the immersion group had greater satisfaction in coping with their pushing efforts than the controls.

One study showed an increase in epidural use and labor augmentation if the water immersion was used early in labor, when compared with use during more advanced labor.

Limitations

Small sample sizes limited all the studies. It is not possible to blind subjects or caregivers to the intervention. Comfort levels with the intervention differ across subjects and caregivers, which can bias pain perception, analgesia use, maternal satisfaction, self-esteem, and postpartum depression. Subjects did not always comply with the protocol to which they were randomized. One study found that 46% of its "immersion" group never got into the water. Reasons included requesting epidurals (which precluded immersion), changing their minds about the immersion, and unavailability of the pool. All studies reported some crossover between groups.

Researchers used different definitions of labor, which can influence length and progression data. Trials varied on their tolerance of ruptured membranes; some required it and some excluded it, which can affect pain perception and analgesia use.

Labor management varied across the trials, as did the presence of a one-to-one caregiver. There were differences in the pool shapes and differences in whether the water was still or moving, which may have affected comfort, position changes, and movement.

Conclusions

Water immersion was associated with a significant decrease in the perception of pain and use of analgesia, and therefore may be of benefit for women in later first-stage labor. There were not enough data to recommend water immersion during second-stage labor.

Implications for Practice

Water immersion can be used to provide comfort in first-stage labor. Use of immersion must occur after labor is well established. Nurses can advocate for equipment in their birthing/labor and delivery units to enable them to offer this option. Having one-to-one caregivers to monitor safety and progress of labor is important.

Implications for Further Research

Standardized definitions, protocols, and outcome measures should be used in future research. Infection, a major concern, was not addressed. Size and shape of the pool and moving versus still water may produce different results. More well-designed trials evaluating water immersion during second-stage labor are needed.

Reference

Cluett E et al: Immersion in water in pregnancy, labour and birth (Cochrane Review). In *The Cochrane Library,* Issue 2, Chichester, UK, 2004, John Wiley & Sons.

usually applied with the heel of the hand, fist, or pads of the thumbs and fingers (Fig. 16-6). Synchronized breathing by the caregiver and the woman is suggested for greater effectiveness. Acupressure points include shoulders, low back, hips, ankles, nails on the small toes, soles of the foot, and sacral points.

Application of Heat and Cold

Warmed blankets, warm compresses, a warm bath or shower, or a moist heating pad can enhance relaxation and reduce pain during labor. Heat relieves muscle ischemia and increases blood flow to the area of discomfort. Heat applica-

Nursing Care Plan

NONPHARMACOLOGIC MANAGEMENT OF DISCOMFORT

NURSING DIAGNOSIS: Anxiety related to lack of confidence in ability to cope effectively with pain during labor

EXPECTED OUTCOME

Woman will express decrease in anxiety and experience satisfaction with her labor and birth performance.

NURSING INTERVENTIONS/*RATIONALES*

Assess whether woman and significant other have attended childbirth classes, her knowledge of labor process, and her current level of anxiety *to plan supportive strategies.*

Encourage support person to remain with woman in labor *to provide support and increase probability of response to comfort measures.*

Teach or review nonpharmacologic techniques available to decrease anxiety and pain during labor (e.g., focusing and feedback, breathing techniques, effleurage, and sacral pressure) *to enhance chances of success in using techniques.*

Explore other techniques that the woman or significant other may have learned in childbirth classes (e.g., hypnosis, yoga, acupressure, biofeedback, therapeutic touch, aromatherapy, imaging, music) *to provide largest repertoire of coping strategies.*

Explore use of hydrotherapy if ordered by physician and if woman meets use criteria (i.e., vital signs within normal limits, cervix 4 to 5 cm dilated, active phase of first stage labor) *to aid relaxation and stimulate production of natural oxytocin.*

Explore use of transcutaneous nerve stimulation per physician order *to provide an increased perception of control over pain and an increase in release of endogenous opiates.*

Assist woman to change positions and to use pillows *to reduce stiffness, aid circulation, and promote comfort.*

Assess bladder for distention and encourage voiding often *to avoid bladder distention and subsequent discomfort.*

Encourage rest between contractions *to minimize fatigue.*

Keep woman and significant other informed about progress *to allay anxiety.*

Guide couple through the labor stages and phases, helping them use and modify comfort techniques that are appropriate to each phase, *to ensure greatest effectiveness of techniques employed.*

Support couple if pharmacologic measures are required to increase pain relief, explaining safety and effectiveness, *to reduce anxiety and maintain self-esteem and sense of control over labor process.*

NURSING DIAGNOSIS: Health-seeking behavior (labor) related to desire for a healthy outcome of labor and birth

EXPECTED OUTCOME

Woman will participate in care planning for labor.

NURSING INTERVENTIONS/*RATIONALES*

Discuss woman's birth plan and knowledge about the birth process *to collect data for plan of care.*

Provide information about the labor process *to correct any misconceptions.*

Inform woman about her labor status and fetus's well-being *to promote comfort and confidence.*

Discuss rationales for all interventions *to incorporate woman into plan of care.*

Incorporate nonpharmacologic interventions into plan of care *to increase woman's sense of control during labor.*

Provide emotional support and ongoing positive feedback *to enhance positive coping mechanisms.*

tion is effective for back pain caused by a posterior presentation or general backache from fatigue.

Cold application such as cool cloths or ice packs may be effective in increasing comfort when the woman feels warm, and may also be applied to areas of pain. Cooling relieves pain by lowering the muscle temperature and relieving muscle spasms.

Heat and cold may be used alternately for a greater effect. Neither heat nor cold should be applied over ischemic or anesthetized areas because tissues can be damaged.

Hypnosis

Hypnosis, although not commonly used for pain management in the United States, is associated with shorter labors and less analgesia. Hypnosis techniques used for labor and birth place an emphasis on relaxation and diminishing fear, anxiety, and perception of pain (see earlier discussion of HypnoBirthing). The woman may be given direct suggestions about pain relief or indirect suggestions that she is experiencing diminished sensations. The woman receives posthypnotic suggestions, such as "you will be able to push the baby out easily," to increase her confidence. To be successful, the woman must be educated regarding hypnosis and practice the techniques during the prenatal period (Gentz, 2001).

Biofeedback

Biofeedback is another relaxation technique that can be used for labor. Biofeedback is based on the theory that if a person can recognize physical signals, certain internal physiologic events can be changed (i.e., whatever signs the woman

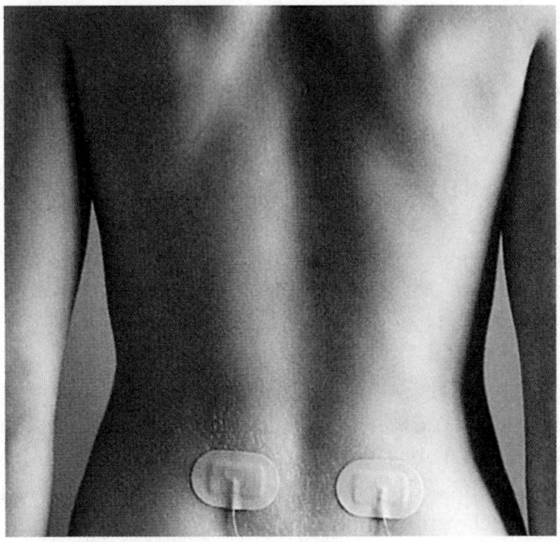

Fig. 16-5 Placement of TENS electrodes on back for relief of labor pain.

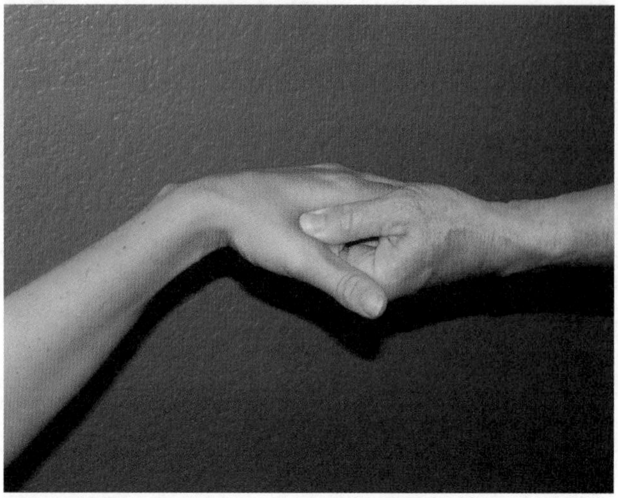

Fig. 16-6 Ho-Ku acupressure point (back of hand where thumb and index finger come together) used to enhance uterine contractions without increasing pain. (Courtesy Julie Perry Nelson, Gilbert, AZ.)

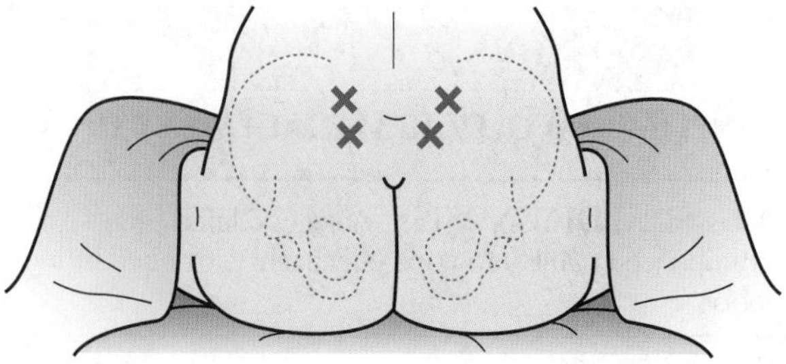

Fig. 16-7 Intradermal injections of 0.1 ml of sterile water in the treatment of women with back pain during labor. Sterile water is injected into four locations on the lower back, two over each posterior superior iliac spine (PSIS) and two 3 cm below and 1 cm medial to the PSIS. The injections should raise a bleb on the skin. Simultaneous injections administered by two clinicians will decrease the pain of the injections. (Adapted from Leeman L et al: The nature and management of labor pain: part I. Nonpharmacologic pain relief, *Am Fam Physician* 68(6): 1109-1112, 2003b.)

has that are associated with her pain). During the prenatal period, the woman must be educated to become aware of her body and its responses and how to relax for biofeedback to be effective. The woman must learn how to use thinking and mental processes (e.g., focusing) to control body responses and functions. Informational biofeedback helps couples develop awareness of their bodies and use strategies to change their responses to stress. If the woman responds to pain during a contraction with tightening of muscles, frowning, moaning, and breath holding, her partner uses verbal and touch feedback to help her relax. Formal biofeedback, which uses machines to detect skin temperature, blood flow, or muscle tension, also can prepare women to intensify their relaxation responses (Gentz, 2001; Snyder & Lindquist, 2000).

Aromatherapy

Aromatherapy uses oils distilled from plants, flowers, herbs, and trees to promote health and well-being and to treat illnesses. The use of herbal teas and vapors is reported to have good effects in pregnancy and labor for some women (Tiran & Mack, 2000). Lavender, clary sage, and bergamot promote relaxation and can be used by adding a few drops to a warm bath, to warm water used for soaking compresses that can be applied to the body, to an aromatherapy lamp to vaporize a room, or to oil for a back massage (Tiran & Mack, 2000).

NURSE ALERT *Caution:* Never apply the essential oils used for aromatherapy full strength directly to the skin. Most oils should be diluted in a vegetable oil base before use. Essential oils vary in terms of safe use during pregnancy (Gentz, 2001). ■

Intradermal Water Block

An intradermal water block involves the injection of small amounts of sterile water (e.g., 0.05 to 0.1 ml) by using a fine needle (e.g., 25 gauge) into four locations on the lower back to relieve back pain. It may be effective in early labor and in an effort to delay the initiation of pharmacologic pain relief measures. Stinging will occur for about 20 to 30 seconds after injection, but back pain will be relieved for approximately 45 minutes to 2 hours. Effectiveness of this method may be related to the mechanisms of counterirritation (i.e., reducing localized pain in one area by irritating the skin in an area nearby), gate control, or an increase in the level of endogenous opioids (endorphins). When the effect wears off, the treatment can be repeated, or another method of pain relief can be used (Gentz, 2001; Simkin & O'Hara, 2002) (Fig. 16-7).

PHARMACOLOGIC MANAGEMENT OF DISCOMFORT

Pharmacologic measures for pain management should be implemented before pain becomes so severe that catecholamines increase and labor is prolonged. Pharmacologic and nonpharmacologic measures, when used together, increase the level of pain relief and create a more positive labor experience for the woman and her family. Nonpharmacologic measures can be used for relaxation and for pain relief, especially in early labor. Pharmacologic measures can be implemented as labor becomes more active and discomfort and pain intensify. Less pharmacologic intervention often is required because nonpharmacologic measures enhance relaxation and potentiate the analgesic's effect (Faucher & Brucker, 2000).

Sedatives

Sedatives such as barbiturates relieve anxiety and induce sleep. They should be used only in prodromal or early latent labor and in the absence of pain. If the woman is having pain, sedatives given without an analgesic may increase apprehension and cause the mother to become hyperactive and disoriented. Undesirable side effects include respiratory and vasomotor depression of both the mother and newborn. These effects are increased if a barbiturate is administered with another central nervous system (CNS) depressant such as an opioid analgesic. Because of these disadvantages, barbiturates are seldom used.

Analgesia and Anesthesia

Nursing management of obstetric analgesia and anesthesia combines the nurse's expertise in maternity care with a knowledge and understanding of anatomy and physiology and of medications and their desired and undesired side effects and methods of administration.

Anesthesia encompasses analgesia, amnesia, relaxation, and reflex activity. Anesthesia abolishes pain perception by interrupting the nerve impulses going to the brain. The loss of sensation may be partial or complete, sometimes with the loss of consciousness.

The term *analgesia* refers to the alleviation of the sensation of pain or the raising of the threshold for pain perception but without loss of consciousness.

The type of analgesic or anesthetic chosen is determined in part by the stage of labor and by the method of birth (Box 16-3).

Systemic Analgesia

Systemic analgesia remains the major method of analgesia for the woman in labor when personnel trained in regional analgesia (i.e., epidural analgesia) are not available (Bricker & Lavender, 2002; Caton et al, 2002). Systemic analgesics cross the blood-brain barrier to provide central analgesic effects. They also cross the placental barrier. Once transferred to the fetus, analgesics cross the fetal blood-brain barrier more readily than the maternal blood-brain barrier. Effects on the fetus and the newborn can be profound (e.g., respiratory depression, decreased alertness, delayed sucking), depending on the characteristics of the specific systemic analgesic used, the dosage given, and the route and timing of administration. Intravenous administration is often preferred to intramuscular (IM) administration because the onset of the medication's effect is faster and more predictable. IV patient-controlled analgesia (PCA) is now available for use during labor. With this method, the woman self-administers small doses of an opioid analgesic by using a pump programmed for dose and frequency. Overall, a lower total amount of analgesic is used, and maternal satisfaction is high (Bricker & Lavender, 2002). Classes of analgesic medications used to relieve the pain of childbirth include opioid (narcotic) agonists, opioid (narcotic) agonist-antagonist compounds, and tranquilizers such as analgesic-potentiating medications (ataractics).

Opioid (Narcotic) Agonist Analgesics

Opioid agonist analgesics such as meperidine (Demerol) and fentanyl (Sublimaze) are especially effective for the relief of severe, persistent, or recurrent pain. They have no amnesic effect but create a feeling of well-being or euphoria (Medication Guide). These analgesics decrease gastric emptying and increase nausea and vomiting. Bladder and bowel elimination can be inhibited.

NURSE ALERT Because heart rate (e.g., bradycardia, tachycardia), blood pressure (e.g., hypotension), and respiratory effort (e.g., depression) can be adversely affected, opioid analgesics should be used cautiously in women with respiratory and cardiovascular disorders. Safety precautions should be taken because sedation and dizziness can occur after administration, increasing the risk for injury. ■

Women who receive opioids for their labor pain have less effective pain relief and are less satisfied with their pain management method than women whose pain is managed by using epidural analgesia. However, opioid use is associated with shorter labors, less oxytocin augmentation, and fewer instrumental vaginal births (e.g., forceps- or vacuum-assisted birth) when compared with epidural analgesia (Bricker & Lavender, 2002; Caton et al, 2002; Leighton & Halpern, 2002).

Meperidine (also known as pethidine) is the most common opioid agonist analgesic used for women in labor throughout the world. It overcomes inhibitory factors in labor and may even relax the cervix. After IV injection, onset is rapid (30 to 60 seconds), peak effect is reached in 5 to 7 minutes, and effects last about 2 to 4 hours. After IM injection, the onset of action is in 10 to 15 minutes; the peak is reached in 30 to 50 minutes; and the duration of action is 2 to 4 hours. Ideally, birth should occur less than 1 hour or more than 4 hours after IM injection to minimize neonatal CNS depression.

NURSE ALERT Because tachycardia is a possible adverse reaction, meperidine is used cautiously in women with cardiac disease. ■

Fentanyl is a potent, short-acting opioid agonist analgesic (Medication Guide). Onset of the drug effect after IV

BOX 16-3

Pharmacologic Control of Discomfort by Stage of Labor and Method of Birth

First Stage
Systemic analgesia
- Opioid agonist analgesics
- Opioid agonist-antagonist analgesics, co-drugs

Epidural (block) analgesia
Combined spinal-epidural (CSE) analgesia
Paracervical block (rarely used)
Nitrous oxide

Second Stage
Nerve block analgesia/anesthesia
- Local infiltration anesthesia
- Pudendal block
- Spinal (block) anesthesia
- Epidural (block) analgesia
- CSE analgesia

Nitrous oxide

Vaginal Birth
Local infiltration anesthesia
Pudendal block
Epidural (block) analgesia/anesthesia
Spinal (block) anesthesia
CSE analgesia/anesthesia
Nitrous oxide

Cesarean Birth
Spinal (block) anesthesia
Epidural (block) anesthesia
General anesthesia

Medication Guide

OPIOID ANALGESICS FOR LABOR

Meperidine (Demerol)

Action

Opioid agonist analgesic; stimulates mu and kappa opioid receptors to decrease transmission of pain impulses

Indication

Labor pain; postoperative pain after cesarean birth

Dosage and Route

25 mg intravenously; 50-75 mg intramuscularly or subcutaneously; may repeat in 1-3 hr; use of co-drugs may potentiate analgesic effect and decrease nausea and vomiting

Adverse Effects

Nausea and vomiting, sedation, confusion, drowsiness, tachycardia or bradycardia, hypotension, dry mouth, pruritis, urinary retention, respiratory depression (woman and newborn), decreased fetal heart rate (FHR) variability, decreased uterine activity if given in early labor

Nursing Considerations

Assess FHR and uterine activity; observe for respiratory depression; if birth occurs within 1-4 hr of dose, observe newborn for respiratory depression; have naloxone available as antidote; keep side rails up; continue use of nonpharmacologic pain relief measures

Butorphanol Tartrate (Stadol)

Action

Mixed agonist-antagonist analgesic; stimulates kappa opioid receptor and blocks mu opioid receptor

Indication

Labor pain; postoperative pain after cesarean birth

Dosage and Route

1 mg intravenously q3-4hr; 2 mg intramuscularly q3-4hr

Adverse Effects

Confusion, sedation, sweating; transient sinusoidal-like fetal heart rhythm; less respiratory depression, nausea and vomiting

Nursing Considerations

See meperidine; may precipitate withdrawal symptoms in opioid-dependent women and their newborns

Nalbuphine (Nubain)

Action

Mixed agonist-antagonist analgesic; stimulates kappa opioid receptor and blocks mu opioid receptor

Indication

Labor pain; postoperative pain after cesarean birth

Dosage and Route

10 mg intravenously; 10-20 mg intramuscularly q3-6hr

Adverse Effects

See butorphanol

Nursing Considerations

See butorphanol

Medication Guide

FENTANYL (SUBLIMAZE) AND SUFENTANIL (SUFENTA)

Action

Opioid analgesics, rapid action with short duration (1-2 hr intramuscularly; 30 min-1 hr intravenously)

Indication

For epidural or intrathecal analgesia, alone or in combination with a local anesthetic

Dosage and Route

Fentanyl–50-100 mcg intramuscularly; 25-50 mcg intravenously

Epidural–fentanyl, 1-2 mcg with 0.125% bupivacaine at rate of 8-10 ml/hr; sufentanil, 1 mcg with 0.125% bupivacaine at rate of 10 ml/hr

Adverse Effects

Dizziness, drowsiness, allergic reactions, rash, pruritus, respiratory depression, nausea and vomiting, urinary retention

Nursing Considerations

Assess for respiratory depression; naloxone should be available as antidote

injection occurs within 2 minutes; the action peaks in 3 to 5 minutes, and the duration of action is 30 to 60 minutes. Onset of the drug effect occurs in 7 to 8 minutes after IM injection, reaches its peak effect in 20 to 30 minutes, and lasts for 1 to 2 hours. Additive CNS and respiratory depression occurs if fentanyl is given with alcohol, antihistamines, antidepressants, or other sedative-hypnotics. Fentanyl is commonly used alone or in combination with a local anesthetic agent for induction of spinal nerve block analgesia (Faucher & Brucker, 2000; Lehne, 2001)

Opioid (Narcotic) Agonist-Antagonist Analgesics

An agonist is an agent that activates or stimulates a receptor to act; an antagonist is an agent that blocks a receptor or a medication designed to activate a receptor. Opioid agonist-antagonist compounds such as butorphanol (Stadol) and nalbuphine (Nubain), in the doses used during labor, provide analgesia without causing respiratory depression in the mother or the neonate (see Medication Guide). They are less likely to cause nausea and vomiting when compared with meperidine, but sedation may be as great or greater. Both IM and IV routes are used for administration. Butorphanol or nalbuphine may be given during the first stage of labor. These opioid analgesics are not suitable for women with an opioid dependence because the antagonist activity could precipitate withdrawal symptoms (abstinence syndrome) in both the mother and her newborn (Hawkins et al, 2002; Lehne, 2001) (Medication Guide; Box 16-4).

Co-Drugs

Medications such as ataractics (tranquilizers) can be used to augment or potentiate the desirable effects but few of the undesirable effects of the opioid analgesics. Ataractics such as the phenothiazines (e.g., promethazine [Phenergan], hydroxyzine [Vistaril]) do not relieve pain but decrease anxiety and apprehension, increase sedation, and potentiate opioid

Medication Guide

NALOXONE (NARCAN)

Action

Opioid antagonist

Indication

Reverses opioid-induced respiratory depression in woman or newborn; may be used to reverse pruritis from epidural opioids

Dosage and Route

Adult–0.1-2 mg intravenously q2-3min until adequate reversal; repeat q1-2hr if needed

Newborn–0.1 mg/kg intravenously, intramuscularly, or subcutaneously q2-3min until adequate reversal; repeat q1-2hr if needed

Adverse Effects

Maternal hypotension and hypertension, tachycardia, nausea and vomiting, sweating, and tremulousness

Nursing Considerations

Woman should delay breastfeeding until medication is out of system; do not give if woman is opioid dependent–may cause abrupt withdrawal; if given to woman for reversal of respiratory depression due to opioid analgesic, pain will return suddenly

BOX 16-4

Signs of Potential Complications

Maternal Opioid Abstinence Syndrome (Opioid/Narcotic Withdrawal)

Yawning, rhinorrhea (runny nose), sweating, lacrimation (tearing), mydriasis (dilation of pupils)
Anorexia
Irritability, restlessness, generalized anxiety
Tremor
Chills and hot flashes
Piloerection ("gooseflesh")
Violent sneezing
Weakness, fatigue, and drowsiness
Nausea and vomiting
Diarrhea, abdominal cramps
Bone and muscle pain, muscle spasm, kicking movements

analgesic effects. This potentiation effect causes the two drugs to work together more effectively, so the opioid dose can be reduced.

Ataractics

Ataractics can be used to reduce the nausea and vomiting that often accompany opioid use. Metoclopramide (Reglan) is an antiemetic that also can be used for this purpose. Benzodiazepines (e.g., diazepam [Valium], lorazepam [Ativan]), when given with an opioid analgesic, seem to enhance pain relief and reduce nausea and vomiting, although the increased sedation experienced may be unacceptable to women in labor (Bricker & Lavender, 2002; Lehne, 2001). Although data are limited, fetal or neonatal problems appear infrequently when women are given therapeutic doses of these co-drugs.

Opioid (Narcotic) Antagonists

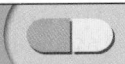

Opioids such as meperidine and fentanyl can cause excessive CNS depression in the mother and newborn. Current practice of giving lower doses of opioids intravenously has reduced the incidence and severity of opioid-induced CNS depression. Opioid antagonists such as naloxone (Narcan) can promptly reverse the CNS depressant effects, especially respiratory depression (see Medication Guide). In addition, the antagonist counters the effect of stress-induced levels of endorphins. An opioid antagonist is especially valuable if labor is more rapid than expected and birth is anticipated when the opioid is at its peak effect. The antagonist may be given through the woman's IV line or it can be administered intramuscularly. Opioid antagonists can counteract maternal and neonatal narcotic effects. The woman should be told that the pain that was relieved with the use of the opioid analgesic will return with the administration of the opioid antagonist.

NURSE ALERT An opioid antagonist must be administered cautiously to an opioid-dependent woman because it may precipitate abstinence syndrome (withdrawal symptoms) in both the mother and the newborn (see Box 16-4). ■

An opioid antagonist can be given to the newborn as part of the treatment for neonatal narcosis, which is a state of CNS depression in the newborn caused by an opioid. Affected infants may exhibit respiratory depression, hypotonia, lethargy, and a delay in temperature regulation. Risk for hypoxia, hypercarbia, and acidosis increases if neonatal narcosis is not treated promptly. Treatment involves ventilation, administration of oxygen, and gentle stimulation. Naloxone is administered, if still required, to reverse CNS depression. Alterations in neurologic and behavioral responses may be evident for 2 to 4 days after birth. Meperidine may be present in the neonate's urine for up to 3 weeks. Some depression of attention and social responsiveness can be evident for up to 6 weeks after birth. The significance of these neurobehavioral changes is unknown (Hawkins et al, 2002; Lehne, 2001)

Nerve Block Analgesia and Anesthesia

A variety of local anesthetic agents are used in obstetrics to produce regional analgesia (some pain relief and motor block) and anesthesia (complete pain relief and motor block). Most of these agents are related chemically to cocaine and end with the suffix *-caine*. This helps identify a local anesthetic.

The principal pharmacologic effect of local anesthetics is the temporary interruption of the conduction of nerve impulses, notably pain. Examples of common agents given in 0.125% to 1% solutions are lidocaine (Xylocaine), bupivacaine (Marcaine), chloroprocaine (Nesacaine), tetracaine (Pontocaine), and mepivacaine (Carbocaine).

Rarely, people are sensitive (allergic) to one or more local anesthetics. Such a reaction may include respiratory depression, hypotension, and other serious adverse effects. Epinephrine, antihistamines, oxygen, and supportive measures should reverse these effects. Sensitivity may be identified by administering minute amounts of the medication to test for an allergic reaction.

Local Infiltration Anesthesia

Local infiltration anesthesia of perineal tissues is commonly used when an episiotomy is to be done and when time or the fetal head position does not permit a pudendal block to be administered. Rapid anesthesia is produced by injecting 1% lidocaine or 2% chloroprocaine into the skin and then subcutaneously into the region to be anesthetized. Epinephrine often is added to the solution to intensify the anesthesia in a limited region and to prevent excessive bleeding and systemic effects by constricting local blood vessels. Repeated injection will prolong the anesthesia as long as needed.

Pudendal Nerve Block

Pudendal nerve block is useful for the second stage of labor, episiotomy, and birth. Although it does not relieve pain from uterine contractions, it does relieve pain in the lower vagina, vulva, and perineum (Fig.16-8, *A*). A pudendal nerve block must be administered 10 to 20 minutes before perineal anesthesia is needed.

The pudendal nerve traverses the sacrosciatic notch just medial to the tip of the ischial spine on each side. Injection of an anesthetic solution at or near these points anesthetizes the pudendal nerves peripherally (Fig. 16-9). The transvaginal approach is generally used because it is less painful for the woman, has a higher success rate, and tends to cause fewer fetal complications. Pudendal block does not change maternal hemodynamic or respiratory functions, vital signs, or FHR. However, the bearing-down reflex is lessened or lost completely.

If all branches of the pudendal nerve are anesthetized, analgesia is sufficient for a spontaneous vaginal birth or for outlet (low) forceps-assisted birth, or a vacuum-assisted birth. A pudendal block does not provide analgesia for uterine exploration or manual removal of the placenta.

Spinal Anesthesia (Block)

In spinal anesthesia/block, an anesthetic solution containing a local anesthetic alone or in combination with fentanyl is injected through the third, fourth, or fifth lumbar interspace into the subarachnoid space (Fig. 16-10, *A*), where the anesthetic solution mixes with cerebrospinal fluid (CSF). This technique is commonly used for cesarean births. A low spinal anesthesia/block may be used for vaginal birth, but it is not suitable for labor. Low spinal anesthesia/block used for cesarean birth provides anesthesia from the nipple (T6) to the feet. If it is used for vaginal birth, the anesthesia level is from the hips (T10) to the feet (Fig. 16-10, *C*).

For spinal anesthesia/block, the woman is sitting or lying on her side (e.g., modified Sims position) with back curved to widen the intervertebral space to facilitate insertion of a small-gauge spinal needle and injection of the anesthetic solution. The nurse supports the woman because she must remain still during the placement of the spinal needle. The insertion is made between contractions. After the anesthetic solution has been injected, the woman may be positioned upright to allow the heavier (hyperbaric) anesthetic solution to flow downward to obtain the lower level of anesthesia suitable for a vaginal birth. She may be positioned supine with head and shoulders slightly elevated and the uterus displaced with a wedge under one of her hips to obtain the higher level of anesthesia desired for cesarean birth. The anesthetic effect usually begins 1 to 2 minutes after the anesthetic solution is injected and lasts 1 to 3 hours, depending on the type of agent used (Hawkins et al, 2002) (see Fig. 16-10).

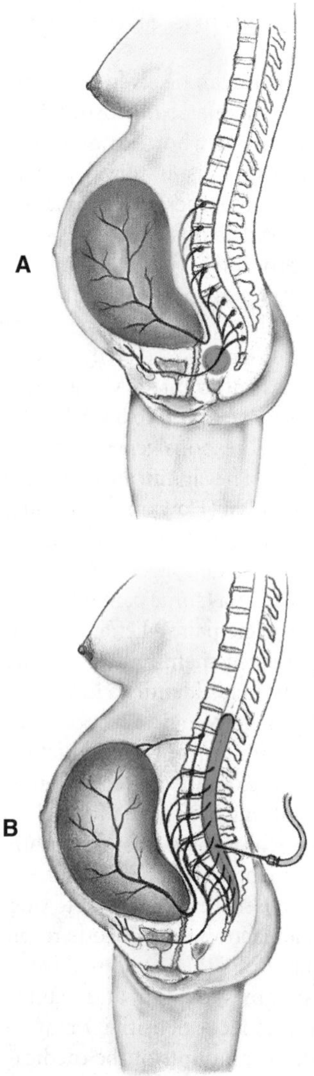

Fig. 16-8 Pain pathways and sites of pharmacologic nerve blocks. **A**, Pudendal block; suitable during second and third stages of labor and for repair of episiotomy. **B**, Epidural block; suitable during all stages of labor and for repair of episiotomy.

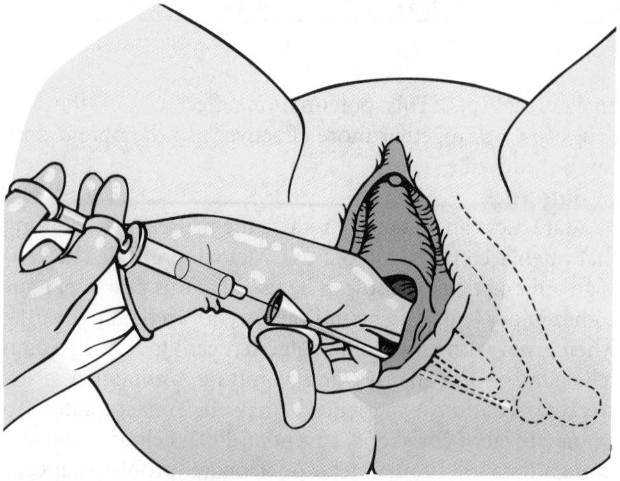

Fig. 16-9 Pudendal block. Use of needle guide ("Iowa trumpet") and Luer-Lok syringe to inject medication.

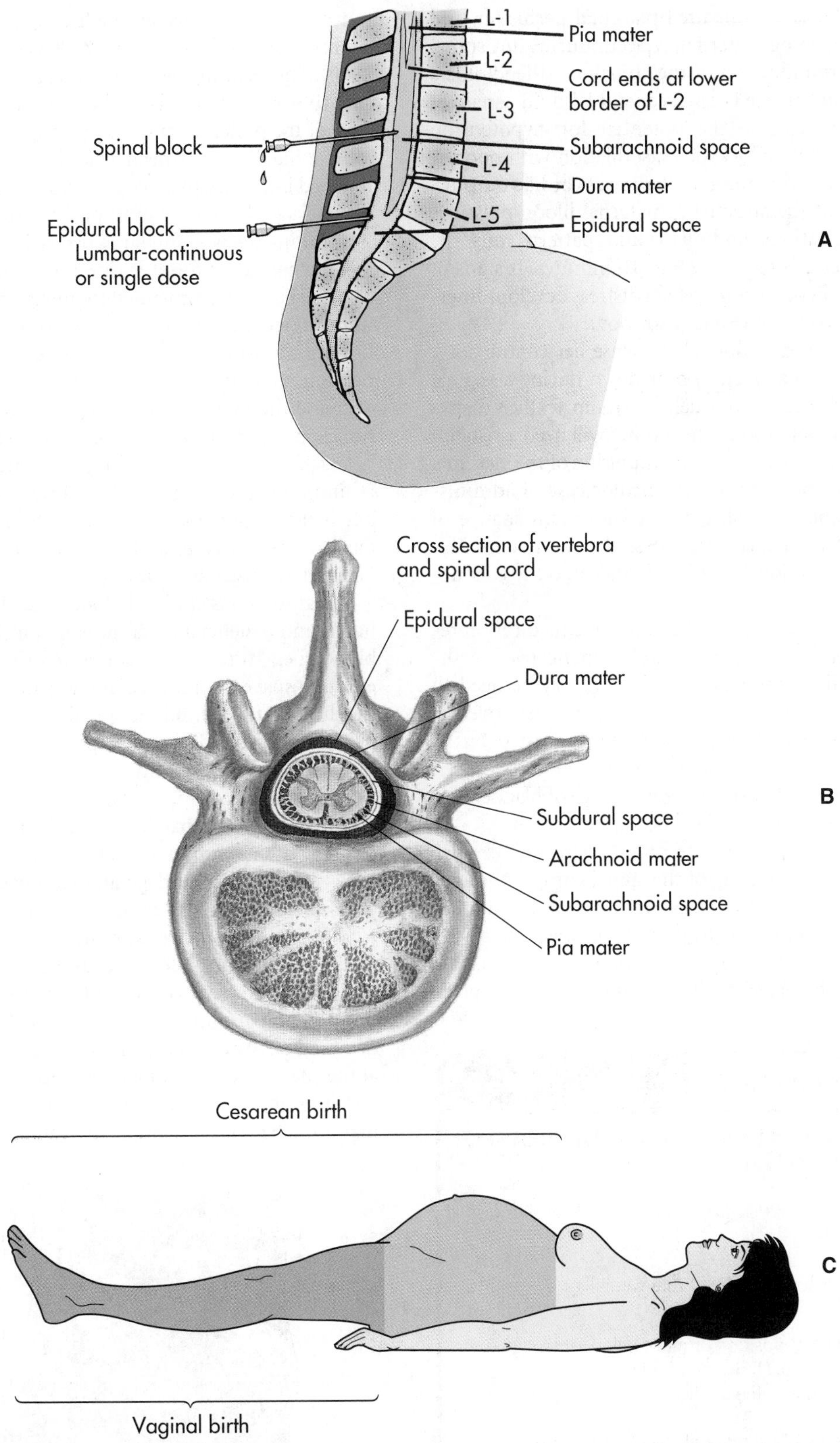

Fig. 16-10 **A,** Membranes and spaces of spinal cord and levels of sacral, lumbar, and thoracic nerves. **B,** Cross section of vertebra and spinal cord. **C,** Levels of anesthesia necessary for cesarean and vaginal births.

Marked hypotension, impaired placental perfusion, and an ineffective breathing pattern may occur during any spinal anesthesia. Before induction of the spinal anesthetic/block, the woman's fluid balance is assessed, and IV fluid usually is administered to decrease the potential for hypotension caused by sympathetic blockade (vasodilation with pooling of blood in the lower extremities decreases cardiac output). After induction of the anesthetic, maternal blood pressure, pulse, and respirations and FHR and pattern must be checked and documented every 5 to 10 minutes. If signs of serious maternal hypotension or fetal distress develop, emergency care must be given (Emergency box).

Because the mother is not able to sense her contractions, she must be instructed when to bear down during a vaginal birth. If the birth occurs in a delivery room (rather than a labor-delivery-recovery room) the mother will need assistance in the transfer to a recovery bed after expulsion of the placenta.

Advantages of spinal anesthesia include ease of administration and absence of fetal hypoxia with maintenance of normotension. Maternal consciousness is maintained, excellent muscular relaxation is achieved, and blood loss is not excessive.

Disadvantages of spinal anesthesia include medication reactions (e.g., allergy), hypotension, and an ineffective breathing pattern; cardiopulmonary resuscitation may be needed. When a spinal anesthetic is given, the need for operative delivery (i.e., episiotomy; forceps- or vacuum-assisted birth) tends to increase because voluntary expulsive efforts are reduced or eliminated. After birth, the incidence of bladder and uterine atony, as well as postspinal headache, is higher.

Leakage of CSF from the site of puncture of the dura mater (membranous covering of the spinal cord) is thought to be the major causative factor in postdural puncture headache (PDPH). Presumably, postural changes cause the diminished volume of CSF to exert traction on pain-sensitive CNS structures. Characteristically, assuming an upright position triggers or intensifies the headache, whereas assuming a supine position achieves relief in 30 minutes or less (Govenar, 2000). The resulting headache and auditory (tinnitus) and visual (blurred vision, photophobia) problems begin within 2 days of the puncture and may persist for days or weeks.

The likelihood of headache after dural puncture can be reduced if the anesthesiologist uses a small-gauge spinal needle and avoids making multiple punctures of the meninges. Positioning the woman flat in bed (with only a small, flat pillow for her head) for at least 8 hours after spinal anesthesia also has been recommended to prevent headache, but no definitive evidence shows that this measure is effective. Positioning the woman on her abdomen, a difficult if not impossible position after a cesarean birth, is thought to decrease the loss of CSF through the puncture site. Hydration is purported to be of value in preventing and treating headache, but no compelling evidence supports its use (Cunningham et al, 2001). Initial treatment for PDPH usually includes oral analgesics; bed rest in a quiet, dimly lit or dark room; caffeine; and increased fluid intake (Govenar, 2000; Hawkins et al, 2002).

An autologous epidural blood patch is the most rapid, reliable, and beneficial relief measure for PDPH. The woman's blood (i.e., 10 to 20 ml) is injected slowly into the lumbar epidural space, creating a clot that patches the tear or hole in the dura mater around the spinal cord. It is considered if the headache does not resolve spontaneously or after use of more conservative, noninvasive techniques (Govenar, 2000) (Fig. 16-11).

After the blood-patch procedure, the woman should be observed for alteration of vital signs, pallor, clammy skin, and leakage of CSF. A bandage and cold pack are placed on the puncture site, and the woman rests in bed for approximately 1 hour. Discharge instructions include resting in bed for 24 to 48 hours, applying cold packs to the site as needed for comfort, avoiding analgesics that affect platelet aggregation (e.g., nonsteroidal antiinflammatory drugs [NSAIDs]) for 2 days, drinking plenty of fluids, and observing for signs of infection at the site and for neurologic symptoms such as pain, numbness and tingling in legs, and difficulty with walking or elimination. The woman should be cautioned to avoid lifting,

Emergency

MATERNAL HYPOTENSION WITH DECREASED PLACENTAL PERFUSION

Signs/Symptoms

Maternal hypotension (20% drop from preblock level or less than 100 mm Hg systolic)
Fetal bradycardia
Decreased beat-to-beat fetal heart rate variability

Interventions

Turn woman to lateral position or place pillow or wedge under hip (see Fig. 18-5, *D*) to deflect uterus.
Maintain IV infusion at rate specified, or increase prn per hospital protocol.
Administer oxygen by face mask at 10-12 L/min or per protocol.
Elevate the woman's legs.
Notify the physician/midwife/anesthesiologist/nurse anesthetist.
Administer IV vasopressor (e.g., ephedrine) per protocol.
Remain with woman; continue to monitor maternal blood pressure and FHR every 5 minutes until her condition is stable or per primary health care provider's order.

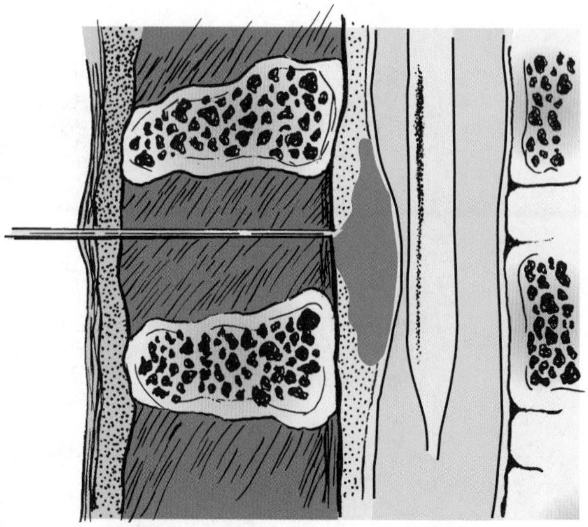

Fig. 16-11 Blood-patch therapy for spinal headache.

straining at stool, coughing, tub bathing, or swimming for at least 2 days (Govenar, 2000; Hawkins et al, 2002).

Epidural Anesthesia/Analgesia (Block)

Pain of uterine contractions and birth (vaginal and abdominal) can be relieved by injecting a suitable local anesthetic agent (e.g., bupivacaine, ropivacaine), an opioid analgesic (e.g., fentanyl, sufentanil), or both into the epidural (peridural) space. Injection is made between the fourth and fifth lumbar vertebrae for a lumbar epidural block (see Figs. 16-8, *B*, and 16-10, *A*). Depending on the type and amount of medication(s) used, an anesthetic or analgesic effect will occur with varying degrees of motor impairment.

Lumbar epidural analgesia is the most effective pharmacologic pain relief method for labor currently available. As a result, it is the most commonly used method for relieving pain during labor in the United States. More than half of the women giving birth each year choose epidural analgesia; some labor and delivery units report rates of 85% to 90% (Lieberman & O'Donoghue, 2002; Mayberry et al, 2003) (Box 16-5; Cultural Awareness). For relieving the discomfort of labor and vaginal birth, a block from T10 to S5 is required. For cesarean birth, a block from at least T8 to S1 is essential. The diffusion of epidural anesthesia depends on the location of the catheter tip, the dose and volume of the anesthetic agent used, and the woman's position (e.g., horizontal or head-up position).

Before placement of the epidural, an IV bolus of 500 to 1000 ml of crystalloids is usually given. The woman is positioned as for a spinal block (i.e., sitting) or in a modified Sims position. For the modified lateral Sims position, the woman is placed on her side with her shoulders parallel, legs slightly flexed, and back arched (Fig. 16-12).

After the epidural has been placed, the woman is preferably positioned on her side so that the uterus does not compress the ascending vena cava and descending aorta, which can impair venous return and decrease placental perfusion. Her position should be alternated from side to side. Upright positions and ambulation may be encouraged, depending on the degree of motor impairment (Mayberry et al, 2003). Oxygen should be available to treat hypotension should it occur despite maintenance of hydration with IV fluid and displacement of the uterus to the side. Ephedrine (a vasopressor used to increase maternal blood pressure) and increased IV fluid infusion may be needed (see Emergency box). The fetal heart rate and pattern, and progress in labor must be monitored carefully because the woman in labor may not be aware of changes in strength of uterine contractions or of descent of the presenting part.

Several methods can be used for an epidural block. The most commonly used method is the continuous block, achieved by using a pump to infuse the anesthetic solution through an indwelling plastic catheter. An intermittent block is achieved by using repeated injections of anesthetic solution; it is the least common method. Patient-controlled epidural analgesia (PCEA) uses an indwelling catheter and a programmed pump that allows the woman to control the dosing.

The advantages of an epidural block are numerous: the woman remains alert and able to participate, good relaxation is achieved, airway reflexes remain intact, only partial motor paralysis develops, gastric emptying is not delayed, and blood loss is not excessive. Fetal complications are rare but may occur in the event of rapid absorption of the medication or marked maternal hypotension. The dose, volume, and type of medication(s) used can be modified to allow the woman to push, to assume upright positions, and to walk; to produce perineal anesthesia; and to permit forceps-assisted, vacuum-assisted, or cesarean birth if required.

The disadvantages of an epidural block also are numerous. The woman's ability to move freely is limited, related to the use of an IV infusion and electronic monitoring, orthostatic hypotension and dizziness, sedation, and weakness of the legs. CNS effects such as excitation, bizarre behavior, tinnitus, disorientation, paresthesia, and convulsions can occur if a solution containing a local anesthetic agent is accidentally injected into a blood vessel. Respiratory arrest can occur if the relatively high dosage used with an epidural block is accidentally injected into the subarachnoid space (Mahlmeister, 2003). Women who receive an epidural have a higher rate of

Critical Thinking Exercise—Patient Receiving Epidural Block

BOX 16-5

Do Women Have a Choice for Labor Analgesia?

"A technologic birthing model that uses labor induction, epidural analgesia, continuous electronic fetal monitoring, and cesarean delivery increasingly dominates labor and delivery wards in the United States and other industrialized countries" (Leeman et al, 2003a). The American Society of Anesthesiologists has suggested that smaller hospitals that cannot support universal access to epidural analgesia should be closed. It is unknown whether the use of epidural analgesia by women in labor in the United States is a true preference or if it is selected because the only other choice is parenteral opioids. For example, nitrous oxide is used rarely in the United States. There is ample evidence of the benefits of the use of doulas and continuous support in labor, yet many women are not offered these options. Research is needed to discover which pain relief methods women would choose if they were offered a wide range of options.

References: Leeman L et al: Editorial: management of labor pain: promoting patient choice, *Am Fam Physician* 68(6):1023-1026, 2003a; Leeman L et al: The nature and management of labor pain: part II. Pharmacologic pain relief, *Am Fam Physician* 68(6):1115-1120, 2003c.

Cultural Awareness

ACCESS TO EPIDURAL ANALGESIA IN LABOR

Epidural analgesia is a highly effective, widely available method of providing pain relief in labor. However, Hispanic women and those on Medicaid are less likely than non-Hispanic women with private insurance or with no insurance to receive epidurals (Atherton, Feeg, & el-Adham, 2004). When Medicaid was introduced in Tennessee, there was a significant decrease in the epidural rate (Johnson & Rosenfeld, 1995). It is not known whether provider preference for type of analgesia is influenced by racial or ethnic considerations. For health care providers to manage labor pain effectively, race, ethnicity, and insurance should not be determining factors.

References: Atherton MJ, Feeg VD, el-Adham AF: Race, ethnicity, and insurance as determinants of epidural use: analysis of a national sample survey, *Nurs Econ* 22(1):6-13, 2004; Johnson S, Rosenfeld JA: The effect of epidural anesthesia on the length of labor, *J Fam Pract*, 40(3):244-247, 1995.

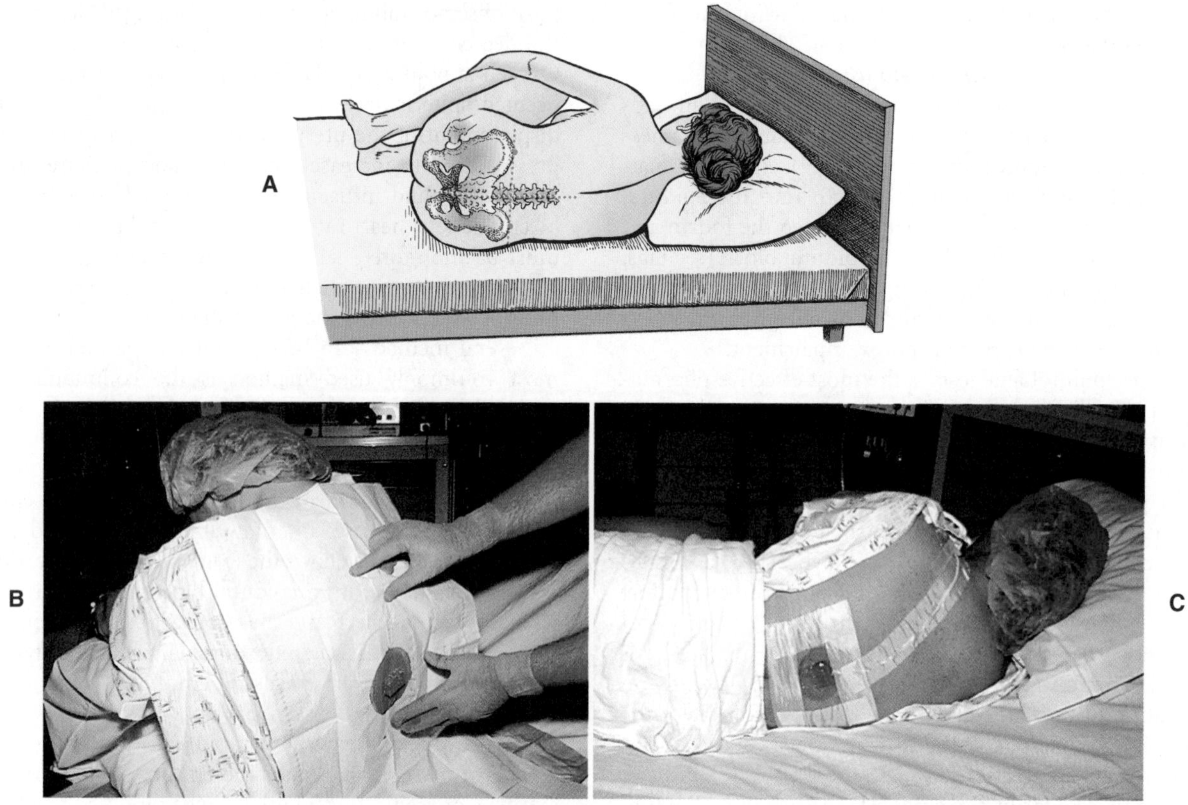

Fig. 16-12 Position for spinal and epidural blocks. **A**, Lateral position. **B**, Upright position. **C**, Catheter is taped to woman's back with port segment located near her shoulder. (*B, C,* Courtesy Michael S. Clement, MD, Mesa, AZ.)

fever (i.e., intrapartum temperature of 38° C or higher), especially when labor lasts longer that 12 hours; the temperature elevation most likely is related to thermoregulatory changes, although infection cannot be ruled out.

The elevation in temperature can result in fetal tachycardia and a neonatal workup for sepsis, whether or not signs of infection are present. Hypotension as a result of sympathetic blockade can be an outcome of an epidural block (see Emergency box). Urinary retention and stress incontinence can occur in the immediate postpartum period. This temporary difficulty in urinary elimination could be related not only to the effects of the epidural block but also to the increased duration of labor and need for instrumental birth associated with the block (Lieberman & O'Donoghue, 2002). Pruritus (itching) is a side effect associated with the use of an opioid, especially fentanyl. A relation between epidural analgesia and longer second-stage labor, increased incidence of fetal malposition, use of oxytocin, and forceps- or vacuum-assisted birth has been documented.

Current research findings have been unable to demonstrate a significant increase in cesarean birth associated with epidural analgesia (Leeman et al, 2003c; Lieberman & O'Donoghue, 2002). Occasionally a PDPH can occur after accidental perforation of the dura mater during the administration of the epidural block. Because a larger needle is used for an epidural block, the risk for severe headache is high as a result of greater CSF loss (Hawkins et al, 2002). For some women, the epidural block is not effective, and a second form of analgesia is required to establish effective pain relief. When women progress rapidly in labor, pain relief may not be obtained before birth occurs (Nursing Care Plan).

"Walking Epidural" Analgesia

Using opioids such as fentanyl and sufentanil to potentiate the effects of local anesthetic agents has resulted in the ability to reduce the amount of the local anesthetic used and thereby reduce motor blockade. Opioids can be used alone, eliminating the effect of a local anesthetic altogether. A combined spinal-epidural (CSE) technique is another approach used to achieve a walking epidural. The opioid is injected into the subarachnoid space for rapid activation of the opioid receptors. Pain transmission is blocked without compromising motor ability. A catheter is left in place in the epidural space to extend the duration of the analgesia by using a lower dose of a local anesthetic agent. Although women can walk, they often choose not to do so because of sedation and fatigue, abnormal sensations perceived in their legs, weakness of the legs, and a feeling of insecurity (Mayberry et al, 2003; Poole, 2003). Often health care providers are reluctant to encourage or assist women to ambulate for fear of injury (Mayberry, Clemmens, & De, 2002). The CSE may be associated with fetal bradycardia, necessitating close assessment of fetal heart rate and pattern (Lieberman & O'Donoghue, 2002).

Epidural and Intrathecal Opioids

The use of epidural or intrathecal opioids without the addition of a local anesthetic agent during labor has several advantages. Opioids administered in this manner do not cause

Nursing Care Plan

EPIDURAL BLOCK DURING LABOR

NURSING DIAGNOSIS: Ineffective coping related to new experience with labor and epidural block

EXPECTED OUTCOME

Woman will perform activities to maintain control over the situation.

NURSING INTERVENTIONS/*RATIONALES*

Assess woman's understanding of the benefits and risks of epidural block procedure *to provide baseline for providing information.*

Encourage woman to express feelings *to provide clarification and verify any needs.*

Reinforce use of positive coping mechanisms *to assist in increasing control over the situation and promote self-esteem.*

Encourage participation of significant other during administration of epidural block and throughout the rest of the labor process *to assist in optimum use of coping mechanisms.*

NURSING DIAGNOSIS: Risk for maternal/fetal injury related to maternal hypotension secondary to epidural block

EXPECTED OUTCOME

No fetal or maternal injury will occur as the result of maternal hypotension for the duration of labor.

NURSING INTERVENTIONS/*RATIONALES*

Assess fetal heart rate and maternal vital signs before initiation of block *to establish baseline data.*

Administer IV bolus solution per physician's orders *to increase circulating blood volume and cardiac output.*

Place the woman in the lateral position *to avoid supine hypotensive syndrome and maintain placental perfusion.*

Monitor fetal heart rate and maternal vital signs *to provide indication of any deviations from the baseline and promote early intervention.*

If hypotension occurs, elevate the woman's legs, increase rate of IV solution per protocol, administer oxygen by mask at 10 to 12 L per minute, notify the primary care provider or anesthesia care provider, and administer vasopressor medication per physician's orders *to quickly increase maternal blood pressure and maintain placental perfusion.*

NURSING DIAGNOSIS: Impaired urinary elimination related to effects of epidural block

EXPECTED OUTCOME

Woman's bladder will show no evidence of distention throughout the labor process.

NURSING INTERVENTIONS/*RATIONALES*

Record and compare intake and output *to observe for decreased output as a result of decreased sensation.*

Palpate the bladder superior to the symphysis pubis frequently *to assess if the bladder is distended as a result of increased fluid intake and decreased sensation.*

Encourage frequent voiding and perform catheterization if unable to empty bladder completely *to avoid interference with labor process and descent of presenting part, as well as potential bladder trauma.*

maternal hypotension or affect vital signs. The woman feels contractions but not pain. Her ability to bear down during the second stage of labor is preserved because the pushing reflex is not lost, and her motor power remains intact.

Fentanyl, sufentanil, or preservative-free morphine may be used. Fentanyl and sufentanil produce short-acting analgesia (i.e., 1.5 to 3.5 hours), and morphine may provide pain relief for 4 to 7 hours. Morphine may be combined with fentanyl or sufentanil. The short-acting opioids are often used with multiparous women, and the morphine may be used with nulliparous women or women with a history of long labor. For most women, intrathecal opioids do not provide adequate analgesia for second-stage labor pain, episiotomy, or birth. Pudendal nerve blocks or local perineal infiltration anesthesia may be necessary.

A more common indication for the administration of epidural or intrathecal analgesics is the relief of postoperative pain. For example, women who give birth by cesarean can receive fentanyl or morphine through a catheter. The catheter may then be removed, and the women are usually free of pain for 24 hours. Occasionally the catheter is left in place in the epidural space in case another dose is needed.

Women who receive epidurally administered morphine after cesarean birth are up soon after surgery with surprising ease and are able to care for their babies. Early ambulation and freedom from pain also facilitate bladder emptying. To those women who have had a previous cesarean birth and experienced the usual postoperative pain, the effects of this approach seem miraculous. However, the mother may not understand why she may experience pain after the narcotic effect wears off.

Side effects of opioids administered by the epidural or intrathecal route include nausea, vomiting, pruritus (itching), urinary retention, and delayed respiratory depression. These side effects are more common when morphine is administered. Antiemetics, antipruritics, and narcotic antagonists are used to relieve these symptoms. For example, naloxone (Narcan), promethazine (Phenergan), or metoclopramide (Reglan) may be administered. Hospital protocols should provide specific instructions for treatment of these side effects. Use of epidural opioids is not without risks. Respiratory depression is a serious concern; for this reason, the woman's respiratory rate should be assessed and documented every hour for 24 hours or per hospital protocol. Naloxone should be readily available for use if the respiratory rate decreases to less than 10 breaths per minute or if the oxygen saturation rate decreases to less than 89%. Administration of oxygen by face mask may also be initiated, and the anesthesia care provider should be notified.

Contraindications to Epidural Blocks

Contraindications to epidural analgesia include the following (Mahlmeister, 2003):

- Maternal refusal or inability to cooperate
- Antepartum hemorrhage
- Anticoagulant therapy or bleeding disorder
- Infection at the injection site
- Allergy to the anesthetic drug
- Refractory maternal hypotension

Effects of Epidural Block on Neonate

Debate persists concerning the effects of epidural anesthesia and analgesia on the newborn's neurobehavioral responses. Findings from studies that examine associations between neurobehavioral outcome and epidural block are far from consistent. For example, studies comparing the neonatal neurobehavioral scores for infants born to mothers who did and mothers who did not receive epidural analgesia either have shown little or no difference in the scores or have shown that the infants of mothers who received epidural anesthesia did not score as well on neurobehavioral tests. In one research study, infants exposed to an epidural block tended to have less muscle tone but were better able to orient and habituate to sound when compared with infants whose mother received opioids during labor (Florence & Palmer, 2003; Lieberman & O'Donoghue, 2002).

Paracervical (Uterosacral) Block

Paracervical block can be used during the first stage of labor to relieve pain from uterine contractions and cervical dilation. It is rarely used for labor because of its association with fetal bradycardia (Leeman et al, 2003c; Rosen, 2002b). Paracervical block may be used for anesthesia during abortion or other gynecologic procedures.

Nitrous Oxide for Analgesia

Nitrous oxide mixed with oxygen can be inhaled in a low concentration to reduce but not eliminate pain during the first and second stages of labor. It is widely used in developed countries except the United States. Entonox, the most commonly used mixture, is a 50:50 blend of nitrous oxide and oxygen (Leeman et al, 2003c). At the doses used for analgesia, the woman remains awake, and the danger of aspiration is avoided because the laryngeal reflexes are unaffected. It can be used in combination with other nonpharmacologic and pharmacologic measures for pain relief.

A face mask or mouthpiece is used to self-administer the gas. The woman should place the mask over her mouth and nose or insert the mouthpiece 30 seconds before the onset of a contraction (if regular) or as soon as a contraction begins (if irregular). When she inhales, a valve opens, and the gas is released. She should continue to inhale the gas slowly and deeply until the contraction starts to subside. When inhalation stops, the valve closes. Onset of action is 50 seconds; therefore beginning the inhalation process 30 seconds before the onset of a contraction provides the best pain relief. During the interval between contractions, the woman should remove the device and breathe normally (Rosen, 2002a).

Most women who use nitrous oxide obtain adequate pain relief and are satisfied with the method. The nurse should observe the woman for nausea and vomiting, drowsiness, dizziness, hazy memory, and loss of consciousness. Loss of consciousness is more likely to occur if opioids are used with the nitrous oxide. The use of nitrous oxide does not appear to depress uterine contractions or cause adverse reactions in the fetus and newborn (Rosen, 2002a).

General Anesthesia

General anesthesia is rarely used for uncomplicated vaginal birth and is infrequently used for cesarean birth. It may be necessary if there is a contraindication to spinal or epidural anesthesia or if indications necessitate a rapid birth (vaginal or cesarean) without sufficient time to perform a block. In addition, being awake and aware during major surgery may be unacceptable for some women having a cesarean birth.

If general anesthesia is being considered, the nurse gives the woman nothing by mouth and sees that an IV infusion is in place. If time allows, the nurse premedicates the woman with a nonparticulate (clear) oral antacid such as sodium citrate (30 ml) to neutralize the acidic contents of the stomach. Some anesthesia care providers and physicians also order the administration of a histamine blocker such as cimetidine (Tagamet) to decrease production of gastric acid and metoclopramide to increase gastric emptying (Hawkins et al, 2002). Before the anesthesia is given, a wedge should be placed under the woman's hip to displace the uterus. Uterine displacement prevents aortocaval compression, which interferes with placental perfusion.

Thiopental, a short-acting barbiturate, is administered intravenously to render the woman unconscious, and then succinylcholine, a muscle relaxer, is administered to facilitate passage of an endotracheal tube. Sometimes the nurse is asked to assist with applying cricoid pressure before intubation as the woman begins to lose consciousness. This maneuver blocks the esophagus and prevents aspiration should the woman vomit or regurgitate (Fig. 16-13). Pressure is released once the endotracheal tube is securely in place.

After the woman is intubated, nitrous oxide and oxygen in a 50:50 mixture are administered. A low concentration of a volatile halogenated agent (e.g., isoflurane) also may be administered to increase pain relief and to reduce maternal

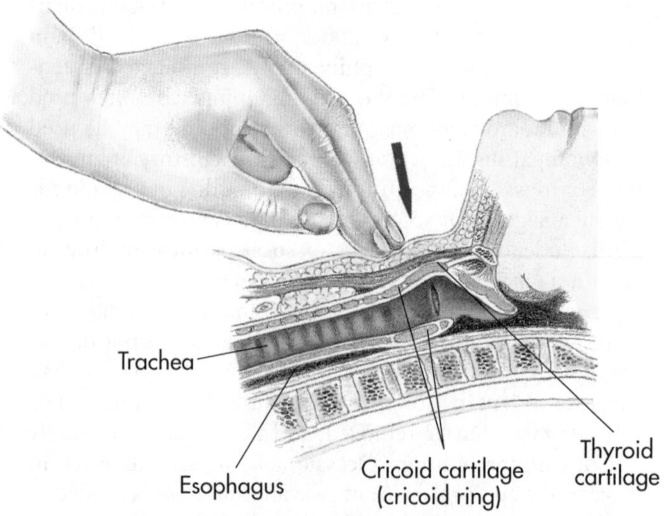

Fig. 16-13 Technique of applying pressure on cricoid cartilage to occlude esophagus to prevent pulmonary aspiration of gastric contents during induction of general anesthesia.

awareness and recall (Hawkins et al, 2002). In higher concentrations, isoflurane or methoxyflurane relaxes the uterus quickly and facilitates intrauterine manipulation, version, and extraction. However, at higher concentrations, these agents cross the placenta readily and can produce narcosis in the fetus and could reduce uterine tone after birth, increasing the risk for hemorrhage.

Priorities for recovery room care are to maintain an open airway, maintain cardiopulmonary functions, and prevent postpartum hemorrhage. Routine postpartum care is organized to facilitate parent-infant interaction as soon as possible and to answer the mother's questions. When appropriate, the nurse assesses the mother's readiness to see the baby, as well as her response to the anesthesia and to the event that necessitated general anesthesia (e.g., cesarean birth when vaginal birth was anticipated).

ENGLISH SPANISH **Guidelines/Guías**

PAIN MANAGEMENT

Do you want to get up and walk?
¿Desea levantarse y caminar?

Do you want pain medication?
¿Quiere medicina para el dolor?

I am going to give you the pain medicine in an injection.
Le voy a dar la medicina para el dolor por inyección.

I am going to give you the pain medicine through an IV.
Le voy a dar la medicina para el dolor por el suero.

This is a pain reliever called Demerol/Stadol/Nubain.
Ésta es una medicina para aliviar el dolor que se llama Demerol/Stadol/Nubain.

The effects of this medicine are relatively short.
Los efectos de esta medicina son de corta duración.

The epidural is a stronger method of pain relief.
La anestesia epidural es un método más potente para aliviar el dolor.

You should not be able to feel the contraction pain.
No debe de sentir el dolor de las contracciones.

Care Management

Assessment

The assessment of the woman, her fetus, and her labor is a joint effort of the nurse and the primary health care providers, who consult with the woman regarding their findings and recommendations. The needs of each woman are different, and many factors must be considered before deciding whether nonpharmacologic methods, pharmacologic methods, or a combination of both will be used to manage labor pain. It is critical that the nurse take note of all pain characteristics, including location, intensity, quality, frequency, duration, and effectiveness of relief measures. The nurse should never assume that because a woman is in labor, her pain must be uterine in origin. Because pain is a subjective phenomenon, the nurse must listen to the woman's description of her pain. A self-assessment tool, such as a visual analog scale, allows the woman to indicate on a line how severe or intense she perceives her pain to be. Pain is rated from "no pain" to "pain as bad as it can possibly be." Self-assessment is recommended to ensure that pain management is based on the subjective nature of the woman's pain rather than just on the nurse's judgment. It is not unusual for a nurse to overestimate or underestimate the pain being experienced by a patient. Baker and colleagues (2001) found that midwives consistently underestimated pain intensity that women described as severe. When there are major cultural differences between the health care provider and the patient, inaccurate interpretation of pain intensity often occurs (Lowe, 2002) (Guidelines/Guías box).

History

The woman's prenatal record is read and relevant information identified. This includes the woman's parity, estimated date of birth, and complications and medications during pregnancy. If the woman has a history of allergies, this is noted, and a warning is displayed in a prominent place. A history of smoking and neurologic and spinal disorders also is noted.

Interview

Interview data consist of the time of the woman's last meal and the type of food and fluid consumed; the nature of any existing respiratory condition (e.g., cold, allergy); and unusual reactions (e.g., allergy) to medications, cleansing agents, or tape. The woman is asked whether she attended childbirth preparation classes, and the extent of her preparation and preferences for management of discomfort are noted. Her knowledge of the options for management of discomfort is assessed. Information on the woman's perception of discomfort and about her expressed need for medication is added to the database. Relevant events that have occurred since the woman's last contact with her primary health care provider also are reviewed (e.g., infections, diarrhea, a change in fetal movement patterns). If verbal and physical signs indicate the existence of substance abuse, the nurse should ask the woman to identify the type of drug used, the last time the drug was taken, and the method of administration.

Physical Examination

The character and status of the labor and fetal response are assessed during a physical examination. The nurse evaluates the woman's hydration status by assessing intake and output measurements, the moistness of the mucous membranes, skin turgor, and concentration of urine. Bladder distention is noted. Any evidence of skin infection near sites of possible needle insertion is recorded and reported. Signs of apprehension such as fist clenching and restlessness also are noted.

If the woman is in labor, the status of maternal vital signs, fetal heart rate and pattern, uterine contractions, amniotic membranes and fluid, cervical effacement and dilation, and fetal descent is determined. The anticipated time until birth is estimated if possible. The length of labor and degree of fatigue are other important considerations. If pharmacologic methods are to be used, the type of analgesia or anesthesia chosen will vary depending on the status of the maternal-fetal unit, the progress of labor, and the method of birth planned (see Box 16-3).

Laboratory Tests

The results of laboratory tests are reviewed to determine whether the woman is experiencing anemia (hemoglobin and hematocrit), a coagulopathy or bleeding disorder (prothrombin time and platelet count), or infection (white blood cell count and differential).

Nursing Diagnoses

The following nursing diagnoses are relevant in the management of discomfort during labor and birth:

- *Acute pain related to*
  —processes of labor and birth
- *Risk for ineffective tissue perfusion related to*
  —effects of analgesia or anesthesia
  —maternal position
- *Situational low self-esteem related to*
  —negative perception of the woman's (or her family's) behavior
- *Anxiety or fear related to deficient knowledge of*
  —procedure for nerve block analgesia
  —expected sensation during nerve block analgesia
- *Risk for injury to fetus related to*
  —maternal hypotension
  —maternal position (aortocaval compression)

Expected Outcomes

The expected outcomes for nursing care in the management of discomfort during labor and birth include the following:

- The woman will promptly report the characteristics of her pain and discomfort.
- The woman will verbalize understanding of her needs and rights with regard to pain relief management that uses a variety of nonpharmacologic and pharmacologic methods reflecting her preferences.
- The woman will experience adequate pain relief without adding to maternal risk (e.g., through the use of appropriate nonpharmacologic methods and appropriate medication, including the appropriate dose, timing, and route of administration).
- The fetus will maintain well-being, and the neonate will adjust to extrauterine life.

Plan of Care and Implementation

A plan of care is developed for each woman to address her particular clinical and nursing problems. The nurse collaborates with the primary health care provider, the anesthesia care provider, and the laboring woman to select those aspects of care relevant to the woman and her family.

Nonpharmacologic Interventions

The nurse supports and assists the woman as she uses nonpharmacologic interventions for pain relief and relaxation. During labor, the nurse should ask the woman how she feels to evaluate the effectiveness of the specific pain management techniques used. Appropriate interventions can then be planned or continued for effective care, such as trying other nonpharmacologic methods or combining nonpharmacologic methods with medications (see Nursing Care Plan).

The woman's perception of her behavior during labor is of utmost importance. If she planned a nonmedicated birth but then needs and accepts medication, her self-esteem may falter. Verbal and nonverbal acceptance of her behavior is given as necessary by the nurse and reinforced by discussion and reassurance after birth. Providing explanations about the fetal response to maternal discomfort, the effects of maternal stress and fatigue on the progress of labor, and the medication itself is a supportive measure. The woman also may experience anxiety and stress related to anticipated or actual pain. Stress can cause increased maternal catecholamine production. Increased levels of catecholamines have been linked to dysfunctional labor and fetal and neonatal distress and illness. Nurses must be able to implement strategies aimed at reducing this stress (Florence & Palmer, 2003; Hodnett, 2002; Leeman et al, 2003b; Lowe, 2002).

Informed Consent

The primary health care provider and anesthesia care provider are responsible for informing women of the alternative methods of pharmacologic pain relief available in the hospital. A description of the various anesthetic techniques and what they entail is essential to informed consent, even if the woman has received information about analgesia and anesthesia earlier in her pregnancy. The discussion of pain management options ideally should take place in the third trimester so the woman has time to consider alternatives. Nurses play a part in the informed consent process by clarifying and describing procedures and by acting as the woman's advocate and asking the primary health care provider for further explanations. The procedure and its advantages and disadvantages must be explained thoroughly.

<u>LEGAL TIP</u> **Informed Consent for Anesthesia** The woman receives (in an understandable manner) all of the following:

- Explanation of the alternative methods of analgesia and anesthesia available
- Description of anesthetic and procedure for administration
- Description of the benefits, discomfort, risks, and consequences of the selected anesthetic for the mother and the fetus
- Explanation of how complications can be treated
- Information that the anesthetic is not always effective
- Indication that the woman may withdraw consent at any time
- Opportunity to have any questions answered
- Opportunity to explain in her own words components of the consent

The consent form will

- Be written or explained in the woman's primary language
- Have the woman's signature
- Have the date of consent
- Carry the signature of anesthesia care provider, certifying that the woman has received and appears to understand the explanation ■

Timing of Administration

It is often the nurse who notifies the primary health care provider that the woman is in need of pharmacologic measures to relieve her discomfort. Orders are often written for the administration of pain medication as needed by the woman and based on the nurse's clinical judgment. Generally, pharmacologic measures for pain relief are not implemented until labor has advanced to the active phase of the first stage of labor and the cervix is dilated approximately 4 to 5 cm to avoid suppressing the progress of labor (see Box 16-3). Nonpharmacologic measures can be used to relieve pain in early labor while relieving stress and enhancing progress (see Box 16-1).

Preparation for Procedures

The nurse reviews the methods of pain relief available to the woman (or validates her choices) and clarifies information as necessary. The procedure and what will be asked of the woman (e.g., to maintain flexed position during insertion of epidural needle) must be explained. The woman can also benefit from knowing the way that the medication is to be given, the degree of discomfort to expect from administration of the medication, the interval before the medication takes effect, and the expected pain relief from the medication. When an indwelling epidural catheter is to be threaded, the woman should be told that she may experience a momentary twinge down her leg, hip, or back and that this feeling is not a sign of injury.

A long needle is used for pudendal blocks (see Fig. 16-8). The sight of this needle may be frightening, and the woman can be reassured that only the tip of the needle will be inserted.

Administration of Medication

Accurate monitoring of the progress of labor forms the basis for the nurse's judgment that a woman needs pharmacologic control of discomfort. Knowledge of the medications used during childbirth is essential. The most effective route of administration is selected for each woman; then the medication is prepared and administered correctly.

Intravenous Route

The preferred route of administration of medications such as meperidine, fentanyl, and nalbuphine is through IV tubing, administered into the port nearest the woman while the infusion of IV solution is stopped. The medication is given slowly in small doses at the beginning of a contraction and over three to five consecutive contractions. Because uterine blood vessels are constricted during contractions, the medication stays within the maternal vascular system for several seconds before the uterine blood vessels reopen. The IV infusion is then restarted slowly to prevent a bolus of medication from being administered. With this method of injection, the amount of medication crossing the placenta to the fetus is minimized. With decreased placental transfer, the mother's degree of pain relief is maximized. The IV route has the following advantages:

- Onset of pain relief is rapid and more predictable.
- Pain relief is obtained with small doses of the drug.
- Duration of effect is more predictable.

Intramuscular Route

IM injections of analgesics, although still used, are not the preferred route of administration for the woman in labor. The advantages of using the IM route are quick administration and no need to site an IV line.

Disadvantages of the IM route include the following:

- Onset of pain relief is delayed.
- Higher doses of medication are required.
- Medication is released at an unpredictable rate from the muscle tissue and is available for transfer across the placenta to the fetus.

IM injections given in the upper portion of the arm (deltoid site) seem to result in more rapid absorption and higher blood levels of the medication than injections given in other sites (Bricker & Lavender, 2002). The deltoid is the preferred site if regional anesthesia is planned later in labor because the autonomic blockage from the regional (e.g., epidural) anesthesia causes blood flow to the gluteal region to be increased and accelerates absorption of the drug. The maternal plasma level of the drug necessary to bring pain relief usually is reached 45 minutes after IM injection, followed by a decline in plasma levels. The maternal drug levels (after IM injections) are unequal because of uneven distribution (maternal uptake) and metabolism.

Spinal Nerve Blocks

An IV line is usually established before induction of nerve blocks such as epidural and spinal blocks. Anesthesia protocols often include the prophylactic administration of a bolus of IV fluid before epidural and spinal anesthesia for blood volume expansion to prevent maternal hypotension. However, routine preloading with IV fluids before epidural analgesia is a form of care with a trade-off between beneficial and adverse effects (Enkin et al, 2000).

Lactated Ringer's solution and normal saline solution are commonly used infusion solutions. Infusion solutions without dextrose are preferred, especially when the solution must be infused rapidly (e.g., to treat dehydration or to maintain blood pressure) because solutions containing dextrose rapidly raise maternal blood glucose levels. The fetus responds to high blood glucose levels by increasing insulin production; fetal or neonatal hypoglycemia may result. In addition, dextrose changes osmotic pressure so that fluid is excreted from the kidneys more rapidly.

Because spinal nerve blocks can reduce bladder sensation, resulting in difficulty in voiding, the woman should empty her bladder before the induction of the block and should be encouraged to void at least every 2 hours thereafter. The nurse should palpate for bladder distention and measure urinary output to ensure that the bladder is being completely emptied. A distended bladder can inhibit uterine contractions and fetal descent, resulting in a slowing of the progress of labor. The status of the maternal-fetal unit and the progress of labor must be established before the block is performed. The nurse or the woman's partner must assist the woman to assume and maintain the correct position for induction of epidural and spinal anesthesia (see Fig. 16-12).

Signs of Potential Problems

Any medication can cause an allergic reaction that may be minor or as severe as anaphylaxis. Minor reactions can consist of a rash, rhinitis, fever, asthma, or pruritus. Management of the less acute allergic response is not an emergency. As part of the assessment for such allergic reactions, the nurse should monitor the woman's vital signs, respiratory status, cardiovascular status, platelet count, and white blood cell count. The woman is observed for side effects of medications, especially drowsiness.

Severe allergic reactions may occur suddenly and lead to shock. The most dramatic form of anaphylaxis is sudden severe bronchospasm, vasospasm, severe hypotension, and death. Signs of anaphylaxis are largely caused by contraction of smooth muscles and may begin with irritability, extreme weakness, nausea, and vomiting. This may then lead to dyspnea, cyanosis, convulsions, and cardiac arrest. An acute allergic reaction—anaphylaxis—must be diagnosed and treated immediately. Treatment usually consists of 1:1000 epinephrine injected subcutaneously or intramuscularly, followed by parenteral administration of antihistamines. Supportive care is given to alleviate symptoms. The type of care is determined by the rapidly assessed cardiovascular and respiratory response of the woman to primary interventions. Cardiopulmonary resuscitation may be necessary. The nurse must also be alert to changes in fetal status: nonreassuring changes in fetal heart rate and pattern should be noted and reported to the primary health care provider.

Safety and General Care

After administration of a spinal nerve block, the woman is protected from injury by raising the side rails and placing a call bell within easy reach when the nurse is not in attendance. Oxygen and suction should be readily available at the bedside. The nurse must make sure that there is no prolonged pressure on an anesthetized part (e.g., lying on one side with weight on one leg; tight bed linen on feet). If stirrups are used for birth, the nurse should pad them, adjust both stirrups at the same level and angle, place both of the woman's legs into them while avoiding putting pressure to the popliteal angle, and apply restraints without restricting circulation.

Depending on the level of motor blockade, the woman should be assisted to remain as mobile as possible. When in bed, her position should be alternated from side to side every hour to ensure adequate distribution of the anesthetic solution and to maintain circulation to the uterus and placenta. Assisting the woman to assume upright positions such as sitting (e.g., modified throne position in which the woman sits on the bed with the bottom part lowered to place her feet below her body) (Fig. 16-14), tug-of-war position (woman tugs on towel or sheet that is tied to the bar on the bed or held by the nurse), and squatting by using the head of the bed or a squatting bar for support (Fig. 16-15) will facilitate fetal descent and enhance bearing-down efforts (Gilder et al, 2002; Mayberry et al, 2003). Ambulation should be encouraged if the woman has received a "walking" epidural. Upright positions are important in the prevention of operative births (e.g., forceps- or vacuum-assisted birth). To prevent injury, the nurse must assess the level of motor function (e.g., three unassisted steps with accompaniment, stand and close eyes noting the degree of unsteadiness, ability to flex legs or rise from a supine position), level of sensation in legs (e.g., degree of numbness), and level of sedation before the woman is assisted out of bed and periodically thereafter (Mayberry et al, 2002). The woman should sit on the side of the bed before standing to determine if orthostatic hypotension occurs. If she is not dizzy or light-headed, she can stand at the side of the bed and finally walk.

The second stage of labor is often prolonged in women who use epidural analgesia for pain management. Research evidence indicates that as long as the well-being of the maternal-fetal unit is established, a period of "laboring down" to allow the fetus to descend and rotate with uterine contractions and the use of open-glottis pushing techniques when the fetus has reached a +1 station and is rotating to an anterior position are the best approaches to use for the management of second-stage labor (Mayberry et al, 2002) (see Chapter 18 for a full discussion of second-stage labor management).

The nurse monitors and records the woman's response to nonpharmacologic pain relief methods and to medication(s). This includes the degree of pain relief, the level of apprehension, the return of sensations and perception of pain, and allergic or untoward reactions (e.g., hypotension, respiratory depression, and hypothermia). The nurse continues to monitor maternal vital signs, blood pressure, strength and frequency of uterine contractions, changes in the cervix and station of the presenting part, presence of the bearing-down reflex, bladder filling, and state of hydration. Determining the fetal response after the administration of analgesia or anesthesia is vital. The woman is asked if she (or the family) has any questions. The nurse assesses the woman's and her family's understanding of the need to ensure her safety (e.g., keeping side rails up, calling for assistance as needed).

The time that elapses between the administration of a narcotic and the baby's birth is noted. Medication given to the newborn to reverse narcotic effects is recorded. After birth, the woman who has had spinal, epidural, or general anesthesia is assessed for return of sensory and motor function, in addition to the usual postpartum assessments.

Anesthesia in the Obese Woman

Obesity is defined as an excess of body fat causing weight to be greater than 20% more than ideal weight. Women who

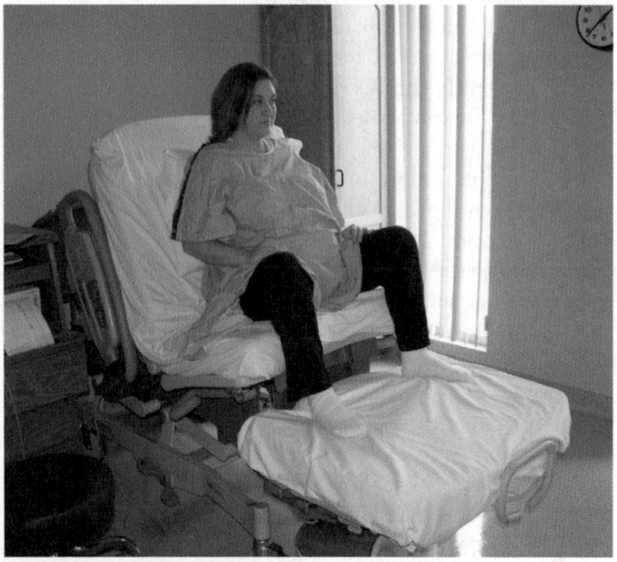

Fig. 16-14 Throne position. (Courtesy Julie Perry Nelson, Gilbert, AZ.)

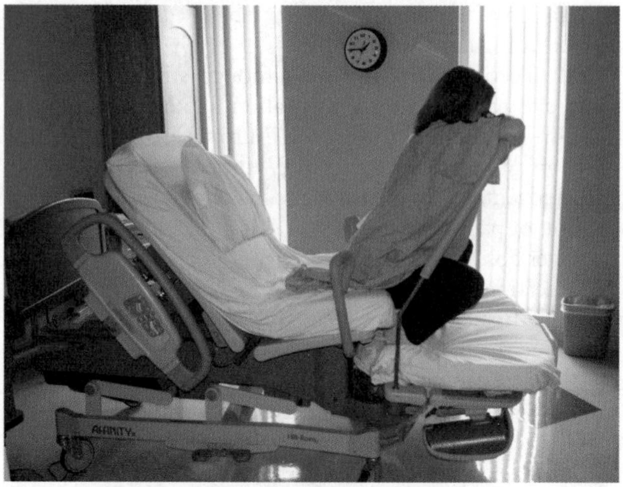

Fig. 16-15 Using squatting bar during labor. (Courtesy Julie Perry Nelson, Gilbert, AZ.)

are obese before pregnancy have an increased risk for cesarean birth when compared with women who are not obese.

Maternal physiologic changes are the product of hormonal influences and mechanical effects. In obese women, the weight of fat tissue and the added metabolic demands this involves also affect maternal physiology. Both pregnancy and obesity cause blood volume and cardiac output to increase, and in the obese woman, they expand in proportion to the amount of fat tissue. During labor and vaginal birth, and in the immediate postpartum period, blood values and cardiac output in obese women can reach levels 80% greater than prelabor values. The enlarged uterus and abdominal fat mass also further increase the possibility of aortocaval compression.

The respiratory system also is stressed in obese pregnant women, and the pulmonary function of an obese laboring woman is in a precarious state. Therefore the woman's oxygenation must be carefully monitored during birth and the immediate postpartum period. Monitoring by pulse oximeter has been suggested.

The gastric emptying time is delayed; the tone of the cardiac sphincter is decreased; and the gastric contents are hyperacidic in all pregnant women. The obese woman also is more likely to have a hiatal hernia and a marked increase in intragastric pressure and volume; therefore these women are at great risk for regurgitation and aspiration.

Management of the obese woman during labor should focus on efforts to minimize oxygen consumption and maximize pulmonary function. Epidural analgesia administered during the first stage of labor can bring about a decreased demand on the metabolic and respiratory systems and improved oxygenation. This is because pain causes the catecholamine levels to increase, which in turn causes cardiac output to increase. Effective epidural analgesia retards this increase in catecholamine levels.

Intravenous opioids may be used during the first stage of labor; however, the doses and the effects must be monitored carefully because obese women are extremely sensitive to the respiratory depressant effects of opioids. An epidural block during the second stage of labor provides complete pain relief and also supports cardiovascular function.

Combined spinal epidural anesthesia is an alternative to epidural anesthesia. Until recently, this option was not available in the morbidly obese pregnant woman because there was not an appropriate long needle manufactured for this purpose; one is currently available (Kuczkowski, 2004).

An epidural block is preferred to general anesthesia in the obese woman who must give birth by cesarean. Problems associated with general anesthesia in obese women include potential difficulties during intubation, a hypertensive effect of laryngoscopy and intubation, and aspiration and pulmonary complications. A spinal block may be used if there is insufficient time to induce an epidural block. Uterine displacement to prevent aortocaval compression is more difficult to achieve in the obese woman in the supine position needed for cesarean birth. If the woman is extremely obese, a wedge may not be able to elevate one hip enough to prevent compression. In this case, it may be necessary to lift the abdominal fat pad off the abdomen manually until the peritoneal cavity has been entered.

??? Critical Thinking Exercise

PAIN MANAGEMENT

You are assigned to a nulliparous woman in active labor who has a history of substance abuse. She is thrashing about in her bed and is requesting something for "this terrible pain." She has the prn orders for pain that are routine on your unit and has an IV line of lactated Ringer's solution in place infusing at 125 ml/hr. She can ambulate and has periodic electronic fetal monitor strips run to check on fetal status.

1. Evidence—Is there sufficient evidence to draw conclusions about what pain relief techniques should be instituted and what medications should be avoided?
2. Assumptions—What assumptions can be made about the following issues?
   a. Reactions to pain of women who abuse substances
   b. Degree of pain relief expected by the woman
   c. Degree of pain relief expected by the nurse
   d. Advisability of giving opioid analgesics to a woman who has a history of addiction to an opioid
3. What implications and priorities for nursing care can be drawn at this time?
4. Does the evidence objectively support your conclusion?
5. Are there alternative perspectives to your conclusion?

Maternal Hypothermia after Analgesia and Anesthesia

Hypothermia is defined as a core body temperature of less than 35° C. During labor and immediately after the birth, women are predisposed to hypothermia because of the combination of the vasodilation that normally occurs during pregnancy and the effects of the analgesia and anesthesia.

Opioids, barbiturates, tranquilizers, and antiemetics are thought to affect thermoregulation by increasing vasodilation and radiant loss; general anesthetic agents are thought to do so by depressing thermoregulation; and epidural and spinal anesthesia are thought to do so by inducing peripheral dilation. During labor, during vaginal or cesarean birth, or immediately after birth, women may have shivering, hypotension, and respiratory distress. The hypothermia may result in cardiovascular, pulmonary, circulatory, hematologic, neurologic, or renal complications. The nurse can minimize these complications by making sure that the birthing areas are warm, wet drapes and towels are removed, women are covered with warm blankets after birth, and hypothermia is recognized early. Explaining these effects to the woman and her support people will help allay concerns.

Evaluation

Evaluation of the effectiveness of care of the woman needing management of discomfort during labor and birth is based on the previously stated outcomes.

Key Points

- The expected outcome of preparation for childbirth and parenting is "education for choice."
- Nonpharmacologic pain and stress management strategies are valuable for managing labor discomfort alone or in combination with pharmacologic methods.

- The gate-control theory of pain and the stress response are the bases for many of the nonpharmacologic methods of pain relief.
- The type of analgesic or anesthetic to be used is determined by maternal and health care provider preference, the stage of labor, and the method of birth.
- Opioid (narcotic) agonist effects can be potentiated with ataractics.
- Naloxone (Narcan) is an opioid (narcotic) antagonist that can reverse narcotic effects, especially respiratory depression.
- Pharmacologic control of discomfort during labor requires collaboration among the health care providers and the woman in labor.
- The nurse must understand medications, their expected effects, potential side effects, and methods of administration.
- Maintenance of maternal fluid balance is essential during spinal and epidural nerve blocks.
- Maternal analgesia or anesthesia potentially affects neonatal neurobehavioral response.
- The use of opioid agonist-antagonist analgesics in women with preexisting opioid dependence may cause symptoms of abstinence syndrome (opioid withdrawal).
- General anesthesia is rarely used for vaginal birth but may be used for cesarean birth or whenever rapid anesthesia is needed in an emergency childbirth situation.

Answer Guidelines to Critical Thinking Exercise

Pain Management

1. Yes, there is sufficient evidence to draw conclusions about what pain relief techniques should be instituted and what medications should be avoided. Many beneficial nonpharmacologic methods of pain relief exist, including massage, music, aromatherapy, and hydrotherapy. The benefits of the use of doulas and continuous support in labor are well known. Although it is usually unnecessary to withhold pain medications, close monitoring for complications associated with each substance is part of the nursing assessment. For example, the nurse should ask the woman to identify the type of substance used, the last time it was taken, and the method of administration. Opioid antagonists or opioid agonist-antagonists should be avoided for women with a history of opioid abuse because abstinence syndrome (withdrawal) may be precipitated in the woman and her newborn (Hawkins et al, 2002). The nurse must know the classification and action of any medications to be administered.
2. (a) Women with a history of substance abuse have as much pain during labor as other women. They may have a low threshold or tolerance of pain. (b) Most women desire pain relief in labor. Satisfaction with their experience of labor is related to how well their expectations met reality, not necessarily how much pain they experienced. Because pain is an individual experience, women should be asked how much pain they have. The nurse would then implement the appropriate intervention, taking into consideration the woman's preference and that of the primary health care provider. (c) Nurses vary in their response to pain and their knowledge of how to manage pain. The response to pain of nurses and patients may be at variance based on experience, race, ethnicity, and culture. For example, in settings where epidurals are common, the nurse may expect all women to request that type of pain relief. A patient with a fear of needles or a belief that birth is natural may plan to go through labor with minimal or no medication. She may or may not find the support for her plan in that setting. (d) The opiates include opium, heroin, meperidine, morphine, codeine, and methadone. Opioid analgesics can be given to a woman who has a history of addiction to an opioid; however, the dose of medication required to achieve pain relief may be greater. Use of nonpharmacologic techniques to augment the effects of pharmacologic methods should be used.
3. The priorities for nursing care are to provide pain relief and ensure the safety of the patient and her fetus. The woman's progress in labor and fetal status are monitored. Instituting nonpharmacologic interventions, providing a calm environment, staying with the patient and responding to her requests and needs, and administering appropriate pharmacologic agents will assist the woman to cope with the pain of labor.
4. Studies of nonpharmacologic and pharmacologic means to assist women to cope with the pain of labor and childbirth are numerous. A variety of techniques and medications are available and effective. Nurses need to keep their knowledge current and use the findings of such studies in their practice; Cochrane Reviews are an excellent source of research evidence to support practice.
5. Pregnant women who abuse substances commonly have little understanding of the ways in which these substances affect them, their pregnancies, or their babies and may not seek prenatal care until labor begins. Many problems of pregnancy are associated with substance abuse. Examples include preeclampsia, intrauterine growth restriction, miscarriage, premature rupture of membranes, infections, breech presentation, and preterm labor. The woman may have poor nutrition, with vitamin, iron, and folic acid deficiencies. She may have medical complications from sexually transmitted infections, hypertension, or frequent use of dirty needles. Fewer than 10% of pregnant women who are substance abusers receive treatment for their addictions. Women often do not seek help because of the fear of losing custody of the child or criminal prosecution.

Resources

Academy for Guided Imagery, Inc.
PO Box 2070
Mill Valley, CA 94942
800-726-2070
www.healthy.net/agi

ALACE—Association of Labor Assistants and Childbirth Educators
PO Box 390436
Cambridge, MA 02139
617-441-2500
888-222-5223 (toll free)
617-441-3167 (fax)
www.alace.org
info@alace.org

American Academy of Husband-Coached Childbirth (Bradley Method of Natural Childbirth)
PO Box 5224
Sherman Oaks, CA 91413
800-422-4784
www.bradleybirth.com

Birthing From Within, Inc.
PO Box 4528
Albuquerque, NM 87196
505-254-4884
www.birthingfromwithin.com

Birthworks, Inc.
PO Box 2045
Medford, NJ 08055
888-862-4784
www.birthworks.org

Childbirth and Postpartum Professional Association (CAPPA)
310 Sweet Ivy Lane
Lawrenceville, GA 30043
888-548-3672
www.childbirthprofessional.com

Cutting Edge Press
Source for information and equipment regarding childbirth support measures by Polly Perez
www.childbirth.org/CEP.html

Healing Touch International, Inc.
12477 W. Cedar Drive, Suite 202
Lakewood, CO 80228
303-989-7982
www.healingtouch.net

HypnoBirthing Institute
PO Box 810
Epsom, NH 03234
603-798-3286
www.hypnobirthing.com

Lamaze International
2025 M Street, Suite 800
Washington, DC 20036-3309
800-368-4404
www.lamaze.org

Maternity Center Association
281 Park Avenue South, 5th Floor
New York, NY 10010
212-777-5000
www.maternitywise.org

Read Natural Childbirth Foundation
PO Box 150956
San Rafael, CA 94915
415-456-8462

Touch Research Institutes
University of Miami School of Medicine (located at Mailman Center for Child Development)
1601 N.W. 12th Avenue, 7th Floor, Suite 7037
Miami, FL 33101
305-243-6781
www.miami.edu/touch-research/home.html

References

Atherton MJ, Feeg VD, el-Adham AF: Race, ethnicity, and insurance as determinants of epidural use: analysis of a national sample survey, *Nurs Econ* 22(1):6-13, 2004.

Baker A et al: Perception of labour pain by mothers and their attending midwives, *J Adv Nurs*, 35(2):171-179, 2001.

Birthing From Within: Internet document available at www.birthingfromwithin.com (accessed September 17, 2004).

Bradley R: *Husband-coached childbirth,* ed 3, New York, 1981, Harper & Collins.

Bricker L, Lavender T: Parenteral opioids for labor pain relief: a systematic review, *Am J Obstet Gynecol* 186(5 suppl Nature):S94-S109, 2002.

Caton D et al: The nature and management of labor pain: executive summary, *Am J Obstet Gynecol* 186(5 suppl Nature):S1-S15, 2002.

Childbirth and Postpartum Professional Association (CAPPA): Internet document available at www.cappa.net (accessed September 17, 2004).

Cluett E et al: Immersion in water in pregnancy, labour and birth (Cochrane Review). In *The Cochrane Library,* Issue 2, Chichester, UK, 2004, John Wiley & Sons.

Cunningham FG et al: *Williams obstetrics,* ed 21, Norwalk, CT, 2001, Appleton & Lange.

Dick-Read G: *Childbirth without fear,* ed 5, New York, 1987, Harper & Collins.

Di Franco JT: Relaxation: music. In Nichols F, Humenick S (eds): *Childbirth education: practice, research and theory,* ed 2, Philadelphia, 2000, WB Saunders.

Enkin M et al: *A guide to effective care in pregnancy and childbirth,* ed 3, Oxford, NY, 2000, Oxford University Press.

Faucher MA, Brucker MC: Intrapartum pain: pharmacologic management, *J Obstet Gynecol Neonatal Nurs* 29(2):169-180, 2000.

Florence DJ, Palmer DG: Therapeutic choices for the discomforts of labor, *J Perinat Neonatal Nurs* 17(4):238-249, 2003.

Gentz BA: Alternative therapies for the management of pain in labor and delivery, *Clin Obstet Gynecol* 44(4):704-732, 2001.

Gilder K et al: Maternal positions in labor with epidural analgesia: results from a multi-site survey, *AWHONN Lifelines* 6(1):40-45, 2002.

Govenar JK: Handling headache after dural puncture, *RN* 63(12):26-30, 2000.

Hawkins JL, Chestnut DH, Gibbs CP: Obstetric anesthesia. In Gabbe SG, Niebyl JR, Simpson JL (eds): *Obstetrics: normal and problem pregnancies,* ed 4, Philadelphia, 2002, Churchill Livingstone.

Hodnett ED: Pain and women's satisfaction with the experience of childbirth: a systematic review, *Am J Obstet Gynecol* 186(5 suppl Nature):S160-S172, 2002.

Hodnett ED et al: Continuous support for women during childbirth, *The Cochrane Library,* Issue 4, Chichester, UK: 2004, John Wiley & Sons.

Hover-Kramer D et al: *Healing touch: a resource for health care professionals,* Albany, NY, 2001, Delmar.

Humenick S, Schrock P, Libresco M: Relaxation. In Nichols F, Humenick S (eds): *Childbirth education: practice, research and theory,* ed 2, Philadelphia, 2000, WB Saunders.

HypnoBirthing: Internet document available at www.hypnobirthing.org (accessed September 17, 2004).

Jiménez SLM: Comfort and pain management. In Nichols F, Humenick S (eds): *Childbirth education: practice, research and theory,* ed 2, Philadelphia, 2000, WB Saunders.

Johnson S, Rosenfeld JA: The effect of epidural anesthesia on the length of labor, *J Fam Pract* 40(3):244-247, 1995.

Karmel M: *Thank you, Dr. Lamaze.* New York, 1959, Dolphin Books.

Kuczkowski KM: Labor analgesia for the morbidly obese parturient: an old problem—new solution, *Arch Gynecol Obstet,* June 2, 2004 (epub ahead of print) (accessed January 17, 2005).

Lamaze Philosophy of Birth. Internet document available at www.lamaze.org/about/PhilosophyofBirth.asp (accessed March 26, 2005).

Lee MC, Essoka G: Continuing education. Patient's perception of pain: comparison between Korean-American and Euro-American obstetric patients, *J Cult Divers* 5(1):29-40, 1998.

Leeman L et al: Editorial: management of labor pain: promoting patient choice, *Am Fam Physician* 68(6):1023-1026, 2003a.

Leeman L et al: The nature and management of labor pain: part I. Nonpharmacologic pain relief, *Am Fam Physician* 68(6):1109-1112, 2003b.

Leeman L et al: The nature and management of labor pain: part II. Pharmacologic pain relief, *Am Fam Physician* 68(6):1115-1120, 2003c.

Lehne RA: *Pharmacology for nursing care,* ed 4, Philadelphia, 2001, WB Saunders.

Leighton BL, Halpern SH: The effects of epidural analgesia on labor, maternal, and neonatal outcomes: a systematic review, *Am J Obstet Gynecol* 186(5 suppl Nature):S69-S77, 2002.

Lieberman E, O'Donoghue C: Unintended effects of epidural anesthesia during labor: a systematic review, *Am J Obstet Gynecol* 186(5 suppl Nature):S31-S68, 2002.

Lowe NK: The nature of labor pain, *Am J Obstet Gynecol* 186(5 suppl Nature):S16-S24, 2002.

Mackey MM: Use of water in labor and birth, *Clin Obstet Gynecol* 44(4):733-749, 2001.

Mahlmeister L: Nursing responsibilities in preventing, preparing for, and managing epidural emergencies, *J Perinat Neonatal Nurs* 17(1):19-32, 2003.

Marks G: Alternative therapies. In Nichols F, Humenick S (eds): *Childbirth education: practice, research and theory,* ed 2, Philadelphia, 2000, WB Saunders.

Mattson S: Striving for cultural competence: providing care for the changing face of the U.S., *AWHONN Lifelines* 4(3):48-52, 2000.

Mayberry LJ, Clemmens D, De A: Epidural analgesia side effects, co-interventions, and care of women during childbirth: a systematic review, *Am J Obstet Gynecol* 186(5 suppl Nature): S81-S93, 2002.

Mayberry LJ et al: Use of upright positioning with epidural analgesia: findings from an observational study, *MCN Am J Matern Child Nurs* 28(3):152-159, 2003.

Poole JH: Neuraxial analgesia for labor and birth: implications for mother and fetus, *J Perinat Neonatal Nurs* 17(4):252-267, 2003.

Righard L: Making childbirth a normal process, *Birth* 28(1):1-4, 2001.

Rosen M: Nitrous oxide for relief of labor pain: a systematic review, *Am J Obstet Gynecol* 186(5 suppl Nature):S110-S126, 2002a.

Rosen M: Paracervical block for labor analgesia: a brief historical review. *Am J Obstet Gynecol* 186(5 suppl Nature):S127-S130, 2002b.

Schuiling KD, Sampselle CM: Comfort in labor and midwifery art, *Image J Nurs Sch* 31(1):77-81, 1999.

Scott J et al: *Danforth's obstetrics and gynecology,* ed 8, Philadelphia, 1999, JB Lippincott.

Simkin P: Reducing pain and enhancing progress in labor: a guide to non-pharmacologic methods of maternity caregivers, *Birth* 22(3):161-191, 1995.

Simkin PP, O'Hara M: Nonpharmacologic relief of pain during labor: systematic reviews of five methods, *Am J Obstet Gynecol* 186(5 suppl Nature):S131-S159, 2002.

Snyder M, Lindquist R (eds): *Complementary/alternative therapies in nursing,* ed 4, New York, 2000, Springer.

Tiran D, Mack S: *Complementary therapies for pregnancy and childbirth,* ed 2, Edinburgh, 2000, Bailliere-Tindall.

Villarruel AM: Mexican-American cultural meanings, expressions, self-care and dependent-care actions associated with experiences of pain, *Res Nurs Health* 18(5):427-436, 1995.

Weber SE: Cultural aspects of pain in childbearing women, *J Obstet Gynecol Neonatal Nurs* 25(1):67-72, 1996.

Wiand N: Relaxation levels achieved by Lamaze-trained pregnant women listening to music and ocean sound tapes, *J Perinatal Educ* 6(4):1-8, 1997.

Fetal Assessment during Labor 17

LEARNING OBJECTIVES

On completion of this chapter the reader will be able to:

- Explain baseline fetal heart rate (FHR) and evaluate periodic changes.
- Identify typical signs of nonreassuring FHR patterns.
- Compare FHR monitoring done by intermittent auscultation (IA) with external and internal electronic methods.
- Describe nursing measures that can be used to maintain FHR patterns within normal limits.
- Differentiate among the nursing interventions used for managing specific FHR patterns, including tachycardia and bradycardia; increased and decreased variability; and late and variable decelerations.
- Review the documentation of the monitoring process necessary during labor.

ELECTRONIC RESOURCES

Additional information related to the content in Chapter 17 can be found on

the companion website at evolve
http://evolve.elsevier.com/Wong/maternal/
- NCLEX Review Questions
- WebLinks

or the interactive student CD-ROM
Activities for Chapter 17 include the following:
- NCLEX Review Questions
- Critical Thinking Exercise—Fetal Monitoring
- Nursing Care Plan—EFM During Labor

The ability to assess the fetus by auscultation of fetal heart tones was initially described more than 300 years ago. With the advent of the fetoscope and stethoscope after the turn of the twentieth century, the listener could hear clearly enough to count the fetal heart rate (FHR). When electronic FHR monitoring made its debut for clinical use in the early 1970s, it was anticipated that its use would effect a decrease in cerebral palsy and be more sensitive than stethoscopic auscultation in predicting and preventing fetal compromise (Simpson & Knox, 2000). Although neither of these possibilities has been realized, electronic fetal monitoring (EFM) is a useful tool for visualizing FHR patterns on a monitor screen or printed tracing.

Pregnant women should be informed about the equipment and procedures used and the risks, benefits, and limitations of intermittent auscultation (IA) and EFM. This chapter discusses the basis for fetal monitoring, the types of monitoring, and nursing assessment and management of nonreassuring fetal status.

BASIS FOR MONITORING

Understanding fetal and uteroplacental circulation is important in understanding FHR and uterine activity monitoring (see Chapter 9).

Fetal Response

Because labor is a period of physiologic stress for the fetus, frequent monitoring of fetal status is part of the nursing care during labor. The fetal oxygen supply must be maintained during labor to prevent fetal compromise and to promote newborn health after birth. The fetal oxygen supply can decrease in a number of ways:

- Reduction of blood flow through the maternal vessels as a result of maternal hypertension (chronic hypertension or pregnancy-induced hypertension), hypotension (caused by supine maternal position, hemorrhage, or epidural analgesia or anesthesia), or hypovolemia (caused by hemorrhage)
- Reduction of the oxygen content in the maternal blood as a result of hemorrhage or severe anemia
- Alterations in fetal circulation, occurring with compression of the umbilical cord (transient: during uterine contractions [UCs]; or prolonged, resulting from cord prolapse), placental separation or complete abruption, or head compression (head compression causes increased intracranial pressure and vagal nerve stimulation with an accompanying decrease in the FHR)
- Reduction in blood flow to the intervillous space in the placenta secondary to uterine hypertonus (generally caused by excessive exogenous oxytocin) or secondary to deterioration of the placental vasculature associated with maternal disorders such as hypertension or diabetes mellitus

Fetal well-being during labor can be measured by the response of the FHR to UCs. In general, reassuring FHR patterns are characterized by the following:

- A baseline FHR in the normal range of 110 to 160 beats/min with no periodic changes and moderate baseline variability
- Accelerations of FHR with fetal movement

Uterine Activity

A normal uterine activity pattern in labor is characterized by contractions occurring every 2 to 5 minutes and lasting less than 90 seconds. Such contractions are moderate to strong in intensity, as evidenced by palpation, or intensity is less than 80 mm Hg, as measured by an intrauterine pressure catheter (IUPC); 30 seconds or more should elapse between the end of one contraction and the beginning of the next contraction. Between contractions, uterine relaxation should be detected by palpation or by an average intrauterine pressure of 20 mm Hg or less (Tucker, 2004).

Fetal Compromise

The goals of intrapartum FHR monitoring are to identify and differentiate reassuring patterns from nonreassuring patterns, which can be indicative of fetal compromise. Nursing care focuses on interventions promoting adequate fetal oxygenation and interventions for nonreassuring patterns if they occur.

Nonreassuring FHR patterns are those associated with fetal hypoxemia, which is a deficiency of oxygen in the arterial blood. If uncorrected, hypoxemia can deteriorate to severe fetal hypoxia, which is an inadequate supply of oxygen at the cellular level. Nonreassuring FHR patterns include the following:

- Progressive increase or decrease in baseline rate
- Tachycardia of 160 beats/min or more
- Progressive decrease in baseline variability
- Severe variable decelerations (FHR less than 60 beats/min lasting longer than 30 to 60 seconds, with rising baseline, decreasing variability, or slow return to baseline)
- Late decelerations of any magnitude, especially those that are repetitive and uncorrectable
- Absence of FHR variability
- Prolonged deceleration (greater than 60 to 90 seconds)
- Severe bradycardia (less than 70 beats/min)

MONITORING TECHNIQUES

The ideal method of fetal assessment during labor continues to be debated. Results from research studies indicate that both intermittent auscultation of the FHR and electronic FHR monitoring are associated with similar fetal outcomes in low risk intrapartum patients (Feinstein, Sprague, & Trepanier, 2000; Thacker, Stroup, & Chang, 2001). Although intermittent auscultation is a high-touch, low-technology method of assessing fetal status during labor that places fewer restrictions on maternal activity, more than 80% of laboring women in the United States are monitored electronically for at least part of their labor (Albers, 2001). The lack of evidence on the efficacy of EFM should be a factor to consider in decision making about which method of fetal assessment is offered to low risk laboring women (Wood, 2003).

Intermittent Auscultation

Intermittent auscultation (IA) uses listening to fetal heart sounds at periodic intervals to assess the FHR. IA of the fetal heart can be performed with a Leff scope, a DeLee-Hillis fetoscope, or an ultrasound device. If a Leff scope is used, the domed side should be opened to the connective tubing to the earpieces. The domed side is then applied to the maternal abdomen. The fetoscope is applied over the listener's head because bone conduction amplifies the fetal heart sounds for counting. The ultrasound device transmits ultrahigh-frequency sound waves reflecting movement of the fetal heart and converts these sounds into an electronic signal that can be counted (Fig. 17-1).

One procedure for performing auscultation is as follows:

1. Perform Leopold maneuvers (see Fig. 18-6) by palpating the maternal abdomen to identify fetal presentation and position.
2. Place the listening device over the area of maximal intensity and clarity of the fetal heart sounds to obtain the clearest and loudest sound, which is easiest to count. Apply ultrasound gel to Doppler ultrasound device if used.
3. Palpate the abdomen for the absence of uterine activity to be able to count the FHR between contractions.
4. Count the maternal radial pulse at the same time as listening to the FHR to differentiate it from the fetal rate.
5. Count the FHR for 30 to 60 seconds between contractions to identify the baseline rate. This rate can be assessed only during the absence of uterine activity.
6. Auscultate the FHR during a contraction and for 30 seconds after the end of the contraction to identify any increases or decreases in FHR in response to the contraction.

By using IA, the nurse can assess the FHR baseline rate, rhythm, and increases and decreases from baseline (Feinstein, 2000). The method and frequency of fetal surveillance during labor will vary depending on maternal-fetal risk factors and the preference of the facility. In the absence of risk factors, one

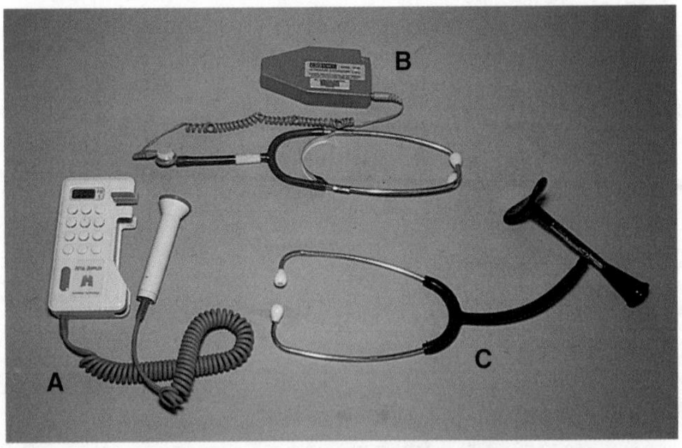

Fig. 17-1 **A,** Ultrasound fetoscope. **B,** Ultrasound stethoscope. **C,** DeLee-Hillis fetoscope. (Courtesy Michael S. Clement, MD, Mesa, AZ.)

recommended practice is to auscultate the FHR as follows (American Academy of Pediatrics/American College of Obstetricians and Gynecologists [AAP/ACOG], 2002; Association of Women's Health, Obstetric, and Neonatal Nurses [AWHONN], 2003):

- First stage
  - Active phase: every 30 minutes
- Second stage
  - Every 15 minutes

If risk factors are present, the FHR is auscultated as follows:

- First stage
  - Active phase: every 15 minutes
- Second stage
  - Every 5 minutes

There is no recommended practice for assessing the FHR in the latent phase of first-stage labor; however, AWHONN (2003) suggests that the FHR be assessed as frequently as maternal vital signs. The FHR also is assessed before and after ambulation, rupture of membranes, administration of medications and anesthesia, and more frequently when nonreassuring FHR patterns are heard (AWHONN, 2003; Tucker, 2004).

NURSE ALERT When the FHR is auscultated and documented, it is inappropriate to use the descriptive terms associated with EFM because most of the terms are visual descriptions of the patterns produced on the monitor tracing. Terms that are numerically defined, however, such as *bradycardia* and *tachycardia,* can be used. ■

Every effort should be made to use the method of fetal assessment the woman desires when possible. However, auscultation of the FHR in accordance with the frequency guidelines just given may be difficult in today's busy labor and birth units. When used as the primary method of fetal assessment, auscultation requires a one-to-one nurse-to-patient staffing ratio. If acuity and census change so that auscultation standards are no longer met, the nurse must inform the physician or nurse-midwife that continuous EFM will be used until staffing can be arranged to meet the standards.

The woman may become anxious if the examiner cannot readily count the fetal heartbeats. It often takes time for the inexperienced listener to locate the heartbeat and find the area of maximal intensity. To allay the mother's concerns, she can be told that the nurse is "finding the spot where the sounds are loudest." If it takes considerable time to locate the fetal heartbeats, the examiner can reassure the mother by offering her an opportunity to listen to them, too. If the examiner cannot locate the fetal heartbeat, assistance should be requested. In some cases, ultrasound can be used to help locate the fetal heartbeat. Seeing the FHR on the ultrasound screen will be reassuring to the mother if there was initial difficulty in locating the best area for auscultation.

When using IA, uterine activity is assessed by palpation. The examiner should keep his or her hand placed over the fundus before, during, and after contractions. The contraction intensity is usually described as mild, moderate, or strong. The contraction duration is measured in seconds, from the beginning to the end of the contraction. The frequency of contractions is measured in minutes, from the beginning of one contraction to the beginning of the next contraction. The examiner should keep his or her hand on the fundus after the contraction is over to evaluate uterine resting tone or relaxation between contractions. Resting tone between contractions is usually described as soft or relaxed (Goodwin, 2000).

Accurate and complete documentation of fetal status and uterine activity is especially important when IA and palpation are being used because no paper tracing record of these assessments is provided as it is by continuous EFM. Labor flow records or computer charting systems that prompt notations of all assessments are useful for ensuring such comprehensive documentation.

Electronic Fetal Monitoring

The purpose of electronic FHR monitoring is the ongoing assessment of fetal oxygenation. FHR tracings are analyzed for characteristic patterns that signify specific hypoxic and nonhypoxic events (King & Parer, 2000; Parer & King, 2000).

The two modes of EFM are (1) the external mode, which uses external transducers placed on the maternal abdomen to assess FHR and uterine activity, and (2) the internal mode, which uses a spiral electrode applied to the fetal presenting part to assess the FHR and an intrauterine pressure catheter to assess uterine activity and pressure. The differences between the external and internal modes of EFM are summarized in Table 17-1.

External Monitoring

Separate transducers are used to monitor the FHR and UCs (Fig. 17-2). The ultrasound transducer works by reflecting high-frequency sound waves off a moving interface: in this case, the fetal heart and valves. Therefore short-term variability and beat-to-beat changes in the FHR cannot be assessed accurately by this method. It is sometimes difficult to reproduce a continuous and precise record of the FHR because of artifacts introduced by fetal and maternal movement. The FHR is printed on specially formatted monitor paper. The standard paper speed is 3 cm/min. Once the area of maximal intensity of the FHR has been located, conductive gel is applied to the surface of the ultrasound transducer, and the transducer is then positioned over this area.

The tocotransducer (tocodynamometer) measures uterine activity transabdominally. The device is placed over the fundus above the umbilicus. UCs or fetal movements depress a pressure-sensitive surface on the side next to the abdomen. The tocotransducer can measure and record the frequency, regularity, and approximate duration of UCs but not their intensity. This method is especially valuable for measuring uterine activity during the first stage of labor in women with intact membranes or for antepartum testing. Because the tocotransducer of most electronic fetal monitors is designed for assessing uterine activity in the term pregnancy, it may not be sensitive enough to detect preterm uterine activity. When monitoring the woman in preterm labor, remember that the fundus may be located below the level of the umbilicus. The nurse may need to rely on the woman to indicate when uterine activity is occurring and to use palpation as an additional way of assessing contraction frequency.

Table 17-1

External and Internal Modes of Monitoring

EXTERNAL MODE	INTERNAL MODE
FETAL HEART RATE	
Ultrasound transducer: High-frequency sound waves reflect mechanical action of the fetal heart. Noninvasive. Does not require rupture of membranes or cervical dilation. Used during both the antepartum and intrapartum periods.	*Spiral electrode:* This electrode converts the fetal ECG as obtained from the presenting part to the FHR via a cardiotachometer. This method can be used only when membranes are ruptured and the cervix is sufficiently dilated during the intrapartum period. The electrode penetrates into fetal presenting part by 1.5 mm and must be attached securely to ensure a good signal.
UTERINE ACTIVITY	
Tocotransducer: This instrument monitors frequency and duration of contractions by means of a pressure-sensing device applied to the maternal abdomen. Used during both the antepartum and intrapartum periods.	*Intrauterine pressure catheter (IUPC):* This instrument monitors the frequency, duration, and intensity of contractions. The two types of IUPCs are a fluid-filled system and a solid catheter. Both measure intrauterine pressure at the catheter tip and convert the pressure into millimeters of mercury on the uterine activity panel of the strip chart. Both can be used only when membranes are ruptured and the cervix is sufficiently dilated during the intrapartum period.

ECG, electrocardiogram; *FHR*, fetal heart rate.

The external transducer is easily applied by the nurse, but it must be repositioned as the woman or fetus changes position (see Fig. 17-2, *B*). The woman is asked to assume a semisitting or lateral position. The equipment is removed periodically to wash the applicator sites and to give back rubs. Use of an external transducer confines the woman to bed. Portable telemetry monitors allow observation of the FHR and uterine contraction patterns by means of centrally located electronic display stations. These portable units permit the woman to walk around during electronic monitoring. Other monitoring equipment can be used when the woman is submerged in water (see Fig. 18-18).

Internal Monitoring

The technique of continuous internal monitoring provides an accurate appraisal of fetal well-being during labor (Fig. 17-3). For this type of monitoring, the membranes must be ruptured, the cervix sufficiently dilated, and the presenting part low enough to allow placement of the electrode. A small spiral electrode attached to the presenting part shows a continuous FHR on the fetal monitor strip.

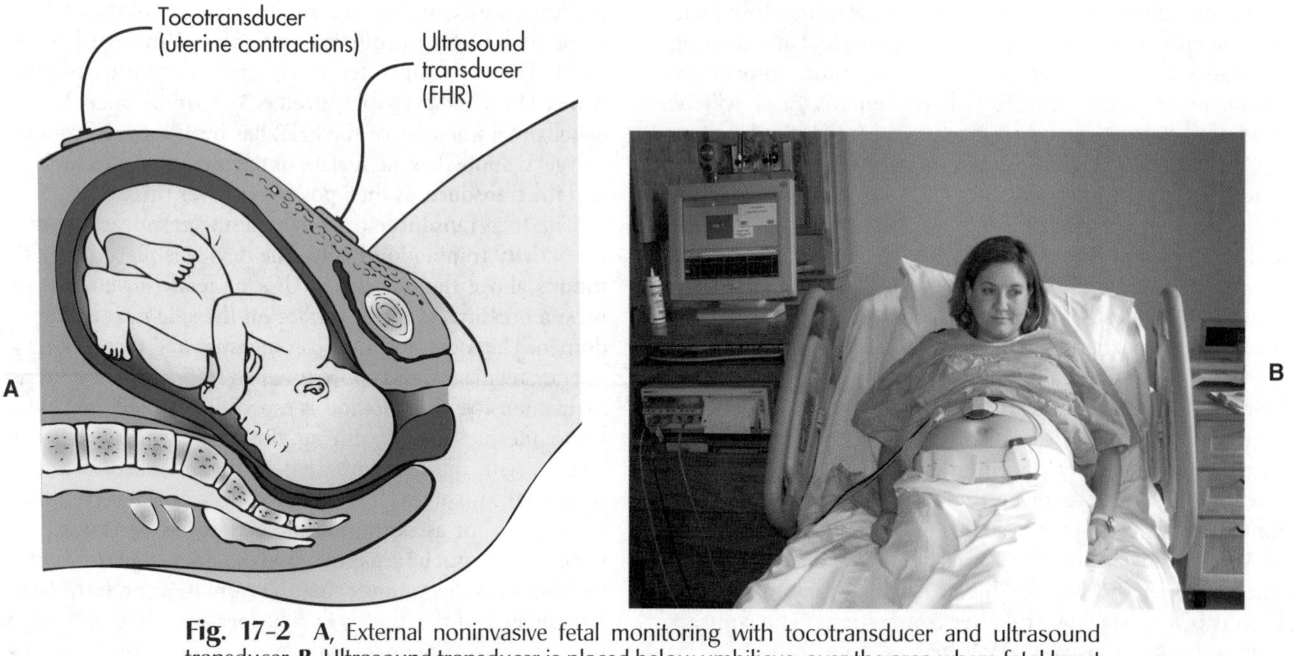

Fig. 17-2 **A,** External noninvasive fetal monitoring with tocotransducer and ultrasound transducer. **B,** Ultrasound transducer is placed below umbilicus, over the area where fetal heart rate is best heard, and tocotransducer is placed on uterine fundus. (*B,* Courtesy Julie Perry Nelson, Gilbert, AZ.)

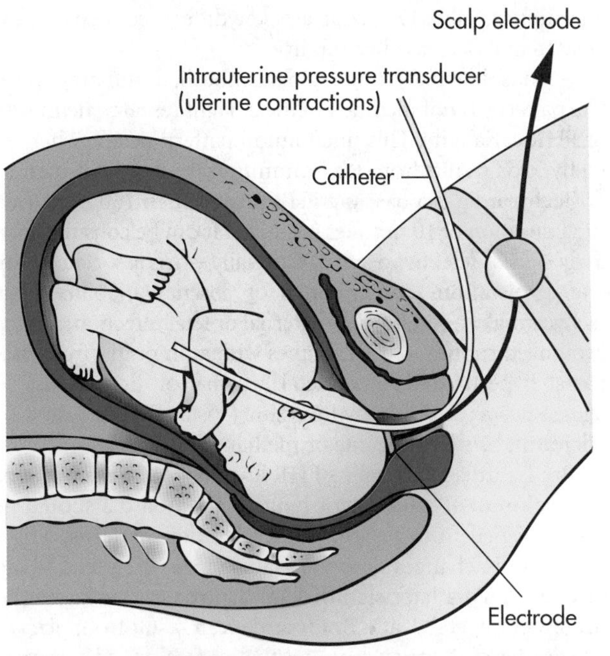

Fig. 17-3 Diagrammatic representation of internal invasive fetal monitoring with intrauterine pressure catheter and spiral electrode in place (membranes ruptured and cervix dilated).

Internal monitoring of the FHR may be implemented without internal monitoring of uterine activity. To monitor uterine activity, a solid or fluid-filled IUPC is introduced into the uterine cavity. A solid catheter has a pressure-sensitive tip that measures changes in intrauterine pressure. Alternatively, a catheter filled with sterile water can be used. As the catheter is compressed during a contraction, pressure is placed on the pressure transducer or strain gauge; this pressure is then converted into a pressure reading in millimeters of mercury. The average pressure during a contraction ranges from 50 to 85 mm Hg. The IUPC can measure the frequency, duration, and intensity of UCs.

The FHR and uterine activity (UA) are displayed on the monitor paper with the FHR in the upper section and UA in the lower section. Figure 17-4 contrasts the internal and external modes of electronic monitoring. Note that each small square represents 10 seconds; each larger box of six squares equals 1 minute (when paper is moving through the monitor at 3 cm/min).

FETAL HEART RATE PATTERNS

Baseline Fetal Heart Rate

The intrinsic rhythmicity of the fetal heart, the central nervous system (CNS), and the fetal autonomic nervous system control the FHR. An increase in sympathetic response results in acceleration of the FHR, whereas an augmentation in parasympathetic response produces a slowing of the FHR. Usually a balanced increase of sympathetic and parasympathetic response occurs during contractions, with no observable change in the baseline FHR.

Baseline fetal heart rate is the average rate during a 10-minute segment that excludes periodic or episodic changes, periods of marked variability, and segments of the baseline that differ by more than 25 beats/min (National Institute of Child Health and Human Development Research Planning Workshop [NICHD], 1997). The normal range at term is 110 to 160 beats/min.

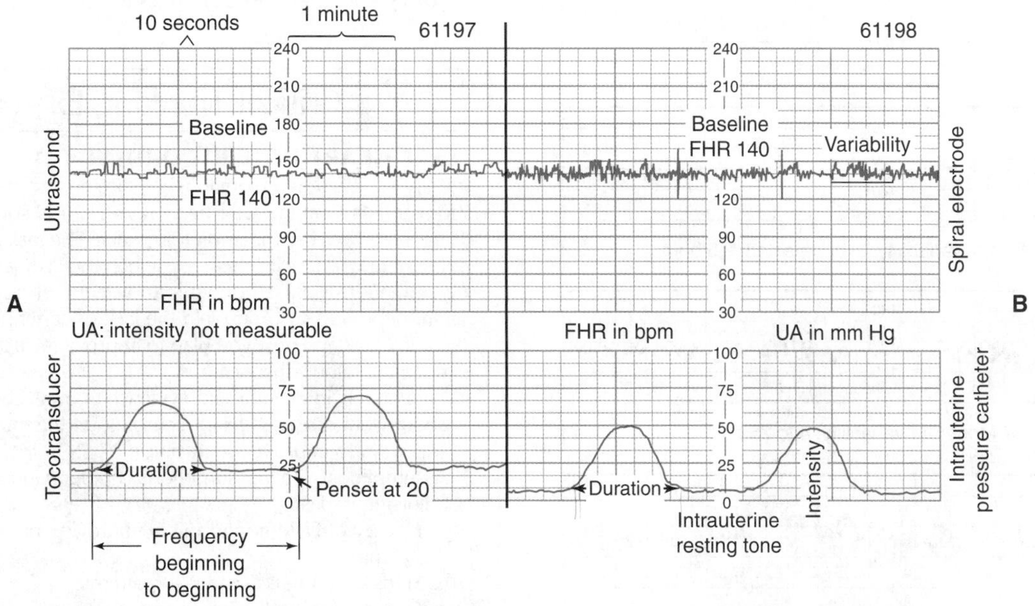

Fig. 17-4 Display of fetal heart rate and uterine activity on monitor paper. **A**, External mode with ultrasound and tocotransducer as signal source. **B**, Internal mode with spiral electrode and intrauterine catheter as signal source. Frequency of contractions is measured from the beginning of one contraction to the beginning of the next. (From Tucker SM: *Pocket guide to fetal monitoring and assessment*, ed 5, St Louis, 2004, Mosby.)

Variability of the FHR can be described as irregular fluctuations in the baseline FHR of two cycles per minute or greater (NICHD, 1997). It is a characteristic of baseline FHR and does not include accelerations or decelerations of the FHR. Variability has been described as short term (beat to beat) or long term (rhythmic waves or cycles from baseline). The current definition for research does not distinguish between short-term and long-term variability because in actual practice, they are viewed together (NICHD, 1997); however, this definition does identify four ranges of variability, as shown in Fig. 17-5. These are based on visualization of the amplitude of the FHR in the peak-to-trough segment in beats per minute and include the following:

- Absent or undetected variability
- Minimal variability (greater than undetected but not more than 5 beats/min)
- Moderate variability (6 to 25 beats/min)
- Marked variability (greater than 25 beats/min)

In many facilities, short-term and long-term variability continue to be used to describe the FHR fluctuations.

Absence of or undetected variability is considered nonreassuring. Diminished variability can result from fetal hypoxemia and acidosis, as well as from certain drugs that depress the CNS, including analgesics, opioids (morphine), barbiturates (secobarbital [Seconal] and pentobarbital [Nembutal]), tranquilizers (diazepam [Valium]), ataractics (promethazine [Phenergan]), and general anesthetics. In addition, a temporary decrease in variability can occur when the fetus is in a sleep state. These sleep states do not usually last longer than 30 minutes. Table 17-2 contrasts key differences between increased and decreased variability.

A sinusoidal pattern (a regular, smooth, undulating wave-like pattern) is not included in the current research definition of FHR variability. This uncommon pattern occurs when fetal hypoxia results from Rh isoimmunization or fetal anemia.

Tachycardia is a baseline FHR greater than 160 beats/min for a duration of 10 minutes or longer. It can be considered an early sign of fetal hypoxemia, especially when associated with late decelerations and minimal or absent variability. Fetal tachycardia can result from maternal or fetal infection, such as prolonged rupture of membranes with amnionitis; from maternal hyperthyroidism or fetal anemia; or in response to drugs such as atropine, hydroxyzine (Vistaril), terbutaline, or illicit drugs such as cocaine or methamphetamines.

Bradycardia is a baseline FHR less than 110 beats/min for a duration of 10 minutes or longer. (Bradycardia should be distinguished from prolonged deceleration patterns, which are periodic changes described later in this chapter.) It can be considered a later sign of fetal hypoxia and is known to occur before fetal death. Bradycardia can result from placental transfer of drugs such as anesthetics, prolonged compression of the umbilical cord, maternal hypothermia, and maternal hypotension. Maternal supine hypotension syndrome, caused by the weight and pressure of the gravid uterus on the vena cava, decreases the return of blood flow to the maternal heart, which then reduces maternal cardiac output and blood pressure. These responses in the mother subsequently result in a decrease in the FHR and fetal bradycardia. Table 17-3 contrasts tachycardia with bradycardia.

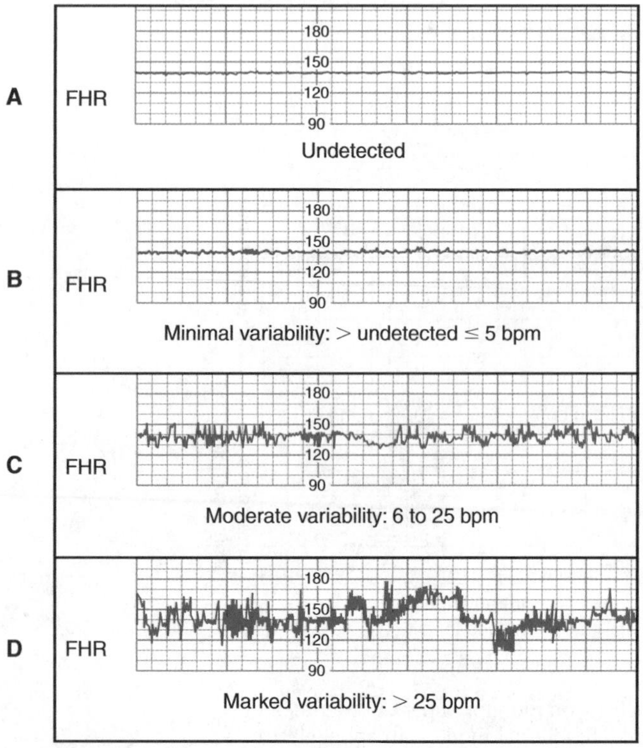

Fig. 17-5 Fetal heart rate variability. **A,** Absent or undetected. **B,** Minimal. **C,** Moderate. **D,** Marked. (Modified from Tucker SM: *Pocket guide to fetal monitoring and assessment,* ed 5, St Louis, 2004, Mosby.)

Changes in Fetal Heart Rate

Changes in FHR from the baseline are categorized as periodic or episodic. Periodic changes are those that occur with

Critical Thinking Exercise

FETAL HEART RATE RECORDING

You are assigned to a woman who is in the first stage of labor. She wonders why the fetal heart rate (FHR) is sometimes not being recorded on the monitor paper. She asks if there is "something wrong with the baby" when the FHR is not recording continuously. Based on your knowledge of how the external monitor works, you explain the lack of continuous recording of the FHR and how you plan to improve the tracing, as well as document your observations.

1. Evidence—Is there sufficient evidence to draw conclusions about what causes gaps in recording on the monitor paper and ways to improve the tracing?
2. Assumptions—What assumptions can be made about the following issues?
   a. Efficacy of FHR monitoring in improving pregnancy outcome
   b. Signs of nonreassuring FHR patterns
   c. Causes of periodic and episodic changes in the FHR
   d. Patient choice in fetal monitoring techniques
3. What implications and priorities for nursing care can be drawn at this time?
4. Does the evidence objectively support your conclusion?
5. Are there alternative perspectives to your conclusion?

Table 17-2

Increased and Decreased Variability

INCREASED VARIABILITY	DECREASED VARIABILITY
CAUSE	
Early mild hypoxemia Fetal stimulation by the following: Uterine palpation Uterine contractions Fetal activity Maternal activity Street drugs (e.g., cocaine and methamphetamines)	Hypoxia/acidosis CNS depressants Analgesics/narcotics Meperidine (Demerol) Alphaprodine (Nisentil) Morphine Pentazocine (Talwin) Barbiturates Secobarbital (Seconal) Pentobarbital (Nembutal) Amobarbital (Amytal) Tranquilizers Diazepam (Valium) Ataractics Promethazine (Phenergan) Propiomazine (Largon) Hydroxyzine (Vistaril) Promazine (Sparine) Parasympatholytics Atropine General anesthetics Prematurity—less than 24 wk Fetal sleep cycles Congenital abnormalities Fetal cardiac dysrhythmias
CLINICAL SIGNIFICANCE	
Significance of marked variability not known; increased variability from a previous average variability is earliest FHR sign of mild hypoxemia	Benign when associated with periodic fetal sleep states, which last 20 to 30 min; if caused by drugs, variability usually increases as drugs are excreted Decreased variability is not reassuring and is considered a sign of fetal stress *unless* it has an identifiable temporary (e.g., fetal sleep) or correctable cause
NURSING INTERVENTION	
Observe FHR tracing carefully for any nonreassuring patterns, including decreasing variability and late decelerations; if using external mode of monitoring, consider using internal mode (spiral electrode) for a more accurate tracing	Dependent on cause; intervention not warranted if associated with fetal sleep states or temporarily associated with CNS depressants; consider performing external stimulation of scalp during a vaginal examination to elicit an acceleration of FHR or return to average variability; consider application of internal mode (spiral electrode); assist health care provider with fetal oxygen saturation monitoring if ordered; prepare for birth if so indicated by the primary health care provider

CNS, central nervous system; *FHR*, fetal heart rate.

UCs. Episodic changes are those that are not associated with UCs. These patterns include accelerations and decelerations (NICHD, 1997).

Accelerations

Acceleration of the FHR is defined as a visually apparent abrupt increase in FHR above the baseline rate. The increase is 15 beats/min or greater and lasts 15 seconds or more, with the return to baseline less than 2 minutes from the beginning of the acceleration. In preterm gestations, the definition of an acceleration is a peak of 10 beats/min or more above baseline for at least 10 seconds. Acceleration of the FHR for more than 10 minutes is considered a change in baseline rate.

Accelerations can be periodic or episodic. Periodic accelerations are caused by dominance of the sympathetic nervous response and are usually encountered with breech presentations (Fig. 17-6, *A*). Pressure of the contraction applied

Table 17-3

Tachycardia and Bradycardia

TACHYCARDIA	BRADYCARDIA
DEFINITION	
FHR >160 beats/min lasting longer than 10 min	FHR <110 beats/min lasting longer than 10 min
CAUSE	
Early fetal hypoxemia Maternal fever Parasympatholytic drugs (atropine, hydroxyzine) Beta-sympathomimetic drugs (ritodrine, isoxsuprine) Intraamniotic infection Maternal hyperthyroidism Fetal anemia Fetal heart failure Fetal cardiac dysrhythmias Street drugs (cocaine, methamphetamines)	Late fetal hypoxia/hypoxemia Beta-adrenergic blocking drugs (propranolol; anesthetics for epidural, spinal, caudal, and pudendal blocks) Maternal hypotension Prolonged umbilical cord compression Fetal congenital heart block Maternal hypothermia Prolonged maternal hypoglycemia
CLINICAL SIGNIFICANCE	
Persistent tachycardia in absence of periodic changes does not appear serious in terms of neonatal outcome (especially true if tachycardia is associated with maternal fever); tachycardia is a nonreassuring sign when associated with late decelerations, severe variable decelerations, or absence of variability.	Bradycardia with moderate variability and absence of periodic changes is not a sign of fetal compromise if FHR remains greater than 80 beats/min; bradycardia caused by hypoxia is a nonreassuring sign when associated with loss of variability and late decelerations.
NURSING INTERVENTIONS	
Dependent on cause; reduce maternal fever with antipyretics as ordered and cooling measures; oxygen at 8 to 10 L/min per face mask may be of some value; carry out health care provider's orders based on alleviating cause.	Dependent on cause; intervention not warranted in fetus with heart block diagnosed by ECG; oxygen at 8 to 10 L/min per face mask may be of some value; carry out health care provider's orders based on alleviating cause. Scalp stimulation may be performed to determine whether the fetus has the ability to compensate physiologically for stress (FHR will accelerate).

ECG, electrocardiogram; *FHR*, fetal heart rate.

to the fetal buttocks results in accelerations, whereas pressure applied to the head results in decelerations. Accelerations may occur, however, during the second stage of labor in cephalic presentations. Episodic accelerations (Fig. 17-6, *B*) of the FHR occur during fetal movement and are indications of fetal well-being.

Decelerations

A deceleration (caused by dominance of parasympathetic response) may be benign or nonreassuring. Three types of decelerations are encountered during labor: *early*, *late*, and *variable*. FHR decelerations are described by their visual relation to the onset and end of a contraction and by their shape.

Early Decelerations

Early deceleration of the FHR is a visually apparent gradual decrease and return to baseline FHR in response to fetal head compression. It is a normal and benign finding (Fig. 17-7, *A*) (NICHD, 1997). The deceleration generally starts before the peak of the UC and returns to the baseline at the same time as the UC returns to its baseline. Early decelerations may also occur during UCs, during vaginal examinations, as a result of fundal pressure, and during placement of the internal mode of fetal monitoring. When present, they usually occur during the first stage of labor when the cervix is dilated 4 to 7 cm. Early decelerations sometimes are seen during the second stage when the woman is pushing.

Because early decelerations are considered to be benign, interventions are not necessary. The value of identifying early decelerations is so that they can be distinguished from late or variable decelerations, which can be nonreassuring and for which interventions are appropriate. The different characteristics of accelerations of the FHR and early decelerations are contrasted in Table 17-4.

Late Decelerations

Uteroplacental insufficiency causes late decelerations. Late deceleration of the FHR is a visually apparent gradual decrease in and return to baseline FHR associated with UCs (NICHD, 1997). The deceleration begins after the contraction has started, and the lowest point of the deceleration occurs after the peak of the contraction. The deceleration usually does not return to baseline until after the contraction is over (Fig. 17-7, *B*).

Persistent and repetitive late decelerations usually indicate the presence of fetal hypoxemia stemming from insufficient placental perfusion. They can be associated with fetal hypoxemia progressing to hypoxia and acidemia progressing to acidosis. They should be considered an ominous sign

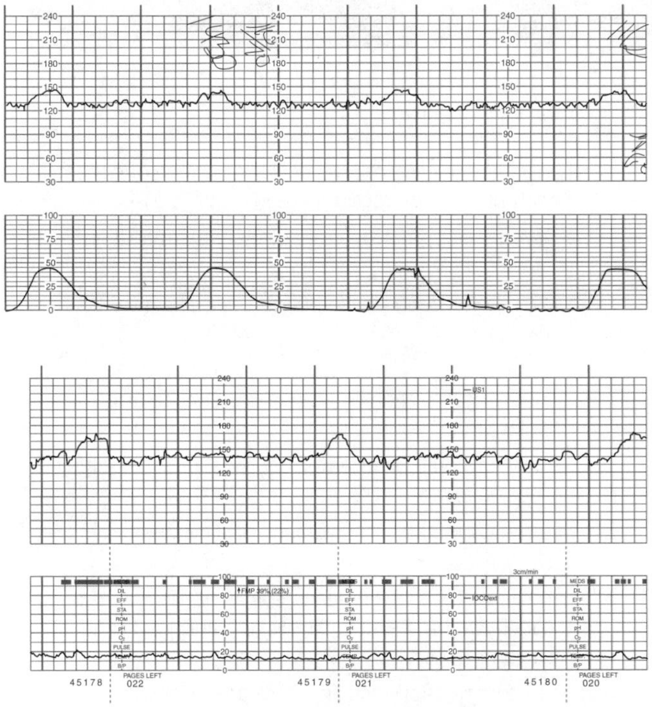

A

B

Fig. 17-6 **A,** Acceleration of fetal heart rate (FHR) with uterine contractions. **B,** Spontaneous (episodic) acceleration of FHR movement. (From Tucker SM: *Pocket guide to fetal monitoring and assessment,* ed 5, St Louis, 2004, Mosby.)

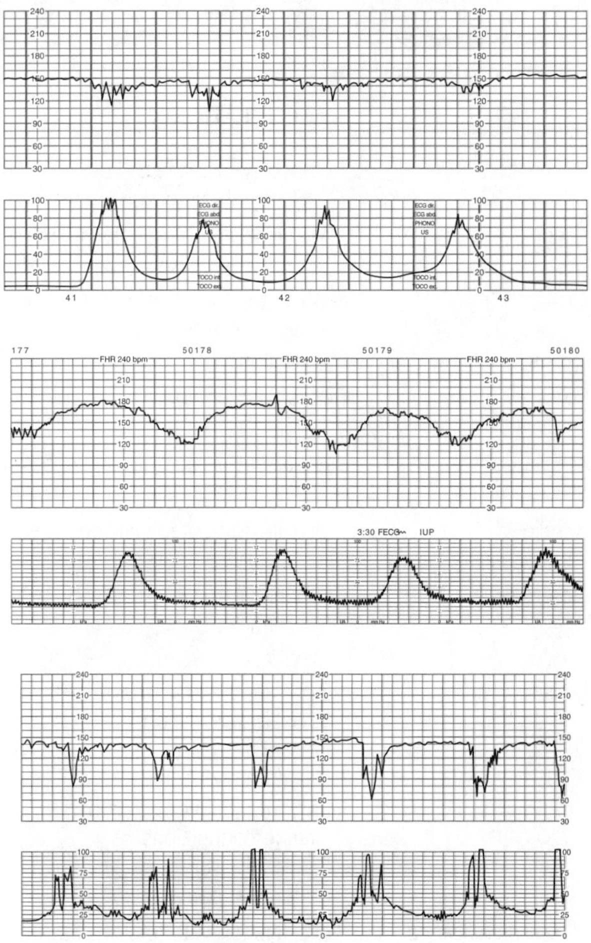

A

B

C

Fig. 17-7 Deceleration patterns. **A,** Early decelerations caused by head compression. **B,** Late decelerations caused by uteroplacental insufficiency. **C,** Variable decelerations caused by cord compression. (From Tucker SM: *Pocket guide to fetal monitoring and assessment,* ed 5, St Louis, 2004, Mosby.)

when they are uncorrectable, especially if they are associated with decreased variability and tachycardia. Late decelerations caused by the maternal supine hypotension syndrome are usually correctable when the woman turns on her side to displace the weight of the gravid uterus off the vena cava. Such lateral positioning allows better return of maternal blood flow to the heart, which in turn increases cardiac output and blood pressure.

Late decelerations caused by uteroplacental insufficiency can result from uterine hyperstimulation with oxytocin, gestational hypertension, postdate or postterm pregnancy, amnionitis, small-for-gestational-age (SGA) fetus, maternal diabetes, placenta previa, abruptio placentae, conduction anesthetics (producing maternal hypotension), maternal cardiac disease, and maternal anemia. The clinical significance of late decelerations and nursing interventions are described in Table 17-5.

Variable Decelerations

Variable deceleration is defined as a visual abrupt decrease in FHR below the baseline. The decrease is 15 beats/min or more, lasts at least 15 seconds, and returns to baseline in less than 2 minutes from the time of onset (NICHD, 1997). Variable decelerations occur any time during the uterine contracting phase and are caused by compression of the umbilical cord. Table 17-5 contrasts late deceleration with variable deceleration.

The pattern of variable decelerations differs from those of early and late decelerations, which closely approximate the shape of the corresponding uterine contraction. Instead, variable decelerations often have a U or V shape, characterized by a rapid descent and ascent to and from the nadir (or depth) of the deceleration (Fig. 17-7, *C*). Some variable decelerations are preceded and followed by brief accelerations of the FHR, known as "shouldering," which is an appropriate compensatory response to compression of the umbilical cord.

Variable decelerations may be related to partial, brief compression of the cord. If encountered in the first stage of labor, they usually can be resolved by changing the mother's position, such as from one side to the other. Oxygen administration by face mask to the mother is sometimes helpful. Variable decelerations are most commonly found during the second stage of labor as a result of umbilical cord compression during fetal descent (Freeman, Garite, & Nageotte, 2003). If repetitive variable decelerations occur during the second stage, it is important to discourage the woman from pushing with every contraction so that the fetus has time to recover. Variable decelerations are associated with neonatal depression only when cord compression is severe or prolonged (i.e., tight nuchal cord, short cord, knot in cord, prolapsed cord). Further descriptions of the types of variable decelerations, their clinical significance, and nursing interventions are given in Table 17-5.

Table 17-4

Accelerations and Early Decelerations

	ACCELERATION	EARLY DECELERATION
Description	Transitory increase of fetal heart rate (FHR) above baseline (see Fig. 17-6)	Transitory decrease of FHR below baseline concurrent with uterine contractions (see Fig. 17-7, *A*)
Shape	May resemble shape of uterine contraction or be spikelike	Uniform shape; mirror image of uterine contraction
Onset	Onset to peak (30 sec; often precedes or occurs simultaneous with uterine contraction)	Early in contraction phase before peak of contraction
Recovery	Less than 2 min from onset	By end of contraction as uterine pressure returns to its resting tone
Amplitude	Usually 15 beats/min above baseline	Usually proportional to amplitude of contraction; rarely decelerates to <100 beats/min
Baseline	Usually associated with average baseline variability	Usually associated with average baseline variability
Occurrence	Variable; may be repetitive with each contraction	Repetitious (occurs with each contraction); usually occurs between 4 and 7 cm dilation and in second stage of labor
Cause	Spontaneous fetal movement Vaginal examination Electrode application Breech presentation Occiput posterior position Uterine contractions Fundal pressure Abdominal palpation	Head compression resulting from the following: Uterine contractions Vaginal examination Fundal pressure Placement of internal mode of monitoring
Clinical significance	Acceleration with fetal movement signifies fetal well-being representing fetal alertness or arousal states	Reassuring pattern not associated with fetal hypoxemia, acidemia, or low Apgar scores
Nursing intervention	None required	None required

Prolonged Decelerations

A prolonged deceleration is a visually apparent decrease in FHR below the baseline 15 beats/min or more and lasting more than 2 minutes but less than 10 minutes. A deceleration lasting more than 10 minutes is considered a baseline change (NICHD, 1997). Generally the benign causes are pelvic examination, application of a spiral electrode, rapid fetal descent, and sustained maternal Valsalva maneuver. Other, less benign causes are progressive severe variable decelerations, sudden umbilical cord prolapse, hypotension produced by spinal or epidural analgesia or anesthesia, paracervical anesthesia, tetanic contraction, and maternal hypoxia, which may occur during a seizure. When the deceleration lasts longer than 1 to 2 minutes, a loss of variability with rebound tachycardia usually occurs. Occasionally a period of late decelerations follows. Prolonged decelerations usually are isolated events that end spontaneously. However, when a prolonged deceleration is seen late in the course of severe variable decelerations or during a prolonged series of late decelerations, the prolonged deceleration may occur just before fetal death.

NURSE ALERT Nurses should notify the physician or nurse-midwife immediately and initiate appropriate treatment of nonreassuring patterns when they see a prolonged deceleration. ■

Care Management

The care given to women being monitored by EFM or auscultation is the same as that given to the woman having a low risk labor. Care of the woman being monitored by internal methods may vary. FHR pattern recognition and intervention may require a nurse to have additional education and clinical experience.

Assessment

The assessment of the woman includes the maternal temperature, pulse, respiratory rate, blood pressure, position, comfort, voiding pattern, status of membranes, uterine contraction pattern, cervical effacement and dilation, and emotional status. The fetal assessment includes the fetal presentation, fetal position, FHR, and identification of both reassuring and nonreassuring FHR patterns. A checklist may be used by the nurse to

Table 17-5

Late Decelerations and Variable Decelerations

	LATE DECELERATION	VARIABLE DECELERATION
Description	Transitory gradual decrease in fetal heart rate (FHR) below baseline rate in contracting phase (see Fig. 17-7, *B*)	Abrupt decrease in FHR that is variable in duration, intensity, and timing related to onset of contractions (see Fig. 17-7, *C*)
Shape	Uniform; mirror images of uterine contraction; may be deep or shallow	Variable; characterized by sudden decrease in FHR in V, U, or W shape
Onset	Late in contraction phase; after peak of contraction; nadir of deceleration occurs after peak of contraction	Onset of deceleration to the beginning of nadir, <30 sec; decrease in FHR baseline is ≥15 beats/min, lasting ≥15 sec; variable times in contracting phase; often preceded by transitory acceleration
Recovery	Well after end of contraction	Return to baseline is rapid and <2 min from onset, sometimes with transitory acceleration or acceleration immediately before and after deceleration (shouldering or "overshoot"); slow return to baseline with severe variable decelerations
Deceleration	Usually proportional to amplitude of contraction; rarely decelerates to <100 beats/min; however, shallow late decelerations have the same significance	*Mild:* decelerates to any level, <30 sec with abrupt return to baseline *Moderate:* decelerates to ≥80 beats/min, any duration, with abrupt return to baseline *Severe:* decelerates to <60 beats/min for >60 sec, with slow return to baseline
Baseline	Often associated with loss of variability and increasing baseline rate	Mild variables usually associated with average baseline variability; moderate and severe variables often associated with decreasing variability and increasing baseline rate
Occurrence	Occurs with each contraction; may be observed at any time during labor	Variable; commonly observed late in labor with fetal descent and pushing
Cause	Uteroplacental insufficiency caused by the following: Uterine hyperactivity or hypertonicity Maternal supine hypotension Epidural or spinal anesthesia Placenta previa Abruptio placentae Hypertensive disorders Postmaturity Intrauterine growth restriction Diabetes mellitus Intraamniotic infection	Umbilical cord compression caused by the following: Maternal position with cord between fetus and maternal pelvis Cord around fetal neck, arm, leg, or other body part Short cord Knot in cord Prolapsed cord
Clinical significance	Nonreassuring pattern associated with fetal hypoxemia, acidemia, and low Apgar scores; considered ominous if persistent and uncorrected, especially when associated with fetal tachycardia and loss of variability	Variable decelerations occur in 50% of all labors and usually are transient and correctable Reassuring variable decelerations last 45 sec; abruptly return to the FHR baseline; normal baseline rate continues; variability does not decrease Nonreassuring variable decelerations decrease to ≤70 beats/min for ≥60 sec; have a prolonged return to baseline; baseline rate increases; variability is absent Nonreassuring variable decelerations are associated with fetal acidemia, hypoxemia, and low Apgar scores; severe variable decelerations with average baseline variability just before birth are usually well tolerated
Nursing interventions	Change maternal position (lateral) Correct maternal hypotension by elevating legs Increase rate of maintenance IV Discontinue oxytocin if infusing Administer oxygen at 8 to 10 L/min with tight face mask Fetal scalp or acoustic stimulation Assist with fetal oxygen saturation monitoring if ordered Assist with birth (cesarean or vaginal assisted) if pattern cannot be corrected	Change maternal position (side to side); if decelerations are severe, proceed with following measures: Discontinue oxytocin if infusing Administer oxygen at 8 to 10 L/min with tight face mask Assist with vaginal or speculum examination If cord is prolapsed, examiner will elevate fetal presenting part with cord between gloved fingers until cesarean birth is accomplished Assist with amnioinfusion if ordered Assist with fetal oxygen saturation monitoring if ordered Assist with birth (vaginal assisted or cesarean) if pattern cannot be corrected

assess the FHR (Box 17-1). All of the assessment information must be documented in the woman's medical record.

Evaluation of the EFM equipment also must be done to ensure that the equipment is working properly and to allow an accurate assessment of the woman and fetus. A checklist for fetal monitoring equipment can be used to evaluate the equipment functions (Box 17-2).

Nursing Diagnoses

Nursing diagnoses for the woman who is being monitored electronically for fetal status are based on assessment findings. Possible diagnoses include the following:

- *Decreased maternal cardiac output related to*
  —supine hypotension secondary to maternal position
- *Anxiety related to*
  —lack of knowledge concerning fetal monitoring during labor
  —restriction of mobility or movement during EFM
- *Impaired fetal gas exchange related to*
  —umbilical cord compression
  —placental insufficiency
- *Acute pain related to*
  —use of belts to position transducers
  —maternal position
  —vaginal examinations associated with application of maternal or fetal internal monitoring equipment or fetal blood sampling
- *Risk for fetal injury related to*
  —unrecognized hypoxemia, hypoxia, or anoxia
  —infection secondary to internal monitoring or scalp blood sampling

BOX 17-1

Checklist for Fetal Heart Rate/Uterine Activity Assessment

Patient's name ________________

Date/time ________________

1. What is the baseline fetal heart rate (FHR)?
   ______ Beats/min
   Check one of the following as observed on the monitor strip:
   ______ Average baseline FHR (110 to 160 beats/min)
   ______ Tachycardia (>160 beats/min)
   ______ Bradycardia (<110 beats/min)
2. What is the baseline variability?
   ______ Absence of variability
   ______ Minimal variability (barely detectable up to 5 beats/min)
   ______ Moderate variability (6 to 25 beats/min)
   ______ Marked variability (>25 beats/min)
3. Are there any periodic or episodic changes in FHR?
   ______ Accelerations with fetal movement
   ______ Repetitive accelerations with each contraction
   ______ Early decelerations (head compression)
   ______ Late decelerations (uteroplacental insufficiency)
   ______ Variable decelerations (cord compression)
   ______ Reassuring (<30 to 45 seconds, abrupt return to baseline, normal baseline, moderate variability)
   ______ Nonreassuring (>60 seconds, slow return to baseline, increasing baseline rate, absence of variability)
   ______ Prolonged deceleration (>2 minutes up to 10 minutes)
4. What is the uterine activity/contraction pattern?
   ______ Frequency (beginning to beginning)
   ______ Duration (beginning to end)
   Abdominal palpation method
   ______ Strength (mild, moderate, strong)
   ______ Resting time (from end of one contraction to beginning of next one)
   Internal monitoring (IUPC)
   ______ Intensity (mm Hg pressure)
   ______ Resting tone (mm Hg pressure)

Comments: ________________

____

Panel number: ________________

What can be or should have been done?

____

____

____

Modified from Tucker SM: *Pocket guide to fetal monitoring and assessment*, ed 5, St Louis, 2004, Mosby.

BOX 17-2

Checklist for Fetal Monitoring Equipment

Preparation of Monitor
1. Is the paper inserted correctly?
2. Are transducer cables plugged into the appropriate outlet of the monitor?
3. Is paper speed set for 3 cm/min?

Ultrasound Transducer
1. Has ultrasound transmission gel been applied to the transducer?
2. Was the FHR tested and noted on the monitor paper?
3. Does a signal light flash or an audible beep occur with each heartbeat?
4. Is the belt secure and snug but comfortable for the laboring woman?

Tocotransducer
1. Is the tocotransducer firmly positioned at the site of the least maternal tissue?
2. Has it been applied without gel or paste?
3. Was the uterine activity (UA) reference knob depressed between contractions?
4. Is the belt secure and snug?

Spiral Electrode
1. Are the wires inserted correctly into the leg plate?
2. Is the spiral electrode attached to the presenting part of the fetus?
3. Is the pre-gelled electrode pad secured to the woman's leg or abdomen?

Intrauterine Pressure Catheter (IUPC)
1. Is the length line on the catheter visible at the introitus?
2. Is it noted on the monitor paper that a UA test or calibration was done?
3. Has the monitor been set to zero according to manufacturer's directions?
4. Is the IUPC properly secured to the woman's thigh?
5. Is baseline resting tone of uterus documented?

Modified from Tucker SM: *Pocket guide to fetal monitoring and assessment*, ed 5, St. Louis, 2004, Mosby.

Expected Outcomes

The primary goals of nursing care are to have healthy fetal and maternal outcomes. The interventions implemented to achieve these outcomes are determined by knowledge of fetal status and by standards for care. The planning process includes accommodating the wishes of the woman and family, answering questions, and explaining nursing interventions.

Expected outcomes for the pregnant woman and family and the fetus include the following:

- The pregnant woman and family will verbalize their understanding of the need for monitoring.
- The pregnant woman and the family will recognize and avoid situations that compromise maternal and fetal circulation.
- The fetus will not have any hypoxemic, hypoxic, or anoxic episodes.
- Should fetal compromise occur, it will be identified promptly, and appropriate nursing interventions such as intrauterine resuscitation will be initiated and the physician or nurse-midwife notified.

Plan of Care and Implementation

It is the responsibility of the nurse providing care to women in labor to assess FHR patterns, implement independent nursing interventions, document observations and actions according to the established standard of care, and report nonreassuring patterns to the primary care provider (e.g., physician, certified nurse-midwife). See Box 17-3 for a sample protocol for FHR monitoring by IA and EFM during labor.

Although the use of EFM can be reassuring to many parents, it can be a source of anxiety to some. Therefore the nurse must be particularly sensitive to and respond appropriately to the emotional, informational, and comfort needs of the woman in labor and those of her family (Fig. 17-8 and Box 17-4).

Electronic Fetal Monitoring Pattern Recognition

Nurses must evaluate many factors to determine whether an FHR pattern is reassuring or nonreassuring. A complete description of FHR tracings includes both qualitative and quantitative descriptions of baseline rate and variability, presence of accelerations, periodic or episodic decelerations, and changes in the FHR pattern over time (NICHD, 1997). Nurses evaluate these factors based on other obstetric complications, progress in labor, and analgesia or anesthesia. They also must consider the estimated time interval until birth. Interventions are therefore based on clinical judgment of a complex, integrated process (Haggerty & Nuttall, 2000).

LEGAL TIP **Fetal Monitoring Standards** Nurses who care for women during childbirth are legally responsible for correctly interpreting FHR patterns, initiating appropriate nursing interventions based on those patterns, and documenting the outcomes of those interventions. Perinatal nurses are responsible for the timely notification of the physician or nurse-midwife in the event of nonreassuring FHR patterns. Perinatal nurses also are responsible for initiating the institutional chain of command should differences in opinion arise among health care providers concerning the interpretation of the FHR pattern and the intervention required. ■

Nursing Management of Nonreassuring Patterns

The term *intrauterine resuscitation* is sometimes used to refer to those interventions initiated when a nonreassuring FHR pattern is noted. These interventions are directed primarily toward improving uterine and intervillous space blood flow and secondarily toward increasing maternal oxygenation and cardiac output (Parilla, 2002). The following preventive interventions are described in this chapter: avoiding the supine position and encouraging maternal position changes; encouraging spontaneous, short bursts of pushing in response to involuntary bearing-down urges; and encouraging pushing with mouth open and glottis open with vocalizing. Previously it was thought that the left lateral maternal position preferentially promoted maternal cardiac output, thereby enhancing blood flow to the fetus. However, it is now known that either the right or left lateral maternal position effectively enhances uteroplacental blood flow. The key issue is to avoid positioning the laboring woman on her back to reduce the risk of supine hypotension leading to decreased placental perfusion.

Compression of the umbilical cord vessels results in variable decelerations. Amnioinfusion is an intervention that can help relieve such pressure on a nonprolapsed umbilical cord. If maternal hypotension caused by acute hemorrhage (hypovolemia) occurs, the rapid infusion of blood volume expanders may be ordered. Until the infusion is established, the nurse can elevate the woman's legs. Blood pooled in the legs, especially that occurring as the result of sympathetic blockade (e.g., epidural anesthesia), will then drain quickly into the central venous circulation, and this will augment the effective intravascular volume (Parilla, 2002).

Oxytocin always should be infused as a piggyback connection near the indwelling needle. If FHR patterns change for any reason, oxytocin stimulation of the uterine muscle must be discontinued. This consists of turning off the intravenous (IV) line from the piggyback (containing oxytocin) and opening the primary infusion line.

Nurses must assign priorities to interventions to maximize the efficacy of the intrauterine resuscitation. The first priority is to open the maternal and fetal vascular systems; the second priority is to increase blood volume; and the third priority is to optimize oxygenation of the circulating blood volume. For example, to relieve an acute FHR deceleration, the nurse can do the following:

- Assist the woman to the side-lying position if she is not already in a lateral position.
- Increase the maternal blood volume by increasing the rate of the primary IV infusion or by raising the woman's legs.
- Provide oxygen by face mask.

Some interventions are specific to the FHR pattern. Nursing interventions appropriate for the management of tachycardia and bradycardia are given in Table 17-2, and those appropriate for the management of increased or decreased variability are given in Table 17-3. No specific nursing interventions are required for the management of FHR acceleration or early deceleration (see Table 17-4). However, late and some types of variable FHR decelerations require aggressive intervention (see Table 17-5). The primary health care provider decides whether medical intervention should be in-

BOX 17-3

Protocol for Fetal Heart Rate Monitoring

Maternal/Fetal Assessments

Obtain a 20-minute strip of EFM for all patients admitted to labor unit

Low Risk Patient

Auscultate or assess tracing every 30 minutes in active phase of first stage of labor

Auscultate or assess tracing every 15 minutes in second stage

High Risk Patient

Auscultate or assess tracing every 15 minutes in active phase and every 5 minutes in second stage

Auscultation: All Patients

Count baseline FHR between contractions

Assess FHR during the contraction and for 30 seconds after the contraction

Note increases or decreases of FHR

Assess FHR before ambulation

Interpret FHR data, nursing interventions, and patient responses

Notify primary health care provider

EFM: All Patients

Assess and interpret baseline FHR, variability of FHR, and presence or absence of decelerations and accelerations

Assessments for All Patients

Assess uterine activity for frequency and duration, the intensity of contractions, and uterine resting tone

Assess FHR immediately after rupture of membranes, vaginal examinations, and any invasive procedure

Maternal Care

Assist woman to a comfortable position other than supine

Change maternal position at least every 2 hours

External Monitoring

Ultrasound Transducer

Function

Monitors FHR with high-frequency sound waves

Nursing Care

Tap transducer before use to ensure sound transmission

Apply ultrasound transmission gel to transducer; clean abdomen and transducer, and reapply gel every 2 hours and as required

Massage reddened skin areas gently and reposition belt or adhesive device every 2 hours and as required

Auscultate FHR with stethoscope or fetoscope if in doubt as to validity of tracing

Position and reposition transducer as required to ensure receipt of clear, interpretable FHR data

Tocotransducer

Function

Monitors uterine activity via a pressure-sensing device placed on the maternal abdomen

Nursing Care

Position and reposition every 2 hours and as required on the fundus, where there is the least maternal tissue

Keep abdominal strap snug but comfortable for the laboring woman

Adjust knob between contractions to print between 10 and 20 mm Hg on the monitor strip paper

Palpate fundus every 30 to 60 minutes to assess strength of contraction; only frequency and duration of contractions can be assessed with tocotransducer

Do not determine woman's need for analgesia based on uterine activity displayed on monitor strip

Gently massage reddened areas under transducer and belt every hour and as required

Internal Monitoring

Spiral Electrode

Function

Obtains fetal electrocardiogram (ECG) from presenting part and converts it into FHR

Nursing Care

Ensure that the connector to the scalp electrode is appropriately attached to leg plate

*If computer charting system is used, follow institutional policies and system guidelines/protocols.

stituted, what intervention is indicated, or whether immediate vaginal or cesarean birth should be performed.

Additional Methods of Assessment and Intervention

Other methods of assessment and intervention are designed to be used in conjunction with EFM in an effort to identify and intervene in the presence of a nonreassuring FHR. These methods include FHR response to stimulation, fetal oxygen saturation monitoring, fetal blood sampling, amnioinfusion, and tocolysis. Umbilical cord acid-base determination is an assessment technique that is a useful adjunct to the Apgar score in assessing the immediate condition of the newborn.

Fetal Heart Rate Response to Stimulation

Stimulation of the fetus is done to elicit an acceleration of the FHR of 15 beats/min for at least 15 seconds (Tucker, 2004). The two methods of fetal stimulation currently in practice are scalp stimulation (using digital pressure during a vaginal examination) and vibroacoustic stimulation (using an artificial larynx or fetal acoustic stimulation device over the fetal head for 1 to 2 seconds). An FHR acceleration usually indicates fetal well-being. If the fetus does not have an acceleration, however, it does not necessarily indicate fetal compromise, but further evaluation of fetal well-being is needed.

Fetal Oxygen Saturation Monitoring

Continuous monitoring of fetal oxygen saturation ($FSpO_2$) or fetal pulse oximetry (FPO) is a method of fetal assessment that was approved for clinical use by the Food and Drug Administration in May 2000 (Porter, 2000). FPO works in a way similar to the pulse oximetry used in children and adults. A specially designed sensor is inserted next to the fetal cheek or temple area to assess oxygen saturation. The sensor is then connected to a monitor, and the data are displayed on the uterine activity panel of the fetal monitor tracing. The normal range of oxygen saturation in the adult is 95% to 100%. The normal range for the healthy fetus is 30% to 70% (Simpson & Porter, 2001) with the cutoff value for the critical threshold of $FSpO_2$ at 30% (Garite et al, 2000).

BOX 17-3

Protocol for Fetal Heart Rate Monitoring—cont'd

Nursing Care—cont'd

Reapply electrode paste to leg plate if needed

Observe FHR tracing on monitor strip for variability

Turn electrode counterclockwise to remove; never pull straight out from presenting part

Administer perineal care after the woman voids during labor and as required

Intrauterine Catheter

Function

Catheter (solid or fluid filled) that monitors intraamniotic pressure internally

Nursing Care

Ensure that the length line on catheter is visible at introitus

For closed-system catheters, set baseline rate between uterine contractions when uterus is relaxed

Flush open-system catheter with sterile water before insertion and as required

For open-system catheters, turn stopcock off to woman, then with pressure valve of strain gauge released, flush strain gauge, remove syringe, and set stylus to 0 line of chart paper; test further according to manufacturer's instructions every 3 to 4 hours and as required

Check proper functioning by tapping catheter, asking woman to cough, or applying fundal pressure; observe appropriate inflection on strip chart

Keep catheter or cable secured to woman's leg to prevent dislodgment

Reportable Conditions

Presence of nonreassuring patterns:

Severe variable decelerations

Late decelerations

Absence of variability

Prolonged deceleration

Severe bradycardia

Worsening of any pattern

Presence of identifiable fetal dysrhythmias

Difficulty in obtaining adequate FHR tracing or inadequate audible FHR

Emergency Measures

Implement the following measures immediately in the event of a nonreassuring pattern:

Reposition woman in lateral position to increase uteroplacental perfusion or relieve cord compression

Administer oxygen at 8 to 10 L/min or per hospital protocol by face mask

Discontinue oxytocin if infusing

Correct maternal hypovolemia by increasing IV rate per protocol or as ordered

Assess for bleeding or other cause of pattern change, such as maternal hypotension

Notify primary health care provider

Assist with other methods of assessment such as fetal oxygen saturation monitoring or interventions such as amnioinfusion

Anticipate emergency preparation for surgical intervention if nonreassuring pattern continues despite interventions

Documentation*

Patient Record: Auscultation

FHR baseline, rate and rhythm, increases or decreases

Patient Record: EFM

Method of monitoring, change in method, and adjustments to equipment

FHR range, variability, presence of decelerations or accelerations

Uterine activity as determined by palpation or by external or internal monitoring

Interpretation of FHR data, nursing interventions, and patient responses

Notification of primary health care provider

Monitor Strip

Patient identification data

Assessments, procedures, and interventions (medications, etc.)

Notification of primary health care provider

Significant occurrences (sterile vaginal examination, rupture of membranes, etc.)

Adjustments of the monitor equipment

FPO may be used if certain criteria are met, including a single fetus at least 36 weeks of gestational age in a vertex presentation with a nonreassuring FHR pattern. The membranes should be ruptured, the cervix dilated at least 2 cm, and the fetal station at least a −2 or less (Garite et al, 2000). The value of $FSpO_2$ monitoring is that in the event of nonreassuring FHR patterns, it can support the decision about whether labor should continue or whether to intervene with an expeditious assisted vaginal or cesarean birth of the fetus (Simpson, 2003).

When the use of FPO becomes more widely practiced, the labor nurse's role will expand to include this type of monitoring in practice (Porter, 2000). Simpson and Porter (2001) suggested that nurses will be involved in identifying potential candidates for monitoring, inserting the sensor (according to state nurse practice acts and institutional policies), interpreting data, documenting findings, and communicating with the primary health care provider.

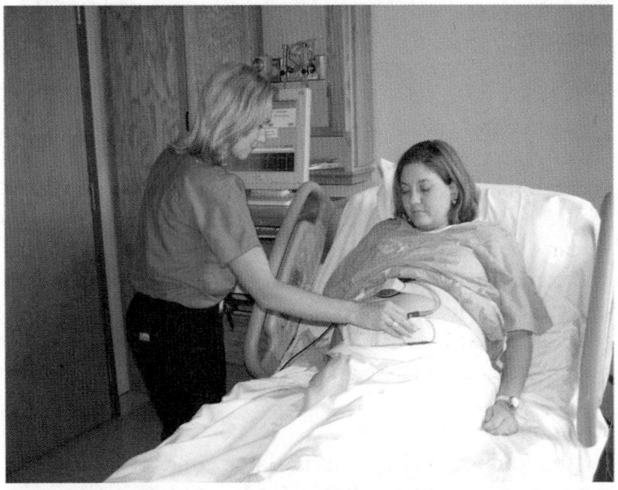

Fig. 17-8 Nurse explains electronic fetal monitoring as ultrasound transducer monitors the fetal heart rate. (Courtesy Julie Perry Nelson, Gilbert, AZ.)

BOX 17-4

Patient/Family Teaching When Electronic Fetal Monitor Is Used

The following guidelines relate to patient teaching and the functioning of the monitor:

Explain the purpose of monitoring.
Explain each procedure.
Provide rationale for maternal position other than supine.
Explain that fetal status can be continuously assessed by electronic fetal monitoring (EFM), even during contractions.
Explain that the lower tracing on the monitor strip paper shows uterine activity; the upper tracing shows the fetal heart rate (FHR).
Reassure woman and partner that prepared childbirth techniques can be implemented without difficulty.
Explain that, during external monitoring, effleurage can be performed on sides of abdomen or upper portion of thighs.
Explain that breathing patterns based on the time and intensity of contractions can be enhanced by the observation of uterine activity on the monitor strip paper, which shows the onset of contractions.
Note peak of contraction; knowing that contraction will not get stronger and is half over is usually helpful.
Note diminishing intensity.
Coordinate with appropriate breathing and relaxation techniques.
Reassure woman and partner that the use of internal monitoring does not restrict movement, although she is confined to bed.*
Explain that use of external monitoring usually requires the woman's cooperation during positioning and movement.
Reassure woman and partner that use of monitoring does not imply fetal jeopardy.
Reassure her that the equipment is removed periodically to permit the applicator sites to be washed and other care to be given.

*Portable telemetry monitors allow the FHR and uterine contraction patterns to be observed on centrally located display stations. These portable units permit ambulation during electronic monitoring.

Fetal Scalp Blood Sampling

Sampling of the fetal scalp blood was designed to assess the fetal pH, Po_2, and Pco_2. The procedure is performed by obtaining a sample of fetal scalp blood through the dilated cervix after the membranes have ruptured. The scalp is swabbed with a disinfecting solution before making the puncture, and the sample is then collected. However, the blood gas values vary so rapidly with transient circulatory changes that fetal blood sampling is seldom performed in the United States (Gilstrap, 2004). When used, it is usually in tertiary centers with the capability for repetitive sampling and rapid report of results. The circulatory changes that cause the variability and thus undermine the utility of this procedure are maternal acidosis or alkalosis, caput succedaneum, the stage of labor, and the time relation of scalp sampling to UCs.

Amnioinfusion

Amnioinfusion is used during labor either to supplement the amount of amniotic fluid to reduce the severity of variable decelerations caused by cord compression or to dilute meconium-stained amniotic fluid with saline or lactated Ringer's solution (Hofmeyr, 2002; Parer & Nageotte, 2004). The procedure to supplement amniotic fluid is indicated for patients with oligohydramnios, secondary to uteroplacental insufficiency, premature rupture of membranes, or postmaturity, who are at risk for variable decelerations because of umbilical cord compression.

Oligohydramnios is an abnormally small amount of amniotic fluid or the absence of amniotic fluid. Without the buffer of amniotic fluid, the umbilical cord can easily become compressed during contractions or fetal movement, diminishing the flow of blood between the fetus and placenta, as evidenced by variable decelerations. Amnioinfusion replaces the "cushion" for the cord and relieves both the frequency and intensity of variable decelerations.

Amnioinfusion also is indicated in the presence of moderate to thick meconium to dilute and flush out the meconium with the intent of avoiding meconium-aspiration syndrome in the neonate (Hofmeyr, 2002).

Risks of amnioinfusion are overdistention of the uterine cavity and increased uterine tone. Techniques of amnioinfusion treatment vary, but usually fluid is administered through an IUPC. The woman's membranes must be ruptured for the IUPC placement. The fluid is administered by attaching plastic (IV) tubing to a liter of normal saline or lactated Ringer's solution through a port in the IUPC. Double-lumen IUPCs are preferred because the intrauterine pressure can be monitored without stopping the procedure. The fluid is usually warmed with a blood warmer before administration for the preterm or SGA fetus (Simpson & Creehan, 2001). The flow rate can be by bolus or continuous flow or by a combination of these two methods.

Intensity and frequency of UCs should be continually assessed during the procedure. The recorded uterine resting tone during amnioinfusion will appear higher than normal because of resistance to outflow and turbulence at the end of the catheter. The true resting tone can be checked by discontinuing the amnioinfusion when using a single-lumen IUPC (Tucker, 2004).

Tocolytic Therapy

Tocolysis (relaxation of the uterus) can be achieved through the administration of drugs that inhibit UCs. This therapy can be used as an adjunct to other interventions in the management of fetal stress when the fetus is exhibiting nonreassuring patterns associated with increased uterine activity. Tocolysis improves blood flow through the placenta by inhibiting UCs. Tocolysis may be considered by the primary health care provider and implemented when other interventions to reduce uterine activity, such as maternal position change and discontinuance of an oxytocin infusion, have no effect on diminishing the UCs. A tocolytic drug such as magnesium sulfate or terbutaline can be administered intravenously to decrease uterine activity (Tucker, 2004). If the FHR pattern improves, the woman may be allowed to continue labor; if there is no improvement, immediate surgical delivery may be needed.

Umbilical Cord Acid-Base Determination

In assessing the immediate condition of the newborn after birth, a sample of cord blood is a useful adjunct to the Apgar score. The procedure is generally done by withdrawing blood from the umbilical artery and having the blood tested for pH, Pco_2, and Po_2. Umbilical cord gas measure-

Evidence-Based Practice

ROUTINE DOPPLER ULTRASOUND

Background

Prenatal diagnosticians have used a noninvasive technique called Doppler ultrasound since 1977 to visualize the movement of blood in a vessel by detecting the change of frequency of reflected sound. Using Doppler ultrasound, the movement of blood in the umbilical artery and the uteroplacental circulation give information about the quality of perfusion to the fetus. This can screen women with high risk pregnancies for conditions leading to intrauterine growth restriction and gestational hypertension perfusion disorders. There is evidence that Doppler ultrasound is a better indicator of fetal well-being than biophysical profile or electronic fetal monitoring.

Use of screening tests in pregnancy should be preceded by questions about the proven clinical effectiveness of testing: sensitivity (ability to detect a problem), specificity (ability to rule out the problem for truly normal subjects), risks of the testing procedure, and what treatments are reasonably available for those with abnormal results. Testing can produce anxiety, inappropriate intervention, and iatrogenic (caused by the caregiver) morbidity and mortality. Questions have been raised in the past about the safety of repeated fetal ultrasound in general. Although it is of unquestionable value in high risk pregnancies, the routine use of Doppler ultrasound in low risk pregnancies deserves answers to these questions, and should be backed up by supportive evidence from randomized, controlled trials.

Objectives

The authors of the review sought to assess the safety and efficacy of Doppler ultrasound in low risk pregnancies. The intervention was the use of Doppler ultrasound on women with low risk pregnancies. Maternal outcomes included fetal monitoring, kick counts, biophysical profile, ultrasound, operative delivery, and psychologic effects. Perinatal outcomes included birth weight, gestational age at birth, preterm birth, respiratory status, Apgar, admission to special care nursery, morbidity, neural development at 2 years, and perinatal death.

Methods

Search Strategy

The authors searched the Cochrane database. Search keywords were not noted.

Five trials, comprising 14,338 women, were selected from France, the United Kingdom, and Australia, dated 1992 to 1997.

Statistical Analyses

Statistical analyses included pooling similar data for meta-analysis and analyzing differences between the Doppler group and controls for each outcome studied. The reviewers accepted results outside the 95% confidence interval as significant.

Findings

No differences between the two groups were found in antenatal admissions or obstetric interventions. One trial found increased perinatal mortality rate in the Doppler group, but when added to the pooled data, the overall difference was not significant. One trial found that the Doppler group was more likely to have repeat tests. No trials evaluated the ability of second trimester Doppler ultrasound to predict preeclampsia, intrauterine growth restriction, or adverse pregnancy outcome. No data were found on acute neonatal problems, long-term neurologic development, or maternal psychologic factors. One trial found that there was an increase in birth weight below the 10th percentile in women who had intensive repeated fetal ultrasound and Doppler ultrasound, when compared with women who only had selected Doppler tests.

Limitations

Interventions varied between trials: some evaluated umbilical artery Doppler alone; others evaluated both umbilical artery and uteroplacental blood flow. One trial compared repeated ultrasound plus Doppler with a group that only had Doppler ultrasounds if they were indicated. Some studies did not allow controls to receive the intervention, and some did allow it. Parameters of measurement differed for the Doppler ultrasound. One trial had differing protocols for high risk and low risk women. The homogeneity of the protocols limits generalizability. Many women dropped out of some studies. No trials included management protocols for abnormal results.

Conclusions

There is no supporting evidence that routine use of Doppler ultrasound in low risk pregnancy is beneficial to mother or baby. The study showing the intrauterine growth restriction (birth weight less than 10th percentile) suggests that repeated ultrasounds may be harmful to the fetus. Doppler ultrasounds remain a valuable tool where indicated for high risk pregnancies.

Implications for Practice

Nurses can question the practice of routine Doppler ultrasound in low risk pregnancy. They can educate patients about the risks and benefits of these routines. As patients become more knowledgeable, they can discuss with their primary health care provider the indications for the test.

Implications for Further Research

Large trials are needed to determine Doppler ultrasound's ability to predict preeclampsia, intrauterine growth restriction, and other adverse outcomes in low risk pregnancies. Outcomes should include maternal psychologic effects, neonatal morbidity, and long-term neurologic development of the baby. Of particular interest is resolving the issue of the safety of ultrasounds.

Reference

Bricker L, Neilson J: Routine Doppler ultrasound in pregnancy (Cochrane Review), 2000. In *The Cochrane Library*, Issue 2, Chichester, UK, 2004, John Wiley & Sons.

ments reflect the acid-base status of the newborn at birth, a measurement not reflected in the Apgar score (Gilstrap, 2004). If acidosis is present (e.g., pH 7.10) the type of acidosis is determined (respiratory, metabolic, or mixed) by analyzing the blood gas values (Table 17-6).

Patient and Family Teaching

Part of the nurse's role includes acting as a partner with the woman to achieve a high-quality birthing experience. In addition to teaching and supporting the woman and her family with understanding of the laboring and birth process, breathing techniques, use of equipment, and pain management techniques, the nurse can assist with two factors that have an effect on fetal status: pushing and positioning. The nurse should provide information and support to the woman in regard to these two factors (Guidelines/Guías box).

Maternal Positioning

Maternal supine hypotensive syndrome is caused by the weight and pressure of the gravid uterus on the ascending vena cava when the woman is in a supine position. This

Table 17-6

Types of Acidosis

BLOOD GASES	RESPIRATORY	METABOLIC	MIXED
pH	↓ (<7.1)	↓ (<7.1)	↓ (<7.1)
Pco_2 (mm Hg)	↑ (>60)	Normal (<60)	↑ (>60)
HCO_3^- (mEq/L)	Normal (16-24)	↓	↓
Base deficit	Normal	↑	↑

Sources: Gilstrap L: Fetal acid-base balance. In Creasy RK, Resnik R, Iams JD (eds): *Maternal-fetal medicine: principles and practice,* ed 5, Philadelphia, 2004, WB Saunders; Pagana KD, Pagana TJ: *Mosby's diagnostic and laboratory test reference,* ed 6, St Louis, 2003, Mosby; Tucker SM: *Pocket guide to fetal monitoring and assessment,* ed 5, St Louis, 2004, Mosby.

ENGLISH SPANISH **Guidelines/Guías**

FETAL MONITORING

I am going to listen to the baby's heartbeat.
Voy a escuchar el latido del corazón del bebé.

I will place my fingers on the top of your uterus to feel your contractions.
Me pondré los dedos sobre su útero para palpar las contracciones.

This equipment records the baby's heartbeat. I will place the belt around your abdomen to monitor the baby's heart rate.
Este equipo graba el latido del corazón del bebé. Pondré el cinturón alrededor de su abdomen para observar el ritmo cardíaco del bebé.

This is a uterine contraction monitor. I will place it on your abdomen to monitor your uterine contractions.
Este es un monitor para las contracciones del útero. Lo pondré sobre su abdomen para observar las contracciones del útero.

Please turn on your side. The blood flows to your uterus better if you do not lie on your back.
Por favor, acuéstese sobre un costado. La sangre corre mejor al útero si no se acuesta de espalda.

If you need to go to the bathroom, we can remove the equipment for a short time.
Si tiene que ir al baño, le podemos quitar el monitor por un rato.

decreases venous return to the woman's heart and cardiac output and subsequently reduces her blood pressure. The low maternal blood pressure decreases intervillous space blood flow during UCs and results in fetal hypoxemia. This is reflected on the fetal monitor as a nonreassuring FHR pattern, usually late decelerations. The nurse should solicit the woman's cooperation in avoiding the supine position. The woman should be encouraged to maintain a side-lying position or semi-Fowler position with a lateral tilt to the uterus.

Discouraging the Valsalva Maneuver

The Valsalva maneuver can be described as the process of making a forceful bearing-down attempt while holding one's breath with a closed glottis and tightening the abdominal muscles. This process stimulates the parasympathetic division of the autonomic nervous system, producing a vagal response, and results in the decrease of the maternal heart rate and blood pressure. Prolonged pushing in this manner can decrease placental blood flow, alter maternal and fetal oxygenation, decrease the fetal pH and Po_2, increase the fetal Pco_2, and increase the likelihood of fetal hypoxemia, as reflected in FHR pattern changes.

During the second stage of labor, when the woman needs to push, an alternative to breath holding with a closed glottis is to perform the open-mouth and open-glottis breathing-pushing technique. The nurse should instruct the woman to keep her mouth and glottis open and to let air escape from the lungs during the pushing process. This may result in an audible grunting sound and will prevent the Valsalva maneuver. Some providers of care prefer the laboring-down process or delayed pushing, which is to refrain from pushing in the early second stage of labor. The natural forces of labor contractions are used to move the fetus down the birth canal, and then focused pushing is used for a short period to expel the fetus from the birth canal.

Documentation

Clear and complete documentation on the woman's monitor strip is started before the initiation of monitoring and consists of identifying information plus other relevant data. This documentation is continued and updated according to institutional protocol as monitoring progresses. In some institutions, observations noted and interventions implemented are recorded on the monitor strip to produce a comprehensive document that chronicles the course of labor and the care rendered. In other institutions, this documentation is confined to the labor flow record or computer chart. Advocates of documenting on both the medical record and the EFM strip cite as advantages of this approach the ease of writing directly on the strip while at the bedside or inputting the data on a computer-based documentation system and the improved accuracy in documenting critical events and the interventions implemented. Others believe that charting on the EFM strip constitutes duplicate documentation of the same information noted in the medical record, and thus it is unnecessary additional paperwork for the nurse.

One way of documenting that frequent maternal-fetal assessments have been done at the bedside is either to initial the EFM strip or to depress the "mark" button during these assessments. Data-entry devices are now available with some EFM systems; assessments are keyed in and subsequently printed on the strip. A disadvantage of documenting on both the EFM strip and the medical record is that frequently the times noted for events and interventions on the EFM strip do not correlate with what is later documented in the medical record. These inaccuracies can lead those involved in the retrospective review process carried out during litigation to infer that documentation errors have occurred. Therefore if institutional policy mandates documentation on both the monitor strip and the medical record, it is critically important for the nurse to make sure the times and notations of events and interventions recorded in each place agree. In some electronic

Fetal Monitor Integration

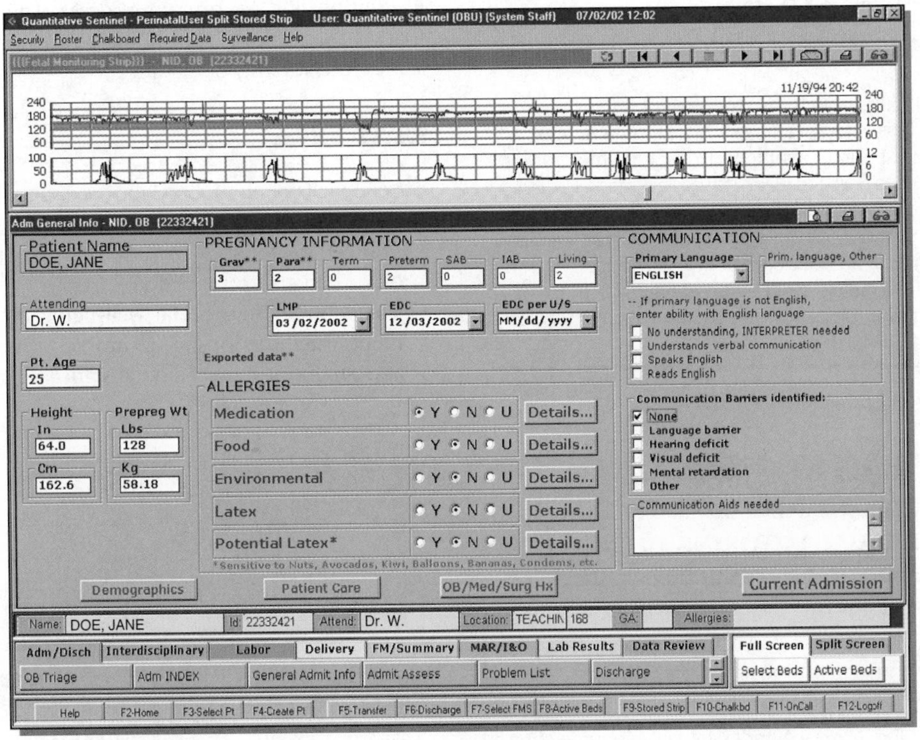

Fig. 17-9 With integration of the fetal monitor tracing into the electronic medical record, the nurse can view the fetal tracing while charting. (Courtesy General Electric Healthcare Technologies, Barrington, IL.).

medical records, the fetal monitor tracing can be integrated into the record and viewed while charting (Fig. 17-9). This assists the nurse in recording events and interventions in a timely manner and accurately. No one method of documentation is right; rather the nurse must be aware of and follow individual institutional policies, as well as participate in formulating such policies (McCartney, 2002). Many of the aspects of care and events that can be documented on the patient's medical record or the monitor strip are listed in Box 17-5.

BOX 17-5

Documentation

Observations

Maternal

Vital signs: blood pressure, temperature, pulse rate, and respiratory rate
Oxygen saturation if monitored
Uterine activity: frequency, duration, intensity, resting tone
Behavior: anxiety, irritability, fear of losing control
Breathing pattern
Position; activity (ambulating, bathroom privileges, use of birthing ball, etc.)
Rupture of membranes: time, color, amount, odor
Voidings; nausea, vomiting
Urge to push; bearing down; pushing

Fetal

FHR, variability, periodic/episodic changes
Fetal movement
Oxygen saturation if monitored
Presentation, position, station

Adjustments

Relocation of transducers
Replacement of electrode
Replacement of IUPC
Adjustment or flushing of IUPC
Testing of monitor
Monitor paper changes; time lapse
Interruption/removal of monitoring equipment

Interventions

Maternal position change
Administration of oxygen
Parenteral fluids; changes in flow rate
Amnioinfusion
Fetal scalp stimulation
Medication administration
Oxytocin
Analgesics
Anesthetics
Tocolytics
Primary health care provider notification, reason, and response
Birth data

Community Focus

EDUCATION ABOUT ELECTRONIC FETAL MONITORING

Interview childbirth educators from two different types of childbirth preparation classes (e.g., Lamaze, Bradley) regarding what they teach expectant parents about electronic fetal monitoring (EFM). Do the educators regard EFM to be "normal"? Do they discuss the advantages and disadvantages of EFM, or do they just describe EFM as a usual intervention? Do they discuss choice in labor; that is, are parents able to select auscultation rather than EFM? Intermittent rather than continuous monitoring? What implications does this information have for your practice as a labor and birth nurse?

Evaluation

Evaluation is a continuous process. The nurse can assume that care was effective when the outcomes for care have been achieved (Nursing Care Plan).

Key Points

- Fetal well-being during labor is gauged by the response of the FHR to UCs.
- FHR characteristics include the baseline FHR and periodic changes in the FHR.
- The monitoring of fetal well-being includes FHR assessment, watching for meconium-stained amniotic fluid, and assessment of maternal vital signs and uterine activity.

Nursing Care Plan

ELECTRONIC FETAL MONITORING DURING LABOR

NURSING DIAGNOSIS: Maternal anxiety related to lack of knowledge about use of electronic monitor

EXPECTED OUTCOMES

The woman will exhibit increased understanding about fetal monitoring and signs of reduced anxiety (i.e., absence of physical indicators, absence of perceived threat, and absence of feelings of dread).

NURSING INTERVENTIONS/*RATIONALES*

Explain and demonstrate to woman and labor support partner how the electronic monitor (internal or external) works in assessing FHR and in detecting and assessing quality of uterine contractions *to remove fear of unknown and ensure that woman can move with the monitor.*

When making adjustment to the monitor, explain to the couple what is being done and why, *because information increases understanding and allays anxiety.*

Explain that although a side-lying position or Fowler's position provides for optimal monitoring, position changes decrease discomfort; therefore encourage frequent changes in position (other than supine) and explain any monitoring adjustments that are being made as a result *to reduce discomfort and allay anxiety.*

NURSING DIAGNOSIS: Risk for fetal injury related to inaccurate placement of transducers/electrodes, misinterpretation of results, or failure to use other assessment techniques to monitor fetal well-being

EXPECTED OUTCOMES

Fetal well-being is adequately assessed, and any fetal compromise is identified immediately.

NURSING INTERVENTIONS/*RATIONALES*

Carefully follow guidelines and checklist for application and initiation of monitoring *to ensure proper placement of monitoring devices and production of accurate output from monitoring device.*

Check placement throughout monitoring process *to ensure that devices remain correctly placed.*

Regularly assess and record results of EFM (FHR and variability, decelerations, accelerations, uterine activity, contractions, uterine resting tone) *to provide consistent and timely evaluation of fetal well-being and progress of labor.*

Auscultate FHR and palpate contractions on a regular basis *to provide a cross-check on the EFM output and ensure fetal well-being.*

NURSING DIAGNOSIS: Risk for maternal injury related to incorrect placement of external or internal monitors or misinterpretation of contraction pattern

EXPECTED OUTCOMES

Maternal well-being is assessed continuously, and any alterations are identified promptly.

NURSING INTERVENTIONS/*RATIONALES*

Palpate uterine contractions *to correlate data with electronic monitoring results.*

Periodically recheck placement *to verify that all monitoring devices are accurately placed.*

Assess uterine activity, contraction pattern, and baseline *to provide ongoing evaluation and basis for further interventions.*

Use correct aseptic technique for insertion of internal monitors *to prevent infection.*

Monitor maternal temperature, as well as color, odor, and amount of amniotic fluid, *to determine indicators of infection.*

NURSING DIAGNOSIS: Risk for impaired physical mobility related to restriction of movement with monitoring devices

EXPECTED OUTCOME

Woman will be able to change positions and ambulate at intervals.

NURSING INTERVENTIONS/*RATIONALES*

Discontinue continuous EFM at intervals *to change position and increase mobility.*

Encourage woman to change position and reposition monitor as needed *to decrease complications of immobility.*

Place external monitor manually at intervals *to collect data while woman is out of bed.*

- It is the responsibility of the nurse to assess FHR patterns, implement independent nursing interventions, and report nonreassuring patterns to the physician or nurse-midwife.
- The Association of Women's Health, Obstetric, and Neonatal Nurses and the American College of Obstetricians and Gynecologists have established and published health care provider standards and guidelines for fetal heart monitoring.
- The emotional, informational, and comfort needs of the woman and her family must be addressed when the mother and her fetus are being monitored.
- Documentation is initiated and updated according to institutional protocol.

Answer Guidelines to Critical Thinking Exercise

Fetal Heart Rate Recording

1. Gaps in recording on the monitor paper are usually caused by inadequate contact with the maternal abdomen over the point of maximal intensity of the fetal heartbeat. Nursing actions to improve the tracing include repositioning the transducer, repositioning the woman, tightening the ultrasound belt if it is too loose, and reapplying gel to the transducer if necessary.
2. (a) FHR monitoring was developed to reduce infant morbidity and mortality rates. However, meta-analyses of clinical trials have not demonstrated improved neonatal outcomes when EFM is compared with IA of the fetal heart rate. It would be unethical to conduct a study comparing outcomes of EFM and IA with those of a control group with no FHR assessment. (b) Nonreassuring patterns of the fetal heart rate include severe variable decelerations, late decelerations, absence of variability, prolonged deceleration, and severe bradycardia. Nurses who work with patients in labor must have education and experience to recognize such patterns and implement interventions designed to correct the problems. These interventions range from changing the position of the mother to setting up for an emergency cesarean birth. (c) Periodic and episodic changes in the FHR have a variety of causes. Head compression, cord compression, and inadequate uterine perfusion are major categories. (d) Patient preference for monitoring should be honored if at all possible. Electronic fetal monitoring is used in 84% of the labors in the United States; IA is used less often. In a low risk pregnancy, intermittent rather than continuous monitoring is common. IA requires a one-to-one nurse-patient ratio. When a unit is busy, this ratio may be impossible to maintain and EFM will be instituted until staffing improves. Some women choose birthing centers or midwifery care to be able to avoid some interventions that are common in a traditional labor and birth unit.
3. Priority for nursing care at this time is to answer the patient's questions and allay her anxiety. She needs some education about EFM and the information that is gained through that mode of assessment and monitoring.
4. Yes, there are many studies of EFM and patient response.
5. Nurses, midwives, physicians, perinatologists, and pregnant women may have varying beliefs about the appropriate means of monitoring the fetus, some opting for more "natural" monitoring of the progress of labor. Medicalization of the birthing process has ensured that a number of interventions will occur. Home birth is an alternative for low risk women. Some physicians (and some nurses) do not consider this option to be safe and do not support a woman's choice of this option.

Resources

American College of Nurse-Midwives
818 Connecticut Ave., NW, Suite 900
Washington, DC 20006
202-728-9860
www.midwife.org

American College of Obstetricians and Gynecologists
409 12th St. SW
Washington, DC 20024
800-762-2264
www.acog.com

Association of Women's Health, Obstetric, and Neonatal Nurses (AWHONN)
2000 L St., NW, Suite 740
Washington, DC 20036
800-673-8499 (United States)
800-245-0231 (Canada)
www.awhonn.org

National Association of Parents and Professionals for Safe Alternatives in Childbirth (NAPSAC)
PO Box 267
Marble Hill, MO 63764
314-238-2010
www.napsac.org

National Institute of Child Health and Human Development (NICHD)
National Institutes of Health
9000 Rockville Pike
Bldg. 31, Room 2A32
Bethesda, MD 20892
301-496-4000
www.nih.gov

References

Albers LL: Monitoring the fetus in labor: evidence to support the methods, *J Midwifery Womens Health* 46(6):366-373, 2001.

American Academy of Pediatrics/American College of Obstetricians and Gynecologists: *Guidelines for perinatal care,* ed 5, Washington, DC, 2002, American Academy of Pediatrics/American College of Obstetricians and Gynecologists.

Association of Women's Health, Obstetric, and Neonatal Nurses: *Fetal heart monitoring principles and practice,* ed 3, Dubuque, IA, 2003, Kendall/Hunt.

Bricker L, Neilson J: Routine Doppler ultrasound in pregnancy (Cochrane Review), 2000. In *The Cochrane Library,* Issue 2, Chichester, UK, 2004, John Wiley & Sons.

Feinstein NF: Fetal heart rate auscultation: current and future practice, *J Obstet Gynecol Neonatal Nurs* 29(3):306-315, 2000.

Feinstein N, Sprague A, Trepanier M: *Fetal heart rate auscultation,* Washington, DC, 2000, Association of Women's Health, Obstetric, and Neonatal Nurses.

Freeman R, Garite T, Nageotte M: *Fetal heart rate monitoring,* ed 3, Philadelphia, 2003, Lippincott Williams & Wilkins.

Garite TJ et al: A multicenter controlled trial of fetal pulse oximetry in the intrapartum management of nonreassuring fetal heart rate patterns, *Am J Obstet Gynecol* 183(5):1049-1058, 2000.

Gilstrap L: Fetal acid-base balance. In Creasy RK, Resnik R, Iams JD (eds): *Maternal-fetal medicine: principles and practice,* ed 5, Philadelphia, 2004, WB Saunders.

Goodwin L: Intermittent auscultation of the fetal heart rate: a review of general principles, *J Perinat Neonatal Nurs* 14(3):53-61, 2000.

Haggerty L, Nuttall R: Experienced obstetric nurses' decision-making in fetal risk situations, *J Obstet Gynecol Neonatal Nurs* 29(5):480-490, 2000.

Hofmeyr G: Amnioinfusion for meconium-stained liquor in labour (Cochrane Review) (2002). In *The Cochrane Library,* Oxford, 2005, Update Software.

King T, Parer J: The physiology of fetal heart rate patterns and perinatal asphyxia, *J Perinat Neonatal Nurs* 14(3):19-39, 2000.

McCartney PR: Electronic fetal monitoring and the legal medical record, *MCN Am J Matern Child Nurs* 27(4):249, 2002.

National Institute of Child Health and Human Development Research Planning Workshop: Electronic fetal heart rate monitoring: research guidelines for interpretation, *Am J Obstet Gynecol* 177(6):1385-1390, 1997.

Pagana KD, Pagana TJ: *Mosby's diagnostic and laboratory test reference,* ed 6, St Louis, 2003, Mosby.

Parer J, King T: Fetal heart rate monitoring: is it salvageable? *Am J Obstet Gynecol* 182(4):982-987, 2000.

Parer JT, Nageotte MP: Intrapartum fetal surveillance. In Creasy RK, Resnik R, Iams JD (eds): *Maternal-fetal medicine: principles and practice,* ed 5, Philadelphia, 2004, WB Saunders.

Parilla B: Estimation of fetal well-being. In Fanaroff AA, Martin RJ (eds): *Neonatal-perinatal medicine: diseases of the fetus and infant,* ed 7, St Louis, 2002, Mosby.

Porter ML: Fetal pulse oximetry: an adjunct to electronic fetal heart rate monitoring, *J Obstet Gynecol Neonatal Nurs* 29(5):537-548, 2000.

Simpson KR: Fetal pulse oximetry update, *AWHONN Lifelines* 7(5): 411-412, 2003.

Simpson KR, Creehan PA: *AWHONN's perinatal nursing,* ed 2, Philadelphia, 2001, Lippincott Williams & Wilkins.

Simpson KR, Knox GE: Risk management and electronic fetal monitoring: decreasing risk of adverse outcomes and liability exposure, *J Perinat Neonatal Nurs* 14(3):40-52, 2000.

Simpson KR, Porter M: Fetal oxygen saturation monitoring: using this new technology for fetal assessment during labor, *AWHONN Lifelines* 5(2):26-33, 2001.

Thacker S, Stroup D, Chang M: Continuous electronic heart rate monitoring for fetal assessment during labor (Cochrane Review). In *The Cochrane Library,* Issue 1, Oxford, 2005, Update Software.

Tucker SM: *Pocket guide to fetal monitoring and assessment,* ed 5, St Louis, 2004, Mosby.

Wood SH: Should women be given a choice about fetal assessment in labor? *MCN Am J Matern Child Nurs* 28(5):292-298, 2003.

Nursing Care during Labor and Birth

18

LEARNING OBJECTIVES

On completion of this chapter the reader will be able to:

- Review the factors included in the initial assessment of the woman in labor.
- Describe the ongoing assessment of maternal progress during each stage of labor.
- Recognize the physical and psychosocial findings indicative of maternal progress during labor.
- Describe fetal assessment during labor.
- Identify signs of developing complications during labor.
- Discuss the nurse's role in managing care for the woman and her significant others (support person[s], family) during each stage of labor.
- Analyze the influence of cultural and religious beliefs and practices on the process of labor and birth.
- Discuss research findings on the importance of support from family, partner, doula, and nurse in facilitating maternal progress during labor and birth.
- Describe the role and responsibilities of the nurse in an emergency childbirth situation.
- Identify the impact of perineal trauma on the woman's reproductive and sexual health.
- Analyze the nurse's role as advocate in reducing the incidence of routine episiotomy.

ELECTRONIC RESOURCES

Additional information related to the content in Chapter 18 can be found on

the companion website at evolve
http://evolve.elsevier.com/Wong/maternal/

- NCLEX Review Questions
- Case Study—First Stage of Labor
- Case Study—Second/Third Stages of Labor
- WebLinks

or the interactive student CD-ROM
Activities for Chapter 18 include the following:

- NCLEX Review Questions
- Case Study—First Stage of Labor
- Case Study—Second/Third Stages of Labor
- Nursing Care Plan—Labor and Birth

The labor process is an exciting and anxious time for the woman and her significant others (support persons, family). In a relatively short period, they experience one of the most profound changes in their lives. For most women, labor begins with the first uterine contraction, continues with hours of hard work during cervical dilation and birth, and ends as the woman and her family begin the attachment process with the infant. Nursing care focuses on assessment and support for the woman and her significant others (support persons, family) throughout labor and birth, with the goal of ensuring the best possible outcome for all involved.

FIRST STAGE OF LABOR

Care Management

The first stage of labor begins with the onset of regular uterine contractions and ends with complete effacement and full cervical dilation. Care begins when the woman reports one or more of the following:

- Onset of progressive, regular uterine contractions that increase in frequency, strength, and duration
- Blood-tinged mucoid vaginal discharge (bloody or pink show) indicating that the mucous plug (operculum) has passed
- Fluid discharge from the vagina (spontaneous rupture of membranes [SROM or SRM])

The first stage of labor consists of three phases: the latent phase (up to 3 cm of dilation), the active phase (4 to 7 cm of dilation), and the transition phase (8 to 10 cm of dilation). Most nulliparous women seek admission to the hospital in the latent phase because they have not experienced labor before and are unsure of the "right" time to come in. Multiparous women usually do not come to the hospital until they are in the active phase. Even though no two labors are identical, women who have given birth before appear less anx-

evolve Case Study—First Stage of Labor

ious about the process, unless their previous experience has been negative.

Involving the woman as a partner in formulating the plan of care helps preserve the woman's sense of control, furthers participation in her own childbirth experience, and enhances her self-esteem and level of satisfaction.

Women often have lingering impressions of their childbirth experiences. Caregivers who are respectful, supportive, available, protective, encouraging, kind, patient, professional, calm, and comforting help these women to remember their childbirth experiences in positive terms. Frustrations women feel regarding their childbirth experiences stem from pain, lack of control, lack of knowledge, or the negative behaviors of some caregivers (Hanson, VandeVusse, & Harrod, 2001; Tumblin & Simkin, 2001).

Assessment

Assessment begins at the first contact with the woman, whether by telephone or in person. Many women call the hospital or birthing center to receive validation that it is all right for them to come in for evaluation or admission. The manner in which the nurse communicates with the woman during this initial contact can set the tone for a positive birth experience. A caring attitude encourages the woman to verbalize her questions and concerns. If possible, the nurse should have the woman's prenatal record in hand when speaking to her or admitting her for evaluation of labor. Copies of records are usually filed on the perinatal unit sometime during the woman's third trimester.

Certain factors are assessed initially to determine if the woman is in true labor and should come for further assessment or admission (Patient Teaching box). The pregnant woman may call the primary health care provider or come to the hospital while in false labor or early in the latent phase of the first stage of labor. She may feel discouraged on learning that the contractions that feel so strong and regular to her are not true contractions because they are not causing cervical dilation or are still not strong or frequent enough for admission.

If the woman lives near the hospital, she may be asked to stay home or return home to allow labor to progress (i.e., until the contractions are more frequent and intense). The ideal setting for low risk women in early labor is the familiar environment of her home. The nurse can use a telephone interview (Box 18-1) to assess the woman's status, give instructions regarding the optimum timing for admission, and reinforce teaching of the signs that require immediate notification of the primary health care provider. Measures the woman and her significant others can use to enhance the

CASE STUDY—FIRST STAGE OF LABOR

Patient Teaching

HOW TO DISTINGUISH TRUE LABOR FROM FALSE LABOR

True Labor

Contractions
- Occur regularly, becoming stronger, lasting longer, and occurring closer together.
- Become more intense with walking.
- Usually felt in lower back, radiating to lower portion of abdomen.
- Continue despite use of comfort measures.

Cervix (by vaginal examination)
- Shows progressive change (softening, effacement, and dilation signaled by the appearance of bloody show).
- Moves to an increasingly anterior position.

Fetus
- Presenting part usually becomes engaged in the pelvis. This results in increased ease of breathing; at the same time, the presenting part presses downward and compresses the bladder, resulting in urinary frequency.

False Labor

Contractions
- Occur irregularly or become regular only temporarily.
- Often stop with walking or position change.
- Can be felt in the back or abdomen above the navel.
- Often can be stopped through the use of comfort measures.

Cervix (by vaginal examination)
- May be soft, but there is no significant change in effacement or dilation or evidence of bloody show.
- Is often in a posterior position.

Fetus
- Presenting part is usually not engaged in the pelvis.

BOX 18-1

Telephone Interview with Woman in Latent Phase of Labor

The perinatal nurse performs the following steps of the nursing process:

Assessment
- Gathers data regarding the woman's status, including signs and symptoms indicative of true or false labor.
- Discusses instructions given by the woman's primary health care provider regarding when to come for admission.

Planning and Implementation
- Decides whether the woman will come for labor assessment and admission or be encouraged to stay at home until contractions increase in duration, frequency, and intensity.
- Assures the woman that she is welcome to call the perinatal unit at any time to discuss her labor status.
- Answers questions the woman and her family may have regarding labor or provides instruction as needed (e.g., which entrance of the hospital to enter).
- Suggests a variety of positions she can assume to maximally enhance uteroplacental and renal blood flow (e.g., side-lying position) and enhance the progress of labor (e.g., upright positions and ambulation).
- Suggests diversional activities, such as walking, reading, watching television, talking to friends.
- Suggests measures to maintain comfort, such as a warm shower, back or foot massage.
- Discusses the oral intake of foods and fluids appropriate for early labor (light foods or fluids or clear liquids depending on the preference of her primary health care provider).
- Instructs the woman to come in immediately if membranes rupture, bleeding occurs, or fetal movements change.

Evaluation
- Evaluates whether instructions and information have been understood by the woman by asking her to verbalize her understanding.

progress of labor, reduce anxiety, and maintain comfort should be described.

A warm shower can be relaxing for the woman in early labor; however, warm baths should be avoided until the cervix is approximately 5 cm dilated, because water immersion in early labor can prolong the labor process and increase the use of oxytocin to stimulate uterine contractions and epidural analgesia for pain reduction (Mackey, 2001). Soothing back, foot, and hand massages, or a warm drink of preferred liquids such as tea or milk, can help the woman to rest and even to sleep, especially if false or early labor is occurring at night. Diversional activities such as walking, reading, watching television, doing needlework, or talking with friends can reduce the perception of early discomfort, help the time pass, and reduce anxiety.

The woman who lives at a considerable distance from the hospital may be admitted in early labor. The same measures used by the woman at home should be offered to the hospitalized woman in early labor.

Admission to Labor Unit

When the woman arrives at the perinatal unit, assessment is the top priority (Fig. 18-1). The nurse first performs a screening assessment, using the techniques of interview and physical assessment, and reviews laboratory and diagnostic test findings to determine the health status of the woman and her fetus and the progress of her labor. The primary health care provider is notified, and if the woman is admitted, a detailed systems assessment is done.

When the woman is admitted, she usually is moved from an observation area to the room where she will labor and give birth: the labor, delivery, and recovery (LDR) room or the labor, delivery, recovery, and postpartum (LDRP) room. Anyone coming in the room should be introduced; women often express concern regarding the number of persons intruding on their labor experience, especially if the role of the person and purpose for his or her presence are not clearly identified (Hanson et al, 2001).

Family-centered care is the trend in maternity today. This approach views labor as wellness and the woman and her support persons as active participants in the process of labor and birth. LDR or LDRP rooms are essential components of family-centered care, and the woman is encouraged to have anyone she wishes present for her support. After birth, the mother, baby, and support persons are permitted to stay together to celebrate the arrival of a new family member.

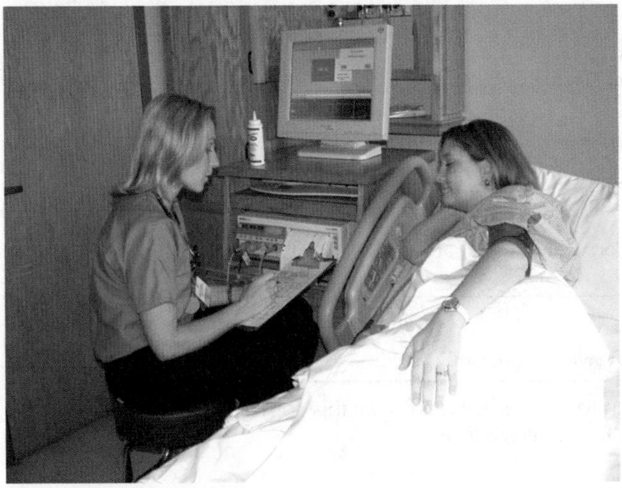

Fig. 18-1 Woman being admitted. (Courtesy Julie Perry Nelson, Gilbert, AZ.)

The woman is asked to undress and put on her own gown or a hospital gown. Her personal belongings are put away safely or given to family members, according to agency policy. Often women who participate in expectant parents classes bring a Birth Bag or Lamaze bag with them. Tennis balls or rolling pins for counterpressure, a pillow for comfort and reminder of home, an object for a focal point (e.g., meaningful picture, stuffed animal), and rice bags for warm packs may be included in her bag.

The nurse orients the woman and her partner to the layout and operation of the unit and room. This includes the use of the call light and telephone system, the location of personal storage areas in the bedside and over-the-bed tables, and how to adjust lighting in the room.

The woman is told how to notify the nurse of her wish to use the bathroom or to ambulate. An admissions bracelet is placed on the woman's wrist, as well as an allergy bracelet (usually colored), when relevant. The nurse should reassure the woman that she is in competent, caring hands; that she and her partner can ask questions related to her care and the status of herself and her fetus at any time during labor; and that questions will be answered.

The nurse can minimize the woman's anxiety by explaining terms commonly used during labor. The woman's interest, response, and prior experience guide the depth and breadth of these explanations.

Admission Data

Admission forms such as the one in Fig. 18-2 can provide guidelines for the acquisition of important assessment information when a woman in labor is being evaluated or admitted. Additional sources of data include the following: (1) the prenatal record, (2) the initial interview, (3) physical examination to determine baseline physiologic parameters, (4) laboratory and diagnostic test results, (5) expressed psychosocial and cultural factors, and (6) the clinical evaluation of labor status.

Prenatal Data

The nurse reviews the prenatal record to identify the woman's individual needs and risks. Incomplete information regarding the woman's prenatal health status could adversely affect the quality and safety of the care provided to her and her fetus or newborn during labor and birth and in the postpartum period. Use of standardized worksheets and flow sheets developed by health care providers and computer access to antepartal health records are strategies to facilitate the gathering of information relevant to the safe and effective management of care during labor.

If the woman has not had any prenatal care or her prenatal record is unavailable, certain baseline information must be obtained. If the woman is having discomfort, the nurse should ask questions between contractions when the woman can concentrate more fully on her responses. At times the partner or support person(s) may need to be secondary sources of essential information.

Obstetric Admitting Record **Page 1 of 2**

Basic Admission Data

Date ___ / ___ / ___ Time ________

☐ Ambulatory ☐ Direct admit ☐ Stretcher
☐ Wheelchair ☐ Transfer from ________

G	T	Pt	A	L	LMP / /	EDD / /	Age

EDD By fetal assessment / /

Race/Ethnicity ________

Occupation ________ Education ________

Marital status S M Sep D W Religion ________

MD/CNM	Tel no	Support person/Relationship	Tel no

Reasons for Admission
☐ **Onset of labor**
☐ Induction of labor
☐ Spontaneous abortion
☐ Cesarean section
 ☐ Primary ☐ Repeat
 (reason for primary________)
☐ VBAC
☐ Tubal ligation
☐ Vaginal bleeding
☐ PROM
☐ Preterm labor

Detail reasons for admission ________

Observation evaluation
☐ Fetal status
 ☐ Ultrasound
 ☐ Amniocentesis
 ☐ NST
 ☐ CST
☐ Medical complications ________
☐ Obstetric complications ________

Patient Triage Data

Contractions ☐ **None** ☐ Palpation ☐ Tocotransducer
 Frequency________ Duration________ Intensity________
 Began on___ / ___ / ___ Time________

Membranes ☐ **Intact** ☐ Bulging
 ☐ Ruptured (Date___ / ___ / ___ Time________)

Fluid ☐ Clear ☐ Bloody ☐ Foul smelling
 ☐ Meconium stained ☐ No foul odor

Vaginal bleeding ☐ **None** ☐ Normal show
 ☐ Bleeding (describe________)

Cervical Exam
 Station________ Effacement________ Dilatation________ cms
 Presentation
 ☐ Vertex ☐ Transverse lie
 ☐ Face/Brow ☐ Compound
 ☐ Breech (type________) ☐ Unknown

Medication allergy/Sensitivity ☐ **None**
 ☐ Identify________

Other allergy/Sensitivity ☐ **None**
 ☐ Identify________

Patient Care Data

Personal Effects	Disposition		
Item	With patient	With support person	Other (describe)

Illness (≤ 14 days prior to admission) ☐ **None**
 ☐ Type/Treatment________

Recent Exposure to Communicable Disease ☐ **None**
 ☐ Type/Date________ ___ / ___ / ___

Last Oral Intake
 Fluids___ / ___ / ___ Time________
 Solids___ / ___ / ___ Time________

Medications ☐ **None**

Type/Dose	Last taken	With patient No	With patient Yes	Disposition
________	________	☐	☐	

Alcohol/Drug use ☐ No ☐ Yes

Substances	Amt/Day	Last used
________	________	___ / ___ / ___ Time________
________	________	___ / ___ / ___ Time________

Plans for Birth and Hospital Stay

Support person present in L&D ☐ No ☐ Yes________
Other family members in L&D ☐ No ☐ Yes________

Anesthesia ☐ **None**
 ☐ Local ☐ Epidural ☐ Spinal ☐ General

Delivery site
 ☐ DR ☐ Birthing room ☐ LDR ☐ LDRP ☐ OR

Personal requests________

Adoption ☐ No
 ☐ Yes Contact with infant ☐ No ☐ Yes
 Adoption contact________

Feeding preference ☐ Breast ☐ Bottle
Room preference ☐ Private ☐ Semi-Private
 ☐ Rooming-In

☐ Tubal ligation Authorization signed ☐ Yes ☐ No
☐ Circumcision Authorization signed ☐ Yes ☐ No

Psychosocial Data

Communication Deficit ☐ **None**
 ☐ Identify________

Other children ☐ No ☐ Yes Age/Sex________
________, ________, ________, ________

Partner involved ☐ Yes ☐ No

Admitting signature________ Time________

Fig. 18-2 Obstetric admitting record. (Permission to use and/or reproduce this copyrighted material has been granted by the owner, Hollister, Inc., Libertyville, IL.)

Obstetric Admitting Record

Page 2 of 2

Psychosocial Data (Cont'd.)

Basic needs met	Yes	No	If no, explain
Housing	☐	☐	________
Clothing	☐	☐	________
Food	☐	☐	________
Transportation	☐	☐	________

Free from apparent physical/emotional abuse ☐ Yes ☐ No

If no, explain________

Life Stress	No	Yes	If yes, explain
Living	☐	☐	________
Working	☐	☐	________
Serious illness	☐	☐	________

Self-Care Needs ☐ None ☐ Needs help with________

Emotional status ☐ Happy ☐ Ambivalent ☐ Anxious ☐ Depressed ☐ Angry

Discharge Planning Data

Discharge planning initiated ☐ **Yes** ☐ No

Discharge needs identified________

Social service referral ☐ No ☐ Yes __ / __ / __

Planned length of stay______days

Significant Prenatal Data

Prenatal Records Available on Admission

☐ **Yes** ☐ No

Source of prenatal data________

First prenatal visit__ / __ / __

Attended prenatal classes ☐ **Yes** ☐ No

Infant care provider:

____

Lab Findings

☐ **None**

Blood type & Rh ____

Rubella titer ____

Serology ____

HbSAg ____

Fetal Assessment Tests

☐ **None**

Date	Test	Result
/		
/		
/		
/		

Maternal Problems Identified ☐ **None**

	Active	Resolved
1.________	☐	☐
2.________	☐	☐
3.________	☐	☐

Fetal Problems Identified ☐ **None**

	Active	Resolved
1.________	☐	☐
2.________	☐	☐
3.________	☐	☐

Physical Assessment

Detail all abnormal findings

Height		Wt pregrav/grav	
Temp	Pulse	Resp	BP

System	Normal	Abnormal
HEENT	☐	☐
Neurologic	☐	☐
Skin	☐	☐
Breasts	☐	☐
Extremities	☐	☐
Cardiovascular	☐	☐
Respiratory	☐	☐
Abdomen	☐	☐
Gastrointestinal	☐	☐
Urinary	☐	☐
Genitalia	☐	☐

Specimens obtained (check all that apply)

Urine test	Time	Results	Blood test	Time	Results
☐ Urinalysis			☐ Hgb		
☐ C + S			☐ Hct		
☐ Glucose			☐ VDRL/RPR		
☐ Albumin			☐ Type/Screen		
☐ Ketones			☐		
☐ pH			☐		
☐ Blood			☐		

Fetal Evaluation Data

Fundal height______cms FHR________

Estimated fetal weight________ ☐ Fetoscope ☐ Doppler ☐ Fetal monitor ☐ Other

Weeks gestation (est)

By dates______wks

By ultrasound______wks

Date__ / __ / __

Multiple gestation ☐ **No** ☐ Yes

	Infant	Presentation	Position
1.			
2.			
3.			

Initial Problems Identified ☐ **None**

1. ________
2. ________
3. ________

Physician/CNM________

Notified by________

Date__ / __ / __Time______

________ Admitting signature

________ Examiner signature

Date__ / __ / __Time______

Fig. 18-2, cont'd For legend see opposite page.

It is important to know the woman's age so that the plan of care can be tailored to the needs of her age group. For example, a 14-year-old and a 40-year-old have different but specific needs, and their ages place them at risk for different problems. Height and weight relationships are important to determine because a weight gain greater than that recommended may place the woman at a higher risk for cephalopelvic disproportion and cesarean birth. This is especially true for women who are petite and have gained 16 kg or more. Other factors to consider are her general health status, current medical conditions or allergies, respiratory status, and previous surgical procedures.

Her past and present pregnancy history are carefully noted. These include gravidity, parity, and problems such as history of vaginal bleeding, gestational hypertension, anemia, gestational diabetes, infections (e.g., bacterial or sexually transmitted), and immunodeficiency.

If this is not the woman's first labor and birth experience, it is important to note the characteristics of her previous experiences. This information includes the duration of previous labors, the type of anesthesia used, the kind of birth (e.g., spontaneous vaginal, forceps- or vacuum-assisted, or cesarean birth), and the condition of the newborn. It is important to confirm the expected date of birth (EDB). Other data in the prenatal record include patterns of maternal weight gain, physiologic measurements such as maternal vital signs (blood pressure; temperature, pulse, respiration), fundal height, baseline fetal heart rate (FHR), and laboratory and diagnostic test results.

Laboratory tests include the woman's blood type and Rh factor, a complete or partial blood cell count (complete blood cell count [CBC], hemoglobin, and hematocrit), the 50 g blood glucose test, determination of the rubella titer, serologic tests (Venereal Disease Research Laboratories [VDRL] or rapid plasma reagin [RPR] test) for syphilis, hepatitis B surface antigen (HBsAg), culture for group B streptococci, and urinalysis. Additional tests may include a tuberculosis screen with purified protein derivative (PPD), screening for the human immunodeficiency virus (HIV), and a screen for sickle cell trait or other genetic disorders (e.g., maternal serum alpha-fetoprotein). Diagnostic tests include amniocentesis, nonstress test (NST), contraction stress test (CST), biophysical profile (BPP), and ultrasound examination.

Questioning about physical abuse and substance abuse should form an integral part of the initial and ongoing assessment.

Interview

The woman's primary complaint or reason for coming to the hospital is determined in the interview. Her primary complaint may be that her bag of waters (BOW, or amniotic membranes) ruptured, with or without contractions. The woman may have come in for an obstetric check, which is a period of observation reserved for women who are unsure about the onset of labor. This allows time on the unit for diagnosis of labor without official admission, and minimizes or avoids cost to the patient when used by the hospital and approved by the woman's health insurance plan.

Even the experienced mother may have difficulty determining the onset of labor. The woman is asked to recall the events of the previous days and to describe the following:

- Time of onset of contractions and progress in terms of frequency and duration
- Location and character of discomfort from the contractions (e.g., back pain, suprapubic discomfort)
- Persistence of contractions despite changes in maternal position and activity (e.g., walking or lying down)
- Presence and character of vaginal discharge or show
- Status of amniotic membranes, such as gush or seepage of fluid (rupture of membranes [ROM])

If there has been a discharge that may be amniotic fluid, the woman is asked the date and time the fluid was first noted and the fluid's characteristics (e.g., amount, color, or unusual odor). In many instances a sterile speculum examination and a nitrazine (pH) or fern test can confirm that the membranes are ruptured (Box 18-2).

These descriptions help the nurse assess the degree of progress in labor. Bloody or pink show is distinguished from bleeding in that it is pink and feels sticky because of its mucoid nature. It is scant to begin with and increases with effacement and dilation of the cervix. A woman may report a scant brownish discharge that may be attributed to cervical trauma resulting from vaginal examination or coitus within the last 48 hours.

In case general anesthesia is required in an emergency, it is important to assess the woman's respiratory status. The nurse determines this by asking the woman if she has a cold or related symptoms (e.g., stuffy nose, sore throat, or cough). The status of allergies is rechecked, including allergies to medications routinely used in obstetrics such as nalbuphine hydrochloride (Nubain), butorphanol tartrate (Stadol), or lidocaine hydrochloride (Xylocaine). Some allergic responses cause swelling of mucous membranes of the respiratory tract, which could interfere with breathing and the administration of inhalation anesthetics.

Because vomiting and subsequent aspiration into the respiratory tract can complicate an otherwise normal labor, the

Community Focus

ETHICAL ISSUES IN PERINATAL CARE IN COMMUNITY SETTINGS

Ethical issues for perinatal nurses are complex; both a mother and fetus are involved. There are at least six areas where ethical conflict may occur: "conflict between the mother and fetus, informed consent, confidentiality, cultural conflicts, conflicts associated with managed care, and conflicts in childbirth education" (Moore, 2000). To resolve ethical issues, the principles of autonomy, beneficence, and justice are used. Perinatal nurses must become informed about ethical principles; they must be willing to advocate for their patients in all settings. Continued dialogue among nurses and other health care providers, attorneys, ethicists, and lay people must take place. There are no easy answers to complex ethical questions.

Does the health care agency where you have your maternity clinical have an ethics committee? Who serves on the committee? If possible, attend a meeting of the committee. What issues were discussed? What ethical principles were addressed? Did you agree with the outcome of the discussion?

Data from Moore M: Ethical issues for nurses providing perinatal care in community settings, *J Perinat Neonatal Nurs* 14(2):25-35, 2000.

BOX 18-2

Procedure: Tests for Rupture of Membranes

Nitrazine Test for pH

Explain procedure to woman/couple.

Procedure

Wash hands.

Use **nitrazine test** paper, a dye-impregnated test paper for determining pH. (Differentiates amniotic fluid, which is slightly alkaline, from urine and purulent material [pus], which are acidic.)

Wearing a sterile glove lubricated with water, place a piece of test paper at the cervical os.

OR

Use a sterile, cotton-tipped applicator to dip deep into vagina to pick up fluid; touch applicator to test paper. (Procedure may be done during speculum examination.)

Read Results:

Membranes probably intact: identifies vaginal and most body fluids that are acidic:

Yellow	pH 5.0
Olive-yellow	pH 5.5
Olive-green	pH 6.0

Membranes probably ruptured: identifies amniotic fluid that is alkaline:

Blue-green	pH 6.5
Blue-gray	pH 7.0
Deep blue	pH 7.5

Realize that false test results are possible because of presence of bloody show, insufficient amniotic fluid, or semen.

Remove gloves and wash hands.

Document Results

Positive or negative.

Test for Ferning or Fern Pattern

Explain procedure to woman/couple.

Wash hands, apply sterile gloves, obtain specimen of fluid (usually during sterile speculum examination).

Spread a drop of fluid from vagina on a clean glass slide with a sterile, cotton-tipped applicator.

Allow fluid to dry.

Examine slide under microscope: observe for appearance of ferning (a frondlike crystalline pattern). (Do not confuse with cervical mucus test, when high levels of estrogen are responsible for causing the ferning.)

Observe for absence of ferning. (Alerts staff to possibility that amount of specimen was inadequate or that specimen was urine, vaginal discharge, or blood.)

Remove gloves and wash hands.

Document Results

Positive or negative.

nurse records the type and time of the woman's last solid food and liquid intake.

Any information not found in the prenatal record is obtained during the admission assessment. Pertinent data include the birth plan (Box 18-3), the choice of infant feeding method, type of pain management, and the name of the pediatrician. A patient profile is obtained that identifies the woman's preparation for childbirth, the support person or family members desired during childbirth and their availability, and ethnic or cultural expectations and needs. The

BOX 18-3

The Birth Plan

The birth plan should include the woman's/couple's preferences related to the following:

- Presence of birth companions such as the partner, older children, parents, friends, a doula, and the role each will play
- Presence of other persons such as students, male attendants, interpreters
- Clothing to be worn
- Environmental modifications such as lighting, music, privacy, focal point, items from home such as pillows
- Labor activities such as preferred positions for labor and for birth, ambulation, birth balls, showers and whirlpool baths, oral food and fluid intake
- Repertoire of comfort and relaxation measures
- Labor and birth medical interventions such as pharmacologic pain relief measures, intravenous therapy, electronic monitoring, induction or augmentation measures, episiotomy
- Care and handling of the newborn immediately after birth such as cutting of the cord, eye care, breastfeeding
- Cultural and religious requirements related to the care of the mother, newborn, and placenta

The Childbirth Organization Web site (www.childbirth.org) provides couples with an interactive birth plan along with examples of birth plans.

woman's use of alcohol, drugs, and tobacco before or during pregnancy should be determined. Screening of the neonate for substances abused by the mother may be required. After birth, the nurse assesses the neonate for signs indicating maternal substance use during pregnancy (e.g., abstinence syndrome, size, and appearance) (Community Focus).

The nurse reviews the birth plan. If no written plan has been prepared, the nurse helps the woman formulate a birth plan by describing options available and finds out the woman's wishes and preferences. The nurse prepares the woman for the possibility that changes may be needed in her plan as labor progresses, and assures her that information will be provided so that she can make informed decisions. The nurse uses the birth plan information to plan individualized care for the woman's labor.

The nurse should discuss with the woman and her family their plans for preserving childbirth memories using photography and videotaping. Health care agencies and insurance companies have voiced concerns that this type of recording of childbirth events could be used in court should the couple sue the health care agency or health care providers. The nurse can promote the appropriate use of cameras during the birth, including who and what will be recorded, the method that will be used, and the person who will perform the task. Protection of privacy and safety and infection control are major concerns. Policies should be in place to address issues such as the use of flash photography in the presence of combustible gases and where the person who is recording the birth can stand. The fact that the birth was recorded should be entered in the patient's record. Consideration should be given to the woman's reaction to viewing the video after birth. She may need help in interpreting the events, behaviors, and reactions she sees depicted in the video, because her impression of her childbirth experience, including her behavior, can have a profound effect on her future labor and birth experiences. Women may have an idealized view of what their birth video will depict, based on childbirth videos viewed during an expectant childbirth class (Cesario, 1998; Hanson et al, 2001).

Psychosocial Factors

The woman's general appearance and behavior (and that of her partner) provide valuable clues to the type of supportive care she will need. However, the nurse should keep in mind that general appearance and behavior may vary depending on the stage and phase of labor.

Women with a History of Sexual Abuse

Memories of sexual abuse can be triggered during labor by intrusive procedures such as vaginal examination; loss of control; being confined to bed and "restrained" by monitors, intravenous (IV) lines, and epidurals; being watched by students; and experiencing intense sensations in the uterus and genital area, especially at the time when the woman must push the baby out. Women who are survivors of abuse may fight the labor process by reacting in panic or anger toward care providers, may take control of everyone and everything related to their childbirth, may surrender by being submissive and dependent, or may retreat by mentally dissociating themselves from the sensations of labor and birth (Rhodes & Hutchinson, 1994).

The nurse can help these women to associate the sensations they are experiencing with the process of childbirth and not with their past abuse. The woman's sense of control should be maintained by explaining all procedures and why they are needed, validating her needs and paying close attention to her requests, proceeding at the woman's pace by waiting for her permission to touch her, accepting her often extreme reactions to labor, and protecting her privacy by limiting the exposure of her body and the number of persons involved in her care. It is recommended that all laboring women be cared for in this manner, because it is not unusual for a woman to choose not to reveal a history of sexual abuse (Heritage, 1998; Waymire, 1997).

Stress in Labor

The way in which women and their support person or family members approach labor is related to the manner in which they have been socialized to the childbearing process. Their reactions reflect their life experiences regarding childbirth—physical, social, cultural, and religious. Society communicates its expectations regarding acceptable and unacceptable maternal behaviors during labor and birth. An idealized perception of labor and birth may be a source of guilt and a sense of failure if the woman finds the process less than joyous, especially when the pregnancy is unplanned or is the product of a shaky or terminated relationship. Often women have heard horror stories or have seen friends or relatives going through labors that appear anything but easy. Multiparous women will often base their expectations of the present labor on their previous childbirth experiences. Feelings a woman has about her pregnancy and fears regarding childbirth should be discussed. Major fears and concerns relate to the process and effects of childbirth, maternal and fetal well-being, and the attitude and actions of the health care staff. Unresolved fears increase a woman's stress and can inhibit the process of labor as a result of the inhibiting effects of catecholamines associated with the stress response on uterine contractions (Melender, 2002).

Women in labor usually have a variety of concerns that they will voice if asked but rarely volunteer. To correct misinformation, it is important for the nurse to ask the woman what she expects or to suggest that the woman ask her primary health care provider about an issue. The following are common concerns that women in labor have: Will my baby be all right? Will I be able to stand labor? Will my labor be long? How will I act? Will I need medication? Will it work for me? Will my partner or someone be there to support me? Do I have to have an IV line?

The nurse's responsibility to the woman in labor in relation to these concerns is to answer her questions or find out the answers, to provide support for her and her support person and family, to take care of her in partnership with those persons the woman wants as her support team, and to serve as their advocate. Women equate emotional support with information giving. Nurses are perceived as supportive when they explain things in detail by using positive terms and provide accurate information and specific directions. Women feel empowered when they are given information they can understand and that reflects support of their efforts. This feeling of empowerment contributes to a positive perception of the birth experience.

The nurse assures the woman that she is not expected to act in any particular way and that the process will end in the birth of her baby, which is the only expectation she should have. Women need to be able to behave in a manner that is natural for them. The woman's views and expectations regarding the nurse's role as caregiver should be determined. The nurse-patient relationship will become increasingly important as labor progresses. Women need to trust in their own innate ability to give birth, and nurses need to support and protect each woman's efforts to achieve this outcome.

The father, coach, or significant other also experiences stress during labor. The nurse can assist and support these individuals by identifying their needs and expectations and by helping make sure these are met. The nurse can ascertain what role the support person intends to fulfill and whether he or she is prepared for that role by making observations and asking herself such questions as the following: Has the couple attended childbirth classes? What role does this person expect to play? Is he or she nervous, anxious, aggressive, or hostile? Does he or she look hungry, tired, worried, or confused? Does he or she watch television, sleep, or stay out of the room instead of paying attention to the woman? Does he or she touch the woman? What is the character of the touch? The nurse should be sensitive to needs of support persons and provide teaching and support as appropriate. Often the support this person is able to give the laboring woman is in direct proportion to the support he or she receives from nurses and other health care providers.

Cultural Factors

It is important to note the woman's ethnic or cultural and religious background to anticipate nursing interventions that may need to be added or eliminated to individualize the plan of care (Fig. 18-3). The woman should be encouraged to request caregiving behaviors and practices that are important to her. If a special request contradicts usual practices in that setting, the woman or nurse can ask the woman's pri-

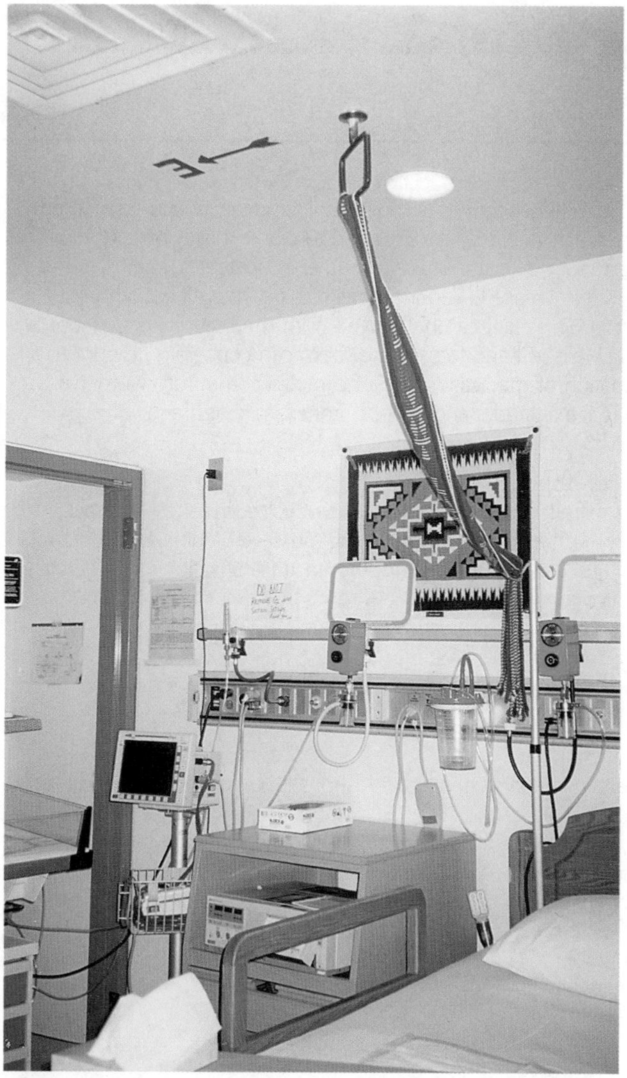

Fig. 18-3 Birthing room specific to a Native American population. Note the arrow pointing east, the rug on the wall, and the cord hanging from the ceiling. (Chinle Comprehensive Health Care Center, Chinle, AZ; photo courtesy Patricia Hess, San Francisco, CA.)

mary health care provider to write an order to accommodate the special request. For example, in many cultures it is unacceptable to have a male caregiver examine a pregnant woman. In some cultures, it is traditional to take the placenta home; in others the woman is given only certain nourishments during labor. Some women believe that cutting her body, as with an episiotomy, allows her spirit to leave her body and that rupturing the membranes prolongs, not shortens, labor. It is important that the rationale for required care measures be carefully explained (Mattson, 2000) (Cultural Awareness box).

When assessing a woman's cultural and religious preferences, Callister (1995) suggested that the nurse ask questions regarding the following:

- The value and meaning placed on the childbirth experience
- The view of childbirth as a wellness or illness experience, and as a private or social event

Cultural Awareness

CULTURAL VARIATIONS IN BIRTH PRACTICES

South Korea
Stoic response to labor pain; fathers usually not present.

Japan
Natural childbirth methods practiced; may labor silently; may eat during labor; father may be present.

China
Stoic response to pain; fathers usually not present; side-lying position preferred for labor and birth, because this position is thought to reduce infant trauma.

India
Natural childbirth methods preferred; father is usually not present; female relatives usually present.

Iran
Father not present, prefers female support and female caregivers.

Mexico
May be stoic about discomfort until second stage, then may request pain relief; fathers and female relatives may be present.

Laos
May use squatting position for birth; fathers may or may not be present; prefers female attendants.

Modified from D'Avanzo CE, Geissler EM: *Pocket guide to cultural health assessment,* ed 3, St Louis, 2003, Mosby.

- Practices regarding diet, medications, activity, and emotional and physical support
- Appropriate maternal and paternal behaviors
- Birth companions—who they should be and what they should do
- Views regarding the newborn and newborn care immediately after birth

Within cultures, women may learn the "right" way to behave in labor and to react to the pain experienced in that way. These behaviors can range from total silence to moaning or screaming, but they are not in and of themselves a gauge of the degree of pain. A woman who moans with contractions may not be in as much physical pain as a woman who is silent but winces during contractions (Table 18-1). Some women feel it is shameful to scream or cry out in pain if a man is present. If the woman's support person is her mother, she may perceive the need to "behave" more strongly than if her support person is the father of the baby. She will perceive herself as failing or succeeding on the basis of her ability to adhere to these "standards" of behavior. Conversely, a woman's behavior in response to pain may influence the support received from significant others. In some cultures women who lose control and cry out in pain may be scolded, whereas in other cultures support persons will become more helpful (Choudhry, 1997; Weber, 1996).

Culture and Father Participation

The choice of birth companion is influenced by the woman's cultural and religious background and by trends in the society in which she lives. For example, in Western societies, the father is viewed as the ideal birth companion; in

Table 18-1

Sociocultural Basis of Pain Experience

WOMAN IN LABOR	NURSE
PERCEPTION OF MEANING	
Origin: Cultural concept of and personal experience with pain; for example: Pain in childbirth is inevitable, something to be endured. Pain in childbirth can be avoided completely. Pain in childbirth is punishment for sin. Pain in childbirth can be controlled.	Origin: Cultural concept of and personal experience with pain; in addition, nurse becomes accustomed to working with certain "expected" pain trajectories. For example, in obstetrics, pain is expected to increase as labor progresses, be intermittent, and have an end point; relief can be derived from medications once labor is well established and fetus or newborn can cope with amount and elimination of medications; relief can also come from woman's knowledge, attitude, and support from family or friends.
COPING MECHANISMS	
Woman may exhibit the following behaviors: Be traditionally vocal or nonvocal; crying out or groaning, or both, may be part of her ritual response to pain. Use counterstimulation to minimize pain (e.g., rubbing, applying heat, or applying counterpressure). Use relaxation, distraction, or autosuggestion as pain-countering techniques. Resist any use of "needles" as modes of administering pain relief agents.	Nurse may respond by: Using self effectively (e.g., using tone of voice, closeness in space, and touch as media for conveying message of interest and caring). Using avoidance, belittling, or other distracting actions as protective device for self. Using pharmacologic resources at hand judiciously. Using comfort measures. Assuming accountability for control and management of pain.
EXPECTATIONS OF OTHERS	
Nurse may be seen as someone who will accept woman's statement of pain and act as her advocate. Medical personnel may be expected to relieve woman of all pain sensations. Nurse may be expected to be interested, gentle, kind, and accepting of behavior exhibited.	Only certain verbal or nonverbal responses to pain may be accepted as appropriate responses. Couple that is prepared for childbirth may be expected to refuse medication and to wish to "do everything on their own." Woman's definition of pain may not be accepted; that is, woman may wish to experience and participate in controlling pain or may not be able to accept any pain as reasonable.

other cultures, the presence of another woman or women is highly desired. For European-American couples, attending childbirth classes together has become a traditional, expected activity. In some other cultures, the father's presence in the labor and birth room is inappropriate, for example, Mexican, Filipino, Chinese, Islamic, and Ethiopian (D'Avanzo & Geissler, 2003). However, among the Hmong, the father plays an important role in the birth. If couples from these cultures immigrate to the United States or Canada, their roles may change. The nurse will need to talk with the woman and her support persons to determine the roles they wish to assume.

The Non–English-Speaking Woman in Labor

A woman's level of anxiety in labor rises when she does not understand what is happening to her or what is being said. Some misunderstanding may occur with English-speaking women and cause some stress; but the effect of misunderstanding on non–English-speaking women is much more dramatic. These women often feel a complete loss of control over their situation if there is no health care provider present who speaks their language. They can panic and withdraw or become physically abusive when someone tries to do something they perceive might harm them or their baby. Sometimes a support person is able to serve as an interpreter. However, this must be done with caution because the interpreter may not be able to convey exactly what the nurse or others are saying or what the woman is saying, and this may raise the woman's stress level even more.

Ideally, a bilingual nurse will care for the woman. Alternatively, an employee or volunteer interpreter may be contacted for assistance. If no one in the hospital is able to translate, a translation service can be called so that a translation can take place over the telephone. For some women, a female interpreter may be more acceptable. If no interpreter is available, the labor and birth staff can prepare a set of cards with graphic depictions that illustrate common situations. These cards then can be used to communicate with non–English-speaking women. Even when the nurse has limited ability to communicate orally with the woman, in most instances the nurse's efforts to communicate are meaningful and appreciated by the woman. Speaking slowly and avoiding complex words and medical terms can help a woman and her partner to understand (Mattson, 2000) (Guidelines/Guías box).

Physical Examination

During the admission process, the physical examination begins with a vaginal examination to rule out imminent birth. The nurse proceeds with the remainder of the initial physical examination to confirm the onset of true labor. The initial physical examination includes a general systems assessment; performance of Leopold's maneuvers to deter-

ENGLISH SPANISH **Guidelines/Guías**

LABOR ASSESSMENT

What time did the contractions begin?
¿A qué hora le empezaron las contracciones?

How far apart are the contractions?
¿Con qué frecuencia tiene las contracciones?

Have the membranes ruptured? When?
¿Se le rompió la fuente? ¿Cuándo?

What color was the fluid? Red? Pink?
¿Qué color tenía el líquido? ¿Rojo? ¿Rosado?

Have you had bleeding?
¿Ha tenido hemorragia?

How much? A cupful? A tablespoonful? A teaspoonful?
¿Cuánto? ¿Una taza? ¿Una cucharada? ¿Una cucharadita?

When was the last time you ate or drank anything?
¿Cuándo fue la última vez que comió o tomó algo?

Have you had any problems with this pregnancy?
¿Ha tenido algún problema con este embarazo?

Are you taking any medications?
¿Toma algún medicamento?

Are you allergic to penicillin or other medicines?
¿Es alérgica a la penicilina u otras medicinas?

Please sign this consent form.
Por favor, firme este formulario de autorización.

mine fetal presentation, position, and point of maximum intensity (PMI) for auscultating the FHR; assessment of fetal status; assessment of uterine contractions; and vaginal examination to assess cervical effacement and dilation, fetal descent, and amniotic membranes and fluid. The most vital aspect of assessment is that of fetal status.

It is important to obtain as many related pieces of information as possible before planning and implementing care. Women often focus on the nature of their contractions as the clearest indicator of how far advanced their labor is. However, the findings from the vaginal examination are more valid indicators of the phase of labor, especially for nulliparous women. ROM significantly affects the woman's plan of care because, once this occurs, the membranes can no longer protect the intrauterine cavity and fetus from infectious organisms that can travel up the birth canal. The risk of umbilical cord prolapse exists once the membranes have ruptured if the presenting part is not engaged.

Expected maternal progress and minimum assessment guidelines during the first stage of labor are presented in Table 18-2 and the Care Path. Standard Precautions should be used for all assessment and care measures (Box 18-4). The assessment findings are explained to the woman whenever possible. Throughout labor, accurate documentation, following agency policy, is done as soon as possible after a procedure has been performed (Fig. 18-4).

General Systems Assessment

A brief systems assessment is performed. This includes assessment of the heart, lungs, and skin; an examination to determine the presence and extent of edema of the legs, face, hands, or sacrum; and testing of deep tendon reflexes and for clonus.

Vital Signs

Vital signs (temperature, pulse, respirations, and blood pressure) are assessed on admission, and initial values are used for comparison with subsequent values. If blood pressure is elevated, it should be reassessed 30 minutes later, between contractions, using a correct-size blood pressure cuff to obtain a reading after the woman has relaxed. To prevent supine hypotension and fetal distress, the woman should be encouraged to lie on her side and not supine (Fig. 18-5 on p. 506). Her temperature is monitored so that signs of infection or fluid deficit (e.g., dehydration associated with inadequate intake of fluids) can be identified. The woman's intake and output should be measured at least every 8 hours. Urinary protein and ketone levels may be determined by using a dipstick each time the woman voids.

Leopold's Maneuvers (Abdominal Palpation)

Leopold's maneuvers are performed with the woman briefly lying on her back (Box 18-5, Fig. 18-6). These maneuvers help identify the following: (1) number of fetuses; (2) presenting part, fetal lie, and fetal attitude; (3) degree of the presenting part's descent into the pelvis; and (4) expected location of the PMI of the fetal heart rate (FHRs) on the woman's abdomen.

BOX 18-4

Standard Precautions during Childbirth

Birth is a time when nurses and other health care providers are exposed to a great deal of maternal and newborn blood and body fluids. Observation of Standard Precautions is necessary to prevent the transmission of infection. Perinatal infections most often are transmitted through contact with body fluids. The Standard Precautions applicable to childbirth include the following:

- Wash hands before and after putting on gloves and performing procedures.
- Wear gloves (clean or sterile, as appropriate) when performing procedures that require contact with the woman's genitalia and body fluids, including bloody show (e.g., during vaginal examination, amniotomy, hygienic care of the perineum, insertion of an internal scalp electrode and intrauterine pressure monitor, and catheterization).
- Wear cap, a mask that has a shield or protective eyewear, shoe covers, and cover gown during the birth. Gowns worn by the primary health care provider who is attending the birth should have a waterproof front and sleeves and should be sterile.
- Drape the woman with sterile towels and sheets as appropriate. Explain to the woman what can and cannot be touched.
- Help the woman's partner put on appropriate coverings for the birth, such as cap, mask, gown, and shoe covers. Show the partner where to stand and what can and cannot be touched.
- Wear gloves and gown when handling the newborn immediately after birth.
- Use an appropriate method to suction the newborn's airway, such as a bulb syringe, mechanical wall suction, or DeLee oral suction device that prevents the newborn's mucus from getting into the user's airway.

Table 18-2

Expected Maternal Progress in First Stage of Labor

	Phases Marked by Cervical Dilation*		
CRITERION	0-3 cm (LATENT)	4-7 cm (ACTIVE)	8-10 cm (TRANSITION)
Duration†	About 6-8 hr	About 3-6 hr	About 20-40 min
Contractions			
• Strength	Mild to moderate	Moderate to strong	Strong to very strong
• Rhythm	Irregular	More regular	Regular
• Frequency	5-30 min apart	3-5 min apart	2-3 min apart
• Duration	30-45 sec	40-70 sec	45-90 sec
Descent			
• Station of presenting part	Nulliparous: 0 Multiparous: 0 to −2 cm	Varies: +1 to +2 cm Varies: +1 to +2 cm	Varies: +2 to +3 cm Varies: +2 to +3 cm
Show			
• Color	Brownish discharge, mucous plug, or pale pink mucus	Pink to bloody mucus	Bloody mucus
• Amount	Scant	Scant to moderate	Copious
Behavior and appearance‡	Excited; thoughts center on self, labor, and baby; may be talkative or silent, calm or tense; some apprehension; pain controlled fairly well; alert, follows directions readily; open to instructions	Becomes more serious, doubtful of control of pain, more apprehensive; desires companionship and encouragement; attention more inner directed; fatigue evidenced; malar (cheeks) flush; has some difficulty following directions	Pain described as severe; backache common; frustration, fear of loss of control, and irritability surface; vague in communications; amnesia between contractions; writhing with contractions; nausea and vomiting, especially if hyperventilating; hyperesthesia; circumoral pallor, perspiration of forehead and upper lips; shaking tremor of thighs; feeling of need to defecate, pressure on anus

*In the nullipara, effacement is often complete before dilation begins; in the multipara, it occurs simultaneous with dilation.
†Duration of each phase is influenced by such factors as parity, maternal emotions, position, level of activity, fetal size, and presentation position. For example, the labor of a nullipara tends to last longer, on average, than the labor of a multipara. Women who ambulate and assume upright positions or change positions frequently during labor tend to experience a shorter first stage. Descent is often prolonged in breech presentations and occiput posterior positions.
‡Women who have epidural analgesia for pain relief may not demonstrate some of these behaviors.

Assessment of Fetal Heart Rate and Pattern

It is important for the nurse to understand the relationship between the location of the PMI of the FHRs and fetal presentation, lie, and position. A high risk for childbirth complications may be revealed by variations in these findings. The PMI of the FHRs is the location on the maternal abdomen where the FHRs are heard the loudest. It is usually directly over the fetal back. The PMI is also an aid in determining the fetal presentation and position (Fig. 18-7 on p. 508). In a vertex presentation, FHRs are heard below the mother's umbilicus in either the right or the left lower quadrant of the abdomen. In a breech presentation, the FHRs are heard above the mother's umbilicus (Fig. 18-7, *A* and Fig. 18-8, *C*). As the fetus descends and rotates internally, the FHRs are heard lower and closer to the midline of the maternal abdomen. The PMI of the fetus in the right occipitoanterior (ROA) position moves to the midline just over the symphysis pubis (Fig. 18-8, *A* and *B*). Just before birth the fetal position is occipitoanterior (OA) and the fetal back is directly above the symphysis pubis. Diagrams of the PMI for different presentations and positions are presented in Fig. 18-7. The assessment recommended for determining fetal status in the low risk woman during each stage of labor is summarized in the Care Paths. The FHR must also be assessed (1) immediately after ROM, because this is the most common time for the umbilical cord to prolapse; (2) after any change in the contraction pattern or maternal status; and (3) before and after medicating the woman or performing a procedure (Tucker, 2004).

Assessment of Uterine Contractions

A general characteristic of effective labor is regular uterine activity; however, uterine activity is not directly related to labor progress. Uterine contractions are the primary powers that act involuntarily to expel the fetus and placenta from the uterus. Several methods are used to evaluate uterine contractions. These include the woman's subjective description, palpation and timing of the contraction by a health care provider, and electronic monitoring.

Care Path

LOW RISK WOMAN IN FIRST STAGE OF LABOR

	Cervical Dilation		
Care Management	**0-3 cm (Latent)**	**4-7 cm (Active)**	**8-10 cm (Transition)**
I. Assessment Measures*	*Frequency*	*Frequency*	*Frequency*
• Blood pressure, pulse, respirations	Every 30-60 min	Every 30 min	Every 15-30 min
• Temperature†	Every 4 hr	Every 4 hr	Every 4 hr
• Uterine activity	Every 30-60 min	Every 15-30 min	Every 10-15 min
• Fetal heart rate (FHR)	Every 30-60 min	Every 15-30 min	Every 15-30 min
• Vaginal show	Every 30-60 min	Every 30 min	Every 15 min
• Behavior, appearance, mood, energy level of woman; condition of partner	Every 30 min	Every 15 min	Every 5 min
• Vaginal examination‡	As needed to identify progress	As needed to identify progress	As needed to identify progress
II. Physical Care Measures§	Stay at home for as long as possible Relaxation measures; rest and sleep if at night Activity–ambulation; emphasize upright positions Diversional activities Nourishment–light foods and full liquids Void every 2 hr Perform basic hygiene measures	Coach breathing techniques Encourage effleurage Assist in using relaxation techniques between contractions Encourage ambulation, upright positions Assist with position changes Use comfort measures desired by woman: massage, hot/cold packs, touch, etc. Initiate hydrotherapy (shower, bath, jacuzzi) Provide nourishment as desired Encourage voiding every 2 hr Assist with hygiene, perineal care Provide pharmacologic pain relief as indicated Provide relief for partner	Coach breathing techniques Reduce touch if increased sensitivity is noted Help to relax between contractions Assist with position changes Use comfort measures according to acceptance level Continue hydrotherapy if effective Provide clear liquids: sips, ice chips Encourage voiding every 2 hr Provide hygiene measures, emphasizing mouth and perineal care Provide pharmacologic pain relief as indicated Prepare for birth
III. Emotional Support	Review birth plan Review process of labor–what to expect, pain management techniques available Redemonstrate breathing techniques Keep informed: progress, procedures	Provide feedback about performance Reduce distractions during contractions Role model comfort measures Reassure, encourage, praise Take charge, talk through contraction until control regained Continue to keep informed	Provide continuous support Reduce distractions Role model care measures to assist partner Continue reassurance, praise, and encouragement Keep informed Take charge as needed

*Full assessment using interview, physical examination, and laboratory testing is performed on admission. Subsequently, frequency of assessment is determined by the risk status of the maternal-fetal unit. More frequent assessment is required in high risk situations. Frequency of assessment and method of documentation are also determined by agency policy, which is usually based on the recommended care standards of medical and nursing organizations.

†If membranes have ruptured, the temperature should be assessed every 1 to 2 hr; assess orally or tympanically between contractions.

‡Perform vaginal examination at admission and thereafter only when signs indicate that progress has occurred (e.g., significant increase in frequency, duration, and intensity of contractions; rupture of membranes; perineal pressure); strict aseptic technique should be used. In the presence of vaginal bleeding, the primary health care provider performs the examination under a double setup in a delivery room, or an ultrasonography is performed to determine placental location.

§Physical care measures are performed by the nurse working together with the woman's partner and significant others. The woman is capable of greater independence in the latent phase but needs more assistance during the active and transition phases.

Each contraction exhibits a wavelike pattern. It begins with a slow increment (the "building up" of a contraction from its onset); gradually reaches an acme (the peak, with intrauterine pressure less than 80 mm Hg); and then diminishes rapidly (decrement, the "letting down" of the contraction). An interval of rest follows (intrauterine pressure less than 20 mm Hg) that ends when the next contraction begins (Tucker, 2004). The outward appearance of the woman's abdomen during and between contractions and the pattern of a typical uterine contraction are shown in Fig. 18-9.

Text continued on p. 506.

Labor Progress Chart

Admit date	Admit time	Blood type and Rh	Age	G	T	P	A	L	EDB __ / __ / __ LMP __ / __ / __	Membranes ☐ **Intact** ☐ Ruptured SROM AROM ☐ Bulging Date __/__/__Time __
__ / __ / __										

Current date __ / __ / __	**Time →**																		
Vital signs	Temperature																		
	Pulse																		
	Respiration																		
	Blood pressure																		
Maternal	Deep tendon reflexes (L/R)	/	/	/	/	/	/	/	/	/	/	/	/	/	/	/	/	/	/
	Urine (Protein/sugar)	/	/	/	/	/	/	/	/	/	/	/	/	/	/	/	/	/	/
	Vaginal bleeding																		
Uterine activity	Monitor mode																		
	Frequency																		
	Duration																		
	Intensity																		
	Resting tone																		
	Peak IUP																		
	MVUs																		
Fetal Assessment	Monitor mode																		
	Baseline (FHR)																		
	STV																		
	LTV																		
	Accelerations																		
	Decelerations																		
	Strip number																		
	Membranes																		
	Fluid																		
Intake/Output (ml's/Hr)	IV																		
	PO																		
	Urine																		
	Emesis																		
Cont meds	Pitocin mU/min																		
	$MgSO_4$ gm/hr																		
	Ritodrine mg/min																		
	Terbutaline mg/hr																		
Intervention	Position change																		
	O_2 L/min																		
	IV bolus																		
Initials																			

Abbreviations/Key	**Vaginal bleeding**	**Monitor mode uterine activity**	**MVUs montevideo units**	**Monitor mode fetal**	**STV short term variability**
	NS = Normal show ABN = Frank vaginal Bleeding	P = Palpation E = External I = Internal	The sum of the peak of each uterine contraction minus resting tone, in a 10 minute period.	A = Auscultation (fetoscope) D = Doppler E = External I = Internal	STV + = Present (roughness of tracing line present) STV Ø = Absent (tracing line is smooth)

Fig. 18-4 Labor progress chart. (Permission to use and/or reproduce this copyrighted material has been granted by the owner, Hollister, Inc., Libertyville, IL.)

Labor Progress Chart

Medication Allergy/Sensitivity ☐ **None**

(Identify)____ Chart________ of________

LTV (long term variability)	Accelerations	Decelerations	Membranes	Fluid
0-2 BPM = Absent 3-5 BPM = Minimal 6-25 BPM = Average >25 BPM = Marked	+ = 15 BPM ↑ × 15 sec 0 = Absent	N = None E = Early V = Variable L = Late P = Prolonged	I = Intact B = Bulging R = Ruptured	C = Clear M = Meconium stained B = Bloody F = Foul smelling NF = Not foul smelling

Fig. 18-4, cont'd For legend see opposite page.

Continued.

Labor Progress Chart

Time →		
Mark X •		10
Station	−4	9
Station	−3	Dilation 8
Station	−2	7
Station	−1	6
Station	0	5
Station	+1	4
Station	+2	3
Station	+3	2
Effacement % and/or position		
Examined by:		

IV Record

Start date	Time	Solution	Amount (mls)	Medication/Dose added	Initials	Infused date	Time	Amount infused

Teaching

Topic	Date time	Comments
Oriented		
Labor review		
Support person		
Pre-Op		
Safety		

Interval Medications

Date time	Medication/Dose	Route	Site	Initials

Initials	Signature

Progress Notes

Date	Time	

Fig. 18-4, cont'd For legend see page 502.

Labor Progress Chart

Progress Notes (Cont'd.)

Date	Time	

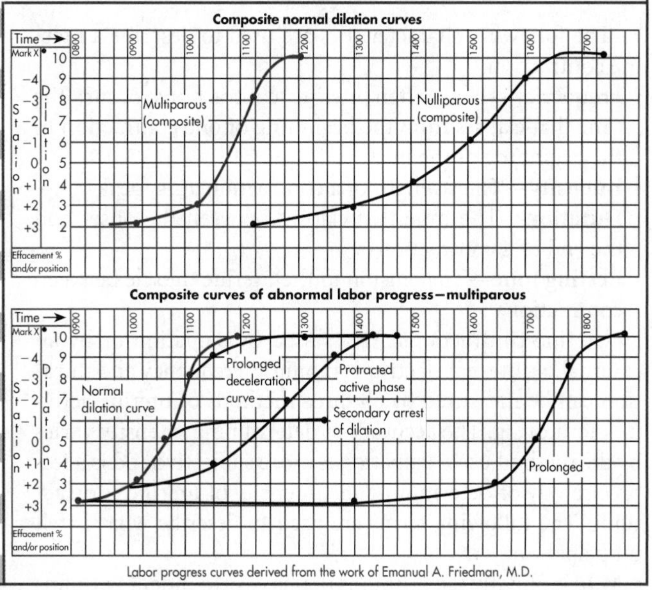

Labor progress curves derived from the work of Emanual A. Friedman, M.D.

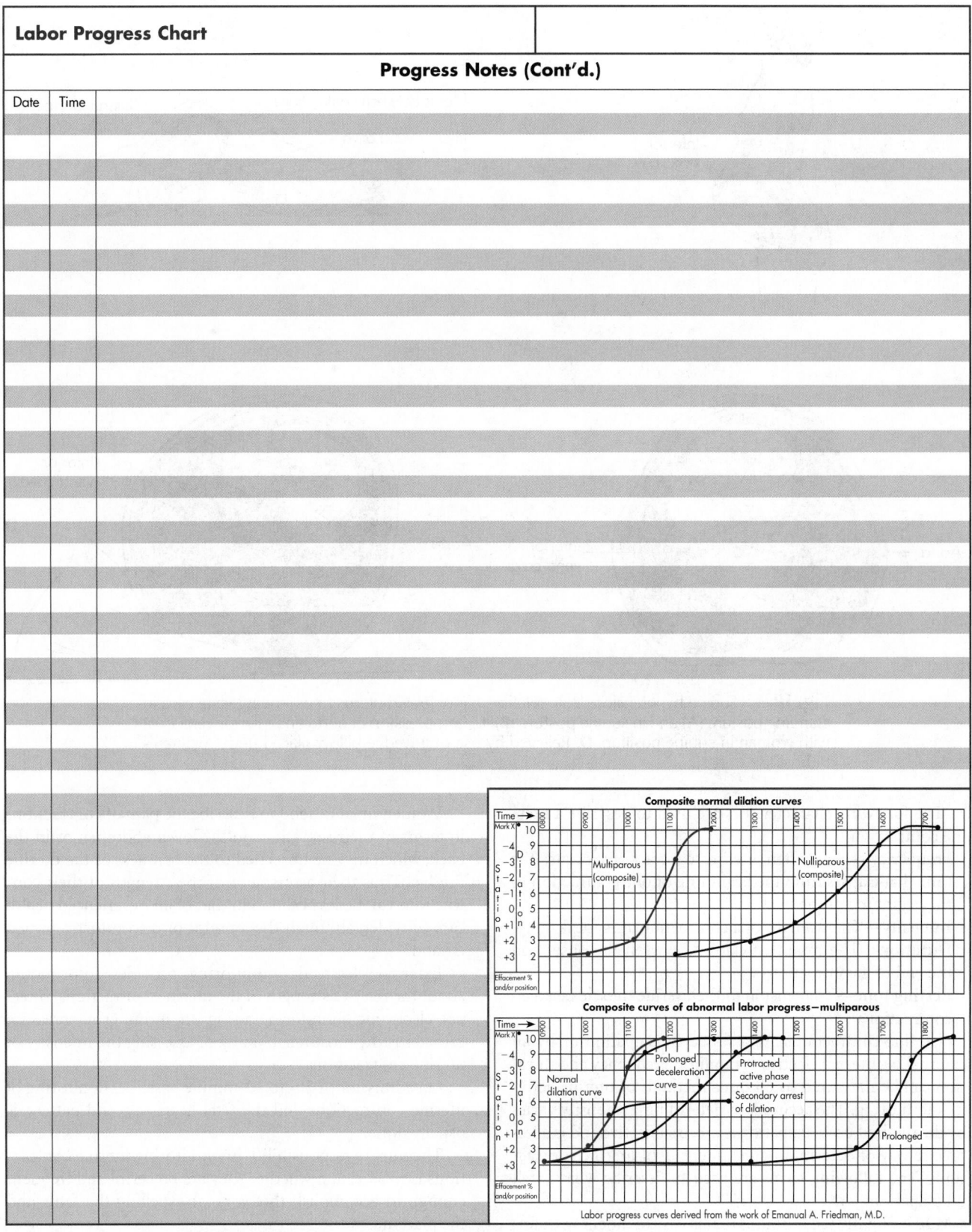

Fig. 18-4, cont'd For legend see page 502.

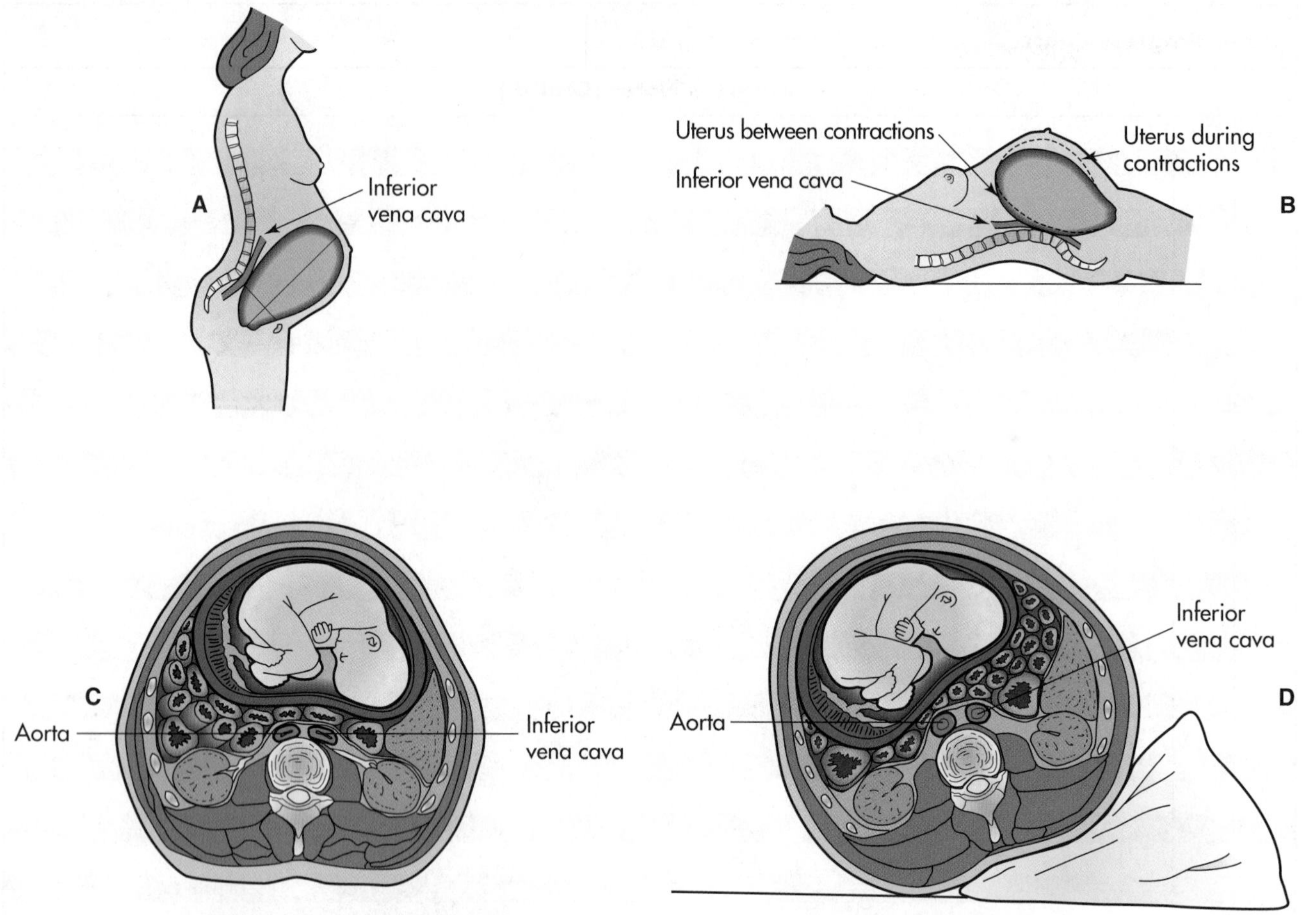

Fig. 18-5 Supine hypotension. Note relationship of gravid uterus to ascending vena cava in standing posture (**A**) and in supine posture (**B**). **C**, Compression of aorta and inferior vena cava with woman in supine position. **D**, Relieved by use of a wedge pillow placed under woman's right side.

The following characteristics are used to describe a uterine contraction:

- **Frequency**—How often uterine contractions occur; the time that elapses from the beginning of one contraction to the beginning of the next
- **Intensity**—The strength of a contraction at its peak
- **Duration**—The time that elapses between the onset and the end of a contraction
- **Resting tone**—The tension in the uterine muscle between contractions

Uterine contractions are assessed by palpation or by an external or internal electronic monitor. Frequency and duration can be measured by all three methods of uterine activity monitoring. The accuracy of determining intensity varies by the method used. Palpation is more subjective and is a less precise way of determining the intensity of uterine contractions. The following terms are used to describe what is felt on palpation:

- **Mild**—Slightly tense fundus that is easy to indent with fingertips (feels like touching finger to tip of nose)
- **Moderate**—Firm fundus that is difficult to indent with fingertips (feels like touching finger to chin)
- **Strong**—Rigid, boardlike fundus that is almost impossible to indent with fingertips (feels like touching finger to forehead)

Women in labor tend to describe the pain of contractions in terms of their sensations in the lower abdomen or in the back, which may be unrelated to the firmness of the uterine fundus. Thus their assessment of the strength of their contractions can be less valid than that of an experienced health care provider, although the amount of discomfort reported is valid.

External electronic monitoring provides information about the relative strength of the uterine contractions. Internal electronic monitoring using an intrauterine pressure catheter is the most reliable way of assessing the intensity of uterine contractions.

On admission, a 20- to 30-minute baseline monitoring of uterine contractions and the fetal heart rate and pattern is usually done.

The nurse's responsibility in monitoring uterine contractions is to ascertain whether they are powerful and frequent enough to accomplish the work of expelling the fetus and the placenta.

NURSE ALERT If the characteristics of contractions are found to be abnormal, either exceeding or falling below what is considered acceptable in terms of the standard characteristics, the nurse should report this to the primary health care provider. ■

BOX 18-5

Procedure: Leopold's Maneuvers and Determination of the Points of Maximum Intensity of the FHR

Leopold's Maneuvers

Wash hands.

Ask woman to empty bladder.

Position woman supine with one pillow under her head and with her knees slightly flexed.

Place small rolled towels under woman's right or left hip to displace uterus off major blood vessels (prevents supine hypotensive syndrome; see Fig. 18-5, *D*).

If right-handed, stand on woman's right, facing her:

1. Identify fetal part that occupies the fundus. The head feels round, firm, freely moveable, and palpable by ballottement; the breech feels less regular and softer. This maneuver identifies fetal lie (longitudinal or transverse) and presentation (cephalic or breech) (see Fig. 18-6, *A*).
2. Using palmar surface of one hand, locate and palpate the smooth convex contour of the fetal back and the irregularities that identify the small parts (feet, hands, elbows). This maneuver helps identify fetal presentation (see Fig. 18-6, *B*).
3. With right hand, determine which fetal part is presenting over the inlet to the true pelvis. Gently grasp the lower pole of the uterus between the thumb and fingers, pressing in slightly (see Fig. 18-6, *C*). If the head is presenting and not engaged, determine the attitude of the head (flexed or extended).
4. Turn to face the woman's feet. Using both hands, outline the fetal head (see Fig. 18-6, *D*) with the palmar surface of the fingertips. When the presenting part has descended deeply, only a small portion of it may be outlined. Palpation of the cephalic prominence helps identify the attitude of the head. If the cephalic prominence is bound on the same side as the small parts, this means that the head must be flexed and the vertex is presenting (see Fig. 18-6, *D*). If the cephalic prominence is on the same side as the back, this indicates that the presenting head is extended and the face is presenting (see Fig. 18-6, *D*).

Document fetal presentation, position, and lie and whether presenting part is flexed or extended, engaged, or free floating. Use hospital's protocol for documentation (e.g., "Vtx, LOA, floating").

Determination of PMI of FHT

Wash hands.

Perform Leopold's maneuvers.

Auscultate FHR based on fetal presentation identified with Leopold's maneuvers. The PMI is the location where the FHT are heard the loudest, usually over the fetal back (see Figs. 18-7 and 18-8).

Chart PMI of FHR using a two-line figure to indicate the four quadrants of the maternal abdomen, as follows: right upper quadrant (RUQ), left upper quadrant (LUQ), left lower quadrant (LLQ), and right lower quadrant (RLQ):

RUQ	LUQ
RLQ	LLQ

The umbilicus is the reference point for the quadrants (point where the lines cross). The PMI for the fetus in vertex presentation, in general flexion with the back on the mother's right side, commonly is found in the mother's right lower quadrant and is recorded with an "X" or with the FHR, as follows:

		or		
X			140	

Vaginal Examination

The vaginal examination reveals whether the woman is in true labor, and enables the examiner to determine whether the membranes have ruptured (Fig. 18-10). Because this examination is often stressful and uncomfortable for the woman, it should be performed only when indicated by the status of the woman and her fetus. For example, a vaginal examination should be performed on admission, when significant change has occurred in uterine activity, on maternal perception of perineal pressure or the urge to bear down, when membranes rupture, or when variable decelerations of the FHR are noted. A full explanation of the examination and support of the woman are important factors in reducing the stress and discomfort associated with the examination.

Cervical Effacement, Dilation, Fetal Descent

Uterine activity must be considered in the context of its effect on cervical effacement and dilation and on the degree of descent of the presenting part. The effect on the fetus must also be considered. Progress of labor can be effectively verified by the use of graphic charts (partograms) on which cervical dilation and station (descent) are plotted. This type of graphic charting assists in early identification of deviations from expected labor patterns. Figure 18-11 provides an example of one type of partogram; however, hospitals and birthing centers

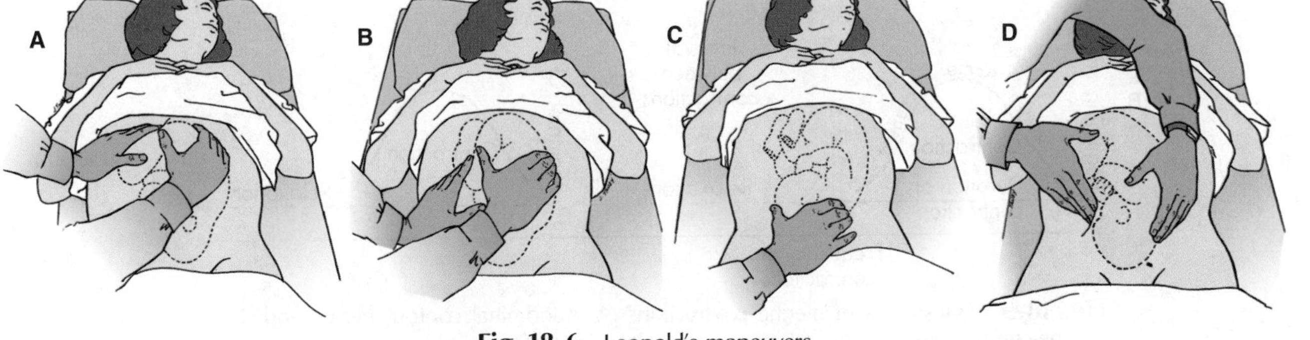

Fig. 18-6 Leopold's maneuvers.

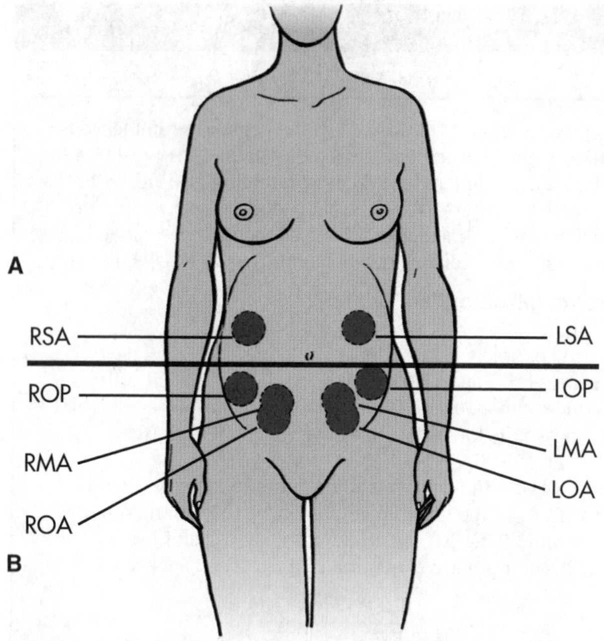

Fig. 18-7 Areas of maximum intensity of FHR for differing positions: *RSA,* right sacrum anterior; *ROP,* right occipitoposterior; *RMA,* right mentum anterior; *ROA,* right occipitoanterior; *LSA,* left sacrum anterior; *LOP,* left occipitoposterior; *LMA,* left mentum anterior; and *LOA,* left occipitoanterior. **A,** Presentation is *breech* if FHT are heard *above* umbilicus. **B,** Presentation is *vertex* if FHT are heard *below* umbilicus.

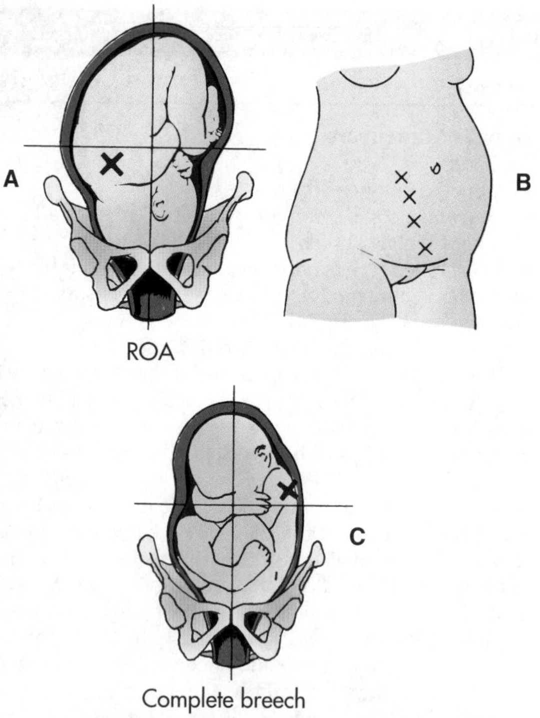

Lie: Vertical
Presentation: Breech (sacrum and feet presenting)
Reference point: Sacrum (with feet)
Attitude: General flexion

Fig. 18-8 Location of the FHR. **A,** With fetus in ROA position. **B,** Changes in location of PMI of FHT as fetus undergoes internal rotation from ROA to OA for birth. **C,** With fetus in left sacrum posterior position. (*A* and *C,* Courtesy Ross Laboratories, Columbus, OH.)

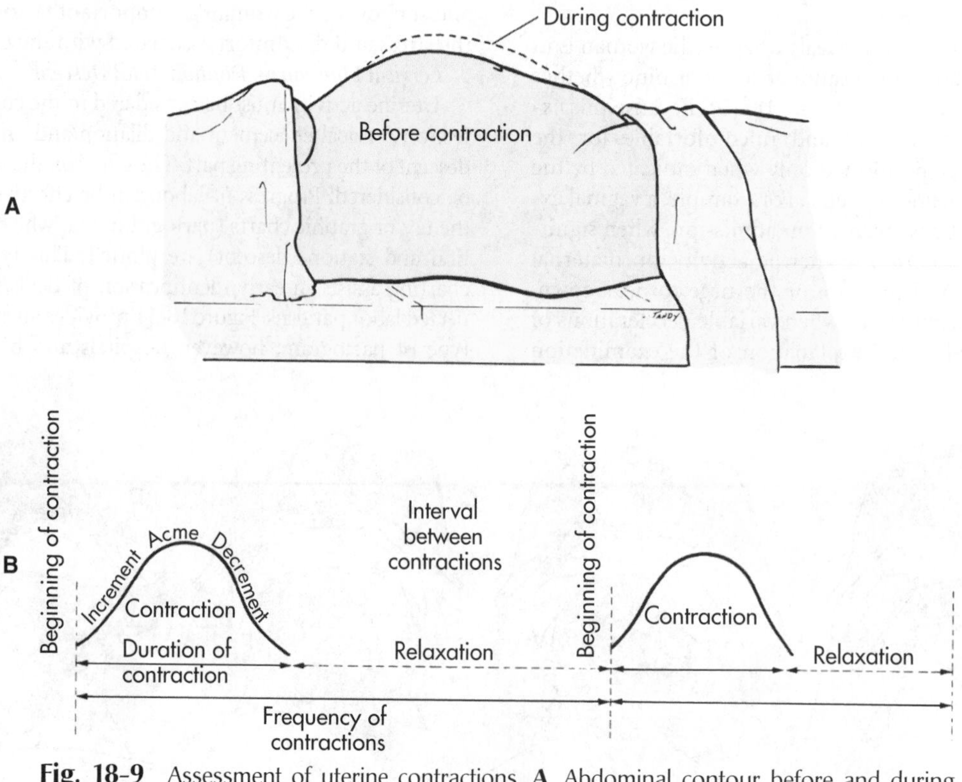

Fig. 18-9 Assessment of uterine contractions. **A,** Abdominal contour before and during uterine contractions. **B,** Wavelike pattern of contractile activity.

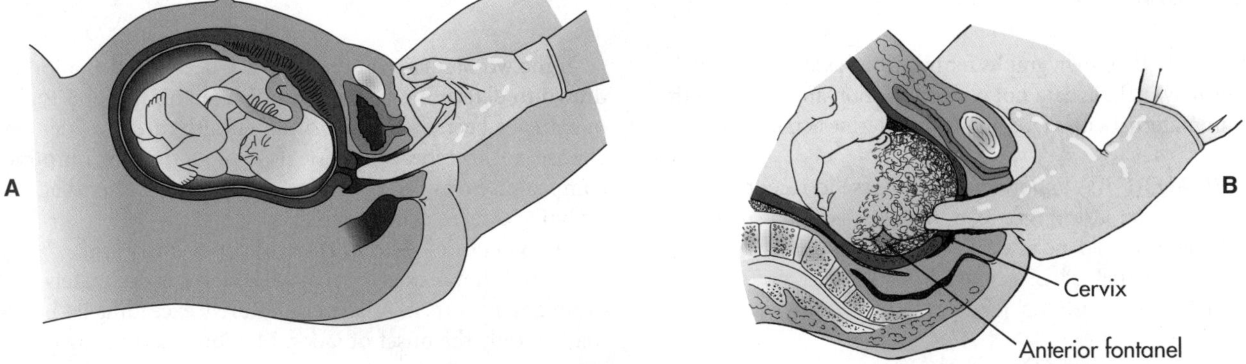

Fig. 18-10 Vaginal examination. **A,** Undilated, uneffaced cervix; membranes intact. **B,** Palpation of sagittal suture line. Cervix effaced and partially dilated.

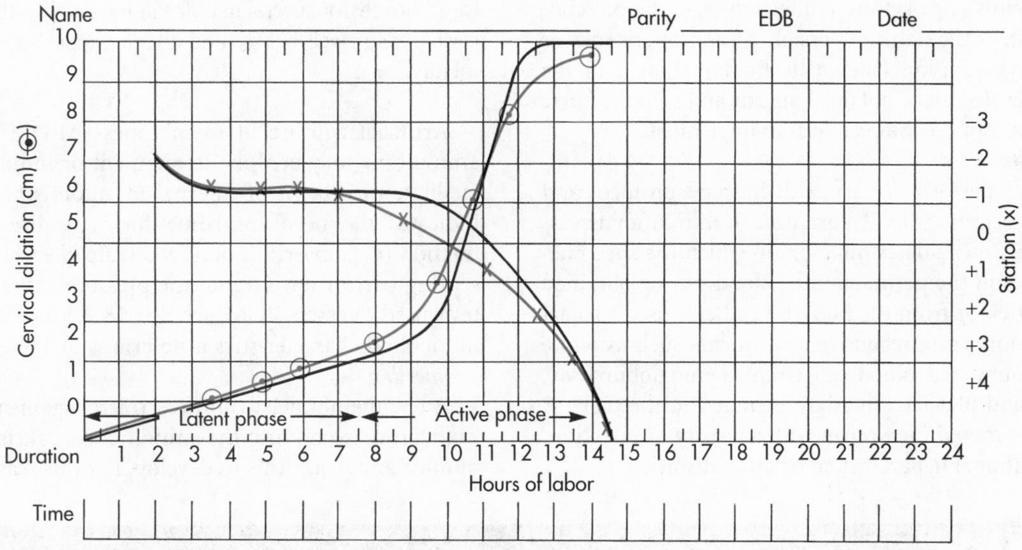

A

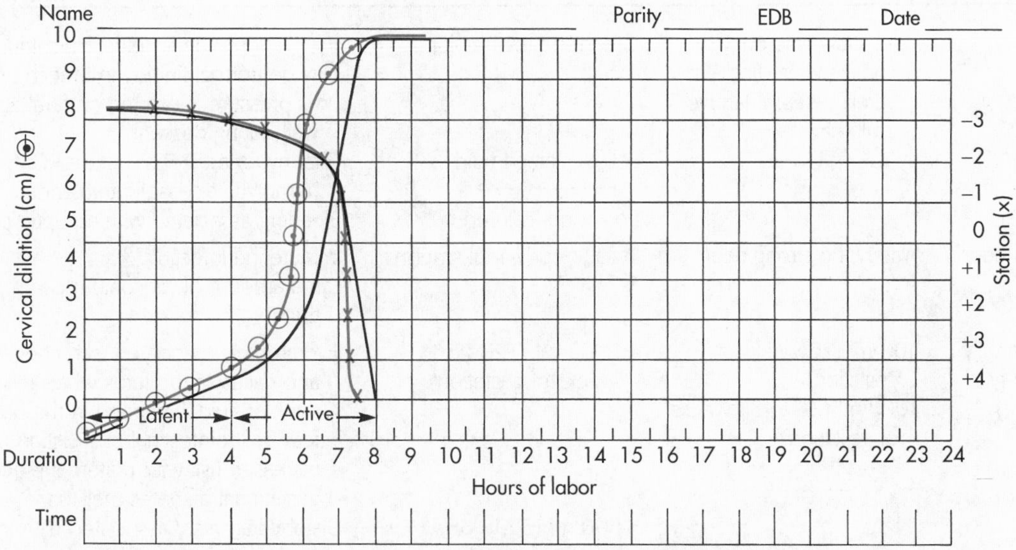

B

Fig. 18-11 Partogram for assessment of patterns of cervical dilation and descent. Individual woman's labor patterns *(colored)* are superimposed on prepared labor graph *(black)* for comparison. **A,** Nulliparous labor. **B,** Multiparous labor. The rate of cervical dilation is indicated by the symbol "O." A line drawn through the symbols depicts the slope of the curve. Station is indicated with an "X." A line drawn through the Xs reveals the pattern of descent.

may develop their own graphs for recording assessments. Such graphs may include data not only on dilation and descent but also on maternal vital signs, FHR, and uterine activity.

NURSE ALERT It is important for the nurse to recognize that active labor can last longer than the expected labor patterns. This finding should not be a cause for concern unless the maternal-fetal unit exhibits signs of distress (e.g., nonreassuring FHR patterns, maternal fever). ■

Laboratory and Diagnostic Tests

Analysis of Urine Specimen

A clean-catch urine specimen may be obtained to gather data about the pregnant woman's health. It is a convenient and simple procedure that can provide information about her hydration status (e.g., by specific gravity, color, and amount), nutritional status (e.g., ketones), infection (e.g., the presence of leukocytes), or the status of possible complications such as gestational hypertension (shown by finding protein in the urine). The results can be obtained quickly and help the nurse determine appropriate interventions to implement.

Blood Tests

Blood tests performed vary with hospital protocol and the woman's health status. An example of minimum assessment is a hematocrit determination, in which the specimen is centrifuged on the perinatal unit. Blood can be obtained by a finger stick or from the hub of a catheter used to start an IV line. More comprehensive assessments such as white blood cell count, red blood cell count, hemoglobin level, hematocrit, and platelet values are included in the CBC. A CBC may be ordered for women with a history of infection, anemia, gestational hypertension, or other disorders.

If the woman's blood type has not been verified, blood is drawn to determine the type and Rh factor. If blood typing has already been done, the primary health care provider may choose not to repeat the test. If obvious signs of immunocompromise or substance abuse are present, other diagnostic blood tests may be ordered.

Assessment of Amniotic Membranes and Fluid

Labor is initiated at term by SROM in approximately 25% of pregnant women. A lag period, rarely exceeding 24 hours, may precede the onset of labor. Membranes (the bag of waters) can also rupture spontaneously at any time during labor but most commonly in the transition phase of the first stage of labor.

NURSE ALERT The umbilical cord may prolapse when the membranes rupture. The FHR and pattern should be monitored closely for several minutes immediately after ROM, to ascertain fetal well-being, and the findings should be documented. ■

Artificial rupture of membranes (AROM or ARM) or amniotomy may be done to augment or induce labor or to facilitate placement of internal monitors when fetal status indicates the need for some form of direct assessment method (e.g., insertion of a fetal scalp electrode to the presenting part or an intrauterine pressure catheter). (For the tests used to assess ROM, see Box 18-2.) Assessment of amniotic fluid characteristics is described in Table 18-3.

Infection

After membranes rupture, microorganisms from the vagina can ascend into the amniotic sac, causing chorioamnionitis and placentitis to develop. For this reason, maternal

Table 18-3

Assessment of Amniotic Fluid

CHARACTERISTIC OF FLUID	NORMAL FINDING	DEVIATION FROM NORMAL FINDING	CAUSE OF DEVIATION FROM NORMAL
Color	Pale, straw colored; may contain white flecks of vernix caseosa, lanugo, scalp hair	Greenish brown color	Hypoxic episode in fetus; meconium in fluid May be normal finding in breech presentation as pressure is exerted on fetal abdominal wall during descent
		Yellow-stained fluid	Fetal hypoxia ≥36 hr before ROM; fetal hemolytic disease; intrauterine infection
		Port wine–colored	Bleeding associated with abruptio placentae
Viscosity and odor	Watery; no strong odor	Thick, cloudy, foul-smelling	Intrauterine infection Large amount of meconium can make fluid thick
Amount (normally varies with gestational age)	400 ml (20 weeks of gestation) 1000 ml (36 to 38 weeks of gestation)	≥2000 ml (32 to 36 weeks of gestation)	Hydramnios; associated with congenital anomalies of the fetus when fetus cannot drink or fluid is trapped in the body (e.g., fetal gastrointestinal obstruction or atresias); increased risk with maternal pregestational or gestational diabetes mellitus
		≤500 ml (32 to 36 weeks of gestation)	Oligohydramnios; associated with incomplete or absent kidney; obstruction of urethra; infant cannot secrete or excrete urine

ROM, rupture of membranes.

temperature and vaginal discharge are assessed frequently (every 1 to 2 hours) so that an infection developing after ROM can be identified early. Even when membranes are intact, however, microorganisms may ascend and cause premature rupture of membranes (PROM). Prophylactic antibiotics for prelabor ROM at term or preterm to protect against infection (chorioamnionitis) that involves both the maternal and fetal sides of the membrane is a form of care of unknown effectiveness (Enkin et al, 2000).

The nurse's responsibility is to report findings promptly to the primary health care provider and to document findings in the labor record and on the monitor strip (if that is agency policy). If abnormal findings are noted, continuous electronic monitoring is usually initiated and maintained for the duration of labor. The presence of meconium-stained amniotic fluid alerts the nurse of the need to observe fetal status more closely. After birth, the newborn may be at high risk for alteration in respiratory status if meconium is aspirated into the lungs with the first breath.

Assessment findings serve as a baseline for evaluating the woman's progress during labor. Although some problems of labor are anticipated, others may appear unexpectedly during the clinical course of labor (Box 18-6).

BOX 18-6

Signs of Potential Complications

Labor

- Intrauterine pressure of more than 75 mm Hg (determined by intrauterine pressure catheter monitoring) or resting tone of more than 15 mm Hg
- Contractions consistently lasting 90 seconds or more
- Contractions consistently occurring 2 minutes or less apart
- Fetal bradycardia, tachycardia, or persistently decreased variability
- Irregular FHR; suspected fetal dysrhythmias
- Appearance of meconium-stained or bloody fluid from the vagina
- Arrest in progress of cervical dilation or effacement, descent of the fetus, or both
- Maternal temperature of 38° C or more
- Foul-smelling vaginal discharge
- Persistent bright-red or dark-red vaginal bleeding

Nursing Diagnoses

Nursing diagnoses appropriate for the woman in first-stage labor include the following:

- *Anxiety related to*
  —negative experience with previous childbirth
  —cultural differences
- *Impaired urinary elimination related to*
  —reduced intake of oral fluids
  —diminished sensation of bladder fullness associated with epidural anesthesia/analgesia
- *Impaired fetal gas exchange related to*
  —maternal hypotension or hypertension
  —intense uterine contractions
  —compression of umbilical cord
- *Situational low self-esteem (maternal) related to*
  —inability to meet self-expectations concerning performance during childbirth
  —loss of control during labor

Nursing diagnoses that represent potential areas for concern during the second stage of labor include the following:

- *Risk for injury to mother and fetus related to*
  —persistent use of Valsalva maneuver
- *Situational low self-esteem related to*
  —deficient knowledge of normal, beneficial effects of vocalization during bearing-down efforts
  —inability to carry out plan for birth without medication
- *Ineffective coping related to*
  —coaching that contradicts woman's physiologic urge to push
- *Anxiety related to*
  —inability to control defecation with bearing-down efforts
  —lack of knowledge of perineal sensations associated with the urge to bear down

Examples of nursing diagnoses relevant to the third stage of labor include the following:

- *Risk for deficient fluid volume related to*
  —blood loss occurring following placental separation and expulsion
  —inadequate contraction of the uterus
- *Anxiety related to*
  —lack of knowledge regarding birth of the placenta
  —occurrence of perineal trauma and the need for repair
- *Fatigue related to*
  —energy expenditure associated with childbirth and the bearing-down efforts of the second stage

Expected Outcomes

The nurse and woman set and prioritize expected outcomes that focus on the woman, the fetus, and the woman's significant others. Expected outcomes for the woman in labor are that the woman will accomplish the following:

- Continue normal progression of labor while the fetal heart rate and pattern remain reassuring and without signs of distress
- Maintain adequate hydration status through oral or IV intake (or both)
- Actively participate in the labor process
- Verbalize discomfort and indicate the need for measures that help reduce discomfort and promote relaxation
- Accept comfort and support measures from significant others and health care providers as needed
- Sustain no injury to herself or the fetus during labor
- Expel the placenta with maternal blood loss of less than 500 ml or less than 1% of body weight
- Initiate, along with the partner and family, the processes of bonding and attachment with the newborn
- Express satisfaction with her performance during labor

Plan of Care and Implementation

Standards of Care

Standards of care guide the nurse in preparing for and implementing procedures with the expectant mother. Protocols for care based on standards include the following:

- Check the primary health care provider's orders

- Assess the orders for appropriateness and correctness (e.g., the dose and route of administration of the analgesic to be administered to relieve discomfort)
- Check labels on IV solutions, medications, and other materials used for nursing care
- Check the expiration date on any packs of supplies used for procedures
- Ensure that information on the woman's identification band is accurate (e.g., the band is the appropriate color for allergies)
- Use an empathic approach when giving care (see Guidelines/Guías box): When explaining procedures, use words the woman can understand; repeat as necessary
  - Respect the woman's individual needs and behaviors
  - Establish rapport with the woman and her significant others
  - Be kind, caring, and competent when performing necessary procedures
  - Be aware that pain and discomfort are as the woman describes them
  - Carry out appropriate comfort measures such as mouth care and back care
  - Include the support persons in the care as desired by the woman and the support persons
  - Recognize that a woman's current childbirth experience and the actions of nurses and other health care providers can have a positive or negative effect on the woman's future childbirth experiences
  - Use Standard Precautions, including precautions for invasive procedures as needed (see Box 18-4)
- Document care according to hospital guidelines and communicate information to the primary health care provider when indicated

ENGLISH SPANISH **Guidelines/Guías**

CARE DURING LABOR

Lie down, please.
Acuéstese, por favor.

I am going to take your vital signs.
Voy a verificar sus signos vitales.

I'm going to listen to the baby's heartbeat.
Voy a escuchar el latido del corazón del bebé.

This is a fetal monitor.
Este es un monitor fetal.

I need to examine you.
Necesito examinarle.

Do you need to use the bathroom?
¿Necesita usar el baño?

Would you like some pain medication?
¿Quisiera medicina para calmar el dolor?

Roll over on your side, please.
Póngase sobre un costado, por favor.

Relax.
Afloje los músculos.

Breathe deeply.
Respire profundamente.

Push.
Puje.

Don't push.
No puje.

Grab your knees and push.
Agárrese las rodillas y puje.

You're doing fine.
Bien. Muy bien.

Congratulations!
¡Felicidades!

You have a beautiful boy.
Usted tiene un niño precioso.

You have a beautiful girl.
Usted tiene una niña preciosa.

Physical Nursing Care during Labor

Physical nursing care of the woman in labor is an essential component of her care. The current emphasis on evidence-based practice supports the management of care by using this approach to enhance the safety, effectiveness, and acceptability of the physical care measures chosen to support the woman during labor and birth (Enkin et al, 2000). The various physical needs, the requisite nursing actions, and the rationale for care are presented in Table 18-4, the Nursing Care Plan, and the Care Paths (see also Table 18-2).

General Hygiene

Women in labor should be offered the use of showers or Jacuzzis, if they are available, to enhance the feeling of well-being and to minimize the discomfort of contractions. Women should also be encouraged to wash their hands after voiding and to perform self-hygiene measures. Linen should be changed if it becomes wet or stained with blood, and linen savers (Chux) should be used and changed as needed.

Nutrient and Fluid Intake

Oral Intake

Traditionally the laboring woman has been offered only clear liquids or ice chips, or given nothing by mouth, during the active phase of labor. This was to minimize the risk of anesthesia complications and their sequelae should general anesthesia be required in an emergency. These sequelae include aspiration of gastric contents and resultant compromise in oxygen perfusion, which may endanger the lives of the mother and fetus. This practice is being challenged today because regional anesthesia is used more often than general anesthesia, even for emergency cesarean births. Women are awake during regional anesthesia and are able to participate in their own care and protect their airway.

Although gastric emptying is slowed as a result of labor, stress, and the use of narcotics or sedatives, fasting does not cause gastric contents to be eliminated and may even cause them to be more acidic. In addition, fasting is identified by many laboring women as a stressor with which they must cope and a source of frustration during labor related to a loss of control with regard to meeting their own nourishment needs.

Adequate intake of fluids and calories is required to meet the energy demands and fluid losses associated with childbirth. The progress of labor slows and ketosis develops if these demands are not met, and fat is metabolized. Reduced energy for bearing-down efforts (pushing) increases the risk

Table 18-4

Physical Nursing Care during Labor

NEED	NURSING ACTIONS	RATIONALE
GENERAL HYGIENE		
Showers/bed baths, Jacuzzi bath	Assess for progress in labor	Determines appropriateness of the activity
	Supervise showers closely if woman is in true labor	Prevents injury from fall; labor may be accelerated
	Suggest allowing warm water to flow over back	Aids relaxation; increases comfort
Perineum	Cleanse frequently, especially after rupture of membranes and when show increases	Enhances comfort and reduces risk of infection
Oral hygiene	Offer toothbrush or mouthwash or wash the teeth with an ice-cold, wet washcloth as needed	Refreshes mouth; helps counteract dry, thirsty feeling
Hair	Brush, braid per woman's wishes	Improves morale; increases comfort
Handwashing	Offer washcloths before and after voiding and as needed	Maintains cleanliness; prevents infection
Face	Offer cool washcloth	Provides relief from diaphoresis; cools and refreshes
Gowns/linens	Change prn; fluff pillows	Improves comfort; enhances relaxation
NUTRIENT AND FLUID INTAKE		
Oral	Offer fluids and solid foods, following orders of primary health care provider and desires of laboring woman	Provides hydration and calories; enhances positive emotional experience and maternal control
Intravenous (IV)	Establish and maintain IV as ordered	Maintains hydration; provides venous access for medications
ELIMINATION		
Voiding	Encourage voiding at least every 2 hr	A full bladder may impede descent of presenting part; overdistention may cause bladder atony and injury, as well as postpartum voiding difficulty
Ambulatory woman	Allow ambulation to bathroom according to orders of primary health care provider, if:	
	The presenting part is engaged	Reinforces normal process of urination
	The membranes are not ruptured	Precautionary measure to protect against prolapse of umbilical cord
	The woman is not medicated	Precautionary measure to protect against injury
Woman on bed rest	Offer bedpan	Prevents complications of bladder distention and ambulation
	Allow tap water to run; pour warm water over the vulva; give positive suggestion	Encourages voiding
	Provide privacy	Shows respect for woman
	Put up side rails on bed	Prevents injury from fall
	Place call bell within reach	
	Offer washcloth for hands	Maintains cleanliness; prevents infection
	Wash vulvar area	Maintains cleanliness; enhances comfort; prevents infection
Catheterization	Catheterize according to orders of primary health care provider or hospital protocol if measures to facilitate voiding are ineffective	Prevents complications of bladder distention
	Insert catheter between contractions	Minimizes discomfort
	Avoid force if obstacle to insertion is noted	"Obstacle" may be caused by compression of urethra by presenting part
Bowel elimination—sensation of rectal pressure	Help the woman ambulate to bathroom or offer bedpan, after careful assessment	Prevents misinterpretation of rectal pressure from the presenting part as the need to defecate
	Perform vaginal examination	Determines degree of descent of presenting part
	Cleanse perineum immediately after passage of stool	Reduces risk of infection and sense of embarrassment

Nursing Care Plan

LABOR AND BIRTH

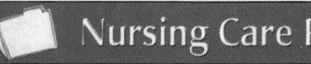

NURSING DIAGNOSIS: Anxiety related to labor and the birthing process

EXPECTED OUTCOME

Woman exhibits decreased signs of anxiety.

NURSING INTERVENTIONS/*RATIONALES*

Orient woman and significant others to labor and birth unit and explain admission protocol *to allay initial feelings of anxiety.*

Assess woman's knowledge, experience, and expectations of labor; note any signs or expressions of anxiety, nervousness, or fear *to establish a baseline for intervention.*

Discuss the expected progression of labor and describe what to expect during the process *to allay anxiety associated with the unknown.*

Actively involve woman in care decisions during labor, interpret sights and sounds of environment (monitor sights and sounds, unit activities), and share information on progression of labor (vital signs, FHR, dilation, effacement) *to increase her sense of control and allay fears.*

NURSING DIAGNOSIS: Acute pain related to increasing frequency and intensity of contractions

EXPECTED OUTCOME

Woman exhibits signs of ability to cope with discomfort.

NURSING INTERVENTIONS/*RATIONALES*

Assess woman's level of pain and strategies that she has used to cope with pain *to establish a baseline for intervention.*

Encourage significant other to remain as support person during labor process *to assist with support and comfort measures, because measures are often more effective when delivered by a familiar person.*

Instruct woman and support person in use of specific techniques such as conscious relaxation, focused breathing, effleurage, massage, and application of sacral pressure *to increase relaxation, decrease intensity of contractions, and promote use of controlled thought and direction of energy.*

Provide comfort measures such as frequent mouth care to prevent dry mouth, application of damp cloth to forehead, and changing of damp gown or bed covers *to relieve discomfort associated with diaphoresis; positioning to reduce stiffness.*

Explain which analgesics and anesthetics are available for use during labor and birth *to provide knowledge to help woman make decisions about pain control.*

NURSING DIAGNOSIS: Risk for impaired urinary elimination related to sensory impairment secondary to labor

EXPECTED OUTCOME

Bladder does not show signs of distention.

NURSING INTERVENTIONS/*RATIONALES*

Palpate the bladder superior to the symphysis on a frequent basis *to detect a full bladder that occurs from increased fluid intake and inability to feel urge to void.*

Encourage frequent voiding (at least every 2 hours) and catheterize if necessary to avoid bladder distention *because it impedes progress of fetus down birth canal and may result in trauma to the bladder.*

Assist to bathroom or commode to void if appropriate and provide privacy *to facilitate bladder emptying with an upright position (natural) and relaxation.*

NURSING DIAGNOSIS: Risk for ineffective individual coping related to birthing process

EXPECTED OUTCOME

Woman actively participates in the birth process with no evidence of injury to her or her fetus.

NURSING INTERVENTIONS/*RATIONALES*

Constantly monitor events of second-stage labor and birth, including physiologic responses of woman and fetus and emotional responses of woman and partner, *to ensure maternal, partner, and fetal well-being.*

Provide ongoing feedback to woman and partner *to allay anxiety and enhance participation.*

Continue to provide comfort measures and minimize distractions *to decrease discomfort and aid in focus on the birth process.*

Encourage woman to experiment with various positions *to assist downward movement of fetus.*

Ensure that woman takes deep cleansing breaths before and after each contraction *to enhance gas exchange and oxygen transport to the fetus.*

Encourage woman to push spontaneously when urge to bear down is perceived during a contraction *to aid descent and rotation of fetus.*

Encourage woman to exhale, holding breath for short periods while bearing down, *to avoid holding breath and triggering a Valsalva maneuver and increasing intrathoracic and cardiovascular pressure and decreasing perfusion of placental oxygen, placing the fetus at risk.*

Have woman take deep breaths and relax between contractions *to reduce fatigue and increase effectiveness of pushing efforts.*

Have mother pant as fetal head crowns *to control birth of head.*

Explain to woman and labor partner what is expected in the third stage of labor *to enlist cooperation.*

Have woman maintain her position *to facilitate delivery of the placenta.*

NURSING DIAGNOSIS: Fatigue related to energy expenditure required during labor and birth

EXPECTED OUTCOME

Woman's energy levels are restored.

NURSING INTERVENTIONS/*RATIONALES*

Educate woman and partner about need for rest and help them plan strategies (e.g., restricting visitors, increasing role of support systems performing functions associated with daily routines) that allow specific times for rest and sleep *to ensure that woman can restore depleted energy levels in preparation for caring for a new infant.*

Monitor woman's fatigue level and the amount of rest received *to ensure restoration of energy.*

NURSING DIAGNOSIS: Risk for deficient fluid volume related to decreased fluid intake and increased fluid loss during labor and birth

EXPECTED OUTCOMES

Fluid balance is maintained, and there are no signs of dehydration.

NURSING INTERVENTIONS/*RATIONALES*

Monitor fluid loss (i.e., blood, urine, perspiration) and vital signs; inspect skin turgor and mucous membranes for dryness *to evaluate hydration status.*

Administer oral/parenteral fluid per physician/nurse-midwife orders *to maintain hydration.*

Monitor the fundus for firmness after placental separation *to ensure adequate contraction and prevent further blood loss.*

for a forceps- or vacuum-assisted birth. This is most likely to occur in women who begin to labor early in the morning after a night without caloric intake. When women are permitted to consume fluids and food freely, they typically regulate their own oral intake, eating light foods (e.g., eggs, yogurt, ice cream, dry toast and jelly, fruit) and drinking fluids during early labor, then tapering off to an intake of clear fluid and sips of water or ice chips as labor intensifies and the second stage approaches. Common practice is to allow clear liquids (e.g., water, tea, apple juice, clear sodas, gelatin, broth) during early labor, tapering off to ice chips and sips of water as labor progresses and becomes more active. Food and fluid consumed orally during labor can meet a laboring woman's hydration and energy demands more effectively and safely than fluid administered intravenously. In addition, the woman's sense of control and level of comfort are enhanced.

Withholding of food and drink from women in labor has been identified as a form of care unlikely to be beneficial; offering oral fluids is demonstrably useful and should be encouraged (Enkin et al, 2000). Nurses should follow the orders of the woman's primary health care provider when offering the woman food or fluids during labor. As advocates, however, nurses can facilitate change by informing others of the current research findings that support the safety and effectiveness of the oral intake of food and fluid during labor and by initiating such research themselves.

Intravenous Intake

Fluids are administered intravenously to the laboring woman to maintain hydration, especially when a labor is long and the woman is unable to ingest a sufficient amount of fluid orally or if she is receiving epidural or intrathecal analgesia. However, routine use of IV fluids during labor is a form of care that is unlikely to be beneficial and may be harmful (Enkin et al, 2000). In most cases, an electrolyte solution without glucose is adequate and does not introduce excess glucose into the bloodstream. The latter is important because an excessive maternal glucose level results in fetal hyperglycemia and fetal hyperinsulinism. After birth, the neonate's high level of insulin will then deplete his or her glucose stores and hypoglycemia will result. If maternal ketosis occurs, the primary health care provider may order an IV solution containing a small amount of dextrose to provide the glucose needed to assist in fatty acid metabolism.

NURSE ALERT Nurses should carefully monitor the intake and output of laboring women receiving IV fluids because they also face an increased danger of hypervolemia as a result of the fluid retention that occurs during pregnancy. ■

Elimination

Voiding

Voiding every 2 hours should be encouraged. A distended bladder may impede descent of the presenting part, inhibit uterine contractions, and lead to decreased bladder tone or atony after birth. Women who receive epidural analgesia or anesthesia are especially at risk for retention of urine, and the need to void should be assessed more frequently in them.

The woman should be assisted to the bathroom to void unless the primary health care provider has ordered bed rest; the woman is receiving epidural analgesia or anesthesia; or, in the nurse's judgment, ambulation would compromise the status of the laboring woman or her fetus. External monitoring can usually be interrupted for the woman to go to the bathroom.

Catheterization

If the woman is unable to void and her bladder is obviously distended, she may need to be catheterized. Most hospitals have protocols that rely on the nurse's judgment concerning the need for catheterization. Before performing the catheterization, the nurse should clean the vulva and perineum because vaginal show and amniotic fluid may be present. During the catheterization, if there appears to be an obstacle that prevents advancement of the catheter, this is most likely the presenting part. If the catheter cannot be advanced, the nurse should stop the procedure and notify the primary health care provider of the difficulty.

Bowel Elimination

Most women do not have bowel movements during labor because of decreased intestinal motility. Stool that has formed in the large intestine often is moved downward toward the anorectal area by the pressure exerted by the fetal presenting part as it descends. This stool is often expelled during second-stage pushing and birth. However, the passage of stool with bearing-down efforts increases the risk of infection and may embarrass the woman, thereby reducing the effectiveness of these efforts. To prevent these problems, the nurse should immediately cleanse the perineal area to remove any stool, while at the same time reassuring the woman that the passage of stool at this time is a normal and expected event, because the same muscles used to expel the baby also expel stool. Routine use of an enema to empty the rectum is considered to be harmful or ineffective and should be eliminated (Enkin et al, 2000).

When the presenting part is deep in the pelvis, even in the absence of stool in the anorectal area, the woman may feel rectal pressure and think she needs to defecate. If the woman expresses the need to defecate, the nurse should perform a vaginal examination to assess cervical dilation and station. When a multiparous woman experiences the urge to defecate, this often means that birth will follow quickly.

Ambulation and Positioning

Freedom of maternal movement and choice of position through labor are forms of care likely to be beneficial for the laboring woman and should be encouraged (Enkin et al, 2000).

The potential advantages of ambulation include enhanced uterine activity, distraction from the discomfort of labor, enhanced maternal control, and an opportunity for close interaction with the woman's partner and care provider as they help her to walk. Ambulation is associated with a reduced rate of operative delivery (i.e., cesarean birth, forceps- and vacuum-assisted birth) and less frequent use of narcotic analgesia.

Walking, sitting, or standing during early labor is more comfortable than lying down and facilitates the progress of labor (Simkin & Ancheta, 2000). Ambulation should be encouraged if membranes are intact, if the fetal presenting part is engaged after rupture of membranes, and if the woman has not received medication for pain (Fig. 18-12). The woman may find it comfortable to stand and lean forward on her partner, doula, or nurse for support at times during labor (Fig. 18-13, *A*). Ambulation may be contraindicated, however, because of maternal or fetal status.

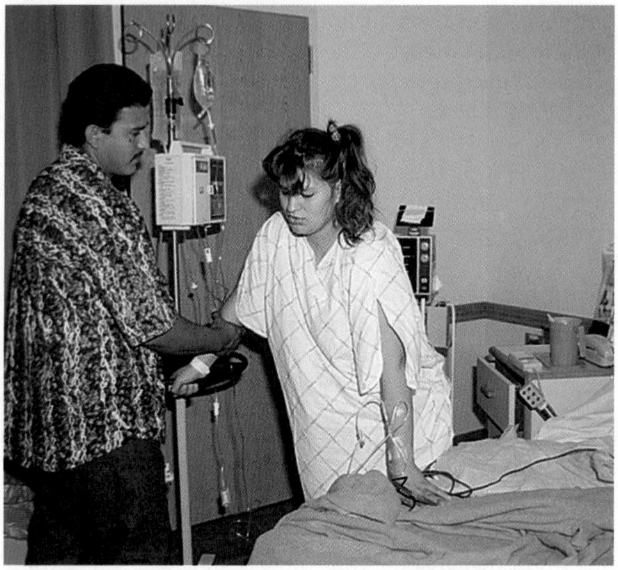

Fig. 18-12 Woman preparing to walk with partner. (Courtesy Marjorie Pyle, RNC, Lifecircle, Costa Mesa, CA.)

When the woman lies in bed she will usually change her position spontaneously as labor progresses. If she does not change position every 30 to 60 minutes, she should be assisted to do so. The side-lying (lateral) position promotes optimal uteroplacental and renal blood flow and increases oxygen saturation (Fig. 18-13, *B*). If the woman wants to lie supine, the nurse may place a pillow under one hip as a wedge to prevent the uterus from compressing the aorta and vena cava. Sitting is not contraindicated unless it adversely affects fetal status, which can be determined by checking the fetal heart rate and pattern. If the fetus is in the occiput posterior position, it may be helpful for the woman to squat during contractions because this position increases pelvic diameter, allowing the head to rotate to a more anterior position (Fig. 18-14, *A*). A hands-and-knees position during contractions is also recommended to facilitate the rotation of the fetal occiput from a posterior to an anterior position as gravity pulls the fetal back forward (Fig. 18-14, *B*). A variety of positions recommended for the laboring woman are described in Box 18-7.

A birth ball (gymnastic ball, also used in physical therapy) can be used to support a woman's body as she assumes a variety of labor and birth positions (Fig. 18-15). The woman can sit on the ball while leaning over the bed, or she can lean over the ball to support her upper body and reduce stress on her arms and hands when she assumes a hands-and-knees position. The birth ball can encourage pelvic mobility and pelvic and perineal relaxation when the woman sits on the firm yet pliable ball and rocks in rhythmic movements. Warm compresses applied to the perineum can maximize this relaxation effect. The birth ball should be large enough so that when the woman sits, her knees are bent at a 90-degree angle and her feet are flat on the floor and approximately 2 feet apart.

Supportive Care during Labor and Birth

Support during labor and birth involves emotional support, physical care and comfort measures, and provision of advice and information (Davies & Hodnett, 2002; Miltner, 2000). Effective physical and emotional support provided to women during labor can result in shorter labors, reduced rates of complications and surgical or obstetric interventions (e.g., cesarean births, labor augmentations and inductions, episiotomies, and forceps-assisted births), and enhanced self-esteem and satisfaction (Gagnon & Waghorn, 1999; Miltner, 2000).

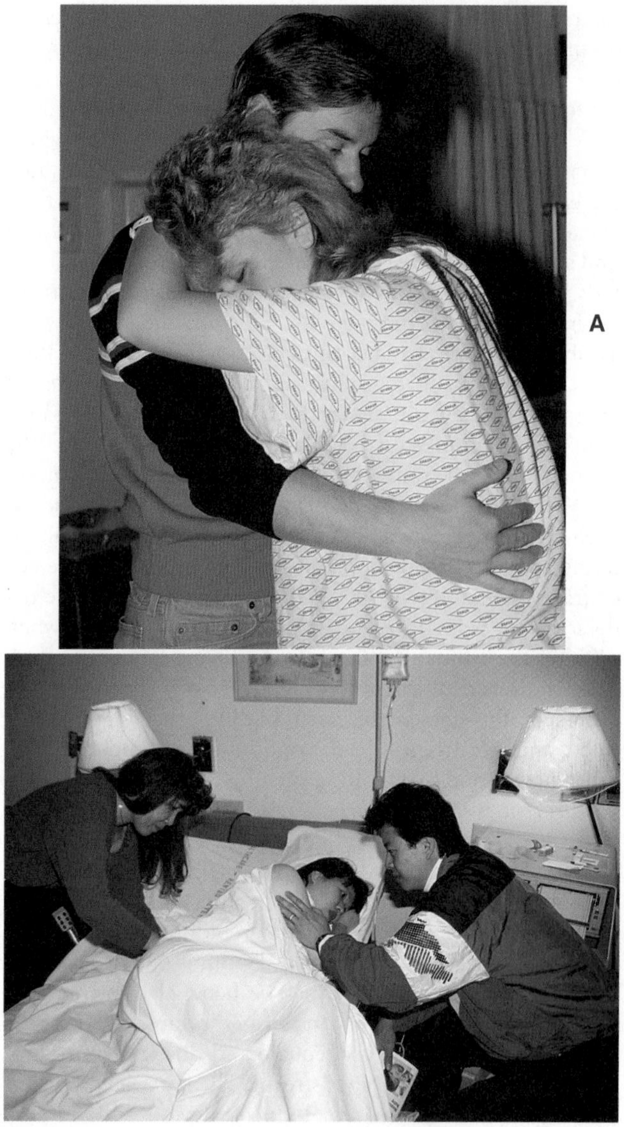

A

B

Fig. 18-13 **A**, Woman standing and leaning forward with support. **B**, Lateral position. Support person is applying sacral pressure while partner provides encouragement. (Courtesy Marjorie Pyle, RNC, Lifecircle, Costa Mesa, CA.)

Labor rooms should be airy, clean, and homelike. The laboring woman should feel safe in this environment and free to be herself and to use the comfort and relaxation measures she prefers. To enhance relaxation, bright overhead lights should be turned off when not needed. Noise and intrusions should be kept to a minimum. The temperature is controlled to ensure the laboring woman's comfort. The room should be large enough to accommodate a comfortable chair for the woman's partner, the monitoring equipment, and hospital personnel. Couples may be encouraged to bring extra pillows to make the hospital surroundings more homelike and to facilitate position changes.

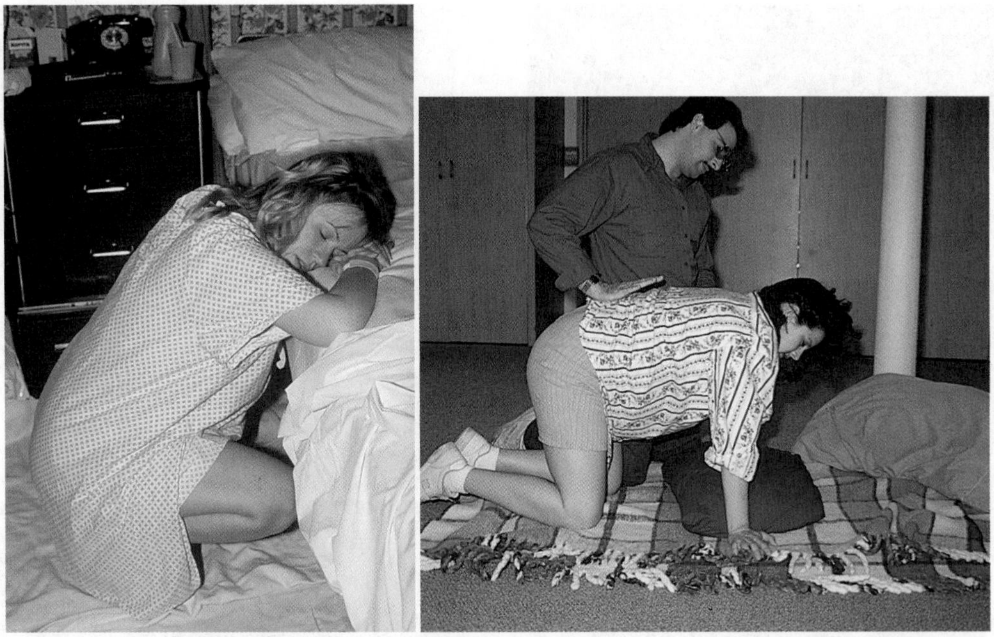

Fig. 18-14 Maternal positions for labor. **A,** Squatting. **B,** Woman in hands-and-knees position. (Courtesy Marjorie Pyle, RNC, Lifecircle, Costa Mesa, CA.)

BOX 18-7

Some Maternal Positions* during Labor and Birth

Semirecumbent Position

With woman sitting with her upper body elevated to at least a 30° angle, place wedge or small pillow under hip to prevent vena caval compression and reduce likelihood of supine hypotension (see Fig. 18-5, *B*).

- The greater the angle of elevation, the more gravity or pressure is exerted, which promotes fetal descent, the progress of contractions, and the widening of pelvic dimensions.
- Convenient for rendering care measures and for external fetal monitoring.

Lateral Position (See Fig. 18-13, *B*)

Have woman alternate between left and right side-lying position, and provide abdominal and back support as needed for comfort.

- Removes pressure from the vena cava and back; enhances uteroplacental perfusion and relieves backache.
- Makes it easier to perform back massage or counterpressure.
- Associated with less frequent, but more intense, contractions.
- Obtaining good external fetal monitor tracings may be more difficult.
- May be used as a birthing position.
- Takes pressure off perineum.

Upright Position

The gravity effect enhances the contraction cycle and fetal descent: the weight of the fetus places increasing pressure on the cervix; the cervix is pulled upward, facilitating effacement and dilation; impulses from the cervix to the pituitary gland increase, causing more oxytocin to be secreted; and contractions are intensified, thereby applying more forceful downward pressure on the fetus, but they are less painful.

- Fetus is aligned with pelvis, and pelvic diameters are widened slightly.
- Effective upright positions include the following:
  - –Ambulation (see Fig. 18-12).
  - –Standing and leaning forward with support provided by coach, end of bed, back of chair, or birth ball; relieves backache and facilitates application of counterpressure or back massage (see Fig. 18-13, *A*).
  - –Sitting up in bed, chair, birthing chair, on toilet or bedside commode.
  - –Squatting (see Fig. 18-14, *A*).

Hands-and-Knees Position—Ideal Position for Posterior Positions of the Presenting Part (see Fig. 18-14, *B*)

Assume an "all-fours" position in bed or on a covered floor; allows for pelvic rocking.

- Relieves backache characteristic of "back labor."
- Facilitates internal rotation of the fetus by increasing mobility of the coccyx, increasing the pelvic diameters, and using gravity to turn the fetal back and rotate the head.

*Assess the effect of each position on the laboring woman's comfort and anxiety level, progress of labor, and fetal heart rate and pattern. Alternate positions every 30 to 60 minutes.

The nurse can alleviate a woman's anxiety by explaining unfamiliar terms, providing information and explanations without her having to ask, and preparing her for sensations she will experience and procedures that will follow. By encouraging the woman or couple to ask questions and by providing honest, understandable answers, the nurse can play a significant role in helping the woman achieve a satisfying birth experience (Miltner, 2002).

Supportive nursing care for a woman in labor includes all of the following:

- Helping the woman maintain control and participate to the extent she wishes in the birth of her infant

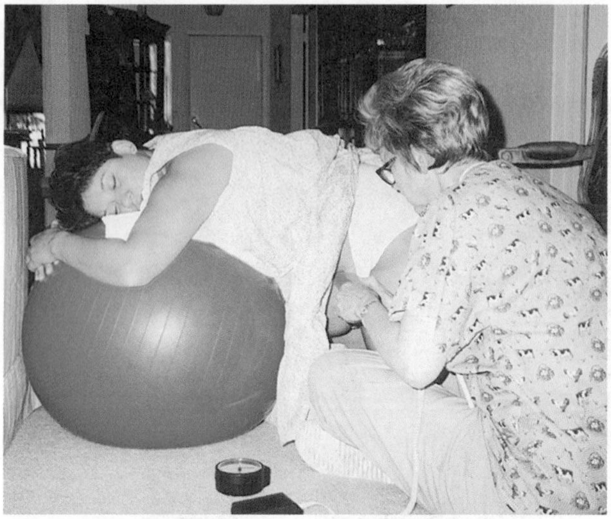

Fig. 18-15 Laboring woman using birth ball. (Courtesy Polly Perez, Cutting Edge Press, Johnson, VT.)

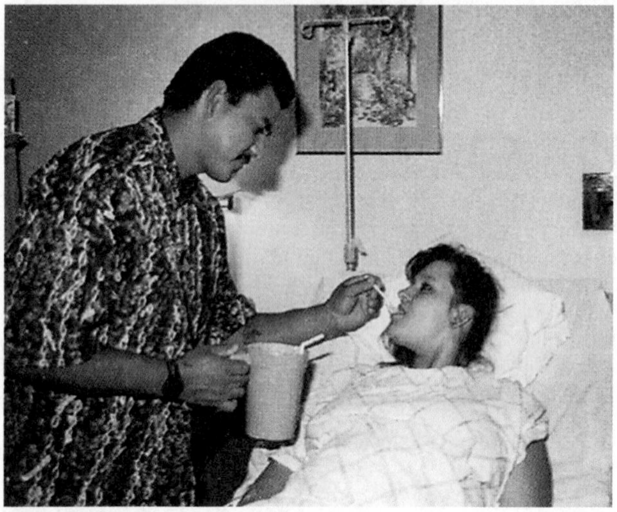

Fig. 18-16 Partner providing comfort measures. (Courtesy Marjorie Pyle, RNC, Lifecircle, Costa Mesa, CA.)

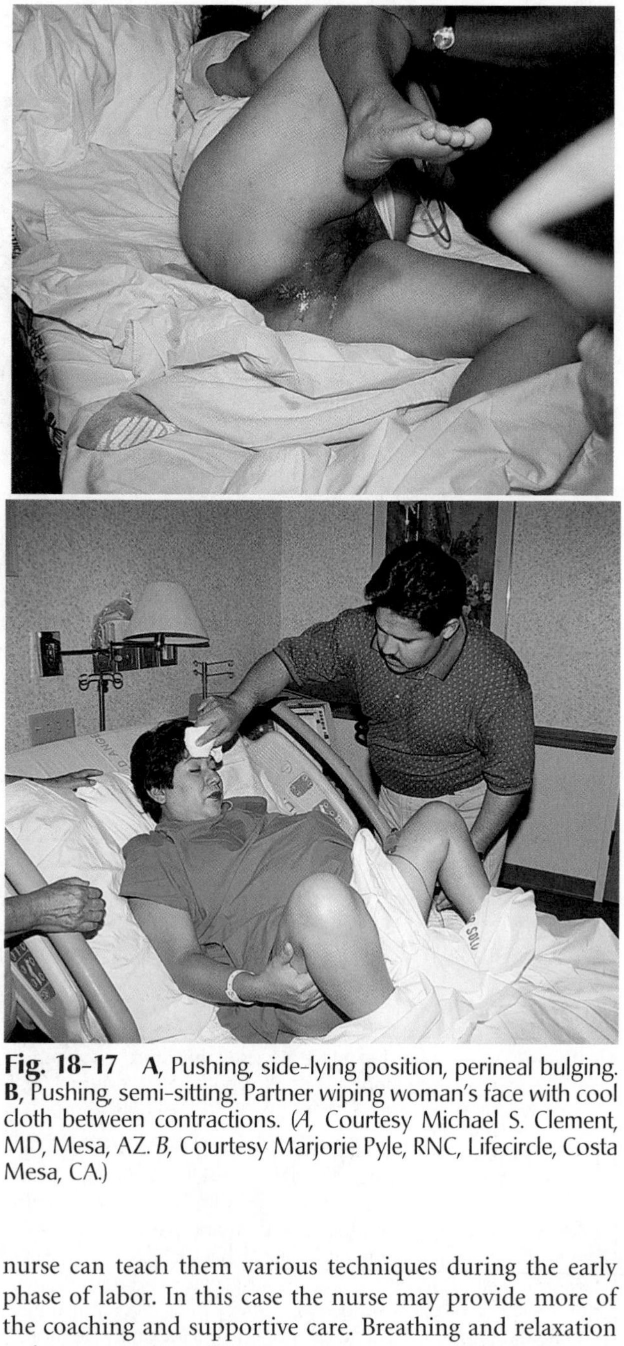

A

B

Fig. 18-17 **A**, Pushing, side-lying position, perineal bulging. **B**, Pushing, semi-sitting. Partner wiping woman's face with cool cloth between contractions. (*A*, Courtesy Michael S. Clement, MD, Mesa, AZ. *B*, Courtesy Marjorie Pyle, RNC, Lifecircle, Costa Mesa, CA.)

- Meeting the woman's expected outcomes for her labor
- Acting as the woman's advocate, supporting her decisions and respecting her choices as appropriate and relating her wishes as needed to other health care providers
- Helping the woman conserve her energy
- Helping control the woman's discomfort
- Acknowledging the woman's efforts, as well as those of her partner, during labor and providing positive reinforcement
- Protecting the woman's privacy and modesty

The nurse serves as a coach to the woman in the absence of other support persons or as an assistant coach to the support persons present. To do this, the nurse must have a thorough knowledge of breathing and relaxation techniques.

Couples who have attended childbirth education programs will know something about the labor process, coaching techniques, and comfort measures. Even when expectant parents have not attended childbirth education classes, the nurse can teach them various techniques during the early phase of labor. In this case the nurse may provide more of the coaching and supportive care. Breathing and relaxation techniques and comfort measures as described in Chapter 16 can be implemented.

Comfort measures vary with the situation (Figs. 18-16 and 18-17, *B*). The nurse can draw on the couple's repertoire of comfort measures learned during the pregnancy. Such measures include maintaining a comfortable, supportive atmosphere in the labor and birth area; using touch therapeutically (e.g., heat or cold applied to the lower back in the event of back labor, a cool cloth applied to the forehead); providing nonpharmacologic measures to relieve discomfort; administering analgesics when necessary; and most of all, just being there (see Tables 18-1 and 18-5; see also the Care Paths on pp. 501 and 526). See Chapter 16 for a full discussion of both pharmacologic and nonpharmacologic comfort measures.

Most women in labor respond positively to touch. They appreciate gentle handling by staff members. Back rubs and counterpressure may be offered, especially if the woman is experiencing back labor. A support person may be taught to exert counterpressure against the woman's sacrum over the occiput of the head of a fetus in a posterior position (see Fig. 18-13, *B*). The back pain is caused by the occiput pressing on spinal nerves, and counterpressure lifts the occiput off these nerves, thereby providing some relief from pain. Once counterpressure is initiated, the woman usually asks her partner to continue doing this for each following contraction. The partner will need to be relieved after a while, however, because exerting counterpressure is hard work. Hand and foot massage also can be soothing and relaxing (Simkin & Ancheta, 2000).

Table 18-5

Woman's Responses and Support Person's Actions during First Stage of Labor

WOMAN'S RESPONSES	NURSE/SUPPORT PERSON'S ACTIONS*
DILATION OF CERVIX 0-3 CM (LATENT) (contractions 10-30 sec long, 5-30 min apart, mild to moderate)	
Mood: alert, happy, excited, mild anxiety	Provides encouragement, feedback for relaxation, companionship
Settles into labor room; selects focal point	Assists to cope with contractions
Rests or sleeps, if possible	Encourages use of focusing techniques
Uses breathing techniques	Helps to concentrate on breathing techniques
Uses effleurage, focusing, and relaxation techniques	Uses comfort measures
	Assists woman into comfortable position
	Informs woman of progress; explains procedures and routines
	Gives praise
	Offers fluids, ice chips as ordered
DILATION OF CERVIX 4-7 cm (ACTIVE) (contractions 30-45 sec long, 3-5 min apart, moderate to strong)	
Mood: seriously labor oriented, concentration and energy needed for contractions, alert, more demanding	Acts as buffer; limits assessment techniques to between contractions
Continues relaxation, focusing techniques	Assists with contractions
Uses breathing techniques	Encourages woman as needed to help her maintain breathing techniques
	Uses comfort measures
	Assists with frequent position changes, emphasizing side-lying and upright positions
	Encourages voluntary relaxation of muscles of back, buttocks, thighs, and perineum; effleurage
	Applies counterpressure to sacrococcygeal area
	Encourages and praises
	Keeps woman aware of progress
	Offers analgesics as ordered
	Checks bladder; encourages her to void
	Gives oral care; offers fluids, ice chips as ordered
DILATION OF CERVIX 8-10 cm (TRANSITION) (contractions 45-90 sec long, 2-3 min apart, strong)	
Mood: irritable, intense concentration, symptoms of transition (e.g., nausea, vomiting)	Stays with woman; provides constant support
Continues relaxation, needs greater concentration to do this	Assists with contractions
Uses breathing techniques	Reminds, reassures, and encourages woman to reestablish breathing pattern and concentration as needed
Uses 4:1 breathing pattern if using psychoprophylactic techniques	Alerts woman to begin breathing pattern before contraction becomes too intense if she is sedated or drowsy
Uses panting to overcome response to urge to push	Prompts panting respirations if woman begins to push prematurely
	Uses comfort measures
	Accepts woman's inability to comply with instructions
	Accepts irritable response to helping, such as counterpressure
	Supports woman who has nausea and vomiting; gives oral care as needed; gives reassurance regarding signs of end of first stage
	Uses relaxation techniques (effleurage and voluntary relaxation)
	Keeps woman aware of progress

*Provided by nurses and by support persons in collaboration with the nurse.

Many women become more sensitive to touch (hyperesthesia) as labor progresses; this is a typical response during transition (see Table 18-2). They may tell their coach to leave them alone or not to touch them. The partner who is unprepared for this normal response may feel rejected and may react by withdrawing active support. The nurse can reassure him or her that this response is a positive indication that the first stage is ending and the second stage is approaching. Women with increased sensitivity to touch may have a positive response when touched on surfaces of the body where hair does not grow, such as the forehead, the palms of the hands, and the soles of the feet.

Although a woman or a man other than the father may be the woman's partner, the father of the baby is usually the support person during labor. He often is able to provide the comfort measures and touch that the laboring woman needs. When the woman becomes focused on her pain, sometimes the partner can persuade her to try nonpharmacologic variations of comfort measures. In addition, he usually is able to interpret the woman's needs and desires to staff members.

The father will be exposed to many sights and smells he may never before have experienced. Therefore it is important to tell him what to expect and to make him feel comfortable about leaving the room to regain his composure should something occur that surprises him. Before he leaves the room, provision should be made for someone else to support the woman during his absence. Staff members should tell the father that his presence is helpful and encourage him to be involved in the care of the woman to the extent to which he is comfortable. They can reassure him that he is not assuming the responsibility for observation and management of his partner's labor, but that his responsibility is to support her as the labor progresses. The nurse can suggest alternative comfort measures when those he is using are no longer helpful or are rejected by his partner (Table 18-5).

Ways in which the nurse can support the father-partner are detailed in Box 18-8. A well-informed father can make an important contribution to the health and well-being of the mother and child, their family interrelationship, and his self-esteem.

Labor Support by Doulas

Continuity of care in labor can be met by a specially trained, experienced female labor attendant called a *doula.* The doula provides a continuous, one-on-one caring presence throughout the labor and birth process of the woman she is attending. This is a beneficial form of care (Enkin et al, 2000) (Evidence-Based Practice). The primary role of the doula is to focus on the laboring woman and provide physical and emotional support by using soft, reassuring words; touching, stroking, and hugging; administering comfort measures to reduce pain and enhance relaxation; and walking with the woman, helping her to change positions, and coaching her bearing-down efforts. Doulas provide information and explain procedures and events. They advocate for the woman's right to participate actively in the management of her labor (Kayne, Greulich, & Albers, 2001).

The doula also supports the woman's partner, who often feels unqualified to be the sole labor support. The doula can encourage and praise the partner's efforts, create a partnership as caregivers, and provide respite care. Doulas also facilitate communication between the laboring woman and her partner, as well as between the couple and the health care team.

Continuous care provided by doulas significantly reduces the cesarean birth rate; duration of labor; use of oxytocin, analgesics, and forceps; and requests for epidural anesthesia. Laboring women also reported a higher level of satisfaction with their childbirth experience and greater success with breastfeeding.

The role of the nurse and the doula are complementary. They should work together as a team, with the doula providing supportive nonmedical care measures. The nurse focuses on monitoring the status of the maternal-fetal unit; implementing clinical care protocols, including pharmacologic interventions; and documenting assessment findings, actions, and responses.

Labor Support by the Grandparents

When grandparents act as labor coaches, it is important to support them and treat them with respect. They may have ways to deal with pain based on their experience. They should be encouraged to help as long as their actions do not compromise the status of the mother or the fetus. One example of an acceptable practice would be giving the woman herbal tea during labor. The nurse acts as a role model for parents by acknowledging the value of the grandparent's contributions to parental support and by recognizing the difficulty parents have in witnessing their child's discomfort or crisis, regardless of the age of that child. If they have never witnessed a birth, the nurse may need to provide explanations about what is happening. Many of the activities used to support fathers also are appropriate for grandparents.

When possible, the nurse offers the grandparents emotional support. A nurse can show such support by offering them liquid refreshment and by initiating discussion with open-ended questions or statements, such as, "It is sometimes hard to watch a daughter in labor." Nursing actions that provide support for the grandparents can have a therapeutic effect on all members of the family. In turn, a strong, supportive family unit is important for the optimal growth and development of its newest member.

Siblings during Labor and Birth

The preparation of siblings for acceptance of the new child helps promote the attachment process. Such preparation and participation during pregnancy and labor may help the older children accept this change. The older child or children who know themselves to be important to the family become active participants. Rehearsal for the event before labor is essential.

The age and developmental level of children influence their responses; therefore preparation for the children to be present during labor is adjusted to meet each child's needs. The child younger than 2 years shows little interest in pregnancy and labor; for the older child, such preparation may reduce fears and misconceptions. Parents need to be prepared for labor and birth themselves and feel comfortable about the process and the presence of their children. Most parents have a "feel" for their children's maturational level and their physical and emotional ability to observe and cope with the events of the labor and birth process.

Preparation can include a description of the anticipated sights, events (e.g., ROM, monitors, IV infusions), smells, and sounds; a labor and birth demonstration; a tour of the birthing unit; and an opportunity to be around a real new-

BOX 18-8

Guidelines for Supporting the Father

- Orient to the labor room and the unit; explain location of the cafeteria, toilet, waiting room, and nursery; visiting hours; names and functions of personnel present.
- Inform him of sights and smells he can expect to encounter; encourage him to leave the room if necessary.
- Respect his or the couple's decision about the degree of his involvement. Offer them freedom to make decisions.
- Tell him when his presence has been helpful and continue to reinforce this throughout labor.
- Offer to teach him comfort measures.
- Inform him frequently of the progress of the labor and the woman's needs. Keep him informed about procedures to be performed.
- Prepare him for changes in the woman's behavior and physical appearance.
- Remind him to eat; offer him snacks and fluids if possible.
- Relieve him of the job of support person as necessary. Offer him blankets if he is to sleep in a chair by the bedside.
- Acknowledge the stress experienced by each partner during labor and birth and identify normal responses.
- Attempt to modify or eliminate unsettling stimuli, such as extra noise and extra light.

born. Children must learn that their mother will be working hard during labor and birth. She will not be able to talk to them during contractions. She may groan, scream, grunt, and pant at times, as well as say things she would not say otherwise (e.g., "I can't take this anymore;" "Take this baby out of me;" or "This pain is killing me"). They can be told that labor is uncomfortable, but that their mother's body is made for the job.

Storybooks about the birth process can be read to or by children to prepare them for the event. Films are available for preparing preschool and school-age children to participate in the labor and birth experience. Most agencies require that a specific person be designated to watch over the children who are participating in their mother's childbirth experience, to provide them with support, explanations, diversions, and comfort as needed. Health care providers involved in attending women during birth must be comfortable with the presence of children and the unpredictability of their questions, comments, and behaviors.

Emergency Interventions

Emergency conditions that require immediate nursing intervention can arise with startling speed. Interventions for nonreassuring FHR, inadequate uterine relaxation, vaginal bleeding, infection, and prolapse of the cord are detailed in the Emergency box.

Preparation for Giving Birth

The first stage of labor ends with complete dilation of the cervix. The nurse begins to prepare for birth when a multiparous woman is 6 to 8 cm dilated because progression through the last few centimeters of dilation can occur rapidly. Factors that influence the process are fetal position and size of the baby in relation to the size of previous babies.

Birth Setting

To prepare for birth in any setting, the birth table or case cart is usually set up during the transition phase of nulliparous women and during the active phase for multiparous

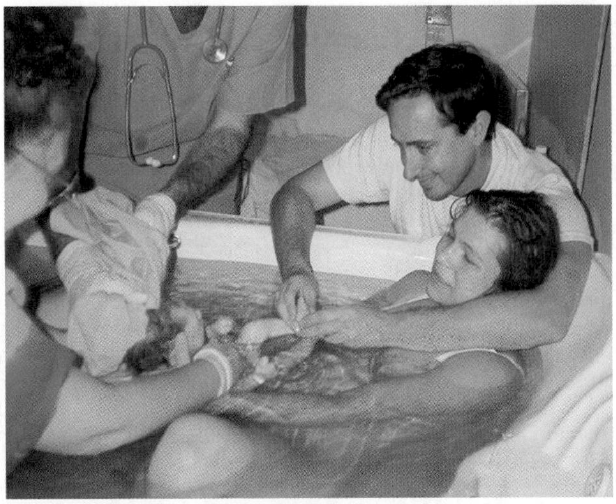

Fig. 18-18 Waterbirth. (Courtesy Global Maternal/Child Health Association, Inc., Wilsonville, OR.)

women. (See Fig. 18-21 for an instrument table setup.) A radiant warmer for the newborn is turned on when crowning begins to occur in the nulliparous woman and when the multiparous woman is 8 to 9 cm dilated. If a traditional delivery room is used, a multiparous woman is usually transferred near the end of the first stage of labor. Transfer of the nulliparous woman takes place when the presenting part begins to distend the perineum between contractions during the second stage of labor (see Fig. 18-17, *A*). Transfer to the delivery room is unnecessary in LDR rooms, LDRP rooms, and birth centers.

Women in labor may use a whirlpool bath for the relaxing effects. Most authorities recommend that birth occur out of the water even though newborns do not begin to breathe until removed from the water. If birth occurs while in the water, the newborn should be removed immediately (Fig. 18-18).

SECOND STAGE OF LABOR

The second stage of labor is the stage in which the infant is born. This stage begins with full cervical dilation (10 cm) and complete effacement (100%) and ends with the baby's birth. The force exerted by uterine contractions, gravity, and maternal bearing-down efforts facilitates achievement of the expected outcome of a spontaneous, uncomplicated, vaginal birth.

The second stage comprises three phases: latent, descent, and transition. These phases are characterized by maternal verbal and nonverbal behaviors, uterine activity, the urge to bear down, and fetal descent.

The latent phase is a period of rest and relative calm (i.e., "laboring down"). During this early phase, the fetus continues to descend passively through the birth canal and rotate to an anterior position as a result of ongoing uterine contractions. The woman is quiet and often relaxes with her eyes closed between contractions. The urge to bear down is not well established and is experienced only during the acme of a contraction or may not be experienced at all. Allowing a woman to rest during this phase, and waiting until the urge

Evidence-Based Practice

CONTINUOUS LABOR SUPPORT

Background

Until the middle of the twentieth century, laboring women of all cultures have had the support of other women to encourage and guide them through birth. Hospital births and the "cascade of medical interventions" have sparked calls for a return to a more humanized culture of birth, with the continuous presence of an emotionally supportive, reassuring woman who dedicates herself to the comfort and well-being of the woman during childbirth. This can include giving advice and praise, labor information, massage, showers, fluids, and advocacy. Labor support may enhance labor physiology and maternal confidence, mitigating the harsh environment of institutional routines, lack of privacy, and high rates of intervention. It may decrease stress and enhance passage of the fetus by encouraging maternal mobility and beneficial positioning. Labor support has frequently been associated with decreased use of pain medication, including epidural anesthesia, which may slow labor and lead to further interventions, such as electronic fetal monitoring and operative birth.

In North America, a trained birth assistant called a *doula* may fill this role. Family members who have given birth themselves may also serve in this role. Observers have questioned the use of hospital staff in this role, because they are technologically oriented and may have conflicting demands on their time and loyalties.

Objectives

The reviewers desired to assess the effects of continuous labor support on mothers and babies, when compared with standard institutional care. Specific influences included the presence of a support person of the woman's own choosing versus a staff member, presence of epidural analgesia, continuous electronic fetal monitoring, and timing of the onset of support during early or late labor.

Outcome measures would ideally include the following:

1. Labor events: amniotomy-augmented labor, electronic fetal monitoring, epidural analgesia, other pain medication, severe pain, and length of labor
2. Birth events: cesarean birth, operative vaginal birth (forceps or vacuum), episiotomy, and perineal trauma
3. Newborn events: 5-minute Apgar score, low cord pH, admission to special care nursery, and prolonged newborn hospital stay
4. Maternal outcomes: anxiety during labor, dissatisfaction, difficulty coping, low coping, postpartum depression, low self-esteem, difficulty mothering, breastfeeding problems, pain, dyspareunia, problems with partner, and urinary or fecal incontinence

Methods

Search Strategy

The reviewers searched Cochrane, MEDLINE, 30 journals, and a weekly awareness service of 37 journals. Keywords were *labor, support, caregiver, doula, labor assistant, birth assistant, childbirth support,* and *labor companion.*

Fifteen randomized, controlled trials, involving 12,791 women, provided high-quality data from hospitals in Australia, Belgium, Botswana, Canada, Finland, France, Greece, Guatemala, Mexico, South Africa, and the United States. All provided continuous presence during active labor as the intervention, and standard care for that institution as the control.

Statistical Analyses

Statistical analyses included pooling of similar data. The reviewers analyzed certain variables, such as epidural analgesia, electronic fetal monitoring, employee or nonemployee support person, and time of support onset. They analyzed how these variables may have influenced specific outcomes, such as pain medication, operative birth or normal spontaneous vaginal delivery (NSVD), low 5-minute Apgar scores, dissatisfaction, and postpartum depression.

Findings

The continuous support groups showed significant decreases in use of any pain medication and regional analgesia, decreased cesarean or operative birth, and maternal dissatisfaction. Reviewers found no difference between groups in augmented labor, low Apgar scores, special care nursery admissions, severe pain, perineal trauma, poor fetal outcomes, incontinence, or postpartum depression.

When influences were compared with outcomes, the greatest benefits (decreased analgesia use, increased NSVD) were derived in settings where the support person was someone of the woman's own choosing and not staff. Benefit from support was dose related: the earlier the onset of support, the greater the effect.

Limitations

This review had few limitations, due to the large numbers and similarities of interventions and outcome measures. There were differences in policies about other family members present, continuous electronic fetal monitoring, and epidural availability. The qualifications of the support people varied, although they were all women. Onset of support varied. Blinding of group randomization was not feasible. Attrition and dropouts were not always noted.

Conclusions

All laboring women need continuous support. The greatest benefit may be early support from a trained or experienced nonstaff support person. The use of nurses or midwives for support may not decrease the cesarean birth rate, due to their interventionist training. Support may provide great benefits to a laboring woman in a resource-poor environment.

Implications for Practice

Childbirth educators can include in their classes the suggestion that a support person be selected to accompany the couple to labor. Nurses in the birthing setting can encourage laboring women to have continuous support and provide support to that person. Laboring women need to be given the choice of their support person.

Implications for Further Research

Further research is needed for maternal and infant health outcomes and longer-term outcomes such as postpartum depression and prolonged pain. Further information about costs, and comparisons of outcomes when support is provided by a trained doula or an experienced female family member or husband, would also be enlightening.

Reference

Hodnett E et al: Continuous support for women during childbirth (Cochrane Review), 2003. In *The Cochrane Library,* Issue 2, Chichester, UK, 2004, John Wiley & Sons.

to push intensifies, has been found to reduce maternal fatigue, conserve energy for bearing-down efforts, and provide optimal maternal and fetal outcomes (Mayberry et al, 1999/2000; Minato, 2000). Coaching a woman to push before her body signals readiness can result in a prolonged period of active pushing with limited to no progress. The woman may become dependent on her coach or nurses to tell her when and how to push (Roberts, 2002). However, women who have epidural analgesia may not feel the urge to bear down and will need coaching.

Emergency

INTERVENTIONS FOR EMERGENCIES

Signs	Interventions*
Nonreassuring Fetal Heart Rate (FHR) Pattern • Fetal bradycardia (FHR <110 beats/min for >10 min)† • Fetal tachycardia (FHR >160 beats/min for >10 min in term pregnancy)§ • Irregular FHR, abnormal sinus rhythm shown by internal monitor • Persistent decrease in baseline FHR variability without any identified cause • Late, severe variable, and prolonged deceleration patterns • Absence of FHR	Notify primary health care provider‡ Change woman to side-lying position Discontinue oxytocin (Pitocin) infusion, if being infused Increase IV fluid rate, if fluid being infused per protocol order Administer oxygen at 8 to 10 L/min by tight face mask Check maternal temperature for elevation Start an IV line if one is not in place Administer amnioinfusion if ordered Stimulate fetal scalp or use acoustic stimulation
Inadequate Uterine Relaxation • Intrauterine pressure >75 mm Hg (shown by intrauterine pressure catheter monitoring) • Contractions consistently lasting >90 sec • Contraction interval <2 min	Notify primary health care provider‡ Discontinue oxytocin infusion, if being infused Change woman to side-lying position Increase IV fluid rate, if fluid is being infused Administer oxygen at 8 to 10 L/min by tight face mask Start an IV line if one is not in place Palpate and evaluate contractions Give tocolytics (terbutaline), as ordered
Vaginal Bleeding • Vaginal bleeding (bright red, dark red, or in amount in excess of that expected during normal cervical dilation) • Continuous vaginal bleeding with FHR changes • Pain; may or may not be present	Notify primary health care provider‡ Anticipate emergency (stat) cesarean birth *Do NOT perform a vaginal examination*
Infection • Foul-smelling amniotic fluid • Maternal temperature >38° C in presence of adequate hydration (straw-colored urine) • Fetal tachycardia >160 beats/min for >10 min	Notify primary health care provider‡ Institute cooling measures for laboring woman Start an IV line if one is not in place Assist with or perform collection of catheterized urine specimen and amniotic fluid sample and send to the laboratory for urinalysis and cultures
Prolapse of Cord • Fetal bradycardia with variable deceleration during uterine contraction • Woman reports feeling the cord after membranes rupture • Cord lies alongside or below the presenting part of the fetus; can be seen or felt in or protruding from the vagina • Major predisposing factors: –Rupture of membranes with a gush –Loose fit of presenting part in lower uterine segment –Presenting part not yet engaged	Call for assistance Have someone notify the primary health care provider immediately Glove the examining hand quickly and insert two fingers into the vagina to the cervix; with one finger on either side of the cord or both fingers to one side, exert upward pressure against the presenting part to relieve compression of the cord Place a rolled towel under the woman's hip Place woman in extreme Trendelenburg or modified Sims' position or knee-chest position Wrap the cord loosely in a sterile towel saturated with warm sterile normal saline if the cord is protruding from the vagina Administer oxygen at 8 to 10 L/min by face mask until birth is accomplished Start IV fluids or increase existing drip rate Continue to monitor FHR by internal fetal scalp electrode, if possible Do not attempt to replace cord into cervix Prepare for immediate birth (vaginal or cesarean)

*Because emergency situations are often frightening events, it is important for the nurse to explain to the woman and her support person what is happening and how it is being managed.
†Practice is to intervene within 2 to 30 min if FHR is <110 beats/min.
‡In most emergency situations, nurses take immediate action, following a protocol and standards of nursing practice. Another person can notify the primary health care provider, or this can be done by the nurse as soon as possible.
§Nonreassuring sign when associated with late decelerations or absence of variability, especially if FHR is >180 beats/min.

The descent phase or phase of active pushing is characterized by strong urges to bear down as the Ferguson reflex is activated by pressure of the presenting part on the stretch receptors of the pelvic floor. At this point, the fetal station is usually 1+, and the position is anterior. This stimulation causes the release of oxytocin from the posterior pituitary gland, which stimulates stronger, expulsive uterine contractions. The woman becomes more focused on bearing-down efforts, which become rhythmic. She changes positions frequently to find a more comfortable pushing position. The woman often announces the onset of contractions and becomes more vocal as she bears down. The urge to bear down intensifies as descent progresses.

In the transition phase the presenting part is on the perineum, and bearing-down efforts are most effective for promoting birth. The woman may be more verbal about the pain she is experiencing; she may scream or swear, and may act out of control (Roberts, 2002).

The nurse encourages the woman to "listen" to her body as she progresses through the phases of the second stage of labor. When a woman listens to her body to tell her when to bear down, her efforts become more effective and she often feels more satisfied with her efforts to give birth to her baby. The woman's trust in her own body and her ability to give birth to her baby should be fostered (Mayberry et al, 1999/2000).

If a woman is confined to bed, especially in a recumbent position, the rhythmic urge to bear down is delayed, because gravity is not being used to press the presenting part against the pelvic floor. Being moved to another room and placed on a delivery table in the lithotomy position, as has been the custom in North America for the past 30 years, also has an inhibiting effect on the urge to bear down. Today, Western societies have adopted the birthing practice of most non-Western societies where labor and birth occur in the same room and women use various positions for bearing down, such as side-lying, kneeling, squatting, sitting, or standing.

The only certain objective sign that the second stage of labor has begun is the inability to feel the cervix during vaginal examination, indicating that the cervix is fully dilated and effaced. The precise moment that this occurs is not easily determined because it depends on when a vaginal examination is performed to validate full dilation and effacement. This makes timing of the actual duration of the second stage difficult (Roberts, 2002). Other signs that suggest the onset of the second stage include the following:

- Sudden appearance of perspiration on upper lip
- An episode of vomiting
- Increased bloody show

Table 18-6

Expected Maternal Progress in Second Stage of Labor

CRITERION	LATENT PHASE (AVERAGE DURATION, 10-30 MIN)	DESCENT PHASE (AVERAGE DURATION VARIES)*	TRANSITION PHASE (AVERAGE DURATION 5-15 MIN)
Contractions	Period of physiologic lull for all criteria; period of peace and rest	Significant increase	Overwhelmingly strong
Magnitude (intensity)			Expulsive
Frequency		2-2.5 min	1-2 min
Duration		90 sec	90 sec
Descent, station	0 to +2	Increases and Ferguson reflex† activated, +2 to +4	Rapid, +4 to birth Fetal head visible in introitus
Show: color and amount		Significant increase in dark-red bloody show	Bloody show accompanies birth of head
Spontaneous bearing-down efforts	Slight to absent, except during acme of strongest contractions	Increased urge to bear down	Greatly increased
Vocalization	Quiet; concern over progress	Grunting sounds or expiratory vocalization; announces contractions	Grunting sounds and expiratory vocalizations continue; may scream or swear
Maternal behavior	Experiences sense of relief that transition to second stage is finished Feels fatigued and sleepy Feels a sense of accomplishment and optimism, because the "worst is over" Feels in control	Senses increased urge to push Alters respiratory pattern: has short 4 to 5 sec breath holds with regular breaths in between, 5 to 7 times per contraction Makes grunting sounds or expiratory vocalizations Frequent repositioning	Describes extreme pain Expresses feelings of powerlessness Shows decreased ability to listen or concentrate on anything but giving birth Describes *ring of fire* (burning sensation of acute pain as vagina stretches and fetal head crowns) Often shows excitement immediately after birth of head

From Anderhold K, Roberts J: Phases of second stage labor: four descriptive case studies, *J Nurse Midwifery* 36(5):267-275, 1991; Mahan C, McKay S: Are we overmanaging second stage labor? *Contemp OB/GYN* 24:37-63, 1984.

*Duration of descent phase can vary depending on maternal parity, effectiveness of bearing-down effort, and presence of spinal anesthesia or epidural analgesia.

†Pressure of presenting part on stretch receptors of pelvic floor stimulates release of oxytocin from posterior pituitary, resulting in more intense uterine contractions.

- Shaking of extremities
- Increased restlessness; verbalization that "I can't go on"
- Involuntary bearing-down efforts

These signs commonly appear at the time the cervix reaches full dilation. However, women with an epidural block may not exhibit such signs. Other indicators for each phase of the second stage are given in Tables 18-6 and 18-7.

Women can begin to experience an irresistible urge to bear down before full dilation; this may occur as early as 5 cm dilation. This is most often related to the station of the presenting part below the level of the ischial spines of the maternal pelvis. This occurrence creates a conflict between the woman, whose body is telling her to push, and her health care providers, who believe that pushing the fetal presenting part against an incompletely dilated cervix will result in cervical edema and lacerations, as well as a slowing down of labor progress. The premature urge to bear down must be evaluated as a phase of labor progress possibly indicating the onset of the second stage of labor. Research is needed to determine the consequences of pushing against a partially dilated cervix. When a woman pushes in relation to the degree of cervical dilation should be based on research evidence rather than on tradition or routine practice. It may be safe and effective for a woman to push with the urge to bear down at the acme of a contraction if her cervix is soft, retracting, and 8 cm or more dilated and if the fetus is at 1+ station and rotating to an anterior position (Roberts, 2002).

Assessment is continuous during the second stage of labor. Professional standards and agency policy determine the specific type and timing of assessments, as well as the way in which findings are documented. The Care Path for the second and third stages of labor (see p. 526) indicates typical assessments and the recommended frequency for their performance. Signs and symptoms of impending birth (see Table 18-2) may appear unexpectedly, requiring immediate action by the nurse (Box 18-9).

Duration of Second Stage

The duration of the second stage of labor is influenced by several factors, such as the effectiveness of the primary and

Table 18-7

Woman's Responses and Support Person's Action during Second Stage of Labor

WOMAN'S RESPONSES	NURSE/SUPPORT PERSON'S ACTIONS*
LATENT PHASE	
Experiences a short period of peace and rest	Encourages woman to "listen" to her body Continues support measures Suggests an upright position to encourage progression of descent if descent phase does not begin after 20 min
DESCENT PHASE	
Senses increased urgency to bear down as Ferguson reflex is activated Notes increase in intensity of uterine contractions—alters respiratory pattern: short 4 to 5 sec breath holds, 5 to 7 times per contraction Makes grunting sounds or expiratory vocalizations	Encourages respiratory pattern of short breath holds Stresses normality and benefits of grunting sounds and expiratory vocalizations Encourages bearing-down efforts with urge to push Encourages/suggests maternal movement and position changes (upright, if descent is not occurring) Encourages woman to "listen" to her body regarding movement and position change if descent is occurring Discourages long breath holds If birth is to occur in a delivery room, transfers woman to delivery room early to avoid rushing or, if permitted, offers her option of walking to delivery room Places woman in lateral recumbent position to slow descent if descent is too fast
TRANSITIONAL PHASE	
Behaves in manner similar to behavior during transition in first stage (8-10 cm) Experiences a sense of severe pain and powerlessness Shows decreased ability to listen Concentrates on birth of baby until head is born Experiences contractions as overwhelming in intensity Reports feeling ring of fire as head crowns Maintains respiratory pattern of three to five 7 sec breath holds per contraction, followed by forced expiration Eases head out with short expirations Responds with excitement and relief after head is born	Encourages slow, gentle pushing Explains that "blowing away the contraction" facilitates a slower birth of the head Provides mirror to help woman see or touch the emerging fetal head (best to extend over two to three contractions) to help her understand the perinatal sensations Coaches woman to relax mouth, throat, and neck to promote relaxation of pelvic floor Applies warm compress to perineum to promote relaxation

*Provided by nurses and by support persons in collaboration with the nurse.

Care Path

LOW RISK WOMAN IN SECOND AND THIRD STAGES OF LABOR

Care Management	Second Stage of Labor	Third Stage of Labor
I. Assessment Measures*	*Frequency*	*Frequency*
• Blood pressure, pulse, respirations	Every 5-30 min	Every 15 min
• Uterine activity	Assess every contraction	Assess for placental separation
• Bearing-down effort	Assess each effort	Perform Apgar at 1 and 5 min
• Fetal heart rate (FHR)	Every 5-15 min	
• Vaginal show	Every 15 min	Assess bleeding until placental expulsion
• Signs of fetal descent: urge to bear down, perineal bulging, crowning	Every 10-15 min	
• Behavior, appearance, mood, energy level of woman; condition of partner	Every 10-15 min	Assess response to completion of childbirth process, reaction to newborn
II. Physical Care Measures†	**Latent phase:** Assist to rest in position of comfort Encourage relaxation to conserve energy Promote urge to push; if delayed: ambulation, shower, pelvic rock, position changes **Descent phase:** Assist to bear down effectively Help to use recommended positions that facilitate descent Encourage correct breathing during bearing-down efforts Help to relax between contractions Provide comfort measures as needed Cleanse perineum immediately if fecal material is expelled **Transition phase:** Assist to pant during contraction to avoid rapid birth of head Coach to gently bear down between contractions	Assist to bear down to facilitate delivery of separated placenta Administer oxytocic medication as ordered Provide pain relief as needed Provide hygiene and comfort measures as needed
III. Emotional Support	Keep informed of progress of fetal descent Provide feedback for bearing-down efforts Explain purpose if medications given Role model comfort measures Provide continuous nursing presence Create a quiet, calm environment Reassure, encourage, praise Take charge as needed, until mother regains confidence in ability to birth her baby Offer mirror to watch birth	Keep informed about progress of placental separation Explain purpose of any medications given Describe status of perineal tissue and inform if repair is needed Introduce parents to their baby Assess and care for newborn within view of parents; delay eye prophylaxis to facilitate eye contact Provide private time for family to bond with their new baby and help them to create memories Encourage breastfeeding if desired

*Frequency of assessment is determined by the risk status of the maternal-fetal unit. More frequent assessment is required in high risk situations. Frequency of assessment and method of documentation are also determined by agency policy, which is usually based on the recommended care standards of medical and nursing organizations.

†Physical care measures are performed by the nurse working together with the woman's partner and significant others.

secondary powers of labor; the type and amount of analgesia or anesthesia used; the physical and emotional condition, position, activity level, parity, and pelvic adequacy of the laboring woman; the size, presentation, and position of the fetus; and the nature and source of support the woman receives.

For many multiparous women, birth occurs within minutes of complete dilation, perhaps only one push later. Nulliparous women usually push for 1 to 2 hours before giving birth. If the woman has been given epidural analgesia, pushing can last more than 2 hours. Epidural analgesia blocks or reduces the urge to bear down and limits the woman's ability to attain an upright position to push. By adjusting dosages to the lowest effective level, allowing the epidural to wear off at full dilation or after 1 hour of pushing, or using mixtures

BOX 18-9

Guidelines for Assistance at the Emergency Birth of a Fetus in the Vertex Presentation

1. The woman usually assumes the position most comfortable for her. A lateral position is often recommended.
2. Reassure the woman that birth is usually uncomplicated and easy in these situations. Use eye-to-eye contact and a calm, relaxed manner. If there is someone else available, such as the partner, that person could help support the woman in the position, assist with coaching, and compliment her on her efforts.
3. Wash your hands and put on gloves, if available.
4. Place under woman's buttocks whatever clean material is available.
5. Avoid touching the vaginal area to decrease the possibility of infection.
6. As the head begins to crown, you should do the following:
   a. Tear the amniotic membrane if it is still intact.
   b. Instruct the woman to pant or pant-blow, thus minimizing the urge to push.
   c. Place the flat side of your hand on the exposed fetal head and apply *gentle* pressure toward the vagina to prevent the head from "popping out." The mother may participate by placing her hand under yours on the emerging head. NOTE: Rapid delivery of the fetal head must be prevented because a rapid change of pressure within the molded fetal skull follows, which may result in dural or subdural tears and may cause vaginal or perineal lacerations.
7. After the birth of the head, check for the umbilical cord. If the cord is around the baby's neck, try to slip it over the baby's head or pull it *gently* to get some slack so that you can slip it over the shoulders.
8. Support the fetal head as restitution (external rotation) occurs. After restitution, with one hand on each side of the baby's head, exert *gentle* pressure downward so that the anterior shoulder emerges under the symphysis pubis and acts as a fulcrum; then, as *gentle* pressure is exerted in the opposite direction, the posterior shoulder, which has passed over the sacrum and coccyx, emerges.
9. Be alert! Hold the baby securely because the rest of the body may emerge quickly. The baby will be slippery!
10. Cradle the baby's head and back in one hand and the buttocks in the other. Keep the head down to drain away the mucus. Use a bulb syringe, if one is available, to remove mucus from the baby's mouth.
11. Dry the baby quickly to prevent rapid heat loss. Keep the baby at the same level as the mother's uterus until the end of the cord stops pulsating. NOTE: It is important to keep the baby at the same level as the mother's uterus to prevent the baby's blood from flowing to or from the placenta and the resultant hypovolemia or hypervolemia. Also, do not "milk" the cord.
12. Place the baby on the mother's abdomen, cover the baby (remember to keep the head warm, too) with the mother's clothing, and have her cuddle the baby. Compliment her (them) on a job well done, and on the baby, if appropriate.
13. *Wait* for the placenta to separate; do *not* tug on the cord. NOTE: Injudicious traction may tear the cord, separate the placenta, or invert the uterus. Signs of placental separation include a slight gush of dark blood from the introitus, lengthening of the cord, and change in the uterine contour from a discoid to globular shape.
14. Instruct the mother to push to deliver the separated placenta. Gently ease out the placental membranes using an up-and-down motion until the membranes are removed. If birth occurs outside a hospital setting, to minimize complications, do not cut the cord without proper clamps and a sterile cutting tool. Inspect the placenta for intactness. Place the baby on the placenta and wrap the two together for additional warmth.
15. Check the firmness of the uterus. Gently massage the fundus and demonstrate to the mother how she can massage her own fundus properly.
16. If supplies are available, clean the mother's perineal area and apply a peripad.
17. In addition to gentle massage of the fundus, the following measures can be taken to prevent or minimize hemorrhage:
   a. Put the baby to the mother's breast as soon as possible. Sucking or nuzzling and licking the nipple stimulates the release of oxytocin from the posterior pituitary. NOTE: If the baby does not or cannot nurse, manually stimulate the mother's nipples.
   b. Do not allow the mother's bladder to become distended. Assess the bladder for fullness and encourage her to void if fullness is found.
   c. Expel any clots from the mother's uterus.
18. Comfort or reassure the mother and her family or friends. Keep the mother and the baby warm. Give her fluids if available and tolerated.
19. If this is a multifetal birth, identify the infants in order of birth (using letters *A*, *B*, etc.).
20. Make notations regarding the following aspects of the birth:
   a. Fetal presentation and position
   b. Presence of cord around neck (nuchal cord) or other parts and number of times cord encircled part
   c. Color, character, and amount of amniotic fluid, if rupture of membranes occurs immediately before birth
   d. Time of birth
   e. Estimated time of determination of Apgar score (e.g., 1 and 5 minutes after birth), resuscitation efforts implemented, and ultimate condition of baby
   f. Sex of baby
   g. Time of placental expulsion, as well as the appearance and completeness of the placenta
   h. Maternal condition: affect, amount of bleeding, and status of uterine tonicity
   i. Any unusual occurrences during the birth (e.g., maternal or paternal response, verbalizations, or gestures in response to birth of baby)

containing an opioid-agonist analgesic and a local anesthetic, the woman is able to perceive more fully the urge to bear down, to move more freely, and to attain an upright position with assistance as a result of increased strength and sensation in her legs. This approach can enhance the ability to bear down effectively and achieve an uncomplicated vaginal birth (Mayberry et al, 1999/2000). However, allowing the analgesia to wear off means that women will have an increase in distress and the severity of pain. This results in an increase in sympathetic activity and the release of catecholamines. Catecholamines inhibit uterine contractions, potentially prolonging the second stage of labor. Allowing these women a "laboring down" period for fetal descent and rotation may result in a more positive outcome (Roberts, 2002).

Commonly, a second stage of more than 2 hours may be considered prolonged in women without regional analgesia and is reported to the primary health care provider. By using assessment findings such as the fetal heart rate and pattern, the descent of the presenting part, the quality of the uterine contractions, and the status of the woman, premature intervention with episiotomy or forceps- or vacuum-assisted birth can be avoided. If the status of the maternal-fetal unit is reassuring and progress is continuing, interventions to end the second stage of labor are unwarranted. Less emphasis should be placed on a definite time limit for the second stage. The duration of active pushing has been found to be more relevant to the newborn's condition at birth than the duration of the second stage of labor itself (d'Entremont, 1996; Minato, 2000; Petersen & Besuner, 1997; Roberts, 2002).

The nurse continues to monitor maternal-fetal status and events of the second stage and provide comfort measures for the mother such as positioning; providing mouth care; maintaining clean, dry bedding; and keeping to a minimum extraneous noise, conversation, or other distractions (e.g., laughing and talking by attending personnel in or outside the labor area). The woman is encouraged to indicate other support measures she would like (see Table 18-5, Care Path: Low Risk Woman in Second and Third Stages of Labor on p. 526, and Nursing Care Plan on pp. 514).

In the hospital, birth may occur in an LDR, LDRP, or delivery room. If the mother is to be transferred to the delivery room for birth, the nurse makes the transfer early enough to avoid rushing the woman. The birth area is readied for the birth.

Maternal Position

There is no single position for childbirth. Labor is a dynamic, interactive process involving the woman's uterus, pelvis, and voluntary muscles. In addition, angles between the baby and the woman's pelvis constantly change as the fetus turns and flexes down the birth canal. The woman may want to assume various positions for childbirth, and she should be encouraged and assisted in attaining and maintaining her positions of choice. Hanson (1998a) found that sitting and side-lying are the two most common positions assumed by women for their bearing-down efforts and birth.

Birth attendants play a major role in influencing a woman's choice of position for birth, with midwives tending to advocate the nonlithotomy positions for the second stage of labor (Hanson, 1998b). Upright positions facilitate birth and fetal descent and reduce the duration of the second stage of labor and the need for episiotomy, forceps, or vacuum extractor in the following ways:

- Straighten the longitudinal axis of the birth canal
- Use gravity to direct the fetal head toward the pelvic inlet, thereby facilitating descent
- Enlarge pelvic dimensions and restrict the encroachment of the sacrum and coccyx into the pelvic inlet
- Increase uteroplacental circulation, resulting in more intense, efficient uterine contractions
- Enhance the woman's ability to bear down effectively, thereby minimizing maternal exhaustion

The upright positions may, however, slightly increase the risk for second-degree lacerations and a blood loss greater than 500 ml. Further investigation is needed to determine the exact mechanism for these outcomes (Shorten, Donsante, & Shorten, 2002).

Squatting is highly effective in facilitating the descent and birth of the fetus (Mayberry et al, 1999/2000; Roberts, 2002). Women should assume a modified, supported squat until the fetal head is engaged, at which time a deep squat can be used. A firm surface is required, and the woman will need side support (see Fig. 18-13, *A*). In a birthing bed, a squat bar is available that she can use to help support herself (see Fig. 16-15). A birth ball can help a woman maintain the squatting position. The fetus will be aligned with the birth canal, and pelvic and perineal relaxation will be facilitated as she sits on the ball or holds it in front of her for support as she squats.

When a woman uses the standing position for bearing down, her weight is borne on both femoral heads, allowing the pressure in the acetabulum to increase the transverse diameter of the pelvic outlet by up to 1 cm. This can be helpful if descent of the head is delayed because the occiput has not rotated from the lateral (transverse diameter of pelvis) to the anterior position. Birthing chairs or rocking chairs may be used to provide women with a good physiologic position to enhance bearing-down efforts during childbirth. The upright position allows the mother to see the birth as it occurs and to maintain eye contact with the attendant. Most birthing chairs are designed so that if an emergency occurs, the chair can be adjusted to the horizontal or Trendelenburg position.

Oversized beanbag chairs and large floor pillows may be used for both labor and birth. They can mold around and support the mother in whatever position she selects. Birthing stools can be used to support the woman in an upright position similar to squatting. Women may want to sit on the toilet to push because they are concerned about stool incontinence during this stage. They must be closely monitored and removed from the toilet before birth is imminent. Because sitting on chairs, stools, toilets, or commodes can increase perineal edema and blood loss, it is important to assist the woman to change her position every 10 to 15 minutes (Shermer & Raines, 1997).

Side-lying is an effective position for the second stage, with the upper part of the woman's leg held by the nurse or coach or placed on a pillow (see Fig. 18-17, *A*). Some women prefer a semi-sitting position. To maintain good uteroplacental circulation and to enhance the woman's bearing-down efforts in this position, the woman's back and shoulders should be elevated to at least a 30-degree angle and a wedge should be placed under one hip (see Fig. 18-17, *B*). The episiotomy rate for nulliparas has been found to be highest in this position (Shorten et al, 2002).

The hands-and-knees position, along with pelvic rocking and abdominal stroking, is an effective position for birth because it enhances placental perfusion, helps rotate a fetus from a posterior to an anterior position, and may facilitate the birth of the shoulders, especially if the fetus is large (see Fig. 18-14, *B*). Perineal trauma may also be reduced (Simkin & Ancheta, 2000).

The birthing bed is commonly used today and can be set for different positions according to the woman's needs (Figs. 18-19 and 18-20). The woman can squat, kneel, sit, recline, or lie on her side, choosing the position most comfortable for her without having to climb into bed for the birth. At the same time, there is excellent exposure for examination, electrode placement, and birth. Squat bars, over-the-bed tables, birth balls, and pillows can be used for support. The bed can be positioned for the administration of anesthesia and is ideal to help women receiving an epidural to assume different positions to facilitate birth. The bed can be used to transport the woman to the operating room if a cesarean birth is necessary.

Bearing-down Efforts

As the fetal head reaches the pelvic floor, most women experience the urge to bear down. Reflexively the woman will begin to exert downward pressure by contracting her abdominal muscles while relaxing her pelvic floor. This bearing down is an involuntary response to the Ferguson reflex, which is activated by the pressure of the presenting part on stretch receptors of the pelvic musculature.

A strong expiratory grunt (vocalization) often accompanies pushing when the woman exhales as she pushes. This natural vocalization by women during open-glottis bearing-down efforts is likely to be discouraged by nurses in part to "conserve the woman's energy" but also as a result of concern that it will seem to other nurses and patients that the woman has lost control or the nurse has lost control of her patient (Petersen & Besuner, 1997).

When coaching women to push, the nurse should encourage them to push as they feel like pushing (instinctive, spontaneous pushing) rather than to give a prolonged push on command. Women will usually begin to push naturally as the contraction increases in intensity and the Ferguson reflex strengthens. The nurse should monitor the woman's breathing so that the woman does not hold her breath for more than 5 to 7 seconds at a time and should remind her to ventilate her lungs fully by taking deep cleansing breaths before and after each contraction. Bearing down while exhaling (open-glottis pushing) and taking breaths between bearing-down efforts help maintain adequate oxygen levels for the mother and fetus and results in approximately five pushes

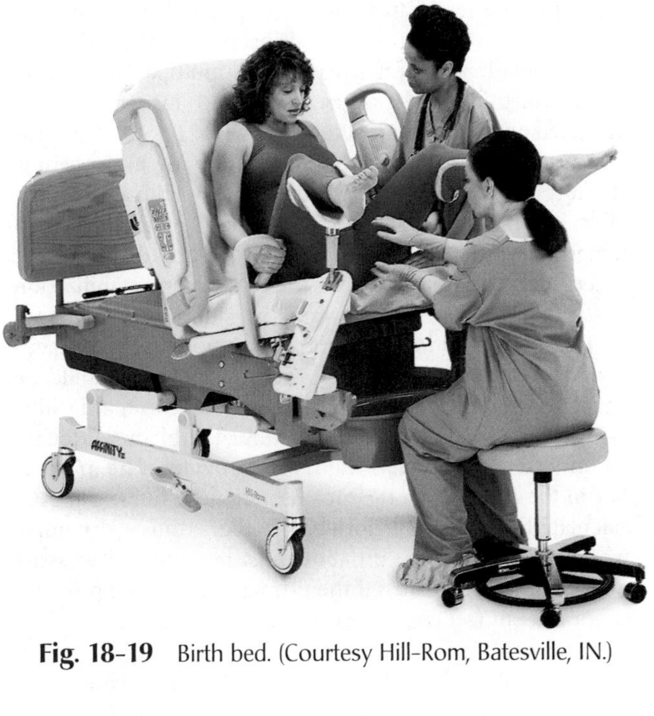

Fig. 18-19 Birth bed. (Courtesy Hill-Rom, Batesville, IN.)

during a contraction, with each push lasting about 5 seconds (Mayberry et al, 1999/2000). Women who use spontaneous pushing are less likely to have second- or third-degree perineal lacerations or episiotomies (Roberts, 2002).

Prolonged breath holding, or sustained, directed bearing down (still a common practice), may trigger the Valsalva maneuver. This maneuver occurs when the woman closes the glottis (closed-glottis pushing), thereby increasing intrathoracic and cardiovascular pressure, reducing cardiac output, and inhibiting perfusion of the uterus and the placenta. Breath holding for more than 5 to 7 seconds causes the perfusion of oxygen across the placenta to be diminished, resulting in fetal hypoxia. This approach to bearing down is harmful or ineffective and should be discouraged (Enkin et al, 2000).

A woman may reach the second stage of labor and then experience a lack of readiness to complete the process and give birth to her child. McKay and Barrows (1991) identified several factors that may inhibit the woman's voluntary bearing-down efforts. These factors include the following:

- Doubts about her readiness to be a mother
- Reluctance to care for another baby
- Desire to wait for support person or primary health care provider to arrive
- Fear or anxiety regarding the unfamiliar or painful sensations of the second stage of labor and pushing
- Embarrassment regarding behaviors during pushing, including sounds made and passage of stool
- Giving up and not wanting to proceed any further toward vaginal birth
- Fear that the baby will be in danger once it emerges from the protective intrauterine environment

By recognizing that a woman may experience a need to hold back the birth of her baby, the nurse can address the woman's concerns and effectively coach her through this stage of labor.

To ensure slow birth of the fetal head, the woman is encouraged to control the urge to bear down by coaching her to take panting breaths or to exhale slowly through pursed lips as the baby's head crowns. At this point, the woman needs simple, clear directions from one person.

Amnesia between contractions is often pronounced in the second stage, and the woman may have to be roused to cooperate in the bearing-down process. Parents who have attended childbirth education classes may have devised a set of verbal cues for the laboring woman to follow. It is helpful for them to have these cues printed on a card that can be attached to the head of the bed so that the nurse can better substitute as coach if the partner has to leave.

Fetal Heart Rate and Pattern

As noted previously, the FHR must be checked. If the rate begins to slow, if there is a loss of variability, or if deceleration patterns develop (e.g., late, variable), prompt treatment must be initiated. The woman can be turned on her side to reduce the pressure of the uterus against the ascending vena cava and descending aorta (see Fig. 18-5), and oxygen can be administered by mask at 8 to 10 L/min (Tucker, 2004). This is often all that is required to restore a reassuring pattern. If the fetal heart rate and pattern do not become reassuring immediately, the primary health care provider should be notified quickly because medical intervention to hasten birth may be indicated.

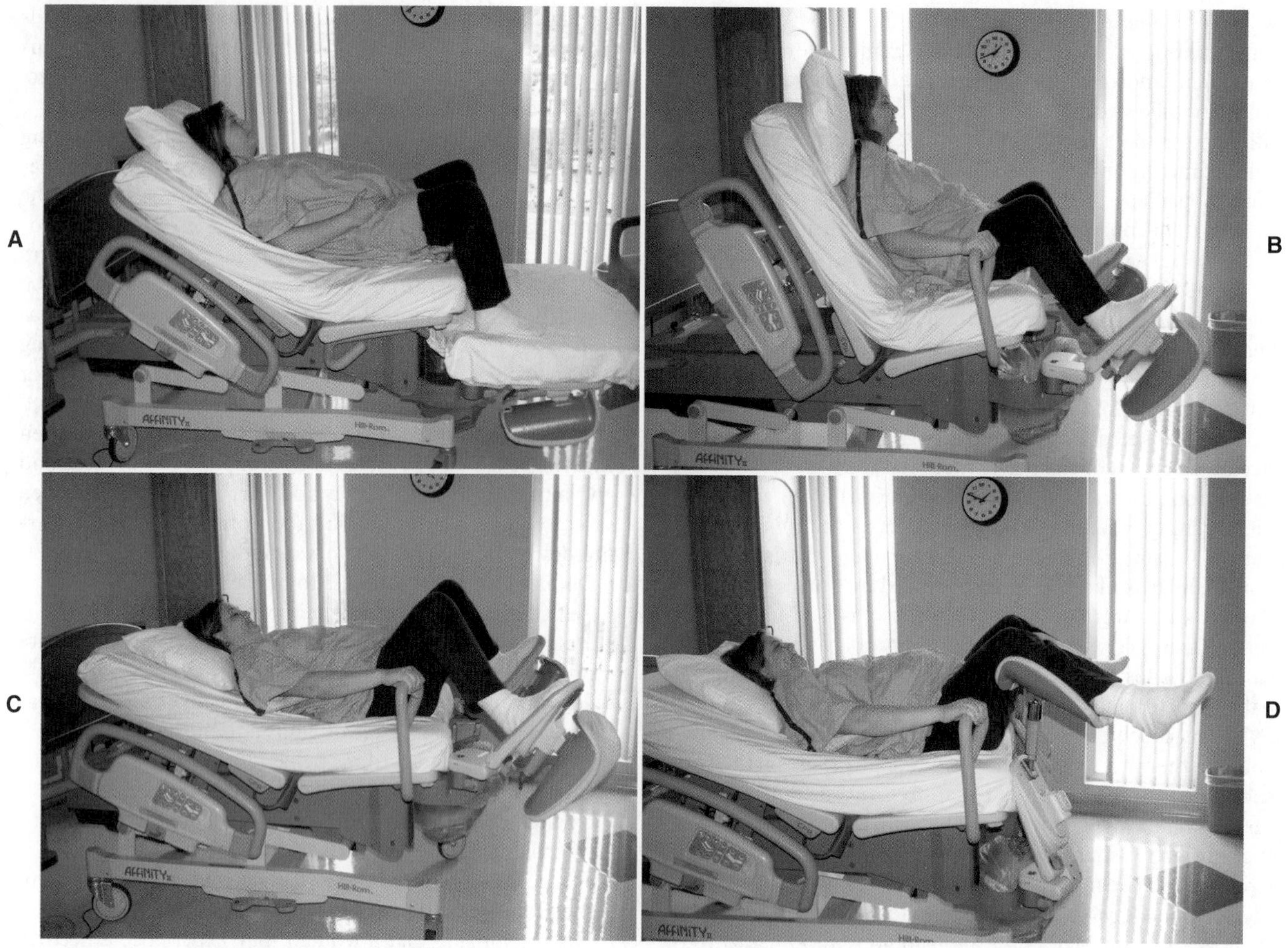

Fig. 18-20 The versatility of today's birthing bed makes it practical in many settings. NOTE: OB table used for lithotomy position. **A**, Labor bed. **B**, Birth chair. **C**, Birth bed. **D**, OB table. (Courtesy Julie Perry Nelson, Gilbert, AZ.)

Support of the Father or Partner

During the second stage, the woman needs continuous support and coaching (see Table 18-7). Because the coaching process can be physically and emotionally tiring for support persons, the nurse offers them nourishment and fluids and encourages them to take short breaks. If birth occurs in an LDR or LDRP room, the partner may be allowed to wear street clothes or be required to wear a clean scrub outfit, cap, and mask (for the birth). The support person who attends the birth in a delivery room is instructed to put on a cover gown or scrub clothes, mask, hat, and shoe covers, as required by agency policy. The nurse also specifies support measures that can be used for the laboring woman and points out areas of the room in which the partner can move freely.

LEGAL TIP Documentation Documentation of all observations (e.g., maternal vital signs, fetal heart rate and pattern, progress of labor) and nursing interventions, including patient response, should be done concurrently with care. The course of labor and maternal-fetal response may change without warning. It is important that all documentation be accurate, complete, timely, and according to agency policy. ■

Supplies, Instruments, and Equipment

To prepare for birth in any setting, the birthing table is usually set up during the transition phase for nulliparous women and during the active phase for multiparous women.

The birthing table is prepared, and instruments are arranged on the instrument table (Fig. 18-21). Standard procedures are followed for gloving, identifying and opening sterile packages, adding sterile supplies to the instrument table, unwrapping sterile instruments, and handing them to the primary health care provider. The crib or radiant warmer and equipment are readied for the support and stabilization of the infant.

The items used for birth may vary among different facilities; therefore each facility's procedure manual should be consulted to determine the protocols specific to that facility.

The nurse estimates the time until the birth will occur and notifies the primary health care provider if he or she is not in the room. Even the most experienced nurse can miscalculate the time left before birth occurs; thus every nurse who attends a woman in labor must be prepared to assist with an emergency birth if the primary health care provider is not present (see Box 18-9).

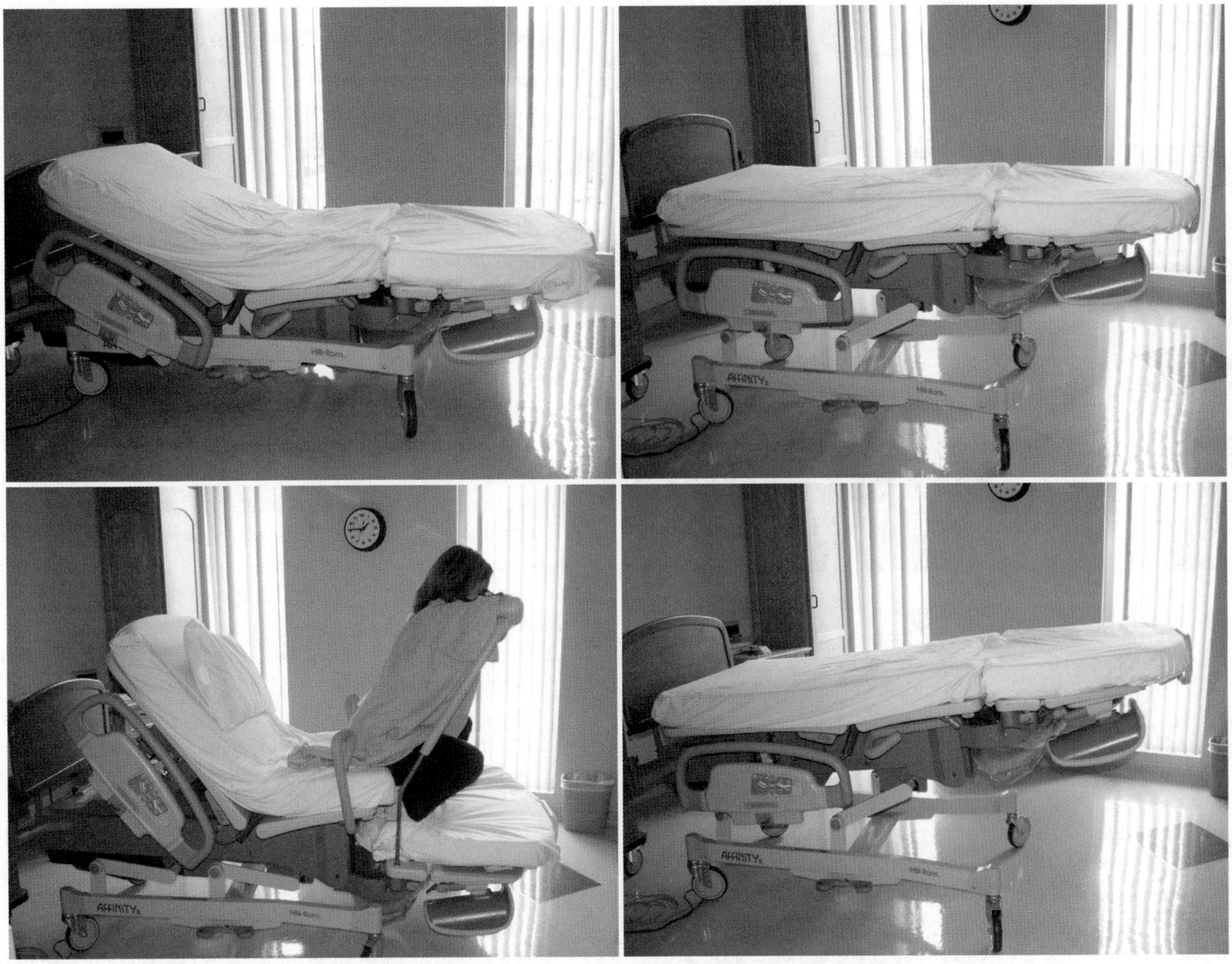

Fig. 18-20, cont'd E, Postpartum. F, Critical care. G, Birth bar. H, Trendelenburg.

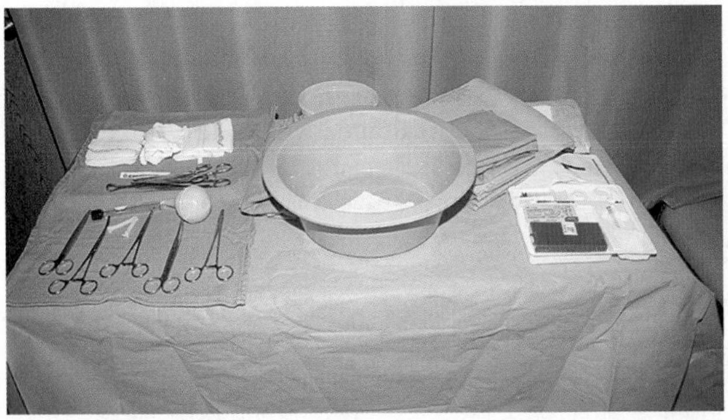

Fig. 18-21 Instrument table. (Courtesy Marjorie Pyle, RNC, Lifecircle, Costa Mesa, CA.)

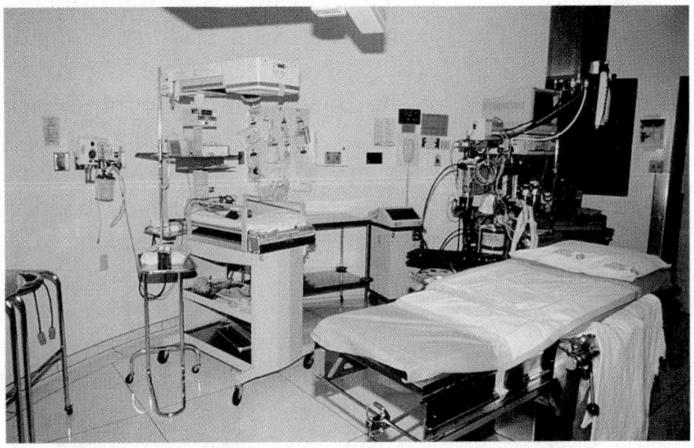

Fig. 18-22 Delivery room. (Courtesy Michael S. Clement, MD, Mesa, AZ.)

Birth in a Delivery Room or Birthing Room

The woman will need assistance if she must move from the labor bed to the delivery table (Fig. 18-22). The woman can help if this is done between contractions, but because of her awkwardness, she cannot be rushed. In a birthing room, no such transfer is necessary (Fig. 18-23). The various positions assumed for birth in a delivery room are the Sims' or lateral position in which the attendant supports the upper part of the woman's leg, the dorsal position (supine position with one hip elevated), and the lithotomy position.

The lithotomy position has been the position most commonly used for birth in Western cultures, although this practice is changing slowly. The lithotomy position makes it more convenient for the primary health care

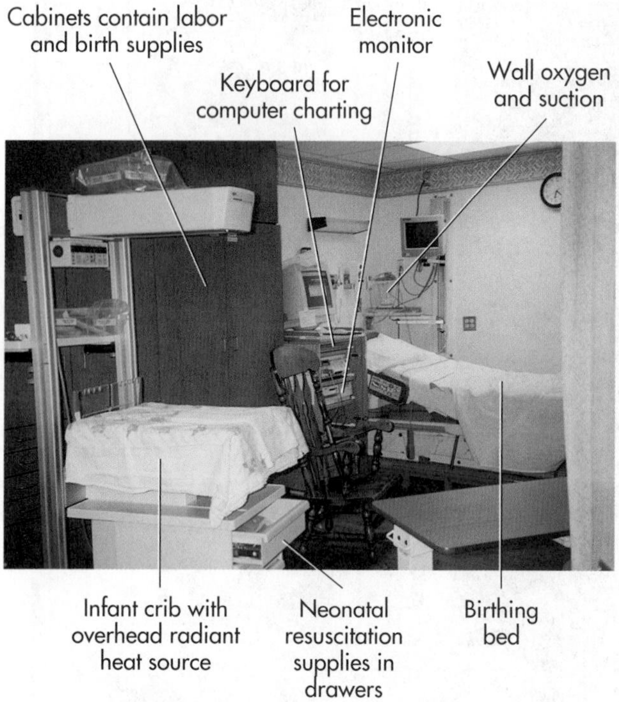

Fig. 18-23 Birthing room. (Courtesy Dee Lowdermilk, Chapel Hill, NC.)

provider to deal with complications that arise. To place the woman in this position, her buttocks are brought to the edge of the table and her legs are placed in stirrups. Care must be taken to pad the stirrups, to raise and place both legs simultaneously, and to adjust the shanks of the stirrups so that the calves of the legs are supported. There should be no pressure on the popliteal space. If the stirrups are not the same height, ligaments in the woman's back can be strained as she bears down, leading to considerable discomfort in the postpartum period. The lower portion of the table may be dropped down and rolled back under the table.

It should be noted that the routine use of a supine or lithotomy position for labor and birth has been identified as a clearly harmful or ineffective practice and should be discouraged (Enkin et al, 2000).

Birth in an LDR or LDRP Room

The maternal position for birth varies from a lithotomy position with the woman's legs in stirrups; to one in which her feet rest on footrests while she holds onto a squat bar; to a side-lying position with the woman's upper leg supported by the coach, nurse, or squat bar. The foot of the bed can be removed so that the primary health care provider attending the birth can gain better perineal access for performing an episiotomy, delivering a large baby, or getting access to the emerging head to facilitate suctioning. Otherwise the foot of the bed is left in place and lowered slightly to form a ledge that allows access for birth and that also serves as a place to place the newborn (see Fig. 18-20).

Once the woman is positioned for birth, the vulva and perineum are cleansed. Hospital protocols and preferences of the primary health care provider for cleansing may vary and can involve washing the area thoroughly with warm soapy water or a soapy povidone-iodine (Betadine) solution and then rinsing the area. Next the area may be sprayed with a disinfectant to prevent bacterial growth.

The circulating nurse (usually the same nurse as the labor nurse) continues to coach and encourage the woman. The nurse auscultates the fetal heart rate or checks the electronic monitor tracing every 5 to 15 minutes, depending on whether the woman is at low or high risk for problems or per protocol of the birthing facility. She keeps the primary health care provider informed of the rate and pattern of the fetal heart (Tucker, 2004). An oxytocic medication such as oxytocin (Pitocin) may be prepared so that it is ready to administer after expulsion of the placenta. Standard Precautions should always be followed while care is administered during the process of labor and birth (see Box 18-4).

In the delivery room, the primary health care provider puts on a cap, a mask that has a shield or protective eyewear, and shoe covers. Hands are scrubbed and a sterile gown (with waterproof front and sleeves) is donned and gloves are put on. Nurses attending the birth may also need to wear caps, protective eyewear, masks, gowns, and gloves. The woman may then be draped with sterile drapes. In the birthing room, Standard Precautions are observed, but the amount and types of protective coverings worn by those in attendance may vary.

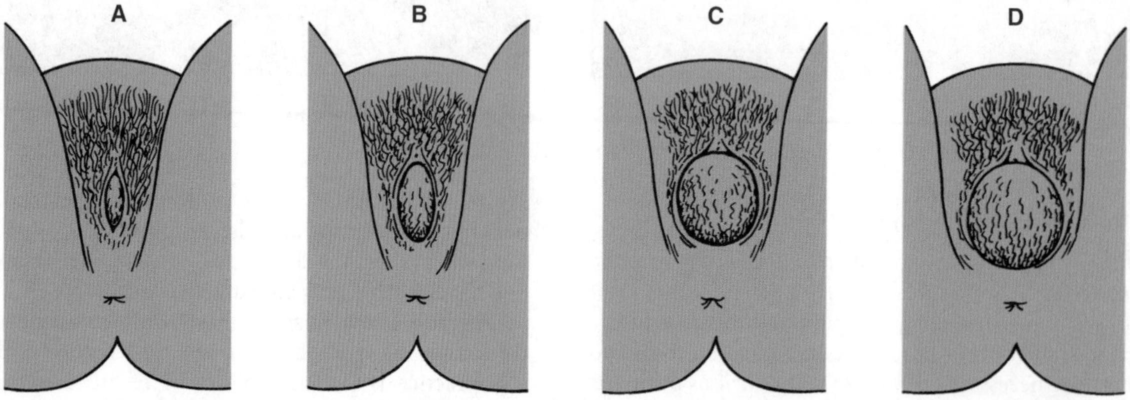

Fig. 18-24 Beginning birth with vertex presenting. **A,** Anteroposterior slit. **B,** Oval opening. **C,** Circular shape. **D,** Crowning.

Nursing contact with the parents is maintained by touching, verbal comforting, explaining the reasons for care, and sharing in the parents' joy at the birth of their child.

Mechanism of Birth: Vertex Presentation

The three phases of spontaneous birth of a fetus in a vertex presentation are (1) birth of the head, (2) birth of the shoulders, and (3) birth of the body and extremities (see Chapter 15).

With voluntary pushing, the head appears at the introitus (Fig. 18-24). Crowning occurs when the widest part of the head (the biparietal diameter) distends the vulva just before birth. The birth attendant may apply mineral oil to the perineum and stretch it as the head is crowning. Immediately before birth, the perineal musculature becomes greatly distended. If an episiotomy (incision into the perineum to enlarge the vaginal outlet) is necessary, it is done at this time to minimize soft tissue damage. Local anesthetic is administered before the episiotomy.

The primary health care provider may use a hands-on approach to control the birth of the head, believing that guarding the perineum results in a gradual birth that will prevent fetal intracranial injury, protect maternal tissues, and reduce postpartum perineal pain. This approach involves (1) applying pressure against the rectum, drawing it downward to aid in flexing the head as the back of the neck catches under the symphysis pubis; (2) then applying upward pressure from the coccygeal region (modified Ritgen maneuver) (Fig. 18-25) to extend the head during the actual birth, thereby protecting the musculature of the perineum; and (3) assisting the mother with voluntary control of the bearing-down efforts by coaching her to pant while letting uterine forces expel the fetus.

Some health care providers use a hands-poised (hands-off) approach when attending a birth. In this approach, hands are prepared to place light pressure on the fetal head to prevent rapid expulsion. Hands are not placed on the perineum or used to assist with birth of the shoulders and body.

The hands-on and hands-poised approaches have similar results in terms of perineal trauma and condition of the newborn. However, perineal pain is slightly less at 10 days postpartum when the hands-on approach is used (McCandlish, 2001). Guarding the perineum is a form of care likely to be beneficial (Enkin et al, 2000).

The umbilical cord often encircles the neck (nuchal cord) but rarely so tightly as to cause hypoxia. After the head is born, gentle palpation is used to feel for the cord. If present, the cord should be slipped gently over the head. If the loop is tight or if there is a second loop, the cord is clamped twice, cut between the clamps, and unwound from around the neck before the birth is allowed to continue. Mucus, blood, or meconium in the nasal or oral passages may prevent the newborn from breathing. To eliminate this problem, moist gauze sponges are used to wipe the nose and mouth. A bulb syringe is then inserted into the mouth and then the oropharynx to aspirate contents. The nares are cleared in the same fashion while the head is supported.

Prevention of Meconium Aspiration

If meconium has been present in the amniotic fluid during labor, preparations are made for wall suction, or in some

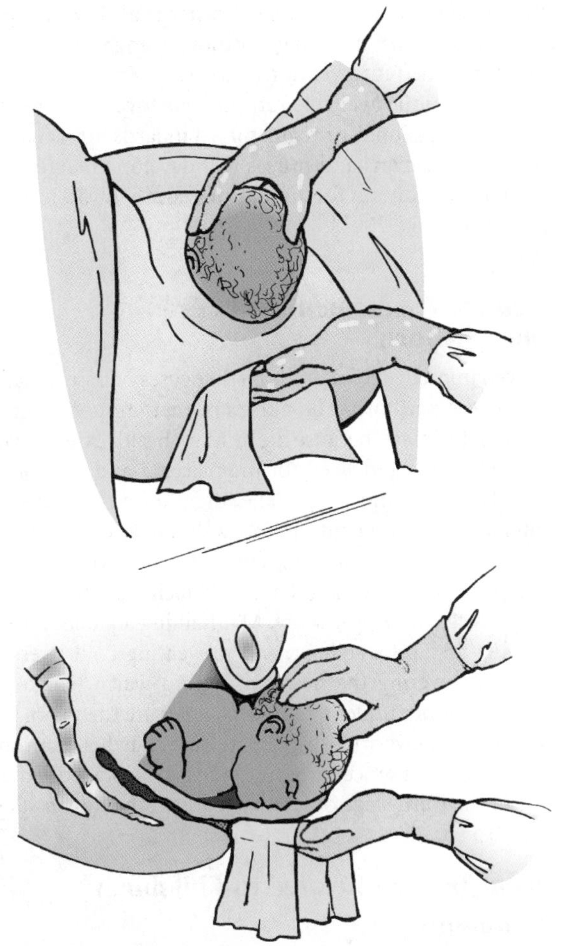

Fig. 18-25 Birth of head with modified Ritgen maneuver. Note control to prevent too rapid birth of head.

cases, a DeLee suction apparatus is placed on the sterile field for use. Fluids are withdrawn from the infant's mouth and nose before the first breath is taken to prevent meconium aspiration. The primary health care provider should refrain from using the DeLee device with oral suction to withdraw fluid from the infant unless the suction device is designed to keep mucus from entering the user's airway.

The time of birth is the precise time when the entire body is out of the mother. This time must be noted on the record.

If the condition of the newborn is not compromised, it may be placed on the mother's abdomen immediately after birth and covered with a warm, dry blanket. The cord may be clamped at this time, and the primary health care provider may ask if the woman's partner would like to cut the cord. If so, the partner is given a sterile pair of scissors and instructed to cut the cord 1 inch (2.5 cm) above the clamp (see Fig. 1-3).

Use of Fundal Pressure

Fundal pressure is the application of gentle, steady pressure against the fundus of the uterus to facilitate vaginal birth. Historically it has been used when the administration of analgesia and anesthesia decreased the woman's ability to push during the birth, for maternal exhaustion, or when second-stage fetal bradycardia or other nonreassuring FHR patterns were present. Fundal pressure is contraindicated in shoulder dystocia. In cases of shoulder dystocia, the all-fours position (the Gaskin maneuver) (Bruner et al, 1998), suprapubic pressure, and maternal position changes are among the recommended interventions (Cosner, 1996). There is no standard technique available for this maneuver, and no current legal, professional, or regulatory standards for its use exist. Ideally, physicians and nurses will develop an agreed-on plan for how requests for fundal pressure will be handled (Simpson & Knox, 2001).

Immediate Assessment and Care of the Newborn

Care given immediately after the birth focuses on assessing and stabilizing the newborn. The nurse's primary responsibility at this time is the infant, because the primary health care provider is involved with the delivery of the placenta and care of the mother. The nurse must watch the infant for signs of distress and initiate appropriate interventions should any appear.

A brief assessment of the infant can be performed while the mother is holding the infant. This includes checking the infant's airway and Apgar score. Maintaining a patent airway, supporting respiratory effort, and preventing cold stress by drying and covering the newborn with a warm blanket or placing him or her under a radiant warmer are the major priorities for the newborn's immediate care. Further examination, identification procedures, and care can be postponed until later in the third stage of labor or early in the fourth stage.

Perineal Trauma Related to Childbirth

Lacerations

Most acute injuries and lacerations of the perineum, vagina, uterus, and their support tissues occur during childbirth. Some injuries to the supporting tissues, whether they were acute or nonacute and whether they were repaired or not, may lead to genitourinary and sexual problems later in life (e.g., pelvic relaxation, uterine prolapse, cystocele, rectocele, dyspareunia, or urinary or bowel dysfunction).

Some damage occurs during every birth to the soft tissues of the birth canal and adjacent structures. The tendency to sustain lacerations varies with each woman because the soft tissue in some women may be less distensible. Heredity may be a factor in this. For example, the tissue of light-skinned women, especially those with reddish hair, is not as readily distensible as that of darker-skinned women, and healing may be less efficient. The perineal skin and vaginal mucosa may appear intact, but numerous small lacerations in underlying muscle and its fascia may be obscured. Damage to pelvic supports usually is readily apparent and is repaired after birth.

Immediate repair promotes healing, limits residual damage, and decreases the possibility of infection. Immediately after birth, the cervix, vagina, and perineum are inspected to look for damage. In addition, during the early postpartum period, the nurse and primary health care provider continue to inspect the perineum carefully and evaluate lochia and symptoms to identify any previously missed damage.

Perineal Lacerations

Perineal lacerations usually occur when the fetal head is being born. The extent of the laceration is defined in terms of its depth:

- **First degree**—Laceration extends through the skin and structures superficial to muscles
- **Second degree**—Laceration extends through muscles of perineal body
- **Third degree**—Laceration continues through anal sphincter muscle
- **Fourth degree**—Laceration also involves the anterior rectal wall

Perineal injury is often accompanied by small lacerations on the medial surfaces of the labia minora below the pubic rami and to the sides of the urethra (periurethral) and clitoris. Lacerations in this highly vascular area often result in profuse bleeding. Such lacerations must be repaired with absorbable suture (Fig. 18-26).

Special attention must be paid to third- and fourth-degree lacerations so that the woman retains fecal continence. Measures are taken to promote soft stools (e.g., roughage, fluid, activity, and stool softeners) for a few days to increase the woman's comfort and to foster healing. Antimicrobial therapy may be used in some cases. Enemas and suppositories are contraindicated for these women.

Vaginal Lacerations

Vaginal lacerations often occur in conjunction with perineal lacerations. Vaginal lacerations tend to extend up the lateral walls (sulci) and, if deep enough, involve the levator ani. Additional injury may occur high in the vaginal vault near the level of the ischial spines. Vaginal vault lacerations may be circular and may result from forceps rotation, especially in the presence of cephalopelvic disproportion, rapid fetal descent, or precipitous birth.

Cervical Injuries

Cervical injuries occur when the cervix retracts over the advancing fetal head. These cervical lacerations occur at the

??? Critical Thinking Exercise

APPLYING FUNDAL PRESSURE

Myra is a gravida 1, para 0 who has been in labor for 18 hours; her cervix has been completely effaced and 10 cm dilated for 2 ½ hours; the station has been at +1 for 45 minutes. She has been pushing for 2 hours and is exhausted. To assist in descent of the fetus, the primary health care provider has asked you to apply fundal pressure while he stretches the vaginal orifice and perineum. What should be your response to this request?

1. Evidence—Is there sufficient evidence to draw conclusions about what your proper action should be?
2. Assumptions—What assumptions can be made about the following issues?
   a. Benefits of fundal pressure
   b. Risks of fundal pressure
   c. Contraindications to fundal pressure
   d. Alternative approaches to the use of fundal pressure
3. What implications and priorities for nursing care can be drawn at this time?
4. Does the evidence objectively support your conclusion?
5. Are there alternative perspectives to your conclusion?

Reference: Simpson KR, Knox GE: Fundal pressure during the second stage of labor: clinical perspectives and risk management issues, *MCN Am J Matern Child Nurs* 26(2):64-71, 2001.

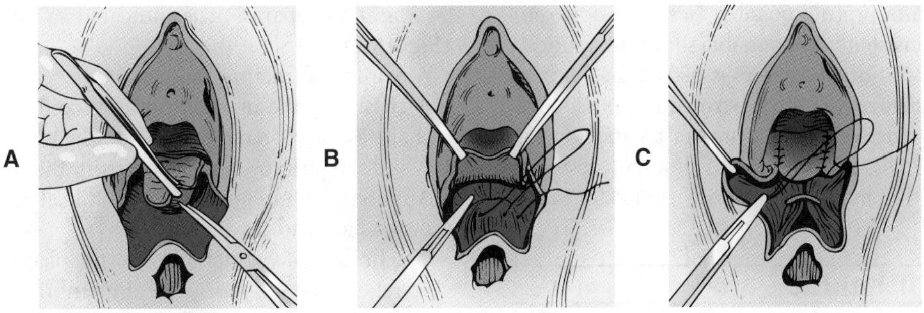

Fig. 18-26 Perineal lacerations. **A,** Bilateral sulcus tears, periurethral tear, and separation of anal sphincter. **B,** Exposure and approximation of levator ani structures. **C,** Approximation of torn bulbocavernous muscle.

lateral angles of the external os; most are shallow, and bleeding is minimal. More extensive lacerations may extend to the vaginal vault or beyond it into the lower uterine segment; serious bleeding may occur. Extensive lacerations may follow hasty attempts to enlarge the cervical opening artificially or to deliver the fetus before full cervical dilation is achieved. Injuries to the cervix can have adverse effects on future pregnancies and childbirths.

Episiotomy

An episiotomy is an incision made in the perineum to enlarge the vaginal outlet. It is performed more commonly in the United States and Canada than in Europe. The side-lying position for birth causes less tension on the perineum, making possible a gradual stretching of the perineum with fewer indications for episiotomies. There is clear evidence that routine or liberal performance of an episiotomy for birth is a form of care that is likely to be harmful or ineffective (Enkin et al, 2000). Currently, the practice in many settings is to manually support the perineum during birth and allow the perineum to tear rather than perform an episiotomy. Tears are often smaller than an episiotomy, are repaired easily, and heal quickly. The pain and discomfort resulting from episiotomies can interfere with mother-infant interaction, breastfeeding, reestablishment of sexual relationship with partner, and even emotional recovery after birth. The rate of episiotomies is lower when nurse-midwives rather than obstetricians attend births.

The type of episiotomy is designated by the site and direction of the incision (Fig. 18-27). Midline (median) episiotomy is most commonly used in the United States. It is effective, easily repaired, and generally the least painful. However, it is associated with a higher incidence of third- and fourth-degree lacerations. Sphincter tone is usually restored following primary healing and a good repair.

Mediolateral episiotomy is used in operative births when the need for posterior extension is likely. Although a fourth-degree laceration may be prevented, a third-degree laceration may occur. The blood loss is greater and the repair more difficult and painful than with midline episiotomies. It is more painful in the postpartum period, and the pain lasts longer.

Alternative measures for perineal management, such as warm compresses, manual support, and massage (e.g., prenatal and intrapartum), have been shown to reduce, to varying degrees, the incidence of episiotomies, but further research is recommended. Use of Kegel exercises in the prenatal and postpartum periods improves and restores the tone and strength of the perineal muscles. Health practices, including good nutrition and appropriate hygienic measures, help maintain the integrity and suppleness of the perineal tissue.

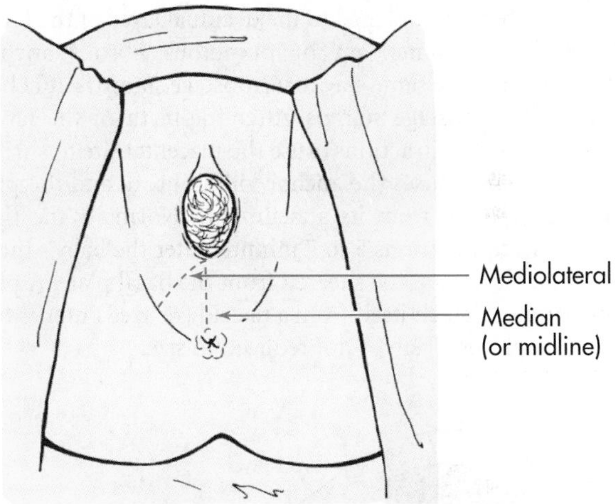

Fig. 18-27 Types of episiotomies.

Nurses acting as advocates can encourage women to use alternative birthing positions that reduce pressure on the perineum (e.g., lateral position) and to use spontaneous bearing-down efforts. In addition, nurses can educate other health care providers about measures to preserve perineal integrity and to be more flexible in defining the maximal limit for the duration of the second stage of labor as long as the maternal-fetal unit is stable.

Emergency Childbirth

Even under the best of circumstances there probably will come a time when the perinatal nurse will be required to assist with the birth of an infant without medical assistance. Because it is neither possible nor desirable to prevent an impending birth, the perinatal nurse must be able to function independently and be skilled in the safe birth of a vertex fetus (see Box 18-9).

A lateral Sims' posture may be the position of choice for birth when (1) the birth is progressing rapidly and there is insufficient time for slow distention of the perineum; (2) the fetal head seems too large to pass through the introitus without laceration, and episiotomy is not possible; or (3) the apparent size of the fetus is consistent with possible shoulder dystocia. In the lateral Sims position, less stress is placed on the perineum and better visualization of the perineum is possible as the upper leg is supported by the woman's partner or the nurse (see Fig. 18-17, *A*). In the event of shoulder dystocia, the lateral Sims' position increases the space needed for birth.

THIRD STAGE OF LABOR

The third stage of labor lasts from the birth of the baby until the placenta is expelled. The goal in the management of the third stage of labor is the prompt separation and expulsion of the placenta, achieved in the easiest, safest manner.

The placenta is attached to the decidual layer of the basal plate's thin endometrium by numerous fibrous anchor villi—much in the same way that a postage stamp is attached to a sheet of postage stamps. After the birth of the fetus, strong uterine contractions cause the placental site to shrink markedly. This causes the anchor villi to break and the placenta to separate from its attachments. Normally the first few strong contractions 5 to 7 minutes after the baby's birth cause the placenta to be sheared from the basal plate. A placenta cannot detach itself from a flaccid (relaxed) uterus because the placental site is not reduced in size.

Placental separation is indicated by the following signs (Fig. 18-28):

- A firmly contracting fundus
- A change in the uterus from a discoid to a globular ovoid shape as the placenta moves into the lower uterine segment
- A sudden gush of dark blood from the introitus
- Apparent lengthening of the umbilical cord as the placenta draws closer to the introitus
- The finding of vaginal fullness (the placenta) on vaginal or rectal examination, or of fetal membranes at the introitus

Depending on the preferences of the primary health care provider, an expectant or active approach may be used to manage the third stage of labor. Expectant management (watchful waiting) involves the natural, spontaneous separation and expulsion of the placenta by efforts of the mother with clamping and cutting of the cord after pulsation ceases. It may involve the use of gravity or nipple stimulation to facilitate separation and expulsion, but no oxytocic (uterotonic) medications are given. A quiet, relaxed environment that supports close skin-to-skin contact between mother and newborn also promotes the release of endogenous oxytocin.

Active management facilitates placental separation and expulsion with administration of one or more oxytocic (uterotonic) medications after the birth of the anterior shoulder of the fetus, clamping and cutting of the umbilical cord immediately, and delivery of the placenta by application of controlled cord

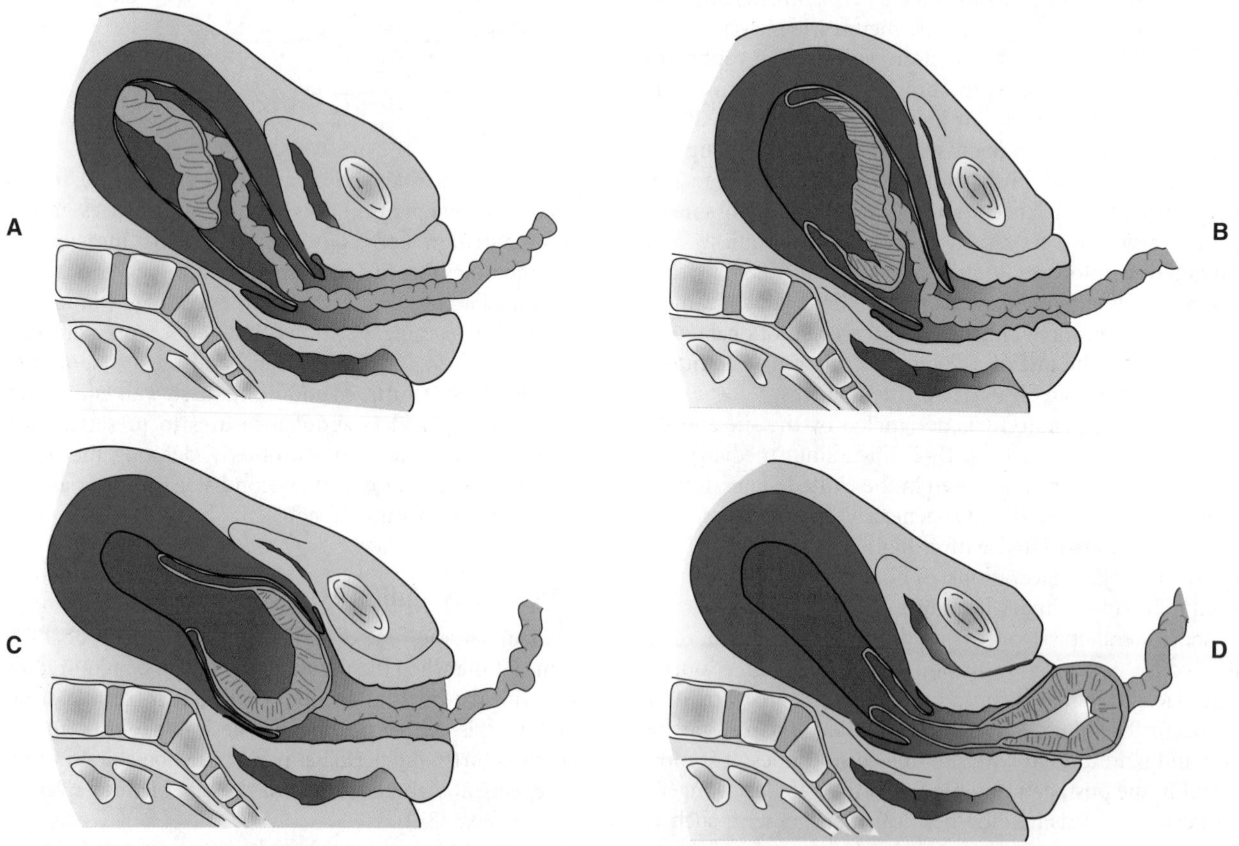

Fig. 18-28 Third stage of labor. **A,** Placenta begins the separation process in central portion with retroplacental bleeding. Uterus changes from discoid to globular shape. **B,** Placenta completes separation and enters lower uterine segment. Uterus is globular in shape. **C,** Placenta enters vagina, cord is seen to lengthen, and there may be increased bleeding. **D,** Expulsion (birth) of placenta and completion of third stage.

traction when signs of separation are noted. Research findings support the superiority of active management in terms of less blood loss and reduced risk of hemorrhage and other complications of the third stage of labor (Brucker, 2001; Prendiville, Elbourne, & McDonald, 2004). Active management of the third stage of labor is a beneficial form of care (Enkin et al, 2000).

To assist in the delivery of the placenta, the woman is instructed to push when signs of separation have occurred. If possible, the placenta should be expelled by maternal effort during a uterine contraction. Alternate compression and elevation of the fundus, plus minimal, controlled traction on the umbilical cord, may be used to facilitate delivery of the placenta and amniotic membranes. Oxytocics may be administered after the placenta is removed because they stimulate the uterus to contract, thereby helping to prevent hemorrhage.

Whether the placenta first appears by its shiny fetal surface (Schultze mechanism) or turns to show its dark roughened maternal surface (Duncan mechanism) is of no clinical importance. After the placenta and the amniotic membranes emerge, the primary health care provider examines them for intactness to ensure that no portion remains in the uterine cavity (i.e., no fragments of the placenta or membranes are retained) (Fig. 18-29).

Some women and their families may have culturally based beliefs regarding the care of the placenta and the manner of its disposal after birth, viewing the care and disposal of the placenta as a way of protecting the newborn from bad luck and illness. Requests by the woman to take the placenta home and dispose of it according to her customs may be at odds with health care agency policies, especially those related to infection control and the disposal of biologic wastes. Many cultures follow specific rules regarding the disposal of the placenta in terms of method (burning, drying, burying, or eating); site for disposal (in or near the home); and timing of disposal (immediately after birth, time of day, or by astrologic signs). If eaten, the placenta can be a means of restoring a woman's well-being after birth or of ensuring quality breast milk (Choudhry, 1997; Howard & Berbiglia, 1997; Lemon, 2002; Molina, 2001; Schneiderman, 1998).

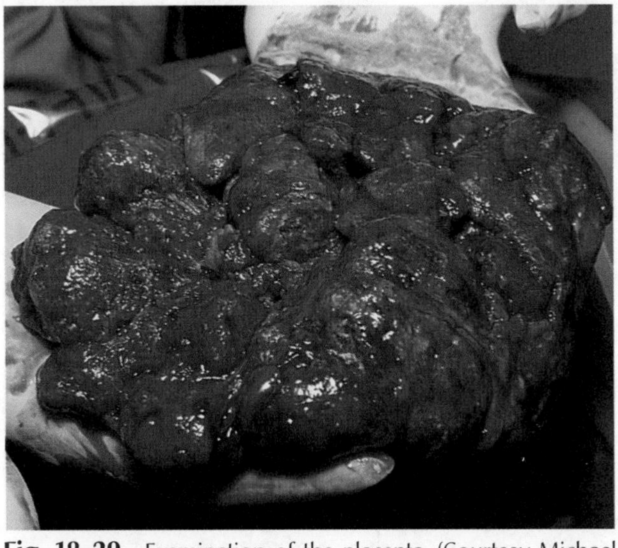

Fig. 18-29 Examination of the placenta. (Courtesy Michael S. Clement, MD, Mesa, AZ.)

Maternal Physical Status

Physiologic changes after birth are profound. The cardiac output increases rapidly as maternal circulation to the placenta ceases and the pooled blood from the lower extremities is mobilized. The pulse rate slows in response to the change in cardiac output and tends to remain slightly slower than before pregnancy for about 1 week.

Soon after the birth the woman's blood pressure usually returns to prepregnancy levels. Several factors contribute to an elevated blood pressure at this time: the excitement of the second stage, certain medications, and the time of day (blood pressure is highest during the late afternoon). Analgesics and anesthetics may also cause hypotension to develop in the hour after birth.

Signs of Potential Problems

The major risk for women during the third stage of labor is postpartum hemorrhage. While the primary health care provider completes the delivery of the placenta, the nurse observes the mother for signs of excessive blood loss, including alteration in vital signs, pallor, light-headedness, restlessness, decreased urinary output, and alteration in level of consciousness and orientation.

Because of the rapid cardiovascular changes taking place (e.g., the increased intracranial pressure during pushing and the rapid increase in cardiac output), the risk of rupture of a preexisting cerebral aneurysm and the risk of formation of pulmonary emboli are greater than usual during this period. Another dangerous, unpredictable problem is amniotic fluid embolism (see Chapter 19).

Women with a history of cardiac disorders are at increased risk for cardiac decompensation and pulmonary edema as a result of circulatory changes associated with the birth of the fetus and expulsion of the placenta. The nurse should carefully assess the woman's respiratory pattern and effort, especially in the early postpartum period.

Care after Placental Delivery

When the third stage is complete, and any lacerations are repaired or an episiotomy is sutured, the vulvar area is gently cleansed with warm, sterile water or normal saline solution and a perineal pad or an ice pack is applied to the perineum (some agencies or primary health care providers may require the use of sterile technique for perineal care immediately after birth). The birthing table or bed is repositioned and the woman's legs are lowered simultaneously if she gave birth in the lithotomy position. Drapes are removed and dry linen is placed under the woman's buttocks; she is provided with a clean gown and a warmed blanket. She is assisted into her bed if she is to be transferred from the birthing area to the recovery area. The side rails are raised during transfer. She may be given the baby to hold during the transfer, or the father or partner may carry the baby or transport it in a crib, either to the recovery area or to the nursery. If the woman labors, gives birth, and recovers in the same bed and room, she is refreshed following the protocol already described. Maternal and neonatal assessments for the fourth stage of labor are instituted. When fourth-stage recovery is complete, the woman may be transferred via wheelchair to a room on the postpartum unit. Box 18-10 summarizes normal vaginal childbirth.

BOX 18-10

Normal Vaginal Childbirth

First Stage

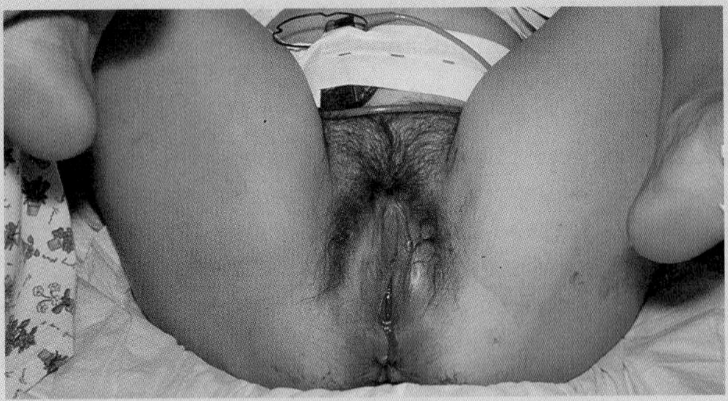

Anteroposterior slit. Vertex visible during contraction.

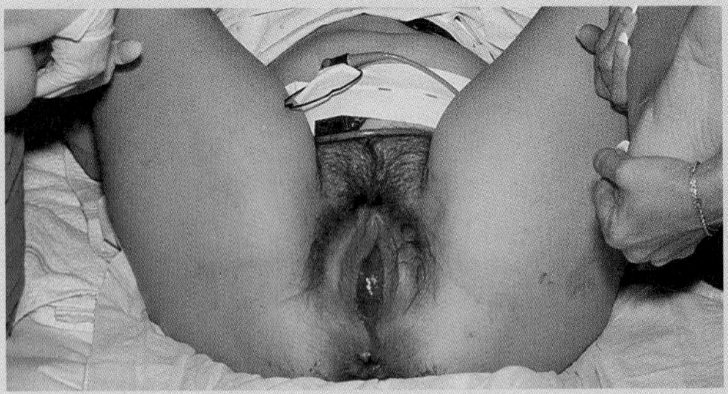

Oval opening. Vertex presenting. NOTE: Nurse *(on left)* is wearing gloves but support person *(on right)* is not.

Second Stage

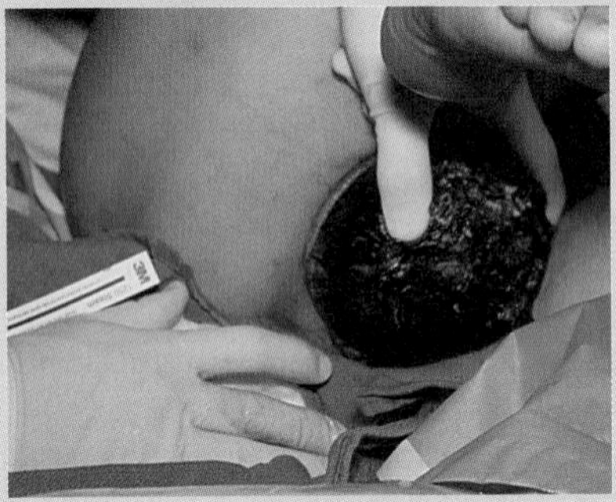

Crowning.

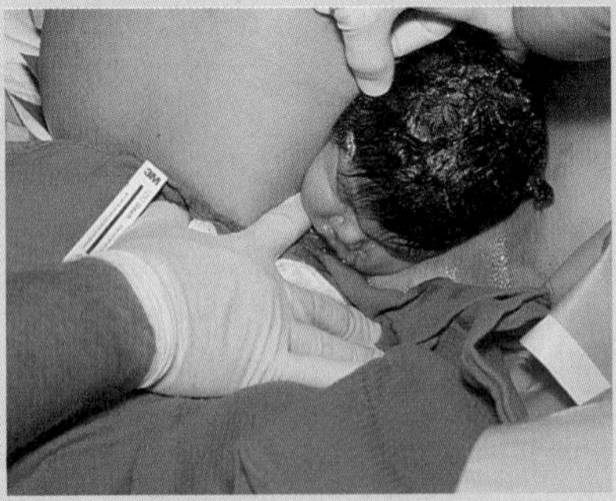

Nurse-midwife using Ritgen maneuver as head is born by extension.

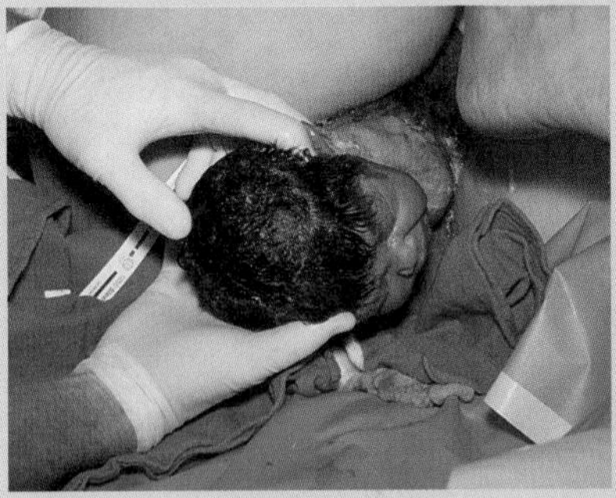

After nurse-midwife checks for nuchal cord, she supports head during external rotation and restitution.

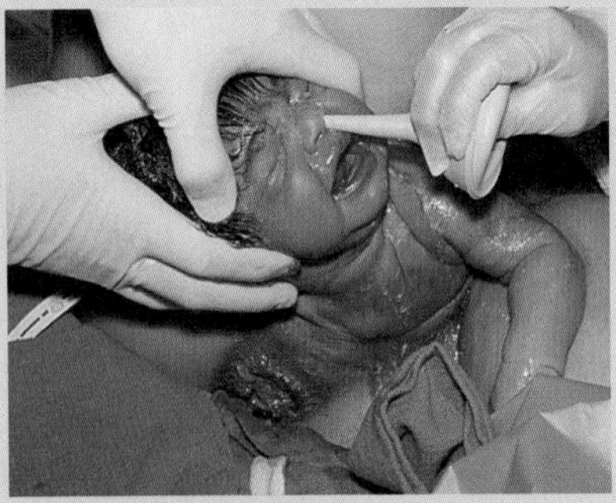

Use of bulb syringe to suction mucus.

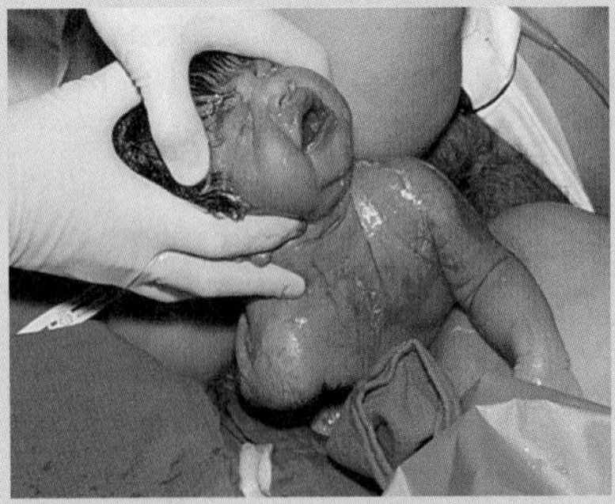

Birth of posterior shoulder.

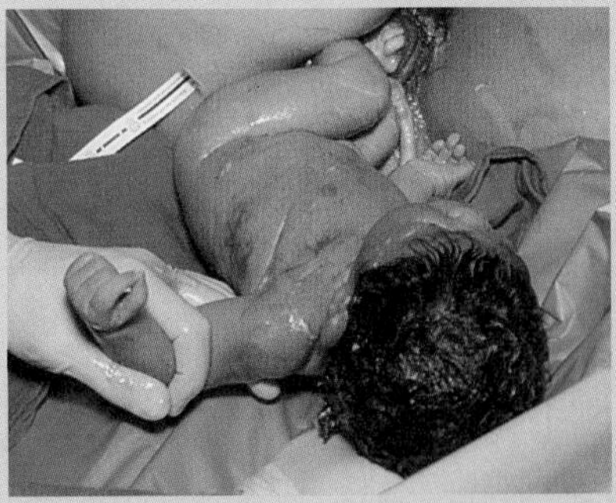

Birth of newborn by slow expulsion.

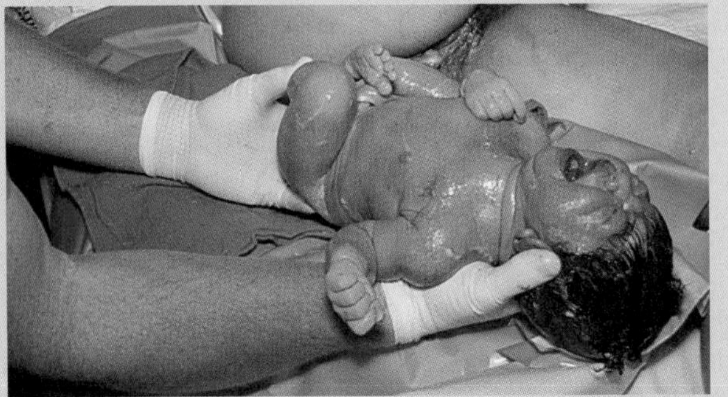

Second stage complete. Note that newborn is not completely pink yet.

Courtesy Michael S. Clement, MD, Mesa, AZ.

BOX 18-10

Normal Vaginal Childbirth—cont'd

Third Stage

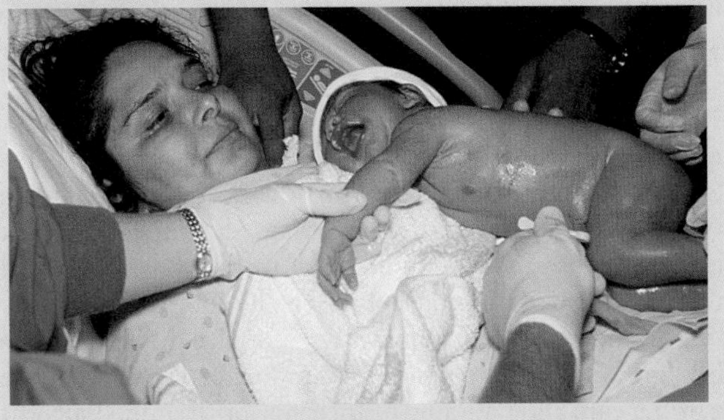

Newborn placed on mother's abdomen while cord is clamped and cut.

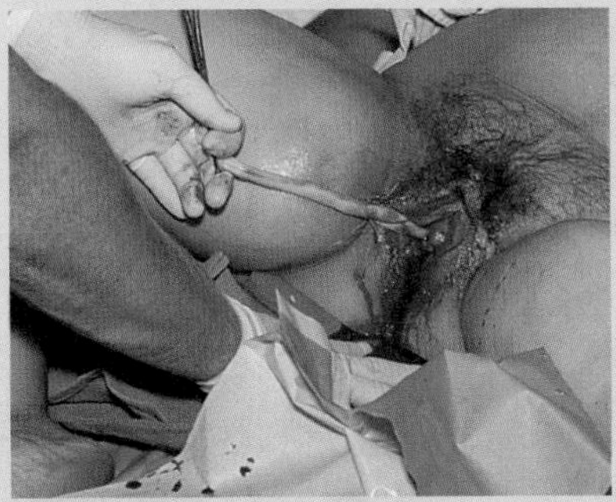

Note increased bleeding as placenta separates.

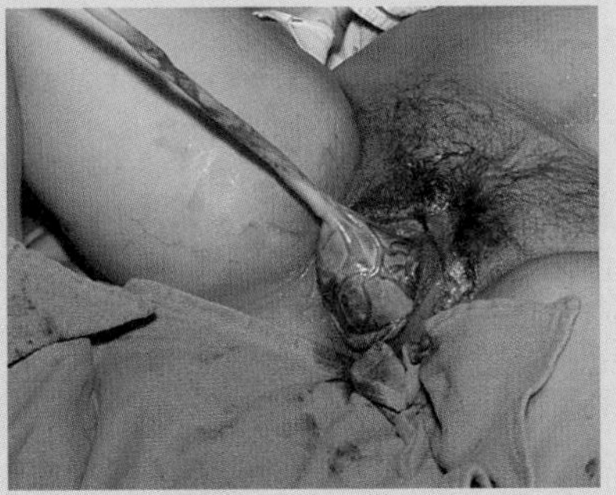

Expulsion of placenta.

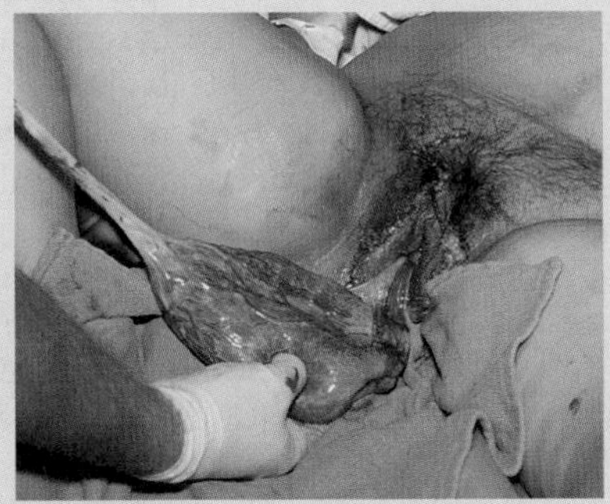

Expulsion is complete, marking the end of the third stage.

The Newborn

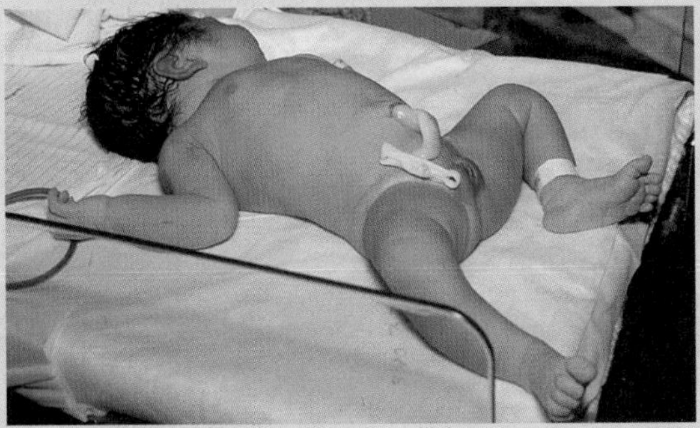

Newborn awaiting assessment. Note that color is almost completely pink.

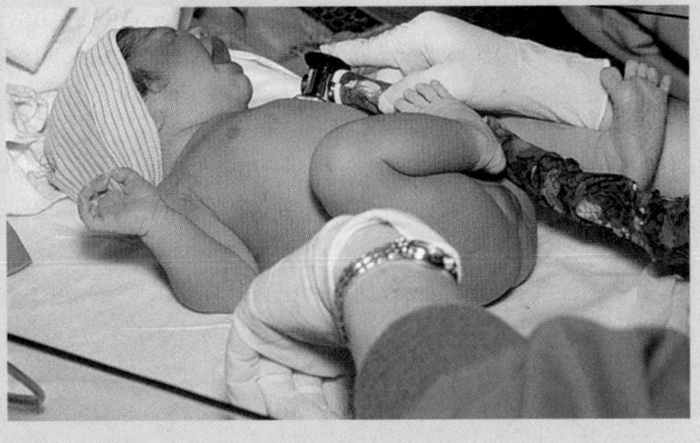

Newborn assessment under radiant warmer.

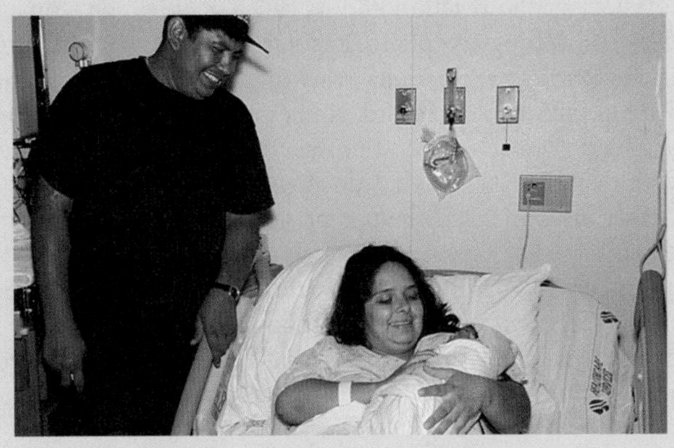

Parents admiring their newborn.

Interactions with the Newborn

Most parents enjoy being able to handle, hold, explore, and examine the baby immediately after birth. Both parents can assist with the thorough drying of the infant. The infant may be wrapped in a receiving blanket and placed on the woman's abdomen. If skin-to-skin contact is desired, the unwrapped infant may be placed on the woman's abdomen and then covered with a warm blanket.

Holding the newborn next to her skin helps the mother maintain the baby's body heat and provides skin-to-skin contact; care must be taken to keep the head warm as well. Stockinette caps are sometimes used to cover the newborn's head.

Many women wish to begin breastfeeding their newborns at this time to take advantage of the infant's alert state (first period of reactivity) and to stimulate the production of oxytocin, which promotes contraction of the uterus. Others prefer to wait until the newborn, parents, and older siblings are together in the recovery area. In some cultures, breastfeeding is not considered acceptable until the milk comes in.

The woman usually feels some discomfort while the primary health care provider carries out the postbirth vaginal examination. The nurse can assist the woman to use breathing and relaxation techniques or distraction techniques to assist her in dealing with the discomfort. During this time, the nurse assesses the newborn's physical condition; the baby can be weighed and measured, given eye prophylaxis and a vitamin K injection, given an identification bracelet, wrapped in warm blankets, and then given to the partner or back to the mother to hold when she is ready.

Family-Newborn Relationships

The woman's reaction to the sight of her newborn may range from excited outbursts of laughing, talking, and even crying to apparent apathy. A polite smile and nod may be her only acknowledgment of the comments of nurses and the primary health care provider. Occasionally the reaction is one of anger or indifference; the woman turns away from the baby, concentrates on her own pain, and may make hostile comments. These varied reactions can arise from pleasure, exhaustion, or deep disappointment. When evaluating parent-newborn interactions after birth, the nurse should also consider the cultural characteristics of the woman and her family and the expected behaviors of that culture. In some cultures, the birth of a male child is preferred, and women may grieve when a female child is born (Choudhry, 1997).

Whatever the reaction and its cause may be, the woman needs continuing acceptance and support from all staff. Notation regarding the parents' reaction to the newborn can be made in the recovery record. Nurses can assess this reaction by asking themselves questions such as the following: How do the parents look? What do they say? What do they do? Further assessment of the parent-newborn relationship can be conducted as care is given during the period of recovery. This is especially important if warning signs (e.g., passive or hostile reactions to newborn, disappointment with sex or appearance of newborn, absence of eye contact, or limited interaction of parents with each other) were noted immediately after birth. The nurse may find it helpful to discuss any warning signs that may have been noted with the woman's primary health care provider.

Siblings, who may have appeared only remotely interested in the final phases of the second stage, tend to experience renewed interest and excitement when the newborn appears. They can then be encouraged to touch or hold the baby (Fig. 18-30).

Parents usually respond to praise of their newborn. Many need to be reassured that the dusky appearance of the baby's extremities immediately after birth is normal until circulation is well established. If appropriate, the nurse should explain the reason for the molding of the newborn's head. Information about hospital routine can be communicated. It is important, however, for nurses to recognize that the cultural background of the parents may influence expectations regarding care and handling of their newborn immediately after birth. For example, some traditional Southeast Asians believe that the head should not be touched because it is the most sacred part of a person's body. They also believe that praise of the baby is dangerous because jealous spirits may cause the baby harm or take it away (D'Avanzo & Geissler, 2003). Hospital staff members, by their interest and concern,

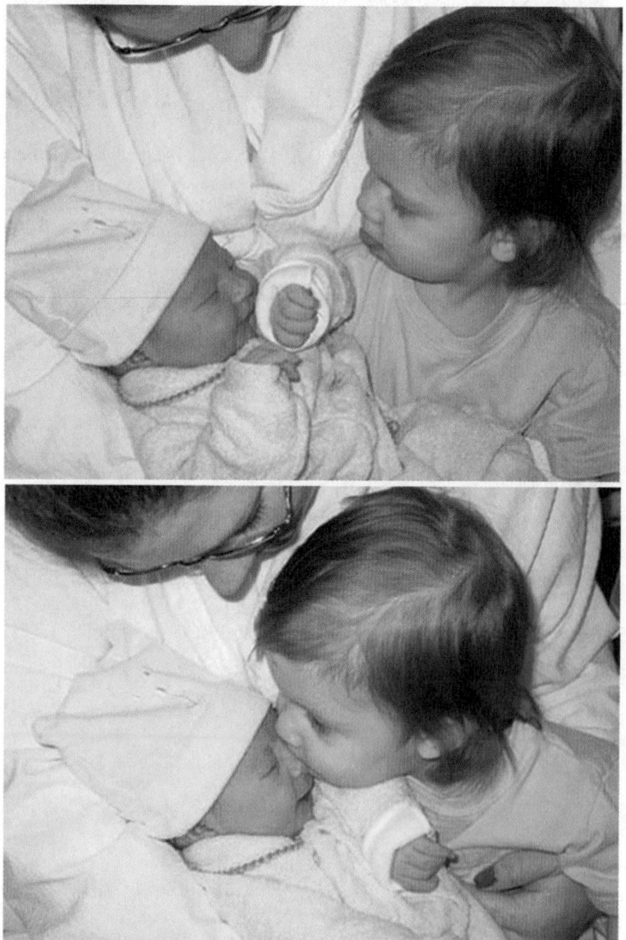

Fig. 18-30 Big sister being introduced to baby brother. **A**, Not sure who this new person is. **B**, A kiss says he is OK. (Courtesy Rebekah Vogel, Ft. Collins, CO.)

can provide an environment for making this time a satisfying experience for parents, family, and significant others.

Determining a woman's satisfaction with and impressions of her childbirth experience is a critical component in the provision of high-quality maternal-newborn health care that meets the individual needs of women and families using these services. Reviewing the childbirth experience with someone who will listen, support, and explain has been found to reduce the degree of postpartum depression experienced by many women during the first week or so after birth (Wessely, 1998).

Evaluation

Evaluation is an ongoing process and is based on expected outcomes of care (see the Nursing Care Plan on pp. 514).

Key Points

- The onset of labor may be difficult to determine for both nulliparous and multiparous women.
- The familiar environment of her home is most often the ideal place for a woman during the latent phase of the first stage of labor.
- The nurse assumes much of the responsibility for assessing the progress of labor and for keeping the primary health care provider informed about progress in labor and deviations from expected findings.
- The fetal heart rate and pattern reveal the fetal response to the stress of the labor process.
- Meconium-stained amniotic fluid is not always indicative of fetal distress associated with hypoxia.
- Regardless of the actual labor and birth experience, the woman's or couple's perception of the birth experience is most likely to be positive when events and performances are consistent with expectations, especially in terms of maintaining control and adequacy of pain relief.
- The woman's level of anxiety may rise when she does not understand what is being said to her about her labor because of the medical terminology used or because of a language barrier.
- Coaching, emotional support, and comfort measures assist the woman to use her energy constructively in relaxing and working with the contractions.
- Doulas provide a continuous supportive presence during labor that can have a positive effect on the process of childbirth and its outcome.
- The cultural beliefs and practices of a woman and her significant others, including her partner, can have a profound influence on their approach to labor and birth.
- Objective signs indicate that the placenta has separated and is ready to be expelled; excessive traction (pulling) on the umbilical cord, before the placenta has separated, can result in maternal injury.
- Siblings present for labor and birth need preparation and support for the event.
- Most parents/families enjoy being able to handle, hold, explore, and examine the baby immediately after birth.
- Nurses should observe progress in the development of parent-child relationships and be alert for warning signs that may appear during the immediate postpartum period.
- Following an emergency childbirth out of the hospital, the neonate sucking on the mother's nipple can stimulate the release of natural oxytocin from the maternal posterior pituitary gland; oxytocin stimulates the uterus to contract, thereby preventing postpartum hemorrhage.
- A woman benefits from reviewing her childbirth experience with the nurse who managed her care during the process of labor and birth.

Answer Guidelines to Critical Thinking Exercise

Applying Fundal Pressure

1. The use of fundal pressure in labor is controversial; clinical disagreements between physicians and nurses can arise when the use of fundal pressure is requested. Nurses may feel pressured to use this technique even when they feel it is not in the best interest of the mother and the fetus. There is no published evidence that fundal pressure is safe or effective. Very little about fundal pressure appears in the literature; often, when it is used, it is not documented in the medical record. To avert clinical disagreements, a plan for how such a request will be handled should be formulated.
2. (a) *Indications for fundal pressure.* Sometimes when artificial rupture of membranes is indicated, pressure is used to guide the head of the fetus into the pelvis against the cervix to reduce the risk of prolapse of the cord. When the FHR is nonreassuring or difficult to trace electronically and a fetal scalp electrode (FSE) is to be placed but the fetal station is high, gentle fundal pressure may move the fetal head down and make it easier to apply the FSE. When the fetal head is crowning, maternal efforts are not enough for birth to occur, and the FHR is nonreassuring (indicating the need for an expeditious birth), fundal pressure may be the quickest way to effect birth. (b) *Risks of fundal pressure.* Fetus/newborn: brachial plexus injury, fractures of the humerus and clavicle, spinal cord injury, subgaleal hemorrhage, and fetal death. Mother: perineal injuries (third- and fourth-degree lacerations), abdominal bruising, fractured ribs, liver rupture, uterine rupture, uterine inversion, possible amniotic fluid embolism. Nurse: back, arm, wrist, and hand injuries have been reported. (c) *Contraindications to fundal pressure.* Fundal pressure should be avoided in the case of shoulder dystocia. If fundal pressure is applied, the anterior shoulder is likely to be further impacted, the birth delayed, and the risk of fetal injury increased. Suprapubic pressure is more commonly used to relieve shoulder dystocia. (d) *Alternatives to the use of fundal pressure.* Provider needs to be patient; pain relief measures should aim for epidural analgesia, not anesthesia; delaying pushing and allowing passive descent to prevent maternal fatigue; directed coaching in pushing efforts.
3. The fetus needs to be assessed. If the fetal heart rate and pattern are reassuring, there is no need to rush to birth and the mother can have a period of rest. Directed coaching in pushing can be provided.

4. There is little evidence in the literature about the risks and benefits of fundal pressure. The literature that exists mainly describes medicolegal problems when fundal pressure to relieve shoulder dystocia was used and it resulted in injury to the fetus/newborn. There is very limited information about the use of fundal pressure to shorten second-stage labor in low risk women.
5. The optimal solution to such requests is to develop an interdisciplinary plan to manage risk before the occasion for the request for application of fundal pressure arises. Each department must develop its own approach. The attorney and professional liability insurance carrier of the agency should be involved in the discussion. If nurses are to apply fundal pressure, they must be trained in the proper application. The use of fundal pressure should be documented.

Resources

American College of Nurse Midwives
818 Connecticut Ave. NW, Suite 900
Washington, DC 20006
202-728-9860
www.midwife.org

Association of Labor Assistants and Childbirth Educators (ALACE)
PO Box 390436
Cambridge, MA 02139
617-441-2500
www.alace.org

Childbirth Graphics
PO Box 21207
Waco, TX 76702-1207
800-299-3366
www.childbirthgraphics.com

Childbirth Organization
www.childbirth.org

Coalition for Improving Maternity Services (CIMS)
c/o ASPO/Lamaze
1200 19th Street NW, S-300
Washington, DC 20036
www.clicked.com/babytime/index.html

Doulas of North America (DONA)
PO Box 626
Jasper, IN 47547
888-788-DONA
www.dona.com

Gentlebirth
www.gentlebirth.org

Global Maternal/Child Health Association and Waterbirth International
PO Box 1400
Wilsonville, OR 97070
503-673-0026
www.waterbirth.org

International Childbirth Education Association, Inc. (ICEA)
PO Box 20048
Minneapolis, MN 55420
952-854-8660
www.icea.org

Journal of Midwifery and Women's Health (formerly *Journal of Nurse-Midwifery*)
Elsevier Science, Inc.
655 Avenue of the Americas
New York, NY 10010
212-989-5800
www.elsevier.com

Journal of Perinatal and Neonatal Nursing
Aspen Publishers, Inc.
7201 McKinney Circle
Frederick, MD 21704
800-234-1660
www.aspenpublishers.com

Midwives Alliance of North America (MANA)
4805 Lawrenceville Hwy.
Suite 116-279
Lilburn, GA 30047
888-923-6262
www.mana.org

National Association of Childbearing Centers (NACC)
3123 Gottschall Road
Perkiomenville, PA 18074
215-234-8068
www.birthcenters.org

National Association of Parents and Professionals for Safe Alternatives in Childbirth (NAPSAC)
Route 4, Box 646
Marble Hill, MO 63764
573-238-2010
www.napsac.org

Online Birth Center (OBC)
www.moonlily.com/obc

References

Anderhold K, Roberts J: Phases of second stage labor: four descriptive case studies, *J Nurse Midwifery* 36(5):267-275, 1991.

Brucker MC: Management of the third stage of labor: an evidence-based approach, *J Midwifery Womens Health* 46(6):381-392, 2001.

Bruner JP et al: All-fours maneuver for reducing shoulder dystocia during labor, *J Reprod Med* 43(5):439-443, 1998.

Callister LC: Cultural meanings of childbirth, *J Obstet Gynecol Neonatal Nurs* 24(4):327-331, 1995.

Cesario SK: Should cameras be allowed in the delivery room? *MCN Am J Matern Child Nurs* 23(2):87-91, 1998.

Choudhry UK: Traditional practices of women from India: pregnancy, childbirth, and newborn care, *J Obstet Gynecol Neonatal Nurs* 26(5):533-539, 1997.

Cosner KR: Use of fundal pressure during second-stage labor: a pilot study, *J Nurse Midwifery* 41(4):334-337, 1996.

D'Avanzo CE, Geissler EM: *Cultural health assessment,* ed 3, St Louis, 2003, Mosby.

Davies BL, Hodnett E: Labor support: nurses' self-efficacy and views about factors influencing implementation, *J Obstet Gynecol Neonatal Nurs* 31(1):48-56, 2002.

d'Entremont M: Directed pushing in the second stage of labour, *Modern Midwife* 6(6):12-16, 1996.

Enkin M et al: *A guide to effective care in pregnancy and childbirth,* ed 3, Oxford, NY, 2000, Oxford University Press.

Gagnon AJ, Waghorn K: One-to-one nurse labor support of nulliparous women stimulated with oxytocin, *J Obstet Gynecol Neonatal Nurs* 28(4):371-376, 1999.

Hanson L: Second stage positioning in nurse midwifery practices. Part 1: position use and preferences, *J Nurse Midwifery* 43(5):320-324, 1998a.

Hanson L: Second stage positioning in nurse midwifery practices. Part 2: factors affecting use, *J Nurse Midwifery* 43(5):326-330, 1998b.

Hanson L, VandeVusse L, Harrod KS: The theater of birth: scenes from women's scripts, *J Perinat Neonatal Nurs* 15(2):18-35, 2001.

Heritage C: Working with childhood sexual abuse survivors during pregnancy, labor, and birth, *J Obstet Gynecol Neonatal Nurs* 27(6):671-677, 1998.

Hodnett E et al: Continuous support for women during childbirth (Cochrane Review, 2003). In *The Cochrane Library,* Issue 4, Chichester, UK, 2004, John Wiley & Sons.

Howard JY, Berbiglia VA: Caring for childbearing Korean women, *J Obstet Gynecol Neonatal Nurs* 26(6):665-671, 1997.

Kayne MA, Greulich MB, Albers LL: Doulas: an alternative yet complementary addition to care during childbirth, *Clin Obstet Gynecol* 44(4):692-703, 2001.

Lemon BS: Exploring Latino rituals in birthing, *AWHONN Lifelines* 6(5):443-445, 2002.

Mackey MM: Use of water in labor and birth, *Clin Obstet Gynecol* 44(4):733-749, 2001.

Mahan C, McKay S: Are we overmanaging second stage labor? *Contemp OB/GYN* 24:37-63, 1984.

Mattson S: Working toward cultural competence: making first steps through cultural assessment, *AWHONN Lifelines* 4(4):41-43, 2000.

Mayberry LJ et al: Managing second stage labor, *AWHONN Lifelines* 3(6):28-34, 1999/2000.

McCandlish R: Perineal trauma: prevention and treatment, *J Midwifery Womens Health* 46(6):396-401, 2001.

McKay S, Barrows T: Holding back: maternal readiness to give birth, *MCN Am J Matern Child Nurs* 16(5):250-254, 1991.

Melender HL: Experiences of fears associated with pregnancy and childbirth: a study of 329 pregnant women, *Birth* 29(2):101-111, 2002.

Miltner RS: Identifying labor support actions of intrapartum nurses, *J Obstet Gynecol Neonatal Nurs* 29(5):491-499, 2000.

Miltner RS: More than support: nursing interventions provided to women in labor, *J Obstet Gynecol Neonatal Nurs* 31(6):753-761, 2002.

Minato JF: Is it time to push? Examining rest in second-stage labor, *AWHONN Lifelines* 4(6):20-23, 2000.

Molina JW: Traditional Native American practices in obstetrics, *Clin Obstet Gynecol* 44(4):661-670, 2001.

Moore M: Ethical issues for nurses providing perinatal care in community settings, *J Perinat Neonatal Nurs* 14(2):25-35, 2000.

Petersen L, Besuner P: Pushing techniques during labor: issues and controversies, *J Obstet Gynecol Neonatal Nurs* 26(6):719-726, 1997.

Prendiville W, Elbourne D, McDonald S: Active versus expectant management in the third stage of labour (Cochrane Review, 2000). *Cochrane Database System Review* (4), 2004.

Rhodes N, Hutchinson S: Labor experiences of childhood sexual abuse survivors, *Birth* 21(4):213-220, 1994.

Roberts JE: The "push" for evidence: management of the second stage, *J Midwifery Womens Health* 47(1):2-15, 2002.

Schneiderman JU: Rituals of placenta disposal, *MCN Am J Matern Child Nurs* 23(3):142-143, 1998.

Shermer RH, Raines DA: Positioning during the second stage of labor: moving back to basics, *J Obstet Gynecol Neonatal Nurs* 26(6):727-734, 1997.

Shorten A, Donsante J, Shorten B: Birth position, accoucheur, and perineal outcomes: informing women about choices for vaginal birth, *Birth* 29(1):18-27, 2002.

Simkin P, Ancheta R: *The labor progress handbook,* Malden, MA, 2000, Blackwell Science.

Simpson KR, Knox GE: Fundal pressure during the second stage of labor: clinical perspectives and risk management issues, *MCN Am J Matern Child Nurs* 26(2):64-71: 2001.

Tucker SM: *Pocket guide to fetal monitoring and assessment,* ed 5, St Louis, 2004, Mosby.

Tumblin A, Simkin P: Pregnant women's perception of their nurse's role during labor and delivery, *Birth* 28(1):52-56, 2001.

Waymire V: A triggering time: childbirth may recall sexual abuse memories, *AWHONN Lifelines* 1(2):47-50, 1997.

Weber SF: Cultural aspects of pain in childbearing women, *J Obstet Gynecol Neonatal Nurs* 25(1):67-72, 1996.

Wessely S: Commentary: reducing distress after normal childbirth, *Birth* 25(4):220-221, 1998.

Unit 4

19 Labor and Birth at Risk

LEARNING OBJECTIVES

On completion of this chapter the reader will be able to:

- Differentiate between *preterm birth* and *low birth weight.*
- Identify risk factors for preterm birth.
- Discuss current interventions to prevent preterm birth.
- Discuss the use of tocolytics and antenatal glucocorticoids in preterm birth.
- Examine the effects of prescribed bed rest on pregnant women and their families.
- Define *preterm premature rupture of membranes* (PPROM).
- Describe nursing management of a trial of labor, induction and augmentation of labor, forceps- and vacuum-assisted birth, cesarean birth, and vaginal birth after a cesarean birth.
- Discuss the criteria for evaluating the nursing care of women experiencing labor and birth complications.
- Describe the care of a woman experiencing postterm pregnancy.
- Discuss obstetric emergencies and their appropriate management.

ELECTRONIC RESOURCES

Additional information related to the content in Chapter 19 can be found on

the companion website at evolve
http://evolve.elsevier.com/Wong/maternal/

- NCLEX Review Questions
- Case Study–Preterm Labor
- Case Study–Postdate Pregnancy
- WebLinks

or the interactive student CD-ROM
Activities for Chapter 19 include the following:

- NCLEX Review Questions
- Case Study–Preterm Labor
- Case Study–Postdate Pregnancy
- Nursing Care Plan–Preterm Labor
- Nursing Care Plan–Dysfunctional Labor

When complications arise during labor and birth, perinatal morbidity and mortality risks increase. Some complications are anticipated, especially if the mother is identified as high risk during the antepartum period; others are unexpected or unforeseen. The woman, her family, and the health care team can feel devastated when things go wrong. Nurses must recognize these feelings if they are to provide effective support. It is crucial for nurses to understand the normal birth process to prevent and detect deviations from normal labor and birth and to implement nursing measures when complications arise. Optimum care of the laboring woman, the fetus, and the family experiencing complications is possible only when the nurse and other members of the obstetric team use their knowledge and skills in a concerted effort to provide care. This chapter focuses on problems of preterm labor and birth, dystocia, and postterm pregnancy and obstetric emergencies.

PRETERM LABOR AND BIRTH

Preterm labor is defined as cervical changes and uterine contractions occurring between 20 weeks and 37 weeks of pregnancy. *Preterm birth* is any birth that occurs before the completion of 37 weeks of pregnancy. Preterm labor and preterm birth are the most serious complications of pregnancy because they lead to about 90% of all neonatal deaths, with more than 75% of these deaths occurring in infants born at fewer than 32 weeks of gestation. Preterm birth is second only to congenital anomalies as a cause of infant death. In 2002, the overall preterm birth rate for all races in the United States was 12.1%. The very low preterm birth rate (birth that occurs before the completion of 32 weeks of pregnancy) was 1.96% in 2002 (Martin et al, 2003).

evolve CASE STUDY–PRETERM LABOR

Preterm Birth vs. Low Birth Weight

Although they have distinctly different meanings, the terms *preterm birth* or *prematurity* and *low birth weight* are often used interchangeably. Preterm birth describes length of gestation (i.e., less than 37 weeks regardless of the weight of the infant), whereas low birth weight describes only weight at the time of birth (i.e., 2500 g or less). Low birth weight is far easier to measure than preterm birth, and thus in many settings and publications, *low birth weight* has been used as a substitute term for *preterm birth.* Preterm birth, however, is a more dangerous health condition for an infant because length of time in the uterus correlates with immaturity of body systems. Low-birth-weight babies can be, but are not necessarily, preterm. Pregnant women who are poorly nourished or who have various complications of pregnancy that interfere with uteroplacental perfusion, such as gestational hypertension, may give birth to a baby at term who is low birth weight because of intrauterine growth restriction (IUGR).

The incidence of preterm birth in the United States is increasing and varies according to race; the 2003 rate for African-Americans (17.8%) was considerable higher than that for Hispanics (11.9%), and Caucasians (11.3%), (Martin et al, 2005). The increase in rates is attributed largely to the increase in multiple births. Sociodemographics may play a part in the race-based differences in preterm birth. Preterm birth rates are higher among socially disadvantaged populations, including minorities, women with low levels of education, and women who receive late or no prenatal care (Martin et al, 2003; Maupin et al, 2004). The preterm birth rate is higher among women younger than 15 years of age or older than 45 years (Martin et al, 2003).

Predicting Preterm Labor and Birth

The known risk factors for preterm birth are shown in Box 19-1. The risk factors most commonly associated with

Critical Thinking Exercise

PRETERM LABOR

You are assigned to Yolanda, who is experiencing preterm labor at 28 weeks of gestation. She has a 2-year-old son at home. This is her third admission for preterm labor during this pregnancy. Her primary health care provider had told her she must remain hospitalized on bed rest until she reaches 37 weeks of gestation or until birth of the baby, whichever comes first. She tearfully asks you why she can't be at home on bed rest, who will help care for her son, and how she will manage to keep from going crazy staying in bed that long. How will you respond to her concerns?

1. Evidence—Is there sufficient evidence to draw conclusions about the benefits of bed rest to prevent preterm birth?
2. Assumptions—What assumptions can be made about the following issues?
   a. The impact her history might have on the medical and nursing care she receives during this pregnancy
   b. The pros and cons of home management vs. hospital management for the prevention of preterm birth for this woman
   c. Ways to reduce the frustration and boredom that the woman will experience if she is restricted to bed rest for the next several weeks
   d. Resources available to assist with care of her 2-year-old son
3. What implications and priorities for nursing care can be drawn at this time?
4. Does the evidence objectively support your conclusion?
5. Are there alternative perspectives to your conclusion?

BOX 19-1

Risk Factors for Preterm Labor

Demographic Risks
- Nonwhite race
- Age (<17 yr, >35 yr)
- Low socioeconomic status
- Unmarried
- Less than high school education

Biophysical Risks
- Previous preterm labor or birth
- Second trimester abortion (more than two spontaneous or therapeutic); stillbirths
- Grand multiparity; short interval between pregnancies (≤1 year since last birth); family history of preterm labor and birth
- Progesterone deficiency
- Uterine anomalies or fibroids; uterine irritability
- Cervical incompetence, trauma, shortened length
- Exposure to DES or other toxic substances
- Medical diseases (e.g., diabetes, hypertension, anemia)
- Small stature (<119 cm in height; <45.5 kg or underweight for height)
- Current pregnancy risks:
  - Multifetal pregnancy
  - Hydramnios
  - Bleeding
  - Placental problems (e.g., placenta previa, abruptio placentae)
  - Infections (e.g., pyelonephritis, recurrent urinary tract infections, asymptomatic bacteriuria, bacterial vaginosis, chorioamnionitis)
  - Gestational hypertension
  - Premature rupture of the membranes
  - Fetal anomalies
  - Inadequate plasma volume expansion; anemia

Behavioral-Psychosocial Risks
- Poor nutrition; weight loss or low weight gain
- Smoking (>10 cigarettes a day)
- Substance abuse (e.g., alcohol; illicit drugs, especially cocaine)
- Inadequate prenatal care
- Commutes of more than 1½ hours each way
- Excessive physical activity (heavy physical work, prolonged standing, heavy lifting, young child care)
- Excessive lifestyle stressors

From Gilbert ES, Harmon JS: *Manual of high risk pregnancy and delivery,* ed 3, St Louis, 2003, Mosby; Iams JD: Preterm birth. In Gabbe SG, Niebyl JR, Simpson JL (eds): *Obstetrics: normal and problem pregnancies,* ed 4, New York, 2002, Churchill Livingstone; Pschirrer E, Monga M: Risk factors for preterm labor, *Clin Obstet Gynecol* 43(4):727-734, 2000; Simpson KR: Preterm birth in the United States: current issues and future perspectives, *J Perinat Neonatal Nurs* 10(4):11-15, 1997; Varney H: *Varney's textbook for midwives,* ed 3, Sudbury, MA, 1997, Jones & Bartlett.
DES, diethylstilbestrol.

preterm labor and birth are a history of preterm birth, race (i.e., African-American), and multiple gestation (Martin et al, 2003). Using these risk factors, researchers have tried to determine which women might go into labor prematurely. No risk scoring system has resulted in lowering the preterm birth rate in the United States, however, because at least 50% of all women who ultimately give birth prematurely have no identifiable risk factors (Martin et al, 2003). The March of Dimes has started a 5 year, $75 million campaign to address the problem of prematurity. The Association of Women's Health, Obstetric, and Neonatal Nurses (AWHONN) is a partner in this project. AWHONN is helping to increase screening for known risk factors and to teach women the signs and symptoms of preterm labor (Nelson, 2004).

Biochemical Markers

The two most common biochemical markers used in an effort to predict who might experience preterm labor are fetal fibronectin and salivary estriol.

Fetal fibronectins are glycoproteins found in plasma and produced during fetal life. They appear in the cervical canal early in pregnancy and then again in late pregnancy. Their appearance between 24 and 34 weeks of gestation predicts labor (Bernhardt & Dorman, 2004; Ramsey & Andrews, 2003). The negative predictive value of fetal fibronectin is high (up to 94%). The positive predictive value is lower (46%) (Iams & Creasy, 2004). This means that it may be possible to predict who will *not* go into preterm labor, but not who will (Bernhardt & Dorman, 2004). The test is done during a vaginal examination.

Salivary estriol is a form of estrogen produced by the fetus that is present in plasma at 9 weeks of gestation. Levels of salivary estriol have been shown to increase before preterm birth. Specimens of salivary estriol are collected by the woman in the home. The testing is done every 2 weeks for about 10 weeks. This marker also has a high negative predictive value (98%) and a lower positive predictive value (7% to 25%) (Bernhardt & Dorman, 2004).

More research is needed before it will be known if these markers offer valuable assistance that is cost effective in the risk assessment for preterm labor.

Endocervical Length

Another possible predictor of imminent preterm labor is endocervical length. Some studies have suggested that a shortened cervix precedes preterm labor and can be determined by ultrasound measurement (Bernhardt & Dorman, 2004; Fuchs et al, 2004). Women whose cervical length is 35 mm at 24 to 28 weeks of gestation are more likely to have a preterm birth than women whose cervical length exceeds 40 mm (Iams & Creasy, 2004). When a woman has a short cervix combined with a positive fetal fibronectin result, her risk for spontaneous preterm birth is substantially higher than that for women positive for only one marker or none at all (Iams & Creasy, 2004).

Causes of Preterm Labor and Birth

The cause of preterm labor is unknown and is assumed to be multifactorial (Iams & Creasy, 2004) (Box 19-2). Infection is thought to be a major etiologic factor in some preterm labors, but trials of antibiotic therapy for all women at risk have not resulted in statistically significant reductions in preterm births (Iams & Creasy, 2004). When cervical, bacterial, or urinary tract infections are present, the risk of preterm birth is increased. Thus early continuous and comprehensive prenatal care, which can detect and treat infection, is essential in dealing with this aspect of preterm birth prevention.

BOX 19-2

Multifactorial Etiology of Preterm Labor and Birth

Maternal Behaviors
Smoking
Substance use (alcohol or illegal drugs)
Poor nutrition
Work/fatigue
Short interpregnancy interval
Sexual activity

Maternal Characteristics
Young or older age
Previous preterm birth
Short stature
Short cervix
Uterine anomalies
Diethylstilbestrol exposure
Prematurely dilated cervix
Low prepregnancy weight
Race (e.g., African-American, Hispanic)
Unmarried
Low socioeconomic status
Victim of domestic violence

Other Factors
Inadequate support systems
Stress
Uterine irritability
Multiple gestation
Late or no prenatal care
Preterm premature rupture of membranes
Anemia
Infection
Catecholamine release
Decreased progesterone production
Decidual cell disruption
Prostaglandin synthesis
Cytokine release

Not all preterm births can or even should be prevented. About 25% of all preterm births are iatrogenic; that is, babies are intentionally delivered prematurely because of pregnancy complications that put the life or health of the fetus or the mother in danger, not because of preterm labor. Another 25% of all preterm births are preceded by spontaneous rupture of membranes (preterm premature rupture of membranes) followed by labor. These births are not known to be preventable. About 50% of preterm births, therefore, are possibly amenable to prevention efforts and are considered idiopathic preterm births (Goldenberg et al, 2001; Iams & Creasy, 2004).

Sociodemographic factors such as poverty, low educational level, lack of social support, smoking, little or no prenatal care, domestic violence, and stress are thought to contribute to the 50% of the preterm births that may be preventable (Iams & Creasy, 2004).

Care Management

Assessment

Because all pregnant women must be considered at risk for preterm labor (as they are for any other pregnancy complication), nursing assessment begins at the time of entry to prenatal care. The onset of preterm labor is often insidious and can be easily mistaken for the normal discomforts of pregnancy; therefore it is essential that nurses teach pregnant women how to detect the early symptoms of preterm labor (Box 19-3) (Witcher, 2002).

The nurse caring for women in a prenatal setting should use known successful modalities for teaching the pregnant woman about early recognition of preterm symptoms and then reassess the woman at each prenatal visit for the symptoms of preterm labor. Pregnant women must be taught what to do if symptoms of preterm labor occur. Some women wait hours or days before contacting a health care provider after preterm labor symptoms have begun. Women may ignore the symptoms because of ignorance regarding their significance or a belief that the symptoms are expected during pregnancy. The symptoms may be attributed to other factors such as the flu, incontinence of urine, or working too hard. Some women will become more vigilant waiting to see if the symptoms subside, go away, or become worse. They may take action by seeking advice about what to do from family or friends, resting more, increasing fluid intake, taking a bath, or rubbing the back or abdomen. Persistence of symptoms and increasing severity finally compel women to seek health care (Weiss, Saks, & Harris, 2002). Waiting too long to see a health care provider could result in inevitable preterm birth without the benefit of the administration of antenatal glucocorticoids (i.e., medication given to accelerate fetal lung maturity). In this event, the infant is born at higher risk for respiratory distress syndrome and intraventricular hemorrhage.

The nurse must assess the psychosocial and emotional status of women in preterm labor and the impact that treatment (e.g., bed rest, hospitalization) can have on family dynamics. Factors influencing the impact of preterm labor treatment include stability of the support system, financial status, and availability of child support and assistance with household maintenance. Pregnant women who have risk factors for preterm birth are often offered special care with more frequent visits. Although there is no evidence in the literature that this enhanced care results in better outcomes, clinically it makes sense to evaluate at-risk women on a more frequent basis. Moore and colleagues (1998) found that telephone support to at-risk women by nurses resulted in a 26% decrease in low-birth-weight births and a 27% decrease in preterm births in African-American women.

BOX 19-3

Signs and Symptoms of Preterm Labor

Uterine Activity
- Uterine contractions more frequent than every 10 minutes persisting for 1 hour or more
- Uterine contractions may be painful or painless

Discomfort
- Lower abdominal cramping similar to gas pains; may be accompanied by diarrhea
- Dull, intermittent low back pain (below the waist)
- Painful, menstrual-like cramps
- Suprapubic pain or pressure
- Pelvic pressure or heaviness
- Urinary frequency

Vaginal Discharge
- Change in character and amount of usual discharge: thicker (mucoid) or thinner (watery), bloody, brown or colorless, increased amount, odor
- Rupture of amniotic membranes

Nursing Diagnoses

Nursing diagnoses relevant for women at risk for preterm birth include the following:
- *Deficient knowledge related to*
  —recognition of preterm labor symptoms
- *Risk for excess maternal fluid volume related to*
  —administration of tocolytics to suppress preterm labor
- *Impaired mobility related to*
  —prescribed bed rest
- *Anticipatory grieving related to*
  —potential for birth of preterm infant

Expected Outcomes

Expected outcomes include that the woman will do the following:
- Learn the symptoms of preterm labor and be able to assess herself and her need for intervention
- Follow teaching suggestions and call her primary health care provider if symptoms occur
- Not experience preterm symptoms, or if she does, take appropriate action
- Maintain her pregnancy for at least 37 completed weeks
- Give birth to a healthy, full-term infant

Plan of Care and Implementation

Prevention

Prevention strategies that address risk factors associated with preterm labor and birth are less costly in human and financial terms than the high-tech and often lifelong care required by preterm infants and their families. With preconception care, maternal risk can be identified and modified (Maloni & Damato, 2004). Programs aimed at health promotion and disease prevention that encourage healthy lifestyles for the population in general and women of childbearing age in particular should be developed to prevent preterm labor and birth (Freda, 2003; Maloni & Damato, 2004; Tiedje, 2003). One of the most important nursing interventions aimed at preventing preterm birth is the education of pregnant women about the early symptoms of preterm labor, so that if symptoms occur the woman can be referred promptly to her care provider for more intensive care (Freda, 2003; Moore, 2003). Box 19-3 identifies the symptoms of preterm labor, and the Guidelines/Guías box identifies what the woman should do if the symptoms appear. Patient education regarding any symptoms of contrac-

ENGLISH SPANISH **Guidelines/Guías**

WHAT TO DO IF SYMPTOMS OF PRETERM LABOR OCCUR

Empty your bladder.
Vacíese la vejiga.

Drink two to three glasses of water or juice.
Tome dos a tres vasos de agua o jugo.

Lie down on your left side for one hour.
Acuéstese del lado izquierdo por una hora.

Palpate for contractions like this.
Palpe por contracciones así.

If symptoms continue, call your health care provider or go to the hospital.
Si continúan los síntomas, llame a su proveedor de los servicios de salud/médico o vaya al hospital.

If symptoms abate, resume light activity, but not what you were doing when the symptoms began.
Si se alivian los síntomas, resuma sus actividades livianas, pero no haga lo que estaba haciendo cuando empezaron los síntomas.

If symptoms return, call your health care provider or go to the hospital.
Si se presentan de nuevo los síntomas, llame a su proveedor de los servicios de salud/médico o vaya al hospital.

If any of the following symptoms occur, call your health care provider immediately:
Si le sucede cualquier de los siguientes síntomas, llame inmediatamente a su proveedor de los servicios de salud/médico:

Uterine contractions every ten minutes or less for one hour or more
Contracciones uterinas cada diez minutos o menos que duran por una hora o más

Vaginal bleeding
Hemorragia vaginal

Odorous vaginal discharge
Flujo vaginal con mal olor

Fluid leaking from the vagina
Flujo que le sale de la vagina

tions or cramping between 20 and 37 weeks of gestation should be directed toward telling the woman that these symptoms are not normal discomforts of pregnancy, and that contractions or cramping which do not go away should prompt the woman to contact her primary health care provider. Because no one can discriminate between Braxton Hicks contractions and the contractions of early preterm labor, Freda and Patterson (1995) suggest that the term *Braxton Hicks contractions* be eliminated from teaching about pregnancy expectations (Fig. 19-1).

Early Recognition and Diagnosis

Early recognition of preterm labor is essential to implement interventions successfully such as tocolytic therapy and administration of antenatal glucocorticoids. The diagnosis of preterm labor is based on three major diagnostic criteria:

- Gestation of 20 to 37 weeks
- Uterine activity (contractions)

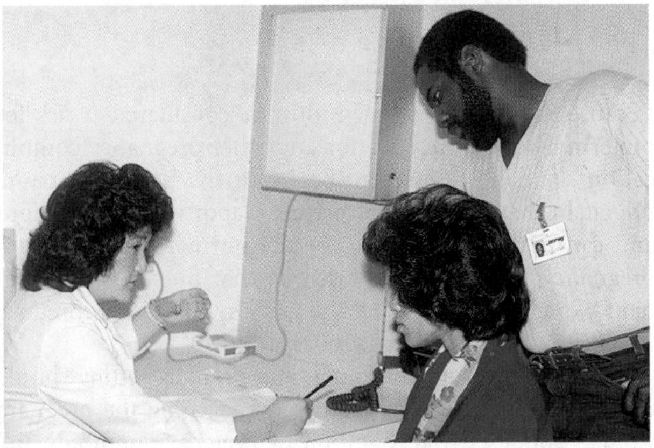

Fig. 19-1 Nurse teaching woman signs and symptoms of preterm labor. (Courtesy Marjorie Pyle, RNC, Lifecircle, Costa Mesa, CA.)

- Progressive cervical change (e.g., cervical effacement of 80% or cervical dilation of 2 cm or greater)

If the presence of fetal fibronectin is used as another diagnostic criterion, a sample of cervical mucus for testing should be obtained before an examination for cervical changes, because the lubricant used to examine the cervix can reduce the accuracy of the test for fetal fibronectin.

The pregnant woman at 30 weeks of gestation with an irritable uterus but no documented cervical change is not in preterm labor. Misdiagnosis of preterm labor can lead to inappropriate use of pharmacologic agents that can be dangerous to the health of the woman, the fetus, or both (Abrahams & Katz, 2002).

Lifestyle Modifications

Nurses caring for women with symptoms of preterm labor should question the women about whether they have symptoms when engaged in any of the following activities:

- Sexual activity
- Riding long distances in automobiles, trains, or buses
- Carrying heavy loads such as laundry, groceries, or a small child
- Standing more than 50% of the time
- Heavy housework
- Climbing stairs
- Hard physical work
- Being unable to stop and rest when tired

If symptoms occur when the woman is engaged in any of these activities, the woman should consider what she was doing when the symptoms began, and then consider stopping those activities until 37 weeks of pregnancy, when preterm birth is no longer a risk. Counseling about lifestyle modifications should be individualized; only women who have symptoms of preterm labor when they are engaged in certain activities need to alter their lifestyles. There are no specific rules for which activities are safe for pregnant women and which are not. Each pregnant woman must understand which lifestyle factors might be contributing to her symptoms and be taught to modify only those factors. Sexual activity, for instance, is not contraindicated during pregnancy. If, however, symptoms of preterm labor occur after sexual activity, such activity may need to be curtailed until 37 weeks of gestation.

Bed Rest

Bed rest is a commonly used intervention for the prevention of preterm labor. Although frequently prescribed, bed rest is not a benign intervention, and there is no evidence in the literature to support the efficacy of this intervention in reducing preterm birth rates. It is a form of care of unknown effectiveness (Enkin et al, 2000; Freda, 2003; Maloni, 1998; Sosa et al, 2004). Maloni and colleagues (1993) described deleterious effects of bed rest on women: after 3 days there is decreased muscle tone, weight loss, calcium loss, and glucose intolerance. Weeks of bed rest lead to bone demineralization, constipation, fatigue, isolation, anxiety, and depression (Box 19-4). Women on bed rest need support and encouragement whether they are at home or are hospitalized. Nurses can create support groups of hospitalized women on bed rest. Internet resources, including chat rooms for women on bed rest at home, as well as family and friends, can be important sources of support for women and reduce the sense of isolation they may feel. Interacting with other women experiencing preterm labor and bed rest has been found to be highly therapeutic (Adler & Zarchin, 2002; Maloni & Kutil, 2000).

Home Care

Women who are at high risk for preterm birth commonly are told that it would be best if they were at home on bed rest for weeks or months. The home care of the woman at risk for preterm birth is a challenge for the nurse, who must assist the woman and her family in dealing with the many difficulties faced by families in which one member is incapacitated. The scope of care given to women in their homes ranges from occasional visits to monitor the maternal and fetal condition to daily telephone consultation and reading of uterine monitoring strips.

Regardless of the frequency of the visits, nursing care for the woman and family in the home demands organization and a sense of just how this family's life has been disrupted by the loss of activity of this essential family member. Families, who are often anxious regarding the health status of the mother and baby, may need help in learning how to organize time and space or to restructure family routines so that the pregnant woman can remain a part of family activity while still maintaining bed rest. It also is important for the nurse to work toward assisting all the family members to explore their feelings regarding the anxieties of preterm labor and help them to share their feelings with each other (Maloni, Brezinski-Tomasi, & Johnson, 2001). The Home Care and Family Focus boxes detail activities for women on bed rest and for their children.

The woman's environment can be modified for convenience by using tables and storage units around her bed to keep essential items within reach (e.g., telephone, television, radio, tape or CD player, computer with Internet access, snacks, books, magazines, newspapers, and items for hobbies) (Fig. 19-2). Ensuring that the bed or couch is near a window and the bathroom is also helpful. Covering the bed with an egg crate mattress can relieve discomfort. Women often find that a daily schedule of meals, activities, and hygiene and grooming (e.g., shower, dressing in street clothes, applying makeup) that they create reduces boredom and

BOX 19-4

Adverse Effects of Bed Rest

Maternal Effects (Physical)

- Weight loss; indigestion; loss of appetite
- Muscle wasting, weakness; aching muscles
- Bone demineralization and calcium loss
- Decreased plasma volume and cardiac output
- Increased clotting tendency; risk for thrombophlebitis
- Alteration in bowel function
- Sleep disturbance, fatigue
- Prolonged postpartum recovery

Maternal Effects (Psychosocial)

- Loss of control associated with role reversals
- Dysphoria—anxiety, depression, hostility, and anger
- Guilt associated with difficulty complying with activity restriction and inability to meet role responsibilities
- Boredom, loneliness
- Emotional lability (mood swings); difficulty concentrating
- Increased stress

Effects on Support System

- Stress associated with role reversals, increased responsibilities, and disruption of family routines
- Financial strain associated with loss of maternal income and cost of treatment
- Fear and anxiety regarding the well-being of the mother and fetus

Home Care

SUGGESTED ACTIVITIES FOR WOMEN ON BED REST

- Set a routine for daily activities (e.g., getting dressed, moving from the bedroom to a "day bed rest place," having social time, eating meals, self-monitoring fetal and uterine activity).
- Do passive exercises as allowed.
- Review childbirth education information or have a childbirth class at home, if this can be arranged.
- Plan menus and make up grocery shopping lists.
- Shop by phone.
- Read books about high risk pregnancy or other topics.
- Keep a journal of the pregnancy.
- Keep a calendar of your progress.
- Reorganize files, recipes, household budget.
- Update address book.
- Do mending, sewing.
- Listen to audiotapes, watch videos or television.
- Do crossword puzzles, jigsaw puzzles, etc.
- Do craft projects; make something for the baby.
- Put pictures in photo albums.
- Call a friend, family member, or support person each day or use e-mail.
- Treat yourself to a facial, manicure, neck massage, or other special treat when you need a lift.

From Bolane J, Furlong J: *Coping with bedrest in pregnancy,* Waco, TX, 1994; Childbirth Graphics; Gilbert ES, Harmon JS: *Manual of high risk pregnancy and delivery,* ed 3, St Louis, 2003, Mosby; Isennock P: *Bed rest before baby: what's a mother to do?* Perry Hall, MD, 1992, Mustard Seed Publications; Maloni JA: *Antepartum bedrest: case studies, research, and nursing care,* Washington, DC, 1998, Association of Women's Health, Obstetric, and Neonatal Nurses.

Family Focus

ACTIVITIES FOR CHILDREN OF WOMEN ON BED REST

- Schedule brief play periods throughout the day.
- Keep a few favorite toys in a box or basket close to the bed or couch.
- Read to the child(ren).
- Put puzzles together.
- Watch videos, play video games (remote control for television is ideal).
- Play cards or board games.
- Color in coloring books.
- Cut out pictures from magazines and paste on cardboard.
- Play bed basketball with a soft (sponge) ball or rolled up sock and a trash can or empty laundry basket.

Adapted from Bolane J, Furlong J: *Coping with bedrest in pregnancy,* Waco, TX, 1994, Childbirth Graphics; Isennock P: *Bed rest before baby: what's a mother to do?* Perry Hall, MD, 1992, Mustard Seed Publications.

helps them maintain control and normalcy. Limiting naps, eating smaller but more frequent meals, and performing gentle range-of-motion exercises can help reduce some of the detrimental effects of bed rest. It is essential that a woman and her family recognize that postpartum recovery will be slower as she works to regain strength and stamina (Maloni, 2002).

Home Uterine Activity Monitoring

Home care companies provide home uterine monitoring services for women diagnosed with preterm labor. Nurses are usually an integral part of the systems developed by companies to educate the patients they serve. However, from the body of research over the past 15 years, researchers have concluded that home uterine activity monitoring does not prevent preterm birth, and its prohibitive cost makes it an unacceptable intervention in the larger scheme of prenatal care

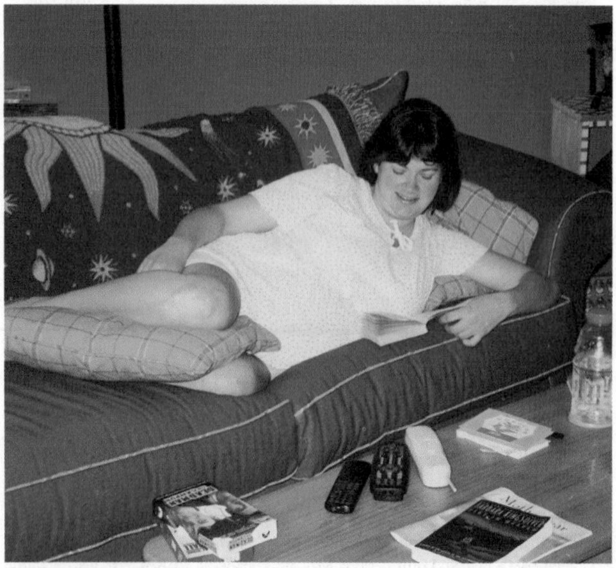

Fig. 19-2 Woman at home on restricted activity for preterm labor prevention. Note how she has arranged her daytime resting area so that needed items are close at hand. (Courtesy Amy Turner, Cary, NC.)

(Maloni, 2000). It is a form of care unlikely to be beneficial in preventing preterm birth (Enkin et al, 2000). Palpation of the uterus is more effective than a monitor for detecting uterine contractions when a woman is obese (e.g., excessive abdominal adipose tissue) or the gestational age is less than 26 weeks (Abrahams & Katz, 2002). Some research suggests that it is the nursing care offered by the home care nurse that helps women the most (Moore, 2003; Moore et al, 1998; Morrison & Chauhan, 2003).

Suppression of Uterine Activity

Tocolytics

Should preterm labor occur, women are usually admitted to the hospital for assessment; fetal monitoring; cervical/vaginal cultures; and assessment of cervical status, amniotic fluid leakage, and maternal temperature (an early sign of chorioamnionitis). The initiation of tocolytic therapy might be considered at this time. Once the pregnancy has progressed beyond 34 weeks of gestation, the benefits of prolonging the pregnancy do not justify the maternal risk of tocolytic therapy (Witcher, 2002). Tocolytic therapy, the administration of pharmaceutical agents that suppress uterine activity, has been studied since the late 1970s. At first it was thought that tocolytic therapy could prolong a threatened pregnancy indefinitely; research has demonstrated that a gain of 48 hours to several days is the best outcome that can be expected if the woman's cervix is less than 6 cm dilated. Once uterine contractions are suppressed, maintenance therapy may be implemented in an attempt to continue the suppression, or tocolytic treatment can be discontinued and resumed only if uterine contractions begin again. Research findings indicate that there is no significant difference in the mean gestational age when the two tocolytic treatment approaches are compared (Maloni, 2000; Witcher, 2002).

It is now thought that the best reason to use tocolytics is that they afford the opportunity to begin administering antenatal glucocorticoids to accelerate fetal lung maturity and reduce the severity of sequelae in infants born preterm (Enkin et al, 2000; Moore, 2003).

The medications most commonly used for this purpose are ritodrine (Yutopar), terbutaline (Brethine), magnesium sulfate, indomethacin (Indocin), and nifedipine (Procardia). Ritodrine and terbutaline, the most commonly used betamimetic medications for tocolysis, work by relaxing smooth muscles. Ritodrine is the only medication approved by the Food and Drug Administration (FDA) specifically for the purpose of cessation of uterine contractions. Other medications are used for this purpose on an "unlabeled" basis (i.e., medications known to be effective for a specific purpose though not specifically developed and tested for this purpose). There are important contraindications to the use of all tocolytics (Box 19-5). Because these medications have the potential for serious adverse reactions for mother and fetus, close nursing supervision during treatment is critical (Lehne, 2001) (Box 19-6; Medication Guide).

Magnesium sulfate is the most commonly used tocolytic agent, because maternal and fetal/neonatal adverse reactions are less common than with other tocolytic agents, especially the β-adrenergic agonists. Although its exact mechanism of action on uterine muscle is unclear, magnesium sulfate does promote relaxation of smooth muscles (Iams, 2002; Witcher, 2002). At the onset of preterm labor, magnesium sulfate is administered via an intravenous infusion. Terbutaline, 0.25 mg, may be injected subcutaneously before the initiation of the magnesium sulfate infusion and then administered again by subcutaneous pump as the infusion is discontinued and the woman prepared for discharge to home care (see Medication Guide).

Ritodrine and terbutaline, β-adrenergic agonist medications for tocolysis, work by relaxing uterine smooth muscle as a result of stimulation of β_2 receptors on uterine smooth muscle. When used, ritodrine is usually administered intravenously as one of the first steps in suppressing preterm labor. Terbutaline is most commonly administered by a subcutaneous injection of 0.25 mg to suppress uterine hyperactivity or by a subcutaneous pump in the home setting. Effectiveness of pump therapy in prolonging gestation is controversial. Terbutaline also may be administered orally. Oral and pump therapy are similar in terms of effectiveness and adverse reactions (Witcher, 2002). β_2-adrenergic agonists have many maternal and fetal cardiopulmonary and metabolic adverse reactions in part related to β_1 stimulation and must always be used with extreme caution and careful, conscientious nursing care. Fewer neonatal adverse reactions occur if the administration of the β-adrenergic agonist is discontinued at least 4 hours before birth (Witcher, 2002). Medication administration and nursing care are aimed at maintaining a therapeutic level of medication and avoiding the most serious side effects while maintaining optimal health of the fetus (see Medication Guide).

NURSE ALERT Caution must be used when administering intravenous fluids to women in preterm labor because this practice can increase the risk for tocolytic-induced pulmonary edema, especially when a β-adrenergic agonist or magnesium sulfate is used. It is recommended that the total oral and intravenous fluid intake in 24 hours should be restricted to 1500 to 2400 ml. Strict intake and output measurement, daily weight determination, and assessment of pulmonary function should be instituted (Gilbert & Harmon, 2003; Witcher, 2002). ■

Nifedipine, a calcium channel blocker, is another tocolytic agent that can suppress contractions. It works by inhibiting calcium from entering smooth muscle cells, thus reducing uterine contractions (Fleming et al, 2004; Lehne, 2001). Mild maternal side effects and ease of administration have increased its use. When the tocolytic effects and maternal tolerance of nifedipine and β-adrenergic agonists were compared, no significant differences in length of delay of birth were found, but significantly fewer maternal side effects occurred with nifedipine. Maternal side effects relate primarily to hypotension that occurs with administration. Concerns regarding adverse fetal effects have been reduced. Safety is achieved by following recommended dosages and maintaining maternal blood pressure, thereby preserving effective uteroplacental perfusion (Iams & Creasy, 2004; Witcher, 2002) (see Medication Guide).

Indomethacin, a nonsteroidal antiinflammatory drug (NSAID), has been shown in some trials to suppress preterm labor by blocking the production of prostaglandins. Two prostaglandins are affected, prostacyclin and thromboxane. The decrease in prostacyclin suppresses uterine contractions, and the decrease in thromboxane suppresses platelet aggregation. However, both of these actions increase the risk for postpartum hemorrhage. The severity of fetal side effects associated with the use of indomethacin for tocolysis makes it less common than other classes of tocolytic drugs. Risk for premature closure of the ductus arteriosus increases if treatment goes beyond 48 hours or if the fetus is 32 or more weeks of gestation. Therefore limiting the use of indomethacin to a short duration of treatment (e.g., 48 hours) or to women at less than 32 weeks of gestation is recommended (Iams & Creasy, 2004; Lehne, 2001; Witcher, 2002).

Promotion of Fetal Lung Maturity

Antenatal Glucocorticoids

Antenatal glucocorticoids given as intramuscular injections to the mother accelerate fetal lung maturity. It is viewed as a form of care likely to be beneficial (Enkin et al, 2000). This class of medications also seems to decrease rates of intraventricular hemorrhage in preterm infants. All

BOX 19-5

Contraindications to Tocolysis

Maternal

Severe pregnancy-induced hypertension or eclampsia
Active vaginal bleeding
Intrauterine infection (chorioamnionitis)
Cardiac disease
Medical or obstetric condition that contraindicates continuation of pregnancy
Dilation >6 cm

Fetal

Estimated gestational age >34 wk
Fetal death
Lethal fetal anomaly
Acute fetal distress
Chronic intrauterine growth restriction

BOX 19-6

Nursing Care for Women Receiving Tocolytic Therapy

- Explain the purpose and side effects of tocolytic therapy to woman and her family.
- Position woman on her side to enhance placental perfusion and reduce pressure on the cervix.
- Monitor maternal vital signs, including lung sounds and respiratory effort, fetal heart rate (FHR) and pattern, and labor status according to hospital protocol and professional standards.
- Assess mother and fetus for signs of adverse reactions related to the tocolytic being administered.
- Determine maternal fluid balance by measuring daily weight and intake and output (I&O).
- Limit fluid intake to 1500-2500 ml/day, especially if a β-adrenergic agonist or magnesium sulfate is being administered.
- Provide psychosocial support and opportunities for women and family to express feelings and concerns.
- Offer comfort measures as required.
- Encourage diversional activities and relaxation techniques.

Medication Guide

TOCOLYTIC THERAPY FOR PRETERM LABOR

Medication	Dosage and Route*	Adverse Reactions	Management Considerations
Ritodrine (Yutopar) β_2-adrenergic agonist Relaxes smooth muscles, inhibiting uterine activity and causing bronchodilation	Mix 150 mg in 500 ml isotonic intravenous solution Attach to controller pump and piggyback to primary infusion Begin infusion at 0.05-0.1 mg/min Increase rate by 0.05 mg q10-20min until contractions stop, intolerable adverse reactions develop, or a maximum dose of 0.35 mg/min is reached Reduce rate gradually to lowest effective rate and maintain effective dose for 12-24 hr Oral dose: 10-20 mg, q3-4hr (maximum oral dose is 120 mg/day)	Maternal: • Shortness of breath (SOB), coughing, tachypnea, pulmonary edema • Tachycardia, palpitations, skipped beats • Chest pain • Hypotension • Fluid retention and decreased urine production • Tremors, dizziness, nervousness • Muscle cramps and weakness • Headache • Hyperglycemia; hypokalemia; hypocalcemia; metabolic acidosis • Nausea and vomiting Fetal/neonatal: • Mild tachycardia, hyperinsulinemia, hyperglycemia (fetal) • Hypoglycemia (neonatal), hyperbilirubinemia, hypotension, ileus	Women should be screened with ECG before therapy begins; maternal heart disease, severe hypertension including preeclampsia, hyperthyroidism, and uncontrolled diabetes mellitus are contraindications Use cautiously if woman has type 1 diabetes, migraines Validate that woman is in PTL and is >20 wk and <35 wk gestation Assess woman and fetus to obtain baseline before beginning therapy and then before and after each increment; follow frequency of agency protocol Discontinue infusion and notify physician if the woman exhibits the following: • Maternal heart rate >120-140 beats/min; dysrhythmias, chest pain • BP <90/60 • Signs of pulmonary edema (e.g., dyspnea, crackles, decreased Sao_2) • Fetal heart rate >180 beats/min Give with meals to reduce GI distress Ensure that propranolol (Inderal) is available to reverse adverse effects related to cardiovascular function
Terbutaline (Brethine)† β_2-adrenergic agonist Relaxes smooth muscles, inhibiting uterine activity and causing bronchodilation	Subcutaneous injection: • 0.25 mg q20-30min for 2 hr; then • Maintenance dose: 0.25 mg q3-4hr Subcutaneous pump: • Maintenance dose 0.03-0.1 mg/hr • Bolus: 0.25 mg q4-6hr according to contraction pattern (peak uterine activity) • Maximum dose: 3 mg/24 hr Oral: 2.5-5 mg q4-6hr	Similar to ritodrine but limited and less severe	Teach woman and family: Assessment measures: pulse, BP, respiratory effort, insertion site for infection, signs of PTL, and adverse reactions of terbutaline Whom to call if problems or concerns arise Site care and pump maintenance Activity restrictions Arrange for follow-up and home care
Magnesium sulfate† Central nervous system depressant; relaxes smooth muscles including uterus	Mix 40 g in 1000 ml intravenous solution, piggyback to primary infusion, and administer using controller pump: • Loading dose of 4-6 g over 15-30 min • Maintenance dose: gradually increase from 2 g/hr to 4 g/hr as needed to suppress contractions; continue until contractions stop (or one contraction or less in 10-15 min) or intolerable adverse reactions develop	Maternal adverse reactions: • Hot flushes, sweating, nausea and vomiting, drowsiness, blurred vision, diplopia, headache, ileus, generalized muscle weakness, dizziness • Hypocalcemia • SOB, transient hypotension • Some may subside when loading dose is completed Fetal/newborn (uncommon): • Decreased breathing movement, reduced FHR variability, nonreactive NST • Hypocalcemia, lethargy, hypotonia, respiratory depression	Assess woman and fetus to obtain baseline before beginning therapy and then before and after each increment; follow frequency of agency protocol Monitor serum magnesium levels with higher doses; therapeutic range is between 4-7.5 mEq/L or 5-8 mg/dl Discontinue infusion and notify physician if intolerable adverse reactions occur Ensure that calcium gluconate (1 g = 10 ml of 10% solution) is available for emergency administration to reverse magnesium sulfate toxicity

BP, blood pressure; *DTRs,* deep tendon reflexes; *ECG,* electrocardiogram; *FHR,* fetal heart rate; *GI,* gastrointestinal; *SOB,* shortness of breath; *PTL,* preterm labor; *NST,* nonstress test.

*NOTE: For variations in recommended administration protocols, always consult agency protocols, which should be evidence based.

†Caution: Not FDA approved for PTL (unlabeled use).

Medication Guide

TOCOLYTIC THERAPY FOR PRETERM LABOR—cont'd

Medication	Dosage and Route*	Adverse Reactions	Management Considerations
Magnesium sulfate—cont'd		Intolerable adverse reactions: • Respiratory rate <12 • Pulmonary edema • Absent DTRs • Chest pain • Severe hypotension • Altered level of consciousness • Extreme muscle weakness • Urine output <25-30 ml/hr or <100 ml/4 hr • Serum magnesium level ≥10 mEq/L (9 mg/dl)	
***Nifedipine (Procardia; Adalat)*†** Calcium channel blocker; relaxes smooth muscles including the uterus by blocking calcium entry	Loading dose: 10-20 mg, po Maintenance dose: 20 mg, po, q6hr for 24 hr; then 20 mg, po, q8hr	Maternal: • Transient tachycardia, palpitations • Hypotension • Dizziness, headache, nervousness • Peripheral edema • Fatigue • Nausea • Facial flushing Fetal/newborn (rare): related to maternal hypotension, which would affect uteroplacental perfusion	Do not use sublingual route Avoid use or use cautiously with magnesium sulfate because severe hypotension can result Assess woman and fetus according to agency protocol, being alert for adverse reactions
***Indomethacin*†** Prostaglandin synthetase inhibitor; relaxes uterine smooth muscle	Loading dose: 50 mg (orally) or 50-100 mg rectally; repeat after 1 hr if no decrease in uterine activity is noted Maintenance dose: 25-50 mg, q4-6hr for 24-48 hr (po or rectal)	Maternal: • Nausea and vomiting, • Dyspepsia, pyrosis • Dizziness • Oligohydramnios • Reduced platelet aggregation increasing risk for hemorrhage Fetal: • Constriction of ductus arteriosus progressing to premature closure Neonate: • Bronchopulmonary dysplasia, respiratory distress syndrome • Intracranial hemorrhage • Necrotizing enterocolitis • Hyperbilirubinemia	Used when other methods fail only if gestational age is <32 wk Administer for ≤48 hr Do not use for women with bleeding potential (coagulopathy), peptic ulcer disease, or oligohydramnios Assess woman and fetus according to agency policy, being alert for adverse reactions Determine amniotic fluid volume and function of ductus arteriosus before initiating therapy and within 48 hr of discontinuing therapy; assessment is critical if therapy continues for >48 hr Administer with food or use rectal route to decrease GI distress Monitor for signs of postpartum hemorrhage

women between 24 and 34 weeks of gestation should be given antenatal glucocorticoids when preterm birth is threatened, unless there is a medical indication for immediate delivery such as cord prolapse, chorioamnionitis, or abruptio placentae (National Institutes of Health, 2000). The regimen for administration of antenatal glucocorticoids is given in the Medication Guide.

NURSE ALERT Nurses need to know that when any woman is admitted to the hospital and is 24 to 34 weeks pregnant, she should receive antenatal glucocorticoids unless she has chorioamnionitis. These drugs require a 24-hour period to become effective, so timely administration is essential. ■

Management of Inevitable Preterm Birth

Labor that has progressed to a cervical dilation of 4 cm is likely to lead to inevitable preterm birth. Preterm births that occur in tertiary care centers lead to better neonatal and maternal outcomes. Women considered at risk for inevitable preterm birth, therefore, should be transferred quickly to such a facility to ensure the best possible outcome.

Maternal transport, while helping to ensure a better health outcome for the mother and the baby, may have its complications. Women may be transported to tertiary centers far from home, making visits by the family difficult and increasing the anxiety levels of the woman and her family. Attention to the needs of the woman and her

Medication Guide

ANTENATAL GLUCOCORTICOID THERAPY WITH BETAMETHASONE, DEXAMETHASONE

Action

Stimulates fetal lung maturation by promoting release of enzymes that induce production or release of lung surfactant. NOTE: The Food and Drug Administration has not approved these medications for this use (i.e., this is an unlabeled use for obstetrics).

Indication

To prevent or reduce the severity of respiratory distress syndrome in preterm infants between 24 and 34 weeks of gestation

Dosage and Route

Betamethasone: 12 mg IM × 2 doses 24 hr apart
Dexamethasone: 6 mg IM × 4 doses 12 hr apart

Adverse Reactions

Possible maternal infection, pulmonary edema (if given with β-adrenergic medications), may worsen maternal condition (diabetes, hypertension)

Nursing Considerations

Give deep IM injection in gluteal muscle. Teach signs of pulmonary edema. Assess blood glucose levels and lung sounds. Do not give if woman has infection. Use in women with PPROM not universally recommended.

IM, intramuscular; *PPROM*, preterm premature rupture of membranes.

Family Focus

IMPACT OF PRETERM BIRTH

Parental concern for the well-being of the infant is apparent during labor. Parents need to be aware of the interest and support of staff members. However, false assurance of fetal health must be avoided. For some parents the reality of the situation is not appreciated until they see their daughter or son in the intensive care unit. For those who experience fetal or neonatal death, the loss intensifies once the stress of labor and childbirth is over.

During the postpartum period, physical care of the mother is similar to that required after any vaginal birth. However, the family will be very anxious concerning the health and prognosis of the infant. Care of the preterm infant involves not only medical and nursing personnel but also participation of the parents. The nurse must be aware of the impact that a preterm birth may have on family dynamics. Parents must accept that the infant has special needs, and they must learn to meet those needs before discharge so that they have more realistic expectations when they are at home.

family before, during, and after the transport is essential to comprehensive nursing care for these families (Family Focus).

Evaluation

Evaluation of the nursing care provided a woman at risk for preterm labor is based on the expected outcomes of care (Nursing Care Plan: Preterm Labor).

PRETERM PREMATURE RUPTURE OF MEMBRANES

Premature rupture of membranes (PROM) is the rupture of the amniotic sac and leakage of amniotic fluid beginning at least 1 hour before the onset of labor at any gestational age. Preterm premature rupture of membranes (PPROM) (i.e., membranes rupture before 37 weeks of gestation) occurs in up to 25% of all cases of preterm labor. Infection often precedes PPROM, but the etiology of PPROM remains unknown. PPROM is diagnosed after the woman complains of either a sudden gush of fluid or a slow leak of fluid from the vagina.

Infection is the serious side effect of PPROM that makes it a major complication of pregnancy. Chorioamnionitis is an intraamniotic infection of the chorion and amnion that is potentially life-threatening for the fetus and the woman. Most cases of intrauterine infection respond well to antibiotics, yet sepsis can occur and can lead to maternal death. Fetal complications from chorioamnionitis include congenital pneumonia, sepsis, and meningitis (Garite, 2004). Even in the absence of infection, PPROM can precipitate cord prolapse or cause oligohydramnios leading to cord compression, potentially life-threatening complications for the fetus.

Care Management: Home vs. Hospital

Whenever PPROM is suspected, strict sterile technique should be used in any vaginal examination to avoid introduction of infection. A nitrazine or fern test is used to determine if the discharge is amniotic fluid or urine (see Box 18-2). A woman with this diagnosis can be cared for at home, with more frequent visits to her primary health care provider (Home Care box). Expectant management will continue as long as there are no signs of infection or fetal distress. Nursing support of the woman and her family is critical at this time. The nurse should encourage expression of feelings and concerns, provide information, and make referrals as needed (Weitz, 2001).

Frequent biophysical profiles are performed to determine fetal health status and estimate amniotic fluid volume. The woman with PPROM also should be taught how to count fetal movements daily, because a slowing of fetal movement has been shown to be a precursor to severe fetal compromise. Several methods are commonly used to count fetal movements; one method for fetal movement counting is described in the Guidelines box. Antenatal glucocorticoids may be administered if chorioamnionitis is absent (Weitz, 2001).

Vigilance for signs of infection is a major part of the nursing care and patient education after PPROM. The woman must be taught how to keep her genital area clean and that nothing should be introduced into her vagina. Signs of infection (e.g., fever, foul-smelling vaginal discharge, rapid pulse) should be reported to the primary health care provider immediately. Prophylactic antibiotic therapy may be ordered in an effort to improve perinatal outcome by preventing infection (Garite, 2004). However, use of prophylactic antibiotics for PROM before labor at term or preterm is a form of care of unknown effectiveness (Enkin et al, 2000).

Nursing Care Plan

PRETERM LABOR

NURSING DIAGNOSIS: Deficient knowledge related to recognition of preterm labor

EXPECTED OUTCOME

Woman and partner delineate the signs and symptoms of preterm labor.

NURSING INTERVENTIONS/*RATIONALES*

Assess what the woman and partner know about abnormal signs and symptoms during pregnancy *to identify areas of deficit.*

Discuss signs and symptoms that serve as warning signs of preterm labor *so that the woman or her partner has adequate information to identify problems early.*

Provide written supplemental materials that include a list of warning signs and instructions regarding what to do if any of the listed signs occur *so that the couple can reinforce and review learning and act swiftly and appropriately should a sign occur.*

Discuss and demonstrate how to assess and time the contractions *to provide needed skills to assess the signs of labor.*

NURSING DIAGNOSIS: Risk for maternal/fetal injury related to recurrence of preterm labor

EXPECTED OUTCOME

Woman demonstrates ability to assess self and fetus for signs of recurring labor; maternal-fetal well-being is maintained.

NURSING INTERVENTIONS/*RATIONALES*

Teach woman/partner how to monitor fetal and uterine contraction activity daily *to provide immediate evidence of a worsening condition.*

Have woman/partner report rupture of membranes, vaginal bleeding, cramping, pelvic pressure, or low backache to appropriate health care resource immediately *because such symptoms are signs of labor.*

If home uterine activity monitoring is to be used, teach woman/partner how to use the monitoring device and how to transmit the data to the health care provider via telephone *to enhance correct use of monitoring device and increase the accuracy of detection of early labor.*

Have woman monitor her weight, diet, fluid intake, and vital signs on a daily basis *to evaluate for potential problems.*

Use a side-lying position *to enhance placental perfusion.*

Teach woman signs and symptoms of thrombophlebitis and encourage gentle exercise of lower extremities *because pregnancy and limited activity increase risk for clot formation.*

Abstain from sexual intercourse and nipple stimulation *because such activities may stimulate uterine contractions.*

Practice relaxation techniques *to decrease uterine tone and decrease anxiety and stress.*

Take tocolytic or other medications per physician's orders *to inhibit uterine contractions.*

Teach woman/partner about and have them report any medication side effects immediately *to prevent medication-induced complications.*

Have family arrange for alternative strategies in carrying out the woman's usual roles and functions *to decrease stress and limit temptations to increase activity.*

If small children are part of the household, encourage family to make alternative arrangements for child care *to enhance woman's adherence to bed rest protocol.*

NURSING DIAGNOSIS: Anxiety related to preterm labor and potentially premature neonate

EXPECTED OUTCOME

Feeling and symptoms of anxiety are reduced.

NURSING INTERVENTIONS/*RATIONALES*

Provide a calm, soothing atmosphere and teach family to provide emotional support *to facilitate coping.*

Encourage verbalization of fears *to decrease intensity of emotional response.*

Involve woman and family in the home management of her condition *to promote a greater sense of control.*

Help the woman identify and use appropriate coping strategies and support systems *to reduce fear/anxiety.*

Explore the use of desensitization strategies such as progressive muscle relaxation, visual imagery, or thought stopping *to reduce fear-related emotions and related physical symptoms.*

NURSING DIAGNOSIS: Deficient diversional activity related to imposed bed rest

EXPECTED OUTCOME

The woman will verbalize diminished feelings of boredom.

NURSING INTERVENTIONS/*RATIONALES*

Assist woman to creatively explore personally meaningful activities that can be pursued from the bed *to ensure activities that have meaning, purpose, and value to the individual.*

Maintain emphasis on personal choices of the woman *because doing so promotes control and minimizes imposition of routines by others.*

Evaluate what support and system resources are available in the environment *to assist in providing diversional activities.*

Explore ways for the woman to remain an active participant in home management and decision making *to promote control.*

Engage support of family and friends in carrying out chosen activities and making necessary environmental alterations *to ensure success.*

Encourage woman to use the Internet to communicate with other women on bed rest *to obtain support and share feelings.*

Teach woman about stress management and relaxation techniques *to help manage tension of confinement.*

Dystocia

Dystocia is defined as long, difficult, or abnormal labor; it is caused by various conditions associated with the five factors affecting labor. It is estimated that dystocia occurs in approximately 8% to 11% of women during the first stage of labor and is the primary cause for cesarean birth (Gregory, 2000; Martin et al, 2003). Dystocia can be caused by any of the following:

- Dysfunctional labor, resulting in ineffective uterine contractions or maternal bearing-down efforts (the powers); the most common cause of dystocia

Home Care

THE WOMAN WITH PPROM

Take your temperature and assess pulse q4hr when awake
Report temperature of more than 38° C
Remain on modified bed rest
Insert nothing in the vagina
Do not engage in sexual activity
Assess for uterine contractions
Do fetal movement counts daily
Do not take tub baths
Watch for foul-smelling vaginal discharge
Wipe front to back after urinating or having a bowel movement
Take antibiotics if prescribed
See primary health care provider as scheduled

PPROM, preterm premature rupture of membranes.

Guidelines

COUNTING FETAL MOVEMENTS (KICK COUNTS)

Choose a time of day when you can sit or lie quietly.
Choices for counting strategies (see Fig. 9-1):

- Starting at 9 AM, count the baby's movements until you have counted 10. If you have not counted 10 movements in 12 hours, notify your primary health care provider immediately.
- Count 4 movements, three times a day after meals. Most people count 4 movements in 1 hour. If you don't, count for 1 more hour. If, at the end of 2 hours, you still have not felt 4 movements, call your primary health care provider immediately.

- Alterations in the pelvic structure (the passage)
- Fetal causes, including abnormal presentation or position, anomalies, excessive size, and number of fetuses (the passenger)
- Maternal position during labor and birth
- Psychologic responses of the mother to labor related to past experiences, preparation, culture and heritage, and support system

These five factors are interdependent. In assessing the woman for an abnormal labor pattern, the nurse must consider the way in which these factors interact and influence labor progress. Dystocia is suspected when there is an alteration in the characteristics of uterine contractions, a lack of progress in the rate of cervical dilation, or a lack of progress in fetal descent and expulsion.

Dysfunctional Labor

Dysfunctional labor is described as abnormal uterine contractions that prevent the normal progress of cervical dilation, effacement (primary powers), or descent (secondary powers). Gilbert and Harmon (2003) list several factors that are suspected to increase a woman's risk for uterine dystocia, including the following:

- Body build (e.g., 30 pounds or more overweight; short stature)
- Uterine abnormalities (e.g., congenital malformations; overdistention, as with multiple gestation or hydramnios)
- Malpresentations and positions of the fetus
- Cephalopelvic disproportion
- Overstimulation with oxytocin
- Maternal fatigue, dehydration and electrolyte imbalance, and fear
- Inappropriate timing of analgesic or anesthetic administration

Dysfunction of uterine contractions can be further described as being hypertonic or hypotonic.

Hypertonic Uterine Dysfunction

The woman experiencing hypertonic uterine dysfunction, or primary dysfunctional labor, is often an anxious first-time mother who is having painful and frequent contractions that are ineffective in causing cervical dilation or effacement to progress. These contractions usually occur in the latent stage (cervical dilation of less than 4 cm) and are usually uncoordinated (Fig. 19-3). The force of the contraction may be in the midsection of the uterus rather than in the fundus, and the uterus is therefore unable to apply downward pressure to push the presenting part against the cervix. The uterus may not relax completely between contractions (Gilbert & Harmon, 2003).

Women with hypertonic uterine dysfunction may be exhausted and express concern about loss of control because of the intense pain they are experiencing and the lack of progress. Therapeutic rest, which is achieved with a warm bath or shower and the administration of analgesics such as morphine, meperidine (Demerol), or nalbuphine (Nubain) to inhibit uterine contractions, reduce pain, and encourage sleep, is usually prescribed for the management of hypertonic uterine dysfunction. After a 4- to 6-hour rest, these women are likely to awaken in active labor with a normal uterine contraction pattern (Gilbert & Harmon, 2003).

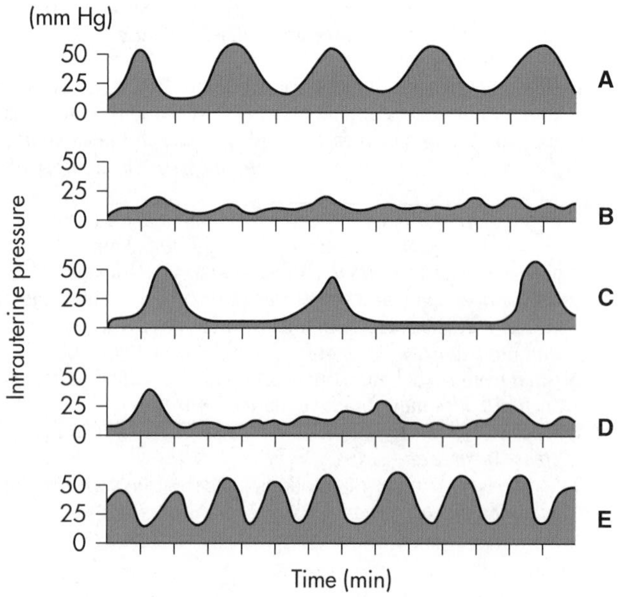

Fig. 19-3 Uterine contractility patterns in labor. **A,** Typical normal labor. **B,** Subnormal intensity, with frequency greater than needed for optimum performance. **C,** Normal contractions but too infrequent for efficient labor. **D,** Incoordinate activity. **E,** Hypercontractility.

Hypotonic Uterine Dysfunction

The second and more common type of uterine dysfunction is hypotonic uterine dysfunction, or secondary uterine inertia. The woman initially makes normal progress into the active stage of labor; then the contractions become weak and inefficient or stop altogether (see Fig. 19-3, *B*). The uterus is easily indented, even at the peak of contractions. Intrauterine pressure during the contraction (usually less than 25 mm Hg) is insufficient for progress of cervical effacement and dilation (Gilbert & Harmon, 2003). Cephalopelvic disproportion and malpositions are common causes of this type of uterine dysfunction.

A woman with hypotonic uterine dysfunction may become exhausted and be at increased risk for infection. Management usually consists of performing an ultrasound or x-ray examination to rule out cephalopelvic disproportion, assessing the fetal heart rate and pattern, characteristics of amniotic fluid if membranes are ruptured, and maternal well-being. If findings are normal, measures such as ambulation, hydrotherapy, enema, stripping or rupture of membranes, nipple stimulation, and oxytocin infusion can be used to augment labor.

Secondary Powers

Secondary powers, or bearing-down efforts, are compromised when large amounts of analgesia are given. Anesthesia may also block the bearing-down reflex and, as a result, alter the effectiveness of voluntary efforts. Exhaustion from lack of sleep or a long labor and fatigue from inadequate hydration and food intake affect the woman's voluntary efforts. Maternal position can work against the forces of gravity and decrease the strength and efficiency of the contraction (Nursing Care Plan). Table 19-1 summarizes the characteristics of dysfunctional labor.

Alterations in Pelvic Structure

Pelvic Dystocia

Pelvic dystocia can occur whenever there are contractures of the pelvic diameters that reduce the capacity of the bony pelvis, including the inlet, midpelvis, outlet, or any combination of these planes.

Disproportion of the pelvis is the least common cause of dystocia. Pelvic contractures may be caused by congenital abnormalities, maternal malnutrition, neoplasms, or lower spinal disorders. An immature pelvic size predisposes some adolescent mothers to pelvic dystocia. Pelvic deformities may also be the result of automobile or other accidents or trauma.

An inlet contracture is diagnosed when the diagonal conjugate is less than 11.5 cm. The incidence of face and shoulder presentation is increased. Because these presentations interfere with engagement and fetal descent, the risk of prolapse of the umbilical cord is increased. Inlet contracture is associated with maternal rickets and a flat pelvis. Weak uterine contractions may be noted during the first stage of labor in affected women.

Midplane contracture, the most common cause of pelvic dystocia, is diagnosed when the sum of the interischial spinous and posterior sagittal diameters of the midpelvis is 13.5 cm or less. Fetal descent is arrested (transverse arrest of the fetal head) because the head cannot rotate internally. These infants are usually born by cesarean, but vacuum-assisted birth has been used safely when the cervix is fully dilated. Midforceps-assisted birth usually is not done because of the increased perinatal morbidity associated with this intervention.

Outlet contracture exists when the interischial diameter is 8 cm or less. It rarely occurs in the absence of midplane contracture. Women with outlet contracture have a long, narrow pubic arch and an android pelvis, and this causes fetal descent to be arrested. Maternal complications include extensive perineal lacerations during vaginal birth because the fetal head is pushed posteriorly.

Soft-Tissue Dystocia

Soft-tissue dystocia results from obstruction of the birth passage by an anatomic abnormality other than that involving the bony pelvis. The obstruction may result from placenta previa (i.e., low-lying placenta) that partially or completely obstructs the internal os of the cervix. Other causes, such as leiomyomas (uterine fibroids) in the lower uterine segment, ovarian tumors, and a full bladder or rectum, may prevent the fetus from entering the pelvis. Occasionally, cervical edema occurs during labor when the cervix is caught between the presenting part and the symphysis pubis or when the woman begins bearing-down efforts prematurely, inhibiting complete dilation. Sexually transmitted infections (e.g., human papillomavirus) can alter cervical tissue integrity and thus interfere with adequate effacement and dilation.

Bandl's ring, a pathologic retraction ring that forms between the upper and lower uterine segments (see Fig. 15-10), is associated with prolonged rupture of membranes, protracted labor, and increased risk of uterine rupture (Cunningham et al, 2001).

Fetal Causes

Dystocia of fetal origin may be caused by anomalies, excessive fetal size and malpresentation, malposition, or multifetal pregnancy. Complications associated with dystocia of fetal origin include neonatal asphyxia, fetal injuries or fractures, and maternal vaginal lacerations. Although spontaneous vaginal birth is possible in these instances, a low-forceps or vacuum-assisted or cesarean birth often is necessary.

Anomalies

Gross ascites, large tumors, and open neural tube defects such as myelomeningocele and hydrocephalus are fetal anomalies that can cause dystocia. The anomalies affect the relationship of the fetal anatomy to the maternal pelvic capacity, with the result that the fetus is unable to descend through the birth canal.

Cephalopelvic Disproportion

Cephalopelvic disproportion (CPD), also called fetopelvic disproportion (FPD), is often related to excessive fetal size (i.e., 4000 g or more). It occurred at the rate of 15.8 per 1000 live births in 2002 (Martin et al, 2003). When CPD is present, the fetus cannot fit through the maternal pelvis to be born vaginally. Excessive fetal size, or macrosomia, is associated with maternal diabetes mellitus, obesity, multiparity, or the large size of one or both parents. If the maternal pelvis is too small, abnormally shaped, or deformed, CPD may be of maternal origin. In this case, the fetus may be of average size or even smaller.

Malposition

The most common fetal malposition is persistent occipitoposterior position (i.e., right occipitoposterior [ROP] or

Nursing Care Plan

DYSFUNCTIONAL LABOR: HYPOTONIC UTERINE DYSFUNCTION WITH PROTRACTED ACTIVE PHASE

NURSING DIAGNOSIS: Risk for injury to mother or fetus (or both) related to oxytocin augmentation secondary to dysfunctional labor

EXPECTED OUTCOMES

Maternal-fetal well-being is maintained; labor progresses and birth occurs.

NURSING INTERVENTIONS/*RATIONALES*

Explain oxytocin protocol to woman and her labor partner *to allay apprehension and enhance participation.*

Encourage woman to void before beginning protocol *to prevent discomfort and remove a barrier to labor progress.*

Apply the electronic fetal monitor per hospital protocol and obtain a 15- to 20-minute baseline strip *to ensure adequate assessment of FHR and contractions.*

Position woman in a side-lying position and administer the oxytocin per physician order using an IV infusion pump *to stimulate uterine activity and provide adequate control of the flow rate.*

Regulate the oxytocin per protocol (e.g., advancing the dose in increments of 1 to 2 milliunits/min every 30 to 60 minutes) *to allow adequate evaluation of the woman's response to stimulation and to prevent hyperstimulation and fetal hypoxia.*

Maintain oxytocin dose and rate when contractions occur every 2 to 3 minutes with a duration of 40 to 90 seconds and intrauterine pressures of 60 to 90 mm Hg (if internal monitoring is used) *to produce effective uterine stimulation without risk of hyperstimulation.*

Monitor maternal vital signs every 30 to 60 minutes *to assess for oxytocin-induced hypertension.*

Monitor contractility pattern and fetal heart rate and pattern every 15 minutes *to assess uterine activity for possible hypertonicity or ineffective uterine response to oxytocin and to detect evidence of fetal distress.*

Monitor intake, output, and specific gravity (limit intake to 1000 ml/8 hr; output should be at least 120 ml/4 hr) *to assess for urinary retention and prevent water intoxication.*

Monitor cervical dilation, effacement, and station *to assess progress of labor.*

If hypertonicity or signs of fetal distress are detected, discontinue oxytocin immediately *to arrest the progress of hypertonicity;* turn woman on her side *to increase placental blood flow;* increase primary IV rate to 200 ml/hr (unless signs of water toxicity are present); administer oxygen per face mask *to enhance placental perfusion;* notify primary health care provider; and continuously monitor maternal vital signs and FHR *to provide ongoing assessment of maternal/fetal status.*

Maintain Standard Precautions and use scrupulous handwashing techniques when providing care *to prevent the spread of infection.*

NURSING DIAGNOSIS: Acute pain related to increasing frequency, regularity, intensity, and prolonged peak of contractions

EXPECTED OUTCOME

The woman exhibits signs of decreased discomfort.

NURSING INTERVENTIONS/*RATIONALES*

Prepare woman and labor partner for the change in the nature of the contractions once the oxytocin drip is initiated *to prepare them and allow for more effective coping.*

Review the use of specific techniques such as conscious relaxation, focused breathing, effleurage, massage, and application of sacral pressure *to increase relaxation, decrease intensity of pain of contractions, and promote use of controlled thought and direction of energy.*

Provide comfort measures such as frequent mouth care *to prevent dry mouth,* application of damp cloth to forehead and changing of damp gown or bed covers *to relieve discomfort of diaphoresis,* and positioning *to reduce stiffness.*

Encourage conscious relaxation between contractions *to prevent fatigue, which contributes to increased pain perceptions.*

Remind woman and labor partner that analgesics are available for use during labor *to provide knowledge to help them make decisions about pain control.*

NURSING DIAGNOSIS: Anxiety related to prolonged labor, increased pain, and fatigue

EXPECTED OUTCOMES

Woman's anxiety is reduced; woman actively participates in the labor process.

NURSING INTERVENTIONS/*RATIONALES*

Provide ongoing feedback to woman and partner *to allay anxiety and enhance participation.*

Present care options when possible *to increase feelings of control.*

Continue to provide comfort measures *to maintain a posture of support and caring and to aid woman in focusing on the labor process.*

Encourage woman and partner to continue to use those mechanisms that promote effective labor (e.g., breathing, activity, positioning) *to keep woman and partner actively involved in process.*

left occipitoposterior [LOP]) (see Fig. 15-2), occurring in about 25% of all labors. Labor, especially the second stage, is prolonged; the woman typically complains of severe back pain from the pressure of the fetal head (occiput) pressing against her sacrum. Box 19-7 identifies suggested measures to relieve back pain and facilitate rotation of the fetal occiput to an anterior position, which will facilitate birth (Gilbert & Harmon, 2003; Simkin & Ancheta, 2000).

Malpresentation

Malpresentation occurred at a rate of 38.1 per 1000 live births in 2002, with the highest rate (58.7) among women 40 to 54 years of age (Martin et al, 2003). Breech presentation is the most common form of malpresentation. The four main types of breech presentation are frank breech (thighs flexed, knees extended); complete breech (thighs and knees flexed); and two types of incomplete breech, one in which the knee extends below the buttocks and the other in which the foot

Table 19-1

Dysfunctional Labor: Primary and Secondary Powers

HYPERTONIC UTERINE DYSFUNCTION	HYPOTONIC UTERINE DYSFUNCTION	INADEQUATE VOLUNTARY EXPULSIVE FORCES
DESCRIPTION		
Usually occurs before 4 cm dilation; cause unknown, may be related to fear and tension (primary powers)	Cause may be pelvic contracture and fetal malposition, overdistention of uterus (e.g., twins), or unknown (primary powers)	Involves abdominal and levator ani muscles Occurs in second stage of labor; cause may be related to nerve block anesthetic/analgesia, exhaustion
CHANGE IN PATTERN OF PROGRESS		
Pain out of proportion to intensity of contraction Pain out of proportion to effectiveness of contraction in effacing and dilating the cervix Contractions increase in frequency Contractions uncoordinated Uterus is contracted between contractions, cannot be indented	Contractions decrease in frequency and intensity Uterus easily indentable even at peak of contraction Uterus relaxed between contractions (normal)	No voluntary urge to push or bear down or inadequate/ineffective pushing
POTENTIAL MATERNAL EFFECTS		
Loss of control related to intensity of pain and lack of progress Exhaustion	Infection Exhaustion Psychologic trauma	Spontaneous vaginal birth prevented
POTENTIAL FETAL EFFECTS		
Fetal asphyxia with meconium aspiration	Fetal infection Fetal and neonatal death	Fetal asphyxia
CARE MANAGEMENT		
Initiate therapeutic rest measures • Administer analgesic (e.g., morphine, nalbuphine, meperidine) if membranes not ruptured or cephalopelvic disproportion not present • Relieve pain to permit mother to rest • Assist with measures to enhance rest and relaxation (e.g., hydrotherapy)	Rule out cephalopelvic disproportion Stimulate labor with oxytocin (augmentation) Perform amniotomy Assist with measures to enhance the progress of labor (e.g., position changes, ambulation, hydrotherapy)	Coach mother in bearing down with contractions; assist with relaxation between contractions Position mother in favorable position for pushing Reduce epidural infusion rate Apply low forceps or vacuum if assistance is needed Perform cesarean birth only if nonreassuring fetal status occurs

extends below the buttocks (Fig. 19-4). Breech presentations are associated with multifetal gestation, preterm birth, fetal and maternal anomalies, hydramnios, and oligohydramnios. Diagnosis is made by abdominal palpation and vaginal examination and usually is confirmed by ultrasound scan (Lanni & Seeds, 2002).

During labor, fetal descent may be slow because the breech is not as good a dilating wedge as the fetal head; the labor itself is usually not prolonged. There is risk of prolapse of the cord if the membranes rupture in early labor. The aftercoming head can be trapped by an incompletely dilated cervix. The presence of meconium in amniotic fluid is not necessarily a sign of fetal distress because it results from pressure on the fetal abdominal wall as it traverses the birth canal. Assessment of fetal heart rate and pattern should be used to determine whether the passage of meconium is an expected finding associated with breech presentation or is a nonreassuring sign associated with fetal hypoxia. The fetal heart tones of infants in a breech position are best heard at or above the umbilicus.

Radiographic pelvimetry is useful to determine which patients are suitable for a trial of labor. Vaginal birth is accomplished by mechanisms of labor that manipulate the buttocks and lower extremities as they emerge from the birth canal. Piper forceps sometimes are used to deliver the head (see Fig. 19-9). External cephalic version (ECV) may be tried to turn the fetus to a vertex presentation. When ECV is performed at 36 weeks of gestation, the success rate is approximately 65%. Cesarean birth may be necessary (Bowes & Thorp, 2004).

BOX 19-7

Back Labor—Occiput Posterior Position

Measures to Relieve Back Pain and Facilitate Rotation of Fetal Head

Measures to Reduce Back Pain during a Contraction

- Counterpressure: apply fist or heel of hand to sacral area
- Heat or cold applications: apply to sacral area
- Double hip squeeze:
  Woman assumes a position with hip joints flexed, such as knee-chest position.
  Partner, nurse, or doula places hands over gluteal muscles and presses with palms of hands up and inward toward the center of the pelvis.
- Knee press:
  Woman assumes a sitting position with knees a few inches apart and feet flat on the floor or on a stool.
  Partner, nurse, or doula cups a knee in each hand with heels of hands on top of tibia, then presses the knees straight back toward the woman's hips while leaning forward toward the woman.

Measures to Facilitate the Rotation of the Fetal Head (May Also Relieve Back Pain)

- Lateral abdominal stroking: stroke the abdomen in direction that the fetal head should rotate
- Hands-and-knees position (all-fours): can also be accomplished by kneeling while leaning forward over a birth ball, padded chair seat, bed, or over-the-bed table
- Squatting
- Pelvic rocking
- Stair climbing
- Lateral position: lie on side toward which the fetus should turn
- Lunges: widens pelvis on side toward which woman lunges
  Woman stands, facing forward, next to/alongside a chair so that she can lunge toward the side the fetal back is on or in the direction of the fetal occiput.
  Woman places foot on seat of chair with toes pointed toward the back of the chair, then lunges.
  Alternative position for lunge: kneeling.

Although opinions vary, a cesarean birth is commonly performed when the fetus is estimated to be larger than 3800 g or smaller than 1500 g, if this is a first pregnancy, if labor is ineffective, or if complications occur. Although cesarean birth reduces the risks to the fetus, the maternal risks are increased. ECV also poses risks and is not always successful. Women whose breech presentation occurs late in pregnancy need to be informed about the options for birth, including the risks associated with each option.

Face and brow presentations are uncommon and are associated with fetal anomalies, pelvic contractures, and CPD. Vaginal birth is possible if the fetus flexes to a vertex presentation, although forceps often are used. Cesarean birth is indicated if the presentation persists, if there is fetal distress, or if labor stops progressing.

Cesarean birth is usually necessary for a fetus in a shoulder presentation (i.e., the fetus is in a transverse lie), although ECV may be attempted after 36 to 37 weeks of gestation (Bowes & Thorp, 2004).

Multifetal Pregnancy

Multifetal pregnancy is the gestation of twins, triplets, quadruplets, or more infants.

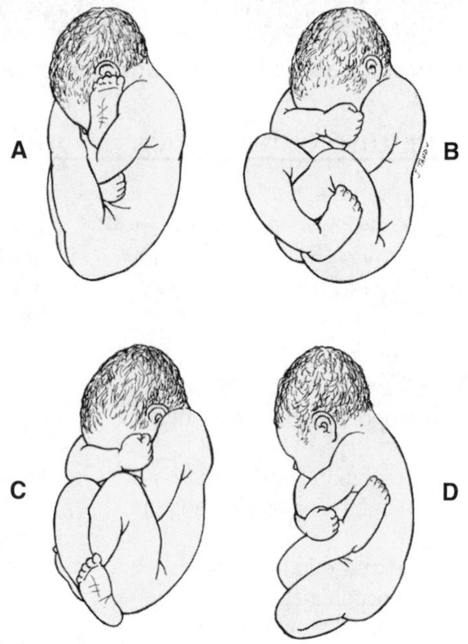

Fig. 19-4 Types of breech presentation. **A**, Frank breech: thighs are flexed on hips; knees are extended. **B**, Complete breech: thighs and knees are flexed. **C**, Incomplete breech: foot extends below the buttocks. **D**, Incomplete breech: knee extends below the buttocks.

The twin birth rate was 31.1 per 1000 live births in 2002. The higher-order multiple birth rate (i.e., triplet and more) was 184 per 100,000 live births in 2002 (Martin et al, 2005). The incidence of multiple births has been increasing since 1980. It is likely that this trend is related to the use of fertility-enhancing medications and procedures and the older age of childbearing women. When compared with younger women, women age 35 years and older are more likely to have a multifetal pregnancy with or without fertility enhancing drugs.

Multiple births are associated with more complications, including dysfunctional labor, than are single births. The high incidence of fetal/newborn complications and higher risk of perinatal death primarily stems from the birth of low-birth-weight infants resulting from preterm birth and intrauterine growth restriction. Fetuses may experience distress and asphyxia during birth as a result of cord prolapse and the onset of placental separation with the birth of the first fetus. As a result, the risk for long-term problems such as cerebral palsy is higher among multiple births.

In addition, fetal complications such as congenital anomalies and abnormal presentations can lead to dystocia and an increased incidence of cesarean birth. For example, in only half of all twin pregnancies do both fetuses present in the vertex presentation, the most favorable for vaginal birth; in one third of pregnancies, one twin may present in the vertex presentation and one in the breech.

The health status of the mother may be compromised by an increased risk for hypertension, anemia, and hemorrhage associated with uterine atony, abruptio placentae, and multiple or adherent placentas. Duration of the phases and stages of labor may vary from the duration experienced with singleton births.

Teamwork and planning are essential in the management of childbirth in multiple pregnancies, especially those of the higher-order multiples. Early detection and effective care of maternal, fetal, and newborn complications associated with multiple births are essential to achieve a positive outcome for mothers and babies. Maternal positioning and active support are used to enhance labor progress and placental perfusion. Emotional support that includes expression of feelings and full explanations of events as they occur and of the status of the mother and the fetuses/newborns is important to reduce the anxiety and stress the mother and her family experience.

Position of the Woman

The functional relationships among the uterine contractions, the fetus, and the mother's pelvis are altered by the maternal position. The position can provide either a mechanical advantage or disadvantage to the mechanisms of labor by altering the effects of gravity and the body part relations important to the progress of labor. For example, the hands-and-knees position facilitates rotation from a posterior occiput position more effectively than does the lateral position. Upright positions such as sitting and squatting facilitate fetal descent during pushing and shorten the second stage of labor (Mayberry et al, 2000; Simkin & Ancheta, 2000). Discouraging maternal movement or restricting labor to the recumbent or lithotomy position may compromise progress. The incidence of dystocia in women confined to these positions is increased, resulting in increased need for augmentation of labor, the use of forceps, and vacuum-assisted or cesarean birth.

Psychologic Responses

Hormones and neurotransmitters released in response to stress (e.g., catecholamines) can cause dystocia. Sources of stress vary for each woman, but pain and the absence of a support person are two recognized factors. Confinement to bed and restriction of maternal movement can be a source of psychologic stress that compounds the physiologic stress caused by immobility in the unmedicated, laboring woman. When anxiety is excessive, it can inhibit normal cervical dilation and result in prolonged labor and increased pain perception. Anxiety also causes increased levels of stress-related hormones (e.g., β-endorphin, adrenocorticotropic hormone, cortisol, and epinephrine). These hormones act on the smooth muscles of the uterus; increased levels can cause dystocia by reducing uterine contractility.

Abnormal Labor Patterns

In 2002, prolonged labor patterns occurred at the rate of 7.0 per 1000 live births, with the incidence highest among women under 20 years of age (8.1 per 1000) (Martin et al, 2003).

Six abnormal labor patterns were identified and classified by Friedman (1989) according to the nature of cervical dilation and fetal descent. The labor patterns seen in normal and abnormal labor are described in Table 19-2.

These patterns may result from a variety of causes that include ineffective uterine contractions, pelvic contractures, CPD, abnormal fetal presentation or position, early use of analgesics, nerve block analgesia/anesthesia, and anxiety and stress. Progress in either the first or second stage of labor can be protracted (prolonged) or arrested (stopped).

Table 19-2

Labor Patterns in Normal and Abnormal Labor

NORMAL LABOR

1. Dilation: continues
   a. Latent phase: <4 cm and low slope
   b. Active phase: >5 cm or high slope
   c. Deceleration phase: ≥9 cm
2. Descent: active at ≥9 cm dilation

ABNORMAL LABOR

PATTERN	NULLIPARAS	MULTIPARAS
Prolonged latent phase	>20 hr	>14 hr
Protracted active phase dilation	<1.2 cm/hr	<1.5 cm/hr
Secondary arrest: no change	≥2 hr	≥2 hr
Protracted descent	<1 cm/hr	<2 cm/hr
Arrest of descent	≥1 hr	≥½ hr
Failure of descent	No change during deceleration phase and second stage	
Precipitous labor	>5 cm/hr	10 cm/hr

Abnormal progress can be identified by plotting cervical dilation and fetal descent on a labor graph (partogram) at various intervals after the onset of labor and comparing the resulting curve with the expected labor curve for a nulliparous or multiparous labor. Figure 19-5, *A*, is a labor graph illustrating progress in a normal labor for a primigravida. Figure 19-5, *B*, illustrates major types of deviation from the normal progress of labor. If a woman exhibits an abnormal labor pattern, the primary health care provider should be notified.

Health care providers must be careful when diagnosing a labor pattern as prolonged and when intervening based on this diagnosis. Criteria defining the differences between false, latent, and active labor should be established. Using hospital or unit admission areas to evaluate a woman's labor status is helpful in preventing the premature implementation of labor interventions such as administration of systemic opioid analgesics or induction of epidural analgesia/anesthesia. If a woman is found to be in false or latent (early) labor, she can be sent home or remain in the admission area until labor becomes active. Women in active labor are admitted to the labor and birth unit.

Maternal morbidity and death may occur as a result of uterine rupture, infection, serious dehydration, and postpartum hemorrhage. The fetus is at increased risk for hypoxia. A long, difficult labor also can have an adverse psychologic effect on the mother, father, and family.

Precipitous Labor

Precipitous labor is defined as labor that lasts less than 3 hours from the onset of contractions to the time of birth. This abnormal labor pattern occurred at a rate of 18.1 per 1000 live births in 2002. Precipitous labor occurred at the highest rate (21.9) among women age 35 to 39 and at the lowest rate (11.7) among women younger than 20 years (Martin et al, 2003).

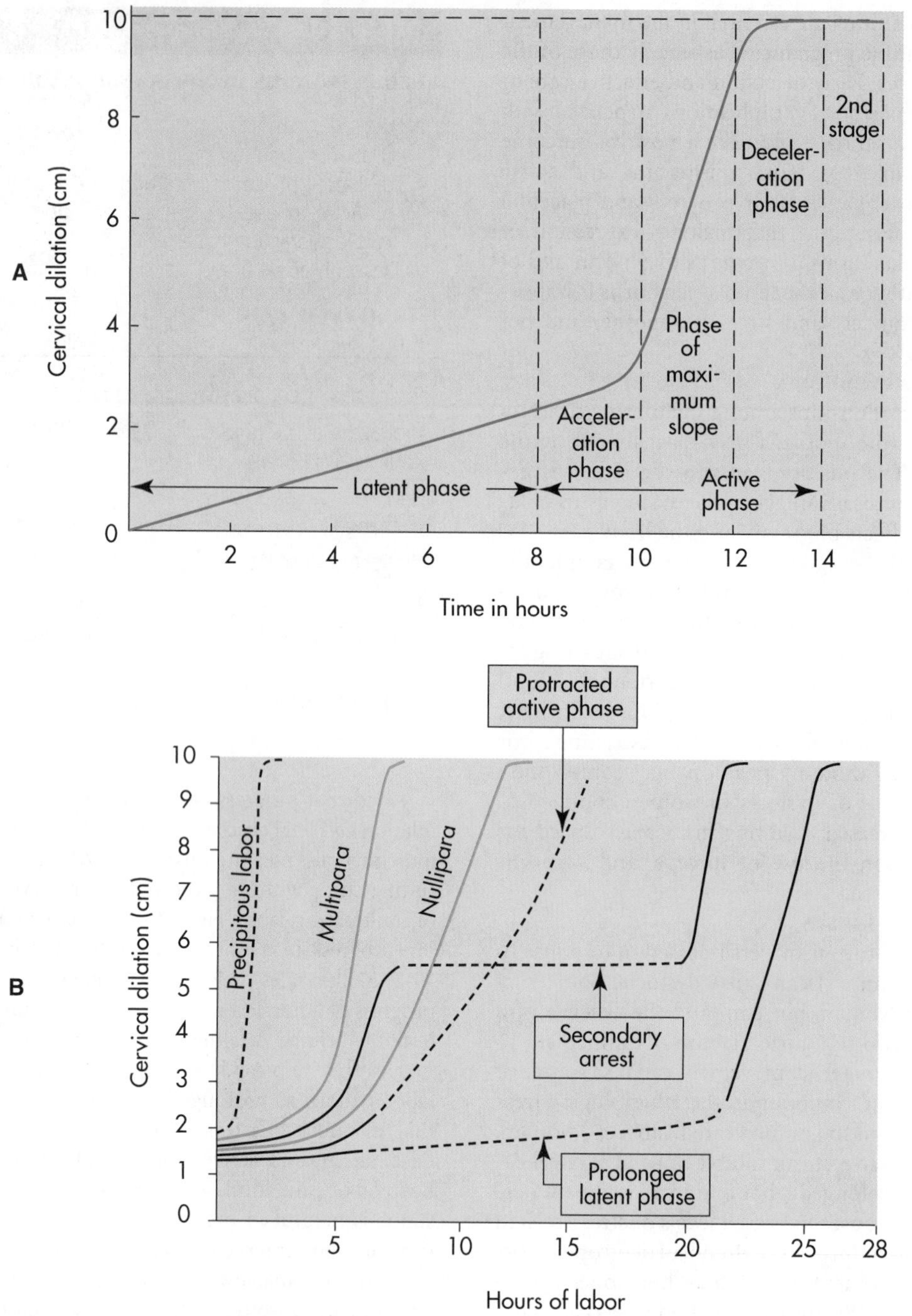

Fig. 19-5 Progress in labor. **A,** Depiction of a normal labor for a primigravida. **B,** Major types of deviation from normal progress of labor may be detected by noting dilation of cervix at various intervals after labor begins. If a woman exhibits an abnormal labor pattern, as depicted by *broken lines,* the primary health care provider should be notified.

Precipitous labor may result from hypertonic uterine contractions that are tetanic in intensity. Maternal and fetal complications can occur as a result. Maternal complications include uterine rupture, lacerations of the birth canal, amniotic fluid embolism, and postpartum hemorrhage. Fetal complications include hypoxia, caused by decreased periods of uterine relaxation between contractions, and intracranial hemorrhage related to rapid birth (Cunningham et al, 2001).

Women who have experienced precipitate labor often describe feelings of disbelief that their labor began so quickly, alarm that their labor progressed so rapidly, panic about the possibility they would not make it to the hospital on time to give birth, and finally relief when they arrived at the hospital. In addition, women have expressed frustration when nurses would not believe them when they reported their readiness to push.

Care Management

Assessment

Risk assessment is a continuous process in the laboring woman. Review of the findings obtained during the initial interview conducted at the woman's admission to the labor unit, and ongoing observations of her psychologic response to labor, may reveal factors that can be a source of dysfunctional labor. These factors may include anxiety or fear, a complication of pregnancy, or previous labor complications. The initial physical assessment and ongoing assessments provide information about maternal well-being; status of labor in terms of the characteristics of uterine contractions and progress of cervical effacement and dilation; fetal well-being in terms of FHR, fetal heart pattern, presentation, station, and position; and status of the amniotic membranes.

Laboratory data such as the scalp pH can be used to identify the degree of fetal distress. Ultrasound scanning can identify potential dysfunctional labor problems related to the fetus or maternal pelvis. All of these assessments contribute to accurate identification of potential and actual nursing diagnoses related to dystocia and maternal-fetal compromise.

Nursing Diagnoses

Nursing diagnoses that might be identified in women experiencing dystocia include the following:

- *Risk for maternal or fetal injury related to*
  —interventions implemented for dystocia
- *Powerlessness related to*
  —loss of control
- *Risk for infection related to*
  —PPROM
  —operative procedures
- *Ineffective individual coping related to*
  —exhaustion
  —inadequate support system

Expected Outcomes

Expected outcomes for the woman who is experiencing dystocia include that the woman will

- Understand the causes and treatment of dysfunctional labor
- Use positive patterns of coping to maintain a positive self-concept
- Express relief of pain
- Experience labor and birth with minimal or no complications such as infection, injury, or hemorrhage
- Give birth to a healthy infant who has not experienced fetal distress or birth injury

ENGLISH SPANISH **Guidelines/Guías**

INDUCTION OF LABOR

Your labor is not progressing.
Su trabajo de parto no está progresando.

We need to stimulate the contractions.
Necesitamos provocar las contracciones.

I'm going to give you some medication to make your contractions stronger.
Le voy a dar una medicina para hacer más fuertes las contracciones.

I'm going to give you Pitocin through your IV.
Le voy a dar pitufina por medio del suero.

Plan of Care and Implementation

Nurses assume many caregiving roles when labor is complicated. They work collaboratively with other health care providers in providing care. Interventions that the nurse may implement or assist with include external cephalic version, trial of labor, induction or augmentation with oxytocin, amniotomy, and operative procedures (e.g., forceps- or vacuum-assisted birth). The nursing role is identified with each of the procedures described.

LEGAL TIP **Standard of Care—Labor and Birth at Risk**

- Document all assessments findings, interventions, and patient responses on patient record and monitor strips according to unit protocols, procedures, and policies and professional standards.
- Assess whether the woman (and family, if appropriate) is fully informed about procedures for which she is consenting.
- Provide full explanations regarding what is happening and what needs to be done to help her and her baby (Guidelines/Guías: Induction of Labor/Cesarean Birth).
- Maintain safety in administering medications and treatments correctly.
- Have verbal orders signed as soon as possible.
- Provide care at the acceptable standard (e.g., according to hospital protocols and professional standards).
- If short staffing occurs in the unit, and the nurse is assigned additional patients, the nurse should document that rejecting the additional assignment would have placed these patients in danger as a result of abandonment.
- Maternal and fetal monitoring continues until birth according to policies, procedures, and protocols of the birthing facility, even when a decision for cesarean birth is made. ■

Version

Version is the turning of the fetus artificially from one presentation to another by the physician. Version may be done externally or internally.

External Cephalic Version

External cephalic version (ECV) is used to attempt to turn the fetus from a breech or shoulder presentation to a

ENGLISH SPANISH **Guidelines/Guías**

CESAREAN BIRTH

You need a cesarean.
Necesita una operación cesárea.

Has your doctor discussed with you the reason for needing a cesarean?
¿Ha hablado el doctor con usted sobre la necesidad de tener una operación cesárea?

Do you understand why you need a cesarean?
¿Entiende usted por qué necesita una operación cesárea?

Your signature on this form will allow us to proceed with the surgery.
Su firma en este formulario nos permitirá seguir adelante con la operación.

Please sign this consent form.
Por favor, firme este formulario de autorización.

vertex presentation for birth. It may be attempted in a labor and birth setting after 37 weeks of gestation. Before it is attempted, ultrasound scanning is done to determine the fetal position; locate the umbilical cord; rule out placenta previa; evaluate the adequacy of the maternal pelvis; and assess the amount of amniotic fluid, the fetal age, and the presence of any anomalies. A nonstress test (NST) is performed to confirm fetal well-being, or the FHR is monitored for a time (usually 10 to 20 minutes). Informed consent is obtained. Contraindications to ECV include uterine anomalies, previous cesarean birth, CPD, placenta previa, multifetal gestation, and oligohydramnios (Cunningham et al, 2001; Lanni & Seeds, 2002). ECV performed at term to avoid breech birth is a beneficial form of care (Enkin et al, 2000).

ECV is accomplished by gentle, constant pressure on the abdomen (Fig. 19-6). A tocolytic agent such as magnesium sulfate or terbutaline often is given to relax the uterus and to facilitate the maneuver. Ultrasound scanning is done to identify potential problems such as cord entanglement and placental separation (Bowes & Thorp, 2004).

During an attempted ECV, the nurse continuously monitors the FHR, especially for bradycardia; checks maternal vital signs; and assesses the woman's level of comfort because the procedure may cause discomfort. After the procedure is completed, the nurse continues to monitor maternal vital signs, uterine activity, fetal heart rate and pattern and assess for vaginal bleeding until the woman's condition is stable. Women who are Rh-negative should receive Rh immune globulin because the manipulation can cause fetomaternal bleeding (Bowes & Thorp, 2004).

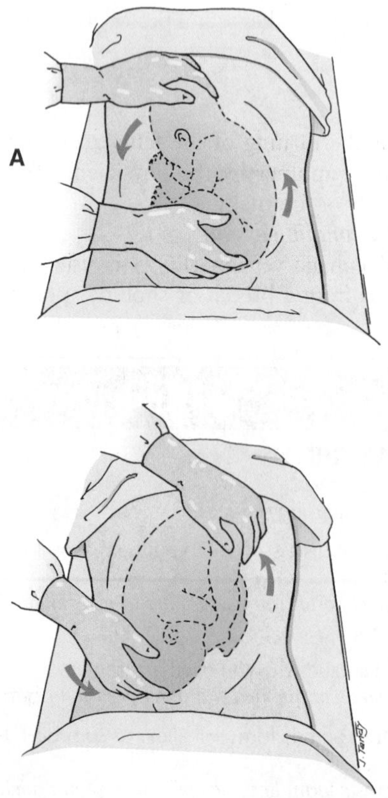

Fig. 19-6 External version of fetus from breech to vertex presentation. This must be achieved without force. **A**, Breech is pushed up out of pelvic inlet while head is pulled toward inlet. **B**, Head is pushed toward inlet while breech is pulled upward.

Internal Version

With internal version, the fetus is turned by the physician, who inserts a hand into the uterus and changes the presentation to cephalic (head) or podalic (foot). Internal version may be used in multifetal pregnancies to deliver the second fetus. The safety of this procedure has not been documented; maternal and fetal injury is possible. Cesarean birth is the usual method for managing malpresentation in multifetal pregnancies. The nurse's role is to monitor the status of the fetus and to provide support to the woman.

Trial of Labor

A trial of labor (TOL) is the observance of a woman and her fetus for a reasonable period (e.g., 4 to 6 hours) of spontaneous active labor to assess the safety of vaginal birth for the mother and infant. TOL may be initiated if the mother's pelvis is of questionable size or shape, if she wishes to have a vaginal birth after a previous cesarean birth, or if the fetus is in an abnormal presentation. It is a form of care likely to be beneficial when implemented after a previous low-segment cesarean birth (Enkin et al, 2000). Fetal sonography or maternal pelvimetry (or both) may be done before a TOL to rule out CPD. The cervix must be ripe (soft and dilatable). During a TOL, the woman is evaluated for the occurrence of active labor, including adequate contractions, engagement and descent of the presenting part, and effacement and dilation of the cervix.

The nurse assesses maternal vital signs, fetal heart rate and pattern and is alert for signs of potential complications. If complications develop, the nurse is responsible for initiating appropriate actions, including notifying the primary health care provider, and for evaluating and documenting the maternal and fetal responses to the interventions. Supporting and encouraging the woman and her partner and providing information regarding progress can reduce stress, enhance the labor process, and facilitate a successful outcome.

Induction of Labor

Induction of labor can be elective (for the convenience of the patient or staff) or indicated for medical, obstetric, or fetal reasons. Induction of labor is the chemical or mechanical initiation of uterine contractions before their spontaneous onset for the purpose of bringing about the birth. In 2002, 20.6% of women who gave birth had their labors induced, more than twice the labor induction rate of 9% in 1989 (Martin et al, 2003). Medical and obstetric reasons include gestational hypertension, diabetes mellitus, chorioamnionitis, and other maternal medical problems; PROM; postdate gestation; suspected fetal jeopardy (e.g., IUGR); logistic factors, such as history of previous rapid birth or distance of the woman's home from the hospital; and fetal death. Under such conditions the risk to the mother or fetus is less than the risk of continuing the pregnancy (Bowes & Thorp, 2004).

Both chemical and mechanical methods are used to induce labor. Intravenous oxytocin and amniotomy are the most common methods used in the United States. Prostaglandins are increasingly used for inducing labor. The most effective protocol (e.g., dose, frequency) to follow when using prostaglandins continues to be investigated (Simpson, 2002).

Less commonly used methods include nipple stimulation (manual or with a breast pump), the ingestion of castor oil or herbal preparations, a soapsuds enema, stripping of membranes, and acupuncture (Bowes & Thorp, 2004). Many folk beliefs exist regarding methods to induce labor. These methods include activity (e.g., walking, exercise, strenuous work, sexual intercourse), fasting, and increasing stress (e.g., frightening the woman). It is important for the nurse to know the practices a woman may believe in and follow, because some of these methods can be harmful (e.g., strenuous activity) (Schaffir, 2002).

Success rates for induction of labor are higher when the cervix is favorable, or inducible. A rating system such as the Bishop score (Table 19-3) can be used to evaluate inducibility. For example, a score of 9 or more on this 13-point scale indicates that the cervix is soft, anterior, 50% or more effaced, and dilated 2 cm or more; and that the presenting part is engaged. Induction of labor is likely to be more successful if the score is 8 or more (Gilbert & Harmon, 2003).

Table 19-3

Bishop Score

	Score			
	0	1	2	3
Dilation (cm)	Closed	1-2	3-4	≥5
Effacement (%)	0-30	40-50	60-70	≥80
Station (cm)	−3	−2	−1, 0	+1, +2
Cervical consistency	Firm	Medium	Soft	
Cervix position	Posterior	Midposition	Anterior	

Cervical Ripening Methods

Chemical Agents

A prostaglandin gel was approved by the FDA in 1993 as a cervical ripening agent. Preparations of prostaglandin E_1 and prostaglandin E_2 can be used before induction to "ripen" (soften and thin) the cervix (Medication Guides). This treatment usually results in a higher success rate for the induction of labor, the need for lower dosages of oxytocin during the induction, and shorter induction times. The use of prostaglandins to increase cervical readiness for induction of labor is a beneficial form of care (Enkin et al, 2000). In some cases, women will go into labor after the application of prostaglandin, thereby eliminating the need to administer oxytocin to induce labor. Prostaglandin E_1, although less expensive and more effective than oxytocin or prostaglandin E_2

Medication Guide

CERVICAL RIPENING USING PROSTAGLANDIN E_2 (PGE_2): DINOPROSTONE (CERVIDIL INSERT; PREPIDIL GEL)

Action

PGE_2 ripens the cervix, making it softer and causing it to begin to dilate and efface; stimulates uterine contractions.

Indications

PGE_2 is used for preinduction cervical ripening (ripen cervix before oxytocin induction of labor when the Bishop score is ≤4), and to induce labor or abortion (abortifacient agent).

Dosage

Place Cervidil insert (10 mg dinoprostone gradually released over 12 hr) intravaginally into the posterior fornix. Insert Prepidil gel (2.5 ml syringe containing 0.5 mg of dinoprostone) into cervical canal just below internal cervical os or into posterior fornix; a shield can be used to prevent insertion past internal os. Repeat gel insertion in 6 hr as needed to a maximum of 1.5 mg in a 24 hr period. Continue treatment until maximum dosage is administered or until an effective contraction pattern is established (three or more uterine contractions in 10 min), cervix ripens (Bishop score of ≥8), or significant adverse reactions occur.

Adverse Reactions

Potential adverse reactions include headache, nausea and vomiting, diarrhea, fever, hypotension, tachysystole (12 or more uterine contractions in 20 min without alteration of fetal heart rate or pattern), hyperstimulation of the uterus (tachysystole with nonreassuring fetal heart rate or patterns), or fetal passage of meconium. Adverse reactions are more common with intracervical administration.

Nursing Considerations

Explain procedure to woman and her family. Ensure that an informed consent has been obtained as per agency policy. Assess maternal-fetal unit before each insertion and during treatment, following agency protocol for frequency. Assess maternal vital signs and health status, fetal heart rate and pattern, and status of pregnancy, including indications for cervical ripening or induction of labor, signs of labor or impending labor, and the Bishop score. Recognize that a nonreassuring fetal heart rate or pattern; maternal fever, infection, vaginal bleeding, or hypersensitivity; and regular, progressive uterine contractions and history of cesarean birth or uterine scar contraindicate the use of dinoprostone. Use caution if the woman has a history of asthma; glaucoma; or renal, hepatic, or cardiovascular disorders. Bring gel to room temperature before administration. Do not force warming process by using a warm water bath or other source of external heat (e.g., microwave). Keep insert frozen until use (no rewarming needed). Have woman void before insertion. Assist woman to maintain a supine position with lateral tilt or a side-lying position for 30 to 60 min after insertion of gel or for 2 hr after placement of insert. Allow woman to ambulate after recommended period of bed rest and observation. Prepare to swab vagina to remove remaining gel using a saline-soaked gauze wrapped around fingers or pull string to remove insert and to administer terbutaline 0.25 mg subcutaneously or intravenously if significant adverse reactions occur. Initiate oxytocin for induction of labor within 6 to 12 hr after last instillation of gel or at least 30 to 60 min after removal of the insert. Follow agency protocol for induction if ripening has occurred and labor has not begun. Document all assessment findings and administration procedures. Dinoprostone is the only FDA-approved medication for cervical ripening or labor induction.

FDA, Food and Drug Administration.

Medication Guide

CERVICAL RIPENING USING PROSTAGLANDIN E_1 (PGE_1): MISOPROSTOL (CYTOTEC)

Action

PGE_1 ripens the cervix, making it softer and causing it to begin to dilate and efface; stimulates uterine contractions.

Indications

PGE_1 is used for preinduction cervical ripening (ripen cervix before oxytocin induction of labor when the Bishop score is ≤ 4) and to induce labor or abortion (abortifacient agent).

Dosage

Insert 25 to 50 mg (¼ to ½ of a 100 mg tablet) intravaginally into the posterior fornix using the tips of index and middle fingers without the use of a lubricant. Repeat every 3 to 6 hr as needed to a maximum of 300 to 400 mg in a 24 hr period or until an effective contraction pattern is established (three or more uterine contractions in 10 min), cervix ripens (Bishop score of ≥ 8), or significant adverse reactions occur. Administer: 50-100 mg po q4-6hr (GI effects increased; there are insufficient data to support effectiveness, therefore oral administration is generally not recommended).

Adverse Reactions

Higher dosages are more likely to result in adverse reactions such as nausea and vomiting, diarrhea, fever, tachysystole (12 or more uterine contractions in 20 min without alteration of fetal heart rate or pattern), hyperstimulation of the uterus (tachysystole with nonreassuring fetal heart patterns), or fetal passage of meconium. Risk for adverse reactions is reduced with lower dosages (i.e., 25 mg) and longer intervals between doses (i.e., q6hr).

Nursing Considerations

Explain procedure to woman and her family. Ensure that an informed consent has been obtained as per agency policy. Assess maternal-fetal unit before each insertion and during treatment, following agency protocol for frequency. Assess maternal vital signs and health status, fetal heart rate and pattern, and status of pregnancy, including indications for cervical ripening or induction of labor, signs of labor or impending labor, and the Bishop score. Recognize that a nonreassuring fetal heart rate or pattern; maternal fever, infection, vaginal bleeding, or hypersensitivity; and regular, progressive uterine contractions and history of cesarean birth or uterine scar contraindicate the use of misoprostol. Use caution if the woman has a history of asthma; glaucoma; or renal, hepatic, or cardiovascular disorders. Have woman void before procedure. Assist woman to maintain a supine position with lateral tilt or a side-lying position for 30 to 40 min after insertion. Prepare to swab vagina to remove unabsorbed medication using a saline-soaked gauze wrapped around fingers and to administer terbutaline 0.25 mg subcutaneously or intravenously if significant adverse reactions occur. Initiate oxytocin for induction of labor at least 4 hr after last dose of misoprostol was administered, following agency protocol, if ripening has occurred and labor has not begun. Document all assessment findings and administration procedures. Misoprostol (Cytotec) has not yet been approved by the FDA for cervical ripening or labor induction. It is a nonscored 100 mg tablet that must be cut in the pharmacy to ensure dosage accuracy.

FDA, Food and Drug Administration.

for inducing labor and birth, is associated with a higher risk for hyperstimulation of the uterus and nonreassuring changes in fetal heart rate and pattern (Goldberg, Greenberg, & Darney, 2001).

Mechanical Methods

Mechanical dilators ripen the cervix by stimulating the release of endogenous prostaglandins. Their use is a form of care with a trade-off between beneficial and adverse effects (Enkin et al, 2000). Balloon catheters (e.g., Foley catheter) can be inserted into the intracervical canal to ripen and dilate the cervix. Hygroscopic dilators (substances that absorb fluid from surrounding tissues and enlarge) also can be used for cervical ripening. Laminaria tents (natural cervical dilators made from seaweed) and synthetic dilators containing magnesium sulfate (Lamicel) are inserted into the endocervix without rupturing the membranes. As they absorb fluid, they expand and cause cervical dilation. These dilators are left in place for 6 to 12 hours before being removed to assess cervical dilation. Fresh dilators are inserted if further cervical dilation is necessary. Synthetic dilators swell faster than natural dilators and become larger with less discomfort (Simpson, 2002). Nursing responsibilities for women who have dilators inserted include documenting the number of dilators and sponges inserted during the procedure, as well as the number removed, and assessment for urinary retention, rupture of membranes, uterine tenderness/pain, contractions, vaginal bleeding, and fetal distress (Gilbert & Harmon, 2003; Norwitz, Robinson, & Repke, 2002; Simpson, 2002).

Amniotomy

Amniotomy (i.e., artificial rupture of membranes [AROM]) can be used to induce labor when the condition of the cervix is favorable (ripe) or to augment labor if progress begins to slow. Labor usually begins within 12 hours of the rupture; the duration of labor is decreased by up to 2 hours, especially if combined with oxytocin administration. However, if amniotomy does not stimulate labor, the resulting prolonged rupture may lead to infection. Once an amniotomy is performed, the woman is committed to giving birth. For this reason, amniotomy often is used in combination with oxytocin induction. Evidence from controlled trials clearly demonstrates that amniotomy combined with oxytocin for induction is more effective than either amniotomy or oxytocin alone and is a beneficial form of care (Enkin et al, 2000). Before the procedure, the woman should be told what to expect; she should also be assured that the actual rupture of membranes is painless for her and the fetus, although she may experience some discomfort when the Amnihook or other sharp instrument is inserted through the vagina and cervix (Box 19-8).

The presenting part of the fetus should be engaged and well applied to the cervix to reduce the risk of cord prolapse. The woman should be free of active infection of the genital tract (e.g., herpes) and human immunodeficiency virus (HIV)

BOX 19-8

Procedure: Assisting with Amniotomy

Procedure

Explain to the woman what will be done.
Assess woman for signs of infection, condition of cervix (e.g., ripeness, dilation), and station of the presenting part.
Assess FHR before procedure begins to obtain a baseline reading.
Place several underpads under the woman's buttocks to absorb the fluid.
Position the woman on a padded bed pan, fracture pan, or rolled-up towel to elevate her hips.
Assist the health care provider who is performing the procedure by providing sterile gloves and lubricant for the vaginal examination.
Unwrap sterile package containing Amnihook or Allis clamp and pass instrument to the primary health care provider, who inserts it alongside the fingers and then hooks and tears the membranes.
Reassess the fetal heart rate and pattern.
Assess the color, consistency, and odor of the fluid.
Assess the woman's temperature every 2 hours or per protocol.
Evaluate the woman for signs and symptoms of infection.

Documentation

Record the following:
Indication for amniotomy
Time of rupture
Color, odor, consistency and clarity of the fluid
Fetal heart rate and pattern before and after the procedure
Maternal status and how well procedure was tolerated

infection (Norwitz et al, 2002). The membranes are ruptured with an Amnihook or other sharp instrument and the amniotic fluid is allowed to drain slowly. The fluid is assessed for color, odor, and consistency (i.e., for the presence or absence of meconium or blood). The time of rupture is recorded.

NURSE ALERT The FHR is assessed before and immediately after the amniotomy to detect any changes (transient tachycardia is common, but bradycardia and variable decelerations are not) that may indicate cord compression or prolapse. ■

The woman's temperature should be checked at least every 2 hours to rule out possible infection. If her temperature is 38° C or greater, the primary health care provider is notified. The nurse assesses for other signs and symptoms of infection such as maternal chills, fetal tachycardia, uterine tenderness on palpation, and foul-smelling vaginal drainage (Simpson, 2002). Comfort measures such as frequently changing the woman's underpads and perineal cleansing are implemented.

Oxytocin

Oxytocin is a hormone normally produced by the posterior pituitary gland; it stimulates uterine contractions. It may be used either to induce labor or to augment a labor that is progressing slowly because of inadequate uterine contractions.

The indications for oxytocin induction of labor may include, but are not limited to, the following:

- Suspected fetal jeopardy (e.g., IUGR)
- Inadequate uterine contractions; dystocia
- Premature rupture of membranes
- Postterm pregnancy
- Chorioamnionitis
- Maternal medical problems (e.g., woman with severe Rh isoimmunization, inadequately controlled diabetes, chronic renal disease, or chronic pulmonary disease)
- Gestational hypertension (e.g., eclampsia)
- Fetal death
- Multiparous women with a history of precipitous labor who live far from the hospital

The management of stimulation of labor is the same regardless of indication. Because of the potential dangers associated with the injection of oxytocin in the prenatal and intranatal periods, the FDA has issued restrictions on its use.

Contraindications to oxytocic stimulation of labor include, but are not limited to, the following:

- CPD, prolapsed cord, transverse lie
- Nonreassurring FHR
- Placenta previa or vasa previa
- Prior classic uterine incision or uterine surgery
- Active genital herpes infection
- Invasive cancer of the cervix

Certain maternal and fetal conditions, although not contraindications to the use of oxytocin to stimulate labor, do require special caution during its administration. These conditions include the following:

- Multifetal presentation
- Breech presentation
- Presenting part above the pelvic inlet
- Abnormal fetal heart rate and pattern not requiring emergency birth
- Polyhydramnios
- Grand multiparity
- Maternal cardiac disease; hypertension

Oxytocin use can present hazards to the mother and the fetus. These hazards are primarily dose related, with most problems caused by high doses that are given rapidly. Maternal hazards include water intoxication and tumultuous labor with tetanic contractions, which may cause premature separation of the placenta, rupture of the uterus, lacerations of the cervix, or postbirth hemorrhage. These complications can lead to infection, disseminated intravascular coagulation, or amniotic fluid embolism. Women may become anxious or fearful if the induction is not successful because they may then have concerns about the method of birth.

Uterine hyperstimulation reduces the blood flow through the placenta and results in FHR decelerations (bradycardia, diminished variability, late decelerations), fetal asphyxia, and neonatal hypoxia. If the estimated date of birth is inaccurate, physical injury, neonatal hyperbilirubinemia, and prematurity are other hazards.

Initiation of induction or augmentation of labor with oxytocin is the responsibility of the primary health care provider, although the medication is usually administered by a nurse through a secondary intravenous line according to

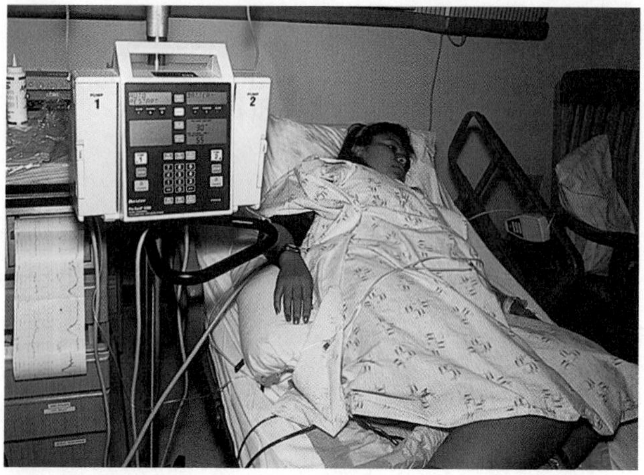

Fig. 19-7 Woman in side-lying position receiving oxytocin. (Courtesy Michael S. Clement, MD, Mesa, AZ.)

agency protocol and professional standards (Fig. 19-7; Box 19-9) (see Guidelines/Guías—Induction of Labor, p. 563).

In the past, the aim of induction was to achieve a contraction pattern that simulates the active phase of labor as quickly as possible. However, research on uterine tolerance to oxytocin has now shown that lower physiologic doses (e.g., initial dose of 0.5 to 1 milliunits/min with increments of 1 to 2 milliunits/min) given over a longer time are as effective as previous protocols. A recommended dosage increment frequency is every 30 to 60 minutes because 30 to 40 minutes is required for a steady state of oxytocin to be reached and for the full effect of a dosage increment to be reflected in more intense, frequent, and longer contractions. Such an approach reduces the amount of oxytocin required to achieve a spontaneous vaginal birth and decreases the risk for uterine hyperstimulation, dysfunctional labor, fetal distress, and other adverse reactions such as water intoxication (Norwitz et al, 2002; Simpson, 2002).

BOX 19-9

Protocol: Induction of Labor with Oxytocin

Patient/Family Teaching

Explain technique, rationale, and reactions to expect:

- Route and rate for administration of medication
- What "piggyback" is for
- Reasons for use: induce labor, improve labor
- Reactions to expect concerning the nature of contractions: the intensity of contraction increases more rapidly, holds the peak longer, and ends more quickly; contractions will come regularly and more often
- Monitoring to anticipate:
  Maternal: blood pressure, pulse, uterine contractions, uterine tone
  Fetal: heart rate, activity/movements
- Success to expect: a favorable outcome will depend on inducibility of the cervix (e.g., Bishop score of 9)
- Keep woman and support person informed of progress

Administration

Position woman in side-lying or upright position

Assess status of maternal-fetal unit

Prepare solution and administer with pump delivery system according to prescribed orders:

- Infusion pump and solution are set up (e.g., 10 units/1000 ml isotonic electrolyte solution)
- Piggyback solution is connected to IV line at proximal port (port nearest point of venous insertion)
- Solution with oxytocin is flagged with a medication label
- Begin induction at 0.5 to 2 milliunits/min
- Increase dose 1 to 2 milliunits/min at intervals of 30 to 60 min until a dose of up to 20 to 40 milliunits/min is reached

Maintain Dose If

- Intensity of contractions results in intrauterine pressures of 40 to 90 mm Hg (shown by internal monitor)
- Duration of contractions is 60 to 90 sec
- Frequency of contractions is 2 to 3 min intervals
- Resting tone of 10 to 15 mm Hg
- Cervical dilation of 1 cm/hr in the active phase

Maternal/Fetal Assessments

- Monitor blood pressure, pulse, and respirations every 30 to 60 min and with every increment in dose
- Monitor contraction pattern and uterine resting tone every 15 min and with every increment in dose
- Assess intake and output; limit IV intake to 1000 ml/8 hr; output should be 120 ml or more every 4 hr
- Perform vaginal examination as indicated
- Monitor for nausea, vomiting, headache, hypotension
- Assess fetal status using electronic fetal monitoring; evaluate tracing every 15 min and with every increment in dose
- Observe emotional responses of woman and her partner

Reportable Conditions

- Uterine hyperstimulation
- Nonreassuring fetal heart rate and pattern
- Suspected uterine rupture
- Inadequate uterine response at 20 milliunits/min

Emergency Measures

Discontinue use of oxytocin per hospital protocol:

- Turn woman on her side
- Increase primary IV rate up to 200 ml/hr, unless woman has water intoxication, in which case the rate is decreased to one that keeps the vein open
- Give woman oxygen by face mask at 8 to 10 L/min or per protocol or primary health care provider's order

Documentation

- Medication: kind, amount, time of beginning, increasing dose, maintaining dose, and discontinuing medication
- Reactions of mother and fetus:
  Pattern of labor
  Progress of labor
  Fetal heart rate and pattern
  Maternal vital signs
  Nursing interventions and woman's response
- Notification of physician or nurse-midwife

From American College of Obstetricians and Gynecologists: *Induction of labor,* ACOG Practice Bulletin no 10, Washington, DC, 1999, American College of Obstetricians and Gynecologists; Pozaic S: Induction and augmentation of labor. In Mandeville L, Troiano N (eds): *High-risk and critical care intrapartum nursing,* ed 2, Philadelphia, 1999, Lippincott; Simpson KR: *Cervical ripening and induction and augmentation of labor,* ed 2, Washington, DC, 2002, Association of Women's Health, Obstetric, and Neonatal Nurses; and Summers L: Methods of cervical ripening and labor induction, *J Nurse Midwifery* 42(2):71-85, 1997.
IV, intravenous.

Nursing Considerations

An evidence-based written protocol for the preparation and administration of oxytocin should be established by the obstetric department (physicians, midwives, nurses) in each institution. The procedure recommended for a woman who is eligible for induction of labor is discussed in Box 19-9.

NURSE ALERT Oxytocin is discontinued immediately and the primary health care provider notified if uterine hyperstimulation or a nonreassuring fetal heart rate and pattern occurs. ■

Other nursing interventions, such as administering oxygen by face mask, positioning the woman on her side, and infusing more intravenous fluids, are implemented immediately (Emergency box). Based on the status of the maternal-fetal unit, the primary health care provider may order that the infusion be restarted once the FHR and uterine activity return to acceptable levels. Depending on the length of time the infusion was discontinued, the induction may be restarted at half the rate that resulted in hyperstimulation (e.g., discontinued for 10 to 20 minutes) or at the same rate as the initial rate (e.g., discontinued for more than 30 to 40 minutes) (Simpson, 2002) (see Nursing Care Plan: Dysfunctional Labor).

Augmentation of Labor

Augmentation of labor is the stimulation of uterine contractions after labor has started spontaneously but progress is unsatisfactory. Augmentation is usually implemented for the management of hypotonic uterine dysfunction resulting in a slowing of labor (protracted active phase). Common augmentation methods include oxytocin infusion, amniotomy, and nipple stimulation. Noninvasive methods such as emptying the bladder, ambulation and position changes, relaxation measures, nourishment and hydration, and hydrotherapy should be attempted before invasive interventions are initiated. The procedures and nursing assessments are similar to those used for oxytocin induction of labor. Protocols for dosage and frequency of increments may vary (e.g., lower dosages may be needed to achieve spontaneous vaginal birth) (Gilbert & Harmon, 2003; Simpson, 2002).

Some physicians advocate *active management* of labor, that is, the augmentation of labor to establish efficient labor with aggressive use of oxytocin so that the woman gives birth within 12 hours of admission to the labor unit. Advocates of active management believe that intervening early (as soon as a nulliparous labor is not progressing at least 1 cm/hr) with use of higher pharmacologic oxytocin doses administered at frequent increment intervals (e.g., a starting dose of 6 milliunits/min with increases of 6 milliunits/min every 15 minutes to a maximum dose of 40 milliunits/min) shortens labor and is associated with a lower incidence of cesarean birth (Norwitz et al, 2002; Simpson, 2002). Active management of labor continues to be under study in the United States to determine effectiveness and impact on perinatal morbidity and mortality rates. Thus far results have been disappointing, especially in terms of reducing the rate of cesarean births. The disappointing results have been attributed, in part, to a greater than one-to-one nurse/patient ratio and the high rate of epidural anesthesia. It is considered to be a form of care of unknown effectiveness (Enkin et al, 2000; Gilbert & Harmon, 2003).

Forceps-Assisted Birth

A forceps-assisted birth is one in which an instrument with two curved blades is used to assist in the birth of the fetal head. The cephalic-like curve of the forceps commonly used is similar to the shape of the fetal head, with a pelvic curve to the blades conforming to the curve of the pelvic axis. The blades are joined by a pin, screw, or groove arrangement. These locks prevent the forceps from compressing the fetal skull. Maternal indications for forceps-assisted birth include the need to shorten the second stage in dystocia (difficult labor), to compensate for the woman's deficient expulsive efforts (e.g., if she is tired or has been given spinal or epidural anesthesia), or to reverse a dangerous condition (e.g., cardiac decompensation).

Fetal indications include the birth of a fetus in distress, certain abnormal presentations, and arrest of rotation, as well as to deliver an aftercoming head in a breech presentation. The use of forceps during childbirth has been decreasing. In 2002, forceps or vacuum were used to assist 5.9% of births (Martin et al, 2003).

Certain conditions are required for a forceps-assisted birth to be successful. The woman's cervix must be fully dilated to avoid lacerations and hemorrhage. The bladder should be empty. The presenting part must be engaged, and a vertex presentation is desired. Membranes must be ruptured so that the position of the fetal head can be determined and the forceps can firmly grasp the head during birth. CPD should not be present.

There are different definitions of forceps applications. Outlet forceps are used when the fetal scalp is visible on the perineum without manually separating the labia. Outlet forceps are used to shorten the second stage of labor (Fig. 19-8). Low forceps refers to the application of forceps to a fetal head that is at least at a +2 cm station. Midforceps is the application of forceps to the fetal head that is engaged (no higher than sta-

Emergency

UTERINE HYPERSTIMULATION WITH OXYTOCIN

Signs

- Uterine contractions lasting >90 sec and occurring more frequently than every 2 min
- Uterine resting tone >20 mm Hg
- Nonreassuring fetal heart rate and pattern:
  - Abnormal baseline (<110 or >160 beats/min)
  - Absent variability
  - Repeated late decelerations or prolonged decelerations

Interventions

- Maintain woman in side-lying position
- Turn off oxytocin infusion; keep maintenance IV line open; increase rate
- Start administering oxygen by face mask, per protocol or physician's order
- Notify primary health care provider
- Prepare to administer terbutaline (Brethine) 0.25 mg subcutaneously if ordered to decrease uterine activity
- Continue monitoring fetal heart rate and pattern, and uterine activity
- Document responses to actions

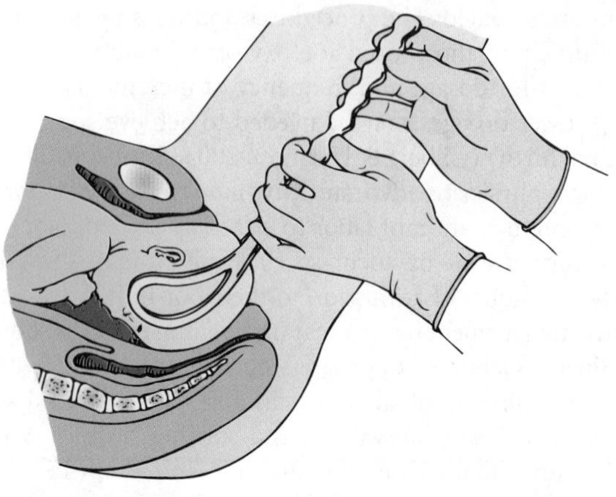

Fig. 19-8 Outlet forceps–assisted extraction of the head.

tion 0) but above the +2 cm station. In no instances should the forceps be applied to an unengaged presenting part.

Nursing Considerations

The nurse obtains the type of forceps requested by the physician (Fig. 19-9). The nurse may explain to the mother that the forceps blades fit like two tablespoons around an egg, with the blades coming over the baby's ears.

NURSE ALERT Because compression of the cord between the fetal head and the forceps would cause a drop in FHR, the fetal heart rate and pattern are checked, reported, and recorded before and after forceps are applied. ■

If a drop in FHR occurs, the physician removes and reapplies the forceps. Ordinarily traction is applied during contractions.

After birth, the mother is assessed for vaginal and cervical lacerations (e.g., bleeding that occurs even with a contracted uterus); urine retention, which may result from bladder injuries or urethral injuries; and hematoma formation in the pelvic soft tissues, which may result from blood vessel damage. The infant should be assessed for bruising or abrasions at the site of the blade applications, facial palsy resulting from pressure of the blades on the facial nerve (cranial nerve VII), and subdural hematoma. Newborn and postpartum caregivers should be told that the birth was forceps assisted.

Vacuum-Assisted Birth

Vacuum-assisted birth, or vacuum extraction, is a birth method involving the attachment of a vacuum cup to the fetal head, using negative pressure to assist in the birth of the head. Indications for use are similar to those for outlet forceps. Prerequisites for use include a vertex presentation, ruptured membranes, and the absence of CPD. When an operative vaginal birth is required, vacuum assistance is preferred as a beneficial form of care when compared with forceps assistance (Enkin et al, 2000).

When the birth is to be vacuum assisted, the woman is prepared for a vaginal birth in the lithotomy position to allow for sufficient traction. The cup is applied to the fetal head, and a caput develops inside the cup as the pressure is initiated (Fig. 19-10). Traction is applied to facilitate descent of the fetal head, and the woman is encouraged to push as

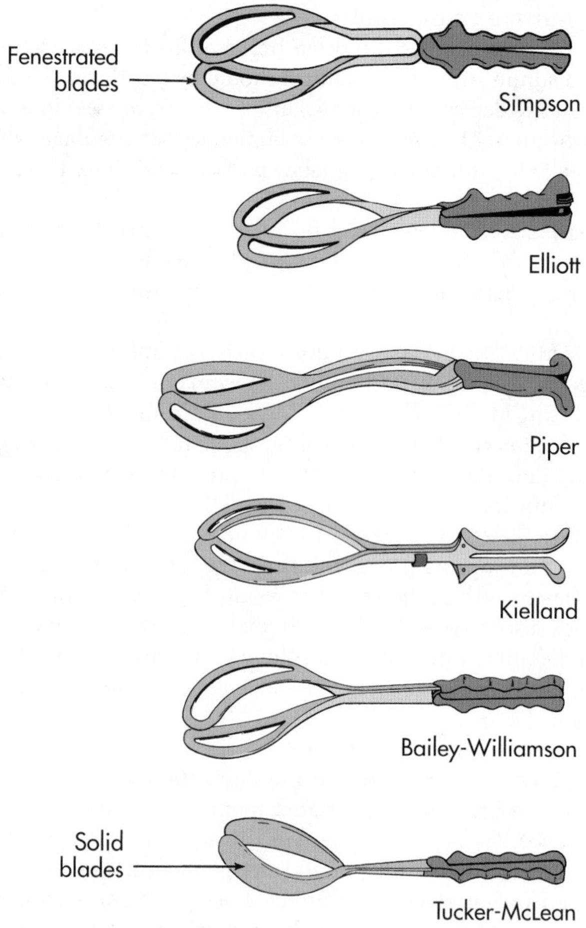

Fig. 19-9 Types of forceps. Piper forceps are used to assist delivery of the head in a breech birth.

suction is applied. As the head crowns, an episiotomy is performed if necessary. The vacuum cup is released and removed after birth of the head. If vacuum extraction is not successful, a forceps-assisted or cesarean birth is performed.

Risks to the newborn include cephalhematoma, scalp lacerations, and subdural hematoma. Fetal complications can be reduced by strict adherence to the manufacturer's recommendations for method of application, degree of suction, and duration of application. Maternal complications are uncommon but can include perineal, vaginal, and cervical lacerations and soft-tissue hematomas.

Nursing Considerations

The nurse's role for the woman who has a vacuum-assisted birth is one of support person and educator. The nurse can prepare the woman for birth and encourage her to remain active in the birth process by pushing during contractions. The FHR should be assessed frequently during the procedure. After birth, the newborn should be observed for signs of trauma at the application site and for cerebral irritation (e.g., poor sucking or listlessness). The newborn may be at risk for cephalhematoma and neonatal jaundice as bruising resolves, as well as for infection at the application site. The parents may need to be reassured that the caput succedaneum will begin to disappear in a few hours. Neonatal caregivers should be told that the birth was vacuum assisted.

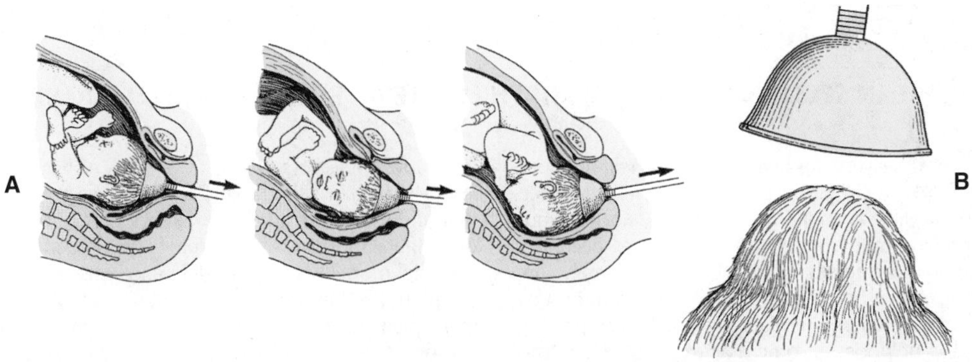

Fig. 19-10 Use of vacuum extraction to rotate fetal head and assist with descent. **A,** *Arrow* indicates direction of traction on the vacuum cup. **B,** Caput succedaneum formed by the vacuum cup.

Cesarean Birth

Cesarean birth is the birth of a fetus through a transabdominal incision of the uterus (Fig. 19-11). Whether a cesarean birth is planned (scheduled) or unplanned (emergency), the loss of the experience of giving birth to an infant in the traditional manner may have a negative effect on a woman's self-concept. An effort is made to maintain the focus on the birth of a child rather than on the operative procedure.

The purpose of cesarean birth is to preserve the life or health of the mother and her fetus; it may be the best choice when there is evidence of maternal or fetal complications. Since the advent of modern surgical methods and care, and the use of antibiotics, maternal and fetal morbidity and mortality rates have decreased. Incisions are made into the lower uterine segment rather than into the muscular body of the uterus and thus promote more effective healing. Despite these advances, cesarean birth still poses threats to the health of both mother and infant.

The incidence of cesarean births increased to 27.6% in 2003, the highest rate ever reported in the United States (Martin et al, 2005). In Canada, the rate was 22.1% in 2001 (Liu et al, 2004). Factors cited in this increase include use of electronic fetal monitoring and epidural anesthesia; an increase in the number of first-time pregnancies, as well as pregnancies at an older age; and the decline in the rate of vaginal birth after cesarean (10.6% in 2003 in the United States; 28.5% in 2001 in Canada) (Liu et al, 2004; Martin et al, 2005). Women 35 to 39 years of age have a cesarean birth rate of 35% and those 40 to 54 years of age have a rate of 40.7%, over twice the rate for teenage women (18.0%) (Martin et al, 2003).

Women who have private insurance, who are of a higher socioeconomic status, or who deliver in a private hospital are more likely to experience cesarean birth than are women who are poor, who have no insurance, who are receiving public assistance (e.g., Medicaid), or who give birth in a public hospital (Gilbert & Harmon, 2003; Moore, 2003).

Approaches for the management of labor and birth to reduce the rate of cesarean births while increasing the rate of vaginal births after cesarean (VBAC) are presented in Box 19-10. However, the rate of VBACs is decreasing. This decline may be due to reports of risks of VBAC, legal pressures, conservative practice guidelines, and debate regarding the relative benefits and risks of cesarean versus vaginal route for births (Martin et al, 2005).

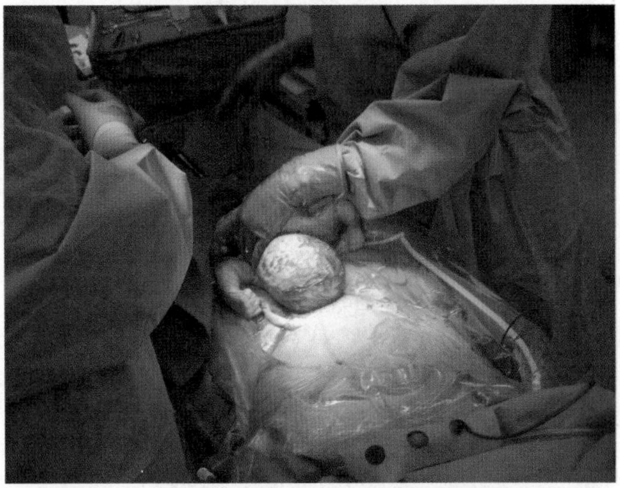

Fig. 19-11 Cesarean birth; lifting the infant out of the uterus. (Courtesy Brian and Mayannyn Sallee, Las Vegas, NV.)

Cesarean Birth on Demand

The decrease in VBACs becomes more complex as women are requesting cesarean births for reasons other than medical, obstetric, or fetal indications. These reasons include the belief that the surgery will prevent future problems with pelvic support or sexual dysfunction and the convenience of planning a date when the father of the baby is available. Some multiparous women may request a cesarean after a previous traumatic birth due to physical injury or psychological trauma (Gardner, 2003). In a committee opinion, the American College of Obstetricians and Gynecologists (ACOG) notes that the right of patients to refuse surgery is well known (ACOG, 2003). It is less clear if they have the right to ask for surgery. The Society of Obstetricians and Gynaecologists of Canada (SOGC) does not promote cesarean on demand and promotes natural childbirth but believes that the final decision as to the safest route for childbirth rests with the woman and her health care provider (SOGC, 2004).

The type of nursing care given may also influence the rate of cesarean births. Radin, Harmon, and Hanson (1993) found that cesarean rates were lower for women whose

Evidence-Based Practice

PLANNED CESAREAN SECTION VS. VAGINAL BIRTH FOR TERM BREECH PRESENTATION

Background

Breech presentation at delivery has been associated with nulliparity, previous breech, uterine or pelvic anomaly, placental malplacement, too much or too little amniotic fluid, extended fetal legs, multiple pregnancy, preterm birth, shortened umbilical cord, decreased fetal activity, intrauterine growth restriction, fetal anomaly, and stillbirth. Commonly, breech presentation is an indication for a cesarean birth. Some researchers speculate that the breech position itself is an indicator of poor outcome. For example, the rate of childhood handicaps among breech babies is high, no matter what method of delivery is employed. In addition, cesarean birth exposes the mother and baby to all the risks of operative procedures: anesthesia problems, infection, pain, delayed recovery, immobility, ileus, uterine rupture in future pregnancies, and neonatal respiratory problems. Length of stay and cost also rise considerably.

Objectives

The reviewers sought to compare the maternal and perinatal outcomes of routine cesarean birth for term breech presentation, compared with term breech presentations delivered vaginally. The perinatal outcomes are death (excluding fatal anomalies), serious neonatal morbidity (Apgar score less than 7, cord blood pH less than 7.0, neonatal intensive care admission, birth asphyxia, birth trauma), and disability in childhood. Maternal outcomes include death, pain, incontinence, instrumental delivery, hemorrhage, infection, depression, self-esteem, relationship with infant and family, problems with future pregnancies and deliveries, satisfaction, and costs. All women should be considered suitable for vaginal delivery.

Methods

Search Strategy

The authors searched the Cochrane database, MEDLINE, 30 journals and conference proceedings, and a weekly current awareness service of 37 journals. Search keyword was *breech.*

Three randomized, controlled trials met the criteria, representing 2396 women. Two trials, dated 1980 and 1983, were from the United States. The other trial, dated 2000, was a large, international multicenter trial, whose countries were not noted in the review.

Statistical Analyses

Similar data were pooled. Reviewers calculated relative risks for dichotomous data, and weighted mean differences for continuous data. Countries with low (20/1000 or less) and high (more than 20/1000) perinatal mortality rates were subgrouped for comparison.

Findings

Of the women with term breech presentation allocated to vaginal delivery, 45% were delivered via cesarean. Those scheduled for cesarean births experienced significantly fewer perinatal deaths (excluding fatal anomalies), decreased short-term neonatal morbidity, fewer low Apgar (less than 7) or very low Apgar (less than 4) scores, less acidotic cord blood, and less cord base excess (15 or more) than did the planned vaginal delivery group. The reduction in risk of perinatal mortality and morbidity was less in countries with high perinatal mortality rates. No difference was noted between groups on infant birth trauma. A small but significant increase was found in the planned cesarean group in short-term maternal morbidity. At 3 months postpartum, the planned cesarean group experienced less urinary incontinence and perineal pain, and more abdominal pain, than the planned vaginal birth group.

Limitations

The two smaller U.S. studies from 1980 and 1983 did not specify the method of randomization. One of those studies had a large discrepancy in numbers between groups. The large multicenter trial used a wide variety of clinical settings and had good follow-up rates, which were strengths.

Conclusions

There is evidence that planned cesarean birth in term breech presentations is associated with decreased perinatal death and morbidity rates and an increase in short-term maternal morbidity.

Implications for Practice

Planned cesarean birth is not always desirable or feasible in all settings. External cephalic version, or the ultrasound-guided process of manually changing the fetal presentation from outside the abdomen, is one alternative. Promising results have been noted in other alternative practices, such as using various positions and moxibustion. (Moxibustion is a method of producing analgesia by holding slow-burning moxa or another substance near the skin without causing pain or burning; sometimes used in conjunction with acupuncture.) Even cesarean birth does not totally eliminate the problems associated with breech presentation. Diagnosis of the presentation before labor is desirable.

Implications for Further Research

Much more evidence is needed on the effects of cesarean births, for breech presentation or other indication, on long-term outcomes, such as reproductive function of women and child development. Researchers need to assess the psychologic impact of cesarean birth on women and their adaptation to parenting. Cost was not addressed in these trials, but remains a primary factor in policy making and decision making.

Reference

Hofmeyr GJ, Hannah ME: Planned caesarean section for term breech delivery (Cochrane Review), 2003. In *The Cochrane Library,* Issue 2, Chichester, UK, 2004, John Wiley & Sons.

nurses provided supportive care during labor. A labor management approach that uses one-to-one support and emphasizes ambulation, maternal position changes, relaxation measures, oral fluids and nutrition, hydrotherapy, and nonpharmacologic pain relief facilitates the progress of labor and reduces the incidence of dystocia (AWHONN, 2000; Miltner, 2000).

Indications

There are few absolute indications for a cesarean birth. Today most are performed primarily for the benefit of the fetus. The complications most closely associated with cesarean births include fetal distress, CPD, malpresentations such as breech or shoulder, placental abnormalities (previa, abruptio), umbilical cord prolapse, dysfunctional labor pattern, and multiple gestation. Medical risk factors most closely associated with cesarean birth include hypertensive disorders, active genital herpes, positive HIV status, and diabetes (Martin et al, 2003).

Forced Cesarean Birth

A woman's refusal to undergo cesarean birth for fetal reasons is often described as a maternal-fetal conflict (Draper, 1997). Health care providers are ethically obliged to protect the well-being of both the mother and the fetus; a decision for one affects the other. If a woman refuses a cesarean birth

BOX 19-10

Selected Measures to Reduce Cesarean Birth Rate and Increase Rate of VBAC

Educate Women Regarding

- Advantages and safety of the home environment for early or latent labor
- Indicators for hospital admission
- Management techniques to use during labor to enhance progress
- Nonpharmacologic measures to reduce pain and discomfort and enhance relaxation
- Safety and effectiveness of TOL and VBAC

Establish Admission Criteria for Women in Labor That

- Distinguish clinical manifestations for false labor, latent/early labor, and active labor
- Conduct admission assessments in a separate admissions area
- Send women in false or early/latent labor home or keep them in the admissions area
- Admit women in active labor to the labor and birth unit

Use Appropriate Assessment Techniques To

- Determine status of the maternal-fetal unit
- Establish an individualized rationale for initiating labor interventions such as epidural anesthesia, induction/augmentation, amniotomy, cesarean birth

Initiate a Doula Program That

- Provides one-to-one support for women in labor

Develop a Philosophy of Labor Management That

- Schedules admission during active labor
- Avoids automatic interventions such as routine induction for spontaneous rupture of membranes at term or postterm pregnancy and cesarean birth for breech presentation, twin gestation, genital herpes, or failure to progress
- Relies on assessment findings reflective of the status of the maternal-fetal unit rather than strict adherence to set ranges for the duration of the stages and phases of labor
- Employs intermittent rather than continuous electronic fetal monitoring of low risk pregnant women
- Focuses on measures that are known to enhance the progress of labor such as upright positions, frequent position changes, ambulation, oral nutrition and hydration, relaxation techniques, hydrotherapy
- Emphasizes nonpharmacologic measures to relieve pain
- Uses nonpharmacologic measures in a manner that reduces their labor-inhibiting effects
- Establishes criteria for elective cesarean birth and TOL
- Encourages women who have had a previous cesarean birth to participate in TOL to attempt a vaginal birth

TOL, trial of labor; *VBAC*, vaginal birth after cesarean.

that is recommended because of fetal jeopardy, health care providers must make every effort to find out why she is refusing and provide information that may persuade her to change her mind. If the woman continues to refuse surgery, the health care providers must decide if it is ethical to get a court order for the surgery; however, every effort should be made to avoid this legal step (Draper, 1997).

Surgical Techniques

The two main types of cesarean operation are the classic and the lower segment cesarean incisions. Classic cesarean birth is rarely performed today, although it may be used when rapid birth is necessary and in some cases of shoulder presentation and placenta previa. The incision is made vertically into the upper body of the uterus (Fig. 19-12, *A*). Because the procedure is associated with a higher incidence of blood loss, infection, and uterine rupture in subsequent pregnancies than is lower-segment cesarean birth, vaginal birth after a classic cesarean is contraindicated.

Lower-segment cesarean birth can be achieved through a vertical or transverse incision into the uterus (Fig. 19-12, *B* and *C*). The transverse incision is more popular, however, because it is easier to perform, is associated with less blood loss and fewer postoperative infections, and is less likely to rupture in subsequent pregnancies (Bowes & Thorp, 2004).

Complications and Risks

Cesarean births are not without risk of complications for both the mother and fetus. Maternal complications include aspiration, pulmonary embolism, wound infection, wound dehiscence, thrombophlebitis, hemorrhage, urinary tract infection, injuries to bladder or bowel, and complications related to anesthesia. The fetus may be born prematurely if gestational age has not been accurately determined; fetal injuries

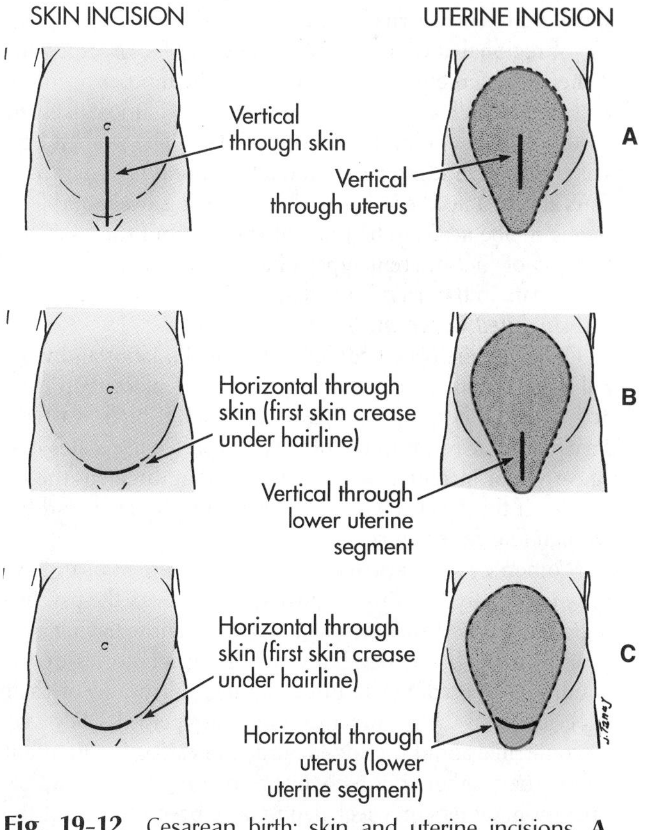

Fig. 19-12 Cesarean birth: skin and uterine incisions. **A**, Classic: vertical incisions of skin and uterus. **B**, Low cervical: horizontal incision of skin; vertical incision of uterus. **C**, Low cervical: horizontal incisions of skin and uterus.

can occur during the surgery (Bowes & Thorp, 2004). Besides these risks, the woman is at economic risk because the cost of a cesarean birth is higher than that of a vaginal birth, and a longer recovery period may require additional expenditures.

Women who experience cesarean birth may feel frustration (at losing control), disappointment, anger, and loss of self-esteem related to a change in body image and perceived inability to give birth as they had expected and hoped. Often women experience a delay in the ability to interact with their newborn after birth. These women are less likely to breastfeed and may even have difficulty expressing positive feelings about their newborns for some time after birth. They often are less satisfied with their childbirth experience and report more fatigue and poor physical functioning during the first few weeks after discharge.

Success at mothering and in the recovery process can do much to restore the self-esteem of these women. Some women see the scar as mutilating, and worries concerning sexual attractiveness may surface. Some men are fearful of resuming intercourse because of the fear of hurting their partner.

Parents may wonder if a cesarean birth was absolutely necessary, and such feelings may surface even years later. They should be given opportunities to discuss the experience to try to understand and resolve concerns after the birth.

Anesthesia

Spinal, epidural, and general anesthetics are used for cesarean births. Epidural blocks are popular because women want to be awake for and aware of the birth experience. However, the choice of anesthetic depends on several factors. The mother's medical history or present condition, such as a spinal injury, hemorrhage, or coagulopathy, may rule out the use of regional anesthesia. Time is another factor, especially if there is an emergency and the life of the mother or infant is at risk. In such a case, general anesthesia will most likely be used unless an epidural is already in place. The woman herself is a factor. She may not know all the options or may have fears about "a needle in her back" or of being awake and feeling pain. She needs to be fully informed about the risks and benefits of the different types of anesthesia so that she can participate in the decision whenever there is a choice.

Scheduled Cesarean Birth

Cesarean birth is scheduled or planned if labor and vaginal birth is contraindicated (e.g., complete placenta previa, active genital herpes, positive HIV status), if birth is necessary but labor is not inducible (e.g., hypertensive states that cause a poor intrauterine environment that threatens the fetus), or if this has been decided on by the physician and the woman (e.g., a repeat cesarean birth).

Women who are scheduled to have a cesarean birth have time to prepare for it psychologically. However, the psychologic responses of these women may vary. Those having a repeat cesarean birth may have disturbing memories of the conditions preceding the initial surgical birth and of their experiences in the postoperative recovery period. They may be concerned about the added burden of caring for an infant and perhaps other children while recovering from a surgical operation. Others may feel glad to have been relieved of the uncertainty about the date and time of birth and to be free from the pain of labor.

Unplanned Cesarean Birth

The psychosocial outcomes of unplanned or emergency cesarean birth are usually more pronounced and negative in nature when compared with the outcomes associated with a scheduled or planned cesarean birth. Women and their families experience abrupt changes in their expectations for birth, postbirth care, and the care of the new baby at home. This may be an extremely traumatic experience for all.

The woman usually approaches the procedure tired and discouraged after an ineffective and difficult labor. Fear predominates as she worries about her own safety and well-being and that of her fetus. She may be dehydrated, with low glycogen reserves. Because preoperative procedures must be done quickly and competently, the time available for explanation of the procedures and operation is often short. Because maternal and family anxiety levels are high at this time, much of what is said may be forgotten or misunderstood. The woman may experience feelings of anger or guilt in the postpartum period. Fatigue is often noticeable in these women, and they need much supportive care.

After surgery, therefore, time must be spent reviewing the events preceding the operation and the operation itself to ensure that the woman understands what has happened and that gaps in her recollections are filled. This approach will help create more realistic memories of the childbirth experience, thereby having a more positive influence on future pregnancies and labors (Ryding, Wijma, & Wijma, 1998).

Prenatal Preparation

Concerned professional and lay groups in the community have established councils for cesarean birth to meet the needs of these women and their families. Such groups advocate that a discussion of cesarean birth be included in all parenthood preparation classes. No woman can be guaranteed a vaginal birth, even if she is in good health and there is no indication of danger to the fetus before the onset of labor. For this reason, every woman needs to be aware of and prepared for this eventuality.

Childbirth educators stress the importance of emphasizing the similarities and differences between a cesarean and vaginal birth. In support of the philosophy of family-centered birth, many hospitals have policies that permit fathers and other partners to share in these births as they do in vaginal ones. Women who have undergone cesarean birth agree that the continued presence and support of their partners helped them respond positively to the entire experience.

In addition to preparing women for the possibility of cesarean birth, childbirth educators should empower women to believe in their ability to give birth vaginally and to seek care measures during labor that will enhance the progress of their labors and reduce their risk for cesarean birth.

Preoperative Care

Family-centered care is the goal for the woman who is to undergo cesarean birth and for her family. The preparation of the woman for cesarean birth is the same as that done for other elective or emergency surgery. The primary health care provider discusses with the woman and her family the need for the cesarean birth and the prognosis for mother and infant. The anesthesiologist assesses the woman's cardiopulmonary system and describes the options for anesthesia. Informed consent is obtained for the procedure (see Guidelines/Guias—Cesarean birth on p. 563).

Blood and urine tests are usually done a day or two before a planned cesarean birth or on admission to the labor unit. Laboratory tests, most commonly ordered to establish baseline data, include a complete blood cell count and chemistry, blood typing and crossmatching, and urinalysis. Maternal vital signs and blood pressure and fetal heart rate and pattern continue to be assessed per hospital routine until the operation begins. Physical preoperative preparation usually includes inserting a retention catheter, to keep the bladder empty, and administering prescribed preoperative medications. Although uncommon, the primary health care provider may order an abdominal-mons shave or a clipping of pubic hair. If general anesthesia is to be used, an antacid is administered orally to neutralize gastric secretions in case of aspiration. This is a beneficial form of care (Enkin et al, 2000). Intravenous fluids are started to maintain hydration and to provide an open line for the administration of blood or medications if needed. Removal of dentures, nail polish, and jewelry may be optional, depending on hospital policies. If the woman wears glasses and is going to be awake, the nurse should make sure her glasses accompany her to the operating room so she can see her infant. If the woman wears contact lenses, the nurse can find out whether they can be worn for the birth.

During preoperative preparation the support person is encouraged to remain with the woman as much as possible to provide continuing emotional support (if this is culturally acceptable to the woman and support person). The nurse provides essential information about the preoperative procedures during this time. Although the nursing actions may be carried out quickly if a cesarean birth is unplanned, verbal communication, particularly explanations, is important. Silence can be frightening to the woman and her support person. The nurse's use of touch can communicate feelings of care and concern for the woman. The nurse can assess the woman's and her partner's perceptions about cesarean birth. As the woman expresses her feelings, the nurse may identify a potential for a disturbance in self-concept during the postpartum period that may need to be addressed. If there is time before the birth, the nurse can teach the woman about postoperative expectations and about pain relief, turning, coughing, and deep breathing measures.

Intraoperative Care

Cesarean births occur in operating rooms in the surgical suite or in the labor and birth unit. Once the woman has been taken to the operating room, her care becomes the responsibility of the obstetric team, surgeon, anesthesiologist, pediatrician, and surgical nursing staff (Fig. 19-13). If possible, the partner, who is gowned appropriately, accompanies the mother to the surgical unit and remains close to her so that continued support and comfort can be provided.

The nurse who is circulating may assist with positioning the woman on the birth (surgical) table. It is important to position her so that the uterus is displaced laterally to prevent compressing the inferior vena cava, which causes decreased placental perfusion. This is usually accomplished by placing a wedge under the hip. A Foley catheter is inserted into the bladder at this time if one is not already in place.

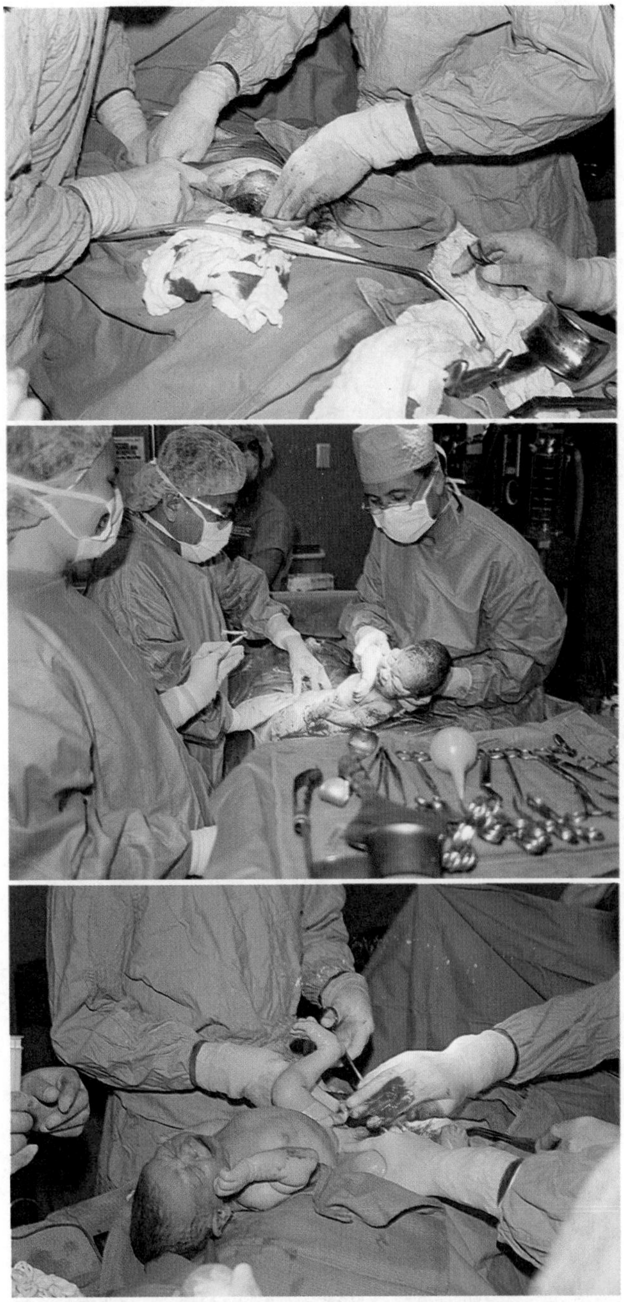
A
B
C

Fig. 19-13 Cesarean birth. **A**, "Bikini" incision has been made, the muscle layer is separated, the abdomen entered, the uterus has been exposed and incised; suctioning of amniotic fluid continues as head is brought up through the incision. Note small amount of bleeding. **B**, The neonate's birth through the uterine incision is nearly complete. **C**, A quick assessment is performed; note extreme molding of head resulting from cephalopelvic disproportion. (Courtesy Marjorie Pyle, RNC, Lifecircle, Costa Mesa, CA.)

If the partner either is not allowed or chooses not to be present, the nurse can stay in communication with him or her and give progress reports whenever possible. If the mother is awake during the birth, the nurse can tell her what is happening and provide support. The mother may be anxious about the sensations she is experiencing, such as the coldness of solutions used to prepare the abdomen, and pressure or pulling during the actual birth of the infant. She also may be apprehensive because of the bright lights or the presence of unfamiliar equipment and masked and gowned personnel in the room. Explanations by the nurse can help decrease the woman's anxiety.

Care of the infant usually is delegated to a pediatrician or a nurse team skilled in neonatal resuscitation, because these infants are considered to be at risk until there is evidence of physiologic stability after the birth.

A crib with resuscitation equipment is readied before surgery. Those responsible for care are expert not only in resuscitative techniques but also in their ability to detect normal and abnormal infant responses. After birth, if the infant's condition permits and the mother is awake, the baby may be placed skin-to-skin on the mother or can be given to the woman's partner to hold (Fig. 19-14). The infant whose condition is compromised is transported after initial stabilization to the nursery for observation and the implementation of appropriate interventions. In some institutions the partner may accompany the infant; if not, personnel keep the family informed of the infant's progress, and parent-infant contacts are initiated as soon as possible.

A

B

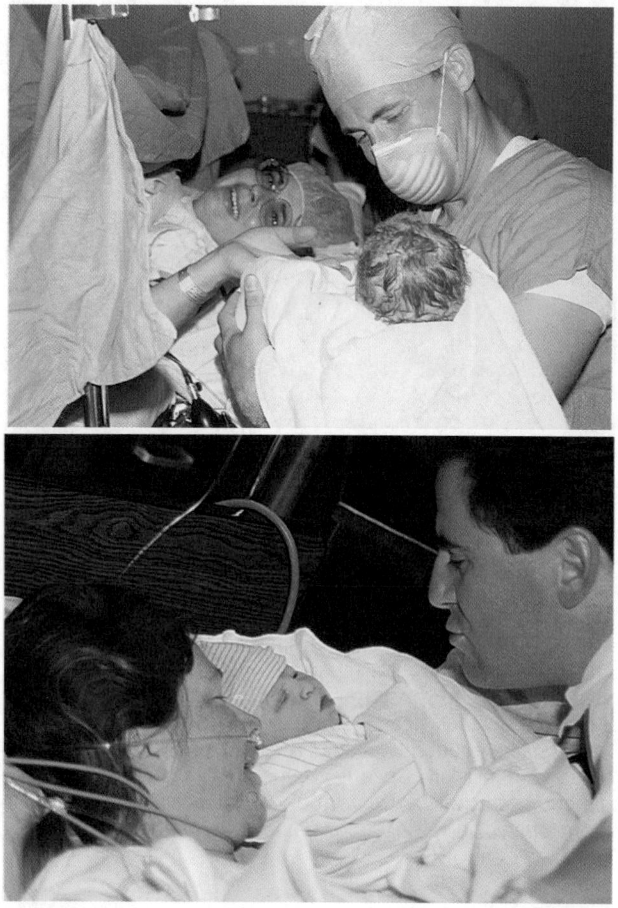

Fig. 19-14 **A,** Parents and their newborn. The physician manually removes the placenta, suctions the remaining amniotic fluid and blood from the uterine cavity, and closes the uterine incision, peritoneum, muscle layer, fatty tissue, and finally the skin, while the new family shares some private time. **B,** Parents become better acquainted with their newborn while mother rests after surgery. (Courtesy Marjorie Pyle, RNC, Lifecircle, Costa Mesa, CA.)

If the family cannot accompany the woman during surgery, the family is directed to the surgical or obstetric waiting room. The physician then reports on the condition of the mother and child to family members after the birth is completed. Family members may accompany the infant as he or she is transferred to the nursery, giving them an opportunity to see and admire the new baby.

NURSE ALERT Some mothers/parents want the privilege of informing family and friends of the sex of the infant (if it was not known before birth). Before responding to requests for such information from people waiting outside the birthing area, the nurse should check with the mother (or ascertain the mother's wishes). ■

Immediate Postoperative Care

Once surgery is completed, the mother is transferred to a recovery room or back to her labor room. Women who have experienced a cesarean birth have both postoperative and postpartum needs that must be addressed. They are surgical patients, as well as new mothers. Nursing assessments in this immediate postbirth period follow agency protocol and include degree of recovery from the effects of anesthesia, postoperative and postbirth status, and degree of pain. A patent airway is maintained, and the woman is positioned to prevent possible aspiration. Vital signs are taken every 15 minutes for 1 to 2 hours, or until stable. The condition of the incisional dressing, the fundus, and the amount of lochia are assessed, as well as intravenous intake and urine output through the Foley catheter. The woman is helped to turn and do coughing, deep breathing, and leg exercises. Medications to relieve pain may be administered.

If the baby is present, the mother and her partner are given some time alone with him or her to facilitate bonding and attachment. Breastfeeding can be initiated if the mother feels like trying. If the woman is in a recovery area or in her labor room, she usually is transferred to the postpartum unit after 1 to 2 hours, or once her condition is stable and the effects of anesthesia have worn off (i.e., she is alert, oriented, and able to feel and move extremities) (Table 19-4).

Postoperative/Postpartum Care

The attitude of the nurse and other health team members can influence the woman's perception of herself after a cesarean birth. The caregivers should stress that the woman is a new mother first and a surgical patient second. This attitude helps the woman perceive herself as having the same problems and needs as other new mothers while at the same time requiring supportive postoperative care.

The woman's physiologic concerns for the first few days may be dominated by pain at the incision site and pain resulting from intestinal gas, and hence the need for pain relief. If epidural anesthesia was used for the surgery, epidural opioids can be given in the immediate postoperative period to provide pain relief for approximately 24 hours. Otherwise, pain medications usually are given every 3 to 4 hours, or patient-controlled analgesia may be ordered. Other comfort measures such as position changes, splinting the incision with pillows, and relaxation techniques may be implemented. Women are often the best judges of what their bodies need and can tolerate, including the postoperative ingestion of foods and fluids. If desired by the woman, early introduction of solid food is safe. Women who eat early have been found to require less analgesia, and gastrointestinal problems do not occur (Abrams, Minassian, & Pickett, 2004; Burrows et al, 1995). Ambulation and rocking in a rocking chair may relieve gas pains, and avoiding consumption of gas-forming foods and carbonated beverages may help minimize them (Thomas et al, 1990) (Patient Teaching box).

Nurses must be alert to a woman's physiologic needs, managing care to ensure adequate rest and pain relief. Mother-baby care (couplet care) for a cesarean birth mother must be modified according to her physiologic limitations as a surgical patient.

Daily care includes perineal care, breast care, and routine hygienic care, including showering after the dressing has been removed (if showering is acceptable according to the woman's cultural beliefs and practices). The nurse assesses the woman's vital signs, incision, fundus, and lochia according to hospital policies, procedures, or protocols. Breath sounds, bowel sounds, circulatory status of lower extremities, and urinary and bowel elimination also are assessed. It is important to note maternal emotional status.

During the postpartum period the nurse can provide care that meets the psychologic and teaching needs of mothers who have had cesarean births. The nurse can explain postpartum procedures to help the woman participate in her recovery from surgery. The nurse can help the woman plan care and visits from family and friends that allow for adequate rest periods. Information and assistance with infant care can facilitate adjustment to her role as a mother. The woman is supported as she breastfeeds her baby by receiving individualized assistance to comfortably hold and position the baby at her breast. The side-lying position or football hold and the use of pillows to support the newborn can enhance comfort and facilitate successful breastfeeding.

The partner can be included in infant teaching sessions and in explanations about the woman's recovery. The couple should be encouraged to express their feelings about the birth experience. Some parents are angry, frustrated, or disappointed that a vaginal birth was not possible. Some women express feelings of low self-esteem or negative self-image. Others express relief and gratitude that the baby is healthy and safely born. It may be helpful for them to have the nurse who was present during the birth visit and help fill in "gaps" about the experience. Other psychologic and lifestyle concerns that have been reported include depression, feeling limited in activities, and changes in family interactions (Ryding et al, 1998).

Discharge after cesarean birth is usually by the third postoperative day. This time is often determined by criteria established by the woman's insurance carrier or the federal government (e.g., diagnosis-related groups).

The Newborn's and Mother's Health Protection Act of 1996 provides for a length of stay of up to 96 hours for cesarean births. These criteria may not coincide with the woman's physical or psychosocial readiness for discharge. Some states have added home care provisions for mothers who meet appropriate criteria for discharge and choose to leave sooner than the allowed length of stay. This policy recognizes that home care is less costly than hospital care and in most cases is more beneficial for recovery (Carpenter, 1998).

The predominant needs at home for women who experienced cesarean birth are for rest and sleep; relief of pain and discomfort; and assistance with household chores, infant care and feeding, and self-care (Eakes & Brown, 1998). The nurse must provide discharge teaching to prepare women for self-care and newborn care in a limited time, while trying to ensure that the woman is comfortable and able to rest. The nurse must assess the woman's information needs and coordinate the health care team's efforts to meet them.

Discharge teaching and planning should include information about nutrition; measures to relieve pain and discomfort (Patient Teaching box); exercise and specific activity restrictions; time management that includes periods of uninterrupted rest and sleep; hygiene, breast, and incision care; timing for resumption of sexual activity and contraception; signs of complications (Home Care box); and infant care. The nurse assesses the woman's need for continued support or counseling to facilitate her emotional recovery from the birth. The woman's family and friends should be educated regarding her needs during the recovery process, and their assistance should be coordinated before discharge. Referrals to support groups or to community agencies may be indicated to further promote the recovery process. A postdis-

Patient Teaching

POSTPARTUM PAIN RELIEF AFTER CESAREAN BIRTH

Incisional Pain

- Splint incision with a pillow when moving or coughing.
- Use relaxation techniques such as music, breathing, and dim lights.

Intestinal Gas

- Walk as often as you can.
- Do not eat or drink gas-forming foods, carbonated beverages, or whole milk.
- Do not use straws for drinking fluids.
- Take antiflatulence medication if prescribed.
- Lie on your left side to expel gas.
- Rock in a rocking chair.

Home Care

SIGNS OF POSTOPERATIVE COMPLICATIONS AFTER DISCHARGE

Report the following signs to your health care provider:

- Temperature exceeding 38° C
- Painful urination
- Lochia heavier than a normal period
- Wound separation
- Redness or oozing at the incision site
- Severe abdominal pain

Table 19-4

Care Path: Cesarean Birth without Complications: Expected Length of Stay–48 to 72 Hours

IMMEDIATE POSTOP CESAREAN	BY 4TH HR AFTER ADMISSION TO PP UNIT	5-24 HR	25-48 HR	BY DISCHARGE
ASSESSMENTS				
Recovery room/ PACU admission assessment completed	PP admission assessment and care plan completed			
VITAL SIGNS				
q15min × 1 hr; q30min × 4 hr, WNL	q1h × 3, WNL	q4-8h, WNL	q8h, WNL	q8h, WNL
POSTPARTUM ASSESSMENT				
q15min × 1 hr, WNL	q1h × 3, WNL	q8h, WNL	q8-12h, WNL	q8-12h, WNL
ABDOMINAL INCISION				
Dressing dry and intact	Dressing dry and intact	Dressing dry and intact	Dressing off or changed, incision intact	Incision intact; staples may be removed and Steri-Strips in place, incision WNL
GENITOURINARY				
Retention catheter output >30 ml/hr	Retention catheter output >30 ml/hr	Retention catheter output >30 ml/hr	Catheter discontinued, output >100 ml/void or 240 ml/8 hr	Urine output >240 ml/8 hr
GASTROINTESTINAL				
	Absent or hypoactive BS	Hypoactive to active BS	Active BS, + flatus	Active BS, + flatus; may or may not have BM
MUSCULOSKELETAL				
Alert or easily aroused, can move legs	Alert and oriented, moving all extremities	Ambulating with help	Ambulating unassisted	Ambulating ad lib
BONDING				
Evidence of parent-infant bonding; first breastfeeding if desired		Parent-infant bonding continues	Parent-infant bonding progressing	
LABORATORY TESTS				
		Intrapartal CBC results on chart/computer; determine Rh status and need for anti-Rh globulin; check for rubella immunity	PP HCT WNL, all lab results on chart, give anti-Rh globulin if indicated	Give rubella vaccine if indicated
INTERVENTIONS				
IV				
IV continues	IV continues	IV continues	IV may be discontinued	
Diet				
NPO	Ice chips, sips of clear liquids	Clear liquids	Regular diet or as tolerated	Regular diet

ADLs, activities of daily living; *BM,* bowel movement; *BS,* bowel sounds; *CBC,* complete blood count; *HCT,* hematocrit; *IM,* intramuscular; *IV,* intravenous; *NPO,* nothing by mouth; *NSAIDs,* nonsteroidal antiinflammatory drugs; *OOB,* out of bed; *PACU,* postanesthesia care unit; *PCA,* patient-controlled analgesia; *PNV,* prenatal vitamins; *PP,* postpartum; *Rx,* prescription; *TCDB,* turn, cough, deep breathe; *WNL,* within normal limits.

Table 19-4

Cesarean Birth without Complications: Expected Length of Stay—48 to 72 Hours—cont'd

IMMEDIATE POSTOP CESAREAN	BY 4TH HR AFTER ADMISSION TO PP UNIT	5-24 HR	25-48 HR	BY DISCHARGE
INTERVENTIONS—cont'd				
Perineal				
	Pericare by nurse	Pericare with help	Self-pericare	
Activity				
Bed rest	Bed rest	OOB × 3 with help, ADLs assisted, assisted to comfortable position to hold and feed baby	Holds baby comfortably, ambulates without assistance, ADLs unassisted	Activity ad lib
Pulmonary Care				
Patent airway; O_2 discontinued	TCDB q2hr with splinting, incentive spirometry q1hr if ordered, lungs clear	TCDB q2hr while awake; lungs clear	TCDB as needed; lungs clear	
Medications				
Oxytocin added to IV Pain control: analgesics, IV, or epidural narcotic	Oxytocin continued Pain control: analgesics—PCA, IM, PO, or epidural narcotic	Oxytocin may be discontinued Pain control: IM, PO, PCA narcotics or analgesics	Oxytocin discontinued Pain control: PO analgesics, NSAIDs; PCA discontinued; stool softener, PNV	Rx filled or given to take home
Teaching, Discharge Plan				
Breastfeeding, positioning, leg exercises	Verbalize understanding/unit routines, how to achieve rest, TCDB, involution, pain control	Self: comfort measures and care; reinforce TCDB and positioning; introduce teaching videos, lactation promotion or suppression Infant: handwashing, infant safety, positioning for feeding and burping; if breastfeeding, then positioning baby, latching on, timing, removing from breast	Self: diet; activity/rest; bowel/bladder function Infant: bonding; parent concerns; feeding; infant bath, cord care; need for car seat; newborn characteristics; circumcision, if requested; answer questions	Self: home care, signs of complications (infections, bleeding), normal psychologic adjustments, normal ADLs; resumption of sexual activities; contraception; identification of support system at home; self-concept issues related to cesarean birth. Inform whom to call if problems; review need to keep follow-up appointment; provide information about community resources; provide copy of home care Infant: parents to demonstrate infant care; reinforce use of booklets for infant care, whom to call if problems; discuss immunization needs; review need to keep follow-up appointments

charge program of telephone follow-up and home visits can facilitate the woman's full recovery after cesarean birth.

Vaginal Birth after Cesarean

Indications for primary cesarean birth, such as dystocia, breech presentation, or fetal distress, often are nonrecurring. Therefore a woman who has had a cesarean birth may subsequently become pregnant and not have any contraindications to labor and vaginal birth in that pregnancy and may attempt a vaginal birth after cesarean (VBAC).

ACOG (1999) encourages a TOL and VBAC attempt in women who have had one previous cesarean birth by low transverse incision. Vaginal birth is relatively safe, but there is risk of uterine rupture through a lower uterine segment scar. Increased reports of uterine rupture in the United States and Canada raised concerns about the safety of VBAC. Recommendations for the use of VBAC are being reevaluated (ACOG, 1999; Bowes & Thorp, 2004). A retrospective cohort analysis of more than 20,000 women who gave birth to a second child after a previous primary cesarean birth found that the incidence of uterine rupture was related to the method of the second labor and birth. The rate of uterine rupture was lowest when the women had a repeat cesarean birth without labor but highest when labor was induced with prostaglandins (Lydon-Rochelle et al, 2001). Labor and a vaginal birth are not recommended if there are contraindications such as a previous fundal classic cesarean scar, a scar from previous surgery, or evidence of CPD.

Women are most often the primary decision makers with regard to choice of birth method. During the antepartal period, the woman should be given information about VBAC and encouraged to choose it as an alternative to a repeat cesarean, as long as no contraindications exist. VBAC support groups and prenatal classes can help prepare the woman psychologically for labor and vaginal birth.

This labor should occur in a hospital facility that has the equipment and personnel available to begin surgery within 30 minutes from the time a decision is made for cesarean birth. Ideally, the woman is admitted to the labor and birth unit at the onset of spontaneous labor. In the latent phase of labor, the nurse encourages her to engage in normal activities such as ambulation. In the active phase of labor, FHR, fetal heart pattern, and uterine activity usually are monitored electronically, and intravenous access such as a saline lock may be established. The physician should be immediately available during active labor.

There is no evidence that administering oxytocin to induce or augment labor or the use of epidural anesthesia is contraindicated, although caution and close monitoring of the laboring woman are urged if these are used (Bowes & Thorp, 2004). However, use of prostaglandins, especially misoprostol (prostaglandin E_1), to ripen the cervix or induce labor is not recommended because they have been associated with an increased risk for uterine rupture.

Attention should be given to the woman's psychologic and physical needs during the TOL. Anxiety increases the release of catecholamines and can inhibit the release of oxytocin, delaying the progress of labor and possibly leading to a repeat cesarean birth. To alleviate anxiety, the nurse can encourage the woman to use breathing and relaxation techniques and to change position to promote labor progress. The woman's partner can be encouraged to provide comfort measures and emotional support. Collaboration among the woman in labor, her partner, the nurse, and other health care providers often results in a successful VBAC. If a trial of labor does not proceed to vaginal birth, the woman will need support and encouragement to express her feelings about having another cesarean birth. It is very important that this outcome not be labeled a failed VBAC.

Evaluation

Evaluation of the effectiveness of nursing care for a woman experiencing dystocia is based on the expected outcomes.

POSTTERM PREGNANCY, LABOR, AND BIRTH

evolve CASE STUDY—POSTDATE PREGNANCY

A postterm or postdate pregnancy is one that extends beyond the end of week 42 of gestation, or more than 294 days from the first day of the last menstrual period. The incidence of postdate pregnancy is estimated to be between 4% and 14% (Resnik & Resnik, 2004). Many pregnancies are misdiagnosed as prolonged. This can occur because (1) the pregnancy is inaccurately dated because the woman has an irregular menstrual cycle pattern, (2) an accurate date of the last menstrual period is unknown, or (3) entry into prenatal care was delayed or did not occur. Although the exact cause of postterm pregnancy is still unknown, a possible cause may be deficiency of placental estrogen and continued secretion of progesterone. Low levels of estrogen may result in a decrease in prostaglandin precursors and reduced formation of oxytocin receptors in the myometrium (Gilbert & Harmon, 2003). A woman who experiences one postterm pregnancy is 30% to 40% more likely to experience it again in subsequent pregnancies (Arulkumarian, 1997).

Clinical manifestations of postterm pregnancy include maternal weight loss, decreased uterine size (because of decreased amniotic fluid), meconium in the amniotic fluid, and advanced bone maturation of the fetal skeleton with an exceptionally hard fetal skull (Gilbert & Harmon, 2003).

Maternal and Fetal Risks

Maternal risks are often related to the birth of an excessively large infant. The woman is at increased risk for dysfunctional labor; birth canal trauma, including perineal lacerations and extension of episiotomy during vaginal birth; postpartum hemorrhage; and infection. Interventions such as induction of labor with prostaglandins or oxytocin, vacuum- or forceps-assisted birth, and cesarean birth are more likely to be necessary. The woman also may experience fatigue and psychologic reactions such as depression, frustration, and feelings of inadequacy as she passes her estimated date of birth (Gilbert & Harmon, 2003).

Fetal risks appear to be twofold. The first is the possibility of prolonged labor, shoulder dystocia, birth trauma, and asphyxia from macrosomia, which is estimated to occur in approximately 25% of prolonged pregnancies (Divon, 2002). The second risk is the compromising effects on the fetus of an "aging" placenta. Placental function gradually decreases after 37 weeks of gestation. Amniotic fluid volume declines to approximately 800 ml by 40 weeks of gestation and to about 400 ml by 42 weeks of gestation. The resulting oligohydramnios can lead to fetal hypoxia related to cord compression. If placental insufficiency is present, there is a high likelihood of fetal distress occurring during labor. Neonatal problems may include asphyxia, meconium aspiration syndrome, dysmaturity syndrome, hypoglycemia, polycythemia, and respiratory distress (Gilbert & Harmon, 2003). Whether an infant born after a postterm pregnancy has neurologic, behavioral, intellectual, or developmental problems must be further investigated.

Care Management

The management of postterm pregnancy is still controversial. The induction of labor at 41 to 42 weeks is suggested by some authorities as a means of reducing the rate of cesarean birth and stillbirth or neonatal death. Others follow a more individualized approach, allowing the pregnancy to proceed to 43 weeks as long as assessment of fetal well-being using a combination of tests is performed and the results of the tests are normal. Tests are usually performed on a weekly or twice-weekly basis (Divon, 2002; Searing, 2001).

Antepartum assessments for postterm pregnancy may include daily fetal movement counts, NSTs, amniotic fluid volume (AFV) assessments, contraction stress tests (CSTs), biophysical profiles (BPPs), and Doppler flow measurements. The woman and her family should be fully informed regarding the tests, including why they are performed and the meaning of the results obtained in terms of the health of the mother and fetus.

The amniotic fluid index (AFI) should be greater than 8 with at least one pocket of amniotic fluid greater than 2 cm. Amniotic fluid should be present throughout the uterine cavity (Gilbert & Harmon, 2003). The BPP may be the best way of gauging fetal well-being because it combines nonstress testing with real-time ultrasound scanning to assess fetal movements, fetal breathing movements, and AFV. Determining the AFV is critical in women with a postterm pregnancy because decreased AFV has been associated with fetal stress.

Cervical checks usually are performed weekly after 40 weeks of gestation to assess whether the condition of the cervix is favorable for induction (see Table 19-3). Vaginal secretions may be assessed for the amount of fetal fibronectin; a low concentration may predict increased risk for prolonged pregnancy, but results of studies have thus far been inconclusive (Divon, 2002; Gilbert & Harmon, 2003). Amniocentesis or amnioscopy may be performed to detect meconium in the amniotic fluid.

During the postterm period the woman is encouraged to assess fetal activity daily, assess for signs of labor, and keep appointments with her primary health care provider (Home Care box). The woman and her family should be encouraged to express their feelings about the prolonged pregnancy. They should be helped to realize that feelings of frustration, anger, impatience, and fear are normal. At times the emotional and physical strain of a postterm pregnancy may seem insurmountable. Referral to a support group or other supportive resource may be needed.

If the woman's cervix is ripe, labor is usually induced with oxytocin. If her cervix is not ripe, fetal surveillance is continued and a cervical ripening agent (e.g., prostaglandin gel or insert) may be administered followed by oxytocin induction (Gilbert & Harmon, 2003).

The fetus of a woman with a postterm pregnancy should be monitored electronically for a more accurate assessment of the fetal heart rate and pattern. Fetal scalp pH sampling or fetal oxygen saturation monitoring may be done to determine whether acidosis is occurring. Inadequate fluid volume leads to compression of the cord, which results in fetal hypoxia that is reflected in variable or prolonged deceleration patterns and passage of meconium. If oligohydramnios is present, amnioinfusion may be performed to restore amniotic fluid volume to maintain a cushioning of the cord. The use of amnioinfusion to treat fetal distress associated with oligohydramnios in labor is a form of care likely to be beneficial.

However, it is likely to be ineffective or harmful to perform an amnioinfusion prophylactically (Enkin et al, 2000). Amnioinfusion may be used to prevent or minimize meconium aspiration syndrome (MAS) by diluting amniotic fluid thickened with meconium passed by a hypoxic fetus. Maternal-fetal risks related to amnioinfusion, although rare, can result from infection and overdistention of the uterine cavity with infused fluid (Gilbert & Harmon, 2003). Accurate assessment of the woman's labor pattern also is important because dysfunctional labor is common.

Emotional support is essential for the woman with a postterm pregnancy and her family. A vaginal birth is anticipated, but the couple should be prepared for a forceps- or vacuum-assisted birth or cesarean birth if complications arise.

> **Home Care**
>
> **POSTTERM PREGNANCY**
> - Perform daily fetal movement counts.
> - Assess for signs of labor.
> - Call your primary health care provider if your membranes rupture, or if you perceive a decrease in or no fetal movement.
> - Keep appointments for fetal assessment tests or cervical checks.
> - Come to the hospital soon after labor begins.

OBSTETRIC EMERGENCIES

Shoulder Dystocia

Shoulder dystocia is an uncommon obstetric emergency that increases the risk for fetal/neonatal and maternal morbidity and mortality during the attempt to deliver the fetus vaginally. It is estimated that 0.24% to 2.0% of all vaginal births are complicated by shoulder dystocia (Bowes & Thorp, 2004).

Shoulder dystocia is a condition in which the head is born but the anterior shoulder cannot pass under the pubic arch. Fetopelvic disproportion due to excessive fetal size (greater than 4000 g) or maternal pelvic abnormalities may be a

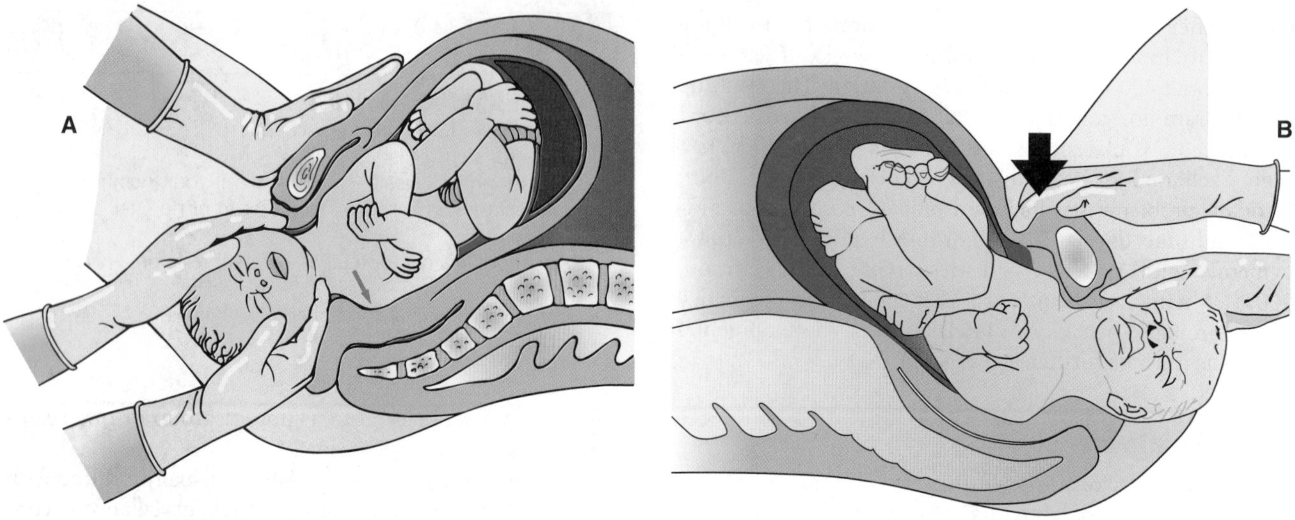

Fig. 19-15 Application of suprapubic pressure. **A**, Mazzanti technique: pressure is applied directly posteriorly and laterally above the symphysis pubis. **B**, Rubin technique: pressure is applied obliquely posteriorly against the anterior shoulder.

cause of shoulder dystocia, although shoulder dystocia can occur in the absence of any known risk factors.

The nurse should be observant for signs that could indicate the presence of shoulder dystocia, including slowing of the progress of labor and formation of a caput succedaneum that increases in size. When the head emerges, it retracts against the perineum (turtle sign), and external rotation does not occur (Hall, 1997).

The fetus/newborn is more likely to experience birth injuries related to asphyxia, brachial plexus damage, and fracture, especially of the humerus or clavicle. The mother's primary risk stems from excessive blood loss as a result of uterine atony or rupture, lacerations, extension of the episiotomy, or endometritis.

Care Management

Many maneuvers such as suprapubic pressure and maternal position changes have been suggested and tried to free the anterior shoulder, although no one particular maneuver has been found to be most effective (Bowes & Thorp, 2004). Suprapubic pressure can be applied to the anterior shoulder using the Mazzanti or Rubin technique (Fig. 19-15) in an attempt to push the shoulder under the symphysis pubis. In the McRoberts maneuver (Fig. 19-16), the woman's legs are flexed apart with her knees on her abdomen. This maneuver causes the sacrum to straighten, and the symphysis pubis rotates toward the mother's head; the angle of pelvic inclination is decreased, freeing the shoulder. Suprapubic pressure can be applied at this time. Having the woman move to a hands-and-knees position (the Gaskin maneuver), a squatting position, or lateral recumbent position also has been used to resolve cases of shoulder dystocia (Bruner et al, 1998). Fundal pressure is contraindicated as a method of relieving shoulder dystocia.

When shoulder dystocia is diagnosed, the nurse helps the woman assume the position(s) that may facilitate birth of the shoulders, and assists the primary health care provider with these maneuvers. The nurse also provides encouragement and support to reduce anxiety and fear.

Newborn assessment should include examination for fracture of the clavicle or humerus, as well as brachial plexus injuries and asphyxia (Bowes & Thorp, 2004). Maternal assessment should focus on early detection of hemorrhage and trauma to the soft tissue of the birth canal.

Prolapsed Umbilical Cord

Prolapse of the umbilical cord occurs when the cord lies below the presenting part of the fetus. In 2000, prolapse of the umbilical cord occurred in 1.9 of 1000 live births (Martin et al, 2002). Umbilical cord prolapse may be occult (hidden,

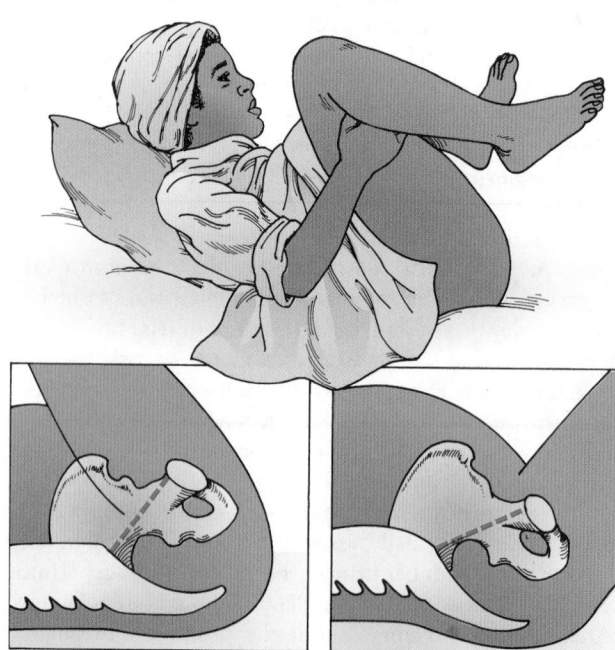

Fig. 19-16 McRoberts maneuver. (Modified from Lanni SM & Seeds JW: Malpresentations. In Gabbe SG, Niebyl JR, Simpson JL: *Obstetrics: normal and problem pregnancies,* ed 4, New York, 2002, Churchill Livingstone.)

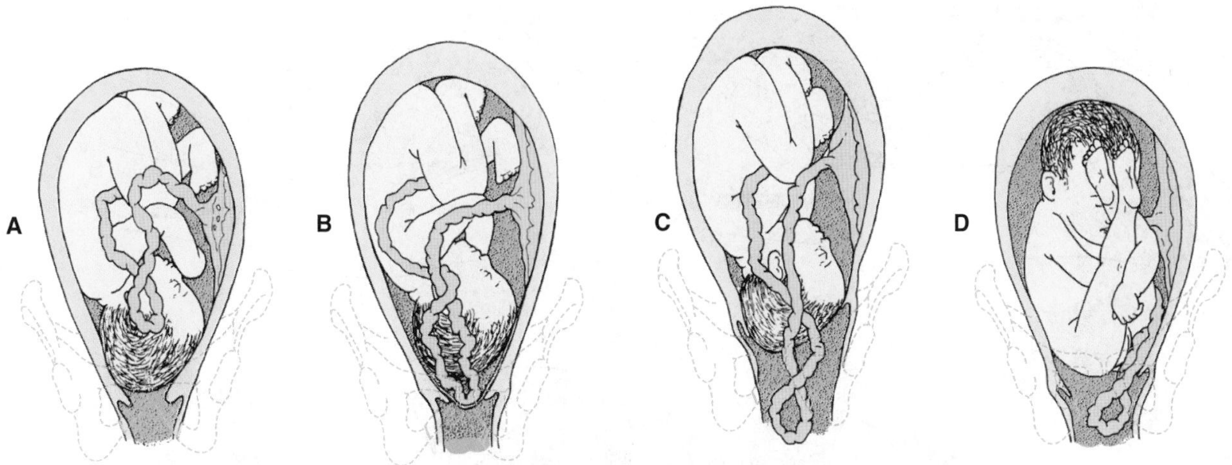

Fig. 19-17 Prolapse of umbilical cord. Note pressure of presenting part on umbilical cord, which endangers fetal circulation. **A,** Occult (hidden) prolapse of cord. **B,** Complete prolapse of cord. Note that membranes are intact. **C,** Cord presenting in front of fetal head may be seen in vagina. **D,** Frank breech presentation with prolapsed cord.

not visible) at any time during labor whether or not membranes are ruptured (Fig. 19-17, *A* and *B*). It is most common to see frank (visible) prolapse directly after rupture of membranes, when gravity washes the cord in front of the presenting part (Fig. 19-17, *C* and *D*). Frank prolapse occurs in 1 out of 400 births. Contributing factors are a long cord (longer than 100 cm), malpresentation (breech), transverse lie, or unengaged presenting part.

If the presenting part does not fit snugly into the lower uterine segment, as in polyhydramnios, when the membranes rupture, a sudden gush of amniotic fluid may cause the cord to be displaced downward. Similarly, the cord may prolapse during amniotomy if the presenting part is high. A small fetus may not fit snugly into the lower uterine segment; as a result, cord prolapse is more likely to occur.

Care Management

Prompt recognition of a prolapsed cord is important because fetal hypoxia resulting from prolonged cord compression (i.e., occlusion of blood flow to and from the fetus for more than 5 minutes) usually results in central nervous system damage or death of the fetus. Pressure on the cord may be relieved by the examiner putting a sterile gloved hand into the vagina and holding the presenting part off of the umbilical cord (Fig. 19-18, *A* and *B*). The woman is assisted into a position such as a modified Sims' (Fig. 19-18, *C*), Trendelenburg, or knee-chest (Fig. 19-18, *D*) position, in which gravity keeps the presenting part off the cord. If the cervix is fully dilated, a forceps- or vacuum-assisted birth can be performed for the fetus in a cephalic presentation; otherwise a cesarean birth is likely to be performed. Nonreassuring fetal heart rate and pattern, inadequate uterine relaxation, and bleeding can also occur as a result of a prolapsed umbilical cord. Indications for immediate interventions are presented in the Emergency box. Ongoing assessment of the woman and her fetus is critical. The woman and her family are often aware of the seriousness of the situation; therefore the nurse must provide support by giving explanations for the interventions being implemented and their effect on the status of the fetus.

Rupture of the Uterus

Rupture of the uterus is a rare but very serious obstetric injury that occurs once in every 1500 to 2000 births. The most common causes of uterine rupture during pregnancy are

Emergency

PROLAPSED CORD

Signs

Fetal bradycardia with variable deceleration during uterine contraction.
Woman reports feeling the cord after membranes rupture.
Cord is seen or felt in or protruding from the vagina.

Interventions

Call for assistance.
Notify primary health care provider immediately.
Glove the examining hand quickly and insert two fingers into the vagina to the cervix. With one finger on either side of the cord or both fingers to one side, exert upward pressure against the presenting part to relieve compression of the cord (see Fig. 19-17, *A* and *B*). Place a rolled towel under the woman's right or left hip.
Place the woman into the extreme Trendelenburg or a modified Sims' position (see Fig. 19-17, *C*), or a knee-chest position (see Fig. 19-17, *D*).
If cord is protruding from vagina, wrap loosely in a sterile towel saturated with warm, sterile normal saline solution.
Administer oxygen to the woman by mask at 8 to 10 L/min until birth is accomplished.
Start IV fluids or increase existing drip rate.
Continue to monitor FHR by internal fetal scalp electrode, if possible.
Explain to woman and support person what is happening and the way it is being managed.
Prepare for immediate vaginal birth if cervix is fully dilated or cesarean birth if it is not.

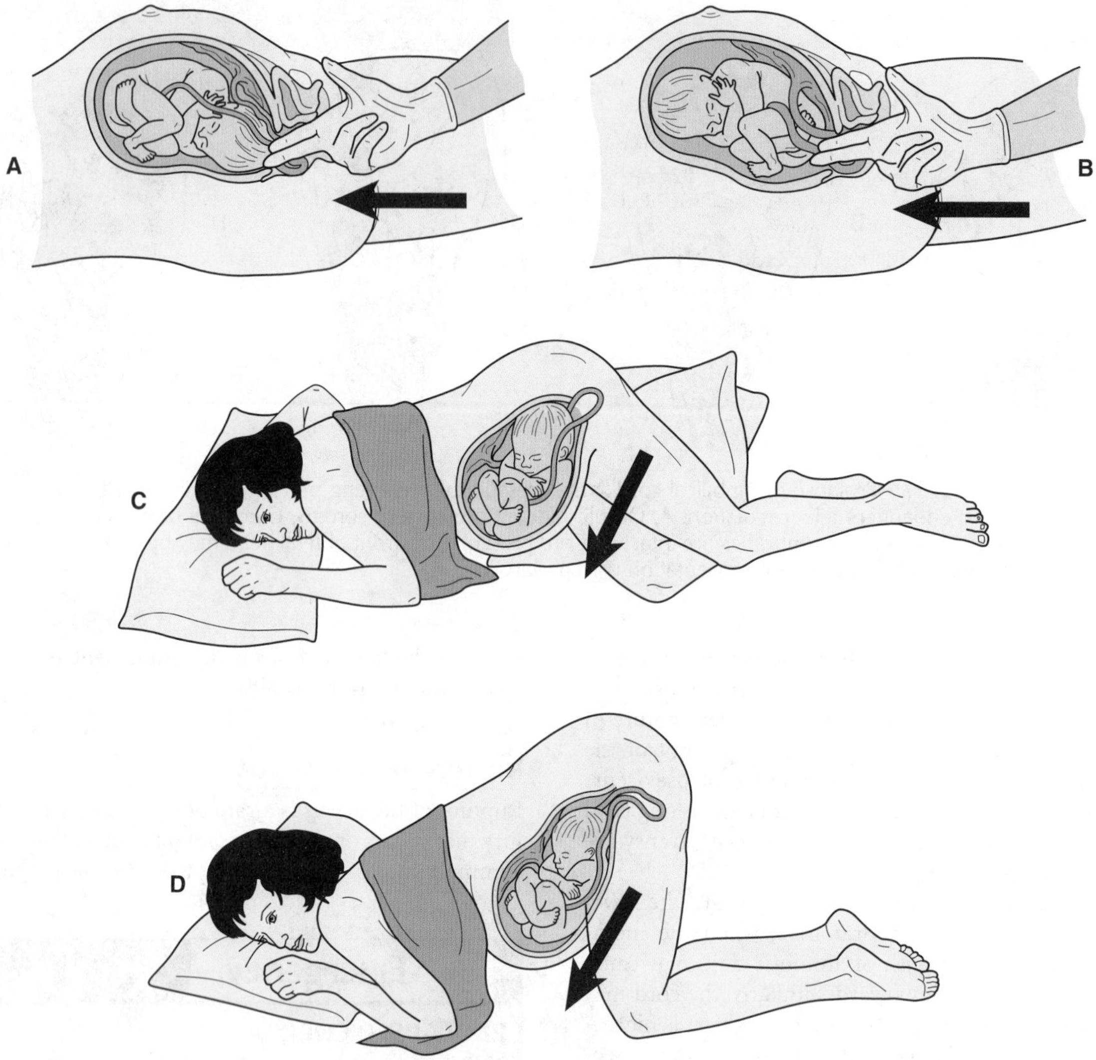

Fig. 19-18 *Arrows* indicate direction of pressure against presenting part to relieve compression of prolapsed umbilical cord. Pressure exerted by examiner's fingers in **A**, vertex presentation, and **B**, breech presentation. **C**, Gravity relieves pressure when woman is in modified Sims' position with hips elevated as high as possible with pillows. **D**, Knee-chest position.

separation of the scar of a previous classic cesarean birth, uterine trauma (e.g., accidents, surgery), and congenital uterine anomaly. During labor and birth, uterine rupture may be caused by intense spontaneous uterine contractions, labor stimulation (e.g., oxytocin, prostaglandin), an overdistended uterus (e.g., multifetal gestation), malpresentation, external or internal version, or a difficult forceps-assisted birth. It occurs more commonly in multigravidas than primigravidas.

A uterine rupture may be classified as complete or incomplete. A complete rupture extends through the entire uterine wall into the peritoneal cavity or broad ligament. An incomplete rupture extends into the peritoneum but not into the peritoneal cavity or broad ligament. Bleeding is usually internal. An incomplete rupture may also be a partial separation of an old cesarean scar and may go unnoticed unless the woman has a subsequent cesarean birth or other uterine surgery.

Signs and symptoms vary with the extent of the rupture and may be silent or dramatic. In an incomplete rupture, pain may not be present. The fetus may or may not have late decelerations, decreased variability, an increased or decreased heart rate, or other nonreassuring signs. The woman may experience vomiting, faintness, increased abdominal tenderness, hypotonic uterine contractions, and lack of progress. Eventually, bleeding and the effects of blood loss will be noted. Fetal heart tones may be lost. In a complete rupture, the woman may complain of a sudden, sharp abdominal pain and may state that "something gave way." If she is in labor, her contractions will cease and pain is relieved. She may exhibit signs of hypovolemic shock caused by hemorrhage (i.e., hypotension; tachypnea; pallor; and cool, clammy skin). If the placenta separates, the fetal heart tones will be absent. Fetal parts may be palpable through the abdomen. The nurse should suspect pulmonary embolism if the woman complains of chest pain.

Care Management

Prevention is the best treatment. Women who have had a previous classic cesarean birth are advised not to attempt vaginal birth in subsequent pregnancies. Women at risk for uterine rupture are assessed closely during labor. Women whose labors are induced with oxytocin or prostaglandin (especially if their previous birth was cesarean) are monitored for signs of uterine hyperstimulation because this can precipitate uterine rupture. If hyperstimulation occurs, the oxytocin infusion is discontinued or decreased and a tocolytic medication may be given to decrease the intensity of uterine contractions. After giving birth, women are assessed for excessive bleeding, especially if the fundus is firm and signs of hemorrhagic shock are present.

If rupture occurs, medical management depends on the severity. A small rupture may be managed with a laparotomy and birth of the infant, repair of the laceration, and blood transfusions if needed. For a complete rupture, hysterectomy and blood replacement is the usual treatment.

The nurse's role may include starting intravenous fluids, transfusing blood products, administering oxygen, and assisting with preparation for immediate surgery. Supporting the woman's family and providing information about the treatment are important during this emergency. The associated fetal mortality rates are high, and the maternal mortality rate may be as high as 50% to 75% if the woman is not treated immediately. Providing information about spiritual support services or suggesting that the family contact their own support system may be warranted.

Amniotic Fluid Embolism (Anaphylactoid Syndrome of Pregnancy)

Amniotic fluid embolism (AFE) occurs when amniotic fluid containing particles of debris (e.g., vernix, hair, skin cells, or meconium) enters the maternal circulation and obstructs pulmonary vessels, causing respiratory distress and circulatory collapse. This can occur because fluid can enter the maternal circulation any time there is an opening in the amniotic sac or maternal uterine veins accompanied by enough intrauterine pressure to force the amniotic fluid into the veins (e.g., if the placenta separates or if there are rapid or strong contractions that cause the uterus to lacerate or rupture). Although uncommon (1 in 20,646 births), this complication is estimated to be the cause of 10% of maternal deaths in the United States (Curran, 2003; Perozzi & Englert, 2004). The maternal mortality rate is approximately 61% and the fetal mortality rate is estimated to be 21% with 50% of the surviving infants having permanent neurologic injury (Perozzi & Englert, 2004). AFE cannot be predicted or prevented.

Amniotic fluid is more damaging if it contains meconium and other particulate matter such as mucus, fat globules, lanugo, bacterial products, or debris from a dead fetus because emboli can then form more readily. Maternal death occurs most often when thick meconium is present in the amniotic fluid, because this clogs the pulmonary veins more completely than other debris does. Even if death does not occur immediately, serious coagulation problems such as disseminated intravascular coagulopathy usually occur. Maternal factors (including multiparity, tumultuous labor, abruptio placentae, and oxytocin induction of labor) and fetal problems (including macrosomia, death, and meconium passage) have been associated with an increased risk for the development of AFE (Cunningham et al, 2001).

In contrast to the mechanical obstruction theory, Clark and colleagues (1995) discovered that 41% of women with exposure to amniotic fluid had a history of allergy. The condition is similar but not identical to anaphylactic shock; hence a new diagnostic title, *anaphylactoid syndrome of pregnancy,* was proposed.

Care Management

To improve the outcome of women with AFE, obstetric and critical care nurses who care for obstetric patients should become familiar with the condition. Increased awareness leads to earlier diagnosis and rapid and aggressive intervention (Perozzi & Englert, 2004). The immediate interventions for AFE are summarized in the Emergency box. Such medical management must be instituted immediately. Cardiopulmonary resuscitation is often needed. The woman is usually placed on me-

Emergency

AMNIOTIC FLUID EMBOLISM

Signs

Respiratory distress
- Restlessness
- Dyspnea
- Cyanosis
- Pulmonary edema
- Respiratory arrest

Circulatory collapse
- Hypotension
- Tachycardia
- Shock
- Cardiac arrest

Hemorrhage
- Coagulation failure: bleeding from incisions, venipuncture sites, trauma (lacerations); petechiae, ecchymoses, purpura
- Uterine atony

Interventions

Oxygenate
- Administer oxygen by face mask (8-10 L/min) or resuscitation bag delivering 100% oxygen
- Prepare for intubation and mechanical ventilation
- Initiate or assist with cardiopulmonary resuscitation. Tilt pregnant woman 30 degrees to side to displace uterus

Maintain cardiac output and replace fluid losses
- Position woman on her side
- Administer IV fluids
- Administer blood: packed cells, fresh frozen plasma
- Insert indwelling catheter, and measure hourly urine output

Correct coagulation failure

Monitor fetal and maternal status

Prepare for emergency birth once woman's condition is stabilized

Provide emotional support to woman, her partner, and her family

chanical ventilation, and blood replacement is initiated; coagulation defects are treated. Although the incidence of possible complications is small, their immediate recognition and the prompt initiation of treatment are important.

NURSE ALERT Automatic blood pressure devices, FHR monitors, and pulse oximeters may be inadequate and inaccurate during extreme clinical conditions. Assessment by a competent nurse is often more accurate than that provided by any one piece of equipment (Curran, 2003). ■

The nurse's immediate responsibility is to assist with the resuscitation efforts. The fetus should be monitored continuously (Perozzi & Englert, 2004). If the woman survives, she is usually moved to a critical care unit where hemodynamic monitoring, blood replacement, and coagulopathy treatment are implemented. If cardiopulmonary arrest occurs, for optimal fetal survival, a perimortum cesarean birth should occur within 5 minutes (Curran, 2003).

Support of the woman's partner and family is needed; they will be anxious and distressed. Brief explanations of what is happening are important during the emergency and can be reinforced after the immediate crisis is over. In many cases, the woman dies and the infant survives; grieving, anger and blame may interfere with parent-infant attachment (Perozzi & Englert, 2004). When both the mother and infant die, it is important that the family has the opportunity to spend time with them. Emotional support and involvement of the perinatal loss support team or other resource for grief counseling including the pastoral care team (if desired by the family), is needed. Referral to grief and loss support groups is appropriate. The nursing staff also may need help in coping with feelings and emotions that result from a maternal death.

Key Points

- Preterm labor is cervical change and uterine contractions occurring between 20 and 37 weeks of pregnancy; preterm birth is any birth that occurs before the completion of 37 weeks of pregnancy.
- The incidence of preterm birth in the United States varies considerably by race.
- The cause of preterm labor is unknown, and is assumed to be multifactorial.
- Beta-mimetics are a class of medications that have many maternal and fetal side effects and must always be used with extreme caution.
- Bed rest, a commonly prescribed intervention for preterm labor, has many deleterious side effects and has never been shown to decrease preterm birth rates.
- Preterm birth that occurs in a tertiary care center leads to better neonatal and maternal outcomes.
- Vigilance for signs of infection is a major part of the care for women with PPROM.
- Dystocia results from differences in the normal relationships among any of the five factors affecting labor.
- Dysfunctional labor occurs as a result of hypertonic uterine dysfunction, hypotonic uterine dysfunction, or inadequate voluntary expulsive forces.
- The functional relationships between the uterine contractions, the fetus, and the mother's pelvis are altered by maternal positioning.
- Uterine contractility is increased by oxytocin and prostaglandin and is decreased by tocolytic agents.
- Cervical ripening using chemical or mechanical measures can increase the success of labor induction.
- Expectant parents benefit from learning about operative obstetrics (e.g., forceps- or vacuum-assisted or cesarean birth) during the prenatal period.
- The basic purpose of cesarean birth is to preserve the life and health of the mother and her fetus.
- Unless contraindicated, a vaginal birth is possible after a previous cesarean birth.
- Labor management that emphasizes one-to-one support of the laboring woman by another woman (doula, nurse, or nurse-midwife) can reduce the rate of cesarean birth and increase the rate of VBACs.
- Postterm pregnancy poses a risk to both the mother and the fetus.
- Obstetric emergencies (e.g., shoulder dystocia, prolapsed cord, rupture of the uterus, and amniotic fluid embolism) occur rarely but require immediate intervention.

Answer Guidelines to Critical Thinking Exercise

Preterm Labor

1. There is no evidence in the literature to support the efficacy of bed rest in reducing preterm birth rates; it is a form of care of unknown effectiveness (Enkin et al, 2000; Maloni, 1998). Deleterious effects of bed rest on women include decreased muscle tone, weight loss, calcium loss, and glucose intolerance. Weeks of bed rest lead to bone demineralization, constipation, fatigue, isolation, anxiety, and depression.
2. (a) Because this is Yolanda's third hospitalization for preterm labor, her risks of giving birth prematurely are increased. Her primary health care provider could choose to have her remain hospitalized until birth to increase the chances of a good outcome for the baby. (b) Bed rest is often ordered as an intervention to prevent preterm birth even though it is of unknown effectiveness. Hospitalization at a facility that can handle high risk or preterm infants increases the chances of a good outcome. Although the home is an ideal location for a pregnant woman, the primary health care provider may have knowledge that Yolanda would be unlikely to remain on bed rest at home because of the need to care for her husband and child. (c) The nurse can coach Yolanda and her family in ways to reduce the frustration and boredom that accompanies restriction to bed rest for the next several weeks. The environment can be modified for convenience and essential items placed within reach (e.g., telephone, television, radio, tape or CD player, computer with Internet access, snacks, books, magazines, newspapers, and items for hobbies). Families, who are often anxious regarding the health status of the mother and baby, may need help in learning how to organize

time and space or to restructure family routines so that the pregnant woman can remain a part of family activity while still maintaining bed rest. (d) The nurse can explore resources available in the community to assist with care of Yolanda's 2-year-old son. Referral to a social worker can be made. Family members can be asked to help; church and social groups can be helpful.

3. The priority for nursing care is to work with Yolanda to prevent preterm birth. Assisting Yolanda to maintain bed rest as ordered, providing diversions, reducing anxiety, and coaching her in exercises she can perform in bed to maintain muscle tone and prevent bone loss are actions to take. Providing explanations and keeping the family informed are essential. The fetus and uterine contractions are monitored as required by protocol or the primary health care provider's orders.
4. Although bed rest has not been shown to be effective in preventing preterm birth, it is a common intervention. Thus the nurse can implement actions to mitigate or prevent the deleterious effects of bed rest. She can work with the family to ensure emotional support and with the social worker to ensure child care for the 2-year-old.
5. Alternatively and importantly, the nurse can also work to ensure that an evidence base exists for care provided. She can work with other health care providers to identify and use the best available evidence on which to base practice. She can provide evidence about the deleterious effects of bed rest and seek to change practice.

Resources

American College of Obstetricians and Gynecologists (ACOG)
409 12th St., SW
PO Box 96920
Washington, DC 20090-6920
800-762-2264
www.acog.org

Birthrites: Healing after Cesarean, Inc.
www.birthrites.org

C/SEC, Inc. (Cesarean/Support Education and Concern)
22 Forest Rd.
Framingham, MA 01701
508-877-8266

A Free Home for Moms on Bedrest
www.momsonbedrest.com

Incompetent Cervix
www.geocities.com/incompetentcervix/

International Cesarean Awareness Network (ICAN)
1304 Kingsdale Ave.
Redondo Beach, CA 90278
310-542-6400
www.ican-online.org

Mothers of Supertwins (MOST)
MOST
PO Box 951
Brentwood, NY 11717
631-859-1110
www.mostonline.org

National Organization of Mothers of Twins Clubs, Inc. (NOMOTC)
PO Box 438
Thompsons Station, TN 37179-0438
615-595-0936
www.nomotc.org

National Perinatal Association
3500 East Fletcher Ave., Suite 205
Tampa, FL 33613-4712
813-971-1008
www.nationalperinatal.org

Preeclampsia
www.preeclampsia.org

Pregnancy Bedrest: A Reading Room to Help You Survive and Thrive during Your Days of Waiting
Amy E. Tracy
445C E. Cheyenne Mtn. Blvd., #194
Colorado Springs, CO 80906
www.pregnancybedrest.com

Pregnancy Bedrest Web: Information on High-Risk Pregnancy for Women, Their Families, and Their Caregivers
Judy Maloni, PhD, RN, FAAN
Case Western Reserve University—Bolton School of Nursing
10900 Euclid Ave.
Cleveland, OH 44106
216-368-2912
fpb.cwru.edu/bedrest

Premature Rupture of Membranes
www.kanalen.org/prom/

Sidelines: High Risk Pregnancy Support Group
PO Box 1808
Laguna Beach, CA 92652
888-447-4754
www.sidelines.org

The Triplet Connection
PO Box 99571
Stockton, CA 95209
209-474-0885
www.tripletconnection.org

VBAC.com—A Woman-Centered Evidence-Based Resource
Nicette Jukelevics
Center for Family
24050 Madison St., Suite 200
Torrance, CA 90505
310-375-3141
www.vbac.com

References

Abrahams C, Katz M: A perspective on the diagnosis of preterm labor, *J Perinat Neonatal Nurs* 16(1):1-11, 2002.

Abrams B, Minassian D, Pickett KE: Maternal nutrition. In Creasy RK, Resnik R, Iams JD (eds): *Maternal-fetal medicine: principles and practice,* ed 5, Philadephia, 2004, WB Saunders.

Adler CL, Zarchin YR: The "Virtual Focus Group": using the Internet to reach pregnant women on home bed rest, *J Obstet Gynecol Neonatal Nurs* 31(4):418-427, 2002.

American College of Obstetricians and Gynecologists: *Vaginal birth after a previous cesarean delivery,* Practice Bulletin no 5, Washington, DC, 1999, American College of Obstetricians and Gynecologists.

American College of Obstetricians and Gynecologists: *New ACOG opinion addresses elective cesarean controversy,* ACOG news release, Washington, DC, October 31, 2003, American College of Obstetricians and Gynecologists.

Arulkumarian S: Prolonged pregnancy. In James D et al (eds): *High risk pregnancy management options,* London, 1997, WB Saunders.

Association of Women's Health, Obstetric, and Neonatal Nurses: *Issue: professional nursing support of laboring women,* Washington, DC, 2000, Association of Women's Health, Obstetric, and Neonatal Nurses.

Bernhardt J, Dorman K: Pre-term birth risk assessment tools. Exploring fetal fibronectin and cervical length for validating risk, *AWHONN Lifelines* 8(1):38-44, 2004.

Bowes WA, Thorp JM: Clinical aspects of normal and abnormal labor. In Creasy RK, Resnik R, Iams JD (eds): *Maternal-fetal medicine: principles and practice,* ed 5, Philadephia, 2004, WB Saunders.

Bruner JP et al: All-fours maneuver for reducing shoulder dystocia during labor, *J Reprod Med* 43(5):439-443, 1998.

Burrows WR et al: Safety and efficacy of early postoperative solid food consumption after cesarean section, *J Reprod Med* 40(6):463-467, 1995.

Carpenter JA: Shortening the short stay, *AWHONN Lifelines* 2(1):28-34, 1998.

Clark SL et al: Amniotic fluid embolism: analysis of the national registry, *Am J Obstet Gynecol* 172(4 pt 1):1158-1167, 1995.

Cunningham F et al: *Williams obstetrics,* ed 21, Stamford, CT, 2001, Appleton & Lange.

Curran CA: Intrapartum emergencies, *J Obstet Gynecol Neonatal Nurs* 32(6):802-813, 2003.

Divon MY: Prolonged pregnancy. In Gabbe SG, Niebyl JR, Simpson JL (eds): *Obstetrics: normal and problem pregnancies,* ed 4, New York, 2002, Churchill Livingstone.

Draper H: Women, forced caesareans and antenatal responsibilities, *Obstet Gynecol Surv* 52(8):475-477, 1997.

Eakes M, Brown H: Home alone—meeting the needs of mothers after cesarean birth, *AWHONN Lifelines* 2(1):36-40, 1998.

Enkin M et al: *A guide to effective care in pregnancy and childbirth,* ed 3, Oxford, NY, 2000, Oxford University Press.

Fleming A et al: Pregnancy and economic outcomes in patients treated for recurrent preterm labor, *J Perinatol* 24(4):223-237, 2004.

Freda MC: Nursing's contribution to the literature on preterm labor and birth, *J Obstet Gynecol Neonatal Nurs* 32(5):659-667, 2003.

Freda MC, Patterson E: *Preterm birth: prevention and nursing management. Nursing Module.* New York, 1995, March of Dimes.

Friedman E: Normal and dysfunctional labor. In Cohen W et al (eds): *Management of labor,* ed 2, Rockville, MD, 1989, Aspen.

Fuchs IB et al: Sonographic cervical length in singleton pregnancies with intact membranes presenting in threatened preterm labor, *Ultrasound Obstet Gynecol* 24(5):554-557, 2004.

Gardner PS: Previous traumatic birth: an impetus for requested cesarean birth, *J Perinat Neonatal Educ* 12(1): 1-5, 2003.

Garite TJ: Premature rupture of the membranes. In Creasy RK, Resnik R, Iams JD (eds): *Maternal-fetal medicine: principles and practice,* ed 5, Philadephia, 2004, WB Saunders.

Gilbert ES, Harmon JS: *Manual of high risk pregnancy and delivery,* ed 3, St Louis, 2003, Mosby.

Goldberg AB, Greenberg MB, Darney PD: Misoprostol and pregnancy, *N Engl J Med* 344(1):38-47, 2001.

Goldenberg RL et al: The Preterm Prediction Study: toward a multiple marker test for spontaneous preterm birth, *Am J Obstet Gynecol* 185(3):643-651, 2001.

Gregory KD: Monitoring, risk adjustment, and strategies to decrease cesarean rates, *Curr Opin Obstet Gynecol* 12(6):481-486, 2000.

Hall SP: The nurse's role in the identification of risks and treatment of shoulder dystocia, *J Obstet Gynecol Neonatal Nurs* 26(1):25-32, 1997.

Hofmeyr GJ, Hannah ME: Planned caesarean section for term breech delivery (Cochrane Review), 2003. In *The Cochrane Library,* Issue 2, Chichester, UK, 2004, John Wiley & Sons.

Iams JD: Preterm birth. In Gabbe SG, Niebyl JR, Simpson JL (eds): *Obstetrics: normal and problem pregnancies,* ed 4, New York, 2002, Churchill Livingstone.

Iams JD, Creasy RK: Preterm labor and delivery. In Creasy RK, Resnik R, Iams JD (eds): *Maternal-fetal medicine: principles and practice,* ed 5, Philadephia, 2004, WB Saunders.

Lanni SM, Seeds JW: Malpresentations. In Gabbe SG, Niebyl JR, Simpson JL (eds): *Obstetrics: normal and problem pregnancies,* ed 4, New York, 2002, Churchill Livingstone.

Lehne R: *Pharmacology for nursing care,* Philadelphia, 2001, WB Saunders.

Liu S et al: Recent trends in caesarean delivery rates and indications for caesarean delivery in Canada, *J Obstet Gynaecol Can* 26(8):735-742, 2004.

Lydon-Rochelle M et al: Risk of uterine rupture during labor among women with a prior cesarean delivery, *N Engl J Med* 345(1):3-8, 2001.

Maloni JA: *Antepartum bedrest: case studies, research, and nursing care,* Washington, DC, 1998, Association of Women's Health, Obstetric, and Neonatal Nurses.

Maloni JA: *The prevention of preterm birth: research-based practice, nursing interventions, and practice scenarios,* Washington, DC, 2000, Association of Women's Health, Obstetric, and Neonatal Nurses.

Maloni JA: Astronauts and pregnancy bed rest: what NASA is teaching us about inactivity, *AWHONN Lifelines* 6(4):318-323, 2002.

Maloni JA, Brezinski-Tomasi JE, Johnson LA: Antepartum bedrest: effect upon the family, *J Obstet Gynecol Neonatal Nurs* 30(2):165-173, 2001.

Maloni JA, Damato EG: Reducing the risk for preterm birth: evidence and implications for neonatal nurses, *Adv Neonatal Care* 4(3):166-174, 2004.

Maloni JA, Kutil RM: Antepartum support group for women hospitalized on bed rest, *MCN Am J Matern Child Nurs* 25(4):204-210, 2000.

Maloni JA et al: Physical and psychosocial side effects of antepartum bed rest, *Nurs Res* 42(4):197-203, 1993.

Martin JA et al: Annual summary of vital statistics-2003, *Pediatrics* 115(3):619-634, 2005.

Martin JA et al: Births: final data for 2000, *Natl Vital Stat Rep* 50(5):1-102, 2002.

Martin JA et al: Births: final data for 2002, *Natl Vital Stat Rep* 52(10):1-113, 2003.

Maupin RM et al: Characteristics of women who deliver with no prenatal care, *J Matern Fetal Neonatal Med* 16(1):45-50, 2004.

Mayberry L et al: *Second stage labor management: promotion of evidence-based practice and a collaborative approach to patient care,* Washington, DC, 2000, Association of Women's Health, Obstetric, and Neonatal Nurses.

Miltner RS: Identifying labor support actions of intrapartum nurses, *J Obstet Gynecol Neonatal Nurs* 29(5): 491-499, 2000.

Moore ML: Preterm labor and birth: what have we learned in the past two decades? *J Obstet Gynecol Neonatal Nurs* 32(5):638-649, 2003.

Moore ML et al: A randomized trial of nurse intervention to reduce preterm and low birthweight births, *Obstet Gynecol* 91(5 pt 1):656-661, 1998.

Morrison JC, Chauhan SP: Current status of home uterine activity monitoring, *Clin Perinatol* 30(4):757-801, 2003.

National Institutes of Health: *Antenatal corticosteroids revisited. Consensus Development Conference Statement,* Bethesda, MD, 2000, National Institutes of Health. Internet document available at http://consensus.nih.gov (accessed February 7, 2005).

Nelson R: Premature births on the rise, *Am J Nurs* 104(6):23-24, 2004.

Norwitz ER, Robinson NJ, Repke JT: Labor and delivery. In Gabbe SG, Niebyl JR, Simpson JL (eds): *Obstetrics: normal and problem pregnancies,* ed 4, New York, 2002, Churchill Livingstone.

Perozzi KJ, Englert NC: Amniotic fluid embolism. An obstetric emergency, *Crit Care Nurse* 24(4): 54-61, 2004.

Pozaic S: Induction and augmentation of labor. In Mandeville L, Troiano N (eds): *High-risk and critical care intrapartum nursing,* ed 2, Philadelphia, 1999, Lippincott.

Pschirrer E, Monga M: Risk factors for preterm labor, *Clin Obstet Gynecol* 43(4):727-734, 2000.

Radin TG, Harmon JS, Hanson DA: Nurses' care during labor: its effects on the cesarean birth rate of healthy nulliparous women, *Birth* 20(1):14-21, 1993.

Ramsey PS, Andrews WW: Biochemical predictors of preterm labor: fetal fibronectin and salivary estriol, *Clin Perinatol* 30(4):701-733, 2003.

Resnik JL, Resnik R: Post-term pregnancy. In Creasy RK, Resnik R, Iams JD (eds): *Maternal-fetal medicine: principles and practice,* ed 5, Philadephia, 2004, WB Saunders.

Ryding EL, Wijma K, Wijma B: Experiences of emergency cesarean section: a phenomenological study of 53 women, *Birth* 25(4): 246-251, 1998.

Schaffir J: Survey of folk beliefs about induction of labor, *Birth* 29(1):47-51, 2002.

Searing KA: Induction vs. post-date pregnancies: exploring the controversy of who's really at risk, *AWHONN Lifelines* 5(2):44-48, 2001.

Simkin P, Ancheta R: *The labor progress handbook,* Malden, MA, 2000, Blackwell Science.

Simpson KR: Preterm birth in the United States: current issues and future perspectives, *J Perinat Neonatal Nurs* 10(4):11-15, 1997.

Simpson KR: *Cervical ripening and induction and augmentation of labor,* ed 2, Washington, DC, 2002, Association of Women's Health, Obstetric, and Neonatal Nurses.

Society of Obstetricians and Gynaecologists of Canada: News. C-sections on demand—SOGC's position, *Birth* 31(2):154, 2004.

Sosa C et al: Bed rest in singleton pregnancies for preventing preterm birth (Cochrane Review), 2003. In *The Cochrane Library,* Issue 1, Chichester, UK, 2005, John Wiley & Sons.

Summers L: Methods of cervical ripening and labor induction, *J Nurse Midwifery* 42(2):71-85, 1997.

Thomas L et al: The effects of rocking, diet modifications, and antiflatulent medication of postcesarean section gas pain, *J Perinat Neonatal Nurs* 4(3):12-24, 1990.

Tiedje LB: Psychosocial pathways to prematurity: changing our thinking toward a lifecourse and community approach, *J Obstet Gynecol Neonatal Nurs* 32(5):650-658, 2003.

Varney H: *Varney's textbook for midwives,* ed 3, Sudberry, MA, 1997, Jones & Bartlett.

Weiss ME, Saks NP, Harris S: Resolving the uncertainty of preterm symptoms: women's experiences with the onset of preterm labor, *J Obstet Gynecol Neonatal Nurs* 31(1):66-76, 2002.

Weitz BW: Premature rupture of the fetal membranes: an update for advanced practice nurses, *MCN Am J Matern Child Nurs* 26(2):86-92, 2001.

Witcher P: Treatment of preterm labor, *J Perinat Neonatal Nurs* 16(1):25-46, 2002.

20 Maternal Physiologic Changes

LEARNING OBJECTIVES

On completion of this chapter the reader will be able to:

- Describe the anatomic and physiologic changes that occur during the postpartum period.
- Identify characteristics of uterine involution and lochial flow and describe ways to measure them.
- List expected values for vital signs and blood pressure, deviations from normal findings, and probable causes of the deviations.

ELECTRONIC RESOURCES

Additional information related to the content in Chapter 20 can be found on

the companion website at evolve
http://evolve.elsevier.com/Wong/maternal/
- NCLEX Review Questions
- WebLinks

or the interactive student CD-ROM
Activities for Chapter 20 include the following:
- NCLEX Review Questions

The postpartum period is the interval between the birth of the newborn and the return of the reproductive organs to their normal nonpregnant state. This period is sometimes referred to as the *puerperium,* or fourth trimester of pregnancy. Although the puerperium has traditionally been considered to last 6 weeks, this time frame varies among women. The physiologic changes that occur during the reversal of the processes of pregnancy, though distinctive, are normal. Many factors, including the mother's energy level and degree of comfort, the health of the newborn, and the care and encouragement given by health professionals, contribute to the mother's response to her infant during this time. To provide care during the recovery period that is beneficial to the mother, her infant, and her family, the nurse must synthesize knowledge of maternal anatomy and physiology of the recovery period, the newborn's physical and behavioral characteristics, infant care activities, and family response to the birth of the infant. This chapter focuses on anatomic and physiologic changes that occur in the mother during the postpartum period.

REPRODUCTIVE SYSTEM AND ASSOCIATED STRUCTURES

Uterus

Involution Process

The return of the uterus to a nonpregnant state following birth is termed *involution.* This process begins immediately after expulsion of the placenta with contraction of the uterine smooth muscle.

At the end of the third stage of labor, the uterus is in the midline, approximately 2 cm below the level of the umbilicus, with the fundus resting on the sacral promontory. At this time, the uterus weighs approximately 1000 g.

Within 12 hours the fundus may rise to approximately 1 cm above the umbilicus (Fig. 20-1). By 24 hours postpartum, the uterus is about the same size it was at 20 weeks of gestation (Resnik, 2004). Involution progresses rapidly during the next few days. The fundus descends 1 to 2 cm every 24 hours. By the sixth postpartum day, the fundus is normally located halfway between the umbilicus and the symphysis pubis. Within 2 weeks after childbirth, the uterus once again lies in the true pelvis.

The uterus, which at full term weighs approximately 11 times its prepregnancy weight, involutes to approximately 500 g by 1 week after birth and to 350 g by 2 weeks after birth. At 6 weeks it weighs 50 to 60 g (see Fig. 20-1). Increased estrogen and progesterone levels are responsible for stimulating the massive growth of the uterus during pregnancy. Prenatal uterine growth results from both hyperplasia, an increase in the number of muscle cells, and from hypertrophy, an enlargement of the existing cells. Postpartally, the decrease in these hormones causes autolysis, the self-destruction of excess hypertrophied tissue. The additional cells laid down during pregnancy remain and account for the slight increase in uterine size after each pregnancy.

Subinvolution is the failure of the uterus to return to a nonpregnant state. The most common causes of subinvolution are retained placental fragments and infection.

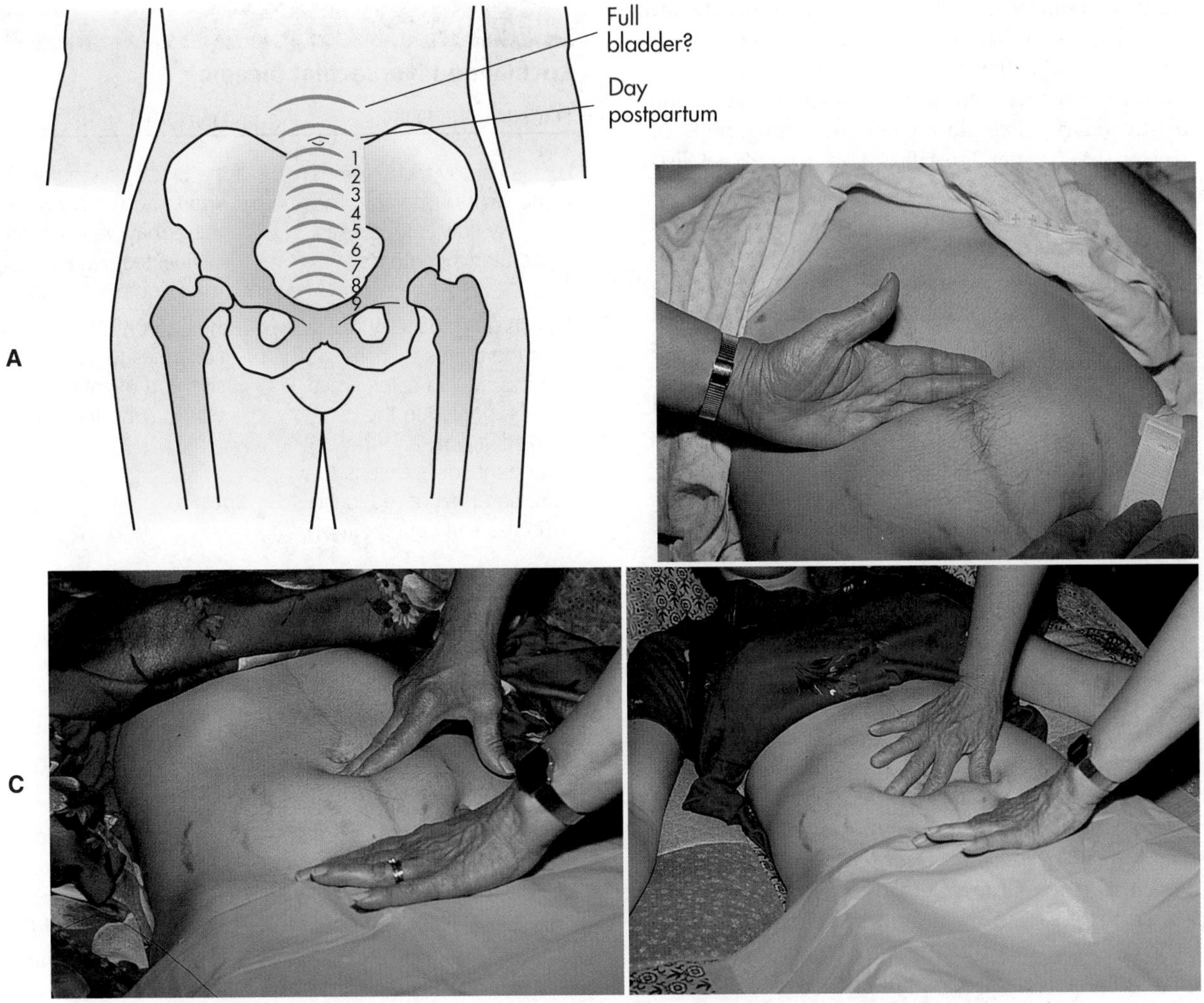

Fig. 20-1 Assessment of involution of uterus after childbirth. **A**, Normal progress, days 1 through 9. **B**, Size and position of uterus 2 hours after childbirth. **C**, Two days after childbirth. **D**, Four days after childbirth. (*B, C,* and *D* courtesy Marjorie Pyle, RNC, Lifecircle, Costa Mesa, CA.)

Contractions

Postpartum hemostasis is achieved primarily by compression of intramyometrial blood vessels as the uterine muscle contracts, rather than by platelet aggregation and clot formation. The hormone oxytocin, released from the pituitary gland, strengthens and coordinates these uterine contractions, which compress blood vessels and promote hemostasis. During the first 1 to 2 postpartum hours, uterine contractions may decrease in intensity and become uncoordinated. Because it is vital that the uterus remain firm and well contracted, exogenous oxytocin (Pitocin) is usually administered intravenously or intramuscularly immediately after expulsion of the placenta. Mothers who plan to breastfeed may be encouraged to put the baby to breast immediately after birth because suckling stimulates oxytocin release.

Afterpains

In first-time mothers, uterine tone is increased, the fundus generally remains firm, and the mother does not perceive uterine cramping. Periodic relaxation and vigorous contractions are more common in subsequent pregnancies and may cause uncomfortable cramping called *afterpains* (afterbirth pains), which persist throughout the early puerperium. Afterpains are more noticeable after births in which the uterus was greatly distended (e.g., large baby, multifetal gestation). Breastfeeding and exogenous oxytocic medication usually intensify these afterpains because both stimulate uterine contractions.

Placental Site

Immediately after the placenta and membranes are expelled, vascular constriction and thromboses reduce the placental site to an irregular nodular and elevated area. Upward growth of the endometrium causes sloughing of necrotic tissue and prevents the scar formation characteristic of normal wound healing. This unique healing process enables the endometrium to resume its usual cycle of changes and to permit implantation and placentation in future pregnancies. Endometrial regeneration is completed by the end of the third postpartum week, except at the placental site (Resnik, 2004). Regeneration at the placental site usually is not complete until 6 weeks after birth.

Lochia

Postbirth uterine discharge, commonly called *lochia*, initially is bright red and changes later to a pinkish red or reddish brown. It may contain small clots.

For the first 2 hours after birth the amount of uterine discharge should be about that of a heavy menstrual period. After that time, the lochia flow should steadily decrease.

Lochia rubra consists mainly of blood and decidual and trophoblastic debris. The flow pales, becoming pink or brown (lochia serosa) after 3 to 4 days. Lochia serosa consists of old blood, serum, leukocytes, and tissue debris. The median duration of lochia serosa discharge is 22 to 27 days (Bowes & Katz, 2002). In most women, about 10 days after childbirth the drainage becomes yellow to white (lochia alba). Lochia alba consists of leukocytes, decidua, epithelial cells, mucus, serum, and bacteria. Lochia alba may continue for 2 to 6 weeks after the birth.

It is difficult to judge the amount of lochial flow based only on observation of perineal pads (see Chapter 21). Any estimation of lochial flow is inaccurate and incomplete without considering the time factor. For example, the woman who saturates a peripad in 1 hour or less is bleeding much more than the woman who saturates a peripad in 8 hours.

If the woman receives an oxytocic medication, the flow of lochia is usually scant until the effects of the medication wear off. The amount of lochia is usually less after cesarean births. Flow of lochia usually increases with ambulation and breastfeeding. Lochia tends to pool in the vagina when the woman is lying in bed; the woman then may experience a gush of blood when she stands. This gush should not be confused with hemorrhage.

Persistence of lochia rubra early in the postpartum period suggests continued bleeding as a result of retained fragments of the placenta or membranes. Recurrence of bleeding 7 to 10 days after birth is from the healing placental site. About 10% to 15% of women will still be having normal lochia serosa discharge at their 6-week postpartum examination (Bowes & Katz, 2002). In the majority of women, however, the continued flow of lochia serosa or lochia alba by 3 to 4 weeks after birth may indicate endometritis, particularly if fever, pain, or abdominal tenderness is associated with the discharge. Lochia should smell like normal menstrual flow; an offensive odor usually indicates infection.

NURSE ALERT Not all postpartal vaginal bleeding is lochia; vaginal bleeding after birth may be due to unrepaired vaginal or cervical lacerations. Table 20-1 distinguishes between lochial and nonlochial bleeding. ■

Cervix

The cervix is soft immediately after birth. Within 2 to 3 postpartum days, however, it has shortened, become firm, and regained its form (Resnik, 2004). The cervix up to the lower uterine segment remains edematous, thin, and fragile for several days after birth. The ectocervix (portion of the cervix that protrudes into the vagina) appears bruised and has some small lacerations—optimal conditions for the development of infection. The cervical os, which dilated to 10 cm during labor, closes gradually. Two fingers may still be introduced into the cervical os for the first 4 to 6 days postpartum; however, only the smallest curette can be introduced by the end of 2 weeks. The external cervical os never regains its prepregnant appearance; it is no longer shaped like a circle but appears as a jagged slit that is often described as a "fish mouth." Lactation delays the production of cervical and other estrogen-influenced mucus and mucosal characteristics.

Table 20-1

Lochial and Nonlochial Bleeding

LOCHIAL BLEEDING	NONLOCHIAL BLEEDING
Lochia usually trickles from the vaginal opening. The steady flow is greater as the uterus contracts.	If the bloody discharge spurts from the vagina, there may be cervical or vaginal tears in addition to the normal lochia.
A gush of lochia may result as the uterus is massaged. If it is dark in color, it has been pooled in the relaxed vagina, and the amount soon lessens to a trickle of bright red lochia (in the early puerperium).	If the amount of bleeding continues to be excessive and bright red, a tear may be the source.

Vagina and Perineum

Postpartum estrogen deprivation is responsible for the thinness of the vaginal mucosa and the absence of rugae. The greatly distended, smooth-walled vagina gradually returns to its prepregnancy size by 6 to 10 weeks after childbirth (Resnik, 2004). Rugae reappear within 3 weeks, but they are never as prominent as they are in the nulliparous woman. Most rugae are permanently flattened. The mucosa remains atrophic in the lactating woman, at least until menstruation resumes. Thickening of the vaginal mucosa occurs with the return of ovarian function. Reduced estrogen levels are also responsible for a decreased amount of vaginal lubrication. Localized dryness and coital discomfort (dyspareunia) may persist until ovarian function returns and menstruation resumes. The use of a water-soluble lubricant to reduce discomfort during sexual intercourse is usually recommended.

Initially the introitus is erythematous and edematous, especially in the area of the episiotomy or laceration repair. It is barely distinguishable from that of a nulliparous woman if lacerations and an episiotomy have been carefully repaired, hematomas are prevented or treated early, and the woman practices good hygiene during the first 2 weeks after birth.

Most episiotomies are visible only if the woman is lying on her side with her upper buttock raised or if she is placed in the lithotomy position. A good light source is essential for visualization of some episiotomies. An episiotomy heals the same way as any surgical incision. Signs of infection (i.e., pain, redness, warmth, swelling, or discharge) or loss of approximation (i.e., separation of the edges of the incision) may occur. Healing should occur within 2 to 3 weeks.

Hemorrhoids (anal varicosities) are commonly seen. Internal hemorrhoids may evert while the woman is pushing during birth. Women often experience associated symptoms such as itching, discomfort, and bright red bleeding upon defecation. Hemorrhoids usually decrease in size within 6 weeks of childbirth.

Pelvic Muscular Support

The supporting structure of the uterus and vagina may be injured during childbirth and may contribute to later gynecologic problems. Supportive tissues of the pelvic floor that are torn or stretched during childbirth may require up to 6 months to regain tone. Kegel exercises, which help strengthen perineal muscles and encourage healing, are recommended after childbirth. Pelvic relaxation refers to the lengthening and weakening of the fascial supports of pelvic structures. These structures include the uterus, upper posterior vaginal wall, urethra, bladder, and rectum. Although relaxation can occur in any woman, it is commonly a direct but delayed complication of childbirth.

ENDOCRINE SYSTEM

Placental Hormones

Significant hormonal changes occur during the postpartal period. Expulsion of the placenta results in dramatic decreases of the hormones produced by that organ. Decreases in human chorionic somatomammotropin (hCS; also called human placental lactogen [hPL]), estrogens, cortisol, and the placental enzyme insulinase reverse the diabetogenic effects of pregnancy, resulting in significantly lower blood sugar levels in the immediate puerperium. Mothers with type 1 diabetes will likely require much less insulin for several days after birth. Because these normal hormonal changes make the puerperium a transitional period for carbohydrate metabolism, it is more difficult to interpret glucose tolerance tests.

Estrogen and progesterone levels drop markedly after expulsion of the placenta, and reach their lowest levels 1 week postpartum. Decreased estrogen levels are associated with breast engorgement and with the diuresis of excess extracellular fluid accumulated during pregnancy. In nonlactating women, estrogen levels begin to increase by 2 weeks after birth and by postpartum day 17 are higher than in women who breastfeed (Bowes & Katz, 2002).

Pituitary Hormones and Ovarian Function

Prolactin levels in blood rise progressively throughout pregnancy. In women who breastfeed, prolactin levels remain elevated (Liu, 2004). Serum prolactin levels are influenced by the frequency of breastfeeding, the duration of each feeding, and the degree to which supplementary feedings are used. Individual differences in the strength of an infant's sucking stimulus probably also affect prolactin levels. In nonlactating women, prolactin levels decline after birth and reach the prepregnant range in 3 to 4 weeks (Liu, 2004).

Lactating and nonlactating women differ considerably in the timing of their first ovulation and when menstruation resumes. The persistence of elevated serum prolactin levels in breastfeeding women appears to be responsible for suppressing ovulation. Because levels of follicle-stimulating hormone (FSH) have been shown to be identical in lactating and nonlactating women, it is thought that ovulation is suppressed in lactating women because the ovary does not respond to FSH stimulation when increased prolactin levels are present (Bowes & Katz, 2002).

Ovulation occurs as early as 27 days after birth in nonlactating women, with a mean time of about 10 weeks. About 70% of nonbreastfeeding women resume menstruating by 12 weeks after birth (Resnik, 2004). The mean time to ovulation in women who breastfeed is about 6 months (Bowes & Katz, 2002), although women who breastfeed for less than 28 days will ovulate at about the same time as women who do not breastfeed at all. In lactating women, both the resumption of ovulation and the return of menses are determined in large part by breastfeeding patterns. Menstruation during the first 6 weeks is anovulatory (Resnik, 2004); however, women may ovulate before their first postpartum menstrual period. Thus discussion of contraceptive options early in the puerperium is necessary.

The first menstrual flow after childbirth is usually heavier than normal. Within three or four cycles the amount of menstrual flow returns to the woman's prepregnancy volume.

Abdomen

When the woman stands during the first days after birth, her abdomen protrudes and gives her a still-pregnant appearance. During the first 2 weeks after birth the abdominal wall is relaxed. It takes about 6 weeks for the abdominal wall to return almost to its prepregnancy state. The skin regains most of its previous elasticity, but some striae may persist. The return of muscle tone depends on previous tone, proper exercise, and the amount of adipose tissue. Occasionally, with or without overdistention because of a large fetus or multiple fetuses, the abdominal wall muscles separate, a condition termed *diastasis recti abdominis* (see Fig. 10-11). Persistence of this separation may be disturbing to the woman, but surgical correction rarely is necessary. With time, the separation becomes less apparent.

Urinary System

The hormonal changes of pregnancy (i.e., high steroid levels) contribute to an increase in renal function; diminishing steroid levels after childbirth may partly explain the reduced renal function that occurs during the puerperium. Kidney function returns to normal within 1 month after birth. From 2 to 8 weeks are required for the pregnancy-induced hypotonia and dilation of the ureters and renal pelves to return to the nonpregnant state. Approximately 20% of women experience incomplete emptying of the bladder; dilation of the urinary tract may persist for 3 months or longer (Resnik, 2004), increasing the chances of developing a urinary tract infection.

Urine Components

The renal glycosuria induced by pregnancy disappears, but lactosuria may occur in lactating women. The blood urea nitrogen (BUN) increases during the puerperium as autolysis of the involuting uterus occurs. This breakdown of excess protein in the uterine muscle cells also results in a mild (+1) proteinuria for 1 to 2 days after childbirth in approximately 50% of women (Simpson & Creehan, 2001). Ketonuria may occur in women with an uncomplicated birth or after a prolonged labor with dehydration.

Postpartal Diuresis

Within 12 hours of birth, women begin to lose excess tissue fluid accumulated during pregnancy. Profuse diaphoresis often occurs, especially at night, for the first 2 or 3 days after childbirth. Postpartal diuresis, caused by decreased estrogen levels, removal of increased venous pressure in the lower extremities, and loss of the remaining pregnancy-induced increase in blood volume, also aids the body to rid itself of excess fluid. Fluid loss through perspiration and increased urinary output accounts for a weight loss of approximately 2.25 kg during the puerperium. This elimination of excess fluid accumulated during pregnancy is sometimes referred to as reversal of the water metabolism of pregnancy.

Urethra and Bladder

Trauma to the urethra and bladder may occur during the birth process as the infant passes through the pelvis, so the bladder wall may be hyperemic and edematous, often with small areas of hemorrhage. Clean-catch or catheterized urine specimens after birth often reveal hematuria from bladder trauma. The urethra and urinary meatus also may be edematous.

Birth-induced trauma, increased bladder capacity following childbirth, and the effects of conduction anesthesia combine to cause a decreased urge to void. In addition, pelvic soreness caused by the forces of labor, vaginal lacerations, or the episiotomy reduces or alters the voiding reflex. Decreased voiding combined with postpartal diuresis may result in bladder distention. Immediately after birth, excessive bleeding can occur if the bladder becomes distended because this pushes the uterus up and to the side and prevents the uterus from contracting firmly. Later in the puerperium, overdistention can make the bladder more susceptible to infection and impede the resumption of normal voiding (Resnik, 2004). With adequate emptying of the bladder, bladder tone is usually restored by 5 to 7 days after childbirth.

GASTROINTESTINAL SYSTEM

Appetite

The mother usually is hungry shortly after the birth and can tolerate a light diet. Most new mothers are very hungry after full recovery from analgesia, anesthesia, and fatigue. Requests for extra portions of food and frequent snacks are not uncommon.

Bowel Evacuation

A spontaneous bowel evacuation may not occur for 2 to 3 days after childbirth. This delay can be explained by decreased muscle tone in the intestines during labor and the immediate puerperium, prelabor diarrhea, lack of food, or dehydration. The mother often anticipates discomfort during the bowel movement because of perineal tenderness as a result of episiotomy, lacerations, or hemorrhoids and resists the urge to defecate. Regular bowel habits should be reestablished when bowel tone returns.

Operative vaginal birth (forceps or vacuum use) and anal sphincter lacerations are associated with an increased risk of postpartum anal incontinence. If it occurs, anal incontinence is often temporary and may resolve within 6 months (Bowes & Katz, 2002). Women should be taught during pregnancy about episiotomy and its possible sequelae. Pelvic floor (Kegel) exercises should be encouraged (see Chapter 4).

BREASTS

Promptly after birth, there is a decrease in the concentrations of hormones that stimulated breast development during pregnancy (i.e., estrogen, progesterone, human chorionic gonadotropin, prolactin, cortisol, and insulin). The time it takes for these hormones to return to prepregnancy levels is determined in part by whether the mother breastfeeds her infant.

Breastfeeding Mothers

As lactation is established, a mass (lump) may be felt in the breast. Unlike the lumps associated with fibrocystic breast disease or cancer, which may be consistently palpated in the same location, a filled milk sac shifts position from day to day. Before lactation begins, the breasts feel soft and a yellowish fluid, colostrum, can be expressed from the nipples. After lactation begins, the breasts feel warm and firm. Tenderness may persist for about 48 hours after the start of lactation. Bluish-white milk with a skim-milk appearance (true milk) can be expressed from the nipples. The nipples are examined for erectility and signs of irritation such as cracks, blisters, or reddening.

Nonbreastfeeding Mothers

The breasts generally feel nodular in contrast to the granular feel of breasts in nonpregnant women. The nodularity is bilateral and diffuse. Prolactin levels drop rapidly. Colostrum is present for the first few days after childbirth. Palpation of the breast on the second or third day, as milk production begins, may reveal tissue tenderness in some women. On the third or fourth postpartum day, engorgement may occur. The breasts are distended (swollen), firm, tender, and warm to the touch (because of vasocongestion). Breast distention is caused primarily by the temporary congestion of veins and lymphatics rather than by an accumulation of milk. Milk is present but should not be expressed. Axillary breast tissue (the tail of Spence) and any accessory breast or nipple tissue along the milk line also may be involved. Engorgement resolves spontaneously, and discomfort decreases usually within 24 to 36 hours. A breast binder or tight bra, ice packs, or mild analgesics may be used to relieve discomfort. Nipple stimulation is avoided. If suckling is never begun (or is discontinued), lactation ceases within a few days to a week.

CARDIOVASCULAR SYSTEM

Blood Volume

Changes in blood volume after birth depend on several factors such as blood loss during childbirth and the amount of extravascular water (physiologic edema) mobilized and excreted. Blood loss results in an immediate but limited decrease in total blood volume. Thereafter, most of the blood volume increase during pregnancy (1000 to 1500 ml) is eliminated within the

Evidence-Based Practice

TIMING OF FLUIDS AND FOOD AFTER CESAREAN BIRTH

Background

Health care is full of assumptions and traditions that do not necessarily stem from evidence. It has long been customary to withhold fluids and food after major abdominal surgery until bowel function returns, evidenced by bowel sounds and passing of flatus and stool. The concern is the occurrence of paralytic ileus, a loss of peristalsis, characterized by abdominal tenderness and distention, nausea and vomiting, and lack of bowel sounds. Some health care providers have a policy of limiting food and fluids to women after cesarean section, even if no handling of the bowel has occurred. Depending on the institution, fluids and food can be withheld up to 24 hours, followed by a transition day from clear to full liquids, and solids by the third day. This is in addition to the time that the woman has already been without food and fluids while in labor.

Critics of this policy find this starvation unnecessary because simple cesarean birth is not associated with bowel manipulation. Indeed, there is some evidence that bowel function continues even after major manipulation, but with altered bowel sounds. Paralytic ileus is thought to be multifactorial, caused by neural and hormonal factors involving the sympathetic and parasympathetic nervous systems, use of narcotics, and type of anesthesia. Some researchers have found that fluids are well-tolerated after cesarean birth, and should be provided unless the operation involved extensive bowel manipulation or sepsis. Some institutions even offer fluids within 90 minutes following birth, and, if well-tolerated, a regular diet soon thereafter.

Objective

Reviewers sought to clarify these different treatment alternatives and question the basis for delaying fluids and foods after cesarean section. They sought to review trials that compared early and delayed reintroduction of fluids and food after cesarean birth. Outcome measures included occurrence of nausea, vomiting, crampy abdominal pain, bloating, and abdominal distention; presence of bowel action on the third postoperative day; delayed return to bowel sounds and action; ketosis; blood sugar values; duration of intravenous fluids; breastfeeding success; women's satisfaction; fatigue; need for analgesia; ambulation; and time spent in the hospital.

Methods

Search Strategy

The reviewers searched the Cochrane Database, MEDLINE, and the journals summarized by ZETOC, the British Library Electronic Table of Contents. Search words were *oral feed, oral fluid, oral hydration, oral intake, eat, drink, food, cesar, Caesar,* and *cesarean section.* Reviewers included six randomized, controlled trials, published from 1993 to 2001. Information about total number of women or number of women per trial was not noted. Countries of origin also were not included in the review.

Statistical Analyses

Statistical analyses of outcomes with early reintroduction of oral fluids and solids (usually within 6 to 8 hours postoperatively) were compared with delayed administration of fluids and solids, as defined by the trial authors. The authors accepted differences between groups that exceeded the 95% confidence interval as significant.

Findings

Early administration of oral fluids was associated with decreased time to first solids, decreased time to bowel sounds, and decreased length of hospitalization in the subgroup that had regional analgesia. Early fluids also led to a trend toward decreased abdominal distention, but this was not significant.

There were no significant differences between early and delayed fluid administration in the following outcomes: nausea, vomiting, time to bowel action, time to passing flatus, paralytic ileus, and number of doses of analgesia taken postoperatively. No adverse outcomes were found with early postcesarean intake of fluids and food.

Limitations

Protocols for times for offering fluids varied. Some trials may have offered clear liquids, some slush, and some fluid and food. Timing of intake varied. Because neither the number of the study participants nor the total number of studies reviewed were reported, it is not possible to assess whether small sample size led to bias. No data were available on intravenous hydration, biochemical changes, patient satisfaction, hunger, fatigue, and breastfeeding.

Conclusions

There is no evidence from randomized trials to justify a policy of delaying fluids or food following uncomplicated cesarean section.

Implications for Practice

Nurses in settings where food and fluid are withheld after cesarean birth should work to change practice.

Implications for Further Research

The reviewers call for larger, well-designed trials. Further information is needed regarding the intake of fluids and food following complicated cesarean birth. It is unknown whether there are any differences in postoperative gastrointestinal recovery between planned and unplanned cesarean births.

Reference

Mangesi L, Hofmeyr G: Early compared with delayed oral fluids and food after caesarean section (Cochrane Review), 2002. In *The Cochrane Library,* Issue 1, Chichester, UK, 2005, John Wiley & Sons.

first 2 weeks after birth, with return to nonpregnancy values by 6 months postpartum (Simpson & Creehan, 2001).

Pregnancy-induced hypervolemia (an increase in blood volume of at least 35% over prepregnancy values near term) (Bowes & Katz, 2002) allows most women to tolerate considerable blood loss during childbirth. Many women lose approximately 500 ml of blood during vaginal birth of a single fetus, and about twice this much during cesarean birth (Resnik, 2004) (Critical Thinking Exercise).

Readjustments in the maternal vasculature after childbirth are dramatic and rapid. The woman's response to blood loss during the early puerperium differs from that in a nonpregnant woman. Three postpartal physiologic changes protect the woman from excessive blood loss: (1) elimination of uteroplacental circulation reduces the size of the maternal vascular bed by 10% to 15%; (2) loss of placental endocrine function removes the stimulus for vasodilation; and (3) mobilization of extravascular water stored during pregnancy increases blood volume. Thus hypovolemic shock usually does not occur in women who experience a normal blood loss during the puerperium.

Cardiac Output

Pulse rate, stroke volume, and cardiac output increase throughout pregnancy. Immediately after the birth, they re-

Critical Thinking Exercise

MATERNAL POSTPARTUM BLOOD LOSS AND FATIGUE

You are caring for four women on the postpartum unit, two of whom had vaginal births and two who had cesarean births. Each of the women has complained about feeling tired and has expressed concern about the amount of blood she lost during birth. Before providing patient education related to fatigue after birth and blood loss, you reviewed the nurses' notes, the intake and output records, and patient records for estimated blood loss and hemoglobin and hematocrit values.

1. Evidence—Is there sufficient evidence to draw conclusions about the relation between tiredness (fatigue) after birth and blood loss?
2. Assumptions—What assumptions can be made about the following factors?
   a. Comparison of amount of blood loss between women who give birth vaginally and by cesarean
   b. Postpartum norms for hematocrit and hemoglobin for women who give birth vaginally and by cesarean
   c. Causes of fatigue after birth
   d. Interventions to alleviate fatigue and replace blood lost at birth
3. What implications and priorities for nursing care can be drawn at this time?
4. Does the evidence objectively support your conclusion?
5. Are there alternative perspectives to your conclusion?

main elevated or rise even higher for 30 to 60 minutes as the blood that was shunted through the uteroplacental circuit suddenly returns to the maternal systemic venous circulation (Bowes & Katz, 2002). Cardiac output remains increased for at least 48 hours after birth. The cardiac output decreases by almost 30% by 2 weeks postpartum. Stroke volume, cardiac output, end-diastolic volume, and systemic vascular resistance remain elevated for 12 weeks postpartum, and left ventricular volume and cardiac output remain elevated for 1 year postpartum (Resnik, 2004).

Vital Signs

Few alterations in vital signs are seen under normal circumstances. There may be a small, transient rise in both systolic and diastolic blood pressure that lasts approximately 4 days after the birth (Table 20-2). Respiratory function returns to nonpregnant levels by 6 to 8 weeks after birth. After the uterus is emptied, the diaphragm descends, the normal cardiac axis is restored, and the point of maximal impulse (PMI) and the electrocardiogram (ECG) are normalized.

Blood Components

Hematocrit and Hemoglobin

During the first 72 hours after childbirth, there is a greater loss of plasma volume than in the number of blood cells. This results in an increase in hematocrit and hemoglobin levels by the seventh day after birth. There is no increased red blood cell (RBC) destruction during the puerperium, but any excess will disappear gradually in accordance with the life span of the RBC. The exact time at which RBC volume returns to prepregnancy values is not known, but it is within normal limits when measured 8 weeks after childbirth (Bowes & Katz, 2002).

White Blood Cell Count

Normal leukocytosis of pregnancy averages approximately 12,000/mm^3. During the first 10 to 12 days after childbirth, values between 20,000 and 25,000/mm^3 are common. Neutrophils are the most numerous white blood cells (WBCs). Leukocytosis, coupled with the normal increase in erythrocyte sedimentation rate that occurs, may obscure the diagnosis of acute infections at this time.

Coagulation Factors

Clotting factors and fibrinogen are normally increased during pregnancy and remain elevated in the immediate puerperium. When combined with vessel damage and immobility, this hypercoagulable state causes an increased risk of thromboembolism (blood clots), especially after a cesarean birth. Fibrinolytic activity also increases during the first few days after childbirth (Bowes & Katz, 2002). Levels of factors I, II, VIII, IX, and X decrease within a few days to nonpregnant levels. Fibrin split products, probably released from the placental site, can also be found in maternal blood.

Varicosities

Varicosities (varices) of the legs and around the anus (hemorrhoids) are common during pregnancy. Varices, even the less common vulvar varices, regress (empty) rapidly immediately after childbirth. Total or nearly total regression of varicosities is expected after childbirth.

NEUROLOGIC SYSTEM

Neurologic changes during the puerperium are those that result from a reversal of maternal adaptations to pregnancy and those resulting from trauma during labor and childbirth.

Pregnancy-induced neurologic discomforts abate after birth. Elimination of physiologic edema through the diuresis that follows childbirth relieves carpal tunnel syndrome by easing compression of the median nerve. The periodic numbness and tingling of fingers that afflict 5% of pregnant women usually disappear after the birth, unless lifting and carrying the baby aggravates the condition. Headache requires careful assessment. Postpartum headaches may be caused by various conditions, including gestational hypertension, stress, and leakage of cerebrospinal fluid into the extradural space during placement of the needle for administration of epidural or spinal anesthesia. Headaches last from 1 to 3 days to several weeks, depending on the cause and effectiveness of the treatment.

MUSCULOSKELETAL SYSTEM

Adaptations of the mother's musculoskeletal system that occur during pregnancy are reversed in the puerperium. These adaptations include the relaxation and subsequent hypermobility of the joints and the change in the mother's center of gravity in response to the enlarging uterus. The joints are completely stabilized by 6 to 8 weeks after birth. However, although all other joints return to their normal prepregnancy state, those in the parous woman's feet do not. The new mother may notice a permanent increase in her shoe size.

Table 20-2

Vital Signs after Childbirth

NORMAL FINDINGS	DEVIATIONS FROM NORMAL FINDINGS AND PROBABLE CAUSES
TEMPERATURE	
During first 24 hours may increase to 38° C as a result of dehydrating effects of labor. After 24 hours, the woman should be afebrile.	A diagnosis of puerperal sepsis is suggested if an increase in maternal temperature to 38° C is noted after the first 24 hours after childbirth and recurs or persists for 2 days. Other possibilities are mastitis, endometritis, urinary tract infections, and other systemic infections.
PULSE	
Pulse, along with stroke volume and cardiac output, remains elevated for the first hour or so after childbirth. It then begins to decrease at an unknown rate. By 8 to 10 weeks after childbirth, the pulse has returned to a nonpregnant rate.	A rapid pulse rate or one that is increasing may indicate hypovolemia as a result of hemorrhage.
RESPIRATIONS	
The respiratory rate should decrease to within the woman's normal prebirth range by 6 to 8 weeks after childbirth.	Hypoventilation may occur after an unusually high subarachnoid (spinal) block or epidural narcotic after a cesarean birth.
BLOOD PRESSURE	
Blood pressure is altered slightly if at all. Orthostatic hypotension, as indicated by feelings of faintness or dizziness immediately after standing up, can develop in the first 48 hours as a result of the splanchnic engorgement that may occur after birth.	A low or decreasing blood pressure may indicate the existence of hypovolemia secondary to hemorrhage; however, it is a late sign, and other symptoms of hemorrhage usually alert the staff. An increased reading may result from excessive use of vasopressor or oxytocic medications. Because gestational hypertension can persist into or occur first in the postpartum period, routine evaluation of blood pressure is needed. If a woman complains of headache, hypertension must be ruled out as a cause before analgesics are administered.

INTEGUMENTARY SYSTEM

Chloasma of pregnancy usually disappears at the end of pregnancy. Hyperpigmentation of the areolae and linea nigra may not regress completely after childbirth. Some women will have permanent darker pigmentation of those areas. Striae gravidarum (stretch marks) on the breasts, abdomen, and thighs may fade but usually do not disappear.

Vascular abnormalities such as spider angiomas (nevi), palmar erythema, and epulis generally regress in response to the rapid decline in estrogens after the end of pregnancy. For some woman, spider nevi persist indefinitely.

Hair growth slows during the postpartum period. Some women may experience hair loss because the amount of hair lost is temporarily more than the amount regrown. The abundance of fine hair seen during pregnancy usually disappears after giving birth; however, any coarse or bristly hair that appears during pregnancy usually remains. Fingernails return to their prepregnancy consistency and strength.

Profuse diaphoresis that occurs in the immediate postpartum period is the most noticeable change in the integumentary system.

IMMUNE SYSTEM

No significant changes in the maternal immune system occur during the postpartum period. The mother's need for a rubella vaccination or for Rh_o (D) immune globulin for prevention of Rh isoimmunization is determined.

Key Points

- Postpartum physiologic changes allow the woman to tolerate considerable blood loss at birth.
- The uterus involutes rapidly after birth and returns to the true pelvis within 2 weeks.
- The rapid decrease in estrogen and progesterone levels after expulsion of the placenta is responsible for triggering many of the anatomic and physiologic changes in the puerperium.
- Assessment of lochia and fundal height is essential to monitor the progress of normal involution and to identify potential problems.
- The time it takes for the hormones that stimulated breast development during pregnancy to return to prepregnancy levels is determined in part by whether the woman breastfeeds her infant.
- Few alterations in vital signs are seen after birth under normal circumstances.
- Activation of blood clotting factors, immobility, and sepsis predispose the woman to thromboembolism.
- Marked diuresis, decreased bladder sensitivity, and overdistention of the bladder can lead to problems with urinary elimination.

Answer Guidelines to Critical Thinking Exercise

Maternal Postpartum Blood Loss and Fatigue

1. Yes, there is evidence of a relationship between tiredness (fatigue) after birth and blood loss. There is an increase in blood loss with an upright position for birth (Gupta & Hofmeyr, 2005). The most common cause of excessive blood loss is uterine atony. Excessive blood loss may also occur in association with placenta previa or abruptio placentae, vaginal or vulvar hematomas, unrepaired lacerations of the vagina or cervix, and retained placental fragments. Active management of the third stage of labor reduces postpartum hemorrhage (Chong, Su, & Arulkumaran, 2004). Factors affecting fatigue after childbirth include length of labor, type of birth, maternal age (Troy & Dalgas-Pelish, 1997), adequacy of sleep (Gay, Lee, & Lee, 2004), type of infant feeding, and anemia. However, effects of anemia may not be felt immediately after birth.
2. (a) Blood volume increases 1000 to 1500 ml during pregnancy. Postpartum hemorrhage (PPH) is difficult to define. Normal blood loss is up to 500 ml after vaginal birth and up to 1000 ml after cesarean birth. Blood loss greater than these amounts or a decrease of 10% in hematocrit from the time of admission for labor to postpartum has been used to define PPH. Close monitoring of lochial flow is important in the postpartum period. The amount of blood loss is commonly underestimated; accurate measurement of amount of blood loss is important (Strand, da Silva, & Bergstrom, 2003). (b) Hemoglobin may decrease to 11 g/dl and hematocrit to 33% during pregnancy. Values return to normal by 6 weeks postpartum. Women who take iron supplements during pregnancy maintain higher hemoglobin and hematocrit values than do those who do not. With cesarean birth and greater blood loss, there is the potential for lower values in the postpartum period. Continued iron supplementation and good nutrition are important to regaining appropriate values. (c) Older mothers, those with a longer length of labor, and those who give cesarean birth are more likely to be fatigued. Breastfeeding, inadequate sleep during the night, anemia, and poor nutrition are additional causes of fatigue after birth. (d) Interventions to alleviate fatigue and replace blood lost at birth include provision for adequate rest and sleep, iron supplementation, good nutrition, adequate fluids, assistance with self- and infant care, and adequate emotional support. If the blood loss was excessive, blood replacement may be necessary.
3. Priorities for nursing care include reviewing the medical records of the women, noting the estimated blood loss during birth, amount of lochia since birth, fundal tone, intake and output, method of infant feeding, amount of sleep and rest, and family support. Laboratory values should be examined. Patient teaching can be done using an individualized plan based on the information gathered.
4. There is evidence of factors affecting blood loss and fatigue. These factors can be related to the information obtained from a review of the medical records to individualize application of the evidence.
5. Fatigue can be related to depression (Bozoky & Corwin, 2002). Nursing assessment should include evidence of postpartum blues and depression. Infection may be associated with anemia and may cause fatigue. Close monitoring of vital signs and evidence of infection are important.

References to Answer Guidelines

Bozoky I, Corwin EJ: Fatigue as a predictor of postpartum depression, *J Obstet Gynecol Neonatal Nurs* 31(4):436-443, 2002.

Chong YS, Su LL, Arulkumaran S: Current strategies for the prevention of postpartum haemorrhage in the third stage of labour, *Curr Opin Obstet Gynecol* 16(2):143-150, 2004.

Gay CL, Lee KA, Lee SY: Sleep patterns and fatigue in new mothers and fathers, *Biol Res Nurs* 5(4):311-318, 2004.

Gupta JK, Hofmeyr GJ: Position in the second stage of labour for women without epidural anaesthesia (Cochrane Review), 2003. In *The Cochrane Library,* Issue 1, Chichester, UK, 2005, John Wiley & Sons.

Strand RT, da Silva F, Bergstrom S: Use of cholera beds in the delivery room: a simple and appropriate method for direct measurement of postpartum bleeding, *Trop Doct* 33(4):215-216, 2003.

Troy NW, Dalgas-Pelish P: The natural evolution of postpartum fatigue among a group of primiparous women, *Clin Nurs Res* 6(2):126-139; discussion 139-141, 1997.

Resources

American College of Nurse-Midwives (ACNM)
818 Connecticut Ave., NW, Suite 900
Washington, DC 20006
202-728-9860
www.midwife.org

American College of Obstetricians and Gynecologists (ACOG)
409 12th St., SW
Washington, DC 20024
800-762-2264
www.acog.org

Association of Women's Health, Obstetric, and Neonatal Nurses (AWHONN)
200 L St., NW, Suite 740
Washington, DC 20036
800-673-8499 (US)
800-245-0231 (Canada)
www.awhonn.org

Coping with the Overall Pregnancy Experience (COPE)
37 Clarendon St.
Boston, MA 02116
617-357-5588

Maternity Center Association, Inc
281 Park Ave., South, 5th Floor
New York, NY 10010
212-777-5000

References

Bowes W, Katz V: Postpartum care. In Gabbe SG, Niebyl JR, Simpson JL (eds): *Obstetrics: normal and problem pregnancies,* ed 4, New York, 2002, Churchill Livingstone.

Liu JH: Endocrinology of pregnancy. In Creasy RK, Resnik R, Iams JD (eds): *Maternal-fetal medicine: principles and practice,* ed 5, Philadelphia, 2004, Saunders.

Mangesi L, Hofmeyr G: Early compared with delayed oral fluids and food after caesarean section (Cochrane Review), 2002. In *The Cochrane Library,* Issue 2, Chichester, UK, 2004, John Wiley & Sons.

Resnik R: The puerperium. In Creasy RK, Resnik R, Iams JD (eds): *Maternal-fetal medicine: principles and practice,* ed 5, Philadelphia, 2004, Saunders.

Simpson KR, Creehan PA: *AWHONN's perinatal nursing,* ed 2, Philadelphia, 2001, JB Lippincott.

Nursing Care during the Fourth Trimester

21

LEARNING OBJECTIVES

On completion of this chapter the reader will be able to:

- Identify the priorities of maternal care given during the fourth stage of labor.
- Identify common selection criteria for safe early postpartum discharge.
- Summarize nursing interventions to prevent infection and excessive bleeding; to promote normal bladder and bowel patterns; and to care for the breasts of women who are breastfeeding or bottle-feeding.
- Explain the influence of cultural expectations on postpartum adjustment.
- Discuss discharge teaching and postpartum care.
- Describe the nurse's role in these postpartum follow-up strategies: home visits, telephone follow-up, warm lines and help lines, support groups, and referrals to community resources.

ELECTRONIC RESOURCES

Additional information related to the content in Chapter 21 can be found on

the companion website at evolve
http://evolve.elsevier.com/Wong/maternal/
- NCLEX Review Questions
- Case Study–Fourth Trimester
- WebLinks

or the interactive student CD-ROM
Activities for Chapter 21 include the following:
- NCLEX Review Questions
- Case Study–Fourth Trimester
- Critical Thinking Exercise–Priority Nursing Care: Postpartum Unit
- Nursing Care Plan–Postpartum Care: Vaginal Birth

The goal of nursing care in the immediate postpartum period is to assist women and their partners during their initial transition to parenting. The approach to the care of women after birth is wellness oriented. Consequently, in the United States most women remain hospitalized no more than 1 or 2 days after giving birth, and some for as few as 6 hours. Because there is so much important information to be shared with these women in a very short time, it is vital that their care be thoughtfully planned and provided. Care is focused on the woman's physiologic recovery, her psychologic well-being, and her ability to care for herself and her new baby. In addition, the nurse considers the needs of other family members and includes strategies in the plan of care to assist the family in adjusting to the new baby.

FOURTH STAGE OF LABOR

The first 1 to 2 hours after birth, sometimes called the fourth stage of labor, is a crucial time for mother and newborn. Both are not only recovering from the physical process of birth but also are becoming acquainted with each other and additional family members. During this time, maternal organs undergo their initial readjustment to the nonpregnant state, and the functions of body systems begin to stabilize. Meanwhile, the newborn continues the transition from intrauterine to extrauterine existence.

The fourth stage of labor is an excellent time to begin breastfeeding because the infant is in an alert state and ready to nurse. Breastfeeding at this time also aids in the contraction of the uterus and the prevention of maternal hemorrhage. In most centers, the mother remains in the labor and birth area during this recovery time. In an institution where labor, delivery, and recovery (LDR) rooms are used, the woman stays in the same room where she gave birth. In traditional settings, women are taken from the delivery room to a separate recovery area for observation. Arrangements for care of the newborn vary during the fourth stage of labor. In many settings, the baby remains at the mother's bedside, and the labor or birth nurse cares for both of them. In other institutions the baby is taken to the nursery for several hours of observation after an initial bonding period with the parents (Fig. 21-1).

Assessment

If the recovery nurse has not previously cared for the new mother, her assessment begins with an oral report from the nurse who attended the woman during labor and birth and

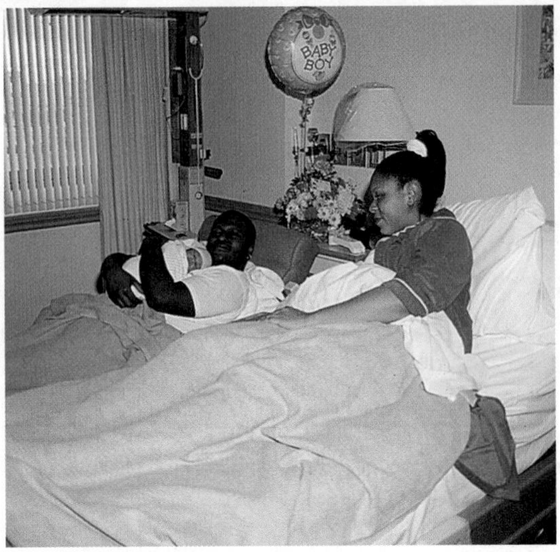

Fig. 21-1 Bonding and attachment begun early after birth are fostered in the postpartum period. (Courtesy Marjorie Pyle, RNC, Lifecircle, Costa Mesa, CA.)

a review of the prenatal, labor, and birth records. Of primary importance are conditions that could predispose the mother to hemorrhage, such as precipitous labor, large baby, grand multiparity (having given birth many times), or induced labor. For healthy women, hemorrhage is probably the most dangerous potential complication.

During the first hour in the recovery room, physical assessments of the mother are frequent. All factors except temperature are assessed every 15 minutes for 1 hour. Temperature is assessed at the beginning and end of the recovery period. After the fourth 15-minute assessment, if all parameters have stabilized within the normal range, assessments are continued every 30 minutes in the second hour. Box 21-1 and Fig. 21-2 describe the physical assessment of the mother during the fourth stage of labor. Fig. 21-3 demonstrates an easy-to-use flow sheet that combines the essential immediate postpartum and anesthesia recovery assessments.

evolve CASE STUDY—FOURTH TRIMESTER

During the fourth stage of labor, many women experience intense tremors that resemble shivering from a chill. They are commonly seen and are not related to infection. Several theories have been offered to explain these tremors or shivering, such as their being the result of a sudden release of pressure on pelvic nerves after birth, a response to a fetus-to-mother transfusion that occurred during placental separation, a reaction to maternal adrenaline production during labor and birth, or a reaction to epidural anesthesia. Warm blankets and reassurance that the chills or tremors are common, self-limiting, and last only a short while are useful interventions.

The nutritional status of the woman is assessed. Restriction of food and fluid intake and the loss of fluids (blood, perspiration, or emesis) during labor cause many women to express a strong desire to eat or drink soon after birth. In the absence of complications, a woman who has given birth vaginally, has recovered from the effects of the anesthetic

BOX 21-1

Assessment during Fourth Stage of Labor

Before beginning the assessment, wash hands thoroughly, assemble necessary equipment, and explain the procedure to the patient.

Blood Pressure

Measure blood pressure per assessment schedule.

Pulse

Assess rate and regularity.

Temperature

Determine temperature.

Fundus

Put on clean examination gloves.

Position woman with knees flexed and head flat.

Just below umbilicus, cup hand and press firmly into abdomen. At the same time, stabilize the uterus at the symphysis with the opposite hand.

If fundus is firm (and bladder is empty), with uterus in midline, measure its position relative to woman's umbilicus. Lay fingers flat on abdomen under umbilicus; measure how many fingerbreadths (fb) or centimeters (cm) fit between umbilicus and top of fundus. If the fundus is above the umbilicus, this is recorded as plus fb or cm; if below, as minus fb or cm.

If fundus is not firm, massage it gently to contract and expel any clots before measuring distance from umbilicus.

Place hands appropriately; massage gently only until firm.

Expel clots while keeping hands placed as in Fig. 21-2. With upper hand, firmly apply pressure downward toward vagina; observe perineum for amount and size of expelled clots.

Bladder

Assess distention by noting location and firmness of uterine fundus and by observing and palpating bladder. Distended bladder is seen as a suprapubic rounded bulge that is dull to percussion and fluctuates like a water-filled balloon. When the bladder is distended, the uterus is usually boggy in consistency, well above the umbilicus, and to the woman's right side.

Assist woman to void spontaneously. Measure amount of urine voided.

Catheterize as necessary.

Reassess after voiding or catheterization to make sure the bladder is not palpable and the fundus is firm and in the midline.

Lochia

Observe lochia on perineal pads and on linen under the mother's buttocks. Determine amount and color; note size and number of clots; note odor.

Observe perineum for source of bleeding (e.g., episiotomy, lacerations).

Perineum

Ask or assist woman to turn on her side and flex upper leg on hip.

Lift upper buttock.

Observe perineum in good lighting.

Assess episiotomy site or laceration repair for intactness, hematoma, edema, bruising, redness, and drainage.

Assess for presence of hemorrhoids.

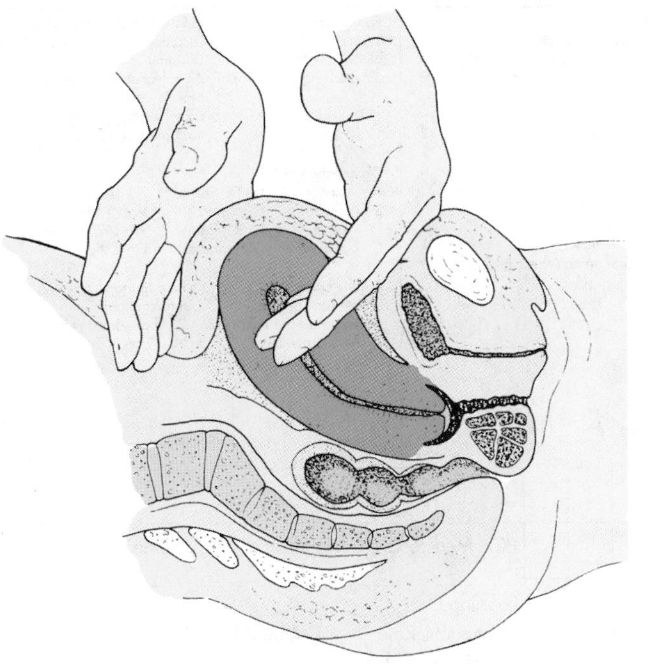

Fig. 21-2 Palpating fundus of uterus during the fourth stage of labor. Note that upper hand is cupped over fundus; lower hand dips in above symphysis pubis and supports uterus while it is massaged gently.

and has stable vital signs, a firm uterus, and small to moderate lochial flow may have fluids and a regular diet as desired.

Postanesthesia Recovery

The woman who has given birth by cesarean or who has received regional anesthesia for a vaginal birth requires special attention during the recovery period. Obstetric recovery areas are held to the same standard of care that would be expected of any other postanesthesia recovery room. A recovery from anesthesia requires the nurse to have available cardiopulmonary support and emergency supplies. A postanesthesia recovery (PAR) score is determined for each patient on her arrival and is updated as part of every 15-minute assessment. Components of the PAR score include activity, respirations, blood pressure, level of consciousness, and color.

CASE STUDY—FOURTH TRIMESTER

NURSE ALERT Regardless of her obstetric status, no woman should be discharged from the recovery area until she has completely recovered from the effects of anesthesia. ■

If the woman received general anesthesia, she should be awake and alert and oriented to time, place, and person. Her respiratory rate should be within normal limits, and her oxygen saturation levels at least 95%, as measured by a pulse oximeter. If the woman received epidural or spinal anesthesia, she should be able to raise her legs, extended at the knees, off the bed; or to flex her knees, place her feet flat on the bed, and raise her buttocks well off the bed. The numb or tingling, prickly sensation should be entirely gone from her legs. Women vary greatly in regard to length of time required to recover from regional anesthesia. Often it takes several hours for these anesthetic effects to disappear.

Transfer from the Recovery Area

After the initial recovery period has been completed, the woman may be transferred to a postpartum room in the same or another nursing unit. In facilities with labor, delivery, recovery, postpartum (LDRP) rooms, the woman stays in the same room, and the nurse who provides care during the recovery period usually continues caring for the woman. Women who have received general or regional anesthesia must be cleared for transfer from the recovery area by a member of the anesthesia care team.

CRITICAL THINKING EXERCISE—PRIORITY NURSING CARE: POSTPARTUM UNIT

In preparing the transfer report, the recovery nurse uses information from the records of admission, birth record, and recovery. Information usually communicated to the postpartum nurse includes identity of the health care provider; gravidity and parity; age; anesthetic used; any medications given; duration of labor and time of rupture of membranes; oxytocin induction or augmentation; type of birth and repair; blood type and Rh status; group B streptococcus (GBS) status; status of rubella immunity; syphilis and hepatitis serology test results (if positive); intravenous infusion of any fluids; physiologic status since birth; description of fundus, lochia, bladder, and perineum; sex and weight of infant; time of birth; pediatrician; chosen method of feeding; any abnormalities noted; and assessment of initial parent-infant interaction.

Most of this information is also documented for the nursing staff in the newborn nursery. In addition, specific information should be provided regarding the infant's Apgar scores, weight, voiding, stooling, and whether fed since birth. Nursing interventions that have been completed (e.g., eye prophylaxis and vitamin K injection) also must be recorded. Table 21-1 gives examples for documenting this information before the transfer of the woman from the recovery area.

Women who give birth in birthing centers may go home within a few hours, after the woman's and infant's conditions are stable.

DISCHARGE—BEFORE 24 HOURS AND AFTER 48 HOURS

Early postpartum discharge, shortened hospital stays, and 1-day maternity stays are all terms for the decreasing length of hospital stays of mothers and their babies after a low risk birth. The trend of shortened hospital stays (24 hours or less for a woman who had an uncomplicated vaginal birth and about 72 hours for a woman who had an uncomplicated cesarean birth) is based largely on efforts to reduce health care costs, coupled with consumer demands to have less medical intervention and more family-focused experiences (Box 21-2).

Laws Relating to Discharge

Health care providers expressed concern with shortened stays because some medical problems do not show up in the first 24 hours after birth, and new mothers may not have had sufficient time to learn to care for their newborns and identify newborn health problems such as jaundice and dehydration related to breastfeeding difficulties. The first day after birth is not a time conducive to learning for many

DIAGNOSIS: ____________________
PHYSICIAN: ____________________
ANESTHESIA: ____________________
ANESTHETIST: ____________________
ARMBANDS: __________ mother __________ infant
CLOTHING: __________ c̄ family __________ c̄ patient
ALLERGIES: ____________________

PAR SCORE: ADM: DC:

ACTIVITY					
RESPIRATION					
BLOOD PRESSURE					
CONSCIOUS LEVEL					
COLOR					
TOTAL					

Activity	
Able to move 4 extremities voluntarily or on command	2
Able to move 2 extremities voluntarily or on command	1
Able to move 0 extremities voluntarily or on command	0
Respiration	
Able to deep breathe and cough freely	2
Dyspnea or limited breathing	1
Apneic	0
Blood Pressure	
BP ± mm Hg of preanesthetic level	2
BP ± 25-50 mm Hg of preanesthetic level	1
BP ± Greater than 50 mm HG of preanesthetic level	0
Conscious Level	
Fully aware	2
Arousable on calling	1
Not responding	0
Color	
Pink	2
Pale, dusky, blotchy, jaundiced, other	1
Cyanotic	0

Pain Scales
Wong Baker = WB
Numeric = N
Simple Descriptive = SD

Pain Characteristics
Location
Duration
Aggravating/Alleviating fx
Nature - dull, gnawing, hot, achy, sharp, burning, throbbing, shooting, stabbing

Observation Codes
A - Anxious D - Depressed H - Relaxed
B - Agitated, Restless E - Crying V - VS Charge
C - Confused R - Restless W - Withdrawn
G - Grimace O - Other

Results Code
0 - No pain present
1 - Improved but still in pain
2 - No improvement

Pain Management Intervention
P - Pharmacological
NP - Non pharmacological

VITAL SIGNS:													
	TIME												
	BP												
	PULSE												
	RESP / O_2 Sat												
	TEMP												
FUNDUS FB-FINGERBREADTH B-BOGGY FM-FIRM MD-MIDLINE	FUNDUS												
LOCHIA CL-CLOTS MOD-MODERATE SM-SMALL LG-LARGE	LOCHIA												
BLADDER D-DISTENDED F-FOLEY ND-NON-DISTENDED	BLADDER												
EPISIOTOMY/INCISION NL-NORMAL D-DRY ABNL-ABNORMAL I-INTACT	EPIS / INC												
CLEAR CL WHEEZING W DIMINISHED	BREATH SOUNDS												
q 1° / q Shift	DTR / PROTEIN												
O_2 liters/min													
JP drain ml/hr													
INTAKE													
OUTPUT													
Pain Scale													
Observation Code													
Pain Management Intervention													
Results Code													
INITIALS													

PCA

PCA Medication, Concentration and Volume
____
Loading Dose ________
Continuous Rate ______ 4 hour limit ________
Lockout Interval ____________
RN ____________ RN ____________
____/____/____ ____:____ am / pm

Meds / IV / Rate	Time / Initial
	/
	/
	/
	/

INTAKE TOTAL
Shift 7A 3P 11P

OUTPUT TOTAL
Shift 7A 3P 11P

IV ______ml LTC
@ D/C

Homans' Sign Pos☐ Neg☐

BONDING
☐ appropriate
☐ inappropriate
☐ NA (explain)

Social Services Notified
___/___/___
___:___ am/pm

TEACHING
☐ fundal massage
☐ TC & DB
☐ breast feeding
☐ assistance on 1st ambulation
☐ pain scale
☐ PCA pump

Signatures/Initials
____

DISCHARGE NOTE

Report Called To: ____________________
ANESTHESIA D/C:
EPIDURAL CATHETER: IN OUT NA

THE MED **Regional Medical Center at Memphis**
MATERNITY RECOVERY ROOM RECORD
FORM NO. 68622 (10/01) White (Chart) Yellow (Pharmacy)

Fig. 21-3 An example of a maternity recovery room record. (Courtesy The Regional Medical Center at Memphis [The Med], Memphis, TN.)

Table 21-1

Recovery Nurse's Report

ITEM	EXAMPLE OF DOCUMENTATION OF MOTHER	EXAMPLE OF DOCUMENTATION OF NEWBORN
Type of labor and birth; unusual observations, if any, of the placenta	Spontaneous or assisted (forceps, vacuum extraction) vaginal birth; vertex presentation; time of ROM	Spontaneous or assisted (forceps) vaginal birth; vertex presentation; time of ROM
Gravidity and parity, age	G1, P1, age 22 yr; 39 wk of gestation	G1, P1, age 22 yr; 39 wk of gestation
Anesthesia and analgesia used	None; epidural, low spinal, local	None; epidural, low spinal, local
Condition of perineum	Episiotomy; repair of lacerations; intact	
Events since birth	Vital signs, BP, fundus, lochia, intake and output, medications (dosage, time of administration, and results), response to newborn, observation of family interactions, including siblings, if present	Vital signs, blood glucose level (if assessed), nursed at breast for ____ min Voided ×1; meconium stool ×1 Eye prophylaxis given Vitamin K injection given Held by siblings who are happy (or have other response to newborn)
Condition and sex of newborn; other information	Time of birth; weight; whether breastfeeding or bottle-feeding; sex of the baby	Time of birth; Apgar at 1 and 5 min; Sex; weight; name of pediatrician; breastfeeding or bottle feeding; mother's hepatitis B status and GBS status; whether mother received magnesium sulfate; time of last systemic analgesia
Relevant information from prenatal record	Need for rubella vaccination; presence of infections; hepatitis B status; HIV status; blood type; Rh status; GBS status and treatment if positive	Unremarkable pregnancy
Miscellaneous information: IV drip	If IV drip is infusing, rate of infusion, medications added (e.g., oxytocin [Pitocin]), whether to keep open or discontinue after completion of bag that is hung	
Social factors	If woman is releasing baby for adoption, whether she wants to see baby, breastfeed, allow visitors, or other preferences she may have	Baby up for adoption; to stay in NBN until discharge

BP, blood pressure; *GBS*, group B streptococcus; *HIV*, human immunodeficiency virus; *NBN*, newborn nursery; *ROM*, rupture of membranes.

BOX 21-2

Advantages and Disadvantages of Early Postpartum Discharge

Advantages

- Reinforces the concept of childbirth as a normal physiologic event.
- Allows shorter separations between mothers and other children.
- Extends a couple's sense of control and participation beyond the birth itself.
- Capitalizes on the security of the home environment during the stressors of early parenting.
- Decreases unnecessary exposure to the pathogens in the hospital environment.
- Allows beds on the maternity service to be used more effectively (i.e., quick turnover in patients or greater availability for patients with a complication).
- Allows more time for mother/father/partner/infant and other family members to bond (see Fig. 21-1).
- Creates less disruption in the daily life of the family.
- Promotes active involvement of family and support persons in assisting the mother and newborn.

Disadvantages

- Complications (maternal or newborn) may go unrecognized.
- Families may be or feel unprepared for the reality they face once the baby is at home.
- The mother is fatigued from the labor and childbirth process.
- The mother is experiencing postpartum pain or discomfort.
- The length of time for learning after the birth in the hospital setting is decreased.
- A vulnerability and crisis potential exists for both women and families.

women. There was also concern that shortened hospital stays would increase maternal hospital readmission for infection, hypertension, and hemorrhage in women who gave birth vaginally.

The widespread concern for the potential increase in adverse maternal-infant outcomes from hospital early discharge practices led the American College of Obstetricians and Gynecologists, the American Academy of Pediatrics, and other professional health care organizations to promote the enactment of federal and various state maternity length-of-stay bills to ensure adequate care for both the mother and the newborn. The passage of the Newborns' and Mothers' Health Protection Act of 1996 provided minimum federal standards for health plan coverage for mothers and their newborns (Ferguson & Engelhard, 1997). Under the Act, all health plans are required to allow the new mother and newborn to remain in the hospital for a minimum of 48 hours after a normal vaginal birth and for 96 hours after a cesarean birth, unless the attending provider, in consultation with the mother, decides upon early discharge.

Research studies to determine the appropriate length of hospital stay for newborns seem to support this legislation. Newborns discharged early (less than 30 hours after birth) were more likely to be rehospitalized for jaundice, dehydration, and infection within 1 month of life than were newborns discharged later (30 to 72 hours after birth) (Liu et al, 1997). Edmonson, Stoddard, and Owens (1997) concluded that readmission was more likely among babies who were firstborn, breastfed, or born to unmarried and poorly educated women. Several early postpartum hospital discharge programs that provided extensive prenatal preparation and postpartum follow-up found it generally safe for mothers who gave birth vaginally and their newborns to be discharged less than 48 hours after birth (Fishbein & Burggraf, 1998; Williams & Cooper, 1996).

The protest against early discharge becomes more powerful in the conventional health care arena in which care does not include a home care visit and there is a long interval between discharge and the first follow-up examination.

Criteria for Discharge

Early discharge and postpartum home care can be a safe and satisfying option for women and their families when it is comprehensive and based on individual needs. However, early discharge is not appropriate for every mother and newborn. Hospital stays need to be long enough to identify problems and to ensure that the woman is sufficiently recovered and prepared to care for herself and the baby at home.

It is essential that nurses consider the medical needs of the woman and her baby and provide care that is coordinated to meet those needs in order to provide timely physiologic interventions and treatment to prevent morbidity and hospital readmission. With predetermined criteria for identifying low risk in the mothers and newborns (Box 21-3), the length of hospitalization can be based on medical need for care in an acute care setting or in consideration of the ongoing care needed in the home environment.

Length of stay is related to sociodemographic variables and readiness for discharge, both clinical and perceived. Earlier discharge is associated with younger age, multiparity, public payer source, low socioeconomic status (SES), bottle-feeding, and absence of a neonatal clinical problem (Weiss et al, 2004). Mothers' perceptions of their readiness for discharge should be considered in discharge planning.

Care paths provide the nurse with an organized approach toward meeting essential maternal-newborn care and teaching goals within a limited time frame (Table 21-2). Care paths can be developed for vaginal or cesarean births. Other methods such as postpartum order sets and maternal-newborn teaching checklists (Fig. 21-4) can be used to accomplish patient care and educational outcomes.

Text continued on p. 608.

BOX 21-3

Criteria for Early Discharge

Mother

- Uncomplicated pregnancy, labor, vaginal birth, and postpartum course
- No evidence of premature rupture of membranes
- Blood pressure, temperature stable and within normal limits
- Ambulating unassisted
- Voiding adequate amounts without difficulty
- Hemoglobin >10 g
- No significant vaginal bleeding; perineum intact or no more than second-degree episiotomy or laceration repair; uterus is firm
- Received instructions on postpartum self-care

Infant

- Term infant (38 to 42 weeks) with weight appropriate for gestational age
- Normal findings on physical assessment
- Temperature, respirations, and heart rate within normal limits and stable for the 12 hours preceding discharge
- At least two successful feedings completed (normal sucking and swallowing)
- Urination and stooling have occurred at least once
- No evidence of significant jaundice in the first 24 hours after the birth
- No excessive bleeding at the circumcision site for at least 2 hours
- Screening tests performed according to state regulations; tests to be repeated at follow-up visit if done before the infant is 24 hours old
- Initial hepatitis B vaccine given or scheduled for first follow-up visit
- Laboratory data reviewed: maternal syphilis and hepatitis B status; infant or cord blood type and Coombs' test results if indicated

General

- No social, family, or environmental risk factors identified
- Family or support person available to assist mother and infant at home
- Follow-up scheduled within 1 week if discharged before 48 hours after the birth
- Documentation of skill of mother in feeding (breast or bottle), cord care, skin care, perineal care, infant safety (use of car seat, sleeping positions), and recognizing signs of illness and common infant problems

Sources: American Academy of Pediatrics: Hospital stay for healthy term infants, *Pediatrics* 96(4):788-790, 1995; Weekly SJ, Neumann ML: Speaking up for baby: the case for individualized neonatal discharge plans, *AWHONN Lifelines* 1(1):24-29, 1997.

Table 21-2

Care Path: 24-Hour Vaginal Birth without Complications

Date of Birth: ______________

Hour of Birth: ______________

The uncomplicated vaginal birth patient's admission/discharge is based on a 24-hour length of stay postbirth based on individual needs.

Time: ________

	Recovery	Adm. to PP Unit–8 Hour	9-16 Hours	17-24 Hours/Discharge
Primary Physiologic Focus	Woman will have normal vital signs (VS) as documented on flowsheet	Woman will have normal VS and moderate lochia rubra	Woman will have normal VS and minimal lochia rubra	Woman will have normal VS and minimal lochia rubra
	NA MET Variance	NA MET Variance	NA MET Variance	NA MET Variance
	Vital signs every 15 min × 1 hour, then hourly Assess perineum/ episiotomy Ice pack prn Assess lochia	Vital signs every 4 hours. Assess perineum/ episiotomy Ice pack prn Assess lochia	Vital signs every shift. Assess perineum/ episiotomy Ice pack prn Assess lochia	Vital signs every shift. Assess perineum/ episiotomy Ice pack prn Assess lochia
	Recovery	**Adm. to PP Unit–8 Hour**	**9-16 Hours**	**17-24 Hours/Discharge**
IVs/Labwork/Medications	Woman will have appropriate lab work done and medication given by time of transfer to mother/ baby unit	Woman will begin to verbalize understanding of hepatitis status and medication requirements	Woman will have appropriate lab work done by 16 hours PP	Woman will have appropriate lab work done and appropriate medications initiated
	NA MET Variance	NA MET Variance	NA MET Variance	NA MET Variance
	CBC, if not done before birth Urine drug screen if ordered U/A–dipstick (Send to lab, if abnormal)	Review hepatitis B status Medication regimen initiated	CBC Review rubella status Review Hgb and Hct	Fe Tab Prenatal vitamin Rubella vaccine, if appropriate Rh immune globulin, if indicated Laxative
	Recovery	**Adm. to PP Unit–8 Hour**	**9-16 Hours**	**17-24 Hours/Discharge**
Nutrition/Elimination	Patient will be up to bathroom before transfer	Woman will resume normal nutritional status and bladder function	Woman will resume normal nutritional status and bladder function	Women will have normal bowel and bladder function
	NA MET Variance	NA MET Variance	NA MET Variance	NA MET Variance
	Assess bladder fullness Assist to bathroom Assess for tolerance of PO intake	Encourage ambulation Encourage PO fluids Assist to bathroom as needed Assess bladder function Encourage PO intake	Encourage ambulation Encourage PO fluids Assist to bathroom as needed Assess bladder function Encourage PO intake	Encourage ambulation Encourage PO fluids Assist to bathroom as needed Laxative prn
	Recovery	**Adm. to PP Unit–8 Hour**	**9-16 Hours**	**17-24 Hours/Discharge**
Psychosocial	Woman/family will begin attachment behaviors with newborn	Woman/family will demonstrate appropriate attachment behaviors	Family will verbalize comfort with new infant	Family will verbalize comfort with new infant
	NA MET Variance	NA MET Variance	NA MET Variance	NA MET Variance
	Encourage mother/family members to hold and touch infant Provide skin-to-skin contact of mother/infant Provide mother the opportunity to breastfeed, if applicable	Offer flexible rooming-in with infant Allow for verbalization of woman's feelings Assess discharge needs and need for Social Service consult	Reinforce interventions	Reinforce interventions Completion of birth certificate Arrange for home visit

Continued

Table 21-2

Care Path: 24-Hour Vaginal Birth without Complications—cont'd

	Recovery	Adm. to PP Unit–8 Hour	9-16 Hours	17-24 Hours/Discharge
Self-Care Activity	Woman will begin self-care activities as tolerated	Woman will be up to bathroom/shower with assistance	Woman will be up to bathroom/shower independently	Woman will be up to bathroom/shower independently
	NA MET Variance	**NA MET Variance**	**NA MET Variance**	**NA MET Variance**
	Instruct woman in pericare and pad changes	Reinforce proper pericare Instruct on use of sitz bath Encourage woman to shower	Reinforce proper pericare. Reinforce use of sitz bath	Reinforce proper pericare Reinforce use of sitz bath
Teaching/Discharge Planning	**Recovery**	**Adm. to PP Unit–8 Hour**	**9-16 Hours**	**17-24 Hours/Discharge**
	Woman will begin to verbalize and/or demonstrate self-care and infant care activities	Woman will begin to verbalize and/or demonstrate infant and self-care activities	Woman/family will demonstrate appropriate infant care activities	Woman/family will demonstrate appropriate infant care activities
	NA MET Variance	**NA MET Variance**	**NA MET Variance**	**NA MET Variance**
	Date: Initials: Teaching to include: Breastfeeding latch-on and positioning, if applicable Appropriate handwashing techniques Cough and deep breathing exercises Instruct in pain relief techniques/medication	Teaching to include: Breastfeeding/formula initial feeding information Breast care Perineal care Proper nutrition Safety issues reviewed	Teaching to include: Attendance at mother/baby care class Breast care or formula information Newborn channel Lactation consult prn Appropriate handwashing techniques	Teaching to include: Reinforcement of teaching from mother/baby class Plans for self/infant follow-up. Review IHSP* Review Baby Net program Telephone number for follow-up questions Home-going meds and purposes
	Additional Topics			
	1.	1.	1.	1.
	2.	2.	2.	2.
	3.	3.	3.	3.
	4.	4.	4.	4.

Variance Documentation:

____

____

____

____

____

____

*IHSP denotes a test done to determine whether follow-up is needed in the Infant Hearing Screening Program (IHSP).
NA, not applicable; *MET*, achieved objective; *VARIANCE*, outcome varied from objective.

Abbott Northwestern Hospital
A HealthSpan™ Organization
SELF/FAMILY LEARNING CHECKLIST

Patient Name, Social Security #, Date of Birth

I learn best by: ☐ *Group classes* ☐ *Individual instruction* ☐ *Video instruction* ☐ *Reading it myself*

Please indicate your desired learning needs by placing a check in one of the columns next to each topic.

KEY *1 = Most important to learn before I go home*
2 = I already know

(Please DATE when learning need is met.)

CARING FOR YOURSELF	1	2	DATE
Episiotomy and perineal care			
Vaginal discharge			
Hemorrhoids/Constipation			
Breast care			
Nutrition			
Activity			
Post partal exercises			
Return of menstruation			
Family planning			
Blood clots			
Post partum emotions			
Post partum warning signs			
Cesarean Birth			
Incisional care			
AFTER DISCHARGE			
When to call health care provider			
OTHER			
Working mothers			
Day care			
Sibling adjustment			
Single parent support			
Time out for parents			
Infant safety and security			
Infant As A Person Class			
New Parent Connection			

CARING FOR BABY	1	2	DATE
Diapering			
Baby bath, skin and cord care			
Circumcised/uncircumcised care			
Burping			
Bowel movements/wet diapers			
Sleeping habits			
Newborn behavior			
Jaundice			
Signs of illness			
Car seat safety			
General infant safety/poison control			
Signs/symptoms of dehydration			
Bulb syringe			
BREAST FEEDING			
Sore nipples			
Positioning			
Frequency of feedings			
Expressing/storing milk			
Engorgement			
Feeding water			
Nursing while working			
Weaning			
BOTTLE FEEDING			
Types of formula			
Preparing formula			
Frequency of feedings			

MEDICATIONS AT HOME

MEDICATIONS	STRENGTH	DOSAGE	FREQUENCY	PURPOSE/SPECIAL INSTRUCTIONS
			times per day	
			times per day	
			times per day	

RESOURCES REFERRALS
☐ *Physician Discharge Instructions* ____
☐ *Home Care Agency* ____
☐ *Other Referrals* ____

VALUABLES: ☐ *Returned* ☐ *None* **MEDICATIONS:** ☐ *Returned* ☐ *None* ☐ *Room checked for belongings*

Patient verbalized understanding of discharge information received.

PATIENT OR SUPPORT PERSON ____ *NURSE'S SIGNATURE* ____ *DATE* ____

SELF/FAMILY LEARNING CHECKLIST

SELF/FAMILY LEARNING CHECKLIST

Fig. 21-4 Self/family learning checklist. (Copyright Abbott Northwestern Hospital of Allina Health System, Minneapolis and St Paul, MN.)

Hospital-based maternity nurses continue to play invaluable roles as caregivers, teachers, and patient and family advocates in developing and implementing effective home care strategies. With coordination, clinical care and education can be planned and provided throughout pregnancy, during the hospital stay, and in the home after discharge to ensure the family's continued well-being.

LEGAL TIP **Early Discharge** Whether or not the woman and her family have chosen early discharge, the nurse and the primary health care provider are held responsible if the woman is discharged before her condition has stabilized within normal limits. If complications occur, the medical and nursing staff could be sued for abandonment. ■

Care Management-Physical Needs

Assessment

A focused physical assessment, including measurement of vital signs, is performed upon admission to the postpartum unit. If the woman's vital signs are within normal limits, they are usually assessed every 4 to 8 hours for the remainder of her hospitalization. Other components of the initial assessment include the mother's emotional status, energy level, degree of physical discomfort, hunger, and thirst. Intake and output assessments should always be included if an intravenous infusion or a urinary catheter is in place. If the woman gave birth by cesarean, her incisional dressing should also be assessed. To some degree, her knowledge level concerning self-care and infant care can also be determined at this time.

ENGLISH / SPANISH Guidelines/Guías

POSTPARTUM PHYSICAL ASSESSMENT

Are you planning to breastfeed or bottle-feed?
¿Piensa darle pecho o biberón al bebé?

Lie down, please.
Acuéstese, por favor.

I am going to take your vital signs.
Le voy a tomar sus signos vitales.

I need to take your blood pressure.
Necesito tomarle la presión sanguínea.

Do you need to use the bathroom?
¿Necesita usar el baño?

I need to examine you.
Necesito examinarle.

Please spread your knees and legs apart.
Por favor, abra las rodillas y las piernas.

Roll over on your side, please.
Póngase sobre un costado, por favor.

Would you like some pain medication?
¿Desea medicina para calmar el dolor?

Would you like to take a sitz bath?
¿Desea tomar un baño de asiento?

Ongoing Physical Assessment

The postpartum woman should be evaluated thoroughly each nursing shift throughout hospitalization (see Guidelines/Guías box). Physical assessments include evaluation of the breasts, uterine fundus, lochia, perineum, bladder and bowel function, vital signs, and legs. If a woman has an intravenous line in place, her fluid and hematologic status should be evaluated before it is removed. Signs of potential problems that may be identified during the assessment process are listed in Box 21-4.

Routine Laboratory Tests

Several laboratory tests may be performed in the immediate postpartum period. Hemoglobin and hematocrit values are often evaluated on the first postpartum day to assess blood loss during childbirth, especially after cesarean birth. In some hospitals a clean-catch or catheterized urine specimen may be obtained and sent for routine urinalysis or culture and sensitivity, especially if an indwelling urinary catheter was inserted during the intrapartum period. In addition, if the woman's rubella and Rh status are unknown, tests to determine her status and need for possible treatment should be performed at this time.

BOX 21-4

Signs of Potential Complications

Physiologic Problems

Temperature
More than 38° C after the first 24 hr

Pulse
Tachycardia or marked bradycardia

Blood Pressure
Hypotension or hypertension

Energy Level
Lethargy, extreme fatigue

Uterus
Deviated from the midline, boggy consistency, remains above the umbilicus after 24 hr

Lochia
Heavy, foul odor; bright red bleeding that is not lochia

Perineum
Pronounced edema, not intact, signs of infection, marked discomfort

Legs
Homans' sign positive; painful, reddened area; warmth on posterior aspect of calf

Breasts
Redness, heat, pain, cracked and fissured nipples, inverted nipples, palpable mass

Appetite
Lack of appetite

Elimination
Urine: inability to void, urgency, frequency, dysuria
Bowel: constipation, diarrhea

Rest
Inability to rest or sleep

Nursing Diagnoses

Although all women experience similar physiologic changes during the postpartum period, certain factors act to make each woman's experience unique. From a physiologic standpoint, the length and difficulty of the labor, type of birth (vaginal or cesarean), presence of episiotomy or lacerations, parity, and whether the mother plans to breastfeed or bottle-feed are factors to be considered with each woman. After analyzing the data obtained during the assessment process, the nurse establishes nursing diagnoses that will provide a guide for planning care. Examples of nursing diagnoses commonly established for the postpartum patient include the following:

- *Risk for deficient fluid volume (hemorrhage) related to*
  —uterine atony after childbirth
- *Urinary retention or constipation related to*
  —postchildbirth discomfort
  —childbirth trauma to tissues
- *Acute pain related to*
  —uterine involution
  —episiotomy or lacerations
  —hemorrhoids
  —engorged breasts
- *Disturbed sleep pattern related to*
  —discomforts of postpartum period
  —long labor process
  —infant care and hospital routine
- *Ineffective breastfeeding related to*
  —maternal discomfort
  —infant positioning

Expected Outcomes

The nursing plan of care includes both the postpartum woman and her infant, even if the nursery nurse retains primary responsibility for the infant. In many hospitals, couplet care (also called *mother and baby care* or *single-room maternity care*) is practiced. Nurses in these settings have been educated in both mother and infant care and function as primary nurses for both mother and infant, even if the infant is kept in the nursery. This approach is a variation of rooming-in, in which the mother and infant room together and mother and nurse share the care of the infant. The organization of the mother's care must take the newborn into consideration. The day actually revolves around the baby's feeding and care times.

Expected outcomes for the postpartum period are based on the nursing diagnoses identified for the individual patient. Examples of common expected outcomes for physiologic needs are that the woman will:

- Remain free from infection
- Demonstrate normal involution and lochial characteristics
- Remain comfortable and injury free
- Demonstrate normal bladder and bowel patterns
- Demonstrate knowledge of breast care, whether breastfeeding or bottle-feeding
- Integrate the newborn into the family

Plan of Care and Implementation

Once the nursing diagnoses are formulated, the nurse plans with the woman what nursing measures are appropriate and which are to be given priority. During her hospital stay the mother is encouraged to assume increasing responsibility for her self-care and her infant's care. As the woman and her partner provide more care for herself and the baby, the nurse's role changes from one of providing direct care to one of teaching, encouragement, and support.

The nursing plan of care includes periodic assessments to detect deviations from normal physical changes, measures to relieve discomfort or pain, safety measures to prevent injury or infection, and teaching and counseling measures designed to promote the woman's feelings of competence in self-care and baby care. Family members are included in the teaching. The nurse evaluates continuously and is ready to change the plan if indicated. Almost all hospitals use standardized care plans as a base. The nurse's adaptation of the standardized plan to meet specific medical and nursing diagnoses results in individualized patient care.

Nurses assume many roles while implementing the nursing plan of care. They provide direct physical care, teach mother and baby care, and provide anticipatory guidance and counseling. Perhaps most important of all, they nurture the woman by providing encouragement and support as she begins to assume the many tasks of motherhood. Nurses who take the time to "mother the mother" do much to increase feelings of self-confidence in new mothers.

The first step in providing individualized care is to confirm the woman's identity by checking her wristband. At the same time, the infant's identification number is matched with the corresponding band on the mother's wrist, and, in some instances, the father's wrist. The nurse determines how the mother wishes to be addressed and then notes her preference in her record and in her nursing care plan.

The woman and her family are oriented to their surroundings. Familiarity with the unit, routines, resources, and personnel reduces one potential source of anxiety—the unknown. The mother is reassured through knowing whom and how she can call for assistance and what she can expect in the way of supplies and services. If the woman's usual daily routine before admission differs from the facility's routine, the nurse works with the woman to develop a mutually acceptable routine.

Infant abduction from hospitals in the United States has increased over the past few years. The mother should be taught to check the identity of any person who comes to remove the baby from her room. Hospital personnel usually wear picture identification badges. On some units, all staff members wear matching scrubs or special badges. Other units use closed circuit television, computer monitoring systems, or fingerprint identification pads. As a rule, the baby is never carried in a staff member's arms between the mother's room and the nursery but rather is always wheeled in a bassinet, which also contains baby care supplies. Patients and nurses must work together to ensure the safety of newborns in the hospital environment (Nursing Care Plan).

Prevention of Infection

One important means of preventing infection is maintenance of a clean environment. Bed linens should be changed as needed. Disposable pads should be changed frequently. Women should wear slippers when walking about to avoid

Nursing Care Plan

POSTPARTUM CARE—VAGINAL BIRTH

NURSING DIAGNOSIS: Risk for deficient fluid volume related to uterine atony/hemorrhage

EXPECTED OUTCOMES

Fundus is firm, lochia is moderate, and there is no evidence of hemorrhage.

NURSING INTERVENTIONS/*RATIONALES*

Monitor lochia (color, amount, consistency) and count and weigh sanitary pads if lochia is heavy *to evaluate amount of bleeding.*

Monitor and palpate fundus for location and tone *to determine status of uterus and dictate further interventions because atonic uterus is most common cause of postpartum hemorrhage.*

Monitor intake and output, assess for bladder fullness, and encourage voiding *because a full bladder interferes with involution of the uterus.*

Monitor vital signs (increased pulse and respirations, decreased blood pressure) and skin temperature and color *to detect signs of hemorrhage/shock.*

Monitor postpartum hematology studies *to assess effects of blood loss.*

If fundus is boggy, apply gentle massage and assess tone response *to promote uterine contractions and increase uterine tone.* (Do not overstimulate because doing so can cause fundal relaxation.)

Express uterine clots *to promote uterine contraction.*

Explain to the woman the process of involution and teach her to assess and massage the fundus and to report any persistent bogginess *to involve her in self-care and increase sense of self-control.*

Administer oxytocic agents per physician/nurse-midwife order and evaluate effectiveness *to promote continuing uterine contraction.*

Administer fluids, blood, blood products, or plasma expanders as ordered *to replace lost fluid and lost blood volume.*

NURSING DIAGNOSIS: Acute pain related to postpartum physiologic changes (hemorrhoids, episiotomy, breast engorgement, cracked/sore nipples)

EXPECTED OUTCOME

Woman exhibits signs of decreased discomfort.

NURSING INTERVENTIONS/*RATIONALES*

Assess location, type, and quality of pain *to direct intervention.*

Explain to the woman the source and reasons for the pain, its expected duration, and treatments *to decrease anxiety and increase sense of control.*

Administer prescribed pain medications *to provide pain relief.*

If pain is perineal (episiotomy, hemorrhoids), apply ice packs in the first 24 hours *to reduce edema and vulvar irritation and reduce discomfort;* encourage sitz baths using cool water first 24 hours *to reduce edema* and warm water thereafter *to promote circulation;* apply witch hazel compresses *to reduce edema;* teach woman to use prescribed perineal creams, sprays, or ointments *to depress response of peripheral nerves;* teach woman to tighten buttocks before sitting and to sit on flat, hard surfaces *to compress buttocks and reduce pressure on the perineum.* (Avoid donuts and soft pillows because they separate the buttocks and decrease venous blood flow, increasing pain.)

If pain is from breasts and woman is breastfeeding, encourage use of a supportive bra *to increase comfort;* ascertain that infant has latched on correctly *to prevent sore nipples;* vary infant position during feeding *to prevent sore nipples.*

If breasts are engorged, have woman use warm compresses or take a warm shower before breastfeeding *to stimulate milk flow and relieve stasis.*

If nipples are sore, have woman air-dry nipples after feeding *to toughen nipples,* apply breast creams as prescribed *to soften nipples and relieve irritation* and wear breast shields in her bra *to relieve irritation.*

If pain is from breast and woman is not breastfeeding, encourage use of a tight supportive bra or breast binder and application of ice packs *to reduce lactation and decrease heaviness.*

NURSING DIAGNOSIS: Disturbed sleep pattern related to excitement, discomfort, and environmental interruptions

EXPECTED OUTCOME

Woman sleeps for uninterrupted periods of time and feels rested after waking.

NURSING INTERVENTIONS/*RATIONALES*

Establish woman's routine sleep patterns and compare with current sleep pattern, exploring things that interfere with sleep, *to determine scope of problem and direct interventions.*

Individualize nursing routines to fit woman's natural body rhythms (i.e., wake/sleep cycles), provide a sleep-promoting environment (i.e., darkness, quiet, adequate ventilation, appropriate room temperature), prepare for sleep using woman's usual routines (i.e., back rub, soothing music, warm milk), teach use of guided imagery and relaxation techniques *to promote optimum conditions for sleep.*

Avoid things or routines (i.e., caffeine, foods that induce heartburn, fluids, strenuous mental/physical activity) *that may interfere with sleep.*

Administer sedation or pain medication as prescribed *to enhance quality of sleep.*

Advise woman/partner to limit visitors and activities *to avoid further taxation and fatigue.*

Teach woman to use infant nap time as a time for her also *to nap and replenish energy and decrease fatigue.*

NURSING DIAGNOSIS: Risk for impaired urinary elimination related to perineal trauma and effects of anesthesia

EXPECTED OUTCOMES

Woman will void within 6 to 8 hours after birth and empty bladder completely.

NURSING INTERVENTIONS/*RATIONALES*

Assess position and character of uterine fundus and bladder *to ascertain if any further interventions are indicated because of displacement of the fundus or distention of the bladder.*

Measure intake and output *to assess any evidence of dehydration and subsequent decreased anticipated urine output.*

Encourage voiding by walking woman to bathroom, running water over perineum, running water in sink, providing privacy *to encourage voiding.*

Encourage oral intake *to replace any fluids lost at delivery and prevent dehydration.*

Catheterize as necessary with indwelling or straight method *to ensure bladder emptying and allow uterine involution.*

contaminating the linens when they return to bed. Supervision of use of equipment to prevent cross-contamination also is necessary. For example, a sitz bath or heat lamp used in common must be scrubbed after each woman's use. Personnel must be conscientious about their handwashing techniques to prevent cross infection. Standard Precautions must be practiced. Staff members with colds, coughs, or skin infections (e.g., a cold sore on the lips [herpes simplex virus type I]) must follow hospital protocol when in contact with postpartum patients. In many hospitals, staff with open herpetic lesions, strep throat, conjunctivitis, upper respiratory infections, or diarrhea are encouraged to avoid contact with mothers and infants by staying home until the condition is no longer contagious.

Proper care of the episiotomy site and any perineal lacerations prevents infection in the genitourinary area and aids the healing process. Educating the woman to wipe from front to back (urethra to anus) after voiding or defecating is a simple first step. In many hospitals, a squeeze bottle filled with warm water or an antiseptic solution is used after each voiding to cleanse the perineal area (Box 21-5). The woman should change her perineal pad from front to back each time she voids or defecates, and wash her hands thoroughly before and after doing so.

Prevention of Excessive Bleeding

The most frequent cause of excessive bleeding after childbirth is uterine atony, or failure of the uterine muscle to contract firmly. The two most important interventions for preventing excessive bleeding are maintaining good uterine tone and preventing bladder distention. If uterine atony occurs, the relaxed uterus distends with blood and clots, blood vessels in the placental site are not clamped off, and excessive bleeding results.

Excessive blood loss after childbirth may be caused by vaginal or vulvar hematomas, unrepaired lacerations of the vagina or cervix, and retained placental fragments.

BOX 21-5

Interventions for Episiotomy, Lacerations, and Hemorrhoids

Explain both procedure and rationale before implementation.

Cleansing

Wash hands before and after cleansing perineum and changing pads.
Wash perineum with mild soap and warm water at least once daily.
Cleanse from symphysis pubis to anal area.
Apply peripad from front to back, protecting inner surface of pad from contamination.
Wrap soiled pad and place in covered waste container.
Change pad with each void or defecation or at least 4 times per day.
Assess amount and character of lochia with each pad change.

Ice Pack

Apply a covered ice pack to perineum from front to back
1. During first 2 hours to decrease edema formation and increase comfort
2. After the first 2 hours following the birth to provide anesthetic effect

Squeeze Bottle

Demonstrate for and assist woman; explain rationale.
Fill bottle with tap water warmed to approximately 38° C (comfortably warm on the wrist).
Instruct woman to position nozzle between her legs so that squirts of water reach perineum as she sits on toilet seat. Explain that it will take whole bottle of water to cleanse perineum.
Remind her to blot dry with toilet paper or clean wipes.
Remind her to avoid contamination from anal area.
Apply clean pad.

Sitz Bath

Built-in Type

Prepare bath by thoroughly scrubbing with cleaning agent and rinsing.
Pad with towel before filling.
Fill one-half to one-third full with water of correct temperature 38° to 40.6° C. Some women prefer cool sitz baths. Ice is added to water to lower the temperature to the level comfortable for the woman.
Encourage woman to use at least twice a day for 20 minutes.
Place call bell within easy reach.
Teach woman to enter bath by tightening gluteal muscles and keeping them tightened and then relaxing them after she is in the bath.
Place dry towels within reach.
Ensure privacy.
Check woman in 15 minutes; assess pulse as needed.

Disposable Type

Clamp tubing and fill bag with warm water.
Raise toilet seat, place bath in bowl with overflow opening directed toward back of toilet.
Place container above toilet bowl.
Attach tube into groove at front of bath.
Loosen tube clamp to regulate rate of flow; fill bath to about one-half full; continue as above for built-in sitz bath.

Surgi-Gator

Assemble Surgi-Gator (Fig. 21-6).
Instruct woman regarding use and rationale.
Follow package directions.
Instruct woman to sit on toilet with legs apart and to put nozzle so tip is just past the perineum, adjusting placement as needed. Remind her to return her applicator to her bedside stand.

Dry Heat

Inspect lamp for defects.
Cover lamp with towels.
Position lamp 50 cm from perineum; use 3 times a day for 20-min periods.
Teach regarding use of 40-W bulb at home.
Provide draping over woman.
If same lamp is being used by several women, clean it carefully between uses.

Topical Applications

Apply anesthetic cream or spray: use sparingly 3 to 4 times per day.
Offer witch hazel pads (Tucks) after voiding or defecating; woman pats perineum dry from front to back, then applies witch hazel pads.

NURSE ALERT A perineal pad saturated in 15 minutes or less, or pooling of blood under the buttocks, are indications of excessive blood loss, requiring immediate assessment, intervention, and notification of the primary health care provider. ■

Accurate visual estimation of blood loss is an important nursing responsibility. Blood loss is usually described subjectively as scant, light, moderate, or heavy (profuse). Figure 21-5 shows examples of perineal pad saturation corresponding to each of these descriptions. Any estimation of lochial flow is inaccurate and incomplete without consideration of the time factor. The woman who saturates a peripad in 1 hour or less is bleeding much more than the woman who saturates one peripad in 8 hours.

It is difficult to judge the amount of lochial flow based only on observation of perineal pads. Postpartal blood loss may be estimated by observing the amount of staining on a perineal pad (see Fig. 21-5). More objective estimates of blood loss include weighing blood clots and items saturated with blood (1 g equals 1 ml), using devices that catch and measure blood flowing from the vagina, and establishing the milliliters it takes to saturate perineal pads being used (Luegenbiehl, 1997). However, these methods are not common in practice.

Luegenbiehl (1997) found that nurses in general tend to overestimate, rather than underestimate, blood loss. Different brands of peripads vary in their saturation volume and soaking appearance. For example, blood placed on some brands tends to soak down into the pad, whereas on other brands it tends to spread outward. Nurses should determine saturation volume and soaking appearance for the peripad brands used in their institution in order to improve accuracy of blood loss estimation.

NURSE ALERT The nurse always checks under the mother's buttocks as well as on the perineal pad. Blood may flow between the buttocks onto the linens under the mother, although the amount on the perineal pad is slight; thus, excessive bleeding goes undetected. ■

Blood pressure is not a reliable indicator of impending shock from early hemorrhage. More sensitive means of identifying shock are provided by respirations, pulse, skin condition, and urinary output (Benedetti, 2002). The frequent physical assessments performed during the fourth stage of labor are designed to provide prompt identification of excessive bleeding (Emergency box).

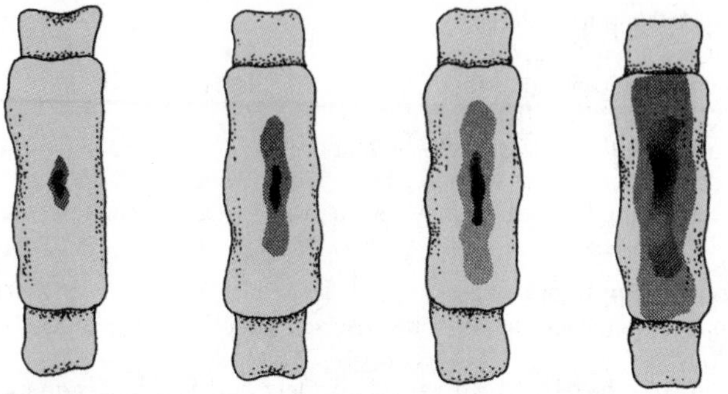

Fig. 21-5 Blood loss after birth is assessed by the extent of perineal pad saturation as *(from left to right)* scant (<2.5 cm); light (<10 cm); moderate (>10 cm); or heavy (one pad saturated within 2 hours).

Maintenance of Uterine Tone

A major intervention to restore good tone is stimulation by gently massaging the uterine fundus until firm (see Fig. 21-2). Fundal massage may cause a temporary increase in the amount of vaginal bleeding seen as pooled blood leaves the uterus. Clots may also be expelled. Fundal massage can be a very uncomfortable procedure. Understanding the causes and dangers of uterine atony and the purpose of fundal massage can help the woman be more cooperative. Teaching the patient to massage her own fundus enables her to maintain some control and decreases her anxiety.

The uterus may remain boggy even after massage and expulsion of clots. If this occurs, it is a major warning sign of uterine atony. The nurse must remain with the woman and summon help, including notifying the primary health care provider immediately. Additional interventions likely to be used are administration of intravenous fluids and oxytocic medications (drugs that stimulate contraction of the uterine smooth muscle). Table 23-1 contains information about common oxytocic medications.

Prevention of Bladder Distention

A full bladder causes the uterus to be displaced above the umbilicus and well to one side of the midline in the abdomen. It also prevents the uterus from contracting normally. Nursing interventions focus on helping the woman

Emergency

HYPOVOLEMIC SHOCK

Signs and Symptoms

- Persistent significant bleeding–perineal pad soaked within 15 minutes; may not be accompanied by a change in vital signs or maternal color or behavior.
- Woman states she feels weak, light-headed, "funny," "sick to my stomach," or "sees stars."
- Woman begins to act anxious or exhibits air hunger.
- Woman's skin turns ashen or grayish.
- Skin feels cool and clammy.
- Pulse rate increases.
- Blood pressure declines.

Interventions

- Notify primary health care provider.
- If uterus is atonic, massage gently and expel clots to cause uterus to contract; compress uterus manually, as needed, using two hands. Add oxytocic agent to IV drip, as ordered.
- Give oxygen by face mask or nasal prongs at 8 to 10 L/min.
- Tilt the woman to her side or elevate the right hip; elevate her legs to at least a 30-degree angle.
- Provide additional or maintain existing IV infusion of lactated Ringer's solution or normal saline solution to restore circulatory volume.
- Administer blood or blood products, as ordered.
- Monitor vital signs.
- Insert an indwelling urinary catheter to monitor perfusion of kidneys.
- Administer emergency drugs, as ordered.
- Prepare for possible surgery or other emergency treatments or procedures.
- Chart incident, medical and nursing interventions instituted, and results of treatments.

empty her bladder spontaneously as soon as possible. The first priority is to assist the woman to the bathroom or onto a bedpan if she is unable to ambulate. Having the woman listen to running water, placing her hands in warm water, or pouring water from a squeeze bottle over her perineum may stimulate voiding. Other techniques include assisting the woman into the shower or sitz bath and encouraging her to void or placing oil of peppermint in a bedpan under the woman. The vapors may relax the urinary meatus and trigger spontaneous voiding. Administering analgesics, if ordered, may be indicated because some women may fear voiding because of anticipated pain. If these measures are unsuccessful, a sterile catheter may be inserted to drain the urine.

Promotion of Comfort, Rest, Ambulation, and Exercise

Comfort

Most women experience some degree of discomfort during the immediate postpartum period. Common causes of discomfort include afterbirth pains, episiotomy or perineal lacerations, hemorrhoids, and breast engorgement. The woman's description of the type and severity of her pain is the best guide in choosing an appropriate intervention. To confirm the location and extent of discomfort, the nurse inspects and palpates areas of pain as appropriate for redness, swelling, discharge, and heat; and observes for body tension, guarded movements, and facial tension. Blood pressure, pulse, and respirations may be elevated in response to acute pain. Diaphoresis may accompany severe pain. A lack of objective signs does not necessarily mean there is no pain, because there may also be a cultural component to the expression of pain. Nursing interventions are intended to eliminate the pain sensation entirely or reduce it to a tolerable level that allows the woman to care for herself and her baby. Nurses may use both nonpharmacologic and pharmacologic interventions to promote comfort. Pain relief is enhanced by using more than one method or route.

Nonpharmacologic Interventions

Afterbirth pains are menstrual-like cramps experienced by many women as the uterus contracts following childbirth. Warmth, distraction, deep breathing, imagery, therapeutic touch, relaxation, and interaction with the infant may decrease the discomfort associated with these uterine contractions.

Simple interventions that can decrease the discomfort associated with an episiotomy or perineal lacerations include encouraging the woman to lie on her side whenever possible and to use a pillow when sitting. Other interventions include application of an ice pack; topical application (if ordered); dry heat; cleansing with a squeeze bottle; and a cleansing shower, tub bath, or sitz bath (Fig. 21-6). Many of these interventions are also effective for hemorrhoids, especially ice packs, sitz baths, and topical applications (such as witch hazel pads). Box 21-5 gives more specific information about these interventions.

The discomfort associated with engorged breasts may be lessened by applying either ice, heat, or cold cabbage leaves to the breasts and wearing a well-fitted support bra. Decisions about specific interventions for relieving engorgement are based on whether the woman chooses breastfeeding or bottle-feeding (see Chapter 26).

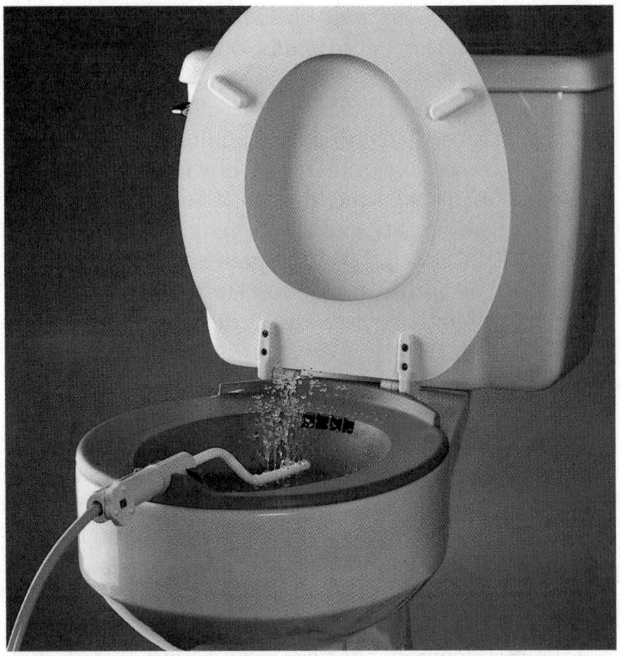

Fig. 21-6 Hygienic sitz bath (Surgi-Gator) for perineal care. (Courtesy Andermac, Inc., Yuba City, CA.)

Pharmacologic Interventions

Most health care providers routinely order a variety of analgesics to be administered as needed. These include both opioid (narcotic) and nonopioid (nonnarcotic) (nonsteroidal antiinflammatory medications) choices, with their dosage and time frequency ranges. Topical application of antiseptic or anesthetic ointments or sprays is a common pharmacologic intervention. Patient-controlled analgesia (PCA) pumps and continuous epidural analgesia infusions are technologies commonly used to provide pain relief after cesarean birth.

NURSE ALERT The nurse should carefully monitor all women receiving opioids because respiratory depression and decreased intestinal motility are side effects. ■

Many women want to participate in decisions about analgesia. Severe pain, however, may interfere with active participation in choosing pain relief measures. If an analgesic is to be given, the nurse must make a clinical judgment of the type, dosage, and frequency from the medications ordered. The woman is informed of the prescribed analgesic and its common side effects; this teaching is documented.

Breastfeeding mothers often have concerns about the effects of an analgesic on the infant. Although nearly all medications present in maternal circulation are also found in breast milk, many analgesics (e.g., ibuprofen, acetaminophen) commonly used during the postpartum period are considered relatively safe for breastfeeding mothers (American Academy of Pediatrics, 2001). Often the timing of medications can be adjusted to minimize infant exposure. A mother may be given pain medication immediately after breastfeeding so that the interval between medication administration and the next nursing period is as long as possible. The decision to administer medications of any type to a breastfeeding mother must always be made by carefully weighing the woman's need against actual or potential risks to the infant.

If acceptable pain relief has not been obtained in 1 hour, and there has been no change in the initial assessment, the nurse may contact the primary care provider for additional pain relief orders or further directions. Unrelieved pain results in fatigue, anxiety, and a worsening perception of the pain. It might also indicate the presence of a previously unidentified or untreated problem. Further assessment and treatment will likely be necessary to determine the cause of the pain and correct it.

Rest

The excitement and exhilaration experienced after the birth of the infant may make rest difficult. The new mother, who is often anxious about her ability to care for her infant or is uncomfortable, may also have difficulty sleeping. The demands of the infant, the hospital environment and routines, and the frequent presence of visitors contribute to alterations in her sleep pattern.

Fatigue

Fatigue is common in the postpartum period (Pugh et al, 1999) and involves both physiologic components associated with long labors, cesarean birth, anemia, and breastfeeding and psychologic components related to depression and anxiety. Infant behavior can also be related to fatigue, particularly for mothers of more difficult infants.

Interventions must be planned to meet the woman's individual needs for sleep and rest. Backrubs, other comfort measures, and medication for sleep for the first few nights may be necessary. Support and encouragement in mothering behaviors help reduce anxiety. Hospital and nursing routines may be adjusted to meet individual needs. In addition, the nurse can help the family limit visitors and provide a comfortable chair or bed for the partner.

Critical Thinking Exercise

FATIGUE AND REST AFTER CHILDBIRTH

Patricia gave birth to her third baby; she has two children at home, ages 3 years and 18 months. Her husband travels frequently with his job. She is breastfeeding the baby without difficulty but is concerned about how she will care for all three of her children, stating "I remember how tired I was after my last baby. I'm not sure I can manage with three children since my husband is gone so much. Do you have any suggestions to help me?"

1. Evidence—Is there sufficient evidence to draw conclusions about whether support would be helpful for Patricia?
2. Assumptions—What assumptions can be made about the following factors?
   a. The relation of breastfeeding and fatigue
   b. Support in the postpartum period
   c. The role of sleep and rest in relation to fatigue and depression
   d. Spacing of pregnancies and fatigue
3. What implications and priorities for nursing care can be drawn at this time?
4. Does the evidence objectively support your conclusion?
5. Are there alternative perspectives to your conclusion?

Ambulation

Early ambulation is successful in reducing the incidence of thromboembolism and in promoting the woman's more rapid recovery of strength. Free movement is encouraged once anesthesia wears off, unless an analgesic has been administered. After the initial recovery period is over, the mother is encouraged to ambulate frequently.

NURSE ALERT Having a hospital staff or family member present the first time the woman gets out of bed after birth is wise because she may feel weak, dizzy, faint, or light-headed. ■

The rapid decrease in intraabdominal pressure after birth results in a dilation of blood vessels supplying the intestines (splanchnic engorgement) and causes blood to pool in the viscera. This condition contributes to the development of orthostatic hypotension and may occur when the woman who has recently given birth sits or stands, first ambulates, or takes a warm shower or sitz bath. The nurse must also consider the baseline blood pressure; amount of blood loss; and type, amount, and timing of analgesic or anesthetic medications administered when assisting a woman to ambulate.

Prevention of thrombus (clot formation) is important. Women who must remain in bed after giving birth are at increased risk for the development of thrombus. If a woman remains in bed longer than 8 hours (e.g., for postpartum magnesium sulfate therapy for preeclampsia), exercise to promote circulation in the legs is indicated using the following routine:

- Alternate flexion and extension of feet
- Rotate ankle in circular motion
- Alternate flexion and extension of legs
- Press back of knee to bed surface; relax

If the woman is susceptible to thromboembolism, she is encouraged to walk about actively and discouraged from sitting immobile in a chair. Women with varicosities are advised to wear support hose. If a thrombus is suspected, as evidenced by a positive Homans' sign (complaint of pain in calf muscles when the foot is dorsiflexed) or warmth, redness, or tenderness in the suspected leg, the primary health care provider should be notified immediately; meanwhile, the woman should be confined to bed, with the affected limb elevated on pillows.

Exercise

Most women who have just given birth are interested in regaining their nonpregnant figures. Postpartum exercise can begin soon after birth, although the woman should be encouraged to start with simple exercises and gradually progress to more strenuous ones. Figure 21-7 illustrates a number of exercises appropriate for the new mother. Abdominal exercises are postponed until about 4 weeks after cesarean birth. Women whose major activities are related to household or infant care or other nonleisure activities may not exercise enough to meet recommendations for moderate or high intensity physical activity (Wilkinson et al, 2004). Follow-up visits may include questions about how much physical activity is undertaken.

Kegel pelvic exercises to strengthen muscle tone are extremely important, particularly after vaginal birth. To

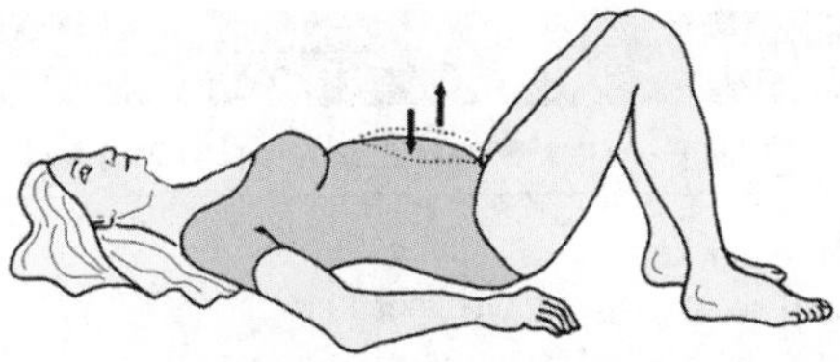

Abdominal Breathing. Lie on back with knees bent. Inhale deeply through nose. Keep ribs stationary and allow abdomen to expand upward. Exhale slowly but forcefully while contracting the abdominal muscles; hold for 3 to 5 seconds while exhaling. Relax.

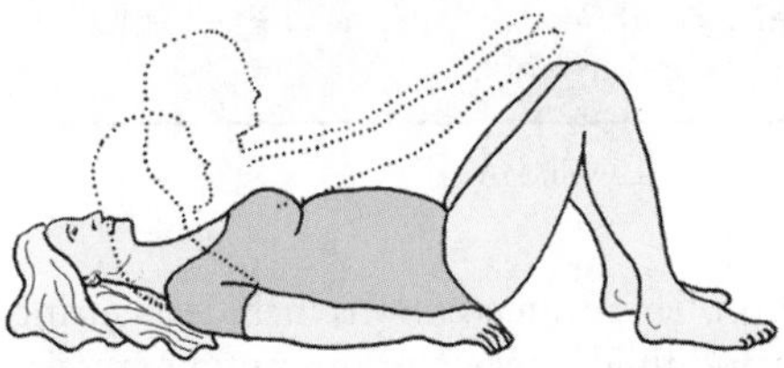

Reach for the Knees. Lie on back with knees bent. While inhaling, deeply lower chin onto chest. While exhaling, raise head and shoulders slowly and smoothly and reach for knees with arms outstretched. The body should only rise as far as the back will naturally bend while waist remains on floor or bed (about 6 to 8 inches). Slowly and smoothly lower head and shoulders back to starting position. Relax.

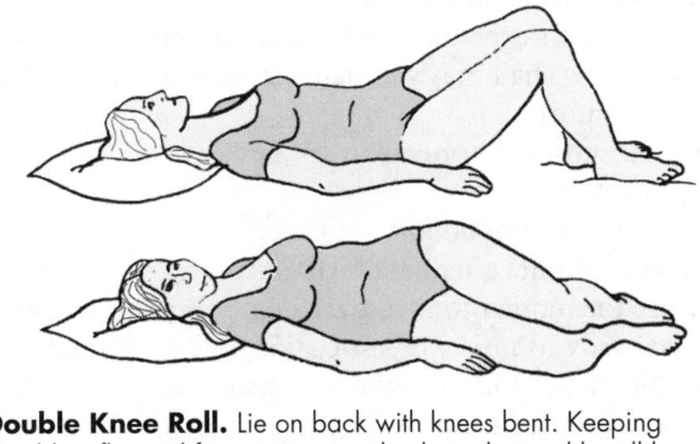

Double Knee Roll. Lie on back with knees bent. Keeping shoulders flat and feet stationary, slowly and smoothly roll knees over to the left to touch floor or bed. Maintaining a smooth motion, roll knees back over to the right until they touch floor or bed. Return to starting position and relax.

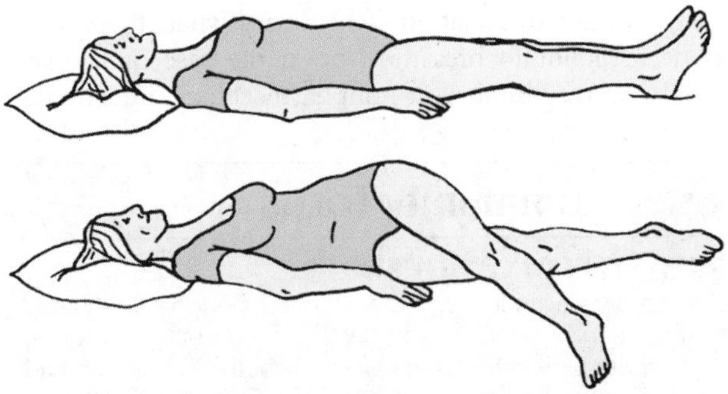

Leg Roll. Lie on back with legs straight. Keeping shoulders flat and legs straight, slowly and smoothly lift left leg and roll it over to touch the right side of floor or bed and return to starting position. Repeat, rolling right leg over to touch left side of floor or bed. Relax.

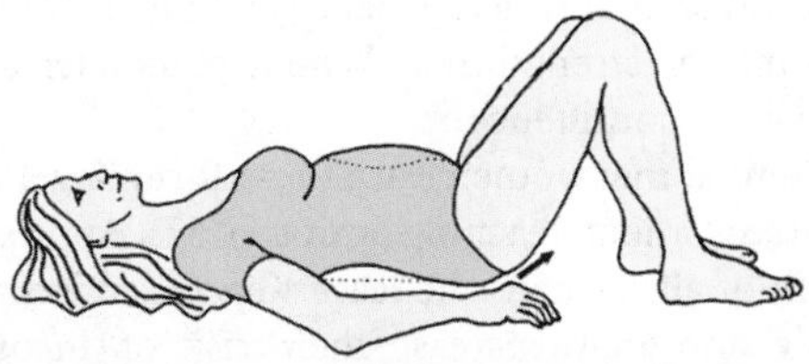

Combined Abdominal Breathing and Supine Pelvic Tilt (Pelvic Rock). Lie on back with knees bent. While inhaling deeply, roll pelvis back by flattening lower back on floor or bed. Exhale slowly but forcefully while contracting abdominal muscles and tightening buttocks. Hold for 3 to 5 seconds while exhaling. Relax.

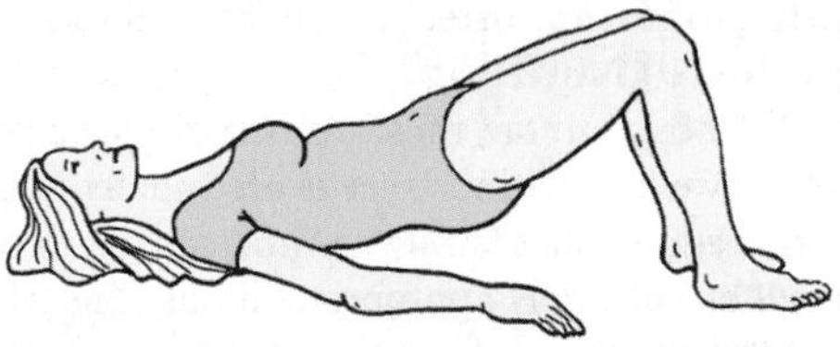

Buttocks Lift. Lie on back with arms at sides, knees bent, and feet flat. Slowly raise buttocks and arch back. Return slowly to starting position.

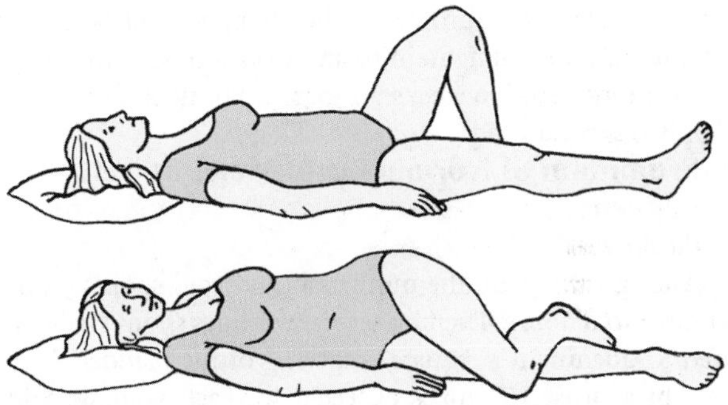

Single Knee Roll. Lie on back with right leg straight and left leg bent at the knee. Keeping shoulders flat, slowly and smoothly roll left knee over to the right to touch floor or bed and then back to starting position. Reverse position of legs. Roll right knee over to the left to touch floor or bed and return to starting position. Relax.

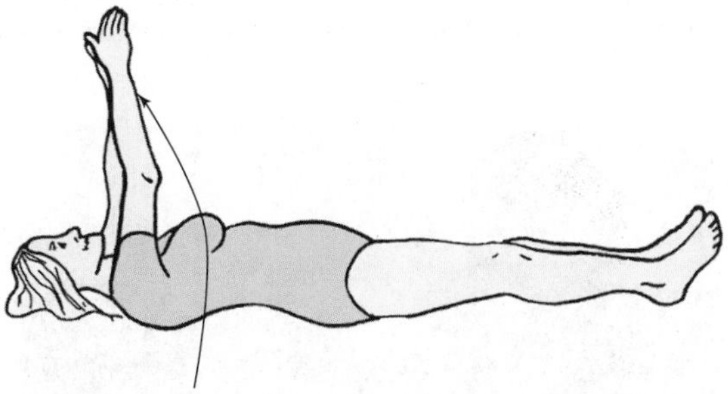

Arm Raises. Lie on back with arms extended at 90-degree angle from body. Raise arms so they are perpendicular and hands touch. Lower slowly.

Fig. 21-7 Postpartum exercise should begin as soon as possible. The woman should start with simple exercises and gradually progress to more strenuous ones.

perform them, the woman alternately contracts and relaxes the muscles around the vagina. Kegel exercises help women regain the muscle tone that is often lost as pelvic tissues are stretched and torn during pregnancy and birth. Women who maintain muscle strength may benefit years later by maintaining urinary continence.

It is essential that women learn to perform Kegel exercises correctly (see Patient Teaching box on p. 67). Approximately one-fourth of all women who learn Kegel exercises do them incorrectly and may increase their risk of incontinence (Sampselle et al, 2000). This may occur when women inadvertently bear down on the pelvic floor muscles, thrusting the perineum outward. The woman's technique can be assessed during the pelvic examination at the 6-week checkup by inserting two fingers intravaginally and checking whether the pelvic floor muscles correctly contract and relax.

Promotion of Nutrition

During the hospital stay, most women display a good appetite and eat well; nutritious snacks are usually welcomed. Women may request that family members bring to the hospital favorite or culturally appropriate foods (Fig. 21-8, Box 21-6). Cultural dietary preferences must be respected. This interest in food presents an ideal opportunity for nutrition counseling on dietary needs after pregnancy, such as for breastfeeding, preventing constipation and anemia, promoting weight loss, and promoting healing and well-being (see Chapter 12). Prenatal vitamins and iron supplements are often continued until 6 weeks postpartum or until the ordered supply has been used.

Promotion of Normal Bladder and Bowel Patterns

Bladder

After giving birth, the mother should void spontaneously within 6 to 8 hours. The first several voidings should be measured to document adequate emptying of the bladder. A volume of at least 150 ml is expected for each voiding. Some women experience difficulty in emptying the bladder, possibly as a result of diminished bladder tone, edema from trauma, or fear of discomfort. Nursing interventions for inability to void and bladder distention are discussed on p. 612-613.

Bowel

Nursing interventions to promote normal bowel elimination include educating the woman about measures to avoid constipation. These interventions include ensuring adequate roughage and fluid intake and promoting exercise. Alerting the woman to side effects of medications such as opioid analgesics (decreased gastrointestinal tract motility) may encourage her to implement measures to reduce the risk of constipation. Stool softeners or laxatives are routinely ordered and may be necessary during the early postpartum period. With early discharge, a new mother may be home before having a bowel movement.

Some mothers experience gas pains. Ambulation or rocking in a rocking chair may stimulate passage of flatus and relief of discomfort.

Breastfeeding Promotion or Lactation Suppression

Breastfeeding Promotion

The first 2 hours after childbirth are an excellent time to encourage the mother to breastfeed. The infant is in an alert state and ready to nurse. Breastfeeding aids in the contraction of the uterus and prevention of maternal hemorrhage. This is an opportune time to instruct the mother in breastfeeding and to assess the physical appearance of the breasts. (See Chapter 26 for further information on assisting the breastfeeding woman.)

Lactation Suppression

Suppression of lactation is necessary when the woman has decided not to breastfeed or in the case of neonatal death. One very important nonpharmacologic intervention

BOX 21-6

Chicken Soup for Postpartum Chinese Women

1 whole chicken
Enough water to cover the chicken
Sliced scallions to taste
1 piece sliced ginger
2 tsp rice wine
White pepper to taste
Mushrooms (optional)

Place in pot. Bring to boil. Reduce temperature and cook for approximately 3 hours or until the chicken is tender and falls from the bones. Serve hot.

Courtesy Lin Zhan, Lowell, MA.

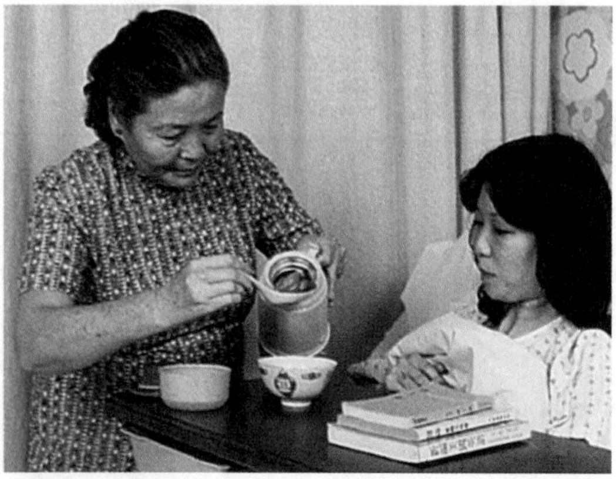

Fig. 21-8 Special foods are considered essential for recovery in the Asian culture. (Courtesy Concept Media, Irvine, CA.)

Community Focus

BREASTFEEDING SUPPORT

Women breastfeed longer if they have support in their breastfeeding efforts. Nurses and lactation consultants provide support during inpatient stays after childbirth. Women can find support in the community in various groups. Social support interventions that include peer support are successful in increasing the duration of exclusive breastfeeding and satisfaction with breastfeeding. Nurses in their discharge planning can refer breastfeeding mothers to community groups for support. Community and home health nurses can facilitate breastfeeding efforts through organizing or facilitating support groups. Mothers experienced in breastfeeding can facilitate these efforts.

Data from Vari P, Camburn J, Henly S: Professionally mediated peer support and early breastfeeding success, *J Perinat Educ* 9(1):22-30, 2000.

is continuously wearing a well-fitted support bra or breast binder for at least the first 72 hours after giving birth. Women should avoid breast stimulation, including running warm water over the breasts, newborn suckling, or pumping of the breasts. A few nonbreastfeeding mothers experience severe breast engorgement (swelling of breast tissue caused by increased blood and lymph supply to the breasts before lactation). If breast engorgement occurs, it can usually be managed satisfactorily with nonpharmacologic interventions.

Ice packs to the breasts are also helpful in decreasing the discomfort associated with engorgement. The woman should use a 15 minutes on, 45 minutes off, schedule (to prevent the rebound swelling that can occur if ice is used continuously), or she can place fresh cold cabbage leaves inside her bra. The leaves are replaced each time they wilt. Cabbage leaves have been used to treat swelling in other cultures for years (Roberts, 1995). The exact mechanism of action is not known, but it is thought that naturally occurring plant estrogens or salicylates may be responsible for the effects. A mild analgesic may also be necessary to help the mother through this uncomfortable time. Medications that were once prescribed for lactation suppression (estrogen, estrogen and testosterone, and bromocriptine) are no longer used.

Health Promotion of Future Pregnancies and Children

Rubella Vaccination

For women who have not had rubella (10% to 20% of all women) or women who are serologically not immune (titer of 1:8 or enzyme immunoassay [EIA] level <0.8), a subcutaneous injection of rubella vaccine is recommended before discharge. Seroconversion occurs in approximately 90% of women vaccinated after birth. The live attenuated rubella virus is not communicable; therefore breastfeeding mothers can be vaccinated. However, because the virus is shed in urine and other body fluids, the vaccine should not be given if the mother or other household members are immunocompromised. Rubella vaccine is made from duck eggs, so women who have allergies to these eggs may develop a hypersensitivity reaction to the vaccine, for which they will need adrenaline. A transient, benign arthralgia or rash is common in vaccinated women. Because the vaccine may be teratogenic, women must be informed about the vaccine.

LEGAL TIP **Rubella Vaccination** Informed consent for rubella vaccination in the postpartum period includes information about possible side effects and the risk of teratogenic effects. Women must understand that they must practice contraception to avoid pregnancy for 2 to 3 months after being vaccinated. ■

Prevention of Rh Isoimmunization

Injection of Rh immune globulin (a solution of gamma globulin that contains Rh antibodies) within 72 hours after birth prevents sensitization in the Rh-negative woman who has had a fetomaternal transfusion of Rh-positive fetal red blood cells (RBCs) (Medication Guide). Rh immune globulin promotes lysis of fetal Rh-positive blood cells before the mother forms her own antibodies against them.

Medication Guide

Rh Immune Globulin, RhoGAM, Gamulin Rh, HypRho-D, Rhophylac

Action

Suppression of immune response in nonsensitized women with Rh-negative blood who receive Rh-positive blood cells because of fetomaternal hemorrhage, transfusion, or accident

Indications

Routine antepartum prevention at 20 to 30 weeks gestation in women with Rh-negative blood; suppress antibody formation after birth, miscarriage/pregnancy termination, abdominal trauma, ectopic pregnancy, amniocentesis, version, or chorionic villi sampling

Dosage/Route

Standard dose: 1 vial (300 mcg) IM in deltoid or gluteal muscle; microdose: 1 vial (50 mcg) IM in deltoid muscle; Rhophylac can be given IM or IV (available in prefilled syringes)

Adverse Effects

Myalgia, lethargy, localized tenderness and stiffness at injection site, mild and transient fever, malaise, headache, rarely nausea, vomiting, hypotension, tachycardia, and allergic response

Nursing Considerations

- Give standard dose to mother at 28 weeks of gestation as prophylaxis, or after an incident or exposure risk that occurs after 28 weeks of gestation (e.g., amniocentesis, second trimester miscarriage or abortion, after version) and within 72 hours after birth if baby is Rh positive.
- Give microdose for first trimester miscarriage or abortion, ectopic pregnancy, chorionic villi sampling.
- Verify that the woman is Rh negative and has not been sensitized, that Coombs' test is negative, and that baby is Rh positive. Provide explanation to the woman about procedure, including the purpose, possible side effects, and effect on future pregnancies. Have the woman sign a consent form if required by agency. Verify correct dosage and confirm lot number and woman's identity before giving injection (verify with another RN or other procedure per agency policy); document administration per agency policy. Observe patient for at least 20 minutes after administration for allergic response.
- The medication is made from human plasma (a consideration if woman is a Jehovah's Witness). The risk of transmitting infectious agents, including viruses, cannot be completely eliminated.

NURSE ALERT After birth, Rh immune globulin is administered to all Rh-negative, antibody (Coombs' test) negative women who give birth to Rh-positive infants. Rh immune globulin is administered to the mother intramuscularly (RhoGAM, Gamulin RH, HypRho-D, Rhophylac) or intravenously (Rhophylac). It should never be given to an infant. ■

The administration of 300 mcg (1 vial) of Rh immune globulin is usually sufficient to prevent maternal sensitization. If a large fetomaternal transfusion is suspected, however, the dosage needed should be determined by performing a Kleihauer-Betke test, which detects the amount of fetal blood in the maternal circulation. If more than 15 ml of fetal blood is present in maternal circulation, the dosage of Rh immune globulin must be increased.

Evidence-Based Practice

PROMOTING BREASTFEEDING

Background

Well-documented benefits of breastfeeding include significantly reduced mortality in preterm infants; reduced morbidity from gastrointestinal, respiratory, urinary tract, and middle ear infections; and less atopic illness. In developing countries, the protective effect against infant and child mortality lasts into the second year of life. Breastfed infants demonstrate significantly higher cognitive abilities and have significantly lower blood pressure through the midteen years.

Women also experience associated health benefits with breastfeeding. A World Health Organization (WHO) review recommends exclusive breastfeeding for 6 months, with introduction of solids and continued breastfeeding thereafter. Yet breastfeeding initiation remains discouragingly low in some areas. In developed countries, the typical breastfeeding mother is advantaged, while mothers who are teenagers with low income and less education are the least likely to initiate or continue breastfeeding. Developing countries, on the other hand, are more likely to see breastfeeding in the lower socioeconomic classes than the educated, advantaged class. Hospitals may be discouraging breastfeeding by dispensing commercial discharge packs with free formula samples, a practice that the UNICEF-WHO Baby Friendly Initiative hopes to make illegal in as many countries as possible, as a standard of good practice. Many interventions, including the "Ten Steps of Successful Breastfeeding" developed by UNICEF-WHO, have been developed to encourage women to initiate and sustain breastfeeding.

Objectives

The reviewers hoped to describe the forms of support for breastfeeding women, the timing, and the settings. They wished to evaluate the effectiveness of the interventions, especially with low-income populations, to determine whether the postnatal intervention is strengthened by an antenatal component, to distinguish the different care providers and training, and to explore whether the background breastfeeding rates of a country influence the success of a breastfeeding intervention. The control group received standard care.

Methods

Search Strategy

Search strategy includes searching Cochrane, MEDLINE, EMBASE, ZETOC, Midwives Information and Resource Service, and asking experts. Search keywords were not noted.

The authors found 20 eligible randomized or quasi-randomized, controlled trials, involving 23,712 women from Brazil, the United States, Nigeria, Canada, Iran, Bangladesh, the United Kingdom, Nelarus, Mexico, and Sweden, dated 1979 to 2000.

Statistical Analyses

Similar data were pooled in a meta-analysis. Reviewers calculated relative risks for dichotomous (categorical) data, and weighted mean differences for continuous data. The authors accepted differences outside the 95% confidence interval as significant.

Findings

Overall, there were significantly beneficial effects on any breastfeeding outcomes in groups that received extra breastfeeding support, and breastfeeding duration was significantly longer. Treatment effect was greater in areas with a greater background breastfeeding rate in the population. The supported groups were significantly more likely to breastfeed exclusively than the controls. Professional support staff were more effective at preventing the cessation of breastfeeding, up to 9 months. Lay support staff were effective at reducing the cessation of breastfeeding in women who were exclusively breastfeeding, compared to controls. Face-to-face contact was more effective than phone calls. Of the training courses for support personnel, the UNICEF-WHO training courses had the most beneficial effect on exclusive and prolonged breastfeeding. Exclusive breastfeeding was especially beneficial to infants with diarrhea. Breastfeeding women expressed greater satisfaction than controls.

In a related review of commercial discharge packs, nine trials of 3720 women found a decrease in exclusive breastfeeding duration when the women were given formula samples by the hospital.

Limitations

The outcomes are measured in myriad ways, such as breastfeeding duration from 2 weeks to 1 year, in a variety of increments. The interventions are not described and therefore not reproducible in many studies. Follow-up was varied. The strengths of the study were the power of the numbers and the consistency of the findings.

Conclusions

Increased support for breastfeeding does increase the initiation, duration of exclusive breastfeeding, and duration of any breastfeeding, with beneficial results for infants. The UNICEF-WHO training courses are effective for personnel. Face-to-face contact is most effective. There is no evidence that antenatal breastfeeding support improves outcomes. Exclusive breastfeeding is very effective in managing infant diarrhea. Finally, a background culture of breastfeeding seems to act synergistically with support to encourage breastfeeding.

Implications for Practice

Nurses can ensure that all mothers receive support for breastfeeding. They can advocate for a hospital discharge pack with breastfeeding related items, such as breast pads and pump, and breastfeeding information. They can strive to have their hospital meet the criteria for Baby Friendly status.

Implications for Further Research

Further research is needed to assess the effectiveness of support personnel and training in a variety of settings, especially in areas of low breastfeeding. Cost-effectiveness is an important outcome. Implementation of the Baby Friendly Initiative needs ongoing monitoring. Qualitative research is needed to identify elements of effective support strategies.

References

Donnelly A et al: Commercial hospital discharge packs for breastfeeding women (Cochrane Review), 2001. In *The Cochrane Library,* Issue 2, Chichester, UK, 2004, John Wiley & Sons.

Indoria S, Wade A: Support for breastfeeding women (Cochrane Review), 2001. In *The Cochrane Library,* Issue 2, Chichester, UK, 2004, John Wiley & Sons.

Sikorski J et al: Support for breastfeeding women (Cochrane Review), 2001. In *The Cochrane Library,* Issue 2, Chichester, UK, 2004, John Wiley & Sons.

A 1:1000 dilution of Rh immune globulin is cross-matched to the mother's RBCs to ensure compatibility. Because Rh immune globulin is usually considered a blood product, precautions similar to those used for transfusing blood are necessary when it is given. The identification number on the patient's hospital wristband should correspond to the identification number found on the laboratory slip. The nurse must also check to see that the lot number of the laboratory slip corresponds to the lot number on the vial. Finally, the expiration date on the vial should be checked to ensure it is a usable product.

Rh immune globulin suppresses the immune response. Therefore the woman who receives both Rh immune globulin and rubella vaccine must be tested in 3 months to see if she has developed rubella immunity. If not, the woman will need another dose of rubella vaccine.

There is some disagreement about whether Rh immune globulin should be considered a blood product. Health care providers need to discuss the most current information about this issue with women whose religious beliefs conflict with having blood products administered to them.

Evaluation

The nurse can be reasonably assured that care was effective when the expected outcomes of care for physical needs have been achieved.

Care Management—Psychosocial Needs

Meeting the psychosocial needs of new mothers involves assessing the parents' reactions to the birth experience, their feelings about themselves, and their interactions with the new baby (Fig. 21-9) and other family members. Specific interventions are then planned to increase the parents' knowledge and self-confidence as they assume the care and responsibility of the new baby and integrate a new member into their existing family structure in a way that meets their cultural expectations.

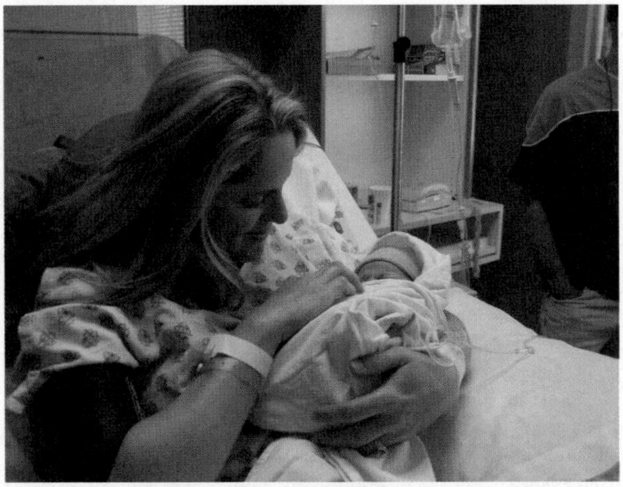

Fig. 21-9 Mother interacting with her new daughter. (Courtesy Tricia Olson, North Ogden, UT.)

Assessment

Impact of the Birth Experience

Many women indicate a need to examine the birth process itself and look at their own intrapartal behavior in retrospect. Their partners may express similar desires. During pregnancy the woman and her partner may have developed a specific birth plan that included a vaginal birth and very little medical intervention. If their birth experience was quite different from that planned (e.g., induction, epidural anesthesia, cesarean birth), both partners may need to mourn the loss of their expectations before they can adjust to the reality of their birth experience. Fathers report not feeling supported by policies (de Montigny & Lacharite, 2004). Inviting them to review the events and describe how they feel helps the nurse assess how well they understand what happened and how well they have been able to put their childbirth experience into perspective. Having control in the experience increases satisfaction (Goodman, Mackey, & Tavakoli, 2004).

Maternal Self-Image

An important assessment concerns the woman's self-concept, body image, and sexuality. How this new mother feels about herself and her body during the puerperium may affect her behavior and adaptation to parenting. The woman's self-concept and body image may also affect her sexuality.

Feelings related to sexual adjustment after childbirth are often a cause of concern for new parents. Women who have recently given birth may be reluctant to resume sexual intercourse for fear of pain, or they may worry that coitus could damage healing perineal tissue. Because many new parents are anxious for information but reluctant to bring up the subject, postpartum nurses should matter-of-factly include the topic of postpartum sexuality during their routine physical assessment. While examining the episiotomy site, for example, the nurse can say, "I know you're sore right now, but it probably won't be long until you (or you and your partner) are ready to make love again. Have you thought about what that might be like? Would you like to ask me questions?" This approach assures the woman and her partner that resuming sexual activity is a legitimate concern for new parents and indicates the nurse's willingness to answer questions and share information.

Maternal Adaptation

The psychosocial assessment includes evaluating adaptation to parenthood, which is a significant stress for many women. The majority (50% to 80%) of new mothers have a psychologic reaction after birth that is often referred to as *maternity* or *postpartum blues* or the *baby blues.* The cause of these baby blues is unknown, but may well be a transient response to the rapid role changes that occur as women adapt to motherhood. Symptoms vary widely from woman to woman, but can include behaviors such as weeping, insomnia, irritability, anxiety, forgetfulness, mood swings, and negative feelings toward the infant. These symptoms, which may be exacerbated by the sleep deprivation that often occurs during the puerperium, usually appear within the first week after birth and generally disappear by postpartum day 10. Extra rest, physical and emotional support, and sympathetic understanding from friends and family are usually sufficient to help women cope with this reaction (Bowes & Katz, 2002). It is important to remember that the baby blues are mild and short-lived.

Parent-Infant Interactions

Adaptation to parenthood can be assessed by evaluating the mother's and father's reactions to and interactions with the new baby. Clues indicating successful adaptation begin to appear early in the postbirth period as parents react positively to the newborn infant and continue the process of establishing a relationship with him or her.

Parents are adapting well to their new role when they exhibit a realistic perception and acceptance of their newborn's needs and his or her limited abilities, immature social responses, and helplessness. Examples of positive parent-infant interactions include taking pleasure in their infant and in the tasks done for and with him or her; understanding their infant's emotional states and providing comfort; and reading their infant's cues for new experiences and sensing his or her fatigue level. See Chapter 22 for a more in-depth discussion of parenting.

Family Structure and Functioning

A woman's adjustment to her role as mother is affected greatly by her relationships with her partner, her mother and other relatives, and any other children. Nurses can help ease the new mother's return home by identifying possible conflicts among family members and helping the woman plan strategies for dealing with these problems before discharge. Such a conflict could arise when couples have very different ideas about parenting. Dealing with the stresses of sibling rivalry and unsolicited grandparent advice can also affect the woman's transition to motherhood. Only by asking about other nuclear and extended family members can the nurse discover potential problems in such relationships and help plan workable solutions for them.

Impact of Cultural Diversity

The final component of a complete psychosocial assessment is the woman's cultural beliefs and values. Much of a woman's behavior during the postpartum period is strongly influenced by her cultural background. In today's world, where travel is commonplace, nurses are likely to come into contact with women from many different countries and cultures. All cultures have developed safe and satisfying methods of caring for new mothers and babies. Only by understanding and respecting the values and beliefs of each woman can the nurse design a plan of care to meet individual needs (Cultural Awareness box).

Sometimes the psychosocial assessment indicates serious actual or potential problems that must be addressed. Box 21-7 lists several psychosocial needs that, at a minimum, warrant ongoing evaluation following hospital discharge. Patients exhibiting these needs should be referred to appropriate community resources for assessment and management.

Cultural Awareness

A CLASH OF CULTURES

A Vietnamese woman who had been in the United States for 4 years requested rooming-in facilities after childbirth. Instead of participating in the care of her infant, she refused to do so, remained in bed, wore a woolen cap, and appeared distressed and angry. The staff were puzzled and upset by her behavior. One nurse decided to put into effect her newly learned concepts concerning cross-cultural nursing. She began by praising the woman's ability to speak English and, after eliciting a smile, remarked, "Every country has developed good ways to look after mothers and babies. Would you tell me about the care in Vietnam?" There was an immediate response. The woman explained that in her country, women remained in bed for at least 10 days after birth, and the biggest danger to their health was getting a cold. The baby was kept in the room with his mother, but either a grandmother or nurse took complete charge of the care.

With this information, the nurse was able to modify her plan of care to make it culturally relevant, and therefore more satisfying for the woman.

Nursing Diagnoses

After analyzing the data obtained during the assessment process, the nurse establishes nursing diagnoses to provide a guide for planning care. Nursing diagnoses related to psychosocial issues that are often established for the postpartum patient include the following:

- *Interrupted family processes related to*
  —unexpected birth of twins
- *Impaired verbal communication related to*
  —patient's hearing impairment
  —nurse's language not the same as patient's
- *Impaired parenting related to*
  —long, difficult labor
  —unmet expectations of labor and birth
- *Anxiety related to*
  —newness of parenting role, sibling rivalry, or response of grandparent
- *Risk for situational low self-esteem related to*
  —body image changes

Expected Outcomes

Expected psychosocial outcomes during the postpartum period are based on the nursing diagnoses identified for the individual woman and her family. Examples of common expected outcomes include that the woman (family) will do the following:

- Identify measures that promote a healthy personal adjustment in the postpartum period.

BOX 21-7

Signs of Potential Complications—Psychosocial

Psychosocial Needs

Unable or unwilling to discuss labor and birth experience
Refers to self as ugly and useless
Excessively preoccupied with self (body image)
Markedly depressed
Lacks a support system
Partner and/or other family members react negatively to the baby
Refuses to interact with or care for baby; (e.g., does not name baby, does not want to hold or feed baby, is upset by vomiting and wet or dirty diapers). (Cultural appropriateness of actions needs to be considered.)
Expresses disappointment over baby's sex
Sees baby as messy or unattractive
Baby reminds mother of family member or friend she doesn't like

- Maintain healthy family functioning based on cultural norms and personal expectations.

Plan of Care and Implementation

The nurse functions in the roles of teacher, encourager, and supporter rather than doer while implementing the psychosocial plan of care for a postpartum woman. Implementation of the psychosocial care plan involves carrying out specific activities to achieve the expected outcome of care planned for each individual woman. Topics that should be included in the psychosocial plan of care include promotion of parenting skills and family member adjustment to the newest member. These topics are discussed in Chapter 22.

Cultural issues must also be considered when planning care. In contrast with allopathic medicine, many traditional health beliefs and practices occur among the different cultures within the North American population. Traditional health practices that are used to maintain health or to avoid illnesses deal with the whole person (body, mind, and spirit) and tend to be culturally based (Kim-Godwin, 2003; White, 2004).

Women from various cultures may view health as a balance between opposing forces (e.g., yin versus yang), being in harmony with nature, or just "feeling good." Traditional practices may include the observance of certain dietary restrictions, clothing, or taboos for balancing the body; participation in certain activities such as sports and art for maintaining mental health; and use of silence, prayer, or meditation for developing spiritually. Practices (e.g., using religious objects or eating garlic) are used to protect oneself from illness and may involve avoiding people who are believed to create hexes, spells, or who have an "evil eye." Restoration of health may involve a person taking folk medicines (e.g., herbs or animal substances) or using a traditional healer (White, 2004).

Childbirth occurs within this sociocultural context. Rest, seclusion, dietary restraints, and ceremonies honoring the mother are all common traditional practices that are followed for the promotion of the health and well-being of the mother and baby (Davis, 2001; Kridli, 2002; Lauderdale, 1999; Mattson, 2000).

Women and their families use several common traditional health practices and hold various beliefs during the postpartum period. In Southeast Asia, for example, the body is thought to be in a "cold" state after birth because of the loss of blood, which is considered a "hot" substance. Therefore balance needs to be restored by increasing the return of yang forces present physically or symbolically in hot food, hot water, and warm air (Davis, 2001; Kim-Godwin, 2003; White, 2004). Vietnamese, Cambodian, and Hmong women believe that if they do not follow the traditional diet or get sufficient rest after childbirth, they will likely become ill or develop serious health problems later in life (Davis, 2001; White, 2004). Khmer women may practice "roasting" in which they lie on a bamboo bed for periods over a wood or charcoal fire to restore heat. Ghosts are attracted to blood, thus Khmer women are vulnerable to attack by ghosts in the postpartum period (White, 2004) (Cultural Awareness box).

Another common belief is that the mother and baby remain in a weak and vulnerable state for a period of several weeks following birth (Davis, 2001; Mattson, 2000; White, 2004). During this time the mother may remain in a passive role, take no baths or showers, and stay in bed to prevent cold air from entering her body. Women who have immigrated to the United States or other Western nations without their extended families may not have much help at home, making it difficult for them to observe these activity restrictions (Davis, 2001).

Box 21-8 lists some common cultural beliefs about the postpartum period and family planning.

It is important that nurses consider all cultural aspects when planning care and not use their own cultural beliefs as the framework for that care. Although the beliefs and behaviors of other cultures may seem different or strange, they should be encouraged as long as the mother wants to conform to them, and she and the baby have no ill effects. The nurse must determine whether a woman is using any folk medicine during the postpartum period because active ingredients in folk medicine may have adverse physiologic effects on the woman when ingested with prescribed medicines (Mattson, 2000). However, the nurse should not assume that a mother desires to use traditional health practices that represent a particular cultural group just because she is a member of that culture. Many young women who are first- generation or second-generation Americans follow their cultural traditions only when older family members are present, or not at all.

Evaluation

The nurse can be reasonably assured that care was effective if expected outcomes of care for psychosocial needs have been met.

Discharge Teaching

Self-Care, Signs of Complications

Discharge planning begins at the time of admission to the unit and should be reflected in the plan of care developed for each individual woman. For example, a great deal of time during the hospital stay is usually spent in teaching about maternal and newborn care, because all women must be capable of providing basic care for themselves and their infants at the time of discharge. It is also crucial that every woman be taught to recognize the physical signs and symptoms that might indicate problems and how to obtain advice and assistance quickly if these signs appear. Boxes 21-4 and 21-8 list several common

> **Cultural Awareness**
>
> **POSTPREGNANCY HERBAL STEAM BATHS**
>
> Traditional Cambodians use a postpregnancy treatment of herbal steams and *aing phleung*. From 80% to 90% of Cambodian women use these treatments. Herbal steams involve sitting in a room or a tent full of hot vapor from boiled herbs and roots. *Aing phleung* involves burning wood and heating rocks under the woman's bed. Both are purported to remove blood from the woman's uterus after birth. Doctors caution use of these treatments. There can be tissue damage from the fire and dehydration if both treatments are used at the same time. If these treatments are used, women should stay in the heat for short periods and turn over every 5 minutes. The newborn should be kept away from the smoke.
>
> Reference: Lebun B: Overuse of post-pregnancy herbal steam baths poses risks, *The Cambodia Daily*, 30(29):16, 2004.

BOX 21-8

Some Cultural Beliefs about the Postpartum Period and Family Planning

Postpartum Care

Chinese, Mexican, Korean, and *Southeast Asian women* may wish to eat only warm foods and drink hot drinks to replace blood loss and to restore the balance of hot and cold in their bodies. These women may also wish to stay warm and avoid bathing, exercises, and hair washing for 7 to 30 days after childbirth. Self-care may not be a priority; care by family members is preferred. The woman has respect for elders and authority. These women may wear abdominal binders. They may prefer not to give their babies colostrum.

Haitian women may request to take the placenta home to bury or burn.

Muslim women follow strict religious laws on modesty and diet. A Muslim woman must keep her hair, body, arms to the wrist, and legs to the ankles covered at all times. She cannot be alone in the presence of a man other than her husband or a male relative. Observant Muslims will not eat pork or pork products and are obligated to eat meat slaughtered according to Islamic laws (halal meat). If halal meat is not available, kosher meat, seafood, or a vegetarian diet is usually accepted.

Family Planning

Birth control is government mandated in mainland *China.* Most *Chinese women* will have an IUD inserted after the birth of their first child. Women do not want hormonal methods of contraception because they fear putting these medications in their bodies.

Saudi Arabian and *Hispanic* women will likely choose the rhythm method because most are Catholic.

(East) Indian men are encouraged to have voluntary sterilization by vasectomy.

Muslim couples may practice contraception by mutual consent as long as its use is not harmful to the woman. Acceptable contraceptive methods include foam and condoms, the diaphragm, and natural family planning.

Hmong women highly value and desire large families, which limits birth control practices.

ENGLISH SPANISH Guidelines/Guías

DISCHARGE TEACHING

When you go to the bathroom, always wipe from front to back.
Cuando vaya al baño, séquese siempre de adelante hacia atrás.

Sit in a warm tub to relieve discomfort.
Siéntese en una bañera con agua tibia para aliviarse.

You will have moderate amounts of vaginal discharge.
Usted tendrá cantidades moderadas de sangrado vaginal.

It may last from 4 to 6 weeks.
Puede durar desde 4 a 6 semanas.

The color may vary from dark brown to red to pink.
El color puede variar entre café oscuro a rojo a rosado.

It may contain blood clots.
Es probable que contenga coágulos.

Use a sanitary pad instead of a tampon.
Use una toalla sanitaria en vez de un tampón.

Your menstrual period will not resume for 4 to 10 weeks.
Su regla no regresará hasta 4 a 10 semanas más tarde.

If you are breastfeeding, it may take a little longer.
Si está amamantando, puede demorar un poco más.

It is possible to become pregnant while you are breastfeeding.
Es posible quedar embarazada mientras amamanta.

Avoid having sexual relations for 2 to 4 weeks after birth.
Evite las relaciones sexuales por 2 a 4 semanas después del parto.

Gradually increase activity to incorporate everyday routines.
Aumente las actividades gradualmente hasta llegar a su rutina normal.

Do your Kegel exercises.
Haga los ejercicios Kegel.

Do not lift heavy objects (>10 pounds).
No levante objetos pesados (de más de 10 libras).

Rest as often as possible.
Descanse mucho.

Rest when your baby sleeps.
Descanse cuando duerma su bebé.

Eat daily:
Cómase diariamente

4 servings of bread/cereals, fruits/vegetables (green), milk or foods made from milk, and 2 servings of meat. You need to drink 8 glasses of fluids a day to support breastfeeding.
4 porciones de pan/cereal, frutas/vegetales (verduras), leche o comidas del grupo de leche, y 2 porciones de carne. Usted necesita tomer beber 8 vasos de líquidos diariamente para soportar el dar de pecho.

Call your doctor (obstetrician) if you have:
Llame al médico de obstétricas si tenga cualquier de lo siguente:

- Fever >38° C
  Fiebre de 38° C
- Increased vaginal bleeding (more than a regular period)
  Aumento de desangre vaginal (más que una regla normal)
- Chills
  Escalofríos
- Painful, burning urination
  Orin que le duele o le quema
- Foul-smelling vaginal discharge
  Desangre vaginal de muy mal olor
- Increased pain or swelling
  Aumento de dolor o hinchazón
- Drainage or separation of incision (cesarean)
  Desangre o deshecho de la herida

indications of maternal physical and psychosocial problems in the postpartum period. (See Chapter 23 for more information on postpartum complications.) Before discharge, women need basic instruction regarding the resumption of sexual intercourse, prescribed medications, routine mother-baby checkups, and contraception (see Guidelines/Guías box).

New mothers may be too overwhelmed physically and emotionally to absorb and retain all this information in the brief time they are in the postpartum unit. Nurses must target their teaching on expressed needs of the woman. Giving the woman a list of topics and asking her to indicate her teaching needs will help the nurse maximize teaching efforts and may increase retention of information by the woman (Ruchala, 2000).

Just before the time of discharge, the nurse reviews the woman's chart to see that laboratory reports, medications, signatures, and other items are in order. Some hospitals have a checklist to use before the woman's discharge. The nurse verifies that medications, if ordered, have arrived on the unit; that any valuables kept secured during the woman's stay have been returned to her and that she has signed a receipt for them; and that the infant is ready to be discharged.

No medication that would make the mother sleepy should be administered if she is the one who will be holding the baby on the way out of the hospital. In most instances, the woman is seated in a wheelchair and is given the baby to hold. Some families leave unescorted and ambulatory, depending on hospital protocol. The woman's possessions are gathered and taken out with her and her family. The woman's and the baby's identification bands are carefully checked. As the woman and the baby are assisted into the car, the nurse should make sure that there is a car seat in which to secure the baby (Fig. 21-10).

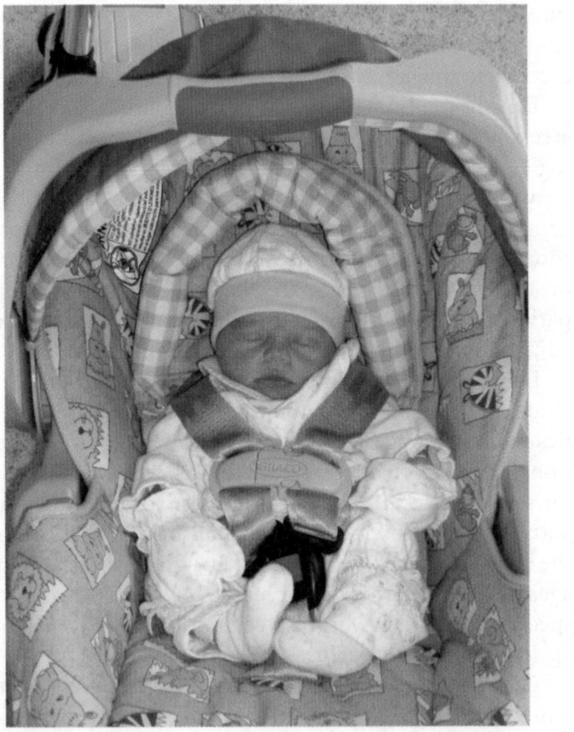

Fig. 21-10 Infant secured in car seat. (Courtesy Tricia Olson, North Ogden, UT.)

Sexual Activity/Contraception

Many couples resume sexual activity before the traditional postpartum checkup 6 weeks after childbirth. Risk of hemorrhage and infection are minimal by approximately 2 weeks postpartum. Couples may be anxious about the topic but uncomfortable and unwilling to bring it up. It is important that the nurse discuss the physical and psychologic effects that giving birth can have on sexual activity (Home Care box). Contraceptive options should be discussed with women (and their partners if present) before discharge so that they can make informed decisions about fertility management before resuming sexual activity. Waiting to discuss contraception at the 6-week checkup may be too late. It is possible, particularly in women who bottle-feed, for ovulation to occur as soon as 1 month after birth. A woman who engages in unprotected sex risks becoming pregnant much sooner than she planned. Current contraceptive options are discussed in detail in Chapter 7. Women who are undecided about contraception at the time of discharge need information about using condoms with foam or creams until the first postpartum checkup.

Prescribed Medications

Women routinely continue to take their prenatal vitamins and iron during the postpartum period. It is especially important that women who are breastfeeding or who are discharged with a lower than normal hematocrit take these medications as prescribed. Women with extensive epi-

Home Care

RESUMPTION OF SEXUAL INTERCOURSE

You can safely resume sexual intercourse by the second to fourth week after birth when bleeding has stopped and the episiotomy has healed. For the first 6 weeks to 6 months, the vagina does not lubricate well.

Your physiologic reactions to sexual stimulation for the first 3 months after birth will be slower and less intense. The strength of the orgasm is reduced.

A water-soluble gel, cocoa butter, or a contraceptive cream or jelly might be recommended for lubrication. If some vaginal tenderness is present, your partner can be instructed to insert one or more clean, lubricated fingers into the vagina and rotate them within the vagina to help relax it and to identify possible areas of discomfort. A position in which you have control of the depth of the insertion of the penis also is useful. The side-by-side or female-on-top position may be more comfortable.

The presence of the baby influences postbirth lovemaking. Parents hear every sound made by the baby; conversely, you may be concerned that the baby hears every sound you make. In either case, any phase of the sexual response cycle may be interrupted by hearing the baby cry or move, leaving both of you frustrated and unsatisfied. In addition, the amount of psychologic energy expended by you in child care activities may lead to fatigue. Newborns require a great deal of attention and time.

Some women have reported feeling sexual stimulation and orgasms when breastfeeding their babies. Breastfeeding mothers often are interested in returning to sexual activity before nonbreastfeeding mothers.

You should be instructed to correctly perform the Kegel exercises to strengthen your pubococcygeal muscle. This muscle is associated with bowel and bladder function and with vaginal feeling during intercourse.

siotomies or vaginal lacerations (third or fourth degree) are usually prescribed stool softeners to take at home. Pain relief medications (analgesics or nonsteroidal antiinflammatory medications) may be prescribed, especially for women who had cesarean birth. The nurse should make certain that the woman knows the route, dosage, frequency, and common side effects of all ordered medications.

Routine Mother and Baby Checkups

Women who have experienced uncomplicated vaginal births are still commonly scheduled for the traditional 6-week postpartum examination. Women who have had a cesarean birth are often seen in the health care provider's office or clinic within 2 weeks after hospital discharge. The date and time for the follow-up appointment should be included in the discharge instructions. If an appointment is not made before the woman leaves the hospital, she should be encouraged to call the health care provider's office or clinic and schedule an appointment herself.

Parents who have not already done so need to make plans for newborn follow-up at the time of discharge. Most offices and clinics like to see newborns for an initial examination within the first week or by 2 weeks of age. If an appointment for a specific date and time was not made for the infant before leaving the hospital, the parents should be encouraged to call the office or clinic right away.

Dealing with Activities of Daily Life at Home

Even the small details of daily life may become stressful, given the demands of a newborn and the discomfort or fatigue associated with birth and a busy homecoming day, or both. The parents may wish to buy disposable diapers for the first hours at home even if they plan to use cloth diapers. During pregnancy, the woman is encouraged to freeze extra casseroles or leftovers to use for the first few meals at home; family, friends, and neighbors can be encouraged to bring prepared food during this time.

Planning for discharge soon after an infant feeding ensures that the couple will have adequate time to get home and relatively settled before the next feeding. Offering a sample carton of premixed bottles for the formula-fed infant prevents need for rushed preparation of formula.

NURSE ALERT Prepackaged formula should not be given to mothers who are breastfeeding. Such "gifts" are associated with earlier cessation of breastfeeding. ■

Dealing with Visitors

A newborn in the family or neighborhood draws visitors. The nurse can help the parents explore ways in which they can assert their needs in such situations. When family or friends ask what they can do to help, the family can respond with "Please bring us a casserole or a meal" or "Could you please pick up some items at the grocery store?" The couple may want to work out a signal for alerting the partner that the new mother is becoming tired or uncomfortable and needs to have the partner invite the visitors into another part of the house. Some new mothers have found that if they remain in their robe and do not appear ready for company, visitors stay for a shorter time. A "Please Do Not Disturb" sign on the front door may be useful when the mother is resting.

Follow-Up after Discharge

Home Visits

The Association of Women's Health, Obstetric, and Neonatal Nurses (AWHONN) (1994) published guidelines for postpartum home care that describe comprehensive perinatal home care follow-up services. The common goal of these services is to ensure that the mother, newborn, and family have an optimal opportunity to prepare for and enjoy safe, comprehensive, and high-quality perinatal care.

Home visits to new mothers and babies within a few days of discharge can help bridge the gap between hospital care and routine visits to health care providers. Nurses are able to assess the mother, infant, and home environment; answer questions and provide education; and make referrals to community resources if necessary. Home visits may also help reduce the need for more expensive health care, such as nonroutine health care visits and rehospitalization, and decrease stress in new families.

A referral form containing information about both mother and baby should be completed at hospital discharge and sent immediately to the home care agency. Figure 21-11 is an example of such a referral form.

The home visit is most commonly scheduled on the woman's second day home from the hospital, but it may be scheduled on any of the first 4 days at home, depending on the individual family's situation and needs. Additional visits are planned throughout the first week, as needed. The home visits may be extended beyond that time if the family's needs warrant it and if a home visit is the most appropriate option for carrying out the follow-up care required to meet the specific needs identified.

A home visit progresses more effectively if it is preplanned and well organized. In advance, the nurse reviews the hospital's discharge summary, teaching plan, and any other records, including the physician's orders; this serves to structure the interview and physical assessment and hence provide continuity of care. Before the visit, the nurse also obtains directions to the family's home and gets a map, if necessary.

During the home visit the nurse conducts a systematic assessment of mother and newborn to determine physiologic adjustment, identify any existing complications, and answer any questions the mother/family has about herself or newborn care. Conducting the assessment in a separate room provides private time for the mother to ask questions on topics such as breast care, family planning, and constipation. The assessment focuses on the mother's emotional adjustment and her knowledge of self- and infant care.

During the newborn assessment, the nurse can demonstrate and explain normal newborn behavior and capabilities and encourage the mother and/or family to ask questions or express concerns each may have. The home care nurse must verify if the newborn screen for phenylketonuria and other inborn errors of metabolism has been drawn. If the baby was discharged from the hospital before 24 hours of age, the home care or clinic nurse will need to collect the specimen for the newborn screening.

Telephone Follow-Up

As part of the routine follow-up of a woman and her infant after discharge from the hospital, many providers are implementing one or more postpartum telephone follow-up calls to their patients for assessment, health teaching, and

OB Homecare
Phone: 612-863-4478
Fax: 612-863-4568

POSTPARTUM HOME CARE REFERRAL

☐PHN Referral Made to ____________ County

Mother's Name: ______________________

Address/Phone where mother will be staying:

Address: ______________________

City: ______________________

Phone #:(_______) ______________________

☐ **Address & Phone Verified**

Language Spoken: ☐ English ☐ Other: ____________

Understands English: ☐ Well ☐ Poor

☐ Mother Needs Interpreter ☐ Hearing Impaired

Who interpreted in hospital: ____________

Phone: (_____) ____________

Mom's MD/Midwife: (Full Name) ____________

Phone #: (_______) ____________

Next Appt: ____________

MOTHER:

Gravida ______ T____ P____ A____ L____

Marital Status: S M W D Sep

Normal Maternal Exam: ☐Yes ☐No (explain below)

☐ Vaginal Birth ☐ C/Birth

Epis/Incision: ____________

Meds: ____________

Allergies: ____________

☐ Needs Large BP Cuff

OTHER ISSUES:

Diabetic: ____________

Hgb pp, if abnormal: ____________

Psycho/Social Issues:

☐ Parent/Child Interaction ☐ Limited Support System
☐ Mental Health Status ☐ Drug Use/Dependency
☐ Previous Losses ☐ Hx of Domestic Violence
☐ Other: ____________

Husband/Significant Other: ____________

Baby's Name: ____________ ☐M ☐F

Delivery Date/Time: __________@__________

Mother's Discharge Date/Time: _________@________

Baby's MD (Full Name): ____________

Phone #: (_______) ____________

Next Appt: ____________

BABY:

Gestation: __________weeks ☐ Fetal Loss

Birth Weight: ____________ Discharge wt: ____________

Apgars: 1" _______ 5" ________

Feedings: ☐ Breast ☐ Bottle ☐ Both

Feeding Issues: ____________

Normal Infant Exam: ☐ Yes ☐ No (explain below)
Circumcised: ☐ Yes ☐ No

Additional Order:

☐ Home care to draw newborn screen
**Must send lab-slip home with family.

ADDITIONAL COMMENTS or
ABNORMAL FINDINGS FOR MOTHER OR BABY:

Mom aware of referral: ☐Yes ☐No **REFERRAL COMPLETED BY:** ____________

☐ ***Faxed to OB Homecare @-612-863-4568:*** ☐ ***Facesheet*** ☐ ***Referral***
☐ ***Faxed to PHN*** ____________ ***County:*** ☐ ***Facesheet*** ☐ ***Referral***
Currently being seen by PHN: ☐ Yes ☐ No

Fig. 21-11 Referral form. (Courtesy OB Homecare of Allina Hospitals and Clinics, Minneapolis, MN.)

identification of complications to effect timely intervention, and referrals. Telephone follow-up may be part of the services offered by the hospital, private physician or clinic, or a private agency; it may be either a separate service, or combined with other strategies for extending postpartum care. If no home care follow-up is provided, then telephone follow-up may take its place. Telephonic nursing assessments are commonly used after a postpartum home care visit to reassess a woman's knowledge about the signs and symptoms of adequate hydration in breastfeeding or, after initiating home phototherapy, to assess the caregiver's knowledge regarding equipment complications.

Warm Lines

The warm line is another type of telephone link between the new family and concerned caregivers or experienced parent volunteers. A warm line is a helpline or consultation service, not a crisis intervention line. The warm line is appropriately used for dealing with less extreme concerns that may seem urgent at the time the call is placed but are not actual emergencies. Calls to warm lines commonly relate to infant feeding, prolonged crying, or sibling rivalry. Often families will be given the telephone number for the nursery or the postpartum unit and encouraged to call if questions or concerns arise after hospital discharge.

Support Groups

A postpartum support group enables mothers and fathers to share with and support each other as they adjust to parenting. Many new parents find it reassuring to discover that they are not alone in their feelings of confusion and uncertainty. An experienced parent can often impart concrete information that can be valuable to other members in a postpartum support group. Inexperienced parents may find themselves imitating the behavior of others in the group whom they perceive as particularly capable.

The woman adjusting to motherhood sometimes seeks a special group experience. Postpartum women who have met earlier in prenatal clinics or on the hospital unit may begin to associate for mutual support. Members of Lamaze classes who attend a postpartum reunion may decide to extend their relationship during the fourth trimester. Realizing the value of group support, nurses may wish to make postpartum support groups available as a strategy for bridging the hospital and home experience.

Referral to Community Resources

At times the nurse will want to refer families needing extra attention for specific problems to appropriate agencies. Health departments and school systems can usually provide information about existing local resources, such as parent or professional support groups. National organizations also can be useful in providing published resource guides and lists of community service agencies specific to the group or condition they represent (see Resources). Individual nurses will find it helpful to develop their own resource file of services that are frequently useful to postpartum families.

Key Points

- Postpartum care is modeled on the concept of health.
- Cultural beliefs and practices affect the patient's response to the puerperium.
- The nursing care plan includes assessments to detect deviations from normal, comfort measures to relieve discomfort or pain, and safety measures to prevent injury or infection.
- Teaching and counseling measures are designed to promote the woman's feelings of competence in self-care and baby care.
- Common nursing interventions in the postpartum period include evaluating and treating the boggy uterus and the full urinary bladder; providing for nonpharmacologic and pharmacologic relief of pain and discomfort associated with the episiotomy, lacerations, or breastfeeding; and instituting measures to promote or suppress lactation.
- Meeting the psychosocial needs of the new mother involves taking into consideration the composition and functioning of the entire family.
- Early postpartum discharge will continue to be the trend as a result of consumer demand, medical necessity, discharge criteria for low risk childbirth, and cost-containment measures.
- The short-stay option in perinatal care is safer when selection criteria are used to determine a woman's eligibility for early discharge and when home care follow-up is available.
- Early discharge classes, telephone follow-up, home visits, warm lines, and support groups are effective means of preventing crisis and facilitating physiologic and psychologic adjustments in the postpartum period.

Answer Guidelines to Critical Thinking Exercise

Fatigue and Rest after Childbirth

1. Tiredness and fatigue are common in the postpartum period. Childbirth educators can foster more realistic expectations for the postnatal period and discuss effective coping strategies for that time. They can legitimate the need for support (McQueen & Mander, 2003). Women with financial worries, lack of social support, and strains after childbirth are more likely to become depressed (Seimyr et al, 2004). Nurses may be able to identify women at risk for problems after childbirth by asking questions about their private and work lives (des Rivieres-Pigeon, Saurel-Cubizolles, & Lelong, 2004).
2. (a) Women who breastfeed may have less sleep and thus experience more tiredness and fatigue. (b) Support from the mother's network of friends, relatives, and caregivers is important for breastfeeding success. Enabling the mother and infant to stay together after birth is important (Ekstrom, Widstrom & Nissen, 2003). (c) Sleep deprivation and inadequate rest may lead to fatigue and depression in the postnatal period. Relevant assessments to identify causes of fatigue should be made. (d) Pregnancies that occur close together prevent the body from recovering completely between pregnancies. Women with closely spaced pregnancies are more likely to be anemic and may have tiredness associated with the anemia. Adequate nutrition and iron supplementation should be provided.
3. The priority for care is to assess Patricia's level of fatigue and mood, and to develop a plan of care with her to promote adequate rest and to enlist support from friends and relatives. Community resources available for Patricia should be identified.
4. There is evidence of the association of childbearing and fatigue and depression. Social support leads to breastfeeding success.
5. It may be necessary to explore further the marital relationship and support provided by Patricia's husband. Contraceptive options should be discussed with the cou-

ple. If more children are desired, increased spacing between pregnancies should be encouraged. Patricia should be assessed for postnatal depression. Follow-up telephone calls and home visits would be useful. Referral to relevant community agencies is appropriate. Further research into postpartum adaptation is warranted.

References for Answer Guidelines

des Rivieres-Pigeon C, Saurel-Cubizolles MJ, Lelong N: Considering a simple strategy for detection of women at risk of psychological distress after childbirth, *Birth* 31(1):34-42, 2004.

Ekstrom A, Widstrom AM, Nissen E: Breastfeeding support from partners and grandmothers: perceptions of Swedish women, *Birth* 30(4):261-266, 2003.

McQueen A, Mander R: Tiredness and fatigue in the postnatal period, *J Adv Nurs* 42(5): 463-469, 2003.

Seimyr L et al: In the shadow of maternal depressed mood: experiences of parenthood during the first year after childbirth, *J Psychosom Obstet Gynaecol* 25(1):23-34, 2004.

Resources

American Red Cross
430 17th St., NW
Washington, DC 20006
202-737-8300
www.redcross.org

Child Welfare League of America
440 First St., NW, Third Floor
Washington, DC 20001-2085
202-638-2952
202-638-4004 (fax)
www.cwla.org/default.htm

Depression after Delivery
PO Box 59973
Renton, WA 98508
206-283-9278
www.behavenet.com

HAND (Helping after Neonatal Death)
PO Box 341
Los Gatos, CA 95031
www.h-a-n-d.org

La Leche League
1400 N. Meacham Rd.
Schaumburg, IL 60168-4079
800-525-3243 (24-hour line)
www.lalecheleague.org

March of Dimes Birth Defects Foundation
National Foundation/March of Dimes
1275 Mamaroneck Ave.
White Plains, NY 10605
914-428-7100
888-663-4637 (MODIMES)
www.modimes.org

National Perinatal Association
101 ½ South Union St.
Alexandria, VA 22314-3323
703-549-5523

Nursing Mothers Council
Consult telephone directory for local chapters

Parent Soup
www.parentsoup.com

Planned Parenthood Federation of America, Inc.
810 Seventh Ave.
New York, NY 10019
800-230-PLAN
www.plannedparenthood.org

Positive Parenting
www.positiveparenting.com

Postpartum Education for Parents
PO Box 6154
Santa Barbara, CA 93160
www.sbpep.org/pepppd.htm

Special Supplemental Nutrition Program for Women, Infants, and Children (WIC)
Food and Consumer Service
3101 Park Center Dr., Room 819
Alexandria, VA 22302
703-305-2286
www.usda.gov/fns/wic.html

References

American Academy of Pediatrics: Hospital stay for healthy term infants, *Pediatrics* 96(4):788-790, 1995.

American Academy of Pediatrics Committee on Drugs: The transfer of drugs and other chemicals into human milk, *Pediatrics* 108(3):776-789, 2001.

Association of Women's Health, Obstetric, and Neonatal Nurses (AWHONN): *Didactic content and clinical skills verification for professional nurse providers of perinatal home care,* Washington, DC, 1994, AWHONN.

Benedetti TJ: Obstetric hemorrhage. In Gabbe SG, Niebyl JR, Simpson JL (eds): *Obstetrics: normal and problem pregnancies,* ed 4, New York, 2002, Churchill Livingstone.

Bowes WA, Katz VL: Postpartum care. In Gabbe SG, Niebyl JR, Simpson JL (eds): *Obstetrics: normal and problem pregnancies,* ed 4, New York, 2002, Churchill Livingstone.

Davis RE: The postpartum experience for Southeast Asian women in the United States, *MCN Am J Matern Child Nurs* 26(4):208-213, 2001.

de Montigny F, Lacharite C: Fathers' perceptions of the immediate postpartal period, *J Obstet Gynecol Neonatal Nurs* 33(3):328-339, 2004.

Donnelly A et al: Commercial hospital discharge packs for breastfeeding women (Cochrane Review), 2001. In *The Cochrane Library,* Issue 2, Chichester, UK, 2004, John Wiley & Sons Ltd.

Edmonson MB, Stoddard JJ, Owens LM: Hospital readmission with feeding-related problems after early postpartum discharge of normal newborns, *JAMA* 278(4):299-303, 1997.

Ferguson SL, Engelhard CL: Short stay: the art of legislating quality and economy, *AWHONN Lifelines* 1(1):17-23, 1997.

Fishbein EG, Burggraf E: Early postpartum discharge: how are mothers managing? *J Obstet Gynecol Neonatal Nurs* 27(2):142-148, 1998.

Goodman P, Mackey MC, Tavakoli AS: Factors related to childbirth satisfaction, *J Adv Nurs,* 46(2):212-219, 2004.

Indoria S, Wade A: Support for breastfeeding women (Cochrane Review), 2001. In *The Cochrane Library,* Issue 2, Chichester, UK, 2004, John Wiley & Sons, Ltd.

Kim-Godwin YS: Postpartum beliefs and practices among non-western cultures, *MCN Am J Matern Child Nurs* 28(2):74-80, 2003.

Kridli SA: Health beliefs and practices among Arab women, *MCN Am J Matern Child Nurs* 27(3):178-182, 2002.

Lauderdale J: Childbearing and transcultural nursing care issues. In Andrews M, Boyle J (eds): *Transcultural concepts in nursing care,* ed 3, Philadelphia, 1999, Lippincott.

Lebun B: Overuse of post-pregnancy herbal steam baths poses risks, *The Cambodia Daily,* 30(29):16, 2004.

Liu LL et al: The safety of newborn early discharge: the Washington State Experience, *JAMA* 278(4):293-298, 1997.

Luegenbiehl D: Improving visual estimation of blood volume on peripads, *MCN Am J Matern Child Nurs* 22(6):294-298, 1997.

Mattson S: Providing culturally competent care: strategies and approaches for perinatal clients, *AWHONN Lifelines* 4(5):37-39, 2000.

Pugh LC et al: Clinical approaches in the assessment of childbearing fatigue, *J Obstet Gynecol Neonatal Nurs* 28(1):74-80, 1999.

Roberts KL: A comparison of chilled cabbage leaves and chilled gelpaks in reducing breast engorgement, *J Hum Lact* 11(1):17-20, 1995.

Ruchala P: Teaching new mothers: priorities of nurses and postpartum women, *J Obstet Gynecol Neonatal Nurs* 29(3):265-273, 2000.

Sampselle CM et al: Continence for women: a test of AWHONN's evidence-based protocol in clinical practice, *J Obstet Gynecol Neonatal Nurs* 29(1):18-26, 2000.

Sikorski J et al: Support for breastfeeding women (Cochrane Review), 2001. In *The Cochrane Library,* Issue 2, Chichester, UK, 2004, John Wiley & Sons, Ltd.

Vari P, Camburn J, Henly S: Professionally mediated peer support and early breastfeeding success, *J Perinat Educ* 9(1):22-30, 2000.

Weekly SJ, Neumann ML: Speaking up for baby: the case for individualized neonatal discharge plans, *AWHONN Lifelines* 1(1):24-29, 1997.

Weiss M et al: Length of stay after vaginal birth: sociodemographic and readiness-for-discharge factors, *Birth* 31(2):93-101, 2004.

White PM: Heat, balance, humors, and ghosts: postpartum in Cambodia, *Health Care Women Int* 25(2):179-194, 2004.

Williams LR, Cooper MK: A new paradigm for postpartum care, *J Obstet Gynecol Neonatal Nurs* 25(9):745-749, 1996.

Wilkinson S et al: Physical activity in low-income postpartum women, *J Nurs Sch* 36(2):109-114, 2004.

Transition to Parenthood 22

LEARNING OBJECTIVES

On completion of this chapter the reader will be able to:

- Discuss ways to facilitate parent-infant adjustment.
- Describe sensual responses that strengthen attachment.
- Identify infant behaviors that facilitate and inhibit parental attachment.
- Differentiate the three periods in parental role change after childbirth.
- Identify behaviors of the three phases of maternal adjustment.
- Discuss paternal adjustment.
- Discuss the effects of the following on parental response: parental age (i.e., adolescence and more than 35 years), social support, culture, socioeconomic conditions, personal aspirations, and sensory impairment.
- Describe sibling adjustment.
- Describe grandparent adaptation.

ELECTRONIC RESOURCES

Additional information related to the content in Chapter 22 can be found on

the companion website at evolve
http://evolve.elsevier.com/Wong/maternal/
- NCLEX Review Questions
- WebLinks

or the interactive student CD-ROM
Activities for Chapter 22 include the following:
- NCLEX Review Questions
- Critical Thinking Exercise—Postpartum Home Care
- Nursing Care Plan—Home Care Follow-up
- Skill—Swaddling

Becoming a parent creates a period of change and instability for men and women who decide to have children. This occurs whether parenthood is biologic or adoptive and whether the parents are married husband-wife couples, cohabiting couples, single mothers, single fathers, lesbian couples with one woman as biologic mother, or gay male couples who adopt a child. This period of developmental change is referred to as the *transition to parenthood. Transition* is a process occurring over time involving development and movement from one state or condition to another. Nurses often encounter patients during times of transition that occur because of developmental, situational, or health-illness events. The transition to parenthood is one such time.

This chapter reviews the transition to parenthood, including the parenting process and the adjustment of parents, siblings, and grandparents.

PARENTING PROCESS

Biologic parenthood begins with the union of ovum and sperm. During the prenatal period, the mother provides an environment in which the unborn child develops and grows. This close symbiotic union ends with birth. At this point, other people assume partial or complete involvement in the infant's care. The biologic or substitute female or male parent then enters into a crucial relationship with the child that persists throughout the life of each. Parenthood can serve as a maturation factor for women and men regardless of whether it is biologically based. For children, parenthood is all-important; their continued existence depends on the quality of care they receive. Sank (1991) described parenting as a process of role attainment and role transition that begins during pregnancy. The transition ends when the parent develops a sense of comfort and confidence in performing the parental role.

Nurses can help inexperienced parents feel confident and competent in their new roles. They can provide opportunities for parents to practice child care tasks in the hospital, birth setting, or in the home, where assistance and feedback are available. Nurses can enhance parents' self-concept by helping them feel more comfortable and confident in their parenting skills.

Parental Attachment, Bonding, and Acquaintance

The process by which a parent comes to love and accept a child, and a child comes to love and accept a parent, is referred to as *attachment.* Using the terms *attachment* and *bonding,* Klaus and Kennell (1997) originally proposed that the period shortly after birth is important to mother-to-infant attachment. They defined the phenomenon of *bonding* as a sensitive period in the first minutes and hours after birth, when mothers and fathers must have close contact with their infants for optimal later development (Klaus & Kennell, 1976). Klaus and Kennell (1982) later revised their theory of parent-infant bonding, modifying their claim of the critical nature of immediate contact with the infant after birth. They acknowledged the adaptability of human parents, stating it took longer than minutes or hours for parents to form an emotional relationship with their infants.

Attachment is developed and maintained by proximity and interaction with the infant; through this the parent becomes acquainted with the infant, identifies the infant as an individual, and claims the infant as a member of the family. Attachment is facilitated by positive feedback (i.e., social, verbal, and nonverbal responses, whether real or perceived, that indicate acceptance of one partner by the other). Attachment occurs through a mutually satisfying experience. A mother commented on her son's grasp reflex, "I put my finger in his hand, and he grabbed right on. It is just a reflex, I know, but it felt good anyway."

The concept of attachment has been extended to include mutuality; that is, the infant's behaviors and characteristics call forth a corresponding set of maternal behaviors and characteristics. The infant displays signaling behaviors such as crying, smiling, and cooing that initiate the contact and bring the caregiver to the child. These behaviors are followed by executive behaviors such as rooting, grasping, and postural adjustments that maintain the contact. The caregiver is attracted to an alert, responsive, cuddly infant and repelled by an irritable, apparently disinterested infant. Attachment occurs more readily with the infant whose temperament, social capabilities, appearance, and sex fit the parent's expectations. If the child does not meet these expectations, resolution of the parent's disappointment can delay the attachment process.

An important part of attachment is acquaintance. Parents use eye contact, touching, talking, and exploring to become acquainted with their infant during the immediate postpartum period. Adoptive parents undergo the same process when they first meet their new child. During this period, families engage in the claiming process, which is the identification of the new baby. The child is first identified in terms of "likeness" to other family members, then in terms of "differences," and finally in terms of "uniqueness." The unique newcomer is thus incorporated into the family. Mother and father scrutinize their infant carefully and point out characteristics that the child shares with other family members and that are indicative of a relationship between them. The claiming process is revealed by maternal comments such as the following: "Russ held him close and said, 'He's the image of his father,' but I found one part like me—his toes are shaped like mine."

On the other hand, some mothers react negatively. They "claim" the infant in terms of the discomfort or pain the baby causes. The mother interprets the infant's normal responses as being negative toward her and reacts to her child with dislike or indifference. She does not hold the child close or touch the child to be comforting; for example, "The nurse put the baby into Marie's arms. She promptly laid him across her knees and glanced up at the television. 'Stay still until I finish watching—you've been enough trouble already.'"

Over the years, attachment research has shown that neither the type of birth (vaginal, planned cesarean, unplanned cesarean) nor the type of infant feeding is related to parental attachment. Parents' perception of their own competence is an important predictor of parental attachment for mothers and fathers. Nurses can use these findings to reassure mothers who have had unplanned cesarean births that they can bond as successfully with their infants as if they had had vaginal births. Through teaching and positive reinforcement, nurses can strengthen parents' sense of competence.

Nurses play an important role in facilitating parental attachment. They can enhance positive parent-infant contacts by heightening parental awareness of an infant's responses and ability to communicate. As the parent attempts to become competent and loving in that role, nurses can bolster the parent's self-confidence and ego. Nurses are in prime positions to identify actual and potential problems and collaborate with other health care professionals who will provide care for the parents after discharge. Nursing interventions related to the promotion of parent-infant attachment are numerous and varied. Table 22-1 lists examples of activities for parent-infant attachment interventions.

Assessment of Attachment Behaviors

One of the most important areas of assessment is careful observation of those behaviors thought to indicate the formation of emotional bonds between the newborn and family, especially the mother. Although the words *bonding* and *attachment* are sometimes referred to as separate phenomena, with *bonding* representing the development of emotional ties from parent to infant, and *attachment* representing the emotional ties from infant to parent, in this discussion, the words are used interchangeably to denote both processes.

Unlike physical assessment of the neonate, which has concrete guidelines to follow, assessment of parent-infant attachment requires much more skill in terms of observation and interviewing. Rooming-in of mother and infant and liberal visiting privileges for father, siblings, and grandparents facilitate recognition of behaviors that demonstrate positive or negative attachment. Guidelines for assessment of attachment behaviors are presented in the Patient Teaching box.

During pregnancy, and often even before conception occurs, parents develop an image of the "ideal" or "fantasy" infant. At birth the fantasy infant becomes the real infant. How closely the dream child resembles the real child influences the bonding process. Assessing such expectations during pregnancy and at the time of the infant's birth allows identification of discrepancies in the parents' view of the fantasy child versus the real child.

The labor process significantly affects the immediate attachment of mothers to their newborn infants. Factors such

Table 22-1

Examples of Parent-Infant Attachment Interventions

INTERVENTION LABEL/DEFINITION	ACTIVITIES
ATTACHMENT PROMOTION	
Facilitation of development of parent-infant relationship	Provide opportunity for parent(s) to see, hold, and examine newborn immediately after birth Encourage parent(s) to hold infant close to body Assist parent(s) to participate in infant care Provide rooming-in in hospitals
ENVIRONMENTAL MANAGEMENT: ATTACHMENT PROCESS	
Manipulation of patient's surroundings to facilitate development of parent-infant relationship	Create environment that fosters privacy Individualize daily routine to meet parent's needs Permit father/significant other to sleep in room with mother Develop policies that permit presence of significant others as much as desired
FAMILY INTEGRITY PROMOTION: CHILDBEARING FAMILY	
Facilitation of growth of individuals or families who are adding infant to family unit	Prepare parent(s) for expected role changes involved in becoming a parent Prepare parent(s) for responsibilities of parenthood Monitor effects of newborn on family structure Reinforce positive parenting behaviors
LACTATION COUNSELING	
Use of interactive helping process to assist in maintenance of successful breastfeeding	Correct misconceptions, misinformation, and inaccuracies about breastfeeding Evaluate parent's understanding of infant's feeding cues (e.g., rooting, sucking, alertness) Determine frequency of feedings in relation to infant's needs Demonstrate breast massage and discuss its advantages to increasing milk supply
PARENT EDUCATION: INFANT	
Instruction on nurturing and physical care needed during first year of life	Determine parent(s) knowledge, readiness, and ability to learn about infant care Provide anticipatory guidance about developmental changes during first year of life Teach parent(s) skills to care for newborn Demonstrate ways in which parent(s) can stimulate infant's development Discuss infant's capabilities for interaction Demonstrate quieting techniques
RISK IDENTIFICATION: CHILDBEARING FAMILY	
Identification of individual or family likely to experience difficulties in parenting and assigning priorities to strategies to prevent parenting problems	Determine developmental stage of parent(s) Review prenatal history for factors that predispose patient to complications Ascertain understanding of English or other language used in community Monitor behavior that may indicate problem with attachment Plan for risk-reduction activities in collaboration with individual or family

Modified from McCloskey JC, Bulechek GM: *Nursing interventions classification*, ed 3, St Louis, 2000, Mosby.

as a long labor, feeling tired or "drugged" after birth, and problems with breastfeeding can delay the development of initial positive feelings toward the newborn.

Because attachment involves a reciprocal interchange, observing the interaction between parent and infant is very important. An excellent opportunity exists during feeding. A useful instrument for systematically describing the parent's and infant's behaviors is the Nursing Child Assessment Feeding Scale (NCAFS) (Barnard, 1994). It consists of 76 behavioral items, 50 of which describe the parent's behavior regarding sensitivity to cues, response to child's distress, social-emotional growth fostering, and cognitive growth

Patient Teaching

ASSESSING ATTACHMENT BEHAVIORS

When the infant is brought to the parents, do they reach out for the infant and call the infant by name? (Recognize that in some cultures, parents may not name the infant in the early newborn period.)

Do the parents speak about the infant in terms of identification? For example, do they surmise whom the infant looks like or identify what appears special about their infant in comparison with other infants?

When parents are holding the infant, what kind of body contact is there? Do parents feel at ease in changing the infant's position? Are fingertips or whole hands used? Are there parts of the body they avoid touching or parts of the body they investigate and scrutinize?

When the infant is awake, what kinds of stimulation do the parents provide? Do they talk to the infant, to each other, or to no one? How do they look at the infant? Do they use direct visual contact, avoid eye contact, or look at other people or objects?

How comfortable do the parents appear in terms of caring for the infant? Do they express any concern regarding their ability or disgust for certain activities, such as changing diapers?

What type of affection do they demonstrate to the newborn, such as smiling, stroking, kissing, or rocking?

If the infant is fussy, what kinds of comforting techniques do the parents use, such as rocking, swaddling, talking, or stroking?

fostering. Twenty-six items focus on the child's behavior in terms of clarity of cues and responsiveness to parent. The results also can be shared with the parent to encourage discussion of feelings about the infant and to highlight behaviors of the dyad that foster successful interaction. The NCAFS is appropriate for use with infants during the first year.

Parent-Infant Contact

Early Contact

Early close contact may facilitate the attachment process between parent and child. This does not mean that a delay will inhibit this process (humans are too resilient for that), but additional psychologic energy may be needed to achieve the same effect. No scientific evidence has demonstrated that immediate contact after birth is essential for the human parent-child relationship.

Parents who desire but are unable to have early contact with their newborn can be reassured that such contact is not essential for optimal parent-infant interactions. Otherwise, adopted infants would not form the usual affectional ties with their parents. Nor does the mode of infant-mother contact after birth (i.e., skin-to-skin versus wrapped) appear to have any important effect. Nurses must counsel parents that the emotional bond to the infant is not necessarily weaker because they missed early contact or because the contact was not skin-to-skin. Opportunities for parents to be with the infant in the intensive care nursery, to touch or hold the baby (if at all possible), and to receive reports of the infant's progress must be part of the nursing plan of care. Nurses need to stress that the parent-infant relationship is a process that occurs over time.

Extended Contact

The provision of rooming-in facilities for the mother and her baby is common in family-centered care. The infant is transferred to the area from the transitional nursery (if the facility uses one) after showing satisfactory extrauterine adjustment. The father is encouraged to participate in the care of the infant, and siblings and grandparents are also encouraged to visit and become acquainted with the infant. Many hospitals have established family birth units such as labor-delivery-recovery (LDR) rooms, labor-delivery-recovery-postpartum (LDRP) rooms, and single-room maternity care (SRMC). The mother is accompanied by her partner during the birth of the infant, and all three may remain together until discharged around 48 hours after birth. Whether the method of family-centered care is rooming-in or a family birth unit, mothers and their partners are considered equal and integral parts of the developing family. Partners are encouraged to take as active a role as they wish (Fig. 22-1). Some hospitals and birth centers arrange for the discharge of the mother and infant any time from 2 to 24 hours after the birth if the parents desire it and the condition of the mother and that of the infant warrant it. Follow-up care with nursing personnel from a home health care agency is usually part of this plan.

Mother-baby care, also called *couplet care,* is another form of family-centered care. Care and teaching for the mother and baby are provided by a primary nurse, fostering family unity. Parents involved in this approach are likely to

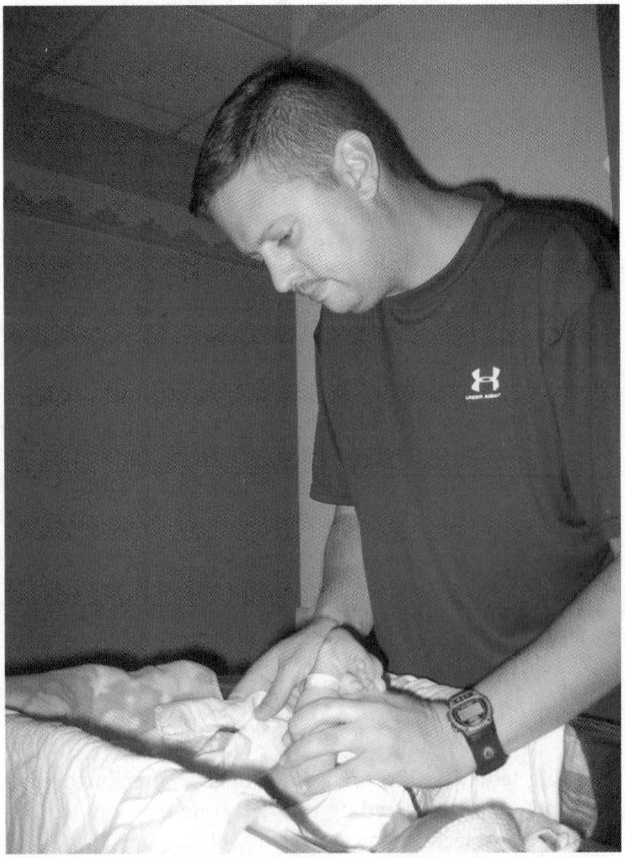

Fig. 22-1 Father changes diaper of his newborn son. (Courtesy Brian and Mayannyn Sallee, Las Vegas, NV.)

be more self-confident in care, and maternal attachment and role attainment are promoted.

Extended contact with the infant should be available for all parents but especially for those at risk for parenting inadequacies, such as adolescents and low-income women. Any activity that optimizes family-centered care is worthy of serious consideration by postpartum nurses. Baby Friendly status for a hospital is one means to promote family-centered care.

The Baby Friendly Hospital Initiative, sponsored by the World Health Organization (WHO) and UNICEF, was founded to encourage institutions to offer optimal levels of care for lactating mothers. When a hospital achieves *The Ten Steps to Successful Breastfeeding for Hospitals,* it is recognized as a Baby Friendly Hospital. The steps include the following: having a written breastfeeding policy, training staff, informing pregnant women about the benefits of breastfeeding, initiating breastfeeding within 1 hour of birth, helping mothers maintain lactation even when separated from their infants, giving newborns only breastmilk to drink, rooming-in 24 hours a day, breastfeeding on demand, avoiding pacifiers, and promoting the establishment of breastfeeding support groups and referring mothers to them.

Communication between Parent and Infant

The parent-infant relationship is strengthened through the use of sensual responses and abilities by both partners in the interaction. The nurse should keep in mind that there may be cultural variations in these interactive behaviors (described later).

Touch

Touch, or the tactile sense, is used extensively by parents and other caregivers as a means of becoming acquainted with the newborn. Many mothers reach out for their infants as soon as they are born and the cord is cut. They lift them to their breasts, enfold them in their arms, and cradle them. Once the infant is close to them, they begin the exploration process with their fingertips, one of the most touch-sensitive areas of the body (Fig. 22-2). Within a short time the caregiver uses the palm to caress the baby's trunk, and eventually enfolds the infant. Gentle stroking motions are used to soothe and quiet the infant. Patting or gently rubbing the infant's back is a comfort after feedings. Infants also pat the mother's breast as they nurse. Both seem to enjoy sharing each other's body warmth. Parents want to touch, pick up, and hold the infant. They comment on the softness of the baby's skin and are aware of milia and rashes. As parents become increasingly sensitive to the infant's like or dislike of different types of touch, they draw closer to their baby.

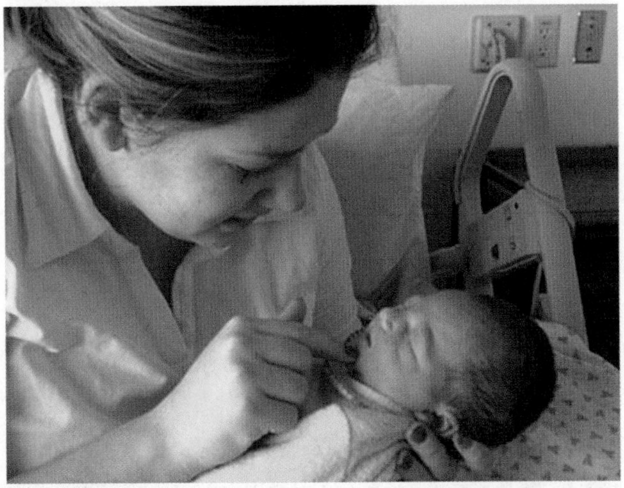

Fig. 22-2 Mother uses fingertip to explore infant. (Courtesy Rebekah Vogel, Ft. Collins, CO.)

Variations in touching behaviors have been noted in mothers from different cultural groups (Galanti, 2003; Inman, 1996; Jambunathan & Stewart, 1995; Jiménez, 1995). For example, minimal touching and cuddling is a traditional Southeast Asian practice thought to protect the infant from evil spirits. Because they hold different traditions and spiritual beliefs, women in India and Bali have practiced infant massage since ancient times.

Eye-to-Eye Contact

Interest in having eye contact with the baby has been demonstrated repeatedly by parents. Some mothers remark that once their babies have looked at them, they feel much closer to them. Parents spend much time getting their babies to open their eyes and look at them. In North American culture, eye contact appears to cement the development of a trusting relationship, and is an important factor in human relationships at all ages (Fig. 22-3). In other cultures, eye-to-eye contact may be perceived differently (see Cultural Awareness box) For example, in Mexican culture, sustained direct eye contact is considered to be rude, immodest, and dangerous for some. This danger may arise from the *mal ojo* ("evil eye"), resulting from excessive admiration. Women and children are thought to be more susceptible to the mal ojo (D'Avanzo & Geissler, 2003).

As newborns become functionally able to sustain eye contact with their parents, time is spent in mutual gazing, often in the *en face* position. In this position, the parent's face and the infant's face are approximately 8 inches apart

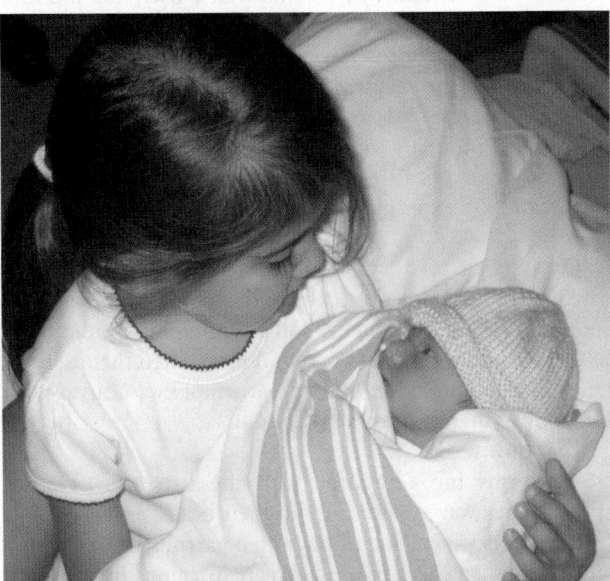

Fig. 22-3 Big sister in eye-to-eye contact with newborn brother. (Courtesy Brian and Mayannyn Sallee, Las Vegas, NV.)

Cultural Awareness

FOSTERING BONDING

Women of Varying Ethnic and Cultural Groups

Childbearing practices and rituals of other cultures may not be congruent with standard practices associated with bonding in the Anglo-American culture. For example, Chinese families traditionally use extended family members to care for the newborn so that the mother can rest and recover, especially after a cesarean birth. Some Native American, Asian, and Hispanic women do not initiate breastfeeding until their breast milk comes in. Haitian families do not name their babies until after the confinement month. Amount of eye contact varies among cultures, too. Yup'ik Eskimo mothers almost always position their babies so that eye contact can be made.

Nurses should become knowledgeable of the childbearing beliefs and practices of diverse cultural and ethnic groups. Because individual cultural variations exist within groups, nurses need to clarify with the patient and family members or friends what cultural norms the patient follows. Incorrect judgments may be made about mother-infant bonding if nurses do not practice culturally sensitive care.

Modified from D'Avanzo C, Geissler E: *Pocket guide to cultural assessment*, ed 3, St Louis, 2003, Mosby.

and on the same plane. Nursing and medical practices need to be implemented that encourage this interaction. Immediately after birth, for example, the infant can be positioned on the mother's abdomen or breasts with the mother's and the infant's faces on the same plane so that they can easily make eye contact. Lights can be dimmed so that the infant's eyes will open. Instillation of prophylactic antibiotic ointment in the infant's eyes can be delayed until the infant and parents have had some time together in the first hour after birth.

Voice

The shared response of parents and infants to each other's voices is also remarkable. Parents wait tensely for the first cry. Once that cry has reassured them of the baby's health, they begin comforting behaviors. As the parents talk in high-pitched voices, the infant is alerted and turns toward them.

The infant responds to higher-pitched voices and can distinguish the mother's voice from others soon after birth. Infants use their cries to signal hunger, pain, boredom, and tiredness. With experience, parents learn to distinguish such cries.

Odor

Another behavior shared by parents and infants is a response to each other's odor. Mothers comment on the smell of their babies when first born, and have noted that each infant has a unique odor. Infants learn rapidly to distinguish the odor of their mother's breast milk.

Entrainment

Newborns move in time with the structure of adult speech. They wave their arms, lift their heads, and kick their legs, seemingly "dancing in tune" to a parent's voice. Culturally determined rhythms of speech are ingrained in the infant long before spoken language is used to communicate. This shared rhythm also gives the parent positive feedback and establishes a positive setting for effective communication.

Biorhythmicity

The fetus is in tune with the mother's natural rhythms, such as heartbeats. After birth, a crying infant may be soothed by being held in a position where the mother's heartbeat can be heard or by hearing a recording of a heartbeat. One of the newborn's tasks is to establish a personal biorhythm. Parents can help in this process by giving consistent loving care and by using their infant's alert state to develop responsive behavior and thereby increase social interactions and opportunities for learning (Fig. 22-4). The more quickly parents become competent in child care activities, the more quickly their psychologic energy can be directed toward observing the communication cues the infant gives them.

Reciprocity and Synchrony

Reciprocity is a type of body movement or behavior that provides the observer with cues. The observer or receiver interprets those cues and responds to them. Reciprocity often takes several weeks to develop with a new baby. For example, when the newborn fusses and cries, the mother responds by picking up and cradling the infant; the baby becomes quiet and alert and establishes eye contact; the mother verbalizes, sings, and coos while the baby maintains eye contact. The baby then averts the eyes and yawns; the mother decreases her active response (Fig. 22-5). If the parent continues to stimulate the infant, the baby may become fussy.

Synchrony refers to the "fit" between the infant's cues and the parent's response. When parent and infant have a synchronous interaction, it is mutually rewarding. Parents need time to interpret the infant's cues correctly. For example, after a certain time the infant develops a specific cry in response to different situations such as boredom, loneliness, hunger, and discomfort. The parent may need assistance in deciphering these cries, along with trial and error interventions, before synchrony develops.

Parental Role after Childbirth

For the biologic parent, the parental role is enlarged and intensified at birth. The care and nurturing of the child were initiated well before birth. The mother who carried out the

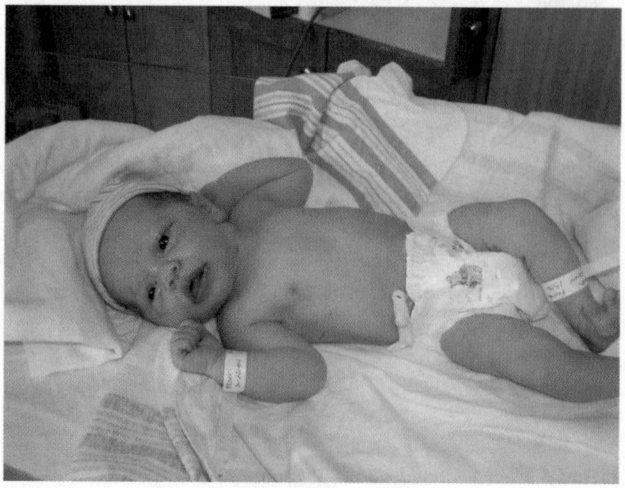

Fig. 22-4 Infant in alert state. (Courtesy Tricia Olson, North Ogden, UT.)

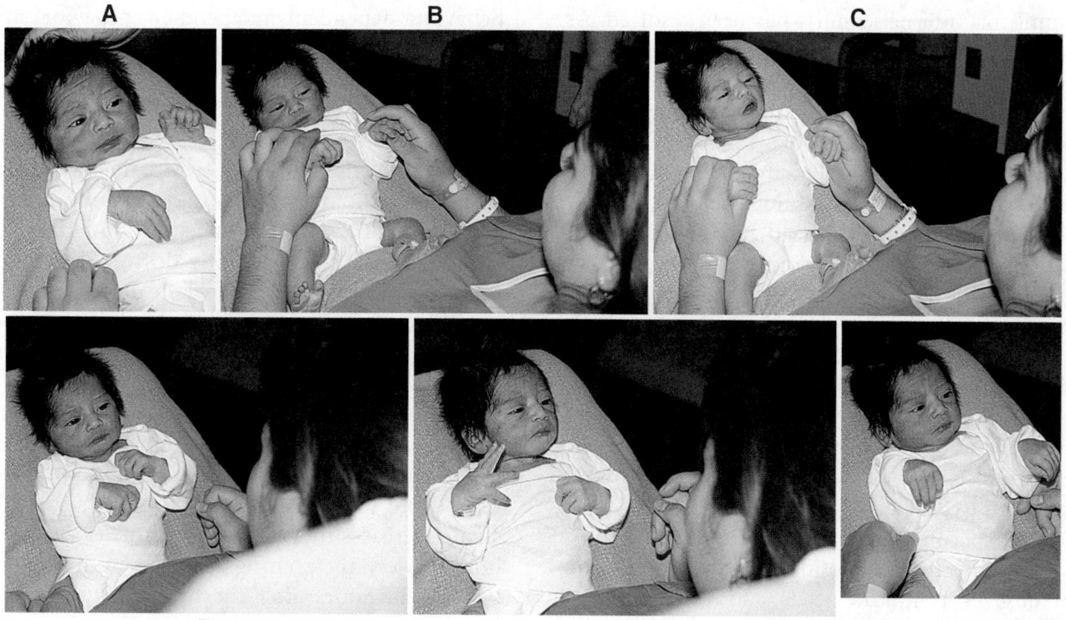

Fig. 22-5 Holding newborn in *en face* position, mother works to alert her daughter, 6 hours old. **A**, Infant is quiet and alert. **B**, Mother begins talking to daughter. **C**, Infant responds, opens mouth like her mother. **D**, Infant gazes at her mother. **E**, Infant waves hand. **F**, Infant glances away, resting. Hand relaxes. (Courtesy Marjorie Pyle, RNC, Lifecircle, Costa Mesa, CA.)

dictates of health (diet, rest, and exercise) for the "good of her baby," the partner who supported and sheltered her, and the parents who became aware of and attached to their unborn child were already functioning in the parental role before the birth. Even preconception decisions about whether and when to have a child influence mothers' and fathers' adjustment to the parental role.

The next few weeks are a time of drawing together and uniting the family unit. This period of consolidation involves negotiations concerning roles (wife-husband, mother-father, mother-partner, parent-child, sibling-sibling). Family integrity and adaptation occur when transactions between spouses regarding roles and role relationships are successful.

Adaptation involves a stabilizing of tasks and a coming to terms with commitments. Parents demonstrate growing competence in child care activities and are more attuned to their infant's behavior. Typically, the period from the decision to conceive through the first months of having a child is termed the *transition to parenthood.*

Transition to Parenthood

Historically, the transition to parenthood was viewed as a crisis. The current perspective is that parenthood is a developmental transition (Tomlinson, 1996) rather than a major life crisis for the majority of families. The transition to parenthood is described as a time of disorder and disequilibrium, as well as satisfaction, for mothers and their partners (Rogan et al, 1997; Tomlinson, 1996). Usual methods of coping often seem ineffective. Some parents can be so distressed that they are unable to be supportive of each other. Since men typically identify their spouses as their primary or only source of support, the transition can be harder for the fathers, who feel deprived because the mothers, who are also experiencing stress, cannot provide their usual level of support. Strong emotions such as the helplessness, inadequacy, and anger that arise when dealing with a crying infant catch many parents unprepared. On the other hand, parenthood allows adults to develop and display a selfless, warm, and caring side that may not be expressed in other adult roles. To view the world through the eyes of a child and to be childlike (not childish) are two rich rewards of parenthood.

For the majority of mothers and their partners, the transition to parenthood is viewed as an opportunity rather than a time of danger. Parents are stimulated to try new coping strategies as they work to master their new roles and reach new developmental levels. As they work through the transition, personal strength and resourcefulness are revealed (Rogan et al, 1997).

Parental Tasks and Responsibilities

Parents need to reconcile the actual child with the fantasy and dream child. This means coming to terms with the infant's physical appearance, sex, innate temperament, and physical status. If the real child differs greatly from the fantasy child, parents may delay acceptance of the child. In some instances, they may never accept the child.

Some parents are startled by the normal appearance of the neonate—the size, color, molding of the head, or bowed appearance of the legs. Many fathers have commented that they thought the odd shape of the infant's head (molding) meant the infant would be mentally retarded.

Many parents know the sex of the infant before birth because of ultrasound assessments; for those who do not have this information, disappointment over the sex of the infant can take time to resolve. The parents may provide adequate physical care but find it difficult to be sincerely involved with the infant until this internal conflict has been resolved. As one mother remarked, "I really wanted a boy. I know it is silly and irrational, but when they said, 'She's a lovely little girl,' I was so disappointed and angry—yes, angry—I could hardly look at her. Oh, I looked after her okay, her feedings and baths and things, but I couldn't feel excited. To tell the truth, I felt like a monster not liking my child. Then one day she was lying there and she turned her head and looked right at me. I felt a flooding of love for her come over me, and we looked at each other a long time. It's okay now. I wouldn't change her for all the boys in the world."

Nursing care plans should include discussion about reconciliation of the real versus the fantasy child. Nurses should provide opportunities for parents to discuss their lack of parental feelings without fear of censure or ridicule. Often the expression of doubts and concerns provides relief and makes it easier for parents to deal with and resolve such feelings.

Parents need to become adept in the care of the infant, including caregiving activities, noting the communication cues the infant gives to indicate needs, and responding appropriately to the infant's needs. Self-esteem grows with competence. Breastfeeding makes mothers feel they are contributing in a unique way to the welfare of the infant. Parents may interpret the infant's response to parental care and attention as a comment on the quality of that care. Infant behaviors that parents interpret as positive responses to their care include being consoled easily, enjoying being cuddled, and making eye contact. Spitting up frequently after feedings, crying, and being unpredictable may be perceived as negative responses to parental care. Continuation of infant responses that are viewed as negative can result in alienation of parent and infant to the detriment of the infant.

Assistance, including advice by husbands, partners, wives, mothers, mothers-in-law, and professional workers, can be seen either as supportive or an indication of how inept these others judge the new parents to be. Criticism, whether real or imagined, of the new parents' ability to provide adequate physical care, nutrition, or social stimulation for the infant can prove devastating. By providing encouragement and praise for parenting efforts, nurses can bolster the new parents' confidence. Parents should feel safe discussing concerns about other peoples' criticisms with the nurses, who can help them practice assertiveness techniques to use with unwanted "critics." The nurses, as patient advocates, can use positive, nonjudgmental approaches to help critics direct their advice constructively.

Parents must establish a place for the newborn within the family group. Whether the infant is the firstborn or the last born, all family members must adjust their roles to accommodate the newcomer. The firstborn child needs support to accept a rival for parental affections. An older child needs help dealing with losing a favored position in the family hierarchy. The parents are expected to negotiate these changes.

Parents need to establish the primacy of their adult relationships to maintain the family as a group. Because this includes reorganizing many roles, such as sexual, childcare, career, and community roles, time and energy must be provided for this vital task (see Guidelines/Guías box).

Maternal Adjustment

Three phases are evident as the mother adjusts to her parental role. These phases are characterized by dependent behavior, dependent-independent behavior, and interdependent behavior (Table 22-2).

Dependent Phase

During the first 24 to 48 hours after childbirth, the mother's dependency needs predominate. To the extent that these needs are met by others, the mother is able to divert her psychologic energy to her infant rather than to focus it on herself. She needs "mothering" herself to "mother." Rubin (1961) aptly described these few days as the taking-in phase, a time when the new mother requires nurturing and protective care. In Rubin's classic description, the taking-in phase lasted 2 to 3 days. Later studies found that women move more rapidly through the taking-in phase (Ament, 1990; Wrasper, 1996). Evans and colleagues (1998), in a study of women giving birth vaginally, found that both taking-in and taking-hold (see next section) were present on the evening of birth. There were small decreases in taking-in and small increases in taking-hold between the evening of birth and the first morning after. For 24 hours after the birth, mature and apparently healthy women appear to suspend their involvement in everyday responsibilities. They rely on others to satisfy their needs for comfort, rest, nourishment, and closeness to their families and newborn.

This dependent phase is a time of great excitement during which parents need to verbalize their experience of pregnancy and birth. Focusing on, analyzing, and accepting these experiences help the parents move on to the next phase. Some parents use staff members or other mothers as an audience, whereas others are more comfortable talking with family and friends about the pregnancy and birth experience.

Because anxiety and preoccupation with her new role often narrow a mother's perceptions, information may have to be repeated. The new mother may require reminders to rest or, conversely, to ambulate enough to promote recov-

ENGLISH SPANISH **Guidelines/Guías**

POSTPARTUM ADJUSTMENT

How do you feel? Happy? Tired? Overwhelmed? Sad?
¿Cómo se siente? ¿Contenta? ¿Cansada? ¿Abrumada? ¿Triste?

Are you able to get enough rest and sleep?
¿Puede descansar y dormir lo suficiente?

Is your appetite good?
¿Tiene buen apetito?

Do you have someone to help you at home?
¿Hay alguien en casa que le pueda ayudar?

Does the baby have fussy periods? Are you able to soothe him/her?
¿Tiene el bebé períodos de nerviosismo? ¿Puede usted calmarlo?

Do you and your family enjoy playing with the baby?
¿Disfrutan usted y su familia de jugar con el bebé?

Does (Do) your other child (children) seem jealous of the baby?
¿Tiene (Tienen) celos del bebé su otro hijo (sus otros hijos)?

Are you and your husband able to spend time together without the baby?
¿Pasan tiempo juntos usted y su esposo sin el bebé?

Table 22-2
Phases of Maternal Postpartum Adjustment

PHASE	CHARACTERISTICS
Dependent: taking-in*	• First 24 hours (range of 1-2 days) • Focus: self and meeting of basic needs • Reliance on others to meet needs for comfort, rest, closeness, and nourishment • Excited and talkative • Desire to review birth experience
Dependent-independent: taking-hold*	• Starts second or third day; lasts 10 days to several weeks • Focus: care of baby and competent mothering • Desire to take charge • Still need for nurturing and acceptance by others • Eagerness to learn and practice—optimal period for teaching by nurses • Handling of physical discomforts and emotional changes • Possible experience with "blues"
Interdependent: letting go*	• Focus: forward movement of family as unit with interacting members • Reassertion of relationship with partner • Resumption of sexual intimacy • Resolution of individual roles

*From Rubin R: Basic maternal behavior, *Nurs Outlook* 9:683-686, 1961.

ery. Hospital or birth center routines may not necessarily be an important priority to the new mother; she may take showers when examinations are scheduled and be involved in a telephone conversation rather than "being ready" for the baby. Regulations seem cumbersome, and sometimes mothers and their families have difficulty accepting rules that interfere with their need to share reactions about their infant.

Physical discomfort from an episiotomy, sore nipples, hemorrhoids, afterpains, and occasionally a sprained coccygeal joint can interfere with the mother's need for rest and relaxation. The selective use of comfort measures and medication depends on the nurse. Many women hesitate to ask for medication, believing that any pain they experience is normal and to be expected. Breastfeeding mothers may fear the effects of medication on the infant. Few have knowledge of the use of heat or cold to relieve local pain.

Dependent-Independent Phase

If the mother has received adequate nurturing in the first few hours or days, by the second or third day, her desire for independent action reasserts itself. In the dependent-independent phase, the mother alternates between a need for extensive nurturing and acceptance by others and the desire to "take charge" once again. She responds enthusiastically to opportunities to learn and to practice baby care or, if she is an accomplished mother, to carry out or direct this care. Rubin (1961) described this phase as the taking-hold phase, and noted that it lasts approximately 10 days. Several studies (Evans et al, 1998; Martell, 1996; Wrasper, 1996) found that contemporary women exhibit taking-hold behaviors sooner than did the women in Rubin's study; however, the peak and duration of the taking-hold phase were not determined. Evans and associates (1998) found that taking-hold behaviors began increasing between the evening of birth and the first morning despite high levels of sleep disturbance. Childbirth preparation classes, early contact with the newborn, rooming-in, and early discharge are some of the current obstetric practices that seem to enhance taking-hold behaviors (Martell, 1996; Wrasper, 1996).

Most mothers are discharged home during this dependent-independent phase. Once home, mothers must continue to cope with physical adaptations and psychologic adjustments. Many mothers identify fatigue as their major physical concern. This fatigue affects various aspects of their lives, such as their relationships with their husbands and other family members and household responsibilities. Because of the relation of fatigue to postpartum depression (PPD), nurses must screen women for psychologic and physical signs and symptoms of fatigue. The Modified Fatigue Screening Checklist (MFSC) (Pugh et al, 1999) is a screening tool with 30 statements to which the mother responds "yes" or "no." Example statements are "My brain feels hot and muddled," and "I can't straighten my posture." Maternity nurses working in hospital postpartum units, birth centers, obstetrics offices, and home care, as well as pediatric nurses who come in contact with mothers during newborn well checks, are in prime positions to screen new mothers for fatigue.

Because fatigue continues to be a major concern of women during the early weeks of parenthood, nurses must provide anticipatory guidance regarding sleep disturbance and fatigue, as well as suggestions for dealing with the fatigue. Another strategy for helping new mothers cope with fatigue is a self-care guide for postpartum fatigue such as the "Tiredness Management Guide" developed by Troy and Dalgas-Pelish (1995). This guide provides a list of eight sources of postpartum fatigue: infection; no chance to rest; inability to get everything done; interrupted sleep; feeling stressed, anxious, or other psychologic changes from demands placed on the mother; low hemoglobin; and social activities. For each source of fatigue, techniques are listed for the mother to use. Two of the techniques, suggested for no chance to rest, are (1) sit or lie in a comfortable position when you feed your baby, and (2) organize your day for rest between tiring activities. The self-care guide is grounded on the principle that adult learners are self-directed, oriented to tasks specific to their social roles, and motivated to learn when immediate application is needed, all of which fit the postpartum woman.

Other physical concerns of mothers are loss of weight or figure, pain from the episiotomy or cesarean incision, sexual relations, and hemorrhoids. Although women express enjoyment during the early postpartum period, most describe the period as hectic and a time of adjustment. Primiparas report feeling uncertain, trapped, and overwhelmed by fatigue and lack of experience in infant care. Many multiparas describe their experience as being better than with previous births, primarily because of their comfort with caring for an infant.

Prenatally and postnatally, nurses can discuss common postpartal concerns that mothers experience. They can provide anticipatory guidance on coping strategies, such as resting when the infant sleeps or planning with an extended family member or friend to do the housework for the first week or two after the baby is born. Once a mother is home, periodic phone calls from a nurse who cared for her in the birth setting can provide the mother with an opportunity to vent her concerns and get support and advice from "her" nurse. First-time mothers inexperienced in child care, women whose careers had provided outside stimulation, women who lack friends or family members with whom to share delights and concerns, and adolescent mothers may need additional supportive counseling. When possible, postpartum home visits are included in the plan of care. Nurses also can discuss the possible stress-diminishing benefit of breastfeeding.

Postpartum Blues

The "pink" period surrounding the first day or two after birth, characterized by heightened joy and feelings of well-being, is often followed by a "blue" period. Approximately 50% to 80% of women of all ethnic and racial groups experience the postpartum blues or "baby blues" (Beeber, 2002; Sutter et al, 1997; Wood et al, 1997). During the blues, women are emotionally labile and often cry easily for no apparent reason. This lability seems to peak around the fifth day, subsiding by the tenth day. Other symptoms of postpartum blues include depression, a let-down feeling, restlessness, fatigue, insomnia, headache, anxiety, sadness, and anger. A reduced level of circulating glucocorticoids or a subclinical hypothyroidism may exist during the puerperium. Biochemical, psychologic, social, and cultural factors have been explored as possible causes of the postpartum depressive state; however, the etiology remains unknown.

Whatever the cause, the early postpartum period appears to be one of emotional and physical vulnerability for new mothers, who may be psychologically overwhelmed by the reality of parental responsibilities. The mother may feel deprived of the supportive care she received from family members and friends during pregnancy. Some mothers regret the loss of the mother-unborn child relationship and mourn its passing. Still others have a let-down feeling when labor and birth are complete. The majority of women experience fatigue after childbirth, which is compounded by the around-the-clock demands of the new baby and can accentuate the feelings of depression (Wood et al, 1997). Postpartum depressive symptoms can have a negative effect on maternal role attainment (Fowles, 1998). To help mothers cope with postpartum blues, nurses can suggest various strategies (Patient Teaching box).

"Am I Blue?" (Johnson & Johnson, 1996), a self-administered questionnaire, can help mothers to assess their level of "blues" and to decide when to seek advice from their nurse, nurse-midwife, or physician (Fig. 22-6). The nurse's home visits and telephone follow-up calls are important to assess the mother's pattern of "blue" feelings and behavior over time. Educating women about normal newborn/infant growth and development can help new mothers develop realistic expectations about infant behavior (Wood et al, 1997), thus decreasing one source of postpartum stress.

Although the postpartum blues are usually mild and short lived, approximately 10% to 15% of women experience a more severe syndrome called postpartum depression (PPD) (Wood et al, 1997) (see Chapter 23). The symptoms can range from mild to severe, with women having "good days" and "bad days." All symptoms can be equally distressing and make the woman feel as if she is "going mad." PPD leaves the woman with feelings of failure, overwhelming guilt, loneliness, and low self-esteem. Nurses need to teach women how to differentiate symptoms of the "blues" and PPD and should urge women to report depressive symptoms promptly if they occur. PPD can go undetected because new mothers generally do not voluntarily admit to this kind of emotional distress out of embarrassment, guilt, or fear. Nurses must be active listeners and compassionate intermediaries in interactions with new mothers so that symptoms of depression can be recognized early, assessed, and treated. Through careful attention to holistic health histories, nurses can identify women who are at high risk for PPD (see Box 23-4).

Interdependent Phase

In this phase, interdependent behavior reasserts itself, and the mother and her family move forward as a unit with interacting members. The relationship of the partners, although altered by the introduction of a baby, resumes many of its former characteristics. A primary need is to establish a lifestyle that both includes and, in some respects, excludes the baby. The couple needs to share interests and activities that are adult in scope.

Patient Teaching

COPING WITH POSTPARTUM BLUES

- Remember that the "blues" are normal.
- Get plenty of rest; nap when the baby does if possible. Go to bed early, and let friends know when to visit.
- Use relaxation techniques learned in childbirth classes (or ask the nurse to teach you and your partner some techniques).
- Do something for yourself. Take advantage of the time your partner or family members care for the baby—soak in the tub or go for a walk.
- Plan a day out of the house—go to the mall with the baby, being sure to take a stroller or carriage, or go out to eat with friends without the baby. Many communities have churches or other agencies that provide child care programs such as Mothers' Morning Out.
- Share your feelings with your partner. For example, talk about feeling tied down, how the birth met your expectations, and things that will help you.
- If you are breastfeeding, give yourself and your baby time to learn.
- Seek out and use community resources such as La Leche League or community mental health centers. One nationally recognized resource is:

  Postpartum Support International
  927 North Kellogg Avenue
  Santa Barbara, CA 93111
  (805) 967-7636

Am I Blue?

Many new mothers feel anxious, sad, or angry about the changes in their lives after the birth of their new baby. It is perfectly normal to feel this way, but sometimes the feelings grow so strong that they make life difficult. This quiz lists many feelings and experiences of "blue" or depressed mothers. Mark how strong each of these feelings or experiences is for you, compared with what is normal for you. For example: Do you feel no anger [0]; mild (very little) anger [1]; moderate (some) anger [2]; or severe (very strong) anger [3] compared with the way you usually feel? Add up your total score when you are finished, and discuss the results with your health care provider.

0 = Not there at all 1 = Mild 2 = Moderate 3 = Severe	0	1	2	3
Anger				
Anxiety attacks: periods of very strong fear, shortness of breath, rapid heartbeat				
Increased or decreased appetite and/or weight gain or loss that doesn't seem normal				
Strong feeling that you need to get away, need more time for your own interests				
Problems in a relationship with a family member, lover, close friend, etc.				
Crying spells				
Less interest in your personal appearance				
Less motivation—less energy or interest in accomplishing goals				
Depression				
Fatigue—feeling tired or exhausted				
Fear of harming yourself or your baby				
Loss of your sense of humor				
Nervousness, feeling tense or edgy				
Feelings of guilt				
Feelings of panic				
Feeling alone or lonely; without the support of others				
Feeling no love, or not enough love, for your baby				
Feeling forgetful, distracted, absent-minded—having trouble concentrating				
Frustration				
Hopelessness				
Insomnia				
Feeling irritable, bad-tempered				
Loss of sexual desire and/or pleasure in sex				
Loss of self-respect or confidence—feeling like you don't count or can't do anything right				
Feeling confused, uncertain				
Mood swings—your moods and emotions change all the time				
Obsessive thoughts—ideas or feelings you can't stop from repeating in your mind				
Odd or frightening thoughts—thoughts or images that scare you or that you can't control				
Thoughts of suicide, feeling like you want to die				
Feeling sad, unhappy				
TOTAL				

SCORE:

0 – 31 = MILD BLUES
This will probably pass, but pay attention to your feelings and needs.

32 – 64 = MODERATE BLUES
You may want to ask for help from a close friend or family member, or ask the advice of your health care provider.

65 – 98 = SEVERE BLUES
You could be depressed; see your health care provider for a check-up and advice as soon as possible.

If you are afraid you might harm yourself or your baby—ask a health care provider you trust for help— you don't have to be alone!

Fig. 22-6 Am I Blue? (Courtesy Johnson & Johnson Consumer Products, Skillman, NJ.)

An important aspect of the adult couple relationship is sexual intimacy. Sexual interest and postpartum resumption of sexual behavior are influenced by biologic, psychologic, and social changes that accompany giving birth. Changes in a woman's sexuality after childbirth are related to hormonal shifts, increased breast size, uneasiness with a body that has yet to return to a prepregnant size, chronic fatigue related to sleep deprivation, and physical exhaustion (Bitzer & Alder, 2000). The early demands of breastfeeding a newborn often can cause the mother not to want to be touched in one more way, especially on her breasts. However, breastfeeding also is a sensual experience for some mothers, promoting relaxation and a sense of being at peace. This may preclude somewhat the woman's need for further sensual experiences.

The couple may begin to engage in sexual intercourse during the second to fourth week after the baby is born. Some couples begin earlier, as soon as it can be accomplished without discomfort, depending on factors such as the presence of an episiotomy, perineal tears, or cesarean incision and amount of vaginal dryness. Regardless of when a couple resumes sexual intercourse, they should consider the prevention of another pregnancy, at least until the woman's body has had time to complete the involution process and until she is emotionally and physically ready for another pregnancy. Before and after birth, nurses should review with new parents their plans for other pregnancies and their preferences for contraception.

Sexual intimacy enhances the adult aspect of the family, and the adult pair shares a closeness denied to other family members. Many new fathers speak of the alienation experienced when they observe the intimate mother-infant relationship, and some are frank in expressing feelings of jealousy toward the infant. The resumption of sexual intimacy seems to bring the parents' relationship back into focus.

The interdependent phase, termed the *letting-go phase,* is often stressful for the parental pair. Interests and needs often diverge during this time. Women and their partners must resolve the effects of their individual roles related to childrearing, homemaking, and careers on their relationship. Mothers (and partners) may take a more traditional role in an effort to adapt to parenthood. A special continuing effort has to be made to strengthen the adult-adult relationship as a basis for the family unit.

Little is known about postpartum maternal adjustment in the lesbian couple. Relationship satisfaction in first-time lesbian parent couples appears related to egalitarianism, commitment, sexual compatibility, and communication skills, as well as to the birth mother's decision for insemination by an anonymous sperm donor (Osterwell, 1991; Reimann, 1997b; Reimann, 1999). Similar to heterosexual parent couples, most lesbian parent couples voice concern about less time and energy for their relationship after the arrival of the baby (Gartrell et al, 1996) and stress occurs when one partner perceives the other as not doing her fair share of the domestic work (Reimann, 1997a). Both partners consider themselves to be equal parents of the baby when they share actively in childrearing (Brewaeys et al, 1995). A primary concern of comothers is the legal vulnerability of lesbian families confounded by their social invisibility (Reimann, 1999).

Lesbian couples face strong social sanctions regarding pregnancy and parenting. Their families may not have resolved the initial dismay and guilt over learning of their daughters' homosexuality, or they may disagree with the lesbian couple's decision to conceive and be parents. Lesbian parents deal with public ignorance, social and legal invisibility, and the lack of biologic connection to the child by using various techniques. These techniques include carefully planning and accomplishing their transition to parenthood, displaying public acts of equal mothering, sharing parenting at home, establishing a distinct parenting role within the family, and supporting each partner's sense of identity as a mother (Reimann, 1997a; 1997b). In situations in which family support is limited or absent, the nurse can help lesbian couples locate more supportive social groups, lesbian or heterosexual.

Paternal Adjustment

Research on paternal adjustment to parenthood indicates that fathers go through predictable phases during their transition to parenthood (Henderson & Brouse, 1991) (Table 22-3). During this period, fathers experience intense emotions. Many fathers acknowledge that their expectations were of limited value once they were immersed in the reality of parenthood. Feelings that often accompany this reality are sadness, ambivalence, jealousy, frustration at not being able to participate in breastfeeding, and an overwhelming desire to be more involved; most of these are different from the feelings mothers report. On the other hand, some fathers are pleasantly surprised at the ease and fun of parenting. In their transition to mastery, fathers take control and become more actively involved in the infant's life (Table 22-4).

First-time fathers perceive the first 4 to 10 weeks of parenthood in much the same way that mothers do, that is, as a

Table 22-3

Transition to Fatherhood: A Three-Stage Process

STAGES	CHARACTERISTICS
Stage 1: Expectations	Father has preconceptions about what life will be like after baby comes home
Stage 2: Reality	Father realizes that expectations are not always based on fact Common feelings experienced are as follows: Sadness Ambivalence Jealousy Frustration Overwhelming desire to be more involved Some fathers are pleasantly surprised at ease and fun of parenting
Stage 3: Transition to mastery	Father makes conscious decision to take control and become more actively involved with infant

period characterized by uncertainty, increased responsibility, disruption of sleep, and inability to control time needed to care for the infant and reestablish the marital dyad. Fathers across cultures believe that fatherhood affects marriage deeply. Generally they feel that the marital quality is enhanced, especially the cohesiveness of the family unit; yet fathers express concerns about (1) decreased attention from their partners relative to their personal relationship, (2) the mother's lack of recognition of the father's desire to participate in decision making for the infant, and (3) limited time available to establish a relationship with their infants (Steinberg, Kruckman, & Steinberg, 2000). These concerns can precipitate feelings of jealousy of the infant. Discussing their needs with the partner and becoming more involved with their infants and partner can help alleviate such feelings of jealousy. A consistent finding in the literature is that fathers who feel affection and support in the relationships with their partners or mates are more involved with infant care, and their involvement is more responsive, affectionate, and developmentally stimulating (Anderson, 1996a; 1996b).

Table 22-4

Development of a Father-Infant Relationship: Process Components

COMPONENT	CHARACTERISTICS
Making a commitment	Willingness to invest in and take responsibility for nurturing the relationship despite difficulties in parenting and other life demands Feel reality of commitment: at confirmation of pregnancy; during pregnancy and birth; when to provide infant care; when infant responds to them Helpless nature of infant affects a felt duty to nurture and protect Desire to get to know and be psychologically involved Rewarded by infant smile, increased self-esteem, gaining a new dimension in life, finding the child within self
Becoming connected	The basic psychologic process in the development of father-infant relationship First meeting with infant: feelings of joy, elation, awe, and wonderment Sense of a bond with the infant: may feel this at first meeting or when first touch/hold the infant or may develop gradually during the first 2 months Turning point: when perceives the infant as more responsive, predictable, and familiar
Making room for baby	Father makes changes in work and social/personal time, in relationship with wife/partner, and within self so more physically and emotionally available to infant

Father-Infant Relationship

In North American culture, neonates have a powerful impact on their fathers, who become intensely involved with their babies (Fig. 22-7). The term used for the father's absorption, preoccupation, and interest in the infant is *engrossment.* Characteristics of engrossment include some of the sensual responses relating to touch and eye-to-eye contact that were discussed earlier, and also the father's keen awareness of features both unique and similar to himself that validate his claim to the infant. An outstanding response is one of strong attraction to the newborn. Fathers spend considerable time "communicating" with the infant and taking delight in the infant's response to them (Fig. 22-8). Fathers experience increased self-esteem and a sense of being proud, bigger, more mature, and older after seeing their baby for the first time.

Fathers spend less time than mothers with infants, and fathers' interactions with their infants tend to be characterized by stimulating social play rather than caretaking. The subtle

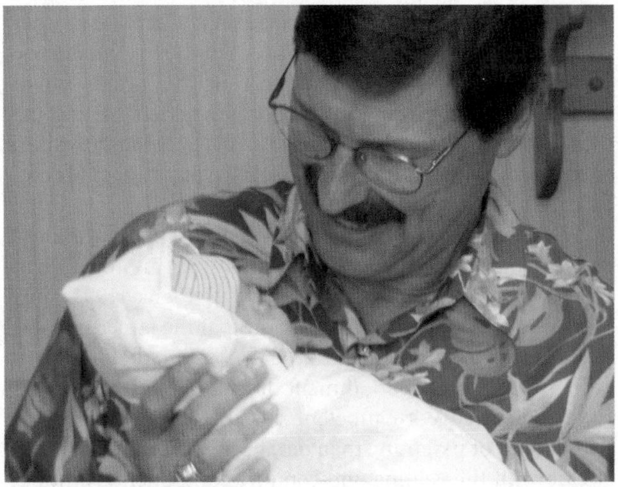

Fig. 22-7 Engrossment. Father absorbed in looking at his newborn. (Courtesy Tricia Olson, North Ogden, UT)

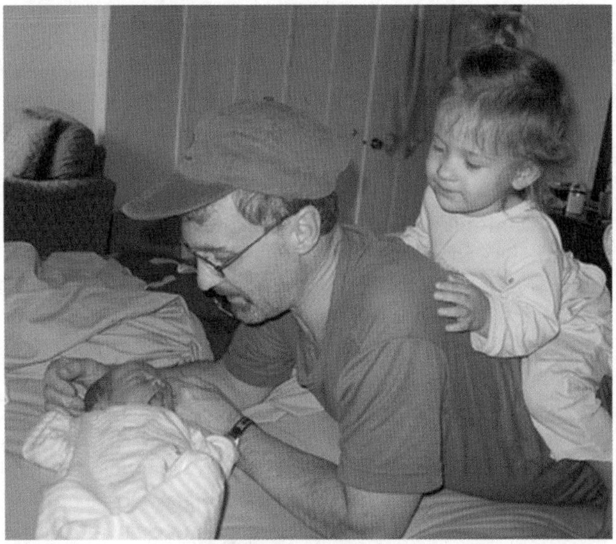

Fig. 22-8 Father interacting with newborn while sibling observes with interest. (Courtesy Christine Brockett, Boulder, CO.)

and more obvious differences in stimulation from two sources, mother and father, provide a wider social experience for the infant.

Impact of Fatherhood

For Caucasian, middle-class, American males, first-time fatherhood is seen as a maturing event during which increased responsibility is assumed. Fathers report taking their work more seriously while also trying to balance work and family demands. These men experience an identity change, developing an image of themselves as fathers. Over time, they develop strong bonds with their infants and feel a sense of fulfillment and purpose in life.

Canadian and Japanese men describe a similar perception of the impact of fatherhood (Steinberg et al, 2000). These men see parenthood as having a major effect on their personal relationship with their wives/partners and on the family's economic status, but they are confused about how to cope. They express concern about providing a sufficient income. Those who considered paternity leave resisted taking it because of financial considerations and, for some, because of workplace discrimination. Many of these Canadian and Japanese fathers perceive society as offering no special status to fatherhood, just added responsibility. They report a lack of health care information and parenting instruction for fathers, stating that they learn to be fathers by trial and error, by living the experience day by day, and turning to their wives/partners for confirmation that they are "fathering" correctly.

Few studies have investigated the impact of fatherhood on African-American men. One study on parental role attainment by African-American parents (Sank, 1991) provides nurses with some understanding of the father's experience. Self-concept was found to be the best predictor of these fathers' parental role attainment during the postpartum period. Fathers felt less competent with the skill and knowledge component of parenting than did the mothers, but they were at ease with the valuing and comfort component. Although these fathers did not see themselves as being as skillful as their partners in caring for infants, they valued parenthood and felt comfortable in the father role.

Despite their active involvement in the perinatal period, fathers tend to gravitate toward a more traditional division of family responsibilities. One reason for this return to more traditional roles may be the new father's concerns about his ability to financially support his new family.

Fathers as well as mothers can experience postpartum depression. The incidence ranges from approximately 1% to 26% in community samples. The incidence is much higher, 24% to 50%, in men whose partners had postnatal depression (Goodman, 2004).

Fathers can benefit from nursing interventions during the postpartum period just as mothers can. Nurses can arrange to teach infant care when the father is present and provide anticipatory guidance for fathers about the transition to parenthood. Separate prenatal and parenting classes and parenting support groups for fathers can provide them with an opportunity to discuss their concerns and have some of their needs met. The nurse's postpartum phone calls and home visits should include time for assessment of the father's adjustment and needs.

Community Focus

FATHERS' EXPERIENCE OF LABOR AND POSTPARTUM

In Western industrialized countries, the trend is for fathers to be present at childbirth. Fathers who attended childbirth classes, and who use avoidance when confronted with threat, experience childbirth as less fulfilling than fathers who cope similarly but do not attend classes. Fathers who reported childbirth as being fulfilling and a delight were less depressed at 6 weeks postpartum. Babies born by cesarean were described more negatively at 6 weeks postpartum when compared with babies born vaginally. More married fathers attended classes and were less depressed than unmarried fathers. Thus it appears that for some fathers, attending prenatal classes is beneficial; for others it may not be. In addition, fathers' experience of childbirth may influence later emotional well-being. Nurses involved in prenatal preparation of families for childbirth need to take into consideration various needs and wishes of individual members. Whereas education may be encouraged to reduce anxiety and fear related to the unknown, attending classes is not the best strategy for some men. For these men, childbirth preparation must be individualized based on expressed needs and wishes.

Data from Greenhalgh R, Slade P, Spiby H: Fathers' coping style, antenatal preparation, and experiences of labor and the postpartum, *Birth* 27(3): 177-184, 2000.

Infant-Parent Adjustment

Newborns participate actively in shaping their parents' reaction to them. The infant and the parent each have unique rhythms, behaviors, and response styles that are brought to every interaction. Infant-parent interactions can be facilitated in at least three ways: (1) modulation of rhythm, (2) modification of behavioral repertoires, and (3) mutual responsivity. Nurses can teach parents about these three aspects of infant-parent interaction through discussions, written materials, and videotapes on infant capabilities (e.g., *The Amazing Newborn*). A creative approach is to videotape the parent-infant pair during an interaction and then use the individualized tape to discuss the pair's rhythm, behavioral repertoire, and responsivity.

Rhythm

To modulate rhythm, both parent and infant must be able to interact. Therefore the infant must be in the alert state, one of the most difficult of the sleep-wake states to maintain. The alert state (see Figs. 22-3 and 22-4) occurs most often during a feeding or in face-to-face play. The parent must work hard to help the infant maintain the alert state long enough and often enough for interactions to take place. The *en face* position (the parent's face is positioned in the same plane as that of the newborn) is usually assumed (Fig. 22-5, *D*). Multiparous mothers in particular are very sensitive and responsive to the infant's feeding rhythms. Mothers learn to reserve stimulation for pauses in sucking activity and not to talk or smile excessively while the infant is sucking because the infant will stop feeding to interact with her. With maturity the infant can sustain longer interactions by modulating activity rhythms, that is, limb movement, sucking, gaze alternation, and habituation. Meanwhile, the parent becomes more attuned to the infant's rhythms and learns to modulate the rhythms, facilitating a rhythmic turn-taking interaction.

Behavioral Repertoires

Both the infant and the parent have a repertoire of behaviors they can use to facilitate interactions. Fathers and mothers engage in these behaviors depending on the extent of contact and caregiving of the infant.

The infant's behavioral repertoire includes gazing, vocalizing, and facial expressions. The infant is able to focus and follow the human face from birth and also is able to alternate the gaze voluntarily, looking away from the parent's face when understimulated or overstimulated (Fig. 22-5, *F*). One of the key responses for the parents to learn is to be sensitive to the infant's capacity for attention and inattention. Developing this sensitivity is especially important when interacting with preterm infants.

Body gestures form a part of the infant's "early language." Babies greet parents with waving hands (Fig. 22-5, *E*) or a reaching out of hands. They can raise an eyebrow or soften their expression to elicit loving attention. Game playing can stimulate them to smile or laugh. Pouting or crying, arching of the back, and general squirming usually signal the end of an interaction.

The parents' repertoire includes various types of interactive behaviors such as constantly looking at the infant and noting the infant's response. New parents often remark that they are exhausted from looking at the baby and smiling. Adults also "infantilize" their speech to help the infant "listen." They do this by slowing the tempo, speaking loudly and rhythmically, and emphasizing key words. Phrases are repeated frequently. Infantilizing does not mean using "baby talk," which involves distortion of sounds.

To communicate emotions to the infant, parents often use facial expressions such as slow and exaggerated looks of surprise, happiness, and confusion. Games such as "peek-a-boo" and imitation of the infant's behaviors are other means of interaction. For example, if the baby smiles, so does the parent; if the baby frowns, the parent responds in kind.

Responsivity

Contingent responses *(responsivity)* are those that occur within a specific time and are similar in form to a stimulus behavior. The adult has the feeling of having an influence on the interaction. Infant behaviors such as smiling, cooing, and sustained eye contact, usually in *en face* position, are viewed as contingent responses. The infant's responses act as rewards to the initiator and encourage the adult to continue with the game when the infant responds positively. When the adult imitates the infant, the infant appears to enjoy it. A progression occurs in the types of behaviors that parents present for the baby to imitate; for example, in early interactions, the parent will grimace rather than laugh, which is in keeping with the infant's developmental level. Such behaviors sustain interactions and promote harmony in the relationship.

Factors Influencing Parental Responses

The way parents respond to the birth of their child is influenced by various factors, including age, social networks, socioeconomic conditions, and personal aspirations of the future.

Age

Maternal age has a definite effect on the outcome of pregnancy. The mother and fetus are at highest risk when the mother is an adolescent or is more than 35 years old.

The Adolescent Mother

Although it is biologically possible for the adolescent female to become a parent, her egocentricity and concrete thinking interfere with her ability to parent effectively. The very young adolescent mother is inexperienced and unprepared to recognize the early signs of illness, potential danger, or household hazards. She may inadvertently neglect her child. The higher mortality rates among the infants of adolescent mothers are attributed to the inexperience, lack of knowledge, and immaturity of the mothers, causing them to be unable to recognize a problem and obtain the necessary resources to rectify the situation. Nevertheless, in most instances, with adequate support and developmentally appropriate teaching, adolescents can learn effective parenting skills.

The transition to parenthood may be difficult for adolescent parents. Coping with the developmental tasks of parenthood is often complicated by the unmet developmental needs and tasks of adolescence. Some young parents may experience difficulty accepting a changing self-image and adjusting to new roles related to the responsibilities of infant care. Other adolescent parents, however, may have higher self-concepts than their nonparenting peers (Alpers, 1998; Dalla & Gamble, 2000). Self-concept of pregnant and parenting teens appears to vary in relation to age, years of schooling, types of schools attended, income sources, and receipt of public assistance (Alpers, 1998). Nurses developing or implementing teen parenting programs should have occasional checkpoints in place throughout their programs to reassess the self-concept of adolescent parents and the types of socioeconomic supports these teens use.

As adolescent parents move through the transition to parenthood, they may feel different from their peers, excluded from fun activities, and prematurely forced to enter an adult social role. The conflict between their own desires and the infant's demands, in addition to the low tolerance for frustration that is typical of adolescence, further contribute to the normal psychosocial stress of childbirth. Lower maternal education is associated with less favorable maternal responses to distress and infant behavior (Dalla & Gamble, 2000; Diehl, 1997).

Maintaining a relationship with the baby's father is beneficial for the teen mother and her infant. A close and satisfying relationship is positively correlated with maternal-fetal and maternal-infant attachment (Bloom, 1998). The involvement of the baby's father is related to appropriate maternal behaviors and positive mother-infant relationship (Diehl, 1997).

Adolescent mothers provide warm and attentive physical care; however, they use less verbal interaction than do older parents, and adolescents tend to be less responsive and to interact less positively with their infants than do older mothers. Interventions emphasizing verbal and nonverbal communication skills between mother and infant are important.

Such intervention strategies must be concrete and specific because of the cognitive level of adolescents. Although some observers suggest that some adolescents may use more aggressive behaviors, a higher incidence of child abuse has not been documented. In comparison with adult mothers, teenage mothers have a limited knowledge of child development. They tend to expect too much of their children too soon and often characterize their infants as being fussy. This limited knowledge may cause teenagers to respond to their infants inappropriately.

Many young mothers pattern their maternal role on what they themselves experienced. Therefore nurses need to determine the kind of support that people close to the young mother are able and prepared to give, as well as the kinds of community aid available to supplement this support. Many teen mothers can identify a source of social support, with the predominant source being their own mothers. Navajo adolescent mothers who had social support (emotional and instrumental) from their own mothers felt able to focus on both the adolescent and the maternal roles without neglecting either role (Dalla & Gamble, 2000). Rural adolescent mothers who reported firm encouragement and resources to pursue their life aspirations had more resilient adjustments to parenthood than did adolescent mothers who did not have this type of support (Camarena et al, 1998).

The need for continued assessment of the new mother's parenting abilities during this postbirth period is essential. Continued support should also be provided by involving the grandparents and other family members, as well as through home visits and group sessions for discussion of infant care and parenting problems. Outreach programs concerned with self-care, parent-child interactions, child injuries, and failure to thrive, in addition to programs that provide prompt and effective community intervention, prevent more serious problems from occurring. As the adolescent performs her mothering role within the framework of her family, she may need to address dependency versus independency issues. The adolescent's family members also may need help adapting to their new roles.

The Adolescent Father

The adolescent father and mother face immediate developmental crises, which include completing the developmental tasks of adolescence, making a transition to parenthood, and sometimes adapting to marriage. These transitions can be stressful. The nurse may initiate interaction with the adolescent father by asking him to be present when postpartum home visits are made and to accompany the mother and the baby to well-baby checks at the clinic or pediatrician's office. With the adolescent mother's agreement, the nurse may contact the father directly. The decision to include the young father in all aspects of the care is based on assessment in the following four areas: (1) the couple's relationship; (2) levels of stress, concern, and coping; (3) educational and vocational goals; and (4) the level of health education knowledge. Adolescent fathers need support to discuss their emotional responses to the pregnancy. The nurse's nonjudgmental attitude is essential for open communication. The father's feelings of guilt, powerlessness, or bravado should be recognized because of their negative consequences for both the parents and the child. Counseling of adolescent fathers needs to be reality oriented. Topics such as finances, child care, parenting skills, and the father's role in the birth experience must be discussed. Teenage fathers also need to know about reproductive physiology and birth control options as well as safer sex practices.

The adolescent father may continue to be involved in an ongoing relationship with the young mother and his baby. In many instances he also plays an important role in the decisions about child care and raising the child. The nurse supports the young father by helping him develop realistic perceptions of his role as father to a child. He is encouraged to use coping mechanisms that are not detrimental to his own, his partner's, or his child's well-being. The nurse enlists support systems, parents, and professional agencies on his behalf.

Maternal Age More Than 35 Years

Women older than 35 years have always continued their childbearing either by choice or because of a lack or failure of contraception during the perimenopausal years. Added to this group are women who have postponed pregnancy because of careers or other reasons, as well as women of infertile couples who finally become pregnant with the aid of technologic advances.

Many mothers 35 years of age and older report having a hard time coping, especially with irregular sleep patterns and the fussy periods babies have in the late afternoon and early evening. Other 35+ mothers, however, found that their preparedness, by delaying motherhood, enhanced their adaptation to parenthood. They felt that midlife mothers had qual-

??? Critical Thinking Exercise

POSTPARTUM ADJUSTMENT FOR THE ADOLESCENT AND THE OLDER MOTHER

You are a home care nurse and have had two patients referred to you. Carol is a 15-year-old first-time mother of a 5-day-old girl; she lives with her mother. The father of the baby, Robert, is 17 years old and attended childbirth classes with Carol. She is breastfeeding the baby, but says that the baby sucks too slowly and takes too much time to eat. She said she thinks the baby should know enough to sleep longer at night. Robert would like to feed the baby some cereal, since he heard that will make a baby sleep longer at night.

Audrey is a 36-year-old attorney who has been practicing law for 7 years. She just gave birth to her first baby; she and her husband delayed parenting by choice until their careers were well established. She had an uneventful pregnancy, labor, and birth. During a telephone call 48 hours after discharge, when she was asked how things were going, Audrey burst into tears and said, "I didn't expect it to be like this! Nothing is going right."

1. Evidence—Is there sufficient evidence to draw conclusions about what teaching and care these new parents need?
2. Assumptions—What assumptions can be made about the following factors:
   a. The relationship of maternal age and postpartum adjustment
   b. The need for social support in the postnatal period
   c. The need for perinatal education
   d. Long-term prognosis for positive outcomes
3. What implications and priorities for nursing care can be drawn at this time?
4. Does the evidence objectively support your conclusion?
5. Are there alternative perspectives to your conclusion?

ities that younger mothers might lack, such as greater life experience, patience and understanding, readiness to settle down, and more mature outlook on life (Garrison et al, 1997; Poelker & Baldwin, 1999; Welles-Nystrom, 1997).

Adjustment of older mothers to changes involved in becoming a parent and seeing themselves as competent is aided by support from their partners. Support from other family members and friends is also important for positive self-evaluation of parenting, for a sense of well-being and satisfaction, and will help in dealing with stress.

Older mothers report having to adjust to changes in the relationships with their partners. Some women regarded the changes as negative (e.g., having less time together), whereas others see the changes as positive (e.g., feeling closer to their partners). Because many of these couples have been together for many years before the baby is born, the loss of the "just-the-two-of-us" aspect of the relationship may be stressful.

Changes in the sexual aspect of a relationship can create a stressor for new midlife parents. Mothers report that finding time and energy for a romantic rendezvous is more difficult. They attribute much of this to the reality of caring for an infant, but also to the decreasing libido that normally accompanies getting older.

Work and career issues are sources of conflict for older mothers (Reece & Harkless, 1996). Conflicts emerge over being disinterested in work, worrying about giving enough attention to work with the distractions of a new baby, and anticipating what it will be like to return to work. Child care is a major factor causing stress about work.

Another major issue for older mothers with careers is the perception of loss of control (Reece & Harkless, 1996). Mothers older than 35, when compared with younger mothers, are at a different stage in their careers, having attained high levels of education, career, and income. The loss of control experienced when going from the consistency of a work role to the inconsistency of the parent role comes as a surprise to many. Helping the older mother have realistic expectations of herself and of parenthood is essential.

New mothers who are also perimenopausal may find it hard to distinguish fatigue, loss of sleep, decreased libido, or other physiologic symptoms as the causes of the change in their sex lives. Although many women view menopause as a natural stage of life, for midlife mothers this cessation of menstruation coincides with the state of parenthood. The changes of midlife and menopause can add more emotional and physical stress to older mothers' lives because of the time- and energy-consuming aspects of raising a young child. Resources that older parents may find helpful are listed in Resources at the end of the chapter.

Paternal Age More Than 35 Years

Literature on the experiences of first-time fathers older than 35 years is sparse. However, in the available literature (Cain, 1994; Poelker & Baldwin, 1999), older fathers describe their experience of midlife parenting as wonderful but not without drawbacks. What they saw as positive aspects of parenthood in older years included increased love and commitment between the spouses, a reinforcement of why one married in the first place, a feeling of being complete, experiencing "the child" in oneself again, more financial stability than in younger years, and more freedom to focus on parenting rather than on career. A common theme expressed was sharing: sharing joy, sharing in raising the child, sharing as a family. These men reported that the main drawback of midlife parenting was the change that it made in the relationships with their partners. They missed the deeper and more selfish couple relationship and looked forward to the time when they could have that again (Cain, 1994).

Social Support

Social support is strongly related to positive adaptation by new parents, including adolescent parents, during the transition to parenthood (Merriwether-deVries, 2000). Social support is multidimensional and includes the number of members in a person's social network, types of support, perceived general support, actual support received, and satisfaction with support available and received. The type and satisfaction of support seem to be more important than the total number of support network members.

Postpartum women who have received social support from a doula, compared with women who did not have a doula, demonstrate a stronger self-esteem, less depression, more positive feelings for their infant, and increased ability to care for their infant during the transition to parenthood (Klaus & Kennell, 1997).

Across cultural groups, families and friends of new parents form an important dimension of the parent's social network. For example, the extended family unit is the single strongest unit in the lives of most Asians. Extended family members also are relied on heavily after childbirth by Jordanians (D'Avanzo & Geissler, 2003). Through seeking help within the social network, new mothers learn culturally valued practices and develop role competency (Pridham, 1997).

Social networks provide a support system on which parents can rely for assistance, but they also can be a source of conflict. Sometimes a large network can cause problems because it results in conflicting advice from numerous people. Grandparents or in-laws are most appreciated when they assist with household responsibilities and do not intrude into the parents' privacy or judge them critically.

Women who have given birth before may have different support needs from those of first-time mothers. First-time mothers may need more follow-up for parenting skills, including referral to community resources. Women with other children may be more realistic in anticipating physical limitations and the changes in roles and relationships. However, these experienced mothers express concerns over separation from their firstborn, loss of the exclusive relationship with the older child or children, and the challenge of caring for two or more children.

Because of the extent of restructuring and reorganization that occurs in a family with the birth of another child, the mothers' moods and fatigue in the postpartum period can be helped more by situation-specific support from family and friends than by general support. General support addresses feeling loved, respected, and valued. Situation-specific support relates to practical concerns such as physical needs and child care. For example, the practical support of a grandparent bathing the infant can help lessen a second-time mother's feelings of loss by providing her time to be with her firstborn child. Second-time mothers report that

Evidence-Based Practice

GROUP PROGRAMS FOR PARENTS OF BABIES AND TODDLERS

Background

Emotional and behavioral problems in young children are predictive of later depression, substance abuse, poor work and marital outcomes, delinquency, and criminal behavior. These outcomes are frequently associated with harsh and inconsistent discipline, little positive parental involvement, and poor supervision. Parenting practices can account for 30% to 40% of the antisocial behavior in children. Praise, encouragement, and loving involvement with a child have a protective effect against later disruptive behavior and substance abuse. Social learning and attachment theories both claim that caregiving accounts for behavior problems in early childhood. Specific behavior problems include low sociability, poor peer relationships, anger, poor self-control, adolescent anxiety, and dissociation. Poor maternal-infant relationships result in cognitive deficits and poor achievement in school. Primary prevention is aimed at stopping the problem before it develops. Secondary prevention screens for early detection and treatment of the problem. Group parenting programs have a dual preventive role, since some of the children already demonstrate troubled behavior, even by 3 to 4 years of age. Group parenting programs have been found effective in improving behaviors in 3- to 10-year-olds and in reducing anxiety, depression, and poor self-esteem.

Objectives

The review authors wished to determine whether group-based parenting programs are effective at improving the emotional and behavioral outcomes of children, 0 to 3 years of age. The intervention was any group-based parenting program. The outcomes could be at least one measure of emotional and behavioral adjustment.

Methods

Search Strategy

The reviewers searched Cochrane, MEDLINE, EMBASE, Biological Abstracts, British Nursing Index, CINAHL, PsycINFO, Sociological Abstracts, Social Science Citation Index, ASSIA, National Research Registry, Dissertation Abstracts, ERIC, and bibliographies. Search keywords were *parent, training, preschool, toddler, infant, baby, babies* and combinations of these terms. Five randomized or quasi-randomized, controlled trials met the criteria, representing 417 parents. Some studies included both mother and father or grandparent/caretaker of the child, and some participants had more than one child in that age group. It is not clear how many children are represented in the studies. The trials, dated 1995 to 2000, were conducted in the United States and the United Kingdom.

Statistical Analyses

Similar data were pooled. The treatment effect for each outcome was calculated and meta-analyzed, where appropriate. The authors accepted differences between groups that exceeded the 95% confidence interval to be significant.

Findings

The five studies measured many outcomes. Some measured child-only behaviors (e.g., parent and teacher questionnaires about behaviors such as inattentiveness, aggression, or excessive crying), while others addressed observable parent-child interactions (e.g., parent affect with child, physical negative behavior causing pain, praise, or critical statements). There was a significant improvement in the observed behavior of the children in the parenting group, when compared with the controls. Parents' report of children's behavior trended in favor of the intervention group, but not to the level of significance. This was interesting, because parents frequently report behavior more favorably than independent observers. Follow-up data showed that improvement in the intervention group persisted, although it no longer reached the level of significance.

Limitations

The reviewers had to compare a variety of scales to measure similar outcomes, which was a challenge. The limited number of studies, their small sizes, and some randomization problems (e.g., using volunteers and cluster data) limit generalizability. The dropout rate, 30% from two trials, was significant. In one of these studies, the dropouts were already using less harsh discipline. In another study, the dropout parents rated their children as significantly less problematic than the group that stayed. In prior studies, dropout rates were higher among subjects with more severe psychosocial problems and stress, and those who dropped out were more likely to be from a lower social class or an ethnic minority. Dropout rates introduce bias; therefore researchers have to account for the dropouts and evaluate the studies' outcomes on "intention-to-treat" basis (i.e., their original randomized allocation), or the remaining data will be skewed.

Conclusions

There is some support of group-based programs for parents of children up to 3 years of age, but conclusions regarding whether benefits are long-term are equivocal. Anecdotally, parenting groups provide peer modeling for parents and networking that can provide support through future stages.

Implications for Practice

Two trials used 10-week Webster-Stratton programs, one called "Incredible Years," and one used a videotape modeling program called "Parent and Child Series." These programs might be useful in parenting programs. Parenting classes during pregnancy and in the postpartum period can help parents know what to expect and prepare them for the challenges of parenting.

Implications for Further Research

The trials did not address the question of primary prevention of mental health problems, and further longer-term research is necessary. Early childhood parenting may provide greater benefits farther out. The researchers' challenge is to capture those follow-up outcomes. Specific programs should be tested for effectiveness, so that the research is reproducible. Therapist credentials and training may account for variable results. (For more information, see "Parenting Groups for Teenage Parents," the Evidence-Based Practice box in Chapter 3).

Reference

Barlow J, Parsons J: Group-based parent-training programmes for improving emotional and behavioral adjustment in 0-3 year old children (Cochrane Review), 2003. In *The Cochrane Library*, Issue 2, Chichester, UK, 2004, John Wiley & Sons.

practical support is the most useful and desirable type of support during the postpartum period.

Nurses must be aware that not all types of support are equally beneficial to mothers after birth, and therefore, should assess the presence and types of practical help available to new mothers. The assumption that second-time (experienced) mothers are "old pros" and therefore do not need help should be avoided. Because second-time mothers may expect this of themselves, nurses can help these mothers explore the differences associated with adding another child to the family and identify the types of support that they need the most.

Culture

Cultural beliefs and practices are important determinants of parenting behaviors. Culture defines what is socially acceptable in terms of eye contact, touch, and space (Lipson, Dibble, & Minarik, 1996). Culture influences the interactions with the baby as well as the parent's or family's caregiving style. For example, the provision for a period of rest and recuperation for the mother after birth is important in several cultures. Asian mothers must remain at home with the baby at least 30 days after birth, and are not supposed to engage in household chores, including care of the baby. Many times the grandmother takes over the baby's care immediately, even before discharge from the hospital (D'Avanzo & Geissler, 2003). An example is the traditional Taiwanese ritual, *Tso-Yueh-Tzu* (translated "doing, within the first month postpartum"). Contemporary Taiwanese women still participate in *Tso-Yueh-Tzu*; however, they express concern over how to use this ritual better in their adaptation to their new role and in transitioning back to contemporary society (Liu-Chiang, 1995). Jordanian mothers have a 40-day lying-in after birth, during which their mothers or sisters care for the baby (D'Avanzo & Geissler, 2003). The Japanese tradition called *Satogairi-Bunben* requires a woman to return to her family of origin for rest during the last month of pregnancy and for the first 2 months after childbirth for recuperation. However, the modern Japanese woman now tends to stay with her husband during the early postpartum period or go to her family for a much shorter time. This change may be due in part to the family of origin living a distance away and, in keeping the tradition, the woman would have to choose between her husband and her family (Steinberg et al, 2000).

Hispanics practice an intergenerational family ritual, *la cuarentena.* For 40 days after birth, the mother is expected to recuperate and get acquainted with her infant. Traditionally this involves many restrictions concerning food (spicy or cold foods, fish, pork, and citrus are avoided; tortillas and chicken soup are encouraged); exercise; and activities, including sexual intercourse. Abdominal binding is a traditional practice, and many women avoid tub bathing and washing their hair. Traditional Hispanic husbands do not expect to see their wives or infants until both have been cleaned and dressed after birth. *La cuarentena* incorporates individuals into the family, instills parental responsibility, and integrates the family during a critical life event (D'Avanzo & Geissler, 2003; Niska, Snyder, & Lia-Hoagberg, 1998).

Desire for and valuing of children is salient in all cultures. In Asian families, children are valued as a source of family strength and stability, are perceived as wealth, and are objects of parental love and affection. Infants almost always are given an affectionate "cradle" name that is used during the first years of life; for example, a Filipino girl might be called "Bong-Bong" and a boy "Ling-Ling." In the Yup'ik culture of the Alaskan Eskimos, where sharing has been necessary for survival throughout their history, children are looked on as security. There is no concept of illegitimacy; whether parents are married does not matter. Every child is welcomed and loved. Adoption is common and is usually within the extended family, for example, by grandparents (MacDonald-Clark & Boffman, 1995).

Differing cultural values can influence parents' interactions with health care professionals. For example, Asians are taught to be humble and obedient; to be outspoken is frowned on. They are brought up to not question authority figures (such as a nurse), to avoid confrontation, and to respect the yin/yang balance in nature. Because of these learned values, an Asian mother might not confront the nurse about the length of time it has taken to receive the medication requested for her episiotomy pain. A mother may nod and say, "Yes," in response to the nurse's directions for using an iced sitz bath but then will not use the sitz bath. The "yes," in this case, is a gesture of courtesy, meaning, "I'm listening"; it is not an indication of agreement to comply. The mother does not use the iced sitz bath because of her traditional avoidance of bathing and cold in the puerperium. Because all members of a cultural group do not necessarily adhere to traditional practices, validating which cultural practices are important to individual parents is important. Also refer to Table 2-3 for examples of some traditional cultural beliefs that may be important to parents from Hispanic, African-American, Asian-American, European American, and Native American cultures.

Knowledge of cultural beliefs can help the nurse make more accurate assessments and diagnoses of observed parenting behaviors. For example, nurses may become concerned when they observe cultural practices that appear to reflect poor maternal-infant bonding. Algerian mothers may not unwrap and explore their infants as part of the acquaintance process because in Algeria, babies are wrapped tightly in swaddling clothes to protect them physically and psychologically (D'Avanzo & Geissler, 2003). The nurse may observe a Vietnamese woman who gives minimal care to her infant but refuses to cuddle or further interact with her baby. This apparent lack of interest in the newborn is this cultural group's attempt to ward off "evil spirits," and actually reflects an intense love and concern for the infant (Galanti, 2003). An Asian mother might be criticized for almost immediately relinquishing the care of the infant to the grandmother and not even attempting to hold her baby when it is brought to her room. However, in Asian extended families, members show their support for a new mother's rest and recuperation by assisting with the care of the baby. Contrary to the guidance given to mothers in the United States about "nipple confusion," a mix of breastfeeding and bottle-feeding is standard practice for Japanese mothers. This is out of concern for the mother's rest during the first 2 to 3 months and does not lead to any problems with lactation; breastfeeding is widespread and successful among Japanese women (Sharts-Hopko, 1995).

Cultural beliefs and values give perspective to the meaning of childbirth for a new mother. Nurses can provide an opportunity for a new mother to talk about her perception of the meaning of childbearing. This may foster self-actualization, promote maternal role attainment, improve her relationship with her partner, and enrich the family perspective. In helping new families adjust to parenthood, nurses must provide culturally sensitive care by following principles that facilitate nursing practice within transcultural situations.

Socioeconomic Conditions

Socioeconomic conditions often determine access to available resources. Parents whose economic condition is made worse with the birth of each child and who choose not to or are unable to use an effective method of fertility management may find childbirth complicated by concern for their own health and a sense of helplessness. Mothers who are single; separated or divorced from their husbands; or without a partner, family, and friends for whatever reason may view the birth of a child with dread. Serious financial problems may override any desire for mothering the infant. Nurses must be sensitive to the stressors that economically disadvantaged mothers have to contend with and consider these in efforts to foster mother-infant bonding (Sharts-Hopko, 1995). Nursing measures designed to help mothers in trying socioeconomic circumstances involve referral to social and economic community service agencies, as well as to health care agencies. A satisfactory outcome for such problems often requires long-term commitments from both the woman or couple and the community. Adequate situational supports must be instituted in the prenatal period.

Personal Aspirations

For some women, parenthood interferes with or blocks their plans for personal freedom or advancement in their careers. Resentment concerning this loss may not have been resolved during the prenatal period, and if it remains unresolved, it will spill over into caregiving activities. This may result in indifference and neglect of the infant, or in excessive concern; the mother may set impossibly high standards for her own behavior or the child's performance.

Role models that assist women in integrating work role and motherhood role may be helpful for new mothers. Mothers returning to work who do not identify with such role models appear to improvise and negotiate relationships to manage their careers and the care of their infants (Miller, 1996). Over time, new mothers progress to nurturing themselves and making new connections, to a time of reclaiming and discovery (Hartrick, 1997). Not all new mothers experience role conflict. Some have less role conflict because their careers provide a sense of self-fulfillment and self-worth, especially when they feel supported by their family and confident in child care arrangements. Other mothers are able to work part time or from home; an employer may provide a place for breastfeeding or day care.

Nursing intervention includes providing opportunities for mothers to express their feelings freely to an objective listener, to discuss measures to permit personal growth, and to learn about the care of their infant.

Nurses also can be proactive in influencing changes in work policies related to maternity and paternity leaves, varying models of work sharing, and "family friendly" work environments. Some corporations already structure their work sites to support new mothers (e.g., by providing on-site day care facilities and breastfeeding rooms).

Parental Sensory Impairment

In the early dialogue between the parent and child, each uses all senses—sight, hearing, touch, taste, and smell—to initiate and sustain the attachment process. A parent who has an impairment of one of the senses needs to maximize use of the remaining senses. Although these parents may need the assistance and support of a sighted or hearing person as well as other accommodations to their disability, they can become skilled parents. It is important for nurses and other health care professionals to remember that these persons are parents living with a disability, not "disabled parents."

Visually Impaired Parent

Visual impairment alone does not seem to have a negative effect on mothers' early parenting experiences. These mothers, just as sighted mothers, express the wonders of parenthood and encourage other visually impaired persons to become parents (Conley-Jung & Olkin, 2001). Mothers with disabilities tend to value the importance of performing parenting tasks in the perceived culturally usual way. Their maternal engagement also is facilitated by self-acceptance of their own unique differences in performing parenting tasks (Farber, 2000).

Although visually impaired mothers initially feel a pressure to conform to traditional, sighted ways of parenting, they soon adapt these ways and develop methods better suited to themselves (Conley-Jung & Olkin, 2001). Examples of activities that visually impaired mothers do differently include preparation of the infant's nursery, clothes, and supplies. Mothers may put an entire clothing outfit together and hang it in the closet rather than keeping the items separately in drawers. They might develop a labeling system for the infant's clothing and put diapering, bathing, and other care supplies where these will be easy to locate with minimal searching (Conley-Jung & Olkin, 2001). A strength that visually impaired parents have is a heightened sensitivity to other sensory outputs. A blind mother can tell when her infant is facing her because she can feel the baby's breath on her face.

Concerns expressed by visually impaired mothers include (1) their infant's safety; (2) the extra planning, time, and effort needed to accommodate their visual limitations beyond those parenting usually requires; (3) transportation; (4) handling other people's reactions; (5) providing proper guidance and discipline as the infant grows; and (5) missing out visually (Conley-Jung & Olkin, 2001). Visually impaired mothers use various strategies to cope with the reactions of others. They suggest being upfront and conveying a sense of openness, making people aware of the nature of the visual impairment early in the relationship, informing and educating people about visual impairment, focusing on the positive and ignoring negative messages, expressing anger, and laughing and joking (Conley-Jung & Olkin, 2001).

One of the major difficulties that visually impaired parents experience is the skepticism, open or hidden, of health care professionals. Blind people sense reluctance on the part of others to acknowledge that they have a right to be parents. All too often, nurses and doctors lack the experience to deal with the childbearing and childrearing needs of visually impaired mothers, as well as mothers with other disabilities (such as the hearing impaired, physically impaired, and mentally challenged). Shyness, fear, or reluctance on the part of nurses can result in visually impaired parents being left alone or being involved in awkward conversations. The nurse's best approach is to assess the mother's capabilities.

From that basis, the nurse can make plans to assist the woman, often in much the same way as for a mother with sight. Visually impaired mothers have made suggestions for providing care for women such as themselves during childbearing (Box 22-1). The nurse's use of this kind of approach can help avoid a sense of increased vulnerability on the mother's part.

Eye-to-eye contact is considered important in North American culture. With a parent who is visually impaired, this critical factor in the parent-child attachment process is obviously missing. However, the blind parent, who may never have experienced this method of strengthening relationships, does not miss it. The infant will need other sensory input from that parent. An infant looking into the eyes of a mother who is blind may not be aware that the eyes are unseeing. Other people in the newborn's environment can also participate in active eye-to-eye contact to supply this need. A problem may arise, however, if the visually impaired parent has an impassive facial expression. Her infant, making repeated unsuccessful attempts to engage in face play with the mother, will abandon the behavior with her and intensify it with the father or other persons in the household. Nurses can provide anticipatory guidance regarding this situation and help the mother learn to nod and smile while talking and cooing to the infant.

Hearing-Impaired Parent

The parent who has a hearing impairment faces another set of problems, particularly if the deafness dates from birth or early childhood. The mother and her partner are likely to have established an independent household. A number of devices that transform sound into light flashes are now marketed and can be fitted into the infant's room to permit immediate detection of crying. Even if the parent is not speech trained, vocalizing can serve as both a stimulus and a response to the infant's early vocalizing. Deaf parents can provide additional vocal training by use of recordings and television, so that from birth, the child is aware of the full range of the human voice. Young children acquire sign language readily, and the first sign used is as varied as the first word.

Section 504 of the Rehabilitation Act of 1973 requires hospitals and other institutions receiving funds from the U.S. Department of Health and Human Services to use various communication techniques and resources with the deaf, including having staff members or certified interpreters who are proficient in sign language. For example, provision of written materials with demonstrations and having nurses stand where the parent can read their lips (if the parent practices lipreading) are two techniques that can be used. A creative approach is for the nursing unit to develop videotapes in which information on postpartum care, infant care, and parenting issues is signed by an interpreter and spoken by a nurse. A videotape in which a nurse signs while speaking would be ideal.

BOX 22-1

Nursing Approaches for Working with Visually Impaired Parents

1. Parents who are blind need verbal teaching by health care providers because printed maternity information is not accessible to blind people.
2. A visually impaired parent needs an orientation to the hospital room that allows the parent to move about the room independently. For example, "Go to the left of the bed and trail the wall until you feel the first door. That is the bathroom."
3. Parents who are blind need explanations of routines.
4. Parents who are blind need to feel devices (e.g., monitors, pelvic models) and to hear descriptions of the devices.
5. Visually impaired parents need a chance to ask questions.
6. Visually impaired parents need the opportunity to hold and touch the baby after birth.
7. Nurses need to demonstrate baby care by touch and to follow with, "Now let me see you do it."
8. Nurses need to give instructions such as, "I'm going to give you the baby. The head is to your left side."

SIBLING ADAPTATION

Because the family is an interactive, open unit, the addition of a new family member affects everyone in the family. Siblings have to assume new positions within the family hierarchy. The older child's goal is to maintain the lead position. Parents are faced with the task of caring for a new child while not neglecting the others. Parents need to distribute their attention in an equitable manner.

Reactions of siblings may result from temporary separation from the mother, changes in the mother's or father's behavior, or the siblings' response to the infant's coming home. Positive behavioral changes of siblings include interest in and concern for the baby (see Figs. 22-3 and 22-9) and increased independence. Regression in toileting and sleep habits, aggression toward the baby, and increased seeking of attention and whining are examples of negative behaviors.

The parents' attitudes toward the arrival of the baby can set the stage for the other children's reactions (Fig. 22-9). Because the baby absorbs the time and attention of the important people in the other children's lives, jealousy is to be expected once the initial excitement of having a new baby in the home is over. However, sibling rivalry, or negative behaviors in siblings, may have been overemphasized in the past. Developmentally appropriate behaviors in siblings are similar before and after the baby arrives. Firstborn children seem to continue their usual routines and are more pleased with the newborns and more understanding of the baby's need for care than the parents predict.

Parents, especially mothers, spend much time and energy promoting sibling acceptance of a new baby. Participating in sibling preparation classes makes a difference in the ability of parents to cope with sibling behavior. Older children are actively involved in preparing for the infant, and this involvement intensifies after the birth of the child. Parents face a number of tasks related to sibling rivalry and adjustment. Parents have to manage their feelings of guilt that the older children are being deprived of parental time and attention. They have to monitor the behavior of older children toward the more vulnerable infant and divert aggressive behavior. Strategies that parents have used to facilitate siblings' acceptance of a new baby are presented in the Family Focus box.

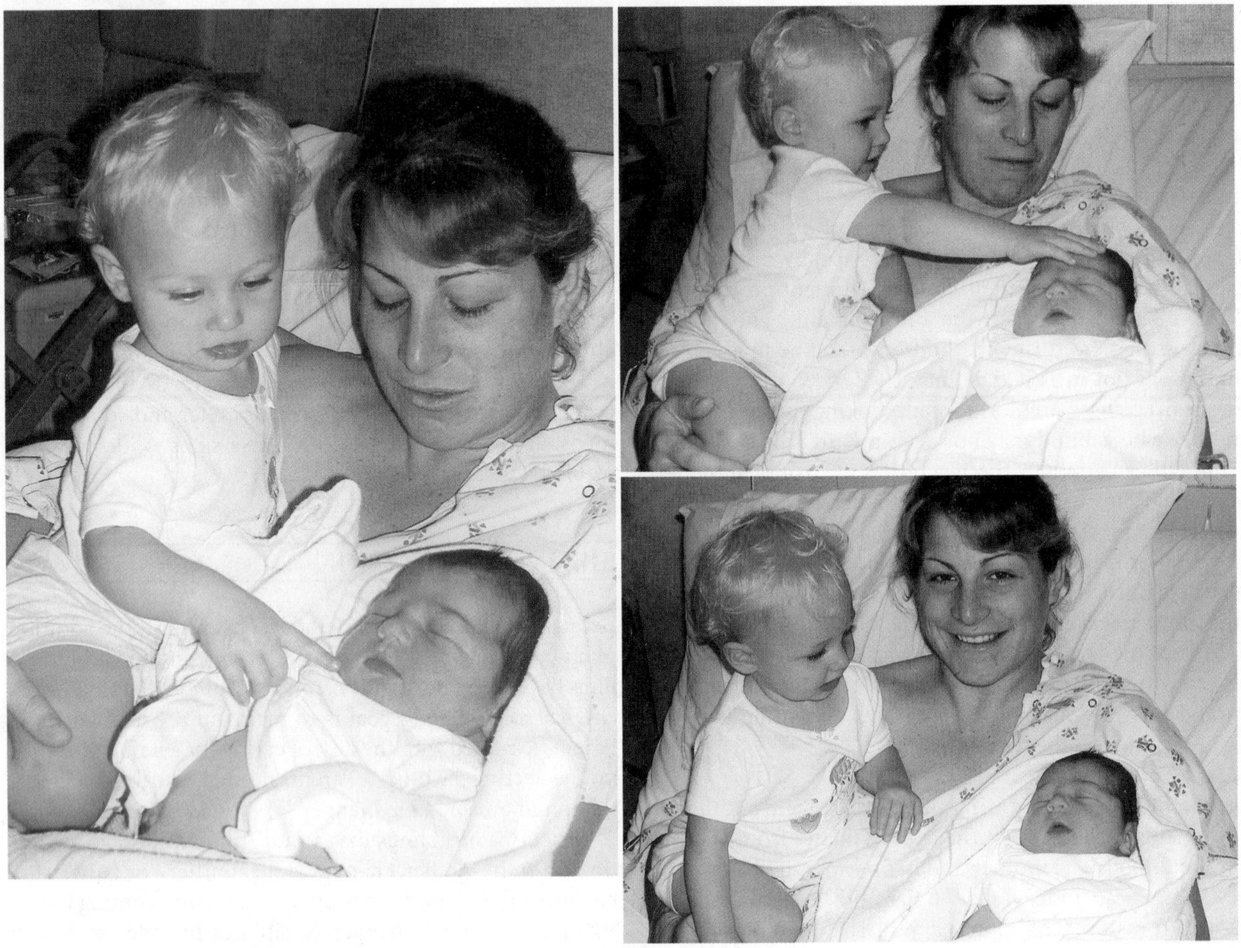

Fig. 22-9 First meeting. **A**, Sister touching new sibling with fingertip. **B**, Touching with whole hand. **C**, Smiles indicate acceptance. (Courtesy Sara Kossuth, Los Angeles, CA.)

Siblings demonstrate acquaintance behaviors with the newborn. The acquaintance process depends on the information given to the child before the baby is born and on the child's cognitive development level. The initial behaviors of siblings with the newborn include looking at the infant and touching the head (Fig. 22-9). The initial adjustment of older children to a newborn takes time, and children should be allowed to interact at their own pace rather than be forced to do so. To expect a young child to accept and love a rival for the parents' affection assumes an unrealistic level of maturity. Sibling love grows as does other love, that is, by being with another person and sharing experiences. The relationship that develops between siblings has been conceptualized as sibling attachment. This bond between siblings involves a secure base in which one child provides support for the other, is missed when absent, and is looked to for comfort and security.

GRANDPARENT ADAPTATION

Grandparents are unique. They contribute to a sense of family continuity and provide maintenance of cultural traditions. They can educate their grandchildren about their roots and relate anecdotes about their parents. In turn, the presence of grandchildren often helps relieve the grandparents' loneliness and boredom. Grandparents who are free to love the grandchild can have a significant positive influence on the child's life (Fig. 22-10).

Grandparents experience a transition to grandparenthood. Intergenerational relationships shift and grandparents must deal with changes in practices and attitudes toward childbirth, childrearing, and men's and women's roles at home and in the workplace. The degree to which grandparents understand and accept current practices can influence how supportive they are perceived to be by their adult children.

At the same time that they are adjusting to grandparenthood, most grandparents are experiencing normative middle- and old-age life transition issues, such as retirement and a move to smaller housing, and need support from their adult children. Some may feel regret about their limited involvement because of poor health or geographic distance. Maternal grandmothers, more so than the other three grandparents, may have high expectations of themselves that cause them to be very self-critical.

The extent of involvement of grandparents in the care of the newborn depends on many factors, for example, the willingness of the grandparents to become involved, the proximity of the grandparents, and ethnic and cultural expecta-

Family Focus

STRATEGIES FOR FACILITATING SIBLING ACCEPTANCE OF A NEW BABY

1. Take your firstborn child on a tour of your hospital room and point out similarities to his or her birth. "This is like the room I was in with you, and the baby is in the same kind of bassinet that you were in."
2. Have a small gift from the baby to give to your older child each day.
3. Give the older child a T-shirt that says, "I'm a big brother" (or "sister").
4. Arrange for your children to be in the first group (grandparents, sister) to see the newborn. Let them hold the baby in the hospital. One mother and father arranged for their firstborn son to be present at the births of his three brothers and to be the first one to hold them.
5. Plan time for both children. "When I get home, I'll arrange my day so that I can have the baby's care done in the morning while Sam (first child) is at school. Maybe the baby will sleep part of the afternoon and I can spend some time with Sam."
6. Fathers can spend time with the older sibling while mothers are taking care of the baby and vice versa. Siblings like to have time and attention from both parents.
7. Give preschool and early school-age siblings a newborn doll as "their baby" to care for. Give the sibling a photograph of the new baby to take to school to show off "his" or "her" baby. Older siblings may enjoy the responsibility of helping care for the newborn, such as learning how to give the baby a bottle or change a diaper. One mother let her preschooler help burp the new baby by patting on the baby's back. She figured her son could pat the baby fairly firmly without harming him and at the same time get out some pent-up aggressive feelings.

tions of the grandparent's role. If the new parents live in the United States, Asian grandparents typically are asked to come to the United States to care for the baby and the mother after birth and to care for the children once the parents return to work. In the United States, paternal grandparents, in contrast to those in other cultures, often consider themselves secondary to the maternal grandparents. Less seems expected of them, and they are initially less involved. Nevertheless, these grandparents are eager to help and express great pleasure in their son's fatherhood and his involvement with the baby. Support that they provide for their son can help the new father in being supportive of the new mother, thus influencing a smoother parental adjustment for the new parents.

For first-time parents, pregnancy and parenthood can reawaken old issues related to dependence versus independence. Some expectant parents may not plan on their parents' help immediately after the baby arrives. They want time "to be a family," inferring a couple-baby unit, not the intergenerational family network. Intergenerational help may be perceived as interference. Contrary to their expectations, however, new parents do call on their parents for help, especially the maternal grandmother (Steinberg et al, 2000). Many grandparents realize their adult children's wishes for autonomy, respect these wishes, and remain available to help when asked.

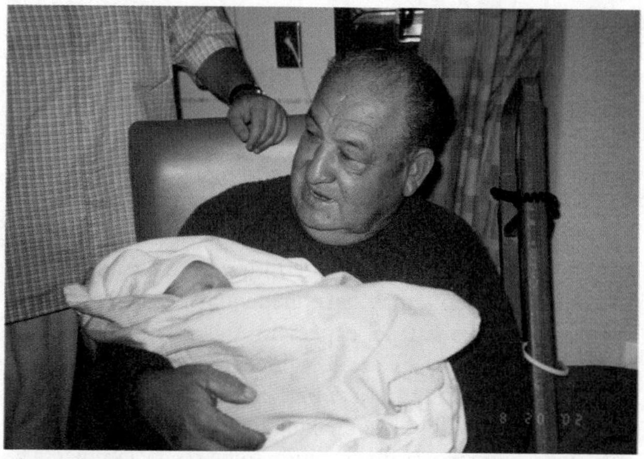

Fig. 22-10 Grandfather and new grandson get acquainted. (Courtesy Shannon Perry, Phoenix, AZ.)

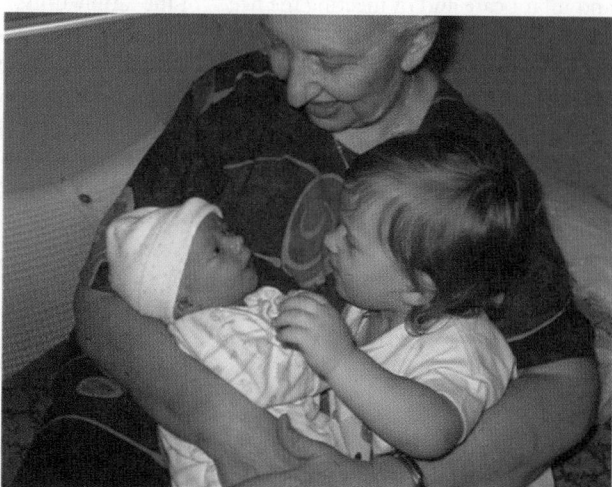

Fig. 22-11 Grandmother and granddaughter becoming acquainted with new grandson/brother. (Courtesy Sharron Humenick, Midlothian, VA.)

The support of grandparents can be a stabilizing influence for families undergoing developmental transitions such as childbearing and new parenthood. Grandparents can foster the learning of parental skills and preserve tradition. The maternal grandmother is an important model for childrearing practices, a source of knowledge, and a support person (Fig. 22-11). With teenage mothers, the regular assistance of grandparents with child care has allowed these young mothers to continue their educations (Dalla & Gamble, 2000).

A simple technique to help people span the generation gap is through a printed "letter to new parents" (written from the grandparents' perspective), which can be included in prenatal kits distributed in childbirth preparation classes and made available to all family members on the postpartum unit. Grandparents' classes can be used to bridge the generation gap and to help the grandparents understand their adult children's parenting concepts. The classes include information on up-to-date childbearing practices; family-centered care; infant care, feeding, and safety (car seats); and exploration of roles that grandparents play in the family unit.

CARE MANAGEMENT: PRACTICAL SUGGESTIONS FOR THE FIRST WEEKS AT HOME

Numerous changes occur during the first weeks of parenthood. Care management should be directed toward helping parents cope with infant care, role changes, altered lifestyle, and change in family structure resulting from the addition of a new baby. Parents may have inadequate or incorrect understanding of what to expect in the early postpartum weeks. Developing skill and confidence in caring for an infant can be especially anxiety provoking.

Nurses, especially those making postpartum visits to parents' homes, are in a prime position to help new families. The nurse's role becomes primarily one of teacher-supporter, focusing on enabling new parents to become capable of self-care and infant care and of meeting the needs of the family unit.

Assessment

Assessment should include a psychosocial assessment focusing on parent-infant attachment, adjustment to the parental role, sibling adjustment, social support, and education needs, as well as mother's and baby's physical adaptation. Early home visits are an excellent opportunity for the nurse to assess beginnings of positive or negative parenting behaviors and to provide positive reinforcement for loving and nurturing behaviors with the infant. Parents who interact in inappropriate or abusive ways with their infants should be followed more closely, and an appropriate mental health practitioner or professional social worker should be notified.

Nursing Diagnoses

Nursing diagnoses pertinent to transition to parenthood include:

- *Readiness for enhanced family coping related to*
  - —positive attitude and realistic expectations for newborn and adapting to parenthood
  - —nurturing behaviors with newborn
  - —verbalizing positive factors in lifestyle change
- *Risk for impaired parenting related to*
  - —lack of knowledge in infant care
  - —feelings of incompetence and/or lack of confidence
  - —unrealistic expectations of newborn/infant
  - —fatigue from interrupted sleep
- *Ineffective parental role performance related to*
  - —role transition and role attainment
  - —unwanted pregnancy
  - —lack of resources to support parenting (e.g., no paid leave)
- *Risk for impaired parent-infant attachment related to*
  - —difficult labor and birth
  - —postpartum complications
  - —neonatal complications/anomalies

Expected Outcomes

A plan of care is formulated in collaboration with the family, incorporating their priorities and preferences, to meet their specific needs. Expected outcomes for effective transition to parenthood include that the parents will:

- Demonstrate behaviors that reflect appreciation of sensory and behavioral capacities of the infant.
- Verbalize increasing confidence and competence in feeding, diapering, dressing, and sensory stimulation of the infant.
- Identify deviations from normal in the infant that should be brought to the immediate attention of the primary health care provider.
- Relate effectively to the newborn's siblings and grandparents.

Plan of Care and Implementation

Instructions for the First Days at Home

Parents, especially first-time parents, must be helped to anticipate what the transition from hospital to home will be like. Anticipatory guidance can help prevent a shock of reality that might negate the parents' joy or cause them undue stress. Even the simplest strategies can provide enormous support. Written information reinforcing education topics is helpful to provide to parents, as is a list of available community resources, both local and national (see Resources at the end of this chapter). Classes in the prenatal period or during the postpartum stay are helpful. Instructions for the first days at home should minimally include activities of daily living, dealing with visitors, and activity and rest.

Infant Care

Providing practical suggestions for infant care can help parents adjust to parenthood. Mothers and fathers want to feel capable and confident in the physical care of their infant. The nurse should assess each parent's need for instruction on care such as bathing, clothing, and safety (see Chapter 25).

Anticipatory Guidance Regarding the Newborn

Anticipatory guidance helps prepare new parents for what to expect as their newborn grows and develops. Parents with realistic expectations of infant needs and behavior are better prepared to adjust to the demands of a new baby and to parenthood itself.

New parents can be overwhelmed by a large volume of information and become anxious. Anticipatory guidance needs to include the following: newborn sleep-wake cycles, interpretation of crying and quieting techniques, infant developmental milestones, sensory enrichment/infant stimulation, recognizing signs of illness, and well-baby follow-up and immunizations.

Development of Day-Night Routines

Nurses can help prepare new parents for the fact that most newborns cannot tell the difference between night and day and must learn the rhythm of day-night routines. Nurses should provide basic suggestions for settling a newborn and for helping him or her develop a predictable routine. Examples of such suggestions include:

- In the late afternoon, bring the baby out to the center of family activity. Keep the baby there for the rest of the evening. If the baby falls asleep, let the baby do so in the infant seat or in someone's arms. Save the crib or bassinet for nighttime sleep.
- Give the baby a bath right before bedtime. This soothes the baby and helps him or her expend energy.
- Feed the baby for the last evening time around 11 PM and put him or her to bed in the crib or bassinet.

- For nighttime feedings and diaper changes, keep a small night light on to avoid turning on bright lights. Talk in soft whispers (if at all) and handle the baby gently and only as absolutely necessary to feed and diaper. Nighttime feedings should be all business and no play! Babies usually go back to sleep if the room is quiet and dark.

A predictable, stable routine gradually develops for most babies; however, some babies will never develop one. New parents will find it easier if they are willing to be flexible and to give up some control during those early weeks.

Interpretation of Crying and Quieting Techniques

Crying is an infant's first social communication. Some babies cry more than others, but all babies cry. They cry to communicate that they are hungry, uncomfortable, wet, ill, or bored, and sometimes for no apparent reason at all. The longer parents are around their infants, the easier it becomes to interpret what a cry means. Many infants have a fussy period during the day, often in the late afternoon or early evening when everyone is naturally tired. Environmental tension adds to the length and intensity of crying spells. Babies also have periods of vigorous crying when no comforting can help. These periods of crying may last for long stretches until the infants seem to cry themselves to sleep. Possibly the infants are trying to discharge enough energy so that they can settle themselves down. The nurse needs to reinforce for new parents that time and infant maturation will take care of these types of cries.

Crying because of colic is a common concern of new parents. Babies with colic cry inconsolably for several hours, pull their legs up to their stomach, and pass large amounts of gas. No one really knows what colic is or why babies get it. Parents can be encouraged to contact their nurse practitioner or pediatrician if they are concerned that their baby has colic.

As their babies develop, some parents are teaching hearing babies sign language to help them communicate their needs before they are able to talk (Acredolo & Goodwyn, 2002).

Certain types of sensory stimulation can calm and quiet infants and help them get to sleep. Important characteristics of this sensory stimulation—whether tactile, vestibular, auditory, or visual—appear to be that the stimulation is mild, slow, rhythmic, and consistently and regularly presented. Tactile stimulation can include warmth, patting, back rubbing, and covering the skin with textured cloth. Swaddling to keep arms and legs close to the body (as in utero) provides widespread and constant tactile stimulation and a sense of security. Vestibular stimulation is especially effective and can be accomplished by mild rhythmic movement such as rocking or holding the infant upright, as on the parent's shoulder.

The nurse can teach parents a number of strategies that help quiet a fussy baby, prevent crying, and induce quiet attention or sleep (Box 22-2 and Guidelines/Guías box).

Developmental Milestones

Knowledge of infant growth and development helps parents have realistic expectations of what an infant can do. When parents understand and appreciate the limitations and developing abilities of their infant, adjustment to parenthood can go more smoothly. Emphasizing the individuality of the infant enhances the family's capacity to offer their infant an optimally nurturing environment.

Brazelton (1995) suggested the concept of "touch-points" for intervention: that is, points at which a change in the sys-

BOX 22-2

How to Swaddle an Infant

1. Fold down the top corner of the blanket. Position the infant on the blanket with the infant's neck near the fold.
2. Bring the blanket around the infant's right side and across the infant, tucking the corner under the left side.
3. Bring the bottom of the blanket up to the infant's chest.
4. Bring the remaining corner of the blanket across the infant, tucking the corner under the infant's right side. The infant should be wrapped securely but not tightly; some room should be left for the infant to move.

SKILL—SWADDLING

ENGLISH SPANISH **Guidelines/Guías**

INFANT QUIETING TECHNIQUES

These suggestions may help to quiet a fussy baby:
Estas sugerencias pueden ayudarle a calmar a un bebé intranquilo:

Let the baby see your face. Talk to the baby in a soothing voice.
Deje que el bebé vea la cara de usted. Hable al bebé con una voz tranquilizante.

Swaddle the baby in a receiving blanket.
Envuelva al bebé con una cobija para bebés.

Babies feel secure in a small, warm, soft place like a bassinet, buggy, or cradle.
Los bebés sienten estables en un lugar pequeño, cálido, y blando como un moisés, cochecito, o cuna.

Some babies need extra sucking to soothe themselves, either at the breast or on a pacifier.
Algunos bebés necesitan amamantar o chupar un chupete un poquito más para tranquilizarse.

A rhythmic, monotonous sound such as a recording of a heartbeat, the dishwasher, or washing machine, helps settle a baby.
Un sonido rítmico y monótono como la grabación de un latido de corazón, el lavavajillas o la lavadora ayuda que el bebé se tranquilice.

Movement such as rocking in a chair, riding in a stroller or a car, often helps quiet a fussy baby.
Tal movimiento como meciendo en una mecedora o andando en cochecito o en coche a menudo ayuda a calmar a un bebé intranquilo.

Carry the baby in a frontpack or backpack.
Lleve al bebé en una mochila de pecho o de espalda.

Place the baby on his/her abdomen across your lap and pat or rub his/her back while bouncing your legs or swaying them from left to right.
Ponga al bebé en la falda acostado de estómago y déle al bebé unas palmaditas en la espalda. Puede masajearlo mientras le hace caballito al bebé o se balancea las piernas de un lado al otro.

Lie in a warm tub of water with the baby on your chest with the baby's body immersed in water.
Acuéstese en una bañera llena de agua tibia con el bebé encima del pecho de usted y con el cuerpo del bebé sumergido en el agua.

tem (i.e., baby, parent, and family) is brought about by the baby's spurts in development (e.g., cognitive, motor, or emotional). Immediately before each spurt in development, there is a predictable short period of disorganization in the baby. Parents are likely to feel disorganized and stressed as well. Because these periods of disorganization are predictable, nurses can offer parents anticipatory guidance to help them understand what happens with infant development and to prepare them for the subsequent spurts in development.

Two touch-points occur during the early postpartum-newborn period: one soon after birth and another at 2 to 3 weeks (Brazelton, 1995). In the hospital or at a home visit during the first week, the nurse can use Brazelton's Neonatal Behavioral Assessment Scale (Brazelton & Nugent, 1996) to demonstrate to parents their baby's amazing repertoire of abilities and to anticipate their infant's response to environmental stimuli (Fowles, 1999). In this way, parents begin to appreciate their baby's individuality and become more sensitive to their baby's behavioral cues. At 2 to 3 weeks, the home care nurse or pediatric office nurse should assess for the regular end-of-the-day fussy period that most infants have between 3 and 12 weeks of age. Helpful topics to include in the anticipatory guidance are the normalcy and positive value of the fussy period, how to settle a fussy baby, and ways to help a baby develop a predictable schedule.

BOX 22-3

Teaching Your Newborn

- Newborns learn things every day. You can teach your newborn by playing with him or her and giving your newborn toys that help him or her learn.
- Talk to your baby a lot. Tell your baby what is going on in the room. ("Listen to the dog barking.") Label objects that you see or use ("Here's the washcloth.") and describe things you are doing ("Let's put the shirt over Kerry's head!").
- Read to your baby and show him or her the pictures in the books. Name the objects in the pictures.
- Look at your baby's face and make eye contact. Play face-making games: smile, stick out your tongue, open your eyes wide. As your baby gets older, he or she will try to imitate these facial expressions.
- Babies like music and rhythmic movement. Rock or swing your baby as you sing to him or her in a gentle voice.
- Acknowledge your baby's attempts to "answer" your talking and singing. He or she will respond to you by looking in your direction, making eye contact, moving his or her arms and legs, and/or making sounds.
- Babies like bright colors and vivid contrasts. Show your baby pictures and objects that are black and white, bright primary colors (red, blue, yellow), and/or large patterns. Keep colorful mobiles and toys where your baby can see them.
- Babies like to be held upright. Holding your newborn on your shoulder lets your baby look around his or her world and provides vestibular stimulation. Let your baby lift his or her head for a few seconds. Keep your hand ready to support your baby's head.

Infant Stimulation

Interacting with their parents is an important way in which infants learn about themselves and their environment. Home health nurses are in a prime position to evaluate the home environment and to make suggestions to parents for promotion of their baby's physical, cognitive, and emotional development. Box 22-3 and Table 22-1 present suggestions for visual, auditory, tactile, and kinetic stimulation.

Another method of sensory enrichment that parents can learn to use is infant massage. This type of nurturing touch can help create a loving bond between the infant and parent and has been shown to contribute to the physical and emotional well-being of both the massage giver and receiver (Schneider, 1996; 1997). Infant massage is a gentle, warm communication done *with* the infant, not *to* the infant. The focus is on reciprocal interaction between infant and parent; the parent talks to the infant, asks permission to start the massage, questions the infant, and facilitates dialogue.

One of the most important benefits of infant massage (Box 22-4) for the parents is the improved ability to read

BOX 22-4

Benefits of Infant Massage

IN THE PSYCHOSOCIAL DOMAIN

Benefits to the Infant of Receiving Massage
- Promotes bonding and attachment
- Promotes body/mind/spirit connection
- Increases self-esteem
- Increases sense of love, acceptance, respect, and trust
- Enhances communication

Benefits to the Parent of Giving Massage
- Improves ability to read infant cues
- Improves synchrony between caregiver and infant
- Promotes bonding
- Increases confidence in parenting
- Increases communication, both verbal and nonverbal
- Improves relaxation
- Provides time to share and quality time
- Promotes parenting skills

IN THE PHYSIOLOGICAL/PHYSICAL GROWTH DOMAIN

Benefits to the Infant of Receiving Massage
- Improves relaxation and release of accumulated stress
- Stimulates circulation
- Strengthens digestive, circulatory, and gastrointestinal systems, which can lead to weight gain
- Reduces discomfort from teething, congestion, gas, colic, and emotional stress
- Improves muscle tone/coordination
- Increases elimination, circulation, and respiration
- Improves sleep patterns
- Increases hormonal function

Benefits to the Parent of Giving Massage
- Improves sense of well-being
- Reduces blood pressure
- Reduces stress
- Improves overall health

From Schneider E: Touch communication: the power of infant massage, *Massage Magazine* 68:40, 1997.

their infant's cues (Schneider, 1997). Positive cues include eye contact, smiling, looking at the parent's face, babbling or cooing, and smooth movements of arms and legs. Negative cues from the infant include pulling away, frowning, grimacing, turning the head away, arching the back, crying, squirming, and flailing the arms and legs. Increased ability to read their infant's cues can increase parental confidence and self-esteem, thereby assisting adaptation to parenthood.

Recognizing Signs of Illness

As well as explaining the need for well-baby follow-up visits, the nurse should discuss with parents the signs of illness in newborns. Of particular importance is the parents' assessment of jaundice in newborns discharged early. Parents should be advised to call their nurse-practitioner or pediatrician immediately if they notice signs of illness or increasing jaundice and to ask about over-the-counter medications, such as Tylenol for infants, to keep at home (Nursing Care Plan).

Evaluation

Evaluation is based on the expected outcomes of care. The plan is revised as needed based on the evaluation findings.

Nursing Care Plan

HOME CARE FOLLOW-UP: TRANSITION TO PARENTHOOD

NURSING DIAGNOSIS: Deficient knowledge of infant care related to lack of experience/lack of support

EXPECTED OUTCOMES

Infant care routines are adequate, and infant appears healthy.

NURSING INTERVENTIONS/*RATIONALES*

Observe infant care routines (bathing, diapering, feeding, play) *to evaluate parental ease with care and adequacy of techniques.*

Observe infant appearance (height-weight ratio, head circumference, fontanels, skin tone and turgor); assess infant's vital signs, overall tone, reflexes, and age-appropriate developmental skills *to evaluate for signs indicative of inadequate care.*

Explore available support systems for infant care *to determine adequacy of existing system.*

Demonstrate care routines and have involved family members return demonstration *to facilitate improvements in care.*

Provide ongoing follow-up as needed *to remediate identified potential and actual care deficits.*

NURSING DIAGNOSIS: Disturbed sleep pattern related to infant demands and environmental interruptions

EXPECTED OUTCOMES

Woman sleeps for uninterrupted periods and feels rested on waking.

NURSING INTERVENTIONS/*RATIONALES*

Discuss woman's routine and specify things that interfere with sleep *to determine scope of problem and direct interventions.*

Explore ways woman and significant others can make environment more conducive to sleep (e.g., privacy, darkness, quiet, back rubs, soothing music, warm milk); teach use of guided imagery and relaxation techniques *to promote optimal conditions for sleep.*

Eliminate things or routines (e.g., caffeine, foods that induce heartburn, strenuous mental/physical activity) *that may interfere with sleep.*

Advise family to limit visitors and activities *to avoid further taxation and fatigue.*

Have family plan specific times to care for the newborn *to allow mother time to sleep;* have mother learn to use infant nap time as a time for her to nap as well *to replenish energy and decrease fatigue.*

NURSING DIAGNOSIS: Risk for impaired home maintenance related to addition of new family member/inadequate resources/inadequate support systems

EXPECTED OUTCOME

Home exhibits signs of safe and functional environment.

NURSING INTERVENTIONS/*RATIONALES*

Observe the home environment (e.g., available living space and sleeping arrangements; adequacy of facilities for food preparation and storage, hygiene and toileting; overall state of repair; cleanliness; presence of safety hazards) *to determine adequacy and effective use of resources.*

Observe arrangements for the newborn, such as sleeping space, care equipment, and supplies (bathing, changing, feeding, transportation) *to determine adequacy of resources.*

Explore who is responsible for cooking, cleaning, child care, and newborn care and determine whether the mother seems adequately rested *to determine adequacy of support systems.*

Identify and arrange referrals to needed social agencies (e.g., Aid to Families with Dependent Children [AFDC], Women, Infants, and Children [WIC] program, food pantries) *to address resource deficits (finances, supplies, equipment).*

NURSING DIAGNOSIS: Risk for interrupted family processes related to inclusion of new family member

EXPECTED OUTCOME

Infant is successfully assimilated into family structure.

NURSING INTERVENTIONS/*RATIONALES*

Explore with family the ways that the birth and neonate have changed family structure and function *to evaluate functional and role adjustment.*

Observe family interaction with the newborn and note degree of bonding, evidence of sibling rivalry, and involvement in newborn care *to evaluate acceptance of newest family member.*

Clarify identified misinformation and misperceptions *to promote clear communication.*

Assist family to explore options for solutions to identified problems *to promote effective problem resolution.*

Support family efforts as they move toward adjusting and incorporating the new member *to reinforce new functions and roles.*

If needed, make referrals to appropriate social services or community agencies *to ensure ongoing support and care.*

Key Points

- The birth of a child necessitates changes in the existing interactional structure of a family.
- Attachment is the process by which the parent and infant come to love and accept each other.
- Attachment is strengthened through the use of sensual responses or interactions by both partners in the parent-infant interaction.
- In adjusting to the parental role, the mother moves from a dependent state (taking in) to an interdependent state (letting go).
- Mothers may exhibit signs of postpartum blues (baby blues) or postpartum depression (PPD).
- Fathers experience emotions and adjustments during the transition to parenthood that are similar to, and also distinctly different from, those of mothers.
- Modulation of rhythm, modification of behavioral repertoires, and mutual responsivity facilitate infant-parent adjustment.
- Many factors (e.g., age, culture, socioeconomic level, and expectations of what the child will be like) influence adaptation to parenthood.
- Parents face a number of tasks related to sibling adjustment that require creative parental interventions.
- Grandparents can have a positive influence on the postpartum family.

Answer Guidelines to Critical Thinking Exercise

Postpartum Adjustment for the Adolescent and the Older Mother

1. Studies of what teaching and care new parents want and need have been conducted. Care providers and new parents may differ on the priority assigned to topics. Nurses should assess parents' preferences when planning teaching. Carol and Robert are exhibiting a knowledge deficit in infant feeding. They need information about breastfeeding, the time it takes, the recommendation for exclusive breastfeeding for 6 months, when to introduce solid foods, sleep patterns of newborn infants, and the fact that adding cereal to milk does not make infants sleep longer. Audrey needs someone to listen to her concerns. Older mothers, used to being in control, are often distressed that they cannot control their infants' behavior (sleeping and eating patterns). In addition, Audrey may be experiencing postpartum blues; further assessment and teaching is warranted.
2. (a) Very young adolescents and older mothers may be at risk for some physiologic problems in pregnancy and childbirth. With adequate support, adolescents can provide appropriate care for the newborn. They tend to have unrealistic expectations for behavior of the infant and need continued education about child development. Older mothers must adjust to the loss of freedom and interruption of a career that care of a newborn entails. (b) Involving the adolescent father in the care of the infant is important. He can provide needed support for the mother. Ordinarily an older mother has more access to financial and other supports than does an adolescent. (c) Education about parenting and recovery from childbirth should begin in the prenatal period to prepare parents for realistic expectations. Education and support should continue after birth and following discharge whenever feasible. (d) With adequate support, the long-term prognosis for positive outcomes is good. The adolescent who becomes a parent is less likely to complete school, is more likely to be a single parent, and to have lower income and receive public assistance. Older mothers need time to adjust to the demands of parenting and support as they make this transition.
3. Carol and Robert have a knowledge deficit in infant feeding (see #1) and Audrey needs support and assessment for postpartum blues. They all need further information about infant development and behavior and support in their transition to parenthood.
4. Yes, there is evidence regarding postpartum teaching needs, adolescent parenting, child development, older mothers, transition to parenthood, and postpartum blues
5. Depending on the receptivity of Carol and Robert to the teaching about infant feeding and child development, the infant may or may not be at risk for child abuse. These parents and infant should participate in follow-up care. Ongoing teaching about child development and support is necessary. Involving Carol's mother in providing support to the young couple may be useful. While Audrey's response appears to be normal, assessment for signs of postpartum depression should continue. Assisting her in obtaining social support from family or friends may assist the transition to parenthood. More involvement of the baby's father would facilitate adjustment.

Resources

At-Home Dad (newsletter for fathers who stay at home)
61 Brightwood Ave.
North Andover, MA 01845-1702
www.athomedad.com

Baby-Friendly USA
327 Quaker Meeting House Rd.
E. Sandwich, MA 02537
508-888-8092
www.babyfriendlyusa.org

The Fatherhood Project at the Families and Work Institute
330 Seventh Ave.
New York, NY 10001
212-465-2044

FEMALE (Formerly Employed Mother at the Leading Edge)
P.O. Box 31
Elmhurst, IL 60126
630-941-3553

Institute for Responsible Fatherhood and Family Revitalization
1146 19th Street NW
Suite 800
Washington, DC 20036
800-7FATHER or 800-732-8437

International Association of Infant Massage (IAIM)
800-248-5432

La Leche League International
1400 North Meacham Road
Schaumburg, IL 60168-4079
847-519-7730
www.lalecheleague.org
(Local La Leche League groups are usually listed in city and town phone books)

Motherhood Maternity Health and Fitness Program
SBI Corporation
1106 Stratford Dr.
Carlisle, PA 17103
717-258-4641

Mothers at Home
8310A Old Courthouse Road
Vienna, VA 22182
703-827-5903

National Council for Adoption
202-328-5903

National Organization of Mothers of Twins Clubs, Inc.
PO Box 23188
Albuquerque, NM 87192
505-275-0955

Pink Inc.! Publishing
PO Box 866
Atlantic Beach, FL 32233-0866
904-731-7120

Postpartum Support International
927 North Kellogg Avenue
Santa Barbara, CA 93111
805-967-7636
www.chss.iup.edu/postpartum

U. S. Department of Transportation
National Highway Traffic Safety Administration (NHTSA)
www.nhtsa.dot.gov
Source for child safety seat information

Single Parent Resource Center
141 West 28th Street
Suite 302
New York, NY 10001
212-947-0221

References

Acredolo L, Goodwyn S: *Baby signs*. Chicago, 2002, Contemporary Books.

Alpers RR: The changing self-concept of pregnant and parenting teens, *J Prof Nurs* 14(2):111-118, 1998.

Ament LA: Maternal tasks of the puerperium re-identified, *J Obstet Gynecol Neonatal Nurs* 19(4):330-335, 1990.

Anderson A: The father-infant relationship: becoming connected, *J Soc Pediatr Nurs* 1(2):83-92, 1996a.

Anderson A: Factors influencing the father-infant relationship, *J Fam Nurs* 2(3):306-324, 1996b.

Barlow J, Parsons J: Group-based parent-training programmes for improving emotional and behavioral adjustment in 0-3 year old children (Cochrane Review), 2003. In *The Cochrane Library,* Issue 2, Chichester, UK, 2004, John Wiley & Sons.

Barnard K: *NCAST feeding manual*. Seattle, 1994, University of Washington.

Beeber L: The pinks and the blues, *Am J Nurs* 102(11):91-98, 2002.

Bitzer J, Alder J: Sexuality during pregnancy and the postpartum period, *J Sex Educ Ther* 25(1):49-58, 2000.

Bloom KC: Perceived relationship with the father of the baby and maternal attachment in adolescents, *J Obstet Gynecol Neonatal Nurs* 27(4): 420-430, 1998.

Brazelton TB: Working with families: opportunities for early intervention, *Pediatr Clin North Am* 42(1):1, 1995.

Brazelton TB, Nugent J: *Neonatal behavioural assessment scale,* ed 3, London, 1996, MacKeith.

Brewaeys A et al: Lesbian mothers who conceived after donor insemination: a follow-up study, *Hum Reprod* 10(10):2731-2735, 1995.

Cain M: *First time mothers, last chance babies: parenting at 35+,* Far Hills, NJ, 1994, New Horizon Press.

Camarena P et al: The nature and support of adolescent mothers' life aspirations, *Fam Relat* 47(2):129-137, 1998.

Conley-Jung C, Olkin R: Mothers with visual impairments who are raising young children, *J Visually Impaired Blind* 95(1):14-30, 2001.

Dalla R, Gamble E: Mother, daughter, teenager—who am I? Perceptions of adolescent maternity in a Navajo reservation community, *J Fam Issues,* 21(2):225-245, 2000.

D'Avanzo C, Geissler E: *Pocket guide to cultural assessment,* ed 3, St Louis, 2003, Mosby.

Diehl K: Adolescent mothers: what produces positive mother-infant interaction? *MCN Am J Matern Child Nurs* 22:89-95, 1997.

Evans ML et al: Postpartum sleep in the hospital: relationship to taking-in and taking-hold, *Clin Nurs Res* 7(4):379-389, 1998.

Farber RS: Mothers with disabilities: in their own voice. *Am J Occup Ther* 54(3):260-268, 2000.

Fowles ER: The Brazelton Neonatal Behavioral Assessment Scale and maternal identity, *MCN Am J Matern Child Nurs* 24(6):287-293, 1999.

Fowles E: The relationship between maternal role attainment and postpartum depression, *Health Care Women Int* 19(1):83-94, 1998.

Galanti G: *Caring for patients from different cultures,* ed 3, Philadelphia, 2003, University of Pennsylvania Press.

Garrison M et al: Delayed parenthood: an exploratory study of family functioning, *Fam Relat* 46:281-290, 1997.

Gartrell N et al: The National Lesbian Family Study: interview with prospective mothers, *Am J Orthopsychiatry* 66(2):272-281, 1996.

Goodman JH: Paternal postpartum depression, its relationship to maternal postpartum depression, and implications for family health, *J Adv Nurs* 45(1):26-35, 2004.

Greenhalgh R, Slade P, Spiby H: Fathers' coping style, antenatal preparation, and experiences of labor and the postpartum, *Birth* 27(3):177-184, 2000.

Hartrick GA: Women who are mothers: the experience of defining self, *Health Care Women Int* 18(3):263-277, 1997.

Henderson AD, Brouse AJ: The experiences of new fathers during the first three weeks of life, *J Adv Nurs* 16(3):293-298, 1991.

Inman M: The power of touch: infant massage therapy, *Childbirth Instructor Magazine* 4th quarter, 1996.

Jambunathan J, Stewart S: Hmong women in Wisconsin: what are their concerns in pregnancy and childbirth? *Birth* 22(4):204-210, 1995.

Jiménez S: The Hispanic culture, folklore, and perinatal health, *J Perinat Educ* 4(1):9, 1995.

Johnson & Johnson: *Compendium of postpartum care,* Skillman, NJ, 1996, Johnson & Johnson Consumer Products.

Klaus M, Kennell J: *Maternal-infant bonding,* St Louis, 1976, Mosby.

Klaus M, Kennell J: *Parent-infant bonding,* ed 2, St Louis, 1982, Mosby.

Klaus M, Kennell J: The doula: an essential ingredient of childbirth rediscovered, *Acta Paediatr* 86:1034-1036, 1997.

Lipson J, Dibble S, Minarik P: *Culture and nursing care: a pocket guide,* San Francisco, 1996, UCSF Nursing Press.

Liu-Chiang CY: Postpartum worries: an exploration of Taiwanese primiparas who participate in the Chinese ritual of tso-yueh-tzu, *Matern Child Nurs J* 23(4):110-122, 1995.

MacDonald-Clark NJ, Boffman JL: Mother-child interaction among the Alaskan Eskimos, *J Obstet Gynecol Neonatal Nurs* 24(5):450-457, 1995.

Martell L: Is Rubin's "taking-in" and "taking-hold" a useful paradigm? *Health Care Women Int* 17(1):1-13, 1996.

McCloskey J, Bulechek G: *Nursing interventions classification,* ed 3, St Louis, 2000, Mosby.

Merriwether-deVries C: Adjustment to the role of motherhood among adolescent African American mothers. *Diss Abs Int, A.: The Humanities and Social Sciences* 61(3):1183-A, 2000.

Miller S: Questioning, resisting, acquiescing, balancing: new mothers' career reentry strategies, *Health Care Women Int* 17(2):109-131, 1996.

Niska K, Snyder M, Lia-Hoagberg B: Family ritual facilitates adaptation to parenthood, *Public Health Nurs* 15(5):329-337, 1998.

Osterwell D: Correlates of relationship satisfaction in lesbian couples who are parenting their first child together. Doctoral dissertation, Berkeley, 1991, California School of Professional Psychology.

Poelker D, Baldwin C: Postponed motherhood and the out-of-sync life cycle, *J Mental Health Couns* 21(2):136-148, 1999.

Pridham KF: Mothers' help seeking as care initiated in a social context, *Image J Nurs Sch* 29(1):65-70, 1997.

Pugh LC et al: Clinical approaches to the assessment of maternal fatigue, *J Obstet Gynecol Neonatal Nurs* 28:74-80, 1999.

Reece SM, Harkless G: Divergent themes in maternal experience in women older than 35 years of age, *Appl Nurs Res* 9(3):148-153, 1996.

Reimann R: Does biology matter? Lesbian couples' transition to parenthood and their division of labor, *Qual Soc* 20(2):153-185, 1997a.

Reimann R: *Will the "real" mother please stand up? Lesbian couples' transition to shared motherhood.* 1997 ASA Conference proceedings: Washington, DC, 1997b, American Sociological Association.

Reimann R: *Becoming lesbian mothers: lesbian couples' transition to parenthood*, 1999 ASA Conference proceedings, Washington, DC, 1999, American Sociological Association.

Rogan F et al: 'Becoming a mother'—developing a new theory of early motherhood, *J Adv Nurs* 25:877-885, 1997.

Rubin R: Basic maternal behavior, *Nurs Outlook* 9:683-686, 1961.

Sank J: *Factors in the prenatal period that affect parental role attainment during the postpartum period in Black American mothers and fathers.* Doctoral dissertation, 1991, University of Texas, Austin.

Schneider E: The power of touch: massage for infants, *Infants Young Child* 8(3):40-55, 1996.

Schneider E: Touch communication: the power of infant massage, *Massage Magazine* 68:40, 1997.

Sharts-Hopko NC: Birth in the Japanese context, *J Obstet Gynecol Neonatal Nurs* 24(14):343-351, 1995.

Steinberg S, Kruckman L, Steinberg S: Reinventing fatherhood in Japan and Canada, *Soc Sci Med* 50:1257-1272, 2000.

Sutter AL et al: Postpartum blues and mild depressive symptomatology at days three and five after delivery: a French cross-sectional study, *J Affect Disord* 44(1):1-4, 1997.

Tomlinson P: Marital relationship change in the transition to parenthood: a reexamination as interpreted through transition theory, *J Fam Nurs* 2(3):286-305, 1996.

Troy NW, Dalgas-Pelish P: Development of a self-care guide for postpartum fatigue, *Appl Nurs Res* 8(2): 92-101, 1995.

Welles-Nystrom B: The meaning of postponed motherhood for women in the United States and Sweden: aspects of feminism and radical timing strategies, *Health Care Women Int* 18(3):279-299, 1997.

Wood AF et al: The downward spiral of postpartum depression: *MCN Am J Matern Child Nurs* 22(6):308-316, 1997.

Wrasper C: Discharge timing and Rubin's concept of puerperal change, *J Perinat Educ* 5(2):13-23, 1996.

Postpartum Complications 23

LEARNING OBJECTIVES

On completion of this chapter the reader will be able to:

- Identify causes, signs and symptoms, possible complications, and medical and nursing management of postpartum hemorrhage.
- Differentiate among the causes of postpartum hemorrhage.
- Describe thromboembolic disorders including incidence, etiology, signs and symptoms, and management.
- Summarize the role of the nurse in assessing potential problems and managing care of women with postpartum complications in the home setting.
- Discuss emotional complications of pregnancy, including management of mood disorders.
- Differentiate among postpartum emotional complications including incidence, risk factors, signs and symptoms, severity, and management.
- Describe emotional, behavioral, cognitive, and physical responses commonly experienced during the grieving process associated with perinatal loss.
- Identify specific nursing interventions to meet the special needs of parents and their families related to perinatal loss and grief.
- Differentiate among helpful and unhelpful responses in caring for parents experiencing loss and grief.

ELECTRONIC RESOURCES

Additional information related to the content in Chapter 23 can be found on

the companion website at evolve
http://evolve.elsevier.com/Wong/maternal/
- NCLEX Review Questions
- WebLinks

or the interactive student CD-ROM
Activities for Chapter 23 include the following:
- NCLEX Review Questions
- Nursing Care Plan–Postpartum Hemorrhage

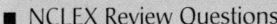

Providing safe and effective care of the woman and family experiencing postpartum physical and psychologic complications, sequelae of childbirth trauma, or grief related to perinatal loss requires a joint effort from all members of the health care team. This chapter focuses on the postpartum complications of hemorrhage and infection, sequelae of childbirth trauma, psychologic complications, and loss and grief.

POSTPARTUM HEMORRHAGE

Postpartum hemorrhage (PPH), traditionally defined as the loss of 500 ml or more of blood after vaginal birth and 1000 ml or more after cesarean birth, is a leading cause of maternal morbidity and mortality in the United States today. Either a 10% change in hematocrit between admission for labor and postpartum or the need for erythrocyte transfusion has been used to define PPH. PPH has been classified as early or late with respect to the birth. Early, acute, or primary PPH occurs within 24 hours of the birth. Late or secondary PPH occurs more than 24 hours but less than 6 weeks postpartum (American College of Obstetricians and Gynecologists [ACOG], 1998). It is a life-threatening event that can occur with little warning and is often unrecognized until the mother has profound symptoms. Shortened hospital stays increase the potential for acute episodes of PPH to occur outside the traditional hospital or birth center setting.

Etiology and Risk Factors

The most common cause of PPH is uterine atony, which complicates approximately 1 in 20 births. Other causes include retained placenta, placenta accreta, cervical or vaginal lacerations, uterine rupture or inversion, lower genital tract lacerations and hematomas, infection, and coagulopathies (Bowes & Thorp, 2004). Excessive bleeding can be considered with reference to the stages of labor. From birth of the fetus until separation of the placenta, the character and quantity of blood passed may suggest excessive bleeding. For example, dark blood is probably of venous origin, perhaps from varices or superficial lacerations of the birth canal. Bright blood is arterial and may indicate deep lacerations of the cervix. Spurts of blood with clots may indicate partial placental separation. Failure of blood to clot or remain clotted indicates coagulopathy.

Excessive bleeding may occur during the period between the separation of the placenta and its expulsion or removal. Commonly such bleeding is the result of incomplete placental separation, undue manipulation of the fundus, or excessive traction on the cord. After the placenta has been expelled, persistent or excessive blood loss most commonly is a result of atony of the uterus (i.e., failure to contract well or maintain contraction) or prolapse of the uterus into the pelvis. Late PPH most commonly is the result of subinvolution of the placental site, retained placental tissue, or endometritis (ACOG, 1998).

Uterine Atony

Uterine atony is marked hypotonia of the uterus. Normally, placental separation and expulsion are facilitated by contraction of the uterus, which also prevents hemorrhage from the placental site. The corpus is in essence a basket weave of strong, interlacing smooth muscle bundles through which many large maternal blood vessels pass (see Fig. 5-3). If the uterus is flaccid after detachment of all or part of the placenta, brisk venous bleeding occurs and normal coagulation of the open vasculature is impaired and continues until the uterine muscle is contracted.

Uterine atony is the leading cause of PPH complicating approximately 1 in 20 births (Gonik & Foley, 2004). It is associated with high parity, hydramnios, a macrosomic fetus, and multifetal gestation. In such conditions the uterus is "overstretched" and contracts poorly after birth. Other causes of atony include traumatic birth, use of halogenated anesthesia (e.g., halothane) or magnesium sulfate, rapid or prolonged labor, chorioamnionitis, and use of oxytocin for labor induction or augmentation (Gonik & Foley, 2004).

Lacerations of the Genital Tract

Lacerations of the cervix, vagina, and perineum are also causes of postpartum hemorrhage. Hemorrhage related to lacerations should be suspected if bleeding continues despite a firm, contracted uterine fundus. This bleeding can be a slow trickle, an oozing, or frank hemorrhage.

Factors that influence the causes and incidence of obstetric lacerations of the lower genital tract include operative birth, precipitous birth, congenital abnormalities of the maternal soft parts, and contracted pelvis. Size, abnormal presentation, and position of the fetus; relative size of the presenting part and the birth canal; previous scarring from infection, injury, or surgery; and vulvar, perineal, and vaginal varicosities can also cause lacerations.

Extreme vascularity in the labia and periclitoral areas often results in profuse bleeding if laceration occurs. Hematomas may also be present.

Lacerations of the perineum are the most common of all injuries in the lower portion of the genital tract. These are classified as first, second, third, and fourth degree (see Chapter 18). An episiotomy may extend to become either a third- or fourth-degree laceration.

Pelvic hematomas (i.e., a collection of blood in the connective tissue) may be vulvar, vaginal, or retroperitoneal in origin. Vulvar hematomas are the most common. Pain is the most common symptom, and most vulvar hematomas are visible. Vaginal hematomas occur more commonly in association with a forceps-assisted birth, an episiotomy, or primigravidity (Benedetti, 2002). Retroperitoneal hematomas are the least common but are life threatening. They are caused by laceration of one of the vessels attached to the hypogastric artery, usually associated with rupture of a cesarean scar during labor. During the postpartum period, if the woman reports a persistent perineal or rectal pain or a feeling of pressure in the vagina, a careful examination is made. However, a retroperitoneal hematoma may cause minimal pain, and the initial symptoms may be signs of shock (Benedetti, 2002).

Cervical lacerations usually occur at the lateral angles of the external os. Most are shallow, and bleeding is minimal. More extensive lacerations may extend into the vaginal vault or into the lower uterine segment.

Retained Placenta

Nonadherent Retained Placenta

Retained placenta may result from partial separation of a normal placenta, entrapment of the partially or completely separated placenta by an hourglass constriction ring of the uterus, mismanagement of the third stage of labor, or abnormal adherence of the entire placenta or a portion of the placenta to the uterine wall. Placental retention because of poor separation is common in very preterm births (20 to 24 weeks of gestation).

Management of nonadherent retained placenta is by manual separation and removal by the primary health care provider. Supplementary anesthesia is usually not needed for women who have had regional anesthesia for birth. For other women, administration of light nitrous oxide and oxygen inhalation anesthesia or intravenous (IV) thiopental facilitates intrauterine exploration and placental separation. After this removal, the woman is at continued risk for PPH and for infection.

Adherent Retained Placenta

Abnormal adherence of the placenta occurs for unknown reasons, but it is thought to result from zygote implantation in an area of defective endometrium so that no zone of separation exists between the placenta and the decidua. Attempts to remove the placenta in the usual manner are unsuccessful, and laceration or perforation of the uterine wall may result, putting the woman at great risk for severe PPH and infection (Cunningham et al, 2001).

Unusual placental adherence may be partial or complete. The following degrees of attachment are recognized:

- *Placenta accreta,* slight penetration of myometrium by placental trophoblast
- *Placenta increta,* deep penetration of myometrium by placenta
- *Placenta percreta,* perforation of uterus by placenta

Bleeding with complete or total placenta accreta may not occur unless separation of the placenta is attempted. With more extensive involvement, bleeding will become profuse when delivery of the placenta is attempted. Treatment includes blood component replacement therapy, and hysterectomy may be indicated (Gonik & Foley, 2004).

Inversion of the Uterus

Inversion (turning inside out) of the uterus after birth is a potentially life-threatening complication. The incidence of uterine inversion is approximately 1 in 2000 to 2500 births (ACOG, 1998) and may recur with a subsequent birth. Uterine inversion may be partial or complete. Complete inversion of the uterus is obvious; a large, red, rounded mass (perhaps with the placenta attached) protrudes 20 to 30 cm outside the introitus. Incomplete inversion cannot be seen but must be felt; a smooth mass will be palpated through the dilated cervix.

Contributing factors to uterine inversion include fundal implantation of the placenta, vigorous fundal pressure, excessive traction applied to the cord, uterine atony, leiomyomas, and abnormally adherent placental tissue (Bowes & Thorp, 2004). Uterine inversion occurs most often in multiparous women and with placenta accreta or increta. The primary presenting signs of uterine inversion are hemorrhage, shock, and pain.

Prevention—always the easiest, cheapest, and most effective therapy—is especially appropriate for uterine inversion. The umbilical cord should not be pulled on unless the placenta has definitely separated.

Subinvolution of the Uterus

Late postpartum bleeding may occur as a result of subinvolution of the uterus (delayed return of the enlarged uterus to normal size and function). Recognized causes of subinvolution include retained placental fragments and pelvic infection.

Signs and symptoms include prolonged lochial discharge; irregular or excessive bleeding; and, sometimes, hemorrhage. A pelvic examination usually reveals a larger-than-normal uterus that may be boggy.

Care Management

Assessment

PPH may be sudden and even exsanguinating. The nurse must be alert to the symptoms of hemorrhage and hypovolemic shock and be prepared to act quickly to minimize blood loss (Box 23-1). The woman's history should be reviewed for factors that predispose the woman to PPH. The fundus is assessed to determine whether it is firmly contracted at or near the level of the umbilicus. Bleeding should be assessed for color and amount. The perineum is inspected for signs of lacerations or hematomas to determine the possible source of bleeding. See the Guidelines/Guías box for assessment questions with translation for a Spanish-speaking person.

Vital signs may not be reliable indicators of shock immediately postpartum because of the physiologic adaptations of this period. However, frequent vital sign measurements in the first 2 hours after birth may identify trends that are related to blood loss (e.g., tachycardia, tachypnea, decreasing blood pressure).

Assessment for bladder distention is important because a distended bladder can displace the uterus and prevent uterine contraction. The skin is assessed for warmth and dryness; nail beds are checked for color and promptness of capillary refill. Laboratory studies include evaluation of hemoglobin and hematocrit levels.

Late PPH develops at least 24 hours after birth or later in the postpartum period. The woman may be at home when the symptoms occur. Discharge teaching should emphasize the signs of normal involution, as well as potential complications.

BOX 23-1

Noninvasive Assessments of Cardiac Output in Postpartum Patients Who Are Bleeding

Palpation of pulses (rate, quality, equality)
- Arterial
- Blood pressure

Auscultation
- Heart sounds/murmurs
- Breath sounds

Inspection
- Skin color, temperature, turgor
- Level of consciousness
- Capillary refill
- Urinary output
- Neck veins
- Pulse oximetry
- Mucous membranes

Presence or absence of anxiety, apprehension, restlessness, disorientation

Nursing Diagnoses

Nursing diagnoses for women experiencing PPH include the following:

- *Deficient fluid volume related to*
  —excessive blood loss secondary to uterine atony, lacerations, or uterine inversion
- *Risk for injury (maternal) related to*
  —attempted manual removal of retained placenta
  —administration of blood products
  —operative procedures

ENGLISH SPANISH Guidelines/Guías

ASSESSING FOR HEMORRHAGE

I am going to palpate (feel) the fundus (top) of your uterus.
Le voy a palpar el fundus (la parte superior) del útero.

Your uterus is not firm; I am going to massage the fundus.
Su útero no está duro. Le voy a masajear el fundus.

Please tell a nurse each time you change your pad; we are monitoring the amount of bleeding.
Por favor, dígale a la enfermera cada vez que cambie su toalla femenina. Queremos observar la cantidad de hemorragia.

Try to urinate every 2 hours. If your bladder is full, it pushes the uterus up and makes it relax and you will have more bleeding.
Trate de orinar cada dos horas. Cuando está llena la vejiga, está empuja el útero para arriba y hace que se afloje, lo cual produce más hemorragia.

- *Risk for impaired parenting related to*
  —separation from infant secondary to treatment regimen
- *Ineffective peripheral tissue perfusion related to*
  —excessive blood loss and shunting of blood to central circulation

Expected Outcomes

Expected outcomes for the woman experiencing PPH include that she will do the following:

- Maintain normal vital signs and laboratory values
- Develop no complications related to excessive bleeding
- Verbalize understanding of her condition, its management, and discharge instructions
- Identify and use available support systems

Plan of Care and Implementation

Medical Management

Early recognition and diagnosis of PPH is critical to care management. The first step is to evaluate the contractility of the uterus. If the uterus is hypotonic, management is directed toward increasing contractility and minimizing blood loss.

The initial management of excessive postpartum bleeding is firm massage of the uterine fundus, expression of any clots in the uterus, eliminating bladder distention, and continuous IV infusion of 10 to 40 units of oxytocin in 1000 ml Ringer's lactate or normal saline solution. If the uterus fails to respond to oxytocin, a dose of 0.2 mg ergonovine (Ergotrate) or methylergonovine (Methergine) may be given intramuscularly (IM) to produce sustained uterine contractions. However, it is more common to administer a 0.25-mg dose of a derivative of prostaglandin $F_{2\alpha}$ (carboprost tromethamine) intramuscularly. It also can be given intramyometrially at cesarean birth or intraabdominally after vaginal birth. See Table 23-1 for a comparison of medications used to manage PPH. In addition to the medications used to contract the uterus, rapid administration of crystalloid solutions and/or blood or blood products will be needed to restore the woman's intravascular volume (Mousa & Walkinshaw, 2001).

NURSE ALERT Use of ergonovine or methylergonovine is contraindicated in the presence of hypertension or cardiovascular disease. Prostaglandin $F_{2\alpha}$ should be used cautiously in women with cardiovascular disease or asthma (Bowes & Thorp, 2004). ■

Hypotonic Uterus

Oxygen can be given to enhance oxygen delivery to the cells. A urinary catheter is usually inserted to monitor urine output as a measure of intravascular volume. Laboratory studies usually include a complete blood count with platelet count, fibrinogen, fibrin split products, prothrombin time, and partial thromboplastin time. Blood type and antibody screen are done if not previously performed.

If bleeding persists, the obstetrician or nurse-midwife may consider bimanual compression. This procedure involves inserting a fist into the vagina and pressing the knuckles against the anterior side of the uterus while placing the other hand on the abdomen and massaging the posterior uterus. If the uterus still does not become firm, manual exploration of the uterine cavity for retained placental fragments is done. If the preceding procedures are ineffective, surgical management may be the only alternative. Surgical management options include vessel ligation (i.e., uteroovar-

Table 23-1

Medications Used to Manage Postpartum Hemorrhage (PPH)

	OXYTOCIN (PITOCIN)	METHYLERGONOVINE (METHERGINE)	PROSTAGLANDIN $F_{2\alpha}$ (PROSTIN/15M; HEMABATE)
ACTION	Contraction of uterus; decreases bleeding	Contraction of uterus	Contraction of uterus
SIDE EFFECT	Infrequent; water intoxication; nausea and vomiting	Hypertension, nausea, vomiting, headache	Headache, nausea, vomiting, fever
CONTRAINDICATIONS	None for PPH	Hypertension, cardiac disease	Asthma, hypersensitivity
DOSAGE; ROUTE	10-40 units/L diluted in lactated Ringer's solution or normal saline at 125-200 milliunits/min IV or 10-20 units IM	0.2 mg IM q2-4hr up to 5 doses; 0.2 mg IV only for emergency	0.25 mg IM or intramyometrially q15-90 min up to 8 doses
NURSING CONSIDERATIONS	Continue to monitor vaginal bleeding and uterine tone	Check blood pressure before giving and do not give if >140/90; continue monitoring vaginal bleeding and uterine tone	Continue to monitor vaginal bleeding and uterine tone

ian, uterine, and hypogastric), angiographic embolization, and hysterectomy (Gonik & Foley, 2004).

Bleeding with a Contracted Uterus

If the uterus is firmly contracted and bleeding continues, the source of bleeding still needs to be identified and treated. Assessment may include visual or manual inspection of the perineum, vagina, cervix, or rectum; and laboratory studies (e.g., hemoglobin, hematocrit, coagulation studies, and platelet count). Treatment depends on the source of the bleeding. Lacerations are usually sutured. Hematomas may be managed with observation, application of cold therapy, ligation of the bleeding vessel, or evacuation. Fluids and or blood replacement may be needed (Benedetti, 2002; Bowes & Thorp, 2004; Gonik & Foley, 2004).

Uterine Inversion

Uterine inversion is an emergency situation requiring immediate recognition, replacement of the uterus within the pelvic cavity, and correction of associated clinical conditions. Tocolytics or halogenated anesthetics may be given to relax the uterus before attempting replacement (Hostetler & Bosworth, 2000). Medical management of this condition includes treating shock, repositioning the uterus, giving oxytocic agents after the uterus is repositioned, and initiating broad-spectrum antibiotics (Benedetti, 2002; Bowes & Thorp, 2004).

Subinvolution

Treatment of subinvolution depends on the cause. Ergonovine 0.2 mg every 4 hours for 2 or 3 days and antibiotic therapy are the most common medications used (Cunningham et al, 2001). Dilation and curettage (D&C) may be needed to remove retained placental fragments or to debride the placental site.

Herbal Remedies

Herbal remedies to control PPH have been used with some success in some settings. Some herbs have homeostatic actions, while others work as oxytocic agents to contract the uterus (Beal, 1998; Schirmer, 1998). Box 23-2 lists herbs that have been used and their actions. However, published evidence of the safety and efficacy of herbal therapy is lacking. Evidence from well-controlled studies is needed before recommendation for practice should be made (Brucker, 2001).

BOX 23-2

Herbal Remedies for Postpartum Hemorrhage

HERBS	ACTION
Witch hazel	Homeostatic
Lady's mantle	Homeostatic
Blue cohosh	Oxytocic
Cotton root bark	Oxytocic
Motherwort	Promotes uterine contraction; vasoconstrictive
Shepherd's purse	Promotes uterine contraction
Alfalfa leaf	Increases availability of vitamin K; increases hemoglobin
Nettle	Increases availability of vitamin K; increases hemoglobin
Red raspberry leaves	Homeostatic, promotes uterine contraction

Source: Schirmer G: *Herbal medicine,* Bedford, TX, 1998, MED2000 Inc; Weed S: *Wise woman herbal for the childbearing years,* Woodstock, NY, 1986, Ash Tree Publishing Co.

Nursing Interventions

Immediate nursing care of the woman with PPH includes assessment of vital signs and uterine consistency and administration of oxytocin or other drugs to stimulate uterine contraction according to standing orders or protocols. The primary health care provider, if not present, is notified.

The woman and her family will be anxious about her condition. The nurse can intervene by calmly providing explanations about interventions being performed and the need to act quickly.

After the bleeding has been controlled, the care of the woman with lacerations of the perineum is similar to that for women with episiotomies (i.e., analgesia as needed for pain and hot or cold applications as necessary). The need for increased roughage in the diet and increased intake of fluids is emphasized. Stool softeners may be used to assist the woman in reestablishing bowel habits without straining and putting stress on the suture lines.

NURSE ALERT To avoid injury to the suture line, a woman with third- or fourth-degree lacerations is not given rectal suppositories or enemas. ■

The care of the woman who has experienced an inversion of the uterus focuses on immediate stabilization of hemodynamic status. This requires close observation of her response to treatment to prevent shock or fluid overload. If the uterus has been repositioned manually, care must be taken to avoid aggressive fundal massage.

Discharge instructions for the woman who has had PPH are similar to those for any postpartum woman. In addition, she should be told that she will probably feel fatigue or even exhaustion and will need to limit her physical activities to conserve her strength. She may need instructions in increasing her dietary iron and protein intake and iron supplementation to rebuild lost red cell volume. She may need assistance with infant care and household activities until she has regained strength. Some women have problems with delayed or insufficient lactation and postpartum depression. Referrals for home care follow-up or to community resources may be needed (see Resources at the end of this chapter).

Evaluation

The nurse can be reasonably assured that care was effective to the extent that the expected outcomes have been achieved (see Nursing Care Plan).

Hemorrhagic (Hypovolemic) Shock

Hemorrhage may result in hemorrhagic (hypovolemic) shock. Shock is an emergency situation in which the perfusion of body organs may become severely compromised; death may occur. Physiologic compensatory mechanisms are activated in response to hemorrhage. The adrenal glands release catecholamines, causing arterioles and venules in the skin, lungs, gastrointestinal tract, liver, and kidneys to con-

Nursing Care Plan

POSTPARTUM HEMORRHAGE

NURSING DIAGNOSIS: Deficient fluid volume related to postpartum hemorrhage

EXPECTED OUTCOME

Woman will demonstrate fluid balance as evidenced by stable vital signs, prompt capillary refill time, and balanced intake and output.

NURSING INTERVENTIONS/*RATIONALES*

Monitor vital signs, oxygen saturation, urine specific gravity, and capillary refill *to provide baseline data.*

Measure and record amount and type of bleeding by weighing and counting saturated pads. If woman is at home, teach her to count pads and save any clots or tissue. If woman is admitted to hospital, save any clots and tissue for further examination *to estimate type and amount of blood loss for fluid replacement.*

Provide quiet environment *to promote rest and decrease metabolic demands.*

Give explanation of all procedures *to reduce anxiety.*

Begin IV access with 18-gauge or larger needle for infusion of isotonic solution as ordered *to provide fluid or blood replacement.*

Administer medications as ordered, such as oxytocin, methergine, or prostin *to increase contractility of the uterus.*

Insert indwelling urinary catheter *to provide most accurate assessment of renal function and hypovolemia.*

Prepare for surgical intervention as needed *to stop the source of bleeding.*

NURSING DIAGNOSIS: Ineffective tissue perfusion related to hypovolemia

EXPECTED OUTCOME

Woman will have stable vital signs, oxygen saturation, arterial blood gases, and adequate hematocrit and hemoglobin.

NURSING INTERVENTIONS/*RATIONALES*

Monitor vital signs, oxygen saturation, arterial blood gases, and hematocrit and hemoglobin *to assess for hypovolemic shock and decreased tissue perfusion.*

Assess for any changes in level of consciousness *to assess for evidence of hypoxia.*

Assess capillary refill, mucous membranes, and skin temperature *to note indicators of vasoconstriction.*

Give supplementary oxygen as ordered *to provide additional oxygenation to tissues.*

Suction as needed, insert oral airway, *to maintain clear, open airway for oxygenation.*

Monitor arterial blood gases *to provide information about acidosis or hypoxia.*

Administer sodium bicarbonate if ordered *to reverse metabolic acidosis.*

NURSING DIAGNOSIS: Anxiety related to sudden change in health status

EXPECTED OUTCOME

Woman will verbalize the anxious feelings are diminished.

NURSING INTERVENTIONS/*RATIONALES*

Using therapeutic communication, evaluate woman's understanding of events *to provide clarification of any misconceptions.*

Provide calm, competent attitude and environment *to aid in decreasing anxiety.*

Explain all procedures *to decrease anxiety about the unknown.*

Allow woman to verbalize feelings *to permit clarification of information and promote trust.*

Continue to assess vital signs or other clinical indicators of hypovolemic shock *to evaluate if psychologic response of anxiety intensifies physiologic indicators.*

strict. The available blood flow is diverted to the brain and heart and away from other organs, including the uterus. If shock is prolonged, the continued reduction in cellular oxygenation results in an accumulation of lactic acid and acidosis (from anaerobic glucose metabolism). Acidosis (lowered serum pH) causes arteriolar vasodilation; venule vasoconstriction persists. A circular pattern is established; that is, decreased perfusion, increased tissue anoxia and acidosis, edema formation, and pooling of blood further decrease the perfusion. Cellular death occurs. See the Emergency box for assessments and interventions for hemorrhagic shock.

Medical Management

Vigorous treatment is necessary to prevent adverse sequelae. Medical management of hypovolemic shock involves restoring circulating blood volume and eliminating the cause of the hemorrhage (e.g., lacerations, uterine atony, or inversion). To restore circulating blood volume, a rapid IV infusion of crystalloid solution is given at a rate of 3 ml infused for every 1 ml of estimated blood loss (e.g., 3000 ml infused for 1000 ml of blood loss). Packed red blood cells (RBCs) are usually infused if the woman is still actively bleeding and no improvement in her condition is noted after the initial crystalloid infusion. Infusion of fresh frozen plasma may be needed if clotting factors and platelet counts are below normal values (Cunningham et al, 2001).

Nursing Interventions

Hemorrhagic shock can occur rapidly, but the classic signs of shock may not appear until the postpartum woman has lost 30% to 40% of blood volume. The nurse must continue to reassess the woman's condition, as evidenced by the degree of measurable and anticipated blood loss, and mobilize appropriate resources.

Most interventions are instituted to improve or monitor tissue perfusion. The nurse continues to monitor the woman's pulse and blood pressure. If invasive hemodynamic monitoring is ordered, the nurse may assist with placement of a central venous pressure (CVP) or pulmonary artery (Swan-Ganz) catheter. The nurse would then monitor CVP, pulmonary artery pressure, or pulmonary artery wedge pressure as ordered.

Additional assessments to be made include evaluation of skin temperature, color, and turgor, as well as assessment of the woman's mucous membranes. Breath sounds should be auscultated before fluid volume replacement, if possible, to

Emergency

HEMORRHAGIC SHOCK

Assessments	**Characteristics**
Respirations	Rapid and shallow
Pulse	Rapid, weak, irregular
Blood pressure	Decreasing (late sign)
Skin	Cool, pale, clammy
Urinary output	Decreasing
Level of consciousness	Lethargy → coma
Mental status	Anxiety → coma
Central venous pressure	Decreased

Intervention

Summon assistance and equipment
Start IV infusion per standing orders
Ensure patent airway; administer oxygen
Continue to monitor status

provide a baseline for future assessment. Inspection for oozing at the sites of incisions or injections and assessment of the presence of petechiae or ecchymosis in areas not associated with surgery or trauma are critical in the evaluation for disseminated intravascular coagulopathy (DIC).

Oxygen is administered, preferably by a nonrebreathing face mask, at 10 to 12 L/min to maintain oxygen saturation. Oxygen saturation should be monitored with a pulse oximeter, although measurements may not always be accurate in a patient with hypovolemia or decreased perfusion. Level of consciousness is assessed frequently and provides additional indications of blood volume and oxygen saturation. In early stages of decreased blood flow, the woman may report "seeing stars" or feeling dizzy or nauseated. She may become restless and orthopneic. As cerebral hypoxia increases, she may become confused and react slowly to stimuli or not at all. Some women complain of headaches. An improved sensorium is an indicator of improved perfusion.

Continuous electrocardiographic monitoring may be indicated for the woman who is hypotensive or tachycardic, who continues to bleed profusely, or who is in shock. A Foley catheter with a urometer is inserted to allow hourly assessment of urine output. The most objective and least invasive assessment of adequate organ perfusion and oxygenation is a urine output of at least 30 ml/hr (Benedetti, 2002). Blood may be drawn and sent to the laboratory for studies that include hemoglobin and hematocrit levels, platelet count, and coagulation profile.

Fluid or Blood Replacement Therapy

Critical to successful management of the woman with a hemorrhagic complication is establishment of venous access, preferably with a large-bore IV catheter. The establishment of two IV lines facilitates fluid resuscitation. Vigorous fluid resuscitation includes the administration of crystalloids (lactated Ringer's, normal saline solution), colloids (albumin), blood, and blood components. Fluid resuscitation must be carefully monitored because fluid overload can occur. Intravascular fluid overload occurs most often with colloid therapy.

Transfusion reactions may follow administration of blood or blood components including cryoprecipitates. Even in an emergency, each unit of fluid should be checked per hospital protocol. Complications of fluid or blood replacement therapy include hemolytic reactions, febrile reactions, allergic reactions, circulatory overloading, and air embolism.

LEGAL TIP **Standard of Care for Bleeding Emergencies** The standard of care for obstetric emergency situations such as PPH or hypovolemic shock is that provision should be made for the nurse to implement nursing actions independently. Policies, procedures, standing orders or protocols, and clinical guidelines should be established by each health care facility in which births occur and should be agreed upon by health care providers involved in the care of obstetric patients. ■

COAGULOPATHIES

When bleeding is continuous and there is no identifiable source, a coagulopathy may be the cause. The woman's coagulation status must be assessed quickly and continuously. The nurse may draw and send blood to the laboratory for studies. Abnormal results depend on the cause and may include increased prothrombin time, increased partial thromboplastin time, decreased platelets, decreased fibrinogen level, increased fibrin degradation products, and prolonged bleeding time. Causes of coagulopathies may be pregnancy complications such as idiopathic thrombocytopenic purpura, von Willebrand disease, or DIC.

Idiopathic Thrombocytopenic Purpura

Idiopathic or immune thrombocytopenic purpura (ITP) is an autoimmune disorder in which antiplatelet antibodies decrease the life span of the platelets. Thrombocytopenia, capillary fragility, and increased bleeding time are diagnostic findings. ITP may cause severe hemorrhage after cesarean birth or from cervical or vaginal lacerations. The incidence of postpartum uterine bleeding and vaginal hematomas is also increased. Neonatal thrombocytopenia, a result of the maternal disease process, occurs in about 50% of cases and is associated with high mortality (Kilpatrick & Laros, 2004).

Medical management focuses on control of platelet stability. If ITP was diagnosed during pregnancy, the woman likely was treated with corticosteroids or intravenous immunoglobulin. Platelet transfusions are usually given when there is significant bleeding. A splenectomy may be needed if the ITP does not respond to medical management.

von Willebrand Disease

von Willebrand disease, a type of hemophilia, is probably the most common of all hereditary bleeding disorders (Strozewski, 2000). Although von Willebrand disease is rare, it is among the most common congenital clotting defects in North American women of childbearing age. It results from a factor VIII deficiency and platelet dysfunction that is transmitted as an incomplete autosomal dominant trait to both sexes. Symptoms include a familial bleeding tendency, previous bleeding episodes, prolonged bleeding time (the most important test), factor VIII deficiency (mild to moderate), and bleeding from mucous membranes. Although factor

VIII increases during pregnancy, there is still a risk for PPH as levels of von Willebrand factor begin to decrease (Kilpatrick & Laros, 2004; Roque, Funai, & Lockwood, 2000).

The woman may be at risk for bleeding for up to 4 weeks postpartum. Treatment of von Willebrand disease may include replacement of factor VIII, and administration of desmopressin or antifibrinolytics (Strozewski, 2000).

NURSE ALERT Cryoprecipitate is no longer recommended by the Medical and Scientific Advisory Council of the National Hemophilia Association as a treatment for von Willebrand disease because it may contain donor viruses (Strozewski, 2000). ■

Disseminated Intravascular Coagulation

Disseminated intravascular coagulation (DIC) is a pathologic form of clotting that is diffuse and consumes large amounts of clotting factors, including platelets, fibrinogen, prothrombin, and factors V and VII. Widespread external bleeding, internal bleeding, or both can result. DIC also causes vascular occlusion of small vessels resulting from small clots forming in the microcirculation. In the obstetric population, DIC may occur as a result of abruptio placentae, amniotic fluid embolism, dead fetus syndrome (i.e., fetus dies but is retained in utero for at least 6 weeks), severe preeclampsia, septicemia, cardiopulmonary arrest, and hemorrhage.

Primary medical management in all cases of DIC involves correction of the underlying cause (e.g., removal of the dead fetus, treatment of existing infection or of preeclampsia or eclampsia, or removal of a placental abruption).

The diagnosis of DIC is made according to clinical findings and laboratory markers. Physical examination reveals unusual bleeding; spontaneous bleeding from the woman's gums or nose may be noted. Petechiae may appear around a blood pressure cuff placed on the woman's arm. Excessive bleeding may occur from the site of a slight trauma (e.g., venipuncture sites, intramuscular or subcutaneous injection sites, nicks from shaving of perineum or abdomen, and injury from insertion of a urinary catheter). Symptoms also may include tachycardia and diaphoresis. Laboratory tests reveal decreased levels of platelets, fibrinogen, proaccelerin, antihemophiliac factor, and prothrombin (the factors consumed during coagulation). Fibrinolysis is increased at first but is later severely depressed. Degradation of fibrin leads to the accumulation of fibrin split products in the blood; these have anticoagulant properties and prolong the prothrombin time. Bleeding time is normal, coagulation time shows no clot, clot-retraction time shows no clot, and partial thromboplastin time is increased. DIC must be distinguished from other clotting disorders before therapy is initiated.

Primary medical management in all cases of DIC involves correction of the underlying cause (e.g., removal of the dead fetus, treatment of existing infection or of preeclampsia or eclampsia, or removal of a placental abruption). Volume replacement, blood component therapy, optimization of oxygenation and perfusion status, and continued reassessment of laboratory parameters are the usual forms of treatment. Plasma levels usually return to normal within 24 hours after birth. Platelet counts usually return to normal within 7 days (Kilpatrick & Laros, 2004).

Nursing interventions include assessment for signs of bleeding and for signs of complications from the administration of blood and blood products, administering fluid or blood replacement as ordered, and protecting from injury. Because renal failure is one consequence of DIC, urinary output is monitored, usually by insertion of an indwelling urinary catheter. Urinary output must be maintained at more than 30 ml/hr.

The woman and her family will be anxious or concerned about her condition and prognosis. The nurse offers explanations about care and provides emotional support to the woman and her family through this critical time.

THROMBOEMBOLIC DISEASE

A thrombosis results from the formation of a blood clot or clots inside a blood vessel and is caused by inflammation (thrombophlebitis) or partial obstruction of the vessel. Three thromboembolic conditions are of concern in the postpartum period:

- Superficial venous thrombosis—Involvement of the superficial saphenous venous system
- Deep venous thrombosis—Involvement varies but can extend from the foot to the iliofemoral region
- Pulmonary embolism—Complication of deep venous thrombosis occurring when part of a blood clot dislodges and is carried to the pulmonary artery where it occludes the vessel and obstructs blood flow to the lungs

Incidence and Etiology

The incidence of thromboembolic disease in the postpartum period varies from about 1 in 1000 to 1 in 2000 women (Cunningham et al, 2001; Lockwood & Silver, 2004). The incidence has declined in the last 30 years because early ambulation after childbirth has become the standard practice. The major causes of thromboembolic disease are venous stasis and hypercoagulation, both of which are present in pregnancy and continue into the postpartum period. Other risk factors include cesarean birth, history of venous thrombosis or varicosities, obesity, maternal age over 35, multiparity, and smoking (Lockwood & Silver, 2004; Weiss & Bernstein, 2000).

Clinical Manifestations

Superficial venous thrombosis is the most common form of postpartum thrombophlebitis. It is characterized by pain and tenderness in the lower extremity. Physical examination may reveal warmth; redness; and an enlarged, hardened vein over the site of the thrombosis. Deep vein thrombosis is more common in pregnancy and is characterized by unilateral leg pain, calf tenderness, and swelling (Fig. 23-1). Physical examination may reveal redness and warmth, but women may also have a large clot with few symptoms (Stenchever et al, 2001). A positive Homans' sign may be present, but further evaluation is needed because the calf pain may be attributed to other causes such as a strained muscle resulting from the birthing position. Pulmonary embolism is characterized by dyspnea and tachypnea. Other

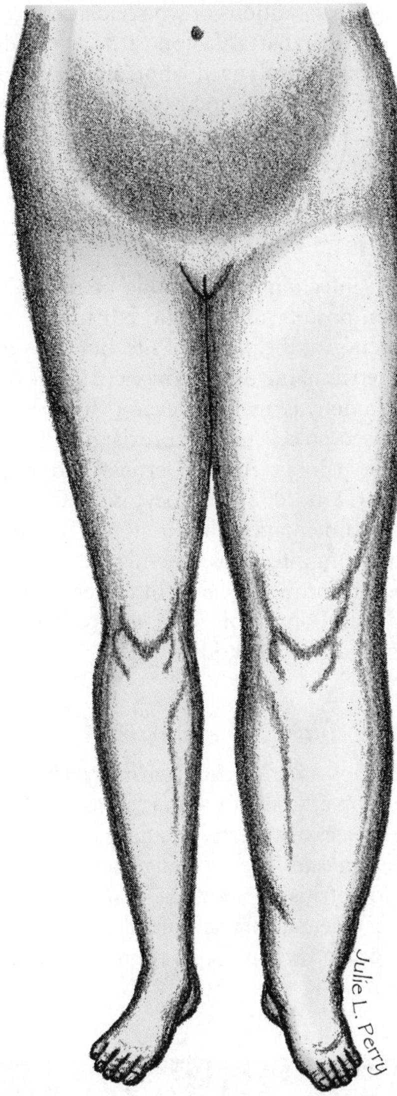

Fig. 23-1 Deep vein thrombophlebitis.

signs and symptoms commonly seen include apprehension, cough, tachycardia, hemoptysis, elevated temperature, and pleuritic chest pain.

Physical examination is not a sensitive diagnostic indicator for thrombosis. Venography is the most accurate method for diagnosing deep venous thrombosis; however, it is an invasive procedure that exposes the woman and fetus to ionizing radiation and is associated with serious complications. Noninvasive diagnostic methods such as real time and color Doppler ultrasound are more commonly used (Cunningham et al, 2001; Laros, 2004). With pulmonary embolism, murmurs may be heard on cardiac auscultation. Electrocardiograms are usually normal. Arterial Po_2 may be lower than normal. A ventilation/perfusion scan, Doppler ultrasound, and pulmonary arteriogram may be used for diagnosis (Laros, 2004).

Medical Management

Superficial venous thrombosis is treated with analgesia (nonsteroidal antiinflammatory agents), rest with elevation of the affected leg, and elastic stockings (Laros, 2004). Local application of heat may also be used. Deep venous thrombosis is initially treated with anticoagulant therapy (usually continuous intravenous heparin), bed rest with the affected leg elevated, and analgesia. After the symptoms have decreased, the woman may be fitted with elastic stockings to use when she is allowed to ambulate. Intravenous heparin therapy continues for 5 to 7 days. Oral anticoagulant therapy (warfarin) is started during this time and will be continued for about 3 months. For pulmonary embolism, continuous intravenous heparin therapy is used until symptoms have resolved. Intermittent subcutaneous heparin or oral anticoagulant therapy is usually continued for 6 months (Laros, 2004).

In the hospital, nursing care of the woman with a thrombosis consists of the following assessments: inspection and palpation of the affected area; palpation of peripheral pulses; checking Homans' sign; measurement and comparison of leg circumferences; inspection for signs of bleeding; monitoring for signs of pulmonary embolism including chest pain, coughing, dyspnea, and tachypnea; and checking respiratory status for presence of crackles. Laboratory reports are monitored for prothrombin or partial thromboplastin times. The woman and her family are assessed for their level of understanding about the diagnosis and their ability to cope during the unexpected extended period of recovery.

Interventions include explanations and education about the diagnosis and the treatment. The woman will need assistance with personal care as long as she is on bed rest. The family should be encouraged to participate in the care if she and they wish. While the woman is on bed rest, she should be encouraged to change positions frequently, but not to place the knees in a sharply flexed position that could cause pooling of blood in the lower extremities. She should also be cautioned not to rub the affected areas because rubbing could cause the clot to dislodge. Once the woman is allowed to ambulate, she is taught how to prevent venous congestion by putting on the elastic stockings before getting out of bed.

Heparin and warfarin are administered as ordered. The physician is notified if clotting times are outside the therapeutic level. If the woman is breastfeeding, she is assured that neither heparin nor warfarin is excreted in significant quantities in breast milk. If the infant has been discharged, the family is encouraged to bring the infant for feedings as permitted by hospital policy; the mother can also express milk to be sent home.

Pain can be managed with a variety of measures. Changing positions, elevating the leg, and applying moist warm heat may decrease discomfort. Administration of analgesics and antiinflammatory medications may be needed.

NURSE ALERT Medications containing aspirin are not given to women on anticoagulant therapy because aspirin inhibits synthesis of clotting factors and can lead to prolonged clotting time and increased risk of bleeding. ■

The woman is usually discharged home on oral anticoagulants and will need an explanation of the treatment schedule and possible side effects. If subcutaneous injections are to be given, the woman and family are taught how to administer the medication and about site rotation. The woman and her family should also be given information about safe care practices to prevent bleeding and injury while she is on anticoagulant therapy, such as using a soft toothbrush and using an electric razor. She will also need information about the need for follow-up with her health care provider to monitor clotting times and to make sure the correct dose of anticoagulant therapy is maintained. The woman should also use a reliable form of contraception if taking warfarin because this medication is considered teratogenic (Laros, 2004).

POSTPARTUM INFECTIONS

Postpartum infection (also known as puerperal sepsis or childbed fever) is any clinical infection of the genital canal that occurs within 28 days after miscarriage, induced abortion, or childbirth. The definition in the United States continues to be the presence of a fever of 38° C or more on 2 successive days of the first 10 postpartum days (not counting the first 24 hours after birth) (Gibbs, Sweet, & Duff, 2004). Puerperal infection is one of the major causes of morbidity and mortality throughout the world; however, in the United States, the incidence is 3% after vaginal births and 5 to 10 times higher after cesarean births (Gibbs et al, 2004). Common postpartum infections include endometritis, wound infections, mastitis, urinary tract infections, and respiratory tract infections. See the Guidelines/Guías box for questions to ask with translations for a Spanish-speaking person.

The most common infecting organisms are the numerous streptococcal and anaerobic organisms. Although less common, *Staphylococcus aureus*, gonococci, coliform bacteria, and clostridia are also serious pathogenic organisms that can cause postpartum infection. Postpartum infections are more common in women who have concurrent medical or immunosuppressive conditions or who had a cesarean or other operative birth. Intrapartal factors such as prolonged rupture of membranes, prolonged labor, and internal maternal or fetal monitoring also increase the risk of infection (Varner, 1998). Factors that predispose the woman to postpartum infection are listed in Box 23-3.

Endometritis

Endometritis (infection of the lining of the uterus) is the most common postpartum infection. It usually begins as a localized infection at the placental site, but can spread to the entire endometrium. Incidence is higher after cesarean birth. Signs of endometritis include fever (usually greater than 38° C); increased pulse; chills; anorexia; nausea; fatigue and lethargy; pelvic pain; uterine tenderness; and foul-smelling, profuse lochia (Duff, 2002). Leukocytosis and a markedly increased RBC sedimentation rate are typical laboratory findings of postpartum infections. Anemia may also be present. Blood cultures or intracervical or intrauterine bacterial cultures (aerobic and anaerobic) should reveal the offending pathogens within 36 to 48 hours.

Wound Infections

Wound infections are also common postpartum infections but often develop after the woman is at home. Sites of infection include the cesarean incision and the episiotomy or repaired laceration site. Predisposing factors are similar to those for endometritis (see Box 23-3). Signs of wound infection include erythema, edema, warmth, tenderness, seropurulent drainage, and wound separation. Fever and pain may also be present.

ENGLISH SPANISH **Guidelines/Guías**

ASSESSING FOR INFECTION

Your temperature is elevated. I am going to palpate your uterus to check for tenderness.
Su temperatura está alta. Le voy a palpar el útero para saber si le molesta.

Has your bleeding increased or changed in color?
¿Ha aumentado de cantidad la hemorragia o ha cambiado de color?

Does your bleeding have an odor?
¿Tiene la hemorragia algún olor?

Please drink more fluids; drink at least 1 glass of water each hour.
Por favor, tome más líquidos; tome cada hora por lo menos un vaso de agua.

Do you have any discomfort when you urinate?
¿Tiene alguna molestia al orinar?

Does the back of your leg hurt when I flex your foot?
¿Le duele la parte de atrás de la pierna cuando yo le doblo el pie?

Are either of your nipples or breasts red or tender?
¿Está rojo o le duele uno de sus pezones o senos?

BOX 23-3

Predisposing Factors for Postpartum Infection

Preconception or Antepartal Factors

History of previous venous thrombosis, urinary tract infection, mastitis, pneumonia
Diabetes mellitus
Alcoholism
Drug abuse
Immunosuppression
Anemia
Malnutrition

Intrapartal Factors

Cesarean birth
Prolonged rupture of membranes
Chorioamnionitis
Prolonged labor
Bladder catheterization
Internal fetal/uterine pressure monitoring
Multiple vaginal examinations after rupture of membranes
Epidural anesthesia
Retained placental fragments
Postpartum hemorrhage
Episiotomy or lacerations
Hematomas

Urinary Tract Infections

Urinary tract infections (UTIs) occur in 2% to 4% of postpartum women. Risk factors include urinary catheterization, frequent pelvic examinations, epidural anesthesia, genital tract injury, history of UTI, and cesarean birth. Signs and symptoms include dysuria, frequency and urgency, low grade fever, urinary retention, hematuria, and pyuria. Costovertebral angle (CVA) tenderness or flank pain may indicate upper UTI. Urinalysis results may reveal *Escherichia coli,* although other gram-negative aerobic bacilli also may cause UTIs.

Mastitis

Mastitis, or breast infection, affects about 1% of women soon after childbirth, most of whom are first-time mothers who are breastfeeding. Mastitis is almost always unilateral and develops well after the flow of milk has been established (Fig. 23-2). The infecting organism generally is the hemolytic *Staphylococcus aureus.* An infected nipple fissure usually is the initial lesion, followed by ductal system involvement. Inflammatory edema and engorgement of the breast soon obstruct the flow of milk in a lobe; regional, then generalized, mastitis follows. If treatment is not prompt, mastitis may progress to a breast abscess.

Symptoms rarely appear before the end of the first postpartum week and are more common in the second to fourth weeks. Chills, fever, malaise, and local breast tenderness are noted first. Localized breast tenderness, pain, swelling, redness, and axillary adenopathy may also occur. Antibiotics are prescribed. Lactation can be maintained by emptying the breasts every 2 to 4 hours by breastfeeding, manual expression, or a breast pump.

Care Management

Prenatal and intrapartal factors that predispose a woman to postpartum infection are listed in Box 23-3. Women with these factors should be assessed carefully. Signs and symptoms associated with postpartum infection were discussed

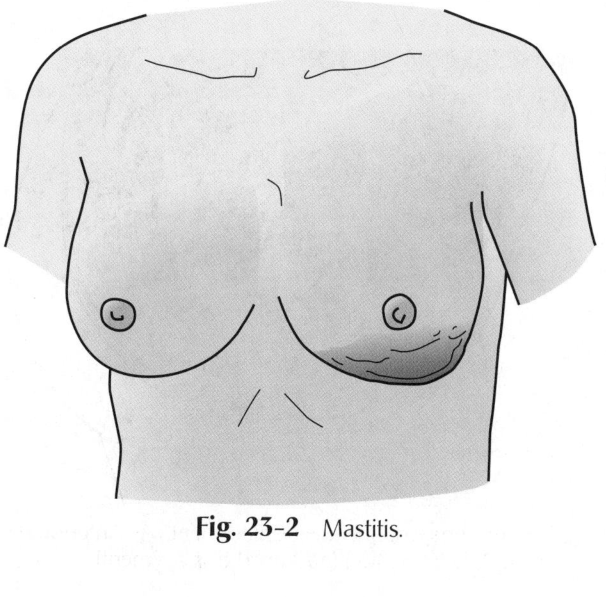

Fig. 23-2 Mastitis.

with each infection. Elevation of temperature, redness and swelling are common signs. The woman may also complain of chills, fever, localized tenderness or pain. Laboratory tests usually performed include a complete blood count, venous blood cultures, and uterine tissue cultures. Review of the history of the woman and the laboratory results should be included in the assessment.

Nursing diagnoses for women experiencing postpartum infection include the following:

- *Deficient knowledge related to*
  —etiology, management, course of infection
  —transmission and prevention of infection
- *Impaired tissue integrity related to*
  —effects of infection process
- *Acute pain related to*
  —mastitis
  —puerperal infection
  —urinary tract infection
- *Interrupted family processes related to*
  —unexpected complication to expected postpartum recovery
  —possible separation from newborn
  —interruption in process of realigning relationships after the addition of the new family member
- *Risk for impaired parenting related to*
  —fear of spread of infection to newborn

The most effective and least expensive treatment of postpartum infection is prevention. Preventive measures include good prenatal nutrition to control anemia and intrapartal hemorrhage. Good maternal perineal hygiene is emphasized. Strict adherence to aseptic techniques by all health care personnel during childbirth and the postpartum period is very important.

Management of endometritis consists of intravenous broad-spectrum antibiotic therapy (cephalosporins, penicillins, or clindamycin and gentamicin) and supportive care, including hydration, rest, and pain relief (French & Smaill, 2002). Antibiotic therapy is usually discontinued 24 hours after the woman is asymptomatic (Gibbs et al, 2004). Assessments of lochia, vital signs, and changes in the woman's condition continue during treatment. Comfort measures depend on the symptoms and may include cool compresses, warm blankets, perineal care, and sitz baths. Teaching should include side effects of therapy, prevention of spread of infection, signs and symptoms of worsening condition, and adherence to the treatment plan and the need for follow-up care. Women may need to be encouraged or assisted to maintain mother-infant interactions and breastfeeding (if allowed during treatment).

Postpartum women are usually discharged to home by 48 hours after birth. This is often before signs of infection are evident. Nurses in birth centers and hospital settings must be able to identify women at risk for postpartum infection and to provide anticipatory teaching and counseling before discharge. After discharge, telephone follow-up, hot lines, support groups, lactation counselors, home visits by nurses, and teaching materials (videos, written materials) are all interventions that can be implemented to decrease the risk of postpartum infections. Home care nurses must be able to recognize signs and symptoms of postpartum infection so that the woman can contact her primary health care provider. These nurses must also be able to provide the appropriate nursing care for women who need follow-up home care.

Treatment of wound infections may combine antibiotic therapy with wound debridement. Wounds may be opened and drained. Nursing care includes frequent assessments of the wound and vital signs, and wound care. Comfort measures include sitz baths, warm compresses, and perineal care. Teaching includes good hygiene techniques (i.e., changing perineal pads front to back, handwashing before and after perineal care), self-care measures, and signs of worsening conditions to report to the primary health care provider. The woman is usually discharged to home for self-care or home nursing care after treatment is initiated in the inpatient setting.

Medical management for UTIs consists of antibiotic therapy, analgesia, and hydration. Postpartum women are usually treated on an outpatient basis; therefore, teaching should include instructions on how to monitor temperature, bladder function, and appearance of urine. The woman should also be taught about signs of potential complications and the importance of taking all antibiotics as prescribed. Other suggestions for prevention of UTIs include proper perineal care, wiping from front to back after urinating or having a bowel movement, and increasing fluid intake.

Because mastitis rarely occurs before the postpartum woman is discharged, teaching should include warning signs of mastitis and counseling about prevention of cracked nipples. Management includes intensive antibiotic therapy (e.g., cephalosporins and vancomycin, which are particularly useful in staphylococcal infections), support of breasts, local heat or cold, adequate hydration, and analgesics.

Almost all instances of acute mastitis can be avoided by using proper breastfeeding technique to prevent cracked nipples. Missed feedings, waiting too long between feedings, and abrupt weaning may lead to clogged nipples and mastitis. Cleanliness practiced by all who have contact with the newborn and new mother also reduces the incidence of mastitis.

SEQUELAE OF CHILDBIRTH TRAUMA

Women are at risk for problems related to the reproductive system from the age of menarche through menopause and the older years. These problems, which include structural disorders of the uterus and vagina related to pelvic relaxation and urinary incontinence, are often the delayed but direct result of childbearing.

With fetopelvic disproportion, prolonged labor, or a precipitous birth, structures of the vesical and vaginal walls are stretched and may be injured. The bladder neck and urethra may be compressed between the presenting part and the pubic bones, or forced downward ahead of the presenting part. Since soft tissue damage usually occurs behind an intact vaginal epithelium, there is nothing visible to repair. However, defects may also occur in women who have never been pregnant.

Structural disorders can have far-reaching effects for the woman and her family. Beyond the obvious physiologic alterations, the woman also experiences threats to her self-concept and her ability to cope. A woman's concept of herself as a sexual being can be affected by the condition and its treatments. A woman's family is also challenged in the way it responds to her diagnosis.

Uterine Displacement and Prolapse

Normally the round ligaments hold the uterus in anteversion, and the uterosacral ligaments pull the cervix backward and upward. Uterine displacement is a variation of this normal placement. The most common type of displacement is posterior displacement, or retroversion, in which the uterus is tilted posteriorly and the cervix rotates anteriorly. Other variations include retroflexion and anteflexion (Fig. 23-3).

By 2 months postpartum, the ligaments should return to normal length; but in about one-third of women, the uterus remains retroverted. This condition is rarely symptomatic, but conception may be difficult because the cervix points toward the anterior vaginal wall and away from the posterior fornix, where seminal fluid pools after coitus. If symptoms occur, they may include pelvic and low back pain, exaggeration of premenstrual tension, and dyspareunia.

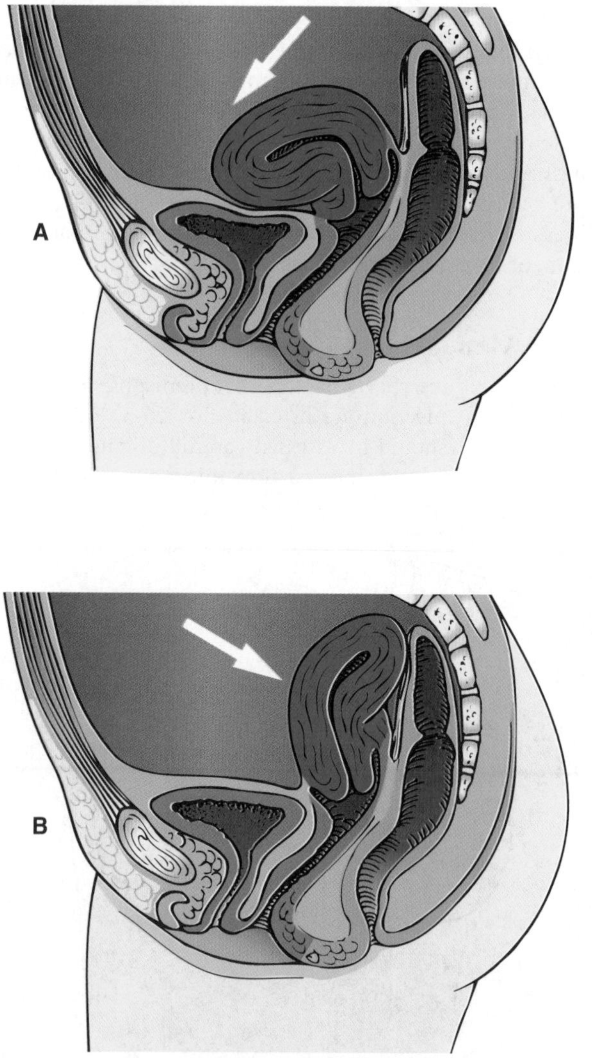

Fig. 23-3 Types of uterine displacement. **A,** Anterior displacement. **B,** Retroversion (backward displacement).

Uterine prolapse is a more serious type of displacement. Degrees of prolapse can vary from mild to complete. In complete prolapse, the cervix and body of the uterus protrude through the vagina and the vagina is inverted (Fig. 23-4).

Uterine displacement and prolapse can be caused by congenital or acquired weakness of the pelvic support structures (often referred to as pelvic relaxation). Although extensive damage may be noted and repaired shortly after birth, symptoms related to pelvic relaxation most often appear during the perimenopausal period, when the effects of ovarian hormones on pelvic tissues are lost and atrophic changes begin. Pelvic trauma, stress and strain, and the aging process are contributing causes. Other causes of pelvic relaxation include reproductive surgery and pelvic radiation.

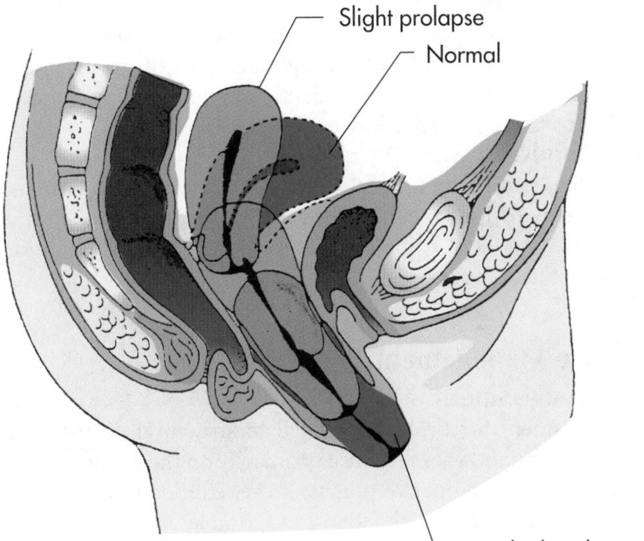

Fig. 23-4 Prolapse of uterus.

Clinical Manifestations

Generally, symptoms of pelvic relaxation relate to the structure involved: urethra, bladder, uterus, vagina, cul-de-sac, or rectum. The most common complaints are pulling and dragging sensations, pressure, protrusions, fatigue, and low backache. Symptoms may be worse after prolonged standing or deep penile penetration during intercourse. Stress urinary incontinence may be present.

Cystocele and Rectocele

Cystocele and rectocele often occur with uterine prolapse (although they can occur independently), causing the uterus to sag even further backward and downward into the vagina. Cystocele (Fig. 23-5, *A*) is the protrusion of the bladder downward into the vagina that develops when supporting structures in the vesicovaginal septum are injured. Anterior wall relaxation develops gradually over time as a result of congenital defects of supports, childbearing, obesity, or advanced age. When the woman stands, the weakened anterior vaginal wall cannot support the weight of the urine in the bladder; the vesicovaginal septum is forced downward, the bladder is stretched, and its capacity is increased. With time the cystocele enlarges until it protrudes into the vagina. Complete emptying of the bladder is difficult because the cystocele sags below the bladder neck. Rectocele is the herniation of the anterior rectal wall through the relaxed or ruptured vaginal fascia and rectovaginal septum; it appears as a large bulge that may be seen through the relaxed introitus (Fig. 23-5, B).

Clinical Manifestations

Cystoceles and rectoceles often are asymptomatic. If symptoms of cystocele are present, they may include complaints of a bearing-down sensation or that "something is in my vagina." Other symptoms include urinary frequency, retention, incontinence, and possible recurrent cystitis and urinary tract infections. On pelvic examination there is a

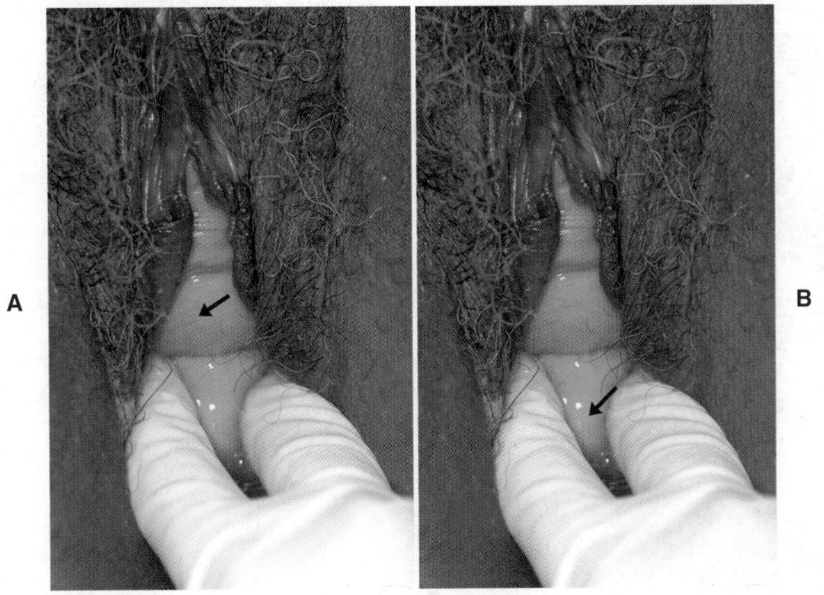

Fig. 23-5 Views of **A**, Cystocele. **B**, Rectocele. (From Seidel HM et al: *Mosby's guide to physical examination,* ed 5, St Louis, 2003, Mosby.)

bulging of the anterior wall of the vagina when the woman is asked to bear down. Unless the bladder neck and urethra are damaged, urinary continence is unaffected. Women with large cystoceles complain of having to push upward on the sagging anterior vaginal wall to be able to void.

Rectoceles may be small and produce few symptoms, but some are so large that they protrude outside of the vagina when the woman stands. Symptoms are absent when the woman is lying down. A rectocele causes a disturbance in bowel function, a sensation of bearing down, or a sensation that the pelvic organs are falling out. With a very large rectocele it may be difficult to have a bowel movement. Each time the woman strains during bowel evacuation, the feces are forced against the thinned rectovaginal wall, stretching it even more. Some women facilitate evacuation by applying digital pressure vaginally to hold up the rectal pouch.

Urinary Incontinence

About 20% of women between ages 25 and 64 years have urinary incontinence (UI) (uncontrollable leakage of urine). Although nulliparous women can have UI, the incidence is higher in women who have given birth and also increases with parity (Sampselle et al, 1997). Conditions that disturb urinary control include stress urinary incontinence, which is due to sudden increases in intraabdominal pressure such as those caused by sneezing or coughing; urge incontinence, caused by disorders of the bladder and urethra such as urethritis and urethral stricture, trigonitis, and cystitis; neuropathies such as multiple sclerosis, diabetic neuritis, and pathologic conditions of the spinal cord; and congenital and acquired urinary tract abnormalities.

Stress urinary incontinence may follow injury to bladder neck structures. A sphincter mechanism at the bladder neck compresses the upper urethra, pulls it upward behind the symphysis, and forms an acute angle at the junction of the posterior urethral wall and the base of the bladder (Fig. 23-6). To empty the bladder, the sphincter complex relaxes and the trigone contracts to open the internal urethral orifice and pull the contracting bladder wall upward, forcing urine out. The angle between the urethra and the base of the bladder is lost or increased if the supporting pubococcygeus muscle is injured; this change, coupled with a urethrocele, causes incontinence. Urine spurts out when the woman is asked to bear down or cough while she is in the lithotomy position.

Genital Fistulas

A fistula is an abnormal communication between one hollow viscus and another, or from one hollow viscus to the outside. Genital fistulas may occur between the bladder and the genital tract (e.g., vesicovaginal); between the urethra and the vagina (urethrovaginal); and between the rectum or sigmoid colon and the vagina (rectovaginal) (Fig. 23-7). Fistulas may be a result of a congenital anomaly, gynecologic surgery, obstetric trauma, cancer, radiation therapy, gynecologic trauma, or infection.

Clinical Manifestations

Signs and symptoms of vaginal fistulas depend on the site but may include the presence of urine, flatus, or feces in the vagina; odors of urine or feces in the vagina; and irritation of vaginal tissues.

Care Management

Assessment

Assessment for problems related to structural disorders of the uterus and vagina focuses primarily on the genitourinary tract, the reproductive organs, bowel elimination, and psychosocial and sexual factors. A complete health history, physical examination, and laboratory tests are done to support the appropriate medical diagnosis. The nurse needs to

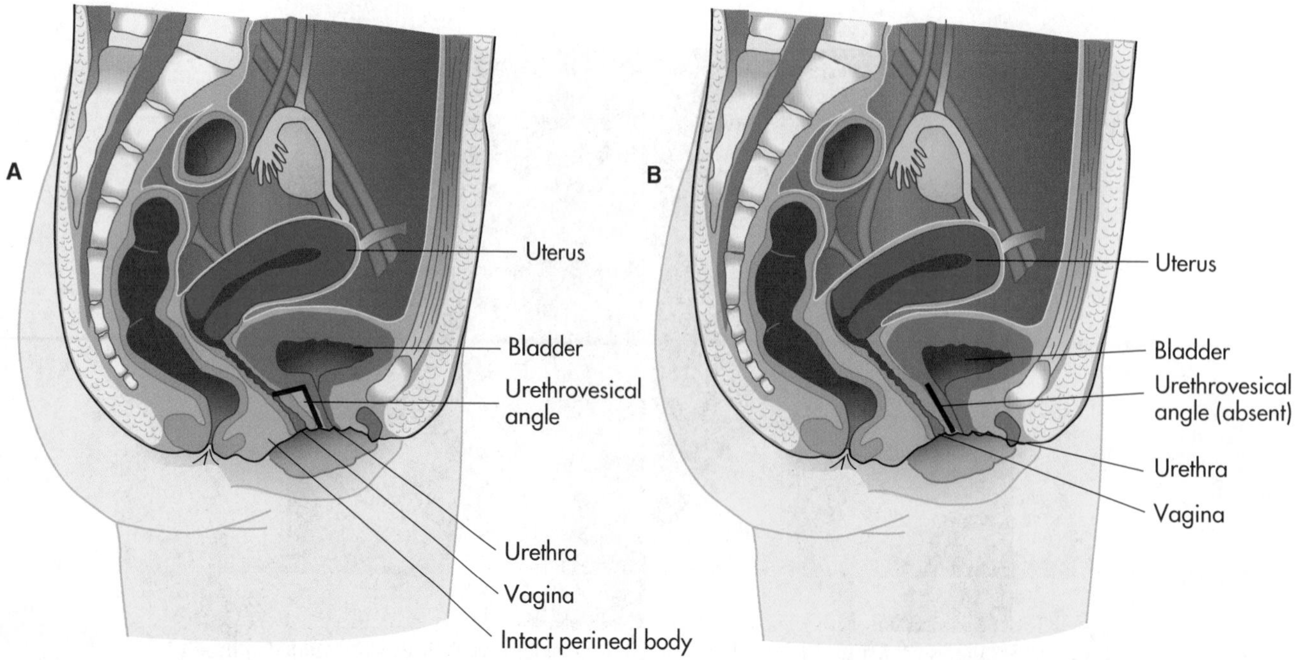

Fig. 23-6 Urethrovesical angle. **A**, Normal angle. **B**, Widening (absence) of angle.

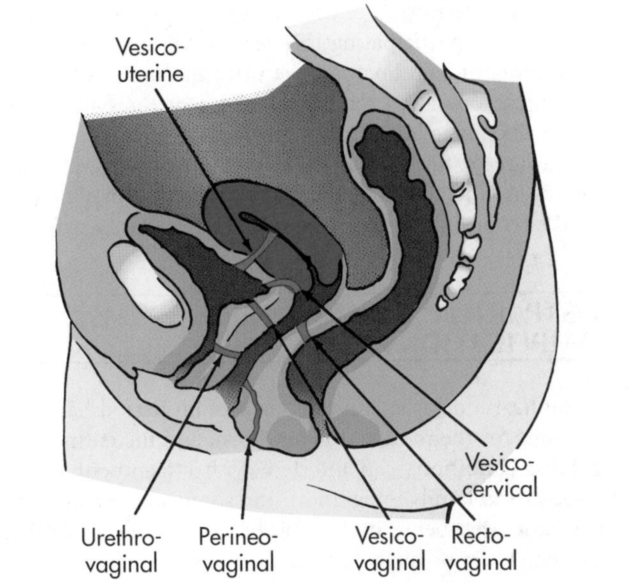

Fig. 23-7 Types of fistulas that may develop in vagina, uterus, and rectum. (From Phipps WJ et al: *Medical-surgical nursing: health and illness perspectives*, ed 7, St Louis, 2003, Mosby.)

assess the woman's knowledge of the disorder, its management, and the possible prognosis.

Nursing Diagnoses

Possible nursing diagnoses for the patient with a structural disorder of the uterus or vagina include the following:

- *Constipation or diarrhea related to*
  —anatomic changes
- *Ineffective coping related to*
  —changes in body image
- *Impaired family processes or interpersonal relationships related to*
  —the woman's anatomic and functional changes
- *Social isolation, spiritual distress, body image disturbance, or self-esteem disturbance related to*
  —changes in anatomy and function
- *Anxiety related to*
  —surgical procedure
  —prognosis

Plan of Care and Implementation

The health care team works together to treat the disorders related to alterations in pelvic support and to assist the woman in management of her symptoms. In general, nurses working with these women can provide information and self-care education to prevent problems before they occur; to manage or reduce symptoms and to promote comfort and hygiene if symptoms are already present; and to recognize when further intervention is needed. This information can be part of all postpartum discharge teaching or can be provided at postpartum follow-up visits in clinics or in physician or midwife offices, during postpartum home visits, or during gynecologic health examinations.

Interventions for specific problems depend on the problem and the severity of the symptoms. If discomfort related to uterine displacement is a problem, several interventions can be implemented to treat uterine displacement. Kegel exercises can be performed several times a day to increase muscular strength. A knee-chest position performed for a few minutes several times a day can correct a mildly retroverted uterus. A pessary to support the uterus and hold it in the correct position may be inserted in the vagina (Fig. 23-8). Usually a pessary is used only for a short time because it can lead to pressure necrosis and vaginitis. Good hygiene is important; some women can be taught to remove the pessary at

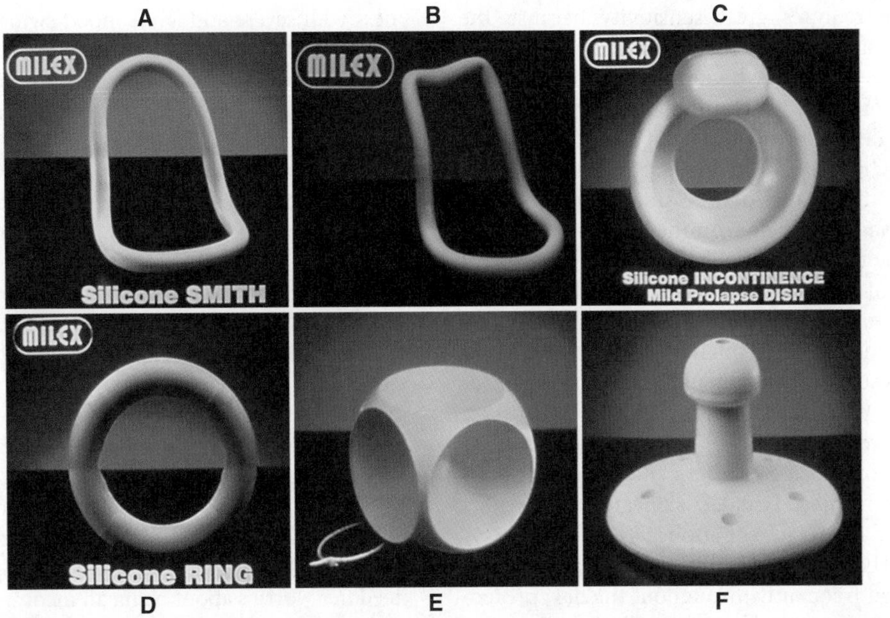

Fig. 23-8 Examples of pessaries. **A,** Smith. **B,** Hodge without support. **C,** Incontinence dish with support. **D,** Ring without support. **E,** Cube. **F,** Gellhorn. (Courtesy Milex Products, Inc., a division of CooperSurgical, Trumbull, CT.)

night, cleanse it, and replace it in the morning. If the pessary is always left in place, regular douching with commercially prepared solutions or weak vinegar solutions (e.g., 1 tablespoon to 1 quart of water) to remove increased secretions and to keep the vaginal pH at 4 to 4.5 is suggested. After a period of treatment, most women are free of symptoms and do not require the pessary. Surgical correction is rarely indicated.

Treatment for uterine prolapse depends on the degree of prolapse. Pessaries may be useful in mild prolapse. Estrogen therapy also may be used in the older woman to improve tissue tone. If these conservative treatments do not correct the problem, or there is a significant degree of prolapse, abdominal or vaginal hysterectomy is usually recommended.

Treatment for a cystocele includes use of a vaginal pessary or surgical repair. Pessaries may not be effective. Anterior repair (colporrhaphy) is the usual surgical procedure and is usually done for large symptomatic cystoceles. This involves a surgical shortening of pelvic muscles to provide better support for the bladder. An anterior repair is often combined with a vaginal hysterectomy.

Small rectoceles may not need treatment. The woman with mild symptoms may get relief from a high-fiber diet and adequate fluid intake, stool softeners, or mild laxatives. Vaginal pessaries usually are not effective. Large rectoceles that are causing significant symptoms are usually repaired surgically. A posterior repair (colporrhaphy) is the usual procedure. This surgery is performed vaginally and involves shortening the pelvic muscles to provide better support for the rectum. Anterior and posterior repairs may be performed at the same time and with vaginal hysterectomy.

Mild to moderate urinary incontinence can be significantly decreased or relieved in many women by bladder training and pelvic muscle (Kegel) exercises (Czarapata & McKillips, 1997; Sampselle et al, 2000). Other management strategies include insertion of a bladder neck support prosthesis, estrogen therapy, and surgery (Stenchever et al, 2001).

Nursing care of the woman with pelvic relaxation problems or a fistula requires great sensitivity because the woman's reactions are often intense. She may become withdrawn or, conversely, hostile because of embarrassment about odors and soiling of her clothing that are beyond her control. Her sexuality is threatened; her partner may refuse sexual intimacy. The nurse should be tactful in suggesting hygienic practices that reduce odor. Commercial deodorizing douches are available, or noncommercial solutions such as diluted chlorine (e.g., 1 teaspoon of chlorine household bleach to 1 quart of water) may be used. The chlorine solution is also useful for external perineal irrigation. Sitz baths and thorough washing of the genitalia with unscented, mild soap and warm water also help. Sparse dusting with deodorizing powders can be useful. If a rectovaginal fistula is present, enemas given before leaving the house may provide temporary relief from oozing of fecal material until corrective surgery is performed. Irritated skin and tissues may benefit from use of a heat lamp or application of vitamins A and D ointment. Hygienic care is time consuming and may need to be repeated frequently throughout the day; protective pads or pants may need to be worn. All of these activities can be demoralizing to the woman and frustrating to her and her family.

Many of the nurse's efforts with these problems are directed toward participating in a team effort to prepare the woman for surgery. Preoperative teaching involves the primary nurse, operating room nurse, surgeon, and anesthesiologist. The nurse in the health promotion setting is usually most aware of the woman's living circumstances, physical limitations, and social problems and therefore may be best suited to coordinate continuity of care after discharge.

POSTPARTUM PSYCHOLOGIC COMPLICATIONS

Mental health disorders in the postpartum period have implications for the mother, the newborn, and the entire family. Such conditions can interfere with attachment to the newborn and family integration, and some may threaten the safety and well-being of the mother, newborn, and other children. Because birth is usually thought to be a happy event, a new mother's emotional distress may puzzle and immobilize family and friends. When she most needs the caring attention of loved ones, they may either criticize or withdraw because of their anxiety.

The Diagnostic and Statistical Manual of Mental Disorders contains the official guidelines for the assessment and diagnosis of psychiatric illness (American Psychiatric Association [APA], 2000). However, specific criteria for postpartum depression (PPD) are not listed. Instead, postpartum onset can be specified for any mood disorder either without psychotic features (i.e., PPD) or with psychotic features (i.e., postpartum psychosis) if the onset occurs within 4 weeks of childbirth (APA, 2000).

Postpartum Depression without Psychotic Features

Postpartum depression (PPD) is an intense and pervasive sadness with severe and labile mood swings and is more serious and persistent than postpartum blues. Intense fears, anger, anxiety, and despondency that persist past the baby's first few weeks are not a normal part of postpartum blues. Occurring in approximately 10% to 15% of new mothers, these symptoms rarely disappear without outside help. The majority of these mothers do not seek help from any source, and only about 20% consult a health professional. The occurrence of PPD among teenage mothers was more than 2.5 times that for older mothers (Herrick, 2002). African-American mothers were twice as likely as white mothers to experience PPD. Younger mothers (younger than 20 years) and those with less than a high school education were significantly less likely to seek help and had higher rates of PPD (Herrick, 2002). Mothers who had no one to talk to about their problems after giving birth had a high rate of PPD and a low rate of help seeking.

The symptoms of postpartum major depression do not differ from symptoms of nonpostpartum mood disorders except that the mother's ruminations of guilt and inadequacy feed her worries about being an incompetent and inadequate parent. In PPD, there may be odd food cravings (often, sweet desserts) and binges with abnormal appetite and weight gain. New mothers report an increased yearning for sleep; sleeping heavily, but awakening instantly with any infant noise; and an inability to go back to sleep after infant feedings.

A distinguishing feature of PPD is irritability. These episodes of irritability may flare up with little provocation, and they may sometimes escalate to violent outbursts or dissolve into uncontrollable sobbing. Many of these outbursts are directed against significant others ("He never helps me.") or the baby ("She cries all the time and I feel like hitting her."). Women with postpartum major depressive episodes often have severe anxiety, panic attacks, and spontaneous crying long after the usual duration of baby blues.

Many women feel especially guilty about having depressive feelings at a time when they believe they should be happy. They may be reluctant to discuss their symptoms or their negative feelings toward the infant. A prominent feature of PPD is rejection of the infant, often caused by abnormal jealousy. The mother may be obsessed by the notion that the baby may take her place in her partner's affections. Attitudes toward the infant may include disinterest, annoyance with care demands, and blaming because of her lack of maternal feeling. When observed, she may appear awkward in her responses to the baby. Obsessive thoughts about harming the infant are very frightening to her. Often she does not share these thoughts because of embarrassment, but when she does, other family members become very frightened.

Medical Management

The natural course is one of gradual improvement over the 6 months after birth. Supportive treatment alone is not efficacious for major postpartum depression. Pharmacologic intervention is needed in most instances. Treatment options include antidepressants, anxiolytic agents, and electroconvulsive therapy. Psychotherapy focuses on her fears and concerns regarding her new responsibilities and roles, as well as monitoring for suicidal or homicidal thoughts. For some women, hospitalization is necessary.

Postpartum Depression with Psychotic Features

Postpartum psychosis is a syndrome most often characterized by depression (as described previously), delusions, and thoughts by the mother of harming either the infant or herself (Kaplan & Sadock, 2000).

A postpartum mood disorder with psychotic features occurs in 1 to 2 per 1000 births (Kaplan & Sadock, 2000). Once a woman has had one postpartum episode with psychotic features, there is a 30% to 50% likelihood of recurrence with each subsequent birth (APA, 2000).

Symptoms often begin within days after the birth, although the mean time to onset is 2 to 3 weeks and almost always within 8 weeks of birth (Kaplan & Sadock, 2000). Characteristically, the woman begins to complain of fatigue, insomnia, and restlessness, and may have episodes of tearfulness and emotional lability. Complaints regarding the inability to move, stand, or work are also common. Later, suspiciousness, confusion, incoherence, irrational statements, and obsessive concerns about the baby's health and welfare may be present (Kaplan & Sadock, 2000). Delusions may be present in 50% of all women and hallucinations in about 25%. Auditory hallucinations that command the mother to kill the infant can also occur in severe cases. When delusions are present, they are often related to the infant. The mother may think the infant is possessed by the devil, has special powers, or is destined for a terrible fate (APA, 2000). Grossly disorganized behavior may be manifested as a disinterest in the infant or an inability to provide care. Some will insist that something is wrong with the baby or accuse nurses or family of hurting or poisoning their child. Nurses are advised to be alert for mothers who are agitated, overactive, confused, complaining, or suspicious.

A specific illness included in depression with psychotic features is bipolar disorder (formerly called manic depressive illness). This mood disorder is preceded or accompanied by manic episodes, characterized by elevated, expansive, or irritable moods. Clinical manifestations of a manic episode include at least three of the following symptoms that have been significantly present for at least 1 week: grandiosity, decreased need for sleep, pressured speech, flight of ideas, distractibility, psychomotor agitation, and excessive involvement in pleasurable activities without regard for negative consequences (APA, 2000). Because these women are hyperactive, they may not take the time to eat or sleep, which leads to inadequate nutrition, dehydration, and sleep deprivation. While in a manic state, mothers will need constant supervision when caring for their infant. Mostly they will be too preoccupied to provide child care.

Medical Management

A favorable outcome is associated with a good premorbid adjustment (before the onset of the disorder) and a supportive family network (Kaplan & Sadock, 2000). Because mood disorders are usually episodic, women may experience another episode of symptoms within a year or two of the birth. Postpartum psychosis is a psychiatric emergency, and the mother will probably need psychiatric hospitalization. Antipsychotics and mood stabilizers such as lithium are the treatments of choice. If the mother is breastfeeding, some sources recommend that no pharmacologic agents should be prescribed (Kaplan & Sadock, 2000), but other sources advise caution while prescribing some agents (Stowe, Strader, & Nemeroff, 2001). Antipsychotics and lithium should be avoided in breastfeeding mothers, but other mood stabilizers may be compatible with breastfeeding (see later discussion in this chapter). It is usually advantageous for the mother to have contact with her baby if she so desires, but visits must be closely supervised. Psychotherapy is indicated after the period of acute psychosis is past.

Care Management

Even though the prevalence of PPD is fairly well established, women are unlikely to seek help from a mental health care provider. Primary health care providers can usually recognize severe PPD or postpartum psychosis but may miss milder forms; even if it is recognized, the woman may be treated inappropriately or subtherapeutically (Gold, 2002; Straub et al, 1998).

Assessment

To recognize symptoms of PPD as early as possible, the nurse should be an active listener and demonstrate a caring attitude. Nurses cannot depend on women to volunteer un-

Evidence-Based Practice

SUPPORT FOR POSTPARTUM DEPRESSION

Background

Clinicians use various definitions of postpartum depression, with ranges of incidence varying from 7% to 30%. Although many define any depression lasting longer than 6 months as chronic, there is no consensus regarding duration. Symptoms can be disabling to the woman, including excessive fatigue, insomnia, inability to cope, suicide ideation, and lack of maternal feelings for the baby. It is distinguished from postpartum psychosis, a psychiatric emergency that may include hallucinations, delusions, and disorganized thoughts and behaviors. Postpartum depression can disrupt relationships, especially with her partner, and her infant can present with attachment disorders and cognitive delays. Causes of postpartum depression are unknown. Hormones may challenge some threshold after birth in the psychologically vulnerable woman. Some factors associated with postpartum depression include age, parity, anxiety, social class, obstetric complications, past psychiatric history, psychosocial and marital stressors, and unplanned pregnancy. Isolation seems to exacerbate the symptoms and support to relieve them. Support has been found to be beneficial to pregnant and laboring women (see "Continuous Labor Support," Evidence-Based Practice box for Chapter 18). A meaningful relationship with a supportive caregiver reinforces the concept that the woman matters to someone, increasing feelings of well-being, control, and positive affect. Although medications are sometimes useful in postpartum depression, researchers have found compliance to be low.

Objective

The authors sought evidence of the effectiveness of professional and/or social support for women who have been diagnosed with postpartum depression. The interventions were any support offering emotional support, counseling, or tangible assistance (childcare, household assistance) via phone, home or clinic visits, individually or in groups, to women with postpartum depression. The controls were women with postpartum depression receiving "usual care" in that setting.

Outcome measures could include unbiased indicators of maternal or family morbidity, duration and resolution of depression, and social functioning.

Methods

Search Strategy

The reviewers searched Cochrane, MEDLINE, and 38 relevant journals via ZETOC, an electronic current awareness service. Search keywords were not noted.

Two randomized, controlled trials met the criteria, representing 137 women from the United Kingdom. In the 1989 trial, the intervention began at 12 weeks postpartum, and was provided by health visitors trained in nondirective counseling who made 8 half-hour home visits. The 1997 trial also began at 12 weeks, and involved 6 sessions with a psychologist trained in cognitive-behavior therapy.

Statistical Analyses

Both trials used the Edinburgh Postnatal Depression Scale, which not only has good evidence of reliability and validity but also allowed pooling of the data. The odds ratio and 95% confidence intervals were calculated for the categorical data.

Findings

At 25 weeks postpartum, the mothers who had received the intervention were significantly less depressed than the controls.

Limitations

Postpartum depression was confirmed by a clinical interview, but the reliability and validity of that was not addressed. The participants were not blinded to the treatment allocation, but the health assessors and outcome assessors were blinded to group. One study had a 30% drop-out rate, which may have introduced bias. Both the number of studies (i.e., both are from one country) and samples are small, limiting generalizability.

Conclusions

Supportive intervention in the postpartum period may be effective in relieving postpartum depression.

Implications for Practice

Isolation may contribute to postpartum depression. Social or professional support may, in theory, help alleviate depression in the vulnerable postpartum woman, but the evidence is too scanty to make policy recommendations.

Implications for Further Research

Larger studies of the benefits suggested by this small review for improving postpartum depression with increased support are needed. Of urgent interest is the optimum timing and duration of such intervention, especially as a preventive measure. The type and training of effective support caregivers, the type of intervention, and the setting are important to determine. Perhaps the family can become involved in the support intervention. Cost is a primary driving factor in mental health services, which need evidence of cost-effectiveness. Long-term follow-up may provide insight into the benefits derived for the mother and the infant and family by alleviating postpartum depression.

Reference

Ray K, Hodnett E: Caregiver support for postpartum depression (Cochrane Review), 2001. In *The Cochrane Library,* Issue 2, Chichester, UK, 2004, John Wiley & Sons.

solicited information about their depression or to ask for help. The nurse should observe for signs of depression and ask appropriate questions to determine moods, appetite, sleep, energy and fatigue levels, and ability to concentrate. Examples of ways to initiate conversation include the following: "Now that you have had your baby, how are things going for you? Have you had to change many things in your life since having the baby?" and "How much time do you spend crying?" If the nurse assesses that the new mother is depressed, she or he must ask if the mother has thought about hurting herself or the baby. The woman may be more willing to answer honestly if the nurse says, "Lots of women feel depressed after having a baby, and some feel so badly that they think about hurting themselves or the baby. Have you had these thoughts?"

Nurses can use screening tools such as the Postpartum Depression Checklist (Beck, 2002) (Box 23-4) and the Edinburgh Postnatal Depression Scale (Cox, Holden, &

BOX 23-4

Suggested Questions to Elicit Responses from the Postpartum Depression Checklist

Lack of Concentration
Are you experiencing difficulty concentrating?
Does your mind seem to be filled with cobwebs?
Does it seem at times like fogginess sets in?

Loss of Interests
Do you feel your life is empty of your previous interests and goals?
Have you lost interest in your hobbies that used to bring you pleasure and enjoyment?

Loneliness
Are you experiencing feelings of loneliness?
Do you feel as though no one really understands what you are experiencing?
Do you feel uncomfortable around other people?
Have you been isolating yourself from other people?

Insecurity
Have you been feeling insecure, fragile, or vulnerable?
Does the responsibility of motherhood seem overwhelming?

Obsessive Thinking
Is your mind constantly filled with obsessive thinking, such as "What's wrong with me?" "Am I going crazy?" "Why can't I enjoy being with my baby?"
When trying to fall asleep at night, is your mind still racing with repetitive thoughts?

Lack of Positive Emotions
Are you experiencing feelings of emptiness?
Do you feel like a robot just going through the motions?
When caring for your infant/child, do you feel any joy or love?

Loss of Self
Do you feel as though you are not the same person you used to be?
Are you afraid that your life will never be normal again?

Anxiety Attacks
Are you experiencing uncontrollable anxiety attacks?
Are you experiencing periods of palpitations, chest pains, sweating, or tingling hands?
When going through an anxiety attack, do you feel as though you're losing your mind?

Loss of Control
Do you feel you are in control of your emotions and thoughts?
Are you experiencing loss of control in any aspects of your life?

Guilt
Are you feeling guilty because you are not giving your infant/child the love and attention he or she needs?
Are you experiencing guilt over thoughts of harming your infant/child?
Do you feel you are a good mother?

Contemplating Death
Have you ever experienced thoughts of harming yourself?
Have you been feeling so low that the thought of leaving this world is appealing to you?

Source: Beck C: Screening methods for postpartum depression, *J Obstet Gynecol Neonatal Nurs* 24(4):308-312, 1995.

Savogsky, 1987) in assessing whether the depressive symptoms have progressed from postpartum blues to PPD. If the initial screening indicates that the woman may be depressed, a formal screening is helpful in determining the urgency of the referral and the type of provider. It is also important to assess the woman's family; they may be able to offer valuable information as well as have a need to express how they have been affected by the woman's emotional disorder (Maley, 2002).

Nursing Diagnoses

Possible nursing diagnoses for the woman experiencing postpartum depression include the following:

- *Risk for violence toward self (mother) or children related to*
  —postpartum depression
- *Ineffective family coping related to*
  —increased care needs of mother and infant
- *Risk for impaired parenting related to*
  —inability of depressed mother to attach to and care for infant
- *Situational low self-esteem in the mother related to*
  —stresses associated with role changes
- *Risk for injury to newborn related to*
  —mother's depression (inattention to infant's needs for hygiene, nutrition, safety) and psychotropic medications via breast milk

Expected Outcomes

Specific measurable criteria can be developed based on the following general outcomes:

- The mother will no longer be depressed.
- The mother's and infant's physical well-being will be maintained.
- The family will cope effectively.
- Family members will demonstrate continued healthy growth and development.
- The infant will be fully integrated into the family.

Plan of Care and Implementation

On the Postpartum Unit

The postpartum nurse must observe the new mother carefully for any signs of tearfulness, and conduct further assessments as necessary. Nurses must discuss PPD to prepare new parents for potential problems in the postpartum period (see Patient Teaching box). The family must be able to recognize the symptoms and know where to go for help. Written materials that explain what the woman can do to prevent depression are useful.

Mothers are often discharged before the blues or depression occurs. If the postpartum nurse is concerned about the mother, a mental health consult should be requested before the mother leaves the hospital. Routine instructions regarding PPD should be given to whoever comes to take the pa-

Patient Teaching

ACTIVITIES TO PREVENT POSTPARTUM DEPRESSION

- Share knowledge about postpartum emotional problems with close family and friends.
- Take care of yourself: eat a balanced diet, exercise on a regular basis, and get enough sleep. Ask someone to take care of the baby so that you can get a full night's sleep.
- Share your feelings with someone close to you; don't isolate yourself at home with the TV.
- Don't overcommit yourself or feel like you need to be a superwoman.
- Don't place unrealistic expectations on yourself.
- Don't be ashamed of having emotional problems after your baby is born. It happens to approximately 15% of women.

tient home; for example, "If you notice that your wife (or daughter) is upset or crying a lot, please call the postpartum care provider immediately. Don't wait for the routine postpartum appointment."

NURSE ALERT Because the newborn may be scheduled for a checkup before the mother's 6-week checkup, nurses in well-baby clinics or pediatrician offices should be alert for signs of PPD in new mothers and be knowledgeable about community referral resources. ■

In the Home and Community

Postpartum home visits can reduce the incidence of or complications from depression. A brief home visit or phone call at least once a week until the new mother returns for her postpartum visit may save the life of a mother and her infant; however, home visits may not be feasible or available. Supervision of the mother with emotional complications may become a prime concern. Because depression can greatly interfere with her mothering functions, family and friends may need to participate in the infant's care. This supervision can be planned by the collaborative efforts of the nurse and family members.

When the woman has PPD, a partner often reacts with confusion, shock, denial, and anger and feels neglected and blamed. The nurse can talk with the woman about how her condition is hard for him too and that he is probably very worried about her. Men oftentimes withdraw or criticize when they are deeply worried about their significant others. The nurse can provide nonjudgmental opportunities for the partner to verbalize feelings and concerns, help the partner identify positive coping strategies, and be a source of encouragement for the partner to continue supporting the woman. Both the woman and her partner need an opportunity to express their needs, fears, thoughts, and feelings in a nonjudgmental environment.

Even if the woman is severely depressed, hospitalization can be avoided if adequate resources can be mobilized to ensure safety for both mother and infant. The nurse in home health care will need to make frequent phone calls or home visits to do assessment and counseling. Community resources that may be helpful are temporary child care or foster care, homemaker service, meals on wheels, parenting guidance centers, mother's-day-out programs, and telephone support groups (see Resources at end of chapter).

Women with moderate to severe cases of PPD should be referred to a mental health therapist, such as an advanced practice psychiatric nurse, for evaluation and therapy. Inpatient psychiatric hospitalization may be necessary. This decision is made when the safety needs of the mother or child are threatened.

When depression is suspected, the nurse asks, "Have you thought about hurting yourself?" If delusional thinking about the baby is suspected, the nurse asks, "Have you thought about hurting your baby?" Four criteria measure the seriousness of a suicidal plan: method, availability, specificity, and lethality. Has the woman specified a method? Is the method of choice available? How specific is the plan? If the method is concrete and detailed, with access to it right at hand, the suicide risk increases. How lethal is the method? The most lethal method is shooting, with hanging a close second. The least lethal is slashing one's wrists. Medication overdose with tricyclic antidepressants (TCAs) does cause death. Avoid TCAs in suicidal women because of their danger in overdose.

PPD is usually treated with antidepressant medications. Women taking mood stabilizers (Box 23-5) must be taught about their many side effects, and those on lithium especially need to be told to have serum lithium levels drawn every 6 months. Women with severe psychiatric syndromes will probably require antipsychotic medications (Box 23-6).

Patient education is important for those taking antipsychotic medications because most of these medications can cause sedation and orthostatic hypotension, both of which could interfere with the mother being able to safely care for her baby. The medications can also cause parasympathetic nervous system (PNS) effects such as constipation, dry mouth, blurred vision, tachycardia, urinary retention, weight gain, and agranulocytosis. Central nervous system (CNS) effects may include akathisia, dystonias, Parkinsonism-like symptoms, tardive dyskinesia (irreversible), and neuroleptic malignant syndrome (potentially fatal).

BOX 23-5

Mood Stabilizers

Carbamazepine (Tegretol)	Divalproex (Depakote)
Clonazepam (Klonopin)	Lithium carbonate (Eskalith)

BOX 23-6

Commonly Used Antipsychotic Medications

Phenothiazines	Other
Chlorpromazine (Thorazine)	Clozapine (Clozaril)
Fluphenazine (Prolixin)	Haloperidol (Haldol)
Perphenazine (Trilafon)	Loxapine (Loxitane)
Thioridazine (Mellaril)	Olanzapine (Zyprexa)
Trifluoperazine (Stelazine)	Pimozide (Orap)
	Quetiapine (Seroquel)
	Risperidone (Risperdal)
	Thiothixene (Navane)

When breastfeeding women have emotional complications and need psychotropic medications, referral to a psychiatrist who specializes in postpartum disorders is preferred. Depressed women who are not breastfeeding will need supervision to take antidepressants as ordered. Because they do not exert any effect before about 2 weeks and usually do not reach full effect before 4 to 6 weeks, many women discontinue taking the medication on their own.

Other Treatments for PPD

Other treatments for PPD include complementary/alternative therapies such as those listed in Box 23-7, electroconvulsive therapy (ECT), and psychotherapy. Alternative therapies may be used alone but often are used with other treatments for PPD. Safety and efficacy studies of these alternative therapies are needed to ensure that care and advice is based on evidence (Tiran & Mack, 2000).

NURSE ALERT St. John's wort is often used to treat depression. It has not been proven safe for women who are breastfeeding. ■

ECT may be used for women with PPD who have not improved with antidepressant therapy. Psychotherapy in the form of group therapy or individual (interpersonal) therapy also has been used with positive results both alone and in conjunction with antidepressant therapy (Beck, 1999); however, more studies are needed to determine what types of professional support are most effective (Ray & Hodnett, 2004).

Evaluation

The nurse can be assured that care has been effective if the physical well-being of the mother and infant is maintained, the mother and family are able to cope effectively, and each family member continues to show a healthy adaptation to the presence of the new member of the family (see Nursing Care Plan).

LOSS AND GRIEF

Situational life crises can be superimposed on the experiences of childbearing. These may include infertility, premature labor/premature birth, a cesarean birth, any perception of loss of control during the birthing experience, birth of a boy when the parents wanted a girl, the birth of a child with handicap, a maternal death, and/or fetal or neonatal death. All of these situations have a common denominator: they are losses of what was hoped for, dreamed about, and/or planned.

From the perspective of health care providers, these crises vary in degree. However, from the perspective of the parents, the perceived loss may be the most terrible thing that has ever happened to them. At the birth they are mourning instead of celebrating life.

The statistics on perinatal loss and death of an infant are grim. Each year, approximately 7 of every 1000 births end in stillbirth or fetal death. Newborn death accounts for almost 27,600 deaths per year in the United States (Arias et al, 2003); 18,000 infants die in the early postpartum period from prematurity, birth defects, and other acute illnesses. Thus parents can experience grief before or during the childbearing experience. In addition, 9 to 10 women per 100,000 die in the United States of childbirth-related causes each year (Minino et al, 2002).

The focus of this section is to prepare the beginning nurse to provide sensitive, supportive, and therapeutic interventions to parents and families experiencing perinatal loss in a variety of settings.

BOX 23-7

Possible Alternative/Complementary Therapies for Postpartum Depression

Acupunture	Healing touch/therapeutic touch
Acupressure	Massage
Aromatherapy	Relaxation techniques
Jasmine	Reflexology
Ylang Ylang	Yoga
Rose	
Herbal	
Lavender tea	

Source: Tiran D, Mack S (eds): *Complementary therapies for pregnancy and childbirth*, ed 2, Edinburgh, 2000, Bailliere Tindall.

Conceptual Model of Parental Grief

Miles (1984) and Miles and Demi (1986; 1997) proposed a conceptual model of parental grief, based on the work of Lindemann (1944), Parkes (1972), Parkes and Weiss (1983), and Worden (1991). The model proposes that the grief responses of a parent are closely linked to that parent's self-image as a mother or father. Parental grief responses occur in three overlapping phases of grief—acute distress, intense grief, and reorganization.

Acute Distress

The loss of a pregnancy or death of an infant is an acute and distressing experience for mothers and fathers who planned for and expected a normal healthy infant as the outcome. The loss encompasses a loss of their identity as a mother or father and the loss of their many dreams related to parenthood. The immediate reaction to news of a perinatal loss or infant death is a period of acute distress. Parents generally are in a state of shock and numbness. They may feel a sense of unreality and confusion, as though they were in a bad dream or in a fog or trancelike state. Disbelief and denial can occur. Parents also feel very sad and depressed; intense outbursts of emotion and crying are common. However, lack of affect, euphoria, and calmness may occur and may reflect numbness, denial, or a personal way of coping with stress.

It is during this time of acute distress that parents face the first task of grief: accepting the reality of the loss. The pregnancy has ended or the baby has died and their lives have changed. While parents are often required to make many decisions, such as naming the infant or making funeral arrangements, normal functioning is impeded and decisions are difficult to make. Grandparents, friends, clergy, or other relatives may be available to help the couple cope. However, it is important that the mother and father ultimately make the decisions that are right for them.

Intense Grief

The phase of intense grief encompasses many difficult emotions, including loneliness, emptiness, and yearning; guilt, anger, and fear; disorganization and depression; and physical symptoms. Being able to adjust to the environment after the loss means learning how to accommodate the changes that the loss has brought. Deciding what to do about the nursery and baby clothes, how to handle comments of co-workers when returning to work, and how to cope with insensitive family members and friends are among the problems bereaved parents face during this phase of grief.

Parents often experience feelings of loneliness, emptiness, and yearning. The mother may report that her arms ache to hold or nurse her baby, and that she wakes to the sound of a baby crying. When her milk comes in, it is particularly poignant when there is no baby to take to breast. Some parents cope with these feelings by avoiding memories and by not talking about the baby, whereas others want to reminisce and discuss their loss over and over.

During this phase of intense grief, guilt may emerge from the deep feelings of helplessness in not somehow preventing the pregnancy loss or the death of the infant. With many perinatal losses, there is no clear cause of the event, leaving the woman to speculate about what she might have done or not done to cause the loss. Guilt may be intense if the mother thinks she is being punished for some unrelated event such as having had a prior induced abortion.

Other common responses during this phase are anger, resentment, bitterness, and irritability. Anger may be focused on the health care team who failed to save the pregnancy or infant; toward a God who allowed the loss to occur; or toward family, friends, or peers when they do not provide the support the bereaved parents need and want.

Deep sadness and depression occur when the parent is faced with the full awareness of the reality of the loss. This may occur several months after the perinatal loss and can continue for some time. Sadness and depression may be accompanied by disorganization and problems with cognitive processing; parents may have difficulty getting things done, be unable to concentrate, be restless, have confused thought processes, have difficulty solving problems, and make poor decisions.

Physical symptoms of grief include fatigue, headaches, dizziness, and backaches. Developing health problems such as colds or hypertension is not uncommon. It may be difficult to sleep; the appetite may be depressed or voracious. Lack of sleep and inadequate nutrition and fluids can complicate other grief responses.

Reorganization

From the time of the pregnancy loss or infant death, parents attempt to understand "why?" This leads to a long and intense search for meaning. At first the "why" is focused on the cause of death. Parents next focus on "why me, why mine?" These questions lead some parents into an existential search about the meaning of life and death. This search continues into the phase of reorganization and may lead to profound changes in the parents' view of the fragility of life.

Time helps to slowly ease the painful feelings of grief. Over time, the pain becomes less frequent. Reorganization occurs when the parent is better able to function at home and work, experiences a return of self-esteem and confidence, can cope with new challenges, and has placed the loss in perspective. Reorganization begins to peak sometime after the first year as parents begin to achieve the task of moving on with their lives. Enjoying the simple pleasures of life without feeling guilty, nurturing self and others, developing new interests, and reestablishing relationships are all signs of moving on. For some women and families, another pregnancy and the birth of a subsequent child is an important step to be able to move on with their lives; however, the term "recovery" is used because the grief related to perinatal loss can continue in varying degrees for life. Parents have shared they will never forget the baby who died, and they are not the same persons as before the loss. The term "bittersweet grief," coined by Kowalski (1984), refers to the grief response that occurs with reminders of the loss. This typically happens on birthdays, death days, and anniversaries; at school events; during changes in the seasons; and during the time of the year when the loss occurred (Box 23-8). Grief feelings also can be triggered after a subsequent live birth.

Anticipatory Grief

Some parents experience anticipatory grief; that is, they have knowledge of an impending loss, such as when a baby is admitted to a neonatal intensive care unit (NICU) with prob-

BOX 23-8

Bittersweet Grief

To Jessica Mayo—on her eleventh birthday
Sunday, November 18, 1990
"The child who is born on the Sabbath day,
Is bonny and blithe and good and gay."
Sundays are special days.
. . . a day of rest, a day to play.
A day to reflect on days past
. . . a day to thank God for all that we bless.
I bless your memory.
I wish you were here.
On your eleventh birthday I still want to share.
. . . Your dreams of the future.
. . . Our memories past.
My baby's first cry.
My daughter's first laugh.
I was told you were an angel in heaven above.
Eleven years later, I'm an expert . . .
At long-distance love.
On your third birthday I wrote my first poem
to you.
Eight years later, it's still true
". . . no birthday cake,
no presents unwrapped . . .
no pictures of you in your party hat.
But the candles are lit,
Never to go out
For they burn forever in my heart.
Love, Mom"
Kathie Rataj Mayo
1990

lems or when a diagnosis of an anencephalic fetus is made by ultrasound examination. The fetus is still alive, but the prognosis is poor. Being able to anticipate the loss gives families an opportunity to plan, feel more in control of their situation, and be able to say good-bye in a special way. However, some individuals or family members may distance or detach themselves from the experience or the baby as a way of protecting themselves or avoiding the pain of loss and grief.

Care Management

Nursing care of mothers and fathers experiencing a perinatal loss begins the first time they are faced with the potential loss of their pregnancy or death of their infant. Supportive interventions are important both at the time of the loss and after the parents have returned home.

Assessment

Assessment of family members' perceptions of the loss and their perceptions of the events surrounding the loss is crucial before intervention. This assessment is as important for families experiencing a miscarriage or ectopic pregnancy as it is for those experiencing stillbirth or neonatal loss.

Support during a perinatal loss is important to most couples. However, it is important to assess the amount and type of support from others that a couple wants. Some prefer to handle the tragedy alone for awhile; others want assistance in calling other family members, friends, and clergy to be with them and to help them with decisions.

Nursing Diagnoses

Examples of nursing diagnoses for a couple experiencing perinatal grief include the following:

- *Interrupted family processes related to*
  - —maternal depression leading to changes in role function
  - —inadequate communication of feelings between the grieving mother and father
  - —lack of attention and support to siblings
- *Fatigue and sleep pattern disturbance related to*
  - —inability to fall asleep because of grief
  - —waking in the night and thinking about the loss
- *Situational low self-esteem related to*
  - —prolonged feelings of poor self-worth because of the loss
  - —feeling unworthy of having a child
- *Spiritual distress related to*
  - —anger with God
  - —confusion about why prayers were not answered
- *Altered thought processes related to*
  - —difficulty making decisions
  - —inability to get organized
  - —poor work performance
  - —confused thinking

Expected Outcomes

Expected outcomes are set and prioritized in patient-centered terms according to the mutual goals chosen by the patient and the nurse. Expected outcomes may include that the woman/ family will do the following:

- Actualize the loss
- Share experiences and verbalize feelings of grief
- Understand the normal grief responses they may experience at the time of and following the loss
- Identify family and community resources for support

Plan of Care and Implementation

Interventions and support for parents from the nursing and medical staff after a perinatal loss or infant death are extremely important in their healing. While parents often cannot recall details of their experiences at the time of death, they may recall vividly a minor event that was perceived as particularly painful or particularly helpful. The interventions provided below are general ideas about what may be helpful to parents. However, care must be individualized to each parent and family.

Communicating and Caring Techniques

Mothers, fathers, and extended families look to the medical and nursing staff for support and understanding during the time of loss. Therapeutic communication and counseling techniques help the mother, father, and other family members express their feelings and emotions, understand their responses to the loss, and make decisions.

The nurse should listen patiently while people tell their story of loss and grief. Asking questions that help people talk about their grief and the experiences surrounding the loss may be needed. However, grief responses in the initial days of crisis make it difficult for individuals to concentrate on what is being asked, to think about what the question means, and to respond to the question. The use of silence often gives the bereaved person the opportunity to collect thoughts and to respond to questions. The nurse should resist the temptation to give advice or to use clichés in offering support (Box 23-9).

Nurses need to become comfortable with their own feelings of grief and loss to effectively support and care for the

BOX 23-9

What to Say and What Not to Say to Bereaved Parents

What to Say

"I'm sad for you."
"How are you doing with all of this?"
"This must be hard for you."
"What can I do for you?"
"I'm sorry."
"I'm here, and I want to listen."

What Not to Say

"God had a purpose for her."
"Be thankful you have another child."
"The living must go on."
"I know how you feel."
"It's God's will."
"You have to keep on going for her sake."
"You're young, you can have others."
"We'll see you back here next year, and you'll be happier."
"Now you have an angel in heaven."
"This happened for the best."
"Better for this to happen now, before you knew the baby."
"There was something wrong with the baby anyway."

Used with permission of Bereavement Services. Copyright Lutheran Hospital-La Crosse, Inc., a Gundersen Lutheran Affiliate, La Crosse, WI.

bereaved. It is appropriate to express feelings with the bereaved families and to share the moment with them.

Worden (1991) identified several counseling techniques the nurse might use in helping the family share and express their grief. These include the following techniques.

Actualize the Loss

Ask the bereaved questions that help them express the experience of the loss. Use the name of their baby, and view the body of the baby before speaking with family members.

Help the survivor identify and express feelings. Expressed grief can be overwhelming to health care professionals. Feelings of anger, guilt, and sadness are paramount in the early days and months following a loss. When the bereaved express feelings of anger, it can be helpful to identify the feeling by simply saying, "You sound angry," or "You look angry. Where is this anger coming from?" Being willing to sit down and talk about their anger can help the survivors move past the anger and identify feelings of powerlessness and helplessness in not being able to control many aspects of the situation.

The bereaved have many questions about their loss. "What did I do?" "What caused this to happen?" "Do you think I should have, could have done . . . ?" Part of the grief process is for the bereaved to figure out what happened and what their role was in the loss. The nurse needs to recognize that the answers to these questions must come from the bereaved. It is part of their healing. When a bereaved mother asks, "Do you think that I shouldn't have painted the baby's room? Did that cause my baby to die?" An appropriate response might be, "I understand you need to find an answer for why your baby died. What are some of the other things you've been thinking about?"

Being with someone who is terribly sad, crying, or sobbing can be extremely difficult. The initial impulse is to touch them and/or hand them a tissue. While this action may seem supportive, it may stop or stifle the expression of emotion. The bereaved will indicate when they are ready for a tissue by beginning to wipe their eyes or nose, raising their head, and looking around or reaching for a tissue.

Careful assessment before using touch as a therapeutic technique is important. If touch is used inappropriately, the bereaved will stiffen, pull away, look at where they were touched, or stop expressing their feelings and emotions.

Provide Time to Grieve

Families become unaware of time frames when they first learn of and come to grips with their loss. They do not care about the change of shifts or the needs that the hospital system might have in "moving things along." When families are pushed or rushed into making decisions, they may make a decision based on the needs of the health care system, not their own. Nurses must be sensitive to the need that families might have to spend time with their baby. Providing time to see and hold their baby in private, making arrangements for their baby to be returned to them for further viewing, and delaying the processing of consent forms for autopsy or removal from the hospital are ways to give the family the opportunity to say good-bye.

Interpret Normal Feelings

Many parents have feelings of losing control when they express the normal feelings and emotions of grief. They may feel like they are "going crazy" because of thoughts that plague them about the baby. It is essential for the nurse to reassure and educate bereaved parents about the grief process, including the physical, social, and emotional responses of individuals and families.

After discharge, providing information/education on the grief process can be done by making follow-up phone calls to bereaved families; offering them the opportunity to talk with other bereaved parents in one-on-one support over the phone; referring them to a mutual, self-help perinatal bereavement support group; or providing a list of publications or websites intended for helping parents who have experienced a perinatal loss. As with any referral, the nurse should read the materials or check out the Websites first.

Allow for Individual Differences

Grief is very personal and private. How people respond to loss and grief depends on such things as age, gender, culture, religion, and socioeconomic status; how others around them respond to their loss; and how they coped with prior losses. Within a family, many different types of responses may occur. Typically, men want to protect their partner from further pain, and parents/grandparents want to protect their children from more hurt. The underlying feelings of powerlessness and helplessness can be hidden behind expressions of anger, resistance to ideas, overcontrol of situations, or blame. These feelings can leave the partner or grandparent feeling isolated and alone, when in fact it is the care and concern for their loved one(s) that perpetuates the expression of the feelings. The nurse can respond to these underlying feelings by recognizing what a difficult time this is for the mother, father, parent, grandparents, and/or child. He or she can acknowledge how hard it must be for them to feel so responsible about making sure everything and everyone is taken care of. The nurse can ask them about their own hopes, dreams, and subsequent feelings of loss. These communication techniques can help the nurse move the resistive person to a position of support where her needs can also be met.

Families need to be given the opportunity to change their minds, to express their needs to each other, and to make decisions based on their needs as individuals and as family members.

Cultural and Spiritual Needs of Parents

Many of the responses to perinatal loss described in this section are based on Euro-American views of perinatal grief and loss. Although there may be no particular differences in individual, intrapersonal experiences of grief based on culture, ethnicity, or religions, there are many differences in

Community Focus

COMMUNITY RESOURCES FOR LOSS AND GRIEF

Investigate what resources and support groups exist in your community to assist parents who have experienced a maternal death; birth of a "less-than-perfect" child; a cesarean birth; or the death of a baby through miscarriage, stillbirth, or newborn death. Are resources available? Are there enough of these resources to assist parents? How difficult was it for you to identify these resources? What could you do to make resources more known to bereaved parents and families?

mourning rituals, traditions, and behavioral expressions of grief (Cowles, 1996; Hebert, 1998). Thus, the practices suggested earlier may not be appropriate for parents from various cultural, ethnic, and religious groups, and the nurse must consider the potential unique responses and needs of parents from different groups (Hebert, 1998). This involves understanding the cultural orientation and beliefs of the individual parent, the partner, the extended family, and the larger community to which they belong.

Cultural and religious differences can affect the way parents respond to a perinatal loss. This includes their way of communicating with health care professionals, as well as their emotional and behavioral responses and family interaction patterns. With perinatal loss, culture and religious beliefs can affect issues such as seeing the infant, naming the infant, taking pictures, allowing autopsies, and baptism or other rituals performed at death.

Physical Comfort

Coping with loss and grief after childbirth can be an overwhelming experience for the woman and her family. Often these families request that the mother be moved off the maternity unit or be discharged to home; the thought of being on the same unit with healthy mothers and babies is more than they can cope with. Other mothers, however, may want to remain on the maternity unit, where the staff nurses are better prepared to meet their physical and emotional needs. It should be the mother's choice as to where she wants to spend her postpartum stay.

The physical needs of a bereaved mother are the same as those of any mother who has given birth, but with an unhappy twist: the milk may come in, but there is no baby to nurse; the afterpains remind the mother of her emptiness; and gas pains feel like there is still a baby moving inside her. Many struggle with the frustration of having to go through all the pain of childbearing, only to return home with empty arms.

Options for Parents

It is sometimes difficult for the nurse to offer the bereaved information about their rights regarding options without making them feel guilty if they do not choose to exercise that right. Communicating with parents that options are their right, not their obligation, is vitally important.

Seeing and Holding

One of the first options to be discussed is whether the family wants to see their baby or, in the case of miscarriage or ectopic pregnancy, the products of conception. A statement such as "Some parents have found it helpful to see their baby" (or "the products of conception") gives the parents permission to do what might seem odd or distasteful. Responses can vary greatly between someone who experiences a miscarriage or ectopic pregnancy and someone who has experienced stillbirth or newborn death, as well as between family members.

Parents appreciate explanations as to how their baby looks (e.g., red, peeling skin like a bad sunburn, dark discoloration similar to bruises, molding of the head that makes the head look soft and swollen, or any defects). This helps them know what to expect. The nurse should make the baby look as normal as possible. Actions such as bathing the baby, applying lotion to the baby's skin, combing the hair, placing identification bands on the arm and leg, dressing the baby in a diaper and special outfit, sprinkling powder in the baby's blanket, and wrapping the baby in a pretty blanket convey to the parents that their baby is cared for as carefully as any baby in the nursery.

Caring for a baby who has died can be a difficult task for the nurse. It can be even more difficult if the fetus has been dead for several days or weeks in utero. In some cases decapitation or dismemberment may have occurred. If the baby has been in the morgue, the baby can be placed underneath a warmer for 20 to 30 minutes and wrapped in a warm blanket before being brought to the parents. Cold cream rubbed over stiffened joints can help in repositioning the baby.

When bringing the baby to the parents, it is important to hold the baby close, touch a hand or cheek, use the baby's name, and talk with the parents about the special features of their child to convey that it is all right for them to do likewise. If a baby has a congenital anomaly, the nurse can have a perfect hand or foot showing.

Parents need to be offered time alone with their baby. They need to know when the nurse will return and how to call should they require anything. It is difficult to predict how much time parents will need to spend with their baby. These moments are the only ones they will have with this child. Some parents need only a few minutes; others need hours. With the current practice of short-stay postpartum care, the nurse may need to advocate for patients who have experienced a loss to give them the time they need to grieve.

Bathing and Dressing

When possible, families should be given the opportunity to bathe, dress, and/or anoint their baby. This can be a very symbolic ritual for many families. The skin of some babies is fragile and may crack or ooze when touched. Parents can still apply lotion with cotton balls, sprinkle powder, tie ribbons, fasten the diaper, and place amulets, medallions, rosaries, or special toys or mementos in their baby's hands or alongside their baby. They may want to do other parenting functions, such as combing hair, wrapping the baby in a blanket, placing the baby in a bassinet, or carrying their baby to the nursery. They may have special clothes for the baby at home, or they may want to purchase a special outfit for the baby.

Privacy

If at all possible, the mother should be admitted to a private room. Marking the door to the room with a special card that denotes to hospital staff that this family has experienced a loss can be helpful (Fig. 23-9).

Visitation with Other Family Members or Friends

Families need to be offered the opportunity to have their children, grandparents, extended family members, and friends visit with them during hospitalization, as well as to see and hold their baby. This affords others the opportunity to become acquainted with the baby, to understand the parents' loss, to offer their support, and to say good-bye. This experience also helps parents explain to their surviving children who their brother or sister was and what death means; it offers the children answers to their questions in a concrete manner and helps them in expressing their grief.

Religious Rituals/Funeral Arrangements

Support from the clergy is an option that should be offered to all parents. Parents may wish to have their own pastor, priest, rabbi, or spiritual leader contacted; they may wish

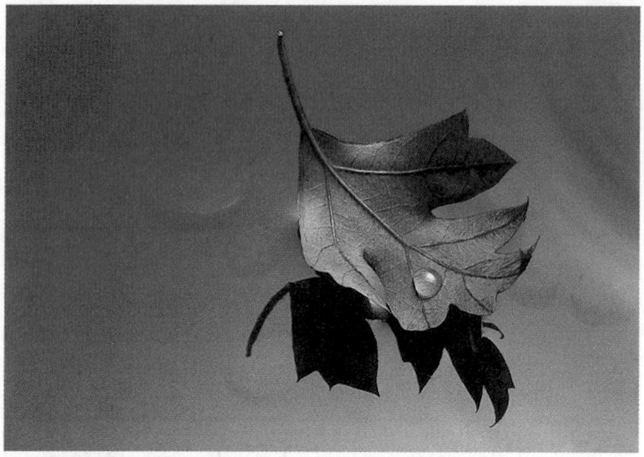

Fig. 23-9 Door card for room of mother who has experienced perinatal loss. (Used with permission of Bereavement Services. Copyright Lutheran Hospital–La Crosse, Inc., a Gundersen Lutheran Affiliate, La Crosse, WI.)

to see the hospital's chaplain; or they may choose neither option. A member of the clergy may offer the parents the opportunity for baptism, when appropriate (Box 23-10). Parents should be given information about the choices for the final disposition of their baby, regardless of gestational age. In the instance of a baby under 20 weeks of gestation, many hospitals offer to make the final disposition arrangements. Babies under 20 weeks of gestation are considered to be products of conception. Embryos, fallopian tubes removed in an ectopic pregnancy, tissue from a pregnancy obtained during a D&C, and fetuses under 20 weeks of gestation are all considered tissue. Should parents want to know what arrangements the hospital makes for their babies, the nurse should answer the parents' questions as honestly as possible. In most states if a baby is over 20 weeks and 1 day of gestation or is born alive, it is the parents' responsibility to make the final arrangements for their baby. Caskets, burial cradles, and burial urns sized for fetuses and infants are available (see Resources at end of chapter). Samples or photographs of such items can be shared with parents (Fig. 23-10).

BOX 23-10

Infant Baptism

In an emergency, baptism may be performed by anyone by pouring water over the forehead (or products of conception) and saying "I baptize you in the name of the Father and of the Son and of the Holy Spirit." The person performing the baptism needs only to have the intention of baptizing and does not necessarily have to believe in infant baptism for the baptism to be valid. If the infant has no signs of life, the person performing the baptism can add "If you are alive, I baptize you. . . ."

In the Greek Orthodox tradition, baptism is only for the living; thus a miscarried or stillborn infant would not be baptized. If the infant is born alive and in serious danger of death, the infant can be lifted up while saying "The servant of God is baptized in the name of the Father and the Son and Holy Spirit."*

*From: Harakas S (RHarakas@aol.com): *E-mail to M. Miles* (mmiles@email.unc.edu), May 17, 1999.

LEGAL TIP Live Birth In all states there are laws that govern what constitutes a live birth. In most states a "live birth" is considered to be any product of conception expelled from a woman that shows any signs of life. Signs of life are considered to be any muscle irritability, respiratory effort, or heart rate regardless of gestational age. Nurses should be knowledgeable about their state laws regarding what constitutes a live birth and what forms need to be completed and filed in the case of fetal death, stillbirth, or newborn death. ■

Special Memories

Parents need tangible mementos of their baby. A lock of hair may be an important keepsake. Parents need to be asked first, for permission, before a lock of hair is cut. Hair can be removed from the nape of the baby's neck, where it is not noticeable. Parents may also bring in a baby book that had already been purchased. In addition, special memory books, cards, and information on grief and mourning are available through national perinatal bereavement organizations for purchase by parents or hospitals/clinics (Fig. 23-11).

The nurse provides information about the baby's weight, length, and head circumference to the family. Footprints and handprints are taken and placed with the other information on a special card or memory/baby book. Sometimes it is difficult to obtain good handprints or footprints. Using alcohol or acetone on the palms or soles first can help the ink adhere to make the prints clearer, especially for small babies.

Any article that comes in contact or is used in caring for the baby should be saved, placed in a sealable bag, and given to the parents. Articles should not be washed or cleaned beforehand, since the parents may want to be able to keep the smell of their baby. Some examples of articles that can be given to parents are the tape measure used to measure the baby, lotions, combs, clothing, hats, blankets, pacifier, crib cards, and identification bands. Identification bands should be placed on the baby before they are given to the parents. These bands help the parents to remember the size of the baby and enable them to touch something their baby touched.

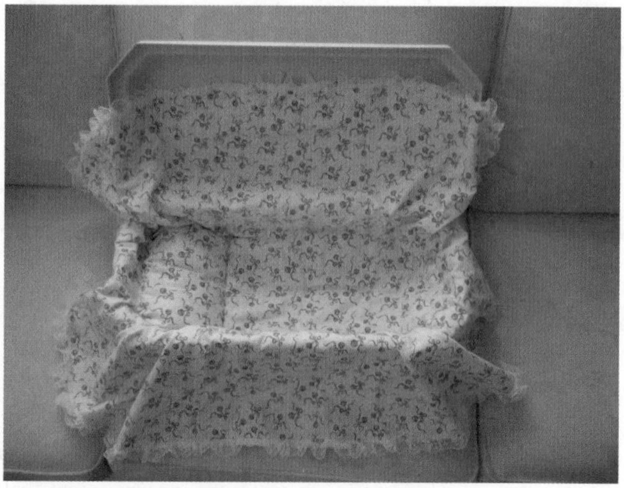

Fig. 23-10 Burial cradle (casket) for newborn infant. (Courtesy Shannon Perry, Phoenix, AZ).

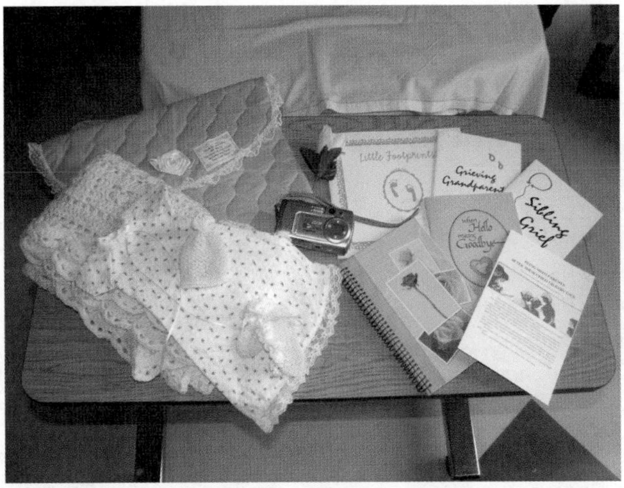

Fig. 23-11 A memory kit assembled at John C. Lincoln Hospital, Phoenix, AZ. Memory kits may include pictures of the infant, clothing, death certificate, footprints, ID bands, fetal monitor printout, and ultrasound picture. (Courtesy Julie Perry Nelson, Gilbert, AZ).

Pictures

Pictures are the most important memento a parent can have. Photographs should be taken whenever there is an identifiable baby. How tiny the baby is, what the baby looks like, or how long the baby has been deceased do not matter.

Pictures can be taken with an instant print camera, as well as with a 35-mm camera. Every effort should be made to make the baby appear special. Pictures should include close-ups of the baby's face, hands, and/or feet. The baby should be clothed or wrapped in a blanket with a hat or gown in some of the pictures and unclothed in other pictures. If there are any congenital anomalies, close-ups of the anomalies should also be taken. Flowers, blocks, stuffed animals, or toys can also be placed in the background to make the picture more special, like a portrait. The parents or siblings may also want to have their picture taken holding the baby. Keeping a camera nearby and taking pictures when parents are spending special time with their baby can provide wonderful memories for later on (Fig. 23-12).

Documentation

Many hospitals have a checklist that is used in providing care, mobilizing members of the multidisciplinary health care team, communicating options the family has chosen, and keeping track of all the details in meeting the needs of bereaved parents (Fig. 23-13). The checklists may or may not be a permanent part of the chart. Documentation in the nursing notes includes primary concerns, grief responses, health teaching, health care advice, and referrals of the mother or any other family members.

Follow-up after Discharge

Follow-up phone calls after a loss occurs are important. The grief of the mother and her family does not end with discharge but really begins once they return home, attend the funeral, and start to live their life without the baby. The calls are made to let the parents know they are still thought of and cared about. The calls are made at predictably difficult times, such as the first week at home; 1 month to 6 weeks later (parents should be invited to attend a support group at this time); 4 to 6 months after the loss; on the due date (for families who experienced a miscarriage, ectopic pregnancy, or death of a premature baby); and/or on the anniversary of the death. The calls are an opportunity for parents to ask questions, share their feelings, seek advice, and receive information to help them in processing their grief.

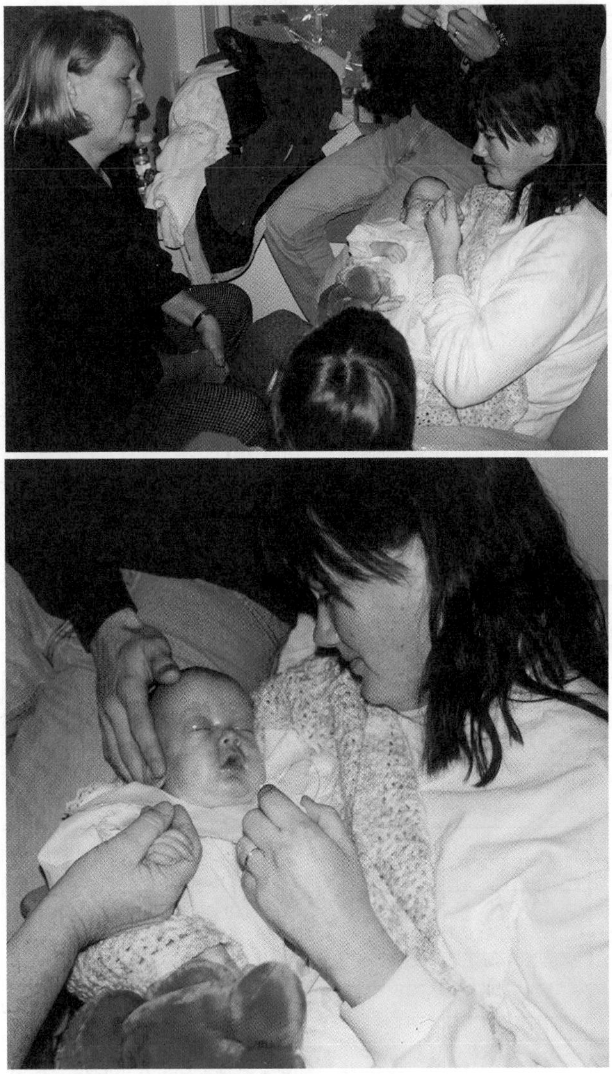

Fig. 23-12 Laura's family members say a special good-bye. (Courtesy Amy and Ken Turner, Cary, NC.)

A grief conference is an opportunity for families to sit down with their health care providers and receive information about the baby's autopsy report or genetic studies, or just to ask questions they have had since their baby's death. Parents appreciate the opportunity to review the events of hospitalization, to go over the baby's and/or mother's chart with their primary health care provider, and to talk with those who cared for them during hospitalization. The grief conference gives health care professionals the opportunity to assess how the family is coping with their loss and to provide additional information/education on grief.

SAMPLE

RTS Bereavement Services
CHECKLIST FOR ASSISTING PARENT(S) EXPERIENCING STILLBIRTH OR NEWBORN DEATH

Mother's discharge date: ______	Age ____ Gr ___ Para ___ L.C. ___ Due date ______
Mother's name: ______	Previous loss: ______
Address: ______	Date/Time delivered: ______
Phone number: ( ) ______	Date/Time death: ______
Father's name: ______	Baby's name: ______ Sex: ______
Address: ______	Children's name(s): ______ Age: ______
Phone number: ( ) ______	______ Age: ______
Optimal call time:	______ Age: ______
RTS Counselor: ______	Support people
Unit: ______ Ext ______	Attending MD &/or Pediatrician
Regular OB MD/Midwife: ______	Notify Peds Nurse Practitioner ______
Religion: ______	

Date	Time		Comments	Initials
		Notify/Assign RTS counselor ☐ Yes ☐ No		
		Pastoral Care notified ☐ Yes ☐ No		
		Funeral Home notified: ☐ Yes ☐ No Family Burial: ☐ Yes ☐ No		
		Saw baby when born and/or after delivery: ☐ Mother ☐ Father		
		Touched and/or held baby: ☐ Mother ☐ Father ☐ Siblings ☐ Grandparents ☐ Friends		
		Offered private time with their baby: ☐ Yes ☐ No		
		Baptism offered: (use seashell as vessel, give to parents) ☐ Yes ☐ No		
		Remembrance of Blessing offered: ☐ Yes ☐ No (can offer for any perinatal loss) ☐ Given to parents		
		Given option to transfer off Maternity Unit: ☐ Yes ☐ No		
		Patient's room flagged with door card ☐ Yes ☐ No		
		Autopsy: ☐ Yes ☐ No Genetic studies: ☐ Yes ☐ No Genetic Associate notified: ☐ Yes ☐ No		
		Regular Physician/Midwife notified of death: ☐ Yes ☐ No Memo sent to Physician/Midwife: ☐ Yes ☐ No		
		Section of Fetal monitor strip: ☐ Given to parents ☐ On file		
		ID Bands/Crib cards/Tape measure: ☐ Given to parents ☐ On file		
		Footprints/Handprints/Weight/Length recorded on "In Memory Of" sheet: ☐ Given to parents ☐ On file		
		Lock of hair offered: (ask permission) ☐ Yes ☐ No ☐ Given to parents ☐ On file		
		Mementos (clothing, hat , blanket, pacifier, crib cards, basin, baby ring, bear, thermometer, silk flower) ☐ Given to parents ☐ On file		
		Complimentary birth keepsake ☐ Given to parents ☐ On file		
		RTS Photos taken: (clothed, unclothed, w. props, family photo) 1) Polaroid - 3 or more ☐ Given to parents ☐ On file 2) 35 mm (6-12 pictures) ☐ Given to parents ☐ On file 3) Medical photos: ☐ Yes ☐ No		

Fig. 23-13 Checklist for assisting parents experiencing stillbirth or newborn death. (Used with permission of Bereavement Services. Copyright Lutheran Hospital–La Crosse, Inc., a Gundersen Lutheran Affiliate, La Crosse, WI.)

Date	Time		Comments	Initials
		Informed about postponing funeral until mother is able to attend: ☐ Yes ☐ No		
		Services/Funeral arrangements, options discussed: ☐ Self-transport ☐ Gravesite service ☐ Visitation ☐ Hospital chapel ☐ Cremation ☐ Funeral home ☐ Burial at foot or head of relative's grave ☐ Specific area for babies in cemetery ☐ Plan own service		
		Funeral arrangements made by: ☐ Mother ☐ Father Discussed: ☐ Seeing baby at funeral home ☐ Taking pictures there ☐ Providing outfit/toy for baby ☐ Dressing baby at funeral home		
		Grief information packet given to: ☐ Mother ☐ Father		
		Discussed grief process/incongruent grief with: ☐ Mother ☐ Father		
		Discussed grief conference: ☐ Yes ☐ No		
		RTS Parents Support Group brochure given to: ☐ Mother ☐ Father		
		RTS business card given to: ☐ Mother ☐ Father		
		Pregnancy & Infant Loss Card sent to RTS secretary: ☐ Yes ☐ No		
		Follow-up calls: 1 week: .... 3 weeks:. .... Due date: .... 6-10 months: .... Anniversary date:		
		Grief conference planned with parents: Date ______ Time ______ Place ______ Letter of confirmation sent: ☐ Yes ☐ No		
		Parent Support Group, first meeting attended: Date: ______ Follow-up meetings attended: Dates ______		
		Would like another parent to call: ☐ Yes ☐ No ☐ Ask later Parent contact: ______		

Forms Needed: Report of fetal death (Photocopy and save for mother.)
Autopsy if ordered
Record of death
Genetics protocol (folder) if ordered
Notice of removal of a human corpse from an institution
Final disposition form
If funeral home involved - Final disposition will be completed by them.
Original certificate of death (for NB death only)

Note: Family Burial - Check with your funeral home.

** You may wish to list your hospital and state forms that are necessary, as required by your state laws and your institution.

Fig. 23-13, cont'd For legend, see opposite page.

MATERNAL DEATH

It is rare for a woman to die in childbirth; the incidence of maternal deaths was 9.8 per 100,000 in 2000 (Minino et al, 2002). The father and extended family, who are faced with not only mourning the death of a wife and mother but also the death of the baby, have a particularly difficult time. On the other hand, the father may be faced with parenting a baby without a surviving mother. Death of a mother disrupts the family structure and leaves the father with the care of a baby at a time when he is greatly distressed. Thus the father and extended family, especially other children and grandparents, need supportive grief counseling at the time of death and following discharge to be able to heal after such a devastating loss.

The nursing care of families at this time is similar to that already described. Options need to be offered, memories made, and mementos obtained and held for the family until they are ready for them. These families are at risk for developing complicated bereavement and altered parenting of the surviving baby and other children in the family. Referral to social services to help the family mobilize support systems, as well as for counseling, can help combat potential problems before they develop and can be beneficial not only at the time of the loss but also in the future.

Critical Thinking Exercise

REDUCING MATERNAL MORTALITY

One of the *Healthy People 2010* objectives is to reduce the maternal mortality rate to no more than 3.3 per 100,000 live births. The maternal mortality rate in the United States was 9.8 in 2000. What is the maternal mortality rate in your community? What efforts are being made in your community to reduce the maternal mortality rate?

1. Evidence–Is there sufficient evidence to draw conclusions about how to reduce the maternal mortality rate?
2. Assumptions–What assumptions can be made about the following factors:
   a. Causes of maternal mortality
   b. Factors associated with increased maternal mortality
   c. Access to prenatal care
   d. Racial disparities in mortality rates.
3. What implications and priorities for nursing care can be drawn at this time?
4. Does the evidence objectively support your conclusion?
5. Are there alternative perspectives to your conclusion?

The emotional toll that a maternal death can take on the nursing and medical staff must also be addressed. Guilt, anger, fear, sadness, and depression are all common responses to a maternal death. The staff may want to review the situation surrounding the events, the medical record, and their responses in the forum of a mortality/morbidity review and a critical incident debriefing to help in coping with the feelings and emotions that result from a maternal death. Attending memorial or funeral services may benefit staff and family.

Evaluation

Evaluation is based on the expected outcomes of care. The plan is revised as needed based on evaluation findings.

Key Points

- Postpartum hemorrhage is the most common and most serious type of excessive obstetric blood loss.
- Hemorrhagic (hypovolemic) shock is an emergency situation in which the perfusion of body organs may become severely compromised and death may ensue.
- The potential hazards of therapeutic interventions may further compromise the woman with hemorrhagic disorders.
- Postpartum infection is a major cause of maternal morbidity and mortality throughout the world.
- Postpartum urinary tract infections are common because of trauma experienced during labor.
- Breast infection affects about 1% of women soon after childbirth.
- Structural disorders of the uterus and vagina related to pelvic relaxation are often the delayed but direct result of childbearing.
- An understanding of grief responses and the bereavement process is fundamental in the implementation of the nursing process.
- Therapeutic communication and counseling techniques can help families in identifying their feelings and in feeling comfortable in expressing their grief.
- Follow-up after discharge is an essential component in providing care to families who have experienced a loss.
- Nurses need to be aware of their own feelings of grief and loss to provide a nonjudgmental environment of care and support for bereaved families.

Answer Guidelines to Critical Thinking Exercise

Reducing Maternal Mortality

1. Causes of maternal mortality are well known and are similar worldwide.
2. (a) The leading causes of maternal mortality are embolism, hemorrhage, and preeclampsia. Ectopic pregnancy is the leading cause of death in the first half of pregnancy. Infection and cardiomyopathy are other causes of maternal death (Chang et al, 2003). (b) Maternal mortality is higher in African-Americans than in Caucasians. Higher maternal mortality is associated with low socioeconomic status, although a cause-effect relationship has not been established. (c) There are racial disparities in access to prenatal care. Women with limited access to care are more likely to experience complications of pregnancy and less likely to seek care for those problems. (d) There are racial disparities in maternal mortality rates with considerably higher rates in African-Americans than in Caucasians. The causes of maternal mortality are multifactorial and racial disparities are not well understood.
3. National and local initiatives to identify causes of complications of pregnancy that result in maternal mortality must be undertaken. Community health nurses can do case finding and work to improve access to care. Education for pregnant women that emphasizes the importance of early prenatal care should be provided. Efforts can be made to influence public policy that supports care for pregnant women. Public health measures to reduce smoking, violence, substance abuse, and other health threats can be supported. Nurses can become involved in political activity in their community and state.
4. Maternal mortality rates have been reduced, although not to the desired level. Approximately 90% of women receive prenatal care. National initiatives and funded research attempt to reduce complications of pregnancy. Research must continue into identifying causes of racial disparities.
5. Increasing the number of health care providers from underrepresented groups and the amount of research into health disparities may improve access to care, compliance with medical regimens and patient education, and may reveal presently unknown causes of maternal mortality and health disparities.

Reference for Answer Guidelines

Chang J et al: Pregnancy-related mortality surveillance—United States, 1991-1999, *MMWR Surveillance Summaries*, 52(SS02):1-8, 2003.

Resources

AAPC
American Association of Pastoral Counselors
www.aapc.org

AHCPR Web site
www.hcfa.gov/medicaid/siq/siqipg/htm

Cherokee Casket Company
P.O. Box 710
Griffin, GA 30223
770-227-4435
800-535-8667
770-229-5356 (fax)
www.cherokeechildcaskets.com
c_casket@bellsouth.net

Growth House, Inc.
Page to grief related to pregnancy, including miscarriage, stillbirth, termination of pregnancy, and neonatal death
www.growthhouse.org

Griefnet
A collection of resources of value to those who are experiencing loss and grief
www.griefnet.org

Hand
Houston's Aid in Neonatal Death: Supporting grieving parents in the greater Houston area with the rest of the world via the Internet
www.hern.org/_hand

Hannah's Prayer
Christian support for fertility challenges
www.hannah.org

Hygeia™
An on-line journal for pregnancy and neonatal loss: Dr. Michael Berman
www.connix.com/_hygeia/

Miscarriage Support and Information Resources
Comprehensive resource list
www.pinelandpress.com/support/miscarriage.html

National Center for Complementary and Alternative Medicine (NCCAM)
PO Box 8218
Silver Spring, MD 20907-8218
888-644-6226
www.nccam.nih.gov

OBGYN.net
List of resources for loss and bereavement
www.obgyn.net/woman/loss/loss.htm

Pen-Parents, Inc.
An international nonprofit support network for bereaved parents
www.penparents.org

A Place to Remember
Uplifting resources for those who have been touched by a crisis in pregnancy or the birth of a baby
www.aplacetoremember.com

Postpartum Support International
927 North Kellog Ave.
Santa Barbara, CA 93111
805-967-7636
www.chss.iup.edu/postpartum

SHARE
Pregnancy and Infant Loss Support, Inc.
www.nationalshareoffice.com

SIDS Network
Sudden infant death syndrome (SIDS) information Web site
www.sids-network.org

The Compassionate Friends
A self-help organization for bereaved parents and siblings
www.compassionatefriends.org

Zerbel's Bay Memorials
321 South 15th Street
Escanaba, MI 49829
906-786-2609
906-786-8148 (fax)
e-mail: allofh@up.net

References

American College of Obstetricians and Gynecologists (ACOG): *Postpartum hemorrhage (ACOG Ed Bull No. 243)*, Washington, DC, 1998, ACOG.

American Psychiatric Association (APA): *Diagnostic and statistical manual of mental disorders,* ed 5, Washington, DC, 2000, American Psychiatric Association Press.

Arias E et al: Annual summary of vital statistics—2002, *Pediatrics* 112(6 pt 1):1215-1230, 2003.

Beal M: Use of complementary and alternative therapies in reproductive medicine, *J Nurse Midwifery* 43(3):224-233,1998.

Beck C: Screening methods for postpartum depression, *J Obstet Gynecol Neonatal Nurs* 24(4):308-312, 1995.

Beck C: Postpartum depression: case studies, research, and nursing care. Washington, DC, 1999, AWHONN.

Beck C: Revision of the postpartum depression predictors inventory, *J Obstet Gynecol Neonatal Nurs* 31(4):394-402, 2002.

Benedetti TJ: Obstetric hemorrhage. In Gabbe SG, Niebyl JR, Simpson JL (eds): *Obstetrics: normal and problem pregnancies,* ed 4, New York, 2002, Churchill Livingstone.

Bowes WA, Thorp JM: Clinical aspects of normal and abnormal labor. In Creasy RK, Resnick R, Iams JD (eds): *Maternal-fetal medicine: principles and practice,* ed 5, Philadelphia, 2004, Saunders.

Brucker M: Management of the third stage of labor: an evidence-based approach, *J Midwifery Women's Health* 46(6): 381-392, 2001.

Cowles KV: Cultural perspectives of grief: an expanded concept analysis, *J Adv Nurs* 23:287-294, 1996.

Cox JL, Holden JM, Sagovsky R: Detection of postnatal depression: development of the 10-item Edinburgh Postnatal Depression Scale, *Br J Psychiatry* 150:782-786, 1987.

Cunningham FG et al: *Williams obstetrics,* ed 21, Stamford, CT, 2001, Appleton & Lange.

Czarapata BJ, McKillips KJ: Silent suffering: helping women find the path to continence, *AWHONN Lifelines* 1(2):28-34, 1997.

Duff P: Maternal and perinatal infection. In Gabbe SG, Niebyl JR, Simpson JL (eds): *Obstetrics: normal and problem pregnancies, ed 4,* New York, 2002, Churchill Livingstone.

French L, Smaill F. Antibiotic regimens for endometritis after delivery (Cochrane Review), 2004. In *The Cochrane Library*, Issue 1. Oxford, 2005, Update Software.

Gibbs RS, Sweet RL, Duff WP: Maternal and fetal infectious disorders. In Creasy RK, Resnick R, Iams JD, (eds): *Maternal-fetal medicine: principles and practice,* ed 5, Philadelphia, 2004, WB Saunders.

Gold L: Postpartum disorders in primary care: diagnosis and treatment, *Prim Care 29*(1):27-41, 2002.

Gonik B, Foley MR: Intensive care monitoring of the critically ill pregnant patient. In Creasy RK, Resnick R, Iams JD (eds): *Maternal-fetal medicine: principles and practice,* ed 5, Philadelphia, 2004, Saunders.

Hebert MP: Perinatal bereavement in its cultural context, *Death Stud* 22(1):61-78, 1998.

Herrick H: *Postpartum depression: who gets help?* Statistical Brief No. 24, Raleigh, NC, 2002, US Department of Health and Human Services.

Hostetler D, Bosworth M: Uterine inversion: a life-threatening obstetric emergency, *J Am Board Fam Practice* 13(2):120-123, 2000.

Kaplan H, Sadock B: *Synopsis of psychiatry,* ed 8, Baltimore, 2000, Williams & Wilkins.

Kilpatrick SJ, Laros RK: Maternal hematologic disorders. In Creasy RK, Resnick R, Iams JD, (eds): *Maternal-fetal medicine: principles and practice,* ed 5, Philadelphia, 2004, Saunders.

Kowalski K: *Perinatal death: an ethnomethodological study of factors influencing perinatal bereavement,* Unpublished doctoral dissertation, Denver, 1984, University of Colorado.

Laros RK: Thromboembolic disease. In Creasy RK, Resnick R, Iams JD (eds): *Maternal-fetal medicine: principles and practice,* ed 5, Philadelphia, 2004, Saunders.

Lindemann E: Symptomatology and management of acute grief, *Am J Psychiatry* 101:141-148, 1944.

Lockwood CJ, Silver RM: Thrombophilias in pregnancy. In Creasy RK, Resnick R, Iams JD (eds): *Maternal-fetal medicine: principles and practice,* ed 5, Philadelphia, 2004, Saunders.

Maley B: Creating a postpartum depression support group: out of the blue, *AWHONN Lifelines* 6(1):62-65, 2002.

Miles M: Helping adults mourn the death of a child. In Wass H, Corr C (eds): *Children and death,* Washington, DC, 1984, Hemisphere Publishing.

Miles M, Demi A: Guilt in bereaved parents. In Rando T (ed): *Parental loss of a child: clinical and research considerations,* Champaign, IL, 1986, Research Press.

Miles M, Demi A: Historical and contemporary theories of grief. In Corless I, Germino B, Pittman-Lindemann M (eds): *Dying, death and bereavement,* Boston, MA, 1997, Jones & Bartlett.

Minino AM et al: Deaths: final data for 2000, *Natl Vital Stat Rep,* 50(15):1-119, 2002.

Mousa HA, Walkinshaw S: Major postpartum haemorrhage, *Curr Opin Obstet Gynecol* 13(6):595-603, 2001.

Parkes C: *Bereavement: studies of grief in adult life,* New York, 1972, International Universities Press.

Parkes C, Weiss R: *Recovery from bereavement,* New York, 1983, Basic Books.

Roque H, Funai R, Lockwood C: von Willebrand disease and pregnancy, *J Matern Fetal Med* 9(5):257-266, 2000.

Sampselle CM et al: Continence for women: evidence-based practice, *J Obstet Gynecol Neonatal Nurs* 26(4):375-385, 1997.

Sampselle CM et al: Continence for women: a test of AWHONN's evidence-based protocol in clinical practice, *J Obstet Gynecol Neonatal Nurs* 29(1):18-26, 2000.

Schirmer G: *Herbal medicine,* Bedford TX, 1998, MED2000 Inc.

Stenchever MA et al: *Comprehensive gynecology,* ed 4, St Louis, 2001, Mosby.

Stowe J, Strader J, Nemeroff C: Psychopharmacology during pregnancy and lactation. In Schartzberg A, Nemeroff C (eds), *Essentials of clinical psychopharmacology*. Washington, DC, 2001, American Psychiatric Publishing, Inc.

Straub H et al: Proactive nursing: the evolution of a task force to help women with postpartum depression, *MCN Am J Matern Child Nurs* 23(5):262-265, 1998.

Strozewski S: Von Willebrand's disease: what you need to know about this inherited bleeding disorder, *Am J Nurs* 100(2):24AA-24DD, 2000.

Tiran D, Mack S (eds): *Complementary therapies for pregnancy and childbirth,* ed 2, Edinburgh, 2000, Bailliere Tindall.

Varner MW: Medical conditions of the puerperium, *Clin Perinatol* 25(2):403-416, 1998.

Weed S: *Wise woman herbal for the childbearing years,* Woodstock, NY, 1986, Ash Tree Publishing Co.

Weiss N, Bernstein P: Risk factor scoring for predicting venous thromboembolism in obstetric patients, *Am J Obstet Gynecol* 182(5):1073-1075, 2000.

Worden W: *Grief counseling and grief therapy: a handbook for the mental health practitioner,* New York, 1991, Springer.

Physiologic Adaptations of the Newborn 24

LEARNING OBJECTIVES

On completion of this chapter the reader will be able to:

- Describe the changes in the biologic system of the neonate during the transition to extrauterine life.
- Describe the sequence to follow in assessment of the newborn.
- Recognize deviations from normal physiologic findings during examination of the newborn.
- Compare and contrast the four types of heat loss in a neonate and describe how to prevent heat loss.
- Describe the behavioral adaptations of the newborn, including periods of reactivity and sleep-wake states.
- Describe the sensory and perceptual functioning of the neonate.

ELECTRONIC RESOURCES

Additional information related to the content in Chapter 24 can be found on

the companion website at evolve
http://evolve.elsevier.com/Wong/maternal/
- NCLEX Review Questions
- Case Study–Newborn Health Problems
- WebLinks

or the interactive student CD-ROM
Activities for Chapter 24 include the following:
- NCLEX Review Questions
- Anatomy Review–Sutures and Fontanels
- Case Study–Newborn Health Problems
- Nursing Care Plan–Immediate Care of Newborn
- Skill–Thermoregulation

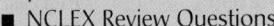

The neonatal period includes the time from birth through the twenty-eighth day of life. By term gestation, the fetus's various anatomic and physiologic systems have reached a level of development and functioning that permits a separate existence from the mother. At birth the newborn infant manifests behavioral competencies and a readiness for social interaction. These adaptations set the stage for future growth and development.

TRANSITION TO EXTRAUTERINE LIFE

Newborns undergo phases of instability during the first 6 to 8 hours after birth. These phases collectively are termed the transition period between intrauterine and extrauterine existence. The first phase of the transition period lasts up to 30 minutes after birth and is called the first period of reactivity. The newborn's heart rate increases rapidly to 160 to 180 beats/min but gradually falls by 30 minutes to a baseline rate between 100 to 120 beats/min. Respirations are irregular, with a rate between 60 and 80 breaths/min. Crackles may be present on auscultation; audible grunting, nasal flaring, and retractions of the chest may also be noted but these should cease within the first hour of birth. The infant is alert and may have spontaneous startles, tremors, crying, and movement of the head from side to side. Bowel sounds are audible and meconium may be passed.

After the first period of reactivity, the newborn either sleeps or has a marked decrease in motor activity. This period of unresponsiveness, often accompanied by sleep, lasts from 60 to 100 minutes and is followed by a second period of reactivity.

The second period of reactivity occurs roughly between 4 and 8 hours after birth and lasts from 10 minutes to several hours. Brief periods of tachycardia and tachypnea occur, associated with increased muscle tone, skin color changes, and mucous production. Meconium is commonly passed at this time. Most healthy newborns experience this transition regardless of type of birth; extremely and very preterm infants do not because of physiologic immaturity.

Physiologic Adjustments

Respiratory System

With the cutting of the umbilical cord, the infant undergoes rapid and complex physiologic changes. The most critical and immediate adjustment a newborn makes at birth is the establishment of respirations. With a vaginal birth some lung fluid is squeezed from the newborn's trachea and lungs; in infants who are born by cesarean birth some lung fluid may be retained within the alveoli. With the first breath of air, the newborn begins a dynamic sequence of cardiopulmonary changes.

Initial breathing is probably the result of a reflex triggered by pressure changes, exposure to cool air temperature, noise, light, and other sensations related to the birth process. In addition, the chemoreceptors in the aorta and carotid bodies initiate neurologic reflexes when arterial oxygen pressure (PO_2) falls, arterial carbon dioxide pressure (PCO_2) rises, and arterial pH falls. In most cases an exaggerated respiratory reaction follows within 1 minute of birth, and the infant takes the first gasping breath and cries.

Once respirations are established, they are shallow and irregular, ranging from 30 to 60 breaths per minute, with periods of periodic breathing that include pauses in respirations lasting less than 20 seconds. These episodes of periodic breathing occur most often during the active (rapid eye movement [REM]) sleep cycle and decrease in frequency and duration with age. Apneic periods lasting 20 seconds or longer are an indication of a pathologic process and should be carefully evaluated.

Signs of Respiratory Distress

Most term infants breathe spontaneously and continue to have normal respiratory patterns. Signs of respiratory distress may include nasal flaring, intercostal or subcostal retractions (i.e., drawing in of tissue between the ribs, or below the rib cage), or grunting with respirations. Suprasternal or subclavicular retractions with stridor or gasping most often represents an upper airway obstruction (Askin, 2003). Seesaw or paradoxical respirations instead of abdominal respirations are abnormal and should be reported. A respiratory rate less than 30 or greater than 60 breaths/min with the infant at rest must be carefully evaluated. The respiratory rate can be negatively influenced (slowed, depressed, or absent) by analgesics or anesthetics administered to the mother during birth. Apneic episodes may be related to a number of events (rapid increase in body temperature, hypothermia, hypoglycemia, and sepsis) that require careful evaluation. Tachypnea may result from inadequate clearance of lung fluid, or it may be an indication of newborn respiratory distress syndrome.

Maintaining Adequate Oxygen Supply

During the first hour of life the pulmonary lymphatics continue to remove large amounts of fluid. Removal of fluid is also a result of the pressure gradient from alveoli to interstitial tissue to blood capillary. Reduced vascular resistance accommodates this flow of lung fluid. Retention of lung fluid may interfere with the infant's ability to maintain adequate oxygenation, especially if other factors (meconium aspiration, congenital diaphragmatic hernia, esophageal atresia with fistula, choanal atresia, congenital cardiac defect, immature alveoli [absent or decreased]) that compromise respirations, are present.

The newborn's chest circumference is approximately 30 to 33 cm at birth. Auscultation of the chest of a newborn infant reveals loud, clear breath sounds that seem very near because there is less chest wall musculature. The ribs of the infant articulate with the spine at a horizontal rather than a downward slope; consequently, the rib cage cannot expand with inspiration as readily as an adult's. Because neonatal respiratory function is largely a matter of diaphragmatic contraction, abdominal breathing is characteristic of newborns. That is, the newborn infant's chest and abdomen rise simultaneously with inspiration, but because of the large size of the abdomen, chest movement is not as visible.

The outer walls of the alveoli are lined with surfactant, a protein manufactured in type II cells of the lungs. Lung expansion is largely dependent on chest wall contraction and adequate presence and secretion of surfactant. Surfactant lowers surface tension, thereby requiring less inspiratory pressure to keep the alveoli open with inspiration, and prevents total alveolar collapse on exhalation, thus maintaining alveolar stability. With absent or decreased surfactant, more pressure must be generated for inspiration, which may soon tire or exhaust preterm or sick term infants. Surfactant may be compared with soapy water on the surface of a group of inflated latex balloons: as air is let out of the balloons (exhalation phase), the soapy water prevents total collapse of the balloons, and conversely, inflation of the balloons occurs readily because of decreased tension (friction) on their surfaces.

Cardiovascular System

The cardiovascular system changes significantly after birth. The infant's first breaths, combined with increased alveolar capillary distention, inflate the lungs and reduce pulmonary vascular resistance to pulmonary blood flow from the pulmonary arteries. Pulmonary artery pressure drops and pressure in the right atrium declines. Increased pulmonary blood flow from the left side of the heart increases pressure in the left atrium, which causes a functional closure of the foramen ovale. During the first few days of life, crying may reverse the flow through the foramen ovale temporarily and lead to mild cyanosis.

In utero, fetal PO_2 is 27 mm Hg. After birth, when the PO_2 level in the arterial blood approximates 50 mm Hg, the ductus arteriosus constricts in response to increased oxygenation. Circulating hormone prostaglandin (PGE_2) levels also have an important role in closure of the ductus arteriosus. Later, the ductus arteriosus occludes and becomes a ligament. With the clamping of the cord, the umbilical arteries, umbilical vein, and ductus venosus close and are converted into ligaments. The hypogastric arteries also occlude and become ligaments.

Heart Rate and Sounds

The heart rate averages 120 to 140 beats/min at birth, with variations noted during sleeping and waking states (Bernstein, 2004). Shortly after the first cry the infant's heart rate may be as high as 175 to 180 beats/min. The range of the heart rate in the full-term newborn is 80 to 90 beats/min during sleep and up to 170+ beats/min while awake. It is not unusual to find a heart rate of 180 beats/min when the infant cries. A heart rate that is either consistently high (>170 beats/min) or low (<80 beats/min) with the newborn at rest should be reevaluated within an hour or when the activity of the infant changes (Bernstein, 2004).

The apical impulse (point of maximal impulse [PMI]) in the newborn is at the fourth intercostal space and to the left of the midclavicular line. The PMI is often visible because of the thin chest wall; this is also called precordial activity.

Apical pulse rates should be obtained on all infants. Auscultation should be for a full minute, preferably when the infant is asleep. An irregular heart rate in newborns is not uncommon in the first few hours of life. After this time an irregular heart rate not attributed to changes in activity or respiratory pattern should be further evaluated.

Heart sounds during the neonatal period are of higher pitch, shorter duration, and greater intensity than during adult life. The first sound (S_1) is typically louder and duller than the second sound (S_2), which is sharp. The third and fourth heart sounds are not auscultated in newborns. Most heart murmurs heard during the neonatal period have no pathologic significance, and more than half of the murmurs disappear by 6 months. However, the presence of a murmur and accompanying signs such as poor feeding, apnea, cyanosis, or pallor are considered abnormal and should be further investigated.

Blood Pressure

The newborn infant's average systolic blood pressure (BP) is 60 to 80 mm Hg, and the average diastolic pressure is 40 to 50 mm Hg. The blood pressure varies from day to day during the first month of life. A drop in systolic blood pressure (about 15 mm Hg) in the first hour of life is common. Crying and movement usually cause increases in the systolic blood pressure. The measurement of BP is best accomplished with an oscillometric device while the infant is at rest. A correctly sized cuff must be used for accurate measurement of an infant's BP. Unless there is a specific indication, blood pressure is not usually measured in the newborn on a routine basis except as a baseline.

Blood Volume

Blood volume in the newborn is about 80 to 85 ml/kg of body weight. Immediately after birth the total blood volume averages 300 ml, but this volume can increase by as much as 100 ml, depending on the length of time to cord clamping and cutting. The infant born prematurely has a relatively greater blood volume than the term newborn. This occurs because the preterm infant has a proportionately greater plasma volume, not a greater red blood cell (RBC) mass.

Early or late clamping of the cord changes circulatory dynamics of the newborn. Late clamping expands the blood volume from the so-called placental transfusion of blood to the newborn. Late cord clamping may result in polycythemia with subsequent clinical signs of hyperviscosity (hematocrit $\geq$ 65%, plethoric or ruddy red appearance, sluggish circulation leading to possible emboli in the microvasculature and organ damage, respiratory distress, and possibly hyperbilirubinemia as a result of red cell breakdown) (Armentrout & Huseby, 2003; Gordon, 2003). There is considerable controversy regarding the timing of cord clamping in the delivery of healthy term newborns and the clinical advantages and disadvantages of the practice.

Hematopoietic System

The hematopoietic system of the newborn exhibits certain variations from that of the adult. Levels of RBCs and leukocytes differ, but platelets levels are relatively the same.

Red Blood Cells and Hemoglobin

At birth the average levels of RBCs and hemoglobin (fetal hemoglobin is predominant) are higher than those in the adult. Cord blood of the term newborn may have a hemoglobin concentration from 14 to 24 g/dl (mean 17 g/dl). The hematocrit ranges from 44% to 64% (mean 55%). The RBC count is correspondingly elevated, ranging from 4.8 to 7.1/mm^3. These values fall and reach the average levels of 11 to 17 g/dl and 4.2 to 5.2/mm^3, respectively, by the end of the first month. The blood values may be affected by delayed clamping of the cord, which results in a rise in hemoglobin, RBCs, and hematocrit. The source of the sample is a significant factor because capillary blood yields higher values than venous blood. When the neonate's blood sample is obtained is also significant; the slight rise in RBCs after birth is followed by a substantial drop. At birth the infant's blood contains about 80% fetal hemoglobin, but because of the shorter life span of the cells containing fetal hemoglobin, the percentage falls to 55% by 5 weeks and to 5% by 20 weeks. Iron stores generally are sufficient to sustain normal RBC production for 4 to 5 months in the term infant, at which time a physiologic anemia that is usually transient may occur.

Leukocytes

Leukocytosis, with a white blood cell (WBC) count of approximately 18,000 per mm^3 (range 9,000 to 30,000 per mm^3), is normal at birth. The number of WBCs increases to 23,000 to 24,000/mm^3 during the first day after birth. The initial high WBC count of the newborn decreases rapidly, and a resting level of 11,500/mm^3 is normally maintained during the neonatal period. Serious infection is not well tolerated by the newborn; leukocytes are slow to recognize foreign protein and to localize and fight infection early in life. Sepsis may be accompanied by a concomitant rise in WBCs (neutrophilia); however, some infants may present with clinical signs of sepsis without a significant elevation in WBCs. In addition, events other than infection—vigorous crying, maternal hypertension, hypoglycemia, hemolytic disease, meconium aspiration syndrome, labor induction with oxytocin, difficult labor, and maternal fever—may cause neutrophilia in the newborn (Weinberg & Powell, 2001).

Platelets

Platelet count ranges between 200,000 and 300,000/mm^3 and is essentially the same in newborns as in adults. The levels of factors II, VII, IX, and X, found in the liver, are decreased during the first few days of life because the newborn cannot synthesize vitamin K. However, bleeding tendencies in the newborn are uncommon, and unless the vitamin K deficiency is great, clotting is sufficient to prevent hemorrhage.

Blood Groups

The infant's blood group is genetically determined and established early in fetal life. However, during the neonatal period there is a gradual increase in the strength of the agglutinogens present in the RBC membrane. Cord blood samples may be used to identify the infant's blood type and Rh status.

Thermogenic System

Next to establishing respirations and adequate circulation, heat regulation is most critical to the newborn's survival. Thermoregulation is the maintenance of balance between heat loss and heat production. Newborns attempt to stabilize their core body temperatures within a narrow range. Hypothermia from excessive heat loss is a common and dangerous problem in neonates. The newborn's ability to produce heat (thermogenesis) often approaches that of the adult; however, the tendency toward rapid heat loss in a cold environment is increased in the newborn and poses a hazard.

SKILL—THERMOREGULATION

Thermogenesis

The shivering mechanism of heat production is rarely operable in the newborn. Nonshivering thermogenesis is accomplished primarily by brown fat, which is unique to the newborn, and secondarily by increased metabolic activity in the brain, heart, and liver. Brown fat is located in superficial deposits in the interscapular region and axillae, as well as in deep deposits at the thoracic inlet, along the vertebral column, and around the kidneys. Brown fat has a richer vascular and nerve supply than ordinary fat. Heat produced by intense lipid metabolic activity in brown fat can warm the neonate by increasing heat production as much as 100%. Reserves of brown fat, usually present for several weeks after birth, are rapidly depleted with cold stress. The less mature the infant, the less reserve of this essential fat is available at birth.

Heat Loss

Heat loss in the newborn occurs by four modes:

1. *Convection* is the flow of heat from the body surface to cooler ambient air. Because of heat loss by convection, the ambient temperature in the nursery is kept at approximately 24°C and newborns in open bassinets are wrapped to protect them from the cold.
2. *Radiation* is the loss of heat from the body surface to a cooler solid surface not in direct contact but in relative proximity. To prevent this type of loss, cribs and examining tables are placed away from outside windows and care is taken to avoid direct air drafts.
3. *Evaporation* is the loss of heat that occurs when a liquid is converted to a vapor. In the newborn, heat loss by evaporation occurs as a result of vaporization of moisture from the skin. This heat loss is intensified by failure to dry the newborn directly after birth or by drying the infant too slowly after a bath. The less mature the newborn, the more severe the evaporative heat loss. Evaporative heat loss, as a component of insensible water loss, is the most significant cause of heat loss in the first few days of life.
4. *Conduction* is the loss of heat from the body surface to cooler surfaces in direct contact. When admitted to the nursery, the newborn is placed in a warmed crib to minimize heat loss. The scales used for weighing the newborn should have a protective cover to minimize conductive heat losses as well.

Loss of heat must be controlled to protect the infant. Control of such modes of heat loss is the basis of caregiving policies and techniques. One method for promoting maternal-newborn interaction is to place the naked healthy newborn next to the mother's skin and cover both with a blanket. This skin-to-skin contact enhances newborn temperature control and interaction (see Evidence-Based Practice box).

Temperature Regulation

Anatomic and physiologic differences among the newborn, child, and adult are notable. The newborn's ability to produce heat initially is less than that of an adult; the blood vessels are closer to the surface of the skin. Newborns have larger body surface to body weight (mass) ratios than children and adults. The flexed position of the newborn helps guard against heat loss because it diminishes the amount of body surface exposed to the environment. Infants can also reduce the loss of internal heat through the body surface by constricting peripheral blood vessels.

Cold stress imposes metabolic and physiologic problems on all infants, regardless of gestational age and condition. The respiratory rate increases in response to the increased need for oxygen. In the cold-stressed infant, oxygen consumption and energy are diverted from maintaining normal brain cell and cardiac function and growth to thermogenesis for survival. If the infant cannot maintain an adequate oxygen tension, vasoconstriction follows and jeopardizes pulmonary perfusion. As a consequence, the partial pressure of arterial oxygen (PaO_2) is decreased, and the blood pH drops. These changes may prompt a transient respiratory distress or may aggravate existing respiratory distress syndrome (RDS). Moreover, decreased pulmonary perfusion and oxygen tension may maintain or reopen the right-to-left shunt across the patent ductus arteriosus.

The basal metabolic rate increases with cold stress (Fig. 24-1). If cold stress is protracted, anaerobic glycolysis occurs, resulting in increased production of acids. Metabolic acidosis develops, and if a defect in respiratory function is present, respiratory acidosis also develops. Excessive fatty acids may displace the bilirubin from the albumin-binding sites and exacerbate hyperbilirubinemia. Another metabolic consequence of cold stress is hypoglycemia. The process of anaerobic glycolysis utilizes approximately three to four times the amount of blood glucose, thereby depleting existing stores; if the infant is sufficiently stressed and low glucose stores are not replaced, hypoglycemia, which can be asymptomatic in the newborn, may ensue.

Hyperthermia develops more rapidly in the newborn than in the adult because of decreased ability to increase

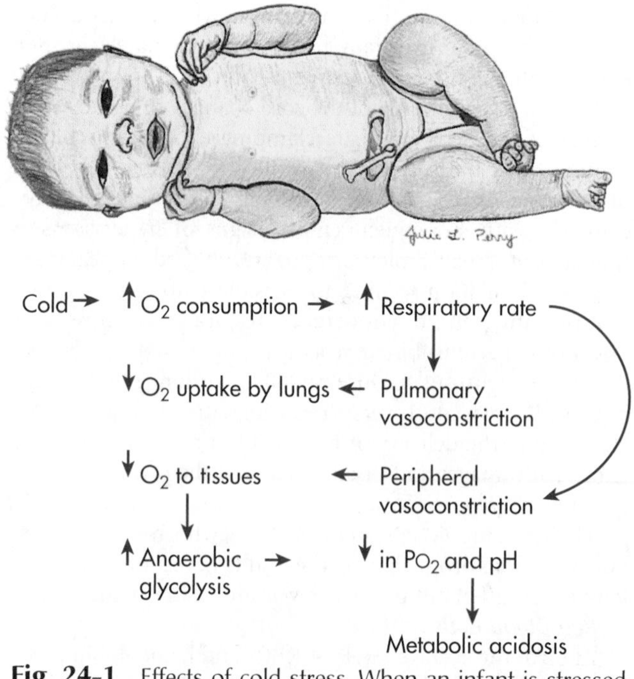

Fig. 24-1 Effects of cold stress. When an infant is stressed by cold, oxygen consumption increases and pulmonary and peripheral vasoconstriction occur, thereby decreasing oxygen uptake by the lungs and oxygen to the tissues; anaerobic glycolysis increases; and there is a decrease in PO_2 and pH, leading to metabolic acidosis.

Evidence-Based Practice

EARLY MATERNAL SKIN-TO-SKIN CONTACT WITH HEALTHY INFANTS

Background

Early, continuous maternal-infant contact after birth is our evolutionary norm. Until comparatively recently, separation of mothers and infants at birth was routine within the Western medical model. For the mother, touch, warmth, and odor are vagal stimulants that release oxytocin, which increases social responsiveness, decreases anxiety, and increases the temperature around the breasts. The newborn in his first awake-alert period has a heightened response to maternal smell. During the sensitive minutes and hours after birth, close contact primes the synchronicity between mother and infant. Skin-to-skin contact (SSC) for more than 50 minutes after birth leads to an eightfold increase in spontaneous nursing and may be a critical component regarding breastfeeding success. Mothers of premature infants benefit from SSC by improved bonding and confidence, and thus duration of breastfeeding is increased. (See "Kangaroo Care for Low-Birth-Weight Infants," Evidence-Based Practice box in Chapter 28).

Objectives

Reviewers sought to examine whether early SSC results in beneficial or adverse maternal and infant outcomes. Specific outcomes to be examined included:

1. Breastfeeding duration and problems
2. Maternal bonding and attachment behaviors (en face [eye-to-eye contact while being held], kissing, smiling, holding, and encompassing)
3. Maternal psychologic changes (anxiety, self-efficacy, parenting competence)
4. Infant physiologic changes (temperature, respiratory rate, heart rate, and blood glucose)
5. Infant behavioral changes (crying and grimacing)
6. Other outcomes, such as length of stay, cost, and long-term morbidity

Methods

Search Strategy

The reviewers searched MEDLINE and Cochrane Central Register of Controlled Trials (CENTRAL). Search keywords were *baby, infant, newborn, neonate, infant care, mother-child relations, mothers, maternal behavior, infant behavior, neonatal, nursing, breastfeeding, lactation, monitoring physiologic, heart rate, respiration, skin temperature, object attachment, touch, therapeutic touch, early contact, immediate contact, kangaroo,* and *skin-to-skin.* Reviewers selected 17 studies, involving a total of 806 women from both upper and lower socioeconomic classes. The studies, dating from 1977 to 1999, were from Canada, Guatemala, Spain, Sweden, Taiwan, and the United States. All were controlled trials. The intervention was some protocol for SSC, with the naked or diapered infant placed on the mother's chest, and covered with a warmed blanket. The controls received standard postpartum care. Sixteen studies used random assignments, while one was quasi-random (assignment not based on patient or clinician preference).

Statistical Analyses

Reviewers performed meta-analyses of studies with comparable outcomes. The reviewers then compared outcomes to see if the outcomes influenced each other.

Findings

There seemed to be a "golden two hours" from immediate postbirth for maximum benefit. Spontaneous, effective suckling occurred at about 55 minutes and lasted through the following hour. More effective suckling was associated with long-term breastfeeding success. Significantly less breast engorgement occurred in the SSC group than with standard care. The SSC group was twice as likely as controls to still be breastfeeding at 3 months. Breastfeeding was also more likely in the SSC group at 1 year, but not significantly so. The benefits to breastfeeding were significant even if SSC was delayed by up to 24 hours, but they were most notable when SSC was instituted immediately after birth. Mothers in the SSC group showed significantly more maternal attachment behavior than controls. Studies found that mothers in the SSC group practiced more affectionate love touch during breastfeeding at 36 to 48 hours, kissed the infant more at 3 months, and increased enface, holding and touching—effects that persisted up to a year later. Newborns in the SSC group had significantly higher temperatures, with less variability, and remained in the thermo-neutral zone. Blood glucose was significantly higher and respiratory rate was significantly lower in the SSC group, demonstrating conservation of energy. Heart rate was also decreased with SSC, but not significantly. Infants in the SCC group showed significantly less crying and grimacing than the controls. This is important for the preterm infant, for whom crying causes hypoxemia, fluctuating cerebral blood flow and risk for hemorrhage, intracranial pressure, and wasted calories.

Limitations

It would be difficult to blind a randomization such as SSC from the staff and patient. Measured outcomes in the studies varied, making comparison challenging. Protocols also varied. Some SSC was initiated immediately, whereas in other studies SSC was delayed as long as 24 hours. Infant physiologic measurements were done on examination tables instead of in the SSC intervention.

Conclusions

By all measures studied, SSC was a beneficial intervention for maternal and infant well-being. No adverse effects of SSC were noted. Our evolutionary norm is strengthened.

Implications for Practice

In particular, SSC during the "golden two hours" immediately after birth seems to strengthen bonding and increase success and duration of breastfeeding. Infant physiology is also more favorable with SSC. Effective latching on and early bonding can strengthen the confidence and decrease the anxiety of a new mother.

Implications for Further Research

More research on SSC effects with preterm and cesarean births would be useful. There is a need to standardize the measures in future trials, especially of maternal emotional well-being and attachment behaviors.

Reference

Anderson G et al: Early skin-to-skin contact for mothers and their healthy newborn infants (Cochrane Review), 2003. In *The Cochrane Library,* Issue 2, Chichester, UK, 2004, John Wiley & Sons.

evaporative skin water losses. Although newborn infants have 6 times as many sweat glands per unit area as adults, in most newborns these glands do not function sufficiently to allow the infant to sweat. Serious overheating of the newborn can cause cerebral damage from dehydration or heat stroke and death.

Renal System

At term the kidneys occupy a large portion of the posterior abdominal wall. The bladder lies close to the anterior abdominal wall and is an abdominal as well as a pelvic organ. In the newborn almost all palpable masses in the abdomen are renal in origin.

At birth, a small quantity (approximately 40 ml) of urine is usually present in the bladder of a full-term infant. The frequency of voiding varies from 2 to 6 times per day during the first and second days of life and from 5 to 25 times during the subsequent 24 hours. About 6 to 8 voidings per day of pale straw-colored urine are indicative of adequate fluid intake. Generally, term infants void 15 to 60 ml of urine per kilogram per day.

Full-term newborns have limited capacity to concentrate urine; therefore, the specific gravity ranges from 1.001 to 1.020. The ability to concentrate urine fully is attained by about 3 months of age. After the first voiding the infant's urine may appear cloudy (because of mucous content) and have a much higher specific gravity. This decreases as fluid intake increases. Normal urine during early infancy is usually straw-colored and almost odorless. Sometimes pink-tinged uric crystal stains appear on the diaper; these stains are normal.

Loss of fluid through urine, feces, lungs, increased metabolic rate, and limited fluid intake results in a 5% to 7% loss of the birth weight. This usually occurs over the first 3 to 5 days of life. If the mother is breastfeeding and her milk supply has not come in yet (which occurs by the third or fourth day after birth), the neonate is somewhat protected from dehydration by its increased extracellular fluid volume. The neonate should regain the birth weight within 10 to 14 days depending on the feeding method.

Because renal thresholds are low in the infant, bicarbonate concentration and buffering capacity are decreased. This may lead to acidosis and electrolyte imbalance.

Fluid and Electrolyte Balance

About 40% of the body weight of the newborn is extracellular fluid. Each day the newborn takes in and excretes roughly 600 to 700 ml of water, which is 20% of the total body fluid or 50% of the extracellular fluid. The glomerular filtration rate (GFR) of a newborn is about 30% to 50% that of an adult. This results in a decreased ability to remove nitrogenous and other waste products from the blood. However, the newborn's ingested protein is almost totally metabolized for growth.

Sodium reabsorption is decreased as a result of a lowered sodium and potassium-activated adenosine triphosphate (ATPase) activity. The decreased ability to excrete excessive sodium results in hypotonic urine compared with plasma. There is a higher concentration of sodium, phosphates, chloride, and organic acids and a lower concentration of bicarbonate ions. The infant has a higher renal threshold for glucose.

Gastrointestinal System

The full-term newborn is capable of swallowing, digesting, metabolizing, absorbing proteins and simple carbohydrates, and emulsifying fats. With the exception of pancreatic amylase, the characteristic enzymes and digestive juices are present even in low-birth-weight neonates.

In the adequately hydrated infant, the mucous membrane of the mouth is moist and pink; the hard and soft palates are intact. The presence of moderate to large amounts of mucus is common in the first few hours after birth. Small whitish areas (Epstein's pearls) may be found on the gum margins and at the juncture of the hard and soft palate. The cheeks are full because of well-developed sucking pads. These, like the labial tubercles (sucking calluses) on the upper lip, disappear around the age of 12 months, when the sucking period is over.

Even though in utero sucking motions have been recorded by ultrasound, these motions are not coordinated with swallowing in any infant born before 32 to 33 weeks of gestation. Sucking behavior is influenced by neuromuscular maturity, maternal medications received during labor and birth, and the type of initial feeding.

A special mechanism present in healthy term newborns coordinates the breathing, sucking, and swallowing reflexes necessary for oral feeding. Sucking in the newborn takes place in small bursts of three or four sucks at a time. The infant is unable to move food from the lips to the pharynx; therefore, placing the nipple (breast or bottle) well inside the baby's mouth is necessary. Peristaltic activity in the esophagus is uncoordinated in the first few days of life. It quickly becomes a coordinated pattern in healthy full-term infants and they swallow easily.

Teeth begin developing in utero with enamel formation continuing until about 10 years of age. Tooth development is influenced by neonatal or infant illnesses, medications, and illnesses of or medications taken by the mother during pregnancy. The fluoride level in the water supply also influences tooth development. Occasionally an infant may be born with one or more teeth.

Bacteria are not present in the infant's gastrointestinal tract at birth. Soon after birth, oral and anal orifices permit entrance of bacteria and air. Generally the highest bacterial concentration is found in the lower portion of the intestine, particularly in the large intestine. Normal colonic bacteria are established within the first week after birth, and normal intestinal flora help synthesize vitamin K, folate, and biotin. Bowel sounds can usually be heard shortly after birth.

Stomach capacity varies from 30 to 90 ml, depending on the size of the infant. Emptying time for the stomach is highly variable. Several factors, such as time and volume of feedings or type and temperature of food, may affect the emptying time. The cardiac sphincter and nervous control of the stomach are immature, so some regurgitation may occur. Regurgitation during the first day or two of life can be decreased by avoiding overfeeding, by burping the infant, and by positioning the infant with the head slightly elevated.

Digestion

The infant's ability to digest carbohydrates, fats, and proteins is regulated by the presence of certain enzymes. Most of these are functional at birth. One exception is amylase, produced by the salivary glands after about 3 months and by the pancreas at about 6 months of age. This enzyme is necessary to convert starch into maltose. The other exception is lipase, which is also secreted by the pancreas; it is necessary for the digestion of fat. Thus the normal newborn is capable of digesting simple carbohydrates and proteins, but has a limited ability to digest fats.

Further digestion and absorption of nutrients occurs in the small intestine in the presence of pancreatic secretions, secretions from the liver through the common bile duct, and secretions from the duodenal portion of the small intestine.

Stools

At birth the lower intestine is filled with meconium. Meconium is formed during fetal life from the amniotic fluid and its constituents, intestinal secretions (including bilirubin), and cells (shed from the mucosa). Meconium is greenish black and viscous and contains occult blood. The first meconium passed is usually sterile, but within hours all meconium passed contains bacteria. The majority of normal term infants pass meconium within 12 hours of life, and almost all do so by 24 hours. The number of stools passed varies during the first week, being most numerous between the third and sixth days. Newborns fed early pass stools sooner. Progressive changes in the stooling pattern indicate a properly functioning gastrointestinal tract (Box 24-1).

Hepatic System

The liver and gallbladder are formed by the fourth week of gestation. In the newborn the liver can be palpated about 1 cm below the right costal margin because it is enlarged and occupies about 40% of the abdominal cavity. The infant's liver plays an important role in iron storage, carbohydrate metabolism, conjugation of bilirubin, and coagulation.

Iron Storage

The fetal liver, which serves as the site for production of hemoglobin after birth, begins storing iron in utero. The infant's iron store is proportional to total body hemoglobin content and length of gestation. At birth the term neonate has an iron store sufficient to last 4 to 6 months; the preterm infant's iron stores are depleted sooner.

Carbohydrate Metabolism

At birth the newborn is cut off from its maternal glucose supply and, as a result, experiences an initial decrease in serum glucose levels. The newborn's increased energy needs, decreased hepatic release of glucose from glycogen stores, increased RBC volume, and increased brain size may initially contribute to the rapid depletion of stored glycogen within the first 24 hours after birth. In most healthy term newborns, blood glucose levels stabilize at 50 to 60 mg/dl during the first several hours after birth; by the third day of life, the blood glucose levels should be approximately 60 to 70 mg/dl. The initiation of feedings assists in the stabilization of the newborn's blood glucose levels.

Jaundice

Jaundice is the manifestation of the pigment bilirubin in the tissues of the body. Jaundice usually does not appear until the bilirubin level reaches 5 mg/dl. Any visible jaundice within the first 24 hours of life or persistence of jaundice beyond 7 to 10 days requires further investigation into the cause as this represents an underlying pathologic process (Fig. 24-2). See Chapter 25 for a further discussion of bilirubin metabolism and hyperbilirubinemia.

Coagulation

Coagulation factors, which are synthesized in the liver, are activated by vitamin K. The lack of intestinal bacteria needed to synthesize vitamin K results in transient blood coagulation deficiency between the second and fifth days of life. The administration of intramuscular vitamin K shortly after birth helps prevent clotting problems.

Immune System

The cells that provide the infant with immunity are developed early in fetal life; however, they are not activated for weeks to months. For the first 3 months of life, the infant is somewhat protected by passive immunity received from the mother. The membrane-protective IgA is missing from the respiratory and urinary tracts and, unless the newborn is breastfed, is also absent from the gastrointestinal tract. The infant begins to synthesize IgG, and levels reach about 40% of adult levels by 1 year of age. Significant amounts of IgM are produced at birth, and adult levels are reached by 9 months of age. The production of IgA, IgD, and IgE is much more gradual, and maximum levels are not attained until early childhood. The infant who is breastfed receives passive immunity through the colostrum and breast milk.

BOX 24-1

Changes in Stooling Patterns of Newborns

Meconium

Infant's first stool; composed of amniotic fluid and its constituents, intestinal secretions, shed mucosal cells, and possibly blood (ingested maternal blood or minor bleeding of alimentary tract vessels).

Passage of meconium should occur within the first 24 to 48 hours, although it may be delayed up to 7 days in very low-birth-weight infants.

Transitional Stools

Usually appear by third day after initiation of feeding; greenish brown to yellowish brown, thin, and less sticky than meconium; may contain some milk curds.

Milk Stool

Usually appears by fourth day.

In *breastfed infants,* stools are yellow to golden, are pasty in consistency, and have an odor similar to that of sour milk.

In *formula-fed infants,* stools are pale yellow to light brown, are firmer in consistency, and have a more offensive odor.

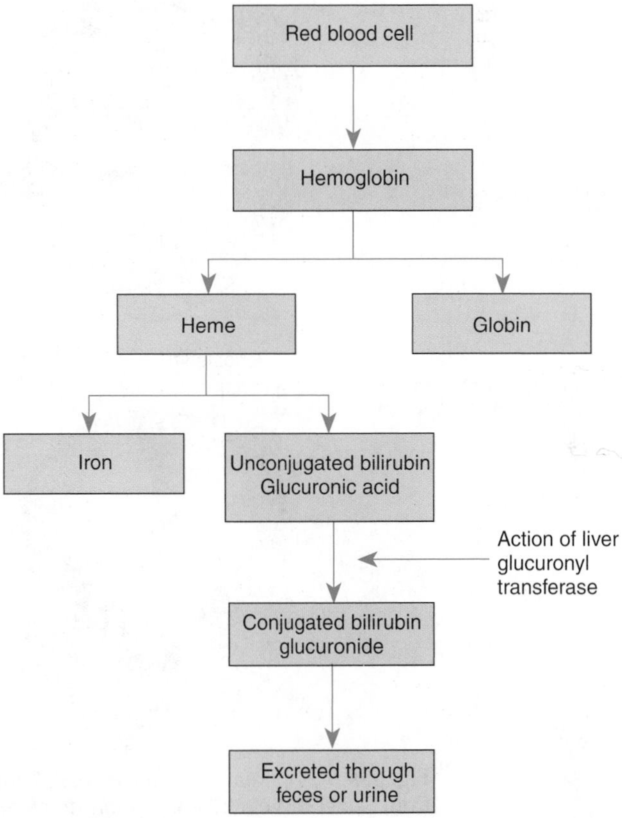

Fig. 24-2 Formation and excretion of bilirubin.

Integumentary System

All skin structures are present at birth. The epidermis and dermis are bound loosely and are very thin. Vernix caseosa (a cheeselike whitish substance) is fused with the epidermis and serves as a protective covering. The infant's skin is very sensitive and can be easily damaged. The term infant has an erythematous (red) skin for a few hours after birth, after which it fades to its normal color. The skin often appears blotchy or mottled, especially over the extremities. The hands and feet appear slightly cyanotic (acrocyanosis); this is caused by vasomotor instability and capillary stasis. Acrocyanosis is normal and appears intermittently over the first 7 to 10 days, especially with exposure to cold.

> **Family Focus**
>
> **NEWBORN SKIN**
>
> A young couple with a healthy newborn girl calls the nurse because they are concerned about the small raised red dots on the baby's face and arms and that her skin is dry and flaky in certain places. The nurse assesses the newborn and draws the conclusion that the spots are not mosquito bites as the family stated but erythema toxicum. What further anticipatory guidance about normal newborn skin appearance could the nurse give the parents to reassure them that the newborn is healthy and "normal"?

The healthy term infant usually has a plump appearance because of large amounts of subcutaneous tissue and extracellular water content. Subcutaneous fat accumulated during the last trimester acts as insulation. Fine lanugo hair may be noted over the face, shoulders, and back. Edema of the face and ecchymosis (bruising) may be noted as a result of face presentation, forceps-assisted birth, or vacuum extraction (see Family Focus box).

Creases can be found on the palms of the hands. The simian line, a single palmar crease, is often found in Asian infants or in infants with Down syndrome

Caput Succedaneum

Caput succedaneum is a generalized, easily identifiable edematous area of the scalp, most commonly found on the occiput (Fig. 24-3, *A*). The sustained pressure of the presenting vertex against the cervix results in compression of local vessels, thereby slowing venous return. The slower venous return causes an increase in tissue fluids within the skin of the scalp, and an edematous swelling develops. This edematous swelling, present at birth, extends across the suture lines of the skull and disappears spontaneously within 3 to 4 days. Infants who are born with the assistance of vacuum extraction usually have a caput in the area where the cup was applied.

Cephalhematoma

Cephalhematoma is a collection of blood between a skull bone and its periosteum. Therefore a cephalhematoma does

evolve CASE STUDY—NEWBORN HEALTH PROBLEMS

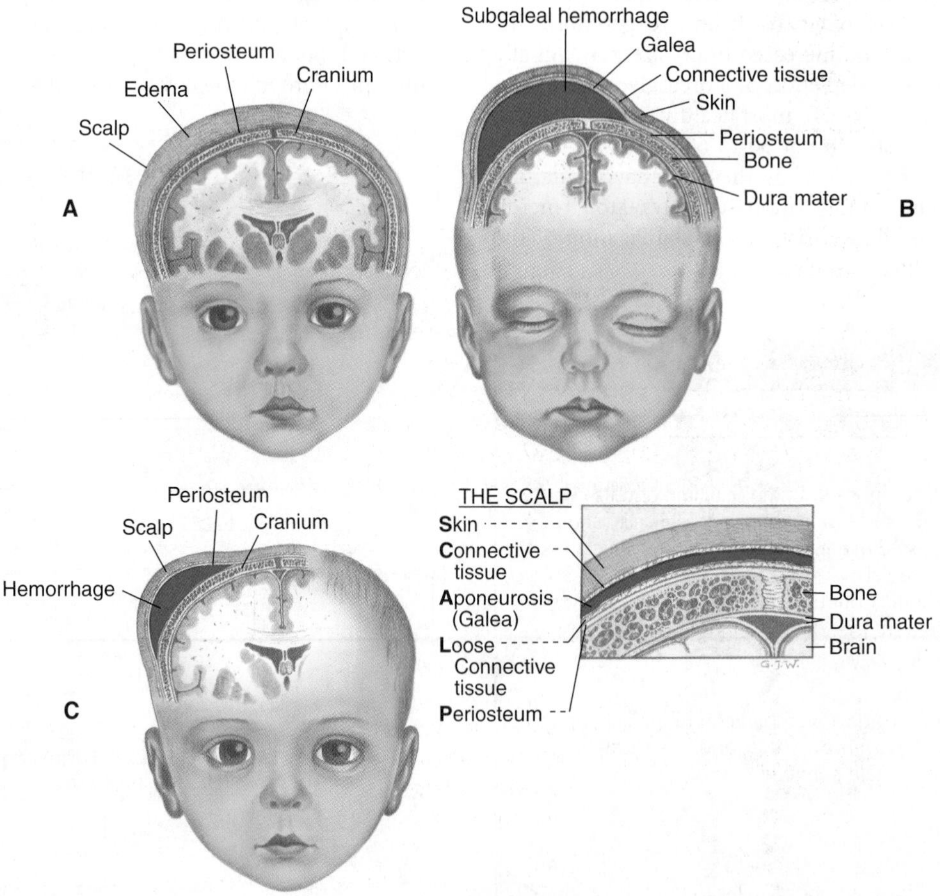

Fig. 24-3 **A**, Caput succedaneum. **B**, Subgaleal hemorrhage. **C**, Cephalhematoma (**A** and **B** from Seidel HM et al: *Mosby's guide to physical examination,* ed 5, St Louis, 2003, Mosby.)

not cross a cranial suture line (Fig. 24-3, *C*). Often caput succedaneum and cephalhematoma occur simultaneously.

Bleeding may occur with spontaneous birth from pressure against the maternal bony pelvis. Low forceps birth and difficult forceps rotation and extraction may also cause bleeding. This soft, fluctuating, irreducible fullness does not pulsate or bulge when the infant cries. It appears several hours or the day after birth and may not become apparent until a caput succedaneum is absorbed. A cephalhematoma is usually largest on the second or third day, by which time the bleeding stops (see Family Focus box). The fullness of a cephalhematoma spontaneously resolves in 3 to 6 weeks. It is not aspirated because infection may develop if the skin is punctured. As the hematoma resolves, hemolysis of RBCs occurs and jaundice may result. Hyperbilirubinemia and jaundice may occur from a cephalhematoma after the newborn is discharged home.

Subgaleal Hemorrhage

Subgaleal hemorrhage is bleeding into the subgaleal compartment (Fig. 24-3, *B*). The subgaleal compartment is a potential space that contains loosely arranged connective tissue; it is located beneath the galea aponeurosis, the tendinous sheath that connects the frontal and occipital muscles and forms the inner surface of the scalp. The injury occurs as a result of forces that compress and then drag the head through the pelvic outlet (Paige & Carney, 2002). There have been reports of concern regarding the increased use of the vacuum extractor at birth and an association with cases of subgaleal hemorrhage, neonatal morbidity, and deaths (Garas et al, 2001; Ross, Fresquez, & El-Haddad, 2001; Uchil & Arulkumaran, 2003). The bleeding extends beyond bone, often posteriorly into the neck, and continues after birth, with the potential for serious complications such as anemia or hypovolemic shock.

Early detection of the hemorrhage is vital; serial head circumference measurements and inspection of the back of the neck for increasing edema and a firm mass are essential. A boggy scalp, pallor, tachycardia, and increasing head circumference may also be early signs of a subgaleal hemorrhage (Putta & Spencer, 2000). Computerized tomography or magnetic resonance imaging is useful in confirming the diagnosis. Replacement of lost blood and clotting factors is required in acute cases of hemorrhage. Another possible early sign of subgaleal hemorrhage is a forward and lateral positioning of the newborn's ears because the hematoma extends posteriorly. Monitoring the infant for changes in level of consciousness and a decrease in the hematocrit are also key to early recognition and management. An increase in serum bilirubin levels may be seen as a result of the degradating blood cells within the hematoma.

> ## Family Focus
>
> **SWELLING ON THE SCALP**
>
> A 2-day-old healthy newborn has a "bump" on the left side of the head. The mother is very concerned that the baby may have somehow fallen out of the crib and sustained an injury to the head. Nursing assessment reveals that the scalp swelling is raised and soft to the touch but does not cross cranial suture lines; there is no apparent bruising or discoloration. The neurologic assessment reveals no significant findings and the newborn's behavior appears to be that of a healthy term infant. How could the nurse explain the condition and reassure the mother that her newborn has a common finding rather than an abnormal condition requiring immediate medical attention?

Sweat Glands

Sweat glands are present at birth but do not respond to increases in ambient or body temperature. Some fetal sebaceous gland hyperplasia and secretion of sebum result from the hormonal influences of pregnancy. Vernix caseosa is a product of the sebaceous glands. Removal of the vernix is followed by desquamation of the epidermis in most infants. Distended, small, white sebaceous glands, noticeable on the newborn face, are known as milia.

Desquamation

Desquamation (peeling) of the skin of the term infant does not occur until a few days after birth. Large generalized areas of skin desquamation present at birth may be an indication of postmaturity.

Mongolian Spots

Mongolian spots, bluish-black areas of pigmentation, may appear over any part of the exterior surface of the body, including the extremities. They are more commonly noted on the back and buttocks (Fig. 24-4). These pigmented areas are most frequently noted in newborns whose ethnic origins are in the Mediterranean area, Latin America, Asia, or Africa. They are more common in dark-skinned individuals, but may occur in 5% to 13% of Caucasians as well (Blackburn, 2003). They fade gradually over months or years.

Nevi

Known as "stork bites," telangiectatic nevi are pink and easily blanched (Fig. 24-5, *A*). They appear on the upper eyelids, nose, upper lip, lower occiput bone, and nape of the neck. They have no clinical significance and fade between the first and second year of life.

A red mark, or nevus vasculosus, is a common type of capillary hemangioma. It consists of dilated, newly formed capillaries occupying the entire dermal and subdermal layers with associated connective tissue hypertrophy. The typical lesion is a raised, sharply demarcated, bright or dark red, rough-surfaced swelling; as the infant grows the heman-

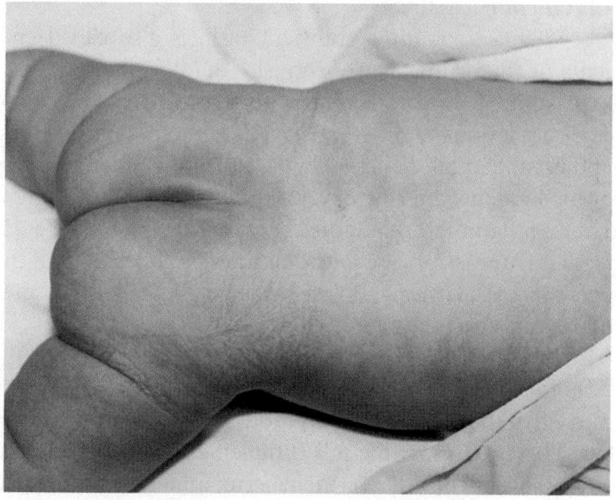

Fig. 24-4 Mongolian spot.

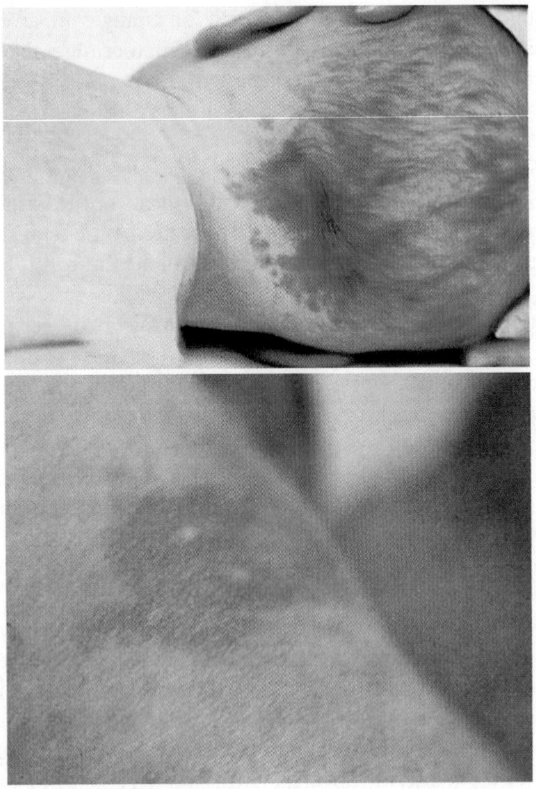

A

B

Fig. 24-5 **A**, Telangiectatic nevus (stork bite). **B**, Erythema toxicum. (Courtesy Mead Johnson & Co., Evansville, IN.)

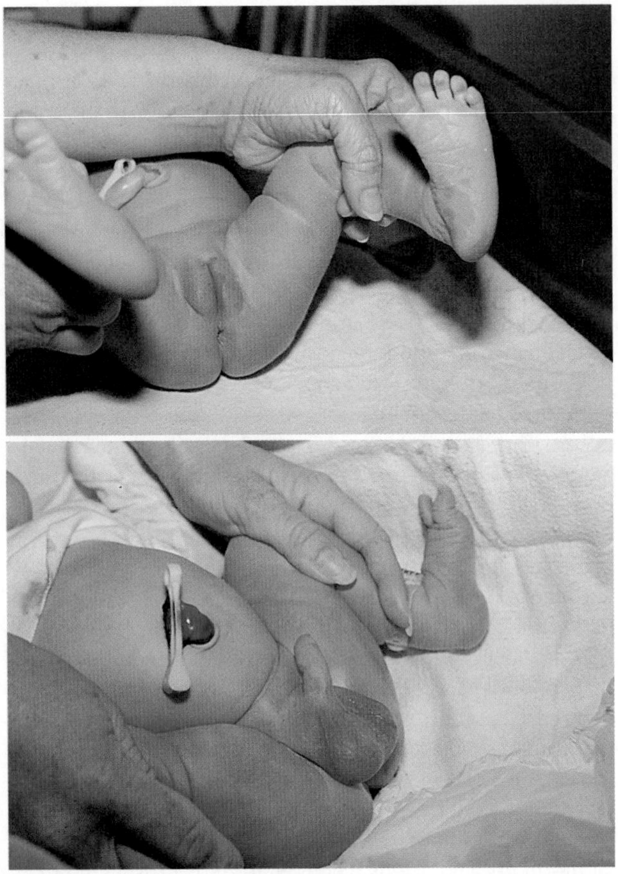

A

B

Fig. 24-6 External genitalia. **A**, Genitalia in female term infant. **B**, Genitalia in uncircumcised male infant. Rugae cover scrotum, indicating term gestation. Cord has been swabbed with ethylene blue to prevent infection. (Courtesy Marjorie Pyle, RNC, Lifecircle, Costa Mesa, CA.)

gioma may proliferate and become more vascular, thereby often being referred to as a strawberry hemangioma. Lesions are usually single but may be multiple, with 75% occurring on the head. These lesions can remain until the child is of school age or sometimes even longer but can be removed successfully with pulsed dye laser therapy, interferon therapy, and prednisone administration.

A port-wine stain, or nevus flammeus, is usually observed at birth and is composed of a plexus of newly formed capillaries in the papillary layer of the corium. It is red to purple; varies in size, shape, and location; and is not elevated. True port-wine stains do not blanch on pressure or disappear. They are most commonly found on the face and neck.

Erythema Toxicum

Erythema toxicum, a transient rash, is also called erythema neonatorum, "newborn rash," or "flea bite" dermatitis. It is found in term neonates during the first 3 weeks of age. It has lesions in different stages: erythematous macules, papules, and small vesicles (Fig. 24-5, *B*). The lesions may appear suddenly anywhere on the body. The rash is thought to be an inflammatory response. Eosinophils, which help decrease inflammation, are found in the vesicles. Although the appearance is alarming, the rash has no clinical significance and requires no treatment.

Reproductive System

Female

At birth the ovaries contain thousands of primitive germ cells. These represent the full complement of potential ova; no oogonia form after birth in term infants. The ovarian cortex, which is made up primarily of primordial follicles, occupies a larger portion of the ovary in the female newborn than in the adult. From birth to sexual maturity, the number of ova decreases by approximately 90%.

An increase in estrogen during pregnancy, followed by a drop after birth, results in a mucoid vaginal discharge and even some slight bloody spotting (pseudomenstruation). External genitals (i.e., labia majora and minora) are usually edematous, with increased pigmentation. In term neonates, the labia majora and minora cover the vestibule (Fig. 24-6, *A*). In preterm infants the clitoris is prominent and the labia majora are small and widely separated. Vaginal or hymenal tags are common findings and have no clinical significance. Vernix caseosa may be present between the labia and should not be forcibly removed during bathing.

If the female was born in the breech position, the labia may be edematous and bruised. The edema and bruising resolve in a few days; no treatment is necessary.

Male

The testes descend into the scrotum by birth in 90% of newborn boys. Although this percentage drops with premature birth, by 1 year of age the incidence of undescended testes in all males is less than 1%.

A tight prepuce (foreskin) is common in newborns. The urethral opening may be completely covered by the prepuce, which may not be retractable for 3 to 4 years. Smegma, a white cheesy substance, is commonly found under the foreskin. Small, white, firm cysts called epithelial pearls may be seen at the tip of the prepuce. In the preterm male of less than 28 weeks of gestation, the testes remain within the abdominal cavity and the scrotum appears high and close to the body. By 28 to 36 weeks of gestation, the testes can be palpated in the inguinal canal, and a few rugae appear on the scrotum. At 36 to 40 weeks of gestation, the testes are palpable in the upper scrotum and rugae appear on the anterior portion. After 40 weeks, the testes can be palpated in the scrotum and rugae cover the scrotal sac. The postterm neonate has deep rugae and a pendulous scrotum. The scrotum is usually more deeply pigmented than the rest of the skin (see Fig. 25-8, *B*) and is especially apparent in darker-skinned infants. This pigmentation is a response to maternal estrogen. A hydrocele, caused by an accumulation of fluid around the testes, may be found. This can be transilluminated with a light and usually decreases in size without treatment.

If the male infant is born in a breech presentation, the scrotum is edematous and may be bruised (see Fig. 28-2). The swelling and discoloration subside within a few days.

Swelling of Breast Tissue

Swelling of the breast tissue in term infants of both sexes is caused by the hyperestrogenism of pregnancy. In a few infants a thin discharge (witch's milk) can be seen. This finding has no clinical significance, requires no treatment, and subsides within a few days as the maternal hormones are eliminated from the infant's body.

The nipples should be symmetric on the chest. Breast tissue and areola size increase with gestation. The areola appears slightly elevated at 34 weeks of gestation. By 36 weeks a breast bud of 1 to 2 mm is palpable and increases to 12 mm by 42 weeks.

Skeletal System

The infant's skeletal system undergoes rapid development during the first year of life. At birth, more cartilage is present than ossified bone. Because of cephalocaudal (head-to-rump) development, the newborn looks somewhat out of proportion.

The head at term is one fourth of the total body length. The arms are slightly longer than the legs. In the newborn the legs are one third of the total body length but only 15% of the total body weight. As growth proceeds, the midpoint in head-to-toe measurements gradually descends from the level of the umbilicus at birth to the level of the symphysis pubis at maturity.

The face appears small in relation to the skull. The skull appears large and heavy. Cranial size and shape can be distorted by molding (the shaping of the fetal head by overlapping of the cranial bones to facilitate movement through the birth canal during labor) (Fig. 24-7).

The bones in the vertebral column of the newborn form two primary curvatures, one in the thoracic region and one in the sacral region. Both are forward, concave curvatures. As the infant gains head control, at approximately 3 months of age, a secondary curvature appears in the cervical region.

In some newborn infants, there is a significant separation of the knees when the ankles are held together, resulting in an appearance of bowlegs. At birth, there is no apparent arch to the foot. The extremities should be symmetric and of equal length. Skin folds should be equal and symmetric. The hips are checked for dysplasia by a trained clinician using

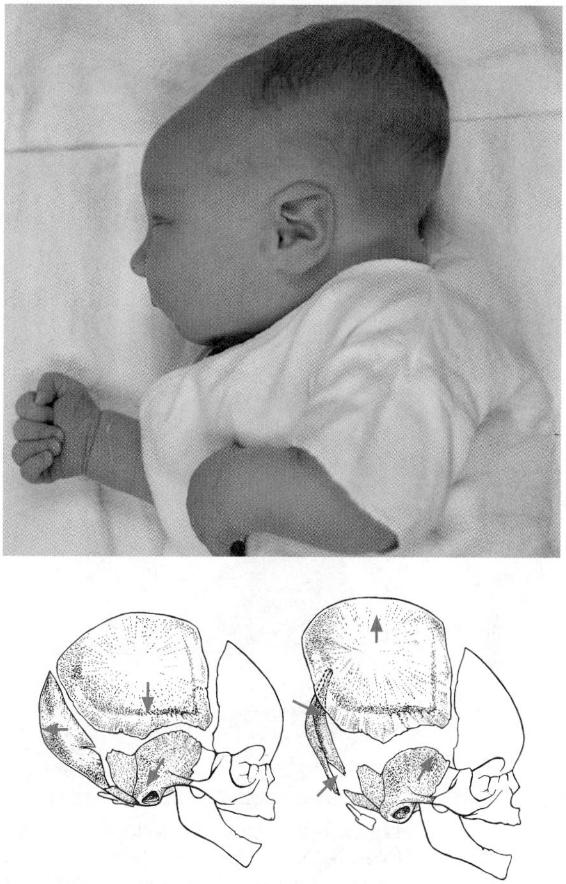

A

B

Fig. 24-7 Molding. **A,** Significant molding after vaginal birth. **B,** Schematic of bones of skull when molding is present. (**A,** Courtesy Kim Molloy, Knoxville, IA.)

Ortolani's maneuver (Fig. 24-8). Fingers and toes should be equal in number and have nails. Extra digits (polydactyly) are sometimes found on the hands and feet. Fingers or toes may be fused (syndactyly). Creases can be found on the palms of the hands and cover the soles of the term newborn's feet. If the infant's presentation was breech, the knees may remain extended and the infant will maintain the in utero position for several weeks.

Two reflexes are elicited, the grasp and the Babinski. To elicit the grasp reflex, touching the palms of the hands or soles of the feet near the base of the digits causes flexion or grasping (Fig. 24-9). To elicit the *Babinski reflex,* stroke the outer sole of the foot upward from the heel across the ball of the foot, which causes the big toe to dorsiflex and the other toes to hyperextend (Table 24-1, p. 705).

The newborn's spine appears straight and can be flexed easily. The vertebrae should appear straight and flat. The base of the spine should be free from a dimple. If a dimple is noted, further inspection is required to determine whether a sinus is present. A pilonidal dimple, especially with a sinus along with a nevus pilosis (hairy nevus), may be associated with spina bifida.

Neuromuscular System

The neuromuscular system is almost completely developed at birth. The term newborn is a vital, responsive, and reactive being with a remarkable capacity for social interaction and self-organization.

ANATOMY REVIEW—SUTURES AND FONTANELS

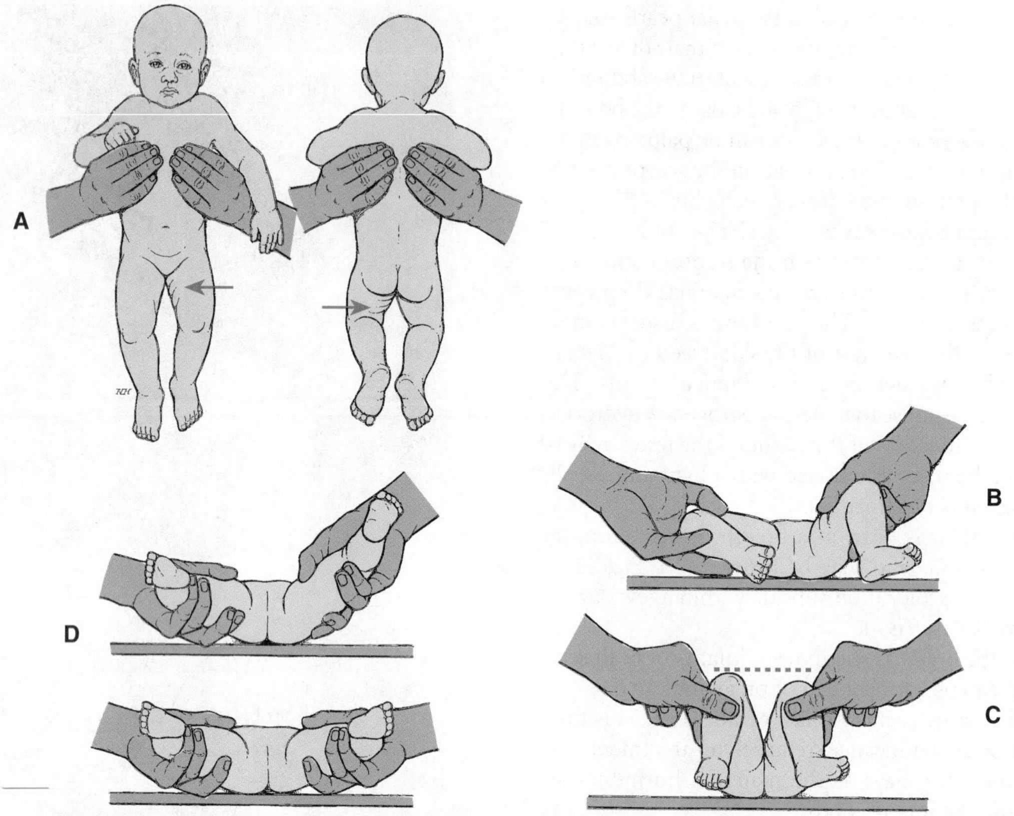

Fig. 24-8 Signs of developmental dysplasia of the hip. **A,** Asymmetry of gluteal and thigh folds. **B,** Limited hip abduction, as seen in flexion. **C,** Apparent shortening of the femur, as indicated by the level of the knees in flexion. **D,** Ortolani click (if infant is under 4 weeks of age). (From Hockenberry et al: *Wong's nursing care of infants and children*, ed 7, St. Louis, 2003, Mosby.)

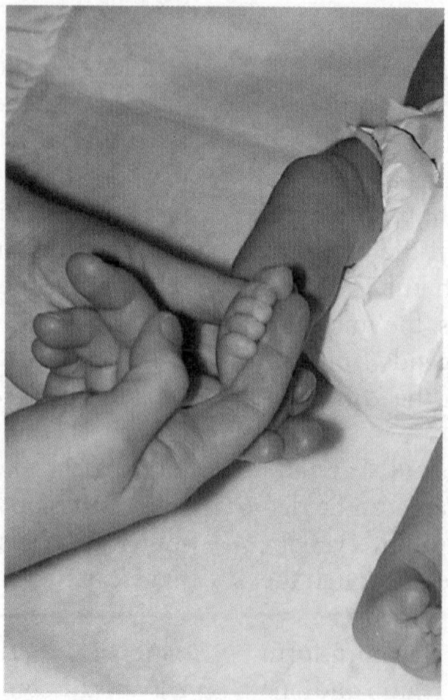

Fig. 24-9 Plantar grasp reflex. (From Zitelli BJ, Davis HW: *Atlas of pediatric physical diagnosis,* ed 4, St Louis, 2002, Mosby.)

Growth of the brain after birth follows a predictable pattern of rapid growth during infancy and early childhood; growth becomes more gradual during the remainder of the first decade and minimal during adolescence. The cerebellum ends its growth spurt, which began at about 30 gestational weeks, by the end of the first year.

The brain requires glucose as a source of energy, and a relatively large supply of oxygen for adequate metabolism. Such requirements signal a need for careful assessment of the infant's respiratory status. The necessity for glucose requires attentiveness to those neonates who are at risk for hypoglycemia (e.g., infants of diabetic mothers, infants

Text continued on p. 707.

Table 24-1

Assessment of Newborn Reflexes

REFLEX	ELICITING THE REFLEX	CHARACTERISTIC RESPONSE	COMMENTS
Rooting	Touch infant's lip, cheek, or corner of mouth with nipple or finger.	Infant turns head toward stimulus and opens mouth. State dependent (i.e., if infant is in deep sleep, reflex may not be elicited)	Response is difficult if not impossible to elicit after infant has been fed; if response is weak or absent, consider prematurity or neurologic defect. Parental guidance: Avoid trying to turn head toward breast or nipple, allow infant to root; response disappears after 3 to 4* mo but may persist up to 1 yr.
Sucking	Elicit rooting reflex as above. May also be elicited by gently stroking tongue with nipple	Infant opens mouth and begins to suck on nipple. A gloved finger may be used to elicit and evaluate suck. State dependent (i.e., if infant is in deep sleep, reflex may not be elicited).	See above.
Swallowing	Feed infant, swallowing usually follows sucking and obtaining fluids.	Swallowing is usually coordinated with sucking and breathing and usually occurs without gagging, coughing, apnea, or vomiting.	If response is weak or absent, this may indicate prematurity, effects of maternal analgesics, or illness that needs investigation. Sucking, swallowing and breathing are often uncoordinated in preterm infant.
Grasp Palmar Plantar (see Fig. 24-9)	Place finger in palm of hand. Place finger at base of toes.	Infant's fingers curl around examiner's fingers, toes curl downward.	Palmar response lessens by 3 to 4 mo, parents enjoy this contact with infant; plantar response lessens by 8 mo.
Extrusion	Touch or depress tip of tongue.	Newborn forces tongue outward.	Response disappears about fourth to fifth month of life
Glabellar (Myerson)	Tap over forehead, bridge of nose, or maxilla of newborn whose eyes are open.	Newborn blinks for first four or five taps.	Continued blinking with repeated taps is consistent with extrapyramidal signs.
Tonic neck or "fencing"	With infant in a supine neutral position, turn head to one side.	With infant facing left side, arm and leg on that side extend; opposite arm and leg flex (turn head to right, and extremities assume opposite postures).	Responses in leg are more consistent. Complete response disappears by 3 to 4 mo, incomplete response may be seen until third or fourth year. After 6 wk, persistent response is sign of an abnormality.

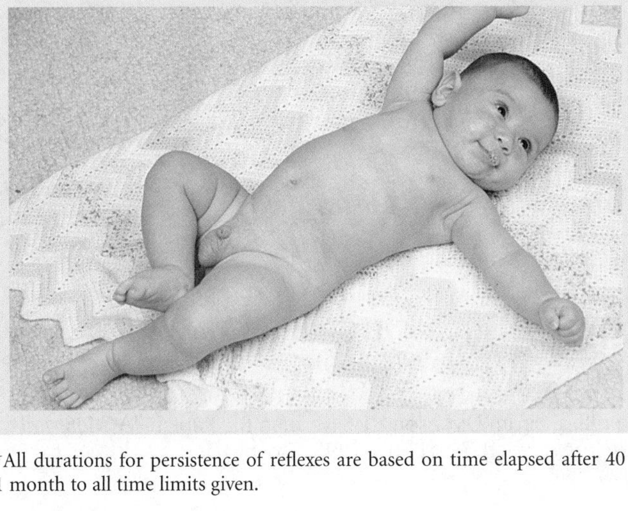

Classic pose in tonic neck reflex. (Courtesy Marjorie Pyle, RNC, Lifecircle, Costa Mesa, CA.)

*All durations for persistence of reflexes are based on time elapsed after 40 weeks of gestation, that is, if newborn was born at 36 weeks of gestation, add 1 month to all time limits given.

Continued

Table 24-1

Assessment of Newborn Reflexes—cont'd

REFLEX	ELICITING THE REFLEX	CHARACTERISTIC RESPONSE	COMMENTS
Moro (or startle)	Hold infant in semisitting position, allow head and trunk to fall backward (with support). Place infant on flat surface, make a loud abrupt noise. State dependent.	Symmetric abduction and extension of arms are seen; fingers fan out and form a C with thumb and forefinger; slight tremor may be noted; arms are adducted in embracing motion and return to relaxed flexion and movement. A cry may accompany or follow motor movement. Legs may follow similar pattern of response. Preterm infant does not complete "embrace"; instead, arms fall backward because of weakness.	Response is present at birth; complete response may be seen until 8 wk; body jerk only is seen between 8 and 18 wk; response is absent by 6 mo if neurologic maturation is not delayed; response may be incomplete if infant is in deep sleep state; give parental guidance about normal response. Asymmetric response may connote injury to brachial plexus, clavicle, or humerus. Persistent response after 6 mo indicates possible neurologic abnormality.
Stepping or "walking"	Hold infant vertically under arms or on trunk, allowing one foot to touch table surface.	Infant will simulate walking, alternating flexion and extension of feet; term infants walk on soles of their feet, and preterm infants walk on their toes.	Response is normally present for 3 to 4 wk.

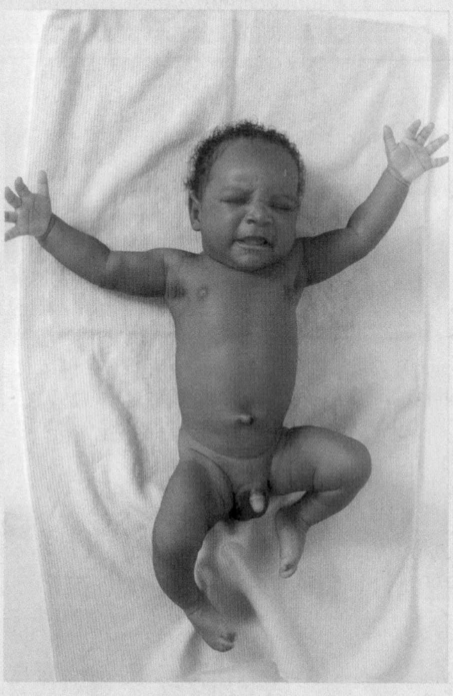

Moro reflex. (Courtesy Paul Vincent Kuntz, Texas Children's Hospital, Houston, TX)

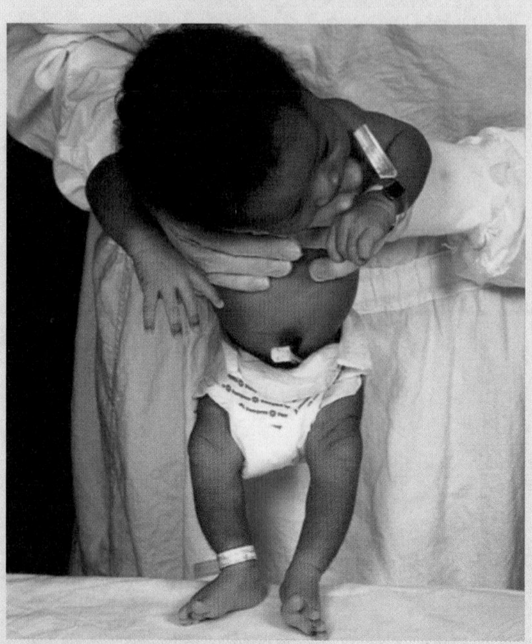

Stepping reflex. (From Dickason EJ, Silverman BL, Kaplan JA: *Maternal-infant nursing care*, ed 3, St Louis, 1998, Mosby.)

Table 24-1

Assessment of Newborn Reflexes—cont'd

REFLEX	ELICITING THE REFLEX	CHARACTERISTIC RESPONSE	COMMENTS
Crawling	Place newborn on abdomen.	Newborn makes crawling movements with arms and legs.	Response should disappear about 6 wk of age.
Deep tendon	Use finger instead of percussion hammer to elicit patellar, or knee jerk, reflex; newborn must be relaxed.	Reflex jerk is present; even with newborn relaxed, nonselective overall reaction may occur.	
Crossed extension	Infant should be supine; extend one leg, press knee downward, stimulate bottom of foot; observe opposite leg.	Opposite leg flexes, adducts, and then extends.	

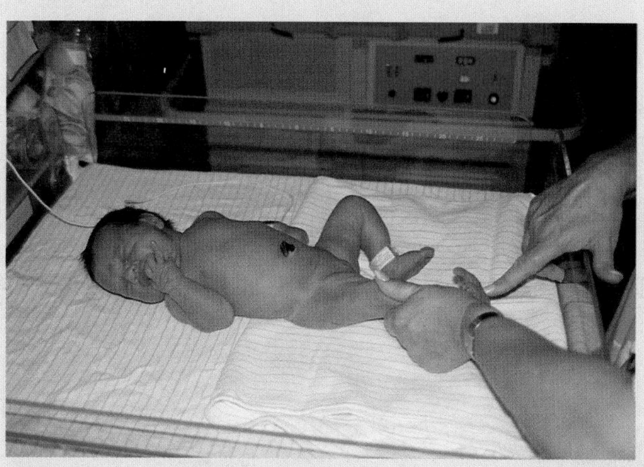

Crossed extension reflex. With infant in supine position, examiner extends one leg of the infant and presses down the knee. Stimulation of sole of foot of fixated limb should cause free leg to flex, adduct, and extend as if attempting to push away stimulating agent. This reflex should be present during newborn period. (Courtesy Marjorie Pyle, RNC, Lifecircle, Costa Mesa, CA.)

REFLEX	ELICITING THE REFLEX	CHARACTERISTIC RESPONSE	COMMENTS
Babinski (plantar)	On sole of foot, beginning at heel, stroke upward along lateral aspect of sole, then move finger across ball of foot.	All toes hyperextend, with dorsiflexion of big toe—recorded as a positive sign.	Absence requires neurologic evaluation, should disappear after 1 yr of age. Response depends on general muscle tone and maturity and condition of infant.

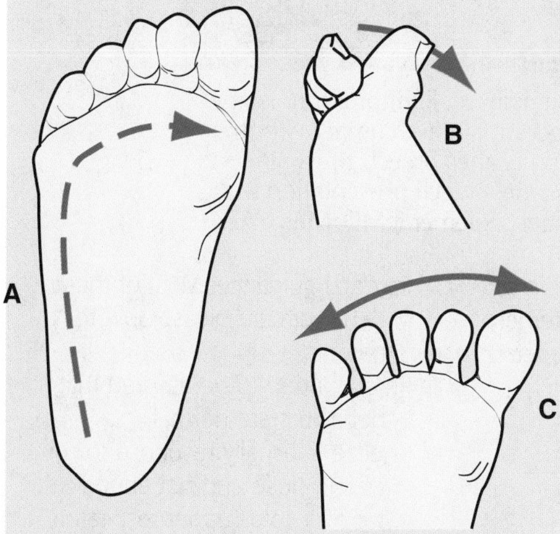

Babinski reflex. **A**, Direction of stroke. **B**, Dorsiflexion of big toe. **C**, Fanning of toes. (From Hockenberry MJ et al: *Wong's nursing care of infants and children*, ed 7, St Louis, 2003, Mosby.)

REFLEX	ELICITING THE REFLEX	CHARACTERISTIC RESPONSE	COMMENTS
Pull-to-sit (traction response); Postural tone	Pull infant up by wrists from supine position with head in midline.	Head comes forward with body with minimal lag; head falls forward when placed in sitting position.	Response disappears by fourth week.

Continued

Table 24-1

Assessment of Newborn Reflexes—cont'd

REFLEX	ELICITING THE REFLEX	CHARACTERISTIC RESPONSE	COMMENTS
Truncal incurvation (Galant)	Place infant prone on flat surface, run finger down back about 4 to 5 cm lateral to spine, first on one side and then down other.	Trunk is flexed and pelvis is swung toward stimulated side.	Absence suggests general depression of nervous system.

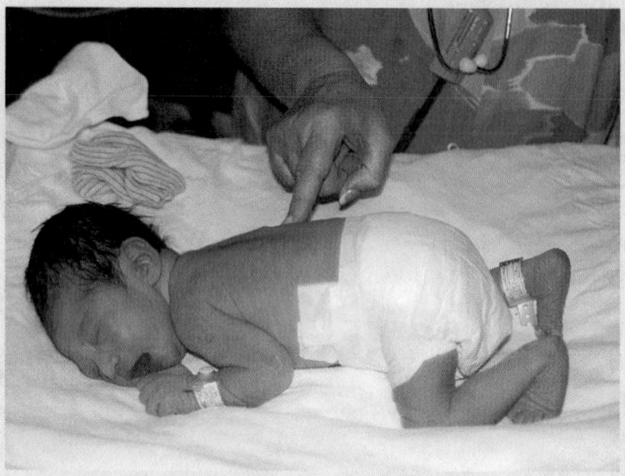

Trunk incurvation reflex. In prone position, infant responds to linear skin stimulus (blunt end of pin or finger) along paravertebral area by flexing the trunk and swinging the pelvis toward stimulus. With transverse lesions of cord, no response below the level of the lesion is present. Response may vary but should be obtainable in all infants, including preterm ones. If not seen in the first few days, it is usually apparent by 5 to 6 days. (Courtesy Marjorie Pyle, RNC, Lifecircle, Costa Mesa, CA.)

REFLEX	ELICITING THE REFLEX	CHARACTERISTIC RESPONSE	COMMENTS
Magnet	Place infant in supine position, partially flex both lower extremities and apply pressure to soles of feet.	Both lower limbs should extend against examiner's pressure.	Absence suggests damage to CNS. Reflex may be weak or exaggerated after breech birth.

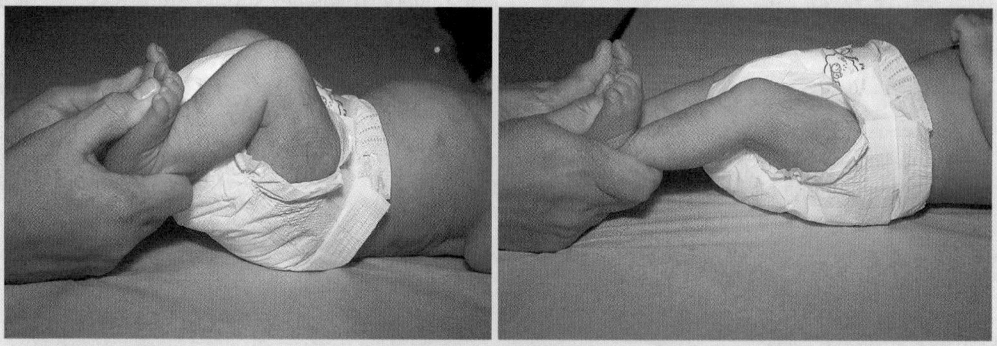

Magnet reflex. With infant in supine position and lower limbs semiflexed, light pressure is applied with fingers to both feet. Normally, while examiner's fingers maintain contact with the soles of the feet, the lower limbs extend. Weak reflex may be seen after breech presentation *without* extended legs or may indicate sciatic nerve stretch syndrome. Breech presentation *with* extended legs may evoke exaggerated response. (Courtesy Michael S. Clement, MD, Mesa, AZ.)

REFLEX	ELICITING THE REFLEX	CHARACTERISTIC RESPONSE	COMMENTS
Additional newborn responses Yawn, stretch, burp, hiccup, sneeze	These are spontaneous behaviors.	May be slightly depressed temporarily because of maternal analgesia or anesthesia, fetal hypoxia, or infection	Parental guidance: Most of these behaviors are pleasurable to parents. Parents need to be assured that behaviors are normal. Sneeze is usually response to mucus, in nose and not an indicator of a cold (upper respiratory infection). No treatment is needed for hiccups; sucking may help. In the preterm infant these are signs of neurodevelopmental immaturity and physiologic stress.

who are macrosomic or small for gestational age, and newborns experiencing prolonged birth, hypoxia, or preterm birth).

Spontaneous motor activity may be seen as transient tremors of the mouth and chin, especially during crying episodes, and of the extremities, notably the arms and hands. Transient tremors are normal and can be observed in nearly every newborn. These tremors should not be present when the infant is quiet and should not persist beyond 1 month of age. Persistent tremors or tremors involving the entire body may indicate pathologic conditions. Normal tremors, tremors of hypoglycemia, and central nervous system (CNS) disorders need to be differentiated so corrective care can be instituted as necessary.

Neuromuscular control in the newborn, although very limited, can be noted. If newborns are placed face down on a firm surface, they will turn their heads to the side. They attempt to hold their heads in line with their bodies if they are raised by their arms. Various reflexes serve to promote safety and adequate food intake.

Newborn Reflexes

The newborn infant has many primitive reflexes. The times at which these reflexes appear and disappear reflect the maturity and intactness of the developing nervous system. The most common reflexes found in the normal newborn are described in Table 24-1.

PHYSICAL ASSESSMENT

The assessment of the newborn should progress in a systematic manner, with evaluation and assessment of each system (e.g., respiratory and cardiovascular). It is recommended that assessment of features (e.g., observe general color, posture, auscultate heart tones and breath sounds), which least disturbs the newborn, be conducted first and then proceed in a head-to-toe manner once the newborn is awake and active. The findings provide a database for implementing the nursing process with newborns, and for providing anticipatory guidance for the parents. An immediate assessment of the newborn is carried out to evaluate the infant's transition to extrauterine life. The Apgar score (see Chapter 25), determined at 1 and 5 minutes, provides information that must be considered in the context of data from the total assessment.

A complete physical examination should be done within 24 hours after birth, after the newborn's temperature stabilizes or under a radiant warmer. The area used for examination should be well-lighted, warm, and free from drafts. The infant is undressed as needed and placed on a firm, warmed, flat surface. The physical assessment should begin with a review of the maternal history and prenatal and intrapartal records. This provides a background for the recognition of any potential problems. This assessment also includes general appearance, behavior, vital signs measurements, and maternal-infant interactions. Descriptions of any variations from normal and all abnormal findings are included (Table 24-2). Ongoing assessments of the newborn are made and an evaluation is performed before discharge.

General Appearance

The neonate's maturity level can be gauged by assessment of general appearance. Features to assess in the general survey include posture, activity, any overt signs of anomalies that may cause initial distress, presence of bruising or other consequences of delivery, and state of alertness. The normal resting position of the neonate is one of general flexion (Fig. 24-10).

Vital Signs

The temperature, heart rate, and respiratory rate are always obtained. BP is assessed as a baseline unless cardiac problems are suspect. An irregular, very slow, or very fast heart rate may indicate a need for BP measurement.

The axillary temperature is a safe, accurate substitute for the rectal temperature. Electronic thermometers have expedited this task and provide a reading within 1 minute. Taking an infant's temperature may cause the infant to cry and struggle against the placement of the thermometer in the axilla. Before taking the temperature the examiner may determine the apical heart rate and respiratory rate while the infant is quiet and at rest. The normal axillary temperature averages 37° C with a range from 36.5° to 37.2° C.

The respiratory rate varies with the state of alertness and activity after birth. Respirations are abdominal in nature and can be counted by observing or by lightly feeling the rise and fall of the abdomen. Neonatal respirations are shallow and irregular. It is important to count the respirations for a full minute to obtain an accurate count because of periods of periodic breathing wherein respirations may cease for seconds (less than 20) and resume again. The examiner should also observe for symmetry of chest movement. The average respiratory rate is 40 breaths/min but will vary between 30 and 60 breaths/min or may be higher than 60 breaths/min if the newborn is very active or crying (see Table 24-2).

An apical pulse rate should be obtained on all newborns. Auscultation should be for a full minute, preferably when the infant is asleep or in a quiet alert state. The infant may need to be held and comforted during assessment. Heart rate

Text continued on p. 720.

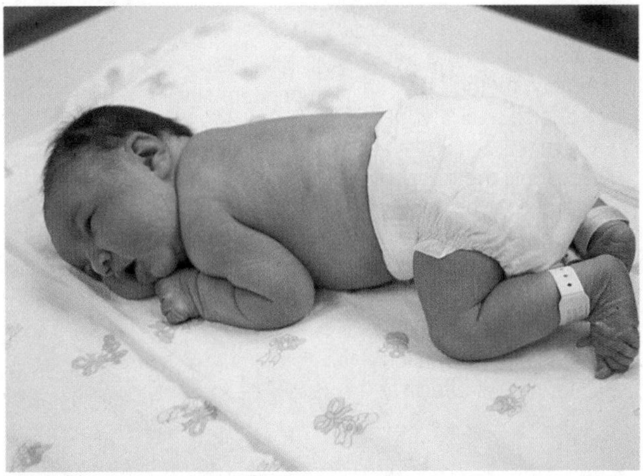

Fig. 24-10 Newborn in position of flexion in prone position while awake. (From Hockenberry MJ et al: *Wong's nursing care of infants and children*, ed 7, St. Louis, 2003, Mosby.)

Table 24-2

Physical Assessment of Newborn

AREA ASSESSED AND APPRAISAL PROCEDURE	Normal Findings: AVERAGE FINDINGS	Normal Findings: NORMAL VARIATIONS	DEVIATIONS FROM NORMAL RANGE: POSSIBLE PROBLEMS (ETIOLOGY)
POSTURE			
Inspect newborn before disturbing for assessment. Refer to maternal chart for fetal presentation, position, and type of birth (vaginal, surgical), since newborn readily assumes in utero position.	Vertex: arms, legs in moderate flexion; fists clenched Resistance to having extremities extended for examination or measurement, crying possible when attempted Cessation of crying when allowed to resume curled-up fetal position Normal spontaneous movement bilaterally asynchronous (legs moving in bicycle fashion) but equal extension in all extremities	Frank breech: legs straighter and stiff, newborn assuming intrauterine position in repose for a few days Prenatal pressure on limb or shoulder possibly causing temporary facial asymmetry or resistance to extension of extremities	Hypotonia, relaxed posture while awake (prematurity or hypoxia in utero, maternal medications) Hypertonia (drug dependence, central nervous system [CNS] disorder) Limitation of motion in any of extremities (see Skeletal System, p. 701)
VITAL SIGNS			
Check heart rate and pulses: Thorax (chest) Inspection Palpation Auscultation Apex: mitral valve Second interspace, left of sternum: pulmonic valve Second interspace, right of sternum: aortic valve Junction of xiphoid process and sternum: tricuspid valve	Visible pulsations in left midclavicular line, fifth intercostal space Apical pulse, fourth intercostal space 100-160 beats/min Quality: *first sound* (closure of mitral and tricuspid valves) and *second sound* (closure of aortic and pulmonic valves) sharp and clear	80-100 beats/min (sleeping) to 180 beats/min (crying); possibly irregular for brief periods, especially after crying Murmur, especially over base or at left sternal border in interspace 3 or 4 (foramen ovale anatomically closing at about 1 yr)	Tachycardia: persistent, ≥180 beats/min (respiratory distress syndrome [RDS]) Bradycardia: persistent, ≤80 beats/min (congenital heart block, maternal lupus) Murmur (possibly functional) Arrhythmias: irregular rate Sounds Distant (pneumopericardium) Poor quality Extra Heart on right side of chest (dextrocardia, often accompanied by reversal of intestines)
Peripheral pulses: femoral, brachial, popliteal, posterior tibial	Peripheral pulses equal and strong		Weak or absent peripheral (decreased cardiac output, thrombus, possible coarctation of aorta if weak on left and strong on right)
Obtain temperature: Axillary: method of choice until 3 yr of age Electronic thermistor probe (avoid taping over bony area) Some temporal and intraauricular thermometers are undergoing evaluation for clinical effectiveness	Axillary: 37° C Temperature stabilized by 8-10 hr of age	36.5° C-37.2° C Heat loss: 200 kcal/kg/min from evaporation, conduction, convection, radiation	Subnormal (prematurity, infection, low environmental temperature, inadequate clothing, dehydration) Increased (infection, high environmental temperature, excessive clothing, proximity to heating unit or in direct sunshine, drug addiction, diarrhea and dehydration) Temperature not stabilized by 6-8 hr after birth (if mother received magnesium sulfate, newborn less able to conserve heat by vasoconstriction; maternal analgesics possibly reducing thermal stability in newborn)

Table 24-2

Physical Assessment of Newborn—cont'd

AREA ASSESSED AND APPRAISAL PROCEDURE	Normal Findings: AVERAGE FINDINGS	Normal Findings: NORMAL VARIATIONS	DEVIATIONS FROM NORMAL RANGE: POSSIBLE PROBLEMS (ETIOLOGY)
VITAL SIGNS—cont'd			
Check respiratory rate and effort: Observe respirations when infant is at rest Count respirations for full minute Listen for sounds audible without stethoscope Observe respiratory effort	40/min Tendency to be shallow and irregular in rate, rhythm, and depth when infant is awake Crackles may be heard after birth No sounds audible on inspiration and expiration Breath sounds: bronchial: loud, clear, near	30-60/min Short periodic breathing episodes and no evidence of respiratory distress or apnea (>20 seconds) First period (reactivity): 50-60/min Second period: 50-70/min Stabilization (1-2 days): 30-40/min	Apneic episodes: >15 sec (preterm infant: "periodic breathing," rapid warming or cooling of infant) Bradypnea: <25/min (maternal narcosis from analgesics or anesthetics, birth trauma) Tachypnea: >60/min (RDS, transient tachypnea of the newborn, congenital diaphragmatic hernia) Sounds Crackles, rhonchi, wheezes (fluid in lungs) Expiratory grunt (narrowing of bronchi) Distress evidenced by nasal flaring, grunting, retractions, labored breathing
Obtain blood pressure (BP) Check oscillometric monitor BP cuff: BP cuff width affects readings, use appropriately sized cuff and palpate brachial, popliteal, or posterior tibial pulse (depending on measurement site)	80s-90s/40s-50s (approximately) At birth Systolic: 60-80 mm Hg Diastolic: 40-50 mm Hg At 10 days Systolic: 95-100 mm Hg Diastolic: slight increase	Variation with change in activity level: awake, crying, sleeping	Difference between upper and lower extremity pressures (coarctation of aorta) Hypotension (sepsis, hypovolemia) Hypertension (coarctation of aorta, renal involvement, thrombus)
WEIGHT*			
Put protective liner cloth or paper in place and adjust scale to 0 grams/pounds/ounces Weigh at same time each day Protect newborn from heat loss	Female 3400 g Male 3500 g Regaining of birth weight within first 2 weeks	2500-4000 g Acceptable weight loss: 10% or less Second baby weighing more than first (on average)	Weight ≤2500 g (prematurity, small for gestational age, rubella syndrome) Weight ≥4000 g (large for gestational age, maternal diabetes, heredity—normal for these parents) Weight loss over 10% to 15% (dehydration)

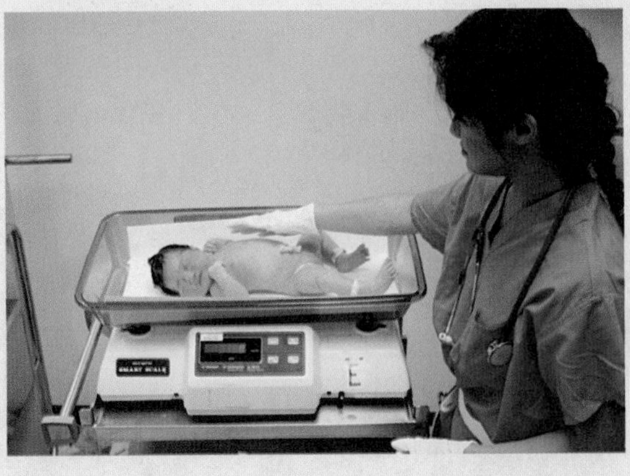

Weighing the infant. Note that a hand is held over infant as a safety measure. The scale is covered to protect against cross infection. (Courtesy Kim Molloy, Knoxville, IA.)

*Note: Weight, length, and head circumference should all be close to the same percentile for any child.

Continued

Table 24-2

Physical Assessment of Newborn—cont'd

AREA ASSESSED AND APPRAISAL PROCEDURE	Normal Findings: AVERAGE FINDINGS	Normal Findings: NORMAL VARIATIONS	DEVIATIONS FROM NORMAL RANGE: POSSIBLE PROBLEMS (ETIOLOGY)
LENGTH			
Measure length from top of head to heel, measuring is difficult in term infant because of presence of molding, incomplete extension of knees	50 cm	45-55 cm	<45 cm or >55 cm (chromosomal abnormality, heredity—normal for these parents); some syndromes present shorter than average limb length (skeletal dysplasias, achondroplasia)

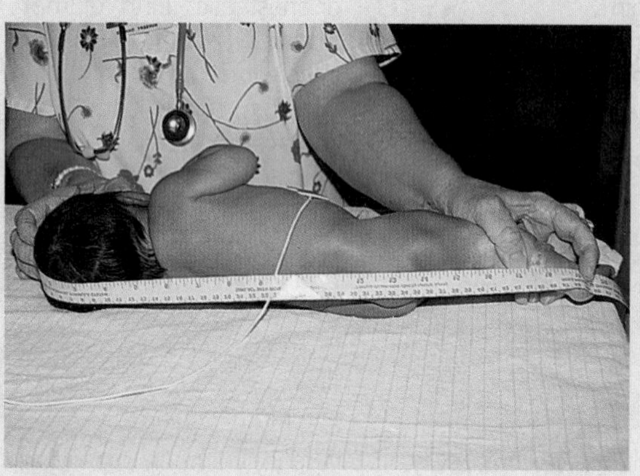

Length, crown to heel. To determine total length, include length of legs. If measurements are taken before the infant's initial bath, wear gloves. (Courtesy Marjorie Pyle, RNC, Lifecircle, Costa Mesa, CA.)

AREA ASSESSED AND APPRAISAL PROCEDURE	Normal Findings: AVERAGE FINDINGS	Normal Findings: NORMAL VARIATIONS	DEVIATIONS FROM NORMAL RANGE: POSSIBLE PROBLEMS (ETIOLOGY)
HEAD CIRCUMFERENCE			
Measure head at greatest diameter: occipitofrontal circumference May need to remeasure on second or third day after resolution of molding and caput succedaneum	33-35 cm Circumference of head and chest approximately the same for first 1 or 2 days after birth	32-36.8 cm	Small head ≤32 cm: microcephaly (maternal rubella, toxoplasmosis, cytomegalovirus, fused cranial sutures [craniosynostosis]) Hydrocephaly: sutures widely separated, circumference ≥4 cm more than chest circumference (maldevelopment, infection) Increased intracranial pressure (hemorrhage, space-occupying lesion)

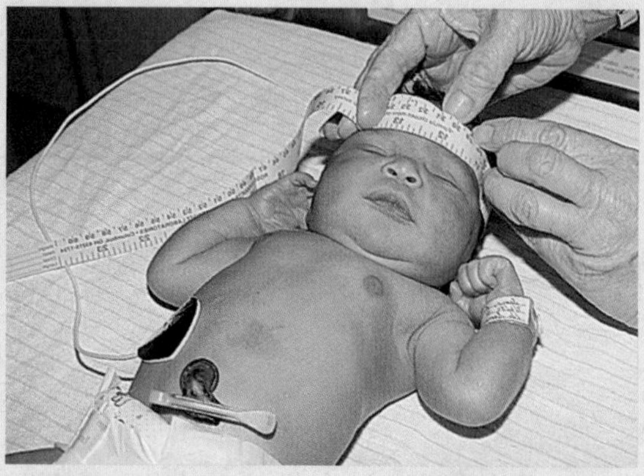

Circumference of head. (Courtesy Marjorie Pyle, RNC, Lifecircle, Costa Mesa, CA.)

Table 24-2

Physical Assessment of Newborn—cont'd

AREA ASSESSED AND APPRAISAL PROCEDURE	Normal Findings: AVERAGE FINDINGS	Normal Findings: NORMAL VARIATIONS	DEVIATIONS FROM NORMAL RANGE: POSSIBLE PROBLEMS (ETIOLOGY)
CHEST CIRCUMFERENCE			
Measure at nipple line	2-3 cm less than head circumference, averages 30-33 cm		≤30 cm (prematurity)

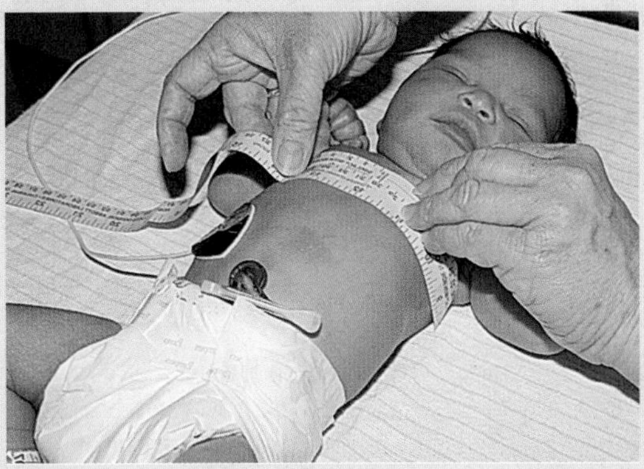

Circumference of chest. (Courtesy Marjorie Pyle, RNC, Lifecircle, Costa Mesa, CA.)

AREA ASSESSED AND APPRAISAL PROCEDURE	Normal Findings: AVERAGE FINDINGS	Normal Findings: NORMAL VARIATIONS	DEVIATIONS FROM NORMAL RANGE: POSSIBLE PROBLEMS (ETIOLOGY)
ABDOMINAL CIRCUMFERENCE			
Measure above umbilicus (not usually measured unless specific indication)	Abdomen enlargement after feeding because of lax abdominal muscles Same size as chest		Enlarging abdomen between feedings (abdominal mass or blockage in intestinal tract)

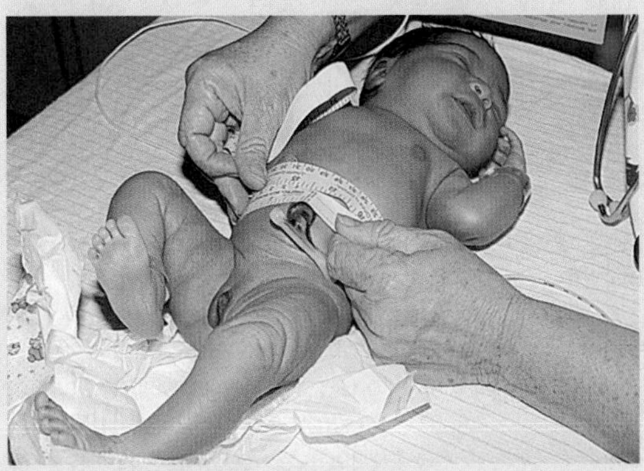

Abdominal circumference. (Courtesy Marjorie Pyle, RNC, Lifecircle, Costa Mesa, CA.)

AREA ASSESSED AND APPRAISAL PROCEDURE	Normal Findings: AVERAGE FINDINGS	Normal Findings: NORMAL VARIATIONS	DEVIATIONS FROM NORMAL RANGE: POSSIBLE PROBLEMS (ETIOLOGY)
SKIN			
Check color: Inspect and palpate Inspect naked newborn in well-lighted, warm area without drafts; natural daylight best Inspect newborn when quiet and alert	Generally pink Varying with ethnic origin, skin pigmentation beginning to deepen right after birth in basal layer of epidermis Acrocyanosis common after birth	Mottling Harlequin sign Plethora Telangiectases ("stork bites" or capillary hemangiomas) (see Fig. 24-5, *A*) Erythema toxicum/neonatorum ("newborn rash") (see Fig. 24-5, *B*) Milia	Dark red (prematurity, polycythemia) Gray (hypotension, poor perfusion) Pallor (cardiovascular problem, CNS damage, blood dyscrasia, blood loss, twin-to-twin transfusion, nosocomial infection) Cyanosis (hypothermia, infection, hypoglycemia, cardiopulmonary diseases, neurologic, or respiratory malformations)
		Petechiae over presenting part	Generalized petechiae (clotting factor deficiency, infection)
		Ecchymoses from forceps in vertex births or over buttocks, genitalia, and legs in breech births	Generalized ecchymoses (hemorrhagic disease)

Continued

Table 24-2

Physical Assessment of Newborn—cont'd

AREA ASSESSED AND APPRAISAL PROCEDURE	Normal Findings: AVERAGE FINDINGS	Normal Findings: NORMAL VARIATIONS	DEVIATIONS FROM NORMAL RANGE: POSSIBLE PROBLEMS (ETIOLOGY)
SKIN—cont'd			
Check for jaundice	None at birth	Physiologic jaundice in up to 80% of term infants in first week of life	Jaundice within first 24 hr (increased hemolysis, Rh isoimmunization, ABO incompatibility)
Check birthmarks or bruises: Inspect and palpate for location, size, distribution, characteristics, color, if obstructing airway or oral cavity		Mongolian spot (see Fig. 24-4) Infants of African-American, Asian, and Native American origin: 70% to 85% Infants of Caucasian origin: 5% to 13%	Hemangiomas Nevus flammeus: port-wine stain Nevus vasculosus: strawberry mark Cavernous hemangioma
Check condition: Inspect and palpate for intactness, smoothness, texture, edema, pressure points if ill or immobilized	No skin edema Opacity: few large blood vessels visible indistinctly over abdomen	Slightly thick; superficial cracking, peeling, especially of hands, feet No visible blood vessels, a few large vessels clearly visible over abdomen Some fingernail scratches	Edema on hands, feet; pitting over tibia (over hydration) Texture thin, smooth, or of medium thickness; rash or superficial peeling visible (prematurity, postmaturity) Numerous vessels very visible over abdomen (prematurity) Texture thick, parchmentlike; cracking, peeling (postmaturity) Skin tags, webbing Papules, pustules, vesicles, ulcers, maceration (impetigo, candidiasis, herpes, diaper rash)
Weigh infant routinely Inspect and palpate Gently pinch skin between thumb and forefinger over abdomen and inner thigh to check for turgor Note presence of subcutaneous fat deposits (adipose pads) over cheeks, buttocks	Dehydration: loss of weight best indicator After pinch released, skin returns to original state immediately	Normal weight loss after birth: up to 10% of birth weight Possibly puffy Variation in amount of subcutaneous fat	Loose, wrinkled skin (prematurity, postmaturity, dehydration: fold of skin persisting after release of pinch) Tense, tight, shiny skin (edema, extreme cold, shock, infection) Lack of subcutaneous fat, prominence of clavicle or ribs (prematurity, malnutrition)
Check voiding	Voiding within 24 hours of birth Voiding six to ten times per day		
Check vernix caseosa: Observe color and odor before bath or removing	Whitish, cheesy, odorless	Usually more found in creases, folds	Absent or minimal (postmaturity) Excessive (prematurity) Green color (possible in utero release of meconium or presence of bilirubin) Odor (possible intrauterine infection)
Assess lanugo: Inspect for this fine, downy hair, amount and distribution	Over shoulders, pinnas of ears, forehead	Variation in amount	Absent (postmaturity) Excessive (prematurity, especially if lanugo abundant, long and thick over back)

Table 24-2

Physical Assessment of Newborn—cont'd

AREA ASSESSED AND APPRAISAL PROCEDURE	Normal Findings: AVERAGE FINDINGS	Normal Findings: NORMAL VARIATIONS	DEVIATIONS FROM NORMAL RANGE: POSSIBLE PROBLEMS (ETIOLOGY)
HEAD			
Palpate skin	(See Skin)	Caput succedaneum, possibly showing some ecchymosis (see Fig. 24-3, *A*)	Cephalhematoma (see Fig. 24-3, *C*)
Inspect shape, size	Making up one fourth of body length Molding (see Fig. 24-7)	Slight asymmetry from intrauterine position Lack of molding (prematurity, breech presentation, cesarean birth)	Molding Severe molding (birth trauma) Indentation (fracture from trauma)
Palpate, inspect, and note status of fontanels (open vs. closed)	Anterior fontanel 5-cm diamond, increasing as molding resolves Posterior fontanel triangle, smaller than anterior	Variation in fontanel size with degree of molding Difficulty in feeling fontanels possible because of molding	Fontanels Full, bulging (tumor, hemorrhage, infection) Large, flat, soft (malnutrition, hydrocephaly, retarded bone age, hypothyroidism) Depressed (dehydration)
Palpate sutures	Palpable and separated sutures	Possible overlap of sutures with molding	Sutures Widely spaced (hydrocephaly) Premature closure (craniosynostosis)
Inspect pattern, distribution, amount of hair; feel texture	Silky, single strands lying flat; growth pattern toward face and neck	Variation in amount	Fine, wooly (prematurity) Unusual swirls, patterns, or hairline; or coarse, brittle (endocrine or genetic disorders)
EYES			
Check placement on face	Eyes and space between eyes each one third the distance from outer-to-outer canthus	Epicanthal folds: characteristic in some ethnicities	Epicanthal folds when present with other signs (chromosomal disorders such as Down, cri-du-chat syndromes)

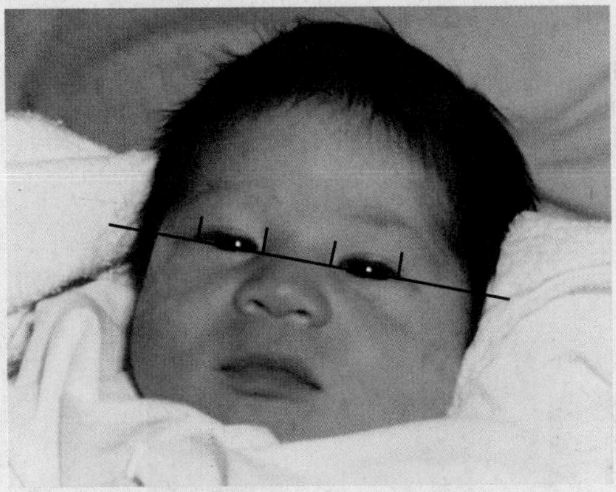

Eyes. In pseudostrabismus, inner epicanthal folds cause the eyes to appear misaligned; however, corneal light reflexes are perfectly symmetric. Eyes are symmetric in size and shape and are well placed.

AREA ASSESSED AND APPRAISAL PROCEDURE	AVERAGE FINDINGS	NORMAL VARIATIONS	DEVIATIONS FROM NORMAL RANGE: POSSIBLE PROBLEMS (ETIOLOGY)
Check for symmetry in size, shape	Symmetric in size, shape		
Check eyelids for size, movement, blink	Blink reflex	Edema if eye prophylaxis drops or ointment instilled;	
Assess for discharge	None	Some discharge if silver nitrate used	Discharge: purulent (infection) Chemical conjunctivitis from eye medication is common—requires no treatment
	No tears	Occasional presence of some tears	
Evaluate eyeballs for presence, size, shape	Both present and of equal size, both round, firm	Subconjunctival hemorrhage	Agenesis or absence of one or both eyeballs

Continued

Table 24-2

Physical Assessment of Newborn—cont'd

AREA ASSESSED AND APPRAISAL PROCEDURE	Normal Findings: AVERAGE FINDINGS	Normal Findings: NORMAL VARIATIONS	DEVIATIONS FROM NORMAL RANGE: POSSIBLE PROBLEMS (ETIOLOGY)
EYES—cont'd			
			Lens opacity or absence of red reflex (congenital cataracts, possibly from rubella) Lesions: coloboma, absence of part of iris (congenital) Pink color of iris (albinism) Jaundiced sclera (hyperbilliru-binemia)
Check pupils	Present, equal in size, reactive to light		Pupils: unequal, constricted, dilated, fixed (intracranial pressure, medications, tumors)
Evaluate eyeball movement	Random, jerky, uneven, focus possible briefly, following to midline	Transient strabismus or nystagmus until third or fourth month	Persistent strabismus Doll's eyes (increased intracranial pressure) Sunset (increased intracranial pressure)
Assess eyebrows: amount of hair, pattern	Distinct (not connected in midline)		Connection in midline (Cornelia de Lange syndrome)
NOSE			
Observe shape, placement, patency, configuration	Midline Some mucus but no drainage Preferential nose breather Sneezing to clear nose	Slight deformity (flat or deviated to one side) from passage through birth canal	Copious drainage (rarely congenital syphilis). Blockage-membranous or bone with cyanosis at rest and return of pink color with crying (choanal atresia). Malformed (congenital syphilis, chromosomal disorder) Flaring of nares (respiratory distress)
EARS			
Observe size, placement on head, amount of cartilage, open auditory canal	Correct placement line drawn through inner and outer canthi of eyes reaching to top notch of ears (at junction with scalp) Well-formed, firm cartilage	Size: small, large, floppy Darwin's tubercle (nodule on posterior helix)	Agenesis Lack of cartilage (prematurity) Low placement (chromosomal disorder, mental retardation, kidney disorder) Preauricular tags Size: possibly overly prominent or protruding ears

A B C

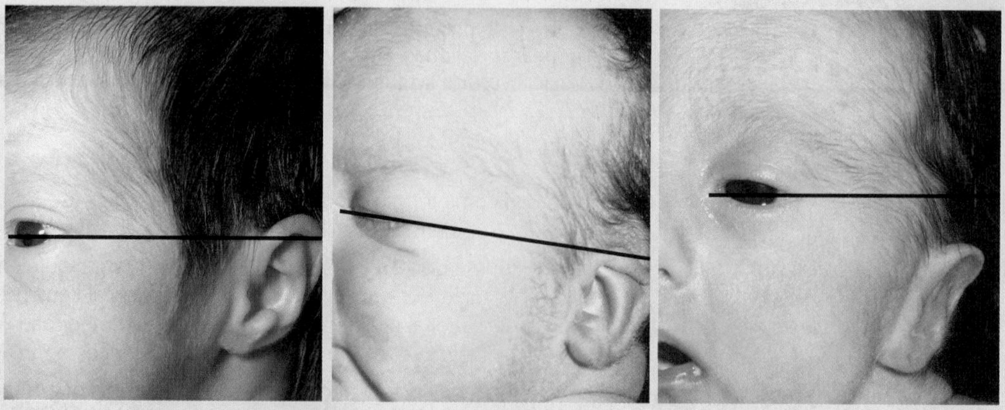

Placement of ears on the head in relation to a line drawn from the inner to the outer canthus of the eye. **A**, Normal position. **B**, Abnormally angled ear. **C**, True low-set ear. (Courtesy Mead Johnson Nutritionals, Evansville, IN.)

Table 24-2

Physical Assessment of Newborn—cont'd

AREA ASSESSED AND APPRAISAL PROCEDURE	Normal Findings: AVERAGE FINDINGS	Normal Findings: NORMAL VARIATIONS	DEVIATIONS FROM NORMAL RANGE: POSSIBLE PROBLEMS (ETIOLOGY)
EARS—cont'd			
Assess hearing	Responds to voice and other sounds	State (e.g., alert, asleep) influencing response	Perform universal newborn hearing screening to identify deficits. Lack of response to loud noise *should not* imply deafness
FACIES			
Observe overall appearance and symmetry of face	Rounded and symmetric; influenced by birth type and/or any molding	Positional deformities	Usually accompanied by other features such as low-set ears, other structural disorders (hereditary, chromosomal aberration)
MOUTH			
Inspect and palpate Assess buccal mucosa Dry or moist Pink Status intact Assess lips for color, configuration, movement	Symmetry of lip movement	Transient circumoral cyanosis	Gross anomalies in placement, size, shape (cleft lip and/or palate, gums) Cyanosis, circumoral pallor (respiratory distress, hypothermia) Asymmetry in movement of lips (seventh cranial nerve paralysis)
Check gums	Pink gums	Inclusion cysts (Epstein's pearls—Bohn's nodules, whitish, hard nodules on gums or roof of mouth)	Teeth: predeciduous or deciduous (hereditary)
Assess tongue for color, mobility, movement, size	Tongue not protruding, freely movable, symmetric in shape, movement Sucking pads inside cheeks	Short lingual frenulum	Macroglossia (prematurity, chromosomal disorder) Thrush: white plaques on cheeks or tongue that bleed if touched *(Candida albicans)*
Assess palate (soft, hard): Arch	Soft and hard palates intact	Anatomic groove in palate to accommodate nipple, disappearance by 3 to 4 yr of age	Cleft hard or soft palate
Uvula	Uvula in midline	Epstein's pearls	
Assess chin	Distinct chin		Micrognathia (Pierre Robin or other syndrome)
Evaluate saliva for amount, character	Mouth moist, pink		Excessive salivation and choking or turning blue (esophageal atresia, tracheoesophageal fistula)
Check reflexes: Rooting Sucking Extrusion	Reflexes present	Reflex response dependent on state of wakefulness and hunger	Absent (prematurity)
NECK			
Inspect and palpate for movement, flexibility, masses, bruising	Short, thick, surrounded by skin folds; no webbing		Webbing (Turner's syndrome)
Check sternocleidomastoid muscles, movement and position of head	Head held in midline (sternocleidomastoid muscles equal), no masses	Transient positional deformity apparent when newborn is at rest: passive movement of head possible	Restricted movement, holding of head at angle (torticollis [wryneck], opisthotonos)

Continued

Table 24-2

Physical Assessment of Newborn—cont'd

AREA ASSESSED AND APPRAISAL PROCEDURE	Normal Findings: AVERAGE FINDINGS	Normal Findings: NORMAL VARIATIONS	DEVIATIONS FROM NORMAL RANGE: POSSIBLE PROBLEMS (ETIOLOGY)
NECK—cont'd			
	Freedom of movement from side to side and flexion and extension, no movement of chin past shoulder		Absence of head control (prematurity, Down syndrome, hypotonia)
Assess trachea for position and thyroid gland	Thyroid not palpable		Masses (enlarged thyroid) Distended veins (cardiopulmonary disorder) Skin tags
CHEST			
Inspect and palpate Shape	Almost circular, barrel shaped	Tip of sternum possibly prominent	Bulging of chest, unequal movement (pneumothorax, pneumomediastinum) Malformation (funnel chest—pectus excavatum)
Check respiratory movements	Symmetric chest movements, chest and abdominal movements synchronized during respirations	Occasional retractions, especially when crying	Retractions with or without respiratory distress (prematurity, RDS)
Evaluate clavicles	Clavicles intact		Fracture of clavicle (trauma); crepitus
Assess ribs	Rib cage symmetrical, intact; moves with respirations		Poor development of rib cage and musculature (prematurity)
Assess nipples for size, placement, number	Nipples prominent, well formed; symmetrically placed		Nipples Supernumerary, along nipple line Malpositioned or widely spaced
Check breast tissue	Breast nodule: approximately 6 mm in term infant	Breast nodule: 3-10 mm Secretion of witch's milk	Lack of breast tissue (prematurity)
Auscultate: Heart sounds and rate and breath sounds (see Vital Signs)			Sounds: bowel sounds (see Abdomen)
ABDOMEN			
Inspect and palpate umbilical cord	Two arteries, one vein Whitish gray Definite demarcation between cord and skin, no intestinal structures within cord Dry around base, drying Odorless Cord clamp in place for 24 hr		One artery (renal anomaly) Meconium stained (intrauterine distress) Bleeding or oozing around cord (hemorrhagic disease) Redness or drainage around cord (infection, possible persistence of urachus)
		Reducible umbilical hernia	Hernia: herniation of abdominal contents through cord opening (e.g., omphalocele); defect covered with thin, friable membrane, possibly extensive
Inspect size of abdomen and palpate contour (see abdominal circumference, p. 711)	Rounded, prominent, dome shaped because abdominal musculature not fully developed	Some diatasis (separation) of abdominal musculature (rectus)	Gastroschisis: herniation of abdominal contents to the side or above the cord, contents not covered by membranous tissue and may include liver

Table 24-2

Physical Assessment of Newborn—cont'd

AREA ASSESSED AND APPRAISAL PROCEDURE	Normal Findings: AVERAGE FINDINGS	Normal Findings: NORMAL VARIATIONS	DEVIATIONS FROM NORMAL RANGE: POSSIBLE PROBLEMS (ETIOLOGY)
ABDOMEN—cont'd			
	Liver possibly palpable 1-2 cm below right costal margin No other masses palpable No distention Few visible veins on abdominal surface		Distention at birth (ruptured viscus, genitourinary masses or malformations: hydronephrosis, teratomas, abdominal tumors) Mild (overfeeding, high gastrointestinal tract obstruction) Marked (lower gastrointestinal tract obstruction, anorectal malformation, anal stenosis), often with bilious emesis Intermittent or transient (overfeeding) Partial intestinal obstruction (stenosis of bowel) Visible peristalsis (obstruction) Malrotation of bowel or adhesions Sepsis (infection)
Auscultate bowel sounds and note number, amount, and character of stools	Sounds present within minutes after birth in healthy term infant Meconium stool passing within 24-48 hr after birth		Scaphoid, with bowel sounds in chest and severe respiratory distress (congenital diaphragmatic hernia)
Assess color		Linea nigra possibly apparent and caused by hormone influence during pregnancy	
Check movement with respiration	Respirations primarily diaphragmatic, abdominal and chest movement synchronous		Decreased abdominal breathing (phrenic nerve palsy, congenital diaphragmatic hernia)
GENITALIA			
Female (see Fig. 24-6, *A*)			
Inspect and palpate			
General appearance	Female genitals	Increased pigmentation caused by pregnancy hormones	Ambiguous genitalia—wide variation
Clitoris	Usually edematous		
Labia majora	Usually edematous, covering labia minora in term newborns	Edema and ecchymosis after breech birth	Virilized female—extremely large clitoris (congenital adrenal hyperplasia)
Labia minora	Possible protrusion over labia majora	Blood-tinged discharge from pseudomenstruation caused by pregnancy hormones	Enlarged clitoris with urinary meatus on tip, absent scrotum, micropenis, fused labia
Discharge	Smegma	Some vernix caseosa between labia possible	Stenosed meatus
Vagina	Open orifice Mucoid discharge Hymenal/vaginal tag		Labia majora widely separated and labia minora prominent (prematurity)
Urinary meatus	Beneath clitoris, difficult to see	Rust-stained urine (uric acid crystals)	Absence of vaginal orifice Fecal discharge (fistula) Bladder exstrophy (bladder outside abdominal cavity and turned inside out)

Continued

Table 24-2

Physical Assessment of Newborn—cont'd

AREA ASSESSED AND APPRAISAL PROCEDURE	Normal Findings: AVERAGE FINDINGS	Normal Findings: NORMAL VARIATIONS	DEVIATIONS FROM NORMAL RANGE: POSSIBLE PROBLEMS (ETIOLOGY)
GENITALIA—cont'd			
Male (see Fig. 24-6, *B*)			
Inspect and palpate			
General appearance	Male genitals	Increased size and pigmentation caused by pregnancy hormones	Ambiguous genitalia
Penis			Micropenis
Urinary meatus appearance—should be at tip of penile shaft	Foreskin covers glans (if uncircumcised), meatus at tip of penis		Urinary meatus not on tip of glans penis (hypospadias, epispadias, foreskin may be retracted or absent)
Prepuce (foreskin)—do not forcibly retract foreskin if uncircumcised	Prepuce covering glans penis and not retractable	Prepuce removed if circumcised Wide variation in size of genitals	Round meatal opening
Scrotum Rugae (wrinkles)	Large, edematous, pendulous in term infant; covered with rugae	Scrotal edema and ecchymosis if breech birth Hydrocele, small, noncommunicating	Scrotum smooth and testes undescended (prematurity, cryptorchidism) Bifid scrotum Hydrocele Inguinal hernia
Testes	Palpable on each side	Bulge palpable in inguinal canal	Undescended (prematurity)
Check urination	Voiding within 24 hr, stream adequate, amount adequate	Rust-stained urine (uric acid crystals)	
Check reflexes:			
Cremasteric	Testes retracted, especially when newborn is chilled		
EXTREMITIES			
Make a general check: Inspect and palpate Degree of flexion Range of motion Symmetry of motion Muscle tone	Assuming of position maintained in utero Attitude of general flexion Full range of motion, spontaneous movements	Transient (positional) deformities	Limited motion (malformations) Poor muscle tone (prematurity, maternal medications, CNS anomalies)
Check arms and hands: Inspect and palpate Color Intactness Appropriate placement	Longer than legs in newborn period Contours and movements symmetric	Slight tremors sometimes apparent Some acrocyanosis	Asymmetry of movement (fracture/crepitus, brachial nerve trauma, malformations) Asymmetry of contour (malformations, fracture) Amelia or phocomelia (teratogens) Palmar creases Simian line with short, incurved little fingers (Down syndrome)
Check number of fingers	Five on each hand Fist often clenched with thumb under fingers		Webbing of fingers: syndactyly Absence or excess of fingers Strong, rigid flexion; persistent fists; positioning of fists in front of mouth constantly (CNS disorder) Yellowed nail beds (meconium staining)
Palpate humerus	Intact		Fractured humerus

Table 24-2

Physical Assessment of Newborn—cont'd

AREA ASSESSED AND APPRAISAL PROCEDURE	Normal Findings: AVERAGE FINDINGS	Normal Findings: NORMAL VARIATIONS	DEVIATIONS FROM NORMAL RANGE: POSSIBLE PROBLEMS (ETIOLOGY)
EXTREMITIES—cont'd			
Evaluate joints Shoulder Elbow Wrist Fingers	Full range of motion, symmetric contour		Increased tonicity, clonus, prolonged tremors (CNS disorder)
Check reflex: grasp (palmar and plantar)			
Check legs and feet: Inspect and palpate Color Intactness Length in relation to arms and body and to each other	Appearance of bowing because lateral muscles more developed than medial muscles	Feet appearing to turn in but can be easily rotated externally, positional defects tending to correct while infant is crying Acrocyanosis	Amelia, phocomelia (chromosomal defect, teratogenic effect) Temperature of one leg differing from that of the other (circulatory deficiency, CNS disorder)
Number of toes	Five on each foot		Webbing, syndactyly (chromosomal defect) Absence or excess of digits (chromosomal defect, familial trait)
Femur	Intact femur		Femoral fracture (difficult breech birth)
Head of femur as legs are flexed and abducted, placement in acetabulum (see Fig. 24-8)			Developmental dysplasia of the hip
Major gluteal folds	Major gluteal folds even		
Soles of feet	Soles well lined (or wrinkled) over two thirds of foot in term infants Plantar fat pad giving flat-footed effect		Soles of feet Few lines (prematurity) Covered with lines (postmaturity) Congenital clubfoot
Evaluate joints Hip Knee Ankle Toes	Full range of motion, symmetric contour		Hypermobility of joints (Down syndrome)
Check reflexes (see Table 24-1)			Asymmetric movement (trauma, CNS disorder)
BACK			
Assess anatomy: Inspect and palpate Spine Shoulders Scapulae Iliac crests	Spine straight and easily flexed Infant able to raise and support head momentarily when prone	Temporary minor positional deformities, correction with passive manipulation	Limitation of movement (fusion or deformity of vertebra)
Base of spine—pilonidal dimple	Shoulders, scapulae, and iliac crests lining up in same plane		Spina bifida cystica (meningocele, myelomeningocele) Pigmented nevus with tuft of hair, location anywhere along the spine, often associated with spina bifida occulta

Continued

Table 24-2

Physical Assessment of Newborn—cont'd

AREA ASSESSED AND APPRAISAL PROCEDURE	Normal Findings: AVERAGE FINDINGS	Normal Findings: NORMAL VARIATIONS	DEVIATIONS FROM NORMAL RANGE: POSSIBLE PROBLEMS (ETIOLOGY)
BACK—cont'd			
Check reflexes (spinal related) Test trunk incurvation reflex	Trunk flexed and pelvis swings to stimulated side	May not be apparent in first few days but is usually present in 5-6 days	If transverse lesion is present, no response below lesion; absence of response: central nervous system abnormality or CNS depression
Test magnet reflex	Lower limbs extend as pressure applied to feet with legs in semiflexed position	Weak or exaggerated response with breech presentation	Absence: suggestive of CNS damage or malformation
ANUS			
Inspect and palpate Placement	One anus with good sphincter tone	Passage of meconium within 48 hr of birth	Imperforate anus without fistula Rectal atresia and stenosis
Patency	Passage of meconium within 24 hr after birth		Absence of anal opening; drainage of fecal material from vagina in female or urinary meatus in male (rectal fistula) or along perineal raphe (midline area between base of penis and anus)—anorectal malformation
Test for sphincter response (active "wink" reflex)	Anal "wink" present, anal opening patent		
Observe for the following: Abdominal distention Passage of meconium from anal opening Fecal drainage from perineum, penis, vagina			
STOOLS			
Observe frequency, color, consistency	Meconium followed by transitional and soft yellow stool		No stool (obstruction) Frequent watery stools (infection, phototherapy)

may range from 80 to 170+ beats/min shortly after birth and, when the infant's condition has stabilized, from 120 to 140 beats/min (Bernstein, 2004). Brachial and femoral pulses are assessed for equality and strength.

If blood pressure is measured, an oscillometric monitor calibrated for neonatal pressures is preferred. An appropriate sized cuff (width-to-arm or calf ratio of 0.45 to 0.70 or approximately ½ to ¾) is essential for accuracy. Neonatal BP usually is highest immediately after birth and falls to a minimum by 3 hours after birth. It then begins to rise steadily and reaches a plateau between 4 and 6 days after birth. This measurement is usually equal to that of the immediate postbirth BP. The BP varies with the neonate's activity; accurate measurement is best obtained while the newborn is at rest.

BP may be measured in both the arms and the legs to detect any discrepancy between the two sides or between the upper and lower body. A discrepancy of 10 mm Hg or more between the arms and legs may signal a cardiac defect such as coarctation of the aorta.

Baseline Measurements of Physical Growth

Baseline measurements are taken and recorded to help assess the progress and determine the growth patterns of the neonate. These may be recorded on growth charts. The following measurements are made when the neonate is assessed.

Weight

The newborn is usually weighed shortly after birth. This may be done in the labor and birthing area, the mother's room, or on admission to the nursery. Care must be taken to ensure the scales are balanced. The totally unclothed neonate is placed in the center of the scale, which is usually covered with a disposable pad or cloth to prevent heat loss via conduction and cross infection. The nurse should place one hand over (but not touching) the neonate to prevent the infant from falling off the scales (p. 709). It is common to weigh the infant at the same time every day during the hospital stay. Birth weight of a term infant typically ranges from 2500g to 4000 g.

Circumferences and Length

The head is measured at the widest part, which is the occipitofrontal diameter (p. 710). The tape measure is placed around the head just above the infant's eyebrows. The term neonate's head circumference ranges from 32 cm to 36.8 cm.

The chest circumference usually measures about 2 cm less than the head circumference. The chest may be the same size as the head but should not exceed it. The tape is placed around the infant's chest at the nipple line (p. 711).

Abdominal circumference is measured by placing the tape around the abdomen just above the umbilicus (p. 711). Measurements vary with the size of the infant. The abdomen should be cylindrical in shape and protrude slightly. Abdominal measurements are not always taken but may be measured when there is suspicion of abdominal distention or pathologic condition.

The length may be difficult to obtain because of the flexed posture of the newborn (p. 710). The examiner places the newborn on a flat surface and extends the leg until the knee is flat against the surface. Placing the head against a perpendicular surface and extending the leg may assist with this measurement. In the term neonate, head-to-heel length ranges from 45 to 55 cm.

Neurologic Assessment

The physical assessment includes a neurologic assessment of newborn reflexes (see Table 24-1). This provides useful information about the infant's nervous system and state of neurologic maturation. Many reflex behaviors (e.g., sucking and rooting) are important for proper development. Other reflexes such as gagging, coughing, and sneezing act as primitive safety mechanisms. The assessment needs to be carried out as early as possible because abnormal signs present in the early neonatal period may require further investigation before the newborn is discharged home.

BEHAVIORAL CHARACTERISTICS

The healthy newborn must accomplish behavioral and biologic tasks to develop normally. Behavioral characteristics form the basis of the social capabilities of the infant. Normal newborns differ in their activity levels, feeding and sleeping patterns, and responsiveness. Parents' reactions to their newborns are often determined by these differences. Showing parents the unique characteristics of their infant assists parents to develop a more positive perception of the infant with increased interaction between infant and parent (see Nursing Care Plan).

Nursing Care Plan

IMMEDIATE CARE OF THE NEWBORN

NURSING DIAGNOSIS: Readiness for enhanced organized infant behavior related to effective transition to extrauterine environment

EXPECTED OUTCOME

Neonate will experience optimal child development.

NURSING INTERVENTIONS/*RATIONALES*

Keep neonate clean, dry, and wrapped securely in blanket *to promote comfort and security.*

Provide parent(s) opportunity for skin-to-skin contact (SSC)[see also Evidence-Based Practice box, p. 695] in birthing room *to promote parent-infant attachment, infant comforting, acquaintance with primary caregiver, and to enhance breastfeeding.*

Discuss infant's individual physical features, characteristics and behavior patterns (sleep/wake states) with parents *to promote parents' knowledge of infant characteristics to enhance family relationship development.*

Encourage father's involvement in infant caretaking activities from birth (such as assisting with breastfeeding, skin-to-skin contact, diaper changing) *to enhance knowledge in caregiving and promote father-infant comfort and familiarity.*

Provide teaching and learning opportunities for parents in regard to infant care (feeding, bathing, holding safely, cord care, circumcision care, car seat safety, jaundice) *to promote parent familiarization with caretaking activities, enhance their knowledge of same, and provide a safe and comfortable environment for infant.*

NURSING DIAGNOSIS: Risk for injury related to infant's total dependence on another for care, transitional events immediately following birth, and environmental factors which may threaten optimal adaptation to extrauterine life

EXPECTED OUTCOME

Neonate will remain free of injury and achieve optimal development.

NURSING INTERVENTIONS/*RATIONALES*

Assign Apgar score at 1 and 5 minutes *to evaluate the newborn's condition and newborn transition to the extrauterine environment.*

Assess neonate thoroughly for any evidence of birth trauma *to provide ongoing identification of potential complications.*

Discuss with parents infant's individual characteristics and any birthmarks or minor trauma occurring as a result of the birth *to promote knowledge and ease anxiety about newborn's appearance.*

Keep neonate clean, dry, and wrapped securely in blanket *to maintain optimal body temperature and promote comfort and security.*

Monitor infant's vital signs and cardiorespiratory function to evaluate transitional events and intervene as necessary *to promote optimal physiologic transition to extrauterine environment.*

Perform a comprehensive physical and gestational age assessment within 24 hours of birth *to identify any risk factors or conditions which require further monitoring and /or intervention.*

Teach parents how to hold infant safely, use a bulb syringe, abduction prevention strategies, supine sleep position, and other physical care (see above Nursing Diagnosis and interventions) *to promote parents' knowledge of caretaking and protect infant from environmental dangers.*

BOX 24-2

Clusters of Neonatal Behaviors in BNBAS

Habituation—Ability to respond to and then inhibit responding to discrete stimulus (e.g., light, rattle, bell, pinprick) while asleep
Orientation—Quality of alert states and ability to attend to visual and auditory stimuli while alert
Motor performance—Quality of movement and tone
Range of state—Measure of general arousal level or arousability of infant
Regulation of state—How infant responds when aroused
Autonomic stability—Signs of stress (e.g., tremors, startles, skin color) related to homeostatic (self-regulator) adjustment of the nervous system
Reflexes—Assessment of several neonatal reflexes

Behavioral responses, as well as physical characteristics, change during the period of transition. The Brazelton Neonatal Behavioral Assessment Scale (BNBAS) can be used to systematically assess the infant's behavior (Brazelton & Nugent, 1996). The BNBAS is an interactive examination that assesses the infant's response to 28 areas organized according to the clusters in Box 24-2. It is generally used as a research or diagnostic tool and requires special training.

In addition to their use as initial and ongoing tools to assess neurologic and behavioral responses, the scales can be used to assess initial parent-infant relationships and as a guide for parents to help them focus on their infant's individuality and to develop a deeper attachment to their child. See Chapter 22 for further discussion of attachment.

Sleep-Wake States

Variations in the state of consciousness of infants are called sleep-wake states. The six states form a continuum from deep sleep to crying (Fig. 24-11). There are two sleep states (i.e., deep sleep and light sleep) and four wake states (i.e., drowsy, quiet alert, active alert, and crying) (Blackburn, 2003). Each state has specific characteristics and state-related behaviors. The optimum state of arousal is the quiet alert state. During this state infants smile, vocalize, move in synchrony with speech, watch their parents' faces, and respond to people talking to them (see Family Focus box). Infants' reactions to internal and external stimuli and ability to control their responses while in these sleep-wake states reflect the ability to organize behavior.

Infants use purposeful behavior to maintain the optimum arousal state as follows: (1) actively withdrawing by increasing physical distance; (2) rejecting by pushing away with hands and feet; (3) decreasing sensitivity by falling asleep or breaking eye contact by turning head; or (4) using signaling behaviors, such as fussing and crying. These behaviors permit infants to quiet themselves and reinstate readiness to interact.

The first 6 weeks of life involve a steady decrease in the proportion of active REM sleep to total sleep. A steady increase in the proportion of quiet sleep to total sleep also occurs. Periods of wakefulness increase. For the first few weeks the wakeful periods seem dictated by hunger, but soon a need for socializing appears as well. The newborn sleeps approximately 16 to 18 hours a day, with periods of wakefulness gradually increasing. By the fourth week of life, some infants stay awake from one feeding to the next.

Family Focus

NEWBORN BEHAVIOR

A first-time single mother asks the nurse about her newborn's activity. She voices concern that the newborn cries when she changes his diaper. "He sleeps a lot and only wakes up to eat or when I change his diaper; is that normal?" Develop a short parent teaching lesson to present newborn behavior and care in relation to the following: sleep-wake states, newborn activities and relationship to crying behaviors in the first few days of life, and how to comfort and console the newborn.

Critical Thinking Exercise

MATERNAL ATTACHMENT

Tara, 16 years old, in labor with her first baby, and Melanie, 38 years old, in labor with her fifth baby, gave birth at approximately the same time. Tara responded excitedly when her baby was placed in her arms but said, "Ugh!" when the nurse suggested placing the infant to breast. Melanie took the baby from the nurse, put him to breast, but said tearfully to the nurse, "I was really hoping for a girl; this is the fifth boy." The nurse determined there was a need to discuss infant feeding with Tara and to promote mother-infant attachment in Melanie. What suggestions would you have for the nurse?

1. Evidence—Is there sufficient evidence to draw conclusions about factors interfering with mother-infant attachment? About appropriate teaching related to breastfeeding and mother-infant attachment? Is age a risk factor in attachment?
2. Assumptions—What assumptions can be made about the following issues?
   a. Method of infant feeding used by adolescent mothers
   b. Attachment in adolescent mothers
   c. Attachment in experienced mothers
   d. Disappointment with the sex of an infant
3. What implications and priorities for nursing care can be drawn at this time?
4. Does the evidence objectively support your conclusion?
5. Are there alternative perspectives to your conclusion?

Other Factors Influencing Behavior of Newborns

Gestational Age

The gestational age of the infant and level of CNS maturity affect the observed behavior. In an infant with an immature CNS (preterm), the entire body responds to a pinprick of the foot although the response may not be observed by an untrained observer; the mature infant withdraws only the foot. CNS immaturity is reflected in reflex development, sleep-wake states, and ability to regulate or modulate a smooth transition between different states. Preterm infants have brief periods of alertness but have difficulty maintain-

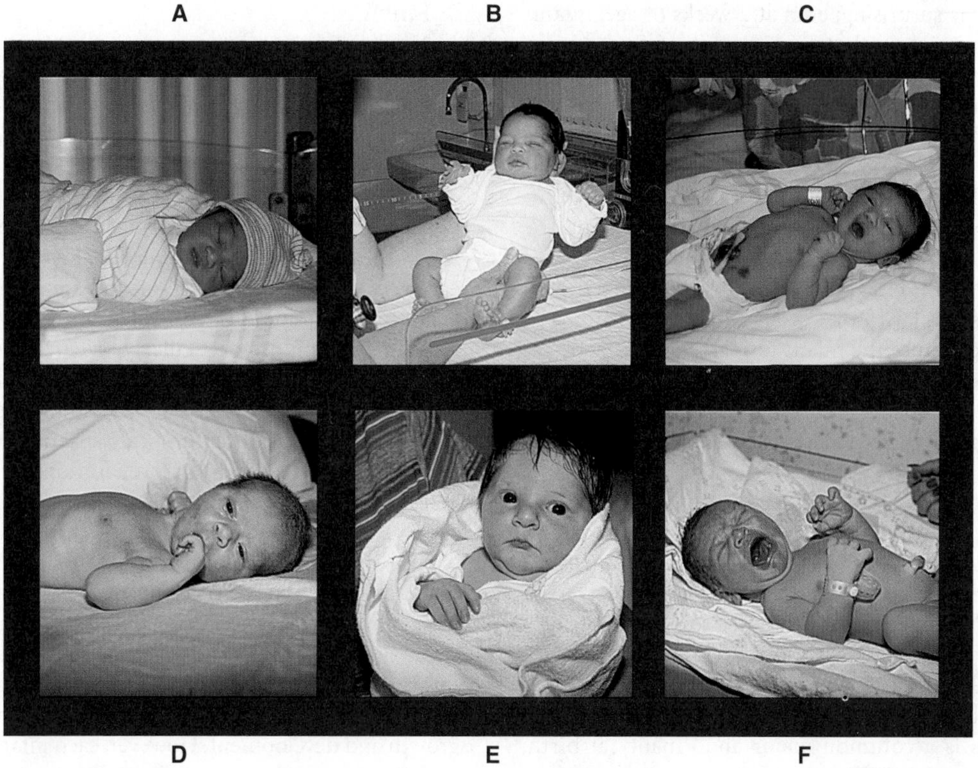

Fig. 24-11 Newborn sleep-wake states. **A**, deep sleep; **B**, light sleep; **C**, drowsy; **D**, quiet alert; **E**, active alert; **F**, crying. (Courtesy Marjorie Pyle, RNC, Lifecircle, Costa Mesa, CA.)

ing the state without becoming overstimulated, which leads to autonomic instability unless intervention is implemented. Preterm or sick infants show signs of fatigue or physiologic stress sooner than full-term healthy infants.

Time

The time elapsed since labor and birth affects the behavior of infants as they attempt to become organized initially. Time elapsed since the previous feeding and time of day may also influence infants' responses.

Stimuli

Environmental events and stimuli affect the behavioral responses of infants. The newborn responds to animate and inanimate stimuli. Nurses in intensive care nurseries observe that infants respond to loud noises, bright lights, monitor alarms, and tension in the unit. If a mother is tense and is nervous or uncomfortable while feeding her infant, the infant may sense her tension and demonstrate difficulty feeding.

Medication

Controversy surrounds the effects on infant behavior of maternal medication (e.g., analgesia and anesthesia) during labor. Some researchers note that infants of mothers given certain analgesic medications may continue to demonstrate poor state organization after the fifth day; medication effects have been noted as long as 30 days after birth. Other researchers maintain that the effect can be beneficial or nonexistent.

Sensory Behaviors

From birth, infants possess sensory capabilities that indicate a state of readiness for social interaction. Infants effectively use behavioral responses in establishing their first dialogues. These responses, coupled with the newborn's "baby appearance" (e.g., facial proportions of forehead and eyes larger than the lower part of the face) and their small size and helplessness, rouse feelings of wanting to hold, protect, and interact with them.

Vision

At birth the eye is structurally incomplete and the muscles are immature. The process of accommodation is not present at birth but improves over the first 3 months of life. The pupils react to light, the blink reflex is easily stimulated, and the corneal reflex is activated by light touch. Term newborns can see objects as far away as 2½ feet. The clearest visual distance is 17 to 20 cm (8 to 12 inches), which is about the distance the infant's face is from the mother's face as she breastfeeds or cuddles. Infants are sensitive to light; they will frown if a bright light is flashed in their eyes, and will turn toward a soft, red light. If the room is darkened, they will open their eyes wide and look about. By 2 months of age, they can detect color; but at 5 days of age and younger, they seem more attracted by black-and-white patterns.

Response to movement is noticeable. If a bright light is shown to newborns (even at 15 minutes of age), they will follow it visually; some will even turn their heads to do so. Because human eyes are bright, shiny objects, newborns will track their parents' eyes. Parents often comment on how exciting this behavior is. The development of eye-to-eye contact is very important for parent-infant attachment. Children of blind parents, and parents who have blind children, must circumvent this obstacle for the formation of a relationship.

Visual acuity is surprising; even at 2 weeks of age, infants can distinguish patterns with stripes 3 mm apart. By 6 months their vision is as acute as that of an adult. They prefer to look at patterns rather than plain surfaces, even if the latter are brightly colored. They prefer more complex patterns to simple ones. They prefer novelty (changes in pattern) by 2 months of age. The infant of a few weeks of age is therefore capable of responding actively to an enriched environment.

Hearing

As soon as the amniotic fluid drains from the ears, the infant's hearing is similar to that of an adult. Loud sounds of about 90 decibels cause the infant to react with a startle reflex. The newborn responds to low frequency sounds such as a heartbeat or lullaby by decreasing motor activity or stopping crying. High-frequency sound elicits an alerting response.

The infant responds readily to the mother's voice. Studies indicate a selective listening to maternal voice sounds and rhythms during intrauterine life that prepares newborns for recognition and interaction with their primary caregivers—their mothers. Newborns are accustomed to hearing the regular rhythm of the mother's heartbeat. As a result, they respond by relaxing and ceasing to fuss and cry if a regular heartbeat simulator is placed in their cribs.

Hearing loss is a common major abnormality at birth; approximately 1 to 3 in 1000 normal term infants have bilateral hearing loss (American Academy of Pediatrics, 2000). To identify affected infants, the hearing of all infants is screened in the newborn nursery (Fig. 24-12).

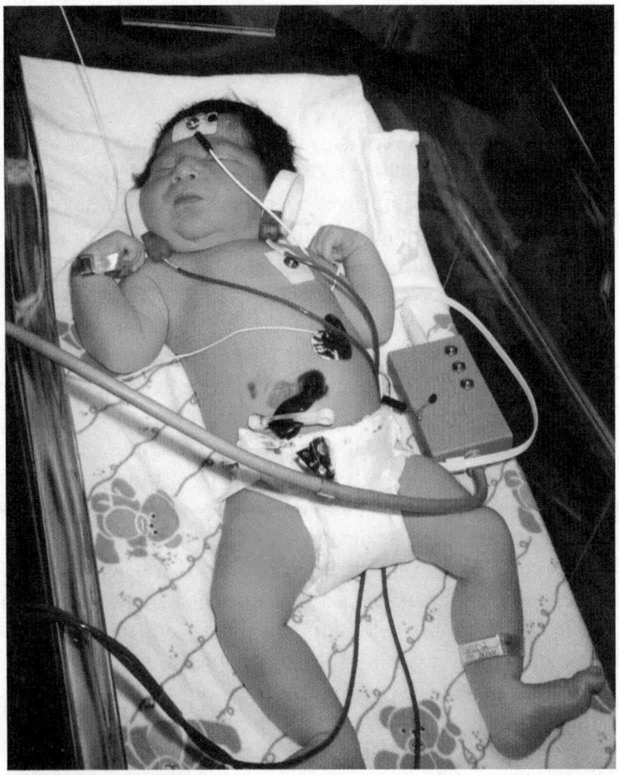

Fig. 24-12 Hearing screening in the newborn nursery. (Courtesy Dee Lowdermilk, Chapel Hill, NC.)

Smell

Newborns react to strong odors such as alcohol or vinegar by turning their heads away. Breastfed infants are able to smell breast milk and can differentiate their mother from other lactating women by the smell (Lawrence & Lawrence, 2005).

Taste

The newborn can distinguish between tastes, and various types of solutions elicit differing facial expressions. A tasteless solution produces no response; a sweet solution elicits eager sucking. A sour solution causes puckering of the lips, and a bitter liquid produces a grimace.

Young infants are particularly oriented toward the use of their mouths, both for meeting their nutritional needs for rapid growth and for releasing tension through sucking. The early development of circumoral sensation, muscle activity, and taste would seem to be preparation for survival in the extrauterine environment.

Touch

The newborn is responsive to touch on all parts of the body. The face (especially the mouth), hands, and soles of the feet seem to be the most sensitive. Reflexes can be elicited by stroking the infant. The newborn's responses to touch suggest this sensory system is well prepared to receive and process tactile messages. Touch and motion are essential to normal growth and development. However, each infant is unique, and variations can be seen in newborns' responses to touch. Birth trauma or stress and depressant drugs taken by the mother decrease the infant's sensitivity to touch or painful stimuli.

Response to Environmental Stimuli

Temperament

Classic studies have identified individual variations in the primary reaction pattern of newborns and described them as temperament. Their style of behavioral response to stimuli is guided by the temperament affecting the newborn's sensory threshold, ability to habituate, and response to maternal behaviors. The newborn possesses individual characteristics that affect selective responses to various stimuli present in the internal and external environments.

The three major patterns of behavioral style or temperament are as follows (Chess, 1969; Chess & Thomas, 1977):

1. The *easy child,* who demonstrates regularity in bodily functions, readily adapts to change, has a predominantly positive mood and moderate sensory threshold, and approaches new situations or objects with a moderate response
2. The *slow-to-warm-up child,* who has a low activity level, withdraws on first exposure to new stimuli, is slow to adapt and low in intensity of response, and is somewhat negative in mood
3. The *difficult child,* who is irregular in bodily functions, intense in reactions, generally negative in mood, and resistant to change or new stimuli and often cries loudly for long periods

Habituation

Habituation is a protective mechanism that allows the infant to become accustomed to environmental stimuli. Habituation is a psychologic and physiologic phenomenon in which the response to a constant or repetitive stimulus is decreased. In the term newborn, this can be demonstrated in several ways. Shining a bright light into a newborn's eyes will cause a startle or squinting the first two or three times. The third or fourth flash will elicit a diminished response, and by the fifth or sixth flash, the infant ceases to respond (Brazelton & Nugent, 1996). The same response pattern holds true for the sounds of a rattle or for a pinprick to the heel.

The ability to habituate allows the healthy term newborn to select stimuli that promote continued learning about the social world, thus avoiding overload. The intrauterine environment seems to have programmed the newborn to be especially responsive to human voices, soft lights, soft sounds, and sweet tastes.

The newborn quickly learns the sounds in a newborn nursery and the home and is able to sleep in their midst. The selective responses of the newborn indicate cerebral organization capable of memory and making choices. The ability to habituate depends on the state of consciousness, hunger, fatigue, and temperament. These factors also affect consolability, cuddliness, irritability, and crying.

Consolability

Barr (1990) described variations in the ability of newborns to console themselves or to be consoled. In the crying state, most newborns initiate one of several ways to reduce their distress. Hand-to-mouth movements are common, with or without sucking, as well as alerting to voices, noises, or visual stimuli.

Cuddliness

Cuddliness is especially important to parents because they often gauge their ability to care for the child by the child's responses to their actions. The degree to which newborns mold into the contours of the person holding them varies. Barr (1990) tested the effect of body contact and vestibular stimulation in both soothing babies and creating alertness. The vestibular stimulation of being picked up and moved had the greater effect.

Irritability

Some newborns cry longer and harder than others. For some the sensory threshold seems low. They are readily upset by unusual noises, hunger, wetness, or new experiences, and thus respond intensely. Others with a high sensory threshold require a great deal more stimulation and variation to reach the active, alert state.

Crying

Crying in an infant may signal hunger, pain, desire for attention, or fussiness. Some mothers state that they learn to distinguish among the cries. The duration of crying is also highly variable in each infant; newborns may cry for as little as 5 minutes or as much as 2 hours or more per day. The amount of crying peaks in the second month and then decreases. There is a diurnal rhythm of crying, with more crying occurring in the evening hours. Crying does not seem to differ with different caretakers.

Key Points

- By full term the newborn's various anatomic and physiologic systems have reached a level of development and functioning that permits a physical existence apart from the mother.
- The healthy term infant has sensory capabilities that indicate a state of readiness for social interaction.
- The appearance of jaundice during the first day of life or persistence of jaundice beyond 7 to 10 days may indicate a pathologic process that requires further investigation.
- Heat loss in the healthy term newborn may exceed the capacity to produce heat; this can lead to metabolic and respiratory complications that threaten the newborn's well-being.
- Assessment of the newborn requires data from the prenatal, intrapartal, and postpartal periods.
- The newborn assessment should proceed systematically so that each system is thoroughly evaluated.
- Some reflex behaviors are important for the newborn's survival.
- Individual personalities and behavioral characteristics of infants play a major role in the ultimate relationship between infants and their parents.
- Each full-term newborn has a predisposed capacity to handle the multitude of stimuli in the external world.

Answer Guidelines to Critical Thinking Exercise

Maternal Attachment

1. Yes. Breastfeeding and mother-infant attachment have been studied extensively. There are various reasons for selecting type of feeding. Women may not be informed about the advantages of breastfeeding for both the baby and the mother; they may have misconceptions about the effects of breastfeeding. Risk factors interfering with attachment and interventions to promote attachment have been identified.
2. (a) Method of infant feeding used by adolescent mothers. Adolescents may have misconceptions about and be unaware of the benefits of breastfeeding. Breastfeeding may be difficult for the adolescent who is trying to complete her education. It may also tie her down when she is trying to achieve the normal developmental task of adolescence of achieving independence. (b) Adolescent mothers become attached to their infants. However, they often overestimate the maturity of the infant and have unrealistic expectations. They need assistance in understanding normal developmental progression of the infant. (c) Experienced mothers may experience "feelings of love" sooner than first-time mothers. Their attachments may be immediate and strong or, in some instances, slow to occur when the newborn does not meet their expectation. Attachment may be facilitated by seeing ultrasound pictures of the baby. (d) Mothers can be disappointed with the sex of an infant. It is sometimes hard for a nurse to understand how a mother can be disappointed with a normal healthy baby. In some cultures, male infants are preferred, and a mother can feel guilt in not producing the male desired by her husband and family.
3. The nurse can discuss with Tara her apparent aversions to breastfeeding and the advantages of breastfeeding to both

the infant and herself. However, Tara must make the feeding choice and the nurse needs to support the choice. Melanie will need time to get over her disappointment and to learn to know her newborn. Providing ample opportunity to interact with the infant is important. In most instances, such disappointments are short-lived and the mother accepts the newborn. In the rare instance that a mother does not accept a child, a social worker or child protective services may need to be involved for the safety of the infant.

4. There is significant literature on methods of feeding, the benefits of breastfeeding, maternal attachment, and factors affecting attachment as well as interventions to promote breastfeeding and to enhance attachment.
5. The significant other/husband of both Tara and Melanie needs to be included in interventions. The support person (who is usually the husband) has a great influence on the success of breastfeeding. Melanie may fear that her husband will be disappointed with a fifth boy or she may be from a culture that favors boys. Family reactions will affect her own reaction. Support from the family is important. Melanie needs time to adjust to the infant.

Resources

The Academy of Neonatal Nursing
2270 Northpoint Parkway
Santa Rosa, CA 95407-7398
707-568-2168
707-569-0786 (fax)
www.academyonline.org

Advances in Neonatal Care
Elsevier
360 Park Avenue South
New York, NY 10010

American Academy of Pediatrics
141 Northwest Point Blvd.
Elk Grove, IL 60007-1098
847-434-4000
847-434-8000 (fax)
www.aap.org

Journal of Perinatal and Neonatal Nursing
Lippincott Williams & Wilkins
530 Walnut St
Philadelphia, PA 19106-3621
215-521-8300
215-521-8902 (fax)
www.lww.com

National Association of Neonatal Nurses (NANN)
4700 W. Lake Avenue Glenview, IL 60025-1485
847-375-3660 or 1-800-451-3795 US/Canada
fax: 888-477-6266, International fax: 732-380-3640
info@nann.org www.nann.org/

Neonatal Network
2270 Northpoint Parkway
Santa Rosa, CA 95407-7398
707-569-1415
707-569-0786 (fax)
www.neonatalnetwork.com

Pediatric Assessment video
Whaley and Wong's Pediatric Nursing Video Series
St Louis, 1996, Mosby
800-426-4545.

References

American Academy of Pediatrics, Joint Committee on Infant Hearing: Year 2000 Position Statement: principle and guidelines for early hearing detection and intervention, *Pediatrics* 106(4):798-824, 2000.

Anderson G et al: Early skin-to-skin contact for mothers and their healthy newborn infants (Cochrane Review), 2003. In *The Cochrane Library,* Issue 2, Chichester, UK, 2004, John Wiley & Sons.

Armentrout DC, Huseby V: Polycythemia in the newborn, *MCN Am J Matern Child Nurs* 28(4):234-239, 2003.

Askin DF: Chest and lungs assessment. In Tappero EP, Honeyfield ME, (eds): *Physical assessment of the newborn,* ed 3, Petaluma, CA., 2003, NICU Ink.

Barr RG: The normal crying curve: what do we really know? *Dev Med Child Neurol* 32(4):356-362, 1990.

Bernstein D: Evaluation of the cardiovascular system. History and physical examination. In Behrman RE, Kliegman R, Jenson HB: *Nelson textbook of pediatrics,* ed 17, St. Louis, 2004, WB Saunders.

Blackburn ST: *Maternal, fetal, and neonatal physiology: a clinical perspective,* ed 2, St Louis, 2003, WB Saunders.

Brazelton T, Nugent J: *Neonatal behavioural assessment scale,* ed 3, London, 1996, MacKeith.

Chess S: Individuality and baby care, *Dev Med Neurol* 11(6):749-754, 1969.

Chess S, Thomas A: Temperament and the parent-child interaction, *Pediatr Ann* 6(9):574-582, 1977.

Dickason EJ, Silverman BL, Kaplan JA: *Maternal-infant nursing care,* ed 3, St Louis, 1998, Mosby.

Garas T et al: Perinatal morbidity: a comparison of vacuum delivery and spontaneous delivery, *Obstet Gynecol* 97(4 suppl 1):S64, 2001.

Gordon EA: Polycythemia and hyperviscosity of the newborn, *J Perinat Neonatal Nurs* 17(3):209-219, 2003.

Hockenberry MJ et al: *Wong's nursing care of infants and children,* ed 7, St Louis, 2003, Mosby.

Lawrence RA, Lawrence RM: *Breastfeeding: a guide for the medical profession,* ed 6, St Louis, 2005, Mosby.

Paige PL, Carney PR: Neurologic disorders. In Merenstein GB, Gardner SL (eds): *Handbook of neonatal intensive care,* ed 5, St Louis, 2002, Mosby.

Putta LV, Spencer JP: Assisted vaginal delivery using the vacuum extractor, *Am Fam Physician* 62(6):1316-1320, 2000.

Ross MG, Fresquez M, El-Haddad MA: Impact of FDA advisory on reported vacuum-assisted delivery and morbidity, *J Fetal Matern Med* 9(6):321-326, 2001.

Seidel HM et al: *Mosby's guide to physical examination,* ed 5, St Louis, 2003, Mosby.

Uchil D, Arulkumaran S: Neonatal subgaleal hemorrhage and its relationship to delivery by vacuum extraction, *Obstet Gynecol Survey* 58(10): 687-693, 2003.

Weinberg JA, Powell KR: Laboratory aids for diagnosis of neonatal sepsis. In Remington JS, Klein JO (eds): *Infectious diseases of the fetus and newborn infant,* ed 5, Philadelphia, 2001, WB Saunders.

Zitelli BJ, Davis HW: *Atlas of pediatric physical diagnosis,* ed 4, St Louis, 2002, Mosby.

Nursing Care of the Newborn 25

LEARNING OBJECTIVES

On completion of this chapter the reader will be able to:

- Identify the purpose and components of the Apgar score.
- Compare and contrast the characteristics of preterm, term, postterm, and postmature neonates.
- Perform a gestational age assessment on a newborn.
- Explain what is meant by a safe environment.
- Discuss phototherapy and the guidelines for teaching parents about this treatment.
- Explain purposes and methods of circumcision, the postoperative care of the circumcised infant, and parent teaching information regarding circumcision.
- Review procedures for a heel stick, collecting urine specimens, and assisting with venipuncture.
- Evaluate pain in the newborn based on physiologic changes and behavioral observations.
- Review anticipatory guidance nurses provide parents before discharge.

ELECTRONIC RESOURCES

Additional information related to the content in Chapter 25 can be found on

the companion website at evolve
http://evolve.elsevier.com/Wong/maternal/

- NCLEX Review Questions
- Case Study–Normal Newborn
- WebLinks

or the interactive student CD-ROM
Activities for Chapter 25 include the following:

- NCLEX Review Questions
- Case Study–Normal Newborn
- Critical Thinking Exercise–Circumcision
- Critical Thinking Exercise–Jaundice
- Nursing Care Plan–Normal Newborn
- Skill–Changing a Diaper
- Skill–Infant Bathing
- Skill–Pain Assessment

Although most infants make the necessary biopsychosocial adjustment to extrauterine existence without undue difficulty, their well-being depends on the care they receive from others. This chapter describes the assessment and care of the infant from immediately after birth until discharge. A discussion of pain in the neonate and its management is included.

BIRTH THROUGH THE FIRST 2 HOURS

Care Management

Care begins immediately after the birth and focuses on assessing and stabilizing the condition of the newborn. The nurse has primary responsibility for the infant during this period, because the physician or midwife is involved with the care of the mother. The nurse must be alert for any signs of distress and initiate appropriate interventions.

With the possibility of transmission of viruses such as hepatitis B virus (HBV) and human immunodeficiency virus (HIV) via maternal blood and blood-stained amniotic fluid, the traditional timing of the newborn's bath has been questioned. The newborn must be considered a potential contamination source until proved otherwise. As part of Standard Precautions, nurses should wear gloves when handling the newborn until blood and amniotic fluid is removed by bathing.

Assessment

Initial Assessment and Apgar Scoring

The first assessment of the newborn is done immediately after birth using the Apgar score (Table 25-1) and a brief physical examination (Box 25-1). A gestational age assessment is done within the first hours of birth in the stable newborn (Fig. 25-1). A more comprehensive physical examination may be completed within 24 hours of birth (see Table 24-2).

Table 25-1

Apgar Score

	Score		
SIGN	0	1	2
Heart rate	Absent	Slow (<100)	Over 100
Respiratory rate	Absent	Slow, weak cry	Good cry
Muscle tone	Flaccid	Some flexion of extremities	Well flexed
Reflex irritability	No response	Grimace	Cry
Color	Blue, pale	Body pink, extremities blue	Completely pink

BOX 25-1

Initial Physical Assessment by Body System

Central Nervous System
- [ ] moves all 4 extremities, flexion, muscle tone good
- [ ] symmetric features, movement
- [ ] Moro, suck, rooting, and grasp reflexes present
- [ ] anterior fontanel soft and flat

Cardiovascular System
- [ ] heart auscultation, regular in rate and rhythm
- [ ] transient acrocyanosis, otherwise pink in color
- [ ] pulses strong/equal bilaterally
- [ ] capillary refill <3 seconds centrally and in peripheral tissues (not nail beds)

Respiratory System
- [ ] lungs auscultated, clear bilaterally with minimal fine crackles shortly after birth
- [ ] respiratory rate <60 breaths/min
- [ ] respiratory effort nonlabored
- [ ] absence of nasal flaring, grunting

Genitourinary System
- [ ] male: urethral opening at tip of penis; testes descended bilaterally; female: labia minora and majora intact; hymenal tag may be visible

Gastrointestinal System
- [ ] abdomen soft, no visible distention
- [ ] cord attached and clamped
- [ ] anus patent

Eyes, Ears, Nose, and Throat
- [ ] eyes clear
- [ ] palates intact
- [ ] nares patent
- [ ] ears in place; correct alignment

Skin
Color [ ] pink [ ] acrocyanotic
- [ ] skin lesions or abrasions documented
- [ ] birthmarks documented
- [ ] caput/molding
- [ ] forceps marks
- [ ] other

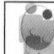

Comments: ______________________________

____

____

Apgar Score

The Apgar score permits a rapid assessment of the newborn's transition to extrauterine existence based on five signs that indicate the physiologic state of the newborn: (1) heart rate based on auscultation with a stethoscope or palpation of the umbilical cord; (2) respiratory rate based on observed movement of respiratory efforts; (3) muscle tone based on degree of flexion and movement of the extremities; (4) reflex irritability based on response to bulb or catheter inserted in nasopharynx; and (5) generalized skin color described as pallid, cyanotic, or pink (see Table 25-1). Evaluations are made at 1 and 5 minutes after birth and can be done by the nurse or birth attendant. Scores of 0 to 3 indicate severe distress, scores of 4 to 6 indicate moderate difficulty, and scores of 7 to 10 indicate that the infant is having minimal or no difficulty adjusting to extrauterine life. Apgar scores do not predict future neurologic outcome, but are useful for describing the newborn's transition to extrauterine environment (Family Focus box). Should resuscitation be required,

Family Focus

SIGNIFICANCE OF THE APGAR SCORE

The Apgar score was developed to provide a systematic method of assessing an infant's condition at birth. Researchers have tried to correlate Apgar scores with various outcomes such as development, intelligence, and neurologic development. In some instances, researchers have attempted to attribute causality to the Apgar score, that is, to suggest that the low Apgar score caused or predicted later problems. This is an inappropriate use of the Apgar score. Instead the score should be used to ensure that infants are systematically observed at birth to ascertain the need for immediate care. Either a physician or a nurse may assign the score; however, to avoid the real or perceived appearance of bias, the person assisting with the birth should not assign the score. Lack of consistency in the assigned scores limits studies of the Apgar's long-term predictive value. Prospective parents and the public need education on the significance of the Apgar, as well as its limits. Because infants often do not receive the maximum score of 10, parents need to know that scores of 7 to 10 are within normal limits. Attorneys involved in litigation related to injury of an infant at birth or negative outcomes, either short term or long term, also need education about the Apgar, its significance, and its limits. This useful tool needs to be used appropriately; health care providers, parents, and the public may need education to ensure appropriate use of the score.

Data from Montgomery K: Apgar scores: examining the long-term significance, *J Perinat Educ* 9(3):5-9, 2000.

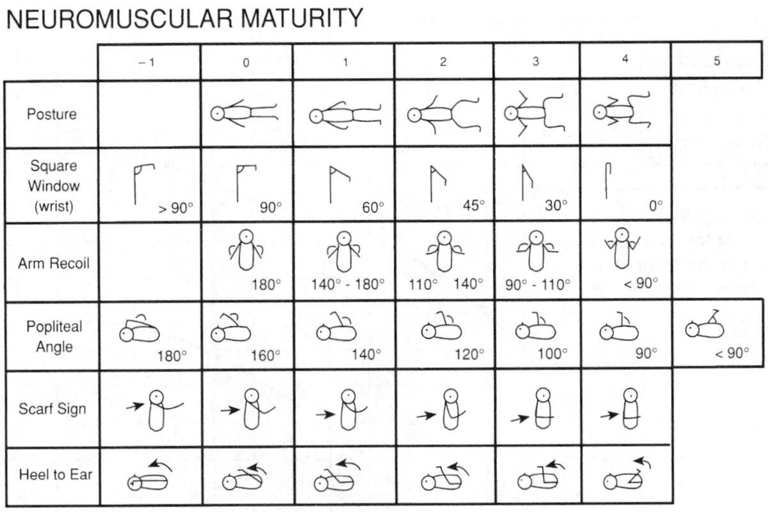
NEUROMUSCULAR MATURITY
−1
0
1
2
3
4
5
Posture
Square Window (wrist)
> 90°
90°
60°
45°
30°
0°
Arm Recoil
180°
140° - 180°
110° 140°
90° - 110°
< 90°
Popliteal Angle
180°
160°
140°
120°
100°
90°
< 90°
Scarf Sign
Heel to Ear

A

PHYSICAL MATURITY

	−1	0	1	2	3	4	5
Skin	sticky friable transparent	gelatinous red, translucent	smooth pink, visible veins	superficial peeling or rash, few veins	cracking pale areas rare veins	parchment deep cracking no vessels	leathery cracked wrinkled
Lanugo	none	sparse	abundant	thinning	bald areas	mostly bald	
Plantar Surface	heel-toe 40-50 mm: -1 <40 mm: -2	>50 mm no crease	faint red marks	anterior transverse crease only	creases ant. 2/3	creases over entire sole	
Breast	imperceptible	barely perceptible	flat areola no bud	stippled areola 1-2 mm bud	raised areola 3-4 mm bud	full areola 5-10 mm bud	
Eye/Ear	lids fused loosely: -1 tightly: -2	lids open pinna flat stays folded	sl. curved pinna; soft; slow recoil	well-curved pinna; soft but ready recoil	formed & firm instant recoil	thick cartilage ear stiff	
Genitals (male)	scrotum flat, smooth	scrotum empty faint rugae	testes in upper canal rare rugae	testes descending few rugae	testes down good rugae	testes pendulous deep rugae	
Genitals (female)	clitoris prominent labia flat	prominent clitoris small labia minora	prominent clitoris enlarging minora	majora & minora equally prominent	majora large minora small	majora cover clitoris & minora	

MATURITY RATING

score	weeks
-10	20
-5	22
0	24
5	26
10	28
15	30
20	32
25	34
30	36
35	38
40	40
45	42
50	44

Fig. 25-1 Estimation of gestational age. **A,** New Ballard scale for newborn maturity rating. Expanded scale includes extremely premature infants and has been refined to improve accuracy in more mature infants. (From Ballard J et al: New Ballard score, expanded to include extremely premature infants, *J Pediatr* 119(3):417, 1991.) *Continued*

it should be initiated before the 1-minute Apgar score (American Academy of Pediatrics and American College of Obstetricians and Gynecologists, 2002).

Initial Physical Assessment

The initial physical assessment includes a brief review of systems (see Box 25-1).

1. **External**—Note skin color, general activity, position; assess nasal patency by closing one nostril at a time while observing respirations; skin: peeling, or lack of subcutaneous fat (dysmaturity or postterm); note meconium staining of cord, skin, fingernails, or amniotic fluid (staining may indicate fetal release of meconium); note length of nails and development of creases on soles of feet
2. **Chest**—Auscultate apical heart for rate and rhythm, heart tones and presence of abnormal sounds; note character of respirations and presence of crackles or other adventitious sounds; note quality of breath sounds by auscultation
3. **Abdomen**—Verify characteristics of abdomen (rounded, flat, concave) and absence of anomalies; auscultate bowel sounds; note number of vessels in cord
4. **Neurologic**—Check muscle tone and assess Moro and suck reflexes; palpate anterior fontanel; note by palpation the presence and size of the fontanels and sutures
5. **Genitourinary**—Note external sex characteristics and any abnormality of same; check anal patency, presence of meconium; note passage of urine
6. **Other observations**—Note gross structural malformation obvious at birth that may require immediate medical attention

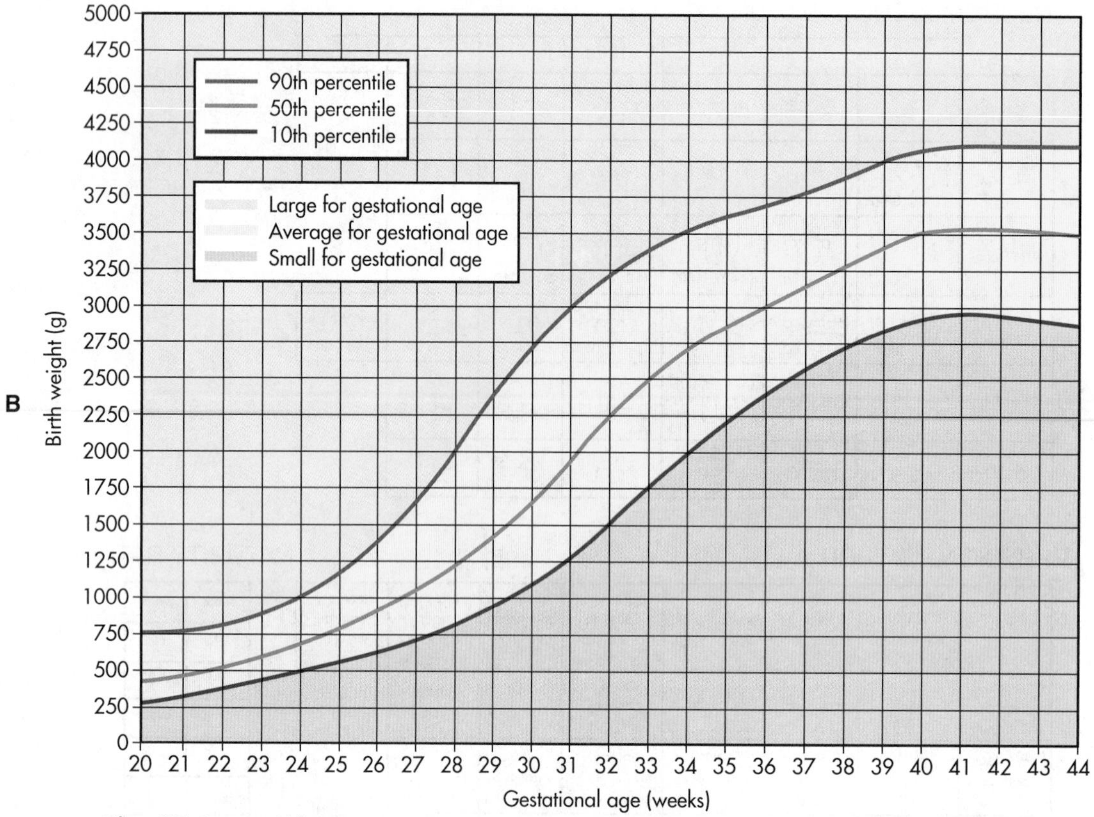

Fig. 25-1—cont'd B, Intrauterine growth: birth weight percentiles based on live single births at gestational ages 20 to 44 weeks. (Data from Alexander GR et al: A United States national reference for fetal growth, *Obstet Gynecol* 87(2):163-168, 1996.)

The nurse responsible for the care of the newborn immediately after birth verifies that respirations have been established, dries the infant, assesses temperature, and places identical identification bracelets on the infant and the mother. In some settings, the father or partner also wears an identification bracelet. The infant may be wrapped in a warm blanket and placed in the arms of the mother, given to the partner to hold, or kept partially undressed under a radiant warmer. In some settings, immediately after birth the infant is placed on the mother's abdomen to allow skin-to-skin contact. This contributes to maintenance of the infant's optimum temperature and parental bonding. The infant may be admitted to a nursery or remain with the parents throughout the hospital stay.

The initial examination of the newborn can occur while the nurse is drying and wrapping the infant, or observations can be made while the infant is lying on the mother's abdomen or in her arms immediately after birth. Efforts should be directed toward minimizing interference in the initial parent-infant acquaintance process. If the infant is breathing effectively, is pink in color, and has no apparent life-threatening anomalies or risk factors requiring immediate attention (e.g., infant of diabetic mother), further examination can be delayed until after the parents have had an opportunity to interact with the infant. Routine procedures and the admission process can be carried out in the mother's room or in a separate nursery. Box 25-2 lists some routine newborn admission orders.

BOX 25-2

Routine Admission Orders

Vital signs on admission and q30min × 2, q1hr × 2, then q8hr
Weight, length, and head and chest circumference on admission; then weigh daily
Tetracycline or erythromycin ophthalmic ointment 5 mg 1 to 2 cm line in lower conjunctiva of each eye (ou) after initial parent-infant contact (but within 2 hours of birth)
Vitamin K 0.5 to 1 mg intramuscularly
Breastfeeding on demand may be initiated immediately after birth
If formula feeding, give formula of mother's choice q3-4hr on demand
Allow rooming-in as desired and infant's condition permits
Newborn screening panel per state health department protocol (phenylketonuria [PKU], thyroxine [T_4], and galactosemia or other newborn screening tests as ordered at least 24 hr after first feeding)
Perform hearing screening and document results before discharge
Serum bilirubin measurement if clinical jaundice evident
Hepatitis B injection if indicated

Nursing Diagnoses

Nursing diagnoses are established after analysis of the findings of the physical assessment. Nursing diagnoses for the newborn include the following:

- *Ineffective airway clearance related to*
  —airway obstruction with mucus, blood, and amniotic fluid

- *Impaired gas exchange related to*
  —airway obstruction
- *Ineffective thermoregulation related to*
  —excess heat loss
- *Risk for infection related to*
  —intrauterine or extrauterine exposure to virulent virus or bacteria
  —multiple sites for opportunistic bacterial/viral entry (e.g., umbilical cord, lesions from fetal scalp electrode or vacuum extraction)

Expected Outcomes

Expected outcomes can apply both to the infant and the parents. Expected outcomes for the newborn during the immediate recovery period include that the infant will achieve the following:

- Maintain effective breathing pattern
- Maintain effective thermoregulation
- Maintain adequate cardiac output/circulation and tissue perfusion
- Remain free from infection
- Receive necessary nutrition for growth

Expected outcomes for the parents include that they will do the following:

- Attain knowledge, skill, and confidence relevant to infant care activities
- State understanding of biologic and behavioral characteristics of the newborn
- Begin to integrate the newborn into the family

Plan of Care and Implementation

Changes can occur rapidly in the newborn immediately after birth. Assessment must be followed by implementation of appropriate care.

Stabilization

Generally, the normal term infant born vaginally has little difficulty clearing the airway. Most secretions are moved by gravity and brought by the cough reflex to the oropharynx to be drained or swallowed. The infant is often maintained in a side-lying position (head stabilized, not in Trendelenburg) with a rolled blanket at the back to facilitate drainage.

If the infant has excess mucus in the respiratory tract, the mouth and nasal passages may be suctioned with a bulb syringe (Fig. 25-2). The nurse may perform gentle percussion over the chest wall using a soft circular mask or a percussion cup to aid in loosening secretions before suctioning (Fig. 25-3). Routine chest percussion is avoided, especially in preterm newborns, because this may cause more harm than good; the head should be kept steady during the procedure and the infant's tolerance to the procedure carefully evaluated (Hagedorn, Gardner, & Abman, 2002). The infant who is choking on secretions should be supported with its head to the side. The mouth is suctioned first to prevent the infant from inhaling pharyngeal secretions by gasping as the nares are touched. The bulb is compressed and inserted into one side of the mouth. The center of the infant's mouth is avoided because this could stimulate the gag reflex. The nasal passages are suctioned one nostril at a time. The bulb syringe should always be kept in the infant's crib. The parents should be given a demonstration of how to use the bulb syringe and asked to perform a return demonstration.

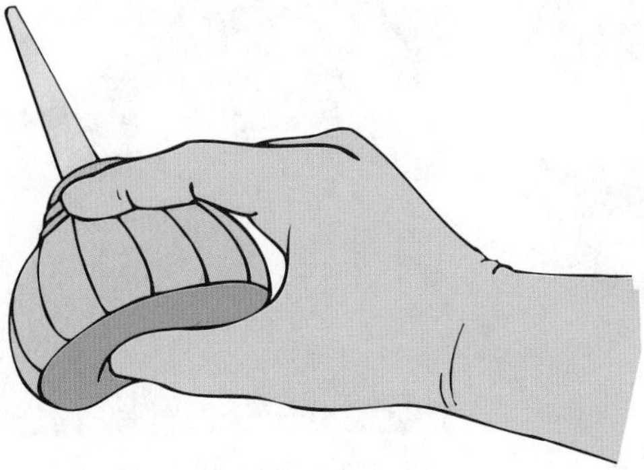

Fig. 25-2 Bulb syringe. Bulb must be compressed before insertion.

Use of Nasopharyngeal Catheter with Mechanical Suction Apparatus

Deeper suctioning may be necessary to remove mucus from the infant's nasopharynx or posterior oropharynx. Proper tube insertion and suctioning 5 seconds or less per tube insertion helps prevent vagal stimulation and hypoxia. If wall suction is used, the pressure should be adjusted to less than 80 mm Hg. After the catheter is properly placed, suction is created by placing one's thumb over the control as the catheter is carefully rotated and gently withdrawn. This procedure may need to be repeated until the infant has a clear airway.

Relieving Airway Obstruction

A choking infant needs immediate attention. Often, simply repositioning the infant and suctioning the mouth and nose with the bulb syringe eliminates the problem. The infant should be positioned to facilitate gravity drainage. The nurse should also listen to the infant's respirations and lung sounds with a stethoscope to determine whether there are crackles, rhonchi, or inspiratory stridor. Fine crackles may be auscultated for several hours after birth. If air movement is adequate, the bulb syringe may be used to clear the mouth and nose. If the bulb syringe does not clear mucus interfering with respiratory effort, mechanical suction can be used.

If the newborn has an obstruction that is not cleared with suctioning, further investigation must occur to determine if

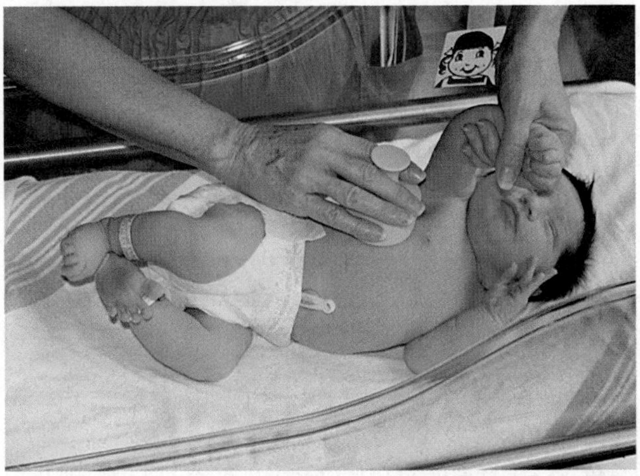

Fig. 25-3 Chest percussion. Nurse performs gentle percussion over the chest wall using a percussion cup to aid in loosening secretions before suctioning. (Courtesy Shannon Perry, Phoenix, AZ.)

there is a mechanical defect (e.g., tracheoesophageal fistula, choanal atresia [see Chapter 28]) causing the obstruction.

Maintaining an Adequate Oxygen Supply

Four conditions are essential for maintaining an adequate oxygen supply:

- A clear airway
- Effective establishment of respirations
- Adequate circulation, adequate perfusion, and effective cardiac function
- Adequate thermoregulation (exposure to cold stress increases oxygen and glucose needs)

Signs of potential complications related to abnormal newborn breathing are listed in Box 25-3.

Maintenance of Body Temperature

Effective neonatal care includes maintenance of an optimal thermal environment (see Chapter 24). Cold stress increases the need for oxygen and may deplete glucose stores. The infant may react to exposure to cold by increasing the respiratory rate and may become cyanotic. Ways to stabilize the newborn's body temperature include placing the infant directly on the mother's abdomen and covering with a warm blanket (skin-to-skin contact); drying and wrapping the newborn in warmed blankets immediately after birth; keeping the head well covered; and keeping the ambient temperature at 23.8° C to 26.1° C (American Academy of Pediatrics and American College of Obstetricians and Gynecologists, 2002).

If the infant does not remain with the mother during the first 1 to 2 hours after birth, the nurse places the thoroughly dried newborn under a radiant warmer or in a warm incubator unit until the body temperature stabilizes. The infant's skin temperature is used as the point of control when using a warmer with a servocontrolled mechanism. The control panel usually is maintained between 36° C and 37° C. This setting should maintain the healthy term infant's skin temperature around 36.5° C to 37° C. A thermistor probe (automatic sensor) is usually placed on the upper quadrant of the abdomen immediately below the right or left costal margin (never over a bone); a reflector adhesive patch may be used over the probe to provide adequate warming. This will ensure detection of minor temperature changes resulting from external environmental factors or neonatal factors (peripheral vasoconstriction, vasodilation, or increased metabolism) before a dramatic change in core body temperature develops; the servocontroller adjusts the warmer temperature to maintain the infant's skin temperature within the preset range. The sensor needs to be checked periodically to make sure that it is securely attached to the infant's skin. The axillary temperature of the newborn is checked every hour (or more often as needed) until the newborn's temperature stabilizes. The time to stabilize and maintain body temperature varies; each newborn should therefore be allowed to achieve thermal regulation as necessary, and care should be individualized.

During all procedures, heat loss must be avoided or minimized for the newborn; examinations and activities are performed with the newborn under a heat panel. The initial bath is postponed until the newborn's skin temperature is stable and can adjust to heat loss from a bath. The exact and optimal timing of the bath for every infant remains unknown.

Even a normal term infant in good health can become hypothermic. Birth in a car on the way to the hospital, a cold birthing room, or inadequate drying and wrapping immediately after birth may cause the infant's temperature to fall below normal range (hypothermia). Warming the hypothermic newborn is accomplished with care. Rapid warming may cause apneic spells and acidosis in an infant. The warming process is therefore monitored to progress slowly over a period of 2 to 4 hours.

BOX 25-3

Newborn Breathing: Signs of Distress

- Bradypnea: respirations (≤30/min)
- Tachypnea: respirations (≥60/min)
- Abnormal breath sounds: crackles, wheezing, rhonchi, expiratory grunting, stridor, diminished or absent air movement
- Respiratory distress: nasal flaring, retractions, labored breathing, apnea ≥20 seconds

Immediate Interventions

It is the nurse's responsibility to perform certain interventions immediately after birth to provide for the safety of the newborn.

Eye Prophylaxis

The instillation of a prophylactic agent in the eyes of all neonates (Fig. 25-4) is mandatory in the United States as a precaution against ophthalmia neonatorum, which is an inflammation of the eyes from gonorrheal or chlamydial infection contracted by the newborn during passage through the mother's birth canal. In the United States, if the family objects to this treatment, the primary care provider may ask that the parents sign an informed refusal form, and their refusal will be noted in the neonate's record. The agent used for prophylaxis varies according to hospital protocols, but usual agents include forms of erythromycin, tetracycline, or

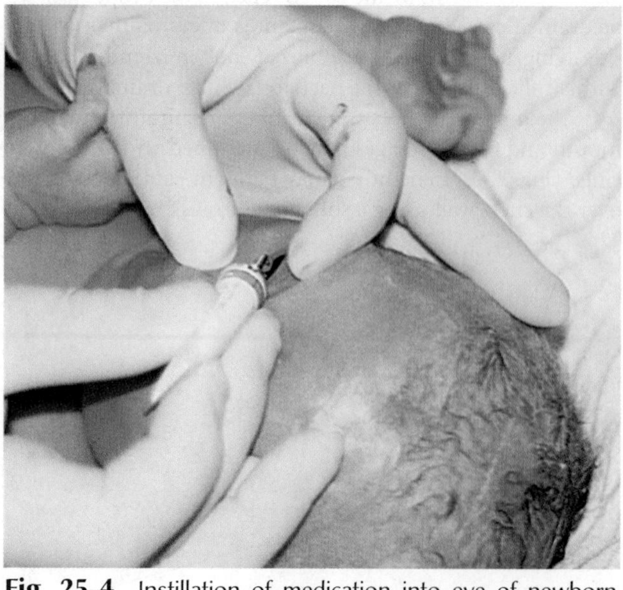

Fig. 25-4 Instillation of medication into eye of newborn. Thumb and forefinger are used to open the eye; medication is placed in the lower conjunctiva from the inner to the outer canthus. (Courtesy Marjorie Pyle, RNC, Lifecircle, Costa Mesa, CA.)

silver nitrate. Canadian hospitals have not recommended the use of silver nitrate since 1986. Its use in the United States is minimal because silver nitrate does not protect against chlamydial infection and can cause chemical conjunctivitis. In some institutions instillation of eye prophylaxis is delayed until an hour or so (up to 2 hours in Canada) after birth so that eye contact and parent-infant attachment and bonding are facilitated.

Topical antibiotics such as tetracycline and erythromycin, silver nitrate, and a 2.5% povidone-iodine solution (currently unavailable in commercial form in the United States) have not proved to be effective in the treatment of chlamydial conjunctivitis.

A 14-day course of oral erythromycin or an oral sulfonamide may be given for chlamydial conjunctivitis (American Academy of Pediatrics and American College of Obstetrician and Gynecologists, 2002) (Medication Guide).

Vitamin K Prophylaxis

Administering vitamin K intramuscularly is routine in the newborn period. A single injection of 0.5 to 1 mg of vitamin K is given soon after birth to prevent hemorrhagic disease of the newborn. Vitamin K is produced in the gastrointestinal tract by bacteria starting soon after microorganisms are introduced. By day 8, normal newborns are able to produce their own vitamin K (Medication Guide).

NURSE ALERT Vitamin K is never administered via the intravenous route for prevention of hemorrhagic disease of the newborn except in some cases of a preterm infant who has no muscle mass. In such cases, the medication should be diluted and given over 10 to 15 minutes with the infant being closely monitored (cardiorespiratory monitor). Rapid bolus administration of vitamin K may cause cardiac arrest. ■

Umbilical Cord Care

The care of the umbilical cord is an important aspect of nursing care and parent teaching. The goal of care is prevention and early detection of hemorrhage or infection. The umbilical cord stump is an excellent medium for bacterial growth and can easily become infected.

Hospital protocol determines the technique for routine cord care. Common methods include the use of an antimicrobial agent such as bacitracin or triple dye. Other methods include the use of soap and water or sterile water alone. The use of antiseptic agents has been shown to prolong cord drying and separation (Zupan & Garner, 2000). Studies regarding bacterial growth and colonization according to the cleansing method used have produced varied results (Dore et al, 1998; Golombek, Brill, & Salice, 2002; Janssen et al, 2003; Zupan & Garner, 2000). Current recommendations for cord care by the Association of Women's Health, Obstetric, and Neonatal Nurses (AWHONN) include cleaning the cord with sterile water or a neutral pH cleanser; subsequent care

Medication Guide

EYE PROPHYLAXIS WITH ERYTHROMYCIN OPHTHALMIC OINTMENT 0.5% AND TETRACYCLINE OPHTHALMIC OINTMENT 1%

Action
These antibiotic ointments are both bacteriostatic and bactericidal. They provide prophylaxis against *Neisseria gonorrhoeae.* Topical treatment of neonatal conjunctivitis caused by *Chlamydia trachomatis* is not indicated; instead the infant should be treated with a 14-day course of either oral erythromycin or ethylsuccinate (American Academy of Pediatrics, 2003).

Indication
These medications are for the prevention of ophthalmia neonatorum in newborns of mothers who are infected with gonorrhea.

Neonatal Dosage
Apply a 1 to 2 cm ribbon of ointment to the lower conjunctival sac of each eye; may also be used in drop form.

Adverse Reactions
May cause chemical conjunctivitis that lasts 24 to 48 hours; vision may be blurred temporarily.

Nursing Considerations
Administer within 1 to 2 hours of birth. Wear gloves. Cleanse eyes if necessary before administration. Open eyes by putting a thumb and finger at the corner of each lid and gently pressing on the periorbital ridges. Squeeze the tube and spread the ointment from the inner canthus of the eye to the outer canthus. Do not touch the tube to the eye. After 1 minute, excess ointment may be wiped off. Observe eyes for irritation. Explain treatment to parents.

Eye prophylaxis for ophthalmia neonatorum is required by law in all states of the United States.

Medication Guide

VITAMIN K: PHYTONADIONE (AQUAMEPHYTON, KONAKION)

Action
This intervention provides vitamin K because the newborn does not have the intestinal flora to produce this vitamin in the first week after birth. Vitamin K promotes formation of clotting factors (II, VII, IX, and X) in the liver.

Indication
Vitamin K is used for prevention and treatment of hemorrhagic disease in the newborn.

Neonatal Dosage
Administer a 0.5 to 1 mg (0.25 to 0.5 ml) dose intramuscularly within 2 hours of birth; may be repeated if newborn shows bleeding tendencies.

Adverse Reactions
Edema, erythema, and pain at injection size may occur rarely; hemolysis, jaundice, and hyperbilirubinemia have been reported, particularly in preterm infants.

Nursing Considerations
Wear gloves. Administer in the middle third of the vastus lateralis muscle using a 25-gauge, 5/8- to 7/8-inch needle. Inject into skin that has been cleaned, or allow alcohol (or other skin antiseptic) to dry on puncture site for 1 minute to remove organisms and prevent infection. Stabilize leg firmly and grasp muscle between the thumb and fingers. Insert the needle at a 90-degree angle; aspirate and inject medication slowly if there is no blood return. After removing needle, rub gently on the injection site with a dry gauze square to decrease the pain. Observe for signs of bleeding from the site.

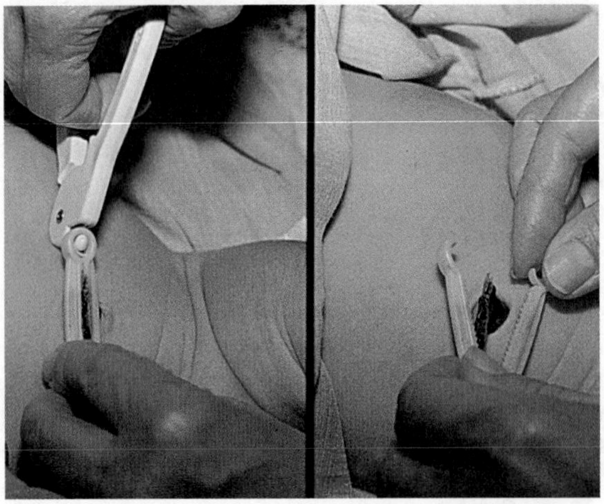

Fig. 25-5 Using special scissors, remove clamp after cord begins drying (about 24 hours). (Courtesy Marjorie Pyle, RNC, Lifecircle, Costa Mesa, CA.)

entails cleansing the cord with water (AWHONN, 2001). The stump and base of the cord should be assessed for edema, erythema, and drainage with each diaper change. The nurse cleanses the cord and skin area around the base of the cord with the prescribed preparation (e.g., sterile water, erythromycin solution, or triple-blue dye). The stump deteriorates through the process of dry gangrene; therefore odor alone is not a positive indicator of omphalitis (infection of the umbilical stump). Cord separation time is influenced by a number of factors, including type of cord care, type of delivery, and other perinatal events. The average cord separation time is 10 to 14 days.

The cord clamp is removed once the stump has started drying and is no longer bleeding (Fig. 25-5), typically in 24 hours.

Promoting Parent-Infant Bonding

Today's childbirth practices strive to promote the family as the focus of care. Parents generally desire to share in the birth process and to have early contact with their infants. Early contact between mother and newborn can be important in developing future relationships. It also has a positive effect on the duration of breastfeeding. There are physiologic benefits of early mother-infant contact. Oxytocin and prolactin levels rise in the mother, and suckling activity is activated in the infant. The process of developing active immunity begins as the infant ingests flora from the mother's colostrum.

Evaluation

Evaluation of the effectiveness of care of the newborn is based on the previously stated outcomes.

FROM 2 HOURS AFTER BIRTH UNTIL DISCHARGE

Care Management

The infant's admission to the nursery may be delayed or may never occur. Depending on the routine of the hospital, the infant often remains in the labor area and is transferred to the nursery/postpartum unit with the mother. Many hospitals have adopted variations of single-room maternity care (SRMC) or mother-baby care. One nurse provides care for both the mother and the newborn. SRMC allows the infant to remain with the parents after the birth. Many of the procedures, such as assessment of weight and measurement, instillation of eye medication, administration of vitamin K, and physical assessment, may be carried out in the labor and birth unit. Nurses who work in an SRMC unit; a labor, delivery, and recovery (LDR) room; or a labor, delivery, recovery, and postpartum (LDRP) room must be educated in intrapartal, neonatal, and postpartum nursing care and be competent in providing it. If the infant is transferred to the nursery, the infant's identification is verified by the nurse receiving the infant, who places the baby in a warm environment and begins the admission process.

Regardless of the physical organization for care, many hospitals have a small holding nursery, which is available for procedures or on request by the mother who wishes her infant to be placed there. This arrangement promotes parent-infant bonding while still allowing the new parents some time to be alone.

Assessment

Assessment of Gestational Age

Assessment of gestational age is an important criterion because perinatal morbidity and mortality rates are related to gestational age and birth weight. A frequently used method of determining gestational age is the simplified Assessment of Gestational Age scale by Ballard, Novak, and Driver (1979) (see Fig. 25-1, *A*). This scale, an abbreviated version of the Dubowitz scale, can be used to measure gestational ages of infants between 35 and 42 weeks. It assesses six external physical and six neuromuscular signs. Each sign has a number score, and the cumulative score correlates with a maturity rating of from 26 to 44 weeks of gestation.

The "new" Ballard scale, a revision of the original scale, can be used with newborns as young as 20 weeks of gestation. The tool has the same physical and neuromuscular sections but includes -1 scores that reflect signs of extremely premature infants, such as fused eyelids; imperceptible breast tissue; sticky, friable, transparent skin; no lanugo; and square-window (flexion of wrist) angle of greater than 90 degrees (see Fig. 25-1, *A*). The examination of infants with a gestational age of 26 weeks or less should be performed at a postnatal age of less than 12 hours. For infants with a gestational age of at least 26 weeks, the examination can be performed up to 96 hours after birth. To ensure accuracy, it is recommended that the initial examination be performed within the first 48 hours of life. Neuromuscular adjustments after birth in extremely immature neonates require that a follow-up examination be performed to further validate neuromuscular criteria. The scale overestimates gestational age by 2 to 4 days in infants younger than 37 weeks of gestation, especially at gestational ages of 32 to 37 weeks (Ballard et al, 1991). See Box 25-4 for specific tests used in gestational age assessment.

Classification of Newborns by Gestational Age and Birth Weight

Classification of infants at birth by both birth weight and gestational age provides a more satisfactory method for predicting mortality risks and providing guidelines for manage-

BOX 25-4

Techniques Used in Assessing Gestational Age

Posture
With infant quiet and in a supine position, observe degree of flexion in arms and legs. Muscle tone and degree of flexion increase with maturity. Full flexion of the arms and legs = score 4.

Square Window
With thumb supporting back of arm below wrist, apply gentle pressure with index and third fingers on dorsum of hand without rotating infant's wrist. Measure angle between base of thumb and forearm. Full flexion (hand lies flat on ventral surface of forearm) = score 4.

Arm Recoil
With infant supine, fully flex both forearms on upper arms and hold for 5 seconds; pull down on hands to fully extend and rapidly release arms. Observe rapidity and intensity of recoil to a state of flexion. A brisk return to full flexion = score 4.

Popliteal Angle
With infant supine and pelvis flat on a firm surface, flex lower leg on thigh and then flex thigh on abdomen. While holding knee with thumb and index finger, extend lower leg with index finger of other hand. Measure degree of angle behind knee (popliteal angle). An angle of less than 90 degrees = score 5.

Scarf Sign
With infant supine, support head in midline with one hand; use other hand to pull infant's arm across the shoulder so that infant's hand touches shoulder. Determine location of elbow in relation to midline. Elbow does not reach midline = score 4.

Heel to Ear
With infant supine and pelvis flat on a firm surface, pull foot as far as possible up toward ear on same side. Measure distance of foot from ear and degree of knee flexion (same as popliteal angle). Knees flexed with a popliteal angle of less than 10 degrees = score 4.

Source: Hockenberry MJ et al: *Wong's nursing care of infants and children*, ed 7, St Louis, 2003, Mosby.

ment of the neonate than estimating gestational age or birth weight alone. The infant's birth weight, length, and head circumference are plotted on standardized graphs that identify normal values for gestational age (see Fig. 25-1, *B*, for weight chart and Box 27-1).

Intrauterine growth curves developed by Battaglia and Lubchenco (1967) have been used to classify infants according to birth weight and gestational age. Since that time, other intrauterine growth charts have emerged to reflect a more heterogeneous sample population than previously described (Cunningham et al, 2001). The primary intrauterine growth charts that provide national reference data include the work of Alexander and colleagues (1996), which is representative of more than 3.1 million live births in the United States; the work of Thomas and colleagues (2000); and the works of Arbuckle, Wilkins, and Sherman (1993) and Kramer and colleagues (2001), which are representative of intrauterine growth among the Canadian population. Thomas and colleagues (2000) concluded that intrauterine growth measured by head circumference, birth weight, and length varies according to race and gender. These researchers also found that altitude did not seem to significantly affect birth weight as has been suggested by other authors. It is recommended that the reader access and use the most current intrauterine growth chart specific to the referent population being evaluated.

Maternal Effects on Gestational Age Assessment

Some maternal conditions can affect the results of the gestational assessment. For example, any infant who has experienced oxygen deprivation during labor will have poor muscle tone. Infants in respiratory distress tend to be flaccid and assume a "frog-leg" posture. Even though an infant may appear large, such as the infant of a diabetic mother, it may respond in the same way as a preterm infant. The infant of a mother who has been on large doses of magnesium sulfate may also be somewhat lethargic if sufficient amounts of the drug were passed in utero.

ASSESSMENT OF COMMON PROBLEMS IN THE NEWBORN

Physical Examination

A complete physical examination is performed within 24 hours, after the infant's condition has stabilized (Guidelines box). See Chapter 24 for a detailed description of this examination.

Physical Injuries

Birth trauma includes any physical injury sustained by a newborn during labor and birth. Many injuries are minor and readily resolve in the neonatal period without treatment. Other types of trauma require some form of intervention. A few are serious enough to be fatal.

Several factors predispose an infant to birth trauma. Maternal factors include uterine dysfunction that leads to prolonged or precipitous labor, preterm or postterm labor, and cephalopelvic disproportion. Injury may result from dystocia caused by fetal macrosomia, multifetal gestation, abnor-

Guidelines

PHYSICAL EXAMINATION OF THE NEWBORN

- Provide a normothermic and nonstimulating examination area.
- Undress only body area to be examined to prevent heat loss.
- Proceed in an orderly sequence (usually head to toe) with the following exceptions:
  - Perform all procedures that require quiet first, such as auscultating the lungs, heart, and abdomen.
  - Perform disturbing procedures, such as testing reflexes, last.
  - Measure head, chest, and length at same time to compare results.
- Proceed quickly to avoid stressing infant.
- Check that equipment and supplies are working properly and are accessible.
- Comfort infant during and after examination; involve parent in the following:
  - Talk softly.
  - Hold infant's hands against chest.
  - Swaddle and hold.
  - Give pacifier or gloved finger to suck.

mal or difficult presentation, and congenital anomalies. Intrapartum events that can result in scalp injury include the use of intrapartum monitoring of the fetal heart rate and fetal scalp blood sampling. Obstetric birth techniques can also cause injury. These include forceps birth, vacuum extraction, external version and extraction, and cesarean birth (see Skeletal Injuries and Peripheral Nervous System Injuries in Chapter 28). Caput succedaneum and cephalhematoma are described in Chapter 24 (see Fig. 24-3).

Soft Tissue Injuries

Subconjunctival and retinal hemorrhages result from rupture of capillaries caused by increased pressure during birth. The hemorrhages clear within 5 days after birth and usually present no further problems. Parents need explanation and reassurance that these injuries are harmless.

Erythema, ecchymoses, petechiae, abrasions, lacerations, or edema of buttocks and extremities may be present. Localized discoloration may appear over presenting parts and may result from application of forceps or the vacuum extractor. Ecchymoses and edema may appear anywhere on the body. Petechiae, or pinpoint hemorrhagic areas, acquired during birth may extend over the upper trunk and face. These lesions are benign if they disappear within 2 or 3 days of birth and no new lesions appear. Ecchymoses and petechiae may be signs of a more serious disorder, such as thrombocytopenic purpura. To differentiate hemorrhagic areas from a skin rash or discoloration, blanch the skin with two fingers. Petechiae and ecchymoses do not blanch because extravasated blood remains within the tissues, whereas skin rashes and discolorations do blanch.

Trauma secondary to dystocia occurs to the presenting fetal part (Fig. 25-6). Forceps injury and bruising from the vacuum cup occur at the site of application of the instruments. In a forceps injury there is commonly a linear mark across both sides of the face that is in the shape of the blades of the forceps. The affected areas are kept clean to minimize risk of infection. These injuries usually resolve spontaneously within several days with no specific therapy. With the increased use of the vacuum extractor and use of padded forceps blades, the incidence of these lesions may be significantly reduced.

Bruises over the face may be the result of face presentation (Fig. 25-7). In a breech presentation, bruising and swelling may be seen over the buttocks or genitalia (Fig. 25-8). The skin over the entire head may be ecchymotic and covered with petechiae caused by a tight nuchal cord. Petechiae, or pinpoint hemorrhagic areas, acquired during birth may extend over the upper portion of the trunk and face. These lesions are usually benign if they disappear within 2 days of birth and no new lesions appear. Ecchymoses and petechiae may be signs of a more serious disorder, such as thrombocytopenia. If the hemorrhagic areas do not disappear spontaneously in 2 days or if the infant's condition changes, the physician is notified. To differentiate hemorrhagic areas from skin rashes and discolorations such as Mongolian spots, the nurse blanches the skin with two fingers as described previously.

Accidental lacerations may be inflicted with a scalpel during cesarean birth. These cuts may occur on any part of the body but are most often found on the scalp, buttocks, and thighs. Usually they are superficial and only need to be kept clean. Butterfly adhesive strips will hold together the edges of more serious lacerations. Rarely are sutures needed.

Physiologic Problems

Conjugation of Bilirubin

Bilirubin is one of the products derived from the hemoglobin released with the breakdown of red blood cells (RBCs) and the myoglobin in muscle cells. The hemoglobin is broken

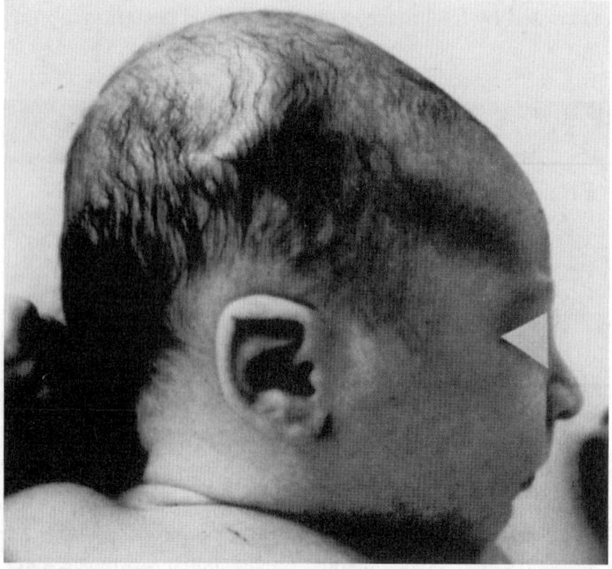

Fig. 25-6 Depressed skull fracture in a full-term male after rapid (1-hour) labor. The infant was delivered by occiput-anterior presentation after rotation from occiput-posterior position. (From Mangurten H: Birth injuries. In Fanaroff AA, Martin RJ: *Neonatal-perinatal medicine: diseases of the fetus and infant,* ed 7, St Louis, 2002, Mosby.)

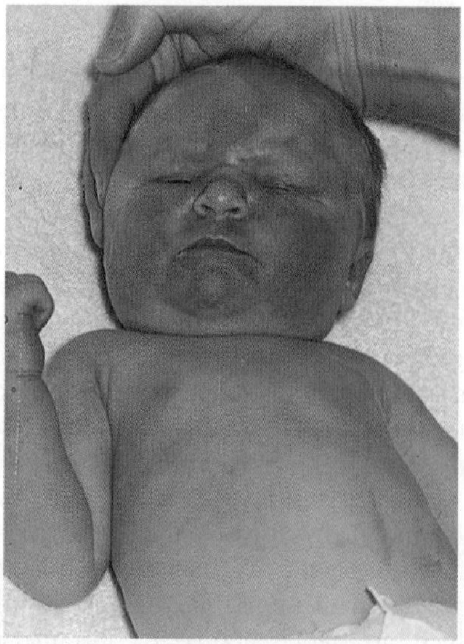

Fig. 25-7 Marked bruising on the entire face of an infant born vaginally after face presentation. Less severe ecchymoses were present on the extremities. Phototherapy was required for treatment of jaundice resulting from the breakdown of accumulated blood. (From O'Doherty N: *Neonatology: micro atlas of the newborn,* Nutley, NJ, 1986, Hoffmann–La Roche.)

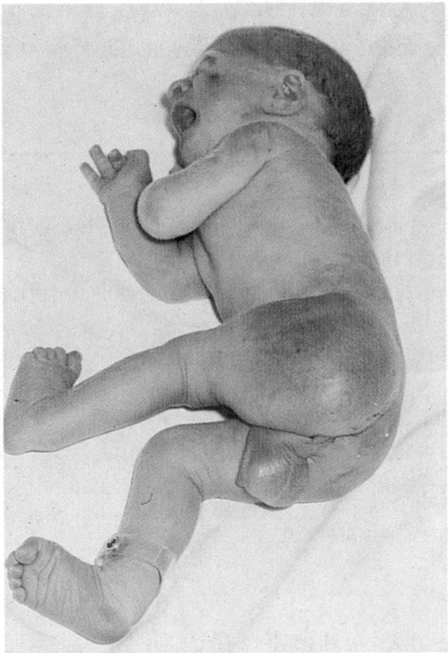

Fig. 25-8 Swelling of genitalia and bruising of the buttocks after a breech delivery. (From O'Doherty N: *Neonatology: micro atlas of the newborn,* Nutley, NJ, 1986, Hoffmann–La Roche.)

down by the reticuloendothelial cells, converted to bilirubin, and released in an unconjugated form. Unconjugated (indirect) bilirubin is relatively insoluble and almost entirely bound to circulating albumin, a plasma protein. The unbound bilirubin can leave the vascular system and permeate other extravascular tissues (e.g., skin, sclera, and oral mucous membranes). The resulting yellow coloring is termed *jaundice.*

In the liver the unbound bilirubin is conjugated with glucuronide in the presence of the enzyme glucuronyl transferase. The conjugated form of bilirubin (direct bilirubin) is soluble and is excreted from liver cells as a constituent of bile. Along with other components of bile, direct bilirubin is excreted into the biliary tract system that carries the bile into the duodenum. Bilirubin is converted to urobilinogen and stercobilinogen within the duodenum through the action of the bacterial flora. Urobilinogen is excreted in urine and feces; stercobilinogen is excreted in the feces (see Fig. 24-2). The total serum bilirubin level is the sum of the levels of both conjugated and unconjugated bilirubin.

Physiologic Jaundice

CRITICAL THINKING EXERCISE—JAUNDICE

Approximately 50% to 80% of all full-term newborns are visibly jaundiced (yellow) during the first 3 days of life. Serum bilirubin levels less than 5 mg/dl usually are not reflected in visible skin jaundice. Although the neonate has the functional capacity to convert bilirubin, physiologic hyperbilirubinemia commonly occurs in infants. Physiologic jaundice or neonatal hyperbilirubinemia occurs in 80% of preterm newborns. The incidence of physiologic jaundice is increased in Asian, Native American, and Eskimo infants. Although neonatal jaundice is considered benign, bilirubin may accumulate to hazardous levels and lead to a pathologic condition. Neonatal jaundice occurs because the newborn has a higher rate of bilirubin production and the reabsorption of bilirubin from the neonatal small intestine is considerable.

Two phases of physiologic jaundice have been identified in term infants. In the first phase bilirubin levels of formula-fed Caucasian and African-American infants gradually increase to approximately 5 to 6 mg/dl by 60 to 72 hours of life, then decrease to a plateau of 2 to 3 mg/dl by the fifth day (Blackburn, 2003). In Asian and Asian-American infants levels reach a peak of 10 to 14 mg/dl around the 3rd to 5th day of life; the levels gradually fall to 2 to 3 mg/dl by the 7th to 10th day. Bilirubin levels maintain a steady plateau state in the second phase without increasing or decreasing until approximately 12 to 14 days, at which time levels decrease to the normal value of 1 mg/dl (Blackburn, 2003; Volpe, 2001). This pattern varies according to racial group, method of feeding (breast vs. bottle), and gestational age. In preterm formula-fed infants, serum bilirubin levels may peak as high as 10 to 12 mg/dl at 5 to 6 days of life and decrease slowly over a period of 2 to 4 weeks (Blackburn, 2003).

Some characteristics of physiologic jaundice include the following:

- The infant is otherwise well in relation to cardiorespiratory status, neurologic status, carbohydrate metabolism, feeding pattern, and elimination.
- In term infants, jaundice first appears *after* 24 hours and disappears by the end of the seventh day.
- In preterm infants, jaundice is first evident after 48 hours and disappears by the ninth or tenth day.
- The infant's predischarge total serum bilirubin falls below the high risk category (<95 percentile) on the hour-specific nomogram (see Fig. 25-9).
- The serum concentration of unconjugated bilirubin usually does not exceed 12 mg/dl in term infants and 15 mg/dl in preterm infants.
- Direct bilirubin does not exceed 1 to 1.5 mg/dl.
- Indirect or unconjugated bilirubin concentration does not increase by more than 5 mg/dl per day.

See Table 25-2 for the varying causes of neonatal indirect hyperbilirubinemia.

NURSE ALERT The appearance of jaundice during the first 24 hours of life or persistence beyond the ages previously delineated usually indicates a potential pathologic process that requires further investigation. ■

In the newborn intestine the enzyme β-glucuronidase is able to convert conjugated bilirubin into the unconjugated form, which is subsequently reabsorbed by the intestinal mucosa and transported to the liver. This process, known as enterohepatic circulation, or enterohepatic shunting, is accentuated in the newborn and is thought to be a primary mechanism in physiologic jaundice (Maisels, 1999). Feeding (1) stimulates peristalsis and produces more rapid passage of meconium, thus diminishing the amount of reabsorption of unconjugated bilirubin, and (2) introduces bacteria to aid in the reduction of bilirubin to urobilinogen. Colostrum, a natural laxative, facilitates meconium evacuation.

Every newborn is assessed for jaundice. To differentiate cutaneous jaundice from normal skin color apply pressure with a finger over a bony area (e.g., nose, forehead, and sternum) for several seconds to empty all the capillaries in that spot. If jaundice is present, the blanched area will look yellow before the capillaries refill. The conjunctiva and buccal mucosa are also assessed, especially in darker-skinned in-

Table 25-2

Causes of Neonatal Indirect Hyperbilirubinemia

BASIS	CAUSES
INCREASED PRODUCTION OF BILIRUBIN	
Increased hemoglobin destruction	Fetomaternal blood group incompatibility (Rh, ABO) Congenital red blood cell abnormalities Congenital enzyme deficiencies (G6PD, galactosemia) Sepsis Enclosed hemorrhage (cephalhematoma, bruising)
Increased amount of hemoglobin	Polycythemia (maternal-fetal or twin-twin transfusion, SGA) Delayed cord clamping
Increased enterohepatic circulation	Delayed passage of meconium, meconium ileus, or plug Fasting or delayed initiation of feeding Intestinal atresia or stenosis
ALTERED HEPATIC CLEARANCE OF BILIRUBIN	
Alteration in glucuronyl transferase production or activity	Immaturity Metabolic/endocrine disorders (e.g., Criglar-Najjar disease, hypothyroidism, disorders of amino acid metabolism)
Alteration in hepatic function and perfusion (and thus conjugating ability)	Sepsis (also causes inflammation) Asphyxia, hypoxia, hypothermia, hypoglycemia Drugs and hormones (e.g., novobiocin, pregnanediol)
Hepatic obstruction (associated with direct hyperbilirubinemia)	Congenital anomalies (biliary atresia, cystic fibrosis) Biliary stasis (hepatitis, sepsis) Excessive bilirubin load (often seen with severe hemolysis)

From Blackburn ST: *Maternal, fetal, and neonatal physiology: a clinical perspective,* ed 2, St Louis, 2003, WB Saunders.
G6PD, glucose-6-phosphate dehydrogenase; *SGA,* small for gestational age.

fants. It is better to assess for jaundice in natural light because artificial lighting and the reflection from nursery walls can distort the actual skin color. Visual assessment of jaundice does not, however, provide an accurate assessment of the level of serum bilirubin.

Jaundice is generally first noticed in the head, especially the sclera and mucous membranes, and then progresses gradually to the thorax, abdomen, and extremities. The most common therapy used to treat a high serum bilirubin level or a rapidly increasing level is phototherapy. The degree of jaundice is determined by serum bilirubin measurements. Normal values of unconjugated bilirubin are 0.2 to 1.4 mg/dl.

It is important to note that the evaluation of jaundice is not based solely on serum bilirubin levels, but also on the timing of the appearance of clinical jaundice; gestational age at birth; age in days since birth; family history, including maternal Rh factor; evidence of hemolysis; feeding method; infant's physiologic status; and the progression of serial serum bilirubin levels.

Kernicterus describes the yellow staining of the brain cells that may result in bilirubin encephalopathy. The damage occurs when the serum concentration reaches toxic levels, regardless of cause. There is evidence that a fraction of unconjugated bilirubin crosses the blood-brain barrier in neonates with physiologic hyperbilirubinemia. When certain pathologic conditions exist in addition to elevated bilirubin levels, there is an increase in the permeability of the blood-brain barrier to unconjugated bilirubin; this creates the potential for irreversible damage. The exact level of serum bilirubin required to cause damage is not yet known. The signs of bilirubin encephalopathy are those of central nervous system depression or excitation. Prodromal symptoms consist of decreased activity, lethargy, irritability, hypotonia, and seizures. Later these subtle findings are followed by development of athetoid cerebral palsy, mental retardation, and deafness. Those who survive may eventually show evidence of neurologic damage, such as mental retardation, attention deficit hyperactivity disorder, delayed or abnormal motor movement (especially ataxia or athetosis), behavior disorders, perceptual problems, or sensorineural hearing loss. The Joint Commission on Accreditation of Healthcare Organizations (2001) has issued a sentinel event alert with guidelines for the prevention of neonatal kernicterus by health care workers and institutions.

Pathologic jaundice is that level of serum bilirubin which, if left untreated, can result in sensorineural hearing loss, mild cognitive delays, and kernicterus, which is the deposition of bilirubin in the brain. With ever-changing medical terminology in the literature there is less emphasis on pathologic jaundice more by omission than anything else. Nonetheless, one might consider any newborn jaundice as being physiologic (see preceding discussion) unless proven otherwise, in which case the condition may be considered pathologic.

Noninvasive monitoring of bilirubin via cutaneous reflectance measurements (transcutaneous bilirubinometry

[TcB]) allows for repetitive estimations of bilirubin. These devices work well on dark- and light-skinned infants and correlate fairly well with serum determinations of bilirubin levels in full-term infants. With shorter maternity stays, the value of transcutaneous bilirubin measurements as an assessment tool in follow-up home care has been demonstrated in a homogeneous population. However, because transcutaneous bilirubin measurements are affected by race, gestational age, and birth weight, their use in heterogeneous populations remains limited for diagnostic purposes (Engle et al, 2002; Maisels, 1999). Also, the intensity of jaundice is not always related to the degree of hyperbilirubinemia. Transcutaneous bilirubin meters have been significantly improved in the last two decades and may reduce or obviate the need for blood sampling in certain healthy neonates (Briscoe, Clark, & Yoxall, 2002). The new TcB monitors provide accurate measurements within 2 to 3 mg/dl in most neonatal populations at serum levels below 15 mg/dl (American Academy of Pediatrics, Subcommittee on Hyperbilirubinemia, 2004). After phototherapy has been initiated, TcB is no longer useful as a screening tool.

The use of hour-specific serum bilirubin levels to predict newborns at risk for rapidly rising levels has now become an official recommendation by the Academy of Pediatrics, Subcommittee on Hyperbilirubinemia (2004), for the monitoring of healthy neonates at 35 weeks of gestation or greater before discharge from the hospital. Using a nomogram (Fig. 25-9) with three levels (high, intermediate, or low risk) of rising total serum bilirubin values assists in the determination of which newborns might need further evaluation after discharge. Universal bilirubin screening based on hour-specific total serum bilirubin may be done at the same time as the routine newborn profile (phenylketonuria [PKU], galactosemia, and others) (American Academy of Pediatrics, Subcommittee on Hyperbilirubinemia, 2004; Bhutani, Johnson, & Sivieri, 1999). In many institutions the hour-specific bilirubin risk nomogram is used to determine the infant's risk for development of hyperbilirubinemia requiring medical treatment or closer screening. Risk factors recognized to place infants in the high risk category include gestational age less than 38 weeks, breastfeeding, previous sibling with significant jaundice, and jaundice appearing before discharge (American Academy of Pediatrics, Subcommittee on Hyperbilirubinemia, 2004). It is now recommended that healthy infants (35 weeks or greater) receive follow-up care and assessment of bilirubin within 3 days of discharge if discharged at less than 24 hours and a risk assessment with tools such as the hour-specific nomogram; likewise, newborns discharged at 24 to 47.9 hours should receive follow-up evaluation within 4 days (96 hours), and those discharged between 48 and 72 hours should receive follow-up within 5 days (American Academy of Pediatrics, Subcommittee on Hyperbilirubinemia, 2004). The newest guidelines for monitoring and treating neonatal hyperbilirubinemia

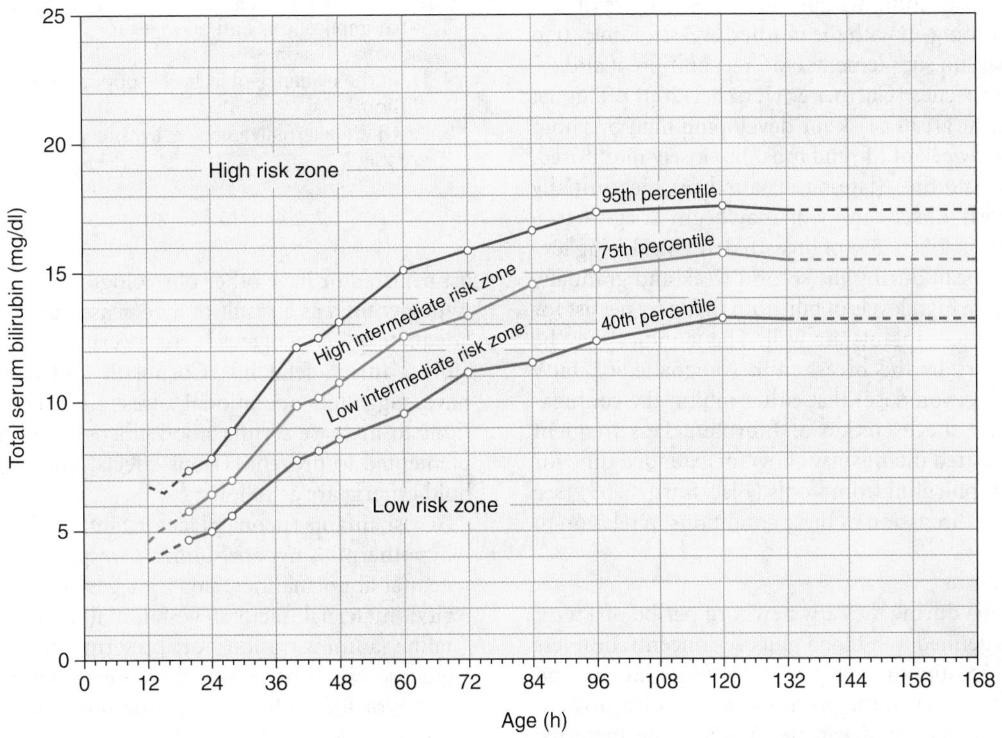

Fig. 25-9 Nomogram for designation of risk in 2840 well newborns at 36 or more weeks of gestational age with birth weight of 2000 g or more or 35 or more weeks of gestational age and birth weight of 2500 g or more based on the hour-specific serum bilirubin values. (This nomogram should not be used to represent the natural history of neonatal hyperbilirubinemia.) (From Bhutani VK, Johnson L, Sivieri EM: Predictive ability of a predischarge hour-specific serum bilirubin for subsequent significant hyperbilirubinemia in healthy term and near-term newborns, *Pediatrics* 103(1):6-14, 1999.)

are published extensively elsewhere (see Resources at end of chapter).

Newer technologies that are currently being evaluated for noninvasive monitoring of neonatal serum bilirubin values. These include carbon monoxide indices (ETCOc) in exhaled breath (carbon monoxide is produced when RBCs are broken down, thus the extent of hemolysis may be appreciated) and the use of transcutaneous bilirubin meters (BiliCheck), that measure the total serum bilirubin and provide a prediction of risk for hyperbilirubinemia in newborns before discharge (Bhutani et al, 2000; Stevens et al, 2001).

Jaundice Associated with Breastfeeding

Breastfeeding is associated with an increased incidence of jaundice. Two types have been identified; however, nomenclature may vary among experts. Breastfeeding-associated jaundice (early-onset jaundice) begins at 2 to 4 days of age and occurs in approximately 10% to 25% of breastfed newborns. The jaundice is related to the process of breastfeeding and probably results from decreased caloric and fluid intake by breastfed infants before the milk supply is well established, because fasting is associated with decreased hepatic clearance of bilirubin (Blackburn, 2003; Porter & Dennis, 2002). The presence of decreased caloric intake (less milk), weight loss of more than 5% to 7% in the first 5 days of life, increasing serum bilirubin (unconjugated) levels, decreased stooling, and increased jaundice is also sometimes referred to as starvation jaundice or nonbreastfeeding jaundice. To prevent this pattern, the following measures are suggested: initiation of breastfeeding within the first few hours of life, continuous rooming-in with the mother, breastfeeding 10 to 12 times per day, no supplements, and recognition of and response to hunger cues (Gartner & Herschel, 2001). This set of newborns is at greater risk for developing high bilirubin levels in the first week of life and must be closely monitored.

Breast milk jaundice (late-onset jaundice) may initially begin as the early-onset variety or may begin at age 4 to 6 days and occurs in 2% to 3% of breastfed infants. Rising levels of bilirubin peak during the second week and gradually diminish. Despite high levels of bilirubin that may persist for 3 to 12 weeks, these infants are well. The jaundice may be caused by factors in the breast milk (pregnanediol, fatty acids, and β-glucuronidase) that either inhibit the conjugation or decrease the excretion of bilirubin. Less frequent stooling by breastfed infants may allow for extended time for reabsorption of bilirubin from stools (Blackburn, 2003) (see Chapter 26 for a discussion of these conditions in relation to nutrition).

Hypoglycemia

Hypoglycemia during the early newborn period of a term infant is often defined as a blood glucose concentration less than adequate to support adequate neurologic, organ, and tissue function; however, the precise level at which this occurs in every neonate is debatable. At birth the maternal source of glucose is cut off with the clamping of the umbilical cord. Most healthy term newborns experience a transient decrease in glucose levels, with a subsequent mobilization of free fatty acids and ketones to help maintain adequate glucose levels (Blackburn, 2003). Insulin does not cross the placental barrier, thus predisposing some infants to low glucose levels as a result of increased insulin activity. Infants who are asphyxiated or have other physiologic stress may experience hypoglycemia as a result of a decreased glycogen supply, inadequate gluconeogenesis, or overutilization of glycogen stored during fetal life. Cornblath and colleagues (2000) have suggested operational thresholds at which interventions to increase serum blood glucose levels should be implemented to prevent serious effects. The suggested threshold criteria are as follows:

- At-risk infants (neonatal factors: infant of diabetic mother, hypothermia, hyperinsulinism, respiratory distress, congenital abnormalities, small for gestational age, prematurity; maternal factors: gestational hypertension, terbutaline administration for preterm labor) should have glucose values of 36 mg/dl or greater within the first few hours of life with a therapeutic objective of 45 mg/dl or greater.

Monitoring blood glucose in the asymptomatic healthy term neonate (not at risk) on a routine basis is not recommended (Cornblath et al, 2000).

Signs of hypoglycemia include jitteriness; irregular respiratory effort; cyanosis; apnea; weak, high-pitched cry; feeding difficulty; lethargy; twitching; eye rolling; and seizures. The signs may be transient but recurrent.

??? Critical Thinking Exercise

JAUNDICE

A full-term, 5-day-old newborn is brought to the minor emergency department late in the evening for evaluation of newborn jaundice. A home health nurse visited earlier in the day and a serum bilirubin was drawn by heel stick with the results of a total bilirubin 14.6, direct bilirubin 0.9. The father is very concerned because a home health care worker mentioned that the newborn might develop brain damage if the bilirubin levels were to increase to high levels. The mother is breastfeeding every 2 to 3 hours, and the newborn has had four wet diapers and three semiliquid stools over the past 18 hours. The newborn's birth weight was 6 lb, 4 oz, and her current weight (nude) is 6 lb. On examination the infant is active and alert, has visibly jaundiced skin and sclerae, and has intact reflexes and strong suck reflex. By history there were no prenatal or delivery complications. Apgar scores at 1 and 5 minutes were 8 and 9, and the initial assessment did not reveal any problems. The mother's blood type is A positive, and the direct Coombs' test is negative. The newborn was discharged from the birth hospital on the second day of life in apparent good health.

1. Evidence—Is there sufficient evidence to draw any conclusions about the newborn's condition at this time?
2. Assumptions—Describe some underlying assumptions about the following:
   a. Newborn jaundice in a healthy term infant
   b. Serum bilirubin levels and the newborn's age in days; other pertinent laboratory values as indicated
   c. Nutritional and excretory function and relation to bilirubin metabolism
   d. Physical status of the infant per assessment data
3. What implications and priorities for nursing care can be drawn at this time?
4. Does the evidence objectively support your argument (conclusion)?
5. Are there alternative perspectives to your arguments? What are they?

Hypoglycemia in the low risk term infant is usually eliminated by feeding the infant a source of carbohydrate (i.e., human milk or formula). Occasionally the intravenous administration of glucose is required for infants with persistently high insulin levels or in those with depleted stores of glycogen.

Hypocalcemia

Hypocalcemia (serum calcium levels less than 7.8 to 8 mg/dl in term infant, 7 mg/dl in preterm infant; ideally, ionized fraction levels reflect the biologically active form and levels range from 3 to 4.4 mg/dl depending on the measurement method [Blackburn, 2003]) may occur in newborns of diabetic mothers, in those who experienced perinatal asphyxia or trauma, and in preterm infants. Early-onset hypocalcemia occurs within the first 72 hours after birth. Although signs of hypocalcemia include jitteriness, tremors, twitching, high-pitched cry, irritability, apnea, and laryngospasm, some infants may be asymptomatic (Blackburn, 2003).

Early-onset hypocalcemia may be self-limiting and resolve within 1 to 3 days, depending on the etiology. Treatment for the condition includes early feeding and, in preterm or asphyxiated infants, the administration of intravenous elemental calcium.

NURSE ALERT Intravenous administration of elemental calcium to any neonate should involve cardiac monitoring to detect bradycardia; the infusion is stopped if bradycardia occurs. Adequate intravenous access should be established because calcium may cause tissue sloughing and necrosis. If intravenous access becomes compromised during administration, discontinue the infusion and procure another site.

Because jitteriness is a symptom of both hypoglycemia and hypocalcemia, the latter must be considered if therapy for hypoglycemia is ineffective. ■

LABORATORY AND DIAGNOSTIC TESTS

Because newborns experience many transitional events in the first 28 days of life, laboratory samples are often gathered to determine adequate physiologic adaptation and to identify disorders that may adversely affect the child's life beyond the neonatal period. Most laboratory tests may be obtained from the neonate with a heel puncture. Tests that may be performed include bilirubin levels, blood glucose, newborn screening tests (e.g., PKU, thyroid [T_4], sickle cell disease, and galactosemia), and drug serum levels. Box 25-5 lists standard laboratory values in a term newborn. Routine screening for hypotension or hypertension, hypoglycemia, polycythemia, or other conditions in the absence of risk factors is not recommended by the American Academy of Pediatrics and American College of Obstetricians and Gynecologists (2002).

Most states have programs for newborn screening, but such programs vary by state. With the increased mobility of the population, newborns at high risk for certain metabolic diseases may not be appropriately screened. It is therefore important that families be educated regarding the availability of tests routinely screened in their state of residence. The advent of tandem mass spectrometry holds promise to increase the number of conditions (30 total) that can be tested

BOX 25-5

Standard Laboratory Values in a Term Newborn*

Hemoglobin	14-24 g/dl
Hematocrit	44%-64%
Glucose	45-65 mg/dl
Leukocytes (WBCs)	9,000-30,000/mm^3
Bilirubin, total serum	<2.0 mg/dl
Blood gases	
Arterial	pH 7.32-7.48
	Pco_2 26-42 mm Hg
	Po_2 60-70 mm Hg
Base excess	−10 to −2 mEq/L (whole blood)
Bicarbonate, serum	21-28 (arterial)
Anion gap	7-16 mEq/L
Venous	pH 7.31-7.41
	Pco_2 40-50 mm Hg
	Po_2 40-50 mm Hg

*These values may change significantly in the first week of life.
WBCs, white blood cells.

with the same minimal amount of blood (Lashley, 2002). Information about which tests are required in a state can be obtained from state health departments (see Resources at end of chapter).

Some of the major disorders for which infants are screened are described in Table 25-3.

Collection of Specimens

Ongoing evaluation and screening of the newborn often requires obtaining blood by heel stick or venipuncture.

Heel Stick

Most blood specimens are drawn by laboratory technicians. However, nurses may be required to perform heel sticks to obtain blood for glucose monitoring or newborn screening. The same technique is needed to complete the PKU form on Guthrie paper or to test for galactosemia and hypothyroidism or other inborn errors of metabolism (see Table 25-3).

It is often helpful to warm the heel before the sample is taken; application of heat for 5 to 10 minutes helps dilate the blood vessels in the area. A cloth soaked with warm water and wrapped loosely around the foot provides effective warming (Fig. 25-10, *A*). Disposable heel warmers are available from a variety of companies; they should be used with care to prevent burns. Nurses should wear gloves when collecting any specimen. The nurse cleanses the area with an appropriate skin antiseptic, restrains the infant's foot with a free hand, and then punctures the site. A spring-loaded automatic puncture device causes less pain and requires fewer punctures than a manual lance blade.

The most serious complication of infant heel stick is necrotizing osteochondritis from lancet penetration of the bone (Meehan, 1998). To prevent this, the penetration should be made at the outer aspect of the heel and should be no deeper than 2.4 mm (Hockenberry et al, 2003). To identify the appropriate puncture site, the nurse should draw an imaginary line running from between the fourth and fifth toes and parallel to the lateral aspect of the foot to the heel

Table 25-3
Newborn Screening Summary

DISORDER/EVIDENCE	SYMPTOMS	SCREENING INCIDENCE	TREATMENT
PKU (classic) Elevated phenylalanine	Severe mental retardation if early detection and treatment not started eczema, seizures, behavior disorders, decreased pigmentation, distinctive musty or mouse-like odor	1:13,500 to 1:19,000 More common in Caucasians and Native Americans	Lifelong dietary management with low-phenylalanine diet; possible tyrosine supplementation
Congenital hypothyroidism (primary) Low T_4, elevated TSH	Mental and motor retardation (although neonatal detection and treatment has decreased incidence of mental retardation), short stature, coarse, dry skin and hair, hoarse cry, constipation	1:3600 to 1 in 5000 live births with some ethnic variation 1:12,000 African-American 1:1000 Native American	Maintain L-thyroxine levels in upper half of normal range; periodic bone age to monitor growth
Galactosemia (transferase deficiency) Elevated galactose; low or absent fluorescence	Hypotonia, lethargy, vomiting, diarrhea, metabolic acidosis, *Escherichia coli* sepsis, or liver dysfunction; mental retardation, jaundice, blindness, cataracts, long-term behavioral problems, and neurologic impairment	1:60,000 to 1:250,000	Eliminate galactose and lactose from the diet; soy formulas in infancy; lactose-free solid foods
Maple syrup urine disease (MSUD) Elevated leucine	Poor feeding, lethargy, hypotonia, ketoacidosis, and seizures; sweet maple syrup odor may occur in urine, cerumen, or sweat,	1:90,000 to 1:100,000; higher in certain Mennonite populations, 1 in 176	Branched-chain amino acid–free formula with added protein-based formula; thiamine supplement in some individuals; lifelong treatment and monitoring necessary
Homocystinuria Elevated methionine	Mental retardation, seizures, behavioral disorders, early-onset thromboses, dislocated lenses, tall lanky body habitus	1:150,000 to 1:200,000; more prevalent in Ireland	Methionine-restricted diet; cystine supplement; vitamin B_6 supplement if responsive
Congenital adrenal hyperplasia (CAH) Elevated 17-hydroxyprogesterone; abnormal electrolytes	Hyponatremia, hyperkalemia, hypoglycemia, dehydration; female virilization; progressive virilization in both sexes	1:10,000 to 1:20,000 ; higher in Native Eskimos, 1 in 300	Reduce excessive corticotropins; replace glucocorticoids and mineral corticoids; corrective surgery for ambiguous genitalia
Sickle cell/hemoglobin SC (thalassemias)	Repeated infections, failure to thrive, pallor, hemolytic anemia; sickle cell crisis	Sickle cell anemia (SCA), 1 in 40,000 to 1 in 60,000 non–African Americans; 1 in 375 African Americans	Preventive care: treatment of meningococcal and pneumococcal infections; hydroxyurea (antisickling agent)
Biotinidase deficiency Deficient or absent activity of biotinidase on colorimetric assay	Myoclonic seizures, hypotonia, feeding difficulties, organic aciduria, fungal infections, ataxia, skin rash, hearing loss, alopecia, optic nerve atrophy, developmental delay, coma, and death	1:60,000 to 1:137,000	5-20 mg biotin daily; less with partial deficiency

Data from Lashley FR: Newborn screening: new opportunities and new challenges, *Newborn Infant Nurs Rev* 2(4):228-242, 2002.
PKU, phenylketonuria; *TSH,* thyroid-stimulating hormone.

A

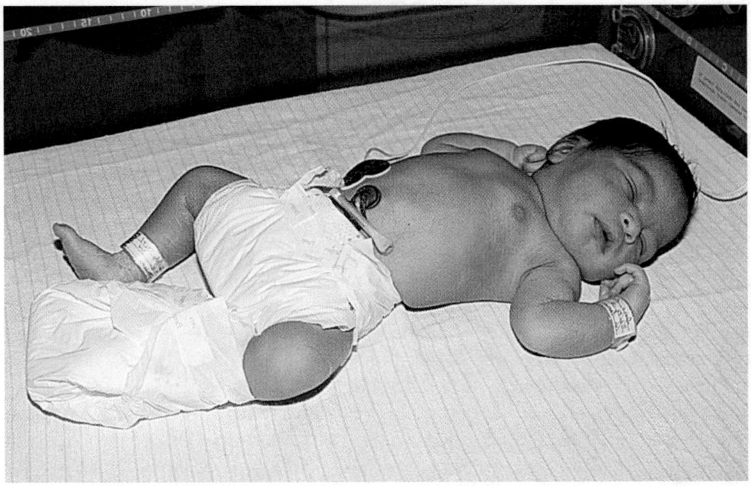

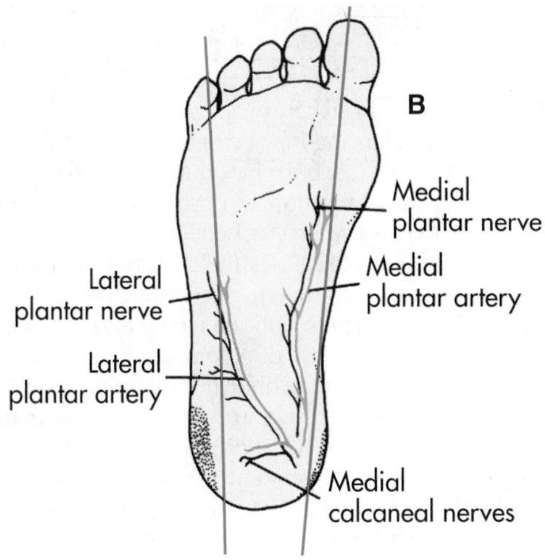

Fig. 25-10 Heel stick. **A**, Newborn with foot wrapped for warmth to increase blood flow to extremity before heel stick. **B**, Heel stick sites *(shaded areas)* on infant's foot for obtaining samples of capillary blood. (*A*, Courtesy Marjorie Pyle, RNC, Lifecircle, Costa Mesa, CA.)

where the stick should be made; a second line can also be drawn from the great toe to the medial aspect of the heel (Fig. 25-10, *B*). Repeated trauma to the walking surface of the heel can cause fibrosis and scarring that may lead to problems with walking later in life.

After the specimen has been collected, pressure is applied with a dry gauze square. No further skin cleanser should be applied because this will cause the site to continue to bleed. The site is then covered with an adhesive bandage. The nurse ensures proper disposal of equipment used, reviews the laboratory slip for correct identification, and checks the specimen for adequate labeling and routing.

A heel stick is traumatic for the infant and causes pain. After several heel sticks, infants have been observed to withdraw their feet when they are touched. To reassure the infant and to promote feelings of safety, the neonate should be cuddled and comforted when the procedure is complete and appropriate pain management measures taken to minimize the pain (Atraumatic Care box).

Venipuncture

Venous blood samples can be drawn from the antecubital, saphenous, superficial wrist, and, rarely, scalp veins. If an existing intravenous site is used to obtain a blood specimen, it is important to consider the type of infusion fluid; contamination of the blood with the fluid can alter results.

When venipuncture is required, positioning of the needle is extremely important. Although regular venipuncture needles may be used, some individuals prefer butterfly needles. A 25-gauge needle is adequate for blood sampling in neonates with minimal hemolysis being observed when the proper procedure is followed. It is necessary to be very patient during the procedure because the blood return from small veins is slow, and consequently the small needle must remain in place longer. A tourniquet is optional but may help increase blood flow with venipuncture. The mummy restraint commonly is used to help secure the infant (see Fig. 45-8).

For blood gas studies, the blood sample container is packed in ice (to reduce blood cell metabolism) and taken immediately to the laboratory for analysis.

Pressure must be maintained over an arterial puncture with a dry gauze square for at least 3 to 5 minutes to prevent bleeding from the site. The nurse should observe the infant frequently for evidence of bleeding or hematoma at the puncture site for at least an hour after any venipuncture. The infant's tolerance of the procedure should be noted and recorded. The infant should be cuddled and comforted (e.g., rocked, given a pacifier) when the procedure is completed and appropriate pain management measures taken to minimize the pain.

NURSE ALERT Only venous or capillary blood samples may be used for newborn screening and genetic studies; cord blood is not used for such samples. ■

Obtaining a Urine Specimen

Examination of urine is a valuable laboratory tool for infant assessment; the way in which the specimen is collected may influence the results. The urine sample should be fresh and examined within 1 hour of collection.

A variety of urine collection bags are available (Fig. 25-11) (see also Fig. 45-14). These are clear plastic, single-use bags with adhesive material around the opening at the point of attachment.

To prepare the infant, the nurse removes the diaper and places the infant in a supine position. The genitalia, perineum, and surrounding skin are washed and thoroughly dried because the adhesive of the bag will not stick to moist, powdered, or oily skin surfaces. The protective paper is removed to expose the adhesive (Fig. 25-11, *A*). In female infants, the perineum is stretched to flatten skin folds; then the adhesive area is pressed firmly to the skin all around the urinary meatus and vagina. (NOTE: Start with the narrow portion of the butterfly-shaped adhesive patch.) The nurse must be sure to start at the bridge of skin separating the rectum from the vagina and work upward (Fig. 25-11, *B*). In male infants the penis (and scrotum, depending on the size of the collection device) is tucked through the opening of the collector before the nurse removes the protective paper from

Atraumatic Care

HEEL PUNCTURES

Repeated heel lancing may be necessary to obtain sufficient blood for a number of newborn blood tests, including newborn screening. It has been anecdotally observed that newborns appear to withdraw the heel when touched for subsequent heel punctures. In fact, Taddio and colleagues (2002) found that infants of diabetic mothers exposed to multiple heel punctures in the first 24 to 36 hours of life learned to anticipate pain and exhibited more intense pain responses. The use of automated lancet devices such as Tenderfoot (International Technidyne, Inc., Edison, NJ) has been found to cause less pain and require fewer punctures than using manual lance blades (Blain-Lewis, 1992; Paes et al, 1993). Additional studies have shown that venipuncture performed by an experienced phlebotomist elicited fewer pain responses (as measured by the Premature Infant Pain Profile) from newborns than did heel punctures (Shah & Ohlsson, 2001). Although maternal anxiety was initially higher in the venipuncture group, mothers who observed the venipuncture reported observing less pain response than mothers who observed heel punctures.

Oral sucrose and nonnutritive sucking have proved effective in decreasing the pain associated with heel punctures in preterm and term infants during the first week of life (Gibbins et al, 2002; Stevens, Yamada, & Ohlsson, 2001); however, the exact effective dose range varies among several studies (Stevens et al, 2001). In one study, infants experiencing venipuncture were either given oral sucrose (30%) and a skin placebo or the eutectic mixture of local anesthetic (EMLA). Pain scores were measured with the Premature Infant Pain Profile, and infants receiving the oral sucrose solution exhibited fewer pain symptoms than those in the EMLA group (Gradin et al, 2002). Giving newborns 2 ml of oral sucrose solution (25% and 50%) significantly demonstrated a reduction in crying time and heart rate after 3 minutes in comparison with controls (given sterile water) during heel stick sampling for serum bilirubin concentrations (Haouari et al, 1995).

Evidence indicates that as little as 2 ml of a 24% oral sucrose solution is effective in decreasing pain in term and preterm infants. In addition, the best analgesic effect is achieved when sucrose is administered 2 minutes before the painful procedure with a pacifier or syringe. In one study protocol wherein oral sucrose was effective, 0.5 ml of 24% oral sucrose solution was administered 2 minutes before the heel puncture, during the heel puncture, and 5 minutes following the heel puncture (Gibbins et al, 2002). Monitoring for adverse effects must accompany each administration (Noerr, 2001).

The mother's holding the infant in skin-to-skin contact has also been shown to significantly reduce the child's distress during the procedure (Blass & Watt, 1999; Gray, Watt, & Blass, 2000). Breastfeeding during heel puncture in term newborns has been shown to be effective in decreasing pain scores when compared with placebo or a 30% oral sucrose solution (Carbajal et al, 2003).

The benefit of applying the topical anesthetic EMLA to reduce the pain of heel lance has produced mixed results in term and preterm infants (Fitzgerald, Millard, & McIntosh, 1989; Stevens et al, 1999; Taddio et al, 1998). There are currently no published studies regarding the use of LMX4 cream, formerly Ela-Max, (4% lidocaine) for newborn heel sticks or circumcision analgesia.

From these studies it is evident that there are a number of effective ways to decrease the pain associated with heel puncture in term and preterm newborns. It is essential that nurses utilize all available resources to advocate for the prevention and management of neonatal pain during such procedures as heel puncture.

A number of commercially available oral sucrose solutions now exist and include, but are not limited to, the following: Ora-Sweet (54% solution; Paddock Labs, Inc.) can be diluted 1:1 to produce a 27% solution; and Sweet-Ease (24% sucrose solution; Children's Medical Ventures, Norwell, MA). When these are not available, the pharmacy may mix an oral sucrose solution to ensure a clean product. An approximate 25% sucrose solution is made by mixing 1 teaspoon of granulated (table) sugar with 4 teaspoons of sterile water; however, this method is the least desirable to prevent contamination of the solution and subsequent problems.

the adhesive; then the protective paper is removed, and the flaps are pressed firmly to the perineum, making sure the entire adhesive coating is firmly attached to skin and the edges of the opening do not pucker (Fig. 25-11, *C*). This helps ensure a leak-proof seal and decreases the chance of contamination from stool. Cutting a slit in the diaper and pulling the bag through the slit may also help prevent leaking.

The diaper is carefully replaced and the bag is checked frequently. When a sufficient amount of urine (this amount varies according to the test done) has been obtained, the bag is removed. The infant's skin is observed for signs of irritation while the bag is in place. The specimen can be aspirated with a syringe or drained directly from the bag. For draining, the bag is held in one hand and tilted to keep urine away from the tab. The tab is then removed and the urine is drained into a clean receptacle.

Collection of a 24-hour specimen can be a challenge; the infant may need to be restrained. The 24-hour urine bag is applied in the manner just described, and the urine is drained into a receptacle. The infant's skin is watched closely for signs of irritation and for lack of a proper seal.

For some types of urine testing, urine can be aspirated directly from the diaper by means of a syringe without a needle. If the diaper has absorbent gelling material that traps urine, a small gauze pad or cotton balls are placed inside the diaper and the urine is aspirated from the cotton or gauze.

Nursing Diagnoses

Possible nursing diagnoses for the newborn include the following:

- *Ineffective breathing pattern related to*
  —obstructed airway
- *Impaired gas exchange related to*
  —ineffective breathing pattern
- *Risk for ineffective thermoregulation related to*
  —excess heat loss to environment
- *Pain related to*
  —circumcision
  —heel stick, venipuncture

Possible nursing diagnoses for the parent(s) are as follows:

- *Readiness for enhanced family coping related to*
  —knowledge of newborn's social capabilities
  —knowledge of newborn's dependency needs
  —knowledge of biologic characteristics of the newborn
- *Situational low self-esteem related to*
  —misinterpretation of newborn's behavioral cues

Examples of nursing diagnoses derived from specific assessment findings are listed in the Nursing Care Plan.

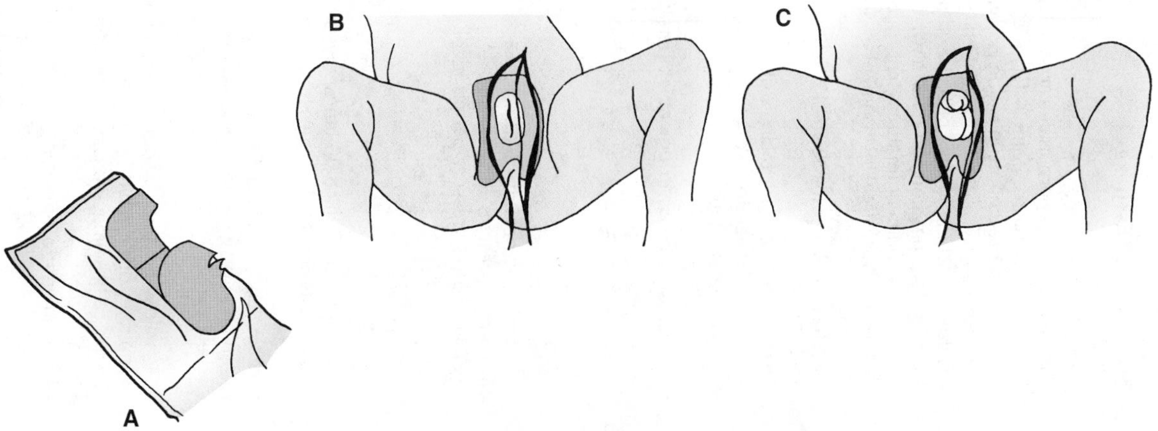

Fig. 25-11 Collection of urine specimen. **A**, Protective paper is removed from the adhesive surface. **B**, Applied to females. **C**, Applied to males. (Permission to use and/or reproduce this copyrighted material has been granted by the owner, Hollister, Inc., Libertyville, IL.)

Expected Outcomes

The expected outcomes for newborn care relate to the infant and to the parents. The expected outcomes for the infant include that the infant will do the following:

- Maintain an effective breathing pattern
- Maintain effective thermoregulation
- Remain free from infection
- Establish adequate elimination patterns
- Receive adequate measures to relieve pain

Expected outcomes for the parents include that they will do the following:

- Attain knowledge, skill, and confidence relevant to infant care activities
- State understanding of biologic and behavioral characteristics of the newborn
- Have opportunities to intensify their relationship with the newborn
- Begin to integrate the infant into the family

Plan of Care and Implementation

In the inpatient setting, priorities of care must be established and a systematic teaching plan for infant care devised. One way to achieve this is to use critical path case management. A care path may be developed that covers the changes expected in the infant during the first few days of life (Care Path). With early discharge (usually within 24 to 48 hours of birth) modifications in the care path to individualize newborn care will be necessary. The existing care path may also be used by nursing staff following the care of the mother-newborn dyad at home in the first few weeks of life to ensure that the infant receives appropriate care and screening, which was once provided in the acute care setting. When variations from the care path occur, further assessment and intervention may be necessary.

Protective Environment

The provision of a protective environment is basic to the care of the newborn. The construction, maintenance, and operation of nurseries in accredited hospitals is monitored by national professional organizations, such as the American Academy of Pediatrics, Joint Commission on Accreditation of Healthcare Organizations, Occupational Health and Safety Administration, and local or state governing bodies. In addition, hospital personnel develop their own policies and procedures for protecting the newborns under their care. Prescribed standards cover areas such as environmental factors, measures to control infection, and safety factors.

Environmental Factors

Environmental factors include provision of adequate lighting, elimination of potential fire hazards, safety of electric appliances, adequate ventilation, and controlled temperature (i.e., warm and free of drafts) and humidity (i.e., 40% to 60%) (American Academy of Pediatrics and American College of Obstetricians and Gynecologists, 2002).

Measures to Control Infection

Measures to control infection include adequate floor space to permit positioning bassinets at least 3 feet apart in all directions, handwashing facilities, and areas for cleaning and storing equipment and supplies. Only those personnel directly involved in the care of mothers and infants are allowed in these areas, thereby reducing the opportunities for the introduction of pathogenic organisms.

NURSE ALERT Personnel are instructed to use good handwashing techniques. The most important single measure in the prevention of neonatal infection is handwashing between handling different infants. ■

Health care workers must wear gloves during the following: when handling the infant before blood and amniotic fluid have been removed from the infant's skin; when drawing blood (e.g., heel stick); when caring for a fresh wound (e.g., circumcision); and during diaper changes.

Visitors and health care providers such as nurses, physicians, parents, brothers and sisters, department supervisors, electricians, and housekeepers are expected to wash their hands before having contact with infants or equipment. Cover gowns are not necessary in such areas but may be worn when holding infants against the health care worker's body as necessary to prevent cross-contamination.

Individuals with infectious conditions are excluded from contact with newborns, or must take special precautions when working with infants. This includes persons with up-

Text continued on p. 749.

Care Path

HEALTHY TERM NEWBORN

Care Aspects	First Hour	2-3 Hr	6 Hr	12 Hr	18 Hr	24 Hr	36-48 Hr to Discharge
Safety	ID band on and verified matching parents'; bulb syringe (for suction) at bedside; newborn safety alarm system activated.‡	ID band on Parent teaching regarding bulb syringe; NB alarm system active	ID band on Bulb syringe in crib; NB alarm system active	ID band on Bulb syringe in crib; NB alarm system active	ID band on Bulb syringe in crib; NB alarm system active	ID band on Bulb syringe in crib; NB alarm system active	ID band on† Remove at discharge only Parents verbalize appropriate car seat in place Discuss and reinforce home safety, including abduction prevention, infection prevention, car seat safety, and falls prevention Reinforce teaching for use of bulb syringe Discuss sleep position—on back, always; sleep environment (mattress, crib rails) Reinforce smoke-free environment around infant Deactivate NB alarm system at discharge
Temperature (axillary)	36.5° C-37.2° C	36.5° C-37.2° C	36.5° C-37.2° C		36.5° C-37.2° C	36.5° C-37.2° C	36.5-37.2° C Reinforce teaching for taking axillary temperature and when to take Thermometer type Normal ranges Discuss home environment temperature
Vital signs	Blood pressure on admission per protocol (not usual unless indicated)						
Heart rate	100-180 beats/min	80-180 beats/min	120-140 beats/min	120-140 beats/min	VS stable	VS stable: 120-140 beats/min	VS stable and documented If murmur present, document Monitor blood pressure per protocol
Respiratory rate	30-50 breaths/min (may be less if asleep)	30-50 breaths/min	30-50 breaths/min	30-50 breaths/min		30-50 breaths/min	
Feeding • Breast	Initiated—latch-on			1 latch-on*	2 latch-ons verified	3-4 successful latch-ons verified*	Feeding successfully 8-10 times/day; discuss and reinforce feeding cues and associated behaviors
• Formula		Sips to verify suck, swallow, and breathing	Sips to verify suck, swallow, and breathing	2 feedings—15-25 ml each	3 successful feedings verified—15-30 ml each	4-5 feedings verified; adequate suck, swallow, and breathing coordination	Feeding successfully 5-6 times/day; discuss and reinforce feeding cues and associated behaviors
Elimination • Voiding		Check		1 void		Minimum of 3 voids/24 hr in first few days	2-3 voids minimum; or number of voids = number of days old Reinforce teaching and care—minimum of 5-6 voids/day 1 meconium documented
• Stooling	Verify anal patency	Check for stool		Check for stool		1 meconium documented	Reinforce teaching and care—approximately 1-2 stools/72-96 hr after first week of life depending on feeding method; more if breastfeeding

Parent interaction	Initiated eye contact and verbalization	Ongoing contact	Exhibit newborn care interest and involvement	Involvement in newborn care		Continued involvement in newborn care	Demonstrates interest in newborn care; participates in newborn care; asks appropriate questions regarding home care; follow-up time and location provided
Cord care	Cord clamped	Cord care per institution protocol		Clamped; no drainage		Cord drying; no drainage	Cord drying; care reinforced to parents; clamp removed before discharge
Circumcision					Pain management—recommend topical anesthesia with DPNB or regional and oral sucrose; verify after procedure	Pain management—recommend topical anesthesia with DPNB or regional and oral sucrose; verify after procedure	Continued evaluation for absence of bleeding and presence of voiding Dressing applied with each diaper change depending on method (Gomco and Mogen clamp) Ring intact if Plastibell Reinforce teaching on care of circumcision at home; pain management care
Bilirubin	<5 mg/dl			<5 mg/dl		≤5-6 mg/dl; color pink; note if jaundice present and documented; transcutaneous bilirubin check per protocol	Note skin color; transcutaneous jaundice meter reading per protocol AND check serum bilirubin at 24-36 hr: <7 mg/dl—low risk <7-11 mg/dl—low intermediate risk <11-13 mg/dl—high intermediate risk >13 mg/dl—high risk
	No visible jaundice; pink	No visible jaundice; pink		No visible jaundice; pink		Check for jaundice	Note color—document Provide parent instruction regarding jaundice and follow-up visit with primary care practitioner within 3-4 days
Newborn screening				Hearing screening completed and documented		Newborn screening completed after 24 hr—document time and method	Verify newborn screening completed, including PKU after 24 hr of oral intake—reschedule if needed
Medications		Eye prophylaxis Vitamin K Maternal HBsAg status verified and documented	Hepatitis B vaccine within 12 hr of birth if mother positive; document			Check eye status; verify free of drainage	Reinforce hepatitis B vaccination at follow-up if not given in birth hospital
Activity	Active, flexed, primitive reflexes present (Moro, suck, tonic neck, Babinski)	May be drowsy but arousable	Active and alert Flexed, strong suck reflex		Active and alert Sleep periods noted Reflexes present Neurologic status intact		Discuss and reinforce sleep-wake patterns with parents; reinforce cues to active engagement with infant (eye contact, socialization); potential signs of danger (decreased activity; not arousable for feedings; color changes [not acrocyanosis], central cyanosis, apnea)

DPNB, dorsal penile nerve block; *HBsAg*, hepatitis B surface antigen; *ID*, identification; *PKU*, phenylketonuria; *VS*, vital signs.
*Minimum observed and documented.
†If still in hospital.
‡NB alarm system is the hospital protocol designed to protect infant from abduction.
Prepared by David Wilson, MS, RNC.

Nursing Care Plan

THE NORMAL NEWBORN

NURSING DIAGNOSIS: Risk for ineffective airway clearance related to excess mucus production/ improper positioning

EXPECTED OUTCOME

Neonate's airway remains patent; breath sounds are clear and no respiratory distress is evident.

NURSING INTERVENTIONS/*RATIONALES*

Suction mouth and nasopharynx with bulb syringe as needed; clean nares of secretions *to clear airway and prevent aspiration and airway obstruction.*

Position neonate on right side after birth *to prevent aspiration* and on back when sleeping *to prevent suffocation.*

Teach parents that gagging, coughing, and sneezing are normal neonatal responses *that assist the neonate in clearing airways.*

Teach parents how to hold, suction, feed, and position the neonate with return demonstration *to ensure parental skill at airway clearance and maintenance.*

NURSING DIAGNOSIS: Risk for imbalanced body temperature related to larger body surface in relationship to mass

EXPECTED OUTCOME

Neonate temperature remains in range of 36.5° C to 37.2° C.

NURSING INTERVENTIONS/*RATIONALES*

Maintain neutral thermal environment *to identify any changes in neonate's temperature that may be related to other causes.*

Monitor neonate's temperature often *to identify any changes promptly and ensure early interventions.*

Sponge bathe neonate when temperature is stable, using warm water, drying carefully, and avoiding exposing neonate to drafts *to avoid heat losses from evaporation and convection.*

Report any alterations in temperature findings promptly *to assess cause and implement interventions to maintain adequate temperature.*

NURSING DIAGNOSIS: Risk for infection related to deficient immunologic defenses, environmental factors

EXPECTED OUTCOME

The neonate will be free from infection.

NURSING INTERVENTIONS/*RATIONALES*

Review maternal record for evidence of any risk factors *to ascertain whether the neonate may be predisposed to viral or bacterial infection.*

Monitor vital signs *to identify early possible evidence of infection, especially temperature instability.*

Have all care providers, including parents, practice good handwashing techniques before handling newborn *to prevent spread of infection.*

Instruct parents to monitor visitors and personnel for evidence of infection and limit contact as needed *to prevent spread of infection.*

Keep genital area clean and dry using proper cleansing techniques *to prevent skin irritation, cross-contamination, and infection.*

Keep umbilical stump clean and dry and keep exposed to air *to allow it to dry and minimize chance of infection.*

Discuss home cord care, bathing and circumcision care with parents *to promote hygiene and prevent infection.*

If circumcised, keep site clean and dressed with prescribed ointment and diaper applied loosely *to prevent trauma and infection and to promote healing.*

Teach parents to keep neonate away from children and adults with colds or infections *to reduce potential sources of infection.*

Evaluate maternal hepatitis B status and implement prophylaxis as recommended (by AAP) *to prevent transmission of hepatitis B to newborn.*

Discuss with parents importance of follow-up well visits with practitioner for immunizations *to promote healthy child care and prevent life-threatening diseases of childhood.*

NURSING DIAGNOSIS: Risk for injury related to sole dependence on caregiver

EXPECTED OUTCOME

Neonate remains safe and free of injury in a protective environment.

NURSING INTERVENTIONS/*RATIONALES*

Monitor environment for hazards such as sharp objects *to prevent injury.*

Ensure that newborn safety system is in place *to protect infant from abduction.* Discuss abduction system precautions with parents *to educate and enlist their support in protecting the newborn from harm.*

Handle neonate gently and support head, transport only in crib, ensure use of car seat by parents, teach parents never to place neonate on high surface unsupervised, and to supervise pet and sibling interactions *to prevent injury.*

Discuss newborn supine sleep position with parents *to prevent sudden infant death syndrome.*

Discuss use of infant tummy time while awake *to prevent plagiocephaly* (misshapen skull).

Assess neonate for any evidence of jaundice *to identify rising bilirubin levels, treat promptly, and prevent kernicterus.*

NURSING DIAGNOSIS: Readiness for enhanced family coping related to anticipatory guidance regarding responses to neonate's crying

EXPECTED OUTCOMES

Parents will verbalize understanding of methods of coping with neonate's crying and describe increased success in interpreting neonate's cries.

NURSING INTERVENTIONS/*RATIONALES*

Discuss with parents crying as neonate's form of communication and that cries can be differentiated to indicate hunger, wetness, pain, and need for comforting *to provide reassurance that crying is not indicative of neonate's rejection of parents and that parents will learn to interpret different cries.*

Differentiate self-consoling behaviors from fussing/crying *to give parents concrete examples of appropriate interventions.*

Discuss methods of consoling a neonate such as changing diapers; showing parent's face to neonate; talking softly to neonate; swaddling; rocking; using a pacifier, feeding, or burping; or going for a car ride *to provide anticipatory guidance.*

Additional nursing diagnoses may be applicable and include but are not limited to:

Breastfeeding, effective
Caregiver Role Strain
Parenting, altered
Infant behavior, Organized, potential for enhanced

per respiratory tract infections, gastrointestinal tract infections, and infectious skin conditions. Most agencies have now coupled this day-to-day self-screening of personnel with yearly health examinations.

Safety Factors

Health care institutions must be proactive in protecting newborns from abduction. Examples of measures taken include placing matching identification bracelets on newborns and their parents; using identification bands with radiofrequency transmitters that set off an alarm if the bracelet is removed or if a certain threshold is crossed (doorway to exit building or floor); and footprinting or taking identification pictures after birth, before the infant leaves the mother's side. In addition, agencies must conduct periodic unit- and hospital-wide drills aimed at preventing newborn abductions. Personnel caring for newborns must be clearly identified by photo identification, and parents must be educated regarding measures to prevent abduction from the mother's room. Parents are also educated before discharge regarding measures to minimize and prevent abduction from the home setting.

SUPPORTING PARENTS IN THE CARE OF THEIR INFANT

The sensitivity of the caregiver to the social responses of the infant is basic to the development of a mutually satisfying parent-child relationship (Leitch, 1999). Sensitivity increases over time as parents become more aware of their infant's social capabilities (Cultural Awareness box).

Social Interactions

The activities of daily care during the neonatal period present the best times for infant and family interactions (Family Focus box) (Community Focus box). While caring for their newborn, the mother and father can talk to the infant, play baby games, caress and cuddle the child, and perhaps use infant massage. In Figure 25-12, a mother, father, and infant are shown engaging in arousal, imitation of facial expression, and smiling. Too much stimulation should be avoided after feeding and before a sleep period. Older siblings' contact with a newborn is encouraged and supervised depending on the developmental level of the child. Parents often keep memento books that record the birth, the hospital stay, and their infant's progress.

Cultural Awareness

CULTURAL BELIEFS AND PRACTICES

Nurses working with childbearing families from other cultures and ethnic groups must be aware of cultural beliefs and practices that are important to individual families. People with a strong sense of heritage may hold on to traditional health beliefs long after adopting other American lifestyle practices. These health beliefs may involve practices regarding the newborn. For example, some Asians, Hispanics, eastern Europeans, and Native Americans delay breastfeeding because they believe that colostrum is "bad." Some Hispanics and African-Americans place a belly band over the infant's navel. The birth of a male child is generally preferred by Asians and Indians, and some Asians and Haitians delay naming their infant.

Source: D'Avanzo C, Geissler E: *Pocket guide to cultural health assessment*, ed 3, St Louis, 2003, Mosby.

Family Focus

FAMILY RELATIONSHIPS AND SOCIAL SUPPORT

The family's ethnic and cultural background is important in determining the health status, genetic or familial risk factors present, and social support available to the woman throughout pregnancy and in the postpartum period. Family relationships, including husband-wife roles, vary among individuals and groups. The husband may be the decision maker, and his consent may be necessary before the woman agrees to prenatal treatment. Female rather than male family members may be involved in the pregnancy and birth. Mothers and mothers-in-law may be present and supportive during pregnancy, birth, and the early postnatal period to provide advice and care. In such instances, they need to be included in teaching sessions. Community and church support may be available. Assessment of family and community resources is an essential component of care.

Community Focus

INFANT CARE CLASS

Prepare and conduct one 20-minute class in infant care for parents. Before class, prepare a written teaching plan that includes assessment of learning needs; a teaching-learning diagnosis; a plan with prioritized patient-centered goals; content and teaching methods with rationales; and evaluative criteria. Take into consideration cultural and ethnic differences among parents. After the class, critique the total experience. What insights have you achieved?

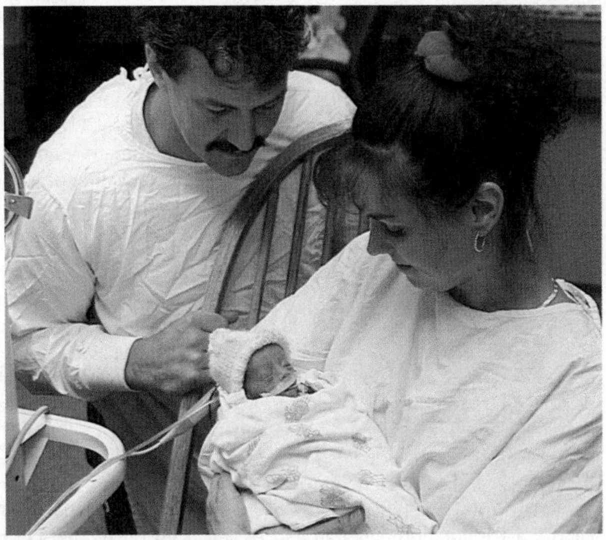

Fig. 25-12 Mother-father-baby interaction. (From Hockenberry MJ et al: *Wong's nursing care of infants and children*, ed 7, St Louis, 2003, Mosby.)

Infant Feeding

The infant may be put to breast shortly after birth, or at least within 4 hours of birth. Newborns are on demand feeding schedules and are allowed to feed when they awaken. Ordinarily mothers are encouraged to breastfeed their infants every 2 to 3 hours (bottle-feed every 3 to 4 hours) during the day and only when the infant awakens during the night in the first few days after birth. Breastfed babies nurse more often than bottle-fed babies because breast milk is digested faster than formulas

Evidence-Based Practice

OPTIMUM DURATION OF EXCLUSIVE BREASTFEEDING: THE SYSTEMATIC WORLD HEALTH ORGANIZATION REVIEW

Background

Breastfeeding unquestionably provides many documented health benefits, and can be lifesaving in developing countries, with a markedly reduced mortality rate that persists into the second year. Breastfeeding has a protective effect against gastrointestinal and respiratory infection, sudden infant death syndrome (SIDS), atopic disease, obesity, diabetes, Crohn's disease, and lymphoma. Breastfeeding may accelerate neurocognitive development and achievement. Maternal health benefits include possible protection against breast cancer, ovarian cancer, and osteoporosis.

An observation of "growth faltering" at about 3 months of age in developing countries has led to questions about the nutritional and energy content of breast milk after 3 or 4 months, the nutritional quality of supplemental foods introduced at about 3 to 4 months, and the risk of infection-caused energy deficit in infants. A debate about the "weanling's dilemma" stemmed from questions about inadequate breast milk nutrition versus nutritionally inadequate or contaminated weaning foods. Growth faltering is relatively uncommon in developed countries, but the more rapid weight gain may not represent a benefit. The debate pitted the World Health Organization (WHO), whose policy was to recommend exclusive breastfeeding for 4 to 6 months, against UNICEF, who recommended "about 6 months" of exclusive breastfeeding. In preparation for a policy reassessment, WHO requested this review of available evidence regarding the optimum duration of breastfeeding.

Objectives

All agreed that exclusive breastfeeding was best for 3 to 4 months. The reviewers were charged with the task of comparing health, growth, and development outcomes for those who continued exclusive breastfeeding until 6 months, versus those who gradually added supplemental liquid or food to breastfeeding. The participants could all be healthy, singleton, term infants (low birth weight accepted, as long as gestationally full term). Infant outcome measures could include weight, length, head circumference, infections, morbidity, mortality, micronutrient status, neuromotor and cognitive developmental milestones, atopic disease, type 1 diabetes, blood pressure, adult chronic illnesses, and inflammatory and autoimmune diseases. Maternal outcome measures include postpartum weight loss, lactational amenorrhea, breast and ovarian cancer, and osteoporosis.

Methods

Search Strategy

An exhaustive search of world literature included Cochrane, MEDLINE, EMBASE, CINAHL, HealthSTAR, EBM Reviews–Best Evidence, SocioFile, CAB Abstracts, EMBASE-Psychology, Econlit, Index Medicus for the WHO Eastern Mediterranean, African Index Medicus, and LILACS Latin American and Caribbean literature. Search keywords included *exclusive breastfeeding* and *growth*.

Twenty studies were reviewed, nine from developing countries (including the Philippines, Peru, Chile, Honduras, Bangladesh, Belarus, East India, and Senegal) and eleven from developed countries (the United States, Sweden, Finland, Australia, and Italy). The studies were published from 1980 to 2000. Two were controlled trials from Honduras, and the rest were observational studies.

Statistical Analyses

Statistical analyses were only possible in the two controlled trials. The observational studies were too heterogeneous and limited by design to pool data.

Findings

The authors found no significant difference in weight, length, or atopic disease in the two groups. Exclusively breastfed infants had significantly decreased gastrointestinal infections, which was consistent with previous evidence. There was a marginally significant decrease in the iron stores of exclusively breastfed infants in developing countries at 6 months, unless they were receiving an iron supplement. Maternal weight loss was accelerated in exclusive breastfeeding, and lactational amenorrhea was prolonged.

Limitations

Observational studies are subject to bias. Confounding by indication refers to the statistical errors that occur because the reason for the treatment (i.e., food supplementation given to a growth-faltering breastfed infant) affects the outcome. Bias can also occur due to reverse causality. For example, an infant with an infection becomes anorectic and reduces milk intake to the point of loss of milk production. Depending on when assessment occurs, the infection might be blamed on the weaning, instead of the reverse. Other unmeasured covariables can also confound the results.

Conclusions

The researchers found no evidence of a "weanling's dilemma," and no benefits from adding supplemental food between 4 and 6 months. The iron deficit of exclusively breastfed babies in developing countries can be corrected with infant drops and does not warrant the loss of protection against gastrointestinal and respiratory infections that exclusive breastfeeding confers. Infants must still be managed individually. Maternal lactational amenorrhea provides contraceptive benefit for child spacing, a clear benefit. Rapid postpartum weight loss may benefit women in developed countries, but may not benefit women with marginal nutritional status. The policy statements of WHO and the World Health Assembly were modified to reflect the recommendation for exclusive breastfeeding for the first 6 months of life.

Implications for Practice

Exclusive breastfeeding should be recommended. Iron supplements for breastfeeding infants are beneficial. The contraceptive benefits of lactational amenorrhea are important.

Implications for Further Research

Public health policy demands information about breastfeeding beyond the observational stage. Large, randomized trials are needed, especially in developing countries, to confirm infection morbidity and infant nutritional status in exclusively breastfed infants of 6 months' duration or longer. Costs are not addressed in these studies. More information on long-term outcomes is needed, particularly neurocognitive achievement, emotional growth, blood pressure, growth, and atopic diseases.

Reference

Kramer M, Kakuma R: Optimal duration of exclusive breastfeeding (Cochrane Review), 2001. In *The Cochrane Library*, Issue 2, Chichester, UK, 2004, John Wiley & Sons.

made from cow's milk and the stomach empties sooner as a result. Water supplements are not recommended. For a thorough discussion of infant feeding, see Chapter 26.

THERAPEUTIC AND SURGICAL PROCEDURES

Intramuscular Injection

As discussed previously, it is routine to administer a single dose of 0.5 to 1 mg of vitamin K intramuscularly (see Medication Guide earlier in this chapter).

Hepatitis B vaccination is recommended for all infants. Infants at highest risk of contracting hepatitis B are those born to women who have hepatitis B or whose hepatitis B status is unknown. If the infant is born to an infected mother or to a mother who is a chronic carrier, hepatitis vaccine and hepatitis B immune globulin (HBIG) should be given within 12 hours of birth (Medication Guides). The hepatitis vaccine is given in one site and the HBIG in another. For infants born to a hepatitis B–negative woman, the first dose of the vaccine may be given at birth or at 1 or 2 months of age. Parental consent should be obtained before administering these medications.

In most cases a 25-gauge, ⅝- to ⅞-inch needle should be used for the vitamin K and hepatitis vaccine injections.

Selection of the site for injection is important. Injections must be given in muscles large enough to accommodate the medication, and major nerves and blood vessels must be avoided. The muscles of newborns may not tolerate more than 0.5 ml per intramuscular injection. The injection site for newborns is the vastus lateralis (Fig. 25-13). The dorsogluteal muscle is very small, poorly developed, and dangerously close to the sciatic nerve, which occupies a larger proportion of space in infants than in older children. Therefore it is not recommended as an injection site until the child has been walking for at least 1 year. The newborn's deltoid muscle has an inadequate amount of muscle for intramuscular administration. An important key factor in preventing and minimizing local reaction to intramuscular injections is adequate deposition of the fluid (medication) deep within the muscle; therefore muscle size, needle length, and amount of medication injected should be carefully considered. The preferred site is the vastus lateralis.

The neonate's leg should be stabilized (see Figure 45-19 for containment method). Gloves are worn for the injection. The nurse cleanses the injection site with an appropriate skin antiseptic. The needle is inserted into the vastus lateralis at a 90-degree angle. The plunger of the syringe is gently withdrawn, and if blood is not aspirated, the medication is injected. If blood is aspirated, the needle is withdrawn and the injection is given in another site. The needle is withdrawn quickly and pressure is maintained at the site to minimize the pain.

Medication Guide

HEPATITIS B VACCINE (RECOMBIVAX HB, ENGERIX-B)

Action
Hepatitis B vaccine induces protective anti–hepatitis B antibodies in 95% to 99% of healthy infants who receive the recommended three doses. The duration of protection of the vaccine is unknown.

Indication
Hepatitis B vaccine is for immunization against infection caused by all known subtypes of hepatitis B virus.

Neonatal Dosage
The usual dosage is Recombivax HB 5 mcg/0.5 ml or Engerix-B 10 mcg/0.5 ml at 0, 1, and 6 months. An alternative dosing schedule is 0, 1, 2, and 12 months and is usually for newborns whose mothers were HBsAg positive. See also Immunizations in Chapter 36.

Adverse Reactions
Common adverse reactions are rash, fever, erythema, swelling, and pain at injection site.

Nursing Considerations
Parental consent must be obtained before administration. Wear gloves. Administer in the middle third of the vastus lateralis muscle using a 25-gauge, ⅝- to ⅞-inch needle. Inject into skin that has been cleaned, or allow alcohol to dry on puncture site for 1 minute to remove organisms and prevent infection. Stabilize leg firmly and grasp muscle between the thumb and fingers. Insert the needle at a 90-degree angle; aspirate and inject medication slowly if there is no blood return. After removing needle, rub gently on the site with a dry gauze square to decrease pain sensation. If the infant was born to an HBsAg-positive mother, hepatitis B immune globulin (HBIG) should be given within 12 hours of birth in addition to the hepatitis B vaccine. Separate sites must be used. Document immunization administration on a vaccination card for parent(s) to have a record.

HBsAg, hepatitis B surface antigen.

Medication Guide

HEPATITIS B IMMUNE GLOBULIN (HBIG)

Action
HBIG provides a high titer of antibody to hepatitis B surface antigen (HBsAg).

Indication
The HBIG vaccine provides prophylaxis against infection in infants born of HBsAg-positive mothers.

Neonatal Dosage
Administer one 0.5 ml dose intramuscularly within 12 hours of birth.

Adverse Reactions
Hypersensitivity may occur.

Nursing Considerations
Must be given within 12 hours of birth. Wear gloves. Administer in the middle third of the vastus lateralis muscle using a 25-gauge, ⅝- to ⅞-inch needle. Inject into skin that has been cleaned, or allow alcohol to dry on puncture site for 1 minute to remove organisms and prevent infection. Stabilize leg firmly and grasp muscle between the thumb and fingers. Insert the needle at a 90-degree angle; aspirate and inject medication slowly if there is no blood return. After removing needle, rub gently on the site with a dry gauze square to decrease pain sensation. May be given at same time as hepatitis B vaccine, but in a separate syringe and at a different site. Document immunization administration on a vaccination card for parent(s) to have a record.

A

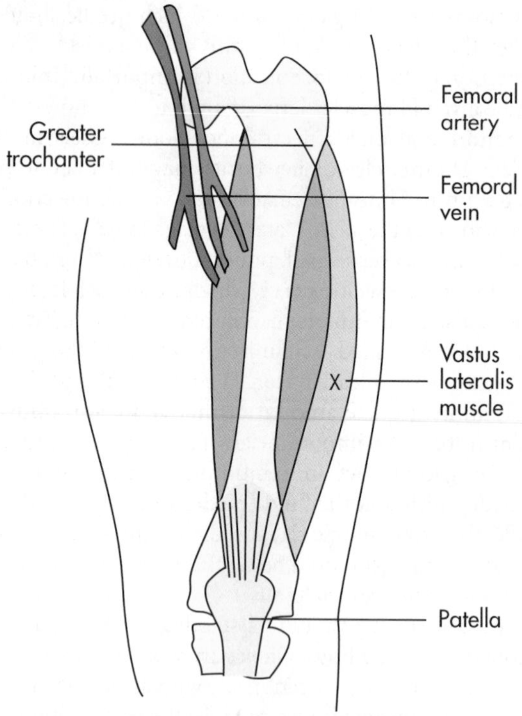

B

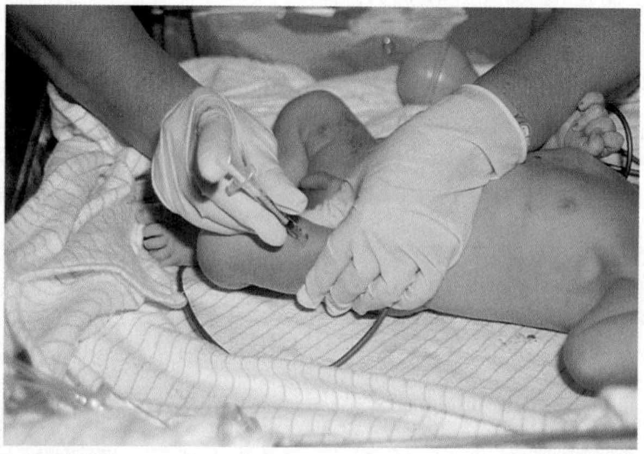

Fig. 25-13 Intramuscular injection. **A**, Acceptable intramuscular injection site *(X)* for newborn infant. **B**, Infant's leg stabilized for intramuscular injection. Nurse is wearing gloves to give injection. (*B*, Courtesy Marjorie Pyle, RNC, Lifecircle, Costa Mesa, CA.)

The nurse should always remember to comfort the infant after an injection and to properly discard equipment. Needles should never be recapped but should be properly discarded in an appropriate safety container. It is important to record medication, date and time, amount, route, and site of injection on the newborn's chart.

Therapy for Hyperbilirubinemia

The best therapy for hyperbilirubinemia is prevention. Because bilirubin is excreted in meconium, prevention can be facilitated by early feeding, which stimulates passage of meconium. However, despite early passage of meconium, the term infant may have trouble conjugating the increased amount of bilirubin derived from disintegrating fetal RBCs. As a result, the serum levels of unconjugated bilirubin may rise beyond normal limits, causing hyperbilirubinemia. The goal of treatment of hyperbilirubinemia is to help reduce the newborn's serum levels of unconjugated bilirubin. There are two ways to reduce unconjugated bilirubin levels: phototherapy and exchange blood transfusion. Exchange transfusion is used to treat those infants whose levels of serum bilirubin are rising rapidly despite the use of intensive phototherapy (see discussion on p. 853).

Phototherapy

During phototherapy the infant is placed, seminude, approximately 45 to 50 cm under a bank of lights. The distance may vary based on unit protocol and type of light used. There should always be a Plexiglas panel or shield between the lights and the infant when conventional lighting is used. The most effective therapy is achieved with lights at 400 to 550 nanometers, and blue-green light spectrum is the most efficient (Steffensrud, 2004). The lamp energy output should be monitored routinely during treatment with a photometer to ensure efficacy of therapy. Phototherapy is carried out until the infant's serum bilirubin level decreases to within acceptable range. The decision to discontinue therapy is based on a definite downward trend in the serum bilirubin values.

Several precautions must be taken while the infant is undergoing phototherapy. The infant's eyes must be protected by an opaque mask to prevent overexposure to the light. The eye shield should cover the eyes completely but not occlude the nares. Before the mask is applied, the infant's eyes should be closed gently to prevent excoriation of the corneas. The mask should be removed periodically and during infant feedings so that the eyes can be checked and cleansed with water and the parents can have visual contact with the infant (Fig. 25-14, *A* and *B* and Family Focus box).

Often a "string bikini" made from a disposable face mask is used instead of a diaper. This allows optimal skin exposure, yet provides sufficient protection to the genitals and bedding. Before its application, the metal strip must be removed from the mask to prevent burning the infant. Lotions and ointments should not be used during phototherapy because they absorb heat and can cause burns.

Family Focus

PHOTOTHERAPY AND PARENT-INFANT INTERACTION

The traditional use of phototherapy has evoked concerns regarding a number of psychobehavioral issues, including parent-infant separation, potential social isolation, decreased sensorineural stimulation, altered biologic rhythms, altered feeding patterns, and activity changes. Parental anxiety is greatly increased, particularly at the sight of the newborn blindfolded and under special lights. The interruption of breastfeeding for phototherapy is a potential deterrent to successful maternal-infant attachment and interaction. Because research has demonstrated that bilirubin catabolism occurs primarily within the first few hours of the initiation of phototherapy, there is increased support for the removal of the infant from treatment for feeding and holding. Intermittent phototherapy may be just as effective as continuous therapy when used correctly. The benefits of stopping phototherapy for short periods of parental feeding and holding the newborn should be carefully weighed by the health care team and the parents.

A

B

C

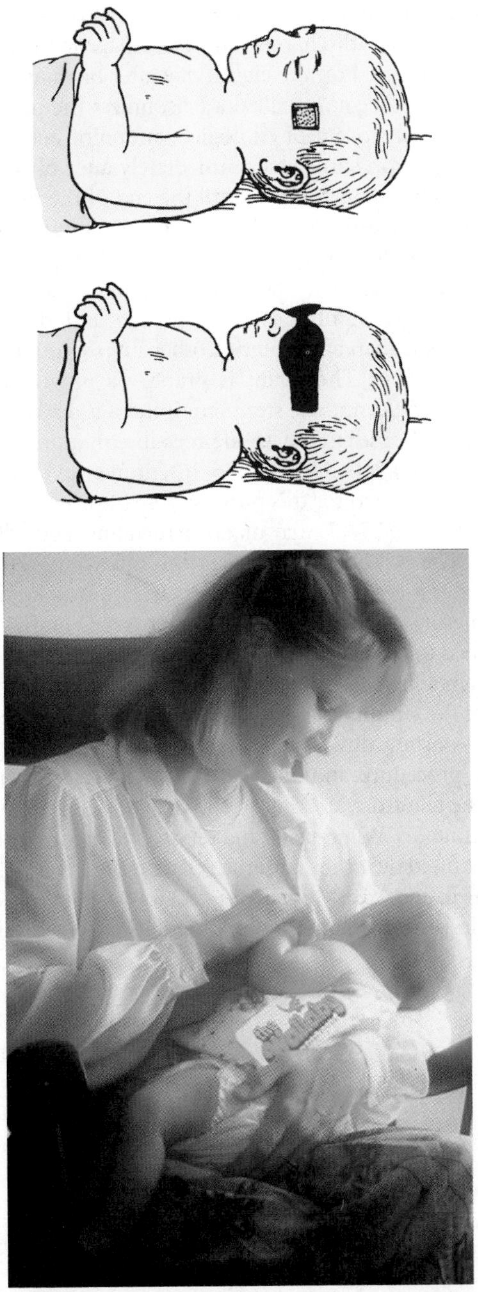

Fig. 25-14 Eye patches for newborns receiving phototherapy. **A,** Small Velcro patch stuck to both sides of head. **B,** Eye cover sticks to Velcro patch, which reduces movement of eye cover and facilitates removal for feedings. **C,** A mother can breastfeed her newborn without interrupting phototherapy when a fiberoptic blanket is used. (*C,* Courtesy Respironics, Inc., Pittsburgh, PA.)

Phototherapy may cause changes in the infant's temperature depending partially on the bed used: bassinet, incubator, or radiant warmer. The infant's temperature should be closely monitored. Phototherapy lights may increase the rate of insensible water loss, making it possible for fluid loss and dehydration to occur. Therefore it is important that the infant be adequately hydrated. Hydration maintenance in the healthy newborn is carried out with human milk or infant formula; there is no advantage or benefit to administering oral glucose or plain water because these do not promote excretion of bilirubin in stools and may in fact perpetuate enterohepatic circulation, thus delaying bilirubin excretion. Urine output may be decreased or unaltered; the urine may have a dark gold or brown appearance.

The number and consistency of stools are monitored. Bilirubin breakdown increases gastric motility, which results in loose stools that can cause skin excoriation and breakdown. The infant's buttocks must be cleaned after each stool to help maintain skin integrity. A fine macropapular rash may appear during phototherapy, but this is transient. Because visualization of the infant's skin color is difficult with blue light, appropriate cardiorespiratory monitoring should be implemented based on the infant's overall condition.

An alternative device for phototherapy that is as safe and effective as traditional phototherapy is a fiberoptic panel attached to an illuminator. The fiberoptic blanket is flexible and may be placed around the newborn's torso or flat in the bed, thus delivering continuous phototherapy. Although fiberoptic lights do not produce heat as do conventional lights, staff should ensure that there is a covering pad between the infant's skin and the fiberoptic device to prevent skin burns, especially in preterm infants. The newborn can remain in the mother's room in an open crib or in her arms during treatment (Fig. 25-14, *C*). Follow unit protocol for the use of eye patches. The blanket may also be used for home phototherapy. In certain situations the infant's bilirubin levels may be increasing rapidly and intensive phototherapy is required; this involves the use of a combination of conventional lights and fiberoptic lights to maximize bilirubin reduction. All aspects of phototherapy should be accurately recorded in the infant's medical record.

Parent Education

Serum levels of bilirubin in the newborn continue to rise until the fifth day of life. Many parents leave the hospital within 24 hours of birth, and some as early as 6 hours after birth. Therefore parents must receive education regarding jaundice and its treatment. They should have written instructions for assessing the infant's condition and the name of a contact person to whom they should report their findings and concerns. Some institutions or third-party providers pay for a home visit to evaluate the infant's condition and to monitor the mother's health as well. If it proves necessary to measure serum bilirubin levels after discharge from the hospital, the home care nurse may draw the blood for the specimen, or the parents may take the baby to a laboratory to have blood drawn for a serum bilirubin. In some cases parents may take the newborn to an outpatient clinic to be evaluated.

CRITICAL THINKING EXERCISE—CIRCUMCISION

Circumcision

Circumcision of male infants is commonly performed in the United States. The American Academy of Pediatrics Task Force on Circumcision (1999) noted that, although there is scientific evidence of potential medical benefits of circumcision, the data are not sufficient to recommend routine circumcision. The Task Force on Circumcision further recommended that if circumcision is performed, analgesia should be used.

Circumcision is a matter of personal parental choice. Parents usually decide to have their newborn circumcised based on one or more of the following factors: hygiene, religious conviction, tradition, culture, or social norms. Regardless of the reason for the decision, parents should be given unbiased information and the opportunity to discuss the benefits and risks (Van Ryzin, 2000).

Expectant parents need to begin learning about circumcision during the prenatal period, but circumcision often is not discussed with the parents before labor. In many instances, it is only when the mother is being admitted to the hospital or birth unit that she is first confronted with the decision regarding circumcision. Because the stress of the intrapartal period makes this a difficult time for parental decision making, this is not an ideal time to broach the topic of circumcision and expect a well-thought-out decision.

Procedure

Circumcision involves removing the prepuce (foreskin) of the glans. The procedure is not usually done immediately after birth because of the danger of cold stress and decreased clotting factors, but it is often performed in the hospital before the infant's discharge. The circumcision of a Jewish male is performed on the eighth day after birth and is done at home in a ceremony called a bris, unless the infant is ill. This is logical from a physiologic standpoint because clotting factors drop somewhat immediately after birth and do not return to prebirth levels until the end of the first week.

Feedings are usually withheld up to 2 to 3 hours before the circumcision to prevent vomiting and aspiration. To prepare the infant for the circumcision, he is positioned on a plastic restraint form (Fig. 25-15) and the penis is cleansed with soap and water or other prep solution such as povidone-iodine. The infant is draped to provide warmth and a sterile field, and the sterile equipment is readied for use.

Although some circumcision procedures require no special equipment or appliances (Fig. 25-16), numerous instruments have been designed for this purpose. Use of the Yellen or Mogen clamp (Fig. 25-17) may make this an almost bloodless operation. The procedure itself takes only a few minutes to perform. After it is completed, a small petrolatum gauze dressing or a generous amount of petrolatum or A & D ointment may be applied to the penis for the first few days to prevent the diaper from adhering to the site. A PlastiBell is another method used for the circumcision. The advantages to its use are that it applies constant direct pressure to prevent hemorrhage during the procedure and afterward protects against infection, keeps the site from sticking to the diaper, and prevents pain with urination. When using the plastic bell for circumcision, it is first fitted over the glans; the suture is tied around the rim of the bell; and excess prepuce is cut away. The plastic rim remains in place for about a week; it falls off after healing has

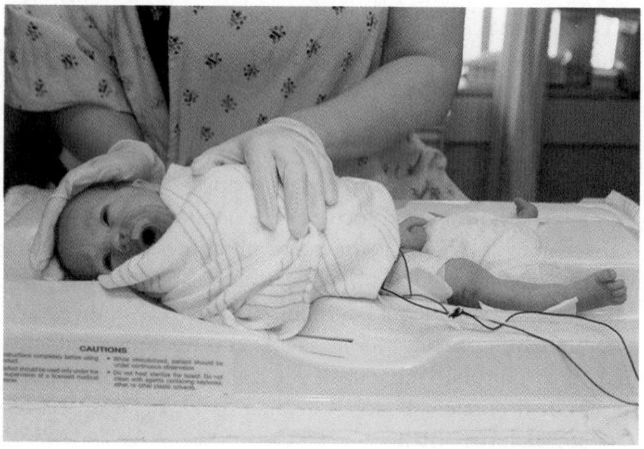

Fig. 25-15 Proper positioning of infant in Circumstraint. (Courtesy Paul Vincent Kuntz, Texas Children's Hospital, Houston, TX.)

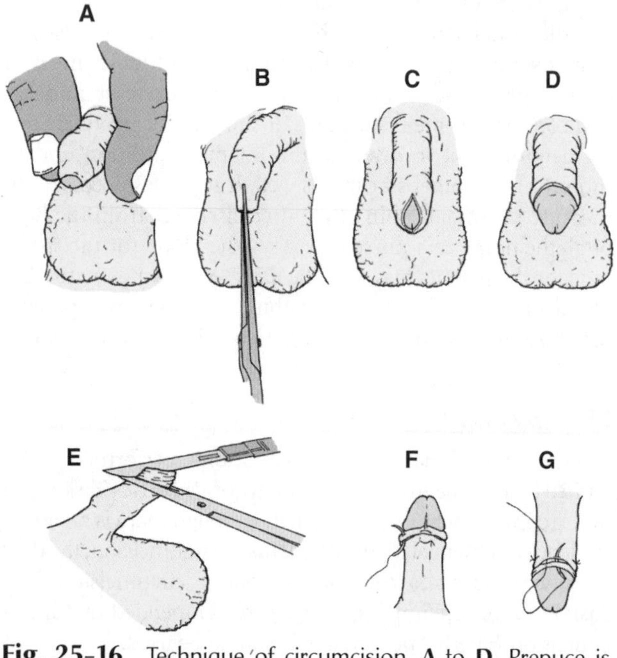

Fig. 25-16 Technique of circumcision. **A** to **D**, Prepuce is stripped and slit to facilitate its retraction behind glans penis. **E**, Prepuce is now clamped and excessive prepuce cut off. **F** and **G**, A very small needle with plain 2-0 or 3-0 catgut is used for suture material; some physicians prefer silk.

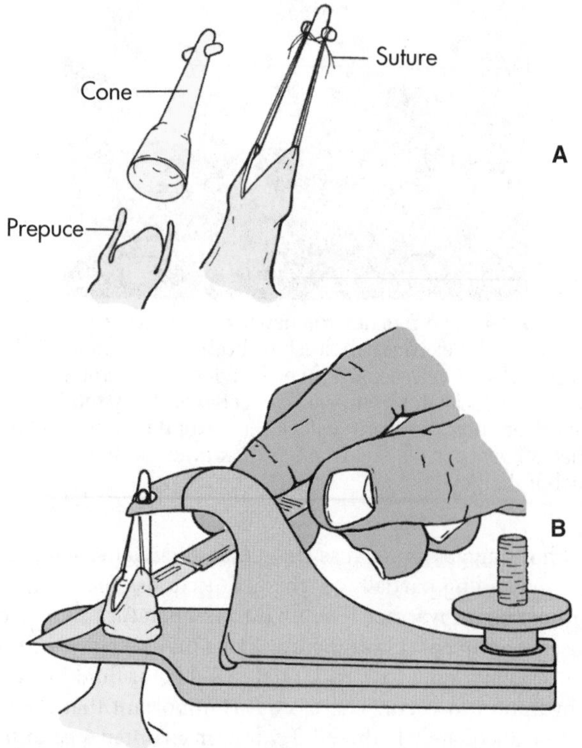

Fig. 25-17 Circumcision with Mogen (Yellen) clamp. **A**, Prepuce drawn over cone. **B**, Mogen clamp is applied, hemostasis occurs, and then prepuce (over cone) is cut away.

taken place, usually within 5 to 7 days (Fig. 25-18). Petrolatum is not usually needed when the bell is used.

Discomfort

Circumcision is painful. The pain is manifested by both physiologic and behavioral changes in the infant (see discussion that follows). Three types of anesthesia/analgesia are used in newborns who undergo circumcision: the ring block, the dorsal penile nerve block (DPNB), and topical anesthetic (Williamson, 1997). Nonpharmacologic methods such as nonnutritive sucking, containment, and swaddling may be used in addition to pharmacologic use of oral acetaminophen and a concentrated oral glucose solution. A combination of ring block or DPNB, topical anesthetic, nonnutritive sucking, oral acetaminophen, concentrated oral sucrose solution (2 ml of a 24% concentration given during the procedure on a pacifier, with a syringe or nipple), and swaddling has been shown to be the most effective at decreasing the pain associated with circumcision.

A ring block is the injection of buffered lidocaine administered subcutaneously on each side of the penile shaft. A DPNB includes subcutaneous injections of buffered lidocaine at the 2 o'clock and 10 o'clock positions at the base of the penis. The circumcision should not be done for at least 5 minutes after these injections.

A topical cream containing prilocaine-lidocaine such as eutectic mixture of local anesthetic (EMLA) can be applied to the base of the penis at least 1 hour before the circumcision. The area where the prepuce attaches to the glans is well coated with 1 g of the cream and then covered with a transparent occlusive dressing or finger cot. The cream is removed just before the procedure. Blanching or redness of the skin may occur.

After the circumcision, the infant is comforted until he is quieted. If the parents were not present during the procedure, the infant is returned to them. The infant may be fussy for several hours and may have disturbed sleep-wake states and disorganized feeding behaviors. Oral acetaminophen may be administered after the procedure every 4 hours (as ordered per practitioner) for a maximum of five doses in 24 hours or a maximum of 75 mg/kg/day (Atraumatic Care box).

Nurses are instrumental in implementing changes in health care practices to effectively manage the pain of neonatal circumcision (Razmus, Dalton, & Wilson, 2004).

Care of the Newly Circumcised Infant

The nurse checks the infant hourly for the next 4 to 6 hours to make sure that no bleeding is occurring and that voiding is normal. If bleeding is noted from the circumcision, the nurse applies gentle pressure to the site of bleeding with a folded sterile gauze pad or sprinkles powdered gel foam on it. If bleeding is not easily controlled, a blood vessel may need to be ligated. In this event, one nurse notifies the physician and prepares the necessary equipment (i.e., circumcision tray and suture materials) while another nurse maintains intermittent pressure until the physician arrives. If the parents take the baby home before the end of the observation period, they must be taught the proper home care (Patient Teaching box). Nursing actions are planned and implemented to prevent infection. Prepackaged commercial wipes for cleaning the diaper area should not be used because they contain alcohol, which delays healing and causes discomfort. Instead, the nurse washes the penis gently with water to remove urine and feces and, if necessary, applies fresh petrolatum around the glans after each diaper change. The glans penis, normally dark red during healing, becomes covered with a yellow exudate in 24 hours. This is part of normal healing, not an infective process. No attempt should be made to remove the exudate, which persists for 2 to 3 days. Parents should be taught to fanfold the diaper so that it does not press on the circumcised area. They should be encouraged to change the diaper at least every 4 hours to prevent it from sticking to the penis.

NEONATAL PAIN

Pain has physiologic and psychologic components. The psychologic component of pain, and the diffuse total body response to pain exhibited by the neonate, led many health care providers to believe that infants, especially preterm infants, do not experience pain (Franck & Gregory, 1993).

A

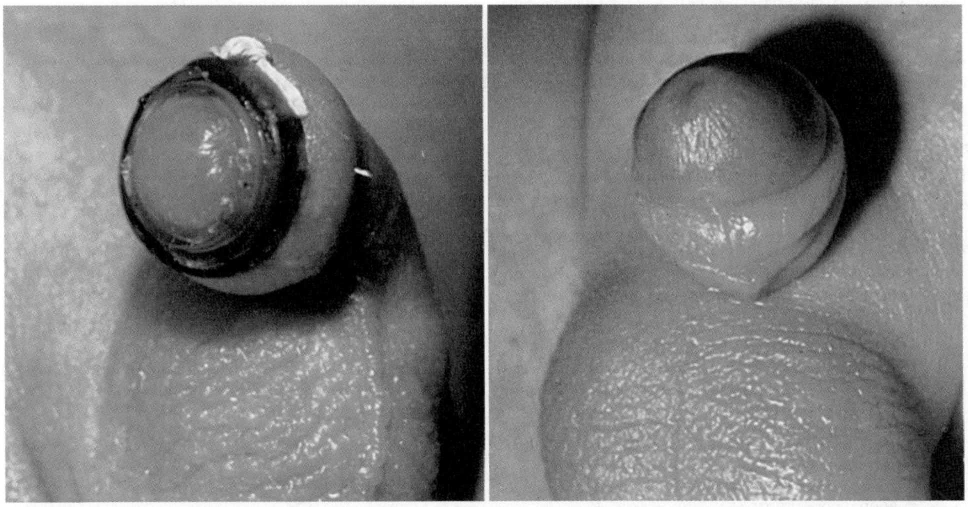

B

Fig. 25-18 Circumcision using Hollister PlastiBell. **A**, Suture around rim of PlastiBell controls bleeding. **B**, Plastic rim and suture drop off in 7 to 10 days. (Permission to use and/or reproduce this copyrighted material has been granted by the owner, Hollister, Inc., Libertyville, IL.)

Atraumatic Care

GUIDELINES FOR PAIN MANAGEMENT DURING NEONATAL CIRCUMCISION

Pharmacologic Interventions

Use of Topical Anesthetic Only

One hour before the procedure, administer acetaminophen (e.g., Tylenol, 15 mg/kg) as ordered by the practitioner and every 4 to 6 hours after the procedure for 24 hours

Place a thick layer (1 g) of eutectic mixture of local anesthetic (EMLA)* cream around the penis where the prepuce (foreskin) attaches to the glans. Avoid placing cream on the tip of the penis where EMLA may come in contact with the urethral opening.

Cover the penis with a "finger cot" that is cut from a vinyl or latex glove or a piece of plastic wrap and secure bottom of covering with tape. Avoid using Tegaderm or large amounts of tape on the skin because removing the adhesive causes pain and can irritate or remove the fragile skin.

If the infant urinates during the time EMLA is applied (1 hour) and a significant amount of EMLA is removed, reapply the cream and covering. The total application of EMLA should not exceed a surface area of $10\ cm^2$ (1.25×1.25 inches).

Remove cream with clean cloth or tissue. Blanching of skin is an expected reaction to EMLA's application under an occlusive dressing; erythema and some edema may occur also.

During the procedure, give the infant a concentrated sucrose solution (24%). Use this solution to coat the pacifier (recoat several times before and during the procedure) or administer 2 ml to the tongue 2 minutes before the procedure.

Following the procedure, apply petrolatum or A & D ointment on a 4×4 dressing before diapering the infant to prevent the wound from adhering to the dressing or diaper.

Administer acetaminophen as ordered by the practitioner (10 to 15 mg/kg) every 4 to 6 hours for 24 hours, not to exceed five doses in 24 hours or a maximum dose of 75 mg/kg/day.

Use of Dorsal Penile Nerve Block (DPNB) or Ring Block

One hour before the procedure, administer acetaminophen as ordered by the practitioner.

One hour before the procedure, apply EMLA. For the DPNB, apply EMLA to the prepuce as described previously and at the penile base. For the ring block, apply EMLA to the prepuce as described previously and to the shaft of the penis. A topical anesthetic should be used in conjunction with the DPNB or ring block to avoid the pain of injecting the anesthetic.

Use a 30-gauge needle to administer the lidocaine.† For the DPNB, 0.4 ml of the lidocaine is infiltrated at the 10:30 o'clock and 1:30 o'clock positions in Buck's fascia at the penile base. For the ring block, 0.4 ml of lidocaine is infiltrated subcutaneously on each side of the shaft of the penis below the prepuce.

For maximum anesthesia, wait 5 minutes following the injection of lidocaine. An alternative anesthesia is chloroprocaine, which is as effective as lidocaine after 3 minutes.

During the circumcision, administer sucrose as described previously.

Apply A & D ointment or petrolatum as described previously.

Administer acetaminophen as described previously.

Nonpharmacologic Interventions (to Accompany Preceding Pharmacologic Interventions)

If Circumstraint board is used, pad with blankets or other thick, soft material such as "lamb's wool." A more comfortable, padded, and physiologic restraint that places the infant in a semireclining position can also decrease distress (Stang et al, 1997).‡

Provide the parents, caregiver, or another staff member with the option to hold the infant during the procedure or to be present during the circumcision.

Swaddle the upper body and legs during the procedure to provide warmth and containment and to reduce movement.

If the patient is not swaddled and is unclothed, use a radiant warmer to prevent hypothermia. Shield the infant's eyes from overhead lights as needed.

Prewarm any topical solutions to be used in sterile preparation of the surgical site by placing in a warm blanket or towel.

Play infant relaxation music§ before, during, and after procedure; allow parents or other caregiver the option to provide the music of choice.

Following the procedure, remove restraints and swaddle. Immediately have the parent, other caregiver, or nursing staff hold the infant. Continue to have the infant suck on pacifier or offer feeding.

Data from Broadman LM et al: Post-circumcision analgesia: a prospective evaluation of subcutaneous ring block of the penis, *Anesthesiology* 67(3):399-402, 1987; Howard CR, Howard FM, Weitzman ML: Acetaminophen analgesia in neonatal circumcision: the effect on pain, *Pediatrics* 93(4):641-646, 1994; Lander J et al: Comparison of ring block, dorsal penile nerve block, and topical anesthesia for neonatal circumcision, *JAMA* 278(24):2157-2162, 1997; Mintz MR, Grillo R: Dorsal penile nerve block for circumcision, *Clin Pediatr* 28(12):590-591, 1989; Serour F, Mandelberg A, Mori J: Slow injection of local anesthetic will decrease pain during dorsal penile nerve block, *Acta Anaesthesiol Scand* 42(8):926-928, 1998; Spencer DM et al: Dorsal penile nerve block in neonatal circumcision: chloroprocaine versus lidocaine, *Am J Perinatol* 9(3):214-218, 1992; Stang H et al: Beyond dorsal penile nerve block: a more humane circumcision, *Pediatrics* 100(2):E3, 1997 (Internet document available at www.pediatrics.org/cgi/content/full/100/2/e3); Stevens B et al: The efficacy of sucrose for relieving procedural pain in neonates—a systematic review and meta-analysis, *Acta Paediatr* 86(8):837-842, 1997; Taddio A et al: Efficacy and safety of lidocaine-prilocaine cream (EMLA) for pain during circumcision, *N Engl J Med* 336(17):1197-1201, 1997; Taddio A: Pain management for neonatal circumcision, *Paediatr Drugs* 3(2):101-111, 2001; Taddio A, Ohlsson K, Ohlsson A: Lidocaine-prilocaine cream for analgesia during circumcision in newborn boys, *Cochrane Syst Rev* 2003(1):CD000496, 2003; Geyer J et al: An evidence-based multidisciplinary protocol for neonatal circumcision pain management, *J Obstet Gynecol Neonatal Nurs* 31(4): 403-410, 2002.

*NOTE: In March 1999 the Food and Drug Administration approved the use of EMLA in infants age 37 weeks of gestation. Although the package insert states, under "Warnings," that patients taking drugs associated with drug-induced methemoglobinemia, such as acetaminophen, are at greater risk for developing methemoglobinemia, there have been no reported cases of this complication occurring in children taking acetaminophen and using EMLA. In fact, there is no evidence that acetaminophen is a methemoglobin-inducing drug in humans (Prescott, 1996). The only reported cases of methemoglobinemia from acetaminophen have been in cats and dogs (Hjelle & Grauer, 1986).

†NOTE: In one study, the use of buffered lidocaine, which normally reduces the stinging sensation of lidocaine, did not provide effective anesthesia for DPNB (Stang et al, 1997). The study on slow injection of the anesthetics lidocaine and bupivacaine compared 40 versus 80 seconds in patients age 15 to 53 years (Serour, Mandelberg, & Mori, 1998).

‡For information on the Stang Circ Chair, contact Pedicraft, 4134 Augustine Rd., Jacksonville, FL 32207; 800-223-7649; e-mail: info@pedicraft.com; Web site: www.pedicraft.com.

§Suggested infant relaxation music: *Heartbeat Lullabies* by Terry Woodford. Available from Baby-Go-To-Sleep Center, Audio Therapy Innovations, Inc., PO Box 550, Colorado Springs, CO 80901; 800-537-7748.

Patient Teaching

CARE OF THE CIRCUMCISED NEWBORN AT HOME

- Wash hands before touching the newly circumcised penis.

Check for Bleeding

- Check circumcision for bleeding with each diaper change.
- If bleeding occurs, apply gentle pressure with a folded sterile gauze square. If bleeding does not stop with pressure, notify primary health care provider.

Observe for Urination

- Check to see that the infant urinates after being circumcised.
- Infant should have a wet diaper 6 to 10 times per 24 hours.

Keep Area Clean

- Change diaper and inspect circumcision at least every 4 hours.
- Wash penis gently with warm water to remove urine and feces. Apply petrolatum to the glans with each diaper change (omit petrolatum if PlastiBell was used).
- Use soap only after circumcision is healed (5 to 6 days).
- Fanfold diaper to prevent pressure on the circumcised area.

Check for Infection

- Glans penis is dark red after circumcision, then becomes covered with yellow exudate in 24 hours. This is normal and will persist for 2 to 3 days. Do not attempt to remove it.
- Redness, swelling, or discharge indicate infection. Notify primary health care provider if you think the circumcision area is infected.

Provide Comfort

- Circumcision is painful. Handle the area gently.
- Provide extra holding, feeding, and opportunities for nonnutritive sucking for a day or two.

However, the central nervous system is well developed as early as 24 weeks of gestation. The peripheral and spinal structures that transmit pain information are present and functional between the first and second trimester. The pituitary-adrenal axis is also well developed at this time, and a fight-or-flight reaction is observed in response to the catecholamines released in response to stress (Franck, 1998).

The physiologic response to pain in the neonate can be life threatening. Pain response can decrease tidal volume, increase demands on the cardiovascular system, and increase metabolism and neuroendocrine imbalance. The hormonal-metabolic response to pain in a term infant has a greater magnitude and shorter duration than in adults. The newborn's sympathetic response to pain is less mature and thus less predictable than an adult's (Franck & Gregory, 1993).

All infants, regardless of gestational age, should receive appropriate analgesia or anesthesia for potentially painful procedures (American Academy of Pediatrics, Committee on Fetus and Newborn, 2000; Anand & International Evidence-Based Group for Neonatal Pain, 2001). Parents are universally concerned that their infants are suffering pain during procedures (Franck, Scurr, & Couture, 2001). Nurses must address these concerns and encourage the parents to speak with the health care professionals involved. Parents have the right to withhold consent for invasive procedures and are entitled to honest answers from those responsible for the infant's care. When feasible, parents may also participate in providing comfort and pain relief for the infant.

Assessment

Pain can be assessed in behavioral, physiologic/autonomic, and metabolic categories.

Behavioral Responses

The most common behavioral sign of pain is a vocalization or cry. The pain cry is distinctive: high pitched and shrill. A cry face is characteristic of an infant experiencing pain. Other facial features exhibited during a pain stimulus include eye squeeze, brow contraction, deepened nasolabial furrows, taut and quivering tongue, and open mouth. The infant will flex and adduct the upper body and lower limbs in an attempt to withdraw from the painful stimulus (Anand, Grunau, & Oberlander, 1997; Hadjistavropoulos et al, 1997). The preterm infant has a lower threshold for initiation of this flex response. An infant who receives a muscle-paralyzing agent such as vecuronium will be unable to mount a behavioral or visible pain response.

SKILL—PAIN ASSESSMENT

Physiologic/Autonomic Responses

Significant changes in heart rate, blood pressure (increased or decreased), intracranial pressure, vagal tone, respiratory rate, and oxygen saturation occur during noxious stimulation (Franck & Gregory, 1993; Lynam, 1995).

Metabolic Responses

Infants release epinephrine, norepinephrine, glucagon, corticosterone, cortisol, 11-deoxycorticosterone, lactate, pyruvate, and glucose in response to pain (Franck & Gregory, 1993; Lynam, 1995).

Several pain assessment tools have been developed for the assessment of pain in the neonate. One pain assessment tool used by nurses who work with neonates is the CRIES (Table 25-4). This tool was developed for use by nurses who work with preterm and full-term infants. CRIES is an acronym for the physiologic and behavioral indicators of pain used in the tool: crying, requiring increased oxygen, increased vital signs, expression, and sleeplessness. Each indicator is scored from 0 to 2. The total possible pain score, which represents the worst pain, is 10. A pain score greater than 4 should be considered significant. This tool can be used on infants between the ages of 32 weeks of gestation and 20 weeks postbirth (Bildner & Krechel, 1996; Krechel & Bildner, 1995).

MANAGEMENT OF NEONATAL PAIN

The goals of management of neonatal pain are to (1) minimize intensity, duration, and physiologic effects of pain, and (2) maximize the neonate's ability to cope with and recover from the pain. Nonpharmacologic and pharmacologic strategies are used to ensure that adequate pain relief is achieved.

Nonpharmacologic Management

Containment, also known as swaddling, is effective in reducing the response to neonatal pain. This may provide comfort through other senses such as thermal, tactile, and propri-

Table 25-4

CRIES Neonatal Postoperative Pain Scale

	0	1	2
Crying	No	High pitched	Inconsolable
Requires O_2 for saturation >95%	No	<30%	>30%
Increased vital signs	Heart rate and blood pressure equal to or less than preoperative state	Heart rate and blood pressure <20% of preoperative state	Heart rate and blood pressure >20% of preoperative state
Expression	None	Grimace	Grimace/grunt
Sleepless	No	Wakes at frequent intervals	Constantly awake

CODING TIPS FOR USING CRIES

Crying	The characteristic cry of pain is *high pitched.* If no cry or cry that is not high pitched, score 0. If cry is high pitched but infant is easily consoled, score 1. If cry is high pitched and infant is inconsolable, score 2.
Requires O_2 for saturation >95%	Look for *changes* in oxygenation. Infants experiencing pain manifest decreases in oxygenation as measured by tCO_2 or oxygen saturation. (Consider other causes of changes in oxygenation, such as atelectasis, pneumothorax, oversedation.) If no oxygen is required, score 0. If <30% O_2 is required, score 1. If >30% O_2 is required, score 2.
Increased vital signs	NOTE: Measure blood pressure last because this may wake child, causing difficulty with other assessments. Use baseline preoperative parameters from a nonstressed period. Multiply baseline HR × 0.2, then add this to baseline HR to determine the HR that is 20% over baseline. Do likewise for BP. Use mean BP. If HR and BP are both unchanged or less than baseline, score 0. If HR or BP is increased but increase is <20% of baseline, score 1. If either one is increased >20% over baseline, score 2.
Expression	The facial expression most often associated with pain is a grimace. This may be characterized by brow lowering, eyes squeezed shut, deepening of the nasolabial furrow, open lips and mouth. If no grimace is present, score 0. If grimace alone is present, score 1. If grimace and noncry vocalization grunt is present, score 2.
Sleepless	This is scored based on the infant's state during the hour preceding this recorded score. If the child has been continuously asleep, score 0. If he or she has awakened at frequent intervals, score 1. If he or she has been awake constantly, score 2.

Neonatal pain assessment tool developed at the University of Missouri–Columbia. From Krechel SW, Bildner J: CRIES: a new neonatal postoperative pain measurement score: initial testing of validity and reliability, *Pediatr Anaesth* 5(1):53-61, 1995.
BP, blood pressure; *HR,* heart rate.

oceptive senses (Franck & Gregory, 1993; Lynam, 1995). Nonnutritive sucking is a common comfort measure used in newborns. However, the effectiveness of nonnutritive sucking on the pain response is limited and confined to the pain caused by certain procedures (Lynam, 1995; Mohan et al, 1998).

Pharmacologic Management

Morphine and fentanyl are the most widely used opioid analgesics for pharmacologic management of neonatal pain. Continuous or bolus intravenous infusion of opioids provides effective and safe pain control (American Academy of Pediatrics, Committee on Fetus and Newborn, 2000). Ketorolac (Toradol) has been shown to be effective in the management of postoperative neonatal pain (Burd & Tobias, 2002). Postoperative neonatal pain should be managed with around-the-clock dosing or use of a continual drip. Dosing as needed (prn) is not considered to be an effective management of chronic or postoperative pain (Hummel & Puchalski, 2001). Traditional belief holds that the continued use of opioids for neonates in the postoperative period results in prolonged intubation. Consequently, traditional practice is to discontinue all opioids several hours before and after extubation, preventing pain relief. Furdon and colleagues (1998) found that continuous opioid infusion in infants without an underlying pulmonary or neurologic pathologic condition actually shortened the time to extubation and caused no problems of respiratory depression that required reintubation.

Other methods for managing neonatal pain are epidural infusion, local and regional nerve blocks, and intradermal or topical anesthetics (American Academy of Pediatrics, Committee on Fetus and Newborn, 2000; Anand & International Evidence-Based Group for Neonatal Pain, 2001; Taddio et al, 1998). Study results vary when EMLA is used in newborns for heel punctures; some find the topical anesthetic to be beneficial in managing heel stick pain whereas others do not. However, EMLA does reduce the pain of circumcision, venous or arterial puncture, and percutaneous venous catheter placement (Taddio et al, 1998). A *concentrated sucrose solution*, especially when administered with a pacifier, can decrease pain associated with heel lance and venipuncture (Blass & Watt, 1999; Gradin et al, 2002; Stevens, Yamada, & Ohlsson, 2001). Oral *acetaminophen* may be administered for painful procedures such as circumcision, venous puncture, and heel stick.

DISCHARGE PLANNING AND TEACHING

Infant care activities can cause much anxiety for the new parent (see the Nursing Care Plan earlier in this chapter). Support from nursing staff members can be an important factor in determining whether new mothers seek and accept help in the future. Whether this is the woman's or couple's first newborn, or an adolescent whose mother will be the primary caregiver, or whether they attended parenthood preparation classes, parents appreciate anticipatory guidance in the care of their infant. The nurse should not try to cover all the content at one time because the parents can be overwhelmed by too much information and become anxious. However, because early discharge of new mothers is currently common practice, it may be a problem for the nurse to teach all the content that is necessary. As a result, many institutions have developed home visitation programs that take the necessary teaching to the new parents, although the hospital nurse still provides most of the essential information for newborn care (see Community Focus box on p. 749).

To set priorities for teaching, the nurse follows parental cues. Deficient knowledge should be identified before beginning to teach. Normal growth and development and the changing needs of the infant (e.g., for stimulation, exercise, and social contacts), as well as the topics that follow, should be included during discharge planning with parents.

Temperature

The following topics should be reviewed:

- The causes of elevation in body temperature (e.g., overwrapping, cold stress with resultant vasoconstriction, or minimal response to infection) and the body's response to extremes in environmental temperature
- Signs to be reported, such as high or low temperatures with accompanying fussiness, lethargy, irritability, poor feeding, and crying
- Ways to promote normal body temperature, such as dressing the infant appropriately for the environmental air temperature and protecting the infant from exposure to direct sunlight
- Use of warm wraps or extra blankets in cold weather
- Technique for taking the newborn's axillary temperature

Respirations

Review the following points:

- Normal variations in the rate and rhythm
- Reflexes such as sneezing to clear the airway
- Need to protect the infant from the following:
  - Exposure to people with upper respiratory tract infections and RSV (respiratory syncytial virus)(see Chapter 46)
  - Exposure to secondhand tobacco smoke
  - Suffocation from loose bedding, water beds, and beanbag chairs; drowning (in bath water); entrapment under excessive bedding or in soft bedding; anything tied around the infant's neck; poorly constructed playpens, bassinets, or cribs
- Sleep position—on back when put to sleep
- Aspiration pneumonia; symptoms of the common cold

A commonly aspirated substance is baby powder, which usually is a mixture of talc (hydrous magnesium silicate) and other silicates. Parents are advised that, if they prefer to use a powder, a cornstarch preparation can be substituted. Whenever a powder is used, it should be placed in the caregiver's hand and then applied to the skin, never sprinkled directly onto the skin.

Symptoms of the common cold include nasal congestion and excess drainage of mucus, coughing, sneezing, difficulty in swallowing or breathing, decreased vigor in feeding, and low-grade fever. Advise the parents on measures to help the infant, such as the following:

- Feeding smaller amounts more often to prevent overtiring the infant
- Holding the baby in an upright position to feed
- For sleeping, raising the infant's head and chest by raising the mattress 30 degrees (do not use pillow)
- Avoiding drafts; not overdressing the baby
- Using only medications prescribed by a physician
- Using nasal saline drops in each nostril and suctioning well with bulb syringe to decrease and relieve secretions

Feeding Schedules

Feeding practices and schedules for newborns are discussed in Chapter 26.

Elimination

A review includes the following reminders:

- Color of normal urine and number of voidings (6 to 10) to expect each day
- Changes to be expected in the color of the stool (i.e., meconium to transitional to soft yellow/golden yellow) and the number of bowel evacuations, plus the odor of stools for breastfed or bottle-fed infants (see Chapter 26)
- Expected pattern of stools in formula-fed infants may be as few as one stool every other day after first few weeks of life

Positioning and Holding

The American Academy of Pediatrics, Task Force on Infant Sleep Position and Sudden Infant Death Syndrome (2000), recommends placing the infant in the supine position during the first few months of life to prevent sudden infant death syndrome (SIDS). The prone position has been associated with an increased incidence of SIDS. Death rates from SIDS have decreased by more than 40% in the United States since the original sleep position statement recommending supine sleeping for all newborns was made in 1992 (Community Focus box–SIDS and Infant Sleep Position).

Anatomically, the infant's shape—a barrel chest and flat, curveless spine—makes it easy for the infant to roll from the side to the prone position; therefore the side-lying position for sleep is not recommended. Care must also be taken to prevent the infant from rolling off flat, unguarded surfaces. When an infant is on such a surface, the parent or nurse who must turn away from the infant even for a moment should always keep one hand placed securely on the infant. The infant is always held securely with its head supported because newborns are unable to maintain an erect head posture for more than a few moments. Figure 25-19 illustrates various positions for holding an infant with adequate support.

Community Focus

SIDS AND INFANT SLEEP POSITION

Prepare a display on SIDS and infant sleep position for a well-baby clinic. Identify the age, education, and ethnicity of patients who come to the clinic. Outline content that is important to include. Describe how you would adapt the display based on the demographics of the patients who come to the clinic.

Critical Thinking Exercise

SIDS AND INFANT SLEEP POSITION

Marlys gave birth to a full-term infant; she and Daniel are being discharged today. The nurse has given her instructions about placing the baby on his back for sleep. Marlys said that she had noticed that the nurses placed Daniel on his side in the nursery and wondered why they did that when she was instructed to place Daniel on his back.

Michelle gave birth to Michael at 32 weeks. During the stay in the nursery, the nurses placed Michael on his abdomen to sleep. At discharge, Michelle was instructed to place Michael on his back to sleep. Michelle asked why she had to place Michael on his back to sleep when he was used to sleeping on his abdomen.

How should the nurses respond to these questions?

1. Evidence–Is there sufficient evidence to draw conclusions about the safety and efficacy of the supine position for sleep in reducing the incidence of SIDS?
2. Assumptions–What assumptions can be made about the following factors related to infant positioning?
   a. Role modeling by nurses
   b. Sleep position in the nursery versus sleep position at home
   c. Sleep position for preterm versus term infants
   d. Nurses' knowledge and use of research evidence
3. What implications and priorities for nursing care can be drawn at this time?
4. Does the evidence objectively support your conclusion?
5. Are there alternative perspectives to your conclusion?

All personnel working with infants must have current infant cardiopulmonary resuscitation (CPR) certification. Many institutions offer infant CPR courses to parents before discharge (see also Chapter 46, Figs. 46-9 and 46-10).

Rashes

Diaper Rash

The warm, moist atmosphere in the diaper area provides an optimal environment for *Candida albicans* growth; dermatitis appears in the perianal area, inguinal folds, and lower abdomen. The affected area is intensely erythematous with a sharply demarcated, scalloped edge, often with numerous satellite lesions that extend beyond the larger lesion. The usual source of infection is from handling by persons who do not practice adequate handwashing. It may also appear 2 to 3 days after an oral infection (thrush).

Therapy consists of applications of an anticandidal ointment, such as clotrimazole or miconazole, with each diaper change. Sometimes the infant also is given an oral antifungal preparation such as nystatin or fluconazole to eliminate any gastrointestinal source of infection.

Washing and drying the wet and soiled area and changing the diaper immediately after voiding or stooling will prevent and help treat diaper rash. Parents can be taught to expose the buttocks to air to help dry up diaper rash. Because bacteria thrive in moist dark areas, exposing the skin to dry air decreases bacterial proliferation. A skin barrier ointment such as zinc oxide may be effective in preventing further excoriation, especially in the presence of loose stools or systemic gastrointestinal candidiasis; the latter will require treatment with a systemic antifungal drug.

Other Rashes

A rash on the cheeks may result from the infant's scratching with long unclipped fingernails or from rubbing the face against the crib sheets, particularly if regurgitated stomach contents are not washed off promptly. The newborn's skin begins a natural process of peeling and sloughing after birth. Dry skin may be treated with a neutral pH lotion, but this should be used sparingly. Newborn rash, erythema toxicum, is a common finding (see Fig. 24-5, *B*, p. 700) and needs no treatment.

Clothing

Parents commonly ask how warmly they should dress their infant. A simple rule of thumb is to dress the child as they dress themselves, adding or subtracting clothes and wraps for the child as necessary. A cotton shirt and diaper may be sufficient clothing for the young infant. A cap or bonnet is needed to protect the scalp and minimize heat loss if the weather is cool, or to protect against sunburn and shade the eyes if it is sunny and hot. Wrapping the infant snugly in a blanket maintains body temperature and promotes a feeling of security. Overdressing in warm temperatures can cause discomfort, as can underdressing in cold weather. Parents are encouraged to dress the infant at all times in flame-retardant clothing. Infant sunglasses are available to protect the infant's eyes when outdoors.

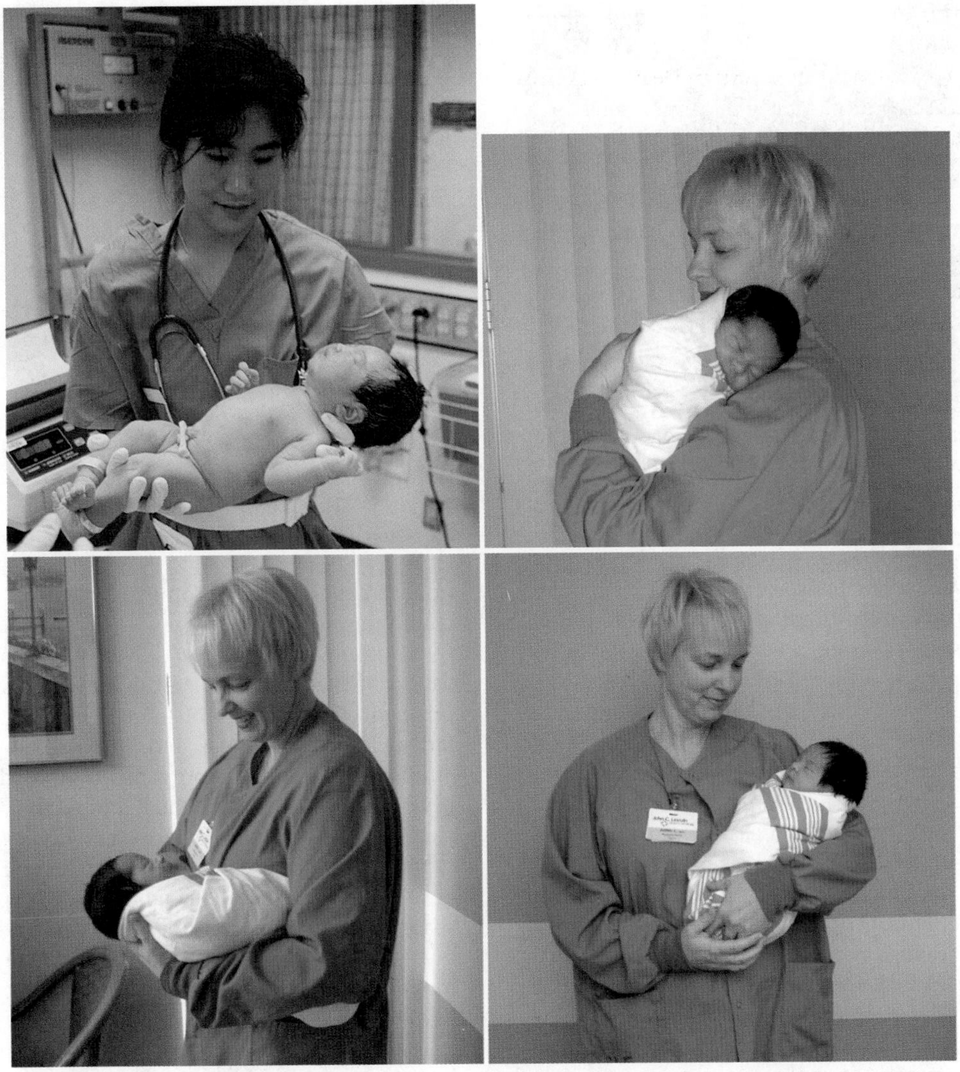

Fig. 25-19 Holding baby securely with support for head. **A,** Holding infant while moving infant from one place to another. Baby is undressed to show posture. **B,** Holding baby upright in "burping" position. **C,** "Football" hold. **D,** Cradling hold. (*A,* Courtesy Kim Molloy, Knoxville. *B, C,* and *D,* Courtesy Julie Perry Nelson, Gilbert, AZ.)

Safety: Use of Car Seat

Infants should travel only in federally approved, rear-facing safety seats secured in the rear seat (Fig. 25-20). The safest area of the car is the back seat. A car seat that faces the rear gives the best protection for the disproportionately weak neck and heavy head of an infant. In this position, the force of a frontal crash is spread over the head, neck, and back; the back of the car seat supports the spine.

NURSE ALERT Infants should use a rear-facing car seat from birth to 20 pounds and to 1 year of age. If the infant reaches the weight limit before the first birthday, the rear-facing position should still be used. ■

The car seat is secured using the vehicle seat belt; the infant is secured using the harness system in the car seat. If the infant must ride in the front seat, the air bag must be turned off to prevent injury from the air bag.*

NURSE ALERT In cars equipped with air bags, rear-facing infant seats must not be placed in the front seat. Serious injury can occur if the air bag inflates because these types of infant seats fit closer to the dashboard. ■

Infants born at less than 37 weeks of gestation and with birthweight less than 2500 grams should be observed in a car seat for a period of time (equal to the length of the car ride home) before discharge. The infant is monitored for apnea, bradycardia, and a decrease in oxygen saturation. It may be necessary to place blanket rolls on either side of the infant for support of the head and trunk. To prevent slumping, the back-to-crotch strap distance should be 14 cm.

---

*Air bag safety sheets are available from the American Academy of Pediatrics, 141 Northwest Point Blvd., Elk Grove Village, IL 60007; phone: 1-800-433-9016; fax: 847-228-1281; or access the Web site at www.aap.org for the latest guidelines for infant car seat restraints.

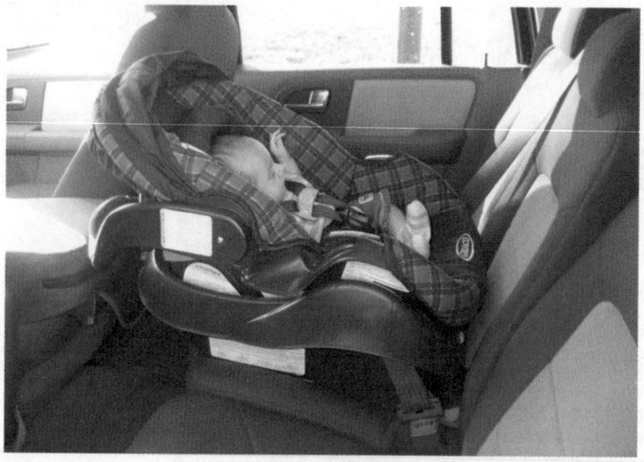

Fig. 25-20 Rear-facing infant seat in rear seat of car. Infant is placed in seat when going home from the hospital. (Courtesy Brian and Mayannyn Sallee, Las Vegas, NV.)

Nonnutritive Sucking

Sucking is the infant's chief pleasure. However, sucking needs may not be satisfied by breastfeeding or bottle-feeding alone. In fact, sucking is such a strong need that infants who are deprived of sucking, such as those with a cleft lip, will suck on their tongues. Some newborns are born with sucking pads on their fingers that developed during in utero sucking. Several benefits of nonnutritive sucking have been demonstrated, such as an increased weight gain in preterm infants, increased ability to maintain an organized state, and decreased crying.

Problems arise when parents are concerned about the sucking of fingers, thumb, or pacifier and try to restrain this natural tendency. Before giving advice, nurses should investigate the parents' feelings and base the guidance they give on the information solicited. For example, some parents may see no problem with the use of a finger but may find the use of a pacifier objectionable. In general, there is no need to restrain either practice, unless thumb sucking persists past 4 years of age or past the time when the permanent teeth erupt. Parents are advised to consult with their pediatrician, pediatric dentist, or pediatric nurse practitioner about this topic.

A parent's excessive use of the pacifier to calm the child should also be explored, however. It is not unusual for parents to place a pacifier in their infant's mouth as soon as it begins to cry, thus reinforcing a pattern of distress-relief.

If parents choose to let their child use a pacifier, they need to be aware of certain safety considerations before purchasing one. A homemade or poorly designed pacifier can be dangerous because the entire object may be aspirated, if it is small, or a portion may become lodged in the pharynx. Improvised pacifiers, such as those commonly made in hospitals from a padded nipple, also pose dangers because the nipple may separate from the plastic collar and be aspirated. Safe pacifiers are made of one piece that includes a shield or flange large enough to prevent entry into the mouth and a handle that can be grasped (Fig. 25-21).

Sponge Bathing, Cord Care, and Skin Care

Bathing serves a number of purposes. It provides opportunities for (1) completely cleansing the infant, (2) observing the infant's condition, (3) promoting comfort, and (4) parent-child-family socializing.

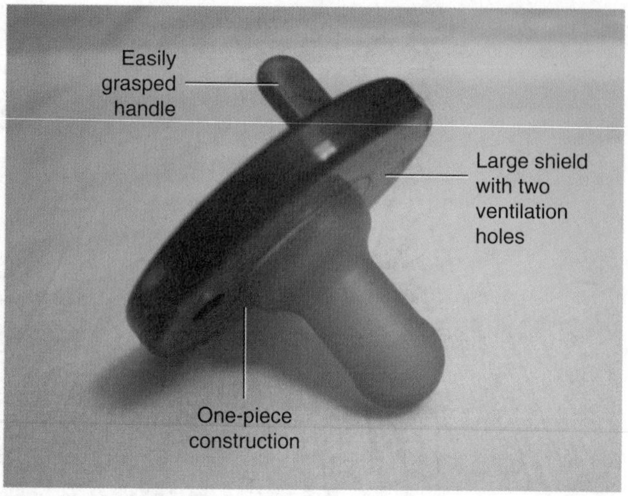

Fig. 25-21 Design of a safe pacifier. (Courtesy Julie Perry Nelson, Gilbert, AZ.)

An important consideration in skin cleansing is preservation of the skin's acid mantle, which is formed from the uppermost horny layer of the epidermis, sweat, superficial fat, metabolic products, and external substances such as amniotic fluid and microorganisms. At birth, the skin has a pH of 6.4. Within 4 days, the pH of the newborn's skin surface falls to within the bacteriostatic range (pH less than 5) (Krebs, 1998). Consequently, only plain, warm water should be used for the bath during that 4-day period. Alkaline soaps (such as Ivory) and oils, powders and lotions should not be used during this time because they alter the acid mantle, thus providing a medium for bacterial growth. Although the sponging technique is generally used, bathing the newborn by immersion has been found to allow less heat loss and provoke less crying; this is not advised, however, until the umbilical cord falls off. A daily bath is not necessary for achieving cleanliness and may do more harm by disrupting the integrity of the newborn's skin; cleansing the perineum after a soiled diaper and daily cleansing of the face may suffice.

Until the initial bath is completed, personnel must wear gloves to handle the newborn.

The umbilical cord begins to dry, shrivel, and blacken by the second or third day of life depending in part on the cleansing method used. The umbilicus should be inspected often for signs of infection (e.g., foul odor, redness, and purulent discharge), granuloma (i.e., small, red, raw-appearing polyp where the umbilical cord separates), bleeding, and discharge. The cord clamp is removed when the cord is dry, in about 24 to 36 hours (see Fig. 25-5). The cord normally falls off in 10 to 14 days after birth but may remain attached for as long as 3 weeks in some cases.

Parents are instructed in appropriate home cord care (per practitioner or institution protocol) and the expected time of cord separation.

The Home Care box contains information regarding sponge bathing, skin care, cord care, cutting nails, and dressing the infant.

Home Care

SPONGE BATHING

Fit Baths into the Family Schedule

Give a bath at any time convenient to you, but not immediately after a feeding period because the increased handling may cause regurgitation.

Prevent Heat Loss

The temperature of the room should be 24° C, and the bathing area should be free of drafts.

Control heat loss during the bath to conserve the infant's energy. Bathing the infant quickly, exposing only a portion of the body at a time, and thorough drying are all important parts of the bathing technique.

Gather Supplies and Clothing before Starting

Clothing suitable for wearing indoors: diaper, shirt; stretch suit or nightgown optional
Unscented, mild soap
Cotton balls
Towels for drying infant and a clean washcloth
Receiving blanket
Tub for water, fill only to 3 to 4 inches of water

Bathe the Baby

Bring infant to bathing area when all supplies are ready.

***Never* leave the infant alone on bath table or in bath water, not even for a second!** If you have to leave, take the infant with you or put back into crib.

Test temperature of the water. It should feel pleasantly warm to the inner wrist (36.6° to 37.2° C).

Do not hold infant under running water—water temperature may change, and infant may be scalded or chilled rapidly.

Wash infant's hair after body to prevent heat loss from prolonged exposure to cold—scalp loses heat rapidly due to size. May wash face, neck, and ears first.

Cleanse the eyes from the inner canthus outward, using separate parts of a clean washcloth for each eye. For the first 2 to 3 days, there may be a discharge resulting from the reaction of the conjunctiva to the ointment (erythromycin) used as a prophylactic measure against infection. Any discharge should be considered abnormal and reported to the health care provider.

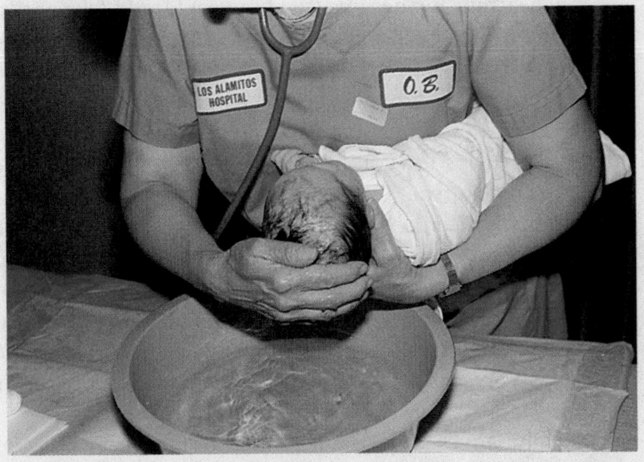

Wash hair with baby wrapped to prevent heat loss from wet scalp. (Courtesy Marjorie Pyle, RNC, Lifecircle, Costa Mesa, CA.)

Wash the scalp with water and mild soap; rinse well and dry thoroughly. Scalp desquamation, called *cradle cap,* often can be prevented by removing any scales with a fine-toothed comb or brush after washing. If condition persists, notify the health care provider.

Creases under the chin and arms and in the groin may need daily cleansing. The crease under the chin may be exposed by elevating the infant's shoulders 5 cm and letting the head drop back.

Cleanse ears and nose with twists of moistened cotton or a corner of the washcloth. Do not use cotton-tipped swabs because they may cause injury.

Undress baby and wash body and arms and legs. Pat dry gently. Baby may be tub bathed after the cord drops off and umbilicus and circumcised penis are completely healed.

Prevent Skin Trauma

The fragile skin can be injured by too vigorous cleansing.

If stool or other debris has dried and caked on the skin, soak the area to remove it. Do not attempt to rub it off, because abrasion may result. Gentleness, patting dry rather than rubbing, and use of a mild soap without perfumes or coloring are recommended. Chemicals in the coloring and perfume can cause rashes on sensitive skin.

Care of the Cord

Use a cotton swab. Dip swab in solution the health care provider has ordered and cleanse around base of the cord where it joins the skin. Notify the health care provider of any odor, discharge, or skin inflammation around the cord. The clamp is removed when the cord is dry (approximately 24 hours). The diaper should not cover the cord because a wet or soiled diaper will slow or prevent drying of the cord and foster infection. When the cord drops off after 10 to 15 days, small drops of blood may be seen when the baby cries. This will heal by itself. It is not dangerous.

Care of Hands and Feet

Wash and dry between the fingers and toes.

Use caution cutting the nails—use blunt scissors. The nails have to grow out far enough from the skin so that the skin is not cut by mistake. If the baby scratches himself or herself, may apply loosely fitted mitts (or baby socks) over each of the baby's hands. Nails should be kept short.

Cleanse Genitals

Cleanse the genitals of infants daily and after voiding or defecating. For girls, the genitals may be cleansed by separating the labia and gently washing from the pubic area to the anus. For uncircumcised boys, do not force (retract) the foreskin. Stop when resistance is felt. Wash and rinse the tip (glans) with soap and warm water and replace the foreskin. The foreskin must be returned to its original position to prevent constriction and swelling. In most newborns, the inner layer of the foreskin adheres to the glans and the foreskin cannot be retracted. By age 3 years in 90% of boys, the foreskin can be retracted easily without causing pain or trauma. For others, the foreskin is not retractable until adolescence. As soon as the foreskin is partly retractable and the child is old enough, he can be taught self-care. Once healed, the circumcised penis does not require any special care other than cleansing with diaper changes.

SKILL—INFANT BATHING

Home Care

NEWBORN HOME CARE FOLLOWING EARLY DISCHARGE*

Wet diapers: 6 to 10 per day
Breastfeeding: successful latch-on and feeding every 1.5 to 3 hours daily
Formula-feeding: successfully, voiding as noted above, taking approximately 3 to 4 ounces every 3 to 4 hours daily
Circumcision: wash with warm water only; yellow exudate forming, nonbleeding, Plastibell intact 48 hours
Stools: at least one every 48 hours (bottle-feeding) or two to three per day (breastfeeding)
Color: pink to ruddy when crying; pink centrally when at rest or asleep
Activity: has four or five wakeful periods per day and alerts to environmental sounds and voices
Jaundice: physiologic jaundice (not appearing in first 24 hours), feeding, voiding, and stooling as noted above or practitioner notification for suspicion of pathologic jaundice (appears within 24 hours of birth, ABO/Rh problem suspected; hemolysis); decreased activity; poor feeding; dark orange skin color persisting beyond fifth day in light-skinned newborn
Cord: kept above diaper line; drying; periumbilical area skin pink (erythematous circle at umbilical site may be sign of omphalitis)
Vital signs: heart rate 120 to 140 beats/min at rest; respiratory rate 30 to 55 breaths/min at rest without evidence of retractions, grunting, or nasal flaring; temperature 36.5° to 37.2° C axillary
Position of sleep: back

From Hockenberry MJ et al: *Wong's nursing care of infants and children*, ed 7, St Louis, 2003, Mosby.
*Any deviation from the above or suspicion of poor newborn adaptation should be reported to the practitioner at once.

Infant Follow-up Care

With shorter hospital stays, the focus and site of infant care are changing. Home care may be provided either by a nurse as part of the routine follow-up care of patients, or through a visiting nurse or community health nurse referral service. For infants discharged early, newborn home care is essential (Home Care box) (see also Chapter 3).

Parents should plan for their infant's follow-up health care at the following ages: within 3 days if early discharge to check for status of jaundice, feeding, and elimination (see also Physiologic Jaundice, pp. 737 to 740 for follow-up guidelines); 2 to 4 weeks of age; then every 2 months until 6 to 7 months of age; then every 3 months until 18 months; at 2 years; at 3 years; at preschool; and every 2 years thereafter.

Immunizations

The schedule for immunizations should be reviewed with the parents. Hepatitis B vaccine is currently administered to newborns before hospital discharge (depending on maternal hepatitis B status) with parental permission. See Chapter 36 for a complete discussion of infant immunizations.

Evaluation

The nurse can be reasonably assured that care was effective to the extent that the expected outcomes for care have been achieved.

Key Points

- Assessment of the newborn requires data from the prenatal, intrapartal, and postnatal periods.
- Knowledge of biologic and behavioral characteristics is essential for guiding assessment and interpreting data.
- Providing a protective environment is a key responsibility of the nurse, and includes such measures as careful identification procedures, protection from abduction, support of physiologic functions, and measures to prevent infection.
- Maintenance of adequate ventilation includes ensuring an open airway and body temperature within the normal range.
- Parent education is a major responsibility of the nurse and includes involvement of parents in all phases of the nursing process.
- The newborn has social as well as physical needs.
- Circumcision is an elective surgical procedure.
- Pain in neonates must be assessed and managed effectively.
- Parents appreciate anticipatory guidance in the care of the newborn.

Answer Guidelines to Critical Thinking Exercises

Jaundice

1. Yes, there are sufficient data to arrive at some possible conclusions.
2. (a) See text, pages 736–740. (b) Levels are within acceptable limits based on available data; based on available data, ABO incompatibility–related hemolysis is not evident but may warrant further investigation. (c) Oral intake is adequate; urine and stool output is appropriate. (d) The assessment of behavior and reflexes indicates no particular concerns; the infant appears to be a healthy newborn.
3. No immediate intervention to reduce bilirubin is warranted at this time, although the treatment is a medical decision. Nursing care should focus on alleviating the parents' concerns regarding the condition of the infant, who appears to be healthy, and address their concerns about the misinformation concerning the potential for brain damage (which is not a problem at this point). Encourage the mother to continue breastfeeding on demand and observe the infant's activity levels, intake, and urine and stool output. Emphasize that jaundice and hyperbilirubinemia are transient conditions of the newborn. At this point a follow-up appointment should be scheduled with the primary practitioner in 24 hours to monitor the bilirubin level, address the parents' concerns, and monitor the infant's weight.
4. Yes—the infant's laboratory data and physical assessment data support these conclusions. Additionally, knowledge

about physiologic hyperbilirubinemia of the newborn supports these conclusions. Phototherapy does not seem warranted at this time based on the available data.

5. One might question the need to interrupt breastfeeding, however, this does not seem necessary at this point. The available data do not point to a pathologic process; however, some may elect to obtain further laboratory data (complete blood count, reticulocyte count).

SIDS and Infant Sleep Position

1. Yes, there is ample evidence that the supine position for sleep reduces the incidence of SIDS. The nurses should cite the evidence and explain that in preterm infants, use of the prone position can assist breathing in the early phases of recovery from respiratory distress. However, as the infant matures, he should be placed on his back to sleep.
2. (a) Role modeling by nurses is a powerful teaching method. Stastny and colleagues (2004) found that only 30% of nursery staff placed babies on their backs to sleep and cited fear of aspiration as the reason. Continued staff education is necessary to promote the use of the supine position for sleep. (b) In the newborn nursery, nurses may place an infant on its side to promote drainage of secretions, although there is no evidence that this is effective. In the neonatal intensive care unit (NICU), infants in respiratory distress may breathe easier in the prone position. As the distress lessens and the infant matures, the infant should be placed on its back for sleep. (c) Parents should be counseled to place infants on their backs for sleep. During waking hours, while the parent is supervising, the infant can be placed on his side or abdomen. (d) Not all nurses read research reports and use research evidence in their practice. Thus they do not place infants on their back to sleep and do not instruct parents in sleep positioning. Continuing education programs for nurses working in nurseries should address the latest findings related to the prevention of SIDS by use of positioning infants on their back to sleep.
3. The nurse needs to reinforce the importance of placing the infant on his back to sleep and discuss with the parents the acceptability of placing the infant on the side or abdomen while the infant is awake. The nurse can also advocate for continuing education programs for the nurses to update their clinical knowledge. Signs could be posted in the nursery to remind nurses of the correct positioning.
4. There is ample evidence of the efficacy of the supine sleep position in prevention of SIDS. There is also documentation that many nurses do not follow these recommendations. Stastny and colleagues (2004) found that Latina and Pacific Islander mothers were less likely than Caucasian mothers to be instructed in the supine sleep position.
5. Nursery nurses may have had experience with babies choking on mucus and used the prone or side-lying position to promote drainage of mucus. Based on that experience, they may fear that the supine position will promote aspiration. They may rely on experience rather than research evidence in their care of infants. Continuing education programs should address utilization of research findings. Nurse managers can implement programs of reward for those nurses who base their practice on evidence.

Reference for Answer Guidelines

Stastny P et al: Infant sleep positioning by nursery staff and mothers in newborn hospital nurseries, *Nurs Res* 53(2):122-129, 2004.

Resources

Academy of Neonatal Nursing
2270 Northpoint Parkway
Santa Rosa, CA 95407-7398
707-568-2168
707-569-0786 (fax)
www.academyonline.org

American Academy of Pediatrics
141 Northwest Point Blvd.
Elk Grove, IL 60007-1098
847-434-4000
847-434-8000 (fax)
www.aap.org

Back to Sleep
PO Box 29111
Washington, DC 20040
800-505-CRIB

First Candle/SIDS Alliance
1314 Bedford Ave., Suite 210
Baltimore, MD
1-800-221-7437
www.firstcandle.org

National Association of Neonatal Nurses (NANN)
4700 W. Lake Avenue
Glenview, IL 60025-1485
847-375-3660 or 800-451-3795
U.S./Canada fax: 888-477-6266
International fax: 732-380-3640
info@nann.org
www.nann.org/

National Healthy Mothers, Healthy Babies Coalition
121 North Washington St., Suite 300
Alexandria, VA 22314
703-836-6110
www.hmhb.org

National Institute of Child Health and Human Development (NICHD)
National Institutes of Health
9000 Rockville Pike
Bldg. 31, Room 2A32
Bethesda, MD 20892
301-496-4000
www.nih.gov

Neonatal Network
2270 Northpoint Parkway
Santa Rosa, CA 95407-7398
707-569-1415
707-569-0786 (fax)
www.neonatalnetwork.com

National Newborn Screening and Genetics Research Center
www.genes-r-us.uthscsa.edu

References

Alexander GR et al: A United States national reference for fetal growth, *Obstet Gynecol* 87(2):163-168, 1996.

American Academy of Pediatrics: Commentary: neonatal jaundice and kernicterus, *Pediatrics* 108(3):763-765, 2001.

American Academy of Pediatrics, Committee on Fetus and Newborn, Committee on Drugs, Section on Anesthesiology, Section on Surgery, Canadian Pediatric Society, Fetus and Newborn Committee: Prevention and management of pain and stress in the neonate, *Pediatrics* 105(2):454-460, 2000.

American Academy of Pediatrics, Committee on Infectious Diseases: Red Book: 2003 report of the Committee on Infectious Diseases, ed 26, Elk Grove Village, IL., 2003, The Academy.

American Academy of Pediatrics, Subcommittee on Hyperbilirubinemia: Clinical practice guideline: management of hyperbilirubinemia in the newborn infant 35 or more weeks of gestation, *Pediatrics* 114(1):297-316, 2004.

American Academy of Pediatrics Task Force on Circumcision: Circumcision policy statement, *Pediatrics* 103(3):686-693, 1999.

American Academy of Pediatrics, Task Force on Infant Sleep Position and Sudden Infant Death Syndrome: Changing concepts of sudden infant death syndrome: implications for infant sleeping environment and sleep position, *Pediatrics* 105(3):650-656, 2000.

American Academy of Pediatrics and American College of Obstetricians and Gynecologists: *Guidelines for perinatal care,* ed 5, Elk Grove Village, IL, 2002, The Academy.

Anand K, Grunau R, Oberlander T: Developmental character and long-term consequences of pain in infants and children, *Child Adolescent Psychiatr Clin North Am* 6(4):703-724, 1997.

Anand KJS, International Evidence-Based Group for Neonatal Pain: Consensus statement for the prevention and management of pain in the newborn, *Arch Pediatr Adolesc Med* 155(2):173-180, 2001.

Arbuckle T, Wilkins R, Sherman G: Birth weight percentiles by gestational age in Canada, *Obstet Gynecol* 81(1):39-48, 1993.

Association of Women's Health, Obstetric, and Neonatal Nurses: *Evidence-based clinical practice guideline: neonatal skin care,* Washington, DC, 2001, The Association.

Ballard J, Novak K, Driver M: A simplified score for assessment of fetal maturity of newly born infants, *J Pediatr* 95(5 pt 1):769-774, 1979.

Ballard J et al: New Ballard score, expanded to include extremely premature infants, *J Pediatr* 119(3):417-423, 1991.

Battaglia FC, Lubchenco LO: A practical classification of newborn infants by weight and gestational age, *J Pediatr* 71(2):159-161, 1967.

Bhutani VK, Johnson L, Sivieri EM: Predictive ability of a predischarge hour-specific serum bilirubin for subsequent significant hyperbilirubinemia in healthy term and near-term newborns, *Pediatrics* 103(1):6-14, 1999.

Bhutani VK et al: Noninvasive measurement of total serum bilirubin in a multiracial newborn population to assess the risk of severe hyperbilirubinemia, *Pediatrics* 106(2):e16, 2000.

Bildner J, Krechel SW: Increasing staff nurse awareness of postoperative pain management in the NICU, *Neonatal Netw* 15(1):11-16, 1996.

Blackburn ST: *Maternal, fetal, and neonatal physiology: a clinical perspective,* ed 2, St Louis, 2003, WB Saunders.

Blain-Lewis N: Comparative studies of bruising and healing after heelstick, *Neonatal Intensive Care* 5(5):18-21, 1992.

Blass EM, Watt LB: Suckling- and sucrose-induced analgesia in human newborns, *Pain* 83(3):611-623, 1999.

Briscoe L, Clark S, Yoxall CW: Can transcutaneous bilirubinometry reduce the need for blood tests in jaundiced full term babies? *Arch Dis Child Fetal Neonatal Ed* 86(3):F190-F192, 2002.

Broadman LM et al: Post-circumcision analgesia: a prospective evaluation of subcutaneous ring block of the penis, *Anesthesiology* 67:339-402, 1987.

Burd RS, Tobias JD: Ketorolac for pain management after abdominal surgical procedures in infants, *South Med* 95(3):331-333, 2002.

Carbajal R et al: Analgesic effect of breast feeding in term neonates: randomized controlled trial, *BMJ* 326(7379):13, 2003.

Cornblath M et al: Controversies regarding operational definition of neonatal hypoglycemia: suggested thresholds, *Pediatrics* 105(5):1141-1145, 2000.

Cunningham FG et al (eds): *Williams obstetrics,* ed 21, New York, 2001, McGraw-Hill.

D'Avanzo C, Geissler E: *Pocket guide to cultural health assessment,* ed 3, St Louis, 2003, Mosby.

Dore S et al: Alcohol versus natural drying for newborn cord care, *J Obstet Gynecol Neonatal Nurs* 27(6):621-627, 1998.

Engle WD et al: Assessment of a transcutaneous device in the evaluation of neonatal hyperbilirubinemia in a primarily Hispanic population, *Pediatrics* 110(1 pt 1):61-67, 2002.

Fitzgerald M, Millard C, McIntosh N: Cutaneous hypersensitivity following peripheral tissue damage in newborn infants and its reversal with topical anaesthesia, *Pain* 3(1):31-36, 1989.

Franck LS: Identification, management, and prevention of pain in the neonate. In Kenner C, Lott JW, Flandermeyer A (eds): *Comprehensive neonatal nursing: a physiologic perspective,* ed 2, Philadelphia, 1998, WB Saunders.

Franck LS, Gregory G: Clinical evaluation and treatment of infant pain in the neonatal intensive care unit. In Schechter M, Berde C, Yaster M (eds): *Pain in infants, children and adolescents,* Baltimore, 1993, Williams & Wilkins.

Franck LS, Scurr K, Couture S: Parent views of infant pain and pain management in the neonatal intensive care unit, *Newborn Infant Nurs Rev* 1(2):106-113, 2001.

Furdon S et al: Outcome measures after standardized pain management strategies in postoperative patients in the NICU, *J Perinat Neonat Nurs* 12(1):58-69, 1998.

Gartner LM: Neonatal jaundice, *Pediatr Rev* 15(11):422-432, 1994.

Gartner LM, Herschel M: Part 2: the management of breastfeeding: jaundice and breastfeeding, *Pediatr Clin North Am* 48(2):389-400, 2001.

Geyer J et al: An evidence-based multidisciplinary protocol for neonatal circumcision pain management, *J Obstet Gynecol Neonatal Nurs* 31(4):403-410, 2002.

Gibbins S et al: Efficacy and safety of sucrose for procedural pain relief in preterm and term neonates, *Nurs Res* 51(6):375-382, 2002.

Golombek SG, Brill PE, Salice AL: Randomized trial of alcohol versus triple dye for umbilical cord care, *Clin Pediatr* 41(6):419-423, 2002.

Gradin M et al: Pain reduction at venipuncture in newborns: oral glucose compared with local anesthetic cream, *Pediatrics* 110(6):1053-1057, 2002.

Gray L, Watt L, Blass EM: Skin-to-skin contact is analgesic in healthy newborns, *Pediatrics* 105(1):110-111, 2000. Internet document available at www.pediatrics.org/cgi/content/full/105/1/e14 (accessed August 22, 2004).

Hadjistavropoulos H et al: Judging pain in infants: behavioural, contextual, and developmental determinants, *Pain* 7(3):319-324, 1997.

Hagedorn ME, Gardner SL, Abman SH: Common systemic diseases of the neonate: respiratory diseases. In Merenstein GB, Gardner SL (eds): *Handbook of neonatal intensive care,* ed 5, St Louis, 2002, Mosby.

Haouari N et al: The analgesic effect of sucrose in full-term infants: a randomised controlled trial, *BMJ* 310(6993):1498-1500, 1995.

Hjelle JJ, Grauer GF: Acetaminophen-induced toxicosis in dogs and cats, *J Am Vet Med Assoc* 188(7):742-749, 1986.

Hockenberry MJ et al: *Wong's nursing care of infants and children,* ed 7, St Louis, 2003, Mosby.

Howard CR, Howard FM, Weitzman ML: Acetaminophen analgesia in neonatal circumcision: the effect on pain, *Pediatrics* 93(4):641-646, 1994.

Hummel P, Puchalski M: Assessment and management of pain in infancy, *Newborn Infant Nurs Rev* 1(2):114-122, 2001.

Janssen PA et al: To dye or not to dye: a randomized, clinical trial of a triple dye/alcohol regime versus dry cord care, *Pediatrics* 111(1):15-20, 2003.

Joint Commission on Accreditation of Healthcare Organizations: Sentinel event alert: kernicterus threatens healthy newborns, Issue 18, April 2001. Internet document available at http://www.jcaho.org/about+

us/news+letters/sentinel+event+alert/sea18.htm (accessed February 21, 2005).

Kramer MS et al: A new and improved population-based Canadian reference for birth weight for gestational age, *Pediatrics* 108(2):e35, 462, 2001.

Krebs T: Cord care: is it necessary? *Mother Baby J* 3(2):5-12, 18-20, 1998.

Krechel SW, Bildner J: CRIES: a new neonatal postoperative pain measurement score: initial testing of validity and reliability, *Pediatr Anaesth* 5(1):53-61, 1995.

Lander J et al: Comparison of ring block, dorsal penile nerve block, and topical anesthesia for neonatal circumcision, *JAMA* 278:2157-2162, 1997.

Lashley FR: Newborn screening: new opportunities and new challenges, *Newborn Infant Nurs Rev* 2(4):228-242, 2002.

Leitch D: Mother-infant interaction: achieving synchrony, *Nurs Res* 48(1):55-58, 1999.

Lynam L: Research utilization: nonpharmacological management of pain in neonates, *Neonatal Netw* 14(5):59-62, 1995.

Maisels MJ: Jaundice. In Avery GB, Fletcher MA, MacDonald MG (eds): *Neonatology: pathophysiology and management of the newborn*, ed 5, Philadelphia, 1999, JB Lippincott.

Meehan R: Heelsticks in neonates for capillary blood sampling, *Neonatal Netw* 17(1):17-24, 1998.

Mintz MR, Grillo R: Dorsal penile nerve block for circumcision, *Clin Pediatr* 28:590-591, 1989.

Mohan C et al: Comparison of analgesics in ameliorating the pain of circumcision, *J Perinat* 18(1):13-14, 1998.

Montgomery K: Apgar scores: examining the long-term significance, *J Perinat Educ* 9(3):5-9, 2000.

Noerr B: Sucrose for neonatal procedural pain, *Neonatal Netw* 20(7):63-67, 2001.

Paes B et al: A comparative study of heel-stick devices for infant blood collection, *Am J Dis Child* 147(3):346-348, 1993.

Porter ML, Dennis BL: Hyperbilirubinemia in the term newborn, *Am Fam Physician* 65(4):599-606, 613-614, 2002.

Prescott LF: *Paracetamol (acetaminophen): a critical bibliographic review*, Bristol, 1996, Taylor & Francis.

Razmus IS, Dalton ME, Wilson D: Pain management for newborn circumcision, *Pediatr Nurs* 30(5):414-417, 427, 2004.

Serour F, Mandelberg A, Mori J: Slow injection of local anesthetic will decrease pain during dorsal penile nerve block, *Acta Anaesthesiol Scand* 42(8):926-928, 1998.

Shah V, Ohlsson A: Venepuncture versus heel lance for blood sampling in term neonates, *Cochrane Database Syst Rev* 2001(2):CD001452, 2001.

Spencer DM et al: Dorsal penile nerve block in neonatal circumcision: chloroprocaine versus lidocaine, *Am J Perinatol* 9(3):214-218, 1992.

Stang H et al: Beyond dorsal penile nerve block: a more humane circumcision, *Pediatrics* 100(2):E3, 1997. (Internet document available at www.pediatrics.org/cgi/content/full/100/2/e3).

Stastny P et al: Infant sleep positioning by nursery staff and mothers in newborn hospital nurseries, *Nurs Res* 53(2):122-129, 2004.

Steffensrud S: Hyperbilirubinemia in term and near-term infants: kernicterus on the rise? *Newborn Infant Nurs Rev* 4(4):191-200, 2004.

Stevens B, Yamada J, Ohlsson A: Sucrose for analgesia in newborn infants undergoing procedures, *Cochrane Database Syst Rev* 2001(4):CD001069, 2001.

Stevens B et al: Management of pain from heel lance with lidocaine-prilocaine (EMLA) cream: is it safe and efficacious in preterm infants? *J Dev Behav Pediatr* 20(4):216-221, 1999.

Stevens B et al: The efficacy of sucrose for relieving procedural pain in neonates—a systematic review and meta-analysis, *Acta Paediatr* 86(8):837-842, 1997.

Stevens DK et al: Prediction of hyperbilirubinemia in near-term and term infants, *J Perinatol* 21(suppl 1):S63-S72, 2001.

Taddio A: Pain management for neonatal circumcision, *Paediatr Drugs* 3(2):101-111, 2001.

Taddio A et al: A systematic review of lidocaine-prilocaine cream (EMLA) in the treatment of acute pain in neonates, *Pediatrics* 101(2):e1, 1998. Internet document available at www.pediatrics.org/cgi/content/full/101/2/e1 (accessed August 22, 2004).

Taddio A et al: Conditioning and hyperalgesia in newborns exposed to repeated heel lances, *JAMA* 288(7):857-861, 2002.

Taddio A et al: Efficacy and safety of lidocaine-prilocaine cream (EMLA) for pain during circumcision, *N Engl J Med* 336(17):1197-1201, 1997.

Taddio A, Ohlsson K, Ohlsson A: Lidocaine-prilocaine cream for analgesia during circumcision in newborn boys, *Cochrane Syst Rev* 2003(1):CD000496, 2003.

Thomas P et al: A new look at intrauterine growth and the impact of race, altitude, and gender, *Pediatrics* 106(2):e21, 2000.

Van Ryzin L: The circumcision debate, *Am J Nurs* 100(7):24A-24B, 2000.

Volpe JJ: *Neurology of the newborn*, ed 4, Philadelphia, 2001, WB Saunders.

Williamson ML: Circumcision anesthesia: a study of nursing implications for dorsal penile nerve block, *Pediatr Nurs* 23(1):59-63, 1997.

Zupan J, Garner P: Topical umbilical cord care at birth, *Cochrane Database Syst Rev* 2000(2):CD001057, 2000.

Unit 6

26 Newborn Nutrition and Feeding

LEARNING OBJECTIVES

On completion of this chapter the reader will be able to:

- Describe current recommendations for feeding infants.
- Discuss benefits of breastfeeding for infants, mothers, families, and society.
- Describe nutritional needs of infants.
- List newborn feeding readiness cues.
- Describe the anatomy and physiology of breastfeeding.
- Identify nursing interventions to facilitate and promote successful breastfeeding.
- List signs of adequate intake in the breastfed infant.
- Identify common problems associated with breastfeeding and nursing interventions to help resolve them.
- Discuss patient teaching for the family using formula-feeding.

ELECTRONIC RESOURCES

Additional information related to the content in Chapter 26 can be found on

the companion website at evolve
http://evolve.elsevier.com/Wong/maternal/
- NCLEX Review Questions
- Case Study–Breastfeeding
- WebLinks

or the interactive student CD-ROM
Activities for Chapter 26 include the following:
- NCLEX Review Questions
- Case Study–Breastfeeding
- Critical Thinking Exercise–Formula Preparation
- Nursing Care Plan–Insufficient Intake of Nutrients
- Skill–Infant Feeding

Good nutrition in infancy fosters optimal growth and development. Infant feeding is more than the provision of nutrition; it represents an opportunity for social and psychologic interactions between parent and infant. It can also establish a basis for lasting development of good eating habits and influence lifelong health habits. The health supervision of infants requires knowledge of their nutritional needs. This chapter focuses on meeting nutritional needs for normal growth and development from birth to 6 months of age, with emphasis on the neonatal period when feeding practices and patterns are being established. Both breastfeeding and formula-feeding are addressed.

RECOMMENDED INFANT NUTRITION

The American Academy of Pediatrics, Section on Breastfeeding (2005), recommends that infants be breastfed exclusively for the first 6 months of life and that breastfeeding continue for at least 12 months (see Evidence-Based Practice box in Chapter 25). If infants are weaned before 12 months, they should receive iron-fortified infant formula. *Healthy People 2010* goals include that 75% of women will breastfeed at birth, 50% will breastfeed for 6 months, and 25% will continue to breastfeed to 1 year of age (Department of Health and Human Services, 2000). Recent figures show that breastfeeding reached an all-time record high of 69.5%, and 32.5% of the women surveyed were still breastfeeding at 6 months (Ryan, Wenjun, & Acosta, 2002).

Benefits of Breastfeeding

Human milk is designed specifically for human infants and is nutritionally superior to any alternative. Breast milk is considered a living tissue because it contains almost as many live cells as blood. It is bacteriologically safe and is always fresh. The nutrients in breast milk are more easily absorbed than those in formula.

Benefits of breastfeeding for the infant include the following:

- Breast milk enhances maturation of the gastrointestinal (GI) tract and contains immune factors that contribute to a lower incidence of gastroenteritis, lymphoma, childhood obesity, Crohn's disease, and celiac disease (Barnard, 1997; Grummer-Strawn, Mei, & Centers for Disease Control and Prevention, 2004; Scariati, Grummer-Strawn, & Fein, 1997).

- Breastfed infants receive specific antibodies and cell-mediated immunologic factors that help protect against otitis media, respiratory illnesses such as respiratory syncytial virus and pneumonia, urinary tract infections, bacteremia, and bacterial meningitis (Bachrach, Schwarz, & Bachrach, 2003; Cushing, 1998; Hanson & Korotkova, 2002).
- There is a lower incidence of certain allergies among breastfed infants from families at high risk. Allergic manifestations occur at a greater rate and are more severe in formula-fed infants (Halken & Host, 1996).
- Breastfed infants are less likely to die from sudden infant death syndrome (SIDS) (Ford et al, 1993).
- Breast milk may have a protective effect against childhood lymphoma and insulin-dependent diabetes (Davis, 1998; Gerstein, 1994).
- Breast milk may enhance cognitive development (Anderson, Johnstone, & Remley, 1999; Horwood & Fergusson, 1998).
- Breastfeeding appears to have an analgesic effect for infants undergoing painful procedures such as venipuncture (Carbajal et al, 2003; Gray et al, 2002).

Maternal benefits include the following:

- Women who have breastfed have a decreased risk of ovarian, uterine, and breast cancer (Enger et al, 1998; Rosenblatt & Thomas, 1995).
- Breastfeeding promotes uterine involution and is associated with a decreased risk of postpartum hemorrhage (Lawrence & Lawrence, 2005).
- Mothers who are breastfeeding tend to return to their prepregnancy weight more quickly (Dewey, Heinig, & Nommsen, 1993).
- Breastfeeding may provide some protection against the development of osteoporosis (Eisman, 1998).
- Breastfeeding provides a unique bonding experience and increases maternal role attainment (Lawrence & Lawrence, 2005).

Benefits to families and society include the following:

- Breastfeeding is convenient; there are no bottles or other equipment to purchase, clean, or dispose of.
- Breastfed babies are portable; when traveling, there are fewer supplies to take along.
- Breastfeeding saves money. The cost of formula far exceeds the cost of extra food for the lactating mother. Breastfeeding families who are eligible for the Special Supplemental Nutrition Program for Women, Infants, and Children (WIC) represent a cost savings to the government. Because breastfed babies have a lower incidence of illness and infection, health care costs are lower for families and federal, state, and local governments. Less time is lost from work because parents do not have to stay home with sick infants, which is a benefit to employers.

Contraindications to Breastfeeding

Contraindications to breastfeeding include the following (American Academy of Pediatrics, Section on Breastfeeding, 2005; Lawrence & Lawrence, 2001):

- Maternal cancer therapy or diagnostic and therapeutic radioactive isotopes
- Active tuberculosis not under treatment in mother
- Human immunodeficiency virus (HIV) infection in mother
- Maternal herpes simplex lesion on a breast
- Galactosemia in infant
- Cytomegalovirus (CMV)—primary risk is to premature infants receiving CMV-infected donor milk, not to infected mother's infant, who already has CMV
- Maternal substance abuse (e.g., cocaine, methamphetamines, marijuana)
- Maternal human T-cell leukemia virus type 1

Mastitis is usually not a contraindication if the discomfort is tolerable. The Centers for Disease Control and Prevention currently does not consider maternal hepatitis C to be a contraindication for breastfeeding (Lawrence & Lawrence, 2001).

Choosing an Infant Feeding Method

Women who elect to breastfeed usually do so because they are aware of the benefits to the infant. Many seek the unique bonding experience between mother and infant that is characteristic of breastfeeding. The support of her partner and family is a major factor in a mother's decision to breastfeed and in her ability to do so successfully. Prenatal preparation ideally includes the father of the baby, providing information about the benefits of breastfeeding and how he can participate in infant care and nurturing.

Prenatal breastfeeding classes are an excellent vehicle to relay important information to expectant parents. Each encounter with an expectant mother is an opportunity to dispel myths, clarify misinformation, and address personal concerns. Connecting expectant mothers with women who are breastfeeding or who have successfully breastfed and are from similar backgrounds may be helpful. Peer counseling programs, such as those instituted by WIC programs, are beneficial, particularly in low socioeconomic groups where bottle-feeding is common. To provide effective support for the mother, health care professionals must be knowledgeable about the benefits of breastfeeding, the basic process of breastfeeding, breastfeeding management, and interventions for common problems (Box 26-1).

Cultural Influences on Infant Feeding

Cultural beliefs and practices are significant influences on infant feeding methods. As many as 50 of 120 cultures studied typically do not give colostrum to newborns and only begin breastfeeding after the milk has "come in." Some Filipinos, Hispanics, Vietnamese, Hmong, Koreans, and Nigerians are among these groups. When breastfeeding is delayed until the milk is in, babies are given prelacteal food. In India, infants may be fed liquids such as honey, tea, water, or sugar water before the initiation of breastfeeding (Choudhry, 1997). Other cultures begin breastfeeding immediately and offer the breast each time the infant cries. Cultural attitudes regarding modesty and breastfeeding are important considerations. Language barriers may also prevent successful breastfeeding and counseling in some situations. Even among Hispanic Spanish-speaking people, terminology used in one country for the act of breastfeeding or describing the breasts may be

BOX 26-1

Guidelines for Breastfeeding Support

- During pregnancy, a breast assessment is performed that includes a breastfeeding history, a breast examination, and a medication use history.
- A prenatal plan of care is developed to prepare the woman for lactation.
- Immediately after birth, the newborn is kept with the mother when possible so that breastfeeding can be initiated when the newborn is most receptive.
- After birth:
  - Assistance with latch-on and positioning are given as needed.
  - Encouragement of frequent feedings is reinforced.
  - Discharge instructions for recognizing signs of successful breastfeeding are given.
  - Information about community resources for breastfeeding is given.
- Especially for premature and low-birth-weight infants, breastfeeding is encouraged.

Adapted from Association of Women's Health, Obstetric and Neonatal Nurses: *Standards and guidelines for professional nursing practice in the care of women and newborns,* ed 5, Washington, DC, 1998, Association of Women's Health, Obstetric and Neonatal Nurses.

offensive in another Spanish-speaking country. Sociocultural values may preclude the mother receiving adequate information regarding breastfeeding; if the family is strongly patriarchal and the father is the only English-speaking person in the family, the necessary information being taught or conveyed to the mother by the health care provider may not be correctly translated. It has been noted that persons immigrating to the United States often tend to acquire the local customs, and, although breastfeeding may have been common in their own country, they may abandon the practice in the United States, considering it "outdated" (Riordan & Gill-Hopple, 2001).

Nutrient Needs

Energy

Infants require adequate caloric intake to provide energy for growth, digestion, physical activity, and maintenance of organ metabolic function. For the first 3 months, the infant needs approximately 110 kcal/kg/day. From 3 months to 6 months, the requirement decreases to approximately 100 kcal/kg/day. This decreases slightly to 95 kcal/kg/day from 6 to 9 months, and increases to 100 kcal/kg/day from 9 months to 1 year.

Human milk provides approximately 67 kcal/100 ml or 20 kcal/oz; the greatest amount of energy is provided by the fat content of breast milk. Infant formulas are made to simulate the caloric content of human milk; standard formulas contain 20 kcal/oz.

Carbohydrate

Because newborns have only small hepatic glycogen stores, carbohydrates should provide at least 40% to 45% of the total calories in the diet. Moreover, newborns may have limited ability for gluconeogenesis (formation of glucose from amino acids and other substrates) and ketogenesis (formation of ketone bodies from fat), which are mechanisms that provide alternative energy sources.

As the primary carbohydrate in human milk, lactose is the most abundant carbohydrate in the diet of infants up to 6 months of age. Lactose provides calories in an easily available form; its slow breakdown and absorption probably also increase calcium absorption. Corn syrup solids or glucose polymers are added to infant formulas to supplement the lactose in cow's milk and provide sufficient carbohydrates.

Fat

For infants to acquire adequate calories from the limited amount of human milk or formula they are able to consume, at least 15% of the calories provided must come from fat (triglycerides). The fat must be easily digestible. Fat in human milk is easier to digest and absorb than that in cow's milk because of the arrangement of the fatty acids on the glycerol molecule and because of the presence of the enzyme lipase.

Modified cow's milk is used to make most infant formulas, but the milk fat is removed and replaced by another fat source, such as corn oil, that can be easily digested and absorbed by the infant. If whole milk or evaporated milk without added carbohydrate is fed to infants, the resulting fecal loss of fat (and therefore loss of energy) may be excessive because the milk moves through the infant's intestines too quickly for adequate absorption to take place. This can lead to poor weight gain. There is evidence that whole milk may also increase the infant's chances for developing allergies from cow milk protein exposure.

In addition to its energy contributions, fat also furnishes essential fatty acids (EFAs), which are required for growth and tissue maintenance. EFAs are components of cell membranes and precursors of some hormones. Inadequate intake of EFAs results in eczema and growth failure. The lack of EFAs in skim and low-fat milk is another reason infants should not be fed these products.

Protein

The protein requirement per unit of body weight is greater in the newborn than at any other time of life. The protein content of human milk, which is lower than that of unmodified cow's milk, is ideal for the newborn. Human milk contains far more lactalbumin in relation to casein than does cow's milk, and lactalbumin is more easily digested than casein. In addition, the amino acid composition of human milk is suited to the newborn's metabolic capabilities. For example, phenylalanine and methionine levels are low, and cystine and taurine levels are high. The protein in some commercial formulas is modified to increase the amount of lactalbumin (or whey protein) and to decrease the relative proportion of casein to more closely approximate human milk. The concentration of protein in infant formula is 1.45 to 1.6 g/dl (American Academy of Pediatrics, 2004).

Fluids

The fluid requirement for healthy term infants is about 100 to 140 ml of water per kilogram of body weight per 24 hours (Kliegman, 2002). Neither breastfed nor formula-fed infants need to be fed water, even those living in very hot climates. Breast milk contains 87% water, which easily meets fluid requirements. Feeding water to infants may cause water toxicity with resulting hyponatremia and seizures. Infants have little room for fluctuation in fluid balance and should be monitored closely for fluid intake and water loss if certain illness factors exist. Infants lose water through excretion of urine and through insensible losses such as respiration. Most healthy infants take in an adequate amount of fluid daily in either breast milk or commercial formula. Conditions that may lead to a decrease in oral intake and subsequent fluid deficit include gastroenteritis (vomiting and diarrhea), poor intake due to illness (congestive heart failure), or conditions affecting the mechanical process of eating (e.g., thrush, viral stomatitis, ankyloglossia [tight lingual frenulum], or poor latch-on early in breastfeeding). Juices are not necessary for proper nutrient intake except perhaps in late infancy when table foods are being consumed.

Vitamins

Human milk contains all the vitamins required for infant nutrition, with individual variations based on maternal diet and genetic differences. Vitamins are added to cow's milk formulas to approximate the levels in breast milk. Cow's milk contains adequate amounts of vitamin A and vitamin B complex; vitamin C (ascorbic acid) and vitamin E must be added.

Vitamin D is also added to commercial infant formulas. Because human milk is somewhat deficient in vitamin D (depending on maternal intake and metabolism), and to prevent vitamin D deficiency rickets, the American Academy of Pediatrics, Section on Breastfeeding (2005), recommends that infants who are exclusively breastfed, who are breastfed and consuming less than 500 ml of vitamin D–fortified formula or milk per day, or who are ingesting less than 500 ml of vitamin D–fortified formula or milk per day be orally supplemented with 200 international units of vitamin D per day.

Vitamin K, required for blood coagulation, is produced by intestinal bacteria. However, the gut is sterile at birth, and a few days are needed for intestinal flora to become established and produce vitamin K. To prevent hemorrhagic problems in the newborn, an injection of vitamin K is routinely given at birth. Oral vitamin K may not provide adequate stores necessary to prevent hemorrhage and is not recommended unless doses are repeatedly given during the first 4 months of life (American Academy of Pediatrics, Section on Breastfeeding, 2005).

Minerals

The mineral content of commercial infant formula is designed to reflect that of breast milk. Whole cow's milk is much higher in mineral content than human milk, which makes it unsuitable for infants in the first year of life. Minerals are typically highest in human milk during the first few days after birth and decrease slightly throughout lactation.

The ratio of calcium to phosphorus in human milk is 2:1, a proportion optimal for bone mineralization. Although cow's milk is high in calcium, the calcium-to-phosphorus ratio is low, resulting in decreased absorption. Consequently, young infants fed whole cow's milk are at risk for hypocalcemia, tetany, and seizures. The calcium-to-phosphorus ratio in commercial infant formulas is between that of human and cow's milk.

Milk of all types is low in iron; however, iron from human milk is better absorbed than that from cow's milk, iron-fortified formula, or infant cereals. Breastfed infants benefit from the high lactose and vitamin C levels in human milk, which facilitate iron absorption. The infant who is totally breastfed normally maintains adequate hemoglobin levels for the first 6 months of life. After that time, iron-fortified cereals and other iron-rich foods are added to the diet. Infants weaned from the breast before 6 months of age and all formula-fed infants should receive an iron-fortified commercial infant formula until 12 months of age. Infants should not be given low-iron formula (American Academy of Pediatrics, 2004).

The fluoride levels in human milk and in commercial formulas are low. This mineral, which is important in the prevention of dental caries, may cause spotting of the permanent teeth (fluorosis) in excess amounts. Fluoride supplementation should be considered for any child over age 6 months whose drinking water is deficient in fluoride. Supplementation based on a fluoride concentration in the water supply of less than 0.3 parts per million is 0.25 mg for a child age 6 months to 3 years (American Academy of Pediatrics, Section on Pediatric Dentistry, 2003).

OVERVIEW OF LACTATION

Milk Production

Each female breast is composed of 15 to 20 segments (lobes) embedded in fat and connective tissue and well supplied with blood vessels, lymphatic tissue, and nerves (Fig. 26-1). Within each lobe are alveoli (the milk-producing cells) surrounded by myoepithelial cells, which contract to send the

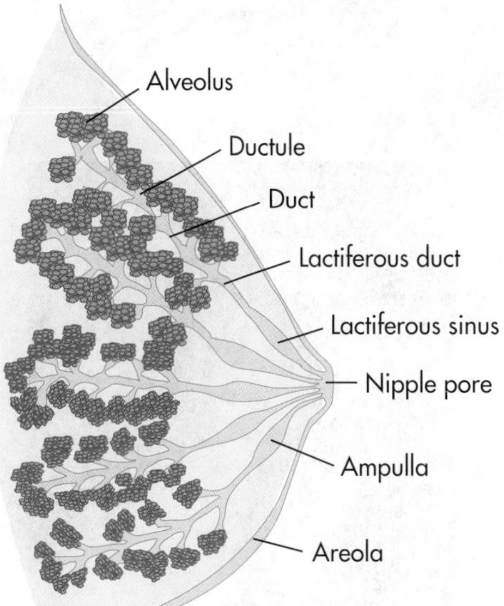

Fig. 26-1 Detailed structural features of human mammary gland.

milk forward into the ductules. Each ductule enlarges into lactiferous ducts and the sinuses, where milk collects just behind the nipple. Each nipple has 15 to 20 pores through which milk is transferred to the suckling infant.

Although nearly every woman can lactate, some mothers have insufficient glandular development to exclusively breastfeed their infants. Typically these women experienced few breast changes during either puberty or early pregnancy. In some cases, women may still be able to breastfeed and offer supplemental nutrition to support optimal infant growth. There are devices available to allow mothers to offer supplements while the baby is at the breast (Fig. 26-2).

After the mother gives birth, there is a precipitous fall in her estrogen and progesterone levels, which triggers release of prolactin from the anterior pituitary. During pregnancy, prolactin prepares the breasts to secrete milk and, during lactation, to synthesize and secrete milk. Prolactin levels are highest during the first 10 days after birth; they gradually decline over time, but remain above baseline levels for the duration of lactation. Prolactin is produced in response to infant suckling and emptying of the breasts (lactating breasts are never completely empty; milk is constantly being produced by the alveoli as the infant feeds) (Fig. 26-3, *A*). Milk production is a supply-meets-demand system; that is, as milk is removed from the breast, more is produced. Incomplete emptying of the breasts with feedings can lead to a decrease in milk production.

Oxytocin is another hormone essential to lactation. As the nipple is stimulated by the suckling infant, the posterior pituitary is prompted by the hypothalamus to produce oxytocin. This hormone is responsible for the milk ejection reflex (MER), or let-down reflex (Fig. 26-3, *B*). The myoepithelial cells surrounding the alveoli respond to oxytocin by contracting and sending the milk forward through the ducts to the nipple. Many "let-downs" can occur with each feeding session. The MER can be triggered by thoughts, sights, sounds, or odors that the mother associates with her baby (or other babies), such as hearing the baby cry. Many women report a tingling "pins and needles" sensation in the breasts

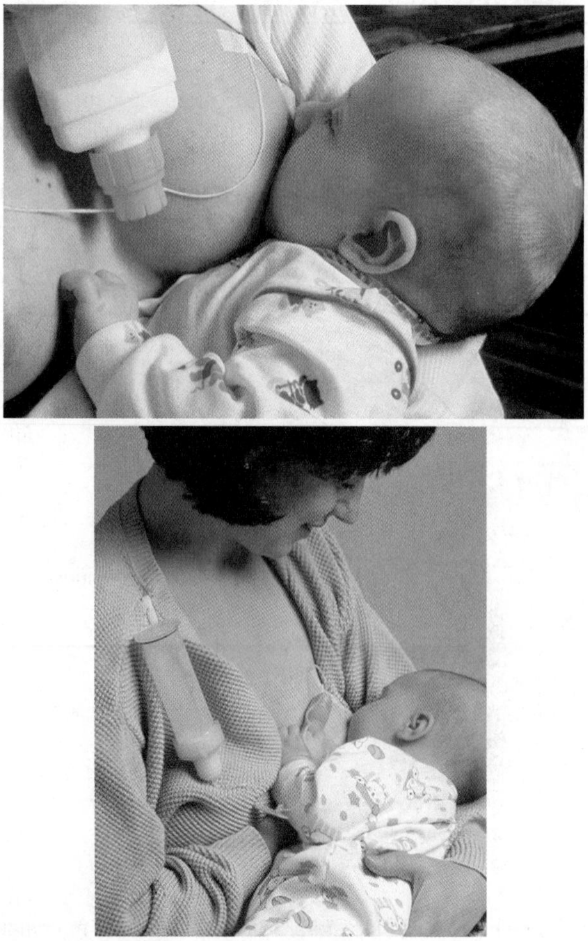

Fig. 26-2 Supplemental nursing system. (Courtesy Medela, Inc., McHenry, IL.)

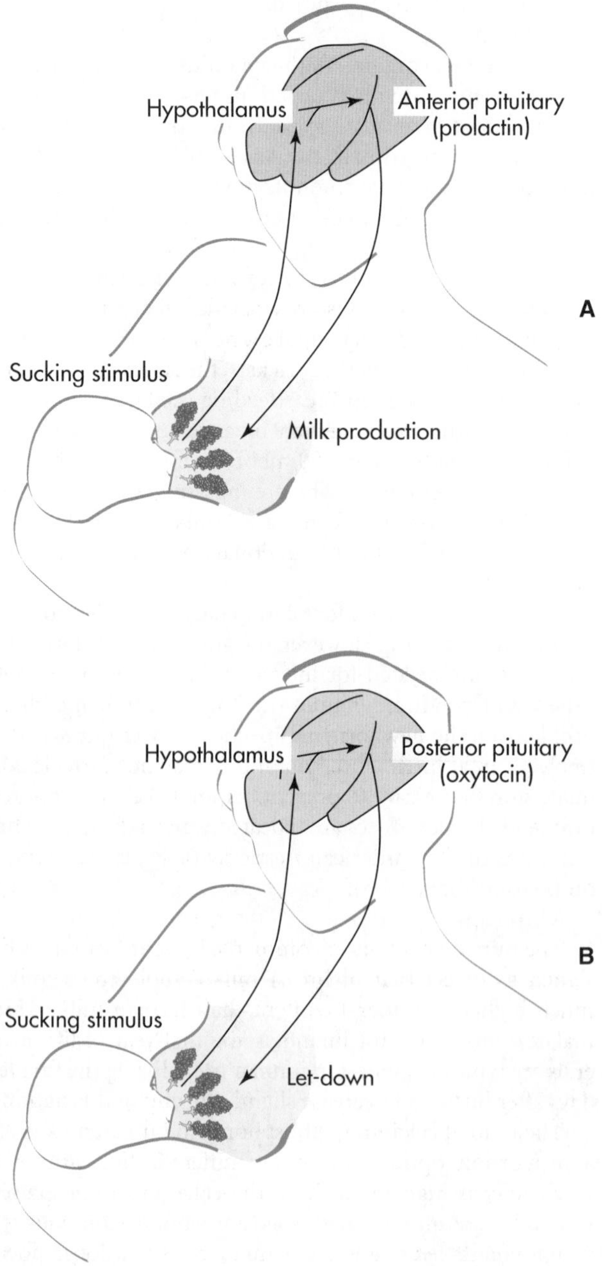

Fig. 26-3 Maternal breastfeeding reflexes. **A,** Milk production. **B,** Let-down.

as let-down occurs, although some mothers can detect milk ejection only by observing the sucking and swallowing of the infant. Let-down may also occur during sexual activity, because oxytocin is released during orgasm.

Oxytocin is the same hormone that stimulates uterine contractions during labor. Oxytocin contracts the mother's uterus after birth to control postpartum bleeding and to promote uterine involution. Thus mothers who breastfeed are at decreased risk for postpartum hemorrhage. The uterine contractions that occur with breastfeeding can be painful during and after the feeding, particularly in multiparas, for 3 to 5 days after giving birth.

Prolactin and oxytocin have been referred to as the "mothering hormones" because they are known to affect the postpartum woman's emotions, as well as her physical state. Many women report feeling thirsty or very relaxed during breastfeeding, probably as a result of these hormones.

The nipple erection reflex is an integral part of lactation. When the infant cries, suckles, or rubs against the breast, the nipple becomes erect. This assists in the propulsion of milk through the lactiferous sinuses to the nipple pores. Nipple size, shape, and ability to become erect vary with individuals. Some women have flat or inverted nipples that do not become erect with stimulation; however, they are usually able to learn to breastfeed successfully. It is important that these infants are not offered bottles or pacifiers until breastfeeding is well established.

Uniqueness of Human Milk

Human milk is a highly complex species-specific fluid uniquely designed to meet the needs of the human infant. It is specific to the needs of each newborn; for example, the milk of the mothers of preterm infants differs in composition from that of mothers who give birth at term.

Human milk contains antibodies that provide some protection against a broad spectrum of bacterial, viral, and protozoan infections. Secretory immunoglobulin A (IgA) is the major antibody in human milk.

Human milk composition and volumes vary according to the stage of lactation. In lactogenesis stage I, beginning in pregnancy, the breasts are preparing for milk production. Colostrum, a clear, yellowish fluid, is present in the breasts at this time. Colostrum is more concentrated than mature milk and is extremely rich in immunoglobulins. It has higher concentrations of protein and minerals, but less fat, than mature milk. The high protein level of colostrum facilitates binding of bilirubin, and the laxative action of colostrum promotes early passage of meconium. Colostrum gradually changes to mature milk; this is referred to as "the milk coming in" or lactogenesis stage II. By the third to fifth day after birth, most women have experienced this onset of copious milk secretion. Breast milk continues to change in composition for approximately 10 days, when the mature milk is established in stage III of lactogenesis (Lawrence & Lawrence, 2005).

Composition of mature milk changes during each feeding. As the infant nurses, the fat content of breast milk increases. Initially there is a release of bluish white foremilk that is part skim milk (about 60% of the volume) and part whole milk (about 35% of the volume). It provides primarily lactose, protein, and water-soluble vitamins. The hindmilk, or cream (about 5%), is usually let down 10 to 20 minutes into the feeding, although it may occur sooner. It contains the denser calories from fat necessary for optimal growth and contentment between feedings. Because of this changing composition of human milk during each feeding, it is important to breastfeed the infant long enough to supply a balanced feeding. Milk production gradually increases, so that by the time her infant is 2 weeks old, the mother produces 720 to 900 ml of milk every 24 hours. Babies experience fairly predictable growth spurts (i.e., at about 10 days, 3 weeks, 6 weeks, 3 months, and 4 to 6 months), when more frequent feedings stimulate increased milk production. These more frequent feedings usually last 24 to 48 hours, and then the infants resume their usual feeding pattern.

Care Management: the Breastfeeding Mother and Infant

Assessment

Infant

Before the initiation of breastfeeding, the nurse needs to consider several factors to effectively assist the breastfeeding infant. Maturity level, experience during labor and birth, any birth trauma or maternal risk factors, congenital defects or physical instability, and state of alertness all affect the readiness and ability of the infant to breastfeed.

During feeding, the infant is assessed by direct observation for latch-on, position and alignment, and suckling and swallowing. After the feeding, the infant is observed for behavior such as contentment or sleepiness. Elimination patterns are noted: within 24 hours after birth, at least one wet diaper and one stool; by day 3, three or four wet diapers and one or two stools that are beginning to change from meconium to yellow; after day 4 (and mother's milk has "come in"), six to eight wet diapers and at least three stools per 24 hours. Other factors to assess include the presence of jaundice, weight loss greater than 5% to 7%, and a regain of birth weight by 10 to 14 days of age.

Mother

Before breastfeeding is begun, the nurse should carefully assess the mother's knowledge of breastfeeding and her physical and psychologic readiness to breastfeed. Factors to include are her previous experience with breastfeeding, knowledge about breastfeeding, cultural factors, physical features of the breasts or nipples or other physical limitations, psychologic readiness (time since birth, mood and energy level), and support of the newborn's father or other family members.

During the time in the hospital, the nurse can help the mother view each breastfeeding session as a "feeding lesson" or "practice session" that will foster maternal confidence and a satisfying breastfeeding experience for mother and infant. Assessment includes condition of nipples, transition to mature milk, breasts feeling lighter or softer after feeding, mother feeling relaxed or sleepy after feeding, uterine cramping or increased lochia flow during and after a feeding, and mother's appearance of comfort with breastfeeding techniques.

Nursing Diagnoses

Nursing diagnoses for the breastfeeding woman include the following:

- *Effective breastfeeding related to*
  - —mother's knowledge of breastfeeding techniques
  - —mother's appropriate response to infant's feeding readiness cues
  - —mother's ability to facilitate efficient breastfeeding
- *Risk for ineffective breastfeeding related to*
  - —insufficient knowledge regarding newborn's reflexes and breastfeeding techniques
  - —lack of support by father of infant, family, friends
  - —lack of maternal self-confidence; presence of anxiety, fear of failure
  - —poor infant suckling reflex
  - —difficulty waking sleepy newborn
- *Risk for imbalanced nutrition: less than body requirements related to*
  - —increased caloric and nutrient needs for breastfeeding (mother)
  - —incorrect latch-on and inability to transfer milk (infant)
- *Risk for deficient fluid volume related to*
  - —ineffective suckling (infant)

Expected Outcomes

The expected outcomes include that the infant will do the following:

- Latch on and feed effectively at least eight times per day
- Gain weight appropriately
- Remain well hydrated (have six to eight wet diapers and at least three bowel movements every 24 hours after day 4)
- Sleep or seem contented between feedings

Examples of expected outcomes for the mother include that she will do the following:

- Verbalize/demonstrate understanding of breastfeeding techniques, including positioning and latch-on, signs of adequate feeding, and self-care
- Report no nipple discomfort with breastfeeding
- Express satisfaction with the breastfeeding experience
- Consume a nutritionally balanced diet with appropriate caloric and fluid intake to support breastfeeding

Plan of Care and Implementation

In the early days after birth, interventions focus on helping the mother and the newborn initiate breastfeeding and achieve some degree of success/satisfaction before discharge from the hospital. Interventions to promote breastfeeding progress from basics such as latch-on and positioning to signs of adequate feeding and self-care measures such as prevention of engorgement. With early discharge from the hospital it is increasingly important to assess the mother-infant dyad in relation to feeding ability. In some cases either a home visit or return to primary practitioner visit is appropriate within 48 to 72 hours after discharge to ensure that adequate latch-on is taking place and that the infant is progressing in feeding, elimination, and jaundice patterns (see also Care Path in Chapter 25). The visit is also an excellent opportunity to evaluate the mother's status, answer any questions about self-care or newborn care, and provide reinforcement of positive parenting and child care abilities.

The ideal time to begin breastfeeding is within 1 hour after birth when the infant is in the quiet, alert state.

Positioning

There are four basic positions for breastfeeding: football hold, cradle, modified cradle or across-the-lap, and side-lying position (Fig. 26-4). Initially it is best to use the position that most easily facilitates latch-on while allowing maximum comfort for the mother. The football hold is usually preferred by mothers who gave birth by cesarean. The modified cradle or across-the-lap hold also works well for early feed-

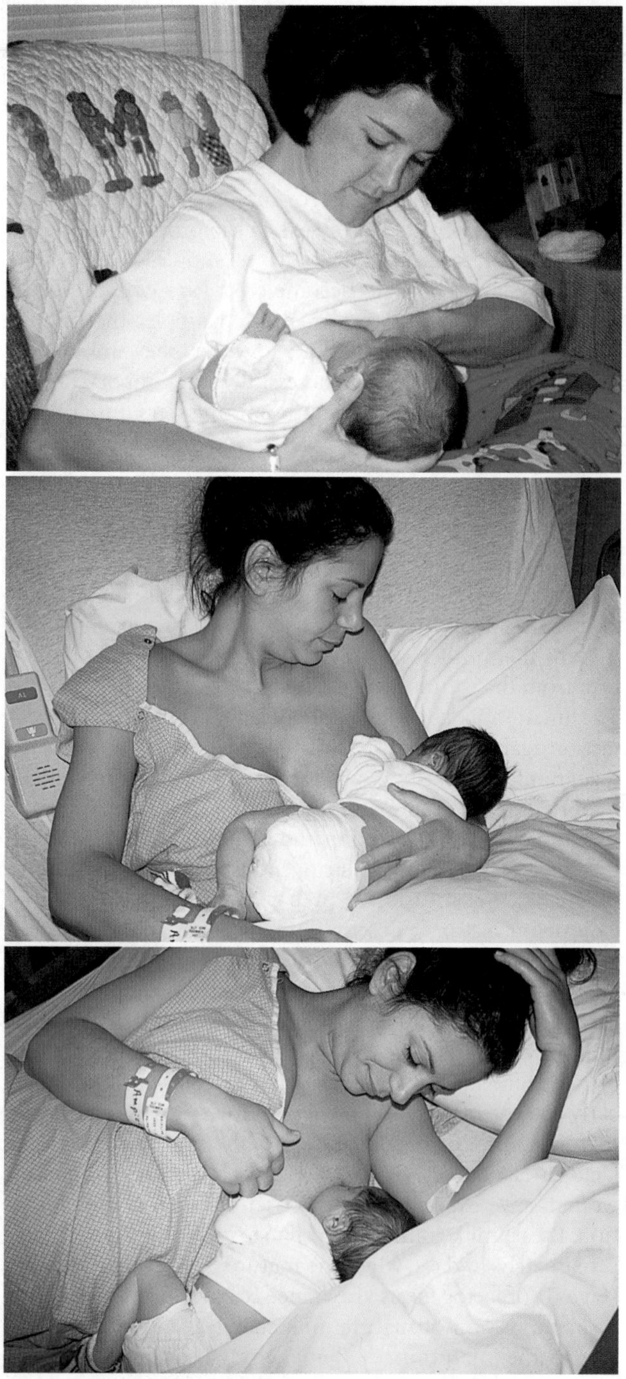

A

B

C

Fig. 26-4 Breastfeeding positions. **A**, Football hold. **B**, Cradling. **C**, Lying down. (*B* and *C*, Courtesy Marjorie Pyle, RNC, Lifecircle, Costa Mesa, CA.)

ings. The side-lying position allows the mother to rest while breastfeeding and is often preferred by women experiencing perineal pain and swelling. Cradling is the most common breastfeeding position for infants who have learned to latch on easily and feed effectively. Before discharge from the hospital, the mother should be assisted to try all of the positions so that she will feel confident in her ability to vary positions at home.

Whichever position is used, the mother should be comfortable, with pillows used as needed to provide support for her back and arms. The infant is placed at the level of the breast, supported by pillows or folded blankets; turned completely on his or her side; and facing the mother so that the infant is "belly to belly" with the arms "hugging" the breast. The newborn's mouth is directly in front of the nipple. It is important that the mother support the newborn's neck and shoulders with her hand and not push on the occiput. The infant's body is held in correct alignment (i.e., ears, shoulders, and hips are in a straight line) during latch-on and feeding (Fig. 26-5).

Latch-on

In preparation for latch-on, it may be helpful for the mother to manually express a few drops of colostrum or milk and spread it over the nipple. This lubricates the nipple and may entice the baby to open the mouth as the milk is tasted.

To facilitate latch-on, the mother supports her breast in one hand with the thumb on top and the fingers underneath at the back edge of the areola. The breast is compressed slightly so that an adequate amount of breast tissue is taken into the mouth with latch-on. Most mothers need to support the breast during feeding for at least the first few weeks until the infant can stay latched on easily.

The mother lightly touches the infant's lower lip with her nipple, stimulating the mouth to open. When the mouth is open wide and the tongue is down, the mother quickly pulls the infant onto the nipple. She brings the infant to the breast, not the breast to the infant. If the breast is pushed into the infant's mouth, the infant often closes the mouth too soon and does not latch on correctly.

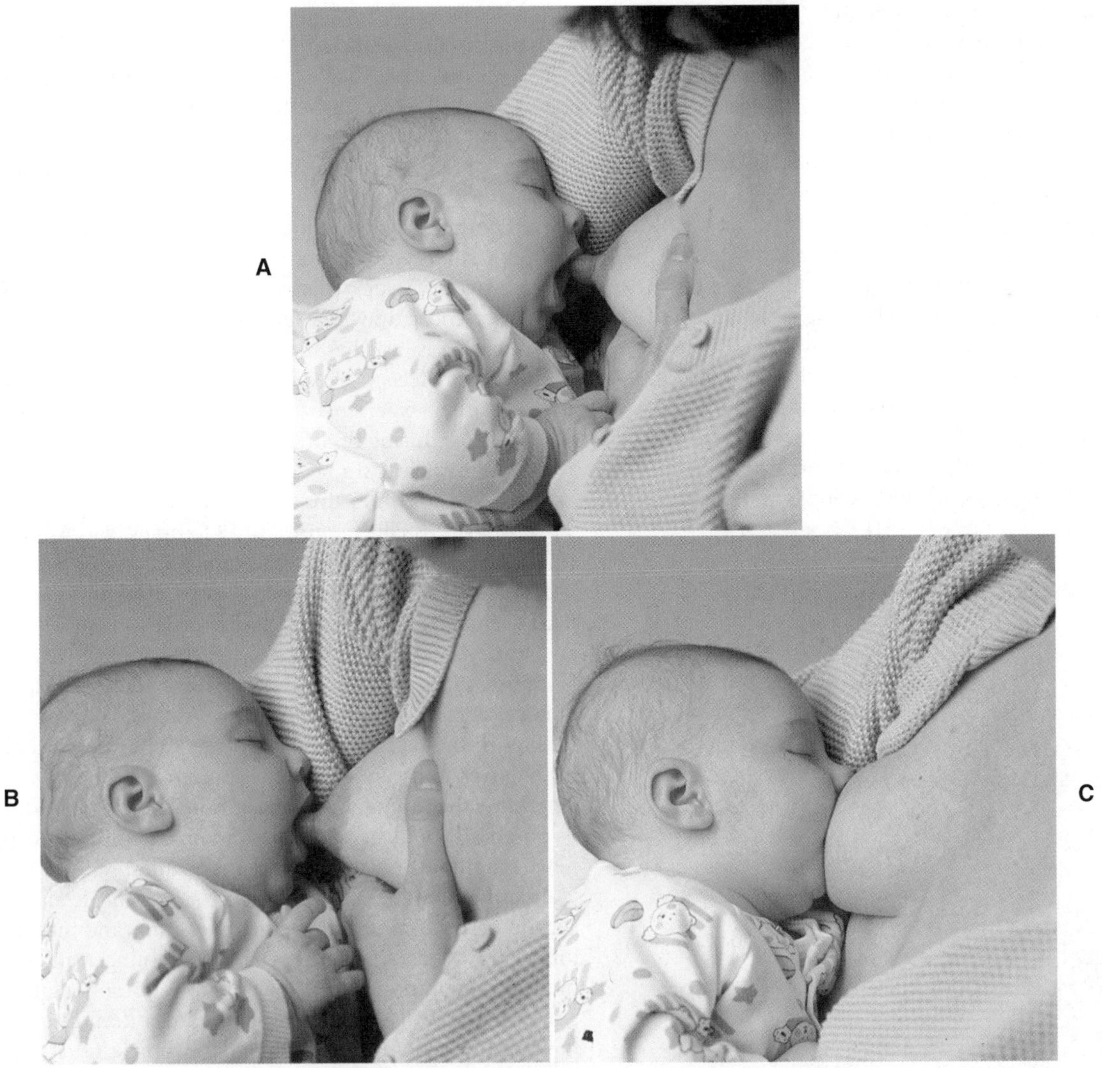

Fig. 26-5 Latching on. **A,** Tickle newborn's lip with your nipple until he or she opens wide. **B,** Once infant's mouth is opened wide, quickly pull infant onto breast. **C,** Infant should have as much areola (dark area around nipple) in his or her mouth as possible, not just the nipple. (Courtesy Medela, Inc., McHenry, IL.)

The amount of the areola in the newborn's mouth with correct latch-on depends on the size of the newborn's mouth and the size of the areola and nipple. In general, the infant's mouth should cover the nipple and an areolar radius of approximately 2 to 3 cm all around the nipple.

When the newborn is latched on correctly, the nose, cheeks, and chin should all be touching the breast (Fig. 26-6). The mother should not pull the nipple out of the mouth when trying to create a breathing space for the newborn's nose. Depressing the breast tissue around the newborn's nose is not necessary. If the mother is worried about the infant's breathing, she can raise the newborn's hips slightly to change the angle of the infant's head at the breast. If the newborn cannot breathe, reflexes will prompt the newborn to move the head and pull back to breathe.

Sucking creates a vacuum in the intraoral cavity as the breast is compressed between the tongue and the palate. If the mother experiences pinching or pain after the first few sucks, or does not feel a firm tugging on the nipple, the latch-on and positioning should be evaluated.

If each suck is painful, the infant may be having difficulty keeping the tongue out over the lower gum ridge. Clicking or smacking may be audible when this occurs. The nurse can place a finger on the side of the newborn's lower jaw, pulling down gently but firmly as the infant sucks, to help stabilize the jaw so that the tongue stays in place.

Any time the signs of adequate latch-on and sucking are not present, the newborn should be taken off the breast and latch-on attempted again. To prevent nipple trauma as the newborn is taken off the breast, the mother is instructed to break the suction by inserting her finger in the side of the infant's mouth between the gums and keeping it there until the nipple is completely out of the newborn's mouth (Fig. 26-7).

When the newborn is latched on correctly and is sucking appropriately, (1) the mother reports a firm tug on her nipple, but no pinching or pain; (2) the newborn sucks with cheeks rounded, not dimpled; (3) the infant's jaw glides smoothly with sucking; and (4) swallowing is audible.

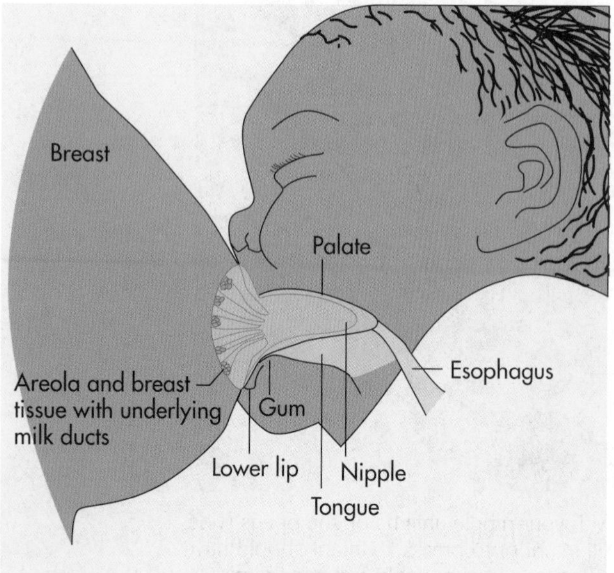

Fig. 26-6 Correct attachment (latch-on) of infant at breast.

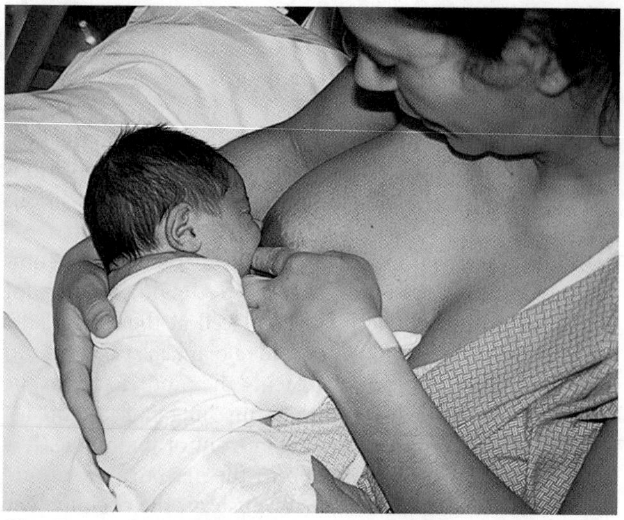

Fig. 26-7 Removing infant from the breast. (Courtesy Marjorie Pyle, RNC, Lifecircle, Costa Mesa, CA.)

Milk Ejection or Let-down

As the newborn begins sucking on the nipple, the let-down, or milk ejection, reflex is stimulated. The hormone oxytocin causes milk to be sent forward from the milk ducts to the nipple. The following signs indicate that let-down has occurred:

- The mother may feel a tingling sensation in the nipples, although many women do not feel their milk let down.
- The newborn's suck changes from quick, shallow sucks to a slower, more drawing, sucking pattern.
- Swallowing is heard as the newborn sucks.
- The mother feels relaxed, even sleepy, during feedings.
- The mother experiences uterine cramping and increased lochia flow during or after the feeding.
- The opposite breast may leak.

Frequency of Feedings

Newborns usually require 8 to 12 feedings in a 24-hour period. During the first 24 to 48 hours after birth, most newborns do not awaken this often to feed. It is important that parents understand that they should awaken the infant to feed at least every 3 hours during the day and at least every 4 hours at night during the first few weeks of life. (Feeding frequency is determined by counting from the beginning of one feeding to the beginning of the next.) Once the newborn is feeding well and gaining weight appropriately, he or she can determine the timing of feedings through demand feedings.

SKILL—INFANT FEEDING

Parents should be cautioned about attempting to place newborn infants on strict feeding schedules.

Infants should be fed whenever they exhibit feeding cues such as hand-to-mouth movements, rooting, and mouth and tongue movements. Crying is a late sign of hunger, and infants may become frantic when they have to wait too long to feed. Some infants will shut down or go into a deep sleep when their needs are not met. Keeping the newborn close is the best way to observe and respond to infant feeding cues. One recent recommendation is that mother and breastfeeding infant sleep in close proximity to promote breastfeeding (American Academy of Pediatrics, Section on Breastfeeding, 2005).

Duration of Feedings

The duration of breastfeeding sessions is highly variable, because the timing of milk transfer differs for each mother-infant pair. Whereas some infants may complete a feeding in 5 or 10 minutes, others may require 45 minutes or longer. The average time for feeding is 30 minutes, or approximately 15 minutes per breast. Instructing mothers to feed for a set number of minutes is inappropriate. It is better to teach mothers how to determine when an infant has finished a feeding: the infant's suck/swallow pattern has slowed, the breast is softened, and the newborn appears content and may fall asleep or release the nipple.

If a newborn seems to be feeding effectively, and is having adequate urine output but not gaining weight well, the mother may be switching to the second breast too soon. The high lactose content in foremilk may cause the newborn to have explosive stools, gas pains, and inconsolable crying. Keeping the infant on the first breast until it is soft ensures that he or she receives the more calorie-dense, high-fat hindmilk, which usually results in increased weight gain.

Supplements, Bottles, and Pacifiers

The American Academy of Pediatrics Section on Breastfeeding (2005) recommends that, unless a medical indication exists, no supplements be given to breastfeeding infants. Situations related to the infant that may necessitate supplemental feedings include low birth weight, hypoglycemia, or an inborn error of metabolism. Mothers may be unable to feed because of severe illness, or they may be taking medications incompatible with breastfeeding.

Offering a bottle after breastfeeding "just to make sure the baby is getting enough" is normally unnecessary and should be avoided. This can contribute to nipple confusion (i.e., difficulty knowing how to latch on to the breast) and to low milk supply because the baby becomes overly full and does not breastfeed often enough. Supplementation interferes with the supply-meets-demand cycle of milk production. The parents may interpret the newborn's willingness to take a bottle to mean that the mother's milk supply is inadequate. They need to know that a newborn will automatically suck from a bottle as the nipple triggers the suck/swallow reflex.

Newborns may become confused going from breast to bottle or bottle to breast when breastfeeding is first initiated. Although there is no research-based evidence to support this idea, there are anecdotal reports of infants who refused the breast once fed formula or even started on a pacifier. Breastfeeding and bottle-feeding require different oral motor skills. The way newborns use their tongues, cheeks, and lips, as well as the swallowing patterns, are very different. Some newborns can transition easily between breast and bottle, but some experience considerable difficulty. It is impossible to predict which infants will adapt well and which ones will not. Therefore it is often recommended by many practitioners to avoid bottles until breastfeeding is well established, usually after 3 to 4 weeks. If supplementation is needed, there are mechanisms such as supplemental nursing systems that allow the infant to breastfeed while being supplemented (see Fig. 26-3). Although some parents combine breastfeeding and bottle-feeding, some infants never take a bottle and go directly from the breast to a cup as they grow.

Studies have linked the early introduction of a pacifier with early termination of breastfeeding, decreased exclusive breastfeeding, and early weaning from the breast; other studies have shown a weak correlation between early weaning from breastfeeding and pacifier use. Biancuzzo (2003) suggests that health care workers maintain a commonsense approach to pacifier usage and breastfeeding. Parents should be informed of the relationship between pacifier use and early termination of breastfeeding so that an informed decision can be made. Furthermore, pacifier use should not replace actual feeding or suckling; prohibiting pacifier use will not ensure an increase in the length of breastfeeding. There should be an emphasis on allowing the infant to control the pace, frequency, and termination of feeding rather than allowing the pacifier (or anything else) to become the focus of the interaction.

The use of a pacifier in infants has also been suggested as a causative factor in the increase in episodes of acute otitis media (Niemela, Uhari, & Mottonen, 1995). However, a later study showed a significant decrease in the incidence of acute otitis media when a pacifier was used only at bedtime (Niemela et al, 2000). The effect of continual pacifier use on early speech and language development is unknown, but the pacifier may decrease the infant's desire to imitate sounds and affect intelligibility. Parents need to be alerted that continual dependency on a pacifier may influence social and speech development.

If the infant uses a pacifier, safety considerations in purchasing one must be stressed. Parents should be cautioned against altering a pacifier, thus making it more dangerous.

At the time of this writing, there is no evidence that pacifier use and nonnutritive sucking in preterm infants has any effect on the initiation and length of breastfeeding. Nonnutritive sucking should not be withheld from preterm infants, especially when performed in conjunction with the use of concentrated sucrose for pain management.

Special Considerations

Sleepy Newborn

During the first few days of life, some newborns need to be awakened for feedings. If the infant is awakened from a sound sleep, attempts at feeding are more likely to be unsuccessful. Unwrapping the newborn, changing the diaper, sitting the infant upright, talking to the newborn with variable pitch, gently massaging the infant's chest or back, and stroking the palms or soles may bring the newborn to an alert state.

Fussy Newborn

Infants sometimes awaken from sleep crying frantically. Although they may be hungry, they cannot focus on feeding until they are calmed. Calming techniques include swaddling, skin-to-skin contact and holding closely, talking soothingly, and allowing the infant to suck on a clean finger.

Some infants cry as soon as they are positioned for feeding. This may be due to a bruised head or previously undetected fractured clavicle. Changing the feeding position may solve the problem.

Fussiness may be related to GI distress (i.e., cramping and gas pains). This may occur in response to an occasional feeding of infant formula, or it may be related to something the mother has ingested. Although most mothers can consume their normal diet without affecting the infant, foods such as cabbage, broccoli, or onions may irritate some infants' stomachs. Others may react to cow's milk products ingested by the mother. There are no standard foods that all mothers should avoid when breastfeeding; each mother/newborn couple responds individually. One rule of thumb is that if the food causes bloating and gas in the mother, there is a strong probability it will do the same for the infant. If gas is a problem, giving the newborn liquid simethicone drops before a feeding may be helpful.

Persistent crying or refusing to breastfeed can indicate illness, and the health care provider should be notified. Ear infections, sore throat, or oral thrush may cause the infant to be fussy and not breastfeed well.

Slow Weight Gain

Commonly newborns lose 7% to 10% of their birth weight during the first 3 to 5 days after birth, which is mostly water weight acquired in utero. Thereafter, they should begin to gain weight at the rate of 110 to 200 g per week or 20 to 28 g per day. The infant who continues to lose weight after 5 days, who does not regain birth weight by 2 weeks, or whose weight is below the 10th percentile by 1 month should be evaluated and closely monitored by a health care provider.

At times, slow weight gain is related to inadequate breastfeeding. Feedings may be short or infrequent, or the infant may be latching on incorrectly or sucking ineffectively or inefficiently. Other causes are illness; infection; malabsorption; or circumstances that increase the newborn's energy needs, such as congenital heart disease, cystic fibrosis, or being small for gestational age. However, newborns gain weight in differing patterns, and one should not assume that the newborn is ill just because weight gain is not the same as that of another breastfed infant.

Maternal factors may contribute to slow weight gain. There may be inadequate emptying of the breasts, pain with feeding, or inappropriate timing of feedings. Inadequate glandular breast tissue or previous breast surgery may affect milk supply. Severe intrapartum or postpartum hemorrhage, illness, or medications may decrease milk supply. Postpartum stress and fatigue may also negatively affect milk production.

Usually the solution to slow weight gain is to improve the feeding technique. Positioning and latch-on are evaluated and adjustments made. It may help to add a feeding or two in a 24-hour period. Massaging alternate breasts during feedings may help increase the amount of milk going to the infant. With this technique, the mother massages her breast from the chest wall to the nipple whenever the baby has sucking pauses. Some think that this technique may also increase the fat content of the milk, which aids in weight gain.

When newborns are calorie deprived and need supplementation, the extra breast milk or formula can be given with a spoon or cup, a nursing supplementer, or a bottle. If there are latch-on problems, it is best to avoid bottles. In most cases, supplementation is needed only for a short time until the newborn gains weight and is feeding adequately. Most breastfeeding problems require simple solutions; a lactation consultant can help solve problems by modifying feeding patterns.

Jaundice

Jaundice and hyperbilirubinemia in the newborn are discussed in detail in Chapter 25. Colostrum has a natural laxative effect and promotes early passage of meconium. Bilirubin is excreted from the body primarily (98%) through the intestines. Infrequent stooling allows bilirubin in the stool to be reabsorbed into the infant's system (enterohepatic shunting), thus promoting hyperbilirubinemia. Infants who receive water or glucose water supplements are more likely to have hyperbilirubinemia, because these do not prevent enterohepatic shunting and only 2% of bilirubin is excreted through the kidneys. The presence of decreased caloric intake (less milk), weight loss of more than 5% to 7% in the first 5 days of life, increasing serum bilirubin (unconjugated) levels, decreased stooling, and increased jaundice is also sometimes referred to as starvation jaundice or "breast non-feeding" jaundice (i.e., the infant is not consuming an adequate amount of breast milk even though breastfeeding). To prevent this pattern, the following are suggested: initiation of breastfeeding within the first few hours of life, continuous rooming-in with the mother, breastfeeding 10 to 12 times per day, no supplements, and recognition of and response to hunger cues (Gartner & Herschel, 2001).

Breast milk jaundice demonstrates a pattern wherein serum bilirubin levels peak around the tenth day of life. High serum levels of bilirubin may still persist at 3 weeks of age, and some infants with breast milk jaundice may remain visibly jaundiced until 3 months. This pattern of jaundice is evidenced in infants of all ethnic origins (Gartner & Herschel, 2001). These infants are typically thriving, gaining weight, and stooling normally, and all pathologic causes of jaundice have been ruled out. It was once postulated that an enzyme in the milk of some mothers caused the bilirubin level to increase. It was previously believed that breastfeeding should be interrupted for 24 to 48 hours to allow bilirubin levels to decrease. However, this is no longer believed to be necessary. The critical element in breastfeeding and jaundice is to encourage early and frequent breastfeeding, which will enhance stooling and decrease the chance for enterohepatic circulation. Achieving a successful latch-on in the first few days of life and a continuation of this pattern will probably do more to decrease jaundice than other medical therapies. The use of oral supplementation of glucose water or water is strongly not recommended.

Preterm Infants

Human milk is the ideal food for preterm infants, with benefits that are unique to the individual preterm infant in addition to those received by healthy term infants. Initially, preterm human milk contains higher concentrations of energy, fat, sodium, and protein; however, by the second or third week of life human milk protein content is less than adequate for preterm infant growth, and supplementation with human milk fortifier is recommended. Human milk fortifier contains minerals (zinc and copper), vitamins (folic acid and vitamins B_2, B_6, C, D, E, and K) and electrolytes (calcium, magnesium, phosphorus, and sodium) necessary to support growth and metabolism in the preterm infant (American Academy of Pediatrics, 2004).

Mothers of preterm infants should begin pumping their breasts as soon as possible after birth with a hospital-grade electric pump. To establish an optimal milk supply, the mother should use a dual collection kit and pump 8 to 10 times daily for 10 to 15 minutes or until the milk flow has ceased for a few minutes (Meier, 1997). These women are taught proper handling and storage of breast milk to minimize bacterial contamination and growth.

See also Chapter 27 for additional information regarding discharge and nutrition of the preterm infant.

Breastfeeding Twins

Caring for twins takes some planning, but breastfeeding means that feedings are always ready instantly; no one has to wash bottles and fix formula; and, for some mothers, both babies can be fed at once. The mother with twins will need extra nourishment (200 to 500 kcal/day for each baby).

Each newborn feeds from one breast per feeding, usually for about 20 to 30 minutes. Some mothers assign each newborn a breast; others switch infants from one breast to the other, either on a schedule or randomly. The mother may find it easiest to use a modified demand feeding schedule; that is, feeding the first infant who wakes up and then waking the second infant for feeding.

During the early weeks, parents may find it helpful to keep a record of feeding times and which breast was used first by which infant. If one twin nurses more vigorously than the other, that infant should be alternated between breasts to equalize breast stimulation.

If the mother wants to feed the newborns simultaneously, she may wish to experiment with positions. For example, one newborn can be held in the football hold and the other in the cradle hold, or the newborns can each be held in a cradling position. Each infant can be supported on firm pillows while in the football hold. At first, some mothers using this position (Fig. 26-8) may require assistance to get the infants off the breasts.

Expressing and Storing Breast Milk

There are situations when expression of breast milk (Fig. 26-9) is necessary or desirable, such as when engorgement occurs, the mother and infant are separated (e.g., preterm or sick infant is in neonatal intensive care), the mother is employed outside the home and wants to maintain her milk supply, the nipples are severely sore or cracked, or the mother leaves the infant with a caregiver and will not be present for feeding.

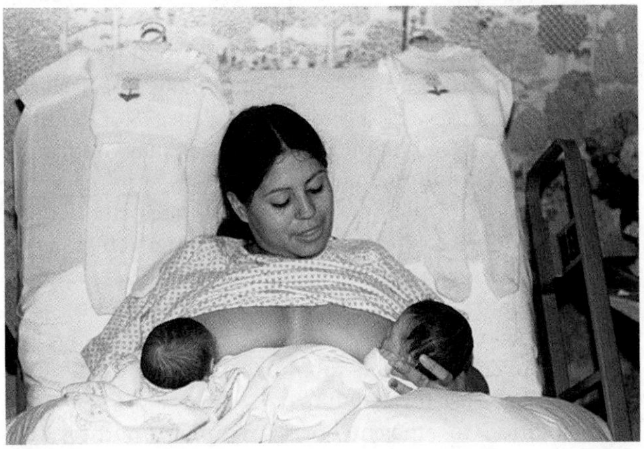

Fig. 26-8 Breastfeeding twins. (Courtesy Marjorie Pyle, RNC, Lifecircle, Costa Mesa, CA.)

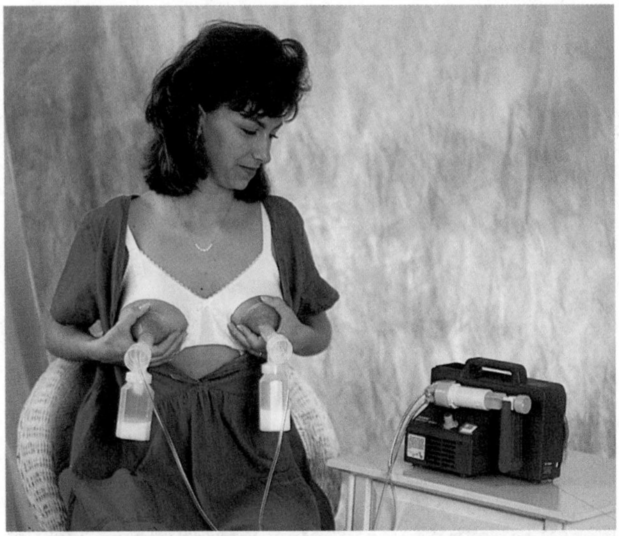

Fig. 26-9 Bilateral breast pumping. (Courtesy Medela, Inc., McHenry, IL.)

Because pumping and hand expression are rarely as effective as an infant in removing milk from the breast, the milk supply should never be judged based on the volume expressed.

Hand Expression

To manually express milk, after thoroughly washing her hands, the mother places one hand on her breast at the edge of the areola. With her thumb above and fingers below, she presses in toward her chest wall and gently compresses the breast while rolling her thumb and fingers forward. These motions are repeated rhythmically until the milk begins to flow. While the milk is flowing easily, the mother maintains a steady, light pressure. The thumb and fingers should not pinch the breast or slip down to the nipple. The hand should be rotated to reach all sections of each breast. After expressing milk from the second breast, she should return to the first breast and then repeat until all readily available milk is expressed.

Pumping

There are numerous ways to approach pumping. Some women pump when they first wake up in the morning or when the baby has fed but did not completely empty the breast. Others prefer to pump just before going to sleep. Some pump one breast while the infant is feeding from the other. Double pumping (pumping both breasts at the same time) saves time (Fig. 26-10).

The amount of milk obtained when pumping depends on the type of pump being used, the time of day, how long it has been since the infant breastfed, the mother's milk supply, how practiced she is at pumping, and her comfort level (pumping is uncomfortable for some women). Breast milk may vary in color and consistency, depending on the time of day, the age of the infant, and foods the mother has eaten (e.g., the milk may appear green after the mother eats spinach).

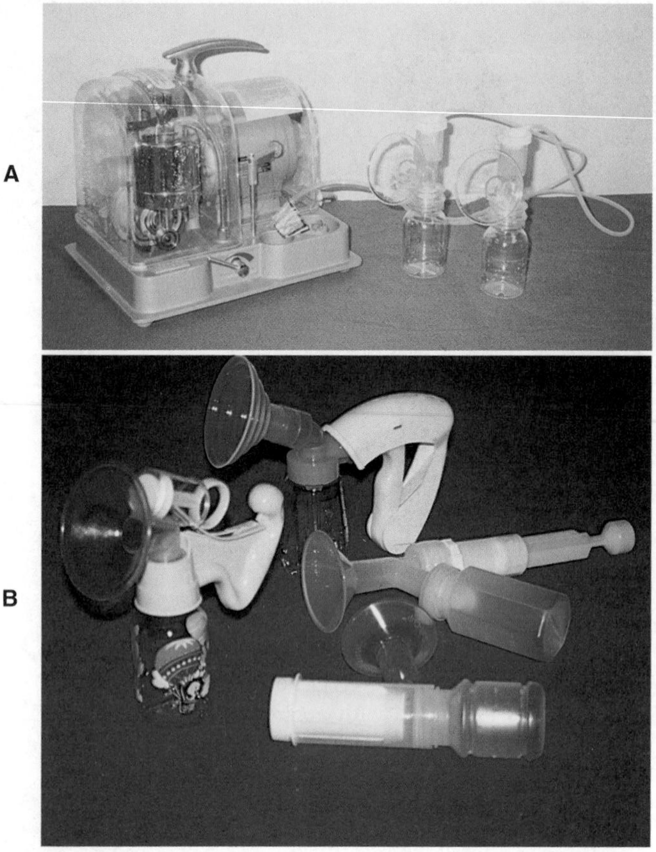

Fig. 26-10 **A,** Hospital-grade electric breast pump. **B,** Manual breast pumps. (*B,* Courtesy Marjorie Pyle, RNC, Lifecircle, Costa Mesa, CA.)

Types of Pumps

There are many types of breast pumps (Fig. 26-10). Some are more effective than others, and they vary in price. Manual pumps are the least expensive and may be the most appropriate where portability and quietness of operation are critical, or when a mother is pumping only for an occasional bottle (see Fig. 26-10, *B*).

Full-service electric pumps, or hospital-grade pumps, are similar to the sucking action and pressure of the breastfeeding infant. These are expensive and therefore are usually rented. When breastfeeding is delayed after birth (e.g., the infant is preterm or ill), or when mother and baby are separated for lengthy periods, these pumps are most appropriate (see Fig. 26-10, *A*). Electric, self-cycling double pumps are efficient and easy to use. Some of these pumps come with carry bags containing coolers to store pumped milk (see Fig. 26-9).

Smaller battery-operated or electric pumps are also available. Some have automatic suck/release cycling and others require use of a finger to regulate strength and speed of suction. These are typically used when pumping is done occasionally, but some models are satisfactory for working mothers or others who pump on a regular basis.

Storage of Breast Milk

Breast milk can be stored safely in any clean glass or plastic container; some suggest plastic containers because cells in breast milk adhere to glass (Lawrence & Lawrence, 2005). Disposable bottle liners are easy and inexpensive to use when storing milk. When using bottle liners, double bagging is recommended to protect the milk most effectively.

Breast milk can be refrigerated safely for 48 hours after it is expressed. If it is not used within that time, it can be frozen (at 0° C) for up to 6 months; it should be kept in the middle or toward the back of the freezer to avoid variations in temperature. Milk can be stored for 1 year in a freezer at −18° C. When storing breast milk, the container should be dated and the oldest milk used first.

Frozen milk is thawed by placing the container in warm water or in the refrigerator. It cannot be refrozen, and should be used within 24 hours. After thawing, the container should be shaken gently to mix the layers that have separated.

NURSE ALERT Do not use microwaving to defrost frozen human milk. High-temperature microwaving (72° C to 98° C) significantly destroys the antiinfective factors and vitamin C content. The safety of low-temperature microwaving (20° C to 53° C) remains questionable. One of the best ways to thaw frozen human milk is to place under a warm flow of tap water until the milk is thawed. Another option is to let the frozen milk thaw overnight in the refrigerator to maintain high levels of secretory IgA (Biancuzzo, 2003). Test the temperature of the milk before feeding. Microwaving does not heat evenly and can cause encapsulated boiling bubbles to form in the center of the liquid. Infants have sustained severe burns to the mouth, throat, and upper GI tract as a result of microwaved milk (Lawrence & Lawrence, 2005). ■

Being Away from the Infant (Maternal Employment)

Many women successfully combine breastfeeding with employment, attending school, or other commitments. If feedings are missed, the milk supply may be affected. Some women's bodies adjust the milk supply to the times she is with the infant for feedings. Other mothers must pump while away or their supply diminishes rapidly. Employed mothers can continue breastfeeding with guidance and encouragement. Mothers are encouraged to set realistic goals for employment and breastfeeding, with accurate information regarding the costs, risks, and benefits of available feeding options. Many mothers may find that a program of breast pumping when away from home and bottle-feeding the infant the expressed milk with or without formula supplementation is successful. Expressed breast milk may be stored in the refrigerator (4° C) without danger of bacterial contamination for up to 5 days (Lawrence & Lawrence, 2005). Although feeding the infant at home may occur on a demand basis, pumping milk away from home may be needed every 3 to 4 hours to maintain adequate supply. Breast milk may be expressed by hand or pump (manual or electric) and stored in an appropriate air-tight glass or plastic container. Expressed breast milk may be frozen (0° F [−18° C] or lower) for up to 12 months. Businesses are increasingly making available rooms where mothers can nurse their infants or use breast pumps.

In addition to efficient breast pumping, mothers also need child care by a trusted individual or agency and support and assistance from significant others. As with all breastfeeding mothers, these women must have proper nutrition and rest for adequate lactation. Maternal fatigue is considered the biggest threat to successful breastfeeding in employed mothers (Corbett-Dick & Bezek, 1997).

Weaning

Typically, weaning is initiated at a time chosen by the mother or the infant. Weaning can be accomplished with little effort and no discomfort when it is done gradually. Abrupt weaning is likely to be distressing for both mother and infant, as well as physically uncomfortable for the mother.

Infant-led weaning means that the infant moves at his or her own pace in omitting feedings. Drinking from a cup and increasing the amount of solid foods substitute for breastfeeding.

Mother-led weaning means that the mother decides which feedings to drop. This is most easily done by omitting the feeding of least interest to the infant or the one the infant is most likely to sleep through. It can also be the feeding most convenient for the mother to omit. After a week or more, another feeding is dropped, and so on, until the infant is weaned from the breast. Allowing time for the milk supply to adjust before omitting another feeding prevents discomfort for the mother as her supply gradually decreases.

Infants can be weaned directly from the breast to a cup. Bottles are usually offered to infants less than 6 months of age. If the infant is weaned before 1 year of age, formula should be offered instead of whole cow's milk.

If abrupt weaning is necessary, breast engorgement often occurs. The mother is instructed to take mild analgesics, wear a supportive bra, apply ice packs or cabbage leaves to the breasts, and pump if needed to increase comfort. The pump should not be used to empty the breasts, because they should remain full enough to promote a decrease in milk production.

Milk Banking

For those infants who cannot be breastfed but who also cannot survive except on human milk, banked donor milk is critically important. Because of the antiinfective and growth-promoting properties of human milk—as well as its superior nutrition—donor milk is used in some neonatal intensive care units for preterm or sick infants when the mother's own milk is not available. Donor milk is also used therapeutically for medical purposes, such as in transplant recipients who are immunocompromised.

The Human Milk Banking Association of North America (HMBANA)(website: www.hmbana.org) has established guidelines for the operation of donor human milk banks (Lawrence & Lawrence, 2005). Donor milk banks collect, screen, process, and distribute milk donated by breastfeeding mothers who are feeding their own infants and pumping a few extra ounces each day for the milk bank. All donors are screened both by interview and serologically for communicable diseases. Donor milk is stored frozen until it is heat processed to kill potential pathogens (bacteria and viruses), and then it is refrozen for storage until it is dispensed for use. The heat processing adds a level of protection for the recipient that is not possible with any other donor tissue or organ. Milk is dispensed only by prescription. A per-ounce fee is charged by the bank for processing, but the HMBANA guidelines prohibit payment to donors.

Care of the Mother

Diet

The composition of human milk varies slightly among women, regardless of their diets. The mother's milk automatically contains everything the baby needs, except in rare cases of maternal nutrient deficiencies. For most women, only 200 to 500 extra calories per day need to be added to the diet to provide adequate nutrients for the infant while also protecting the mother's body stores.

There are no specific foods or drinks that all breastfeeding mothers must either consume or avoid. Lactating mothers should ideally consume a balanced diet of nutrient-dense foods. Adequate amounts of calcium, minerals, and fat-soluble vitamins are important.

If the breastfeeding mother is drinking enough fluids to quench her thirst, she is likely drinking enough to support lactation. Typically, women find that they are drinking as much as 2 to 3 quarts of fluid each day, with the choice of fluid depending on the mother's preference. Because of her increased need for fluids, the breastfeeding mother may wish to keep a drink within reach during breastfeeding. An indicator of adequate fluid intake is the color of the mother's urine. If she is drinking enough fluids, her urine should be clear to light yellow throughout the day.

Weight Loss

Because it takes energy to produce milk, many mothers experience a gradual weight loss while breastfeeding as fat stores deposited during pregnancy are used. For the mother who is overweight, this fact can present an added incentive for breastfeeding. However, the mother who wants to diet while lactating should avoid losing large amounts of weight quickly because fat-soluble environmental contaminants to which she has been exposed are stored in her body's fat reserves, and these may be released into her milk. In addition, some mothers find that their milk supply decreases when caloric intake is severely restricted. Most mothers find that they can lose about 1 kg per week without affecting their milk supply.

Exercise

There is no reason for a breastfeeding woman to restrict her physical activity. Women continue activities such as hiking, jogging, swimming, and aerobics with no detrimental effect on milk supply or composition. Women often find that they are more comfortable if they engage in exercise soon after breastfeeding when their breasts are as empty as possible. Wearing a well-designed, supportive bra may also be helpful.

Rest

It is important for the breastfeeding mother to rest as much as possible, especially in the first 1 to 2 weeks after birth. Fatigue, stress, and worry can interfere with milk production and let-down. The nurse can encourage the mother to sleep when the baby sleeps. Breastfeeding in a side-lying position promotes rest for the mother. Assistance with household chores and caring for other children can be done by the father, grandparents or other relatives, and friends.

Breast Care

The breastfeeding mother's normal bathing routine is all that is required to keep her breasts clean. Soap can have a drying effect on nipples, so she should be instructed to avoid washing the nipples with soap. The small amount of soap that runs down her breasts while washing her face and neck or shampooing her hair is of no concern.

Breast creams should not be used routinely because they may block the natural oil secreted by the Montgomery glands on the areola. Some breast creams contain alcohol, which may dry the nipples. Vitamin E oil or cream is not recommended for use on nipples because it is a fat-soluble vitamin and a breastfeeding infant might consume enough vitamin E from the nipple to reach toxic levels. In addition, some people are allergic to vitamin E oil.

Modified lanolin with reduced allergens can be used safely on dry or sore nipples. Lanolin is beneficial in moist wound healing of sore nipples (Brent et al, 1998; Huml, 1995). Because lanolin is made from sheep's wool, the nurse should ask the mother if she is allergic to wool before applying the ointment. Lanolin is not recommended if it is suspected that nipple soreness may be due to a monilial infection (see Family Focus box). Antifungal creams are used to treat yeast infections on nipples.

The mother with flat or inverted nipples will likely benefit from wearing breast shells in her bra. These hard plastic devices exert mild pressure around the base of the nipple to encourage nipple eversion. They are also useful for sore nipples to keep the mother's bra or clothing from touching the nipples (Fig. 26-11).

If a mother needs breast support, she will be uncomfortable unless she wears a bra, because the ligament that supports the breast (Cooper's ligament) will otherwise stretch and be painful. If she is comfortable without a bra, there is no reason for her to wear one. If a woman prefers to wear a bra, it should fit well, offer nonbinding support, and feel comfortable. Underwire bras or improperly fitting bras may contribute to clogged milk ducts. Mothers should be encouraged to breastfeed at least once daily without a bra on so that all milk ducts can empty well.

Leakage of milk between feedings is a problem for some women. Using breast pads (washable or disposable) inside a bra and wearing layered or printed tops can help camouflage the leakage. Plastic-lined pads are not recommended because they trap moisture and may lead to sore nipples. To stop leakage, the mother can be alert to any sensation, such as tingling, that her milk is letting down. If this happens, she can usually stop the let-down by pressing straight back on her nipples. In public the mother can fold her arms across her chest to apply pressure unobtrusively.

Breast Self-Examination

Although only 1% to 2% of cases of breast cancer are diagnosed during pregnancy or lactation, the breastfeeding woman should perform breast self-examination (BSE) (see Chapter 5). The woman who is not menstruating should choose a convenient date on which to do her BSE every month. She needs to become familiar with the normal nodularity of her lactating breasts so that she can detect anything unusual on examination. Nodules that match in location in both breasts are almost always breast tissue. Nodules that increase and decrease in size are probably milk glands or ducts. Because lactating breasts are very dense, mammography is of limited diagnostic value. Should a suspicious nodule be discovered, a biopsy can usually be done without interrupting breastfeeding.

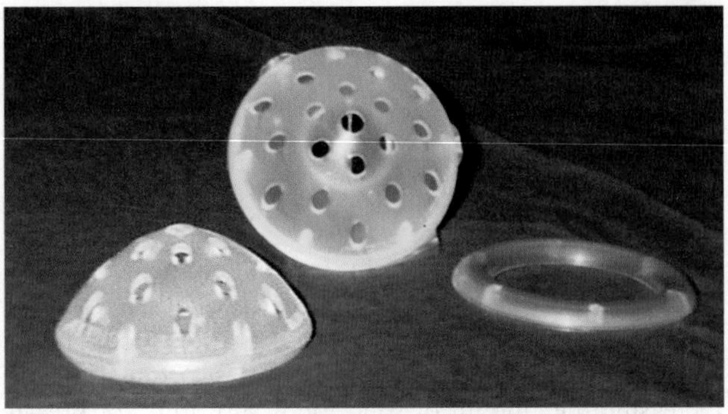

Fig. 26-11 Breast shells.

> ## Family Focus
> **SORE NIPPLES IN BREASTFEEDING MOTHER**
>
> Role play how you could determine whether a mother's telephone call for help with sore nipples requires teaching about positioning and correct latch-on or if she might have a monilial infection on her nipples. What specific questions would you ask? To whom might you refer her?

Effect of Menstruation

The return of menstrual periods varies among lactating women. The majority will resume menstruation by 6 months postpartum. Menstruation has no effect on breastfeeding. There are no hormonal effects on the infant, although some babies may seem fussy for the first day. The quality of milk is not affected (Lawrence & Lawrence, 2005).

Sexual Sensations

Some women experience rhythmic uterine contractions during breastfeeding. Such sensations are not unusual because uterine contractions and milk ejection are both triggered by oxytocin; but they may be disturbing to some mothers who perceive them to be similar to orgasm.

Breastfeeding and Contraception

Although breastfeeding confers a period of infertility, it is not considered an effective method of contraception. Breastfeeding delays the return of ovulation and menstruation; however, ovulation may occur before the first menstrual period after birth. Thus the breastfeeding woman who is relying on the lactational amenorrhea method of birth control needs to be knowledgeable about ways to determine when ovulation occurs (i.e., basal body temperature, presence of cervical mucus, and cervical position). Hormonal contraceptives, including pills, injectables, and implants, may cause a decrease in the milk supply and are best avoided during the first 6 weeks postpartum. Oral contraceptives containing estrogen are not recommended for breastfeeding mothers. Progestin-only birth control pills are less likely to interfere with the milk supply. Some mothers find that the progestin-only injection (Depo-Provera) interferes with milk production, although others notice no alteration in the milk supply. Nonhormonal contraceptive methods (e.g., foam, condom, nonhormonal intrauterine device [IUD], natural family planning, sterilization) are less likely to have a detrimental effect on breastfeeding.

Breastfeeding during Pregnancy

It is possible for a breastfeeding woman to conceive and continue breastfeeding throughout the subsequent pregnancy if there are no medical contraindications (e.g., risk of preterm labor). When the second baby is born, colostrum is produced. The practice of breastfeeding a newborn and an older child is called *tandem nursing.* The nurse should remind the mother to always feed the newborn first to ensure that the newborn is receiving adequate nutrition. The supply-meets-demand principle works just as with breastfeeding multiple babies.

Diabetic Mother

The diabetic mother is encouraged to breastfeed. In addition to benefits for the infant and maternal satisfaction, breastfeeding has an antidiabetogenic effect. Blood glucose levels and insulin requirements are lower because of the carbohydrate used in milk production. During lactation, the diabetic woman may be able to eat more food and still take less insulin. However, insulin dosage must be adjusted as the infant is weaned. Some diabetic women are at increased risk for sore nipples caused by monilial infections and may have an increased risk for mastitis (Lawrence & Lawrence, 2005).

Breastfeeding and Drugs

Although there is much concern about the compatibility of drugs and breastfeeding, there are in fact few drugs that are contraindicated during lactation (see Appendix A). Considerations in evaluating the safety of a specific medication during breastfeeding include the pharmacokinetics of the drug in the maternal system, as well as the absorption, metabolism, distribution, storage, and excretion in the infant. The gestational and chronologic age of the infant, body weight, and breastfeeding pattern are also considered (Lawrence & Lawrence, 2005). Most medications do not cause problems for the infant, but breastfeeding mothers should be cautioned about taking any but essential ones. In certain instances (e.g., radioactive diagnostic agents) the mother is instructed to pump her breasts and discard the pumped milk until the drug has cleared her body.

Smoking may impair milk production; it also exposes the infant to the risks of secondhand smoke. Mothers who continue to smoke tobacco when lactating should be advised not to smoke within 2 hours before breastfeeding and to never smoke in the same room with the infant. If a mother chooses to consume alcohol, she should be advised to minimize its effects by having only one drink and consuming it immediately after a feeding or waiting for 2 hours after drinking to breastfeed. Alcoholic beverages may impair the milk ejection reflex. The mother who is pumping for a preterm or sick infant should avoid alcohol until her baby is healthy.

Coffee intake may lead to a reduced iron concentration in milk, and consequently contribute to the development of anemia in the infant. The caffeine concentration in milk is only about 1% of the level in the mother's plasma.

The infant's immature renal system limits the ability to excrete the caffeine; caffeine accumulates in the infant's system and can cause irritability and poor sleeping patterns. Some infants are sensitive to even small amounts of caffeine; mothers of such infants should limit caffeine intake. Caffeine is found in coffee, tea, chocolate, and many soft drinks (Lawrence & Lawrence, 2005).

Herbs and herbal teas are becoming more widely used during lactation. Although some are considered safe, others contain pharmacologically active compounds that may have detrimental effects, particularly on the neonate. A thorough history should include the composition of any herbal remedies. Each remedy should then be evaluated for its compatibility with breastfeeding. Herbal teas which are considered safe during lactation include rose hips, orange spice, chicory, peppermint, raspberry, and red brush tea (Lawrence & Lawrence, 2005). A regional poison control center may provide information on the active properties of herbs. Consult Resources at end of chapter and Appendix A for more information about drugs in breast milk.

Environmental Contaminants

Except under unusual circumstances, breastfeeding is not contraindicated because of exposure to environmental contaminants such as DDT (an insecticide) and tetrachloroethylene (used in dry cleaning) (Lawrence & Lawrence, 2005). It is recommended that breastfeeding mothers not expose their infant to secondhand smoke; this often leads to an increase in the incidence of reactive airway disease, wheezing, and upper respiratory infections. Mothers who must smoke should change clothes before breastfeeding because tobacco residue may adhere to most clothes and the infant is thus exposed to the effects of nicotine and smoke even in the absence of active smoking.

Special Considerations

The breastfeeding mother may experience some common problems. In the majority of cases, these complications are preventable if the mother receives appropriate education about breastfeeding. Early recognition and resolution of these problems is important to prevent interruption of breastfeeding and to promote the mother's comfort and sense of well-being. Emotional support provided by the nurse or lactation consultant is essential to help allay the mother's frustration and anxiety and to prevent early cessation of breastfeeding.

Engorgement

Engorgement is a common response of the breasts to the sudden change in hormones and the presence of increased volume of milk. It usually occurs on the third to fifth day postpartum when the milk comes in and lasts about 24 hours. Blood supply to the breasts increases and causes swelling of tissues surrounding the milk ducts. The duct may be pinched shut, so that the milk does not flow. The breasts are firm, tender, swollen, and hot, and they may appear shiny and red. The tenderness and swelling extend into the axilla. The areolae are firm and the nipples may flatten, making it difficult for the newborn to latch on. Because back pressure on full milk glands inhibits milk production, if milk is not removed from the breasts, the milk supply may diminish.

When engorgement occurs, the nurse should assure the mother that this is a temporary condition usually resolved within 24 hours. The mother is instructed to feed every 2 hours, softening at least one breast, and pumping the other breast to soften. Pumping during engorgement will not cause a problematic increase in milk supply.

Because of the swelling of breast tissue surrounding the milk glands' ducts, ice packs are recommended in a 15 to 20 minutes on, 45 minutes off rotation between feedings.

The ice packs should cover both breasts. Large bags of frozen peas or corn make easy packs and can be refrozen between uses.

Fresh raw cabbage leaves placed over the breasts in between feedings may help reduce the swelling (Roberts, 1995). The mother washes the cabbage leaves and places them in her freezer until they are cold, then places them over her breasts. The leaves are replaced when they begin to wilt. Although the exact mechanism of action of cabbage leaves in treatment of engorgement is not understood, it is thought that continuous application might decrease milk supply. Raw cabbage leaves are often very effective for formula-feeding mothers who want their milk to "dry up."

Antiinflammatory medications such as ibuprofen may help reduce pain and swelling associated with engorgement. Mothers often have an elevated temperature and experience achiness in their breasts; ibuprofen can help remedy this.

Because heat increases blood flow, application of heat to an already congested breast is usually counterproductive. Occasionally, however, standing in a warm shower will start the milk leaking or the mother may be able to manually express enough milk to soften the areola enough for the baby to be able to latch on and feed.

Sore Nipples

Mild nipple discomfort at the beginning of feedings or mild nipple tenderness during the first few days of breastfeeding is common. Severe soreness and abraded, cracked, or bleeding nipples are not normal and most often result from poor positioning, incorrect latch-on, improper suck, or a monilial infection. Many women expect breastfeeding to be painful based on stories they have heard from family and friends; however, breastfeeding is not supposed to be painful. Limiting the time at the breast will not prevent sore nipples; the key to preventing sore nipples is correct breastfeeding technique.

evolve CASE STUDY—BREASTFEEDING

For the first few days after birth, the mother may experience some tenderness with the infant's initial sucks. This should quickly dissipate as the milk begins to flow and acts as a lubricant. To make the initial sucks less painful, the mother can express a few drops of milk to moisten the nipple and areola before latch-on. The mother should ensure that the newborn is well supported, is in straight body alignment, and has no pressure on the back of her or his head. The newborn's nose, cheeks, and chin should be touching the breast, and the mother should be supporting the breast with her hand during the early feedings. The nurse helps to reposition as necessary to try to resolve the nipple discomfort.

If the mother reports a pinching sensation of the nipple as the infant sucks, it may be helpful to gently pull down on the side of the newborn's jaw while he or she is sucking to increase the amount of breast tissue in the infant's mouth. If the nipple pain continues, the mother needs to remove the infant from the breast, breaking suction with her finger in the infant's mouth. She then attempts latch-on again, making sure the infant's mouth is open wide before the infant is pulled quickly to the breast (see Fig. 26-5).

The infant's suck can be assessed by the nurse or lactation consultant by inserting a clean gloved finger in the newborn's mouth and stimulating the newborn to suck. If the newborn is not extruding his tongue over the lower gum, and the mother reports pain or pinching with sucking, the newborn may have a short frenulum (commonly referred to as being "tongue-tied"). Sometimes this is corrected surgically to free the tongue for less painful, more effective breastfeeding.

The treatment for sore nipples is first to correct the cause. Once the problem is identified and corrected, sore nipples should heal within a few days, even though the baby continues to breastfeed regularly.

When sore nipples occur, it is more comfortable to start the feeding on the least sore nipple. Applying ice to the nipple for 2 to 3 minutes provides a numbing effect that increases comfort with latch-on. After feeding, the nipples are wiped with water to remove the baby's saliva. A few drops of milk can be expressed, rubbed into the sore area, and allowed to air dry. It is usually soothing to apply a cooled, steeped caffeinated tea bag to sore nipples (tannic acid may help promote healing). The tea bag is "dabbed" on the nipples, and should not be left in place for longer than 1 to 2 minutes. Warm water compresses may also be comforting (Lavergne, 1997).

If nipples are extremely sore or damaged and the mother cannot tolerate breastfeeding, she may be advised to use an electric breast pump for 24 to 48 hours to allow the nipples to begin healing before resuming breastfeeding. It is important that the mother use a pump that will effectively empty the breasts.

Sore nipples should be open to air as much as possible. Breast shells worn inside the bra allow for air to circulate while keeping clothing off sore nipples.

CASE STUDY—BREASTFEEDING

Flexible nipple shields have been marketed as a treatment for sore nipples; however, they do not protect the nipples and can actually chafe the nipple as the infant sucks. There is also danger of the infant not receiving adequate milk flow through the shield because it is difficult for most infants to get far enough back on the breast to adequately compress the lactiferous sinuses and get the milk to flow. There are special situations in which nipple shields are useful; however, they should be used only by trained lactation consultants who closely monitor the infant's intake of milk and growth.

Monilial Infections

Sore nipples that occur after the newborn period are often due to a monilial (yeast) infection. The mother usually reports severe nipple pain and tenderness, burning, or stinging, and she may have sharp, shooting, burning pains in the breasts during and after feedings. The nipples appear somewhat pink and shiny or may be scaly or flaky; there may be a visible rash, small blisters, or thrush. Most often, the pain is out of proportion to the appearance of the nipple. Yeast infections of the nipples and breast can be excruciatingly painful and can lead to early cessation of breastfeeding if not recognized and treated promptly.

Infants may or may not exhibit symptoms of monilial infection. Oral thrush and a red, raised diaper rash are common indications of a yeast infection. An affected infant is often very fussy and gassy. When feeding, the infant is likely to pull off the breast soon after starting to feed, crying with apparent pain. The infant may be biting or gumming at the breast.

The most common predisposing factors for yeast infections of the breast include previous antibiotic use, vaginal yeast infections, and nipple damage.

Mothers and infants must be treated simultaneously, even if the infant has no visible signs of infection. Treatment for mother is typically an antifungal cream applied to the nipples after feedings and in some cases, a systemic antifungal medication such as fluconazole. Most pediatricians prescribe an oral antifungal medication, such as nystatin or fluconazole, for infants. Treatment should continue for at least 7 days after symptoms begin to improve. Careful handwashing is essential to prevent the spread of yeast.

Plugged Milk Ducts

A milk duct may become plugged or clogged, causing an area of the breast to become swollen and tender. This area typically does not empty or soften with feeding or pumping. There may also be a small white pearl on the tip of the nipple; this is the curd of milk blocking the flow. The mother is afebrile and has no generalized symptoms.

Plugged ducts are most often the result of inadequate emptying of the breast. This may be due to clothing that is too tight, a poorly fitting or underwire bra, or always using the same position for feeding. Application of warm compresses to the affected area and to the nipple before feeding helps promote emptying of the breast and release of the plug. (A disposable diaper filled with warm water makes an easy compress.)

Frequent feeding is recommended, with the infant beginning the feeding on the affected side to foster more complete emptying. The mother is advised to massage the affected area while the infant nurses or while she is pumping. Varying feeding positions and feeding without wearing a bra may be useful in resolving a plugged duct.

If the mother develops fever or flu-like symptoms, she may have developed mastitis and should notify her health care provider. Plugged milk ducts do not necessarily cause mastitis, but milk stasis may increase susceptibility to breast infection.

Mastitis

A breast infection, or mastitis, is characterized by the sudden onset of flu-like symptoms, including fever, chills, body aches, and headache. (Flu-like symptoms in a breastfeeding mother should be considered indicative of mastitis, until proven otherwise.) There is localized breast pain and tenderness and a hot, reddened area on the breast, often resembling the shape of a pie wedge. Mastitis most commonly occurs in the upper outer quadrant of the breast; it may affect one or both breasts.

Certain factors may predispose a woman to mastitis. Inadequate emptying of the breasts is common, related to engorgement, plugged ducts, a sudden decrease in the number of feedings, abrupt weaning, or wearing underwire bras. Sore, cracked nipples may lead to mastitis by providing a portal of entry for causative organism (*Staphylococcus, Streptococcus,* and *Escherichia coli* are most common). Stress and fatigue, ill family members, breast trauma, and poor maternal nutrition are also predisposing factors for mastitis (Fetherston, 1998).

Breastfeeding mothers should be taught the signs of mastitis before they are discharged from the hospital, and they need to know to call the health care provider promptly if the symptoms occur. Treatment includes antibiotics such as cephalexin or dicloxacillin and analgesics/antipyretic medications such as ibuprofen. Rest is extremely important; the mother is advised to sleep whenever the baby sleeps. The mother should feed the baby or pump frequently, striving to adequately empty the affected side. Warm compresses to the breast before feeding or pumping may be useful. Adequate fluid intake and a balanced diet are important for the mother with mastitis.

Complications of mastitis include breast abscess, chronic mastitis, and fungal infections of the breast. Most complications can be prevented by early recognition and treatment.

Hepatitis C

The infection rate of infants born to mothers with hepatitis C is 5% to 6% in both bottle-fed and breastfed infants. There is no evidence that HCV is transmitted in breast milk and therefore the Centers for Disease Control and Prevention guidelines maintain there is no increased risk of transmission with breastfeeding as long as the mother is also HIV negative (American Academy of Pediatrics, Committee on Infectious Diseases, 2003) (see Contraindications to Breastfeeding earlier in this chapter).

Role of the Nurse in Promoting Successful Lactation

Nurses play a major role in breastfeeding education and support for new parents. Nurses often work with lactation consultants in hospitals, physicians' offices, or community settings. Although the vast majority are registered nurses, lactation consultants come from a variety of educational backgrounds such as nutrition, physical and occupational therapy, home economics, psychology, social work, education, or the basic sciences. Lactation consultants have had specialized postbaccalaureate education, training, and clinical experience working with breastfeeding mothers, and they have passed a certifying examination that requires meeting defined academic and clinical experience criteria.

Nurses in prenatal settings can educate the mother and her partner about the advantages of breastfeeding and explore reasons why they may prefer bottle-feeding. They can provide expectant parents with current reading materials and information about prenatal classes. At each encounter, the nurse can answer questions and provide additional information as needed.

Assessment of the mother's breasts and nipples during pregnancy is important. Flat or inverted nipples are identified. The mother may be offered breast shells (see Fig. 26-11) to wear during the last trimester of pregnancy to encourage eversion of the nipples, although antepartal use may be ineffective. These breast shells can also be worn postpartum between feedings.

The nurse should determine if the woman has had any breast surgery. Breast reduction or augmentation may interfere with the ability to produce milk and transfer it successfully to the baby.

No special nipple preparation is necessary during pregnancy. Efforts to "toughen" the nipples by pulling on them or rubbing them with a rough towel are to be avoided. Such stimulation can cause release of oxytocin and result in preterm labor; or damage the outer layer of protective skin cells, which may increase the risk of sore nipples.

In the immediate postpartum period, the nurse is instrumental in helping the mother initiate breastfeeding as soon as possible after birth. Encouraging parents to keep the baby in the mother's room (rooming-in) allows the opportunity for the mother to learn to recognize feeding cues and to feed the baby when these cues are present. The nurse provides help with positioning and latch-on until the mother can accomplish this independently. Explanations are given early regarding frequency and duration of feedings, how to wake a sleepy baby, and how to determine if the baby is getting enough milk. Information about the transition to mature milk (milk coming in) and how to prevent or deal with engorgement is needed. The mother is informed about the prevention and treatment of sore nipples and about signs of mastitis (including the importance of contacting the primary health care provider if these occur).

Parents often expect that because breastfeeding is "natural" it will come naturally for both mother and baby. This misconception needs to be clarified early so that parents may view breastfeeding as a learning process and not have unrealistic expectations. All health care providers who are knowledgeable about breastfeeding can offer needed support and encouragement to parents, helping to instill a sense of confidence.

The Baby-Friendly Hospital Initiative (BFHI) is a joint effort of the World Health Organization and the United Nations Children's Fund (Unicef) to encourage, promote, and support breastfeeding as the model for optimum infant nutrition. Ten research-supported practices were developed by BFHI as a guideline for maternity facilities worldwide to promote breastfeeding (Kyenkya-Isabirye, 1992; Wright, Rice, & Wells, 1996) (Box 26-2).

BOX 26-2

Ten Steps to Successful Breastfeeding

Every facility providing maternity services and care for newborns should

1. Have a written breastfeeding policy that is routinely communicated to all health care staff.
2. Train all health care staff in skills necessary to implement this policy.
3. Inform all pregnant women about the benefits and management of breastfeeding.
4. Help mothers initiate breastfeeding within a half-hour of birth.
5. Show mothers how to breastfeed and how to maintain lactation, even if they are separated from their newborns.
6. Give newborns no food or drink other than breast milk, unless medically indicated.
7. Practice rooming-in—allow mothers and newborns to remain together—24 hours a day.
8. Encourage breastfeeding on demand.
9. Give no artificial teats or pacifiers (also called dummies or soothers) to breastfeeding newborns.
10. Foster the establishment of breastfeeding support groups and refer mothers to them on discharge from the hospital or clinic.

From Kyenkya-Isabirye M: UNICEF launches the Baby-Friendly Hospital Initiative, *MCN Am J Matern Child Nurs* 17(4):177-179, 1992; Wright A, Rice S, Wells C: Changing hospital practices to increase the duration of breastfeeding, *Pediatrics* 97(5):669-675, 1996.

Institutions that provide care of the mother and newborn have been challenged to adopt the 10 practices spelled out in the BFHI to demonstrate support for mothers and their breastfeeding infant. Currently, there are 42 Baby Friendly Hospitals in the United States and three in Canada.

Concern has been voiced that the increasingly early discharge of new mothers from hospitals, more aggressive marketing of infant formulas to the public, and more employed mothers will contribute to the decline of breastfeeding. There is evidence that hospital practices intended to provide optimum maternal-newborn health may instead undermine breastfeeding. Early separation of mother and newborn, delays in initiating breastfeeding, provision of formula in the hospital and in discharge packs, conflicting information by health care workers, and formula coupons given at discharge have been implicated in the decline of breastfeeding following discharge. Rooming-in has correlated positively with successful breastfeeding, whereas the use of a pacifier has sometimes been associated with earlier weaning from breast to bottle. Changing hospital practices that were perceived as detrimental to breastfeeding significantly improved the overall duration of breastfeeding in one study (Wright et al, 1996). Although some studies have shown that the availability of commercial formula from hospital "discharge packs" may influence mothers to bottle-feed, other studies have found no such effect (Donnelly et al, 2000; Dungy et al, 1997).

A survey of breastfeeding mothers indicated that the determining factors for changing to bottle-feeding included the mother's perception of the father's attitude toward breastfeeding and the mother's uncertainty regarding the amount of milk the infant would receive (Arora et al, 2000). These findings have important implications for involving fathers in education and discussion regarding breastfeeding before and during the pregnancy. Fathers may express concerns of feeling left out during the newborn period if they have little involvement other than diapering and holding the infant. Encouraging fathers regarding their positive role in supporting the mother to breastfeed may help decrease feelings of isolation, benefit mother-infant interaction, and decrease a sense of helplessness and isolation.

Follow-up after Hospital Discharge

Problems with sore nipples, engorgement, and jaundice are likely to occur after discharge. Thus it is the role of the hospital nurse to educate and prepare the mother for problems she may encounter once she is home. It is critical that the mother be given a list of resources for help with breastfeeding concerns, and that she realizes when to call for assistance. Community resources for breastfeeding mothers include lactation consultants in hospitals, physicians' offices, or in private practice; nurses in pediatric or obstetric offices; support groups such as La Leche League; and peer counseling programs (such as those offered through WIC).

Telephone follow-up by hospital or office nurses within the first day or two after discharge can provide a means to identify

Nursing Care Plan

THE NEWBORN WITH INSUFFICIENT INTAKE OF NUTRIENTS

NURSING DIAGNOSIS: Ineffective breastfeeding related to deficient knowledge of mother as evidenced by ongoing incorrect latch-on technique

EXPECTED OUTCOMES

Mother will express increased satisfaction with breastfeeding, and neonate will exhibit satisfaction of hunger and sucking needs.

NURSING INTERVENTIONS/*RATIONALES*

Assess mother's knowledge and motivation for breastfeeding *to acknowledge mother's desire for effective outcome and provide starting point for teaching.*

Observe a breastfeeding session *to provide database for positive reinforcement and problem identification.*

Describe and demonstrate ways to stimulate the sucking reflex, various positions for breastfeeding, and the use of pillows during a session *to promote maternal and neonatal comfort and effective latch-on.*

Monitor neonatal position of mouth on areola and position of head and body *to give positive reinforcement for correct latch-on position or to correct poor latch-on position.*

Teach mother ways to stimulate neonate to maintain an awake state by diapering, unwrapping, massaging, or burping *to complete a breastfeeding thoroughly and satisfactorily.*

Give mother information regarding lactation diet, expression of milk by hand or pump, and storage of expressed breast milk *to provide basic information.*

Make sure mother has written information on all aspects of breastfeeding *to reinforce verbal instructions and demonstrations.*

Refer to support group and lactation consultant if needed *to provide further information and group support.*

any problems and offer needed advice and support. The American Academy of Pediatrics, Subcommittee on Hyperbilirubinemia (2004) recommends that infants discharged before 48 hours of age be seen by a health care provider within 48 hours. In some settings and circumstances, home care follow-up is available for mothers after hospital discharge.

Evaluation

Evaluation is based on the expected outcomes, and the plan of care is revised as needed based on the evaluation (Nursing Care Plan).

FORMULA-FEEDING

Rationale for Formula-Feeding

The decision to feed a baby infant formula may be the result of the mother's or partner's personal preference, the influence of other significant family members, or simply a lack of familiarity with breastfeeding. Occasionally there is no other option: the mother may have extensive breast scarring or may have had a bilateral mastectomy; the mother may be taking medications that preclude breastfeeding; or the baby may be adopted. Some mothers are able to induce lactation for an adopted baby. Rarely, an infant may have galactosemia and must be fed a lactose-free formula.

Infant formula may be used to supplement breastfeeding if the mother's milk supply is inadequate. It may also be fed to the baby if the mother will be away from the home and wishes to leave a bottle of formula instead of expressed breast milk.

Formula-feeding is also recommended for mothers who have HIV.

Parent Education

Inexperienced mothers and fathers who are formula-feeding their infants usually need teaching, counseling, and support. They may need assistance with the feeding process and with any problems they may experience. Some parents who are formula-feeding express concern that the baby will suffer as a result of their decision. Emphasis on the beneficial use of feeding times for close contact and socializing with the infant can help relieve some of this concern.

Readiness for Feeding

The first feeding of formula is ideally given after the initial transition to extrauterine life is made. Feeding readiness cues include such things as stability of vital signs, presence of bowel sounds, an active sucking reflex, an effective breathing pattern, and those cues described earlier for breastfed babies.

Feeding Patterns

Typically a newborn at first will take 10 to 15 ml of formula at a feeding. Intake gradually increases during the first week of life. Most newborns are drinking 90 to 150 ml at a feeding by the end of the second week, or sooner. The newborn infant should be fed at least every 3 to 4 hours, even if that requires waking the newborn for the feedings. The infant showing an adequate weight gain can be allowed to sleep at night and be fed only on awakening. Most newborns need six to eight feedings in 24 hours, and the number of feedings decreases as the infant matures. Usually by 3 to 4 weeks after birth a fairly predictable feeding pattern has developed. Scheduling feedings arbitrarily at predetermined intervals may not meet a newborn's needs, but initiating feedings at convenient times often moves the newborn's feedings to times that work for the family.

Mothers will usually notice an increase in the infant's appetite at ages 7 to 10 days, 3 weeks, 6 weeks, 3 months, and 6 months. These appetite spurts correspond to growth spurts. The amount of formula per feeding should be increased by about 30 ml at these times to meet the baby's needs.

Feeding Techniques

Parents who choose formula-feeding often need education regarding feeding techniques. Formula can be fed at room temperature or warmed. Formula should never be heated in a microwave oven. Microwaving does not heat evenly and can cause encapsulated boiling bubbles to form in the center of the liquid. This may not be detected when checking drops of milk for temperature. Babies have sustained severe burns to the mouth, throat, and upper GI tract as a result of microwaved milk (Lawrence & Lawrence, 2005). If it is warmed, the formula's temperature should be tested before it is given to the infant.

During feedings parents should be encouraged to sit comfortably, holding the infant closely in a semi-upright position. Feedings provide an opportunity to bond with the infant through touching, talking, singing, or reading to the infant. Parents should consider feedings, whether breast or bottle, as a time of peaceful relaxation with their newborn (Figs. 26-12 and 26-13).

The bottle should never be propped with a pillow or other inanimate object and left with the infant. Likewise, small children should not be given charge of bottle-feeding the infant unless there is close adult supervision. This practice may result in choking, and it deprives the infant of important interaction during feeding. Moreover, propping the bottle has been implicated in causing nursing bottle caries, or decay of the first teeth resulting from continuous bathing of the teeth with carbohydrate-containing fluid as the infant sporadically sucks the nipple.

The bottle should be held so that fluid fills the nipple and none of the air in the bottle is allowed to enter the nipple (see Fig. 26-13). After the newborn period the infant who falls asleep, turns aside the head, or ceases to suck usually is signaling that enough formula has been taken. Parents should be taught to look for these cues and avoid overfeeding, which could contribute to obesity.

Most infants swallow air when fed from a bottle and should be given a chance to burp several times during a feeding (Fig. 26-14).

Bottles and Nipples

Various brands and styles of bottles and nipples are available to parents. Most babies will feed well with any bottle and nipple. It is important that the bottles and nipples be washed in warm, soapy water using a bottle and nipple brush to facilitate thorough cleansing. Careful rinsing is necessary. Boiling of bottles and nipples is not needed unless there is some question about the safety of the water supply. An angled bottle is preferable to a straight bottle, because it encourages more physiologic positioning of the infant, improves the infant's comfort level, and decreases the need for burping (Farber, Van Fossen, & Koontz, 1995).

Infant Formulas

Commercial Formulas

Because human milk is species specific to meet the needs of the human infant, it is used as the standard for all infant formulas. Commercial infant formulas are designed to resemble human milk as closely as possible, although none has ever duplicated it.

Infants who are not breastfed should be given commercial formulas. If this is too expensive, the family may be eligible for services through the WIC program, which provides iron-fortified infant formula.

Commercially prepared formulas are cow's milk–based formulas that have been modified to closely resemble the nutritional content of human milk. These formulas are altered from cow's milk by removing butterfat, decreasing the protein content, and adding vegetable oil and carbohydrate. Some cow's milk–based formulas have demineralized whey added to yield a whey:casein ratio of 60:40. The standard cow's milk–based formulas, regardless of the commercial brand, have essentially the same compositions of vitamins, minerals, protein, carbohydrates, and essential amino acids, with minor variations such as the source of carbohydrate;

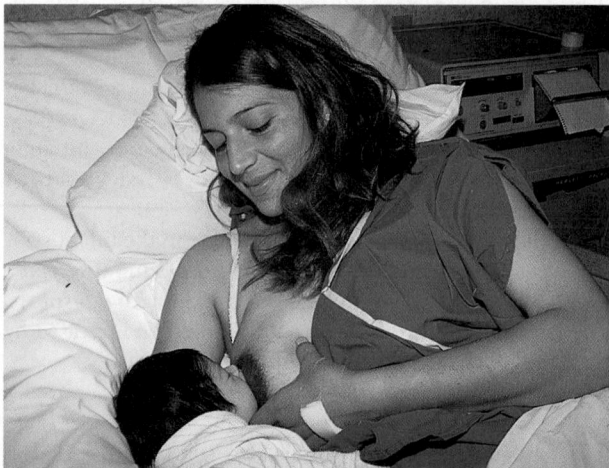

Fig. 26-12 Mother and infant enjoying breastfeeding. (Courtesy Marjorie Pyle, RNC, Lifecircle, Costa Mesa, CA.)

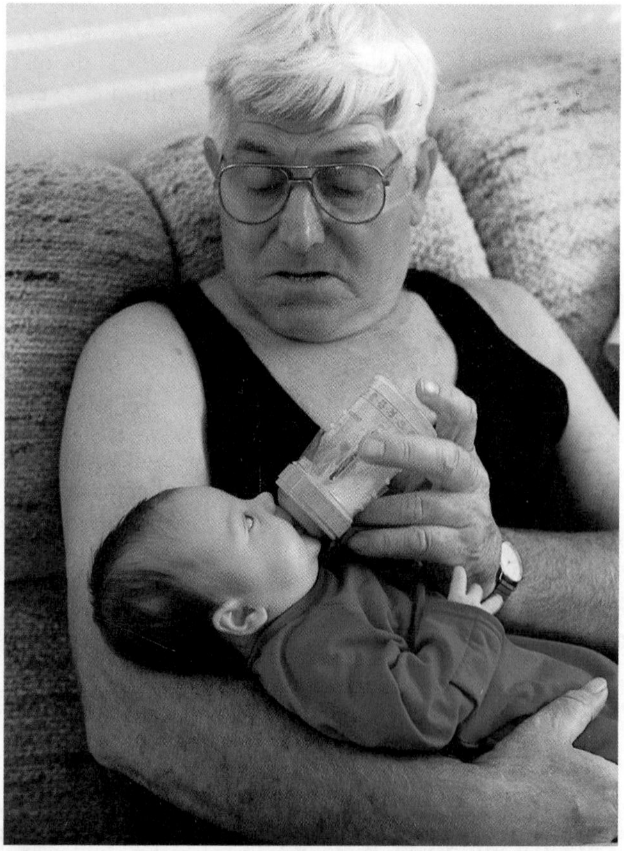

Fig. 26-13 Grandfather feeding infant granddaughter. Note angle of bottle, which ensures milk covers nipple area. (Courtesy Kim Molloy, Knoxville, IA.)

A

B

C

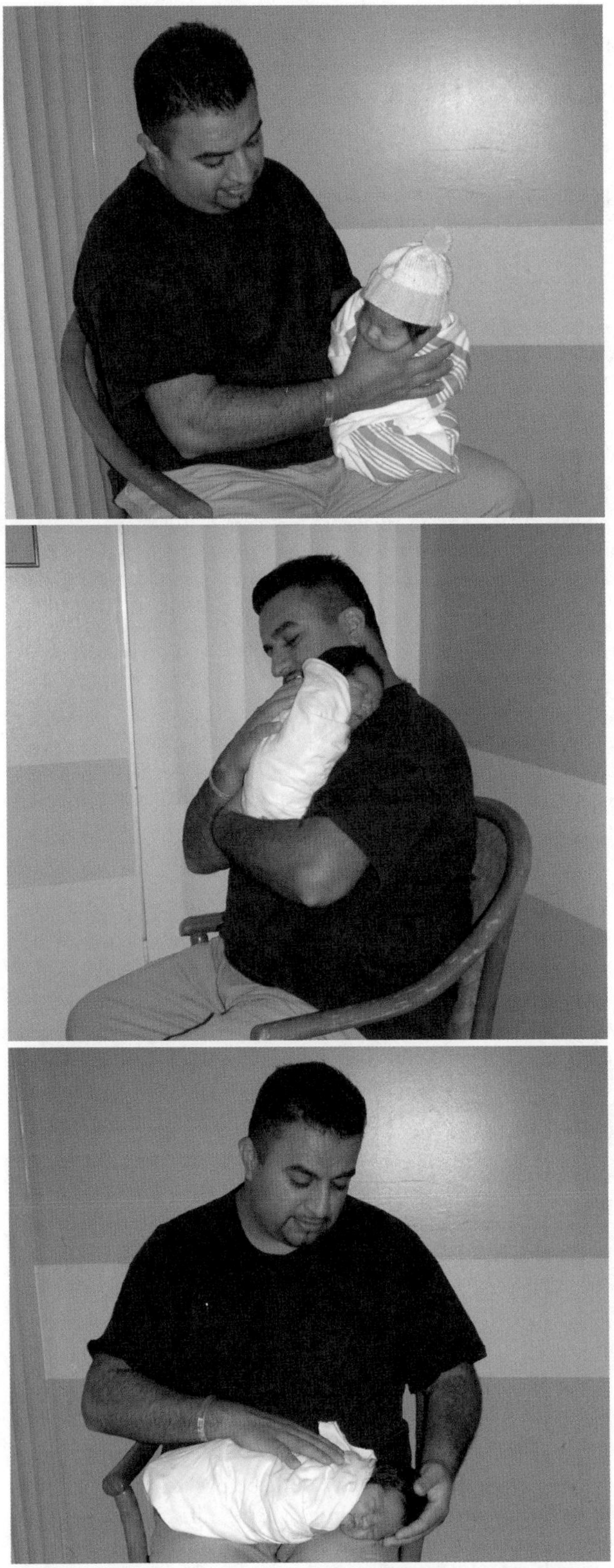

Fig. 26-14 Positions for burping an infant. **A**, Sitting. **B**, On the shoulder. **C**, Across the lap. (Courtesy Julie Perry Nelson, Gilbert, AZ.)

nucleotides to enhance immune function; and long-chain polyunsaturated fatty acids, docosahexaenoic acid (DHA), and arachidonic acid (AA), which are thought to improve CNS, visual and cognitive function (Georgieff, 2001: Gil, Ramirez, & Gil, 2003). Furthermore, the Food and Drug Administration (FDA) regulates the manufacture of infant formula in the United States to ensure product safety. Standard cow's milk–based formulas are sold as low-iron and iron-fortified formulas; however, only the iron-fortified formulas meet the requirements of infants.

There are four main categories of commercially prepared infant formulas: (1) *cow's milk–based formulas,* available in 20 kcal/fl oz as liquid (ready to feed), as powder (requires dilution with water), or as a concentrated liquid (requires dilution with water); (2) *soy-based formulas,* available commercially in ready-to-feed 20 kcal/fl oz powder and concentrated liquid forms, commonly used for children who are lactose or cow's milk protein intolerant; (3) *casein-* or *whey-hydrolysate formulas,* commercially available in ready-to-feed and powder forms and used primarily for children who cannot tolerate or digest cow's milk or soy-based formulas; and (4) *amino acid formulas.*

The American Academy of Pediatrics (2004) recommends the use of soy protein–based formulas for infants with galactosemia, hereditary lactase deficiency, documented IgE allergies caused by cow's milk, and documented evidence of lactose intolerance. Soy protein–based formulas, however, have not been proved to be effective against colic or in the prevention of allergy in healthy or high risk infants (Evidence-Based Practice box).

Commercial formulas are available in three forms: powder, concentrate, and ready-to-feed. All are equivalent in nutritional content, but they vary considerably in price. Powdered formulas are least expensive and are convenient because they are lightweight and require no refrigeration before mixing with water. Concentrated liquid formula is more expensive than powder. It is diluted with water and can be stored in the refrigerator for 24 hours after opening. Ready-to-feed formula is most expensive but easiest to use. The desired amount is poured into the bottle. The opened can is safely refrigerated for 24 hours. This type of formula can also be purchased in individual disposable bottles for the most convenient feeding.

Formula Preparation

The commercial infant formula must include label directions for preparation and use of the formula with pictures and symbols for the benefit of individuals who cannot read. Some manufacturers translate the directions into languages such as Spanish, French, Vietnamese, Chinese, and Arabic to prevent misunderstanding and errors in formula preparation. It is important to impress on families that the proportions must not be altered—that is, neither diluted to extend the amount of formula nor concentrated to provide more calories.

Although manufacturers of commercial formulas include directions for preparing their products, the nurse should review formula preparation with the mother or primary caretaker. It is especially important that formula be mixed properly. The newborn's kidneys are immature; giving the infant overly concentrated formula may provide protein and min-

CRITICAL THINKING EXERCISE—FORMULA PREPARATION

Evidence-Based Practice

HYDROLYZED PROTEIN INFANT FORMULA FOR PREVENTION OF ALLERGIES

Background

Allergies are the specific immunoglobulin E (IgE) response to normally benign substances (allergens). Twenty percent of the population suffer from allergies, including allergic rhinitis (hay fever), asthma, eczema or atopic dermatitis, and food allergies. Half of all childhood asthma and 80% of all hay fever persists into adulthood. The risk of atopy (inherited allergy) is 33% if one parent has allergies, and 70% if both parents are atopic. There is evidence that the longer the duration of exclusive breastfeeding, the less likely the baby will suffer childhood allergies. Food intolerance is an adverse reaction that is due to an enzyme error, irritation, toxicity, or pharmacologic effect. It is diagnosed when the cause is eliminated from the diet with subsequent symptom relief, and recurs with a challenge of the substance. Cow's milk allergy is often associated with exposure to cow's milk in the first month of life. Prevention of allergies can include maternal avoidance of allergens during pregnancy and lactation, and avoiding infant sensitization to allergens. Cow's milk and soy milk infant formulas may have their allergenic properties decreased by partially or completely hydrolyzing the protein. This may decrease childhood allergies in vulnerable children.

Objectives

The reviewers sought to compare allergy and food intolerance in infants fed hydrolyzed formula. Of interest was whether there was a difference between partially or completely hydrolyzed milk or soy formula, the most effective onset and duration of feeding, and the type of infant likely to benefit from hydrolyzed formula. The intervention is the hydrolyzed formula. The control group received human breast milk or cow's milk–based infant formula. The subjects are infants up to 6 months of age without evidence of allergy. The outcomes could include any type of diagnosed atopy (asthma, eczema, allergic rhinitis, and food allergy), food intolerance, growth parameters, cost, and infant refusal.

Methods

Search Strategy

The authors searched Cochrane, MEDLINE, CINAHL, EMBASE, references, and conferences. Search keywords were *infant, newborn, neonatal, pediatric, paediatric, plus feed, food, formula, hydrolysed, allergies, diet, protein,* and *milk.* Eighteen randomized or quasi-randomized trials were included in the review, dated 1989 to 2001, representing 7453 infants. Countries were not always noted in the review, but included Canada, Belgium, The Netherlands, and the United Kingdom.

Statistical Analyses

Similar data were pooled. Reviewers calculated relative risks for categorical data and weighted mean differences for continuous data, all with a 95% confidence interval. Results outside the confidence interval represent significant differences.

Findings

None of the trials compared the development of allergies in infants fed human milk with prolonged hydrolyzed formula-fed infants. Short-term hydrolyzed formula groups showed no significant difference in allergies with human milk–fed groups in two trials. In high risk infants, meta-analysis revealed a significant reduction in infant and childhood allergies, including asthma, eczema, allergic rhinitis, and cow's milk allergy in the hydrolyzed formula group, when compared with the cow's milk formula. These benefits seem to persist at least until 5 years of age. When completely hydrolyzed formula was compared with partially hydrolyzed formula, the differences in allergy symptoms were equivocal. The reviewers found no adverse effects from hydrolyzed formulas, and no difference in weight gain or length at 6 months of age.

Limitations

The trial criteria limited studies to less than a 10% loss to follow-up/dropout rate, which is a strength. Some trials were quasi-randomized, limiting generalizability. Some trials did not address allocation concealment, suggesting the possibility of bias by the clinical allergy assessors. Several trials were sponsored by infant formula manufacturers, suggesting possible conflict of interest.

Conclusions

For prevention of allergies and many other reasons, breast milk is still best. For high risk infants who cannot breastfeed, the prolonged use of hydrolyzed formula seems to be less allergenic than cow's milk formula. Partially hydrolyzed formula is more cost-effective than completely hydrolyzed formula, but evidence about their allergenic differences is inconclusive.

Implications for Practice

Breastfeeding should be encouraged, especially among infants at risk for allergies. When breastfeeding is not possible, hydrolyzed formula should be used.

Implications for Further Research

Much more research is needed about allergies beyond childhood. Cost, which was not addressed in these trials, can be a daily struggle for parents trying to provide the more expensive hydrolyzed formula. The question of the benefits of partially versus completely hydrolyzed formula persists.

Reference

Osborn D, Sinn J: Formulas containing hydrolysed protein for prevention of allergy and food intolerance in infants (Cochrane Review), 2003. In *The Cochrane Library,* Issue 2, Chichester, UK, 2004, John Wiley & Sons.

erals in amounts that exceed the kidneys' excretory ability. In contrast, if the formula is diluted too much (sometimes done to save money), the infant does not consume sufficient calories and does not grow well (see Critical Thinking Exercise).

Sterilization of formula rarely is recommended when families have access to a safe public water supply. Instead, formula is prepared with attention to cleanliness. When water from a private well is used, parents should be advised to contact the health department to have a chemical and bacteriologic analysis of the water done before using the water in formula preparation. The presence of nitrates, excess fluoride, or bacteria may be harmful to the infant.

If the sanitary conditions in the home appear unsafe, it would be better to recommend the use of ready-to-feed formula or to teach the mother to sterilize the formula. The two traditional methods for sterilization are terminal heating and the aseptic method. In the terminal heating method, the prepared formula is placed in the bottles, which are topped with the nipples placed upside down and covered with the

Home Care

FORMULA PREPARATION AND FEEDING

Your newborn will be hungry about every 2.5 to 3 hours, but sometimes may go 3 to 4 hours between feedings. The newborn should not go longer than 4 hours between feedings until a weight gain pattern is established–usually in about 2 weeks. Your newborn needs to be awake before being fed. If your newborn is sleepy, massage the newborn's back and chest and talk to him or her.

Your infant's feedings will change a lot in the first week after birth. The first day, most newborns drink only 15 to 25 ml (roughly 3 to 5 teaspoons) of formula at a feeding. By the time they are 1 week old, most infants drink 30 to 60 ml (1 to 2 oz) at a feeding and then gradually increase their intake as they grow. If you do not use all of the formula at a feeding, throw away what is left because it spoils once it has mixed with the infant's saliva.

You may want to write down how many ounces your infant drinks each day. When you take the infant in for a checkup, the physician or nurse will ask you about how much formula the infant drinks. By 1 to 2 weeks of age, most infants who weigh 3 to 4.5 kg (7 to 9 lb) are drinking about 840 ml in 24 hours (roughly 28 ounces or 3 to 3.5 ounces per feeding, based on eight feedings per day). Smaller infants may drink a little less because their stomach capacity is less. These figures, however, are approximations only, and infants will consume the amount necessary for growth provided they are healthy. Parents should not force feed an infant if less amounts are consumed unless directed by the primary care practitioner.

To feed your newborn, place the nipple in the newborn's mouth on the tongue. It should touch the top of the tongue to stimulate the infant's sucking reflex. Hold the bottle like a pencil. Keep the bottle tipped so that the nipple stays filled with milk and the newborn does not suck in air. With most bottles you will notice air bubbles in the bottle as the infant sucks on the nipple; this means the infant is getting formula from the bottle. The plastic bag bottles will not have as many air bubbles as hard plastic or glass bottles. A curved bottle decreases the amount of air being swallowed during a feeding.

Hold your newborn close for feedings. This should be a pleasant time for social interaction and cuddling. Some newborns take longer to feed than others; be patient. It may be necessary to keep the infant awake and encourage continued sucking. Moving the nipple gently in the infant's mouth may stimulate more sucking.

Some newborns swallow air when sucking. Give your infant a chance to burp several times during early feedings. As your infant gets older and you get more experienced, you will know when to stop for burping.

If your infant fusses or cries between feedings, check the diaper to see if he or she needs to be changed and see if the infant needs to be picked up and cuddled. If the child continues to cry and acts hungry, he or she needs to be fed. Infants do not get hungry on a schedule.

Place your baby on his or her back to sleep. Do not use the side-lying position for sleep because the infant may roll forward onto his or her face and stomach. In the event that the infant does not usually sleep after a feeding, he or she may be placed on the tummy provided there is adult supervision; this does not occur until the infant is older because most infants sleep approximately 18 hours per day.

The stools (bowel movements) of a formula-fed newborn are yellow and soft but formed. The newborn will probably have a stool during or after each feeding in the first 2 weeks, but this will then gradually decrease to one or two stools each day.

Safety Tips

- Infants should be held and never left alone while feeding. Do not prop the bottle: The infant could inhale formula or choke on any that was spit up.
- Know how to use the bulb syringe in case your infant should choke.
- Drinking bottles of formula or juice while falling asleep can cause tooth decay (nursing bottle caries) in young children.
- Juice is not recommended in infants for nutritional purposes.

Formula Preparation

- Wash your hands and clean the bottle, nipple, and can opener carefully before preparing formula.
- If new nipples seem too hard, they can be softened by boiling them in water for 5 minutes before use.
- Read the label on the container of formula and mix it exactly according to the directions.
- Use tap water to mix concentrated or powdered formula unless directed otherwise by your infant's physician or nurse. Some manufacturers sell bottles of distilled or fluoridated water for formula preparation; however, neither of these is necessary for preparation of infant formulas unless prescribed by the primary care practitioner.
- Test the size of the nipple hole by holding a prepared bottle upside down. The formula should drip slowly from the nipple. If it runs in a stream, the hole is too big and should not be used. If it has to be shaken for the formula to come out, the hole is too small. You can either buy a new nipple or enlarge the hole by boiling the nipple for 5 minutes with a sewing needle inserted in the hole.
- If a nipple collapses when your infant sucks, loosen the nipple ring a little to let in air.
- Opened cans of ready-to-feed or concentrated formula should be covered and refrigerated. Any unused portions must be discarded after 48 hours.
- Unopened (sealed) bottles or cans of formula can be stored at room temperature.
- If the formula is refrigerated, warm it by placing the bottle in a pan of hot water. Never use a microwave to warm any food to be given to a baby. Test the temperature of the formula by letting a few drops fall on the inside of your wrist. If the formula feels comfortably warm to you, it is the correct temperature.

caps, and then sealed loosely with the rings. The bottles are then boiled together in a water bath for 25 minutes. In the aseptic method, the bottles, rings, caps, nipples, and any other necessary equipment, such as a funnel, are boiled separately, after which the formula is poured into the bottles. Any formula left in the bottle after the feeding should be discarded because the infant's saliva has mixed with it. (Instructions for formula preparation and feeding are provided in the Home Care box.)

Vitamin and Mineral Supplementation

Commercial iron-fortified formula contains all the nutrients needed by the infant for the first 6 months of life. After 6 months, fluoride supplementation of 0.25 mg of fluoride per day is required if the local water supply is not fluori-

Critical Thinking Exercise

BOTTLE-FEEDING MOTHER–SLOW WEIGHT GAIN

Donna brought her infant daughter in for a 1-month well-baby examination. She mentions to you that her mother-in-law told her the baby looks "skinny," so she has been putting less water in the formula to increase the caloric intake of each feeding. The infant weighed 3515 g (7 lb 12 oz) at birth. The infant now weighs 4115 g (9 lb 1 oz). What should you do with this information you have obtained?

1. Evidence–Is there sufficient evidence to draw conclusions about what information Donna needs about infant feeding and appropriate weight gain for infants?
2. Assumptions–What assumptions can be made about the following factors?
   a. Appropriate weight gain for newborn infants
   b. Correct formula preparation
   c. Advice from well-meaning relatives
   d. Seeking advice from medical practitioners
3. What implications and priorities for nursing care can be drawn at this time?
4. Does the evidence objectively support your conclusion?
5. Are there alternative perspectives to your conclusion?

dated. Vitamin D supplementation is discussed earlier in this chapter.

Weaning

The bottle-fed infant will gradually learn to use a cup, and the parents will find that they are preparing fewer bottles. Commonly the feeding before bedtime is the last one to remain. Infants have a strong need to suck, and the infant who has had the bottle taken away too early or abruptly will compensate with nonnutritive sucking on his or her fingers or thumb, a pacifier, or even his or her own tongue. Weaning from a bottle should therefore be done gradually because the infant has learned to rely on the comfort that sucking provides.

Key Points

- Human milk is species specific and is the recommended form of nutrition for infants. It provides immunologic protection against many infections and diseases.
- Breast milk changes in composition with each stage of lactation, during each feeding, and as the infant grows.
- During the prenatal period, parents should be informed of the benefits of breastfeeding for infants, mothers, families, and society.
- Infants should be breastfed as soon as possible after birth and at least 8 to 12 times per day thereafter.
- There are objective, measurable indicators that the infant is breastfeeding effectively.
- Breast milk production is based on a supply-meets-demand principle; the more the infant nurses, the greater the milk supply.
- Commercial infant formulas provide satisfactory nutrition for most infants.
- All infants should be held for feedings.
- Parents should be instructed about the types of commercial infant formulas, proper preparation for feeding, and correct feeding technique.
- Unmodified (whole) cow's milk is not appropriate for feeding the infant during the first year of life.

Answer Guidelines to Critical Thinking Exercise

Bottle-Feeding Mother—Slow Weight Gain

1. Yes. Donna is preparing formula incorrectly. This can pose a problem for the infant. The kidneys of a newborn are immature. Giving the infant formula that is overconcentrated may provide protein and minerals in amounts that exceed the kidneys' excretory ability. If the formula is diluted too much (sometimes done to save money), the infant does not receive enough calories and does not gain weight adequately. The nurse can consult growth charts to see whether the weight gain is appropriate.
2. (a) For the first months of life, infants should gain 150 to 210 g (5 to 7 oz) per week. (b) The manufacturer specifies the correct way to prepare formula on the label. The directions may be included in several languages. When teaching formula preparation, the nurse should ascertain the parents' ability to read, as well as the language that the parents use. (c) Well-meaning relatives and friends may give unsolicited advice based on their past experience or their own ideas of health and wellness. For example, fat babies may be considered to be healthy. Parents must be prepared to use their own common sense and judgment when deciding what advice to accept. It is helpful to have written materials from the health care providers for the parent to consult when given conflicting advice from relatives and friends. (d) Parents should be counseled about when to seek advice from medical practitioners. For example, if there is a concern about appropriate weight gain, the practitioner could teach about appropriate rate of growth and weigh the infant to ascertain whether the infant is following norms for growth. Reinforcement about patterns and amounts of feeding is also helpful. Increase in intake during growth spurts can be explained. Questioning about formula preparation may also be appropriate.
3. The priority for nursing care is to ascertain whether the infant is urinating in appropriate amounts and concentration, and teaching Donna about formula preparation and the hazards of not following manufacturer's directions. She also needs some education about normal patterns of weight gain.
4. There is evidence about normal patterns of weight gain and appropriate formula preparation and the hazards of formula that is either too concentrated or too dilute.
5. It may also be useful or necessary to coach Donna in how to deal with advice from her mother-in-law or others who provide advice. She can be assisted in learning how to differentiate good from inappropriate advice, how to seek additional information from a variety of sources, and how to trust her own judgment.

Resources

American Academy of Pediatrics
141 Northwest Point Blvd.
Elk Grove, IL 60007-1098
847-434-4000
847-434-8000 (fax)
www.aap.org

Baby-Friendly USA
327 Quaker Meeting House Road
E. Sandwich, MA 02537
508-888-8092
508-888-8050 (fax)

Breastfeeding and Human Lactation Study Center
University of Rochester School of Medicine and Dentistry
Department of Pediatrics, Box 777
601 Elmwood Avenue
Rochester, NY 14642
716-275-0088
716-461-3614 (fax)

Breastfeeding Committee of Canada
www.breastfeedingcanada.ca

Breastfeeding resources
www.parentsplace.com/expert/lactation/

Bright Future Lactation Resource Centre
www.bflrc.com

Dr. Thomas Hale (medications and breastfeeding)
neonatal.ama.ttuhsc.edu/lact/

Human Milk Banking Association of North America (HMBANA)
www.hmbana.org

International Lactation Consultant Association
4101 Lake Boone Trail, Suite 201
Raleigh, NC 27607
919-787-5181
919-787-4916 (fax)
users.erols.com/ilca

Journal of Human Lactation
Sage Publications
2455 Teller Road
Thousand Oaks, CA 91320
805-499-9774
805-375-1700
www.sagepub.com

Lact-Aid (provides information and services to promote breastfeeding)
PO Box 1066
Athens, TN 37303
614-744-9090

Lactation Education Resources
www.leron-line.com

La Leche League
1400 N. Meacham Rd.
Schaumburg, IL 60168-4079
800-525-3243 (24-hour line)
www.lalecheleague.org

La Leche League Canada
National Office
18C Industrial Drive
PO Box 29
Chesterville, Ontario
K0C 1H0
613-448-1842
613-448-1845 (fax)
E-mail: ofm@LLC.ca
www.lalecheleaguecanada.ca

Mothers' Milk Banks

Lactation Support Service
Children's and Women's Milk Bank
British Columbia Children's Hospital
Vancouver, British Columbia, Canada V6H 3V4
604-875-2345, ext. 7607

Mothers' Milk Bank
Presbyterian/St. Luke's Medical Center
Denver, CO 80218
303-869-1888

Mothers' Milk Bank
Valley Medical Center
San Jose, CA 95128
408-998-4550

Mothers' Milk Bank
WakeMed
3000 New Bern Avenue
Raleigh, NC 27610
919-350-8599
919-350-8923 (fax)

Special Care Nursery Mothers' Milk Bank
Christiana Care Health Services
4755 Ogletown Stanton Rd.
PO Box 6001
Newark, DE 19718
302-733-2340

National Healthy Mothers, Healthy Babies Coalition
121 S. Washington St., Suite 300
Alexandria, VA 22314
703-836-6110
www.hmhb.org.

Nursing Mothers Advisory Council
E-mail: nmac@phillyburbs.com
www.nursingmoms.net

Special Supplemental Nutrition Program for Women, Infants, and Children (WIC)
Food and Consumer Service
3103 Park Center Dr., Room 819
703-305-2286

UNICEF—The Americas and Caribbean Regional Office (TACRO)
Apartado 3667
Balboa Ancón
Panamá City
República de Panamá
507-317-0257
E-mail: unicef@sinfo.net
www.uniceflac.org

References

American Academy of Pediatrics: *Pediatric nutrition handbook,* ed 5, Elk Grove Village, IL, 2004, The Academy.

American Academy of Pediatrics, Committee on Infectious Diseases: *Red book: 2003 report of the Committee on Infectious Diseases,* ed 26, Elk Grove Village, IL, 2003, The Academy.

American Academy of Pediatrics, Section on Breastfeeding: Breastfeeding and the use of human milk, *Pediatrics* 115(2):496-506, 2005.

American Academy of Pediatrics, Section on Pediatric Dentistry: Oral health risk assessment timing and establishment of the dental home, *Pediatrics* 111(5):1113-1116, 2003.

American Academy of Pediatrics, Subcommittee on Hyperbilirubinemia: Clinical practice guideline: Management of hyperbilirubinemia in the newborn infant 35 or more weeks of gestation, *Pediatrics* 114(1):297-316, 2004.

Anderson JW, Johnstone BM, Remley DT: Breastfeeding and cognitive development: a meta-analysis, *Am J Clin Nutr* 70(4):525-535, 1999.

Arora S et al: Major factors influencing breastfeeding rates: mother's perception of father's attitude and milk supply, *Pediatrics* 106(5):E67, 2000.

Association of Women's Health, Obstetric and Neonatal Nurses: *Standards and guidelines for professional nursing practice in the care of women and newborns,* ed 5, Washington, DC, 1998, Association of Women's Health, Obstetric and Neonatal Nurses.

Bachrach VR, Schwarz E, Bachrach LR: Breastfeeding and the risk of hospitalization for respiratory disease in infancy, *Arch Pediatr Adolesc Med* 157(3):237-243, 2003.

Barnard J: Gastrointestinal disorders due to cow's milk consumption, *Pediatr Ann* 26(4):244-250, 1997.

Biancuzzo M: *Breastfeeding the newborn: clinical strategies for nurses,* ed 2, St Louis, 2003, Mosby.

Brent N et al: Sore nipples in breastfeeding women: a clinical trial of wound dressings vs. conventional care, *Arch Pediatr Adolesc Med* 152(11):1077-1082, 1998.

Carbajal R et al: Analgesic effect of breast feeding in term neonates: randomized controlled trial, *BMJ* 326(7379):13, 2003.

Choudhry UK: Traditional practices of women from India: pregnancy, childbirth, and newborn care, *J Obstet Gynecol Neonatal Nurs* 26(5):533-539, 1997.

Corbett-Dick P, Bezek SK: Breastfeeding promotion for the employed mother, *J Pediatr Health Care* 11(1):12-19, 1997.

Cushing AH et al: Breastfeeding reduces risk of respiratory illness in infants, *Am J Epidemiol* 147(9):863-870, 1998.

Davis M: Review of the evidence for an association between infant feeding and childhood cancer, *Int J Cancer Suppl* 11: 29-33, 1998.

Department of Health and Human Services: *Healthy people 2010,* conference edition, vol 2, *Objectives for improving health,* Washington, DC, 2000, Department of Health and Human Services. Internet document available at www.health.gov/healthypeople/document/default.htm (accessed February 18, 2005).

Dewey KG, Heinig MJ, Nommsen LA: Maternal weight-loss patterns during prolonged lactation, *Am J Clin Nutr* 58:162-166, 1993.

Donnelly A et al: Commercial hospital discharge packs for breastfeeding women, *Cochrane Database Syst Rev* 2000(2):CD002075, 2000.

Dungy CI et al: Hospital infant formula discharge packages: do they affect the duration of breast-feeding? *Arch Pediatr Adolesc Med* 151(7):724-729, 1997.

Eisman J: Relevance of pregnancy and lactation to osteoporosis, *Clin Perinatol* 25(2):303-326, 1998.

Enger S et al: Breastfeeding experience and breast cancer risk among postmenopausal women, *Cancer Epidemiol Biomarkers Prev* 7(5):365-369, 1998.

Farber SD, Van Fossen RL, Koontz SW: Quantitative and qualitative video analysis of infants feeding: angled- and straight-bottle feeding systems, *J Pediatr* 126(6):S118-S124, 1995.

Fetherston C: Risk factors for lactational mastitis, *J Hum Lact* 14(2):101-109, 1998.

Ford R et al: Breastfeeding and the risk of sudden infant death syndrome, *Int J Epidemiol* 22(5):885-890, 1993.

Gartner LM, Herschel M: Part 2. The management of breastfeeding: jaundice and breastfeeding, *Pediatr Clin North Am* 48(2):389-400, 2001.

Georgieff MK: Taking a rational approach to the choice of formula, *Contemp Pediatr* 18(8):112-130, 2001.

Gerstein HC: Cow's milk exposure and type I diabetes mellitus, *Diabetes Care* 17:13-19, 1994.

Gil A, Ramirez M, Gil M: Role of long-chain polyunsaturated fatty acids in infant nutrition, *Eur J Clin Nutr* 57 (Suppl 1):S31-S34, 2003.

Gray L et al: Breastfeeding is analgesic in healthy newborns, *Pediatrics* 109(4):590-593, 2002.

Grummer-Strawn LM, Mei Z, Centers for Disease Control and Prevention Pediatric Nutrition Surveillance System: Does breastfeeding protect against pediatric overweight? Analysis of longitudinal data from the Centers for Disease Control and Prevention Pediatric Nutrition Surveillance System, *Pediatrics* 113(2):E81-E86, 2004.

Halken S, Host A: Prevention of allergic disease: exposure to food allergens and dietetic intervention, *Pediatr Allergy Immunol* 7(9 suppl):102-107, 1996.

Hanson LA, Korotkova M: The role of breastfeeding in prevention of neonatal infection, *Semin Neonatol* 7(4):275-281, 2002.

Horwood L, Fergusson D: Breastfeeding and later cognitive and academic outcomes, *Pediatrics* 101(1):E9, 1998.

Huml S: Cracked nipples in the breastfeeding mother, *Adv Nurse Pract,* 1, April 1995.

Kliegman R: Fetal and neonatal medicine. In Behrman R, Kliegman R, (eds): *Nelson essentials of pediatrics,* Philadelphia, 2002, W. B. Saunders.

Kyenkya-Isabirye M: UNICEF launches the Baby-Friendly Hospital Initiative, *MCN Am J Matern Child Nurs* 17(4):177-179, 1992.

Lavergne NA: Does application of tea bags to sore nipples while breastfeeding provide effective relief? *J Obstet Gynecol Neonatal Nurs* 26(1):53-58, 1997.

Lawrence RA, Lawrence RM: The evidence for breastfeeding: given the benefits of breastfeeding, what contraindications exist? *Pediatr Clin North Am* 48(1):235-251, 2001.

Lawrence RA, Lawrence RM: *Breastfeeding: A guide for the medical profession,* ed 6, St Louis, 2005, Mosby.

Meier P: *Professional guide to breastfeeding premature infants,* Columbus, OH, 1997, Ross Products Division, Abbott Laboratories.

Niemela M, Uhari M, Mottonen M: A pacifier increases the risk of recurrent acute otitis media in children in day care centers, *Pediatrics* 96(5 pt 1):884-888, 1995.

Niemela M et al: Pacifier as a risk factor for acute otitis media: a randomized, controlled trial of parental counseling, *Pediatrics* 106(3):483-488, 2000.

Riordan J, Gill-Hopple K: Breastfeeding care in multicultural populations, *J Obstet Gynecol Neonatal Nurs* 30(2):216-223, 2001.

Roberts KL: A comparison of chilled cabbage leaves and chilled gelpaks in reducing breast engorgement, *J Hum Lact* 11(1):17-20, 1995.

Rosenblatt KA, Thomas DB: Prolonged lactation and endometrial cancer. WHO collaborative study of neoplasia and steroid contraceptives, *Int J Epidemiol* 24:499-503, 1995.

Ryan AS, Wenjun Z, Acosta A: Breastfeeding continues to increase in the new millennium, *Pediatrics* 110(6):1103-1109, 2002.

Scariati PD, Grummer-Strawn LM, Fein SB: A longitudinal analysis of infant morbidity and the extent of breastfeeding in the United States, *Pediatrics* 99(6):E5, 1997.

Wright A, Rice S, Wells S: Changing hospital practices to increase the duration of breastfeeding, *Pediatrics* 97(5):669-675, 1996.

Infants with Gestational Age-Related Problems

27

LEARNING OBJECTIVES

On completion of this chapter the reader will be able to:

- Compare and contrast the characteristics of preterm, term, and postterm neonates.
- Discuss respiratory distress syndrome and the approach to treatment.
- Compare methods of oxygen therapy for the sick infant.
- Describe nursing interventions for nutritional care of the preterm infant.
- Discuss the pathophysiology of retinopathy of prematurity and chronic lung disease (bronchopulmonary dysplasia), and identify risk factors that predispose preterm infants to these problems.
- Describe the treatment of the infant with meconium aspiration.
- Describe risk factors associated with the birth and transition of an infant of a diabetic mother.
- Plan developmentally appropriate care for high risk infants.
- Develop a plan to meet the needs of parents of high risk infants.

ELECTRONIC RESOURCES

Additional information related to the content in Chapter 27 can be found on

the companion website at evolve
http://evolve.elsevier.com/Wong/maternal/
- NCLEX Review Questions
- WebLinks

or the interactive student CD-ROM
Activities for Chapter 27 include the following:
- NCLEX Review Questions
- Critical Thinking Exercise–Patent Ductus Arteriosus
- Nursing Care Plan–Infant of Mother with Diabetes Mellitus
- Nursing Care Plan–High Risk Preterm Newborn

Modern technology and expert nursing care have made important contributions to improving the health and overall survival of high risk infants. However, infants who are born considerably before term and survive are particularly susceptible to the development of sequelae related to their preterm birth. These conditions include necrotizing enterocolitis, bronchopulmonary dysplasia, intraventricular and periventricular hemorrhage, and retinopathy of prematurity. The focus of this chapter is on care of the preterm infant, but care of other high risk infants with gestational age–related problems is also discussed. Infants born of mothers with diabetes are included because they may experience problems that place them at risk for proper function and development.

High risk infants are most often classified according to birth weight, gestational age, and predominant pathophysiologic problems (Box 27-1). Intrauterine growth rates are not the same for all infants, and other factors (e.g., heredity, placental insufficiency, and maternal disease) influence intrauterine growth and birth weight. The classification system in the box encompasses birth weight and gestational age.

THE PRETERM INFANT

Preterm infants, those born before 37 weeks of gestation, are at risk because their organ systems are immature and they lack adequate physiologic reserves to function in an extrauterine environment. The range of birth weight and physiologic problems varies widely among preterm infants as a result of increased survivability among those who weigh less than 1000 g. However, one general concept is that the lower the weight and the gestational age, the fewer chances of survival exist among infants born preterm. Preterm birth is responsible for almost two thirds of infant deaths. The cause of preterm birth is largely unknown; however, the incidence of preterm birth is highest among low socioeconomic groups. This is likely a result of the lack of comprehensive prenatal health care. Other factors found to be associated with preterm birth include gestational hypertension; maternal infection; multifetal pregnancy; HELLP syndrome (*h*emolysis, *e*levated *l*iver enzymes, and *l*ow *p*latelet count occurring in association with preeclampsia); premature dilation of the

BOX 27-1

Classification of High Risk Infants

Classification According to Size

Low-birth-weight (LBW) infant—An infant whose birth weight is less than 2500 g, regardless of gestational age

Very-low-birth-weight (VLBW) infant—An infant whose birth weight is less than 1500 g

Extremely-low-birth-weight (ELBW) infant—An infant whose birth weight is less than 1000 g

Appropriate-for-gestational-age (AGA) infant—An infant whose birth weight falls between the 10th and 90th percentiles on intrauterine growth curves

Small-for-date (SFD) or small-for-gestational-age (SGA) infant—An infant whose rate of intrauterine growth was restricted and whose birth weight falls below the 10th percentile on intrauterine growth curves

Large-for-gestational-age (LGA) infant—An infant whose birth weight falls above the 90th percentile on intrauterine growth charts

Intrauterine growth restriction (IUGR)—Found in infants whose intrauterine growth is restricted (sometimes used as a more descriptive term for the SGA infant)

Symmetric IUGR—Growth restriction in which the weight, length, and head circumference are all affected

Asymmetric IUGR—Growth restriction in which the head circumference remains within normal parameters while the birth weight falls below the 10th percentile

Classification According to Gestational Age

Premature (preterm) infant—An infant born before completion of 37 weeks of gestation, regardless of birth weight

Full-term infant—An infant born between the beginning of 38 weeks and the completion of 42 weeks of gestation, regardless of birth weight

Postmature (postterm) infant—An infant born after 42 weeks of gestational age, regardless of birth weight

Classification According to Mortality

Live birth—Birth in which the neonate manifests any heartbeat, breathes, or displays voluntary movement, regardless of gestational age

Fetal death—Death of the fetus after 20 weeks of gestation and before delivery, with absence of any signs of life after birth

Neonatal death—Death that occurs in the first 27 days of life; early neonatal death occurs in the first week of life; late neonatal death occurs at 7 to 27 days

Perinatal mortality—Total number of fetal and early neonatal deaths per 1000 live births

cervix; and placental or umbilical cord conditions that affect the fetus' reception of nutrients.

The potential problems and care needs of the preterm infant weighing 2000 g differ from those of the term, postterm, or postmature infant of equal weight. The presence of physiologic disorders and anomalies affects the infant's response to treatment. In general, the closer infants are to term, the easier their adjustment to the external environment.

There are varying opinions about the practical and ethical dimensions of resuscitation of extremely-low-birth-weight (ELBW) infants (those infants whose birth weight is 1000 g or less). Ethical issues associated with resuscitation of these infants include whether to resuscitate, who should make that decision, whether the cost of resuscitation is justified, and whether the benefits of technology outweigh the burdens on the infant, family, and society in relation to quality of life.

CARE MANAGEMENT

Assessment

For the high risk infant, an accurate assessment of gestational age (see Chapter 25) is critical in helping the nurse identify the potential problems the newborn is likely to experience. The response of the preterm or postterm infant to extrauterine life is different from that of the term infant. By understanding the physiologic basis of these differences, the nurse can assess these infants, determine the response of the preterm or postterm infant, and discern which of the potential problems are most likely to occur.

Respiratory Function

Pink color, adequate tissue perfusion, and respiratory patterns are quickly established in nonstressed newborns, and they are soon vigorous and show appropriate muscle tone. However, infants with a potential for respiratory depression at birth because of asphyxia, maternal analgesia or illness, immaturity, prematurity, or congenital malformations may exhibit cyanosis, decreased tissue perfusion, retractions, nasal flaring, tachypnea, or a combination of these problems.

The preterm infant is likely to have difficulty making the pulmonary transition from intrauterine to extrauterine life. Numerous problems may affect the respiratory system of preterm infants and may include the following:

- Decreased number of functional alveoli
- Deficient surfactant levels
- Smaller lumen in the respiratory system
- Greater collapsibility or obstruction of respiratory passages
- Insufficient calcification of the bony thorax
- Circulating hormones that may affect cardiovascular function
- Immature and fragile capillaries in the lungs
- Greater distance between functional alveoli and capillary bed

In combination, these deficits severely hinder the infant's respiratory efforts and can produce respiratory distress or apnea. Early signs of respiratory distress include flaring of the nares and expiratory grunting. Depending on the severity of respiratory distress and cause, retractions may begin as subcostal, intercostal, or suprasternal. Increasing respiratory effort (e.g., paradoxical breathing patterns, retractions, nasal flaring, expiratory grunting, tachypnea, or apnea) indicates increasing distress. Initially, a compromised infant's color may be cyanotic centrally or pale. Acrocyanosis is a normal finding in the neonate, but central cyanosis indicates the existence of an underlying problem.

Periodic breathing is a respiratory pattern commonly seen in premature infants. Such infants exhibit 5- to 10-second respiratory pauses followed by 10 to 15 seconds of compensatory rapid respirations. Such periodic breathing should not be confused with apnea, which is a cessation of respirations of 20 seconds or more. The nurse must be prepared to provide oxygen and artificial ventilation as necessary when the newborn demonstrates an inability to initiate or maintain adequate respiratory function.

Cardiovascular Function

Evaluation of heart rate and rhythm, color, blood pressure, perfusion, pulses, oxygen saturation, and acid-base status provides information on cardiovascular status. The nurse must be prepared to intervene if symptoms of hypovolemia, shock, or both are found. These symptoms include hypotension, prolonged capillary refill (>3 seconds), tachycardia initially then bradycardia, and continued respiratory distress despite the provision of oxygen and ventilation.

Blood pressure (BP) is monitored routinely in the sick neonate by either internal or external means. Direct recording with arterial catheters is often used but carries the risks inherent in any procedure in which a catheter is introduced into an artery. An umbilical venous catheter may also be used to monitor the neonate's central venous pressure. Oscillometry (Dinamap) and Doppler transcutaneous apparatus are simple, effective means for detecting alterations in systemic BP (hypotension or hypertension).

Maintaining Body Temperature

Preterm infants are susceptible to temperature instability as a result of numerous factors. Preterm infants are at high risk for heat loss because of the large surface area in relation to body weight. Other factors that place preterm infants at risk for temperature instability include the following:

- Minimal insulating subcutaneous fat
- Limited stores of brown fat (an internal source for the generation of heat present in normal term infants)
- Decreased or absent reflex control of skin capillaries (vasoconstriction)
- Inadequate muscle mass activity (therefore the preterm infant is unable to produce its own heat)
- Poor muscle tone, resulting in more body surface area being exposed to the cooling effects of the environment
- An immature temperature regulation center in the brain
- Increased insensible water losses
- Decreased ability to increase oxygen consumption
- Decreased caloric intake

The goal of thermoregulation is a neutral thermal environment (NTE), which is the environmental temperature at which oxygen consumption and metabolic rate are minimal but adequate to maintain the body temperature (Horns, 2002). The NTE for preterm infants weighing less than 1000 g is very narrow, and the prediction of NTE for each infant is impossible. With knowledge of the four mechanisms of heat transfer (i.e., convection, conduction, radiation, and evaporation), the nurse can create an environment for the preterm infant that prevents temperature instability (see Chapter 24). The infant is kept in a radiant warmer or incubator with control settings at a temperature to maintain the NTE. Since overheating produces an increase in oxygen and calorie consumption, the infant is also jeopardized if he or she becomes hyperthermic (apnea and flushed color may indicate hyperthermia). Unlike older children, the preterm infant is not able to sweat and thus dissipate heat.

Skin-to-skin (kangaroo) contact between the stable preterm infant and parent is also a viable option for interaction because of the maintenance of appropriate body temperature by the infant.

Central Nervous System Function

The preterm infant's central nervous system (CNS) is susceptible to injury as a result of the following problems:

- Birth trauma with damage to immature structures
- Bleeding from fragile capillaries
- Impaired coagulation process, including prolonged prothrombin time
- Recurrent anoxic and hyperoxic episodes
- Predisposition to hypoglycemia
- Fluctuating systemic blood pressure with concomitant variation in cerebral flow and pressure

In the preterm neonate neurologic function is dependent on gestational age, associated illness factors, and predisposing factors such as intrauterine asphyxia, which may have caused neurologic damage. Clinical signs of neurologic dysfunction may be subtle, nonspecific, or specific; however, five categories of clinical manifestations should be carefully evaluated in the preterm infant. These clinical signs include seizure activity, hyperirritability, CNS depression, elevated intracranial pressure, and abnormal movements such as decorticate posturing (Blackburn, 1998). Primary and tendon reflexes are generally present in preterm infants by 28 weeks of gestation and should be part of the neurologic examination. Ongoing assessment and documentation of these neurologic signs are needed both for the purposes of discharge teaching and making follow-up recommendations, as well as for their predictive value.

Maintaining Adequate Nutrition

The initial goal of neonatal nutrition in the preterm infant is to prevent catabolism and excess fluid losses. Once the infant has been stabilized in regard to respiratory and cardiac function, the goal of nutrition is to promote normal growth and development. However, the maintenance of adequate nutrition in the preterm infant is complicated by problems with intake and metabolism of nutrients adequate to promote physical and brain growth. The preterm infant has the following disadvantages with regard to intake: weak or absent suck, swallow, and gag reflexes; a small stomach capacity; and immature digestive enzymes. The preterm infant's metabolic functions are compromised by a limited store of nutrients, a decreased ability to digest proteins and absorb nutrients, and immature enzyme systems.

The nurse must continuously assess the infant's nutritional status. Some preterm infants require gavage or intravenous (IV) feedings instead of oral feedings, depending on the gestational age and birth weight and existing illness factors such as respiratory distress.

Maintaining Renal Function

The preterm infant's immature renal system is unable to (1) adequately excrete metabolites and drugs; (2) concentrate urine; or (3) maintain acid-base, fluid, or electrolyte balance. Therefore intake and output, as well as specific gravity, must be assessed. Laboratory tests must be performed to assess acid-base and electrolyte balance. Medication levels are also monitored in preterm infants because metabolism via renal and hepatic routes is often hindered. Because of great variability in drug metabolism, serum levels are obtained to ensure adequate therapeutic range for treatment and to prevent toxicity.

Maintaining Hematologic Status

The preterm infant is predisposed to hematologic problems because of the following conditions:

- Increased capillary fragility
- Increased tendency to bleed (prolonged prothrombin time and partial thromboplastin time)
- Decreased production of red blood cells (RBCs) resulting from physiologic rapid decrease in erythropoiesis after birth
- Large amount of fetal hemoglobin
- Loss of blood attributable to frequent blood sampling for laboratory tests
- Decreased RBC survival related to the relatively larger size of the RBC and its increased permeability to sodium and potassium
- Decreased levels of circulating albumin

The nurse assesses such infants for any evidence of bleeding from puncture sites and the gastrointestinal (GI) tract. Infants are also examined for signs of anemia (e.g., decreased hemoglobin and hematocrit levels, pale skin, increased apnea, lethargy, tachycardia, and poor weight gain). The amount of blood withdrawn for laboratory testing is monitored.

Resisting Infection

Preterm infants are at increased risk for infection because they have a shortage of stored maternal immunoglobulins, an impaired ability to make antibodies, and a compromised integumentary system (i.e., thin skin). Preterm and term infants exhibit various nonspecific signs and symptoms of infection (Box 27-2). Early identification and treatment of sepsis is essential.

BOX 27-2

Signs and Symptoms of Neonatal Infection

Many are subtle and nonspecific
- Temperature instability
- Hypothermia—most common
- Hyperthermia—rarely

CNS changes
- Lethargy
- Irritability
- Altered LOC (level of consciousness)

Changes in color
- Cyanosis, pallor
- Mottling (marbling)
- Jaundice

Cardiovascular instability
- Poor perfusion
- Hypotension
- Bradycardia/tachycardia
- Prolonged capillary refill (>3 seconds)

Respiratory distress
- Tachypnea/bradypnea
- Apnea
- Retractions, nasal flaring, grunting

GI problems
- Feeding intolerance, increased residuals
- Vomiting
- Diarrhea
- Bloody stools (frank or occult positive)
- Abdominal distention

Metabolic instability
- Glucose instability
- Metabolic acidosis

Other
- Electrolyte imbalance
- Decreased urinary output

Protection from Infection

Protection from infection is an integral part of all newborn care, but preterm and sick infants are particularly susceptible to infectious organisms. As with all aspects of care, strict handwashing is the single most important measure to prevent nosocomial infections. Personnel with known infectious disorders are barred from the unit until they are no longer infectious. Standard Precautions are instituted in all nursery areas as a method of infection control to protect the infants and staff.

Skin Care

The skin of preterm infants is characteristically immature relative to that of full-term infants. Because of its increased sensitivity and fragility, the use of alkaline-based soap that might destroy the acid mantle of the skin is avoided. The increased permeability of the skin facilitates absorption of ingredients that may become toxic. All skin products (e.g., alcohol or povidone-iodine) are used with caution, and the skin is rinsed with water afterward because these substances may cause severe irritation and chemical burns in low-birth-weight (LBW) infants. Adhesives used after heel sticks or to secure monitoring equipment or intravenous infusions may excoriate the skin or adhere to the skin surface so firmly that the epidermis can be separated from understructures and pulled away with the tape. The use of pectin barriers and hydrocolloid adhesives may be useful because these products mold well to skin contours and adhere in moist conditions. Recommendations for protecting the integrity of premature skin include using minimal adhesive tape, backing the tape with cotton, and delaying adhesive and pectin barrier removal until adherence is reduced (Lund & Kuller, 2003). An emollient such as Eucerin or Aquaphor may also be used to promote skin integrity and prevent dry, cracking, and peeling skin in infants at risk for skin breakdown (Horii & Lane, 2001; Lund et al, 1999). Solvents used to remove tape are avoided because they tend to dry and burn the delicate skin. Guidelines for skin care are listed in the Guidelines box.

Guidelines

NEONATAL SKIN CARE

General Skin Care

Assessment

Assess skin every day or once a shift for redness, dryness, flaking, scaling, rashes, lesions, excoriation, or breakdown.

Evaluate and report abnormal skin findings and analyze for possible causation.

Intervene according to interpretation of findings or physician order.

Bathing

Initial bath

Assess for stable temperature a minimum of 2 to 4 hours before first bath.

Use cleansing agents with neutral pH or minimal dyes or perfume in water.

Do not completely remove vernix.

Bathe preterm infant (<32 weeks) in sterile water only.

Routine

Decrease frequency of baths to every second or third day by daily cleansing of eye, oral, and diaper areas and pressure points.

Use cleanser or soaps no more than 2 to 3 times a week.

Avoid rubbing skin during bathing or drying.

Immerse stable infants fully (except head) in an appropriately sized tub.

Use swaddled immersion bathing technique: slow unwrapping after gently lowering into water for sensitive, but stable, infants needing assistance with motor system reactivity.

Emollients

Follow hospital protocol or consider the following:

Apply petroleum-based ointment without preservative sparingly to body (avoid face, head) every 6 to 12 hours during the first 2 to 4 weeks for infants <32 weeks (except when neonate is in radiant heat source).

Apply emollient as needed to infants >32 weeks for dry, flaking skin.

Adhesives

Decrease use as much as possible.

Use transparent adhesive dressings to secure IVs, catheters, and central lines.

Use hydrogel or limb electrodes.

Consider pectin barriers (Hollihesive,* Duoderm†) beneath adhesives to protect skin.

Secure pulse oximeter probe or electrodes with elasticized dressing material (carefully avoid restricting blood flow). Change pulse oximeter site at least every 8 hours or more often, especially with compromised circulation.

Do not use adhesive remover, solvents, and bonding agents.

Avoid removing adhesives for at least 24 hours after application.

Adhesive removal can be facilitated using water, mineral oil, or petrolatum.

Remove adhesives or skin barriers slowly, supporting the skin underneath with one hand and gently peeling away the product from the skin with the other hand.‡

Antiseptic Agents

Apply before invasive procedures.

Apply povidone-iodine two times, air dry for 30 seconds; remove completely with sterile water or sterile saline solution following procedure.

Avoid use of alcohol.

Transepidermal Water Loss (TEWL)

Minimize TEWL and heat loss in small premature infants <30 weeks by:

- Measuring ambient humidity during first weeks of life.
- Considering an increase in humidity to >70% by using one or more of the following options or hospital guidelines:
  Transparent dressings.
  Emollient application every 6 to 8 hours or according to hospital protocol.
  Servocontrolled humidifying incubator.

Skin Breakdown

Prevention

Decrease pressure from externally applied forces using water, air, or gel mattresses, sheepskin, or cotton bedding.

Provide adequate nutrition, including protein, fat, and zinc.

Apply transparent adhesive dressings to protect arms, elbows, and knees from friction injury.

Use tracheostomy and gastrostomy dressings for drainage and relief of pressure from trach or G tube (Hydrasorb or Lyofoam).†

Use emollient in the diaper area (groin and thighs) to reduce urine irritation.

Treating Skin Breakdown

Irrigate wound every 4 to 8 hours with warm half-strength normal saline (NS) using a 30-ml or larger syringe and 20-gauge Teflon catheter.

Culture wound and treat if signs of infection (excessive redness, swelling, pain on touch, heat, or resistance to healing) are present.

Use transparent adhesive dressing for uninfected wounds.

Apply hydrogel with or without antibacterial or antifungal ointments (as ordered) for infected wounds (may need to moisten before removal).

Use hydrocolloid for deep, uninfected wounds (leave in place for 5 to 7 days) or as an ostomy barrier and to improve appliance adhesion; warm barrier in hand for several minutes to soften before applying to skin.

Avoid use of antiseptic solutions for wound cleansing (used for intact skin only).

Treating Diaper Dermatitis

Maintain clean, dry skin; use absorbent diapers; and change often.

If mild irritation occurs, use petrolatum barrier.

For developing dermatitis, apply a generous quantity of zinc-oxide barrier.

Modified from Kuller JM: Skin breakdown: risk factors, prevention, and treatment, *NINR* 1(1):33-42, 2001; Johnson FE, Maikler VE: Nurses' adoption of the AWHONN/NANN Neonatal Skin Care Project, *NINR* 1(1):59-67, 2001; Lund CH, Kuller J, Lott JW: Neonatal skin care: clinical outcomes of the AWHONN/NANN evidence-based clinical practice guideline, *J Obstet Gynecol Neonatal Nurs* 30(1):41-51, 2001; Taquino LT: Promoting wound healing in the neonatal setting: process versus protocol, *J Perinat Neonatal Nurs* 14(1):108-118, 2000; Lund C, Lane A, Raines DA: Neonatal skin care: the scientific basis for practice, *J Obstet Gynecol Neonatal Nurs* 28(3):241-254, 1999; Malloy MB, Perez-Woods R: Neonatal skin care: prevention of skin breakdown, *Pediatr Nurs* 17(1):41-48, 1991.

*Hollister, Libertyville, IL.

†ConvaTec/Bristol-Myers Squibb Co, Princeton, NJ.

‡Caution: Scissors are not to be used for tape or dressing removal because of hazard of cutting skin or amputating tiny digits.

Continued

Guidelines

NEONATAL SKIN CARE—cont'd

Treating Diaper Dermatitis—cont'd

For severe dermatitis, identify cause (frequent stooling from spina bifida, severe opiate withdrawal, or malabsorption syndrome) and treat.

Treat *Candida albicans* with antifungal ointment or cream.

Avoid powders and antibiotic ointments (not recommended).

(See Cord and Circumcision Care, Chapter 25.)

Other Skin Care Concerns

Use of Substances on Skin

Evaluate all substances that come in contact with infant's skin.

Before using any topical agent, analyze components of preparation and:

- Use sparingly and only when necessary.
- Confine use to smallest possible area.
- Whenever possible and appropriate, wash off with water.
- Monitor infant carefully for signs of toxicity and systemic effects.

Use of Thermal Devices

Avoid heat lamps because of increased potential for burns. If needed, measure actual temperature of exposed skin every 15 minutes.

When using heating pads (Aqua-K pads):

- Change infant's position every 15 minutes initially and then every 1 to 2 hours.
- Preset temperature of heating pads <40° C (104° F).

When using preheated transcutaneous electrodes:

- Avoid use on infants weighing less than 1000 g.
- Set at lowest possible temperature (<44° C [111.2° F]) and secure with plastic wrap.
- Use pulse oximetry rather than transcutaneous monitoring whenever possible.

When prewarming heels before phlebotomy, avoid temperatures >40° C.

Warm ambient humidity, direct away from infant; use aerosolized sterile water and maintain ambient temperature so as not to exceed 40° C.

Document use of all heating devices.

Use of Fluid Therapy/Hemodynamic Monitoring

Be certain fingers or toes are visible whenever extremity is used for IV or arterial line.

Assess extremity distal to insertion site hourly for signs of poor circulation, edema, or inadequate perfusion.

Secure catheter or needle with transparent dressing/tape to promote easy visualization of site.

Assess site hourly for signs of ischemia, infiltration, and inadequate perfusion (check capillary refill).

Avoid use of restraints (e.g., arm boards); if used, check that they are secured safely and not restricting circulation or movement (check for pressure areas).

Use commercial IV protector (i.e., I.V. House) with minimal tape.

Growth and Development Potential

Although it is impossible to predict with complete accuracy the growth and development potential of each preterm newborn, some findings support an anticipated favorable outcome in the absence of ongoing medical sequelae that can affect growth, such as chronic lung disease (CLD) (formerly bronchopulmonary dysplasia), necrotizing enterocolitis, and CNS problems. The lower the birth weight, the greater the likelihood of negative sequelae. The growth and development milestones (e.g., motor milestones, vocalization, and growth) are corrected for gestational age until the child is approximately 2½ years of age.

The age of a preterm newborn is corrected by adding the gestational age and the postnatal age. For example, an infant born at 32 weeks of gestation 4 weeks ago would now be considered 36 weeks of age. The infant's corrected age 6 months after the birth date is then 4 months, and the infant's responses are accordingly evaluated against the norm expected for a 4-month-old infant.

Certain measurable factors predict normal growth and development. The preterm infant experiences catch-up body growth during the first 2 to 3 years of life, with maximum growth occurring between 36 and 40 weeks of postconceptional age. The head is the first to experience catch-up growth, followed by a gain in weight and height. An effective discharge plan should include frequent outpatient follow-up with a primary care practitioner and developmental specialist for monitoring growth and achievement of developmental milestones.

Parental Adaptation to Preterm Infant

Parents who experience the preterm birth of their infant have a much different experience from parents giving birth to a full-term infant. Because of this difference, parental attachment and adaptation to the parental role may differ as well.

Parental Tasks

Parents must accomplish a number of psychologic tasks before effective relationships and parenting patterns can evolve. These tasks include the following:

- Experiencing anticipatory grief over the potential loss of an infant. The parent grieves in preparation for the infant's possible death, although the parent clings to the hope that the infant will survive. This begins during labor and lasts until the infant dies or shows evidence of surviving.
- Acceptance by the mother of her failure to give birth to a healthy, full-term infant. Grief and depression typify this phase, which persists until the infant is out of danger and is expected to survive.
- Resuming the process of relating to the infant. As the infant's condition begins to improve and the infant gains weight, feeds by nipple, and is weaned from the incubator, the parent can begin the process of developing an attachment to the infant that was interrupted by the infant's critical condition at birth.
- Learning how this infant differs in special needs and growth patterns, caregiving needs, and growth and development expectations.
- Adjusting the home environment to the needs of the new infant. Visitors may be limited to reduce the risk of expo-

Critical Thinking Exercise

PRETERM INFANT

After having two full-term pregnancies, Charlotte gave birth to her third baby at 28 weeks of gestation. The infant was transported to a tertiary center that could provide the care the infant needed. Charlotte lives 60 miles from the city in which the tertiary center is located, and she is to be discharged tomorrow. It is anticipated that the infant will require a stay in the NICU for at least 8 more weeks. You have been caring for Charlotte and are preparing her for discharge. You have spoken to the nurse caring for the baby. The infant is stable at present, in a small amount of oxygen, and has started gavage feeding. The IV is to be discontinued when the infant can tolerate adequate amounts of milk. The nursery has asked for breast milk from Charlotte to feed the baby.

1. Evidence—Is there sufficient evidence to draw conclusions about what to tell Charlotte about her own recovery and the expected progress of the baby?
2. Assumptions—What assumptions can be made about the following?
   a. Charlotte's postpartum recovery
   b. The infant's expected progress
   c. The possibility of Charlotte furnishing breast milk for the baby
   d. The long-term outcome for the baby
3. What implications and priorities for nursing care can be drawn at this time?
4. Does the evidence objectively support your conclusion?
5. Are there alternative perspectives to your conclusion?

sure to pathogens, and the environmental temperature may be altered to optimize conditions for the infant.

Grandparents and siblings also react to the birth of the preterm infant. Parents must deal with the grief of grandparents and the bewilderment and anger of the infant's siblings at the apparent disproportionate amount of parental time spent with the newborn.

Parental Responses

Parents progress through stages as they interact with their infants, from maintaining an *en face* position and stroking and touching their infant (Fig. 27-1) to assuming some child care activities such as feeding, bathing, and diapering the infant.

Parenting Disorders

The incidence of physical and emotional abuse is greater in infants who, because of preterm birth or illness, are separated from their parents for a time after birth. Physical abuse includes varying degrees of poor nutrition, poor hygiene, and bodily harm. Emotional abuse ranges from subtle disinterest to outright dislike of the infant. Appropriate resources should be made available to assess the parent's feelings regarding the preterm infant's birth. In addition, proper guidance and counseling are made available, including posthospital discharge, to help families adjust to and care for the preterm infant. The ultimate goal is for the family to incorporate the infant as a regular family member (Critical Thinking Exercise).

Factors surrounding the birth may predispose parents to subconsciously or overtly reject the infant. These factors might include parental pain and anxiety, a heavy financial burden because of the cost of the infant's care, unresolved anticipatory grief, threat to self-esteem, or the fact that the infant was the product of an unwanted pregnancy. The goal of health professionals is early identification of inadequate coping skills and potentially dysfunctional parenting so that further problems can be prevented and early intervention accessed.

Nursing Diagnoses

Potential nursing diagnoses for high risk infants and their parents include the following:

- *Ineffective breathing pattern related to*
  —decreased number of functional alveoli
  —surfactant deficiency
  —immature respiratory control
  —increased pulmonary vascular resistance
- *Ineffective thermoregulation related to*
  —immature CNS thermoregulatory control
  —increased heat loss to environment and inability to produce heat
  —greater body surface exposed to environment
  —decreased brown fat reserves to produce body heat

A

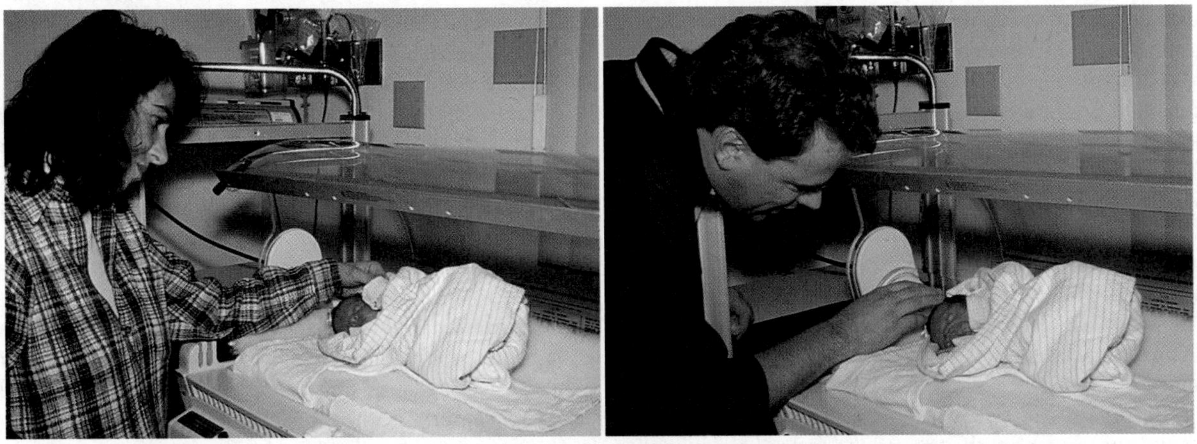

B

Fig. 27-1 **A,** Mother interacts with her preterm infant by touch. **B,** Father interacts with his newborn by stroking and touching infant with fingertips. (Courtesy Michael S. Clement, MD, Mesa, AZ.)

- *Risk for infection related to*
  - —invasive procedures
  - —decreased immune response
  - —ineffective skin barrier
- *Parental anxiety related to*
  - —lack of knowledge about infant's condition
  - —lack of knowledge regarding infant's prognosis (uncertain outcome)
  - —inability to perform expected caregiving activities
  - —neonatal intensive care unit (NICU) environment noise and high-tech care

Expected Outcomes

The nursing plan of care for the preterm infant is dictated by the physiologic needs of the infant's immature systems and often involves emergency treatments and procedures. Nursing care is a critical element in the infant's chances for survival. In addition to meeting the infant's physical needs, nursing care is planned in conjunction with parents to promote parent-infant attachment and interaction. Expected outcomes are presented in patient-centered terms and include that the infant will do the following:

- Maintain adequate physiologic functioning (airway, breathing, circulation)
- Receive adequate nutrition
- Maintain body temperature
- Remain free of infection
- Experience appropriate parent-infant interactions

Expected outcomes for the parents include that they will do the following:

- Perceive the infant as potentially normal (if this is medically substantiated)
- Provide care comfortably
- Experience pride and satisfaction in the care of the infant
- Organize their time and energies to meet the love, attention, and care needs of the other members of the family as well as their own needs.

Plan of Care and Implementation

The best environment for fetal growth and development is in the uterus of a healthy, well-nourished woman. The goal of care for the preterm infant is to provide an extrauterine environment that approximates a healthy intrauterine environment in order to promote normal growth and development. Medical and nursing personnel, respiratory therapists, occupational and physical therapists, dietitians, and pharmacists work as a team to provide the intensive care needed.

The admission of a preterm newborn to the intensive care nursery is usually an emergency situation. Resuscitation is started in the birthing unit, and warmth and oxygen are provided during transport to the nursery. A rapid initial assessment is done to determine the infant's need for lifesaving treatment.

The nurse uses many technologic support systems to monitor body responses and maintain body functions in the infant. Technical skill needs to be combined with a gentle touch and concern about the traumatic effects of harsh lighting and the volume of machinery noise. The NICU environment may be a major contributing factor to learning and behavioral problems in preterm infants (Blackburn, 1998).

Physical Care

The preterm infant's environmental support typically consists of the following equipment and procedures:

- Incubator or radiant warmer to control body temperature (NTE)
- Oxygen administration, depending on infant's pulmonary and circulatory status
- Electronic monitors as needed for observation of respiratory and cardiac functions
- Assistive devices for positioning the infant
- Clustering of care and minimization of stimulation

Various metabolic support measures that may be instituted consist of the following:

- Parenteral fluids to support nutrition and hydration
- IV access to facilitate antibiotic therapy if sepsis is a concern
- Blood work to monitor arterial blood gases (ABGs), blood glucose level, electrolytes, and other diagnostic studies (C-reactive protein, white count with differential, hemoglobin and hematocrit) as indicated

Maintaining Body Temperature

The high risk infant is susceptible to heat loss and its complications (see Fig. 24-1). In addition, LBW infants may be unable to increase their metabolic rate because of impaired gas exchange, caloric intake restrictions in relation to high expenditure, or poor thermoregulation. Transepidermal water loss is greater because of skin immaturity in ELBW and very-low-birth-weight (VLBW) infants (i.e., those weighing less than 1000 g and 1500 g, respectively) and can contribute to temperature instability.

High risk infants are cared for in the thermoneutral environment created by use of an external heat source. A probe applied to the infant is attached to an external heat source supplied by a radiant warmer or a servocontrolled incubator. Studies indicate that optimum thermoneutrality cannot be predicted for every high risk infant's needs. Guidelines for providing an optimum thermal environment for the VLBW infant suggest maintaining the infant's core temperature at rest within a range of 36.7° to 37.3° C, with core and mean temperatures changing less than 0.2° and 0.3° C an hour (Sauer, Dane, & Visser, 1984). Standard guidelines for maintaining NTE in the LBW infant are published (Blake & Murray, 2002). Further research is needed to define an NTE for the ELBW infant.

Warming the Hypothermic Infant

Rapid changes in body temperature may cause apnea and acidosis in the neonate. Therefore the warming of a hypothermic infant should occur over a period of hours; rapid rewarming may cause apnea and too slow rewarming increases metabolic distress and oxygen consumption. Rewarming must therefore be individualized for each infant according to illness and ability to produce heat. To accomplish this, the infant is placed either under a radiant warmer or in an incubator with a servocontrol mechanism. It has been suggested that rewarming proceed at a rate of 1° to 2° C per hour. Another approach is to gradually increase the environmental temperature of the incubator and increase the humidity (above 70%) (Blackburn, 2003). Appropriate guidelines for rewarming the hypothermic infant should be consulted for further information.

Weaning the Infant from the Incubator

To wean the infant from the incubator, the incubator heat is decreased slowly over at least several hours. On average, infants who are medically stable, gaining weight, and tolerating enteral feedings and weigh 1300 g to 1500 g may be weaned (depending on institution protocol). The following general guidelines may be followed to wean the infant from the incubator:

- Disconnect the Servo control probe (if still in use)
- Dress the infant in a diaper, shirt, and cap
- Lower the incubator temperature by no more than 0.5° C per each 2-hour period
- Record the temperature of both the infant and the incubator
- Assess the infant's responses to the changes every hour until four stable readings are obtained
- Monitor the infant's temperature and other vital signs

This procedure is repeated until the incubator temperature is the same as the room temperature, and the infant's body temperature consistently remains in the range of 36° to 37° C. The infant is placed in an open bassinet when the body temperature is stable, after which it is reassessed in conjunction with the delivery of routine care. If necessary, the infant may be returned to the incubator and weaning repeated once the infant is able to regulate its temperature.

Oxygen Therapy

The goals of oxygen therapy are to provide adequate oxygen to the tissues, prevent lactic acid accumulation resulting from hypoxia, and at the same time avoid the potentially negative effects of oxygen barotrauma. Numerous methods have been devised to improve oxygenation. All require that the gas be warmed and humidified before entering the respiratory tract. If the infant does not require mechanical ventilation, oxygen can be supplied to a plastic hood placed over the infant's head to supply variable concentrations of humidified oxygen. Because oxygen therapy is not without inherent hazards, each infant must be carefully monitored to prevent hyperoxemia and hypoxemia.

Infants who require oxygen should have their respiratory status assessed accurately every 1 to 2 hours; this includes a continuous pulse oximetry reading and, as warranted, ABG measurement. Vital signs including heart rate and blood pressure are monitored to ensure not only adequate respiratory function but also adequate circulation and perfusion of tissues. The interventions implemented range from hood oxygen administration to ventilator therapy.

Interest in the resuscitation of asphyxiated newborns with 21% oxygen rather than 100% oxygen has increased; preliminary studies demonstrate no significant neurologic morbidities at 18 to 24 months in newborns resuscitated with 21% oxygen (Saugstad et al, 2003). Proponents for room air resuscitation suggest fewer complications are associated with oxidative stress and hyperoxemia when room air is administered (Vento et al, 2003). Large multicenter studies are currently in progress to determine the optimum concentration of oxygen for resuscitation.

Oxygen Hood

Oxygen in a specified concentration can be administered by hood to infants who do not require mechanical pressure support. The hood is a clear plastic cover that is sized to fit over the head and neck of the infant (Fig. 27-2, *A*). The oxygen level is checked every 1 to 2 hours and the concentration adjusted in response to the infant's condition.

Nasal Cannula

Low-flow amounts of oxygen can be administered by nasal cannula (Fig. 27-2, *B*). Nasal cannula are used for infants who are out of the acute phase of illness and recuperating but still require supplemental oxygen; they are the preferred method for home oxygen administration. The infant receives an adequate, continuous flow of oxygen while allowing optimal vision, positioning, and parental holding. Infants can also breastfeed while receiving oxygen by this method. The nasal prongs must be inspected often to ensure that they are not partially obstructed by milk or secretions.

Continuous Distending Pressure

Infants who are unable to maintain an adequate PaO_2 despite the administration of oxygen by hood or nasal cannula may require the delivery of oxygen using continuous distending airway pressure via continuous positive airway pressure (CPAP) or continuous negative pressure. CPAP delivers oxygen at a preset pressure (Fig. 27-3, *A*) by means of nasal prongs, nasal pharyngeal tubes, endotracheal tube, or face mask. Nasal prongs are the most common method of CPAP delivery. An

A

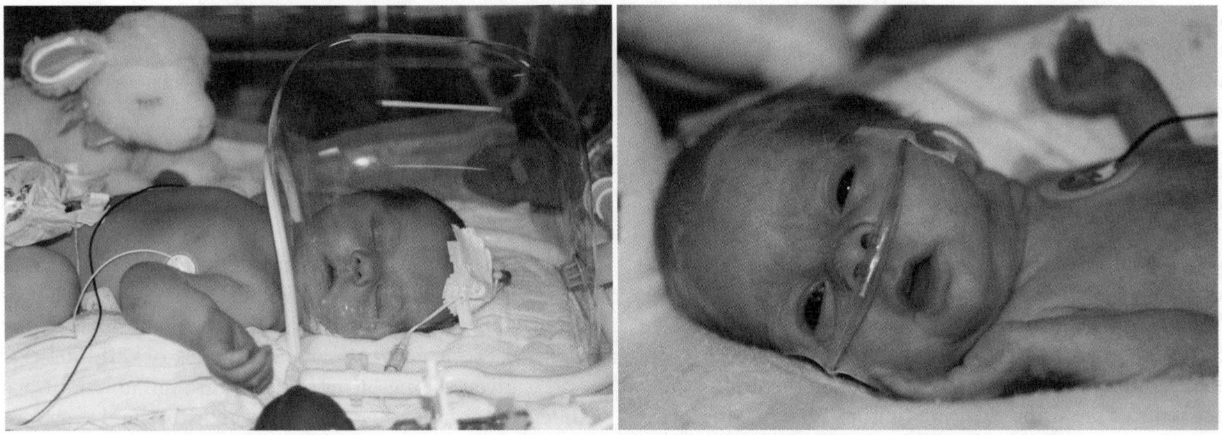

B

Fig. 27-2 **A,** Infant under hood. **B,** Infant with nasal cannula. (Courtesy Victoria Langer, RNC, MSN, NNP.) From Dickason E, Silverman B, Kaplan J: *Maternal-infant nursing care,* ed 3, St Louis, 1998, Mosby.)

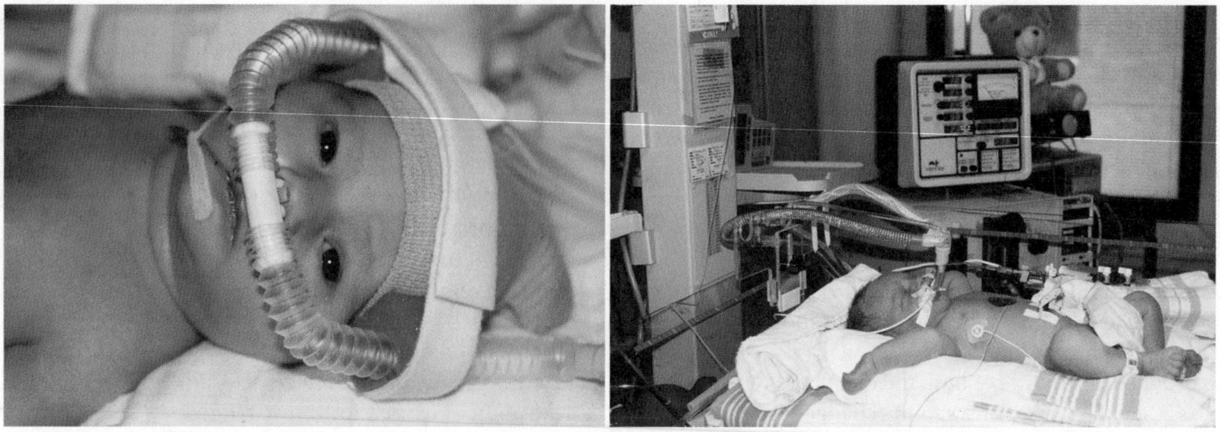

A B

Fig. 27-3 **A,** Infant receiving ventilatory assistance with nasal continuous positive airway pressure (CPAP). **B,** Infant intubated and on ventilator. (Courtesy Victoria Langer, RNC, MSN, NNP.) From Dickason E, Silverman B, Kaplan J: *Maternal-infant nursing care,* ed 3, St Louis, 1998, Mosby.)

orogastric tube may be necessary for decompression of the stomach during use of nasal prongs. CPAP increases the functional residual capacity; improves the diffusion time of pulmonary gases, including oxygen; and can decrease pulmonary vascular resistance and intrapulmonary shunting. If implemented early enough, CPAP may preclude the need for mechanical ventilation. CPAP is the preferred mode for infants who require minor distending pressure without the trauma associated with endotracheal intubation and its inherent complications (Hagedorn, Gardner, & Abman, 2002).

Mechanical Ventilation

Mechanical ventilation must be implemented if other methods of therapy cannot correct abnormalities in oxygenation. Its use is indicated whenever blood gas values reveal the existence of severe hypoxemia or severe hypercapnia (Fig. 27-3, *B*). The condition of the infant experiencing apnea with bradycardia, ineffective respiratory effort, shock, asphyxia, infection, meconium aspiration syndrome, respiratory distress syndrome (RDS), or congenital defects that affect ventilation may also deteriorate and require intubation to reverse the process. Ventilator settings are determined by the infant's particular needs. The ventilator is set to provide a predetermined amount of oxygen to the infant during spontaneous respirations and also to provide mechanical ventilation in the absence of spontaneous respirations. Newer technologies in ventilation allow oxygen to be delivered at lower pressures and in assist modes, thereby preventing the overriding of the infant's spontaneous breathing and providing distending pressures within a physiologic range, decreasing barotrauma and associated complications such as pneumothorax and pulmonary interstitial emphysema. See Table 27-1 for an explanation of types of mechanical ventilation used in newborns.

Surfactant Replacement Therapy

Surfactant is a surface-active phospholipid secreted by the alveolar epithelium. Acting much like a detergent, this substance reduces the surface tension of fluids that line the alveoli and respiratory passages, resulting in uniform expansion and maintenance of lung expansion at low intraalveolar pressure. Immature development of these functions produces consequences that seriously compromise respiratory efficiency. Deficient surfactant production causes unequal inflation of alveoli on inspiration and the collapse of alveoli on end expiration. Without surfactant, infants are unable to keep their lungs inflated and therefore exert a great deal of effort to reexpand the alveoli with each breath. With increasing exhaustion, infants are able to open fewer and fewer alveoli. This inability to maintain lung expansion produces widespread atelectasis.

In the absence of alveolar stability (normal functional residual capacity) and with progressive atelectasis, pulmonary vascular resistance (PVR) increases, whereas with normal lung expansion PVR decreases. Consequently, there is hypoperfusion to the lung tissue, with a decrease in effective pulmonary blood flow. The increase in PVR causes partial reversion to the fetal circulation, with a right-to-left shunting of blood through the persisting fetal communications—the ductus arteriosus and foramen ovale. Inadequate pulmonary perfusion and ventilation produce hypoxemia and hypercapnia. Pulmonary arterioles, with their thick muscular layer, are markedly reactive to diminished oxygen concentration. Thus, a decrease in oxygen tension causes vasoconstriction in the pulmonary arterioles that is further enhanced by a decrease in blood pH. This vasoconstriction contributes to a significant increase in PVR. In normal ventilation with increased oxygen concentration, the ductus arteriosus constricts, and the pulmonary vessels dilate to decrease PVR.

Surfactant can be administered as an adjunct to oxygen and ventilation therapy. Generally, infants born before 32 weeks of gestation do not have adequate amounts of pulmonary surfactant to survive extrauterine life. In many centers the use of prophylactic surfactant is reserved for infants younger than 29 weeks who will likely have RDS (Hagedorn et al, 2002). Exogenous surfactant is manufactured artificially or extracted from bovine, porcine, or calf lung extract and is given as one or more doses through an endotracheal tube. The infant must be monitored for the occurrence of potential side effects such as patent ductus arteriosus and pulmonary hemorrhage. Although use of this medication has been associated with a significantly reduced length of

Table 27-1

Common Methods for Assisted Ventilation in Neonatal Respiratory Distress*

METHOD	DESCRIPTION	HOW PROVIDED
Continuous distending pressure—continuous positive airway pressure (CPAP)	Provides constant distending pressure to airway in spontaneously breathing infant	Nasal prongs Endotracheal tube Face mask Nasal cannula or nasopharyngeal tubes Bubble CPAP uses water resistance
Intermittent mandatory ventilation (IMV)	Allows infant to breathe spontaneously at own rate but provides mechanical cycled respirations and pressure at regular preset intervals; infant may maintain asynchronous ventilation efforts, which diminishes effective gas exchange, air leaks, and air trapping; uses positive end-expiratory pressure (PEEP)	Endotracheal intubation
Synchronized intermittent mandatory ventilation (SIMV)	Mechanically delivered breaths are synchronized to the onset of spontaneous patient breaths; assist/control mode facilitates full inspiratory synchrony; involves signal detection of onset of spontaneous respiration from abdominal movement, thoracic impedance, and airway pressure or flow changes; *pressure support ventilation* provides an inspiratory pressure assist when spontaneous breathing is detected to decrease infant's work of breathing	Patient-triggered infant ventilator with signal detector and assist/control (A/C) mode; endotracheal tube; SIMV, A/C, and pressure support are also referred to as patient-triggered ventilation
Volume guarantee ventilation	Delivers a predetermined volume of gas using an inspiratory pressure that varies according to the infant's lung compliance (often used in conjunction with SIMV)	Volume guarantee ventilator with flow sensor; endotracheal tube
High-frequency oscillation (HFO)	Application of high-frequency, low-volume, sine-wave flow oscillations to airway at rates between 480 and 1200 breaths/min	Variable-speed piston pump (or loudspeaker, fluidic oscillator); endotracheal tube
High-frequency jet ventilation (HFJV)	Uses a separate, parallel, low-compliant circuit and injector port to deliver small pulses or jets of fresh gas deep into airway at rates between 250 and 900 breaths/min	May be used alone or with low-rate IMV; endotracheal tube

*This is not a comprehensive list of available ventilation modes. For more information, consult specific references on mechanical ventilation such as Donn SM, Sinha SK: Invasive and noninvasive neonatal mechanical ventilation, *Respir Care* 48(4):426-441, 2003.

time on mechanical ventilation and oxygen therapy and an increased survival rate in premature infants, it has not significantly decreased the incidence of CLD, intraventricular hemorrhage, or patent ductus arteriosus. The administration of antenatal steroids to the mother and surfactant replacement has decreased the incidence of RDS and concomitant morbidities.

Inhaled nitric oxide (INO), extracorporeal membrane oxygenation (ECMO), and liquid ventilation are additional therapies used in the treatment of respiratory distress and respiratory failure in neonates. INO is used in term and near-term infants with conditions such as persistent pulmonary hypertension, meconium aspiration syndrome, pneumonia, sepsis, and congenital diaphragmatic hernia to decrease or reverse pulmonary hypertension, pulmonary vasoconstriction, acidosis, and hypoxemia. Nitric oxide is a colorless, highly diffusable gas that can be administered through the ventilator circuit blended with oxygen. INO therapy may be used in conjunction with surfactant replacement therapy, high-frequency ventilation, or ECMO. INO has not proved to be significantly effective in decreasing RDS or in improved survival rates in preterm infants, although clinical trials are still ongoing (Kinsella & Abman, 2000; Kinsella et al, 1999). Clinical trials have demonstrated, however, that the use of INO improved ventilatory status in infants with pulmonary hypertension, decreased requirements for ventilatory support (Sadiq et al, 2003), and decreased the need for ECMO (Kinsella & Abman, 2000).

ECMO may be used in the management of term infants with acute severe respiratory failure for the same conditions as those mentioned for INO. This therapy involves a modified heart-lung machine, although in ECMO the heart is not stopped, and blood does not entirely bypass the lungs. Blood is shunted from a catheter in the right atrium or right internal jugular vein by gravity to a servo-regulated roller pump, pumped through a membrane lung where it is oxygenated, through a small heat exchanger where it is warmed, and then returned to the systemic circulation via a major artery such as the carotid artery to the aortic arch. ECMO provides oxygen to the circulation, allowing the lungs to "rest," and decreases pulmonary hypertension and hypoxemia in such conditions as persistent pulmonary hypertension of the newborn, congenital diaphragmatic hernia, sepsis, meconium aspiration, and severe pneumonia. ECMO is not used in preterm infants younger than 34 weeks of gestation because of the anticoagulant therapy required in the pump and circuits; this may increase the potential for intraventricular hemorrhage in such infants. In some centers the success of high frequency ventilation and INO has greatly decreased the demand for and use of ECMO.

Liquid ventilation has been used experimentally in various neonatal clinical trials to increase pulmonary compliance, decrease lung surface tension, and decrease inflating pressures and subsequent barotrauma in newborn respiratory failure. This therapy involves the use of *perfluorocarbons,* which are inert liquids derived by replacing all the carbon-bound hydrogen atoms on organic compounds with fluorine. Oxygen delivery in the compromised neonate is significantly improved with perfluorocarbons; antibiotics and surfactant may be administered directly into the lungs with liquid ventilation (LV) and removal of debris such as meconium is facilitated.

The use of permissive hypercapnia to decrease lung damage and the incidence of CLD in neonates has had varying results, and trial studies to date have not produced a significant decrease in outcomes of decreased mortality, decreased lung tissue damage, or pulmonary and neurodevelopmental morbidity (Thome & Carlo, 2002; Woodgate & Davies, 2001). In permissive hypercapnia, the $PaCO_2$ is allowed to reach levels in the range of 45 to 55 mm Hg, whereas the previous goal was to maintain the $PaCO_2$ in the range of 35 to 45 mm Hg. Hypercapnia has been linked with an increased incidence of intraventricular hemorrhage.

High-Frequency Ventilation

Other modes of ventilator therapy include high-frequency oscillator ventilation and jet ventilation (see Table 27-1). These methods of high-frequency ventilation work by providing smaller volumes of oxygen at a significantly more rapid rate (more than 300 breaths/min) than traditional mechanical ventilators. As a result, the intrathoracic pressure and the risk of barotrauma are decreased.

Weaning from Respiratory Assistance

The infant is ready to be weaned from respiratory assistance when the ABG and oxygen saturation levels are maintained within normal limits (WNL) and the infant is able to establish spontaneous ventilation sufficient to maintain acid-base balance. A spontaneous, adequate respiratory effort must be present, and the infant must show improved muscle tone during increased activity. Weaning is done in a stepwise and gradual manner. This may consist of the infant being extubated, placed on nasal CPAP, and then weaned to oxygen by means of a hood or nasal cannula. Throughout the weaning process the infant's oxygen levels are monitored by pulse oximetry, $tcPO_2$ monitoring, and blood gas levels.

Some infants are not able to be weaned from all oxygen support by the time of discharge from the hospital and may require home oxygen therapy for several months. CLD (bronchopulmonary dysplasia), or congenital anomalies such as repaired congenital diaphragmatic hernia or tracheoesophageal fistula, or a neurologic insult with resultant dysfunction may prevent weaning.

The parents need to be given consistent information and be reassured about the infant's respiratory progress. Decisions regarding the nature of continued interventions should be included in a multidisciplinary plan of care, and the therapy should be explained frequently to the family.

Nutritional Care

Optimum nutrition is critical in the management of LBW and preterm infants, but there are difficulties in providing for their nutritional needs. The various mechanisms for ingestion and digestion of foods are not fully developed; the more immature the infant, the greater the problem. In addition, the nutritional requirements for this group of infants are not known with certainty. It is known that all preterm infants are at risk because of poor nutritional stores and several physical and developmental characteristics.

An infant's need for rapid growth and daily maintenance must be met in the presence of several anatomic and physiologic disabilities. Although some sucking and swallowing activities are demonstrated before birth and in premature infants, coordination of these mechanisms does not occur until approximately 32 to 34 weeks of gestation, and they are not fully synchronized until 36 to 37 weeks. Initial sucking is not accompanied by swallowing, and esophageal contractions are uncoordinated. The gag reflex may not be developed until 36 weeks of gestation. Consequently, infants are highly prone to aspiration and its attendant dangers. As infants mature, the suck-swallow pattern develops but is slow and ineffectual, and these reflexes may also become easily exhausted.

The amount and method of feeding are determined by the size and condition of the infant. Nutrition can be provided by either the parenteral or enteral route or by a combination of the two. Infants who are ELBW, VLBW, or critically ill are often fed exclusively by the parenteral route because of their inability to digest and absorb enteral nutrition. Illness factors resulting in hypoxia and major organ immaturity further preclude the use of enteral feeding until the infant's condition has stabilized; necrotizing enterocolitis has previously been associated with enteral feedings in acutely ill or distressed infants (see Necrotizing Enterocolitis, p. 818). Total parenteral nutrition (TPN) support of acutely ill infants may be accomplished quite successfully with commercially available IV solutions specifically designed to meet the infant's nutritional needs, including protein, amino acids, trace minerals, vitamins, carbohydrates (dextrose), and fat (lipid emulsion).

Studies have shown that the early introduction of small amounts of enteral feedings in metabolically stable preterm infants is beneficial. These minimal enteral or trophic feedings have been shown to stimulate the infant's GI tract, preventing mucosal atrophy and subsequent enteral feeding difficulties. Minimal enteral feedings with as little as 0.1 to 4 ml/kg preterm formula or breast milk may be given by gavage as early as the second or third postnatal day. Parenteral hydration and nutrition is continued until the infant is able to tolerate an amount of enteral feeding sufficient to sustain growth. An increased incidence of necrotizing enterocolitis in those VLBW infants fed enterally has not been substantiated (Evans & Thureen, 2001). In fact, minimal enteral feedings increase mineral absorption, increase serum calcium and alkaline phosphatase activity, and substantially decrease the incidence of bilious gastric residuals and feeding intolerance in preterm infants (Schanler et al, 1999). Minimal enteral feedings have been recommended as the standard of care for feeding VLBW infants (Kliegman, 1999).

Type of Nourishment

The types of formulas used, the mode and volume of feeding, and the infant's feeding schedule are based on the findings yielded by assessment of the following variables:

- Weight of the infant
- Pattern of weight gain or loss (infants weighing less than 1500 g require more energy for growth and thermoregulation)
- Presence or absence of suck and swallow reflexes
- Behavioral readiness to take oral feedings
- Physical condition, including presence or absence of bowel sounds, abdominal distention, or bloody stools, as well as presence and degree of respiratory distress or apneic episodes
- Residual from previous feeding, if being gavage fed
- Malformations (especially GI defects)
- Renal function, including urinary output and laboratory values (e.g., nitrogen balance, electrolyte balance, and glucose level)

Sufficient evidence now indicates that human milk is the best source of nutrition for term and preterm infants. Studies indicate that even small preterm infants are able to breastfeed, if they have adequate sucking and swallowing reflexes and no other contraindications, such as respiratory complications, or concurrent illness are present (Morton, 2002). Mothers who wish to breastfeed their preterm infants are encouraged to pump their breasts until their infants are sufficiently stable to tolerate breastfeeding. Appropriate guidelines for the storage of expressed mother's milk (EMM) should be followed to decrease the risk of milk contamination and destruction of its beneficial properties.

Preterm infants may be able to successfully breastfeed earlier than previously believed (28 to 36 weeks); in addition, preterm infants who are breastfed rather than bottle-fed demonstrate fewer oxygen desaturations, absence of bradycardia, warmer skin temperature, and better coordination of breathing, sucking, and swallowing (Gardner, Snell, & Lawrence, 2002).

Commercially available preterm formulas are cow's milk–based; whey-predominant; and have a higher concentration of protein, calcium, and phosphorus than term formulas to meet the unique needs of the preterm infant (American Academy of Pediatrics, 2004). Most preterm formulas are either 22 cal/oz or 24 cal/oz. The preparation of powdered formula in preterm infants should be carefully performed under strict aseptic technique, preferably in a pharmacy, and the formula properly refrigerated to prevent infection (American Academy of Pediatrics, 2004).

NURSE ALERT Contamination of powdered infant formula in hospitals by *Enterobacter sakazakii* has been associated with serious neonatal infections, necrotizing enterocolitis, and mortality (*Morbidity and Mortality Weekly Report* [MMWR], 2002; van Acker et al, 2001). When possible, alternatives to powdered formula should be chosen; otherwise, such formula should be carefully mixed in a designated preparation room using aseptic technique. Continuous infusion of powdered formula should not exceed 4 hours (MMWR, 2002). ■

Hydration

High risk infants often receive supplemental parenteral fluids to supply additional calories, electrolytes, or water. Adequate hydration is particularly important in preterm infants because their extracellular water content is higher (70% in full-term infants and up to 90% in preterm infants), their body surface is larger, and the capacity for osmotic diuresis is limited in preterm infants' underdeveloped kidneys. Therefore, these infants are highly vulnerable to fluid depletion.

Infants who are ELBW, tachypneic, receiving phototherapy, or in a radiant warmer have increased insensible water losses that require appropriate fluid adjustments. Nurses must monitor fluid status by daily (or more frequent) weights and accurate intake and output of all fluids, including medications and blood products. Urine-specific gravity and dipstick measurements are monitored per unit protocol, and serum electrolytes are obtained as warranted by the infant's condition. ELBW infants often require more frequent monitoring of these parameters because of their inordinate transepidermal fluid loss, immature renal function, and propensity to dehydration or overhydration. Intolerance of even dextrose 5% is not uncommon in the ELBW infant, with subsequent glycosuria and osmotic diuresis. Alterations in behavior, alertness, or activity level in these infants receiving IV fluids may signal an electrolyte imbalance, hypoglycemia, or hyperglycemia. The nurse is also observant for tremors or seizures in the VLBW or ELBW infant, because these may be a sign of hyponatremia or hypernatremia. Weight gain from fluid overload in the sick preterm infant may occur as a result of fluid retention (renal failure), inappropriate fluid administration (parenteral), or congestive heart failure. An increased fluid gain may result in the opening of a previously closed patent ductus arteriosus (PDA), thus exacerbating associated illness. Growing preterm infants, especially those with CLD, on oral electrolyte supplements should be carefully monitored for rapid weight gain that may result in pulmonary congestion, PDA, and electrolyte imbalance. See Box 27-3 for calculation of a weight loss or gain.

Elimination Patterns

Frequency of urination, as well as the amount, color, pH, and specific gravity of the urine is assessed. The assessment of bowel movements includes frequency of stooling and

BOX 27-3

Calculation of a Weight Loss or Gain

Example 1

Day 1	1,750 g (birth weight)	$\frac{70}{1{,}750} = \frac{X\%}{100\%}$
Day 3	1,680 g	1,750X = 7,000
	70 g loss	$1{,}750\overline{)7{,}000.0}$ = 4.0
		X = 4.0% weight loss

Example 2

Day 3	1,680 g	$\frac{40}{1{,}680} = \frac{X\%}{100\%}$
Day 4	1,720 g	1,680X = 4,000
	40 g gain	$1{,}680\overline{)4{,}000.00}$ = 2.38
		X = 2.4% weight gain

character of the stool, as well as whether there is constipation, diarrhea, or loss of fats (steatorrhea). Infants with unexplained abdominal distention are assessed carefully to rule out the presence of necrotizing enterocolitis or obstruction of the GI tract.

Oral Feeding

Nourishment by the oral route is preferred for the infant who has adequate strength and GI function. The best milk for an infant is human milk. Breast milk may be fed by breast, bottle, or gavage. Formula may be fed by bottle or gavage.

Many high risk infants cannot suck well enough to breastfeed or bottle-feed until they have recovered from their initial illness or matured physically. Infants may be put to breast for practice feeds as soon as medically stable. Mothers of high risk infants are encouraged to continue pumping breast milk. Because of the significant breastfeeding attrition rates among these mothers, they need support and frequent encouragement to continue pumping while their infant is not yet able to nurse.

Gavage Feeding

Gavage feeding is a method of providing breast milk or formula through a nasogastric or orogastric tube (Fig. 27-4). Gavage feeding can be accomplished either with a tube inserted at each feeding (bolus) or continuously through an indwelling feeding tube. Breast milk or formula can be supplied intermittently using a syringe with gravity-controlled flow, or can be given continuously using an infusion pump. The type of fluid instilled is recorded with every syringe change. The volume of the continuous feedings is recorded hourly, and the residual gastric aspirate is measured before each feeding. Residuals of less than a quarter of a feeding can be refed to the infant, depending largely on unit protocol. Feeding may be stopped if the residual is greater than 2 to 4 ml/kg or a 1-hour volume and is not resumed until the infant can be assessed for a possible feeding intolerance (Anderson et al, 2002).

The orogastric route of gavage feedings may be preferred because most infants are preferential nose breathers. However, some infants do not tolerate oral tube placement. The procedure for inserting a gavage feeding tube is described in Box 27-4.

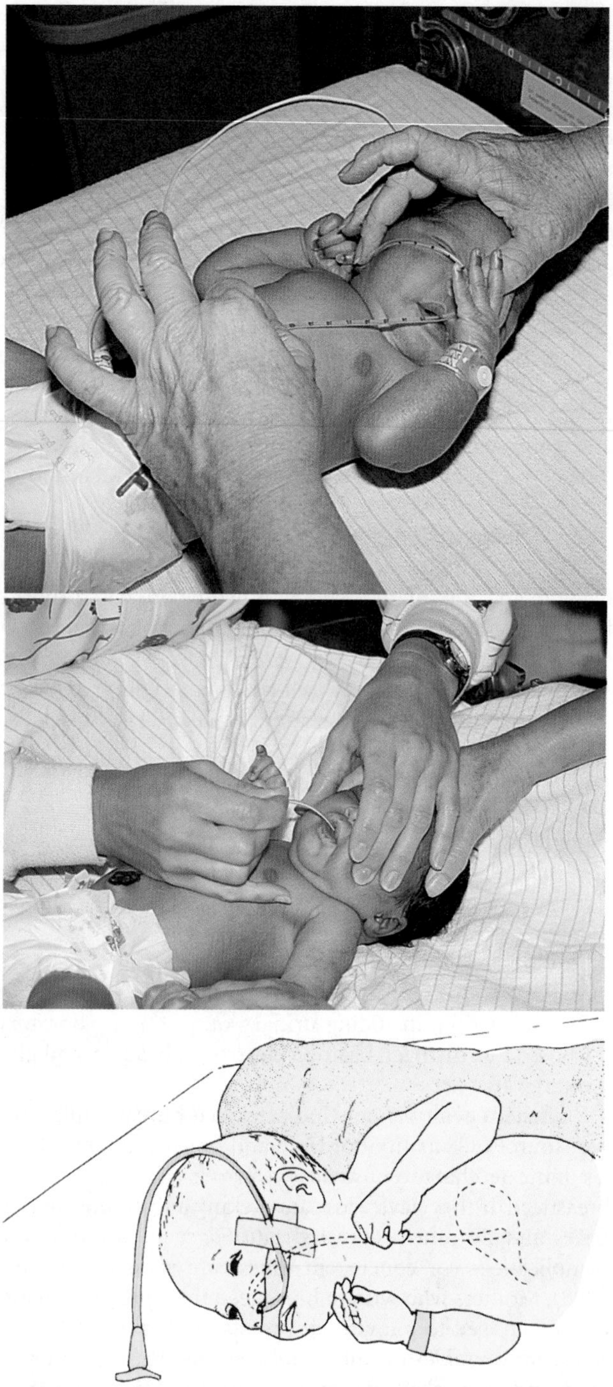

A

B

C

Fig. 27-4 Gavage feeding. **A,** Measurement of gavage feeding tube from tip of nose to earlobe and to midpoint between end of xiphoid process and umbilicus. Tape may be used to mark correct length on tube. **B,** Insertion of gavage tube using orogastric route. **C,** Indwelling gavage tube, nasogastric route. After feeding by orogastric or nasogastric tube, infant is propped on right side or placed prone (preterm infant) for 1 hour to facilitate emptying of stomach into small intestine. Note rolled towel for support. (**A** and **B,** courtesy Marjorie Pyle, RNC, Lifecircle, Costa Mesa, CA.)

To begin the feeding, the nurse connects the barrel of a syringe to the gavage tube. While crimping the feeding tube, the nurse pours the specified amount of breast milk or formula into the syringe. The crimp in the tube is then released

BOX 27-4

Procedure: Inserting a Gavage Feeding Tube

1. Measure the length of the gavage tube from the tip of the nose to the lobe of the ear to the midpoint between the xiphoid process and the umbilicus (Fig. 27-4, *A*). Mark the tube with a piece of tape.
2. Lubricate the tip of the tube with sterile water and insert gently through the nose or mouth (Fig. 27-4, *B*) until the predetermined mark is reached. Placement of the tube in the trachea will cause the infant to gag, cough, or become cyanotic.
3. Check correct placement of the tube by:
   a. Pulling back on the plunger to aspirate stomach contents. Lack of stomach aspirate or fluid is not necessarily evidence of improper placement. Aspiration of respiratory secretions may be mistaken for stomach contents; however, the pH of the stomach contents is much lower (more acidic) than the pH of respiratory secretions.
   b. Injecting a small amount of air (1 to 3 ml) into the tube while listening for gurgling by using a stethoscope placed over the stomach. Ensure that the tube is inserted to the mark; it is possible to hear air entering the stomach even if the tube is positioned above the gastroesophageal (cardiac) sphincter.
4. Tape the tube in place and also tape it to the cheek to prevent accidental dislodgement and incorrect positioning (Fig. 27-4, *C*).
   a. Assess the infant's skin integrity before taping the tube.
   b. Edematous or very preterm infants should have a pectin barrier placed under the tape to prevent abrasions, or use a hydrocolloid adhesive to prevent epidermal stripping.*
5. Tube placement *must* be assessed before each feeding.

*Lund CH, Durand DJ: Skin and skin care. In Merenstein GB, Gardner SL (eds): *Handbook of neonatal intensive care*, ed 5, St Louis, 2003, Mosby.

and the feeding allowed to flow by gravity at a rate that approximates that of an oral feeding (about 1 ml/min). The infant can be held or swaddled to help the infant associate the feeding with positive interactions.

Once the prescribed volume has been delivered, the tube is crimped or pinched and the syringe removed. The gavage tube is capped (or the nurse continues to pinch it) while removing it in one steady motion. Capping or pinching the tube prevents breast milk or formula from leaking from the tube and being aspirated during removal of the tube.

After the feeding, the infant is positioned to prevent aspiration. The documentation of the procedure includes the size of the feeding tube, the amount and quality of the residual from the previous feeding, the type and quantity of fluid instilled, and the infant's response to the procedure.

Gastrostomy Feeding

Gastrostomy feeding involves the surgical placement of a tube through the skin of the abdomen into the stomach. With percutaneous gastrostomy insertion, feedings are often started within hours of insertion. Feedings by gravity are done slowly over 20 to 30 minutes. Special care must be taken to prevent rapid bolusing of the fluid because this may lead to abdominal distention, GI reflux into the esophagus, diarrhea with malabsorption, or respiratory compromise. Meticulous skin care at the tube insertion site is necessary to prevent skin breakdown or infection. Intake and output is carefully monitored to ensure adequate fluid and calorie intake and adequate renal function.

Advancing Infant Feedings

Feedings are advanced from passive (parenteral and gavage) to active (nipple and breastfeeding) as assessment data and the infant's ability to tolerate feedings warrant. The infant's sucking patterns and demonstration of a quiet alert state can also be used to determine readiness to nipple feed.

The infant receiving nutrition parenterally is gradually weaned off this type of nutrition. The nourishment given by gavage feedings is increased as parenteral fluids are decreased, depending on the infant's tolerance of enteral feeding. Feedings are advanced slowly and cautiously; if feedings are advanced too rapidly, vomiting, diarrhea, abdominal distention, and apneic episodes may result.

The infant receiving gavage feedings progresses to bottle-feeding or breast milk feedings. Gavage feedings are decreased as the infant's ability to suckle breast milk or formula improves. Often the infant is fed by both nipple and gavage feeding during this transition; this ensures intake of the prescribed volumes of both fluid and nutrients. The parents should be encouraged to interact by talking and making eye contact with the infant during feedings.

Because preterm infants are often being discharged at weights equal to 1500 g, the need to continue nutritional intake and growth to match intrauterine growth remains. A concern in recent years has been the delayed growth of preterm infants discharged home after neonatal intensive care. To address these growth needs, it is now recommended that formerly preterm infants receive either human breast milk with a preterm human milk fortifier or a 22 cal/oz formula until the postnatal age of 9 months (Evidence-Based Practice).

Nonnutritive Sucking

For the infant who requires gavage or parenteral feedings, nonnutritive sucking on a pacifier during the gavage procedure may improve oxygenation and facilitate earlier transition to nipple feeding (Fig. 27-5). Such nonnutritive sucking may lead to decreased energy expenditure with less restlessness.

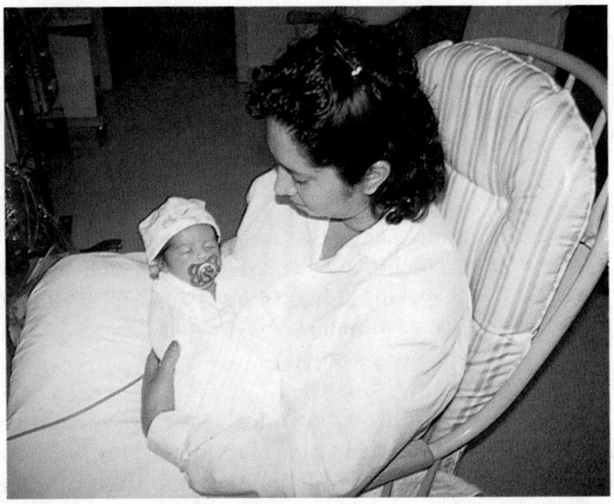

Fig. 27-5 Nonnutritive sucking by infant. (Courtesy Marjorie Pyle, RNC, Lifecircle, Costa Mesa, CA.)

Evidence-Based Practice

EARLY DISCHARGE OF GAVAGE-FED PRETERMS

Background

Preterm babies (<37 weeks of gestation) typically remain hospitalized until full oral feeding is established. Stable preterm infants could be discharged 1 to 2 weeks earlier, if the transition from gavage feeding to oral feeding could happen at home. The benefits of such a policy include uniting the family sooner, decreased nosocomial (hospital-acquired) infections, and considerable cost savings. Possible adverse outcomes include extra care burden for the family and complications such as aspiration pneumonia or growth failure. Health care support offered to families of preterm infants discharged while still on gavage feeding has included outpatient clinic visits, professional home visits, phone contact, and emergency room visits. Several studies of early discharge with home gavage infants show no evidence of inadequate weight gain or increase of readmissions.

Objectives

To establish safety, the reviewers compared the effects of early discharge of stable, gavage-fed preterm infants to the usual practice of hospitalizing preterm infants until full oral feeding is established. Also of interest was any difference in outcomes dependent upon the type of support (home versus clinic). The infants could not have intravenous supplementation. Outcomes could include number of days to transition to full sucking, breastfeeding prevalence, weight gain, length of hospitalization, neurodevelopment, readmission, milk aspiration, infection, death, satisfaction, cost, and health service use.

Methods

Search Strategy

The authors searched MEDLINE, Cochrane, CINAHL, and EMBASE for trials relating to early discharge. Search keywords included *early discharge, hospital in the home, gavage, tube, feed, low birth weight, preterm, premature infant, premature infant diseases, patient discharge, length of stay,* and *enteral nutrition.* Only one quasi-randomized trial met the criteria for the review. It was a 1999 Swedish trial of 88 infants from 75 families. The intervention group ($n = 45$) received early discharge with home visits by a registered nurse. The control group ($n = 43$) stayed in the hospital until full oral feeding was established.

Statistical Analyses

Reviewers calculated relative risks for dichotomous (categoric) data, and mean differences for continuous data. Results outside the 95% confidence intervals were accepted as significantly different.

Findings

The early discharge group had mean reductions in lengths of stay of 9.3 days. During that time, the intervention group had significantly fewer infections than the hospitalized controls. While the controls were still hospitalized, 8 of the 45 intervention group infants were readmitted during the home gavage program (2 for jaundice, 2 for blood transfusions, 1 for inguinal herniorrhaphy and cryotherapy for retinopathy, 1 for removal of apnea monitor, 1 for skin condition and maternal anxiety, and 1 for respiratory syncytial virus). No differences were found in duration or exclusivity of breastfeeding, weight gain, readmission, health care use, maternal anxiety, or maternal confidence. Intervention mothers did score higher on feeling prepared to care for their infant, but the difference did not meet the level of significance. Cost was not measured directly, but the reviewers estimated the hospitalization costs of the control group exceeded the cost of health care support used by the intervention group. One infant in the control group died of sudden infant death syndrome (SIDS).

Limitations

The trial is quasi-randomized and small, limiting generalizability. The paucity of trials led to this single study being included, even though 9 of the 45 infants in the intervention (20%) never actually received home gavage feedings, but were hospitalized until full oral feedings were established. Their data were included in the intervention group statistics, which follows the usual statistical guidelines of keeping subjects in "intention-to-treat" grouping. Nevertheless, one out of five in the intervention group actually received the control protocol.

Conclusions

While the early discharge group had mean reductions in lengths of stay of 9.3 days and the intervention group had significantly fewer infections than the hospitalized controls, no conclusions can be drawn because of the inclusion of only one study.

Implications for Practice

Policy changes for early versus usual discharge for stable preterm gavage-fed infants cannot be made on the basis of one small, quasi-randomized trial.

Implications for Further Research

Large randomized, controlled trials are needed to be able to suggest safety and efficacy of early discharge of stable gavage-fed preterm infants. Outcomes need to include growth, infection rates, costs, family impact, complications, and long-term outcomes. Of great interest to community health nurses are the types of support most effective to families with special-needs infants.

Reference

Collins C, Makrides M, McPhee A: Early discharge with home support of gavage feeding for stable preterm infants who have not established full oral feeds (Cochrane Review), 2003. In *The Cochrane Library,* Issue 2, Chichester, UK, 2004, John Wiley & Sons.

Mothers of premature infants should be encouraged to let their infant start sucking at the breast during kangaroo care; some infant's suck and swallow reflexes may be coordinated as early as 32 weeks of gestation.

Environmental Concerns

Infants in NICUs are exposed to high levels of auditory input from the various machine alarms, and this can have adverse effects (Fig. 27-6). Continuous noise levels of 45 to 85 decibels (db) are common in NICUs. An incubator produces a constant noise level of 60 to 80 db (Haubrich, 1998), and each new piece of life-support equipment used adds another 20 db to the background noise. The infant's hearing may be damaged if it is exposed to a constant decibel level of 90 db or frequent decibel swings higher than 110 db.

The infant's vision may be altered by the overhead lights or a phototherapy mask, making it difficult for the infant to interact with caregivers and family members. The infant may be unable to establish diurnal and nocturnal rhythms be-

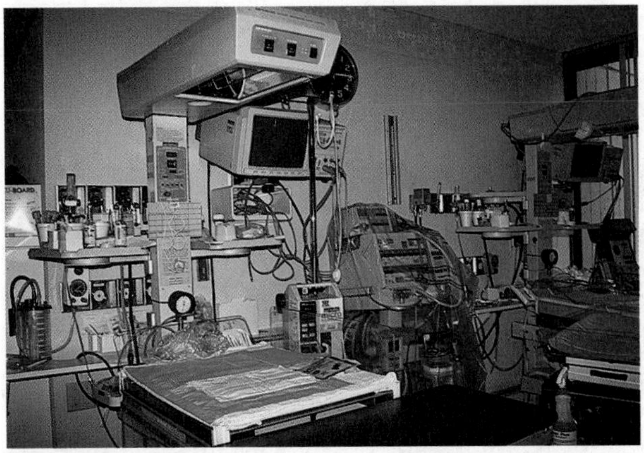

Fig. 27-6 NICU equipment, which, although necessary, may contribute to significant environmental stimulation. Note bed, wall oxygen attachments, monitor, ventilator, incubator, and pumps, all of which have alarm systems. (Courtesy Marjorie Pyle, RNC, Lifecircle, Costa Mesa, CA.)

cause of the continuous exposure to overhead lighting. In addition, sedation or pain medications affect the way in which the infant perceives the environment.

Effects of environmental hazards can be potentiated by some drugs used for infant therapy. Diuretics (especially furosemide [Lasix]), antibiotics (gentamicin), and antimalarial agents can potentiate noise-induced hearing loss. Routine hearing screening should be performed on all infants before discharge (see Fig. 24-14).

Nurses can modify the environment to provide a developmentally supportive milieu. In that way, the infant's neurobehavioral and physiologic needs can be better met, the infant's developing organization can be supported, and growth and development fostered (Blackburn, 1998).

In one study, preterm infants less than 32 weeks of gestation grew faster than similar cohorts when cycled lighting was provided instead of continuous near darkness (Brandon, Holditch-Davis, & Belyea, 2002). Other studies have found varying results regarding the provision of near darkness by dimming NICU lights and the incidence of retinopathy of prematurity (ROP) in NICUs.

Developmental Care

The goal of developmental care is to support each infant's efforts to become as well-organized, competent, and stable as possible. Developmental care includes all care procedures and the physical and social aspects of care in the NICU (Als, 1998). The caregiver uses the infant's own behavior and physiologic functioning as the basis for planning care and providing interventions. Through caregiver observation, the infant's strengths, thresholds for disorganization, and areas in which the infant is vulnerable can be identified (Als, 1998). The family is included in developmental care as the primary co-regulators (Als, 1998; Heermann & Wilson, 2000). Working together, the family and other caregivers provide opportunities to enhance the strengths of the family and the infant and to reduce the stress associated with the birth and care of high risk infants.

Lowering light and noise levels by instituting "quiet hours" during each 8-hour shift and positioning are just two of the ways in which nurses can support infants in their development (Gray et al, 1998). Sleep interruptions are minimized, and positioning and bundling the infant help promote self-regulation and prevent disorganization (Petryshen et al, 1997).

Positioning

The motor development of preterm infants permits less flexion than their full-term counterparts. Caregivers can provide a variety of positions for infants; side-lying and prone are preferred to supine. Body containment with use of blanket rolls, swaddling, holding the infant's arms in a crossed position, and secure holding provide boundaries and promote self-regulation during feeding, procedures, and other stressful interventions (Gardner & Goldson, 2002). The prone position encourages flexion of the extremities; a sling or hip roll assists in maintenance of flexion. Holding the limbs close to the body (containment) when the infant is moved decreases stimulation that produces jerky, uncoordinated movements. Proper body alignment is necessary to prevent developmental problems that may affect the ability to walk as the child matures.

Reducing Inappropriate Stimuli

Staff can reduce unnecessary noise by closing doors or portholes on incubators quietly, avoiding placing objects on top of incubators, avoiding radios, speaking quietly, and handling equipment noiselessly.

Nursing care affects sleep-wake behaviors in preterm infants (Brandon, Holditch-Davis, & Belyea, 1999). Infants can be protected from light by dimming the lights during the night or placing a blanket over the incubator (Fig. 27-7). Sleep-wake cycles can be induced with such measures. Infants need periods when they are completely undisturbed.

Infant Communication

Infants communicate their needs and ability to tolerate sensory stimulation through physiologic responses. The nurses and parents of high risk infants must therefore be alert to such cues. Although full-term infants may thrive on stimulation, this same stimulation in high risk infants can instead provoke physical symptoms of stress and anxiety (Blackburn, 1998; Gardner & Goldson, 2002).

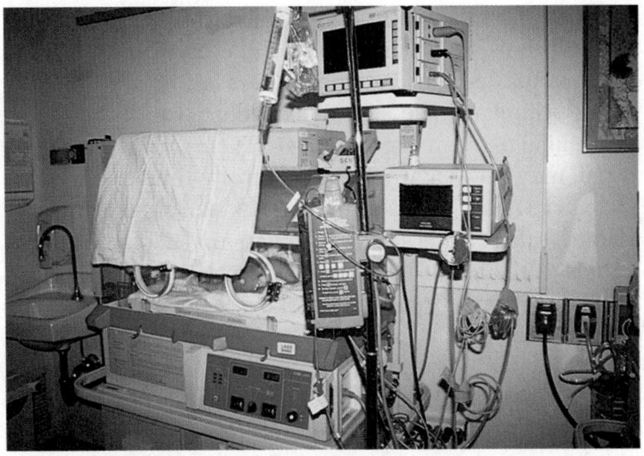

Fig. 27-7 Infant in double-walled incubator with a blanket for a light shield. (Courtesy Marjorie Pyle, RNC, Lifecircle, Costa Mesa, CA.)

Problems with noxious stimuli and barriers to normal contact may cause anxiety and tension. Clues to overstimulation include gaze aversion, hiccupping, gagging, or regurgitating food. Term infants exhibit a startle reflex, and premature infants move all of their limbs in an uncoordinated fashion in response to noxious stimuli. An irregular respiratory rate or an increased heart rate may develop in severely distressed infants, and they may then be unable to regain a calm state.

A relaxed infant state is indicated by stabilization of vital signs, closed eyes, and a relaxed posture. Nonintubated infants may make soothing verbal sounds when they are relaxed. Infants requiring artificial ventilation cannot cry audibly and often show their distress through posturing; they then relax once their needs are met. As high risk infants heal and mature, they increasingly respond to stimuli in a self-regulated manner rather than with a dissociated response. Infants who do not demonstrate ability for self-regulation should be further evaluated for potential neurologic problems.

Infant Stimulation

A Neonatal Individualized Development Care and Assessment Program (NIDCAP) routinely integrates aspects of neurodevelopmental theory with caregivers' observations, environmental interventions, and parental support (Gardner & Goldson, 2002). Routine reassessment is built into the program's design. Developmental stimuli may consist of such simple measures as placing a waterbed on top of the infant's mattress, or kangaroo (skin-to-skin) holding by the parents. The simplest calming technique is to contain the infant's extremities close to the body using both hands. The care of the infant is organized to allow extended periods of undisturbed rest and sleep. Pain medications or sedatives should be administered consistently per the unit's protocol.

Infants acquire a sense of trust as they learn the feel, sound, and smell of their parents (Gardner & Goldson, 2002). High risk infants must also learn to trust their caregivers to obtain comfort. However, caregivers in the nursery may inflict pain as part of the care they must give. For this reason, it is important for both the parents and the caregivers to employ comforting interventions such as removing painful stimuli, stopping hunger, and changing wet or soiled clothing to foster trust.

When the infant is ready for interaction, the nurse has many options. All infants can tolerate being held, even if only for short periods. Additional ways for the nurse or parents to stimulate infants include cuddling, rocking, singing, and talking to the infant (Fig. 27-8). These activities are beneficial, increase weight gain, and decrease time to discharge (Standley, 1998). Stroking the infant's skin during medical therapy can provide tactile stimulation. The caregiver responds to the infant's cues by offering reassurance, providing for nonnutritive sucking, stroking the infant's back, and talking to the infant.

Mobiles and decals that can be changed frequently may also be placed within the infant's visual range to stimulate the infant visually. Wind-up musical toys provide rhythmic distractions as long as they are not too loud. If the infant is receiving phototherapy, the protective eye patches are removed periodically (e.g., during feeding) so that the infant can see the caregiver's face for short, comforting sessions. Although much beneficial infant interaction with caregivers may be desired, it is important to continually assess the infant's response to interactions designed to improve neurodevelopment. The caregivers cannot assume that the infant likes the mobile because the arms are extended and fingers splayed; this is actually a "time out" signal indicating stress. It is particularly important to help parents understand the infant's neurodevelopmental cues as not being a rejection of their caretaking abilities; at times preterm infants who are still disorganized need a time out from parental interaction in order to fully recover. The nurse can promote feelings of parental involvement by jointly developing an individualized plan of care for the infant. This may involve a written sign at the bedside with a brief message such as "Hello Mom. This is Josh. I just had blood drawn at 1:00 PM so I need a 1-hour nap. I will see you at 2:00 PM. Love, Josh."

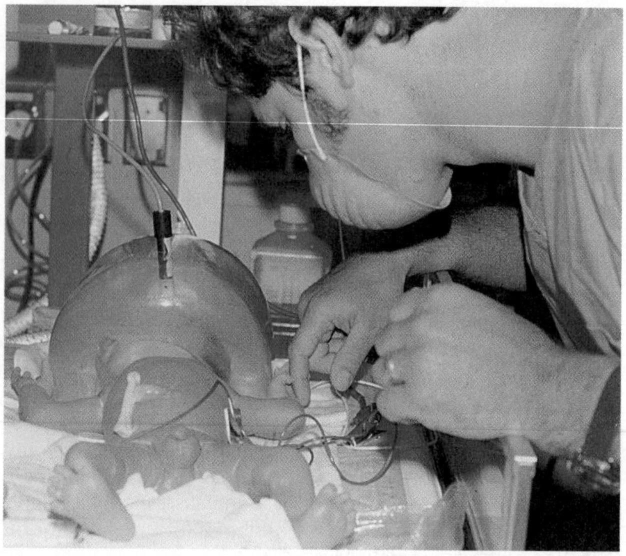

Fig. 27-8 A father caresses his tiny preterm infant receiving oxygen by hood in the NICU. (Courtesy Marjorie Pyle, RNC, Lifecircle, Costa Mesa, CA.)

Kangaroo Care

Kangaroo care (skin-to-skin holding) helps infants to directly interact with their parents (Gale & VandenBerg, 1998). In this technique the infant, dressed only in a diaper, is placed directly on the parent's bare chest and then covered with the parent's clothing, a warmed blanket, or an overhead warmer lamp (Fig. 27-9). In this way, the parent's body temperature also functions as an external heat source that enhances the infant's temperature regulation. Even ventilator-dependent infants weighing less than1 kg have been found to benefit from this measure, although they usually tolerate it for 30 minutes or less at a time (Neu, 1999).

Preterm infants experiencing kangaroo care recover rapidly from birth-related fatigue (Ludington-Hoe et al, 1999). Infants and parents who participate in kangaroo care have been observed to have dramatically better outcomes. The mothers report increased breast milk output and fewer feelings of helplessness related to their experiences in the NICU. Infants have been found to maintain their temperatures and

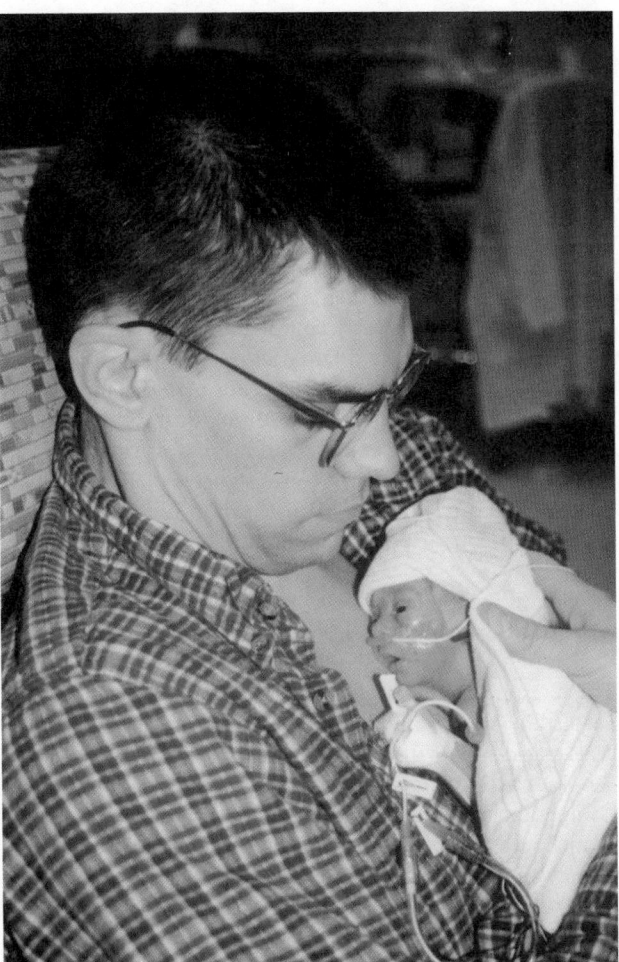

Fig. 27-9 Father providing kangaroo care. (Courtesy Judy Meyr, St. Louis, MO.)

oxygenation levels better and to experience fewer episodes of crying, apnea, and periodic respirations (Neu, Browne, & Vojir, 2000). They have also been observed to be alert and quiet longer and to have slightly higher heart rates. Kangaroo care also meets developmental needs by fostering neurobehavioral development.

Parental Support

The nurse as support person and teacher shapes the environment and makes caregiving more responsive to the needs of parents and infant. Nurses are instrumental in helping parents learn who their infant is and to recognize behavioral cues in his or her development (VandenBerg, 1999).

If a high risk birth is anticipated, the family can be given a tour of the NICU or shown a video to prepare them for the sights and activities of the unit. After the birth, the parents can be given a booklet, be shown a video, or have someone describe what they will see when they go to the unit to see their infant. As soon as possible, the parents should see and touch their infant so that they can begin to acknowledge the reality of the birth and the infant's true appearance and condition. They will need encouragement to begin to accomplish the psychologic tasks imposed by the preterm birth. A nurse and primary health care provider should be present during the parent's first visit to see the infant for the following reasons:

- To help them "see" the infant rather than focus on equipment. The significance and function of the apparatus that surrounds the infant should be explained.
- To explain the characteristics normal for an infant of their baby's gestational age. In this way, parents do not compare their infant with a full-term healthy baby.
- To encourage the parent to express feelings about the pregnancy, labor, and birth and the experience of having a preterm infant.
- To assess the parent's perceptions of the infant and determine the appropriate time for them to become actively involved in care.

As soon after the birth as possible, the parents are given the opportunity to meet the infant in the *en face* position, to touch the infant, and to see his or her favorable characteristics. Both parents, but especially the mother are encouraged to visit the nursery as desired and help with the infant's care. When the family cannot be present physically, staff members devise appropriate methods to keep the family in frequent touch with the newborn, such as daily phone calls, notes written as if from the infant, video or photographs of the baby (Family Focus box).

Some hospitals have support groups for parents of infants in intensive care nurseries. These groups encourage parents experiencing anxiety and grief to share their feelings. A parent with NICU experience often makes contact with a new member and provides additional support. These parents provide support for the new NICU parent through hospital visits, phone contact, and home visits.

In one testimonial, parents of infants in NICU identified the following four central themes for NICU staff to consider when caring for the NICU family: (1) nurturing the parents; (2) providing accurate and consistent information; (3) clarifying NICU policies for neonatal treatment and family interaction; and (4) helping parents of NICU neonates connect with other parents in the NICU and graduates of NICU care (Woodwell, 2002). Ward (2001) developed a 20-item NICU Family Needs Inventory to help identify the particular needs of parents with an infant in the NICU. Perceived needs identified in the initial study included providing information about the infant's condition and treatment plan,

Family Focus

PRETERM INFANT

A multiparous, single woman has a preterm infant who was born at 28 weeks of gestation and subsequently transported to a special care nursery. The woman does not live in the city where the tertiary center is located, and she is to be discharged tomorrow. It is anticipated that the infant will require a stay in the NICU for at least 6 to 7 more weeks. What information should the transport team provide the parents? What methods of assistance will this mother need now? Identify resources in the community with services that may be beneficial for the woman. Use your community or town as a guide to such resources.

answering parents' questions honestly, actively listening to parents' fears and concerns, assisting parents in understanding the infant's responses, and providing assurance.

Some high risk infants can be discharged earlier than expected. Criteria for early discharge require the infant to be physiologically stable, receiving adequate nutrition and gaining weight daily, and to have a stable body temperature in an open bassinet. The parents or other caregivers must exhibit physical, emotional, and educational readiness to assume care of the infant. Ideally, the home environment is adequate for meeting the needs of the infant. The parents need to show that they know the way to take the infant's temperature, signs and symptoms to report, and that they understand the dietary needs of the infant.

Parent Education

Cardiopulmonary Resuscitation

Sudden infant death syndrome (SIDS) is more likely to occur in preterm infants than in term infants; infants discharged from an NICU are about twice as likely to die unexpectedly during the first year of life as infants in the general population. Instruction in cardiopulmonary resuscitation (CPR) is essential for parents of all infants but especially for parents of infants at risk for life-threatening events. Risk factors include prematurity, apnea and/or bradycardia spells, and the tendency to choke. Before taking the infant home, parents must be able to administer infant CPR. All parents should be encouraged to obtain instruction in CPR at the hospital, local Red Cross, or other community agency. It should be emphasized that CPR knowledge does not preclude or substitute for proper positioning of the infant in the crib (i.e., supine) when put to sleep, unless otherwise directed by the primary care physician. In addition the bed should have a firm mattress and be free of extra blankets, stuffed animals, or toys, which may cause the infant to become entangled and subsequently smothered.

Evaluation

The nurse uses the previously stated outcomes of care to evaluate the effectiveness of the physical and psychosocial aspects of care (Nursing Care Plan—The High-Risk Preterm Newborn).

Complications of Prematurity

Respiratory Distress Syndrome

Respiratory distress syndrome (RDS) is a lung disorder usually affecting preterm infants, although a small percentage of term or near term infants may also be affected. Maternal and fetal conditions associated with a decreased incidence and severity of RDS include female infant; African-American race; maternal steroid (betamethasone) therapy; and stressors such as maternal gestational hypertension, maternal drug abuse, chronic retroplacental abruption, prolonged rupture of membranes, and IUGR (Hagedorn et al, 2002). The incidence and severity of RDS increase with a decrease in gestational age. Perinatal asphyxia, hypovolemia, male infant, Caucasian race, maternal diabetes, second-born twin, familial predisposition, maternal hypotension, cesarean birth without labor, hydrops fetalis, and third-trimester bleeding are all factors that place an infant at increased risk for RDS (Hagedorn et al, 2002).

RDS is caused by a lack of pulmonary surfactant, which leads to progressive atelectasis, loss of functional residual capacity, and ventilation-perfusion imbalance with an uneven distribution of ventilation. Surfactant deficiency may be caused by insufficient surfactant production, abnormal composition and function, disruption of surfactant production, or a combination of these factors. The sequence of events that occurs is further compromised by weak respiratory muscles and an overly compliant chest wall, which are common to premature infants. Lung capacity is compromised by the presence of proteinaceous material and epithelial debris in the airways. The resulting decreased oxygenation, cyanosis, and metabolic or respiratory acidosis can increase pulmonary vascular resistance (PVR). This increased PVR can lead to right-to-left shunting and a reopening of the ductus arteriosus and foramen ovale (Hagedorn et al, 2002).

Clinical symptoms of RDS include tachypnea; grunting; nasal flaring; intercostal, or subcostal retractions; hypercapnia; respiratory or mixed acidosis; hypotension; and shock. These respiratory symptoms usually present immediately after birth or within 6 hours of birth. Physical examination reveals crackles, poor air exchange, pallor, use of accessory muscles (retractions), and occasionally apnea. Radiographic findings include uniform reticulogranular appearance and air bronchograms. The infant's clinical course is variable. There is usually an increased oxygen requirement and increased respiratory effort as atelectasis, loss of functional residual capacity, and ventilation-perfusion imbalance worsen.

Severe RDS is often associated with a shocklike state, as manifested by diminished cardiac inflow and low arterial blood pressure. The ELBW or VLBW infant, as a result of extreme pulmonary immaturity, decreased glycogen stores, and lack of accessory muscles, may have severe RDS at birth.

RDS is a self-limiting disease with respiratory symptoms abating after 72 hours. The disappearance of respiratory symptoms coincides with the production of surfactant in type II cells of the alveoli.

The treatment for RDS is supportive. Adequate ventilation and oxygenation must be established and maintained in an attempt to prevent ventilation-perfusion mismatch and atelectasis. Exogenous surfactant, which alters the typical course of RDS, may be administered at or shortly after birth. Positive-pressure ventilation, CPAP, and oxygen therapy may be needed during the respiratory illness. Prevention of complications associated with mechanical ventilation is critical. These complications include pulmonary interstitial emphysema (PIE), pneumothorax, pneumomediastinum, and pneumopericardium.

Acid-base balance is evaluated by monitoring ABG values (Table 27-2 on p. 817). Frequent blood sampling requires arterial access either by umbilical artery catheter (UAC) or by a peripheral arterial line. Pulse oximetry and transcutaneous carbon dioxide and oxygen monitors document trends in ventilation and oxygenation. Capillary blood gas values may be used to evaluate pH and P_{CO_2} in infants whose condition is more stable.

Nursing Care Plan

THE HIGH RISK PRETERM NEWBORN

NURSING DIAGNOSIS: Ineffective breathing pattern related to pulmonary, cardiovascular, and neuromuscular immaturity, decreased energy reserves as evidenced by assessment findings (e.g., nasal flaring, tachypnea, grunting)

EXPECTED OUTCOME

Infant exhibits adequate oxygenation (i.e., ABG levels and acid-base balance WNL for age, oxygen saturations 92% or greater, respiratory rate and pattern WNL for age, breath sounds clear, absence of grunting, nasal flaring, minimal retractions, skin color appropriate).

NURSING INTERVENTIONS/*RATIONALES*

Position neonate prone or supine, avoiding neck hyperextension *to promote optimum air exchange.* Use a side-lying position after feeding or in cases of excessive mucous production *to avoid aspiration.* Avoid Trendelenburg position *because it can cause increased intracranial pressure and reduce lung capacity.*

Suction nasopharynx, trachea, and endotracheal tube only as necessary *to remove mucus/secretions.* Avoid oversuctioning because *it can cause bronchospasm, bradycardia, hypoxia, and predispose neonate to intraventricular hemorrhage.*

Administer percussion, vibration, and postural drainage only as necessary *to facilitate drainage of secretions.*

Administer oxygen and monitor neonatal response *to maintain oxygen saturation.*

Maintain a neutral thermal environment *to conserve oxygen and glucose use.*

Monitor ABG levels, acid-base balance, oxygen saturation, respiratory rate and pattern, breath sounds, and airway patency; observe for grunting, nasal flaring, retractions, and cyanosis *to detect signs of respiratory distress.*

NURSING DIAGNOSIS: Ineffective thermoregulation related to immature CNS temperature regulation, decreased brown fat, inability to produce body heat, and minimal subcutaneous fat stores as evidenced by assessment findings (e.g., absent or decreased subcutaneous tissue, body temperature less than 36.5° C)

EXPECTED OUTCOME

Infant exhibits maintenance of stable body temperature within normal range for postconceptional age (36.5° C to 37.2° C).

NURSING INTERVENTIONS/*RATIONALES*

Place neonate in a prewarmed radiant warmer *to maintain stable temperature.*

Place temperature probe over tissue (not bone) such as abdomen *to control heat levels delivered by radiant warmer.*

Take axillary temperature periodically *to monitor temperature and cross-check functioning of warmer unit.*

Avoid infant exposure to cool air and drafts, cold scales, cold stethoscopes, cold examination tables, and prolonged bathing *that predispose the infant to heat loss.*

Use additional shield or cover in warmer (plastic wrap) *to prevent further heat loss from exposure to drafts and air currents and minimize insensible water loss.*

Monitor probe function and status frequently *because detachment can cause overheating or warmer-induced hyperthermia.*

Transfer infant to a servocontrolled incubator *when temperature has stabilized.*

NURSING DIAGNOSIS: Risk for infection related to immature immune system, exposure to multiple sources of infection (invasive procedures, maternal infection) as evidenced by assessment findings (e.g., feeding intolerance, apnea, temperature instability)

EXPECTED OUTCOME

Infant exhibits no evidence of infection.

NURSING INTERVENTIONS/*RATIONALES*

Institute scrupulous handwashing techniques before and after handling neonate; ensure all supplies and/or equipment are clean before use; and ensure strict aseptic technique with invasive procedures *to minimize exposure to infective organisms.*

Prevent contact with persons who have communicable infections and instruct parents in infection control procedures *to minimize infection risk.*

Administer prescribed antibiotics *to provide coverage for infection during sepsis workup.*

Continuously monitor vital signs for stability *because instability, hypothermia, or prolonged temperature elevations serve as indicators of infection.*

NURSING DIAGNOSIS: Risk for imbalanced nutrition: less than body requirements related to inability to ingest adequate nutrients for growth secondary to GI immaturity, decreased stomach capacity, and associated illness factors as evidenced by inadequate weight gain

EXPECTED OUTCOMES

Infant receives adequate amount of nutrients with sufficient caloric intake to maintain positive nitrogen balance; demonstrates steady weight gain (as appropriate to acuity).

NURSING INTERVENTIONS/*RATIONALES*

Administer parenteral fluid/TPN as prescribed *to provide adequate nutrition and fluid intake.*

Monitor for signs of intolerance to TPN, which can interfere with effective replenishment of nutrients.

Periodically assess readiness to orally feed (i.e., strong suck, swallow, and gag reflexes) *to provide appropriate transition from TPN to oral feeding as soon as neonate is ready.*

Advance volume and concentration of formula when orally feeding per unit protocol *to avoid overfeeding and feeding intolerance.*

Provide expressed breast milk (including colostrum) when stable *to enhance GI development, provide natural immunity and other benefits of human milk (digestive enzymes)*

If mother desires to breastfeed when neonate is stable, demonstrate how to express milk *to establish and maintain lactation until infant can breastfeed.*

Continued

Nursing Care Plan

THE HIGH RISK PRETERM NEWBORN—cont'd

NURSING DIAGNOSIS: Risk for imbalanced (specify if deficient or excess) fluid volume related to large ECF volume, decreased ability to regulate fluid shifts, renal immaturity, permeable skin, and insensible and TEWL (transepidermal water losses) as evidenced by excessive weight gain or loss

EXPECTED OUTCOME

Infant exhibits evidence of fluid homeostasis.

NURSING INTERVENTIONS/*RATIONALES*

Administer parenteral fluids as prescribed and regulate carefully *to maintain fluid balance.* Avoid hypertonic fluids such as undiluted medications and concentrated glucose *because they can cause excess solute load on immature kidneys.*

Implement strategies (e.g., use of plastic covers and increase of ambient humidity) *that minimize insensible water loss.*

Monitor hydration status (i.e., skin turgor, blood pressure, edema, weight, mucous membranes, fontanels, urine specific gravity, and electrolytes) and intake and output *to evaluate for evidence of dehydration or overhydration.*

NURSING DIAGNOSIS: Risk for impaired skin integrity related to immature skin structure, poor perfusion, immobility, and invasive procedures as evidenced by epidermal stripping with adhesive removal or placement and translucent skin, erythema, abrasions

EXPECTED OUTCOME

Infant's skin remains intact with no evidence of irritation or injury.

NURSING INTERVENTIONS/*RATIONALES*

Cleanse skin as needed with plain warm water and apply moisturizing agents to skin *to prevent dryness and reduce friction across skin surface.*

When performing procedures: minimize use of tape and apply a skin barrier between tape and skin; use transparent elastic film for securing central and peripheral lines; use limb electrodes for monitoring or attach with hydrogel and rotate electrodes often; remove adhesives with soap and water rather than alcohol or acetone-based adhesive removers *to minimize skin damage.*

Monitor carefully use of thermal devices such as pulse oximeter probes, biliblankets or thermal heating pads *to prevent burns.*

Monitor skin closely for evidence of redness, rash, irritation, bruising, breakdown, ischemia, and infiltration *to detect and treat potential complications early.*

NURSING DIAGNOSIS: Risk for CNS injury related to fluctuating systemic and intracranial pressures, immature vascular bed, immature state regulatory ability, environmental stimuli, and episodes of hyperoxia and hypoxia as evidenced by episodes of hypoxia associated with handling, fluctuating blood pressure readings

EXPECTED OUTCOME

Infant will exhibit normal intracranial pressure (ICP) with no evidence of intraventricular hemorrhage.

NURSING INTERVENTIONS/*RATIONALES*

Institute minimum stimulation protocol (i.e., minimal handling, clustering care techniques, avoidance of sudden head movements to one side, undisturbed sleep periods, light variations to simulate day and night, limiting personnel and equipment noise in environment) *to decrease stress responses, which can increase ICP.*

Institute ordered pharmacologic and nonpharmacologic pain control methods *to manage pain and reduce physical stress.*

Avoid hypertonic solutions and medications *because they increase cerebral blood flow.*

Elevate head of bed 15 to 20 degrees *to decrease ICP.*

Monitor vital signs *for evidence of increased ICP.*

Recognize signs of overstimulation (i.e., flaccidity, yawning, irritability, crying, staring, and active averting) *so stimulation can be stopped to allow rest.*

NURSING DIAGNOSIS: Risk for impaired parenting related to separation and interruption of parent/infant attachment secondary to premature birth, severity of infant's illness, high-tech NICU environment, and anticipatory grieving over loss of perfect newborn as evidenced by physical separation from parents, verbalization of shock and disbelief at appearance of infant, lack of contact between infant and parent

EXPECTED OUTCOMES

Parents establish contact with neonate; demonstrate competent parenting skills and willingness to care for neonate.

NURSING INTERVENTIONS/*RATIONALES*

Before parents' first visit to the NICU, prepare them by explaining what the neonate will look like, what the equipment will look like, and its function *to diminish fear and decrease sense of shock.*

Keep parents informed about infant's condition (e.g., improvements and setbacks) and important aspects of infant's care; encourage and answer parental questions; actively listen to parent concerns *to establish trust, open communication, and caring atmosphere to aid in coping.*

Encourage parents to contact NICU staff any time, day or night, for concerns regarding the infant's condition *to maintain open channels of communication regarding infant's status and decrease parents' fear of unknown.*

Encourage parents to visit the NICU often; to name infant; to touch, hold, or caress infant as physical condition permits; to be actively involved in infant's care; to bring personal items (e.g., clothing, stuffed animals, or pictures of family) *to allow formation of emotional bond.*

Reinforce parent involvement and praise care endeavors *to increase self-confidence in their contribution.*

Encourage parents to bring other siblings to visit preterm infant as age-appropriate; explain to siblings what they are seeing; encourage siblings to draw pictures or write letters for infant and place in or near infant's crib *to promote family involvement, help ease sibling fears, and let them contribute to infant's care.*

Refer parents to social services as needed *to ensure comprehensive care.*

Provide consistent and frequent information regarding infant's condition through multidisciplinary conferences *to promote parent trust in caregivers and provide consistent information.*

Table 27-2

Normal Arterial Blood Gas Values for Neonates

VALUE	RANGE
pH	7.35-7.45
Arterial oxygen pressure (Pao_2)	60-80 mm Hg
Carbon dioxide pressure ($Paco_2$)	35-45 mm Hg
Bicarbonate (HCO^-_3)	22-26 mEq/L
Base excess	(−4) to (+4)
Oxygen saturation	92%-94%

From Parry WH, Zimmer J: Acid-base homeostasis and oxygenation. In Merenstein GB, Gardner SL (eds): *Handbook of neonatal intensive care*, ed 5, St Louis, 2002, Mosby.

The maintenance of an NTE continues to be of critical importance in infants with RDS; infants with hypoxemia are unable to increase their metabolic rate when cold stressed.

The clinical and radiographic presentation of neonatal pneumonia may be similar to that of RDS. Therefore sepsis evaluation, including blood culture, complete blood count (CBC) with differential, and occasionally a lumbar puncture, is done in infants with RDS to rule out systemic infection; laboratory and radiographic tests rarely confirm the diagnosis of neonatal pneumonia, rather it is the clinical history and presenting clinical signs that provide a basis for the diagnosis and treatment (Stoll, 2004). Broad-spectrum antibiotics are begun while the results of cultures are awaited.

Fluid and nutrition must be maintained for the infant critically ill with RDS. Parenteral nutrition can provide protein and fat to promote a positive nitrogen balance. Daily monitoring of electrolytes, urine output, specific gravity, and weight assists in the evaluation of hydration status.

Respiratory distress of a nonpulmonary origin in neonates may also be caused by sepsis, cardiac defects (structural or functional), exposure to cold, airway obstruction (atresia), intraventricular hemorrhage, hypoglycemia, metabolic acidosis, acute blood loss, and drugs. Pneumonia in the neonatal period may present as respiratory distress caused by bacterial or viral agents and may occur alone or as a complication of RDS.

CRITICAL THINKING EXERCISE—PATENT DUCTUS ARTERIOSUS

Patent Ductus Arteriosus

The ductus arteriosus is a muscular contractile structure in the fetus connecting the left pulmonary artery and the dorsal aorta. The ductus constricts after birth as oxygenation, the levels of circulating prostaglandins, and the muscle mass increase. Other factors that promote ductal closure include catecholamines, low pH, bradykinin, and acetylcholine. When the fetal ductus arteriosus fails to close after birth, patent ductus arteriosus (PDA) occurs. Ductal closure usually occurs within hours or days in the term infant but may be delayed in preterm infants as a result of oxygenation and circulating hormones (prostaglandins).

The clinical presentation in an infant with a PDA includes systolic murmur, active precordium, bounding peripheral pulses, tachycardia, tachypnea, crackles, and hepatomegaly. The systolic murmur is heard best at the second or third intercostal space at the upper left sternal border. An active precordium is caused by an increased left ventricular stroke volume. A widened pulse pressure may result in an increase in peripheral pulses.

Radiographic studies of infants with a large shunting PDA typically show cardiac enlargement and pulmonary edema; with a smaller PDA, the radiograph may appear normal for the infant's age (Montoya & Washington, 2002). ABG findings reveal hypercarbia and metabolic acidosis. A color flow Doppler echocardiograph can demonstrate a PDA, identify the direction of the shunting (left-to-right, right-to-left, or both) and can quantitate the amount of blood shunting across the PDA.

The PDA can be managed medically or surgically. Medical management consists of ventilatory support, fluid restriction, and the administration of diuretics and indomethacin. Indomethacin is a prostaglandin synthetase inhibitor that blocks the effect of the arachidonic acid products on the ductus and causes the PDA to constrict. Ventilatory support is adjusted based on ABG levels. Fluid restriction is implemented to decrease cardiovascular volume overload in association with the diuretic therapy. Surgical ligation is performed when PDA is clinically significant and medical management has failed. The nonsteroidal anti-inflammatory drug (NSAID), ibuprofen, has been used with some success in the medical closure of PDA in preterm infants. This drug has fewer side effects than indomethacin and acts by inhibiting prostaglandin formation (Flores, 2003).

Nursing care of the infant with PDA focuses on supportive care. The infant needs an NTE, adequate oxygenation, meticulous fluid balance, and parental support.

Periventricular-Intraventricular Hemorrhage

Periventricular-intraventricular hemorrhage (PV-IVH) is one of the most common types of brain injury that occurs in neonates and is among the most severe in both short-term and long-term outcomes. The true incidence of PV-IVH is unknown, but the general estimate is 15% in infants less than 32 weeks of gestation or under 1501 g (Volpe, 2001). PV-IVH occurs in approximately 3.5% to 5% of term infants, with 50% of those cases caused by asphyxia or trauma. In term infants the symptoms appear within 48 hours of birth (Paige & Carney, 2002).

The pathogenesis of PV-IVH includes intravascular factors (e.g., fluctuating or increasing cerebral blood flow, increases in cerebral venous pressure, and coagulopathy), vascular factors, extravascular factors (hypoglycemia, acidosis), and routine nursery care (rapid volume expansion, blood transfusion). PV-IVH events typically occur within the first week of life. PV-IVH is classified according to severity, which determines long-term neurodevelopmental outcomes.

Nursing care focuses on recognition of factors that increase the risk of PV-IVH, interventions to decrease the risk of bleeding, and supportive care to infants who have bleeding episodes. The infant is positioned with the head in midline and the head of the bed elevated slightly to prevent or minimize fluctuations in intracranial blood pressure. NTE is maintained, as well as oxygenation. Rapid infusions of fluids should be avoided. Blood pressure is monitored closely for fluctuations. The infant is monitored for signs of pneumothorax because it often precedes PV-IVH.

Necrotizing Enterocolitis

Necrotizing enterocolitis (NEC) is an acute inflammatory disease of the GI mucosa, commonly complicated by perforation. This often fatal disease occurs in about 2% to 5% of newborns in NICUs. Three factors appear to play an important role in the development of NEC: intestinal ischemia, colonization by pathogenic bacteria, and substrate (formula feeding) in the intestinal lumen. The precise cause of NEC is still uncertain, but it appears to occur in infants whose gastrointestinal tract has suffered vascular compromise. Intestinal ischemia of unknown etiology, immature gastrointestinal host defenses, bacterial proliferation, and feeding substrate are now believed to have a multifactorial role in the etiology of NEC. Prematurity remains the most prominent risk factor in the development of NEC.

The onset of NEC in the full-term infant usually occurs between 4 and 10 days after birth. In the preterm infant the onset may be delayed for up to 30 days. Signs of developing NEC are nonspecific, which is characteristic of many neonatal disease processes. Some generalized signs include decreased activity, hypotonia, pallor, recurrent apnea and bradycardia, decreased oxygen saturation, respiratory distress, metabolic acidosis, oliguria, hypotension, decreased perfusion, temperature instability, and cyanosis. GI symptoms include abdominal distention, increasing or bile-stained residual gastric aspirates, vomiting (bile or blood), grossly bloody stools, abdominal tenderness, and erythema of the abdominal wall (Bensard et al, 2002).

Diagnosis of NEC is confirmed by radiographic examination that reveals bowel loop distention, pneumatosis intestinalis, pneumoperitoneum, portal air, or a combination of these findings. The abnormal radiographic findings are caused by the bacterial colonization of the GI tract associated with NEC, resulting in an ileus. Pneumatosis intestinalis, pneumoperitoneum, and portal air are caused by gas produced by the bacteria that invade the wall of the intestines and escape into the peritoneum and portal system when perforation occurs. Laboratory evaluation includes a complete blood cell count with differential, coagulation studies, ABG analysis, serum electrolyte levels, and blood culture. The white blood cell (WBC) count may be either increased or decreased. The platelet count and coagulation studies may be abnormal, with thrombocytopenia and disseminated intravascular coagulation (DIC). Electrolyte levels may be abnormal, with leaking capillary beds and fluid shifts with the infection.

Treatment of infants with NEC is supportive and preventive for bowel perforation. Oral or tube feedings are discontinued to rest the GI tract. A nasogastric tube is inserted and placed to low suction to provide gastric decompression. Parenteral therapy (often by TPN) is begun. NEC is an infectious disease; control of infection is imperative, with an emphasis on careful handwashing before and after infant contact. Systemic antibiotic therapy is instituted, and surgical resection is performed if perforation or clinical deterioration occurs.

With early recognition and treatment, medical management is increasingly successful. If there is progressive deterioration under medical management or evidence of perforation, surgical resection and anastomosis are performed. Extensive involvement may necessitate surgical intervention and establishment of an ileostomy, jejunostomy, or colostomy. Sequelae in surviving infants include short-gut syndrome, colonic stricture with obstruction, fat malabsorption, and failure to thrive secondary to intestinal dysfunction. Various surgical interventions for NEC are available and depend on the extent of bowel necrosis, associated illness factors, and infant stability. Intestinal transplantation has been successful in some former preterm infants with NEC-associated short-gut syndrome who had already developed life-threatening TPN-related complications. Transplantation may be a lifesaving option for infants who previously faced high morbidity and mortality (Vennarecci et al, 2000). Therapy may be prolonged and recovery may be delayed by adhesions, complications of bowel resection, short-gut syndrome (especially if the ileocecal valve is removed), and intolerance of oral feedings.

NURSE ALERT Observe for indications of early development of NEC by checking the appearance of the abdomen for distention (measuring abdominal girth, measuring residual gastric contents before feedings, and listening for the presence of bowel sounds) and performing all routine assessments for high risk neonates. ■

Minimal enteral feedings (trophic feeding, GI priming) have gained acceptance with no evidence of increased incidence of NEC. Early experience indicates such feedings may in fact be protective against NEC in nonasphyxiated preterm infants in addition to exerting other potential benefits. There is evidence that human milk may have a protective effect against the development of NEC (Diehl-Jones & Askin, 2004).

Complications of Oxygen Therapy

Retinopathy of Prematurity

Retinopathy of prematurity (ROP) is a complex, multicausal disorder that affects the developing retinal vessels of premature infants. The normal retinal vessels begin to form in utero at approximately 16 weeks of gestation in response to an unknown stimulus. The retinal vessels continue to develop until they reach maturity at approximately 42 to 43 weeks after conception. Once the retina is completely vascularized, the retinal vessels are not susceptible to ROP. The mechanism of injury in ROP is unclear. Oxygen tensions that are too high for the level of retinal maturity initially result in vasoconstriction. After oxygen therapy is discontinued, neovascularization occurs in the retina and vitreous, with capillary hemorrhages, fibrotic resolution, and possible retinal detachment. Scar tissue formation and consequent visual impairment may be mild or severe. The entire disease process in severe cases may take as long as 5 months to evolve. Examination by an ophthalmologist before discharge and a schedule for repeat examinations thereafter are recommended for the parents' guidance.

The key to management of ROP is prevention and early detection of premature birth.

Although exposure to bright light has not proven to contribute to ROP, such exposure is nevertheless undesirable from a neurobehavioral developmental perspective. All caregivers should use supplemental oxygen judiciously, monitor oxygen blood levels carefully, promptly attend to saturation monitor alarms, and prevent wide fluctuations in oxygen blood levels (hyperoxemia and hypoxemia).

Circumferential cryopexy, laser photocoagulation, vitamin E therapy, and decreasing the intensity of ambient light are used in the treatment of ROP with varying results. Early screening and detection should be provided in infants born at less than 28 weeks of gestation and whose weight is less than1500 g and in infants weighing between 1500 g and 2000 g who are believed to be at high risk for development of ROP (American Academy of Pediatrics, 2001).

Chronic Lung Disease (Formerly Bronchopulmonary Dysplasia)

Chronic lung disease (CLD) is a chronic pulmonary iatrogenic condition caused by barotrauma from pressure ventilation and oxygen toxicity (Hagedorn et al, 2002). The etiology of CLD is multifactorial and includes pulmonary immaturity, surfactant deficiency, lung injury and stretch, barotrauma, inflammation caused by oxygen exposure, fluid overload, ligation of a patent ductus arteriosus, and genetic predisposition (Hagedorn et al, 2002). The incidence of CLD in infants weighing less than 1500 g who require mechanical ventilation for RDS ranges from 23% to 80% (Berger et al, 2004; Gracey et al, 2002). In some institutions, the overall incidence of CLD has decreased over the past decade (Byrne et al, 2002).

Clinical symptoms of CLD include tachypnea, retractions, nasal flaring, increased work of breathing, exercise intolerance (to handling and feeding), and tachycardia (Hagedorn et al, 2002). Auscultation of lung fields in affected infants reveals crackles, decreased air movement, and occasionally expiratory wheezing.

Treatment for CLD includes oxygen therapy, nutrition, fluid restriction, and medications (e.g., diuretics, corticosteroids, and bronchodilators). The use of corticosteroids to prevent or treat CLD is controversial because of the side effects and varied results in clinical trials; however, corticosteroids are used in many centers to treat or prevent CLD (American Academy of Pediatrics, 2002).The key to the management of CLD is prevention by reducing the incidence of prematurity and RDS and by using surfactant, antenatal steroids, and minimizing lung trauma from mechanical ventilation and high oxygen concentrations.

The prognosis for infants with CLD depends on the degree of pulmonary dysfunction. Most deaths occur within the first year of life as a result of cardiorespiratory failure, sepsis, or respiratory infection; in some infants the deaths are sudden and unexplained.

THE POSTMATURE INFANT

Postterm infants are those whose gestation is prolonged beyond 42 weeks, regardless of birth weight; the infant is called postmature. These infants may be large-for-gestational-age (LGA) or small-for-gestational-age (SGA), but most often their weight is appropriate-for-gestational-age (AGA). It is important to determine whether the pregnancy is actually prolonged and also whether there is any evidence of fetal jeopardy as a result. The cause of prolonged pregnancy is unknown. Postmaturity can be associated with placental insufficiency, resulting in a newborn who has a thin, emaciated appearance (dysmature) at birth because of loss of subcutaneous fat and muscle mass. There may be meconium staining of the fingernails, the hair and nails may be long, and vernix may be absent. The skin may peel off. Not all postmature infants show signs of dysmaturity; some continue to grow in utero and are large at birth.

Perinatal mortality is significantly higher in the postmature fetus and neonate. During labor and birth, increased oxygen demands of the postmature fetus may not be met. Insufficient gas exchange in the postmature placenta increases the likelihood of intrauterine hypoxia, which may result in the passage of meconium in utero, thereby increasing the risk for meconium aspiration syndrome. Of all the deaths of postmature newborns, one-half occur during labor and birth, about one-third occur before the onset of labor, and one-sixth occur in the newborn period.

Meconium Aspiration Syndrome

Meconium staining of the amniotic fluid can be indicative of nonreassuring fetal status, especially in a vertex presentation. It appears in 8% to 20% of all births. Many infants with meconium staining exhibit no signs of depression at birth; however, the presence of meconium in the amniotic fluid necessitates careful supervision of labor and close monitoring of fetal well-being. The presence of a team skilled in neonatal resuscitation is required at the birth of any infant with meconium-stained amniotic fluid. The mouth and nares of the infant are routinely suctioned on the perineum before the infant's first breath. However, Vain et al (2005) in a multicentered randomized, controlled trial found no difference in outcomes between those infant who were suctioned and those who were not. The current practice needs further study.

If meconium is not removed from the airway at birth, it can migrate down to the terminal airways, causing mechanical obstruction leading to meconium aspiration syndrome (MAS). The fetus may have aspirated meconium in utero, which can cause a chemical pneumonitis. These infants may develop persistent pulmonary hypertension of the newborn (PPHN), further complicating their management. Infants with moderate-to-severe MAS may receive surfactant replacement to improve alveolar function.

Persistent Pulmonary Hypertension of the Newborn

PPHN is a term applied to the combined findings of pulmonary hypertension, right-to-left shunting, and a structurally normal heart. PPHN may present either as a single entity or as the main component of MAS, congenital diaphragmatic hernia, RDS, hyperviscosity syndrome, or neonatal pneumonia or sepsis. PPHN is also called persistent fetal circulation (PFC) because the syndrome includes reversion to fetal pathways for blood flow.

A brief review of fetal blood flow can help in the visualization of the problems with PPHN (see Fig. 8-11). In utero, oxygen-rich blood leaves the placenta via the umbilical vein, goes through the ductus venosus, and enters the inferior vena cava. From there, it empties into the right atrium and is mostly shunted across the foramen ovale to the left atrium, effectively bypassing the lungs. This blood enters the left ventricle, leaves through the aorta, and preferentially perfuses the carotid and coronary arteries. Thus the heart and brain receive the most oxygenated blood. Blood drains from the brain into the superior vena cava, reenters the right atrium, proceeds to the right ventricle, and exits through the main pulmonary artery. The lungs are a high-pressure circuit, needing only enough perfusion for growth and nutrition. The ductus arteriosus (connecting the main pulmonary artery and the aorta) is the path of least resistance for the blood leaving the right side of the fetal heart, shunting most of the cardiac output away from the lungs and toward the systemic system. This right-to-left shunting is the key to fetal circulation.

After birth, both the foramen ovale and the ductus arteriosus close in response to various biochemical processes, pressure changes within the heart, and dilation of the pulmonary vessels. This dilation allows virtually all of the cardiac output to enter the lungs, become oxygenated, and provide oxygen-rich blood to the tissues for normal metabolism. Any process that interferes with this transition from fetal to neonatal circulation may precipitate PPHN. PPHN characteristically proceeds into a downward spiral of exacerbating hypoxia and pulmonary vasoconstriction. Prompt recognition and aggressive intervention are required to reverse this process.

The infant with PPHN is typically born at term or postterm and presents with tachycardia and cyanosis and within minutes or hours progresses to severe respiratory compromise with concomitant acidosis, which further compromises pulmonary perfusion and deteriorating oxygenation. Management depends on the underlying etiology of the persistent pulmonary hypertension. The use of INO and ECMO (see previous discussion) has improved the chances of survival of these infants.

Another mode of treatment for PPHN and other respiratory disorders of the newborn is high-frequency ventilation, an assisted-ventilation method that delivers small volumes of gas at high frequencies and limits the development of high airway pressure, thus theoretically reducing barotrauma.

OTHER PROBLEMS RELATED TO GESTATION

Small-for-Gestational-Age Infants and Intrauterine Growth Restriction

Infants who are small for gestational age (i.e., weight is below the 10th percentile expected at term) or infants who have intrauterine growth restriction (IUGR) (i.e., rate of growth does not meet expected growth pattern) are considered high risk, with the perimortality rate 5 to 20 times greater than that for the normal term infant (Kliegman & Das, 2002).

Various conditions can affect and impede growth in the developing fetus. Conditions occurring in the first trimester that affect all aspects of fetal growth (e.g., infections, teratogens, and chromosomal abnormalities) or extrinsic conditions early in pregnancy result in symmetric IUGR (i.e., head circumference, length, and weight are all less than the 10th percentile). Conditions causing symmetric growth restriction result in an SGA infant, usually with a smaller head circumference and reduced brain capacity. Growth restriction in later stages of pregnancy, as a result of maternal or placental factors, results in asymmetric growth restriction (with respect to gestational age, weight will be less than the 10th percentile, whereas length and head circumference will be greater than the 10th percentile). Infants with asymmetric IUGR have the potential for normal growth and development. Abnormal fetal size may indicate an adaptive response, with diminished fetal weight-sparing brain growth.

Care of the SGA infant is based on the clinical problems present and is the same given to preterm infants with similar problems. Gas exchange is supported by maintaining a clear airway and preventing cold stress. Hypoglycemia is treated with oral feedings (e.g., breast, formula, or intravenous dextrose) as the infant's condition warrants. An external heat source (radiant warmer or incubator) is used until the infant is able to maintain an adequate body temperature. Nursing support of parents is the same as that given to parents of preterm infants.

Common problems that affect small-for-gestational-age IUGR infants are perinatal asphyxia, meconium aspiration (discussed previously), immunodeficiency, hypoglycemia, polycythemia, and temperature instability.

Perinatal Asphyxia

Commonly, IUGR infants have been exposed to chronic hypoxia for varying periods before labor and birth. Labor is a stressor to the normal fetus; it is an even greater stressor for the growth-restricted fetus. The chronically hypoxic infant is severely compromised by a normal labor and has difficulty compensating after birth. The alert, wide-eyed appearance of the newborn is attributed to prolonged fetal hypoxia. Appropriate management and resuscitation are essential for the depressed infant.

The birth of the SGA newborn with perinatal asphyxia may be associated with a maternal history of heavy cigarette smoking; gestational hypertension; low socioeconomic status; multifetal gestation; gestational infections such as rubella, cytomegalovirus, and toxoplasmosis; advanced diabetes mellitus; and cardiac problems. Sequelae to perinatal asphyxia include MAS and hypoglycemia.

Hypoglycemia

All high risk infants are at risk for the development of hypoglycemia. Infants who are asphyxiated or have other physiologic stress may experience hypoglycemia as a result of a decreased glycogen supply, inadequate gluconeogenesis, or overutilization of glycogen stored during fetal life. The concept of hypoglycemia as being a single cutoff value has received criticism because of the wide variability of glucose values from one newborn to another, expressed along a continuum of falling blood glucose values (Blackburn, 2003).

Preterm infants with plasma glucose values equal to 47 mg/dl on 5 different days in the first 2 months of life showed significant yet transient abnormal neuromotor and cognitive performance (Lucas, Morley, & Cole, 1988). Because hypoglycemia is often asymptomatic in newborns, dependence on clinical signs or a single blood glucose value alone is inadequate.

Symptoms of hypoglycemia include poor feeding, hypothermia, and diaphoresis. CNS symptoms can include tremors and jitteriness, weak cry, lethargy, floppy posture, seizures, or coma. Diagnosis is confirmed by laboratory blood glucose determinations or glucose reflectance meter. The use of reagent strips alone is reported to be unreliable, especially at values lower than 40 to 50 mg/dl, and may be affected by the hematocrit (Blackburn, 2003).

Cornblath and others (2000) have suggested operational thresholds at which interventions to increase serum blood glucose levels should be implemented to prevent serious effects. The threshhold criterion that applies is as follows:

- At-risk infants (*neonatal factors:* infant of diabetic mother, hypothermia, hyperinsulinism, respiratory distress, congenital abnormalities, SGA, prematurity; *maternal factors:* gestational hypertension, terbutaline administration for preterm labor) should have glucose values equal to 36 mg/dl within the first few hours of life with a therapeutic objective of 45 mg/dl.

  In these infants it is recommended that close observation and blood glucose levels be monitored within 2 to 3 hours of birth. If the newborn has a blood glucose below 36 mg/dl (2.0 mmol/L), intervention such as breast or bottle feeding should be instituted; if levels remain low despite feeding, intravenous dextrose is warranted.
- Blood glucose levels for infants with severe hyperinsulinism may need to be higher (60 mg/dl; 3.3 mmol/L) to prevent serious effects.
- Hypoglycemia in preterm infants requires further studies, but it has been suggested that values be maintained above 47 mg/dl (2.6 mmol/L) (Cornblath et al, 2000).

Heat Loss

SGA infants are particularly susceptible to temperature instability as a result of decreased brown fat deposit; decreased adipose tissue; large body surface exposure and, often, poor flexion; as well as decreased glycogen storage in major organs such as the liver and heart. Therefore, close attention must be given to maintain a thermoneutral environment. Nursing considerations focus on maintenance of thermoneutrality to promote recovery from perinatal asphyxia because cold stress jeopardizes such recovery.

Large-for-Gestational-Age Infants

The large-for-gestational-age (LGA) infant is defined as an infant weighing 4000 g or more at birth. An infant is considered LGA despite gestation when the weight is above the 90th percentile on growth charts or two standard deviations above the mean weight for gestational age. Certain fetal disorders, including transposition of the great vessels and Beckwith-Wiedemann syndrome, can also result in LGA infants.

Maternal pelvic diameters have not kept pace with the better maternal health and nutrition that results in larger newborns; thus, fetopelvic disproportion may occur, particularly in obese women, women who gain 16 kg or more during gestation, and women with undiagnosed and/or uncontrolled diabetes who are prone to have large newborns. Birth trauma, especially associated with breech or shoulder presentation, is a serious hazard for the oversized neonate. Asphyxia, CNS injury, or both may occur.

All pregnancies of longer than 42 weeks of gestation must be carefully evaluated. All large fetuses are monitored during a trial of labor, and preparation is made for a cesarean birth if nonreassuring fetal status or poor progress of labor occurs. LGA newborns may be preterm, term, or postdate; they may be infants of diabetic mothers; or they may be postmature. Each of these problems carries special concerns. Regardless of coexisting potential problems, the LGA infant is at risk by virtue of size alone.

The nurse assesses the LGA infant for hypoglycemia and trauma resulting from vaginal or cesarean birth. The blood glucose levels of LGA infants are monitored, and hypoglycemia is corrected. Any specific birth injuries are identified and treated appropriately.

Infants of Diabetic Mothers

All infants born to mothers with diabetes are at some risk for complications. The degree of risk is influenced by the severity and duration of maternal disease. Problems seen in infants of diabetic mothers (IDMs) include congenital anomalies, macrosomia, birth trauma and perinatal asphyxia, RDS, hypoglycemia, hypocalcemia and hypomagnesemia, cardiomyopathy, hyperbilirubinemia, and polycythemia. Because some of these problems are also seen in infants with gestational age–related problems, discussion of infants of mothers with diabetes is included here.

Pathophysiology

The mechanisms responsible for the problems seen in IDMs are not fully understood. Congenital anomalies are believed to be caused by fluctuations in blood glucose levels and episodes of ketoacidosis in early pregnancy. Later in pregnancy, when the mother's pancreas cannot release sufficient insulin to meet increased demands, maternal hyperglycemia results. The high levels of glucose cross the placenta and stimulate the fetal pancreas to release more insulin. The combination of the increased supply of maternal glucose and other nutrients, the inability of maternal insulin to cross the placenta, and increased fetal insulin results in excessive fetal growth called macrosomia (see the discussion that follows).

Hyperinsulinemia accounts for many of the problems the fetus or infant develops. In addition to fluctuating glucose levels, maternal vascular involvement or superimposed maternal infection adversely affect the fetus. Normally, maternal blood has a more alkaline pH than does carbon dioxide–rich fetal blood. This phenomenon encourages the exchange of oxygen and carbon dioxide across the placental membrane. When the maternal blood is more acidotic than the fetal blood, such as during ketoacidosis, little carbon dioxide or oxygen exchange occurs at the level of the placenta. The mortality for the unborn infant resulting from an episode of maternal ketoacidosis may be as high as 50% or more (Kalhan & Parimi, 2002).

There are indications that some neonatal conditions (e.g., macrosomia, hypoglycemia, polyhydramnios, preterm birth, and perhaps fetal lung immaturity) may be eliminated, or the incidence decreased, by maintaining tight control over maternal glucose levels within narrow limits (Reece et al, 1998). Tight glucose control is defined as the maintenance of maternal blood glucose levels between 100 and 120 mg/dl.

Congenital Anomalies

Congenital anomalies occur in about 7% to 10% of IDMs. Their incidence is two to four times that for infants born to mothers without diabetes. The incidence is greatest among SGA newborns. IUGR leading to SGA infants is seen in IDMs with severe vascular disease. The most commonly occurring anomalies involve the cardiac, musculoskeletal, and central nervous systems. In most defects associated with diabetic pregnancies, the structural abnormality occurs before the eighth week after conception. This reinforces the importance of control of blood glucose both before conception and in the early stages of pregnancy.

The incidence of congenital heart lesions in these infants is five times higher than that in the general population. Coarctation of the aorta, transposition of the great vessels, and atrial or ventricular septal defects are the most common lesions encountered in the IDM. Maternal diabetic control is correlated with the incidence of defects; that is, the better the control, the fewer the defects.

CNS anomalies include anencephaly, encephalocele, meningomyelocele, and hydrocephalus. The musculoskeletal system may be affected by caudal regression syndrome (i.e., sacral agenesis, with weakness or deformities of the lower extremities, malformation and fixation of the hip joints, and shortening or deformity of the femurs). Hypertrichosis on the pinnae (excessive hair growth on the external ear) has been added to the list of characteristic clinical features. Other defects noted in this population include GI atresia and urinary tract malformations.

Macrosomia

Despite improvements in the control of maternal blood sugar levels, the incidence of macrosomia in the insulin-dependent diabetic is higher than in infants born of mothers who are not diabetic. At birth the typical LGA infant has a round, cherubic ("tomato" or cushingoid) face, chubby body, and a plethoric or flushed complexion (Fig. 27-10). The infant has enlarged internal organs (i.e., hepatosplenomegaly, splanchnomegaly, and cardiomegaly) and increased body fat, especially around the shoulders. The placenta and umbilical cord are larger than average. The brain is the only organ that is not enlarged. IDMs may be LGA but physiologically immature.

The macrosomic infant is at risk for hypoglycemia, hypocalcemia, hyperviscosity, and hyperbilirubinemia. The excessive shoulder size in these infants often leads to dystocia, particularly because the head may be smaller in proportion to the shoulders than in a nonmacrosomic infant. Macrosomic infants born vaginally or by cesarean birth after a trial of labor may incur birth trauma.

Birth Trauma and Perinatal Asphyxia

Birth injury (resulting from macrosomia or method of birth) and perinatal asphyxia occur in 20% of infants of gestational diabetic mothers (IGDMs) and 35% of IDMs. Examples of birth trauma include cephalhematoma; paralysis of the facial nerve (seventh cranial nerve) (see Fig. 28-3); fracture of the clavicle or humerus; brachial plexus paralysis, usually Erb-Duchenne (right upper arm) palsy (see Figs. 28-1 and 28-2); and phrenic nerve paralysis, invariably associated with diaphragmatic paralysis.

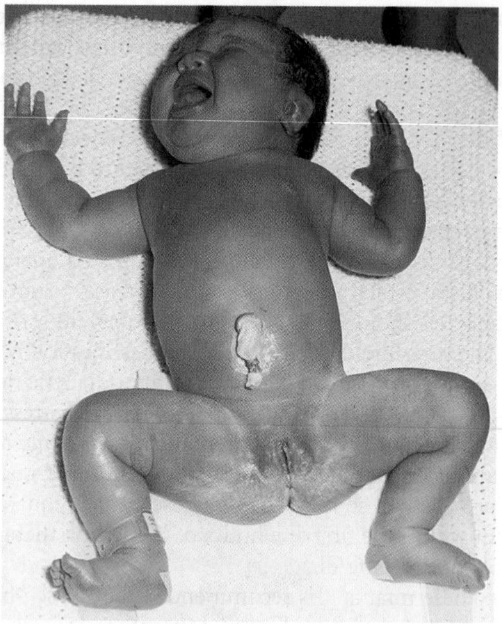

Fig. 27-10 Macrosomic newborn. (From O'Doherty N: *Neonatology: micro atlas of the newborn,* Nutley, NJ, 1986, Hoffmann-La Roche.)

Respiratory Distress Syndrome

IDMs are four to six times more likely than normal infants to develop RDS. With improved maternal glucose control, this risk has been substantially reduced. In the fetus exposed to high levels of maternal glucose, synthesis of surfactant may be delayed because of the high fetal serum level of insulin. Fetal lung maturity, as evidenced by a lecithin/sphingomyelin (L/S) ratio of 2:1, is not reassuring if the mother has diabetes mellitus or gestation-induced diabetes mellitus. For the infants of such mothers, an L/S ratio of 3:1 or more or the presence of phosphatidylglycerol in the amniotic fluid is more indicative of adequate lung maturity.

Hypoglycemia

Hypoglycemia affects many IDMs. After constant exposure to high circulating levels of glucose, hyperplasia of the fetal pancreas occurs, resulting in hyperinsulinemia. Disruption of the fetal glucose supply occurs with the clamping of the umbilical cord, and the neonate's blood glucose level falls rapidly in the presence of fetal hyperinsulinism. Hypoglycemia is most common in the macrosomic or SGA infant, but blood glucose levels should be monitored in all infants of known or suspected diabetic mothers.

Asymptomatic or symptomatic hypoglycemia most commonly presents within the first 1 to 3 hours after birth. Signs of hypoglycemia include jitteriness, apnea, tachypnea, and cyanosis. Significant hypoglycemia may result in seizures. Hypoglycemia is worsened by the presence of hypothermia or respiratory distress.

Hypocalcemia and Hypomagnesemia

Hypocalcemia occurs in as many as 50% of IDMs. A number of these cases are related to hypoxia or prematurity; however, the overall incidence of hypocalcemia is higher than in nondiabetic pregnancies. Hypomagnesemia is believed to develop because of maternal renal losses that occur in diabetes. Hypocalcemia is associated with preterm birth,

birth trauma, and perinatal asphyxia. Signs of hypocalcemia, a prevalent finding in IDMs, are similar to those of hypoglycemia, but they occur within the first 24 hours of age.

Cardiomyopathy

All IDMs need careful observation for cardiomyopathy because an increased heart size is often found among these infants. Two types of cardiomyopathy can occur. Clinicians must be alert to identify correctly the type of lesion so that appropriate therapy is instituted. Both types of lesions are associated with respiratory symptoms and congestive heart failure.

Hypertrophic cardiomyopathy (HCM) is characterized by a hypercontractile and thickened myocardium. The ventricular walls are thickened, as is the septum, which in severe cases results in outflow tract obstructions. The mitral valve is poorly functioning. In nonhypertrophic cardiomyopathy (non-HCM) the myocardium is poorly contractile and overstretched. The ventricles are increased in size, and there is no outflow obstruction. Most infants are asymptomatic, but severe outflow obstruction may cause left ventricular heart failure. HCM may be treated with a beta-adrenergic blocker (such as propranolol to decrease contractility and heart rate). A cardiotonic agent is used to treat non-HCM (such as digoxin to increase contractility and decrease heart rate). The abnormality usually resolves in 3 to 12 months.

Hyperbilirubinemia and Polycythemia

IDMs are at increased risk of developing hyperbilirubinemia. Many IDMs are also polycythemic. Polycythemia increases blood viscosity, thereby impairing circulation. In addition, this increased number of RBCs to be hemolyzed increases the potential bilirubin load that the neonate must clear. The excessive RBCs are produced in extramedullary foci (liver and spleen) in addition to the usual sites in bone marrow. Therefore both liver function and bilirubin clearance may be adversely affected. Bruising associated with birth of a macrosomic infant will contribute further to high bilirubin levels.

Nursing Care

Ideally, planning for the IDM begins during the antenatal period. Pediatric staff members are present at the birth. Implementation of care depends on the neonate's particular problems. If the maternal blood glucose level was well controlled throughout the pregnancy, the infant may require only monitoring. Because euglycemia is not always possible, the nurse must promptly recognize and treat any consequences of maternal diabetes that arise (Nursing Care Plan).

Nursing Care Plan

THE INFANT OF MOTHER WITH DIABETES MELLITUS

NURSING DIAGNOSIS: Risk for injury related to hypoglycemia secondary to hyperinsulinemia and maternal diabetes

EXPECTED OUTCOME

Infant will exhibit serum blood glucose levels that are WNL.

NURSING INTERVENTIONS/*RATIONALES*

Monitor blood glucose levels in infants at known risk for hypoglycemia (e.g., SGA, preterm [ELBW, VLBW], infant of diabetic mother) *to assess and detect early onset to prevent complications.*

Observe for signs of hypoglycemia (e.g., jitteriness, twitching, lethargy, apathy, seizures, cyanosis, sweating, eye rolling, and refusal to eat) *to assess and detect signs of onset to prevent complications.*

Institute early feeding of breast milk or infant formula *to prevent or treat early hypoglycemia.*

Reduce adverse environmental factors (e.g., cold stress, hypoxia, and respiratory distress) *that can predispose infant to hypoglycemia.*

NURSING DIAGNOSIS: Ineffective breathing pattern related to lung immaturity secondary to maternal gestational diabetes

EXPECTED OUTCOME

Infant will exhibit breathing pattern adequate to maintain oxygenation (i.e., respiratory rate, rhythm, and amplitude).

NURSING INTERVENTIONS/*RATIONALES*

Monitor infant vital signs and patency of airway *to evaluate pulmonary and circulatory status.*

Avoid activities that may lower body temperature and lead to cold stress, *which can induce respiratory distress.*

Suction as needed *to keep airway patent and prevent aspiration.*

Position infant on side initially *to facilitate mucous drainage.*

Have resuscitation equipment and oxygen available *for quick treatment of respiratory distress.*

NURSING DIAGNOSIS: Risk for imbalanced body temperature related to physiologic immaturity

See the Nursing Plan of Care for the term newborn in Chapter 25.

NURSING DIAGNOSIS: Anxiety (risk for powerlessness, situational low self-esteem, ineffective coping) related to neonate's condition, management, and prognosis

EXPECTED OUTCOME

Parents demonstrate understanding of prognosis and therapy for infant.

NURSING INTERVENTIONS/*RATIONALES*

Explain potential effects of maternal diabetic condition on newborn *to relieve fear of unknown and support ability to cope.*

Encourage open communication (e.g., inform parents of ongoing condition, procedures, and treatment; answer questions; correct misperceptions; actively listen to parental concerns) *to provide support and help provide sense of control.*

Encourage parents to interact with infant and to become involved in care routines *to foster emotional connection.*

Arrange for return demonstration of care by parents *to assess competence, provide positive reinforcement, and decrease their anxiety.*

DISCHARGE PLANNING

Discharge planning for the high risk newborn begins early in the hospitalization. Throughout the infant's hospitalization, the nurse gathers information from the health care team members and the family. This information is used to determine the infant's and family's readiness for discharge.

As home care needs of the infant's parents are assessed, steps are taken to eliminate any knowledge deficits. Discharge teaching for the high risk newborn family is extensive, requires time, and cannot be adequately accomplished on the day of discharge. Information is provided about infant care, especially as it pertains to the particular infant's home needs (e.g., supplemental oxygen, gastrostomy feedings). Parent education includes having them give return demonstrations of their infant care skills to show whether they are becoming increasingly independent in the provision of this care. Parents of infants who have special needs or who were born at less than 34 weeks of gestation should be given the opportunity to spend a night or two in a predischarge room providing care for the infant away from the NICU to become better acquainted with the necessary care and to have a time of transition in which questions may be answered regarding home care. Additional parent teaching should include bathing and skin care; requirements for meeting nutritional needs following discharge; safety in the home, including supine sleep position and prevention of infection (e.g., RSV); and medication administration. Preterm infants have a high rate of readmission to acute care centers and emergency room visits; it is imperative that the family have a health professional they may contact for questions regarding infant care and behavior once they are home. Parents should obtain an age-appropriate car seat before the discharge of their infant and demonstrate its use with the infant; in many cases the preterm infant will require adjustments and it is recommended that a period of time be used to monitor the infant in the car seat for oxygen desaturations so adjustments can be made. Before discharge all high risk or preterm infants should receive the appropriate immunizations, metabolic screening, hematology assessment (bilirubin risk as appropriate), and evaluation of hearing (American Academy of Pediatrics, 1998).

Successful discharge of high risk infants to their homes requires a multidisciplinary approach. Medical, nursing, social services, and other professionals (physical therapy, occupational therapy, developmental follow-up specialist) are crucial to the smooth transition of these infants and their families to the community and home. If the infant is transported back to the community hospital that referred either the mother before birth or the infant after birth, interfacility communication is essential to continuity of care.

Discharge to home for high risk infants does not mean they can be treated like healthy term newborns. Follow-up by a specialized practitioner familiar with the complications common to the high risk newborn is essential. Further follow-up of specific complications by qualified specialists and referral to centers for developmental interventions can help ensure the best outcome possible for these infants.

Referrals for appropriate resources also need to be made. Infants with developmental disabilities, or those infants who may be at risk for further problems (preterm infants), are referred to appropriate community programs. Social service involvement is especially important for young or psychosocially high risk parents (e.g., substance abusers or those with a mental illness).

For the family of the child who is technology dependent, special education needs are discussed before discharge. For further discussion of home care, see Chapter 43.

TRANSPORT TO A REGIONAL CENTER

If a hospital is not equipped to care for a high risk mother and fetus or a high risk infant, transfer to a specialized perinatal or regional tertiary care center is arranged. Maternal transport ideally occurs with the fetus in utero because this has two distinct advantages: (1) neonatal morbidity and mortality are decreased, and (2) the mother and infant are not separated at birth.

For a variety of reasons, it is not always possible to transport the mother before the birth. Therefore, physicians and nurses in all facilities must have the skills and equipment necessary for making an accurate diagnosis and implementing emergency interventions to stabilize the infant's condition until transport can occur (Pettett, Sewell, & Merenstein, 2002). The goal of these interventions is to maintain the infant's condition within the normal physiologic range. Specific attention is given to vital signs, oxygenation and ventilation, thermoregulation, acid-base balance, fluid and electrolyte status, blood glucose, and developmental interventions.

Arrangements for transport to an intensive care facility are made as soon as the high risk infant is identified (see Community Focus box). Each hospital that delivers infants should be able to provide for appropriate neonatal stabilization and arrange for transport to a tertiary care facility. The infant must be kept warm and adequately oxygenated (including intubation and surfactant replacement as indicated); have vital signs and oxygen saturation monitored; and, when indicated, receive an intravenous infusion. The infant is transported in a specially designed incubator unit containing a complete life-support system and other emergency equipment that can be carried by ambulance, van, or helicopter (Fig. 27-11).

The transport team may consist of physicians, nurse-practitioners, nurses, and respiratory therapists. Commonly

Community Focus

NEONATAL TRANSPORT

During a scheduled clinical experience in the NICU or a special care nursery, observe a transport team leaving to pick up an infant from a referring hospital or bringing in an infant to the special care nursery. Who are the transport team members? What equipment are they using? How was the referral made? What communication links are there between the special care nursery and the community hospitals in the surrounding area? How are parents kept informed of the infant's condition?

BOX 27-5

Information for Parents about the Tertiary Center

- Exact location of the unit–address, map, waiting area for relatives and friends
- Visiting hours and hospital rules
- Telephone numbers
- Names of individuals likely to be involved with the newborn's care (e.g., primary nurse, neonatologist, clinical manager)
- Information about the special care unit–what it is, what it does
- Location of parking facilities, nearby lodging, and rules regarding visitation by young children (siblings)
- Any particular rules or regulations regarding the special care unit

From Pettett G, Sewell S, & Merenstein GB: Regionalization and transport in perinatal care. In Merenstein GB, Gardner SL (eds): *Handbook of neonatal intensive care,* ed 5, St Louis, 2002, Mosby.

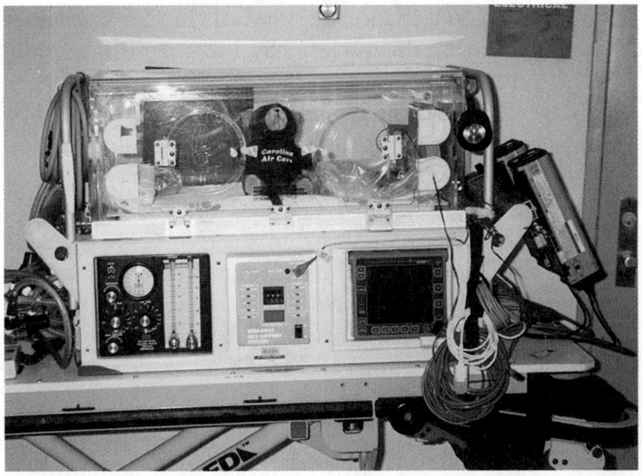

Fig. 27-11 Total life support system for transport of high risk newborns. (Courtesy UNC Hospitals, Carolina Air Care, Chapel Hill, NC.)

a nurse trained in neonatal intensive care and a respiratory therapist constitutes the team. The team must have experience in resuscitation, stabilizations, and provision of critical care during the transport. Teams provide information for the parents about the tertiary center (Box 27-5).

The birth of any high risk infant can cause profound parental stress. Parents can grieve the loss of the ideal infant. They are fearful of the possible eventual outcomes for the infant. They must also deal with the technologic world surrounding their infant. Amid all the equipment, it is sometimes difficult for them to perceive the infant and respond to its needs. Parents of high risk infants who have been transported to regional centers therefore need special support.

TRANSPORT FROM A REGIONAL CENTER

Infants may need to be transferred back to the referring facility; however, in many cases the infant is discharged home from the tertiary center. Often premature infants who require thermoregulation and gavage feedings can be cared for in community hospitals closer to the parents' home. This allows parents to visit their infant more easily and to work with their personal health care provider on the long-range expected outcomes for the infant. Specialized incubators make these trips possible (see Fig. 27-11). However, parents may express mixed feelings about such return transports and may be reluctant to adapt to a different facility and group of caregivers. To minimize some of these concerns, it is important to give the parents very clear information about return transports during the initial discharge planning.

Although at the time of discharge parents may not recognize the need for information on the various resources available to help them in the care of their infant, they can be given such lists of agencies and telephone numbers for later use. Providing them with a patient-specific directory covering special programs, social support, community, and funding resources can help them make the transition to the home care of their infants. As the nurse continually reinforces the idea that the infant will go home, this prompts the parents to plan for the days ahead and therefore be ready to take their infant home when the time comes.

Key Points

- Preterm infants are at risk for problems related to the immaturity of their organ systems.
- Respiratory distress syndrome, retinopathy of prematurity, and chronic lung disease (bronchopulmonary dysplasia) are associated with prematurity.
- High risk infants must be observed for respiratory distress and other early signs of physiologic distress.
- Metabolic abnormalities of diabetes mellitus in pregnancy adversely affect embryonic and fetal development.
- The adaptation of parents to preterm or high risk infants differs from that of parents of full-term infants.
- Parents need special instruction (e.g., CPR, oxygen therapy, suctioning, developmental care) before they take a high risk infant home.
- Infants born to diabetic mothers are at risk for hypoglycemia and RDS.
- SGA infants are considered to be at risk because of fetal growth restriction.
- Nonreassuring fetal status among postmature infants is related to the progressive placental insufficiency that can occur in a postterm pregnancy.
- Specially trained nurses may transport high risk infants to and from special care units.

Answer Guidelines to Critical Thinking Exercise

Preterm Infant

1. Yes, there is sufficient evidence. The normal progress in recovery from childbirth is well documented. Because the baby was born preterm, Charlotte was not prepared for the birth at this time nor for the probability of a long-term stay in the NICU for the infant. At 28 weeks, the in-

fant has a good chance for survival. In the absence of problems during the nursery stay, the prognosis is good. If Charlotte chooses to breastfeed, she will have to pump regularly for a considerable amount of time before she can actually nurse the baby. In addition, she has the problem of transporting the milk to the nursery.

2. (a) Charlotte's physical recovery should progress easily. However, her emotional/psychologic recovery may be difficult. She is likely to ask herself what she did to cause the preterm birth and feel guilt, particularly if the infant develops problems. The relationship between her husband and herself and the other two children may be strained by the worry about the baby and the time she spends traveling to see the infant. (b) Barring complications, the infant can be expected to progress and develop normally. However, the infant's hospitalization and separation from the family will likely put a strain on family members, who will be worried about the infant as long as it is in the NICU and until the baby is home. (c) Charlotte can be informed that the cause of the majority of preterm births is unknown and that she need not feel guilt for having the baby early. Charlotte can pump and freeze her breast milk and transport it to the hospital in a cooler; however, she will likely not be able to travel that distance to see the infant every day. Obtaining breast milk at 28 weeks takes perseverance and regular pumping. Although this puts a burden on Charlotte, it is important for the infant's well-being. (d) Infants born at 28 weeks with no concomitant problems can develop normally. However, they are at risk for nosocomial infections, and some infants have developmental delays.
3. Charlotte and her family need information about postpartum recovery, the possibility of postpartum "blues" or depression associated with a preterm birth, and stresses associated with a preterm birth and neonatal transport. They may need assistance in talking to their two older children about the baby and the need for the baby to be in the hospital. They need to be informed about how to contact the NICU and care providers, usual care in that setting, directions to the hospital, and be prepared for back transport to their local hospital when the infant's condition improves such that NICU care is no longer required. They need to be kept informed daily about the progress of the baby.
4. Phases of postpartum recovery and the stresses associated with preterm birth and neonatal transport are well documented. Long-term outcomes for preterm infants, parental responses to preterm birth, and integration of the infant into the family have been studied extensively. The nurse can use those studies and patient education materials to assist the family.
5. The above recommendations assume the infant is progressing normally with no problems. If the infant has or develops problems, additional support for the family will be necessary. Participation in parent groups is helpful. They may be referred to the clergy of their choice for additional support. If the infant does not survive, the bereavement service at the hospital can provide information and support.

Resources

American Academy of Pediatrics
141 Northwest Point Blvd.
Elk Grove, IL 60007-1098
847-228-5005
www.aap.org

The Academy of Neonatal Nursing
2270 Northpoint Parkway
Santa Rosa, CA 95407-7398
707-568-2168
707-569-0786 (fax)
www.academyonline.org

Advances in Neonatal Care
Elsevier
360 Park Avenue South
New York, NY 10010

Journal of Perinatal and Neonatal Nursing
Lippincott Williams & Wilkins
530 Walnut St.
Philadelphia, PA 19106-3621
215-521-8300
215-521-8902 (fax)
www.lww.com

National Association of Neonatal Nurses
4700 W. Lake Ave.
Glenview, IL 60025-1485
800-451-3795
888-477-6266 (fax)
www.nann.org
info@nann.org

Neonatal Network
2270 Northpoint Parkway
Santa Rosa, CA 95407-7398
707-569-1415
707-569-0786 (fax)
www.neonatalnetwork.com

Parents of Prematures
13613 NE 26th Place
Bellevue, WA 98005
206-283-7466

Recommended Standards for NICU Design
www.nd.edu/~kkolberg/frmain.htm

Special Care Nursery Mothers' Milk Bank
Christiana Care Health Services
4755 Ogletown Stanton Rd.
PO Box 6001
Newark, DE 19718
302-733-2340

References

Als H: Developmental care in the newborn intensive care unit, *Curr Opin Pediatr* 10(2):138-142, 1998.

American Academy of Pediatrics, Committee on Fetus and Newborn: Hospital discharge of the high-risk neonate—proposed guidelines, *Pediatrics* 102(2):411-417, 1998.

American Academy of Pediatrics, Committee on Fetus and Newborn: Postnatal corticosteroids to treat or prevent chronic lung disease in preterm infants, *Pediatrics* 109(2):330-337, 2002.

American Academy of Pediatrics, Committee on Nutrition: *Pediatric nutrition handbook*, ed 5, Elk Grove Village, IL, 2004, The Academy.

American Academy of Pediatrics, Section on Ophthalmology: Screening examination of premature infants for retinopathy of prematurity, *Pediatrics* 108(3):809-811, 2001.

Anderson MS et al: Enteral nutrition. In Merenstein GB, Gardner SL (eds): *Handbook of neonatal intensive care,* ed 5, St Louis, 2002, Mosby.

Bensard DD et al: Neonatal surgery. In Merenstein GB, Gardner SL (eds): *Handbook of neonatal intensive care,* ed 5, St Louis, 2002, Mosby.

Berger TM et al: Impact of improved survival of very low-birth-weight infants on incidence and severity of bronchopulmonary dysplasia, *Biol Neonate* 86(2):124-130, 2004.

Blackburn ST: Environmental impact of the NICU on developmental outcomes, *J Pediatr Nurs* 13(5):279-289, 1998.

Blackburn ST: *Maternal, fetal, and neonatal physiology: a clinical perspective,* ed 2, St. Louis, 2003, WB Saunders.

Blake WW, Murray JA: Heat balance. In Merenstein GB, Gardner SL: *Handbook of neonatal intensive care,* ed 5, St Louis, 2002, Mosby.

Brandon DH, Holditch-Davis D, Belyea M: Nursing care and the development of sleeping and waking behaviors in preterm infants, *Res Nurs Health* 22(3):217-219, 1999.

Brandon DH, Holditch-Davis D, Belyea M: Preterm infants born at less than 31 weeks' gestation have improved growth in cycled light compared with continuous near darkness, *J Pediatr* 140(2):192-199, 2002.

Byrne BJ et al: Is the BPD epidemic diminishing? *Semin Perinatol* 26(6):461-466, 2002.

Collins C, Makrides M, McPhee A: Early discharge with home support of gavage feeding for stable preterm infants who have not established full oral feeds (Cochrane Review), 2003. In *The Cochrane Library,* Issue 2, Chichester, UK, 2004, John Wiley & Sons.

Cornblath M et al: Controversies regarding operational definition of neonatal hypoglycemia: suggested thresholds, *Pediatrics* 105(5):1141-1145, 2000.

Dickason E, Silverman B, Kaplan J: *Maternal-infant nursing care,* ed 3, St Louis, 1998, Mosby.

Diehl-Jones WL, Askin DF: Nutritional modulation of neonatal outcomes, *AACN Clin Issues* 15(1):83-96, 2004.

Donn SM, Sinha SK: Invasive and noninvasive neonatal mechanical ventilation, *Respir Care* 48(4):426-441, 2003.

Evans RA, Thureen PJ: Early feeding strategies in preterm & critically ill neonates, *Neonatal Netw* 20(7):7-18, 2001.

Flores M: Ibuprofen: alternative treatment for patent ductus arteriosus, *Neonatal Netw* 22(2):27-31, 2003.

Gale G, VandenBerg KA: Kangaroo care, *Neonatal Netw* 17(5):69-71, 1998.

Gardner SL, Goldson E: The neonate and the environment: impact on development. In Merenstein GB, Gardner SL (eds): *Handbook of neonatal intensive care,* ed 5, St Louis, 2002, Mosby.

Gardner SL, Snell BJ, Lawrence RA: Breastfeeding the neonate with special needs. In Merenstein GB, Gardner SL (eds): *Handbook of neonatal intensive care,* ed 5, St Louis, 2002, Mosby.

Gracey K et al: The changing face of bronchopulmonary dysplasia: Part 1, *Adv Neonatal Care* 2(6):327-338, 2002.

Gray K et al: Developmentally supportive care in a neonatal intensive care unit: a research utilization project, *Neonatal Netw* 17(2):33-38, 1998.

Hagedorn MIE, Gardner SL, Abman H: Respiratory diseases. In Merenstein GB, Gardner SL (eds): *Handbook of neonatal intensive care,* ed 5, St Louis, 2002, Mosby.

Haubrich K: Assessment and management of auditory dysfunction. In Kenner C, Lott JW, Flandermyer A (eds): *Comprehensive neonatal nursing: a physiologic perspective,* ed 2, Philadelphia, 1998, WB Saunders.

Heermann JA, Wilson ME: Nurses' experiences working with families in an NICU during implementation of family-focused developmental care, *Neonatal Netw* 19(4):23-29, 2000.

Horii KA, Lane AT: Evidence-based use of emollients in neonates, *Newborn Infant Nurs Rev* 1(1):21-24, 2001.

Horns KM: Comparison of two microenvironments and nurse caregiving on thermal stability of ELBW infants, *Adv Neonatal Care* 2(3):149-160, 2002.

Johnson FE, Maikler VE: Nurses' adoption of the AWHONN/NANN Neonatal Skin Care Project, *NINR* 1(1):59-67, 2001.

Kalhan SC, Parimi PS: Disorders of carbohydrate metabolism. In Fanaroff AA, Martin RJ (eds): *Neonatal-perinatal medicine: diseases of the fetus and infant,* ed 7, St Louis, 2002, Mosby.

Kinsella JP, Abman SH: Inhaled nitric oxide: current and future uses in neonates, *Semin Perinatol* 24(6):387-395, 2000.

Kinsella JP et al: Inhaled nitric oxide in premature infants with severe hypoxaemic respiratory failure: a randomised controlled trial, *Lancet* 354(9184):1047-1048, 1999.

Kliegman RM, Das UG : Intrauterine growth retardation. In Fanaroff A, Martin RJ (eds): *Neonatal-perinatal medicine:diseases of the fetus and infant,* ed 7, St. Louis, 2002, Mosby.

Kliegman RM: Commentaries: experimental validation of neonatal feeding practices, *Pediatrics* 103(2):492-493, 1999.

Kuller JM: Skin breakdown: risk factors, prevention, and treatment, *NINR* 1(1):33-42, 2001.

Lucas A, Morley R, Cole JJ: Adverse neurodevelopmental outcome of moderate neonatal hypoglycemia, *Br J Med* 297:1304-1308, 1988.

Ludington-Hoe S et al: Birth-related fatigue in 34-36 week preterm neonates: rapid recovery with very early kangaroo (skin-to-skin) care, *J Obstet Gynecol Neonatal Nurs* 28(1):94-103, 1999.

Lund CH, Kuller JM: Assessment and management of the integumentary system. In Kenner C, Lott JW (eds): *Comprehensive neonatal nursing: a physiologic perspective,* ed 5, Philadelphia, 2003, Saunders.

Lund CH et al: Neonatal skin care: the scientific basis for practice, *J Obstet Gynecol Neonatal Nurs* 28(3):241-254, 1999.

Lund CH, Durand DJ: Skin and skin care. In Merenstein GB, Gardner SL (eds): *Handbook of neonatal intensive care,* ed 4, St Louis, 1998, Mosby.

Lund CH, Kuller J, Lott JW: Neonatal skin care: clinical outcomes of the AWHONN/NANN evidence-based clinical practice guideline, *J Obstet Gynecol Neonatal Nurs* 30(1):41-51, 2001.

Lund C, Lane A, Raines DA: Neonatal skin care: the scientific basis for practice, *J Obstet Gynecol Neonatal Nurs* 28(3):241-254, 1999.

Malloy MB, Perez-Woods R: Neonatal skin care: prevention of skin breakdown, *Pediatr Nurs* 17(1):41-48, 1991.

Montoya KD, Washington RL: Cardiovascular disease and surgical interventions. In Merenstein GB, Gardner SL (eds): *Handbook of neonatal intensive care,* ed 5, St Louis, 2002, Mosby.

Morbidity and Mortality Weekly Report: *Enterobacter sakazakii* infections associated with the use of powdered infant formula-Tennessee, 2001, *MMWR Morb Mortal Wkly Rep* 51(14):297-300, 2002.

Morton JA: Strategies to support extended breastfeeding of the premature infant, *Adv Neonatal Care,* 2(5):267-282, 2002.

Neu M: Parents' perception of skin-to-skin care with their preterm infants requiring assisted ventilation, *J Obstet Gynecol Neonatal Nurs* 28(2):157-164, 1999.

Neu M, Browne J, Vojir C: The impact of two transfer techniques used during skin-to-skin care on the physiologic and behavioral responses of preterm infants, *Nurs Res* 49(4):215-223, 2000.

O'Doherty N: *Neonatology: micro atlas of the newborn,* Nutley, NJ, 1986, Hoffmann-La Roche.

Paige PL, Carney PR: Neurologic disorders. In Merenstein GB, Gardner SL (eds): *Handbook of neonatal intensive care,* ed 5, St Louis, 2002, Mosby.

Parry WH, Zimmer J: Acid-base homeostasis and oxygenation. In Merenstein GB, Gardner SL (eds): *Handbook of neonatal intensive care,* ed 5, St Louis, 2002, Mosby.

Petryshen P et al: Comparing nursing costs for preterm infants receiving conventional vs. developmental care, *Nurs Econ* 15(3):138-145, 150, 1997.

Pettett G, Sewell S, Merenstein GB: Regionalization and transport in perinatal care. In Merenstein GB, Gardner SL (eds): *Handbook of neonatal intensive care,* ed 5, St Louis, 2002, Mosby.

Reece EA et al: Pregnancy outcomes among women with and without diabetic microvascular disease (White's classes B to FR) versus nondiabetic controls, *Am J Perinatol* 15(9):549-555, 1998.

Sadiq HF et al: Inhaled nitric oxide in the treatment of moderate persistent pulmonary hypertension of the newborn: a randomized controlled, multicenter trial, *J Perinatol* 23(2):98-103, 2003.

Sauer PJ, Dane HJ, Visser HK: New standards for neutral thermal environment of healthy very low birthweight infants in one week of life, *Arch Dis Child* 59(1):18-22, 1984.

Saugstad OD et al: Resuscitation of newborn infants with 21% or 100% oxygen: follow-up at 18 and 24 months, *Pediatrics* 112(2):296-300, 2003.

Schanler RJ et al: Feeding strategies for premature infants: randomized trial of gastrointestinal priming and tube-feeding method, *Pediatrics* 103(2):434-439, 1999.

Standley J: The effect of music and multimodal stimulation on responses of premature infants in neonatal intensive care, *Pediatr Nurs* 24(6):532-538, 1998.

Stoll BJ: Infections in the neonatal infant. In Behrman RE, Kliegman RM, Jenson HB (eds): *Nelson textbook of pediatrics*, ed 17, Philadelphia, 2004, Saunders.

Taquino LT: Promoting wound healing in the neonatal setting: process versus protocol, *J Perinat Neonatal Nurs* 14(1):108-118, 2000.

Thome UH, Carlo W: Permissive hypercapnia, *Semin Neonatol* 7(5):409-419, 2002.

Vain NE et al: Oropharyngeal and nasopharyngeal suctioning of meconium-stained neonates before delivery of their shoulders: multicenter, randomized, controlled trial, *Obstet Gynecol Surv* 60(2):88-89, 2005.

van Acker J et al: Outbreak of necrotizing enterocolitis associated with *Enterobacter sakazakii* in powdered milk formula, *J Clin Microbiol* 39(1):293-297, 2001.

VandenBerg K: What to tell parents about the developmental needs of their baby at discharge, *Neonatal Netw* 18(1):57-59, 1999.

Vennarecci G at al: Intestinal transplantation for short gut syndrome attributable to necrotizing enterocolitis, *Pediatrics* 105(2):1-5, 2000.

Vento M et al: Oxidative stress in asphyxiated term infants resuscitated with 100% oxygen, *J Pediatr* 142(3):240-246, 2003.

Volpe JJ: *Neurology of the newborn,* ed 4, Philadelphia, 2001, WB Saunders.

Ward K: Perceived needs of parents of critically ill infants in a neonatal intensive care unit (NICU), *Pediatr Nurs* 27(3):281-286, 2001.

Woodgate PG, Davies MW: Permissive hypercapnia for the prevention of morbidity and mortality in mechanically ventilated newborn infants, *Cochrane Database Syst Rev* (2):CD002061, 2001.

Woodwell WH: The long road home: perspectives on parenting in the NICU, *Adv Neonatal Care* 2(3):161-169, 2002.

The Newborn at Risk: Acquired and Congenital Problems

28

LEARNING OBJECTIVES

On completion of this chapter the reader will be able to:

- Summarize assessment and care of the newborn with soft tissue, skeletal, and nervous system injuries due to birth trauma.
- Identify maternal conditions that place the newborn at risk for infection.
- Describe methods used to identify infection in the newborn.
- Identify the effects of maternal use of alcohol, heroin, methadone, marijuana, methamphetamine, cocaine, and smoking tobacco on the fetus and newborn.
- Describe the assessment of a newborn exposed to recreational drugs in utero.
- Identify clinical signs of infection in the newborn.
- Describe the role of the nurse in the diagnosis of neonatal sepsis.
- Compare neonatal Rh and ABO incompatibility.
- Describe preoperative and postoperative nursing care of the newborn.
- Describe congenital disorders presented in this chapter and identify the priority of nursing care for each.

ELECTRONIC RESOURCES

Additional information related to the content in Chapter 28 can be found on

the companion website at evolve
http://evolve.elsevier.com/Wong/maternal/
- NCLEX Review Questions
- WebLinks

or the interactive student CD-ROM
Activities for Chapter 28 include the following:
- NCLEX Review Questions
- Critical Thinking Exercise–Fetal Alcohol Syndrome
- Nursing Care Plan–Drug-Exposed Newborn

A challenge for the nurse is the birth of an infant at risk because of conditions or circumstances that are superimposed on the normal course of events associated with birth and the adjustment to extrauterine existence. The infant may be considered high risk because of birth trauma, maternal substance abuse, infection, or congenital anomalies. Birth trauma includes physical injuries a neonate sustains during labor and birth. Congenital anomalies include such conditions as gastrointestinal (GI) malformations, neural tube defects, abdominal wall defects, and cardiac defects.

At times, the nurse is able to anticipate problems, such as when a woman is admitted in premature labor or a congenital anomaly is diagnosed by ultrasound before birth. At other times, the birth of a high risk infant is unanticipated. In either case, the personnel and equipment necessary for immediate care of the infant must be available.

BIRTH TRAUMA

Birth trauma (injury) is physical injury sustained by a neonate during labor and birth. It remains an important source of neonatal morbidity.

In theory, most birth injuries may be avoidable, especially if careful assessment of risk factors and appropriate planning of birth occur. The use of fetal ultrasonography allows antepartum diagnosis of many conditions that may be treated in utero or shortly after birth. Elective cesarean birth can be chosen for some pregnancies to prevent significant birth injury. A small percentage of significant birth injuries are unavoidable despite skilled and competent obstetric care, such as in especially difficult or prolonged labor or when the infant is in an abnormal fetal presentation. Some injuries cannot be anticipated until the specific circumstances are encountered during childbirth. Emergency cesarean birth may provide a last-minute salvage, but in these circumstances the injury may be truly unavoidable. The same injury might be caused in several ways; for example, a cephalhematoma could result from an obstetric technique such as forceps birth or vacuum extraction or from pressure of the fetal skull against the maternal pelvis.

Many injuries are minor and resolve readily in the neonatal period without treatment. Other trauma requires some degree of intervention; few are serious enough to be fatal. The nurse's contributions to the welfare of the newborn begin with early observation of the newborn's transition. The prompt reporting of signs that indicate deviations from normal permits early initiation of appropriate therapy. Table 28-1 provides an overview of neurologic birth injuries and the sites in which they occur.

Care Management

When the newborn is born the nurse makes a rapid inspection and physical assessment to determine if there are any life-threatening conditions requiring immediate medical or surgical attention. A comprehensive physical assessment of the newborn is performed after the parents have had the opportunity to interact with the newborn. Because evidence of some birth injuries may not be apparent at the initial examination, assessment continues during each contact with the neonate.

Table 28-1

Types of Birth Injuries

SITE OF INJURY	TYPE OF INJURY
Scalp	Caput succedaneum Subgaleal hemorrhage Cephalhematoma
Skull	Linear fracture Depressed fracture Occipital osteodiastasis
Intracranial	Epidural hematoma Subdural hematoma (laceration of falx, tentorium, or superficial veins) Subarachnoid hemorrhage Cerebral contusion Cerebellar contusion Intracerebellar hematoma
Spinal cord (cervical)	Vertebral artery injury Intraspinal hemorrhage Spinal cord transection or injury
Plexus	Erb palsy Klumpke paralysis Total (mixed) brachial plexus injury Horner syndrome Diaphragmatic paralysis Lumbosacral plexus injury
Cranial and peripheral nerve	Radial nerve palsy Medial nerve palsy Sciatic nerve palsy Laryngeal nerve palsy Diaphragmatic paralysis Facial nerve palsy

From Paige PL, Carney PR: Neurologic disorders. In Merenstein GB, Gardner SL (eds): *Handbook of neonatal intensive care,* ed 5, St Louis, 2002, Mosby.

Soft tissue injuries that commonly occur at birth are discussed at length in Chapter 25. Caput succedaneum and cephalhematoma are discussed in Chapter 24.

Skeletal Injuries

The newborn's immature, flexible skull can withstand a great degree of deformation (molding) before fracture results. Considerable force is required to fracture the newborn's skull. Two types of skull fractures typically are identified in the newborn: linear fractures and depressed fractures. The location of the fracture and involvement of underlying structures determine its significance.

If an artery lying in a groove on the undersurface of the skull is torn as a result of the fracture, increased intracranial pressure (ICP) will follow. Unless a blood vessel is involved, linear fractures, which account for 70% of all fractures for this age group, heal without special treatment. The soft skull may become indented without laceration of either the skin or the dural membrane. These depressed fractures, or ping-pong ball indentations, may occur during difficult births from pressure of the head on the bony pelvis. They also can occur as a result of injudicious application of forceps.

The clavicle is the bone most often fractured during birth. Generally the break is in the middle third of the bone (Fig. 28-1). Dystocia, particularly shoulder impaction, may be the predisposing problem. Limitation of motion of the arm, crepitus over the bone, and the absence of the Moro reflex on the affected side are diagnostic. Except for use of gentle rather than vigorous handling, no accepted treatment for fractured clavicle exists, and the prognosis is good. The humerus and femur are other bones that may be fractured during a difficult birth. Fractures in newborns generally heal rapidly. Immobilization is accomplished with slings, splints, swaddling, and other immobilization devices.

The parents need support in handling these infants because they often are fearful of hurting them. Parents are en-

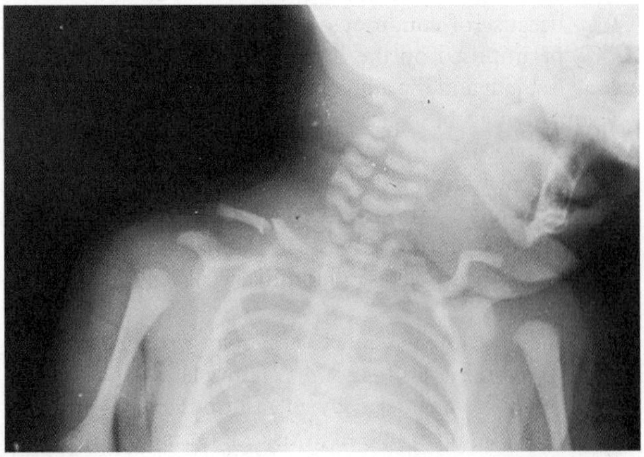

Fig. 28-1 Fractured clavicle after shoulder dystocia. (From O'Doherty N: *Neonatology: micro atlas of the newborn,* Nutley, NJ, 1986, Hoffmann-La Roche.)

couraged to practice handling, changing, and feeding the affected neonate under the guidance of nursery personnel. This increases their confidence and knowledge and facilitates attachment. A plan for follow-up therapy is developed with the parents so that the times and arrangements for therapy are acceptable to them.

Peripheral Nervous System Injuries

Plexus injury results from forces that alter the normal position and relationship of the arm, shoulder, and neck. Erb palsy (Erb-Duchenne paralysis) is caused by damage to the upper plexus and usually results from a stretching or pulling away of the shoulder from the head such as might occur with shoulder dystocia or with a difficult vertex or breech delivery. The less common lower plexus palsy, or Klumpke palsy, results from severe stretching of the upper extremity while the trunk is relatively less mobile.

The clinical manifestations of Erb palsy are related to the paralysis of the affected extremity and muscles. The arm hangs limp alongside the body. The shoulder and arm are adducted and internally rotated. The elbow is extended, and the forearm is pronated, with the wrist and fingers flexed; a grasp reflex may be present because finger and wrist movement remain normal (Tappero, 2003) (Fig. 28-2). In lower plexus palsy, the muscles of the hand are paralyzed, with consequent wrist drop and relaxed fingers. In a third and more severe form of brachial palsy, the entire arm is paralyzed and hangs limp and motionless at the side. The Moro reflex is absent on the affected side for all of the forms of brachial palsy. Total plexus is the second most common type of plexus injury (Dunham, 2003).

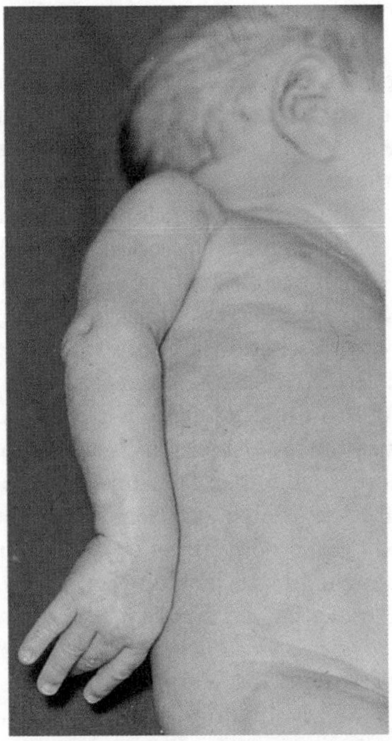

Fig. 28-2 Erb-Duchenne paralysis in newborn infant. Moro reflex is absent in right upper extremity. Recovery was complete. (From O'Doherty N: *Neonatology: micro atlas of the newborn,* Nutley, NJ, 1986, Hoffmann-La Roche.)

Treatment of the affected arm is aimed at preventing contractures of the paralyzed muscles and maintaining correct placement of the humeral head within the glenoid fossa of the scapula. Complete recovery from stretched nerves usually takes 3 to 6 months. However, avulsion of the nerves (complete disconnection of the ganglia from the spinal cord that involves both anterior and posterior roots) results in permanent damage. For those injuries that do not improve spontaneously by 3 months, surgical intervention may be needed to relieve pressure on the nerves or to repair the nerves with grafting (Volpe, 2001). In some cases injection of botulinum toxin A into the triceps muscle may be effective in reducing muscle contractures after birth-related brachial plexus injuries (Rollnik et al, 2000).

Nursing care of the newborn with brachial palsy is concerned primarily with proper positioning of the affected arm. The affected arm should be gently immobilized on the upper abdomen. Passive range-of-motion exercises of the shoulder, wrist, elbow, and fingers are initiated in the latter part of the first week (Volpe, 2001). Wrist flexion contractures may be prevented with the use of supportive splints. In dressing the infant, preference is given to the affected arm. Undressing begins with the unaffected arm, and redressing begins with the affected arm to prevent unnecessary manipulation and stress on the paralyzed muscles. Parents are taught to use the "football" position when holding the infant and to avoid picking the child up from under the axillae or by pulling on the arms.

Pressure on the facial nerve during delivery may result in injury to cranial nerve VII. The primary clinical manifestations are loss of movement on the affected side, such as an inability to completely close the eye, drooping of the corner of the mouth, and absence of wrinkling of the forehead and nasolabial fold (Fig. 28-3). Facial palsy or paralysis is most noticeable when the infant cries. The mouth is drawn to the

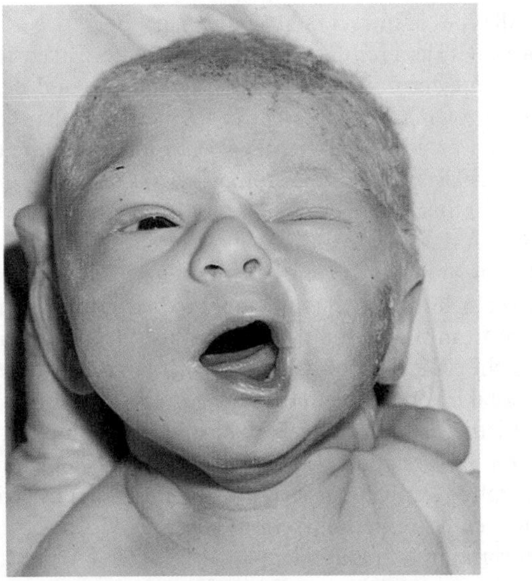

Fig. 28-3 Facial paralysis 15 minutes after forceps birth. Absence of movement on affected side is especially noticeable when infant cries. (From O'Doherty N: *Neonatology: micro atlas of the newborn,* Nutley, NJ, 1986, Hoffmann-La Roche.)

unaffected side, the wrinkles are deeper on the normal side, and the eye on the involved side remains open. Often the condition is temporary, resolving within hours or days of birth. Permanent paralysis is rare.

Nursing care of the infant with facial nerve paralysis involves aiding the infant in sucking and helping the mother with feeding techniques. The infant may require gavage feeding to prevent aspiration. Breastfeeding is not contraindicated, but the mother will need additional assistance in helping the infant grasp and compress the areolar area.

If the lid of the eye on the affected side does not close completely, artificial tears can be instilled daily to prevent drying of the conjunctiva, sclera, and cornea. The lid is often taped shut to prevent accidental injury. If eye care is needed at home, the parents are taught the procedure for administering eyedrops before the infant is discharged from the nursery.

Phrenic nerve paralysis results in diaphragmatic paralysis as demonstrated by ultrasonography, which shows paradoxic chest movement and an elevated diaphragm. Initially, radiography may not demonstrate an elevated diaphragm if the neonate is receiving positive pressure ventilation (Volpe, 2001). The injury sometimes occurs in conjunction with brachial palsy. Respiratory distress is the most common and important sign of injury. Because injury to the phrenic nerve is usually unilateral, the lung on the affected side does not expand, and respiratory efforts are ineffectual. The infant is positioned on the affected side to facilitate maximum expansion of the uninvolved lung. Breathing is primarily thoracic, and cyanosis, tachypnea, or complete respiratory failure may be seen. Pneumonia and atelectasis on the affected side may also occur.

The infant with phrenic nerve paralysis requires the same nursing care as any infant with respiratory distress. As with other birth injuries, the emotional needs of the family are similar to those discussed for soft-tissue injury (see Chapter 25). Follow-up is also essential because of the extended length of recovery.

Central Nervous System Injuries

All types of intracranial hemorrhage (ICH) occur in newborns. ICH as a result of birth trauma is more likely to occur in the full-term, large infant. The frequency and degree of severity of ICH are different in the newborn than in older children or adults. In the newborn, more than one type of hemorrhage can and does commonly occur.

A subdural hematoma, or life-threatening collection of blood in the subdural space, most often is produced by the stretching and tearing of the large veins in the tentorium of the cerebellum, the dural membrane that separates the cerebrum from the cerebellum. When this type of bleeding occurs, the typical history includes a primiparous mother, with the total labor and birth occurring in less than 2 or 3 hours; a difficult birth involving high or midforceps application; or a large-for-gestational-age infant. Subdural hematoma occurs infrequently because of improvements in obstetric care. However, it is especially serious because of its inaccessibility to aspiration by subdural tap.

Subarachnoid hemorrhage, the most common type of ICH, occurs in term infants as a result of trauma and in preterm infants as a result of hypoxia. Small hemorrhages are the most common. Bleeding is of venous origin, and underlying contusion also may occur.

The clinical presentation of hemorrhage in the full-term infant can vary considerably. In many infants, signs are absent, and hemorrhaging is diagnosed only because of abnormal findings on lumbar puncture, for example, red blood cells (RBCs) in the cerebrospinal fluid (CSF) or a hemorrhage is seen on a computerized tomography (CT) scan. The initial clinical manifestations of neonatal subarachnoid hemorrhage may be the early onset of alternating central nervous system (CNS) depression and irritability, with refractory seizure. Poor feeding, apnea, and unequal pupils may suggest an intracranial insult. Occasionally the infant appears normal initially then has seizures on the second or third day of life, followed by no apparent sequelae.

In general, nursing care of an infant with ICH is supportive and includes monitoring neurologic signs and intravenous therapy, observation and management of seizures, and prevention of increased ICP.

Spinal cord injuries almost always result from breech births, especially difficult ones in which version and extraction are used. This type of injury is rarely seen today because cesarean birth is often used for breech presentation (Paige & Carney, 2002).

NEONATAL INFECTIONS

Sepsis

Sepsis (the presence of microorganisms or their toxins in the blood or other tissues) continues to be one of the most significant causes of neonatal morbidity and mortality. Maternal immunoglobulin M (IgM) does not cross the placenta. Immunoglobulin A (IgA) and IgM require time to reach optimum levels after birth. Phagocytosis is less efficient. Serum complement levels are inadequate; serum complement (C1 through C6) is involved in immunologic reactions, some of which kill or lyse bacteria and enhance phagocytosis. Dysmaturity seen with intrauterine growth restriction (IUGR) and preterm and postdate birth further compromises the neonate's immune system.

Table 28-2 outlines risk factors for neonatal sepsis. Special precautions for preventing infection, as well as prompt recognition when it occurs, are necessary for optimum newborn care. Neonatal infections may be acquired in utero, during birth or resuscitation, and nosocomially.

Neonatal bacterial infection is classified into two patterns according to the time of presentation. Early-onset or congenital sepsis usually manifests within 24 to 48 hours of birth, progresses more rapidly than later-onset infection, and carries a mortality rate as high as 50%. Early-onset infection is usually caused by microorganisms from the normal flora of the maternal vaginal tract, including group B streptococci, *Haemophilus influenzae, Listeria monocytogenes, Escherichia coli,* and *Streptococcus pneumoniae* (Merenstein, Adams, & Weisman, 2002). With the widespread use of intrapartum penicillin for group B streptococci, *E. coli* has been reported to be the most common offending pathogen in early-onset sepsis (Stoll et al, 2002). *Coagulase negative staphylococcus* (CONS) has also been reported in some centers as the most common pathogen (Edwards et al, 2003), but this is debatable because some consider it to be a contaminant (Polak,

Table 28-2

Risk Factors for Neonatal Sepsis

SOURCE	RISK FACTORS
Maternal	Low socioeconomic status Poor prenatal care Poor nutrition Substance abuse
Intrapartum	Premature rupture of fetal membranes Maternal fever Chorioamnionitis Prolonged labor Rupture of membranes >12 to 18 hr Premature labor Maternal urinary tract infection
Neonatal	Twin or multiple gestation Male Birth asphyxia Meconium aspiration Congenital anomalies of skin or mucous membranes Galactosemia Absence of spleen Low birth weight or prematurity Malnourishment Prolonged hospitalization

Ringler, & Daugherty, 2004). Early onset sepsis is associated with a history of obstetric events such as preterm labor, prolonged rupture of membranes (>18 hours), maternal fever during labor, and chorioamnionitis (Merenstein et al, 2002).

Nosocomial infection (late-onset) is most commonly seen after 2 weeks of age and is slower in progression. Bacteria responsible for late-onset sepsis are varied, may be acquired from the birth canal or from the external environment, and include *Staphylococcus aureus, Staphylococcus epidermidis, Pseudomonas* organisms, and group B streptococci.

Viral infections may cause miscarriage, stillbirth, intrauterine infection, congenital malformations, and acute neonatal disease. These pathogens also may cause chronic infection, with subtle manifestations that may be recognized only after a prolonged period. It is important to recognize the manifestations of infections in the neonatal period to be able to treat the acute infection, to prevent nosocomial infections in other infants, and to anticipate effects on the infant's subsequent growth and development.

Fungal infections are of greatest concern in the immunocompromised or premature infant. Occasionally, fungal infections such as thrush are found in otherwise healthy term infants.

Septicemia refers to a generalized infection in the bloodstream. Pneumonia, the most common form of neonatal infection, is one of the leading causes of perinatal death. Bacterial meningitis affects 1 in 2500 live-born infants. Gastroenteritis is sporadic, depending on epidemic outbreaks. Local infections such as conjunctivitis and omphalitis occur commonly. Infection continues to be a significant factor in fetal and neonatal morbidity and mortality.

Care Management

Assessment

The prenatal record is reviewed for risk factors associated with infection and the signs and symptoms suggestive of infection. Maternal vaginal or perineal infection may be transmitted directly to the infant during passage through the birth canal. Psychosocial history and history of sexually transmitted infections (STIs) may indicate possible human immunodeficiency virus (HIV), hepatitis B virus (HBV), herpes (HSV 2), or cytomegalovirus (CMV) infection.

Perinatal events also are reviewed. Premature rupture of membranes (PROM) may be caused by maternal or intrauterine infection. Ascending infection may occur after prolonged PROM, prolonged labor, or intrauterine fetal monitoring. In some cases infection may occur with intact membranes or contribute to early rupture. A maternal history of fever during labor or the presence of foul-smelling amniotic fluid may also indicate the presence of infection. Antibiotic therapy initiated during labor should be noted. The neonate's gestational age, maturity, birth weight, and sex all affect the incidence of infection. Sepsis occurs about twice as often and results in a higher mortality in male than in female infants. The neonate is assessed for respiratory distress, skin abscesses, rashes, and other indications of infection.

During the postnatal period, the time of onset of suspicious signs is noted. Onset within the first 48 hours of life is more often associated with prenatal or perinatal predisposing factors. Onset after 2 or 3 days more often reflects disease acquired at or subsequent to birth.

The earliest clinical signs of neonatal sepsis are characterized by a lack of specificity. The nonspecific signs include lethargy, poor feeding, poor weight gain, and irritability. The nurse or parent may simply note that the infant is just not doing as well as before. Differential diagnosis may be difficult because signs of sepsis are similar to signs of noninfectious neonatal problems such as hypoglycemia and stress. Additional clinical and laboratory information and appropriate cultures supplement the findings described. Table 28-3 outlines the clinical signs associated with neonatal sepsis.

Laboratory studies are important. Specimens for cultures include blood, CSF, stool, and urine. Fluids such as urine and CSF may be evaluated by counterimmune electrophoresis (CIE) or latex agglutination (LA) to assist in the identification of the bacteria. A complete blood cell count with differential is performed to determine the presence of bacterial infection or increased or decreased WBC count (the latter is an ominous sign). The total neutrophil count, immature to total neutrophil (I:T) ratio, absolute neutrophil count (ANC), and C-reactive protein may be used to determine the presence of sepsis (Table 28-4). Advances in technology include detection of viral DNA or antibodies by polymerase chain reaction (PCR) amplification in fluids (Frenkel, 2005). Detection of antepartal infection can now be successfully treated with a number of antiviral medications to decrease viral replication and fetal transmission of disease; neonates may also be treated with antiviral medications such as ganciclovir. Treatment with antibiotics is initiated after cultures are obtained in neonates; in high risk infants with significant illness antiviral or antibiotic treatment may begin once cul-

Table 28-3

Signs of Sepsis*

SYSTEM	SIGNS
Respiratory	Apnea, bradycardia Tachypnea Grunting, nasal flaring Retractions Decreased oxygen saturation Metabolic acidosis
Cardiovascular	Decreased cardiac output Tachycardia Hypotension Decreased perfusion
Central nervous	Temperature instability Lethargy Hypotonia Irritability, seizures
Gastrointestinal	Feeding intolerance (decreased suck strength and intake; increasing residuals) Abdominal distention Vomiting, diarrhea
Integumentary	Jaundice Pallor Petechiae Mottling

Adapted from Askin DF: Bacterial and fungal sepsis in the neonate, *J Obstet Gynecol Neonatal Nurs* 24(7):635-643, 1995.
*Laboratory findings include neutropenia, increased bands, hypoglycemia or hyperglycemia, metabolic acidosis, and thrombocytopenia.

tures are obtained and once the pathogen is identified antibiotic therapy may be modified.

Vigilant assessment continues during and after treatment. The newborn continues to be assessed for sequelae to septicemia, which include meningitis, disseminated intravascular coagulation (DIC), necrotizing enterocolitis, pneumonia, and septic shock. Septic shock results from the toxins released into the bloodstream. The most common signs include decreasing oxygen saturations, poor perfusion, tachycardia, respiratory distress, and hypotension.

Nursing Diagnoses

Various nursing diagnoses are possible, depending on the infant's gestational age and birth weight, the organ systems involved, and the nature of the infection. Examples of nursing diagnoses related to neonatal infections include the following:

Newborn

- *Risk for infection related to*
  —maternal vaginal (or other) infection
  —indwelling umbilical catheters, parenteral fluids (invasive procedures)
  —intrauterine electronic fetal monitoring
  —dysmaturity, IUGR, gestational age
- *Ineffective thermoregulation related to*
  —systemic infection
- *Impaired skin integrity related to*
  —use of multiple supportive invasive measures (e.g., physiologic monitoring, parenteral fluid therapy, inhalation therapy)
- *Acute pain related to*
  —multiple supportive invasive measures

Table 28-4

Suspected Neonatal Sepsis

ASSESSMENTS	1. Potential maternal risk factors and unstable vital signs, especially temperature instability 2. Sepsis screen in first hour (CBC with differential, platelets, and CRP level) if there are significant maternal risk factors (prolonged rupture of membranes, maternal temperature) or if infant demonstrates physiologic signs of sepsis
TREATMENT	1. Start IV administration of antibiotics by peripheral IV 2. Provide other treatments as needed for additional physiologic problems (supplemental oxygen or ventilator for respiratory distress, incubator for temperature instability)
POSSIBLE CONSULTATIONS	1. Neonatologists and advanced practice nurses for care of unstable infants 2. Medical specialists for care of infants with additional problems (congenital deformities) 3. Lactation consultant, interpreter, social worker, and chaplain as needed or requested
ADDITIONAL ASSESSMENTS	1. Weight and measurements 2. Blood culture, chest x-ray, urinalysis, and lumbar puncture, if infant is symptomatic or CRP level is positive 3. Repeat determination of CRP level in the morning for 2 days; if negative and infant not symptomatic, stop antibiotic treatment 4. Continuous cardiac and oxygen saturation monitor assessment if infant's condition is unstable
DIRECT INFANT CARE	1. Vital signs every 1 to 2 hr for the first 4 hr, then every 4 hr 2. Advance oral feedings as tolerated (infant NPO only if condition is physiologically unstable) 3. Bath and cord care done per unit protocols
TEACHING AND DISCHARGE PLANNING	1. Initiate on admission. Provide parents with written and oral information on suspected sepsis 2. Reinforce information and determine parents' understanding of information before discharge. Include information on well-baby care and community follow-up with the family's primary health care provider

From Lucile Salter Packard Children's Hospital at Stanford, CA.
CRP, C-reactive protein.

Parents and Family

- *Anxiety, fear, or anticipatory grieving related to*
  —uncertainty about infant's prognosis
  —therapy (invasive)
- *Risk for impaired parent-infant attachment related to*
  —separation of parent and newborn
  —feelings of inadequacy in caring for infant
- *Powerlessness or spiritual distress related to*
  —perinatal events or newborn's condition beyond parents' control

Expected Outcomes

Planning begins with the development of standards for preventive measures in nurseries, and protocols for the diagnosis and treatment of infections. Individual assessment findings are used to plan care for each infant. Parents and family are encouraged to participate in planning. Expected outcomes include the following:

- The newborn will remain free of infection.
- The newborn's early signs of sepsis will be recognized, and appropriate therapy will be instituted.
- If therapy is necessary, the newborn will suffer no harmful sequelae.
- Parents will begin interacting and caring for newborn and be involved in his or her care.
- Parents will maintain self-esteem by understanding that their role as parents is important to the infant's well-being.

Plan of Care and Implementation

Prevention

Virtually all controlled clinical trials have demonstrated that effective handwashing is responsible for the prevention of nosocomial infection in nursery units. Nursing is directly or indirectly responsible for minimizing or eliminating environmental sources of infectious agents in the nursery. Measures to be taken include Standard Precautions, careful and thorough cleaning of contaminated equipment, frequent replacement of used equipment (e.g., changing intravenous and nasogastric tubing per hospital protocol, and cleaning resuscitation, ventilation equipment, intravenous pumps, and incubators), and disposal of contaminated linens and diapers in an appropriate manner. Overcrowding must be avoided in nurseries. Guidelines for space, visitation, and general infection control in areas where newborns receive care have been established and published (American Academy of Pediatrics [AAP] and American College of Obstetricians and Gynecologists [ACOG], 2002).

Infants cared for in NICUs are at high risk for infection. In a study of infants cared for in the National Institute for Child Health and Human Development's Neonatal Research Network, of those who survived beyond 3 days, 25% had 1 or more instances of blood culture-proven sepsis. Of those infants with sepsis, 17% died. There is center to center variability with infection rates from 11.5% to 34% (Buus Frank, 2004). Handwashing is the single most effective measure to reduce nosocomial infection. However, the rate of compliance with standards for hand hygiene is only 22%. The combined use of alcohol, hand hygiene, and gloves is effective in reducing the incidence of systemic infection (Buus-Frank, 2004). It is incumbent upon caregivers to strictly adhere to recommended guidelines for hand hygiene.

Antibiotic is instilled into newborns' eyes 1 to 2 hours after birth to prevent infection (see Fig. 25-4). The skin, its secretions, and normal flora are natural defenses that protect against invading pathogens. Warm water may be used to remove blood and meconium from the neonate's face, head, and body. A mild nonmedicated soap (in single-use container or in a small bar reserved for a single newborn) can be used with careful water rinsing. Vernix caseosa is not scrubbed vigorously for removal as this further disrupts the skin barrier properties (see Skin Care Guidelines box in Chapter 27). No single method of cord care has been shown to be more effective in the promotion of drying and separation and prevention of colonization. Alcohol, triple dye, or an antimicrobial agent are typically used. Studies indicate that cords cleaned with sterile water or those left to dry naturally separate more quickly than those cleaned with alcohol, and neither method resulted in an increased number of infections (Dore et al, 1998; Medves & O'Brien, 1997). Current recommendations for cord care by the Association of Women's Health, Obstetric and Neonatal Nursing (AWHONN) include cleaning the cord with sterile water or a neutral pH cleanser; subsequent care entails cleansing the cord with water (AWHONN, 2001). Nurses must follow agency protocols for cord care, but they can recommend revision of protocols based on research.

NURSE ALERT Artificial and long natural fingernails worn by nurses and other caregivers have been associated with serious neonatal infection and morbidity from *Pseudomonas aeruginosa* in the neonatal intensive care unit (NICU) (Moolenaar et al, 2000). ■

Care Management

Breastfeeding or feeding the newborn breast milk from the mother is encouraged. Breast milk provides protective mechanisms. Colostrum contains IgA, which offers protection against infection in the GI tract. Human milk contains iron-binding protein that exerts a bacteriostatic effect on *E. coli.* Human milk also contains macrophages and lymphocytes. The vulnerability of infants to common mucosal pathogens such as respiratory syncytial virus (RSV) may be reduced by passive transfer of maternal immunity in the colostrum and breast milk. Some evidence indicates that early enteral feedings (trophic or minimal enteral feedings) may be beneficial in establishing a natural barrier to infection in extremely-low-birth-weight (ELBW) and very-low-birth-weight (VLBW) infants; further studies are needed to make general recommendations and establish protocols (Strodtbeck, 2003). Human milk is thought to provide some degree of protection from the occurrence of necrotizing enterocolitis (Diehl-Jones & Askin, 2004).

Administering medications, taking precautions when performing treatments, and following isolation procedures are also interventions to be considered in the prevention and treatment of neonatal sepsis.

Monitoring the intravenous infusion rate and administering antibiotics are nursing responsibilities. It is important to administer the prescribed dose of antibiotic within 1 hour after it is prepared to avoid loss of drug stability. If the intravenous fluid the infant is receiving contains electrolytes, vitamins, or other medications, the nurse should check with the hospital pharmacy before adding antibiotics. The antibiotic (or other medication) may be deactivated or may form a precipitate when combined with other medications. In that case a piggyback solution of the prescribed fluid is attached with a three-way stopcock at the infusion site.

Care must be taken in suctioning secretions from any newborn's oropharynx or trachea. Routine suctioning is not recommended and may further compromise the infant's immune status as well as cause hypoxia and increase ICP. Isolation procedures are implemented as indicated according to hospital policy. Isolation protocols are changing rapidly, and the nurse is urged to participate in continuing education and in-service programs to remain up to date.

Evaluation

The nurse can be reasonably assured that care was effective if the outcomes established for care are met.

TORCH Infections

The occurrence of certain maternal infections during early pregnancy is known to be associated with various congenital malformations and disorders. The most common and best understood infections are represented by the acronym TORCH, for *t*oxoplasmosis, *o*ther (gonorrhea, hepatitis B, syphilis, varicella-zoster virus, parvovirus B19, and HIV), *r*ubella, *c*ytomegalovirus, and *h*erpes simplex virus [HSV]) (Box 28-1). One of the problems with these viral infections is the lack of maternal symptomatology, resulting in lack of treatment and thus often producing an affected newborn at birth. With the advent of newer diagnostic methods these viral infections may be diagnosed in utero and interventions planned based on the availability of intrauterine treatments. HSV may result in a severe, often fatal systemic illness in neonates. Survivors of herpetic infection may have residual CNS damage (encephalitis) and chorioretinitis. The other congenital infections also may result in encephalopathy with various anomalies, including microcephaly, chorioretinitis, intracranial calcifications, microphthalmus, and cataracts. To a certain extent, the varied clinical manifestations of these infections overlap, but a specific diagnosis can be made by the clustering of clinical findings, as well as specific antibody studies.

BOX 28-1

TORCH Infections Affecting Newborns

T	Toxoplasmosis
O	Other: gonorrhea, syphilis, varicella, hepatitis B virus (HBV), human parvovirus B19, human immunodeficiency virus (HIV)
R	Rubella
C	Cytomegalovirus (CMV) infections
H	Herpes simplex virus (HSV) infection

Toxoplasmosis

Toxoplasmosis is a multisystem disease caused by the protozoan *Toxoplasma gondii.* Cats who hunt infected birds and mice harbor the parasite and excrete the infective oocysts in their feces. Human infection follows hand-to-mouth contact, such as after disposal of cat litter or after handling or ingesting raw meat from cattle or sheep that grazed in contaminated fields. About 30% of women who contract toxoplasmosis during gestation transmit the disease (transplacental) to their offspring (Lynfield & Guerina, 1997). First trimester exposure to the protozoan is more serious for the fetus than third trimester or perinatal transmission. Intrauterine detection of the condition may occur as early as 18 weeks using polymerase chain reaction (PCR) of the gene (B1) of the protozoa in amniotic fluid. The detection of intrauterine infection and subsequent maternal treatment with spiramycin may prevent fetal infection (Boyer & Boyer, 2004). More than 70% of affected infants are free of symptoms. The clinical features of toxoplasmosis resemble cytomegalic inclusion disease (CMID) in the infant. Both diseases are responsible for serious perinatal mortality and morbidity: 10% to 15% die, 85% have severe psychomotor problems or mental retardation by age 2 to 4 years, and 50% have visual problems by age 1 year.

Severe toxoplasmosis is associated with preterm birth, growth restriction, microcephaly or hydrocephaly, microphthalmus, chorioretinitis, CNS calcification, thrombocytopenia, jaundice, and fever. Petechiae or a maculopapular rash may also be evident. Some clinical manifestations do not develop until later in life. The affected infant may be treated with pyrimethamine, as well as oral sulfadiazine, but folic acid supplement will be required to prevent anemia.

Gonorrhea

The incidence of gonococcal infection in pregnant women ranges from 2.5% to 7.3%. With this high incidence, it is not surprising that neonatal infection with *Neisseria gonorrhoeae* often occurs. After rupture of membranes, ascending infection can result in orogastric contamination of the fetus. The organism also may invade mucosal surfaces such as the conjunctiva (ophthalmia neonatorum), rectal mucosa, and pharynx. Contamination may occur as the infant passes through the birth canal, or it may occur postnatally from an infected adult. Neonatal gonococcal arthritis, septicemia, meningitis, vaginitis, and scalp abscesses can also develop.

Eye prophylaxis (e.g., with 0.5% erythromycin ointment) is administered at or shortly after birth to prevent ophthalmia neonatorum. The infant with a mild infection often recovers completely with appropriate treatment (e.g., single dose of intramuscular [IM] or intravenous [IV] ceftriaxone). Occasionally, infants die of overwhelming infection in the early neonatal period. The newborn with clinical disease should be admitted to a hospital for treatment (AAP & ACOG, 2002).

Syphilis

Congenital and neonatal syphilis have reemerged in recent years as significant health problems. It is estimated that for every 100 women diagnosed with primary or secondary disease, two to five infants will contract congenital syphilis. If syphilis during pregnancy is untreated, 40% to 50% of neonates born to these women will have symptomatic congenital syphilis. Treatment failure can occur, particularly when treatment is given in the third trimester; therefore, infants born to women treated after 20 weeks of gestation should be investigated for congenital syphilis.

Fetal infestation with the spirochete *Treponema pallidum* is blocked by Langhans' layer in the chorion until this layer begins to atrophy between 16 and 18 weeks of gestation. If spirochetemia is untreated, it will result in fetal death by midtrimester, miscarriage, or stillbirth (in 1 in 4 cases). All neonates in whom the infection occurs before 7 months of gestation are affected. Only 60% are affected if the infection occurs late in pregnancy. If maternal infection is treated adequately before the eighteenth week, neonates seldom demonstrate signs of the disease. Although treatment after the eighteenth week may cure fetal spirochetemia, pathologic changes may not be prevented completely.

Because the fetus becomes infected after the period of organogenesis (first trimester), organs develop normally. Congenital syphilis may stimulate preterm labor, but no evidence indicates that it causes IUGR. Organs affected later by congenital syphilis may include the liver, spleen, kidneys, adrenal glands, and bone covering and marrow. Disorders of the CNS, teeth, and cornea may not become evident until several months after birth.

The most severely affected infants occur in untreated mothers, and the newborn may be hydropic (edematous) and anemic, with enlarged liver and spleen. Hepatosplenomegaly probably results from extramedullary hematopoietic activity stimulated by the severe anemia. In some infants, signs of congenital syphilis do not appear until late in the neonatal period. In these newborns, early signs such as poor feeding, slight hyperthermia, and snuffles may be nonspecific. *Snuffles* refers to the copious, clear, serosanguineous mucus discharge from the neonate's nose. A mucopurulent discharge indicates secondary infection, usually by streptococci or staphylococci.

By the end of the first week of life, a copper-colored maculopapular dermal rash appears in untreated newborns. The rash is characteristically first noticeable on the palms of the hands, soles of the feet (Fig. 28-4), the diaper area, and around the mouth and anus. The maculopapular lesions may become vesicular and confluent and extend over the trunk and extremities. Condylomata (i.e., elevated, wartlike lesions) may be seen around the anus. Rough, cracked, mucocutaneous lesions of the lips heal to form circumoral radiating scars known as *rhagades.*

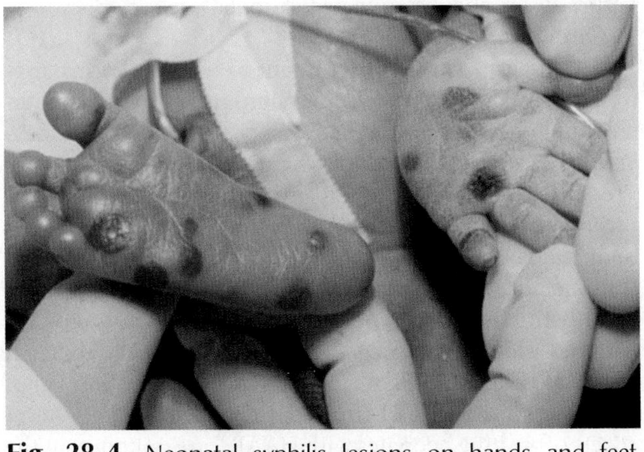

Fig. 28-4 Neonatal syphilis lesions on hands and feet. (Courtesy Mahesh Kotwal, MD, Phoenix, AZ.)

If the mother was adequately treated before giving birth, and serologic testing of the infant does not show syphilis, generally the infant is not treated with antibiotics. The infant is checked for antibody titer (received from the mother via the placenta) every 2 weeks for 3 months, at which time the test result should be negative. Some physicians recommend antibiotic therapy for asymptomatic or inconclusive cases.

A 10-day course of aqueous penicillin G or procaine penicillin G (consult drug references for dosage and administration route for each) is the usual treatment for congenital syphilis (Boyer & Boyer, 2004). Erythromycin is the substitute antibiotic of choice for infants sensitive to penicillin.

NURSE ALERT The infant with congenital syphilis may be entirely asymptomatic until after discharge from the birth hospital. It is therefore imperative that caregivers use Standard Precautions with all newborns. ■

In general, treatment of syphilis is more effective if it is begun early rather than later in the course of the disease. However, a recurrence rate of 5% can be expected. Even adequate treatment of congenital syphilis after birth does not always prevent late complication (e.g., 5 to 15 years after initial infection). Potential complications include neurosyphilis, deafness, Hutchinson's teeth (notched incisors), saber shins, joint involvement, saddle nose (depressed bridge), gummas (soft, gummy tumors) over the skin and other organs, and interstitial keratitis (inflammation of the cornea).

Varicella Zoster

The varicella zoster virus responsible for chickenpox and shingles is a member of the herpes family. About 90% of women in their childbearing years are immune; therefore, the risk of infection in pregnancy is low, 0.7 to 3 per 1000 births (Birthistle & Carrington, 1998; Chapman, 1998).

Varicella transmission to the fetus may occur across the placenta when the disease is contracted in the first half of pregnancy, but this is relatively infrequent. When transmission to the fetus does occur in the early part of pregnancy, the effects on the fetus include limb atrophy, neurologic abnormalities, eye abnormalities, and IUGR.

When maternal infection occurs in the last few days of pregnancy, 20% of infants born to these mothers will develop clinical varicella (Boyer & Boyer, 2004). The severity of the infant's illness increases greatly if maternal infection occurred within 5 days before or 2 days after birth. The mortality in severe illness is 30% (Chapman, 1998).

Infants born to mothers who develop chickenpox between 5 days before birth and 48 hours after birth should be given varicella-zoster immune globulin (VZIG) at birth because of the risk of severe disease. Acyclovir can be used to treat infants with generalized involvement and pneumonia (Myers, Stanberry, & Seward, 2004).

Term infants exposed to chickenpox after birth will have either a mild infection or no infection if they are born to immune mothers. Those born to nonimmune mothers may develop chickenpox, but the course is not usually severe. Experts are divided as to whether this group of infants should receive VZIG. Infants less than 28 weeks of age are at risk regardless of their mother's status and probably benefit from VZIG if exposed to chickenpox.

Hepatitis B Virus

Hepatitis B virus (HBV) infection during pregnancy is not associated with an increase in malformations, stillbirths, or IUGR; however, about a 32% increase in risk exists for preterm birth. The transmission rate of HBV to the newborn is as high as 90% when the mother is seropositive for both hepatitis B surface antigen (HbsAg) and hepatitis B e antigen (HbeAg) (Duff, 1998). Transmission occurs transplacentally; serum to serum; and by contact with contaminated blood, urine, feces, saliva, semen, or vaginal secretions during birth. Infants are most commonly infected during birth or in the first few days of life. The rate of transmission is highest when the mother contracts the virus immediately before birth. These mothers will be positive for HBsAg. Transmission may occur through breast milk, but antigens also develop in formula-fed infants at the same or higher rate. Diagnosis is made by viral culture of amniotic fluid as well as the presence of HBsAg and IgM in the cord blood or newborn's serum.

Neonatal and fetal effects are serious. Preterm birth exposes the neonate to the problems of prematurity. Infants may be symptom free at birth or show evidence of acute hepatitis with changes in liver function. The mortality for full-blown hepatitis is 75%. Infants who become carriers are at high risk for chronic hepatitis, cirrhosis of the liver, or liver cancer even years later (Cowles & Gonik, 2002).

Infants whose mothers have antibodies for HBsAg or who have developed hepatitis during pregnancy or the postpartum period should be treated with hepatitis B immunoglobulin (HBIG), 0.5 ml IM, as soon as possible after birth or within the first 12 hours of life. The hepatitis B vaccine should also be given concurrently, but at a different site (AAP Committee on Infectious Diseases, 2003). The second dose of vaccine is given at 1 month and the third dose at 6 months. The vaccine should protect the child for up to 9 years. After the infant has been cleansed thoroughly and has received the vaccine, breastfeeding may be initiated. Vaccination for infants not exposed to maternal HBV is recommended before discharge from the birth hospital; breastfeeding for these infants may begin before the vaccine is given.

Human Immunodeficiency Virus (Type 1)

It is estimated that globally, more than 1 million children born to HIV-infected women will acquire the virus (Mofenson, 1997). The total number of children with active viral infection decreased by 81% between 1992 and 2000 as a result of decreased perinatal transmission of the virus (AAP Committee on Infectious Diseases, 2003). The majority of cases of pediatric AIDS (90% or more) result from maternal-to-fetal transmission. Universal counseling and screening of pregnant women is recommended in the United States and Canada.

Transmission of HIV from the mother to the infant may occur transplacentally at various gestational ages. The risk of infection in an infant born to an HIV-positive mother (not treated) is approximately 13% to 39% (AAP Committee on Infectious Diseases, 2003). Globally the rate of maternal transmission of the virus is estimated to be 25%. With antepartum, intrapartum, and neonatal zidovudine treatment the incidence of neonatal HIV infection is decreased to 5% to 8%, and compliance with highly active antiretroviral therapy (HAART) is said to further reduce newborn infection rates to 1% to 2% (Cooper et al, 2002; Kriebs, 2002). A critical factor in perinatal transmission is the maternal viral load; a high viral load creates a greater chance for perinatal transmission of the virus. Postpartum transmission may also occur with an additional risk of 14% attributed to breast milk contact (Scarlatti, 1996; Weinberg, 2000).

Diagnosis of HIV infection in the neonate is complicated by the presence of maternal IgG antibodies, which cross the placenta after 32 weeks of gestation. The most accurate test for newborns and infants younger than 18 months is the HIV DNA PCR assay, which is performed on neonatal blood, not cord blood; results may be obtained by 24 hours (AAP Committee on Infectious Diseases, 2003). Follow-up testing for infants born to HIV-positive mothers is recommended at several intervals within the first year of life.

Typically the HIV-infected neonate is asymptomatic at birth. Early-onset illness (i.e., virus detected within 48 hours of birth) is attributed to prenatal infection and occurs in 10% to 15% of infected infants. These infants develop opportunistic infections (*Candida* and *pneumocystis carinii* pneumonia [PCP]) and rapid progression of immunodeficiency, which progresses to death in the first 1 to 2 years of life.

The remainder of infants seroconvert over a period of months to years. By 1 year of life, 80% to 90% of perinatally infected infants show signs of infection. Some children infected at birth show no signs of disease 8 to 10 years later. The age of onset of symptoms predicts the length of survival.

The presenting signs and symptoms of HIV infection vary from severe immunodeficiency to nonspecific findings such as failure to thrive, parotitis, and recurrent or persistent upper respiratory infections. In the first year of life, lymphadenopathy and hepatosplenomegaly are common. The infant may have fever, chronic diarrhea, chronic dermatitis, interstitial pneumonitis, persistent thrush, and AIDS-defining secondary infections. Common secondary infections include PCP, candidiasis, CMV infection, cryptosporidiosis, herpes simplex or herpes zoster, and disseminated varicella.

Care Management

Although it is rare for an infant to be born with symptoms of HIV infection, all infants born to seropositive mothers should be presumed to be HIV positive until proven otherwise. Management begins by implementing Standard Precautions. Measures should also be undertaken to protect the infant from further exposure to maternal blood and body fluids. Regimens for the prevention of HIV transmission include antepartum, intrapartum, and neonatal treatment with HAART. Neonates may be treated with a combination of zidovudine (ZDV), didanosine, and nevirapine. In some cases lamivudine or stavudine may be used instead of didanosine for neonatal treatment (Bell, 2004). Long-term effects of treating neonates with HAART are unknown at the time of this writing, but initial studies demonstrated a decrease in viral load in most infants (although sample sizes were small) at 16 and 56 months (Bell, 2004). Another study demonstrated improved long-term viral load suppression in infants younger than 3 months when antiviral treatment (stavudine, lamivudine, nevirapine, and nelfinavir) was started early (Luzuriaga et al, 2004). If the infant is diagnosed with HIV infection, the family should be counseled about conventional and investigational treatment options.

Counseling regarding the care of the mothers themselves, the family's care of the infant, and future pregnancies should be provided. The risk for transmission among members of the same household is minimal. Social services are required in these cases. If the parent chooses to keep the infant, home health care may be arranged. For more information and updated information, parents are offered the following resource: the National AIDS hotline, 1-800-342-AIDS.

In the United States, breastfeeding in the HIV-positive mother is contraindicated; however, in developing countries, the issue of risks versus benefits in relation to number of infant deaths attributed to poor sanitary conditions and availability of an appropriate food supply for infants and the theoretic risk of HIV transmission via breast milk is less clear (Kriebs, 2002). The World Health Organization (WHO) (2001) has published recommendations for HIV-positive women and breastfeeding in developing countries.

The family must be counseled about vaccinations. Children with symptomatic or asymptomatic HIV infection should receive all routine vaccines. Although data regarding children with HIV and varicella vaccine are limited, the AAP Committee on Infectious Diseases (2003) recommends that children with no or mild symptoms be immunized for varicella.

Rubella Infection

Since rubella vaccination was begun in 1969, cases of congenital rubella have been reduced dramatically; however, it is still seen occasionally in the newborn. Vaccination failures, lack of compliance, and the immigration of nonimmunized persons result in periodic outbreaks of rubella, also known as German or 3-day measles.

The risk for congenital anomalies varies with the gestational age of the fetus at the time maternal infection occurs. Abnormalities are most severe if the mother contracts the virus during the first trimester.

More than two-thirds of infected infants have no symptoms apparent at birth, but sequelae may develop years later. Hearing loss, the most common result, appears to be progressive after birth. Initially the newborn may present with hepatosplenomegaly, lymphedema, IUGR, jaundice, hepatitsis, thrombocytopenic purpura with petechiae, and the characteristic blueberry muffin lesions. Congenital rubella syndrome often includes chronic problems such as cataracts or glaucoma, sensorineural hearing impairment, hypogammaglobulinemia, peripheral pulmonary stenosis, and diabetes mellitus type 1 (Boyer & Boyer, 2004). The rubella virus has been cultured in infants for up to 18 months after their birth. These infants are a serious source of infection to susceptible individuals, particularly women in the childbearing years. Extended pediatric isolation is mandatory until the noncontagious stage of rubella has been reached (i.e., the infant should be isolated until pharyngeal mucus and the urine are free of virus).

Cytomegalovirus Infection

CMV infection during pregnancy may result in miscarriage, stillbirth, or congenital illness. It is the most common cause of congenital viral infections in the United States (Boyer & Boyer, 2004). Most (90% to 95%) of the affected infants are asymptomatic at birth; however, sensorineural hearing impairment and learning disabilities have been reported in previously asymptomatic infants.

The neonate with classic, full-blown CMV displays IUGR and has microcephaly. The neonate may also have a rash, jaundice, and hepatosplenomegaly (Fig. 28-5). Anemia, thrombocytopenia, and hyperbilirubinemia are common in the early stages of the illness. Intracranial, periventricular calcification often is noted on radiography. Inclusion bodies ("owl's eye" figures) in cells sedimented from freshly voided urine or in liver biopsy specimens are typical.

The virus may be isolated from urine or saliva of the newborn using the PCR assay. Differential diagnosis includes other causes of jaundice, syphilis (positive Venereal Disease Research Laboratories [VDRL] findings), toxoplasmosis (positive Sabin-Feldman dye test result), hemolytic disease of the newborn (positive Coombs' test reaction), or coxsackievirus infection (positive culture).

Despite the extensive, endemic nature of the disease in women and men and its potential for havoc in perinatal life, only occasionally are critically affected newborns seen. Milder forms of the disease often result when the fetus is affected late in pregnancy. CMV can be transmitted through breast milk while the mother is experiencing acute CMV syndrome. CMV infections acquired after birth are often asymptomatic and have no sequelae. Exceptions to this occur in preterm infants, in whom postnatal acquisition of CMV can result in pneumonia, hepatitis, thrombocytopenia, and long-term neurologic sequelae.

Antenatally infected infants who are asymptomatic at birth are at risk for late sequelae. Hearing loss may not be apparent until after the first year of life. Chorioretinitis, microcephaly, mental retardation, and neuromuscular deficits may occur by 2 years of age. Some children are at risk for a defect in tooth enamel, resulting in severe caries.

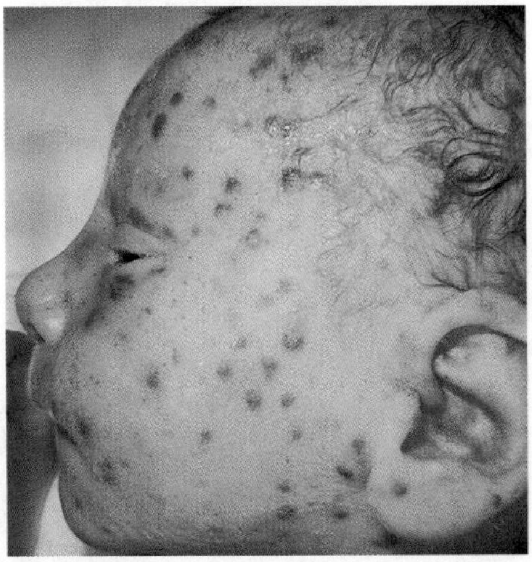

Fig. 28-5 Neonatal cytomegalovirus (CMV) infection. Typical rash seen in a severely affected infant. (Courtesy David A. Clarke, Philadelphia, PA.)

Treatment of the infected newborn with ganciclovir demonstrated a decrease in viral replication and severity of neurologic damage. Such treatment demands careful monitoring of the infant because the drug is toxic to bone marrow (Modlin et al, 2003).

Herpes Simplex Virus

HSV infections among newborns are being diagnosed more frequently and are estimated to occur in as many as 1 in 3000 to 1 in 20,000 births (AAP Committee on Infectious Diseases, 2003).

The neonate may acquire the virus by any of four modes of transmission:

- Transplacental infection
- Ascending infection by way of the birth canal
- Direct contamination during passage through an infected birth canal
- Direct transmission from infected personnel or family

Congenital infection is rare and is characterized by in utero destruction of normally formed organs. Affected infants are growth restricted. They have severe psychomotor restriction, with intracranial calcifications, microcephaly, hypertonicity, and seizures. They suffer eye involvement, including microphthalmus, cataracts, chorioretinitis, blindness, and retinal dysplasia. Some infants have patent ductus arteriosus, limb anomalies, and recurrent skin vesicles, with a short life expectancy.

Most infants are infected directly during passage through the birth canal. The risk of infection during vaginal birth in the presence of genital herpes has not been clearly delineated. It may be as high as 33% to 50%, with active primary infection at term. Primary maternal infections after 32 weeks of gestation carry a higher risk for the fetus and newborn than do recurrent infections (Baley & Toltzis, 2002). The transmission rate of chronic vaginal herpes from the pregnant woman to her newborn is low. Passive intrauterine immunity to herpes may be responsible.

Postnatal acquisition of the virus and spread within a nursery have been documented by deoxyribonucleic acid (DNA) analysis. Both mother and father, as well as maternal breast lesions, have been implicated in neonatal infections. There also is concern regarding symptomatic and asymptomatic shedding among hospital personnel. Nursery personnel with cold sores should practice strict handwashing and wear a mask, but no evidence indicates they should be removed from the nursery unless they have a herpetic whitlow (primary HSV infection of the terminal segment of a finger).

Clinically, neonatal HSV infections are classified as disseminated infection; localized CNS disease; or localized infection of the skin, eye, or mouth. Disseminated infections may involve virtually every organ system, but those primarily involved are the liver, adrenal glands, and lungs. Affected infants exhibit initial symptoms usually in the first week of life but sometimes in the second week, with signs of bacterial sepsis or shock. Clinical manifestations include skin vesicles in about 33% of infants (Fig. 28-6). Death results from progression of CNS involvement, respiratory distress and pneumonitis, shock, DIC, and bleeding. Overall, the mortality without antiviral therapy is 57% (Riley, 1998).

Care Management

Standard Precautions should be observed when caregivers have contact with these infants. The neonate's eyes, oral cavity, and skin are inspected carefully for the presence of any lesions (Fig. 28-7). Cultures are obtained from the mouth, eyes, and any lesions. Circumcision, if performed, is delayed until the infant is ready to be discharged. The infant may be discharged with the mother if the infant's cultures are negative for the virus. As long as no suspicious lesions are on the mother's breasts, breastfeeding is allowed. For the infant at risk, a prophylactic topical eye ointment (vidarabine

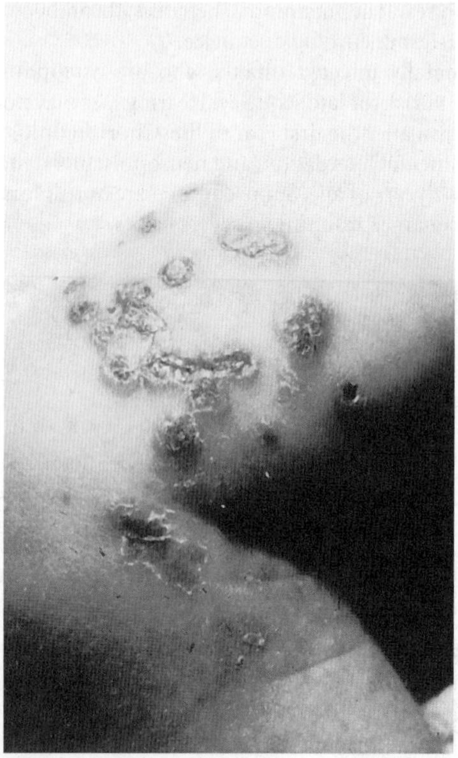

Fig. 28-6 Neonatal herpes simplex virus (HSV) skin infection. (From Behrmann R: *Neonatology: diseases of the fetus and infant,* St Louis, 1973, Mosby.)

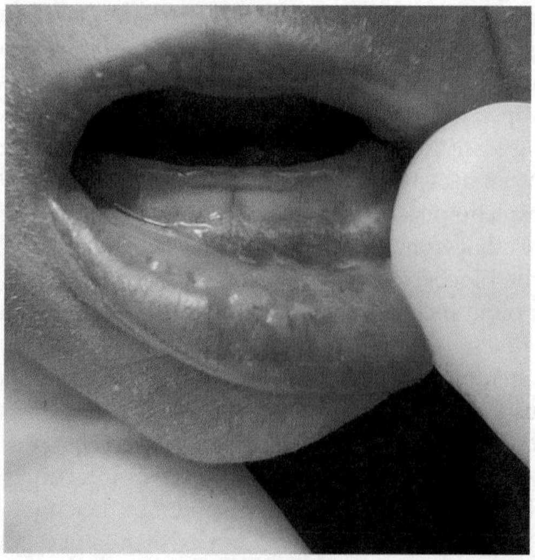

Fig. 28-7 HSV oral lesions. (Courtesy David A. Clarke, Philadelphia, PA.)

or trifluridine) is administered for 5 days to prevent keratoconjunctivitis. Acyclovir should also be given to infants with ocular manifestation. No current recommendations exist for prophylactic systemic therapy; each case should be considered individually. Blood, urine, and CSF specimens should be cultured when indicated clinically. If herpetic lesions first occur after 6 weeks of life, the risk of dissemination and severe illness is very low (Baley & Toltzis, 2002).

Therapy includes general supportive measures, as well as treatment with IV acyclovir. Acyclovir is the most commonly used and recommended drug for treatment of HSV. It is considered safe because only viral replication is inhibited, although long-term sequelae are not yet known. Although acyclovir is easier to administer than vidarabine, there is no difference between the two drugs regarding treatment of HSV. Continuing therapy may be required in recurrences. Ophthalmic ointment should be administered simultaneously.

Parvovirus B 19

Parvovirus B 19 is well-known in older children as fifth disease or "slapped cheek illness" because of the characteristic facial appearance of the affected child. During pregnancy infection may result in fetal miscarriage or the development of nonimmune fetal hydrops. The estimated risk of transplacental transmission is approximately 30%, and fetal death may occur in about 9% of those affected (Boyer & Boyer, 2004). Protocols for intrauterine management have not been well developed, but intrauterine transfusion has offered limited success. Serial ultrasounds to detect fetal hydrops are possible. The virus may be isolated from amniotic fluid, fetal blood, or tissues using DNA PCR assay (Boyer & Boyer, 2004). Pericardial, pleural, and peritoneal effusions are common and fatal if not treated immediately, with cardiac failure from anemia being the most common cause of death.

Bacterial Infections

Group B Streptococcus

Until recently GBS has been the most common cause of neonatal sepsis and meningitis in the United States; however, antepartum maternal screening and administration of penicillin has significantly decreased the incidence of GBS. The Centers for Disease Control and Prevention (CDC) (2002) reported that, as a result of screening and treatment of maternal GBS in the 1990s, the incidence of GBS decreased by 70% to a low of 0.5 per 1000 live births in 1999. Early-onset GBS infection in the neonate occurs in the first 7 days of life but most commonly manifests in the first 24 hours following birth. Risk factors for the development of early-onset GBS include low birth weight, preterm birth, rupture of membranes of more than 18 hours, maternal fever, previous GBS infant, maternal GBS bacteriuria, and multiple gestation. Usually resulting from vertical transmission from the birth canal, early-onset disease results in a respiratory illness that mimics the symptoms of severe respiratory distress syndrome. The infant may rapidly develop septic shock, which has a significant mortality rate.

Late-onset GBS infection presents between 1 week and 3 months of age with an average age of onset of 24 days. Eighty-five percent of infants with late-onset GBS have meningitis; this population has a mortality rate of 0% to 23%. Fifty percent of the survivors develop neurologic damage.

Escherichia Coli

E. coli is the second most common cause of neonatal sepsis and meningitis in the United States, although some preliminary reports suggest that this organism has increased in some NICUs (Stoll et al, 2002). *E. coli* is found in the GI tract soon after birth and makes up the bulk of human fecal flora. In addition to meningitis, *E. coli* can also cause infections in other body systems, including the urinary tract. There is concern that increasing the use of ampicillin in labor as prophylaxis against GBS infection will result in more virulent *E. coli* infection due to ampicillin-resistant organisms.

Tuberculosis

The incidence of tuberculosis (TB), which is caused by *Mycobacterium tuberculosis,* is increasing in Canada and the United States. Congenitally acquired TB, although rare, can cause otitis media, pneumonia, hepatosplenomegaly, enlarged lymph glands, or disseminated disease. After birth, exposed infants contract TB through droplets expelled by infected individuals, which results in pneumonia and necrosis of lung tissue. Untreated neonatal tuberculosis is almost always fatal.

Chlamydia Infection

Chlamydia trachomatis is an intracellular bacterium that causes neonatal conjunctivitis and pneumonia. The conjunctivitis, with minimal watery discharge, develops 5 days to 2 weeks after birth. Inclusion conjunctivitis is usually self-limiting, but if untreated, chronic follicular conjunctivitis (trachoma) with conjunctival scarring and corneal microgranulations has been reported. The organism may spread to the lungs from nasal secretions if left untreated, causing chlamydia pneumonia in about 33% of infected infants with symptoms of a repetitive staccato cough, tachypnea, rales, hyperinflation and bilateral diffuse infiltrates on radiographic examination (Popovich & McAlhany, 2004).

Ophthalmic silver nitrate, 0.5% erythromycin, and 1% tetracycline are not effective against *C. trachomatis;* therefore, it is recommended that infants born to mothers who are positive for *Chlamydia* be followed closely for the development of symptoms. The neonate with positive cultures should be treated with oral erythromycin (AAP Committee on Infectious Diseases, 2003) or oral sulfonamide for 2 to 3 weeks. Erythromycin administration in infants younger than 6 weeks has been associated with an increased risk of infantile hypertrophic pyloric stenosis (IHPS); therefore, parents should be educated regarding the symptoms of the condition (feeding intolerance, projectile vomiting, and abdominal distention).

Fungal Infections

Candidiasis

Candida infections, formerly known as moniliasis, may occur in the newborn. *Candida albicans,* the organism usually responsible, may cause disease in any organ system. It is a yeastlike fungus (producing yeast cells and spores) that can be acquired from a maternal vaginal infection during birth; by person-to-person transmission; or from contaminated hands, bottles, nipples, or other articles. It usually is a benign disorder in the neonate, often confined to the oral and diaper regions. Diaper dermatitis caused by *Candida* presents as a moist, erythematous eruption with small white or yellow pebbly pustules. Small areas of skin erosion may also be seen.

Candidal diaper dermatitis appears on the perianal area, inguinal folds, and lower portion of the abdomen. The affected area is intensely erythematous, with a sharply demarcated, scalloped edge, often with numerous satellite lesions that extend beyond the larger lesion. The source of the infection can be through the GI tract or caretakers' hands. Topical application of 1 ml nystatin (Mycostatin) over the surfaces of the oral cavity 4 times a day, or every 6 hours, is usually sufficient to prevent spread of the disease or prolongation of its course. Several other drugs may be used, including amphotericin B (Fungizone), clotrimazole (Lotrimin, Mycelex), fluconazole (Diflucan), or miconazole (Monistat, Micatin) given intravenously, orally, or topically. To prevent relapse, therapy should be continued for at least 2 days after the lesions disappear (Zenk, 2000). Gentian violet solution may be used in addition to one of the antifungal drugs in chronic cases of oral thrush; however, the former does not treat GI *Candida* and may be irritating to the oral mucosa.

NURSE ALERT Nystatin is best absorbed when given either 1 hour before feeding or after a feeding. Using a needleless syringe or medicine dropper, apply the medication to each side of the infant's mouth for optimal absorption. ■

Oral candidiasis (thrush or mycotic stomatitis) is characterized by the appearance of white plaques on the oral mucosa, gums, and tongue. The white patches are easily differentiated from milk curds; the patches cannot be removed and tend to bleed when touched. In most cases the infant does not seem to be in discomfort from the infection; however, some will pull away from the breast or bottle and cry. The child may be brought to the primary care provider with a complaint of poor oral intake.

Infants who are sick, debilitated, or receiving prolonged antibiotic therapy are more susceptible to thrush. Those with conditions such as cleft lip or palate, neoplasms, and hyperparathyroidism seem to be more vulnerable to mycotic infection.

Care Management

The objectives of management are to eradicate the causative organism and to control exposure to *C. albicans*. Interventions include maintenance of scrupulous cleanliness (by nursing personnel, parents, and others) to prevent reinfection. Good handwashing technique is always essential. Clean surfaces should be provided for neonates. Proper cleanliness of the equipment and environment is critical. Diaper dermatitis is treated with a topical fungicide at each diaper change. When possible, exposing the perineal area to dry air is recommended because yeast prefers a moist environment.

Infants who are breastfed may acquire thrush from the mother. In the event that the mother is colonized, treatment for mother and infant is recommended. There is no need to stop breastfeeding even if the mother is receiving systemic antifungal medications (Lawrence & Lawrence, 1999).

SUBSTANCE ABUSE

Certain maternal behaviors result in perinatal risk. Maternal habits hazardous to the fetus and neonate include recreational drug abuse, smoking, and alcohol abuse. Physiologic signs of withdrawal have been reported in neonates of mothers who use to excess such drugs as barbiturates, alcohol, or amphetamines. Prescription opioids such as oxycodone (Percodan) have been identified as increasingly popular drugs of abuse which may cause withdrawal symptoms in neonates (Rao & Desai, 2002). Serious withdrawal reactions are seen in neonates whose mothers abuse psychoactive drugs. Mothers in substance abuse treatment receiving methadone may give birth to an infant who exhibits withdrawal symptoms requiring treatment. Almost 50% of pregnancies of women addicted to opioids result in low-birth-weight (LBW) infants who are not necessarily preterm. Alcohol is a teratogen that produces CNS effects that may not be evident for years. Maternal ethanol abuse during gestation can lead to a readily identifiable fetal alcohol syndrome (FAS or ARBD [alcohol-related birth defect]) or a constellation of neurobehavioral and cognitive problems which may only be identified by maternal history and behavioral characteristics.

It is important to note that the term *addiction* is often associated with behaviors whereby the person seeks the drug(s) to experience a high, euphoria, escape from reality, or satisfy a personal need. Newborns who have been exposed to drugs in utero are not addicted in a behavioral sense, yet they may experience mild to strong physiologic signs as a result of the exposure. Therefore, to say that an infant born to a mother who uses substances is addicted is incorrect; *drug-exposed newborn,* which implies intrauterine drug exposure, is a better term.

The adverse effects of exposure of the fetus to drugs are varied. They include transient behavioral changes such as fetal breathing movements and irreversible effects such as fetal death, IUGR, structural malformations, cognitive and motor delay, and behavioral problems. Critical determinants of the effect of the drug on the fetus include the specific drug, the dosage, the route of administration, the genotype of the mother or fetus, and the timing of the drug exposure. Fig. 28-8 shows critical periods in human embryogenesis and the teratogenic effects of drugs. Table 28-5 summarizes the effects of commonly abused substances on the fetus and neonate.

Critical Thinking Exercise—Fetal Alcohol Syndrome

Alcohol

The incidence of FAS (also known as alcohol-related birth defects [ARBD]) in the United States is about 0.2 to 1.5 per 1000 live births (CDC, 2004). According to Abel (1997), FAS is based on minimum criteria of signs in each of three categories: prenatal and postnatal growth restriction; CNS malfunctions, including mental retardation; and craniofacial features such as microcephaly, small eyes or short palpebral fissures, thin upper lip, flat midface, and an indistinct philtrum. Neurologic problems in FAS children include some degree of intelligence quotient (IQ) deficit, attention deficit disorder, diminished fine motor skills, and poor speech (Jones & Bass, 2003). Infants exposed prenatally to alcohol who are affected but do not meet the criteria for FAS may be said to have alcohol-related neurodevelopmental disorder (ARND), previously referred to as *fetal alcohol effects* (FAE)

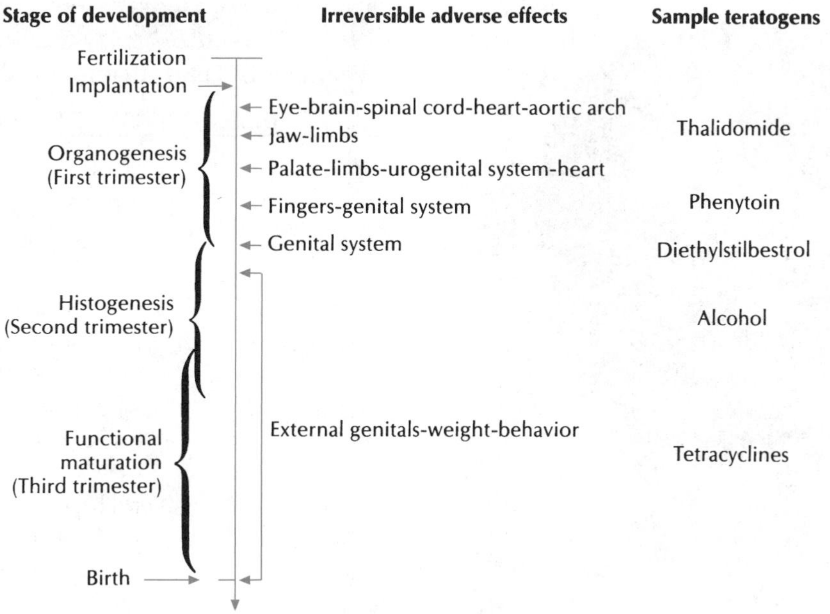

Fig. 28-8 Critical periods in human embryogenesis. (From Aranda JV et al: Developmental pharmacology. In Fanaroff AA, Martin RJ: *Neonatal-perinatal medicine: diseases of the fetus and infant,* ed 7, St Louis, 2002, Mosby.)

(CDC, 2004). These effects range from learning disabilities and behavioral problems to speech or language problems and hyperactivity. Often these problems are not detected until the child goes to school and learning problems become evident. Predictable abnormal patterns of fetal and neonatal morphogenesis are often attributed to severe, chronic alcoholism in women who continue to drink heavily during pregnancy; however, the amount of alcohol consumption does not always correlate with identifiable features. Rather, it is the amount of alcohol consumed in excess of the maternal liver's ability to detoxify alcohol that defines what manifestations or effects will be evidenced from one child to another. The pattern of growth restriction begun in prenatal life persists after birth, especially in the linear growth rate, rate of weight gain, and growth of head circumference.

Ocular structural anomalies are common findings (Fig. 28-9). Limb anomalies and various cardiocirculatory anomalies, especially ventricular septal defects, pose problems for the child. Table 28-6 outlines physical findings in FAS. Mental retardation (e.g., IQ of 79 or below at 7 years of age), hyperactivity, and fine motor dysfunction (e.g., poor hand-to-mouth coordination, weak grasp) add to the

Table 28-5

Summary of Neonatal Effects of Commonly Abused Substances

SUBSTANCE	NEONATAL EFFECTS
Alcohol	*Fetal alcohol syndrome* (FAS): craniofacial features vary, may include short eyelid opening, flat midface, flat upper lip groove, thin upper lip; microcephaly; hyperactivity; developmental delays; attention deficits
	Alcohol-related neurodevelopmental disorder (ARND): varying forms of FAS, cognitive, behavioral and psychosocial problems without typical physical features
Cocaine	Prematurity, small for gestational age, microcephaly, poor feeding, irregular sleep patterns, diarrhea, visual attention problems, hyperactivity, difficult to console, hypersensitivity to noise and external stimuli, irritability, developmental delays, congenital anomalies such as prune belly syndrome (i.e., distended, flabby, wrinkled abdomen caused by lack of abdominal muscles)
Heroin	Low birth weight, small for gestational age, irritability, tachypnea, feeding difficulties, vomiting, high-pitched cry, seizures
Methamphetamine	Small for gestational age, prematurity, poor weight gain, lethargy, behavioral problems later in childhood
Tobacco	Prematurity; low birth weight; increased risk for sudden infant death syndrome; increased risk for bronchitis, pneumonia, developmental delays
Marijuana	Possible neonatal tremors, low birth weight, growth restriction

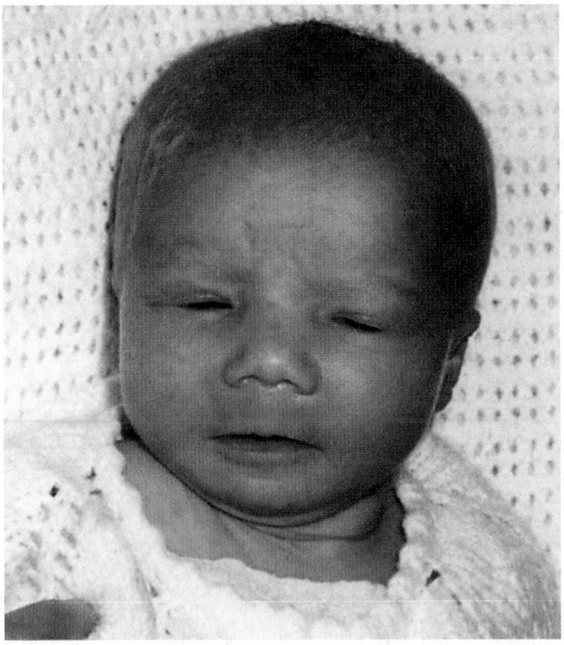

Fig. 28-9 Infant with fetal alcohol syndrome. (From Markiewicz M, Abrahamson E: *Diagnosis in color: neonatology,* St Louis, 1999, Mosby.)

handicapping problems that maternal alcoholism can impose. Genital abnormalities are seen in daughters of alcohol-addicted mothers. Two-thirds of newborns with FAS are girls; the cause of this altered fetal sex ratio is unknown. Severe and chronic alcoholism (ethanol toxicity), not maternal malnutrition, is responsible for the severity and consistency of postnatal performance problems. High alcohol levels are lethal to the developing embryo. Lower levels cause brain and other malformations. Long-term prognosis is discouraging even in an optimum psychosocial environment, when one considers the combination of growth failure and mental retardation.

Alcohol effects depend not only on the amount of alcohol consumed but also on the interaction of quantity, frequency, type of alcohol, and other drug abuse (polydrug use). Other drugs, such as cigarettes (nicotine), caffeine, opiates and marijuana, may potentiate the fetal effects of alcohol consumption during gestation.

The infant of a mother who abuses alcohol is faced with many clinical problems. Identification of the problems leads to the medical diagnosis of FAS. The infant may suffer respiratory distress related to preterm birth, neurologic damage, and a "floppy" epiglottis and small trachea. Tracheoepiglottal anomalies may cause cardiopulmonary arrest. Other disorders include recurrent otitis media and hearing loss. Craniofacial features may be important in diagnosing craniofacial and oral anomalies, dental development abnormalities, and long-term body growth patterns. Feeding difficulties are related to preterm birth, poor sucking ability, and possible cleft palate. The infant may exhibit CNS dysfunction, microcephaly, and irritability.

Long-term effects into childhood may include impaired visualmotor perception and performance, lowered IQ scores, and delayed receptive and expressive language, as well as reduced capacity to process and store factual data (Church & Abel, 1998). FAS is now recognized as one of the leading, yet entirely preventable, causes of mental retardation in the United States. Although the distinctive facial features of the infant tend to become less evident, the mental capacities never become normal.

Nursing care involves many of the same strategies used for the care of preterm infants or drug exposed infants, depending on the clinical manifestations. Special efforts are made to involve the parents in their child's care and to encourage opportunities for parent-child attachment.

Placing infants in a warm, caring environment with understanding caregivers who can deal with the infant's hyperirritability can lead to improved emotional development and social functioning. These caregivers provide extensive cuddling and human contact and can deal with the eating problems that typically lead to a diagnosis of failure to thrive. However, these infants may not go home to an optimal environment because many such families are dysfunctional.

Table 28-6

Features of Fetal Alcohol Syndrome

AFFECTED PART	CHARACTERISTICS
Eyes	Epicanthal folds, strabismus, ptosis, hypoplastic retinal vessels
Mouth	Poor suck, cleft lip, cleft palate, small teeth
Ears	Sensorineural hearing deficits
Skeleton	Radioulnar synostosis, fusion of cervical vertebrae, restricted bone growth
Heart	Atrial and ventricular septal defects, tetralogy of Fallot, patent ductus arteriosus
Kidney	Renal hypoplasia, hydronephrosis, urogenital sinus
Liver	Extrahepatic biliary atresia, hepatic fibrosis
Immune system	Increased infections: otitis media, upper respiratory infections, immune deficiencies
Tumors	Nonspecific neoplasms
Skin	Abnormal palmar creases, irregular hair, whorls

From Weiner L, Morse B: FAS: clinical perspectives and prevention. In Chasnoff I (ed): *Drugs, alcohol, pregnancy and parenting,* Boston, 1991, Kluwer.

Tobacco

Cigarette smoking in pregnancy is associated with birth weight deficits of up to 250 g for a full-term neonate (Aranda et al, 2002). Maternal cigarette smoking is implicated in 21% to 39% of LBW infants. Passive exposure to secondhand

Evidence-Based Practice

KANGAROO CARE FOR LOW-BIRTH-WEIGHT INFANTS

Background

Low-birth-weight (LBW) babies (<2500 g, regardless of gestational age) are at greater risk for diseases; mortality; and possibly, diseases as adults. Most infant deaths occur in this group worldwide. Medical care is costly and scarce in developing countries. A low-technologic, low-cost intervention to improve the outcomes for LBW infants would be an important advance. Kangaroo mother care (KMC) combines skin-to-skin contact between mother and infant, frequent breastfeeding, and early discharge from the hospital. Skin-to-skin contact has been shown to significantly increase and stabilize infant temperature, decrease respirations, increase blood glucose, and improve breastfeeding duration and lasting maternal-infant bonding. (See "Early Maternal Skin-to-Skin Contact with Healthy Infants," the Evidence-Based Practice box in Chapter 24.) Babies in KMC are secured between their mother's breasts in an upright position, day and night. Infants are not eligible for this intervention until they have demonstrated respiratory, temperature, and feeding stabilization (exclusive breastfeeding or a combination of gavage and breastfeeding).

Objectives

The review committee sought evidence that would assess the beneficial and adverse effects of KMC on infants born weighing less than 2500 g, regardless of gestational age. Specific research questions included the effect of KMC on mortality, illness, infant growth, infection, admission to NICUs, breastfeeding, length of stay, costs, and satisfaction of parents and staff.

Methods

Search Strategy

The reviewers searched the Cochrane Library, MEDLINE, EMBASE, LILACS, POPLINE, and CINAHL databases. Keywords were *kangaroo mother care, skin-to-skin, infants,* and *low-birth-weight infants.* The reviewers found three randomized, controlled trials, involving 1362 infants from Ecuador, Colombia, Ethiopia, Indonesia, and Mexico, published from 1994 to 1998. All three studies used skin-to-skin contact and exclusive or nearly exclusive breastfeeding. Early hospital discharge was considered in only one study. Controls received standard neonatal care, including incubator use.

Statistical Analysis

Statistical analyses allowed comparison of data at 41 weeks corrected gestational age, discharge, 6 months corrected age, and 12 months corrected age. Discharge may have occurred before 41 weeks corrected gestational age. "Corrected age" is counted not from the preterm birth, but from 41 weeks corrected gestational age, which would have been the term due date. Reviewers calculated relative risks for dichotomous (categoric) data, and weighted mean differences for continuous data. The authors accepted differences outside the 95% confidence intervals as significant.

Findings

No difference was found in infant mortality between the KMC and control groups. Most mortality occurred during the stabilization process before eligibility for the study.

Reviewers found a significant decrease in nosocomial (hospital acquired) infection at 41 weeks corrected gestational age. There was significantly less severe illness and lower respiratory tract disease in the KMC group at 6 months. There was no difference in other severe infections at 41 weeks corrected gestational age, or 12 months. Breastfeeding was significantly better established as exclusive, or nearly exclusive, at discharge from hospital, but no difference was noted at term, 1, 6, or 12 months corrected age. No difference in readmissions between groups was noted. Weight and head circumference at discharge were significantly higher in the KMC group, but the difference was lost by term and 12 months. There was no difference between psychomotor skills at 12 months. Mothers felt competent and significantly more satisfied with their caregiving in the KMC group, but felt less social support regarding the NICU, although both groups were similar in perception of social support from the hospital, worry, stress, sensitivity, and infant responsiveness from mother. Infant temperatures were more stable in the KMC group. Hospital length of stay was variable, with one study reporting the KMC group had a shorter stay, and another study reporting longer stays than controls. Cost was lower for KMC, but there was not enough information to determine if this was significant. Most of the cost came during the stabilization period before enrollment in the study.

Limitations

Patients, staff, and evaluators were fully aware of the group into which they were randomized, which could introduce bias or some other confounding influence. The definition of stabilization was not clarified. This could affect the outcomes because a more immature infant is more fragile. Missing and incomplete information regarding costs limited the ability to analyze this important outcome. All three studies were carried out in developing countries.

Conclusions

The authors conclude that KMC appears to both reduce severe infant morbidity and to have no adverse outcomes, but the available research has methodologic problems that limit its usefulness.

Implications for Practice

The reviewers conclude that evidence to recommend the routine use of KMC in LBW infants is insufficient.

Implications for Further Research

Well-designed, randomized controlled trials that account for lack of concealment and dropouts can provide higher quality evidence to recommend this promising intervention. While developing countries stand to benefit from evidence that this low-technologic, low-cost method can benefit LBW infants, it would be informative to have data from developed countries for comparison.

Reference

Conde-Agudelo A, Diaz-Rosello J, Belizan J: Kangaroo mother care to reduce morbidity and mortality in low birth weight infants (Cochrane Review), 2003. In *The Cochrane Library*, Issue 2, Chichester, UK, 2004, John Wiley & Sons.

smoke by a pregnant woman may also result in the birth of an LBW infant. The rate of miscarriage and preterm birth is increased in the smoking population (Lee, 1998). Nicotine and cotinine, the two pharmacologically active substances in tobacco, are found in higher concentrations in infants whose mothers smoke. These substances can be secreted in breast milk for up to 2 hours after the mother has smoked. Cigarette smoke contains more than 2000 compounds, including carbon monoxide, dioxin, cyanide, and cadmium. Deficits in growth, intellectual and emotional development, poor auditory responsiveness, increased fine motor tremors, hypertonicity, and decreased verbal comprehension have been observed in infants exposed to smoke. There is also a positive dose-response relationship between the amount of tobacco exposure and newborn neurobehavior; increased tobacco exposure in utero is related to increasing negative neurobehavioral effects (Law et al, 2003). In addition, it is now recognized that neonates may experience withdrawal symptoms following exposure to nicotine. Pregnant women must be informed about the harmful effects of smoking on their unborn baby's health. These include IUGR, miscarriage, PROM, placenta previa, perinatal death, LBW, deficits in learning and behavior, and sudden infant death syndrome (SIDS) (Bennett, 1999; Lee, 1998).The positive association between maternal smoking and SIDS (Lee, 1998; Milerad et al, 1998) reflects in utero exposure and passive exposure postnatally. Mothers and all others should refrain from smoking near the infant. Smoking cessation during pregnancy greatly decreases the chance of fetal complications; therefore, women should be counseled regarding smoking cessation programs.

Marijuana

Marijuana has replaced cocaine as the most common illicit drug used by women ages 18 to 44 years (nonpregnant and pregnant) in the United States (Ebrahim & Gfoerer, 2003). Marijuana crosses the placenta. Its use during pregnancy may result in a shortened gestation and a higher incidence of IUGR (Wagner et al, 1998). A strong association has been reported between the use of marijuana and a decrease in fetal growth and infant birth weight and length (Hurd et al, 2005). Other investigators have found a higher incidence of meconium staining (Rosen & Bateman, 2002). Compounding the issue of the effects of marijuana, especially among women ages 18 to 30 years (Ebrahim & Gfoerer, 2003), is multidrug use, which combines the harmful effects of marijuana, tobacco, alcohol, opiates and cocaine. Long-term follow-up studies on exposed infants are needed.

Cocaine

Cocaine, a common illicit drug used in the United States, has multiple modes of use. However, use of the relatively inexpensive and easily administered "crack" form is increasingly common, especially among women of childbearing age (Eyler & Behnke, 1999). Because crack vaporizes at relatively low temperatures, it is smoked and absorbed in large quantities through pulmonary vasculature. The drug readily crosses the placenta, placing the fetus at risk (Malanga & Kosofsy, 1999).

Cocaine is a CNS stimulant and peripheral sympathomimetic. Legally it is classified as a narcotic, but it is not an opioid. The effects on the fetus are secondary to maternal effects—increased BP, decreased uterine blood flow, and increased vascular resistance. Consequently, the fetus suffers decreased blood flow and oxygenation because of placental and fetal vasoconstriction. The difficulties encountered by cocaine-exposed infants are compounded when the mother is taking the drug in conjunction with other illicit drugs (Askin & Diehl-Jones, 2001). Researchers have concluded that variables such as the mother's lack of prenatal care; poor nutrition; and use of tobacco, alcohol, and other drugs during pregnancy compound the effects of cocaine exposure in the infant (Tronick & Beeghly, 1999).

Infants may appear normal, or they may show neurologic problems at birth that may continue during the neonatal period. Fortunately, these findings are transient, and there has been little evidence of permanent sequelae. Either of two types of behavior may emerge as a result of cocaine effects on fetal development: neurobehavioral depression or excitability. The behaviors of the depressed infant include lethargy, poor suck, hypotonia, weak cry, and difficulty in arousing. The behaviors of the excitable neonate may include a high-pitched cry, hypertonicity, rigidity, irritability, inability to be consoled, and intolerance to a change in routine (Chiriboga et al, 1999; Richardson, Hamel, & Goldschmidt, 1996). Other behaviors may include frequent startling, poor awake state, sleeping difficulties, and persistent primitive reflexes. Some infants develop late onset of symptoms (2 to 8 weeks). They may become irritable and hypertonic, experience sleep-awake disruptions, and demonstrate an inability to tolerate change; they may also be slightly febrile. However, these findings have been refuted in other studies (Eyler & Behnke, 1999; Tronick & Beeghly, 1999).

The adverse effects on the cocaine-exposed neonate are related to dose-response. The higher the dose, the more effects such as IUGR, hypertonia, and decreased fetal head growth are noted (Chiriboga et al, 1999).

Sequelae of prenatal cocaine exposure include a smaller head circumference, decreased birth length, and decreased weight. Head growth may be one of the best predictors of long-term development (Bateman & Chiriboga, 2000). Other neonatal effects of cocaine exposure include increased incidence of gastroschisis, genitourinary anomalies, and periventricular and intraventricular hemorrhage. Long-term sequelae for newborns exposed to cocaine include lower language, motor, and cognitive scores in some studies (Koren et al, 1998; Singer et al, 2002); however, in one study there were no significant differences in the expressive, receptive, and total language scores (Hurt et al, 1997). Arendt and others (1999) noted that the fine and gross motor development indices in 2-year-old children who were exposed to cocaine prenatally were lower than in the control group. Some researchers noted that the exposed children may be affected emotionally rather than intellectually. In a study of first-grade students, Delaney-Black and others (1998) concluded that the children who were exposed to cocaine prenatally were rated by their teachers as having more behavior problems than the control group. A recent study however seems to refute these findings. In a large controlled study of children exposed to cocaine and opiates in utero, only subtle deficiencies in mental and psychomotor functioning were noted at 3 years of age (Messinger et al, 2004). No significant differences were noted in mental, psychomotor, or behavioral functioning. The environmental factors to which these children were exposed were perceived as an important factor in their development. Further long-term studies of exposed infants were recommended (Messinger et al, 2004).

Scores on the Brazelton Neonatal Behavioral Assessment Scale have shown infants to be low in responding appropriately to arousal, auditory, and visual stimuli (Eyler, Behnke, & Conlon, 1998). However, other studies have not found significant differences (Frank et al, 1998; Richardson et al, 1996; Tronick et al, 1996).

Nursing care of cocaine-exposed infants is the same as that for other drug-exposed infants. Because they have increased flexor tone, these infants respond to swaddling in a semiflexed position (Askin & Diehl-Jones, 2001). Positioning, infant massage, and limited tactile stimulation have been shown to be effective interventions. Effects of the drug from breast milk have been reported (Kandall, 1999); therefore, mothers should be cautioned about this hazard to their infants.

Referral to early intervention programs, including child health care, parental drug treatment, individualized developmental care, and parenting education, is essential in promoting the optimum outcome for these children. Many studies indicate that there is little or no significance between the cocaine-exposed and nonexposed groups. However, both groups score significantly lower than published norms. Because these children often live in an impoverished environment, both groups are at high risk for cognitive delays, lack of child health care, and inadequate nutrition and would benefit from an early intervention program (Tronick & Beeghly, 1999). A "one-stop shopping" model affords comprehensive care for mothers and children at one location, not only for drug treatment, but also for the social and medical problems that exist (Tanney & Lowenstein, 1997).

Phencyclidine ("Angel Dust")

Phencyclidine (PCP) increases the risk of injury to the pregnant woman and therefore also to her fetus. The user may be unaware that she is ingesting PCP because it often is misrepresented as another drug of abuse or is mixed with other drugs.

PCP crosses the placenta and is found in breast milk. Literature about the effects on infants is limited. Infants exposed to PCP may exhibit abnormal motor behavior such as irritability, jitteriness, and hypertonicity (D'Apolito, 1999).

Heroin

Heroin crosses the placenta and often results in IUGR. Heroin may have a direct growth-inhibiting effect on the fetus, but the exact mechanisms of growth inhibition are not clear. There is an increased rate of stillbirths but not of congenital anomalies.

Many of the medical complications attributed to heroin ingestion result from prematurity. Other risks include physical dependence in the fetus and the risk of exposure to infections, including hepatitis B and C virus and HIV.

Drug withdrawal in the mother is accompanied by fetal withdrawal, which can lead to fetal death (Kaltenbach, Berghella, & Finnegan, 1998; Wagner et al, 1998). Maternal detoxification in the first trimester carries an increased risk of miscarriage. Detoxification is not recommended after the thirty-second week because of possible withdrawal-induced fetal distress (Kaltenbach et al, 1998).

Heroin withdrawal occurs in 50% to 80% of infants born to addicted mothers, usually within the first 24 to 72 hours of life (Wagner et al, 1998). The signs depend on the length of maternal addiction, the amount of drug taken, and the time of injection before birth. The infant whose mother is taking methadone may not demonstrate signs of withdrawal until a week or so after birth. The symptoms of infants whose mothers used heroin or methadone are similar. Initially the infant may be depressed. The withdrawal syndrome may manifest as a combination of any of the following signs:

- Infant may be jittery and hyperactive
- Cry is shrill and persistent
- Infant may yawn or sneeze frequently
- Tendon reflexes are increased, but the Moro reflex is decreased
- Neonate may exhibit poor feeding and sucking, tachypnea, vomiting, diarrhea, hypothermia or hyperthermia, and sweating
- Infant may exhibit abnormal sleep cycle, with absence of quiet sleep and disturbance of active sleep

The risk of SIDS is 5 to 10 times higher for infants with significant withdrawal problems than for infants in the general population.

If withdrawal is not treated, vomiting, diarrhea, dehydration, apnea, and convulsions may develop. Death may follow. Therapy is individualized. Dehydration and electrolyte imbalance are prevented or treated. Usually the following drugs are given, singly or in combination: phenobarbital, diluted tincture of opium (paregoric), methadone, or morphine.

NURSE ALERT The use of naloxone (Narcan) is contraindicated in infants born to narcotic addicts because it may exacerbate narcotic abstinence syndrome and cause seizures. ■

Methadone

Methadone, a synthetic opiate, has been the therapy of choice for heroin addiction since 1965. Methadone crosses the placenta. An increasing number of infants have been born to methadone-maintained mothers, who seem to have better prenatal care and a somewhat better lifestyle than those taking heroin.

Some question exists concerning the benefits of methadone therapy during pregnancy because of its effect on the fetus. Methadone withdrawal resembles heroin withdrawal but tends to be more severe and prolonged. Signs of methadone withdrawal include tremors, irritability, state lability, hypertonicity, hypersensitivity, vomiting, mottling, and nasal stuffiness (Jansson, Velez, & Harrow, 2004). These infants exhibit a disturbed sleep pattern similar to that seen in heroin withdrawal. They have a higher birth weight than those infants in heroin withdrawal, usually AGA. No increased incidence of congenital anomalies is seen. The American Academy of Pediatrics (2001) has revised its statement regarding breastfeeding for mothers who are in a methadone treatment program suggesting such mothers be allowed to breastfeed regardless of the methadone treatment dosage; follow-up counseling and monitoring of the mother and infant is recommended.

Late-onset withdrawal occurs at age 2 to 4 weeks and may continue for weeks or months. A higher incidence of SIDS also has been reported in these infants (Wagner et al, 1998). This factor is important for perinatal nurses who coordinate follow-up care for the infant and education for the mother or other caregiver. Community health nurses must know about the potential for withdrawal symptoms to occur.

Therapy for methadone withdrawal is similar to that for heroin withdrawal. The few available follow-up studies of these infants reveal a high incidence of hyperactivity, learning and behavior disorders, and poor social adjustment.

Miscellaneous Substances

Methamphetamines

The fetal and neonatal effects of maternal use of methamphetamines in pregnancy are not well known but appear to be dose related (Smith et al, 2003). LBW, preterm birth, and perinatal mortality may be consequences of higher doses used throughout pregnancy. In addition, a higher incidence of cleft lip and palate and cardiac defects has been reported in infants exposed to methamphetamines in utero (Plessinger, 1998).

Methamphetamine use has increased significantly in the past 10 years in certain regions of the United States. In Smith and colleagues' (2003) study, 63% of pregnant women reported using methamphetamine throughout the pregnancy. A higher incidence of preterm delivery and placental abruption was associated with methamphetamine use. In addition, fetal growth restriction (small for gestational age [SGA]) was slightly higher in methamphetamine-exposed offspring; however, 80% of these neonates' mothers also had significant intake of alcohol and tobacco use (Smith et al, 2003).

Study reports vary in the time of clinical manifestations of withdrawal from this drug; one study did not identify any signs of withdrawal in the first 3 days after birth, but long-term data were not collected (Smith et al, 2003). Following birth, infants may experience bradycardia or tachycardia that resolves as the drug is cleared from the infant's system. Lethargy may continue for several months, along with frequent infections and poor weight gain. Emotional disturbances and delays in gross and fine motor coordination may be seen during early childhood.

Phenobarbital

Phenobarbital crosses the placenta readily and is subsequently found in high levels in the fetal liver and brain. Because of its slow metabolic rate, withdrawal onset is generally 2 to 14 days after birth and duration is about 2 to 4 months. Irritability, crying, hiccups, and sleepiness mark the initial response. During the second stage, the infant is extremely hungry, regurgitates and gags frequently, and demonstrates episodic irritability, sweating, and a disturbed sleep pattern.

Caffeine

Caffeine has not been implicated as a teratogen in humans. Fernandes and colleagues (1998) reported that caffeine consumption greater than 150 mg per day was associated with IUGR and LBW. Santos and co-workers (1998) reported no adverse effects in the fetus with consumption of less than 300 mg of caffeine a day.

D'Apolito and Hepworth (2001) studied a small group (14) of infants exposed to multiple drugs (polydrug) in utero; these included opioids, stimulants, depressants, and sedatives. The most common symptoms observed were increased tone, increased respiratory rate, disturbed sleep, fever, frantic and increased sucking, and loose or watery stools. These findings are significant for nurses working in neonatal and obstetric areas; the presence of such findings may alert the nurse so documentation of events (per NAS scoring tool or other objective measure) may take place and therapy promptly implemented. Initial nursing interventions such as providing a quiet environment and offering a pacifier for frantic and excessive sucking may be implemented independently. It is important not to overfeed infants who demand frequent sucking as part of the withdrawal process.

Care Management

Assessment

Assessment of the newborn requires a review of the mother's prenatal record. A medical and social history of drug abuse and detoxification is noted. The infant may have IUGR or be preterm with LBW.

The woman who is abusing chemical substances may have infections that compound the risk to the infant, including hepatitis B; septicemia; and STIs, including HIV-positive status.

The nurse often is the first to observe the signs of drug withdrawal in the infant. In many cases the newborn may be discharged before the appearance of any manifestations of withdrawal. The infant is assessed by means of the guidelines discussed in Chapter 25. The infant's gestational age and maturity are noted. In utero exposure to some drugs results in observable malformations or dysmorphism (abnormality of shape). Neonatal behavior may arouse suspicion. Neonatal abstinence syndrome (NAS) is the term used to describe the set of behaviors exhibited by the infant exposed to chemical substances in utero (Table 28-7). Fig. 28-10 provides an example of a Neonatal Abstinence Scoring system for assessing withdrawal symptoms. Because many women are multidrug users, the newborn initially may exhibit a variety of withdrawal manifestations.

Another scoring tool has been recently developed specifically aimed at measuring neurologic behavior and resultant effects on the neonate when substances are used during pregnancy. The NICU Network Neurobehavioral Scale

Table 28-7

Signs of Neonatal Abstinence Syndrome

SYSTEM	SIGNS
Gastrointestinal	Poor feeding, vomiting, regurgitation, diarrhea, excessive sucking
Central nervous	Irritability, tremors, shrill cry, incessant crying, hyperactivity, little sleep, excoriations on face, convulsions
Metabolic, vasomotor, respiratory	Nasal congestion, tachypnea, sweating, frequent yawning, increased respiratory rate >60/min, fever >37.2° C

NEONATAL ABSTINENCE SCORING SYSTEM

SYSTEM	SIGNS AND SYMPTOMS	SCORE	AM	PM	COMMENTS
CENTRAL NERVOUS SYSTEM DISTURBANCES	Excessive High Pitched (Or Other) Cry Continuous High Pitched (Or Other) Cry	2 3			Daily Weight:
	Sleeps <1 Hour After Feeding Sleeps <2 Hours After Feeding Sleeps <3 Hours After Feeding	3 2 1			
	Hyperactive Moro Reflex Markedly Hyperactive Moro Reflex	2 3			
	Mild Tremors Disturbed Moderate-Severe Tremors Disturbed	1 2			
	Mild Tremors Undisturbed Moderate-Severe Tremors Undisturbed	3 4			
	Increased Muscle Tone	2			
	Excoriation (Specific Area)	1			
	Myoclonic Jerks	3			
	Generalized Convulsions	5			
METABOLIC/VASOMOTOR/RESPIRATORY DISTURBANCES	Sweating	1			
	Fever <101° (99-100.8° F./37.2-38.2° C.) Fever >101° (38.4° C. and Higher)	1 2			
	Frequent Yawning (>3 or 4 Times/Interval)	1			
	Mottling	1			
	Nasal Stuffiness	1			
	Sneezing (>3 or 4 Times/Interval)	1			
	Nasal Flaring	2			
	Respiratory Rate >60/min Respiratory Rate >60/min with Retractions	1 2			
GASTROINTESTINAL DISTURBANCES	Excessive Sucking	1			
	Poor Feeding	2			
	Regurgitation Projectile Vomiting	2 3			
	Loose Stools Watery Stools	2 3			
	TOTAL SCORE				
	INITIALS OF SCORER				

Fig. 28-10 Neonatal Abstinence Scoring (NAS) system, developed by L. Finnegan. (From Nelson N: *Current therapy in neonatal-perinatal medicine,* ed 2, St Louis, 1990, Mosby.)

(NNNS) was developed by the NIH and provides an assessment of neurologic, behavioral, and stress/abstinence function in the neonate. The test combines items from other tests such as the Neonatal Behavioral Assessment Scale (NBAS), stress/abstinence items developed by Finnegan (see Fig. 28-10), and a complete neurologic examination, which includes primitive reflexes and active and passive tone (Law et al, 2003).

Newborn urine, hair, or meconium sampling may be required to identify drug exposure and implement appropriate early interventional therapies aimed at minimizing the consequences of intrauterine drug exposure. Meconium sampling for fetal drug exposure is reported to provide more screening accuracy than urine, since drug metabolites accumulate in meconium (Kandall, 1999; Ostrea, 2001). Urine toxicology screening has less accuracy because it only reflects recent substance intake by the mother (Huestis & Choo, 2002). Meconium and hair testing for drug metabolites have the advantages of ease of collection, being noninvasive, and providing greater accuracy.

Nursing Diagnoses

Nursing diagnoses, which depend on the assessment findings, are tailored to the individual needs of the neonate and the family. Following are examples of nursing diagnoses:

Neonate

- *Risk for infection related to*
  —Maternal risk behaviors that include sexual activity
  —Prolonged rupture of membranes
  —IUGR, preterm birth
- *Risk for disorganized infant behavior related to*
  —Chemical effects of maternal substance abuse
  —Caregiver cue misreading
  —Caregiver cue knowledge deficit
  —Sensory overstimulation
- *Disturbed sleep pattern related to*
  —Drug, chemical withdrawal

Parents

- *Risk for impaired parenting related to*
  —Continuation of substance abuse or detoxification program
  —Guilt about infant's condition
  —Inability to cope with care needs of a special infant
- *Anxiety related to deficient knowledge regarding*
  —Care needs of an affected infant
- *Violence: self-directed or directed toward infant related to*
  —Drug-dependent lifestyle

Expected Outcomes

Examples of expected outcomes for neonates and parents are as follows:

Neonate

- The neonate will remain free of infection
- Early manifestations of infection (viral or bacterial) will be recognized and appropriate therapy to minimize effects of disease will be implemented
- Newborn manifestation of withdrawal (NAS) will be recognized and appropriate therapy implemented to provide infant state regulation
- Infant will receive appropriate physical and emotional care to minimize effects of maternal chemical substance use
- Neonate will have steady patterns of uninterrupted sleep throughout the day
- Neonate will demonstrate appropriate growth and development

Parent(s)

- Parent(s) will demonstrate ability to consistently meet basic caregiving needs of neonate
- Parent(s) will continue to participate in substance abuse program to enhance ability to cope with life and effectively parent the newborn
- Parent(s) will receive counseling and information from health care staff regarding infant behavior, cues requiring comfort and feeding, signs of withdrawal, and general baby care
- Parent(s) will recognize pattern of self destructive behavior (substance abuse) and seek intervention

Plan of Care and Implementation

Planning for care of the infant born to a substance-abusing mother presents a challenge to the health care team. Parents are included in the planning for the newborn's care and are also encouraged to plan for their own care. A multidisciplinary approach is needed that includes home health or community resource personnel (e.g., regulatory agencies such as child protective services). Education and social support to prevent the abuse of drugs provide the ideal approach. However, given the scope of the drug abuse problem, total prevention is unrealistic.

Nursing care of the drug-exposed neonate involves supportive therapy for fluid and electrolyte balance, nutrition, infection control, and respiratory care. Swaddling, holding, reducing environmental stimuli, and feeding as necessary may be helpful in easing withdrawal (Nursing Care Plan). Specific suggestions for providing care to infants experiencing withdrawal are listed in the Patient Teaching box.

Pharmacologic treatment is usually based on the severity of withdrawal symptoms, as determined by an assessment tool (see Fig. 28-10). Drug therapies to decrease withdrawal side effects include administration of phenobarbital, morphine, diluted tincture of opium, or methadone (Coyle et al, 2002; Johnson, Gerada, & Greenough, 2003).

Patient Teaching

CARE OF THE INFANT EXPERIENCING WITHDRAWAL

- Place the infant in a side-lying position with the spine and legs flexed.
- Position the infant's hands in midline with the arms at the side.
- Carry the infant in a flexed position.
- When interacting with the infant, introduce one stimulus at a time when the infant is in a quiet, alert state. Watch for time-out or distress signals (e.g., gaze aversion, yawning, sneezing, hiccups, arching, mottled color).
- When the infant is distressed, swaddle in a flexed position and rock in a slow, rhythmic fashion.
- Put the infant in a sitting position with chin tucked down for feeding.

Nursing Care Plan

THE DRUG-EXPOSED NEWBORN

NURSING DIAGNOSIS: Risk for injury related to hyperactivity, irritability, and disorganized state

EXPECTED OUTCOME

Infant exhibits age-appropriate state modulation regulation and stability (i.e., quiet alert state, deep sleep state, drowsy) with minimal irritability and inability to modulate state.

NURSING INTERVENTIONS/*RATIONALES*

Use an objective measure/tool such as the Neonatal Abstinence Scoring system, *to verify and document behaviors associated with withdrawal.*

Perform a comprehensive neurobehavioral assessment of the infant, *to gather individual assessment data to assist in planning individualized care appropriate for the infant experiencing withdrawal as a result of intrauterine drug exposure.* NOTE: These first two interventions take precedence over all others because manifestations of withdrawal may vary from one infant to another.

Administer medications *to decrease CNS irritability.*

Decrease environmental stimuli *that may trigger irritability and hyperactive behaviors*.

Plan care activities carefully *to allow for appropriate interaction as per infant's behavioral clues.*

Wrap infant snugly and hold infant tightly *to reduce self-stimulation behaviors.*

Position to avoid eye contact, swaddle infant, use vertical rocking techniques, and use a pacifier *to counter poor organizational response to stimuli and depressed interactive behaviors.*

Monitor activity level, note the relationship between activity level and external stimulation, and stop external stimulation *if it causes activity increase.*

Provide scheduled periods of rest, decreased overhead lighting, and no physical care *to allow time for recovery of quiet state after periods of care*.

Help mother understand that infant behavioral cues are not a sign of rejection of her caretaking abilities, *to facilitate long-lasting maternal-infant interaction, decrease maternal guilt, and enhance environment conducive to infant growth (promote infant's sense of trust).*

NURSING DIAGNOSIS: Imbalanced nutrition: less than body requirements related to CNS irritability, disorganized sucking pattern, vomiting, and loose/watery stools

EXPECTED OUTCOME

Infant exhibits appropriate weight gain.

NURSING INTERVENTIONS/*RATIONALES*

Observe for feeding cues indicating readiness for interaction (quiet alert, rooting) and feed frequent small amounts and burp well *to diminish vomiting and aspiration.*

Monitor weight daily and maintain strict intake and output *to evaluate success of feeding.*

If intake is insufficient, feed by gavage order *to ensure ingestion of needed nutrients.*

Modify environment of feeding area as necessary, *to decrease stimuli that detract from feeding process and interaction with caregiver.*

NURSING DIAGNOSIS: Risk for impaired skin integrity related to hyperactivity, rubbing knees, elbows and face against linen, and loose, watery stools

EXPECTED OUTCOME

Infant exhibits evidence of intact skin.

NURSING INTERVENTIONS/*RATIONALES*

Position infant supine with knees and arms flexed and place a blanket role at front and back, *to promote containment and comfort and minimize frantic irritable activity.*

Monitor hydration and nutritional status (i.e., skin turgor, weight, mucous membranes, fontanels, urine specific gravity, electrolytes) *to evaluate for evidence of poor skin integrity.*

Administer medications intended to decrease hyperactivity, irritability and frantic posturing, *to decrease exposure of skin to surfaces that may cause skin breakdown.*

Cleanse face and diaper area promptly after regurgitation or stooling *to prevent skin breakdown.*

Wrap infant snugly in blanket and place hands in midline next to face *to promote self comforting and decrease frantic activity.*

Cuddle infant *to promote quiet and relaxation.*

NURSING DIAGNOSIS: Ineffective maternal coping, anxiety, powerlessness, related to drug use, infant distress during withdrawal, and single-parent status

EXPECTED OUTCOME

Mother will accept newborn's condition and participate in care activities, showing evidence of maternal-infant bonding process.

NURSING INTERVENTIONS/*RATIONALES*

Explain effects of maternal drug use on newborn and the withdrawal process *to provide understanding and reality concerning effects of drug use.*

Encourage open communication (e.g., inform mother of ongoing condition, procedures, and treatment; answer questions; correct misperceptions; actively listen to her concerns) *to provide a sense of respect, provide support, and encourage a sense of control.*

Encourage mother to interact with infant and to become involved in care routines *to foster emotional connection.*

Explain how to do care procedures, how to avoid excess stimulation, and how to hold and comfort infant *to enhance mother's care abilities and her sense of confidence and control.*

If the infant demonstrates signs of withdrawal, explain to mother the infant's inability to interact, gaze aversion, arching back, and lack of response to cuddling *to enhance understanding of infant behaviors.*

Make appropriate referrals to social agencies for treatment of maternal substance abuse, infant development programs, and other needed support services *to ensure adequate resources for care of self and infant.*

Encourage maternal participation in a substance abuse counseling (and methadone maintenance, as appropriate) program *to enhance maternal coping skills for effective caretaking of affected newborn.*

A combination of these drugs may be necessary to treat infants exposed to multiple drugs in utero and careful attention should be given to possible adverse effects of the treatment drugs (Johnson, Gerada, & Greenough, 2003).

After the presence of NAS is identified in an infant, nursing care is directed toward treatment of the presenting signs, decreasing stimuli that may precipitate hyperactivity and irritability (e.g., dimming the lights, decreasing noise levels), providing adequate nutrition and hydration, and promoting maternal-infant relationships. Appropriate individualized developmental care is implemented to facilitate self-consoling and self-regulating behaviors. Irritable and hyperactive infants have been found to respond to physical comforting, movement, and close contact. Wrapping infants snugly and rocking and holding them tightly limits their ability to self-stimulate. The infant's arms should remain flexed with hands in close proximity of the mouth for sucking as is appropriate; sucking on fingers or hands is a form of self-control and comfort. Arranging nursing activities to reduce the amount of disturbance helps decrease exogenous stimulation.

Rocking infants with signs of drug withdrawal in a bed designed to mimic the soothing intrauterine environment did not prove to be effective in decreasing withdrawal symptoms; the rocking bed was thought to be too stimulating for the infants studied (D'Apolito, 1999). Loose stools, poor intake, and regurgitation after feeding predispose these infants to malnutrition, dehydration, and electrolyte imbalance. Frequent weighing to detect fluid losses or caloric intake, careful monitoring of intake and output, electrolytes, and additional caloric supplementation may be necessary. In addition, these infants burn up energy with continual activity and increase oxygen consumption at the cellular level. It takes considerable time and patience to ensure that they receive a sufficient caloric and fluid intake.

Hyperactive infants must be protected from skin abrasions on the knees, toes, and cheeks that are caused by rubbing on bed linens while in a prone position while awake. The incidence of SIDS in such children is high and parents should be reminded that the supine position for sleep is preferred. Monitoring and recording the activity level and its relationship to other activities, such as feeding and preventing complications, are important nursing functions.

Breastfeeding is encouraged in mothers who are not using illicit substances, are negative for HIV infection, and are compliant with a methadone program; breastfeeding promotes maternal-infant bonding, and the small amount of methadone passed through breast milk has not proved to be harmful to the neonate (Berghella et al, 2003; Hale, 2002; Philipp, Merewood, & O' Brien, 2003). Because many new drugs are being manufactured, it is recommended that the reader consult with updated references regarding the safety of medications for breastfeeding infants (see also AAP, [2001] for a complete list of drugs that should be avoided with breastfeeding). It is reasonable to expect that the pregnant mother should abstain from the so-called recreational drugs mentioned above because none of these are safe in any given quantity for any given fetus.

Evaluation

Evaluation is based on the expected outcomes of care. The plan is revised as needed based on evaluation findings.

HEMOLYTIC DISORDERS

Hyperbilirubinemia, physiologic jaundice, pathologic jaundice, and kernicterus are discussed in Chapter 25.

Hemolytic Disease of the Newborn

Hemolytic disease occurs when the blood groups of the mother and newborn are different; the most common of these are RhD factor and ABO incompatibilities. Hemolytic disorders occur when maternal antibodies are present naturally or form in response to an antigen from the fetal blood crossing the placenta and entering the maternal circulation. The maternal antibodies of the IgG class cross the placenta, causing hemolysis of the fetal RBCs, resulting in fetal anemia and often neonatal jaundice and hyperbilirubinemia.

Rh Incompatibility

Rh incompatibility, or isoimmunization, occurs when an RhD-negative mother has an RhD-positive fetus who inherits the dominant Rh-positive gene from the father. The Rh blood group consists of several antigens (since D is the most prevalent Rh antigen the following discussion focuses on RhD isoimmunization). If the mother is Rh-negative, and the father is Rh-positive and homozygous for the Rh factor, all the offspring will be Rh-positive. If the father is heterozygous for the factor, there is a 50% chance that each infant born of the union will be Rh-positive and a 50% chance that each will be Rh-negative. An Rh-negative fetus is in no danger because it has the same Rh factor as the mother. An Rh-negative fetus with an Rh-positive mother is also in no danger. Only the Rh-positive offspring of an Rh-negative mother is at risk. From 10% to 15% of all Caucasian couples and about 5% of African-American couples have Rh incompatibility. Incompatibility is rare in Asian couples. The incidence of Rh sensitization and resulting hemolytic disease of the newborn have decreased dramatically since the development of Rh_o(D) immune globulin in 1968.

The pathogenesis of Rh incompatibility is as follows: hematopoiesis in the fetus, or the formation of blood cells, begins as early as the eighth week of gestation; in up to 40% of pregnancies, these cells pass through the placenta into the maternal circulation. When the fetus is Rh-positive and the mother Rh-negative, the mother forms antibodies against the fetal blood cells: first IgM antibodies that are too large to pass through the placenta and then IgG antibodies that can cross the placenta. The process of antibody formation is called maternal sensitization. Sensitization may occur during pregnancy, birth, induced abortion or miscarriage, or amniocentesis. Usually women become sensitized in their first pregnancy with an Rh-positive fetus but do not produce enough antibodies to cause lysis (destruction) of the fetal blood cells. In subsequent pregnancies, antibodies form in response to repeated contact with the antigen from the fetal blood, and lysis results. In approximately 10% to 15% of sensitized mothers, there is no hemolytic reaction in the newborn. In addition, some Rh-negative women, even though exposed to Rh-positive fetal blood, are immunologically unable to produce antibodies to the foreign antigen (Neal, 2001).

Severe Rh incompatibility results in marked fetal hemolytic anemia because the fetal erythrocytes are destroyed by maternal Rh-positive antibodies. Although the placenta usually clears the bilirubin generated by the RBC breakdown, in extreme cases fetal bilirubin levels increase. The fetus compensates for the anemia by producing large numbers of immature erythrocytes to replace those hemolyzed, thus the name for this condition: erythroblastosis fetalis. In hydrops fetalis, the most severe form of this disease, the fetus has marked anemia, as well as cardiac decompensation, cardiomegaly, and hepatosplenomegaly. Hypoxia results from the severe anemia. In addition, because of the decreased intravascular oncotic pressure involved, fluid leaks out of the intravascular space, resulting in generalized edema as well as effusions into the peritoneal (ascites), pericardial, and pleural (hydrothorax) spaces. The placenta is often edematous, which, along with the edematous fetus, can cause the uterus to rupture.

Intrauterine or early neonatal death may occur as a result of hydrops fetalis, although intrauterine transfusions and early delivery of the fetus may avert this. Intrauterine transfusion involves the infusion of Rh-negative, type O blood into the umbilical vein. The frequency of intrauterine transfusions may vary according to institution and fetal hydropic status, but it may be as often as every 2 weeks until the fetus reaches pulmonary maturity at approximately 37 to 38 weeks of gestation (Moise, 2002).

ABO Incompatibility

ABO incompatibility is more common than Rh incompatibility, but causes less severe problems in the affected infant. It occurs if the fetal blood type is A, B, or AB and the maternal type is O. It occurs rarely in infants with type B blood born to mothers with type A blood. The incompatibility arises because naturally occurring anti-A and anti-B antibodies are transferred across the placenta to the fetus. Unlike the situation that pertains to Rh incompatibility, first-born infants may be affected because mothers with type O blood already have anti-A and anti-B antibodies in their blood. Such a newborn may have a weakly positive direct Coombs' test (also referred to as a direct antiglobulin test [DAT]). The cord bilirubin level usually is less than 4 mg/dl, and any resulting hyperbilirubinemia usually can be treated with phototherapy. Exchange transfusions are required only occasionally. Although ABO incompatibility is a common cause of hyperbilirubinemia, it rarely precipitates significant anemia resulting from the hemolysis of RBCs.

Other

It is not within the scope of this text to discuss the many potential causes of hemolytic jaundice in childhood. However, in some populations there is a high incidence of glucose-6-phosphate dehydrogenase deficiency (G-6-PD), which may cause an exaggerated jaundice in a newborn within 24 to 48 hours of birth. G-6-PD red cells hemolyze at a greater rate than healthy red cells, thus overwhelming the immature neonatal liver's ability to conjugate the indirect bilirubin. Some of the triggers that potentiate hemolysis include vitamin K, acetaminophen, aspirin, sepsis, and exposure to certain chemicals (Reiser, 2004). Treatment is the same as for any newborn with rapidly rising serum bilirubin levels. Other metabolic and inherited conditions that increase hemolysis and may cause jaundice in the infant include galactosemia, Criglar-Najjar disease, and hypothyroidism.

Care Management

At the first prenatal visit of an Rh-negative woman with a fetus who may be Rh-positive, an indirect Coombs' test should be done to determine whether she has antibodies to the Rh antigen. In this test the maternal blood serum is mixed with Rh-positive RBCs. If the Rh-positive RBCs agglutinate or clump, this indicates that maternal antibodies are present or that the mother has been sensitized. The dilution of the specimen of blood at which clumping occurs determines the titer, or level, of maternal antibodies. This titer indicates the degree of maternal sensitization. A level of 1:8 rarely results in fetal jeopardy. If the titer reaches 1:16, amniocentesis is performed to determine the delta optical density (ΔOD) of the amniotic fluid to estimate fetal hemolytic process. Rising bilirubin levels may indicate the need for an intrauterine transfusion. Genetic testing allows early identification of paternal zygosity at the RhD gene locus, thus allowing earlier detection of the potential for isoimmunization and precluding further maternal or fetal testing (Moise, 2002).

The indirect Coombs' test is repeated at 28 weeks. If the result remains negative, indicating that sensitization has not occurred, the woman is given an intramuscular injection of $Rh_o(D)$ immune globulin. If the test result is positive, showing that sensitization has occurred, the test is repeated at 4- to 6-week intervals to monitor the maternal antibody titer as just described.

At birth, the neonate's cord blood is sent to the laboratory to determine the infant's blood type and Rh status. A direct Coombs' test is performed on this cord blood to determine whether there are maternal antibodies in the fetal blood. If antibodies are present, the titer, which indicates the degree of maternal sensitization, is measured. If the titer is 1:64, an exchange transfusion is indicated. In addition, the prevention of or prompt therapy for perinatal asphyxia, acidosis, cold stress, sepsis, and hypoglycemia will decrease the newborn's risk for severe hemolytic disease and his or her susceptibility to kernicterus. Early feeding is also initiated to stimulate stooling and thus facilitate the removal of bilirubin.

If jaundice is present, the cause is determined and therapeutic management is begun. Phototherapy is used to reduce rapidly increasing serum bilirubin levels. See Chapter 25 for a discussion of phototherapy.

Exchange transfusions are needed infrequently because of the decrease in the incidence of severe hemolytic disease in newborns resulting from isoimmunization. Other factors must always be considered as well, particularly the clinical condition of the infant, because it is a procedure with potential complications. Guidelines for the initiation of exchange transfusion in relation to serum bilirubin levels in infants of ≥35 weeks gestation may be found in the 2004 AAP, Subcommittee on hyperbilirubinemia: Clinical Practice Guideline.

Exchange transfusion is accomplished by alternately removing a small amount of the infant's blood and replacing it with an equal amount of donor blood. If the infant has Rh incompatibility, type O Rh-negative blood is used for transfusion, so the maternal antibodies still present in the infant do not hemolyze the transfused blood. Depending on the infant's size, maturity, and condition, amounts of 5 to 20 ml of the infant's blood are removed at one time and replaced with warmed donor blood. The total amount of blood exchanged approximates 170 ml/kg of body weight, or 75% to 85% of the infant's total blood volume. Preservatives in donor blood lower the infant's serum calcium level; therefore, calcium gluconate is often given during the exchange transfusion. The neonate is monitored closely for signs of a blood transfusion reaction as well as hypotension, temperature instability, and cardiorespiratory compromise.

CONGENITAL ANOMALIES

Congenital defects occur in 2% to 3% of all live births (Steele, 1997), but this number increases to about 6% by 5 years, when more anomalies are diagnosed. In addition, the incidence of congenital malformations in fetuses that are aborted is higher than that in infants who are born alive, thus also adding to the overall incidence. Major congenital defects are the leading cause of death in infants younger than 1 year of age in the United States and account for 20% of neonatal deaths. Although the incidences of other causes of neonatal mortality have decreased, the death rate associated with most congenital anomalies has essentially remained stable since 1932.

The most common major congenital anomalies that cause serious problems in the neonate are congenital heart disease, choanal atresia, neural tube defects (NTDs), cleft lip or palate, clubfoot, and developmental dysplasia of the hip. These are thought to result from the interaction of multiple genetic and environmental factors. Some of the most common malformations include lack of a helical fold of the pinna, complete or incomplete simian creases, and a capillary hemangioma other than on the face or posterior aspect of the neck.

Ways of detecting and preventing some of these anomalies are being improved continuously, as are some surgical techniques for the care of the fetus with certain anomalies. Promoting the availability of these services to populations at risk challenges community health care systems. An interdisciplinary team approach is vital for providing holistic care: the surgical treatment, rehabilitation, and education of the child, as well as psychosocial and financial assistance for the parents. Parental disappointment and disillusion add to the complexity of the nursing care needed for these infants.

Central Nervous System Anomalies

Most congenital anomalies of the CNS result from defects in the closure of the neural tube during fetal development. Although the cause of NTDs is unknown, they are thought to stem from the interaction of many genes that may be influenced by factors in the fetal environment. Environmental influences such as treatment with valproic acid (an anticonvulsant), methotrexate (a chemotherapeutic agent), and alcohol and tobacco consumption have been implicated. Maternal folic acid deficit has a direct bearing on failure of the neural tube to close; therefore, folic acid supplementation is recommended for women of childbearing age. In the United States, rates of NTDs have declined from 1.3 per 1000 births (1970) to 0.3 per 1000 births after the introduction of mandatory food fortification with folic acid in 1998 (Honein, 2001). Increased use of prenatal diagnostic techniques and termination of pregnancies have also impacted the overall incidence of NTDs. Although a neural tube defect is usually an isolated defect, it can occur with some chromosomal abnormalities and syndromes and also with other defects such as cleft palate, ventricular septal defect, tracheoesophageal fistula, congenital diaphragmatic hernia, imperforate anus, and renal anomalies.

Encephalocele and Anencephaly

Encephalocele and anencephaly are abnormalities resulting from failure of the anterior end of the neural tube to close. An encephalocele is a herniation of the brain and meninges through a skull defect. Treatment consists of surgical repair and shunting to relieve hydrocephalus, unless a major brain malformation is present. Some of these infants will have some degree of cognitive deficit. Anencephaly is the absence of both cerebral hemispheres and of the overlying skull. It is a condition that is incompatible with life; many of the infants are stillborn or die within a few days of birth. Comfort measures are provided until the infant eventually dies of temperature instability and respiratory failure.

Spina Bifida

Spina bifida, the most common defect of the CNS, results from failure of the neural tube to close at some point. There are two categories of spina bifida: spina bifida occulta and spina bifida cystica. Spina bifida occulta is a malformation in which the posterior portion of the laminas fails to close but the spinal cord or meninges do not herniate or protrude through the defect. It is usually asymptomatic and may not be diagnosed unless there are associated problems. Spina bifida cystica includes meningocele and myelomeningocele. A meningocele is an external sac that contains meninges and CSF and that protrudes through a defect in the vertebral column. A myelomeningocele is similar, except that it also contains nerves; therefore the infant has motor and sensory deficits below the lesion. A myelomeningocele is visible at birth, most often in the lumbosacral area. It is usually covered with a very fragile, thin membrane (Fig. 28-11). The sac can tear easily, allowing CSF to leak out and providing an entry for infectious agents into the CNS (Fig. 28-11, *B*). Myelomeningocele usually is associated with an Arnold-Chiari malformation, which results from the improper development and downward displacement of part of the brain into the cervical spinal canal. This in turn results in the development of hydrocephalus, which affects about 90% of children with myelomeningocele, although it is usually not present at birth. The long-term prognosis in an affected infant can be determined to a large extent at birth, with the degree of neurologic dysfunction related to the level of the lesion, which determines the nerves involved. Many physicians recommend that treatment be instituted regardless of the level of the lesion unless there is a severe CNS anomaly, advanced hydrocephalus at birth, severe anoxic brain damage, active CNS infection, or a malformation or syndrome incompatible with long-term survival. Prenatal diagnosis makes possible a scheduled cesarean birth allowing for more

A

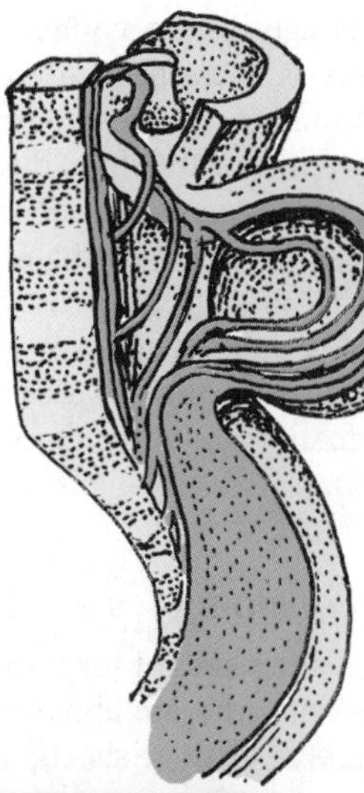

B

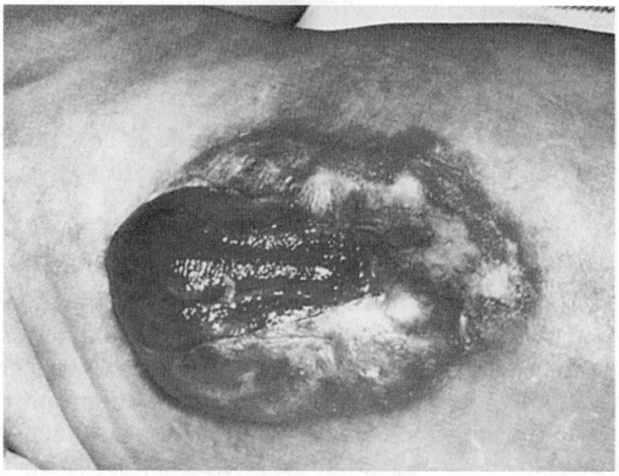

Fig. 28-11 **A**, Myelomeningocele. Note absence of vertebral arches. **B**, Myelomeningocele (ruptured sac exposing defect). (From Zitelli BJ, Davis HW: *Atlas of pediatric physical diagnosis*, ed 4, St Louis, 2002, Mosby.)

careful delivery of the infant's back to try to prevent rupture of the meningeal sac.

A major preoperative nursing intervention for a neonate with a myelomeningocele is to protect the protruding sac from injury, rupture, and resultant risk of CNS infection. Such infants should be positioned in a side-lying or prone position to prevent pressure on the sac until surgical repair is done. If the infant is able to be held, the nurse or parent must be careful to keep the defect from being injured. The sac should be covered with a sterile, moist, nonadherent dressing and cared for using sterile technique. The skin around the defect must be cleansed and dried carefully to prevent breakdown, which would establish a portal of entry for infectious agents. A major nursing intervention is providing support and needed information to parents as they begin to learn to cope with an infant who has immediate needs for intensive care and who probably will have long-term needs as well. Surgical repair is performed in the neonatal period, often within the first 24 to 48 hours. Very early closure can prevent CNS infection and trauma to the exposed nerves. It can also prevent stretching of other nerve roots, which can occur as the sac continues to enlarge after birth. Surgical shunt procedures to prevent increasing hydrocephalus may be needed. Other problems, such as infection, are treated as they occur.

Hydrocephalus

Hydrocephalus is a condition in which the ventricles of the brain are enlarged as a result of an imbalance between the production and absorption of the CSF. Congenital hydrocephalus usually arises as a result of a malformation in the brain or an intrauterine infection. About one-third of all cases of congenital hydrocephalus result from stenosis of the aqueduct of Sylvius in the brain. Hydrocephalus often occurs in conjunction with a myelomeningocele, which blocks the flow of CSF.

An infant with congenital hydrocephalus initially has a bulging anterior fontanel and a head circumference that increases at an abnormal rate, resulting from the increase in CSF pressure. Enlargement of the forehead with depressed eyes that are rotated downward, causing a "setting sun" sign, occurs as the condition worsens. If the surgical shunting of excess CSF from the brain is not done soon after birth, the resulting increasing ICP will lead to irreversible neurologic damage, as evidenced by palpably widening sutures and fontanels, distended scalp veins; lethargy; poor feeding; vomiting; irritability; opisthotonic positioning; and a high-pitched, shrill cry.

Nursing actions appropriate to the needs of a newborn with hydrocephalus include care similar to any high risk newborn. Measurement of the head circumference and neurologic assessments are done frequently. If the infant's head is large, the placement of sheepskin or a special pressure-sensitive air mattress under the infant and frequent position changes are necessary to prevent skin breakdown. Chapter 51 contains a more detailed description of the evaluation and management of the child with hydrocephalus.

Microcephaly

Microcephaly refers to a head circumference that measures more than three standard deviations below the mean for age and sex. Brain growth is usually restricted and thus mental retardation is common. Microcephaly can be the result of an autosomal-dominant disorder; a chromosomal abnormality; fetal exposure to teratogens such as radiation; and congenital infections such as rubella, toxoplasmosis, or cytomegalovirus. Infants with microcephaly require supportive nursing care and medical observation to determine the extent of the psychomotor retardation that almost always accompanies this abnormality. There is no treatment. Parents need support to learn to care for a child with cognitive impairment.

Cardiovascular System Anomalies

Congenital heart defects (CHDs) are anatomic abnormalities of the heart that are present at birth, although they may not be diagnosed immediately. Some type of congenital cardiovascular problem is present in approximately 3.7 to 8 of every 1000 live births (Carey, 2002) and about 2 to 3 newborns will be symptomatic with heart disease in the first year of life (Bernstein, 2004). Ventricular septal defects, constituting more than 20% to 25% of all CHDs, are the most common type of acyanotic lesion. Tetralogy of Fallot, constituting 5% to 7% of all CHDs, is the most common type resulting in cyanosis. After prematurity, CHDs, often in association with other congenital anomalies, are the next major cause of death in the first year of life.

The etiology of CHDs is unknown in more than 90% of the cases. Maternal factors associated with a higher incidence of CHD include maternal rubella, alcohol intake, diabetes mellitus, systemic lupus erythematosus, phenylketonuria, poor nutrition, or antiepileptic medication (AED) use.

Genetic factors are implicated in the pathogenesis of CHD. As a general rule, these defects are thought to be multifactorial in origin, involving both genetic and environmental influences; however, a familial occurrence of virtually all forms of CHD has been noted.

Chromosomal abnormalities may also be associated with CHDs. For example, 50% of children with trisomy 21, or Down syndrome, have a cardiac defect. Most children who have trisomy 18, the second most common chromosomal abnormality, have a cardiac anomaly. See Chapter 48 for a discussion of classifications of CHDs.

Some CHDs are often evident immediately after birth, especially those defects that cause central cyanosis (e.g., transposition of the great vessels) despite 100% oxygen administration. Infants with these anomalies are transferred directly to an intensive care nursery or pediatric intensive care unit.

Affected newborns may be cyanotic and unrelieved by oxygen treatment, with the cyanosis increasing whenever the child cries. Pulse oximetry readings which remain low (below 89%) despite oxygen administration are not unusual and respiratory distress may or may not be present. In many cases the infant's color is unrelated to the severity of the defect. Other infants may be acyanotic and pale, with or without mottling upon exertion, such as crying, feeding, or stooling.

The affected newborn's activity level varies from restlessness to lethargy and possible unresponsiveness, except to pain. Persistent bradycardia (i.e., resting heart rate of <80 to 100 beats/min) or tachycardia (i.e., rate exceeding 160 to 180 beats/min) may be noted. The infant born to a mother with systemic lupus may exhibit bradycardia with normal sinus rhythm and good perfusion; eventually cardioversion may be required if the rhythm persists. The cardiac rhythm may be abnormal, and a murmur may or may not be heard. In many cases, however, ductal (ductus arteriosus) dependent defects or large shunts will not present with a murmur. Signs of congestive heart failure, diminished cardiac output, and poor tissue perfusion may be evident.

Because the cardiac and respiratory systems function together, cardiac disease may also be manifested by respiratory signs and symptoms. The respiratory rate should be determined when the newborn is in a resting state. Abnormal findings may include tachypnea, which is a rate of 60 breaths/min or more; retractions with nasal flaring; grunting occurring with or without exertion; and dyspnea, which may worsen with crying and activity.

A major role of the nurse is to assess infants for abnormal findings such as central cyanosis and poor perfusion. Newborns exhibiting these symptoms require prompt attention and appropriate therapy in a neonatal or pediatric intensive care unit. Interventions planned when a nursing diagnosis of decreased cardiac output is made include administering oxygen as ordered, although oxygen content is usually decreased once the defect is identified; administering cardiotonic medications to increase cardiac output, and medications designed to prevent closure of the ductus arteriosus (prostaglandin), and diuretic agents as needed for CHF; decreasing the work load of the heart by maintaining a thermoneutral environment; and feeding using the gavage method if necessary. Various diagnostic tests such as echocardiography and cardiac catheterization are performed to obtain specific information about the defect and the need for surgical intervention.

Respiratory System Anomalies

Screening for congenital anomalies of the respiratory system is necessary even in infants who are apparently normal at birth. Respiratory distress at birth or shortly thereafter may be the result of lung immaturity or anomalous development. Congenital laryngeal web and bilateral choanal atresia are readily apparent at birth. Respiratory distress caused by congenital diaphragmatic hernia and tracheoesophageal fistula may appear immediately or be delayed, depending on the severity of the defect.

Laryngeal Web and Choanal Atresia

A laryngeal web, which is uncommon, results from the incomplete separation of the two sides of the larynx and is most often between the vocal cords. Choanal atresia (Fig. 28-12) is the most common congenital anomaly of the nose; it is a bony or membranous septum located between the nose and the pharynx. Inability to pass a suction catheter through the nose into the pharynx or cyanosis without obvious respiratory distress usually leads to its detection. Nearly half of the infants with choanal atresia have other

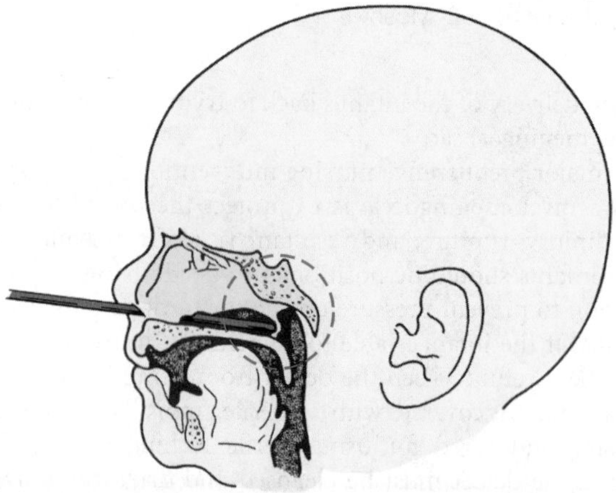

Fig. 28-12 Choanal atresia. Posterior nares are obstructed by membrane or bone, either bilaterally or unilaterally. Infant becomes cyanotic at rest. With crying, newborn's color improves. Nasal discharge is present. Snorting respirations often are observed with increased respiratory effort. Newborn may be unable to breathe and eat at the same time. Diagnosis is made by noting inability to pass small feeding tube through one or both nares. (Used with permission of Ross Products Division, Abbott Laboratories, Inc., Columbus, OH 43216. From Clinical Education Aid No. 6, Copyright 1963, Ross Products Division, Abbott Laboratories, Inc.)

anomalies. Infants with either a laryngeal web or choanal atresia require emergency surgery.

Congenital Diaphragmatic Hernia

Congenital diaphragmatic hernia (CDH) results from a defect in the formation of the diaphragm, allowing the abdominal organs to be displaced into the thoracic cavity. It occurs in approximately 1 in 5000 live births. However, if stillbirths resulting from this defect are included, the incidence increases to 1 in 2000 (Hartman, 2004). Herniation of the abdominal viscera into the thoracic cavity may cause severe respiratory distress and represent a neonatal emergency (Fig. 28-13). The defect and herniation may be minimal and easily repaired, or the defect may be so extensive that the viscera present in the thoracic cavity during embryonic life have prevented the normal development of pulmonary tissue. The defect is usually on the left because that is the side of the diaphragm that fuses last.

Most congenital diaphragmatic hernias are discovered prenatally on ultrasound. Hernias may be repaired by fetal surgery in some research institutions. Intrauterine surgical correction of CDH has met with poor neonatal outcomes in many cases, primarily as a result of tocolysis failure and early delivery. At birth, most affected infants have severe respiratory distress, and respiratory assessment reveals worsening distress as the bowel fills with air. Typically the breath sounds are diminished and bowel sounds are heard in the chest. Heart sounds may be heard on the right side of the chest because the heart has been displaced there by the abdominal contents. Physical examination reveals a flat or scaphoid abdomen and a prominent ipsilateral chest. Diagnosis can be made on the basis of the x-ray finding of loops of intestine in the thoracic cavity and the absence of intestine in the abdominal cavity.

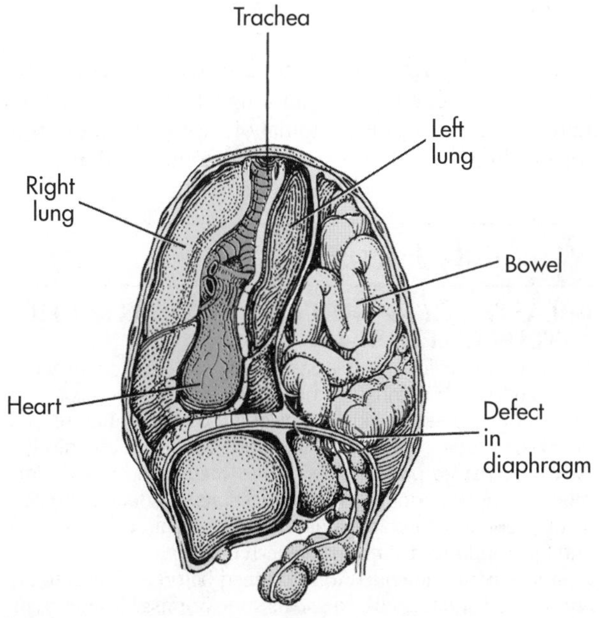

Fig. 28-13 Congenital diaphragmatic hernia. (Used with permission of Ross Products Division, Abbott Laboratories, Inc., Columbus, OH 43216. From Clinical Education Aid No. 6, Copyright 1963, Ross Products Division, Abbott Laboratories, Inc.)

Preoperative nursing interventions include participating in the stabilization of the infant's condition until surgical repair can be done. Inhaled nitric oxide (NO) has been used in many centers with moderate success to treat the accompanying persistent pulmonary hypertension (Bradshaw, 2004). Gastric contents are aspirated and suction applied to decompress the GI tract and prevent further cardiothoracic compromise. Oxygen therapy, mechanical ventilation, and the correction of acidosis are necessary in infants with early clinical respiratory distress from CDH. Extracorporeal membrane oxygenation (ECMO) may be used in infants with severe circulatory and respiratory complications.

The prognosis depends largely on the degree of fetal pulmonary development, but the prognosis in severe cases is often poor. The overall survival rate for infants who are symptomatic within the first few hours of life is about 50%, although it has improved recently with the advent of inhaled NO, improved management of high frequency ventilation, and ECMO.

Gastrointestinal System Anomalies

Anomalies in the GI system can occur anywhere along the GI tract, from the mouth to the anus. Some anomalies, such as cleft lip, omphalocele, and gastroschisis, are apparent at birth. Others, including cleft palate, esophageal atresia, intestinal obstruction, and imperforate anus become apparent as the infant is further assessed or becomes symptomatic.

Cleft Lip and Palate

Cleft lip or palate is a commonly occurring congenital midline fissure, or opening, in the lip or palate resulting from failure of the primary palate to fuse (Fig. 28-14). One or both deformities may occur. Multiple genetic and, to a lesser extent, environmental factors (e.g., maternal infection, radiation exposure, alcohol ingestion, and treatment with medications such as corticosteroids, some tranquilizers, and antiepileptics) appear to be involved in their development. Pathophysiology, evaluation, and treatment are addressed in Chapter 47.

Feeding is difficult because the cleft lip renders the newborn unable to maintain a seal around a nipple; the cleft palate renders the infant unable to form a vacuum to maintain suction when feeding. In addition, the inability to suck and swallow normally allows milk to pool in the nasopharynx, which increases the likelihood of aspiration. Furthermore, as the infant attempts to suck, milk often comes out through the cleft and out of the nares. Although the degree of difficulty depends on the size of the cleft, feeding problems are greater in infants with a cleft palate than in those with a cleft lip alone (See Fig. 28-14). Breastfeeding can be successful in some infants. There are special nipples, bottles, and appliances available to aid in feeding (Fig. 28-15) (see Family Focus box). In general, parents of infants with these defects need a great deal of education and support as they learn to feed their baby, to prevent what should be a normal part of infant care from becoming a very frustrating experience.

Parents of infants with a cleft lip or palate need much support, particularly in the case of a cleft lip because this is both a cosmetic and functional defect. Recognizing that this

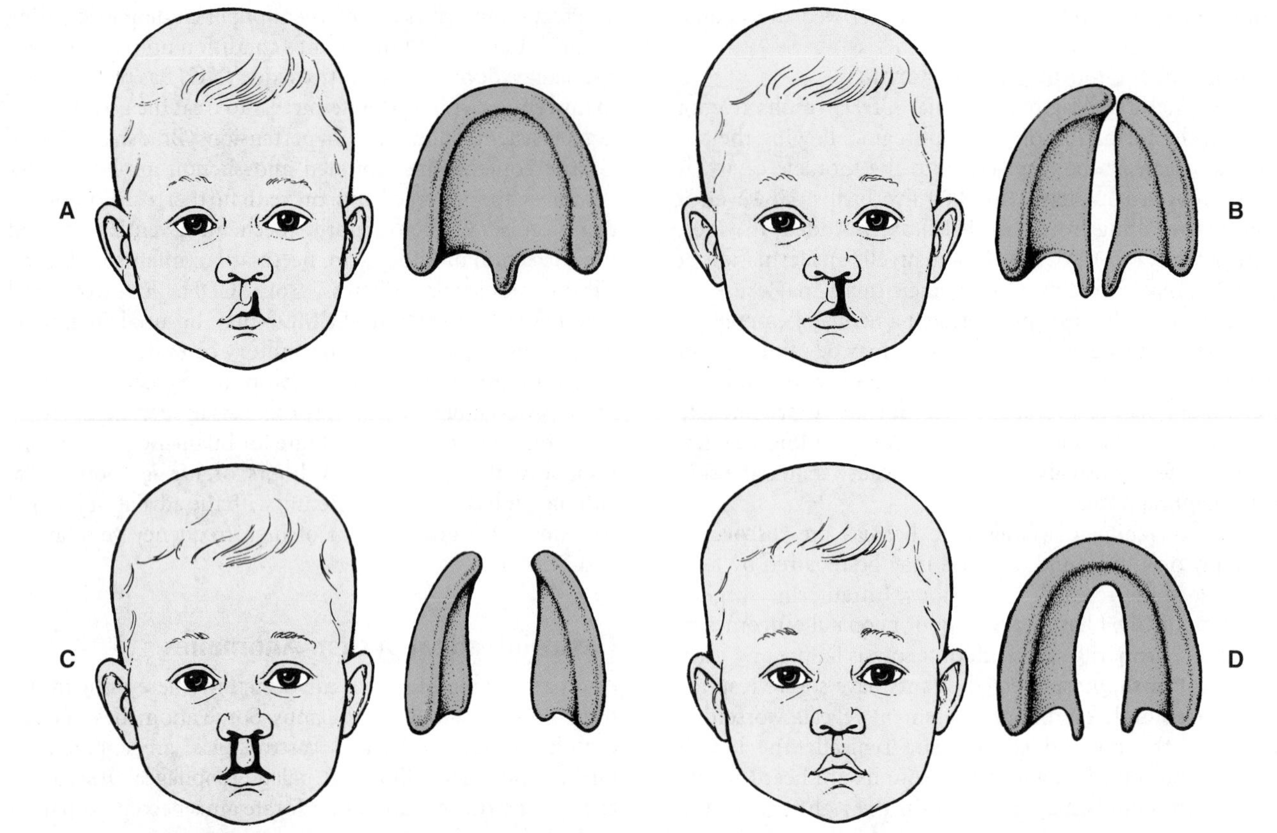

Fig. 28-14 Variations in clefts of lip and palate at birth. **A**, Notch in vermilion border. **B**, Unilateral cleft lip and cleft palate. **C**, Bilateral cleft lip and cleft palate. **D**, Cleft palate.

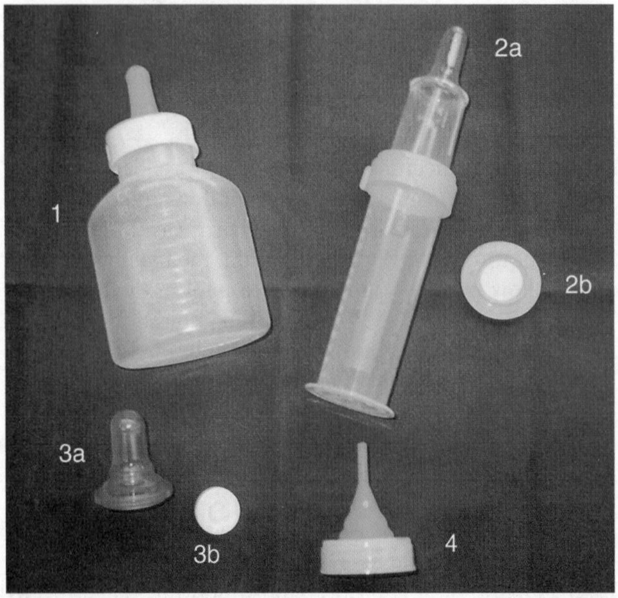

Fig. 28-15 *1*, Mead Johnson bottle and nipple for cleft palate. Cleft palate nipple system *(2a)* with valve *(2b)* to regulate flow. Haberman feeder *(3a)* with disc *(3b)* to control flow of milk. *4*, Ross cleft palate assembly. Nipple can be trimmed to accommodate palate size. (Courtesy Shannon Perry, Phoenix, AZ.)

may interfere with normal parent-infant bonding in the neonatal period, the nurse must assess for this and intervene appropriately (Critical Thinking Exercise).

Esophageal Atresia and Tracheoesophageal Fistula

Esophageal atresia (EA) and tracheoesophageal fistula (TEF) often occur together although they can also occur singly. EA is a congenital anomaly in which the esophagus ends in a blind pouch or narrows into a thin cord, thus fail-

Family Focus

BREASTFEEDING THE INFANT WITH CLEFT LIP AND/OR CLEFT PALATE

Many health professionals assume that successful breastfeeding is impossible because of the cleft lip and/or cleft palate. On the contrary, breastfeeding is not only possible, it has several benefits, including the normal integration of the infant into the family, decreased problems with otitis media, and passive immunity to upper respiratory tract infections. In addition, breastfeeding enhances normal muscular movements of the mouth and face, and benefits normal speech development.*

If the mother intended to breastfeed before delivery, she is encouraged and helped to do so as soon as possible after birth. When available, the services of a lactation expert should be used.

*Danner S: Breastfeeding the infant with a cleft palate, *NAACOG Clin Issues Perinat Womens Health Nurs* 3:634, 1992.

Critical Thinking Exercise

BIRTH OF A CHILD WITH A CONGENITAL ANOMALY

Emilie, an 18-year-old single mother, has just given birth to a son, John, who has a unilateral cleft lip and palate. You are bringing the baby to the mother for the first time. Emilie knows that John has a cleft lip and palate but has not yet seen him. How will you introduce John to Emilie? How will you describe his defect and its treatment?

1. Evidence—Is there sufficient evidence to draw conclusions about what you should tell Emilie?
2. Assumptions—What assumptions can be made about the following factors:
   a. Your feelings about the infant and his physical defect
   b. Emilie's initial reaction to the sight of her son
   c. Surgical treatment of the defect
   d. Long-term outcome for John
3. What implications and priorities for nursing care can be drawn at this time?
4. Does the evidence objectively support your conclusion?
5. Are there alternative perspectives to your conclusion?

ing to form a continuous passageway to the stomach (Fig. 28-16). TEF is an abnormal connection between the esophagus and trachea.

Maternal hydramnios is a common finding, particularly if the fetus has an EA without TEF. The infant with EA or TEF may also show some fetal growth restriction and will thus be SGA. In addition, the presence of a midline defect such as EA or TEF is often accompanied by another significant embryonic defect such as a cardiac anomaly, cleft lip and /or palate, vertebral, genitourinary, or abdominal wall defect (Bensard et al, 2002). Variations of the anomalies are possible, depending on the presence or absence of a TEF, the site of the fistula, and the location and degree of the esophageal obstruction (see Fig. 28-16).

Infants with EA and TEF may show significant respiratory difficulty immediately after birth. EA with or without TEF results in excessive oral secretions, drooling, and feeding intolerance. When fed, the infant may swallow, but then cough and gag and return the fluid through the nose and mouth. Respiratory distress can result from aspiration or from the acute gastric distention produced by the TEF. Choking, coughing, and cyanosis occur after even a small amount of fluid is taken by mouth.

Nursing interventions are supportive until surgery is performed. Any infant with excessive oral secretions and respiratory distress should not be fed orally until further evaluation is carried out. The infant is placed in the position least likely to cause aspiration of either mouth or stomach secretions. A double-lumen catheter is placed in the proximal esophageal pouch and attached to continuous suction to remove secretions and decrease the possibility of aspiration. Other supportive measures include maintaining thermoregulation, fluid and electrolyte balance intravenously, acid-base balance and prevention of any further complications as a result of an associated defect. Surgical correction, done in one stage if possible, consists of ligating the fistula and anastomosing the two segments of the esophagus. The chances for survival in those infants in a good-risk category exceed 95% depending on the presence of associated defects and the infant's birth weight. Many EA and TEF infants will have postoperative issues related to feeding difficulties such as gastroesophageal reflux (GER) and esophageal strictures requiring periodic dilation. (See Chapter 47 for further discussion of surgical treatment and nursing care.)

Omphalocele and Gastroschisis

Omphalocele and gastroschisis are two of the more common congenital defects that occur in the abdominal wall. They are rare, however, with omphalocele occurring in approximately 1 in 3000 to 10,000 live births whereas the incidence of gastroschisis is 1 in 6000 live births (Blackburn, 2003).

An omphalocele is a covered defect of the umbilical ring into which varying amounts of the abdominal organs may herniate (Fig. 28-17). Although it is covered with a peritoneal sac, the sac may rupture during or after birth. Many infants born with an omphalocele are preterm, and more than half have other serious syndromes or defects involving the GI, cardiac, genitourinary, musculoskeletal, and nervous systems.

Gastroschisis is the herniation of the bowel through a defect in the abdominal wall to the right of the umbilical cord. No membrane covers the contents, as occurs with an omphalocele. Unlike infants with omphalocele, these infants have less than 10% to 15% likelihood of associated anomalies, most of which are cardiac.

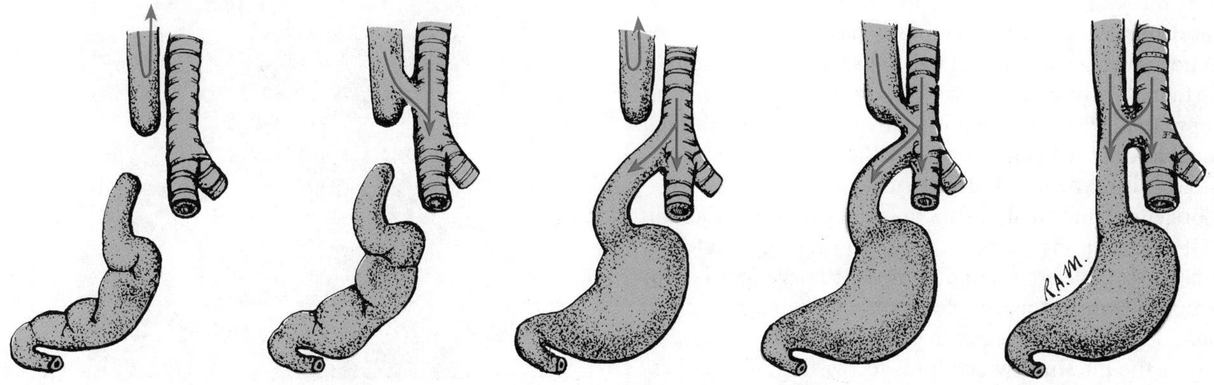

Fig. 28-16 Five most common types of esophageal atresia (EA) and tracheoesophageal fistula (TEF).

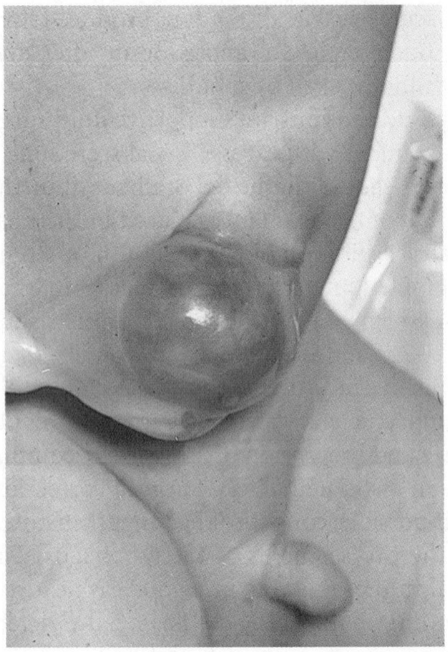

Fig. 28-17 Omphalocele. (From O'Doherty N: *Neonatology: micro atlas of the newborn,* Nutley, NJ, 1986, Hoffmann-La Roche.)

The preoperative nursing care is similar for infants with either defect. Exposure of the viscera causes problems with thermoregulation and fluid and electrolyte balance. Before closure is performed, the exposed viscera are covered with moistened saline gauze and plastic wrap. In some cases the infant may be placed in an impermeable, clear plastic bowel bag to decrease insensible water losses, maintain thermoregulation, and prevent contamination of the exposed viscera (Bensard et al, 2002). Antibiotics, fluid and electrolyte replacement, gastric decompression, and thermoregulation are needed for physiologic support. If complete closure is impossible because of the small size of the abdominal cavity and the large amount of viscera to be replaced, a Silastic silo pouch (Dow Corning, Midland, MI) is created and sewn to the fascia of the abdominal defect. The defect is closed surgically after the reduction of contents is complete, which usually takes 7 to 10 days. Gastric decompression is necessary preoperatively to prevent aspiration pneumonia and to allow as much bowel as possible to be placed into the abdomen during surgery. Surgery is usually performed soon after birth. With surgical treatment, nutritional support, and medical management, the prognosis has improved for infants born with an abdominal wall defect. It is estimated that more than 80% of infants born with omphalocele survive, as do more than 90% of those born with gastroschisis although residual feeding difficulties such as GER are not uncommon.

Gastrointestinal Obstruction

Congenital intestinal obstruction can occur anywhere in the GI tract and takes one of the following forms: atresia, which is a complete obliteration of the passage; partial obstruction, in which the symptoms may vary in severity and sometimes not be detected in the neonatal period; or malrotation of the intestine, which leads to twisting of the intestine (volvulus) and obstruction. EA, discussed previously, is a type of GI obstruction. Meconium ileus is an obstruction caused by impacted meconium and is the earliest symptom of cystic fibrosis, a life-threatening chronic illness. Infants with this type of obstruction should be tested for cystic fibrosis because 95% of infants with meconium ileus have cystic fibrosis.

In addition to polyhydramnios in the pregnant woman, the infant shows the following cardinal signs and symptoms: bilious vomiting, abdominal distention, and failure to pass normal amounts of meconium in the first 24 hours.

Nursing care is aimed at supporting the infant until surgical intervention can be carried out to eliminate the obstruction. Oral feedings are withheld, a nasogastric tube is placed for suction, and intravenous therapy is initiated to provide needed fluid and electrolytes. In infants with an intestinal obstruction, surgery consists of resecting the obstructed area of bowel and anastomosing the nonaffected bowel. In recent years the survival rate for these infants has risen to 90% to 95% as a result of better treatments, improved neonatal intensive care, and an increased understanding of the total problem.

Imperforate Anus

Imperforate anus is a term used to describe a wide range of congenital disorders involving the anus and rectum and genitourinary system in many cases (Fig. 28-18). These anomalies are relatively common, with an incidence of approximately 1 in 5000 live births (Bensard et al, 2002). Occurring more in male than in female infants, they result from the failure of anorectal development in weeks 7 and 8 of gestational life. Such infants have no anal opening, and commonly there is also a fistula from the rectum to the perineum or genitourinary system. Types of anorectal malformations include the typical cloaca in females, which involves the vagina, colon, and urethra forming a single common passage in the perineum. Others include the low rectovaginal fistula (female) and rectourethral bulbar fistula (male). Extensive surgical repair is often required in stages for the more complex types of anorectal malformations. In some cases the anomaly may involve stenotic areas, or there may be a thin translucent membrane covering the anal opening. Treatment for such a membrane is excision followed by daily dilation,

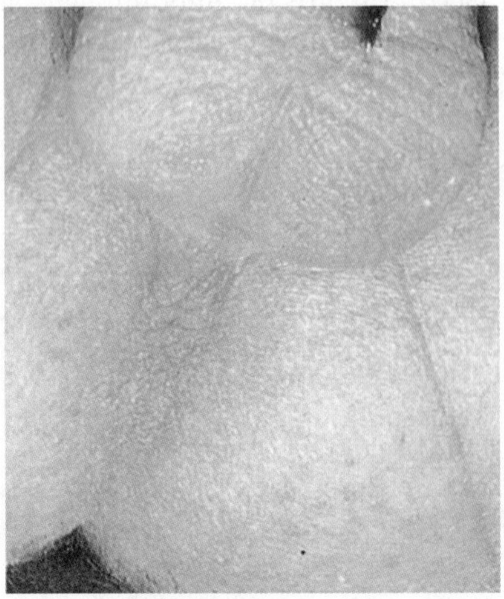

Fig. 28-18 Imperforate anus. (From Chessell G et al: *Diagnostic picture tests in clinical medicine* (vol 2), St Louis, 1984, Mosby.)

which parents are taught to do. See Chapter 47 for further discussion of surgical treatment.

Musculoskeletal System Anomalies

Developmental Dysplasia of the Hip

The broad term *developmental dysplasia of the hip* (DDH) describes a spectrum of disorders related to abnormal development of the hip that may develop at any time during fetal life, infancy, or childhood. A change in terminology from congenital hip dysplasia (CHD) and congenital dislocation of the hip (CDH) to DDH more properly reflects a variety of hip abnormalities in which there is a shallow acetabulum, subluxation, or dislocation.

The incidence of hip instability of some kind is approximately 10 per 1000 live births. The incidence of frank dislocation or a dislocatable hip is 1 per 1000 live births (Wall, 2000), and approximately 30% to 50% of infants with DDH are born breech (Thompson, 2004).

The cause of DDH is unknown, but certain factors such as sex, birth order, family history, intrauterine position, birth type, joint laxity, and postnatal positioning are believed to affect the risk of DDH. Predisposing factors associated with DDH may be divided into three broad categories: (1) physiologic factors, which includes maternal hormone secretion and intrauterine positioning; (2) mechanical factors, which involves breech presentation, multiple fetus, oligohydramnios, and large infant size; other mechanical factors may include continued maintenance of the hips in adduction and extension that will in time cause a dislocation; and (3) genetic factors, which entail a higher incidence (6%) of DDH in siblings of affected infants, and an even greater incidence (36%) of recurrence if a sibling and one parent were affected.

Three degrees of DDH are illustrated in Fig. 28-19 and are described as follows:

Acetabular dysplasia (or preluxation)—mildest form of DDH in which there is neither subluxation nor dislocation. There is a delay in acetabular development evidenced by osseous hypoplasia of the acetabular roof that is oblique and shallow, although the cartilaginous roof is comparatively intact. The femoral head remains in the acetabulum.

Subluxation—The largest percentage of DDH, subluxation, implies incomplete dislocation of the hip and is sometimes regarded as an intermediate state in the development from primary dysplasia to complete dislocation. The femoral head remains in contact with the acetabulum, but a stretched capsule and ligamentum teres cause the head of the femur to be partially displaced. Pressure on the cartilaginous roof inhibits ossification and produces a flattening of the socket.

Dislocation—The femoral head loses contact with the acetabulum and is displaced posteriorly and superiorly over the fibrocartilaginous rim. The ligamentum teres is elongated and taut.

DDH is often not detected at the initial examination after birth; thus, all infants should be carefully monitored for hip dysplasia at follow-up visits throughout the first year of life. In the newborn period dysplasia usually appears as hip joint laxity rather than as outright dislocation. Subluxation and the tendency to dislocate can be demonstrated by the Ortolani or Barlow tests. The Ortolani and Barlow tests are most reliable from birth to 2 or 3 months of age. Other signs of DDH are shortening of the limb on the affected side (Galeazzi sign, Allis sign), asymmetric thigh and gluteal folds, and broadening of the perineum (in bilateral dislocation) (see also Fig. 24-8).

NURSE ALERT The Ortolani and Barlow tests must be performed by an experienced clinician to prevent fracture or other damage to the hip. If these tests are performed too vigorously in the first 2 days of life, when the hip subluxates freely, persistent dislocation may occur. ■

Treatment is begun as soon as the condition is recognized, because early intervention is more favorable to the restoration of normal bony architecture and function. The longer treatment is delayed, the more severe the deformity, the more difficult the treatment, and the less favorable the prognosis. The treatment varies with the age of the child and the extent of the dysplasia. The goal of treatment is to obtain and maintain a safe, congruent position of the hip joint to promote normal hip joint development and ambulation.

The hip joint is maintained by dynamic splinting in a safe position with the proximal femur centered in the acetabu-

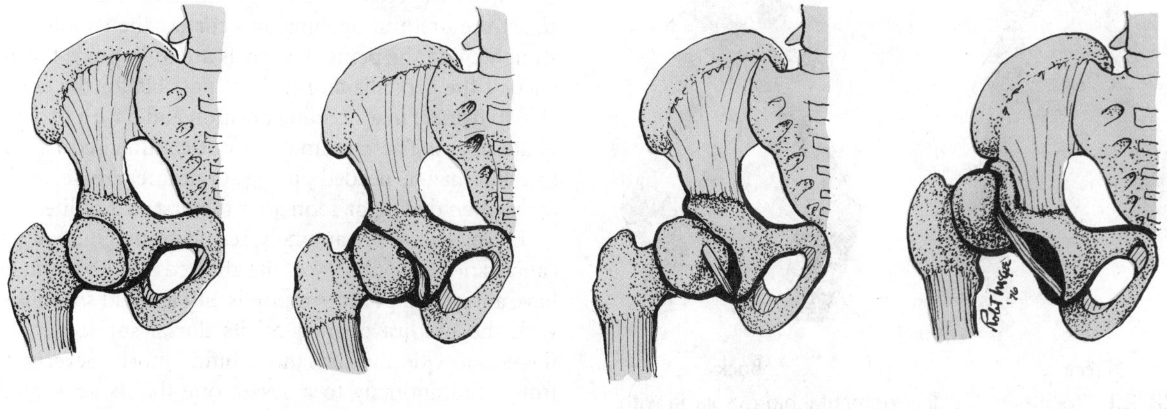

Fig. 28-19 Configuration and relationship of structures in developmental dysplasia of the hip.

lum in an attitude of flexion. Of the numerous devices available, the Pavlik harness is the most widely used, and with time, motion, and gravity, the hip works into a more abducted, reduced position (Fig. 28-20). The harness is worn continuously until the hip is proved stable on clinical and radiographic examination, usually in about 3 to 5 months.

NURSE ALERT The former practice of double- or triple-diapering for DDH is not recommended because it promotes hip extension, thus worsening proper hip development. ■

See Chapter 54 for more detailed discussion of developmental dysplasia of the hip.

Clubfoot

Congenital ***clubfoot*** is a complex deformity of the ankle and foot that includes forefoot adduction, midfoot supination, hindfoot varus, and ankle equinus. Deformities of the foot and ankle are described according to the position of the ankle and foot. The more common positions involve the following variations:

Talipes varus—An inversion or a bending inward
Talipes valgus—An eversion or bending outward
Talipes equinus—Plantar flexion in which the toes are lower than the heel
Talipes calcaneus—Dorsiflexion, in which the toes are higher than the heel

Most cases of clubfoot are a combination of these positions, and the most frequently occurring type of clubfoot (approximately 95%) is the composite deformity talipes equinovarus (TEV), in which the foot is pointed downward and inward in varying degrees of severity (see Fig. 54-13 on p. 1820). Unilateral clubfoot is somewhat more common than bilateral clubfoot and may occur as an isolated defect or in association with other disorders or syndromes, such as chromosomal aberrations, arthrogryposis (a generalized immobility of the joints), cerebral palsy, or spina bifida.

The goal of treatment for clubfoot is to achieve a painless, plantigrade (able to walk on the sole of the foot with the heel on the ground), and stable foot. Treatment of clubfoot involves three stages: (1) correction of the deformity, (2) maintenance of the correction until normal muscle balance is regained, and (3) follow-up observation to avert possible recurrence of the deformity. Some feet respond to treatment readily; some respond only to prolonged, vigorous, and sustained efforts; and the improvement in others remains disappointing even with maximum effort on the part of all concerned.

Serial casting is begun shortly after birth, before discharge from the nursery. Successive casts allow for gradual stretching of skin and tight structures on the medial side of the foot. Manipulation and casting are repeated frequently (every week) to accommodate the rapid growth of early infancy. In some cases daily manipulation and stretching of tissues is accomplished with taping and splinting of the affected extremity; a continuous passive motion (CPM) machine may be used several hours daily to stretch and strengthen muscle groups involved (Faulks & Luther, 2005). The extremity or extremities are often casted or splinted until maximum correction is achieved, usually within 8 to 12 weeks. A Denis Browne splint may be used to manage feet that correct with casting and manipulation.

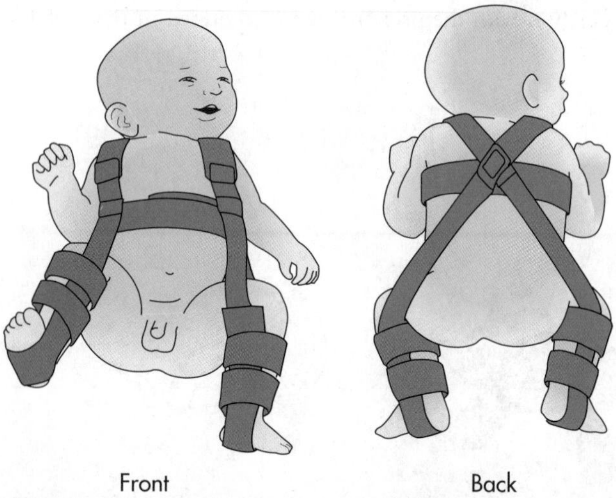

Fig. 28-20 Treatment for developmental hip dysplasia with Pavlik harness. (From Ball J: *Mosby's pediatric patient teaching guides,* St Louis, 1998, Mosby.)

Polydactyly

Occasionally hands or feet are seen with extra digits. In some instances, polydactyly is hereditary. If there is little or no bone involvement, the extra digit is tied with silk suture soon after birth. The finger falls off within a few days, leaving a small scar. When there is bone involvement, surgical repair is indicated.

Genitourinary System Anomalies

Hypospadias and Epispadias

Hypospadias constitutes a range of penile anomalies associated with an abnormally located urinary meatus. The meatus can open below the glans penis or anywhere along the ventral surface of the penis, the scrotum, or the perineum. It is the most common anomaly of the penis, affecting approximately 1 in 300 infants (Bukowski & Zeman, 2001). It is classified according to the location of the meatus and the presence or absence of chordee, which is a ventral curvature of the penis.

Mild cases of hypospadias (Fig. 28-21) are often repaired for cosmetic reasons and involve a single surgical procedure. In more severe cases, several operations are required to reconstruct the urethral opening and correct the chordee, thereby straightening the penis. The goals are to improve the appearance of the genitalia and make it possible for the child to be able to urinate in a standing position and have a sexually adequate organ. These infants are not circumcised because the foreskin may be needed during surgical repair. Repair is done early, often during or soon after the first year of life.

Epispadias, a rare anomaly, results from failure of urethral canalization. About 55% of the affected infants are males who have a widened pubic symphysis and a broad spadelike penis with the urethra opened on its dorsal surface. In females there is a wide urethra and a bifid clitoris. Severity ranges from mild anomaly to a severe one that is associated with exstrophy of the bladder. Surgical correction is necessary, and affected male infants should not be circumcised.

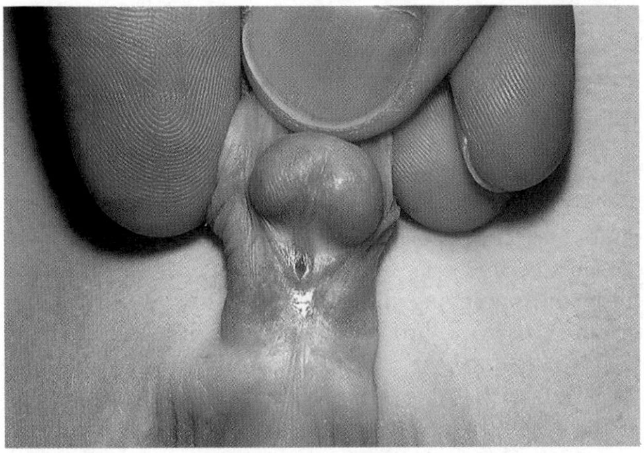

Fig. 28-21 Hypospadias. (Courtesy H. Gil Rushton, MD, Children's National Medical Center, Washington, DC.)

Exstrophy of the Bladder

The most common bladder anomaly is exstrophy (Fig. 28-22), which often occurs in conjunction with epispadias. It is rare, occurring only in about 1 in 35,000 to 40,000 live births (Elder, 2004). It results from the abnormal development of the bladder, abdominal wall, and the symphysis pubis that causes the bladder, urethra, and ureteral orifices to all be exposed. The bladder is visible in the suprapubic area as a red mass with numerous folds, with urine draining from it onto the infant's skin.

Immediately after birth the exposed bladder is covered with a sterile, nonadherent dressing to protect it until closure can be performed. It is recommended that reconstructive surgery be started in the neonatal period, preferably with the bladder being closed during the first or second day of life.

Ambiguous Genitalia

Ambiguous genitalia in the newborn (Fig. 28-23) often is discovered by the nurse during a physical assessment. Erroneous or abnormal sexual differentiation may be a genetic defect, such as congenital adrenal hypoplasia, which can be life-threatening because it involves deficiency of all adrenocortical hormones. Other possible causes of sexual ambiguity include chromosomal abnormalities, defective sex hor-

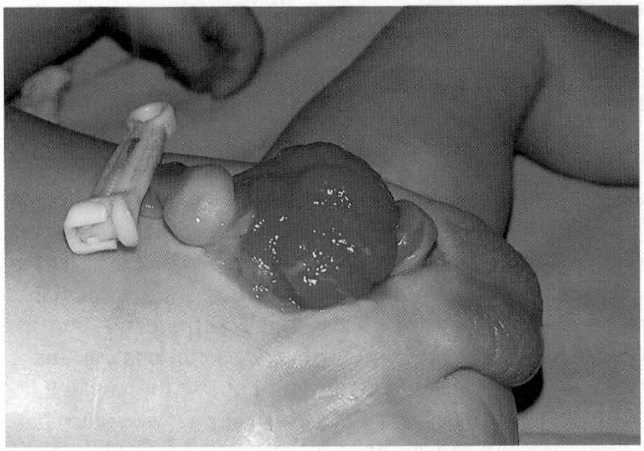

Fig. 28-22 Exstrophy of bladder. (Courtesy H. Gil Rushton, MD, Children's National Medical Center, Washington, DC.)

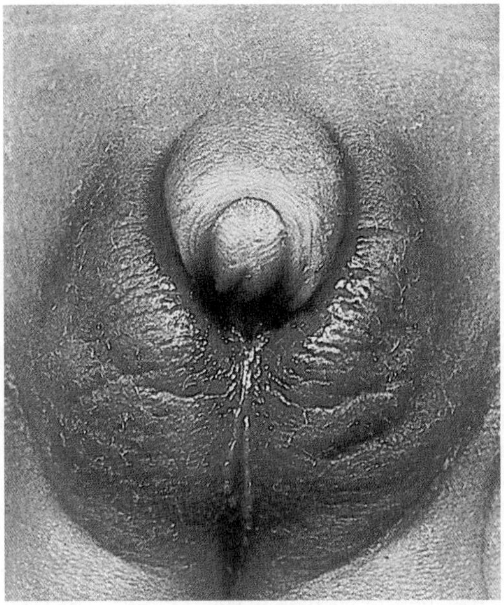

Fig. 28-23 Ambiguous external genitalia (i.e., structure may be enlarged clitoral hood and clitoris or micropenis and bifid scrotum). (Courtesy Edward S. Tank, MD, Division of Urology, Oregon Health Sciences University, Portland, OR.)

mone synthesis in males, and the placental transfer of masculinizing agents to female fetuses. Gender assignment should be based on data gathered from the following sources: maternal and family history, including the ingestion of steroids during pregnancy and relatives with ambiguous genitalia or who died during the neonatal period; physical examination; chromosomal analysis (results are available in 2 to 3 days); endoscopy, ultrasonography, and radiographic contrast studies; biochemical tests, such as analysis of urinary steroid excretion, which helps detect several of the adrenal cortical syndromes; and, in some instances, laparotomy or gonad biopsy.

Therapeutic intervention, including any counseling and surgery, should be started as soon as possible. Any child born with ambiguous genitalia should not receive gender assignment until the appropriate gender of rearing may be properly assessed and assigned. An appropriate gender assignment should be based on the following: age at presentation, potential for mature sexual function, potential fertility, and the long-term psychologic and intellectual impact on the child and family. Parents need much support as they learn to deal with this very challenging situation.

Teratoma

A teratoma is an embryonal tumor that may be solid, cystic, or mixed. It is composed of at least two and usually three types of embryonal tissue: ectoderm, mesoderm, and endoderm. A teratoma in the newborn may occur in the skull, mediastinum, abdomen, or sacral area; more than half are located in the sacrococcygeal area. The treatment of choice for such neonates is complete surgical resection. Approximately 80% of all teratomas are benign, and no additional therapy is needed after complete resection done in the neonatal period. If the tumor is not surgically resected before the infant is 1 to 2 months old, the likelihood of the teratoma becoming malignant increases rapidly.

Care Management

Any deviations from normal are reported to the primary health provider immediately. A thorough assessment of all body systems follows, with identification of both visible anomalies and those that might not be visible.

Some infants have multiple congenital anomalies. A recognized pattern of malformations is referred to as a syndrome. The most common is Down syndrome, with the diagnosis confirmed early in the neonatal period.

Genetic Diagnosis

Diagnostic procedures for the detection of genetic disorders are performed after birth at any time from the postnatal period through adulthood. Many tests are available for various disorders; only the most commonly used ones are discussed here.

Newborn Screening

The most widespread use of postnatal testing for genetic disease is the routine screening of newborns for inborn errors of metabolism such as phenylketonuria (PKU), galactosemia, hemoglobinopathy (sickle cell disease and thalassemias) and hypothyroidism; these are the minimum mandatory newborn screening tests in most states in the United States. An inborn error of metabolism (IEM) is the term applied to a large group of disorders caused by a metabolic defect that results from the absence of or change in a protein, usually an enzyme, and mediated by the action of a certain gene. These defects can involve any substrate produced from protein, carbohydrate, or fat metabolism. Inborn errors of metabolism are recessive disorders, and a person must receive a defective gene from each parent for them to occur. The parents usually are unaffected because their normal dominant gene directs the synthesis of sufficient protein to meet their metabolic needs under normal circumstances. With the advent of new biochemical techniques, it is now possible to detect the abnormal gene responsible for causing an increasing number of these disorders early in the neonatal period so appropriate therapies to prevent further morbidity may be implemented. A new screening test, tandem mass spectrometry, has the potential for identifying more than 20 inborn errors of metabolism, in addition to the standard IEMs. With tandem mass spectrometry earlier identification of IEMs may prevent further developmental delays and morbidities in affected children.

Phenylketonuria

PKU results from a deficiency of the enzyme phenylalanine dehydrogenase. The test for PKU is not reliable until the newborn has ingested an ample amount of the amino acid phenylalanine, a constituent of both human and cow's milk. The nurse must document the initial ingestion of milk and perform the test at least 24 hours after that time. The current trend toward early infant discharge from the hospital has the potential to cause neonates with a disorder such as PKU not to be screened as often as in the past. In response to this, the AAP (1996) made the following recommendations:

- Obtain a subsequent sample before 2 weeks of age if the initial specimen is collected before the newborn is 24 hours old.
- Designate a primary care provider for all newborns before discharge for adequate newborn screening follow-up.
- Collect the initial specimen as close as possible to discharge and no later than 7 days after birth.

If the infant is found to have PKU, a diet low in phenylalanine is begun soon after birth. Breastfeeding or partial breastfeeding may be possible for some infants if the phenylalanine levels are monitored carefully and remain within acceptable limits (Kirby, 1999). Many affected children have some intellectual impairment. Successful management and outcome is largely dependent on early identification of the condition, modifying the diet, and compliance with the treatment regimen throughout the entire life cycle.

Galactosemia

Galactosemia, caused by a deficiency of the enzyme galactose-1-phosphate uridyltransferase, results in the inability to convert galactose to glucose. Galactosemia can be detected by measuring the blood levels of galactose in the urine of newborns suspected of having the disease who have ingested formula containing galactose. Early symptoms are vomiting, weight loss, and CNS symptoms, including poor feeding, drowsiness, and seizures. If the disorder goes untreated, the galactose levels will continue to increase and the affected infant will show failure to thrive, mental retardation, cataracts, jaundice, hepatomegaly, and cirrhosis of the liver, with death possibly occurring in the first month of life. Therapy consists of eliminating lactose from the diet; this condition precludes breastfeeding since lactose is present in breast milk.

Hypothyroidism

Congenital hypothyroidism results from a deficiency of thyroid hormones; it affects approximately 1 of every 3600 to 5000 newborns (AAP, 1996). All states in the United States routinely screen for hypothyroidism. This involves measuring thyroxine (T_4) in a drop of blood obtained from a heel stick at 2 to 5 days of age. At this time the normally expected increase in T_4 would be lacking in newborns with hypothyroidism. It is more often included as part of the newborn screen done in the first 24 to 48 hours or before discharge. Neonatal screening consists of an initial filter paper blood spot thyroxine (T_4) measurement followed by measurement of thyroid-stimulating hormone (TSH) in specimens with low T_4 values. Early screening may have false-positive results. Treatment is thyroid replacement. In the newborn, thyroid function studies are elevated in comparison with values in older children; therefore, it is important to document the timing of the tests. In preterm and sick full-term infants thyroid function tests are usually lower than in the healthy full-term infant; a repeat T_4 and TSH may be evaluated after 30 weeks (corrected age) in newborns born before that time and after resolution of the acute illness in the sick full-term infant.

Cytogenetic Studies

Abnormalities can occur in either the autosomes or the sex chromosomes. Chromosomal disorders may sometimes be diagnosed on the basis of the clinical manifestations alone. However, an infant may have a clinical appearance that is only suggestive of a problem. Cytogenetic studies then need to be done to confirm or rule out a suspected diagnosis. Newer techniques in molecular cytogenetic analysis make possible a more precise identification of risk for having a fetus affected with a genetic defect such as phenylketonuria.

Disorders in the number or structure of chromosomes can be diagnosed by a karyotype (see Fig. 8-1, *B*), which is a photographic enlargement of the chromosomes arranged by their numbered pairs.

Dermatoglyphics

Dermatoglyphics is the study of the patterns formed by the ridges in the skin on the digits, palms, and soles. These patterns, formed early in development, are strongly correlated with the effects of chromosomes. Many disorders that affect multiple body systems also affect these dermal ridges. The addition or deletion of genetic material produces alterations in the loops, swirls, and arches of the finger and toe prints, in the palm lines, and in the flexion creases on the palms of the hands and soles of the feet. Characteristic dermatoglyphic patterns have been noted for almost all the chromosomal abnormalities, such as Down syndrome.

An infant with Down syndrome may have a single, palmar crease; a single flexion crease of the fifth digit; and an increased distance between the first and second toes (Matthews & Robin, 2002). The characteristic dermatoglyphic feature in a child with Turner syndrome is the large size of the dermal patterns on the fingers and toes. Certain fingerprint patterns may also be found in those people who have cardiac valvular problems later in life. Asymmetry of palmar ridges has been reported in congenital anomalies such as cleft lip and palate and congenital vertebral anomaly (Goldberg et al, 1997).

Nursing Care

Newborn

A collaborative health team approach that includes specialists and community service representatives is needed in the care of infants with some disorders. Surgical intervention in the neonatal period may be necessary for the infant requiring either immediate correction or a palliative procedure to relieve the symptoms of the anomaly until definitive correction can be done. There is also a higher morbidity and mortality in neonates than in older children or adults undergoing similar procedures. However, despite these problems unique to neonates, advances in surgical techniques, anesthesia, and the nursing care given in intensive care nurseries have together been responsible for decreasing the risk of surgery in neonates.

The health care team must be highly skilled to meet the needs of these infants. These needs are similar to those of other high risk infants. In addition to stabilization of the infant's condition (oxygenation and perfusion of tissues), other preoperative interventions, such as nasogastric tube placement for abdominal decompression, pain management, and the maintenance of fluid and electrolyte balance, are implemented to manage specific problems.

Postoperatively, the infant is returned to the intensive care nursery, where close monitoring is maintained. The infant's respiratory efforts are supported; this often requires mechanical ventilation. Constant surveillance is necessary to detect any respiratory complications resulting from the anesthesia. A pulse oximeter is attached to measure the oxygen saturation in hemoglobin, which closely correlates with arterial oxygen saturation. Oxygen is provided as needed. An indwelling gastric catheter attached to intermittent suction is placed to remove gastric secretions, thereby preventing aspiration and distention of the abdomen. The infant's fluid, electrolyte, and acid-base balances are monitored and adjusted as needed. Urinary output is monitored and should equal 1 to 2 ml/kg/hr. Other nursing interventions are focused on caring for the surgical site, maintaining thermoregulation, pain management, and promoting comfort.

Parents and Family

While the infant is receiving optimal care, the parents also have needs that must be met as they deal with the crisis of having an infant with an abnormal condition. Their reactions are carefully assessed and are likely to be those typical of a grief response. Facilitating their understanding of the information given them about their infant's condition is a vital nursing intervention. A newly diagnosed disorder often implies the need for the implementation of a therapeutic regimen. For example, the disorder may be an inborn error of metabolism, such as PKU, which requires consistent and rigid adherence to a diet. The family may need help with securing the required formula and in receiving counseling from a clinical dietitian. The importance of maintaining the diet, keeping an adequate supply of special preparations, and avoiding the use of unauthorized substitutions must be impressed on the family.

Referral to appropriate agencies is another essential component of the follow-up management, and the nurse should make the parents aware of all possible sources of aid, including pertinent literature, parent groups, and national organizations. Many organizations and foundations, such as the March of Dimes provide services and counseling for families of affected children. There are also numerous parent groups the family can join. There they can share experiences and derive mutual support in coping with problems similar to those of other group members. Nurses must be familiar with the services available in their community that provide assistance and education to families with these special problems.

A major nursing function is providing emotional support to the family during all aspects of the care of the child born with a defect or disorder. The feelings stemming from the real or imagined threat posed by a congenital anomaly are as varied as the people being counseled. Responses may include apathy, denial, anger, hostility, fear, embarrassment, grief, and loss of self-esteem.

Parents benefit from seeing before-and-after pictures of other babies born with the same defect. Coupled with other verbal and nonverbal supportive care, this visual reassurance may be effective in allaying their concerns.

Families need much information, guidance, and support as they make decisions regarding the care of their infant. Once they have been given the facts and possible consequences and all the assistance they need in problem solving, the final decision regarding a course of action must be their own. It is then incumbent on health care providers to support the decision of the family.

Nurses frequently encounter children with genetic diseases and families in which there is a risk that a disorder may be transmitted to or occur in an offspring. It is a responsibility of nurses to be alert to situations in which persons could benefit from a genetic evaluation and counseling to be aware of the local genetic resources, to aid the family in finding services, and offer support and care for children and families affected by genetic conditions. Local genetic clinics can be located through several sites, such as the Gene Tests (www.genetests.org), a publicly funded medical genetics information resource developed for physicians and other health care providers, is available at no cost to all interested persons. Another resource is the National Society of Genetic Counselors (www.nsgc.org), which lists genetic counselors by states in the United States. See also Chapter 8.

Key Points

- The identification of maternal and fetal risk factors in the antepartum and intrapartum periods is vital for planning adequate care of high risk infants.
- A small percentage of significant birth injuries may occur despite skilled and competent obstetric care.
- Metabolic abnormalities of diabetes mellitus in pregnancy adversely affect embryonic and fetal development.
- Infection in the newborn may be acquired in utero, at birth, in breast milk, and from within the nursery.
- The most common maternal infections during early pregnancy that are associated with various congenital malformations are represented by the acronym TORCH.
- HIV transmission from mother to infant occurs transplacentally at various gestational ages, perinatally by maternal blood and secretions, and by breast milk.
- Preterm infants are at risk for problems related to the immaturity of organ systems.
- Hyperbilirubinemia has a variety of etiologic factors, including maternal-fetal Rh and ABO incompatibility.
- The injection of $Rh_o(D)$ immune globulin in Rh-negative and Coombs' test–negative women minimizes the possibility of isoimmunization.
- The nurse often first observes signs of newborn drug withdrawal (neonatal abstinence syndrome) and acquires information from the maternal history.
- Major congenital defects are now the leading cause of death in term neonates.
- The curative and rehabilitative problems of a child with a congenital disorder are often complex, requiring a multidisciplinary approach to care.
- Parents often need special instruction (e.g., cardiopulmonary resuscitation [CPR], oxygen therapy, or meeting nutrition requirements) before they take a high risk infant home.
- The supportive care given to the parents of infants with an abnormal condition must begin at birth or at the time of diagnosis and continue for years.

Answer Guidelines to Critical Thinking Exercise

1. Yes, evidence is sufficient to draw conclusions about what you should tell Emilie about the treatment and prognosis for John. Although the defect is disfiguring, it is correctable with surgery. The lip will be repaired early, and the palate will be repaired later once John has grown some. Breastfeeding may be possible if Emilie desires. Emilie will be taught to feed John by breast, using a special nipple, or by gavage, if that is more appropriate. A surgeon should meet with her soon to discuss the repair. She should be told about the possibility of the need for speech therapy as John starts to talk.
2. (a) An open cleft lip and palate is disfiguring. A nurse may be able to more readily accept the appearance of the defect knowing that it can be repaired in a way that will leave little evidence of the original defect. (b) Emilie may find it hard to look at or accept her son and think that the disfigurement is more serious than it is (i.e., although a heart defect may be life threatening, it may seem less serious because it is not visible). The nurse can assist Emilie to look for the positive features of John and assure her that surgery can correct the defect. (c) The lip will be repaired at 6 to 12 weeks of age, whereas the palate will be repaired at 12 to 18 months of age when the palate has grown but before faulty speech habits have developed. (d) Many children with cleft lip and palate have some speech impairment that requires speech therapy. Some problems may result from improper tooth alignment and improper drainage of the eustachian tube leading to recurrent otitis media and varying degrees of hearing loss. Orthodontic treatment may be required.
3. Priority for nursing care at this time is to point out positive aspects of John, to explain the physical defects and the treatment, and to assure Emilie that she will be helped to learn how to feed and care for John. It is important to ascertain any support available from the father of the baby or her family. Reassurance and support is essential. Referral to a social worker may be useful if Emilie does not have the resources to pay for the necessary surgical treatment.
4. Treatment of the child with cleft lip and palate is surgical and usually does not require long-term intervention. However, successful management of cleft lip and palate requires a multidisciplinary team.
5. Emilie may not be able to manage care of John. Additional family support should be sought. There may be long-term difficulties with the child's social adjustment related to low self-esteem from the scar and any speech abnormalities. (See Chapter 47 for a more detailed discussion of the child with a cleft lip and palate.)

Resources

Advances in Neonatal Care
Elsevier
360 Park Avenue South
New York, NY 10010

AIDS Network Hotline
800-342-2437

American Academy of Pediatrics
141 Northwest Point Blvd.
Elk Grove, IL 60007-1098
847-228-5005
www.aap.org

American Cleft Palate Association
1218 Grandview Ave.
Pittsburgh, PA 15211
412-681-1376
800-242-5338 (800-24-CLEFT)
www.cleftline.org

American Society of Plastic Surgeons
Plastic Surgery Educational Foundation
Plastic Surgery Information Service: FAQs
www.plasticsurgery.org/faq/cleft.htm

Birth Defect Research for Children, Inc. (BDRC)
930 Woodcock Rd, Suite 225
Orlando, FL 32803
800-313-2232
www.birthdefects.org

Brachial Plexus Palsy Foundation
210 Spring Haven Circle
Rayersford, PA 19468
www.membrane.com/bpp/index.html

Centers for Disease Control and Prevention
1600 Clifton Rd. NE
Atlanta, GA 30333
404-329-1819
404-329-3286
www.cdc.gov

Gene Tests (funded by the NIH)
9725 Third Avenue NE
Suite 602
Seattle, WA 98115
206-616-4033
206-221-4679 (fax)
genetests@genetests.org
www.genetests.org

HEST (Helga's European Specialty Toys)
www.downsyndromedolls.com
(Down syndrome dolls used to teach children about disabilities and for children with Down syndrome)

Journal of Genetic Counseling
Kluwer Academic Publishers
PO Box 322
3300 AH Dordrecht
The Netherlands
+31 (0) 78 657 60 50
+31 (0) 78 657 64 74 (fax)
frontoffice@wkap.nl
www.wkap.nl

Journal of Perinatal and Neonatal Nursing
Lippincott Williams & Wilkins
530 Walnut St.
Philadelphia, PA 19106-3621
215-521-8300
215-521-8902 (fax)
www.lww.com

March of Dimes Birth Defects Foundation
National Foundation/March of Dimes
1275 Mamaroneck Ave.
White Plains, NY 10605
914-663-4637 (800-MODIMES)
www.modimes.org

National AIDS Information Clearinghouse
PO Box 6003
Rockville, MD 20849-6003
800-458-5231 (English and Spanish)

National Association of Neonatal Nurses
4700 W. Lake Ave.
Glenview, IL 60025-145
800-451-3795
888-477-6266 (fax)
www.nann.org
E-mail: info@nann.org

National Clearinghouse for Alcohol and Drug Abuse Information
PO Box 426
Dept. DQ
Kensington, MD 20795
800-729-6686
www.health.org

National Down Syndrome Congress
1800 Dempster St.
Park Ridge, IL 60069-1146
708-823-7550
800-232-6372
www.ndsccenter.org

National Down Syndrome Society Hotline
666 Broadway
New York, NY 10012
800-221-4602
www.ndss.org

National Society of Genetic Counselors
233 Canterbury DR.
Wallingford, PA 19086-6617
610-872-7608
FYI@nsgc.org
www.nsgc.org

Neonatal Network
2270 Northpoint Parkway
Santa Rosa, CA 95407-7398
707-569-1415
707-569-0786 (fax)
www.neonatalnetwork.com

Spina Bifida Association of America
4590 McArthur Blvd. NW, Suite 250
Washington, DC 20007-4226
800-621-3141
www.sbaa.org

References

Abel E: *Fetal alcohol abuse syndrome revisited*, New York, 1997, Plenum Press.

American Academy of Pediatrics and American College of Obstetricians and Gynecologists: *Guidelines for perinatal care,* ed 5, Elk Grove Village, IL, 2002, The Academy.

American Academy of Pediatrics, Committee on Drugs: The transfer of drugs and other chemicals into human milk, *Pediatrics* 108(3):776-789, 2001.

American Academy of Pediatrics, Committee on Genetics: Newborn screening fact sheet, *Pediatrics* 98(3 Pt 1):473-501, 1996.

American Academy of Pediatrics, Committee on Infectious Diseases: *Red book: 2003 report of the committee on infectious diseases*, ed 26, Elk Grove Village, IL, 2003, The Academy.

American Academy of Pediatrics, Subcommittee on hyperbilirubinemia: Clinical Practice Guideline: management of hyperbilirubinemia in the newborn infant 35 or more weeks of gestation, *Pediatrics* 114(1): 297-316, 2004.

Aranda JV et al: Developmental pharmacology. In Fanaroff AA, Martin RJ (eds): *Neonatal-perinatal medicine: diseases of the fetus and infant*, ed 7, St Louis, 2002, Mosby.

Arendt R et al: Motor development of cocaine-exposed children at age two years, *Pediatrics* 103(1):86-92, 1999.

Askin DF: Bacterial and fungal sepsis in the neonate, *J Obstet Gynecol Neonatal Nurs* 24(7):635-643, 1995.

Askin DF, Diehl-Jones B: Cocaine: effects of in utero exposure on the fetus and newborn, *J Perinat Neonat Nurs* 14(4):83-102, 2001.

Association of Women's Health, Obstetric and Neonatal Nursing (AWHONN): *Evidence-based clinical practice guideline: neonatal skin care*, Washington, DC, 2001, The Association.

Baley JE, Toltzis P: Viral infections. In Fanaroff AA, Martin RJ (eds): *Neonatal-perinatal medicine: diseases of the fetus and infant*, ed 7, St Louis, 2002, Mosby.

Ball J: *Mosby's pediatric patient teaching guides*, St Louis, 1998, Mosby.

Bateman DA, Chiriboga CA: Dose-response effect of cocaine on newborn head circumference, *Pediatrics* 106(3):e33, 2000.

Behrmann R: *Neonatology: diseases of the fetus and infant*, St Louis, 1973, Mosby.

Bell SG: Pointers in practical pharmacology: highly active antiretroviral therapy in neonates and young infants, *Neonatal Netw* 23(2):55-64, 2004.

Bennett AD: Perinatal substance abuse and the drug-exposed neonate, *Adv Nurse Pract* 7(5):32-36, 1999.

Bensard D et al: Neonatal surgery. In Merenstein GB, Gardner SL (editors), *Handbook of neonatal intensive care*, ed. 5, St. Louis, 2002, Mosby.

Berghella V et al: Maternal methadone dose and neonatal withdrawal, *Am J Obstet Gynecol* 189(2), 312-317, 2003.

Bernstein D: Congenital heart disease, In Behrman RE, Kliegman RM, Jenson HB (eds): *Nelson textbook of pediatrics*, ed 17, St Louis, 2004, Mosby.

Birthistle K, Carrington D: Fetal varicella syndrome—a reappraisal of the literature, *J Infect* 36(suppl 1):25-29, 1998.

Blackburn S: *Maternal, fetal, & neonatal physiology: a clinical perspective*, ed 2, St. Louis, 2003, Saunders.

Boyer SG, Boyer KM: Update on TORCH infections in the newborn infant, *Newborn Infant Nurs Rev* 4(1):70-80, 2004.

Bradshaw WT: The use of nitric oxide in neonatal care, *Crit Care Nurs Clin N Am* 16:249-255, 2004.

Bukowski TP, Zeman PA: Hypospadias: of concern but correctable, *Contemp Pediatr* 18(2):89-109, 2001.

Buus-Frank M: Hands that heal—hands that harm, *Adv Neonatal Care* 4(5): 251-255, 2004.

Carey BE: Incidence and epidemiology of congenital cardiovascular malformation in the newborn infant, *Newborn Infant Nurs Rev* 2(2):54-59, 2002.

Centers for Disease Control and Prevention: *Fetal alcohol syndrome, fetal alcohol information*. Internet document available at www.cdc.gov/ncbdd/fas/fasak.htm (accessed June 15, 2004).

Centers for Disease Control and Prevention: Prevention of perinatal group B streptococcal disease, *MMWR Morb Mortal Wkly Rep* 51(RR-11): 1-231, 2002.

Chapman SJ: Varicella in pregnancy, *Semin Perinatol* 22(4):339-346, 1998.

Chessell G et al: *Diagnostic picture tests in clinical medicine* (vol. 2), St Louis, 1984, Mosby.

Chiriboga C et al: Dose-response of fetal cocaine exposure on newborn neurologic function, *Pediatrics* 103(6):79-85, 1999.

Church MW, Abel EL: Fetal alcohol syndrome: hearing, speech and vestibular disorders, *Obstet Gynecol Clin North Am* 25(1):85-97, 1998.

Conde-Agudelo A, Diaz-Rosello J, Belizan J: Kangaroo mother care to reduce morbidity and mortality in low birth weight infants (Cochrane Review), 2003. In *The Cochrane Library*, Issue 2, Chichester, UK, 2004, John Wiley & Sons.

Cooper ER et al: Combination antiretroviral strategies for the treatment of pregnant HIV-1 infected women and prevention of perinatal HIV-1 transmission, *J AIDS* 29:484-494, 2002.

Cowles TA, Gonik B: Perinatal infections. In Fanaroff AA, Martin RJ (eds): *Neonatal-perinatal medicine: diseases of the fetus and infant*, ed 7, St Louis, 2002, Mosby.

Coyle MG et al: Diluted tincture of opium (DTO) and Phenobarbital versus DTO alone for neonatal opiate withdrawal in term infants, *J Pediatr* 140(5):561-564, 2002.

Danner S: Breastfeeding the infant with a cleft palate, *NAACOG Clin Issues Perinat Womens Health Nurs* 3:634, 1992.

D'Apolito K: Comparison of a rocking bed and standard bed for decreasing withdrawal symptoms in drug-exposed infants, *MCN Am J Matern Child Nurs* 24(3):138-144, 1999.

D'Apolito K, Hepworth JT: Prominence of withdrawal symptoms in polydrug-exposed infants, *J Perinat Neonatal Nurs* 14(4):46-60, 2001.

Delaney-Black V et al: Prenatal cocaine exposure and child behavior, *Pediatrics* 102(4 pt 1):945-950, 1998.

Diehl-Jones W, Askin DF: Nutritional modulation of neonatal outcomes, *AACN Clin Issues* 15(1):83-96, 2004.

Dore S et al: Alcohol versus natural drying for newborn cord care, *J Obstet Gynecol Neonatal Nurs* 27(6):621-627, 1998.

Duff P: Hepatitis in pregnancy, *Semin Perinatol* 22(4):277-283, 1998.

Dunham EA: Obstetrical brachial plexus palsy, *Orthop Nurs* 22(2):106-116, 2003.

Ebrahim SH, Gfoerer J: Pregnancy-related substance use in the United States during 1996-1998, *Obstet Gynecol* 101(2):374-379, 2003.

Edwards RK et al: Intrapartum antibiotic prophylaxis and early-onset neonatal sepsis patterns, *Infect Dis Obstet Gynecol* 11(4):221-224, 2003.

Elder JS: Urologic disorders in infants and children: anomalies of the bladder. In Behrman RE, Kliegman RM, Jenson HB (eds): *Nelson textbook of pediatrics*, ed 17, St Louis, 2004, Mosby.

Eyler FD, Behnke M: Early development of infants exposed to drugs prenatally, *Clin Perinatol* 26(1):107-150, 1999.

Eyler FD, Behnke M, Conlon M: Birth outcome from a prospective, matched study of prenatal crack/cocaine use. II. Interactive and dose effects on neurobehavioral assessment, *Pediatrics* 101(2):237-241, 1998.

Faulks S, Luther B: Changing paradigm for the treatment of clubfeet, *Orthop Nurs* 24(1):25-30, 2005.

Fernandes O et al: Moderate to heavy caffeine consumption during pregnancy and relationship to spontaneous abortion and abnormal fetal growth: a meta-analysis, *Reprod Toxicol* 12(4):435-444, 1998.

Frank DA et al: Heavily cocaine exposed children show positive effects of early intervention on Bayley Scales of Infant Development (abstract), *Pediatr Res* 43:214A, 1998.

Frenkel L: Challenges in the diagnosis and management of neonatal herpes simplex virus encephalitis, *Pediatrics* 115(3): 795-797, 2005.

Goldberg CJ et al: Fluctuating asymmetry and vertebral malformation: a study of dermatoglyphics in congenital spine deformities, *Spine* 22(7):775-779, 1997.

Hale TW: *Medications and mothers' milk*, Amarillo, TX, 2002, Pharmasoft Medical Publishing.

Hartman GE: Diaphragmatic hernia. In Behrman RE, Kliegman RM, Jenson HB (eds): *Nelson textbook of pediatrics*, ed 17, St Louis, 2004, Mosby.

Honein MA: Impact of folic acid fortification of the US food supply and occurrence of neural tube defects, *JAMA* 285(23):2981-2986, 2001.

Huestis MA, Choo RE: Drug abuses's smallest victims: in utero drug exposure, *Forensic Sci Int* 128(1-2):20-30, 2002.

Hurd YL et al: Marijuana impairs growth in mid-gestation fetuses, *Neurotoxicol Teratol* 27(2): 221-229, 2005.

Hurt H et al: A prospective education of early language development in children with in utero cocaine exposure and in control subjects, *J Pediatr* 130(2):310-312, 1997.

Jansson LM, Velez M, Harrow C: Methadone maintenance and lactation: a review of the literature and current management guidelines, *J Hum Lact* 20(1):62-71, 2004.

Johnson K, Gerada C, Greenough A: Treatment of neonatal abstinence syndrome, *Arch Dis Child Fetal Neonatal Ed* 88(1):F2-F5, 2003.

Jones MW, Bass WT: Fetal alcohol syndrome, *Neonatal Netw* 22(3):63-70, 2003.

Kandall SR: Treatment strategies for drug-exposed neonates, *Clin Perinatol* 26(1):231-243, 1999.

Kaltenbach K, Berghella V, Finnegan L: Opioid dependence during pregnancy. Effects and management, *Obstet Gynecol Clin North Am* 25(1):139-151, 1998.

Kirby R: Maternal phenylketonuria: a new cause for concern, *J Obstet Gynecol Neonatal Nurs* 28(3):227-234, 1999.

Koren G et al: Long-term neurodevelopmental risks in children exposed in utero to cocaine: the Toronto adoption study, *Ann NY Acad Sci* 846: 306-312, 1998.

Kriebs JM: The global reach of HIV: Preventing mother-to-child transmission, *J Perinat Neonatal Nurs* 16(3):1-10, 2002.

Law KL et al: Smoking during pregnancy and newborn neurobehavior, *Pediatrics* 111(6):1318-1323, 2003.

Lawrence RA, Lawrence RM: *Breastfeeding: a guide for the medical profession,* ed 5, St Louis, 1999, Mosby.

Lee M: Marihuana and tobacco use in pregnancy, *Obstet Gynecol Clin North Am* 25(1):65-83, 1998.

Luzuriaga K et al: A trial of three antiretroviral regimens in HIV-infected children, *N Engl J Med* 350(24):2471-2480, 2004.

Lynfield R, Guerina N: Toxoplasmosis, *Pediatr Rev* 18(3):75-83, 1997.

Malanga CJ, Kosofsy BE: Mechanism of action of drugs of abuse on the developing fetal brain, *Clin Perinatol* 26(1):17-37, 1999.

Markiewicz M, Abrahamson E: *Diagnosis in color: neonatology,* St. Louis, 1999, Mosby Ltd.

Matthews AL, Robin NH: Genetic disorders, malformations, and inborn errors of metabolism. In Merenstein GB, Gardner SL (eds): *Handbook of neonatal intensive care,* ed 5, St. Louis, 2002, Mosby.

Medves J, O'Brien B: Cleaning solutions and bacterial colonization in promoting healing and early separation of the umbilical cord in healthy newborns, *Can J Public Health* 88(6):380-382, 1997.

Merenstein GB, Adams KM, Weisman LE: Infection in the neonate. In Merenstein GB, Gardner SL (eds): *Handbook of neonatal intensive care,* ed 5, St Louis, 2002, Mosby.

Messinger DS et al: The maternal lifestyle study: cognitive, motor, and behavioral outcomes of cocaine-exposed and opiate-exposed infants through three years of age, *Pediatrics* 113(6):1677-1685, 2004.

Milerad J et al: Objective measurements of nicotine exposure in victims of sudden infant death syndrome and in other unexpected child deaths, *J Pediatr* 133(2):232-236, 1998.

Modlin JF et al: Case records of the Massachusetts General Hospital. Weekly clinicopathological exercises. Case 25-2003. A newborn boy with petechiae and thrombocytopenia, *N Engl J Med* 349(16):1575-1576, 2003.

Mofenson L: Mother-child HIV-1 transmission: timing and determinants, *Obstet Gynecol Clin North Am* 24(4):759-784, 1997.

Moise KJ: Management of rhesus alloimmunization in pregnancy, *Obstet Gynecol* 100(3):600-611, 2002.

Moolenaar RL et al: A prolonged outbreak of *Pseudomonas aeruginosa* in a neonatal intensive care unit: did staff fingernails play a role in disease transmission? *Infect Control Hosp Epidemiol* 21(2):80-85, 2000.

Myers MG, Stanberry LR, Seward JF: Varicella-zoster virus. In Behrman RE, Kliegman RM, Jenson HB (eds): *Nelson textbook of pediatrics,* ed 17, Philadelphia, 2004, Saunders.

Neal JL: RhD isoimmunization and current management modalities, *J Obstet Gynecol Neonatal Nurs* 30(6):589-607, 2001.

Nelson N: *Current therapy in neonatal-perinatal medicine,* ed 2, St Louis, 1990, Mosby.

O'Doherty N: *Neonatology: micro atlas of the newborn,* Nutley, NJ, 1986, Hoffmann-La Roche.

Ostrea E: Understanding drug testing in the neonate and the role of meconium analysis, *J Perinat Neonatal Nurs* 14(4):61-82, 2001.

Paige PL, Carney PR: Neurologic disorders. In Merenstein GB, Gardner SL (eds): *Handbook of neonatal intensive care,* ed 5, St Louis, 2002, Mosby.

Philipp BL, Merewood A, O'Brien S: Commentary: Methadone and breastfeeding: new horizons, *Pediatrics* 111(6 Pt 1):1429-1430, 2003.

Plessinger M: Prenatal exposure to amphetamines, *Obstet Gynecol Clin North Am* 25(1):119-138, 1998.

Polak JD, Ringler N, Daugherty B: Unit based procedures: impact on the incidence of nosocomial infections in the newborn intensive care unit, *Newborn Infant Nurs Rev* 4(1):38-45, 2004.

Popovich DM, McAlhany A: Practitioner care and screening guidelines for infants born to Chlamydia-positive mothers, *Newborn Infant Nurs Rev* 4(1):51-55, 2004.

Rao R, Desai NS: OxyContin and neonatal abstinence syndrome, *J Perinatol* 22(4):324-325, 2002.

Reiser DJ: Neonatal jaundice: physiologic variation or pathologic process, *Crit Care Nurs Clin N Am* 16:257-269, 2004.

Richardson GA, Hamel SC, Goldschmidt L: The effects of cocaine use on neonatal neurobehavioral status, *Neurotoxicol Teratol* 18(5):519-528, 1996.

Riley L: Herpes simplex virus, *Semin Perinatol* 22(4):284-292, 1998.

Rollnik JD et al: Botulinum toxin treatment of cocontractions after birth-related brachial plexus lesions, *Neurology* 55(1):112-114, 2000.

Rosen TS, Bateman DA: Infants of addicted mothers. In Fanaroff AA, Martin RJ (eds): *Neonatal-perinatal medicine: diseases of the fetus and infant,* ed 7, St Louis, 2002, Mosby.

Santos I et al: Caffeine intake and low birth weight: a population-based case-control study, *Am J Epidemiol* 147(7):620-627, 1998.

Scarlatti G: Pediatric HIV infection, *Lancet* 348(9031):863-867, 1996.

Singer LT et al: Cognitive and motor outcomes of cocaine-exposed infants, *JAMA* 287(15):1952-1960, 2002.

Smith L et al: Effects of prenatal methamphetamine exposure on fetal growth and drug withdrawal symptoms in infants born at term, *J Devel Behav Pediatr* 24(1):17-23, 2003.

Steele M: Common chromosomal disorders. In Zitelli B, Davis H (eds): *Atlas of pediatric physical diagnosis,* ed 3, St Louis, 1997, Mosby.

Stoll BJ et al: Changes in pathogens causing early-onset sepsis in very-low-birth-weight infants, *N Engl J Med* 347(4):240-247, 2002.

Strodtbeck F: The role of early enteral nutrition in protecting premature infants from sepsis, *Crit Care Nurs Clin North Am* 15(1):79-87, 2003.

Tanney MR, Lowenstein V: One-stop shopping: description of a model program to provide primary care to substance-abusing women and their children, *J Pediatr Health Care* 11(1):20-25, 1997.

Tappero E: Musculoskeletal system assessment. In Tappero E, Honeyfield MA (eds): *Physical assessment of the newborn,* ed 3, Santa Rosa, CA, 2003, NICU Ink.

Thompson GH: The hip. In Behrman RE, Kliegman RM, Jenson HB (eds), *Nelson textbook of pediatrics,* ed 17, Philadelphia, 2004, WB Saunders.

Tronick EZ et al: Late dose-response effects of prenatal cocaine exposure on neurobehavioral performance, *Pediatrics* 98(1):78-83, 1996.

Tronick EZ, Beeghly M: Prenatal cocaine exposure, child development, and the compromising effects of cumulative risk, *Clin Perinatol* 26(1): 151-171, 1999.

Volpe JJ: *Neurology of the newborn,* ed 4, Philadelphia, 2001, WB Saunders.

Wagner C et al: The impact of prenatal drug exposure on the neonate, *Obstet Gynecol Clin North Am* 25(1):169-194, 1998.

Wall EJ: Practical primary pediatric orthopaedics, *Nurs Clin North Am* 35(1):95-113, 2000.

Weinberg GA: The dilemma of postnatal mother-to-child transmission of HIV: to breastfeed or not? *Birth* 27(3):199-205, 2000.

Weiner L, Morse B: FAS: clinical perspectives and prevention. In Chasnoff I (ed): *Drugs, alcohol, pregnancy and parenting,* Boston, 1991, Kluwer.

World Health Organization: *Effect of breastfeeding on mortality among HIV-infected women, WHO Statement,* 7 June, 2001. Internet document available at http://www.who.int/reproductive-health/rtis/MTCT/WHO_Statement_on_breast_feeding_June.htm (accessed June 16, 2004).

Zenk KE: *Neonatal medications and nutrition,* Petaluma, CA, 2000, NICU Ink.

Zitelli BJ, Davis HW: *Atlas of pediatric physical diagnosis,* ed 4, St Louis, 2002, Mosby.

PART II
Pediatric Nursing

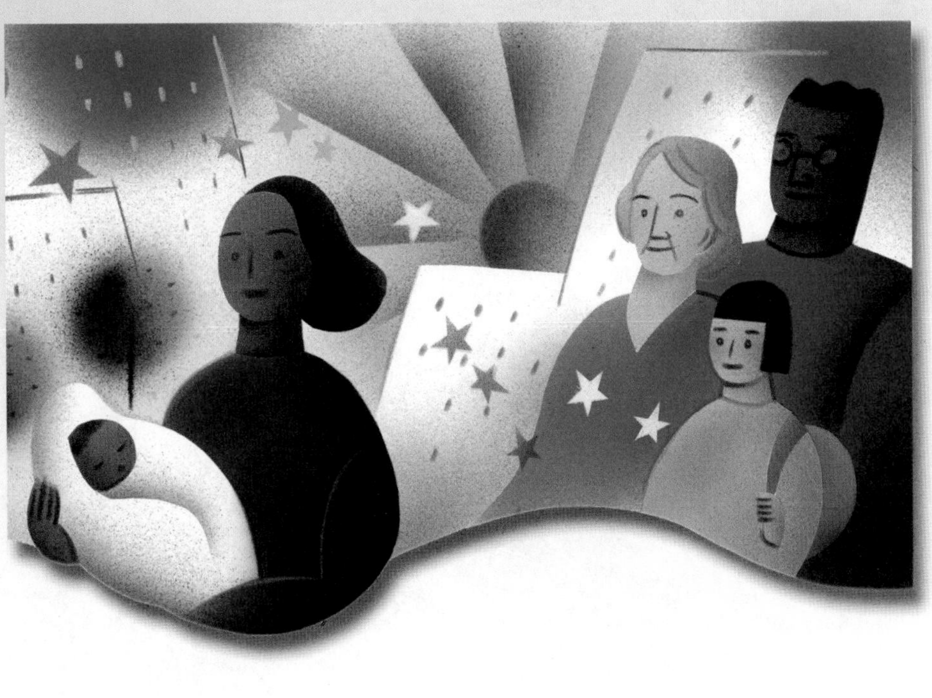

Contemporary Pediatric Nursing 29

LEARNING OBJECTIVES

On completion of this chapter the reader will be able to:

- Define the terms *mortality* and *morbidity*.
- Identify two ways that knowledge of mortality and morbidity can improve child health.
- List three major causes of death during infancy, early childhood, later childhood, and adolescence.
- List two major causes of illness during childhood.
- Outline four events that were significant in the evolution of child health care in the United States.
- Describe five broad functions of the pediatric nurse in promoting the health of children.
- Define the term *critical thinking*.
- Identify the five steps of the nursing process.
- Define the term *nursing diagnosis*.
- Differentiate among the three domains of nursing practice: dependent, independent, and interdependent.
- Differentiate a standard care plan from an individualized care plan.

ELECTRONIC RESOURCES

Additional information related to the content in Chapter 29 can be found on

the companion website at evolve
http://evolve.elsevier.com/Wong/maternal/
- NCLEX Review Questions
- WebLinks

or the interactive student CD-ROM
Activities for Chapter 29 include the following:
- NCLEX Review Questions

HEALTH DURING CHILDHOOD

The World Health Organization (WHO) has defined *health* as "a state of complete physical, mental, and social well-being and not merely the absence of disease." This is an abstract definition that does not lend itself to concrete, specific observations. In reality, information about health is gained by observing *mortality* (death) and *morbidity* (illness) among groups of individuals over specific periods of time. The balance between physical, mental, and social well-being and the presence of disease is inferred from analysis of data relating to mortality and morbidity.

Mortality and morbidity data also provide information about (1) the causes of death and illness, (2) high risk age groups for certain disorders or hazards, (3) advances in treatment and prevention, and (4) specific areas of health counseling. Such information is valuable to nurses because it guides the planning and delivery of nursing care.

Healthy People 2000 and *Healthy People 2010*

Although the health of children in the United States improved dramatically during the twentieth century, several areas of concern remain. Serious domestic problems such as acquired immunodeficiency syndrome (AIDS), drug abuse, violence, and unwanted pregnancies have direct effects on the health of children. Solutions to these problems lie in their prevention.

In the last two decades, documents such as *Healthy People 2000 (www.healthypeople.gov)* and *National Health Promotion and Disease Prevention Objectives* established national health objectives and served as the basis for the development of state and community plans. *Healthy People 2010,* released in 2000, contains two overriding goals: (1) to increase the quality and length of healthy life and (2) to eliminate health disparities. The document also contains 10 leading health indicators relating to issues such as substance abuse, injury and violence, and other priority areas for the nation's health. The health indicators serve as focus areas for health improvement efforts. Many states have worked with community coalitions to develop their own versions of *Healthy People 2010.* The *Healthy People Toolkit** found on the Internet provides examples of state and national experiences using the objectives of *Healthy People 2010.*

Mortality

Figures describing rates of occurrence for events such as death in children are referred to as *vital statistics.* In the United States, the National Center for Health Statistics (NCHS) is responsible for the collection, analysis, and dissemination of health data. Since 1991, several changes have occurred in the reporting of health statistics. Figures for birth and death are currently based on the person's state of residence, not the state in which the event occurred. In addition, tabulation of race for live births has changed from the race of the child to the race of the mother. As a result of these changes, figures for births, deaths, and infant mortality rates by race cannot be compared with statistics reported before 1991. *Mortality statistics* describe the incidence or number of individuals who have died over a specific period. These statistics are usually presented as rates per 100,000 and are calculated from a sample of death certificates.

Infant Mortality

The *infant mortality rate* is the number of deaths during the first year of life per 1000 live births. Infant mortality is divided into *neonatal mortality* (less than 28 days of life) and *postneonatal mortality* (28 days to 11 months). In the United States, there has been a dramatic decrease in infant mortality rate. At the beginning of the twentieth century, the rate was approximately 200 infant deaths per 1000 live births. In 2002, infant mortality rate was 6.9 per 1000 live births (provisional data; Arias et al, 2003). This decrease resulted primarily from improvements in perinatal care, such as treatment of respiratory distress syndrome, and fewer deaths from sudden infant death syndrome (SIDS). The mortality rate in 2001 for white infants was 5.7, and the rate for African-American infants was 14.0 (Arias et al, 2003). The challenge for this century is to reduce the gap between infant mortality rates for white and African-American infants.

From a global perspective, the United States lags behind other developed countries. In 2000, the United States ranked last among nations with the lowest infant death rates. Singapore had the lowest infant death rate (Arias et al, 2003). Although the exact reason for the low ranking of the United States is unknown, one explanation may be that many countries with lower infant death rates have national health programs.

Birth weight is considered the major determinant of neonatal death in technologically developed countries. There is a definite relationship between birth weight and mortality (Guyer et al, 2000). The high incidence of *low birth weight (LBW)* (less than 2500 g) in the United States is a key factor in its higher neonatal mortality rates when compared with other countries. Access to and use of high-quality prenatal care is the single most important preventive strategy to decrease early delivery and infant mortality rates. Other factors that increase the risk of infant mortality include African-American race, male gender, short or long gestation, maternal age, and a low level of maternal education (Guyer et al, 2000).

Although there has been a steady and significant decline in infant mortality rate, the number of deaths in the first year of life is still proportionately high when compared with death rates at other ages (Table 29-1). Serious health conditions in preterm LBW infants occur most often during the first 6 months after hospital discharge. In the United States, the death rate for infants under 1 year of age is greater than the rate for individuals ages 1 through 54 years. It is not until age 55 and over that the death rate begins to exceed the rate for infants.

In the 1960s attention was focused on perinatal health care in an effort to decrease the number of neonatal deaths. Neonatal mortality rate declined from 20.5 per 1000 live births in 1950 to 4.5 per 1000 live births in 2001 (Arias et al, 2003). This decline resulted from advances in neonatal intensive care and better treatment of perinatal illnesses. However, many of the leading causes of death during infancy continue to occur during the perinatal period (Table 29-2). The first four causes—congenital anomalies, disorders related to short gestation and unspecified LBW, SIDS, and newborn affected by maternal complications of pregnancy—account for just under half of all deaths of infants under 1 year of age (Anderson & Smith, 2003).

Although a number of perinatal problems have benefited from improved treatment, congenital anomalies continue to be a leading cause of infant mortality. The incidence of the majority of birth defects has remained substantially the same. Heart defects have been rising, but the increase is the result of improved methods of detection, not increased births of affected infants. Anencephaly and spina bifida are

Table 29-1

Death Rates by Age and Sex: United States, 2001, Preliminary Data (Rates per 100,000 Population)

	All Races		
AGE (YEARS)	BOTH SEXES	MALE	FEMALE
All ages*	848.5	846.4	850.4
<1†	684.8	752.1	614.4
1-4	33.3	37.0	29.5
5-9	15.3	16.7	13.9
10-14	19.2	22.8	15.3
15-19	66.9	93.7	38.5

Modified from Anderson RN, Smith BL: Deaths: leading causes for 2001, *Natl Vital Stat Rep* 52(9):1-85, 2003.

*Figures for ages not stated are included in "All ages" but not distributed among age groups.

†Death rates for "<1 year" (based on population estimates) differ from infant mortality rates (based on live births).

*www.health.gov/healthypeople/state/toolkit.

Table 29-2

Mortality Rates and Percentage of Total Deaths for 10 Leading Causes of Infant Death in 2001 (Rate Per 1000 Live Births)

RANK	CAUSE OF DEATH (BASED ON TENTH REVISION, INTERNATIONAL CLASSIFICATION OF DISEASES)	PERCENT	RATE
—	*ALL RACES, ALL CAUSES*	*100.00*	*684.8*
1	Congenital anomalies	20.0	136.9
2	Disorders relating to short gestation and unspecified low birth weight	16.0	109.5
3	Sudden infant death syndrome	8.1	55.5
4	Newborn affected by maternal complications of pregnancy	5.4	37.2
5	Newborn affected by complications of placenta, cord, and membranes	3.7	25.3
6	Respiratory distress syndrome	3.7	25.1
7	Accidents (unintentional injuries)	3.5	24.2
8	Bacterial sepsis of newborn	2.5	17.3
9	Diseases of the circulatory system	2.3	15.4
10	Intrauterine hypoxia and birth asphyxia	1.9	13.3

Modified from Anderson RN, Smith BL: Deaths: leading causes for 2001, *Natl Vital Stat Rep* 52(9):1-85, 2003.

expected to decrease with the recommendation of folic acid supplementation for all women of childbearing age (see Spina Bifida [Myelomeningocele], Chapter 55). Reducing LBW will also prevent congenital anomalies. Infant mortality resulting from human immunodeficiency virus (HIV) infection has decreased significantly; in 2000, HIV/AIDS accounted for less than 0.04% of all deaths in children younger that 1 year of age (Minino et al, 2002).

When infant death rates are categorized according to race, the infant mortality rate for whites is lower than that for all other races in the United States, and the infant mortality rate for African-Americans is twice the rate for whites. The gap between these two racial groups has remained fairly constant. The LBW rate is also higher for African-American infants than for any other group. Reasons for these high rates are unknown. One encouraging note is that the gap in mortality rates between white and nonwhite races other than African-Americans is narrowing. Infant mortality rates for Hispanics and Asians/Pacific Islanders decreased dramatically during the last 20 years (Minino et al, 2002).

Childhood Mortality

Death rates for children older than 1 year of age have always been less than the rate for infants. Children ages 5 to 14 years have the lowest rate of death (Table 29-3). However, a sharp rise occurs during later adolescence, primarily from injuries, homicide, and suicide. In 2000, these conditions were responsible for approximately 72% of deaths in teenagers and young adults 15 to 19 years old (Minino & Smith, 2001). The trend in racial differences that occurs in infant mortality is also seen in childhood deaths for all ages and for both sexes. Whites have fewer deaths for all ages, and male deaths outnumber female deaths.

After 1 year of age there is a dramatic change in the cause of death. Unintentional injuries (accidents) are the leading cause of death from the youngest ages to the adolescent years. In addition, *violent deaths* are increasing among young

Table 29-3

Five Leading Causes of Death in Children in the United States: Selected Age Intervals, 2000, Preliminary Data (Rates per 100,000)

RANK	AGES 1-4	RATE	AGES 5-9	RATE	AGES 10-14	RATE	AGES 15-19	RATE
	All causes	33.3	All causes	15.3	All causes	19.2	All causes	66.9
1	Accidents	11.2	Accidents	6.4	Accidents	7.4	Accidents	32.8
2	Congenital anomalies	3.6	Cancer	2.4	Cancer	2.5	Homicide	9.4
3	Cancer	2.7	Congenital anomalies	0.9	Suicide	1.3	Suicide	7.9
4	Homicide	2.7	Homicide	0.7	Congenital anomalies	0.9	Cancer	3.6
5	Heart disease	1.5	Heart disease	0.5	Homicide	0.9	Heart disease	1.7

Modified from Anderson RN, Smith BL: Deaths: leading causes for 2001, *Natl Vital Stat Rep* 52(9):1-85, 2003.

people ages 10 through 25 years, especially among African-American males. Homicide is the second leading cause of death in the 15- to 19-year-old age group (see Table 29-3). Children 12 years of age and older are more likely to be killed by non–family members (acquaintances and gangs, typically of the same race) and most frequently by firearms. Firearm homicide is the leading cause of death among African-American males ages 15 to 19 years. *Suicide* is the third leading cause of death among adolescents and young adults 15 to 19 years old (see Table 29-4).

The causes of increased violence against children and self-inflicted violence are not fully understood. In young children the increase in homicide may represent more accurate identification of child abuse. The problem of child homicides is complex and involves psychologic, social, and economic factors. Nurses need to be aware of young people who are depressed, repeatedly in trouble with the criminal justice system, or associated with groups known to be violent. Prevention requires identification of these individuals and therapeutic intervention by qualified professionals. Pediatric nurses can also assess children and adolescents for risk factors related to violence (such as the presence of a gun in a household) and educate families, teachers, and community leaders about the importance of maintaining safe, nonviolent homes, schools, and neighborhoods.

The major declines in death rates during childhood have occurred in deaths caused by gastrointestinal diseases, infectious diseases, perinatal conditions, neoplasms, and injuries. The absence of infectious diseases as a leading cause of death is related to the use of antibacterial agents and immunizations. Deaths caused by infectious diseases have decreased considerably in recent years. In particular, deaths from HIV infection have decreased, and HIV is no longer one of the 10 leading causes of death (Anderson & Smith, 2003). Other disorders

Table 29-4

Mortality from Leading Types of Unintentional Injuries, United States, 1997 (Rates per 100,000 Population in Each Age Group)

	Age (Years)			
TYPE OF ACCIDENT	UNDER 1	1-4	5-14	15-24
MALES				
All causes	818.0	39.8	24.0	124.4
Unintentional injuries (all types)	22.3	15.2	10.6	52.3
Motor vehicle	4.4 (2)	5.3 (1)	5.8 (1)	38.3 (1)
Drowning	1.8 (4)	3.9 (2)	1.6 (2)	3.2 (2)
Fires and burns	1.5 (5)	2.5 (3)	0.8 (3)	—
Firearms	—	—	0.5 (4)	1.5 (4)
Ingestion of food/object	2.5 (3)	0.5 (5)	—	—
Falls	—	—	—	1.2 (5)
Mechanical suffocation	9.1 (1)	0.6 (4)	0.4 (5)	—
Poisoning	—	—	—	2.8 (3)
All other unintentional injuries	3.1	2.3	1.4	5.3
*Accidents as a percent of all deaths	2.7%	38.2%	44.3%	42.0%
FEMALES				
All causes	662.9	31.8	17.4	46.0
Unintentional injuries (all types)	18.1	10.9	6.7	20.0
Motor vehicle	4.4 (2)	4.7 (1)	4.3 (1)	17.1 (1)
Drowning	1.4 (4)	2.0 (2)	0.6 (3)	0.4 (3)
Fires and burns	1.2 (5)	2.0 (2)	0.7 (2)	—
Firearms	—	—	0.1 (4)	0.1 (5)
Ingestion of food/object	1.5 (3)	0.4 (4)	—	—
Falls	—	—	—	0.2 (4)
Mechanical suffocation	6.9 (1)	0.3 (5)	0.1 (4)	—
Poisoning	—	—	—	0.8 (2)
All other unintentional injuries	2.7	1.5	0.9	1.5
*Accidents as a percent of all deaths	2.7%	34.2%	38.2%	43.4%

Modified from National Safety Council: *Injury facts, 2000 edition*, Itaska, IL, 2000, National Safety Council. Data source: National Center for Health Statistics.
*Indicates rank among the leading types of accidents.

such as neoplasms have become more prominent causes of death, although childhood deaths from cancer are currently less frequent than ever before (see Leukemias, Chapter 49).

Injuries

Injuries, the leading cause of death in children over 1 year of age, are responsible for more childhood deaths and disabilities than all causes of disease combined. As children grow older, the percentage of deaths from injuries increases (Table 29-4). Injuries have not shown the dramatic declines seen in other areas of childhood mortality because injuries have traditionally been regarded as unavoidable accidents or behavioral problems, rather than health problems. The term *accident* suggests a chaotic, random event related to "luck" or "chance." The term *injury* is now preferred because this term indicates a sense of responsibility and control.

The pattern of deaths caused by unintentional injuries, especially from motor vehicles, drowning, and burns, is consistent in Western societies. However, the United States exceeds other countries in the number of violent deaths. The leading causes of deaths from injuries for each age group according to sex are presented in Table 29-4. The majority of deaths from injuries occur in males. It is important to note that accidents account for more teen deaths than any other source (Annie E. Casey Foundation, 2001). Fortunately, prevention strategies such as the use of car restraints, bicycle helmets, and smoke detectors have resulted in a significant decrease in fatalities for younger children. Currently, all states have legislation requiring young children to be properly restrained in motor vehicles. Despite safety efforts, the overwhelming cause of death in children over 1 year of age is motor vehicle (MV)–related fatalities, including occupant, pedestrian, bicycle, and motorcycle deaths (Fig. 29-1). Even though the *percentage* of infants dying from MV injuries is small compared with the total number of deaths in infancy, children under 1 year of age continue to have a high death rate from MV-occupant deaths because they are not properly restrained.

When deaths from injuries are compared according to sex and age, the causes of death differ. The developmental stage of the child determines the type of injury that is most likely to occur at a specific age. For example, a child between ages 1 and 4 years is equally likely to die as an occupant or as a pedestrian in MV injuries. However, children ages 5 to 9 years are more likely to die from pedestrian crashes, and adolescents are more likely to die from occupant crashes. Children ages 5 to 14 are at greatest risk of bicycling fatalities. The majority of bicycling deaths are from head injuries. Helmets reduce the risk of head injury by 85%, but few children wear helmets (National Safety Council, 2000).

Drowning and burns are the second and third leading causes of death in males ages 1 to 14, but the order is reversed in females (Fig. 29-2). Drowning is a significant cause of death in older teenagers. In addition, improper use of firearms is a major cause of death in males (Fig. 29-3). Dur-

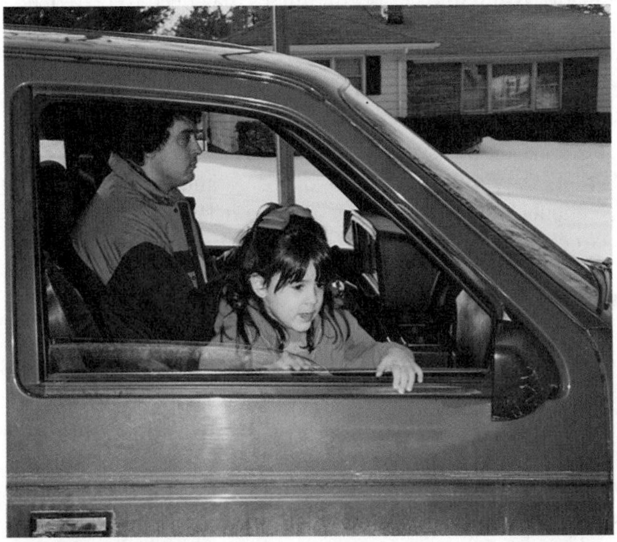

Fig. 29-1 Motor vehicle injuries are the leading cause of death in children over 1 year of age. The majority of the fatalities involve occupants who are unrestrained.

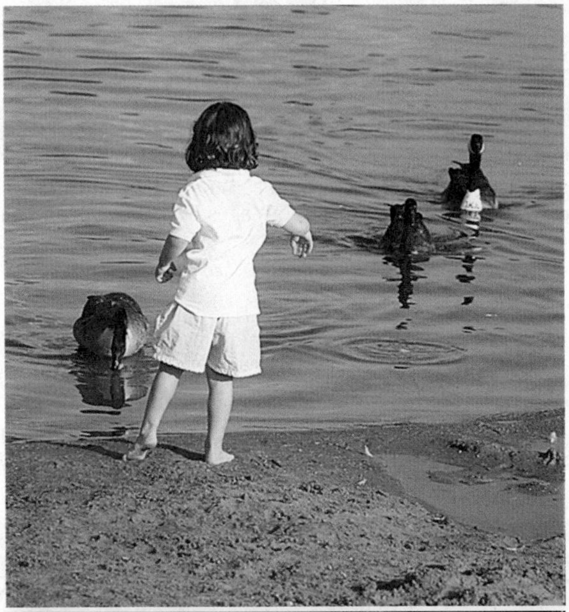

A

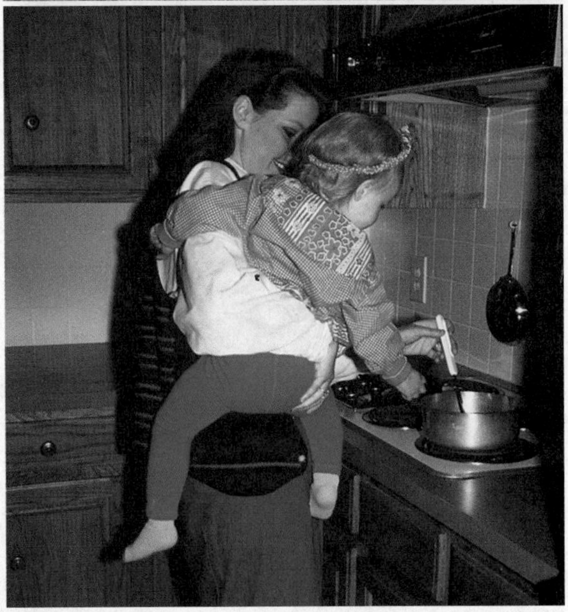

B

Fig. 29-2 **A,** Drowning is the second leading cause of death from injury in boys and the third in girls ages 5 to 14 years. **B,** Burns are the second leading cause of death from injury in girls and the third in boys ages 1 to 14 years.

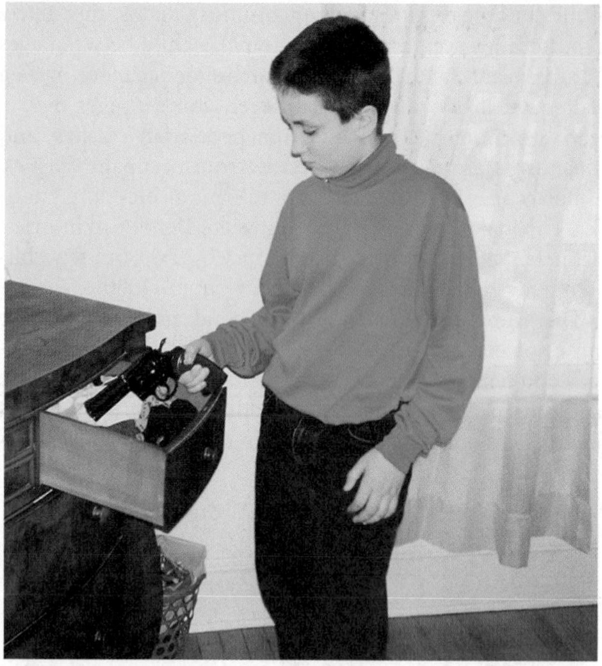

Fig. 29-3 Improper use of firearms is the fourth leading cause of death from injury in boys ages 5 to 24 years and girls ages 5 to 14 years.

ing infancy, more males die from aspiration or suffocation than do females (Fig. 29-4). More than half of all poisonings occur in children under 2 years of age (Fig. 29-5). By ages 4 to 5 years, unintentional poisonings are uncommon. Another increase occurs in the 15- to 24-year-old age group, when poisoning is the third leading cause of death in males and the second leading cause of death in females. Poisoning in this age group is often intentional and represents death from suicide (especially females) or drug abuse.

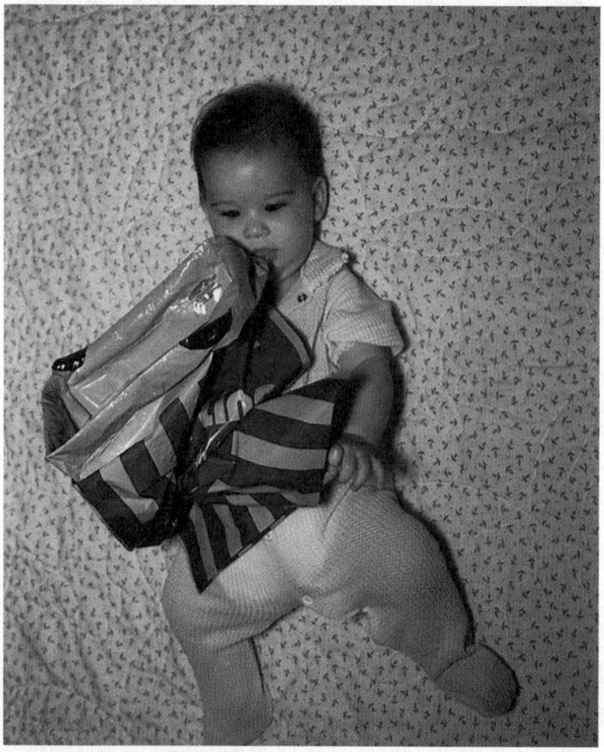

Fig. 29-4 Mechanical suffocation is often the leading cause of death from injury in infants.

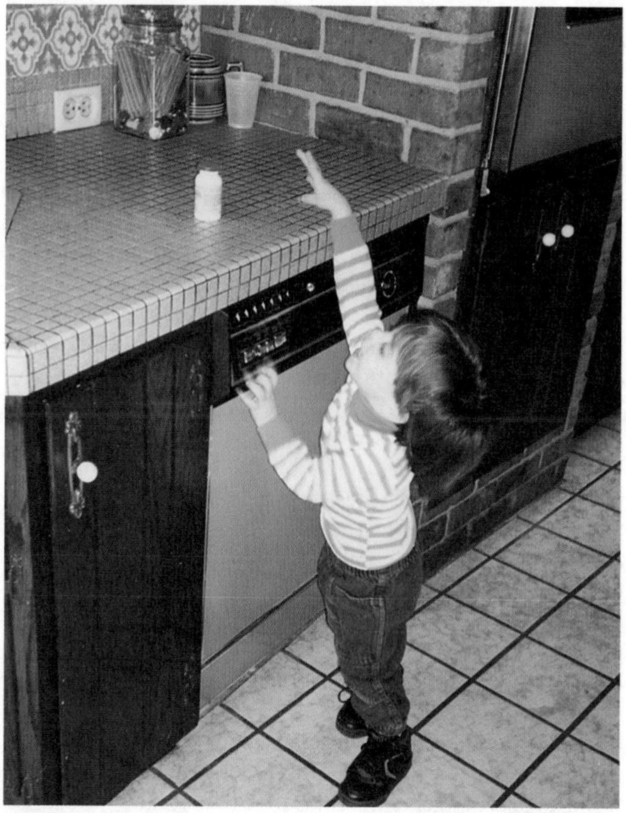

Fig. 29-5 Poisoning causes a considerable number of injuries in children under 4 years of age, but it is the third leading cause of death from injury in males and second in females (usually from suicide) ages 15 to 24 years.

It is important to remember that not all injuries are unintentional; some may be intentional and represent abuse or suicide. When injuries occur, nurses may need to help determine if they were intentional.

NURSE ALERT The history of the injury is essential in assessing intentional injury from abuse or neglect. The following questions are important:

When—Did the parent or guardian seek immediate medical attention, or has there been a long delay?

Where—Does the reported location of the accident correlate with the nature of the injury?

How—Are the circumstances surrounding the injury logical? ■

Injury Prevention

When comparing deaths from injuries with other causes of childhood mortality, it is clear that preventing injuries is the best strategy to improve survival. Nurses play a major role in providing anticipatory guidance to parents and older children regarding hazards during each age period.

Theoretically all injuries are preventable. Injury prevention is an ongoing part of health promotion for all age groups. Anticipatory guidance regarding developmental expectations serves to alert parents to the types of injuries most common at any given age. Early in the parent-child relationship, parents need advice on how to provide a safe environment. It cannot be assumed that parents of one or more children are familiar with all areas of child safety. The addition of a new infant may cause sibling rivalry, and the new infant may be at risk from a jealous sibling. The American Academy of Pediatrics has developed The Injury Prevention Program (TIPP) that provides useful information and anticipatory guidance on safety issues for parents and health care providers.* Another resource is the Consumer Product Safety Commission (CPSC) of the U.S. government, which provides publications that recommend areas of safety for children.†

Morbidity

The prevalence of specific illnesses in the population at a particular time is known as *morbidity statistics.* These are generally presented as rates per 1000 population because of their greater frequency of occurrence. Unlike mortality, morbidity is difficult to define and may denote acute illness, chronic disease, or disability. Sources of data for morbidity statistics include reasons for visits to physicians, diagnoses for hospital admission, and household interviews. Unlike death rates, which are updated annually, morbidity statistics are revised less frequently and may not represent the general population.

Acute illness is defined as symptoms severe enough to limit activity or require medical attention. Respiratory illness accounts for about 50% of all acute conditions; infections and parasitic disease cause 11%, and injuries cause 15%. The chief illness of childhood is the common cold.

The types of diseases that children contract during childhood vary according to age. For example, upper respiratory tract infections and diarrhea decrease with age, but other disorders such as acne and headaches increase. Children who have had a particular type of problem are more likely to have that problem again. Morbidity is not distributed randomly in children. Children from poor families tend to have more health problems. This finding suggests a need for heightened efforts to improve access to health care for low-income children.

Recent concern has focused on specific groups of children who have increased morbidity—homeless children, children living in poverty, LBW children, children with chronic illnesses, foreign-born adopted children, and children in day care centers. Several factors place these groups at risk for poor health. One factor is barriers to health care, especially for the homeless, the poor, and children with chronic health problems. Other factors include improved survival of children with chronic health problems, particularly infants of very low birthweight (VLBW). Children living in or exposed to at-risk environments such as the country of origin for adopted children and day care centers may be more likely to have medical problems such as infections (Lears, Guth, & Lewandowski, 1998).

Injuries are an additional factor influencing morbidity. Each year 40,000 to 50,000 children are injured permanently and one million children receive medical care because of unintentional injuries.

The most important aspect of morbidity is the degree of disability it produces. *Disability* can be measured in days absent from school or days confined to bed. On average, a child loses 5.3 days per year because of injury or illness. (The incidence of chronic conditions is discussed in Chapter 41.)

For many children childhood is a time of relative health, but it is the rare child who never becomes ill. Education of parents regarding the usual types of childhood illnesses and recognition of symptoms that require treatment is an important part of nursing care. Health promotion and health education are important roles for pediatric nurses.

In addition to disease and injury, children face behavioral, social, family, and educational problems that are referred to as the *new morbidity* or *pediatric social illness.* These problems (e.g., poverty, violence, school failure) interfere with children's social and academic development. Estimates of the incidence of these problems vary from 5% to 30%. Although no conclusive characteristics have been identified, several findings appear to define at-risk groups. These include (1) children from low socioeconomic status, (2) children of the male gender, and (3) children with a sibling who has had a previous injury (Altemeier, 2000).

Evolution of Child Health Care in the United States

Children in colonial America were born into a world with many hazards to their health and survival. Epidemics were common. Physicians were few, and only a small number had formal training. Midwives were untrained, and they based their practice on past experiences. Books providing information on child care and feeding were scarce and, when available, were helpful only to literate parents.

Medical care by physicians was limited to wealthy families who lived in or could travel to more developed cities. Children who lived on farms were cared for by another family member or by a competent neighbor. Traveling medicine men and various forms of quackery were common. Children who were bought as slaves or born to slaves had only as much care as their owner was able or willing to provide. Native American children were treated according to the tradition of their tribe, which was often a mixture of medicine, magic, and religion. With the colonization of America, Native Americans were exposed to new, often fatal, diseases.

Reliable statistics on childhood mortality rates during the colonial period are unavailable. Epidemic diseases included smallpox, measles, mumps, chickenpox, influenza, diphtheria, yellow fever, cholera, and whooping cough. Dysentery was the most common cause of childhood death. Other diseases that contributed to childhood illness were the "slow epidemics" of tuberculosis, nutritional diseases, and injuries.

Although scientific knowledge was accumulating in the colonial period, there were no organized efforts in the United

*For more information contact the American Academy of Pediatrics, 141 Northwest Point Boulevard, Elk Grove Village, IL 60007; phone: 888-227-1770; fax: 847-228-1281; Web site: www.aap.org.

†For more information call 800-638-CPSC or 800-638-2272.

States to apply this knowledge to the sick until the nineteenth century. At this time, the consequences of childhood illness and injury and the effects of child labor, poverty, and neglect became widely recognized.

The study of pediatrics began in the 1800s, under the influence of a Prussian-born physician, Abraham Jacobi (1830-1919), who is referred to as the "father of pediatrics." Jacobi broke new ground in the scientific and clinical investigation of childhood diseases. One outstanding achievement of this time was the establishment of "milk stations," where mothers could bring sick children for treatment and learn the importance of pure milk and its proper preparation.

The crusade for pure milk helped bring the dairy industry under legal control and led to the establishment of infant welfare stations. The remarkable decline in infant mortality rates since 1900 has been achieved through health-promoting measures such as improved sanitation and pasteurization of milk. Before these regulations existed, unsanitary milk was a source of infantile diarrhea and bovine tuberculosis. Cows were often kept in filthy stables and fed garbage and distillery wastes. Milk from these cows was reported to make infants "tipsy."

At this time, increasing concern developed for the social welfare of children, especially those who were homeless or employed as factory laborers. The work of one reformer, Lillian Wald (1867-1940), had far-reaching effects on child health and nursing. Wald founded the Henry Street Settlement in New York City, which eventually provided nursing service, social work, and an organized program of social, cultural, and educational activities. She is regarded as the "founder of public health or community nursing" and was instrumental in establishing the role of the first full-time school nurse, Lina Rogers. Soon other nurses were employed to teach parents and children about the prevention or need for treatment of minor skin conditions, malnutrition, and other illnesses identified in the school. An outgrowth of this nursing involvement in school health was the development of pediatric courses and clinical experience in schools of nursing.

As causes of disease were identified, emphasis on isolation and asepsis occurred. In the early 1900s, children with contagious diseases were isolated from adult patients. Parents were prohibited from visiting because they might transmit disease to and from the home. Even toys and personal articles of clothing were kept from the child. In the1940s, the investigations of Spitz and Robertson highlighted the effects of isolation and maternal deprivation on institutionalized children. Their research stimulated interest in the psychologic health of children and resulted in changes for hospitalized children, such as rooming-in, sibling visitations, child life programs, prehospitalization preparation, parent education, and hospital schooling.

Influenced by social reformers such as Lillian Wald, national leaders took action to improve children's living conditions. In 1909 President Theodore Roosevelt convened the first White House Conference on Children, which focused on the care of dependent children and addressed the deplorable working conditions of youngsters. As a result of this conference, the U.S. Children's Bureau was established in 1912. This marked the beginning of a period of studies of economic and social factors related to infant mortality, maternal deaths, and maternal and infant care in rural settings. These studies stimulated the creation of better standards of care for mothers and children, and led to the first Maternity and Infancy Act. This act provided grants to states to develop a division of maternal and child health (MCH) as a unit of the health department, and influenced the creation of the American Academy of Pediatrics.

In 1935 Title V of the Social Security Act (SSA) was passed and a federal-state partnership was established under the administration of the Children's Bureau. Title V included federal grants-in-aid to states (matched by state funds), for three types of work: maternal and child health (MCH), Crippled Children's Services (CCS), and child welfare services. The first programs provided by Title V were prenatal, postnatal, and child health clinics. Another focus of the CCS was orthopedic care. With the recognition that a child's ability to function could be limited by a chronic illness, state CCS programs became involved with children with developmental, behavioral, and educational problems and more recently with home care of children with complex medical conditions. This broadened concept was reflected in the 1985 passage of legislation that changed the name of the CCS to the Program for Children with Special Health Needs (CSHN).

Other federal programs that have had a major impact on maternal and child health include the following:

Medicaid. Medicaid was created in 1965 under Title XIX of the Social Security Act to reduce financial barriers to health care for the poor. It is the largest maternal-child health program. A major project under Medicaid is the Child Health Assessment Program (CHAP), which provides services for pregnant women and children. Financial eligibility varies from state to state.

Aid to Families with Dependent Children (AFDC). The SSA of 1935 established AFDC as a cash grant program to enable states to aid needy children without fathers.

MCH Services Block Grant. MCH Services Block Grant provides health services to mothers and children, particularly those with low income or limited access to health services. Its primary purposes are (1) to reduce infant mortality rates and the incidence of preventable disease and handicapping conditions among children and (2) to increase the availability of prenatal, delivery, and postpartum care to eligible mothers.

Alcohol, Drug Abuse, and Mental Health Block Grant. Established by the Omnibus Budget Reconciliation Act of 1981, this block grant provides funds to states for (1) projects to support prevention, treatment, and rehabilitation related to substance abuse and (2) grants to community mental health centers for the identification, assessment, and treatment of severely mentally disturbed children and adolescents.

Social Services Block Grant. Established under Title XX of the SSA, this grant provides states with funds for child day care, protective and emergency services, counseling, family planning, home-based services, information and referral, and adoption and foster care services.

Women, Infants, and Children (WIC). The WIC Special Supplemental Food Program was started in 1974. It provides nutritious food and nutrition education to low-income, pregnant, postpartum, and lactating women and to infants and children up to age 5 years. Other nutrition programs include Food Stamps, the National School Lunch Program, the School Breakfast Program, and the Child Care Food Program, which provides financial assistance for nutritious meals to children in day care centers, family and group day care homes, and Head Start centers.

Education for All Handicapped Children Act (Public Law [PL] 94-142). In 1975 PL 94-142 was passed to provide free public education to all handicapped children ages 3 to 21 years and to provide supportive services (such as speech and counseling) that ensure the benefit of special education.

Education of the Handicapped Act Amendments of 1986 (PL 99-457). In 1986 PL 99-457 was passed to allow federal funding to states to develop and implement a statewide, comprehensive, coordinated, and multidisciplinary program of early intervention services for handicapped infants and toddlers and their families.

Omnibus Budget Reconciliation Act of 1990. This act required states to extend Medicaid coverage to all children ages 6 to 18 years with family incomes below 133% of the poverty level.

Family and Medical Leave Act (FMLA). FMLA was signed into law in 1993. This Act allows eligible employees to take up to 12 weeks of unpaid leave from their jobs every year to care for newborn or newly adopted children; to care for children, parents, or spouses who have serious health conditions; or to recover from their own serious health conditions. After the leave, the law entitles employees to return to their previous jobs or equivalent jobs with the same pay, benefits, and other conditions.

Health Insurance Portability and Accountability Act (HIPAA). The first-ever federal privacy standards to protect patients' medical records and other health information provided to health plans, doctors, hospitals, and other health care providers took effect on April 14, 2003. HIPAA, developed by the U.S. Department of Health and Human Services (USDHHS), established new standards that provide patients with access to their medical records and more control over how their personal health information is used and disclosed. For further information see the USDHHS Web site at www.hhs.gov/ocr/hipaa.

Despite federal and state programs available to assist children and families, serious barriers to health care remain. These include (1) *financial barriers,* such as not having insurance, having insurance that does not cover certain services, or being unable to pay for services; (2) *system barriers,* such as having to travel great distances for health care or state-to-state variations in Medicaid benefits; and (3) *knowledge barriers,* such as a lack of understanding of the need for prenatal or child health supervision or an unawareness of the services available. The current thrust in health care is to improve access to health care for all children and their families.

Another major change in health care delivery has been the establishment of a *prospective payment system* based on *diagnosis-related groups (DRGs).* The DRG categories define *pretreatment (prospective) billing* for U.S. hospitals reimbursed by Medicare. When hospitals are held financially responsible if Medicare patients exceed the allotted admission stay, patients are discharged early. Early discharges have created a need for home care and community-based services. Health care cost containment remains a national priority; currently, many children are enrolled in *managed care companies* and *health maintenance organizations (HMOs).** In some instances, these companies and organizations have improved access to preventive health care for children, but in other cases, they have reduced access to specialty care for children with chronic conditions (Szilagy, 1998).

PEDIATRIC NURSING

Philosophy of Care

Nursing of infants and children is consistent with the revised *definition of nursing* proposed by the Social Policy Task Force of the American Nurses Association in 2003. This definition states that "nursing is the prevention of illness, the alleviation of suffering, and the protection, promotion, and restoration of health in the care of individuals, families, groups, communities, and populations" (American Nurses Association, 2001; 2003). This definition incorporates the four essential features of nursing practice:

1. Attention to the full range of human experiences and responses to health and illness without restriction to a problem-focused orientation
2. Integration of objective data with knowledge gained from an understanding of the patient's or group's subjective experience
3. Application of scientific knowledge to the processes of diagnosis and treatment
4. Provision of a caring relationship that facilitates health and healing (American Nurses Association, 2003)

Family-Centered Care

The philosophy of *family-centered care* recognizes the family as the one constant in a child's life. Three key components of family-centered care are respect, collaboration, and support (Galvin et al, 2000). Families are supported in their caregiving and decision making when health care professionals build on their unique strengths and acknowledge their expertise in caring for their child both within and outside the hospital setting (Newton, 2000). Patterns of living at home and in the community are promoted, and the needs of all family members, not just the child's, are considered (Box 29-1). The philosophy of family-centered care acknowledges diversity among family structures and backgrounds; family goals, dreams, strategies, and actions; and family support, service, and information needs.

Two basic concepts in family-centered care are enabling and empowerment. Professionals *enable* families by creating opportunities for all family members to display their current abilities and competencies and to acquire new ones that are necessary to meet the needs of the child and family. *Empow-*

*For information on managed care references and resources, see www.nursingworld.org.

BOX 29-1

Key Elements of Family-Centered Care

Incorporating into policy and practice the recognition that the *family is the constant* in a child's life while the service systems and support personnel within those systems fluctuate

Facilitating *family/professional collaboration* at all levels of hospital, home, and community care:
- Care of an individual child
- Program development, implementation, and evaluation
- Policy formation

Exchanging complete and unbiased information between family members and professionals in a supportive manner at all times

Incorporating into policy and practice the *recognition and honoring of cultural diversity,* strengths, and individuality within and across all families, including *ethnic, racial, spiritual, social, economic, educational, and geographic diversity*

Recognizing and respecting *different methods of coping* and implementing comprehensive policies and programs that provide *developmental, educational, emotional, environmental, and financial support* to meet the diverse needs of families

Encouraging and facilitating *family-to-family support* and networking

Ensuring that *home, hospital,* and *community service* and *support systems* for children needing specialized health and developmental care and their families are *flexible, accessible,* and *comprehensive* in responding to diverse family-identified needs

Appreciating families as families and children as children, recognizing that they possess a wide range of strengths, concerns, emotions, and aspirations beyond their need for specialized health and developmental services and support

From Shelton TL, Stepanek JS: *Family-centered care for children needing specialized health and developmental services,* Bethesda, MD, 1994, Association for the Care of Children's Health.

erment describes the interaction of professionals with families in such a way that families maintain or acquire a sense of control over their lives and make positive changes that result from helping behaviors that foster their own strengths, abilities, and actions.

The *parent-professional partnership* is a powerful mechanism for enabling and empowering families.* Parents serve as respected equals with professionals and have the right to decide what is important for themselves and their family. The professional supports and strengthens the family's ability to nurture and promote family development. Professionals must also work together as a team to benefit children and their families.

Partnerships imply the belief that partners are capable individuals who become more competent by sharing knowledge, skills, and resources in a manner that benefits all participants. Collaboration is viewed as a continuum. Families have the option of being anywhere along the continuum, depending on their strengths and needs and their relationships with professionals. The nurse can help *every* family, including those with a previous history of serious personal or family problems, to identify their strengths, build on them, and assume a comfortable level of participation. Although caring for the family is strongly emphasized throughout the text, it is highlighted in features such as Cultural Awareness, Family Focus, and Home Care boxes.

Atraumatic Care

Although tremendous advances have been made in pediatric care, many changes that have cured illnesses and prolonged life are traumatic, painful, upsetting, and frightening. Unfortunately, minimizing the trauma of medical interventions has not kept pace with the technologic advances. Health professionals must be aware of the stresses facing ill children and their families, and strive to provide interventions that are safe, effective, and helpful. Health professionals must also attempt to provide atraumatic care.

Atraumatic care is the provision of therapeutic care in settings, by personnel, and through the use of interventions that eliminate or minimize the psychologic and physical distress experienced by children and their families in the health care system. *Therapeutic care* encompasses the prevention, diagnosis, treatment, or palliation of chronic or acute conditions. *Setting* refers to whatever place that care is given—the home, the hospital, or any other health care setting. *Personnel* includes anyone directly involved in providing therapeutic care. *Interventions* range from psychologic approaches, such as preparing children for procedures, to physical interventions, such as providing space for a parent to room in with a child. *Psychologic distress* may include anxiety, fear, anger, disappointment, sadness, shame, or guilt. *Physical distress* may range from sleeplessness and immobilization to the experience of disturbing sensory stimuli such as pain, temperature extremes, loud noises, bright lights, or darkness. Atraumatic care is concerned with the who, what, when, where, why, and how of any procedure performed on a child for the purpose of preventing or minimizing psychologic and physical stress (Wong, 1989).

The overriding goal in providing atraumatic care is *first, do no harm.* Three principles provide the framework for achieving this goal: (1) prevent or minimize the child's separation from the family; (2) promote a sense of control; and (3) prevent or minimize bodily injury and pain. Examples of atraumatic care include fostering the parent-child relationship during hospitalization, preparing the child before any unfamiliar treatment or procedure, controlling pain, allowing the child privacy, providing play activities for expression of fear and aggression, providing choices to children, and respecting cultural differences.

Atraumatic care is an integral part of nursing care discussions in the text. Atraumatic Care boxes highlight selected examples, and several boxes focusing on culture, family teaching, research, and critical thinking incorporate atraumatic care. Chapter 44, Reaction to Illness and Hospitalization, is organized according to principles of atraumatic care.

Case Management

Case management developed as an approach to coordinate care and control costs. The benefits of case management include improved patient/family satisfaction, decreased frag-

*For information about parent-professional partnerships, a free pamphlet, *Equals in This Partnership,* is available from the National Center for Infants, Toddlers and Families, 200 M St., NW, Suite 200, Washington, DC 20036; phone: 202-638-1144.

mentation of care, and the ability to describe and measure outcomes for a homogeneous group of patients.

Case managers are responsible and accountable for particular groups of patients and often use timelines derived from standards of care. Timelines have a variety of names: critical paths, guidelines for care, case management plans, Caremaps,* coordinated care plans, or other titles agreed on within a specific agency. Regardless of their name, timelines are multidisciplinary plans that include all the components of care for an episode or multiple episodes of illness, as well as the expected outcomes or result of care. Timelines can be confined to inpatient care or the entire continuum of care, including home care (see also Chapter 43).

In addition to providing care in a systematic manner, professional and government organizations often follow *clinical practice guidelines* for the care of an illness, disease, or problem. Care timelines are developed within an institution and reflect local practice patterns, but clinical practice guidelines are developed on a national level and reflect research related to a specific disease or illness. The Agency for Healthcare Research and Quality (AHRQ) is a federal agency that has developed several clinical practice guidelines relevant to pediatrics (e.g, acute pain management, management of otitis media with effusion, and diagnosis and treatment of sickle cell disease) (Box 29-2).

Role of the Pediatric Nurse

Therapeutic Relationship

A therapeutic relationship is the essential foundation for quality nursing care. Pediatric nurses must relate to children and their families in a meaningful way, and yet remain separate enough to distinguish their own feelings and needs. In a *therapeutic relationship,* caring, well-defined boundaries separate the nurse from the child and family (Peternelj-Taylor, 2002). These boundaries are positive and professional and promote the family's control over the child's health care (Rushton, McEnhill, & Armstrong, 1996). Within a therapeutic relationship, both the nurse and the family are empowered, and open communication is maintained. In a *nontherapeutic relationship* boundaries are blurred, and many of the nurse's actions may serve personal needs, such as a need to feel wanted and involved, rather than the family's needs. Some settings make the establishment of boundaries more difficult than others. For example, in the home care setting several factors challenge the definition of boundaries. The informal home environment, the casual social conversations among family members, the participation by family members in the care of the child, and the attempt by some families to incorporate the home care nurse into the family all present major challenges to establishing and maintaining clear boundaries.

Exploring whether relationships with patients are therapeutic or nontherapeutic helps nurses to identify problem areas early in their interactions with children and families. Although questions for exploring types of involvement can be labeled negative or positive, no one action makes a relationship therapeutic or nontherapeutic. For example, nurses may spend additional time with the family but still recognize their own needs and maintain professional separateness. An important clue to nontherapeutic relationships is the staff's concerns about their peer's actions with the family.

Family Advocacy/Caring

Although nurses are responsible to themselves, the profession, and the institution of employment, their primary responsibility is to the consumer of nursing services—the child and the family. The nurse must work with family members, identify *their* goals and needs, and plan interventions that meet the defined problems. As an advocate, the nurse assists children and their families in making informed choices and acting in the child's best interest. Advocacy involves ensuring that families are aware of all available health services, informed of treatments and procedures, involved in the child's care, and encouraged to change or support existing health care practices. The United Nations Declaration of the Rights of the Child (Box 29-3) provides guidelines for nursing practice to ensure that every child receives optimum

BOX 29-2

AHRQ Clinical Practice Guidelines Relevant to Pediatric Practice

- Acute pain management: operative or medical procedures and trauma
- Urinary incontinence
- Pressure ulcers: prediction and intervention
- Treatment of pressure ulcers
- Diagnosis and treatment of depressed outpatients in primary care settings
- Diagnosis and treatment of sickle cell disease
- Initial evaluation and early treatment of the HIV-infected individual
- Management of cancer-related pain
- Diagnosis and treatment of heart failure
- Otitis media with effusion

Modified from Agency for Health Care Policy and Research (AHCPR; now known as Agency for Healthcare Research and Quality [AHRQ]). To order guidelines contact AHRQ Publications Clearinghouse, PO Box 8547, Silver Spring, MD 20907; phone: 800-358-9295; Web site: www.ahcpr.gov.

BOX 29-3

United Nations Declaration of the Rights of the Child

All children need:
- To be free from discrimination
- To develop physically and mentally in freedom and dignity
- To have a name and nationality
- To have adequate nutrition, housing, recreation, and medical services
- To receive special treatment if handicapped
- To receive love, understanding, and material security
- To receive an education and develop their abilities
- To be the first to receive protection in disaster
- To be protected from neglect, cruelty, and exploitation
- To be brought up in a spirit of friendship among people

*Caremap is a registered trademark of the Center for Case Management, Inc., South Natick, MA 01760; phone: 508-651-2600.

care. The nurse uses this knowledge to adapt care for the child and the family.

As nurses care for children and families, they must demonstrate *caring,* compassion, and empathy for others. Aspects of caring include atraumatic care and the development of a therapeutic relationship. Parents perceive caring as a sign of quality nursing care, which is often focused on the nontechnical needs of the child and family. Parents describe "personable" care as nursing actions that include acknowledging the parent's presence, listening, making the parent feel comfortable, involving both the parent and the child in care, showing interest and concern for their welfare, communicating with them, and individualizing the nursing care. Parents perceive "personable" nursing care as an integral of a positive relationship.

The nurse is aware of the needs of children and works with all caregivers to ensure that these needs are met. This often requires the nurse to expand the boundaries of practice to less traditional settings. The nurse may be involved in education, political or legislative change, rehabilitation, screening, administration, and even engineering and architecture. Regardless of how removed from direct patient care nurses become, they must continue to foster health care practices that promote the well-being of children and that incorporate knowledge of child growth and development. For example, as educators, nurses are responsible for helping others learn about and care for children. Their audience may be other nurses, parents, teachers, other members of the health team, or the community at large.

Disease Prevention/Health Promotion

Current health care focuses on prevention of illness and maintenance of health, rather than treatment of disease or disability. Nursing has kept pace with this change. In 1965 pediatric nurse practitioner (PNP) programs were developed and led to several specialized ambulatory or primary care roles for nurses. Today, these programs provide education for nurses beyond the basic undergraduate preparation in areas of child health maintenance. Practitioner programs now prepare PNPs in areas such as school health, acute care, and oncology. Although the curriculum varies, the course content includes history-taking, physical diagnosis, growth and development, health education, pharmacology, counseling, common childhood problems, and care planning for individuals and groups. These programs are an integral part of graduate nursing education, and graduates from these programs provide high-quality care to children.

The clinical nurse specialist (CNS) role was developed in an attempt to provide expert nursing care. Today, the CNS serves as a role model for clinical practice, a researcher to validate nursing observations and interventions, a change agent within the health care system, and a consultant/teacher to the health care team. The CNS is competent in providing nursing care during all stages of illness or wellness and functions in any setting where patients are found—the hospital, home, community, clinic, or long-term care facility. The CNS role has developed within each of the traditional specialty areas, as well as subspecialties, such as cardiovascular, oncology, and neurology. Like the PNP role, the educational preparation for the CNS includes a graduate degree in nursing. Some graduate programs combine the PNP and CNS roles. Both PNPs and CNSs are commonly called advanced nurse practitioners (ANPs) or advanced registered nurse practitioners (ARNPs).

Every nurse who is involved with caring for children must practice preventive health. The best approach to prevention is education and anticipatory guidance. In this text, each chapter on health promotion also includes sections on anticipatory guidance. An appreciation of the hazards of each developmental period enables the nurse to guide parents regarding childrearing practices that are aimed at preventing potential problems. One significant example is safety. Because children of every age are at risk for injury, education of the parents is essential to decrease disability and prevent death.

Prevention also involves less obvious aspects of care such as promoting mental health. For example, it is not sufficient to administer immunizations without regard for the psychologic trauma associated with administering them.

Health Teaching

Health teaching is inseparable from family advocacy and prevention. Health teaching may be direct, as during parenting classes, or indirect, as when nurses help parents and children to understand a diagnosis or treatment, encourage children to ask questions about their bodies, refer families to health-related professional or lay groups, supply appropriate literature, and provide anticipatory guidance. To be effective health teachers, nurses need preparation and practice with competent role models. Health education involves transmitting information at the child's and family's level of understanding. Effective educators also focus on giving appropriate feedback and evaluation to promote learning.

Support/Counseling

Attention to emotional needs requires support and sometimes counseling. The role of child advocate or health teacher is supportive because this role requires an individualized approach. Support can be offered by listening, by touching, and through physical presence. Touching and physical presence are helpful with children because these interventions facilitate nonverbal communication.

Counseling involves a mutual exchange of ideas and opinions that provides the basis for mutual problem solving. It involves support, teaching, fostering expression of feelings or thoughts, and helping families to cope with stress. Optimally, counseling not only helps to resolve a crisis or problem but also enables the family to attain a higher level of functioning, greater self-esteem, and closer relationships. Although advanced practice nurses frequently do most of the formal counseling of parents and children, counseling techniques are discussed in this text to help students and nurses cope with immediate crises and refer families for additional professional assistance.

Coordination/Collaboration

The nurse, as a member of the health team, collaborates and coordinates nursing services with the activities of other professionals. Working in isolation does not serve the child's best interest. The concept of "holistic care" can only be realized through a unified interdisciplinary approach. Being aware of individual contributions and limitations to the child's care, the nurse collaborates with other specialists to provide high-quality health services. Failure to recognize limitations can be nontherapeutic and perhaps destructive. For example, the nurse who feels competent in counseling but who is really inadequate in this area may not only prevent the child from dealing with a crisis but also impede future success with a qualified professional.

Even nurses who practice in isolated geographic areas separated from other health professionals are not totally independent. Every nurse works interdependently with the child and family, collaborating on needs and interventions so the final care plan is one that truly meets the child's needs. Unfortunately, collaboration and coordination with the child and the family is sometimes lacking in health care planning. Numerous disciplines often work together to formulate a comprehensive approach without consulting the child and the family. The nurse is in a vital position to include the child and family members in their care, either directly or indirectly, by communicating their thoughts to the health team.

Ethical Decision Making

Ethical dilemmas arise when competing moral considerations underlie various alternatives. Parents, nurses, physicians, and other health care team members may reach different but morally defensible decisions by assigning different weight to the competing moral values. These competing moral values may include *autonomy,* the patient's right to be self-governing; *nonmaleficence,* the obligation to minimize or prevent harm; *beneficence,* the obligation to promote the patient's well-being; and *justice,* the concept of fairness (Cornelison, 1998; Salvatore & Baxter, 1998). Nurses must determine the most beneficial or least harmful action within the framework of societal mores, professional practice standards, the law, institutional rules, religious traditions, the family's value system, and the nurse's personal values.

When ethical conflicts occur, nurses may experience conflicting loyalties to their profession, colleagues, patients and families, institutions, and society. The nurse's role in ethical decision making can be ambiguous. A nurse may be obliged to carry out procedures that are based on physician orders or hospital policy but inconsistent with the patient's best interest. Often members of the health care team do not seek the nurse's input, leaving the nurse with incomplete information or without a voice in clinical decision making.

The role of nurses as members of the health care team justifies their participation in collaborative ethical decision making. Nurses routinely use a systematic problem-solving method, the *nursing process,* to resolve clinical problems. Using the nursing process, the nurse collects pertinent physiologic and psychosocial data, assesses relevant values held by the patient and family, and incorporates data into a plan of care. Each of these activities is a crucial component of ethical decision making.

Nurses spend most of their time in direct patient care, and are in a unique position to provide insight about the child's condition and response to therapy. They also assist families by interpreting information about the child's condition, prognosis, and treatment options, and by facilitating informed decisions. Because of their relationship to families, nurses represent children's and parents' values, beliefs, and preferences. Nurses also serve as the liaison between the family and other health team members.

In their practice, nurses use a professional code of ethics for guidance and professional self-regulation. The Code of Ethics for Nurses with Interpretive Statements (American Nurses Association, 2001) focuses on the nurse's accountability and responsibility to the client and emphasizes the nurse's role as an independent professional with legal liability (Box 29-4).

Nurses must prepare themselves for collaborative ethical decision making. This is accomplished through formal coursework, continuing education, and contemporary literature and by working in environments that are conducive to ethical discourse. Nurses must be aware of mechanisms for conflict resolution, case review by ethics committees, procedural safeguards, state statutes, and case law.

Research and Evidence-Based Practice

Practicing nurses should contribute to research because they are the individuals observing human responses to health and illness. Unfortunately, few nurses systematically analyze their observations. Pediatric nurses often devise innovative methods to encourage children to comply with treatments. When nurses evaluate these clinical interventions and share them with other nurses in research publications, nursing practice becomes based on empirical data or science, not tradition or trial and error.

The emphasis on promoting evidence-based practice by developing measurable outcomes to determine the efficacy of interventions (often in relation to the cost) demands that nurses know whether clinical interventions result in positive outcomes for their clients. The current trend toward *evidence-based practice* also necessitates that nurses question *why* an intervention is effective and *if* there is a better approach. The concept of evidence-based practice involves analyzing and translating published clinical research into everyday nursing practice. When nurses base their practice

BOX 29-4

Standard 12: American Nurses Association: Ethics

The nurse integrates ethical provisions in all areas of practice.

Measurement Criteria

The nurse:

1. Delivers care in a manner that preserves/protects patient autonomy, dignity, and rights.
2. Maintains patient confidentiality within legal and regulatory parameters.
3. Serves as a patient advocate, assisting patients in developing skills for self-advocacy.
4. Maintains a therapeutic and professional patient-nurse relationship with appropriate professional role boundaries.
5. Demonstrates a commitment to practicing self-care, managing stress, and connecting with self and others.
6. Contributes to resolving ethical issues of patients, colleagues, or systems.
7. Reports illegal, incompetent, or impaired practices.

Modified from American Nurses Association. *Nursing: scope and standards of practice,* Washington, DC, 2004, American Nurses Association.

on science and research and document clinical outcomes, they validate their contributions to health not only for clients, third-party payers, and institutions, but also for the nursing profession (Freda, 1998). Evaluation is essential to the nursing process, and research is one of the best ways to accomplish it.

Health Care Planning

Today, the nurse's role has expanded beyond the nucleus of the family to include the community-based health-driven system. Traditionally, nurses were involved in public health either on a continuous or an episodic basis. Nurses were involved in health care planning on a political or legislative level less frequently. Future nurses will need to incorporate a political component into their professional identity and attempt to influence the decision-making body of government.*

As the largest health care profession, nursing has a valuable voice, especially as family/consumer advocate. Nurses must become aware of community needs, interested in the formulation of bills, and supportive of politicians to ensure passage (or rejection) of significant legislation. Nurses also need to become actively involved with groups that are dedicated to the welfare of children (e.g., professional nursing societies, parent-teacher organizations, parent support groups, and volunteer organizations).

Health care planning involves not only providing new services to children and their families but also promoting the highest quality in existing services. In addition to following the Code of Ethics for Nurses, nurses ensure excellence in their profession by following standards of practice. A *standard of practice* is the level of performance that is expected of a professional. In the past, pediatric nursing has not had national or international standards of care or education. Most pediatric nurses often merged with other specialties within nursing and followed the Standards of Maternal-Child Health Nursing or the standards of several of the pediatric specialties, such as pediatric oncology nursing or school nursing.† However, as the theoretic, practice, and research bases for pediatric nursing mature, the need for standards of practice for all basic pediatric nurses and for advanced practice registered nurses has become more evident. In 2003, the Society of Pediatric Nurses and the American Nurses Association published the *Scope and Standards of Pediatric Nursing*. This document identifies standards of practice that are congruent with current professional policy for both the nurse generalist and the advanced pediatric nurse.‡

Throughout the text the highest standards of nursing practice are reflected in the emphasis on thorough assessment, the focus on scientific rationale as the basis for care, the summary of nursing care goals and responsibilities, and the comprehensive discussion of growth and development.

Future Trends

The present shift from treatment of disease to promotion of health has expanded nurses' roles in ambulatory care and highlighted the prevention and health teaching aspects of nursing practice. Prospective payment and the need for home care and community health services require nurses to be more independent and to acquire skills that are useful in settings beyond the hospital. These trends are illustrated throughout the text, with increased emphasis on prevention through anticipatory guidance, child health and family assessment, and discharge planning and care in the home and community. As changing social policy shapes the expanding health care arena, the focus of nursing care is no longer on what we do *for* families, but what we do *in partnership with* them. The philosophy of family-centered care is no longer an option, but a mandate.

Today, technologic advances and the demand for computer knowledge in the work setting are obvious. The current shortage of nurses will persist into the future, and the pressure to create positions in the health care system that do not require a nursing background will become more intense. As new categories of workers enter the health care field, nurses must continue to update their knowledge of technology and prove their unique contribution to health care. Nurses must utilize technology and learn to work collaboratively with unlicensed assistive personnel. *Unlicensed assistive personnel (UAP)* "are individuals who are trained to function in an assistive role to the registered professional nurse in the provision of [student] care activities as delegated by and under the supervision of the registered professional nurse" (American Nurses Association, 1994).

NURSE ALERT When the registered nurse (RN) determines that someone who is not licensed to practice nursing can safely provide a selected nursing activity or task for a patient and delegates that activity to the individual, the RN remains responsible and legally accountable for the care provided. ■

Changing demographics will also influence pediatric nursing. Although the actual number of children under age 18 years will increase to an estimated 78 million in 2020, their relative importance in terms of the proportion of the total population will decrease from 26% to 24%. In the future, the adult population will grow faster than the pediatric population. The number of younger children will decrease, but the number of older children will increase. Racial composition of the population will also change. The number of whites in the population will decrease, whereas the number of individuals in minority groups will increase. The largest increases will occur in the number of Hispanic and Asian births. The impact of these changes will be an increase in the problems of adolescents and minority groups. Because the elderly will make up a larger percentage of the population, health care dollars will be split between the youngest and oldest groups, with shrinking resources to meet the needs of both. Nurses will

---

*The following are sources of information on government issues: White House Comment Line: 202-456-1111, 9 AM–5 PM eastern standard time; White House fax: 202-456-2461; White House e-mail: president@whitehouse.gov.

†Available from the Association of Pediatric Oncology Nurses, 4700 W. Lake Ave, Glenview, IL 60025-1485; phone: 847-375-4724; fax: 877-734-8755; and the National Association of School Nurses, Lamplighter Lane, PO Box 1300, Scarborough, ME 04074; phone: 207-883-2117; Web site: www.nasn.org.

‡For more information on the *Scope and Standards of Pediatric Nursing*, contact the Society of Pediatric Nurses, 7794 Grow Drive, Pensacola, FL 32514-7172; phone: 1-800-723-2902; fax: 850-484-8762; Web site: www.pedsnurses.org.

need to be aware of developments in adolescent medicine and to continually adapt their care to the cultural milieu in which they practice. Finally, cost containment will present an ever-present challenge to providing quality care.

Key Points

- *Healthy People 2010* broadened the health care objectives of the past and focuses on prevention as the method to accomplish health goals.
- Infant mortality rate in the United States is at an all-time low, but the nation continues to lag behind other major countries.
- Low birth weight, which is closely related to early gestational age, is the leading cause of neonatal death in the United States.
- Injuries are the leading cause of death in children over age 1 year, with the majority being motor vehicle injuries.
- Childhood morbidity encompasses acute illness, chronic disease, and disability.
- Eighty percent of childhood illness is attributable to infections, with respiratory tract infections occurring two to three times as often as all other illnesses combined.
- The "new morbidity" refers to behavioral, social, and educational problems that can significantly alter a child's health.
- Developmental stage and environment are important factors in the prevalence of injuries at every age and should guide injury preventive measures.
- During the early 1900s public health initiatives such as environmental strategies to control infection and the development of antibiotics were the major advances leading to decreased childhood deaths.
- During the late 1900s the advancement and application of medical knowledge and technology, specifically in the care of high risk and low-birth-weight newborns, lowered the number of deaths in children, especially the neonatal mortality rate.
- The work of Lillian Wald, a social reformer, had far-reaching effects on child health and nursing. She started visiting nurse services in New York City and was instrumental in establishing the role of the first full-time school nurse.
- The philosophy of family-centered care recognizes the family as the constant in a child's life and that service systems and personnel must support, respect, encourage, and enhance the strength and competence of the family.
- Atraumatic care is the provision of therapeutic care in settings, by personnel, and through the use of interventions that eliminate or minimize the psychologic and physical distress experienced by children and their families in the health care system.
- Managed care is a health care delivery system that attempts to balance cost and quality through a network of health care providers and predetermined prospective payment for services.
- Roles of the pediatric nurse include establishing a therapeutic relationship, family advocacy, disease prevention/health promotion, health teaching, support-counseling, coordination/collaboration of care, ethical decision making, research, and health care planning.
- With the shift in focus from treatment of disease to promotion of health, nurses' roles are expanding beyond traditional health care facilities into ambulatory care centers, schools, the family's home, and the community.
- Changing demographics in the United States will result in greater significance of adolescents' and minority groups' problems and decreasing resources for health care.
- Critical thinking is purposeful, goal-directed thinking based on rational and deliberate thought.
- The process of nursing children and families includes accurate and complete *assessment,* analysis of assessment data to arrive at a *nursing diagnosis, planning* of care, *implementation* of the plan, and *evaluation* of interventions.

References

Altemeier WA: Prevention of pediatric injuries: so much to do, so little time, *Pediatr Ann* 29(6):324-325, 2000.

American Nurses Association: *Registered professional nurses and unlicensed assistive personnel,* Washington, DC, 1994, American Nurses Association Publishing.

American Nurses Association: *Code of ethics for nurses with interpretive statements,* Washington, DC, 2001, American Nurses Association Publishing.

American Nurses Association, Nursing's Social Policy Statement Revision Task Force: *Nursing's social policy statement, 2003,* Washington, DC, 2003, American Nurses Association Publishing.

Anderson RN, Smith BL: Deaths: leading causes for 2001, *Natl Vital Stat Rep* 52(9):1-85, 2003.

Annie E Casey Foundation: *Kids count data book: state profiles of child well-being,* Washington, DC, 2001, Center for the Study of Social Policy.

Arias E et al: Annual summary of vital statistics—2002, *Pediatrics* 112(6):1215-1230, 2003.

Cornelison AH: A profile of ethical principles, *J Pediatr Nurs* 13(6):383-386, 1998.

Freda MC: Toward evidence-based practice, *MCN* 23:177, 1998.

Galvin E et al: Challenging the precepts of family-centered care: testing a philosophy, *Pediatr Nurs* 26(6):625-632, 2000.

Guyer B et al: Annual summary of vital statistics: trends in the health of Americans during the 20th century, *Pediatrics* 106(6):1307-1317, 2000.

Lears MK, Guth KJ, Lewandowski L: International adoption: a primer for pediatric nurses, *Pediatr Nurs* 24:578-586, 1998.

Minino AM, Smith BL: Deaths, preliminary data for 2000, *Natl Vital Stat Rep* 49(12): 1-40, 2001.

Minino AM et al: Deaths: final data for 2000, *Natl Vital Stat Rep* 50(15): 1-119, 2002.

National Safety Council: *Injury facts, 2000 edition,* Itaska, IL, 2000, National Safety Council.

Newton MS: Family-centered care: current realities in parent participation, *Pediatr Nurs* 26(2):164-168, 2000.

Peternelj-Taylor C: Professional boundaries. a matter of therapeutic integrity, *J Psychosoc Nurs Ment Health Serv* 40(4):22-29, 2002.

Rushton CH, McEnhill M, Armstrong L: Establishing therapeutic boundaries as patient advocates, *Pediatr Nurs* 22(3):185-189, 1996.

Salvatore T, Baxter T: *Administrative ethics: a guide for home care providers,* Springfield, PA, 1998, HCMA Ltd.

Szilagy P: Managed care for children: effect on access to care and utilization of health, *Future Child* 8(2, summer):39-60, 1998.

Wong D: Principles of atraumatic care. In Feeg V (ed): *Pediatric nursing: forum on the future: looking toward the 21st century,* Pitman, NJ, 1989, Anthony J Jannetti.

30 Community-Based Nursing Care of the Child and Family

LEARNING OBJECTIVES

On completion of this chapter the reader will be able to:

- Define *community nursing.*
- Describe community health nursing.
- Identify the roles and functions of the community health nurse.
- Discuss selected aspects of the epidemiologic process.
- Explain the purpose of an economic evaluation.
- Discuss the components of the community nursing process.

ELECTRONIC RESOURCES

Additional information related to the content in Chapter 30 can be found on

the companion website at evolve
http://evolve.elsevier.com/Wong/maternal/
- NCLEX Review Questions
- WebLinks

or the interactive student CD-ROM
Activities for Chapter 30 include the following:
- NCLEX Review Questions

NURSING IN THE COMMUNITY

The health of children and their families is greatly influenced by their community, and nurses can make a significant contribution by working with the community to promote children's heath. Nurses working with pediatric populations in the community need an understanding of the concepts and processes critical to address pediatric concerns from a community health perspective. Healthy communities provide not only excellent medical care; they also provide children a nurturing, safe place in which to live and grow. Healthy communities address concerns through collaboration between and among citizens, health care providers, businesses, and governmental and private agencies (Flynn & Ivanov, 2000).

In this chapter, community health nursing is discussed as it relates to children. First it identifies and defines the concepts and principles that serve as the basis of community health nursing. Then it describes the community health nursing process, step by step. It concludes by using the process to address a very real child health concern, immunization status.

COMMUNITY CONCEPTS

There are several ways to define a community. A *community* is a group of individuals with shared characteristics or interests who interact with each other (Allender & Spradley, 2001). A community is a system that includes children and families, the physical environment, educational facilities, safety and transportation resources, political and governmental agencies, health and social services, communication resources, economic resources, and recreational facilities. The community is also the client of the community health nurse (Anderson & McFarlane, 2000). Community health initiatives are directed at either the general health of the community as a whole or at specific populations within the community that have unique needs. In this context, *populations* can be described as groups of people who live in a community, for example, school-age children. *Target populations* or *subpopulations* are more narrowly defined groups (e.g., nonimmunized preschoolers, or obese middle school children) toward whom nurses direct activities in order to improve the health status of individuals in the group. Common values often guide behaviors of populations and subpopulations in relation to health promotion and disease prevention (Williams, 2000).

Community care involves a collaboration of individuals and groups including health care providers, advocates, government, managed care organizations, businesses, children, and families within a specific community. The goal of the collaborative effort is to provide services that promote the child health initiatives of *Healthy People 2010* (see the *Healthy People 2010* Web site at www.healthypeople.gov). Community care is "without walls" in that the services of the health care system are frequently redesigned to meet the changing needs of the community. Those involved in community care partner with the community to identify, plan, intervene, and evaluate activities that improve the health of the community (Anderson & McFarlane, 2000).

Community health nursing focuses on promoting and maintaining the health of individuals, families, and groups in the community setting. Community health nursing is a synthesis of nursing and public health. It collaborates with other disciplines to assess, plan, and implement care that emphasizes personal responsibility for health and self-care by community members (Allender & Spradley, 2001; Williams, 2000). Community health nursing, at its best, empowers communities by enabling community members to gain the knowledge and skills needed to fulfill their own needs.

Although community health concepts can be used to address health concerns in any setting, traditional community health settings include the following: home health agencies, schools, doctors' offices, ambulatory health clinics, emergency rooms, triage call centers, insurance agencies, health departments, international relief agencies, health education agencies, juvenile detention facilities, camps, day care centers, foster care facilities, and rehabilitation agencies. The American Nurses Association (1986) has established nine standards for community health nursing to guide practice across settings. They include the following categories: theory, data collection, diagnosis, planning, intervention, evaluation, quality assurance and professional development, interdisciplinary collaboration, and research.

The *roles and functions* of the community health nurse continue to evolve. In the future, more pediatric nurses will be working in community settings. The Health Resources and Services Administration (2001) reported that 18.3% of the total registered nurse workforce was employed in a community or public health setting and 9.5% in ambulatory care. Only 59% of registered nurses were employed in hospital settings.

Traditionally, the roles and functions of community health nurses included caregiver, advocate, case manager, case finder, counselor, educator, epidemiologist, group process leader, health planner, and manager (Clemen-Stone, McGuire, & Eigsti, 1998). For example, the nurse employed in a pediatric outpatient clinic will function in a number of roles to provide care to a child with type 2 diabetes. The nurse provides case management by coordinating care between the disciplines, provides counsel by supporting the child and family through developmental crises, and acts as a case finder by identifying risk factors in the child's siblings.

The Institute of Medicine developed a list of *core functions* to guide the work of public health professionals, including nurses. The core functions are directed to population-wide services and to personal and home services for people at risk (Institute of Medicine, 1988). The population-wide service is based on assessment of health status monitoring and disease *surveillance, policy development,* and *assurance* that policies are translated into service. A certain skill set has been identified as important for the nurse in a public health setting. Some of the skills needed include the ability to analyze data, measure health status, connect people to organizations, bring about change in organizations, build strength in diversity, build coalitions, develop interdisciplinary teams, and devise approaches to quality improvement (Gebbie & Hwang, 2000). Consequently, the pediatric nurse employed in a managed care environment may be asked to develop a creative approach to teaching children with asthma about peak flow meters during an emergency department visit. Included in the request may be a mechanism for evaluating the cost of the approach and the occurrence of repeated emergency department visits.

NURSE ALERT Nurses must be able to communicate and work with professionals from other disciplines. This includes being able to understand the terms used by demographers, epidemiologists, and economists. ■

Demography

Demography is the study of population characteristics. *Demographic characteristics* include age, gender, race/ethnicity, socioeconomic status, and education. Individuals, families, and communities may have demographic characteristics that affect their health risks (Anderson & McFarlane, 2000). *Risk* is an increased probability of developing a disease, injury, or illness. Age is one of the most important risk factors for disease prevention and certain health conditions. For example, children under age 5 years are more likely to have respiratory infections than children ages 5 to 17, and those of the older age group are more likely to suffer fractures and dislocations than children under age 5 years (Institute of Medicine, 1998). Gender also plays an important role. Males are at much greater risk of having hemophilia A and B than females. Race/ethnicity has long been associated with increased risk for disease and disability, but it is now thought that, aside from genetic predisposition, there is a complicated relationship between minority status and socioeconomic status that increases the risk for disease and disability (Smith, 2000). Low socioeconomic status predisposes children to a variety of problems. Poor children are more likely to be hospitalized for pneumonia, asthma, dehydration, and gastroenteritis than children from affluent families (Institute of Medicine,1998). They are less likely to be immunized against childhood illnesses (Ortega et al, 2000).

Epidemiology

Epidemiology is the science of population health applied to the detection of morbidity and mortality in a population. The epidemiologic process identifies the distribution and causes of disease or injury across a population (Anderson & McFarlane, 2000). It also serves as an important component in developing health programs. For example, *Healthy People 2010* incorporated the process to develop a set of health objectives for the United States. Health professionals in community, state, and national health care organizations use the objectives as a guide to develop programs that have the greatest impact on the health of children.

Distribution of Disease, Injury, or Illness

Morbidity rates are used to measure disease and injury, and, along with *natality and mortality rates,* they present an objective picture of the health status of a community. There are two types of morbidity rates: incidence and prevalence. *Incidence* measures the occurrence of new events in a population during a period of time. *Prevalence* measures existing events in a population during a period of time (Hennekens & Buring, 1987). For example, the incidence of type 1 diabetes in a community is estimated by counting the new cases of type 1 diabetes in a population and dividing that figure by the population at risk. The prevalence of type 1 diabetes is estimated by counting the existing cases of type 1 diabetes in a population and dividing that figure by the population at risk. Both incidence and prevalence are usually given as rates per 1000, 10,000, or 100,000 population, depending on their frequency. Box 30-1 presents frequently used mortality and morbidity rates.

Epidemiologic Triangle

Three factors form the epidemiologic triangle, and their interrelationship alters the risk of acquiring a disease or condition (McKeown & Weinrich, 2000). These factors are agent, host, and environment (Fig. 30-1).

An *agent* is responsible for causing a disease and may be an infectious agent, such as *Mycobacterium tuberculosis;* a chemical agent, such as lead in paint; or a physical agent, such as fire. *Host factors* are those that are specific to an individual or group. These may be genetic factors, which cannot be controlled, or they can be lifestyle factors, such as food selections or exercise patterns. *Environmental factors* provide a setting for the host and include the climatic conditions in which the host lives, as well as factors related to the home, neighborhood, and school.

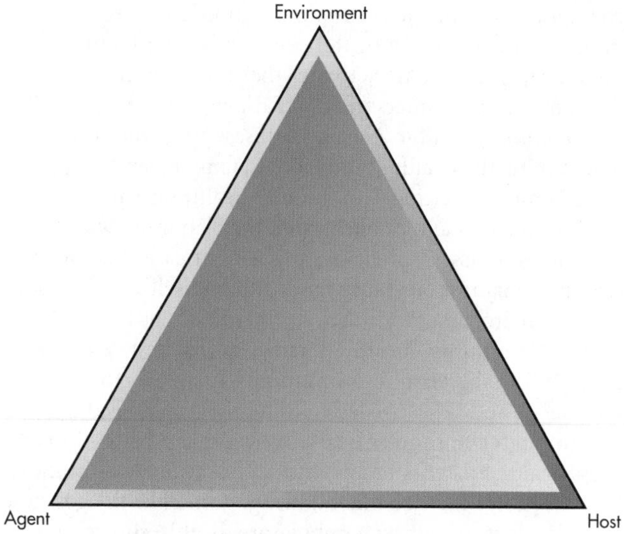

Fig. 30-1 The epidemiologic triangle.

BOX 30-1

Frequently Used Mortality and Morbidity Rates

Crude Birth Rate

$$\frac{\text{Number of births in a population}}{\text{Total population}} \text{ within a time period} \times 1000$$

Crude Death Rate

$$\frac{\text{Number of deaths in a population}}{\text{Total population}} \text{ within a time period} \times 1000$$

Cause-specific Death Rate

$$\frac{\text{Number of deaths in a population due to a certain disease}}{\text{Total population}} \text{ within a time period} \times 1000$$

Age-specific Death Rate

$$\frac{\text{Number of deaths in a population in a certain age group}}{\text{Total population in that age group}} \text{ within a time period} \times 1000$$

Incidence of Disease

$$\frac{\text{Number of new events in a population}}{\text{Total at-risk population}} \text{ within a time period} \times 1000$$

Prevalence of Disease

$$\frac{\text{Number of existing events in a population}}{\text{Total at-risk population}} \text{ within a time period} \times 1000$$

From National Center for Health Statistics: www.cdc.gov/nchs.

Levels of Prevention

Community health programs are based on three classic levels of prevention (Leavell & Clark, 1965). *Primary prevention* focuses on health promotion and prevention of disease or injury. Examples of primary prevention activities include well-child care clinics, immunization programs, safety programs (bike helmets, car seats, seat belts, childproof containers), nutrition programs, environmental efforts (clean air programs), sanitation measures (chlorinated water, garbage removal, sewage treatment), and community parenting classes. *Secondary prevention* focuses on screening and early diagnosis of disease. Examples of secondary interventions include tuberculosis and lead screening programs and mental health counseling for stressful events such as separation, divorce, death, or community natural disasters (e.g., earthquakes, floods, and hurricanes). *Tertiary prevention* focuses on optimizing function for children with a disability or chronic disease. Tertiary interventions include rehabilitation and disease management programs for asthma, sickle cell disease, cancer, anorexia, and special education programs for children.

Screening

Community health nurses are frequently involved in *screening,* a secondary prevention activity. The purpose of screening is to detect and treat disease early in the period of pathogenesis in order to prevent the spread and progression of the disease (Wilson & Jungner, 1968). However, screening is not appropriate for every condition. In a classic article, Wilson and Jungner (1968) described 10 principles that will help the nurse determine whether or not a screening program will be useful (Box 30-2). Although screening may bring benefit there is a certain amount of risk associated with any intervention. In the case of screening, there is the psy-

BOX 30-2

Principles of Early Disease Detection

1. The condition sought should be an important health problem.
2. There should be an accepted treatment for patients with recognized disease.
3. Facilities for diagnosis and treatment should be available.
4. There should be a recognizable latent or early symptomatic stage.
5. There should be a suitable test or examination.
6. The test should be acceptable to the population.
7. The natural history of the condition, including development from latent to declared disease, should be adequately understood.
8. There should be an agreed policy on whom to treat as patients.
9. The cost of case finding (including diagnosis and treatment of patients diagnosed) should be economically balanced in relation to possible expenditures on medical care as a whole.
10. Case finding should be a continuing process and not a "once and for all" project.

From Wilson JMG, Jungner G: *Principles and practice of screening for disease: public health papers 34,* Geneva, 1968, World Health Organization. Reprinted with permission.

chologic risk associated with false-positive results, as well as the danger that a parent may treat a child differently because of early identification of a disease (Clayton, 1999; Kwon & Farrell, 2000). A great deal of planning is required to ensure that the benefits of screening exceed the risks and cost.

Economics

A basic understanding of the *economics* of health care is essential because it enables the nurse to participate in decision making about the worth of children's health programs. Economists theorize that individuals and societies view health as a basic utility, that is, something that is perceived as valuable (Gold et al, 1996). Other basic utilities are food, shelter, and clothing. People are willing to trade resources, such as money and time, for a program or intervention that will improve their health. Economists measure the amount of resources individuals and communities are willing to pay for good health. They also examine how different groups prioritize health care needs and allocate health care dollars. Methods for defining and estimating cost have been well described, as has the need for a standardized approach to the measurement of cost and effects (Brosnan & Swint, 2001; Drummond et al, 1997).

Economic evaluation provides objective information to establish the value of a program to the community. An example is the evaluation of a school-based hepatitis B vaccination program by Wilson (2000). He concluded that the percentage of vaccinated sixth graders increased from 8% without the program to 82% with the program. The higher vaccination rate potentially saved money that might have eventually been spent to treat these children for hepatitis, cirrhosis, or cancer in the future. The program resulted in potential cost savings of $24 million when compared with the no-program alternative.

COMMUNITY NURSING PROCESS

In community nursing, the focus of the nursing process shifts from the individual child and family to the community or target population (Box 30-3). The stages of the process (assessment and diagnosis, planning, intervention, and evaluation) are similar whether the client is one child or a population of children; only the type of interventions and indicators of wellness and illness differ (Anderson & McFarlane, 2000). *Assessment* is focused on collecting subjective and objective information about the target population in order to *diagnose* problems based on community needs. *Planning* involves the development of community-centered goals. During the *intervention* stage the nurse works with the community to implement a program that enables members to reach their goals. Finally, the nurse *evaluates* whether or not the goals were met. Community nursing is collaborative, and the nurse is one member of a community team that includes other health professionals, educators, politicians, religious leaders, members of public and voluntary organizations, and consumers. The role of the nurse depends on the scope of the project, the target population, and the expertise of team members. For instance, the school nurse may assume a leadership role in planning for the health needs of elementary school children and serve as a panel member on a citywide committee assessing environmental pollution.

Community Needs Assessment

The assessment phase of the community nursing process is called a *community needs assessment.* Assessment involves the collection of *subjective and objective information* about a community. Subjective information indicates what community members say are their most important needs and can be determined in a number of ways. One way is to distribute questionnaires to a sample of people living in the community. Another way is to interview community members directly, phoning or meeting with individuals who represent the group or who have a special role in the group. Community leaders are an example of people who have a special role.

Objective information is data that the nurse collects either by direct observation or through written sources. A "windshield tour" is one method of direct observation. Nurses drive through a neighborhood and take notes about

BOX 30-3

The Community Nursing Process

Assessment and diagnosis: The nurse collects subjective and objective information about a community and develops a diagnosis based on community needs and problems.
Planning: The nurse develops community-centered goals to address the identified needs and problems.
Intervention: The nurse implements a program that enables community members to reach their goals.
Evaluation: The nurse conducts a systematic evaluation to determine that goals and program objectives were met.

the environment, including the appearance of houses, the presence of sidewalks and gutters, the number of public areas, and so on. Objective information about the health status of the community can also be obtained from such sources as the the local chamber of commerce, the U.S. Census Bureau, libraries, state health departments, and the Internet sites of voluntary health organizations or government agencies. Information about service agencies can be found in resource directories. Resource directories include the local telephone book, community resource directories compiled by such organizations as the United Way, and population-specific books provided by public and voluntary agencies.

One way to organize an assessment is to use a guide that lists community systems that need to be examined. This process is similar to using a physical assessment guide to examine the different body systems in an individual patient. Anderson and McFarlane (2000) described eight community systems that the nurse should examine: health and social services, communication, recreation, physical environment, education, safety and transportation, politics and government, and economics. During the assessment the nurse studies how well each component in the community functions and interacts to meet the health needs of children, identifies the strengths of the community, and determines whether any barriers disrupt the components and prevent access to care for children and their families.

Once the assessment is completed the community nurse collaborates with team members to analyze the results of surveys and questionnaires, determine if the needs described by community members can be met by existing community agencies, and identify individuals at highest risk. During the analysis the demographic characteristics, the morbidity rates, and the mortality rates in the community are compared with a standard. Comparisons can be made on the basis of time or place. In time comparisons, the nurse contrasts the rates in the current year with the rates during an earlier period. In comparisons of place, the nurse contrasts the rates in the community with a standard population. Standard rates may come from another community or from city, state, or national rates. For example, the rate of tuberculosis in a group of preschool children in the community in 2002 could be compared with the rate of tuberculosis in preschool children in the state in 2002.

A *community health diagnosis* is the reflection of health status, risks, or needs as determined by a causative agent. The format of a community diagnosis is similar to an individual nursing diagnosis with a problem (need) and an etiology related to that problem (causative agent). An example of a community nursing diagnosis is "Child abuse related to a violent environment" (Visiting Nurse Association of Omaha, 1986).

NURSE ALERT All communities have strengths and limitations. The community health nurse draws on the strengths of a community to solve problems. ■

Community Planning

The nurse collaborates with community members in developing a plan that addresses the needs and problems of the target population. To maximize the use of community resources, problems should first be prioritized on the basis of their severity, the felt needs of the community, and the ability of the community nurse to bring about change. Once the problems are prioritized, the nurse works with community members to develop at least one goal for each problem the members will address. *Goals* are outcomes that give direction to interventions and provide a measure of the change the interventions produced. Community interventions frequently take the form of *health programs* for improving the health status of the target population. Community health programs are based on the three levels of prevention: primary, secon-cxdary, and tertiary. For example, a goal for preventing bicycle injuries is, "Within 1 year all students in the first grade will wear bicycle helmets." The nurse and community members then plan a program that includes a health education program about bicycle safety for students and their parents (primary prevention).

The planning group considers the resources that are already available in the community and resources that will be needed for implementing a health program, including personnel, supplies and equipment, office space, phones, and computers. Decisions are made about the timeline of the program, the budget, and strategies that can be used to obtain funding. The nurse may also contact health professionals who have implemented successful programs in other communities; they can provide valuable, time-saving tips and suggestions. Program descriptions are found through professional contacts, in online resources, and by reviewing the literature. An example of a community assessment and planning project is presented in Box 30-4.

Community Intervention

During program implementation the nurse and community members carry out the intervention. Whether the program is simple or complex, oversight is needed to ensure that everyone involved is communicating with each other, following the guidelines of the plan, keeping within the timeline, and documenting daily activities and expenses. The documentation will prove invaluable during the evaluation phase of the process.

Community Evaluation

Evaluation identifies whether the goals and program objectives were met. There are various models of program evaluation. The structure, process, and outcomes method is commonly used by health care organizations. Donabedian (1980) described this approach as follows:

1. *Structure:* Where and by whom is the care delivered in a program?
2. *Process:* Was the care delivered using operational standards and within the financial guidelines of the program?
3. *Outcomes:* What was the effect on health status? Was there an improvement?

Structure focuses on the qualifications of personnel; the adequacy of buildings and offices, supplies, and equipment; and the characteristics of the target population.

BOX 30-4

An Example of Community Assessment and Planning

Meadowlark is an elementary school with 500 children in prekindergarten to sixth-grade classes. The school nurse has been asked to conduct a community assessment and develop a plan of care. The children who attend the school and their families are the target population.

Community Needs Assessment

The school nurse formed an alliance of community members, including parents, school faculty and staff, health care professionals, local religious leaders, and politicians. The group met at regularly scheduled intervals. Their first task was to complete the community assessment. The alliance members mailed questionnaires to a random sample of families and held focus groups with community members to obtain subjective information about the needs of the community. Alliance members obtained objective data from the local health department, school records, and the U.S. Census Bureau. The nurse also conducted a windshield tour of the neighborhood surrounding the school. The following information was collected:

People: Meadowlark is located in an ethnically diverse community composed of 30% Hispanics, 30% African-Americans, 30% non-Hispanic whites, and 10% Asians. It is located in a large southwestern city.

Safety and transportation: School bus service was rated very good to excellent by a majority of those surveyed. Transportation records indicated that the last school bus accident occurred 10 years ago.

Economics: Although at least one member was fully employed in 94% of the families living in the community, 25% of the families lived below the poverty level. The number below poverty had not changed in 10 years.

Education: Of the adult population, 60% had a high school diploma, and 10% had at least 1 year of college. School attendance was higher than overall state attendance rates.

Communication: 95% of homes had telephones compared with 85% 10 years ago. An estimated 10% of the target population did not speak English, and Spanish was the primary language spoken in this group.

Recreation: There were few places where small children were able to play. The focus groups recommended more parks and playgrounds.

Politics and government: The school system was strongly centralized and headed by a school superintendent. The city had a mayor and city council.

Social: Of families living below the poverty level, 60% received some type of welfare assistance, including food stamps.

Health: Immunization levels for children under 2 years of age were 60%, a decrease of 20% in 10 years. *Healthy People 2000* recommended that 90% of children in this group be fully immunized. Immunization levels of children under 4 years of age were 70%, a decrease of 5% in 10 years. The incidence rate of vaccine-preventable disease was 30 per 100,000 children less than 5 years of age compared with the national rate of 24 per 100,000 children less than 5 years of age (Teitelbaum & Edmunds, 1999). Responses from questionnaires and focus groups indicated that parents were not always aware of the importance of immunizations, that clinic locations were not well publicized, and that clinic hours were not convenient.

On the basis of this assessment, the following community diagnoses were made:

1. Decreased immunization levels related to knowledge deficit and barriers to access
2. Lack of safe play areas related to an insufficient number of community parks

Planning

Alliance members agreed that decreased immunization levels were a priority problem and developed the following goals:

1. Within 2 years immunization levels among children under 2 years of age will be 80%.
2. Within 4 years immunization levels of children under 4 years of age will be 90%.
3. Within 5 years the incidence of vaccine-preventable disease in the Meadowlark community will be 24 per 100,000 children under 5 years of age.

The alliance members searched the literature for communities that had experienced similar problems, contacted school and health department officials in other areas of the country, examined the results of successful programs, and planned a health program that addressed the unique needs of the target population. Program objectives were as follows:

1. Within 6 months each new mother will receive a pamphlet about the importance of immunizations before hospital discharge. Pamphlets will be available in Spanish and English.
2. Within 1 year auxiliary immunization sites will be established around the community at shopping centers and churches. Clinic hours will be expanded to include evenings and weekends.
3. Each September the nurse will address the school's parent association about the importance of timely immunizations.

The alliance members determined the amount of resources needed to implement the program, including personnel, supplies, and equipment. They estimated the total cost of setting up the program and maintaining it for 5 years and applied for funding to the city and state health departments. The school nurse and other alliance members assumed responsibility for the timely implementation of the health program and the evaluation of program objectives and goals.

Process focuses on the interaction of patients and providers. Process indicators include the number of people who attended a health education program, the number of pamphlets distributed, and the efficiency of the program. Outcome focuses on whether program objectives and community goals were met. Program evaluation should be ongoing so that performance improvement initiatives are monitored and so that an improvement in the way health care is delivered will affect the health status of the target population.

Key Points

- Caring for children within a community requires a multidisciplinary approach.
- Healthy communities provide children with not only quality medical care, but also a nurturing, safe place in which to live and grow.
- Community health nursing focuses on promoting and maintaining the health of individuals, families, and groups in the community setting.

- Individual families and communities may have demographic characteristics that affect their risk for disease or injury.
- Epidemiology is the science of population health applied to the detection of morbidity and mortality in a population.
- Community health programs are based on three levels of intervention: primary, secondary, and tertiary intervention.
- Economic evaluations provide objective information to establish the value of a program to society.
- A community needs assessment involves collection of subjective and objective information about the community.
- A community health diagnosis is a problem with a defined etiology related to a community problem.
- Program planning and implementation in the community require collaboration between the nurse and community members who are in positions to promote change.
- Evaluation of effective community programs includes consideration of the structure, process, and outcomes related to the program.

References

Allender JA, Spradley BW: *Community health nursing: concepts and practice,* Philadelphia, 2001, Lippincott Williams & Wilkins.

American Nurses Association: *Standards of community health nursing practice,* Kansas City, MO, 1986, American Nurses Association.

Anderson ET, McFarlane J: *Community as partner: theory and practice in nursing,* Phiadelphia, 2000, JB Lippincott.

Brosnan CA, Swint JM: Cost analysis: concepts and application, *Public Health Nurs* 18(1):13-18, 2001.

Clayton EW: What should be the role of public health in newborn screening and prenatal diagnosis? *Am J Prev Med* 16(2):111-115, 1999.

Clemen-Stone S, McGuire SL, Eigsti DG: *Comprehensive community health nursing,* St Louis, 1998, Mosby.

Donabedian A: *The definition of quality and approaches to its assessment,* Ann Arbor, MI, 1980, Health Administration Press.

Drummond MF et al: *Methods for the economic evaluation of health care programmes,* ed 2, New York, 1997, Oxford University Press.

Flynn BC, Ivanov LL: Health promotion through healthy cities. In Stanhope M, Lancaster J: *Community and public health nursing,* St Louis, 2000, Mosby.

Gebbie KM, Hwang I: Preparing currently employed public health nurses for changes in the health system, *Am J Public Health* 90(5): 716-721, 2000.

Gold MR et al: Identifying and valuing outcomes. In Gold MR et al (eds): *Cost-effectiveness in health and medicine,* New York, 1996, Oxford University Press.

Health Resources and Services Administration: *The registered nurse population,* Rockville, MD, 2001, US Department of Health and Human Services.

Hennekens CH, Buring JE: *Epidemiology in medicine,* Boston, 1987, Little, Brown.

Institute of Medicine: *The future of public health,* Washington, DC, 1988, National Academy Press.

Institute of Medicine: *America's children. Health insurance and access to care,* Washington, DC, 1998, National Academy Press.

Kwon C, Farrell PM: The magnitude and challenge of false-positive newborn screening test results, *Arch Pediatr Adolesc Med* 154:714-718, 2000.

Leavell HR, Clark EG: *Preventive medicine for the doctor in his community: an epidemiologic approach,* New York, 1965, McGraw-Hill.

McKeown RE, Weinrich SP: Epidemiologic applications. In Stanhope M, Lancaster J: *Community and public health nursing,* St Louis, 2000, Mosby.

Ortega NA et al: The impact of a pediatric medical home on immunization coverage, *Clin Pediatr* 39:89-96, 2000.

Smith GD: Learning to live with complexity: ethnicity, socioeconomic position, and health in Britain and the United States, *Am J Public Health* 90:1694-1698, 2000.

Teitelbaum MA, Edmunds M: Immunization and vaccine-preventable illness, United States, 1992 to 1997, *Stat Bull Metrop Insur Co* 80(2):13-20, 1999.

Visiting Nurse Association of Omaha: *Client management information system for community health nursing agencies,* Rockville, MD, 1986, US Department of Health and Human Services.

Williams CA: Community-oriented population-focused practice: The foundation of specialization in public health nursing. In Stanhope M, Lancaster J: *Community and public health nursing,* St Louis, 2000, Mosby.

Wilson JMG, Jungner G: *Principles and practice of screening for disease: public health papers 34,* Geneva, 1968, World Health Organization.

Wilson T: Economic evaluation of a metropolitan-wide, school-based hepatitis B vaccination program, *Public Health Nurs* 17(3):222-227, 2000.

Internet Resources

Children Now—Report Card Guide: www.childrennow.org/report_guide.html
Healthy People 2010: www.healthypeople.gov
Kids Count Data, Annie E. Casey Foundation: www.kidscount.org/
National Center for Health Statistics: www.cdc.gov/nchs
National Institute of Environmental Health Sciences: www.niehs.nih.gov
National Safe Kids Web site: www.safekids.org
National Safety Council: www.nsc.org
Office of Disease Prevention: www.odphp.osophs.dhhs.gov
U.S. Census Bureau, U.S. and State Census Information: www.census.gov/
U.S. Department of Education: www.ed.gov/
U.S. Department of Health and Human Services: www.os.dhhs.gov/
World Health Organization: www.who.int/

Family Influences on Child Health Promotion

31

LEARNING OBJECTIVES

On completion of this chapter the reader will be able to:

- Discuss definitions of *family.*
- Describe three major family theories.
- Identify different family structures found in the United States.
- Discuss the effect of family size and configuration on personality development.
- Discuss the role transition experienced by new parents.
- Explain various parenting behaviors such as parenting styles, disciplinary patterns, and communication skills.
- Demonstrate an understanding of special parenting situations such as adoption, divorce, single parenting, parenting in reconstituted families, and dual-earner families.

ELECTRONIC RESOURCES

Additional information related to the content in Chapter 31 can be found on

the companion website at evolve
http://evolve.elsevier.com/Wong/maternal/
- NCLEX Review Questions
- WebLinks

or the interactive student CD-ROM
Activities for Chapter 31 include the following:
- NCLEX Review Questions
- Case Study—Family Functioning

GENERAL CONCEPTS

Definition of Family

The term *family* has been defined in a number of ways and for a number of purposes according to the individual's own frame of reference, value judgment, or discipline. For example, biology describes the family as fulfilling the biologic function of perpetuation of the species. Psychology emphasizes the interpersonal aspects of the family and its responsibility for personality development. Economics views the family as a productive unit providing for material needs, and sociology depicts it as the social unit that reacts with the larger society. Others define family in relation to the persons who make up the family unit; the most common type of relationships are *consanguineous* (blood relationships), *affinal* (marital relationships), and *family of origin* (family unit a person is born into).

Traditionally, a family has been conceptualized as a group of individuals with the belief that both a mother and father are needed to rear a child. Nearly all societies grant a very high rank to the married status, but in today's society a broad definition of the family is needed, such a group of individuals who live together or are in close, supportive relationships that provide guidance for their dependents Most important for any given patient, "family" is whatever the patient considers it to be. A family can be defined as an institution where individuals, related through biology or enduring commitments, and representing similar or different generations and genders, participate in roles involving mutual socialization, nurturance, and emotional commitment (Friedman, 1999). Considerable emotion has been generated about the newer concepts of family, such as communal families, single-parent families, and homosexual families. To accommodate these and other varieties of family styles, the descriptive term *household* is being used more frequently (Critical Thinking Exercise). These important people in the family's life may be related, unrelated, immediate family, or extended family members.

Nursing of infants and children is intimately involved with care of the child *and* the family. Consequently, nurses must be aware of the functions of the family, various types of family structures, and theories that provide a foundation for understanding the changes within a family and for directing family-oriented interventions.

Family Nursing Interventions

In working with children, nurses must include family members in their plan of care. In essence, *the patient is the family.* To discover family dynamics and the unit's strengths and

Critical Thinking Exercise

FAMILY STRUCTURE

As the nurse, you are interviewing the mother of John, a school-age boy. John's mother states that their family consists of herself, her son, a female friend, and two foster children. John's father lives in another state and has no contact with him. John has one grandparent, who lives in another city in a nursing home. As you plan care for John and his family, what type of family structure do you think John's family represents?

1. Evidence—Is there sufficient evidence to draw any conclusions about the structure of this family?
2. Assumptions—Describe the underlying assumption about each of the following types of family structure:
   a. Traditional nuclear family
   b. Single-parent family
   c. Extended family
   d. Gay or lesbian family
3. What implications for nursing care can be drawn from this situation?
4. Does the evidence support your conclusion?
5. What alternative perspectives might you have?

weaknesses, a thorough family assessment is needed (see Chapter 34). The interventions that nurses use with families depend on their theoretic model of the family. In family systems theory, for example, the focus is on the interactions of the members rather than on an individual member. In this case, using group dynamics to involve all members in the intervention process and being a skillful communicator are essential (Critical Thinking Exercise). Systems theory also presents an excellent opportunity for anticipatory guidance. Because each member of the family reacts to every stress experienced by that system (e.g., the birth of a child), nurses can intervene to help the family prepare for and cope with the change.

Critical Thinking Exercise

FAMILY THEORIES

As the school nurse, you are working with a family that consists of a mother, a father, and their 10-year-old son and 16-year-old daughter. The daughter, Jenny, has stopped going to school this week.

Although she has had many conflicts with her parents, her relationship with her father is very strained. He recently took away her driving privileges because of curfew violations. Jenny says she is quitting school if she cannot drive. Which family theory would you find most helpful in guiding your nursing care when working with this family?

1. Evidence—Is there sufficient evidence to make a decision about which theory to use?
2. Assumptions—Describe an underlying assumption about each of the following theories:
   a. Family systems theory
   b. Family stress theory
   c. Developmental theory
3. What implications for nursing care can be drawn at this time?
4. Does the evidence support your conclusion?
5. What alternative perspectives might you have?

BOX 31-1

Family Nursing Interventions

Behavior modification
Contracting
Case management, including coordination and advocacy
Collaboration
Consultation
Counseling, including support, cognitive reappraisal (reframing), crisis intervention, and group work
Empowerment strategies
Environmental modification
Family advocacy
Lifestyle modification, including stress management
Networking, including use of self-help groups and social support
Referring
Role modeling
Role supplementation
Teaching strategies
Values clarification

From Friedman MM: *Family nursing: theory and practice,* ed 4, Norwalk, CT, 1999, Appleton & Lange.

In the family stress theory, crisis intervention strategies are employed, and the chief focus is on helping members cope with the challenging event. In the developmental theory, a primary nursing function is to provide anticipatory guidance that prepares members for transition to the next family stage.

Nurses use a variety of strategies when working with families (Box 31-1). It is important for nurses to be aware of their degree of professional competence in using family nursing interventions. An important nursing role is to recognize situations where referral to more specialized services is required.

FAMILY ROLES, RELATIONSHIPS, AND STRENGTHS

Each individual has a position, or status, in the family structure, and plays culturally and socially defined roles in interactions within the family group. Each family has its own traditions and values, and sets its own standards for interaction within and outside the group. Each family determines the experiences its children should have, those experiences they are to be shielded from, and how each of these experiences meets the needs of family members. Where family ties are strong, social control is highly effective, and most members conform to their roles willingly and with commitment. Conflicts arise when people do not fulfill their roles in ways that meet other family members' expectations, either because they are unaware of the expectations or because they choose not to meet them.

Parental Roles

In all family groups the socially recognized status of father and mother exists with socially sanctioned roles that prescribe appropriate sexual behavior and childrearing responsibilities. The guides for behavior in these roles serve to control sexual conflict in society and provide for prolonged care of children. The degree to which parents are committed and the way they play their roles are influenced by their unique socialization experience.

Role definitions are changing as a result of the changing economy and the women's liberation movement. Women are achieving equality with men in education; more are entering the labor force; and the number of women who choose to have fewer children, or none at all, is increasing. During childhood, particularly in the upper and middle classes, the trend is toward deemphasizing the basic male-female characteristics of aggression, dependence, and achievement. As the role of the woman changes, there must necessarily be a change in the complementary role of the man. Fathers are taking a more active role in childrearing and household activities, particularly in middle-class families. Marital roles remain most segregated in the lower classes. Redefinition of sex roles in the American family is taking place, but a cultural lag of the persisting traditional role definitions creates conflicts in many of these families.

Role Learning

Roles are learned through the socialization process. During all stages of development children learn and practice, through interaction with others and in their play, a set of social roles and something of the characteristics of the roles of others. They behave in patterned and more or less predictable ways because they learn roles that define mutual expectations in typical and recurring social relationships. Although role definitions are changing, the basic determinants of parenting remain the same. These three determinants of parenting infants and young children are (1) the parental personality and psychologic well-being, (2) contextual subsystems of support, and (3) child characteristics (Foss, 1996). These determinants have been consistent measurements in determining a person's success in fulfilling the parental role.

Role conceptions are transmitted by socializing agents (e.g., parents, peers, and authority figures) who use positive and negative sanctions to ensure conformity to their norms. Role behaviors positively reinforced by rewards such as love, affection, friendship, and honors are strengthened. Negative reinforcement takes the form of ridicule, withdrawal of love, expressions of disapproval, or banishment.

In some cultures the role behavior expected of children conflicts with desirable adult behavior. For example, in the United States, children are expected to be submissive in childhood but dominant as adults. This conflict of expectations is known as *role discontinuity.* Other cultures value the same behaviors, such as courage and aggression, both in children and in adults; this provides *role continuity.*

One responsibility of the family is to develop culturally appropriate role behavior in the children. At a very early age children learn to perform in expected ways consistent with their position in the family and culture. The observed behavior of each child is a single manifestation—a combination of social influences and individual psychologic processes. In this way the uniting of the child's intrapersonal system (the self) with the interpersonal system (the family) is simultaneously understood as the conduct of the child.

Role structuring initially takes place within the family unit, where the children fulfill a set of roles and respond to the complementary roles of their parents and other family members. The roles of the children are shaped primarily by the parents, who apply direct or indirect pressures in an attempt to induce or force children into the desired patterns of behavior or direct their efforts toward modification of the role responses of the child on a mutually acceptable basis. Parents have their own techniques and will determine the course that the process of socialization is to follow (see Guidelines box on p. 903).

Children respond to life situations according to behaviors learned in reciprocal transactions. As they acquire important role-taking skills, their relationships with others change. For instance, when a teenager is also the mother but lives in a household where the grandmother is a co-resident, the adolescent mother may experience more support for the adolescent role than for the parenting role.

Children become proficient at understanding others as they acquire the ability to discriminate their own perspectives from those of others. Children who get along well with others and attain status in the peer group have well-developed role-taking skills.

Family Size and Configuration

Parenting practices differ between small and large families. In small families more emphasis is placed on the individual development of the children. Parenting is intensive rather than extensive, and there is constant pressure to measure up to family expectations. Children's development and achievement are measured against that of other children in the neighborhood and social class. In small families there is more democratic participation by the children than in larger families. Adolescents in small families identify more strongly with their parents and rely more on their parents for advice. They have well-developed, autonomous inner controls as contrasted with adolescents from larger families, who rely more on adult authority.

Children in a large family are able to adjust to a variety of changes and crises. There is more emphasis on the group and less on the individual (Fig. 31-1). Cooperation is essential, often because of economic necessity. The large number of persons sharing a limited amount of space requires a greater degree of organization, administration, and authoritarian control. The control is wielded by a dominant family member—a parent or an older child. The number of children reduces the intimate, one-to-one contact between the parent and any individual child. Consequently, children turn to each other for what they cannot get from their parents. The reduced parent-child contact encourages individual children to adopt specialized roles in an attempt to gain recognition in the family.

Discipline is often administered by older siblings in large families. Siblings are usually better attuned to what constitutes misbehavior, and sibling disapproval or ostracism is often a more meaningful disciplinary measure than parental interventions. In situations such as the death or illness of a parent, an older sibling assumes responsibility for the family at considerable personal sacrifice. Large families seem to

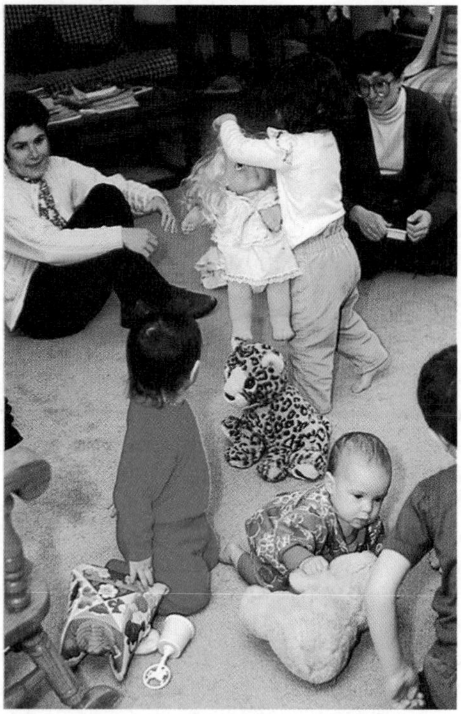

Fig. 31-1 Innumerable relationships and activities are possible in a large family.

generate a sense of security in the children that is fostered by sibling support and cooperation. However, adolescents from a large family are more peer oriented than family oriented.

Spacing of Children and Ordinal Position

Age differences between siblings affect the childhood environment, but to a lesser extent than does the sex of the siblings. The arrival of a sibling has the greatest impact on the older child, and a 2- to 4-year difference in age appears to be most threatening to the older child. When the older child is very young, the self-image is too immature to be threatened. At an older age the child is better able to understand the situation and therefore is less likely to see the newcomer as a threat, although the child does feel the loss of the only-child status. Children who are less than 2 years apart have more conflict then children who are spaced further apart (American Academy of Pediatrics, 1996). In general, the narrower the spacing between siblings, the more the children influence one another, especially in emotional characteristics. The wider the spacing, the greater the influence of the parents.

For a number of years, sibling relationships were viewed from a Freudian perspective that emphasizes the concept of sibling rivalry; however, researchers in recent decades have viewed siblings through developmental or ecologic frameworks and have focused on interactions within family systems. Results of these broader perspectives reveal rich and varied sibling interaction.

Perhaps the sibling relationship's most unique feature is its duration. Likely the longest relationship one will share with another human being, the sibling relationship lasts through a lifetime, often 50 to 80 years, as compared with the child-parent relationship of approximately 30 to 50 years. Siblings spend long periods together and come to know each other—at their best and worst—extremely well.

It has been observed for some time that the birth position of children affects their personalities. Parents treat children differently, and sibling interactions are different depending on the children's position within the family. Also, power is unequally distributed among siblings. Older siblings attempt to dominate younger ones; therefore younger siblings develop interpersonal skills, the ability to negotiate, and an ability to accept unfavorable outcomes to a greater extent than older siblings. Later-born children are obliged to interact with other siblings from birth and seem to be more outgoing and make friends more easily than firstborns. However, children vary tremendously; these generalizations represent averages and do not apply in all situations. General characteristics of children in the various ordinal positions are presented in Box 31-2.

BOX 31-2

Influence of Ordinal Position on Children

Firstborn Children

Are more achievement oriented
Are more dominant
Receive more physical punishment
Are allowed to show more aggression toward siblings
Have stronger consciences; are more self-disciplined and inner directed
Are more socially anxious
Are prone to feelings of guilt
Identify more with parents than with peers
Are more conservative
Are subject to greater parental expectations
Begin to speak earlier in life
Demonstrate higher intellectual achievement
Plan better and experience fewer frustrations
Are likely to be most wanted

Middle Children

Have more demands made on them for household help
Are praised less often
Receive less of the parents' time
Learn to compromise and be adaptable
Are less stimulated toward achievement
Are more difficult to characterize because of a variety of positions in the family

Youngest Children

Are less dependent than firstborn children
Are less tense, more affectionate, and more good-natured
Tend to identify more with peer group than with parents
Are more flexible in their thinking
Are popular with classmates
Have fewer demands placed on them for household help

Only Children

Resemble firstborn children
Are more mature and cultivated
Experience greater parental pressure for mature behavior and achievement
Demonstrate superiority in language facility
Rarely develop into the stereotype of a spoiled, selfish child
Often enjoy a rich fantasy life as a result of isolation

Sibling Functions

Siblings exert power, exchange services, and express feelings in reciprocal ways that are often not revealed explicitly in the presence of parents. They see themselves in their brother or sister, experience life vicariously through their sibling's behavior, and begin to expand on their own possibilities. Siblings can also be touchstones for what the other would not like to be, and they tend to use each other as yardsticks for comparison. They are sounding boards for one another; they offer a safe forum for experimenting with new behaviors and roles before using either with parents or nonfamily peers.

Brothers and sisters provide each other with tangible services (e.g., lending money, clothing, toys, sports equipment; or teaching a skill), help each other with childhood problems, provide support for each other in dealing with parents or others outside the family, and may provide introductions for each other to new friendship groups. Children learn to negotiate and bargain, and sometimes to manipulate. Many opportunities arise for conflict and conflict resolution. Siblings learn about sharing, competition, rivalry, and compromise. They can also protect one another from parental-executive abuse of power and can form a coalition to deal with the issues of authority, power, and emotional support. Negotiating with parents is stronger when siblings act together rather than singly.

Siblings interpret the outside world for each other and perform genuine educative functions for the parents. A related function is *pioneering,* wherein one sibling initiates a process, thereby giving permission to the others to follow accordingly. Patterns may include breaking explicit family rules, taking new developmental pathways (such as leaving the family), or adopting different moral/political codes and lifestyles.

Tattling can be an important lever in sibling interactions; on the other hand, there is often a conspiracy of silence among siblings that can leave the parents feeling isolated and excluded. A willingness to make and maintain each other's privacy often serves as a powerful bond of loyalty among the children. It is this loyalty that often distinguishes the relationship between siblings from that between friends.

More Active Sibling Relationships

Sibling relationships vary among cultures. Certain factors, however, may be giving the sibling relationship greater significance in North America than in the past. Shrinking family size, longer life spans, divorce and remarriage, geographic mobility, maternal employment and alternative sources of child care, competitive pressures, stress, and various forms of parental insufficiency may be propelling siblings into greater contact and emotional interdependence than ever before.

For example, siblings often join forces to confront the trauma of divorce. They often rely on each other for support when parents remarry. The large number of working mothers means that many young siblings today have large amounts of time when their relationship is not monitored by a personally committed adult. Often an older sibling is required to baby-sit, resulting in children spending more and more time together unsupervised. In a worried, mobile, small-family, high-stress, fast-paced, parent-absent society, children often turn to a brother or sister to meet their needs for contact, constancy, and permanency.

Multiple Births

A deviation in early development that occurs with variable frequency is multiple births. Twins are not uncommon in the population, but triplets are rare and quadruplets or quintuplets are extremely unusual. In any of these situations the offspring can be of the like or unlike gender (i.e., derived from a single ovum; from multiple ova; or a combination of the two, which can involve one or more cell divisions). The cause of twinning is unknown, but the increase in the number of larger multiples (e.g., quintuplets and sextuplets) during recent years has been associated with fertility-enhancing techniques (i.e., ovulation-inducing drugs and assisted reproductive techniques such as in vitro fertilization) (Ventura et al, 1997). Because women in their thirties are almost 2.5 times as likely as women in their twenties to have higher-order plural births, the rise in the multiple-birth ratio has been associated with increased childbearing among older women, as well as the expanded use of fertility drugs (Guyer et al, 1999).

Twins are of two distinct type: *identical,* or *monozygotic (MZ);* and *fraternal,* or *dizygotic (DZ)* (Box 31-3). In the United States the overall twinning rate is approximately 1 in 80 pregnancies; one third are MZ twins, and two thirds are DZ twins.

A special kind of sibling relationship is observed in twins, although getting along with each other and quarreling are not much different from those behaviors in any other two siblings, especially if they are different-sex fraternal twins. Twins generally tend to work out a relationship that is reasonably satisfactory to both and demonstrate early inde-

BOX 31-3

Characteristics of Twins

Monozygotic (MZ, Identical Twins)	Dizygotic (DZ, Fraternal Twins)
Result of one fertilized ovum that became separated early in development	Result of fertilization of two ova
Alike physically and genetically	Differ physically and genetically
Same sex	May be same or opposite sex
Frequency: occurs uniformly in all populations	Frequency: varies among races (highest—blacks; lowest—Asians; intermediate—whites)
Unaffected by maternal age	More common with advancing maternal age (maximum at age 35-39, then decreases rapidly)
Tendency unaffected by heredity	Marked familial tendency Expressed only in the female Fathers appear to transmit disposition toward double ovulation to daughters
Similar behavior	Dissimilar behavior; more sibling rivalry

pendence from parental attention. They develop a remarkable capacity for cooperative play and considerable loyalty and generosity toward each other. It is not uncommon for them to evolve a private language between themselves that may interfere with development of the family language.

In a twinship, one member of the pair, to a greater or lesser extent, is more dominant, outgoing, and assertive than the other, often to the consternation of their parents. However, the seemingly more passive twin is able to accomplish as much and get his or her way as often as the more assertive twin.

It has also been observed that there is a difference in behavior between identical and fraternal twins. Whereas there is near unison in the actions of identical twins (although they alternate in assuming the leadership), fraternal twins, even of the same sex, do not display this quality. Sibling rivalry can be quite pronounced in fraternal twins, especially in different-sex twins.

Identical twins also differ in their response to the tendency of some parents to treat twins exactly alike. The present philosophy is to determine the degree to which the children demonstrate an inclination toward togetherness. Some twins thrive best when they are constantly in each other's company; others prefer more individuality and separateness. The conservative approach is to allow the children to follow their natural inclinations. Early years of togetherness are often the basis of the twins' security; to separate them too early may produce unnecessary stresses. The tendency is to foster individual differences as they are evidenced in order to ease the process of separation when it becomes advisable.

Parental Adjustment

The entrance of any new member into a household creates a number of stresses, but with multiple births two or more new members must be incorporated into the family at the same time. The problems are obvious. Two infants must be provided with physical care, including twice the feeding, diapering, and all of the purchasing and preparation that accompany the care of an infant. Scheduling becomes crucial, and each advancement in development brings new problems and adjustments (e.g., space and sleeping arrangements, selecting a stroller and other equipment). Care must be observed in selecting toys. As play becomes a serious business, some toys that would be safe and appropriate for a single child become weapons when two infants share a playpen. It is a good idea to select different toys for the children as they grow older, and encourage sharing.

PARENTING

Motivation for Parenthood

A dominant characteristic in all societies is that adults are expected to become parents and to be gratified by the experience. Pressures of tradition, sentiment regarding the state of parenthood, and religious exhortations to fulfill divine commands of fertility profoundly influence decision making, because conformity to social-role expectations is a strong influence in family planning.

Factors that are likely to influence family size include social class, religion, race, financial stability, type of conjugal-role relationships, and the social-psychologic aspects of sexual relations. Of course, how effectively the couple practices contraception may determine whether the family size remains as planned. Also, in the case of divorce and remarriage, an individual may decide to have more children with the new spouse.

Preparation for Parenthood

The basic goals of parenting are to promote the physical survival and health of the children, to foster the skills and abilities necessary to be a self-sustaining adult, and to foster behavioral capabilities for maximizing cultural values and beliefs. However, new parents approach parenthood with meager experience and scant knowledge, although no other task can compare, in overall consequences, with that of rearing a human being. Parents learn by trial and error, committing the same mistakes that have been committed by countless other parents; but they somehow manage to accomplish the task, becoming more skilled with each additional child. Tradition, rather than rational planning, furnishes the chief norms for childrearing. Experience in having been nurtured as a child is an essential component of successful parenting.

Their own parents are probably the only persons who parents observe intimately in the parental role; this results in a *generational continuity*—parents rear their own children in much the same way as they themselves were reared. Other essential skills and knowledge parents need in order to feel more comfortable in the parenting role include a basic understanding of childhood growth and development, bathing, feeding, use of play, and interpersonal communication skills. All of this information is integrated throughout this text.

Transition to Parenthood

Although there is disagreement as to whether or not the birth of a couple's first child should be labeled a crisis, the early weeks of an infant's life call for a couple to make drastic adjustments. Although the parents have anticipated and perhaps prepared for the child's arrival, the birth means the sudden imposition of totally dependent care 24 hours a day for the new member of the family. It may very well be a crisis if the event is perceived as disturbing old habits and relationships and eliciting new responses. It requires role changes, destroys or significantly modifies former relationships, and means adjusting to new role realignments. Whereas previously the roles of a couple were husband and wife, they now become, in addition, father and mother. It is difficult to adjust to being parents, but it is a normal human experience and a tool for personal growth.

The advent of a new family member requires that the family cope with greater financial responsibilities, a possible loss of income, changes in sleeping habits, and less time for the husband and wife to spend with each other (especially if it is a firstborn) or with other children. If the events are perceived as aversive, it could well disrupt the couple's bond. Some investigators find that the birth of a first child results in a reduction of the couple's intimacy and affection, whereas others report that the adjustment to parenthood is only mildly stressful.

Other factors influencing the transition to the parental role include the following:

- Parents with previous experience, such as another child, appear to be more relaxed and have less conflict in disciplinary relationships, and they are more aware of normal growth and development expectations.
- The amount of stress experienced by one or both parents may interfere with their ability to exhibit patience and understanding or otherwise cope with their children's behavior.
- Special characteristics of the infant, such as being temperamentally difficult, can cause the parents to lose confidence and doubt their abilities. Also, an infant with special care needs, such as those associated with a disability, can be a significant source of added stress.
- Fathers who are highly involved with their child often feel more comfortable in the parenting role (Fig. 31-2).
- Marital relationships can have a negative effect on parental transition, because marital tension or strife can alter caregiving routines and interfere with enjoyment of the infant. Conversely, parents who support and encourage one another serve as a positive influence on establishing a satisfying parental role.

Support Systems

Successful adaptation to the stress of transition to parenthood involves at least two types of family resources (McCubbin & McCubbin, 1989). First are the *internal resources* of the family, such as adaptability and integration. Changing from an orderly, predictable life to a relatively disordered, unpredictable one is a universal adaptation that families must make. Rigid schedules are impossible to maintain, and former activities must be curtailed or abandoned. *Adaptation* is reflected in learning to be patient, becoming better organized, and becoming more flexible. *Integration* involves an attempt of the couple to continue some activities they engaged in before they became parents. In this way couples are able to maintain a sense of continuity and appreciate the importance of the husband-wife relationship.

The second kind of resource for coping with stress is the use of *coping strategies* that strengthen the organization and functioning of the family. These include the use of community resources, the use of social support, and the adoption of a future orientation. Interpersonal supports that provide information, advice, and caretaking are derived from friends, relatives, and neighbors. Relationships with family, friends, and community are essential. Arranging for time away from the child or children is beneficial. Fathers can assume care of the family to allow the mother some time to herself at home or away from the home, even if just for an afternoon or evening. Adoption of a future orientation provides reassurance to parents that things will get better, that they will cope, and that it is realistic to plan for the time when they will be able to engage in self-fulfilling activities.

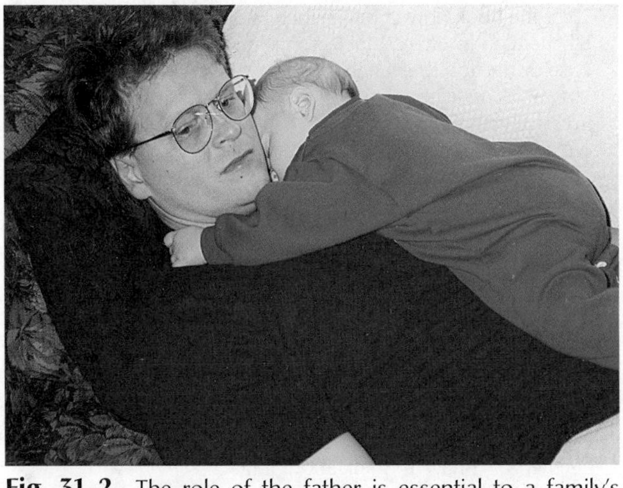

Fig. 31-2 The role of the father is essential to a family's health and well-being.

It is also reassuring to know that others experience ambivalent feelings toward parenthood and share the same difficulties and frustrations. Exchanging ideas and experiences with other parents provides an opportunity to voice concerns and to learn new ways of coping with the multiple problems of childrearing. Whether it is family, friends, or community resources, parents need persons to whom they can turn for advice, comfort, and assistance—persons with whom they can share the joys and difficulties of childrearing.

Parenting Behaviors

Parental Styles of Control

Parenting behaviors are directly linked to personality characteristics in children (Reti et al, 2002). Although there are variations and degrees in parenting styles, they can generally be described as either authoritarian, permissive, or authoritative. *Authoritarian,* or *dictatorial,* parents try to control their children's behavior and attitudes through unquestioned mandates. They establish rules and regulations or a standard of conduct that they expect to be followed rigidly and unquestioningly. They value and reward absolute obedience, mute acceptance of their word, and unfailing respect for the family's principles and beliefs. They forcefully punish any behavior that is contrary to parental standards. Parental authority is exercised with little explanation and little involvement of the child in decision making. The message is, "Do it because I say so."

Punishment need not be corporal but may be stern, such as withdrawal of love and approval. Careful training often results in rigidly conforming behavior in the children, who tend to be sensitive, shy, self-conscious, retiring, and submissive. They are more apt to be courteous, loyal, honest, and dependable—but docile. These behaviors are more typically observed when parental arbitrary power assertion is accompanied by close supervision and a reasonable level of affection. If not, arbitrary power assertion is more likely to be associated with both defiant and antisocial behavior.

Permissive, or *laissez faire,* parents exert little or no control over their children's actions. These well-meaning parents sometimes confuse permissiveness with license. They avoid imposing their own standards of conduct and allow their children to regulate their own activity as much as possible. These parents consider themselves to be resources for the children, not role models. If rules do exist, the parents explain the underlying reason, encourage the children's opinions, and consult them in decision-making processes.

They employ lax, inconsistent discipline, do not set sensible limits, and do not prevent the children from upsetting the home routine. The parents rarely punish the children, because most behavior is considered acceptable. Consequently, the children, in effect, control the parents. Children of permissive parents are often disobedient, disrespectful, irresponsible, aggressive, and generally defiant of authority.

Authoritative, or *democratic,* parents combine some childrearing practices from both the foregoing extremes. They direct their children's behavior and attitudes by emphasizing the reason for rules and by negatively reinforcing deviations. They respect the individuality of each of their children, and allow them to voice their objections to family standards or regulations. Parental control is firm and consistent but tempered with encouragement, understanding, and security. Control is focused on the issue, not on withdrawal of love or the fear of punishment. These parents foster "inner-directedness," a conscience that regulates behavior based on feelings of guilt or shame for wrongdoing, not on fear of being caught or punished. Parents' realistic standards and reasonable expectations produce children with high self-esteem who are self-reliant, assertive, inquisitive, content, and highly interactive with other children.

Limit Setting and Discipline

In its broadest sense, *discipline* means to teach or it simply refers to a set of rules governing conduct. In a narrower sense, it refers to the actions taken to enforce the rules following noncompliance. *Limit setting* refers to establishing the rules or guidelines for behavior. Generally, the clearer the limits that are set and the more consistently they are enforced, the less need there is for disciplinary action. For example, it is often suggested that parents should set limits on the amount of time children spend watching television (Bar-on, 2000).

Therefore the initial goal for the family is for the nurse to help parents establish realistic and concrete "rules." Limit setting and discipline are positive, necessary components of childrearing and serve several useful functions as they help children do the following:

- Test their limits of control
- Achieve in areas appropriate for mastery at their level
- Channel undesirable feelings into constructive activity
- Protect themselves from danger
- Learn socially acceptable behavior

Children want and need limits. Unrestricted freedom is a tremendous threat to their security and safety. Through testing the limits imposed on them, children learn the extent to which they can manipulate their environment, as well as gain reassurance from knowing that others will be there to protect them from potential harm.

Minimizing Misbehavior

The goals of or reasons for misbehavior may include attention, power, defiance, and a display of inadequacy (e.g., the child misses classes because of a fear that he or she is unable to do the work). Children may also misbehave because the rules are not clear or consistently applied. Acting-out behavior, such as a temper tantrum, may represent uncontrolled frustration, anger, depression, or pain.

The best approach is to structure interactions with children so that unacceptable behavior is prevented or minimized. Although many parents devise strategies that are most effective for their child, general guidelines include those listed in the Home Care box.

Types of Discipline

To deal with misbehavior, parents need to implement appropriate disciplinary action. Numerous approaches are available, and some have definite advantages over others (Guidelines box).

Reasoning involves explaining why an act is wrong; it is usually appropriate for older children, especially when moral issues are involved. However, young children cannot be expected to "see the other side" because of their egocentrism. Children in the preoperative stage of cognitive development (i.e., toddlers and preschoolers) have a limited ability to distinguish between their point of view and those of others.

Sometimes children use "reasoning" as a way of gaining attention; for example, they may misbehave in order for the parents to give them a lengthy explanation of the wrongdoing, because negative attention is better than none. When children use this technique, parents may have to end the ex-

Home Care

MINIMIZING MISBEHAVIOR

Set realistic goals for acceptable behavior and expected achievements.
Structure opportunities for small successes to lessen feelings of inadequacy.
Praise children for desirable behavior with attention and verbal approval.
Structure the environment to prevent unnecessary difficulties (e.g., place fragile objects in inaccessible area).
Set clear and reasonable rules; expect the same behavior regardless of the circumstances, and if exceptions are made, clarify that the change is for one time only.
Teach desirable behavior through own example, such as using a quiet, calm voice rather than screaming.
Review expected behavior before special or unusual events, such as visiting a relative or having dinner in a restaurant.
Phrase requests for appropriate behavior positively, such as "Put the book down," rather than "Don't touch the book."
Call attention to unacceptable behavior as soon as it begins; use distraction to change the behavior or offer alternatives to annoying actions, such as a quiet toy for one that is excessively noisy.
Give advance notice or "friendly reminders," such as "When the TV program is over, it is time for dinner" or "I'll give you to the count of three and then we have to go."
Be attentive to situations that increase the likelihood of misbehaving, such as overexcitement or fatigue, or decreased personal tolerance to minor infractions.
Offer sympathetic explanations for not granting a request, such as "I am sorry I can't read you a story now, but I have to finish dinner. Then we can spend time together."
Keep any promises made to children.
Avoid outright conflicts; temper discussions with statements such as "Let's talk about it and see what we can decide together" or "I have to think about it first."
Provide children with opportunities for power and control.

Guidelines

IMPLEMENTING DISCIPLINE

Consistency. Implement disciplinary action exactly as agreed on and for each infraction.

Timing. Initiate discipline as soon as child misbehaves; if delays are necessary, such as to avoid embarrassment, verbally disapprove of the behavior and state that disciplinary action will be implemented.

Commitment. Follow through with the details of the discipline, such as timing of minutes; avoid distractions that may interfere with the plan, such as telephone calls.

Unity. Make certain that all caregivers agree on the plan and are familiar with the details to prevent confusion and alliances between child and one parent.

Flexibility. Choose disciplinary strategies that are appropriate to child's age, temperament, and the severity of the misbehavior.

Planning. Plan discipline strategies in advance and prepare child if feasible (e.g., explain use of time-out); for unexpected misbehavior, try to discipline when you are calm.

Behavior-orientation. Always disapprove of the behavior, not the child, with such statements as "That was a wrong thing to do. I am unhappy when I see behavior like that."

Privacy. Administer discipline in private, especially with older children, who may feel ashamed in front of others.

Termination. Once the discipline is administered, consider child as having a "clean slate" and avoid bringing up the incident or lecturing.

planation by stating, "This is the rule, and this is how I expect you to behave. I won't explain it any further."

Unfortunately, reasoning is often combined with *scolding,* which sometimes takes the form of shame or criticism. For example, the parent may state, "You are a bad boy for hitting your brother." Children take such remarks seriously and personally, believing that *they* are bad.

NURSE ALERT When reprimanding children, focus only on the misbehavior, not on the child. Use of "I" messages rather than "you" messages expresses personal feelings without accusation or ridicule. For example, an "I" message attacks the behavior ("I am upset when Johnny is punched; I don't like to see him hurt"), not the child.* ■

Positive and negative reinforcement is the basis of *behavior modification* theory—behavior that is rewarded will be repeated; behavior that is not rewarded will be extinguished. Using *rewards* is a positive approach; by encouraging children to behave in specified ways, the tendency to misbehave is lessened. With young children, using paper stars is a very effective method. For older children the "token system" is appropriate, especially if a certain number yields a special reward, such as a trip to the movies or a new book. For a reward system to be effective, the expected behaviors must be explained to the child and the rewards must be reinforcing. A chart should be used to record the stars or tokens, and every earned reward should be promptly given. Verbal approval should always accompany material rewards.

Consistently *ignoring* behavior will eventually extinguish or minimize the act. Although this approach sounds very simple, it is often difficult to implement consistently. Parents often "give in" and resort to previous patterns of discipline. Consequently, the behavior is actually reinforced because the child learns that persistence gains parental approval.

For ignoring to be effective, health professionals must devote a fair amount of time toward (1) explaining the approach in detail; (2) recording behavior before the extinction process is instituted to see if a problem exists and to compare results after ignoring is begun; (3) making certain that the parent's attention is the reinforcer; and (4) warning parents of a phenomenon called "response burst," which refers to an *increase* in the child's behavior soon after the process is initiated because the child is testing the parents to see if they are serious about the plan.

The strategy of *consequences* involves allowing children to experience the results of their misbehavior and includes three types:

1. **Natural**—those that occur without any intervention, such as being late and missing dinner
2. **Logical**—those that are directly related to the rule, such as not being allowed to play with another toy until the used ones are put away
3. **Unrelated**—those that are imposed deliberately, such as no playing until homework is completed or the use of time-out

Natural or logical consequences are preferred but are effective only when they are meaningful to children. For example, the natural consequence of living in a messy room may do little to encourage cleaning up, but allowing no friends over until the room is neat can be very motivating! Withdrawing privileges is often an unrelated consequence. After the child experiences the consequence, the parent should refrain from any comment, because the usual tendency is for the child to try to place blame for imposing the rule.

Time-out is actually a refinement of the common practice of "sending the child to his or her room" and is a type of unrelated consequence. It is also based on the premise of removing the reinforcer (i.e., the satisfaction or attention the child is receiving from the activity). When placed in an unstimulating and isolated place, children become bored and consequently agree to behave in order to reenter the family group (Fig. 31-3). Time-out avoids many of the problems of other disciplinary approaches, because no physical punishment is involved, no reasoning or scolding is given, and the parent is usually not present for all of the time-out, facilitating his or her ability to consistently apply the punishment. It also offers both the child and the parent a "cooling off" time. To be effective, time-out must be planned in advance (Home Care box).

Corporal punishment, or *physical punishment,* most often takes the form of spanking. Based on the principles of aver-

*For more information contact Active Parenting Publishers, 810 Franklin Ct., Suite B, Marietta, GA 30067; phone: 1-800-825-0060; Web site: www.active-parenting.com. For parents of adolescents, the pamphlet *Parents* can point out what to look for and where to seek help with emotional and behavior issues. It can be ordered from Parents, PO Box 9538, Washington, DC 20016.

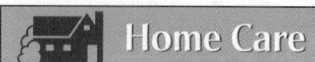

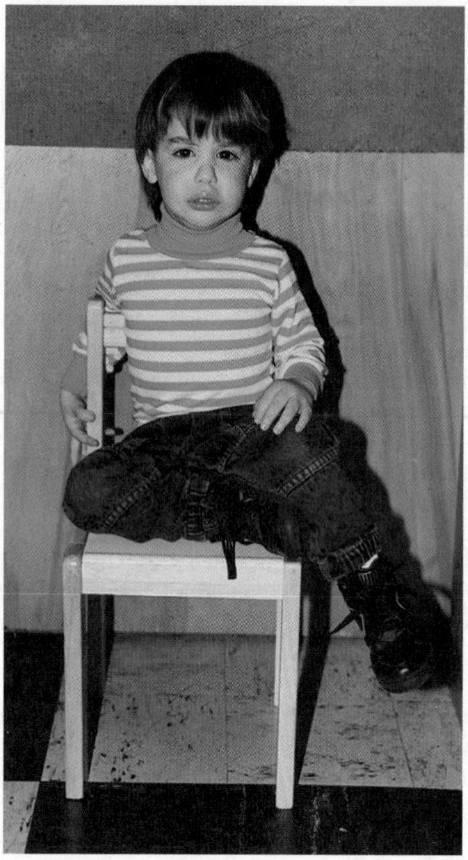

Fig. 31-3 Time-out is an excellent disciplinary strategy for young children.

sive therapy, inflicting pain through spanking causes a dramatic short-term decrease in the behavior. However, there are some serious flaws in this approach: (1) it teaches children that violence is acceptable; (2) many times the spanking is the result of parental rage and may physically harm the child; and (3) children become "accustomed" to spanking, requiring more severe corporal punishment each time (American Academy of Pediatrics, Committee on Psychosocial Aspects of Child and Family Health, 1998).

Spanking can result in severe physical injury. Nevertheless, corporal punishment is often exempted from the category of assault, even when it produces specific injuries, which may be treated as "accidental" or "incidental" to discipline.

Even when corporal punishment does not involve serious physical damage to children, the psychologic impact may be great (Bauman & Friedman, 1998; Smith & Brooks-Gunn, 1997). It can also interfere with effective parent-child interaction; children who receive corporal punishment are less likely to learn what they *should* do, because the focus is on what they should *not* do (American Academy of Pediatrics, Committee on Psychosocial Aspects of Child and Family Health, 1998). In addition, when the parent is not around, the misbehavior is likely to occur, because children have not learned to behave well for their own sake. Parental use of corporal punishment may also interfere with the child's development of moral reasoning.

Home Care

USING TIME-OUT

Select an area for time-out that is safe, convenient, and unstimulating, but where the child can be monitored, such as the bathroom, hallway, or laundry room; avoid frightening areas such as a cellar or a dark closet.

Determine what behaviors warrant a time-out.

Make sure children understand the "rules" and how they are expected to behave.

Explain to children the process of time-out:
- When they misbehave, they will be given one warning.
- If they do not obey, they will be sent to the place designated for time-out.
- They are to sit there for a specified period of time.
- If they cry, refuse, or display any disruptive behavior, the time-out period will begin after they quiet down.
- When they are quiet for the duration of the time, they can then leave the room.

A rule for the length of time-out is *1 minute per year of age;* use a kitchen timer with an audible bell to record the time rather than a watch.

Implement time-out in a public place by selecting a suitable area or explain to children that time-out will be spent immediately on returning home.

SPECIAL PARENTING SITUATIONS

Parenting is a demanding task under the most ideal circumstances, but when parents and children are faced with situations that deviate from what is considered to be the norm, the potential for family disruption is increased. Some of the issues that are encountered frequently are divorce, single parenthood, blended families, adoption, and dual-career families. The problems associated with children of alcoholic parents, parents with physical disabilities, homeless parents, or incarcerated parents are ones that are not addressed in the following discussions but may be topics that the reader may wish to investigate.

Parenting the Adopted Child

Adoption establishes the legal relationship of parent and child between persons who are not so related by birth, with the same rights and obligations that exist between children and their biologic parents. In the past the biologic mother alone made the decision to relinquish the rights to her child. In recent years, however, the courts have acknowledged the legal rights of the biologic father regarding the decision. Concerned child advocates have questioned decisions that honor the father's rights when the decision may not be in the best interests of the child. As the rights of the child have become recognized, older children have successfully dissolved their legal bond with their biologic parents to pursue adoption by adults of their choice. Furthermore, there is a growing interest and demand within the gay and lesbian community to adopt. Agencies have developed few specific policies in this regard and face questions about the legal and social ramifications of adopting in a relationship not based on marriage, as well as possible consequences of not developing policies (Bilchik, 2005).

Unlike biologic parents who prepare for their child's birth with prenatal classes and the support of friends and relatives, adoptive parents have few sources of support and preparation for the new addition to their family. Nurses who offer services to adoptive parents can provide the information, support, and reassurance needed to reduce parental anxiety regarding the adoptive process, and make referrals to state parental support groups that provide guidance for adoptive parents. Such sources can be contacted through a state or county welfare office. Prospective parents seeking information on international adoptions can contact Families Adopting Children Everywhere, Inc. (FACE).*

Most problems faced by adoptive parents are no different from those encountered by natural parents. All parents want to be good parents, but this desire is often intensified in adoptive parents. Adoptive parents have been portrayed as being more apprehensive and insecure than biologic parents and in need of more assistance. However, adoptive parents may feel the need for less assistance than biologic parents. This feeling is probably due to the adoptive parents' completely voluntary decision to become parents, the relatively long time they have to prepare for parenting, and the maturity associated with adopting.

The sooner infants enter their adoptive home, the better for purposes of parent-infant attachment; the more caregivers the infant has before adoption, the more problems are likely to be encountered in attachment. The infant must break the bond with the previous caregiver and form a new bond with the adoptive parents. The difficulties in forming an attachment will depend on the amount of time the infant has spent with earlier caregivers, such as the birth mother, nurse, or adoption agency personnel.

Siblings, adopted or biologic, who are old enough to understand should be included in decisions regarding the commitment to adopt, with reassurance that they are not being replaced. Ways that the siblings can interact with the adopted child should be stressed (Fig. 31-4).

Issues of Origin

The task of telling children that they are adopted is a cause of deep concern and anxiety. There are no clear-cut guidelines for parents to follow in determining precisely when and at what age children are ready for the information, and parents are naturally reluctant to present the children with such unsettling news. However, it is an important aspect of their parental responsibilities, and although they may be tempted to withhold the fact from the child, it is an essential component of the child's identity.

The timing seems to arise naturally as parents become aware of the child's readiness. Most authorities believe that children should be informed at an age young enough so that as they grow older, they do not remember a time when they did not know that they were adopted. The time must be right for both the parents and the child and is highly individual; it may be when children ask where babies come from, at which time children can also be told the facts of their adoption. If they are told in such a way as to convey the idea that they were active participants in the selection process, they will be less apt to feel that they were abandoned victims in a helpless situation. For example, parents can tell children that their personal qualities drew the parents to them. It is wise for parents who have not previously discussed adoption to tell children that they are adopted before the children enter school to avoid third parties inadvertently telling the children before the parents have had the opportunity to do so. Complete honesty between parents and children usually strengthens the relationship.

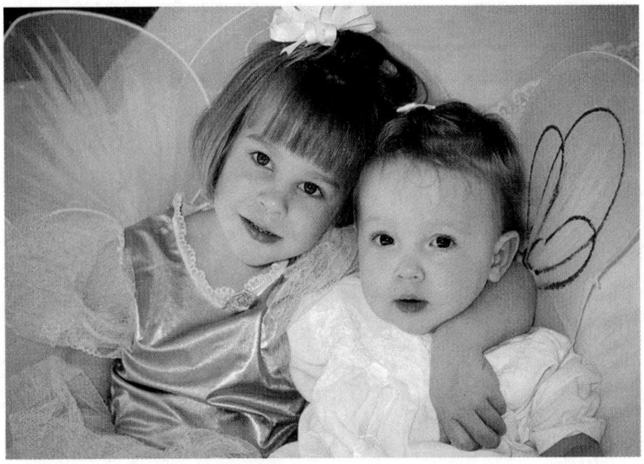

Fig. 31-4 An older sister lovingly embraces her adopted sister.

Parents can anticipate some behavior changes following the disclosure—especially in children who are older. One study found that children who were adopted were two to five times more likely to be referred for psychologic treatment than nonadopted peers (Grotevant & McRoy, 1996). Children may use the fact of their adoption as a weapon to manipulate and threaten parents. There is the inevitable "My real mother would not treat me like this," or "You don't love me as much because I'm adopted." Statements such as these hurt parents and increase their feelings of insecurity, so that as parents they may become overly permissive. Adopted children need the same undemanding love, combined with firm discipline and limit setting, as any other child.

Adolescence may be an especially trying time for parents of adopted children. The normal confrontations between adolescents and parents may assume more painful aspects in adoptive families. Adolescents may use their adoption as a tool in defying parental authority, or as a justification for aberrant behavior. As they attempt to master the task of identity formation, the feeling of abandonment by their biologic parents may come to awareness or may be intensified. The children fantasize about their biologic parents, and may feel the need to discover their identity in order to define themselves and their own identity—one of the major tasks of adolescent development. It is important for adoptive parents to keep lines of communication open and to reassure the youngsters that they understand the feelings of needing to search for their identities. In some states birth certificates

*PO Box 28058, Northwood Station, Baltimore, MD 21239; phone: 410-488-2656.

are made legally available to adopted children when they come of age. It is important for parents to be honest with questioning adolescents and to tell them of this possibility (the parents themselves are unable to obtain the birth certificate; it is the child's responsibility if he or she desires it).

Cross-Racial and International Adoption

Adoption of children of racial backgrounds different from that of the family is relatively commonplace. The number of orphans entering the United States has more than doubled in the last 10 years (U.S. State Department, 2004). In addition to the problems faced by adopted children of any age, children of a cross-racial adoption must deal with their uniqueness. It is advised that parents who adopt such children do everything to preserve the adopted children's racial heritage.

NURSE ALERT As a health care provider, it is important not to ask the wrong questions, such as "Is she yours, or is she adopted?" "What do you know about the 'real' mother?" "Are they really brother and sister?" or "How much did she cost?" ■

Although the children are full-fledged members of an adopting family and citizens of the adopted country, if they have a foreign appearance or other decided racial characteristics, problems may be encountered outside the family. Bigotry may appear among relatives and friends. Strangers may make thoughtless comments and talk about the children as though they were not members of the family. It is vital that the family make it clear to others that this is their child and a cherished member of the family.

In international adoptions* the medical information the parents receive may be either quite complete or very sketchy: weight, height, and head circumference are often the only objective information present in the child's medical record (Monsen, 2004). Tuberculosis organisms, hepatitis A and B viruses, and measles viruses have been transmitted from adopted children to family and community members. Intestinal parasites, *Bordetella pertussis,* and other infectious diseases can also be transmitted (Chen, Barnett, & Wilson, 2003; Stauffer, Kamat, & Walker, 2002). Many internationally adopted children were born prematurely, and common health problems such as infant diarrhea and malnutrition may delay growth and development. Some children may have serious or multiple health problems, and this can be very stressful for the parents.

Parenting and Divorce

In 1999 (June 1998 to June 1999) the divorce rate for the United States was 4.2 per 1000 total population (U.S. Department of Health and Human Services, 2000). The divorce rate has changed very little since 1987. In the previous decade the rate increased almost yearly, with a peak in 1979. Although almost half of all divorcing couples are childless, over 1 million children experience divorce each year, and most of the children are very young (Wallerstein, 2005).

The process of divorce begins with a period of marital conflict of varying length and intensity, followed by a separation, the actual legal divorce, and the reestablishment of different living arrangements. Because a function of parenthood is to provide for the security and emotional welfare of children, disruption of the family structure often engenders strong feelings of guilt in the parents.

During a divorce, parents' coping abilities may be compromised. The parents may be much too preoccupied with their own feelings, needs, and life changes to be available and supportive to their children. Newly employed parents, usually mothers, are likely to leave children with new caregivers, in strange settings, or alone after school. The parent may also spend more time away from home, searching for or establishing new relationships. Sometimes, however, the adult feels frightened and alone and begins to depend on the child as a substitute for the absent parent. This dependence places an enormous burden on the child.

Common characteristics in the custodial household following separation and divorce include disorder, coercive types of control, inflammable tempers in both parents and children, reduced parental competence, a greater sense of parental helplessness, poorly enforced discipline, and diminished regularity in enforcing household routines. Noncustodial parents also are seldom prepared for the role of visitor, may assume the role of recreational and "fun" parent, and may not have a residence suitable for children's visits. They may be concerned about maintaining the arrangement over the years to follow.

Impact of Divorce on Children

The results of numerous studies show that divorce has a profound effect on children. Long-term studies indicate that many youngsters suffer from psychologic and social difficulties associated with continuing or new stresses in the postdivorce family. A main outcome is heightened anxiety about forming enduring relationships as young adults (Wallerstein, 2005). Even when a divorce is amiable and open, children may recall parental separation with the same emotions felt by victims of a natural disaster: loss, grief, and vulnerability to forces beyond their control.

The impact of divorce on children depends on a variety of factors, including the age and sex of the children, the outcome of the divorce, and the quality of the parent-child relationship and parental care during the years following the divorce. Family characteristics appear to be more crucial to children's well-being than specific child characteristics, such as age or sex. The most damaging factor is continuing conflict between the divorced parents. The quality of the child's relationship with the father is important for child adjustment (Dunn et al, 2004). High levels of ongoing family conflict are related to problems of social development, emotional stability, and cognitive skills for the child.

Complications sometimes associated with divorce include efforts on the part of one parent to subvert the child's loyalties to the other, abandonment to other caregivers, and adjustment to a stepparent. A major problem occurs when children become the middle person between the divorced

*For more information contact the International Adoption Clinic, Fairview University Medical Center, PO Box 211, 420 Delaware St., SE, Minneapolis, MN 55455; phone: 1-800-688-5252.

parents. They become the message bearer between the parents, are often quizzed about the activities of the other parent, and have to listen to criticisms from one parent about the other. A nurse may be able to intercede by helping the child get out of the middle by stating "I messages" based on the formula of "I feel…" This approach may empower the child to feel more in control. For example, the "I message" may be, "I feel uncomfortable when you ask me all those questions about Mom. I would like it if you would talk to her yourself."

Children may feel a sense of shame and embarrassment concerning the family situation. Feelings experienced by children of different ages are listed in Box 31-4. Such feelings cause children to see themselves as different, inferior, or unworthy of love, especially if they feel any responsibility for the family dissolution. Although the social stigma attached to divorce no longer produces the emotions it did in the past, it may still exist in some areas and can reinforce children's negative self-image. The lasting effects of divorce depend on the children's and the parents' adjustment to the transition from an intact family to a single-parent family and, often, to a reconstituted family.

Although most studies have concentrated on the negative effects of divorce on youngsters, positive outcomes of divorce have been reported. A successful postdivorce family, either as a single-parent or as a reconstituted family, can improve the quality of life for adults and children. Living with conflict is resolved, and a better relationship with one or both parents may result. Children may also have less contact with a disturbed parent.

Age- and Sex-Related Responses to Divorce

Previously it was believed that divorce had a greater impact on younger children, but more recent observations indicate that divorce constitutes a major disruption for children in all age groups. The feelings and behaviors of children may differ according to age (see Box 31-4) and sex, but all suffer stresses second only to the stress produced by the death of a parent.

Telling the Children

Parents are understandably hesitant to tell children about their decision to divorce. A vast majority of parents neglect to discuss with their preschool children either the divorce or the inevitable changes it brings. Without preparation, even children who remain in the family home may be confused by the parental separation.

Most likely, the children are already experiencing vague, uneasy feelings that are more difficult to cope with than be-

BOX 31-4

Feelings and Behaviors of Children Related to Divorce

Infancy
- Effects of reduced mothering or lack of mothering
- Increased irritability
- Disturbance in eating, sleeping, and elimination
- Interference with attachment process

Early Preschool Children (Ages 2-3 Years)
- Frightened and confused
- Blame themselves for the divorce
- Fear of abandonment
- Increased irritability, whining, tantrums
- Regressive behaviors (e.g., thumb-sucking, loss of elimination control)
- Separation anxiety

Later Preschool Children (Ages 3-5 Years)
- Fear of abandonment
- Blame themselves for the divorce; decreased self-esteem
- Bewilderment regarding all human relationships
- Become more aggressive in relationships with others (e.g., siblings, peers)
- Engage in fantasy to seek understanding of the divorce

Early School-Age Children (Ages 5-6 Years)
- Depression and immature behavior
- Loss of appetite and sleep disorders
- May be able to verbalize some feelings and understand some divorce-related changes
- Increased anxiety and aggression
- Feel abandoned by departing parent

Middle School-Age Children (Ages 6-8 Years)
- Panic reactions
- Feelings of deprivation—loss of parent, attention, money, and secure future
- Profound sadness, depression, fear, and insecurity
- Feelings of abandonment and rejection
- Fear regarding the future
- Difficulty expressing anger at parents
- Intense desire for reconciliation of parents
- Impaired capacity to play and enjoy outside activities
- Decline in school performance
- Altered peer relationships—become bossy, irritable, demanding, and manipulative
- Frequent crying, loss of appetite, sleep disorders
- Disturbed routine, forgetfulness

Later School-Age Children (Ages 9-12 Years)
- More realistic understanding of divorce
- Intense anger directed at one or both parents
- Divided loyalties
- Able to express feelings of anger
- Ashamed of parental behavior
- Feel the need for revenge; may wish to punish the parent they hold responsible
- Feel lonely, rejected, and abandoned
- Altered peer relationships
- Decline in school performance
- May develop somatic complaints
- May engage in aberrant behavior such as lying, stealing
- Temper tantrums
- Dictatorial attitude

Adolescents (Ages 12-18 Years)
- Able to disengage themselves from parental conflict
- Feel a profound sense of loss—of family, childhood
- Feelings of anxiety
- Worry about themselves, parents, siblings
- Express anger, sadness, shame, embarrassment
- May withdraw from family and friends
- Disturbed concept of sexuality
- May engage in acting-out behaviors

ing told truthfully about the situation. If possible, the initial disclosure should include both parents and siblings, followed by later discussions with each child individually. Ample time should be set aside for the discussions, and they should take place during a period of calm, not after an argument. Parents who physically hold or touch their children provide them with a feeling of warmth that is reassuring. The discussions should include the reason for the divorce—while minimizing blame—and reassurance that the divorce is not the fault of the children. Children may feel guilty, as though they have somehow failed or are being punished for misbehavior. They wonder what role they played in the divorce or failure to keep the family together.

Parents need not fear crying in front of the children; it gives the children permission to cry also. Children need to ventilate their feelings. They normally feel anger and resentment and should be allowed to communicate these feelings without punishment. They also have feelings of terror and abandonment and long for consistency and order in their lives. They need to know where they will live, who will take care of them, if they will be with their siblings, and if there will be enough money to live on. The children may also fear that if the parents stopped loving each other, they could stop loving them as well. Their need for assurance of love is tremendous at this time.

Further issues a child may ponder include questions about what will happen on special days such as birthdays and holidays, whether both parents will come to school events, and whether the child will still have the same friends.

Custody and Parenting Partnerships

Traditionally, when parents separated, the mother was given custody of the children. Now both parents and the courts are seeking alternatives. The present belief is that neither fathers nor mothers should be awarded custody automatically. Rather, custody should be awarded to the parent who is best able to provide for the children's welfare. In certain situations children experience severe stress when living or spending time with a parent. In most divorce cases the mother still receives custody of the child with visitation agreements for the father. However, more courts are now awarding custody to fathers. Men usually make more money and can offer more material benefits than many women are able to provide. The incidence of delinquent support payments to custodial mothers is a matter of universal knowledge and concern.

Often overlooked are the changes that may occur in the children's relationships with other relatives, especially grandparents. Grandparents on the noncustodial side are often kept from their grandchildren; those on the custodial side may be overwhelmed by their adult child's return to the household with grandchildren.

Two other, less common, custody arrangements are divided custody and joint custody. *Divided custody,* or *split custody,* means that each parent is awarded custody of one or more of the children, thereby separating siblings. For example, sons might live with the father and daughters with the mother. Joint custody takes one of two forms. In *joint physical custody* the parents alternate the physical care and control of the children on a reasonably equitable basis while maintaining shared parenting responsibilities legally. This type of custody arrangement works well for families who live close to each other and whose occupations allow an active role in the care and rearing of the children. In *joint legal custody* the children reside with one parent but both parents are the children's legal guardians and both participate in childrearing.

Co-parenting offers substantial benefits for the family: children can be close to both parents, and life with each parent can be more normal as opposed to a disciplinarian mother and a recreational father. However, to be successful, the parents must place a high value on the commitment to provide parenting that is as normal as possible and be able to separate their marital conflicts from the parenting roles. No matter what type of custody arrangement is awarded, the primary consideration is the welfare of the children.

Single Parenting

Single-parent status is acquired by means of divorce, separation, or death, or through birth or adoption of a child by a single person. Although divorce rates have stabilized, the number of single-parent households continues to rise. Approximately 3 of 10 children younger than 18 years of age live in single-parent families, and the majority of single parents are women (U.S. Census Bureau, 2003). It is estimated that at least half of the children born during the 1990s will spend part of their life in a family headed by a divorced, separated, widowed, or never-married mother. Although some women are single parents by choice, most of these women never planned on being single parents, and many feel pressure to marry or remarry.

Managing shortages of money, time, and energy are major concerns for single parents. Studies repeatedly confirm the financial difficulties of single-parent families, particularly in the case of single mothers. Approximately 41% of female-headed families lived in poverty in 1999. Only 31% of mother-headed households receive any child support or alimony (Annie E. Casey Foundation, 2001). Divorced mothers from marriages in which the father assumed the breadwinning role and the mother the household maintenance and parenting roles have been found to have the most difficulty in adjusting to becoming the breadwinner for the family (Youngblut et al, 2000). Many single parents have trouble arranging for adequate child care, and care for sick children is especially difficult to obtain.

Fathers who have custody of their children have many of the same problems as divorced mothers (Dunn et al, 2004). They feel overburdened by the responsibility, are depressed, and are concerned about their ability to cope with the emotional needs of the children, especially the needs of the girls. A lack of homemaking skills is characteristic of most fathers. They find it difficult at first to coordinate household tasks, school visits, and other activities associated with managing a household alone. Fathers often demand more assistance with household tasks and more independence from their children than custodial mothers do, and they are likely to make use of alternative caregiving and support systems.

Supports and resources for single-parent families include health care services that are open evenings and weekends;

high-quality child care; respite child care to relieve parental exhaustion and burnout; and parent enhancement centers for advancing education and job skills, providing recreational activities, and offering parenting education. Groups for single-parent fathers and grandparents who are primary caregivers are also important. There is a need on the part of the parent for social contacts and a life separate from the children for the emotional growth of both parent and child. The single parent can find support and encouragement from Parents Without Partners, Inc.,* an organization designed to meet the needs of this increasingly important group.

Parenting in Reconstituted Families

In the United States, approximately one in eight dependent children in homes where parents have divorced will experience yet another major change in their lives after divorce—a return to a nuclear family and the sudden acquisition of a stepparent when the custodial parent remarries. The entry of a stepparent into a ready-made family requires adjustments for all of the family members. Some obstacles to the role adjustments and family problem solving include disruption of previous lifestyles and interaction patterns, complexity in the formation of new ones, and lack of social supports. Despite these problems, most children from divorced families want to live in a two-parent home.

Cooperative parenting relationships can allow more time for each set of parents to be alone to establish their own relationships with the children. Under ideal circumstances, power conflicts between the two households can be reduced, and tension and anxiety can be lessened for all family members. In addition, the children's self-esteem can be increased, and there is a greater likelihood of continued contact with grandparents. Flexibility, mutual support, and open communication are critical in successful relationships in stepfamilies and stepparenting situations.

Unfortunately, stepfamilies usually do not seek help to prevent problems from arising. Typically, information and counseling are sought only when problems have surfaced and can no longer be ignored. A preventive rather than remedial approach to stepfamilies and stepparenting is needed (Family Focus box).

Parenting in Dual-Earner Families

No change in family lifestyle has had more impact than the large numbers of women entering the workplace. As women moved away from the traditional homemaker pattern, the numbers of dual-earner families increased dramatically. This trend is unlikely to diminish. As a result, the family is subjected to considerable stress as members attempt to meet the challenge of the often competing demands of occupational needs and those regarded as necessary for a rich family life.

Role definitions are often altered to arrange an equitable division of time and labor, as well as to resolve conflicts between earlier and later norms, especially those related to the traditional norms of the culture. Overload is a common source of stress in a dual-earner family, and social activities are significantly curtailed. Time demands and scheduling are major problems, and when there are children, the demands can be even more intense; dual-earner couples may increase the strain on themselves to avoid creating stress for their children, although there is no evidence to indicate that the dual-earner lifestyle, as such, is stressful to children. However, the stress experienced by the parents may affect the children indirectly.

Working Mothers

Working mothers have become the norm in the United States. However, disapproving attitudes from some health care workers and child care books, lack of a national policy on child care, and memories from their own childhood experience with an at-home mother contribute to the sense of stress and guilt that many working mothers experience (Youngblut et al, 2000).

Child care is critical to the working mother's well-being. The quality of child care is a persistent concern for all working parents. Determinants of child care quality are based on health and safety requirements, responsive and warm interaction between staff and children, developmentally appropriate activities and trained staff, limited group size, age-appropriate caregivers, child ratios, and adequate indoor and outdoor space (American Academy of Pediatrics, 2002; Scarr, 1998). In general, the quality of child care is affected by lower ratios, smaller group sizes, and better-qualified teachers.

Any research on the effects of day care must be examined carefully; the characteristics of the day care setting and the measures used for child outcomes, such as attachment, must be taken into consideration. Also, the economic background of the family interacts with the effects of the type of child care and its psychologic outcomes.

Nurses play an important role in helping families to find suitable sources of child care and to prepare children for this experience. Although many types of families exist, it is more important to know and understand how a particular family functions (Acock & Demo, 1996).

Family Focus

BLENDED FAMILIES AND LIVING "IN STEP"

Let relationships develop slowly and naturally. Don't expect too much too soon, from the children, from your spouse, or from yourself.

Don't criticize or belittle lost (or new) parents, or try to erase or replace them. Stepparents are additional parents.

Expect confused feelings, anxieties, competition for attention, bids for loyalty. Decide on standards of discipline and behavior and stick to them.

Communicate. Don't pretend everything is fine if it isn't. Look at problems squarely and deal with them openly.

If you need help, admit it and get it. Read a book, get counseling, join a support group, call a family meeting.

From Stein B: Yours, mine, and ours: a look at stepfamilies, *Growing Parent* 12(9):1-5, 1984.

*International Headquarters, 401 N. Michigan Ave., Chicago, IL 60611-4267; phone: 312-644-6610; or Web site: www.parentswithoutpartners.org.

Key Points

- Because there is no agreement about the definition of family, a family is what a patient considers it to be.
- Although the traditional family structure has been nuclear or extended, in recent years other forms, such as the single-parent family, have emerged.
- Family size and positioning within the family structure have a strong impact on a child's development.
- Interpersonal skills and a basic understanding of childhood growth and development are two essential areas of focus for parents.
- Parental control tends to be predominantly one of three types: authoritarian, permissive, or authoritative.
- Three areas of special concern to adoptive families are the initial attachment process, the task of telling the children they are adopted, and identity formation during adolescence.
- Marital factors within the home significantly influence a child's development. The impact of divorce on a child depends on the child's age and sex, and the quality of the parent-child relationship and parental care following the divorce.
- Single parenting and stepparenting create adjustment difficulties and stress that is added to the already-demanding parental role. Significant numbers of children will live in a single-parent or reconstituted family at some point.

Answer Guidelines to Critical Thinking Exercises

Family Structure

1. It is difficult to categorize or draw a definite conclusion about the structure of this family. At first glance, the nurse might think that this family is a gay or lesbian family. However, the nurse does not have enough information to draw this conclusion. The nurse needs to gather more data to determine if the mother's female friend is a lesbian and if there is a common-law tie between the mother and this friend. At this point in time, this family does not fit into any of the definitions of typical family structures.
2. (a) The traditional nuclear family consists of a married couple and their biologic children. (b) The single-parent family exists when a single woman has a child, but does not choose to have a husband. (c) An extended family includes at least one parent, one or more children, and one or more members (related or unrelated) other than a parent or sibling. (d) A gay or lesbian family is one in which there is a common-law tie between two persons of the same sex who have children.
3. The implication for nursing care is that John's family consists of those people who live in his home at the present time. The nurse needs to recognize that not all families are traditional in their membership or easy to define. Many alternative family structures such as John's occur.
4. The evidence does not support identifying a specific structure for John's family. John's family is whatever John's mother says it is.
5. In the assessment of this family, the nurse should be aware of his or her own thoughts and feelings about family structure. Many alternative family structures such as John's occur, and any preconceived or negative ideas about this family on the part of the nurse could have a negative effect on the nurse's interactions with the family.

Family Theories

1. Yes, the nurse has information about a specific situation and the interactions of specific in members of a family. The nurse also has information about a specific change that has occurred within this family.
2. (a) Family systems theory views the family as a system whose members continually interact with each other. An action of one family member affects other members. (b) Family stress theory is used to explain how a family reacts to stressful events and suggests factors that promote adaptation to stress. (c) Developmental theory addresses family change over time using family life-cycle stages.
3. The nurse can help this family by applying family systems theory to examine the interactions that are occurring between the father and the daughter. In this situation, the interactions between the father and daughter are the source of the problem. The first priority is to try to promote better communication between the father and daughter to get the daughter back into school. The nurse might call a family conference at the school in an attempt to get the father, mother, and daughter to communicate. If this approach is unsuccessful, the nurse could refer the family for counseling.
4. There is no evidence to support the use of family stress theory because the family is not experiencing a stress-related problem, and there is no evidence to support crisis intervention. Developmental theory is not appropriate because the family is not entering a new stage. The daughter is in the middle of adolescence and the conflicts with her parents have been an ongoing problem.
5. The school nurse should perform a thorough assessment of this family to determine whether any other events are influencing the daughter's behavior and interactions. For example, is the daughter experimenting with drugs? Has she recently joined a peer group that is influencing her behavior?

References

Acock A, Demo D: Family structure, family process, and adolescent well-being, *J Res Adolesc* 6(4):457-488, 1996.

American Academy of Pediatrics: Child care—finding high-quality care. 2002. Internet document available at www.medem.com/medlb/article_detaillb.cfm?article_ID=ZZZ3IIGC44D&sub_cat=13 (accessed September 6, 2003).

American Academy of Pediatrics, Committee on Psychosocial Aspects of Child and Family Health: Guidance for effective discipline, *Pediatrics* 101(4):723-728, 1998.

American Academy of Pediatrics: *Sibling relationships: guidelines for parents*, Elk Grove Village, Il, 1996, AAP Publications.

Annie E Casey Foundation: *Kids count 2001*, Washington, DC, 2001, Center for the Study of Social Policy.

Bar-on ME: The effects of television on child health: implications and recommendations, *Arch Dis Child* 83:289-292, 2000.

Bauman LJ, Friedman SB: Corporal punishment, *Pediatr Clin North Am* 45(2):403-415, 1998.

Bilchik S: Children and the law. In Cosby A. G., Greenberg R. E., Southward L. H., & Weitzman M. (Eds.) *About children: An authoritative resource on the state of childhood today* (pp. 172-175), 2005, American Academy of Pediatrics.

Chen LH, Barnett ED, Wilson ME: Preventing infectious diseases during and after international adoption, *Ann Intern Med* 139(5 pt 1):371-378, 2003.

Dunn H et al: Children's perspectives on their relationships with their nonresident fathers: influences, outcomes and implications, *J Child Psychol Psychiatry* 45(3):553-566, 2004.

Foss G: A conceptual model for studying parenting behaviors in immigrant populations, *Adv Nurs Sci* 19(2):74-87, 1996.

Friedman MM: *Family nursing: theory and practice,* ed 4, Norwalk, CT, 1999, Appleton & Lange.

Grotevant H, McRoy R: Emotional disorders in adopted children and youth. In McManus M (ed): Adoption: a lifelong journey for children and families, *Focal Point: A National Bulletin on Family Support and Children's Mental Health,* 10(1), 1996.

Guyer B et al: Annual summary statistics—1998, *Pediatrics* 104(8): 1229-1245, 1999.

McCubbin M, McCubbin H: Theoretical orientation to family stress and coping. In Figley C (ed): *Treating families under stress,* New York, 1989, Brunner/Mazel.

Monsen BR: Adopting children, *J Pediatr Nurs* 19(3):214-216, 2004.

Patterson J: Promoting resilience in families experiencing stress, *Pediatr Clin North Am* 42(1):47-63, 1995.

Reti IM et al: Influences of parenting on normal personality traits, *Psychiatry Res* 111(1):55-64, 2002.

Scarr S: American child care today, *Am Psychol* 53(2):95-108, 1998.

Smith J, Brooks-Gunn J: Correlates and consequences of harsh discipline for young children, *Arch Pediatr Adolesc Med* 15(8):777-786, 1997.

US Census Bureau: *Two married parents the norm*, Washington, DC, 2003, Department of Commerce News, Available online: www.census.gov.

US Department of Health and Human Services: Births, marriages, divorces, and deaths: provisional data for June 1999, *Natl Vital Stat Rep* 48(8):1-2, 2000.

US State Department: Immigrant visas issued to orphans coming to the US. Internet document available at http://travel.state.gov/family/adoption/stats/stats_451.html (accessed February 23, 2005).

Ventura SJ et al: Advance report of final natality statistics, 1995, *Monthly Vital Stat Rep* 44(3) suppl, 1997.

Wallerstein J: The consequences of divorce. In Cosby A. G., Greenberg R. E., Southward L. H., & Weitzman M. (Eds.) *About children: An authoritative resource on the state of childhood today* (pp. 64-67), 2005, American Academy of Pediatrics.

Youngblut JM et al: Factors influencing single mothers' employment status, *Health Care Women Int* 21:125-136, 2000.

32 Social, Cultural, and Religious Influences on Child Health Promotion

LEARNING OBJECTIVES

On completion of this chapter the reader will be able to:

- Define *culture, culture shock, ethnicity,* and *race.*
- Describe the subcultural influences on child development in the areas of socialization, education, and aspiration.
- Compare and contrast the advantages and disadvantages encountered in the educational system by children from lower- and middle-class backgrounds.
- Characterize family life in present-day America.
- Identify common diseases or disorders that affect certain ethnic or cultural groups.
- Identify areas of potential conflict of values and customs for a nurse interacting with a family from a different cultural/ethnic group.
- Describe three religious groups whose beliefs significantly affect their health practices.

ELECTRONIC RESOURCES

Additional information related to the content in Chapter 32 can be found on

the companion website at evolve
http://evolve.elsevier.com/Wong/maternal/
- NCLEX Review Questions
- Case Study—Cultural Considerations
- WebLinks

or the interactive student CD-ROM
Activities for Chapter 32 include the following:
- NCLEX Review Questions
- Skill—Providing Culturally Sensitive Care

CULTURE

The future of any society depends on its children; therefore society must provide for their care, nurture, and socialization. Culture plays a critical role in the socialization agenda of children through particular views of parenting and child development. The customs and values of the culture help to organize a society's childrearing system and are transmitted from one generation to the next through the medium of the family.

Culture is the context of the child's experience of health and illness, wellness and sickness (White et al, 2004). A holistic view of any child requires that nurses develop some understanding of the ways that culture contributes to the development of social and emotional relationships and influences childrearing practices and attitudes toward health.

Transcultural nursing knowledge has become imperative during the past decade because of the increased migration of people worldwide. Professional nurses are providing care to diverse populations from almost every point of the globe (Lipson, Dibble, Minarik, 2003). This orientation to transcultural nursing includes an awareness of the nurse's own culture. The nurse who is becoming culturally competent learns about, becomes able to assess from, and shares the culture of others (Dunn, 2002).

Culture is a pattern of assumptions, beliefs, and practices that unconsciously frames or guides the outlook and decisions of a group of people. Culture differs from both race and ethnicity. *Race* is defined as a division of mankind possessing traits that are transmissible by descent and that are sufficient to characterize it as a distinct human type. One classification of race, based on skin color, is Caucasian (white), Negroid (African-American), and Mongoloid (yellow). *Ethnicity* is the affiliation of a set of persons who share a unique cultural, social, and linguistic heritage. *Socialization* is the process by which society imparts its competencies, values, and expectations to children (Trawick-Smith, 2000).

Culture is a complex whole in which each part is interrelated. It provides the lens through which all facets of human behavior can be interpreted (Spector, 2000). A culture is composed of individuals who share a set of values, beliefs, practices (language, dress, diet, health care), social relationships, laws, politics, economics, and norms of behavior that are learned, integrative, social, and satisfying (Lipson et al, 2003). Culture is not a surface veneer that covers a basic outlook shared by all human beings; rather, it is an ingrained orientation to life that serves as a frame of reference for individual perception and judgment. People from one culture differ from those in other cultures in the ways they think, solve problems, and perceive and structure the world. Culture is, essentially, the way of life of a group of people that incorporates experiences of the past, influences thought and action in the present, and transmits these traditions to future group members. Adaptation is necessary, however, for the culture to survive in an ever-changing world. Consciously and unconsciously, the members abandon, modify, or assume new patterns to meet the needs of the group.

The observable components of a culture, such as material objects (dress, art, utensils, and other artifacts) and actions, are sometimes termed the *material overt* or *manifest culture; nonmaterial covert culture* refers to those aspects that cannot be observed directly, such as the ideas, beliefs, customs, and feelings of the culture. Related to the large culture are many *subcultures,* each with an identity of its own. Children are socialized into a particular subculture rather than into the culture as a whole. Subcultural influences, such as ethnicity and social class, are discussed in more detail later in this chapter.

The culture in which children are reared determines the type of food they will eat, the language they will speak, the ideals of behavior they will follow, and the way they will conduct themselves in social roles. To be acceptable members of the culture, children must learn how the culture expects them to behave toward others in the group. In turn, they learn how they can expect others to behave toward them.

Cultures and subcultures contribute to the uniqueness of child members in such a subtle way and at such an early age that children grow up to feel that their beliefs, attitudes, values, and practices are the "correct" or "normal" ones. By age 5 years, children can identify persons who belong to their own race or cultural background. During later primary years, children are able to identify people from different cultures (Trawick-Smith, 2000). A set of values learned in childhood is apt to characterize children's attitudes and behavior for life, guiding their long-range strivings and monitoring their short-range, impulsive inclinations. Thus every ongoing society socializes each succeeding generation to its cultural heritage.

The manner and sequence of the growth and development phenomenon are universal and fundamental features of all children; however, the variations in behavioral responses that children display to similar events are believed to be determined by their culture. Inborn temperament and modes of behavior that prompt children to behave in their own preferred and highly individual manner may be in harmony or in conflict with the culture. Such forces as heredity and maturation impose limits on the influence that parents and other social groups may bring to bear.

The culture fosters and reinforces those behaviors deemed desirable and appropriate; it attempts to depress or extinguish those at conflict with cultural norms. Some cultures encourage aggressive behaviors in their children; others favor amiability and compliance. Some foster individual resourcefulness and competition; others emphasize cooperation and submission to group interest. The child from a culture that values cooperation will not respond to a challenge such as "I'll bet you can get dressed faster than Johnny can," whereas a child from a culture that emphasizes individual achievement will be stimulated by the challenge.

Cultures may also differ in whether status in the group is based on age or on skill. Even children's play and their types of games are culturally determined. In some cultures children play in groups composed of members of the same sex; in others, they play in mixed-sex groups. In some cultures team games predominate; in others, most play is limited to individual games.

Standards and norms vary from culture to culture and from location to location; a practice that is accepted in one area may meet with disapproval or create tension in another. The extent to which cultures tolerate divergence from the established norm varies among cultures and subcultural groups. Although conformity provides a degree of security, it is a decided deterrent to change.

Social Roles

Much of children's self-concept is derived from their ideas about their social roles. *Roles* are cultural creations; therefore the culture prescribes patterns of behavior for persons in a variety of social positions. All persons who hold similar social positions have an obligation to behave in a particular manner. A role prohibits some behaviors and allows others. Because it delineates and clarifies roles, the culture is a significant influence on the development of children's self-concept (i.e., attitudes and beliefs they have about themselves).

A social group consists of a system of roles carried out in both primary and secondary groups. A *primary group* is characterized by intimate, continued, face-to-face contact; mutual support of members; and the ability to order or constrain a considerable proportion of individual members' behavior. Two such groups are the family and the peer group, both of which exert a great deal of influence on the child.

Secondary groups are groups that have limited, intermittent contact and in which there is generally less concern for members' behavior. These groups offer little in terms of support or pressure toward conformity except in rigidly limited areas. Examples of secondary groups are professional associations and church organizations (also considered in relation to subgroups). The childrearing orientation in a secondary-group environment, such as urban communities, differs considerably from that of a primary-group community. An urban community is dynamic and rapidly changing; therefore many of the traditional behaviors and values do not meet its needs. Consequently, parents are often uncertain about what to teach their children. They may wish to rear their children with values consistent with their own, but the differences in experience between the generations are too great. As a result, they often grant their children autonomy in some areas of decision making early in the developmental process, and other secondary groups assume a greater influence. The children are exposed to an assortment of social groups with diverse sets of values and expectations. None of the groups is highly dominant in its influence; therefore the children are exposed to an eclectic set of values, some in agreement and some at conflict with the others. From these they must ultimately select those that they determine to be best for them and adopt them to form a consistent set of roles and behaviors to be incorporated into the self-concept.

Self-Esteem and Culture

A child's sense of self-esteem is influenced by his or her culture (Trawick-Smith, 2000). Some cultures are more collective in thought and action. A child from a collective culture will hold an inclusive view of self. Self-evaluation is related to the accomplishments or competencies of the entire family or community. School experiences that focus on personal achievement may promote positive self-esteem in some children but not in others who are more dependent on the success of a whole family or peer group. A child's sense of control may come not from individual self-reliance but rather from a feeling of worth in one's family or community (Trawick-Smith, 2000).

Families and culture also influence the criteria children use to evaluate their own abilities. Additionally, cultures vary in whether they instill an *internal locus of control* (a belief in the ability to regulate one's own life). Effects on self-esteem are minimal if these beliefs are directed by parents and are in accordance with cultural customs (Trawick-Smith, 2000). What is damaging to emotional health is helplessness that stems from prejudice. A factor that has helped maintain positive self-image and protect against the damage that prejudice can cause is ethnic pride (Trawick-Smith, 2000).

Subcultural Influences

Except in rare situations, children grow and develop in a blend of cultures and subcultures. In a large, complex society such as that of the United States, different groups have their own sets of standards, values, and expectations within the collective ways of the large culture. Although many cultural differences are related to geographic boundaries, subcultures are not always restricted by location.

Children's membership in a cultural subgroup is, for the most part, involuntary. They are born into a family with a specific ethnic or racial heritage, socioeconomic level, and religious beliefs. Although in the complex North American society there are countless subcultures and considerable variation in the way of life, those subcultures that seem to exert the greatest influence on childrearing are ethnicity, social class, and occupational role. In addition, schools and peer-group subcultures are strong influences in the socialization of the child.

Ethnicity

Ethnicity is the classification of or affiliation with any of the basic groups or divisions of mankind or any heterogeneous population differentiated by customs, characteristics, language, or similar distinguishing factors. Ethnic differences extend to many areas and include such manifestations as family structure, language, food preferences, moral codes, and expression of emotion. Some standards of behavior result from the cultural heritage of the specific ethnic group. The term *ethnic* has aroused strong negative feelings and is often rejected by the general population (Spector, 2000).

To establish their place in the group, children learn how to adhere to a mode of behavior that is in accordance with standards distinctive to the group and learn how they can expect others to behave toward them. They take their cues from observing and imitating those to whom they are exposed. For example, children of a racial minority form a perception of their role as a group member by observing the manner in which role models within the subgroup respond to treatment by people outside the subgroup. When they see group members display an attitude of inferiority, they assume this to be the appropriate behavior. These perceptions are then incorporated into their own self-concept.

In the United States, the cross-cultural lines are becoming blurred as subcultures are assimilated and blended into the larger culture (Fig. 32-1). It is particularly difficult for persons to attempt to maintain an identity with a subculture while living in and conforming to the requirements of the dominant culture. Universal customs and language used in commercial and educational systems are different from those of the minority culture. Consequently, children reared in this environment are confused about roles and values, and they usually adopt those of the more influential or higher-status culture. Youths, in particular, are influenced by the locally dominant group.

Ethnocentrism is the emotional attitude that one's own ethnic group is superior to others; that one's values, beliefs, and perceptions are the correct ones; and that the group's ways of living and behaving are the best way (Spector, 2000). *Ethnic stereotyping* or labeling stems from ethnocentric views of people. Ethnocentrism implies that all other groups are inferior and that their ways are not in the best interests of the group. It is a common attitude among a dominant ethnic group and strongly influences the ability of one person to evaluate the beliefs and behaviors of others objectively. This inherent viewpoint of individuals tends to bias their inter-

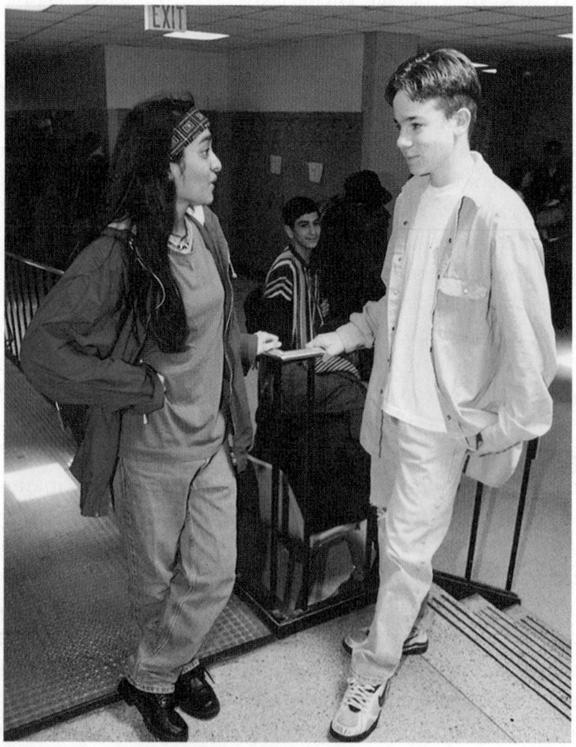

Fig. 32-1 Youngsters from different cultural backgrounds interact within the larger culture.

pretation and understanding of the behavior of others. The culturally competent nurse, however, has empathy for others, an openness to feeling what the other feels, an attitude of curiosity, a willingness to ask questions to better understand, an attitude of basic respect for self and other, and an acknowledgment of the intrinsic value of all humans (Carrillo, Green, & Belancourt, 1999).

Socioeconomic Class

It is important to recognize that family relationships may be stronger among some ethnic or cultural groups than others. However, the influence of socioeconomic class cannot be overlooked.

Socioeconomic class relates to the family's economic and education levels. Strong family relationships exist among those of lower socioeconomic class who have few resources and must rely on the support of a family network to meet physical and emotional needs. Middle- and upper-class people often have resources that reach beyond the extended family. They are able to access physical and emotional support in the community (Giger & Davidhizar, 1999).

The term *socioeconomic class* should not be confused with cultural or ethnic diversity. Children of a specific race are not necessarily of low socioeconomic status. Additionally, children of poverty do not automatically have developmental delays (Trawick-Smith, 2000).

Poverty

A subcultural influence closely related to, but different from, social class is the condition known as poverty. It is a relative concept and is usually associated with the general standards of a population. The term *poverty* implies both visible and invisible impoverishment. It is a condition in which families live without adequate resources (Trawick-Smith, 2000). *Visible poverty* refers to lack of money or material resources, which includes insufficient clothing, poor sanitation, and deteriorating housing. *Invisible poverty* refers to social and cultural deprivation, such as limited employment opportunities, inferior educational opportunities, lack of or inferior medical services and health care facilities, and an absence of public services.

An *absolute standard* of poverty attempts to delimit some basic set of resources needed for adequate existence; a *relative standard* reflects the median standard of living in a society and is the term used in referring to childhood poverty in the United States. That is, what appears to be substandard living conditions in one area may be a standard or norm in another.

An important development affecting the American family since the end of World War II is the widening disparity in income status among generations. Research indicates that the safety net (federal financial support) is working less effectively for children than for elderly people and poor adults (Ozawa & Yat-sang, 1996). Growth in the ranking of poor children over the last decade has not been due to an increase in the number of welfare-dependent families. It is because the ranks of the working poor have been growing. Between 1976 and 2000, the number of poor children living in families with income from earnings but no public assistance increased from 4.4 million to 6.9 million. Data on poverty are based on the official poverty measure of $14,494 in 1992 for a family of one adult and two children. These low-income working families are struggling to raise 10.2 million children, or about 15% of America's children. Forty-two percent of the children are non-Hispanic Caucasian, 22% are non-Hispanic African-American, 31% are Hispanic, 4% are non-Hispanic Asian/Pacific Islander, and 1% are non-Hispanic American Indian/Alaskan Native. Two-thirds of these children live with married parents. These low-income working parents also lack crucial benefits such as health insurance and sick leave. Their irregular work schedules, child care needs, and lack of basic benefits prevent an escape from poverty. Parents who must work during evening, nights, and weekends may leave children unsupervised and vulnerable (Annie E. Casey Foundation, 2003).

Homelessness

One of the most pressing problems in the United States is the growing number of homeless families. *Homeless individuals* are those who lack resources and community ties necessary to provide for their own adequate shelter. In the past the homeless population traditionally included single adults, mostly men. Currently, 50% of today's homeless are families with children, most of which are headed by single parents (Tropello, 2000).

Homeless children have increased in numbers as poverty has become feminized, minorities have become poorer, and low-income housing has become less accessible. Estimates on the number of homeless children in the United States at any given time range from 68,000 to 100,000. The majority of children are younger than 5 years of age and predominantly from minority groups.

Most homelessness is a direct result of the increasing number of people in poverty combined with a lack of decent, affordable housing. Government housing subsidies have decreased, whereas the number of working poor has increased (Tropello, 2000). Other reasons include job layoffs, low income, parental mental illness, domestic conflict, and unexpected family or economic crises. Many families move into homelessness gradually after family members and friends are no longer willing to provide housing.

Another group of homeless children are the "runaway" and "throwaway" adolescents. Many runaways are victims of physical and sexual abuse and leave home because of long-term family or school problems. Poor parent-child relationships, extreme family conflict, feelings of alienation from parents, inconsistency in supervision, and unpredictability in discipline are other factors often cited.

Lack of a permanent dwelling deprives children of the most basic necessities for proper growth and development. Homelessness disrupts a child's friendships and schooling (Strehlow & Amos-Jones, 1999). Homeless children suffer from physical and mental disorders that exceed those found in poor children who have a permanent residence.

Migrant Families

One of the most disadvantaged groups is migrant farm workers and their children. Indications suggest that in the United States there are between 3 million and 5 million migrant and seasonal workers and their dependents, whose average yearly income is well below the poverty level. In addition, most of these families have no health care insurance.

The low position of these families on the economic scale and their rootless, mobile existence subject them to inadequate sanitation, substandard housing, social isolation, and lack of educational and medical facilities (Sandhaus, 1998). This lifestyle is especially deleterious to the children. Schooling and health care are inadequate. Children are apt to live in a number of localities and attend a variety of schools in the course of a year, with no continuity in either education or health care. Because both parents work in the fields, children receive little adult supervision; therefore injury rates are high, and meals are erratic. Except where prohibited and enforced by law, children are even recruited to work in the fields along with the adults.

Some migrants have a home base to which they return at the end of growing season; others travel continuously, migrating north in summer and south in winter. With most, there is little if any integration into the dominant culture; therefore migrant groups suffer social isolation. Groups who travel together, especially those with the same ethnic background, develop a cohesiveness and form their own set of values and customs. Sometimes a migrant family will leave the migration stream and became a part of a permanent community. However, this involves adaptation to a new environment and lifestyle that can be stress provoking to these families.

Religion

Probably the most influential factor in shaping the culture of the United States is the Judeo-Christian faith. Many immigrants came to the United States for religious freedom and established a religious and moral atmosphere that persists today. However, there are individual differences that are part of the general culture.

The religious orientation of the family dictates a code of morality and influences the family's attitudes toward education, male and female role identity, and beliefs regarding their ultimate destiny (Fig. 32-2). It may also determine the school that the children attend, the companions with whom they associate, and often their mate selection. In a few instances, such as in the Mennonite and Amish communities, religion is the basis for a common way of life that determines where children are reared and their lifestyle. (See also Religious Beliefs, p. 927)

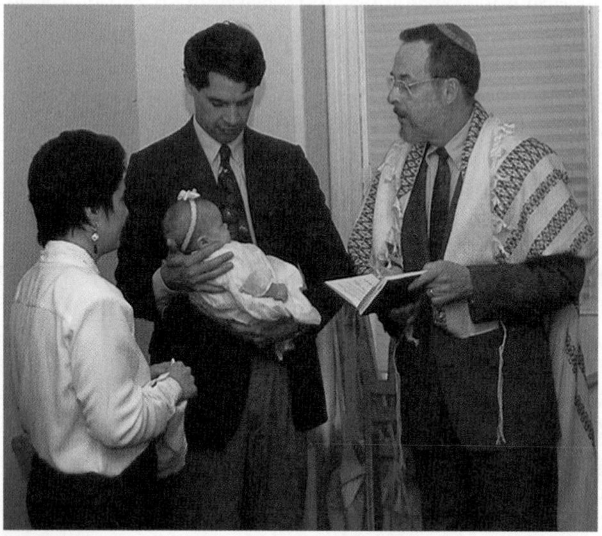

Fig. 32-2 Soon after an infant is born, many families have special religious ceremonies.

Schools

Next to the family, schools exert the major force in providing continuity between generations by conveying a vast amount of culture from the older members to the young. In this way children are prepared to carry out the traditional social roles they are expected to assume as adults in society. School rules and regulations regarding attendance, authority relationships, and the system of sanctions and rewards based on achievement transmit to the child the behavioral expectations of the adult world of employment and relationships. School is often the only institution in which children systematically learn about the negative consequences of behaviors that deviate from social expectations. Teachers are expected to stimulate and guide the intellectual development of children and their sense of esthetics and to foster their capacity for creative problem solving. Through education, individuals in the lower classes are offered the opportunity for further education and the capacity to move up in the social strata.

Traditionally, the socialization process of school has begun when the child enters kindergarten or first grade. Today, with more than 60% of mothers of preschool children working outside the home, this socialization process begins much earlier for a significant number of children in a variety of child care settings.

Children of some cultural groups fare less well in school. They come from underrepresented groups, including African-American, Mexican-American, Puerto Rican, and Native-American children (Trawick-Smith, 2000). These cultural variations can be attributed to high rates of poverty, as well as different cognitive styles, ineffective schools, and parental viewing of schools as oppressive to cultural and traditional values (Trawick-Smith, 2000).

Communities

Surveys of more than 1 million young persons in the United States grades 6 through 12 have shown that those who experience a higher number of specific assets in their lives are more likely to make healthy choices and avoid high risk behaviors. These assets offer a framework for positive child and adolescent development. The child's or adolescent's community is made up of the family, school, neighborhood, youth organization, and other members. They all contribute to the young person's experience within any culture (Search Institute, 2003).

Categories of external assets that youths receive from the community include the following:

Support. Young people need to feel support, care, and love from their families, neighbors, and others. They also need organizations and institutions that offer positive, supportive environments.

Empowerment. Young people need to feel valued by their community and be able to contribute to others. They need to feel safe and secure.

Boundaries and expectations. Young people need to know what is expected of them and what activities and behaviors are within the community boundaries and what are outside of them.

Constructive use of time. Young people need opportunities for growth through constructive, enriching opportunities and quality time at home.

Internal assets must also be nurtured in the community's young members. These internal qualities guide choices and create a sense of centeredness, purpose, and focus. The four categories of internal assets are as follows (Search Institute, 2003):

Commitment to learning. Young people need to develop a commitment to education and lifelong learning.

Positive values. Youths need to have a strong sense of values that direct their choices.

Social competencies. Young people need competencies that help them make positive choices and build relationships.

Positive identity. Young people need a sense of their own power, purpose, worth, and promise.

Peer Cultures

Peer groups also have an impact on the socialization of children (Fig. 32-3). Peer relationships become increasingly important and influential as children proceed through school. In school, children have what can be regarded as a culture of their own. It is most apparent in the school and in the unsupervised play group. The play group presents this culture in a much purer form than does the school, which is partly produced by adults.

During their lives children are exposed to value systems such as those of the family, ethnic group, and social class. In peer-group interaction they are confronted with a variety of these sets of values. The values imposed by the peer group are especially compelling because children must accept and conform to them to be accepted as members of the group. When the peer values are not too different from those of family and teachers, the mild conflict created by these small differences serves to separate children from the adults in their lives and to strengthen the feeling of belonging to the peer group.

The kind of socialization provided by the peer group depends on the special subculture that develops from the background, interests, and capabilities of its members. Some groups support school achievement, others focus on athletic prowess, and still others are decidedly antithetic to educative goals. Scholastic achievement is strongly related to the value system of the peer groups. Many conflicts between teachers and students and between parents and students can be attributed to fear of rejection by peers. A conflict between what is expected from parents regarding academic achievement and what is expected from the peer culture is especially pronounced in high school.

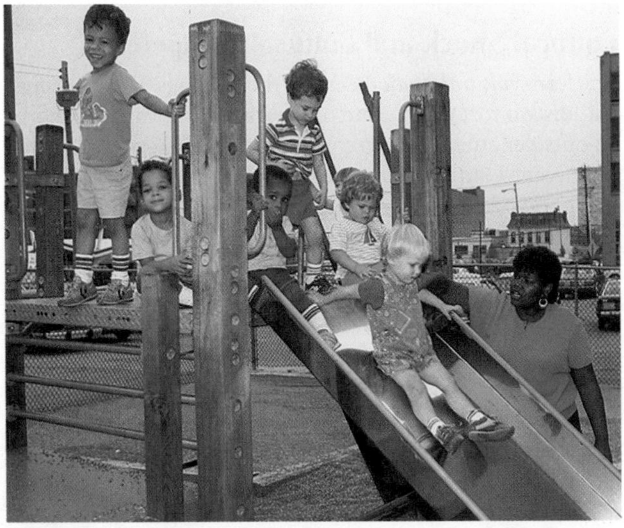

Fig. 32-3 Children from a variety of cultural and ethnic backgrounds begin to socialize in the child care setting.

Biculture

Some children are exposed to the values, role relationships, and lifestyles of two or more cultures. The virtual "straddling" of two cultures is referred to as *biculturation* and involves the ability to efficiently bridge the gap between an individual's culture of origin and the dominant culture (Rogers, 1995). This may occur because the child's parents are from two or more different cultures. In Hawaii, for example, it is common for children to be of four or more cultures. Other children straddle cultures as members of a minority culture within the dominant culture. This biculture is sometimes observed in the play group but usually is not a significant factor until children enter school. Then they must unlearn some of the established practices of one culture in order to become socialized in the other, especially in role relationships. For example, children from Hispanic and Asian cultures are taught to look away when scolded; in U.S. schools, the teacher expects direct eye contact—"Look at me when I speak to you." Children learn new roles and social behavior more rapidly than their adult counterparts.

This biculture is particularly marked in language differences. The bilingual child is said to be at a disadvantage in school situations of the dominant culture, in which there is controversy over bilingual education. Those supporting bilingual education adhere to the principle that children will understand more readily and perform more realistically (especially in testing situations) if learning is directed in their own language; others contend that children living in a dominant culture should adopt the ways of that culture, including language. There is less conflict for children when their language and culture are supported by the school, even if the dominant language is used.

The Child and Family in North America

Family life in North America is characterized by increasing geographic and economic mobility. There is less reliance on tradition, families are fragmented, and there is limited opportunity to transmit and acquire the traditional and accepted customs of a culture. Consequently, young adults rely to a greater extent on the professed experts, peers, and the mass media for acquisition of acceptable patterns of behavior, including childrearing practices. Conflicting information can be a source of confusion and frustration as parents attempt to determine the comparatively stable, essential components of the culture and transmit these to their children.

Children in North America grow up with a number of adults who differ from one another but who all provide input as role models, teachers, and standards for behavior.

Most children live in some form of nuclear family located in sharply differentiated neighborhoods determined by income and ethnic status within a highly technical, largely urban society. Class differences in childrearing persist, but they are becoming less divergent as a result of the increased homogeneity of the culture.

Minority-Group Membership

The United States has more racial, ethnic, and religious minority groups than any other country as a result of high immigration rates and high birthrates among these groups. Ethnic minority groups are becoming increasingly important because it is anticipated that these groups will produce children at a faster rate than will the majority Caucasian population. Consequently, the minority population is increasing, whereas the majority Caucasian population is decreasing. The term *cultural diversity* refers to the differences that exist among these various groups of people (O'Hare, 2005).

The 2000 U.S. census found that there were more than 280 million people in the United States, with 6.8 million reporting more than two races. There were 35 million African-Americans (alone or in combination with another race) and more than 35 million Hispanics or Latinos of any race. The Hispanic population increased 58%, or 13 million people, from 1990 to 2000 (Murdock, U.S. Census Bureau, 2000; 2005) (Cultural Awareness box).

NURSE ALERT Because American cultures and subcultures can be so diverse, it is essential that nurses be aware of and knowledgeable about the predominant groups in their work community and apply the knowledge in their practice. ■

Cultural Awareness

OVERVIEW OF RACE AND HISPANIC ORIGIN IN THE 2000 U.S. CENSUS

The federal government defines *race* and *Hispanic origin* as two separate and distinct concepts. In the 2000 U.S. census, responders were first asked if they were of Spanish/Hispanic/Latino origin. The second question asked respondents to report the race or races they considered themselves to be. The definitions of racial groups included the following:

- Caucasians are people having "origins in any of the original peoples of Europe, the Middle East, or North Africa."
- African-Americans are referred to as *blacks* and defined as "any persons whose lineage included ancestors who originated from any of the black racial groups of Africa."
- An *Asian* or *Pacific Islander* is any person with "origins in any of the original peoples of the Far East, Southeast Asia, or the Indian subcontinent."
- *Native Hawaiians* and *Other Pacific Islanders* are "people having origins in any of the original peoples of Hawaii, Guam, Samoa, or other Pacific Islands."
- Native Americans are referred to as *American Indians* and *Alaska Natives* and defined as "persons having origins in the original peoples of North America, and who maintain cultural identification through tribal affiliations or community attachment."

US Census Bureau: Overview of race and Hispanic origin census 2000 brief, 2000. Internet document available at www.census.gov/main/www/cen2000.html (accessed March 4, 2005).

NURSE ALERT Generalizations made about an ethnic group may not apply to certain groups and individuals. ■

When minority groups immigrate to another country, a certain degree of cultural/ethnic blending occurs through the involuntary process of *acculturation,* those gradual changes produced in a culture by the influence of another culture that cause one or both cultures to be more similar to the other. This process is involuntary in nature; the minority group member is forced to learn the new culture to survive (Spector, 2000). However, the changes occur to various degrees in different families and groups. Many groups continue to identify with their traditional heritage while adapting to the ill-defined concept of the "American way." Acculturation may be referred to as *assimilation,* which is the process of developing a new cultural identity (Spector, 2000).

Evidence indicates that changes in attitudes are slowly taking place in some groups and in some places. *Cultural pluralism* supports the rights of group differences and promotes a mutual respect for the existence of cultural differences (Culley, 1996; Rogers, 1995). With growing awareness, interest, and understanding by increasing numbers of the majority group, which have accompanied the recent emergence of racial and ethnic pride, minority-group children are becoming more secure and confident in their racial or ethnic identity. Individuals vary in their reactions to membership in a minority group, and much of this variation can be attributed to familial factors. As with all children, the most important influences on development of a positive self-image are warm, understanding parents who take an active interest in fostering their children's growth. Parents who accept their children and react positively and constructively rather than in a negative and self-defeating manner will help their children develop feelings of self-worth, self-esteem, and self-acceptance. The more adequate children feel, the more positive will be their attitudes toward both majority and minority children, the greater will be their ability to withstand prejudice and intolerance, and the less will be their need for counteraggressive behavior.

Cultural Shock and Cultural Competence

The term *cultural shock* describes the "feelings of helplessness and discomfort and a state of disorientation experienced by an outsider attempting to comprehend or effectively adapt to a different cultural group because of differences in cultural practices, values, and beliefs" (Leininger, 1978). This state occurs with both patients and health care providers who move from one cultural setting to another. It can happen to persons who immigrate to a new country (such as Asian refugees) or to those from a subcultural group who must adjust to the ways of an unfamiliar subgroup (such as children entering the school subculture or consumers who enter the hospital subculture). Cultural shock is characterized by the inability to respond to or function in a new or strange situation (Critical Thinking Exercise).

Numerous factors influence reactions to a new environment. Language barriers, including dialects and jargon (such as medical language) specific to a subcultural group,

Critical Thinking Exercise

REDUCING CULTURAL SHOCK

A woman from the Middle East is visiting her child, who is hospitalized for a serious illness. Her husband left for home a short time ago to wash and change clothes. She speaks little English. You need to obtain consent from her for an emergency procedure. She is hesitant and refuses to sign the consent form. What should you do?

1. Evidence—Do sufficient data exist to draw any conclusions about this woman's actions?
2. Assumptions—Describe any underlying assumptions about each of the following:
   a. Arab culture
   b. Need for interpreter
   c. Approval for emergency procedures
   d. Documentation of the need for the emergency procedure
3. What priorities for nursing care should be established at this time?
4. Does the evidence support your nursing intervention(s)?
5. What alternative perspectives might you have?

inhibit effective communication. Habits and customs (such as different role behaviors or etiquette) and differences in attitudes and beliefs are puzzling to the stranger in the new environment. The outsider experiences an intense sense of isolation and feelings of loneliness and nonrelatedness.

Nurses are challenged to overcome cultural shock and develop the dynamics of *cultural sensitivity,* an awareness of cultural similarities and differences. In doing so, the nurse is helped to practice *culturally competent* care. This requires changing the way people think about, understand, and interact with the world around them. Cultural competence is an ongoing process that is interactive and without end (Dunn, 2002). Six elements are included in the process of developing cultural competence (Dunn, 2002):

- Working on changing one's worldview through examining one's own values and behaviors and working to reject racism and institutions that support it
- Becoming familiar with core cultural issues by recognizing these issues and exploring them with patients
- Becoming knowledgeable about the cultural groups nurses work with while learning about each individual patient's unique history
- Becoming familiar with core cultural issues related to health and illness and communicating in a way that encourages patients to explain what an illness means to them
- Developing a relationship of trust with the patient and creating a welcoming atmosphere in the health care setting
- Negotiating for mutually acceptable and understandable interventions of care

NURSE ALERT Because American cultures and subcultures can be so diverse, it is essential that nurses be aware of and knowledgeable about the predominant groups in their work community and apply the knowledge in their practice. ■

CULTURAL/RELIGIOUS INFLUENCES ON HEALTH CARE

Susceptibility to Health Problems

Some groups of people are more susceptible than others to certain illnesses. An innate susceptibility is acquired through generations of evolutionary changes that take place within constrained or segregated populations. The proximity to disease, environmental factors, and the general physical status are significant factors associated with health problems.

Hereditary Factors

Historically, the increased health risks associated with ethnicity have been explained in terms of genetic differences or related factors such as socioeconomic status (Scribner, 1996). The genetic constitution of individuals as groups influences the degree to which they are susceptible to a specific disorder. It may be a result of an inherent lack of resistance to a disease organism; it may be a trait that is an advantage in one environment, but places the possessor at a disadvantage in another; or it may be a consequence of intermarriage within a relatively narrow range of geographic, ethnic, or religious restrictions.

A classic example of a geographic constraint is the common communicable disease rubeola (measles). The rubeola virus, or the populations that were continually exposed to it, became altered in such a way that the disease was considered to be a universal disease of childhood from which the majority of children suffered without ill effects. When other populations (e.g., the inhabitants of the Hawaiian Islands) were exposed to the virus by explorers and missionaries, they experienced a violent response that resulted in high mortality rates.

A number of conditions show ethnic or racial differences. For example, Tay-Sachs disease, characterized by early neurologic deterioration and mental retardation, affects primarily Ashkenazi Jewish families, particularly those of northeastern European origin, whereas Sephardic Jewish families appear to be no more at risk for the disease than are other populations. The incidence of cystic fibrosis is highest in Caucasians and almost nonexistent in Asians, and the rare affected African-Americans are usually in areas where there is apt to be mixed ancestry. A classic disorder of African-Americans is sickle cell disease; however, the incidence of cardiovascular disease, pneumonia, and diabetes is also high among African-Americans. Native Americans are at risk for type 2 diabetes and lactose intolerance. Racial and ethnic differences are further considered in relation to diseases and defects as they are discussed throughout the book.

Common food items and drugs may cause health problems in certain ethnic groups. For example, persons of Mediterranean, African, Near Eastern, and Asian origin frequently have glucose-6-phosphate dehydrogenase deficiency. They may develop acute hemolytic anemia after they ingest fava (horse or broad) beans or certain drugs such as aspirin preparations, sulfonamides, or primaquine. Other groups, especially southern Europeans, Jews, Arabs, African-Americans, Asians, and Native Americans, have a deficiency of lactase, the enzyme needed to metabolize lactose. Ingestion of lactose can cause abdominal distention, flatus, and diarrhea. Unknowing but well-meaning health workers may be responsible for these symptoms in their patients when they prescribe foods or food supplements containing lactose as sources of nutrients.

Physical Characteristics

Among racial groups there are observable differences in physical appearance. The most obvious are skin and hair coloring and texture. Skin color is determined by the amount of melanin pigment present in the skin. Persons from countries located near the equator have darkly pigmented skin, which serves to protect the skin from the year-round exposure to the sun's rays; persons from the northern countries have very light skin, which provides for maximum exposure to the sun's rays (necessary for vitamin D metabolism) during the short daylight hours. There can be wide variations in skin color between these two extremes in terms of geographic origin or from intermixing of dark and light skin color. As a consequence of the dark pigmentation, the detection of skin color changes (e.g., vasomotor alterations, cyanosis, jaundice) can be difficult and requires modification of assessment techniques (see Table 7-8).

Variations in the newborn are often related to racial or ethnic origin. For example, newborn infants of Asian-American and African-American parents are often smaller than infants of Caucasian parentage, and bluish pigmented areas (mongolian spots) on the sacral region are a common observation in Asian-American, African-American, Native-American, and Mexican-American infants. It is important that health care providers be familiar with these birthmarks. They should be documented at newborn examinations and subsequent visits so that they are not misinterpreted as bruises (Garwick & Auger, 2000).

Evaluation of stature and body build reveals some racial tendencies. Children from Asian countries are commonly smaller, falling below the 10th percentile on weight and height charts used for children in the United States. This difference in stature can lead to misinterpretation of health status and capabilities. A small child may appear very intelligent for body size but be of average mental ability for age.

Socioeconomic Factors

The most overwhelming adverse influence on health is socioeconomic status. A higher percentage of lower-class individuals suffer from some health problem at any one time than those in any other group. The sum of all aspects of their situation contributes to and compounds health problems; this includes crowded living conditions and poor sanitation, which facilitate transfer of disease (e.g., tuberculosis). There is a higher incidence of lead poisoning in children from families from the lower socioeconomic classes because there is more ready access to lead in the environment, especially lead-based paint in old housing (Centers for Disease Control and Prevention, 1997).

In the lower classes children are less likely to be immunized against preventable diseases than are children in the upper and middle classes. Lack of funds or inaccessibility to health services inhibits treatment for any but severe illness or injury. Sometimes health care is inadequate because of lack of information. In some areas a disorder is so commonplace that it is looked on as unavoidable; it is not recognized as something that requires (or is amenable to) treatment. The parents may not have information regarding causes, treatment, outcome of the illness, or preventive measures. The nurse can use the limited opportunities when the family does come into contact with the health care system to inquire about immunizations, screen for vision problems, provide nutritional information, and offer additional prevention and health promotion resources.

Poverty

A high correlation between poverty and the prevalence of illness has long been observed. Impoverished families suffer from poor nutrition; without medical insurance, they have little if any preventive health care, inadequate health maintenance, and very limited access to medical treatment. One of the most significant health problems related to poverty is a high infant mortality rate. Although the infant mortality rate in the United States is at an all-time low, it remains higher than that of most industrialized nations (Annie E. Casey Foundation, 2003). Day-to-day needs of food, clothing, and lodging take precedence over health care as long as the ailing person feels able to perform activities of daily living.

Poor families are denied access to many health institutions for emergency or other hospital care. Frequently they must travel long distances to service centers that are willing to assume their care. In an emergency they must find money for taxi fare, borrow an automobile, or seek other means of transportation. They must find care for dependents, such as other infants and small children, or have them accompany them when taking the ill child for care. Families tend to delay preventive care indefinitely unless health services are relatively accessible. They are more likely to consult folk practitioners or other persons within their community.

Poor nutrition accounts for many health problems in the lower classes. Lack of funds and knowledge results in a diet that may be seriously lacking in essential food substances, especially protein, vitamins, and iron. This inadequate diet often leads to nutritional deficiency disorders and growth retardation in children. In many, the total intake is insufficient to support normal growth. Unstructured eating patterns and irregularly scheduled mealtimes can also contribute to erratic food intake and a proportionately larger consumption of nonnourishing snacks, which can result in excessive weight gain.

Because of deficient preventive care, dental problems are more prevalent. Lack of standard immunizations, together with reduced resistance from poor nutrition, renders the exposed children in poor segments of the population vulnerable to communicable diseases. Poor sanitation and crowded living conditions also contribute to the higher incidence and perpetuation of illness. In general, poor people become ill more frequently and remain ill for longer periods of time than do persons in the general population.

Homelessness

Research indicates that families are the fastest-growing subgroup of the homeless population. Rural homeless families have been found to be similar to other homeless families in that the majority are headed by women. Unfortunately, rural families are less likely to escape from poverty (Wagner, Menke, & Cicconi, 1995).

Homeless children experience all of the health problems associated with poverty, as well as other types of disorders. Their families have fewer resources with which to control the environment or to promote rehabilitation and prevent disease. Preventive health care, especially immunization and dental care, is seriously lacking. Impaired vision is common among homeless children, perhaps reflecting missed opportunities for vision screening. Homeless children have been found to experience poorer health status and more emergency department visits than low-income housed children (Weinreb et al, 1998).

Children who are homeless have double the health problems, developmental delays, hunger, depression, and behavioral problems (Lewit & Baker, 1996). High rates of iron deficiency among homeless children have also been reported (Fierman et al, 1993; Page, Ainsworth, & Pett, 1993). Lack of adequate food is only part of the problem; homeless families may believe they are meeting nutritional needs when actually the reverse is true. They may also lack knowledge about how to safely prepare and store food.

Estimates of the number of homeless adolescents in the United States range from 500,000 to 2 million (Ensign & Santelli, 1998). Studies indicate that homeless adolescents have poor health compared with the general youth population. Homeless youths have high rates of sexually transmitted diseases, including human immunodeficiency virus (HIV) infection, pregnancy, depression, and injuries (Ensign & Santelli, 1998).

Migrant Families

Migrants generally suffer more illness, both acute and chronic, than the general population. They are subject to unhealthy environments, poverty, and insufficient medical care; their health-seeking behavior in general is an illness- or injury-oriented recourse to medical care. Affected persons will postpone seeking care for themselves or their children until physical pain or suffering is almost unbearable. Health problems common among migrant children include dental caries, upper respiratory tract infections, tuberculosis, otitis media, scabies and lice, intestinal parasites, pesticide exposure, injuries, teenage pregnancy, and growth and development delay.

Tuberculosis rates among migrant families are high. A risk factor for the increased incidence of tuberculosis in children has been the migration of families from high risk prevalence areas of tuberculosis, such as Asia, Africa, and Latin America (Castiglia, 1997). Also, farm workers are approximately six times more likely to develop the disease than the general population of employed adults. Drug-resistant tuberculosis is an important consideration among this population; it requires altered treatment regimens, and higher rates of resistance have been found. In addition to the migrant farm workers, the homeless have an increased risk for tuberculosis (MMWR, 2005).

When medical care is provided to migrant families, follow-up care is usually impossible because of their transient lifestyle. Compliance with medical therapies is primarily related to accessibility and availability. For example, medications provided by health workers are more likely to be taken than those that must be obtained at a pharmacy. In addition, medications are often discontinued following self-perceived recovery.

Customs and Folkways

Nurses must be aware of the need to consider cultural differences in patients when providing health care. An understanding of the various beliefs regarding the causation of illness and disease, as well as traditional health practices, is essential to successful intervention. The more nurses know about the values, beliefs, and customs of other ethnic groups, the better able they are to meet the needs of these families and to gain their cooperation and compliance.

evolve CASE STUDY—CULTURAL CONSIDERATIONS

NURSE ALERT Develop a cultural reference manual that includes a brief description of the culture; views on health, illness, diet, and other matters; and how to access interpreters, ethnic community services, or other sources for quick reference. ■

Cultural Relativity

Although clinical characteristics of a disease or condition are essentially the same across cultures, how a child or family interprets or experiences it varies. Culture as an influence is one obvious explanation for variance. *Cultural relativity* is the concept that any behavior must be judged first in relation to the context of the culture in which it occurs. Nurses must first relate to the family's perceptions and interpretations of experiences from the family's background and cultural belief system before they can effectively intervene.

Some cultures, for example, may view a chronic illness or disability as affecting only particular aspects of a child's life, and the child as a whole is viewed as normal. In contrast, Chinese families frequently describe the illness as having global effects on many aspects of the child's present and future life (Martinson, Armstrong, & Qiao, 1997). These contrasting views may result in a difference in goals and expectations that parents have for their children.

In some cultures the child's gender may influence a family's perception of the implications of an illness or disability. For example, in the Arabic and Asian cultures the male child is held in higher esteem than the female child. This also holds true for some families of Jewish, Italian, Greek, and Indian origin. The male child may receive better health care and more food, because this is the child who will take care of his parents in their old age.

Defining disease or signs and symptoms of illness is also influenced by culture. Some cultures, for example, perceive diarrhea as a cleansing of the body that is essential for health maintenance and illness prevention or cure. Furthermore, signs or symptoms resulting from diarrhea and ensuing dehydration, such as malaise, fever, anorexia, and irritability, may be viewed as separate illness entities.

Nurses can often recognize a family's health-related cultural perceptions and interpretations through discussion and observation. Implications of these perceptions should be explored and considered when planning effective culturally appropriate interventions.

Relationships with Health Care Providers

The manner of relating with health care providers differs considerably among cultural groups. One area of conflict to some nurses is the attitude toward time and waiting that is part of some cultures. For example, African-Americans are very flexible in their time orientation; an African-American family may be late for or miss appointments because other issues take precedence over the appointment, and the family may not communicate this to the health agency. Hispanics, too, have a very relaxed view of time. Whereas the dominant culture in the United States says that "time flies," the Hispanic says, "time walks." The Japanese, on the other hand, consider time to be valuable and to be used wisely. They tend to be punctual for medical appointments and persistent in following prescribed regimens. A Vietnamese family will subordinate time to values considered to be more significant, such as propriety. They may be late for an appointment because of an overextended visit by a friend in their home. In general, Asian-Americans view the American focus on time as offensive. They spend hours getting to know people and view predetermined, abrupt endings as rude. Introductory small talk is considered good manners.

In many cultural groups the mother assumes the responsibility for health care; in others, both parents are involved equally in relationships with health workers. A somewhat different approach is apparent in some Asian cultures. For example, the father in Vietnamese families, as unquestioned head of the family, is traditionally the family member who interacts with persons, including health care providers, outside the family unit (Fig. 32-4).

In the Hispanic family the father, as head of the house, makes decisions regarding illness and treatment of family members, but the grandmother in the extended family is consulted regarding child care. Usually the family confers with other members before reaching a decision regarding treatment or hospitalization of a child. The Arab family also relies on others to give advice and guidance in a time of crisis. A Japanese father may appear to be passive and uninvolved but actually is involved according to his own cultural standards.

NURSE ALERT In working with families, it is essential for nurses to identify key members. Failure to include these significant individuals in teaching can seriously hinder adherence to the plan of care. ■

Nurses should make themselves aware of any specific attitudes regarding the manner of approach to a child in a given culture. Navajo Indians do not like a stranger near their infants. It is feared that the stranger may "witch" the child and cause him or her harm. On the other hand, if a stranger, particularly a woman, lavishes attention on a Latino infant but fails to touch the child, the child will develop symptoms of the "evil eye" (see p. 925). Vietnamese and Korean families may become upset if a newborn is admired at length for fear that the evil spirits will overhear and desire the infant.

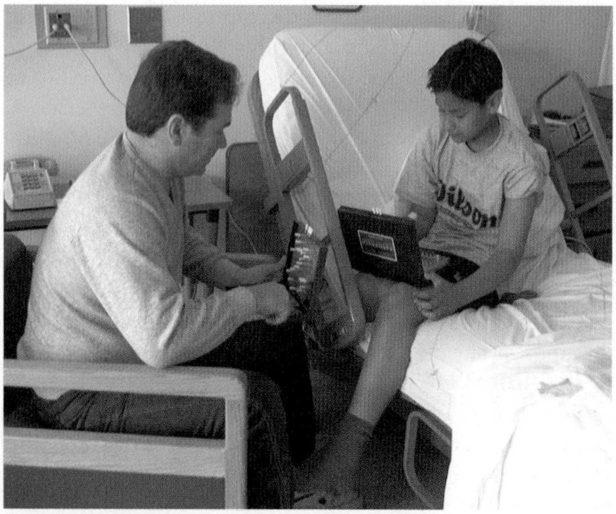

Fig. 32-4 A father with his hospitalized child.

Some ethnic groups, such as the Amish, consider a child's admission to the hospital a family affair, with all members gathering to support and console the child and parents. In others, such as the Samoan family, the family is willing to relinquish the care of the child to the hospital authority without interference. Their visits with the child are short, although intense, but this behavior may be misinterpreted by the hospital staff as disinterest or abandonment.

Nurses who are members of a majority culture may encounter tension and distrust in a child from a minority culture as a result of the child's learned perception or relationships with other persons in the majority group. Based on these perceptions, minority children often suspect that nurses may have hostile feelings toward them and fear ill treatment. When such children are hospitalized, this feeling compounds the feelings of loneliness, helplessness, and retribution that accompany fearful happenings and separation from families. The reverse situation may be encountered by a nurse from a minority culture attempting to meet the needs of a child who has been conditioned to view the nurse's cultural or ethnic group as inferior.

Communication

Communication may be a source of distress and misunderstanding between persons from different ethnic groups, especially if the languages are different. Also, prejudice has been found to be one of the biggest barriers to cross-cultural communication (Taylor, 1998). The Office of Minority Health of the U.S. Department of Health and Human Services has established national standards on culturally and linguistically appropriate services in health care. Health care organizations must ensure the competence of language assistance provided to persons with limited English proficiency (LEP) by interpreters and bilingual staff. Family and friends should not be used for interpretation services except on request by the patient (Shaw-Taylor, 2002).

Some persons with poor or limited language comprehension may simply smile and nod in agreement if they do not understand the questions or directives. It is vital that the family fully understand all implications of a child's care and management before they sign permits for special procedures or assume responsibility for the child's care. It is not uncommon for a Vietnamese or a Japanese family to indicate "yes" when in fact they mean "no" in order to avoid social disharmony. They tend to use indirectness rather than confrontation and may become evasive when direct questioning makes them feel uncomfortable.

NURSE ALERT *Helpful Communication Tools*

- Have a series of audio and audiovisual recordings in several languages designed to greet and familiarize the family with the hospital.

- In the event that an interpreter is not available, develop a multilingual booklet containing illustrations of commonly used phrases and hospital routines.
- Have legal consent forms and explanations of common diagnostic tests available in several languages.
- Keep cards with common greetings, phrases, and names of body parts in the family's language with the patient's chart (e.g., miseries [pain] and locked bowels [constipation] in African-Americans and caida de la mollera [fallen fontanel from dehydration], susto [fright], dolor, duele, or lele [pain], and la diarrhea [diarrhea] in Hispanics).

Nonverbal communication is a practiced art in many Native-American tribes, and the members are highly sensitive to body language. They emphasize periods of silence to formulate thoughts in preparation for speech and often remain silent after listening to statements by others to properly assimilate what has been said. Interruption, interjection, or haste to arrive at abrupt conclusions is perceived as immature behavior.

The level of comfort with body space or distance from others varies among cultures. For example, Hispanics tend to get closer, whereas Asians prefer a greater distance.

Eye contact is viewed differently in different cultures. Although Anglos are advised to look people straight in the eye, it is not uncommon for persons in some ethnic groups to avoid eye contact and become uncomfortable when conversing with health workers. A Vietnamese patient may not look directly into the nurse's eyes as a sign of respect. Some Native Americans will make eye contact during the initial greeting, but continued, unwavering eye contact is considered insulting and disrespectful. Asians may consider eye contact a sign of hostility or impoliteness.

Gestures also may have different meanings. For example, some Asians consider finger or foot pointing disrespectful. Native Americans consider vigorous handshaking a sign of aggression, whereas to Anglos the gesture is a sign of good will.

Families may be reluctant to question or otherwise initiate contact with health professionals. In the Asian cultures, for example, it is considered a sign of disrespect to question those who are viewed as persons of authority. A Japanese family may wait silently rather than ask or question. They believe that the health professionals know best and will meet their needs without being asked. It is also important to avoid criticism. Criticism can cause Asians to "lose face," to feel ashamed, which is highly undesirable.

Language has been considered the biggest barrier to the use of health care services by many families, especially Southeast Asians (Mattson, 1995). Often families may have poor language comprehension, so it is necessary to speak slowly and carefully, not loudly, when conversing with them. Many persons are able to read and write English better than they can speak or understand it. Also, the dominant language usually takes over in anxiety-provoking situations, even in those who are able to communicate satisfactorily under ordinary circumstances.

Terms of address and use of first and last names vary among cultures and can create confusion. For example, in Asian cultures the family name is given first in respect for the family and the given name follows. Therefore all siblings in a family have the same first name. Ethiopians have a very complex system whereby women retain their last names after marriage and the paternal grandfather's name becomes the child's last name.

The expression of emotion also varies ethnically. In some cultures (e.g., Hispanic or Jewish) emotions are expressed openly and members are accustomed to sharing their sorrows and joys with family and friends. Conversely, Nordic and Asian groups are more restrained.

Health care providers generally ask questions and use handouts, booklets, and—particularly with children—dolls and pictures as communication aids. This is uncommon in some cultures. For example, Native-American healers ask few questions and do not use forms. In some cultures it is inappropriate or considered taboo to look at the inside of the body, even in pictures, or to use dolls or puppets (Malach & Segel, 1990). Nurses need to consider both verbal and nonverbal communication techniques to interact effectively with children from different cultures and their families (Guidelines box).

Guidelines

CULTURALLY SENSITIVE INTERACTIONS

Nonverbal Strategies

Invite family members to choose where they would like to sit or stand, allowing them to select a comfortable distance.
Observe interactions with others to determine which body gestures (e.g., shaking hands) are acceptable and appropriate. Ask when in doubt.
Avoid appearing rushed.
Be an active listener.
Observe for cues regarding appropriate eye contact.
Learn appropriate use of pauses or interruptions for different cultures.
Ask for clarification if nonverbal meaning is unclear.

Verbal Strategies

Learn proper terms of address.
Use a positive tone of voice to convey interest.
Speak slowly and carefully, not loudly, when families have poor language comprehension.
Encourage questions.
Learn basic words and sentences of the family's language, if possible.
Do not use jargon or professional terms.
When asking questions, tell the family why the questions are being asked, the way in which the information they provide will be used, and how it might benefit their child.
Repeat important information more than once.
Always give the reason or purpose for a treatment or prescription.
Use information written in the family's language.
Offer the services of an interpreter when necessary
Learn, from families and representatives of their culture, methods of communicating information without creating discomfort.
Address intergenerational needs (e.g., family's need to consult with others).
Be sincere, open, and honest. When appropriate, share personal experiences, beliefs, and practices to establish rapport and trust.

Food Customs

Food customs and symbolism are an integral part of various cultural, ethnic, and religious groups. Although in a large country such as the United States most persons have adopted the eclectic food habits that have evolved over countless generations, many ethnic and geographic food traditions and preferences are retained. Special holidays, ceremonies, and life experiences such as births, birthdays, weddings, and deaths are often marked by special food items or feasts. In many cultures specific food practices are followed during pregnancy in the belief that certain foods damage the developing fetus.

The distinctive food customs of ethnic groups are a product of their native environment, determined by availability. Fish is a staple food of persons living near the ocean, such as people from Japan, Polynesia, southern Europe, and Scandinavia. Fruit and vegetable preferences are directly related to the climate in which they grow naturally or can be cultivated. The types of grain that are ethnically associated are also those that grow best in the native lands. For example, wheat and basmati rice are the staple grains of South Asians, and roti (unleavened bread) is the most commonly eaten bread in the home (Sekhon, 1996). The diet of the Eskimo is predominantly fish and meat, depending on which is the most easily procured in the area. Even in the continental United States there are regional favorites, such as rice, hominy grits, and okra in the Southern states. In some cultures food is highly spiced; in others, foods tend to be bland. Table 32-1 lists the food items common to most cultures and can be used to select foods that most children know and like.

There are a number of restrictions related to food items. Some have a physiologic origin, such as lack of dairy foods in the diets of some persons of African or Asian ancestry in whom a hereditary lactase deficiency prevents digestion of foods containing lactose. Others have religious restrictions, such as kosher foods and food preparation of the Orthodox Jewish faith and the vegetarian diet of Seventh-Day Adventists.

Children in a strange environment, such as the hospital, feel much more comfortable when they are served familiar foods (Fig. 32-5). Hospital food often tastes strange and bland. The family may be concerned that their child is not receiving foods appropriate to their culture and beliefs. Where possible, it is advisable to provide children's ethnic foods or allow families to bring favorite foods. Concern for differences in food habits and patterns projects an attitude of respect for the family's ethnic or religious heritage.

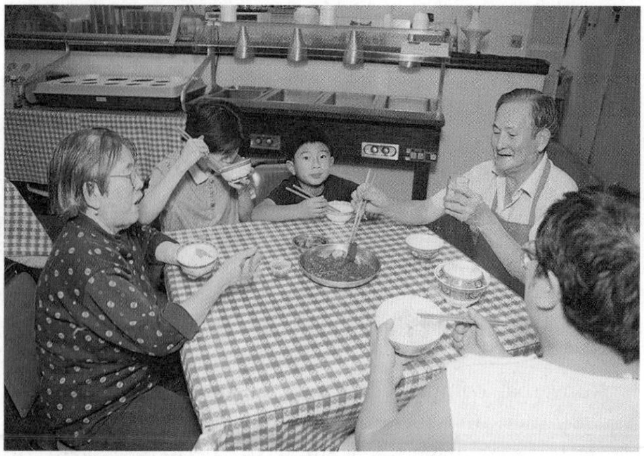

Fig. 32-5 Food customs outside the home can differ significantly from traditional cultural practices.

Health Beliefs and Practices

Health Beliefs

Beliefs related to the cause of illness and the maintenance of health are an integral part of the cultural heritage of families. Often inseparable from religious beliefs, they influence the way that families cope with health problems and the way that they respond to health care providers. Predominant among most cultures are beliefs related to natural forces, supernatural forces, and imbalance between forces.

Natural Forces

The most common natural forces held responsible for ill health if the body is not adequately protected include cold air entering the body, impurities in the air, or other natural sources. For example, a Chinese mother may overdress her infant in an effort to keep cold wind from entering the

Table 32-1

Foods Common to Most Ethnic Food Patterns

MEAT AND ALTERATIONS	MILK AND MILK PRODUCTS	GRAIN PRODUCTS	VEGETABLES	FRUITS	OTHERS
Pork*	Milk	Rice	Carrots	Apples	Fruit juices
Beef	Ice cream	White bread	Cabbage	Bananas	
Chicken	Yogurt	Noodles, macaroni, spaghetti	Green beans	Oranges	
Eggs		Dry cereal	Greens (especially spinach)	Peaches	
Beans			Sweet potatoes or yams	Pears	
			Tomatoes		

From Endres JB, Rockwell RE: *Food, nutrition, and the young child,* St Louis, 1980, Mosby.
*May be restricted because of religious custom.

child's body. The Chinese believe that cold weather, rain, and wind are responsible for "cold" conditions.

In the African-American culture, natural phenomena such as phases of the moon, seasons of the year, and planet positions are believed to affect the body and its processes; therefore health maintenance is strongly associated with the ability to read "the signs." Most Native Americans consider health to be a state of harmony with nature and the universe.

Supernatural Forces

High on the list of causes of illness are forces beyond comprehension and logical explanation. Evil influences such as voodoo, witchcraft, or evil spirits are viewed in some cultures as causes of adverse health, especially those illnesses that cannot be explained by other means.

A health belief that is common among people from Latin American, Mediterranean, Near Eastern, some Asian, and some African societies is the concept of the *evil eye* (*malojo* is the Hispanic term) (Leininger, 1995). It is part of the concept of health as a state of balance; illness is a state of imbalance (see Imbalance of Forces, following). Strength and power are associated with the evil eye. Therefore as long as an individual's strength and weakness remain in balance, he or she is unlikely to become a victim of the evil eye. Weaknesses are not necessarily physical. For example, an excess of some emotion, such as envy, can create a weakness. Infants and small children, because of immature development of their internal strength-weakness states, are especially vulnerable to the gaze of the evil eye. Consequently, the evil eye concept serves to rationalize an inexplicable onset of illness in children who display such symptoms as restlessness, crying, diarrhea, vomiting, and fever.

Although seldom expressed to health care providers, the belief that a witch can cast a spell over others at the request of someone who wishes them ill is found in Caribbean, African, and Australian aboriginal cultures. The victim is often tortured in effigy by pins driven into a doll at the location where the intended victim is to be hurt. "Voodoo deaths" have occurred from the victim's belief in the curse and may result from dehydration as the victim gives up the will to live and refuses to drink (Chidester, 2001).

Imbalance of Forces

The concept of balance or equilibrium is widespread throughout the world. One of the most common imbalances supported by the Hispanic, Filipino, Chinese, and Arab cultures is that which exists between "hot" and "cold." This belief is reputedly derived from the Hippocratic theory of humoral pathology, which states that illness is caused by an imbalance of the four humors: phlegm, blood, black bile, and yellow bile. Hot and cold describe certain properties and conditions completely unrelated to temperature. Diseases, areas of the body, foods, and illnesses are classified as either "hot" or "cold." In Chinese health belief the forces are termed *yin* (cold) and *yang* (hot). To maintain health, these hot and cold forces must be kept in balance.

Illness is treated by restoring normal balance through the application of appropriate "hot" or "cold" remedies. A "cold" condition such as a respiratory disease is believed to be caused by exposure to cold weather, rain, or cold wind entering the body; it is treated by administration of "hot" foods, herbs, or drugs. Menstruation is considered to be a "hot" condition; therefore women are cautioned against ingesting "hot" foods, which might increase menstrual flow or produce cramping. Ingesting too much of either "hot" or "cold" foods can also be interpreted as a cause of illness.

Health care workers who are aware of this belief are better able to understand why some persons refuse to eat certain foods. It is possible to help families devise a diet that contains the necessary balance of basic food groups prescribed by the medical subculture while conforming to the beliefs of the ethnic subculture.

The hot-cold food classification may have adverse effects. For example, newborn infants are often started on evaporated milk formulas. Evaporated milk is considered to be a "hot" food, whereas whole milk is viewed as a "cold" food. Infants tend to develop rashes, which are believed to be caused by "hot" foods; in such cases, parents may decide to switch to whole milk. However, parents fear that it is dangerous to change too rapidly, so they often feed the child some type of neutralizing substance, which may create additional health problems. Such a problem might be averted if the family's preference is determined before discharge from the hospital, with a formula prescribed that is agreeable to both the family and the practitioner.

Health Practices

There are numerous similarities among cultures regarding prevention and treatment of illness. All cultures have some types of home remedies that they apply before seeking help from other persons. Within the ethnic community, folk healers who are endowed with the ability to "cure" maladies are sought for special situations and when home remedies are unsuccessful. There is the *curandero* (male) or *curandera* (female) of the Mexican-American community, whose healing powers are believed to be a gift from God. The Asian consults an herbalist, knowledgeable in medicines, or an ethnic practitioner practiced in Asian therapies, including *acupuncture* (insertion of needles), *acupressure* (application of pressure), and *moxibustion* (application of heat). Native Americans consult a variety of healers with specific skills and knowledge. Specialized medicine persons diagnose illness, provide nonsacred treatments (usually by way of massage and herbs), and care for souls. Other specialists perform services or affect cures through spiritual means. Native Hawaiians consult *kahunas* and practice *ho' oponopono* to heal family imbalance or disputes.

The folk healers are very powerful persons in their community. They "speak the language" of the family who seeks help and often combine their rituals and potions with prayer and entreaties to God. They also are able to create an atmosphere conducive to successful management. Furthermore, they exhibit a sincere interest in the family and their problem.

Some folk remedies are compatible with the medical regimen and can be used to reinforce the treatment plan. For example, most of the foods contraindicated for persons with peptic ulcers are "hot" foods and would be avoided because of their belief systems. Also, aspirin (a "hot" medication) is an appropriate therapy for "cold" diseases such as the common cold and arthritis. It is not uncommon to discover that a folk prescription has a scientific basis. However, numerous health remedies or preventive practices have no scientific basis, such as the use of garlic or *asafetida* (a piece of rotten flesh that looks like a dried sponge), which is worn around the neck to prevent contagious diseases. Also, the wearing of copper or silver bracelets to protect the wearer as he or she grows has no scientific basis. Practices that do no harm should be respected.

Overcoming the effect of the evil eye usually requires specialized rituals conducted by the appropriate practitioner. For example, the Chicano *curandera* ascertains that the condition is truly the result of the evil eye by performing an assessment ritual and then, with a confirmed diagnosis, performs a curative ritual. Sometimes the faith in the folk practitioner results in a delay in obtaining needed medical treatment, although the practitioner will usually suggest medical care if his or her ministrations are unsuccessful.

Health practices of different cultures may also present problems in assessment and interpretation. For example, certain cultural practices or remedies can be misdiagnosed as evidence of "child abuse" by uninformed professionals (Box 32-1). It is important to explain why these and other familiar remedies may now be considered harmful. Families need to understand how such practices can place them in jeopardy with child protective services and to explore alternative measures that are more acceptable to the dominant culture (Hayes & Dreher, 1991).

BOX 32-1

Cultural Practices Possibly Considered Abusive by the Dominant Culture

Burning. A practice of some Southeast Asian groups whereby small areas of skin are burned to treat enuresis and temper tantrums.

Coining. A Vietnamese practice that may produce weltlike lesions on the child's back when a coin, held on edge, is repeatedly rubbed lengthwise on the oiled skin to rid the body of a disease.

Cupping. An Old World practice (also practiced by the Vietnamese) of placing a container (e.g., tumbler, bottle, jar) containing steam against the skin surface to "draw out the poison" or other evil element. When the heated air within the container cools, a vacuum is created that produces a bruiselike blemish on the skin directly beneath the mouth of the container.

Female genital mutilation (female circumcision). Removal of or injury to any part of the female genital organ; practiced in Africa, the Middle East, Latin America, India, the Far East, North America, Australia, and Western Europe (Wright, 1996).

Forced kneeling. A child discipline measure of some Caribbean groups in which a child is forced to kneel for a long period of time.

Topical garlic application. A practice of Yemenite Jews in which crushed garlic cloves or garlic-petroleum jelly plaster is applied to the wrists to treat infectious disease; the practice can result in blisters or garlic burns.

Traditional remedies that contain lead. *Greta* and *azarcon* (Mexico; used for digestive problems), *paylooah* (Southeast Asia; used for rash or fever), and *surma* (India; used as a cosmetic to improve eyesight).

Cultural health remedies that are detrimental to health include eating clay, excessive amounts of salt, or compounds that contain lead or mercury. A careful history can reveal these remedies, but it may require the collaboration of a folk healer to convince a user to stop the practice.

Haitian folk medicine considers it essential to rid the newborn of meconium to ensure neonatal survival. The newborn's first food is a *lok,* or purgative, prepared by cooking a mixture of castor oil, grated nutmeg, sour orange juice, garlic, unrefined sugar, and water. It may be administered several times until the color of the newborn's bowel movement changes from black to yellow. All other oral intake may be restricted until this occurs, which may result in dehydration (DeSantis, 1988).

Faith healing and religious rituals are closely allied with many folk-healing practices. Wearing of amulets, medals, and other religious relics believed by the culture to protect the individual and facilitate healing is a common practice. It is important for health workers to recognize the value of this practice and keep the items where the family has placed them or nearby. It offers comfort and support and rarely impedes medical and nursing care. If an item must be removed during a procedure, it should be replaced, if possible, when the procedure is completed. The reason for its temporary removal is explained to the family, and they are reassured that their wishes will be respected (Family Focus box).

Family Focus

ON CULTURAL AWARENESS

I am a pediatric emergency nurse with a high regard for cultural diversities and a respect for healing practices and beliefs. I even made a manual for my emergency department that contains some of the information needed to help us to understand and communicate with subcultures in the urban community that we serve. Although I learned a great deal putting this manual together, it doesn't come close to the lesson I learned with the following experience.

A 15-month-old Bosnian child in status epilepticus was carried in by her parents. They were very frightened and spoke very little English. I learned that the child had received a measles, mumps, and rubella (MMR) immunization the day before. As I proceeded to unwrap her from the blanket she was in, I quickly assessed the ABCs (airway, breathing, and circulation). I noticed that she was very warm (probably a febrile seizure) and that a rag soaked in alcohol was tied around each thigh. Focusing on her potential airway compromise and trying to calm the parents, I proceeded to put an oxygen mask on her, undress her for a full assessment, and remove the alcohol rags. I spoke to the parents all the while in a calm, soothing voice. Once an IV was established and I gave her Ativan, the seizures stopped. So did the communication between her parents and me. I noticed that they would no longer give me eye contact, and the mother would not even speak to me after the seizures stopped. It wasn't until I was returning to the department from admitting her that I realized why they might have stopped communicating with me . . . I had removed the rags! Had I only thought to ask their permission to remove the rags, things may have been different.

Laura L. Kuensting, MSN(R), RN
Cardinal Glennon Children's Hospital
St. Louis, Missouri

Nurses can be most effective by operating from a multicultural perspective. Adopting a multicultural perspective means using appropriate aspects of each health cultural orientation under consideration to develop culturally acceptable health care interventions.

NURSE ALERT Avoid directly criticizing traditional health cultural beliefs and practices as wrong or harmful or implying that biomedical measures are uniformly correct and effective, and the only way to prevent illness or treat sickness. Such criticisms usually result in rejection of both biomedical health care practitioners and their health teaching. When folk practices do not interfere with the welfare of the patient, they need not be discouraged. Often a compromise can be reached that accomplishes the goal of the nurse while maintaining the dignity and self-esteem of the child and family. ■

Folklore Related to Prenatal Influences

The processes of pregnancy and birth have been surrounded by strongly held beliefs and superstitions that involve taboos and prescriptions for behavior directed toward ensuring the well-being of the unborn child.

It has been a widespread belief that the appearance of the unborn child will be improved if the pregnant woman looks at beautiful people or things. The same concept in reverse has been used to explain birth defects. For example, if a pregnant woman was frightened by a rabbit, it was believed that her child would be born with a cleft lip (harelip); a microcephalic infant was attributed to the mother's seeing a monkey during pregnancy; and the mother's viewing a person with missing limbs would cause the unborn child to be similarly affected. Activities such as a mother reaching her arms above her head, walking in circles, or tying knots were believed to cause the umbilical cord to be knotted or twisted around the neck of the fetus. Even the shape of birthmarks and other skin defects is sometimes believed to reflect maternal impressions. For example, eating strawberries by the mother is associated with nevi. Articles of apparel or adornment, food cravings, emotions such as fright and anger, undesirable thoughts, and the time and manner of announcing the pregnancy are all believed to influence the well-being of the unborn child.

In most instances these customs are relatively harmless and are not in conflict with sound health practices. However, in some situations conformity to cultural or subcultural beliefs may compromise the health and well-being of the mother or fetus (e.g., the practice of eating clay). Nurses and other health care workers must be understanding and take care to explore with the mother all of the ramifications of the practice without creating undue stress and guilt.

Religious Beliefs

Religious and spiritual dimensions of life are among the most important influences in many people's lives. The terms *religion* and *spirituality* are often used interchangeably; however, spirituality subsumes religion. Both religion and spirituality give meaning to life and provide a source of love and relatedness between individuals and their God (Lukoff, Lu, & Turner, 1995). Holistic nursing care is promoted through an integration of spiritual and psychosocial care. The care focuses on activities that support a person's system of beliefs and worship, such as prayer, reading religious materials, and assisting with religious rituals. Meeting the spiritual needs of the child and family can provide strength, whereas unmet spiritual needs can result in spiritual distress and debilitation (Fulton & Moore, 1995). In practice, application of the nursing process for spiritual care (Box 32-2) can provide for the spiritual well-being of the child and family.

Religion affects the way people interpret and respond to illness (Spector, 2000). Among many groups, illness, injury, and death are believed to be sent by God as a punishment for sin. Some may believe that health workers will be unable to help a person whom God is punishing and may express a fatalistic attitude toward treatment, stating that it is the "will of God." Others view it as a test of strength, like the testing of Job in the Bible, and strive to remain faithful and overcome the conflicts.

Religious affiliation has implications for many health-related functions and procedures. It is comforting for the family of an ill child to have this need recognized and re-

BOX 32-2

Application of the Nursing Process for Spiritual Care

Assessment

Observe the environment for religious articles.
Observe if the child uses religious rituals, such as prayers or stories, or receives visits from spiritual leaders.
Ask open-ended questions to elicit the importance of religion.
Assess physical and psychosocial behaviors that are indicators of spiritual distress (anger, guilt, fear, alienation, sleeplessness, regression); assess family interactions and relationships.

Planning

Be aware of needs related to specific religious beliefs.
Consider the developmental stage of the child, particularly with regard to lack of abstract thinking and the need for a sense of accomplishment and control.
Develop a trusting relationship and include family members in the process.
Teach family interventions to promote spiritual well-being.

Implementation

Offer opportunities for religious rituals and expressions if they are part of the child's spiritual life.
Offer use of self by listening to the concerns of the child and family.
Explore the spiritual dimension through the use of therapeutic play, bibliotherapy, and other forms of artistic expression while involving family members; provide direction and choices to support management of the chronic condition.

Outcomes

Use of religious practices, if relevant
Positive statements about meaning and purpose in life
Statements that reflect forgiveness of self and others
Restored relationships with significant others

From Fulton RA, Moore CM: Spiritual care of the school-age child with a chronic condition, *J Pediatr Nurs* 10(4):224-231, 1995.

spected. Nurses need to determine if there are any special considerations, including dietary restrictions, related to spiritual practices that are important to the family. Family members are asked whether they want a clergy member present and whether they prefer hospital staff to call or prefer to do this on their own.

It is also important to determine the wishes of the family regarding baptism, rites or practices related to death, and other religious rituals (such as circumcision, communion, or use of amulets or icons). Religion, which offers families understanding and spiritual support, is a valuable asset to health care. Characteristics of selected religions with beliefs that affect health care are outlined in Table 32-2.

Importance of Culture and Religion to Nurses

A general agreement exists among nurses to raise the cultural competence of professional nursing practice. To begin to understand and to deal effectively with families in a multicultural community or in a unicultural community that is different from one's own, nurses must be aware of their own attitudes and values regarding a way of life, including health practices (Lipson, Dibble, Minarik, 2003). Nurses, too, are a product of their own cultural background. They also need to recognize that they are part of the "nursing culture." Nurses function within the framework of a professional culture with its own values and traditions and, as such, become socialized into their professional culture in their educational program and later in their work environments and professional associations.

Frequently, nurses and other health care workers are not aware of their own cultural values and how those values influence their thoughts and actions. A model for self-examination on cultural competence is the ASKED model (Box 32-3). Recognizing that a behavior may be characteristic of a culture rather than an "abnormal" behavior places nurses at an advantage in their relationships with families. When nurses respect the cultural differences of a family, they are better able to determine whether the behavior is distinctive to the individual or a characteristic of the culture.

BOX 32-3

Exploring Your Cultural Competence

ASKED Model of Cultural Competence

Awareness: Am I aware of my personal biases and prejudices toward cultural groups different than mine?

Skill: Do I have the skill to conduct a cultural assessment and perform a culturally based physical assessment in a sensitive manner?

Knowledge: Do I have knowledge of the patient's worldview and the field of biocultural ecology?

Encounters: How many face-to-face encounters have I had with patients from diverse cultural backgrounds?

Desire: What is my genuine desire to "want to be" culturally competent?

Data from Campinha-Bacote J: Many faces: addressing diversity in health care, *Online J Issues Nurs* 8:1, 2003. Internet document available at www.nursingworld.org/ojin/topic20/tpc20_2.htm (accessed March 3, 2005).

Cultural standards and values, the family structure and function, and experience with health care influence a family's feelings and attitudes toward health, their children, and health care delivery systems. It is often difficult for nurses to be nonjudgmental and objective in working with families whose behaviors and attitudes differ from or conflict with their own. The nurse needs to understand how one's own cultural background influences the way care is delivered (Lipson, Dibble, Minarik, 2003). Relying only on one's own values and experiences for guidance may result in frustration and disappointment. It is one thing to know what is needed to deal with a health problem; it is often quite another to implement a fruitful course of action unless nurses work within the cultural and socioeconomic framework of the family.

It is beneficial to adapt ethnic practices to the health needs of the family rather than attempt to change longstanding beliefs. To aid their efforts to understand and respect the cultural beliefs of families, nurses should have a readily available resource file containing pertinent information about the cultural and subcultural characteristics of the community in which they practice (e.g., traditional practices related to infant feeding practices and the time and manner of weaning and toilet training). The nurse needs to develop knowledge on how cultural groups understand life processes, define health and illness, view the causes of illness, and have their healers care for the cultural group's members (Lipson et al, 2003).

Some characteristics of selected cultures are outlined in Table 32-3. Tables 32-2 and 32-3 are presented as beginning frameworks for practicing transcultural nursing. Nurses must assess the cultural and religious practices of families to identify how these practices are similar to and different from those of their own cultural and religious backgrounds.

NURSE ALERT These generalizations are presented to help nurses learn the unique beliefs and practices of various groups and are not meant to be stereotypes of any group. It is critical to remember that no cultural group is homogeneous; every racial and ethnic group contains great diversity, and knowledge of a culture may not reflect an individual member's beliefs (Nance, 1995). ■

Key Points

- Culture is the sum total of mores, traditions, and beliefs about how people function and encompasses other products of human works and thoughts specific to members of an intergenerational group, community, or population.
- Nurses have a responsibility to continually develop cultural competence. This includes understanding and respecting the influence of culture, race, and ethnicity on the development of social and emotional relationships, childrearing practices, and attitudes toward health.
- A child's self-concept evolves from ideas about his or her social roles.
- Important subcultural influences on children include ethnicity, socioeconomic class, occupation, poverty, religion, schools, community, peers, and biculture.

Text continued on p. 934.

Table 32-2

Religious Beliefs that Affect Nursing Care

BIRTH AND DEATH	DIET AND FOOD PRACTICES	MEDICAL CARE
BUDDHIST		
Birth: No baptism Infant presentation **Death:** Last rite chanting is often practiced at bedside soon after death; the deceased's family or Buddhist priest should be contacted **Organ donation/transplantation:** Believe that organ donation is a matter of individual conscience	No requirements or restrictions Some sects are strictly vegetarian Discourage use of alcohol and drugs	Illness is believed to be a trial to aid development of soul; illness resulting from karmic causes May be reluctant to have surgery or certain treatments on holy days Cleanliness is believed to be of great importance Family may request Buddhist priest for counseling
CHURCH OF CHRIST SCIENTIST (CHRISTIAN SCIENCE)		
Birth: No baptism **Death:** No last rites; autopsy is not permitted except in cases of sudden death; it is an individual's decision to choose burial or cremation **Organ donation/transplantation:** Church takes no specific position on transplantation or donation as distinct from other medical or surgical procedures	No requirements or restrictions	Oppose human intervention with drugs or other therapies, however, accept legally required immunizations Many adhere to belief that disease is human mental concept that can be dispelled by spiritual truth
CHURCH OF JESUS CHRIST OF LATTER DAY SAINTS (MORMON)		
Birth: No baptism Infant is blessed by church official at first opportunity after birth (in church) Baptism by immersion at 8 years of age **Death:** Believe that it is proper to bury the dead in the ground; cremation is discouraged **Organ donation/transplantation:** Question of whether one should will his or her organs to be used as transplants is left to the individual	Prohibits tea, coffee, and alcohol Some individuals avoid chocolate and other products that contain caffeine Encourage sparing use of meats Fasting for 24 hours each month	Devout adherents believe in divine healing Medical therapy is not prohibited
HINDU		
Birth: No baptism **Death:** Certain prescribed rites are followed after death; priest may tie thread around neck or wrist to signify blessing; family will wash the body; are particular about who touches their dead; bodies are to be cremated **Organ donation/transplantation:** No religious laws prohibiting donation; individual decision	Many dietary restrictions Beef and veal are not eaten Some are strict vegetarians	Illness or injury is believed to represent sins committed in previous life Accept most modern medical practices
ISLAM (MUSLIM/MOSLEM)		
Birth: At birth, the first words said to the infant in his or her right ear are Allah-o-Akbar (Allah is great) and the remainder of the Call for Prayer is recited. An Aqeeqa (party) to celebrate the birth of the child is arranged by the parents. Circumcision of the male child is practiced.	Prohibits all pork products; fasting is practiced during the ninth month of the Islamic year (Ramadan)	Believers are encouraged in the Qu'ran to seek treatment. It is taught that only Allah cures; however, Muslims are taught not to refuse treatment in the belief that Allah will take care of them because he also chooses at times to work through the efforts of humans.

McQueay JE: Cross cultural customs and beliefs related to health crisis, death, and organ donation/transplantation, *Crit Care Nurs Clin North Am* 7(3): 581-594, 1995; Lipson JG, Dibble SL, Minarik PA: *Culture and nursing care: a pocket guide*, San Francisco, 2003, UCSF Nursing Press; Spector RE: *Cultural diversity in health and illness*, ed 5, Upper Saddle River, NJ, 2000, Prentice-Hall.

Continued

Table 32-2

Religious Beliefs That Affect Nursing Care—cont'd

BIRTH AND DEATH	DIET AND FOOD PRACTICES	MEDICAL CARE
ISLAM (MUSLIM/MOSLEM)—cont'd		
Death: At the time of death, there are specific rituals (e.g., bathing, wrapping the body in cloth) that must be done. Before moving and handling the body, it is preferable to contact someone from the person's mosque or the local Islamic Society to perform these rituals. **Organ donation/transplantation:** Permitted; however, there are some stipulations depending on the type of transplant/donation and its effect on the donor and recipient.		
JEHOVAH'S WITNESS		
Birth: No baptism **Death:** No official last rites practiced when death occurs **Organ donation/transplantation:** No definite statement related to this issue	No ingestion of blood of any kind; can eat animal flesh that has been drained	Adherents are generally absolutely opposed to transfusions, including banking of own blood May be opposed to use of albumin, globulin, factor replacement (hemophilia), vaccines Not opposed to non–blood plasma expanders
JUDAISM (ORTHODOX AND CONSERVATIVE)		
Birth: No baptism Ritual circumcision of male infants on eighth day; performed by Mohel (ritual circumciser familiar with Jewish law and aseptic technique) **Death:** According to tradition, during last moments of life, relatives and close friends remain with the deceased **Organ donation/transplantation:** Amputated limbs or surgically removed tissues should be made available to family for burial. Autopsy and organ donation are discouraged but may be permitted if it may save a life or where local law requires it. Cremation is not allowed.	Numerous dietary kosher laws exist Are allowed only meat from animals that are vegetable eaters and are ritually slaughtered; fish that have scales and fins Milk products served first can be followed by meat in a few minutes, but milk may not be consumed for several hours after eating meat Fasting is part of Yom Kippur observance Matzo replaces leavened bread during Passover week	May resist surgical procedures during Sabbath, which extends from sundown Friday until sundown Saturday Seriously ill and pregnant women are exempt from fasting Illness is grounds for violating dietary laws (e.g., patient with congestive heart failure does not have to use kosher meats, which are high in sodium)
ROMAN CATHOLIC		
Birth: Infant baptism; especially urgent if poor prognosis, when it may be performed by anyone **Death:** Sacrament of the Sick is performed if prognosis is poor while patients is alive **Organ donation/transplantation:** Transplantation of organs is viewed by Catholics as ethically and morally acceptable to Vatican; organ donation is viewed as an act of charity	Fasting (eating only one full meal and no eating between meals) and abstaining from meat are practiced on Ash Wednesday and Good Friday; fasting is optional during Lent; no meat on Fridays during Lent as a general rule. Children and most hospital patients are exempt from fasting	Encourage anointing of the sick Traditional church teaching does not approve of contraceptives or abortion

Table 32-3

Cultural Characteristics Related to Health Care of Children and Families

CULTURAL GROUP	HEALTH BELIEFS	HEALTH PRACTICES	FAMILY RELATIONSHIPS	COMMUNICATION
African	Illness classified as *natural* or *unnatural:* **Natural**—affected by forces of nature without adequate protection (e.g., cold air, pollution, food and water) **Unnatural**—God's punishment for improper behavior May see illness as the "will of God"	Self-care and folk medicine very prevalent Folk therapies usually religious in origin Folk therapies often not shared with the medical provider Prayer is common means for prevention and treatment	Strong kinship bonds in extended family; members come to aid of others in crisis Less likely to view illness as a burden Place strong emphasis on work and ambition Elders cared for and respected	Alert to any evidence of discrimination Place importance on nonverbal behavior Affection shown by touching and hugging Silence may indicate lack of trust Eye contact important to establish trust Best to use direct, but caring, approach
American Indian	Believe health is state of harmony with nature and universe Respect of bodies through proper management Depend on individual belief in traditional culture Traditional health beliefs holistic and wellness oriented Health practices include self-sufficiency and harmonious living Participation in religious ceremonies and prayer promotes health	Distinction made between indigenous health problem requiring native healer or practice and Western disease requiring other medical care	Cultures vary in kinship structure Extended family structure—usually includes relatives from both sides of family Elder members assume leadership roles	Most continue to speak their Indian language as well as English Nonverbal communication Individuals usually speak for themselves
Chinese	A healthy body viewed as gift from parents and ancestors and must be cared for Health is one of the results of balance between the forces of *yin* (cold) and *yang* (hot)—energy forces that rule the world Illness caused by imbalance Believe blood is source of life and is not regenerated *Chi* is innate energy	Goal of therapy is to restore balance of yin and yang Acupuncturist applies needles to appropriate meridians identified in terms of yin and yang Acupressure and *tai chi* replacing acupuncture in some areas *Moxibustion* is application of heat to skin over specific meridians Wide use of medicinal herbs procured and applied in prescribed ways Meals may or may not be planned to balance hot and cold	Extended family pattern common Strong concept of loyalty of young to old Respect for elders taught at early age—acceptance without questioning or talking back Children's behavior a reflection on family Family and individual honor and "face" important Self-reliance and self-esteem highly valued; self-expression repressed	Open expression of emotions unacceptable Often smile when they do not comprehend

Data from Lipson JG, Dibble SL, Minarik PA: *Culture and nursing care: A pocket guide,* San Francisco, CA, 2003, UCSF Nursing Press; Spector RE: *Cultural diversity in health and illness,* ed 5, Upper Saddle River, NJ, 2000, Prentice-Hall.

Continued

Table 32-3

Cultural Characteristics Related to Health Care of Children and Families—cont'd

CULTURAL GROUP	HEALTH BELIEFS	HEALTH PRACTICES	FAMILY RELATIONSHIPS	COMMUNICATION
Vietnamese	Good health considered to be balance between yin and yang Concept of health based on harmony and balance Many use rituals to prevent illness	Family uses all means possible before using outside agencies for health care Regard health as family responsibility; outside aid sought when resources run out Use herbal medicine, spiritual practices, and acupuncture May use cupping, coin rubbing, or pinching skin May use inhaling aromatic oils, herbal teas, or wearing strings tied on body	Family is revered institution Multigenerational families Family is chief social network Children highly valued Individual needs and interests are subordinate to those of a family group Father is main decision maker Woman taught submission to men Parents expect respect and obedience from children	Many immigrants are not proficient in speaking and understanding English May hesitate to ask questions Questioning authority is sign of disrespect; asking questions considered impolite May avoid eye contact with health professionals as a sign of respect
Filipino	Health is a result of balance Illness is a result of imbalance To be able to be healthy again is to correct an evil deed	May not respond to illness until it is advanced May use herbal medicine Eating well, not necessarily eating right, promotes good health Physical ailment may be caused by the supernatural	Family is highly valued, with strong family ties Multigenerational family structure common, often including collateral members Members avoid any behavior that would bring shame on the family	Immigrants and older persons may not be able to speak or understand English Sensitive to tone and manner of speaker Limited direct eye contact
Haitian	Illness is a punishment **Natural** cause (*maladi bone die*—disease of the Lord) caused by environmental factors, movement of blood within the body, changes between hot and cold, and bone displacement **Supernatural** (*loa*—spirits' anger) Good health is the maintenance of equilibrium Prayer and good spiritual habits very important	Health is a personal responsibility Foods have properties of "hot"/"cold" and "light"/"heavy" and must be in harmony with one's life cycle and bodily states Natural illnesses treated by home and folk remedies first May use religious medallions, rosary beads, or figure of saint to pray with	Maintenance of family reputation paramount Lineal authority supreme; children in a subordinate position in family hierarchy Children valued for parental social security in old age and expected to contribute to family welfare at an early age	Recent immigrants and older persons may speak only Haitian Creole Often smile and nod in agreement when do not understand Quiet and gentle communication style and lack of assertiveness lead health care providers to falsely believe they comprehend health teaching and are compliant May not ask questions if health care provider is busy or rushed

Japanese	*Shinto* religious influence Human inherently good Evil caused by outside spirits Illness caused by contact with polluting agents (e.g., blood, corpses, skin diseases) Health achieved through harmony and balance between self and society Disease caused by disharmony with society and not caring for body	Energy restored by means of acupuncture, acupressure, massage, and moxibustion along affected meridians *Kampō* medicine—use of natural herbs Believe in removal of diseased parts Trend is to use both Western and Asian healing methods Care for disabled viewed as family's responsibility Take pride in child's good health Seek preventive care, medical care for illness	Close intergenerational relationships Generational categories: *Issei*—first generation to live in United States *Nisei*—second generation *Sansei*—third generation *Yonsei*—fourth generation Family tends to keep problems to self Value self-control and self-sufficiency Concept of *haji* (shame) imposes strong control; unacceptable behavior of children reflects on family	Issei—born in Japan; usually speak Japanese only Nisei, Sansei, and Yonsei have few language difficulties Make significant use of nonverbal communication with subtle gestures and facial expression Tends to suppress emotions Will often wait silently
Mexican-American	Health controlled by environment fate and by will of God Certain illnesses considered hot and cold states and are treated with food that complement those states Disease based on imbalance between individual and environment	Seek help from *curandero* or *curandera,* especially in rural areas *Curandero(a)* receives position by birth, apprenticeship, or a "calling" via dream or vision Treatments involve use of herbs, rituals, and religious artifacts Practice for severe illness—make promises, visit shrines, offer medals and candles, offer prayers Adhere to "hot" and "cold" food prescriptions and prohibitions for prevention and treatment of illness	Strong kinship extended families include *compadres* (godparents) established by ritual kinship Children valued highly and desired, taken everywhere with family Elderly treated with respect	Spanish speaking or bilingual May have a strong preference for native language and revert to it in times of stress May shake hands or engage in introductory embrace Interpret prolonged eye contact as disrespectful Relaxed concept of time—may be late to appointments
Puerto Rican	Subscribe to the "hot-cold" theory of causation of illness Believe some illness caused by evil forces Destiny (*Si Dios quiere*—if God wants) is in control of health	Infrequent use of health care system Seek folk healers *(Espiritistas)*—use of herbs, rituals Treatment classified as "hot" or "cold" Many varieties of herbal teas used to treat illness and promote healing	Family usually large and home centered—the core of existence Father has authority in family Great respect for elders Children valued—seen as a gift from God Children taught to obey and respect parents	Spanish speaking or bilingual Strong sense of family privacy—may view questions regarding family as impudent

Data from Lipson JG, Dibble SL, Minarik PA: *Culture and nursing care: A pocket guide,* San Francisco, CA, 2003, UCSF Nursing Press; Spector RE: *Cultural diversity in health and illness,* ed 5, Upper Saddle River, NJ, 2000, Prentice-Hall.

- A trend that has significantly influenced the American family is increasing geographic and economic mobility.
- Membership in a minority group presents special challenges for children, although changes in societal attitudes are slowly taking place.
- A child's physical characteristics and susceptibility to health problems are strongly related to ethnic and cultural variations of hereditary and socioeconomic forces.
- Hereditary and socioeconomic forces play an important role in a child's susceptibility to health problems.
- Groups of children suffering from greater physical and mental health problems are those living in poverty, those who are homeless, and those who have migrant families.
- Because verbal and nonverbal communication is an important cultural consideration, nurses need to acknowledge and respect their patient's practices for productive interaction to occur.
- Cultural beliefs related to cause of illness and maintenance of health may focus on natural forces, supernatural forces, or imbalance of forces.
- In planning and implementing patient care, nurses need to strive to adapt ethnic practices to the family's health needs rather than attempt to change long-standing beliefs.
- No cultural group is homogeneous; every racial and ethnic group contains great diversity.

Answer Guidelines to Critical Thinking Exercise

Reducing Cultural Shock

1. An understanding of the Arab culture provides insight into the woman's hesitancy to make decisions in her husband's absence.
2. (a) Typically, in the Arab culture men make the decisions and women are expected to support these decisions. (b) The need for an interpreter is evident to make sure the mother understands the seriousness of the situation. (c) Knowledge of the procedures for obtaining approval for emergency procedures without informed consent will facilitate the best care for the child. (d) Appropriate documentation of how approval was obtained without parental consent is essential.
3. The first priority is to make sure the child is receiving the best care possible and that the necessary procedure is performed as soon as possible. The next priority is to make sure the mother understands the urgency of the situation by using an interpreter.
4. The health status of the child is most important at this time.
5. Attempts should continue to try to reach the father by phone, and continued support of the mother during this stressful time is important.

References

Annie E. Casey Foundation: *Kids count data book: state profiles of child well-being; available online:* http://www.aecf.org/kidscount/kc2003/pdfs/entire_book.pdf. accessed March 3, 2005.

Campinha-Bacote J: Many faces: addressing diversity in health care, *Online J Issues Nurs* 3:2, 2003. Internet document available at www.nursingworld.org/ojin/topic20/tpc20_2.htm (accessed March 3, 2005).

Carrillo JE, Green AR, Belancourt JR: Cross-cultural primary care: a patient-based approach, *Ann Intern Med* 130:829-834, 1999.

Castiglia PT: Tuberculosis: a pediatric concern, *J Pediatr Health Care* 11(2):75-77, 1997.

Centers for Disease Control and Prevention: *Preventing lead poisoning in young children,* Atlanta, 1997, Centers for Disease Control and Prevention.

Chidester D: *Patterns of transcendence: religion, death, and dying,* ed 2, Belmont, CA, 2001, Wadsworth.

Gulley L: A critique of multiculturalism in health care: the challenge for nurse education, *J Adv Nurs* 23:564-570, 1996.

DeSantis L: Cultural factors affecting newborn and infant diarrhea, *J Pediatr Nurs* 3(6):391-398, 1988.

Dunn AM: Culture competence and the primary care provider, *J Pediatr Health Care* 16:105-111, 2002.

Ensign J, Santelli J: Health status and service use: comparison of adolescents at a school-based health clinic with homeless adolescents, *Arch Pediatr Adolesc Med* 152(1):20-24, 1998.

Fierman A et al: Status of immunization and iron nutrition in New York City homeless children, *Clin Pediatr* 32(3):151-155, 1993.

Fulton RA, Moore CM: Spiritual care of the school-age child with a chronic condition, *Pediatr Nurs* 10(4):224-231, 1995.

Garwick A, Auger S: What do providers need to know about American Indian culture? Recommendations from urban Indian family caregivers, *Fam Systems Health* 18:177-189, 2000.

Giger JN, Davidhizar RE: *Transcultural nursing: assessment and intervention,* ed 3, St Louis, 1999, Mosby.

Hayes J, Dreher C: Providing culturally sensitive care. In Smith D (ed): *Comprehensive child and family nursing skills,* St Louis, 1991, Mosby.

Leininger M: *Transcultural nursing,* New York, 1978, John Wiley & Sons.

Leininger M: *Transcultural nursing: concepts, theories, research and practices,* ed 2, New York, 1995, McGraw-Hill.

Lewit EM, Baker LS: Homeless families and children, *Future Children* 6(2):146-158, 1996.

Lipson JG, Dibble SL, Minarik PA: *Culture and nursing care: A pocket guide,* San Francisco, CA, 2003, UCSF Nursing Press.

Lukoff D, Lu FG, Turner R: Cultural considerations in the assessment and treatment of religious and spiritual problems, *Psychiatr Clin North Am* 18(3):467-485, 1995.

Malach F, Segel N: Perspectives on health care delivery systems for American Indian families, *Child Health Care* 19(4):219-228, 1990.

Martinson IM, Armstrong V, Qiao J: The experience of the family of children with chronic illness at home in China, *Pediatr Nurs* 23(4):371-375, 1997.

Mattson S: Culturally sensitive perinatal care for Southeast Asians, *J Obstet Gynecol Neonatal Nurs* 24(4):335-341, 1995.

MMWR Morb Mortal Wkly Rep. Tuberculosis transmission in a homeless shelter population—New York, 2000-2003. 54(6):149-52, 2005.

Murdock SH: Minority child population growth. In Cosby A.G., Greenberg R.E., Southward L.H., & Weitzman M. (Eds.) *About children: An authoritative resource on the state of childhood today* (pp. 178-181), 2005, American Academy of Pediatrics.

Nance TA: Intercultural communications: finding common ground, *J Obstet Gynecol Neonatal Nurs* 24(3):249-255, 1995.

O'Hare WP: Changes in the well-being of children. In Cosby A.G., Greenberg R.E., Southward L.H., & Weitzman M. (Eds.) *About children: An authoritative resource on the state of childhood today* (pp. 178-181), 2005, American Academy of Pediatrics.

Ozawa MN, Yat-sang L: How safe is the safety net for poor children? *Soc Work Res* 20(4):238-254, 1996.

Page A, Ainsworth A, Pett M: Homeless families and their children's health problems: a Utah urban experience, *West J Med* 158(1):30-35, 1993.

Rogers G: Educating case managers for culturally competent practice, *J Case Manage* 4(2):60-65, 1995.

Sandhaus S: Migrant health: a harvest of poverty, *Am J Nurs* 98(9):52-54, 1998.

Scribner R: Paradox as paradigm: the health outcomes of Mexican Americans, *Am J Public Health* 86(3):303-304, 1996.

Search Institute: Developmental assets: an overview, 2003. Internet document available at www.search-institute.org/assets/ (accessed March 4, 2005).

Sekhon SK: Insights into South Asian culture: food and nutritional values, *Top Clin Nutr* 11(4):47-56, 1996.

Shaw-Taylor Y: Culturally and linguistically appropriate health care for racial or ethnic minorities: analysis of the US Office of Minority Health's recommended standards, *Health Policy* 62:211-221, 2002.

Spector RE: *Cultural diversity in health and illness,* ed 5, Upper Saddle River, NJ, 2000, Prentice-Hall.

Strehlow AJ, Amos-Jones T: The homeless as a vulnerable population, *Nurs Clin North Am* 34(2):261-274, 1999.

Taylor R: Check your cultural competence, *Nurs Manage* 29(8):30-32, 1998.

Trawick-Smith J: *Early childhood development: a multicultural perspective,* ed 2, Upper Saddle River, NJ, 2000, Prentice-Hall.

Tropello PD: The many faces of homelessness. In Kelley ML, Fitzsimons VM (eds): *Understanding cultural diversity,* Sudbury, MA, 2000, Jones & Bartlett.

US Census Bureau: Overview of race and Hispanic origin census 2000 brief, 2000. Internet document available at www.census.gov/prod/2001pubs/c2kbr01-1pdf (accessed March 4, 2005).

Wagner J, Menke EM, Cicconi MA: What is known about the health of rural homeless families, *Public Health Nurs* 12(6):400-408, 1995.

Weinreb L et al: Determinants of health and service use patterns in homeless and low-income housed children, *Pediatrics* 102(3):554-562, 1998.

White L, Chalmers S, Litchfield K et al: Cultural diversity and child health, *J Paediatr Child Health* 40(9-10):589, 2004.

Wright J: Female genital mutilation: an overview, *J Adv Nurs* 24:251-259, 1996.

Unit 7

33 Developmental Influences on Child Health Promotion

LEARNING OBJECTIVES

On completion of this chapter the reader will be able to:

- Describe the major trends in growth and development.
- Explain the alterations in the major body systems that take place during the process of growth and development.
- Discuss personality, cognitive, language, moral, spiritual, and self-concept development and the relationships among them.
- Describe the role of play in the growth and development of children.
- Demonstrate an understanding of the roles of innate and environmental factors in the physical and emotional development of children.

ELECTRONIC RESOURCES

Additional information related to the content in Chapter 33 can be found on

the companion website at evolve
http://evolve.elsevier.com/Wong/maternal/
- NCLEX Review Questions
- WebLinks

or the interactive student CD-ROM
Activities for Chapter 33 include the following:
- NCLEX Review Questions
- Critical Thinking Exercise–Growth Trends during Infancy

GROWTH AND DEVELOPMENT

Foundations of Growth and Development

Growth and development is usually referred to as a unit; it expresses the sum of the numerous changes that take place during the lifetime of an individual. The entire course is a dynamic process that encompasses several interrelated dimensions:

Growth—An increase in number and size of cells as they divide and synthesize new proteins; results in increased size and weight of the whole or any of its parts

Development—A gradual change and expansion; advancement from lower to more advanced stages of complexity; the emerging and expanding of the individual's capacities through growth, maturation, and learning

Maturation—An increase in competence and adaptability; aging; usually used to describe a qualitative change; a change in the complexity of a structure that makes it possible for that structure to begin functioning; to function at a higher level

Differentiation—Processes by which early cells and structures are systematically modified and altered to achieve specific and characteristic physical and chemical properties; sometimes used to describe the trend of mass to specific; development from simple to more complex activities and functions

All of these processes are interrelated, simultaneous, and ongoing; none occurs apart from the others. The processes depend on a sequence of endocrine, genetic, constitutional, environmental, and nutritional influences (Seidel et al, 2003). The child's body becomes larger and more complex; the personality simultaneously expands in scope and complexity. Very simply, growth can be viewed as a *quantitative* change, and development as a *qualitative* change.

Stages of Development

Most authorities in the field of child development conveniently categorize child growth and behavior into approximate age stages or in terms that describe the features of an age group. The age ranges of these stages are admittedly arbitrary and, because they do not take into account individual differences, cannot be applied to all children with any degree of precision. However, this categorization affords a convenient means to describe the characteristics associated with the majority of children at periods when distinctive developmental changes appear and specific developmental tasks must be accomplished. (A *developmental task* is a set of skills and competencies specific to each developmental stage that children must accomplish or master in order to deal effectively with their environment.) It is also significant for nurses to know that there are characteristic health problems specific to each major phase of development. The sequences of descriptive age periods and subperiods that are used here, and that are elaborated in subsequent chapters, are listed in Box 33-1.

Patterns of Growth and Development

There are definite and predictable patterns in growth and development that are continuous, orderly, and progressive. These patterns or trends are universal and basic to all human beings, but each human being accomplishes them in a manner and time unique to that individual.

Directional Trends

Growth and development proceed in regular, related directions or gradients and reflect the physical development and maturation of neuromuscular functions (Fig. 33-1). The first pattern is the *cephalocaudal*, or *head-to-tail*, direction. The head end of the organism develops first and is very large and complex, whereas the lower end is small and simple and takes shape at a later period. The physical evidence of this trend is most apparent during the period before birth, but it also applies to postnatal behavior development. Infants achieve structural control of the head before they have control of the trunk and extremities, hold their backs erect before they stand, use their eyes before their hands, and gain control of their hands before they have control of their feet.

Second, the *proximodistal*, or *near-to-far*, trend applies to the midline-to-peripheral concept. A conspicuous illustration is the early embryonic development of limb buds, which is followed by rudimentary fingers and toes. In the infant, shoulder control precedes mastery of the hands, the whole hand is used as a unit before the fingers can be manipulated, and the central nervous system develops more rapidly than the peripheral nervous system.

These trends or patterns are bilateral and appear symmetric—each side develops in the same direction and at the same rate as the other. For some of the neurologic functions, this symmetry is only external because of unilateral differentiation of function at an early stage of postnatal development. For example, by approximately 5 years of age the child has demonstrated a decided preference for the use of one hand over the other, although previously either one had been used.

The third trend, differentiation, describes development from simple operations to more complex activities and functions. From very broad, global patterns of behavior, more specific, refined patterns emerge. All areas of development (i.e., physical, mental, social, and emotional) proceed in this direction. Through the process of development and differentiation, early embryonal cells with vague, undifferentiated functions progress to an immensely complex organism composed of highly specialized and diversified cells, tissues, and organs. Generalized development precedes specific or specialized development; gross, random muscle movements take place before fine muscle control.

Critical Thinking Exercise: Growth Trends During Infancy

Sequential Trends

In all dimensions of growth and development there is a definite, predictable sequence, with each child normally passing through every stage. Children crawl before they creep, creep before they stand, and stand before they walk. Later facets of the personality are built on the early foundation of trust. The child babbles, then forms words and, finally, sentences; writing emerges from scribbling.

BOX 33-1

Developmental Age Periods

Prenatal period: Conception to birth

Germinal: Conception to approximately 2 weeks
Embryonic: 2 to 8 weeks
Fetal: 8 to 40 weeks (birth)

A rapid growth rate and total dependency make this one of the most crucial periods in the developmental process. The relationship between maternal health and certain manifestations in the newborn emphasizes the importance of adequate prenatal care to the health and well-being of the infant.

Infancy period: Birth to 12 months

Neonatal: Birth to 27 or 28 days
Infancy: 1 to approximately 12 months

The infancy period is one of rapid motor, cognitive, and social development. Through mutuality with the caregiver (parent), the infant establishes a basic trust in the world and the foundation for future interpersonal relationships. The critical first month of life, although part of the infancy period, is often differentiated from the remainder because of the major physical adjustments to extrauterine existence and the psychologic adjustment of the parent.

Early childhood: 1 to 6 years

Toddler: 1 to 3 years
Preschool: 3 to 6 years

This period, which extends from the time the children attain upright locomotion until they enter school, is characterized by intense activity and discovery. It is a time of marked physical and personality development. Motor development advances steadily. Children at this age acquire language and wider social relationships, learn role standards, gain self-control and mastery, develop increasing awareness of dependence and independence, and begin to develop a self-concept.

Middle childhood: 6 to 11 or 12 years

Frequently referred to as the "school age," this period of development is one in which the child is directed away from the family group and centered around the wider world of peer relationships. There is steady advancement in physical, mental, and social development, with emphasis on developing skill competencies. Social cooperation and early moral development take on more importance with relevance for later life stages. This is a critical period in the development of a self-concept.

Later childhood: 11 to 19 years

Prepubertal: 10 to 13 years
Adolescence: 13 to approximately 18 years

The tumultuous period of rapid maturation and change known as adolescence is considered to be a transitional period that begins at the onset of puberty and extends to the point of entry into the adult world—usually high school graduation. Biologic and personality maturation are accompanied by physical and emotional turmoil, and there is redefining of the self-concept. In the late adolescent period the young person begins to internalize all previously learned values and to focus on an individual, rather than a group, identity.

Developmental Pace

Although there is a fixed, precise order to development, it does not progress at the same rate or pace. There are periods of accelerated growth and periods of decelerated growth in

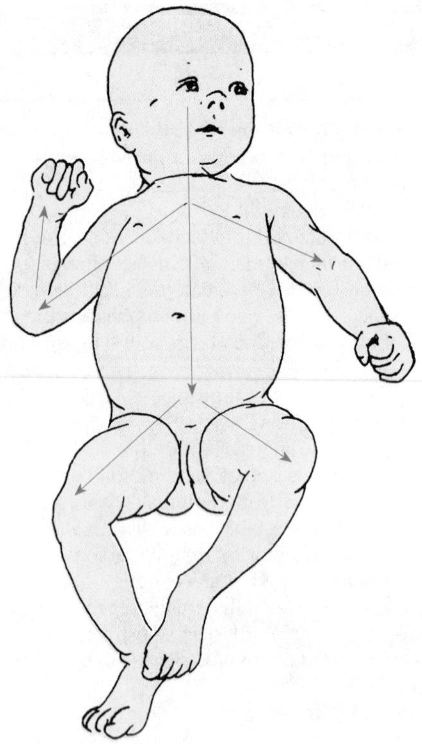

Fig. 33-1 Directional trends in growth.

both total body growth and the growth of subsystems. The rapid growth before and after birth gradually levels off throughout early childhood. Growth is relatively slow during middle childhood, increases markedly at the beginning of adolescence, and levels off in early adulthood. Each child grows at his or her own pace. Marked differences are observed between children as they reach and surmount developmental milestones.

Sensitive Periods

There are limited times during the process of growth when the organism will interact with a particular environment in a specific manner. Periods termed *critical, sensitive, vulnerable,* and *optimal* are those times in the lifetime of an organism when it is more susceptible to positive or negative influences.

The quality of interactions during these sensitive periods determines whether the effects on the organism will be beneficial or harmful. For example, physiologic maturation of the central nervous system is influenced by adequacy and timing of contributions from the environment such as stimulation and nutrition. The first 3 months of prenatal life are sensitive periods for physical growth of the fetus.

Psychologic development also appears to have sensitive periods when an environmental event has maximal influence on the developing personality. For example, primary socialization occurs during the first year when the infant makes the initial social attachments and establishes a basic trust in the world. A warm relationship with a parent figure is fundamental to a healthy personality. The same concept might be applied to readiness for learning skills such as toilet training or reading. In these instances there appears to be an opportune time when the skill is best learned.

Individual Differences

Each child grows in his or her own unique and personal way. Great individual variation exists in the age at which developmental milestones are reached. The sequence is predictable; the exact timing is not. Rates of growth vary, and measurements are defined in terms of ranges to allow for individual differences. Some children are fast growers, others are moderate, and still others are slower to reach maturity. Periods of fast growth, such as the pubescent growth spurt, may begin earlier or later in some children. Children may grow quickly or slowly during the spurt, and may finish sooner or later than others. Gender is an influential factor because girls seem to be more advanced in physiologic growth at all ages.

Biologic Growth and Physical Development

As children grow, their external dimensions change. These changes are accompanied by corresponding alterations in structure and function of internal organs and tissues that reflect the gradual acquisition of physiologic competence. Each part has its own rate of growth, which may be directly related to alterations in the size of the child (e.g., the heart rate). Skeletal muscle growth approximates whole body growth; brain, lymphoid, adrenal, and reproductive tissues follow distinct and individual patterns. When there has been a secondary cause of growth deficiency, such as severe illness or acute malnutrition, recovery from the illness or the establishment of an adequate diet will produce a dramatic acceleration of the growth rate that usually continues until the child's individual growth pattern is resumed.

External Proportions

Variations in the growth rate of different tissues and organ systems produce significant changes in body proportions during childhood. The cephalocaudal trend of development is most evident in total body growth as indicated by these changes (Fig. 33-2). During fetal development the head is the fastest growing body part, and at 2 months of gestation the head constitutes 50% of total body length. During infancy growth of the trunk predominates; the legs are the most rapidly growing part during childhood; in adolescence the trunk once again elongates. In the newborn infant the lower limbs are one third of the total body length but only 15% of the total body weight; in the adult the lower limbs constitute one half of the total body height and 30% or more of the total body weight. As growth proceeds, the midpoint in head-to-toe measurements gradually descends from a level even with the umbilicus at birth to the level of the symphysis pubis at maturity.

Biologic Determinants of Growth and Development

The most prominent feature of childhood and adolescence is physical growth. Throughout development various tissues in the body undergo changes in growth, composition, and structure. In some tissues the changes are continuous (e.g., bone growth and dentition); in others, significant alterations occur at specific stages (e.g., appearance of secondary sex characteristics). When these measurements are compared with standardized norms, a child's developmental progress can be determined with a high degree of confidence (Table 33-1).

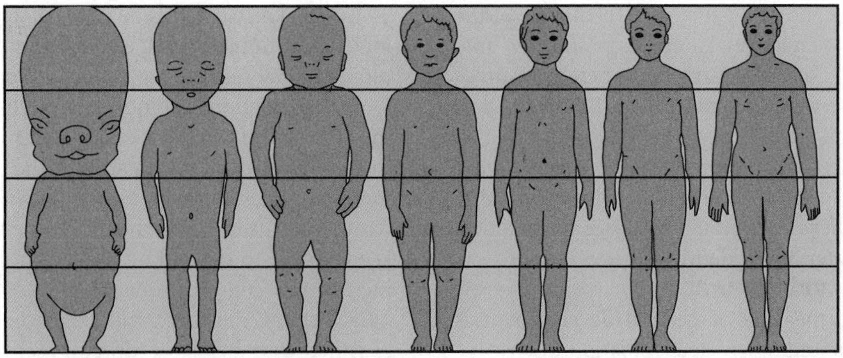

Fig. 33-2 Changes in body proportions from before birth to adulthood. (From Crouch JE, McClintic JR: *Human anatomy and physiology,* ed 2, New York, 1976, Wiley & Sons.)

Table 33-1

General Trends in Height and Weight Gain during Childhood

AGE GROUP	WEIGHT*	HEIGHT*
Infants		
Birth to 6 months	Weekly gain: 140-200 g (5-7 oz) Birth weight doubles by end of first 4-7 months	Monthly gain: 2.5 cm (1 inch)
6-12 months	Weight gain: 85-140 g (3-5 oz) Birth weight triples by end of first year	Monthly gain: 1.25 cm (½ inch) Birth length increases by approximately 50% by end of first year
Toddlers	Birth weight quadruples by age 2½ Yearly gain: 2-3 kg (4½-6½ lb)	Height at age 2 years is approximately 50% of eventual adult height Gain during second year: about 12 cm (4¾ inches) Gain during third year: about 6-8 cm (2⅜-3¼ inches)
Preschoolers	Yearly gain: 2-3 kg (4½-6½ lb)	Birth length doubles by age 4 years Yearly gain: 5-7.5 cm (2-3 inches)
School-age children	Yearly gain: 2-3 kg (4½-6½ lb)	Yearly gain after age 7: 5 cm (2 inches) Birth length triples by about age 13 years
PUBERTAL GROWTH SPURT		
Females—10-14 years	Weight gain: 7-25 kg (15-55 lb) Mean: 17.5 kg (38⅛ lb)	Height gain: 5-25 cm (2-10 inches); approximately 95% of mature height achieved by onset of menarche or skeletal age of 13 years Mean: 20.5 cm (8¼ inches)
Males—11-16 years	Weight gain: 7-30 kg (15-65 lb) Mean: 23.7 kg (52⅛ lb)	Height gain: 10-30 cm (4-12 inches); approximately 95% of mature height achieved by skeletal age of 15 years Mean: 27.5 cm (11 inches)

*Yearly height and weight gains for each age group represent averaged estimates from a variety of sources.

Linear growth, or *height,* occurs almost entirely as a result of skeletal growth and is considered a stable measurement of general growth. Growth in height is not uniform throughout life, and it ceases when maturation of the skeleton is complete. The maximum growth in length occurs before birth, but the newborn continues to grow at a rapid, though slower, rate.

NURSE ALERT Double the child's height at age 2 years to estimate how tall he or she may be as an adult. ■

At birth, *weight* is more variable than height and is, to a greater extent, a reflection of the intrauterine environment. The average newborn weighs from 3175 to 3400 g (7 to 7.5 pounds). In general, the birth weight doubles by 4 to 7 months of age and triples by the end of the first year. By the end of the second year it usually quadruples. After this point the "normal" rate of weight gain, just as the growth in height, assumes a steady annual increase of approximately 2 to 2.75 kg (4.4 to 6 pounds) per year until the adolescent growth spurt.

Both *bone age* determinants and state of *dentition* are used as indicators of development. Because both are discussed elsewhere, neither is elaborated here (see next section for bone age; see Chapter 36 for dentition).

Skeletal Growth and Maturation

The most accurate measure of general development is *skeletal* or *bone age,* the radiologic determination of osseous maturation. Skeletal age appears to correlate more closely with other measures of physiologic maturity (e.g., onset of menarche) than with chronologic age or height. Bone age is determined by comparing the mineralization of ossification centers and advancing bony form with age-related standards.

Bone formation begins during the second month of fetal life when calcium salts are deposited in the intracellular substance (matrix) to form first calcified cartilage and then true bone. There are some differences in this bone formation. In small bones the bone continues to form in the center and cartilage continues to be laid down on the surfaces. In long bones the ossification begins in the *diaphysis* (the long central portion of the bone) and continues in the *epiphysis* (the end portions of the bone). Between the diaphysis and the epiphysis, an *epiphyseal cartilage plate* unites with the diaphysis by columns of spongy tissue, the *metaphysis.* Active growth in length takes place in the epiphyseal growth plate. Interference with this growth site by trauma or infection can result in deformity.

The first centers of ossification appear in the 2-month-old embryo, and at birth the number is approximately 400, or about half the number at maturity. New centers appear at regular intervals during the growth period and provide the basis for assessment of bone age. Postnatally the earliest centers to appear (at 5 to 6 months of age) are those of the capitate and hamate bones in the wrist. Therefore radiographs of the hand and wrist provide the most useful areas for screening to determine skeletal age, especially before age 6 years. These centers appear earlier in girls than in boys.

Nurses must understand that the growing bones of children possess many unique characteristics. Bone fractures occurring at the growth plate may be difficult to discover and may significantly affect subsequent growth and development (Cutler et al, 2004). Factors that may influence skeletal muscle injury rates and types in children and adolescents include the following (Kaczander, 1997):

- Less protective sports equipment for children
- Less emphasis on conditioning, especially flexibility
- In adolescents, fractures are more common than ligamentous ruptures because of the rapid growth rate of the physeal zone of hypertrophy (i.e., the segment of tubular bone that is concerned mainly with growth)

Neurologic Maturation

In contrast to other body tissues, which grow rapidly after birth, the nervous system grows proportionately more rapidly before birth. Two periods of rapid brain cell growth occur during fetal life: a dramatic increase in the number of neurons between 15 and 20 weeks of gestation, and another increase at 30 weeks, which extends to 1 year of age. The rapid growth of infancy continues during early childhood and then slows to a more gradual rate during later childhood and adolescence.

It is believed that no new nerve cells appear after the sixth month of fetal life. Postnatal growth consists of increasing the amount of cytoplasm around the nuclei of existing cells, increasing the number and intricacy of communications with other cells, and advancing their peripheral axons to keep pace with expanding body dimensions. This allows for increasingly complex movement and behavior. Neurophysiologic changes also provide the foundation for language, learning, and behavior development. Neurologic or electroencephalographic development is sometimes used as an indicator of maturational age in the early weeks of life.

Lymphoid Tissues

Lymphoid tissues contained in the lymph nodes, thymus, spleen, tonsils, adenoids, and blood lymphocytes follow a growth pattern unlike that of other body tissues. These tissues are small in relation to total body size, but they are well developed at birth. They increase rapidly to reach adult dimensions by 6 years of age and continue to grow. At about age 10 to 12 years they reach a maximum development that is approximately twice their adult size. This is followed by a rapid decline to stable adult dimensions by the end of adolescence.

Development of Organ Systems

All tissues and organ systems undergo changes during development. Some are striking; others are more subtle. Many have implications for assessment and care. Because the major importance of these changes relates to their dysfunction, the developmental characteristics of various systems and organs are discussed throughout the book as they relate to these areas. Physical characteristics and physiologic changes that vary with age are included in age-group descriptions.

Physiologic Changes

Physiologic changes that take place in all organs and systems are discussed as they relate to dysfunction. Others, such as pulse and respiratory rates and blood pressure, are an integral part of physical assessment (see Chapter 35). In addition, there are changes in basic functions, including metabolism, temperature, and patterns of sleep and rest.

Metabolism

The rate of metabolism when the body is at rest—the *basal metabolic rate* (BMR)—demonstrates a distinctive change throughout childhood. Highest in the newborn infant, the BMR closely relates to the proportion of surface area to body mass, which changes as the body increases in size. In both sexes the proportion decreases progressively to maturity. The BMR is slightly higher in boys at all ages and during pubescence further increases over that in girls.

The rate of metabolism determines the caloric requirements of the child. The basal energy requirement of infants is about 108 kcal/kg of body weight and decreases to 40 to 45 kcal/kg at maturity (Table 33-2). Water requirements remain at approximately 1.5 ml per calorie of energy expended throughout life. Children's energy needs vary considerably at different ages and with changing circumstances. The energy requirement to build tissue steadily decreases with age, following the general growth curve; however, energy needs vary

Table 33-2

Recommended Calories and Protein through Adolescence

AGE (YEARS)	ENERGY ALLOWANCE (kcal/kg)	PROTEIN (g)
INFANTS		
0-½	108	13
½-1	98	14
CHILDREN		
1-3	102	16
4-6	90	24
7-10	70	28
MALES		
11-14	55	45
15-18	45	49
FEMALES		
11-14	47	46
15-18	40	44

Adapted from Sizer F, Whitney E: *Nutrition concepts and controversies,* ed 9, Belmont, CA, 2003, Thomson Learning Inc.

with the individual child and may be considerably higher. For short periods (e.g., during strenuous exercise) and more prolonged periods (e.g., illness), the needs can be very high.

Temperature

Body temperature, reflecting metabolism, displays the same decrement from infancy to maturity (see Appendix H). Thermoregulation is one of the most important adaptation responses of the infant during the transition from intrauterine to extrauterine life. Following the unstable regulatory ability in the neonatal period, heat production steadily declines as the infant grows into childhood. Individual differences of 0.5° to 1° F are normal, and occasionally a child normally displays an unusually high or low temperature. Beginning at approximately 12 years of age, girls display a temperature that remains relatively stable, whereas the temperature in boys continues to fall for a few more years. Females maintain a temperature slightly above that of males throughout life.

Even with improved temperature regulation, infants and young children are highly susceptible to temperature fluctuations. Body temperature responds to changes in environmental temperature and is increased with active exercise, crying, and emotional upset. Infections can cause a higher and more rapid temperature increase in infants and young children than in older children. In relation to body weight, an infant produces more heat per unit than children near maturity. Consequently, during active play or when heavily clothed, an infant or small child is likely to become overheated.

Sleep and Rest

Sleep, a protective function in all organisms, allows for repair and recovery of tissues following activity. As in most aspects of development, there is wide variation among individual children in the amount and distribution of sleep at various ages. As children mature, there is a change in the total time they spend in sleep and the amount of time they spend in deep sleep.

Newborn infants sleep much of the time that is not occupied with feeding and other aspects of their care. As infants grow older, the total time spent in sleep gradually decreases, they remain awake for longer periods, and they sleep longer at night. For example, the length of a sleep cycle increases from approximately 50 to 60 minutes in the newborn infant to approximately 90 minutes in adolescence (Anders, Sadeh, & Appareddy, 1995). During the latter part of the first year, most children sleep through the night and take one or two naps during the day. By the time they are 12 to 18 months old, most children have eliminated the second nap. After the preschool years the child has usually given up daytime naps, except in cultures in which an afternoon nap or siesta is customary (Davis, Parker, & Montgomery, 2004). During ages 4 to 10 years, sleep time declines slightly and then increases somewhat during the pubertal growth spurt. The changes in length of sleep at different ages are shown in Fig. 33-3.

There is a change in the quality of sleep as children mature. The time spent in deep, restful sleep increases from 50% in infancy to 80% in the older child.

Temperament

Temperament is defined as "the manner of thinking, behaving, or reacting characteristic of an individual" (Shiner & Caspi, 2003) and refers to the way in which a person deals with life. From the time of birth, children exhibit marked individual differences in the way that they respond to their environment and the way others, particularly the parents, respond to them and their needs. A genetic basis has been suggested for some differences in temperament. Nine characteristics of temperament have been identified through interviews with parents (Box 33-2). Temperament refers to behavioral tendencies, not to discrete behavioral acts. There are no implications of good or bad. Most children can be placed into one of three common categories based on their overall pattern of temperamental attributes (Chess & Thomas, 1985):

The easy child. Easygoing children are even-tempered, are regular and predictable in their habits, and have a positive approach to new stimuli. They are open and adaptable to change and display a mild to moderately intense mood that is typically positive. Approximately 40% of children fall into this category.

The difficult child. Difficult children are highly active, irritable, and irregular in their habits. Negative withdrawal responses are typical, and they require a more structured environment. These children adapt slowly to new routines, people, or situations. Mood expressions are usually intense and primarily negative. They exhibit frequent periods of crying, and frustration often produces violent tantrums. This group makes up about 10% of children.

The slow-to-warm-up child. Slow-to-warm-up children typically react negatively and with mild intensity to new stimuli and, unless pressured, adapt slowly with repeated contact. They respond with only mild but passive resistance to novelty or changes in routine. They are quite inactive and moody, but show only moderate irregularity in functions. Fifteen percent of children demonstrate this temperament pattern.

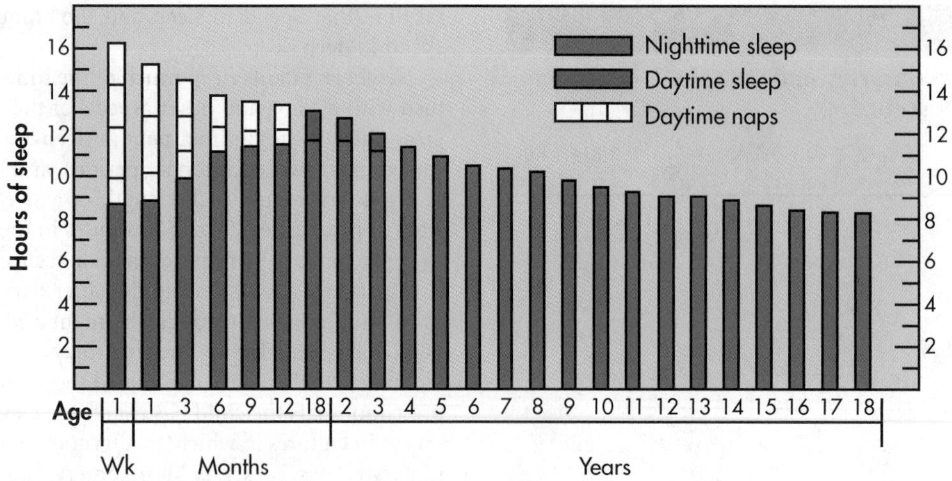

Fig. 33-3 Changes in number of hours of sleep with increasing age. (Modified from Ferber R: *Solve your child's sleep problems,* New York, 1985, Simon & Schuster.)

BOX 33-2

Attributes of Temperament

Activity—level of physical motion during activity such as sleep, eating, play, dressing, and bathing

Rhythmicity—regularity in the timing of physiologic functions such as hunger, sleep, and elimination

Approach-withdrawal—nature of initial responses to a new stimulus such as people, situations, places, foods, toys, and procedures (*Approach* responses are positive and are displayed by activity or expression; *withdrawal* responses are negative expressions or behaviors.)

Adaptability—ease or difficulty with which the child adapts or adjusts to new or altered situations

Threshold of responsiveness (sensory threshold)—amount of stimulation, such as sounds or light, required to evoke a response in the child

Intensity of reaction—energy level of the child's reactions, regardless of quality or direction

Mood—amount of pleasant, happy, friendly behavior compared with unpleasant, unhappy, crying, unfriendly behavior exhibited by the child in various situations

Distractibility—ease with which a child's attention or direction of behavior can be diverted by external stimuli

Attention span and persistence—length of time a child pursues a given activity *(attention)* and the continuation of an activity in spite of obstacles *(persistence)*

Thirty-five percent of children either have some, but not all, of the characteristics of one of the categories or are inconsistent in their behavioral responses. Many normal children demonstrate this wide range of behavioral patterns.

Significance of Temperament

Observations indicate that children who display the difficult or slow-to-warm-up patterns of behavior are more vulnerable to the development of behavior problems in early and middle childhood. Any child can develop behavior problems if there is dissonance between the child's temperament and the environment. Demands for change and adaptation that are in conflict with the child's capacities can become excessively stressful. However, authorities emphasize that it is not the temperament patterns of children that place them at risk; it is the *degree of fit* between children and their environment, specifically their parents, that determines the degree of vulnerability. The potential for optimum development exists when environmental expectations and demands fit with the individual's style of behavior and the parents' ability to navigate this period (see Failure to Thrive, Chapter 36).

Early identification of temperament provides a useful tool for caregivers in anticipating probable areas of difficulty or risk associated with development (McClowry, 2002). For example, "difficult" children may be prone to colic in infancy; active children require more vigilance to prevent injury; and school entry requires different approaches for children with different temperaments.

Research indicates that irritable and unadaptable infants can raise doubts in mothers about their competence (Beck, 1996). Studies on the relationship between temperament and the ability to perform a task successfully (mastery motivation) have found that infants with high mastery are more cooperative and less difficult (Shiner & Caspi, 2003).

DEVELOPMENT OF PERSONALITY AND MENTAL FUNCTION

Personality and cognitive skills develop in much the same manner as biologic growth—new accomplishments build on previously mastered skills. Many aspects depend on physical growth and maturation. This is not a comprehensive account of the multiple facets of personality and behavior development. Many aspects are integrated with the child's emotional and social development in later discussion of various age groups. Table 33-3 summarizes some of the developmental theories.

Theoretic Foundations of Personality Development

Psychosexual Development (Freud)

Freud considered the sexual instincts to be significant in the development of the personality. However, he used the term *psychosexual* to describe any *sensual pleasure.* During childhood certain regions of the body assume a prominent

Table 33-3

Summary of Personality, Cognitive, and Moral Development Theories

STAGE/AGE	PSYCHOSEXUAL STAGES (FREUD)	PSYCHOSOCIAL STAGES (ERIKSON)	COGNITIVE STAGES (PIAGET)	MORAL JUDGMENT STAGES (KOHLBERG)
I INFANCY				
Birth to 1 year	Oral-sensory	Trust vs. mistrust	Sensorimotor (birth to 2 years)	
II TODDLERHOOD				
1-3 years	Anal-urethral	Autonomy vs. shame and doubt	Preoperational thought, preconceptual phase (transductive reasoning, e.g., specific to specific) (2-4 years)	Preconventional (premoral) level Punishment and obedience orientation
III EARLY CHILDHOOD				
3-6 years	Phallic-locomotion	Initiative vs. guilt	Preoperational thought, intuitive phase (transductive reasoning) (4-7 years)	Preconventional (premoral) level Naive instrumental orientation
IV MIDDLE CHILDHOOD				
6-12 years	Latency	Industry vs. inferiority	Concrete operations (inductive reasoning and beginning logic) (7-11 years)	Conventional level Good-boy, nice-girl orientation Law-and-order orientation
V ADOLESCENCE				
12-18 years	Genitality	Identity and repudiation vs. identity confusion	Formal operations (deductive and abstract reasoning) (11-15 years)	Postconventional or principled level Social-contract orientation Universal ethical principle orientation (no longer included in revised theory)

psychologic significance; this source of new pleasures and new conflicts gradually shifts from one part of the body to another at particular stages of development:

Oral stage (birth to 1 year)—During infancy the major source of pleasure seeking is centered on oral activities such as sucking, biting, chewing, and vocalizing. Children may prefer one of these over the others, and the preferred method of oral gratification can provide some indication of the personality they develop.

Anal stage (1 to 3 years)—Interest during the second year of life centers in the anal region as sphincter muscles develop and children are able to withhold or expel fecal material at will. At this stage the climate surrounding toilet training can have lasting effects on children's personalities.

Phallic stage (3 to 6 years)—During the phallic stage the genitals become an interesting and sensitive area of the body. Children recognize differences between the sexes and become curious about the dissimilarities. This is the period around which the controversial issues of the Oedipus and Electra complexes, penis envy, and castration anxiety are centered.

Latency period (6 to 12 years)—During the latency period children elaborate on previously acquired traits and skills. Physical and psychic energy are channeled into acquisition of knowledge and vigorous play.

Genital stage (age 12 and over)—The last significant stage begins at puberty with maturation of the reproductive system and production of sex hormones. The genital organs become the major source of sexual tensions and pleasures, but energies are also invested in forming friendships and preparation for marriage.

Psychosocial Development (Erikson)

The most widely accepted theory of personality development is that advanced by Erikson (1963). Although built on Freudian theory, it is known as *psychosocial* development and emphasizes a healthy personality as opposed to a pathologic approach. Erikson also uses the biologic concepts of critical periods and epigenesis, describing key conflicts or core problems that the individual strives to master during critical periods in personality development. Successful completion or mastery of each of these core conflicts is built on the satisfactory completion or mastery of the previous core problem.

Each psychosocial stage has two components (i.e., the favorable and the unfavorable aspects of the core conflict), and progress to the next stage depends on resolution of this conflict. No core conflict is ever mastered completely but remains a recurrent problem throughout life. No life situation is ever secure. Each new situation presents the conflict in a new form. For example, when children who have satisfactorily achieved a sense of trust encounter a new experience (e.g., hospitalization), they must again develop a sense of trust in those responsible for their care in order to master the situation. Erikson's life span approach to personality development consists of eight stages; however, only the first five relating to childhood are included here:

Trust vs. mistrust (birth to 1 year)—The first and most important attribute to develop for a healthy personality is a basic trust. Establishment of basic trust dominates the first year of life and describes all of the child's satisfying experiences at this age. Corresponding to Freud's oral stage, it is a time of "getting" and "taking in" through all the senses. It exists only in relation to something or someone; therefore consistent, loving care by a nurturing person is essential to development of trust. *Mistrust* develops when trust-promoting experiences are deficient or lacking or when basic needs are inconsistently or inadequately met. Although shreds of mistrust are sprinkled throughout the personality, from a basic trust in parents stems trust in the world, other people, and oneself. The result is *faith* and *optimism*.

Autonomy vs. shame and doubt (1 to 3 years)—Corresponding to Freud's anal stage, the problem of *autonomy* can be symbolized by the holding on and letting go of the sphincter muscles. The development of autonomy during the toddler period is centered around children's increasing ability to control their bodies, themselves, and their environment. They want to do things for themselves, using their newly acquired motor skills of walking, climbing, and manipulating and their mental powers of selection and decision making. Much of their learning is acquired through imitating the activities and behavior of others. Negative feelings of *doubt* and *shame* arise when children are made to feel small and self-conscious, when their choices are disastrous, when others shame them, or when they are forced to be dependent in areas in which they are capable of assuming control. The favorable outcomes are *self-control* and *willpower.*

Initiative vs. guilt (3 to 6 years)—The stage of *initiative* corresponds to Freud's phallic stage and is characterized by vigorous, intrusive behavior; enterprise; and a strong imagination. Children explore the physical world with all their senses and powers. They develop a conscience. No longer guided only by outsiders, there is an inner voice that warns and threatens. Children sometimes undertake goals or activities that are in conflict with those of parents or others, and being made to feel that their activities or imaginings are bad produces a sense of *guilt.* Children must learn to retain a sense of initiative without impinging on the rights and privileges of others. The lasting outcomes are *direction* and *purpose.*

Industry vs. inferiority (6 to 12 years)—The stage of industry is the latency period of Freud. Having achieved the more crucial stages in personality development, children are ready to be workers and producers. They want to engage in tasks and activities that they can carry through to completion; they need and want real achievement. Children learn to compete and cooperate with others, and they learn the rules. It is a decisive period in their social relationships with others. Feelings of *inadequacy* and *inferiority* may develop if too much is expected of them, or if they believe that they cannot measure up to the standards set for them by others. The ego quality developed from a sense of industry is *competence.*

Identity vs. role confusion (12 to 18 years)—Corresponding to Freud's genital period, the development of *identity* is characterized by rapid and marked physical changes. Previous trust in their bodies is shaken, and children become overly preoccupied with the way they appear in the eyes of others as compared with their own self-concept. Adolescents struggle to fit the roles they have played and those they hope to play with the current roles and fashions adopted by their peers, to integrate their concepts and values with those of society, and to come to a decision regarding an occupation. Inability to solve the core conflict results in *role confusion.* The outcome of successful mastery is *devotion* and *fidelity* to others and to values and ideologies.

Theoretic Foundations of Mental Development

Cognitive Development (Piaget)

Cognitive development consists of age-related changes that occur in mental activities. The best-known theory regarding children's thinking, and a more comprehensive developmental theory than those already described, was developed by the Swiss psychologist Jean Piaget (1969). According to Piaget, intelligence enables individuals to make adaptations to the environment that increase the probability of survival, and through their behavior individuals establish and maintain equilibrium with the environment.

Piaget proposed three stages of reasoning: (1) intuitive, (2) concrete operational, and (3) formal operational. When they enter the stage of concrete logical thought at about age 7 years, children are able to make logical inferences, classify, and deal with quantitative relationships about concrete things. Not until adolescence are they able to reason abstractly with any degree of competence. Each stage is derived from and builds on the accomplishments of the previous stage in a continuous, orderly process. The course of intellectual development is both maturational and invariant and is divided into the following stages (ages are approximate):

Sensorimotor (birth to 2 years)—The sensorimotor stage of intellectual development consists of six substages (see Chapters 36 and 37) that are governed by sensations in which simple learning takes place. Children progress from reflex activity through simple repetitive behaviors to imitative behavior. They develop a sense of "cause and effect" as they direct behavior toward objects. Problem solving is primarily trial and error. They display a high level of curiosity, experimentation, and enjoyment of novelty, and begin to develop a sense of self as they are able to differentiate themselves from their environment. They become aware that objects have *permanence*—that an object exists even though it is no longer visible. Toward the end of the sensorimotor period children begin to use language and representational thought.

Preoperational (2 to 7 years)—The predominant characteristic of the preoperational stage of intellectual development is *egocentrism,* which in this sense does not mean selfishness or self-centeredness, but the inability to put oneself in the place of another. Children interpret objects and events not in terms of general properties, but in terms of their relationships or their use to them. They are unable to see things from any perspective other than their own; they cannot see another's point of view, nor can they see any reason to do so (see Cognitive Development [Piaget], Chapter 38).

Preoperational thinking is concrete and tangible. Children cannot reason beyond the observable, and they lack the ability to make deductions or generalizations. Thought is dominated by what they see, hear, or otherwise experience. However, they are increasingly able to use language and symbols to represent objects in their environment. Through imaginative play, questioning, and other interacting, they begin to elaborate concepts and to make simple associations between ideas. In the latter stage of the period their reasoning is intuitive (e.g., the stars have to go to bed just as they do) and they are only beginning to deal with problems of weight, length, size, and time. Reasoning is also transductive—because two events occur together, they cause each other, or knowledge of one characteristic is transferred to another (e.g., all women with big bellies have babies).

Concrete operations (7 to 11 years)—At this age thought becomes increasingly logical and coherent. Children are able to classify, sort, order, and otherwise organize facts about the world to use in problem solving. They develop a new concept of permanence—conservation (see Cognitive Development [Piaget], Chapter 39). That is, they realize that physical factors such as volume, weight, and number remain the same even though outward appearances are changed. They are able to deal with a number of different aspects of a situation simultaneously. They do not have the capacity to deal in abstraction; they solve problems in a concrete, systematic fashion based on what they can perceive. Reasoning is inductive. Through progressive changes in thought processes and relationships with others, thought becomes less self-centered. They can consider points of view other than their own. Thinking has become socialized.

Formal operations (11 to 15 years)—Formal operational thought is characterized by adaptability and flexibility. Adolescents can think in abstract terms, use abstract symbols, and draw logical conclusions from a set of observations. For example, they can solve the following question: If A is larger than B, and B is larger than C, which symbol is the largest? (The answer is A.) They can make hypotheses and test them; they can consider abstract, theoretic, and philosophic matters. Although they may confuse the ideal with the practical, most contradictions in the world can be dealt with and resolved.

Language Development

Children are born with the mechanism and capacity to develop speech and language skills. However, they will not speak spontaneously. The environment must provide a means for them to acquire these skills. Speech requires intact physiologic structure and function (including respiratory, auditory, and cerebral) plus intelligence, a need to communicate, and stimulation.

The rate of speech development varies from child to child and is directly related to neurologic competence and cognitive development. Gesture precedes speech, and in this way a small child communicates satisfactorily. As speech develops, gesture recedes but never disappears entirely. At all stages of language development, children's comprehension vocabulary (what they understand) is greater than their expressed vocabulary (what they can say), and this development reflects a continuing process of modification that involves both the acquisition of new words and the expanding and refining of word meanings previously learned. By the time they begin to walk, children are able to attach a name to objects and persons.

The first parts of speech used are nouns, sometimes verbs (e.g., "go"), and combination words (such as "bye-bye"). Responses are usually structurally incomplete during the toddler period, although the meaning is clear. Next they begin to use adjectives and adverbs to qualify nouns, followed by adverbs to qualify nouns and verbs. Later, pronouns and gender words are added (such as "he" and "she"). By the time children enter school, they are able to use simple, structurally complete sentences that average five to seven words.

Moral Development (Kohlberg)

Children also acquire moral reasoning in a developmental sequence. Moral development, as described by Kohlberg (1968), is based on cognitive developmental theory and consists of the following three major levels, each of which has two stages:

Preconventional level—The preconventional level of moral development parallels the preoperational level of cognitive development and intuitive thought. Culturally oriented to the labels of good/bad and right/wrong, children integrate these in terms of the physical or pleasurable consequences of their actions. At first children determine the goodness or badness of an action in terms of its consequences. They avoid punishment and obey without question those who have the power to determine and enforce the rules and labels. They have no concept of the basic moral order that supports these consequences. Later children determine that the right behavior consists of that which satisfies their own needs (and sometimes the needs of others). Although elements of fairness, give and take, and equal sharing are evident, they are interpreted in a very practical, concrete manner without loyalty, gratitude, or justice.

Conventional level—At the conventional stage children are concerned with conformity and loyalty. They value the maintenance of family, group, or national expectations regardless of consequences. Behavior that meets with approval and pleases or helps others is considered to be good. One earns approval by being "nice." Obeying the rules, doing one's duty, showing respect for authority, and maintaining the social order is the correct behavior. This level is correlated with the stage of concrete operations in cognitive development.

Postconventional, autonomous, or principled level—At the postconventional level the individual has reached the cognitive stage of formal operations. Correct behavior tends to be defined in terms of general individual rights and standards that have been examined and agreed on by the entire society. Although procedural rules for reaching consensus become important with emphasis on the legal point of view, there is also emphasis on the possibility for changing law in terms of societal needs and rational considerations.

The most advanced level of moral development is one in which self-chosen ethical principles guide decisions of conscience (Dunsmore, 2001). These are abstract and ethical but universal principles of justice and human rights with respect for the dignity of persons as individuals. It is believed that few persons reach this stage of moral reasoning.

Spiritual Development

Spiritual beliefs are closely related to the moral and ethical portion of the child's self-concept and, as such, must be considered as part of the child's basic needs assessment. Children need to have meaning, purpose, and hope in their lives. Also, the need for confession and forgiveness is present, even in very young children. Extending beyond religion (an organized set of beliefs and practices), spirituality affects the whole person: mind, body, and spirit (Houskamp, Fisher, & Stuber, 2004). Fowler (1974) has identified seven stages in the development of faith, four of which are closely associated with and parallel cognitive and psychosocial development in childhood:

Stage 0: Undifferentiated—This stage of development encompasses the period of infancy during which children have no concept of right or wrong, no beliefs, and no convictions to guide their behavior. However, the beginnings of a faith are established with the development of basic trust through their relationships with the primary caregiver.

Stage 1: Intuitive-projective—Toddlerhood is primarily a time of imitating the behavior of others. Children imitate the religious gestures and behaviors of others without comprehending any meaning or significance to the activities. During the preschool years children assimilate some of the values and beliefs of their parents. Parental attitudes toward moral codes and religious beliefs convey to children what they consider to be good and bad. Children still imitate behavior at this age and follow parental beliefs as part of their daily lives rather than through an understanding of their basic concepts.

Stage 2: Mythical-literal—Through the school-age years, spiritual development parallels cognitive development and is closely related to children's experiences and social interactions. Most children have a strong interest in religion during the school-age years. The existence of a deity is accepted, and petitions to an omnipotent being are important and expected to be answered; good behavior is rewarded, and bad behavior is punished. Their developing conscience bothers them when they disobey. They have a reverence for thoughts and matters and are able to articulate their faith. They may even question its validity.

Stage 3: Synthetic-convention—As children approach adolescence, they become increasingly aware of spiritual disappointments. They recognize that prayers are not always answered (at least on their own terms) and may begin to abandon or modify some religious practices. They begin to reason, to question some of the established parental religious standards, and to drop or modify some religious practices.

Stage 4: Individuating-reflexive—Adolescents become more skeptical and begin to compare the religious standards of their parents with those of others. They attempt to determine which to adopt and incorporate into their own set of values. They also begin to compare religious standards with the scientific viewpoint. It is a time of searching rather than reaching. Adolescents are uncertain about many religious ideas but will not achieve profound insights until late adolescence or early adulthood.

Development of Self-Concept

Self-concept is how an individual describes himself or herself (Willoughby, King, & Polatajko, 1996). The term *self-concept* includes all the notions, beliefs, and convictions that constitute an individual's relationships with others. It is not present at birth but develops gradually as a result of unique experiences within the self, with significant others, and with the realities of the world. However, an individual's self-concept may or may not reflect reality.

In infancy the self-concept is primarily an awareness of one's independent existence learned in part as a result of social contacts and experiences with others. The process becomes more active during toddlerhood as children explore the limits of their capacities and the nature of their impact on others. School-age children are more aware of differences among people, are more sensitive to social pressures, and become more preoccupied with issues of self-criticism and self-evaluation. During early adolescence children focus more on physical and emotional changes taking place and on peer acceptance. The self-concept is crystallized during later adolescence as young people organize their self-concept around a set of values, goals, and competencies acquired throughout childhood.

Body Image

A vital component of self-concept, *body image* refers to the subjective concepts and attitudes that individuals have toward their own bodies. It consists of the physiologic (the perception of one's physical characteristics), psychologic (values and attitudes toward the body, abilities, and ideals), and social nature of one's image of self (the self in relation to others). All three of the components interrelate with each other. Body image is a complex phenomenon that evolves and changes during the process of growth and development. Any actual or perceived deviation from the "norm" (no matter how this is interpreted) is cause for concern. The extent to which a characteristic, defect, or disease affects children's body image is influenced by the attitudes and behavior of those around them.

The significant others in their lives exert the most important and meaningful impact on children's body image. Labels that are attached to them (such as "skinny," "pretty," or "fat") or body parts (such as "ugly mole," "bug eyes," or "yucky skin") are incorporated into the body image. Because they lack the understanding of deviations from the physical standard or norm, children notice prominent differences in others and unwittingly make "rude" and often cruel remarks about such minor deviations as large or widely spaced front teeth, large or small eyes, moles, or extreme variations in height.

Infants receive input about their bodies through self-exploration and sensory stimulation from others. As they begin to manipulate their environment, they become aware of their bodies as separate from others. Toddlers learn to identify the various parts of their bodies and are able to use symbols to represent objects. Preschoolers become aware of the wholeness of their bodies and discover the genitals. Exploration of the genitals and the discovery of differences between the sexes become important. There is only a vague concept of internal organs and function (Stuart & Sundeen, 1998).

School-age children begin to learn about internal body structure and function and become aware of differences in body size and configuration. They are highly influenced by the cultural norms of society and current fads. Children whose bodies deviate from the norm are often criticized or ridiculed.

Adolescence is the age when children become most concerned about the physical self. The unfamiliar body changes and the new physical self must be integrated into the self-concept. Adolescents face conflicts over what they see and what they visualize as the ideal body structure. Body image formation during adolescence is a crucial element in the shaping of identity, the psychosocial crisis of adolescence.

The term *self-esteem* refers to a personal, subjective judgment of one's worthiness derived from and influenced by the social groups in the immediate environment and individuals' perceptions of how they are valued by others. Self-esteem changes with development. Highly egocentric toddlers are unaware of any difference between competence and social approval. On the other hand, preschool and early school-age children are increasingly aware of the discrepancy between their competencies and the abilities of more advanced children. Being accepted by adults and peers outside the family group becomes more important to them. Positive feedback enhances their self-esteem; they are vulnerable to feelings of worthlessness and are anxious about failure.

As children's competencies increase and they develop meaningful relationships, their self-esteem rises. This self-esteem is again at risk during early adolescence when they are defining an identity and sense of self in the context of their peer group. Unless children are continually made to feel incompetent and of little worth, any decrease in self-esteem during vulnerable times is only temporary. Children assess the following aspects of themselves in forming an overall evaluation of their self-esteem (Sieving & Zirbel-Donisch, 1990):

Competence—How adequate are my cognitive, physical, and social skills?

Sense of control—How well can I complete tasks needed to produce desired actions? Is someone or something specific or is luck or chance responsible for my successes and failures?

Moral worth—How closely do my actions and behaviors meet moral standards that have been set?

Worthiness of love and acceptance—How worthy am I of love and acceptance from my parents, other significant adults, siblings, and peers?

Factors that influence the formation of a child's self-esteem include (1) the child's temperament and personality, (2) abilities and opportunities available to accomplish age-appropriate developmental tasks, (3) significant others, and (4) social roles assumed and the expectations of these roles (see also Psychosocial History, Chapter 34).

ROLE OF PLAY IN DEVELOPMENT

Through the universal medium of play children learn what no one can teach them. They learn about their world and how to deal with this environment of objects, time, space, structure, and people. They learn about themselves operating within that environment—what they can do, how to relate to things and situations, and how to adapt themselves to the demands society makes on them. Play is the *work* of the child. In play children continually practice the complicated, stressful processes of living, communicating, and achieving satisfactory relationships with other people.

Classification of Play

From a developmental point of view, patterns of children's play can be categorized according to content and social character. In both there is an additive effect; each builds on past accomplishments, and some element of each is maintained throughout life. At each stage in development the new predominates.

Content of Play

The content of play involves primarily the physical aspects of play, although social relationships cannot be ignored. The content of play follows the directional trend of the simple to the complex:

Social-affective play—Play begins with social-affective play, wherein infants take pleasure in relationships with people. As adults talk, touch, nuzzle, and in various ways elicit a response from an infant, the infant soon learns to provoke parental emotions and responses with such behaviors as smiling, cooing, or initiating games and activities. The type and intensity of the adult behavior with children varies among cultures.

Sense-pleasure play—Sense-pleasure play is a nonsocial stimulating experience that originates from without. Objects in the environment—light and color, tastes and odors, textures and consistencies—attract children's attention, stimulate their senses, and give pleasure. Pleasurable experiences are derived from handling raw materials (e.g., water, sand, and food), from body motion (e.g., swinging, bouncing, and rocking), and from other uses of senses and abilities (e.g., smelling and humming) (Fig. 33-4).

Skill play—Once infants have developed the ability to grasp and manipulate, they persistently demonstrate and exercise their newly acquired abilities through skill play, repeating an action over and over again. The element of sense-pleasure play is often evident in the practicing of a new ability; but all too often the determination to conquer the elusive skill produces pain and frustration (e.g., learning to ride a bicycle).

Unoccupied behavior—In unoccupied behavior children are not playful, but focus their attention momentarily on anything that strikes their interest. Children daydream, fiddle with clothes or other objects, or walk aimlessly. This role differs from that of onlookers, who actively observe the activity of others.

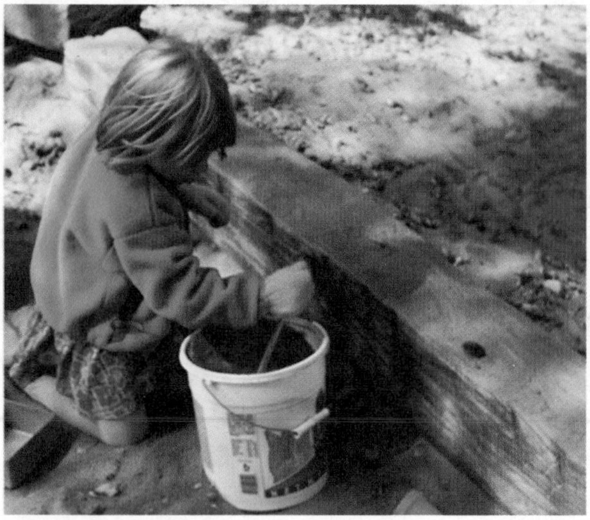

Fig. 33-4 Children derive pleasure from handling raw materials.

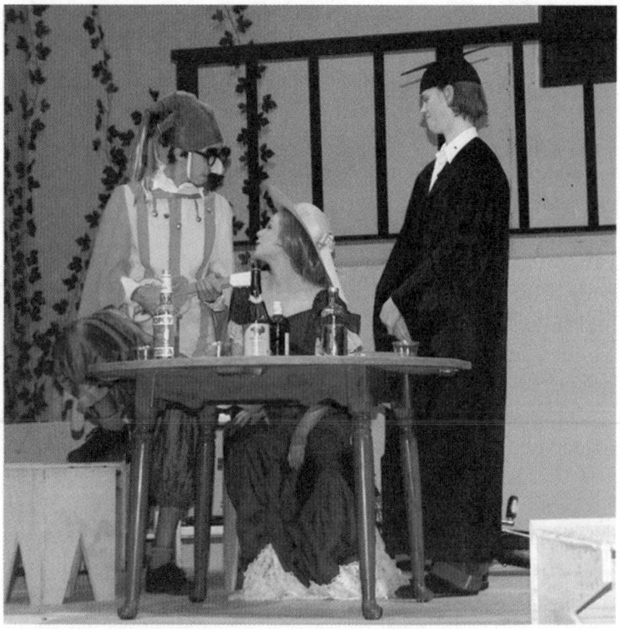

Fig. 33-5 Older children enjoy being in plays.

Dramatic, or pretend, play—One of the vital elements in children's process of identification is dramatic play, also known as symbolic or pretend play. It begins in late infancy (11 to 13 months) and is the predominant form of play in the preschool child. Once children begin to invest situations and people with meanings and to attribute affective significance to the world, they can pretend and fantasize almost anything. By acting out events of daily life, children learn and practice the roles and identities modeled by the members of their family and society. Children's toys, replicas of the tools of society, provide a medium for learning about adult roles and activities that may be puzzling and frustrating to them. Interacting with the world is one way children get to know it. The simple, imitative, dramatic play of the toddler, such as using the telephone, driving a car, or rocking a doll, evolves into the more complex, sustained dramas of the preschooler, which extend beyond common domestic matters to the wider aspects of the world and the society, such as playing police officer, storekeeper, teacher, or nurse. Older children work out elaborate themes, act out stories, and compose plays (Fig. 33-5).

Games—Children in all cultures engage in games, alone and with others. Solitary activity involving games begins as very small children participate in repetitive activities and progress to more complicated games that challenge their independent skills, such as puzzle solving, solitaire, and computer or video games. Very young children participate in simple, *imitative games* such as pat-a-cake and peekaboo. Preschool children learn and enjoy *formal games* that begin with ritualistic, self-sustaining games such as ring-around-a-rosy and London Bridge. With the exception of some simple board games, preschool children do not engage in competitive games. Preschoolers hate to lose and will try to cheat, want to change rules, or demand exceptions and opportunities to change their moves. School-age children and adolescents enjoy *competitive games,* including cards, checkers, chess, and physically active games such as baseball.

Social Character of Play

The play interactions of infancy are between the child and an adult. Children continue to enjoy the company of an adult but are increasingly able to play alone. As age advances, interaction with age-mates increases in importance and becomes an essential part of the socialization process. Through interaction, highly egocentric infants, unable to tolerate delay or interference, ultimately acquire concern for others and the ability to delay or even reject their own gratification needs at the expense of another. A pair of toddlers engage in considerable combat because their personal needs cannot tolerate delay or compromise. By the time they reach age 5 or 6 years, children are able to arrive at a compromise or make use of arbitration, usually after they have attempted and failed to gain their own way. Through continued interaction with peers and the growth of conceptual abilities and social skills, children are able to increase participation with others in the following types of play:

Onlooker play—During onlooker play children watch what other children are doing but make no attempt to enter into the play activity. There is an active interest in observing the interaction of others but no movement toward participating. Watching an older sibling bounce a ball is a common example of the onlooker role.

Solitary play—During solitary play children play alone with toys different from those used by other children in the same area. They enjoy the presence of other children but make no effort to get close to or speak to them. Their interest is centered on their own activity, which they pursue with no reference to the activities of the others.

Parallel play—During parallel activities children play independently but among other children. They play with toys like those the children around them are using, but play as each child sees fit, neither influencing nor being influenced by the other children. Each plays beside, but not with, other children (Fig. 33-6). There is no group association. Parallel play is the characteristic play of toddlers, but it may also

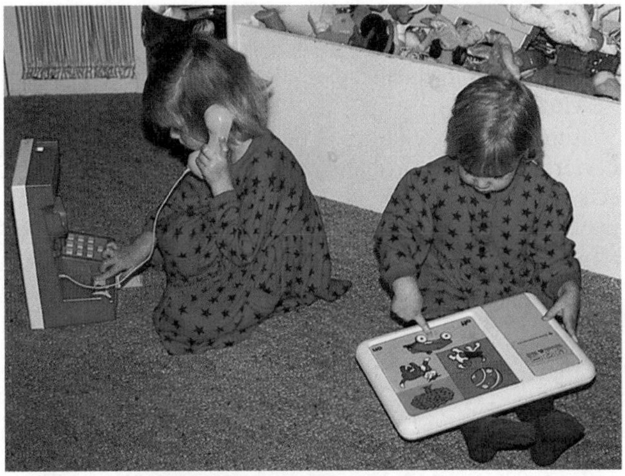

Fig. 33-6 Parallel play.

occur in other groups of any age. Individuals involved in a creative craft, with each person separately working on an individual project, are engaged in parallel play.

Associative play—In associative play children play together and are engaged in a similar or even identical activity, but there is no organization, division of labor, leadership assignment, or mutual goal. Children borrow and lend play materials, follow each other with wagons and tricycles, and sometimes attempt to control who may or may not play in the group. Each child acts according to his or her own wishes; there is no group goal (Fig. 33-7). For example, two children play with dolls, borrowing articles of clothing from each other and engaging in similar conversation, but neither directs the other's actions or establishes rules regarding the limits of the play session. There is a great deal of behavioral contagion: when one child initiates an activity, the entire group follows the example.

Cooperative play—Cooperative play is organized, and children play in a group *with* other children (Fig. 33-8). They discuss and plan activities for the purposes of accomplishing an end—to make something, to attain a competitive goal, to dramatize situations of adult or group life, or to play formal games. The group is loosely formed, but there is a marked sense of belonging or not belonging. The goal and its attainment require organization of activities, division of labor, and playing roles. The leader-follower relationship is definitely established, and the activity is controlled by one or two members who assign roles and direct the activity of the others. The activity is organized to allow one child to supplement another's function in order to complete the goal.

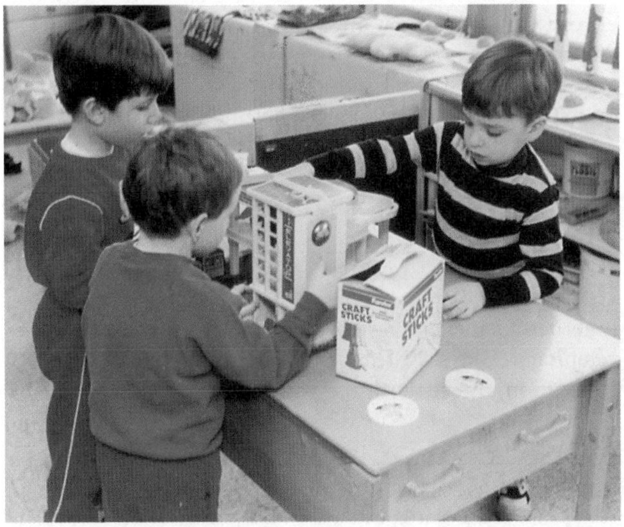

Fig. 33-7 Associative play.

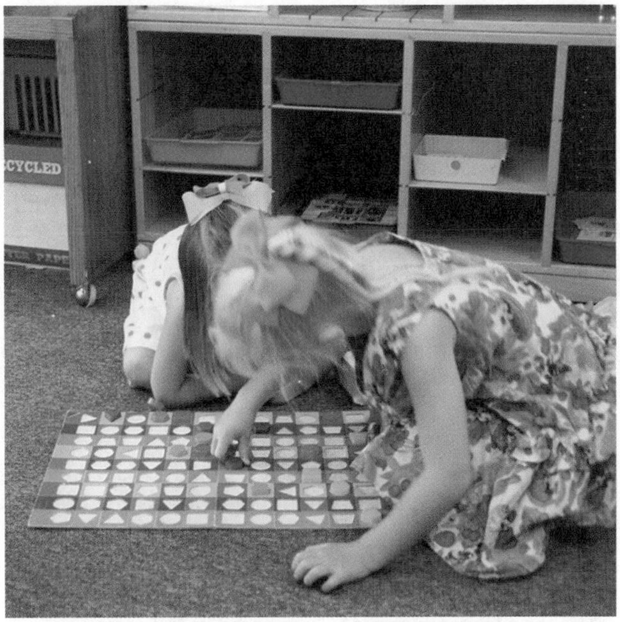

Fig. 33-8 Cooperative play.

Functions of Play

Sensorimotor Development

Sensorimotor activity is a major component of play at all ages and is the predominant form of play in infancy. Active play is essential for muscle development and serves a useful purpose as a release for surplus energy. Through sensorimotor play children explore the nature of the physical world. Infants gain impressions of themselves and their world through tactile, auditory, visual, and kinesthetic stimulation. Toddlers and preschoolers revel in body movement and exploration of things in space. With increasing maturity, sensorimotor play becomes more differentiated and involved. Whereas very young children run for the sheer joy of body movement, older children incorporate or modify the motions into increasingly complex and coordinated activities such as races, games, roller-skating, and bicycle riding.

Intellectual Development

Through exploration and manipulation, children learn colors, shapes, sizes, textures, and the significance of objects. They learn the significance of numbers and how to use them; they learn to associate words with objects; and they develop an understanding of abstract concepts and spatial relationships, such as *up, down, under,* and *over.* Activities such as puzzles and games help them develop problem-solving skills. Books, stories, films, and collections expand knowledge and provide enjoyment as well. Play provides a means to practice and expand language skills. Through play children continually rehearse past experiences to assimilate them into new perceptions and relationships. Play helps children comprehend the world in which they live and distinguish between fantasy and reality.

The availability of play materials and the quality of parental involvement are two of the most important variables related to cognitive development during infancy and preschool (Chase, 1994).

NURSE ALERT Toys need to have several levels of challenge to keep from becoming obsolete too quickly. ■

Socialization

From very early infancy children show interest and pleasure in the company of others. Their initial social contact is with the nurturing person, but through play with other children they learn to establish social relationships and to solve the problems associated with these relationships. They learn to give and take, which is more readily learned from critical peers than from the more tolerant adults. They learn the sex role that society expects them to fulfill, as well as approved patterns of behavior and conduct. Closely associated with socialization is development of moral values and ethics. Children learn right from wrong, the standards of the society, and to assume responsibility for their actions.

Creativity

In no other situation is there more opportunity to be creative than in play. Children can experiment and try out their ideas in play through every medium at their disposal, including raw materials, fantasy, and exploration. Creativity is stifled by pressure toward conformity; therefore striving for peer approval may inhibit creative endeavors in the school-age or adolescent child. Creativity is primarily a product of solitary activity; yet creative thinking is often enhanced in group settings where listening to others' ideas stimulates further exploration of one's own ideas. Once children feel the satisfaction of creating something new and different, they transfer this creative interest to situations outside the world of play.

Self-Awareness

Beginning with active explorations of their bodies and awareness of themselves as separate from the mother, the process of self-identity is facilitated through play activities. Children learn who they are and their place in the world. They become increasingly able to regulate their own behavior, to learn what their abilities are, and to compare their abilities with those of others. Through play children are able to test their abilities, to assume and try out various roles, and to learn the effect their behavior has on others.

Therapeutic Value

Play is therapeutic at any age. It provides a means for release from the tension and stress encountered in the environment. In play children can express emotions and release unacceptable impulses in a socially acceptable fashion. Children are able to experiment and test fearful situations and can assume and vicariously master the roles and positions that they are unable to perform in the world of reality. Children reveal much about themselves in play. Through play children are able to communicate to the alert observer the needs, fears, and desires that they are unable to express with their limited language skills. Throughout their play children need the acceptance of adults and their presence to help them control aggression and to channel their destructive tendencies.

Moral Value

Although children learn at home and at school those behaviors considered right and wrong in the culture, the interaction with peers during play contributes significantly to their moral training. Nowhere is the enforcement of moral standards so rigid as in the play situation. If they are to be acceptable members of the group, children must adhere to the accepted codes of behavior of the culture (e.g., fairness, honesty, self-control, and consideration for others). Children soon learn that their peers are less tolerant of violations than are adults, and that to maintain a place in the play group they must conform to the standards of the group.

Toys

The types of toys chosen by or provided for children can facilitate their development in the areas just described. Toys that are small replicas of the culture and its tools help them assimilate their culture. Toys that require pushing, pulling, rolling, and manipulating teach them about physical properties of the items and help develop muscles and coordination. Rules and the basic elements of cooperation and organization are learned through board games.

Because they can be used in a variety of ways, raw materials with which children can exercise their own creativity and imaginations are sometimes superior to ready-made items. For example, building blocks can be used to construct a variety of things, to count, and to learn shapes and sizes.

Toy Safety

Selection of toys and play equipment is a joint effort between parents and children, but evaluation of their safety is the responsibility of the adult. Government agencies do not inspect and police all toys on the market. Therefore adults who purchase, supervise purchases, or allow children to use play equipment need to evaluate such equipment for its safety, including toys that are gifts or those that are purchased by the children themselves (Home Care box). They should also be alert to notices of toys determined to be defective and recalled by the manufacturers. Parents and health care workers can obtain information on a variety of recalled products and can report potentially dangerous toys and child products to the U.S. Consumer Product Safety Commission (CPSC)* or, in Canada, the Canadian Toy Testing Council.†

SELECTED FACTORS THAT INFLUENCE DEVELOPMENT

Heredity

Inherited characteristics have a profound influence on development. The sex of the child, determined at the time of conception, directs both the pattern of growth and the be-

*CPSC hotline: 1-800-638-CPSC; Web site: www.cpsc.gov.

†22 Hamilton Ave North, Ottowa, Ontario, Canada K1Y 1V6; phone: 613-729-7101.

Home Care

TOY SAFETY*

Selection

Select toys that suit the skills, abilities, and interests of children.

Select toys that are safe for the specific child; look for a label that indicates the intended age group. Toys that are safe for one age may not be safe for another.

For infants, toddlers, and all children who still mouth objects, avoid toys with small parts that may pose a fatal choking or aspiration hazard. Toys in this category are usually labeled, "Not recommended for children under 3 years."

For infants avoid toys with strings or cords that are 7 inches or longer because they may cause strangulation.

For all children under 8 years avoid electric toys with heating elements.

For children under 5 years avoid arrows or darts.

Check for safety labels such as "flame retardant" or "flame resistant."

Select toys durable enough to survive rough play; look for sturdy construction such as tightly secured eyes, nose, or any small parts.

Select toys light enough that they will not cause harm if one falls on a child.

Look for toys with smooth, rounded edges. Avoid toys with sharp edges that can cut or that have sharp points. Points on the inside of the toy can puncture if the toy is broken.

Avoid toys with any shooting or throwing objects that can injure eyes.

This includes toys with which other missiles such as sticks or pebbles might be used as substitutes for the intended projectiles.

Arrows and darts used by children should have blunt tips and be manufactured from resilient materials; make certain the tips are securely attached.

Make certain that materials in toys are nontoxic.

Avoid toys that make loud noises that might be damaging to a child's hearing.

Even some squeaking toys are too loud when held close to the ear.

If selecting caps for cap guns, look for the label required by federal law to be on boxes or packages of caps, which states: "Warning—Do not fire closer than 1 foot to the ear. Do not use indoors."

If selecting a toy gun, be certain that the barrel or the entire gun is brightly colored to avoid being mistaken for a real gun.

Check toy instructions for clarity. They should be clear to an adult and, when appropriate, to the child.

Supervision

Maintain a safe play environment.

Remove and discard plastic wrappings on toys immediately; they could suffocate a child.

Remove large toys, bumper pads, and boxes from playpens; an adventuresome child can use such items as a means of climbing or falling out.

Set "ground rules" for play.

Supervise young children closely during play.

Teach children how to use toys properly and safely.

Instruct older children to keep their toys away from younger brothers, sisters, and friends.

Keep children who are playing with riding toys away from stairs, hills, traffic, and swimming pools.

Establish and enforce rules regarding protective gear.

Insist that children wear helmets when using bicycles, skateboards, or in-line skates.

Insist that children wear gloves and wrist, elbow, and knee pads when using skateboards or in-line skates.

Instruct children on electrical safety.

Teach children the proper way to unplug an electric toy—pull on the plug, not the cord.

Teach children to beware of electrical appliances and even electrically operated playthings; often children are unfamiliar with the hazards of electricity in association with water.

Teach children the safe use of utensils that under certain circumstances can cause injury—scissors, knives, needles, heating elements, or loops, long string, or cord.

Maintenance

Inspect old and new toys regularly for breakage, loose parts, and other potential hazards.

Look for jagged or sharp edges or broken parts that might constitute a choking hazard.

Check moveable parts to make certain they are attached securely to the toys; sometimes pieces that are safe when attached to the toy become a danger when detached.

Examine all outdoor toys regularly for rust and weak or sharp parts that could become a danger to a child.

Check electrical cords and plugs for cracked or fraying parts.

Maintain toys in good repair, without signs of possible hazards such as sharp edges, splinters, weak seams, or rust.

Make repairs immediately, or discard out of reach of children.

Sand sharp wooden toys or splintered surfaces so they are smooth.

Use only paint labeled "nontoxic" to repaint toys, toy boxes, or children's furniture.

Storage

Provide a safe place for children to store toys.

Select a toy chest or toy box that is ventilated, is free of self-locking devices that could trap a child inside, and has a lid designed not to pinch a child's fingers or fall on a child's head.

To avoid entrapment and suffocation, containers other than toy chests used for storage purposes should be fitted with spring-loaded support devices if they have a hinged lid.

Teach children to store toys safely to prevent accidental injury from stepping, tripping, or falling on a toy.

Playthings meant for older children and adults should be safely stowed away on high shelves, in locked closets, or in other areas unavailable to younger children.

*Another helpful resource is *Toy safety: guidelines for parents,* from American Academy of Pediatrics, Division of Publications, 141 Northwest Point Blvd, Elk Grove Village, IL, 60007; phone: 888-227-1770; fax: 847-228-1281; Web site: www.aap.org.

havior of others toward the child. In all cultures, attitudes and expectations are different with respect to the sex of the child. Sex and other hereditary determinants strongly affect the end result of growth and the rate of progress toward it. There is a high correlation between parent and child with regard to traits such as height, weight, and rate of growth. Most physical characteristics, including shape and form of features, body build, and physical peculiarities, are inherited and can influence the way in which children grow and interact with their environment. Many dimensions of personality, such as temperament, activity level, responsiveness, and a tendency toward shyness, are believed to be inherited.

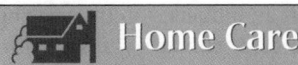

Differences in health and vigor of children may be attributed to hereditary traits. An inherited physical or mental disorder will alter or modify a child's physical and/or emotional growth and interactions. The extent to which disabling conditions interfere with the child's growth and well-being is considered in relation to numerous disabilities throughout the remainder of the text.

Neuroendocrine Factors

It has been suggested there may be a growth center in the hypothalamic region responsible for maintaining genetically determined growth patterns. Some functional relationship is believed to exist between the hypothalamus and the endocrine system that influences growth. There is also evidence, based on observations of denervated skeletal muscles, that the peripheral nervous system may influence growth, because muscles deprived of nerve supply degenerate. Many of these effects are not sufficiently explained by disuse or diminished blood supply.

Probably all hormones affect growth in some fashion. Three hormones (i.e., growth hormone, thyroid hormone, and androgens), when given to persons deficient in these hormones, stimulate protein anabolism and thereby produce retention of elements essential for building protoplasm and bony tissue. It appears that each of the hormones that has a significant influence on growth manifests its major effect at a different period of growth (see Chapter 52).

Nutrition

Nutrition is probably the single most important influence on growth. Dietary factors regulate growth at all stages of development, and their effects are exerted in numerous and complex ways. During the rapid prenatal growth period, poor nutrition may influence development from the time of implantation of the ovum until birth. During infancy and childhood the demand for calories is relatively great, as evidenced by the rapid increase in both height and weight. At this time protein and caloric requirements are higher than at almost any period of postnatal development. As the growth rate slows with its concomitant decrease in metabolism, there is a corresponding reduction in caloric and protein requirements (see Table 33-2).

Growth is uneven during the periods of childhood between infancy and adolescence when there are plateaus and small growth spurts. The child's appetite will fluctuate in response to these variations until the turbulent growth spurt of adolescence, when adequate nutrition is extremely important but may be subjected to numerous emotional influences. Adequate nutrition is closely related to good health throughout life, and an overall improvement in nourishment is evidenced by the gradual increase in size and early maturation of children in the last century.

Interpersonal Relationships

Relationships with significant others play a critical role in development, particularly in emotional, intellectual, and personality development. Not only do the quality and quantity of contacts with other persons exert an influence on the growing child, but also the widening range of contacts is essential to learning and the development of a healthy personality.

The nurturing person is unquestionably the single most influential person during early infancy. This person is the one who meets the infant's basic needs of food, warmth, comfort, and love. He or she provides stimulation for the child's senses, and facilitates his or her expanding capacities. Through this person the child learns to trust the world and to feel secure to venture in increasingly wider relationships.

It is generally the parents who are most influential in helping the child to assume sex-role identification. Parents define and reinforce acceptable sex-role behavior and provide sex-appropriate role models for the child. In the absence of a sex-role model in the family setting, the child may adopt some characteristics of the opposite-sex parent or sibling. Often the child identifies with a teacher or other significant person of the same sex.

Siblings are children's first peers, and the way in which they learn to relate to each other affects later interactions with peers outside the family group. The sphere of persons from whom children seek approval widens to include other members of their family, their peers, and, to a lesser extent, other authority figures (e.g., teachers). The increasing importance of the peer group in determining the behavior of school-age children and adolescents is well documented (Fig. 33-9).

When children fail to have quality interpersonal relationships with nurturing persons, they experience *emotional deprivation.* The most prominent feature of emotional deprivation, particularly during the first year, is developmental delays. Much of the information regarding the adverse effects of interpersonal influences on development has been acquired through retrospective studies of gross deprivation and trauma. The most notable instances involved homeless infants who were placed in institutions for care. Those infants who did not receive a mother's consistent care failed to gain weight even with an adequate diet; they were pale, listless, and immobile, and were unresponsive to stimuli that usually elicit a response such as smiling or cooing in the

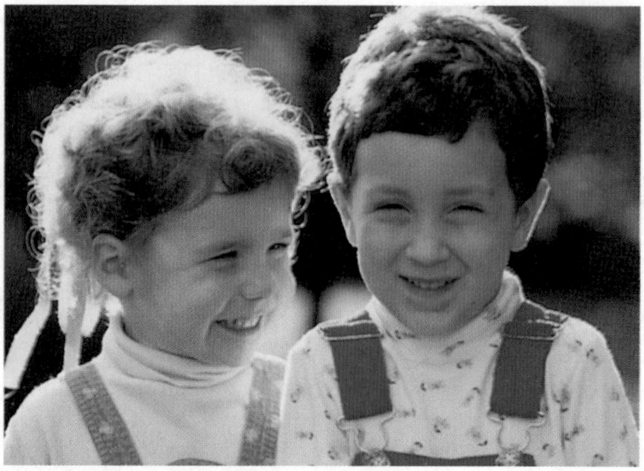

Fig. 33-9 Peers become increasingly important as children develop friendships outside the family group.

normal infant. If emotional deprivation continues for a sufficient length of time, the child may not survive infancy.

Although the most remarkable examples of emotional deprivation were first recognized among infants in institutions, the term *masked deprivation* has been used to describe children reared in homes where there is a distorted parent-child relationship or otherwise disordered home environment. Infants do not thrive if the caregiving person is hostile, fearful of handling them, or indifferent to them and their needs. Such children exhibit poor growth even though they are apparently free of physical disease. Growth delays in these children are believed to be caused by a psychologically induced endocrine imbalance that interferes with growth. These same infants and children display "catch-up" growth in a changed environment (see Failure to Thrive, Chapter 36).

Socioeconomic Level

Evidence indicates that the socioeconomic level of a child's family has a significant impact on growth and development. At all ages children from upper- and middle-class families are taller than comparative children of families in the lower socioeconomic strata. The cause of these differences is less definite, although the poorer health and nutrition of lower socioeconomic levels are probably significant factors. Nutritious food sources (especially proteins) are scarce, and other factors (e.g., larger family size and irregularity in eating, sleeping, and exercise) may play a role.

Families from lower socioeconomic groups may lack the knowledge or resources needed to provide the safe, stimulating, and enriched environment that fosters optimum development for children. They may be unable to move from unsafe neighborhoods where drug traffic and drive-by shootings are the norm. The effects on the emotional development of children living under these conditions have been compared with those experienced by children living in war zones.

Disease

Altered growth and development is one of the clinical manifestations in a number of hereditary disorders. Growth impairment is particularly marked in skeletal disorders, such as the various forms of dwarfism and at least one of the chromosomal anomalies (i.e., Turner syndrome). Many of the disorders of metabolism (e.g., vitamin D–resistant rickets, the mucopolysaccharidoses, and the numerous endocrine disorders) interfere with the normal growth pattern. In other disorders the tendency for growth is toward the upper percentile of height (e.g., Klinefelter and Marfan syndromes).

Many chronic illnesses that are associated with varying degrees of growth failure are congenital cardiac anomalies and respiratory disorders such as cystic fibrosis. Any disorder characterized by the inability to digest and absorb body nutrients will have an adverse effect on growth and development.

Environmental Hazards

Hazards in the environment are a source of concern to health care providers and others interested in health and safety. Physical injuries are the most prevalent consequences of environmental dangers; these are discussed extensively throughout the text as they apply in relation to age, specific hazards, and selected physical disabilities.

Children are at a high risk for harm resulting from the chemical residues of modern life present in the environment. The hazards of these chemical residues relate to their potential carcinogenicity, enzymatic effects, and accumulation (Holland et al, 2000; Kaiser, 2000). The harmful agents most often associated with health risks are chemicals and radiation. Water, air, and food contamination from a variety of origins is well documented. Significant sources of exposure are substances in the immediate environment such as lead and asbestos; chemicals secreted in breast milk (especially prescribed drugs and nicotine); and contamination within well-insulated homes (especially from disinfectants or burning of substances that produce toxic fumes). Passive inhalation of tobacco smoke by infants and children is a hazard at all stages of development. The harmful effects of large doses of radiation are unquestioned, although the effects of low-dose or short-term radiation are debatable, as are the safe vs. harmful dosage levels.

Stress in Childhood

Although all children experience stress, some youngsters appear to be more vulnerable than others. Children's age, temperament, life situation, and state of health affect their vulnerability, reactions, and ability to handle stress. Also, the responses to a stressor can be behavioral, psychologic, or physiologic. It is impossible, unrealistic, and undesirable to protect children from stress; but providing them with interpersonal security helps them develop coping strategies for dealing with stress.

Parents and other caregivers can try to recognize signs of stress to help children deal with stresses before they become overwhelming. Signs of stress take many forms but are typically the same ones seen in children who are abused (see Chapter 37) or depressed (see Chapter 39). If a number of stresses are imposed on children at the same time, the children are more vulnerable. When a succession of stresses produces an excessive stress load, children may experience a serious change in health or behavior.

It is most important that parents and persons working with children understand the nature of childhood stress and the ways it can be recognized or anticipated. Caregivers must *listen* to children so they are aware of children's fears and concerns, and must let them know that they are important and that what they say matters. Physical contact is comforting and reassuring to children. Simply holding, touching, or hugging children is both relaxing and comforting and facilitates communication. Spending unhurried time with children; family outings and vacations; and exposing children to positive influences all help build children's strength and security. Supportive interpersonal relationships are essential to the psychologic well-being of children.

Coping

Coping refers to a special class of individual reactions to stressors: specifically, a reaction to a stressor that resolves, reduces, or replaces the affect state classified as stressful. *Coping strategies* are the specific ways in which children cope with stressors, as distinguished from *coping styles*, which are relatively unchanging personality characteristics or outcomes of coping (Boyd & Hunsberger, 1998). Research indicates that as children age they tend toward a more internal locus of control and use more vigilant modes of coping (LaMontagne et al, 1996). Children, like adults, respond to everyday stress by trying to change the circumstances or by trying to adjust to circumstances the way they are. Any strategy that provides relaxation is effective in reducing stress, and most children have their own natural methods such as withdrawal, physical activity, reading, listening to music, working on a project, or taking a nap. Some turn to parents to solve their problems, or they may develop socially unacceptable strategies, such as cheating, stealing, or lying.

Children can be taught stress-reduction techniques to use in coping. First, they must be helped to recognize signs of tension in themselves; they can then be taught any of a variety of appropriate strategies—special exercises, relaxation and breathing, mental imagery, and numerous other simple activities. Also, parents and other caregivers can anticipate possible stress-provoking events and prepare children for coping by role playing a scenario or by "talking it through" beforehand. Most of the stress-reducing strategies discussed in Chapter 44 in relation to managing pain are effective for any stress situation.

Probably the most useful tool that children can learn is how to solve problems. When children can view any new situation as a problem to be solved and an opportunity to learn, they are not vulnerable to the control of others. It provides them with a sense of mastery over their own lives and reinforces the fact that they have within themselves the ability and information to handle whatever comes their way. Problem-solving skills give them the confidence to know where and how to seek help when they need it.

Influence of the Mass Media

Media can have an enormous influence on the developing child. There is no doubt that the media provide children with a means for extending their knowledge about the world in which they live, and have contributed to narrowing the differences between classes. However, there is growing concern regarding the enormous influence the media can have on the developing child, because today's children are just as captivated as they were decades ago. Linkages have been established between mass media use and risk-taking behaviors in adolescents (Strasburger & Donnerstein, 1999). The images of risky behavior presented by the media may serve to establish or reinforce teenagers' perceptions of their social environment. Also, media content may directly influence risk perception; media protagonists seldom suffer adverse consequences of their behaviors despite their grossly distorted experiences with violence, illness, or crime (Cheng et al, 2004; Walma van der Molen, 2004). Children may identify closely with people or characters portrayed in reading materials, movies, videos, and television programs and commercials.

Reading Materials

Books, newspapers, and magazines are the oldest forms of mass media. They contribute to children's competence in almost every direction and also provide enjoyment. Recognition of the impact that reading matter used in the schools has on the value system and socialization processes has prompted reevaluation of the content of textbooks in terms of the biased presentation of male and female role models, the sugar-coated view of life situations, and the biased history of minority groups.

Fairy tales, for generations the mainstay of young children's literature, for a time suffered condemnation as being sexist; overly violent in content; and riddled with unfavorable stereotypes, such as the wicked stepmother, dwarfs, and physical unattractiveness associated with evil. They are now believed to provide an excellent medium for explaining puzzling and important topics such as death, stepparents, and inner feelings and turmoils. Although they do not provide solutions, fairy tales confront children with emotional predicaments and offer suggestions for dealing with them.

Comic books and other "pulp" reading materials have been popular in every generation, usually at the expense of literature provided by schools, libraries, and parents. Many children have nothing else to read. The easy reading, quick action, and adventure in brief episodes seem to fulfill a need for children who are striving to understand both aggression in others and their own impulses. Reading ability, intelligence, and school adjustment apparently have no relationship to the number and type of comic books read. Most comic books appear to be relatively harmless to the majority of children and may be beneficial. Comic books seem to have only a minor influence on acquisition of beliefs, values, and behaviors. The popularity of this medium has prompted some educators to encourage translations of literature into comic book form to stimulate students' interest in the classics.

Movies

Movies that are closely bound to reality and often portray an assortment of socially approved behaviors perhaps make a contribution to children's value systems and do provide opportunities for desirable social learning. On the other hand children, especially adolescents, flock to the "macho" movies in which heroes resort to violent resolution of problems, such as karate and wild automobile chases. The carry-over of these influences into daily life and relationships may account in part for the increase in violent behavior of young persons. Also, research indicates that videos may desensitize the viewer to violence (Rowitz, 1996).

Another concern is the plethora of "slasher" and R-rated movies available to children and teenagers in theaters and through cable television and videocassettes. The content of movies has changed markedly during the past few years, with violence and mutilation being major themes. To children who are unable to distinguish between reality and fantasy, these films play on their deepest fears and result in bedtime fears, nightmares, and a fearful view of the world.

Young children can be frightened by some of the movies considered safe for family viewing. For example, *Bambi* can be frightening to young children, and the villainous witches in *Snow White* and the *Wizard of Oz* are terrifying figures. Also, certain classic Disney movies, such as *Snow White* and

Cinderella, depict stepmothers as evil, destructive persons; such portrayals can have a deleterious effect on children-stepmother relationships or can be confusing to children who have developed a positive relationship with a stepmother.

Television

The medium with the most impact on children in North America today is television, which has become one of the most significant socializing agents in the lives of young children. The content of programs and commercials provides multiple sources for acquiring information, modeling behaviors, and observing value orientations. Besides producing a leveling effect on class differences in general information and vocabulary, TV exposes children to a wider variety of topics and events than they encounter in day-to-day life. Television always has time to talk to children and is a form of access to the adult world.

NURSE ALERT It has been reported that the television is on for more than 6 hours per day in more than half of American homes, and that children watch an average of 21 to 28 hours of television per week (Clarke-Pearson, 1997; Vessey, Yim-Chiplis, & MacKenzie, 1998). ■

Controversy continues to be generated regarding the favorable vs. deleterious influence of television on child development and behavior. The American Academy of Pediatrics (2001) states that television has a powerful influence on the development of unhealthy behaviors and negative attitudes in children. Several factors encourage the learning or performing of television-influenced behaviors (Box 33-3).

BOX 33-3

Factors that Encourage Learning or Performing Television-Influenced Behaviors

Age. Younger children focus on behaviors rather than on motives or consequences. They view alternatives in a concrete manner, and they are unable to differentiate between central and peripheral plot information. Small children remember various assorted items in the program; for example, they remember the act, not the motive or consequences.

Identification with characters or situations. Children will more often imitate behaviors of persons and situations similar to those in their own lives.

Reward and punishment syndrome. Children will imitate behaviors they see rewarded or *not* punished when it is expected. They are less likely to repeat an act they see punished; their attention is immediately attracted when they see an act committed that they know should be punished but is not.

Opportunity to reproduce behaviors. Children will imitate behaviors when given the right environment or when violence seems an accepted solution. When children see a situation on television, they will use this information when they encounter a similar situation that requires a solution.

Motivation to reproduce behaviors. Children will imitate behavior when given the appropriate incentives: expectation of reward or lack of punishment. Some children have self-control; others do not.

Researchers have concluded that the amount of young children's (1 to 3 years of age) television exposure is related to later attention problems (Christakis et al, 2004). Increased verbal and physical aggressive behavior, reduced persistence at problem solving, greater sex-role stereotyping, and reduced creativity have been reported repeatedly.

The passive activity associated with television watching is often accompanied by eating—in many cases, high-caloric snacks. Furthermore, children may expend tremendous mental energy processing the audiovisual messages from television, which may be very exhausting and make them less likely to engage in physical activity later. Television viewing has a fairly profound effect of lowering the metabolic rate and may be a mechanism for the relationship between obesity and the amount of television viewing. Andersen and colleagues (1998) found that the incidence of body fat increased in direct proportion to the amount of hours of television watched by children in the United States; as the number of hours of television viewing increased, children were less likely to participate in vigorous physical activities.

Television programs and commercials, like movies, contain many implicit and explicit messages that promote alcohol consumption, smoking, violence, and promiscuous or unsafe sexual activity. An area of increasing concern is Music Television (MTV), especially when heavy metal rock groups, whose lyrics and videos sensationalize violent sex, suicide, and satanism, are featured. There is now clear evidence documenting a relationship between television viewing and the use of alcohol or tobacco, violence and aggressive behavior, the use of guns to commit violent acts, and early sexual activity (Strasburger & Donnerstein, 1999). Media advertisement has increasingly been scrutinized out of concern for its effects in encouraging young people to purchase and use alcohol and tobacco.

On the positive side, television has been shown to be a positive influence on children's abilities to deal with a variety of social issues such as divorce, the arrival of a new baby, discrimination, honesty, and helpfulness. Children who view educational programming (e.g., *Mister Rogers' Neighborhood* and *Sesame Street*) for a long period become more affectionate, considerate, cooperative, and helpful toward their playmates. The ways that minority and ethnic characters are portrayed on television can have an impact on the way the majority culture views minority persons and on the self-image of minority children.

Many parents are concerned about the effects of television viewing on their children, and most would like information regarding its use. Parents need to supervise the amount and type of TV programs their children watch, and to teach their children how to watch TV (Home Care box).

Computers/Internet

The use of computers in both the classroom and the home has affected childhood learning and development. Schools offer a variety of computer programs that enable children of all ages to broaden their worldviews. Computers offer the advantage of interactive learning and hand-eye coordination. Parents have a wide variety of computer software choices for learning and gaming.

Although computer technology has enhanced many forms of learning and recreation, there are potential dan-

Home Care

TELEVISION VIEWING

Provide a positive role model by developing television substitutes such as reading, athletics, physical conditioning, and hobbies.

Construct a time chart of child's activities (homework, television viewing, scheduled outside activities, playing with a friend).

Discuss with child what you both believe to be a balanced set of activities.

At the beginning of each week, select appropriate programs for television schedules.

Allow child to select programs from this approved list.

Limit child's viewing to 2 hours or less per day.

Rule out television at specific times (e.g., before breakfast or on school nights).

Make a list of alternative activities (e.g., riding a bicycle, reading a book, or working on a hobby).

Require that child choose to do something from this list before watching television.

Watch programs with child.

Discuss program and commercial content with child:

- Distinguish between the real and the unreal.
- Correlate consequences with actions.
- Point out subtle messages.
- Explore alternatives to aggressive conflict resolution.
- Stress purpose of program (e.g., entertainment, education).
- Explain likes and dislikes.

Turn the television off after the selected program is over.

Monitor cable and pay television selections; use a lockbox if necessary.

Limit use of television as a safe distraction to potentially stressful times (e.g., keeping the children occupied while the parent gets organized after a difficult day).

gers to children. The Internet and electronic mailing have made correspondence and information available to children from around the world in minutes. Some activities such as "cybersex" and "kiddie porn," as well as some "chat rooms," may expose children to individuals who may attempt to take advantage of the child's naiveté for illicit purposes. Government officials are working to curb illegal activities on the Internet that involve children, yet at the same time maintain freedom of speech. Filtered Internet service providers are available that may serve to protect children from objectionable sites.* Nurses must be involved in encouraging parents to be knowledgeable of their children's Internet activities while providing appropriate learning activities unique to computers. One helpful strategy is to locate the computer in a public area of the home such as the kitchen or family room, which enables parents to easily monitor its use.

*FamilyConnect, Inc., provides a filtering system that prevents access to pornographic and illegal Web sites. For more information call 888-400-0239 or visit the Web site at www.familyconnect.com. An excellent book that explains the dangers of the Internet and strategies to protect children is *Wicked Wild Web* by J. R. Robison and C. Ophus (2000), Autumn Sky Publishing, PO Box 702252, Tulsa, OK 74170; phone: 888-400-0239 (then dial 0 for operator); Web site: www.wickedwildweb.com.

Key Points

- Growth describes a change in quantity and occurs when cells divide and synthesize new proteins.
- Maturation, a qualitative change, describes the aging process or an increase in competence and adaptability.
- Differentiation refers to a biologic description of the processes by which early cells and structures are modified and altered to achieve specific and characteristic physical and chemical properties.
- Development involves change from a lower to a more advanced stage of complexity.
- The five major developmental periods are prenatal, infancy, early childhood, middle childhood, and later childhood (pubescence and adolescence).
- Growth and development proceed in predictable patterns of direction, sequence, and pace.
- The directional trends in growth and development are cephalocaudal, proximodistal, and mass to specific.
- Physical development includes increase in height and weight and changes in body proportion, dentition, and some body tissues.
- The three broad classifications of child temperament are the easy child, the difficult child, and the slow-to-warm-up child.
- The developmental theories most widely used in explaining child growth and development are Freud's psychosexual stages, Erikson's stages of psychosocial development, Piaget's stages of cognitive development, and Kohlberg's stages of moral development.
- To develop a positive self-concept, children need recognition for their achievements and the approval of others.
- Through play, children learn about their world and how to relate to things, people, and situations.
- Play provides a means of development in the areas of sensorimotor and intellectual progress, socialization, creativity, self-awareness, and moral behavior; it serves as a means for release of tension and expression of emotions.
- Growth and development are affected by a variety of conditions and circumstances, including heredity, physiologic function, gender, disease, physical environment, nutrition, and interpersonal relationships.
- Children's vulnerability and reactions to stress depend to a large extent on their age, coping behaviors, and support systems.
- The mass media can be influential in children's learning and behavior.

References

American Academy of Pediatrics: Committee on Publication Education. Media violence, *Pediatrics* 108:1222-1226, 2001.

Anders TF, Sadeh A, Appareddy V: Normal sleep in neonates and children. In Ferber R, Kryger M (eds): *Principles and practice of sleep medicine in the child,* Philadelphia, 1995, WB Saunders.

Andersen RE et al: Relationship of physical activity and television watching with body weight and level of fatness among children, *JAMA* 279(12): 938-943, 1998.

Beck CT: A meta-analysis of the relationship between postpartum depression and infant temperament, *Nurs Res* 45(4):225-230, 1996.

Boyd JR, Hunsberger M: Chronically ill children coping with repeated hospitalizations: their perceptions and suggested interventions, *J Pediatr Nurs* 13(6):330-341, 1998.

Chase RA: Toys, play, and infant development, *J Perinat Educ* 3(2):7-19, 1994.

Cheng TL et al: Children's violent televion viewing: are parents monitoring? *Pediatrics* 114(1):94-98, 2004.

Chess S, Thomas A: Temperamental differences: a critical concept in child health care, *Pediatr Nurs* 11:167-171, 1985.

Christakis DA et al: Early television exposure and subsequent attentional problems in children, *Pediatrics* 113:708-713, 2004.

Clarke-Pearson KM: Children—media violence—solutions, *N C Med J* 58(4):265-268, 1997.

Cutler L et al: Do CT scans aid assessment of distal tibial physeal fractures? *J Bone Joint Surg Br* 86(2):239-243, 2004.

Davis KF, Parker KP, Montgomery GL: Sleep in infants and young children. Part one: normal sleep, *J Pediatr Health Care* 18(2):65-71, 2004.

Dunsmore JC: Moral development and bioethics, *Psychiatric Annals* 31(2):93-101, 2001.

Erikson EH: *Childhood and society,* ed 2, New York, 1963, WW Norton.

Fowler JW: Toward a developmental perspective on faith, *Relig Educ* 69: 207-219, 1974.

Holland P et al: Life course accumulation of disadvantage: childhood health and hazard exposure during adulthood, *Soc Sci Med* 50: 1285-1295, 2000.

Houskamp BM, Fisher LA, Stuber ML: Spirituality in children and adolescents: research findings and implications for clinicians and researchers, *Child Adolesc Psychiatr Clin North Am* 13(1):221-230, 2004.

Kaczander BI: Pediatric sports medicine: a unique perspective, *Pediatr Manage* 16(2):53-60, 1997.

Kaiser J: Hazards of particles, PCBs focus of Philadelphia meeting, *Science* 288:424-425, 2000.

Kohlberg L: Moral development. In Sills DL (ed): *International encyclopedia of the social sciences,* New York, 1968, Macmillan.

LaMontagne LL et al: Children's preoperative coping and its effects on postoperative anxiety and return to normal activity, *Nurs Res* 45(3):141-147, 1996.

McClowry SG: The temperament profiles of school-age children, *J Pediatr Nurs* 17(1):3-10, 2002.

Piaget J: *The theory of stages in cognitive development,* New York, 1969, McGraw-Hill.

Rowitz M: Heavy metal: do videos and lyrics alter attitudes? *AAP News* 12(1):20-21, 1996.

Seidel HM et al: *Mosby's guide to physical examination,* ed 5, St Louis, 2003, Mosby.

Shiner R, Caspi A: Personality differences in childhood and adolescence: measurement, development, and consequences, *J Child Psychol Psychiatry* 44(1):2-32, 2003.

Sieving R, Zirbel-Donisch S: Development and enhancement of self-esteem in children, *J Pediatr Health Care* 4(6):290-296, 1990.

Strasburger VC, Donnerstein E: Children, adolescents, and the media: issues and solution, *Pediatrics* 103(1):129-139, 1999.

Stuart GW, Sundeen SJ: *Principles and practice of psychiatric nursing,* ed 6, St Louis, 1998, Mosby.

Vessey JA, Yim-Chiplis PK, MacKenzie NR: Effects of television viewing on children's development, *Pediatr Nurs* 23(5):483-486, 1998.

Walma van der Molen JH: Violence and suffering in television news: toward a broader conception of harmful television content for children, *Pediatrics* 113(6):1771-1774, 2004.

Willoughby C, King G, Polatajko H: A therapist's guide to children's self-esteem, *Am J Occup Ther* 50(2):124-132, 1996.

34 Communication and Health Assessment of the Child and Family

LEARNING OBJECTIVES

On completion of this chapter the reader will be able to:
- Describe guidelines for communication and interviewing.
- Identify communication strategies for interviewing parents.
- Formulate guidelines for using an interpreter.
- Identify communication strategies for communicating with children of different age groups.
- Describe four communication techniques that are useful with children.
- State the components of a complete health history.
- Describe two strategies for structural and functional assessment of the family.
- List three areas that are evaluated as part of nutritional assessment.

ELECTRONIC RESOURCES

Additional information related to the content in Chapter 34 can be found on

the companion website at evolve
http://evolve.elsevier.com/Wong/maternal/
- NCLEX Review Questions
- WebLinks

or the interactive student CD-ROM
Activities for Chapter 34 include the following:
- NCLEX Review Questions
- Case Study–Communicating with Adolescents
- Critical Thinking Exercise–The Interview
- Skill–Communicating with Children

COMMUNICATION

Communication may be verbal, nonverbal, or abstract. *Verbal communication* may involve language and its expression; vocalizations in the form of laughs, moans, or squalls; or the implications of what is not said in light of what has been said. *Nonverbal communication* is often called *body language* and includes gestures, movements, facial expressions, postures, and reactions. *Abstract communication* takes the form of play, artistic expression, symbols, photographs, and choice of clothing. Because it is possible to exert greater conscious control over verbal communication, it is a less reliable indicator of true feelings, especially with children.

Many factors influence the communication process. To be successful (gratifying), communication must be appropriate to the situation, properly timed, and clearly delivered. This implies that nurses understand and use techniques of effective communication, including listening. Verbal and nonverbal messages must be congruent; that is, two or more messages sent via different levels must not be contradictory.

Verbal Communication—The Power of Words

Words shape reality, and thus they hold tremendous power. A person can change another's perception of reality by the choice of words that are used. For example, if the diagnosis of cancer is always referred to as a tumor, cyst, malignancy, or carcinoma, patients may never really know that they have cancer. Consequently, they may assume less responsibility for their care than if they were aware of the seriousness of the condition. By learning to recognize how patients and health professionals use language to manipulate reality, one can also learn how to change perceptions and communicate more effectively.

Avoidance Language

The most common way that people try to alter reality is by avoiding words that truly describe it. For example, euphemisms such as "passed on" are used instead of "death." Avoidance language indicates that a person wants to hide something, particularly feelings. As a rule, accepting a person's use of euphemisms only serves to perpetuate the fears and never helps the person deal with them. In contrast, use of straightforward, precise, descriptive language lends perspective to the situation and allows the person to discuss the fears. Most often, imagined fears are much worse than reality.

Distancing Language

People may use impersonal words, such as "it" or "others," to shield themselves from the painful reality of a situation. For example, parents may state that they know *someone* with a child who is slow, when they may actually be talking about personal fears regarding *their* child. By realizing that the parents may need to talk about this difficult subject, the nurse can provide sensitive statements that ease them into discussing their situation.

Sometimes distancing is desirable because the topic may be too painful to discuss directly. The use of the third-person technique (see Box 34-3) may be therapeutic in allowing an individual the opportunity to indirectly approach a subject and receive feedback but still remain in control.

Nonverbal Communication–Paralanguage

In addition to the spoken word, messages are also relayed through nonverbal means, or *paralanguage*—the pitch, pause, intonation, rate, volume, and stress apparent in speech. Young children become very adept at understanding paralanguage; long before they know the meaning of words, they sense anxiety or fear by the rise in pitch or the accelerated rate of the parent's voice. By careful observation of the spoken word, nurses can better understand the meaning of another's verbal message and more accurately control their own paralanguage.

Because most people do not exert conscious control over their paralanguage, it is a valuable clue to feelings and concerns. For example, *pausing* may signify a need to formulate thoughts, recall information, or fabricate a story. Frequent pauses often make the speaker sound unsure. Long pauses may mean that the individual needs more information.

Rate is another characteristic that gives unspoken messages. Talking too fast usually makes the speaker sound glib and insensitive. Talking slowly with a firm tone and appropriate pauses conveys authority. Therefore a person is much more likely to "hear" instructions if the latter approach is used. Children in particular respond attentively to a slow, even, steady voice.

Confirming and Disconfirming Behaviors

People respond to each other through *confirming behaviors,* such as nodding the head, using direct eye contact, repeating or requesting clarification, and making appropriate comments, or *disconfirming behaviors,* such as tapping fingers or a foot, turning away from the speaker, avoiding eye contact, and interrupting. Because there is a reciprocal relationship between such behaviors, nurses need to use confirming behaviors to receive confirmation in return. This "mirroring" effect is particularly evident in children because of their sensitivity to nonverbal cues.

GUIDELINES FOR COMMUNICATION AND INTERVIEWING

The most widely used method of communicating with parents on a professional basis is the interview process. Unlike social conversation, interviewing is a specific form of goal-directed communication. As nurses converse with children and adults, they focus on the individuals to determine the kind of person they are, their usual mode of handling problems, whether help is needed, and the way in which they react to counseling. Developing interviewing skills requires time and practice, but following some guiding principles can facilitate this process. An organized approach is most effective when using interviewing skills in patient teaching.

Establishing a Setting for Communication

Appropriate Introduction

Introduce yourself to, and ask the name of, each family member who is present. Address parents or other adults by their appropriate titles, such as "Mr." and "Mrs.," unless they specify a preferred name. Record the preferred name on the medical record. Using formal address or their preferred names, rather than using first names or "mother" or "father," conveys respect and regard for the parents or other caregivers (Seidel et al, 2003).

At the beginning of the visit, include children in the interaction by asking them their name, age, and other information. Nurses often direct all questions to adults, even when children are old enough to speak for themselves. This serves to terminate an extremely valuable source of information: the patient. When the child is included, follow the general rules for communicating with children in the Guidelines box on p. 964.

Role Clarification and Explanation of the Interview

During the introduction it is also necessary to clarify the nurse's particular role in the health setting. For example, nurses performing interviews may be pediatric nurse practitioners, inpatient staff nurses, clinic nurses, office nurses, visiting nurses, or school nurses. A parent is much more likely to reveal personal information about the child and family if the relevance and importance of the interview are stressed. If this is not done, parents may refuse to elaborate on certain areas because they feel it has no bearing on the "problem." In addition, because more than one member of the health team may take a history during the course of a hospital admission, it is important to clarify the reason for each interview (Seidel et al, 2003).

Another reason for role clarification is education of the health consumer. With expanded roles in nursing, it is not unusual for families to think that the examiner is a physician rather than a nurse. Role clarification is especially important because some parents may feel deceived if they later are made aware of the nurse's identity. The general consumer acceptance of pediatric nurse practitioners (PNPs) has been very favorable, so it is also important to acknowledge their expertise by emphasizing the PNP's role.

Preliminary Acquaintance

To make the family feel at ease and to develop rapport, begin the interview with some general conversation. The opening statements should be general but still informative. Comments such as "How have things been since your last visit?" "Tell me about Johnny," or (to the child) "What do you think is going to happen today?" allow the parent or child to express the main concern in a casual, relaxed atmosphere.

The preliminary acquaintance conversation also reveals how responsive the informant may be to questions. For example, using open-ended statements, such as "Tell me about the baby," may lead the parent into a lengthy, detailed discussion. In this case, direct questions toward specific answers to avoid irrelevant remarks. At other times a parent may respond to open-ended questions with only minimal information, in which case continue to use open-ended questions rather than questions with "yes" or "no" answers.

Assurance of Privacy and Confidentiality

The place where the interview is conducted is almost as important as the interview itself. The physical environment should allow for as much privacy as possible, with distractions, such as interruptions, noise, or other visible activity, kept to a minimum. At times it is necessary to turn off a television or radio. The environment should also have some play provision for young children to keep them occupied during the parent-nurse interview (Fig. 34-1). Parents who are constantly interrupted by their children are unable to concentrate fully and tend to give short, brief answers to terminate the interview as quickly as possible.

Confidentiality is also an essential component of the initial phase of the interview. Because the interview is usually shared with other members of the health team or the teacher (as in the case of students), be sure to inform the family of the limits regarding confidentiality. If there is concern regarding confidentiality in a situation, such as talking to a parent suspected of child abuse or a teenager contemplating suicide, deal with this directly and inform the person that in such instances confidentiality cannot be ensured. However, the nurse judiciously protects information of a confidential nature (Sullivan, 1997).

NURSE ALERT In 2003, the Health Insurance Portability and Accountability Act was implemented to further ensure patient privacy and limit access to sensitive health information. Nurses and students should become familiar with their institution's policy regarding HIPAA compliance (see www.hhs.gov/ocr/hipaa). ■

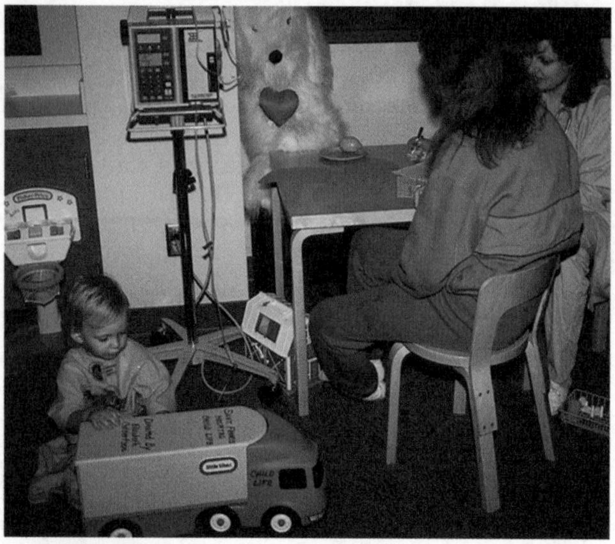

Fig. 34-1 Child plays while nurse interviews parent.

Computer Privacy and Applications in Nursing

The use of computer technology to store and retrieve health information has become widespread. The privacy and security of this health information has generated a growing concern throughout the health care community. Any person accessing health information of a confidential nature is charged with managing safeguards for disclosures, because violations might incur civil damages.

In 1994 a committee of the Institute of Medicine recommended a national code of fair health information practices. The suggestion was made that health data organizations (HDOs) should establish data protection units to develop privacy policies and security practices for manual and automated data processing systems. Technologic safeguards, such as encryption and managerial security procedures, can be applied to computer hardware across a network to ensure that individual patient privacy is protected.

Computer and information applications in nursing *(nursing informatics)*, such as electronic medical records, are used by many institutions to record care and access information. Two important health care applications are record transmission, including facsimile (fax) and electronic mail (e-mail), and telemedicine. The telemedicine application is capable of two-way video conferencing, transmission of radiographs, and clinical consultation between remote sites and centralized resources.*

Telephone Triage and Counseling

Nurses are increasingly becoming responsible for assessment of children's symptoms and clinical judgment for further medical care *(triage)* via telephone report. Most often, health problems are assessed and prioritized according to urgency, and treatment is judiciously provided via telephone services. Successful outcomes are based on the consistency and accuracy of the information provided, and parents are empowered to participate in their child's medical care. Telephone triage care management has increased access to quality health care services, and patient satisfaction has significantly improved. Unnecessary emergency department and clinic visits have decreased, saving medical costs and time (less work absence) for families in need of health care. The most common telephone triage call is for a fever (see Chapter 45). Approximately 37% of the triage calls related to fever require emergency care, and nearly 50% benefit from home management (Deadrick & Boggess, 1996).

NURSE ALERT Legal issues can emerge from errors in telephone triage care management. Always advise the caller that the child should be seen if there is any doubt as to the seriousness of the illness. ■

A well-designed telephone triage program is essential for safe, prompt, and consistent-quality health care (Rutenberg,

*Resources: Nicoll LH, *Nurses' guide to the Internet,* ed 3, Philadelphia, 2001, JB Lippincott. Also available is a bimonthly publication, *Computers, Informatics, Nursing.* To order, call 800-638-3030; fax: 301-714-2300; e-mail: CustomerService@LWW.com; Web site: www.cinjournal.com.

2000). Telephone triage is more than "just a phone call," because a child's life is an unacceptably high price to pay for poorly managed or incompetent telephone assessment skills. Typically, general guidelines for telephone triage include screening questions; determining when to immediately refer to emergency medical services (EMS) (dial 911); and determining when to refer to same-day appointments, appointments in 24 to 72 hours, appointments in 4 days or more, or home care.

COMMUNICATING WITH FAMILIES

Communicating with Parents

Although the parent and child are separate and distinct individuals, relationships with the child are frequently mediated via the parent, particularly in the case of younger children. For the most part, information about the child is acquired by direct observation or is communicated to the nurse by the parents. Usually it can be assumed that because of the close contact with the child, the parent gives reliable information. Making an assessment of the child requires input from the child (verbal and nonverbal), information from the parent, and the nurse's own observations of the child and interpretation of the relationship between the child and the parent. Counseling and guidance must be directed to the caregiver of infants and small children; when children are old enough to be active participants in their own health maintenance, the parent becomes a collaborator in health care.

Encouraging the Parent to Talk

Interviewing parents not only offers the opportunity to determine the health and developmental status of the child, but also offers information about factors that influence the child's life. Whatever the parent sees as a problem should be a concern of the nurse. These problems are not always easy to identify. Nurses need to be alert for clues and signals by which a parent communicates worries and anxieties. Careful phrasing with broad, open-ended questions such as "What is Jimmy eating now?" provides more information than several single-answer questions such as "Is Jimmy eating what the rest of the family eats?"

Critical Thinking Exercise: The Interview

Sometimes the parent will take the lead without prompting. At other times it may be necessary to direct another question on the basis of an observation, such as "Connie seems unhappy today" or "How do you feel when David cries?" If the parent appears to be tired or distraught, consider asking, "What do you do to relax?" or "What help do you have with the children?" A comment such as "You handle the baby very well. What kinds of experience have you had with babies?" to new parents who appear comfortable with their first child gives positive reinforcement and provides an opening for any questions they might have regarding the care of the infant. Often all that is required to keep parents talking is a nod or saying "yes" or "uh-huh."

When attempting to elicit feelings and covert problem areas, avoid closed-ended questions that begin with "Does . . .," "Did . . .," or "Is . . .," which usually require only a single response. In addition, asking questions such as "Does your son have any problems at school?" subtly implies a lack of parental skills and evokes defensiveness. Instead, say, "What . . .," "How . . .," or "Tell me about . . .," and encourage elaboration with "You were saying . . .," "You say that . . .," or reflecting back a key word. Open-ended questions are nonthreatening and encourage description.

Directing the Focus

The ability to direct the focus of the interview while allowing for maximum freedom of expression is one of the most difficult goals in effective communication. One approach is the use of open-ended or broad questions, followed by guiding statements. For example, if the parent proceeds to list the other children by name, say, "Tell me their ages, too." If the parent continues to describe each child in depth, which is not the purpose of the interview, redirect the focus by stating, "Let's talk about the other children later. You were beginning to tell me about Paul's activities at school." This approach conveys interest in the other children but focuses the assessment on the patient.

In the event that the parent has suggested that a problem exists with one of the other children, reintroduce this subject at the end of the interview to assess the need for further family follow-up. Saying to the parent, "Before, you were mentioning that your older son is having trouble in school. Tell me what you see as the problem," reintroduces this subject but only in terms of the possible problem.

Listening and Cultural Awareness

Listening is the most important component of effective communication. When listening is truly aimed at understanding the patient, it is an active process that requires concentration and attention to all aspects of the conversation—verbal, nonverbal, and abstract. Major blocks to listening are environmental distraction and premature judgment.

The attitudes and feelings of the nurse are easily injected into an interview. Often nurses' perceptions of a parent's behavior are influenced by their own perceptions, prejudices, and assumptions, which may include racial, religious, and cultural stereotypes. What may be interpreted as passive hostility or disinterest in a parent may be shyness or an expression of anxiety. For example, in Western cultures eye contact and directness are signs of paying attention. However, in many non-Western cultures, including that of Native Americans, directness, such as looking someone in the eye, is considered rude. Children are taught to avert their gaze and to look down when being addressed by an adult, especially one with authority (Seidel et al, 2003). Therefore judgments about "listening," as well as verbal interactions, need to be made with an appreciation of cultural differences (see Guidelines box in Chapter 32).

Although it is necessary to make some preliminary judgments, listen with as much objectivity as possible by clarifying meanings and attempting to see the situation from the parent's point of view. Effective interviewers use conscious control over their reactions, responses, and the techniques they use.

Minimum verbal activity with active listening facilitates parent involvement. It is tempting to spend time explaining, describing, and interpreting health information when the opportunity presents itself. However, it is possible to provide effective health education by timing the information properly and presenting only as much as is necessary at the moment.

Careful listening facilitates the use of clues, verbal leads, or signals from the interviewee to move the interview along. Frequent references to an area of concern, repetition of certain key words, and a special emphasis on something or someone serve as cues to the interviewer for the direction of inquiry. Concerns and anxieties are usually mentioned in a casual, offhand manner. Even though they are casual, they are important and deserve careful scrutiny to identify problem areas. For example, a parent who is concerned about a child's habit of bed-wetting may casually mention that the child's bed was "wet this morning."

Because the interview is almost always triangular—between the nurse, parent, and child—the parent may wish to convey information in such a way as to prevent the child from hearing it. This requires active listening on the part of the nurse to hear the unspoken message. The following example illustrates this point:

> During a routine health visit, the nurse performed a complete history and physical examination on a 4-year-old girl. The child was accompanied by her mother, who appeared to be a reliable, well-informed, and talkative informant. During the child's birth history, the mother gave all the information asked. However, during the family history, the mother stated to the nurse, "I had a hysterectomy 6 years ago." Because the nurse gave no indication of acknowledging the significance of this statement, the mother repeated it, only this time she stressed the "6 years." The nurse, who had not been listening as attentively as she should have, realized that the mother was telling her something very important. The mother raised her eyebrows and gently shook her head "no," warning the nurse not to explore this area too openly. The nurse correctly read the cues and stated, "Let's return to your health history later."
>
> At the completion of the physical examination, the nurse took the child to the health center's playroom and took the opportunity to investigate this contradictory information of a "4-year-old child born to a woman with a hysterectomy 6 years ago." The mother revealed that the child was adopted. The mother was greatly concerned about the fact that the child was unaware of this and requested the nurse's advice.
>
> Fortunately, the nurse had "listened" carefully enough to realize the significance of this woman's concern and allowed her the opportunity to discuss it in private.

Listening is also helpful in assessing reliability. For example, the answers elicited at the beginning of the interview may differ from those at the end, when the parent feels more confident in revealing problems. It is important to identify any discrepancies and reintroduce those topics for further investigation.

Using Silence

Silence as a response is often one of the most difficult interviewing techniques to learn. It requires a sense of confidence and comfort on the part of the interviewer to allow the interviewee space in which to think without interruptions. Silence permits the interviewee to sort out thoughts and feelings and search for responses to questions. It also allows for sharing of feelings in which two or more people absorb the emotion to its depth. Silence can also be a clue for the interviewer to go slower, reexamine his or her approach, and not push too hard (Seidel et al, 2003).

Sometimes it is necessary to break the silence and reopen communication. Do this in a way that encourages the person to continue talking about what is considered important. Breaking a silence by introducing a new topic or by prolonged talking essentially terminates the interviewee's opportunity to use the silence. Suggestions for breaking the silence include statements such as "Is there anything else you wish to say?" "I see you find it difficult to continue; how may I help?" or "I don't know what this silence means. Perhaps there is something you would like to put into words but find difficult to say."

Being Empathic

Empathy is the capacity to understand what another person is experiencing from within that person's frame of reference; it is often described as the ability to put oneself in another's shoes. The essence of empathic interaction is accurately understanding another's feelings (Price & Archbold, 1997; Reynolds, Scott, & Jessiman, 1999; White, 1997). Empathy differs from *sympathy,* which is having feelings or emotions in common with another person, rather than understanding those feelings. Sympathy is not therapeutic in the helping relationship, because it leads to feeling emotionally overinvolved, and potentially leads to professional burnout (Yegdich, 1999).

Defining the Problem

To arrive at a solution to a problem, the nurse and the parent must agree that a problem exists. Sometimes the parent may believe that there is a problem that the nurse is unable to see. For example, a mother was overly concerned about every small sniffle, sneeze, or cough in her infant, who had been carefully examined and found to be healthy with no evidence of a respiratory problem. On careful questioning, the nurse discovered that a previous child had died of pneumonia in infancy. Consequently, the nurse was better able to understand the mother's concern and could help the mother deal with her anxieties about her infant; the nurse could also teach her how to recognize any need for concern.

Occasionally the nurse identifies a problem that the parent denies exists. In this case pursue the situation and either find a way to deal with it or enlist the aid of other health team members. For example, the parents of a child with Down syndrome may refuse to believe that their child is different from any other child of the same age. They may say, "He is just a little slow," or "All the child needs to do is to try harder." A child with an obvious behavior problem may be described by the parents as "stubborn." Such statements may be clues that the parents have not progressed past the stage of denial in adjusting to the condition.

Solving the Problem

Once the problem is identified and agreed on by the parent and the nurse, they can begin to arrive at a solution. A parent who is included in the problem-solving process is more apt to follow through with a course of action. Such questions as "What have you tried so far?" or "What have you thought about doing?" provide leads for exploration and give the parents the feeling that their ideas and solutions are worthwhile. These can be followed by "What prevents you from trying that?" "That sounds like a good plan," and "You seem to be stumped. Have you considered trying this?" Such approaches encourage active participation and reinforce rather than belittle parents' efforts to solve their problems.

Sometimes the parents arrive at a solution that the nurse does not consider the best alternative. If it can be ascertained that it will do no harm and if the parents are convinced of its merits, it is usually best to allow them to continue with the plan. A course of action is more likely to be carried out when parents can reach their own conclusions. However, when parental decisions may be hazardous, nurses are obligated to discuss the risks with the family and try to reach a more beneficial solution. Whenever possible, decisions should be theirs, with the nurse serving as a *facilitator* in problem solving.

Providing Anticipatory Guidance

The ideal way to handle a situation is to deal with it *before* it becomes a problem. The best preventive measure is anticipatory guidance. Traditionally, anticipatory guidance has focused on providing families with information on normal growth and development, as well as nurturing childrearing practices. For example, one of the most significant areas in pediatrics is injury prevention. Beginning prenatally, parents need specific instructions on home safety. Because of the child's maturing developmental skills, home safety changes must be implemented early to minimize risks to the child.

Many normal developmental changes can disturb unprepared parents, such as a toddler's diminished appetite, negativism, altered sleeping patterns, and anxiety toward strangers. Such topics are discussed in the chapters on health promotion to provide the nurse with knowledge to counsel parents.

However, anticipatory guidance should extend beyond giving information to empowering families to use the information as a means of building competence in their parenting abilities. To achieve this level of anticipatory guidance, do the following (Desselle & Pearlmutter, 1997):

- Base interventions on needs identified by the family, not by the professional.
- View the family as competent or as having the ability to be competent.
- Provide opportunities for the family to achieve competence.

Avoiding Blocks to Communication

A number of blocks to communication can adversely affect the quality of the helping relationship. Many of these blocks are initiated by the interviewer, such as giving unrestricted advice or forming prejudged conclusions. Another type of block occurs primarily with the interviewees and deals with information overload. When individuals are presented with too much information or information that is overwhelming, they will often demonstrate signals of increasing anxiety or decreasing attention. Such signals should alert the interviewer to give less information or to clarify what has been said. Some of the more common blocks to communication, including signs of information overload, are listed in Box 34-1.

Communication blocks can be corrected by careful analysis of the interview process. One of the best methods for improving interviewing skills is audiotape or videotape feedback. With supervision and guidance, the interviewer can recognize the blocks and consciously avoid them.

Communicating with Families through an Interpreter

Sometimes communication is impossible because two people speak different languages. In this case it is necessary to obtain information through a third party, the interpreter. When an interpreter is used, the same guidelines for interviewing are used. Specific guidelines for using an adult interpreter are presented in the Guidelines box.

BOX 34-1

Blocks to Communication

Socializing
Giving unrestricted and sometimes unasked for advice
Offering premature or inappropriate reassurance
Giving overready encouragement
Defending a situation or opinion
Using stereotyped comments or cliches
Limiting expression of emotion by asking directed, closed-ended questions
Interrupting and finishing the person's sentence
Talking more than the interviewee
Forming prejudged conclusions
Deliberately changing the focus

Signs of Information Overload

Long periods of silence
Wide eyes and fixed facial expression
Constant fidgeting or attempting to move away
Nervous habits (e.g., tapping, playing with hair)
Sudden disruptions (e.g., asking to go to the bathroom)
Looking around
Yawning, eyes drooping
Frequently looking at a watch or clock
Attempting to change topic of discussion

Communicating with families through an interpreter requires sensitivity to cultural, legal, and ethical considerations. For example, in some cultures using a child as an interpreter is considered an insult to an adult, because children are expected to show respect by not questioning their elders. In some cultures class differences between the interpreter and the family may cause the family to feel intimidated and less inclined to offer information. Therefore choose the translator carefully, and provide time for the interpreter and family to establish rapport.

Issues of legal and ethical concerns may also arise. For example, in obtaining informed consent through an interpreter, it is important that the family be fully informed of all aspects of the particular procedure that they are consenting to. Issues of confidentiality may arise when family members related to another patient are asked to interpret for the family, thus revealing sensitive information that may be shared with other families on the unit. With increased sensitivity toward patient rights and confidentiality, many institutions now require consent forms to be produced in the primary language of the patient.

When no one else is available to translate, children within the family are often asked to assume this role. In this situation it is important to stress *literal* translation of parent responses. To maximize correct translations, it may be necessary to interrupt the parent and ask the child to translate every few sentences. When using children as interpreters, ask questions directed at specific answers and assess the interpreted translation in terms of nonverbal expressions of communication. It should be noted that some institutions prohibit or discourage the use of children as interpreters; check institutional policy for compliance.*

*Interpreting services are also available through American Telephone and Telegraph (AT&T) by calling 800-628-8486 or 800-752-6096.

Guidelines

USING AN INTERPRETER

Explain to interpreter the reason for the interview and the type of questions that will be asked.
Clarify whether a detailed or brief answer is required and whether the translated response can be general or literal.
Introduce interpreter to family and allow some time before the actual interview so that they can become acquainted.
Communicate directly with family members when asking questions to reinforce interest in them and to observe nonverbal expressions, but do not ignore interpreter.
Pose questions to elicit only one answer at a time, such as "Do you have pain?" rather than "Do you have any pain, tiredness, or loss of appetite?"
Refrain from interrupting family member and interpreter while they are conversing.
Avoid commenting to interpreter about family members, because they may understand some English.
Be aware that some medical words, such as "allergy," may have no similar word in another language; avoid medical jargon whenever possible.
Respect cultural differences; it is often best to pose questions about sex, marriage, or pregnancy indirectly–ask about "child's father" rather than "mother's husband."
Allow time following the interview for interpreter to share something that he or she felt could not be said earlier; ask about interpreter's impression of nonverbal clues to communication and family members' reliability or ease in revealing information.
Arrange for family to speak with same interpreter on subsequent visits whenever possible.

NURSE ALERT When using translated materials, such as a health history form, be sure the informant is literate in the foreign language. ■

Communicating with Children

Although the greatest amount of verbal communication may usually be carried out with the parent, do not exclude the child during the interview. Pay attention to infants and younger children through play or by occasionally directing questions or remarks to them. Include older children as active participants.

In communication with children of all ages, the nonverbal components of the communication process convey the most significant messages. It is difficult to disguise feelings, attitudes, and anxiety when relating to children. They are very alert to surroundings and attach meaning to every gesture and move that is made; this is particularly true of very young children.

Active attempts to make friends with children before they have had an opportunity to evaluate an unfamiliar person tend to increase their anxiety. It is helpful to continue to talk to the child and parent but go about activities that do not involve the child directly, thus allowing the child to observe from a safe position. If the child has a special toy or doll, "talk" to the doll first. Ask simple questions such as "Does your teddy bear have a name?" to ease the child into conversation. Other guidelines for communicating with children are presented in the Guidelines box. Specific guidelines for preparing children for procedures, a common nursing function, are discussed in Chapter 45.

SKILL: COMMUNICATING WITH CHILDREN

Communication Related to Development of Thought Processes

The normal development of language and thought offers a frame of reference in knowing how to communicate with children. Thought processes progress from sensorimotor to perceptual to concrete and finally to abstract, formal operations. The early social communicative development of children has been divided into three stages: (1) *perlocutionary stage*—unintentional communication behavior; (2) *illocutionary stage*—true intent in communication efforts; and (3) *locutionary stage*—intentional communication behaviors and use of symbols (Hoge & Parette, 1995). An understanding of the typical characteristics of these stages provides the nurse with a framework to facilitate social communication (Box 34-2).

Guidelines

COMMUNICATING WITH CHILDREN

Allow children time to feel comfortable.
Avoid sudden or rapid advances, broad smiles, extended eye contact, or other gestures that may be seen as threatening.
Talk to the parent if child is initially shy.
Communicate through transition objects such as dolls, puppets, stuffed animals before questioning a young child directly.
Give older children the opportunity to talk without the parents present.
Assume a position that is at eye level with child (Fig. 34-2).
Speak in a quiet, unhurried, and confident voice.
Speak clearly; be specific; use simple words and short sentences.
State directions and suggestions positively.
Offer a choice only when one exists.
Be honest with children.
Allow them to express their concerns and fears.
Use a variety of communication techniques.

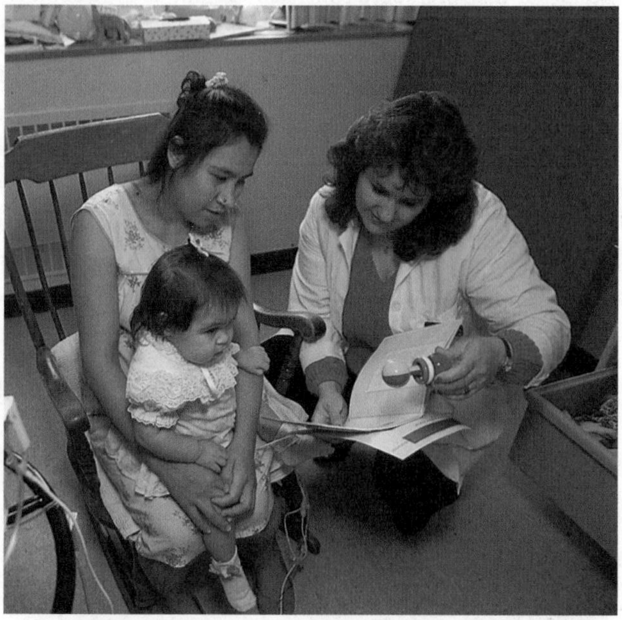

Fig. 34-2 Nurse assumes position at child's level.

BOX 34-2

Stages of Communicative Development in Young Children

Perlocutionary Stage (Birth to 8-9 Months)
Characteristics
Child is reflexive to stimuli
Increasing purpose in action

Emerging Illocutionary Stage (8-9 to 12-15 Months)
Characteristics
Communicates intentionally with signals and gestures

Conventional Illocutionary/Emerging Locutionary Stage (12-15 to 18-24 Months)
Characteristics
Communicates intentionally with gestures, vocalizations, and verbalizations

Modified from Hoge DR, Parette HP: Facilitating communicative development in young children with disabilities, *Transdisciplinary J* 5(2):113-130, 1995.

Infancy

Because they are unable to use words, infants primarily use and understand nonverbal communication. Infants communicate their needs and feelings through nonverbal behaviors and vocalizations that can be interpreted by someone who is around them for a sufficient amount of time. Infants smile and coo when content and cry when distressed. Crying is provoked by unpleasant stimuli from inside or outside, such as hunger, pain, body restraint, or loneliness. Adults interpret this to mean that an infant needs something and consequently try to alleviate the discomfort and reduce tension. Crying (or the desire to cry) persists as a part of everyone's communication repertoire.

Infants respond to adults' nonverbal behaviors. They become quiet when they are cuddled, patted, or receive other forms of gentle, physical contact. They derive comfort from the sound of a voice, even though they do not understand the words that are spoken. Until infants reach the age at which they experience stranger anxiety, they readily respond to any firm, gentle handling and quiet, calm speech. Loud, harsh sounds and sudden movements are frightening.

Older infants' attentions are centered on themselves and their parents; therefore any stranger is a potential threat until proved otherwise. Holding out the hands and asking the child to "come" is seldom successful, especially if the infant is with the parent. If infants must be handled, simply pick them up firmly without gestures. Observe the position in which the parent holds the infant. Most infants have learned to prefer a particular position and manner of handling. In general, infants are more at ease upright than horizontal. Also, hold infants so that they can see their parents. Until they have developed the understanding that an object (in this case the parent) removed from sight can still be present, they have no way of knowing that the object is still there.

Early Childhood

Children under 5 years of age are egocentric. They see things only in relation to themselves and from their point of view. Therefore focus communication on *them.* Tell them what they can do or how they will feel. Experiences of others are of no interest to them. It is futile to use another child's experience as an attempt to gain the cooperation of very small children. Allow them to touch and examine articles that will come in contact with them. A stethoscope bell will feel cold; palpating a neck might tickle. Although they have not yet acquired sufficient language skills to express their feelings and wants, toddlers are able to communicate effectively with their hands to transmit ideas without words. They push an unwanted object away, pull another person to show them something, point, and cover the mouth that is saying something they do not wish to hear.

Everything is direct and concrete to small children. They are unable to work with abstractions and interpret words literally. Analogies escape them because they are unable to separate fact from fantasy. For example, they attach literal meaning to such common phrases as "two-faced," "sticky fingers," or "coughing your head off." Children who are told they will get "a little stick in the arm" may not be able to envision an injection (Fig. 34-3). Therefore avoid using a phrase that might be misinterpreted by a small child (see Home Care box under Preparation for Procedures, Chapter 45).

Use language that is consistent with the child's developmental level. For example, in talking with a toddler, use simple, *short* sentences; repeat words that are *familiar* to the child; and limit descriptions to *concrete* explanations. Be certain that nonverbal messages are consistent with words and actions. For example, do not smile while doing something painful; children may think you enjoy hurting them.

Young children assign human attributes to inanimate objects. Consequently, they fear that objects may jump, bite,

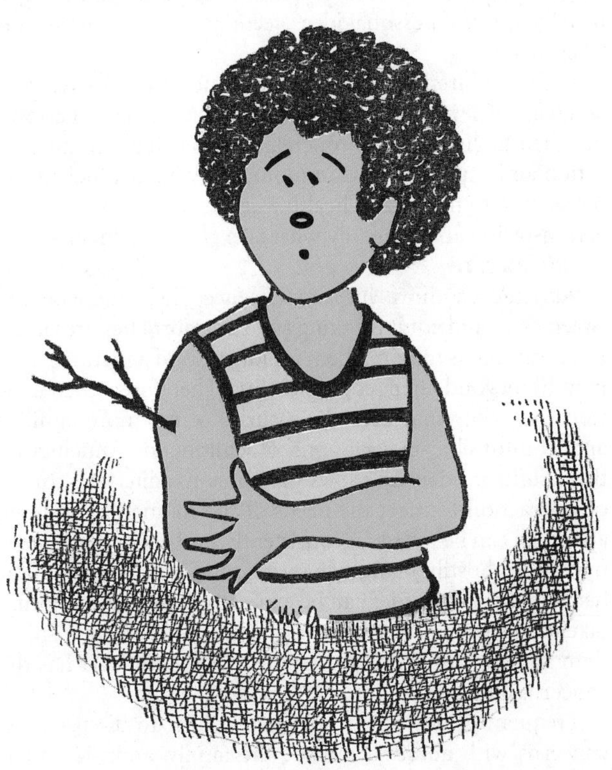

Fig. 34-3 A young child may take the expression "a little stick in the arm" literally.

cut, or pinch all by themselves. Children do not know that these devices are unable to perform without human direction. To minimize their fear, keep unfamiliar equipment out of view until it is needed.

School-Age Years

Younger school-age children rely less on what they see and more on what they know when faced with new problems. They want explanations and reasons for everything but require no verification beyond that. They are interested in the functional aspect of all procedures, objects, and activities. They want to know why an object exists, why it is used, how it works, and the intent and purpose of its user. They need to know what is going to take place and why it is being done to *them* specifically. For example, to explain a procedure such as taking a blood pressure, show the child how squeezing the bulb pushes air into the cuff and makes the "silver" in the tube go up. Let the child operate the bulb. An explanation for the reason might be as simple as "I want to see how far the silver goes up when the cuff squeezes your arm." Consequently, the child becomes an enthusiastic participant.

School-age children have a heightened concern about body integrity. Because of the special importance and value they place on their body, they are overly sensitive to anything that constitutes a threat or suggestion of injury to it. This concern extends to their possessions also, so that they may appear to overreact to loss or threatened loss of treasured objects. Helping children to voice their concerns enables the nurse to provide reassurance and to implement activities that reduce their anxiety. For example, if a shy child dislikes being the center of attention, ignore that particular child by talking and relating to other children in the family or group. When children feel more comfortable, they will usually interject personal ideas, feelings, and interpretations of events.

Older children have an adequate and satisfactory use of language. They still require relatively simple explanations, but their ability to think concretely can facilitate communication and explanation. Commonly, they have sufficient experience with health and health workers to understand what is transpiring and generally what is expected of them.

Adolescence

CASE STUDY: COMMUNICATING WITH ADOLESCENTS

As children move into adolescence, they fluctuate between child and adult thinking and behavior. They are riding a current that is moving them rapidly toward a maturity that may be beyond their coping ability. Therefore, when tensions rise, they may seek the security of the more familiar and comfortable expectations of childhood. Anticipating these shifts in identity allows the nurse to adjust the course of interaction to meet the needs of the moment. No single approach can be relied on consistently, and encountering cooperation, hostility, anger, bravado, and a variety of other behaviors and attitudes can be expected. It is as much a mistake to regard the adolescent as an adult with an adult's wisdom and control as it is to assume that the teenager has the concerns and expectations of a child.

Frequently adolescents are more willing to discuss their concerns with an adult outside the family, and they often welcome the opportunity to interact with a nurse outside of the presence of their parents. They are accepting of anyone who displays a genuine interest in them. However, adolescents are quick to reject persons who attempt to impose their values on them, whose interest is feigned, or who appear to have little respect for who they are and what they think or say.

As with all children, adolescents need to express their feelings. Generally, they talk quite freely when given an opportunity. However, what adolescents say cannot always be taken at face value. When emotional factors are involved, the feelings that are interjected into words are as significant as the words that are used. To give support, be attentive, try not to interrupt, and avoid comments or expressions that convey disapproval or surprise. Avoid prying and asking embarrassing questions, and resist any impulse to give advice. Frequently adolescents reveal their feelings or a source of concern or ask a question when they are involved in routine matters such as a physical assessment.

Teenagers characteristically have a language and culture all their own that further sets them apart. To avoid misinterpretation, clarify terms frequently. Occasionally adolescents refuse to answer or answer only in monosyllables. Usually this happens when they are opposed to the contact or do not yet feel safe enough to reveal themselves. In this instance confine discussions to neutral topics to reduce the element of threat until such time as they feel more secure. Be alert for signals indicating that they are ready to talk. The major sources of concern for adolescents are attitudes and feelings toward sex, substance abuse, relationships with parents, peer-group acceptance, and developing a sense of identity.

Interviewing the adolescent presents some special situations. The first may be whether to talk with the adolescent alone, with the adolescent and parents together, or with each person individually. Of course, if the adolescent is alone, there is no question, except whether to suggest to the teenager that the parents may be interviewed at another time. If the parents and teenager are together, talking with the adolescent first has the advantage of immediately identifying with the young person, thus fostering the interpersonal relationship. However, talking with the parents initially may provide insight into the family relationship. In either case, give both parties an opportunity to be included in the interview. If time constraints are important, such as during history taking, clarify these at the onset to avoid appearing to "take sides" by talking more with one person than with the other.

Confidentiality is of great important when interviewing adolescents. Explain to parents and teenagers the limits of confidentiality, specifically that young persons' disclosures will not be shared unless they indicate a need for intervention, as in the case of suicidal behavior.

Another dilemma in interviewing adolescents is that two views of a problem frequently exist—the teenager's and the parents'. Clarification of the problem is a major task. However, providing both parties with an opportunity to discuss their perceptions in an open and unbiased atmosphere can, by itself, be therapeutic. Demonstrating positive communication skills can help families communicate more effectively (Guidelines box).

Guidelines

COMMUNICATING WITH ADOLESCENTS

Build a Foundation

Spend time together.
Encourage expression of ideas and feelings.
Respect their views.
Tolerate differences.
Praise good points.
Respect their privacy.
Set a good example.

Communicate Effectively

Give undivided attention.
Listen, listen, listen.
Be courteous, calm, and open-minded.
Try not to overreact. If you do, take a break.
Avoid judging or criticizing.
Avoid the "third degree" of continuous questioning.
Choose important issues when taking a stand.
After taking a stand:
- Think through all options.
- Make expectations clear.

Communication Techniques

In addition to such conventional interviewing methods as reflection and open-ended questions, a number of techniques encourage family members to express their thoughts and feelings in a less directive and confrontational manner. Several approaches are *projective*—they present nonspecific material that enables individuals to externalize or project inner aspects of themselves to others.

A variety of verbal techniques can be used to encourage communication. Some of these techniques can be used to pose questions or explore concerns in a less threatening manner. Others can be presented as "word games," which are often well received by children. However, for many children and adults, talking about feelings is difficult and verbal communication may be more stressful than supportive. In such instances several nonverbal techniques can be used to encourage communication.

Both verbal and nonverbal techniques are described in Box 34-3. Because of the importance of play in communicating with children, play is discussed more extensively in

BOX 34-3

Creative Communication Techniques with Children

Verbal Techniques

"I" Messages

Relate a feeling about a behavior in terms of "I."
Describe effect behavior had on the person.
Avoid use of "you."
- "You" messages are judgmental and provoke defensiveness.
- ***Example:*** "You" message—"You are being very uncooperative about doing your treatments."
- ***Example:*** "I" message—"I am concerned about how the treatments are going because I want to see you get better."

Third-Person Technique

Involves expressing a feeling in terms of a third person ("he," "she," "they").
Is less threatening than directly asking children how they feel because it gives them an opportunity to agree or disagree without being defensive.
- ***Example:*** "Sometimes when a person is sick a lot, he feels angry and sad because he cannot do what others can." Either wait silently for a response or encourage a reply with a question such as, "Did you ever feel that way?"

Approach allows children three choices: (1) to agree and, hopefully, express how they feel; (2) to disagree; or (3) to remain silent, in which case they probably have such feelings but are unable to express them at this time.

Facilitative Responding

Involves careful listening and reflecting back to patients the feelings and content of their statements.
Responses are empathic and nonjudgmental, and legitimize the person's feelings.
Formula for facilitative responses: "You feel ___________ because ___________."
- ***Example:*** If child states, "I hate coming to the hospital and getting needles," a facilitative response is, "You feel unhappy because of all the things that are done to you."

Storytelling

Uses the language of children to probe into areas of their thinking while bypassing conscious inhibitions or fears.
Simplest technique is asking children to relate a story about an event, such as "being in the hospital."
Other approaches:
- Show children a picture of a particular event, such as a child in a hospital with other people in the room, and ask them to describe the scene.
- Cut out comic strips, remove words, and have child add statements for scenes.

Mutual Storytelling

Reveals child's thinking and attempts to change child's perceptions or fears by retelling a somewhat different story (more therapeutic approach than storytelling).
Begins by asking child to tell a story about something, followed by another story told by the nurse that is similar to child's tale but with differences that help child in problem areas.
- ***Example:*** Child's story is about going to the hospital and never seeing his or her parents again. Nurse's story is also about a child (using different names but similar circumstances) in a hospital whose parents visit every day, but in the evening after work until the child is better and goes home with them.

Bibliotherapy

Uses books in a therapeutic and supportive process.
Provides children with an opportunity to explore an event that is similar to their own but sufficiently different to allow them to distance themselves from it and remain in control.
General guidelines for using bibliotherapy:
- Assess child's emotional and cognitive development in terms of readiness to understand the book's message.
- Be familiar with the book's content (intended message or purpose) and the age for which it is written.
- Read the book to the child if child is unable to read.

Continued

BOX 34-3

Creative Communication Techniques with Children—cont'd

Verbal Techniques—cont'd

Bibliotherapy—cont'd

Explore the meaning of the book with the child by having child do the following:

- Retell the story
- Read a special section with the nurse or parent
- Draw a picture related to the story and discuss the drawing
- Talk about the characters
- Summarize the moral or meaning of the story

Dreams

Often reveal unconscious and repressed thoughts and feelings.

Ask child to talk about a dream or nightmare.

Explore with child what meaning dream could have.

"What If" Questions

Encourage child to explore potential situations and to consider different problem-solving options.

Example: "What if you got sick and had to go the hospital?" Children's responses reveal what they know already and what they are curious about, provide opportunity for helping children learn coping skills, especially in potentially dangerous situations.

Three Wishes

Involves asking, "If you could have any three things in the world, what would they be?"

If child answers, "That all my wishes come true," ask child for specific wishes.

Rating Game

Uses some type of rating scale (numbers, sad to happy faces) to rate an event or feeling.

Example: Instead of asking youngsters how they feel, ask how their day has been "on a scale of 1 to 10, with 10 being the best."

Word Association Game

Involves stating key words and asking children to say the first word they think of when they hear the word.

Start with neutral words and then introduce more anxiety-producing words, such as "illness," "needles," "hospitals," and "operation."

Select key words that relate to some event in child's life that is relevant.

Sentence Completion

Involves presenting a partial statement and having child complete it. The following are some sample statements:

The thing I like best (least) about school is ______________.

The best (worst) age to be is ______________.

The most (least) fun thing I ever did was ______________.

The thing I like most (least) about my parents is ______________.

The one thing I would change about my family is ______________.

If I could be anything I wanted, I would be ______________.

The thing I like most (least) about myself is ______________.

Pros and Cons

Involves selecting a topic, such as "being in the hospital," and having child list "five good things and five bad things" about it.

Is an exceptionally valuable technique when applied to relationships, such as things family members like and dislike about each other.

Nonverbal Techniques

Writing

Is an alternative communication approach for older children and adults.

Specific suggestions include the following:

Keep a journal or diary.

Write down feelings or thoughts that are difficult to express.

Write "letters" that are never mailed (a variation is making up a "pen pal" to write to).

Keep an account of child's progress from both a physical and an emotional viewpoint.

Drawing

Is one of the most valuable forms of communication—both nonverbal (from looking at the drawing) and verbal (from child's story of the picture).

Children's drawings tell a great deal about them because they are projections of their inner selves.

Spontaneous drawing involves giving child a variety of art supplies and providing the opportunity to draw.

Directed drawing involves a more specific direction, such as "draw a person" or the "three themes" approach (state three things about child and ask child to choose one and draw a picture).

Guidelines for Evaluating Drawings

Use spontaneous drawings and evaluate more than one drawing whenever possible.

Interpret drawings in light of other available information about child and family.

Interpret drawings as a whole rather than on specific details of the drawing.

Consider individual elements of the drawing that may be significant:

Sex of figure drawn first—Usually relates to child's perception of own sex role.

Size of individual figures—Expresses importance, power, or authority.

Order in which figures are drawn—Expresses priority in terms of importance.

Child's position in relation to other family members—Expresses feelings of status or alliance.

Exclusion of a member—May denote feeling of not belonging or desire to eliminate.

Accentuated parts—Usually express concern for areas of special importance (e.g., large hands may be a sign of aggression).

Absence of or rudimentary arms and hands—Suggest timidity, passivity, or intellectual immaturity; tiny, unstable feet may be an expression of insecurity, and hidden hands may mean guilt feelings.

Placement of drawing on the page and type of stroke—Free use of paper and firm, continuous strokes express security, whereas drawings restricted to a small area and lightly drawn in broken or wavering lines may be a sign of insecurity.

Erasures, shading, or cross-hatching—Expresses ambivalence, concern, or anxiety with a particular area.

Magic

Uses simple magic tricks to help establish rapport with child, encourage compliance with health interventions, and provide effective distraction during painful procedures.

Although "magician" talks, no verbal response from child is required.

Play

Is universal language and "work" of children.

Tells a great deal about children because they project their inner selves through the activity.

Spontaneous play involves giving child a variety of play materials and providing the opportunity to play.

Directed play involves a more specific direction, such as providing medical equipment or a dollhouse for focused reasons, such as exploring child's fear of injections or exploring family relationships.

the following paragraphs. Any of the verbal or nonverbal techniques can give rise to strong feelings that surface unexpectedly. Be prepared to handle them or to recognize when issues go beyond your ability to deal with them. At that point, consider an appropriate referral.

Play

Play is a universal language of children. It is one of the most important forms of communication and can be an effective technique in relating to them. Clues about physical, intellectual, and social developmental progress can often be gleaned from the form and complexity of a child's play behaviors. Play requires a minimum of equipment or none at all. Therapeutic play is often used to reduce the trauma of illness and hospitalization (see Chapter 44) and to prepare children for therapeutic procedures (see Chapter 45).

Because their ability to perceive precedes their ability to transmit, small infants respond to activities that register on their senses. Patting, stroking, and other skin play convey messages. Repetitive actions, such as stretching infants' arms out to the side while they are lying on their back and then folding them across the chest or raising and revolving the legs in a bicycling motion, will elicit pleasurable sounds. Colorful items to catch the eye or interesting sounds, such as a ticking clock, chimes, bells, or singing, can be used to attract children's attention.

Older infants respond to simple games. The old game of peekaboo is an excellent means of initiating communication with infants while maintaining a "safe," nonthreatening distance. After this intermittent eye-to-eye contact, the nurse is no longer viewed as a stranger but as someone who is a friend. This can be followed by touch games. Clapping an infant's hands together for pat-a-cake or wiggling the toes for "this little piggy" delights an infant or small child. Much of the nursing assessment can be carried out with the use of games and simple play equipment while the infant remains in the safety of the parent's arms or lap. Talking to a foot or other part of the child's body is an effective tactic.

The nurse can capitalize on the natural curiosity of small children by playing games such as "Which hand do you take?" and "Guess what I have in my hand" or by manipulating items such as a flashlight or stethoscope. Finger games are very useful. More elaborate materials, such as puppets and replicas of familiar or unfamiliar items, serve as excellent means of communicating with small children. The variety and extent are limited only by the nurse's imagination.

Through play, children reveal their perceptions of interpersonal relationships with their family, their friends, or hospital personnel. Children may also reveal the wide scope of knowledge they have acquired from listening to others around them. For example, through needle play, children may disclose how carefully they have watched each procedure by precisely duplicating the technical skills. They may also reveal how well they remember those who performed procedures. One child who painstakingly reenacted every detail of a tedious medical procedure also played the role of the physician who had repeatedly shouted at her to be still for the long ordeal. Her anger at him was most evident during the play session and revealed the cause for her abrupt withdrawal and passive hostility toward the medical and nursing staff following the test.

Play sessions serve not only as assessment tools for determining children's awareness and perception of their illness, but also as methods of intervention and evaluation. In the previous example, when the child revealed anger toward the physician, the nurse acted the part of the patient but this time did not accept the physician's harsh commands to stay still. Instead, the nurse said to the physician all the things the child had wished she could say.

Subsequent play sessions can also be used to evaluate the child's progress. A change in the type of drawing or the theme of the play may indicate progression toward or away from the ability to deal with anxiety.

HISTORY TAKING

Performing a Health History

The format used for history taking may be (1) *direct*—the nurse asks for information via direct interview with the informant—or (2) *indirect*—the informant supplies the information by completing some type of questionnaire. The direct method is superior to the indirect approach or a combination of both. However, in view of time constraints, the direct approach is not always practical. If the direct approach cannot be used, review parents' written responses and question them regarding any unusual answers. The categories listed in Box 34-4 encompass children's current and past health status and information about their psychosocial environment.

Identifying Information

Much of the identifying information may already be available from other recorded sources. However, if the parent and youngster seem anxious, use this opportunity to ask about such information to help them feel more comfortable.

Informant

One of the important elements of identifying information is the *informant,* the person(s) who furnished the information. Record (1) who the person is (child, parent, or other); (2) an impression of the informant's reliability and willingness to communicate; and (3) any special circumstances, such as the use of an interpreter or conflicting answers by more than one person.

Chief Complaint

The chief complaint is the specific reason for the child's visit to the clinic, office, or hospital. It may be viewed as the theme with the present illness as the description of the problem. The chief complaint is elicited by asking open-ended, neutral questions such as "What seems to be the matter?" "How may I help you?" or "Why did you come here today?" Avoid labeling-type questions such as "How are you sick?" or "What is the problem?" because it is possible that the reason for the visit is not an illness or problem.

Occasionally it is difficult to isolate one symptom or problem as the chief complaint because the parent may identify many. In this situation be as specific as possible when asking questions. For example, asking informants to state which *one* problem or symptom prompted them to seek help now may help them focus on the most immediate concern.

BOX 34-4

Outline of a Pediatric Health History

Identifying Information

1. Name
2. Address
3. Telephone number
4. Birthdate and place
5. Race/ethnic group
6. Sex
7. Religion
8. Date of interview
9. Informant

Chief Complaint (CC)

To establish the major specific reason for the child's and parents' seeking professional health attention

Present Illness (PI)

To obtain all details related to the chief complaint

Past History (PH)

To elicit a profile of the child's previous illnesses, injuries, or operations

1. Birth history (pregnancy, labor and delivery, perinatal history)
2. Previous illnesses, injuries, or operations
3. Allergies
4. Current medications
5. Immunizations
6. Growth and development
7. Habits

Review of Systems (ROS)

To elicit information concerning any potential health problem

1. General
2. Integument
3. Head
4. Eyes
5. Ears
6. Nose
7. Mouth
8. Throat
9. Neck
10. Chest
11. Respiratory
12. Cardiovascular
13. Gastrointestinal
14. Genitourinary
15. Gynecologic
16. Musculoskeletal
17. Neurologic
18. Endocrine

Family Medical History

To identify the presence of genetic traits or diseases that have familial tendencies and to assess exposure to a communicable disease in a family member and family habits that may affect the child's health, such as smoking and other chemical use

Psychosocial History

To elicit information about the child's self-concept

Sexual History

To elicit information concerning the child's sexual concerns or activities and any pertinent data regarding adults' sexual activity that influence the child

Family History

To develop an understanding of the child as an individual and as a member of a family and a community

1. Family composition
2. Home and community environment
3. Occupation and education of family members
4. Cultural and religious traditions
5. Family function and relationships

Nutritional Assessment

To elicit information on the adequacy of the child's nutritional intake and need

1. Dietary intake
2. Clinical examination

Present Illness

The history of the present illness* is a narrative of the chief complaint from its earliest onset through its progression to the present. Its four major components are (1) the details of *onset*, (2) a complete *interval* history, (3) the *present* status, and (4) the reason for seeking help *now*. The focus of the present illness is on all factors relevant to the main problem, even if they have disappeared or changed during the onset, interval, and present.

Analyzing a Symptom

Because pain is often the most characteristic symptom denoting the onset of a physical problem, it is used as an example for analysis of a symptom. Assessment includes (1) type, (2) location, (3) severity, (4) duration, and (5) influencing factors (Guidelines box) (see also Pain Assessment, Chapter 44).

*The term *illness* is used in its broadest sense to denote any problem of a physical, emotional, or psychosocial nature. It is actually a history of the chief complaint.

Guidelines

ANALYZING THE SYMPTOM: PAIN

Type

Be as specific as possible. With young children, asking the parents how they know the child is in pain may help describe its type, location, and severity. For example, a parent may state, "My child must have a severe earache because she pulls at her ears, rolls her head on the floor, and screams. Nothing seems to help." Help older children describe the "hurt" by asking them if it is sharp, throbbing, dull, or stabbing. Record whatever words they use in quotes.

Location

Be specific. "Stomach pains" is too general a description. Children can better localize the pain if they are asked to "point with one finger to where it hurts" or to "point to where Mommy or Daddy would put a Band-Aid." Determine if the pain radiates by asking, "Does the pain stay there or move? Show me with your finger where the pain goes."

Severity

Severity is best determined by finding out how it affects the child's usual behavior. Pain that prevents a child from playing, interacting with others, sleeping, and eating is most often severe. Assess pain intensity using a rating scale, such as a numeric scale or "faces" scale (see Table 44-2).

Duration

Include the duration, onset, and frequency. Describe this in terms of activity and behavior, such as "pain lasted all night, because child refused to sleep and cried intermittently."

Influencing Factors

Include anything that causes a change in the type, location, severity, or duration of the pain: (1) precipitating events (those that cause or increase the pain), (2) relieving events (those that lessen the pain, such as medications), (3) temporal events (times when the pain is relieved or increased), (4) positional events (standing, sitting, lying down), and (5) associated events (meals, stress, coughing).

Past History

The past history contains information relating to all previous aspects of the child's health status and concentrates on several areas that are ordinarily deleted in the history of an adult, such as birth history, detailed feeding history, immunizations, and growth and development. Because a great deal of information is included in this section, use a combination of open-ended and fact-finding questions. For example, begin interviewing for each section with an open-ended statement such as "Tell me about your child's birth" in order to provide the informants with the opportunity to relate what they think is most important. Ask fact-finding questions related to specific details whenever necessary to focus the interview on certain topics.

Birth History

The birth history includes all data concerning (1) the mother's health during pregnancy, (2) the labor and delivery, and (3) the infant's condition immediately after birth. Prenatal influences have significant effects on a child's physical and emotional development; therefore a thorough investigation of the birth history is essential. Because parents may question what relevance pregnancy and birth have on the child's present condition, particularly if the child is past infancy, explain why such questions are included. An appropriate statement may be, "I will be asking you some questions about your pregnancy and . . . (refer to child by name) birth. Your answers will give me a more complete picture of his (or her) overall health."

Because emotional factors also affect the outcome of pregnancy and the subsequent parent-child relationship, investigate (1) concurrent crises during pregnancy and (2) prenatal attitudes toward the fetus. It is best to approach the topic of parental acceptance of pregnancy through indirect questioning. Asking parents if the pregnancy was planned is a leading statement because they may respond affirmatively for fear of criticism if the pregnancy was unexpected. Rather, encourage parents to disclose their true reactions by referring to specific facts relating to the pregnancy, such as the spacing between offspring, an extended or short interval between marriage and conception, or the concurrent experience of pregnancy and adolescence. The parent can choose to explore such statements with further explanations or, for the moment, may not be able to reveal such feelings. If the parent remains silent, refocus on this topic later in the interview.

Dietary History

Because parental concerns are common and nursing interventions are important in ensuring optimum nutrition, the dietary history is discussed in detail at the end of this chapter under Nutritional Assessment.

Previous Illnesses, Injuries, and Operations

When inquiring about past illnesses, begin with a general question such as "What other illnesses has your child had?" Because parents are most likely to recall serious health problems, ask specifically about colds; earaches; and childhood diseases such as measles, rubella (German measles), chickenpox, mumps, pertussis (whooping cough), diphtheria, tuberculosis, scarlet fever, strep throat, tonsillitis, or allergic manifestations.

In addition to illnesses, ask about injuries that required medical intervention, operations, and any other reason for hospitalization, including the dates of each incident. It is important to focus on injuries such as accidental falls, poisonings, chokings, or burns, because this may be a potential area for parental guidance.

Allergies

Ask about commonly known allergic disorders such as hay fever and asthma, as well as unusual reactions to drugs, food, or latex products, or other contact agents such as poisonous plants, animals, household products, or fabrics. If asked appropriate questions, most people can give reliable information about drug reactions. The accompanying Guidelines box describes how to take an allergy history.

NURSE ALERT Information about allergic reactions to drugs or other products is essential. Failure to document a serious reaction places the child at risk if the agent is given. ■

Current Medications

Inquire about current drug regimens, including vitamins, antipyretics (especially aspirin), antibiotics, antihistamines, decongestants, and antitussives. List all medications, including name, dose, schedule, duration, and reason for administration. Often, parents are unaware of the actual name of the drug. Whenever possible, ask parents to bring the containers with them to the next visit, or ask them for the name of the pharmacy and call for a list of all the child's recent prescription medications. However, this list will not include over-the-counter medications, which are important to know.

Immunizations

A record of all immunizations is essential. Because many parents are unaware of the exact name and date of each immunization, the most reliable source of information is a hospital, clinic, or private practitioner's record. All immunizations and "boosters" are listed, stating (1) the name of the specific disease, (2) the number of injections, (3) the dosage (sometimes lesser amounts are given if a reaction is antici-

Guidelines

TAKING AN ALLERGY HISTORY

Has your child ever taken any drugs or tablets that have disagreed with your child or caused an allergy? If yes, can you remember the name(s) of these drugs?
Can you describe the reaction?
Was the drug by mouth (as a tablet or medicine), or was it an injection?
How soon after starting the drug did the reaction happen?
How long ago did this happen?
Did anyone tell you it was an allergic reaction, or did you decide for yourself?
Has your child ever taken this drug, or a similar one, again? If yes, did your child experience the same problems?
Have you told the doctors or nurses about your child's reaction or allergy?

Modified from Cantrill JA, Cottrell WN: Accuracy of drug allergy documentation, *Am J Health Syst Pharm* 54:1627-1629, 1997.

pated), (4) the ages when administered, and (5) the occurrence of any reaction following the immunization.

NURSE ALERT Inquire about previous administration of any horse or other foreign serum, recent administration of gamma globulin or blood transfusion, and anaphylactic reactions to neomycin or chicken eggs. ■

Growth and Development

The most important previous growth patterns to record are (1) approximate weight at 6 months, 1 year, 2 years, and 5 years of age; (2) approximate length at ages 1 and 4 years; and (3) dentition, including age of onset, number of teeth, and symptoms during teething. Developmental milestones include (1) age of holding up head steadily; (2) age of sitting alone without support; (3) age of walking without assistance; (4) age of saying first words with meaning; (5) present grade in school; (6) scholastic grades; and (7) interaction with other children, peers, and adults.

Use specific and detailed questions when inquiring about each developmental milestone. For example, "sitting up" can mean many different activities, such as sitting propped up, sitting in someone's lap, sitting with support, sitting up alone but in a hyperflexed position for assisted balance, or sitting up unsupported with the back slightly rounded. A clue to misunderstanding of the requested activity may be an unusually early age of achievement (see Developmental Assessment, Chapter 35).

Habits

Habits are an important area to explore (Box 34-5). Parents frequently express concerns during this part of the history. Encourage their input by saying, "Please tell me any concerns you have about your child's habits, activities, or development." Investigate further any concerns that are expressed.

One of the most common concerns relates to sleep. Many children develop a normal sleep pattern, and all that is required during the assessment is a general overview of nighttime sleep and nap schedules. However, a number of children also develop sleep problems (see Sleep Problems, Chapters 36 and 38). When sleep problems occur, a more detailed sleep history is required in order to guide appropriate interventions.*

*A sleep history and a sleep chart for the family to record the child's daily sleep and wake activities is available in Hockenberry M: *Wong's clinical manual of pediatric nursing,* ed 6, St Louis, 2004, Mosby.

BOX 34-5

Habits to Explore during Health Interview

Behavior patterns such as nail-biting, thumb-sucking, pica (habitual ingestion of nonfood substances), rituals ("security" blanket or toy), and unusual movements (head banging, rocking, overt masturbation, and walking on toes)
Activities of daily living, such as hour of sleep and arising, duration of nighttime sleep and naps, type and duration of exercise, regularity of stools and urination, age of toilet training, and occurrences of daytime or nighttime bed-wetting
Unusual disposition, as well as response to frustration
Use or abuse of alcohol, drugs, coffee, or tobacco

Habits related to use of chemicals apply primarily to older children and adolescents. If a youngster admits to smoking, drinking, or drug use, ask about the quantity and frequency. Questions such as "Have you ever had a drinking or drug problem?" or "When was the last time you had a drink or took drugs?" may yield more reliable data than questions such as "How much do you drink?" or "How often do you drink or take drugs?" Clarify that "drinking" includes all types of alcohol, such as beer and wine. When quantities such as a "glass" of wine or a "can" of beer are given, ask about the size of the container.

If older children deny use of chemical substances, inquire about past experimentation. Asking, "You mean you never tried to smoke or drink?" implies that the nurse expects some such activity, and the youngster may be more inclined to answer truthfully. Be aware of the confidential nature of such questioning, of the adverse effect that the parents' presence may have on the adolescent's willingness to answer, and that self-report may not be an accurate account of chemical abuse.

Review of Systems

The review of systems is a specific review of each body system, similar to the order of the physical examination (Box 34-6). Often the history of the present illness provides a complete review of the system involved in the chief complaint. Because asking questions about other body systems may appear unrelated and irrelevant to the parents or child, precede the questioning with an explanation of why the data are needed (similar to the explanation concerning the relevance of the birth history) and reassure the parents that the child's main problem has not been forgotten.

Begin the review of a specific system with a broad question such as "How has your child's general health been?" or "Has your child had any problems with his eyes?" If the parent states that there have been past problems with some bodily function, pursue this with an encouraging statement such as "Tell me more about that." If the parent denies any problems, query for specific symptoms (e.g., "No headaches, bumping into objects, or squinting?"). If the parent reconfirms the absence of such symptoms, record positive statements in the history, such as "Mother denies headaches, bumping into objects, or squinting." In this way, anyone who reviews the health history is aware of exactly what symptoms were investigated.

Family Medical History

The family medical history is used primarily for the purpose of discovering the potential existence of hereditary or familial diseases in the parents and child. In general, it is confined to first-degree relatives (parents, siblings, grandparents, and immediate aunts and uncles). Information for each family member includes age, marital status, state of health if living, cause of death if deceased, and any evidence of the following conditions: heart disease, hypertension, cancer, diabetes mellitus, obesity, congenital anomalies, allergy, asthma, seizures, tuberculosis, sickle cell disease, mental retardation, mental disorders such as depression or psychosis, emotional problems, syphilis, or rheumatic fever. Confirm the accuracy of the reported disorders by inquiring about the symptoms, course, treatment, and sequelae of each diagnosis.

BOX 34-6

Guidelines for Review of Systems

General—Overall state of health, fatigue, recent or unexplained weight gain or loss (period of time for either), contributing factors (change of diet, illness, altered appetite), exercise tolerance, fevers (time of day), chills, night sweats (unrelated to climatic conditions), frequent infections, general ability to carry out activities of daily living

Integument—Pruritus, pigment or other color changes, acne, eruptions, rashes (location), tendency for bruising, petechiae, excessive dryness, general texture, disorders or deformities of nails, hair growth or loss, hair color change (for adolescent, use of hair dyes or other potentially toxic substances, such as hair straighteners)

Head—Headaches, dizziness, injury (specific details)

Eyes—Visual problems (ask about behaviors indicative of blurred vision, such as bumping into objects, clumsiness, sitting very close to television, holding a book close to face, writing with head near desk, squinting, rubbing the eyes, bending head in an awkward position), cross-eye (strabismus), eye infections, edema of lids, excessive tearing, use of glasses or contact lenses, date of last optic examination

Nose—Nosebleeds (epistaxis), constant or frequent runny or stuffy nose, nasal obstruction (difficulty in breathing), alteration or loss of sense of smell

Ears—Earaches, discharge, evidence of hearing loss (ask about behaviors, such as need to repeat requests, loud speech, inattentive behavior), results of any previous auditory testing

Mouth—Mouth breathing, gum bleeding, toothaches, toothbrushing, use of fluoride, difficulty with teething (symptoms), last visit to dentist (especially if temporary dentition is complete), response to dentist

Throat—Sore throats, difficulty in swallowing, choking (especially when chewing food—may be from poor chewing habits), hoarseness, or other voice irregularities

Neck—Pain, limitation of movement, stiffness, difficulty in holding head straight (torticollis), thyroid enlargement, enlarged nodes or other masses

Chest—Breast enlargement, discharge, masses, enlarged axillary nodes (for adolescent female, ask about breast self-examination)

Respiratory—Chronic cough, frequent colds (number per year), wheezing, shortness of breath at rest or on exertion, difficulty in breathing, sputum production, infections (pneumonia, tuberculosis), date of last chest x-ray examination, and skin reaction from tuberculin testing

Cardiovascular—Cyanosis or fatigue on exertion, history of heart murmur or rheumatic fever, anemia, date of last blood count, blood type, recent transfusion

Gastrointestinal (much of this in regard to appetite, food tolerance, and elimination habits has been asked elsewhere)—Nausea, vomiting (not associated with eating, may be indicative of brain tumor or increased intracranial pressure), jaundice or yellowing skin or sclera, belching, flatulence, recent change in bowel habits (blood in stools, change of color, diarrhea, or constipation)

Genitourinary—Pain on urination, frequency, hesitancy, urgency, hematuria, nocturia, polyuria, unpleasant odor to urine, force of stream, discharge, change in size of scrotum, date of last urinalysis (for adolescent, sexually transmitted disease, type of treatment; for male adolescent, ask about testicular self-examination)

Gynecologic—Menarche, date of last menstrual period, regularity or problems with menstruation, vaginal discharge, pruritus, date and result of last Pap smear (include obstetric history as discussed under birth history when applicable); if sexually active, type of contraception, sexually transmitted disease and type of treatment

Musculoskeletal—Weakness, clumsiness, lack of coordination, unusual movements, back or joint stiffness, muscle pains or cramps, abnormal gait, deformity, fractures, serious sprains, activity level

Neurologic—Seizures, tremors, dizziness, loss of memory, general affect, fears, nightmares, speech problems, any unusual habits

Endocrine—Intolerance to weather changes, excessive thirst or urination, excessive sweating, salty taste to skin, signs of early puberty

Geographic Location

One of the important areas to explore when assessing the family health history is geographic location, including the birthplace and travel to different areas in or outside of the country, for identification of possible exposure to endemic diseases. Although the primary interest focuses on the child's temporary residence in various localities, also inquire about close family members' travel, especially during tours of military service or business trips. Children are especially susceptible to parasitic infestation in areas of poor sanitary conditions and to vector-borne diseases, such as those from mosquitoes or ticks in warm and humid or heavily wooded regions.

Psychosocial History

The traditional medical history includes a personal and social section that concentrates on children's personal status, such as school adjustment and any unusual habits, and the family and home environment. Because several personal aspects are covered under Development and Habits, and the social aspects are discussed in detail under Family Assessment, only those issues related to children's ability to cope and their general view of themselves in terms of self-concept are presented here (see Development of Self-Concept, Chapter 33).

Through observation, obtain a general idea of how children handle themselves in terms of confidence in dealing with others, ability to answer questions, and coping with new situations. Observe the parent-child relationship for the types of messages sent to children about their coping skills and self-worth. Do the parents treat the child with respect, focusing on strengths, or is the interaction one of constant reprimands, with emphasis on weaknesses and faults? Do the parents help the child learn new coping strategies or support the ones the child uses?

Messages about body image are also conveyed through the parent-child interaction. Do the parents label the child and body parts, such as "bad boy," "skinny legs," or "ugly scar"? Do the parents handle the child gently, using soothing touch to calm an anxious child, or do they treat the child roughly, using slaps or restraint to force compliance? If the child touches certain parts of the body, such as the genitals, do the parents make comments that suggest a negative connotation?

With older children, many of the communication strategies discussed earlier in the chapter are useful in eliciting more definitive information about their coping and self-concept. Children can write down five things they like and dislike about themselves. Sentence completion statements such as "The thing I like best (or worst) about myself is ____________," "If I could change one thing about myself, it would be ____________," or "When I am scared, I ____________," can be used.

Sexual History

The sexual history is an essential component of adolescents' health assessment. The history uncovers areas of concern related to sexual activity, alerts the nurse to circumstances that may indicate screening for sexually transmitted diseases or testing for pregnancy, and provides information related to the need for sexual counseling, such as safe sex practices.

One approach toward initiating a conversation about sexual concerns is to begin with a history of peer interactions. Open-ended statements such as "Tell me about your social life," or "Who are your closest friends?" generally lead into a discussion of dating and sexual issues. To probe further, include questions about the adolescent's attitudes on such topics as sex education, "going steady," "living together," and premarital sex. Phrase questions to reflect concern rather than judgment or criticism of sexual practices.

In any conversation regarding sexual history, be aware of the language that is used in either eliciting or conveying sexual information. For example, avoid asking if the adolescent is "sexually active," because this term is broadly defined. "Are you having sex with anyone?" is probably the most direct and best understood question. Because homosexual experimentation may occur, refer to all sexual contacts in nongender terms, such as "anyone" or "partners," rather than "girlfriends" or "boyfriends."

A detailed account of sexual partners is needed if the patient has a history of, displays any of the symptoms of, or asks for treatment of a sexually transmitted disease. A difficult but necessary part of the interview is to determine the sites of possible infection. Because sexual diseases can be contracted at any of the body orifices, inform the adolescent that a sexually transmitted disease can be acquired without visible signs of disease at nongenital sites.

FAMILY ASSESSMENT

Assessment of the family, both its structure and function, is an important component of the history-taking process. Because the quality of the functional relationship between the child and family members is a major factor in emotional and physical health, family assessment is discussed separately and in greater detail apart from the more traditional health history.

Family assessment is the collection of data about the composition of the family and the relationships among its members. In its broadest sense, *family* refers to all those individuals who are considered by the family member to be significant to the nuclear unit, including relatives, friends, and other social groups such as the school and church. Although family assessment is not family therapy, it can and frequently is therapeutic. Involving family members in discussing family characteristics and activities often stimulates productive discussion and insight into family dynamics and relationships.

Because of the time involved in performing an in-depth family assessment as presented here, be selective in deciding when knowledge of family function may facilitate nursing care. During brief contacts with families, a full assessment is not appropriate, and screening with one or two questions from each category may reflect the health of the family system or the potential need for additional assessment.

Assessment of Family Structure

Family structure refers to the composition of the family—who lives in the home and those social, cultural, religious, and economic characteristics that influence the child's and family's overall psychobiologic health (see also Chapters 31 and 32). Because the information elicited in this part of the history is often the most personal and confidential, include it toward the end of the interview when rapport is well established.

The most common method of eliciting information on the family structure is to interview family members. The principal areas of concern (Box 34-7) are (1) family composition, (2) home and community environment, (3) occupation and education of family members, and (4) cultural and religious traditions.

NURSE ALERT In assessing family composition, it is sometimes difficult to ascertain the status of the adult relationships. If the parent fails to mention the other parent, ask, "Where is the child's father (or mother)?" Avoid saying "husband" or "wife" because this assumes that only marital relationships exist. ■

Several structural assessment tools can be used to collect and record data about the family composition and environment. Like the interview method, such tools also provide information about relationships, although several additional methods should be used to assess family function.

A *sociogram* is a drawing of circles that indicates the significant persons in an individual's life; its use is appropriate for adults and children as young as 5 years of age. The person is given blank paper and a pencil with the following instructions: "Draw a circle to represent you. Around the circle draw circles to represent the most significant persons in your life and label each. Draw the circles in proximity to your circle to represent closeness. For example, the person who is most significant is the circle closest to you." Family members can label the relationships as supportive with a plus sign or negative with a minus sign.

Not only is the sociogram a portrait of the person's significant relationships, it may also uncover unresolved relationships (Fig. 34-4). After completing the sociogram, encourage the family to explore their feelings further with questions such as the following:

- How would you change the circles to improve relationships?
- How do you think you could accomplish these changes?
- If one person in the circle were to change, what effect do you think that would have on others in the circle?

BOX 34-7

Family Assessment Interview

General Guidelines for Family Interview

Schedule the interview with the family at a time that is most convenient for all parties; include as many family members as possible; clearly state the purpose of the interview.

Begin the interview by asking each person's name and their relationship to each other.

Restate the purpose of the interview and the objective.

Keep the initial conversation general to put members at ease and to learn the "big picture" of the family.

Identify major concerns and reflect these back to the family to be certain that all parties perceive the same message.

Terminate the interview with a summary of what was discussed and a plan for additional sessions if needed.

Structural Assessment Areas

Family Composition

Immediate members of the household (names, ages, and relationships)

Significant extended family members

Previous marriages, separations, death of spouses, or divorces

Home and Community Environment

Type of dwelling, number of rooms, occupants

Sleeping arrangements

Number of floors, accessibility of stairs, elevators

Adequacy of utilities

Safety features (fire escape, smoke and carbon monoxide detectors, guardrails on windows, use of car restraint)

Environmental hazards (e.g., chipped paint, poor sanitation, pollution, heavy street traffic)

Availability and location of health facilities, schools, play areas

Relationship with neighbors

Recent crises or changes in home

Child's reaction/adjustment to recent stresses

Occupation and Education of Family Members

Types of employment

Work schedules

Work satisfaction

Exposure to environmental/industrial hazards

Sources of income and adequacy

Effect of illness on financial status

Highest degree or grade level attained

Cultural and Religious Traditions

Religious beliefs and practices

Cultural/ethnic beliefs and practices

Language spoken in home

Assessment Questions

Does the family identify with a particular religious/ethnic group? Are both parents from that group?

How is religious/ethnic background part of family life?

What special religious/cultural traditions are practiced in the home (e.g., food choices and preparation)?

Where were family members born, and how long have they lived in this country?

What language does the family speak most frequently?

Do they speak/understand English?

What do they believe causes health or illness?

What religious/ethnic beliefs influence the family's perception of illness and its treatment?

What methods are used to prevent/treat illness?

How does the family know when a health problem needs medical attention?

Who is the person the family contacts when a member is ill?

Does the family rely on cultural/religious healers or remedies? If so, ask them to describe the type of healer or remedy.

Who does the family go to for support (clergy, medical healer, relatives)?

Does the family experience discrimination because of their race, beliefs, or practices? Ask them to describe.

Functional Assessment Areas

Family Interactions and Roles

Interactions refer to ways family members relate to each other.

Chief concern is amount of intimacy and closeness among the members, especially spouses.

Roles refer to behaviors of people as they assume a different status or position.

Observations

Family members' responses to each other (cordial, hostile, cool, loving, patient, short-tempered)

Obvious roles of leadership versus submission

Support and attention shown to various members

Assessment Questions

What activities do the family members perform together?

To whom do family members talk when something is bothering them?

What are members' household chores?

Who usually oversees what is happening with the children, such as at school or concerning their health?

How easy or difficult is it for the family to change or accept new responsibilities for household tasks?

Power, Decision Making, and Problem Solving

Power refers to individual member's control over others in family; manifested through family decision making and problem solving.

Chief concern is clarity of boundaries of power between parents and children.

One method of assessment involves offering a hypothetic conflict or problem, such as a child failing school, and asking family how they would handle this situation.

Assessment Questions

Who usually makes the decisions in the family?

If one parent makes a decision, can the child appeal to the other parent to change it?

What input do children have in making decisions or discussing rules?

Who makes and enforces the rules?

What happens when a rule is broken?

Communication

Communication is concerned with clarity and directness of communication patterns.

Further assessment includes periodically asking family members if they understood what was just said and to repeat the message.

Observations

Who speaks to whom

If one person speaks for another or interrupts

If members appear disinterested when certain individuals speak

If there is agreement between verbal and nonverbal messages

Continued

BOX 34-7

Family Assessment Interview—cont'd

Assessment Questions

How often do family members wait until others are through talking before "having their say?"

Do parents or older siblings tend to lecture and preach?

Do parents tend to talk "down" to the children?

Expression of Feelings and Individuality

Expressions are concerned with personal space and freedom to grow with limits and structure needed for guidance.

Observing patterns of communication offers clues to how freely feelings are expressed.

Assessment Questions

Is it OK for family members to get angry or sad?

Who gets angry most of the time? What do they do?

If someone is upset, how do other family members try to comfort this person?

Who comforts specific family members?

When someone wants to do something, such as try out for a new sport or get a job, what is the family's response (offer assistance, discouragement, or no advice)?

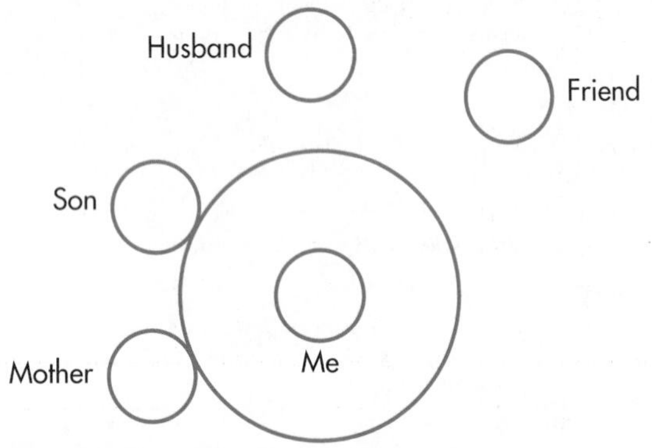

Fig. 34-4 Sociogram of mother with strong, unresolved grief feelings regarding loss of child.

Assessment of Family Function

Family function is concerned with how the family members behave toward one another and with the quality of the relationships (see also Chapter 31). It is considered the most important component in determining "family health." Assessment of function requires more skill on the part of the interviewer than does assessment of structure and is best approached after structure is assessed. As in assessment of family structure, the more traditional method of eliciting information on family function is by interviewing family members. The principal areas of concern are discussed in Box 34-7.

In addition to observing and interviewing the family to assess family function, several other methods are available and should be used as needed to obtain a comprehensive assessment. The following section discusses selected instruments that are reliable and valid but require little or no formal training and minimal time to administer.

The *Family APGAR* is a brief screening questionnaire designed to reflect a family member's satisfaction with the functional state of the family (Smilkstein, Ashworth, & Montano, 1982) (see Appendix B). The acronym APGAR is for *A*daptation, *P*artnership, *G*rowth, *A*ffection, and *R*esolve (commitment). The acronym was chosen because it is familiar to health professionals, but it bears no relationship to the Apgar scoring system for newborns.

The questions in Box 34-8 can be used in the interview without the Family APGAR ratings to elicit similar types of information. It can be completed in about 5 minutes, can be used by families with traditional and alternative lifestyles and from different cultures, and is appropriate for children 10 years of age or older. Separate forms have been designed to assess relationships with friends and fellow workers, because these groups represent other significant sources of support.

The responses to the five questions are scored as follows: "Almost always"—2; "Some of the time"—1; and "Hardly ever"—0. Each score is totaled. Scores of 7 to 10 suggest a highly functional family; 4 to 6, a moderately dysfunctional family; and 0 to 3, a severely dysfunctional family. Also, a low score in any single item could signal family dysfunction. The Family APGAR is not recommended for use with individuals from enmeshed (overly close) or "psychosomatic" families. Persons with health problems, such as asthma, atopic dermatitis, or irritable bowel syndrome, may report falsely high scores (Smilkstein, 1993).

The *Feetham Family Functioning Survey* provides information about family members' *perception* of relationships that contribute to or are affected by family functioning* (Feetham, Perkins, & Carroll, 1993). Although recommended primarily as a research instrument, it can be used clinically without scoring the items to identify areas that may be of concern to the family. The survey consists of 25 ratings of family functioning (household tasks; child care; sexual and marital relationships; interaction with family, children, and friends; community involvement; and sources of emotional support) and two open-ended questions. Each of the questions on family functioning is rated on three 7-point scales of "How much is there now?" "How much should there be?" and "How important is this to me?" Discrepancy between the first two ratings, together with the rating of importance, contributes to an assessment of the members' perceptions of family functioning. The survey takes less than 10 minutes to complete and can be used with single-parent and two-parent families (Feetham et al, 1993).

*The survey is available for a fee from Nursing Systems and Research, Children's National Medical Center, 111 Michigan Ave. NW, Washington, DC 20010; phone: 202-939-4980.

BOX 34-8

Family APGAR

Definition

Adaptation is the use of intrafamilial and extrafamilial resources for problem solving when family equilibrium is stressed during a crisis.

Partnership is the sharing of decision-making and nurturing responsibilities by family members.

Growth is the physical and emotional maturation and self-fulfillment that is achieved by family members through mutual support and guidance.

Affection is the caring or loving relationship that exists among family members.

Resolve is the commitment to devote time to other members of the family for physical and emotional nurturing. It also usually involves a decision to share wealth and space.

Functions Measured by the Family APGAR

How resources are shared, or the degree to which a member is satisfied with the assistance received when family resources are needed

How decisions are shared, or the member's satisfaction with mutuality in family communication and problem solving

How nurturing is shared, or the member's satisfaction with the freedom available within the family to change roles and attain physical and emotional growth or maturation

How emotional experiences are shared, or the member's satisfaction with the intimacy and emotional interaction that exists in the family

How time (and space and money) is shared, or the member's satisfaction with the time commitment that has been made to the family by its members

Relevant Open-Ended Questions

How have family members aided each other in time of need?

In what way have family members received help or assistance from friends and community agencies?

How do family members communicate with each other about such matters as vacations, finances, medical care, large purchases, and personal problems?

How have family members changed during the past years?

How has this change been accepted by family members?

In what ways have family members aided each other in growing or developing independent lifestyles?

How have family members reacted to your desire for change?

How have members of your family responded to emotional expressions, such as affection, love, sorrow, or anger?

How do members of your family share time, space, and money?

Modified from Smilkstein G: The Family APGAR: a proposal for a family function test and its use by physicians, *J Fam Pract* 6(6):1231-1239, 1978.

Undoubtedly the richest environment for observing a child's development and interactions with family members is the home. Two tools that can be used to assess the child's home environment are the *Home Observation for Management of the Environment (HOME) Inventory** (Caldwell & Bradley, 1984) and the *Home Screening Questionnaire (HSQ)** (Frankenburg & Coons, 1986). Both are divided into two age groups: birth to 3 years of age and 3 to 6 years of age. HOME has an additional inventory for children ages 6 to 10 years. Forms are also available for children with moderate to severe disabilities in each of the three age groups for visual, auditory, orthopedic, and cognitive impairments.

Some of the HOME items require direct observation, whereas others necessitate questioning of the parents. Each item receives a "yes" or "no" response. The number of "yes" responses correlates with the amount of appropriate environmental stimulation. Any "no" responses indicate possible areas for intervention and counseling. Use of HOME requires about a 1-hour home visit with both the child and the major caregiver.

The HSQ was developed using HOME as a guide. The 0- to 3-year form consists of 30 items plus a checklist of toys available to the child in the home. The 3- to 6-year form has 34 items and a similar toy checklist. The questions are written at approximately a third- to sixth-grade reading level and, unlike the HOME, can be completed by the parents in any setting in about 15 to 20 minutes. Scoring directions are detailed in the manual and are based on credits for different answers. For each age group there is a minimum score for determining suspect or nonsuspect results.

NUTRITIONAL ASSESSMENT

Dietary Intake

Knowledge of the child's dietary intake is a useful and practical component of a nutritional assessment. However, it is also one of the most difficult factors to assess. Individuals' recall of food consumption, especially amounts eaten, is frequently unreliable. In addition, people may be hesitant to reveal their eating patterns if they sense criticism from the nurse. People from different cultures may have difficulty adequately describing the types of food they eat. Despite these obstacles, a food intake record is essential. Several methods are available.

Regardless of the format used in recording food intake, every nutritional assessment should begin with a *dietary history.* The exact questions used to elicit a dietary history vary with the child's age. In general, the younger the child, the more specific and detailed the history should be. Box 34-9 provides a sample dietary history for children and includes additional questions regarding infant feeding.

The broad overview elicited from the dietary history can be helpful in evaluating food frequency records. It also is concerned with financial and cultural factors that influence food selection and preparation (Cultural Awareness box).

The most common and probably easiest method of assessing daily intake is the *24-hour recall.* The child or parent recalls every item eaten in the past 24 hours and the approximate amounts. The 24-hour recall is most beneficial when it represents a typical day's intake. Some of the difficulties with

*The forms and an administration manual are available for a fee from the Center for Research on Teaching and Learning, College of Education, University of Arkansas at Little Rock, 2801 S. University Ave., Little Rock, AK 72204; phone: 501-569-3422.

*The forms and manual are available for a fee from Denver Developmental Materials, Inc., PO Box 371075, Denver, CO 80237-5075; phone: 303-355-4729 or 800-419-4729.

BOX 34-9

Dietary History

What are the family's usual mealtimes?
Do family members eat together or at separate times?
Who does the family grocery shopping and meal preparation?
How much money is spent to buy food each week?
How are most foods prepared—baked, broiled, fried, other?
How often does the family or your child eat out?
 What kinds of restaurants do you go to?
 What kinds of food does your child typically eat at restaurants?
Does your child eat breakfast regularly?
Where does your child eat lunch?
What are your child's favorite foods, beverages, and snacks?
 What are the average amounts eaten per day?
 What foods are artificially sweetened?
 What are your child's snacking habits?
 When are sweet foods usually eaten?
 What are your child's toothbrushing habits?
What special cultural practices are followed? What ethnic foods are eaten?
What foods and beverages does your child dislike?
How would you describe your child's usual appetite (hearty eater, picky eater)?
What are your child's feeding habits (breast, bottle, cup, spoon, eats by self, needs assistance, any special devices)?
Does your child take vitamins or other supplements? Do they contain iron or fluoride?
Are there any known or suspected food allergies? Is your child on a special diet?
Has your child lost or gained weight recently?
Are there any feeding problems (excessive fussiness, spitting up, colic, difficulty sucking or swallowing)? Are there any dental problems or appliances, such as braces, that affect eating?
What types of exercise does your child do regularly?
Is there a family history of cancer, diabetes, heart disease, high blood pressure, or obesity?

Additional Questions for Infants

What was the infant's birth weight? When did it double? Triple?
Was the infant premature?
Are you breastfeeding or have you breastfed your infant? For how long?
If you use a formula, what is the brand?
 How long has the infant been taking it?
 How many ounces does the infant drink a day?
Are you giving the infant cow's milk (whole, low fat, skim)?
 When did you start?
 How many ounces does the infant drink a day?
Do you give your infant extra fluids (water, juice)?
If the infant takes a bottle to bed at nap or nighttime, what is in the bottle?
At what age did you start cereal, vegetables, meat or other protein sources, fruit, fruit juice, finger food, table food?
Do you make your own baby food or use commercial foods, such as infant cereal?
Does the infant take a vitamin/mineral supplement? If so, what type?
Has the infant shown an allergic reaction to any food(s)? If so, list the foods and describe the reaction.
Does the infant spit up frequently, have unusually loose stools, or have hard, dry stools? If so, how often?
How often do you feed your infant?
How would you describe your infant's appetite?

Cultural Awareness

FOOD PRACTICES

Because cultural practices are very prevalent in food preparation, consider carefully the kinds of questions that are asked and the judgments made in regard to counseling. For example, some cultures, such as Hispanic, black, and Native American, include many vegetables, legumes, and starches in their diet that together provide sufficient essential amino acids, even though the actual amount of meat or dairy protein is low. (See Chapter 32 for cultural food practices.)

a daily recall are the family's inability to remember exactly what was eaten and inaccurate estimation of portion size. To increase accuracy of reporting portion sizes, the use of food models and additional questioning are recommended. In general, this method is most useful in providing *qualitative* information about the child's diet.

To improve the reliability of the daily recall, the family can complete a *food diary* by recording every food and liquid consumed for a certain number of days. A 3-day record consisting of 2 weekdays and 1 weekend day is representative for most people. Providing specific charts to record intake can improve compliance. The family should record items immediately after eating.

A *food frequency questionnaire* or *record* (Box 34-10) provides information about the number of times in a day, week, or month a child consumes items from the different food groups. In general, it provides a qualitative overview but has the advantage of avoiding recall based on a "typical" day. It can be especially useful when verifying a food history or diary.

Clinical Examination

A significant amount of information regarding nutritional deficiencies is elicited from a clinical examination, especially from assessing the skin, hair, teeth, gums, lips, tongue, and eyes. Hair, skin, and mouth are vulnerable because of the rapid turnover of epithelial and mucosal tissue. Table 34-1 summarizes clinical signs of possible nutritional deficiency or excess. Few are diagnostic for a specific nutrient, and if suspicious signs are found, they must be confirmed with dietary and biochemical data. Generally, the clinical examination does not reveal children *at risk* for a deficiency or excess.

Anthropometry, an essential parameter of nutritional status, is the measurement of height, weight, head circumference, proportions, skinfold thickness, and arm circumference in young children. Height and head circumference reflect past nutrition, whereas weight, skinfold thickness, and arm circumference reflect present nutritional status, especially of protein and fat reserves. Skinfold thickness is a measurement of the body's fat content because approximately one half of the body's total fat stores are directly beneath the skin. The upper arm muscle circumference is correlated with measurements of total muscle mass. Because muscle serves as the body's major protein reserve, this measurement is considered an index of the body's protein stores. Ideally, growth measurements are recorded over a period of time, and comparisons are made regarding the *velocity* of growth based on previous and present values. Techniques for anthropometric measurement are discussed in Chapter 35.

BOX 34-10

Food Frequency Record*

FOOD GROUP	NUMBER OF SERVINGS (DAY, WEEK)	SERVING SIZE (IN CUP, TABLESPOON, OR OUNCE PORTIONS)
Breads/Cereals/Rice/Pasta		
Bread, tortilla		
Cooked pasta, rice, hot cereal		
Dry cereal (not pre-sweetened)		
Crackers		
Muffins		
Other		
Vegetables		
Yellow or orange		
Green/leafy		
Other		
Fruits/Fruit Juices		
Citrus (orange, grapefruit, strawberries, lemon, lime, tangerine)		
Noncitrus		
Other		
Milk/Cheese/Yogurt		
Milk		
Cheese		
Yogurt		
Pudding		
Ice cream		
Other		
Other Protein Foods		
Meat		
Fish		
Poultry		
Egg		
Peanut butter		
Legumes (dried beans, peas, soy beans)		
Nuts		
Other		
Fats/Oils/Sweets		
Butter, oil, margarine, mayonnaise, salad dressing		
Soda, punch		
Cake/cookie, etc.		
Candy		
Presweetened cereal		

*For comparison of actual intake with recommended intake, see Food Guide Pyramid, Fig. 47-1.

Numerous *biochemical tests* are available for assessing nutritional status and include analysis of plasma, blood cells, urine, or tissues from liver, bone, hair, and fingernails. Many of these tests are complicated and are not performed routinely. Common laboratory procedures for nutritional status include measurement of hemoglobin, hematocrit, transferrin, albumin, creatinine, and nitrogen. Laboratory values for these tests and more specific nutrient measurements are given in Appendix I.

Evaluation of Nutritional Assessment

After collecting the data needed for a thorough nutritional assessment, evaluate the findings to plan appropriate counseling. From the data, assess if the child is (1) malnourished, (2) at risk for becoming malnourished, or (3) well nourished with adequate reserves.

Analyze the daily food diary for the variety and amounts of foods suggested in the Food Guide Pyramid (see Fig. 47-1). For example, if the list includes no vegetables, inquire about this rather than assuming that the child dislikes vegetables, because it could be that none were served on that day. Also, evaluate the information in terms of the family's ethnic practices and financial resources. Encouraging increased protein intake with additional meat may be unfeasible for families on a limited budget or may be in conflict with food practices that use meat sparingly, such as in Asian meal preparation.

Compare findings from clinical examination and anthropometry with the data obtained from the dietary intake. For example, signs of anemia and a dietary record of iron-poor foods suggest laboratory analysis of hemoglobin, hematocrit, and transferrin. Refer any suspicious findings for further evaluation.

Key Points

- Communication, the most important skill nurses must possess in the care of children, has verbal, nonverbal, and abstract components.
- To effectively establish a setting for communication, nurses must make an appropriate introduction, clarify their role and the purpose of the interview, and ensure privacy and confidentiality.
- When communicating with parents, nurses need to encourage parental involvement, listen carefully, use silence, and be empathic.
- Communication with children must reflect their developmental stage.
- Verbal communication techniques that have proved to be effective include the third-person technique, facilitative responding, storytelling, bibliotherapy, the use of "what if" questions, and other word games.
- The objectives of performing a health history are to identify pertinent information, determine the chief complaint, analyze the present illness, secure the past history, review biologic systems, and record a family medical history and child psychosocial and sexual history.
- Family assessment is the collection of data about family composition and relationships among its members; it also focuses on home and community environment, occupation and education, and cultural and religious traditions.
- The family function interview examines interaction and roles, power, decision making, problem solving, communication, and expression of feelings and individuality.
- Nutritional assessment is performed by determining dietary intake, clinical examination, and biochemical analysis.

Table 34-1

Clinical Assessment of Nutritional Status

EVIDENCE OF ADEQUATE NUTRITION	EVIDENCE OF DEFICIENT OR EXCESS NUTRITION	DEFICIENCY/EXCESS*
GENERAL GROWTH		
Within 5th and 95th percentiles for height, weight, and head circumference	Below 5th or above 95th percentiles for growth	Protein, calories, fats, and other essential nutrients, especially vitamin A, pyridoxine, niacin, calcium, iodine, manganese, zinc
Steady gain with expected growth spurts during infancy and adolescence	Absence of or delayed growth spurts; poor weight gain	
Sexual development appropriate for age	Delayed sexual development	Excess vitamin A, vitamin D
SKIN		
Smooth, slightly dry to touch	Hardening and scaling	Vitamin A
Elastic and firm	Seborrheic dermatitis	Excess niacin
Absence of lesions	Dry, rough, petechiae	Riboflavin
Color appropriate to genetic background	Delayed wound healing	Vitamin C
	Scaly dermatitis on exposed surfaces	Riboflavin, vitamin C, zinc Niacin
	Wrinkled, flabby	Protein, calories, zinc
	Crusted lesions around orifices, especially nares	
	Pruritus	Excess vitamin A, riboflavin, niacin
	Poor turgor	Water, sodium
	Edema	Protein, thiamine Excess sodium
	Yellow tinge (jaundice)	Vitamin B_{12} Excess vitamin A, niacin
	Depigmentation	Protein, calories
	Pallor (anemia)	Pyridoxine, folic acid, vitamin B_{12}, vitamin C, vitamin E (in premature infants), iron Excess vitamin C, zinc
	Paresthesia	Excess riboflavin
HAIR		
Lustrous, silky, strong, elastic	Stringy, friable, dull, dry, thin	Protein, calories
	Alopecia	Protein, calories, zinc
	Depigmentation	Protein, calories, copper
	Raised areas around hair follicles	Vitamin C
HEAD		
Even molding, occipital prominence, symmetric facial features	Softening of cranial bones, prominence of frontal bones, skull flat and depressed toward middle	Vitamin D
Fused sutures after 18 months	Delayed fusion of sutures	Vitamin D
	Hard tender lumps in occiput	Excess vitamin A
	Headache	Excess thiamine
NECK		
Thyroid not visible, palpable in midline	Thyroid enlarged; may be grossly visible	Iodine
EYES		
Clear, bright	Hardening and scaling of cornea and conjunctiva	Vitamin A
Good night vision		
Conjunctiva—Pink, glossy	Night blindness	
	Burning, itching, photophobia, cataracts, corneal vascularization	Riboflavin
EARS		
Tympanic membrane—Pliable	Calcified (hearing loss)	Excess vitamin D

*Nutrients listed are deficient unless specified as excess.

Table 34-1

Clinical Assessment of Nutritional Status

EVIDENCE OF ADEQUATE NUTRITION	EVIDENCE OF DEFICIENT OR EXCESS NUTRITION	DEFICIENCY/EXCESS*
NOSE		
Smooth, intact nasal angle	Irritation and cracks at nasal angle	Riboflavin Excess vitamin A
MOUTH		
Lips—Smooth, moist, darker color than skin	Fissures and inflammation at corners	Riboflavin Excess vitamin A
Gums—Firm, coral pink color, stippled	Spongy, friable, swollen, bluish red or black color, bleed easily	Vitamin C
Mucous membranes—Bright pink, smooth, moist	Stomatitis	Niacin
Tongue—Rough texture, no lesions, taste sensation	Glossitis Diminished taste sensation	Niacin, riboflavin, folic acid Zinc
Teeth—Uniform white color, smooth, intact	Brown mottling, pits, fissures Defective enamel Caries	Excess fluoride Vitamin A, vitamin C, vitamin D, calcium, phosphorus Excess carbohydrates
CHEST		
In infants, shape is almost circular In children, lateral diameter increases in proportion to anteroposterior diameter	Depressed lower portion of rib cage Sharp protrusion of sternum	Vitamin D
Smooth costochondral junctions	Enlarged costochondral junctions	Vitamin C, vitamin D
Breast development—Normal for age	Delayed development	See under General Growth; especially zinc
CARDIOVASCULAR SYSTEM		
Pulse and blood pressure (BP) within normal limits	Palpitations Rapid pulse Arrhythmias Increased BP Decreased BP	Thiamine Potassium Excess thiamine Magnesium, potassium Excess niacin, potassium Excess sodium Thiamine; excess niacin
ABDOMEN		
In young children, cylindric and prominent Older children, flat Normal bowel habits	Distended, flabby, poor musculature Prominent, large Potbelly, constipation Diarrhea Constipation	Protein, calories Excess calories Vitamin D Niacin Excess vitamin C Excess calcium, potassium
MUSCULOSKELETAL SYSTEM		
Muscles—Firm, well developed, equal strength bilaterally	Flabby, weak, generalized wasting Weakness, pain, cramps Muscle twitching, tremors Muscular paralysis	Protein, calories Thiamine, sodium, chloride, potassium, phosphorus, magnesium Excess thiamine Magnesium Excess potassium
Spine—Cervical and lumbar curves (double S curve)	Kyphosis, lordosis, scoliosis	Vitamin D
Extremities—Symmetric; legs straight with minimum bowing	Bowing of extremities, knock-knees Epiphyseal enlargement Bleeding into joints and muscles, joint swelling, pain	Vitamin D, calcium, phosphorus Vitamin A, vitamin D Vitamin C

Continued

Table 34-1

Clinical Assessment of Nutritional Status—cont'd

EVIDENCE OF ADEQUATE NUTRITION	EVIDENCE OF DEFICIENT OR EXCESS NUTRITION	DEFICIENCY/EXCESS*
MUSCULOSKELETAL SYSTEM—CONT'D		
Joints—Flexible, full range of motion, no pain or stiffness	Thickening of cortex of long bones with pain and fragility, hard tender lumps in extremities	Excess vitamin A
	Osteoporosis of long bones	Calcium; excess vitamin D
NEUROLOGIC SYSTEM		
Behavior—Alert, responsive, emotionally stable	Listless, irritable, lethargic, apathetic (sometimes apprehensive, anxious, drowsy, mentally slow, confused)	Thiamine, niacin, pyridoxine, vitamin C, potassium, magnesium, iron, protein, calories Excess vitamin A, vitamin D, thiamine, folic acid, calcium
Absence of tetany, convulsions	Masklike facial expression, blurred speech, involuntary laughing	Excess manganese
		Thiamine, pyridoxine, vitamin D, calcium, magnesium
	Convulsions	Excess phosphorus (in relation to calcium)
Intact peripheral nervous system	Peripheral nervous system toxicity (unsteady gait, numb feet and hands, fine motor clumsiness)	Excess pyridoxine
Intact reflexes	Diminished or absent tendon reflexes	Thiamine, vitamin E

*Nutrients listed are deficient unless specified as excess.

References

Bradley RH et al: A reexamination of the association between HOME scores and income, *Nurs Res* 43(5):260-266, 1994.

Caldwell B, Bradley R: *Home observation for measurement of the environment,* rev ed, Little Rock, 1984, University of Arkansas.

Campbell-Heider N, Hart CA: Updating the nurse's bedside manner, *Image J Nurse Sch* 25(2):133-139, 1993.

Cantrill JA, Cottrell WN: Accuracy of drug allergy documentation, *Am J Health Syst Pharm* 54:1627-1629, 1997.

Deadrick D, Boggess P: *Pediatrics on telephone line.* Paper presented at the First Annual National Conference for Advanced Practice Nurses, Rutgers University, Nov 6-8, 1996.

Desselle DD, Pearlmutter L: Navigating two cultures: deaf children, self-esteem, and parents' communication patterns, *Soc Work Educ* 19(1): 23-30, 1997.

Feetham S, Perkins M, Carroll R: Exploratory analysis: a technique for analysis of dyadic data in research of families. In Feetham S et al (eds): *The nursing of families: theory/research/education/practice,* Newbury Park, CA, 1993, Sage.

Frankenburg W, Coons C: Home Screening Questionnaire: its validity in assessing home environment, *J Pediatr* 108(4):624-626, 1986.

Hoge DR, Parette HP: Facilitating communicative development in young children with disabilities, *Transdisciplinary J* 5(2):113-130, 1995.

McBurney BH, Schultz C: Defining quality services in a general pediatric unit, *J Nurs Care Qual* 7(3):51-60, 1993.

Price V, Archbold J: What's it all about, empathy? *Nurs Educ Today* 17(2):106-110, 1997.

Reynolds WH, Scott B, Jessiman WC: Empathy has not been measured in clients' terms or effectively taught: a review of the literature, *J Adv Nurs* 30(5):1117-1185, 1999.

Rutenberg CD: Telephone triage, *Am J Nurs* 100(3):77-78, 80-81, 2000.

Seidel HM et al: *Mosby's guide to physical examination,* ed 5, St Louis, 2003, Mosby.

Smilkstein G: Family APGAR analyzed, *Fam Med* 25(5):293-294, 1993 (letter).

Smilkstein G, Ashworth C, Montano D: Validity and reliability of the Family APGAR as a test of family function, *J Fam Pract* 15(2):303-311, 1982.

Spinetta J et al: The kinetic family drawing in childhood cancer. In Spinetta J, Deasy-Spinetta P (eds): *Living with childhood cancer,* St Louis, 1981, Mosby.

Sullivan GH: Protecting patient's privacy, *RN* 60(6):55-56, 58-59, 1997.

Thompson JM, Wilson SF: *Health assessment for nursing practice,* St Louis, 1996, Mosby.

White SJ: Empathy: a literature review and concept analysis, *J Clin Nurs* 6(4):253-257, 1997.

Wissow LS, Roter DL, Wilson MEH: Pediatrician interview style and mother's disclosure of psychosocial issues, *Pediatrics* 93(2):289-295, 1994.

Yegdich T: On the phenomenology of empathy in nursing: empathy or sympathy? *J Adv Nurs* 30(1):83-93, 1999.

Physical and Developmental Assessment of the Child

35

LEARNING OBJECTIVES

On completion of this chapter the reader will be able to:

- Prepare a child for a physical examination based on his or her developmental needs.
- Perform a comprehensive physical examination in a sequence appropriate to the child's age.
- Recognize expected normal findings for children at various ages.
- Record the physical examination according to the head-to-toe format.
- Perform a developmental assessment using a standard screening test.

ELECTRONIC RESOURCES

Additional information related to the content in Chapter 35 can be found on

the companion website at evolve
http://evolve.elsevier.com/Wong/maternal/

- NCLEX Review Questions
- WebLinks

or the interactive student CD-ROM
Activities for Chapter 35 include the following:

- NCLEX Review Questions
- Anatomy Review—Superficial Lymph Nodes
- Anatomy Review—Location of Sinuses
- Anatomy Review—Structures in the Neck
- Anatomy Review—Structures of the Eye
- Anatomy Review—Landmarks of the Pinna
- Anatomy Review—External and Internal Structures of the Nose
- Anatomy Review—Interior Structures of the Mouth
- Anatomy Review—Rib Cage
- Anatomy Review—Imaginary Landmarks of the Chest
- Anatomy Review—Percussion Sounds in Thorax
- Anatomy Review—Location of Pulses
- Anatomy Review—Direction of Heart Sounds
- Anatomy Review—Location of Hernias
- Case Study—Pediatric Assessment
- Critical Thinking Exercise—Cardiovascular Assessment
- Skill—Measuring Physical Growth

GENERAL APPROACHES TOWARD EXAMINING THE CHILD

Sequence of the Examination

Ordinarily, the sequence for examining patients follows a head-to-toe direction. The main function of such a systematic approach is to provide a general guideline for assessment of each body area to minimize omitting segments of the examination. The standard recording of data also facilitates exchange of information among different professionals. The typical organization of a physical examination is indicated in the chapter outline. In examining children, this orderly sequence is frequently altered to accommodate the child's developmental needs, although the examination is recorded following the head-to-toe model. Using developmental and chronologic age as the main criteria for assessing each body system accomplishes several goals:

- Minimizes stress and anxiety associated with assessment of various body parts
- Fosters a trusting nurse-child-parent relationship
- Allows for maximum preparation of the child
- Preserves the essential security of the parent-child relationship, especially with young children
- Maximizes the accuracy and reliability of assessment findings

Preparation of the Child

Although the physical examination consists of painless procedures, to a child the use of a tight arm cuff, probes in the ears and mouth, pressing on the abdomen, and listening to the chest with a cold piece of metal can be considerably stressful. General guidelines related to the examining process are presented in Box 35-1. The physical examination should be as pleasant as possible, as well as educational. For example, the nurse can use a detailed drawing or an anatomically correct doll to help preschoolers and older children learn about their bodies (Vessey, 1995). The paper-doll technique is a useful approach to teaching children about the part of the body that is being examined (Fig. 35-1). At the conclu-

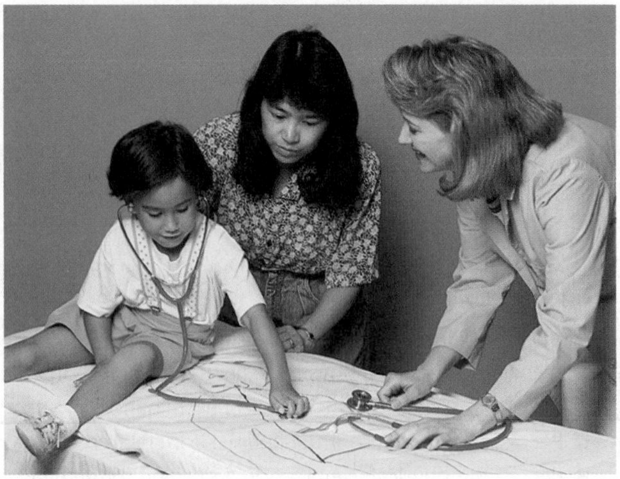

Fig. 35-1 Using paper-doll technique to prepare child.

BOX 35-1

General Guidelines for Performing Pediatric Physical Examination

- Perform examination in appropriate, nonthreatening area.
  - Have room well lit and decorated with neutral colors.
  - Have room temperature comfortably warm.
  - Place all strange and potentially frightening equipment out of sight.
  - Have some toys, dolls, stuffed animals, and games available for child.
  - If possible, have rooms decorated and equipped for different-age children.
  - Provide privacy, especially for school-age children and adolescents.
- Provide time for play and becoming acquainted.
- Observe behaviors that signal child's readiness to cooperate:
  - Talking to the nurse
  - Making eye contact
  - Accepting the offered equipment
  - Allowing physical touching
  - Choosing to sit on examining table rather than parent's lap
- If signs of readiness are not observed, use the following techniques:
  - Talk to parent while essentially "ignoring" child; gradually focus on child or a favorite object, such as a doll.
  - Make complimentary remarks about child, such as appearance, dress, or a favorite object.
  - Tell a funny story or play a simple magic trick.
  - Have a nonthreatening "friend" available, such as a hand puppet to "talk" to child for the nurse (see Fig. 35-22, *A*).
- If child refuses to cooperate, use the following techniques:
  - Assess reason for uncooperative behavior; consider that a child who is unduly afraid may have had a previous traumatic experience.
  - Try to involve child and parent in process.
  - Avoid prolonged explanations about examining procedure.
  - Use a firm, direct approach regarding expected behavior.
  - Perform examination as quickly as possible.
  - Have attendant gently restrain child.
  - Minimize any disruptions or stimulation.
  - Limit number of people in room.
  - Use isolated room.
  - Use quiet, calm, confident voice.
- Begin examination in a nonthreatening manner for young children or children who are fearful:
  - Use activities that can be presented as games, such as test for cranial nerves (see Table 35-11) or parts of developmental screening tests (p. 1023).
  - Use approaches such as Simon Says to encourage child to make a face, squeeze a hand, stand on one foot, and so on.
  - Use paper-doll technique.
  - Lay child supine on an examining table or floor that is covered with a large sheet of paper.
  - Trace around child's body outline.
  - Use body outline to demonstrate what will be examined, such as drawing a heart and listening with stethoscope before performing activity on child.
- If several children in the family will be examined, begin with most cooperative child to provide modeling of desired behavior.
- Involve child in examination process:
  - Provide choices, such as sitting on table or in parent's lap.
  - Allow child to handle or hold equipment.
  - Encourage child to use equipment on a doll, a family member, or the examiner.
  - Explain each step of the procedure in simple language.
- Examine child in a comfortable and secure position:
  - Sitting in parent's lap
  - Sitting upright if in respiratory distress
- Proceed to examine the body in an organized sequence (usually head to toe) with the following exceptions:
  - Alter sequence to accommodate needs of different-age children (see Table 35-1).
  - Examine painful areas last.
  - In emergency situation, examine vital functions (airway, breathing, and circulation) and injured area first.
- Reassure child throughout examination, especially about bodily concerns that arise during puberty.
- Discuss findings with family at end of examination.
- Praise child for cooperation during examination; give reward such as a small toy or sticker.

sion of the visit, the child can bring home the paper doll as a memento of the experience.

In most instances children cooperate best when their parents remain with them. There are occasions, however, when older children, particularly adolescents, prefer to be examined alone, such as during the genital examination. Frequently, the child being examined is also accompanied by a sibling, who may be disruptive because of boredom. It is a helpful tactic to involve the sibling in the examination by allowing the child to hold the stethoscope or a tongue blade and praising the child for the "help" during the assessment.

Table 35-1 summarizes guidelines for positioning, preparing, and examining children at various ages. Because no child fits precisely into one age category, it may be necessary to vary the approach after a preliminary assessment of the child's developmental achievements and needs. Even when the best approach is used, many toddlers are uncooperative and unable to be consoled for much of the physical examination. However, some seem intrigued by the new surroundings and unusual equipment and respond more like preschoolers than toddlers. Likewise, some early preschoolers may require more of the "security measures" employed with younger children, such as continued parent-child contact, and less of the preparatory measures used with preschoolers, such as playing with the equipment before and during the actual examination (Fig. 35-2).

Although the variations in the general approaches are numerous, some of them are elaborated on here because they are more common. For example, the suggested sequence may change considerably when the child is in pain or when obvious physical defects are present. In either situation, examine the affected area last to minimize distress early in the examination and to focus on normal, healthy, or functioning body parts.

Positioning may also be altered because of physical distress. For example, the child who is having difficulty breathing may not be able to lie down; in this situation, perform as much of the physical examination as possible with the child in a sitting or slightly reclining position, or complete the examination at another time.

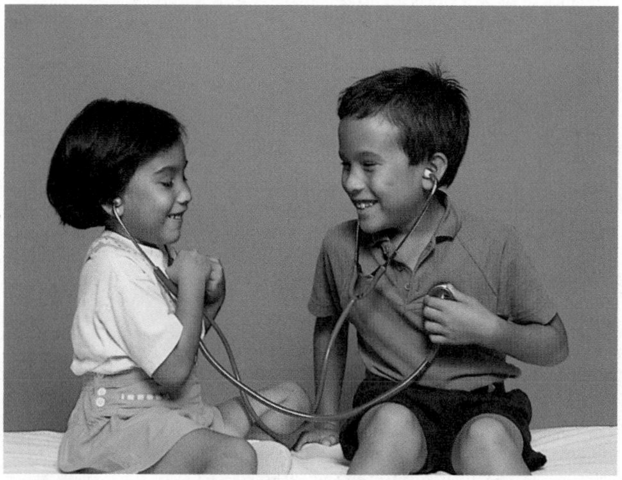

Fig. 35-2 Preparing children for physical examination.

PHYSICAL EXAMINATION

Although the approach to and sequence of the physical examination differ according to the child's age, the following discussion outlines the traditional model for physical assessment. Although the focus includes all pediatric age groups, the reader is referred to Chapter 36 for a detailed discussion of a newborn assessment. Because the physical examination is a vital part of preventive pediatric care, a schedule for periodic health visits is given in Box 35-2.

Growth Measurements

Measurement of physical growth in children is a key element in evaluating their health status. Physical growth parameters include weight, height (length), skinfold thickness, arm circumference, and head circumference. Values for these growth parameters are plotted on percentile charts, and the child's measurements in percentiles are compared with those of the general population.

Growth Charts

The most commonly used growth charts in the United States are from the National Center for Health Statistics (NCHS). The growth charts have been revised to include the body mass index–for–age (BMI-for-age) charts, 3rd and 97th smoothed percentiles for all charts, and the 85th percentile for the weight-for-stature and BMI-for-age charts (see Appendix E). The data were collected from five national surveys between 1963 and 1994. The revised charts have eliminated the disjunctions between the curves for infants and other children and have been extended for children and adolescents to 20 years (NCHS, 2000).

The weight-for-age percentile distributions are now continuous between the infant and the older child charts at 24 to 36 months. The length-for-age to stature-for-age and weight-for-length to weight-for-stature curves are parallel in the overlapping ages of 24 to 36 months. The revised weight-for-stature charts provide a smoother transition from the weight-for-length charts for preschool-age children.

The most prominent change to the complement of growth charts for older children and adolescents is the addition of the BMI-for-age growth curves. The BMI-for-age charts were developed with national survey data (1963–1994), excluding data from the 1988–1994 National Health and Nutrition Examination Survey III (NHANES III) for children older than 6 years because an increase in body weight and BMI occurred between NHANES III and previous national surveys. Without this exclusion, the 85th and 95th percentile curves would have been higher, and fewer children and adolescents would have been classified as at risk or overweight. Therefore the BMI-for-age growth curves do not represent the current population of children older than 6 years of age.

NURSE ALERT The sex-specific BMI-for-age charts for ages 2 to 20 years replace the 1977 NCHS weight-for-stature charts that were limited to prepubescent boys younger than 11.5 years of age and statures less than 145 cm, and to prepubescent girls younger than 19 years of age and statures less than 137 cm. ■

Table 35-1

Age-Specific Approaches to Physical Examination During Childhood

POSITION	SEQUENCE	PREPARATION
INFANT		
Before sits alone: supine or prone, preferably in parent's lap; before 4 to 6 months: can place on examining table After sits alone: use sitting in parent's lap whenever possible If on table, place with parent in full view	If quiet, auscultate heart, lungs, abdomen Record heart and respiratory rates Palpate and percuss same areas Proceed in usual head-to-toe direction Perform traumatic procedures last (eyes, ears, mouth [while crying]) Elicit reflexes as body part is examined Elicit Moro reflex last	Completely undress if room temperature permits Leave diaper on male infant Gain cooperation with distraction, bright objects, rattles, talking Smile at infant; use soft, gentle voice Pacify with bottle of sugar water or feeding Enlist parent's aid for restraining to examine ears, mouth Avoid abrupt, jerky movements
TODDLER		
Sitting or standing on or by parent Prone or supine in parent's lap	Inspect body area through play: "count fingers," "tickle toes" Use minimal physical contact initially Introduce equipment slowly Auscultate, percuss, palpate whenever quiet Perform traumatic procedures last (same as for infant)	Have parent remove outer clothing Remove underwear as body part is examined Allow to inspect equipment; demonstrating use of equipment is usually ineffective If uncooperative, perform procedures quickly Use restraint when appropriate; request parent's assistance Talk about examination if cooperative; use short phrases Praise for cooperative behavior
PRESCHOOL CHILD		
Prefer standing or sitting Usually cooperative prone/supine Prefer parent's closeness	If cooperative, proceed in head-to-toe direction If uncooperative, proceed as with toddler	Request self-undressing Allow to wear underpants if shy Offer equipment for inspection; briefly demonstrate use Make up story about procedure: "I'm seeing how strong your muscles are" (blood pressure) Use paper-doll technique Give choices when possible Expect cooperation; use positive statements: "Open your mouth"
SCHOOL-AGE CHILD		
Prefer sitting Cooperative in most positions Younger child prefers parent's presence Older child may prefer privacy	Proceed in head-to-toe direction May examine genitalia last in older child Respect need for privacy	Request self-undressing Allow to wear underpants Give gown to wear Explain purpose of equipment and significance of procedure, such as otoscope to see eardrum, which is necessary for hearing Teach about body functioning and care
ADOLESCENT		
Same as for school-age child Offer option of parent's presence	Same as older school-age child	Allow to undress in private Give gown Expose only area to be examined Respect need for privacy Explain findings during examination: "Your muscles are firm and strong" Matter-of-factly comment about sexual development: "Your breasts are developing as they should be" Emphasize normalcy of development Examine genitalia as any other body part; may leave to end

BOX 35-2

Child Preventive Care Time Line

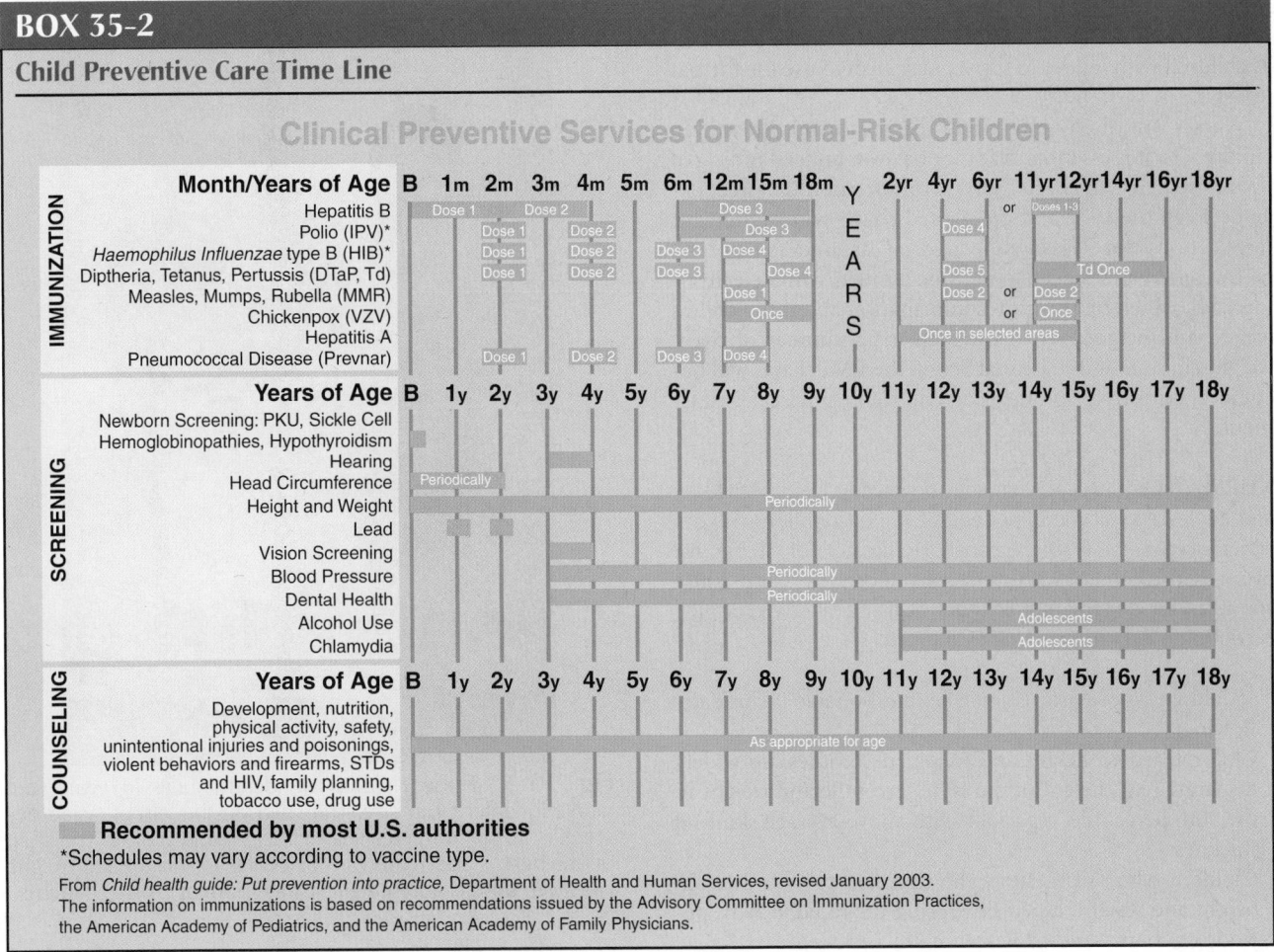

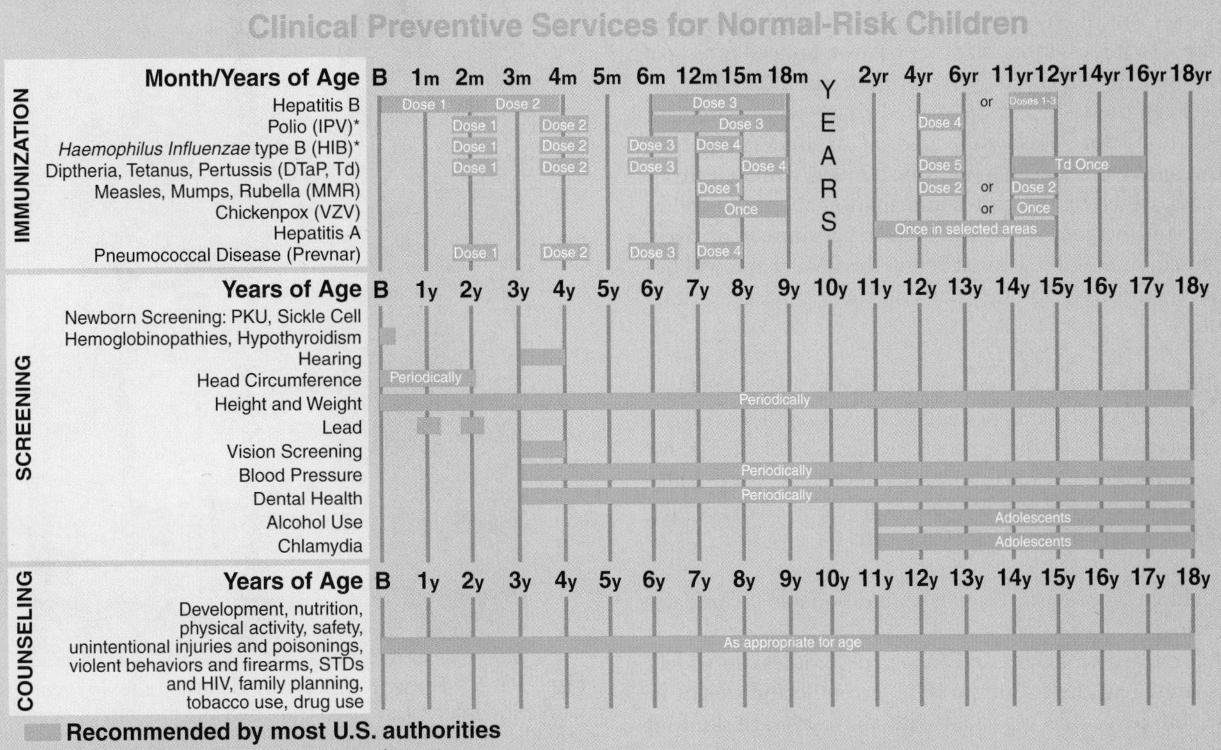

*Schedules may vary according to vaccine type.

From *Child health guide: Put prevention into practice,* Department of Health and Human Services, revised January 2003. The information on immunizations is based on recommendations issued by the Advisory Committee on Immunization Practices, the American Academy of Pediatrics, and the American Academy of Family Physicians.

Breastfed and Formula-Fed Infants

The national survey data better represent the combined size and growth patterns of the general U.S. population (1971 to 1994). Over the past two decades in the United States, approximately half of all infants were reported ever to have been breastfed, and approximately one third were breastfed for 3 months or more. Therefore, compared with the 1977 NCHS growth charts, the nationally representative data on which the revised infant growth charts are based will better represent the combined growth patterns of breastfed and formula-fed infants in the U.S. population.

With regard to differences in the growth of breastfed or formula-fed infants, other research efforts are currently in progress to address this issue. A working group of the World Health Organization (WHO) is collecting data at seven international study centers to develop a new set of international growth charts for infants and preschoolers through age 5 years. These charts will be based on the growth of exclusively or predominantly breastfed infants. The basic assumption is that infants from healthy populations, following the current WHO feeding recommendations, are growing optimally.

Special Groups

Although there are differences in size and growth among the major racial and ethnic groups in the United States, these appear to be small and inconsistent. Therefore the revised growth charts include all infants and children whatever their race or ethnicity. Because the growth patterns of preterm, very-low-birth-weight (VLBW) (less than 1500 g) infants are considerably different from those of higher-birth-weight term infants, and because specialized growth charts exist to track the growth of VLBW infants, data for VLBW infants were excluded from the revised charts.

Version of the Growth Charts

Three different versions of the charts are available at www.cdc.gov/growthcharts. The first set contains all nine smoothed percentile lines (3rd, 5th, 10th, 25th, 50th, 75th, 90th, 95th, 97th), and the second and third sets contain seven smoothed percentile lines. The second set contains the 5th and 95th percentile lines, and the third set contains the 3rd and 97th percentile lines at the extremes of the distribution. In addition, the charts for weight-for-stature and BMI-for-age contain the 85th percentile. In all the growth charts, age is truncated to the nearest full month, for example, 1 month (1.0 to 1.9 months), 11 months (11.0 to 11.9 months), 23 months (23.0 to 23.9 months), and so forth.

The three sets of charts are provided to meet the needs of various users. Set 1 shows all of the major percentile curves but may have limitations when the curves are close together, especially at the youngest ages. Most users in the United States may wish to used the format shown in Set 2 for the majority of routine clinical applications. Pediatric endocrinologists and others dealing with special populations, such as children with failure to thrive, may wish to use the format in Set 3.

Nurses are often responsible for measuring growth in children, so it is essential that they have an understanding of the revised growth charts. Several important differences exist between the 1977 and the revised charts with significant implications for classifying children as underweight or overweight. Nurses need to become familiar with determining BMI, which only requires information about the child's weight and height.* With the increasing number of overweight children in the United States, the BMI charts will become a critical component of children's physical assessment.

NURSE ALERT BMI-for-age may be used to identify children and adolescents at the upper end of the distribution who are either overweight (95th percentile or greater) or at risk for overweight (85th to 95th percentile) (Roche & Guo, 2001). Formulas for determining BMI are available at www.cdc.gov/nccdphp/dnpa/bmi/bmi-definiton.htm. ■

Children whose growth may be questionable include the following:

- Children whose height and weight percentiles are widely disparate (e.g., height in the 10th percentile and weight in the 90th percentile, especially with above-average skinfold thickness)
- Children who fail to show the expected growth rates in height and weight, especially during the rapid growth periods of infancy and adolescence (Table 35-2)
- Children who show a sudden increase (except during puberty) or decrease in a previously steady growth pattern

Because growth is a continuous but uneven process, the most reliable evaluation lies in comparing growth measurements over time. It is important to remember that normal growth patterns vary among children of the same age (Fig. 35-3).

*BMI = (Weight in pounds ÷ Height in inches ÷ Height in inches) × 703.

Table 35-2

Expected Growth Rates at Various Ages

AGE	EXPECTED GROWTH RATE (cm/yr)
1-6 months	18-22
6-12 months	14-18
Second year	11
Third year	8
Fourth year	7
Fifth-tenth years	5-6

From *Human growth and growth disorders: an update,* South San Francisco, 1989, Genentech.

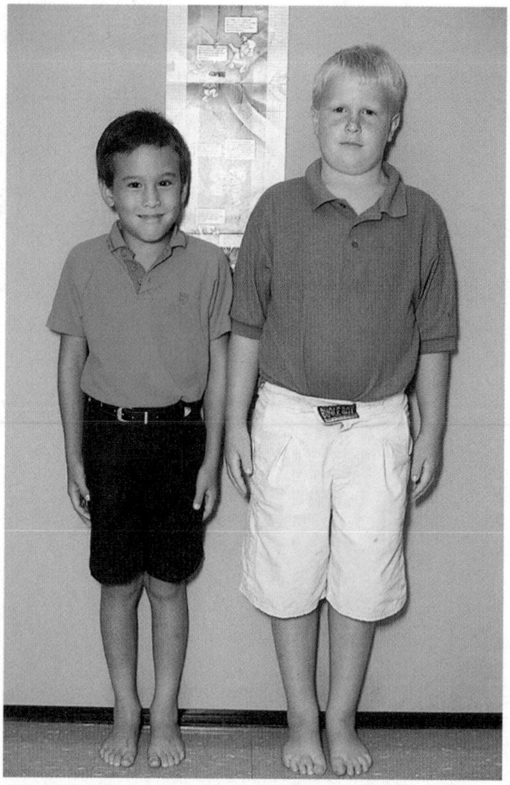

Fig. 35-3 These children of identical age (8 years) are markedly different in size. The child on the left, of Asian descent, is at the 5th percentile for height and weight. The child on the right is above the 95th percentile for height and weight. However, both children demonstrate normal growth patterns.

Ethnic Differences in Growth

A potential concern with the U.S. growth charts is their accuracy in evaluating the growth of children from different ethnic and socioeconomic backgrounds. Research findings indicate that these growth charts can serve as a reference guide for all racial or ethnic groups if used from the perspective that different groups of children have varying normal distributions on the growth curves. The NCHS charts are accurate for U.S. African-American children because this group was included in the sample population. Special growth charts for Chinese children are included in Appendix E.

Length

The term *length* refers to measurements taken when children are supine (also referred to as *recumbent length*). Until children are 24 months old (36 months if the birth to 36-month chart is used), measure recumbent length. Because of the normally flexed position during infancy, fully extend the body by (1) holding the head in midline, (2) grasping the knees together gently, and (3) pushing down on the knees until the legs are fully extended and flat against the table. If using a measuring board, place the head firmly at the top of the board and the heels of the feet firmly against the footboard.

If such a measuring device is not available, measure length by placing the child on a paper-covered surface, marking the end points of the top of the head and the heels of the feet, and measuring between these two points (Fig. 35-4). For accurate measurement, hold the writing utensil at

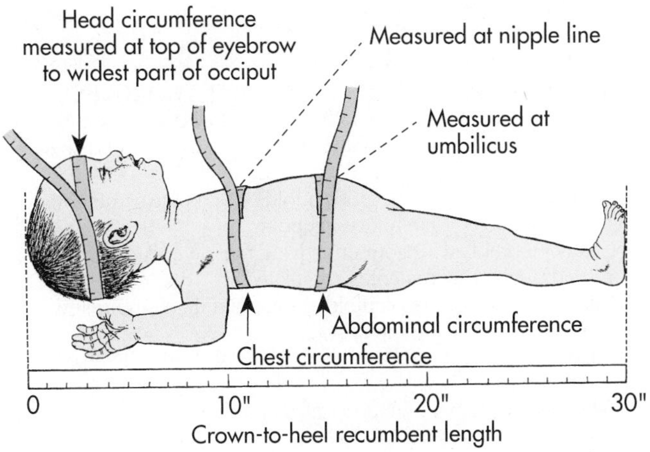

Fig. 35-4 Measurement of head, chest, and abdominal circumference and crown-to-heel (recumbent) length.

a right angle to the table when marking the cephalic point; position the feet with the toes pointing directly to the ceiling when marking the heel point. Regardless of the method used, have someone assist in holding the child's head in midline while you extend the legs and take the measurements.

Height

The term *height* (or *stature*) refers to the measurement taken when children are standing upright. Measure height by having the child, with shoes removed, stand as tall and straight as possible, with the head in midline and the line of vision parallel to the ceiling or floor. Be sure the child's back is to the wall or other vertical flat surface, with the heels, buttocks, and back of the shoulders touching the wall and the medial malleoli touching if possible (Fig. 35-5). Check for and correct bending of the knees, slumping of the shoulders, or raising of the heels of the feet.

NURSE ALERT Normally, height is less if measured in the afternoon than in the morning. To minimize this variation, apply modest upward pressure under the jaw or the mastoid processes behind the ears. ■

For the most accurate measurement, use a wall-mounted unit (*stadiometer;* see Fig. 35-5). The movable measuring rod of platform scales is accurate only if it maintains a parallel position to the floor and rests securely on the topmost part of the head. To improvise a flat surface for measuring length, attach a paper or metal tape or yardstick to the wall, position the child adjacent to the tape, and place a three-dimensional object, such as a thick book or box, on top of the head. Rest the side of the object firmly against the wall to form a right angle. Measure length or stature to the nearest 1 mm or 1/8 inch.

Weight

Weight is measured with an appropriately sized beam balance scale, which measures weights to the nearest 10 g or 0.5 ounce for infants and 100 g or 0.25 pound for children. Before the child is weighed, the scale is balanced by setting it at zero and noting if the balance registers exactly in the middle of the mark. If the end of the balance beam rises to the top or bottom of the mark, more or less weight, respectively, is

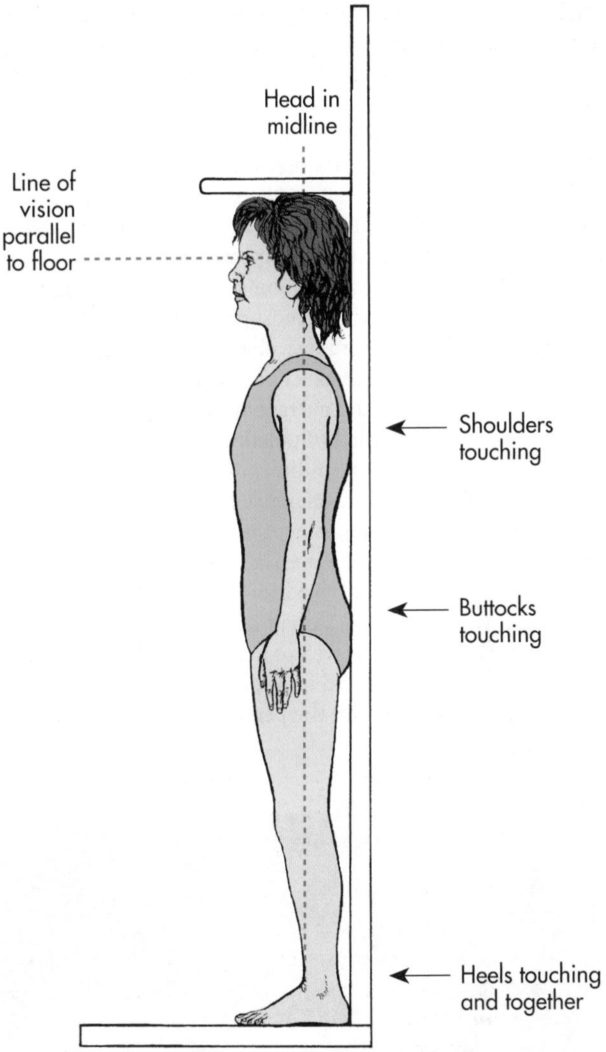

Fig. 35-5 Measurement of height. (Redrawn from *Human growth and growth disorders: an update*, South San Francisco, 1989, Genentech.)

added. Some scales are designed to allow for self-correction, but others need to be recalibrated by the manufacturer. Scales vary in their accuracy; infant scales tend to be more accurate than adult platform scales, and newer scales tend to be more accurate than older ones, especially at the upper levels of weight measurement. When precise measurements are needed, two nurses should take the weight independently, and if there is a discrepancy, a third reading should be taken.

Take measurements in a comfortably warm room. When the birth to 36-month growth charts are used, children should be weighed nude. Older children are usually weighed while wearing their underpants or a light gown. However, always respect the privacy of all children. If the child must be weighed wearing some article of clothing or some type of special device, such as a prosthesis or an armboard for an intravenous device, note this when recording the weight. Children who are measured for recumbent length are usually weighed on an infant platform scale and placed in a lying-down or sitting position. When weighing children, place your hand lightly above the body of the infant to prevent the child from accidentally falling off the scale (Fig. 35-6, *A*) or stand close to the toddler, ready to prevent a fall (Fig. 35-6, *B*). For maximum asepsis, cover the scale with a clean sheet of paper between each child's measurement.

Skinfold Thickness and Arm Circumference

Measures of relative weight and stature cannot distinguish between adipose (fat) tissue or muscle. One convenient measure of body fat is *skinfold thickness,* which is increasingly recommended as a routine measurement. Skinfold thickness is measured with special calipers, such as the Lange calipers. The most common sites for measuring skinfold thickness are the triceps (most practical for routine clinical use), subscapula, suprailiac, abdomen, and upper thigh. For greatest reliability, the exact procedure for measurement must be followed and the average of at least two measurements of one site recorded (Guidelines box).

Arm circumference is an indirect measure of muscle mass. Measurement of arm circumference follows the same procedure for skinfold thickness except the midpoint is measured with a paper or steel tape. Place the tape vertically, along the posterior aspect of the upper arm to the acromial process and to the olecranon process; half the measured length is the midpoint. Percentiles for triceps skinfold and arm circumference in children are listed in Appendix E and may be used as reference data. However, the percentiles are not standards or norms, because values between the 5th and 95th percentiles are not ranges of normal.

Guidelines

MEASURING TRICEPS SKINFOLD THICKNESS

With child's right arm flexed 90 degrees at elbow, mark midpoint between acromion and olecranon on posterior aspect of arm.
With arm hanging freely, grasp a fold of skin between thumb and forefinger 1 cm above midpoint.
Gently pull fold away from underlying muscle and continue to hold until measurement is completed.
Place caliper jaws over skinfold at midpoint mark and follow directions for using the device.
Estimate reading to nearest 1 mm, 2 to 3 seconds after applying pressure.
Take measurements until duplicates agree within 1 mm.

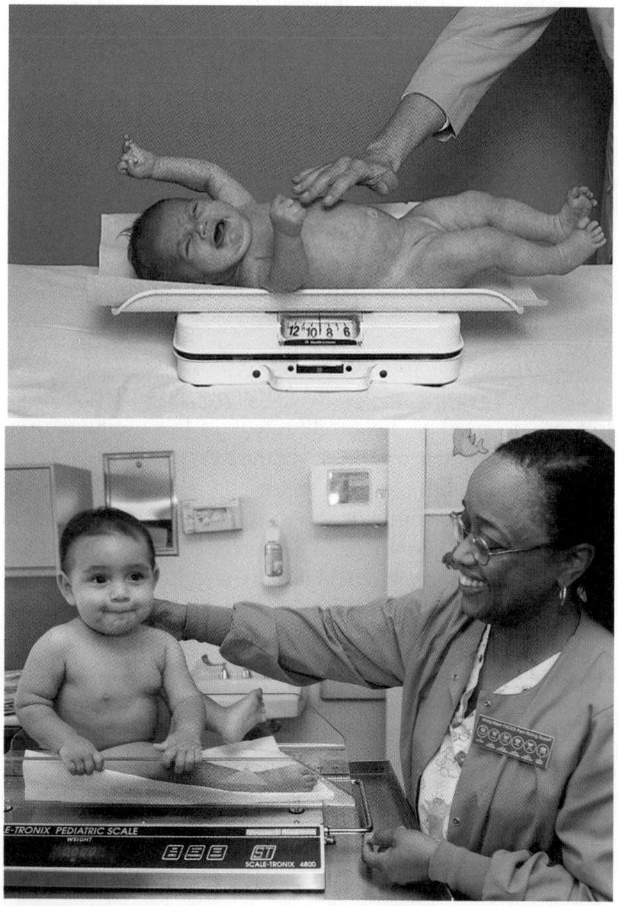

A

B

Fig. 35-6 **A,** Infant on scale. **B,** Toddler on scale. Note presence of nurse to prevent falls. (*B,* Courtesy Paul Vincent Kuntz, Texas Children's Hospital.)

Head Circumference

Measure head circumference in children up to 36 months of age and in any child whose head size is questionable. Measure the head at its greatest circumference, usually slightly above the eyebrows and pinna of the ears and around the occipital prominence at the back of the skull (see Fig. 35-4). Because head shape can affect the location of the maximum circumference, more than one measurement at points above the eyebrows may need to be taken to obtain the most accurate measure. Use a paper or metal tape because a cloth tape can stretch and give a falsely small measurement. For greatest accuracy, use devices with tenths of a centimeter, because the percentile charts have only 0.5 cm increments.

Plot the head size on the appropriate growth chart under head circumference. Generally, head and chest circumferences are equal at about 1 to 2 years of age. During childhood, chest circumference exceeds head size by about 5 to 7 cm (2 to 3 inches). (For newborns see Physical Assessment, Chapter 25.)

Physiologic Measurements

Physiologic measurements, key elements in evaluating physical status of vital functions, include temperature, pulse, respiration, and blood pressure. Compare each physiologic recording with normal values for that age group (see Appendix J). In addition, compare the values taken on preceding health visits with present recordings. For example, a falsely elevated blood pressure reading may not indicate hypertension if previous recent readings have been within normal limits. The isolated recording may indicate some stressful event in the child's life.

As in most procedures carried out with children, older children and adolescents are treated much the same as are adults. However, special consideration must be given to preschool children (Atraumatic Care box).

For best results in taking vital signs of infants, count respirations first (before the infant is disturbed), take the pulse next, and measure temperature last. If vital signs cannot be taken without disturbing the child, record the child's behavior (e.g., crying) along with the measurement.

Atraumatic Care

REDUCING YOUNG CHILDREN'S FEARS

Young children, especially preschoolers, fear intrusive procedures because of their poorly defined body boundaries. Therefore avoid invasive procedures, such as measuring rectal temperature, whenever possible. Also, avoid using the word "take" when measuring vital signs, because young children interpret words literally and may think that their temperature or other function will be taken away. Instead, say, "I want to know how warm you are."

Temperature

Temperature in healthy or ill children can easily be measured at several body sites via the oral, rectal, axillary, ear canal, or skin route. Substitutes for the no-longer-used mercury glass thermometer are electronic thermometers, infrared ear-based thermometers, chemical indicator thermometers, plastic strips, and digital thermometers, all of which offer advantages (rapid temperature taking, minimal intrusion, and reduced cross-contamination) and some disadvantages (Table 35-3). The accuracy of these instruments may differ, and variations in results may occur if the correct technique is not ap-

Table 35-3

Comparison of Body Temperature and Site Techniques*

TEMPERATURE TYPES	COMMENTS
ORAL TEMPERATURE	
Device to be placed under tongue in right or left posterior sublingual pocket, not in front of tongue. Have child keep mouth closed, without biting on thermometer.	Oral site indicates rapid changes in core body temperature, but accuracy may be an issue when compared with rectal site (Jensen et al, 2000). Several factors affect mouth temperature: eating/mastication, hot/cold beverages, smoking, open-mouth breathing, ambient temperature (Hooker & Houston, 1996, Rabinowitz et al, 1996).
AXILLARY TEMPERATURE	
Place tip under arm in center of axilla and keep close to skin, not clothing. Child's arm must be held firmly against side (see Fig. 35-7, *A*).	Recommended for children objecting to rectal measurement and for whom oral temperature is not feasible. May be affected by poor peripheral perfusion (results in lower value) or use of radiant warmers or brown fat in cold-stress neonates (results in higher value) (Bliss-Holtz, 1995; Haddock, Merrow, & Swanson, 1996). Advantage: avoids intrusive procedure and eliminates risk of rectal perforation.
RECTAL TEMPERATURE	
Place well-lubricated tip at maximum 2.5 cm (1 inch) into rectum; securely hold thermometer close to anus. Child may be placed in side-lying, supine, or prone position (i.e., supine with knees flexed toward abdomen); cover penis because procedure may stimulate urination. A small child may be placed prone across parent's lap.	Although very reliable, only recommended when no other route or device can be used (children whose mental age or temperament prevents cooperation, agitated children, and those who have oral/axillary injuries or surgery) (Barone & Rowe, 1999; Jensen et al, 2000). Accuracy is affected by stool in rectum (higher value) (Loveys et al, 1999). Contraindicated in the following patients: children with recent rectal surgery, children with diarrhea or anorectal lesions, and children receiving chemotherapy (cancer treatment usually affects mucosa and causes neutropenia) (Hockenberry-Eaton & Kline, 2001). Rectal temperature technique (see Fig. 35-7, *B*)
ELECTRONIC THERMOMETER	
Senses temperature with an electronic component called *thermistor* mounted at tip of plastic and stainless steel probe, which is connected to an electronic recorder. Temperature measurement appears on digital display within 60 seconds. Probe can be placed in mouth, axilla, or rectum.	Ideally suited to pediatric use. Devices are safe because of unbreakable plastic sheath. Child's mouth can remain open when oral temperature is taken. Accuracy for axillary temperature is supported by some research but not by other studies (Greyling, Viljoen, & Joubert, 2000; Haddock et al, 1996; Wilshaw et al, 1999).

Continued

Table 35-3

Comparison of Body Temperature and Site Techniques—cont'd

THERMOMETER TYPES	COMMENTS
ELECTRONIC THERMOMETER—cont'd	Studies recommend that electronic rectal measurements are more accurate than the electronic measurements at axillary, oral, or tympanic sites (Jensen et al, 2000). The Penguin electronic thermometer measures rectal temperature in term and near-term infants (Dollberg, Lahav, & Mimouni, 2001).
INFRARED THERMOMETER Infrared thermometers measure thermal radiation from axilla, ear canal, or tympanic membrane. Temperature measurement appears on digital display in approximately 1 second.	Three types of infrared thermometers are available for ear-based use: tympanic, ear-canal, and arterial heat balance via the ear canal (AHBE); often these devices are all inappropriately referred to as "tympanic thermometers." Temperatures measured in this way reflect arterial (bloodstream) temperature (Pompei & Pompei, 1996; Wilshaw et al, 1999).
EAR-BASED TEMPERATURE SENSOR Insert covered tip of probe gently in ear canal, pointing toward midpoint between opposite eyebrow and sideburns (Childs, Harrison, & Hodkinson, 1999). For most accurate results: straighten ear canal for sensor to measure heat appropriately (see Fig. 35-7, C); take three measurements and record highest reading. Most models use "offsets" for internal calculations that transform ear temperature into supposedly equivalent oral or rectal temperatures.	Although frequently used in pediatric settings (especially ambulatory clinics) debate still continues on the reliability of ear-based thermometry in screening of febrile children (Jean-Mary et al, 2002; Lanham et al, 1999; Modell et al, 1998; Saxena et al, 2001). Studies suggest that ear-based thermometry does not show sufficient agreement with an established method of temperature measurement to be used in situations where body temperature needs to be assessed with precision (Banitalebi & Bangstad, 2002; Craig et al, 2002; Sganga et al, 2000). Although correct probe placement is difficult in an infant's ear, accuracy may be affected for this age group as well (Blackburn et al, 2001; Houlder, 2000; Robinson et al, 1998).
EAR SENSOR (LighTouch LTX)† Measures the infrared heat energy radiating from canal opening, scans canal for highest temperature reading, and then calculates arterial temperature (correlates highly with core or internal body temperature). Insert hemispheric probe in ear opening; ear tug is not necessary.	Available in two sizes; smaller size of LighTouch Pedi-Q is for infants and toddlers (Wilshaw et al, 1999). Does not calculate offsets; therefore reading is only for arterial temperature (not equivalent to other sites).
AXILLARY SENSOR (LighTouch LTN)† Measures the infrared heat energy radiating from axilla. Touch covered probe to axilla, depress and release button, remove, and read.	Can be used on wet skin, in incubators, or under radiant heaters, warming pads, or other heat sources. Research suggests that reliability of axillary site may be a general issue when nonmercury thermometers are used (Craig et al, 2000; Haddock et al, 1996; Zengeya & Blumenthal, 1996).
DIGITAL THERMOMETER Consists of probe that connects to microprocessor chip, which translates signals into degrees and sends temperature measurement to digital display. Used in the same manner as an oral electronic thermometer.	More accurate and easier to read, but somewhat more expensive than plastic strip thermometer.
LIQUID CRYSTAL SKIN CONTACT THERMOMETER (CHEMICAL DOT THERMOMETER) Single-use, disposable, flexible thermometer with specific chemical mixture in each circle that changes color to measure temperature increments of two tenths of a degree. Two types: • Used in the same manner as mercury thermometer; kept in mouth (1 minute), axilla (3 minutes), or rectum (3 minutes); color change is read 10-15 seconds after removing thermometer.	May underestimate oral temperature and overestimate axillary temperature (Erickson, Meyer, & Woo, 1996). When compared with mercury glass thermometer, offers less reliable results (Kongpanichkul & Bunjongpak, 2000; Molton, Blacktop, & Hall, 2001). Skin temperature is influenced by clothing, swaddling, and probe placement, especially in neonates and infants (Leick-Rude & Bloom, 1998).

†Manufactured by Exergen Corporation, 51 Water St., Watertown, MA 02172; phone: 800-422-3006, 617-923-9911; Web site: www.exergen.com.

Table 35-3

Comparison of Body Temperature and Site Techniques—cont'd

THERMOMETER TYPES	COMMENTS
LIQUID CRYSTAL SKIN CONTACT THERMOMETER (CHEMICAL DOT THERMOMETER)—cont'd	
• Wearable, continuous-use thermometer, which is placed under axilla; may be read within 2-3 minutes after placement and continuously thereafter; discard and replace every 48 hours	Easier to read than plastic strip thermometer (Macqueen, 2001). Tempa.DOT single-use clinical thermometer can be used for routine temperature taking (Macqueen, 2001). Read thermometer away from heat source (e.g., radiant warmer). For older chemical dot thermometers, if unused thermometer changes color from storage in a warm area (above 35° C [95° F]), place in freezer for 1 hour and then at room temperature for 24 hours before using (Py Ma H Corporation, 1994); newer types do not require special storage (Medical Indicators, Inc., 1999). Wearable, continuous-reading thermometer may be preferred by parents because it requires minimal disturbance to child (i.e., nurse can just lift child's arm to get a temperature reading) (Riveral et al, 1997).
PLASTIC STRIP THERMOMETER (THERMOGRAPH)	
Changes color in response to temperature changes. Place strip on forehead until color change occurs; usually takes less than 15 seconds. Some strips are used in the same manner as oral mercury thermometer.	Accuracy is variable; may be used for screening (Shann & Mackenzie, 1996). Advantages for home and community use include simple instructions and minimal cost (Valadez, Elmore-Meegan, & Morley, 1995).

plied (Fig. 35-7), if the child is febrile, or if the child's age is not appropriately considered (Erickson, 1999; Loveys et al, 1999; Robinson et al, 1998; Romanovsky et al, 1997).

The most frequently used temperature measurement devices in children are as follows (Healthcare Product Comparison System, 1996a, 1996b, 1996c):

1. *Electronic continuous thermometers* measure the patient's temperature during the administration of general anesthesia, treatment of hypothermia or hyperthermia, and other situations that require continuous monitoring.
2. *Electronic intermittent thermometers* measure the patient's temperature at oral, rectal, and axillary sites and are used as primary diagnostic indicators.
3. *Infrared thermometers* measure the patient's temperature by collecting emitted thermal radiation from a particular site (e.g., ear canal).

NURSE ALERT Mercury thermometers should not be used because if they are broken, inhaled vapors can cause significant toxicity (Goldman & Shannon, 2001). ■

The routine sites for taking temperature are the sublingual pocket, the rectum, the axilla, and the ear canal. As a general rule in children, temperature is currently taken in the axilla or rectum in infants and young children, and by mouth after age 4 to 5 years when the child understands how to hold the thermometer. Ear-based temperature devices may also be a convenient option (Barone & Rowe, 1999).

The time of the device's placement at the measurement site should be noted. No universal agreement exists regarding the length of time mercury thermometers should be kept in place. Recommendations based on research vary from 8 to 10 minutes for an oral reading, 4 minutes for a rectal reading, and 5 minutes for an axillary reading, but some researchers recommend longer placements for oral and axillary routes (Barone & Rowe, 1999). These times may also vary widely within practice settings. Electronic devices considerably lower the measurement time to the range of seconds. However, all efforts should be made to obtain an accurate reading, and devices should be kept in place long enough to achieve this.

Based on the classical literature, the normal core body temperature is 99° to 100° F (actually assessed for research for surgical and intensive care purposes). The peripheral temperature considered normal in the clinical setting registers as 37.0° C (98.6° F) via the oral route. Temperatures taken at different sites may present small variations from the value of a given reference-criterion site (i.e., oral or rectal) (Childs, Harrison, & Hodkinson, 1999; Cretel et al, 1999; Irvin, 1999; Wilshaw et al, 1999). Traditionally it has been assumed that rectal temperatures are around 1° C higher (mean) and axillary temperatures around 1° C lower (mean) than oral temperatures. Recent research reinforces that differences among these sites (rectal, axillary, ear, and oral) may show wide and significant variation across studies (Craig et al, 2000).

A

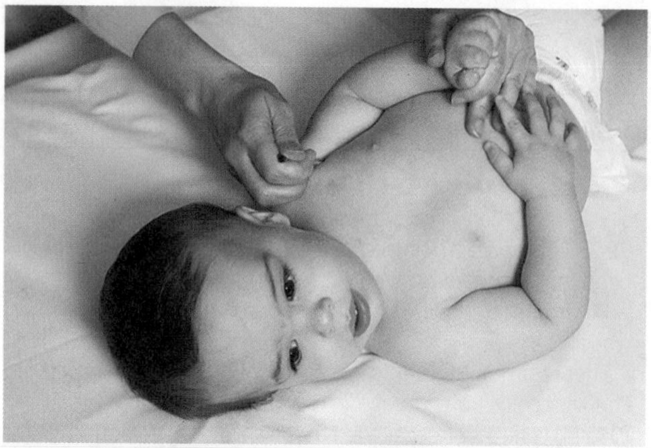

B

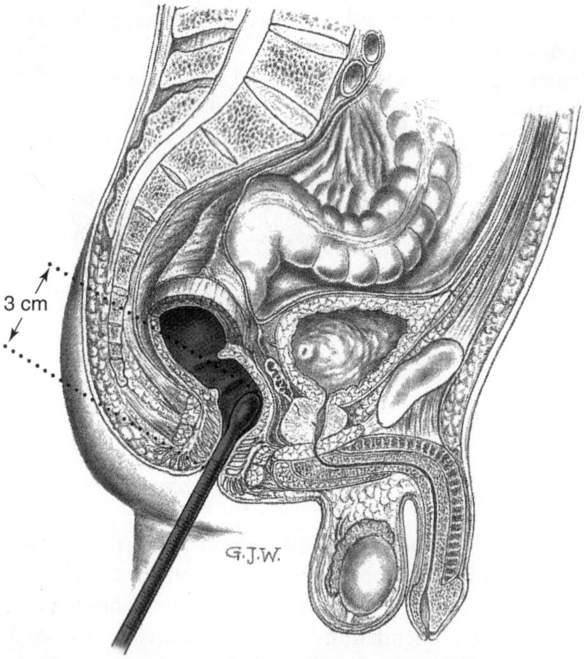

C

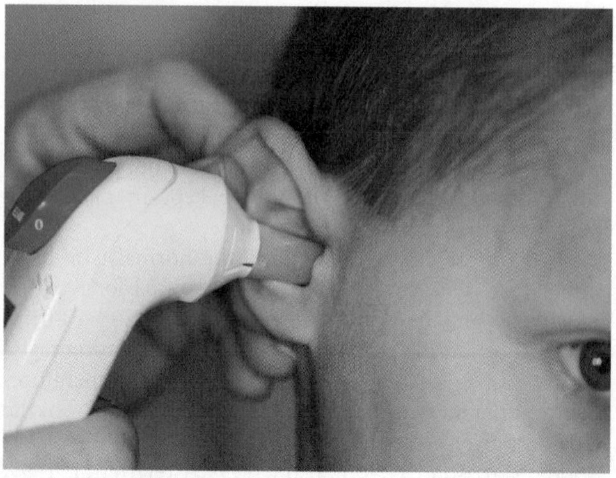

Fig. 35-7 A, Position for taking axillary temperature. **B,** Cross section of rectum illustrates curve approximately 3 cm from anus, where risk of perforation from thermometer is greatest in infants under 3 months of age. **C,** Position for tympanic temperature measurement. Note ear tug to help straighten the canal for the infrared sensor to focus on the eardrum.

NURSE ALERT Because of variations in temperature among rectal, axillary, oral, and ear sites, it is necessary to chart the route along with the recorded temperature reading and to consistently use one route if possible. ■

Pulse

A satisfactory pulse can be taken radially in children older than 2 years of age. However, in infants and young children, the apical impulse (heard through a stethoscope held to the chest at the apex of the heart) is more reliable (see Fig. 35-29 for location of pulses). Count the pulse for 1 full minute in infants and young children because of possible irregularities in rhythm. However, when frequent apical rates are needed, use shorter counting times (e.g., 15- or 30-second intervals). For greater accuracy, measure the apical rate while the child is asleep; record the child's behavior along with the rate. Pulses may be graded according to the criteria in Table 35-4. Compare radial and femoral pulses at least once during infancy to detect the presence of circulatory impairment, such as coarctation of the aorta.

Respiration

Count the respiratory rate in the same manner as for the adult patient. However, in infants observe abdominal movements because respirations are primarily diaphragmatic. Because the movements are irregular, count them for 1 full minute for accuracy (see Appendix J).

Blood Pressure

Blood pressure (BP) measurement by noninvasive methods is part of a routine vital sign determination. BP should be measured annually in children 3 years of age through adolescence and in children with symptoms of hypertension, children in emergency departments and intensive care units, and high risk infants (National Institutes of Health [NIH], 1996; Seidel, Rosenstein, & Pathak, 1997). Ambulatory BP monitoring in children and adolescents is a valuable method for the assessment and management of suspected hypertension (Bald, 2002).

Measurement Devices

BP can also be measured using electronic devices that employ oscillometric or Doppler techniques. In *oscillometry,* pressure changes are transmitted through the arterial wall to the pressure cuff, and the oscillations are detected by a pressure-sensitive indicator. Oscillometers have digital readouts for systolic BP, diastolic BP, mean arterial pressure

Table 35-4

Grading of Pulses

GRADE	DESCRIPTION
0	Not palpable
+1	Difficult to palpate, thready, weak, easily obliterated with pressure
+2	Difficult to palpate, may be obliterated with pressure
+3	Easy to palpate, not easily obliterated with pressure (normal)
+4	Strong, bounding, not obliterated with pressure

(MAP), and pulse. The MAP is not the same as the mean BP (arithmetic average of systolic and diastolic pressures). Rather, it is a value somewhat lower than the arithmetic mean. BP readings using oscillometry, such as Dinamap, are generally higher and correlate better with direct radial artery values than measurements using auscultation (Amoore, 1998; Gillman & Cook, 1995; Ling et al, 1995; Wattigney et al, 1996) (see Table 35-7). Oscillometry also eliminates common problems found with the auscultation method, such as deflating the cuff too rapidly, not hearing the softest sounds, and rounding numbers for the Korotkoff sounds.

Doppler ultrasound translates changes in ultrasound frequency caused by blood movement within the artery to audible sound by means of a transducer in the cuff. This technique is useful for systolic pressure measurement but is unreliable for diastolic pressure measurement. Oscillometric and Doppler instruments are very useful in measuring BP in infants and have largely replaced the flush method, which reflects only the mean BP, and the auscultatory method.

Selection of Cuff

No matter what type of noninvasive technique is used, the most important factor in accurately measuring BP is the use of an appropriately sized cuff (*cuff size* refers only to the inner inflatable bladder, not the cloth covering). A technique to establish an appropriate cuff size is to choose a cuff having a bladder width that is approximately 40% of the arm circumference midway between the olecranon and the acromion. This will usually be a cuff bladder that covers 80% to 100% of the circumference of the arm (Fig. 35-8) (Beevers, Lip, & O'Brien, 2001; NIH, 1996). Researchers have found that cuff selection of a bladder width to equal 40% of the upper arm circumference most accurately reflects directly measured radial arterial pressure (Clark et al, 2002).

Using limb circumference for selecting cuff width more accurately reflects direct arterial BP than using limb length, because this method takes into account the variations in thickness of the arm and the amount of pressure required to compress the artery (Gillman & Cook, 1995). For measurement sites other than the upper arms, the limb circumference guidelines can be used, although the shape of the limb (i.e., conical shape of the thigh) may prevent appropriate placement of the cuff and inaccurately reflect intraarterial BP (Table 35-5).

Cuffs that are either too narrow or too wide affect the accuracy of BP measurements. If the cuff size is too small, the reading on the device is falsely high. If the cuff size is too large, the reading is falsely low (Clark et al, 2002).

When another site is used, BP measurements using noninvasive techniques may differ. Generally, systolic pressure in the lower extremities (thigh or calf) is greater than pressure in the upper extremities, and systolic BP in the calf is higher than that in the thigh (Fig. 35-9). These differences are listed in Table 35-6 and apply to oscillometric measurements taken on the right extremities with the child supine and the cuff size based on the circumference method (Park, Lee, & Johnson, 1993).

NURSE ALERT Compare BP in the upper and lower extremities at least once to detect abnormalities, such as coarctation of the aorta, in which the lower extremity pressure is less than the upper extremity pressure. ■

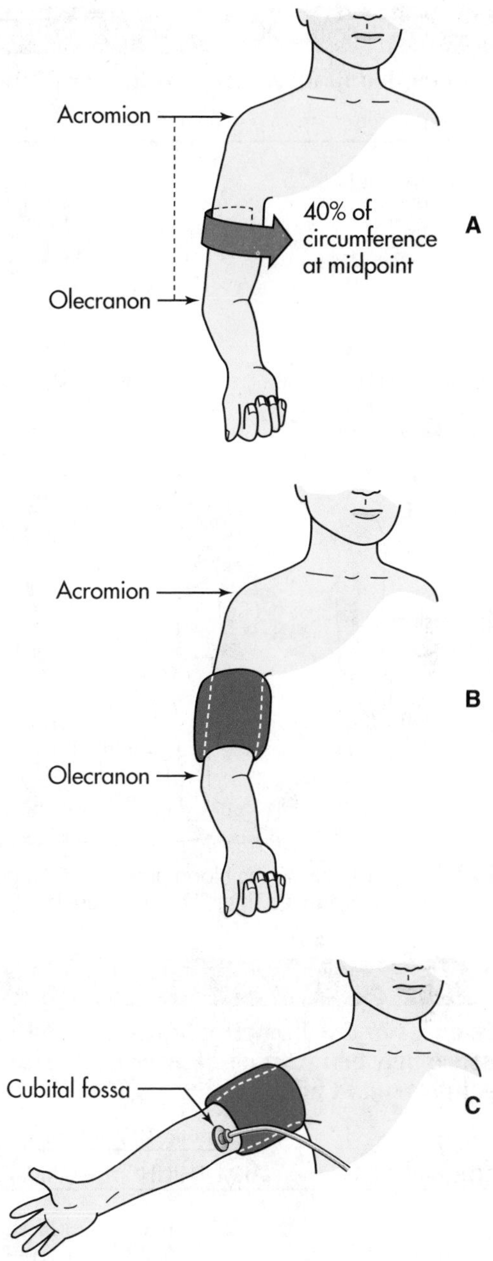

Fig. 35-8 Determination of proper cuff size. **A,** The cuff bladder width should be approximately 40% of the circumference of the arm measured at a point midway between the olecranon and acromion. **B,** The cuff bladder length should cover 80% to 100% of the circumference of the arm. **C,** Blood pressure should be measured with the cubital fossa at heart level. The arm should be supported. The stethoscope bell is placed over the brachial artery pulse, proximal and medial to the cubital fossa and below the bottom edge of the cuff. (From National Institutes of Health, National Heart, Lung, and Blood Institute: *Update on the Task Force Report [1987] on high blood pressure in children and adolescents: a working group report from the National High Blood Pressure Education Program,* NIH pub no 96-3790, Bethesda, MD, September 1996.)

Table 35-5

Recommended Bladder Dimensions for Blood Pressure Cuffs

ARM CIRCUMFERENCE AT MIDPOINT (CM)	CUFF NAME*	BLADDER WIDTH (CM)	BLADDER LENGTH (CM)
5-7.5	Newborn	3	5
7.5-13	Infant	5	8
13-20	Child	8	13
24-32	Adult	13	24
32-42	Wide adult	17	32
42-50	Thigh	20	42

From Frohlich ED et al: Recommendations for human blood pressure determination by sphygmomanometers: report of a special task force appointed by the Steering Committee, American Heart Association, *Circulation* 77:501A, 1988.
*Cuff name does not guarantee that cuff will be appropriate size for a child within that age range.

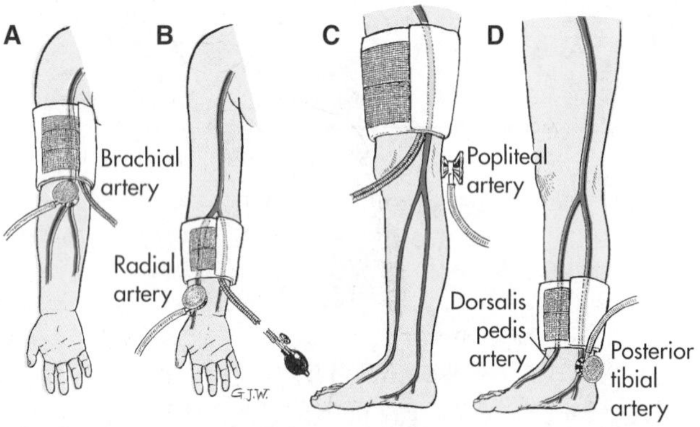

Fig. 35-9 Sites for measuring blood pressure. **A,** Upper arm. **B,** Lower arm or forearm. **C,** Thigh. **D,** Calf or ankle.

Table 35-6

Differences in Oscillometric Systolic Blood Pressure between Arm and Lower Extremity Sites in Normal Children

	Systolic BP × (Mean ± SD)	
AGE GROUP (YEARS)	ARM-THIGH	ARM-CALF
4-8	−7.1 ± 6.8	−9.3 ± 7.4
9-16	−2.4 ± 7.7	−5.0 ± 26.9

From Park M, Lee D, Johnson GA: Oscillometric blood pressures in the arm, thigh, and calf in healthy children and those with aortic coarctation, *Pediatrics* 91(4):761-765, 1993.
BP, blood pressure; *SD,* standard deviation.

NURSE ALERT In choosing cuff sizes, use an appropriately sized cuff. When the correct size is not available, use an oversized cuff rather than an undersized one or use another site that more appropriately fits the cuff size. Do not choose a cuff based on the name of the cuff (e.g., an "infant" cuff may be too small for some infants). ■

Measurement and Interpretation

Measuring and interpreting BP in infants and children requires additional attention to correct procedure because (1) limb sizes vary and cuff selection must accommodate the circumference; (2) excessive pressure on the antecubital fossa affects the Korotkoff sounds; (3) children easily become anxious, which can elevate BP; and (4) BP values change with age and growth.

Age, height, weight, and body mass have been shown to be highly correlated with BP (NIH, 1996). Studies indicate that height is a more appropriate index of maturation than weight for use with normative BP data and should be considered when evaluating BP in children. Tables are now available that indicate—when height is taken into account—that more short children (10th percentile for age-sex–specific height) and fewer tall children (90th percentile for age-sex–specific height) are likely to be classified as hypertensive (see Appendix J for BP tables).

Although the technique of BP measurement in children is generally the same as that used for adults (Guidelines box), some aspects of the procedure are especially important. Because children are easily upset by unfamiliar procedures, prepare them for BP measurement. For children of preschool age and above, explain each step of the procedure and tell them how the cuff will feel, such as a tight feeling or an arm hug. Use explanations such as "I want to see how strong your muscle is" or "Let's watch the silver rise in the tube." Because the child should be quiet and relaxed during the procedure, measure BP before performing any anxiety-producing procedures. Infants and small children may be more quiet if the reading is taken while they are sitting in the parent's lap.

Use a pediatric stethoscope and bell for hearing BP sounds in small children and infants. If auscultation is not possible, obtain a systolic reading by palpation; measure the point at which the pulse at the radial or brachial artery reappears as the cuff is deflated. BP should be measured twice, and the average measurement should be recorded (NIH, 1996).

The average BP readings at various ages throughout childhood using sphygmomanometry are listed in Appendix J, and readings using oscillometry are listed in Table 35-7. A *normal* BP is defined as a systolic and diastolic BP less than the 90th percentile for age and sex.

NURSE ALERT Published norms for BP, such as those in Appendix J, are valid only if the same method of measurement (auscultation and limb length for cuff size) is used in clinical practice. ■

Guidelines

MEASURING BLOOD PRESSURE

Use an appropriately sized cuff.
Use same position, preferably sitting, and right arm for brachial artery site (see Figs. 35-8 and 35-9, *A*)
Use alternative site as needed to accommodate available cuff sizes.
- Use smaller size on forearm: place cuff above wrist and auscultate radial artery (see Fig. 35-9, *B*).
- Use larger size on thigh: place cuff above knee and auscultate popliteal artery (see Fig. 35-9, *C*).
- Use larger size on calf: place cuff above malleoli or at midcalf and auscultate posterior tibial or dorsal pedal artery (see Fig. 35-9, *D*).

Position limb at level of heart.
Rapidly inflate cuff to about 20 mm Hg above point at which radial pulse disappears.
Release cuff pressure at a rate of about 2 to 3 mm Hg/sec during auscultation of artery.
Read mercury-gravity manometer at eye level.
Record systolic value as onset of a clear tapping sound (first Korotkoff sound [K1]).
Record diastolic pressure as follows:
- Fourth Korotkoff sound (K4) (low-pitched, muffed sound) for children up to age 12 years
- Fifth Korotkoff sound (K5) (disappearance of all sound) for children ages 13 to 18 years

Record also limb, position, cuff size, and method of measurement.
If using electronic monitor, follow manufacturer's instructions and guidelines for correct cuff size.
- With oscillometric device (i.e., Dinamap), all four limb sites can be used, but reserve the thigh for last, because it is the most uncomfortable.
- Stabilize limb during cuff deflation, because movement interferes with the device's ability to measure blood pressure accurately.

Table 35-7

Normative Dinamap Blood Pressure Values (Systolic/Diastolic; Mean Arterial Pressure in Parentheses)

AGE GROUP	MEAN	90TH PERCENTILE	95TH PERCENTILE
Newborn (1-3 days)	65/41 (50)	75/49 (59)	78/52 (62)
1 month-2 years	95/58 (72)	106/68 (83)	110/71 (86)
2-5 years	101/57 (74)	112/66 (82)	115/68 (85)

From Park M, Menard S: Normative oscillometric blood pressure values in the first 5 years in an office setting, *Am J Dis Child* 143(7):860-864, 1989.

NURSE ALERT Use the following quick formula for average *systolic BP* using auscultation:
- 1 to 7 years: age in years + 90
- 8 to 18 years: (2 × age in years) + 83

Use the following formula for average *diastolic BP* using auscultation:
- 1 to 5 years: 56
- 6 to 18 years: age in years + 52 ■

General Appearance

The general appearance of the child is a cumulative, subjective impression of the child's physical appearance, state of nutrition, behavior, personality, interactions with parents and nurse (also siblings if present), posture, development, and speech. Although general appearance is recorded at the beginning of the physical examination, it encompasses all of the observations of the child during the interview and physical assessment.

Note the *facies,* the facial expression and appearance of the child. For example, the facies may give clues to children who are in pain; have difficulty breathing; feel frightened, discontented, or happy; are mentally deficient; or are acutely ill.

Observe the *posture, position,* and types of *body movement.* The child with hearing or vision loss may characteristically tilt the head in an awkward position to hear or see better. The child in pain may favor a body part. The child with low self-esteem or a feeling of rejection may assume a slumped, careless, and apathetic pose or posture. Likewise, a child with confidence, a feeling of self-worth, and a sense of security usually demonstrates a tall, straight, well-balanced posture. While observing such "body language," do not interpret too freely but rather record objectively.

Note the child's *hygiene* in terms of cleanliness; unusual body odor; the condition of the hair, neck, nails, teeth, and feet; and the condition of the clothing. Such observations are excellent clues to possible instances of neglect, inadequate financial resources, housing difficulties (e.g., no running water), or lack of knowledge concerning children's needs.

General appearance includes an overall impression of the child's state of *nutrition.* This impression is more than a statement describing body weight or stature, such as "slender and tall." It is an estimation of the quality, as well as the quantity, of nutritional intake. For example, two children can be of the same height and weight, yet one can appear overweight because of flabby, loose skin, whereas the other child appears strong, robust, and well built because of firm, well-defined musculature. Likewise, a small, slender child may be well nourished with no signs of chronic undernutrition, such as bony prominences, a protuberant abdomen, flat buttocks, gaunt facies, and poor muscle tone with evidence of wasting.

Compare your impression of the nutritional state with the parents' history of feeding practices. Discrepancies between the two "impressions" may be a valuable area for nutritional counseling. For example, parents who believe that their child is too thin and eats too little, despite evidence of adequate growth and physical signs of proper nutrition, may find it helpful to keep a daily diary to calculate the child's cumulative food intake. Many parents are surprised at the quantity of food ingested, even though the amounts at each meal or snack are small.

Behavior includes the child's personality, level of activity, reaction to stress, requests, frustration, interactions with others (primarily the parent and nurse), degree of alertness, and response to stimuli. Mental questions that serve as reminders for observing behavior include the following: What is the child's overall personality? Does the child have a long attention span or is he or she easily distracted? Can the child follow two or three commands in succession without the need for repetition? What is the youngster's response to delayed gratification or frustration? Is eye-to-eye contact used during conversation? What is the child's reaction to the nurse and family members? Is the child quick or slow to grasp explanations?

Development can be assessed by carefully observing the child, but verify your impressions with screening tests. Various tests for assessing development, speech, vision, and hearing are discussed later in this chapter and in Chapter 42 .

Record an overall estimate of the child's speech development, motor skills, degree of coordination, and recent area of achievement under general appearance. For example, the following statement may apply to an 18-month-old child: "Motor development advanced for age; climbs, runs, jumps (most recent motor skill), manipulates small objects with ease; excellent coordination and balance; beginning to name many objects; uses two-word phrases; and enjoys 'talking' to self and others."

Skin

Skin is assessed for color, texture, temperature, moisture, and turgor. Examination of the skin and its accessory organs primarily involves inspection and palpation. Touch allows the nurse to assess the texture and turgor of the skin, as well as the temperature (Turnbull, 2000). The normal *color* in light-skinned children varies from a milky white and rose color to a deeply hued pink color. Dark-skinned children, such as those of Native American, Hispanic, or black descent, have inherited various brown, red, yellow, olive green, and bluish tones in their skin. Asian persons have skin that is normally of a yellow tone.

Several variations in skin color can occur, some of which warrant further investigation. The types of color change and their appearance in children with light or dark skin are summarized in Table 35-8.

Normally the skin *texture* of young children is smooth, slightly dry, and not oily or clammy. Evaluate skin *temperature* by symmetrically feeling each part of the body and comparing upper areas with lower ones. Note any difference in temperature.

Determine *tissue turgor,* or the amount of elasticity in the skin, by grasping the skin on the abdomen between the thumb and index finger, pulling it taut, and quickly releasing it. Elastic tissue immediately assumes its normal position without residual marks or creases. In children with poor skin turgor, the skin remains suspended or tented for a few seconds before

Table 35-8

Differences in Color Changes of Racial Groups

DESCRIPTION	APPEARANCE IN LIGHT SKIN	APPEARANCE IN DARK SKIN
CYANOSIS		
Bluish tone through skin; reflects reduced (deoxygenated) hemoglobin	Bluish tinge, especially in palpebral conjunctiva (lower eyelid), nail beds, earlobes, lips, oral membranes, soles, and palms	Ashen gray lips and tongue
PALLOR		
Paleness may be a sign of anemia, chronic disease, edema, or shock	Loss of rosy glow in skin, especially face	Ashen gray appearance in black skin More yellowish brown color in brown skin
ERYTHEMA		
Redness may be result of increased blood flow from climatic conditions, local inflammation, infection, skin irritation, allergy, or other dermatoses or may be caused by increased numbers of red blood cells as a compensatory response to chronic hypoxia	Redness easily seen anywhere on body	Much more difficult to assess; rely on palpation for warmth or edema
ECCHYMOSES		
Large, diffuse areas, usually black and blue in color, caused by hemorrhage of blood into skin; are typically result of injuries	Purplish to yellow-green areas; may be seen anywhere on skin	Very difficult to see unless in mouth or conjunctiva
PETECHIAE		
Same as ecchymosis except for size: small, distinct pinpoint hemorrhages 2 mm or less in size; can denote some type of blood disorder, such as leukemia	Purplish pinpoints most easily seen on buttocks, abdomen, and inner surfaces of the arms or legs	Usually invisible except in oral mucosa, conjunctiva of eyelids, and conjunctiva covering eyeball
JAUNDICE		
Yellow staining of the skin usually caused by bile pigments	Yellow staining seen in sclerae of eyes, skin, fingernails, soles, palms, and oral mucosa	Most reliably assessed in sclerae, hard palate, palms, and soles

slowly falling back on the abdomen. Skin turgor is one of the best estimates of adequate hydration and nutrition.

Accessory Structures

Inspection of the accessory structures of the skin may be performed while the skin is being examined or when the scalp and extremities are being assessed.

Inspect the *hair* for color, texture, quality, distribution, and elasticity. Children's scalp hair is usually lustrous, silky, strong, and elastic. Genetic factors affect the appearance of hair. For example, the hair of black children is usually curlier and coarser than that of white children. Hair that is stringy, dull, brittle, dry, friable, and depigmented may suggest poor nutrition. Record any bald or thinning spots. Loss of hair in infants may indicate lying in the same position and may be a clue for counseling parents concerning the child's stimulation needs.

Inspect the hair and scalp for general cleanliness. Various ethnic groups condition their hair with oils or lubricants, which, if not thoroughly washed from the scalp, clog the sebaceous glands, causing scalp infections. Also examine the area for lesions; scaliness; evidence of infestation, such as lice or ticks; and signs of trauma, such as ecchymoses, masses, or scars.

In children who are approaching puberty, look for growth of secondary hair as a sign of normally progressing pubertal changes. Note precocious or delayed appearance of hair growth because, although not always suggestive of hormonal dysfunction, it may be of great concern to the early- or late-maturing adolescent.

Inspect the *nails* for color, shape, texture, and quality. Normally the nails are pink, convex, smooth, and hard but flexible (not brittle). The edges, which are usually white, should extend over the fingers. Dark-skinned individuals may have more deeply pigmented nail beds. Short, ragged nails are typical of habitual biting. Uncut, dirty nails are a sign of poor hygiene.

Each individual has a distinct set of handprints and footprints. The patterns, or *dermatoglyphics,* are unique to the individual and vary a great deal in detail and complexity.

The palm normally shows three flexion creases (Fig. 35-10, *A*). In some situations such as Down syndrome, the two distal horizontal creases are fused to form a single horizontal crease (the *single palmar crease,* or *transpalmar crease*) (Fig. 35-10, *B*). If grossly abnormal lines or folds are observed, sketch a picture to describe them and refer the finding to a specialist for further investigation.

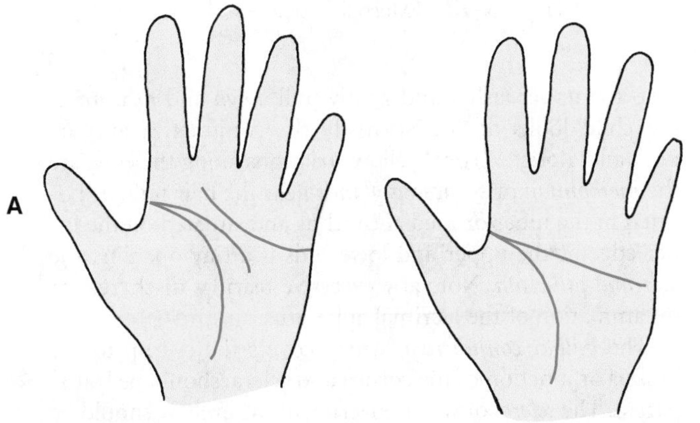

Fig. 35-10 Examples of flexion creases on palm. **A,** Normal. **B,** Transpalmar crease.

Lymph Nodes

Lymph nodes are usually assessed when the part of the body in which they are located is examined. The body's lymphatic drainage system is extensive; the usual sites for palpating accessible lymph nodes are shown in Fig. 35-11.

Palpate nodes by using the distal portion of the fingers and gently but firmly pressing in a circular motion along the regions where nodes are normally present. During assessment of the nodes in the head and neck, tilt the child's head upward slightly but without tensing the sternocleidomastoid or trapezius muscles. This position facilitates palpation of the *submental, submaxillary, tonsillar,* and *cervical nodes.* Palpate the *axillary nodes* with the arms relaxed at the sides but slightly abducted. Assess the *inguinal nodes* with the child in the supine position. Note size, mobility, temperature, and tenderness, as well as reports by the parents regarding any visible change of enlarged nodes. In children, small, nontender, movable nodes are usually normal. Tender, enlarged, warm lymph nodes generally indicate infection or inflammation close to their location. Report such findings for further investigation.

Anatomy Review: Superficial Lymph Nodes

Head and Neck

Observe the head for general *shape* and *symmetry.* A flattening of one part of the head, such as the occiput, may indicate that the child continually lies in this position. Marked asymmetry is usually abnormal and may indicate premature closure of the sutures (craniosynostosis).

NURSE ALERT Significant head lag after 6 months of age strongly indicates cerebral injury and is referred for further evaluation. ■

Note *head control* in infants and *head posture* in older children. Most infants by 4 months of age should be able to hold the head erect and in midline when in a vertical position.

Evaluate range of motion by asking the older child to look in each direction (to either side, up, and down) or manually putting the younger child through each position. Limited range of motion may indicate *wryneck,* or *torticollis,* a result of injury to the sternocleidomastoid muscle in which the child holds the head to one side with the chin pointing toward the opposite side.

Anatomy Review: Location of Sinuses

NURSE ALERT Hyperextension of the head (opisthotonos) with pain on flexion is a serious indication of meningeal irritation and is referred for immediate medical evaluation. ■

Palpate the *skull* for patent sutures, fontanels, fractures, and swellings. Normally the posterior fontanel closes by the second month of life and the anterior fontanel fuses between 12 and 18 months of age. Early or late closure is noted, because either may be a sign of a pathologic condition. (For a more detailed discussion of the cranial bones, see Chapter 36.)

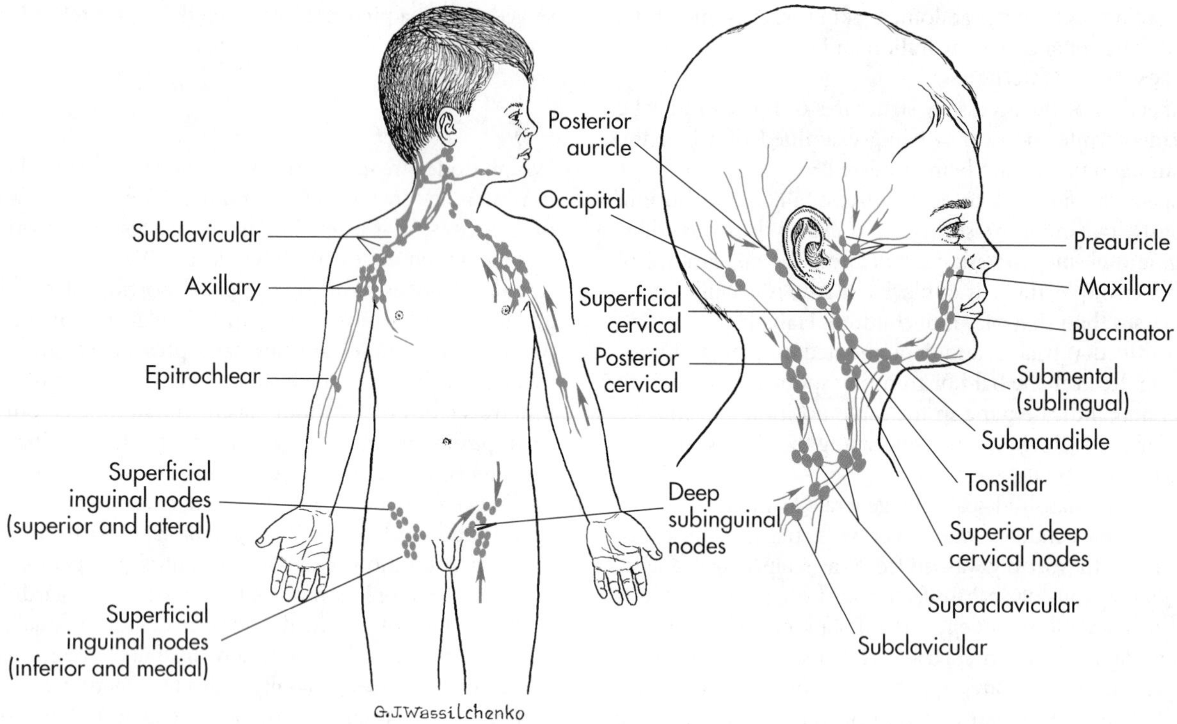

Fig. 35-11 Location of superficial lymph nodes. *Arrows* indicate directional flow of lymph.

ANATOMY REVIEW: STRUCTURES IN THE NECK

While examining the head, observe the *face* for symmetry, movement, and general appearance. Ask the child to "make a face" to assess symmetric movement and disclose any degree of paralysis. Note any unusual facial proportion, such as an unusually high or low forehead, wide- or close-set eyes, or a small, receding chin.

In addition to assessment of the head and neck for movement, inspect the neck for size and palpate it for associated structures. The neck is normally short, with skinfolds between the head and shoulders during infancy; however, it lengthens during the next 3 to 4 years.

NURSE ALERT If any masses are detected in the neck, report them for further investigation. Large masses can block the airway. ■

ANATOMY REVIEW: STRUCTURES OF THE EYE

Eyes

Inspection of External Structures

Inspect the *lids* for proper placement on the eye. When the eye is open, the upper lid should fall near the upper iris. When the eyes are closed, the lids should completely cover the cornea and sclera (Fig. 35-12).

Determine the general slant of the *palpebral fissures* or lids by drawing an imaginary line through the two points of the medial canthus and across the outer orbit of the eyes and aligning each eye on the line. Usually the palpebral fissures lie horizontally. However, in Asians, the slant is normally upward.

Also inspect the inside lining of the lids, the *palpebral conjunctiva.* To examine the lower conjunctival sac, pull the lid down while the patient looks up. To evert the upper lid, hold the upper lashes and gently pull *down* and *forward* as the child looks down. Normally the conjunctiva appears pink and glossy. Vertical yellow striations along the edge are the *meibomian* or *sebaceous glands* near the hair follicle. Located in the inner or medial canthus and situated on the inner edge of the upper and lower lids is a tiny opening, the *lacrimal punctum.* Note any excessive tearing, discharge, or inflammation of the lacrimal apparatus.

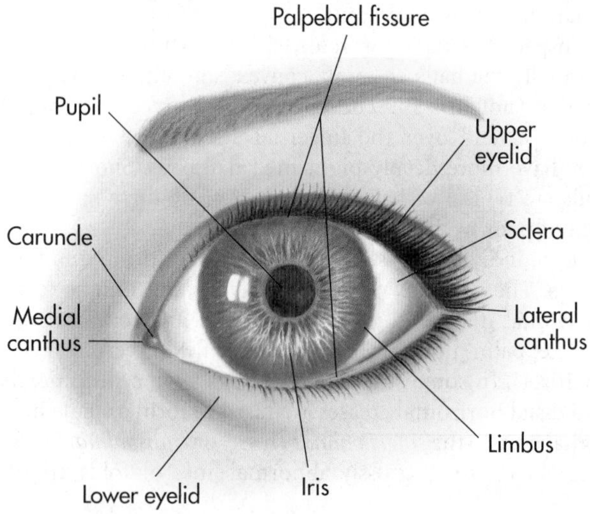

Fig. 35-12 External structures of eye.

The *bulbar conjunctiva,* which covers the eye up to the limbus or junction of the cornea and sclera, should be transparent. The *sclera,* or white covering of the eyeball, should be clear. Tiny black marks in the sclera of heavily pigmented individuals are normal.

The *cornea,* or covering of the iris and pupil, should be clear and transparent. Record opacities because they can be signs of scarring or ulceration, which can interfere with vision. The best way to test for opacities is to illuminate the eyeball by shining a light at an angle (obliquely) toward the cornea.

Compare the *pupils* for size, shape, and movement. They should be round, clear, and equal. Test their *reaction to light* by quickly shining a source of light toward the eye and removing it. As the light approaches, the pupils should constrict; as the light fades, the pupils should dilate. Test the pupillary response of *accommodation* by having the child look at a bright, shiny object at a distance and quickly moving the object toward the face. The pupils should constrict as the object is brought near the eye. Normal findings on examination of the pupils may be recorded as *PERRLA,* which means "*P*upils *E*qual, *R*ound, *R*eact to *L*ight and *A*ccommodation."

Inspect the *iris* and pupil for color, size, shape, and clarity. Permanent eye color is usually established by 6 to 12 months of age. As the iris and pupil are inspected, look for the *lens.* Normally the lens is not visible through the pupil.

Inspection of Internal Structures

The ophthalmoscope permits visualization of the interior of the eyeball with a system of lenses and a high-intensity light. The lenses permit clear visualization of eye structures at different distances from the nurse's eye and correct visual acuity differences in the examiner and child. Use of the ophthalmoscope requires practice to know which lens setting produces the clearest image.

The ophthalmic and otic head are usually interchangeable on one "body" or handle, which encloses the power source, either disposable or rechargeable batteries. The nurse should practice changing the heads, which snap on and are secured with a quarter turn, and replacing the batteries and light bulbs. Nurses who are not directly involved in physical assessment are often responsible for ensuring that the equipment functions properly.

Preparing the Child

The nurse can prepare the child for the ophthalmoscopic examination by showing the child the instrument, demonstrating the light source and how it shines in the eye, and explaining the reason for darkening the room. For infants and young children who do not respond to such explanations, it is best to try to use distraction to encourage them to keep their eyes open. Forcibly parting the lids results in an uncooperative, watery-eyed child and a frustrated nurse. Usually, with some practice, the nurse can elicit a red reflex almost instantly while approaching the child and may also gain a momentary inspection of the blood vessels, macula, or optic disc.

Funduscopic Examination

Fig. 35-13 shows the structures of the back of the eyeball, or the *fundus.* The fundus is immediately apparent as the *red reflex.* The intensity of the color increases in darkly pigmented individuals.

NURSE ALERT A brilliant, uniform red reflex is an important sign because it rules out many serious defects of the cornea, aqueous chamber, lens, and vitreous chamber. Any dark shadows or opacities are recorded because they indicate some abnormality in any of these structures. ■

As the ophthalmoscope is brought closer to the eye, the most conspicuous feature of the fundus is the *optic disc,* the area where the blood vessels and optic nerve fibers enter and exit from the eye. The color of the disc is creamy pink; it is lighter in color than the surrounding fundus. Normally it is round or vertically oval.

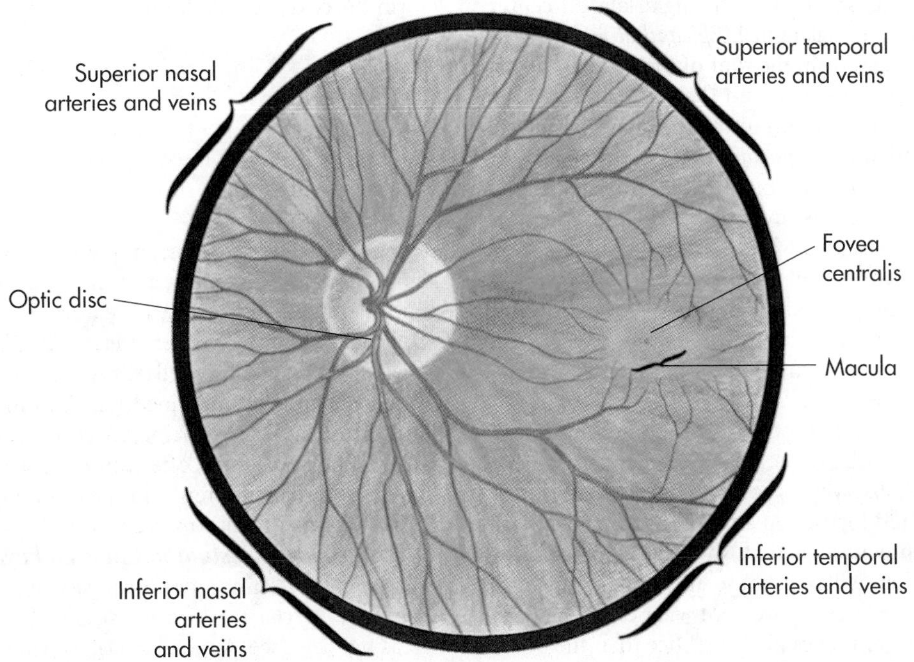

Fig. 35-13 Structures of fundus. (From Seidel HM et al: *Mosby's guide to physical examination,* ed 4, St Louis, 1999, Mosby.)

After the optic disc is located, the area is inspected for *blood vessels.* The central retinal artery and vein appear in the depths of the disc and emanate outward with visible branching. The *veins* are darker in color and about one fourth larger in size than the *arteries.* Normally the branches of the arteries and veins cross each other.

Other structures that may be seen are the *macula,* the area of the fundus with the greatest concentration of visual receptors, and, in the center of the macula, a minute glistening spot of reflected light called the *fovea centralis;* this is the area of most perfect vision.

Vision Testing

Several tests are available for assessing vision. This discussion focuses on four areas: (1) ocular alignment, (2) visual acuity, (3) peripheral vision, and (4) color vision. Vision screening should be performed at the earliest possible age and at regular intervals (American Academy of Pediatrics [AAP], Committee on Practice and Ambulatory Medicine, Section on Ophthalmology, 2003; Wall et al, 2002).

Ocular Alignment

Normally, by age 3 to 4 months, children achieve the ability to fixate on one visual field with both eyes simultaneously (binocularity). One of the most important tests for binocularity is alignment of the eyes to detect nonbinocular vision, or *strabismus* (Halle, 2002). In strabismus, or cross-eye, one eye deviates from the point of fixation. If the malalignment is constant, the weak eye becomes "lazy," and the brain eventually suppresses the image produced by that eye. If strabismus is not detected and corrected by age 4 to 6 years, blindness from disuse, known as *amblyopia,* may result.

Tests commonly used to detect malalignment are the corneal light reflex and the cover tests. To perform the *corneal light reflex test,* or *Hirschberg test,* shine a flashlight or the light of the ophthalmoscope directly into the patient's eyes from a distance of about 40.5 cm (16 inches). If the eyes are *orthophoric,* or normal, the light falls symmetrically within each pupil (Fig. 35-14, *A*). If the light falls off center in one eye, the eyes are malaligned. *Epicanthal folds,* excess folds of skin that extend from the roof of the nose to the inner termination of the eyebrow and that partially or completely overlap the inner canthus of the eye, may give a false impression of malalignment *(pseudostrabismus)* (Fig. 35-14, B). Epicanthal folds are often found in Asian children.

In the *cover test,* one eye is covered, and the movement of the *uncovered* eye is observed while the child looks at a near (33 cm, or 13 inches) or distant (6 m, or 20 feet) object. If the uncovered eye does not move, it is aligned. If the uncovered eye moves, a malalignment is present because when the stronger eye is temporarily covered, the misaligned eye attempts to fixate on the object.

In the *alternate cover test,* occlusion is shifted back and forth from one eye to the other, and movement of the eye that was *covered* is observed as soon as the occluder is removed while the child focuses on a point in front of him or her. If normal alignment is present, shifting the cover from one eye to the other will not cause the eye to move. If malalignment is present, eye movement will occur when the cover is moved. This test takes more practice than the other cover test because the occluder must be moved back and forth quickly and accurately to see the eye move. Because deviations can occur at different ranges, it is important to perform the cover tests at both close and far distances.

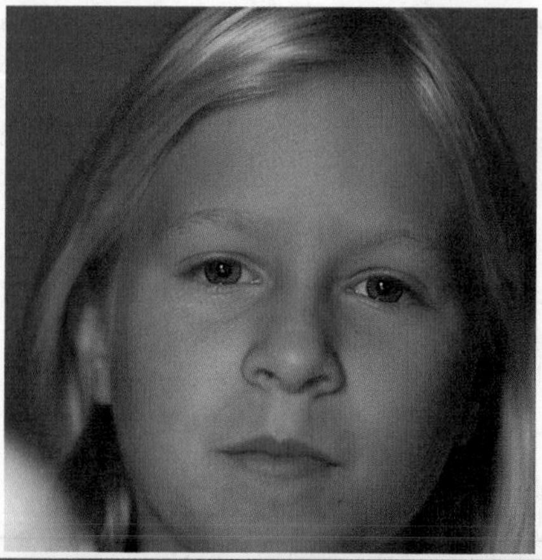
A

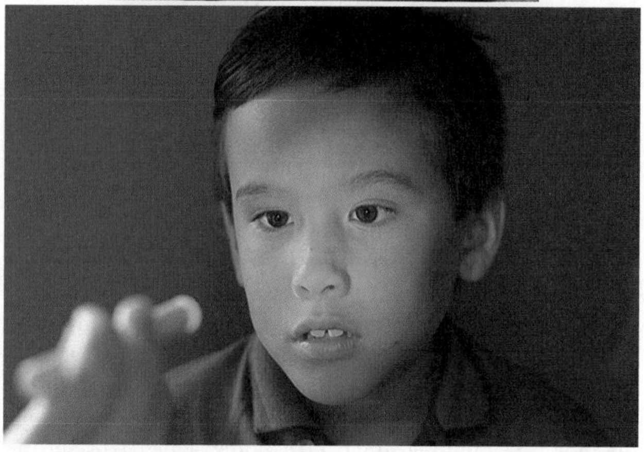
B

Fig. 35-14 **A,** Corneal light reflex test demonstrating orthophoric eyes. **B,** Pseudostrabismus. Inner epicanthal folds cause eyes to appear malaligned; however, corneal light reflexes fall perfectly symmetrically.

NURSE ALERT The cover test is usually easier to perform if the examiner uses his or her own hand rather than a card-type occluder (Fig. 35-15). Attractive occluders fashioned like an ice cream cone or happy-face lollipop cut from cardboard are also well received by young children.

Photoscreening is a technique used to screen for amblyopia, refractive disorders, and media opacities (AAP, Committee on Practice and Ambulatory Medicine, Section on Ophthalmology, 2003; Berry et al, 2001). Using a camera, images of the papillary reflexes (reflections) and red reflexes (Bruckner test) are obtained (AAP, Committee on Practice and Ambulatory Medicine, Section on Ophthalmology, 2003). Photoscreening offers an effective way to screen infants, preverbal children, and those with developmental delays who are difficult to screen.

Visual Acuity Testing in Children beyond Infancy

The most common test for measuring visual acuity is the *Snellen letter chart,* which consists of lines of letters of decreasing size (see Appendix D). During testing, the AAP, Committee on Practice and Ambulatory Medicine, Section

A

B

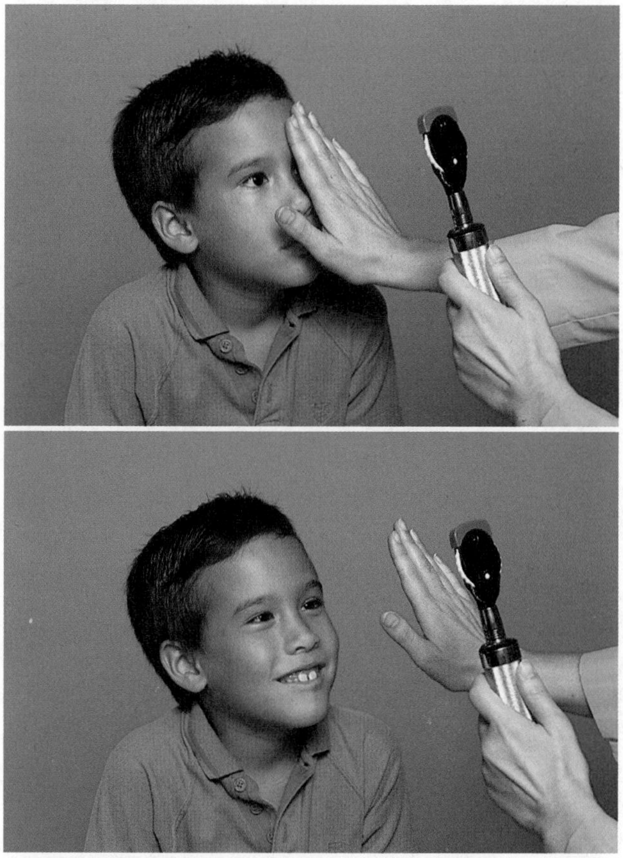

Fig. 35-15 Alternate cover test to detect amblyopia in patients with strabismus. **A,** Eye is occluded, and child is fixating on light source. **B,** If eye does not move when uncovered, eyes are aligned.

on Ophthalmology (2003), now recommends that children stand 10 feet from the chart with their heels at the 10-foot line. When screening for visual acuity in children, the child's right eye is tested first by covering the left. Children who wear glasses should be screened wearing the lenses. Tell the child to keep both eyes open during the examination. If the child fails the current line, move up the chart to the next larger line. Continue up the chart until a line is found that the child can pass. Then begin moving down the chart again until the child fails to read the line. To pass each line, the child must correctly identify four of six symbols on the line. Repeat the procedure, covering the right eye. Table 35-9 provides a list of visual screening tests for children and guidelines for referral recommended by the AAP, Committee on Practice and Ambulatory Medicine, Section on Ophthalmology (2003).

For children unable to read letters and numbers, the *tumbling E* or *HOTV test* is useful (Coats & Jenkins, 1997). The tumbling E test uses the capital letter E to point in four different directions. The child is then asked to point in the direction the E is facing. The HOTV test consists of a wall chart composed of *H*'s, *O*'s, *T*'s, and *V*'s. The child is given a board containing a large H, O, T, and V. The examiner points to a letter on the wall chart, and the child matches the correct letter on the board held in his or her hand. The tumbling E and HOTV are excellent tests for preschool-age children.

When a child is unable to perform the tumbling E or HOTV test, the LH symbol or Allen card test may be used. The Allen card test uses common figures to test the child's vision. It is important to assess whether the child is able to identify the pictures before actual vision testing. The examiner walks backward slowly, flipping through the cards and presenting different pictures to the child. The examiner continues to move backward as the child correctly calls out the figures. When the child begins to miss the figure on the cards, the examiner moves forward to confirm that the child is able to identify the figures at that point. All Allen card figures are 20/30 in size. The farthest distance at which the child is able to accurately identify the pictures becomes the numerator, and 30 becomes the denominator. For example, if the child is able to identify the pictures accurately at 15 feet, the visual acuity is recorded as 15/30. This is equivalent to 20/40 or 10/20 visual acuity. The LH symbol test is somewhat different from the Allen card test because it is a spiral-bound set of flash cards. The flash cards contain large pictures of a house, an apple, a circle, and a square. The LH symbol cards contain the symbol size and visual acuity value for a 10-foot testing distance. The visual acuity is determined by the smallest symbols the child is able to identify at 10 feet.

Visual Acuity Testing in Infants and Difficult-to-Test Children

In newborns, vision is tested mainly by checking for *light perception* by shining a light into the eyes and noting responses such as pupillary constriction, blinking, following the light to midline, increased alertness, or refusal to open the eyes after exposure to the light. Although the simple maneuver of checking light perception and eliciting the pupillary light reflex indicates that the anterior half of the visual apparatus is intact, it does not confirm that the infant can see. In other words, this test does not assess whether the brain receives the visual message and interprets the signals.

Another test of visual acuity is the infant's ability to fix on and follow a target. Although any brightly colored or patterned object can be used, the human face is excellent. Hold the infant upright while moving your face slowly from side to side.

NURSE ALERT If visual fixation and following are not present by 3 to 4 months of age, further ophthalmologic evaluation is needed. ■

Other signs that may indicate visual loss or other serious eye problems include fixed pupils, strabismus, constant nystagmus, the setting-sun sign, and slow lateral movements. Unfortunately, it is very difficult to test each eye separately; the presence of such signs in one eye could indicate unilateral blindness.

Special tests are available for testing infants and other difficult-to-test children to assess acuity or confirm blindness. For example, in *visually evoked potentials,* the eyes are stimulated with a bright light or pattern, and electrical activity to the visual cortex is recorded through scalp electrodes. Acuity is assessed by using progressively smaller patterns.

Table 35-9

Eye Examination Guidelines*

FUNCTION	RECOMMENDED TESTS	REFERRAL CRITERIA	COMMENTS
AGES 3-5 YEARS			
Distance visual acuity	Snellen letters Snellen numbers Tumbling E HOTV Picture test • Allen figures • LEA symbols	1. Fewer than 4 of 6 correct on 20-ft line with either eye tested at 10 ft monocularly (i.e., less than 10/20 or 20/40) or 2. Two-line difference between eyes, even within the passing range (i.e., 10/12.5 and 10/20 or 20/25 and 20/40)	1. Tests are listed in decreasing order of cognitive difficulty; the highest test that the child is capable of performing should be used; in general, the tumbling E or the HOTV test should be used for children 3-5 years of age and Snellen letters or numbers for children 6 years and older. 2. Testing distance of 10 ft is recommended for all visual acuity tests. 3. A line of figures is preferred over single figures. 4. The nontested eye should be covered by an occluder held by the examiner or by an adhesive occluder patch applied to the eye; the examiner must ensure that it is not possible to peek with the nontested eye.
Ocular alignment	Cross-cover test at 10 ft (3 m) Random dot E stereo test at 40 cm Simultaneous red reflex test (Bruckner test)	Any eye movement Fewer than 4 of 6 correct Any asymmetry of pupil color, size, brightness	Child must be fixing on a target while cross-cover test is performed. Direct ophthalmoscope used to view both red reflexes simultaneously in a darkened room from 2 to 3 feet away; detects asymmetric refractive errors as well.
Ocular media clarity (cataracts, tumors, etc.)	Red reflex	White pupil, dark spots, absent reflex	Direct ophthalmoscope, darkened room. View eyes separately at 12 to 18 inches; white reflex indicates possible retinoblastoma.
6 YEARS AND OLDER			
Distance visual acuity	Snellen letters Snellen numbers Tumbling E HOTV Picture test • Allen figures • LEA symbols	1. Fewer than 4 of 6 correct on 15-ft line with either eye tested at 10 ft monocularly (i.e., less than 10/15 or 20/30) or 2. Two-line difference between eyes, even within the passing range (i.e., 10/10 and 10/15 or 20/20 and 20/30)	1. Tests are listed in decreasing order of cognitive difficulty; the highest test that the child is capable of performing should be used; in general, the tumbling E or the HOTV test should be used for children 3-5 years of age and Snellen letters or numbers for children 6 years and older. 2. Testing distance of 10 ft is recommended for all visual acuity tests. 3. A line of figures is preferred over single figures. 4. The nontested eye should be covered by an occluder held by the examiner or by an adhesive occluder patch applied to eye; the examiner must ensure that it is not possible to peek with the nontested eye.
Ocular alignment	Cross-cover test at 10 ft (3 m) Random dot E stereo test at 40 cm Simultaneous red reflex test (Bruckner test)	Any eye movement Fewer than 4 of 6 correct Any asymmetry of pupil color, size, brightness	Child must be fixing on a target while cross-cover test is performed. Direct ophthalmoscope used to view both red reflexes simultaneously in a darkened room from 2 to 3 ft away; detects asymmetric refractive errors as well.
Ocular media clarity (cataracts, tumors, etc)	Red reflex	White pupil, dark spots, absent reflex	Direct ophthalmoscope, darkened room. View eyes separately at 12 to 18 inches; white reflex indicates possible retinoblastoma.

From American Academy of Pediatrics: Eye examination in infants, children, and young adults by pediatricians, *Pediatrics* 111(4):902-907, 2003.

*Assessing visual acuity (vision screening) represents one of the most sensitive techniques for the detection of eye abnormalities in children. The American Academy of Pediatrics Section on Ophthalmology, in cooperation with the American Association for Pediatric Ophthalmology and Strabismus and the American Academy of Ophthalmology, has developed these guidelines to be used by physicians, nurses, educational institutions, public health departments, and other professionals who perform vision evaluation services.

Peripheral Vision

In children who are old enough to cooperate, estimate *peripheral vision,* or the visual field of each eye, by having children fixate on a specific point directly in front of them as an object, such as a finger or a pencil, is moved from beyond the field of vision into the range of peripheral vision. Check each eye separately and for each quadrant of vision. As soon as children see the object, have them say "stop." At that point measure the angle from the anteroposterior axis of the eye (straight line of vision) to the peripheral axis (point at which the object is first seen). Normally children see about 50 degrees upward, 70 degrees downward, 60 degrees nasalward, and 90 degrees temporally. Limitations in peripheral vision may indicate blindness from damage to structures within the eye or to any of the visual pathways.

Color Vision

Another important test is for color vision. It is estimated that 8% to 10% of white males and less than half that percentage of black males inherit the X-linked disorder known as *color vision deficit* (or *color blindness,* a less acceptable term). From 0.5% to 1% of white females are affected. Although the severity of impaired perception of color varies considerably, the two most common types are *protanomaly,* in which the child confuses gray with pink or pale blue with green, and *deuteranomaly,* in which the child confuses gray with pale purple or green. In most of these individuals the color vision deficit causes no major problems. However, some of the difficulties encountered by individuals with more severe deficits may be inability to distinguish amber or red traffic lights, failure to see a red brake light on the rear of a car, difficulty in distinguishing green traffic lights from certain types of incandescent street lamps, and a poor sense of color coordination of clothing. For school-age children the greatest difficulty lies in performance of academic skills that use color as a visual aid. Adolescents may be ineligible for certain vocational opportunities, such as electronics, photography, printing, interior decorating, pharmaceuticals, textiles, police work, and several types of military service.

The tests available for color vision include the *Ishihara test* and the *Hardy-Rand-Rittler (HRR) test.* Each consists of a series of cards (pseudoisochromatic) on which is printed a color field composed of spots of a certain "confusion" color. Against the field is a number or symbol similarly printed in dots but of a color likely to be confused with the field color by the person with a color vision deficit. As a result, the figure or letter is invisible to an affected individual but is clearly seen by a person with normal vision.

Ears

Inspection of External Structures

The entire external earlobe is called the *pinna,* or *auricle,* and is located on each side of the head. Measure the *height* alignment of the pinna by drawing an imaginary line from the outer orbit of the eye to the occiput, or most prominent protuberance of the skull. The top of the pinna should meet or cross this line. Low-set ears are commonly associated with renal anomalies or mental retardation. Measure the *angle* of the pinna by drawing a perpendicular line from the imaginary horizontal line and aligning the pinna next to this mark. Normally the pinna lies within a 10-degree angle of the vertical line (Fig. 35-16). If it falls outside this area, record the deviation and look for other anomalies.

ANATOMY REVIEW: LANDMARKS OF THE PINNA

Normally the pinna extends slightly outward from the skull. Except in newborn infants, ears that are flat against the head or protruding away from the scalp may indicate problems. Flattened ears in infants may suggest a frequent side-lying position and, just as with isolated areas of hair loss, may be a clue to investigating parents' understanding of the child's stimulation needs.

Inspect the *skin* surface around the ear for small openings, extra tags of skin, or sinuses. If a sinus is found, note this because it may represent a fistula that drains into some area of the neck or ear. Cutaneous tags represent no pathologic process but may cause parents concern in terms of the child's appearance.

Also assess the ear for *hygiene.* An otoscope is not necessary for looking into the external canal to note the presence of *cerumen,* a waxy substance produced by the ceruminous glands in the outer portion of the canal. Cerumen is usually yellow-brown and soft. If an otoscope is used and any discharge is seen, its color and odor are noted. Prevent transmitting potentially infectious material to the other ear or to another child through handwashing and using disposable specula or sterilizing reusable specula between each examination.

Inspection of Internal Structures

The head of the otoscope permits visualization of the tympanic membrane by use of a bright light, a magnifying glass, and a speculum. Some otoscopes have an attachment for a pneumonic device to insert air into the canal to determine membrane compliance (movement). The speculum, which is inserted into the external canal, comes in a variety of sizes to accommodate different canal widths. The largest speculum that fits comfortably into the ear is used to achieve the greatest area of visualization. The lens, or magnifying glass, is movable, allowing the examiner to insert an object, such as a curette, into the ear canal through the speculum while still viewing the structures through the lens.

Positioning the Child

Before beginning the otoscopic examination, position the child properly and restrain if necessary. Older children usually cooperate and do not need restraint. However, prepare

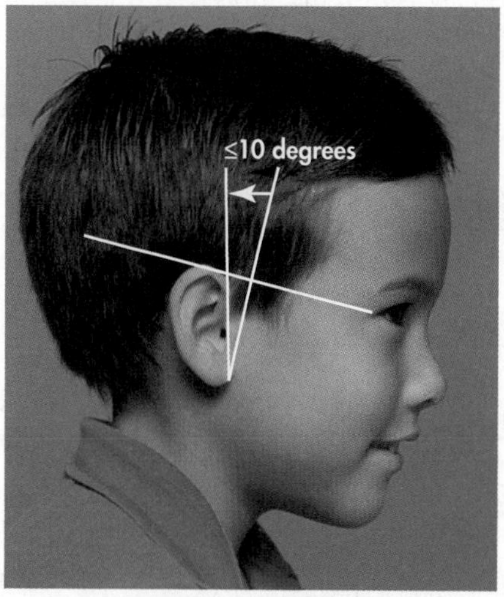

Fig. 35-16 Ear alignment.

them for the procedure by allowing them to play with the instrument, demonstrating how it works, and stressing the importance of remaining still. A helpful suggestion is to let them observe you examining the parent's ear. Restraint is needed for younger children because the ear examination upsets them (Atraumatic Care box).

As you insert the speculum into the meatus, move it around the outer rim to accustom the child to the feel of something entering the ear. If examining a painful ear, touch a nonpainful part of the affected ear, then examine the unaffected ear, and finally return to the painful ear. By this time the child is usually less fearful of anything causing discomfort to the ear and will cooperate more.

For their protection and safety, infants and toddlers must be restrained for the otoscopic examination. There are two general positions of restraint. In one the child is seated sideways in the parent's lap with one arm "hugging" the parent and the other arm at the side. The ear to be examined is toward the nurse. With one arm the parent holds the child's head firmly against his or her chest, and with the other arm "hugs" the child, thereby securing the child's free arm. The ear is examined using the same procedure for holding the otoscope as described later (Fig. 35-17, *A*).

The other position involves placing the child on the side, back, or abdomen with the arms at the side and the head turned so that the ear to be examined points toward the ceiling. Lean over the child and use the upper part of the body to restrain the arms and upper trunk movements, and the examining hand to stabilize the head. This position is practical for young infants or for older children who need minimal restraining, but it may not be feasible for other children who protest vigorously. For safety enlist the parent's or an assistant's help in immobilizing the head by firmly placing one hand above the ear and the other on the child's side, abdomen, or back (Fig. 35-17, *B*).

With cooperative children examine the ear with the child in a side-lying, sitting, or standing position. One disadvantage to standing is that the child may "walk away" as the otoscope enters the canal. If the child is standing or sitting, tilt the head slightly toward the child's opposite shoulder to achieve a better view of the drum (Fig. 35-18).

With the thumb and forefinger of the free (usually nondominant) hand, grasp the auricle. For the two positions of restraint, hold the otoscope upside down at the junction of its head and handle with the thumb and index finger. Place the other fingers against the skull to allow the otoscope to move with the child in case of sudden movement. In examining a cooperative child, hold the handle with the otic head upright or upside down. Use the dominant hand to examine both ears or reverse hands for each ear, whichever is more comfortable.

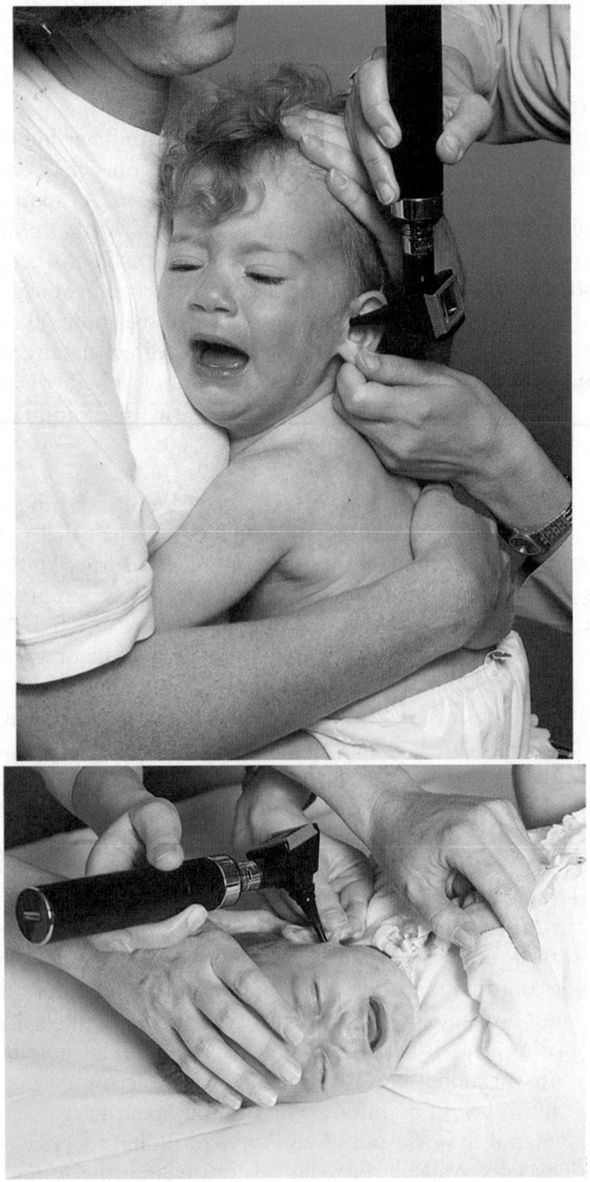

A

B

Fig. 35-17 Position for restraining child, **A**, and infant, **B**, during otoscopic examination.

Before using the otoscope, visualize the external ear and the tympanic membrane as being superimposed on a clock (Fig. 35-19). The numbers become important geographic landmarks. Introduce the speculum into the meatus between the 3 and 9 o'clock positions in a *downward* and *forward* position. Because the canal is curved, the speculum does not permit a panoramic view of the tympanic membrane unless the canal is straightened. In infants the canal curves upward. Therefore pull the pinna *down* and *back* to the 6 to 9 o'clock range to straighten the canal (Fig. 35-20, *A*).

With older children, usually those older than 3 years of age, the canal curves downward and forward. Therefore pull the pinna *up* and *back* toward a 10 o'clock position (Fig.

Atraumatic Care

REDUCING DISTRESS FROM OTOSCOPY IN YOUNG CHILDREN

Make examining the ear a game by explaining that you are looking for a "big elephant" in the ear. This kind of make-believe is an absorbing distraction and usually elicits cooperation. After the ear has been examined, clarify that "looking for elephants" was only pretend and thank the child for letting you look in his or her ear. You can also ask the child to put a finger on the opposite ear to keep the light from getting out, which is a great distraction technique.

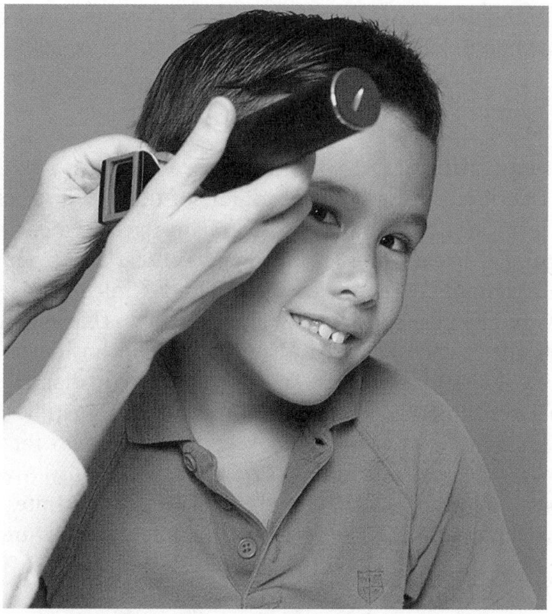

Fig. 35-18 Positioning head by tilting it toward opposite shoulder for full view of tympanic membrane.

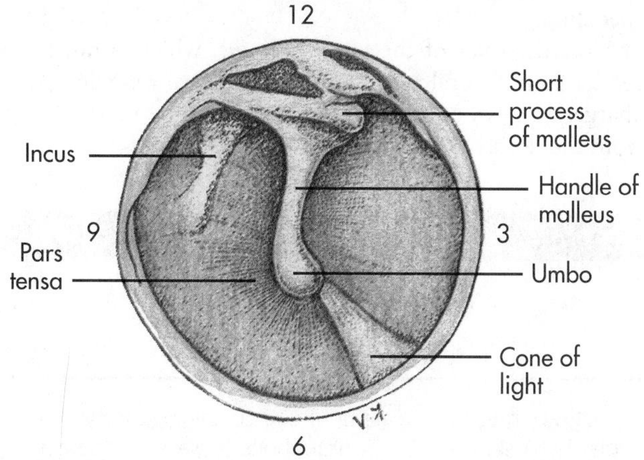

Fig. 35-19 Landmarks of tympanic membrane with "clock" superimposed. (Modified from Potter PA, Perry AG: *Basic nursing: theory and practice,* ed 2, St Louis, 1991, Mosby.)

35-20, *B*). If there is difficulty in visualizing the membrane, try repositioning the head, introducing the speculum at a different angle, and pulling the pinna in a slightly different direction. Do not insert the speculum past the cartilaginous (outermost) portion of the canal, usually a distance of 0.60 to 1.25 cm (0.25 to 0.5 inch) in older children. Insertion of the speculum into the posterior or bony portion of the canal causes pain.

In neonates and young infants the walls of the canal are pliable and floppy because of the underdeveloped cartilaginous and bony structures. Therefore the very small 2 mm speculum usually needs to be inserted deeper into the canal than in older children. Great care must be exercised not to damage the walls or drum. For this reason, only an experienced examiner should insert an otoscope into the ears of very young infants.

Otoscopic Examination

As you introduce the speculum into the external canal, inspect the walls of the canal, the color of the tympanic

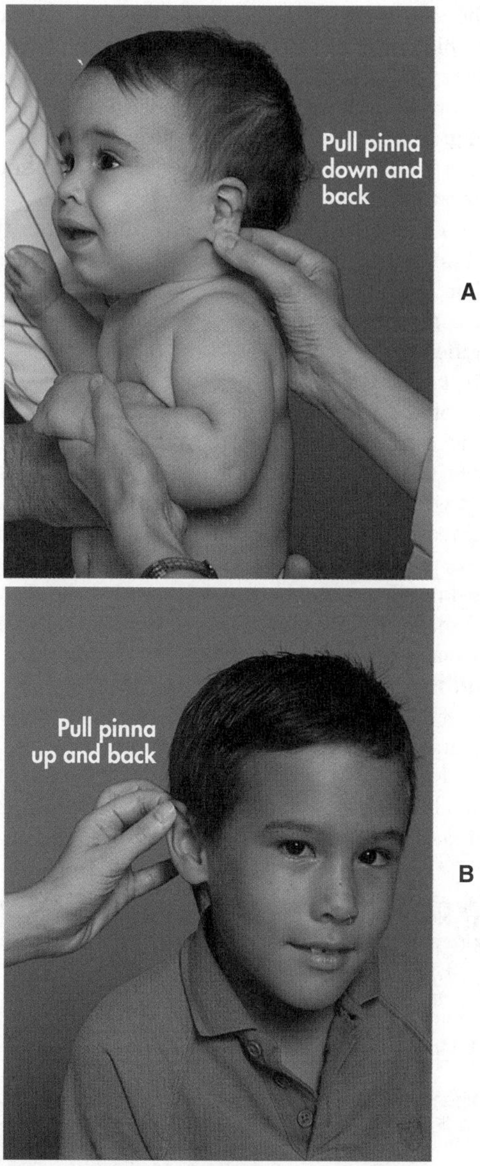

Fig. 35-20 Positioning of eardrum **A,** in infant, and **B,** in child older than 3 years of age.

membrane, the light reflex, and the usual landmarks of the bony prominences of the middle ear.

The *walls* of the external auditory canal are pink, although they are more pigmented in dark-skinned children. Minute hairs are evident in the outermost portion, where cerumen is produced. Note signs of irritation, foreign bodies, or infection.

Foreign bodies in the ear are not uncommon in children and range from erasers to beans. Symptoms may include pain, discharge, and affected hearing. Soft objects, such as paper or insects, can be removed with forceps. Small, hard objects, such as pebbles, can be removed with a suction tip, a hook, or irrigation. However, irrigation is contraindicated if the object is vegetative matter, such as beans or pasta, which swells when in contact with fluid.

NURSE ALERT If there is any doubt about the type of object in the ear and the appropriate method to remove it, refer the child to the appropriate practitioner. ■

The *color* of the *tympanic membrane* is a translucent, light pearly pink or gray. Note marked erythema (which may indicate suppurative otitis media), a dull nontransparent grayish color (sometimes suggestive of serous otitis media), or ashen gray areas (signs of scarring from a previous perforation). A black area usually suggests a perforation of the membrane that has not healed.

The characteristic tenseness and slope of the tympanic membrane cause the light of the otoscope to reflect at about the 5 or 7 o'clock position. The *light reflex* is a fairly well defined cone-shaped reflection, which normally points away from the face.

The *bony landmarks* of the drum are formed by the *umbo,* or tip of the malleus bone. It appears as a small, round, opaque concave spot near the center of the drum. The *manubrium* (long process or handle) of the malleus appears to be a whitish line extending from the umbo upward to the margin of the membrane. At the upper end of the long process near the 1 o'clock position (in the right ear) is a sharp, knoblike protuberance, representing the *short* process of the malleus. Note the absence of the light reflex or loss or abnormal prominence of any of these landmarks.

Auditory Testing

Several types of hearing tests are available (Table 35-10). The nurse must operate under a high index of suspicion for those children who may have conditions associated with hearing loss and who may have developed behaviors that indicate auditory impairment (AAP, Committee on Practice and Ambulatory Medicine, Section on Otolaryngology and Bronchoesophagology, 2003; Cunningham & Cox, 2003).

Nose

Inspection of External Structures

The nose is located in the middle of the face just below the eyes and above the lips. Compare its placement and alignment by drawing an imaginary vertical line from the center point between the eyes down to the notch of the upper lip. The nose should lie exactly vertical to this line, with each side exactly symmetric. Note its location, any deviation to one side, and asymmetry in overall size and in diameter of the nares (nostrils). The *bridge* of the nose is sometimes flat in Asian and black children. Observe the *alae nasi* for any sign of flaring, which indicates respiratory difficulty. Always report any flaring of the alae nasi. Fig. 35-21 illustrates the usual landmarks used in describing the external structures of the nose.

Inspection of Internal Structures

Inspect the *anterior vestibule* of the nose by pushing the tip upward, tilting the head backward, and illuminating the cavity with a flashlight or otoscope without the attached ear speculum.

Note the *color* of the *mucosal lining,* which is normally redder than the oral membranes, as well as any swelling, discharge, dryness, or bleeding. There should be no discharge from the nose.

Anatomy Review: External and Internal Structures of the Nose

Table 35-10

Audiologic Tests for Infants and Children

AGE OF CHILD	AUDITORY TEST/AVERAGE TIME	TYPE OF MEASUREMENT	PROCEDURE
All ages	Evoked otoacoustic emissions, 10-minute test	Physiologic test specifically measuring cochlear (outer hair cell) response to presentation of a stimulus	Small probe containing a sensitive microphone is placed in the ear canal for stimulus delivery and response detection
Birth-9 mo	Auditory brainstem response, 15-minute test	Electrophysiologic measurement of activity in auditory nerve and brainstem pathways	Placement of electrodes on child's head detects auditory stimuli presented though earphones one ear at a time
9 mo-2.5 yr	Conditioned oriented responses or visual reinforced audiometry, 30-minute test	Behavioral tests measuring responses of the child to speech and frequency-specific stimuli presented through speakers	Both techniques condition the child to associate speech or frequency-specific sound with a reinforcement stimulus, such as a lighted toy
2.5-4 yr	Play audiometry, 30-minute test	Behavioral test measuring auditory thresholds in response to speech and frequency-specific stimuli presented through earphones or bone vibrator (or both)	Child is conditioned to put a peg in a peg board or drop a block in a box when stimulus tone is heard
4 yr-adolescence	Conventional audiometry, 30-minute test	Behavioral test measuring auditory thresholds in response to speech and frequency-specific stimuli presented through earphone or bone vibrator (or both)	Patient is instructed to raise his or her hand when stimulus is heard

Adapted with permission from Bachmann KR, Arvedson JC: Early identification and intervention for children who are hearing impaired, *Pediatr Rev* 19:155-165, 1998.

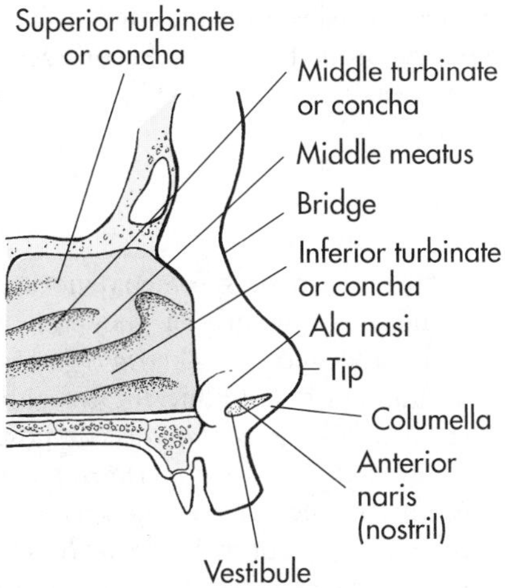

Fig. 35-21 External landmarks and internal structures of nose.

On looking deeper into the nose, inspect the *turbinates* or *concha,* plates of bone that jut into the nasal cavity and are enveloped by mucous membrane. The turbinates greatly increase the surface area of the nasal cavity as air is inhaled. The spaces or channels between the turbinates are called *meatus* and correspond to each of the three turbinates. Normally the front end of the inferior and middle turbinate and the middle meatus are seen. They should be the same color as the lining of the vestibule.

Inspect the *septum,* which should divide the vestibules equally. Note any deviation, especially if it causes an occlusion of one side of the nose. A perforation may be evident within the septum. If this is suspected, shine the light of the otoscope into one naris and look for admittance of light. Because olfaction is an important function of the nose, testing for smell may be done at this point or as part of cranial nerve assessment (see Table 35-11).

Mouth and Throat

With a cooperative child, almost the entire examination of the mouth and throat can be accomplished without the use of a tongue blade. Ask the child to open the mouth wide, to move the tongue in different directions for full visualization, and to say "ahh," which depresses the tongue for full view of the back of the mouth (tonsils, uvula, and oropharynx). For a closer look at the buccal mucosa, or lining of the cheeks, ask children to use their fingers to move the outer lip and cheek to one side (Atraumatic Care box).

Infants and toddlers, however, usually resist attempts to keep the mouth open. Because inspecting the mouth is an upsetting part of the examination, leave it for the end of the physical examination (along with examination of the ears) or do it during episodes of crying. However, the use of a tongue blade (preferably flavored) to depress the tongue is necessary. Place the tongue blade along the *side* of the tongue, not in the center back area where the gag reflex is elicited. Fig. 35-22, *B,* illustrates proper positioning of the child for the oral examination.

The major structure of the exterior of the mouth is the *lips.* The lips should be moist, soft, smooth, and pink, the color of a deeper hue than the surrounding skin. The lips should be symmetric when relaxed or tensed. Assess symmetry when the child talks or cries.

Atraumatic Care

ENCOURAGING OPENING THE MOUTH FOR EXAMINATION

Perform the examination in front of a mirror.
Let child first examine someone else's mouth, such as the parent, the nurse, or a puppet (Fig. 35-22, *A*) and then examine child's mouth.
Instruct child to tilt the head back slightly, breathe deeply through the mouth, and hold the breath; this action lowers the tongue to the floor of the mouth without the use of a tongue blade.
Lightly brushing the palate with a cotton swab also may open the mouth for assessment.

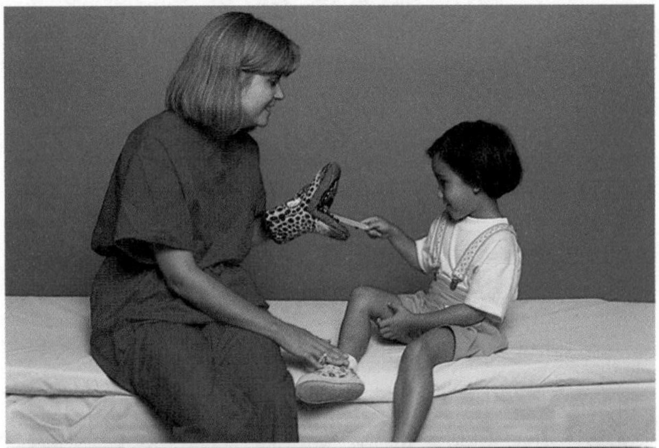

A

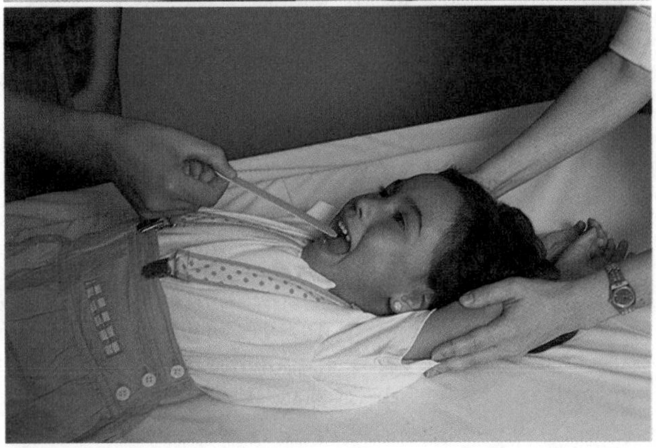

B

Fig. 35-22 **A,** Encouraging child to cooperate. **B,** Positioning child for examination of mouth.

Inspection of Internal Structures

The major structures that are visible within the oral cavity and oropharynx are the mucosal lining of the lips and cheeks, gums or gingiva, teeth, tongue, palate, uvula, tonsils, and posterior oropharynx (Fig. 35-23). Inspect all areas lined with *mucous membranes* (inside the lips and cheeks, gingiva, underside of the tongue, palate, and back of the pharynx) for color, any areas of white patches or ulceration, bleeding, sensitivity, and moisture. The membranes should be bright pink, smooth, glistening, uniform, and moist.

Inspect the *teeth* for number in each dental arch, for hygiene, and for occlusion or bite. Discoloration of tooth

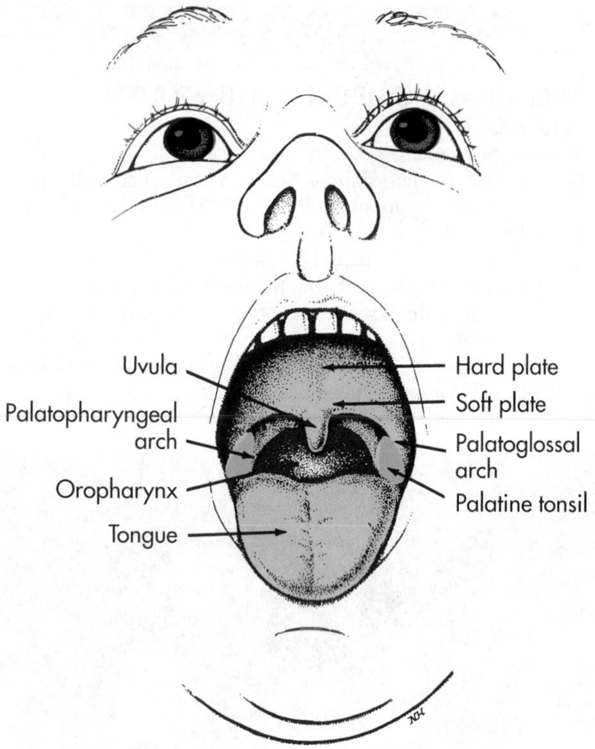

Fig. 35-23 Interior structures of mouth.

enamel with obvious plaque (whitish coating on the surface of the teeth) is a sign of poor dental hygiene and indicates a need for counseling. Brown spots in the crevices of the crown of the tooth or between the teeth may be caries (cavities). Chalky white to yellow or brown areas on the enamel may indicate fluorosis (excessive fluoride ingestion). Teeth that appear greenish black may be stained temporarily from ingestion of supplemental iron.

Examine the *gums (gingiva)* surrounding the teeth. The color is normally coral pink, and the surface texture is stippled, similar to the appearance of orange peel. In dark-skinned children, the gums are more deeply colored, and a brownish area is often observed along the gum line.

Inspect the *tongue* for the presence of papillae, small projections that contain several taste buds and give the tongue its characteristic rough appearance. Note the size and mobility of the tongue. Normally the tip of the tongue should extend to the lips or beyond.

The roof of the mouth consists of the *hard palate,* which is located near the front of the oral cavity, and the *soft palate,* which is located toward the back of the pharynx and which has a small midline protrusion called the *uvula.* Carefully inspect the palates to be sure that they are intact. The arch of the palate should be dome shaped. A narrow, flat roof or a high, arched palate affects the placement of the tongue and can cause feeding and speech problems. Test movement of the uvula by eliciting a gag reflex. It should move upward to close off the nasopharynx from the oropharynx.

Examine the oropharynx and note the size and color of the *palatine tonsils.* They are normally the same color as the surrounding mucosa; glandular, rather than smooth in appearance; and barely visible over the edge of the palatoglossal arches. The size of the tonsils varies considerably during childhood. However, report any swelling, redness, or white areas on the tonsils.

Chest

Anatomy Review: Rib Cage

Inspect the *chest* for size, shape, symmetry, movement, breast development, and the presence of the bony landmarks formed by the ribs and sternum. The *rib cage* consists of 12 ribs and the sternum, or breast bone, located in the midline of the trunk (Fig. 35-24). The *sternum* is composed of three main parts. The *manubrium,* the uppermost portion, can be felt at the base of the neck at the *suprasternal notch.* The largest segment of the sternum is the *body,* which forms the *sternal angle (angle of Louis)* as it articulates with the manubrium. At the end of the body is a small, movable process called the *xiphoid.* The angle of the costal margin as it attaches to the sternum is called the *costal angle* and is normally about 45 to 50 degrees. These bony structures are important landmarks in the location of ribs and intercostal spaces.

Intercostal spaces (ICSs) are the spaces between the ribs. They are numbered according to the rib directly *above* the space. For example, the space immediately below the second rib is the second ICS.

Anatomy Review: Imaginary Landmarks of the Chest

The *thoracic cavity* is also divided into segments by drawing imaginary lines on the chest and back. Fig. 35-25 illustrates the anterior, lateral, and posterior divisions.

Measure the *size* of the chest by placing the measuring tape around the rib cage at the nipple line (see Fig. 35-4). For greatest accuracy, take two measurements—one during inspiration and the other during expiration—and record the average. Chest size is important, mainly in comparison with its relationship to head circumference, which is discussed on p. 989. Always report marked disproportions because most are caused by abnormal head growth, although some may be a result of altered chest shape, such as *barrel chest* (chest is round) or *pigeon chest* (sternum protrudes outward).

During infancy the *shape* of the chest is almost circular, with the anteroposterior (front-to-back) diameter equaling the transverse, or lateral (side-to-side), diameter. As the child grows, the chest normally increases in the transverse direction, causing the anteroposterior diameter to be less than the lateral diameter. Note the *angle* made by the lower costal margin and the sternum, and palpate the junction of the ribs with the costal cartilage (costochondral junction) and sternum, which should be fairly smooth.

Movement of the chest wall should be symmetric bilaterally and coordinated with breathing. During inspiration the chest rises and expands, the diaphragm descends, and the costal angle increases. During expiration the chest falls and decreases in size, the diaphragm rises, and the costal angle narrows (Fig. 35-26). In children younger than 6 or 7 years of age, respiratory movement is principally abdominal or diaphragmatic. In older children, particularly girls, respirations are chiefly thoracic. In either type, the chest and abdomen should rise and fall together. Always report any asymmetry of movement.

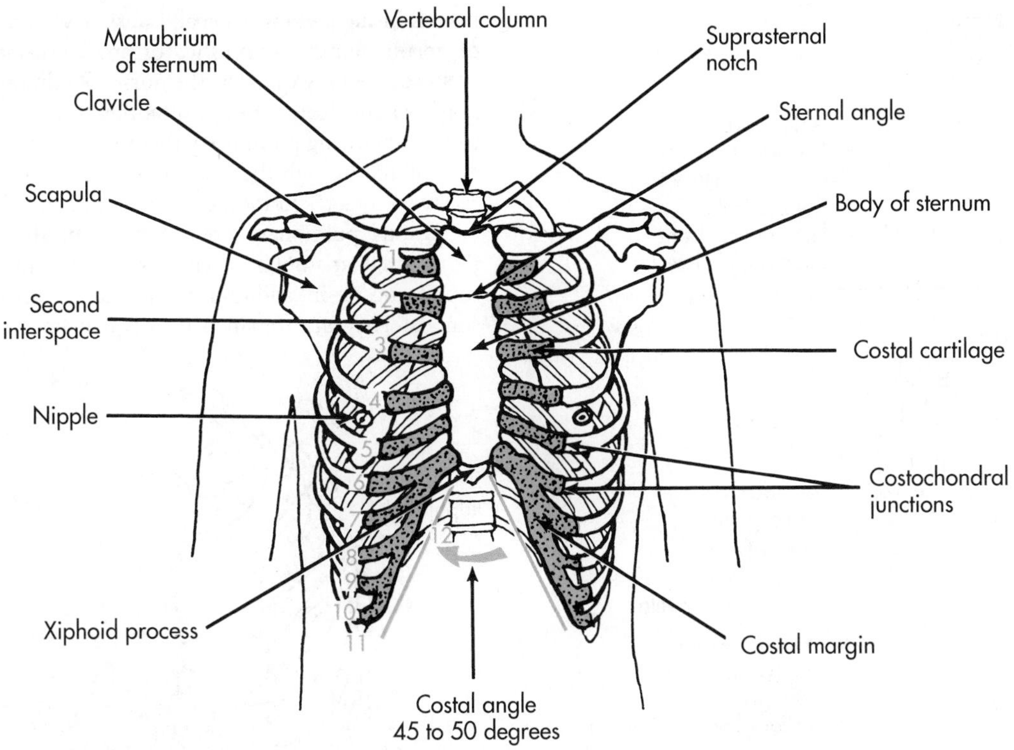

Fig. 35-24 Rib cage.

While inspecting the skin surface of the chest, observe the position of the *nipples,* as well as any evidence of *breast development.* Normally the nipples are located slightly lateral to the midclavicular line between the fourth and fifth ribs. Note symmetry of nipple placement and normal configuration of a darker pigmented areola surrounding a flat nipple in the prepubertal child.

Pubertal breast development usually begins in girls between 10 and 14 years of age. Record early (precocious) or delayed breast development, as well as evidence of any other secondary sexual characteristics. In males, *breast enlargement (gynecomastia)* may be caused by hormonal or systemic disorders, but more commonly it is a result of adipose tissue from obesity or a transitory body change during early puberty. In either situation investigate the child's feelings regarding breast enlargement.

In adolescent females who have achieved sexual maturity, palpate the breasts for evidence of any masses or hard nodules. Use this opportunity to discuss the importance of routine breast self-examination. Emphasize that most palpable masses are benign to decrease any fear or concern that results when a mass is felt.

Lungs

The *lungs* are situated inside the thoracic cavity, with one lung on each side of the sternum. Each lung is divided into an *apex,* which is slightly pointed and rises above the first rib; a *base,* which is wide and concave and rides on the dome-shaped diaphragm; and a body, which is divided into *lobes.* The right lung has three lobes: the upper, middle, and lower. The left lung has only two lobes, the upper and lower, because of the space occupied by the heart (Fig. 35-27).

Inspection of the lungs primarily involves observation of respiratory movements, which were discussed previously. Evaluate respirations for rate (number per minute), rhythm (regular, irregular, or periodic), depth (deep or shallow), and quality (effortless, automatic, difficult, or labored). Note the character of breath sounds, such as noisy, grunting, snoring, or heavy.

Evaluate respiratory movements by placing each hand flat against the back or chest with the thumbs in midline along the lower costal margin of the lungs. The child should be sitting during this procedure and, if cooperative, should take several deep breaths. During respiration your hands will move with the chest wall. Assess the amount and speed of respiratory excursion and note any asymmetry of movement.

Experienced examiners may percuss the lungs. The anterior lung is percussed from apex to base, usually with the child in the supine or sitting position. Each side of the chest is percussed in sequence to compare the sounds. When the posterior lung is percussed, the procedure and sequence are the same, although the child should be sitting. Resonance is heard over all the lobes of the lungs that are not adjacent to other organs. Any deviation from the expected sound is recorded and reported.

Auscultation

Auscultation involves using the stethoscope to evaluate breath sounds (Guidelines box). Breath sounds are best heard if the child inspires deeply (Atraumatic Care box). In the lungs, breath sounds are classified as vesicular, bronchovesicular, or bronchial (Box 35-3).

Absent or *diminished breath sounds* are always an abnormal finding warranting investigation. Fluid, air, or solid

ANATOMY REVIEW: PERCUSSION SOUNDS IN THORAX

masses in the pleural space all interfere with the conduction of breath sounds. Diminished breath sounds in certain segments of the lung can alert the nurse to pulmonary areas that may benefit from chest physiotherapy. Increased breath sounds following pulmonary therapy indicate improved passage of air through the respiratory tract. Terms used to describe various respiration patterns are defined in Box 35-4.

Various pulmonary abnormalities produce *adventitious sounds* that are not normally heard over the chest. These sounds occur in addition to normal or abnormal breath sounds. They are classified into two main groups: *crackles,*

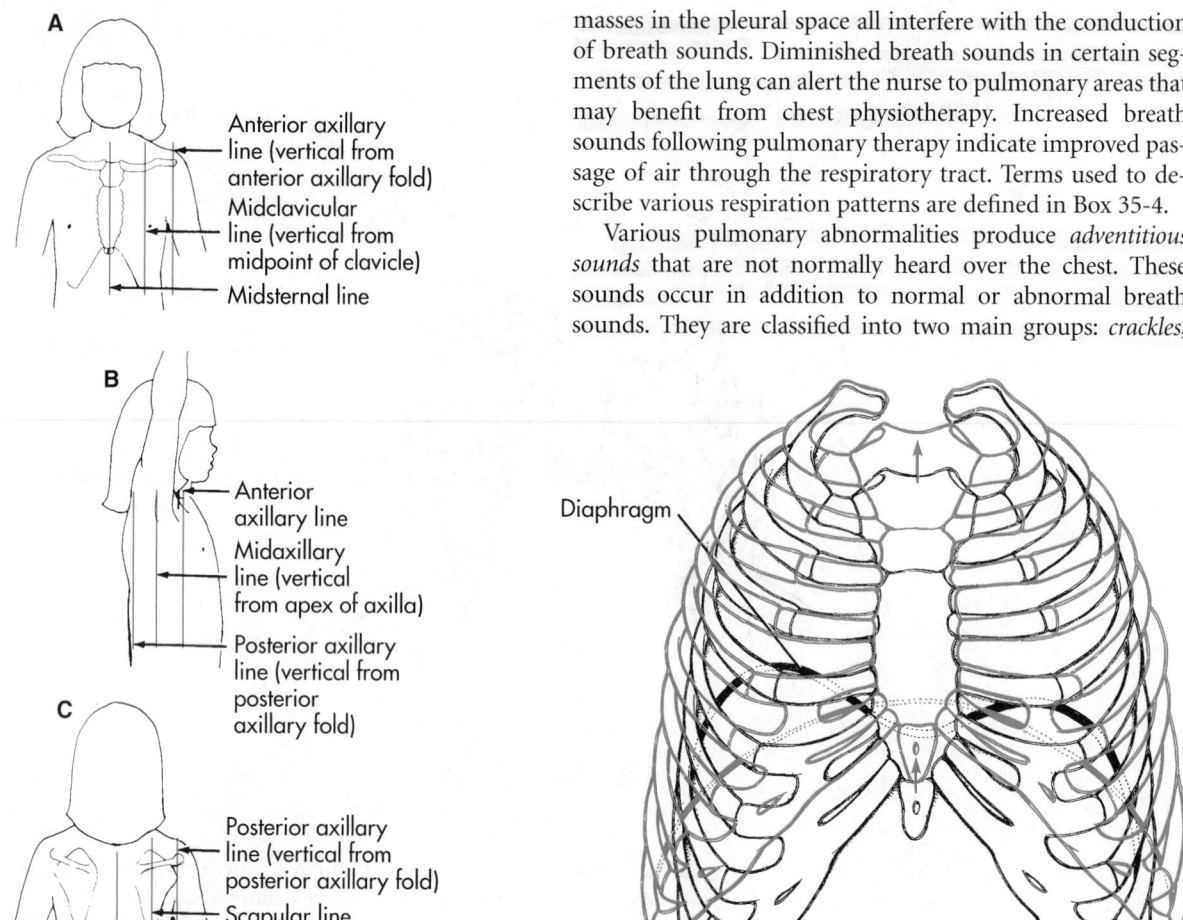

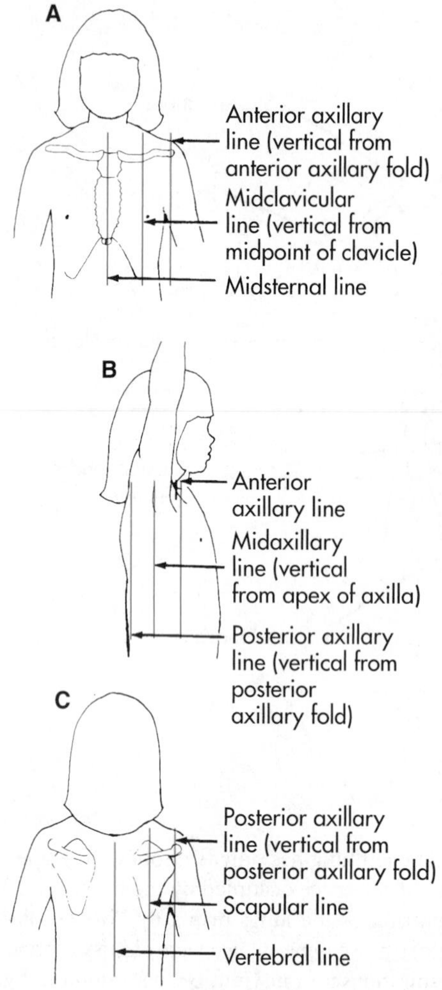

Fig. 35-25 Imaginary landmarks of chest. **A,** Anterior. **B,** Right lateral. **C,** Posterior.

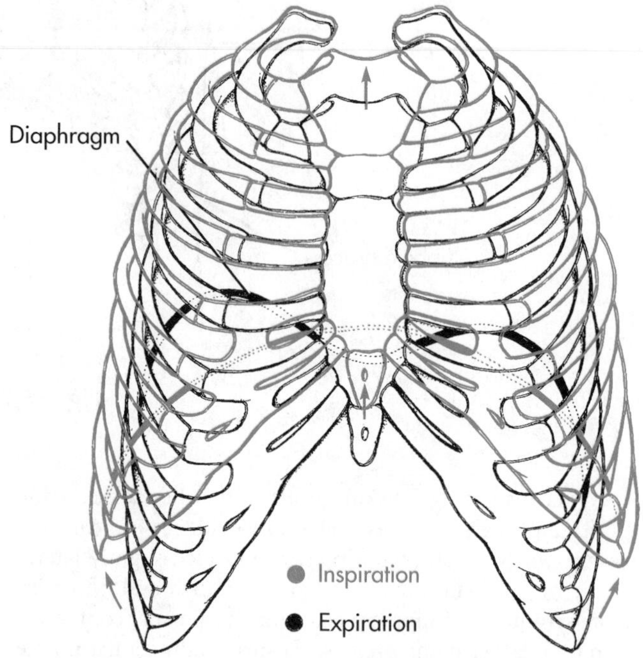

Fig. 35-26 Movement of chest during respiration.

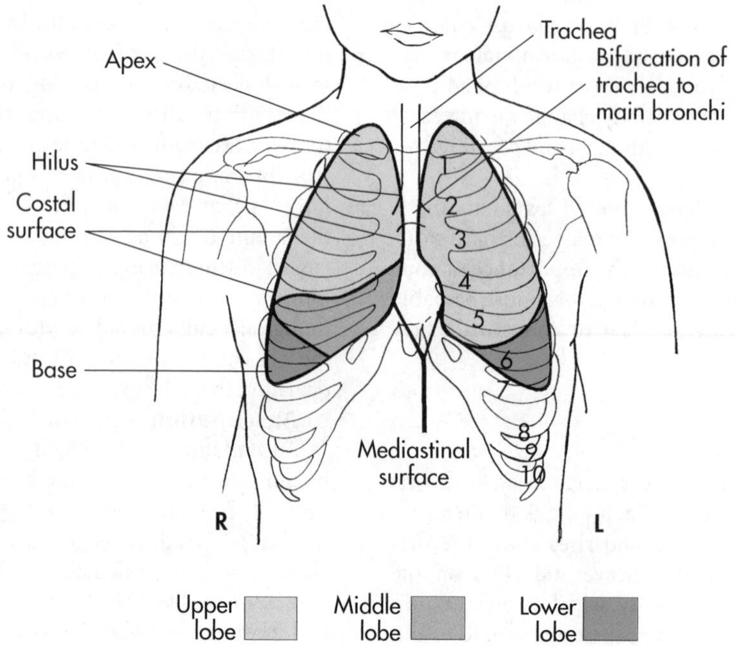

Fig. 35-27 Location of lobes of lungs within thoracic cavity.

which result from the passage of air through fluid or moisture, and *wheezes,* which are produced as air passes through narrowed passageways, regardless of the cause, such as exudate, inflammation, spasm, or tumor. Considerable practice with an experienced tutor is necessary to differentiate the various types of lung sounds. Often it is best to describe the type of sound heard in the lungs rather than trying to label it. Always report any abnormal sounds for further medical evaluation.

Heart

The heart is situated in the thoracic cavity between the lungs in the mediastinum and above the diaphragm (Fig. 35-28).

Guidelines

EFFECTIVE AUSCULTATION

Make sure child is relaxed and not crying, talking, or laughing. Record if child is crying.
Check that room is comfortable and quiet.
Warm stethoscope before placing it against skin.
Apply firm pressure on chestpiece but not enough to prevent vibrations and transmission of sound.
Avoid placing stethoscope over hair or clothing, moving it against skin, breathing on tubing, or sliding fingers over chestpiece, which may cause sounds that falsely resemble pathologic findings.
Use a symmetric and orderly approach to compare sounds.

Atraumatic Care

ENCOURAGING DEEP BREATHS

Ask child to "blow out" the light on an otoscope or pocket flashlight; discreetly turn off the light on the last try so that the child feels successful.
Place a cotton ball in child's palm; ask child to blow the ball into the air and have parent catch it.
Place a small tissue on the top of a pencil and ask child to blow the tissue off.
Have child blow a pinwheel, a party horn, or bubbles.

BOX 35-3

Classification of Normal Breath Sounds

Vesicular Breath Sounds
Heard over entire surface of lungs, with exception of upper intrascapular area and area beneath manubrium.
Inspiration is louder, longer, and higher pitched than expiration.
Sound is soft, swishing noise.

Bronchovesicular Breath Sounds
Heard over manubrium and in upper intrascapular regions where trachea and bronchi bifurcate.
Inspiration is louder and higher in pitch than in vesicular breathing.

Bronchial Breath Sounds
Heard only over trachea near suprasternal notch.
Inspiratory phase is short, and expiratory phase is long.

BOX 35-4

Various Patterns of Respiration

Tachypnea—Increased rate
Bradypnea—Decreased rate
Dyspnea—Distress during breathing
Apnea—Cessation of breathing
Hyperpnea—Increased depth
Hypoventilation—Decreased depth (shallow) and irregular rhythm
Hyperventilation—Increased rate and depth
Kussmaul breathing—Hyperventilation, gasping and labored respiration, usually seen in diabetic coma or other states of respiratory acidosis
Cheyne-Stokes respirations—Gradually increasing rate and depth with periods of apnea
Biot breathing—Periods of hyperpnea alternating with apnea (similar to Cheyne-Stokes except that depth remains constant)
Seesaw (paradoxic) respirations—Chest falls on inspiration and rises on expiration
Agonal—Last gasping breaths before death

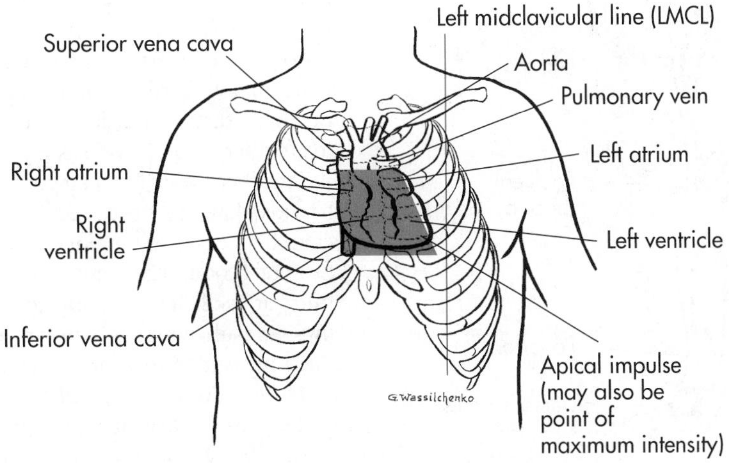

Fig. 35-28 Position of heart within thorax.

About two thirds of the heart lies within the left side of the rib cage, with the other third on the right side as it crosses the sternum. The heart is positioned in the thorax like a trapezoid:

Vertically along the right sternal border (RSB) from the second to the fifth rib

Horizontally (long side) from the lower right sternum to the fifth rib at the left midclavicular line (LMCL)

Diagonally from the left sternal border (LSB) at the second rib to the LMCL at the fifth rib

Horizontally (short side) from the RSB and LSB at the second ICS—base of the heart

Inspection is best done with the child sitting in a semi-Fowler position. Look at the anterior chest wall from an angle, comparing both sides of the rib cage with each other. Normally they should be symmetric. In children with thin chest walls, a pulsation may be visible. Because comprehensive evaluation of cardiac function is not limited to the heart, also consider other findings such as the presence of all pulses (especially the femoral pulses) (Fig. 35-29), distended neck veins, clubbing of the fingers, peripheral cyanosis, edema, blood pressure, and respiratory status.

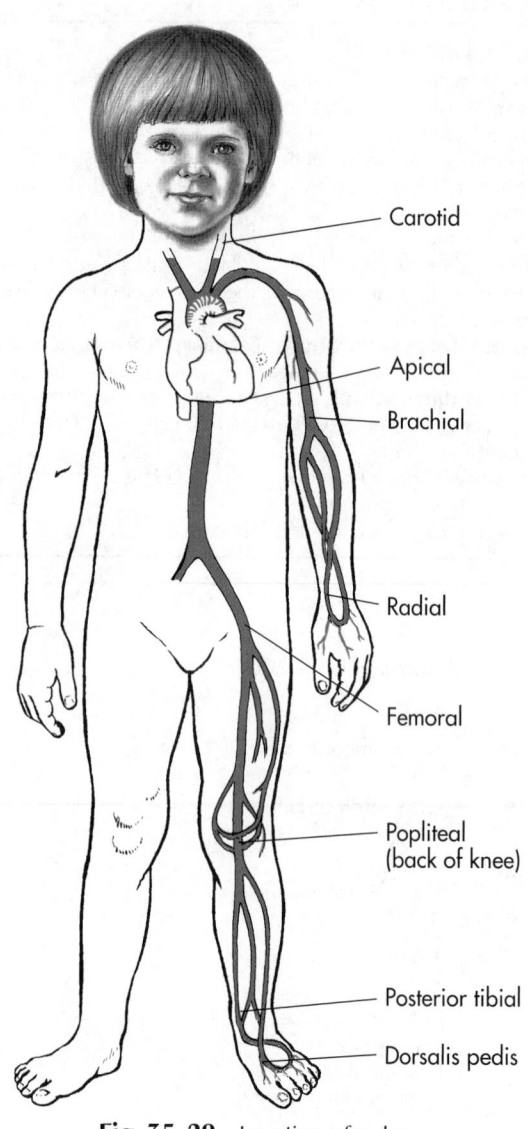

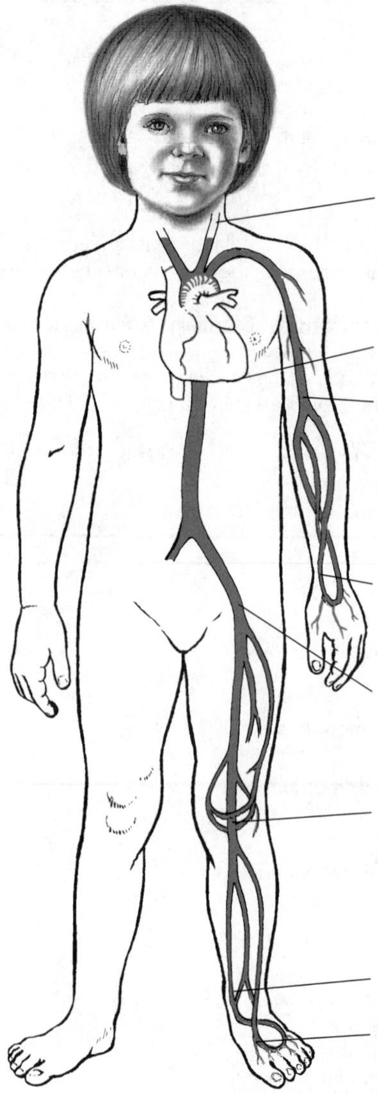

Fig. 35-29 Location of pulses.

Use palpation to determine the location of the *apical impulse (AI)*, the most lateral cardiac impulse that may correspond to the apex. The AI is found

- Just lateral to the left MCL and fourth ICS in children younger than 7 years of age
- At the left MCL and fifth ICS in children 7 years of age and older

Although the AI gives a general idea of the size of the heart (with enlargement, the apex is lower and more lateral), its normal location is quite variable, making it an unreliable indicator of heart size.

The *point of maximum impulse (PMI)*, as the name implies, is the area of most intense pulsation. Usually the PMI is located at the same site as the AI, but it can occur elsewhere. For this reason, the two terms should not be used synonymously.

Assess *capillary filling time*, an important test for peripheral circulation, by pressing the skin lightly on a central site, such as the forehead, or a peripheral site, such as the top of the hand, to produce a slight blanching. The time it takes for the blanched area to return to its original color is the *capillary refill time.*

NURSE ALERT Capillary refill should be brisk–in less than 2 seconds; prolonged refill may be associated with poor systemic perfusion, as well as a cool ambient temperature. ■

Auscultation

Origin of Heart Sounds

The heart sounds are produced by the opening and closing of the valves and the vibration of blood against the walls of the heart and vessels. Normally two sounds—S_1 and S_2—are heard, which correspond, respectively, to the familiar "lubb" and "dubb" often used to describe the sounds. S_1 is caused by closure of the *tricuspid* and *mitral valves* (sometimes called the *atrioventricular valves*). S_2 is the result of closure of the *pulmonic* and *aortic valves* (sometimes called *semilunar valves*). Normally the split of the two sounds in S_2 is distinguishable and widens during inspiration. *Physiologic splitting* is a significant normal finding.

NURSE ALERT "Fixed splitting," in which the split in S_2 does not change during inspiration, is an important diagnostic sign of atrial septal defect. ■

Two other heart sounds—S_3 and S_4—may be produced. S_3 is normally heard in some children. S_4 is rarely heard as a normal heart sound; if heard, it usually indicates the need for further cardiac evaluation.

Another important category of heart sounds is *murmurs,* sounds that are produced by vibrations within the heart chambers or in the major arteries from the back-and-forth flow of blood. The description and classification of murmurs are skills that require considerable practice and training. Consult with an experienced practitioner whenever a murmur is identified or suspected.

Differentiating Normal Heart Sounds

Fig. 35-30 illustrates the approximate anatomic position of the valves within the heart chambers. Note that the anatomic location of valves does not correspond to the area

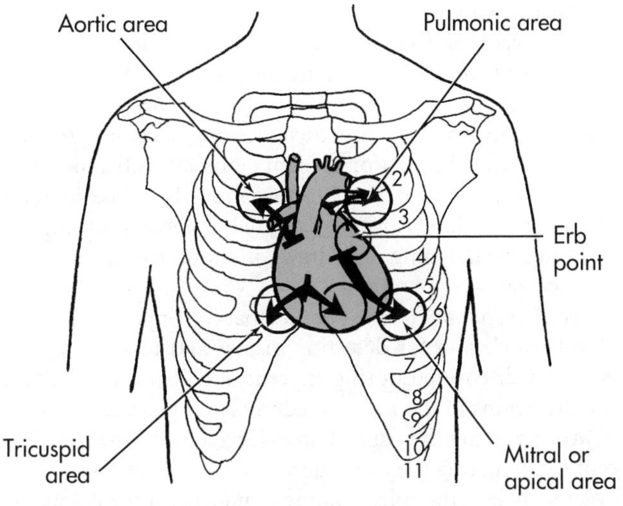

Fig. 35-30 Direction of heart sounds for anatomic valve sites and areas *(circled)* for auscultation.

where the sounds are heard best. The auscultatory sites are located in the direction of the blood flow through the valves.

Normally S_1 is louder at the apex of the heart in the mitral and tricuspid area, and S_2 is louder near the base of the heart in the pulmonic and aortic area. Listen to each sound by inching down the chest. The following areas should also be auscultated for sounds, such as murmurs, which may radiate to these sites: sternoclavicular area above the clavicles and manubrium, area along the sternal border, area along the left midaxillary line, and area below the scapulae.

NURSE ALERT To distinguish between S_1 and S_2 heart sounds, simultaneously palpate the carotid pulse with the index and middle fingers and listen to the heart sounds; S_1 is synchronous with the carotid pulse. ■

Auscultate the heart with the child in at least two positions: sitting and reclining. If adventitious sounds are detected, further evaluate them with the child standing, sitting and leaning forward, and lying on the left side. For example, atrial sounds such as S_4 are heard best with the person in a recumbent position and usually fade if the person sits or stands.

Evaluate heart sounds for (1) *quality* (should be clear and distinct, not muffled, diffuse, or distant); (2) *intensity*, especially in relation to the location or auscultatory site (should not be weak or pounding); (3) *rate* (should be the same as the radial pulse); and (4) *rhythm* (should be regular and even). A particular arrhythmia that occurs normally in many children is *sinus arrhythmia*, in which the heart rate increases with inspiration and decreases with expiration. Differentiate this rhythm from a truly abnormal arrhythmia by having children hold their breath. In sinus arrhythmia, cessation of breathing causes the heart rate to remain steady.

Abdomen

Examination of the abdomen involves inspection, followed by auscultation and then palpation. Perform palpation last because it may distort the normal abdominal sounds. Knowledge of the anatomic placement of the abdominal organs is essential to differentiate normal, expected findings from abnormal ones (Fig. 35-31).

For descriptive purposes the abdominal cavity is divided into four quadrants by drawing a vertical line midway from the sternum to the pubic symphysis and a horizontal line across the abdomen through the umbilicus. Each section is named as follows:

- Left upper quadrant
- Left lower quadrant
- Right upper quadrant
- Right lower quadrant

Inspection

Inspect the *contour* of the abdomen with the child erect and supine. Normally the abdomen of infants and young children is quite cylindric and, in the erect position, fairly prominent because of the physiologic lordosis of the spine. In the supine position the abdomen appears flat. A midline protrusion from the xiphoid to the umbilicus or pubic symphysis is usually *diastasis recti*, or failure of the rectus abdominis muscles to join in utero. In a healthy child a midline protrusion is usually a variation of normal muscular development.

NURSE ALERT A tense, boardlike abdomen is a serious sign of paralytic ileus and intestinal obstruction. ■

The *skin* covering the abdomen should be uniformly taut, without wrinkles or creases. Sometimes silvery, whitish striae ("stretch marks") are seen, especially if the skin has been stretched as in obesity. Superficial veins are usually visible in light-skinned, thin infants, but distended veins are an abnormal finding.

Observe *movement* of the abdomen. Normally chest and abdominal movements are synchronous. In infants and thin children *peristaltic waves* may be visible through the abdominal wall; they are best observed by standing at eye level to and across from the abdomen. Always report this finding.

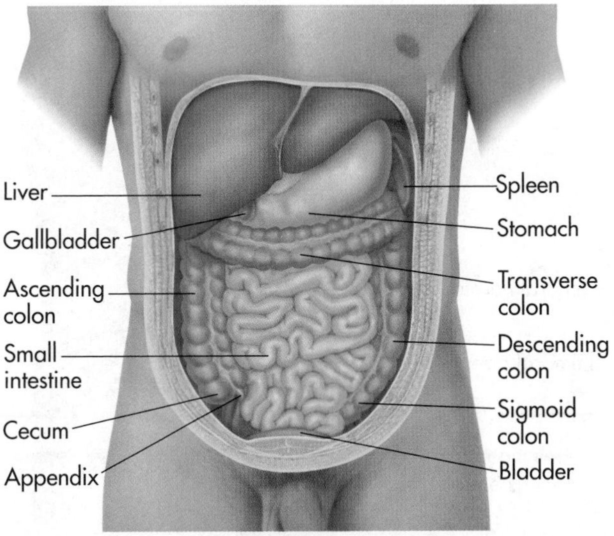

Fig. 35-31 Location of structures in abdomen. (From Seidel HM et al: *Mosby's guide to physical examination*, ed 5, St Louis, 2003, Mosby.)

Examine the *umbilicus* for size, hygiene, and evidence of any abnormalities, such as hernias. The umbilicus should be flat or only slightly protruding. If a herniation is present, palpate the sac for abdominal contents and estimate the approximate size of the opening. *Umbilical hernias* are common in infants, especially in black children.

Hernias may exist elsewhere on the abdominal wall (Fig. 35-32). An *inguinal hernia* is a protrusion of peritoneum through the abdominal wall in the inguinal canal. It occurs mostly in males, is frequently bilateral, and may be visible as a mass in the scrotum. To locate a hernia, slide the little finger into the external inguinal ring at the base of the scrotum and ask the child to cough. If a hernia is present, it will hit the tip of the finger.

NURSE ALERT If the child is too young to cough, have the child blow up a balloon or laugh to raise the intraabdominal pressure sufficiently to demonstrate the presence of an inguinal hernia. ■

A *femoral hernia,* which occurs more frequently in girls, is felt or seen as a small mass on the anterior surface of the thigh just below the inguinal ligament in the femoral canal (a potential space medial to the femoral artery). Feel for a hernia by placing the index finger of your right hand on the child's right femoral pulse (left hand for left pulse) and the middle ring finger flat against the skin toward the midline. The ring finger lies over the femoral canal, where the herniation occurs. Palpation of hernias in the pelvic region is often part of the examination of genitalia.

Auscultation

The most important finding to listen for is *peristalsis,* or *bowel sounds,* which sound like short metallic clicks and gurgles. Their frequency per minute should be recorded (e.g., 5 sounds/min). Bowel sounds may be stimulated by stroking the abdominal surface with a fingernail. Report absence of bowel sounds or hyperperistalsis because either usually denotes an abdominal disorder.

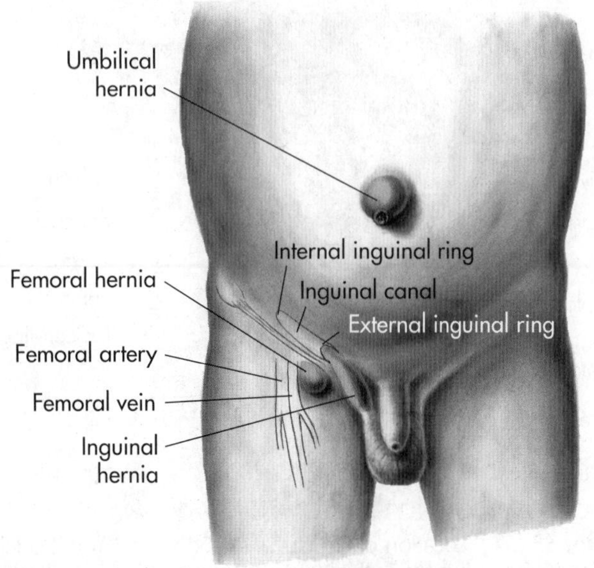

Fig. 35-32 Location of hernias.

Palpation

Two types of palpation are performed: superficial and deep. In *superficial palpation,* lightly place your hand against the skin and feel each quadrant, noting any areas of tenderness, muscle tone, and superficial lesions, such as cysts. Because superficial palpation is often perceived as tickling, several techniques can be used to minimize this sensation and provide relaxation (Atraumatic Care box). Admonishing the child to stop laughing only draws attention to the sensation and decreases cooperation.

Deep palpation is used for palpating organs and large blood vessels and for detecting masses and tenderness that were not discovered during superficial palpation. Palpation usually begins in the lower quadrants and proceeds upward to avoid missing the edge of an enlarged liver or spleen. Except for palpating the liver, successful identification of other organs, such as the spleen, kidney, and part of the colon, requires considerable practice with tutored supervision. Report any questionable mass.

The lower edge of the *liver* is sometimes felt in infants and young children as a superficial mass 1 to 2 cm (0.4 to 0.8 inch) below the right costal margin (the distance is sometimes measured in fingerbreadths). Normally, the liver descends during inspiration as the diaphragm moves downward. Do not mistake this downward displacement as a sign of liver enlargement.

NURSE ALERT If the liver is palpable 3 cm below the right costal margin or the spleen is palpable more than 2 cm below the left costal margin, these organs are enlarged—a finding that is always reported for further medical investigation. ■

Palpate the *femoral pulses* by placing the tips of two or three fingers (index, middle, or ring) along the inguinal ligament about midway between the iliac crest and pubic sym-

Atraumatic Care

PROMOTING RELAXATION DURING ABDOMINAL PALPATION

- Position child comfortably, such as in a semireclining position in the parent's lap, with knees flexed.
- Warm the hands before touching the skin.
- Use distraction, such as telling stories or talking to child.
- Teach child to use deep breathing and to concentrate on an object.
- Give infant a bottle or pacifier.
- Begin with light, superficial palpation and gradually progress to deeper palpation.
- Palpate any tender or painful areas last.
- Have child hold the parent's hand and squeeze it if palpation is uncomfortable.
- Use the nonpalpating hand to comfort child, such as placing the free hand on the child's shoulder while palpating the abdomen.
- To minimize sensation of tickling during palpation:
  - Have children "help" with palpation by placing their hand over the palpating hand.
  - Have them place their hand on the abdomen with the fingers spread wide apart, and palpate between their fingers.

physis. Feel both pulses simultaneously to make certain that they are equal and strong (Fig. 35-33).

NURSE ALERT Absence of femoral pulses is a significant sign of coarctation of the aorta and is referred for medical evaluation. ■

Genitalia

Examination of genitalia conveniently follows assessment of the abdomen while the child is still supine. In adolescents inspection of the genitalia may be left to the end of the examination. The best approach is to examine the genitalia matter-of-factly, placing no more emphasis on this part of the assessment than on any other segment. It helps to relieve children's and parents' anxiety by telling them the results of the findings; for example, the nurse might say, "Everything looks fine here."

If it is necessary to ask questions, such as about discharge or difficulty in urinating, respect the child's privacy by covering the lower abdomen with the gown or underpants. To prevent embarrassing interruptions, keep the door or curtain closed and post a "do not disturb" sign. Have a drape ready to cover the genitalia if someone enters the room.

In examining the genitalia, wear gloves whenever touching body substances. It might be helpful for the adolescent to know that wearing gloves also prevents skin-to-skin contact.

The genital examination is an excellent time for eliciting questions of concern about body functioning or sexual activity. Also use this opportunity to increase or reinforce the child's knowledge of reproductive anatomy by naming each body part and explaining its function. This part of the health assessment is an opportune time to teach testicular self-examination to boys.*

Male Genitalia

Note the external appearance of the glans and shaft of the penis, the prepuce, the urethral meatus, and the scrotum (Fig. 35-34). The *penis* is generally small in infants and young boys until puberty, when it begins to increase in both length and width. In an obese child the penis often looks abnormally small because of the folds of skin partially covering it at the base. Be familiar with normal pubertal growth of the external male genitalia to compare the findings with the expected sequence of development.

*For free information on testicular cancer, contact Jason A. Struble Memorial Cancer Fund, Inc., 624 Kehrs Mill Rd., Ballwin, MO 63011.

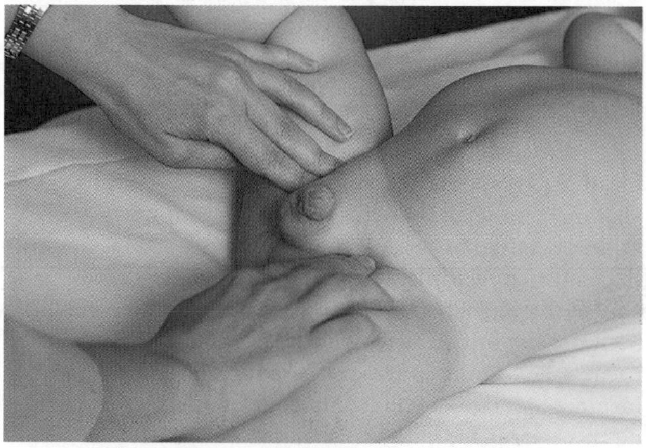

Fig. 35-33 Palpating for femoral pulses.

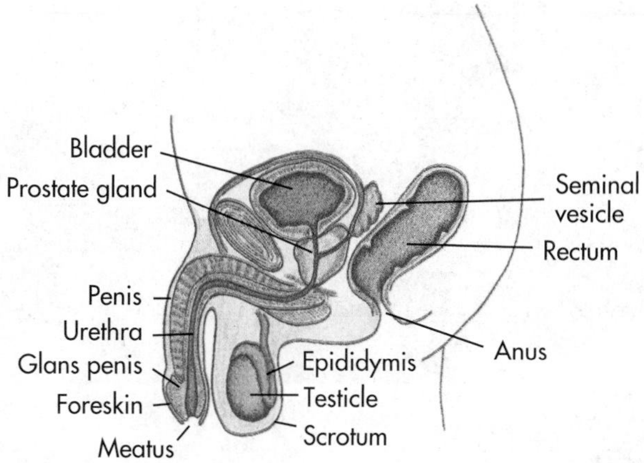

Fig. 35-34 Major structures of genitalia in uncircumcised postpubertal male. (From Potter PA, Perry AG: *Basic nursing: theory and practice,* ed 3, St Louis, 1995, Mosby.)

Examine the *glans* (head of the penis) and *shaft* (portion between the perineum and prepuce) for signs of swelling, skin lesions, inflammation, or other irregularities. Any of these signs may indicate underlying disorders, especially sexually transmitted diseases.

The *urethral meatus* is carefully inspected for location and evidence of discharge. Normally it is centered at the tip of the glans.

Hair distribution is also noted. Normally, before puberty, no pubic hair is present. Soft, downy hair at the base of the penis is an early sign of pubertal maturation. In older adolescents hair distribution is diamond shaped from the umbilicus to the anus.

The location and size of the *scrotum* are noted. The scrotum hangs freely from the perineum behind the penis, and the left side of the scrotum normally hangs lower than the right. In infants the scrotum appears large in relation to the rest of the genitalia. The skin of the scrotum is loose and highly rugated (wrinkled). During early adolescence the skin normally becomes redder and coarser. In dark-skinned children the scrotum is usually more deeply pigmented.

Palpation of the scrotum includes identification of the testes, epididymis, and, if present, inguinal hernias. The two *testes* are felt as small ovoid bodies about 1.5 to 2 cm (0.6 to 0.8 inch) long—one in each scrotal sac. They do not enlarge until puberty, when they approximately double in size.

When palpating for the presence of the testes, avoid stimulating the *cremasteric reflex,* which is stimulated by cold, touch, emotional excitement, or exercise. This reflex pulls the testes higher into the pelvic cavity. Several measures are useful in preventing the cremasteric reflex during palpation of the scrotum. First, warm the hands. Second, if the child is old enough, examine him in a tailor or "Indian" position, which stretches the muscle, preventing its contraction (Fig. 35-35, *A*). Third, block the normal pathway of ascent of the testes by placing the thumb and index finger over the upper part of the scrotal sac along the inguinal canal (Fig. 35-35, *B*). If there is

A

B

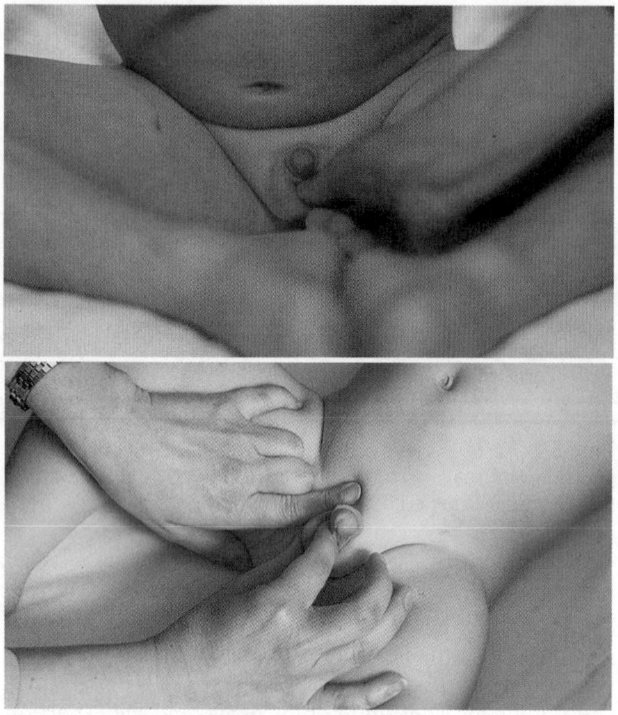

Fig. 35-35 **A,** Preventing cremasteric reflex by having child sit in "tailor" position. **B,** Blocking inguinal canal during palpation of scrotum for descended testes.

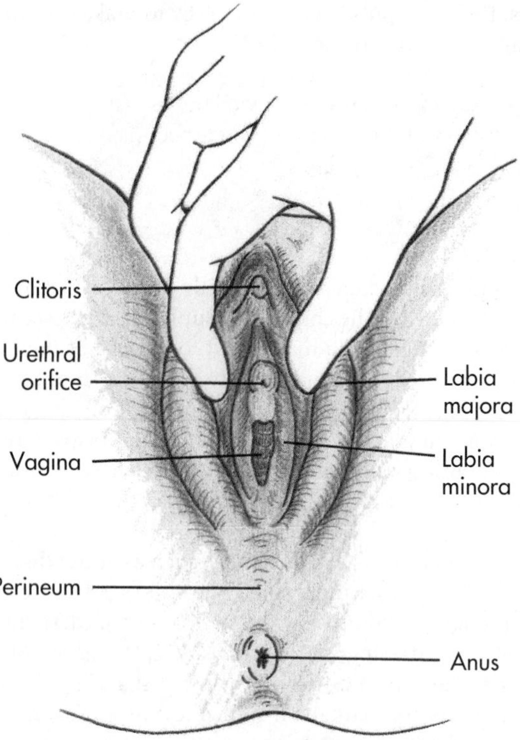

Fig. 35-36 External structures of genitalia in postpubertal female. Labia are spread to reveal deeper structures. (From Potter PA, Perry AG: *Basic nursing: theory and practice,* ed 4, St Louis, 1999, Mosby.)

any question concerning the existence of two testes, place the index and middle fingers in a scissors fashion to separate the right and left scrotum. If after using these techniques the testes have not been palpated, feel along the inguinal canal and perineum to locate masses that may be undescended testes. Although undescended testes may descend at any time during childhood and are checked at each visit, failure to palpate testes is reported.

Female Genitalia

The examination of female genitalia is limited to inspection and palpation of external structures. If a vaginal examination is required, an appropriate referral is made unless the nurse is qualified to perform the procedure. A convenient position for examination of the genitalia involves placing the young child supine on the examining table or in a semireclining position on the parent's lap with the feet supported on your knees as you sit facing the child. Divert the child's attention from the examination by instructing her to try to keep the soles of her feet pressed against each other. Separate the labia majora with the thumb and index finger and retract outward to expose the labia minora, urethral meatus, and vaginal orifice.

Examine the female genitalia for size and location of the structures of the *vulva* or *pudendum* (Fig. 35-36). The *mons pubis* is a pad of adipose tissue over the symphysis pubis. At puberty the mons is covered with hair, which extends along the labia. The usual pattern of female *hair distribution* is an inverted triangle. The appearance of soft, downy hair along the labia majora is an early sign of sexual maturation. Note the size and location of the *clitoris.* It is a small erectile organ located at the anterior end of the labia minora. It is covered by a small flap of skin, the *prepuce.*

The *labia majora* are two thick folds of skin running posteriorly from the mons to the posterior commissure of the vagina. Internal to the labia majora are two folds of skin called the *labia minora.* Although the labia minora are usually prominent in the newborn, they gradually atrophy, which makes them almost invisible until their enlargement during puberty.

The inner surface of the labia should be pink and moist. Note the size of the labia and any evidence of fusion, which may suggest the male scrotum. Normally no masses are palpable within the labia.

The *urethral meatus* is located posterior to the clitoris and is surrounded by Skene glands and ducts. Although not a prominent structure, the meatus appears as a small V-shaped slit. Note its location, especially if it opens from the clitoris or inside the vagina. Gently palpate the glands, which are common sites of cysts and sexually transmitted lesions.

The *vaginal orifice* is located posterior to the urethral meatus. Its appearance varies depending on individual anatomy and sexual activity. Ordinarily, examination of the vagina is limited to inspection. In virgins a thin crescent-shaped or circular membrane, called the *hymen,* may cover part of the vaginal opening. In some instances it completely occludes the orifice. After rupture, small rounded pieces of tissue called *caruncles* remain. Although an imperforate hymen denotes lack of penile intercourse, a perforate one does not necessarily indicate sexual abuse.

NURSE ALERT In females who have been circumcised, the genitalia will appear different. Do not show surprise or disgust, but note the appearance and discuss the procedure with the young woman. ■

Surrounding the vaginal opening are *Bartholin glands,* which secrete a clear, mucoid fluid into the vagina for lubrication during intercourse. Palpate the ducts for cysts. Also note the discharge from the vagina, which is usually clear or white.

Anus

After examination of the genitalia, the anal area is easily examined, although the child should be placed on the abdomen. Note the general firmness of the *buttocks* and symmetry of the *gluteal folds.* Assess the tone of the anal sphincter by eliciting the *anal reflex.* Gently scratching the anal area results in an obvious quick contraction of the external anal sphincter.

Back and Extremities

Spine

The general *curvature* of the spine is noted. Normally the back of a newborn is rounded or C shaped from the thoracic and pelvic curves. The development of the cervical and lumbar curves approximates development of various motor skills, such as cervical curvature with head control, and gives the older child the typical double S curve.

Marked curvatures in posture are abnormal. *Scoliosis,* lateral curvature of the spine, is an important childhood problem, especially in girls. Although scoliosis may be identified by observing and palpating the spine and noting a sideways displacement, more objective tests include the following:

- With the child standing erect, clothed only in underpants (and bra if older girl), observe from behind, noting asymmetry of the shoulders and hips.
- With the child bending forward so that the back is parallel to the floor, observe from the side, noting asymmetry or prominence of the rib cage.

A slight limp, a crooked hemline, or complaints of a sore back are other signs and symptoms of scoliosis.

Inspect the *back,* especially along the spine, for any tufts of hair, dimples, or discoloration. *Mobility* of the vertebral column is easily assessed in most children because of their propensity for constant motion during the examination. However, mobility can be tested by asking the child to sit up from a prone position or to do a modified sit-up exercise.

Movement of the cervical spine is an important diagnostic sign of neurologic problems, such as meningitis. Normally movement of the head in all directions is effortless.

NURSE ALERT Hyperextension of the neck and spine, or *opisthotonos,* which is accompanied by pain when the head is flexed, is always referred for immediate medical evaluation. ■

Extremities

Inspect each extremity for symmetry of length and size; refer any deviation for orthopedic evaluation. Count the fingers and toes to be certain of the normal number. This is so often taken for granted that an extra digit *(polydactyly)* or fusion of digits *(syndactyly)* may go unnoticed.

Inspect the arms and legs for *temperature* and *color,* which should be equal in each extremity, although the feet may normally be colder than the hands.

Assess the *shape* of bones. Several variations of bone shape may be observed in children. Although many of them cause parents concern, most are benign and require no treatment. *Bowleg,* or *genu varum,* is lateral bowing of the tibia. It is clinically present when the child stands with the medial malleoli (rounded prominence on either side of the ankle) opposite each other and the space between the knees is greater than approximately 5 cm (2 inches) (Fig. 35-37). Toddlers are usually bowlegged after beginning to walk until all of their lower back and leg muscles are well developed. Unilateral or asymmetric bowlegs that are present beyond age 2 to 3 years, particularly in black children, may represent pathologic conditions requiring further investigation.

Knock-knee, or *genu valgum,* appears as the opposite of bowleg, in that the knees are close together but the feet are spread apart. It is determined clinically by using the same method as for genu varum but by measuring the distance between the malleoli, which normally should be less than 7.5 cm (3 inches) (Fig. 35-38). Knock-knee is normally present in children from about 2 to 7 years of age. Knock-knee that is excessive, asymmetric, accompanied by shortened stature, or evident in a child nearing puberty requires further evaluation.

Next inspect the *feet.* Infants' and toddlers' feet appear flat because the foot is normally wide and the arch is covered by a fat pad. Development of the arch occurs naturally from the action of walking. Normally, at birth the feet are held in a valgus (outward) or varus (inward) position. To determine whether a foot deformity at birth is a result of intrauterine position or development, scratch the outer, then inner, side of the sole. If the foot position is self-correctable, it will assume a right angle to the leg. As the child begins to walk, the feet turn outward less than 30 degrees and inward less than 10 degrees.

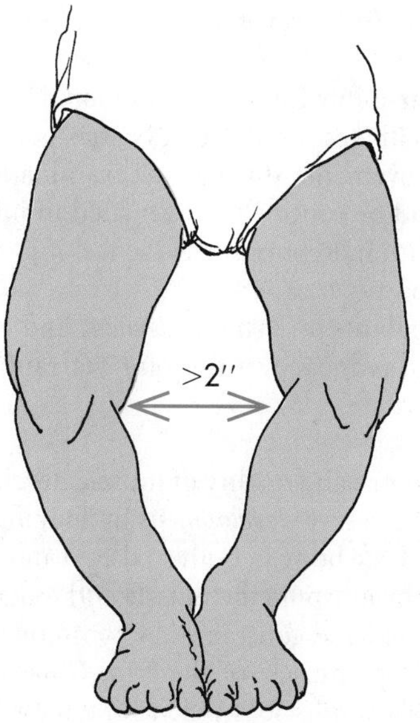

Fig. 35-37 Bowleg.

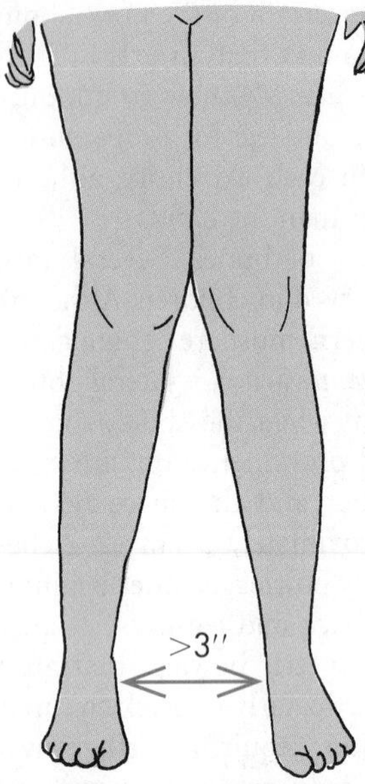

Fig. 35-38 Knock-knee.

Toddlers have a "toddling" or broad-based gait, which facilitates walking by lowering the center of gravity. As the child reaches preschool age, the legs are brought closer together. By school age the walking posture is much more graceful and balanced.

The most common gait problem in young children is *pigeon toe,* or *toeing in,* which usually results from torsional deformities, such as internal tibial torsion (abnormal rotation or bowing of the tibia). Tests for tibial torsion include measuring the thigh-foot angle, which requires considerable practice for accuracy.

Elicit the *plantar* or *grasp reflex* by exerting firm but gentle pressure with the tip of the thumb against the lateral sole of the foot from the heel upward to the little toe and then across to the big toe. The normal response in children who are walking is flexion of the toes. *Babinski sign,* dorsiflexion of the big toe and fanning of the other toes, is normal during infancy but abnormal after about 1 year of age or when locomotion begins.

Joints

Evaluate the joints for *range of motion.* Normally this requires no specific testing if the nurse has been observant of the child's movements during the examination. However, the hips should be routinely investigated in infants for congenital dislocation. Report any evidence of joint immobility or hyperflexibility.

Palpate the joints for *heat, tenderness,* and *swelling.* These signs, as well as redness over the joint, warrant further investigation.

Muscles

Note symmetry and quality of muscle development, tone, and strength. Observe *development* by looking at the shape and contour of the body in both a relaxed and a tensed state. Estimate *tone* by grasping the muscle and feeling its firmness when it is relaxed and contracted. A common site for testing tone is the biceps muscle of the arm. Children are usually willing to "make a muscle" by clenching their fist.

Estimate *strength* by having the child use an extremity to push or pull against resistance, as in the following examples:

Arm strength. Child holds the arms outstretched in front of the body and tries to raise the arms while downward pressure is applied.

Hand strength. Child shakes hands with nurse and squeezes one or two fingers of the nurse's hand.

Leg strength. Child sits on a table or chair with the legs dangling and tries to raise the legs while downward pressure is applied.

Note symmetry of strength in the extremities, hands, and fingers, and report evidence of paresis or weakness.

Neurologic Assessment

The assessment of the nervous system is the broadest and most diverse part of the examining process, because every human function, both physical and emotional, is controlled by neurologic impulses. Much of the neurologic examination has already been discussed, such as assessment of behavior, sensory testing, and motor functioning. The following focuses on a general appraisal of cerebellar functioning, deep tendon reflexes, and the cranial nerves.

Cerebellar Functioning

The cerebellum controls balance and coordination. Much of the assessment of cerebellar functioning is included in observing the child's posture, body movements, gait, and development of fine and gross motor skills. Tests such as balancing on one foot and the heel-to-toe walk assess balance. Test *coordination* by asking the child to reach for a toy, button clothes, tie shoes, or draw a straight line on a piece of paper, provided that the child is old enough to do these activities. Coordination can also be tested by any sequence of rapid successive movements, such as quickly touching each finger with the thumb of the same hand.

Several tests for cerebellar function are described in Box 35-5 and can be performed as games. When the Romberg test is done, stay beside the child if there is a possibility that the child may fall. School-age children should be able to perform these tests, although, in the finger-to-nose test, preschoolers normally can only bring the finger within 5 to 7.5 cm (2 to 3 inches) of the nose. Difficulty in performing these exercises indicates poor sense of position (especially with the eyes closed) and incoordination (especially with the eyes opened).

Reflexes

Testing reflexes is an important part of the neurologic examination. Persistence of primitive reflexes, loss of reflexes, or hyperactivity of deep tendon reflexes is usually a result of a cerebral insult.

BOX 35-5

Tests for Cerebellar Function

Finger-to-nose test. With child's arm extended, ask child to touch the nose with the index finger with eyes open and then closed.

Heel-to-shin test. While standing, have child run the heel of one foot down the shin or anterior aspect of the tibia of the other leg, both with eyes opened and then closed.

Romberg test. With eyes closed, have child stand with heels together; falling or leaning to one side is abnormal and is called *Romberg sign.*

Elicit reflexes by using the rubber head of the reflex hammer, flat of the finger, or side of the hand. If the child is easily frightened by equipment, use your hand or finger. Although testing reflexes is a simple procedure to perform, the child may inhibit the reflex by unconsciously tensing the muscle. To avoid tensing, distract younger children with toys or talk to them. Older children can concentrate on the exercise of grasping their two hands in front of them and trying to pull them apart. This diverts their attention away from the testing and causes involuntary relaxation of the muscles.

Deep tendon reflexes are stretch reflexes of a muscle. The most common deep tendon reflex is the *knee jerk*, or *patellar, reflex* (this is sometimes called the *quadriceps reflex*). The reflexes normally elicited are described in Figs. 35-39 to 35-42. Report any diminished or hyperreflexic response for further evaluation.

Cranial Nerves

Assessment of the cranial nerves is an important area of neurologic assessment (Table 35-11). With young children, present the tests as games to encourage trust and security at the beginning of the examination. Or include the cranial

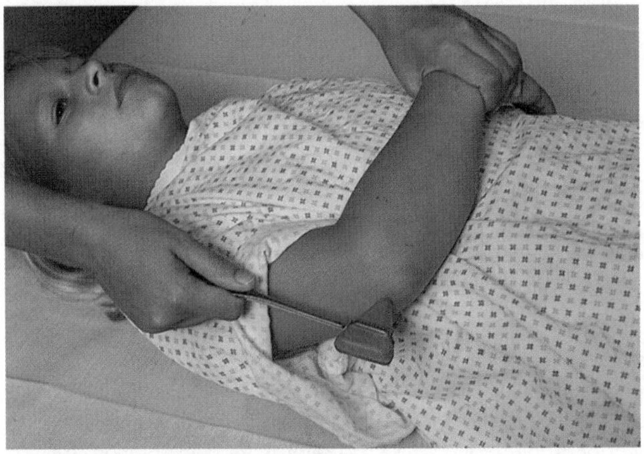

Fig. 35-39 Testing for triceps reflex. Child is placed supine, with forearm resting over chest, and triceps tendon is struck. Alternative procedure: child's arm is abducted, with upper arm supported and forearm allowed to hang freely. Triceps tendon is struck. Normal response is partial extension of forearm.

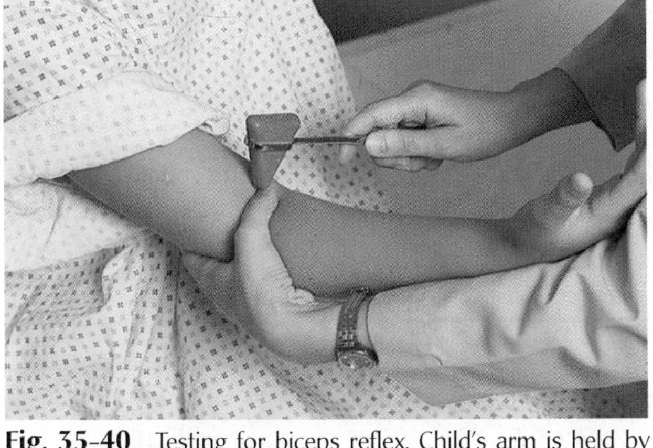

Fig. 35-40 Testing for biceps reflex. Child's arm is held by placing partially flexed elbow in examiner's hand with thumb over antecubital space. Examiner's thumbnail is struck with hammer. Normal response is partial flexion of forearm.

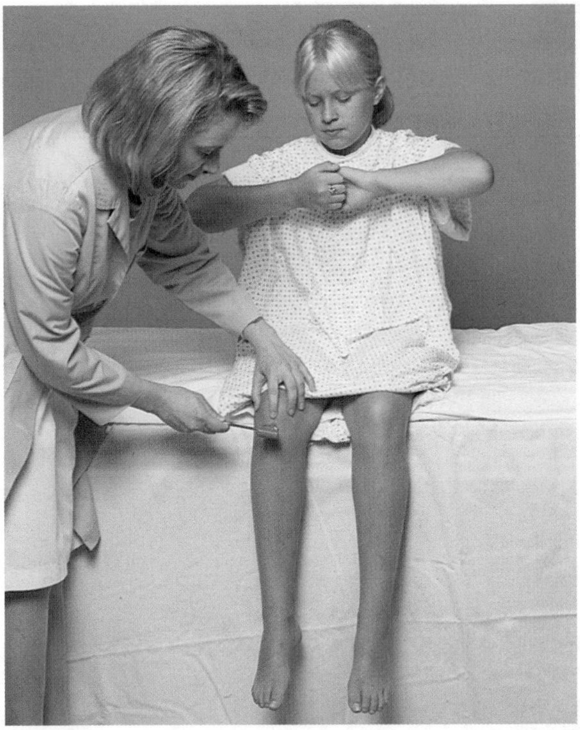

Fig. 35-41 Testing for patellar, or knee jerk, reflex, using distraction. Child sits on edge of examining table (or on parent's lap) with lower legs flexed at knee and dangling freely. Patellar tendon is tapped just below kneecap. Normal response is partial extension of lower leg.

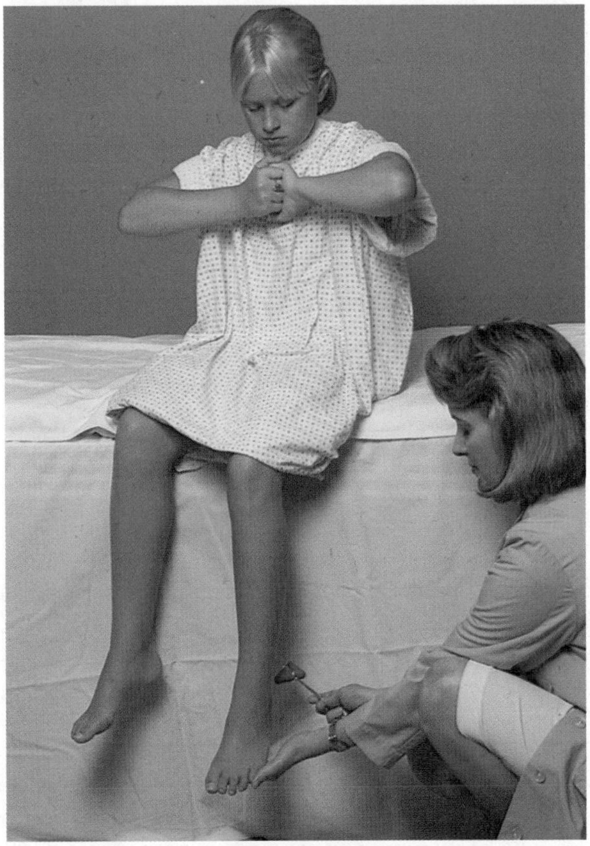

Fig. 35-42 Testing for Achilles reflex. Child should be in same position as for knee jerk reflex. Foot is supported lightly in examiner's hand, and Achilles tendon is struck. Normal response is plantar flexion of foot (foot pointing downward).

Table 35-11

Assessment of Cranial Nerves

DESCRIPTION/FUNCTION	TESTS
I–OLFACTORY NERVE	
Olfactory mucosa of nasal cavity Smell	With eyes closed, have child identify odors such as coffee, alcohol from a swab, or other smells; test each nostril separately.
II–OPTIC NERVE	
Rods and cones of retina, optic nerve Vision	Check for perception of light, visual acuity, peripheral vision, color vision, and normal optic disc.
III–OCULOMOTOR NERVE	
Extraocular muscles (EOMs) of eye: Superior rectus (SR)—moves eyeball up and in Inferior rectus (IR)—moves eyeball down and in Medial rectus (MR)—moves eyeball nasally Inferior oblique (IO)—moves eyeball up and out	Have child follow an object (toy) or light in the six cardinal positions of gaze (see Fig. 35-43).
Pupil constriction and accommodation	Perform PERRLA.
Eyelid closing	Check for proper placement of lid.
IV–TROCHLEAR NERVE	
Superior oblique (SO) muscle Moves eye down and out	Have child look down and in (see Fig. 35-43).
V–TRIGEMINAL NERVE	
Muscles of mastication	Have child bite down hard and open jaw; test symmetry and strength.
Sensory: face, scalp, nasal and buccal mucosa	With child's eyes closed, see if child can detect light touch in mandibular and maxillary regions. Test corneal and blink reflex by touching cornea lightly (approach from side so that child does not blink before cornea is touched).
VI–ABDUCENS NERVE	
Lateral rectus (LR) muscle Moves eye temporally	Have child look toward temporal side (see Fig. 35-43).
VII–FACIAL NERVE	
Muscles for facial expression	Have child smile, make funny face, or show teeth to see symmetry of expression.
Anterior two thirds of tongue (sensory)	Have child identify a sweet or salty solution; place each taste on anterior section and sides of protruding tongue; if child retracts tongue, solution will dissolve toward posterior part of tongue.
VIII–AUDITORY, ACOUSTIC, OR VESTIBULOCOCHLEAR NERVE	
Internal ear Hearing/balance	Test hearing; note any loss of equilibrium or presence of vertigo.
IX–GLOSSOPHARYNGEAL NERVE	
Pharynx, tongue	Stimulate posterior pharynx with a tongue blade; child should gag.
Posterior one third of tongue (sensory)	Test sense of sour or bitter taste on posterior segment of tongue.
X–VAGUS NERVE	
Muscles of larynx, pharynx, some organs of gastrointestinal system, sensory fibers of root of tongue, heart, lung, and some organs of gastrointestinal system	Note hoarseness of voice, gag reflex, and ability to swallow. Check that uvula is in midline; when stimulated with a tongue blade, should deviate upward and to stimulated side.
XI–ACCESSORY NERVE	
Sternocleidomastoid and trapezius muscles of shoulder	Have child shrug shoulders while applying mild pressure; with examiner's hands placed on shoulders, have child turn head against opposing pressure on either side; note symmetry and strength.
XII–HYPOGLOSSAL NERVE	
Muscles of tongue	Have child move tongue in all directions; have child protrude tongue as far as possible; note any midline deviation. Test strength by placing tongue blade on one side of tongue and having child move it away.

PERRLA, pupils equal, round, react to light, accommodation.

nerve test when each "system" is examined, such as tongue movement and strength, gag reflex, swallowing, cardinal positions of gaze (Fig. 35-43), and position of the uvula during examination of the mouth.

DEVELOPMENTAL ASSESSMENT

One of the most essential components of a complete health appraisal is assessment of developmental functioning. *Screening* procedures are designed to identify quickly and reliably those children whose developmental level is below normal for their age and who therefore require further investigation. They also provide a means of recording objective measurements of present developmental functioning for future reference. Since the passage of P.L. 99-457, the Education of the Handicapped Act Amendments of 1986, much greater emphasis is placed on developmental assessment of children with disabilities, and nurses can play a vital role in providing this service. All of the procedures discussed in this section can be administered in a variety of settings—home, school, day care center, hospital, practitioner's office, or clinic.

Denver II

The most widely used developmental screening tests for young children has been the series of tests developed by Dr. William Frankenburg and his colleagues in Denver, Colorado. The oldest and best known, the *Denver Developmental Screening Test (DDST)* and its revision, the *DDST-R,* have been revised, restandardized, and renamed the *Denver II.* Before administering the Denver II, the examiner should be trained by, and receive a certificate from, a master instructor who has been trained by the Denver faculty.* The Denver II differs from the DDST in items, test form, interpretation, and referral (see Appendix D). The previous total of 105 items has been increased to 125, including an increase from 21 DDST to 39 Denver II language items. Previous items that were difficult to administer or interpret have been either modified or eliminated. Many items that were previously tested by parental report now require observation by the examiner.

*Forms and complete instructions are available from Denver Developmental Materials, Inc., PO Box 6919, Denver, CO 80206-9019; phone: 303-355-4729. The DDST and DDST-R are no longer available because they have been replaced by the Denver II.

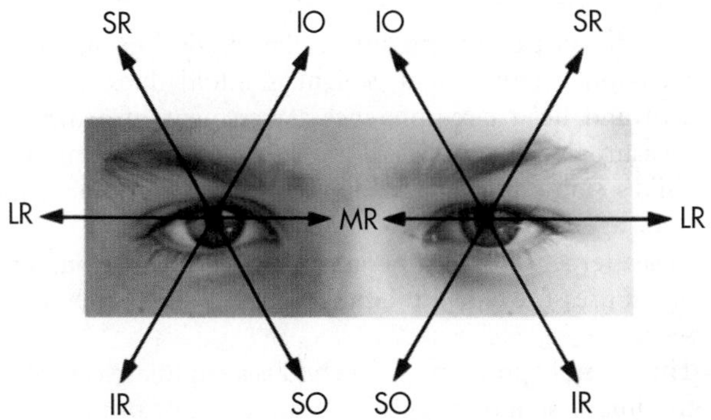

Fig. 35-43 Testing cardinal positions of gaze.

Each item was evaluated to determine if significant differences exist on the basis of sex, ethnic group, maternal education, and place of residence. Items for which clinically significant differences exist were replaced or, if retained, are discussed in the *Technical Manual.* When evaluating children delayed on one of these items, the examiner can look up norms for the subpopulations to consider if the delay may be caused by sociocultural or environmental differences.

The items on the test form are arranged in the same format as the DDST-R. The norms for the distribution bars were updated with the new standardization data but retain the 25th, 50th, 75th, and 90th percentile divisions. The test form contains a place to rate the child's behavioral characteristics (compliance, interest in surroundings, fearfulness, and attention span).

To determine relative areas of advancement and areas of delay, sufficient items should be administered to establish the basal and ceiling levels in each sector. By scoring appropriate items as "pass," "fail," "refusal," or "no opportunity," and relating such scores to the age of the child, each item can be interpreted as described in the accompanying box. To identify cautions, all items intersected by the age line are administered. To screen solely for developmental delays, only the items located totally to the *left* of the child's age line are administered. Criteria for referral are based on the availability of resources in the community (Box 35-6).

Research on the Denver II's validity and accuracy continues. One study found that most children with even subtle developmental problems were identified. However, almost

BOX 35-6

Denver II Scoring

Interpretation of Denver II Scores

Advanced–Passed an item completely to the right of the age line (passed by less than 25% of children at an age older than the child)

OK–Passed, failed, or refused an item intersected by the age line between the 25th and 75th percentiles

Caution–Failed or refused items intersected by the age line on or between the 75th and 90th percentiles

Delay–Failed an item completely to the left of the age line; refusals to the left of the age line may also be considered delays, because the reason for the refusal may be inability to perform the task

Interpretation of Test

Normal–No delays and a maximum of one caution

Suspect–One or more delays or two or more cautions

Untestable–Refusals on one or more items completely to the left of the age line or on more than one item intersected by the age line in the 75% to 90% area

Recommendations for Referral for Suspect and Untestable Tests

Rescreen in 1 to 2 weeks to rule out temporary factors.

If rescreen is suspect or untestable, use clinical judgment based on the following: number of cautions and delays; which items are cautions and delays; rate of past development; clinical examination and history; availability of referral resources.

half of the children without developmental problems received suspect scores, resulting in a high rate of overreferrals (Glascoe et al, 1992). To minimize overreferrals, a decision for referral depends not only on the results of the Denver II, but also on the practitioner's clinical judgment after considering the child's developmental history; general health status; social, cultural, and emotional environment; and the availability of local resources for diagnosis and treatment (Frankenburg, 1994a; 1994b).

Although it is not the purpose of this discussion to detail the instruction manual, some points concerning preparation, administration, and interpretation of the Denver II are important to stress. Before beginning the screen, ask if the child was born prematurely and correctly calculate the adjusted age. Up to 24 months of age, allowances are made for infants born prematurely by subtracting the number of weeks of missed gestation from their present age and testing them at the adjusted age. For example, a 16-week-old infant who was born 4 weeks early is tested at a 12-week adjusted age level. Explain to the parents and child, if appropriate, that the screenings are *not* intelligence tests but rather are a method of showing what the child can do at a particular age. Emphasize that the child is *not* expected to perform each item on the test.

Tell the parent before the screening begins that the results of the child's performance will be explained after all of the items have been concluded. It is the nurse's responsibility to properly inform parents of any testing or screening procedure before its administration so that they are fully aware of its purpose and intent.

Prepare toddlers and preschoolers for the procedure by presenting it as a game. Frequently, the Denver II is an excellent way to begin a health appraisal because it is nonthreatening, requires no painful or unfamiliar procedures, and capitalizes on the child's natural activity of play. Because children are easily distracted, perform each item quickly and present only one toy from the kit at a time. After that toy's purpose is concluded, such as building a tower of blocks or identifying its color, replace the toy in the bag and take out another one. Other temporary factors that may interfere with the child's performance include fatigue, illness, fear, hospitalization, separation from the parent, or general unwillingness to perform the activities. In addition, undiagnosed mental retardation, hearing loss, vision loss, neurologic impairment, or a familial pattern of slow development greatly influences the child's performance.

After completion of the Denver II, ask the parent if the child's performance was typical of behavior at other times. If the parent replies affirmatively and the child's cooperation was satisfactory, explain the results, emphasizing all successful items first; then those items failed but that the child was not expected to pass; and finally those items that were delays. If the parent replies that the child's performance was not typical of usual behavior, it is best to defer any scoring or discussion of results, especially if the refusals yield a suspect score. In this situation reschedule testing for a time when the child is more likely to cooperate.

In explaining a normal score, focus on how well the child performed and reinforce the parents' efforts in satisfactorily stimulating their child. In addition to assessing the child's present developmental level, the Denver II can be used to guide parents toward those activities that are appropriate, although not necessarily expected, for the child's age. By testing for items to the right of the age line (ones the child is not expected to perform), children with advanced development, who may be gifted, can be identified.

In explaining delays, carefully note the parent's response, especially casual acceptance such as "He'll catch up" or questions such as "Does this mean my child is retarded?" Be aware of personal anxieties during these situations and refrain from giving glib reassurances such as "I'm sure he will do better next time." Rather, respond honestly to parents' questions, yet with appropriate flexibility and concern, stressing the need for further developmental testing.

Denver II Prescreening Developmental Questionnaire

The Denver II Prescreening Developmental Questionnaire (PDQ-II) is a further revision of the PDQ and the R-PDQ. This version uses the norms (90th and 75th percentiles) from the Denver II. The PDQ-II is a parent-answered prescreen consisting of 91 questions from the Denver II, although only a subset of questions are asked for each age group. The form may need to be read to parents and caregivers who are less educated.

Four different forms are available and are selected based on age: orange (0 to 9 months), purple (9 to 24 months), cream (2 to 4 years), and white (4 to 6 years). The caregiver answers questions until (1) three "nos" are circled (they do not have to be consecutive) or (2) all the questions on both sides of the form have been answered. Scoring is based on the number of delays or cautions (see Box 35-6). Children who have no delays or cautions are considered to be developing normally. If a child has one delay or two cautions, the caregiver is provided with age-appropriate developmental activities to pursue with the child, and a rescreen with the PDQ-II is done 1 month later. If on rescreening the child has one or more delays, the Denver II is administered as soon as possible. If a child has two or more delays or three or more cautions on the first screening with the PDQ-II, the Denver II is administered as soon as possible.

Key Points

- The most common approach to examining children follows a head-to-toe sequence.
- Growth measurements during the physical examination focus on length, height, weight, skinfold thickness, and arm and head circumference. Assessment of growth is measured against standard growth charts to determine a child's status in comparison with other children of the same age.
- Measurements of temperature, pulse, respiration, and blood pressure constitute the physiologic approach to assessment.
- The general appearance of a child is a cumulative, subjective impression of physical appearance, state of nutrition,

behavior, personality, interactions with parents and nurse, posture, development, and speech.
- Assessment of the skin, which primarily involves inspection and palpation, focuses on color, texture, temperature, moisture, and turgor. The nurse needs to be aware of both physiologic and ethnic factors that may affect these areas.
- In assessment of the lymph nodes, the nurse examines, by palpation, the part of the body in which the glands are located.
- The head is inspected for shape, symmetry, mobility, and muscle control.
- Examination of the eyes includes placement and alignment, inspection of external and internal structures, and vision testing.
- The ears are examined for placement and alignment, inspection of external and internal structures, and auditory testing.
- The lungs are examined by methods of inspection, palpation, percussion, and auscultation.
- Auscultation is the most important procedure for examining the heart.
- Abdominal assessment follows an orderly sequence of inspection, auscultation, and palpation, because palpation may distort normal abdominal sounds.
- Examination of the genitalia may provoke anxiety in the child, and the nurse must avoid any transference of anxiety.
- Neurologic assessment addresses behavior; motor, sensory, and cerebellar functioning; reflexes; and cranial nerves.
- The Denver II, a major revision and restandardization of the DDST, differs from the DDST in items included in the test, the test form, and the interpretation of scoring.

References

American Academy of Pediatrics, Committee on Practice and Ambulatory Medicine, Section on Ophthalmology: Eye examination in infants, children, and young adults by pediatricians, *Pediatrics* 111(4):902-907, 2003.

American Academy of Pediatrics, Committee on Practice and Ambulatory Medicine, Section on Otolaryngology and Bronchoesophagology: Hearing assessment in infants and children: recommendations beyond neonatal screening, *Pediatrics* 111(2):436-440, 2003.

Amoore JN: A comparative evaluation of the Dinamap 8100 and Dinamap Compact TS using a non-invasive blood pressure simulator, *Blood Press Monit* 3(5):309-314, 1998.

Bald M: Ambulatory blood pressure monitoring in children and adolescents, *Minerva Pediatr* 54(1):13-24, 2002.

Banitalebi H, Bangstad HJ: Measurement of fever in children—is infrared tympanic thermometry reliable? *Tidsskr Nor Laegeforen* 122(28):2700-2701, 2002.

Barone MA, Rowe PC: Pediatric procedures. In McMillan JA, DeAngelis CD, Feigin RD (eds): *Oski's pediatrics—principles and practice,* ed 3, Philadelphia, 1999, Lippincott Williams & Wilkins.

Beevers G, Lip GYH, O'Brien E: ABC of hypertension blood pressure measurement part I—sphygmomanometry: factors common to all techniques, *BMJ* 322(7292):981-985, 2001.

Berry BE et al: Preschool vision screening using the MTI-Photoscreener, *Pediatr Nurs* 27(1):27-34, 2001.

Blackburn S et al: Neonatal thermal care, part III: the effect of infant position and temperature probe placement, *Neonatal Netw* 20(3):25-30, 2001.

Bliss Holtz J: Methods of newborn infant temperature monitoring: a research review, *Issues Compr Nurs* 18(4):287-298, 1995.

Childs C, Harrison R, Hodkinson C: Tympanic membrane temperature as a measure of core temperature, *Arch Dis Child* 80(3):262-266, 1999.

Clark JA et al: Discrepancies between direct and indirect blood pressure measurements using various recommendations for arm cuff selection, *Pediatrics* 110(5):920-923, 2002.

Coats DK, Jenkins RH: Vision assessment of the pediatric patient: refinements, *Am Acad Ophthalmol* 1(1):1-12, 1997.

Craig JV et al: Temperature measured at the axilla compared with rectum in children and young people: systematic review, *BMJ* 320(7243):1174-1178, 2000.

Craig JV et al: Infrared ear thermometry compared with rectal thermometry in children: a systematic review, *Lancet* 360:603-609, 2002.

Cretel E et al: A comparative study of body temperature using rectal and tympanic measurement, *Rev Med Intern* 20(11):981-984, 1999.

Cunningham M, Cox EO: Hearing assessment in infants and children: recommendations beyond neonatal screening, *Pediatrics* 111(2):436-440, 2003.

Dollberg S, Lahav S, Mimouni FB: Precision of a new thermometer for rapid rectal temperature measurement in neonates, *Am J Perinatol* 18(2):103-105, 2001.

Erickson RS: The continuing question of how best to measure body temperature, *Crit Care Med* 27(10):2307-2310, 1999.

Erickson RS, Meyer LT, Woo TM: Accuracy of chemical dot thermometers in critically ill adults and children, *Image J Nurs Sch* 28(1):23-28, 1996.

Frankenburg WK: Preventing developmental delays: is developmental screening sufficient? I. Developmental screening and the Denver II, *Pediatrics* 93(4):586-589, 1994a.

Frankenburg WK: Preventing developmental delays: is developmental screening sufficient? II. Partners in health care, *Pediatrics* 93(4):589-593, 1994b.

Gillman MW, Cook NR: Blood pressure measurement in childhood epidemiological studies, *Circulation* 92(4):1049-1057, 1995.

Glascoe FP et al: Accuracy of the Denver-II in developmental screening, *Pediatrics* 89:1221-1225, 1992.

Goldman LR, Shannon MW: Technical report: mercury in the environment: implications for pediatricians, *Pediatrics* 108(1):197-205, 2001.

Greyling G, Viljoen MJ, Joubert G: Axillary temperature compared to tympanic membrane temperature in children, *Curationis* 23(3):54-61, 2000.

Haddock BJ, Merrow DL, Swanson MS: The falling grace of axillary temperatures, *Pediatr Nurs* 22(2):121-125, 1996.

Halle C: Achieve new vision screening objectives, *Nurse Pract* 27(3):15-35, 2002.

Healthcare Product Comparison System: *Thermometers, electronic, continuous,* Plymouth Meeting, PA, 1996a, ECRI.

Healthcare Product Comparison System: *Thermometers, electronic, intermittent,* Plymouth Meeting, PA, 1996b, ECRI.

Healthcare Product Comparison System: *Thermometers, infrared, ear,* Plymouth Meeting, PA, 1996c, ECRI.

Hockenberry-Eaton M, Kline NE: Nursing support of the child with cancer. In Pizzo PA, Poplack DP (eds): *Principles and practices of pediatric oncology,* vol 4, Philadelphia, 2001, JB Lippincott.

Hooker EA, Houston H: Screening for fever in an adult emergency department: oral vs tympanic thermometry, *South Med J* 89(2):230-234, 1996.

Houlder LC: The accuracy and reliability of tympanic thermometry compared to rectal and axillary sites in young children, *Pediatr Nurs* 26(3):311-314, 2000.

Irvin SM: Comparison of the oral thermometer versus the tympanic thermometer, *Clin Nurs Spec* 13(2):85-89, 1999.

Jean-Mary MB et al: Limited accuracy and reliability of infrared axillary and aural thermometers in a pediatric outpatient population, *J Pediatr* 141(5):671-676, 2002.

Jensen BN et al: Accuracy of digital tympanic, oral, axillary, and rectal thermometers compared with standard rectal mercury thermometers, *Eur J Surg* 166(11):848-851, 2000.

Kongpanichkul A, Bunjongpak S: A comparative study on accuracy of liquid crystal forehead, digital electronic axillary, infrared tympanic with glass-mercury rectal thermometer in infants and young children, *J Med Assoc Thai* 83(9):1068-1076, 2000.

Lanham DM et al: Accuracy of tympanic temperature readings in children under 6 years of age, *Pediatr Nurs* 25(1):39-42, 1999.

Leick-Rude MK, Bloom LF: A comparison of temperature-taking methods in neonates, *Neonatal Netw* 17(5):21-37, 1998.

Ling J et al: Clinical evaluation of the oscillometric blood pressure monitor in adults and children based on the 1992 AAMI SP-10 standards, *J Clin Monit* 11(2):123-130, 1995.

Loveys AA et al: Comparison of ear to rectal temperature measurements in infants and toddlers, *Clin Pediatr (Phila)* 38(8):463-466, 1999.

Macqueen S: Clinical benefits of 3M Tempa.DOT thermometer in paediatric settings, *Br J Nurs* 10(1):55-58, 2001.

Medical Indicators, Inc: NexTemp™ single-use clinical thermometers: the quick, accurate, "no-hassle" way to take a temp, NCF1, January 1999, Pennington, NJ.

Modell JG et al: Unreliability of the infrared tympanic thermometer in clinical practice: a comparative study with oral mercury and oral electronic thermometers, *South Med J* 91(7):649-654, 1998.

Molton AH, Blacktop J, Hall CM: Temperature taking in children, *J Child Health Care* 5(1):5-10, 2001.

National Center for Health Statistics: CDC growth charts: United States, *Advance Data* No. 314, 2000.

National Institutes of Health, National Heart, Lung, and Blood Institute: *Update on the Task Force Report (1987) on high blood pressure in children and adolescents: a working group report from the National High Blood Pressure Education Program,* NIH pub no 96-3790, Bethesda, MD, September 1996.

Park M, Lee D, Johnson GA: Oscillometric blood pressures in the arm, thigh and calf in healthy children and those with aortic coarctation, *Pediatrics* 92(4):761-765, 1993.

Pompei F, Pompei M: *Physicians reference handbook on temperature,* Watertown, MA, 1996, Exergen.

Py Ma H Corporation: *Tempa Dot single use thermometer: technical information,* Flemington, NJ, 1994, The Corporation.

Rabinowitz RP et al: Effects of anatomic site, oral stimulation, and body position on estimates of body temperature, *Arch Intern Med* 156(7):777-780, 1996.

Riveral AY et al: Evaluation of a liquid crystal contact thermometer in children with fever, *J Investig Med* 45(1):93A, 1997.

Robinson JL et al: Comparison of esophageal, rectal, axillary, bladder, tympanic, and pulmonary artery temperatures in children, *J Pediatr* 133:553-556, 1998.

Roche AF, Guo S: The new growth charts, *Pediatr Basics* 94:2-13, 2001.

Romanovsky AA et al: A difference of 5 degrees C between ear and rectal temperatures in a febrile patient, *Am J Emerg Med* 15(4):383-385, 1997.

Saxena AK et al: Application criteria for infrared ear thermometers in pediatric surgery, *Technol Health Care* 9(3):281-285, 2001.

Seidel HM, Rosenstein BJ, Pathak A: *Primary care of the newborn,* ed 2, St Louis, 1997, Mosby.

Sganga A et al: A comparison of four methods of normal newborn temperature measurement, *MCN Am J Matern Child Nurs* 25(2):76-79, 2000.

Shann F, Mackenzie A: Comparison of rectal, axillary and forehead temperatures, *Arch Pediatr Adolesc Med* 150:74-78, 1996.

Turnbull R: Skin assessment in children: a methodical approach, *Nursing Times* 96(41):33-34, 2000.

Valadez JJ, Elmore-Meegan M, Morley D: Comparing liquid crystal thermometer readings and mercury thermometer readings of infants and children in a traditional African setting, *Trop Geogr Med* 47(3):130-133, 1995.

Vessey JA: Developmental approaches to examining young children, *Pediatr Nurs* 21(1):53-56, 1995.

Wall TC et al: Compliance with vision-screening guidelines among a national sample of pediatricians, *Ambulatory Pediatrics* 2(6):449-455, 2002.

Wattigney WA et al: Utility of an automatic instrument for blood pressure measurement in children: the Bogalusa Heart Study, *Am J Hypertens* 9(3):256-262, 1996.

Wilshaw R et al: A comparison of the use of tympanic, axillary, and rectal thermometers in infants, *J Pediatr Nurs* 14(2):88-93, 1999.

Zengeya ST, Blumenthal I: Modern electronic and chemical thermometers used in the axilla are inaccurate, *Eur J Pediatr* 155(12):1005-1008, 1996.

The Infant and Family 36

LEARNING OBJECTIVES

On completion of this chapter the reader will be able to:

- Identify the major biologic, psychosocial, cognitive, and social developments during the first year of life.
- Relate parent-child attachment, separation anxiety, and stranger fear to developmental achievements during infancy.
- Provide anticipatory guidance to parents regarding common parental concerns during infancy.
- Provide anticipatory guidance to parents regarding recommendations for feeding infants.
- Outline immunization requirements during infancy and early childhood.
- List general contraindications, precautions, and administration routes for immunizations.
- Provide anticipatory guidance to parents regarding injury prevention based on the infant's developmental achievements.
- Provide principles of anticipatory guidance in the care of the family with an infant who is experiencing colic.
- Plan nursing care that meets the physical and emotional needs of the nonorganic failure-to-thrive child and family.
- Provide nursing care that meets the immediate and long-term needs of the family who lost a child from sudden infant death syndrome.
- Provide anticipatory guidance for the prevention of sudden infant death syndrome.
- Identify the needs of the family whose child is home monitored for apnea.

ELECTRONIC RESOURCES

Additional information related to the content in Chapter 36 can be found on

the companion website at evolve
http://evolve.elsevier.com/Wong/maternal/
- NCLEX Review Questions
- Case Study—Infant Growth and Development
- Case Study—Child Abuse
- WebLinks

or the interactive student CD-ROM
Activities for Chapter 36 include the following:
- NCLEX Review Questions
- Case Study—Immunizations
- Case Study—Health Problems of Infants
- Critical Thinking Exercise—Infant Safety

PROMOTING OPTIMUM GROWTH AND DEVELOPMENT

Biologic Development

At no other time in life are physical changes and developmental achievements so dramatic as during infancy. All major body systems undergo progressive maturation, and there is concurrent development of skills that increasingly allows infants to respond to and cope with the environment. Acquisition of these fine and gross motor skills occurs in an orderly head-to-toe and center-to-periphery (cephalocaudal and proximodistal) sequence.

Proportional Changes

During the first year growth is very rapid, especially during the initial 6 months. Infants gain 150 to 210 g (5 to 7 ounces) weekly until approximately age 5 to 6 months, when the birth weight has at least doubled. An average weight for a 6-month-old child is 7.26 kg (16 pounds). Weight gain slows during the second 6 months. By 1 year of age the infant's birth weight has tripled, for an average weight of 9.75 kg (21.5 pounds). Infants who are breastfed beyond 4 to 6 months of age typically gain less weight than those who are bottle-fed. Because breastfed infants grow at a different rate than those who are bottle-fed, growth charts that reflect both patterns of infant weight gain should be used.

Height increases by 2.5 cm (1 inch) a month during the first 6 months and also slows during the second 6 months. Increases in length occur in sudden spurts, rather than in a slow, gradual pattern. Average height is 65 cm (25½ inches) at 6 months and 74 cm (29 inches) at 12 months. By 1 year the birth length has increased by almost 50%. This increase occurs mainly in the trunk, rather than in the legs, and contributes to the characteristic physique of the infant.

Head growth is also rapid. During the first 6 months head circumference increases approximately 1.5 cm (6/10 inch) a month but decreases to only 0.5 cm (2/10 inch) monthly during the second 6 months. The average size is 43 cm (17 inches) at 6 months and 46 cm (18 inches) at 12 months. By 1 year, head size has increased by almost 33%. Closure of the cranial sutures occurs, with the posterior fontanel fusing by 6 to 8 weeks of age and the anterior fontanel closing by 12 to 18 months of age (the average age being 14 months).

Expanding head size reflects the growth and differentiation of the *nervous system.* By the end of the first year the brain has increased in weight about 2½ times. Maturation of the brain is exhibited in the dramatic developmental achievements of infancy (see Table 36-2). Primitive reflexes are replaced by voluntary, purposeful movement, and new reflexes that influence motor development appear.

The *chest* assumes a more adult contour, with the lateral diameter becoming larger than the anteroposterior diameter. The chest circumference approximately equals the head circumference by the end of the first year. The heart grows less rapidly than does the rest of the body. Its weight is usually doubled by 1 year of age; in comparison, body weight triples during the same period. The size of the heart is still large in relation to the chest cavity; its width is approximately 55% of the chest width.

Maturation of Systems

Other organ systems also change and grow during infancy. The *respiratory* rate slows somewhat (see Appendix J) and is relatively stable. Respiratory movements continue to be abdominal. Several factors predispose the infant to more severe and acute respiratory problems. The close proximity of the trachea to the bronchi and its branching structures rapidly transmits infectious agents from one anatomic location to another. The short, straight eustachian tube closely communicates with the ear, allowing infection to ascend from the pharynx to the middle ear. In addition, the inability of the immune system to produce *immunoglobulin A (IgA)* in the mucosal lining provides less protection against infection in infancy than during later childhood.

The *heart rate* slows (see Appendix J), and the rhythm is often *sinus arrhythmia* (i.e., rate increases with inspiration and decreases with expiration). Blood pressure also changes during infancy (see Appendix J). Systolic pressure rises during the first 2 months as a result of the increasing ability of the left ventricle to pump blood into the systemic circulation. Diastolic pressure decreases during the first 3 months, then gradually rises to values close to those at birth. Fluctuations in blood pressure occur during varying states of activity and emotion.

Significant *hemopoietic changes* occur during the first year (see Appendix F). Fetal hemoglobin (HgbF) is present for the first 5 months, with adult hemoglobin steadily increasing through the first half of infancy. Fetal hemoglobin results in a shortened survival of red blood cells (RBCs) and thus a decreased number of RBCs. A common result at 2 to 3 months of age is *physiologic anemia.* High levels of HgbF are thought to depress the production of erythropoietin, a hormone released by the kidney that stimulates RBC production.

Maternal iron stores are present for the first 5 to 6 months and gradually diminish, which also accounts for lowered hemoglobin levels toward the end of the first 6 months. The occurrence of physiologic anemia is not affected by an adequate supply of iron. However, when erythropoiesis is stimulated, iron supplies are necessary for the formation of hemoglobin.

The *digestive processes* are immature at birth. Saliva is secreted in small amounts, but the majority of the digestive processes do not begin functioning until age 3 months, when drooling is common because of the poorly coordinated swallowing reflex. The enzyme *ptyalin* (also called *amylase*) is present in small amounts but usually has little effect on the foodstuffs because of the small amount of time the food stays in the mouth. Gastric digestion in the stomach consists primarily of the action of hydrochloric acid and rennin, an enzyme that acts specifically on the casein in milk to cause the formation of curds (i.e., coagulated semisolid particles of milk). The curds cause the milk to be retained in the stomach long enough for digestion to occur.

Digestion also takes place in the duodenum, where pancreatic enzymes and bile begin to break down protein and fat. Secretion of the pancreatic enzyme *amylase,* which is needed for digestion of complex carbohydrates, is deficient until about the fourth to sixth month of life. *Lipase* is also limited, and infants do not achieve adult levels of fat absorption until 4 to 5 months of age. *Trypsin* is secreted in sufficient quantities to catabolize protein into polypeptides and some amino acids.

The immaturity of the digestive processes is evident in the appearance of stools. During infancy, solid foods (e.g., peas, carrots, corn, and raisins) are passed incompletely broken down in the feces. An excess quantity of fiber easily disposes the child to loose, bulky stools.

During infancy the stomach enlarges to accommodate a greater volume of food. By the end of the first year the infant is able to tolerate three meals a day and an evening bottle and may have one or two bowel movements daily. With any type of gastric irritation, however, the infant is vulnerable to diarrhea, vomiting, and dehydration (see Chapter 47).

The *liver* is the most immature of all the gastrointestinal organs throughout infancy. The ability to conjugate bilirubin and secrete bile is achieved after the first couple of weeks of life. However, the capacities for gluconeogenesis, formation of plasma protein and ketones, storage of vitamins, and deaminization of amino acids remain relatively immature for the first year of life.

Maturation of the suckling, sucking, and swallowing reflexes and the eruption of teeth (see Teething, p. 1047) parallel the changes in the gastrointestinal tract and prepare the infant for the introduction of solid foods.

The *immunologic system* undergoes numerous changes during the first year. IgA is present in large amounts in colostrum; this is believed to have a protective role in the gastrointestinal tract against many bacteria such as *Escherichia coli* and viruses such as poliovirus. The function and quantity of T-lymphocytes, lymphokines, and complement is reduced in early infancy, thus preventing optimal response to certain bacteria and viruses.

The full-term newborn receives significant amounts of maternal IgG, which for approximately 3 months confers immunity against antigens to which the mother was exposed. During this time the infant begins to synthesize IgG; approximately 40% of adult levels are reached by 1 year of age. Significant amounts of IgM are produced at birth, and adult levels are reached by 9 months of age. The production of IgA, IgD, and IgE is much more gradual, and maximum levels are not attained until early childhood.

During infancy, *thermoregulation* becomes more efficient; the ability of the skin to contract and of muscles to shiver in response to cold increases. The peripheral capillaries respond to changes in ambient temperature to regulate heat loss. The capillaries constrict in response to cold, conserving core body temperature and decreasing potential evaporative heat loss from the skin surface. The capillaries dilate in response to heat, decreasing internal body temperature through evaporation, conduction, and convection. Shivering *(thermogenesis)* causes the muscles and muscle fibers to contract, generating metabolic heat that is distributed throughout the body. Increased adipose tissue during the first 6 months insulates the body against heat loss.

A shift in the *total body fluid* occurs. At birth 75% of the term infant's body weight is water, and there is an excess of extracellular fluid (ECF). As the percentage of body water decreases, so does the amount of ECF—from 40% at term to 20% in adulthood. The high proportion of ECF, which is composed of blood plasma, interstitial fluid, and lymph, predisposes the infant to a more rapid loss of total body fluid and, consequently, dehydration.

The immaturity of the *renal structures* also predisposes the infant to dehydration. Complete maturity of the kidney occurs during the latter half of the second year, when the cuboidal epithelium of the glomeruli becomes flattened. Before this time the filtration capacity of the glomeruli is reduced. Urine is voided frequently and has a low specific gravity (i.e., 1.000 to 1.010).

Auditory acuity is at adult levels during infancy. Visual acuity begins to improve, and binocular fixation is established. *Binocularity,* or the fixation of two ocular images into one cerebral picture *(fusion),* begins to develop by 6 weeks of age and should be well established by age 4 months. *Depth perception (stereopsis)* begins to develop by age 7 to 9 months but may exist earlier as an innate safety mechanism against accidental falling.

Fine Motor Development

Fine motor behavior includes the use of the hands and fingers in the prehension (grasp) of an object. Grasping occurs during the first 2 to 3 months as a reflex and gradually becomes voluntary. At 1 month of age the hands are predominantly closed, and by 3 months they are mostly open. By this time infants demonstrate a desire to grasp an object, but they "grasp" it more with the eyes than with the hands. If a rattle is placed in the hand, the infant will actively hold onto it. By 4 months of age the infant regards both a small pellet and the hands and then looks from the object to the hands and back again. By 5 months the infant is able to voluntarily grasp an object.

Gradually the palmar grasp (using the whole hand) is replaced with a pincer grasp (using the thumb and index finger). By 8 to 9 months of age the infant uses a crude pincer grasp and by 11 months has progressed to a neat pincer grasp (Fig. 36-1).

By 6 months of age infants have increased manipulative skill: they hold their bottle, grasp their feet and pull them to their mouth, and feed themselves a cracker. By 7 months they transfer objects from one hand to the other, use one hand for grasping, and hold a cube in each hand simultaneously. They enjoy banging objects and will explore the moveable parts of a toy.

By 10 months of age the pincer grasp is sufficiently established to enable infants to pick up a raisin and other finger foods. They can deliberately let go of an object and will offer it to someone. By 11 months they put objects into a container and like to remove them. By age 1 year, infants try to build a tower of two blocks but fail.

Gross Motor Development

Head Control

The full-term newborn can momentarily hold the head in midline and parallel when the body is suspended ventrally and can lift and turn the head from side to side when prone. This is not the case when the infant is lying prone on a pillow or soft surface; infants do not have the head control to lift their head out of the depression of the object and therefore risk suffocation in the prone position early in infancy (see Sudden Infant Death Syndrome, p. 1080). Marked head lag is evident when the infant is pulled from a lying to a sitting position. By 3 months of age infants can hold their head well beyond the plane of the body. By 4 months of age infants can lift the head and front portion of the chest approximately 90 degrees above the table, bearing their weight on the forearms. Only slight head lag is evident when the infant is pulled from

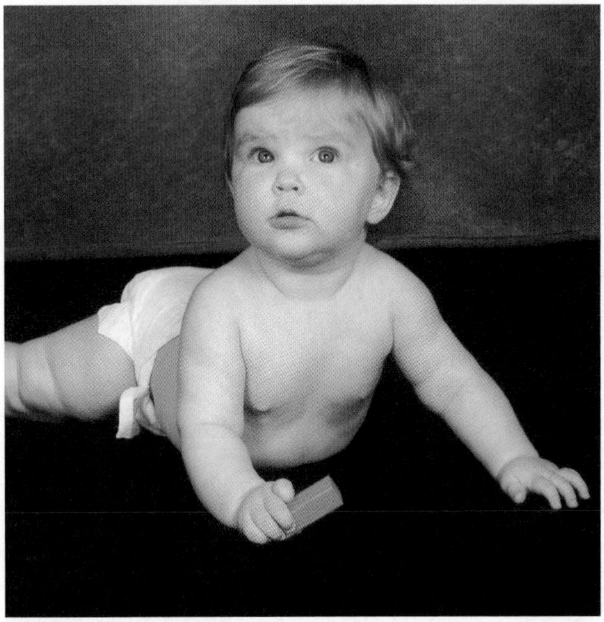

Fig. 36-1 Crude pincer grasp at 8 to 10 months. (Photo by Paul Vincent Kuntz, Texas Children's Hospital, Houston, Texas.)

a lying to a sitting position, and by 4 to 6 months head control is well established (Figs. 36-2 and 36-3).

NURSE ALERT Any child who displays head lag at 6 months of age should have a developmental/neurologic evaluation. ■

Rolling Over

Newborns may roll over accidentally because of their rounded back. The ability to willfully turn from the abdomen to the back occurs at 5 months, and the ability to turn from the back to the abdomen occurs at 6 months. Infants put to sleep on their sides may easily roll over to a prone (face-down) position, thus placing them at higher risk for sudden infant death syndrome (SIDS). It is therefore important to place infants in a supine position for sleep. While the infant is awake, a prone position is acceptable to enhance achievement of milestones such as head control, crawling, creeping, and turning over. It is noteworthy that the parachute reflex (Fig. 36-4), which elicits a protective response to falling, appears at 7 months.

Sitting

The ability to sit follows progressive head control and straightening of the back (Fig. 36-5). For the first 2 to 3 months the back is uniformly rounded. The convex cervical curve forms at approximately 3 to 4 months of age, when head control is established. The convex lumbar curve appears when the child begins to sit, at about age 4 months. As the spinal column straightens, the infant can be propped in

A

B

C

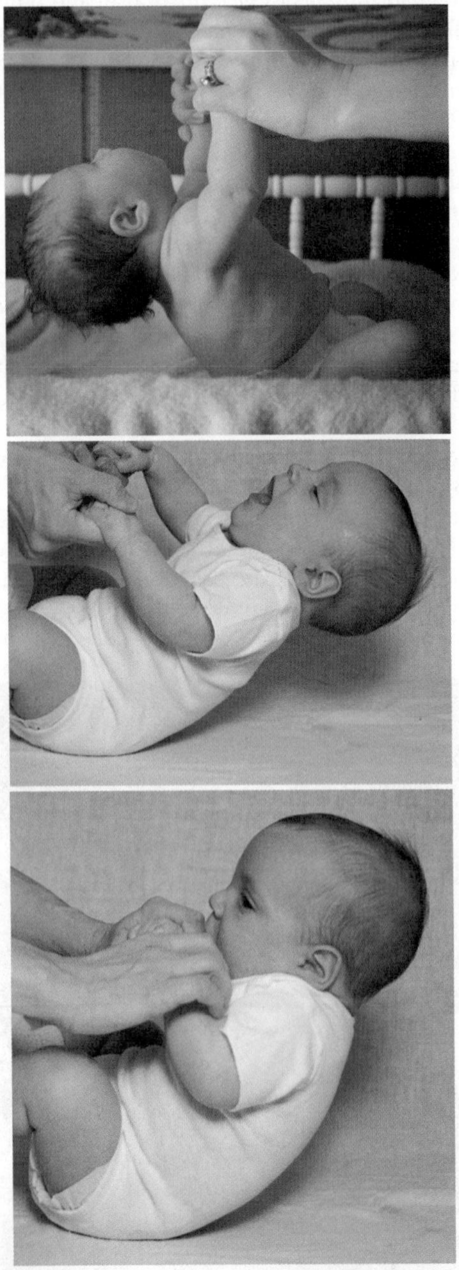

Fig. 36-2 Head control while pulled to sitting position. **A,** Complete head lag at 1 month. **B,** Partial head lag at 2 months. **C,** Almost no head lag at 4 months.

A

B

C

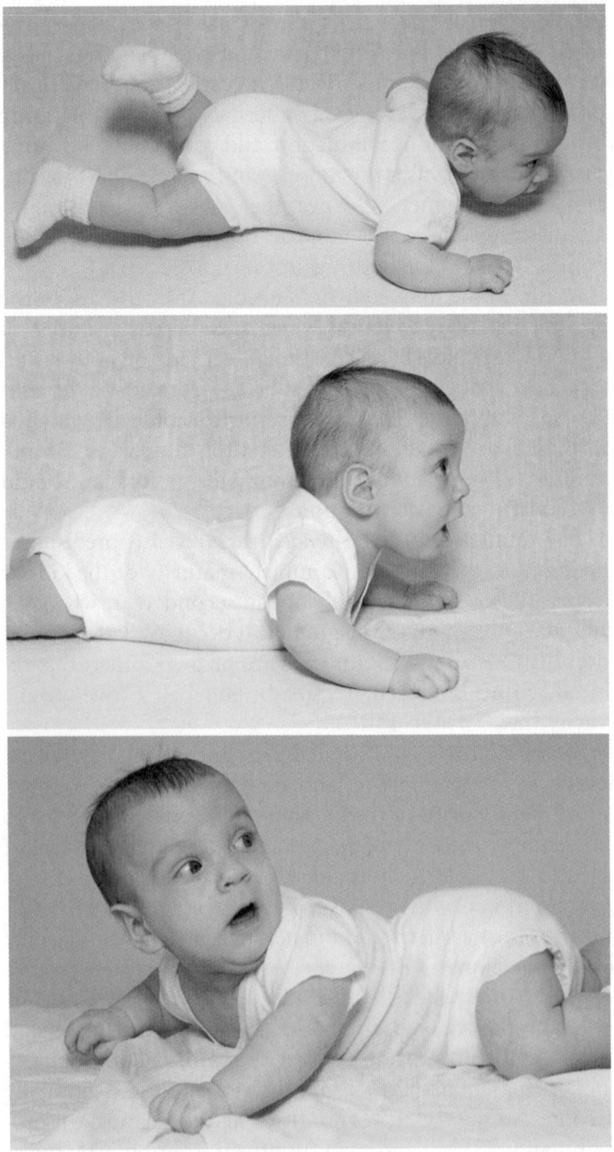

Fig. 36-3 Head control while prone. **A,** Infant momentarily lifts head at 1 month. **B,** Infant lifts head and chest 90 degrees and bears weight on forearms at 4 months. **C,** Infant lifts head, chest, and upper abdomen and can bear weight on hands at 6 months. Note how this position facilitates turning from abdomen to back.

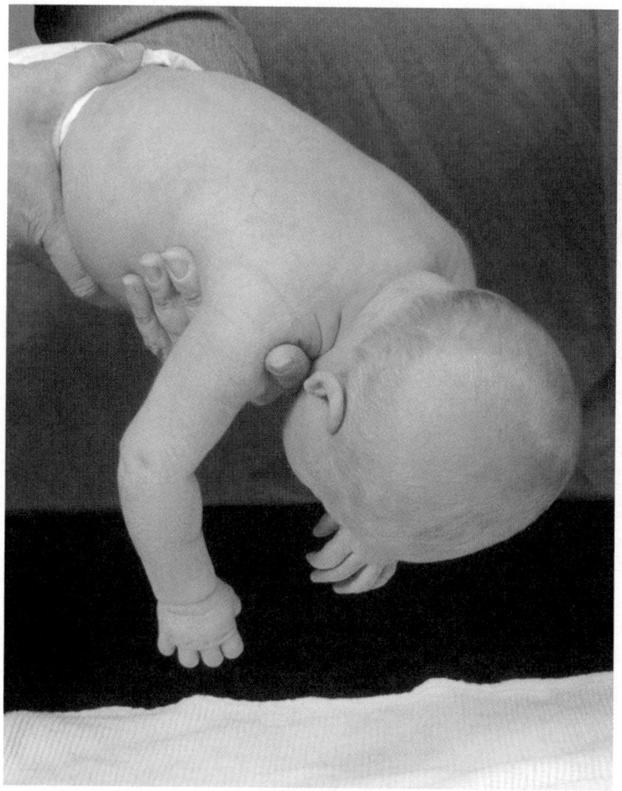

Fig. 36-4 Parachute reflex. (Photo by Paul Vincent Kuntz, Texas Children's Hospital, Houston, Texas.)

a sitting position. By age 7 months infants can sit alone, leaning forward on their hands for support. By age 8 months they can sit well while unsupported and begin to explore their surroundings in this position rather than in a lying position. By 10 months they can maneuver from a prone to a sitting position.

Locomotion

Locomotion involves acquiring the ability to bear weight, propel forward on all four extremities, stand upright with support, and, finally, walk alone (Fig. 36-6). Following a cephalocaudal pattern, infants 4 to 6 months old have increasing coordination in their arms. Initial locomotion results in infants propelling themselves backward by pushing with the arms. By 6 to 7 months of age they are able to bear all their weight on their legs with assistance. *Crawling* (propelling forward with belly on floor) progresses to *creeping* (on hands and knees with belly off floor) by 9 months. At this time they stand while holding onto furniture and can pull themselves to the standing position, but they are unable to maneuver back down except by falling. By 11 months they walk while holding onto furniture or with both hands held, and by age 1 year they may be able to walk with one hand held. A number of infants attempt their first independent steps by their first birthday.

NURSE ALERT An infant who does not pull to a standing position by 11 to 12 months of age should be further evaluated for possible developmental dysplasia of the hip. Although there is considerable variation among infants for the achievement of these milestones, they provide guidelines for early intervention. ■

Psychosocial Development

Developing a Sense of Trust (Erikson)

Erikson's (1963) phase I (birth to 1 year) is concerned with *acquiring a sense of trust* while *overcoming a sense of mistrust.* The trust that develops is a trust of self, of others, and of the world. Infants "trust" that their feeding, comfort, stimulation, and caring needs will be met. The crucial element for the achievement of this task is the quality of both the parent-child (or caregiver-child) relationship and the care the infant receives. The provision of food, warmth, and shelter by itself is inadequate for the development of a strong sense of self. The infant and parent must jointly learn to satisfactorily meet their needs in order for mutual regulation of frustration to occur. When this synchrony fails to develop, mistrust is the eventual outcome.

Failure to learn "delayed gratification" leads to mistrust. Mistrust can result either from too much or too little frustration. If parents always meet their children's needs before the children signal their readiness, infants will never learn to test their ability to control the environment. If the delay is prolonged, infants experience constant frustration and eventually mistrust others in their efforts to satisfy them. Therefore consistency of care is essential.

The trust acquired in infancy provides the foundation for all succeeding phases. Trust allows infants a feeling of physical comfort and security, which assists them in experiencing unfamiliar, unknown situations with a minimum of fear. Erikson has divided the first year of life into two oral/social stages. During the first 3 to 4 months, food intake is the most important social activity in which the infant engages. The newborn can tolerate little frustration or delay of gratification. Primary *narcissism* (total concern for oneself) is at its height.

However, as bodily processes such as vision, motor movements, and vocalization become better controlled, infants use more advanced behaviors to interact with others. For example, rather than cry, infants may put their arms up to signify a desire to be held.

The next social modality involves a mode of reaching out to others through *grasping.* Grasping is initially reflexive, but even as a reflex it has a powerful social meaning for the parents. The reciprocal response to the infant's grasping is the parents' holding on and touching. There is pleasurable tactile stimulation for both the child and the parents.

Tactile stimulation is extremely important in the total process of acquiring trust. The degree of mothering skill, the quantity of food, or the length of sucking does not determine the quality of the experience. Rather, it is the total nature of the quality of the interpersonal relationship that influences the infant's formulation of trust.

During the second stage the more active and aggressive modality of *biting* occurs. Infants learn that they can hold onto what is their own and can more fully control their environment. During this stage infants may be confronted with one of their first conflicts. If they are breastfeeding, they quickly learn that biting causes the mother to become upset and withdraw the breast. Yet biting also brings internal relief from teething discomfort and a sense of power or control.

This conflict may be solved in a variety of ways. The mother may wean the infant from the breast and begin

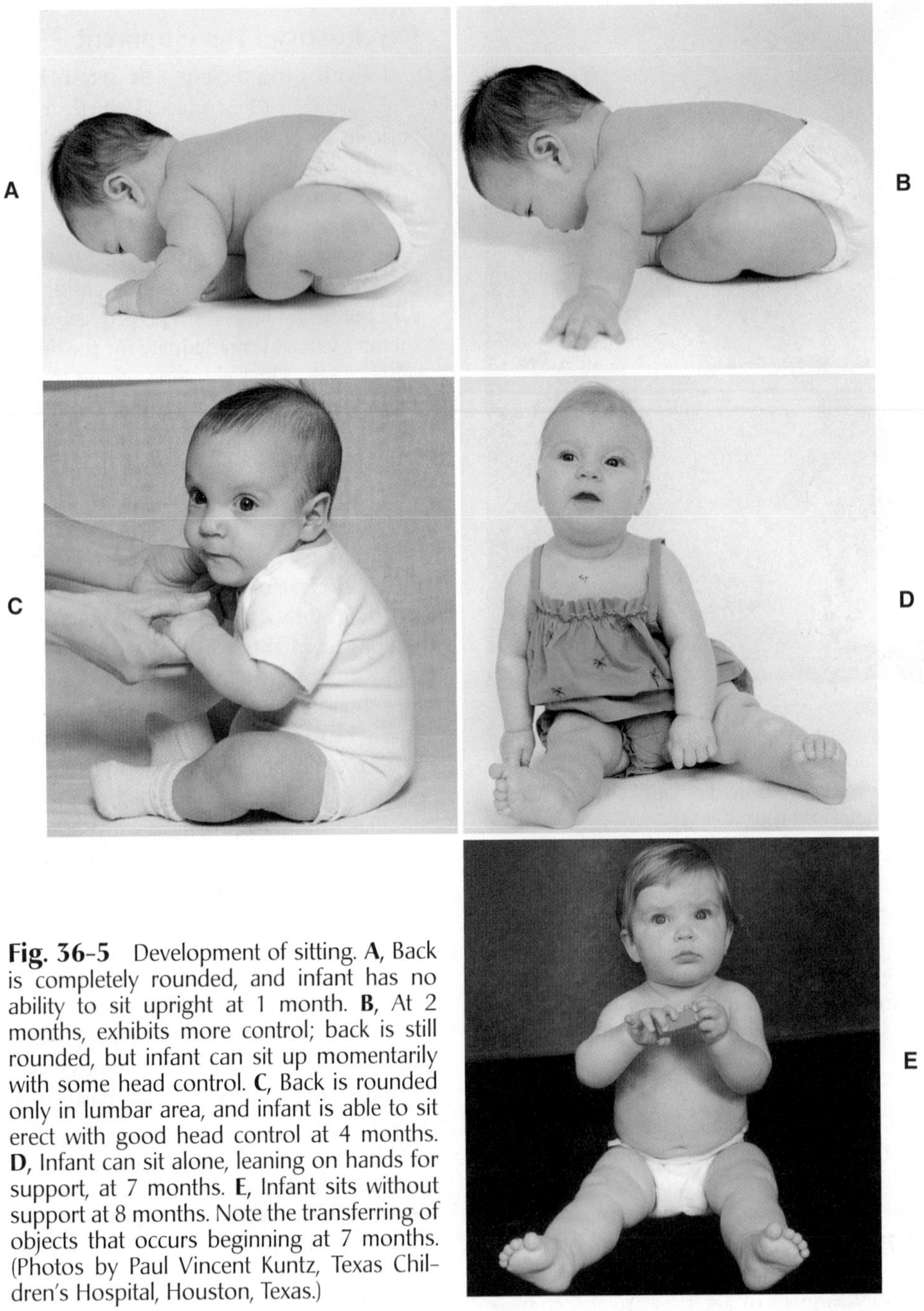

Fig. 36-5 Development of sitting. **A,** Back is completely rounded, and infant has no ability to sit upright at 1 month. **B,** At 2 months, exhibits more control; back is still rounded, but infant can sit up momentarily with some head control. **C,** Back is rounded only in lumbar area, and infant is able to sit erect with good head control at 4 months. **D,** Infant can sit alone, leaning on hands for support, at 7 months. **E,** Infant sits without support at 8 months. Note the transferring of objects that occurs beginning at 7 months. (Photos by Paul Vincent Kuntz, Texas Children's Hospital, Houston, Texas.)

bottle-feeding, or the infant may learn to bite substitute "nipples," such as a pacifier, and retain pleasurable breast-feeding. The successful resolution of this conflict strengthens the mother-child relationship because it occurs at a time when infants are recognizing the mother as the most significant person in their life.

Cognitive Development

Sensorimotor Phase (Piaget)

The theory most commonly used to explain *cognition,* or the ability to know, is that of Piaget (1952). The period from birth to 24 months is termed the *sensorimotor phase* and is composed of six stages; however, because this discussion is concerned with ages birth to 12 months, only the first four stages are discussed. The last two stages occur during the toddler period of 12 to 24 months and are discussed in Chapter 37.

During the sensorimotor phase infants progress from reflex behaviors to simple repetitive acts to imitative activity. Three crucial events take place during this phase. The first event involves *separation,* in which infants learn to separate themselves from other objects in the environment. They realize that others besides themselves control the environment and that certain readjustments must take place for mutual satisfaction to occur. This coincides with Erikson's concept of the formation of trust.

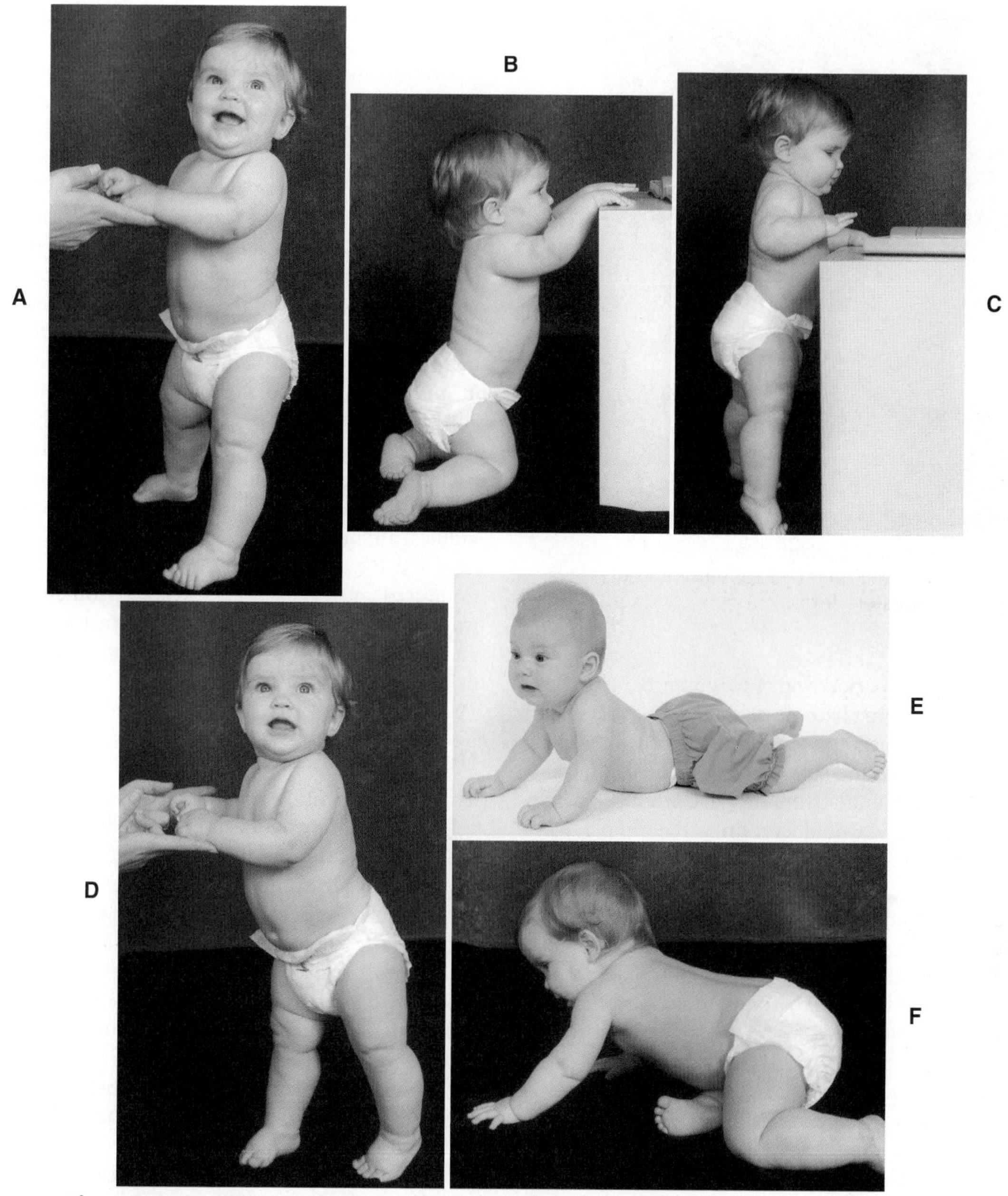

Fig. 36-6 Development of locomotion. **A,** Infant bears full weight on feet by 7 months. **B,** Infant can maneuver from sitting to kneeling position. **C,** Infant can stand holding onto furniture at 9 months. **D,** While standing, infant takes deliberate step at 10 months. **E,** Infant crawls with abdomen on floor and pulls self forward, and then, **F,** creeps on hands and knees at 9 months. (Photos by Paul Vincent Kuntz, Texas Children's Hospital, Houston, Texas.)

The second major accomplishment is achieving the concept of *object permanence,* or the realization that objects that leave the visual field still exist. A typical example of the development of object permanence is when infants are able to pursue objects they observe being hidden under a pillow or behind a chair (Fig. 36-7). This skill develops at approximately 9 to 10 months of age, which corresponds to the time of increased locomotion skills.

The last major intellectual achievement of this period is the ability to use *symbols,* or *mental representation.* The use of symbols allows the infant to think of an object or situation without actually experiencing it. The recognition of symbols is the beginning of the understanding of time and space.

Piaget's first stage, from birth to 1 month, is identified by the infant's *use of reflexes.* At birth the infant's individuality and temperament are expressed through the physiologic reflexes of sucking, rooting, grasping, and crying. The repetitious nature of the reflexes is the beginning of associations between an act and a sequential response. When infants cry because they are hungry, a nipple is put in the mouth, and they suck, feel satisfaction, and sleep. They are assimilating this experience while perceiving auditory, tactile, and visual cues. This experience of perceiving certain patterns, or "ordering," provides a foundation for the subsequent stages.

The second stage, *primary circular reactions,* marks the beginning of the replacement of reflexive behavior with vol-

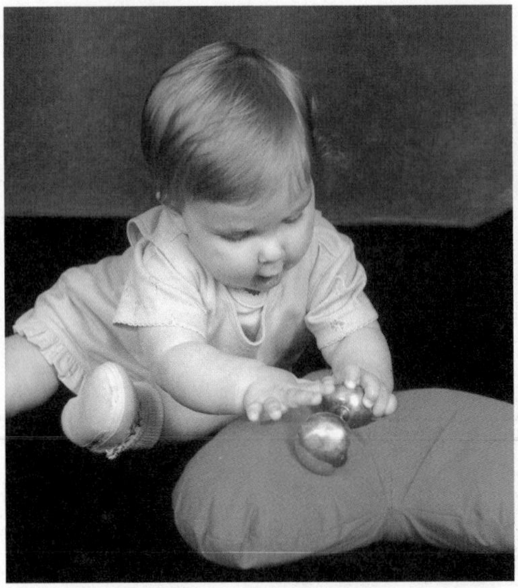

Fig. 36-7 Nine-month-old infant actively searches for object hidden behind pillow. (Photo by Paul Vincent Kuntz, Texas Children's Hospital, Houston, Texas.)

untary acts. During the period from 1 to 4 months, activities such as sucking or grasping become deliberate acts that elicit certain responses. The beginning of accommodation is evident. Infants incorporate and adapt their reactions to the environment and recognize the stimulus that produced a response. Previously they would cry until the nipple was brought to the mouth. Now they associate the nipple with the sound of the parent's voice. They accommodate this new piece of information and adapt by ceasing to cry when they hear the voice—before receiving the nipple. What is taking place is a realization of causality and a recognition of an orderly sequence of events. The environment is taken in with all of the senses and with whatever motor ability is present.

The *secondary circular reactions* stage is a continuation of primary circular reactions and lasts until 8 months of age. In this stage the primary circular reactions are repeated and prolonged for the response that results. Grasping and holding now become shaking, banging, and pulling. Shaking is performed to hear a noise, not solely for the pleasure of shaking. The quality and quantity of an act become evident. More or less shaking produces different responses. Causality, time, deliberate intention, and separateness from the environment begin to develop.

Three new processes of human behavior occur. *Imitation* requires the differentiation of selected acts from several events. By the second half of the first year, infants can imitate sounds and simple gestures. *Play* becomes evident as they take pleasure in performing an act after they have mastered it. Many of the infant's waking hours are absorbed in sensorimotor play. *Affect* (the outward manifestation of emotion and feeling) is seen as infants begin to develop a sense of permanency. During the first 6 months infants believe that an object exists only for as long as they can visually perceive it. In other words, out of sight—out of mind. Affect to external objects is evident when the object continues to be present or remembered even though it is beyond the range of perception. Object permanence is a critical component of parent-child attachment and is seen in the development of separation anxiety at 6 to 8 months of age (see p. 1035).

During the fourth sensorimotor stage, *coordination of secondary schemas and their application to new situations,* infants use previous behavioral achievements primarily as the foundation for adding new intellectual skills to their expanding repertoire. This stage is largely transitional. Increasing motor skills allow for greater exploration of the environment. They begin to discover that hiding an object does not mean that it is gone but that removing an obstacle will reveal the object. This marks the beginning of intellectual reasoning. Furthermore, they can experience an event by observing it, and they begin to associate symbols with events (e.g., "bye-bye" with "Daddy goes to work"), but the classification is purely their own. In this stage they learn from the object itself; this is in contrast to the second stage, in which infants learn from the type of interaction between objects or individuals. Intentionality is further developed in that infants now actively attempt to remove a barrier to the desired (or undesired) action (see Fig. 36-7). If something is in their way, they attempt to climb over it or push it away. Previously an obstacle would cause them to give up any further attempt to achieve the desired goal.

Development of Body Image

The development of body image parallels sensorimotor development. Infants' kinesthetic and tactile experiences are the first perceptions of their body, and the mouth is the principal area of pleasurable sensations. Other parts of the body are primarily objects of pleasure—the hands and fingers to suck and the feet to play with. As physical needs are met, they feel comfort and satisfaction with their body. Messages conveyed by the caregivers reinforce these feelings. For example, when infants smile, they receive emotional satisfaction from others who smile back.

Achieving the concept of object permanence is basic to the development of self-image. By the end of the first year infants recognize that they are distinct from their parents. At the same time, there is increasing interest in their image, especially in the mirror (Fig. 36-8). As motor skills develop, they learn that parts of the body are useful; for example, the hands bring objects to the mouth, and the legs help them move to different locations. All of these achievements transmit messages to them about themselves. Therefore it is important to transmit positive messages to infants about their bodies.

Social Development

Infants' social development is initially influenced by their reflexive behavior, such as the grasp, and eventually depends primarily on the interaction between them and the principal caregivers. *Attachment* to the parent is increasingly evident during the second half of the first year. In addition, tremendous strides are made in communication and personal-social behavior. Whereas crying and reflexive behavior are methods to meet one's needs in the neonatal period, the so-

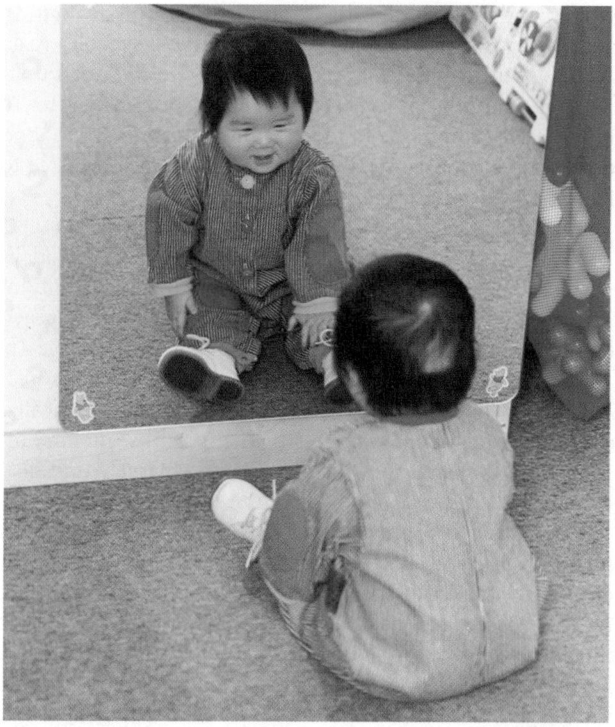

Fig. 36-8 Nine-month-old infant enjoying own image in mirror.

cial smile is an early step in social communication. This has a profound effect on family members and is a tremendous stimulus for evoking continued responses from others. By 4 months infants laugh aloud.

Play is a major socializing agent and provides stimulation needed to learn from and interact with the environment. By age 6 months infants are very personable. They play games such as peekaboo when their head is hidden in a towel, they signal their desire to be picked up by extending their arms, and they show displeasure when a toy is removed or their face is washed.

Attachment

The importance of human physical contact to infants cannot be overemphasized. Parenting is not an instinctual ability but a learned, acquired process. The attachment of parent and child, which begins before birth and assumes even more importance at birth, continues during the first year. In the following discussion of attachment, the term *mother* is used in the broad context of the consistent caregiver with whom the child relates more than anyone else. However, in society's changing social climate and sex-role stereotypes, this person may very well be the father or a grandparent. Studies on paternal-infant attachment demonstrate that stages similar to maternal attachment occur and that fathers are more involved in child care when mothers are employed (although mothers continue to do the majority of infant care). Additional research has shown that inexperienced, first-time fathers are as capable as experienced fathers of developing a close attachment with their infants.

Attachment progresses during infancy, with the child assuming an increasingly significant role. Two components of cognitive development are required for attachment: (1) the ability to discriminate the mother from other individuals, and (2) the achievement of object permanence. Both of these processes prepare the infant for an equally important aspect of attachment—separation from the parent. Separation-individuation should occur as a harmonious, parallel process with emotional attachment.

During the formation of attachment to the parent, the infant progresses through four distinct but overlapping stages. For the first few weeks infants respond indiscriminately to anyone. Beginning at approximately 8 to 12 weeks of age, they cry, smile, and vocalize more to the mother than to anyone else but continue to respond to others, whether familiar or not. At approximately 6 months of age, infants show a distinct preference for the mother. They follow her more, cry when she leaves, enjoy playing with her more, and feel most secure in her arms. About 1 month after showing attachment to the mother, many infants begin attaching to other members of the family, most often the father.

Infants acquire other developmental behaviors that influence the attachment process. These include (1) differential crying, smiling, and vocalization (more to the mother than to anyone else); (2) visual-motor orientation (looking more at the mother, even if she is not close); (3) crying when the mother leaves the room; (4) approaching through locomotion (crawling, creeping, or walking); (5) clinging (especially in the presence of a stranger); and (6) exploring away from the mother while using her as a secure base.

Reactive attachment disorder is a psychologic and developmental problem that stems from maladaptive or absent attachment between the infant and parent and may persist into childhood and even adulthood. Signs of reactive attachment disorder are usually seen before age 5 in infants who had insecure attachments to the mother or other primary caretaker. The child may manifest behaviors such as not being cuddly with parents, failing to make eye contact with significant others, having poor impulse control, and being destructive to self and others. Maltreated and orphaned children often are diagnosed with this complex disorder. Without early intervention, some of these children fail to develop a conscience and suffer from an antisocial personality disorder that may lead to criminal acts.

Separation Anxiety

Between ages 4 and 8 months the infant progresses through the first stage of separation-individuation and begins to have some awareness of self and mother as separate beings. At the same time, object permanence is developing, and the infant is aware that the parent can be absent. Therefore separation anxiety develops and is manifested through a predictable sequence of behaviors.

During the early second half of the first year, infants protest when placed in their crib, and a short time later they object when the mother leaves the room. Infants may not notice the mother's absence if they are absorbed in an activity. However, when they realize her absence, they protest. From this point on, they become very alert to her activities and whereabouts. By 11 to 12 months they are able to anticipate her imminent departure by watching her behaviors, and they begin to protest before she leaves. At this point many parents learn to postpone alerting the child to their departure until just before leaving.

Stranger Fear

As infants demonstrate attachment to one person, they correspondingly exhibit less friendliness to others. Between ages 6 and 8 months, fear of strangers and stranger anxiety become prominent and are related to infants' ability to discriminate between familiar and nonfamiliar people. Behaviors such as clinging to the parent, crying, and turning away from the stranger are common (Fig. 36-9).

Language Development

The infant's first means of verbal communication is crying. Crying as a biologic sign conveys a message of urgency and signals displeasure, such as hunger. However, crying is also a social event that affects the development of the parent-infant relationship—either by its absence, which usually has a positive effect on parents, or its presence, which may involve a negative response or persuade parents to minister to the child's physical or emotional needs.

In the first few weeks of life, crying has a reflexive quality and is mostly related to physiologic needs. Infants cry for 1 to 1½ hours a day up to 3 weeks of age; then build up to 2 and even 4 hours by 6 weeks. Crying tends to decrease by 12 weeks of age. It is thought that the increase in crying for no apparent reason during the first few months may be related to the discharge of energy and the maturational changes in the central nervous system. During the end of the first year, infants cry for attention; from fear (especially stranger fear); and from frustration, usually in response to their developing but inadequate motor skills.

NURSE ALERT Be alert to parents' reports about maternal postpartum depression and infant crying, because these concerns may indicate a stressed mother-infant relationship. ■

Vocalizations heard during crying eventually become syllables and words (e.g., the "mama" heard during vigorous crying). Infants vocalize as early as 5 to 6 weeks of age by making small throaty sounds. By 2 months they make single vowel sounds such as *ah, eh,* and *uh.* By 3 to 4 months the consonants *n, k, g, p,* and *b* are added, and the infants coo, gurgle, and laugh aloud. By 8 months they imitate sounds, add the consonants *t, d,* and *w,* and combine syllables (e.g., "dada"), but they do not ascribe meaning to the word until 10 to 11 months of age (Family Focus box). By 9 to 10 months they comprehend the meaning of the word "no" and obey simple commands. By age 1 year they can say three to five words with meaning.

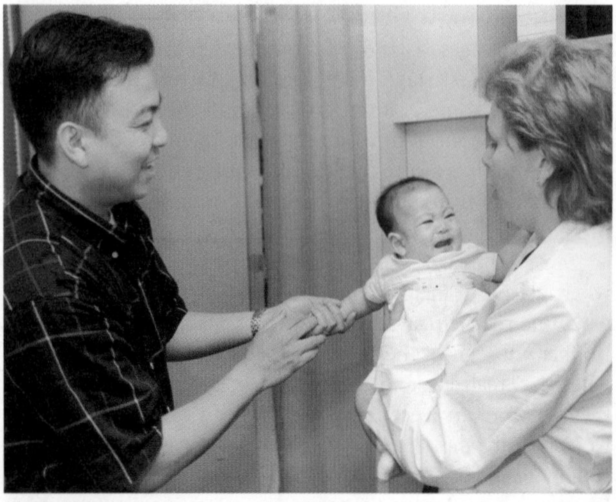

Fig. 36-9 Behaviors related to fear of strangers include clinging to the parent and turning away from the stranger. (Photo by Paul Vincent Kuntz, Texas Children's Hospital, Houston, Texas.)

Play

Play during infancy represents the various social modalities observed during cognitive development. The activity of infants is primarily narcissistic and revolves around their own body. As discussed under Development of Body Image (p. 1034), body parts are primarily objects of play and pleasure.

During the first year, play becomes more sophisticated and interdependent. From birth to 3 months, infants' responses to the environment are global and largely undifferentiated. Play is dependent; pleasure is demonstrated by a quieting attitude (1 month), a smile (2 months), or a squeal (3 months). From 3 to 6 months, infants show more discriminate interest in stimuli and begin to play alone with a rattle or a soft stuffed toy or with someone else. There is much more interaction during play. By 4 months of age they laugh aloud, show preference for certain toys, and become excited when food or a favorite object is brought to them. They recognize an image in a mirror, smile at it, and vocalize to it.

By 6 months to 1 year, play involves sensorimotor skills. Actual games such as peekaboo and pat-a-cake are played. Verbal repetition and imitation of simple gestures occurs in response to demonstration. Play is much more selective, not only in terms of specific toys, but also in terms of "playmates." Although play is solitary or one-sided, infants choose with whom they will interact. At 6 to 8 months they usually refuse to play with strangers. Parents are definite favorites, and infants know how to attract their attention. At 6 months they extend the arms to be picked up, at 7 months cough to make their presence known, at 10 months pull the parent's clothing, and at 12 months call them by name. This represents a tremendous advance from the newborn who signaled biologic needs by crying to express displeasure.

Stimulation is as important for psychosocial growth as food is for physical growth. Knowledge of developmental milestones allows nurses to guide parents regarding proper play for infants. It is not sufficient to place a mobile over a crib and toys in a playpen for a child's optimum social, emotional, and intellectual development. Play must provide interpersonal contact and recreational and educational stimu-

Family Focus

CHILD'S DEVELOPING LANGUAGE SKILLS

During the acquisition of new language skills the child temporarily may stop using other recently learned sounds or words. This is often distressing for parents, who have waited in anticipation for the words "dada" or "mama," because these sounds are commonly replaced by other vocalizations and may not be repeated for several weeks. Nurses can reassure parents that the child will again say these special words, and with increased meaning.

lation. Infants need to be *played with*, not merely *allowed to play*. Although the type of play infants engage in is called *solitary*, this is a figurative, not literal, term to denote one-sided play. The type of toys given to the child is much less important than the quality of personal interaction that occurs.

Table 36-1 lists play activities appropriate for the developmental level of the infant in view of motor, language, and personal-social achievements. Although the activities are grouped according to the major mode of stimulation provided, there is overlap in many instances. In addition, play

Table 36-1

Play During Infancy

AGE (MONTHS)	VISUAL STIMULATION	AUDITORY STIMULATION	TACTILE STIMULATION	KINETIC STIMULATION
SUGGESTED ACTIVITIES				
Birth-1	Look at infant at close range Hang bright, shiny object within 20-25 cm (8-10 inches) of infant's face and in midline Hang mobiles with black-and-white designs	Talk to infant; sing in soft voice Play music box, tape, or CD Have ticking clock or metronome nearby	Hold, caress, cuddle Keep infant warm May like to be swaddled	Rock infant; place in cradle Use stroller for walks
2-3	Provide bright objects Make room bright with pictures or mirrors Take infant to various rooms while doing chores Place infant in infant seat for vertical view of environment	Talk to infant Include in family gatherings Expose to various environmental noises other than those of home Use rattles, wind chimes	Caress infant while bathing, at diaper change Comb hair with a soft brush Give massage	Use infant swing Take in car for rides Exercise body by moving extremities in swimming motion Use cradle gym
4-6	Place infant in front of unbreakable mirror Give brightly colored toys to hold (small enough to grasp)	Talk to infant; repeat sounds infant makes Laugh when infant laughs Call infant by name Crinkle different papers by infant's ear Place rattle or ball in hand	Give infant soft squeeze toys of various textures Allow to splash in bath Place nude on soft, furry rug and move extremities	Use swing or stroller Bounce infant in lap while holding in standing position Support infant in sitting position; let infant lean forward to balance self Place infant on floor to crawl, roll over, sit
6-9	Give infant large toys with bright colors, moveable parts, and noisemakers Place unbreakable mirror where infant can see self Play peekaboo, especially hiding face in a towel Make funny faces to encourage imitation Give ball of yarn or string to pull apart	Call infant by name Repeat simple words such as "dada," "mama," "bye-bye" Speak clearly Name parts of body, people, and foods Tell infant what you are doing Use "no" only when necessary Give simple commands Show how to clap hands, bang a drum	Let infant play with fabrics of various textures Have bowl with foods of different sizes and textures to feel Let infant "catch" running water Encourage "swimming" in large bathtub or shallow pool Give wad of sticky tape to manipulate	Hold upright to bear weight and bounce Pick up, say "up" Put down, say "down" Place toys out of reach; encourage infant to get them Play pat-a-cake
9-12	Show infant large pictures in books Take infant to places where there are animals, many people, different objects (shopping center) Play ball by rolling it to child, demonstrate "throwing" it back Demonstrate building a two-block tower	Read infant simple nursery rhymes Point to body parts and name each one Imitate sounds of animals	Give infant finger foods of different textures Let infant mess and squash food Let infant feel cold (ice cube) or warm objects, say what temperature each is Let infant feel a breeze (fan blowing)	Give large push-pull toys Place furniture in a circle to encourage cruising Turn in different positions

Continued

Table 36-1

Play During Infancy—cont'd

AGE (MONTHS)	VISUAL STIMULATION	AUDITORY STIMULATION	TACTILE STIMULATION	KINETIC STIMULATION
SUGGESTED TOYS				
Birth-6	Nursery mobiles Unbreakable mirrors See-through crib bumpers Contrasting colored sheets	Music boxes Musical mobiles Crib dangle bells Small-handled, clear rattle	Stuffed animals Soft clothes Soft or furry quilt Soft mobiles	Rocking crib/cradle Weighted or suction toy Infant swing
6-12	Various colored blocks Nested boxes or cups Books with rhymes and bright pictures Strings of big beads Simple take-apart toys Large ball Cup and spoon Large puzzles Jack-in-the-box	Rattles of different sizes, shapes, tones, and bright colors Squeaky animals and dolls Light, rhythmic music	Soft, different-texture animals and dolls Sponge toys, floating toys Squeeze toys Teething toys Books with textures/objects, such as fur and zipper	Activity box for crib Push-pull toys Wind-up swing

activities suggested for one age group may be appropriate for older infants but inappropriate for younger infants.

Temperament

The infant's temperament or behavioral style influences the type of interaction that occurs between the child and parents, especially the mother, and other family members (see general discussion of temperament in Chapter 33). In assessing a child's temperament, it is the parents' perception of the child and the degree of fit between their expectations and the child's actual temperament that are important. The more dissonance or lack of harmony between the child's temperament and the parent's ability to accept and deal with the behavior, the more risk for subsequent parent-child conflicts.

Although most behavioral researchers agree that there is a strong biologic component to temperament, researchers also suggest that temperament may be modified by the environment, particularly the family (Wilson et al, 2000). Family interaction with the infant is perceived as a circular process wherein each family member affects each other and the family as a unit. With these concepts in mind, the nurse has an important role in helping the family understand the infant's temperament as it relates to family dynamics and the eventual well-being of the child and family unit (Wilson et al, 2000).

The Revised Infant Temperament Questionnaire (RITQ) (Carey & McDevitt, 1978) can be used as a screening tool with parents. The questionnaire focuses on nine temperament variables, but the 95 questions relate specifically to activities such as sleep, feeding, play, diapering, and dressing. The scores from the RITQ help identify the child's temperamental style. Use of the RITQ is well accepted by parents and should be accompanied by an adequate explanation of the results. In discussing the results, it is best to avoid descriptors such as "difficult" by describing such infants in terms of characteristics such as "intense" or "less predictable." The Early Infancy Temperament Questionnaire is a 76-item parent questionnaire that was adapted from the RITQ to specifically evaluate temperament characteristics of infants 1 to 4 months old, whereas the RITQ is best suited for infants 4 months old and older (Medoff-Cooper, Carey, & McDevitt, 1993).

With knowledge of the infant's temperament, nurses are better able to (1) provide parents with background information that will help them see their child in a better perspective, (2) offer a more organized picture of their child's behavior and possibly reveal distortions in their perceptions of the behavior, and (3) guide parents regarding appropriate childrearing techniques.

Childrearing Practices Related to Temperament

Most parents realize that their infant is born with unique characteristics, and few parents of difficult infants need to be told of the challenge of caring for them. However, very few parents are aware of the significance of the temperamental characteristics and of constructive approaches to dealing with them. The following are examples of interventions that promote more positive parenting of infants with different temperament styles.*

"Difficult" children may respond better to scheduled feedings and structured caregiving routines than to demand feedings and frequent changes in daily routines.

*Recommended resources for parents are *The Difficult Child* by S. K. Turecki and L. Tonner (2000, Bantam Books; www.randomhouse.com) and *Know Your Child: An Authoritative Guide for Today's Parents* by S. Chess and A. Thomas (1996, Jason Aronson, Inc.; www.aronson.com).

These children sleep less and may need more structured approaches to bedtime to prevent bedtime problems. "Highly distractible" children may require additional soothing measures such as swinging, rocking, or being carried in a pack that the parent wears across the chest or back. Children with "high activity" levels require vigilant watching, and parents need to take extra precautions in safeguarding the home. These children benefit from increased opportunities for gross motor activity to constructively channel their energy.

The child who is "slow to warm up" may demonstrate more stranger fear than other children and may require gradual and frequent preparation for new situations, such as substitute child care. Even the "easy child" can present problems in that the parents may need reminders to feed the child who sleeps for prolonged intervals and rarely cries. They may need to "retrain" the child because of the ease of developing habits such as keeping the child up late or sleeping with the youngster, which may later become troublesome.

Appropriate counseling based on awareness of the child's temperament can greatly enhance the quality of interaction between parents and infant. Even just letting parents know that "difficult" traits are innate can relieve feelings of guilt and incompetence (Family Focus box).

Because of the complexity of the developmental process during the first 12 months, Table 36-2 is presented to help organize and clarify the data already discussed. Although all milestones are important, some represent essential integrative aspects of development that lay the foundation for achievement of more advanced skills. These essential milestones are designated by an asterisk in the table. The table represents the average monthly age at which various skills are attained. It must be remembered that although the sequence is the same, the rate will vary among children.

Coping with Concerns Related to Normal Growth and Development

Separation and Stranger Fear

A number of fears can appear during infancy. However, the fear that causes parents the most concern is fear related to strangers and separation. Although erroneously interpreted by some as a sign of undesirable, antisocial behavior, stranger fear and separation anxiety are important components of a strong, healthy, parent-child attachment. Nevertheless, this period can present difficulties for the parent and child. Parents may be more confined to the home because baby-sitters are violently protested by the infant. To accustom the infant to new people, parents are encouraged to have close friends or relatives visit often. This provides for other persons with whom the child is comfortable and who can give parents time for themselves.

Infants also need opportunities to safely experience strangers. Usually toward the end of the first year, infants begin to venture away from the parent and demonstrate curiosity about strangers. If allowed to explore at their own rate, many infants eventually "warm up." If parents hold the child away from their face, the infant can observe while maintaining close physical contact.

The best approach for the stranger (who may be the nurse) is to talk softly, meet the child at eye level (to appear smaller), maintain a safe distance from the infant, and avoid sudden, intrusive gestures, such as holding the arms out and smiling broadly.

Parents also may wonder whether they should encourage the child's clinging, dependent behavior, especially if there is pressure from others who view this as "spoiling" (see the following discussion). Parents need to be reassured that such behavior is healthy, desirable, and necessary for the child's optimum emotional development. If parents can reassure the infant of their presence, the infant will learn to realize that they are still there even if not physically present. Talking to infants when leaving the room, allowing them to hear one's voice on the telephone, and using transitional objects (e.g., a favorite blanket or toy) reassures them of the parent's continued presence.

Alternative Child Care Arrangements

For many parents, especially working mothers, the need for locating safe and competent child care facilities for the infant is an increasingly difficult problem—one that is compounded by the number of mothers working outside the home. Over the past 30 years there has been a marked shift in child care arrangements, with fewer children being cared

Text continued on p. 1044.

Family Focus

DIFFICULT TEMPERAMENT AND PRETERM INFANTS

Parents typically rate preterm, low-birth-weight infants as being more difficult than full-term infants (Hughes et al, 2002; Langkamp, Kim, & Pasco, 1998). Parents are often concerned that the difficult temperament is permanent and results from the many negative and painful hospital experiences. The family can be reassured that although these infants may be difficult to parent for the first 6 months of corrected age (chronologic age minus amount of prematurity), over time the infants tend to become less difficult (Medoff-Cooper, 1995). In one study, preterm infants were rated by their mothers at 4 and 9 months of age in relation to temperament. The preterm infants at 9 months were still significantly perceived as more difficult in comparison with full-term infants at the same age (Langkamp & Pascoe, 2001). Further research is needed to clarify the relationship between preterm infant temperament, extent of illness at birth, and family and environmental influences. Many of the studies indicating that preterm infants are more difficult to console were performed before wide-scale implementation of individualized developmental care for such infants; kangaroo care and assisting the infant in self-regulation behaviors may change current thought. One study found that healthy low-birth-weight infants who experienced kangaroo care (skin-to-skin contact) versus infants who received standard medical/nursing care had higher scores for consolability and state orientation and lower intensity ratings (Ohgi et al, 2002). By enabling the preterm infant to experience more positive caretaking and less stressful stimuli, such infants may be found in the future to be less temperamental.

Table 36-2

Growth and Development during Infancy

AGE (MONTHS)	PHYSICAL	GROSS MOTOR	FINE MOTOR
1	Weight gain of 150-210 g (5-7 ounces) weekly for first 6 months Height gain of 2.5 cm (1 inch) monthly for first 6 months Head circumference increases by 1.5 cm (6/10) inch) monthly for first 6 months Primitive reflexes present and strong Doll's eye reflexes and dance reflex fading Obligatory nose breathing (most infants)	Assumes flexed position with pelvis high but knees not under abdomen when prone (at birth, knees flexed under abdomen)* Can turn head from side to side when prone; lifts head momentarily from bed (see Fig. 36-3, *A*)* Has marked head lag, especially when pulled from lying to sitting position (see Fig. 36-2, *A*) Holds head momentarily parallel and in midline when suspended in prone position Assumes asymmetric tonic neck reflex position when supine When held in standing position, body is limp at knees and hips In sitting position, back is uniformly rounded, absence of head control	Hands predominantly closed Grasp reflex strong Hand clenches on contact with rattle
2	Posterior fontanel closed Crawling reflex disappears	Assumes less flexed position when prone—hips flat, legs extended, arms flexed, head to side* Less head lag when pulled to sitting position (see Fig. 36-2, *B*) Can maintain head in same plane as rest of body when held in ventral suspension When prone, can lift head almost 45 degrees off table When moved to sitting position, head is held up but bends forward (see Fig. 36-5, *B*) Assumes asymmetric tonic neck reflex position intermittently	Hands often open Grasp reflex fading
3	Primitive reflexes fading	Able to hold head more erect when sitting, but still bobs forward Has only slight head lag when pulled to sitting position Assumes symmetric body positioning Able to raise head and shoulders from prone position to a 45- to 90-degree angle from table; bears weight on forearms When held in standing position, able to bear slight fraction of weight on legs Regards own hand	Actively holds rattle but will not reach for it* Grasp reflex absent Hands kept loosely open Clutches own hand; pulls at blankets and clothes
4	Drooling begins Moro, tonic neck, and rooting reflexes have disappeared*	Has almost no head lag when pulled to sitting position (see Fig. 36-2, *C*)* Balances head well in sitting position (see Fig. 36-5, *C*)* Back less rounded, curved only in lumbar area Able to sit erect if propped up Able to raise head and chest off surface to angle of 90 degrees (see Fig. 36-3, *B*) Assumes predominant symmetric position Rolls from back to side*	Inspects and plays with hands; pulls clothing or blanket over face in play* Tries to reach objects with hand but overshoots Grasps object with both hands Plays with rattle placed in hand, shakes it, but cannot pick it up if dropped Can carry objects to mouth

*Milestones that represent essential integrative aspects of development that lay the foundation for the achievement of more advanced skills.

SENSORY	VOCALIZATION	SOCIALIZATION/COGNITION
Able to fixate on moving object in range of 45 degrees when held at a distance of 20-25 cm (8-10 inches) Visual acuity approaches 20/100† Follows light to midline Quiets when hears a voice	Cries to express displeasure Makes small, throaty sounds Makes comfort sounds during feeding	Is in sensorimotor phase—stage I, use of reflexes (birth-1 month), and stage II, primary circular reactions (1-4 months) Watches parent's face intently as parent talks to infant
Binocular fixation and convergence to near objects beginning When supine, follows dangling toy from side to point beyond midline Visually searches to locate sounds Turns head to side when sound is made at level of ear	Vocalizes, distinct from crying* Crying becomes differentiated Coos Vocalizes to familiar voice	Demonstrates social smile in response to various stimuli*
Follows object to periphery (180 degrees)* Locates sound by turning head to side and looking in same direction* Begins to have ability to coordinate stimuli from various sense organs	Squeals aloud to show pleasure* Coos, babbles, chuckles Vocalizes when smiling "Talks" a great deal when spoken to Less crying during periods of wakefulness	Displays considerable interest in surroundings Ceases crying when parent enters room Can recognize familiar faces and objects, such as feeding bottle Shows awareness of strange situations
Able to accommodate to near objects Binocular vision fairly well established Can focus on a 1.25 cm (½-inch) block Beginning eye-hand coordination	Makes consonant sounds *n, k, g, p, b* Laughs aloud* Vocalization changes according to mood	Is in stage III, secondary circular reactions Demands attention by fussing; becomes bored if left alone Enjoys social interaction with people Anticipates feeding when sees bottle or mother if breastfeeding Shows excitement with whole body, squeals, breathes heavily Shows interest in strange stimuli Begins to show memory

†Degree of visual acuity varies according to vision measurement procedure used.

Continued

Table 36-2

Growth and Development during Infancy—cont'd

AGE (MONTHS)	PHYSICAL	GROSS MOTOR	FINE MOTOR
5	Beginning signs of tooth eruption Birth weight doubles	No head lag when pulled to sitting position When sitting, able to hold head erect and steady Able to sit for longer periods when back is well supported Back straight When prone, assumes symmetric positioning with arms extended Can turn over from abdomen to back* When supine, puts feet to mouth	Able to grasp objects voluntarily* Uses palmar grasp, bidextrous approach Plays with toes Takes objects directly to mouth Holds one cube while regarding a second one
6	Growth rate may begin to decline Weight gain of 90-150 g (3-5 ounces) weekly for next 6 months Height gain of 1.25 cm (½ inch) monthly for next 6 months Teething may begin with eruption of two lower central incisors* Chewing and biting occur*	When prone, can lift chest and upper abdomen off surface, bearing weight on hands (see Fig. 36-3, *C*) When about to be pulled to a sitting position, lifts head Sits in high chair with back straight Rolls from back to abdomen When held in standing position, bears almost all of weight Hand regard absent	Resecures a dropped object Drops one cube when another is given Grasps and manipulates small objects Holds bottle Grasps feet and pulls to mouth
7	Eruption of upper central incisors	When supine, spontaneously lifts head off surface Sits, leaning forward on hands (see Fig. 36-5, *D*)* When prone, bears weight on one hand Sits erect momentarily Bears full weight on feet (see Fig. 36-6, *A*) When held in standing position, bounces actively	Transfers objects from one hand to the other (see Fig. 36-5, *E*)* Has unidextrous approach and grasp Holds two cubes more than momentarily Bangs cube on table Rakes at a small object
8	Begins to show regular patterns in bladder and bowel elimination Parachute reflex appears (see Fig. 36-4)	Sits steadily unsupported (see Fig. 36-5, *E*)* Readily bears weight on legs when supported; may stand holding onto furniture Adjusts posture to reach an object	Has beginning pincer grasp using index, fourth, and fifth fingers against lower part of thumb Releases objects at will Rings bell purposely Retains two cubes while regarding third cube Secures an object by pulling on a string Reaches persistently for toys out of reach
9	Eruption of upper lateral incisor may begin	Creeps on hands and knees Sits steadily on floor for prolonged time (10 minutes) Recovers balance when leans forward but cannot do so when leaning sideways Pulls self to standing position and stands holding onto furniture (see Fig. 36-6, *B* and *C*)*	Uses thumb and index fingers in crude pincer grasp (see Fig. 36-1)* Preference for use of dominant hand now evident Grasps third cube Compares two cubes by bringing them together

*Milestones that represent essential integrative aspects of development that lay the foundation for the achievement of more advanced skills.

SENSORY	VOCALIZATION	SOCIALIZATION/COGNITION
Visually pursues a dropped object Is able to sustain visual inspection of an object Can localize sounds made below ear	Squeals Makes cooing vowel sounds interspersed with consonant sounds (e.g., *ah-goo*)	Smiles at mirror image Pats bottle or breast with both hands More enthusiastically playful, but may have rapid mood swings Is able to discriminate strangers from family Vocalizes displeasure when object is taken away Discovers parts of body
Adjusts posture to see an object Prefers more complex visual stimuli Can localize sounds made above ear Will turn head to the side, then look up or down	Begins to imitate sounds* Babbling resembles one-syllable utterances—*ma, mu, da, di, hi** Vocalizes to toys, mirror image Takes pleasure in hearing own sounds (self-reinforcement)	Recognizes parents; begins to fear strangers Holds arms out to be picked up Has definite likes and dislikes Begins to imitate (cough, protrusion of tongue) Excites on hearing footsteps Laughs when head is hidden in a towel Briefly searches for a dropped object (object permanence beginning)* Frequent mood swings—from crying to laughing with little or no provocation
Can fixate on very small objects* Responds to own name Localizes sound by turning head in a curving arch Beginning awareness of depth and space Has taste preferences	Produces vowel sounds and chained syllables—*baba, dada, kaka** Vocalizes four distinct vowel sounds "Talks" when others are talking	Increasing fear of strangers; shows signs of fretfulness when parent disappears* Imitates simple acts and noises Tries to attract attention by coughing or snorting Plays peekaboo Demonstrates dislike of food by keeping lips closed Exhibits oral aggressiveness in biting and mouthing Demonstrates expectation in response to repetition of stimuli
	Makes consonant sounds *t, d,* and *w* Listens selectively to familiar words Utterances signal emphasis and emotion Combines syllables, such as *dada,* but does not ascribe meaning to them	Increasing anxiety over loss of parent, particularly mother, and fear of strangers Responds to word "no" Dislikes dressing, diaper change
Localizes sounds by turning head diagonally and directly toward sound Depth perception increasing	Responds to simple verbal commands Comprehends "no-no"	Parent (mother) is increasingly important for own sake Shows increasing interest in pleasing parent Begins to show fears of going to bed and being left alone Puts arms in front of face to avoid having it washed

Continued

Table 36-2

Growth and Development during Infancy—cont'd

AGE (MONTHS)	PHYSICAL	GROSS MOTOR	FINE MOTOR
10	Labyrinth-righting reflex is strongest—when infant is in prone or supine position, is able to raise head	Can change from prone to sitting position Stands while holding onto furniture, sits by falling down Recovers balance easily while sitting While standing, lifts one foot to take a step (see Fig. 36-6, *D*)	Crude release of an object beginning Grasps bell by handle
11	Eruption of lower lateral incisor may begin	When sitting, pivots to reach toward back to pick up an object Cruises or walks holding onto furniture or with both hands held*	Explores objects more thoroughly (e.g., clapper inside bell) Has neat pincer grasp Drops object deliberately for it to be picked up Puts one object after another into a container (sequential play) Able to manipulate an object to remove it from tight-fitting enclosure
12	Birth weight tripled* Birth length increased by 50%* Head and chest circumference equal (head circumference 46 cm [18 inches]) Has total of six to eight deciduous teeth Anterior fontanel almost closed Landau reflex fading Babinski reflex disappears Lumbar curve develops; lordosis evident during walking	Walks with one hand held* Cruises well May attempt to stand alone momentarily; may attempt first step alone* Can sit down from standing position without help	Releases cube in cup Attempts to build two-block tower but fails Tries to insert a pellet into a narrow-necked bottle but fails Can turn pages in a book, many at a time

*Milestones that represent essential integrative aspects of development that lay the foundation for the achievement of more advanced skills.

for at home and more children being cared for in group centers or other settings.

The basic types of care are in-home care, either in the parents' or caregivers' home (family day care), and center-based care, usually in a day care center. *In-home care* may consist of a full-time baby-sitter who lives in the home, a full-time baby-sitter who comes to the home, cooperative arrangements such as exchange baby-sitting, and family day care. A licensed *family day care home* typically provides care and protection for up to five children for part of a day and does not include informal arrangements such as exchange baby-sitting or caregivers in the child's own home. The five children include the family day care provider's own children younger than 5 years of age living in the home. Unfortunately, many family day care homes operate without a license and may care for large numbers of infants without adequate staff and facilities.

Center-based care usually refers to a licensed day care facility that provides care for six or more children, for 6 or more hours in a day. *Work-based group care* is another op-

Table 36-2

Growth and Development during Infancy

SENSORY	VOCALIZATION	SOCIALIZATION/COGNITION
	Says "dada," "mama" with meaning* Comprehends "bye-bye" May say one word (e.g., "hi," "bye," "no")	Inhibits behavior to verbal command of "no-no" or own name Imitates facial expressions; waves bye-bye Extends toy to another person but will not release it Develops object permanence* Repeats actions that attract attention and cause laughter Pulls clothes of another to attract attention Plays interactive game such as pat-a-cake Reacts to adult anger; cries when scolded Demonstrates independence in dressing, feeding, locomotive skills, and testing of parents Looks at and follows pictures in a book
	Imitates definite speech sounds	Experiences joy and satisfaction when a task is mastered Reacts to restrictions with frustration Rolls ball to another on request Anticipates body gestures when a familiar nursery rhyme or story is being told (e.g., holds toes and feet in response to "This little piggy went to market") Plays game up-down, "so big," or peekaboo Shakes head for "no"
Discriminates simple geometric forms (e.g., circle) Amblyopia may develop with lack of binocularity Can follow rapidly moving object Controls and adjusts response to sound; listens for sound to recur	Says three to five words besides "dada," "mama"* Comprehends meaning of several words (comprehension always precedes verbalization) Recognizes objects by name Imitates animal sounds Understands simple verbal commands (e.g., "Give it to me," "Show me your eyes")	Shows emotions such as jealousy, affection (may give hug or kiss on request), anger, fear Enjoys familiar surroundings and explores away from parent Is fearful in strange situation; clings to parent May develop habit of "security blanket" or favorite toy Has increasing determination to practice to locomotor skills Searches for an object even if it has not been hidden, but searches only where object was last seen*

tion that is becoming increasingly popular as employers recognize the benefit of providing quality and convenient child care to their employees. *Sick-child care* may also be available for times when the youngster is ill. Such programs are often located in community hospitals or in work settings.

A major nursing responsibility is guiding parents in locating suitable facilities that have a well-qualified staff. State licensing agencies can help parents identify day care centers that accept children of specific age groups and that are convenient to home and work. Their records are available to the public and provide reports from the health, safety, and fire departments; periodic evaluations from the licensing agency; complaints filed against the center; and qualifications of the center's employees. State-licensed programs are supposed to abide by established standards, which represent the minimum requirements and safeguards; however, enforcement of the standards is sometimes inadequate. Early childhood programs may also belong to a voluntary accreditation system, the National

Academy of Early Childhood Programs, which serves as a model for optimum care.* References from other parents are also helpful, provided that they have investigated the center carefully and have remained involved with the agency's activities.

The same attention should be applied to locating competent baby-sitters. References from other employers are essential, and there is no substitute for observing the interaction between the individual and the child. Although very young infants need little if any preparation for the introduction of a new caregiver, older infants may benefit from a gradual placement to reduce stranger anxiety. At all times the parent should have the right to visit the child, and regular conferences should be established to review the child's progress. With computer technology some child care centers provide a service whereby the parent may log on to the Internet from work and view the child's activity at the center for reassurance that the child is well.

Limit Setting and Discipline

As infants' motor skills advance and mobility increases, parents are faced with the need to set safe limits to protect the child and establish a positive and supportive parent-child relationship (see Nurse's Role in Injury Prevention, p. 1073). Although there are numerous disciplinary techniques, some are more appropriate for this age than others. An effective approach used in disciplining a child is the use of "time-out." The basic principles are the same as those discussed in Chapter 31, except that the place for time-out needs to be commensurate with the child's abilities. For example, the playpen is better for most infants than a chair. Although parents may be concerned with instituting discipline during infancy, it is important to stress that the earlier effective disciplinary methods are employed, the easier it is to continue these approaches.

Parents must recognize the child's cognitive and behavioral limitations; adequate protection from hazards must be implemented because infants and toddlers do not understand a cause-effect relationship between dangerous objects and physical harm. Children will innately test limits and explore during the exploratory phase of growth; instead of discouraging exploration, safe alternatives should be provided, dangerous household items should be put away, and children should be given consistent discipline and nurturing.

*Information about the accreditation criteria and procedures of the National Academy of Early Childhood Programs is available from the National Association for the Education of Young Children, 1509 16th St. NW, Washington, DC 20036; phone: 800-424-2460 or 202-232-8777; fax: 202-328-1846; Web site: www.naeyc.org. These criteria are excellent guidelines for evaluating child care facilities. Other resources are *Child Care: Choosing the Best for Your Family,* available from the American Academy of Pediatrics, 141 Northwest Point Blvd., Elk Grove Village, IL 60007; phone: 888-227-1770, fax: 847-228-1281; Web site: www.medem.com, then enter Medical Library for pamphlet titles; and *Parent's Guide to Day Care,* available from the National Association of Pediatric Nurse Associates and Practitioners (NAPNAP), 1101 Kings Highway North, Suite 206, Cherry Hill, NJ 08034-1912; phone: 877-662-7627 or 856-667-1773; fax: 856-667-7187; Web site: www.napnap.org.

Thumb-Sucking and Use of a Pacifier

Sucking is the infant's chief pleasure and may not be satisfied by breastfeeding or bottle-feeding. It is such a strong need that infants who are deprived of sucking, such as those with a cleft lip repair, will suck on their tongue. Some newborns are born with sucking blisters on their hands from in utero sucking activity. The benefits of nonnutritive sucking in preterm infants have been documented, such as increased weight gain, decreased length of stay, and improved pain management (Pickler & Frankel, 1995; Pinelli & Symington, 2000; Pinelli, Symington, & Ciliska, 2002).

Problems arise when parents are concerned about the sucking of the fingers, thumb, or pacifier and attempt to restrain this natural tendency. Before giving advice, nurses should investigate the parents' feelings and base guidance on this information.

During infancy and early childhood there is no need to restrain nonnutritive sucking of the fingers. Malocclusion may occur if thumb-sucking persists past 4 years of age, or 6 years as indicated by some authorities (Johns, Miller, & Hochstetler, 1998; Van Norman, 2001), or when the permanent teeth erupt. Others have linked pacifier use in infancy and higher incidence of malocclusion regardless of pacifier type (regular or orthodontic) (Nowak & Warren, 2000). Pacifiers may be relinquished earlier than thumbs because they are less readily available.

There are studies linking the early introduction of a pacifier with early termination of breastfeeding, decreased exclusive breastfeeding, and early weaning from the breast; other studies have shown a weak correlation between early weaning from breastfeeding and pacifier use. Biancuzzo (1999) suggests that health care workers maintain a commonsense approach to pacifier usage and breastfeeding. Parents should be informed of the relationship between pacifier use and early termination of breastfeeding so that an informed decision can be made. Furthermore, pacifier use should not replace actual feeding or suckling; prohibiting pacifier use will not ensure an increase in the length of breastfeeding, and there should be an emphasis on allowing the infant to control the pace, frequency, and termination of feeding rather than allowing the pacifier (or anything else) to become the focus of the interaction.

The use of a pacifier in infants has also been suggested as a causative factor in the increase in episodes of acute otitis media (Niemela, Uhari, & Mottonen, 1995); however, a later study showed a significant decrease in the incidence of acute otitis media when a pacifier was used only at bedtime (Niemela et al, 2000). The effect of continual pacifier use on early speech and language development is unknown, but the pacifier may decrease the child's desire to imitate sounds and affect intelligibility. Parents need to be alerted that continual dependency on a pacifier may influence social and speech development.

If the child uses a pacifier, safety considerations in purchasing one must be stressed. Parents should be cautioned against altering a pacifier, thus making it more dangerous (see Aspiration of Foreign Objects, p. 1065-1066). To decrease dependence on nonnutritive sucking in young infants, sucking pleasure can be increased by prolonging feeding time. A small-holed, firm nipple causes stronger sucking and slower feeding. Also, the parent's excessive use of the pacifier to calm the child should be explored. It is not unusual for parents to place a pacifier in the infant's mouth as soon as crying begins, thus reinforcing a pattern of distress-relief.

At the time of this writing, there is no evidence that pacifier use and nonnutritive sucking in preterm infants has any effect on the initiation and length of breastfeeding. Nonnutritive sucking should not be withheld from preterm infants, especially when performed in conjunction with the use of concentrated sucrose for pain management.

Thumb-sucking reaches its peak at age 18 to 20 months and is most prevalent when the child is hungry or tired.

Persistent thumb-sucking in a listless, apathetic child always warrants investigation. It may be a sign of an emotional problem between parent and child or of boredom, isolation, and lack of stimulation.

Teething

One of the more difficult periods in the infant's (and parents') life is the eruption of the deciduous (primary) teeth, often referred to as *teething.* The age of tooth eruption shows considerable variation among children, but the order of their appearance is fairly regular and predictable (Fig. 36-10). The first primary teeth to erupt are the lower central incisors, which appear at approximately 6 to 8 months of age. These are followed closely by the upper central incisors. The following is a quick guide to assessment of deciduous teeth during the first 2 years:

Age of the child in months – 6 = Number of teeth
For example: 8 months of age – 6 = 2 teeth

Teething is a physiologic process; some discomfort is common as the crown of the tooth breaks through the periodontal membrane. Some children show minimum evidence of teething, such as drooling, increased finger sucking, or biting on hard objects. Others are very irritable, have difficulty sleeping, and refuse to eat. Generally, signs of illness such as fever (higher than 102° F), vomiting, or diarrhea are not symptoms of teething but of illness and may warrant further investigation. However, as many parents report, a low-grade temperature is common in the 4- to 19-day period before and on the day of tooth eruption.

Because teething pain is a result of inflammation, cold is soothing. Giving the child a frozen teething ring helps relieve the inflammation. Several nonprescription topical anesthetic ointments (e.g., Baby Ora-Jel) are available. The active ingredient in most of these is benzocaine. If such products are used, parents are advised to apply them correctly. In the event of persistent irritability that affects sleeping and feeding, systemic analgesics such as acetaminophen or ibuprofen (age-appropriate dose) can be given; however, parents should know that this is a temporary measure.

NURSE ALERT The use of teething powders or procedures, such as cutting the gums or rubbing them with aspirin, is discouraged because ingestion of the powder, infection or irritation of the tissue, or aspiration of the aspirin can occur. Hard candy may cause accidental choking or aspiration and should be avoided at this age. ■

Infant Shoes

Many parents are unaware of the type of shoes that are appropriate for the older infant and buy expensive infant shoes because of misleading advertising claims. Inflexible shoes that have hard soles can be detrimental. They can delay walking, aggravate intoeing or outtoeing, and impede the development of supportive foot muscles. Therefore the counseling of parents regarding footwear should begin when infants are 6 months old—well before they are walking.

It is helpful to begin by explaining to parents that changes in the feet occur during infancy and early childhood as locomotion and weight bearing progress. At birth the feet are flat because the arches are protected by fat pads on the soles of the feet. As the bones in the arches develop, the pads disappear and the feet begin to assume a mature shape. A normal arch is determined by proper alignment of all the bones and development of the surrounding musculature, not by the height of the arch.

When children begin walking, the main reason for shoes is protection. To provide protection, the shoe should retain its fit; be made of durable material with a smooth interior and few construction seams to irritate the skin; and be soft and flexible, especially in the toe area. A high-top shoe is not necessary for support but may be helpful in keeping the foot in the shoe.

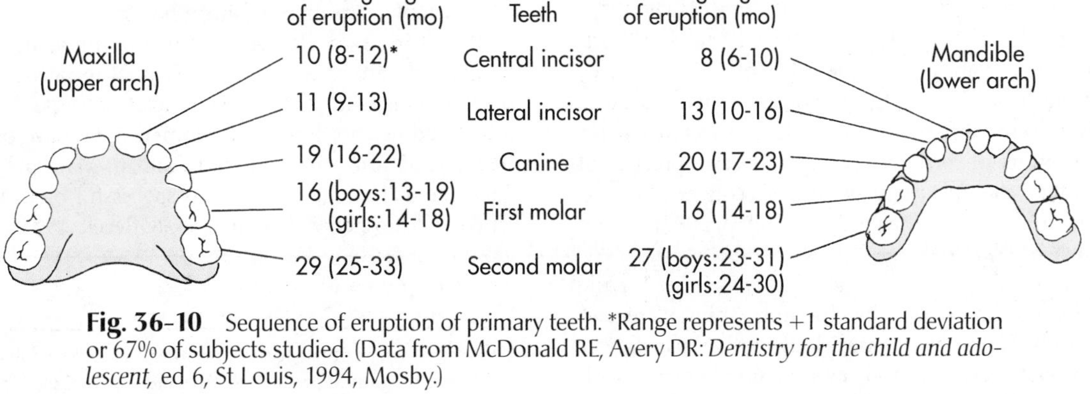

Fig. 36-10 Sequence of eruption of primary teeth. *Range represents +1 standard deviation or 67% of subjects studied. (Data from McDonald RE, Avery DR: *Dentistry for the child and adolescent,* ed 6, St Louis, 1994, Mosby.)

A good shoe conforms to the anatomic shape of the foot, with a rounded toe and sufficient toe room. During weight bearing there should be at least the space of half the width of the thumbnail, or 1.25 cm (roughly ½ inch), between the end of the longest toe and the shoe. Roomy and square-toed socks allow for proper growth and alignment. Inexpensive but well-constructed sneakers or soft-leather moccasin-type shoes are suggested as adequate footgear for walking infants.

Even if the shoes are fitted properly, frequent changes are needed to accommodate the infant's rapidly growing feet. Shoe size changes at approximately 3-month intervals between 12 and 36 months; during this time the child's foot should be measured every 3 months. Curled toes when shoes are removed, and redness and irritation of the skin on the bottom of the toes, indicate the need for a larger shoe size.

PROMOTING OPTIMUM HEALTH DURING INFANCY

Nutrition

Ideally, discussion of optimum nutrition should begin prenatally with the decision to breastfeed or bottle-feed the infant. The choice for either is highly individual and is discussed in Chapter 26. This section is primarily concerned with infant nutrition during the next 12 months, when growth needs and developmental milestones ready the child for the introduction of solid foods. There is concern that, despite adequate availability of optimal nutrient sources, infants are not being fed appropriately. These practices may have far-reaching, long-term health consequences for infants. It has been shown that infant health practices have an impact on the child's life. Certain chronic health conditions have been linked to feeding practices in infancy (Calamaro, 2000; Hobbie, Baker, & Bayerl, 2000). Nurses must continue to be proactive in teaching parents about what constitutes appropriate infant nutrition and nutritional habits, which provide the opportunity to grow and develop into a healthy child and adult.

The use of *complementary and alternative medicine* has recently gained increased awareness by health professionals, particularly in relation to therapies used in children that may not be as beneficial as touted in various media sources. One concern is the intake of megavitamins and herbs by children; parents may assume that the word "natural" in reference to ingredients means the product is safe, when this may not be the case. One report recently cited the home administration of star anise tea as the cause of adverse neurologic reactions in seven infants (Ize-Ludlow et al, 2004). The tea was given to the infants to treat colic. It is important for nurses to be aware of the effects, availability, and practice of complementary therapies and be able to cogently discuss their use in children with the parents (Loman, 2003).

The First 6 Months

Human milk is the most desirable complete diet for the infant during the first 6 months. The normal infant receiving breast milk from a well-nourished mother usually requires no specific vitamin and mineral supplements, with the exception of iron by 4 to 6 months of age (when fetal iron stores are depleted). Daily supplements of vitamin D and vitamin B_{12} may be indicated if the mother's intake of these vitamins is inadequate. The American Academy of Pediatrics (2003a) recently issued a recommendation that all infants (including those exclusively breastfed) receive a daily supplement of 200 international units of vitamin D beginning in the first 2 months of life to prevent rickets and vitamin D deficiency. If the infant is being exclusively breastfed after 4 to 6 months, iron supplementation is recommended to offset the decrease in iron available in human milk at this time and to enhance erythropoiesis. Infants, whether breastfed or bottle-fed, do not require additional fluids, especially water or juice, during the first 4 months of life. Excessive intake of water in infants may result in water intoxication, failure to thrive, and hyponatremia.

Employed mothers can continue breastfeeding with guidance and encouragement. Mothers are encouraged to set realistic goals for employment and breastfeeding, with accurate information regarding the costs, risks, and benefits of available feeding options. The working mother is also encouraged to develop and implement a strategic plan, such as a set routine for feeding and pumping and a backup contingency for successful feeding. Barriers encountered by working breastfeeding mothers include lack of employer or coworker support, unavailable or inadequate facilities for pumping and storing milk, and insufficient time allowed during work time to pump (Rojjanasrirat, 2004). Important themes that emerged in the study by Rojjanasrirat (2004) of working breastfeeding mothers included support (emotional, informational, and instrumental), attitude, and psychologic distress. Many mothers may find that a program of breast pumping when away from home and bottle-feeding the infant the expressed milk with or without formula supplementation is successful.

Expressed breast milk may be stored in the refrigerator (4° C [39° F]) without danger of bacterial contamination for up to 5 days (Lawrence & Lawrence, 2005). Although feeding the infant at home may occur on a demand basis, pumping milk away from home may be needed every 3 to 4 hours to maintain adequate supply. Breast milk may be expressed by hand or pump (manual or electric) and stored in an appropriate air-tight glass or plastic container. Expressed breast milk may be frozen (–18° C [0° F] or lower) for up to 12 months, but care should be taken to prevent the typical freezer burn. Health care workers and new mothers may find the booklet *Working and Breastfeeding—Can You Do It? Yes, You Can!* by Johnson & Johnson helpful.*

In addition to efficient breast pumping, mothers also need child care by a trusted individual or agency and support and assistance from significant others. As with all breastfeeding mothers, these women must have proper nutrition and rest for adequate lactation. Maternal fatigue is considered the biggest threat to successful breastfeeding in employed mothers (Corbett-Dick & Bezek, 1997).

*Developed by National Healthy Mothers, Healthy Babies Coalition, 121 S. Washington St., Suite 300, Alexandria, VA, 22314; phone: 703-836-6110; Web site: www.hmhb.org.

NURSE ALERT To prevent oral burns from uneven warming of the milk, breast milk should never be thawed or rewarmed in a microwave oven. To thaw the frozen milk, either place the container under a lukewarm water bath (less than 40.5° C [105° F]) or place it in the refrigerator overnight. ■

An acceptable alternative to breastfeeding is commercial iron-fortified formula. Like human milk, it supplies all of the nutrients needed by the infant for the first 6 months.

Unmodified whole cow's milk, low-fat cow's milk, skim milk, other animal milks, and imitation milks are not acceptable as a major source of nutrition for infants because of their altered ability to be digested, an increased risk of contamination, and a lack of components needed for appropriate growth. Whole milk can cause iron deficiency anemia in infants, possibly as a result of occult gastrointestinal blood loss. Pasteurized whole cow's milk is deficient in iron, zinc, and vitamin C and has a high renal solute load, which makes it undesirable for infants less than 12 months of age (American Academy of Pediatrics, 2004a).

NURSE ALERT Whole milk should not be introduced to infants until after 1 year of age (American Academy of Pediatrics, 2004a). ■

NURSE ALERT Dietary fat should not be restricted in infancy. Substituting skim or low-fat milk is unacceptable, because the essential fatty acids are inadequate and the solute concentration of protein and electrolytes, such as sodium, is too high. ■

NURSE ALERT Although microwaving of bottles and baby food is not recommended, it remains a common practice. Guidelines have been developed for microwave heating of refrigerated formula, and these should be given to the family (Home Care box). ■

The amount of formula per feeding and the number of feedings per day vary among infants. Infants on demand feeding usually determine their own feeding schedule, but some infants may need a more planned schedule based on average feeding patterns to ensure sufficient nutrients. In general, the number of feedings decreases from six at 1 month of age to four to five at 6 months. Regardless of the number of feedings, the total amount of formula ingested will usually level off at about 32 ounces (960 ml/day). Parents should be cautioned concerning the excessive use of juices and nonnutritive drinks such as fruit-flavored drinks or carbonated beverages (soda or pop) during this period. Many juices and nonnutritive drinks, although readily available to consumers, do not provide sufficient caloric intake for infants less than 12 months of age; such drinks may replace the nutrients in milk (formula) and lead to growth or health problems. Also, water supplementation is not recommended for healthy infants, because it may lead to water intoxication (American Academy of Pediatrics, 2004a).

Home Care

MICROWAVE HEATING OF REFRIGERATED INFANT FORMULA

Before heating:
- Heat only 4 ounces or more.
- Heat only *refrigerated* formula.
- Always *stand* the bottle up.
- Always leave the bottle top *uncovered* to allow heat to escape.

Heating instructions (full power):
- Heat 4-ounce bottles for no more than 30 seconds.
- Heat 8-ounce bottles for no more than 45 seconds.

Serving instructions:
- Always replace nipple assembly; *invert* 10 times (vigorous shaking is unnecessary).
- Formula should be cool to the touch; formula warm to the touch may be too hot to serve.
- Always *test* formula; place several drops on your tongue or on the back of the hand (not the inside wrist).

Modified from Sigman-Grant M, Bush G, Anantheswaran R: Microwave heating of infant formula: a dilemma resolved, *Pediatrics* 90(3):414, 1992.

NURSE ALERT If infants are being fed powdered or concentrated formula, they may receive a substantial amount of lead from tap water, placing them at risk for lead poisoning. Bottled water for mixing powdered or concentrated formula is a relatively safe alternative to tap water if available tap water has a high lead content. Fluoridated bottled water is not necessary for mixing powdered formula unless the local water source is low in fluoride, in which case fluoride supplementation is recommended after age 6 months (see Dental Health, p. 1054). ■

The addition of solid foods before 4 to 6 months of age is not recommended. During the early months solid foods are not compatible with the ability of the gastrointestinal tract and nutritional needs of the infant. Feeding solids to young infants exposes them to food antigens that may produce food protein allergy. Developmentally, infants are not ready for solid food. The extrusion (protrusion) reflex is strong and causes food to be pushed out of the mouth. Despite these recommendations, and lacking evidence-based information to support such practices, many parents introduce solids as early as 2 weeks of age. In such cases, rice cereal is often added to the formula to help the infant sleep better at night or to enhance weight gain (Calamaro, 2000; Wilson & Bowman, 2000); however, this practice is not substantiated by any scientific evidence (American Academy of Pediatrics, 2004a; Morin, 2004). Fruit juices are not required during the first 6 months of life; there are no studies demonstrating benefits of giving fruit juices, yet parents may perceive this practice as beneficial.

The Second 6 Months

During the second half of the first year, human milk or formula continues to be the primary source of nutrition. Fluoride supplementation should begin, depending on the infant's intake of fluoridated tap water (see Dental Health, p. 1054). If breastfeeding is discontinued, a commercial iron-fortified formula should be substituted. Follow-up or transition formulas specially marketed for older infants offer no special advantages over other infant formulas (American Academy of Pediatrics, 2004a).

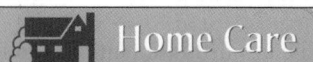

The major change in feeding habits is the addition of solid foods to the infant's diet. Physiologically and developmentally, the infant 4 to 6 months of age is in a transition period. By this time the gastrointestinal tract has matured sufficiently to handle more complex nutrients and is less sensitive to potentially allergenic foods. Tooth eruption is beginning and facilitates biting and chewing. The extrusion reflex has disappeared, and swallowing is more coordinated to allow the infant to accept solids easily. Head control is well developed, which permits infants to sit with support and purposely turn the head away to communicate disinterest in food. Voluntary grasping and improved eye-hand coordination gradually allow infants to pick up finger foods and feed themselves. Their increasing sense of independence is evident in their desire to hold the bottle and try to "help" during feeding.

Selection and Preparation of Solid Foods

The choice of solid foods to introduce first is variable but should meet the reasons for feeding solids, such as supplying nutrients not found in formula or breast milk. Iron-fortified infant cereal is generally introduced first because of its high iron content (7 mg/3 tablespoons of prepared dry cereal). Commercially prepared ready-to-serve dry cereals for infants include rice, barley, oatmeal, and high-protein cereals; rice is usually suggested as an initial food because of its easy digestibility and low allergenic potential. Cereals such as cream of farina are not used, because infant commercial cereals are a better source of iron. Some of the commercial baby cereals are combined with fruit. There is little nutritional benefit from these preparations, and they are more expensive. New foods should be added one at a time; therefore parents should avoid cereal combinations when beginning a new grain.

Infant cereal (iron fortified) is mixed with formula until whole milk is given. If the infant is breastfed, the cereal is mixed with expressed breast milk or water. After 6 months of age, fruit juices can be mixed with the dry cereal; the vitamin C content of the juice enhances the absorption of iron in the cereal. Because of their benefit as a source of iron, infant cereals should be continued until the child is 18 months of age.

The addition of solid foods to the exclusively breastfed infant's diet does not significantly increase overall caloric intake or weight gain (Dewey, 2001).

Fruit juice can be offered from a cup for its rich source of vitamin C and as a substitute for milk for one feeding a day. Large quantities of certain juices (e.g., apple, pear, prune, sweet cherry, peach, grape) are avoided because they may cause abdominal pain, diarrhea, or bloating in some children. White grape juice is reported to be better absorbed and safe for infants this age (less than 6 oz/day) without causing gastrointestinal distress. Some studies have shown that excessive fruit juice consumption (12 or more oz/day) in young children increases the likelihood of short stature and childhood obesity (Dennison, Rockwell, & Baker, 1997) and nonorganic failure to thrive (Smith & Lifshitz, 1994); however, Skinner and colleagues (1999) found no association between growth failure and the consumption of 12 ounces or more of 100% fruit juices in children 24 to 36 months of age. In addition, some researchers have found fruit juice, particularly apple juice, to exacerbate colic and diarrhea, possibly because of carbohydrate malabsorption (Duro et al, 2002; Moukarzel, Lesicka, & Ament, 2002). It is recommended that fruit juice intake not exceed 4 to 6 ounces per day and that juices not be given to infants less than 4 to 6 months old (American Academy of Pediatrics, 2004a). Because vitamin C is naturally destroyed by heat, juice is not warmed. Juice containers are always kept covered and refrigerated to prevent further vitamin loss.

NURSE ALERT Offer fruit juice from a cup, rather than a bottle, to prevent the development of nursing caries (see Low-Cariogenic Diet, Chapter 37). ■

The addition of other foods is arbitrary. A common sequence is to introduce strained fruits, followed by vegetables, and finally meats. If foods are introduced early, citrus fruits, meats, and eggs are delayed until after 6 months of age because of their potential to result in allergy. At 6 months, foods such as a cracker or zwieback can be offered as a type of finger and teething food. By 8 to 9 months, junior foods and nutritious finger foods such as a firmly cooked vegetable, raw pieces of fruit (except grapes), or cheese can be given. By 1 year, well-cooked table foods are served.

Commercially prepared baby foods are the most commonly used types of food served to infants in the United States. They are convenient and usually contain no added salt or sugar, but they are relatively expensive. An alternative is to prepare baby foods at home, which is a simple and inexpensive process. Fruits and vegetables can be steamed in a small amount of water and pureed in a blender or food processor. Many of them, such as ripe banana, can be mashed fine with a fork. Fruits such as apples or pears require little or no water in the cooking process. Vegetables such as carrots, potatoes, or string beans require additional water in the cooking and blending process.

Preferably, home-prepared infant foods should be fresh or frozen, because canned foods, other than those prepared for infants, may contain excessive sodium or sugar or be a source of lead from the container. If sweetening is needed, refined sugar can be used, but honey and corn syrup are avoided because of the risk of infant botulism. There is no evidence that the addition of salt to foods such as vegetables increases the infant's acceptance of the new food. Additional guidelines for the home preparation of baby foods are provided by Morin (2005).

Low-calorie foods should be avoided in infants and toddlers unless a strict, medically prescribed diet is required. The infant's growth during this phase is crucial to future development, and curtailing dietary fat should be done with great caution. Many parents may be concerned that their child is getting too much dietary fat; in such cases the primary practitioner should be consulted before dietary substitutions are made. On the other hand, making an infant or toddler finish a bottle or "clean up the plate" may lead to unhealthy eating habits (see Obesity, Chapter 40).

Introduction of Solid Foods

When the spoon is first introduced, infants often push it away and appear dissatisfied. Patience and skill are required to overcome this initial response. A small-bowled, straight, long-handled spoon, similar to a demitasse spoon, allows a small portion of food to be placed toward the back of the tongue. Food that is placed on the front of the tongue and pushed out is simply scooped up and refed. As infants become accustomed to the spoon, they more eagerly accept the food and eventually will open the mouth in anticipation (or keep it closed in dislike). Because the first introduction of food is a new experience, spoon feeding should be attempted after ingestion of some breast milk or formula to associate this activity with a pleasurable and satisfying experience. Trying to introduce a food *after* the entire milk feeding is usually useless because the infant is satiated and has no inclination to try something new.

After several spoon feedings, food can be introduced at the beginning of a meal. It is best to introduce many foods during the first year, when the infant is more likely to eat them because of a hearty appetite resulting from a rapid growth rate. During the toddler years eating becomes less of an adventure, and strong food preferences become evident.

One food item is introduced at intervals of 4 to 7 days to allow for identification of food allergies. New foods are fed in small amounts, from 1 teaspoon to a few tablespoons. As the amount of solid food increases, the quantity of milk is decreased to less than 1 L daily to prevent overfeeding.

Because feeding is a learning process, as well as a means of nutrition, new foods are given alone to allow the child to learn new tastes and textures. Food should not be mixed in the bottle and fed through a nipple with a large hole; this deprives the child of the pleasure of learning new tastes and of developing a discriminating palate. It can also cause problems with poor chewing of food later in life because of lack of experience. Guidelines for the introduction of new foods are given in the Home Care box.*

The infant's first, second, and often twentieth try at self-feeding or cup feeding is a sloppy experience. Finger foods such as soft fruits or vegetables are just as good playthings as food; they can be squeezed, smeared, squashed, and thoroughly painted on oneself, others, and the surrounding environment. However, all of this is part of learning, and mastery follows many accidents.

*A recommended resource is *Starting Solids: A Guide for Parents and Child Care Providers,* available from the National Association of Pediatric Nurse Associates and Practitioners (NAPNAP), 1101 Kings Highway North, Suite 206, Cherry Hill, NJ 08034-1912; phone: 877-662-7627 or 856-667-1773; fax: 856-667-7187; Web site: www.napnap.org.

Home Care

INTRODUCING SOLID FOODS TO INFANTS

- Introduce solids when infant is hungry.
- Begin spoon feeding by pushing food to back of tongue because of infant's natural tendency to thrust the tongue forward.
- Use a small spoon with a straight handle; begin with 1 or 2 teaspoons of food; gradually increase to a couple of tablespoons per feeding.
- Introduce one food at a time, usually at intervals of 4 to 7 days to allow for identification of food allergies.
- As the amount of solid food increases, decrease the quantity of milk to prevent overfeeding.
- Do not introduce foods by mixing them with formula in the bottle.

If parents find this experience distressing, a few suggestions may prove helpful. The feeding area should have a floor that can be easily wiped and is relatively far from walls, upholstered furniture, or drapes. A handheld portable vacuum is helpful in cleaning up crumbs. Messes are confined to one area if the child is seated in a high chair rather than allowed to crawl or walk around while drinking or eating. Infants should be expected to get themselves covered with food; therefore a large bib (plastic can be wiped easily but needs to be removed after feeding) should be used, as well as washable clothes that are easily removed. In a carpeted eating area, a bedsheet or washable drop cloth can be spread under the high chair to save on cleanup time and avoid frustration; the infant can be expected to drop food at this stage. High chairs can be thoroughly cleaned in a shower. Outdoor dining provides an excellent opportunity for practicing with a cup, spoon, or fingers because accidents are simple to hose or sweep away. Children cannot be pressured into eating neatly or into developing table manners before manipulative skill is acquired.

Parents are encouraged to interpret the infant's signals of discomfort and intervene in ways other than through feeding. Crying, fussiness, and sucking do not necessarily indicate hunger. Rocking, stroking, holding, and offering a toy or a pacifier may be more appropriate than automatically responding with food.

Weaning

Defined as the process of giving up one method of feeding for another, *weaning* usually refers to relinquishing the breast or bottle for a cup. In Western societies this is generally regarded as a major task for infants and is often seen as a potentially traumatic experience. It is psychologically significant because the infant is required to give up a major source of oral pleasure and gratification.

There is no one time for weaning that is best for every child, but generally most infants show signs of readiness during the second half of the first year. They have learned that good things come from a spoon. Their increasing desire for freedom of movement may lessen their desire to be held close for feedings. They are acquiring more control over their actions and can easily manipulate a cup to their lips (even if it is held upside down!). Imitation becomes a powerful motivator by age 8 or 9 months, and they enjoy using a cup or glass like others do.

Weaning should be gradual, replacing one bottle-feeding or breastfeeding at a time. The nighttime feeding is usually the last feeding to be discontinued. It is advisable never to begin allowing a child to take a bottle of milk to bed—this is a major cause of nursing caries in deciduous teeth. If breastfeeding is terminated before 5 or 6 months of age, weaning should be to a bottle to provide for the infant's continued sucking needs. If discontinued later, weaning can be directly to a cup, especially by age 12 to 14 months. Any sweet liquid, such as fruit juice, should be given in a cup.

Sleep and Activity

Sleep patterns vary among infants, with active infants typically sleeping less than placid children. Generally, by 3 to 4 months of age most infants have developed a nocturnal pattern of sleep that lasts 9 to 11 hours. The total daily sleep is approximately 15 hours. The number of naps per day varies, but infants may take one or two naps by the end of the first year. Breastfed infants usually sleep for less prolonged periods, with more frequent waking, especially during the night, than do bottle-fed infants. Because of the trend toward breastfeeding, sleep norms such as those previously described, which were based primarily on bottle-fed infants, may not be relevant.

Most infants are naturally active and need no encouragement to be mobile. However, problems can arise when devices such as playpens, strollers, commercial swings, and walkers are used excessively. These items restrict movement and prevent infants from exploring and developing gross motor skills. Contrary to popular belief, walkers do not enhance coordination and are dangerous if tipped over or placed near stairs. The American Academy of Pediatrics (2001) recommended a ban on the sale of infant walkers because of the large number of injuries. Newer models of infant walkers have been designed without wheels to decrease infant injuries (see Falls, p. 1070).

NURSE ALERT Formal infant exercise programs do not provide any long-term benefit to normal infants, and the possibility for damage to the infant's skeletal system exists. For these reasons, such programs are not recommended (American Academy of Pediatrics, 1988). ■

Sleep Problems

Concerns regarding sleep are common during infancy. Sometimes these concerns are as basic as parents' questioning if the infant needs additional sleep. In this case it is best to investigate the reason for their concern, stressing the individual needs of each child. Infants who are active during wakeful periods and growing normally are sleeping a sufficient amount of time.

However, there are a number of more serious concerns that require intervention. The more common sleep disturbances are a learned pattern or developmental characteristic of some infants (Table 36-3). Although many families may report sleep problems typical of these patterns, interventions are offered only when the pattern is disruptive to the family (Cultural Awareness box).

Sleep problems in early infancy have also been positively correlated with higher maternal depression scores (Hawkins-Walsh, 2003; Hiscock & Wake, 2001); therefore nurses must discuss infant sleep problems with the mother (and family) in addition to other developmental aspects of newborn care.

When a sleeping problem exists, a careful assessment is essential. Charting sleep habits both before and after interventions is also an important strategy. Questions regarding the frequency and duration of waking, the usual bedtime routine, the number of nighttime feedings, the perceived problem (e.g., how much disruption the behavior generates), and the attempted interventions are important in planning effective approaches designed for the specific sleep problem. A common suggestion given for any type of sleep problem—"let the child cry until he or she falls asleep"—is very difficult to implement and is inappropriate for certain conditions. Once the parents relent and console the child, they have only reinforced the crying.

An equally effective and more atraumatic approach to night crying, known as *graduated extinction,* is to let the child cry for progressively longer times between brief parental interventions that consist only of reassurance—not rocking, holding, or using a bottle or pacifier. For example, the parents may check on the child every 5 minutes during

Cultural Awareness

THE FAMILY BED

Co-sleeping, or sharing the "family bed," in which parents allow the children to sleep with them, is a relatively common and accepted practice, especially among African-American, Hispanic, and Asian families, such as the Japanese (Schachter et al, 1989). A recent survey indicates the practice is growing in some parts of the United States, especially among young (<18 years of age) African-American and Asian females in the Southern states; infants in the survey who co-slept with an adult were less than 8 weeks old (Willinger et al, 2003). Other groups who practice co-sleeping include (1) single parents, whose need for company may encourage this practice; (2) working parents, who desire the closeness at night that was lost during the day; and (3) parents who have had an issue about sleep or separation in their own past (Brazelton, 1990). Ball (2003) reported a positive relationship between parent-infant bed sharing and increased frequency of breastfeeding in the United Kingdom. Despite initial popular belief that co-sleeping would prevent SIDS there is no scientific evidence to support infant co-sleeping with the mother as a preventive measure against the occurrence of SIDS (American Academy of Pediatrics, 2000b). There is evidence of an increase in the number of infant deaths by suffocation associated with bed sharing and the use of adult beds, particularly in infants less than 3 months old (Drago & Dannenberg, 1999). Other studies have correlated higher incidences of SIDS and infant co-sleeping with maternal smoking, co-sleeping with multiple family members, soft bedding, and unintentional asphyxiation resulting from adult intoxication (overlaying) (American Academy of Pediatrics, 2000b; Hauck et al, 2003; McGarvey et al, 2003; Person, Lavezzi, & Wolf, 2002).

Population-based studies of infant co-sleeping and SIDS are currently in progress; until there is evidence-based data to support or abandon the practice, parents should carefully evaluate the options available for sharing the family bed with infants, particularly under known high risk conditions that place the infant at risk for asphyxia, whether intentional or otherwise. One of the difficulties in interpreting the available data on the studies of infant-parent co-sleeping to date is the interpretation of the terminology used to define co-sleeping (Mesich, 2005). At times parents may place the infant to sleep in the adult bed then carry the child to her/his own bed after a given period of time. In some cases a breastfeeding mother may wish to have the infant with her in an adult bed for feeding and comfort, and then place the child in a crib or bassinette. Whether these incidents constitute co-sleeping in the larger studies finding co-sleeping as a risk factor for SIDS is not clear. Further studies must clearly define the terminology of co-sleeping. As Willinger and colleagues (2003) point out, further studies on infant co-sleeping are needed to clarify the issues because the practice is not only growing but also has cultural meaning in some populations. In a recent article, Mesich (2005) encouraged nurses to become familiar with the various studies and terminology regarding parent co-sleeping in order to counsel parents effectively.

Table 36-3

Selected Sleep Disturbances during Infancy and Early Childhood

DISORDER/DESCRIPTION	MANAGEMENT
NIGHTTIME FEEDING	
Child has a prolonged need for middle-of-night bottle-feeding or breastfeeding Child goes to sleep at breast or with a bottle Awakenings are frequent (may be hourly) Child returns to sleep after feeding; other comfort measures (e.g., rocking or holding) are usually ineffective	Increase daytime feeding intervals to 4 hours or more (may need to be done gradually) Offer last feeding as late as possible at night; may need to gradually reduce amount of formula or length of breast-feeding Offer no bottles in bed Put to bed *awake* When child is crying, check at progressively longer intervals each night; reassure child but do not hold, rock, take to parent's bed, or give bottle or pacifier
DEVELOPMENTAL NIGHT CRYING	
Child age 6-12 months with undisturbed nighttime sleep now awakes abruptly; may be accompanied by nightmares	Parents should be reassured that this phase is temporary Enter room immediately to check on child but keep reassurances *brief* Avoid feeding, rocking, taking to parent's bed, or any other routine that may initiate trained night crying
TRAINED NIGHT CRYING (INAPPROPRIATE SLEEP ASSOCIATIONS)	
Child typically falls asleep in place other than own bed (e.g., rocking chair or parent's bed) and is taken to own bed while asleep; on awakening, cries until usual routine is instituted (e.g., rocking)	Put child in own bed when *awake* If possible, arrange sleeping area separate from other family members When child is crying, check at progressively longer intervals each night; reassure child but do not resume usual routine
REFUSAL TO GO TO SLEEP	
Child resists bedtime and comes out of room repeatedly Nighttime sleep may be continuous, but frequent awakenings and refusal to return to sleep may occur and become a problem if parent allows child to deviate from usual sleep pattern	Evaluate if hour of sleep is too early (child may resist sleep if not tired) Parents should be assisted in establishing consistent before-bedtime routine and enforcing consistent limits regarding child's bedtime behavior If child persists in leaving bedroom, close door for progressively longer periods Use reward system with child to provide motivation
NIGHTTIME FEARS	
Child resists going to bed or wakes during the night because of fears Child seeks parent's physical presence and falls asleep easily with parent nearby, unless fear is overwhelming	Evaluate if hour of sleep is too early (child may fantasize when nothing to do but think in dark room) Calmly reassure the frightened child; keeping a night light on may be helpful Use reward system with child to provide motivation to deal with fears Avoid patterns that can lead to additional problems (e.g., sleeping with child or taking child to parent's room) If child's fear is overwhelming, consider desensitization (e.g., progressively spending longer periods of time alone; consult professional help for protracted fears) Distinguish between nightmares and sleep terrors (confused partial arousals)

Modified from Ferber R: Behavioral "insomnia" in the child, *Psychiatr Clin North Am* 10(4):641-653, 1987.

the first night and progressively extend this interval by 5 minutes on successive nights.

Families who cannot tolerate unexpected crying spells while everyone else is asleep can try the two-step approach. Graduated extinction is used during naps and at bedtime until the parents retire. If the child cries during the night, the parents use comforting measures. However, once the child is partially trained, step 2 is initiated—the use of graduated extinction at all times.

The best way to prevent sleep problems is to encourage parents to establish bedtime rituals that do not foster problematic patterns. One of the most constructive is placing infants *awake* in their own crib. When infants are accustomed to falling asleep somewhere else, such as in their parent's arms, and then being transferred to their crib, they awaken in unfamiliar surroundings and are unable to fall asleep until the routine is repeated. Also, the bed should be used for sleeping only—not as a playpen. It is advisable not to hang playthings over or on the bed; in this way the child associates the bed with sleep, not with activity. Although the interventions described previously and in Table 36-3 are usually successful, it is much easier to prevent the problem with appropriate counseling during the early months of the infant's life.*

Dental Health

Good dental hygiene begins with appropriate maternal dental health and counseling during early infancy regarding dietary intake for the promotion of optimal oral hygiene (Douglass, Douglass, & Silk, 2004). Parents are counseled early regarding the risk of feeding practices which increase the risk of poor dental health. Some of these have been previously mentioned and include avoiding propping the milk bottle or giving the milk bottle in the bed, and avoiding fruit juices in a bottle, especially before six months of age. Once the primary teeth erupt cleaning should begin. The teeth and gums are initially cleaned by wiping with a damp cloth; toothbrushing is too harsh for the tender gingiva. The caregiver can stabilize the infant by cradling the child with one arm and using the free hand to cleanse the teeth. Oral hygiene can be made pleasant by singing or talking to the infant. There are no clear guidelines regarding when toothbrushing should begin; however, it is recommended that the infant have an oral health examination by 6 months of age from a qualified pediatric health practitioner. Infants at high risk for dental caries should be seen by a dentist between 6 months and 1 year of age (American Academy of Pediatrics, 2003b). It is generally recommended that a small, soft-bristled toothbrush be used as more teeth erupt and the infant adjusts to the routine of cleaning. Water is preferred to toothpaste, which the infant will swallow (and if the toothpaste is fluoridated, the infant will ingest excessive amounts of fluoride).

Fluoride, an essential mineral for building caries-resistant teeth, is needed beginning at 6 months of age if the infant does not receive water with an adequate fluoride content. The American Academy of Pediatrics and the American Academy of Pediatric Dentists no longer recommend fluoride supplementation from birth to 6 months. The fluoride dosage has been decreased from earlier recommendations because of an increased occurrence of dental fluorosis from excessive fluoride ingestion. The latest recommendation is to give children 6 months to 3 years of age 0.25 mg of fluoride daily if water fluoride content is less than 0.3 parts per million (ppm) (American Academy of Pediatrics, 2004a).

Dietary considerations are also important because habits begun during infancy tend to continue into later years. Foods with added concentrated sugar are used sparingly (if at all) in the infant's diet. The practice of coating pacifiers with honey or using commercially available hard-candy pacifiers is discouraged. Besides being cariogenic, honey also may cause infant botulism, and parts of the candy pacifier can be aspirated (see Aspiration of Foreign Objects, pp. 1065-1066). Parents need to be counseled regarding the detrimental effects of frequent and prolonged bottle-feeding or breastfeeding during sleep, when the sweet milk or other fluid, such as juice, bathes the teeth, producing nursing caries. In addition, carbonated beverages should be avoided in infancy.

(See Chapter 37 for a more extensive discussion of dental care, including nursing caries.)

Immunizations

One of the most dramatic advances in pediatrics has been the decline of infectious diseases during the twentieth century because of the widespread use of immunization for preventable diseases. Although many of the immunizations can be given to individuals of any age, the recommended primary schedule begins during infancy and, with the exception of boosters, is completed during early childhood. Therefore the discussion of childhood immunizations for diphtheria, tetanus, pertussis (DTaP using acellular pertussis); polio; measles, mumps, rubella (MMR); *Haemophilus influenzae* type b (Hib); hepatitis B virus (HBV); pneumococcal conjugate vaccine (PCV); influenza; and chickenpox is included under health promotion during infancy. Selected vaccines generally reserved for children considered at high risk for the disease are discussed here and as appropriate throughout the text. (See also Communicable Diseases, Chapter 38, for a discussion of several of the diseases for which vaccines are available.)

CASE STUDY: IMMUNIZATIONS

Schedule for Immunizations

In the United States, two organizations—the Advisory Committee on Immunization Practices (ACIP) of the Centers for Disease Control and Prevention (CDC) and the Committee on Infectious Diseases of the American Academy of Pediatrics (AAP)—govern the recommendations for immunization policies and procedures. In Canada, recommendations are from the National Advisory Committee on Immunization under the authority of the Minister of National Health and Welfare. The policies of each committee are *recommendations,* not rules, and they change as a result of advances in the field of immunology. Nurses need to keep informed of the latest advances and changes in policy.

In the United States the recommended age for beginning primary immunizations of infants is within 2 weeks of birth or, in special circumstances, at birth (Table 36-4). Children born prematurely should receive the full dose of each vaccine at the appropriate chronologic age. Catch-up immunizations for children who do not receive vaccines according to the recommended schedule in Table 36-4 are included in Table 36-5. Table 36-6 describes immunization schedules for Canadian children.

*An excellent resource for parents is *Solve Your Child's Sleep Problems,* by Richard Ferber (1986, Simon & Schuster Trade; phone: 800-223-2336; Web site: www.simonsays.com). Also available in Spanish. Another resource is *Guide to Your Child's Sleep,* American Academy of Pediatrics, 2000, www.aap.org.

Children who began primary immunization at the recommended age, but fail to receive all of the doses, do not need to begin the series again but instead receive only the missed doses. For situations in which there is doubt that the child will return for immunization according to the optimum schedule, any of the recommended vaccines can be administered simultaneously. Parenteral vaccines are given in separate syringes in different injection sites (American Academy of Pediatrics, 2003c).

Recommendations for Routine Immunizations

Hepatitis B Virus

Hepatitis B virus (HBV) is a significant pediatric disease because HBV infections that occur during childhood and adolescence can lead to fatal consequences from cirrhosis or liver cancer during adulthood. Up to 90% of infants infected perinatally and 25% to 50% of children infected before age 5 years become HBV carriers. In addition, the incidence of HBV infection increases rapidly during adolescence (American Academy of Pediatrics, 2003c). It is recommended that newborns receive the vaccine before hospital discharge if the mother is hepatitis B surface antigen (HBsAg) negative. Monovalent Hep B should be given as the birth dose, whereas combination vaccine containing Hep B may be given for subsequent doses in the series. Both full-term and preterm infants born to mothers whose HBsAg status is positive or unknown should receive hepatitis B vaccine and hepatitis B immune globulin (HBIG), 0.5 ml, within 12 hours of birth at two different injection sites. In the event that the preterm infant is given a dose at birth, the current recommendation is that the infant be given the full series (three additional doses) at 1, 2, and 6 months of age. The American Academy of Pediatrics (2003c) also encourages immunization of all children by age 11 years.

The vaccine is given intramuscularly in the vastus lateralis in newborns or in the deltoid for older infants and children. Regardless of age, the dorsogluteal site is avoided because it has been associated with low antibody seroconversion rates, indicating a reduced immune response (Zuckerman, Cockcroft, & Zuckerman, 1992). No data exist regarding the seroconversion when the ventrogluteal site is used. The vaccine can be safely administered simultaneously at a separate site with DTaP, MMR, and Hib vaccines.

Hepatitis A Virus

Hepatitis A virus (HAV) is now recognized as a significant child health problem, particularly in communities with unusually high infection rates. HAV is spread by the fecal-oral route and from person-to-person contact, by ingestion of contaminated food or water, and rarely by blood transfusion. The illness has an abrupt onset with fever, malaise, anorexia, nausea, abdominal discomfort, dark urine, and jaundice being the most common clinical signs of infection. In children younger than 6 years of age, who represent approximately one third of all cases of HAV, the disease may be asymptomatic, and jaundice is rarely evident. Children living in communities with high infection rates should be immunized with either HAVRIX or VAQTA vaccine, given by the intramuscular route in the deltoid. These vaccines are recommended for children 2 years of age and older, in two doses administered at least 6 months apart. States in which reporting of hepatitis A is mandatory are Arizona, Oklahoma, Alaska, New Mexico, South Dakota, Idaho, Nevada, Oregon, Utah, California, and Washington (Prevention of Hepatitis A, 1999). For further information see Table 36-4, footnote 8.

Diphtheria

Diphtheria vaccine is commonly administered (1) in combination with tetanus and pertussis vaccines (DTaP) or DTaP and Hib vaccines for children younger than 7 years of age; (2) in combination with a conjugate *H. influenzae* type B vaccine (see Table 36-4); (3) in a combined vaccine with tetanus (DT) for children younger than 7 years of age who have some contraindication to receiving pertussis vaccine; (4) in smaller doses (15% to 20% of that in DTaP or DT) with tetanus vaccine (Td) for use in children age 7 years and older; (5) in a combined vaccine with hepatitis B, tetanus, pertussis, and inactivated poliovirus vaccine for use during the primary series in infants; or (6) as a single antigen when combined antigen preparations are not indicated. Although the diphtheria vaccine does not produce absolute immunity, protective antitoxin persists for 10 years or more when given according to the recommended schedule, and boosters are given every 10 years for life.

Tetanus

Two forms of tetanus vaccine—tetanus toxoid and tetanus immune globulin (TIG) (human)—are available (Tetanus antitoxin is not available in the U.S.). Tetanus toxoid is used for routine primary immunization, usually in one of the combinations listed for diphtheria, and provides protective antitoxin levels for 10 years or more.

For wound management, passive immunity is available with TIG. In persons with a history of two previous doses of tetanus toxoid, a booster dose of the toxoid can be given. Separate syringes and different sites are used when tetanus toxoid and TIG are given concurrently. Table 36-7 presents a summary of the recommended procedure for tetanus prophylaxis in wound management.

Pertussis

Pertussis vaccine is recommended for all children 6 weeks through 6 years of age (up to the seventh birthday) who have no neurologic contraindications to its use. It is not given to children age 7 years or older because the risk of receiving the vaccine increases as the incidence, severity, and risk of fatality of the disease decrease.

Two forms of pertussis vaccine are available in the United States. The whole-cell pertussis vaccine is prepared from inactivated cells of *Bordetella pertussis* and contains multiple antigens. In contrast, the acellular pertussis vaccine contains one or more immunogens derived from the *B. pertussis* organism. The highly purified acellular vaccine is associated with fewer local and systemic reactions than those occurring with the whole-cell vaccine in children of similar age. The acellular pertussis vaccine is recommended by the American Academy of Pediatrics (2003c) for the first three immunizations and is usually given at 2, 4, and 6 months of age with DTaP. Several forms of acellular pertussis vaccine are currently licensed for use in infants: Daptacel, Tripedia, Infanrix (diphtheria, tetanus toxoid, and acellular pertussis conjugate), and PEDIARIX (diphtheria, tetanus, hepatitis B, and inactivated poliovirus vaccine).

Text continued on p. 1059.

Table 36-4

Recommended Childhood and Adolescent Immunization Schedule UNITED STATES • 2005

Vaccine ▼ / Age ▶	Birth	1 month	2 months	4 months	6 months	12 months	15 months	18 months	24 months	4–6 years	11–12[9] years	13–18 years
Hepatitis B[1]	HepB #1		HepB #2			HepB #3				HepB Series		
Diphtheria, Tetanus, Pertussis[2]			DTaP	DTaP	DTaP		DTaP			DTaP	Td	Td
Haemophilus influenzae type b[3]			Hib	Hib	Hib	Hib						
Inactivated Poliovirus			IPV	IPV		IPV				IPV		
Measles, Mumps, Rubella[4]						MMR #1				MMR #2	MMR #2	
Varicella[5]							Varicella			Varicella		
Pneumococcal[6]			PCV	PCV	PCV	PCV			PCV	PPV		
Influenza[7]						Influenza (Yearly)				Influenza (Yearly)		
Vaccines below red line are for selected populations												
Hepatitis A[8]										Hepatitis A Series		

This schedule indicates the recommended ages for routine administration of currently licensed childhood vaccines, as of December 1, 2004, for children through age 18 years. Any dose not administered at the recommended age should be administered at any subsequent visit when indicated and feasible.

■ Indicates age groups that warrant special effort to administer those vaccines not previously administered. Additional vaccines may be licensed and recommended during the year. Licensed combination vaccines may be used whenever any components of the combination are indicated and other components of the vaccine are not contraindicated. Providers should consult the manufacturers' package inserts for detailed recommendations. Clinically significant adverse events that follow immunization should be reported to the Vaccine Adverse Event Reporting System (VAERS). Guidance about how to obtain and complete a VAERS form are available at **www.vaers.org** or by telephone, **800-822-7967**.

- **Range of recommended ages**
- **Preadolescent assessment**
- **Only if mother HBsAg(−)**
- **Catch-up immunization**

DEPARTMENT OF HEALTH AND HUMAN SERVICES
CENTERS FOR DISEASE CONTROL AND PREVENTION

The Childhood and Adolescent Immunization Schedule is approved by:
Advisory Committee on Immunization Practices www.cdc.gov/nip/acip
American Academy of Pediatrics www.aap.org
American Academy of Family Physicians www.aafp.org

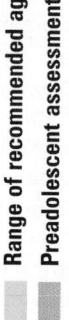

1. **Hepatitis B (HepB) vaccine.** All infants should receive the first dose of HepB vaccine soon after birth and before hospital discharge; the first dose may also be administered by age 2 months if the mother is hepatitis B surface antigen (HBsAg) negative. Only monovalent HepB may be used for the birth dose. Monovalent or combination vaccine containing HepB may be used to complete the series. Four doses of vaccine may be administered when a birth dose is given. The second dose should be administered at least 4 weeks after the first dose, except for combination vaccines which cannot be administered before age 6 weeks. The third dose should be given at least 16 weeks after the first dose and at least 8 weeks after the second dose. The last dose in the vaccination series (third or fourth dose) should not be administered before age 24 weeks.

   Infants born to HBsAg-positive mothers should receive HepB and 0.5 mL of hepatitis B immune globulin (HBIG) at separate sites within 12 hours of birth. The second dose is recommended at age 1-2 months. The final dose in the immunization series should not be administered before age 24 weeks. These infants should be tested for HBsAg and antibody to HBsAg (anti-HBs) at age 9-15 months.

   Infants born to mothers whose HBsAg status is unknown should receive the first dose of the HepB series within 12 hours of birth. Maternal blood should be drawn as soon as possible to determine the mother's HBsAg status; if the HBsAg test is positive, the infant should receive HBIG as soon as possible (no later than age 1 week). The second dose is recommended at age 1-2 months. The last dose in the immunization series should not be administered before age 24 weeks.

2. **Diphtheria and tetanus toxoids an acellular pertussis (DTaP) vaccine.** The fourth dose of DTaP may be administered as early as age 12 months, provided 6 months have elapsed since the third dose and the child is unlikely to return at age 15-18 months. The final dose in the series should be given at age ≥4 years. **Tetanus and diphtheria toxoids (Td)** is recommended at age 11-12 years if at least 5 years have elapsed since the last dose of tetanus and diphtheria toxoid-containing vaccine. Subsequent routine Td boosters are recommended every 10 years.

3. ***Haemophilus influenzae* type b (Hib) conjugate vaccine.** Three Hib conjugate vaccines are licensed for infant use. If PRP-OMP (PedvaxHIB® or ComVax® [Merck]) is administered at ages 2 and 4 months, a dose at age 6 months is not required. DTaP/Hib combination products should not be used for primary immunization in infants at ages 2, 4 or 6 months but can be used as boosters after any Hib vaccine. The final dose in the series should be administered at age ≥12 months.

4. **Measles, mumps, and rubella vaccine (MMR).** The second dose of MMR is recommended routinely at age 4-6 years but may be administered during any visit, provided at least 4 weeks have elapsed since the first dose and both doses are administered beginning at or after age 12 months. Those who have not previously received the second dose should complete the schedule by age 11-12 years.

5. **Varicella vaccine.** Varicella vaccine is recommended at any visit at or after age 12 months for susceptible children (i.e., those who lack a reliable history of chickenpox). Susceptible persons aged ≥13 years should receive 2 doses administered at least 4 weeks apart.

6. **Pneumococcal vaccine.** The heptavalent **pneumococcal conjugate vaccine (PCV)** is recommended for all children aged 2-23 months and for certain children aged 24-59 months. The final dose in the series should be given at age ≥12 months. **Pneumococcal polysaccharide vaccine (PPV)** is recommended in addition to PCV for certain high-risk groups. See *MMWR* 2000;49(RR-9): 1-35.

7. **Influenza vaccine.** Influenza vaccine is recommended annually for children aged ≥6 months with certain risk factors (including, but not limited to, asthma, cardiac disease, sickle cell disease, human immunodeficiency virus [HIV], and diabetes), healthcare workers, and other persons (including household members) in close contact with persons in groups at high risk (see *MMWR* 2004;53(RR-6):1-40). In addition, healthy children aged 6-23 months and close contacts of healthy children aged 0-23 months are recommended to receive influenza vaccine because children in this age group are at substantially increased risk for influenza-related hospitalizations. For healthy persons aged 5-49 years, the intranasally administered, live, attenuated influenza vaccine (LAIV) is an acceptable alternative to the intramuscular trivalent inactivated influenza vaccine (TIV). See *MMWR* 2004;53(RR-6):1-40. Children receiving TIV should be administered a dosage appropriate for their age (0.25 mL if aged 6-35 months or 0.5 mL if aged ≥3 years). Children aged ≤8 years who are receiving influenza vaccine for the first time should receive 2 doses (separated by at least 4 weeks for TIV and at least 6 weeks for LAIV).

8. **Hepatitis A vaccine.** Hepatitis A vaccine is recommended for children and adolescents in selected states and regions and for certain high-risk groups; consult your local public health authority. Children and adolescents in these states, regions, and high-risk groups who have not been immunized against hepatitis A can begin the hepatitis A immunization series during any visit. The 2 doses in the series should be administered at least 6 months apart. See *MMWR* 1999;48(RR-12):1-37.

9. **Meningococcal vaccine.** In May 2005 the American Academy of Pediatrics issued a recommendation that young adolescents receive the quadrivalent conjugate vaccine MCV4 (Menactra; manufactured by Sanofi Pasteur) at the 11- to 12-year visit. The quadrivalent vaccine protects against meningococcal disease caused by serogroups A, C, Y and W-135 and should also be administered to adolescents at high school entry or 15 years of age (whichever comes first) who have not been previously immunized for meningococcal disease, college freshmen living in dormitories, and for pediatric patients 11 years and older who are at increased risk of meningococcal disease (adolescents with asplenia or complement deficiencies) (AAP News, 2005). MCV4 is administered as an intramuscular injection (0.5 mL). The Advisory Committee on Immunization Practices (ACIP) of the Centers for Disease Control and Prevention has issued a similar recommendation in late May, 2005 (MMWR, 2005).

AAP News: AAP issues recommendations on use of meningococcal vaccines, *AAP News* 26(5):2005. www.aapnews. aappublications.org/cgi/content/full/e2005176v1 (accessed May 27, 2005).

MMWR: Prevention and control of meningococcal disease, *MMWR* 54(RR07):1-21, 2005.

Table 36-5

Recommended Immunization Schedule for Children and Adolescents Who Start Late or Who Are More Than 1 Month Behind UNITED STATES • 2005

The tables below give catch-up schedules and minimum intervals between doses for children who have delayed immunizations. There is no need to restart a vaccine series regardless of the time that has elapsed between doses. Use the chart appropriate for the child's age.

CATCH-UP SCHEDULE FOR CHILDREN AGED 4 MONTHS THROUGH 6 YEARS

VACCINE	MINIMUM AGE FOR DOSE 1	MINIMUM INTERVAL BETWEEN DOSES: DOSE 1 TO DOSE 2	DOSE 2 TO DOSE 3	DOSE 3 TO DOSE 4	DOSE 4 TO DOSE 5
Diphtheria, Tetanus, Pertussis	6 wks	4 weeks	4 weeks	6 months	6 months[1]
Inactivated Poliovirus	6 wks	4 weeks	4 weeks	4 weeks[2]	
Hepatitis B[3]	Birth	4 weeks	8 weeks (and 16 weeks after first dose)		
Measles, Mumps, Rubella	12 mo	4 weeks[4]			
Varicella	12 mo				
Haemophilus influenzae type b[5]	6 wks	**4 weeks:** if first dose given at age <12 months **8 weeks (as final dose):** if first dose given at age 12-14 months **No further doses needed:** if first dose given at age ≥15 months	**4 weeks**[6]: if current age <12 months **8 weeks (as final dose)**[6]: if current age ≥12 months and second dose given at age <15 months **No further doses needed:** if previous dose given at age ≥15 mo	**8 weeks (as final dose):** This dose only necessary for children aged 12 months–5 years who received 3 doses before age	
Pneumococcal[7]	6 wks	**4 weeks:** if first dose given at age <12 months and current age <24 months **8 weeks (as final dose):** if first dose given at age ≥12 months or current age 24–59 months **No further doses needed:** for healthy children if first dose given at age ≥24 months	**4 weeks:** if current age <12 months **8 weeks (as final dose):** if current age ≥12 months **No further doses needed:** for healthy children if previous dose given at age ≥24 months	**8 weeks (as final dose):** This dose only necessary for children aged 12 months–5 years who received 3 doses before age 12 months	

CATCH-UP SCHEDULE FOR CHILDREN AGED 7 YEARS THROUGH 18 YEARS

VACCINE	MINIMUM INTERVAL BETWEEN DOSES: DOSE 1 TO DOSE 2	DOSE 2 TO DOSE 3	DOSE 3 TO BOOSTER DOSE
Tetanus, Diphtheria	4 weeks	6 months	**6 months**[8]: if first dose given at age <12 months and current age <11 years **5 years**[8]: if first dose given at age ≥12 months and third dose given at age <7 years and current age ≥11 years **10 years**[8]: if third dose given at age ≥7 years
Inactivated Poliovirus[9]	4 weeks	4 weeks	IPV[2,9]
Hepatitis B	4 weeks	8 weeks (and 16 weeks after first dose)	
Measles, Mumps, Rubella	4 weeks		
Varicella[10]	4 weeks		

Children and Adolescents Catch-up Schedules UNITED STATES • 2005

1. **DTaP:** The fifth dose is not necessary if the fourth dose was administered after the fourth birthday.
2. **IPV:** For children who received an all-IPV or all-oral poliovirus (OPV) series, a fourth dose is not necessary if third dose was administered at age ≥4 years. If both OPV and IPV were administered as part of a series, a total of 4 doses should be given, regardless of the child's current age.
3. **HepB:** All children and adolescents who have not been immunized against hepatitis B should begin the HepB immunization series during any visit. Providers should make special efforts to immunize children who were born in, or whose parents were born in, areas of the world where hepatitis B virus infection is moderately or highly endemic.
4. **MMR:** The second dose of MMR is recommended routinely at age 4–6 years but may be administered earlier if desired.
5. **Hib:** Vaccine is not generally recommended for children aged ≥5 years.
6. **Hib:** If current age <12 months and the first 2 doses were PRP-OMP (PedvaxHIB® or ComVax® [Merck]), the third (and final) dose should be administered at age 12–15 months and at least 8 weeks after the second dose.
7. **PCV:** Vaccine is not generally recommended for children aged ≥5 years.
8. **Td:** For children aged 7–10 years, the interval between the third and booster dose is determined by the age when the first dose was administered. For adolescents aged 11–18 years, the interval is determined by the age when the third dose was given.
9. **IPV:** Vaccine is not generally recommended for persons aged ≥18 years.
10. **Varicella:** Administer the 2-dose series to all susceptible adolescents aged ≥13 years.

Report adverse reactions to vaccines through the federal Vaccine Adverse Event Reporting System. For information on reporting reactions following immunization, please visit www.vaers.org or call the 24-hour national toll-free information line 800-822-7967. Report suspected cases of vaccine-preventable diseases to your state or local health department.

For additional information about vaccines, including precautions and contraindications for immunization and vaccine shortages, please visit the National Immunization Program Web site at www.cdc.gov/nip or call the National Immunization Information Hotline at 800-232-2522 (English) or 800-232-0233 (Spanish).

Table 36-6

Routine Immunization Schedule for Infants and Children: Canada, 2002

AGE AT VACCINATION	DTaP[1]	IPV	Hib[2]	MMR	Td[3] OR dTap[10]	Hep B[4] (3 DOSES)	V	PC	MC
Birth						Infancy or			
2 months	X	X	X			preadolescence		X[8]	X[9]
4 months	X	X	X			(9-13 years)		X	X
6 months	X	(X)[5]	X					X	X
12 months				X			X[7]	X	
18 months	X	X	X	(X)[6] or					or
4-6 years				(X)[6]					
14-16 years					X[10]				X[9]

ROUTINE IMMUNIZATION SCHEDULE FOR CHILDREN <7 YEARS OF AGE NOT IMMUNIZED IN EARLY INFANCY

TIMING	DTaP[1]	IPV	Hib	MMR	Td[3] OR dTAP[10]	Hep B[4] (3 DOSES)	V	P	M
First visit	X	X	X[11]	X[12]		X	X[7]	X[8]	X[9]
2 months later	X	X	X	(X)[6]		X		(X)	(X)
2 months later	X	(X)[5]						(X)	
6-12 months later	X	X	(X)[11]			X			
4-6 years of age[13]	X	X							
14-16 years of age					X				

ROUTINE IMMUNIZATION SCHEDULE FOR CHILDREN ≥7 YEARS OF AGE NOT IMMUNIZED IN EARLY INFANCY

TIMING	DTaP[10]	IPV	MMR	Hep B[4] (3 DOSES)	V	M
First visit	X	X	X	X	X	X[9]
2 months later	X	X	X[6]	X	(X)[7]	
6-12 months later	X	X		X		
10 years later	X					

From *Canadian immunization guide* ed 6, 2002, Health Canada. Reproduced with permission of the Minister of Public Works and Government Services, Canada, 2004.

NOTES:

1. DTaP (diphtheria, tetanus, acellular or component pertussis) vaccine is the preferred vaccine for all doses in the vaccination series, including completion of the series in children who have received ≥1 dose of DPT (whole-cell) vaccine.
2. Hib schedule shown is for PRP-T or HbOC vaccine. If PRP-OMP is used, give at 2, 4, and 12 months of age.
3. Td (tetanus and diphtheria toxoid), a combined absorbed "adult type" preparation for use in people ≥7 years of age, contains less diphtheria toxoid than preparations given to younger children and is less likely to cause reactions in older people.
4. Hepatitis B vaccine can be routinely given to infants or preadolescents, depending on the provincial/territorial policy; three doses at 0, 1, and 6 month intervals are preferred. The second dose should be administered at least 1 month after the first dose, and the third at least 2 months after the second dose. A two-dose schedule for adolescents is also possible.
5. This dose is not needed routinely, but can be included for convenience.
6. A second dose of MMR is recommended, at least 1 month after the first dose for the purpose of better measles protection. For convenience, options include giving it with the next scheduled vaccination at 18 months of age or with school entry (4 to 6 years) vaccinations (depending on the provincial/territorial policy), or at any intervening age that is practicable. The need for a second dose of mumps and rubella vaccine is not established but may benefit (given for convenience as MMR). The second dose of MMR should be given at the same visit as DTaP IPV (±Hib) to ensure high uptake rates.
7. Children aged 12 months to 12 years should receive one dose of varicella vaccine. Individuals ≥13 years of age should receive two doses at least 28 days apart.
8. Recommended schedule, number of doses, and subsequent use of 23 valent polysaccharide pneumococcal vaccine depend on the age of the child when vaccination is begun.
9. Recommended schedule and number of doses of meningococcal vaccine depend on the age of the child.
10. dTap adult formulation with reduced diphtheria toxoid and pertussis component.
11. Recommended schedule and number of doses depend on the product used and age of the child when vaccination is begun. Not required past age 5.
12. Delay until subsequent visit if child is <12 months of age.
13. Omit these doses if the previous doses of DTaP and polio were given after the fourth birthday.

DTaP, Diphtheria, tetanus, pertussis (acellular) vaccine; *IPV,* inactivated poliovirus vaccine; *Hib, Haemophilus influenzae* type b conjugate vaccine; *MMR,* measles, mumps, and rubella vaccine; *Td,* tetanus and diphtheria toxoid, adult type with reduced diphtheria toxoid; *dTap,* tetanus and diphtheria toxoid, acellular pertussis, adolescent/adult type with reduced diphtheria and pertussis components; *Hep B,* hepatitis B vaccine; *V,* varicella; *PC,* pneumococcal conjugate vaccine; *MC,* meningococcal C conjugate vaccine; *P,* pneumonococcal vaccine; *M,* meningococcal vaccine.

Polio

An all–inactivated poliovirus (all-IPV) schedule for routine childhood polio vaccination is now recommended; oral poliovirus (OPV) is no longer used in the United States. All children should receive four doses of IPV at 2 months, 4 months, 6 to 18 months, and 4 to 6 years of age (American Academy of Pediatrics, 2003c).

The change from the exclusive use of OPV to the exclusive use of IPV is related to the rare risk of vaccine-

Table 36-7

Guide to Tetanus Prophylaxis in Routine Wound Management

	Clean, Minor Wounds		All Other Wounds*	
HISTORY OF ABSORBED TETANUS TOXOID (DOSES)	Td†	TIG¶	Td†	TIG¶
Unknown or less than three	Yes	No	Yes	Yes
Three or more‡	No§	No	No‖	No

Data from American Academy of Pediatrics, Committee on Infectious Diseases, Pickering L (ed): *2003 Red Book: report of the Committee on Infectious Diseases,* ed 26, Elk Grove Village, IL, 2003, The Academy.

Td, adult-type diphtheria and tetanus toxoids vaccine; *TIG,* tetanus immune globulin.

*Such as, but not limited to, wounds contaminated with dirt, feces, soil, and saliva; puncture wounds; avulsions; and wounds resulting from missiles, crushing, burns, and frostbite.

†For children <7 years old: DTaP (DT, if pertussis vaccine is contraindicated) is preferred to tetanus toxoid alone. For persons ≥7 years of age, Td is preferred to tetanus toxoid alone.

‡If only three doses of fluid toxoid have been received, a fourth dose of toxoid, preferably an adsorbed toxoid, should be given.

§Yes, if >10 years since last dose.

‖Yes, if >5 years since last dose. (More frequent boosters are not needed and can accentuate side effects.)

¶Equine tetanus antitoxin should be used, if available, when TIG is not available (not available in the U.S.).

associated polio paralysis from OPV. The exclusive use of IPV eliminates the risk of this paralysis.

Measles

The measles (rubeola) vaccine is given at 12 to 15 months of age. During the course of measles outbreaks, the vaccine can be given any time after 6 months of age, followed by a second inoculation after age 12 months.

Because of continued outbreaks of measles among unvaccinated preschool-age children and among vaccinated school-age children and college students, a second measles immunization is recommended at 4 to 6 years of age (at school entry) but may be administered at any time as long as 4 weeks have passed since the first dose and provided that both doses are administered at or after age 12 months. Otherwise the child may be revaccinated by 11 to 12 years of age.

Mumps

Mumps virus vaccine is recommended for children at 12 to 15 months of age and is typically given in combination with measles and rubella. It should not be administered to infants younger than 12 months because persisting maternal antibodies can interfere with the immune response.

Because of recent outbreaks of the disease, especially in children 10 to 19 years of age, mumps immunization is recommended for all individuals born after 1957 who may be susceptible to mumps (i.e., those who have no history of having had the disease or vaccine and when there is no laboratory evidence of immunity).

Rubella

Rubella is a relatively mild infection in children, but in a pregnant woman the actual infection presents serious risks to the developing fetus. Therefore, the aim of rubella immunization is actually protection of the unborn child rather than the recipient of the immunization.

Rubella immunization is recommended for all children at 12 to 15 months of age and is administered in a combined form with measles and mumps vaccine. Increased emphasis should also be placed on vaccinating all unimmunized prepubertal children and susceptible adolescents and adult women in the childbearing age group.

Because the live attenuated virus may cross the placenta and theoretically present a risk to the developing fetus, rubella vaccine is not given to any pregnant woman. Although this is standard practice, current evidence from women who received the vaccine while pregnant and delivered unaffected offspring indicates that the risk to the fetus is negligible. In addition, there is no reported danger of administering rubella vaccine to a child if the mother is pregnant.

Pneumococcal (Prevnar)

A seven-valent *Streptococcus pneumoniae* conjugate vaccine (PCV7 or PCV) has now been approved for use in all children 2 months to 23 months old. Streptococci pneumococci are responsible for a number of bacterial infections in children younger than age 2 years; these infections may cause death or serious morbidity. Among these are generalized infections such as septicemia and meningitis, or localized infections such as otitis media, sinusitis, and pneumonia. The vaccine is administered at 2, 4, and 6 months, with a fourth dose at 12 months of age or older. The vaccine is also recommended for children 24 to 59 months with conditions such as cardiac disease, pulmonary diseases (excluding asthma), immunodeficiency (human immunodeficiency virus, asplenia, sickle cell), diabetes mellitus, renal failure, leukemia, and malignancies (Preventing pneumococcal disease among infants, 2000). PCV is also recommended for children 24 to 59 months old who attend group day care. The vaccine may be administered at the same time as other vaccines but in a separate syringe and at a separate site; it is given as an intramuscular injection (Preventing pneumococcal disease among infants, 2000).

The pneumococcal polysaccharide vaccine (PPV) is also recommended after two doses of PCV (2 months apart and PPV given no sooner than 2 months after second dose of PCV) in children 24 to 59 months old with cardiac disease, pulmonary disease, immunodeficiencies, renal failure, sickle cell disease, nephrotic syndrome, asplenia, leukemia, and solid organ transplantation (Preventing pneumococcal disease among infants, 2000).

NURSE ALERT The use of meningococcal and diphtheria proteins in combination vaccines does not mean the child has received adequate immunization for meningococcal or diphtheria illnesses; the child must be given the appropriate vaccine for that specific disease. ■

Haemophilus influenzae Type B

Haemophilus influenzae type B (Hib) conjugate vaccines provide protection against a number of serious infections caused by Hib, especially bacterial meningitis, epiglottitis, bacterial pneumonia, septic arthritis, and sepsis (Hib is not associated with the viruses that cause influenza, or "flu"). Several Hib vaccines are available, three of which may be given to infants (PRP-OMP [PedvaxHIB], ComVax, and

ActHIB). Some Hib vaccines are combination vaccines, such as Comvax (Hib and HBV). These conjugate vaccines connect Hib to a nontoxic form of another organism, such as meningococcal protein or diphtheria protein. There is no antibody response to these nontoxic proteins, but they significantly improve the antibody response to Hib, especially in infants. The use of combination vaccines provides equivalent immunogenicity and decreases the number of injections an infant receives; however, it is important that they be given to the appropriate-age child.

The DTaP/Hib combination vaccine (TriHIBit) should not be used for the first three doses at 2, 4, and 6 months but may be used as a booster thereafter. When PRP-OMP or ComVax is administered at 2 and 4 months, a dose at 6 months is not required (American Academy of Pediatrics, 2004b).

When possible, the Hib conjugate vaccine used at the first vaccination should be used for all subsequent vaccinations in the primary series. All Hib vaccines are administered by intramuscular injection using a separate syringe and at a separate site from any concurrent vaccinations.

Varicella

Administration of the cell-free live-attenuated varicella vaccine (Varivax) is recommended for healthy children 12 months of age or older who are susceptible. A single dose of 0.5 ml should be given by subcutaneous injection. Children 13 years of age or older who are susceptible should receive two doses administered at least 4 weeks apart (American Academy of Pediatrics, 2004b). The vaccine should be kept frozen in the lyophilized form (stable particles that readily go into solution) and used within 30 minutes of being reconstituted to ensure viral potency (American Academy of Pediatrics, 2003c).

Varicella vaccine may be administered simultaneously with MMR. However, separate syringes and injection sites should be used. If they are not administered simultaneously, the interval between administration of varicella vaccine and MMR should be at least 1 month. Varicella vaccine may also be given simultaneously with DTaP, IPV, HBV, or Hib (American Academy of Pediatrics, 2003c).

Influenza

The influenza vaccine is now recommended for children 6 months and older with risk factors including but not limited to the following: asthma, cardiac disease, human immunodeficiency virus, sickle cell disease, diabetes, and household members with individuals at high risk. Influenza vaccine (trivalent inactivated influenza vaccine) may be given to any healthy children 6 to 23 months old because this age group is at particular risk for influenza-related hospitalizations (American Academy of Pediatrics, 2004b). The vaccine is usually started in the fall before the flu season begins and is repeated yearly because different strains of influenza may be predominant each year. The intramuscular vaccine is administered as two separate doses 2 weeks apart in first-time recipients younger than 8 years old. The dose is 0.25 ml for children 6 to 35 months old and 0.5 ml for those over 3 years. The vaccine may be given at the same time as other immunizations but in a separate syringe and at a separate site (American Academy of Pediatrics, 2003c). A new preparation of the vaccine, FluMist, a live attenuated influenza vaccine, has been released by the Food and Drug Administration (Bechtel, 2003). The vaccine is given nasally as two doses 6 weeks apart in healthy persons age 5 to 49 years. Although it is an alternative to the injection, there is a cost increase, and insurance companies may not cover the cost of the nasal vaccine.

Recommendations for Selected Immunizations

Several additional vaccines are recommended for children at high risk for particular diseases. Most of these children have chronic disorders or impaired immune systems that make them more susceptible to certain infections than the general population. Selected immunizations are presented in Table 36-8. Others, such as the rabies vaccine, are discussed elsewhere in this text.

Reactions

Vaccines used for routine immunizations are among the safest and most reliable drugs available. However, minor side effects do occur following many of the immunizations and, rarely, a serious reaction may result from the vaccine.

With inactivated antigens, such as DTaP, side effects are most likely to occur within a few hours or days of adminis-

Table 36-8

Recommendations for Selected Nonmandated Vaccines

DESCRIPTION	ADMINISTRATION/PRECAUTIONS
MENINGOCOCCAL POLYSACCHARIDE VACCINE (MENOMUNE)	
Affords protection against *Neisseria meningitidis:* sero-groups A, C, Y, and W-135. Recommended for children 2 years of age and older with terminal complement deficiencies and anatomic or functional asplenia.	Subcutaneous injection Duration of protection unknown Safety during pregnancy not established
LYME DISEASE VACCINE	
Affords protection against infection with the spirochete *Borrelia burgdorferi,* which causes Lyme disease (LD). Recommended for individuals 15 to 70 years of age who are at high risk for LD from significant exposure to tick habitats in endemic areas (northeast and north-central United States) and for those who have been infected with LD.	Intramuscular injection in deltoid muscle Administered on 0-, 1-, and 12-month schedule. Doses 2 and 3 should be given several weeks before *B. burgdorferi* season, which usually begins in April.

tration and are usually limited to local tenderness, erythema, and swelling at the injection site; low-grade fever; and behavioral changes (e.g., drowsiness, fretfulness, eating less, and prolonged or unusual cry). Local reactions tend to be less severe when the deltoid (except in small infants) rather than the vastus lateralis site is used and when a needle of sufficient length to deposit the vaccine in the muscle is used (Atraumatic Care box). Rarely, more severe reactions may occur, especially with pertussis (see Table 36-9). Reactions to DTaP tend to be more severe if they occurred with a previous immunization.

Hib vaccine is one of the safest vaccines available but may be associated with low-grade fever and mild local reactions at the site of injection, which resolve rapidly. Fever (temperature higher than 38.5° C [101.3° F]) may rarely occur.

Unlike the inactivated antigens, live attenuated virus vaccines such as MMR multiply for days or weeks, and unfavorable reactions and "vaccine-associated" disorders can occur for 30 to 60 days. These reactions are usually mild, although reactions to rubella tend to be more troublesome in older children and adults.

Studies in the United States and in various European countries (Denmark, Finland) have found no association between the MMR vaccine and the incidence of autism (Campion, 2002; Dales, Hammer, & Smith, 2001; Hviid et al, 2003).

Atraumatic Care

IMMUNIZATIONS

To minimize local reactions from vaccines:

- Select a needle of adequate length (1 inch [2.5 cm] in infants) to deposit the antigen deep in the muscle mass.
- Inject into the vastus lateralis or ventrogluteal muscle; the deltoid may be used in children 18 months of age or older or in infants receiving HBV vaccine.
- Use an air bubble to clear the needle after injecting the vaccine (theoretically beneficial but unproved).

To minimize pain:

- Apply the topical anesthetic EMLA to the injection site and cover with an occlusive dressing for $2\frac{1}{2}$ hours.
- Apply a vapocoolant spray (ethyl chloride or Fluori-Methane) directly to the skin or to a cotton ball, which is placed on the skin for 15 seconds immediately before the injection.*
- In preschool children use distraction, such as telling the child to "take a deep breath and blow and blow and blow until I tell you to stop."

NOTE: Changing the needle on the syringe after drawing up the vaccine and before injecting it has not been shown to decrease local reactions. In children 4 to 6 years of age, the administration of sequential injections or simultaneous injections of vaccines did not alter their perceptions of distress, but parents preferred the simultaneous method.†

*Reis EC, Holubkov R: Vapocoolant spray is equally effective as EMLA cream in reducing immunization pain in school-aged children, *Pediatrics* 100(6):1025, 1997.

†Horn MI, McCarthy AM: Children's responses to sequential versus simultaneous immunization injections, *J Pediatr Health Care* 13(1):18-23, 1999.

Contraindications/Precautions

Nurses need to be aware of the reasons for withholding immunizations—both for the child's safety in terms of avoiding reactions and for the child's maximum benefit from receiving the vaccine. Unfounded fears and lack of knowledge regarding contraindications can needlessly prevent a child from having protection from life-threatening diseases. Issues that have surfaced regarding vaccines include the misconception that administering combination vaccines may overload the child's immune system; the combined vaccines have undergone rigorous study in relation to side effects and immunogenicity rates following administration. Parents must be given appropriate information regarding vaccine safety, benefits, and risks so they can make informed decisions regarding vaccinations for their children (Koslap-Petraco & Parsons, 2003). The advantage of widespread media via television and the Internet is that information is readily available at any given moment; the disadvantage is that some of this information may be incorrect, incomplete, or misleading and may influence parents to make decisions that may have deleterious consequences on their children's health.

For the contraindications to the usual childhood vaccines, see Table 36-9.

Administration

The principal precautions in administering immunizations include proper storage of the vaccine to protect its potency and institution of recommended procedures for injection. The nurse must be familiar with the manufacturer's directions for storage and reconstitution of the vaccine. For example, if the vaccine is to be refrigerated, it should be stored on a center shelf and not in the door, where frequent temperature increases from opening the refrigerator can alter the vaccine's potency. For protection against light, the vial can be wrapped in aluminum foil. Periodic checks are established to ensure that no vaccine is used after its expiration date.

The DTaP vaccines contain the adjuvant alum to retain the antigen at the injection site and prolong the stimulatory effect. One of the most important features of injecting vaccines is adequate penetration of the muscle for deposition of the drug intramuscularly and not subcutaneously. The use of appropriate needle length is an essential component of administering vaccines. In one study, the use of a longer needle (25 versus 16 mm; 23 versus 25 gauge, respectively) significantly decreased the incidence of localized edema and tenderness when vaccines were administered to a group of infants (Diggle & Deeks, 2000). Because subcutaneous or intracutaneous injection of the adjuvant can cause local irritation, inflammation, or abscess formation, attention to excellent intramuscular injection technique must be used (see Atraumatic Care box).

The total series requires several injections, and every attempt is made to rotate the sites and administer the injections as painlessly as possible (see discussion on intramuscular injections in Chapter 45). When two or more injections are given at separate sites, the order of injections is arbitrary. Some practitioners suggest injecting the less painful one first. Some believe this is DTaP, whereas others

Table 36-9

Contraindications and Precautions to Vaccinations[a]

TRUE CONTRAINDICATIONS AND PRECAUTIONS	NOT CONTRAINDICATIONS (VACCINES MAY BE ADMINISTERED)
GENERAL FOR ALL VACCINES (DTAP, IPV, MMR, HIB, HEPATITIS B, VARICELLA, PCV, HEPATITIS A, INFLUENZA)	
Contraindications Anaphylactic reaction to a vaccine contraindicates further doses of that vaccine Anaphylactic reaction to a vaccine constituent contraindicates the use of vaccines containing that substance Moderate or severe illnesses with or without a fever	**Not Contraindications** Mild to moderate local reaction (soreness, redness, swelling) following a dose of an injectable antigen Mild acute illness with or without low-grade fever Current antimicrobial therapy Convalescent phase of illnesses Prematurity (same dosage and indications as for normal, full-term infants) Recent exposure to an infectious disease History of penicillin or other nonspecific allergies or family history of such allergies
DIPHTHERIA, TETANUS, PERTUSSIS OR ACELLULAR PERTUSSIS (DTAP)	
Contraindications Encephalopathy within 7 days of administration of previous dose of DTaP	**Not Contraindications** Temperature of <40.5° C (105° F) following a previous dose of DTaP Family history of seizures[b] Family history of sudden infant death syndrome Family history of an adverse event following DTaP administration
Precautions[b] Fever of ≥40.5° C (105° F) within 48 hours after vaccination with a prior dose of DTaP Collapse or shocklike state (hypotonic-hyporesponsive episode) within 48 hours of receiving a prior dose of DTaP Seizures within 3 days of receiving a prior dose of DTaP[c] Persistent, inconsolable crying lasting ≥3 hours within 48 hours of receiving a prior dose of DTaP	
INACTIVATED POLIO (IPV)	
Contraindication Anaphylactic reaction to neomycin or streptomycin	**Not Contraindications** Breastfeeding Diarrhea
Precaution[b] Pregnancy	
MEASLES, MUMPS, RUBELLA (MMR)[e]	
Contraindications Pregnancy Known altered immunodeficiency (hematologic and solid tumors, congenital immunodeficiency, and long-term immunosuppressive therapy)	**Not Contraindications[d]** Tuberculosis or positive PPD skin test Simultaneous TB skin testing[d] Breastfeeding Pregnancy of mother of recipient Immunodeficient family member or household contact Infection with HIV Nonanaphylactic reactions to eggs or neomycin

Modified from American Academy of Pediatrics, Committee on Infectious Diseases, Pickering L (ed): *2003 Red Book: report of the Committee on Infectious Diseases,* ed 26, Elk Grove Village, IL, 2003, The Academy.

[a]This information is based on the recommendations of the Advisory Committee on Immunization Practices (ACIP) and those of the Committee on Infectious Diseases (*Red Book* Committee) of the American Academy of Pediatrics (AAP). Sometimes these recommendations vary from those contained in the manufacturer's package inserts. For more detailed information, providers should consult the published recommendations of the ACIP, AAP, and the manufacturer's package inserts.

[b]The events or conditions listed as precautions, although not contraindications, should be carefully reviewed. The benefits and risks of administering a specific vaccine to an individual under the circumstances should be considered. If the risks are believed to outweigh the benefits, the vaccination should be withheld; if the benefits are believed to outweigh the risks (e.g., during an outbreak or foreign travel), the vaccination should be administered. Whether and when to administer DTaP to children with proven or suspected underlying neurologic disorders should be decided on an individual basis. It is prudent on theoretic grounds to avoid vaccinating pregnant women.

[c]Acetaminophen given before administering DTaP and thereafter every 4 hours for 24 hours should be considered for children with a personal or family history of convulsions in siblings or parents.

[de]Measles vaccination may temporarily suppress tuberculin reactivity. If testing cannot be done the day of MMR vaccination, the test should be postponed for 4 to 6 weeks.

Continued

Table 36-9

Contraindications and Precautions to Vaccinations—cont'd

TRUE CONTRAINDICATIONS AND PRECAUTIONS	NOT CONTRAINDICATIONS (VACCINES MAY BE ADMINISTERED)
MEASLES, MUMPS, RUBELLA (MMR)[e]—cont'd	
Precautions[b]	
Recent immune globulin (IG) administration	
Immune globulin products and MMR should not be given simultaneously; if unavoidable, give at different sites and revaccinate or test for seroconversion in 3 months; if IG is given first, MMR should not be given for at least 3-6 months, depending on dose; if MMR is given first, IG should not be given for 2 weeks	
Thrombocytopenia/thrombocytopenia purpura	
***HAEMOPHILUS INFLUENZAE* TYPE B (HIB)**	
Contraindication	**Not a Contraindication**
Nonidentified	History of Hib disease
HEPATITIS B VIRUS (HBV)	
Contraindication	**Not a Contraindication**
Anaphylactic reaction to common baker's yeast	Pregnancy
VARICELLA	
Contraindications	**Not a Contraindication**
Immunocompromised individuals (e.g., HIV, acute lymphocytic leukemia)	Breastfeeding
Pregnancy	
PNEUMOCOCCAL	**Not a Contraindication**
Allergy to vaccine components	Minor illneses with or without a fever
Acute, moderate, or severe illness with or without fever	Mild upper respiratory tract infection
	Allergic rhinitis
INFLUENZA*	
Acute febrile illness	
Egg hypersensitivity	

*See James JM et al: Safe administration of influenza vaccine to patients with egg allergies, *J Pediatr* 133:624-628, 1998.

suggest the MMR or Hib vaccine. Still others advocate injecting at two sites simultaneously (which requires two operators).

One study found that children age 4 to 6 years rated sequential injections for immunizations versus simultaneous injections as being equally successful (Horn & McCarthy, 1999). Parents in the study preferred simultaneous immunization injections.

Because allergic reactions can occur after injection of vaccines, appropriate precautions are taken (see Anaphylaxis, Chapter 48).

Because nurses often administer vaccines, they have the responsibility for adequately informing parents of the nature, prevalence, and risks of the disease; the type of immunization product to be used; the expected benefits and the risk of side effects of the vaccine; and the need for accurate immunization records. Referring to immunizations as "baby shots" and limiting the discussion to vague statements about the vaccines are unacceptable practices.

Another important nursing responsibility is accurate documentation. Each child should have an immunization record for parents to keep, especially for families who move often. A survey of the accuracy of parental recall of children's immunizations found that parents underestimated the number of polio, DTaP, and MMR vaccines. The accuracy rate was not related to ethnic background, education level, or insurance coverage. Although immunization rates have increased significantly, health professionals should use every opportunity to encourage complete immunization of all children (see Community Focus box). Blank immunization records may be downloaded from a number of Web sites, including the Immunization Action Coalition (www.immunize.org), which has vaccine information and records in a number of languages.

The following information is documented on the medical record: day, month, and year of administration; manufacturer and lot number of vaccine; expiration date of vaccine; and the name, address, and title of the person administering the vaccine. Additional data to record are the site and route of administration and evidence that the parent or legal guardian gave informed consent before the immunization was administered. Any adverse reactions after the administration of any vaccine are reported to the Vaccine Adverse Event Reporting System (VAERS).*

*For information call 800-822-7967; Web site: www.fda.gov/cber/vaers/vaers.htm.

Community Focus

IMPROVING IMMUNIZATION AMONG CHILDREN AND ADOLESCENTS

Strategies that may increase compliance include giving parents vaccine information at the time of the newborn's discharge, mailing reminder cards, making immunization services readily available, removing barriers to vaccination (such as long waiting times and appointment-only systems), and taking every opportunity to immunize children when they enter a health care facility (such as emergency departments, clinics, private offices, and hospitals).

Despite improving vaccination rates among infants and young children, *adolescents* are often incompletely immunized. An immunization update is an important part of adolescent preventive care, especially at 11 to 12 years of age. With the exception of pregnant teenagers, all adolescents should receive a second dose of the *measles, mumps, and rubella (MMR) vaccine* unless they have documentation of two MMR vaccinations after the first 12 months of life. All adolescents who have not previously completed the three-dose series of the *hepatitis B (HBV) vaccine* should initiate or complete the series at age 11 to 12 years.

Adolescents age 11 to 12 years should receive a booster dose of *diphtheria-tetanus (Td) vaccine* if they have received the primary series of vaccinations and if no dose has been received during the previous 5 years. Unvaccinated adolescents who lack a reliable history of chickenpox should receive the *varicella virus vaccine* at age 11 to 12 years.

Hepatitis A vaccine should be given to

- Adolescents who are traveling or living in countries where the hepatitis A virus is endemic
- Adolescents who live in communities with high rates of hepatitis A
- Adolescents who have chronic liver disease
- Adolescents who are intravenous drug users
- Adolescent males who have sex with other males

Adolescents who have chronic disorders or underlying medical conditions that place them at high risk for complications associated with the disease, such as influenza, should receive the appropriate vaccines (see p 1064).

An additional source of vaccine information that must be given to parents (by law; National Childhood Vaccine Injury Act, 1986) before the administration of given vaccines is the *vaccine information statement* (VIS) for the particular vaccine being administered. Practitioners are required to fully inform families of the risks and benefits of the vaccines. VISs are designed to provide updated information to the adult vaccinee or parents/legal guardians of children being vaccinated regarding the risks and benefits of each vaccine. Questions regarding the information in the VISs should be answered by the practitioner. VISs are available for the following vaccines: anthrax, DTaP, Td, MMR, IPV, varicella, Hib, influenza, meningococcal, pneumococcal (PCV and PPV), and hepatitis A and B. An updated VIS should be provided, and documentation in the patient's chart should include that the VIS was given and the publication of the VIS. VISs are available from state or local health departments and the following Web sites:

Immunization Coalition—www.immunize.org/vis/
Centers for Disease Control and Prevention—www.cdc.gov/nip/publications/vis/

In response to the concerns of manufacturers, practitioners, and parents of children with serious vaccine-associated injuries, the National Childhood Vaccine Injury Act (NCVIA) of 1986 and the Vaccine Compensation Amendments of 1987 were passed. These laws are designed to provide fair compensation for children who are inadvertently injured and provide greater protection from liability for vaccine manufacturers and providers.

Injury Prevention

Injuries are a major cause of death during infancy, especially for children 6 to 12 months old. According to recent surveys (Agran et al, 2003; Pickett et al, 2003) the leading causes of injury to infants are falls, ingestion injuries (poison and medications), and burns. Constant vigilance, awareness, and supervision are essential as the child gains increased locomotor and manipulative skills that are coupled with an insatiable curiosity about the environment. Table 36-10 lists the major developmental achievements of each period during infancy and the appropriate injury prevention plan.

Aspiration of Foreign Objects

Asphyxiation by foreign material in the respiratory tract, combined with mechanical suffocation, is one of the leading causes of fatal injury in children younger than 1 year of age. In at least one study, choking was the fourth leading cause of death in infants (Brenner et al, 1999). The size, shape, and consistency of foods or objects are important determinants of fatal obstruction. For example, small spheric or cylindric and pliable objects (less than 3.2 cm, or 1.25 inches) are more likely to completely obstruct the airway. Unfortunately, common household items can be deadly to infants.

As soon as infants have the ability to find their mouth, they are vulnerable to aspiration of small objects, such as those left within reach or removeable parts of objects that may on initial inspection appear safe. All toys must be carefully inspected for potential danger. Rattles, for example, have small beads in them to produce noise. A broken or cracked rattle can be dangerous because the beads can easily be aspirated while the infant has the toy in the mouth. Stuffed animals are another potentially dangerous toy if any of the parts, such as the eyes or nose, are removeable buttons or plastic pieces. An active infant can grab a low-hanging mobile and quickly chew off a small piece. As soon as the infant crawls or plays on the floor, the floor must be kept free of any small articles that can be picked up and swallowed, such as coins, buttons or batteries.

When infant *clothes* are purchased, the type of closure is important. A front button can easily be pulled off and swallowed. Safety pins for diapers are kept closed and away from the dressing table. Even though a young infant may not search for them, practicing this good habit from the beginning prevents future injuries.

Table 36-10

Injury Prevention during Infancy

AGE: BIRTH–4 MONTHS

Major Developmental Accomplishments

Involuntary reflexes, such as the crawling reflex, may propel infant forward or backward, and the startle reflex may cause the body to jerk

May roll over

Increasing eye-hand coordination with voluntary grasp reflex

Injury Prevention

Aspiration

Not as great a danger to this age group, but should begin practicing safeguarding early (see under Age: 4-7 Months)

Never shake baby powder directly on infant; place powder in hand and then on infant's skin; store container closed and out of infant's reach

Hold infant for feeding; do not prop bottle

Know emergency procedures for choking

Use pacifier with one-piece construction and loop handle

Suffocation/drowning

Keep all plastic bags stored out of infant's reach; discard large plastic garment bags after tying in a knot

Do not cover mattress with plastic

Use firm mattress and loose blankets; no pillows

Make sure crib design follows federal regulations and mattress fits snugly—crib slats <2⅜ inches (6 cm) apart

Position crib away from other furniture and away from radiators

Do not tie pacifier on a string around infant's neck

Remove bibs at bedtime

Never leave infant alone in bath

Do not leave infant younger than 12 months alone on adult or youth mattress or "beanbag" type pillows

Falls

Always raise crib rails

Never leave infant on a raised, unguarded surface

When in doubt as to where to place child, use floor

Restrain child in infant seat and *never* leave child unattended while the seat is resting on a raised surface

Avoid using a high chair until child can sit well with support

Poisoning

Not as great a danger to this age group, but should begin practicing safeguards early (see under Age: 4-7 Months)

Burns

Install smoke detectors in home

Use caution when warming formula in microwave oven; always check temperature of liquid before feeding

Check bathwater—never leave unattended.

Do not pour hot liquids when infant is close by; such as sitting on lap

Beware of cigarette ashes that may fall on infant

Do not leave infant in sun for more than a few minutes; keep exposed areas covered

Wash flame-retardant clothes according to label directions

Use cool-mist vaporizers

Do not leave child in parked car

Check surface heat of car restraint before placing child in seat

Motor vehicles

Transport infant in federally approved, rear-facing car seat, preferably in back seat

Do not place infant on seat (of car) or in lap

Do not place child in a carriage or stroller behind a parked car

Do not place infant or child in front passenger seat with an air bag

Bodily damage

Avoid sharp, jagged objects

Keep diaper pins closed and away from infant

AGE: 4–7 MONTHS

Major Developmental Accomplishments

Rolls over

Sits momentarily

Grasps and manipulates small objects

Resecures a dropped object

Has well-developed eye-hand coordination

Can focus on and locate very small objects

Mouthing is very prominent

Can push on hands and knees

Crawls backward

Injury Prevention

Aspiration

Keep buttons, beads, syringe caps, and other small objects out of infant's reach

Keep floor free of any small objects

Do not feed infant hard candy, nuts, food with pits or seeds, or whole or circular pieces of hot dog

Exercise caution when giving teething biscuits, because large chunks may be broken off and aspirated

Do not feed infant while child is lying down

Inspect toys for removeable parts

Keep baby powder, if used, out of reach

Suffocation

Keep all latex balloons out of reach

Remove all crib toys that are strung across crib or playpen when child begins to push up on hands or knees or is 5 months old

Falls

Restrain in a high chair

Keep crib rails raised to full height

Table 36-10

Injury Prevention during Infancy—cont'd

AGE: 4-7 MONTHS—cont'd	
Injury Prevention—cont'd	
Burns Keep faucets out of reach Place hot objects (cigarettes, candles, incense) on high surface Limit exposure to sun; apply sunscreen ***Motor vehicles*** See under Age: Birth-4 Months	***Poisoning*** Avoid storing large quantities of cleaning fluid, paints, pesticides, and other toxic substances Discard used containers of poisonous substances Do not store toxic substances in food containers Make sure that paint for furniture or toys does not contain lead Place toxic substances on a high shelf or in locked cabinet Hang plants or place on high surface rather than on floor Discard used button-sized batteries; store new batteries in safe area Know telephone number of local poison control center (usually listed in front of telephone directory) ***Bodily damage*** Give toys that are smooth and rounded, preferably made of wood or plastic Avoid long, pointed objects as toys Avoid toys that are excessively loud Keep sharp objects out of infant's reach
AGE: 8-12 MONTHS	
Major Developmental Accomplishments	
Crawls/creeps Stands, holding onto furniture Stands alone Cruises around furniture Walks Climbs Pulls on objects	Throws objects Is able to pick up small objects; has pincer grasp Explores by putting objects in mouth Dislikes being restrained Explores away from parent Increasing understanding of simple commands and phrases
Injury Prevention	
Aspiration Keep lint and small objects off floor, off furniture, and out of reach of children Take care in feeding solid table food to ensure that very small pieces are given Do not use beanbag toys or allow child to play with dried beans See also under Age: 4-7 Months ***Suffocation/drowning*** Keep doors of ovens, dishwashers, refrigerators, coolers, and front-loading clothes washers and dryers closed at all times If storing an unused appliance, such as a refrigerator, remove the door Supervise contact with inflated balloons; immediately discard popped balloons, and keep uninflated balloons out of reach Fence swimming pools Always supervise when near any source of water, such as cleaning buckets, drainage areas, toilets Keep bathroom door closed Eliminate unnecessary pools of water Keep one hand on child at all times when in tub	***Falls*** Fence stairways at top and bottom if child has access to either end* Dress infant in safe shoes and clothing (soles that do not "catch" on floor, tied shoelaces, pant legs that do not touch floor) Avoid walkers, especially near stairs Ensure that furniture is sturdy enough for child to pull self to standing position and cruise ***Poisoning*** Administer medications as a drug, not as a candy Do not administer medications unless so prescribed by a practitioner Replace medications and poisons immediately after use; replace caps properly if a child-protector cap is used Have telephone number for local Poison Control Center readily available ***Burns*** Place guards in front of or around any heating appliance, fireplace, or furnace Keep electrical wires hidden or out of reach Place plastic guards over electrical outlets; place furniture in front of outlets Keep hanging tablecloths out of reach (child may pull down hot liquids or heavy or sharp objects) Avoid placing hair curling irons on cabinet edge where child can reach

*Information on many items, such as cribs and walkers, is available from the U.S. Consumer Product Safety Commission; phone: 1-800-638-CPSC; Web site: www.cpsc.gov/.

Food items are the second most common cause of aspiration, and the most common offenders are hot dogs, candy, nuts, and grapes. When new foods are given to the child, nuts, hard candies, marshmallows, large amounts of peanut butter, and fruits with pits or seeds are avoided. When traveling (especially in airplanes) or entertaining, snack foods such as peanuts and popcorn are kept away from young children. If given to young children, hot dogs must be cut into small, irregular pieces rather than served whole or sliced into sections, because their size (diameter), round shape, and consistency allow for complete occlusion of the airway. Perhaps the most dangerous foods are dried beans, which, if aspirated, enlarge when they come in contact with the wet mucosa and block the airway.

Pacifiers can also be dangerous because the entire object may be aspirated if it is small, or the nipple and shield may become detached from the handle and become lodged in the pharynx. Improvised pacifiers, such as those made in hospitals from a padded nipple, also present dangers. The nipple may separate from the plastic collar and be aspirated. In addition, parents may continue to offer this pacifier to the infant at home. To eliminate the hazards of improvised pacifiers, hospitals should use only safe, commercial types. Pacifiers should not be altered from their original shape to encourage or discourage usage. Candy pacifiers pose dangers because the candy portion can dislodge from the circular base and be aspirated. To be safe, pacifiers should have the following:

- Sturdy, one-piece construction with material that is nontoxic, flexible, and firm but not brittle
- An easily grasped handle
- A mouthguard that cannot be separated from the nipple, that has two ventilating holes, and that is too large to be aspirated
- No detachable ribbon or string
- A label warning against tying the pacifier around the infant's neck

Using a syringe to accurately measure and dispense oral liquid medications to young children has become common practice. However, the *syringe cap* is a potential aspiration hazard. As a precaution, keep parts of medication devices out of the reach of children and be certain the cap is removed before dispensing medication. Medication administration syringes without caps are now readily available; syringes with caps should not be used for medication administration.

Another hazardous substance if aspirated is *baby powder,* which is usually a mixture of talc (hydrous magnesium silicate) and other silicates. Although the use of talc has been discouraged, it is a common baby care product that can cause severe and often fatal aspiration pneumonia. One of the factors involved in talc aspiration is the similar appearance of baby powder containers and nursing bottles. Talc containers often become favorite playthings and are placed in the mouth. Improperly using powder by sprinkling it directly on the skin creates a cloud of talc dust that is easily inhaled. Parents are advised of the danger of baby powder and are discouraged from using it. If they prefer to use a powder, a cornstarch preparation can be substituted (see Diaper Dermatitis, Chapter 53). Whenever a powder is used, it should be placed in the hand and then applied to the skin, never shaken directly from the container onto the skin. The container is kept closed and immediately stored in a safe place, especially away from curious toddlers, who often imitate caregiving activities and may accidentally shake it on the infant.

Suffocation

Mechanical suffocation includes suffocation by covering of the airway (i.e., mouth and nose); by pressure on the throat and chest; and by exclusion of air, such as by refrigerator entrapment. Nonfood items cause the majority of deaths in young children. *Latex balloons,* whether partially inflated, uninflated, or popped, are a leading cause of pediatric choking deaths from children's products. They should be kept away from infants and young children. Even the practice of inflating latex gloves to amuse children in health care settings may pose a danger, especially if the child is latex sensitive.

NURSE ALERT Encourage adults to
Blow up balloons for children
Supervise children's balloon play
Pick up and dispose of broken balloon pieces
Warn older children of dangers of chewing or sucking on balloons
Substitute Mylar or paper balloons for latex balloons ■

In addition, the accessibility of the plastic linings of diapers used on the infant or on dolls is especially dangerous to young children.

The *bed* or *crib* poses a number of hazards. An infant who is placed in a bed under tucked-in blankets and sheets can be caught under them and unable to wriggle free. Baby pillows filled with plastic foam beads that make them resemble small beanbags are dangerous; very young infants are suffocated when the pillow contours to the face and blocks the airway. There are potential dangers when adults sleep with a small infant because of the possibility of rolling over and smothering the child (overlaying). The incidence of infant suffocation by a bed-sharing adult increased between 1980 and 1997 (Drago & Dannenberg, 1999). The most common causes of infant suffocation are wedging between a bed or mattress and a wall and oronasal obstruction by a plastic bag.

Infant strangulation may occur if the infant's head becomes caught between the crib slats and mattress or other objects close to the crib. Suffocation deaths are not confined to cribs; ill-fitting mattresses in adult or youth beds, bunk beds, and waterbeds have also been reported. According to U.S. federal regulation, the distance between crib slats should not be more than 2⅜ inches (approximately 6 cm), roughly the width of three adult fingers. Mattresses and bumper pads should fit snugly against the slats. A general rule is that the mattress is too small if two adult fingers can be placed between the mattress and crib or bed side. A temporary solution is to place large, rolled towels in the space to create a snug fit.

Corner post extensions on cribs are another source of strangulation. Children have died when their clothing caught on raised corner posts as they climbed out of the crib.

Voluntary manufacturing standards state that corner post extensions must not exceed $\frac{1}{16}$ inch; however, the safety of any extension is questionable. Decorative extensions need to be removed from cribs. Ideally, information regarding correct crib design should be given prenatally, before parents have purchased or borrowed a crib.*

Mesh-sided playpens and cribs can result in death if the sides are left in the lowered position. Infants have suffocated when they fell off the edge of the mattress and the head or chest was compressed between the floorboard and mesh side. Parents should be advised of this danger and encouraged to always keep the sides locked securely in the up position whenever the child is in the playpen or crib.

The crib should be positioned away from large furniture, because children who crawl out of the crib may become caught between the two objects. Cribs should also be located away from windows, where drape or blind cords can become wrapped around the infant's neck.

Another cause of suffocation is *plastic bags.* Plastic bags are very lightweight and can easily and quickly be wrapped around the head of an active infant or pressed against the face. For this reason, pillows and mattresses should not be covered with plastic. Older infants may play with a plastic bag and accidentally pull it over their heads. Because plastic is nonporous, suffocation occurs in a matter of minutes.

Cords (e.g., drapery or window blinds) located near the infant are a potential cause of strangulation. Bibs are removed at bedtime, and objects such as pacifiers are never hung on a string around the infant's neck. This is a common practice in some cultures that can be remedied by tying a *short* string to a pacifier and clipping the string to the child's shirt.

Toys that have strings attached (e.g., a telephone) or toys that are tied to cribs or playpens can be hazards because the string can become wrapped around the child's neck or the child can become entrapped in the toy. As a precaution, all cords should be less than 30 cm (12 inches) long. Crib toys should be hung high enough that the infant cannot become entangled in them and should no longer be used once the child is able to reach them.

CRITICAL THINKING EXERCISE: INFANT SAFETY

If applied too loosely or left unfastened, restraining straps can be a hazard. For example, a child may slide off a high chair beneath the tray and become strangled on the loose strap. All straps should be fastened securely.

Motor Vehicle Injuries

Automobile injuries are the leading cause of accidental death in children older than 1 year of age (Motor-vehicle occupant injury, 2001). However, a significant number of infants are injured or die from improper restraint within the vehicle, most often from riding on the lap of another occupant. Reports indicate that child restraint use decreases with increasing age of children and increasing number of occupants. Lack of proper child restraint continues to be a major factor in fatal accidents involving children. All infants must be secured in a U.S. federally approved restraint rather than held or placed on the seat of the car. There is no safe alternative.

Infant restraints are designed either as an infant-only model (Fig. 36-11) or as a convertible infant-toddler model. Either restraint is a semireclined seat that faces the rear of the car. A rear-facing car seat provides the best protection for the disproportionately heavy head and weak neck of a young child. This position minimizes the stress on the neck by spreading the forces of a frontal crash over the entire back, neck, and head; the spine is supported by the back of the car seat. If the seat were faced forward, the head would whip forward because of the force of the crash, creating enormous stress on the neck.

The restraint is anchored to the vehicle with the vehicle's seat belt, and the restraint has a harness system for securing the infant. Some harness systems require a clip to keep the

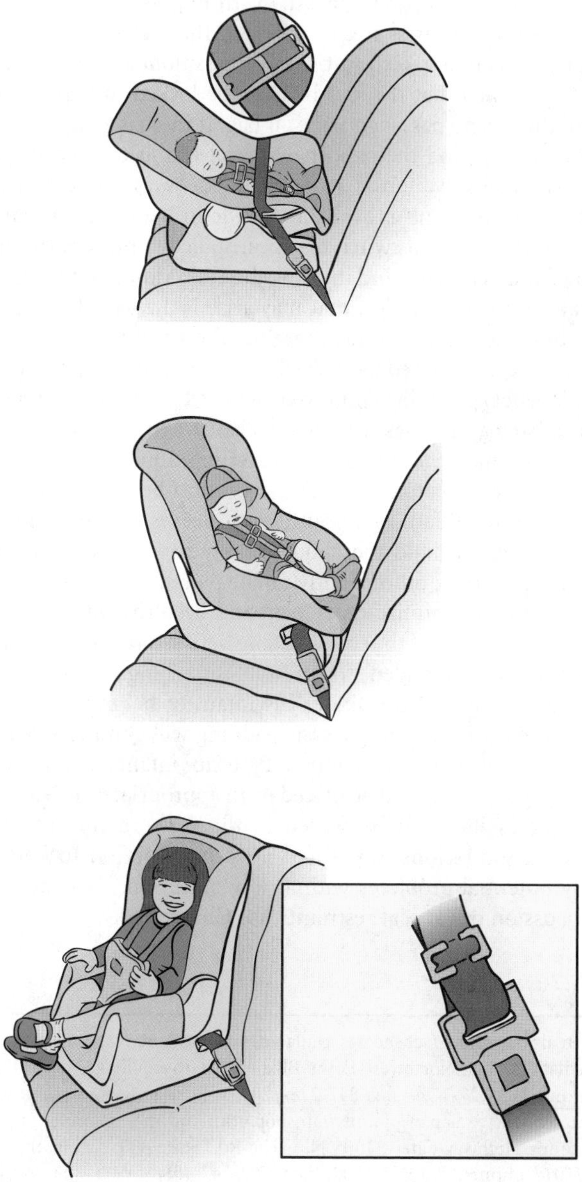

Fig. 36-11 Federally approved infant car restraint. Note placement in middle of back seat and use of car lap/shoulder belt for older child.

*A number of parent education pamphlets—such as *Crib Safety Tips* and *Is Your Used Crib Safe?*—are available in English and Spanish from the U.S. Consumer Product Safety Commission, Publication Request, Washington, DC 20207; phone: 800-638-2772; Web site: www.cpsc.gov. Additional free information is available from the Danny Foundation, 3158 Danville Blvd., PO Box 680, Alamo, CA 94507; phone: 800-83-DANNY; Web site: www.dannyfoundation.org.

shoulder straps correctly positioned. Newer vehicles (manufactured after 1999) have tether straps or anchors that attach to the top of a car seat to better anchor the seat and minimize forward movement in the event of an accident. The LATCH (lower anchor and tether for children) system provides car seat anchors between the front cushion and backrest so that the seat belt does not have to be used. Some automobiles have tether anchors for rear-facing infant-only seats as well (see Chapter 37). Although many infant restraints can be recliners, they are used in the car only in the position specified by the manufacturer.

NURSE ALERT Infants should face the rear from birth to 20 pounds and as close to 1 year of age as possible. If the child weighs 20 pounds but is not 1 year old, the rear-facing position is still recommended. ■

Severe injuries and deaths in children have occurred from air bags deploying on impact in the front passenger seat. The back seat is the safest area of the car. If the back seat is not an option, an infant restraint may be positioned in the front seat provided that the seat belt can be locked into position and there is no passenger-side air bag. If there is a passenger-side air bag, and the child has special health care needs or constant observation is recommended by the practitioner and no other adult is available to ride in the back seat with the child, an on/off switch may be installed to prevent the air bag from deploying and injuring the child riding in the front seat. Another condition that may arise is the use of vehicles without a back seat; in such cases it is best that the front passenger seat be placed as far back as possible and appropriate child safety restraint employed. With advanced technology, new, "smart" air bags will include features that make them a safer alternative for children (Kamerling, 2002).*

For restraints to be effective, they must be used properly. Dressing the infant in an outfit with sleeves and legs allows the harness to hold the child securely in the seat. A small blanket or towel rolled tightly can be placed on either side of the head to minimize movement and keep the infant's hips against the back of the seat. Padding between the infant's legs and crotch is added to prevent slouching. Thick, soft padding is not placed under the infant or behind the back because during the impact the padding will compress, leaving the harness straps loose. Preterm infants being discharged home should be placed in an appropriate car seat restraint as it would be placed in the car and the infant's oxygen saturations monitored for a brief period to detect any potential problems with airway occlusion. (For further discussion of car seat restraints, see Chapter 37.)

*An air bag safety fact sheet is available from the American Academy of Pediatrics, 141 Northwest Point Blvd., Elk Grove Village, IL 60009; phone: 888-227-1770; fax: 847-228-1281; Web sites: www.aap.org; for car seats, www.aap.org/family/famshop.htm; and the Insurance Institute for Highway Safety, 1005 N. Glebe Rd., Suite 800, Arlington, VA 22201; phone: 703-247-1500; fax: 703-247-1588; Web site: www.highwaysafety.org. The National Highway Traffic Safety Administration also contains child passenger safety and air bag safety information for parents; Web site: www.nhtsa.org.

NURSE ALERT Rear-facing infant safety seats must not be placed in the front seats of cars equipped with an air bag on the passenger side. If an infant safety seat is placed in the passenger seat with an air bag, the child could be seriously injured if the air bag is released, because rear-facing infant seats extend closer to the dashboard. ■

Another automobile-related hazard for infants is *overheating* (hyperthermia) and subsequent death when left in a vehicle in hot weather (over 80° F [26.4° C]). Infants dissipate heat poorly, and an increase in body temperature may cause death in a few hours. Parents are cautioned against leaving infants in a vehicle alone for *any reason.* A small sign or placard has been designed to hang in the rear-view mirror to remind the parent that there is a child in the back seat. Busy parents may easily forget the child in the back when preoccupied with errands, children's school and extracurricular activities, and busy work schedules.

Falls

Trauma is the leading cause of accidental death in children and falls are the leading cause of traumatic injury in children (Agran et al, 2003; Patterson, 1999; Pickett et al, 2003). A recent study of childhood injuries found that beginning at the age of 3 to 5 months the incidence of falls increased dramatically with increasing age, peaking at 15 to 17 months of age. Most falls were from heights such as furniture, stairs and buildings (Agran et al, 2003). A large percentage of infants were noted to have fallen as a result of being dropped, from car seats, down stairs and in child walkers (Dedoukou et al, 2004; Pickett et al, 2003). Most childhood injuries in these studies correlated with developmental achievements such as increased independent mobility, exploratory behavior and increased hand-to-mouth activity, with a decreased awareness of hazards in the environment (Agran et al, 2003).

The best advice for prevention of falls is to never place a child of any age unattended on a raised surface that is not designed to protect the child from accidentally falling. When in doubt, the safest place is the floor. Even though young infants cannot climb over a partially raised crib rail, it is best to form a habit of raising the rail all the way, because someday that infant will be able to climb out. Crib sides should have a latching device that cannot be easily released. The welds attaching the crib corner locks to the corner posts should not be cracked or broken. If the welds are damaged, the bedspring could fall to the floor. Ideally, cribs should be placed on carpeted, not hard, floors.

Another danger area for falling is the *changing table,* which is usually high and narrow. Although these tables have a restraining belt, children are never left unattended, even when restrained. The best way to avoid needing to leave is to arrange the area with all necessary articles within easy reach so that the child is always in full sight of the caregiver. It takes only a fraction of a second for an infant to fall off. During the latter half of the first year, infants usually resist dressing and diapering and may be difficult to manage. If there is danger that the child is strong enough to resist restraining, the infant should be changed on a safer surface, such as a clean floor.

Infant seats, high chairs, walkers, and swings present additional opportunities for falls. If the *infant seat* is placed on a table, the child should never be left unrestrained or unattended. The same rule is essential for other baby equipment, particularly when the child has learned to crawl and to stand up. *High chairs* are designed for older infants who can sit well and who are tall enough to have the tray at the level of their chest or abdomen. Small infants can slip through a high chair if a protective harness is not used. *Infant walkers* are responsible for a number of different types of injuries that occur because the walker tipped over or fell down stairs. Parents need to be warned of these dangers and encouraged to keep a constant vigil on their child's activities. The American Academy of Pediatrics (2001) does not recommend the use of mobile infant walkers. In response to the large number of accidents and deaths associated with mobile infant walkers, several manufacturers made modifications on these products to prevent falls down stairs. The new models should have a label or sign indicating "meets new safety standard," must be wider than 36 inches, or must have a braking mechanism to stop the walker. Mobile infant walkers may still pose a risk for climbing up to reach dangerous objects and should be carefully supervised. One alternative is to use a stationary play station with a seat similar to a walker. There is no evidence that use of infant walkers helps infants walk sooner.

Once infants are mobile, they should not be allowed to crawl unsupervised on any raised surface, near stairs, or near any water reservoir. Gates should be used at the *bottom* and *top of stairs,* because both present dangers to the crawling and climbing infant. However, certain types of gates can present hazards. Freestanding enclosures constructed of crisscrossed wood slats that expand and contract can trap the head or neck when children attempt to climb over them. If these types of gates are used, they must be securely fastened to prevent mobility of the slats.

As children begin to pull themselves to a standing position, *heavy objects,* such as unsturdy furniture or any freestanding item (e.g., wrought iron fish tank stands or televisions), can be extremely dangerous if pulled down on top of the child. To prevent such injury, televisions should be placed on lower furniture and as far back as possible, and angle braces or anchors can secure furniture to walls.

Even when the environment is made safe, infants may sometimes literally trip over their own feet from *clothing.* Slippery socks; hard, slick soles on shoes or rubber soles that can catch, especially on a carpet; and long pants or pajama bottoms can easily upset a child's balance. Such dangers need to be pointed out to parents, especially when infants are taking their first steps.

An alarming number of small children fall out of windows and are hurt; this is especially common with window ledges such as bay windows that have wide ledges for children to sit on. Window screens should not be perceived as fall-prevention devices; rather, window guards should be installed to prevent falls from any window, regardless of the height. Furniture should be kept away from windows so children cannot climb onto the furniture and access the window (Feury, 2003).

Poisoning

Poisoning is one of the major causes of death in children younger than 5 years of age. The highest incidence occurs in the 2-year-old group, with the second highest incidence occurring in 1-year-old children. Infants who do not crawl are relatively free from danger of poisonous agents by virtue of immobility. However, once locomotion begins, danger from poisoning is present almost everywhere. There are more than 500 toxic substances in the average home, and approximately one third of all poisonings occur in the kitchen.

The major reason for ingestion of poisons is *improper storage.* To protect the infant, toxic agents should not be placed on a low shelf, a low table, or the floor. Drugs that are kept in a purse pose additional dangers; if the handbag is given to infants to play with, they may open it and ingest the drug. Another unrecognized hazard occurs during diaper changes, when infants are near many toxic substances such as ointments, creams, oils, and talc. Parents may even hand infants a potentially poisonous object to quiet them. Such dangers need to be stressed to parents, and toys need to be kept at diapering areas to minimize risks.

Plants are another source of poisoning for infants. Plants are commonly placed on the floor, and the leaves or flowers are attractive and easy to pull off. More than 700 species of plants are known to have caused illness or death.

Another danger is ingestion of the *button-sized batteries* used in devices such as hearing aids, calculators, watches, and cameras. Because they are bright and shiny, they are attractive to children. However, they can cause severe morbidity, even death, if lodged in the esophagus. The strong alkali in a battery can leak and cause a severe caustic burn. As a precaution, small batteries must be safely stored and discarded where young children cannot easily retrieve them.

Not all poisonings result from ingestion—*inhalation* is another possible route, such as inhaling chlorine vapors from household cleaning or pool supplies. Passive cocaine toxicity has occurred in young children exposed to freebase cocaine ("crack") smoking by adults. Children should be protected from environments in which airborne toxins exist. (For a discussion of passive secondhand tobacco smoke, see Chapter 46.)

The production of methamphetamines, a common central nervous system stimulant also known as ice, speed, or crystal, involves the use of a number of chemicals that may be toxic alone (contact or ingestion) or during the production (cooking) of the drug itself. Methamphetamine labs are common in household areas where children may be exposed to harmful inhalants. Mobile methamphetamine labs are also common, and children may be similarly exposed to dangerous chemicals. Methamphetamine use and exposure has been shown to cause developmental problems and short- and long-term permanent brain damage, particularly in children. Reports of the number of children exposed daily to methamphetamine labs in the United States and Canada are alarming; such children are also at high risk for abuse and neglect because their caretakers are preoccupied with production, sale, and use of the drug (Mecham & Melini, 2002). Children should be protected from environments in which inhaled toxins exist.

The only sure way to prevent poisoning is to remove toxic agents; this means placing containers out of the infant's reach or contact. Because crawling infants soon become climbing toddlers, it is best to keep all toxic agents, especially drugs, in a locked cabinet. Special plastic hooks can be attached to the inside of cabinet doors to keep them securely closed (Fig. 36-12). Firm thumb pressure is required to unlatch the hook, and small children are usually unable to manipulate them. Locks are best, but for frequently used cleaning agents, such as those often kept under a kitchen sink, hooks are a practical alternative.

With several hundred toxic substances in each house, locking up all potentially toxic substances can present a problem; however, careful planning can help. A large surplus of cleaning agents, furniture polishes, laundry additives, paints, insecticides, and solvents should be avoided. Used poison containers should be promptly discarded and not used to store another poison without adequately marking the package. Potentially hazardous substances should not be stored in any type of food container. A popular container used to store toxic liquids is a soda, or pop, bottle. A child unaware of the dangerous contents is vulnerable to poisoning. Parents should know the location of local poison control centers and call one in the event of a suspected poisoning. Ipecac syrup, used to induce vomiting, is no longer a standard recommendation. Emergency measures for poisoning are discussed in Chapter 47.

Burns

Scalding from water that is too hot; excessive sunburn; and burns from house fires, electrical wires, sockets, and heating elements such as radiators, registers, and floor furnaces cause a significant number of deaths and many more injuries in infants. The infant's skin is particularly sensitive to irritation, and the mechanisms for temperature perception are not completely developed. As a general precaution, all homes should have smoke alarms installed near the bedroom areas and on each level of the building.

Scald burns from *hot tap water* can be prevented by lowering the water heater to a safe temperature of 49° C (120° F). In addition, the bathwater should be checked before the infant is immersed. The two most common types of scald injury are from the infant pulling a hot pan of water off a stove or elevated surface and the child overturning a container of hot water on her-himself (Drago, 2005). Scalds can also occur from bathing infants in the kitchen sink when the garbage disposal, occluded with debris, causes the draining dishwasher effluent to back up into the sink. The temperature of the effluent from a dishwasher is typically that of the maximum water temperature of the household water heater, but many dishwashers are equipped with heating elements that heat water to a temperature that is even higher. As a precaution, instruct caregivers to avoid bathing small children in the kitchen sink while the dishwasher is running.

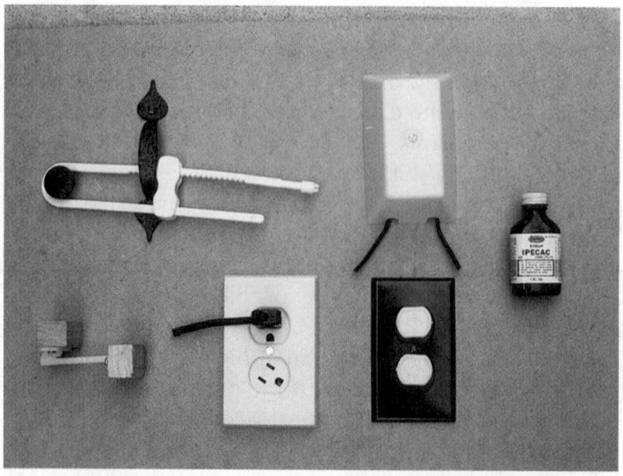

Fig. 36-12 Safety demonstration board. *Clockwise from lower left:* two types of cabinet latches; a shock guard for an electrical outlet in use; syrup of ipecac; and two types of outlet covers (the one with the white cover has passive devices that automatically cover the outlet when a plug is removed).

If formula or food is warmed in a *microwave oven,* it must be checked before feeding because the container may remain cool while the contents are hot. Another danger is explosion of the container from the buildup of steam. Because of these dangers, microwaving infant formula or food should be avoided or done using the guidelines in the Home Care box on p. 1049. The handles of cooking utensils should be turned toward the back of the stove. When the infant is underfoot, pouring hot liquids and cooking with hot oil are avoided. Hanging tablecloths are also placed out of the infant's reach to prevent pulling hot items off the table.

Sunburn can be a source of a first- or second-degree burn. Exposure to direct sunlight should be avoided for the first 6 months. When infants are in the sun, the body, especially the face and head, should be covered. Sunscreen can be used on older infants, but should be used on small areas of the body and only sparingly in infants under 6 months (American Academy of Pediatrics, 1999) (see Sunburn, Chapter 53). Although infants burn less readily, their thin skin can become sunburned and needs protection.

Electrical outlets should be covered with protective plastic caps that prevent the child from sucking on the outlet or putting objects such as hairpins into it (see Fig. 36-12). Live wires are placed out of reach so that curious infants cannot chew on them and break the rubber coating (Fig. 36-13). Infants should not be allowed to play near television sets, stereo units, or other appliances.

Any *heat-producing element* should have a guard placed in front of it. Fireplaces should be well screened because they are very appealing and within easy access. Small, portable heaters should be placed on a high surface. Floor furnaces should have barrier gates to prevent children from crawling or walking over them. Burning cigarettes, candles, and incense should be kept out of reach, and infants should not be held by a smoking adult because falling ashes are a hazard, especially to the eyes. Heated-mist vaporizers are a source of burns and should not be used. If humidity is needed, only cool-mist vaporizers are safe. Handheld curling irons are also a common source of hand burns in small children.

By law, all infant sleepwear must be flame retardant. Unfortunately, this does not apply to all *infant clothing.* Flame-retardant fabric must never be viewed as the ultimate protection against burns. Repeated washing reduces the flame-retardant properties, and the use of soap or bleach destroys the protection. If sleepwear is home sewn, parents are advised to look for specially treated, flame-retardant fabric.

Children can also be burned by overheated metal hardware and vinyl seats in cars parked in the sun. As a precaution, the surface heat of car restraints should be determined

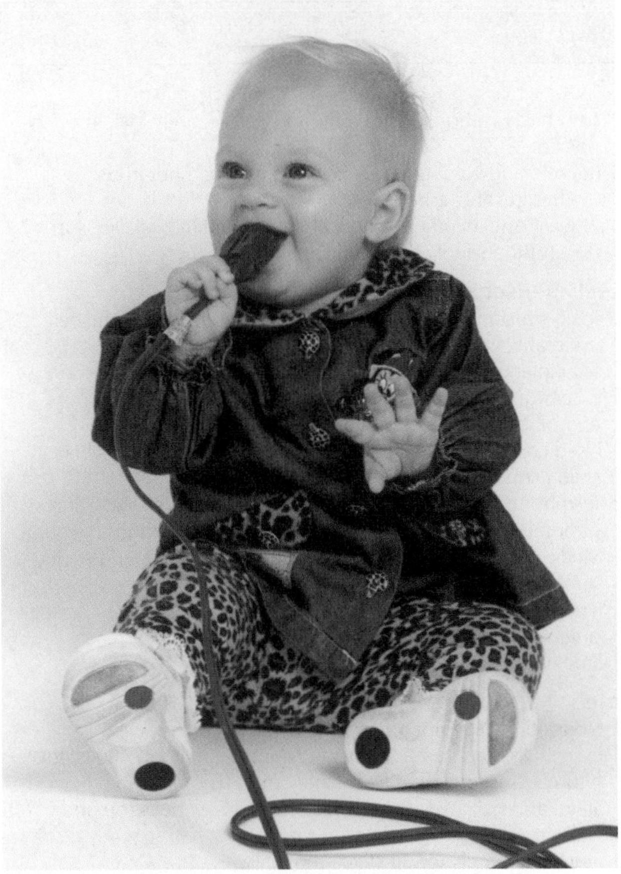

Fig. 36-13 Infants can find hazardous electrical wires. (Photo by Paul Vincent Kuntz, Texas Children's Hospital.)

before placing children in them. Covering the restraints and hardware (such as metal latches on seat belts) may be necessary to prevent skin burns. An additional safeguard is buying a light-colored restraint, which absorbs less heat.

Drowning

Drowning in this age group can occur in just an inch or two of water. Consequently, infants should always be supervised in a bathtub, in a hot tub, and near a source of water such as a swimming pool, lake, toilet, or bucket. A survey of drownings found that most infants younger than age 1 year drowned in a toilet, bathtub, or bucket (Lassman, 2002); 5-gallon buckets are particularly dangerous because the child may inadvertently fall in head first and, because of the weight of the upper body at this age, cannot withdraw from the bucket. Organized swimming instruction is not recommended for children younger than 4 years of age, because it may lead to a false sense of security (American Academy of Pediatrics, 2000a). No infant can be expected to learn the elements of water safety or to react appropriately in an emergency. Therefore all young children need to be considered at risk when near water. Infants and toddlers are also at increased risk of infection and seizures from swallowing large amounts of water.

Bodily Damage

Injuries can occur in numerous ways. Sharp, jagged-edged objects can cause wounds in the skin. Long, pointed articles, such as the common toothpick or fork, can be poked into the eye or ear, causing serious damage. Such articles should be safely stored away from the infant's reach; forks are best avoided for self-feeding until the child has mastered the spoon, usually by age 18 months.

In addition to hazards such as aspiration, small articles can be placed in the ear or nose, and excessive noise from toys can result in sensorineural hearing loss. Although toys with the highest noise levels are model airplanes, air guns, and toy cap guns, even common squeaking toys used by young children may be harmful if placed close to the ear.

Even clothes and hair can present dangers to infants who cannot call attention to the problem. For example, constriction injuries can occur from excessively tight bands on socks, as well as fibers of hair or thread wrapped tightly around appendages, usually toes or fingers.

A disturbing trend is the increasing amount of infant deaths attributed to homicide. In one study 6.4% of 10,370 infant injury deaths occurred as a result of homicide (Brenner et al, 1999). A high rate of battering injury has been reported in infants 0 to 5 months (Agran et al, 2003). Specific interventions must be set in place to protect infants from harm, especially in preventable situations.

evolve CASE STUDY: CHILD ABUSE

Another commonly unrecognized danger to infants is animal attacks. As newcomers to the home, helpless infants can provoke jealousy in animals, especially dogs and cats. Parents must be constantly vigilant to protect the child from household pets and farm animals (see Animal Bites, Chapter 53).

Nurse's Role in Injury Prevention

The task of injury prevention begins to be appreciated only when the potential environmental dangers to which infants are vulnerable are considered. Nurses must be aware of the possible causes of injury in each age group in order for anticipatory preventive teaching to occur. For example, the guidelines for injury prevention during infancy presented in Table 36-10 should be discussed before the child reaches the susceptible age group. Preventive teaching ideally occurs during pregnancy. Two thirds of all injuries to children occur in the home, and therefore the importance of safety cannot be overemphasized. The Home Care box summarizes a home safety checklist that can be presented to parents to increase their awareness of danger areas in the home and assist them in implementing safety devices and practices before their absence can inflict injury on infants. In addition, displays such as a safety demonstration board can be helpful in familiarizing parents with inexpensive commercial devices that can be used in the home to prevent injuries. To help parents appreciate the dangers present in their home to young children, suggest that they get eye level with the floor to survey the environment from a child's viewpoint.

Injury prevention requires protection of the child and education of the caregiver. Nurses in ambulatory care settings, health maintenance centers, or visiting nurse agencies are in a favorable position for injury education. This does not exclude nurses in inpatient facilities, who could use visiting times as an excellent opportunity for discussing this topic.

One approach to teaching injury prevention is to relate why children in various age groups are prone to specific types of injuries. Stressing prevention is just as important as emphasizing the why of the injury. However, injury preven-

Home Care

CHILD SAFETY HOME CHECKLIST

Safety: Fire, Electrical, Burns

- ☐ Guards in front of or around any heating appliance, fireplace, or furnace (including floor furnace)*
- ☐ Electrical wires hidden or out of reach*
- ☐ No frayed or broken wires; no overloaded sockets
- ☐ Plastic guards or caps over electrical outlets, furniture in front of outlets*
- ☐ Hanging tablecloths out of reach, away from open fires*
- ☐ Smoke detectors tested and operating properly
- ☐ Kitchen matches stored out of child's reach*
- ☐ Large, deep ashtrays throughout house (if used)
- ☐ Small stoves, heaters, and other hot objects (cigarettes, candles, coffee pots, slow cookers) placed where they cannot be tipped over or reached by children
- ☐ Hot water heater set at 49° C (120° F) or lower
- ☐ Pot handles turned toward back of stove, center of table
- ☐ No loose clothing worn near stove
- ☐ No cooking or eating hot foods or liquids with child standing nearby or sitting in lap
- ☐ All small appliances, such as iron, turned off, disconnected, and placed out of reach when not in use
- ☐ Cool, not hot, mist vaporizer used
- ☐ Fire extinguisher available on each floor and checked periodically
- ☐ Electrical fuse box and gas shutoff accessible
- ☐ Family escape plan in case of a fire practiced periodically; fire escape ladder available on upper-level floors
- ☐ Telephone number of fire or rescue squad and address of home with nearest cross street posted near phone

Safety: Suffocation and Aspiration

- ☐ Small objects stored out of reach*
- ☐ Toys inspected for small removeable parts or long strings*
- ☐ Hanging crib toys and mobiles placed out of reach
- ☐ Plastic bags stored away from young child's reach, large plastic garment bags discarded after tying in knots*
- ☐ Mattress or pillow not covered with plastic or in manner accessible to child*
- ☐ Crib design according to federal regulations (crib slats less than 2⅜ inches [6 cm] apart) with snug-fitting mattress*†
- ☐ Crib positioned away from other furniture or windows*
- ☐ Portable playpen gates up at all times while in use*
- ☐ Accordion-style gates not used*
- ☐ Bathroom doors kept closed and toilet seats down*
- ☐ Faucets turned off firmly*
- ☐ Pool fenced with locked gate
- ☐ Proper safety equipment at poolside
- ☐ Electric garage door openers stored safely and garage door adjusted to rise when door strikes object
- ☐ Doors of ovens, trunks, dishwashers, refrigerators, and front-loading clothes washers and dryers kept closed*
- ☐ Unused appliance, such as a refrigerator, securely closed with lock or doors removed*
- ☐ Food served in small, noncylindric pieces*
- ☐ Toy chests without lids or with lids that securely lock in open position*
- ☐ Buckets and wading pools kept empty when not in use*
- ☐ Clothesline above head level
- ☐ At least one member of household trained in basic life support (CPR) including first aid for choking

Safety: Poisoning

- ☐ Toxic substances, including batteries, placed on a high shelf, preferably in locked cabinet
- ☐ Toxic plants hung or placed out of reach*
- ☐ Excess quantities of cleaning fluids, paints, pesticides, drugs, and other toxic substances not stored in home
- ☐ Used containers of poisonous substances discarded where child cannot obtain access
- ☐ Telephone number of local poison control center and address of home with nearest cross street posted near phone
- ☐ Medicines clearly labeled in childproof containers and stored out of reach
- ☐ Household cleaners, disinfectants, and insecticides kept in their original containers, separate from food and out of reach
- ☐ Smoking in areas away from children

Safety: Falls

- ☐ Nonskid mats, strips, or surfaces in tubs and showers
- ☐ Exits, halls, and passageways in rooms kept clear of toys, furniture, boxes, or other items that could be obstructive
- ☐ Stairs and halls well lighted, with switches at both top and bottom
- ☐ Sturdy handrails for all steps and stairways
- ☐ Nothing stored on stairways
- ☐ Treads, risers, and carpeting in good repair
- ☐ Glass doors and walls marked with decals
- ☐ Safety glass used in doors, windows, and walls
- ☐ Gates on top and bottom of staircases and elevated areas, such as porch, fire escape*
- ☐ Guardrails on upstairs windows with locks that limit height of window opening and access to areas such as fire escape*
- ☐ Crib side rails raised to full height; mattress lowered as child grows*
- ☐ Restraints used in high chairs or other baby furniture; preferably walkers with wheels not used*
- ☐ Scatter rugs secured in place or used with nonskid backing
- ☐ Walks, patios, and driveways in good repair

Safety: Bodily Injury

- ☐ Knives, power tools, and unloaded firearms stored safely or placed in locked cabinet
- ☐ Garden tools returned to storage racks after use
- ☐ Pets properly restrained and immunized for rabies
- ☐ Swings, slides, and other outdoor play equipment kept in safe condition
- ☐ Yard free of broken glass, nail-studded boards, other litter
- ☐ Cement birdbaths placed where young child cannot tip them over*

*Safety measures are specific for homes with young children. All safety measures should be implemented in homes where children reside and visit frequently, such as those of grandparents or baby-sitters.
†Federal regulations are available from U.S. Consumer Product Safety Commission; phone: 1-800-638-CPSC; Web site: www.cpsc.gov.

tion must also be practical. Asking parents for their ideas leads to realistic suggestions that can be followed. For instance, bathroom cleaning agents, cosmetics, and personal care items can be placed on a top shelf in the linen closet, and towels or sheets can be stored on the lower shelves and floor.

If an injury has occurred, the nurse should not be too quick to admonish the parent; injuries do not always indicate neglect. It is a difficult task to watch children carefully without overprotecting or unnecessarily confining them. Allowing children to explore while maintaining consistent, age-appropriate limits is sound advice.

Parents need to remember that infants and young children cannot anticipate danger or understand when it is or is not present. A dead electrical wire may present no actual harm; but if the child is allowed to play with it, a poor behavior is enforced and will be practiced when the child encounters a live wire. Although it is always wise to explain why something is dangerous, it must be remembered that small children need to be physically removed from the situation.

It is not easy to teach safety, supervise closely, and refrain from saying "no" a hundred times a day. Parents become acutely aware of this dilemma as soon as the infant learns to crawl. Preventing injuries to children is usually the first reason for limit setting and discipline, but limits are also set to prevent danger to valuable household objects. When small children are in the home, dangerous objects must be removed or guarded and valuable articles placed out of reach.

When children are taught the meaning of "no," they should also be taught what "yes" means. Children should be praised for playing with suitable toys, their efforts at behaving or listening should be reinforced, and innovative and creative recreational toys should be provided for them. Infants love to tear paper and avidly pursue books, magazines, or newspapers left on the floor. Instead of always scolding them for destroying a valued book, child-safe books (such as those constructed of fabric) can be kept available for them to play with. If they enjoy pots and pans, a cabinet can be arranged with safe utensils for them to explore.

One additional factor must be stressed concerning injury prevention and education. Children are imitators; they copy what they see and hear. *Practicing safety teaches safety.* This applies to parents and their children and to nurses and their patients. Saying one thing but doing another confuses children and can lead to difficulties as the child grows older.

Home Care

GUIDANCE DURING INFANT'S FIRST YEAR

First 6 Months

- Teach car safety with use of federally approved restraint, facing rearward, in the middle of the back seat—not in a front seat with an air bag.
- Understand each parent's adjustment to newborn, especially mother's postpartal emotional needs.
- Teach care of infant and help parents to understand his or her individual needs and temperament and that the infant expresses wants through crying.
- Reassure parents that infant cannot be spoiled by too much attention during the first 4 to 6 months.
- Encourage parents to establish a schedule that meets needs of child and themselves.
- Help parents understand infant's need for stimulation in environment.
- Support parents' pleasure in seeing child's growing friendliness and social response, especially smiling.
- Plan anticipatory guidance for safety.
- Stress need for immunizations.
- Prepare for introduction of solid foods.

Second 6 Months

- Prepare parents for child's "stranger anxiety."
- Encourage parents to allow child to cling to them and avoid long separation from either.
- Guide parents concerning discipline because of infant's increasing mobility.
- Encourage use of negative voice and eye contact rather than physical punishment as a means of discipline.
- Encourage showing most attention when infant is behaving well, rather than when infant is crying.
- Teach injury prevention because of child's advancing motor skills and curiosity.
- Encourage parents to leave child with suitable caregiver to allow some free time.
- Discuss readiness for weaning.
- Explore parents' feelings regarding infant's sleep patterns.

Anticipatory Guidance—Care of Families

Childrearing is no easy task; it presents challenges to both new and "seasoned" parents. With society's changing roles and mores, combined with a highly mobile population, there is little stability for additional role models and time-honored methods of raising children. As a result, parents look to professionals for guidance. Nurses are in an advantageous position to render assistance and offer suggestions. Every phase of a child's life has its particular traumas—toilet training for toddlers, unexplained fears for preschoolers, and identity crises for adolescents. For parents of an infant, some challenges center around dependency, discipline, increased mobility, and safety. Major areas for parental guidance during the first year are listed in the Home Care box.

Special Health Problems

FEEDING DIFFICULTIES

Regurgitation and "Spitting Up"

The return of small amounts of food after a feeding is a common occurrence during infancy. It should not be confused with actual vomiting, which can be associated with a number of disturbances that may be insignificant or serious. It is usually benign, although persistent regurgitation necessitates medical evaluation to rule out gastroesophageal reflux. For clarification the following terms are defined:

Regurgitation—Return of undigested food from the stomach, usually accompanied by burping

Spitting up—Dribbling of unswallowed formula from the infant's mouth immediately after a feeding

The normal occurrence of regurgitation or spitting up should be explained to parents, especially to those who are unduly concerned about it. Regurgitation can be reduced by some simple measures, such as frequent burping during and after feeding, minimum handling during and after feeding, and positioning the child on the right side with the head slightly elevated after feeding. The inconvenience of spitting up can be managed with the use of absorbent bibs on the infant and protective cloths on the parent.

Sometimes frequent dribbling of formula causes excoriation of the corners of the mouth, the chin, and the neck.

Keeping the area dry promotes healing but can be difficult to maintain. Helpful suggestions include applying a thin film of a moisture barrier cream such as A and D emollient ointment to the affected areas after cleansing and using absorbent, nonplastic-lined terry cloth bibs, which are changed often.

Paroxysmal Abdominal Pain (Colic)

Colic is reported to occur in 5% to 30% of all infants (Neu & Robinson, 2003) yet has no particular affinity with regard to the gender, race, or socioeconomic status of the infant and family (Ellett, 2003). The condition is generally described as paroxysmal abdominal pain or cramping that is manifested by loud crying and drawing the legs up to the abdomen. Other definitions include variables such as duration of cry greater than 3 hours a day, occurring more than 3 days per week, and parental dissatisfaction with the child's behavior. Some studies report an increase in symptoms (fussiness and crying) in the late afternoon or evening; however, in some infants the onset of symptoms occurs at another time. Colic is more common in infants under 3 months of age than in older infants, and infants with the so-called "difficult" temperaments are more likely to be colicky. Despite the obvious behavioral indications of pain, the child tolerates breast milk or some type of infant formula well, gains weight, and usually thrives. There is no evidence of a residual effect of colic on older children, except perhaps a strained parent-child relationship in some cases; in other words, infants who are colicky grow up to be normal children and adults.

Among the theories that have been investigated as potential causes are too rapid feeding, overeating, swallowing excessive air, improper feeding technique (especially in positioning and burping), and emotional stress or tension between parent and child. Although all of these may occur, there is no evidence that one factor is consistently present. In some infants colic may be a sign of cow's milk allergy or intolerance, and eliminating cow's milk products from the infant's diet and the diet of lactating mothers can reduce the symptoms. Parental smoking, strained parent-infant interaction, lactase deficiency, difficult infant temperament, difficulty regulating emotions, central nervous system immaturity, and neurochemical dysregulation in the brain have also been proposed as potential causes of colic (Ellett, 2003; Friedman, 1996; Neu & Robinson, 2003). A positive association between consumption of fruit juices (carbohydrate malabsorption) and colic has been demonstrated in some cases (Duro et al, 2002). The final consensus of most experts who study colic is that it is multifactorial in nature and that no single treatment for every colicky infant will be effective in alleviating the symptoms.

Therapeutic Management

Management of colic should begin with an investigation of possible organic causes, such as cow's milk protein allergy. If a sensitivity to cow's milk is strongly suspected, a trial substitution of another formula such as a casein hydrolysate (Nutramigen, Alimentum, Pregestimil), whey hydrolysate, or amino acid (Neocate; EleCare) is warranted. Soy formulas are avoided because of the possibility of sensitivity to soy protein as well.

The use of drugs, including sedatives, antispasmodics, antihistamines, and antiflatulents, is sometimes recommended. The most commonly used sedatives are phenobarbitol, hydroxyzine hydrochloride (Atarax), and chloral hydrate. Simethicone (Mylicon) may also help allay the symptoms of colic. However, in most controlled studies none of these drugs completely reduces the symptoms of colic. Herbal (chamomile) tea offered at the onset of crying and up to three times daily has been proved to be effective in relieving the symptoms of colic (Weizman et al, 1993). The addition of lactase to infant formula has produced mixed results as far as abatement of overall symptoms.

Nursing Considerations

The initial step in managing colic is to take a thorough, detailed history of the usual daily events. Areas that should be stressed include the following: (1) the infant's diet; (2) the diet of the breastfeeding mother; (3) the time of day when crying occurs; (4) the relationship of the crying to feeding time; (5) the presence of specific family members during the crying and habits of family members, such as smoking; (6) activity of the mother or usual caregiver before, during, and after the crying; (7) characteristics of the cry (e.g., duration, intensity); (8) measures used to relieve the crying and their effectiveness; and (9) the infant's stooling, voiding, and sleeping patterns. Of special emphasis is a careful assessment of the feeding process via demonstration by the parent.

If milk sensitivity is suspected, breastfeeding mothers should follow a milk-free diet for a minimum of 3 to 5 days in an attempt to reduce symptoms in the infant. Mothers need to be cautioned that some nondairy creamers may contain calcium caseinate, a cow's milk protein. If a milk-free diet is helpful, lactating mothers may need calcium supplements to meet the body's requirement. Bottle-fed infants may improve with the same dietary modifications as for the child with cow's milk allergy.

One important and appropriate nursing intervention (before and after organic cause has been eliminated) is reassurance of both parents that they are not doing anything wrong and that the infant is not experiencing any physical or emotional harm. Parents, especially mothers, become easily frustrated with the infant's crying and perceive this as a sign that there is something horribly wrong. An empathetic, gentle, and reassuring attitude, in addition to suggestions about remedies for treatment, will help allay parents' anxieties, which are usually exacerbated by loss of sleep and preoccupation over the infant's welfare. Other support persons and extended family members may be enlisted to help support the parents during this time of difficulty.

When no cause can be identified, helping parents understand the infant's crying behavior and modifying parent interventions to promptly attend to the infant's needs can decrease the length of fussiness and crying (Dihigo, 1998). Other approaches for relieving colic are listed in the Home Care box. Parents are encouraged to try as many of these approaches as possible, because not all are effective for every infant. Research is in progress on an Infant Colic Scale, which will assist in narrowing the cause of infant colic (Ellett, 2003). Meanwhile, the researcher suggests that a problem-solving discussion with the parents, in addition to acknowledgment that the infant has colic, is an optimal strategy for helping parents manage the infant with colic until a cure is found (Ellett, 2003).

Failure to Thrive

Failure to thrive (FTT) is a sign of inadequate growth resulting from inability to obtain or use calories required for growth. FTT has no universal definition, although one of the more common parameters is a weight (and sometimes height) that falls below the 5th percentile for the child's age. Growth measurements alone are not used to diagnose children with FTT; rather, the finding of a persistent deviation from an established growth curve is cause for concern.

Three general categories of failure to thrive are the following:

1. *Organic failure to thrive (OFTT)*—Result of a physical cause, such as congenital heart defects, neurologic lesions, microencephaly, chronic renal failure, gastroesophageal reflux, malabsorption syndrome, endocrine dysfunction, cystic fibrosis, or acquired immunodeficiency syndrome (AIDS).

Home Care

MANAGING THE COLICKY INFANT

Place infant prone over a covered hot-water bottle, heated towel, or covered heating pad.
Massage infant's abdomen.
Respond immediately to the crying.
Change infant's position frequently; walk with child's face down and with body across parent's arm, with parent's hand under infant's abdomen, applying gentle pressure (Fig. 36-14).
Use a front carrier for transporting infant.
Swaddle infant tightly with a soft, stretchy blanket.
Place infant in a wind-up swing.
Take infant for car rides or outside for a change in environment.
Use bottles that minimize air swallowing (curved bottle or inner collapsible bag).
Use a commercial device* in the crib that stimulates the vibration and sound of a car ride or plays soothing "noise," in utero sounds, or music.†
Provide smaller, frequent feedings; burp infant during and after feedings using the shoulder position or sitting upright, and place infant in an upright seat after feedings.
Introduce a pacifier for added sucking.
In breastfed infants, mother should avoid all milk products for a trial period.
If household members smoke, avoid smoking near infant; preferably confine smoking activity to outside of home.
Give appropriate dose of acetaminophen elixir or suppository if suggested by health professional; not recommended for daily use.
If nothing reduces the crying, place infant in crib and allow to cry; periodically hold and comfort child and put down again.

*Sweet Dreems, Inc., Sleep Tight Order Department, 4710 E. Walnut St., Westerville, OH 43081; phone: 1-800-NO COLIC, 1-800-662-6542.
†Suggested infant relaxation music: *Heartbeat Lullabies*, by Terry Woodford. Available from Baby-Go-To-Sleep Center, Audio Therapy Innovations, Inc., PO Box 550, Colorado Springs, CO 80901; phone: 1-800-537-7748; Web site: www.babygotosleep.com.

2. *Nonorganic failure to thrive (NFTT)*—Has a definable cause that is unrelated to disease. NFTT is most often the result of psychosocial factors, such as inadequate nutritional information by the parent; deficiency in maternal care or a disturbance in maternal-child attachment; or a disturbance in the child's ability to separate from the parent, leading to food refusal to maintain attention.
3. *Idiopathic failure to thrive*—Unexplained by the usual organic and environmental etiologies but may also be classified as NFTT. Both categories of NFTT account for the majority of cases of FTT.

Traditionally the category of NFTT has implied a disturbance in the parent-child interaction; however, this is not always the case. Many other factors can lead to inadequate feeding of the infant, such as the following:

Poverty—Lack of finds to buy sufficient food; may dilute formula to extend available supply
Health or childrearing beliefs—Use of fad diets; excessive concern with preventing conditions (e.g., obesity, hypercholesterolemia, or nursing caries); strict use of scheduled feedings
Inadequate nutritional knowledge—Confusion of newly arrived immigrants who are unaware of appropriate food selections in American markets; parents with cognitive impairment
Family stress—Involvement with another chronically ill child; any number of other stresses (e.g., financial, marital, excessive parenting and employment responsibilities, depression, chemical abuse, acute grief)

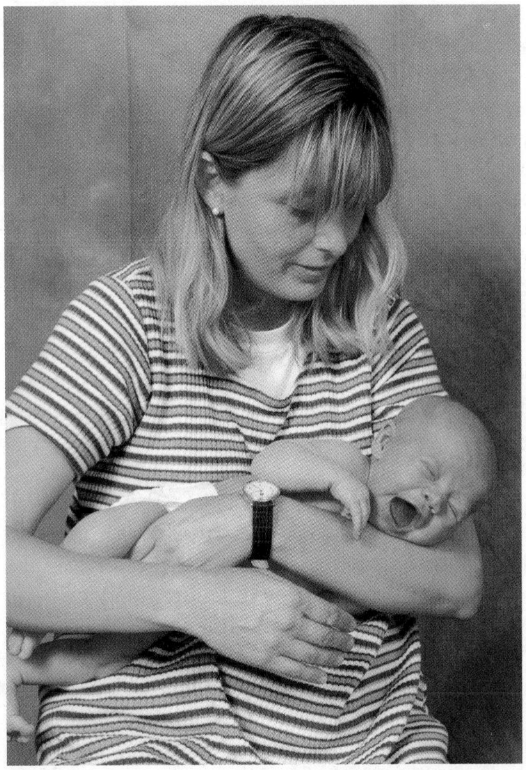

Fig. 36-14 The "colic carry" may be comforting to an infant with colic. (Photo by Paul Vincent Kuntz, Texas Children's Hospital.)

Feeding resistance—Result of nonoral nutritional therapy early in life

Insufficient breast milk—Result of a number of different causes (e.g., fatigue, illness, poor release of milk, insufficient glandular tissue, lack of maternal confidence)

In these instances parent education and provision of necessary supports (e.g., financial or psychosocial) are successful in correcting the reason for the malnutrition. It has also been suggested that growth failure in childhood may be a combination of both NFTT (possibly disturbed parent-infant interaction or nonnurturing environment) and OFTT (child's difficult disposition) and that malnutrition itself often makes the child's behavior less interactive, thus further contributing to the ongoing paradigm of growth failure (Careaga & Kerner, 2000).

Dealing with families in which a child has NFTT because of a parent-child disturbance is much more difficult and is the focus of the nursing care discussion.

Diagnostic Evaluation

Diagnosis is initially made from evidence of growth retardation. If FTT is recent, the weight, but not the height, is below accepted standards (usually the 5th percentile); if FTT is long-standing, both weight and height are depressed, indicating chronic malnutrition. Additional diagnostic procedures include a complete health and dietary history, physical examination for evidence of organic causes, developmental assessment, and family assessment. Other tests are selected only as indicated to rule out organic problems. To prevent the overuse of diagnostic procedures, NFTT should be considered early in the differential diagnosis. To avoid the social stigma of NFTT during the early investigative phase, many health care workers use the term *growth delay* (or *growth failure*) until the actual cause is established.

Therapeutic Management

Regardless of the cause of FTT, the treatment is directed at reversing the malnutrition. The goal is to provide sufficient calories to support "catch-up" growth—a rate of growth greater than the expected rate for age. Any coexisting medical problems are treated.

In most cases of NFTT a multidisciplinary team consisting of a physician, nurse, dietitian, child-life specialist, and social worker or mental health professional is needed to deal with the multiple psychologic problems. Efforts are made to relieve any additional stresses on the family, such as referrals to welfare agencies or supplemental food programs.

Prognosis

The prognosis for NFTT is related to the cause. If the parents have simply been ignorant of the infant's needs, teaching may remedy the child's limited caloric intake and permanently reverse the growth failure. Inadequate or decreased feeding periods by the infant's primary caretaker are often observed to be the cause of NFTT in conjunction with family disorganization. When the family dysfunction is extensive, the prognosis is uncertain. Factors related to poor prognosis are severe feeding resistance, lack of awareness in and cooperation from the parent(s), low family income, low maternal educational level, and early age of onset of NFTT.

Nursing Care Management

Assessment

Nurses play a critical role in the diagnosis of NFTT through their assessment of the child, parents, and family interaction. Knowledge of the characteristics of children with NFTT and their families is essential in helping identify these children and hastening the confirmation of a correct diagnosis (Box 36-1). Accurate assessment of initial weight and height and daily weight, as well as recording of all food intake, is mandatory. The feeding behavior of the child is documented, as well as the parent-child interaction during feeding, other caregiving activities, and play.

An excellent feeding observation instrument is the Nursing Child Assessment Satellite Training (NCAST) Feeding Scale, which is designed to assess the feeding interaction of infants up to 12 months of age (Barnard et al, 1993).*

A 25-item observational scale, the *Feeding Checklist,* was developed specifically for the purpose of observing mother-infant dyads with NFTT. The checklist has helped nurses and other health care professionals in the objective assessment of key aspects of infant and toddler feeding situations related to NFTT (MacPhee & Schneider, 1996).

A feature of many children with NFTT is their irregularity (low rhythmicity) in activities of daily living. Some of these children typify the "difficult" temperament pattern. However, another type is the passive, sleepy, lethargic infant who does not wake up for feedings. Parents who have been advised of "demand feeding schedules" may be unsure of whether to wake the child or let the child sleep. Because of their inexperience and lack of guidance, parents may develop a pattern of infrequent feeding that is inadequate to meet the infant's nutritional needs. Such a pattern is particularly detrimental with the breastfeeding infant, in whom frequent nursing is essential to an adequate milk supply.

*Training is required to use the NCAST Feeding Scale; information on the training program is available from Jean F. Kelly, PhD, Director, NCAST, WJ-10, University of Washington, Seattle, WA 98195; phone: 206-543-8528; www.ncast.org; e-mail: ncast@u.washington.edu.

BOX 36-1

Clinical Manifestations of Nonorganic Failure to Thrive

Growth failure–below 5th percentile in weight only or weight and height
Developmental retardation–social, motor, adaptive, language
Apathy
Poor hygiene
Withdrawn behavior
Feeding or eating disorders, such as vomiting, anorexia, pica, rumination
No fear of strangers (at age when stranger anxiety is normal)
Avoidance of eye contact
Wide-eyed gaze and continual scan of the environment ("radar gaze")
Stiff and unyielding or flaccid and unresponsive
Minimal smiling

Some parents are at increased risk for attachment problems because of (1) isolation and social crisis; (2) inadequate support systems, such as teenage and single mothers; and (3) poor parenting role models as a child. Other factors that should be considered are lack of education; physical and mental health problems, such as physical and sexual abuse, depression, or drug dependence; immaturity, especially in adolescent parents; and lack of commitment to parenting, such as giving priority to other ventures such as entertainment or employment. Often these parents and their families are under stress and in multiple chronic emotional, social, and financial crises.

Nursing Diagnoses

A number of nursing diagnoses are prominent in the nursing care of the child with NFTT. The most common nursing diagnoses are as follows:

- *Altered nutrition: less than body requirements related to*
  —deprivation of necessities
  —emotional deprivation
- *Altered growth and development related to*
  —socially restricted environment (infant deprivation)
  —physical neglect
- *Altered parenting related to*
  —specify (e.g., knowledge deficit, poverty)

If an organic cause is found, additional nursing diagnoses may be related to care specific for that disorder, such as heart disease.

Plan of Care and Implementation

It is now more common for children with NFTT to be treated on an outpatient basis unless socioeconomic factors place the infant at risk in the home setting. The infant may be hospitalized until a diagnosis is established and then sent home for further care on an outpatient basis. The highest-priority nursing goal is providing the infant with sufficient nutrients for growth. More specific nursing care depends on the identified cause of FTT. If an organic cause is confirmed, care is related primarily to management of the disorder. If the problem is one of inadequate knowledge regarding child feeding, parental education is required. When serious psychosocial factors are involved, hospitalization is needed and additional interventions are required to meet the needs of both the child and the family. The following are goals for the hospitalized child with NFTT and the child's family:

1. The child will experience weight gain.
2. The child will demonstrate positive response to developmental stimulation.
3. The family will demonstrate ability to provide appropriate care to the child.
4. The family will receive adequate support and home services.

Because part of the difficulty between parent and child is dissatisfaction and frustration, the child should have a primary core of nurses (Fig. 36-15). The nurses caring for the child can learn to perceive the child's cues and reverse the cycle of dissatisfaction, especially in the area of feeding. Depending on the cause of NFTT, children may be treated on an outpatient basis.

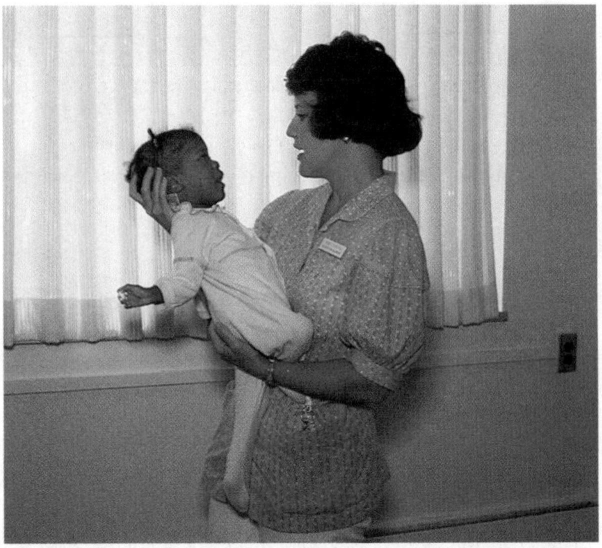

Fig. 36-15 Consistent nursing contact is important in developing trust in infants with nonorganic failure to thrive.

Because many of these children are responding to stimuli that have led to the negative feeding patterns, the first goal is to structure the feeding environment to encourage eating. General guidelines for the feeding process are outlined in the Guidelines box.

Four primary goals in the nutritional management of growth failure (FTT) are to (1) correct nutritional deficiencies and achieve ideal weight for height; (2) allow for catch-up growth; (3) restore optimum body composition; and (4) educate the parents or primary caregivers regarding the child's nutritional requirements and appropriate feeding methods (Maggioni & Lifshitz, 1995). To increase caloric intake in formula-fed infants, supplements such as Polycose or medium-chain triglycerides (MCTs) may be added slowly (Corrales & Utter, 1999). Other carbohydrate additives may include rice cereal and vegetable oil. Breastfed infants with NFTT may require caloric supplementation, which may be accomplished by adding 1 teaspoon of 24 kcal/oz formula to 3 ounces of breast milk. The consumption of fruit juices is not recommended in infants under 6 months. Because vitamin and mineral deficiencies may occur, multivitamin supplementation, including zinc and iron, is recommended. Usually only in extreme cases of malnourishment are tube feedings or intravenous therapy required.

Besides attending to the physical needs of the child, the interdisciplinary team must plan care for appropriate developmental stimulation. Once an approximate developmental age is established, a planned program of play is begun. Ideally a child-life specialist is involved to implement and supervise the stimulation program. Every effort is made to teach the parent how to play and interact with the child.

Nursing care of these children involves a "family systems" approach. In other words, for the entire family to become healthy, each member must be helped to change. Care of the parents is aimed at helping them increase their feelings of self-esteem through positive, successful parenting skills. Initially this necessitates providing an environment in which they feel welcomed and accepted. Because these parents are often distrustful of authority figures, it may take some time

Guidelines

FEEDING CHILDREN WITH NONORGANIC FAILURE TO THRIVE

Provide a primary core of staff to feed the child. The same nurses are able to learn the child's cues and respond consistently.

Provide a quiet, unstimulating atmosphere. A number of these children are very distractable, and their attention is diverted with minimal stimuli. Older children do well at a feeding table; younger children should always be held.

Maintain a calm, even temperament throughout the meal. Negative outbursts may be commonplace in this child's habit formation. Limits on eating behavior definitely need to be provided, but they should be stated in a firm, calm tone. If the nurse is hurried or anxious, the feeding process will not be optimized.

Talk to the child by giving directions about eating. "Take a bite, Lisa" is appropriate and directive. The more distractible the child, the more directive the nurse should be to refocus attention on feeding. Positive comments about feeding are actively given.

Be persistent. This is perhaps one of the most important guidelines. Parents often give up when the child begins negative feeding behavior. Calm perseverance through 10 to 15 minutes of food refusal will eventually diminish negative behavior. Although forced feeding is avoided, "strictly encouraged" feeding is essential.

Maintain a face-to-face posture with the child when possible. Encourage eye contact and remain with the child throughout the meal.

Introduce new foods slowly. Often these children have been exclusively bottle-fed. If acceptance of solids is a problem, begin with pureed food and, once accepted, advance to junior and regular solid foods.

Follow the child's rhythm of feeding. The child will set a rhythm when the previous conditions are met.

Develop a structured routine. Disruptions in their other activities of daily living have great impact on feeding responses, so bathing, sleeping, dressing, and playing, as well as feeding, are structured. The nurse should feed the child in the same way and place as often as possible. The length of the feeding should also be established (usually 30 minutes).

before they develop any trust toward the nurse. One approach is to empathize with the parent about the difficulties of childrearing. For example, the nurse may state that many parents find adjusting to parenthood a trying time or that the demands of caring for an infant can become overwhelming.

Teaching infant care techniques to the parents is begun through *example* and *demonstration,* not by lecturing.

As the nurse perceives the infant's cues, these are emphasized to the parents. For example, during a feeding the nurse might comment that the infant is still hungry because the child sucks vigorously and looks at the nurse. When the infant is satisfied, the nurse points out that the infant is signaling this by releasing the strong suck, closing the eyes, and breathing deeply and more slowly. By example, the child is placed in the crib for a nap.

Plans are made to implement these interventions at home. A home health referral is made, and if a foster grandparent was included, this person should also visit the family. Social agencies that can provide financial or housing assistance to lessen the stress of everyday life are also contacted.

Evaluation

The effectiveness of nursing interventions is determined by continual reassessment and evaluation of care, based on the following observational guidelines and expected outcomes:

1. Record weight and caloric intake daily; document child's reaction to feeding environment; review notes to see whether changes were made as necessary to improve eating and whether consistent group of nurses fed the child.
2. Perform developmental screening tests as needed.
3. Document parents' relationship with the child, staff, and other supportive individuals. Note length of time parents visit, appointments kept with referral services, and any requests for help.
4. Keep a record of all patient teaching and note whether outcome behaviors were met.

Expected outcomes include the following:

1. Child gains weight (specify; usually a minimum of 1 to 2 oz/day).
2. Child displays a positive response to interventions (e.g., social smile).
3. Family demonstrates ability to provide appropriate care to child.
4. Family experiences reduction of anxiety and follows through on programs and activities.

DISORDERS OF UNKNOWN ETIOLOGY

Sudden Infant Death Syndrome

Sudden infant death syndrome (SIDS) is defined as the sudden death of an infant under 1 year of age that remains unexplained after a complete postmortem examination, including an investigation of the death scene and a review of the case history. In the United States the mortality rate from SIDS has declined more than 40% since 1992; there were 1.3 deaths per 1000 live births in 1991 versus 0.65 deaths per 1000 live births in 1999 (American Academy of Pediatrics, 2000b; CDC, 2001). The dramatic decrease is attributed to the "Back to Sleep" campaign* (see following section). SIDS is the third leading cause of death in children between 1 month and 1 year of age and claimed the lives of almost 2295 infants in 2002 (Anderson & Smith, 2005). Table 36-11 summarizes the major epidemiologic characteristics of SIDS.

Etiology

Numerous theories have been proposed regarding the etiology of SIDS; however, the cause remains unknown. The most compelling hypothesis is that SIDS is related to a brainstem abnormality in the neurologic regulation of cardiorespiratory control. Abnormalities include prolonged sleep apnea, increased frequency of brief inspiratory pauses, excessive periodic breathing, and impaired arousal respon-

*"Back to Sleep" materials may be ordered by calling 800-505-CRIB; faxing requests to 301-496-7101; or writing to NICHD/Back to Sleep, 31 Center Drive, Room 2A32, Bethesda, MD 20892-2425; Web site: www.nichd.nih.gov/publications/pubskey.cfm?from=sids.

Table 36-11

Epidemiology of SIDS

FACTORS	OCCURRENCE
Incidence	0.55:1000 live births (2001)
Peak age	2 to 4 months; 95% occur by 6 months
Sex	Higher percentage of males affected
Time of death	During sleep
Time of year	Increased incidence in winter
Racial	Greater incidence in Native Americans, African-Americans, and Hispanics
Socioeconomic	Increased occurrence in lower socioeconomic class
Birth	Higher incidence in the following: Premature infants, especially infants of low birth weight; Multiple births*; Neonates with low Apgar scores; Infants with central nervous system disturbances and respiratory disorders such as bronchopulmonary dysplasia (chronic lung disease); Increasing birth order (subsequent siblings as opposed to firstborn child); Infants with a recent history of illness
Sleep habits	Prone position; use of soft bedding; overheating (thermal stress); co-sleeping with adult, especially on sofa
Feeding habits	Lower incidence in breastfed infants
Siblings	May have greater incidence
Maternal	Young age; cigarette smoking, especially during pregnancy; poor prenatal care; substance abuse (heroin, methadone, cocaine)

*Although a rare event, simultaneous death of twins from SIDS can occur.

siveness to increased carbon dioxide or decreased oxygen. However, sleep apnea is not the cause of SIDS. The vast majority of infants with apnea do not die, and only a minority of SIDS victims have documented *apparent life-threatening events (ALTEs)* (see Apnea of Infancy, p. 1084). Numerous studies indicate that there is no association between SIDS and diphtheria, tetanus, and pertussis vaccines.

Maternal smoking, both prenatally and postnatally, has been proposed as a possible cause of SIDS, as has poor prenatal care and low maternal age (Leach et al, 1999). Increased nicotine concentrations were found in infants who died of SIDS compared with a group of controls, regardless of whether smoking was reported (McMartin et al, 2002). Co-sleeping, or bed sharing, has been reported to have an association with the incidence of SIDS, especially in cases of maternal smoking (McGarvey et al, 2003). The American Academy of Pediatrics (2000b) recommends that adults follow the same safeguards in the bed as in the crib. In addition, the bed sharer (which should only be parents) should not smoke or use substances such as alcohol or drugs that may impair arousal. Unlike cribs, which are designed to meet safety standards for infants, adult beds or sofas are not so designed and may carry a risk of accidental entrapment and suffocation. One survey found a high association between infant deaths, nonstandard beds, and bed sharing; a large percentage of infants were found dead on their backs when bedsharing was in effect, suggesting suffocation by an adult (overlaying) (Unger et al, 2003).

Suffocation hazards included wedging between a mattress or bed and wall and oronasal obstruction by a plastic bag (Drago & Dannenberg, 1999). The prone sleeping position was found to be higher among African-American infants dying of SIDS in Chicago than Caucasians (Hauck et al, 2003). Another survey revealed that non–college educated, lower-income families and Hispanics were less likely to place the infant to sleep on the back at age 3 months (Corwin et al, 2003). Another postulated cause of SIDS is prolonged Q-T interval; however, at this time there is no strong evidence to support this as a cause. Overheating has been proposed as a potential cause of SIDS; therefore infants should be dressed in light clothing and the room temperature kept at a comfortable range for a lightly dressed adult. Overbundling the infant should be avoided.

The most compelling data come from studies that link sleep habits with an increased risk of SIDS. Sleeping in the prone position may cause oropharyngeal obstruction or affect the thermal balance or arousal state.

The American Academy of Pediatrics (2000b) recommends that healthy infants be placed to sleep in the supine (on the back) position. There is an increased risk of SIDS in infants placed in the side-lying position, primarily because of their ability to turn to a prone position. Soft bedding such as pillows or quilts should not be used under the infant for bedding. Bedding items such as stuffed animals or towels should be removed from the crib while the infant is asleep to prevent possible asphyxia. In the event that the side sleeping position is used, the infant's dependent arm should be placed forward to prevent rolling over onto the prone position. Most preterm infants being discharged from the hospital should be placed in the supine sleep position unless there are factors that predispose to airway obstruction.

Although the etiology is unknown, autopsies reveal consistent pathologic findings such as pulmonary edema and intrathoracic hemorrhages that confirm the diagnosis of SIDS. Consequently, autopsies should be performed on all infants suspected of dying of SIDS, and the findings should be shared with the parents as soon as possible after the death.

Whether subsequent siblings of one SIDS infant are at increased risk for SIDS is unclear. Even if the increased risk is correct, families have a 99% chance that their subsequent child will not die of SIDS. Home monitoring is not recommended for this group of children, but it is often used by practitioners and may even be requested by parents. Monitoring is best initiated on an individual basis.

Nursing Considerations

Nurses have a vital role in the prevention of SIDS by educating families about the risk of prone sleeping position in infants from birth to 6 months of age, using appropriate bedding surfaces, parental smoking around the infant, and the dangers in sharing an adult bed with the infant. It has been reported that as many as 20% of all infants this age are still placed to sleep in the prone position (Willinger et al, 2000). Nurses must be proactive in further decreasing the incidence of prone sleeping and other potential threats to healthy infants; postpartum discharge planning, newborn discharge teaching and newborn-care classes, follow-up home visits, well-baby clinic visits, and immunization visits provide an excellent opportunity to educate parents and caregivers in these matters (Home Care box).

A concern of many health care workers has been that infants placed on the back to sleep will aspirate emesis or mucus; one survey found no increase in infant deaths, aspiration, asphyxia, or respiratory failure as a result of supine sleep positioning over a 3-year period (Malloy, 2002). One study indicated that 20% of SIDS cases occurred in day care settings out of the home; therefore it is important that infant sleep position be discussed with day care workers as well (Moon, Patel, & Shaefer, 2000).

Home Care

INFANT SLEEP POSITION AND SIDS

For decades nurses have been taught to place newborns and infants on their tummies or sides to sleep in order to prevent aspiration and subsequent asphyxia. Nurses instructed parents to do the same. In the early 1990s, however, research data from New Zealand suggested that infants placed prone to sleep were more likely to die of SIDS than those who were placed in a nonprone (supine) position. In 1992 the Back to Sleep campaign was initiated to encourage physicians, nurses, and other health professionals to inform parents about placing newborns and infants in a side-lying or nonprone position to sleep in order to decrease the risk of SIDS. This recommendation was later amended to propose that infants be placed only in a supine sleep position because infants placed in the side-lying position might role over to a prone position and be at greater risk for SIDS. Since 1992, the incidence of SIDS in the United States has decreased by more than 40% to an all-time low of 0.7 per 1000 live births (American Academy of Pediatrics, 2000b). In 1992 SIDS was the leading cause of death in infants less than 1 year old; SIDS is now the third leading cause of death, preceded by congenital anomalies and prematurity (Moon, 2001). Yet research indicates that approximately 20% of all infants under 6 months of age are still being placed in a side-lying or prone position to sleep despite findings in New Zealand, Great Britain, Australia, and the United States that the supine sleeping position has not been associated with an increase in the number of asphyxiation events or deaths in this age group (American Academy of Pediatrics, 2000b). Additional research from Australia supports the theory that supine sleeping does not increase the incidence of mortality as a result of gastric contents being aspirated into the trachea (Byard & Beal, 2000).

Research from 90 Iowa hospitals indicates that a large number of newborns are still being placed in side-lying sleep positions; 51.4% of those surveyed indicated that the rationale for placing the newborn on the side was out of fear of asphyxiation (Hein & Pettit, 2001). Parents encouraged by physicians and nurses to place the infant supine at home may be confused by witnessing hospital workers placing infants prone or in side-lying positions in the nursery or mother-infant care unit. It is imperative that research be evaluated carefully, and it is time for nurses to be the front-line proponents for saving the lives of thousands of infants yearly by helping parents and caregivers understand the importance of preventing SIDS by putting infants to sleep on their back—at home, in hospital nurseries, and in day care facilities.

Loss of a child from SIDS presents several crises with which the parents must cope. In addition to grief and mourning for the death of their child, the parents must face a tragedy that was sudden, unexpected, and unexplained. The psychologic intervention for the family must deal with these additional variables. This discussion focuses primarily on the objectives of care for families experiencing SIDS, rather than on the process of grief and mourning, which is explored in Chapter 41.

NURSE ALERT Research findings have important implications for practices that may reduce the risk of SIDS, such as avoiding smoking during pregnancy, postnatally, and near the infant; encouraging the supine sleeping position; avoiding soft, moldable mattresses, blankets, and pillows; discouraging bed sharing in conditions which may increase the risk of SIDS; encouraging breastfeeding; and avoiding overheating during sleep. The infant's head position should be varied to prevent flattening of the skull (positional plagiocephaly) (Family Focus box and Fig. 36-16). ■

Finding the Infant

Usually it is the mother who finds the child dead in the crib. Typically the child is in a disheveled bed, with blankets over the head, and huddled in a corner. Frothy, blood-tinged fluid fills the mouth and nostrils, and the infant may be lying face down in the secretions, suggesting that he or she bled to death. The diaper is wet and full of stool, which is consistent with a cataclysmic type of death. The hands may be clutching the sheets, as if the child were in distress before death. The initial appearance of the child, combined with the shock of such an unexpected event, adds to the horror that the parents must face.

Often the mother is alone and must deal with her initial shock, panic, grief, questions of the other siblings, and the decision of where to find help. The first persons to arrive may be the police and ambulance attendants. Ideally, they will handle the situation by asking few questions; giving no indication of wrongdoing, abuse, or neglect; making sensitive judgments concerning any resuscitation efforts for the child; and comforting the members of the family as much as possible. These individuals should be properly informed about SIDS in order to recognize its characteristic signs and tell parents that their child probably died of a disease called sudden infant death syndrome, which cannot be predicted or prevented. A compassionate, sensitive approach to the family during the very first few minutes can help spare them some of the overwhelming guilt and anguish that commonly follow this type of death.

Arriving at the Emergency Department

The first contact that nurses typically have with these families is in the emergency department, when the infant is seen by a physician in order to be pronounced dead. Usually there is no attempt at resuscitation. During the time in the emergency department several aspects warrant special consideration. Parents are asked only factual questions, such as when they found the infant, how he or she looked, and whom they called for help. Any remarks that may suggest re-

Family Focus

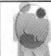

THE MISSHAPEN HEAD

Since the Back to Sleep campaign in 1992 advocating nonprone sleeping for infants, an increase in the incidence of positional *plagiocephaly* has been observed. Because the infant's sutures are not closed, the skull is very pliable, and when the infant is placed on the back to sleep the posterior occiput flattens over time; a typical bald spot will develop, which is usually transient. As a result of prolonged pressure on one side of the skull, that side becomes misshapen; facial asymmetry may develop. The sternocleidomastoid muscle may tighten on the preferential side and torticollis may also develop. Treatment of torticollis and plagiocephaly initially involves exercises to loosen the tight muscle and alternating head position from one side to another during feeding, carrying, and sleep. If the plagiocephaly is not resolved after 4 to 8 weeks of physical therapy, a customized helmet may be worn to decrease the pressure on the affected side of the skull (Biggs, 2003). Minor skull flattening is not considered significant, but efforts should be taken to educate parents regarding changing head positions during sleep. To prevent plagiocephaly it is recommended that the infant's head position be altered during sleep time. Infants should be placed prone during awake time, which is encouraged to prevent plagiocephaly and to encourage development of upper shoulder girdle strength; the latter helps in the progressive development of movements such as rolling over and starting to rise up on all fours, which are precursors to crawling and eventually walking. Since the supine sleeping position has resulted in a significant decrease in loss of infant lives from SIDS, no changes in this stance appear to be on the horizon. The increased incidence of misshapen heads in infants as a result of supine sleeping can easily be prevented by changing certain infant care habits so that the infant's skull shape remains intact and subsequent development progresses. Parents should not become so alarmed at the development of plagiocephaly that they abandon supine sleeping position for the infant but should consult with the practitioner for further advice.

sponsibility, such as why didn't they go in earlier, didn't they hear the infant cry out, was the head buried in a blanket, or were the other siblings jealous of this child, are avoided.

If statements were made that were misguided, such as "This looks like suffocation," they can be corrected before parents harbor them in their minds as indications of their guilt. The discussion of an autopsy should be presented at this time, emphasizing that a diagnosis cannot be confirmed until the postmortem examination is completed. If the mother was breastfeeding, she needs information about abrupt discontinuation of lactation.

Another important aspect of compassionate care for these parents is allowing them to say good-bye to their child. Because the parents leave the hospital without their infant, it is helpful to accompany them to the car or arrange for someone else to take them home. A debriefing session may help health care workers who dealt with the family and deceased infant to deal with feelings that are often engendered when a SIDS victim is brought into the acute care facility.

Returning Home

When the parents return home, they should be visited by a competent, qualified professional as soon after the death as possible. Printed material that contains excellent informa-

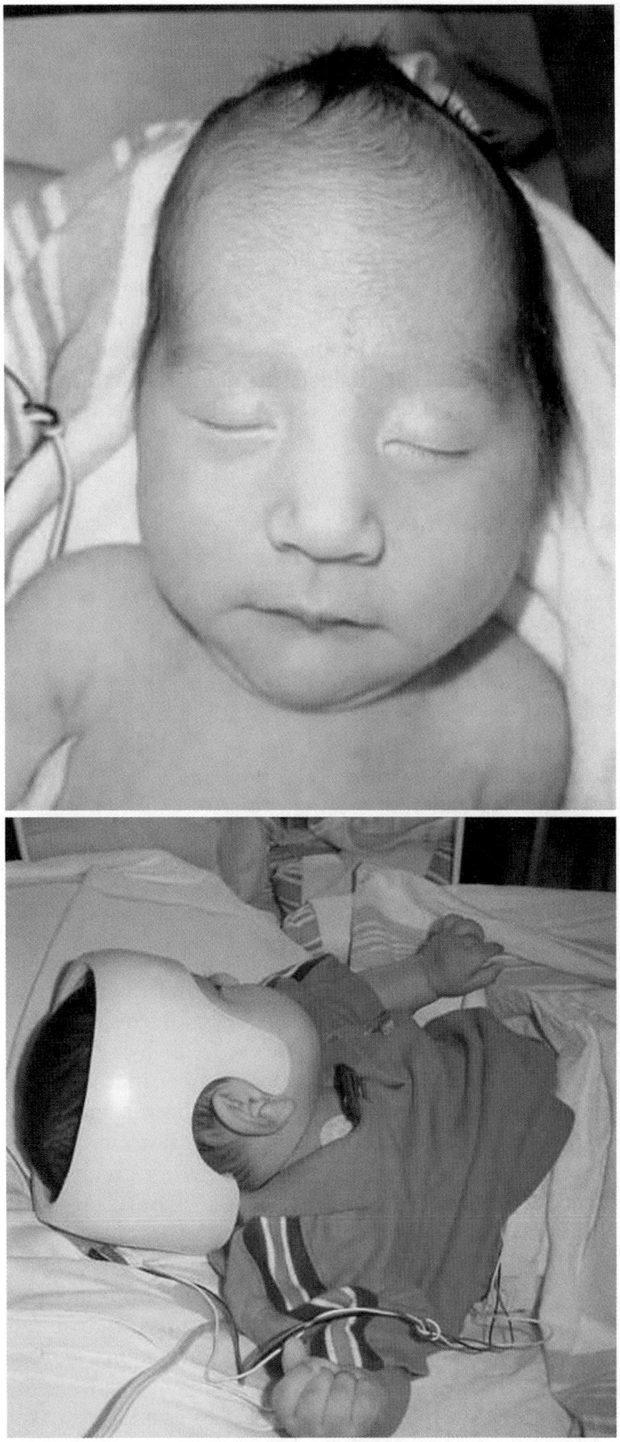

A

B

Fig. 36-16 **A**, Plagiocephaly. **B**, Helmet used to correct plagiocephaly. (Courtesy Dr. Gerardo Cabrera-Meza, Department of Neonatology, Baylor College of Medicine, Houston, TX.)

tion about SIDS (available from the national organizations*) should be provided.

*American Sudden Infant Death Syndrome (SIDS) Institute, 6065 Roswell Rd., Suite 876, Atlanta, GA 30328; phone: 800-232-SIDS (in Georgia, 800-847-SIDS); Web site: www.sids.org. The Sudden Infant Death Syndrome Alliance, 1314 Bedford Ave., Suite 210, Baltimore, MD 21208; phone: 800-221-SIDS; Web site: www.sidsalliance.org. National SIDS Resource Center, 2070 Chain Bridge Rd., Suite 450; phone: 866-866-7437 (free) or 703-821-8955; Web site: www.sidscenter.org.

Ideally, the number of visits and plans for subsequent intervention need to be flexible. For example, the siblings may initially appear accepting of the explanation and well adjusted, but may later refuse to go to sleep or ask questions about graves or funerals, indicating their need for further help in dealing with the death. Parents facing the question of a subsequent child will need support. Both the birth of a subsequent child and the survival of that child, especially past the age of death of the previous child, are important transitional stages for parents.

Because the mourning process continues *for at least a year,* and because most health plans do not cover periodic visits to the family to evaluate their progress, referrals to other parents who have lost a child to SIDS should be considered.

Apnea of Infancy

Apnea of infancy (AOI) generally refers to pathologic apnea in infants older than 37 weeks of gestation. The clinical presentation of AOI is an apparent life-threatening event (ALTE) (previously referred to by the inaccurate and misleading expression, "near-miss SIDS") that is described as

- Frightening to the observer, who fears the child died or would have died without vigorous intervention
- Some combination of
  - *Apnea*—cessation of breathing for 20 seconds or more
  - *Color change*—cyanosis or pallor, but sometimes plethora
  - *Marked change in muscle tone*—usually marked hypotonia
  - *Choking or gagging*

AOI can be a symptom of many disorders, including sepsis, seizures, upper airway abnormalities, gastroesophageal reflux, hypoglycemia or other metabolic problems, impaired regulation of breathing during sleep or feeding, or a result of intentional poisoning by a caregiver. Abnormal physical properties of pulmonary surfactant have been identified in some children with recurrent ALTE (Silvestri & Weese-Mayer, 1996). However, in about half the cases no cause is identified. Infants with a history of ALTEs are at increased risk for SIDS, but these children constitute less than 7% of all SIDS victims. A diagnosis of AOI is made when no identifiable cause for the ALTE is found. Results from the Collaborative Home Infant Monitoring Evaluation study found that apnea and bradycardia occurred at conventional and extreme alarm thresholds in all groups of infants studied: siblings of SIDS infants, infants with ALTEs, symptomatic (of apnea and bradycardia) and asymptomatic preterm infants weighing less than 1750 g at birth, and healthy term infants. The researchers concluded that many infants experience apnea and bradycardia in each of these groups but do not die. Furthermore, it was reported that apnea does not appear to be an immediate precursor to SIDS and that cardiorespiratory monitoring is not an effective tool for identifying infants at greater risk for SIDS (American Academy of Pediatrics, 2003d).

Diagnostic Evaluation

It is currently recommended that any infant experiencing an ALTE be admitted to an appropriate acute care center for evaluation of the event, which involves a detailed history and physical examination. The most widely used test is continuous recording of cardiorespiratory patterns (cardiopneumogram or pneumocardiogram). Four-channel (or multichannel pneumogram) pneumocardiograms monitor heart rate, respirations (chest impedance), nasal airflow, and oxygen saturation. A more sophisticated test, polysomnography ("sleep study"), also records brain waves, eye and body movements, esophageal manometry, and end-tidal carbon dioxide measurements. However, none of these tests can predict risk. Some children with normal results may still have subsequent apneic episodes.

Therapeutic Management

Treatment usually involves continuous home monitoring of cardiorespiratory rhythms. The criteria for discontinuing the monitoring are based on the infant's clinical condition. A general guideline for discontinuation is when infants with ALTEs have gone 1 or 2 months without a significant number of episodes requiring intervention. Newer home apnea monitors allow download of information that assists the practitioner in the decision about when home monitoring may be discontinued. It is imperative to keep in mind, however, that the home apnea monitor will not predict or prevent SIDS deaths (Home Care box).

Home Care

USING APNEA MONITORS

Use the monitor as instructed by the practitioner.
Do not adjust the monitor to eliminate false alarms. Adjustments could compromise the monitor's effectiveness.
Place the monitor on a firm surface away from the crib and drapes; plug power cord directly into a wall socket with a three-pronged outlet.
Do not sleep in the same bed as a monitored infant.
Keep pets and children away from the monitor and infant.
Keep the monitor away from possible electrical interferences such as appliances (e.g., electric blankets, televisions, air conditioners, remote telephones [including cellular phones]).
Check the monitor several times a day to be sure the alarm is working and that it can be heard from room to room. Be sure the caregiver can reach the monitor quickly (in less than 30 seconds).
Periodically check the monitor's breath detection indicator and battery or charger connections.
Be aware that strong signals from nearby radio and television stations, airports, ham radios, cellular phones, or police stations could interfere with the monitor. Check for interference if the monitor is to be operated in these areas.
Read the monitor's user manual carefully; report problems promptly.
Inform community utility and rescue squads of home monitoring as appropriate.
Keep emergency rescue numbers near phones in the home.
Practice safety precautions:
- Remove leads when infant is not attached to the monitor.
- Unplug the power cord from the electrical outlet when the cord is not plugged into the monitor.
- Use safety covers on electrical outlets to prevent children from inserting objects into a socket.

Data primarily from *FDA safety alert: important tips for apnea monitor users,* Rockville, MD, 1990, US Department of Health and Human Services.

Nursing Considerations

The diagnosis of AOI engenders great anxiety and concern in parents, and the implementation of home monitoring presents additional physical and emotional burdens. Parents of infants on home apnea monitors report experiencing emotional distress, especially depression and hostility, during the first few weeks following hospital discharge (Abendroth et al, 1999). If monitoring is required, the nurse can be a major source of support to the family in terms of education about the equipment, observation of the infant's status, and immediate intervention during apneic episodes, including cardiopulmonary resuscitation (CPR). To help the family cope with the numerous procedures they must learn, adequate preparation before discharge and written instructions are essential. In the first few weeks following discharge, parents may benefit by having a practitioner readily available to answer questions regarding false alarms and for other technical assistance.

Several types of home monitors are available, and most hospitals select the model that the infant will use at home. Nurses, especially those involved in the care at home, must become familiar with the equipment, including its advantages and disadvantages. Safety is a major concern because monitors can cause electrical burns and electrocution. The following precautions are recommended:

- Remove leads from infant when not attached to monitor.
- Unplug power cord from electrical outlet when cord is not plugged into monitor.
- Use safety covers on electrical outlets to discourage children from inserting objects into a socket.

Siblings should also be supervised when near the infant and taught that the monitor is not a toy. Other safety practices include informing local utility and rescue squads of the home monitoring in case of an emergency. Telephone numbers for these services should be posted near all telephones in the home.

Caregivers need detailed information regarding proper attachment of the electrodes to the infant's chest with impedance monitors that detect chest movement. The electrodes are placed in the midaxillary line, at a space one or two fingerbreadths below the nipple (Fig. 36-17). Adhesive electrodes are attached directly to the skin. For home use, electrodes attached to a belt that is placed around the child's trunk are preferred. The belt is positioned so that the electrodes contact the skin in the same area as shown in Fig. 36-17. Monitors may have memory chips that allow for event recording, which can be an effective tool in evaluating the use of the monitor and reported frequency of alarms.

Monitors are effective only if they are used. They do not prevent death but alert the caregiver to the ALTE in time to intervene. The need to use the monitor and to respond appropriately to alarms must be stressed. Noncompliance can result in the infant's death.

NURSE ALERT If the infant is apneic, gently stimulate the trunk by patting or rubbing it. If the infant is prone, turn to the back and flick the feet. If there is still no response, begin CPR. Never vigorously shake the child. No more than 15 to 20 seconds are spent on stimulation before implementing CPR. ■

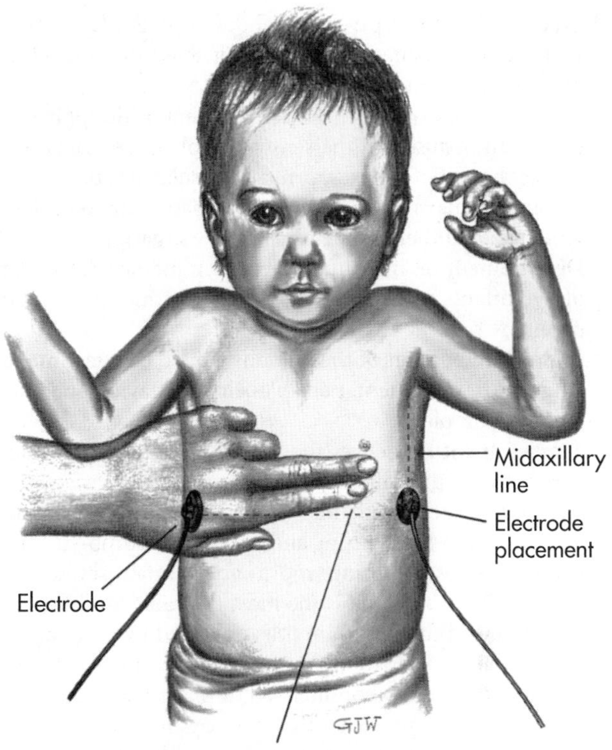

Fig. 36-17 Electrode placement for apnea monitoring. In small infants one fingerbreadth may be used.

Family Support

Although AOI is not a chronic illness, many of the stresses observed during the monitoring period are characteristic of those of families with chronically ill children. Parents report increased stress, including concern for the child's survival, fear of incompetency in assuming home responsibility, inadequate respite care, social isolation, constant work, and fatigue. Siblings are affected, as well as the child with AOI, who may be characterized as "spoiled" and have developmental delays. To deal with these potential effects, nurses need to use the same interventions as those discussed for children with chronic illness (see Chapter 41) and be aware of the need for referral when difficulties are suspected.

To lessen the continuous responsibility of monitoring, other family members such as grandparents should be taught how to manipulate the equipment, read and interpret the signals, and administer CPR. They are encouraged to stay with the infant for regular periods to allow parents respite. Support groups of other families who have successfully completed monitoring can also be of benefit. Because baby-sitters are difficult to locate, support group members or nursing students may be potential sources of qualified caregivers.

Key Points

- Biologic development of the child encompasses proportional changes; sensory changes, including binocularity, depth perception, and visual preference; maturation of biologic systems; fine motor development; and gross motor development.

- Erikson's theory of psychosocial development (birth to 1 year) is concerned with acquiring a sense of trust while overcoming a sense of mistrust.
- Piaget's theory of cognitive development, as it applies to the infant, focuses on the sensorimotor phase, which includes the use of reflexes, primary circular reactions, secondary circular reactions, and coordination or secondary schemata and their application to new situations.
- Development of body image begins in infancy; by 1 year of age infants recognize that they are distinct from their parents.
- Social development of the infant is guided by attachment, language development, personal-social behavior, and participation in play.
- Temperament influences the type of interaction that occurs between the child and parents and siblings.
- Parents are faced with many concerns, including infant fears, day care, limit setting and discipline, thumb-sucking and pacifier use, teething, and choice of infant shoes.
- Breast milk or formula is the most desirable food for the infant during the first 6 months, followed by gradual introduction of solid food during the second 6 months. Whole milk is not recommended until after 12 months.
- Common sleep problems that develop during infancy—and that are easily prevented—are associated with night crying and feeding. Nurses should instruct the parents, after careful assessment, in strategies to deal with the specific problem.
- Cleaning the teeth regularly and appropriate dietary intake promote good dental health.
- Recommended routine immunizations include those for hepatitis B virus, hepatitis A virus (in some states), diphtheria, influenza, tetanus, pertussis, polio, measles, mumps, rubella, pneumoccoccus, chickenpox, and *Haemophilus influenzae* type b.
- Recommended immunizations for selected groups of children are hepatitis A, Lyme, and pneumococcal and meningococcal vaccines.
- Because injuries are a major cause of death during infancy, parents should be alerted to aspiration of foreign objects, suffocation, falls, poisoning, burns, motor vehicle injuries, and bodily damage, as well as preventive actions needed to make the environment safe for infants.
- Treatment of colic may involve change in feeding practices, correction of a stressful environment, behavior modification, and support of the parent.
- Failure to thrive may be classified as organic, resulting from some physical cause; or nonorganic, resulting from psychosocial factors involving the child and caregiver (e.g., maternal deprivation), environmental causes (e.g., inadequate parental knowledge of child feeding), or unexplained causes.
- Sudden infant death syndrome is the third leading cause of death in children between 1 month and 1 year of age.
- Evidence linking SIDS to the prone sleeping position has led to the recommendation that healthy infants sleep supine.
- The primary nursing responsibility in care associated with sudden infant death and other conditions of unknown etiology is emotional support of the family.
- Children with apnea of infancy receive home monitoring to alert the family to an apparent life-threatening event.

References

Abendroth D et al: Do apnea monitors decrease emotional distress in parents of infants at high risk for cardiopulmonary arrest? *J Pediatr Health Care* 13(2):50-57, 1999.

Agran PF et al: Rates of pediatric injuries by 3-month intervals for children 0 to 3 years of age, *Pediatrics* 111(6):e683-e692, 2003.

American Academy of Pediatrics, Committee on Sports Medicine: Infant exercise programs, *Pediatrics* 82(5):800, 1988.

American Academy of Pediatrics, Task Force on Infant Positioning and SIDS: Does bed sharing affect the risk of SIDS? *Pediatrics* 109(2):272-273, 1997.

American Academy of Pediatrics, Committee on Environmental Health: Ultraviolet light: a hazard to children, *Pediatrics* 104(2):328-333, 1999.

American Academy of Pediatrics, Committee on Sports Medicine and Committee on Injury and Poison Prevention: Swimming programs for infants and toddlers, *Pediatrics* 105(4, pt 1 of 2):868-869, 2000a.

American Academy of Pediatrics, Task Force on Infant Sleep Position and Sudden Infant Death Syndrome: Changing concepts of sudden infant death syndrome: implications for infant sleeping environment and sleep position, *Pediatrics* 105(3):650-656, 2000b.

American Academy of Pediatrics, Committee on Injury and Poison Prevention: Injuries associated with infant walkers, *Pediatrics* 108(3):790-792, 2001.

American Academy of Pediatrics: Prevention of rickets and vitamin D deficiency: new guidelines for vitamin D intake, *Pediatrics* 111(4):908-910, 2003a.

American Academy of Pediatrics, Section on Pediatric Dentistry: Oral health risk assessment timing and establishment of the dental home, *Pediatrics* 111(5):1113-1116, 2003b.

American Academy of Pediatrics, Committee on Infectious Diseases, Pickering L (ed): *2003 red book: report of the Committee on Infectious Diseases,* ed 26, Elk Grove Village, IL, 2003c, The Academy.

American Academy of Pediatrics, Committee on Fetus and Newborn: Apnea, sudden infant death syndrome, and home monitoring, *Pediatrics* 111(4):914-917, 2003d.

American Academy of Pediatrics, Committee on Nutrition: *Pediatric nutrition handbook,* ed 5, Elk Grove Village, IL, 2004a, The Academy.

American Academy of Pediatrics, Committee on Infectious Diseases: Recommended childhood and adolescent immunization schedule—United States, July-December 2004, *Pediatrics* 113(5):1448-1449, 2004b.

Anderson RN, Smith BL: Deaths: Leading causes for 2002, *Natl Vital Stat Rep* 53(17):1-89, 2005.

Ball HL: Breastfeeding, bed sharing, and infant sleep, *Birth* 30(3):181-188, 2003.

Barnard K et al: Measurement and meaning of parent-child interaction. In Morrison F, Lord C, Keating D (eds): *Applied developmental psychology,* vol 3, New York, 1993, Academic Press.

Bechtel B: Intranasal influenza vaccine granted approval by FDA, *Infect Dis Children* 3:3, 2003.

Biancuzzo M: *Breastfeeding the newborn: clinical strategies for nurses,* St Louis, 1999, Mosby.

Biggs WS: Diagnosis and management of positional head deformity, *Am Family Physician* 67(9):1953-1956, 2003.

Brazelton T: Parent-infant cosleeping revisited, *The Brazelton Center Newsletter,* vol 2, Boston, 1990.

Brenner RA et al: Deaths attributable to injuries in infants, United States, 1983-1991, *Pediatrics* 103(5):968-974, 1999.

Byard RW, Beal SM: Gastric aspiration and sleeping position in infancy and early childhood, *J Paediatr Child Health* 36(4):403-405, 2000.

Calamaro CJ: Infant nutrition in the first year of life: tradition or science? *Pediatr Nurs* 26(2):211-215, 2000.

Campion EW: Suspicions about the safety of vaccines, *N Engl J Med* 347(19):1474-1475, 2002.

Careaga MG, Kerner JA: A gastroenterologist's approach to failure to thrive, *Pediatr Ann* 29(9):558-567, 2000.

Carey WB, McDevitt SC: Revision of the infant temperament questionnaire, *Pediatrics* 61(5):735-739, 1978.

Centers for Disease Control and Prevention: Deaths: final data for 1999, Centers for Disease Control and Prevention, National Center for Health Statistics, *Natl Vital Stat Rep* 49(8):1-114, 2001.

Corbett-Dick P, Bezek SK: Breastfeeding promotion for the employed mother, *J Pediatr Health Care* 11(1):12-19, 1997.

Corrales KM, Utter SL: Failure to thrive. In Samoor PQ, Helm KKI, Lang CE (eds): *Handbook of pediatric nutrition,* ed 2, Gaithersburg, MD, 1999, Aspen.

Corwin MJ et al: Secular changes in sleep position during infancy: 1995-1998, *Pediatrics* 111(1):52-60, 2003.

Dales L, Hammer SJ, Smith NJ: Time trends in autism and in MMR immunization coverage in California, *JAMA* 285(9):1183-1185, 2001.

Dedoukou X et al: Incidence and risk factors of fall injuries among infants, *Arch Pediatr Adolesc Med* 158(10):1002-1006, 2004.

Dennison BA, Rockwell HL, Baker SL: Excess fruit juice consumption by preschool-aged children is associated with short stature and obesity, *Pediatrics* 99(1):15-22, 1997.

Dewey KG: Nutrition, growth, and complementary feeding of the breastfed infant, *Pediatr Clin North Am* 48(1):87-104, 2001.

Diggle L, Deeks J: Effect of needle length on incidence of local reactions to routine immunizations in infants aged 4 months: randomized controlled trial, *BMJ* 321(7266):931-993, 2000.

Dihigo SK: New strategies for the treatment of colic: modifying the parent/infant interaction, *J Pediatr Health Care* 12(5):256-262, 1998.

Douglass JM, Douglass AB, Silk HJ: A practical guide to infant oral health, *American Family Physician* 70(11):2113-2120, 2004.

Drago DA: Kitchen scalds and thermal burns in children five years and younger, *Pediatrics* 115(1): 10-16, 2005.

Drago DA, Dannenberg AL: Infant mechanical suffocating deaths in the United States, 1980-1997, *Pediatrics* 103(5):e59, 1999.

Duro D et al: Association between infantile colic and carbohydrate malabsorption from fruit juices in infancy, *Pediatrics* 109(5):797-805, 2002.

Ellett MLC: What is known about colic? *Gastroenterol Nurs* 26(2):60-65, 2003.

Erikson EH: Childhood and society, ed 2, New York, 1963, W.W. Norton.

Feury KJ: Injury prevention: where are the resources? *Orthop Nurs* 22(2):124-130, 2003.

Friedman EH: Infantile colic, *Arch Pediatr Adolesc Med* 150(6):770-771, 1996.

Guyer B et al: Annual summary of vital statistics—1998, *Pediatrics* 104(6):1229-1246, 1999.

Hauck FR et al: Sleep environment and the risk of sudden infant death syndrome in an urban population: the Chicago Infant Mortality Study, *Pediatrics* 111(5 pt 2):1207-1214, 2003.

Hawkins-Walsh E: A behavioural infant sleep intervention resolved sleep problems, *Evidence-Based Nurs* 6(1):10-12, 2003.

Hein HA, Pettit SF: Back to sleep: good advice for parents but not for hospitals? *Pediatrics* 107(3):537-539, 2001.

Hiscock H, Wake M: Infant sleep problems and postnatal depression: a community-based study, *Pediatrics* 107(6):1317-1322, 2001.

Hobbie C, Baker S, Bayerl C: Parental misunderstanding of basic infant nutrition: misinformed feeding choices, *J Pediatr Health Care* 14(1):26-31, 2000.

Horn MI, McCarthy AM: Children's responses to sequential versus simultaneous immunization injections, *J Pediatr Health Care* 13(1):18-23, 1999.

Hughes MB et al: Temperament characteristics of premature infants in the first year of life, *J Dev Behav Pediatr* 23(6):430-435, 2002.

Hviid A et al: Association between thimerosal-containing vaccine and autism, *JAMA* 290(13):1763-1766, 2003.

Ize-Ludlow D et al: Neurotoxicites in infants seen with the consumption of star anise tea, *Pediatrics* 114(5):e653, 2004.

Johns RM, Miller L, Hochstetler I: Mother and baby dental care, *Mother Baby J* 3(3):15-22, 1998.

Kamerling SN: Airbags and children: making correct choices in child passenger restraints, *MCN* 27(5):264-273, 2002.

Koslap-Petraco MB, Parsons T: Communicating the benefits of combination vaccines to parents and health care providers, *J Pediatr Health Care* 17(2):53-57, 2003.

Langkamp DL, Kim Y, Pascoe JM: Temperament of preterm infants at 4 months of age: maternal ratings and perceptions, *J Dev Behav Pediatr* 19(6):391-396, 1998.

Langkamp DL, Pascoe JM: Temperament of pre-term infants at 9 months of age, *Amb Child Health* 7(3/4):203-212, 2001.

Lassman J: Water safety, *J Emerg Nurs* 28(3):241-243, 2002.

Lawrence RA, Lawrence RM: *Breastfeeding: a guide for the medical profession,* ed 6, St Louis, 2005, Mosby.

Leach CEA et al: Epidemiology of SIDS and explained sudden infant deaths, *Pediatrics* 104(4):e43, 1999.

Loman DG: The use of complementary and alternative health care practices among children, *J Pediatr Health Care* 17(2):58-63, 2003.

MacPhee M, Schneider J: A clinical tool for nonorganic failure-to-thrive feeding interactions, *J Pediatr Nurs* 11(1):29-39, 1996.

Maggioni A, Lifshitz F: Nutritional management of failure to thrive, *Pediatr Clin North Am* 42(4):791-810, 1995.

Malloy MH: Trends in postneonatal aspiration deaths and reclassification of sudden infant death syndrome: impact of the "Back to Sleep" program, *Pediatrics* 109(4):661-665, 2002.

McGarvey C et al: Factors relating to the infant's last sleep environment in sudden infant death syndrome in the Republic of Ireland, *Arch Dis Child* 88(12):1058-1064, 2003.

McMartin KI et al: Lung tissue concentrations of nicotine in sudden infant death syndrome, *J Pediatr* 140(2):205-209, 2002.

Mecham N, Melini J: Unintentional victims: development of a protocol for the care of children exposed to chemicals at methamphetamine laboratories, *Pediatr Emerg Care* 18(4):327-332, 2002.

Medoff-Cooper B: Infant temperament: implications for parenting from birth through 1 year, *J Pediatr Nurs* 10(3):141-145, 1995.

Medoff-Cooper B, Carey WB, McDevitt SC: The early infancy temperament questionnaire, *J Dev Behav Pediatr* 14(4):230-235, 1993.

Mesich HM: Mother-infant co-sleeping: Understanding the debate and maximizing infant safety, *MCN* 30(1):30-37, 2005.

Moon RY: Are you talking to parents about SIDS? *Contemp Pediatr* 18(3):122-129, 2001.

Moon RY, Patel KM, Shaefer SJM: Sudden infant death syndrome in child care settings, *Pediatrics* 106(2):295-300, 2000.

Morin K: Infant nutrition: solids—when and why, *MCN* 29(4):259, 2004.

Morin K: Infant nutrition: Preparing baby food at home safely, *MCN* 30(1): 67, 2005.

Motor-vehicle occupant injury: strategies for increasing use of child safety seats, increasing use of safety belts, and reducing alcohol-impaired driving, *MMWR* 50(RR7):1-13, 2001.

Moukarzel AA, Lesicka H, Ament ME: Irritable bowel syndrome and nonspecific diarrhea in infancy and childhood—relationship with juice carbohydrate malabsorption, *Clin Pediatr* 41(3):145-150, 2002.

Neu M, Robinson JA: Infants with colic: their childhood characteristics, *J Pediatr Nurs* 18(1):12-20, 2003.

Niemela M, Uhari M, Mottonen M: A pacifier increases the risk of recurrent acute otitis media in children in day care centers, *Pediatrics* 96(5, pt 1):884-888, 1995.

Niemela M et al: Pacifier as a risk factor for acute otitis media: a randomized, controlled trial of parental counseling, *Pediatrics* 106(3):483-488, 2000.

Nowak AJ, Warren JJ: Infant oral health and oral habits, *Pediatr Clin North Am* 47(5):1043-1066, 2000.

Oghi S et al: Comparison of kangaroo care and standard care: behavioral organization, development, and temperament in healthy, low-birth-weight infants through 1 year, *J Perinatol* 22(5):374-379, 2002.

Patterson MM: Prevention: The only cure for pediatric trauma, *Orthopaedic Nursing* 18(4):16-20, 1999.

Person TL, Lavezzi WA, Wolf BC: Cosleeping and sudden unexpected death in infancy, *Arch Pathol Lab Med* 126(3):343-345, 2002.

Piaget J.: *The origins of intelligence in children.* New York, 1952, International Universities Press.

Pickett W et al: Injuries experienced by infant children: a population-based epidemiological analysis, *Pediatrics* 111 (4 pt 1):e365-e370, 2003.

Pickler R, Frankel H: The effect of non-nutritive sucking on preterm infants' behavioral organization and feeding performance, *Neonatal Network* 14(2):83, 1995.

Pinelli J, Symington A: Non-nutritive sucking for promoting physiologic stability and nutrition in preterm infants, *Cochrane Database Syst Rev* 2000(2):CD001071, 2000.

Pinelli J, Symington A, Ciliska D: Nonnutritive sucking in high-risk infants: benign intervention or legitimate therapy? *J Obst Gynecol Neonatal Nurs* 31(5):582-591, 2002.

Preventing pneumococcal disease among infants: recommendations of the Advisory Committee on Immunization Practices, *MMWR* 49(RR09): 1-38, 2000.

Prevention of hepatitis A through active or passive immunization: recommendations of the Advisory Committee on Immunization Practices (ACIP), *MMWR* 48(RR12):1-37, 1999.

Rojjanasrirat W: Working women's breastfeeding experiences, *MCN* 29(4):222-227, 2004.

Schachter F et al: Cosleeping and sleep problems in Hispanic-American urban young children, *Pediatrics* 84(3):522-530, 1989.

Silvestri JM, Weese-Mayer DE: Respiratory control disorders in infancy and childhood, *Curr Opin Pediatr* 8(3):216-220, 1996.

Skinner JD et al: Fruit juice is not related to children's growth, *Pediatrics* 103(1):58-64, 1999.

Smith MM, Lifshitz F: Excess fruit juice consumption as a contributing factor in nonorganic failure to thrive, *Pediatrics* 93(3):438-443, 1994.

Unger B et al: Racial disparity and modifiable risk factors among infants dying suddenly and unexpectedly, *Pediatrics* 111(2):E127-E131, 2003.

Van Norman RA: Why we can't afford to ignore prolonged digit-sucking, *Contemp Pediatr* 18(6):61-81, 2001.

Weizman Z et al: Efficacy of herbal tea preparation in infantile colic, *J Pediatr* 122(4):650-652, 1993.

Willinger M et al: Factors associated with caregiver's choice of infant sleep position, 1994-1998: the National Infant Sleep Position study, *JAMA* 283(16):2135-2142, 2000.

Willinger M et al: Trends in infant bed sharing in the United States, 1993-2000: the National Infant Sleep Position Study, *Arch Pediatr Adolesc Med* 157(1): 43-49, 2003.

Wilson D, Bowman C: Infant nutrition: building blocks for the future, *Mother Baby J* 5(4):17-21, 2000.

Wilson ME et al: Family dynamics, parental-fetal attachment and infant temperament, *J Advanced Nurs* 31(1):204-210, 2000.

Zuckerman JN, Cockcroft A, Zuckerman AJ: Site of injection for vaccination, *BMJ* 305(6862):1158, 1992.

The Toddler and Family 37

LEARNING OBJECTIVES

On completion of this chapter the reader will be able to:

- Identify the major biologic, psychosocial, cognitive, and social developments during the toddler years.
- Relate separation anxiety and negativism to developmental tasks.
- Recognize readiness for toilet training and offer parents guidelines.
- Prepare toddlers for the birth of a sibling.
- Provide parents with guidelines for handling temper tantrums.
- Provide parents with feeding recommendations.
- Outline a preventive dental hygiene plan for toddlers.
- Provide anticipatory guidance to parents regarding injury prevention based on the toddler's developmental achievements.

ELECTRONIC RESOURCES

Additional information related to the content in Chapter 37 can be found on

the companion website at evolve
http://evolve.elsevier.com/Wong/maternal/
- NCLEX Review Questions
- Case Study–Salicylate Ingestion
- Case Study–Ingestion of an Injurious Agent
- WebLinks

or the interactive student CD-ROM
Activities for Chapter 37 include the following:
- NCLEX Review Questions
- Case Study–Toilet Training/Toddler Development
- Case Study–Heavy Metal Poisoning
- Skill–Car Seat Safety

PROMOTING OPTIMUM GROWTH AND DEVELOPMENT

The term *terrible twos* has often been used to describe the toddler years, the period from 12 to 36 months of age. It is a time of intense exploration of the environment as children attempt to find out how things work and how to control others through temper tantrums, negativism, and obstinacy. Although this can be a challenging time for parents and child as each learns to know the other better, it is an extremely important period for developmental achievement and intellectual growth.

Biologic Development

Proportional Changes

Growth slows considerably during toddlerhood. The average *weight* gain is 1.8 to 2.7 kg (4 to 6 pounds). The birth weight is quadrupled by 2½ years of age. The rate of increase in height also slows. The usual increment is an addition of 7.5 cm (3 inches) per year and occurs mainly in elongation of the legs rather than the trunk. The average *height* of a 2-year-old is 86.6 cm (34 inches). In general, adult height is about twice the 2-year-old child's height. Accurate measurement of height and weight during the toddler years should reveal a steady growth curve that is *steplike* in nature rather than linear (straight), which is characteristic of the growth spurts during the early childhood years.

The rate of increase in *head circumference* slows somewhat by the end of infancy, and head circumference is usually equal to chest circumference by 1 to 2 years of age. The usual total increase in head circumference during the second year is 2.5 cm (1 inch). Then the rate of increase slows until at age 5 years the increase is less than 1.25 cm (½ inch) per year. The anterior fontanel closes between 12 and 18 months of age.

Chest circumference continues to increase in size and exceeds head circumference during the toddler years. Its shape also changes as the transverse, or lateral diameter exceeds the anteroposterior diameter. After the second year the chest circumference exceeds the abdominal measurement; this, in addition to the growth of the lower extremities, gives the child a taller, leaner appearance. However, the toddler retains a squat, "pot-bellied" appearance because of the less well-developed abdominal musculature and short legs. The legs retain a slightly bowed or curved appearance during the second year from the weight of the relatively large trunk.

Sensory Changes

Visual acuity of 20/40 is considered acceptable during the toddler years. Full binocular vision is well developed, and any evidence of persistent strabismus requires professional attention as early as possible to prevent amblyopia. Depth perception continues to develop but, because of the child's lack of motor coordination, falls from heights continue to be a persistent danger.

The senses of *hearing, smell, taste,* and *touch* become increasingly well developed, coordinated with each other, and associated with other experiences. All of the senses are used to explore the environment. Toddlers will visually inspect an object by turning it over; they may taste it, smell, it, and touch it several times before they are satisfied with their investigation. They will shake it to see if it makes noise and vigorously test its durability.

Another example of the integrated function of the senses is the toddler's development of specific *taste preferences.* The child is much less likely than infants to try a new food because of its appearance or smell, not just its taste.

Maturation of Systems

Most of the physiologic systems are relatively mature by the end of toddlerhood. Volume of the *respiratory tract* and growth of associated structures continue to increase during early childhood, lessening some of the factors that predisposed the child to frequent and serious infections during infancy. The internal structures of the ear and throat continue to be short and straight, and the lymphoid tissue of the tonsils and adenoids continues to be large. As a result, otitis media, tonsillitis, and upper respiratory tract infections are common. The respiratory and heart rates slow, and the blood pressure increases (see Appendix J). Respirations continue to be abdominal.

Under conditions of moderate variation in temperature, the toddler rarely has the difficulties of the young infant in maintaining *body temperature.* The mature functioning of the renal systems serves to conserve fluid under times of stress, decreasing the risk of dehydration.

The *digestive processes* are fairly complete by the beginning of toddlerhood. The acidity of the gastric contents continues to increase and has a protective function, since it is capable of destroying many types of bacteria. Stomach capacity increases to allow for the usual schedule of three meals a day.

One of the more prominent changes of the gastrointestinal system is the voluntary control of elimination. With complete myelination of the spinal cord, control of the anal and urethral sphincters is gradually achieved. The physiologic ability to control the sphincters probably occurs somewhere between ages 18 and 24 months. Bladder capacity also increases considerably, and by 14 to 18 months of age the child is able to retain urine for up to 2 hours or longer.

The *defense mechanisms* of the skin and blood, particularly phagocytosis, are much more efficient in toddlers than in infants. The production of antibodies is well established. However, many young children demonstrate a sudden increase in colds and minor infections when they enter preschool or other group situations, such as day care, because of their exposure to pathogens.

Gross and Fine Motor Development

The major *gross motor skill* during the toddler years is the development of locomotion. By 12 to 13 months of age toddlers walk alone using a wide stance for extra balance and by 18 months they try to run but fall easily (Fig. 37-1). Between 2 and 3 years of age, refinement of the upright, biped position is evident in improved coordination and equilibrium. At age 2 years, toddlers can walk up and down stairs; by age 2½ years they can jump using both feet, stand on one foot for a second or two, and manage a few steps on tiptoe. By the end of the second year they can stand on one foot, walk on tiptoe, and climb stairs with alternate footing.

Fine motor development is demonstrated in increasingly skillful manual dexterity. For example, by age 12 months toddlers are able to grasp a very small object but are unable to release it at will. At 15 months they can drop a pellet into a narrow-necked bottle. Casting or throwing objects and retrieving them become almost obsessive activities at about 15 months. By 18 months of age toddlers can throw a ball overhand without losing their balance.

Mastery of gross and fine motor skills is evident in all phases of the child's activity, such as play, dressing, language comprehension, response to discipline, social interaction, and propensity for injuries. Activities occur less in isolation and more in conjunction with other physical and mental abilities to produce a purposeful result. For example, the toddler walks to reach a new location, releases a toy to pick it up or to choose a new one, and scribbles to look at the im-

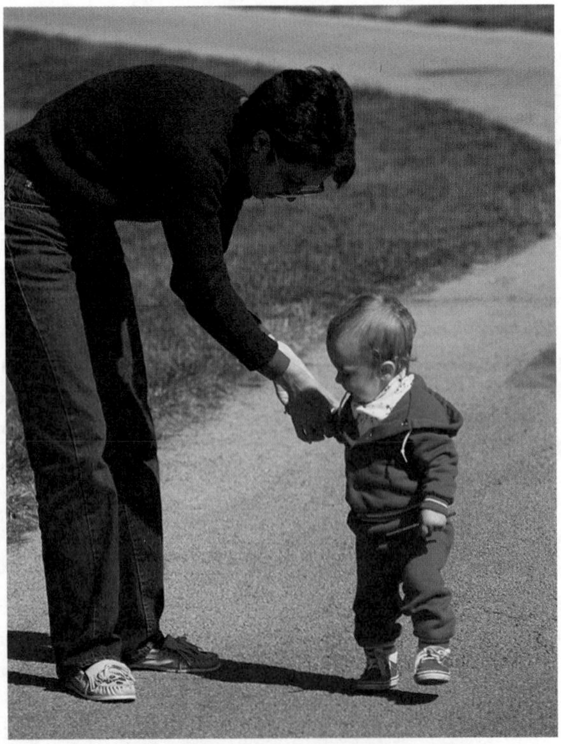

Fig. 37-1 Typical toddling gait.

age produced. The possibilities of the exploration, investigation, and manipulation of the environment—and its hazards—are endless.

Psychosocial Development

Toddlers are faced with the mastery of several important tasks. If the need for basic trust has been satisfied, they are ready to give up dependence for control, independence, and autonomy. Some of the specific tasks to be dealt with include:

- Differentiation of self from others, particularly the mother
- Toleration of separation from parent
- Ability to withstand delayed gratification
- Control over bodily functions
- Acquisition of socially acceptable behavior
- Verbal means of communication
- Ability to interact with others in a less egocentric manner

Mastery of these goals is only begun during late infancy and the toddler years, and such tasks as developing interpersonal relationships with others may not be completed until adolescence. However, crucial foundations for successful completion of such developmental tasks are established during these early formative years.

Developing a Sense of Autonomy (Erikson)

According to Erikson, the developmental task of toddlerhood is acquiring a sense of *autonomy* while overcoming a sense of *doubt* and *shame.* As infants gain trust in the predictability and reliability of their parents, environment, and interaction with others, they begin to discover that their behavior is their own and that it has a predictable, reliable effect on others. However, although they realize their will and control over others, they are confronted with the conflict of exerting autonomy and relinquishing the much-enjoyed dependence on others. Exerting their will has definite negative consequences, whereas retaining dependent, submissive behavior is generally rewarded with affection and approval. However, continued dependency creates a sense of doubt regarding their potential capacity to control their actions. This doubt is compounded by a sense of shame for feeling this urge to revolt against others' will and a fear that they will exceed their own capacity for manipulating the environment.

Just as the infant has the social modalities of grasping and biting, the toddler has the newly gained modality of holding on and letting go. To hold on and let go is evident with the use of the hands, mouth, eyes, and eventually the sphincters, when toilet training is begun. These social modalities are expressed constantly in the child's play activities, such as casting or throwing objects; taking objects out of boxes, drawers, or cabinets; holding on tighter when someone says, "No, don't touch"; and spitting out food as taste preferences become very strong.

Several characteristics, especially negativism and ritualism, are typical of toddlers in their quest for autonomy. As toddlers attempt to express their will, they often act with *negativism,* the persistent negative response to requests. The words "no" or "me do" can be the sole vocabulary. Emotions become very strongly expressed, usually in rapid mood swings. One minute, toddlers can be engrossed in an activity, and the next minute they might be extremely angry because they are unable to manipulate a toy or open a door. If scolded for doing something wrong, they can have a temper tantrum and almost instantaneously pull at the parent's legs to be picked up and comforted. Understanding and coping with these swift changes is often difficult for parents. Many parents find the negativism exasperating and, instead of dealing constructively with it, give in to it, which further threatens children in their search for learning acceptable methods of interacting with others (see Temper Tantrums and Negativism, p. 1097).

In contrast to negativism, which often disrupts the environment, *ritualism,* the need to maintain sameness and reliability, provides a sense of comfort. Toddlers can venture out with security when they know that familiar people, places, and routines still exist. One can easily understand why change such as hospitalization represents such a threat to these children. Without the comfortable rituals, there is little opportunity to exert autonomy. Consequently, dependency and regression occur (see Regression, p. 1098).

Erikson focuses on the development of the *ego,* which may be thought of as reason or common sense, during this phase of psychosocial development. There is a struggle as the child deals with the impulses of the *id* and attempts to tolerate frustration and learn socially acceptable ways of interacting with the environment. The *ego* is evident as the child is able to tolerate delayed gratification.

There is also a rudimentary beginning of the *superego,* or conscience, which is the incorporation of the morals of society and the process of acculturation. With the development of the ego, children further differentiate themselves from others and expand their sense of trust within themselves. But as they begin to develop awareness of their own will and capacity to achieve, they also become aware of their ability to fail. This ever-present awareness of potential failure creates doubt and shame. Successful mastery of the task of autonomy necessitates opportunities for self-mastery while withstanding the frustration of necessary limit setting and delayed gratification. Opportunities for self-mastery are present in appropriate play activities, toilet training, the crisis of sibling rivalry, and successful interactions with significant others.

Cognitive Development

Sensorimotor and Preconceptual Phase (Piaget)

The period from 12 to 24 months of age is a continuation of the final two stages of the sensorimotor phase. During this time the cognitive processes develop rapidly and at times seem similar to those of mature thinking. However, reasoning skills are still quite primitive and need to be understood to effectively deal with the typical behaviors of a child of this age.

Tertiary Circular Reactions

In the fifth stage of the sensorimotor phase (13 to 18 months of age), the child uses active experimentation to achieve previously unattainable goals. Newly acquired physical skills are increasingly important for the function they serve rather than for the acts themselves. The child incorporates the old learning of secondary circular reactions with new skills and applies the combined knowledge to new situations, with emphasis on the results of the experimentation.

In this way there is the beginning of rational judgment and intellectual reasoning. During this stage there is further differentiation of one's self from objects. This is evident in the child's increasing ability to venture away from the parent and to tolerate longer periods of separation.

Awareness of a causal relationship between two events is apparent. After flipping a light switch, toddlers are aware that a reciprocal response occurs. However, they are not able to transfer that knowledge to new situations. Therefore, every time they see what appears to be a light switch, they must reinvestigate its function. Such behavior demonstrates the beginning of categorizing data into distinct classes and subclasses. Examples of this type of behavior are innumerable as toddlers continuously explore the same object each time it appears in a new place.

Because classification of objects is still rudimentary, the appearance of an object denotes its function. For example, if the child's toys are stored in a paper bag or large container, that toy receptacle is no different from the garbage pail or laundry basket. If allowed to turn over the toy receptacle, the child will just as quickly do the same to other similar containers because, in the child's mind, there is no difference. Expecting the child to judge which receptacles are permissible to explore and which are not is inappropriate for this age group. Instead, the forbidden object, such as the garbage pail, should be placed out of reach.

The discovery of objects as objects leads to the awareness of their spatial relationships. Children are able to recognize different shapes and their relationship to each other. For example, they can fit slightly smaller boxes into each other (nesting) and can place a round object into a hole, even if the board is turned around, upside down, or reversed. Children are also aware of space and the relationship of their body to dimensions such as height. They will stretch, stand on a low stair or stool, and pull a string to reach an object.

Object permanence has also advanced. Although they still cannot find an object that has been invisibly displaced or moved from under one pillow to another without their seeing the change, toddlers are increasingly aware of the existence of objects behind closed doors, in drawers, and under tables. Parents are usually acutely aware of this developmental achievement and find high places and locked cabinets the only places inaccessible to toddlers.

Invention of New Means through Mental Combinations

From ages 19 to 24 months the child is in the final sensorimotor stage. During this stage the child completes the more primitive, autistic thought processes of infancy and is prepared for the more complex mental operations that occur during the phase of preoperational thought. One of the most dramatic achievements of this stage is in the area of object permanence. Children will now actively search for an object in several potential hiding places. In addition, they can infer a cause when only experiencing the effect. They can infer that an object was hidden in any number of places even if they only saw the original hiding place.

Imitation displays deeper meaning and understanding. There is greater symbolization to imitation. The child is acutely aware of others' actions and attempts to copy them in gestures and in words. *Domestic mimicry* (imitating household activities) and gender-role behavior become increasingly common during this period and during the second year. Identification with the parent of the same gender becomes apparent by the second year and represents the child's intellectual ability to differentiate different models of behavior and to imitate them appropriately (Fig. 37-2).

The concept of time is still embryonic, but children have some sense of timing in terms of anticipation, memory, and the limited ability to wait. They may listen to the command, "Just a minute," and behave appropriately. However, their sense of timing is exaggerated—1 minute can seem like an hour. Toddlers' limited attention spans also indicate their sense of immediacy and concern for the present.

Preconceptual Phase

At approximately 2 years of age the child enters the preconceptual phase of cognitive development, which lasts until about age 4 years. The preconceptual phase is a subdivision of the preoperational phase, which spans ages 2 to 7 years. The preconceptual phase is primarily one of transition that bridges the purely self-satisfying behavior of infancy and the rudimentary socialized behavior of latency. *Preoperational thought* implies that children cannot think in terms of *operations*—the ability to manipulate objects in relation to each other in a logical fashion. Rather, toddlers think primarily on the basis of their perception of an event. Problem solving is based on what they see or hear directly rather than on what they recall about objects and events. Several characteristics are unique to preoperational thought (Box 37-1).

Within the second year the child increasingly uses language symbolically and is concerned with the "why" and "how" of things. For example, a pencil is "something to write with," and food is "something to eat." However, such mental symbolization is closely associated with prelogical reasoning. For instance, a needle is "something that hurts." Such

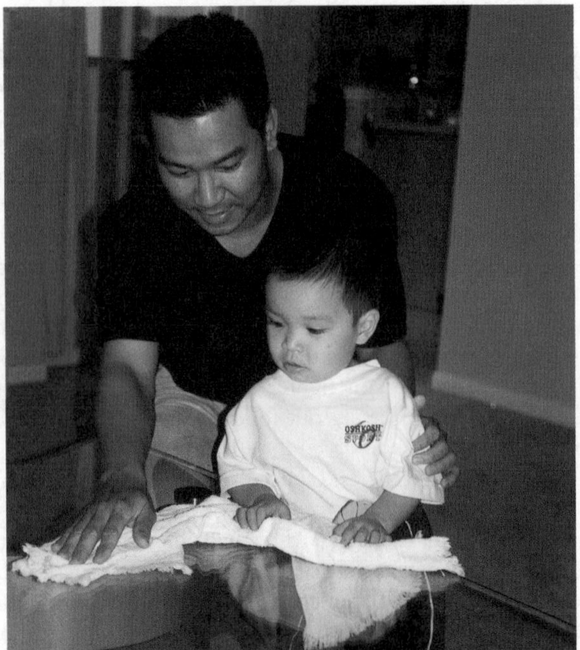

Fig. 37-2 Domestic mimicry and sex-role behavior are common during toddlerhood.

BOX 37-1

Characteristics of Preoperational Thought

Egocentrism—Inability to envision situations from perspectives other than one's own

Example: If a person is positioned between the toddler and another child, the toddler, who is facing the person, will explain that both children can see the middle person's face. The young child is unable to realize that the other person views the middle person from a different perspective, the back.

Implication: Avoid moralizing about "why" something is wrong if it requires an understanding of someone else's feelings or opinion. Telling a child to stop hitting because hitting hurts the other person is often ineffective because, to the aggressor, it feels good to hit someone else. Instead, emphasize that hitting is not allowed.

Transductive—Reasoning from the particular to the particular

Example: Child refuses to eat a food because something previously eaten did not taste good.

Implication: Accept child's reasoning; offer refused food at different time.

Global organization—Reasoning that changing any one part of the whole changes the entire whole

Example: Child refuses to sleep in room because location of bed is changed.

Implication: Accept child's reasoning; use same bed position or introduce change slowly.

Centration—Focusing on one aspect rather than considering all possible alternatives

Example: Child refuses to eat a food because of its color, even though its taste and smell are acceptable.

Implication: Accept child's reasoning.

Animism—Attributing lifelike qualities to inanimate objects

Example: Child scolds stairs for making child fall down.

Implication: Join child in the "scolding." Keep frightening objects out of view.

Irreversibility—Inability to undo or reverse the actions initiated physically

Example: When told to stop doing something, such as talking, child is unable to think of positive activity.

Implication: State requests or instructions *positively* (e.g., "Be quiet.")

Magical—Believing that thoughts are all-powerful and can cause events

Example: Child wishes someone died; then if the person dies, child feels at fault because of the "bad" thought that made the death happen.

Calling children "bad" because they did something wrong makes children feel as if they are bad.

Implication: Clarify that thoughts do not make things happen and that child is not responsible.

Use "I" messages rather than "you" messages to communicate thoughts, feelings, expectations, or beliefs without imposing blame or criticism. Emphasize that the act is bad, not the child.

Inability to conserve—Inability to understand the idea that a mass can be changed in size, shape, volume, or length without losing or adding to the original mass (instead, children judge what they see by the immediate perceptual clues given to them)

Example: If two lines of equal length are presented in such a way that one appears longer than the other, child will state that one line is longer even if child measures both lines with a ruler or yardstick and finds that each has the same length.

Implication: Change the most obvious perceptual clue to reorient child's view of what is seen. For example, give medicine in a small medicine cup, rather than a large cup, since child will imagine that the large vessel contains more liquid. If child refuses the medicine in the small cup, pour it into a large cup, because the liquid will appear to be less in a tall, wide container.

Give a large, flat cookie rather than a thick, small one, or do the reverse with meat or cheese; child will usually eat larger size of favorite food and smaller size of less favorite food.

painful experiences take on new significance because memory is associated with the specific event, and fears are likely to develop, such as resistance to people who wear a uniform or rooms that look like the practitioner's office. Because of the vulnerability of these early years, it is essential to prepare children for any new experience, whether it is a new babysitter or a visit to the dentist.

Spiritual Development

Toddlers learn about God through the words and the actions of those closest to them. They have only a vague idea of God and religious teachings because of their immature cognitive processes; however, if spoken about with reverence young children associate God with something special. They begin to assimilate behaviors associated with the divine (folding hands in prayer). Routines such as saying prayers before meals or at bedtime can be very important and comforting. Near the end of toddlerhood, when children use preoperational thought, there is some advancement of their understanding of God. Religious teachings, such as reward or fear of punishment (heaven or hell) and moral development (see Chapter 32), may influence their behavior (Fosarelli, 2003).

Development of Body Image

As in infancy, the development of body image closely parallels cognitive development. With increasing motor ability, toddlers recognize the usefulness of body parts and gradually learn their respective names. They also learn that certain parts of the body have various meanings; for example, during toilet training the genitals become significant and cleanliness is emphasized. By 2 years of age there is recognition of gender differences and reference to self by name and then by pronoun. Gender identity is developed by age 3 years. Also by this time the child begins to remember events with reference to their personal significance, forming an autobiographic memory that helps establish a continuous identity throughout life's events (Thompson, 2001).

Once they begin preoperational thought, toddlers can use symbols to represent objects, but their thinking may lead to inaccuracies. For example, if someone who is pregnant is called "fat," they will describe all "fat" women as having babies. There is a beginning recognition of words used to describe physical appearance, such as "pretty," "handsome," or "big boy." Such expressions eventually influence how children view their own bodies.

Although little research has been done on body-image development in young children, it is evident that body integrity is poorly understood and that intrusive experiences are threatening (Dahlquist et al, 2002). For example, toddlers forcefully resist procedures such as examining the ear or mouth and taking a rectal temperature. Toddlers also have unclear body boundaries and may associate nonviable parts, such as feces, with essential body parts. This can be seen in a toddler who is upset by flushing the toilet and watching the stool disappear.

Nurses can assist parents in fostering a positive body image in their child by encouraging them to avoid negative labels, such as "skinny arms" or "chubby legs," self-perceptions that can last a lifetime. Body parts, especially those related to elimination and reproduction, should be called by their correct names. Respect for the body should be practiced.

Development of Gender Identity

Just as toddlers explore their environment, they also explore their bodies and find that touching certain body parts is pleasurable. Genital fondling (masturbation) can occur and involves manual stimulation, as well as posturing movements (especially in young girls) such as tightening of the thighs or mechanical pressure applied to the pubic or suprapubic area. Other demonstrations of pleasurable activities include rocking, swinging, and hugging people and toys. During the activity the child may perspire and the activity may be difficult to interrupt. If performed in public the behavior should be ignored. The child should be taught that it is more acceptable to perform the behavior in private (Meyer, 2002).

Children in this age group are learning vocabulary associated with anatomy, elimination, and reproduction. Certain associations between words and functions become significant and can influence future sexual attitudes. For example, if parents refer to the genitals as dirty, especially in the context of elimination, this association between "genitals" and "dirty" may be transferred to sexual functions. Sex-role differences become obvious to children and are evident in much of their imitative play. A sense of maleness or femaleness, *gender identity,* is formed by age 3 years. Early attitudes are formed about affectionate behaviors between adults from observing parental and other adult sexual/sensual activities (see also Sex Education, Chapter 38). The quality of relationships with parents is important to the child's capacity for sexual and emotional relationships later in life (DeLamater & Friedrich, 2002).

Social Development

A major task of the toddler period is differentiation of self from significant others, usually the mother. The differentiation process consists of two phases: *separation,* the child's emergence from a symbiotic fusion with the mother; and *individuation,* those achievements that mark the child's assumptions of his or her individual characteristics in the environment. Although the process begins during the latter half of infancy, the major achievements occur during the toddler years.

Toddlers have an increased understanding and awareness of object permanence and some ability to withstand delayed gratification and tolerate moderate frustration. As a result, toddlers react differently to strangers than do infants. The appearance of unfamiliar persons does not represent such a significant threat to their attachment to mother. They have learned from experience that parents still exist when physically absent. Repetition of events such as going to bed without the parents, but waking to find them there again reinforces the reliability of such brief separations. Consequently, toddlers are able to venture away from their parents for brief periods of time because of the security of knowing that the parents will be there when they return.

Transitional objects, such as a favorite blanket or toy, provide security for children, especially when they are separated from parents, dealing with a new stress, or just fatigued (Fig. 37-3). Security objects often become so important to toddlers that they refuse to have them taken away. Such behavior is normal; there is no need to discourage this tendency. During separations such as day care, hospitalization, or even staying overnight with a relative, transitional objects should be provided to minimize any feelings of fear or loneliness.

Learning to tolerate and master brief periods of separation is an important developmental task of children in this age group. In addition, it is a necessary component of parenting, since brief periods of separation allow parents to recuperate their energy and patience and to minimize directing their irritations and frustrations at the children.

Language

The most striking characteristic of language development during early childhood is the increasing level of comprehension. Although the number of words acquired—from about 4 at 1 year of age to approximately 300 at age 2 years—is notable, *the ability to comprehend and understand speech is much greater than the number of words the child can say.* Bilingual children can also achieve their early linguistic milestones in each of the languages at the same time and produce a substantial number of semantically corresponding words in each of their two languages from the very first words or signs (Petitto et al, 2001).

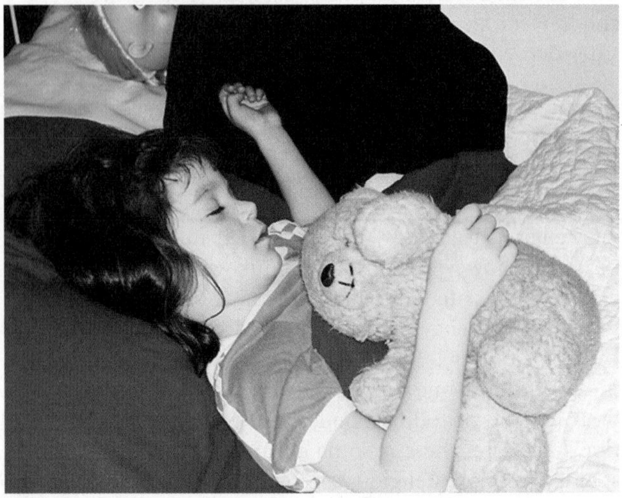

Fig. 37-3 Transitional objects, such as a fuzzy stuffed animal, are sources of security to a toddler.

At age 1 year the child uses one-word sentences or holophrases. The word "up" can mean "pick me up" or "look up there." For the child, the one word conveys the meaning of a sentence, but to others it may mean many things or nothing. At this age about 25% of the vocalizations are intelligible. By the age of 2 years the child uses multiword sentences by stringing together two or three words, such as the phrases, "mama go bye-bye" or "all gone," and approximately 65% of the speech is understandable. By 3 years the child puts words together into simple sentences, begins to master grammatical rules, and acquires 5 to 6 new words daily.

Gestures precede or accompany each of the language milestones up to 30 months of age (putting phone to ear, pointing). Once language is sufficiently mastered, gestures phase out and the pace of word learning increases (Bates & Dick, 2002).

Personal-Social Behavior

One of the most dramatic aspects of development in the toddler is personal-social interaction. Parents often wonder why their manageable, docile, lovable infant has turned into a determined, strong-willed, volatile-tempered little tyrant. In addition, the tyrant of the terrible twos can swiftly and unpredictably revert back to the adorable infant. All of this is part of "growing up" and is evident in such areas as dressing, feeding, playing, and establishing self-control.

Toddlers are developing skills of independence, and these are evident in all areas of behavior. By 15 months children feed themselves, drink well from a covered cup, and manage a spoon with considerable spilling. By 24 months they use a spoon well and by 36 months may be using a fork. Between ages 2 and 3 years they eat with the family and like to help with chores such as setting the table or removing dishes from the dishwasher; however, they lack table manners and may find it difficult to sit through the family's entire meal.

In dressing, toddlers also demonstrate strides in independence. The 15-month-old child helps by putting the arm or foot out for dressing and pulls shoes and socks off. The 18-month-old child removes gloves, helps with pullover shirts, and may be able to unzip. By age 2 years the toddler removes most articles of clothing and puts on socks, shoes, and pants without regard for right or left and back or front. Help is still needed to fasten clothes.

Toddlers also begin to develop concern for the feelings of others and develop an understanding of how adult expectations for behavior apply to specific situations (causing a sibling to cry while playing rough) (Thompson, 2001). As their understanding is fostered, they are able to develop control. Age-appropriate discipline contributes to healthy social and emotional development. Positive reinforcement, redirecting, and time-out are appropriate for most toddlers. It is recognized that social and emotional problems can develop in the youngest children. Early screening and intervention promotes more positive developmental outcomes as the young child grows and develops.

Play

Play magnifies the toddler's physical and psychosocial development. Interaction with people becomes increasingly important. The solitary play of infancy progresses to *parallel play*—the toddler plays alongside, not with, other children. Although sensorimotor play is still prominent, there is much less emphasis on the exclusive use of one sensory modality. The toddler inspects the toy, talks to the toy, tests it strength and durability, and invents several uses for it. Imitation is one of the most distinguishing characteristics of play and enriches the child's opportunity to engage in fantasy. With less emphasis on gender-stereotyped toys, play objects such as dolls, carriages, dollhouses, dishes, cooking utensils, child-size furniture, trucks, and dress-up clothes (Fig. 37-4) are suitable for both genders; however, boys may be more interested than girls in activities related to trucks, trailers, men, and logs, whereas girls may prefer doll-related activities.

Increased locomotive skills make push-pull toys, straddle trucks or cycles, a small gym and slide, balls of various sizes, and rocking horses appropriate for the energetic toddler. Finger paints; thick crayons; chalk; a blackboard; paper; and puzzles with large, simple pieces use the child's developing fine motor skills. Interlocking blocks in various sizes and shapes provide hours of fun and, during later years, are useful objects for creative and imaginative play. The most educational toy is the one that fosters the interaction of an adult with a child in supportive, unconditional play. Toys are never substitutes for the attention of devoted caregivers, but toys can enhance these interactions (Glassy & Romano, 2003).

Certain aspects of play are related to emerging linguistic abilities. Talking is a form of play for toddlers who enjoy musical toys such as age-appropriate cassette tape players, "talking" dolls and animals, and toy telephones. Appropriate children's television programs are excellent for children in this age group, who learn to associate words with visual images. However, total media time should be limited to 1 to 2 hours of quality programming per day (American Academy of Pediatrics [AAP], Committee on Public Health, 2001). Toddlers also enjoy "reading" stories from a picture book and imitating the sounds of animals.

Tactile play is also important for the exploring toddler. Water toys, a sandbox with pail and shovel, finger paints, soap bubbles, and clay provide excellent opportunities for creative and manipulative recreation. Adults sometimes forget the fascination of feeling slippery cream, such as whipped cream or pudding; catching airy bubbles; squeezing and reshaping clay; or smearing paints. These types of unstructured activities are as important as educational play to allow children freedom of expression.

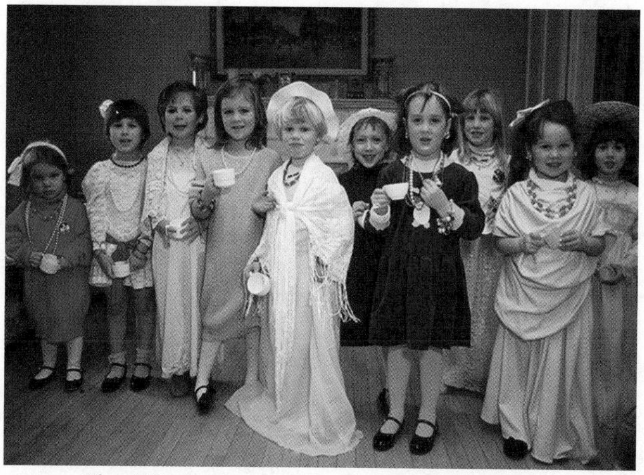

Fig. 37-4 Young children enjoy dressing up.

Selection of appropriate toys must involve safety factors, especially in relation to size and sturdiness. The oral activity of toddlers puts them at risk for aspirating small objects or for ingesting toxic substances. Parents need to be especially vigilant of toys of older siblings, or those played with in other children's homes. Toys are a potential source of serious bodily damage to toddlers who may have the physical strength to manipulate them but not the knowledge to appreciate their danger (see the Home Care box on p. 951).

The major features of growth and development for the age groups of 15, 18, 24, and 30 months are summarized in Table 37-1.

Coping with Concerns Related to Normal Growth and Development

Toilet Training

CASE STUDY: TOILET TRAINING/TODDLER DEVELOPMENT

One of the major tasks of toddlerhood is toilet training. Voluntary control of the anal and urethral sphincters is achieved sometime after the child is walking, probably between ages 18 and 24 months. However, complex psychophysiologic factors are required for readiness. The child must be able to recognize the urge to let go and hold on and be able to communicate this sensation to the parent. In addition, there may be some necessary motivation in the desire to please the parent by holding on, rather than pleasing oneself by letting go.

Usually, physiologic and psychologic readiness for toilet training is not complete until 18 to 24 months of age. By this time, the child has mastered the majority of essential gross motor skills, can communicate intelligibly, is less in conflict with self-assertion and negativism, and is aware of the ability to control the body and please the parent. Helping parents identify the right time to initiate training can alleviate stress and anxiety for the child that could prolong the toilet training process. There is not a universal right age to begin toilet training or an absolute deadline to complete training. One of the most important responsibilities of nurses is to help parents identify the readiness signs in their child (Guidelines box).*

Nighttime bladder control normally takes several months to years after daytime training. This is because the sleep cycle needs to mature so the child can awake in time to urinate. Few children will have night wetting episodes after daytime dryness is achieved; however, those children that do not have nighttime dryness by the age of 6 years are likely to require intervention (Mercer, 2003).

Bowel training is usually accomplished before bladder training because of its greater regularity and predictability. There is a stronger sensation for defecation than for urination, and the sensation of defecation can be brought to the child's attention. A well-balanced diet that includes dietary fiber helps keep stool soft and supports the development and maintenance of regular bowel movements.

A number of techniques can be helpful when initiating training. One is the selection of a potty chair and/or use of the toilet. A freestanding potty chair allows children a feeling of security. Planting the feet firmly on the floor also facilitates defecation. Another option is a portable seat attached to the regular toilet, which may ease the transition from potty chair to regular toilet. Placing a small bench under the feet helps to stabilize the child's position. It is probably best to keep the potty chair in the bathroom and to let the child observe the excreta being flushed down the toilet to associate these activities with usual practices. If a potty chair seat is not available, having the child sit facing the toilet tank provides added support. Boys may begin toilet training in the stand-up position or by sitting on a potty chair or toilet (Fig. 37-5).

Practice sessions should be limited to 5 or 10 minutes; a parent should stay with the child, and sanitary habits should be employed after every session. Children should be praised for cooperative behavior and/or successful evacuation. Dressing children in easily removed clothing; using training pants, "pull-on" diapers, or panties; and encouraging imitation by watching others are other helpful suggestions.

When the child begins to show regular daytime dryness, parents may experiment with underwear during the day. Daytime accidents are common, particularly during periods of intense activity. Young children become so engrossed in play activity that if they are not reminded, they will wait until it is too late to reach the bathroom. Therefore, frequent reminders and trips to the toilet are necessary.

As the child develops each step of toileting (discussion, undressing, going, wiping, dressing, flushing, and handwashing), he or she gains a sense of accomplishment that should be reinforced by parents. If the parent-child relation-

> **Guidelines**
>
> **ASSESSING TOILET TRAINING READINESS**
>
> **Physical Readiness**
>
> Voluntary control of anal and urethral sphincters, usually by 18 to 24 months of age
> Ability to stay dry for 2 hours; decreased number of wet diapers; waking dry from nap
> Regular bowel movements
> Gross motor skills of sitting, walking, and squatting
> Fine motor skills to remove clothing
>
> **Mental Readiness**
>
> Recognizes urge to defecate or urinate
> Verbal or nonverbal communicative skills to indicate when wet or has urge to defecate or urinate
> Cognitive skills to imitate appropriate behavior and follow directions
>
> **Psychologic Readiness**
>
> Expresses willingness to please parent
> Able to sit on toilet for 5 to 10 minutes without fussing or getting off
> Curiosity about adults' or older sibling's toilet habits
> Impatience with soiled or wet diapers; desire to be changed immediately
>
> **Parental Readiness**
>
> Recognizes child's level of readiness
> Willing to invest the time required for toilet training
> Absence of family stress or change, such as a divorce, moving, new sibling, or imminent vacation

*A helpful book is *Guide to Toilet Training,* available from American Academy of Pediatrics, 888-227-1770; Web site: www.aap.org/bookstore.

ship becomes strained, both may need a break to focus on enjoyable activities together. Regression may coincide with a stressful family situation or if the child is being pushed too hard and too fast. Regression is a normal part of toilet training and does not mean failure but should be viewed as a temporary setback to a more comfortable place for the child.

Day care providers also play a role in the support and education of parents regarding toilet training practices. It is important for parents to inform all caregivers of their individual family values and the child's specific needs when planning for training away from home. Ensuring consistency in care of the toddler as well as ensuring healthy practices in a sanitary environment allow for safe and effective toilet practices in all settings.

Sibling Rivalry

The natural jealousy and resentment of children to a new child in the family is referred to as *sibling rivalry.* The arrival of a new infant represents a crisis for even the best-prepared toddlers. It is not the infant that toddlers resent but the changes that this additional sibling produces, especially the separation from mother during the birth. The parents now share their love and attention with someone else, the usual routine is disrupted, and toddlers may lose their crib and/or room, all at a time when they thought they were in control of their world. Sibling rivalry tends to be most pronounced in the firstborn, who experiences *dethronement* (i.e., loss of sole parental attention). It also seems to be most difficult for young children, particularly in terms of mother-child interaction.

Preparation of children for the birth of a sibling is quite individual, but age dictates some important considerations. Time for toddlers is a vague concept. Tomorrow could be yesterday or next week, and a month from now could be never. Preparing children too soon for the birth may lessen their interest by the time the event occurs. A good time to start talking about the new baby is when the toddler becomes aware of the pregnancy and the changes taking place in the home in anticipation of the new member.

Toddlers need to have a realistic idea of what the newborn will be like. Telling them that a new playmate will come home soon sets up unrealistic expectations. Rather, parents should stress the activities that will take place when the baby arrives home, such as diapering, bottle- or breastfeeding, bathing, and dressing. At the same time, parents should emphasize which routines will stay the same, such as reading stories or going to the park. If toddlers have had no contact with an infant, it is a good idea to introduce them to one, if feasible.

A new sibling in the home is stressful, so any additional stresses for the toddler should be avoided or minimized. For example, moving the toddler to a regular bed or to a different room should be done well in advance of the infant's arrival.

Pregnancy is an abstraction for toddlers. They need concrete illustrations of how the baby is growing inside the mother. It is an excellent opportunity for introducing aspects of reproduction and sexuality. Seeing simple pictures of the uterus and fetus and feeling the fetus move help the child feel involved in the experience (see Fig. 11-3). Children also benefit from classes for siblings that may be part of prenatal sessions (see Fig. 11-4).

When the newborn arrives, toddlers keenly feel the changed focus of attention. Visitors may initiate problems when they inadvertently shower the infant with attention and presents while neglecting the older child. Parents can minimize this by alerting visitors to the toddler's needs, by having small presents on hand for the toddler, and by including the child in the visits as much as possible. The toddler can also help with the care of the newborn by getting diapers and doing other small tasks (Fig. 37-6).

How children exhibit jealousy is complex. Some will overtly hit the infant, push the child off the mother's lap, or pull the bottle or breast from the infant's mouth. More often the expressions of hostility and resentment are more subtle and covert. Toddlers may verbally express a wish that the infant "go back inside mommy," or they will revert to more infantile forms of behavior, such as demanding a bottle, soiling their underpants, clinging for attention, using baby talk, or aggressively acting out toward others. For this reason, infants must be protected by parental supervision of the interaction between the siblings.

Temper Tantrums

Toddlers may assert their independence by violently objecting to discipline. They may lie down on the floor, kick their feet, and scream as loud as possible. Some have learned the effectiveness of holding their breath until the parent relents. Although holding one's breath may cause fainting from lack of oxygen, the accumulation of carbon dioxide will stimulate the respiratory control center, resulting in no physical harm.

The best approach toward tapering temper tantrums requires consistency and developmentally appropriate expectations and rewards. Ensuring consistency among all caregivers in expectations, prioritizing what rules are important, and developing consequences that are reasonable for the child's level of development help manage the behavior. For example, a popular time for a tantrum is before bed. Active toddlers often have trouble slowing down and, when placed in bed, resist staying there. Parents can reinforce consistency and expectations by stating, "After this story it is bedtime." Starting at 18 months, time-outs work well for managing temper tantrums.

During tantrums ignore the behavior, provided the behavior is not injurious to the child, such as violently banging the head on the floor. Continue to be present to provide a feeling of control and security to the child once the tantrum has subsided. At this time a toy or a favorite activity can be substituted for the request. (See also Limit Setting and Discipline, Chapter 31.) During periods of no tantrums, practice developmentally appropriate positive reinforcement.

Negativism

One of the more difficult aspects of rearing children in this age group is their persistent "no" response to every request. The negativism is not an expression of being stubborn or insolent, but a necessary assertion of self-control. One method of dealing with the negativism is to reduce the opportunities for a "no" answer. Asking the child, "Do you want to go to sleep now?" is an almost certain example of a question that will be answered with an emphatic "no." Instead, tell the child that it is time to go to sleep and proceed accordingly.

Table 37-1

Growth and Development during Toddler Years

AGE (MONTHS)	PHYSICAL	GROSS MOTOR	FINE MOTOR
15	Steady growth in height and weight Head circumference 48 cm (19 in) Weight 11 kg (24 lb) Height 78.7 cm (31 in)	Walks without help (usually since age 13 mo) Creeps up stairs Kneels without support Cannot walk around corners or stop suddenly without losing balance Assumes standing position without support Cannot throw ball without falling	Constantly casting objects to floor Builds tower of two cubes Holds two cubes in one hand Releases a pellet into a narrow-necked bottle Scribbles spontaneously Uses cup well but rotates spoon
18	Physiologic anorexia from decreased growth needs Anterior fontanel closed Physiologically able to control sphincters	Runs clumsily; falls often Walks up stairs with one hand held Pulls and pushes toys Jumps in place with both feet Seats self on chair Throws ball overhand without falling	Builds tower of three or four cubes Release, prehension, and reach well developed Turns pages in a book two or three at a time In drawing, makes stroke imitatively Manages spoon without rotation
24	Head circumference 49-50 cm (19.5-20 in) Chest circumference exceeds head circumference Lateral diameter of chest exceeds anteroposterior diameter Usual weight gain of 1.8-2.7 kg (4-6 lb) Usual gain in height of 10-12.5 cm (4-5 in) Adult height approximately double height at 2 years of age May have achieved readiness for beginning daytime control of bowel and bladder Primary dentition of 16 teeth	Goes up and down stairs alone with two feet on each step Runs fairly well, with wide stance Picks up object without falling Kicks ball forward without overbalancing	Builds tower of six or seven cubes Aligns two or more cubes like a train Turns pages of book one at a time In drawing, imitates vertical and circular strokes Turns doorknob; unscrews lid
30	Birth weight quadrupled Primary dentition (20 teeth) completed May have daytime bowel and bladder control	Jumps with both feet Jumps from chair or step Stands on one foot momentarily Takes a few steps on tiptoe	Builds tower of eight cubes Adds chimney to train of cubes Good hand-finger coordination; holds crayon with fingers rather than fist Moves fingers independently In drawing, imitates vertical and horizontal strokes; makes two or more strokes for cross

In their attempt to exert control, children like to make choices. When confronted with appropriate choices, such as "You may have a peanut-butter-and-jelly sandwich or chicken-noodle soup for lunch," they are more likely to choose one rather than automatically say no. However, if their response is negative, parents should make the choice for the child.

Regression

The retreat from one's present pattern of functioning to past levels of behavior is referred to as regression. It usually occurs in instances of discomfort or stress when one attempts to conserve psychic energy by reverting to patterns of behavior that were successful in earlier stages of development.

SENSORY	LANGUAGE	SOCIALIZATION
Able to identify geometric forms; places round object into appropriate hole Binocular vision well developed Displays an intense and prolonged interest in pictures	Uses expressive jargon Says four to six words, including names "Asks" for objects by pointing Understands simple commands May use head-shaking gesture to denote "no" Uses "no" even while agreeing to the request	Tolerates some separation from parent Less likely to fear strangers Beginning to imitate parents, such as cleaning house (sweeping, dusting), folding clothes May discard bottle Manages spoon but rotates it near mouth Kisses and hugs parents; may kiss pictures in a book Expresses emotions; has temper tantrums
	Says 10 or more words Points to a common object, such as a shoe or ball, and to two or three body parts	Great imitator (domestic mimicry) Takes off gloves, socks, and shoes and unzips Temper tantrums may be more evident Beginning awareness of ownership ("my toy") May develop dependency on transitional objects, such as "security blanket"
Accommodation well developed In geometric discrimination, able to insert square block into oblong space	Has vocabulary of approximately 300 words Uses 2- or 3-word phrases Uses pronouns "I," "me," "you" Understands directional commands Gives first name; refers to self by name Verbalizes need for toileting, food, or drink Talks incessantly	Stage of parallel play Has sustained attention span Temper tantrums decreasing Pulls people to show them something Increased independence from parent Dresses self in simple clothing
	Gives first and last name Refers to self by appropriate pronoun Uses plurals Names one color	Separates more easily from parent In play, helps put things away; can carry breakable objects; pushes with good steering Begins to notice sex differences; knows own sex May attend to toilet needs without help except for wiping

Regression is common in toddlers because almost any additional stress hinders their ability to master present developmental tasks. Any threat to their autonomy, such as illness, hospitalization, separation, or adjustment to a sibling, represents a need to revert to earlier forms of behavior, such as increased dependency; refusal to use the potty chair; temper tantrums; demand for the bottle, stroller, or crib; and loss of newly learned motor, language, social, and cognitive skills.

At first, such regression appears acceptable and comfortable for children. The loss of newly acquired achievements is actually frightening and threatening because children are aware of their helplessness. Parents become concerned about

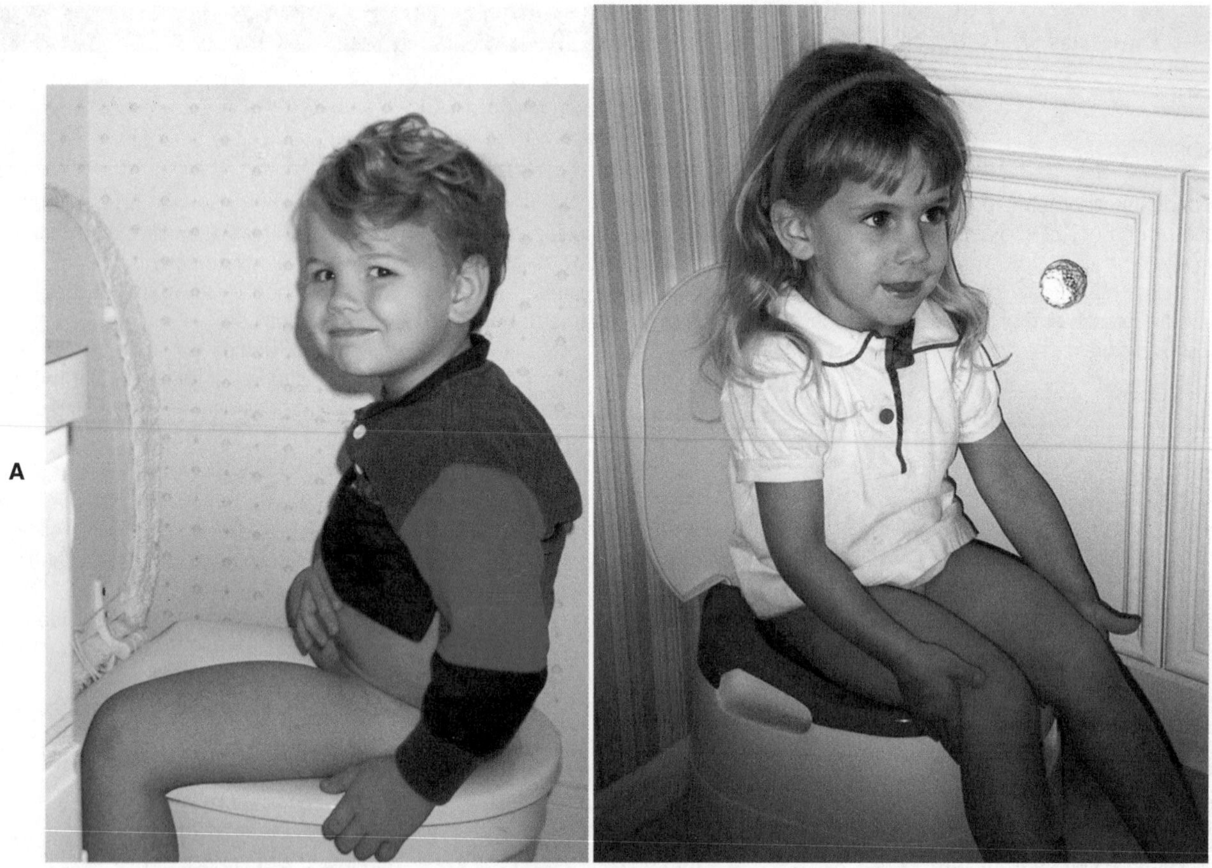

Fig. 37-5 **A,** Sitting in reverse fashion on a regular toilet provides additional security to a young child. **B,** Children may begin toilet training sitting on a small toilet.

regressive behavior and often, in their efforts to deal with it, force the child to cope with an additional source of stress—the pressure to live up to expected standards. Brazelton (1999) suggests that these predictable times of regression, or *touchpoints,* are an opportunity to prepare parents for the next step in their child's development.

When regression does occur, the best approach is to ignore it while praising existing patterns of appropriate behavior. Regression is a child's way of saying, "I can't cope with this present stress and perfect this skill as well, but I will if given patience and understanding." For this reason, it is advisable not to attempt new areas of learning when an additional crisis is present or expected, such as beginning toilet training shortly before a sibling is born or attempting new areas of learning during a brief period of hospitalization.

PROMOTING OPTIMUM HEALTH DURING TODDLERHOOD

Nutrition

During the period from 12 to 18 months of age, the growth rate slows, decreasing the child's need for calories, protein, and fluid. However, the protein (1.2 g/kg) and caloric (102 kcal/kg) requirements are still relatively high to meet the demands for muscle tissue growth and high activity level (Picciano et al, 2000). The need for minerals such as iron, calcium, and phosphorus is still high, particularly when one considers the poor food habits of children in this age group and the increased mineralization within bones.

At approximately 18 months of age, most toddlers manifest this decreased nutritional need with a decrease in appetite, a phenomenon known as *physiologic anorexia.* They become picky, fussy eaters with strong taste preferences. Toddlers are increasingly aware of the nonnutritive function of food: the pleasure of eating, the social aspect of mealtime, and the control of refusing food. They are influenced by factors other than taste when choosing food. If a family member refuses to eat something, toddlers are likely to imitate that response. If the plate is overfilled, they are likely to push it away, overwhelmed by its size. In essence, mealtime is more closely associated with psychologic components than with nutritional ones.

Many authorities consider this period of picky eating to be a developmental phase and stress that most toddlers will consume the necessary amount of food required for growth (Cathey & Gaylord, 2004).

Developmentally, by 12 months of age most children are eating the same food prepared for the rest of the family. Some may have mastered using a cup with occasional spilling, although most cannot adeptly use a spoon until 18 months of age or later and generally prefer using their fingers.

Nutritional Counseling

Eating habits established in the first 2 or 3 years of life tend to have lasting effects on subsequent years. If food is

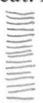

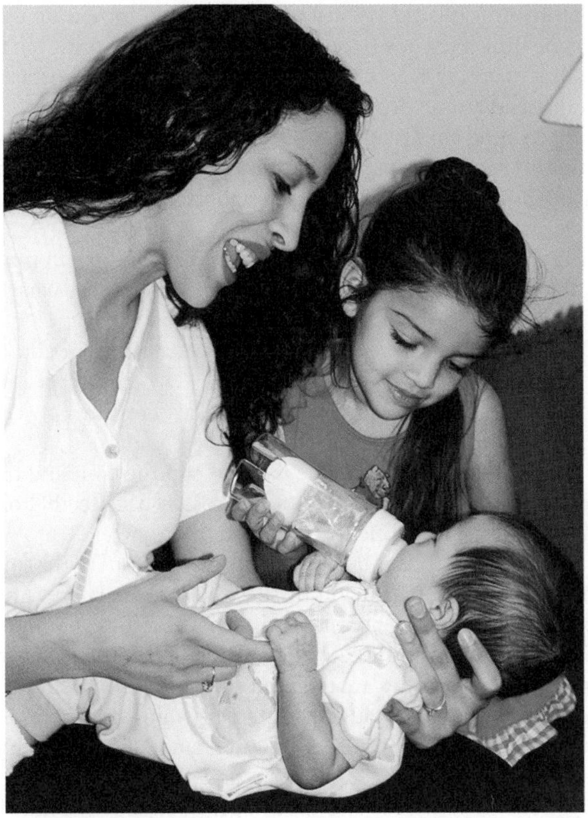

Fig. 37-6 To minimize sibling rivalry, parents should include the toddler during caregiving activities.

used as a reward or sign of approval, a child may overeat for nonnutritive reasons. If food is forced and mealtime is consistently unpleasant, the usual pleasure associated with eating may not develop. Mealtimes should be enjoyable rather than times for discipline or family arguments. The social aspect of mealtime may be distracting for young children; therefore, an earlier feeding hour may be appropriate. Young children are unable to sit through a long meal and become restless and disruptive. This is particularly common when children are brought to the table just after active play.

The method of serving food also takes on more importance during this period. Toddlers need to have a sense of control and achievement in their abilities. Giving them large, adult-size portions can be overwhelming. In general, what is eaten is much more significant than how much is consumed. Small amounts of meat and vegetables supply greater food value than a large consumption of bread or potato. Serving sizes need to be appropriate for age (Box 37-2). See also Chapter 47 pp. 1486-1487 regarding the new Dietary Guidelines for Americans and the MyPyramid food guide, which applies to children as young as 2 years of age.

Substitutions can be provided for foods that they do not enjoy, although this practice should not cater to all of their desires. Providing frequent nutritious *planned* snacks may provide adequate caloric intake at this age. *Planned grazing*—nibbling and snacking—is a good way to ensure proper nutrition, provided that appropriate foods are offered; giving the child something to eat merely to pacify is not recommended.

BOX 37-2

Sample Menu for Toddlers Based on Dietary Guidelines for Americans–2005*

Breakfast	½ cup dry, unsweetened cereal
	½ cup orange juice
	4 oz low-fat milk†
Snack	½-1 whole banana
Lunch	1 tbsp peanut butter
	2 tsp all-fruit preserves
	1 slice whole-wheat bread
	2 tbsp peas
	4 oz low-fat milk†
Snack	2 graham crackers
	4 oz low-fat milk†
Dinner	1 chicken leg, roasted without skin
	¼-½ cup macaroni and cheese
	2 tbsp green beans, cooked
	2 tbsp carrots, cooked
	4-6 oz low-fat milk†
Snack	½ cup frozen yogurt

Daily Amount‡

Bread, cereal, rice, pasta	5-6 oz
Vegetables	1.5 cups
Fruits	1.5 cups
Milk, yogurt, cheese	2 cups
Meat, poultry, dried beans, eggs, fish, nuts	4 oz

*Use fats, oils, and sweets sparingly. Increase fluids with servings of water. Serving sizes are minimums for nutritional adequacy. Many children eat more.

†Substitute whole milk if child is younger than 24 months.

‡Based on a 2-3 year old, active lifestyle, 1400 cal/day intake (www.mypyramid.gov)

NURSE ALERT To determine serving size for young children, use the following guidelines:
- A general guide to the serving size of food is 1 tablespoon of solid food per year of age or one-fourth to one-third of the adult portion size.
- Use the tablespoon guide for easily measured foods such as vegetables or rice.
- Use the fraction guide for bread or milk. ■

The ritualism of this age also dictates certain principles in feeding practices. Toddlers like the same dish, cup, or spoon every time they eat. They may reject a favorite food simply because it is served in a different utensil. If one food touches another, they often refuse to eat it. For some children a regular mealtime schedule also helps satisfy their desire and need for predictability and ritualism.

Most children by 12 months of age are eating the same food prepared for the rest of the family. However, appetite and food preferences are sporadic. Often the interest in food parallels a growth spurt, so that periods of good eating are interspersed with phases of poor eating. Food "jags" are common.

This period can be a trying one for parents and child alike. Because eating habits are established in early life and affect not only the child's future eating habits but also the child's health as an adolescent and adult, it is recommended that toddlers not be forced to eat foods they are reluctant to eat. Evidence indicates that toddlers are able to regulate their hunger and satiety needs internally and that forcing foods during this period may exacerbate or lead to future eating problems (Cathey & Gaylord, 2004).

Sleep and Activity

Total sleep decreases only slightly during the second year and averages about 12 hours a day. Most children take one nap a day, and by the end of the second or third year many relinquish this habit. Children reach an adult pattern of sleep by 3 years of age (Howard & Wong, 2001).

The activity level is high, and too little physical exercise is rarely a problem provided inappropriate restrictions are not instituted. With increasing numbers of young children being cared for outside the home, attention to the kinds of activity provided is important. For example, children with high activity levels may benefit from an environment in which outdoor play is encouraged.

Sleep problems are common, especially going to bed and falling asleep, and are probably related to fears of separation. Bedtime rituals (e.g., same hour of sleep, snack, and quiet activity) are helpful; and transitional objects, such as a favorite stuffed animal or blanket, can help ease the child's insecurity at bedtime (see Fig. 37-3).

Dental Health

Regular Dental Examinations

The AAP Section on Pediatric Dentistry (2003) now recommends that every child have an oral health examination by a practitioner by 6 months of age. If the child is in a high risk category for caries, an initial visit to a dentist or pedodontist (pediatric dentist) by age 6 months or within 6 months of the eruption of the first tooth is recommended. Initial visits to the dentist should be nontraumatizing. Because toddlers react negatively to new and potentially frightening experiences, the initial visit can center around meeting the dentist, seeing the equipment, and sitting in the chair. If the child is cooperative, the dentist may just look at the teeth but reserve a more thorough examination for another visit. Modeling, in which the child observes procedures performed on the parent or a cooperative sibling, can also be effective.

Removal of Plaque

Oral hygiene measures should be implemented as noted above to remove plaque, soft bacterial deposits that adhere to the teeth and cause *dental caries* (decay or cavities) and *periodontal* (gum) *disease*. Poor oral hygiene and poor dietary habits are associated with the development of caries in children. The most effective methods for plaque removal are brushing and flossing. Several brushing techniques exist, although there is no universal agreement regarding the best method. One that is suitable for cleaning the primary teeth is the scrub method. The tips of the bristles are placed firmly at a 45-degree angle against the teeth and gums and moved back and forth in a vibratory motion. The ends of the bristles should be wiggling but not moving forcefully back and forth, which can damage the gums and enamel. All the surfaces of the teeth are cleaned in this manner except the lingual (inner) surfaces of the anterior teeth. To clean these surfaces, the toothbrush is placed vertical to the teeth and moved up and down. Only a few teeth are brushed at one time, using six to eight strokes for each section. A systematic approach is used so that all surfaces are thoroughly cleaned (Fig. 37-7).

For young children, the most effective cleaning is done by parents (Fig. 37-8). Several positions can be used that facilitate access to the mouth and help stabilize the head for comfort:

- Stand with child's back toward adult. (When done in front of a bathroom mirror, both child and adult can see what is being done in the mirror.)
- Sit on a couch or bed with child's head resting in adult's lap.
- Sit on the floor or a stool with child's head resting between adult's thighs.

With all positions, use one hand to cup the chin and the other to brush the teeth. For easier access to back teeth, hold the mouth partially open.

For effective cleaning, a small toothbrush with soft, rounded, multitufted nylon bristles that are short and uniform in length is recommended. Nylon bristles dry more rapidly after use and retain their shape better than natural bristles. Toothbrushes are replaced as soon as the bristles are frayed or bent. With young children, brushing may be more easily accomplished using only water, since many children dislike the foam from toothpaste and the foam interferes with visibility. There is also the danger of swallowing fluoridated toothpaste (see following discussion under Fluoride). When using toothpaste, children should select the flavor they like to encourage the brushing habit.

After the teeth have been cleaned, flossing with dental floss is done to remove plaque and debris from between the teeth and below the gum margin, where brushing is ineffective. Since young children do not have the dexterity to manipulate the floss, parents are taught the procedure.

A disclosing agent is helpful in identifying those areas of the teeth where plaque accumulates. It also helps motivate children to clean their teeth because plaque is difficult to see. After cleaning, the mouth is inspected to ensure that all traces of plaque have been removed. Where plaque remains, the teeth are rebrushed.

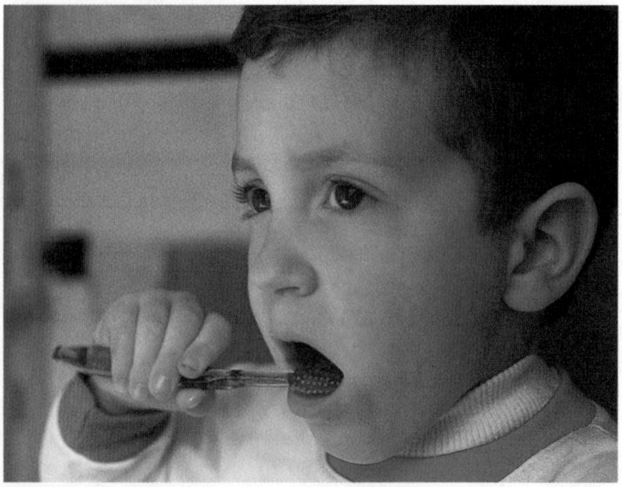

Fig. 37-7 Young children can participate in toothbrushing, but parents need to brush all the child's teeth thoroughly.

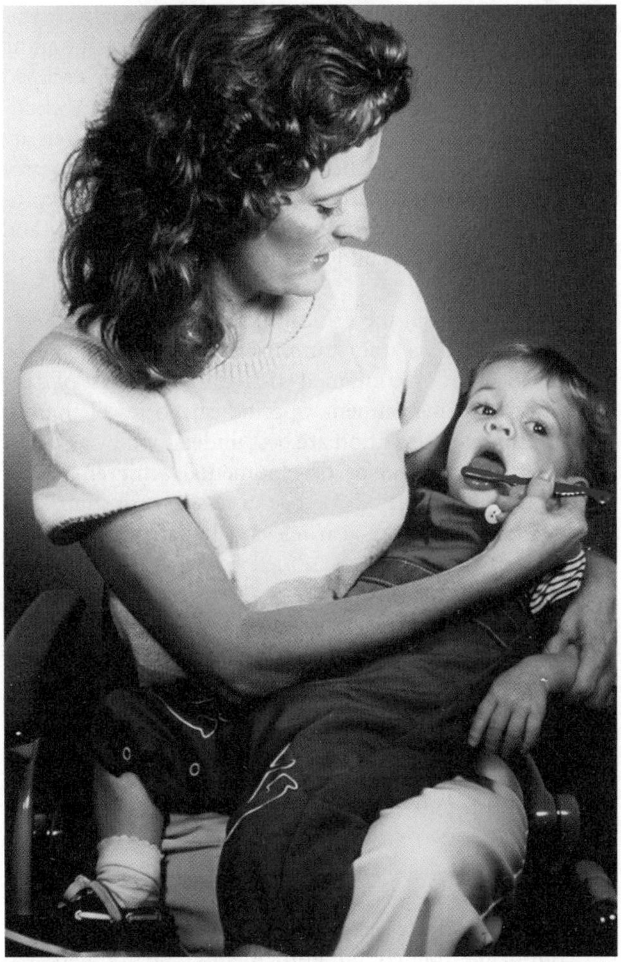

Fig. 37-8 The most effective cleaning of the teeth is done by parents.

Ideally, the teeth should be cleaned after each meal and especially before bedtime, and the child should be given nothing to eat or drink after the night brushing except water. At those times when brushing is impractical, the "swish-and-swallow" method of cleaning the mouth is taught: with a mouthful of water the child rinses the mouth and swallows, repeating the procedure three or four times.*

Fluoride

Fluoride supplementation should be considered for any child over the age of 6 months whose drinking water is deficient in fluoride. Supplementation based on fluoride concentration of water supply <0.3 parts per million is 0.25 mg for a child age 6 months to 3 years of age (American Academy of Pediatric Dentistry, 1999).

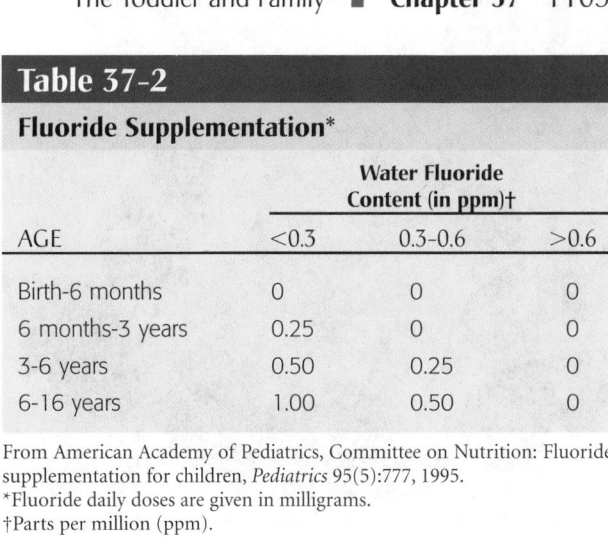

Fluoride, a mineral, is found in water, foods, or drinks in which fluoridated water was used as part of the processing system. Because the water fluoridation process and manufacturing of fluoride toothpaste are almost impossible to standardize in the United States, the dosage of fluoride supplements has been lowered to reduce the incidence of fluorosis (Table 37-2). Increased fluoride ingestion leads to enamel protein retention, hypomineralization of the enamel and dentin, and disturbance of crystal formation. The effects caused by this change range from barely discernible white fiberlike lines or spots to gray-brown stains or pitted areas.

Nurses have a responsibility to ensure an optimal fluoride regimen for children and to counsel families regarding correct use of supplements. The nurse should have knowledge of the fluoride content of the community water supply and provide instruction to parents regarding correct administration of fluoride drops or tablets. Supplements should remain in the mouth for 30 seconds before swallowing and be taken on an empty stomach. Afterward the child should not drink or eat for 30 minutes. All fluoride products (toothpaste, supplements, and rinse) need to be stored away from young children to prevent poisoning. If the water supply is fluoridated, parents are encouraged to use water to prepare drinks and foods.

*More detailed information can be obtained by contacting the American Academy of Pediatric Dentistry Web site: www.aapd.org.

Table 37-2

Fluoride Supplementation*

	Water Fluoride Content (in ppm)†		
AGE	<0.3	0.3-0.6	>0.6
Birth-6 months	0	0	0
6 months-3 years	0.25	0	0
3-6 years	0.50	0.25	0
6-16 years	1.00	0.50	0

From American Academy of Pediatrics, Committee on Nutrition: Fluoride supplementation for children, *Pediatrics* 95(5):777, 1995.
*Fluoride daily doses are given in milligrams.
†Parts per million (ppm).

Low-Cariogenic Diet

Diet is critical to developing good teeth because carious development depends primarily on fermentable sugars, especially sucrose. Refined table sugar, honey, molasses, corn syrup, and dried fruits such as raisins are highly cariogenic.

Ideally, such foods should be eliminated. However, since this is impractical, some suggestions can be helpful. First, *the frequency with which sugar is consumed is more important than the total amount eaten.* Therefore, when sweets are eaten, they are less damaging if consumed immediately after a meal rather than as a snack between meals. When sweets are served as the dessert, the teeth can be cleaned afterward, decreasing the amount of time the sugar is in the mouth.

Second, the form of sugar is important. The more cariogenic foods are those that are sticky or hard, since they remain in the mouth longer. Consequently, sucking on lollipops is more cariogenic than eating a chocolate bar. Sometimes the source of the sugar is "hidden," such as in numerous prescription and nonprescription drugs and in many popular cereals, including the "all-natural" variety. Reading food labels is essential in identifying and eliminating sources of sucrose.

A special form of tooth decay in children between 18 months and 3 years of age is *nursing caries* (also called *nursing bottle caries* or *bottle-mouth caries*); this occurs when the child is routinely given a bottle of milk or juice at nap- or

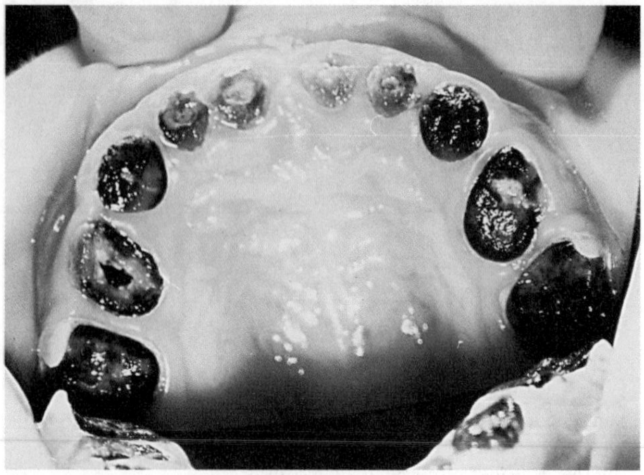

Fig. 37-9 Nursing caries. Note extensive carious involvement of maxillary primary incisors. (Courtesy Bruce Carter, DDS, Texas Children's Hospital, Houston, Texas.)

bedtime or uses the bottle as a pacifier while awake. Frequent nocturnal breastfeeding for prolonged periods also leads to extensive destruction of the teeth. The practice of coating pacifiers in honey can also contribute to caries and may be a potential source of botulism poisoning. As the sweet liquid pools in the mouth, the teeth are bathed for several hours in this cariogenic environment. The maxillary (upper) incisors and molars are affected most, since the mandibular (lower) incisors are protected by the lower lip, tongue, and saliva (Fig. 37-9). Severely decayed teeth may require the application of stainless steel bands to preserve the spacing until the permanent teeth erupt.

Prevention involves eliminating the bedtime bottle completely, feeding the last bottle before bedtime, substituting a bottle of water for milk or juice, not using the bottle as a pacifier, and never coating pacifiers in sweet substances. Putting juice in bottles, especially commercially available ready-to-use bottles, is discouraged: the beverage is especially damaging because the sugar is more readily converted to acid. Juice should always be offered in a cup to avoid prolonging the bottle-feeding habit. Toddlers should be encouraged to drink from a cup at the first birthday and weaned from a bottle by 14 months of age. Nurses are in an excellent position to counsel parents regarding the dangers of this habit and other aspects of dental care.*

Injury Prevention

Injuries cause more deaths in children between the ages of 1 to 4 years than in any other childhood age group except adolescence. The injury death rate has remained relatively unchanged during the past decade; however, the corresponding rates from all other causes of death combined have declined significantly. Traumatic injury is the leading cause of childhood hospitalization, and infants and younger children are at higher risk because of their small size and inability to protect themselves (Dowd, Keenan, & Bratton 2002). Child protection (adapting environment, society regulations and laws) and parent and child education are key determinants in injury prevention.

A major factor in the critical increase of injuries during early childhood is the unrestricted freedom achieved through locomotion combined with an unawareness of danger within the environment. Specific categories of injuries and appropriate prevention are best understood by associating them with the major developmental achievements of young children (Table 37-3). The discussions of injuries in Chapters 29 and 36 are also relevant to safety concerns at this age.

Motor Vehicle Injuries

Motor vehicle injuries cause more accidental deaths in all pediatric age groups after age 1 year than any other type of injury or disease and are responsible for almost one-half of all accidental deaths among children ages 1 to 4 years. Many of the deaths are caused by injuries within the car when restraints have not been used or have been used improperly. Approved restraints properly installed and applied can reduce the majority of fatalities and injuries (AAP, 2005).

SKILL: CAR SEAT SAFETY

Nurses have a responsibility for educating parents regarding the importance of car restraints and their proper use. Five types of restraints are available: (1) infant-only devices, (2) convertible models for both infants and toddlers, (3) boosters, (4) safety belts, and (5) devices for children with special needs (see Chapter 41). Infant-type restraints are discussed in Chapter 36; convertible restraints and boosters are included here. The *convertible restraint* is suitable for infants in the rearward-facing position and for toddlers in the forward-facing position (Fig. 37-10).

The transition point for switching to the forward-facing position is defined by the manufacturer but is generally at a body weight of at least 9 kg (20 pounds) and 1 year of age. Infants who weigh 20 pounds before 1 year of age should continue to ride in rear-facing position (AAP, 2005). A convertible safety seat is positioned semireclined and facing the rear of the car for a child younger than 1 year weighing less than 20 pounds. The seat is positioned upright and facing forward for an older and heavier child (up to 40 pounds). Convertible safety seats should be used until the child weighs at least 40 pounds. Convertible restraints use different types of harness systems: a five-point harness that consists of a strap over each shoulder, one on each side of the pelvis, and one between the legs (all five come together at a common buckle); a padded shield that uses shoulder straps attached to a shield that is held in place by a crotch strap; and a T-shield that has retracting shoulder straps attached to a flat chest shield with a rigid stalk that attaches to a restraint between the legs.

Booster seats, also known as belt-positioning devices, allow proper use of the shoulder harness and provide an artificial pelvis to serve as the anchor points for the lap belt.

*Sources of information about nursing caries and other aspects of child dental health include the National Institute of Dental and Craniofacial Research, Building 31, 31 Center Dr., MFC-2290, Bethesda, MD 20892-2290; 301-496-4261; Web site: www.nidr.nih.gov; Academy of Pediatric Dentistry, 211 E. Chicago Ave., Suite 700, Chicago, IL 60611; 312-337-2169 or 800-544-2174 (outside Illinois); Web site: www.aapd.org; American Dental Association, 211 E. Chicago Ave., Chicago, IL 60611; 312-440-2500 or 800-621-8099 (outside Illinois); Web site: www.ada.org; and Canadian Dental Association, 1815 Alta Vista Dr., Ottawa, Ontario K1G 3Y6; 613-523-1770 or 800-267-6354; Web site: www.cda-adc.ca/.

Table 37-3

Injury Prevention during Early Childhood

DEVELOPMENTAL ABILITIES RELATED TO RISK OF INJURY	INJURY PREVENTION
Walks, runs, and climbs Able to open doors and gates Can ride tricycle and other toy vehicles Can throw ball and other objects	***Motor vehicles*** Use federally approved car restraint Supervise child while playing outside Do not allow child to play on curb or behind a parked car Do not permit child to play in pile of leaves, snow, or large cardboard container in trafficked area Supervise tricycle riding Lock fences and doors if not directly supervising children Teach child to obey pedestrian safety rules Obey traffic regulations; cross only at crosswalks and only when traffic signal indicates it is safe Stand back a step from the curb until it's time to cross Look left, right, and left again and check for turning cars before crossing street Use sidewalks; when there is no sidewalk, walk on the left, facing traffic Wear light colors at night and attach fluorescent material to clothing
Able to explore if left unsupervised Has great curiosity Helpless in water; unaware of its danger; depth of water has no significance	***Drowning*** Supervise closely when near any source of water, including buckets Keep bathroom doors closed and lid down on toilet (or install latch) Have fence around swimming pool and lock gate Teach swimming and water safety (this is, however, not a substitute for safety)
Able to reach heights by climbing, stretching, and standing on toes Pulls objects Explores any holes or opening Can open drawers and closets Unaware of potential sources of heat or fire Plays with mechanical objects	***Burns*** Turn pot handles toward back of stove Place electrical appliances, such as coffee maker and popcorn machine, toward back of counter Place guardrails in front of radiators, fireplaces, or other heating elements Store matches and cigarette lighters in locked or inaccessible area; discard carefully Place burning candles, incense, hot foods, and cigarettes out of reach Do not let tablecloth hang within child's reach Do not let electric cord from iron, curling iron or other appliance hang within child's reach Cover electrical outlets with protective plastic caps Keep electrical wires hidden or out of reach Do not allow child to play with electrical appliance, wires, or lighters Stress danger of open flames; teach what "hot" means Always check bathwater temperature; adjust water heater temperature to 120° F (48.9° C) or lower; do not allow children to play with faucets Apply a sunscreen when child is exposed to sunlight
Explores by putting objects in mouth Can open drawers, closets, and most containers Climbs Cannot read labels Does not know safe dose or amount	***Poisoning*** Place all potentially toxic agents out of reach or in a locked cabinet Caution against eating nonedible items, such as plants Replace medications or poisons immediately; replace child-guard caps properly Administer medications as a drug, not as a candy Do not store large surplus of toxic agents Promptly discard empty poison containers; never reuse to store a food item or other poison Teach child not to play in trash containers Never remove labels from containers of toxic substances Do not store toxic liquids in containers not specifically intended for their storage e.g., empty soda bottle that child may drink (unaware of difference in contents) Have Poison Control Center number telephone next to phone or readily available (usually listed in front of telephone directory)
Able to open doors and some windows Goes up and down stairs	***Falls*** Keep screen in window, fasten securely, and use guardrail Place gates at top and bottom of stairs

Continued

Table 37-3

Injury Prevention during Early Childhood—cont'd

DEVELOPMENTAL ABILITIES RELATED TO RISK OF INJURY	INJURY PREVENTION
	Falls—cont'd
Depth perception unrefined Climbs on higher surfaces	Keep doors locked or use child-proof doorknob covers at entry to stairs, high porch, or other elevated area, including laundry chute Remove unsecured or scatter rugs Apply nonskid decals in bathtub or shower Keep crib rails fully raised and mattress at lowest level Place carpeting under crib and in bathroom Keep large toys and bumper pads out of crib or playpen (child can use these as "stairs" to climb out), then move to youth bed when child is able to climb out of crib Avoid using wheeled walkers, especially near stairs and floor furnace Dress in safe clothing (soles that do not "catch" on floor, tied shoelaces, pant legs that do not touch floor) Keep child restrained in vehicles; never leave unattended in shopping cart Supervise at playgrounds; select play areas with soft ground cover and safe equipment
	Choking and suffocation
Puts things in mouth May swallow hard or nonedible pieces of food	Avoid large, round chunks of meat, such as whole hot dogs (slice lengthwise into short pieces) Avoid fruit with pits, fish with bones, dried beans, hard candy, chewing gum, nuts, popcorn, grapes, marshmallows Choose large, sturdy toys without sharp edges or small removeable parts Discard old refrigerators, ovens, and so on; if storing an old appliance, remove the door Keep automatic garage door transmitter in inaccessible place; check pressure safety release periodically Select safe toy boxes or chests without heavy, hinged lids Keep venetian blind (or shades) cords out of child's reach Remove drawstrings from clothing
	Bodily damage
Still clumsy in many skills Easily distracted from tasks Unaware of potential danger from strangers or other people	Avoid giving sharp or pointed objects—such as knives, scissors, or toothpicks—especially when walking or running Do not allow lollipops or similar objects in mouth when walking or running Teach safety precautions (e.g., to carry knife or scissors with pointed end away from face) Store all dangerous tools, garden equipment, and firearms in locked cabinet Be alert to danger of supervised animals and household pets Use safety glass and decals on large glassed areas, such as sliding glass doors Teach child name, address, and phone number and to ask for help from appropriate people (cashier, security guard, policeman) if lost; have identification on child (sewn in clothes, inside shoe) Teach stranger safety Avoid personalized clothing in public places Never go with a stranger Tell parents if anyone makes child feel uncomfortable in any way Always listen to child's concerns regarding others' behavior Teach child to say "no" when confronted with uncomfortable situations

Booster seats are used for children who are less than 4 feet, 9 inches, and weigh more than 40 pounds, typically between 4 and 8 years old. A booster seat should be used until the child is able to sit against the back of the seat with feet hanging down and legs bent at the knees. The belt positioning booster model raises a child higher in the seat, moving the shoulder part of the belt off the neck and the lap portion of the belt off the abdomen onto the pelvis. Booster seats must be used with the lap and shoulder belts and should never be used in a position with an active front airbag; rear seat use is recommended (Ebel & Grossman, 2003) (Fig 37-11). A shield booster model uses a large plastic shield slipped into

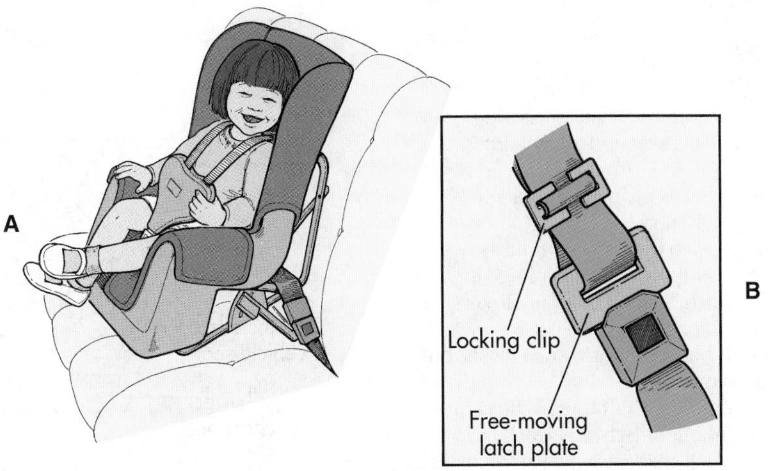

Fig. 37-10 **A,** Convertible seat in forward-facing position for older infants and children. **B,** Use of locking clip.

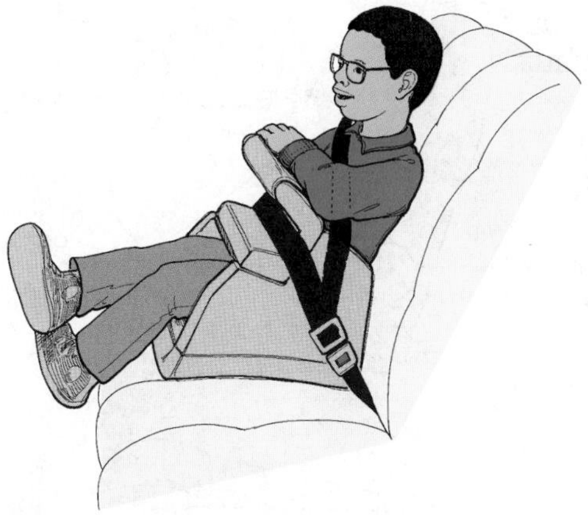

Fig. 37-11 Automobile booster seat. Note placement of shoulder strap (away from neck or face).

place in front of the child. The shields have been found to be unsafe for children weighing more than 40 pounds and must be removed when the child reaches this weight. Both the National Highway Traffic Safety Administration and the AAP (2005) recommend that children use a harness-type seat instead of a shield booster when possible; however, if used, the plastic shield must be removed.

Some older model restraints require the use of a top anchor (tether) strap to prevent the child from pitching forward in a crash. If the tether strap is not used, up to 90% of the restraint's protection is lost. Instructions for proper installation of the tether strap and permanent bracket are included with the car restraint. Cars with free-sliding latch-plates on the lap/shoulder belt require the use of a metal locking clip to keep the belt in a tight-holding position. The locking clip is threaded onto the belt above the latch plate (see inset, Fig. 37-10). If parents have newer cars with automatic lap/shoulder belts, they need to have additional lap belts installed to properly secure the restraint.

Children should use specially designed car restraints until they weigh at least 60 pounds or are 8 years old (AAP, 2005). Children who outgrow the convertible restraint may still be able to ride safely in a booster seat until the midpoint of the head is higher than the vehicle seat back. If a car safety seat is not available, the lap belt provides more protection than no restraint (except for infants, for whom there is no safe alternative to approved restraint devices). Shoulder-only automatic belts are designed to protect adults. Children should use the manual shoulder belts in the rear seat. Air bags do not take the place of child safety seats or seat belts and can be lethal to young children. The safest area of the car for children is the back seat. Children who must ride in the passenger side of the front seat with an air bag should be positioned as far back as possible.

NURSE ALERT Safety belts should be worn low on the hips, snug, and not on the abdominal area. Children should be taught to sit up straight to allow for proper fit. The shoulder belt is used *only* if it does not cross the child's neck or face. ■

Built-in seats are available in some cars and vans. They may be used for children who are at least 1 year of age and weight at least 20 pounds. Built-in seats eliminate installation problems. However, weight and height limits vary. Reinforce that owners verify with vehicle manufacturers details about built-in seats.

For any restraint to be effective, it must be used consistently and properly. Examples of misuse include misrouting the vehicle seat belt through the restraint; failing to use the vehicle seat belt to secure the restraint; failing to use a tether strap; failing to use the restraint's harness system; and incorrectly positioning the child, especially facing infants forward instead of rearward. To address these issues, nurses must stress correct use of car restraints and rules that ensure compliance (see Home Care box). Children riding in car safety seats are generally much better behaved than children left unrestrained, which can be a major benefit to parents and should be emphasized as an additional advantage of restraints.*

*American Academy of Pediatrics, 141 Northwest Point Blvd., PO Box 927, Elk Grove Village, IL 60007; 888-227-1770; Web site: www.aap.org; and local division of traffic safety or U.S. Department of Transportation, National Highway Traffic Safety Administration, 400 Seventh St., SW, Washington, DC 20590; 800-424-9393; Web site: www.nhtsa.dot.gov.

Home Care

USING CAR SAFETY SEATS

Read manufacturer's directions and follow them exactly.
Anchor safety seat securely to car's seat and apply harness snugly to child.
Do not start the car until everyone is properly restrained.
Always use the restraint, even for short trips.
If child begins to climb out or undo the harness, firmly say, "No." It may be necessary to stop the car to reinforce the expected behavior. Use rewards, such as stars or stickers, to encourage cooperative behavior.
Encourage child to help attach buckles, straps, and shields, but always double-check fastenings.
Decrease boredom on long trips. Keep soft toys in the car for quiet play; talk to child; point out objects and teach child about them. Stop periodically. If child wishes to sleep, make sure child stays in the restraint.
Insist that others who transport children also follow these safety rules.

NURSE ALERT The LATCH (Lower Anchors and Tethers for Children) universal child safety seat system was implemented as a requirement starting in the fall of 2002 for all new automobiles and child safety seats. This system provides a uniform anchorage consisting of two lower anchorages and one upper anchorage in the rear seat of the vehicle. New child safety seats will have a hook, buckle, strap, or other tether that attaches to the anchorage (Fig. 37-12). Seat belts will no longer be used to anchor child safety seats in newer vehicles. The first phase requires all new cars to have an upper anchorage. By fall of 2002, all new cars must have had the entire LATCH system installed.* ■

Injuries may also occur during sudden stops when objects are left unrestrained. On sudden impact, a loose ball becomes a projectile missile. Therefore all items should be secured or stored in the trunk.

Children over 3 years of age are often involved in pedestrian traffic injuries. Because of their gross motor skills of walking, running, and climbing, and their fine motor skills of opening doors and fence gates, they are likely to be in hazardous areas when unsupervised. Unaware of danger and unable to approximate the speed of a car, they are often hit by moving vehicles. Running after a ball, riding a tricycle, and playing behind a parked car are common activities that may result in a vehicular tragedy. A precaution when children are playing in driveways is attaching to the tricycle a pole with a bright flag that is high enough to be visible through an automobile's back window. Another safeguard is the use of a device that beeps when the vehicle is driven in reverse to alert children to the oncoming car, van, or truck.

One type of injury that has become more commonplace occurs when children crawl into an open trunk and pull it closed; asphyxia may occur in such cases; therefore, car trunks should not be left open when children are not being supervised. Some cars are equipped with a safety switch that can be activated from inside the trunk to open a closed trunk door.

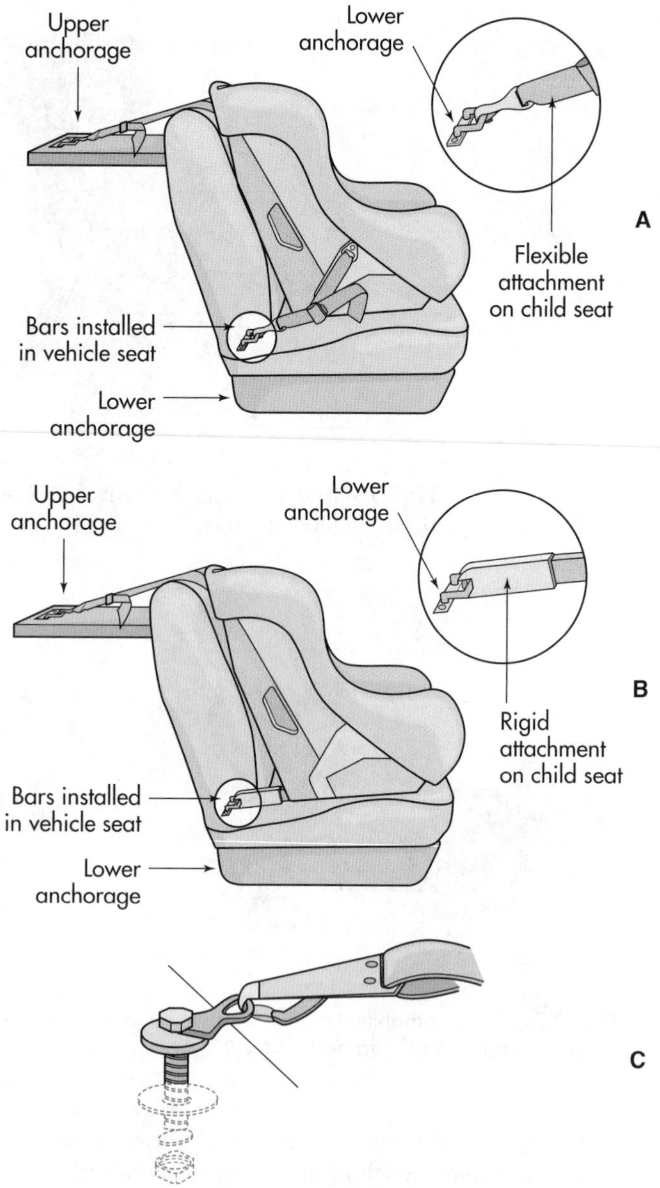

Fig. 37-12 Lower anchors and tethers for children (LATCH). **A**, Flexible 2-point attachment with top tether. **B**, Rigid 2-point attachment with top tether. **C**, Top tether. (Courtesy: U.S. Dept. of Transportation, National Highway Traffic Safety Administration.)

Preventing vehicular injuries involves protecting and educating children about the danger of moving or parked vehicles. Although preschool children are too young to be trusted to always obey, the parent should emphasize looking for moving vehicles before crossing the street, recognizing the stop and go colors of traffic lights, and following traffic officers' signals. Physical barriers limiting children from playing near vehicles help prevent these injuries (Mayr et al, 2001). Most important, what is preached must be practiced. Children learn through imitation, and consistency reinforces learning.

*U.S. Department of Transportation, National Highway Traffic Safety Administration, 400 Seventh St., SW, Washington, DC 20590; 800-424-9393; Web site: www.nhtsa.dot.gov.

Another automobile-related hazard for toddlers is *overheating* (hyperthermia) and subsequent death when left in a vehicle in hot weather (>80° F [26.4° C]). Small children dissipate heat poorly and an increase in body temperature may cause death in a few hours. Parents are cautioned against leaving infants in a vehicle alone for *any reason.* A small sign or placard has been designed to hang in the rearview mirror to remind the parent that there is a child in the back seat.

Drowning

Drowning, not including drowning from water transportation, ranks second among boys and third among girls ages 1 to 4 years as a cause of accidental death. With well-developed skills of locomotion, toddlers are able to reach potentially dangerous areas, such as bathtubs, toilets, buckets, swimming pools, hot tubs, and lakes. Their intense drive for exploration and investigation, combined with an unawareness of the danger of water and their helplessness in water, makes drowning always a viable threat. It is also one category of injuries that results in death within minutes, diminishing the chance for rescue and survival. Adult supervision of children when near any source of water is essential; teaching swimming and water safety can be helpful but cannot be regarded as sufficient protection.

Burns

Burns rank second among girls and third among boys in this age group as a cause of accidental death. Toddlers' ability to climb, stretch, and reach objects above their heads makes any hot surface a potential source of danger. Scalds from children pulling pots on top of themselves are a major source of burns. As a precaution, pot handles should be turned toward the back of the stove. Ideally, the knobs for controlling the range burners should be out of reach, not on the front panel where nimble fingers can turn them on and accidentally touch the hot burner. Oven doors should be closed whenever the oven is turned on or when it is cooling. The outside of doors of automatic self-cleaning ovens may become hot and, if touched, could cause a burn. Microwave ovens present much less of a burn hazard to toddlers because the outside remains cool, and they are often inaccessible, although foods heated in microwaves can scald children (Wolf, Adler, & Hauben, 2001).

Other sources of heat, such as radiators, fireplaces, accessible furnaces, kerosene heaters, or wood-burning stoves, should have a guard placed in front of them. The tops of some of these heaters are designed to become hot enough to boil water to provide humidity; thus, they are hazardous if touched or if the pan of water is spilled. Portable electrical heaters must be placed in a high area, well out of reach of climbing young children. Hair curling irons may easily burn the hands of curious toddlers when left within easy reach.

Hot objects such as candles, incense, cigarettes, pots of tea or coffee, or irons must be placed away from children. The flame of a candle and the smoke of a cigarette invite investigation. Ashtrays with a center well are preferred to prevent the cigarette from falling off the rim, and adults should try not to smoke, cook, or drink hot liquids when children are physically close. If tablecloths are used, the edges should be placed out of reach to prevent injuries from both burns and falling objects.

Flame burns represent one of the most fatal types of burns and commonly occur when children play with matches and accidentally set themselves (and the home) on fire. To prevent flame burns, matches and lighters must be stored safely away from children, and parents need to teach children the dangers of playing with such objects. In addition, all homes should have smoke detectors installed to alert the occupants to a fire. A safety plan for immediate escape is also essential.

Electrical burns also represent an immediate danger to children. With preschoolers' ability to manipulate small, thin objects, they are able to insert hairpins or other conductive articles into electrical sockets. Young toddlers may explore outlets and wires by mouthing them. Since water is an excellent conductor, the chance for a severe circumoral electrical burn is great. Electrical outlets should have protective guards plugged into them when not in use (Fig. 37-13) or be made inaccessible by having furniture placed in front of them when feasible. Children should not be allowed to play with electrical cords or appliances, which should be kept out of reach as much as possible.

Scald burns are the most common type of thermal injury in children. A scalding burn is often caused by high-temperature tap water, which children come in contact with either as a result of turning on the hot-water faucet, falling into a bathtub of hot water, or deliberate abuse. Always supervising youngsters when they are near tap water and checking bathwater temperatures are methods of prevention. Limiting household water temperatures to less than 49° C (120° F) is also recommended. At this temperature it takes 10 minutes of exposure to the water to cause a full-thickness burn. Conversely, water temperatures of 54° C (130° F), the

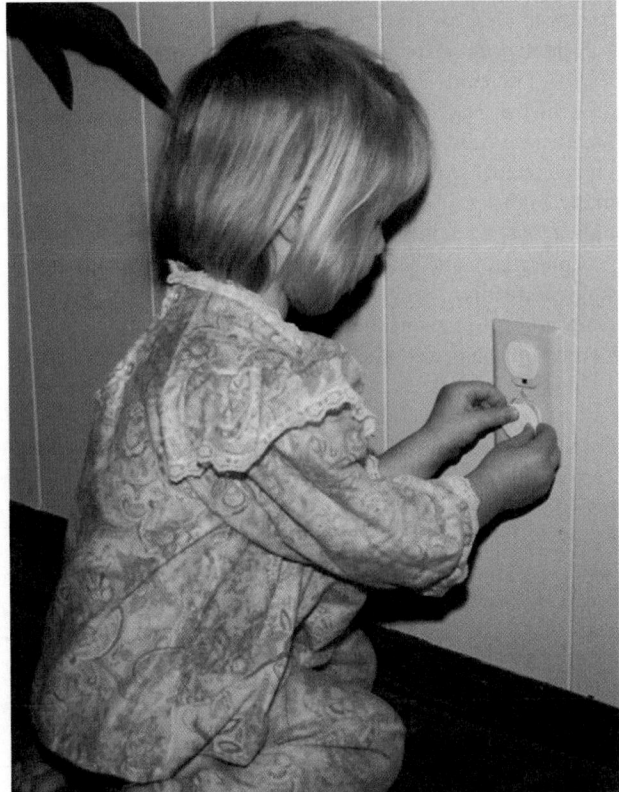

Fig. 37-13 Special plastic caps in electrical sockets prevent young fingers from exploring dangerous areas.

usual setting of most water heaters, expose household members to the risk of full-thickness burns within 30 seconds. Nurses can help prevent such burns by advising parents of this common household danger and recommending that they readjust the water heater to a safe temperature. A meat or candy thermometer is a convenient way to measure water temperature. An easy-to-read hot-water gauge that changes color to show water temperatures between 120° and 150° F [49° C and 54° C] is also available; it shows a "hot," "cool," or "OK" water temperature. A special device can also be added to the faucet that reduces the water flow once the set temperature is reached. Scalding also often occurs when a curious child tries to sip a parent's coffee or tea and spills the boiling liquid down the chin and chest.

Poisoning

evolve CASE STUDY: SALICYLATE INGESTION

CASE STUDY: HEAVY METAL POISONING

Toddlers are at the highest risk for poisoning. Mouthing activity continues to be prevalent after 1 year of age, and exploring objects by tasting them is part of children's curious investigation. Many household products, medications, and plants can be poisonous if swallowed, if in contact with the skin or eyes, or if inhaled (Shannon, 2003). Although in many instances poisoning does not result in mortality, it may cause significant morbidity, such as esophageal stricture from lye ingestion. Toddlers are able to climb most heights, open most drawers or closets, and unscrew most lids. By trial and error, younger children also manage to undo tops of bottles, plastic containers, aerosol cans, and jars, including those with child-resistant lids. In addition, drugs are often transferred to regular containers for the elderly, who may have difficulty with child-resistant lids. Newer forms of drugs, such as transdermal patches and cough-suppressant lozenges, have created additional dangers, since they are not packaged with safety caps and the lozenges look like candy.

The major reason for poisoning is improper storage (Fig. 37-14). The guidelines suggested in Chapter 36 apply to children in this age group as well. However, unlike the infant, who was confined to certain heights and unable to unlatch inventive locks, young children manage to find access to many high-level, tight-security places. For this age group, only a locked cabinet is safe.

Emergency and preventive measures for accidental poisoning are discussed in Chapter 36. Parents should have ready access to the telephone number for the Poison Control Center and be prepared to act on the advice of the Center.*

Falls

Falls are still a hazard to children in this age group, although by the later part of early childhood, gross and fine motor skills are well developed, decreasing the incidence of falls down stairs or from chairs. However, playground injuries are common. Children need to be taught safety at play areas, such as no horseplay on high slides or jungle gyms, *sitting* on swings, and staying away from moving swings

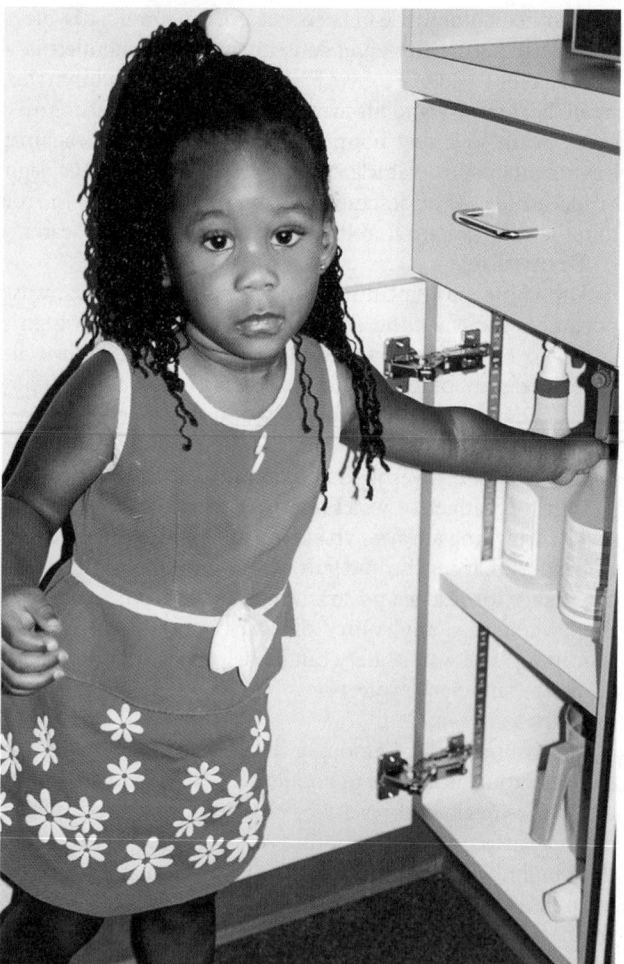

Fig. 37-14 Children are most likely to ingest substances that are on their level, such as cleaning agents stored under sinks, rat poison, plants, or diaper pail deodorants.

(Purvis & Hirsch, 2003). Passive prevention includes placement of grass, sand, or wood chips under play equipment. Swing seats should be made of plastic, canvas, or rubber and have smooth or rounded edges. Slides should not exceed an incline of 30 degrees, and should have evenly spaced rungs for climbing and protective "tunnels."

The climbing and running of the typical toddler are complicated by the child's total neglect for and lack of appreciation of danger. Gates must be placed at both ends of stairs. Accessible windows that are left open during warm weather must be screened or guarded with a rail. Falling from open windows is a major cause of accidental death in children from urban, lower socioeconomic groups; parents are advised that a screened window is not a safety device to prevent falls. Doors leading to stairwells or porches must be locked because preschoolers can easily open them. A convenient type of lock is a sliding bar or hook that can be attached to the door and frame at a level higher than the child can reach.

Cribs and vehicles are other sources of falls. To avoid injury, crib rails should be fully raised, the mattress should be kept at the lowest position, and toys or bumper pads that may be used as steps to climb out should be removed. Ideally, the floor should be carpeted. Once children reach a height of 89 cm (35 inches), they should sleep in a bed rather

*The national toll-free telephone number for Poison Control Centers is 800-222-1222. This number provides everyone in the United States with free access, 24 hours a day, 7 days a week, to their regional Poison Center. For some tips on preventing poisoning in your home, see the TIPP® slip, "*Protect your Child . . . Prevent Poisoning,*" available online at www.aap.org/family/poistipp.htm.

than a crib. If a bunk bed is selected, parents should be aware of possible dangers such as falls and head entrapment between the mattress and guardrail or between the supporting mattress slats. If the beds are constructed of tubular metal, parents should check for breaks or cracks in the metal and welds that may lead to collapse and injury. Children who sleep on the top bunk should be 6 years or older.

Children who are unrestrained can fall from high chairs, shopping carts, carriages, car seats, and strollers if not properly restrained or because of a change in balance created with weighing the object down with heavy objects (Powell, Jovtis, & Tanz, 2002). Therefore, proper restraint and adequate supervision are essential. Children, especially older infants who are mobile, should not be placed in an infant seat on top of a shopping cart because the infant seat may fall off the cart; the safest place for an infant seat is inside the cart's bed.

Clothing can also increase the chance of falling. Simple safety measures, such as checking clothing and shoes and keeping shoelaces tied with double knots or using self-adhering closures, can prevent accidents.

Aspiration and Suffocation

evolve Case Study: Ingestion of an Injurious Agent

Usually by 1 year of age children chew well, but they may have difficulty with large pieces of food, such as meat and whole hot dogs, and with hard foods, such as nuts or dried beans. Young children cannot discard pits from fruit or bones from fish. It takes practice to learn how to chew gum without swallowing it. Therefore, the same precautions as discussed for infants regarding food selection must be implemented (see Chapter 36).

Play objects for toddlers must still be chosen with an awareness of danger from small parts. Large, sturdy toys without sharp edges or removeable parts are safest. Coins, paper clips, pins, bells, button batteries, pull-tabs on cans, thumbtacks, nails, screws, jewelry (especially pierced earrings), and all types of pins are common household objects that can cause significant harm if swallowed or aspirated. Because of the danger of aspiration, parents should be taught emergency procedures for choking (see Airway Obstruction, Chapter 46).

Another cause of death by traumatic injury is from electrically operated garage doors. Young children playing in the garage may become trapped under the door. Although the automatic doors (only models built since 1993) should reverse when striking an object, they may not do so when hitting a flexible object or one that is very close to the ground. Precautions include placing controls where they are inaccessible to children, such as high on a wall and in a locked car and instructing children not to run under a closing garage door. Periodically the door should be checked to determine if it returns after striking an object and if the limit settings meet manufacturer recommendations. Additional safety precautions include having an automatic eye near ground level of the door frame, which prevents the door from closing when an object is detected at the door opening.

Suffocation from causes seen during infancy is less frequent, but old refrigerators, ovens, and other large appliances are an ever-present threat. Toddlers can climb inside these appliances and, if they close the door behind them, can be trapped inside. Discarding old appliances or removing all doors during storage prevents such tragic deaths. Toddlers may also suffocate when unsafe toy box lids accidentally close on their head or neck. Parents should be advised of this danger and encouraged to buy storage chests with lightweight, removable covers.

Hollow, semirigid hemispherical or ellipsoidal objects (toys, compartments of toys, containers) can form suction and cupping around a small child's face causing complete airway obstruction. Several different types of objects have been involved with choking incidents, including toys, components of toys, and containers (Nakamura, Pollack-Nelson, & Chidekel, 2003).

Bodily Damage

Toddlers are still clumsy in many of their skills and can seriously harm themselves by walking while holding a sharp or pointed object or by having food or objects such as spoons in their mouths. Preventing such occurrences is the best approach with toddlers. With preschoolers, teaching safety is most important. The child should be taught that when walking with a pointed object such as a knife or scissors, the pointed end is held away from the face. Dangerous garden or workshop equipment and all firearms should be stored in a locked cabinet. Power lawnmowers are especially dangerous, and young children should not be allowed in an area where a mower is being used; nor should they be taken for a ride on a mower or allowed to operate that device. Safety education should include respect for firearms and their proper and appropriate use, including nonpowder guns, such as air guns and rifles, which cause serious penetrating injuries. In addition, the child should be warned of and protected against potential danger from animals (see Animal Bites, Chapter 53).

Toys can be a source of danger, and safety must be a prime consideration when selecting toys (see Home Care box, p. 951). Most toys have age ranges written on them to designate their safety, but this information must be used with knowledge of the specific child's readiness.

Household safety should be practiced and includes the usual precautions recommended for any age group (see Home Care box, p. 1074). An additional safeguard for young children is the use of safety glass in doors, windows, and tabletops; and the application of decals on glassed areas to lessen the likelihood of running through glass. Also, children should not be allowed to run, jump, wrestle, or play ball near glass structures.

Anticipatory Guidance—Care of Families

Understanding toddlers is fundamental to successful childrearing. Nurses, particularly those in ambulatory or child health centers, are in a favorable position to assist parents in meeting the tasks and needs of children in this age group. Prevention yields better results than treatment. Anticipatory guidance is paramount if one wishes to prevent future problems (Home Care box). Advice is sometimes not the sole answer. Actual assistance, such as being available for home visits or telephone consulting, should be part of the nurse's flexible repertoire of interventions. Whether parents are experiencing the childrearing dilemmas of a first or a subsequent child, they benefit from sharing their feelings, frustrations, and satisfactions. They need adult companionship,

Home Care

GUIDANCE DURING TODDLER YEARS

Ages 12 to 18 Months

Prepare parents for expected behavioral changes of toddler, especially negativism and ritualism.

Assess present feeding habits and encourage gradual weaning from bottle and increased intake of solid foods.

Stress expected feeding changes of picky eating habits, presence of food fads and strong taste preferences, need for scheduled routine at mealtimes, inability to sit through an entire meal, and lack of table manners.

Assess sleep patterns at night, particularly the habit of a bedtime bottle, which is a major cause of dental caries, and procrastination behaviors that delay hour of sleep.

Prepare parents for potential dangers of the home, particularly motor vehicle injuries, poisoning, and falling injuries; give appropriate suggestions for safety proofing the home.

Discuss need for firm but gentle discipline and ways in which to deal with negativism and temper tantrums; stress positive benefits of appropriate discipline.

Emphasize importance for both child and parents of brief, periodic separations.

Discuss new toys that use developing gross and fine motor, language, cognitive, and social skills.

Emphasize need for dental supervision, types of basic dental hygiene at home, and food habits that predispose to caries; stress importance of supplemental fluoride (according to age [>6 mo] and fluoride content of local water supply).

Ages 18 to 24 Months

Stress importance of peer companionship in play.

Explore need for preparation for additional sibling; stress importance of preparing child for new experiences.

Discuss present discipline methods, their effectiveness, and parents' feelings about child's negativism; stress that negativism is important aspect of developing self-assertion and independence and is not a sign of spoiling.

Discuss signs of readiness for toilet training; emphasize importance of waiting for physical and psychologic readiness.

Discuss development of fears, such as darkness or loud noises, and of habits, such as security blanket or thumb sucking; stress normalcy of these transient behaviors.

Prepare parents for signs of regression in time of stress.

Assess child's ability to separate easily from parents for brief periods of separation under familiar circumstances.

Allow parents opportunity to express their feelings of weariness, frustration, and exasperation; be aware that it is often difficult to love toddlers at times when they are not asleep!

Point out some of the expected changes of the next year, such as longer attention span, somewhat less negativism, and increased concern for pleasing others.

Ages 24 to 36 Months

Discuss importance of imitation and domestic mimicry and need to include child in activities.

Discuss approaches toward toilet training, particularly realistic expectations and attitude toward accidents.

Stress uniqueness of toddlers' thought processes, especially through their use of language, poor understanding of time, causal relationships in terms of proximity of events, and inability to see events from another's perspective.

Stress that discipline still must be quite structured and concrete and that relying solely on verbal reasoning and explanation leads to injuries, confusion, and misunderstanding.

Discuss investigation of preschool or day care center toward completion of second year.

freedom from childrearing responsibilities, and periodic separations from their children. Part of a nurse's responsibility is to provide opportunities for parents to express their feelings and to meet their physical, mental, and spiritual needs.

Key Points

- The toddler stage, extending from 12 to 36 months, is a period of intense exploration of the environment.
- Biologic development during the toddler years is characterized by the acquisition of fine and gross motor skills that allow children to master a wide range of activities.
- Although most of the physiologic systems are mature by the end of toddlerhood, development of certain areas of the brain is still occurring, allowing for greater intellectual capacity.
- Locomotion is the major gross motor skill acquired during toddlerhood, followed by increased eye-hand coordination.
- Specific tasks in the psychosocial development of a toddler include differentiating self from others, tolerating separation from parent, coping with delayed gratification, controlling bodily functions, acquiring socially acceptable behavior, communicating verbally, and interacting with others in a less egocentric manner.
- According to Erikson the major developmental task of toddlerhood is acquiring a sense of autonomy while overcoming a sense of doubt and shame.
- In Piaget's sensorimotor and preconceptual phases of development, the toddler experiments by incorporating the old learning of secondary circular reactions with new skills and applies this knowledge to new situations. There is the beginning of rational judgment, an understanding of causal relationships, and discovery of objects as objects.
- Preconceptual thought is characterized by egocentricism, centration, global organization of thought processes, animism, and irreversibility.
- Language is the major cognitive achievement in toddlerhood.
- The most striking characteristic of language development during early childhood is the increasing level of comprehension.
- Development of body image occurs with increasing motor ability, at which point toddlers recognize the importance and capacity of body parts.
- The two phases of differentiation of self from significant others are separation and individuation.
- Parental concerns during the toddler years include toilet training; coping with sibling rivalry; limit setting and discipline; and dealing with temper tantrums, negativism, and regression.

- Effective discipline techniques for toddlers include reward, ignoring or extinction, and time-out.
- Nutrition is important at this stage because eating habits established in toddlerhood tend to have lasting effects in subsequent years.
- Regular dental examinations, fluoride supplementation, removal of plaque, and provision of a low-cariogenic diet promote optimum dental health.
- Because of increased locomotion, toddlers are at high risk for sustaining injuries. Fatal injuries are primarily a result of motor vehicle accidents, drownings, and burns.

References

American Academy of Pediatric Dentistry: Oral health policies, *Pediatr Dent* 21(5 Spec. no.):18-37, 1999.

American Academy of Pediatrics: Car safety seats: a guide for families 2005. Internet document available at www.aap.org/family/carseatguide.htm (accessed May 29, 2005).

American Academy of Pediatrics, Committee on Public Health: Children, adolescents, and television, *Pediatrics* 107(2):423-426, 2001.

American Academy of Pediatrics, Section on Pediatric Dentistry: Oral health risk assessment timing and establishment of the dental home, *Pediatrics* 111(5):1113-1116, 2003.

Bates E, Dick F: Language, gesture, and the developing brain, *Dev Psychobiol* 40 (3):293-310, 2002.

Brazelton TB: How to help parents of young children: the touchpoints model, *J Perinatol* 19(6 part 2):S6-7, 1999.

Cathey M, Gaylord N: Picky eating: a toddler's approach to mealtime, *Pediatric Nursing* 30(2):101-107, 2004.

Dahlquist LM et al: Distraction for children of different ages who undergo repeated needle sticks, *J Pediatr Oncol Nurs* 19(1):22-34, 2002.

DeLamater J, Friedrich WN: Human sexual development, *J Sex Res* 39(1):10-14, 2002.

Dowd DM, Keenan HT, Bratton SL: Epidemiology and prevention of childhood injuries, *Crit Care Med* 30(11):S385-S392, 2002.

Ebel BE, Grossman DC: Crash proof kids? An overview of current motor vehicle child occupant safety strategies, *Curr Prob Pediatr Adolesc Health Care* 33 (2):38-55, 2003.

Fosarelli P: Children and the development of faith: implications for pediatric practice, *Contemporary Pediatr* 20(1):85-98, 2003.

Glassy D, Romano J, and the Committee on Early Childhood, Adoption, and Dependent Care: Selecting appropriate toys for young children: the pediatrician's role, *Pediatrics* 111(4):911-913, 2003.

Howard BJ, Wong J: Sleep disorders, *Pediatr Rev* 22(10):327-342, 2001.

Lyytinen P et al: The development and predictive relations of play and language across the second year, *Scand J Psych* 40:177-186, 1999.

Mayr JM et al: Vehicles reversing or rolling backwards: an underestimated hazard, *Inj Prev* 7(4):327-328, 2001.

Mercer R: Treating nocturnal enuresis, *Adv Nurs Pract* 11(2):26-31, 2003.

Meyer TL: Unveiling the secrecy behind masturbation, *Pediatr Rev* 23(4):148-149, 2002.

Nakamura SW, Pollack-Nelson C, Chidekel AS: Suction-type suffocation incidents in infants and toddlers, *Pediatrics* 111(1):e12-e16, 2003.

Petitto LA et al: Bilingual signed and spoken language acquisition from birth: implications for the mechanisms underlying early bilingual language acquisition, *J Child Lang* 28(2):453-496, 2001.

Picciano MF et al: Nutritional guidance is needed during dietary transition in early childhood, *Pediatrics* 106(1):109-114, 2000.

Powell EC, Jovtis E, Tanz RR: Incidence and description of stroller related injuries to children, *Pediatrics* 110(5):e62, 2002.

Purvis JM, Hirsch SA: Playground injury prevention, *Clin Orthop* April (409):11-19, 2003.

Shannon M: Primary care: ingestion of toxic substances by children, *N Engl J Med* 342(3):186-191, 2003.

Thompson RA: Caring for infants and toddlers, *Future Child* 11(1):21-33, 2001.

Wolf Y, Adler N, Hauben DJ: Exploding microwaved eggs-revisited, *Burns* 27(8):853-855, 2001.

38 The Preschooler and Family

LEARNING OBJECTIVES

On completion of this chapter the reader will be able to:

- Identify the major biologic, psychosocial, cognitive, moral, spiritual, and social developments that occur during the preschool years.
- List the benefits of imaginary playmates.
- Prepare preschoolers for preschool or day care experience.
- Provide parents with guidelines for sex education.
- Provide parents with guidelines for dealing with a child's fears, stresses, aggression, and sleep problems.
- Recognize the causes of stuttering during the preschool years.
- Offer parents suggestions for preventing speech problems.
- Recognize feeding patterns of preschoolers.
- Provide anticipatory guidance to parents regarding injury prevention based on the preschooler's developmental achievements.
- State three factors thought to be associated with child abuse.
- State four areas of the history that should arouse suspicion of abuse.
- Describe the nursing care of the abused child.

ELECTRONIC RESOURCES

Additional information related to the content in Chapter 38 can be found on

the companion website at evolve
http://evolve.elsevier.com/Wong/maternal/
- NCLEX Review Questions
- Case Study–Sleep Problems
- Case Study–Varicella in Spite of Vaccine
- Case Study–Bacterial Conjunctivitis
- WebLinks

or the interactive student CD-ROM
Activities for Chapter 38 include the following:
- NCLEX Review Questions
- Case Study–Chickenpox (Varicella)
- Critical Thinking Exercise–Imitative Play
- Critical Thinking Exercise–Conjunctivitis
- Nursing Care Plan–The Child with a Communicable Disease
- Nursing Care Plan–The Child Who Is Maltreated

PROMOTING OPTIMUM GROWTH AND DEVELOPMENT

The combined biologic, psychosocial, cognitive, spiritual, and social achievements during the *preschool period* (3 to 5 years of age) prepare preschoolers for their most significant change in lifestyle—entrance into school. Their control of bodily functions, experience of brief and prolonged periods of separation, ability to interact cooperatively with other children and adults, use of language for mental symbolization, and increased attention span and memory ready them for the next major period—the school years. Successful achievement of previous levels of growth and development is essential for preschoolers to refine many of the tasks that were mastered during the toddler years.

Biologic Development

The rate of physical growth slows and stabilizes during the preschool years. The average *weight* is 14.6 kg (32 pounds) at 3 years, 16.7 kg (36.75 pounds) at 4 years, and 18.7 kg (41.25 pounds) at 5 years. The average weight gain per year remains approximately 2.3 kg (5 pounds).

Growth in *height* also remains steady at a yearly increase of 6.75 to 7.5 cm (2.5 to 3 inches) and generally occurs in elongation of the legs rather than of the trunk. The average height is 95 cm (37.25 inches) at 3 years, 103 cm (40.5 inches) at 4 years, and 110 cm (43.25 inches) at 5 years.

Physical proportions no longer resemble those of the squat, potbellied toddler. The preschooler is slender but sturdy, graceful, agile, and posturally erect. There is little difference in physical characteristics according to gender, except as dictated by such factors as dress and hairstyle.

Most organ systems can adjust to moderate stress and change. During this period most children are toilet trained. For the most part, motor development consists of increases in strength and refinement of previously learned skills, such as walking, running, and jumping. However, muscle development and bone growth are still far from mature. Excessive activity and overexertion can injure delicate tissues. Good posture, appropriate exercise, and adequate nutrition and rest are essential for optimum development of the musculoskeletal system.

Gross and Fine Motor Behavior

Walking, running, climbing, and jumping are well established by age 36 months. Refinement in eye-hand and muscle coordination is evident in several areas. At age 3 the preschooler rides a tricycle, walks on tiptoe, balances on one foot for a few seconds, and broad jumps. By age 4 the child skips and hops proficiently on one foot (Fig. 38-1) and catches a ball reliably. By age 5 the child skips on alternate feet, jumps rope, and begins to skate and swim.

Fine motor development is evident in the child's increasingly skillful manipulation, such as in drawing and dressing. These skills provide readiness for learning and independence for entry into school.

Psychosocial Development

Developing a Sense of Initiative (Erikson)

Once preschoolers have mastered the tasks of the toddler period, they are ready to face the developmental endeavors of the preschool period. Erikson asserts that the chief psychosocial task of this period is acquiring a sense of *initiative.* Children are in a stage of energetic learning. They play, work, and live to the fullest and feel a real sense of accomplishment and satisfaction in their activities. Conflict arises when children overstep the limits of their ability and inquiry and experience a sense of *guilt* for not having behaved appropriately. Feelings of guilt, anxiety, and fear may also result from thoughts that differ from expected behavior.

A particularly stressful thought is wishing one's parent dead. As a sense of rivalry or competition develops between the child and same-sex parent, the child may think of ways to get rid of the interfering parent. In most situations this rivalry is resolved by strongly identifying with the same-sex parent and peers during the school years. However, if that parent dies before the identification process is completed, the preschooler can be overwhelmed with feelings of guilt for having wished and therefore "caused" the death. Clarifying for children that wishes cannot and do not make events occur is essential in helping them overcome their guilt and anxiety.

Development of the *superego,* or *conscience,* has its beginnings toward the end of the toddler years and is a major task for preschoolers (Cultural Awareness box). Learning right from wrong and good from bad is the beginning of morality (see Moral Development later in this chapter).

Cognitive Development

One of the tasks related to the preschool period is readiness for school and scholastic learning. Many of the thought processes of this period are crucial for achieving such readi-

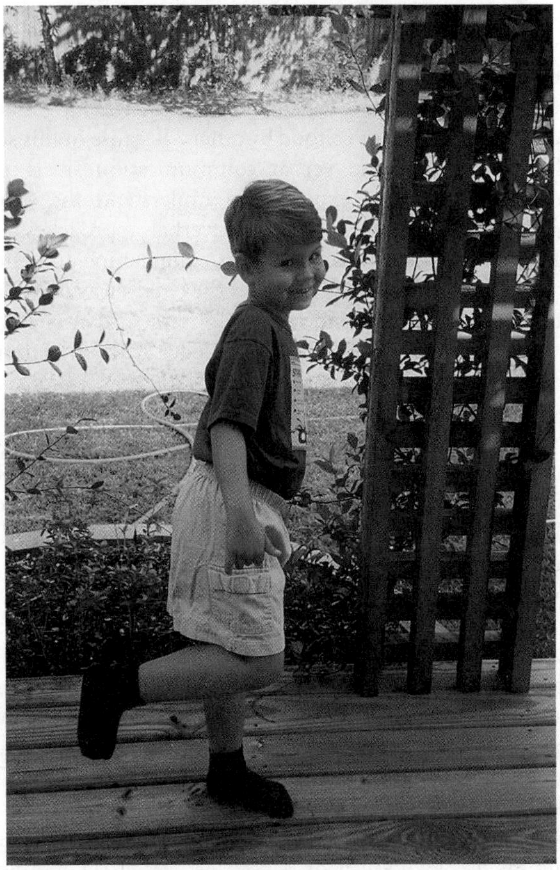

Fig. 38-1 A 4-year-old child has sufficient balance to walk or hop on one foot.

> **Cultural Awareness ▸▸**
>
> **LEARNING SOCIOCULTURAL MORES**
>
> Developing a conscience implies learning the sociocultural mores of the family's heritage. Depending on the type of attitudes conveyed, children will learn not only appropriate behaviors, but also tolerant, biased, or prejudicial values concerning their ethnic, religious, and social background and those of other groups. Much of this influence may remain dormant until they associate with children or adults of a different heritage. Then, depending on the particular group, they may be accepted or ostracized for their attitudes.

ness, and it is intentional that the child begins school between ages 5 and 6 rather than at an earlier age.

Preoperational Phase (Piaget)

Piaget's cognitive theory actually does not include a period specifically for children 3 to 5 years old. The *preoperational phase* comprises the age span from 2 to 7 years and is divided into two stages: the *preconceptual phase,* ages 2 to 4, and the phase of *intuitive thought,* ages 4 to 7. One of the main transitions during these two phases is the shift from totally egocentric thought to social awareness and the ability to consider other viewpoints. However, egocentricity is still evident. (For a review of the characteristics of preoperational thought, see Chapter 37.)

Language continues to develop during the preschool period. Speech remains primarily a vehicle of egocentric communication. Preschoolers assume that everyone thinks as they do and that a brief explanation of their thinking makes the entire thought understood by others. Because of this self-referenced, egocentric verbal communication, it is frequently necessary to explore and understand the young child's thinking through other nonverbal approaches. For children in this age group, the most enlightening and effective method is *play,* which becomes the child's way of understanding, adjusting to, and working out life's experiences.

Preschoolers increasingly use language without comprehending the meaning of words, particularly concepts of right and left, causality, and time. Children may use the concepts correctly but only in the circumstances in which they have learned them. For example, they may know how to put on shoes by remembering that the buckle is always on the outside of the foot. However, if different shoes have no buckles, they cannot reason which shoe fits which foot. In other words, they do not understand the concept of *right and left.*

Superficially, *causality* resembles logical thought. Preschoolers explain a concept as they heard it described by others, but their understanding is limited. An example is the concept of time. Because *time* is still incompletely understood, the child interprets it according to his or her own frame of reference, such as "A long time means until Christmas." Consequently, time is best explained in relationship to an event, such as "Your mother will visit you after you finish your lunch." Avoiding words such as "yesterday," "tomorrow," "next week," or "Tuesday" to express when an event is expected to occur and associating time with usual expected daily occurrences help children learn about temporal relationships while increasing their trust in others' predictions.

Preschoolers' thinking is often described as *magical thinking.* Because of their egocentrism and transductive reasoning, they believe that thoughts are all-powerful. Such thinking places them in the vulnerable position of feeling guilty and responsible for bad thoughts, which may coincide with the occurrence of a wished event. Their inability to logically reason the cause and effect of illness or an injury makes it especially difficult for them to understand such events.

Preschoolers believe in the power of words and accept their meaning literally. An example of this type of thinking occurs when a child is called "bad" because the child did something wrong. In the preschooler's mind, being called "bad" means the child is a bad person; thus it is better to say that the child's *actions* were bad, rather than calling the *child* bad, so that this does not become ingrained into the child's sense of self-worth.

Moral Development

Preconventional or Premoral Level (Kohlberg)

Young children's development of moral judgment is at the most basic level. There is little, if any, concern for why something is wrong. They behave because of the freedom or restriction that is placed on actions. In the *punishment and obedience orientation,* children (ages about 2 to 4 years) judge whether an action is good or bad depending on whether it results in reward or punishment. If children are punished for it, the action is bad. If they are not punished, the action is good, regardless of the meaning of the act. For example, if parents allow hitting, the child will perceive that hitting is good because it is not associated with punishment.

From approximately 4 to 7 years of age children are in the stage of *naive instrumental orientation,* in which actions are directed toward satisfying their needs and less frequently the needs of others. They have a very concrete sense of justice. Reciprocity or fairness involves the philosophy of "You scratch my back, and I'll scratch yours," with no thought of loyalty or gratitude (Thomas, 1996).

Spiritual Development

Children's knowledge of faith and religion is learned from significant others in their environment, usually from the parents and their religious practices (Kenny, 1999). However, young children's understanding of spirituality is influenced by their cognitive level. Preschoolers have a concrete concept of a God with physical characteristics, who is often like an imaginary friend. They understand simple Bible stories and memorize short prayers, but their understanding of the meaning of these rituals is limited. Preschoolers benefit from concrete representations of religious practices, such as picture Bible books and small statues (e.g., those of the Nativity scene). They imitate the religious practices of their parents without fully understanding the significance of these acts.

Development of the conscience is strongly linked to spiritual development. At this age children are learning right from wrong and behave correctly to avoid punishment. Wrongdoing provokes feelings of guilt, and preschoolers often misinterpret illness as a punishment for real or imagined transgressions. When children feel an overwhelming sense of guilt about their wrongdoings, it affects their concept of who they are in relation to God. If they perceive themselves as being unloved and unaccepted by parents or their environment, they in turn will not be able to perceive God as a loving God (Steen & Anderson, 1995); instead they will perceive God as a strict disciplinarian. Thus it is important that parents discipline the child consistently yet demonstrate unconditional love to help the preschooler lay a healthy foundation for faith and spirituality. It is important that children view God as one who bestows unconditional love, rather than as a judge of good or bad behavior. Praying to God and observing religious traditions (e.g., prayers before meals or bedtime) can help children through stressful periods, such as hospitalization. In many religious faiths, cultural practices and religion are closely intertwined (McEvoy, 2003) and are an important part of the child's and the family's life (Community Focus box).

Development of Body Image

The preschool years play a significant role in the development of body image. With increasing comprehension of language, preschoolers recognize that individuals have undesirable and desirable appearances. They recognize differences in skin color and racial identity and are vulnerable to learning prejudices and biases. They are aware of the meaning of words such as "pretty" or "ugly," and they reflect the opinions

Community Focus

SPIRITUAL ASSESSMENT

The mnemonic BELIEF was developed by McEvoy (2000) for pediatric nurses to initiate discussions with parents and children about their faith or religious values and beliefs. The components of the assessment tool are as follows:

B–Belief system
E–Ethics or values
L–Lifestyle
I–Involvement in a spiritual community (church, synagogue, mosque)
E-Education
F–Future events

The tool may be used to develop a culturally sensitive dialog regarding spiritual matters and practices that affect the child and family.

of others regarding their own appearance. By 5 years of age children compare their size with their peers' and can become conscious of being large or short, especially if others refer to them as "so big" or "so little" for their age. In one study, negative associations between weight status and self-concept were identified in girls as young as 5 years (Davison & Birch, 2001).

Despite their advances in body-image development, preschoolers have poorly defined body boundaries and little knowledge of their internal anatomy. Intrusive experiences are frightening, especially those that disrupt the integrity of the skin, such as injections and surgery. There is a fear that if the skin is "broken," all of their blood and "insides" can leak out. Therefore bandages are critical to "keeping everything from coming out."

Development of Sexuality

Sexual development during these years is a very important phase to a person's overall sexual identity and beliefs. Preschoolers are forming strong attachments to the opposite-sex parent while identifying with the same-sex parent. *Sex-typing,* or the process by which an individual develops the behavior, personality, attitudes, and beliefs appropriate for his or her culture and sex, occurs through several mechanisms during this period. Probably the most powerful mechanisms are childrearing practices and imitation. Studies increasingly demonstrate that gender identification is a result of complex prenatal and postnatal psychologic factors, as well as biologic or genetic factors, and that most children are aware of their gender and the expected sets of related behaviors by 1 to 2 years of age.

As sexual identity is developing beyond gender recognition, modesty may become a concern, as well as fears of mutilation. There is sex-role imitation, and "dressing up like Mommy (or Daddy)" is an important activity. Attitudes and responses of others to role-playing can condition the child to views of self or others. For example, comments such as "Boys shouldn't play with dolls" can influence a boy's self-concept of masculinity (Finan, 1997).

Sexual exploration may be more pronounced now than ever before, particularly in terms of exploring and manipulating the genitals. Questions about sexual reproduction may come to the forefront in the preschooler's search for understanding (see Chapters 39 and 40).

Social Development

During the preschool period the *individuation-separation process* is completed. Preschoolers have overcome much of the anxiety associated with strangers and the fear of separation of earlier years. They relate to unfamiliar people easily and tolerate brief separations from parents with little or no protest. However, they still need parental security, reassurance, guidance, and approval, especially when entering preschool or elementary school. Prolonged separation, such as that imposed by illness and hospitalization, is difficult, but preschoolers respond very well to anticipatory preparation and concrete explanation. They can cope with changes in daily routine much better than toddlers; however, they may develop more imaginary fears. Preschoolers gain security and comfort from familiar objects, such as toys, dolls, or photographs of family members. They are able to work through many of their unresolved fears, fantasies, and anxieties through play, especially if guided with appropriate play objects (e.g., dolls or puppets) that represent family members, medical and nursing staff, and other children.

Language

During the preschool years language becomes more sophisticated and complex. Both cognitive ability and environment (in particular, consistent role models) influence vocabulary, speech, and comprehension (Huttenlocher, 1998). Language becomes a major mode of communication and social interaction, and its development during the preschool period sets the stage for later success in school (Needlman, 2004) (Fig. 38-2). Vocabulary increases dramatically, from 300 words at age 2 to more than 2100 words at the end of 5 years. Sentence structure, grammatical usage, and intelligibility also advance to a more adult level. Through language, preschool children learn to express feelings of frustration or anger without acting them out.

Children between ages 3 and 4 form sentences of about three to four words and include only the most essential words to convey a meaning. Such speech is often termed *tel-*

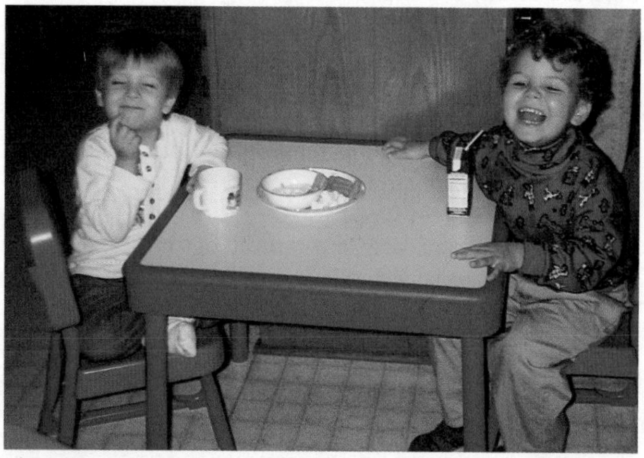

Fig. 38-2 Preschool children enjoy friends and often use nonverbal messages to communicate.

egraphic for its brevity in length. Three-year-old children ask many questions and use plurals, correct pronouns, and the past tense of verbs. They name familiar objects, such as animals, parts of the body, relatives, and friends. They can give and follow simple commands. They talk incessantly, regardless of whether anyone is listening or answering them. They enjoy musical or talking toys or dolls and imitate new words proficiently.

From ages 4 to 5 years preschoolers use longer sentences of four to five words and use more words to convey a message, such as prepositions, adjectives, and a variety of verbs. They follow simple directional commands, such as "Put the ball on the chair," but can carry out only one request at a time. They answer questions such as "What do you do when you are hungry?" by describing the appropriate action. The pattern of asking questions is at its peak, and children usually repeat the question until they receive an answer.

By the end of age 5 years children can use all parts of speech correctly, except for deviations from the rule. They can define simple things by describing their use, shape, or general category of classification, rather than simply describing their outward appearance. For example, they define a ball as "round, something you bounce, or a toy," rather than by its color. They can give some opposites, such as "If Mommy is a woman, Daddy is a man." By the time they are 6 years old, they can describe an object according to its composition, such as "A spoon is made of metal."

Personal-Social Behavior

The pervasive ritualism and negativism of toddlerhood gradually diminish during the preschool years. Although self-assertion is still a major theme, preschoolers demonstrate their sense of autonomy differently. They are able to verbalize their request for independence and perform independently because of their much-refined physical and cognitive development. By 4 or 5 years of age they need little if any assistance with dressing, eating, or toileting (Fig. 38-3). They can also be trusted to obey warnings of danger, although 3- or 4-year-old children may exceed their boundaries at times.

They are also much more sociable and willing to please. They have internalized many of the standards and values of the family and culture. However, by the end of early childhood they begin to question parental values and compare them with those of their peer group and other authority figures; as a result, they may be less willing to abide by the family's code of conduct. Preschoolers become increasingly aware of their position and role within the family. Although this is a more secure age for experiencing the addition of another sibling, relinquishing the position of first or youngest is still difficult and requires appropriate preparation (see Sibling Rivalry, Chapter 37).

Play

Various types of play are typical of this period, but preschoolers especially enjoy *associative play*—group play in similar or identical activities but without rigid organization or rules. Play should provide for physical, social, and mental development.

Play activities for physical growth and refinement of motor skills include jumping, running, and climbing. Tricycles, scooter trucks, wagons, gym and sports equipment, sandboxes, wading pools, and winter sleds can help develop muscles and coordination. Activities such as swimming and skating teach safety, as well as muscle development and coordination. Children involved in the work of play do not require expensive toys and gadgets to keep them entertained but often find common household items such as a broom handle or even items adults consider junk (sticks, rocks, dirt, and sand) to play with. The imaginative mind of the preschooler enjoys play for its own sake.

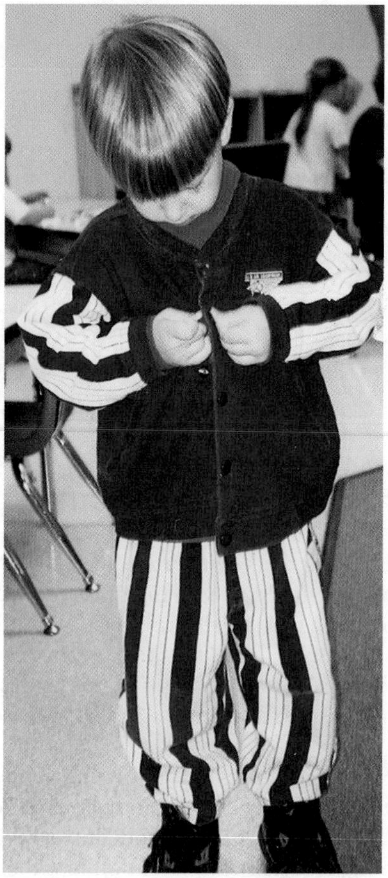

Fig. 38-3 Most preschoolers are able to dress themselves but need help with more difficult items of clothing.

Manipulative, constructive, creative, and educational toys provide for quiet activities, fine motor development, and self-expression. Easy construction sets, large blocks of various sizes and shapes, a counting frame, alphabet or number flash cards, paints, crayons, simple carpentry tools, musical toys, illustrated books, simple sewing or handicraft sets, large puzzles, and clay are suitable toys (Fig. 38-4). Electronic games and computer programs are especially valuable in helping children learn basic skills, such as letters and simple words.

CRITICAL THINKING: IMITATIVE PLAY

Probably the most characteristic and pervasive preschool activity is *imitative, imaginative,* and *dramatic play.* Dress-up clothes, dolls, housekeeping toys, dollhouses, playstore toys, telephones, farm animals and equipment, village sets, trains, trucks, cars, planes, hand puppets, and doctor and nurse kits provide hours of self-expression (Fig. 38-5). Probably at no other time is the reproduction of adult behavior so faithful and absorbing as in 4- and 5-year-old children. During this time gender-stereotyping is also part of the child's develop-

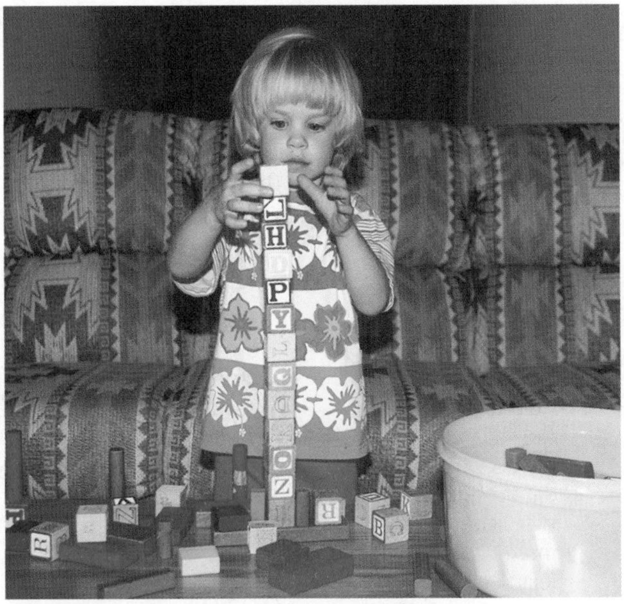

Fig. 38-4 Preschoolers enjoy a sense of accomplishment from activities such as building blocks.

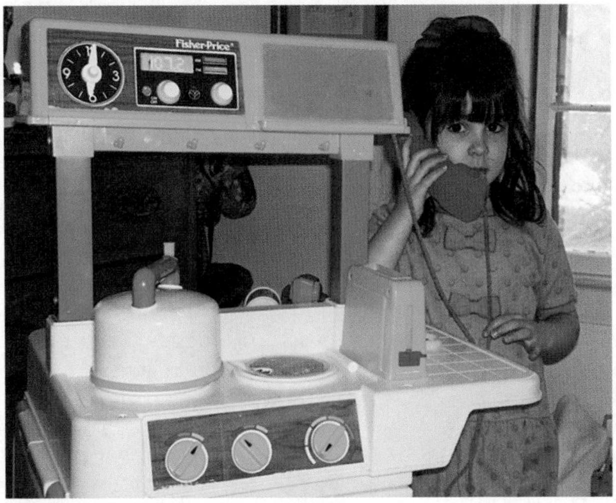

Fig. 38-5 Imaginative and dramatic play is typical of preschoolers, who enjoy fantasy.

ment; the notion that men can become nurses, women can become doctors, and so on becomes ingrained in the child's set of life expectations, especially if such notions are reinforced by the parents or significant-other adults. Toward the end of the preschool period, children are less satisfied with make-believe or pretend objects and enjoy actually doing the activity, such as cooking and carpentry.

Television and videotapes also have their places in children's play, although each should be only one part of children's total repertoire of social and recreational activities. Parents and other caregivers should supervise selection of programs, preview programs for appropriateness, and schedule hours for television viewing (Vessey, Yim-Chiplis, & MacKenzie, 1998). Children also enjoy and learn from educational programs; television can become an interactive activity when adults view programs with children and discuss program content (see discussion on television, including Parent Guidelines, in Chapter 33). In one study, viewing educational programs as preschoolers was associated with higher grades, reading more books, greater emphasis on achievement, increased creativity, and less aggression in adolescent years (Anderson et al, 2001). The researchers emphasize that the quality of television viewing is thought to be more important than the amount viewed.

Play is so much a part of the young child's life that reality and fantasy become blurred. The make-believe is reality during play and only becomes fantasy when the toys are put away or the dress-up clothes are removed. It is no wonder that *imaginary playmates* are so much a part of this age period.

The appearance of imaginary companions usually occurs between ages 2½ and 3 years, and for the most part such playmates are relinquished when the child enters school. There seems to be a relationship between the level of intelligence and the presence of the imaginary companion. More intelligent children tend to have more vivid and complex pretend playmates.

Imaginary companions serve many purposes: They become friends in times of loneliness, they accomplish what the child is still attempting, and they experience what the child wants to forget or remember. It is not unusual for the "friend" to have a myriad of vices and to be blamed for wrongdoing. Sometimes the child hopes to escape punishment by saying, "My friend George broke the glass." At other times the child may fantasize that the companion misbehaved and play the role of parent. This becomes a way of assuming control and authority in a safe situation.

Parents often worry about the imaginary playmates, not realizing how normal and useful they are. They need to be reassured that children's fantasy is a sign of health that helps them differentiate between make-believe and reality. Parents can acknowledge the presence of the imaginary companion by calling him or her by name and even agreeing to simple requests such as setting an extra place at the table, but they should not allow the child to use the playmate to avoid punishment or responsibility. For example, if the child blames the companion for messing a room, parents need to state clearly that the child is the only one they see and therefore the child is responsible for cleaning up.

Children also benefit from play that occurs between them and a parent. *Mutual play* fosters development from birth through the school years and provides enriched opportunities for learning. Through mutual play parents can provide tactile and kinesthetic experiences, can maximize verbal and language abilities, and can offer praise and encouragement for exploration of the world. In addition, mutual play encourages positive interactions between the parent and child, strengthening their relationship (Gottesman, 1999).* Table 38-1 summarizes the major developmental achievements for children 3, 4, and 5 years old.

*Recommended books for suggestions on mutual play include *Quick and fun learning activities* books, by Teacher Created Material, Inc., 6421 Industry Way, Westminster, CA 92683; phone: 714-891-7895, 800-858-7339; Web site: www.teachercreated.com.

Table 38-1

Growth and Development during Preschool Years

AGE (YEARS)	PHYSICAL	GROSS MOTOR	FINE MOTOR	LANGUAGE
3	Usual weight gain of 1.8-2.7 kg (4-6 pounds) per year Average weight of 14.6 kg (32 pounds) Usual gain in height of 7.5 cm (3 inches) per year Average height of 95 cm (37¼ inches) May have achieved nighttime control of bowel and bladder	Rides tricycle Jumps off bottom step Stands on one foot for a few seconds Goes up stairs using alternate feet; may still come down using both feet on step Broad jumps May try to dance, but balance may not be adequate	Builds tower of 9 or 10 cubes Builds bridge with three cubes Adeptly places small pellets in narrow-necked bottle In drawing, copies a circle, imitates a cross, names what has been drawn, cannot draw stick figure but may make circle with facial features	Has vocabulary of about 900 words Uses primarily "telegraphic" speech Uses complete sentences of three or four words Talks incessantly regardless of whether anyone is paying attention Repeats sentence of six syllables Asks many questions
4	Pulse and respiration rates decrease slightly Growth rate is similar to that of previous year Average weight of 16.7 kg (36¾ pounds) Average height of 103 cm (40½ inches) Length at birth is doubled Maximum potential for development of amblyopia	Skips and hops on one foot Catches ball reliably Throws ball overhand Walks down stairs using alternate footing	Uses scissors successfully to cut out picture following outline Can lace shoes but may not be able to tie bow In drawing, copies a square, traces a cross and diamond, adds three parts to stick figure	Has vocabulary of 1500 words or more Uses sentences of four or five words Questioning is at peak Tells exaggerated stories Knows simple songs May be mildly profane if associates with older children Comprehends up to four prepositional phrases, such as "under," "on top of," "beside," "in back of," or "in front of" Names one or more colors Comprehends analogies, such as, "If ice is cold, fire is ___"
5	Pulse and respiration rates decrease slightly Average weight of 18.7 kg (41¼ pounds) Average height of 110 cm (43¼ inches) Eruption of permanent dentition may begin Handedness is established (about 90% are right-handed)	Skips and hops on alternate feet Throws and catches ball well Jumps rope Skates with good balance Walks backward with heel to toe Jumps from height of 12 inches and lands on toes Balances on alternate feet with eyes closed	Ties shoelaces Uses scissors, simple tools, or pencil very well In drawing, copies a diamond and triangle; adds seven to nine parts to stick figure; prints a few letters, numbers, or words, such as first name	Has vocabulary of about 2100 words Uses sentences of six to eight words, with all parts of speech Names coins (e.g., nickel, dime) Names four or more colors Describes drawing or pictures with much comment and enumeration Knows names of days of week, months, and other time-associated words Knows composition of articles, such as "A shoe is made of ___" Can follow three commands in succession

SOCIALIZATION	COGNITION	FAMILY RELATIONSHIPS
Dresses self almost completely if helped with back buttons and told which shoe is right or left Pulls on shoes Has increased attention span Feeds self completely Can prepare simple meals, such as cold cereal and milk Can help set table; can dry dishes without breaking any May have fears, especially of dark and going to bed Knows own gender and gender of others Play is parallel and associative; begins to learn simple games but often follows own rules; begins to share	Is in preconceptual phase Is egocentric in thought and behavior Has beginning understanding of time; uses many time-oriented expressions, talks about past and future as much as about present, pretends to tell time Has improved concept of space, as demonstrated by understanding of prepositions and ability to follow directional command Has beginning ability to view concepts from another perspective	Attempts to please parents and conform to their expectations Is less jealous of younger sibling; may be opportune time for birth of additional sibling Is aware of family relationships and sex-role functions Boys tend to identify more with father or other male figure Has increased ability to separate easily and comfortably from parents for short periods
Very independent Tends to be selfish and impatient Aggressive physically as well as verbally Takes pride in accomplishments Has mood swings Shows off dramatically, enjoys entertaining others Tells family tales to others with no restraint Still has many fears Play is associative Imaginary playmates are common Uses dramatic, imaginative, and imitative devices Sexual exploration and curiosity demonstrated through play, such as being "doctor" or "nurse"	Is in phase of intuitive thought Causality is still related to proximity of events Understands time better, especially in terms of sequence of daily events Unable to conserve matter Judges everything according to one dimension, such as height, width, or order Immediate perceptual clues dominate judgment Is beginning to develop less egocentrism and more social awareness May count correctly but has poor mathematic concept of numbers Obeys because parents have set limits, not because of understanding of right or wrong	Rebels if parents expect too much, such as impeccable table manners Takes aggression and frustration out on parents or siblings Do's and don'ts become important May have rivalry with older or younger siblings; may resent older sibling's privileges and younger sibling's invasion of privacy and possessions May "run away" from home Identifies strongly with parent of opposite sex
Less rebellious and quarrelsome than at age 4 years More settled and eager to get down to business Not as open and accessible in thoughts and behavior as in earlier years Independent but trustworthy; not foolhardy; more responsible Has fewer fears; relies on outer authority to control world Eager to do things right and to please; tries to "live by the rules" Has better manners Cares for self totally, occasionally needing supervision in dress or hygiene Not ready for concentrated close work or small print because of slight farsightedness and still unrefined eye-hand coordination Play is associative; tries to follow rules but may cheat to avoid losing	Begins to question what parents think by comparing them with age-mates and other adults May notice prejudice and bias in outside world Is more able to view other's perspective, but tolerates differences rather than understanding them May begin to show understanding of conservation of numbers through counting objects regardless of arrangement Uses time-oriented words with increased understanding Very curious about factual information regarding world	Gets along well with parents May seek out parent more often than at age 4 years for reassurance and security, especially when entering school Begins to question parents' thinking and principles Strongly identifies with parent of same sex, especially boys with their fathers Enjoys activities such as sports, cooking, and shopping with parent of same sex

Coping with Concerns Related to Normal Growth and Development

Preschool and Kindergarten Experience

Some children are home-schooled, but many children attend some type of early childhood program, usually preschool or a day care center. Group care has become commonplace with the large number of mothers presently employed outside the home (see Alternate Child Care Arrangements, Chapter 36). The effects of early education and stimulation on children have increasingly gained recognition and importance. (For a discussion of the effects of day care on young children, see Working Mothers, Chapter 31.) Because social development widens to include age-mates and other significant adults, preschool provides an excellent vehicle for expanding children's experiences with others. It also is an excellent preparation for entrance into elementary school.

In preschool or day care centers children are exposed to opportunities for learning group cooperation, adjusting to various sociocultural differences, and coping with frustration, dissatisfaction, and anger. If activities are tailored to provide mastery and achievement, children increasingly have feelings of success, self-confidence, and personal competence. Whether or not structured learning is imposed is less important than the social climate, type of guidance, and attitude toward the children that is fostered by the teacher or leader. With a teacher who is aware of preschoolers' developmental abilities and needs, children will learn from the activity that is provided. Most programs incorporate a daily schedule of quiet play, active outdoor play, group activities such as games and projects, creative or free play, and snack and rest periods. Preschool is particularly beneficial for children who lack a peer-group experience, such as an only child, and for children from impoverished homes. It also is an excellent preparation for kindergarten.

One of the issues that parents face is the child's readiness for preschool or kindergarten. There are no absolute indicators for school readiness, but the child's social maturation, especially attention span, is as important as his or her academic readiness. Using a developmental screening tool that addresses cognitive (especially language), social, and physical milestones can help identify children who may benefit from diagnostic testing. Developmental screening focuses on the potential to learn and differs from readiness testing, which stresses the specific skills the child has acquired (Glascoe, 2001).

Nurses and other health care workers can be helpful in guiding parents in selecting enriched social and educational early intervention programs and schools. Careful selection of early childhood education is intrinsic to future learning and development. Licensed and regulated programs are mandated to abide by established standards, which represent minimum requirements and safeguards. The importance of regulation is to protect children from harm, to promote the conditions essential for children's healthy development and learning, and to provide a variety of firsthand experiences and learning activities either directly to children or through parent participation (National Association for the Education of Young Children, 1995). The National Association for the Education of Young Children (NAEYC) serves as the model for optimum care of small children.*

Areas for parents to evaluate include the facility's daily program, teacher qualifications, staff-to-student ratio, discipline policy, environmental safety precautions, provision of meals, sanitary conditions, adequate indoor/outdoor space per child, and fee schedule. References from other parents help evaluate a facility, but personal observation of the facility is recommended. Encourage parents to meet the director and some of the employees at a few facilities to make an informed choice.

Important in selecting child care centers is an evaluation of the facility's health practices. Substantial evidence shows that children in day care centers, especially those under 3 years of age, have more illnesses, especially diarrhea, hepatitis A, meningitis, otitis media, respiratory tract infections, and cytomegalovirus, than children not in day care centers (Rovers et al, 1999).

Nurses play an important role in infection control. Not only can they advise parents regarding the evaluation of a facility's sanitary practices, but they can also take an active part in educating staff in measures to minimize transmission of infection (Lafontaine & Bedard, 1997). For example, in centers caring for children who are not toilet trained, reducing environmental contamination with urine and feces is an important infection control issue (Fig. 38-6).

Children need preparation for the preschool or kindergarten experience. For young children it represents a change from their usual home environment and prolonged separation from parents.

Before the child begins the school experience, the parents should present the idea as exciting and pleasurable. Talking to the child about activities such as painting, building with blocks, or enjoying swings and other outdoor equipment allows the child to fantasize about the forthcoming event in a positive manner. When the first day of school arrives, the parents should behave confidently. Such behavior requires parents to have resolved their own feelings regarding the experience.

Parents should introduce their child to the teacher and the facility. In some instances it is helpful to remain for at least some part of the first day until the child is comfortable and at ease. Other specific actions that can help lessen separation anxiety include providing the school with detailed information about the child's home environment, such as familiar routines, favorite activities, food preferences, names of siblings or pets, and personal habits. Such information helps the child feel familiar in the strange surroundings. When schools automatically request this information, the parent has a valuable clue to evaluating the quality of the program, because the request represents the staff's awareness

*Information about the accreditation criteria and procedures of the National Academy of Early Childhood Programs is available from the National Association for the Education of Young Children, 1509 16th Street, NW, Washington, DC 20036; phone: 202-232-8777 or 800-424-2460; Web site: www.naeyc.org. These criteria are excellent guidelines for evaluating preschools and day care centers.

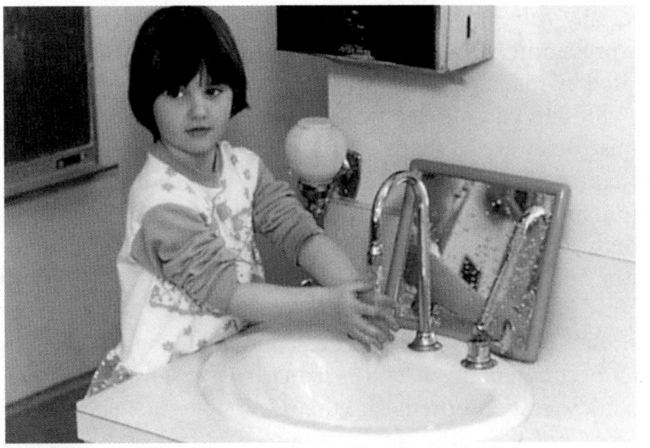

Fig. 38-6 Thorough handwashing is the single most effective method of preventing infection.

of each child's needs. Transitional objects, such as a favorite toy, may also help the child bridge the gap from home to school.

Sex Education

Preschoolers have experienced a tremendous amount of information during their short lifetimes. Although their thinking may not be mature, they search constantly for explanations and reasons that are logical and reasonable to them. The word "why" seems to supplant the word "no," which was common in toddlerhood. It is only natural that as they learn about "me," they will also want to know "why me" and "how me." Questions such as "Where do babies come from?" are as casual as "What makes it rain?" or "Who is that?" It is the *way* in which questions about procreation are answered that conditions children, even the youngest, to separate these questions from others about their world.

Two rules govern answering sensitive questions about topics such as sex. The first is to *find out what children know and think.* By investigating the theories children have produced as a reasonable explanation, parents not only give correct information, but also help children understand why their explanation is inaccurate. Another reason for ascertaining what the child thinks before offering any information is that the "unasked for" answer may be given. For example, 4-year-old Sally asked her father, "Where did I come from?" Both parents quickly took this inquiry as a clue for offering sex education. After the explanation, Sally exclaimed, "I don't know about all that! All I know is Mary came from New York and I want to know where I was born."

The second rule for giving information is to *be honest.* It is true that much of the correct information will be forgotten or misunderstood by the preschooler, but what is more important is that the correct information can be restated until the child absorbs and comprehends the facts. Even though the correct anatomic words may be hard to pronounce or even more difficult to remember, they become foundational content for explaining other concepts later on.

Honesty does not imply imparting to children every fact of life or allowing excessive permissiveness in sexual curiosity. When children ask one question, they are looking for one answer. When they are ready, they will ask about the other "unfinished" parts of the story. Sooner or later they will wonder how the "sperm meets the egg" and "how the baby gets out," but it is best to wait until they ask (during this period).

Regardless of whether children are given sex education, they will engage in games of sexual curiosity and exploration. At about 3 years of age children are aware of the anatomic differences between the sexes and are very concerned with how the other sex "works." This is not really "sexual" curiosity, because many children are still unaware of the reproductive function of the genitals. Their curiosity is for the eliminative function of the anatomy. Little boys wonder how girls can urinate without a penis, so they watch girls go to the bathroom. Because they cannot see anything but the stream of water coming out, they want to observe further for what makes it come out. "Doctor play" is often a game invented for just such investigation. Little girls are no less curious about boys' anatomy. It is very intriguing to have a closer inspection of this "thing" that girls do not have.

One question that parents often have is how to handle such sexual curiosity. A positive approach is to neither condone nor condemn the sexual curiosity but to express that if children have questions, they should ask the parents; then the parents should encourage them to engage in some other activity. In this way children can be helped to understand that there are ways that their sexual curiosity can be satisfied other than through playing investigative games. This in no way condemns the act but stresses alternative methods to seek solutions and answers. Allowing children unrestricted permissiveness only intensifies their anxiety and concern, because exploring and searching usually yield little evidence to satisfy their curiosity.

Many excellent books on sex education are available for preschool children at public libraries, and the Sexuality Information and Education Council of the United States (SIECUS),* local chapters of the Planned Parenthood Federation of America,† and the American Academy of Pediatrics‡ have bibliographies of suggested reading material. Parents should read the book themselves *before* giving or reading it to a child.

Another concern for some parents is *masturbation,* or self-stimulation of the genitals. This occurs at any age for a variety of reasons and, if not excessive, is normal and healthy. It is most common at 4 years of age and during adolescence. For preschoolers it is a part of sexual curiosity and exploration. If parents are concerned about masturbation in their children, it is essential for nurses to investigate the circumstances associated with the activity, because it may be an expression of anxiety, boredom, or unresolved conflicts. For example, a boy who repeatedly touches his penis is not masturbating for pleasure but may be reassuring himself that it is intact. Also, children who openly and publicly masturbate are inviting a reaction, such as discipline, punishment, or criticism. They

---

*130 W. 42nd St., Suite 350, New York, NY 10036; phone: 212-819-9770; Web site: www.siecus.org.

†National office: 434 West 33rd St., New York, NY 10001; phone: 212-541-7800 or 800-829-7732; Web site: www.plannedparenthood.org.

‡141 Northwest Point Blvd., Elk Grove Village, IL 60007; phone: 888-227-1770; fax: 847-228-1281; Web site: www.aap.org.

may be overwhelmed by their sexual feelings and asking others to help them channel them into more constructive outlets. Because masturbation, like other forms of sex play, is a private act, parents should emphasize this to children as part of teaching them socially acceptable behavior.

Fears

The greatest number and variety of real and imagined fears are present during the preschool years and include fear of the dark, being left alone (especially at bedtime), animals (particularly large dogs and snakes), ghosts, sexual matters (castration), and objects or persons associated with pain (Muris, Merckelbach, & Prins, 2000). The exact cause of children's fears is unknown. Parents often become perplexed about handling the fears because no amount of logical persuasion, coercion, or ridicule will send away the ghosts, boogeymen, monsters, and devils. Prolonged or inappropriate television viewing by preschoolers may increase fears and anxieties because of the inability to separate reality-based experiences from fantasy, which is often portrayed in television and video game media. Preschool boys are known to imitate and act out violent behavior viewed on television (Krug & Mikus, 1999; Villani, 2001). The preschooler who fears sitting on the toilet seat may relate to a television program in which a toilet became a monster and swallowed a child. This, of course, is fantasy, or *animism,* yet preschoolers may not be able to separate fantasy from reality or to adequately verbalize their fears. Fear of annihilation is common in preschoolers. Their fear of losing body parts with certain medical procedures such as insertion of an intravenous line or cast application on a limb is a very real threat to their existence.

The best way to help children overcome their fears is by actively involving them in finding practical methods to deal with the frightening experience. This may be as simple as keeping a night light on in the child's bedroom for assurance that no monsters lurk in the dark. Exposing children to the feared object in a safe situation also provides a type of conditioning, or *desensitization.* For instance, children who are afraid of dogs should never be forced to approach or touch one, but they may be gradually introduced to the experience by watching other children play with the animal. This type of modeling, demonstrating fearlessness in others, can be very effective if the child is allowed to progress at his or her own rate.

Usually by 5 or 6 years of age children relinquish these old fears. Explaining the developmental sequence of fears and their gradual disappearance may help parents feel more secure in handling preschoolers' fears. Sometimes fears do not subside with simple measures or developmental maturation. When children experience severe fears that disrupt family life, professional help is required.

Stress

Although for parents the preschool years generally are less troublesome than toddlerhood, this period of life presents children with many unique stresses. Some are innate and stem from preschoolers' unique understanding of the world, such as fears. Others are imposed, such as beginning school. Although minimum amounts of stress are beneficial during the early years to help children develop effective coping skills, excessive stress is harmful. Young children are especially vulnerable because of their limited capacity to cope. Expression of frustration, fear, or anxiety is further exacerbated by inadequate expressive language.

To help parents deal with stress in their child's life, they must be aware of signs of stress (see Stress in Childhood, Chapter 33) and be helped to identify the source. In addition, any number of other stresses may be present, such as the birth of a sibling, marital discord, divorce and separation, relocation, or illness. The best approach to dealing with stress is prevention—monitoring the amount of stress in children's lives so that levels exceeding their coping ability do not occur. In many instances structuring children's schedules to allow rest and preparing them for change, such as entering school, are sufficient measures.

Aggression

The term *aggression* refers to behavior that attempts to hurt a person or destroy property. Aggression differs from anger, which is a temporary emotional state, but anger may be expressed through aggression. Aggression is influenced by a complex set of biologic, sociocultural, and familial variables. Factors that tend to increase aggressive behavior are gender, frustration, modeling, and reinforcement. Hyperaggressive behavior in preschoolers is characterized by unprovoked physical attacks on other children and adults, destruction of others' property, frequent intense temper tantrums, extreme impulsivity, disrespect, and noncompliance.

There is evidence that males are more overtly aggressive than females (Stormshak et al, 2000). *Frustration,* or the continual thwarting of self-satisfaction by disapproval, humiliation, punishment, and insults, can lead children to act out against others as a means of release. Especially if they fear parents, these children will displace their anger on others, particularly peers and other authority figures. This type of aggression often applies to the child who is well behaved at home but a discipline problem at school or a bully among playmates.

Modeling, or imitating the behavior of significant others, is a powerful influencing force in preschoolers. Children who see their parents as verbally or physically abusive are observing behavior that they come to know as acceptable (Hart et al, 1998). Another aspect of modeling is the "double standard" for acceptable conduct. For example, in some families, aggression is synonymous with masculinity, and boys are encouraged to defend themselves. Television is also a significant source for modeling at this age. Therefore parents need encouragement to supervise television programs viewed by their preschool children. The American Academy of Pediatrics (AAP), Committee on Public Education (2001), offers a list of recommendations for healthy television viewing.

Reinforcement can also shape aggressive behavior. Sometimes the reward for aggression is negative (e.g., punishment) yet reinforcing because it brings attention. For example, children who are ignored by a parent until they hit a sibling or the parent learn that this act garners attention.

When extreme behaviors such as aggression are present in children, parents are concerned about the need for professional help. Generally the difference between "normal" and "problematic" behavior is not the behavior itself but its *quantity* (number of occurrences), *severity* (interference with social or cognitive functioning), *distribution* (different manifestations), *onset* (when behavior started), and *duration* (at least 4 weeks).*

Speech Problems

The most critical period for speech development occurs between 2 and 4 years of age. During this period children are using their rapidly growing vocabulary faster than they can produce the words. This failure to master sensorimotor integrations results in *stuttering* or *stammering* as children try to say the word they are already thinking about. This dysfluency in speech pattern is a *normal* characteristic of language development (Ambrose & Yairi, 1999) and usually resolves provided caregivers speak clearly and do not complete the child's sentences and overcorrect mistakes. When parents or other significant persons place undue emphasis or stress on this pattern of dysfluency, an abnormal speech pattern may develop. The best therapy for speech problems is prevention and early detection. Common causes of speech problems are hearing loss, developmental delay, and a lack of verbal stimulation (AAP, 2003). Referral for further evaluation and treatment may be necessary to prevent a problem from interfering with learning. Anticipatory preparation of parents for expected developmental norms may allay caregiver concerns.

Children pressured into producing sounds ahead of their developmental level may develop *dyslalia* (articulation problems) or revert to using infantile speech. Prevention involves discussing with parents the usual achievement of speech production during childhood. The *Denver Articulation Screening Examination (DASE)* is an excellent tool for assessing articulation skills in the child and for explaining to parents the expected progression of sounds (see Appendix D).

PROMOTING OPTIMUM HEALTH DURING THE PRESCHOOL YEARS†

Nutrition

Nutritional requirements for preschoolers are fairly similar to those for toddlers. The requirement for calories per unit of body weight continues to decrease slightly to 90 kcal/kg, for an average daily intake of 1800 calories. Fluid requirements may also decrease slightly to about 100 ml/kg daily but depend on activity level, climatic conditions, and state of health. The protein requirements are 1.2 g/kg, for an average daily consumption of 24 g. A diet that is moderately reduced in fat may be recommended for healthy preschool children (Williams et al, 2002). The AAP, Committee on Nutrition (1998), recommends that by 5 years of age saturated fatty acid consumption should be less than 10% of total caloric intake. There is increasing evidence that the incidence of coronary heart disease, obesity, and chronic health problems such as diabetes mellitus can be influenced by early eating patterns. Preschoolers may have a decreased fat intake with substitutes such as soy-enriched foods without affecting overall growth (Endres et al, 2003; Johnson, 2000). In a Healthy Start intervention study, a group of preschool children consumed meals with 10% less saturated fat and maintained adequate total energy intake; interventions were aimed at counseling cooks in the Head Start centers to prepare foods with less saturated fats (Williams et al, 2002). Parents and others who provide soy substitutes should ensure that the products are vitamin enriched and low in fat content because some soy products may not have a lower fat content and may be deficient in some nutrients (Endres et al, 2003). It is important that the diet contain adequate nutrients such as calcium. Milk and dairy products are excellent sources of calcium and vitamin D (fortified). Low-fat milk may be substituted so that the quantity of milk may remain the same but fat intake limited overall.

In children over 2 years of age, intake of fiber, fruits, and vegetables should equal the child's age plus 5 in grams per day. This translates into five servings of fruits and vegetables each day (Johnson, 2000). The amount of fruit juice intake should not exceed 6 ounces per day (approximately one serving) for children ages 1 to 6 (AAP, Committee on Nutrition, 2001). Intake of carbonated beverages in young children is known to contribute large amounts of nonnutritive calories, which may displace or preclude intake of nutrients necessary for growth. In one study, 5-year-olds consumed more carbonated beverages and fruit drinks (non-100% fruit juice) than the recommended 4 to 6 oz/day of 100% fruit juice (Rampersaud, Bailey, & Kauwell, 2003). Parents should be educated regarding the association of nonnutritious fruit drinks, which usually contain less than 10% fruit juice yet are often advertised as healthy and nutritious; sugar content is increased dramatically and often precludes an adequate intake of milk by the child. Nutritious midmorning and midafternoon snacks may be given to preschoolers without affecting their overall daily intake of protein and energy or mealtime intake (Wilson, 1999). The U.S. Department of Agriculture, Center for Nutrition Policy and Promotion (2005), Food Guide Pyramid for Young Children (see Fig. 47-1) is appropriate for preschoolers. The foods depicted are those commonly eaten by children in this age group, and the illustrations emphasize the importance of physical activity. Parents and caregivers can provide opportunities for children to learn to like a variety of nutritious foods by exposing them to these foods (Fig. 38-7). The importance of role modeling by parents cannot be overemphasized in regard to food intake and dietary habits; if the parent will not eat a particular food or if dietary habits are poor in the adults, they will be in the child as well.

NURSE ALERT Obesity has increased over the last two decades in young children. Efforts to provide a healthy diet and to encourage physical activity should begin early to help children achieve optimal health. ■

Some preschoolers still have food habits that are typical of toddlers, such as food fads and strong taste preferences. When children reach 4 years of age, they seem to enter another period of finicky eating, which is generally character-

*A helpful site for resources dealing with child behavior is the Developmental-Behavioral Pediatrics Online Community Web site at www.dbpeds.org.

†For a more comprehensive understanding, the reader is urged to review the material presented in Chapter 37 under Promoting Optimum Health during Toddlerhood.

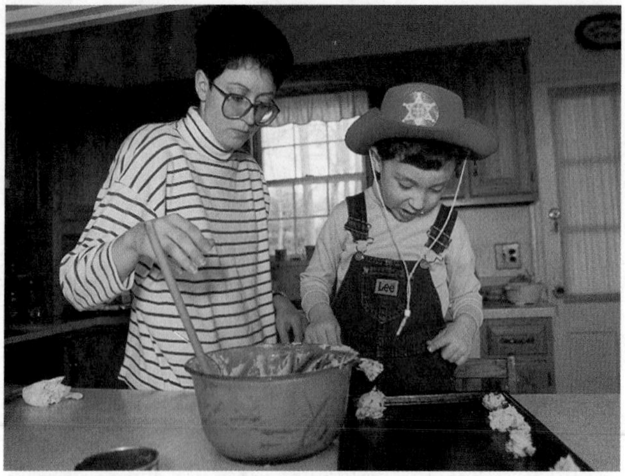

Fig. 38-7 Preschool-age children enjoy helping adults and are more likely to try new foods if they can assist in the preparation.

istic of the more rebellious and rowdy behavior of children in this age group. Just as with the toddler, small portions should be offered of each item being served. Large portions tend to overwhelm the child and lead to less intake. The practice of having the child remain at the table until the "plate is clean" should be avoided because this may contribute to overeating and the development of poor eating habits, which may contribute to poor health later in life. By age 5 years children are more willing to try new foods, especially if they are encouraged by an adult who allows them to help with food preparation or experiment with a new taste or different dish (see Fig. 38-7). Mealtimes can become battlegrounds if parents expect perfect table manners. Usually the 5-year-old child is ready for the "social" side of eating, but the 3- or 4-year-old child still has difficulty sitting quietly through a long family meal.

The amount and variety of foods consumed by young children vary greatly from day to day. Consequently, parents sometimes worry about the quantity of food preschoolers consume. In general, the quality is much more important than the quantity, a fact that should be stressed during nutritional counseling. Some evidence suggests that children self-regulate their caloric intake. If they eat less at one meal, they will compensate at another meal or will snack.

One approach toward lessening this parental concern is advising parents to keep a weekly record of everything the child eats. In particular, the need for measuring the amount of food, such as setting aside ½ cup of vegetables, and serving the child from this premeasured amount is stressed to provide a more accurate estimate of food intake at each meal. When parents look at the food chart at the end of the week they are usually amazed at how much the child has consumed. In general, preschoolers consume only slightly more than toddlers, or about half an adult's portion.

Sleep and Activity

Sleep patterns vary widely, but the average preschooler sleeps about 12 hours a night and infrequently takes daytime naps. Waking during the night is common throughout early childhood and may be related to social rather than developmental factors (Thiedke, 2001). Motor activity levels continue to be high and allow preschoolers to explore their environment, begin learning physical games and sports, and interact with others. Passive activities, such as television, are increasingly appealing and can become an unhealthy substitute for active play. Preschoolers' increased gross motor abilities and coordination provide them with the opportunity to engage in many physical activities, if only at a novice level. Whether young children should begin formalized training in an activity at this early age is controversial. Training programs must consider the child's physical and psychologic immaturity. Readiness to participate in organized sports should be determined individually. The decision should be based on the child's (not the parent's) motivation and enjoyment. The AAP, Committee on Sports Medicine and Fitness and Committee on School Health (2000), encourages free play, a variety of physical activities, a noncompetitive atmosphere, and emphasis on fun and safety.

Sleep Problems*

evolve CASE STUDY: SLEEP PROBLEMS

The preschool years are a prime time for sleep disturbances. As toddlers and preschoolers cope with autonomy, separation, and object permanence, they begin to have more sleep problems (Thiedke, 2001). Some have trouble going to sleep, especially after so much activity and stimulation during the day. Others may develop bedtime fears, wake during the night, or have nightmares or sleep terrors. Still others may prolong the inevitable through elaborate rituals.

Recommendations for handling a sleep disturbance are offered only *after* a thorough assessment of the problem has been completed. Cultural traditions may dictate sleep practices that are contrary to certain well-accepted professional recommendations. Therefore parents may not perceive a particular sleep practice as a problem (Cultural Awareness box).

Interventions differ greatly; for example, *nightmares* (frightening dreams that are followed by full waking) and *sleep terrors* (partial arousal from deep, nondreaming sleep) require very different approaches.

For children who delay going to bed, a recommended approach involves counseling parents about the importance of a consistent bedtime ritual. Attention-seeking behavior is ignored, and the child is not taken into the parents' bed or allowed to stay up past a reasonable hour. Other measures that may be helpful include keeping a light on in the room, providing transitional objects such as a favorite toy, or leaving a drink of water by the bed.

Helping children slow down *before* bedtime also contributes to less resistance to going to bed. One approach is to establish limited rituals that signal readiness for bed, such as a bath or story. Parents can reinforce the pattern by stating, "After this story it is bedtime," and consistently carrying out the routine. If extra stimulation, such as having visitors arrive at bedtime, is disruptive to children's routine, it is advisable to settle children in bed beforehand. Television viewing before bedtime may cause bedtime resistance and delay sleep onset.

*Guidelines for helping parents deal with sleep problems are available in Hockenberry MH: *Wong's clinical manual of pediatric nursing*, ed 6, St Louis, 2004, Mosby.

Cultural Awareness

CO-SLEEPING

Although many experts recommend that infants and children be trained to always sleep in their own crib or bed, *co-sleeping,* or the "family bed" (in which parents allow the children to sleep with them or the siblings to sleep together in one bed), is a relatively common and accepted cultural practice, especially among African-American, Hispanic, and Asian families, such as the Japanese (Latz, Wolf, & Lozoff, 1999). Other groups that are adopting co-sleeping include (1) single parents, whose need for company may encourage this practice; (2) working parents, who desire the closeness at night that was lost during the day; and (3) parents who have had an issue about sleep or separation in their own past (Anderson, 2000). There is some concern among health care professionals that the incidence of sudden infant death syndrome (SIDS) may be increased with bedsharing, especially when parental smoking, maternal obesity, and use of an atypical adult bed are involved. However, co-sleeping and breastfeeding are not believed to be effective in preventing SIDS. Co-sleeping may be a practical solution to limited numbers of bedrooms or beds in lower socioeconomic families. In a longitudinal study measuring the effects of co-sleeping at 6 and 18 years, bedsharing in early childhood was found to correlate positively with increased cognitive competence in 6-year-olds. Co-sleeping was not associated with sleep problems, sexual pathology, or any other problematic consequences at 6 and 18 years. At 18 years children who had practiced bedsharing experienced no particular measurable positive effects of the experience. The researchers caution health care workers about warning parents to avoid bedsharing to prevent SIDS and further question the safety of solitary sleep (Okami, Weisner, & Olmstead, 2002). Parents who are considering adopting the practice of bedsharing should be made aware that this is a difficult habit for the child to break in the future.

Dental Health

By the beginning of the preschool period the eruption of the deciduous teeth is complete. Dental care is essential to preserve these temporary teeth and to teach good dental habits (see Chapter 37). Although preschoolers' fine motor control is improved, they still require assistance and supervision with brushing twice daily, and flossing should be performed by parents. Professional care and prophylaxis, especially fluoride supplements, should be continued. Routine dental care should be well established during preschool years and is recommended at 6- to 12-month intervals depending on the family history, the child's dental development, and the presence or absence of dental caries (Martof, 2001). For children cared for away from home, parents are encouraged to monitor the dental care provided by others, including keeping cariogenic foods to a minimum in the diet. Trauma to teeth during this period is not uncommon, and prompt evaluation by a dentist is warranted if oral trauma occurs. Preservation of the space previously occupied by an avulsed tooth is necessary for proper eruption of the secondary tooth.

Injury Prevention

Because of improved gross and fine motor skills, coordination, and balance, preschoolers are less prone to falls than are toddlers. They tend to be less reckless, listen more to parental rules, and are aware of potential dangers, such as hot objects, sharp instruments, and dangerous heights. Putting objects in the mouth as part of exploration has all but ceased, although accidental poisoning is still a danger and playground injuries increase. Pedestrian motor vehicle injuries increase because of activities such as playing in the parking lot, driveway, or street; riding tricycles and running after balls; or forgetting safety regulations when crossing streets.

In general, the guidelines suggested for injury prevention in Table 37-3 apply to children in this age group as well. However, emphasis is now on *education* for safety and potential hazards, in addition to appropriate protection. This period is an excellent time to start enforcing the use of safety items such as bicycle helmets to prevent head trauma; children are less likely to warm to the idea later in life because of peer pressure. Because preschoolers are great imitators, it is essential that parents set a good example by "practicing what they preach." Children quickly observe discrepancies in what they are told to do and what they see others do. Establishing habits at this time, such as wearing bicycle helmets, can create long-term safety behaviors.

Anticipatory Guidance–Care of Families

The preschool years present fewer childrearing difficulties than earlier years, and this stage of development is facilitated by appropriate anticipatory guidance in the areas already discussed (Home Care box). There is a shift in childrearing practices from protection to education. Whereas injury prevention previously focused on safeguarding the immediate environment, with less emphasis on reasoning, now the protective guardrails or electrical outlet caps may be substituted with verbal explanations of why danger exists and how to avoid it with appropriate judgment and understanding.

During this period an emotional transition between parent and child is also occurring. Although children are still attached to their parents and accepting of all parental values and beliefs, they are nearing the period of life when they will question previous teachings and prefer the companionship of peers. Entry into school marks a separation from home for parents, as well as for children. Parents need help in adjusting to this change, particularly if the mother has focused her daily activity primarily on home responsibilities. All family members must adjust to changes, which is part of the process of growth and development.

SPECIAL HEALTH PROBLEMS

Communicable Diseases

The incidence of childhood communicable diseases has declined greatly since the advent of immunizations. Serious complications resulting from such infections have been further reduced with the use of antibiotics and antitoxins. However, infectious diseases do occur, and nurses must be familiar with the infectious agent to recognize the disease and to institute appropriate preventive and supportive interventions (Table 38-2). (See also Chapter 53 for a discussion of nursing care for dermatologic conditions.)

Home Care

GUIDANCE DURING PRESCHOOL YEARS

Age 3 Years

Prepare parents for child's increasing interest in widening relationships.
Encourage enrollment in preschool.
Emphasize importance of setting limits.
Prepare parents to expect exaggerated tension reduction behaviors, such as need for "security blanket."
Encourage parents to offer child choices when child vacillates.
Prepare parents to expect marked changes at 3½ years, when child becomes less coordinated (motor and emotional), becomes insecure, and exhibits emotional extremes.
Prepare parents for normal dysfluency in speech and advise them to avoid focusing on the pattern.
Prepare parents to expect extra demands on their attention as a reflection of child's emotional insecurity and fear of loss of love.
Warn parents that equilibrium of 3-year-old will change to aggressive, out-of-bounds behavior of 4-year-old.
Inform parents to anticipate more stable appetite with more food selections.
Stress need for protection and education of child to prevent injury (see Injury Prevention, Chapter 37).

Age 4 Years

Prepare parents for more aggressive behavior, including motor activity and offensive language.
Prepare parents to expect resistance to parental authority.
Explore parental feelings regarding child's behavior.
Suggest some kind of respite for primary caregivers, such as placing child in preschool for part of the day.
Prepare parents for child's increasing sexual curiosity.
Emphasize importance of realistic limit setting on behavior and appropriate discipline techniques.
Prepare parents for highly imaginative 4-year-old who indulges in "tall tales" (to be differentiated from lies) and for child's imaginary playmates.
Prepare parents to expect nightmares or an increase in them and suggest that parents make sure child is fully awakened from a frightening dream.
Provide reassurance that a period of calm begins at 5 years of age.

Age 5 Years

Inform parents to expect tranquil period at 5 years.
Help parents to prepare child for entrance into school environment.
Make sure immunizations are up to date before entering school.
Suggest that nonemployed mothers (or fathers if appropriate) consider own activities when child begins school.
Suggest swimming lessons for child.

Nursing Care Management

Assessment

Identification of the infectious agent is of primary importance to prevent exposure to susceptible individuals. Nurses in ambulatory care settings, child care centers, and schools are often the first persons to see signs of a communicable disease, such as a rash or sore throat. The nurse must operate under a high index of suspicion for common childhood diseases in order to identify potentially infectious cases and to recognize diseases that require medical intervention. An example is the common complaint of sore throat. Although most often a symptom of a minor viral infection, it can signal diphtheria or a streptococcal infection, such as scarlet fever. Each of these bacterial conditions requires appropriate medical treatment to prevent serious sequelae.

When a communicable disease is suspected, it is important to assess the following: (1) recent exposure to a known case; (2) *prodromal symptoms* (symptoms that occur between early manifestations of the disease and its overt clinical syndrome) or evidence of constitutional symptoms, such as a fever or rash (see Table 38-2); (3) immunization history; and (4) history of having the disease. Immunizations are available for many diseases, and infection usually confers lifelong immunity; therefore the possibility of many infectious agents can be eliminated based on these two criteria.

Nursing Diagnoses

Several nursing diagnoses are prominent in the nursing care of the child with a communicable disease. Others specific to individual cases may also be evident. The most common nursing diagnoses are presented in the Nursing Care Plan on p. 1138.

Plan of Care and Implementation

The principal nursing goals, in addition to identification of the communicable disease (see Assessment), are as follows:

1. Child will not spread the infection to others.
2. Child will not experience complications.
3. Child will have minimal discomfort.
4. Child and family will receive adequate emotional support.

Prevent Spread

Prevention consists of two components: prevention of the disease and control of its spread to others. Primary prevention rests almost exclusively on immunization. (The nurse's role in immunization of children is discussed in Chapter 36.)

Control measures to prevent spread of disease should include techniques to reduce risk of cross-transmission of infectious organisms between patients and to protect health care workers from organisms harbored by patients. If the child is hospitalized, the facility's policies for infection control are followed (see Chapter 45). The most important procedure is handwashing. Persons directly caring for the child or handling contaminated articles must wash their hands before care of another patient. The child is instructed to practice good handwashing technique after toileting and before eating. For those diseases spread by droplets, the nurse instructs parents in measures to reduce airborne transmission. The child who is old enough should use a tissue to cover the face during coughing or sneezing; otherwise the parent should cover the child's mouth with a tissue and then discard it. The usual hygiene measures of not sharing eating and drinking utensils are stressed to the family.

NURSE ALERT If a child is admitted to the hospital with an undiagnosed exanthema, strict isolation is instituted until a diagnosis is confirmed. Childhood communicable diseases re-

Critical Thinking Exercise: Conjunctivitis

evolve Case Study: Bacterial Conjunctivitis

Nursing Care Plan: The Child with a Communicable Disease

quiring isolation are diphtheria, chickenpox, measles, tuberculosis, adenovirus, *Haemophilus influenzae* type b, influenza, mumps, *Mycoplasma pneumoniae*, pertussis, plague, streptococcal pharyngitis, pneumonia, and scarlet fever (AAP, Committee on Infectious Diseases, 2003). ■

Prevent Complications

evolve CASE STUDY: VARICELLA IN SPITE OF VACCINE

Although most children recover without difficulty, certain groups are at risk for serious, even fatal, complications from communicable diseases, especially the viral diseases of chickenpox and erythema infectiosum (EI). Children with immunodeficiency—those receiving steroid or other immunosuppressive therapy, those with a generalized malignancy such as leukemia or lymphoma, or those with an immunologic disorder—are at risk for viremia from replication of the *varicella-zoster virus (VZV)** in the blood. VZV is so named because it causes two distinct diseases: *varicella (chickenpox)* and *zoster* (*herpes zoster* or *shingles*). Varicella occurs primarily in children under 15 years of age. However, it leaves the threat of herpes zoster, an intensely painful varicella that is localized to a single dermatome (body area innervated by a particular segment of the spinal cord). Immunocompromised patients and healthy infants under 1 year of age (who also have reduced immunity) are at a higher risk for reactivation of VZV, causing herpes zoster, probably as a result of a deficiency in cellular immunity (Chen et al, 2002).

Children with hemolytic disease, such as sickle cell disease, are at risk for aplastic anemia from EI. The *human parvovirus (HPV)* infects and lyses red blood cell precursors, thus interrupting the production of red blood cells. Therefore the virus may precipitate a severe aplastic crisis in patients who need increased red blood cell production to maintain normal red blood cell volumes. Because the fetus depends on a high rate of red blood cell production and has an immature immune system, the fetus may develop severe anemia as a result of HPV infection in the mother.

NURSE ALERT High risk children who have signs of these communicable diseases are referred to the practitioner immediately. School nurses are responsible for warning parents about recent outbreaks of these communicable diseases in order to prevent susceptible children's exposure to known cases. ■

Prevention of complications from diseases such as diphtheria and scarlet fever necessitates compliance with antibiotic therapy. With oral preparations the need to complete the entire course of therapy is stressed (see Compliance, Chapter 45). The use of varicella-zoster immune globulin (VZIG) should be strongly considered in high risk children after exposure to chickenpox to prevent the development of varicella. The antiviral agent acyclovir (Zovirax) may be used to treat varicella infections; it is effective in decreasing the number of lesions, shortening the duration of fever, and decreasing itching, lethargy, and anorexia. Acyclovir should be considered for otherwise healthy, nonpregnant individuals over 12 years of age; children with chronic cutaneous or pulmonary conditions; those receiving chronic salicylate therapy; and those receiving short, intermittent, or aerosolized courses of corticosteroids (AAP, Committee on Infectious Diseases, 2003). Immunocompromised children should receive acyclovir by intravenous infusion (AAP, Committee on Infectious Diseases, 2003).

Recent evidence suggests that vitamin A supplementation reduces both morbidity and mortality rates in measles and that all children with severe measles should be given vitamin A supplements (Stalkup, 2002). A single oral dose of 200,000 international units for children at least 1 year old (half that dose for children 6 to 12 months of age) is recommended. The higher dose may be associated with vomiting and headache for a few hours. The dose should be repeated the next day and at 4 weeks for children with ophthalmologic evidence of vitamin A deficiency (AAP, Committee on Infectious Diseases, 2003).

NURSE ALERT Although the risk of vitamin A toxicity from these doses (they are 100 to 200 times the recommended dietary allowance) is very low, nurses should instruct parents on safe storage of the drug. Ideally, vitamin A should be dispensed in the age-appropriate unit dose to prevent excessive administration and possible toxicity. ■

Provide Comfort

Many communicable diseases cause skin manifestations that are bothersome to the child. The chief discomfort from most rashes is itching, and measures such as cool baths (usually without soap) and lotions (e.g., calamine) are helpful.

NURSE ALERT When lotions with active ingredients such as diphenhydramine in Caladryl are used, they are applied sparingly, especially over open lesions, where excessive absorption can lead to drug toxicity. These lotions should be avoided in children who are simultaneously receiving oral diphenhydramine. ■

To avoid overheating, which increases itching, children should wear lightweight, loose, nonirritating clothing and keep out of the sun. If the child persists in scratching, the nails are kept short and smooth; mittens and clothes with long sleeves or legs may be needed. For severe itching, antipruritic medication, such as diphenhydramine (Benadryl) or hydroxyzine (Atarax), may be required, especially when the child desires to sleep.

An elevated temperature is common, and both antipyretic medicine (acetaminophen or ibuprofen) and environmental manipulation are implemented (see Controlling Elevated Temperature, Chapter 45). The acetaminophen is effective in lowering the fever but does not significantly reduce the symptoms of itching, anorexia, abdominal pain, fussiness, or vomiting.

A sore throat, another frequent symptom, is managed with lozenges, saline rinses (if the child is old enough to cooperate), and analgesics. Because most children are anorectic during an illness, bland foods and increased liquids are usually preferred. During the early stages of the disease, children

Text continued on p. 1136.

*Educational materials may be obtained from the Varicella Zoster Virus Research Foundation, 40 East 72nd St., New York, NY 10021; or GlaxoSmithKline, 3030 Cornwallis Rd., Research Triangle Park, NC 27709; phone: 919-248-3000 or 888-825-5249; Web site: www.gsk.com.

Table 38-2

Communicable Diseases of Childhood

DISEASE

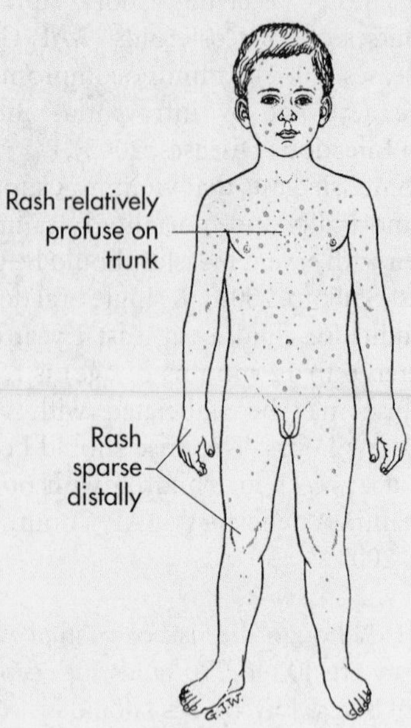

CHICKENPOX (VARICELLA) (Fig. 38-8)
Agent: Varicella-zoster virus (VZV)
Source: Primary secretions of respiratory tract of infected persons; to a lesser degree, skin lesions (scabs not infectious)
Transmission: Direct contact, droplet (airborne) spread, and contaminated objects
Incubation period: 2-3 weeks, usually 14-16 days
Period of communicability: Probably 1 day before eruption of lesions (prodromal period) to 6 days after first crop of vesicles when crusts have formed

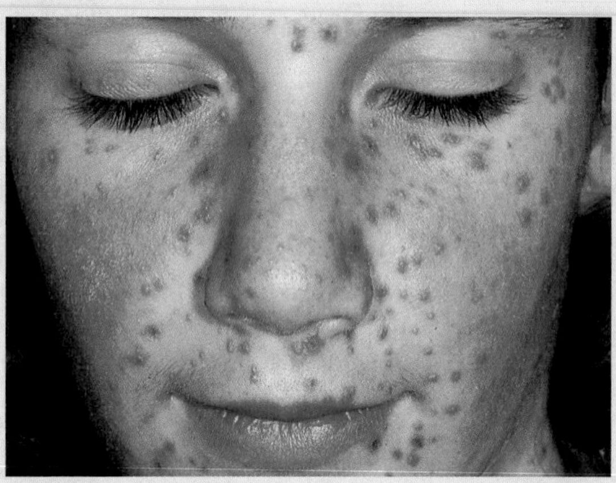

Fig. 38-8 Chickenpox (varicella). (Clinical view from Habif TP: *Clinical dermatology: a color guide to diagnosis and therapy*, ed 3, St Louis, 1996, Mosby.)

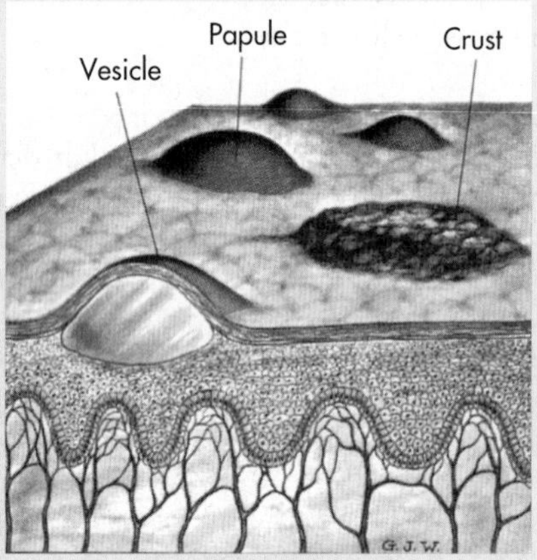

Simultaneous stages of lesions in chickenpox

DIPHTHERIA
Agent: *Corynebacterium diphtheriae*
Source: Discharges from mucous membranes of nose and nasopharynx, skin, and other lesions of infected person
Transmission: Direct contact with infected person, a carrier, or contaminated articles
Incubation period: Usually 2-5 days, possibly longer
Period of communicability: Variable; until virulent bacilli are no longer present (identified by three negative cultures); usually 2 weeks but as long as 4 weeks

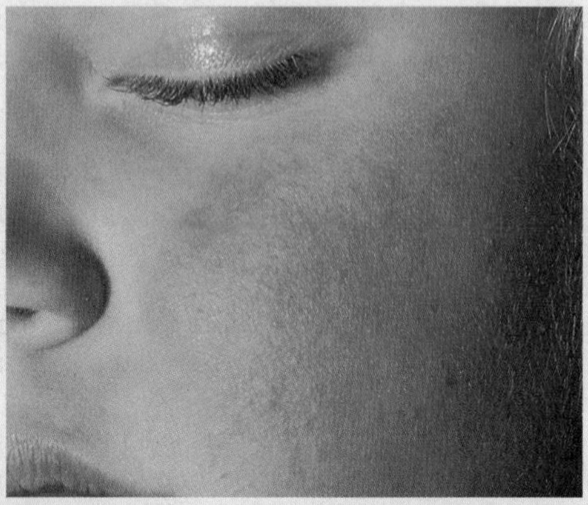

Fig. 38-9 Erythema infectiosum. (From Habif TP: *Clinical dermatology: a color guide to diagnosis and therapy,* ed 3, St Louis, 1996, Mosby.)

ERYTHEMA INFECTIOSUM (Fifth disease) (Fig. 38-9)
Agent: Human parvovirus B19 (HPV)
Source: Infected persons
Transmission: Unknown; possibly respiratory secretions and blood
Incubation period: 4-14 days, may be as long as 21 days
Period of communicability: Uncertain but before onset of symptoms in most children; also for about 1 week after onset of symptoms in children with aplastic crisis

CLINICAL MANIFESTATIONS	THERAPEUTIC MANAGEMENT/ COMPLICATIONS	NURSING CONSIDERATIONS
Prodromal stage: Slight fever, malaise, and anorexia for first 24 hours; rash highly pruritic; begins as macule, rapidly progresses to papule and then vesicle (surrounded by erythematous base, becomes umbilicated and cloudy, breaks easily and forms crusts); all three stages (papule, vesicle, crust) present in varying degrees at one time **Distribution:** Centripetal, spreading to face and proximal extremities but sparse on distal limbs and less on areas not exposed to heat (i.e., from clothing or sun) **Constitutional signs and symptoms:** Elevated temperature from lymphadenopathy, irritability from pruritus	**Specific:** Antiviral agent acyclovir (Zovirax); varicella-zoster immune globulin (VZIG) after exposure in high risk children **Supportive:** Diphenhydramine hydrochloride or antihistamines to relieve itching; skin care to prevent secondary bacterial infection **Complications:** Secondary bacterial infections (abscesses, cellulitis, necrotizing fasciitis, pneumonia, sepsis) Encephalitis Varicella pneumonia (rare in normal children) Hemorrhagic varicella (tiny hemorrhages in vesicles and numerous petechiae in skin) Chronic or transient thrombocytopenia	Maintain strict isolation in hospital Isolate child in home until vesicles have dried (usually 1 week after onset of disease), and isolate high risk children from infected children Administer skin care: give bath and change clothes and linens daily; administer topical calamine lotion; keep child's fingernails short and clean; apply mittens if child scratches Keep child cool (may decrease number of lesions) Lessen pruritus; keep child occupied Remove loose crusts that rub and irritate skin Teach child to apply pressure to pruritic area rather than scratching it If older child, reason with child regarding danger of scar formation from scratching Avoid use of aspirin
Vary according to anatomic location of pseudomembrane **Nasal:** Resembles common cold, serosanguineous mucopurulent nasal discharge without constitutional symptoms; may be frank epistaxis **Tonsillar/pharyngeal:** Malaise; anorexia; sore throat; low-grade fever; pulse increased above expected for temperature within 24 hours; smooth, adherent, white or gray membrane; lymphadenitis possibly pronounced ("bull's neck"); in severe cases, toxemia, septic shock, and death within 6-10 days **Laryngeal:** Fever, hoarseness, cough, with or without previous signs listed; potential airway obstruction, apprehensive, dyspneic retractions, cyanosis	Antitoxin (usually intravenously); preceded by skin or conjunctival test to rule out sensitivity to horse serum Antibiotics (penicillin or erythromycin) Complete bed rest (prevention of myocarditis) Tracheostomy for airway obstruction Treatment of infected contacts and carriers **Complications:** Myocarditis (second week) Neuritis	Maintain strict isolation in hospital Participate in sensitivity testing; have epinephrine available Administer antibiotics; observe for signs of sensitivity to penicillin Administer complete care to maintain bed rest Use suctioning as needed Observe respiration for signs of obstruction Administer humidified oxygen if prescribed
Rash appears in three stages: I—Erythema on face, chiefly on cheeks, "slapped face" appearance; disappears by 1-4 days II—About 1 day after rash appears on face, maculopapular red spots appear, symmetrically distributed on upper and lower extremities; rash progresses from proximal to distal	**Symptomatic and supportive:** Antipyretics, analgesics, antiinflammatory drugs Possible blood transfusion for transient aplastic anemia **Complications:** Self-limited arthritis and arthralgia (arthritis may become chronic)	Isolation of child not necessary, except hospitalized child (immunosuppressed or with aplastic crisis) suspected of HPV infection is placed on respiratory isolation and Standard Precautions Pregnant women: need not be excluded from workplace where HPV infection is present; should not care

Continued

Table 38-2

Communicable Diseases of Childhood—cont'd

DISEASE

ERYTHEMA INFECTIOSUM (Fifth disease)—cont'd

EXANTHEMA SUBITUM (ROSEOLA) (Fig. 38-10)
Agent: Human herpesvirus type 6 (HHV-6)
Source: Unknown
Transmission: Unknown (virtually limited to children between 6 months and 3 years of age)
Incubation period: Usually 5-15 days
Period of communicability: Unknown

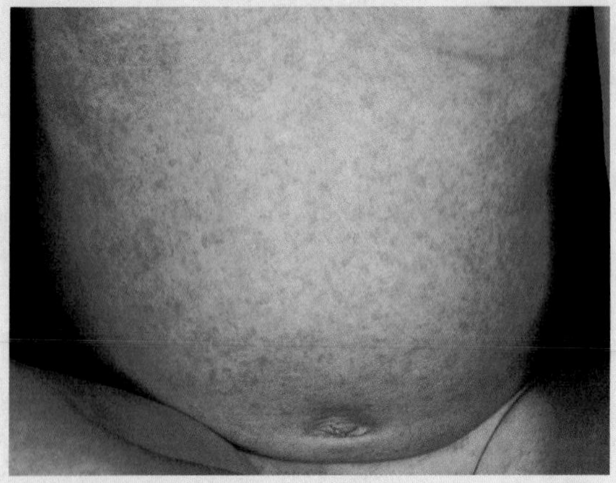

Fig. 38-10 Roseola infantum. (From Habif TP: *Clinical dermatology: a color guide to diagnosis and therapy,* ed 3, St Louis, 1996, Mosby.)

MEASLES (RUBEOLA) (Fig. 38-11)
Agent: Virus
Source: Respiratory tract secretions, blood, and urine of infected person
Transmission: Usually by direct contact with droplets of infected person
Incubation period: 10-20 days
Period of communicability: From 4 days before to 5 days after rash appears but mainly during prodromal (catarrhal) stage

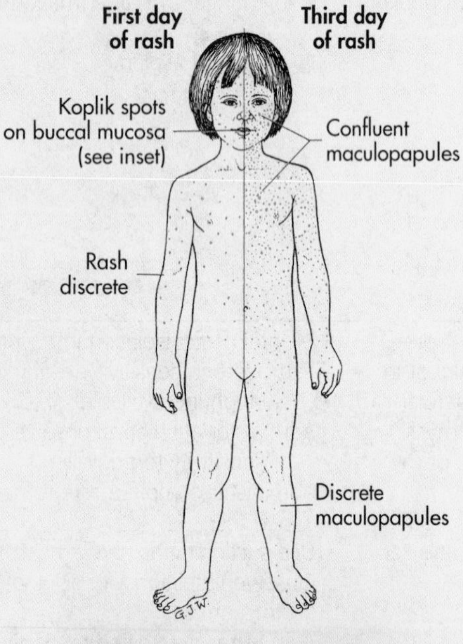

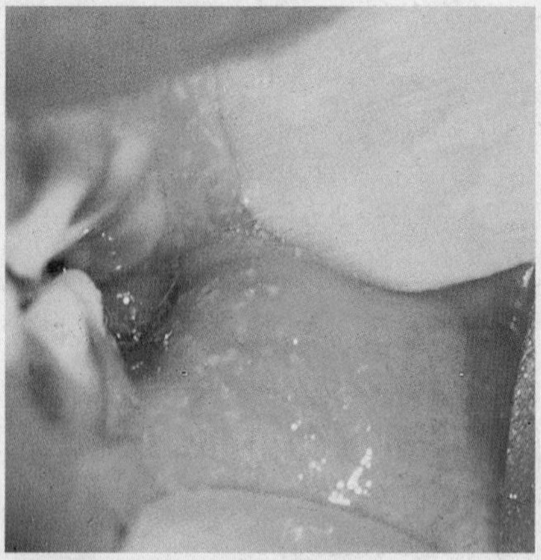

Koplik spots

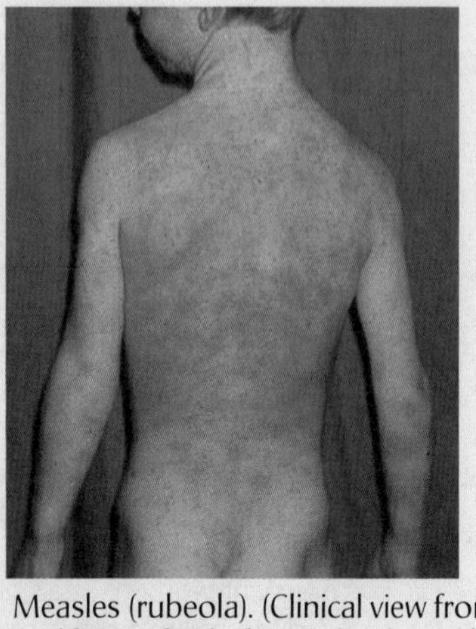

Fig. 38-11 Measles (rubeola). (Clinical view from Seidel HM et al: *Mosby's guide to physical examination,* ed 4, St Louis, 1999, Mosby. Koplik spots from Zitelli BJ, Davis HW: *Atlas of pediatric physical diagnosis,* ed 3, St Louis, 1997, Mosby.)

MUMPS
Agent: Paramyxovirus
Source: Saliva of infected persons
Transmission: Direct contact with or droplet spread from an infected person
Incubation period: 14-21 days
Period of communicability: Most communicable immediately before and after swelling begins

CLINICAL MANIFESTATIONS	THERAPEUTIC MANAGEMENT/ COMPLICATIONS	NURSING CONSIDERATIONS
surfaces and may last a week or more III—Rash subsides but reappears if skin is irritated or traumatized (sun, heat, cold, friction) In children with aplastic crisis, rash is usually absent and prodromal illness includes fever, myalgia, lethargy, nausea, vomiting, and abdominal pain	May result in fetal death if mother infected during pregnancy, but no evidence of congenital anomalies Aplastic crisis in children with hemolytic disease or immunodeficiency Myocarditis (rare)	for patients with aplastic crisis; explain low risk of fetal death to those in contact with affected children
Persistent high fever for 3-4 days in child who appears well Precipitous drop in fever to normal with appearance of rash **Rash:** Discrete rose-pink macules or maculopapules appearing first on trunk, then spreading to neck, face, and extremities; nonpruritic, fades on pressure, lasts 1-2 days **Associated signs and symptoms:** Cervical/postauricular lymphadenopathy, inflamed pharynx, cough, coryza	Nonspecific Antipyretics to control fever **Complications:** Recurrent febrile seizures (possibly from latent infection of central nervous system that is reactivated by fever) Encephalitis (rare)	Teach parents measures for lowering temperature (antipyretic drugs) If child is prone to seizures, discuss appropriate precautions, possibility of recurrent febrile seizures.
Prodromal (catarrhal) stage: Fever and malaise, followed in 24 hours by coryza, cough, conjunctivitis, Koplik spots (small, irregular red spots with a minute, bluish white center first seen on buccal mucosa opposite molars 2 days before rash); symptoms gradually increase in severity until second day after rash appears, when they begin to subside **Rash:** Appears 3-4 days after onset of prodromal stage; begins as erythematous maculopapular eruption on face and gradually spreads downward; more severe in earlier sites (appears confluent) and less intense in later sites (appears discrete); after 3-4 days assumes brownish appearance, and fine desquamation occurs over areas of extensive involvement **Constitutional signs and symptoms:** Anorexia, malaise, generalized lymphadenopathy	Vitamin A supplementation **Supportive:** Bed rest during febrile period; antipyretics Antibiotics to prevent secondary bacterial infection in high risk children **Complications:** Otitis media Pneumonia Bronchiolitis Obstructive laryngitis and laryngotracheitis Encephalitis	Isolation until fifth day of rash; if hospitalized, institute respiratory precautions Maintain bed rest during prodromal stage; provide quiet activity **Fever:** Instruct parents to administer antipyretics; avoid chilling; if child is prone to seizures, institute appropriate precautions **Eye care:** Dim lights if photophobia present; clean eyelids with warm saline solution to remove secretions or crusts; keep child from rubbing eyes; examine cornea for signs of ulceration **Coryza/cough:** Use cool-mist vaporizer; protect skin around nares with layer of petrolatum; encourage fluids and soft, bland foods **Skin care:** Keep skin clean; use tepid baths as necessary
Prodromal stage: Fever, headache, malaise, and anorexia for 24 hours, followed by "earache" that is aggravated by chewing **Parotitis:** By third day, parotid glands (or gland) (either bilateral or unilateral) enlarge(s) and reach(es) maximum size in 1-3 days; accompanied by pain and tenderness	**Symptomatic and supportive:** Analgesics for pain and antipyretics for fever Intravenous fluid may be necessary for child who refuses to drink or vomits because of meningoencephalitis **Complications:** Sensorineural deafness Postinfectious encephalitis	Isolation during period of communicability; institute respiratory precautions during hospitalization Maintain bed rest during prodromal phase until swelling subsides Give analgesics for pain; if child is unwilling to chew medication, use elixir form Encourage fluids and soft, bland foods; avoid foods requiring chewing

Continued

Table 38-2

Communicable Diseases of Childhood—cont'd

DISEASE

MUMPS—cont'd

PERTUSSIS (WHOOPING COUGH)

Agent: *Bordetella pertussis*

Source: Discharge from respiratory tract of infected persons

Transmission: Direct contact or droplet spread from infected person; indirect contact with freshly contaminated articles

Incubation period: 6-20 days, usually 7-10 days

Period of communicability: Greatest during catarrhal stage before onset of paroxysms and may extend to fourth week after onset of paroxysms

POLIOMYELITIS

Agent: Enteroviruses, three types: type 1—most frequent cause of paralysis, both epidemic and endemic; type 2—least frequently associated with paralysis; type 3—second most frequently associated with paralysis

Source: Feces and oropharyngeal secretions of infected persons, especially young children

Transmission: Direct contact with persons with apparent or inapparent active infection; spread is via fecal-oral and pharyngeal-oropharyngeal routes

Incubation period: Usually 7-14 days, with range of 5-35 days

Period of communicability: Not exactly known; virus is present in throat and feces shortly after infection and persists for about 1 week in throat and 4-6 weeks in feces

RUBELLA (GERMAN MEASLES) (Fig. 38-12)

Agent: Rubella virus

Source: Primarily nasopharyngeal secretions of person with apparent or inapparent infection; virus also present in blood, stool, and urine

Transmission: Direct contact and spread via infected person; indirectly via articles freshly contaminated with nasopharyngeal secretions, feces, or urine

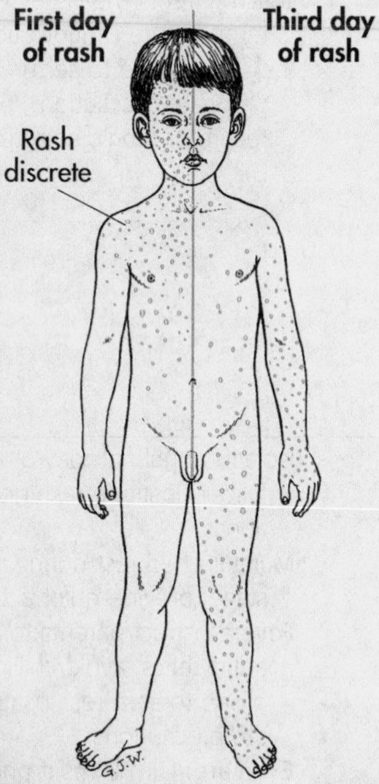

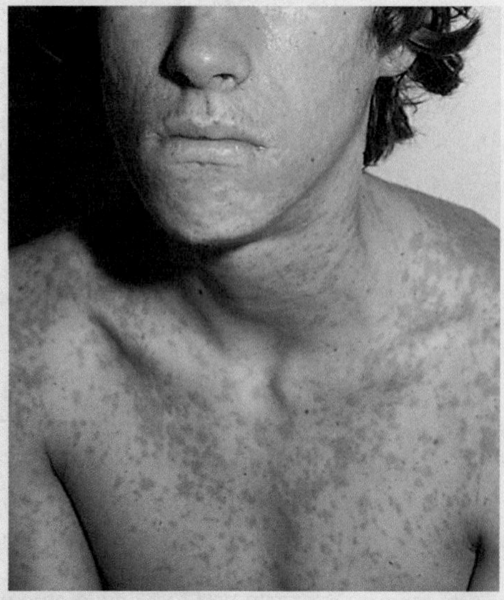

Fig. 38-12 Rubella (German measles). **A**. Progression of rash. **B**, Clinical view. (From Zitelli BJ, Davis HW: *Atlas of pediatric physical diagnosis,* ed 3, St Louis, 1997, Mosby; courtesy Dr. Michael Sherlock.)

CLINICAL MANIFESTATIONS	THERAPEUTIC MANAGEMENT/ COMPLICATIONS	NURSING CONSIDERATIONS
	Myocarditis Arthritis Hepatitis Epididymo-orchitis Sterility (extremely rare in adult males) Meningitis	Apply hot or cold compresses to neck, whichever is more comforting To relieve orchitis, provide warmth and local support with tight-fitting underpants (stretch bathing suit works well)
Catarrhal stage: Begins with symptoms of upper respiratory tract infection, such as coryza, sneezing, lacrimation, cough, and low-grade fever; symptoms continue for 1-2 weeks, when dry, hacking cough becomes more severe **Paroxysmal stage:** Cough most often occurs at night and consists of short, rapid coughs followed by sudden inspiration associated with a high-pitched crowing sound or "whoop"; during paroxysms, cheeks become flushed or cyanotic, eyes bulge, and tongue protrudes; paroxysm may continue until thick mucous plug is dislodged; vomiting frequently follows attack; stage generally lasts 4-6 weeks, followed by convalescent stage	Antimicrobial therapy (e.g., erythromycin) Administration of pertussis immune globulin **Supportive treatment:** Hospitalization required for infants, children who are dehydrated, or those who have complications Bed rest Increased oxygen intake and humidity Adequate fluids Intubation possibly necessary **Complications:** Pneumonia (usual cause of death) Atelectasis Otitis media Seizures Hemorrhage (subarachnoid, subconjunctival, epistaxis) Weight loss and dehydration Hernia Prolapsed rectum	Isolation during catarrhal stage; if hospitalized, institute respiratory precautions Maintain bed rest as long as fever present Provide restful environment and reduce factors that promote paroxysms (dust, smoke, sudden change in temperature, chilling, activity, excitement); keep room well ventilated Encourage fluids; offer small amount of fluids frequently; refeed child after vomiting Provide high humidity (humidifier or tent); suction gently but often to prevent choking on secretions Observe for signs of airway obstruction (increased restlessness, apprehension, retractions, cyanosis) Involve public health nurse if child cared for at home
May be manifested in three different forms: **Abortive or inapparent**—Fever, uneasiness, sore throat, headache, anorexia, vomiting, abdominal pain; lasts a few hours to a few days **Nonparalytic**—Same manifestations as abortive but more severe, with pain and stiffness in neck, back, and legs **Paralytic**—Initial course similar to nonparalytic type, followed by recovery and then signs of central nervous system paralysis	Treatment is supportive Complete bed rest during acute phase Assisted respiratory ventilation in case of respiratory paralysis Physical therapy for muscles following acute stage **Complications:** Permanent paralysis Respiratory arrest Hypertension Kidney stones from demineralization of bone during prolonged immobility	Maintain complete bed rest Administer mild sedatives as necessary to relieve anxiety and promote rest Participate in physiotherapy procedures (use of moist hot packs and range-of-motion exercises) Position child to maintain body alignment and prevent contractures or decubiti; use footboard Encourage child to move; administer analgesics for maximum comfort during physical activity Observe for respiratory paralysis (difficulty in talking, ineffective cough, inability to hold breath, shallow and rapid respirations); report such signs and symptoms to practitioner; have tracheostomy tray at bedside
Prodromal stage: Absent in children, present in adults and adolescents; consists of low-grade fever, headache, malaise, anorexia, mild conjunctivitis, coryza, sore throat, cough, and lymphadenopathy; lasts 1-5 days, subsides 1 day after appearance of rash	No treatment necessary other than antipyretics for low-grade fever and analgesics for discomfort **Complications:** Rare (arthritis, encephalitis, or purpura); most benign of all childhood communicable diseases; greatest danger is teratogenic effect on fetus	Reassure parents of benign nature of illness in affected child Use comfort measures as necessary Isolate child from pregnant women

Continued

Table 38-2

Communicable Diseases of Childhood—cont'd

DISEASE
RUBELLA (GERMAN MEASLES)—cont'd **Incubation period:** 14-21 days **Period of communicability:** 7 days before to about 5 days after appearance of rash **Constitutional signs and symptoms:** Occasionally low-grade fever, headache, malaise, and lymphadenopathy
SCARLET FEVER (Fig. 38-13) **Agent:** Group A β-hemolytic streptococci **Source:** Usually from nasopharyngeal secretions of infected persons and carriers **Transmission:** Direct contact with infected person or droplet spread; indirectly by contact with contaminated articles or ingestion of contaminated milk or other food **Incubation period:** 2-5 days, with range of 1-7 days **Period of communicability:** During incubation period and clinical illness, approximately 10 days; during first 2 weeks of carrier phase, although may persist for months

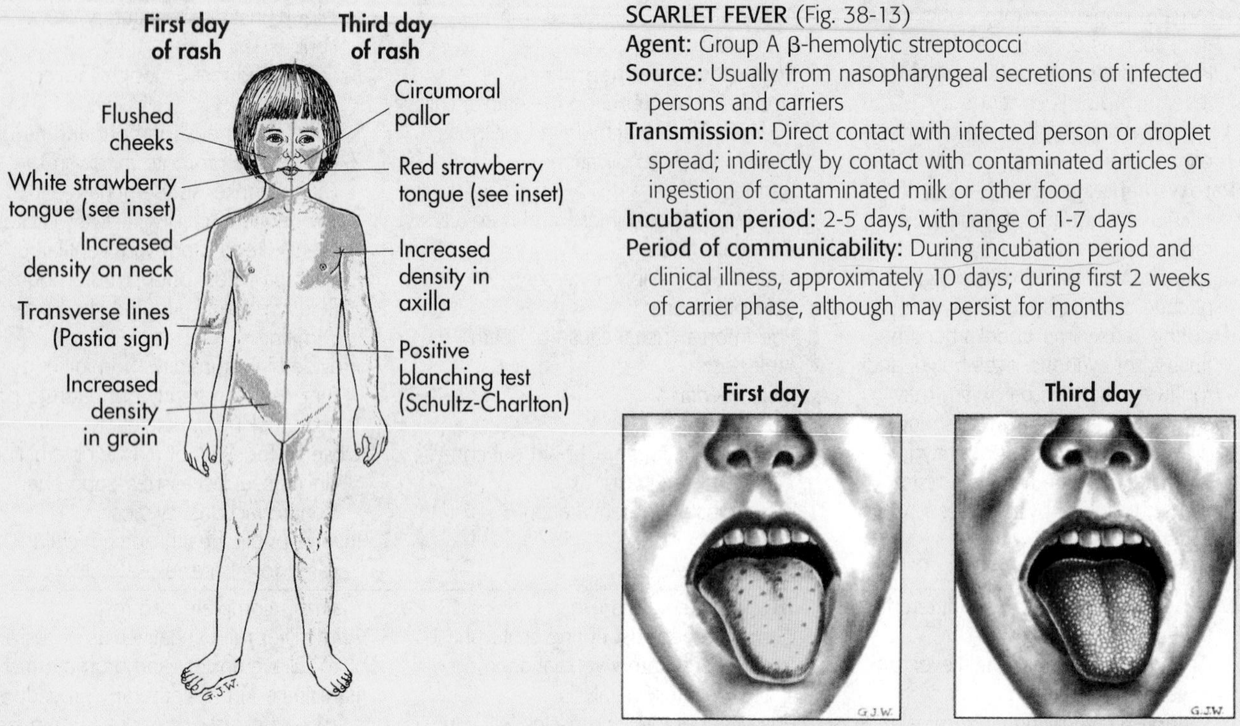

Fig. 38-13 Scarlet fever.

voluntarily curtail their activity, and although bed rest is beneficial, it should not be imposed unless specifically indicated (e.g., with pertussis). During periods of irritability, quiet activity (e.g., reading, music, television, videos, puzzles, and coloring) helps distract children from the discomfort.

Support Child and Family

Most communicable diseases are benign, but may produce considerable concern and anxiety for parents. Often the occurrence of a disease such as chickenpox is the first time the child is acutely uncomfortable. Parents need assistance to cope with manifestations of the illness, such as intense itching. Sometimes a visiting nurse may be beneficial to help the family develop a plan of care and encourage compliance with treatments.

The family and child need reassurance that recovery is generally rapid. However, visible signs of the dermatosis may be present for some time after the child is well enough to resume usual activities. When the disease involves noticeable signs, such as the crusts of chickenpox, the child may benefit from preparation before returning to school. For example, the parent can discuss the child's physical appearance with the teacher, the school nurse, or both and request that they explain the child's condition to classmates.

NURSE ALERT The occurrence of a communicable disease provides the opportunity to ask parents about the child's immunization status and reinforce the benefits of vaccines for children. ■

CLINICAL MANIFESTATIONS	THERAPEUTIC MANAGEMENT/ COMPLICATIONS	NURSING CONSIDERATIONS
Rash: First appears on face and rapidly spreads downward to neck, arms, trunk, and legs; by end of first day, body is covered with discrete, pinkish red maculopapular exanthema; disappears in same order as it began and is usually gone by third day		
Prodromal stage: Abrupt high fever, pulse increased out of proportion to fever, vomiting, headache, chills, malaise, abdominal pain **Enanthema:** Tonsils enlarged, edematous, reddened, and covered with patches of exudate; in severe cases appearance resembles membrane seen in diphtheria; pharynx is edematous and beefy red; during first 1-2 days tongue is coated and papillae become red and swollen (white strawberry tongue); by fourth or fifth day white coat sloughs off, leaving prominent papillae (red strawberry tongue); palate is covered with erythematous punctate lesions **Exanthema:** Rash appears within 12 hours after prodromal signs; red pinhead-sized punctate lesions rapidly become generalized but are absent on face, which becomes flushed with striking circumoral pallor; rash is more intense in folds of joints; by end of first week desquamation begins (fine, sandpaper-like on torso; sheetlike sloughing on palms and soles), which may be complete by 3 weeks or longer	Treatment of choice is full course of penicillin (or erythromycin in penicillin-sensitive children); antibiotic therapy for newly diagnosed carriers (nose or throat cultures positive for streptococci) **Supportive measures:** Bed rest during febrile phase, analgesics for sore throat **Complications:** Otitis media Peritonsillar and retropharyngeal abscess Sinusitis Glomerulonephritis Carditis, polyarthritis (uncommon)	Institute respiratory precautions until 24 hours after initiation of treatment Ensure compliance with oral antibiotic therapy (intramuscular benzathine penicillin G [Bicillin] may be given if parents' reliability in giving oral drugs is questionable) Maintain bed rest during febrile phase; provide quiet activity during convalescent period Relieve discomfort of sore throat with analgesics, gargles, lozenges, antiseptic throat sprays, and inhalation of cool mist Encourage fluids during febrile phase; avoid irritating liquids (citrus juices) or rough foods; when child is able to eat, begin with soft diet Advise parents to consult practitioner if fever persists after beginning therapy Discuss procedures for preventing spread of infection

Evaluation

The effectiveness of nursing interventions is determined by continual reassessment and evaluation of care based on the following observational guidelines and expected outcomes:

1. Observe or inquire about family members' use of control measures; observe for signs of disease in household contacts.
2. Monitor vital signs, especially temperature; inquire about the identification of high risk contacts and appropriate isolation of the contact; observe or inquire about compliance with antibiotic or antiviral therapy.
3. Inquire about effectiveness of comfort measures.
4. Interview family and child regarding their feelings and concerns, especially when child returns to school.

The *expected outcomes* are described in the Nursing Care Plan on pp. 1138.

CHILD MALTREATMENT

The broad term *child maltreatment* includes intentional physical abuse or neglect, emotional abuse or neglect, and sexual abuse of children, usually by adults. It is one of the most significant social problems affecting children. In 2002, Child Protective Service (CPS) agencies in the United States

Nursing Care Plan

THE CHILD WITH A COMMUNICABLE DISEASE

NURSING DIAGNOSIS: Risk for infection related to susceptible host and infectious agents

EXPECTED OUTCOME
Infection remains confined to original source.

NURSING INTERVENTIONS/*RATIONALES*

Institute appropriate infection control practices as recommended by the Centers for Disease Control and Prevention (see Chapter 45) *to prevent spread of microorganisms.* (**Scrupulous handwashing by all who have contact with the infected child is critical in control of the disease.**)

Work with family and public health nurse *to ensure adherence to infection control practices and therapeutic regimens if individual is treated in the home.*

Report disease to health department *to monitor outbreak.*

Identify susceptible individuals in community (e.g., high risk children, close contacts of infected child) who may require prophylactic treatment or need to practice careful avoidance and close monitoring practices *to prevent contracting the disease.*

Promote public education and service programs (e.g., immunization, food handling, animal control, screening) *that aim at prevention/spread of communicable disease on community level.*

NURSING DIAGNOSIS: Risk for injury related to disease complications, trauma to skin from scratching

EXPECTED OUTCOME
Patient will show no evidence of complications; skin remains intact.

NURSING INTERVENTIONS/*RATIONALES*

Involve child and parents in planning and carrying out therapeutic regimen (e.g., bed rest, hydration, feeding, prescribed medications) *to increase compliance.*

Monitor vital signs and appropriate laboratory values and make ongoing assessments of appropriate systems *to detect early signs of potential complications (ear, eye, respiratory infections; seizures, central nervous system involvement; myocarditis, arthritis, hepatitis).* Observe skin *to detect signs of scratching, trauma, infection.*

Institute seizure precautions *if febrile convulsions are a possible complication.*

Maintain good body hygiene; use antipruritics, lotions as needed; keep child's fingernails trimmed, use mittens or restraints, cover affected areas; keep skin cool *to prevent scratching, relieve itching, and reduce risk of trauma and secondary infection of lesions.*

Offer small, frequent sips of child's favorite liquids and water *to ensure hydration* and frequent small feedings of favorite soft, bland foods (soups, ice cream, pudding, gelatin) *to reduce anorexia, nausea, and vomiting.*

NURSING DIAGNOSIS: Pain related to skin lesions, malaise

EXPECTED OUTCOME
Patient will exhibit minimum signs of discomfort.

NURSING INTERVENTIONS/*RATIONALES*

Use comfort measures such as vaporizer, gargles, and lozenges *to keep membranes moist;* petrolatum *for chapped lips;* saline *to cleanse crusted eyes;* cool moist cloths, tepid baths, and lotion *to relieve itching skin.*

Use nonpharmacologic techniques (e.g., distraction, relaxation, guided imagery, positive self-talk, thought stopping) *for pain reduction.*

Administer analgesics, antipyretics, and antipruritics per physician order *to relieve pain, fever, itching.* (**Do not use salicylates because of possible risk of Reye syndrome.**)

NURSING DIAGNOSIS: Social isolation related to environmentally imposed constraints secondary to communicable disease

EXPECTED OUTCOME
Patient will interact in socially acceptable and developmentally appropriate manner and participate in meaningful diversional activity.

NURSING INTERVENTIONS/*RATIONALES*

Explain reasons for confinement *to enhance child's understanding.*

Enlist child's assistance with enforcing restrictions *to provide increased sense of control.*

Allow child to examine and play with any needed isolation supplies (e.g., gown, gloves, mask) *to relieve fears, increase sense of control.*

Have staff identify themselves to child before donning any required protective clothing *to increase child's trust in caregivers.*

Encourage parents to remain with child during hospitalization *to decrease separation and feelings of isolation.*

Encourage contact with peers and siblings by telephone *to maintain social interaction and reduce sense of isolation.*

Plan specific periods of developmentally appropriate diversional activity suited to child's physical condition and energy level *to decrease feelings of boredom and negative self-absorption.*

confirmed that just under one million children were victims of child maltreatment. Of the confirmed cases, 20% suffered physical abuse, 10% sexual abuse, 60% neglect, 7% emotional abuse, and 20% other forms of maltreatment (these percentages add up to more than 100% because some children were victims of more than one type of maltreatment). In 2002, estimates indicated that 1400 children died as a result of child abuse and neglect (National Clearinghouse on Child Abuse and Neglect Information, 2004). Reported statistics only partially represent the actual incidence of child maltreatment, because many cases are believed to go unreported.

Child Neglect

Child neglect is the most common form of maltreatment. About one half of all reported cases are associated with deprivation of necessities, and more than one third of deaths from maltreatment are in this group. *Neglect* is generally defined as the failure of a parent or other person legally responsible for the child's welfare to provide for the child's basic needs and an adequate level of care.

Little is known about the etiology of neglect, although it is thought that many of the risk factors identified in physical abuse apply to neglect as well (see following discussion). Ignorance of the child's needs and a lack of resources are important contributing factors. For example, neglectful parents often demonstrate poor parenting skills. They may be unaware that an infant needs to be fed every 3 to 4 hours, may not know what to feed the child, and may have insufficient funds to buy food. The most serious lack of knowledge is failure to recognize emotional nurturing as an essential need of children. (See also Failure to Thrive, Chapter 36.)

Types of Neglect

Neglect takes many forms and can be classified broadly as physical or emotional maltreatment. *Physical neglect* involves the deprivation of necessities, such as food, clothing, shelter, supervision, medical care, and education. *Emotional neglect* generally refers to failure to meet the child's needs for affection, attention, and emotional nurturance. It may also include lack of intervention for or fostering of maladaptive behavior, such as delinquency or substance abuse. *Emotional abuse,* an even more difficult aspect of maltreatment to define, refers to the deliberate attempt to destroy or significantly impair a child's self-esteem or competence. Emotional abuse may take the following forms: rejecting, isolating, terrorizing, ignoring, corrupting, verbally assaulting, and overpressuring the child (Nelms, 2001).

Physical Abuse

The deliberate infliction of physical injury on a child, usually by the child's caregiver, is termed *physical abuse.* Minor physical injury is responsible for more reported cases of maltreatment than major physical injury, but major physical abuse causes more deaths. Despite the importance of the problem, a universally accepted definition of what constitutes minor and major physical abuse does not exist. Rather, each state in the United States defines abuse according to its individual reporting laws.

Munchausen Syndrome by Proxy

One of the more unusual and perplexing types of abuse, usually physical, is Munchausen syndrome by proxy (MSP), which refers to illness that one person fabricates or induces in another person (Hall et al, 2000; Paulk, 2001). In children it is usually the mother who fabricates signs and symptoms of illness in her child, the proxy, to gain attention from the medical staff. MSP can take many forms, such as adding maternal blood to the child's urine to simulate hematuria, presenting a fictitious medical history, chronic poisoning of the child, or suffocating the child to cause apnea and seizures. Alleging that the child has been sexually abused by someone else to gain recognition as the child's protector is another form of MSP.

Such cases are often very difficult to confirm and require a high index of suspicion to protect the children. Warning signs of MSP include the following:

- Unexplained, prolonged, recurrent, or extremely rare illness
- Discrepancies between clinical findings and history
- Illness unresponsive to treatment
- Signs and symptoms occurring only in parent's presence
- Parent knowledgeable about illness, procedures, and treatments
- Parent very interested in interacting with health team members
- Parent very attentive toward child (refuses to leave hospital)
- Family members with similar symptoms

Consequences for children with MSP can be serious. They often undergo needless and painful medical procedures and treatments. The parent's actions may induce a serious illness in children—one that is fatal in almost 10% of the cases (Hall et al, 2000; Souid, Keith, & Cunningham, 1998). Children may develop chronic invalidism, accepting the illness story and believing themselves to be ill. Finally, they may develop MSP as an adult. Even when some of these children are removed from the home, they continue to suffer severe psychologic trauma. Other siblings remaining in the home may become substitute victims.

Factors Predisposing to Physical Abuse

The exact cause of child abuse is not known, although three factors—parental characteristics, characteristics of the child, and environmental characteristics—influence the potential for abuse. However, no single factor or group of factors is predictive of abuse. Rather, the interaction of these factors is thought to increase the risk of abuse occurring in a particular family.

Parental Characteristics

Extensive research has focused on parental characteristics that distinguish abusive parents from nonabusive parents. Although some studies provide conflicting evidence, it is not generally recognized that parental history of abuse or neglect during childhood is a significant risk factor for child abuse (Johnson, 2004; Murray, Baker, & Lewin, 2000). Although physical punishment tends to occur in abusive parents' childhood, most of the parents were not physically abused as children. However, abusive parents who report that they were severely punished as children are much more likely to injure their own children. If the abuse was not overt physical violence, abusive parents typically recall their punishment as unfair and severe, and they characterize their relationship with their parents as negative. Abusive parents tend to have difficulty coping with stress and in controlling anger expression (Rodriguez & Green, 1997).

Another finding is that abusive families are often more socially isolated and have fewer supportive relationships than nonabusive parents. Children of teenage mothers are more at risk of abuse than those of older mothers (McCullough & Scherman, 1998; Murray et al, 2000). With little or no available support system and the presence of concurrent stresses imposed by the child or environment, these parents are extremely vulnerable to additional crises of any nature and literally strike out at the child as a method of releasing their increasing frustration and anxiety.

Other factors identified in abusive parents include low self-esteem and less adequate maternal functioning. Although inadequate knowledge of childrearing is often cited as a characteristic of abusive parents, research findings do not consistently support this belief. However, this does not mean that these parents cannot benefit from learning more constructive ways of rearing their children, especially nonviolent discipline methods.

Characteristics of the Child

The child also unintentionally contributes to the abusive situation. In families of two or more children, usually only one child is the victim of abuse. This child's temperament, position in the family, additional physical needs if ill or disabled, activity level, or degree of sensitivity to parental needs all contribute to the potential for physical abuse. For example, one child may not be abused if he or she fits into the "easy-child pattern," whereas another sibling with a difficult temperament may add to the parent's stress sufficiently to precipitate an abusive act. However, temperament alone is not the critical factor; rather, it is the "fit" or compatibility between the child's temperament and the parent's ability to deal with that behavioral style.

Occasionally the abused child is illegitimate, unwanted, brain damaged (especially in situations where the parents cannot accept the retardation), hyperactive, or physically disabled. Sometimes children are abused because they remind the parent of someone the parent dislikes, such as a younger brother or sister who received all of the attention from their own parents. Premature infants may be at risk for maltreatment because of the failure of parent-child bonding during early infancy. Often a difficult pregnancy, labor, or delivery is a predisposing factor in abuse, especially when the infant is born prematurely or with congenital anomalies.

Although one child is usually the victim in an abusive family, removing that child from the home often places the other siblings at risk for abuse. Child maltreatment usually is not confined to one child because of a disturbed parent-child relationship but is a result of a family in distress. Therefore no child is safe if left in the abusive environment unless the parents can be helped to learn new parenting skills and to meet their needs and release their frustration through alternatives other than attacking their children.

Environmental Characteristics

The environment is a significant part of the potential abusive situation. Typically the environment is one of chronic stress, including problems of divorce, poverty, unemployment, poor housing, frequent relocation, alcoholism, and drug addiction. Increased exposure between children and parents, such as that which occurs in crowded living conditions, also increases the likelihood of abuse.

Although most reporting of abuse has been from lower socioeconomic populations, child abuse is not a problem of any one societal group. It spans all educational, social, and economic levels. Stresses imposed by poverty predispose lower socioeconomic families to abusive situations, and abuse in these groups is more apt to be reported. However, concealed crises may also be present in upper-class families. For example, a wealthy family experiencing major life changes, such as rehousing, the birth of an additional child, or marital discord, may have sufficient environmental stressors imposed on them to produce a potentially abusive situation. Wealthy families may be so overinvolved with commitments outside the home that abuse may be inflicted by substitute caregivers. Nurses need to be aware of all these factors to identify the less obvious examples of child abuse and neglect.

Sexual Abuse

Sexual abuse is one of the most devastating types of child maltreatment, and current estimates indicate that it has increased significantly during the past decade. Child sexual abuse constitutes approximately 10% of officially substantiated child maltreatment cases. Some of the apparent increase can be attributed to increased awareness (Putnam, 2003).

As with all forms of child maltreatment, no universal definition for sexual abuse exists. The Child Abuse and Prevention Act (Public Law 100-235) defines *sexual abuse* as "the use, persuasion, or coercion of any child to engage in sexually explicit conduct (or any simulation of such conduct) for producing any visual depiction of such conduct, or rape, molestation, prostitution, or incest with children."

Sexual abuse includes the following types of sexual maltreatment:

Incest—Any physical sexual activity between family members; blood relationship is not required (abusers can include stepparents, nonrelated siblings, grandparents, uncles, and aunts); does not include sexual relations between legally sanctioned partners, such as spouses

Molestation—A vague term that includes "indecent liberties," such as touching, fondling, kissing, single or mutual masturbation, or oral-genital contact

Exhibitionism—Indecent exposure, usually exposure of the genitals by an adult male to children or female adults

Child pornography—Arranging and photographing, in any media, sexual acts involving children, alone or with adults or animals, regardless of consent by the child's legal guardian; also may denote distribution of such material in any form with or without profit

Child prostitution—Involving children in sex acts for profit and usually with changing partners

Pedophilia—Literally means "love of child" and does not denote a type of sexual activity but the preference of an adult for prepubertal children as the means of achieving sexual excitement

Characteristics of Abusers and Victims

Anyone, including siblings and mothers, can be sexual abusers, but a typical abuser is a male whom the victim knows. Offenders come from all levels of society. Some are prominent persons in the community, and some, especially in the case of pedophiles (also called "child molesters"), are in positions where they work closely with children, such as teaching or coaching.

Pornography and prostitution may involve strangers, as well as the children's own parents. There are no typical characteristics of these offenders, although the abused children tend to be runaways—young adolescents who engage in these activities to obtain money for food, shelter, drugs, and alcohol. Incestuous relationships between father or stepfather and daughter are generally prolonged, and the victims are usually reluctant to report the situation because of fear of retaliation and fear that they will not be believed. Typically, incestuous relationships begin later than other forms of child abuse. The eldest daughter is usually abused, but in her absence another sister is substituted. Sibling incest may also occur (Adler & Schutz, 1995). Sexual abuse by relatives with a strong emotional bond with the victim is the most devastating to the child (Fischer & McDonald, 1998).

Boys are also victims of both intrafamilial and extrafamilial abuse. Male victims are much less likely to report abuse, and they may suffer much greater emotional harm from incestuous relationships, especially between mother and son, than female victims (Moody, 1999). Boys are likely to be subjected to anal penetration and oral-genital contact; to have subtle physical findings; and to be abused by a father, stepfather, or mother's boyfriend.

Initiation and Perpetuation of Sexual Abuse

The cycle of sexual abuse often starts innocently unless it involves an isolated attack, such as rape. Often offenders spend time with the victims to gain their trust before initiating any sexual contact. Most victims are then pressured into being an accessory to the sexual activity through various means (Box 38-1) and may be unaware that sexual activity is part of the offer. Children may not reveal the truth for fear that their parents would not believe them if they told, especially if the offender is a trusted member of the family. Some fear that they will be blamed for the situation, and many young children with limited vocabulary have difficulty describing the activity when they do have the courage or opportunity to reveal the abuse.

Seductiveness by the child does not initiate incest. Most young girls experiment in seduction, especially during the preschool years, but the father's response normally differentiates this playfulness from overt sexual invitation. Although the reasons for incest are complicated and can occur in various family types, it does not occur in healthy families. Most incestuous relationships are directly tied to sexual maladjustment and estrangement between husband and wife. Most begin following the cessation of sexual relationships with the usual partner. Most fathers experience little guilt, and many wives at some level are aware of the incestuous affair. The wife may react by tolerating the situation or may resort to use of denial; some remain unaware of the activity. Consequently, the home offers little protection to young victims, because abusers have easy access to their victims and the children feel they cannot reveal their secret to other family members. However, not all incestuous relationships follow this pattern of silence. Currently, reports of father-daughter incest during child custody conflicts have become more common and have raised serious concerns regarding the possibility of false accusation. Rather than tolerating or denying the child's sexual abuse, the other parent (usually the mother) is typically the chief accuser.

Nursing Care of the Maltreated Child

Assessment

A critical responsibility of health professionals is identifying abusive situations as early as possible. The characteristics that may predispose members of some families to commit abuse can serve as a framework for assessing vulnerability but are never predictive of actual abuse. A thorough physical examination and a careful, detailed history are the diagnostic tools needed to identify abuse. Nurses have a special role because they may be the first person to see the child and parent and are the consistent caregivers if the child is hospitalized (Guidelines box).

NURSE ALERT Nurses must be aware of their biases regarding child abuse. Studies show that nurses are less likely to report abuse when the child is female and from a middle-income, as opposed to lower-income, family (Pillitteri et al, 1992); are significantly less comfortable dealing with sexual abuse, abuse of infants, and fathers as the abusers (Seidl et al, 1993); and experience greater discomfort when dealing with abusers of children with disabilities than with abusers of children without disabilities (Stanton et al, 1994). ■

Evidence of Maltreatment

Recognition of abuse or neglect necessitates a familiarity with both physical and behavioral signs that suggest maltreatment (Box 38-2). No one indicator can be used to diagnose maltreatment. It is a pattern or combination of indicators that should arouse suspicion and further investigation. In addition, signs of possible abuse must be coupled with an understanding of diseases, such as bleeding disorders, osteogenesis imperfecta, or sudden infant death syndrome (SIDS), and cultural practices, such as cupping or coin rub-

BOX 38-1

Methods Used to Pressure Children into Sexual Activity

- The child is offered gifts or privileges.
- The adult misrepresents moral standards by telling the child that it is "okay to do."
- Isolated and emotionally and socially impoverished children are enticed by adults who meet their needs for warmth and human contact.
- The successful sex offender pressures the victim into secrecy regarding the activity by describing it as a "secret between us" that other people may take away if they find out.
- The offender plays on the child's fears, including fear of punishment by the offender, fear of repercussions if the child tells, and fear of abandonment or rejection by the family.

Guidelines

TALKING WITH CHILDREN WHO REVEAL ABUSE

- Provide a private time and place to talk.
- Do not promise not to tell; tell them that you are required by law to report the abuse.
- Do not express shock or criticize their family.
- Use their vocabulary to discuss body parts.
- Avoid using any leading statements that can distort their report.
- Reassure them that they have done the right thing by telling.
- Tell them that the abuse is not their fault, that they are not bad or to blame.
- Determine their immediate need for safety.
- Let the child know what will happen when you report.

BOX 38-2

Warning Signs of Abuse

Physical evidence of abuse or neglect, including previous injuries
Conflicting stories about the "accident" or injury from the parents or others
Cause of injury blamed on sibling or other party
An injury inconsistent with the history, such as a concussion and broken arm from falling off a bed
History inconsistent with child's developmental level, such as a 6-month-old turning on the hot water
A complaint other than the one associated with signs of abuse (e.g., a chief complaint of a cold when there is evidence of first- and second-degree burns)
Inappropriate response of caregiver, such as an exaggerated or absent emotional response; refusal to sign for additional tests or agree to necessary treatment; excessive delay in seeking treatment; absence of the parents for questioning
Inappropriate response of child, such as little or no response to pain; fear of being touched; excessive or lack of separation anxiety; indiscriminate friendliness to strangers
Child's report of physical or sexual abuse
Previous reports of abuse in the family
Repeated visits to emergency facilities with injuries

bing (see Health Practices, Chapter 32), that may mimic physical abuse. Unintentional injuries may also be wrongly diagnosed as abuse, such as burns from metal buckles on car seats, lacerations from seat belts, or retinal hemorrhage after cardiopulmonary resuscitation. Normal variants, such as mongolian spots and congenital anomalies of genitalia, can be mistaken for abuse.

Not all forms of physical abuse have obvious signs. Violent shaking of children *(shaken baby syndrome [SBS])* can cause fatal intracranial trauma without signs of external head injury (Castiglia, 2001). Nurses should suspect SBS in infants less than 1 year of age who have subdural or retinal (or both) hemorrhages in the absence of external signs of trauma (Castiglia, 2001).

NURSE ALERT Stress to parents the dangers of shaking infants (shaking can cause SBS). Advise against shaking as a method of burping or waking the infant, against tossing the infant in the air, and against shaking the infant when feeling angry or tense. ■

If abuse is suspected, nurses play an important role in monitoring the parent's activities to identify instances of causing the children's symptoms. Using a hidden video camera to document the parent's behavior is becoming a more common diagnostic procedure, but the parent's right of privacy must be considered (Hall et al, 2000).

Neglect and Emotional Abuse

Neglect from deprivation of necessities is easier to identify than emotional neglect or abuse because physical signs are usually evident. Emotional maltreatment may be readily suspected, but it is very difficult to substantiate. Physical signs are often nonspecific, and nurses must rely on behavioral indicators, which range from depression to acting-out behavior, to help identify a possibly abusive situation. Any persistent and unexplained change in the child's behavior is an important clue to possible emotional abuse.

Sexual Abuse

Identifying instances of sexual abuse is particularly difficult because frequently few if any obvious physical indications of the activity exist. Also, many individuals are hesitant to believe children and are unwilling to report incidents. Even health professionals are sometimes at fault when they perform cursory physical examinations of the genitalia and ignore behavior or verbal comments that suggest abuse. When sexual abuse is suspected, other children in the family should be evaluated, because multiple victims are not uncommon.

Unfortunately, there is no typical profile of the victim, and there must be a high index of suspicion to identify these children. Physical signs vary and may include any of those listed for sexual abuse. The victim may exhibit various behavioral manifestations. Unfortunately, none of these behaviors is diagnostic. When abused children exhibit these behaviors, the signs may be incorrectly attributed to the normal stresses of childhood, especially in older school-age children or adolescents. Even signs considered most predictive of sexual abuse, such as certain genital findings, sexually inappropriate behavior for age, enactment of adult sexual activity, and intense focus on sexual activity (e.g., masturbation), do not always indicate that sexual abuse has occurred. Conversely, abused children may not demonstrate more knowledge of sexual activity than nonabused children. However, one difference in the abused children's explanation of sexual activity may be unusual affective responses. For example, abused children may have an increased incidence of sleep disorders, temper tantrums, and depression (Calam et al, 1998).

Many genital findings that have been reported as conclusive or highly suspect for sexual abuse, such as vaginal opening greater than 4 mm, hymenal tears and synechiae (tissue bands) inside the vagina, reflex anal dilation, and condylomata acuminata (anogenital or venereal warts), may be found in unabused prepubertal children (Brodeur & Monteleone, 1994). Results of a physical examination are normal in 80% of child victims of sexual abuse (Lahoti et al, 2001).

History Pertaining to the Incident

In addition to observable evidence of abuse, the type of history revealed by the parents or other caregiver, such as the baby-sitter or mother's boyfriend, is a significant factor. Areas of the history that should arouse suspicion of abuse are summarized in Box 38-3.

NURSE ALERT Incompatibility between the history and the injury is probably the most important criterion on which to base the decision to report suspected abuse. ■

An important point to remember when taking a history is that maltreated children rarely betray their parents by admitting to the abuse they received. If questioned, they will repeat the same story as the parents and try to defend their parents' actions. If the interviewer directly accuses the par-

BOX 38-3

Clinical Manifestations of Potential Child Maltreatment

Physical Neglect

Suggestive Physical Findings

Failure to thrive
Signs of malnutrition, such as thin extremities, abdominal distention, lack of subcutaneous fat
Poor personal hygiene
Unclean or inappropriate dress
Evidence of poor health care, such as delayed immunization, untreated infections, frequent colds
Frequent injuries from lack of supervision

Suggestive Behaviors

Dull and inactive; excessively passive or sleepy
Self-stimulatory behaviors, such as finger sucking or rocking
In older children:
- Begging or stealing food
- Absenteeism from school
- Drug or alcohol addiction
- Vandalism or shoplifting

Emotional Abuse and Neglect

Suggestive Physical Findings

Failure to thrive
Feeding disorders
Enuresis
Sleep disorders

Suggestive Behaviors

Self-stimulatory behaviors, such as biting, rocking, sucking
During infancy, lack of social smile and stranger anxiety
Withdrawal
Unusual fearfulness
Antisocial behavior, such as destructiveness, stealing, cruelty
Extremes of behavior, such as overcompliant and passive, or aggressive and demanding
Lags in emotional and intellectual development, especially language
Suicide attempts

Physical Abuse

Suggestive Physical Findings

Bruises and welts (may be in various stages of healing)
- On face, lips, mouth, back, buttocks, thighs, or areas of torso
- Regular patterns descriptive of object used, such as belt buckle, hand, wire hanger, chain, wooden spoon, squeeze or pinch marks
- May be present in various stages of healing

Burns
- On soles of feet, palms of hands, back, or buttocks
- Patterns descriptive of object used, such as round cigar or cigarette burns; sharply demarcated areas from immersion in scalding water; rope burns on wrists or ankles from being bound; burns in the shape of an iron, a radiator, or an electric stove burner
- Absence of "splash" marks and presence of symmetric burns
- Stun gun injury: lesions circular, fairly uniform (up to 0.5 cm), and paired about 5 cm apart (Frechette & Rimsza, 1992)

Fractures and dislocations
- Skull, nose, or facial structures
- Injury may denote type of abuse, such as spiral fracture or dislocation from twisting of an extremity or whiplash from shaking the child
- Multiple new or old fractures in various stages of healing

Lacerations and abrasions
- On backs of arms, legs, torso, face, or external genitalia
- Unusual symptoms, such as abdominal swelling, pain, and vomiting from punching
- Descriptive marks such as from human bites or pulling out of hair

Chemical
- Unexplained repeated poisoning, especially drug overdose
- Unexplained sudden illness, such as hypoglycemia from insulin administration

Suggestive Behaviors

Wary of physical contact with adults
Apparent fear of parents or going home
Lying very still while surveying environment
Inappropriate reaction to injury, such as failure to cry from pain
Lack of reaction to frightening events
Apprehensive when hearing other children cry
Indiscriminate friendliness and displays of affection
Superficial relationships
Acting-out behavior, such as aggression, to seek attention
Withdrawal behavior

Sexual Abuse

Suggestive Physical Findings

Bruises, bleeding, lacerations, or irritation of external genitalia, anus, mouth, or throat
Torn, stained, or bloody underclothing
Pain on urination or pain, swelling, and itching of genital area
Penile discharge
Sexually transmitted disease, nonspecific vaginitis, or venereal warts
Difficulty in walking or sitting
Unusual odor in the genital area
Recurrent urinary tract infections
Presence of sperm
Pregnancy in young adolescent

Suggestive Behaviors

Sudden emergence of sexually related problems, including excessive or public masturbation, age-inappropriate sexual play, promiscuity, or overtly seductive behavior
Withdrawn behavior, excessive daydreaming
Preoccupied with fantasies, especially in play
Poor relationships with peers
Sudden changes, such as anxiety, loss or gain of weight, clinging behavior
In incestuous relationships, excessive anger at mother for not protecting daughter
Regressive behavior, such as bed-wetting or thumb-sucking
Sudden onset of phobias or fears, particularly fears of the dark, men, strangers, or particular settings or situations (e.g., undue fear of leaving the house or staying at the day care center or the baby-sitter's house)
Running away from home
Substance abuse, particularly of alcohol or mood-elevating drugs
Profound and rapid personality changes, especially extreme depression, hostility, and aggression (often accompanied by social withdrawal)
Rapidly declining school performance
Suicidal attempts or ideation

ents of abuse, the child may accept responsibility for the act in an attempt to vindicate the parents. Whether children respond in this way out of fear is uncertain. However, children do fear losing whatever security and love they have. Between abusive acts, children may receive some measure of attention and love from the parents. If they betray the parents, they may lose this and be uncertain or fearful of the consequences, such as foster care. Preserving the present situation may be less frightening than the unknown future.

The *disclosure of sexual abuse* occurs in several ways: it is observed by others, resulting in a direct confrontation; the child tells someone; visible clues are observed (such as an accumulation of coins, gifts, or candy); or the child appears disheveled, demonstrates physical or behavioral signs and symptoms, or becomes pregnant. Children usually describe the experience in terms of whether it was unpleasant or hurt or was pleasurable (usually a response to hand-genital contact); some indicate no reaction. Young children often feel no guilt or shame because the act is pleasurable and they are unaware of its inappropriateness.

NURSE ALERT When children report potentially sexually abusive experiences, their reports need to be taken seriously, but also cautiously to avoid alarming the child or falsely accusing someone. ■

Children's reports of sexual abuse may vary from contradictory stories to unwavering versions of the experience. Stories that sound contradictory may reflect the child's experiences in several instances of abuse. Also, children who repeatedly tell identical facts may have been prompted to do so. Increasing evidence suggests that the types of interrogation children are exposed to following reports of sexual abuse shape their thinking. To avoid biasing the interaction, nurses must be very skillful interviewers when questioning children who may be victims of abuse. Medical records should include verbatim statements made by the child and interviewer that reflect appropriate, nonleading questions and statements (Hornor, 2001; McClain et al, 2000).

Parental Behaviors

Certain behavioral responses of the parents to their child and to the interviewer should alert the nurse to the possibility of maltreatment. Although no one pattern of behavior is characteristic of these parents, some responses include the following. Abusive parents have difficulty in showing concern toward their child. They are unable to comfort the child and give no indication of realizing how the child may feel, physically or emotionally. Instead, they are critical of and angry with the child for being injured. They maintain that the child is responsible for the injury, and if asked any question regarding their responsibility of protecting or supervising the child, they become hostile and aggressive. They act as if the child's injury is an assault on them. Their entire perception of the incident is in terms of how it affects them, not the child, which is an indication of their preoccupation with their own needs and of their inability to give any support to others.

During the child's hospitalization they may not become involved in the child's care and may show little concern for his or her progress, eventual discharge, or need for follow-up care. However, if they are pressured during interrogation, they immediately demand to take the child home, regardless of the child's readiness for discharge.

Families respond to sexual abuse with a wide variety of emotional reactions, which range from not believing the child to being very supportive. Parents and other family members may display the same type of emotional responses as the victim, such as inability to eat or sleep, and somatic complaints, such as headache. In the acute emotional phase, parents have a need to blame someone. The three common targets are the offender, the child, and themselves. The parents frequently express anger at the child for "stupid" behavior and may even restrict the child's privileges as punishment. When the victim is a girl, the parents may question her sexual provocation of the event. Self-blaming parents assume full responsibility, believing that they have been inadequate parents or should not have allowed the child to go out. When a baby-sitter or trusted relative is involved in the assault and the child's complaint has not been believed until gross evidence is presented, the parents are often devastated by guilt.

Child Behaviors

Abused children's responses to their parents or the injury may also support the suspicion of abuse. Although no one pattern is typical, extremes of behavior may be observed. Children may be very unresponsive to the parent or excessively clinging and intolerant of separation. They may be overattached to the abusive parent, possibly in the hope of preventing any upset that may precipitate anger and another attack. During care of the injury, children may be passive and accepting of the discomfort or uncooperative and fearful of any physical contact. Some children maintain a wary watchfulness of all strangers; some shy away from strangers as if frightened; others are unusually affectionate and outgoing.

Nursing Diagnoses

A number of nursing diagnoses are prominent in the nursing care of the maltreated child and family, and others specific to individual cases become evident. The most common nursing diagnoses are outlined in the Nursing Care Plan on p. 1147.

Plan of Care and Implementation

The main nursing goals related to child maltreatment are as follows:

1. Child will be protected from further abuse.
2. Child and family will receive adequate support.
3. Hospitalized child and family, including foster parents if appropriate, will be prepared for discharge.
4. Child will not experience any maltreatment.

Protect Child from Further Abuse

Initially, identification of instances of suspected abuse or neglect is essential. The nurse may come in contact with abused children in an emergency department, practitioner's office, home, day care center, or school.

NURSE ALERT The priority is to remove the child from the abusive situation to prevent further injury. ■

All states and provinces in North America have laws for mandatory reporting of child maltreatment. Suspected child abuse is reported to the local authorities.* Referrals usually come to the state child welfare department and are assigned to a caseworker in an agency such as CPS. Once a referral has been made, a caseworker is assigned to investigate the report. Based on the findings, the child is left in the home or temporarily removed.

A court proceeding may be necessary before the child can be placed outside the home or when parental rights are to be terminated. When the courts are involved, they usually require firsthand testimony by the referring parties. Nurses may be subpoenaed to appear in court, or their notes may be introduced as evidence in court hearings. Accurate and factual documentation is essential. Behaviors are described, not interpreted, and are recorded daily to establish a progress record (Guidelines box). Conversations among the nurse, child, and parent are recorded verbatim as much as possible.

Support Child

Frequently children suspected of abuse are hospitalized for medical management of their injuries. The type of care needed by the sexually abused child depends on the circumstances of the abuse. It varies from reassurance and support when the abuse involves exhibitionism to long-term counseling in incestuous situations. In interviewing these children, the nurse must be very careful to avoid biasing the child's retelling of the events. Some experts suggest that health professionals limit the interview to the child's physical and mental health concerns and leave topics of the family's social, legal, or other problems to the police or CPS personnel (McClain et al, 2000). When the sexually abused child has been physically harmed, the care is consistent with that provided to a rape victim. Regardless of the type of abuse, the child's needs are the same as those of any hospitalized child. The child should be treated as a child with the usual physical needs, developmental tasks, and play interests, not as a dramatic victim of abuse. The nurse is the child's advocate in this goal. The nurse also encourages the child's relationship with the parents.

The nurse does not become a substitute parent to the exclusion of the child's natural parents. Such behavior only intensifies the parents' feelings of inadequacy, worthlessness, and isolation. It does not help them understand their child or promote their trust in health professionals. The goal of the *consistent* nurse-child relationship is to provide a role model for the parents in helping them to relate positively and constructively to their child and to foster a therapeutic environment for the child in his or her reprieve from the abusing situation.

Support Family

One of the most difficult, yet essential, components of success with abusive parents is the quality of the *therapeutic relationship.* It must be one of genuine concern and treatment, not one of accusation and punishment. Nurses must examine their personal feelings toward these parents, particularly when sexual abuse is present. A therapeutic approach is to view the parent as the patient and the child as the victim of abuse. Unless the nurse's attitude is positive, abusive parents will not be motivated to change, because they will not be working with a trusting person who demonstrates the kind of behavior that is being asked of them.

When parental ignorance of childrearing practices has played a part in the abuse, the nurse can educate the parent regarding children's physical and emotional needs. Because of the parents' own childrearing, they may not be aware of nonviolent methods of discipline, such as time-out. They may also need help in dealing with their frustration so that they do not vent anger on the child. Because these parents may be sensitive to criticism or domination and already possess a very low self-esteem, teaching is implemented through demonstration and example rather than through lecturing. Any competent parenting abilities they demonstrate are praised to promote their sense of parental adequacy.

Care of the family also depends on the circumstances of the *sexual abuse.* With a nonparent offender the family may be more able to support the child than if incest were involved. Family members are encouraged to express their feelings of anger, guilt, shame, or embarrassment but are also cautioned to avoid displacing such feelings on the child. For example, it is easy for parents to admonish the child with a statement such as "We told you never to go with strangers," which makes the child feel responsible.

Family members are advised to encourage the child to resume normal activities and observe the child for signs of distress (see Posttraumatic Stress Disorder, Chapter 39). Chil-

*Telephone numbers are usually listed under "Child Abuse" in the business white pages of the local directory, or call the emergency child abuse hotline: 800-422-4453 (800-4-A-CHILD).

Guidelines

RECORDING ASSESSMENT DATA IN SUSPECTED ABUSE

History of Injury

1. Date, time, and place of occurrence
2. Sequence of events with recorded times
3. Presence of witnesses, especially person caring for child at time of incident
4. Time lapse between occurrence of injury and initiation of treatment
5. Interview with child when appropriate, including verbal quotations and information from drawing or other play activities
6. Interview with parent, witnesses, or other significant persons, including verbal quotations
7. Description of parent-child interactions (verbal interactions, eye contact, touching, parental concern)
8. Name, age, and condition of other children in home (if possible)

Physical Examination

1. Location, size, shape, and color of bruises; approximate location, size, and shape on drawing of body outline
2. Distinguishing characteristics, such as a bruise in the shape of a hand; round burn (possibly caused by cigarette)
3. Symmetry or asymmetry of injury; presence of other injuries
4. Degree of pain; any bone tenderness
5. Evidence of past injuries; general state of health and hygiene
6. Developmental level of child; perform screening test (see Developmental Assessment, Chapter 35)

dren express their feelings primarily through behavior. Parents should be alert for changes in behavior that indicate distress resulting from the incident, such as remaining in the house, refusing to go to school, changes in sleeping patterns, and frequency of dreams and nightmares. Children are encouraged to talk about these feelings and nightmares, because the more they talk about the experience, the more they are able to gain control over it.

Referral to appropriate agencies is also essential. Most abusive parents tend to live in poverty, and the daily stresses imposed by their lifestyle are overwhelming. Resources for financial aid, improved housing, and child care should be sought. Self-help groups also provide important services. Groups such as Parents Anonymous* (a group for parents who have abused or fear that they may abuse their child, but only in terms of physical abuse, not sexual abuse) and Parents United International, Inc.† (a group devoted to helping sexually abused families), are very accepting and nonjudgmental.

There is no way to predict which families will be successfully rehabilitated. With father-daughter incest, however, the best results occur when the father accepts full responsibility for the act, the mother acknowledges her role in failing to protect the child, and the child is able to understand and forgive the parents and develop a positive self-image despite the traumatic experience.

Plan for Discharge

Discharge planning should begin as soon as the legal disposition for placement has been decided, which may be temporary foster home placement, return to the parents, or permanent termination of parental rights. The latter is the most drastic solution, but it is necessary in situations of repeated, life-threatening abuse. Whenever children are sent to a foster home or juvenile institution, they must be allowed an opportunity to express their feelings. No matter how severe the abuse, they usually mourn the loss of their parents. They need help to understand why they must not return home and that this new home is in no way a punishment. Whenever possible, foster parents are encouraged to visit in the hospital, and the nurse should take an active role in helping these new parents understand the child. It is unfortunate that some abused children live in torment as they are sent from one foster home to another, sometimes enduring worse circumstances than those that existed in their original home. Only through constant evaluation of the placement residence and the child's adjustment to a new environment can the vicious circle of abuse, abandonment, and neglect be stopped.

Prevent Abuse

Prevention of child maltreatment has been an extremely difficult goal. Programs aimed at identifying potential abusers and instituting supportive intervention before the occurrence of an abusive act have met with variable success (Flournoy, 1996). However, nurses have played an important role in such programs. For example, home visiting by nurses to primiparas who were either teenagers, unmarried, or of low socioeconomic status was noted to be an effective preventive measure (Eckenrode et al, 2000; McMillian, 2000). The nurses provided information on normal child growth and development and routine health care needs, served as informal support persons, and referred families to appropriate services when a need for assistance was identified.

Such programs provide models that can be used to reduce factors that increase the risk of abuse. Nurses in a variety of settings can implement similar activities. For example, nurses in prenatal clinics can prepare expectant families for adjustment to parenthood. Nursery and postpartum nurses can foster the attachment process by encouraging parents to hold and look at their infant. Nurses in neonatal intensive care units can minimize the effects of separation by encouraging parents to visit and can help parents to become comfortable caring for their child. Nurses in ambulatory settings can teach parents appropriate methods of bathing, feeding, toileting, disciplining, and preventing injuries, while stressing the normal needs and developmental characteristics of children. Nurses must be sensitive to parental needs for attention, reassurance, and reinforcement, and refer parents to community services and self-help groups.

Unlike preventive efforts for neglect and physical abuse, which have been aimed at the potential offender, *prevention of child sexual abuse* has centered on education of children to protect themselves. Currently, much controversy surrounds the effectiveness of these programs. The main issue is whether young children should be expected to participate in their own protection. Clearly, sexual abuse prevention is more than teaching children to say "no" or to recognize their right not to be touched in "private places." It is equally important to teach children safety in terms of potential risk situations. Several suggestions for parents regarding protecting and educating children against possible molestation are presented in the Home Care box.

The nurse is frequently in a position to discuss this topic with parents and to provide guidelines. Books are available for parents that describe sexual abuse and its prevention.* Supporting parental qualities of respect, affection, empathy, and ability to set boundaries, and providing quality child care and education, constitute the true preventive approach to sexual abuse (Flournoy, 1996). Helpful games such as "What if the baby-sitter wants to wrestle

*675 W. Foothill Blvd., Suite 220, Claremont, CA 91711; phone: 909-621-6181; Web site: www.parentsanonymous/natl.org.

†PO Box 952, San Jose, CA 95108; phone: 408-453-7616.

*Sources of information include the following: Prevent Child Abuse America, Publishing Department, 200 S. Michigan Ave., Suite 1700, Chicago, IL 60604-4357; phone: 312-663-3520 or 800-CHILDREN; Web site: www.childabuse.org; Kempe Children's Center, 1825 Marion St., Denver, CO 80218; phone: 303-864-5250; Web site: www.kempecenter.org. American Association for Protecting Children, American Humane Association, 63 Inverness Dr., E., Englewood, CO 80112; phone: 800-227-4645 (outside Colorado) or 303-792-9900; National Clearinghouse on Child Abuse and Neglect Information, 330 C St., SW, Washington, DC 20447; phone: 800-394-3366; Web site: http://nccanch.acf.hhs.gov/.

Home Care

PREVENTING OR DEALING WITH SEXUAL ABUSE OF CHILDREN

Sexual assault of children is much more common than most people realize. It may be preventable if children have good preparation.

To provide protection and preparation:

- Pay careful attention to who is around children. (Unwanted touch may come from someone liked and trusted.)
- Back up a child's right to say "no."
- Encourage communication by taking seriously what children say.
- Take a second look at signals of potential danger.
- Refuse to leave children in the company of those not trusted.
- Include information about sexual assault when teaching about safety.
- Provide specific definitions and examples of sexual assault.
- Remind children that even "nice" people sometimes do mean things.
- Urge children to tell about *anybody* who causes them to be uncomfortable.
- Prepare children to deal with bribes and threats, as well as possible physical force.
- Virtually eliminate secrets between children and parents.
- Teach children how to say "no," ask for help, and control who touches them and how.
- Model self-protective and limit-setting behavior for children.

Should it ever become necessary to help a child recover from a sexual assault:

- Listen carefully to understand children.
- Support the child for telling through praise, belief, sympathy, and lack of blame.
- Know local resources and choose help carefully.
- Provide opportunities to talk about the assault.
- Provide opportunities for the entire family to go through a recovery process.

Sexual assault affects everyone. To help deal with this social problem:

- Provide care and support to those who have been victimized.
- Recognize that offenders do not change without intervention.
- Organize neighborhood programs to support each other's efforts to protect children.
- Encourage schools to provide information about sexual assault as a problem of health and safety.
- Organize community groups to support educational treatment and law enforcement programs.

Modified from Adams C, Fay J: *No more secrets: protecting your child from sexual assault,* San Luis Obispo, CA, 1981, Impact.

Nursing Care Plan

THE CHILD WHO IS MALTREATED

NURSING DIAGNOSIS: Risk for trauma related to characteristics of environment, child, caregiver(s)

EXPECTED OUTCOME

Patient will exhibit no evidence of further injury or neglect.

NURSING INTERVENTIONS/*RATIONALES*

Identify children at risk for potential abuse *to initiate preventive measures.*

Identify signs of maltreatment and implement measures *to prevent further maltreatment* (e.g., report suspicions to appropriate authorities; assist in removing child from unsafe environment and establishing in a safe environment; institute strict supervision if child is hospitalized).

Keep factual records (e.g., child's physical condition, behavioral responses; family responses; description of environment) *for documentation of maltreatment.*

Help child to recognize situations that place child at risk for sexual abuse and teach assertive responses *to discourage abuse.*

Refer family to appropriate social agencies for assistance with finances, food, shelter, clothing, and health care *to help prevent neglect.*

Participate in multidisciplinary team efforts *to assess for continued abuse or neglect and make decisions about removal from and return to the environment.*

NURSING DIAGNOSIS: Fear/anxiety related to repeated maltreatment, powerlessness, potential loss of parents

EXPECTED OUTCOME

Patient will exhibit decreasing evidence of distress.

NURSING INTERVENTIONS/*RATIONALES*

Provide consistent caregivers and therapeutic environment during hospitalization *to build trust and relieve stress.*

Provide support to child (e.g., treat child as someone with the usual age-appropriate physical, developmental, and social needs; avoid interrogation; ask permission to touch child; show attention to praise child's abilities and appropriate behaviors; give child opportunity to talk and ask questions without pressure to do so; use play to promote self-expression) *to decrease anxieties and increase confidence.*

Continued

Nursing Care Plan

THE CHILD WHO IS MALTREATED—cont'd

NURSING DIAGNOSIS: Altered parenting related to child, caregiver, or situational characteristics that precipitate abusive behavior

EXPECTED OUTCOME

Patient will exhibit evidence of changing parenting behaviors.

NURSING INTERVENTIONS/*RATIONALES*

Provide support to family (e.g., interactions with parents that reflect care and concern rather than accusation and punishment; encourage parent-child relationship; do not usurp parental role but rather provide a role model for constructive interaction with the child) *to establish trust and provide motivation for change.* Assess parenting-childrearing beliefs and practices *to establish baseline for teaching.*

Teach realistic expectations of child behavior and capabilities, emphasizing alternative methods of discipline such as reward, time-out, *to give parents alternatives to verbal or physical abusive behavior.*

Identify appropriate developmental issues (e.g., toilet training, toddler negativism, independence seeking) that may trigger abuse and help parents work out specific methods for management of the issue *to provide concrete approaches to timely issues.*

Use demonstration, role-modeling approaches rather than lecture or authoritarian approach *to overcome lack of self-esteem and sensitivity to criticism and establish trust.*

Praise competent parenting behaviors *to increase confidence in parenting abilities.*

Refer parent(s) to appropriate sources for classes on how to parent; counseling to explore abuse patterns; support groups *to decrease chances of repeat abuse.*

and hug but tells you to keep it a secret?" can be used to explore dangerous situations in advance and help children learn the importance of saying "no." They need reassurance that no matter what the other person says or does, the parents want to know about it and will not punish them. Even if children do participate in the activity before telling the parents, they must be reassured that it was not their fault.

In addition, parents need to be made aware that "nice" people, including friends and relatives, can be offenders; parents should carefully observe how others act toward the child. A sudden change in the child's behavior and a response such as "I don't like Uncle anymore" are clues to investigate the relationship. In the event of any doubt, further solitary encounters with this person and the child should be prevented. It is sometimes to the child's great misfortune that parents do not take certain comments seriously, such as "He hugs me too tight" or "I don't want to go with him." Casual parental statements such as "He just loves you" or "You do whatever adults tell you to do" can place children in jeopardy. Health professionals must alert parents to such dangers and guide them toward an appreciation of the problem, providing concrete guidelines toward child education and protection.

Evaluation

Continual reassessment and evaluation of care based on the following observational guidelines determine the effectiveness of nursing interventions:

1. Observe child for additional physical and behavioral evidence of abuse; observe child's reactions to health professionals; if child is hospitalized, check staffing patterns for schedule of consistent group of nurses caring for child.
2. Interview parents regarding their knowledge of children's physical and development needs.
3. Interview child regarding feelings about returning home or placement outside the home.
4. Investigate community programs aimed at preventing child maltreatment.

The *expected outcomes* are described in the Nursing Care Plan on pp. 1147.

Key Points

- The preschool years comprise the period from 3 to 5 years of age, a time that is considered critical for emotional and psychologic development.
- Biologic development in the preschool period is characterized by mature body systems and refinement in gross and fine motor behavior, as evidenced by participation in activities such as running, riding a tricycle, and drawing.
- According to Erikson, acquiring a sense of initiative is the chief psychosocial task of the preschooler. Development of the superego occurs during this period, and conscience begins to emerge.
- According to Piaget, the preschool age is characterized by intuitive or prelogical thinking and a move toward logical thought processes through advanced, complex learning, language, and understanding of causality.
- The seeds of moral development are planted during the preschool period. According to Kohlberg, children are in the stage of naive instrumental orientation, in which they are concerned with satisfying their own needs and less frequently the needs of others.
- Social development includes further individuation-separation; more sophisticated language; greater independence; and more complex, imaginative forms of play.
- Areas of special concern to parents during the preschool period are preschool and kindergarten experience, sex education, fears, stress, and speech problems.
- In selecting an early learning program, parents should inquire about daily programs, teacher qualifications, accreditation, student-staff ratio, safety, meals, fees, and health practices.

- Two rules that govern answering questions about sex and other sensitive issues are to find out what the child knows and to be honest.
- Fears constitute a great part of the preschool period; objects, potential annihilation, and parent-induced fears are common sources.
- Preschool aggression may result from frustration, modeling behavior, and reinforcement.
- Hesitancy or dysfluency in speech patterns is a normal characteristic of language development. Speech problems can occur when parents express excessive concern over this pattern.
- Health promotion continues to be directed toward proper nutrition, adequate sleep, proper dental care, and injury prevention.
- Child maltreatment may take the form of physical abuse or neglect, emotional abuse or neglect, or sexual abuse.
- Parental, child, and environmental characteristics are criteria that may predispose children to maltreatment.
- Identification of abuse entails securing evidence of maltreatment, taking a history pertaining to the incident, and assessing parental and child behaviors.
- The reported incidence of sexual abuse has increased in the last decade; common forms are incest, molestation, rape, exhibitionism, child pornography, child prostitution, and pedophilia.

References

Adler NA, Schutz J: Sibling incest offenders, *Child Abuse Negl* 19(7):811-819, 1995.

Ambrose NG, Yairi E: Normative disfluency data for early childhood stuttering, *J Speech Lang Hear Res* 42(4):895-909, 1999.

American Academy of Pediatrics: Hearing assessment in infants and children: recommendations beyond neonatal screening, *Pediatrics* 111(2):436-440, 2003.

American Academy of Pediatrics, Committee on Infectious Diseases, Pickering L (editor): *2003 red book: report of the Committee on Infectious Diseases,* ed 26, Elk Grove Village, IL, 2003, The Academy.

American Academy of Pediatrics, Committee on Nutrition: *Pediatric nutrition handbook,* ed 4, Elk Grove Village, IL, 1998, The Academy.

American Academy of Pediatrics, Committee on Nutrition: The use and misuse of fruit juices in pediatrics, *Pediatrics* 107(5):1210-1213, 2001.

American Academy of Pediatrics, Committee on Public Education: Children, adolescents, and television, *Pediatrics* 107(2):423-426, 2001.

American Academy of Pediatrics, Committee on Sports Medicine and Fitness and Committee on School Health: Physical fitness and activity in schools, *Pediatrics* 105(5):1156-1157, 2000.

Anderson DR et al: Early childhood television viewing and adolescent behavior: the recontact study, *Monogr Soc Res Child Dev* 66(1):I-VIII, 1-147, 2001.

Anderson JE: Co-sleeping: can we ever put the issue to rest? *Contemp Pediatr* 107(6):98-120, 2000.

Brodeur AE, Monteleone JA: *Child maltreatment, a clinical guide and reference,* St Louis, 1994, Mosby.

Calam R et al: Psychological disturbances and child sexual abuse: a follow-up study, *Child Abuse Negl* 22(9):901-913, 1998.

Castiglia R: Shaken baby syndrome, *J Pediatr Health Care* 15(2):78-80, 2001.

Chen TM et al: Clinical manifestations of varicella-zoster virus infection, *Dermatol Clin* 20(2):267-282, 2002.

Davison KK, Birch LL: Weight status and self-concept in young girls, *Pediatrics* 107(1):46-53, 2001.

Eckenrode J et al: Preventing child abuse and neglect with a program of nurse home visitation: the limiting effects of domestic violence, *JAMA* 284(11):1385-1391, 2000.

Endres J et al: Soy-enhanced lunch acceptance by preschoolers, *J Am Diet Assoc* 103(3):346-351, 2003.

Finan SL: Promoting healthy sexuality: guidelines for infancy through preschool, *Nurse Pract* 22(10):79-80, 83-86, 88, 1997.

Fischer DG, McDonald WL: Characteristics of intrafamilial and extrafamilial child sexual abuse, *Child Abuse Negl* 22(9):915-929, 1998.

Flournoy J: Incest prevention: the role of the pediatric nurse practitioner, *J Pediatr Health Care* 10(6):246-254, 1996.

Frechette A, Rimsza ME: Stun gun injury: a new presentation of the battered child syndrome, *Pediatrics* 89(5):898-901, 1992.

Gottesman MM: Playing to learn: the work of children and their parents, *J Pediatr Health Care* 13(5):259-262, 1999.

Hall D et al: Evaluation of covert video surveillance in the diagnosis of Munchausen by proxy: lessons from 41 cases, *Pediatrics* 105(6):1305-1312, 2000.

Hart CH et al: Overt and relational aggression in Russian nursery-school-aged children: parenting style and marital linkages, *Dev Psychol* 34(4):687-697, 1998.

Hornor G: Repeated sexual abuse allegations: a problem for primary care providers, *J Pediatr Health Care* 15(2):71-76, 2001.

Huttenlocher J: Language input and language growth, *Prev Med* 27(2):195-199, 1998.

Johnson RK: Changing eating and physical activity patterns of U.S. children, *Proc Nutr Soc* 59(2):295-301, 2000.

Kenny G: Assessing children's spirituality: what is the way forward? *Br J Nurs* 8(1):28, 30-32, 1999.

Krug EF, Mikus KC: The preschool years. In Levine MD, Carey WB, Crocker AC (eds): *Developmental-behavioral pediatrics,* ed 3, Philadelphia, 1999, WB Saunders.

Lahoti SL et al: Evaluating the child for sexual abuse, *Am Fam Physician* 63(5):883-892, 2001.

Latz S, Wolf AW, Lozoff B: Cosleeping in context: sleep practices and problems in young children in Japan and the United States, *Arch Pediatr Adolesc Med* 153(4):339-346, 1999.

Martof A: Consultation with the specialist: dental care, *Pediatr Rev* 22(1):13-15, 2001.

McClain N et al: Evaluation of sexual abuse in the pediatric patient, *J Pediatr Health Care* 14(3):93-102, 2000.

McEvoy M: An added dimension to the pediatric health maintenance visit: the spiritual history, *J Pediatr Health Care* 14(5):216-220, 2000.

McEvoy M: Culture and spirituality as an integrated concept in pediatric care, *MCN* 28(1):39-43, 2003.

McMillian H: Child maltreatment: what we know in the year 2000, *Can J Psychiatr* 45(8):702-709, 2000.

Moody CW: Male child sexual abuse, *J Pediatr Health Care* 13(3):112-119, 1999.

Muris P, Merckelbach H, Prins E: How serious are common childhood fears? II. The parents' point of view, *Behav Res Ther* 38(3):813-818, 2000.

National Clearinghouse on Child Abuse and Neglect Information: Child maltreatment 2002: summary of key findings, 2004. Internet document available at http://nccanch.acf.hhs.gov/general/stats/index.cfm (Accessed March 23, 2005).

Needlman R: Growth and development: preschool years. In Behrman RE, Kliegman RM, Jenson HB (eds): *Nelson textbook of pediatrics,* ed 17, Philadelphia, 2004, WB Saunders.

Nelms BC: Emotional abuse: helping prevent the problem, *J Pediatr Health Care* 15(3):103-104, 2001.

Okami P, Weisner T, Olmstead R: Outcome correlates of parent-child bed-sharing: An eighteen-year longitudinal study, *J Dev Behav Pediatr* 23(4):244-253, 2002.

Paulk D: Munchausen syndrome by proxy, *Clin Rev* 11(8):51-56, 2001.

Pillitteri A et al: Parent gender, victim gender, and family socioeconomic level influences on the potential reporting by nurses of physical child abuse, *Issues Compr Pediatr Nurs* 15:239-247, 1992.

Putnam FW: Ten year update review: child sexual abuse, *J Am Acad Child Adolesc Psychiatry* 42(3):269-278, 2003.

Rampersaud GC, Bailey LB, Kauwell GPA: National survey beverage consumption data for children and adolescents indicate the need to encourage a shift toward more nutritive beverages, *J Am Diet Assoc* 103(1): 97-100, 2003.

Rovers MM et al: Day-care and otitis media in young children: a critical review, *Eur J Pediatr* 158(1):1-6, 1999.

Seidl AH et al: Nurses' attitudes toward the child victims and the perpetrators of emotional, physical, and sexual abuse, *Issues Child Abuse Accus* 5(1):28-38, 1993.

Stalkup JR: A review of measles virus, *Dermatol Clin* 20(2):209-215, 2002.

Stanton M et al: Nurses' attitudes toward emotional, sexual, and physical abusers of children with disabilities, *Rehabil Nurs* 19(4):214-218, 1994.

Steen S, Anderson B: Ages and stages of spiritual development, *J Christ Nurs* 12(2):6-11, 1995.

Stormshak EA et al: Parenting practices and child disruptive behavior problems in early elementary school, *J Clin Child Psychol* 29(1):17-29, 2000.

Thiedke CC: Sleep disorders and sleep problems in childhood, *Am Fam Physician* 63(2):277-284, 2001.

Thomas RM: *Comparing theories of child development,* ed 4, Pacific Grove, CA, 1996, Brooks-Cole.

US Department of Agriculture, Center for Nutrition Policy and Promotion: My pyramid—The New Food Guidance System, 2005. Internet document available at www.usda.gov/cnpp (accessed June 6, 2005).

Vessey JA, Yim-Chiplis PK, MacKenzie NR: Effects of television viewing on children's development, *Pediatr Nurs* 23(5):483-485, 1998.

Villani S: Impact of media on children and adolescents: a 10-year review research, *J Am Acad Child Adolesc Psychiatry* 40(4):392-401, 2001.

Williams CL et al: Healthy Start: outcome of an intervention to promote a heart healthy diet in preschool children, *J Am Coll Nutr* 21(1):62-71, 2002.

Wilson JF: Preschoolers' mid-afternoon snack intake is not affected by lunchtime food consumption, *Appetite* 33(3):319-327, 1999.

The School-Age Child and Family 39

LEARNING OBJECTIVES

On completion of this chapter the reader will be able to:

- Describe the physical, cognitive, and moral changes that take place during the middle childhood years.
- Describe ways to help a child develop a sense of accomplishment.
- Demonstrate an understanding of the changing interpersonal relationships of school-age children.
- Discuss the role of the peer group in the socialization of the school-age child.
- Discuss the role of schools in the development and socialization of the school-age child.
- Demonstrate an understanding of the types, causes, and prevention of sports injuries in middle childhood.
- Describe the most common causes of growth and maturation failure in later childhood.
- Discuss the manifestations and nursing management of selected emotional and behavioral problems.
- Outline an appropriate health teaching plan for the school-age child.
- Plan a sex education session for a group of school-age children.
- Identify the causes and discuss the preventive aspects of injury in middle childhood.

ELECTRONIC RESOURCES

Additional information related to the content in Chapter 39 can be found on

the companion website at evolve
http://evolve.elsevier.com/Wong/maternal/
- NCLEX Review Questions
- Case Study—Attention Deficit/Hyperactivity Disorder
- Weblinks

or the interactive student CD-ROM
Activities for Chapter 39 include the following:
- NCLEX Review Questions
- Case Study—Injury Prevention
- Critical Thinking Exercise—Turner Syndrome

PROMOTING OPTIMUM GROWTH AND DEVELOPMENT

The segment of the life span that extends from age 6 to approximately age 12 has a variety of labels, each of which describes an important characteristic of the period. These middle years are most often referred to as the *school-age years* or the *school years.* This period begins with entrance into the school environment, which has a significant impact on development and relationships.

Physiologically the middle years begin with the shedding of the first deciduous tooth and end at puberty with the acquisition of the final permanent teeth (with the exception of the wisdom teeth). Before 5 or 6 years of age, children have progressed from helpless infants to sturdy, complicated individuals with an ability to communicate, conceptualize in a limited way, and become involved in complex social and motor behaviors. Physical growth is also rapid during the preschool-age years. In contrast, the period of middle childhood, between the rapid growth of early childhood and the prepubescent growth spurt, is a time of gradual growth and development with more even progress in both physical and emotional aspects.

Biologic Development

During middle childhood, growth in height and weight assumes a slower but steady pace as compared with the earlier years. Between ages 6 and 12, children will grow an average of 5 cm (2 inches) per year to gain 30 to 60 cm (1 to 2 feet) in height and will almost double their weight, increasing 2 to 3 kg (4½ to 6½ pounds) per year. The average 6-year-old child is about 116 cm (45 inches) tall and weighs about 21 kg (46 pounds); the average 12-year-old child is about 150 cm (59 inches) tall and weighs approximately 40 kg (88 pounds). During this period, girls and boys differ very little in size, although boys tend to be slightly taller and somewhat heavier than girls. Toward the end of the school-age years, both boys and girls begin to increase in size, although most girls begin to surpass boys in both height and weight, to the acute discomfort of both girls and boys.

Proportional Changes

School-age children are more graceful than they were as preschoolers, and they are steadier on their feet. Their body proportions take on a slimmer look, with longer legs, varying body proportion, and a lower center of gravity. Posture improves over that of the preschool period to facilitate locomotion and efficiency in using the arms and trunk. These proportions make climbing, bicycle riding, and other activities easier. Fat gradually diminishes, and its distribution patterns change, contributing to the thinner appearance of the child during the middle years.

Accompanying the skeletal lengthening and fat diminution is an increase in the percentage of body weight represented by muscle tissue. By the end of this age period, both boys and girls double their strength and physical capabilities, and their steady and relatively consistent development of coordination increases their poise and skill. However, this increased strength can be misleading. Although strength increases, muscles are still functionally immature when compared with those of the adolescent, and they more readily suffer muscular injury caused by overuse.

The most pronounced changes that indicate increasing maturity in children are a decrease in head circumference in relation to standing height, a decrease in waist circumference in relation to height, and an increase in leg length related to height. These observations often provide a clue to a child's degree of physical maturity and have proved useful in predicting readiness for meeting the demands of school. There appears to be a correlation between physical indications of maturity and success in school.

Facial Changes

Specific physiologic and anatomic characteristics are typical of children in middle childhood. Facial proportions change as the face grows faster in relation to the remainder of the cranium. The skull and brain grow very slowly during this period and increase little in size. Because all of the primary (deciduous) teeth are lost during this age span, middle childhood is sometimes known as the *age of the loose tooth* (Fig. 39-1). The early years of middle childhood, when the new secondary (permanent) teeth appear too large for the face, are known as the *ugly duckling stage.*

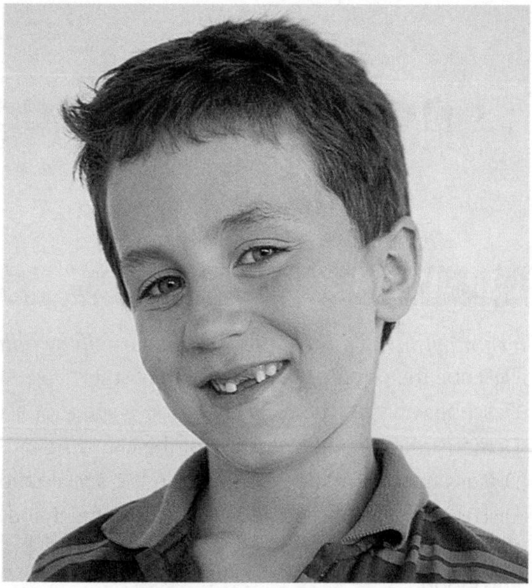

Fig. 39-1 Middle childhood is the stage of development when deciduous teeth are shed.

Maturation of Systems

Maturity of the gastrointestinal system is reflected in fewer stomach upsets, better maintenance of blood glucose levels, and an increased stomach capacity, which permits retention of food for longer periods. The school-age child does not need to be fed as carefully, as promptly, or as frequently as the preschool-age child. Caloric needs are less than they were in the preschool years.

Physical maturation is evident in other body tissues and organs. *Bladder capacity,* although differing widely among individual children, is generally greater in girls than in boys. The *heart* grows more slowly during the middle years and is smaller in relation to the rest of the body than at any other period of life. Heart and respiratory rates steadily decrease and blood pressure increases during ages 6 to 12 (see Appendix J).

The *immune system* becomes more competent in its ability to localize infections and to produce an antibody-antigen response. However, children may have several infections in the first 1 to 2 years of school because of increased exposure to other children.

Bones continue to ossify throughout childhood but yield to pressure and muscle pulls more readily than mature bones. Children need ample opportunity to move around, but they should observe caution in carrying heavy loads. For example, they should shift books or tote bags from one arm to the other. Backpacks distribute weight more evenly than tote bags.

Wider differences between children are observed at the end of middle childhood than at the beginning. These differences become increasingly apparent, and, if they are extreme or unique, they may create emotional problems. The associated characteristics of height and weight relationships, rapid or slow growth, and other important features of development should be explained to children and their families. Physical maturity is not necessarily correlated with emotional and social maturity. Seven-year-old children who look like 10-year-old children will, in fact, think and act like 7-year-old children. To expect behaviors appropriate for the older age is unrealistic and can be detrimental to their development of competence and self-esteem. Conversely, to treat 10-year-old children who look young physically as though they were younger is an equal disservice to them.

Prepubescence

Preadolescence is the period of approximately 2 years that begins at the end of middle childhood and ends with the thirteenth birthday. Because puberty signals the beginning of the development of secondary sex characteristics, *prepubescence* typically occurs during preadolescence.

Toward the end of middle childhood the discrepancies in growth and maturation between boys and girls become apparent. There is an average difference of approximately 2 years between girls and boys in the age of onset of pubescence. This is a period of rapid growth in height and weight, especially for girls.

There is no universal age at which children assume the characteristics of prepubescence. The first physiologic signs appear at about 9 years of age (particularly in girls) and are usually clearly evident in 11- to 12-year-old children. Although preadolescent children do not want to be different, variability in physical growth and physiologic changes between children of the same sex and between the two sexes is often striking at this time. This variability, especially in relation to the onset of secondary sexual characteristics, is of great concern to the preadolescent. Either early or late appearance of these characteristics is a source of embarrassment and uneasiness to both sexes.

Preadolescence is a period of time when considerable overlapping of developmental characteristics of both middle childhood and early adolescence occurs. However, several unique characteristics set this period apart from others. Generally, the earliest age at which puberty begins is 10 years in girls and 12 years in boys, although there has been an increase in the number of girls reaching puberty at age 9. The average age of puberty is 12 years in girls and 14 years in boys. Boys experience little visible sexual maturation during preadolescence.

Psychosocial Development

Freud described middle childhood as the *latency period,* a time of tranquility between the Oedipal phase of early childhood and the eroticism of adolescence. During this time children experience relationships with same-sex peers following the indifference of earlier years and preceding the heterosexual fascination that occurs for most boys and girls in puberty.

Developing a Sense of Industry (Erikson)

Successful mastery of Erikson's first three stages of psychosocial development are important in terms of development of a healthy personality (Erikson, 1963). Successful completion of these stages requires a loving environment within a stable family unit. These experiences prepare the child to engage in experiences and relationships beyond the intimate family group.

A *sense of industry,* or a *stage of accomplishment,* is achieved somewhere between age 6 and adolescence. School-age children are eager to develop skills and participate in meaningful and socially useful work. They acquire a sense of personal and interpersonal competence, receive the systematic instruction prescribed by their individual cultures, and develop the skills needed to become useful, contributing members of their social communities.

Interests expand in the middle years, and with a growing sense of independence, children want to engage in tasks that can be carried through to completion (Fig. 39-2). They gain satisfaction from independent behavior in exploring and manipulating their environment and from interaction with peers. Often the acquisition of skills provides a way to achieve success in social activities. Reinforcement in the form of grades, material rewards, additional privileges, and recognition provides encouragement and stimulation.

A sense of accomplishment also involves the ability to cooperate, to compete with others, and to cope effectively with people. Middle childhood is the time when children learn the value of doing things with others and the benefits derived from division of labor in the accomplishment of goals. Peer approval is a strong motivating power.

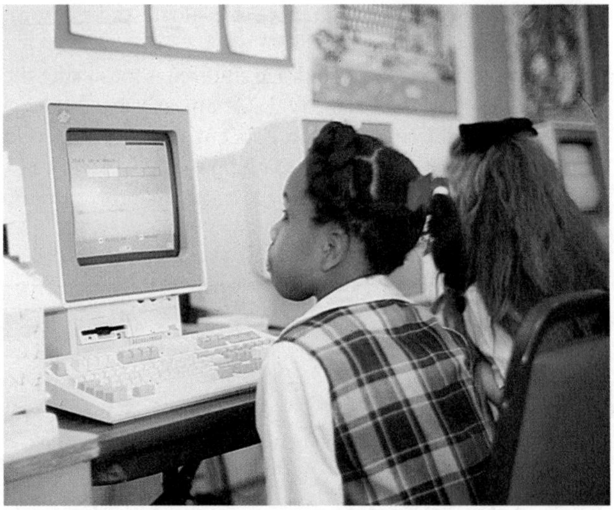

Fig. 39-2 School-age children are motivated to complete tasks working alone.

The danger inherent in this period of development is the occurrence of situations that might result in a sense of *inferiority.* Children with physical and mental limitations may be at a disadvantage for acquisition of certain skills. When the reward structure is based on evidence of mastery, children who are incapable of developing these skills are at risk for feeling inadequate and inferior. However, even children without chronic disabilities may experience feelings of inadequacy in some areas. No child is able to do everything well, and children must learn that they will not be able to master every skill that they attempt. All children, even children who usually have positive attitudes toward work and their own abilities, will feel some degree of inferiority when they encounter specific skills that they cannot master.

Children need and want real achievement. When they have access to tasks that need to be done, that they are able to do well despite individual differences in their innate capacities and emotional development, and for which they are suitably rewarded, children achieve a sense of industry.

Cognitive Development (Piaget)

When children enter the school years, they begin to acquire the ability to relate a series of events to mental representations that can be expressed both verbally and symbolically. This is the stage that Piaget describes as *concrete operations,* when children are able to use thought processes to experience events and actions. The rigid, egocentric view of the preschool years is replaced by mental processes that allow children to see things from another's point of view.

During this stage, children develop an understanding of relationships between things and ideas. They progress from making judgments based on what they see *(perceptual thinking)* to making judgments based on what they reason *(conceptual thinking).* They are able to master symbols and to use their memories of past experiences to evaluate and interpret the present.

One cognitive task of school-age children is mastering the concept of *conservation* (Fig. 39-3). At an early age (about 5 to 7 years), children grasp the concept of reversibility of numbers as a basis for simple mathematics problems (e.g., 2 + 4 = 6 and 6 − 4 = 2). They learn that simply altering their arrangement in space does not change certain properties of the environment, and they are able to resist perceptual cues that suggest alterations in the physical state of an object. For example, they recognize that changing the shape of a substance such as a lump of clay does not alter its total mass. They no longer perceive a tall, thin glass of water as containing a greater volume than a short, wide glass; they can dis-

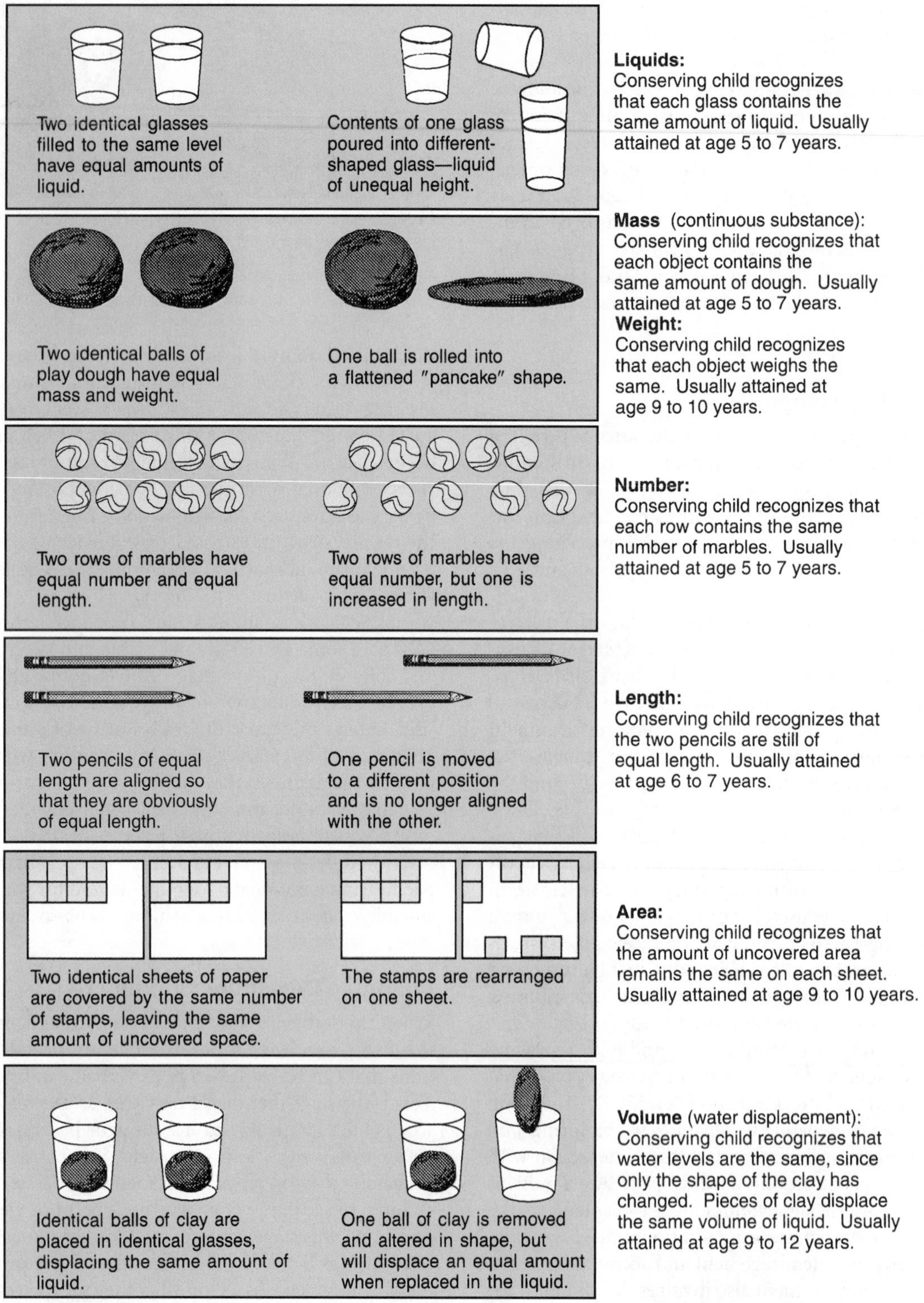

Fig. 39-3 Common examples that demonstrate the child's ability to conserve (ages are only approximate).

tinguish between the weight of items regardless of their size. They recognize that size is not necessarily related to weight or volume. There is a developmental sequence in children's capacity to conserve matter. Conservation of mass usually is accomplished first, weight some time later, and volume last.

School-age children also develop *classification* skills. They can group and sort objects according to the attributes that they share, place things in a sensible and logical order, and hold a concept in mind while making decisions based on that concept. Another characteristic of middle childhood that children derive enjoyment from is classifying and ordering their environment. They become occupied with collections of objects, such as stickers, stamps, shells, dolls, cars, and stones. They may even begin to order friends and relationships (e.g., first best friend, second best friend).

They develop the ability to understand relational terms and concepts, such as bigger and smaller; darker and paler; heavier and lighter; to the right of and to the left of; first, last, and intermediate relationships; and more than and less than. They view family relationships in terms of reciprocal roles (e.g., in order to be a brother, one must have a sibling).

School-age children learn the alphabet and the world of symbols called words that can be arranged in terms of structure and their relationship to the alphabet. They learn to tell time, to see the relationship of events in time (history) and places in space (geography), and to combine time and space relationships (geology and astronomy).

The *ability to read* is acquired during the school years and becomes the most significant and valuable tool for independent inquiry. Children's capacity to explore, imagine, and expand their knowledge is enhanced by reading.

Moral Development (Kohlberg)

As children move from egocentrism to more logical patterns of thought, they also move through stages in the development of conscience and moral standards. Young children do not believe that standards of behavior come from within themselves but that rules are established and set down by others. During the preschool years children adopt and internalize the moral values of their parents. They learn standards for acceptable behavior, act according to these standards, and feel guilty when they violate them.

Although children of 6 or 7 years of age know the rules and behaviors expected of them, they do not understand the reasons behind them. Rewards and punishments guide their judgment; a "bad act" is one that breaks a rule or does harm. Young children believe that what other people tell them to do is right and that what they themselves think is wrong. Consequently, children 6 or 7 years old may interpret accidents or misfortunes as punishment for "bad" acts.

Older school-age children are able to judge an act by the intentions that prompted it rather than just its consequences. Rules and judgments become less absolute and authoritarian, and begin to be founded on the needs and desires of others. For older children, a rule violation is likely to be viewed in relation to the total context in which it appears. The situation, as well as the morality of the rule itself, influences reactions. Although younger children judge an act only according to whether it is right or wrong, older children take into account a different point of view. They are able to understand and accept the concept of treating others as they would like to be treated.

Spiritual Development

Children at this age think in concrete terms, but are avid learners and have a great desire to learn about their God. They picture God as human and use adjectives such as "loving" and "helping" to describe their deity. They are fascinated by the concepts of hell and heaven, and with a developing conscience and concern about rules. They may fear going to hell for misbehavior. School-age children want and expect to be punished for misbehavior and, when given the option, tend to choose a punishment that "fits the crime." However, they may view illness or injury as a punishment for a real or imagined misdeed. The beliefs and ideals of family and religious persons are more influential than those of their peers in matters of faith.

School-age children begin to learn the difference between the natural and the supernatural but have difficulty understanding symbols. Consequently, religious concepts must be presented to them in concrete terms. Prayer or other religious rituals comfort them, and if these activities are a part of their daily lives, they can help them cope with threatening situations. Their petitions to their God in prayers tend to be for tangible rewards. Although younger children expect their prayers to be answered, as they get older, they begin to recognize that this does not always occur and become less concerned when prayers are not answered. They are able to discuss their feelings about their faith and how it relates to their lives (Cultural Awareness box).

Social Development

One of the most important socializing agents in the school-age years is the peer group. In addition to parents and the schools, the peer group conveys a substantial amount of material to its members. Peer groups have a culture of their own, with secrets, mores, and codes of ethics that promote feelings of solidarity and detachment from adults. Through peer relationships children learn ways to deal with dominance and hostility, how to relate to persons in positions of leadership and authority, and how to explore ideas and the physical environment.

Peer group identification is an important factor in gaining independence from parents. The aid and support of the group provides the child with enough security to risk the

Cultural Awareness

RELIGIOUS ORIENTATION

Many schools and communities have a Judeo-Christian orientation toward prayer, holidays, and values. This may result in conflict and discomfort for children of other religious/ethnic groups. Sensitivity must be exercised so as not to offend and confuse children from other religious backgrounds, such as the Buddhist, Hindu, and Muslim faiths.

moderate parental rejection brought about by small victories in the development of independence.

A child's concept of the appropriate sex role is influenced by relationships with peers. During the early school years there are few gender differences in the play experiences of children. Both girls and boys share games and other activities. However, in the later school years the differences in the play of boys and girls becomes more marked.

Social Relationships and Cooperation

Daily relationships with peers provide important social interactions for school-age children. For the first time, children join group activities with unrestrained enthusiasm and steady participation. Previous interactions were limited to short periods under considerable adult supervision. With increased skills and wider opportunities, children become involved with one or more peer groups in which they can gain status as respected members.

Valuable lessons are learned from daily interaction with age-mates. First, children learn to appreciate the numerous and varied points of view that are represented in the peer group. As children interact with peers who see the world in ways that are somewhat different from their own, they become aware of the limits of their own point of view. Because age-mates are peers and are not forced to accept each other's ideas as they are expected to accept those of adults, other children have a significant influence on decreasing the egocentric outlook of the child. Consequently, children learn to argue, persuade, bargain, cooperate, and compromise to maintain friendships.

Second, children become increasingly sensitive to the social norms and pressures of the peer group. The peer group establishes standards for acceptance and rejection, and children are often willing to modify their behavior to be accepted by the group. The need for peer approval becomes a powerful influence toward conformity. Children learn to dress, talk, and behave in a manner acceptable to the group. A variety of roles, such as class joker or class hero, may be assumed by individual children to gain approval from the group.

Third, the interaction among peers leads to the formation of intimate friendships between same-sex peers. The school-age period is the time when children have "best friends" with whom they share secrets, private jokes, and adventures; they come to one another's aid in times of trouble. In the course of these friendships children also fight, threaten each other, break up, and reunite. These relationships, in which the child experiences love and closeness for a peer, may be important as a foundation for relationships in adulthood (Fig. 39-4).

Clubs and Peer Groups

One of the outstanding characteristics of middle childhood is the formation of formalized groups, or clubs. A prominent feature of these groups is the rigid rules imposed on the members. There is exclusiveness in the selection of persons who have the privilege of joining. Acceptance in the group is often determined on a pass-fail basis according to social or behavioral criteria. Conformity is the core of the group structure. There are often secret codes, shared interests, and special modes of dress, and each child must abide by a standard of behavior established by the members. Conforming to the rules provides children with feelings of security and relieves them of the responsibility of making decisions. By merging their identities with those of their peers, children are able to move from the family group to an outside group as a step toward seeking further independence. Peer groups and clubs allow children to substitute conformity to a peer group for conformity to a family at a time when children are still too insecure to function independently.

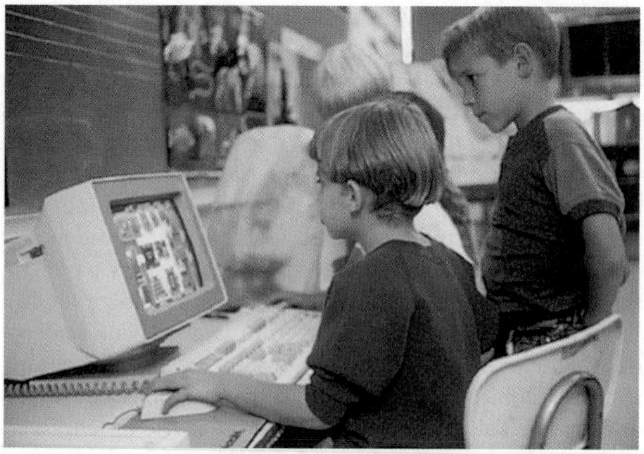

Fig. 39-4 School-age children enjoy engaging in activities with a "best friend."

During the early school years, groups are usually small and loosely organized, with changing membership and no formal structure. The prolonged cohesiveness characteristic of groups or cliques in later school years is not obvious. In general, girls' groups are less formalized than boys' are, and although there may be a mixture of both sexes in the early school years, the groups of later school years are composed predominantly of children of the same sex. Common interests are the basis around which the group is structured.

Peer-group identification and association are essential to a child's socialization. Poor relationships with peers and a lack of group identification can contribute to bullying. *Bullying* is the repetitive, persistent use of verbal or nonverbal behaviors by one or more peers to inflict physical or psychologic abuse (Olweus, 1997). Bullying occurs most frequently at school during unstructured times such as recess or lunch. Bullies may be from any ethnic, racial, or socioeconomic group. They are generally defiant toward adults, antisocial, and likely to break school rules. They have little anxiety, have strong self-esteem, and may come from homes in which physical punishment is used and parental involvement and warmth are lacking. Boys who bully tend to use physical force, whereas girls who bully may employ psychologic methods such as ostracism or rumors. Bullying by boys is more common than by girls. Children who are targeted for bullying often have characteristics different from the group norm (e.g., children who are short; who are obese; or who have facial deformities, attention-deficit/hyperactivity disorder, mental retardation, or other developmental disabilities) (Vessey, Carlson, & David, 2003). The long-term consequences of bullying are significant. Chronic bullies seem to continue their behaviors into adulthood, negatively influencing their ability to develop and maintain relationships. Victims of bullying often fear school and can develop school phobia or long-term problems of depression and low self-esteem (Muscari, 2002). School personnel play an important role in developing proactive strategies to deal with bullies and by promoting a safe environment where bullying is not tolerated (Cavendish & Salomone, 2001).

There are also dangers in peer-group attachments that are too strong. Peer pressures force some children to take risks or engage in behaviors that are against their better judgment. Peer-group activities that result in unlawful or criminal *gang violence* are increasing in the United States, and gang violence is an important factor contributing to the problem of school violence (Kettl, 2001).

Relationships with Families

Although the peer group is influential and necessary to normal child development, parents are the primary influence in shaping the child's personality, setting standards for behavior, and establishing value systems. Family values usually take precedence over peer value systems. Although children may reject parental values while testing the new values of the peer group, ultimately they retain and incorporate into their own value systems the parental values they have found to be of worth.

In the middle school years, children want to spend more time in the company of peers, and they often prefer peer-group activities to family activities. This can be very disturbing to parents. Children become intolerant and critical of parents and their ways when they deviate from those of the group. They discover that parents can be wrong, and they begin to question their knowledge and authority. Parents are no longer considered to be all-knowing or all-powerful.

Although increased independence is the goal of middle childhood, children are not ready to abandon parental control. They need and want restrictions placed on their behavior; and they are not prepared to cope with all the problems of their expanding environment. They feel more secure knowing that there is an authority figure to implement controls and restrictions. Children may complain loudly about restrictions and try to break down parental barriers, but they are uneasy if they succeed in doing so. They respect adults who prevent them from acting on every urge. Children view this behavior as an expression of love and concern for their welfare.

Children also need their parents as adults, not as pals. Sometimes parents, hurt at their children's rejection, attempt to maintain their love and gratitude by assuming the role of "pals." Children need the stable, secure strength provided by mature adults to whom they can turn during troubled relationships with peers or stressful changes in their world. With a secure base in a loving family, children are able to develop the self-confidence and maturity needed to break loose from the group and stand independently.

Play

Play takes on new dimensions that reflect a new stage of development in the school years. Play involves increased physical skill, intellectual ability, and fantasy. Children form groups and cliques and develop a sense of belonging to a team or club.

Rules and Rituals

The need for conformity in middle childhood is strongly manifested in the activities and games of school-age children. In the preschool years, children's games were either invented for them or played in the company of a friend or an adult. Now children begin to see the need for rules, and their games have fixed and unvarying rules that may be bizarre and extraordinarily rigid (especially those made up by the group). Conformity and ritual permeate their play; and are also evident in their behavior and language. Childhood is full of chants and taunts, such as "Eeeny, meeny, miney, mo," "Last one is a rotten egg," and "Step on a crack, break your mother's back." Children derive a sense of pleasure and power from such sayings, which have been handed down with few changes through generations.

Team Play

A more complex form of play that evolves from the need for peer interaction is the team game and sports. The rules of team games may require the presence of a referee, an umpire, or a person of authority so that the rules can be followed more accurately. Team play teaches children to modify or exchange personal goals for the goals of the group; it also teaches them that division of labor is an effective strategy for attaining a goal. Children learn about competition and the importance of winning—an attribute highly valued in the United States.

Team play can also contribute to children's social, intellectual, and skill growth. Children will work hard to develop the skills needed to become team members, to improve their contribution to the group, and to anticipate the consequences of their behavior for the group. Team play helps stimulate cognitive growth as children are called on to learn many complex rules, make judgments about those rules, plan strategies, and assess the strengths and weaknesses of members of their own team and members of the opposing team.

Quiet Games and Activities

Although play at this age is highly active, school-age children also enjoy quiet and solitary activities. The middle years are the time for collections, which constitute another ritual. Young school-age children's collections are an odd assortment of unrelated objects in messy, disorganized piles. Collections of later school years are more orderly, selective, and organized in scrapbooks, on shelves, or in boxes.

School-age children become fascinated with complex board, card, or computer games that they can play alone, with a best friend, or with a group. As in all games, adherence to the rules is fanatic. There is usually much discussion and argument, but any disagreements are easily resolved through reading the rules of the game.

The newly acquired skill of reading becomes increasingly satisfying as school-age children expand their knowledge of the world through books (Fig. 39-5). School-age children never tire of stories, and like preschool children, they love to have stories read aloud. Sewing, cooking, carpentry, gardening, and creative activities such as painting are other activities enjoyed. Many creative skills, such as music and art, as well as athletic skills, such as swimming, horseback riding, dancing, and skating, are learned during these years and continue to be enjoyed into adolescence and adulthood (Fig. 39-6).

Ego Mastery

Play affords children the means to acquire mastery over themselves, their environment, and others. Through play

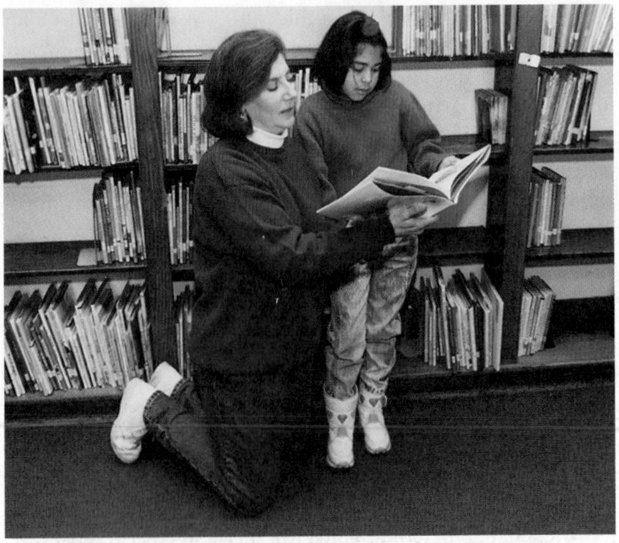

Fig. 39-5 Selecting a book with the assistance of an adult.

children can feel as big, as powerful, and as skillful as their imaginations will allow. They can also feel in control and attain vicarious mastery and power over whomever and whatever they choose. Schoolchildren still need the opportunity to use large muscles in exuberant outdoor play and the freedom to exert their newfound autonomy and initiative. They need space in which to exercise large muscles and to deal with tensions, frustrations, and hostility. Physical skills practiced and mastered in play help them to develop a feeling of personal competence, which contributes to a sense of accomplishment and provides status in their peer group.

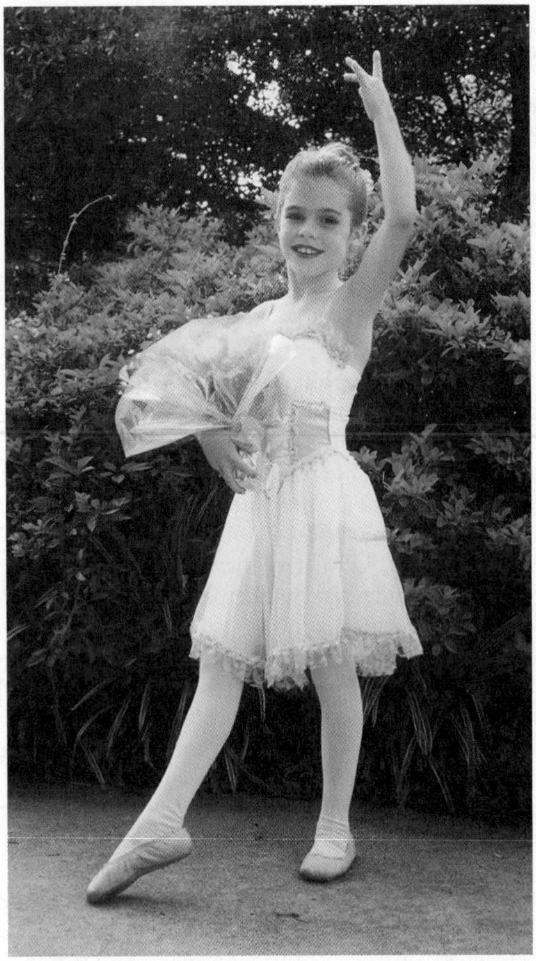

Fig. 39-6 School-age children take pride in learning new skills.

Developing a Self-Concept

The term *self-concept* refers to a conscious awareness of a variety of self-perceptions, such as one's physical characteristics, abilities, values, self-ideals and expectancy, and an idea of self in relation to others. It also includes one's body image, sexuality, and self-esteem. Although primary caregivers continue to exert influence on children's self-evaluation, the opinions of peers and teachers provide valuable input during middle childhood. With the emphasis on skill building and broadened social relationships, children are continually engaged in the process of self-evaluation.

Significant adults can often manage to unobtrusively manipulate the environment so that children experience success. Each small success increases a child's self-image. The more positive children feel about themselves, the more confident they will be in trying for success in the future. All children profit from feeling that they are in some way special to a significant adult. A positive self-concept makes children feel likable, worthwhile, and capable of significant contributions. These feelings lead to self-respect, self-confidence, and happiness. Negative feelings lead to self-doubt.

Developing a Body Image

School-age children have a relatively accurate and positive perception of their physical selves, but in general they like their physical selves less as they grow older. The head appears to be the most important part of the school-age child's perceived image of self, with hair and eye color the characteristics used most frequently to describe the physical self.

Body image is influenced, but not solely determined, by significant others. The number of significant others influencing one's perception of the physical self increases with age. Children are acutely aware of their own body, the bodies of their peers, and those of adults. They are also aware of deviations from the norm. It is important that children learn about bodily functions and that adults provide correct information.

Physical impairments, such as hearing or visual defects, ears that "stick out," or birthmarks, assume great importance. Increasing awareness of these differences, especially when accompanied by unkind comments and taunts from others, may cause a child to feel inferior and less desirable. This is especially true if the defect interferes with the child's ability to participate in games and activities. Table 39-1 summarizes the major developmental achievements of the school-age years.

Coping with Concerns Related to Normal Growth and Development

School Experience

The school serves as the agent for transmitting the values of the society to each succeeding generation of children. School is also the setting for relationships with peers. After

Table 39-1

Growth and Development during the School-Age Years

AGE (YEARS)	PHYSICAL AND MOTOR	MENTAL	ADAPTIVE	PERSONAL-SOCIAL
6	Height and weight gain continues slowly Weight: 16-23.6 kg (35½-58 pounds); height: 106.6-123.5 cm (42-48 inches) Central mandibular incisors erupt Loses first tooth Gradual increase in dexterity Active age; constant activity Often returns to finger feeding More aware of hand as a tool Likes to draw, print, color Vision reaches maturity	Develops concept of numbers Counts 13 pennies Knows whether it is morning or afternoon Defines common objects such as fork and chair in terms of their use Obeys triple commands in succession Knows right and left hands Says which is pretty and which is ugly of a series of drawings of faces Describes the objects in a picture rather than simply enumerating them Attends first grade	At table, uses knife to spread butter or jam on bread At play, cuts, folds, pastes paper toys; sews crudely if needle is threaded Takes bath without supervision; performs bedtime activities alone Reads from memory; enjoys oral spelling game Likes table games, checkers, simple card games Giggles a lot Sometimes steals money or attractive items Has difficulty owning up to misdeeds Tries out own abilities	Can share and cooperate better Has great need for children of own age Will cheat to win Often engages in rough play Often jealous of younger brother or sister Does what adults are seen doing May have occasional temper tantrums Is a boaster Is more independent, probably influence of school Has own way of doing things Increases socialization
7	Begins to grow at least 5 cm (2 inches) in height per year Weight: 17.7-30 kg (39-66½ pounds); height: 111.8-129.7 cm (44-51 inches) Maxillary central incisors and lateral mandibular incisors erupt More cautious in approaches to new performances Repeats performances to master them Jaw begins to expand to accommodate permanent teeth	Notices that certain parts are missing from pictures Can copy a diamond Repeats three numbers backward Develops concept of time; reads ordinary clock or watch correctly to nearest quarter hour; uses clock for practical purposes Attends second grade More mechanical in reading; often does not stop at the end of a sentence, skips words such as "it," "the," and "he"	Uses table knife for cutting meat; may need help with tough or difficult pieces Brushes and combs hair acceptably without help May steal Likes to help and have a choice Is less resistant and stubborn	Is becoming a real member of the family group Takes part in group play Boys prefer playing with boys; girls prefer playing with girls Spends a lot of time alone; does not require a lot of companionship
8-9	Continues to gain 5 cm (2 inches) in height per year Weight: 19.6-39.6 kg (43-87 pounds); height: 117-141.8 cm (46-56 inches) Lateral incisors (maxillary) and mandibular cuspids erupt Movement fluid; often graceful and poised Always on the go; jumps, chases, skips	Gives similarities and differences between two things from memory Counts backward from 20 to 1; understands concept of reversibility Repeats days of the week and months in order; knows the date Describes common objects in detail, not merely their use Makes change out of a quarter	Makes use of common tools such as hammer, saw, screwdriver Uses household and sewing utensils Helps with routine household tasks such as dusting, sweeping Assumes responsibility for share of household chores Looks after all of own needs at table	Is easy to get along with at home Likes the reward system Dramatizes Is more sociable Is better behaved Is interested in boy-girl relationships but will not admit it Goes about home and community freely, alone or with friends Likes to compete and play games

Continued

Table 39-1

Growth and Development during the School-Age Years—cont'd

AGE (YEARS)	PHYSICAL AND MOTOR	MENTAL	ADAPTIVE	PERSONAL-SOCIAL
8-9—cont'd	Increased smoothness and speed in fine motor control; uses cursive writing Dresses self completely Likely to overdo; hard to quiet down after recess More limber; bones grow faster than ligaments	Attends third and fourth grades Reads more; may plan to wake up early just to read Reads classic books, but also enjoys comics More aware of time; can be relied on to get to school on time Can grasp concepts of parts and whole (fractions) Understands concepts of space, cause and effect, nesting (puzzles), conservation (permanence of mass and volume) Classifies objects by more than one quality; has collections Produces simple paintings or drawings	Buys useful articles; exercises some choice in making purchases Runs useful errands Likes pictorial magazines Likes school; wants to answer all the questions Is afraid of failing a grade; is ashamed of bad grades Is more critical of self Takes music and sport lessons	Shows preference in friends and groups Plays mostly with groups of own sex but is beginning to mix Develops modesty Compares self with others Enjoys organizations, clubs, and group sports
10-12	**Boys:** Slow growth in height and rapid weight gain; may become obese in this period Weight: 24.3-58 kg (54-128 pounds); height: 127.5-162.3 cm (50-64 inches) Posture is more similar to an adult's; will overcome lordosis **Girls:** Pubescent changes may begin to appear; body lines soften and round out Remainder of teeth will erupt and tend toward full development (except wisdom teeth)	Writes brief stories Attends fifth to seventh grades Writes occasional short letters to friends or relatives on own initiative Uses telephone for practical purposes Responds to magazine, radio, or other advertising Reads for practical information or own enjoyment—stories or library books of adventure or romance, animal stories	Makes useful articles or does easy repair work Cooks or sews in small way Raises pets Washes and dries own hair Is responsible for a thorough job of cleaning hair, but may need reminding to do so Is sometimes left alone at home for an hour or so Is successful in looking after own needs or those of other children left in his or her care	Loves friends; talks about them constantly Chooses friends more selectively; may have a "best friend" Enjoys conversation Develops beginning interest in opposite sex Is more diplomatic Likes family; family really has meaning Likes mother and wants to please her in many ways Demonstrates affection Likes father, who is admired and may be idolized Respects parents

the family, schools are the second most important socializing agent in the lives of children.

Entrance into school causes a sharp break in the structure of the child's world. For many children it is their first experience in conforming to a group pattern imposed by an adult who is not a parent and who has responsibility for too many children to be constantly aware of each child as an individual. Children want to go to school and usually adapt to the new conditions with little difficulty. Successful adjustment is related to the physical and emotional maturity of the child and to the parent's readiness to accept the separation associated with school entrance. Unfortunately, some parents express their unconscious attempts to delay the child's maturity by clinging behavior, particularly with their youngest child.

By the time they enter school, most children have a fairly realistic concept of what school involves. They receive information regarding the role of a student from parents, siblings, playmates, and the media. In addition, most children have had some experience with day care, preschool, or kindergarten. Middle-class children have fewer adjustments to make and less to learn about expected behavior, because schools tend to reflect dominant middle-class customs and values. If the child has attended a preschool program, the focus of the preschool program also affects the child's adjustment. Some preschool programs provide custodial care only, whereas others emphasize emotional, social, and intellectual development.

Classmates have a significant impact on the socialization of children. School is the first time that most children become members of a large group of individuals their own age. Peer relationships become increasingly important and influential as children proceed through school. The specific influence exerted by the peer group depends on the background, interests, and abilities of the individual child.

Teachers

Children respond best to teachers who possess the characteristics of a warm, loving parent. Teachers in the early grades perform many of the activities formerly assumed by the parent, such as recognizing the child's personal needs (e.g., the need to go to the bathroom or a need for help with clothing) and helping to develop their social behavior (e.g., manners).

Teachers, like parents, are concerned about the psychologic and emotional welfare of the child. Although the functions of teachers and parents differ, both place constraints on behavior and both are in a position to enforce standards of conduct. However, the teacher's primary responsibility involves stimulating and guiding children's intellectual development, as opposed to providing for their physical welfare beyond the school setting.

Teachers serve as models that children try to emulate. Children seek their teacher's approval and avoid their disapproval. The teacher is a very significant person in the life of the early schoolchild, and hero worship of a teacher may extend into late childhood and preadolescence. Teachers who make supportive statements that reassure or commend children, use accepting and clarifying statements that help children refine ideas and feelings, and provide assistance that aids children with their own problem solving contribute to the development of a positive self-concept in the school-age child.

Parents

Parents share responsibility for helping children achieve their maximum potential. There are numerous ways that parents can supplement the school program (Home Care box). Cultivating responsibility is the goal of parental assistance. Being responsible for schoolwork helps children learn to keep promises, meet deadlines, and succeed at their jobs as adults. Responsible children may occasionally ask for help (e.g., with a spelling list), but usually they prefer to think through their work by themselves. Excessive pressure or lack of encouragement from parents may inhibit the development of these desirable traits.

Home Care

HELPING CHILDREN IN SCHOOL

General Guidelines

Be supportive—through companionship, share ideas and thoughts.
Be positive—every child should experience some success each day.
Share an interest in reading—use the library; discuss books they are reading.
Support and encourage activity rather than passivity.
Encourage originality—help children make their own projects from discarded articles or other available materials.
Foster the development of hobbies and collections.
Encourage children to wonder and reflect during free time.
Encourage family experiences and trips to places of interest.
Encourage questions—help children discover sources for information or places to explore and investigate.
Stimulate creative thinking and problem solving—help children try out new solutions to problems without fear of making mistakes.
Use rewards rather than punishment.

Specific Guidelines

Meet the teacher at the beginning of school and plan to visit the school to see what is taught and expected.
Send the child to school every day—teachers are concerned when parents make other plans for their children; it conveys the impression that school is unimportant.
Demonstrate an interest in what the child is learning.
Demonstrate an interest in content and growth more than in grades.
Make it clear to the child that schoolwork is between the child and the teacher; teacher and child should set goals for better school performance to allow the child to feel responsible for school successes and failures.
Take advantage of situations that support and reinforce school learning.
Share information with teachers that will help them understand the child better.
Communicate with the teacher if there appears to be a problem—do not wait for a scheduled conference.
Provide a quiet, well-lighted area for study that is safe from interruption; do not allow television or radio.
Avoid dictating a study time, but do enforce rules, such as no television until homework is done; accept the child's word that work is complete.
Help with homework should focus on explaining the question, not giving the answer.
Teach the child to break large tasks (e.g., a report) into smaller, manageable tasks spread over the allotted time rather than attempt the entire project the night before it is to be completed.
Limit home tutoring to special circumstances, such as when the teacher requests parental assistance after a child's prolonged absence.
Request special help for children with learning problems.
Support the school staff by showing respect for both the school system and the teacher, at least in the child's presence.

Latchkey Children

The term *latchkey children* is used to describe children in elementary school who are left to care for themselves before or after school without the supervision of an adult. The increasing numbers of single-parent families and working mothers, together with the lack of available child care, have created a stress-provoking situation for many school-age children. Some of these children may have a chronic illness as well.

Inadequate adult supervision after school leaves children at greater risk for injury and delinquent behavior. In some instances outside activities are curtailed and relationships with peers may be significantly diminished. Latchkey children may feel more lonely, isolated, and fearful than children who have someone to care for them. To cope with their fears and anxieties while alone, these children may devise strategies such as hiding, playing the television at loud volume, or using pets as a comfort.

Many communities and persons concerned about the welfare of latchkey children are trying to help these children and their parents deal with this potentially serious problem. Some communities and employers have implemented after-school programs or telephone "hotlines" that provide check-in and reassurance for children. Nurses should be aware of these community services and also encourage parents to teach self-help skills to these children.

Limit Setting and Discipline

Many factors influence the amount and manner of discipline and limit setting imposed on school-age children, including the psychosocial maturity of the parents, the childhood and childrearing experiences of the parents, the temperament of the children, the context of the children's misconduct, and the response of the children to rewards and punishments. When children develop an ability to see a situation from the point of view of another, they are also able to understand the effects of their reactions on others and themselves.

Disciplinary techniques should help children control their own behavior. Reasoning is an effective technique for middle school–age children. With advancing cognitive skills they are able to benefit from more complex disciplinary strategies. For example, withholding privileges, requiring compensation, imposing penalties, and contracting can be used with great success. Problem solving is the best approach to limit setting, and children themselves can be included in the process of determining appropriate disciplinary measures.

Dishonest Behavior

During middle childhood children may engage in what is considered to be antisocial behavior. Lying, stealing, and cheating may become manifest in previously well-behaved children. Such behaviors are disturbing and challenging to parents.

Lying can occur for a number of reasons. By the time children enter school, they still "tell stories," and often they exaggerate a story or situation as a means of impressing their family or friends. However, during middle childhood, children become able to distinguish between fact and fantasy. If children do not develop this characteristic, parents need to teach them what is real and what is make-believe.

Young children may lie to escape punishment or to get out of some difficulty even when their misbehavior is very evident. Older children may lie to meet expectations set by others to which they have been unable to measure up. However, most children know that lying and cheating are wrong, and they are very concerned when it is observed in their friends. They are quick to tell on others when they detect cheating.

Parents need to be reassured that all children lie sometimes and that sometimes they may have difficulty separating fantasy from reality. Parents should be helped to understand the importance of being truthful in their relationships with children.

Cheating is most common in young children 5 to 6 years of age. They find it difficult to lose at a game or contest, and so they cheat to win. They have not yet acquired the realization that this behavior is wrong, and they do it almost automatically. This behavior usually disappears as they mature. However, because children model observed behaviors, parents need to be aware of their own behavior. When parents set examples of honesty, children are more likely to conform to these standards.

As with other ethically related behavior, *stealing* is not an unexpected event in the younger child. Between 5 and 8 years of age, children's sense of property rights is limited, and they tend to take something simply because they are attracted to it or to take money for what it will buy. They are equally likely to give away something valuable that belongs to them. When young children are caught and punished, they are penitent—they "didn't mean to" and "promise never to do it again"—but it is quite likely that they will repeat the performance the following day. Often they not only steal but also lie about their behavior or attempt to justify it with excuses. It is seldom helpful to trap children into admission by asking directly if they committed the offense. Children do not take responsibility for these behaviors until the end of middle childhood.

Children steal for several reasons. Young children may lack a sense of property rights or attempt to acquire a specific object to bribe favors from other children. A strong desire to own a coveted item, or a desire for revenge (to "get back at someone," usually a parent for unfair treatment) are additional reasons for stealing. Older children may steal to supplement an inadequate allowance. However, stealing can be an indication that something is seriously wrong or lacking in the child's life. For example, children may steal to make up for love or another satisfaction that they feel is lacking. In most situations it is wise not to attempt to find a hidden or deep meaning to the stealing. An admonition, together with an appropriate and reasonable punishment, such as having the older child pay back the money or return the stolen items, usually takes care of most cases. Most children can be taught to respect the property rights of others with little difficulty despite numerous temptations and opportunities. If children's personal rights are respected, they are likely to respect the rights of others. Some children simply need more time to learn the rules regarding private property.

Stress and Fear

Children today experience significant amounts of stress, and for some children, this stress can cause long-term adjustment and health problems. Stress in childhood comes from a variety of sources, such as conflict within the family, interpersonal relationships, poverty, and chronic illness. The school environment itself may be a source of stress. Competing with classmates for grades and teacher recognition, test anxiety, and performance anxiety are common sources of school-related stress (Lau, 2002). When parents and teachers stress achievement and performance extensively, children experience emotional distress, and some children may actually develop school phobia (an exaggerated fear associated with attending school).

The increasing violence in society has also spilled over into the school setting. In the present information age, when tragedy is broadcast daily in the media, children come to school knowing more about the latest world events than any previous generation of children. In addition, today's children are often personally aware of violence in their families or communities. Many children know other children who have been killed, or children who have brought weapons to school. School-age children are also the victims of teasing, bullying, and physical abuse in the school environment (Nansel et al, 2003).

To help children cope with stress, parents, teachers, and health care providers must recognize signs that indicate a child is undergoing stress, promptly identify the source of the stress, and refer those children who need specialized treatment.

NURSE ALERT The nurse who observes the following signs of stress in a child should explore the situation further:

- Stomach pains or headache
- Sleep problems
- Bed-wetting
- Changes in eating habits
- Aggressive or stubborn behavior
- Reluctance to participate
- Regression to earlier behaviors (e.g., thumb-sucking) ■

Children 7 to 12 years of age are capable of identifying their own physiologic responses to stress with terms that have meaning to them. Words or phrases used by children to describe their body's reaction to stress include "tight muscles," "hot or red in the face," "tingling," "chills or goose bumps," "shakiness," "heart beating fast," "headache," and "stomachache" (Sharrer & Ryan-Wenger, 2002). Children should be taught to recognize these signs as indicators of stress and to use techniques to manage their stress. Parents can help children to problem solve and to develop a plan to cope with stress. When an effective strategy has been developed for one situation, parents can show the child how to transfer the coping strategy or technique to other situations. Age-appropriate chores are an excellent way to teach children to face problems and learn to solve them (Lau, 2002). As children accept responsibility for chores and accomplish specific tasks, they develop strength of character, a sense of personal competence, and a willingness to accept new challenges.

In addition to stress, school-age children experience a wide variety of fears, including fear of the dark, excessive worry about past behavior, self-consciousness, social withdrawal, and an excessive need for reassurance. These fears are considered normal for children at this age. During the middle school years, children become less fearful of body safety than they were as preschoolers, but they still fear being hurt, being kidnapped, or having to undergo surgery. They also fear death and are fascinated by all aspects of death and dying. The fears of noises, darkness, storms, and dogs lessen, but new fears related predominantly to school and family bother children during this time.

Nutrition

Although caloric needs are diminished in relation to body size during middle childhood, resources are being laid down at this time for the increased growth needs of adolescence. Parents, as well as children, need to be aware of the value of a balanced diet to promote growth, because children usually eat what their family members eat. The quality of the child's diet depends on the family's pattern of eating.

Likes and dislikes established at an early age continue in middle childhood, although preferences for single foods subside, and children develop a taste for a variety of foods. However, the easy availability of fast-food restaurants, the influence of the mass media, and the temptation of "junk food" make it easy for children to fill up on empty calories. Foods that do not promote growth, such as sugars, starches, and excess fats, are common in the school-age child's diet. The easy availability of high-calorie foods, combined with the tendency toward more sedentary activities, has also contributed to an epidemic of childhood obesity. This problem is discussed further in Chapter 40.

Parents are unable to monitor what their children eat when they are away from home. A parent may pack a lunch for school but be unaware of how much is eaten, traded, sold, or thrown away. Nutrition education can and should be integrated in the curriculum throughout the school years. The Food Guide Pyramid, elements of a wholesome diet, and how food products are grown, processed, and prepared are important aspects of nutrition education. However, the school cafeteria may not always provide healthy, nutritious meals. The school nurse can take an active role in nutrition education by working with teachers to plan and implement units on nutrition instruction and by working with parents and children to give nutritional guidance.

Sleep and Rest

The amount of sleep and rest required during middle childhood is highly individualized. The amount of sleep depends on the child's age, activity level, and state of health. The growth rate slows in the school-age years, and less energy is expended in growth than during preceding years.

School-age children usually do not require a nap, and they sleep approximately 9½ hours at night. Although fewer bedtime problems occur during these years, occasional difficulties are still associated with the bedtime ritual. Usually children 6 or 7 years old exhibit few problems, and encouraging quiet activity before bedtime, such as coloring or reading, facilitates the task of going to bed. However, most children in middle childhood must be reminded frequently to go to bed; 8- to 9-year-old children and 11-year-old children are particularly resistant. Often these children are unaware that they are tired. However, if they are allowed to remain up later than usual, they are fatigued the following day. Sometimes, bedtime resistance can be resolved by allowing a later bedtime as the child gets older. Twelve-year-old children usually offer no resistance at bedtime; some even retire early to read a book or listen to music.

Exercise and Activity

The improved capabilities and adaptability of the school-age child permit greater speed and effort in motor activities. Larger, stronger muscles permit longer and increasingly strenuous play without exhaustion. School-age children acquire the coordination, timing, and concentration that are required to participate in adult-type activities, but they may lack the strength, stamina, and control of the adolescent and adult. They can engage in a greater amount of physical activity during the school years. However, parents, teachers, and coaches must remember that although children this age are large and appear to be strong, they may not be ready for strenuous competitive athletics.

All growing children need regular exercise and opportunities for satisfying experiences that meet individual likes and dislikes. Appropriate activities during the school-age years include running, jumping rope, swimming, roller skating, in-line skating, ice skating, dancing, and bicycle riding. Positive reinforcement achieved by experiencing increasingly smooth, rhythmic, and efficient use of the body conditions the child toward regular physical activity. Exercise is essential for muscle development and tone, refinement of balance and coordination, increased strength and endurance, and stimulation of body functions and metabolic processes. Children need ample space to run, jump, skip, and climb and safe indoor and outdoor facilities and equipment. Most children have abundant energy and need little encouragement to engage in physical activity. Children with disabling conditions or those who hesitate to become involved in active play (such as obese children) require special assessment and help so that activities that appeal to them, and that are compatible with their limitations while also meeting their developmental needs, can be determined.

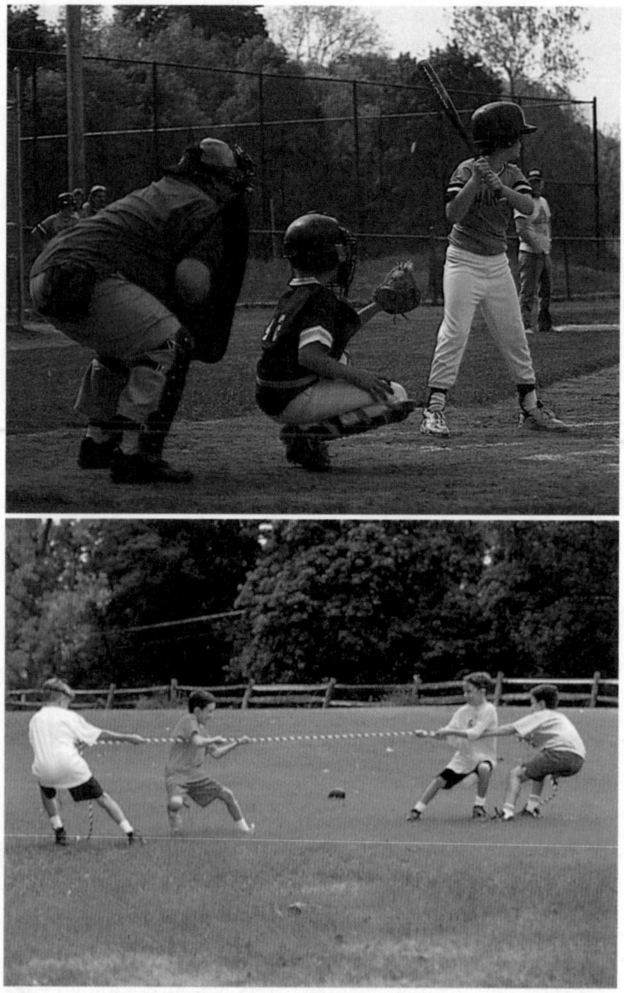

A

B

Fig. 39-7 The activities engaged in by school-age children vary according to interest and opportunity. **A,** Little League competitors. **B,** Playing tug-of-war.

Sports

Considerable controversy surrounds the trend toward early participation in competitive athletics and the amount and type of competitive sports that are appropriate for children in the elementary grades. The current view is that virtually every child is suited for some sport, and authorities do not discourage participation if children are matched to the type of sport appropriate to their abilities and to their physical and emotional constitution. School-age children enjoy competition. However, teachers and coaches must understand the physical limitations of school-age children and teach them the proper techniques and safety measures needed to avoid injuries. Even the most unskilled and noncompetitive child can participate in safe, appropriate activities (Fig. 39-7). Common activities for school-age children include baseball, soccer, gymnastics, and swimming. Equipment must be maintained in safe condition, and protective apparatus should be worn to prevent serious injury (see Traumatic Injury, Chapter 54).

During the school-age years, girls have the same basic body structure as boys and have a similar response to systematic exercise training. However, at puberty, boys become larger and have more muscle mass; therefore it is usually recommended that girls compete only against other girls at this age. Before puberty there is no essential difference in strength and size between girls and boys, making these precautions unnecessary.

Preadolescence is a time to teach fundamental motor skills; develop fitness in a practical, safe, and gradual manner; and promote healthy attitudes and values. Activities should include both practice sessions and unstructured play; the actual game or event should be managed in a manner that stresses mastery of the sport and enhancement of self-image rather than winning or pleasing others. All children should have an opportunity to participate, and special ceremonies should recognize all participants, not just individuals who excel in sports or athletics.

Acquisition of Skills

School-age children demonstrate increasing fine motor abilities and complex artistic skills. Handedness is well established by the beginning of the school years, and children make great strides in writing and drawing during this age period. It is a time of energetic and vibrant creative productivity. With the tools of language and reading, children create poems, stories, and plays. With more advanced fine motor skills, they are able to master an unlimited variety of handicrafts, such as ceramics, needlework, wood carving, and beadwork. They avidly pursue these skills in solitude, with a friend, or in programs offered through organized groups such as boys' or girls' clubs or special interest groups that use crafts or other activities as a means to occupy, entertain, and educate children.

School-age children are capable of assuming responsibility for their own needs, although their distaste for soap and water and "dress" clothes is legendary. School-age children can and want to assume their share of household tasks, which usually are related to the male and female roles that have been defined by their culture. Many children also assume responsibility for tasks outside the home, such as baby-sitting, mowing lawns, or paper routes.

Dental Health

The first permanent (secondary) teeth erupt at about 6 years of age, beginning with the 6-year molar, which erupts posterior to the deciduous molars. Other permanent teeth appear in approximately the same order as eruption of the primary teeth (see Teething, Chapter 36) and follow shedding of the deciduous teeth (Fig. 39-8). With the appearance of the second permanent (12-year) molar, most permanent teeth are present. Permanent dentition is more advanced in girls than in boys.

Because the permanent teeth erupt during the school-age years, dental hygiene and regular attention to dental caries are important parts of health supervision during this period (see Dental Health, Chapter 36). Correct brushing techniques should be taught or reinforced, and the role that fermentable carbohydrates play in production of dental caries should be emphasized. It is important to be alert to possible malocclusion problems that may result from irregular eruption of permanent teeth and that may impair function. Regular dental supervision and continued fluoride supplementation are essential parts of the health maintenance program.

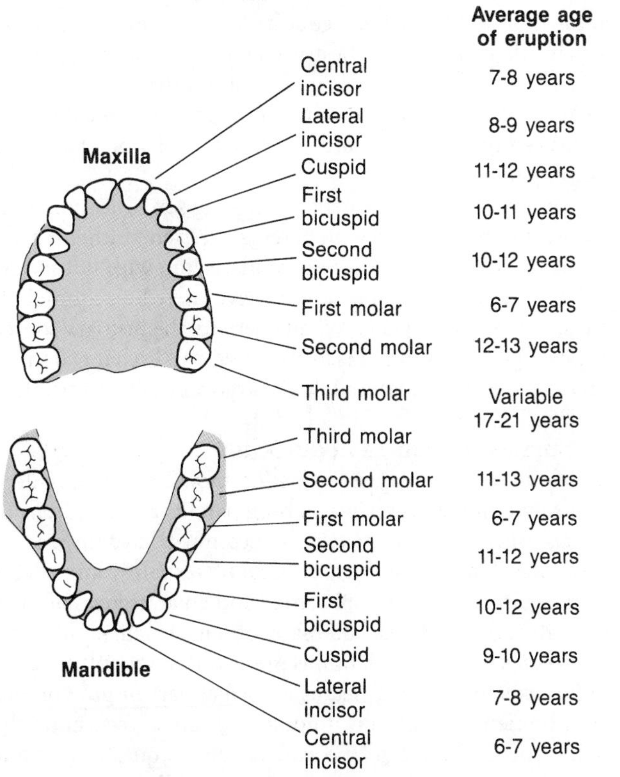

Fig. 39-8 Sequence of eruption of secondary teeth. (Data from McDonald RE, Avery DR: *Dentistry for the child and adolescent,* ed 6, St Louis, 1994, Mosby.)

The most effective means of preventing dental caries is proper oral hygiene. Children should be taught to perform their own dental care with the supervision and guidance of the parents. Parents should learn the correct brushing technique with their children, and they should monitor their child's efforts until the child can assume full responsibility.

Teeth should be brushed after meals, after snacks, and at bedtime. Children who brush their teeth frequently and become accustomed to the feel of a clean mouth at an early age usually maintain the habit throughout life. For the school-age child with mixed and permanent dentition, the best toothbrush is one with soft nylon bristles and an overall length of about 21 cm (6 inches). Several methods of brushing have been described and recommended for children, but there is no conclusive evidence that one method is superior to another. Thorough cleaning is more important than the specific technique used. The dentist should assess factors, such as the manipulative skills and special needs of the child, and suggest the most appropriate brushing technique and regimen. Flossing follows brushing. Parents should perform the flossing until children acquire the manual dexterity required for flossing (usually at about 8 or 9 years of age).

Dental Problems

Limited or inadequate dental care results in the most common dental problems (dental caries, malocclusion, and periodontal disease). Trauma, especially tooth evulsion, is another important dental problem. All of these conditions benefit from early intervention to prevent tooth loss.

Dental caries (cavities) is the principal oral problem in children and adolescents. Reducing the incidence and consequences of dental caries is extremely importance in childhood. If untreated, dental caries can result in total destruction of the involved teeth. The ages of greatest vulnerability are 4 to 8 years for the primary dentition and 12 to 18 years for the secondary, or permanent, dentition.

Dental caries is a multifactorial disease involving susceptible teeth, cariogenic microflora, and an appropriate oral environment. The incidence of lesions and the likelihood of progressive invasion vary considerably and depend on a number of factors being present in the right combination. Oral inspection is an integral part of the nursing assessment of the child. If there is any evidence of dental caries or other unhealthy dental state, the child should be referred for dental services. An alarming number of children do not receive regular dental supervision, and a significant number reach adulthood without dental examinations or treatment by a dentist.

Periodontal disease, an inflammatory and degenerative condition involving the gums and tissues supporting the teeth, often begins in childhood and accounts for a significant amount of tooth loss in adulthood. The more common periodontal problems are *gingivitis* (simple inflammation of the gums) and *periodontitis* (inflammation of the gums and loss of connective tissue and bone in the supporting structures of the teeth).

Gingivitis, the most prevalent peridontal disease, is a reversible inflammatory disease that begins in early childhood. It is most often associated with the buildup of plaque on the teeth. Changes take place in the plaque bacteria, in both the type and number of organisms, causing them to release destructive exotoxins, enzymes, and other noxious agents. These substances produce an inflammatory reaction in the gingival tissues, causing the gums to become red, edematous, tender, and subject to bleeding at the slightest irritation. Management is directed toward prevention by conscientious brushing and flossing, including the use of fluoride. The child should see the dentist at any signs of inflammation or irritation.

Malocclusion occurs when teeth of the upper and lower dental arches do not approximate in the proper relationships. As a result, the physiologic function of chewing is less effective and the cosmetic effect is displeasing. Teeth that are uneven, crowded, or overlapping are unable to meet their counterparts in the opposite jaw in the appropriate relationships and may be predisposed to disease in later years.

Orthodontic treatment is most successful when it is started in the later school-age or early teenage years, after the last primary teeth have been shed and before growth ceases. However, referral should be made as soon as malocclusion is evident, because some deformities can be corrected at an earlier age.

Dental injury may occur in childhood and includes fractures of varying degrees of severity, chipping, dislocation, or evulsion. All tooth injuries require prompt treatment by a competent dentist to prevent permanent displacement or loss. Delayed examination and diagnosis of tooth damage can result in infection or pulp involvement. Because it can affect the remaining teeth, replacement of the lost tooth is needed to maintain normal alignment and position of the other teeth.

Emergency

EVULSED TOOTH

Recover tooth.
Hold tooth by crown; do not touch root area.
If tooth is dirty, rinse it gently under running water or saline; be sure to insert stopper in sink or basin (to prevent tooth loss).
Insert tooth into socket.
Have child maintain tooth in place.
Transport child to dentist immediately.
Avoid sudden stops or sharp turns to prevent dislodging tooth.

If Reluctant to Reimplant Tooth:

Place evulsed tooth in suitable medium for transport:
- Cold milk
- Saliva—under child's or parent's tongue

If child is holding tooth in the mouth, avoid sudden stops to prevent swallowing tooth.
DO NOT FORGET TO TAKE TOOTH.

A tooth that is *evulsed* (exarticulated, or "knocked out") should be replanted by the child, parent, or nurse and stabilized as soon as possible so that the blood supply to the tooth can be reestablished and the tooth kept alive (Emergency box). If the tooth is replaced within 30 minutes, there is a 70% chance that it will become reattached and the roots will not resorb or the crown exfoliate. Evulsed primary teeth are usually not reimplanted.

As with all injuries to the mouth, an evulsed tooth causes a large amount of bleeding, which is frightening to children and their families. Therefore the nurse or anyone faced with dental trauma should be prepared to cope with the emotionality that accompanies tooth evulsion. A calm approach and gentle reassurance to the child are successful strategies to reduce anxiety.

Sex Education

Many children experience some form of sex play during or before preadolescence as a response to normal curiosity, not as a result of love or sexual urges. Children are experimentalists by nature, and sex play is incidental and transitory. Any adverse emotional consequences or guilt feelings depend on how the behavior is managed by the parents, if it is discovered, or whether children view their actions as wrong in the eyes of significant persons, particularly the parents.

The child's attitude toward sex is acquired indirectly at a very early age. Initial curiosity about differences in body structure between boys and girls and between children and adults arises in the preschool years. Middle childhood is an ideal time for formal sex education, and many authorities believe that the topic is best presented from a life-span approach. Information about sexual maturation and the process of reproduction helps minimize the child's uncertainty, embarrassment, and feelings of isolation that often accompany puberty.

An important component of ongoing sex education is effective communication with parents. If parents either repress the child's sexual curiosity or avoid dealing with it, the sexual information that the child receives may be acquired almost entirely from peers. When peers are the primary source of sexual information, it is transmitted and exchanged in secret conversation and contains a large amount of misinformation.

Nurse's Role in Sex Education

No matter where nurses practice, they can provide information on human sexuality to both parents and children. To discuss the topic adequately, nurses must have an understanding of the physiologic aspects of sexuality, knowledge of the cultural and societal values, and an awareness of their own attitudes, feelings, and biases about sexuality.

When sexual information is presented to school-age children, sex should be treated as a normal part of growth and development. Questions should be answered honestly, matter-of-factly, and to the same extent as questions about other topics. Answers should be at the child's level of understanding. There may be times when boys and girls should be taught content separately.

Children need help to differentiate sex and sexuality. Exercises on clarifying values, identifying role models, engaging in problem-solving skills, and practicing responsibility are important to prepare children for early adolescence and puberty. In addition, children need explanations of sexual information that is provided via the media or jokes. Information concerning human immunodeficiency virus (HIV) infection should be presented in simple, accurate terms and should focus on how HIV is transmitted.

Preadolescents need precise and concrete information that will allow them to answer questions such as "What if I start my period in the middle of class?" or "How can I keep people from telling I have an erection?" It is important to tell children what they want to know and what they can expect to happen as they become mature sexually.

During encounters with parents, nurses can be open and available for questions and discussion. They can set an example by the language they use in discussing body parts and their function and by the way in which they deal with problems that have emotional overtones, such as exploratory sex play and masturbation. Parents need help to understand normal behaviors and to view sexual curiosity in their children as a part of the developmental process. Assessing the parents' level of knowledge and understanding of sexuality provides cues to their need for supplemental information that will prepare them for the increasingly complex explanations they will need to provide as their children grow older.

School Health

Child health maintenance is ultimately the responsibility of the parents; however, the public schools and health departments in the United States have contributed to the improvement of child health by providing a healthful school environment, health services, and health education that emphasizes sound health practices. Most of these functions constitute major components of community health services and involve large amounts of public funds and large numbers of health professionals, including nurses.

A school health program is involved in ongoing health maintenance through assessment, screening, and referral activities. Routine health services provided by most schools include health appraisal, emergency care, safety education, communicable disease control, counseling, and follow-up care. Health education of schoolchildren is directed toward providing knowledge of health and influencing habits, attitudes, and conduct in relation to health and injury prevention.

Traditionally, school nurses were viewed as the person who detected diseases, applied bandages, and cared for students who were ill or injured. Although these functions remain important parts of the school nurse's job, the role of the school nurse has expanded considerably in recent years. Today, school nurses manage and coordinate all the care required by regular students and students with special health care needs. In many settings, school health services have enlarged into family health centers that meet the needs of not only school-age children, but also their families and the community. In these settings, school nurse practitioners provide health care that includes assessment of physical, psychomedical, psychoeducational, behavioral, and learning problems, as well as comprehensive well-child care (American Academy of Pediatrics [AAP], Committee on School Health, 2001).

The passage of Public Laws 94-142 and 99-457 mandated the integration of children with chronic illness or disability into regular classrooms. School nurses are responsible for the medical and nursing needs of these children while they are in the school setting. School nurses develop, implement, and evaluate individualized health care plans for these children. Unfortunately, not all schools have a school nurse, and the use of unlicensed assistive personnel (UAP) is increasing. In many schools, nurses are faced with the task of delegating to and supervising UAP (Delegation of school health services to unlicensed assistive personnel, 1995; Rhodes, 1997). Delegation and supervision of UAP requires skillful nursing assessment and professional judgment.

Injury Prevention

CASE STUDY: INJURY PREVENTION

Because school-age children have developed more refined muscular coordination and control and can apply their cognitive capacities to their behavior, the number of injuries in middle childhood is diminished compared with the number in early childhood. The most common cause of severe injury and death in school-age children is motor vehicle accidents—either as pedestrian or passenger. It is important that nurses continue to emphasize three automobile safety measures that have been found to reduce the severity of injuries: effective car restraint systems, door-lock mechanisms, and appropriate passenger-seating locations in the motor vehicle. The AAP, Committee on Injury and Poison Prevention (2002), advises health professionals and parents that the rear vehicle seat is the safest place for children of any age to ride in an automobile.

The school-age child's desire for riding bicycles increases the risk of injury on streets. Other serious injuries include accidents on skateboards, roller skates, in-line skates, skis, and other sports equipment. All-terrain vehicles (ATVs), popular with children under 16 years of age, are unstable, difficult to handle, and responsible for an increasing number of childhood injuries. The AAP, Committee on Injury and Poison Prevention (2000), views ATVs as a major health hazard for children and opposes their use by children less than 16 years of age.

Most injuries occur in or near the home or school. The most effective means of prevention is education of the child and family regarding the hazards of risk taking and the improper use of equipment. Safety helmets, protective eye and mouth shields, and protective padding are strongly recommended for children engaging in active sports, even though they may not be required equipment. Falls from bicycles, ATVs, and skating devices are the cause of a significant number of head injuries in school-age children. Because head injury is the major cause of bicycle-related fatalities, the most important aspect of bicycle safety is to encourage the rider to wear a protective helmet (Fig. 39-9) (AAP, Committee on Injury and Poison Prevention, 2001).

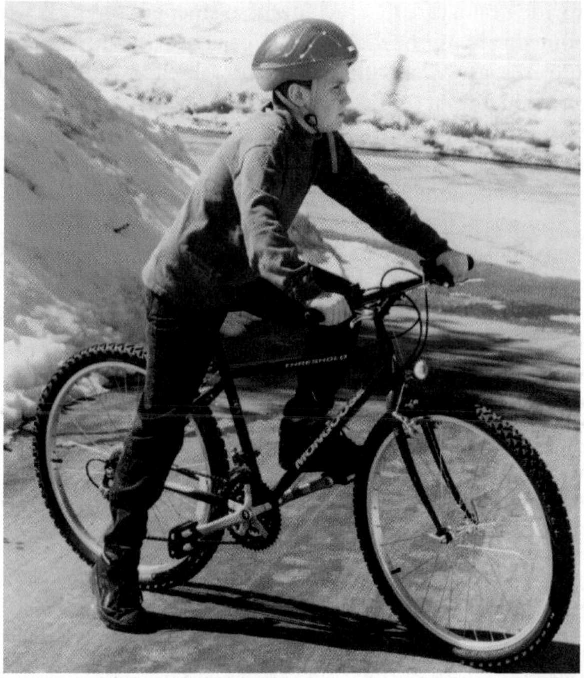

Fig. 39-9 The right-size bike is important; the child should be able to sit on the bike and place the balls of both feet on the ground. The foot should comfortably reach and manipulate the pedal in the down position. Wearing a protective helmet is mandatory. The helmet should be positioned on the head so that it sits low on the forehead and parallel to the ground when the head is held upright. It should not rock back and forth or shift from side to side. The strap should be fastened securely under the chin.

Physically active school-age children are also highly susceptible to cuts and abrasions, and the incidence of childhood fractures, strains, and sprains is high. Trampoline injuries are highest in children ages 5 through 14 years and account for numerous fractures, sprains, and head injuries. The AAP, Committee on Injury and Poison Prevention and Committee on Sports Medicine and Fitness (1999), recommends against the use of trampolines in the home environment, routine physical education classes, or outdoor playgrounds. Injuries of a serious nature are discussed elsewhere in this book—burns (Chapter 53), eye trauma (Chapter 42), near-drowning (Chapter 51), and head injuries (Chapter 51). The prevalence of injuries depends on the dangers present in the environment, the protection offered by adults, and the behavior patterns of the children. Table 39-2 lists characteristics of school-age children that make them prone to injury and suggestions for injury prevention. Home Care boxes provide guidelines for bicycle, skateboard, and in-line skate safety and guidance during the school years.

Home Care

BICYCLE SAFETY

Always wear a properly fitted bicycle helmet that is approved by the U.S. Consumer Product Safety Commission (CPSC); encourage parents to look for the CPSC approval sticker on the inside liner of the helmet.
Replace a helmet every 5 years or sooner if manufacturer recommends it. **Never use a damaged or outgrown helmet.**
Ride bicycles with traffic and away from parked cars.
Ride single file.
Walk bicycles through busy intersections only at crosswalks.
Give hand signals well in advance of turning or stopping.
Keep as close to the curb as practical.
Watch for drain grates, potholes, soft shoulders, and loose dirt or gravel.
Keep both hands on handlebars, except with signaling.
Never ride double on a bicycle.
Do not carry packages that interfere with vision or control; do not drag objects behind bike.
Watch for and yield to pedestrians.
Watch for cars backing up or pulling out of driveways; be especially careful at intersections.
Look left, right, and then left again before turning into traffic or roadway.
Never hitch a ride on a truck or other vehicle.
Learn rules of the road and respect for traffic officers.
Obey all local ordinances.
Wear shoes that fit securely while riding.
Wear light colors at night and attach fluorescent material to clothing and bicycle.
Be certain the bicycle is the correct size for rider.
Equip bicycle with proper lights and reflectors.
Have bicycle inspected to ensure good mechanical condition.
Children riding as passengers must wear appropriate-size helmets in specially designed protective seats.

Modified from American Academy of Pediatrics, Committee on Injury and Poison Prevention: Bicycle helmets, *Pediatrics* 108(4):1030-1032, 2001.

Home Care

SKATEBOARD AND IN-LINE SKATE SAFETY

Children younger than 5 years of age should not use skateboards or in-line skates. They are not developmentally prepared to protect themselves from injury.
Children who ride skateboards or in-line skates should wear helmets and other protective equipment, especially on knees, wrists, and elbows, to prevent injury.
Skateboards and in-line skates should never be used near traffic. Their use should be prohibited on streets and highways. Activities that bring skateboards together (e.g., "catching a ride") are especially dangerous.
Some types of use, such as riding homemade ramps on hard surfaces, may be particularly hazardous.

Modified from American Academy of Pediatrics, Committee on Injury and Poison Prevention: Skateboard injuries, *Pediatrics* 95(4):611-612, 1995.

Anticipatory Guidance–Care of Families

Parents of the school-age child must share their child's time with the increasingly important peer group. Experiences with the peer group prepare school-age children for the broader world of relationships and increased independence from their parents. Parents must learn to provide support as unobtrusively as possible without feeling rejected, hurt, or angry. The nurse can help parents of the school-age child by providing anticipatory guidance and reassurance throughout this period (Home Care box).

Table 39-2

Injury Prevention during the School-Age Years

DEVELOPMENTAL ABILITIES RELATED TO RISK OF INJURY	INJURY PREVENTION
Is increasingly involved in activities away from home Is excited by speed and motion Is easily distracted by environment Can be reasoned with	**Motor vehicle accidents** Educate child regarding proper use of seat belts while a passenger in a vehicle Maintain discipline while a passenger in a vehicle (e.g., keep arms inside, do not lean against doors or interfere with driver) Remind parents and children that no one should ride in the bed of a pickup truck Emphasize safe pedestrian behavior Insist on wearing safety apparel (e.g., helmet) when applicable, such as riding bicycle, motorcycle, moped, or all-terrain vehicle (see Home Care box, p. 1168)
Is apt to overdo May work hard to perfect a skill Has cautious, but not fearful, gross motor actions Likes swimming	**Drowning** Teach child to swim Teach basic rules of water safety Select safe and supervised places to swim Check sufficient water depth for diving Swim with a companion Use an approved flotation device in water or boat Advocate for legislation requiring fencing around pools Learn cardiopulmonary resuscitation (CPR)
Has increasing independence Is adventuresome Enjoys trying new things	**Burns** Make sure smoke detectors are in homes Set water heaters to 48.9° C (120° F) to avoid scald burns Instruct child in behavior in areas involving contact with potential burn hazards (e.g., gasoline, matches, bonfires or barbecues, lighter fluid, firecrackers, cigarette lighters, cooking utensils, chemistry sets); avoid climbing or flying kite around high-tension wires Instruct child in proper behavior in the event of fire (e.g., fire drills at home and school) Teach child safe cooking (use low heat; avoid any frying; be careful of steam burns, scalds, or exploding foods, especially from microwaving)
Adheres to group rules May be easily influenced by peers Has strong allegiance to friends	**Poisoning** Educate child regarding hazards of taking nonprescription drugs and chemicals, including aspirin and alcohol Teach child to say "no" if offered illegal or dangerous drugs or alcohol Keep potentially dangerous products in properly labeled receptacles, preferably out of reach
Has increased physical skills Needs strenuous physical activity Is interested in acquiring new skills and perfecting attained skills Is daring and adventurous, especially with peers Frequently plays in hazardous places Confidence often exceeds physical capacity Desires group loyalty and has strong need for friends' approval Attempts hazardous feats Accompanies friends to potentially hazardous facilities Delights in physical activity Is likely to overdo Growth in height exceeds muscular growth and coordination	**Bodily damage** Help provide facilities for supervised activities Encourage playing in safe places Keep firearms safely locked up except during adult supervision Teach proper care of, use of, and respect for devices with potential danger (e.g., power tools, firecrackers) Teach children not to tease or surprise dogs, invade their territory, take dogs' toys, or interfere with dogs' feeding Stress eye, ear, or mouth protection when using potentially hazardous objects or devices or when engaged in potentially hazardous sports Do not permit use of trampolines except as part of supervised training Teach safety regarding use of corrective devices (glasses); if child wears contact lenses, monitor duration of wear to prevent corneal damage Stress careful selection, use, and maintenance of sports and recreation equipment, such as skateboards and in-line skates (see Home Care box, p. 1168) Emphasize proper conditioning, safe practices, and use of safety equipment for sports or recreational activities Caution against engaging in hazardous sports, such as those involving trampolines Use safety glass and decals on large glassed areas, such as sliding glass doors Use window guards to prevent falls Teach name, address, and phone number and emphasize that child should ask for help from appropriate people (e.g., cashier, security guard, police) if lost; have identification on child (e.g., sewn in clothes, inside shoe) Teach stranger safety: • Avoid personalized clothing in public places • Caution child to never go with a stranger • Have child tell parents if anyone makes child feel uncomfortable in any way • Always listen to child's concerns regarding others' behavior • Teach child to say "no" when confronted with uncomfortable situations.

Home Care

GUIDANCE DURING SCHOOL YEARS

Age 6 Years

Prepare parents to expect strong food preferences and frequent refusal of specific food items.
Prepare parents to expect increasingly ravenous appetite.
Prepare parents for emotionality as child experiences erratic mood changes.
Help parents anticipate continued susceptibility to illness.
Teach injury prevention and safety, especially bicycle safety.
Encourage parents to respect child's need for privacy and to provide a separate bedroom for child, if possible.
Prepare parents for child's increasing interests outside the home.
Help parents understand the need to encourage child's interactions with peers.

Ages 7 to 10 Years

Prepare parents to expect improvement in health with fewer illnesses, but warn them that allergies may increase or become apparent.
Prepare parents to expect an increase in minor injuries.
Emphasize caution in selecting and maintaining sports equipment and reemphasize safety.
Prepare parents to expect increased involvement with peers and interest in activities outside the home.
Emphasize the need to encourage independence while maintaining limit setting and discipline.
Prepare mothers to expect more demands at 8 years.
Prepare fathers to expect increasing admiration at 10 years; encourage father-child activities.
Prepare parents for prepubescent changes in girls.

Ages 11 to 12 Years

Help parents prepare child for body changes of pubescence.
Prepare parents to expect a growth spurt in girls.
Make certain child's sex education is adequate with accurate information.
Prepare parents to expect energetic but stormy behavior at 11 years, to become more even-tempered at 12 years.
Encourage parents to support child's desire to "grow up" but to allow regressive behavior when needed.
Prepare parents to expect an increase in masturbation.
Instruct parents that the amount of rest the child needs may increase.
Help parents educate child regarding experimentation with potentially harmful activities.

Health Guidance

Help parents understand the importance of regular health and dental care for the child.
Encourage parents to teach and model sound health practices, including diet, rest, activity, and exercise.
Stress the need to encourage children to engage in appropriate physical activities.
Emphasize providing a safe physical and emotional environment.
Encourage parents to teach and model safety practices.

Special Health Problems

HEALTH PROBLEMS RELATED TO SPORTS PARTICIPATION

Every sport has the potential for injury to the participant—whether the youngster engages in serious competition or participates for enjoyment. Serious injury occurs most often during rough contact sports or to persons who are not physically prepared for the activity. Injuries also occur to children or adolescents when their body is not suited to the sport, when their muscles and body systems (respiratory and cardiovascular) are not conditioned to endure physical stress, or when they lack the insight and judgment to recognize that an activity exceeds their physical abilities. More injuries occur during recreational sports participation than during organized athletic competition.

The environment and the sports or recreational equipment can also present risks (Fig. 39-10). Children who participate in physical activity or sports do so in many different environments: indoors and outdoors, on floors, on the ground and snow, on or beneath water surfaces, and sometimes in free air space. Most of these activities also involve equipment.

Acute overload injuries are those that occur suddenly during an activity and produce immediate symptoms. A blow or overstretching, twisting, or sudden stress to tissues can cause these injuries. For descriptions and management of traumatic injuries, see Chapter 54.

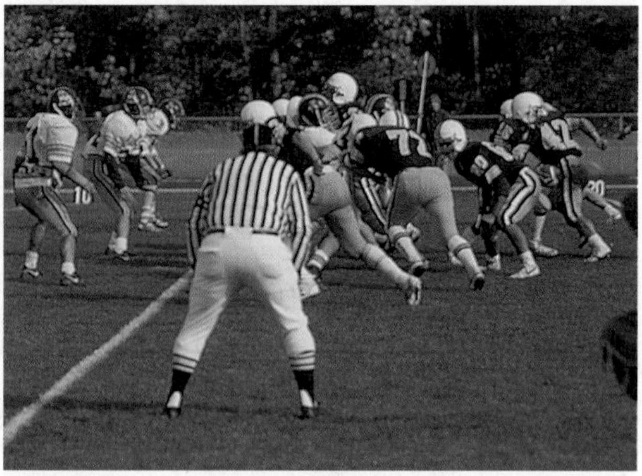

Fig. 39-10 Football is an example of a strenuous collision sport.

Overuse Syndromes

To excel in sports, the young athlete is forced to train longer, harder, and earlier in life than previously. The rewards are an increased level of fitness, better performances, faster times, and the satisfaction of attaining a personal goal. However, the risk of overuse injury is always present and is related to several factors: training errors, muscle-tendon imbalance, anatomic malalignment, incorrect footwear or playing surface, an associated disease state, and growth.

A common feature in overuse injuries is the *repetitive microtrauma* that occurs to a particular anatomic structure when the same movements are performed over a long period of time. The result is inflammation of the involved structure with complaints of chronic pain, tenderness, swelling, and disability. Examples of overuse syndromes include "Little League elbow" (tendinitis and osteochondritis from repetitive throwing), "tennis elbow" (lateral epicondylitis from repetitive elbow strain), and Osgood-Schlatter disease (traction apophysitis of the tibial tubercle).

Stress Fractures

Stress fractures occur as a result of repeated muscle contraction and are seen most often in repetitive weight-bearing sports such as running, gymnastics, and basketball. They occur less often in swimmers. The most common symptoms are a sharp, persistent, progressive pain or a deep, persistent, dull ache located over the bone. Sometimes there is pain on impact (heel strike), but the most important clinical sign is pain over the involved bony surface. Diagnosis is established on the basis of clinical observation, but occasionally a bone scan is performed.

Therapeutic Management

Inflammation is common in all overuse syndromes, and management is directed toward rest or alteration of activities, physical therapy, and medication. Rest is the primary therapy and is usually interpreted as reduced activity and the use of alternative exercise—*not* bed rest or immobilization with casting. The primary purpose is to alleviate the repetitive stress that initiated the symptoms. It is important to keep the youngster mobile, and training can be continued. Alternative exercise that maintains conditioning without aggravating the injury is selected. For example, pool running (treading water in the deep end of a pool) is an excellent alternative to running. Pool running uses the same movements as running without weight bearing. Other therapies include cryotherapy; cold whirlpools; and sometimes taping, bracing, splinting, or other orthoses. Treatment is specific to the injury. Nonsteroidal antiinflammatory medications are prescribed to reduce pain and inflammation. Topical medications are of questionable value.

Nurse's Role in Sports for Children and Adolescents

Nurses are often involved in sports activities in the areas of preparation and evaluation for activities, prevention of injury, treatment of injuries, and rehabilitation after injury. Selecting an appropriate sport for both recreation and competition is a joint effort of the youngster, parents, and health professionals. The best approach to counseling children and parents regarding sports participation is to encourage activities that are most likely to provide pleasure and physical benefits throughout childhood and into adulthood. Exposure to a variety of activities is better for young children than limiting them to one sport. Parents should be cautioned against overcommitting children to sports activities so that they have time for other activities.

When children sustain athletic injuries, nurses are often responsible for instructions regarding care. Instructions (e.g., schedule for appointments, application of ice, and any restrictions in activity) should be clear and accompanied by written directions. The importance of taking medications as prescribed is emphasized, especially if medications are needed for an extended period of time and if adherence is an issue. Medications given an hour before practice or competition may be advantageous to children continuing their activities.

Prevention of sports injuries is the most important aspect of athletic programs. Children should be suited to the activity; the environment and the equipment must be safe. Children should be prepared for the sport, especially if it requires strenuous or continuous physical exertion. Nurses, coaches, and athletic trainers must collaborate to ensure that safety measures are implemented. Stretching exercises, warm-up and cool-down activities, and appropriate training are requirements for safe participation. Protective measures such as pads, taping, and wrapping are also important to prevent injury. Finally, nurses must be aware of environmental safety risks.

ALTERED GROWTH AND MATURATION

The absence of physical or sexual maturation at a time when other children are experiencing positive evidence of sexual development and its associated spurt in growth and physical strength is an important concern to both the parents and their affected child. Fortunately, in most instances the delay in development is a simple physiologic or *constitutional delay* that represents one end of the normal genetically influenced variation of pubertal growth. These children will go through a delayed but normal puberty and finally catch up, in their late teens, with their more rapidly developing agemates. Less benign causes of delayed development may be the result of endocrine disorders or chromosomal abnormalities. Delayed development can also be a result of chronic diseases (such as malabsorption or chronic asthma) that are serious enough to retard development or a result of environmental factors (such as stress or poor nutrition).

The rate of maturation is important during the school years, but at puberty it assumes gigantic proportions to both teens and their parents. Girls or boys who lag behind their peers in physical maturation are painfully aware of their difference in growth. Adolescent girls with delayed maturation feel out of place among companions whose hips and breasts are developing, feel cheated if they have not yet menstruated, and feel left out when their friends giggle and talk about boys. Adolescent boys with delayed maturation feel weak and small compared to their more muscular companions, with whom they can no longer compete. Slow-maturing youngsters need support and reassurance that they are not abnormal and that they will develop the physical characteristics they desire.

Serial measurements of growth are plotted periodically on standard growth charts to determine the pattern of growth and to compare the individual child with the norms for his or her age group. When children are in the extremes of height ranges, it is important to compare their height with that of their parents and siblings.

Tall or Short Stature

Tall Stature

Despite the fact that the average height of both boys and girls is steadily increasing, there is a small group of children who, because of some organic disorder or a familial tendency, are excessively tall when compared with their peers. To boys, this may be a source of pride; to girls, it may cause intense anxiety and be a severe social handicap.

When the rate of height change before puberty suggests the probability of excessive adult height, treatment with hormones may be considered, although there is considerable controversy regarding the use of hormones for this purpose. The use of estrogens is effective in controlling height when therapy is initiated before menarche and before the end of the adolescent growth spurt that normally precedes menarche. The selection of children for hormonal therapy is made on the basis of a careful evaluation of physical, psychologic, and social factors.

Short Stature

Short stature is a nonspecific finding that may be the first manifestation of a serious disorder, or it may be of no consequence medically. On a worldwide scale, the most common cause of short stature or delayed development is inadequate nutrition. The major physical disorders that produce delayed development are chronic diseases, endocrine dysfunction, and syndromes of primary gonadal failure.

Chronic diseases can interfere with growth, but unless the illness is unduly prolonged, catch-up growth occurs. Diseases and disorders that cause some degree of growth delay include asthma, cystic fibrosis, gastrointestinal diseases (such as parasitic infections), malabsorption syndromes, cardiac anomalies, and chronic renal disturbances. The duration of the illness is more significant than the intensity in terms of the effect on growth, although the precise length of time necessary to affect growth permanently has not been determined.

Skeletal disorders that affect growth in stature are those described as dwarfism. Most disorders are caused by congenital defects and disorders, such as achondroplasia, and by inborn errors of metabolism, such as Hurler syndrome or Hunter syndrome.

Psychosocial, or *deprivation, dwarfism* is a stress-induced growth failure. It is defined as growth retardation in children over 2 years of age that is caused by environmental (emotional) stress and is associated with a marked delay in physical growth, delayed developmental skills, and immature behavior. When these children are removed from the deprived environment, their growth proceeds at a normal or increased rate. (See also Failure to Thrive, Chapter 36, and Child Maltreatment, Chapter 38.)

Management involves continued medical observation, attention to general health and nutrition, and psychologic support. When growth delay is accompanied by poor self-esteem, many authorities recommend hormonal therapy. Testosterone in carefully regulated doses is effective in some cases. Growth hormone is capable of increasing height and is used to treat growth hormone deficiency (see Hypopituitarism, Chapter 52). Its use with children who have constitutional delay is highly controversial.

Nursing Care Management

Deviation from the normal course of puberty is a significant concern for affected adolescents. For some teens, this concern assumes monumental proportions. Most cases of delayed development are caused by simple constitutional delay of puberty, and the child can be assured that normal development will eventually take place.

One difficulty related to a size that is incongruent with chronologic and mental age is the manner in which others relate to the child. People often respond to children with short stature as though they are younger than their age. Consequently, these children may react with babyish or juvenile behavior, thus establishing a circular pattern of behavior and response. Conversely, children who are tall or physically advanced for their age are frequently treated as though they are more advanced than their years. They are often considered to be retarded or immature when they perform according to the normal behavioral expectations for their age.

Listening to distressed adolescents and conveying interest and concern are important interventions for these children and adolescents. Counseling and therapy are individualized for each youth. Encouraging these children to focus on the positive aspects of their bodies and personalities and to adopt sound health practices and practice good grooming fosters a more positive self-image.

Sex Chromosome Abnormalities

Most sex chromosome abnormalities are caused by an alteration in sex chromosome number (Table 39-3). The majority of these conditions are due to nondisjunction. An alteration in the number of sex chromosomes usually does not produce the profound defects that are associated with the autosomal trisomies. Intelligence may be normal or low normal or the child may have some learning disabilities. Moderate or severe mental retardation is less common.

Turner Syndrome

Turner syndrome is caused by absence of one of the X chromosomes. Most girls who have this disorder have one X chromosome missing from all cells (45,X). This disorder is often recognized at birth if the newborn has a webbed neck, low posterior hairline, widely spaced nipples, and edema of the hands and feet. It can also be diagnosed at puberty because of three features: short stature, sexual infantilism, and amenorrhea. Girls with Turner syndrome are generally infertile. They may also have difficulty with peer relationships and understanding social cues. They frequently exhibit behavioral problems, especially in relation to their immature, socially isolated behavior. Diagnosis is confirmed on the basis of a negative sex chromatin test.

Critical Thinking Exercise: Turner Syndrome

Therapy is individualized for these girls and consists primarily of hormone treatment and psychologic counseling for both the child and the parents. Linear growth can be increased by the administration of growth hormone if therapy is begun early. Estrogen therapy is initiated during the usual time for puberty to promote the development of secondary sex characteristics. Responses to estrogen therapy vary from girl to girl, but gradual feminization is accomplished to some degree in most individuals.

Klinefelter Syndrome

Klinefelter syndrome, the most common of all sex chromosome abnormalities, is caused by the presence of one or more additional X chromosomes. Most males with this syndrome have a chromosome complement of 47,XXY. The disorder is seldom seen before puberty, at which time varying degrees of failure of adolescent virilization occur. Some males are not diagnosed until they appear for evaluation for

Table 39-3

Common Sex Chromosome Abnormalities

SYNDROME	CHROMOSOMAL NOMENCLATURE	PHENOTYPE	INCIDENCE (LIVE BIRTHS)	CLINICAL MANIFESTATIONS
Turner	45,X or 45XO	Female	1:2500 female births*	Short stature; webbed neck; low posterior hairline; shield-shaped chest with widely spaced nipples; sterile; no development of secondary sex characteristics
Triple X, or superfemale	47,XXX (can also be 48,XXXX or 49,XXXXX)	Female	1:850-1250 female births	Normal female characteristics; usually tall; variable mental capacity and behavior; at risk for impaired language, learning difficulties; fertile
XYY male	47,XYY (can also be 48,XYYY or mosaic)	Male	1:900 male births*	Usually normal sexual development; tendency to be tall with long head; poor coordination; may demonstrate aberrant behavior
Klinefelter	47,XXY (48,XXYY, 48,XXXY, 49,XXXXY, and so on, mosaics)	Male	1:850 male births*	Tall with long legs; hypogenitalism; sterile; male secondary sex characteristics may be deficient; may demonstrate aberrant behavior; learning disabled; possible gynecomastia

*Data from Nora JJ, Fraser FC: *Medical genetics: principles and practice,* ed 3, Philadelphia, 1989, Lea & Febiger.

infertility. All have absence of sperm in the semen (azoospermia), small testes, and defective development of secondary sex characteristics. In 80% of these boys there is a chromatin-positive buccal smear, and the extra chromosome is apparent on chromosome analysis.

Cognitive impairment is a frequent clinical finding and appears to be related to the number of X chromosomes. Boys may also have gross motor skill difficulties, a developmental language delay, poor verbal skills, reduced auditory memory, shyness, passivity, behavioral problems, and school difficulties. Therapy is directed toward enhancing the masculine characteristics through administration of testosterone.

Nursing Care Management

The nursing care of children with Turner syndrome or Klinefelter syndrome is primarily supportive. Nurses assist in diagnosis, explain tests and therapies, and provide support and encouragement to the child and the family. Because both disorders render the individual unable to reproduce, psychologic counseling is an important aspect of care. Marriage and sexual relationships are possible, but alternative reproductive options, such as artificial insemination and adoption, should be discussed.

DISORDERS WITH BEHAVIORAL COMPONENTS

Attention-Deficit/Hyperactivity Disorder and Learning Disability

evolve CASE STUDY: ATTENTION DEFICIT/HYPERACTIVITY DISORDER

Attention-deficit/hyperactivity disorder (ADHD) refers to developmentally inappropriate degrees of inattention, impulsiveness, and hyperactivity. To be diagnosed as ADHD, the symptoms must have been present before age 7 years and must be present in at least two settings. In addition, the persistence of developmentally inappropriate and marked inattention must not be a symptom of another disorder (American Psychiatric Association, 2000). A *learning disability (LD)* refers to a heterogeneous group of disorders manifested by significant difficulties in the acquisition and use of listening, speaking, reading, writing, reasoning, or mathematic skills.

ADHD and LDs affect every aspect of the child's life but are most obvious in the classroom. Early identification of affected children is important because the characteristics of these disorders significantly interfere with the normal course of emotional and psychologic development. Many children develop maladaptive behavior patterns that impede psychosocial adjustment while they try to cope with cognitive dysfunction. Their behavior evokes negative responses from others, and repeated exposure to negative feedback adversely affects their self-concept. The characteristics of ADHD affect the child's written and adaptive skills, social status, and self-esteem (Myers, Eisenhauer, & Ryan, 2003).

Diagnostic Evaluation

The behaviors exhibited by the child with ADHD are not unusual aspects of behavior. The difference lies in the quality of motor activity and developmentally inappropriate inattention, impulsivity, and hyperactivity that the child displays. The manifestations may be numerous or few, mild or severe, and will vary with the developmental level of the child. Any given child will not have every symptom of the condition. The basic characteristics of ADHD are outlined in Box 39-1.

A comprehensive battery of tests is needed to confirm a learning disability. These include intelligence tests (many children have normal or above average intelligence quotients [IQs]); hand-eye coordination tests; and measurements of auditory and visual perception, comprehension, and memory. Often there is a wide gap between verbal and performance scores on IQ tests.

Therapeutic Management

Management of the child with ADHD usually involves multiple approaches that include family education and counseling, medication, proper classroom placement, envi-

BOX 39-1

Diagnostic Criteria for Attention-Deficit/Hyperactivity Disorder

A. Either (1) or (2):
  (1) Six (or more) of the following symptoms of *inattention* have persisted for at least 6 months to a degree that is maladaptive and inconsistent with developmental level:
  Inattention
    (a) Often fails to give close attention to details or makes mistakes in schoolwork, work, or other activities
    (b) Often has difficulty sustaining attention in tasks or play activities
    (c) Often does not seem to listen when spoken to directly
    (d) Often does not follow through on instructions and fails to finish schoolwork, chores, or duties in the workplace (not because of oppositional behavior or failure to understand instructions)
    (e) Often has difficulty organizing tasks and activities
    (f) Often avoids, dislikes, or is reluctant to engage in tasks that require sustained mental effort (such as schoolwork or homework)
    (g) Often loses things necessary for tasks or activities (e.g., toys, school assignments, pencils, books, or tools)
    (h) Is often easily distracted by extraneous stimuli
    (i) Is often forgetful in daily activities
  (2) Six (or more) of the following symptoms of *hyperactivity-impulsivity* have persisted for at least 6 months to a degree that is maladaptive and inconsistent with developmental level:
  Hyperactivity
    (a) Often fidgets with hands or feet or squirms in seat
    (b) Often leaves seat in classroom or in other situations in which remaining seated is expected
    (c) Often runs about or climbs excessively in situations in which it is inappropriate (in adolescents or adults, may be limited to subjective feelings of restlessness)
    (d) Often has difficulty playing or engaging in leisure activities quietly
    (e) Is often "on the go" or often acts as if "driven by a motor"
    (f) Often talks excessively
  Impulsivity
    (g) Often blurts out answers before questions have been completed
    (h) Often has difficulty awaiting turn
    (i) Often interrupts or intrudes on others (e.g., butts into conversations or games)

B. Some hyperactive-impulsive or inattentive symptoms that caused impairment were present before age 7 years.
C. Some impairment from the symptoms is present in two or more settings (e.g., at school, at work, and at home).
D. There must be clear evidence of clinically significant impairment in social, academic, or occupational functioning.
E. The symptoms do not occur exclusively during the course of or are not accounted for by another mental disorder.

From American Psychiatric Association: *Diagnostic and statistical manual of mental disorders,* ed 4 (DSM-IV), Washington, DC, 1994, The Association.

ronmental manipulation, and sometimes behavioral therapy or psychotherapy for the child. Interventions for children with LDs are primarily educational.

Medication

Stimulant medications and behavioral therapy are appropriate for the school-age child with ADHD (Clinical Practice Guideline, 2001). The most frequently prescribed medications are the psychostimulants methylphenidate hydrochloride (Ritalin) and dextroamphetamine sulfate (Dexedrine). These medications increase dopamine and norepinephrine levels, which leads to stimulation of the inhibitory system of the central nervous system. Tricyclic antidepressants, bupropion, and the α_2-adrenergic agonists (clinidine and guanfacine) are second-line medications.

Recently, atomoxetine, a presynaptic norepinephrine transport inhibitor, became available for use in children (Aschenbrenner, 2003; Michelson et al, 2001). Regularly scheduled evaluations of the child are essential with all of these medications. Children taking stimulant medication may have side effects that include nervousness, insomnia, increased blood pressure, and decreased appetite with subsequent weight loss (Critical Thinking Exercise). Long-term use of dextroamphetamine may result in suppression of growth.

Environmental Manipulation

In ADHD the child's environment is simplified by decreasing external stimuli and distractions, reducing alternatives, increasing consistency in routines, and encouraging desired patterns of behavior. Parents need to develop firm

Critical Thinking Exercise

ATTENTION-DEFICIT/HYPERACTIVITY DISORDER

Johnnie, age 8 years, is a third-grader who was recently diagnosed with attention-deficit/hyperactivity disorder (ADHD). He has been taking the drug methylphenidate (Ritalin) for about a month. In the short time that Johnnie has been on this medication, his math teacher has noticed an improvement in his performance in math class. He is receiving a grade of B instead of his previous grades of D on most math quizzes. The math teacher has also noted that Johnnie is socializing more with his classmates and that he now has a "best friend" in math class. Johnnie usually receives his Ritalin from the school nurse before lunch. Yesterday Johnnie's mother told the school nurse that he has not eaten his lunch for the past week and that he is not hungry.

What important issues regarding Johnnie's medication should the nurse consider in her discussions with Johnnie's mother?

1. Evidence—Is there sufficient evidence to draw conclusions about Johnnie's medication from his behavior?
2. Assumptions—Describe some underlying assumptions about the following:
   a. Pharmacologic action of methylphenidate in ADHD
   b. Side effects of methylphenidate
   c. Management of side effects
3. What implications for nursing care can be drawn at this time?
4. Does the evidence objectively support your conclusion?
5. Are there alternative perspectives to your arguments?

but reasonable limits and to provide a stable and predictable environment with regular routines of sleeping, eating, working, and playing.

Classroom Education

Special activities are designed to address learning deficits that involve visual perception, auditory perception, and other areas involving integration and coordination. The purpose of programs for children with LDs is to assist them to move toward more successful achievement and personal adjustment in the regular classroom. According to Public Law 94-142, the Education for All Handicapped Children's Act, children with ADHD or LDs must receive free public education in the least restrictive environment (see Chapters 29 and 41).

Prognosis

ADHD is relatively stable through early adolescence for most children. Some children experience decreased symptoms during late adolescence and adulthood, but a significant number of these children carry their symptoms into adulthood. The goal for children with LDs is to help them identify their areas of weakness and learn to compensate for them.

Nursing Care Management

Nurses are active participants in all aspects of management of the child with ADHD or LD. Nurses in the community work with families and school personnel on a long-term basis to help plan and implement therapeutic regimens and to evaluate the effectiveness of therapy. They should teach parents and children to take stimulant medication in the morning to maximize its effectiveness in the classroom and to decrease its insomnia-producing potential. If decreased appetite is a concern, giving the psychostimulant with or after meals rather than before is helpful. Parents also benefit from practical, specific strategies that help children with ADHD, such as the need for structure and consistency in dressing, meals, sleep, and discipline.

Nurses must understand which type of LD a child has to provide direction for the child, parents, and teachers. Children with an auditory perceptual deficit are often unable to follow directions or to comprehend large amounts of verbal teaching. These children need diagrams, pictures, demonstration, and written lists. Children with visual perceptual deficits may have difficulty reading, lining up numbers for mathematic operations, or judging distance. These children may have dyslexia (letter reversals) and do better with demonstration and a verbal approach. Children with an integrative deficit may have difficulty sequencing data or storing and retrieving sensory data. Multisensory techniques should be used, and comprehension should be checked frequently throughout instruction. Children with dysgraphia often benefit from computers in the classroom, because their handwriting will *not* improve. They need to find an alternative to physical competition that requires coordination of movement (Selekman & Snyder, 2000).

Enuresis

Enuresis (bed-wetting) is a common and troublesome disorder that is defined as intentional or involuntary passage of urine into bed (usually at night) or into clothes during the day in children who are beyond the age when voluntary bladder control should normally have been acquired. The inappropriate voiding of urine must occur are least twice a week for at least 3 months, and the chronologic or developmental age of the child must be at least 5 years (Cultural Awareness box). The predominant symptom is urgency that is immediate and accompanied by acute discomfort, restlessness, and urinary frequency. Enuresis is more common in boys; nocturnal bedwetting usually ceases between 6 and 8 years of age.

Organic causes that may be related to enuresis should be ruled out before psychogenic factors are considered. These include structural disorders of the urinary tract; urinary tract infection; neurologic deficits; disorders that increase the normal output of urine, such as diabetes; and disorders that impair the concentrating ability of the kidneys, such as chronic renal failure or sickle cell disease. A bladder volume of 300 to 350 ml is sufficient to hold a night's urine. (To determine a child's bladder capacity, have the child void in a measuring cup after holding urine for as long as possible. Normal bladder capacity [in ounces] is the child's age plus 2 [e.g., a 6-year-old's normal capacity is 8 ounces].) In other cases the enuresis is influenced by emotional factors, although it is doubtful that they are causative factors. Parents report that these children sleep more soundly than other children; however, the depth of sleep has not been identified as the cause of nocturnal enuresis. Enuresis has a strong familial tendency.

Therapeutic techniques used to manage enuresis include medications, bladder training, restriction or elimination of fluids after the evening meal, interruption of sleep to void, and various devices designed to establish a conditioned reflex response to waken the child at the initiation of voiding.

Three types of drugs are used to treat enuresis: tricyclic antidepressants, antidiuretics, and antispasmodics. The drug used most frequently to inhibit urination is the tricyclic antidepressant imipramine (Tofranil). Another anticholinergic drug, oxybutynin, reduces uninhibited bladder contractions and may be helpful for children with daytime urinary frequency. Desmopressin (DDAVP) nasal spray, an analog of vasopressin, reduces nighttime urine output to a volume less than functional bladder capacity.

Nursing Care Management

No matter what techniques are used, the nurse can help both children and parents to understand the problem of enuresis, the treatment plan, and the difficulties they may encounter in the process. The nurse can also provide consis-

Cultural Awareness ▸▸

ENURESIS

The age at which children attain urinary continence varies widely. For example, white children in the United States tend to achieve continence earlier than African-American children. In addition, children in Great Britain and Sweden appear to attain continence slightly earlier than children in the United States, and in the extreme, the East African Digos often achieve bladder control by age 12 months. Therefore practitioners must be sensitive to the differences among groups before labeling a child enuretic (Rappaport, 1992).

tent support and encouragement to help sustain both the child and the parents through the inconsistent and unpredictable treatment process. Parents need to understand that punishment is contraindicated because of its negative emotional impact and limited success in reducing the behavior. Children need to believe that they are helping themselves, and they need to sustain feelings of confidence and hope.

Encopresis

Encopresis is the repeated voluntary or involuntary passage of feces of normal or near-normal consistency into places not appropriate for that purpose according to the individual's own sociocultural setting. The event must occur at least once a month for at least 3 months, and the chronologic or developmental age of the child must be at least 4 years. The fecal incontinence must not be caused by any physiologic effect, such as a laxative, or a general medical condition.

Primary encopresis is identified by age 4 when the child has not achieved fecal continence. *Secondary encopresis* is fecal incontinence occurring in a child over 4 years of age after a period of established fecal continence. The disorder is more common in boys than in girls.

One of the most common causes of encopresis is constipation, which may be precipitated by environmental change. Chronic, severe constipation has a tendency to impair the usual movement and contractions of the colon, which can lead to fecal obstruction. Abnormalities in the digestive tract can also lead to encopresis.

Children with encopresis often feel ashamed and may wish to avoid situations that might lead to embarrassment. School performance and attendance are affected as the child's offensive odor becomes a target for scorn and ridicule from classmates. Therapeutic management consists of determining the cause of the soiling and using appropriate interventions to correct the problem. Interventions may involve dietary changes, relief of a fecal impaction, or behavioral therapy. Psychotherapeutic intervention with the child and the family is often necessary.

Nursing Care Management

The nursing care of the child with encopresis involves education and support of the family, as well as treatment of existing constipation. Education regarding the physiology of normal defecation, toilet training as a developmental process, and the treatment outlined for the particular family is essential to a successful outcome. Family counseling is directed toward reassurance that most problems resolve successfully, although relapses during periods of stress are possible (Family Focus box).

> **Family Focus**
>
> **HELPING FAMILIES UNDERSTAND ENCOPRESIS**
>
> The prevailing attitude of nurses toward the family of a child with encopresis should be one of "no-fault," thus relieving the guilt of both parents and child. Because parents and children are often reluctant to volunteer information, direct questioning about the soiling is more successful. Parents are usually relieved to know that other parents share this problem and are surprised to know that functional changes that take place as the condition develops make control of seepage impossible. Many parents complain that their children soil because they do not take time from play for a bowel movement. Actually, the children may be unaware of a prior sensation and unable to control the urge once it begins. They may be so accustomed to bowel accidents that they are unable to smell or feel it and even deny soiling when it occurs.

Posttraumatic Stress Disorder

Posttraumatic stress disorder (PTSD) refers to the development of characteristic symptoms following exposure to an extremely traumatic experience or catastrophic event. The traumatic experience is typically life-threatening to self or a significant other and may involve grotesque mutilation or death, serious injury, or physical coercion (e.g., an assault, a natural disaster, sexual abuse, or witnessing violence). It is important to note that PSTD is not limited to children who have lived in "war-torn" countries. Events such as automobile, school, or recreational accidents and bullying have been identified as causes of PTSD (Sundelin-Wahlsten, Ahmad, & von Knorring, 2001). The characteristic symptoms are persistent reexperiencing of the traumatic event, avoidance of stimuli associated with the event or trauma, numbing of general responsiveness, and increased arousal.

The response to the event takes place in three stages. The *initial response* involves intense arousal, which usually lasts for a few minutes to 1 or 2 hours. The stress hormones are at the maximum as the individual prepares for "fight" or "flight." A prolonged arousal phase may indicate psychosis.

The *second phase,* which lasts approximately 2 weeks, is one in which defense mechanisms are mobilized. It is a period of quiescence in which the event appears to have produced no impression. The child feels numb, and stress hormone secretion is absent. Defense mechanisms are less adaptive to specific situations and may not be what the situation demands. Denial that anything is wrong is a frequently observed defense mechanism.

The *third phase* is one of coping and consciously directed inquiry, which normally extends over 2 to 3 months. The victims want to know what happened and appear to be getting worse, when actually they are getting better. Numerous psychologic symptoms, such as depression, phobia, anxiety, and conversion reactions, may be present. Children frequently display repetitive actions. They play out the situation over and over again in an attempt to come to terms with their fear. Flashbacks are common. This phase can be self-perpetuating, and a prolonged reaction can develop into an obsession with the traumatic event. Some traumatic effects remain indefinitely.

Nursing Care Management

Children need to deal with any traumatic event. Their reactions depend heavily on their social environment and the way in which their caretaking adults react to the event. In the second phase of the PTSD, the appropriateness of the defense mechanism must be assessed, and children must be assisted in application of their defense. If children do not engage in some catharsis, or if their defense phase is prolonged, they need referral for special psychologic help.

Coping is a learned response, and children in the third phase can be helped to deal with their fear. Children usually are willing to accept reasoning. Those who are assisted in their catharsis and allowed expression will survive without serious lasting effects. They should be encouraged to play out the stress and to discuss their feelings about the event. If they are unable to do this, they may become obsessed with the traumatic event and require professional help. Conversion reactions are common obsessive behaviors in children suffering from PTSD.

Children need professional help if any of the phases of PTSD are prolonged. Boys tend to have a prolonged defense phase more often than girls. Occasionally the event will be unrecognized, and the affected child will engage in what is considered to be unusual behavior. Children exhibiting any sudden change in behavior need to be assessed for a traumatic event. When the change in behavior is traced to a traumatic event, treatment can be implemented.

School Phobia

Children, other than beginning students, who resist going to school or who demonstrate extreme reluctance to attend school for a sustained period of time as a result of severe anxiety or fear of school-related experiences are said to have *school phobia.* The terms *school refusal* and *school avoidance* are also used to describe this behavior. School-avoidance behaviors occur in both boys and girls and in children from all socioeconomic levels.

Physical symptoms are prominent and may affect any part of the body (e.g., anorexia, nausea, vomiting, diarrhea, dizziness, headache, leg pains, abdominal pains, or even a low-grade fever). A striking feature of school phobia is the prompt subsiding of symptoms when it is evident that the child can remain at home. Another significant observation is absence of symptoms on weekends and holidays unless they are related to other places such as Sunday school or parties. Occasional mild reluctance is not uncommon among schoolchildren, but if the fear continues for longer than a few days it must be considered a serious problem.

Nursing Care Management

Treatment for school phobia depends on the cause. The primary goal is to *return the child to school.* The longer a child is permitted to stay out of school, the more difficult it is for the child to reenter. Parents must be convinced gently but firmly that *immediate* return is essential and that it is their responsibility to insist on school attendance.

A school reentry protocol may be necessary for the child with severe symptoms. In reentry programs, the child role-plays routines involved in getting ready for school and that occur at school. Relaxation techniques are also used. The child usually goes to school initially for a half day and then progresses to a full day. Often the school nurse is asked to provide support to the parents and the teacher during the reentry process. If the problem persists, professional help is recommended.

Recurrent Abdominal Pain

Recurrent abdominal pain (RAP) is a complaint that is often attributed to a psychogenic etiology, although it can be a symptom of either psychosomatic or organic disease. RAP is defined as three or more separate episodes of abdominal pain during a 3-month period similar to the "spastic" or "irritable" colon syndrome of adulthood. Children with RAP have real pain that is usually located in the periumbilical or epigastric area (or both). On palpation the pain is likely to be experienced in the epigastric area or in the lower right or left quadrant and is accompanied by vague tenderness without muscle guarding. The pain is irregular in time, duration, and intensity and associated with either loose or pellet-formed stools. Other symptoms that may accompany the pain are headache, pallor, dizziness, dysuria, flushing, vomiting, diarrhea, and fatigue.

Children at risk for RAP tend to be high achievers who have extensive personal goals or whose parents have unusually high expectations. They are described as sensitive and overly concerned about what others think of them. They are uncomfortable with expressions of anger or argument, especially in those persons who are significant in their life. School attendance is adversely affected, and these children may exhibit poor learning performance. It is not uncommon for symptoms to be aggravated during school days.

Treatment involves providing reassurance and reducing or eliminating the symptoms. Hospitalization may be necessary, and the child frequently shows improvement in the hospital. Initial efforts are directed toward ruling out organic causes of the pain, relieving discomfort, and attempting to determine the situations that precipitate attacks. A high-fiber diet, psyllium bulk agents, lubricants such as mineral oil, and bowel training are emphasized. Other therapies include cognitive-behavioral therapy, biofeedback, and medications such as famotidine and propantheline bromide (an antispasmodic).

Nursing Care Management

Once the diagnosis has been established, the parents and the child need an explanation of the pain, which can be compared to a skeletal muscle cramp or "charley horse." Reassurance that the symptoms are not unique to their child and that the pain can be expected to subside is helpful in relieving parental fears and anxieties.

The simple measure of having the child rest in a peaceful, quiet environment and providing comfort will often relieve the symptoms in a short time. A heating pad may also help ease the discomfort (see Nonpharmacologic Pain Management, Chapter 44). When pain is not relieved by these simple measures, the parents are taught how to administer antispasmodics, if prescribed. For example, if pain is precipitated by meals, having the child take the medication 20 to 30 minutes before mealtime may prevent an episode.

The most valuable assistance that the nurse can provide is support and reassurance to the family. When open communication is established and families appreciate the relationship between stress-provoking situations and the child's symptoms, the chance for remedial action is enhanced. Follow-up care and continued support are essential, because the symptoms tend to remit and exacerbate. The availability of a supportive health professional is a source of comfort to the child and family.

Conversion Reaction

Conversion reaction, also known as *hysteria, hysterical conversion reaction,* and *childhood hysteria,* is a psychophysiologic disorder with a sudden onset that can usually be traced to a precipitating environmental event. In childhood the disorder is observed with equal frequency in both sexes, but girls outnumber boys during adolescence.

The manifestations involve primarily the voluntary musculature and special senses. Symptoms include abdominal pain, fainting, pseudoseizures, paralysis, headaches, and visual field restriction. The most common symptom is seizure activity, which can be differentiated from symptoms of neurogenic origin by formal tests. A normal electroencephalogram indicates that the origin is not neurogenic. Many children with a conversion reaction have experienced a major family crisis (such as the loss of a parent or other significant person through death, divorce, or moving) before the onset of symptoms.

Nursing Care Management

Nursing care is similar to that for the child with recurrent abdominal pain. If significant personality problems are evident, psychiatric consultation is indicated.

Childhood Depression

Depression in childhood is often difficult to detect because children may be unable to express their feelings and tend to act out their problems and concerns. Some states of depression are of a temporary nature (e.g., acute depression precipitated by a traumatic event). This might include a period of hospitalization; loss of a parent through death or separation; or loss of a significant relationship with something (a pet), someone (a friend or family member), or a place (move from a familiar home, neighborhood, or city). Children with depression may demonstrate a variety of behaviors (Box 39-2). Most responses in children are not sustained and can be modified with social and family support.

BOX 39-2

Characteristics of Children with Depression

Behavior

- Predominantly sad facial expression with absence or diminished range of affective response
- Solitary play or work; tendency to be alone; disinterest in play
- Withdrawal from previously enjoyed activities and relationships
- Lowered grades in school; lack of interest in doing homework or achieving in school
- Diminished motor activity; tiredness
- Tearfulness or crying
- Dependent and clinging or aggressive and disruptive

Internal States

- Utterance of statements reflecting lowered self-esteem, sense of hopelessness, or guilt
- Suicidal ideations

Physiology

- Constipation
- Nonspecific complaints of not feeling well
- Change in appetite resulting in weight loss or gain
- Alterations in sleeping pattern, sleeplessness, or hypersomnia

More serious and less common are the depressive responses to chronic stress and loss; these are frequently observed in children with chronic illness or disability when other family members are in denial and often depressed. There is no apparent precipitating event, but there is often a history of frequent disruptions in important relationships. Often, there is also a history of depressive illness in one or both parents. Manifestations in the child are similar to those observed in acute depression, but they occur more frequently and extend over a longer period of time.

Nursing Care Management

Depressed children are managed by a health team especially prepared in the care of children with mental disorders. Treatment is highly individualized and undertaken in the least restrictive environment. Suicidal children are admitted to the hospital for protection if the family is unable to provide constant monitoring. Pharmacotherapy may involve tricyclic antidepressants or serotonin reuptake inhibitors (SRIs) such as fluoxetine (Prozac), trazodine (Desyrel), sertraline (Zoloft), paroxetine (Paxil), bupropion (Wellbutrin), and venlafaxine (Effexor). Nurses should be aware that depression is a problem that can easily be overlooked in the child and one that can interrupt normal growth and development. Recognizing depression and suicidal tendencies in depressed adolescents and making appropriate referrals is an important nursing function. Identification of the depressed child requires a careful history (health, growth and development, social, and family health); interviews with the child; and observations by the nurse, parents, and teachers. (See also Suicide, Chapter 40).

Childhood Schizophrenia

Childhood schizophrenia is a term that refers to severe deviations in ego functioning and is generally reserved for psychotic disorders that appear in children younger than 15 years of age. Childhood schizophrenia is a very rare illness among children in the general population, and among children with mental illness, only about 2 in every 1000 have childhood schizophrenia.

Childhood schizophrenia is characterized by symptoms that last for at least 6 months and that seriously interfere with the child's functioning in school, at home, or in social situations. The basic disturbance is a lack of contact with reality and the subsequent development of a world of the child's own. Other areas of development that may be impaired include cognition, perception, emotion, language, and physical motor control. The most common manifestations involve language disturbances, impaired interpersonal relationships, and inappropriate affect (outward expression of emotion). Treatment involves management of the symptoms, prevention of relapse, and social and occupational rehabilitation of the young person. Antipsychotic drugs that are used to treat schizophrenia include haloperidol, chlorpromazine, and risperidone.

Nursing Care Management

Nursing care of psychotic children is a highly specialized area. However, nurses should be alert to the possibility that schizophrenia can occur in children, and refer children who consistently demonstrate abnormal behavior to a psychiatrist for evaluation. In addition, nurses will need to teach family members of children taking antipsychotic drugs to observe for possible side effects.

Key Points

- Middle childhood, also known as the school years, is the period of life that extends from 6 to 12 years of age.
- Although growth is slower than in previous years, there is a steady gain in height and weight with maturation of body systems; primary teeth are lost and replaced by permanent teeth.
- A major task during the middle school years is developing a sense of industry or accomplishment (Erikson).
- Piaget's period of concrete operations refers to the school-age period, when children are able to use their thought processes to experience events and actions and make judgments based on what they reason.
- The child develops a conscience and is able to understand and adhere to rules and standards set by others.
- Entertaining different points of view, becoming sensitive to social norms, and forming peer friendships are important features of social development during the school years.
- Cooperative play, team activities, and the acquisition of skills are prime elements of play during the school years; rules and rituals assume greater importance.
- Parental concerns during middle childhood are beginning separation from the family unit, dishonest behavior, and school achievement.
- The availability of junk foods, irregular family meals, and schedules of working parents often hamper optimum nutrition.
- Dental care is important during this time; dental problems include caries, periodontal disease, malocclusion, and dental injury.
- Increased socialization and media exposure make the school years an ideal time for sex education.
- School health ideally offers programs that include health appraisal, emergency care, safety education, communicable disease control, counseling, guidance, and health education with adjustment to individual student needs.
- Injury prevention is directed toward safety education, provision of safe play areas and equipment, and well-supervised sports activities.
- Participation in sports predisposes children and adolescents to both acute injuries and overuse syndromes.
- Alterations in growth and maturation may be manifested as short or tall stature, precocious puberty, or delayed sexual development.
- Tools for assessment of growth include a family history, previous growth patterns, physical examination, bone age determination, and endocrine studies.
- Behavior problems in middle childhood can result from attention-deficit/hyperactivity disorder, enuresis, encopresis, school phobia, recurrent abdominal pain, childhood depression, conversion reaction, and childhood schizophrenia.

Answer Guidelines to Critical Thinking Exercise

Attention-Deficit/Hyperactivity Disorder

1. Yes, there are sufficient data to arrive at a possible conclusion.
2. (a) Methylphenidate is a stimulant that increases dopamine and norepinephrine levels, which leads to stimulation of the inhibitory system of the central nervous system. (b) Common side effects of methylphenidate include nausea, anorexia, decreased appetite, and insomnia. (c) Although the absorption rate of methylphenidate is increased when the drug is taken with meals, side effects such as decreased appetite may become more pronounced with this schedule of administration. Side effects can be alleviated by changing the times that the drug is administered or by switching to a sustained time-release form of the drug that is taken once a day in the morning.
3. Although Johnnie seems to have responded favorably to his medication and has demonstrated several positive effects of methylphenidate (improvement in math class and increasing self-confidence in social skills), the nurse should be concerned about the fact that Johnnie has not eaten his lunch for the past week and that he is not hungry. Decreased appetite is a negative side effect of methylphenidate.
4. Yes, the data indicate that Johnnie is currently experiencing a decrease in his appetite. Because decreased appetite is a common side effect of methylphenidate, there is a high probability that this symptom is related to Johnnie's medication. However, adjusting or changing the times the medication is administered can often alleviate this side effect. Another option is to ask Johnnie's doctor to switch his medication to a sustained time-release form of methylphenidate that can be given once a day in the morning.
5. It is possible that Johnnie's decreased appetite is due to some other factor and not related to his medication. Therefore the nurse should encourage the mother to communicate information about this side effect to Johnnie's primary care physician so that a more complete evaluation can be made.

References

American Academy of Pediatrics, Committee on Injury and Poison Prevention: All terrain vehicle injury prevention: two- three- and four-wheeled unlicensed motor vehicles, *Pediatrics* 105(6):1352-1354, 2000.

American Academy of Pediatrics, Committee on Injury and Poison Prevention: Bicycle helmets, *Pediatrics* 108(4):1030-1032, 2001.

American Academy of Pediatrics, Committee on Injury and Poison Prevention: Selecting and using the most appropriate car safety seats for growing children: guidelines for counseling parents, *Pediatrics* 109(3):550-553, 2002.

American Academy of Pediatrics, Committee on Injury and Poison Prevention and Committee on Sports Medicine and Fitness: Trampolines at home, school, and recreational centers, *Pediatrics* 103(5, pt 1):1053-1056, 1999.

American Academy of Pediatrics, Committee on School Health: School health centers and other integrated school health services, *Pediatrics* 107(1):198-201, 2001.

American Psychiatric Association: *Diagnostic and statistical manual of mental disorders,* ed 4 (DSM-IV TR), Washington, DC, 2000, The Association.

Aschenbrenner DS: New drug for ADHD, *Am J Nurs* 103(4):63, 2003.

Cavendish R, Salomone C: Bullying and sexual harassment in the school setting, *J Sch Nurs* 17(1):25-31, 2001.

Clinical Practice Guideline: Treatment of the school-aged child with attention-deficit/hyperactivity disorder, *Pediatrics* 108(4):1033-1044, 2001.

Delegation of school health services to unlicensed assistive personnel: a position paper of the National Association of State School Nurse Consultants, *J Sch Nurs* 11(4):13-16, 1995.

Erikson EH: *Childhood and society,* ed 2, New York, 1963, Norton.

Kettl P: Biological and social causes of school violence. In Shafii M, Shafii S (eds): *School violence: assessment, management, prevention,* Washington, DC, 2001, American Psychiatric Publishing.

Lau BWK: Stress in children: can nurses help? *Pediatr Nurs* 28(1):13-19, 2002.

Michelson D et al: Atomoxetine in the treatment of children and adolescents with attention-deficit/hyperactivity disorder: a randomized, placebo-controlled, dose-response study, *Pediatrics* 108:E83, 2001.

Muscari ME: Sticks and stones: the NP's role with bullies and victims, *J Pediatr Health Care* 16(1):22-28, 2002.

Myers SM, Eisenhauer NJ, Ryan ME: ADHD: it is real, and it can be treated, *Clinical Advisor* 6(3):15-25, 2003.

Nansel TR et al: Relationships between bullying and violence among US youth, *Arch Pediatr Adolesc Med* 157(4):348-353, 2003.

Olweus D: Bully/victim problems in school: facts and intervention, *Eur J Psych Educ* 12:495-510, 1997.

Rappaport LA: Enuresis. In Levine M and others: *Developmental-behavioral pediatrics,* ed 2, Philadelphia, 1992, WB Saunders.

Rhodes AM: Liability for unlicensed assistive personnel, part I, *MCN* 22:269, 1997.

Selekman J, Snyder M: Learning disabilities and/or attention deficit disorder. In Jackson P, Vessey JA (eds): *Primary care of children with chronic conditions,* ed 3, St Louis, 2000, Mosby.

Sharrer VW, Ryan-Wenger NA: School-age children's self-reported stress symptoms, *Pediatr Nurs* 28(1):21-27, 2002.

Sundelin-Wahlsten V, Ahmad A, von Knorring AL: Traumatic experiences and post-traumatic stress reactions in children from Kurdistan and Sweden, *Acta Paediatr* 90:563-568, 2001.

Vessey JA, Carlson K, David J: Helping children who are being teased and bullied, *Nursing Spectrum* 13:16-18, 2003.

The Adolescent and Family 40

LEARNING OBJECTIVES

On completion of this chapter the reader will be able to:

- Describe the physical changes that occur at puberty.
- Discuss the reactions of the adolescent to physical changes that take place at puberty.
- Demonstrate an understanding of the processes by which the adolescent develops a sense of identity.
- Discuss the significance of the changing interpersonal relationships and the role of the peer group during adolescence.
- Outline a health teaching plan for adolescents.
- Identify the causes and discuss the preventive aspects of injuries during adolescence.
- Demonstrate an understanding of common disorders of the male and female reproductive systems.
- Demonstrate an understanding of health problems related to sexuality.
- Outline a plan of care for the child or adolescent with an eating disorder.
- Discuss the manifestations and nursing management of selected emotional and/or behavioral problems.

ELECTRONIC RESOURCES

Additional information related to the content in Chapter 40 can be found on

the companion website at evolve
http://evolve.elsevier.com/Wong/maternal/

- NCLEX Review Questions
- Case Study–Teen Smoking
- Case Study–Interviewing Adolescents
- WebLinks

or the interactive student CD-ROM
Activities for Chapter 40 include the following:

- NCLEX Review Questions
- Case Study–Behaviors Indicative of Future Child Abuse
- Critical Thinking Exercise–Obesity

PROMOTING OPTIMUM GROWTH AND DEVELOPMENT

Adolescence is a period of transition between childhood and adulthood—a time of rapid physical, cognitive, social, and emotional maturing as the boy prepares for manhood and the girl prepares for womanhood (Cultural Awareness box). The precise boundaries of adolescence are difficult to define, but this period is customarily viewed as beginning with the gradual appearance of secondary sex characteristics at about 11 or 12 years of age and ending with cessation of body growth at 18 to 20 years.

Several terms are used to refer to this stage of growth and development. *Puberty* refers to the maturational, hormonal, and growth process that occurs when the reproductive organs begin to function and the secondary sex characteristics develop. This process is sometimes divided into three stages: *prepubescence,* the period of about 2 years immediately before puberty when the child is developing preliminary physical changes that herald sexual maturity; *puberty,* the point at which sexual maturity is achieved, marked by the first menstrual flow in girls but by less obvious indications in boys; and *postpubescence,* a 1- to 2-year period following puberty during which skeletal growth is completed and reproductive functions become fairly well established. *Adolescence,* which literally means "to grow into maturity," is generally regarded as the psychologic, social, and maturational process initiated by the pubertal changes. It involves three distinct subphases: *early adolescence* (ages 11 to 14), *middle adolescence* (ages 15 to 17), and *late adolescence* (ages 18 to 20). The term *teenage years* is used synonymously with *adolescence* to describe ages 13 through 19.

Biologic Development

The physical changes of puberty are primarily the result of hormonal activity under the influence of the central nervous system, although all aspects of physiologic functioning are mutually interacting. The obvious physical changes are

Cultural Awareness ▸▸

THE ADOLESCENT YEARS

Other societies in which adolescence is seen as part of the life cycle may differ from American culture regarding how the adolescent years are to be spent. For example, some societies discourage contact between adolescent males and females. Sexual experimentation is outlawed, and all grown children, males and females, remain in the home of their parents until they wed. In America we tend to believe that the way our culture is organized is the way all cultures are or should be organized, but of course this is not so. Each society is unique. The way we describe adolescence, the way we experience it, and the predisposition of our adolescents toward violence are peculiar to our American culture.

Modified from Prothrow-Stith D: *Deadly consequences: how violence is destroying our teenage population and a plan to begin solving the problem,* New York, 1993, HarperCollins.

noted in increased physical growth and in the appearance and development of secondary sex characteristics; less obvious are physiologic alterations and neurogonadal maturity, accompanied by the ability to procreate. Physical distinction between the sexes is made on the basis of distinguishing characteristics. *Primary sex characteristics* are the external and internal organs that carry out the reproductive functions (e.g., ovaries, uterus, breasts, penis). *Secondary sex characteristics* are the changes that occur throughout the body as a result of hormonal changes (e.g., voice alterations, development of facial and pubertal hair, fat deposits) but which play no direct part in reproduction.

Hormonal Changes of Puberty

The events of puberty are caused by hormonal influences and controlled by the anterior pituitary (adenohypophysis) in response to a stimulus from the hypothalamus. Stimulation of the gonads has a dual function: (1) production and release of gametes—production of sperm in the male and maturation and release of ova in the female—and (2) secretion of sex-appropriate hormones—estrogen and progesterone from the ovaries (female) and testosterone from the testes (male).

Sex Hormones

The ovaries, testes, and adrenals secrete sex hormones. These hormones are produced in varying amounts by both sexes throughout the life span. The adrenal cortex is responsible for the small amounts secreted before the pubescent years, but the sex hormone production that accompanies maturation of the gonads is responsible for the biologic changes observed during puberty.

Estrogen, the feminizing hormone, is found in low quantities during childhood. This hormone is secreted in slowly increasing amounts until about age 11 years. In males this gradual increase continues through maturation. In females the onset of estrogen production in the ovary causes a pronounced increase that continues until about 3 years after the onset of menstruation, at which time it reaches a maximum level that continues throughout the reproductive life of the female.

Androgens, the masculinizing hormones, are also secreted in small and gradually increasing amounts up to about 7 or 9 years of age, at which time there is a more rapid increase in both sexes, especially boys, until about age 15 years. These hormones appear to be responsible for most of the rapid growth changes of early adolescence. With the onset of testicular function, the level of androgens (principally *testosterone*) in males increases over that in females and continues to increase until a maximum is attained at maturity.

Sexual Maturation

The visible evidence of sexual maturation is achieved in an orderly sequence, and the state of maturity can be estimated on the basis of the appearance of these external manifestations. The age at which these changes are observed and the time required to progress from one stage to another may vary among children. The time from the appearance of breast buds to full maturity may be 1½ to 6 years for adolescent girls. It may take 2 to 5 years for male genitalia to reach adult size. The stages of development of secondary sex characteristics and genital development have been defined as a guide for estimating sexual maturity and are referred to as the *Tanner stages.* The usual sequence of appearance of maturational changes is presented in Box 40-1.

Sexual Maturation in Girls

In most girls the initial indication of puberty is the appearance of breast buds, an event known as *thelarche,* which occurs between 9 and 13½ years of age (Fig. 40-1). This is followed in approximately 2 to 6 months by growth of pubic hair on the mons pubis, known as *adrenarche* (Fig. 40-2). In a minority of normally developing girls, however, pubic hair may precede breast development.

The initial appearance of menstruation, or *menarche,* occurs about 2 years after the appearance of the first pubescent changes, approximately 9 months after attainment of peak height velocity and 3 months after attainment of peak weight velocity. Menarche has been related to a critical gain in body fat content (more fat content, earlier menarche), although this is controversial. The normal age range of menarche is usually 10½ to 15 years, with the average age being 12 years 9½ months for North American girls. Ovulation and

BOX 40-1

Usual Sequence of Maturational Changes

Girls
- Breast changes
- Rapid increase in height and weight
- Growth of pubic hair
- Appearance of axillary hair
- Menstruation (usually begins 2 years after first signs)
- Abrupt deceleration of linear growth

Boys
- Enlargement of testicles
- Growth of pubic hair, axillary hair, hair on upper lip, hair on face and elsewhere on body (facial hair usually appears about 2 years after appearance of pubic hair)
- Rapid increase in height
- Changes in the larynx and consequently the voice (usually take place along with growth of penis)
- Nocturnal emissions
- Abrupt deceleration of linear growth

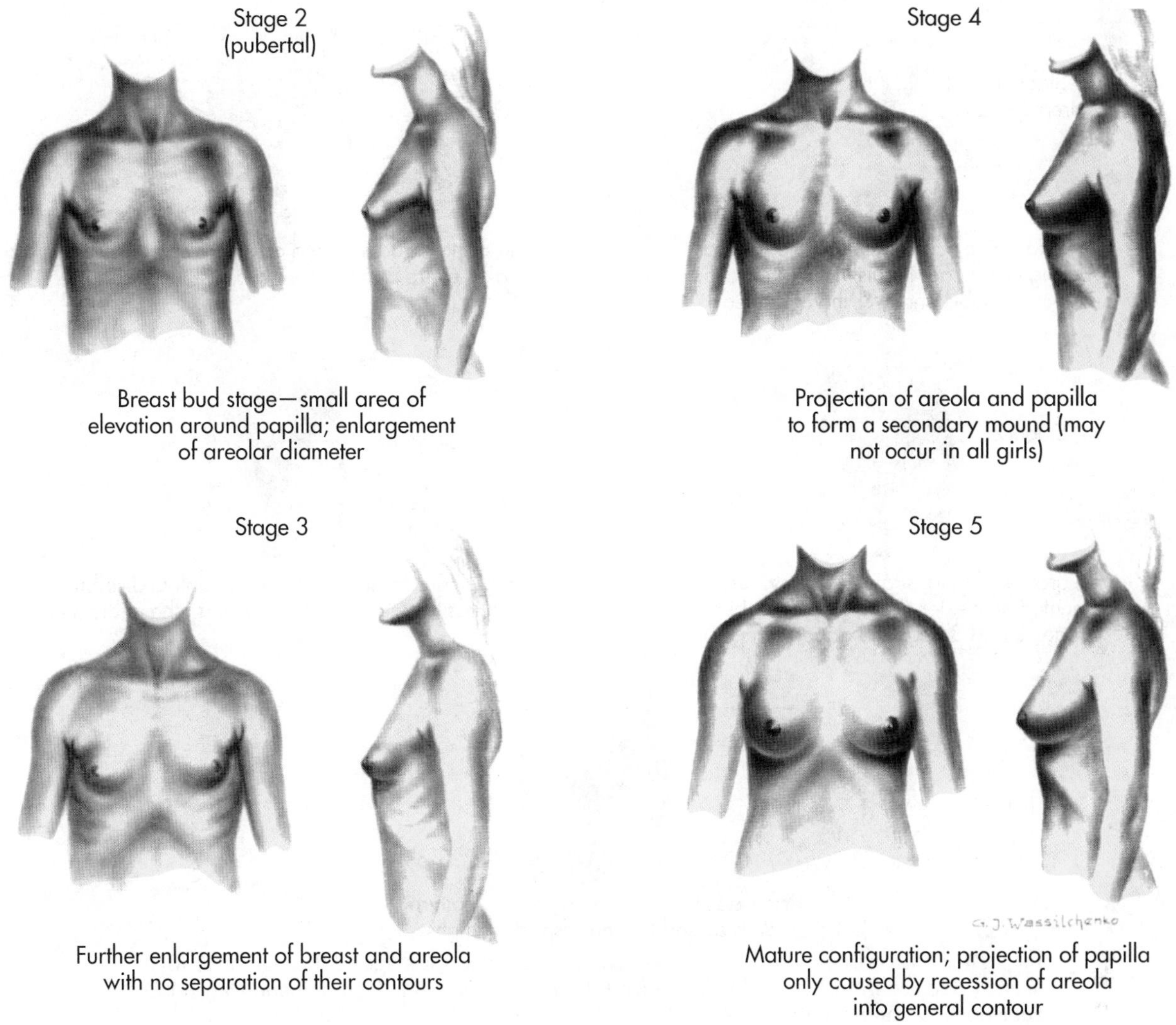

Fig. 40-1 Development of the breast in girls–average age span: 11 to 13 years. Stage 1 (prepubertal–elevation of papilla only) is not shown. (Modified from Marshall WA, Tanner JM: *Arch Dis Child* 44:291, 1969; and Daniel WA, Paulshock BZ: *Patient Care*, pp 122-124, May 13, 1979.)

regular menstrual periods usually occur 6 to 14 months after menarche. Girls may be considered to have *pubertal delay* if breast development has not occurred by age 13 or if menarche has not occurred within 4 years of the onset of breast development.

Sexual Maturation in Boys

The first pubescent changes in boys are testicular enlargement accompanied by thinning, reddening, and increased looseness of the scrotum (Fig. 40-3). These events usually occur between 9½ and 14 years of age. Early puberty is also characterized by the initial appearance of pubic hair. Penile enlargement begins, and testicular enlargement and pubic hair growth continue throughout midpuberty. During this period there is also increasing muscularity, early voice changes, and development of early facial hair. Temporary breast enlargement and tenderness, *gynecomastia,* are common during midpuberty, occurring in up to one-third of boys. The spurts in height and weight occur concurrently toward the end of midpuberty. For most boys, breast enlargement disappears within 2 years. By late puberty there is a definite increase in the length and width of the penis, testicular enlargement continues, and first ejaculation occurs. Axillary hair develops, and facial hair extends to cover the anterior neck. Final voice changes occur secondary to the growth of the larynx. Concerns about *pubertal delay* should be considered for boys who exhibit no enlargement of the testes or scrotal changes by 13½ to 14 years of age, or if genital growth is not complete 4 years after the testicles begin to enlarge.

Physical Growth

A constant phenomenon associated with sexual maturation is a dramatic increase in growth. The final 20% to 25% of height is achieved during puberty, and most of this growth occurs during a 24- to 36-month period—the adolescent *growth spurt.* This accelerated growth occurs in all children but, as in other areas of development, is highly variable in age of onset, duration, and extent. The growth spurt begins earlier in girls, usually between ages 9½ and 14½ years; on the average it begins between ages 10½ and 16 years in boys. During this period, the average boy gains 10 to 30

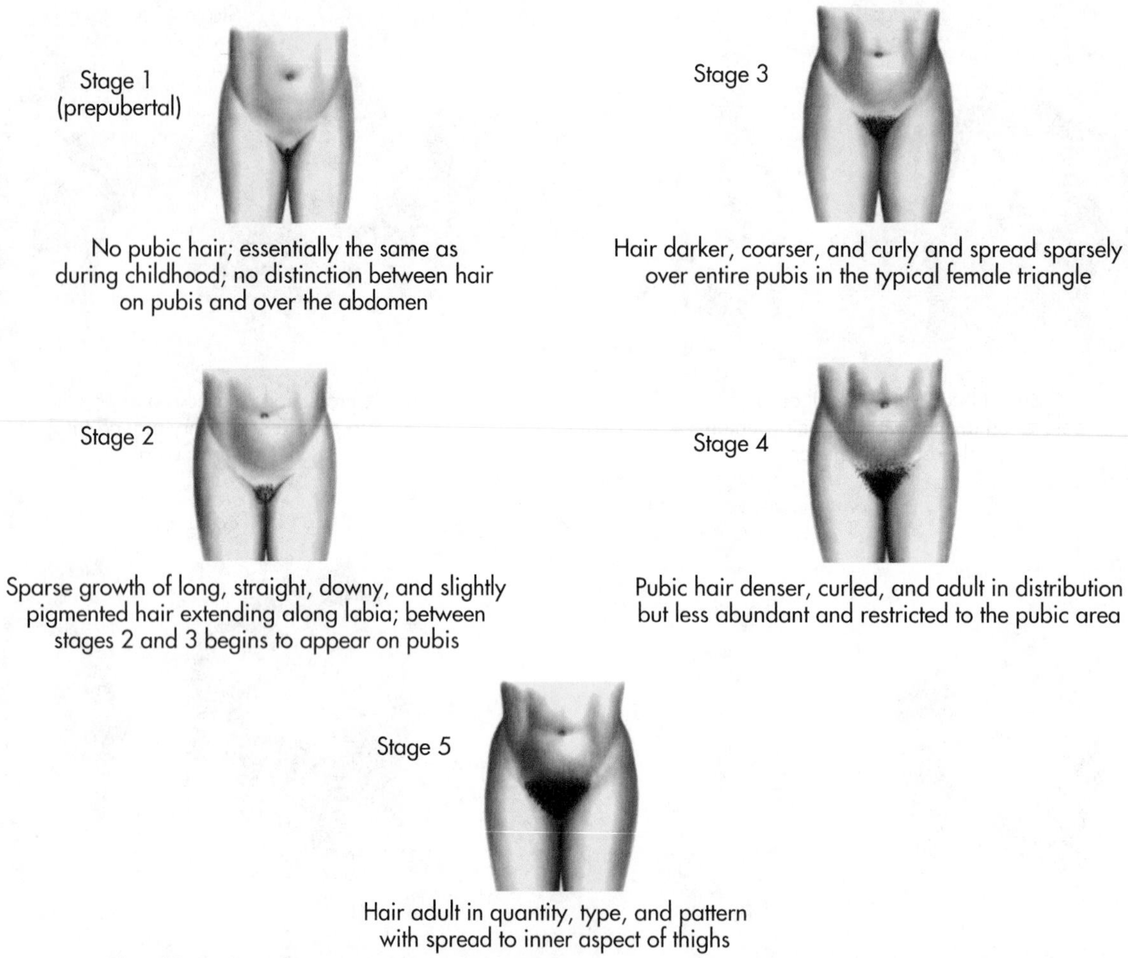
Stage 1
(prepubertal)
No pubic hair; essentially the same as during childhood; no distinction between hair on pubis and over the abdomen
Stage 3
Hair darker, coarser, and curly and spread sparsely over entire pubis in the typical female triangle
Stage 2
Sparse growth of long, straight, downy, and slightly pigmented hair extending along labia; between stages 2 and 3 begins to appear on pubis
Stage 4
Pubic hair denser, curled, and adult in distribution but less abundant and restricted to the pubic area
Stage 5
Hair adult in quantity, type, and pattern with spread to inner aspect of thighs

Fig. 40-2 Growth in pubic hair in girls—average age span for stages 2 through 5: 11 to 14 years. (Modified from Marshall WA, Tanner JM: *Arch Dis Child* 44:291, 1969; and Daniel WA, Paulshock BZ: *Patient Care*, pp 122-124, May 13, 1979.)

cm (4 to 12 inches) in height and 7 to 30 kg (15 to 65 pounds) in weight. The average girl, in whom the growth spurt is slower and less extensive, gains 5 to 20 cm (2 to 8 inches) in height and 7 to 25 kg (15 to 55 pounds) in weight. Growth in height typically ceases 2 to 2½ years after menarche in girls and at age 18 to 20 years in boys.

This increase in size is acquired in a characteristic sequence. Growth in length of the extremities and neck precedes growth in other areas, and since these parts are the first to reach adult length, the hands and feet appear larger than normal during adolescence. Increases in hip and chest breadth take place in a few months, followed several months later by an increase in shoulder width. These changes are followed by increases in length of the trunk and depth of the chest. This sequence of changes is responsible for the characteristic long-legged, gawky appearance of the early adolescent child.

Sex Differences in General Growth Patterns

Sex differences in general growth and distribution patterns are apparent in skeletal growth, muscle mass, adipose tissue, and skin. Skeletal growth differences between boys and girls are apparently a function of hormonal effects at puberty and are evident primarily in limb length. The earlier cessation of growth in girls is caused by epiphyseal unity under the potent effect of estrogen secretion, and the hormonal effect on female bone growth is much stronger than the similar effect of testosterone in boys. In boys the prolonged growth period before puberty and the less rapid epiphyseal closure are reflected in their greater overall height and longer arms and legs. Other skeletal differences are increased shoulder width in boys and broader hip development in girls.

Hypertrophy of the laryngeal mucosa and enlargement of the larynx and vocal cords occur in both boys and girls to produce voice changes. Girls' voices become slightly deeper and considerably fuller, but the effect in boys is striking. The change in the voice of adolescent boys occurs between Tanner stages 3 and 4, with the voice often shifting uncontrollably from deep to high tones in the middle of a sentence. The change is associated with not only a lengthening of the vocal cords, but also an increase in the structure and mass of the vocal folds (Harries et al, 1998).

Growth of lean body mass, principally muscle, which tends to occur after the bone growth spurt, takes place steadily during adolescence. Lean body mass is both quantitatively and qualitatively greater in boys than in girls at comparable stages of pubertal development. Muscle development, under the influence of androgenic hormones, increases steadily. Muscles become remarkably well devel-

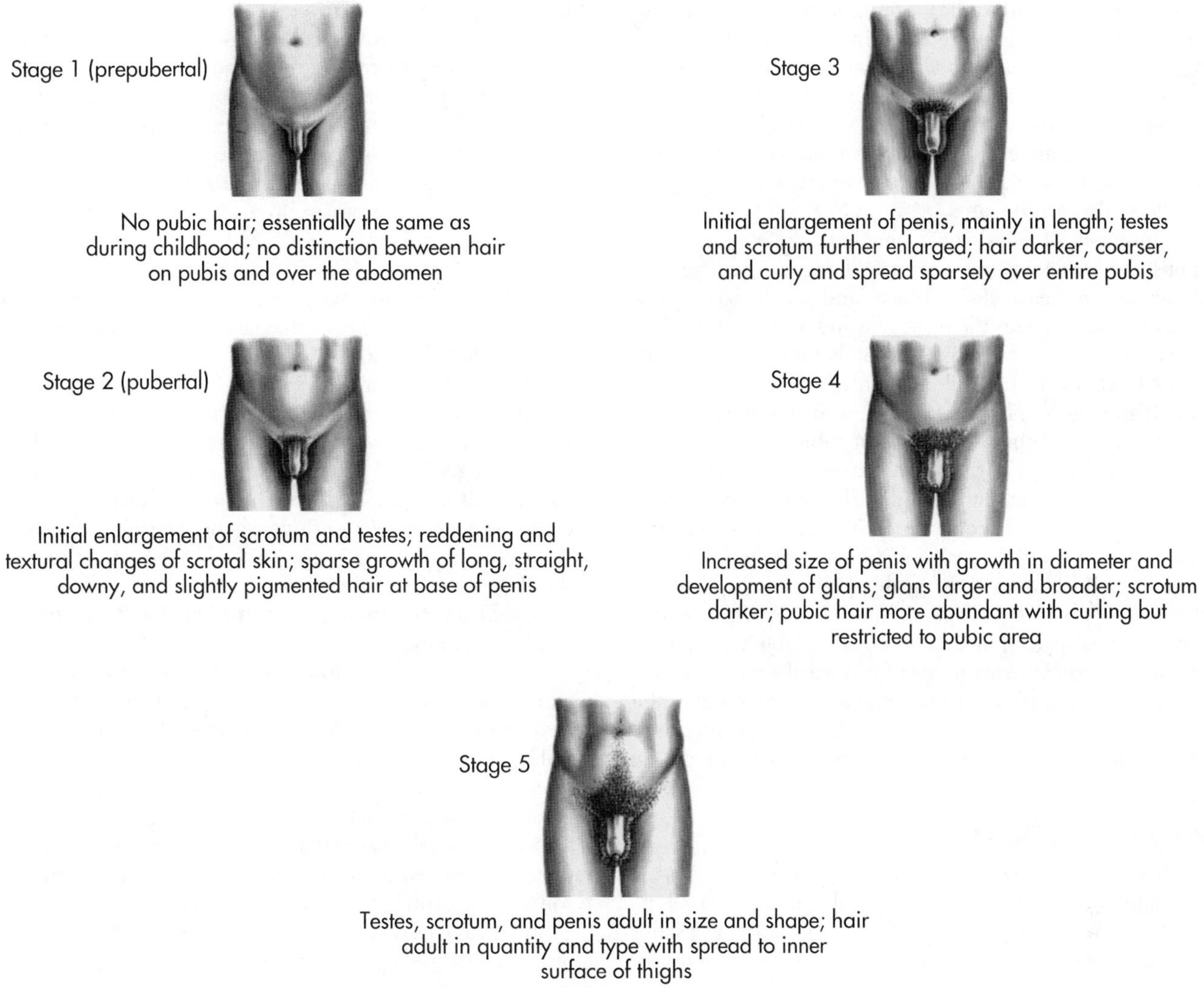
Stage 1 (prepubertal)
No pubic hair; essentially the same as during childhood; no distinction between hair on pubis and over the abdomen
Stage 2 (pubertal)
Initial enlargement of scrotum and testes; reddening and textural changes of scrotal skin; sparse growth of long, straight, downy, and slightly pigmented hair at base of penis
Stage 3
Initial enlargement of penis, mainly in length; testes and scrotum further enlarged; hair darker, coarser, and curly and spread sparsely over entire pubis
Stage 4
Increased size of penis with growth in diameter and development of glans; glans larger and broader; scrotum darker; pubic hair more abundant with curling but restricted to pubic area
Stage 5
Testes, scrotum, and penis adult in size and shape; hair adult in quantity and type with spread to inner surface of thighs

Fig. 40-3 Developmental stages of secondary sex characteristics and genital development in boys—average age span, 12 to 16 years. (Modified from Marshall WA, Tanner JM: *Arch Dis Child* 44:291, 1969; and Daniel WA, Paulshock BZ: *Patient Care*, pp 122-124, May 13, 1979.)

oped in boys, whereas in girls, muscle mass increase is proportionate to general tissue growth.

Nonlean body mass, primarily fat, is also increased but follows a less orderly pattern. There may be a transient increase in subcutaneous fat just before the skeletal growth spurt, especially in boys. This is followed 1 to 2 years later by a modest-to-marked decrease, which is again more notable in boys. Later, variable amounts of fat are deposited to fill out and contour the mature physique in patterns characteristic of the adolescent's sex, particularly in the regions over the thighs, hips, and buttocks and around the breast tissue. It should be noted, however, that pediatric obesity is steadily on the increase in the United States, and obesity can change the timing of puberty. Early maturers (beginning puberty 1.5 to 3.3 years earlier) are shorter and have a greater body mass index than mid-onset or late maturers (Biro et al, 2001).

Hormonal influences during puberty cause acceleration in growth and maturation of the skin and its structural appendages. Sebaceous glands become extremely active at this time, especially those on the genitals and in the "flush areas" of the body (i.e., face, neck, shoulders, upper back, and chest). This increased activity and the structural nature of the glands are extremely important in the pathogenesis of a common problem of puberty: acne (see Chapter 53). The eccrine sweat glands, present almost everywhere on the human skin, become fully functional and respond to emotional as well as thermal stimulation. Heavy sweating appears to be more pronounced in boys than in girls. The apocrine sweat glands, nonfunctional in childhood, reach secretory capacity during puberty. Unlike the eccrine sweat glands, the apocrine glands are limited in distribution and grow in conjunction with hair follicles in the axillae, around the areola of the breast, around the umbilicus, on the external auditory canal, and in the genital and anal regions. Apocrine glands secrete a thick substance as a result of emotional stimulation that, when acted on by surface bacteria, becomes highly odoriferous.

Body hair assumes very characteristic distribution patterns and changes texture during puberty. Under the influence of gonadal and adrenal androgens, hair coarsens, darkens, and lengthens at sites related to secondary sex characteristics. Pubic and axillary hair appears in both sexes, although pubic hair is more extensive in males than in females. Beard, mustache, and body hair on the chest, upward along the linea alba, and sometimes on other areas (e.g., back and shoulders) appears in males and is androgen dependent. Extremity hair appears in varying amounts in both males and females but is also more prolific in the male.

Physiologic Changes

A number of physiologic functions are altered in response to some of the pubertal changes. The size and strength of the heart, blood volume, and systolic blood pressure increase, whereas the pulse rate and basal heat production decrease (see Appendix J). Blood volume, which has increased steadily during childhood, reaches a higher value in boys than in girls, a fact that may be related to the increased muscle mass in pubertal boys. Adult values are reached for all formed elements of the blood. Respiratory rate and basal metabolic rate, decreasing steadily throughout childhood, reach the adult rate in adolescence. Respiratory volume and vital capacity are increased and to a far greater extent in males than in females. During this period, physiologic responses to exercise change drastically: performance improves, especially in boys, and the body is able to make the physiologic adjustments needed for normal functioning after exercise is completed. These capabilities are a result of the increased size and strength of muscles and the increased level of cardiac, respiratory, and metabolic functioning.

Psychosocial Development

Developing a Sense of Identity (Erikson)

Traditional psychosocial theory holds that the developmental crisis of adolescence leads to the formation of a sense of identity (Erikson, 1963). Throughout childhood, individuals have been going through the process of identification as they concentrate on various parts of the body at specific times. During infancy children identify themselves as being separate from the mother; during early childhood they establish a gender-role identification with the appropriate-sex parent; and in later childhood they establish who they are in relation to others. In adolescence they come to see themselves as distinct individuals, somehow unique and separate from every other individual.

The early period of adolescence begins with the onset of puberty and extends to relative physical and emotional stability at or near graduation from high school. During this time the adolescent is faced with the crisis of *group identity vs. alienation.* In the period that follows, the individual strives to attain autonomy from the family and develop a sense of *personal identity* as opposed to *role diffusion.* A sense of group identity appears to be essential to the development of a sense of personal identity. Young adolescents must resolve questions concerning relationships with a peer group before they are able to resolve questions about who they are in relation to family and society.

Group Identity

During the early stage of adolescence, pressure to belong to a group is intensified. Teenagers find it essential to have a group to which they feel they can belong and that provides them with status. Belonging to a crowd helps adolescents establish the differences between themselves and their parents. They dress as the group dresses and wear makeup and hairstyles according to group criteria, all of which are different from those of the parental generation. Language, music, and dancing reflect a culture that is exclusive to the adolescent. When adults begin to emulate these fashions and interests, the style changes immediately. The evidence of adolescent conformity to the peer group and nonconformity to the adult group provides teenagers with a frame of reference in which they can display their own self-assertion while they reject the identity of their parents' generation. To be different is to be unaccepted and alienated from the group.

Individual Identity

The quest for personal identity is part of the ongoing identification process. As youngsters establish identity within a group, they also attempt to incorporate multiple body changes into a concept of the self. Body awareness is part of self-awareness. In their search for identity, adolescents consider the relationships that have developed between themselves and others in the past, as well as the directions they hope to take in the future.

Significant Others Hold Expectations for the Behavior of the Adolescent

Often these expectations or demands are persistent enough to result in certain decisions that might be made differently or not at all if the individual could be solely responsible for identity formation. It is all too easy to slip into the roles that are expected by these external influences without incorporating personal goals or questioning these decisions. Thus, individuals may become what parents or others wish them to be, based on these premature decisions. Young persons might form a negative identity when society or their culture provides them with a self-image that is contrary to the values of the community. Labels such as "juvenile delinquent," "hoodlum," or "failure" are applied to certain adolescents, who then accept and live up to these labels with behaviors that validate and strengthen them.

The process of evolving a personal identity is time-consuming and fraught with periods of confusion, depression, and discouragement. Determining an identity and a place in the world is a critical and perilous feature of adolescence (Critical Thinking Exercise). However, as the pieces are gradually shifted and settled into place, a positive identity eventually emerges. Role diffusion results when the individual is unable to formulate a satisfactory identity from the multiplicity of aspirations, roles, and identifications.

Case Study: Behaviors Indicative of Future Child Abuse

Sex-role Identity

Adolescence is the time for consolidation of a sex-role identity. During early adolescence the peer group begins to communicate expectations regarding heterosexual relationships, and as development progresses, adolescents encounter expectations for mature sex-role behavior from both peers and adults. Expectations vary from culture to culture, among geographic areas, and among socioeconomic groups.

Emotionality

Adolescents vacillate in their emotional states between considerable maturity and childlike behavior. One minute they are exuberant and enthusiastic; the next minute they are depressed and withdrawn. Unpredictable, but essentially normal, mood swings are common during this time period.

Critical Thinking Exercise

DISCUSSING THE FUTURE

Jeremy, age 17, will be graduating from high school in the spring. His mother, a single parent, tells you that she is concerned because graduation is quickly approaching and Jeremy has made no plans for what he will do with his life after graduation. Whenever Jeremy mentions the topic, his mother tells him, "This is what you must do," and begins to outline the steps he must take. Jeremy just walks away. She asks, "What should I do?" What advice should you give Jeremy's mother?

1. Evidence—Is there sufficient evidence to draw any conclusions about what advice the nurse should give Jeremy's mother?
2. Assumptions—Describe an underlying assumption about each of the following issues:
   a. Adolescents and the search for personal identity
   b. The influence of others on the adolescent's search for personal identity
   c. Ways to communicate with adolescents
3. What implications and priorities for nursing care can be drawn at this time?
4. Does the evidence objectively support your argument (conclusion)?
5. Are there alternative perspectives to your arguments? What are they?

As the tension is relieved, emotion is brought under control and individuals retreat to review what has happened, to attempt to master their anger, and to grow in their ability to control their emotions and gain from the new experience. Because of these mood swings, adolescents are frequently labeled as unstable, inconsistent, and unpredictable. Little things can cause an emotional upheaval and, depending on the teenager's interpretation can mean a great deal.

Teenagers are better able to control their emotions in later adolescence. They can approach problems more calmly and rationally, and although they are still subject to periods of sadness, their feelings are less vulnerable and they begin to demonstrate the more mature emotions of later adolescence. Whereas early adolescents react immediately and emotionally, older adolescents can control their emotions until socially acceptable times and places for expression present themselves. They are still subject to heightened emotion, and when it is expressed, their behavior reflects feelings of insecurity, tension, and indecision.

Cognitive Development (Piaget)

Cognitive thinking culminates with the capacity for *abstract thinking.* This stage, the period of *formal operations,* is Piaget's fourth and last stage. Adolescents are no longer restricted to the real and actual, which was typical of the period of concrete thought; they are also concerned with the possible. They now think beyond the present. Without having to center attention on the immediate situation, they can imagine a sequence of events that might occur, such as college and occupational possibilities; how things might change in the future, such as relationships with parents; and the consequences of their actions, such as dropping out of school. At this time their thoughts can be influenced by logical principles rather than just their own perceptions and experiences. They become increasingly capable of scientific reasoning and formal logic.

Adolescents are capable of mentally manipulating more than two categories of variables at the same time. For example, they can consider the relationship between speed, distance, and time in planning a trip. They can detect logical consistency or inconsistency in a set of statements and evaluate a system or set of values in a more analytic manner. For instance, they question the parent who insists on honesty in the youngster but at the same time cheats on an income tax report or expense account.

In adolescence, young people begin to think about both their own thinking and the thinking of others. They wonder what opinion others have of them, and they are able to imagine the thoughts of others. With this capacity comes the ability to differentiate between others' thoughts and their own and to interpret the thoughts of others more accurately. They are able to understand that few concepts are absolute or independent of other influencing factors. As they become aware that other cultures and communities have different norms and standards from their own, it becomes easier for them to accept members of these other cultures, and the decision to behave in their own culture in an accepted manner becomes a more conscious commitment.

Moral Development (Kohlberg)

Although younger children merely accept the decisions or point of view of adults, adolescents, to gain autonomy from adults, must substitute their own set of morals and values. When old principles are challenged but new independent values have not yet emerged to take their place, young people search for a moral code that preserves their personal integrity and guides their behavior, especially in the face of strong pressure to violate the old beliefs. Their decisions involving moral dilemmas must be based on an *internalized set of moral principles* that provides them with the resources to evaluate the demands of the situation and to plan actions that are consistent with their ideals.

Late adolescence is characterized by serious questioning of existing moral values and their relevance to society and the individual. Adolescents can easily take the role of another. They understand duty and obligation based on reciprocal rights of others, as well as the concept of justice that is founded on making amends for misdeeds and repairing or replacing what has been spoiled by wrongdoing. However, they seriously question established moral codes, often as a result of observing that adults verbally ascribe to a code but do not adhere to it.

Spiritual Development

As youngsters move toward independence from parents and other authorities, some begin to question the values and ideals of their families. Others cling to these values as a stable element in their lives as they struggle with the conflicts of this turbulent period. Adolescents need to work out these conflicts for themselves, but they also need support from authority figures and/or peers for their resolution.

Adolescents are capable of understanding abstract concepts and of interpreting analogies and symbols. They are able to empathize, philosophize, and think logically. Most teens search for ideals and speculate about illogical statements and conflicting ideologies. Their tendency toward introspection and emotional intensity often makes it difficult for others to know what they are thinking. They tend to keep their thoughts private, fearing that no one will understand these feelings that they perceive to be unique and special. However, they may reveal deep spiritual concerns. They need support and encouragement in their struggle for understanding and the freedom to question without censure.

Greater levels of religiosity and spirituality are associated with fewer high-risk behaviors and more health promoting behaviors (Brown, 2001). Nurses play an important role for teens by providing an opportunity to discuss issues regarding spirituality.

Social Development

To achieve full maturity, adolescents must free themselves from family domination and define an identity independent of parental authority. However, this process is fraught with ambivalence on the part of both teenagers and their parents. Adolescents want to grow up and to be free of parental restraints, but they are fearful as they try to comprehend the responsibilities that are linked with independence. Feelings of immortality and exemption from the consequences of risk-taking behavior, although viewed as negative, can serve an important developmental function at this time. These feelings give adolescents the courage to separate from their parents and become independent. Part of this emancipation involves developing social relationships outside the family that help teenagers identify their role in society. Adolescence is a time of intense sociability and often a time of equally intense loneliness. Acceptance by peers, a few close friends, and the secure love of a supportive family are requisites for interpersonal maturation.

Relationships with Parents

During adolescence the parent-child relationship changes from one of protection-dependency to one of *mutual affection and equality.* The process of achieving independence often involves turmoil and ambiguity as both parent and adolescent learn to play new roles and work toward this end while, at the same time, resolving the often painful series of rifts essential to establishing the ultimate relationship.

Most behavior observed in the adolescent is related to the struggle for independence and the external restrictions and checks that are placed on this spontaneous maturation process. On the one hand, adolescents are accepted as maturing preadults. They are allowed privileges heretofore denied, and they are provided with increasing responsibilities. On the other hand, because of their unpredictability and insecurity in evaluating situations and making sound judgments, they must conform to regulations and restrictions set by adults. This state of affairs is particularly exemplified by the struggle between parents and adolescents concerning the nightly curfew.

As teenagers assert their rights for grown-up privileges, they frequently create tensions within the home. They resist parental control, and conflicts can arise from almost any situation or any subject. Favorite topics of dispute include use of the telephone, manners, dress, chores and duties, homework, disrespectful behavior, friendships, dating, money, automobiles, drinking and/or drugs, and time schedules. Present in these areas of conflict is the overriding argument that "Everyone else has one" or is allowed the desired item or privilege and the ever-present assertions that "You don't understand me or trust me" and "You always treat me like a baby." Spoken or unspoken, parents' reactions consist of "Is this all the thanks I get for what I have done for you?"

The teenager's earliest attempts to achieve emancipation from parental controls are manifested in a period of rejection of the parents. They absent themselves from home and family activities and spend an increasing amount of time with the peer group. They confide less in their parents, but parents continue to play an important role in the personal and health-related decision making of adolescents.

With advancing adolescence, teenagers become more competent, and with this competence comes a need for more autonomy. Although they may be psychologically prepared for independence, they are often thwarted in their efforts by lack of money or other parental barriers. Conflict arises in relation to the teenager's outside activities and the elements of privacy and trust. Parental supervision remains important throughout adolescence and may have a direct influence on adolescent sexual and substance use behavior. Parents should be guided toward an authoritative style of parenting in which authority is used to guide the adolescent while allowing developmentally appropriate levels of freedom and providing clear, consistent messages regarding expectations (Baker et al, 1999). However, to gain the trust of adolescents, parents must respect their youngster's privacy, as well as show an honest and sincere interest in what the adolescent believes and feels (Family Focus box).

Relationships with Peers

Although parents remain the primary influence in their lives, for the majority of teenagers, peers assume a more significant role in adolescence than they did during childhood. The peer group serves as a strong support to teenagers, individually and collectively, providing them with a sense of belonging and a feeling of strength and power. The peer group forms the transitional world between dependence and autonomy.

Peer Group

Adolescents are usually social, gregarious, and group minded. Thus the peer group has an intense influence on adolescents' self-evaluation and behavior. To gain acceptance by a group, younger teenagers tend to conform completely in such things as mode of dress, hairstyle, taste in music, and vocabulary. Teenagers use the peer group as a yardstick of what is normal.

The school is psychologically important to adolescents as a focus of social life. Teenagers usually distribute themselves into a relatively predictable social hierarchy. They know to which groups they and others belong. A sense of school connectedness has been found to predict decreased risk-taking

Family Focus

COMMUNICATION WITH TEENS: THE ART OF LISTENING

Conflicts between parents and their adolescents are often a result of a very natural characteristic of parenthood: the desire to protect one's offspring from harm or from simply doing something "stupid" or embarrassing or something they may later regret. Teenagers sometimes "bounce" their thoughts and ideas off adults. At times they really want some feedback; at other times they simply want to elicit a reaction.

I found it easy to listen openly, thoughtfully, and without interrupting when my teenagers' friends discussed troublesome topics. However, one day, when one of my own teenagers had a similar conversation with me, the parent part kicked in. I felt responsible and spoke my piece on the spot. This brought communication to a halt and resulted in defensiveness. It was a long time before my child tried to talk to me about anything controversial again. The next time one of my teenagers started a similar conversation, I decided to try to trick myself.

Throughout the entire conversation, I told myself over and over again to act as if this were not my teenager, but rather someone else's child. I found this actually worked quite well, and I was able to listen without interrupting. I continued to use the system, sometimes with more success than at other times.

Mother of four

behaviors in adolescents (Resnick et al, 1997). School connectedness is correlated with caring teachers and the absence of prejudice or discrimination from peers. A sense of school connectedness is less dependent upon class size, attendance, academic preparation, and parental involvement (Maes & Lievens, 2003).

Within the larger groups are smaller, distinct, and rather exclusive crowds or cliques of selected close friends who are emotionally attached to each other. The selection is based on common tastes, interests, and background. Although cliques may become formalized, most remain informal and small. However, each has an identifying feature that proclaims its difference from others and its solidarity within itself, in much the same manner as the adolescent generation as a whole sets itself apart from the adult generation. Cliques are usually made up of one sex, and girls tend to be more cliquish than boys and to have a greater need for close friendships (Fig. 40-4). Within the intimacy of the group, adolescents gain support in learning about themselves, consideration for the feelings of others, and increased ego development and self-reliance.

To belong is of utmost importance; thus adolescents behave in a way that will ensure their establishment in a group. Adolescents are highly susceptible to social approval, acceptance, and demands. To be ignored or criticized by peers creates feelings of inferiority, inadequacy, and incompetence.

Best Friends

Personal friendships of the one-on-one variety usually develop between same-sex adolescents. This relationship is closer and more stable than it is in middle childhood, and it is important in the quest for identity. A best friend is the best audience on whom to try out possible roles and identities that an adolescent wants to test. Best friends may try a role

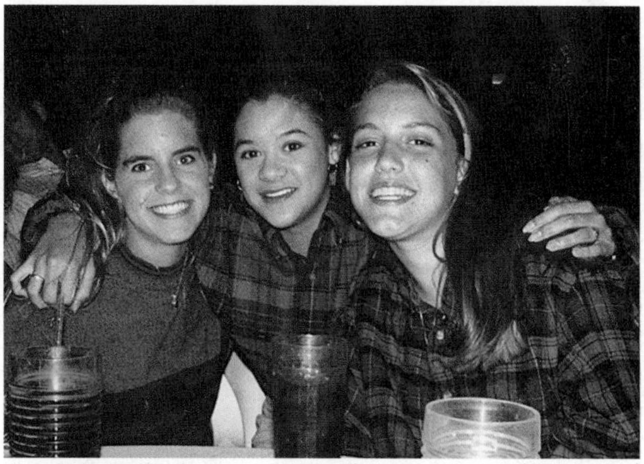

Fig. 40-4 Teenagers like to gather in small groups.

together, each providing support for the other. Each cares about what the other thinks and feels. Since a sense of intimacy grows within a permanent relationship, the stability of this same-sex friendship is an important link in the progress toward an intimate relationship in young adulthood.

Heterosexual Relationships

During adolescence, relationships with members of the opposite sex take on new importance (Fig. 40-5). Although there seems to be a trend toward earlier dating, on the *average,* dating activities begin in the seventh and eighth grades and are usually "crowd" dates at organized school functions.

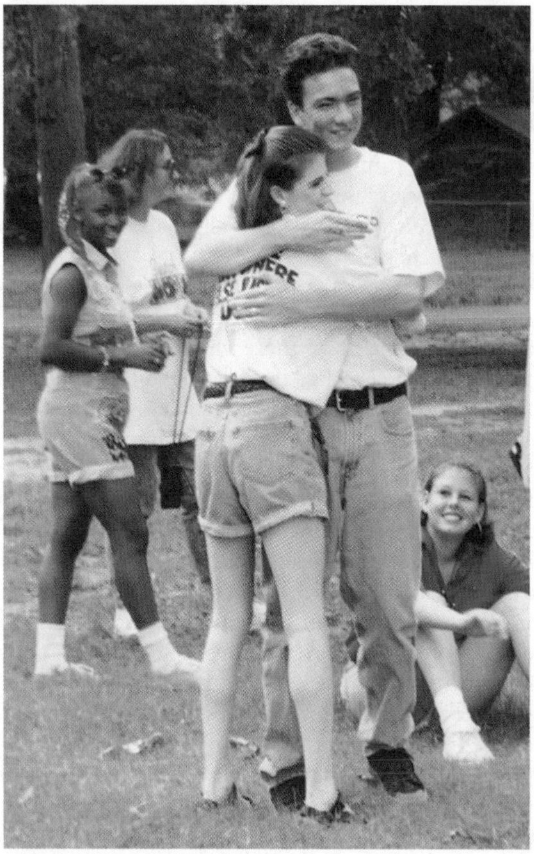

Fig. 40-5 Heterosexual relationships are an important part of adolescence.

For example, a group of girls just happen to be around a certain group of boys at most activities. During high school, crowd dates are still popular, but there is more pairing off of couples. Double-dating and then single-pair dating follow group dating. Most adolescents are dating to some degree by the time they leave high school.

The type and degree of seriousness of heterosexual relationships vary. The initial stage is usually noncommittal, extremely mobile, and seldom characterized by any deep romantic attachments. Crushes, those strong feelings of attachment to an important or well-liked adult who embodies the qualities considered most valuable by the adolescent, are common in early adolescence and constitute one of the earliest "love" attachments. The behavioral sequencing in sexual development is from less to more intimate forms of behavior with another person.

Middle adolescence is the time when teenagers begin to develop romantic relationships and when most teenagers begin sexual experimentation. Early and middle adolescents choose their partners based on physical and personality characteristics that are acceptable to their peer group. Through these relationships and experimentation, early and middle adolescents begin to explore and understand romantic feelings and experiences. As teenagers move into late adolescence, the partner choice is more likely to be based on individual characteristics and interests.

Sexual Activity

Sexuality and sexual activity is an area that should be addressed with each adolescent in a confidential manner. Messages to postpone sexual involvement must begin by the middle school period. Although sexual activity rates have decreased for older teens, the percentage of teens under 15 years of age who are engaging in sexual activity has increased. Among teenagers who have initiated sexual intercourse at an age younger than 14 years, the incidence of sexual abuse is very high. However, by 17 years of age, more than 50% of teenagers have had volitional sexual intercourse (Alan Guttmacher Institute, 1998).

Adolescents report the pressure to have sex is exceeded only by the pressure to drink. This pressure to engage in sexual activity is strongest for those who have already been sexually active and for males. Teens engage in a wide range of sexual activity including kissing and petting, oral sex, and vaginal and rectal sex. Teens remain uninformed about sexually transmitted disease transmission, contraception, and access to confidential care (Hoff, Greene, & Davis, 2003). Many adolescents feel uncomfortable bringing up sexual health issues with their health care provider. They prefer to have the provider approach the subject in a clear and direct manner. Discomfort about sexuality issues on the part of the provider presents a barrier for teens in need of accurate health information.

Adolescents become involved in sexual relationships for a wide variety of reasons: to obtain pleasurable sensations, to satisfy sexual drives, to satisfy curiosity, as a conquest, as an expression of affection, or because they are not able to withstand pressures to conform. Often the urge to belong to and gain reassurance from a group and the wish to really belong to someone provoke a series of increasingly intimate physical contacts with a favored boyfriend or girlfriend.

Homosexuality in Adolescents

During adolescence, youths develop a sexual identity. This process becomes incredibly complicated when the sexual identity is not heterosexual. Retrospective studies of gay men and lesbians indicate that adolescence is when individuals become aware of same-sex attraction. Gay men become aware of same-sex attraction at a younger mean age than women. Homosexual and bisexual youths face tremendous challenges to growing up and becoming mentally and physically healthy when confronted with antihomosexual attitudes and values. These adolescents are at increased risk for health-damaging behaviors, not because of the sexual behavior itself, but because of society's reaction to the behavior (Saewyc et al, 1998). Behaviors that place homosexual and bisexual youths at risk for poor health outcomes include early initiation of sexual activity (usually heterosexual), substance abuse, suicide and suicidal ideation, running away from home, and engaging in behaviors that result in sexually transmitted diseases. Nurses should view gay and lesbian youth within the broader context of general adolescent development. The goal is not to identify all gay and lesbian youth but to provide a safe environment for appropriate health care (Garofalo & Katz, 2001) (Critical Thinking Exercise).

Interests and Activities

Adolescents spend a large amount of time engaging in leisure-time activities. As teenagers progress through the developmental stages of adolescence, these leisure-time activities move from being family centered to being peer centered. In addition to providing teenagers with fun and enjoyment, leisure-time activities assist in the development of social, physical, and cognitive skills. Leisure-time activities also allow teenagers the opportunity to learn to set priorities and structure their time (Fig. 40-6).

Today, many adolescents must learn to juggle their time between school, leisure-time activities, and the responsibilities of a job. Adolescent work experiences provide many benefits, including time management, teamwork skills, and

??? Critical Thinking Exercise

DISCUSSING SEXUAL ORIENTATION WITH ADOLESCENTS

John, a 17-year-old adolescent, comes into the school-based clinic and tells the nurse practitioner that he thinks he is homosexual. What is the most appropriate response for the nurse practitioner?

1. Evidence—Is there sufficient evidence to draw any conclusions about John's sexual orientation at this time?
2. Assumptions—Describe an underlying assumption about each of the following issues:
   a. Sexual orientation in adolescents
   b. Society's reaction to homosexuality
   c. Health care professionals and sexuality
3. What implications and priorities for nursing care can be drawn at this time?
4. Does the evidence support your argument (conclusion)?
5. Are there alternative perspectives to your arguments? What are they?

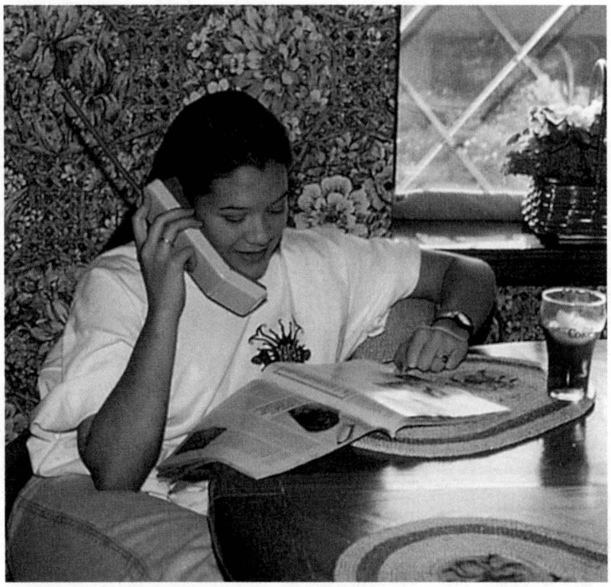

Fig. 40-6 The telephone, especially the portable phone, provides teenagers with hours of conversation with same-sex and opposite-sex friends.

increased income. However, many jobs available to teenagers do not provide opportunities to apply the skills they learn in school, and jobs often have high demands for quick work with low rewards. Very few apprentice opportunities are available for teenagers. It is generally recommended that adolescents limit their work to no more than 20 hours per week during the school year.

Development of Self-Concept and Body Image

The sudden growth that takes place in early adolescence creates feelings of confusion for adolescents. They have lost the security of a familiar body and feel uncomfortable with their altered body. Consequently, they may try to either hide their body or advertise it, or they may alternate between the two extremes. Teenagers are acutely aware of their appearance as they begin to acquire images of themselves as adults, but they see discrepancies between their ideal and actual skills and abilities.

Adolescents are continually comparing themselves with their peers and making judgments about their own normality based on these observations. Pubertal children feel most comfortable when they are just like their friends and agemates. Perceived defects or deviations from the group average are threatening to their idealized image. Any blemish is likely to be magnified out of proportion, and any delay of the visible evidence of maturity is cause for worry. Unfortunately, this is also the time when the hormonal effect of the sebaceous glands produces acne, which creates problems for many youngsters. To the adolescent, even the most insignificant pimple may be viewed as a gross disfigurement. The advent of chronic disease or a permanent physical disability has very special significance during adolescence and creates additional stresses for both youngsters with the condition and health care providers.

It has been determined that the body image established during adolescence is the one that individuals retain throughout life. Much of adolescents' search for identity takes place before a mirror as they try to read from the reflected features just who they are and what they look like to other people. Adolescents practice facial expressions and postures, try out hair arrangements, worry about a pimple, and in other ways attempt to assess the best means to achieve a maximum effect—to reveal the "true self."

The self-concept becomes more differentiated as adolescents acquire a more complex picture of themselves, one that takes situational factors into account. The self-concept gradually becomes more individualized and more distinct from the concepts of others. Although younger teenagers describe themselves in terms of similarities with peers, as adolescence advances, young people describe themselves in terms of their special characteristics.

Responses to Puberty

The response to the physical changes of pubertal growth and development is manifested differently depending on the stage of development. During early adolescence, young adolescents become preoccupied with the rapid changes in their body and are very interested in the anatomy, physiology, and function of their sexual organs. Boys must also confront the sexual feelings and tensions that accompany puberty, and the appearance of nocturnal emissions may be puzzling, troublesome, or embarrassing events. Unless the boy has been prepared in advance, he may find it difficult to discuss his feelings with his parents and may turn to his friends for information and guidance. Many girls also find the rapid changes in their body to be sources of concern. Some girls perceive the increase in weight and associated fat deposition as evidence of obesity and may indulge in fad diets. Although many girls look forward to menstruation and take this event in stride, others may find the first menstrual period a distressing and frightening event. All teenagers, regardless of gender, are very concerned with the question, "Am I normal?" To answer this question, they compare their body with the bodies of their peers and with images in the media. This leads to a great deal of uncertainty about their appearance and attractiveness.

If an adolescent does not enter puberty at the same time as his or her peers, considerable inner conflict may occur. Early-maturing girls and boys, as well as late-maturing boys, have higher rates of risk-taking behaviors than their on-time peers (Graber et al, 1997; Hayward et al, 1997). Nurses who work with adolescents must provide teaching and health care interventions that are appropriate for the chronologic and cognitive development of the adolescent rather than the physical maturation.

As growth and development proceed through middle adolescence, the rapid body changes diminish, and the adolescent has time to try to make the body more attractive. Adolescents strive to achieve the perfect body within their own cultural norms. The "right" clothes and hairstyle become very important. By late adolescence the heightened concern with body image has ended and is replaced with a general comfort with the body.

The changes that occur during the early, middle, and late phases of adolescence are summarized in Table 40-1.

Table 40-1

Growth and Development during Adolescence

EARLY ADOLESCENCE (11-14 YEARS)	MIDDLE ADOLESCENCE (15-17 YEARS)	LATE ADOLESCENCE (18-20 YEARS)
GROWTH		
Rapidly accelerating growth Reaches peak velocity Secondary sex characteristics appear	Growth decelerating in girls Stature reaches 95% of adult height Secondary sex characteristics well advanced	Physically mature Structure and reproductive growth almost complete
COGNITION		
Explores newfound ability for limited abstract thought Clumsy groping for new values and energies Comparison of "normality" with peers of same sex	Developing capacity for abstract thinking Enjoys intellectual powers, often in idealistic terms Concern with philosophic, political, and social problems	Established abstract thought Can perceive and act on long-range options Able to view problems comprehensively Intellectual and functional identity established
IDENTITY		
Preoccupied with rapid body changes Trying out of various roles Measurement of attractiveness by acceptance or rejection of peers Conformity to group norms	Modifies body image Very self-centered; increased narcissism Tendency toward inner experience and self-discovery Has a rich fantasy life Idealistic Able to perceive future implications of current behavior and decisions; variable application	Body image and gender-role definition nearly secured Mature sexual identity Phase of consolidation of identity Stability of self-esteem Comfortable with physical growth Social roles defined and articulated
RELATIONSHIPS WITH PARENTS		
Defining independence-dependence boundaries Strong desire to remain dependent on parents while trying to detach No major conflicts over parental control	Major conflicts over independence and control Low point in parent-child relationship Greatest push for emancipation; disengagement Final and irreversible emotional detachment from parents; mourning	Emotional and physical separation from parents completed Independence from family with less conflict Emancipation nearly secured
RELATIONSHIPS WITH PEERS		
Seeks peer affiliations to counter instability generated by rapid change Upsurge of close, idealized friendships with members of the same sex Struggle for mastery takes place within peer group	Strong need for identity to affirm self-image Behavioral standards set by peer group Acceptance by peers extremely important—fear of rejection Exploration of ability to attract opposite sex	Peer group recedes in importance in favor of individual friendship Testing of romantic relationships against possibility of permanent alliance Relationships characterized by giving and sharing
SEXUALITY		
Self-exploration and evaluation Limited dating, usually group Limited intimacy	Multiple plural relationships Internal identification of heterosexuality, homosexual, or bisexual attractions Exploration of "self appeal" Feeling of "being in love" Tentative establishment of relationships	Forms stable relationships and attachment to another Growing capacity for mutuality and reciprocity Dating as a romantic pair May publicly identify as gay, lesbian, or bisexual Intimacy involves commitment rather than exploration and romanticism
PSYCHOLOGIC HEALTH		
Wide mood swings Intense daydreaming Anger outwardly expressed with moodiness, temper outbursts, and verbal insults and name-calling	Tendency toward inner experiences; more introspective Tendency to withdraw when upset or feelings are hurt Vacillation of emotions in time and range Feelings of inadequacy common; difficulty in asking for help	More constancy of emotion Anger more apt to be concealed

PROMOTING OPTIMUM HEALTH DURING ADOLESCENCE

The major causes of morbidity and mortality in adolescence are not diseases, but health-damaging behaviors. New sources of morbidity in adolescence include injury, depression, violence, sexually transmitted infections, and pregnancy. Health promotion for this age group consists mainly of teaching and guidance to avoid risk-taking activities and health-damaging behaviors. Adolescence provides an opportunity for teenagers to incorporate healthy lifestyle behaviors that will benefit them not only during the teenage years, but also throughout the life span.

Effective health education for adolescents should incorporate a developmentally appropriate, multifaceted approach, but education alone is not enough to change behavior. Effective programs must include opportunities for skill building and must be comprehensive rather than problem focused and include a community-wide approach (Hamburg, 1997).

As teenagers progress through adolescence, they are able to assume additional responsibility for their own health, including maintaining health practices, taking prescribed medications, keeping appointments, and performing procedures when necessary. Health professionals who work with adolescents should consider the adolescent's increasing independence and responsibility while maintaining privacy and ensuring confidentiality (Guidelines box and Critical Thinking Exercise). Parents should also respect their teenager's independence and move toward the role of consultant about health issues while also maintaining some level of parental involvement throughout adolescence.

In response to changes in adolescent morbidity and mortality, the American Medical Association developed the Guidelines for Adolescent Preventive Services (GAPS), which provide a framework for health care providers to use in their clinical practice. The following discussion provides information on specific GAPS topics and recommendations related to screening, guidance, and immunizations.

evolve CASE STUDY: INTERVIEWING ADOLESCENTS

Guidelines

INTERVIEWING ADOLESCENTS

Ensure confidentiality and privacy; interview adolescent without parents.

Show concern for adolescent's perspective: "First, I'd like to talk about your main concerns" and "I'd like to know what you think is happening."

Offer a nonthreatening explanation for the questions you ask: "I'm going to ask a number of questions to help me better understand your health."

Maintain objectivity; avoid assumptions, judgments, and lectures.

Ask open-ended questions when possible; move to more directive questions if necessary.

Begin with less sensitive issues and proceed to more sensitive ones.

Use language that both the adolescent and you understand. Clarify terms, such as "having sex."

Restate: reflect back to adolescents what they have said, along with feelings that may be associated with their descriptions.

Critical Thinking Exercise

RESPECTING PRIVACY

Jamie, a 17-year-old girl, arrives at the adolescent clinic with her mother, Mrs. S, for a routine history and physical examination with the nurse practitioner. As the nurse practitioner walks with Jamie to an examination room, Mrs. S whispers to the nurse practitioner, "I need to speak with you in private." How should the nurse practitioner respond to Mrs. S's request?

1. Evidence—Is there sufficient evidence to formulate a response to Jamie's mother?
2. Assumptions—Describe an underlying assumption about each of the following topics:
   a. The role of the adolescent in health care
   b. The role of the parents in the health of their adolescent
   c. Adolescents and confidentiality
3. What implications for nursing care should be established at this time?
4. Does the evidence support your conclusion?
5. Are there alternative perspectives that you should consider?

Immunizations

An immunization update is an important part of adolescent preventive care. Obtaining a record of the teenager's prior immunizations is important. Adolescents should receive a tetanus-diphtheria (Td) vaccine at the age of 11 to 12 years if a period of at least 5 years has elapsed since the last dose of diphtheria-tetanus-pertussis or acellular pertussis, or diphtheria-tetanus (DTP, DTaP, or DT) vaccine. Subsequent routine Td boosters are recommended every 10 years. With the exception of pregnant teenagers, all adolescents should receive a second measles-mumps-rubella (MMR) vaccine unless they have documentation of two MMR vaccinations during childhood but not before 12 months of age. All adolescents who have not previously received three doses of hepatitis B vaccine should be vaccinated against hepatitis B virus. All adolescents should also be assessed for previous history of varicella infection or vaccination. Vaccination with the varicella vaccine is recommended for those with no previous history. For adolescents over age 13 years, the varicella vaccine is given in 2 doses 4 or more weeks apart. Hepatitis A vaccine should be given to adolescents living in communities with high rates of hepatitis A or those with risk factors for hepatitis A such as injectable drug use or high-risk sexual activity (American Academy of Pediatrics [AAP], Committee on Infectious Diseases, 2003). College freshmen living in dormitories are at increased risk for meningococcal disease. Discussions for incoming college students and their parents should include encouragement to obtain the meningococcal immunization (Rosenstein, Fischer, & Tappero, 2001) (See also Immunizations, Chapter 36.)

Nutrition

The rapid and extensive increase in height, weight, muscle mass, and sexual maturity of adolescence is accompanied by increased nutritional requirements. Because nutritional needs are closely related to the increase in body mass, the peak requirements occur in the years of maximum growth, during which the body mass almost doubles. The caloric and protein requirements during this time are higher than at almost any other time of life. As a result of this increased anabolic need, the adolescent is highly sensitive to caloric restrictions.

The nutritional needs of adolescents are difficult to determine because of meager nutrition information on members of this age group. This difficulty is further complicated by the influence of emotional and other stress factors affecting nutrient utilization and the psychologic factors that influence eating habits. In addition, the wide variations in growth rates during adolescence and the equally wide variations in ages at which these changes take place complicate attempts to set minimum dietary standards.

Adolescents usually have sufficient intake of protein to meet their needs, except those who limit their food intake because of economic problems or in an attempt to lose weight. The need for the minerals calcium, iron, and zinc substantially increases during periods of rapid growth: calcium for skeletal growth, iron for expansion of muscle mass and blood volume, and zinc for the generation of both skeletal and bone tissue. Girls with very heavy or frequent menses may be especially susceptible to iron deficiency due to blood loss. Calcium intake from food sources is essential during adolescence to assist in the prevention of osteoporosis. Eventual bone mass is a balance between the amount of bone laid down during adolescence and the amount later lost with aging. Overall, osteoporosis is a result of genetic and environmental factors such as nutrition and exercise (Ralston, 1997). Dietary intervention should promote the regular consumption of breakfast and a balanced intake of a variety of foods.

Eating Habits and Behavior

Eating and attitudes toward food are primarily family centered during early and middle childhood, and food habits are largely related to cultural and individual family preferences and patterns. With adolescence and the move toward independence, family influences on the child change. Children's interests, attitudes, and routines are altered as an increasing number of meals are eaten away from home. These changes are largely a result of the high value that teenagers place on peer acceptability and sociability. Their peers easily influence their eating habits.

Pressure for time and commitments to activities adversely affect the teenager's eating habits. Omitting breakfast or eating a breakfast that is nutritionally poor in quality is frequently a problem. Snacks, usually selected on the basis of accessibility rather than nutritional merit, become more and more a part of the habitual eating pattern during adolescence (Fig. 40-7). Adolescents often eat an insufficient amount of fresh fruits and vegetables, especially those that are rich in ascorbic acid. Milk is usually passed over in favor of soft drinks.

Overeating or undereating during adolescence presents special problems. When they experience the normal increase in weight and fat deposition of the growth spurt, teenage girls often resort to dieting. The desire for a slim figure and a fear of becoming "fat" prompt teenage girls to embark on

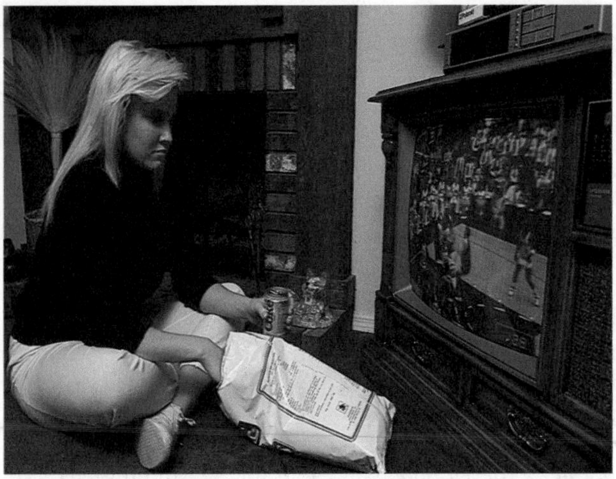

Fig. 40-7 Snacking on empty calories is common among adolescents, especially during inactivity.

nutritionally inadequate reducing regimens that drain their energy and deprive their growing bodies of essential nutrients. They resort to diets on their own or with peers in an effort to conform. Many adopt current fad diets and are victims of food misinformation. Boys are less inclined to undereat. They are more concerned about gaining size and strength. However, they tend to eat foods high in calories but low in other essential nutrients.

Obesity is increasing among both children and adolescents in the United States. The obesity currently seen is not a result of metabolic disturbances, but of poor dietary habits and increased sedentary lifestyles. Childhood obesity often results in obesity in adulthood. The last two decades have revealed an increase in the overall portion size for foods. The largest portions for most foods are found at fast food restaurants. However, portion sizes for desserts and hamburgers are the largest at home (Nielsen & Popkin, 2003). Lifestyle changes necessary for adolescents to lose weight require the involvement of family members who provide support and encourage active participation.

Nursing Care Management

Healthy dietary habits should be discussed with all adolescents. Adolescents need to learn about the Food Guide Pyramid; the relationships among dietary fat, weight status, and health; and food sources of fat, salt, and fiber (Seidell, 1999). Their food habits must be considered when planning nutrition education and guidance because they reflect many influences and conditions. Nurses in the school setting can assist in advocating for comprehensive nutrition services for preschool through grade twelve students. Comprehensive nutrition education with access to nutritious meals and snacks and physical activity at school will begin to reverse the trend of childhood obesity (Briggs, Safaii, & Beall, 2003).

To help teenagers select a nutritious diet, it is best to begin with their present diet and actively involve them in the process. Teenagers do not respond well to judgmental attitudes and dislike lectures, but they do respond when their independence is respected, and they are given the opportunity to make their own decisions regarding food choices.

In general, adolescents are body conscious and concerned about their appearance. Concrete messages about the relationship between an attractive appearance and the benefits of a healthy lifestyle are most effective. However, helping young persons arrive at a decision for change is more difficult than providing information. They respond best when the counselor provides straightforward information, uses instructional methods that actively involve them, talks *with* them and not at them, and listens to what they have to say.

Sleep and Rest

Teenagers vary in their need for sleep and rest. Rapid physical growth, the tendency toward overexertion, and the overall increased activity of this age contribute to fatigue in adolescents. During growth spurts the need for sleep is increased. Their propensity for staying up late makes it very difficult to arise in the morning, and they may sleep late at every opportunity. Adequate sleep and rest at this time are important to a total health regimen.

Exercise and Activity

Although today's youth are less fit than children 20 years ago, adolescents probably spend more time and energy practicing and participating in sports activities than members of any other age group. Many adolescents participate in sports within school settings (Fig. 40-8). School-based, health-oriented physical education may provide both immediate effects of the activity and sustained effects through encouragement of lifelong activity patterns. Although daily physical education classes have decreased in schools in the last 10 years, the physical education classes that are held include more time spent in actual physical activity (Centers for Disease Control and Prevention [CDC], 2000).

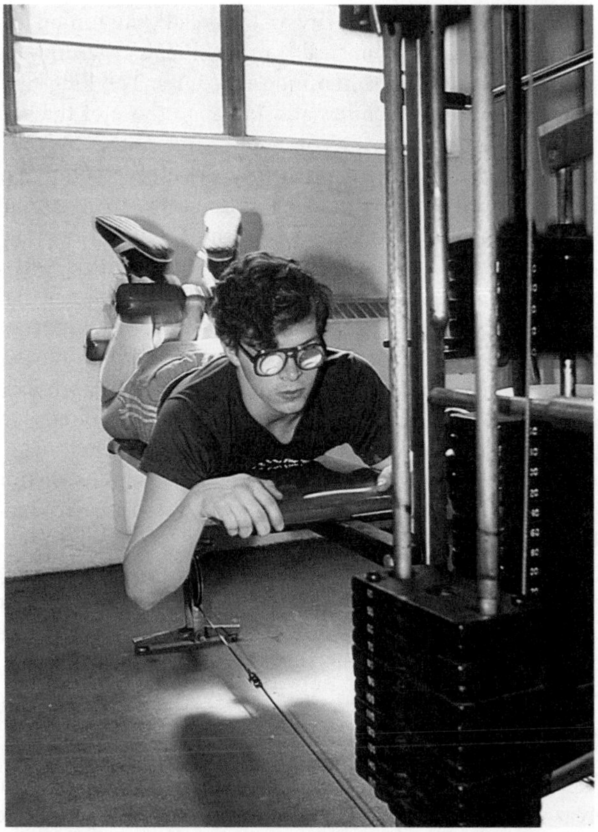

Fig. 40-8 Adolescents should be encouraged to participate in activities that contribute to lifelong physical fitness.

The practice of sports, games, and even dancing contributes significantly to growth and development, the education process, and better health. These activities provide exercise for growing muscles, interactions with peers, and a socially acceptable means of enjoying stimulation and conflict. In addition, competitive activities help the teenager in the process of self-appraisal, the development of self-respect, and concern for others. Because physical fitness appears to be a major influence on one's lifelong health status, children should be encouraged to participate in activities that contribute to lifelong physical fitness. Nurses can encourage participation as a way to promote health and build self-esteem. However, youngsters should not be encouraged to engage in physical activities that are beyond their physical or emotional capacity (see Health Problems Related to Sports Participation, Chapter 39).

Dental Health

Dental health should not be neglected during adolescence, although the rate of caries formation is not as great as in childhood. Dental care is an aspect of preventive care that substantial proportions of children in the United States do not receive. Pit and fissure sealants are an underutilized safe and effective technique for dental caries prevention (Simonsen, 2002). Early adolescence is usually when corrective orthodontic appliances are worn, and these are commonly a source of embarrassment and concern to the youngster. Reassurance regarding the temporary nature of the annoyance and anticipation of an improved appearance help make the inconvenience tolerable. It is also important to reinforce the orthodontist's directions regarding use and care of the appliances and to emphasize careful attention to toothbrushing during this time (see also Chapters 37 and 39).

Personal Care

The body-conscious teenager is highly amenable to discussion and counseling about personal care and hygiene. Body changes associated with puberty bring special needs for cleanliness. The hyperactive sebaceous glands and newly functioning apocrine glands make frequent bathing or showering a necessity, and underarm deodorants assume an important place in personal care. The adolescent discovers that hair requires more frequent shampooing, and girls often have questions about hair removal, use of cosmetics, and menstrual hygiene. Peer group discussions center on the advantages of particular products or methods. Adolescents are continually bombarded with messages from the media regarding the best way to enhance their popularity and attractiveness. Nurses are in a position to help them evaluate the relative merits of commercial products.

Vision

Regular vision testing is an important part of health care and supervision during adolescence. During adolescence, visual refractive difficulties reach a peak that is not exceeded until the fifth decade of life. The increased demands of schoolwork make adequate vision essential for academic success. Consequently, teenagers are more likely to be referred for visual evaluation. The need for corrective lenses can create psychologic problems for teenagers if they believe that glasses spoil their appearance or do not fit their body image. For those who can afford them, contact lenses are a preferred solution. For some, the impact of a visual defect, no matter how slight, may be stressful.

Hearing

Considerable concern has focused on current teenage practices that cause hearing damage. Cochlear damage from relatively continuous exposure to the loud sound levels of rock music has been documented. The popularity of portable radios, stereo cassettes, and compact disc (CD) players with lightweight earphones are of particular concern to health care professionals. When these units are used for extended periods, permanent hearing loss can occur. Although appeals for more judicious use are not always successful, teenagers should be informed of the risk. Efforts directed toward legislating legal limits to the noise exposure that can be achieved through the sets may be another possible solution. (See Chapter 42 for a discussion of noise-related hearing loss.)

Posture

Many adolescents demonstrate altered posture. Rapid skeletal growth is often associated with slower muscular growth, and as a result, some teenagers may appear awkward or slump and fail to stand or sit upright. However, some postural defects of adolescence require early medical intervention. Scoliosis is a defect of the spine that occurs frequently in adolescence and is more common in girls than in boys (see Scoliosis, Chapter 54). The majority of the cases are idiopathic, and the defect presents as a painless curvature of the spine. Fortunately, most of these spinal curvatures will not require treatment. However, because there is no way to predict which curvatures will progress, all curvatures of the spine should be referred for further evaluation.

Body Art

Body art (piercing and tattooing) is utilized to assist with adolescent identity formation. The skin has become the latest source of parent-adolescent conflict. The adolescent often seeks body art as an expression of his or her personal identity and style. Tattoos are often obtained to mark significant life events such as new relationships, births, and deaths. Piercing the ear, nose, nipple, navel, penis, or tongue may sometimes create a health problem in the uninformed teenager. It is a nursing responsibility to caution girls and boys against the practice of having piercing performed by friends, mothers, or themselves. Although most cases of piercing are accompanied by few if any serious side effects, there is always a danger of complications such as infection, cyst or keloid formation, bleeding, dermatitis, or metal allergy. Using the same unsterilized needle to pierce body parts of multiple teenagers presents the same risk of human immunodeficiency virus (HIV) and hepatitis B virus transmission as occurs with other needle-sharing activities.

A qualified operator using proper sterile technique should perform the procedure. This is especially important if a youngster has a history of diabetes, allergies, or skin disorders. Adolescents should be informed about the approximate time for healing after body piercing and the care of the pierced area during and after healing. Some body sites require extra precautions. For example, cartilage (ear, nose) has a poor blood supply and heals slowly and scars easily; nipple piercing puts the adolescent at risk for breast abscess. Finally, migration of the piercing is common with naval and other flat skin surface piercing. Piercing guns should not be used for piercing anything other than the earlobe because guns place the piercing too deeply.

Nearly 15% of adolescents have at least one tattoo (Carroll et al, 2002). Professionals as well as amateur artists administer tattoos. The risk to the adolescent receiving a tattoo is low. The greatest risk is for the tattoo artist who comes in contact with the client's blood. Adolescents who are amateur tattoo artists benefit from discussions about universal precautions and the hepatitis B vaccination. Many states either have no regulations or do not enforce existing regulations of piercing and tattooing facilities. The state health department is a source of information about local regulatory requirements.

Suntanning

The quest for an attractive appearance leads many teenagers to excessive sunbathing and artificial means for suntanning. However, this practice has serious long-term risks, and the adolescent should be educated regarding the detrimental effects of sunlight on the skin (see Sunburn, Chapter 53). Long-term effects include premature aging of the skin; increased risk of skin cancer; and, in susceptible individuals, phototoxic reactions.

The increasing popularity of artificial suntanning has prompted concern from health professionals regarding the use of sunlamps and suntanning machines. The long-term effects of tanning machines are similar to those of the sun; dermatologists do not recommend suntanning by these means. Those who insist on using suntanning equipment should be warned that goggles must be worn in tanning booths to prevent serious corneal burning. Education on the use of sunscreens, including hypoallergenic products, with a sun protective factor (SPF) of at least 15 and a nonalcohol base without lanolin, parobens, or fragrance is important (Starr, 1999). Self-tanning creams safely simulate the appearance of a tan; however, teens using these products should be cautioned that sun protection is still required. Targeting health education messages to adolescents and incorporating educational components relating to sun protection behaviors in school health curricula are essential (Hoffman, Rodrique, & Johnson, 1999). A large cross-sectional study of 12- to 18-year-olds in the United States found that teens are not following these recommendations; 34% used sunscreen routinely in the past summer and 14% used a tanning bed at least once (Geller et al, 2002).

Stress Reduction

The multiple changes occurring in adolescence can result in great stress (Fig. 40-9 and Box 40-2). Adolescents are faced with pressures from peers that often involve flaunting adult

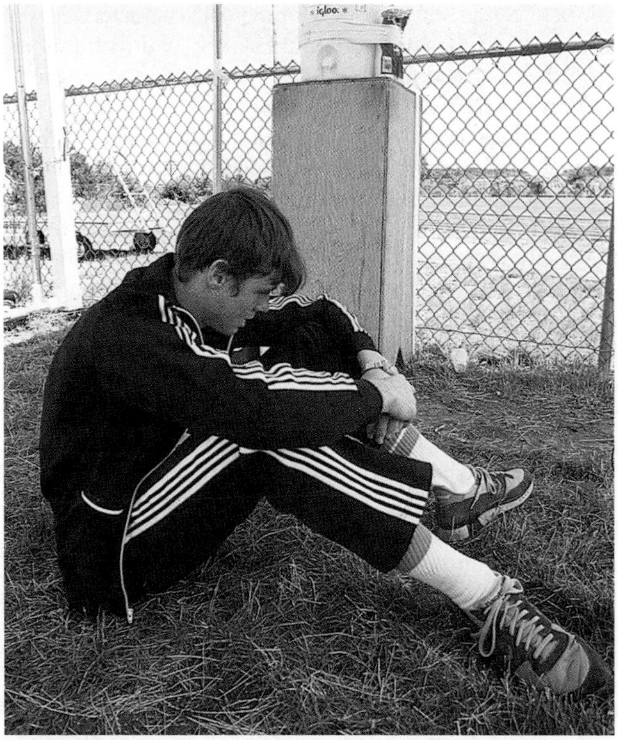

Fig. 40-9 Adolescents use being alone as a method of coping with stress.

BOX 40-2

Areas of Stress in Adolescence

Body image
Sexuality conflicts
Scholastic pressures
Competitive pressures
Relationships with parents
Relationships with siblings
Relationships with peers
Finances
Decisions about present and future roles
Career planning
Ideologic conflicts

authority and taking serious health risks. Health risks include pressures for sexual experimentation and use of drugs, alcohol, and cigarettes, as well as potentially dangerous physical activities.

Early-maturing girls and late-maturing children are especially sensitive to the stresses of being different from their peers. Many feel intense anxiety over their identity. Both early- and late-maturing children feel out of place among their classmates, but slow-maturing children appear to suffer the most pronounced inner turmoil and may be hesitant to voice their concerns. Slow-maturing youngsters need support and reassurance that they are not abnormal and need only be patient until the time comes when they, too, will develop the characteristics for which they yearn.

Sexuality Education and Guidance

Contemporary adolescents are constantly exposed to sexual symbolism and erotic stimulation from the mass media. At the same time, the development of primary and secondary sex characteristics and the increased sensitivity of the genitals produce thoughts and fantasies about sexual relationships. Sexual aspects of interpersonal relationships become particularly important. Societal expectations push adolescents toward dating, and their own inner sex drive urges them toward exploration.

Our society continues to do a poor job of educating adolescents about pubertal growth and development. Omar, McElderry, and Zakharia (2003) found that 36% of males and 2% of females never were spoken to about pubertal development or sexuality issues. Girls received education at a mean age of 13 years and boys at an average age of 15 years. A large portion of their knowledge relating to sex is acquired from their peers, television, the movies, and magazines. In addition, some information obtained from their parents may be inaccurate. As a result, the information they accumulate may be incomplete, inaccurate, riddled with cultural and moral judgments, and not very helpful.

The responsibility for providing sexuality education has been assumed by parents, schools, churches, community agencies such as Planned Parenthood Federation of America, Inc.*, and health professionals, especially nurses. Many adolescents perceive nurses, especially school nurses, as individuals who possess important information and who are willing to discuss sex with them. To be able to discuss the topic adequately, nurses must have not only an understanding of the physiologic aspects of sexuality and a knowledge of cultural and societal values, but also an awareness of their own attitudes, feelings, and biases about sexuality.

Comprehensive information about sexuality education is offered by the Sexuality Information and Education Council of the United States (SIECUS)† and the Sex Information and Education Council of Canada (SIECCAN).‡ SIECUS maintains that every sexuality education program should present the topic from six aspects: biologic, social, health, personal adjustments and attitudes, interpersonal associations, and the establishment of values.

Whether nurses counsel young people on an individual basis, in mixed groups, or in groups segregated by gender makes little difference. Ideally, boys and girls should be able to discuss sexuality objectively with one another and in groups, but this is not always possible. The differences in the rate of maturation between boys and girls and between different members of the same sex often make it desirable to discuss certain aspects of sexuality in segregated groups. As a general rule, the need for separate discussion groups diminishes as young people progress toward maturity.

*810 Seventh Ave., New York, NY 10019; phone: 800-230-PLAN; Web site: www.plannedparenthood.org.

†130 W. 42nd St., Suite 350, New York, NY 10036; phone: 212-819-9770; Web site: www.siecus.org.

‡850 Coxwell Ave., East York, Ontario M4C 5R1; phone: 416-466-5304.

Sexuality education should consist of instruction concerning normal body functions and should be presented in a straightforward manner using correct terminology. When discussing sex and sexual activities, nurses should use simple but correct language, not street language, highly scientific terminology, or evasive jargon. Once the meanings of biologic terms such as *uterus, testicles,* and *vagina* are understood, most teenagers prefer to use them in their discussions.

Many girls arrive at menarche with ambivalent attitudes, myths, and illogical beliefs. Even girls adequately prepared for menstruation do not always understand its relationship to the total process of reproduction. Many are under the incorrect impression that the "safe" time for sexual intercourse is midway between menstrual periods.

Teenagers' curiosity and desire for information extend beyond the need for anatomic and physiologic knowledge. They need to know more than the mechanics of conception, pregnancy, and birth. Adolescents, girls in particular, want answers to questions such as "What is it like?" "Does it hurt?" "What happens when . . . ?" and "Is it all right if you . . . ?" Boys are often concerned about the fallacy that a relationship exists between penis size and sexual function. They need reassurance that masturbation is a normal and common practice, that some degree of homosexuality is not unusual in early adolescence, and that oral-genital relations can be normal substitutes for intercourse.

Teenagers need to discuss intercourse, alternative methods of sexual satisfaction, and how to resist peer pressure. With the increased incidence of sexually transmitted diseases, especially HIV infection, the topic of "safe sex," especially abstinence or the use of condoms and abstinence, is essential. Role-playing can help teenagers learn effective approaches to dealing with difficult situations. Sex and sexuality cannot be taught without discussions of mature decision making, sexual responsibility, and values clarification.

Adolescents need role models and life experiences with delayed gratification. Most important, they need problem-solving experience and decision-making skills so that they can anticipate the positive and negative outcomes of a decision. With these types of assistance, teenagers can become sexually responsible young adults.

Injury Prevention

Physical injuries are the greatest single cause of death in the adolescent age group and claim more lives than all other causes combined. The most vulnerable ages are the years 15 to 24, when accidental injuries account for about 60% of deaths in boys and 40% of deaths in girls. These figures remain fairly constant from year to year and are significant because almost all fatal injuries are preventable.

During adolescence, peak physical, sensory, and psychomotor function gives teenagers a feeling of strength and confidence that they have never experienced before, and the physiologic changes of puberty give impetus to many basic instinctual forces. One manifestation of this is an increase in energy that simply must be discharged through action, often at the expense of logical thinking and other control mechanisms. Their propensity for risk-taking behavior plus feelings of indestructibility make adolescents especially prone to injuries. Some of the developmental characteristics of teenagers and the common injuries associated with this age group are outlined in Table 40-2.

Vehicle-Related Injuries

The adolescent's newly acquired ability to drive and the normal developmental need for independence and freedom make the automobile an attractive part of an adolescent's life. Forty percent of all teen deaths in the United States are the result of motor vehicle crashes (CDC, 1999). Many factors contribute to the higher rate of crashes among teen drivers including lack of driving experience and maturity, following too closely, driving too fast, having other teen passengers in the car, and using alcohol (Williams & Ferguson, 2002). Because the number of accidents significantly increase when adolescents drive at night, many states have effectively enacted driving curfews to curtail this risk. Nurses should educate teenagers and their parents about the risk of driving while drinking alcohol or when intoxicated, or of riding in an automobile with a drunk driver. Many families have developed a plan to arrange a no-questions-asked ride home to prevent an adolescent from riding with a drunk driver. Families should also require adolescents to log several hours of supervised practice driving before taking the car out alone. The major risk for death in a motor vehicle accident is failure to use a safety restraint. Teenage seat belt use, especially among males is lower than adult seat belt usage. Belt use as a passenger is low for teens even when the driver is an adult. Continued efforts to ensure teenage seat belt use should be focused at the individual educational level as well as through tough enforcement laws (Williams, McCartt, & Geary, 2003).

Nonautomotive Vehicle Injuries

The increasing use of motorized bicycles, all-terrain vehicles (ATVs), jet skis, and snowmobiles has caused an increase in injuries among youngsters below the legal age for driving automobiles. Many adolescents ride bicycles without helmets and without lights at night, and the overwhelming majority of deaths from bicycle injuries (primarily head injuries) involve teenagers.

Firearms

Firearms are the major cause of intentional fatal injuries in the United States. Adolescence is the peak age for being either a victim or an offender in an injury involving a firearm. Gun carrying among adolescents is on the rise and is not limited to the stereotypic inner-city youth. Family members and acquaintances are a common source of guns for young people. Gun availability in the general population is linked to increased gun death among children (Miller, Azrael, & Hemenway, 2002). Having a gun in the home increases the risk of adolescent suicide and homicide. All families should be assessed for the presence of a gun in the home and informed of the increased risk for suicide and homicide. When guns are present in the home, families must take preventive action to be sure that the guns are never loaded, that they are locked up in a safe place, and that ammunition is stored and locked up separately in a location where only appropriate adults have access to it.

Nonpowder Firearms

Guns that do not use powder (e.g., air rifles, BB guns), although viewed as toys by many, account for almost as many

Table 40-2

Injury Prevention during Adolescence

DEVELOPMENTAL ABILITIES RELATED TO RISK OF INJURY	INJURY PREVENTION
Need for independence and freedom Testing independence Age permitted to drive a motor vehicle (varies) Inclination for risk taking Feeling of indestructibility Need for discharging energy, often at expense of logical thinking and other control mechanisms Strong need for peer approval May attempt hazardous feats Peak incidence for practice and participation in sports Access to more complex tools, objects, and locations Can assume responsibility for own actions	**MOTOR/NONMOTOR VEHICLES** *Pedestrian*—Emphasize and encourage safe pedestrian behavior At night, walk with a friend If someone is following you, go to nearest place with people Do not walk in secluded areas; take well-traveled walkways *Passenger*—Promote appropriate behavior while riding in a motor vehicle *Driver*—Provide competent driver education; encourage judicious use of vehicle; discourage drag racing, "playing chicken"; maintain vehicle in proper condition (brakes, tires, etc.) Teach and promote safety and maintenance of two-wheeled vehicles Promote and encourage wearing of safety apparel such as helmet, long trousers Reinforce the dangers of drugs, including alcohol, when operating a motor vehicle ***Drowning*** Teach nonswimmer to swim Teach basic rules of water safety Judicious selection of place to swim Sufficient water depth for diving Swimming with companion ***Burns*** Reinforce proper behavior in areas involving contact with burn hazards (gasoline, electric wires, fires) Advise regarding excessive exposure to natural or artificial sunlight (ultraviolet burn) Discourage smoking Encourage use of sunscreen ***Poisoning*** Educate in hazards of drug use, including alcohol ***Falls*** Teach and encourage general safety measures in all activities ***Bodily damage*** Promote acquisition of proper instruction in sports and use of sports equipment Instruct in safe use of and respect for firearms and other devices with potential danger (e.g., power tools, firecrackers) Provide and encourage use of protective equipment when using potentially hazardous devices Promote access to and/or provision of safe sports and recreational facilities Be alert for signs of depression (potential suicide) Discourage use of and/or availability of hazardous sports equipment (e.g., trampoline, surfboards) Instruct regarding proper use of corrective devices (e.g., glasses, contact lenses, hearing aids) Encourage and foster judicious application of safety principles and prevention

injuries as powder guns. The regulations regarding nonpowder guns are relaxed; they can be purchased legally by youngsters and are labeled as suitable for children as young as 8 years of age. Few states regulate their use. Nurses should act as child advocates and urge passage of laws to regulate the sale of these potentially dangerous "toys."

Sports Injuries

Because the degree of physical maturation, size, coordination, and endurance varies greatly among adolescents of the same age, sports competition among young people who differ greatly in strength and agility is unfair and hazardous. Matching candidates for sports should be done relative to physical maturity, height, weight, and physical fitness and skills, particularly in a sport involving rigorous body contact. Age is a less important consideration.

Every sport has some potential for injury, whether one participates in serious competition or is actively engaged in the activity for pure enjoyment. Overuse injuries are common in adolescents and result in more time missed from the activity than fractures. A large number of severe or fatal injuries occur to youths who are not physically prepared for the activity. The increase in strength and vigor in adolescence may tempt youngsters to overextend themselves, especially boys who are urged on by teammates or are stimulated by the admiration of female observers. The range of injuries sustained in sports or recreational activities can involve any part of the body and extend from relatively minor cuts, bruises, and abrasions to totally incapacitating central nervous system injuries or death. The leading cause of serious sports injuries among boys is participation in football, whereas most girls are injured while participating in gymnastics.

Nursing Care Management

Injury prevention is an ongoing part of nursing responsibility throughout the childhood years. Anticipatory guidance to parents and children regarding the expected problems and hazards related to growth and development does not end as children approach maturity. They need education in basic safety precautions, as well as instruction in skills required in the performance of activities such as sports, instruction in handling motor vehicles, proper protective equipment, and instruction in proper maintenance of equipment. During adolescence, however, health and safety education and guidance are more effective when the young people are involved directly. Parents and health professionals can emphasize the importance of safety during performance of activities and the proper conditioning and preparation for sports.

Prevention can occur on a variety of levels. Safety advocacy, changing public policy, and legislation can curtail injuries. Examples of such approaches are laws that mandate wearing seat belts, mandatory helmet use while driving moving vehicles other than automobiles, keeping the legal drinking age at 21 years, and instituting curfews for teen drivers. In addition to improving the environment, health education for teenagers and significant adults is essential. Helping adolescents understand their need for engaging in risky behavior, exploring possible negative outcomes, and weighing possible alternatives are critical components of injury prevention.

Anticipatory Guidance—Care of Families

Both adolescents and their parents are often confused and perplexed about the changes and behavior of this stage of development. Parents need support and guidance to help them through this trying time. They need to understand the changes taking place and to accept the expected behaviors that accompany the process of detachment. Parents may need help to "let go," and to promote the changed relationship from one of dependence to one of mutuality (Home Care box).

Home Care

GUIDANCE DURING ADOLESCENCE

Encourage Parents to:

- Accept adolescent as a unique individual.
- Respect adolescent's ideas, likes and dislikes, and wishes.
- Be involved with school functions and attend adolescent's performances, whether it be a sporting event or a school play.
- Listen and try to be open to teenager's views, even when they disagree with parental views.
- Avoid criticism about no-win topics.
- Provide opportunity for choosing options and accept natural consequences of these choices.
- Allow young person to learn by doing, even when choices and methods differ from those of adults.
- Provide adolescent with clear, reasonable limits.
- Clarify house rules and consequences for breaking them.
- Let society's rules and consequences teach responsibility outside the home.
- Allow increasing independence within limitations of safety and well-being.
- Be available but avoid pressing teenager too far.
- Respect adolescent's privacy.
- Try to share adolescent's feelings of joy or sorrow.
- Respond to feelings, as well as words.
- Be available to answer questions, give information, and provide companionship.
- Try to make communication clear.
- Avoid comparisons with siblings.
- Assist adolescent in selecting appropriate career goals and preparing for adult role.
- Welcome adolescent's friends into the home and treat them with respect.
- Provide unconditional love.
- Be willing to apologize when mistaken.

Be Aware that Adolescents:

- Are subject to turbulent, unpredictable behavior.
- Are struggling for independence.
- Are extremely sensitive to feelings and behavior that affect them.
- May receive a different message than what was sent.
- Consider friends extremely important.
- Have a strong need to belong.

Special Health Problems

DISORDERS RELATED TO THE REPRODUCTIVE SYSTEM

Amenorrhea

Menarche, or the first menstrual period, occurs relatively late in female pubertal development. Although there is variation among girls in the onset and rate of progression of pubertal development, the sequence and tempo should be the same. When an adolescent presents with a complaint of absence of menses, a careful history of the timing of her pubertal development will help determine if there is a need for further evaluation or if reassurance is all that is necessary.

Primary amenorrhea is an absence of secondary sex characteristics and no uterine bleeding by 14 to 15 years of age, or absence of uterine bleeding with secondary sex characteristics by 16 to 16½ years of age. No uterine bleeding after attaining sexual maturity rating 5 (SMR 5) for 1 year, or after breast development for 4 years, is also considered primary amenorrhea (Neinstein, 2002). The etiology of primary amenorrhea may be anatomic, hormonal, genetic, or idiopathic. A thorough history and physical examination will provide clues to the etiology.

Secondary amenorrhea is defined as the absence of menses for 6 months or at least three cycles after menstruation was previously established. Irregular menstrual cycles are common within the first year or two after menarche. These early cycles may be anovulatory resulting in regular, irregular or absent bleeding; however, cycle lengths greater than 90 days are rare and should be investigated (Timmreck & Reindollar, 2003). Girls with a later onset of menarche will take longer to establish regular ovulatory cycles. Pregnancy is the most common cause of secondary amenorrhea and should be ruled out in both types of amenorrhea, even if the adolescent denies sexual activity. When pregnancy has been ruled out, the history should be evaluated for evidence of stress, weight changes, and changes in the environment. Other common causes of amenorrhea in adolescents include hyperandrogenism, eating disorders, and exercise-induced amenorrhea (Hillard & Nelson, 2003).

Dysmenorrhea

A certain amount of discomfort during the first day or two of the menstrual flow is extremely common. Most girls experience cramping, abdominal pain, backache, and leg ache, but in a few the pain is intolerable and incapacitating. *Primary* dysmenorrhea is painful menses not related to any pelvic disease. When the discomfort is related to endometriosis, infection, adhesions from peritonitis, or other pelvic disease, the complaint is termed *secondary dysmenorrhea.*

Primary dysmenorrhea usually begins at the time of menarche or within 6 to 12 months. The pain begins with menstrual flow or hours before the onset of bleeding each month, usually continuing for 48 to 72 hours. The exact etiology is widely debated. The pain is clearly related to ovulatory cycles. The overproduction of uterine prostaglandins has been implicated, and women with dysmenorrhea have higher levels of prostaglandins. Overproduction of vasopressin (a hormone that stimulates the contraction of muscular tissue) may also contribute to dysmenorrhea.

A careful history should include the onset of symptoms, the duration, type of pain and relationship to menstrual flow, age at menarche, family history of dysmenorrhea and sexual history. The nurse should also ask about previous treatment that has been tried including dosages of medications. Associated symptoms such as nausea, vomiting, diarrhea, and leg and back pain are helpful for diagnosis and treatment. Depending on the results of the history, the physical exam may include a gynecologic examination.

Therapeutic Management

First-line treatment for adolescents with dysmenorrhea is the administration of nonsteroidal antiinflammatory drugs that block the formation of prostaglandins for 2 to 3 days of the menstrual cycle. The girl should be instructed to begin the medication at the first sign of cramping or bleeding. Girls with vomiting at the time of menstruation benefit from beginning the medication 1 to 2 days before the onset of their menses. The medications should be taken with food.

Cyclic estrogen therapy and oral contraceptives are also effective. Simple exercises such as pelvic rocking, assuming the knee-chest position, and breathing exercises may be beneficial. Encouraging adequate personal hygiene, participation in regular activities, and methods to decrease stress should be discussed with the adolescent.

A balanced diet and specific dietary changes that may be helpful include the elimination of caffeine from the diet and the addition of herbal teas. Many dietary and herbal treatments have been tried including vitamins B_1, B_6 and E, omega-3 fatty acids, and magnesium. Vitamin B_1, 100 mg daily, is the only dietary treatment with a large clinical trial to demonstrate its effectiveness. Use of magnesium has shown promise in smaller studies (Wilson & Murphy, 2001).

Nursing Care Management

All adolescent girls need reassurance that menstruation is a normal function. When nurses are asked for advice regarding menstrual problems, they have a valuable opportunity to engage in health teaching concerning menstrual physiology and hygiene, as well as the importance of a well-balanced diet, exercise, and general health maintenance. Health teaching can dispel myths about menstruation and femininity. When assessment indicates a potential problem and the need for evaluation, referral to an appropriate practitioner, health service, or clinic may be necessary.

One of the most difficult experiences facing the adolescent girl is the gynecologic examination. Whether it is her first experience or not, she is often filled with apprehension. Almost all adolescents are extremely self-conscious about their bodies and the changes taking place. They need continuing support in the form of anticipatory guidance regarding what to expect and suggestions of what to do to relax during the procedure. Usually the stressful experience of being placed in stirrups for the pelvic examination can be avoided. The adolescent girl who is relaxed may be examined in the supine position with hips and knees flexed and legs abducted. If a female nurse is not the examiner, it is essential for her to remain with the patient during the examination to offer support and guidance.

Vaginitis

Vaginitis can be caused by physical, chemical, or infectious agents. Physical causes may include a forgotten tampon; chemical irritants include bubble bath, douching, deodorant pads, and tampons. Removal of the offending material or discontinuing use of the irritating substance is usually all that is necessary to treat physical or chemical vaginitis. Infectious vaginitis can be caused by *Candida* fungi (yeast), *Trichomonas* protozoa parasites, or bacteria. Diagnosis is confirmed with microscopic evaluation of vaginal secretions. Treatment varies depending on the infectious agent.

Health teaching is important in the prevention and management of vaginitis. Adolescent girls need reassurance that increased vaginal mucus can occur at the time of ovulation, before menstruation, or with sexual excitement. Many teenage girls mistake these variations as signs of infection. Girls should be taught to wipe from front to back after toileting and to realize that vaginitis can result from irritation, foreign objects, and sexual activity. Nurses should stress the importance of an evaluation to determine the exact cause.

Disorders of the Male Reproductive System

Most obvious anomalies, such as hypospadias, hydrocele, phimosis, and cryptorchidism, have been identified, and corrective measures have been instituted during early childhood. The most frequent problems related to the reproductive organs in later childhood are (1) infections, such as urethritis (see Urinary Tract Infection, Chapter 50); (2) hematuria; (3) penile problems, such as nonretractable foreskin in uncircumcised males, carcinoma, and trauma; (4) scrotal conditions, such as varicocele (elongation, dilation, and tortuosity of the veins superior to the testicle); and (5) testicular torsion (a condition in which the testicle hangs free from its vascular structures, which can result in partial or complete venous occlusion with rotation). Tumors of the testes are not common, but when manifested in adolescence, they are generally malignant and demand immediate evaluation.

The usual presenting symptom for testicular cancer is a heavy, hard painless mass (either smooth or nodular) that is palpated on the testis. Treatment involves surgical removal of the affected testicle (orchiectomy) and possibly chemotherapy and radiation if metastasis has occurred.

Nursing Care Management

The adolescent boy is extremely self-conscious about his changing body and needs preparation for a genital examination. The most successful approach is to assume a matter-of-fact attitude toward the examination, explain precisely what will take place, and maintain a continuous commentary about what is being done and the findings at each phase of the examination.

The routine health assessment of every adolescent boy should include teaching about testicular cancer and how to perform a testicular self-examination (TSE) every month. This rare malignancy is curable if detected early. Nurses are in an ideal position to teach TSE, in a manner that is respectful of the adolescent boy's anxieties and promotes early treatment (Critical Thinking Exercise).

> **Critical Thinking Exercise**
>
> **TESTICULAR SELF-EXAMINATION**
>
> At a recent faculty meeting, Paul, the pediatric nurse practitioner who runs the school-based health clinic, presented his plan for a class on testicular self-examination (TSE) to be delivered to the sophomore boys. Several teachers questioned the value of providing such a class when time to deliver content relating to "routine academic subjects" is limited. What important issues regarding testicular cancer and TSE should Paul use to justify providing this class to the sophomore boys?
>
> 1. Evidence—Is there sufficient evidence to justify teaching sophomore boys about TSE?
> 2. Assumptions—Describe the underlying assumption about each of the following:
>   a. Detection of testicular cancers in adolescence
>   b. Usual presenting symptom of testicular cancer
>   c. Knowledge of genital anatomy among adolescent boys
>   d. Ways to teach adolescent boys about their anatomy
> 3. What priorities for nursing care can be drawn at this time?
> 4. Does the evidence support your nursing intervention?
> 5. What alternative perspectives might you have?

The normal testicle is a firm organ with a smooth, egg-shaped contour; the epididymis is palpated as a raised swelling on the superior aspect of the testicle and should not be confused as an abnormality.

Gynecomastia

The male breast, although not strictly part of the male reproductive system, responds to hormonal changes. Some degree of bilateral or unilateral breast enlargement occurs frequently in boys during puberty. It is estimated that approximately half of adolescent boys have transient gynecomastia, usually lasting less than 1 year that subsides spontaneously with achievement of male development. A careful assessment of the pubertal stage at the onset of gynecomastia; medication history including anabolic steroids; and the exclusion of renal, liver, thyroid, and endocrine disorders or dysfunction allow the examiner to reassure the adolescent that the changes are pubertal gynecomastia and no further assessment is indicated.

If the condition persists or is extensive enough to cause embarrassment or to produce doubts about gender identity in the young boy, plastic surgery may be indicated for cosmetic and psychologic considerations. Administration of testosterone has no effect on breast development or regression and may aggravate the condition.

Nursing Care Management

Treatment usually consists of assurance to the adolescent and his parents that this is a benign and temporary situation. Adolescents who are distressed about physical integrity and masculinity may benefit from the knowledge that this condition occurs in more than 50% of all adolescent boys.

EATING DISORDERS

Obesity

Critical Thinking Exercise: Obesity

Few problems in childhood and adolescence are so obvious to others, so difficult to treat, and have such long-term effects on health as obesity. Several different definitions exist for obesity and overweight. *Obesity* is currently defined as an excessively high amount of body fat or adipose tissue in relation to lean body mass (CDC, 2002). *Overweight* refers to the state of increased body weight in relation to height. Currently, authorities recommend that the body mass index (BMI) measurement be used to screen for childhood obesity. The BMI measurement is strongly associated with subcutaneous and total body fat and also with skinfold thickness (SFT) measurements. The CDC has standards available for tracking children's BMI from 2 to 20 years of age (Lindeke, Rogers, & Finley, 2002).* Children with a BMI between the 85th and 95th percentile are considered overweight, and obesity is defined by a BMI greater than the 95th percentile (Moran, 2003).

Regardless of the definition used, the number of overweight children in the United States is increasing and may be

*Centers for Disease Control growth charts as well as instruction for nurses on accurate measurement and interpretation of children's growth can be found at www.cdc.gov/growthcharts.

approaching epidemic status. In the 1999-2000 National Health and Nutrition Examination Survey, data indicated that 15% of children and teens between 6 to 19 years were overweight (Ogden et al, 2002). The prevalence of childhood obesity in the United States is estimated to be 25% to 30% (Moran, 1999). Although obesity occurs across gender, racial, ethnic, and socioeconomic lines, obesity rates are higher among low-income youths and among African American, Hispanic, and Native American population groups. Increases in the number of overweight children and adolescents pose serious problems for society. Obesity is associated with numerous physical complications including type 2 diabetes mellitus, coronary artery disease, pulmonary dysfunction, arthritis, ischemic stroke, and some forms of cancer (National Task Force on the Prevention and Treatment of Obesity, 2000). Obesity is also a serious handicap to the social well-being of children and adolescents. Common emotional consequences of obesity include poor body image, low self-esteem, social isolation, and feelings of depression and rejection.

Etiology/Pathophysiology

Obesity in childhood and adolescence occurs as the result of several interrelated influences such as hypothalmic, hereditary, metabolic, social, cultural, and psychologic factors (Fig. 40-10). The complex interrelationships between hunger, satiety, the central nervous system, and metabolism continue to be investigated. Underlying diseases such as hypothyroidism, adrenal hypercorticoidism, hyperinsulinism, or dysfunction of the central nervous system are responsible for only a small number of cases of childhood obesity. Heredity is an important factor in the development of obesity. Identical twins reared apart tend to resemble their natural parents to a greater extent than they do their adoptive parents. However, it is impossible to distinguish between hereditary and environmental factors because both may be operating in any situation when other family members are obese.

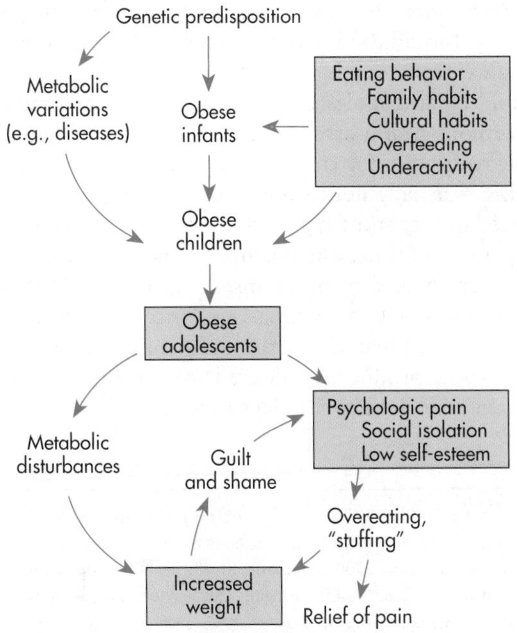

Fig. 40-10 Complex relationships in obesity

Investigators have proposed the following theories to explain the development of obesity:

Adipose cell theory. Obese children have larger adipose tissue cells that stay the same size once they reach a maximum, and their fat cells appear to increase in number during childhood.

Set point theory. Individuals have a programmed level or set point for body weight that remains relatively stable during adulthood. With increased caloric intake the metabolic rate increases to burn the excess; when intake is reduced, metabolism decreases to conserve energy.

Sociocultural factors also play a role in weight gain. Patterns of eating are learned in the culture, and the food preferences of the culture may contribute to the development of obesity. Many mothers consider plumpness a sign of health, view obesity as evidence of well-being, and foster weight gain as a desirable feature (Baughcum et al, 2000).

Psychologic factors may influence weight. In infancy, children experience relief from discomfort through feeding and learn to associate eating with feelings of security and the comforting presence of the nurturing person. Eating is often associated with the feeling of being loved. Many parents use food as a positive reinforcer for desired behavior. This practice may become a habit, and the child may continue to use food as a reward; a comfort; and a means to deal with feelings of depression, hostility, boredom, or loneliness.

Decreased physical activity is clearly related to body fatness and an increased risk of obesity. Our society has changed to include more sedentary lifestyles. Currently, children between 6 and 11 years of age spend an average of 26 hours per week watching television. This is as much time as they spend attending school (McArdle, Katch, & Katch, 2000). Other factors that lead to a sedentary lifestyle among children include apartment living, unsafe neighborhood environments, a limited time spent with parents in recreational activities, limited finances to participate in recreational activities, and limited opportunities to participate in extracurricular events that involve physical activity (McWhorter, Wallmann, & Alpert, 2003).

Diagnostic Evaluation

Methods to determine weight status such as magnetic resonance imaging, bioelectric impedance, and underwater weighing are accurate but expensive and invasive. Currently, clinicians rely on SFT measurements, body fat distribution, and weight-height indices, especially the BMI, to assess weight. The BMI measurement expresses the relationship between height and weight (i.e., kilograms divided by meters squared [kg/m^2]). BMI is easily calculated using growth charts available from the CDC. These charts are considered more accurate than the older weight-for-stature charts. Appropriate diagnostic tests should also be performed to rule out metabolic or endocrine disorders that can cause obesity.

Nursing Care Management

Assessment

Obtaining an accurate measurement of the child or adolescent's height and weight is an essential part of assessment. These measurements are necessary to calculate the BMI measurement. Children with a BMI greater than or equal to the 95th percentile for age and sex should receive an in-depth medical assessment. Children with a BMI in the 85th to 95th percentile range should be evaluated for secondary complications such as hypertension and hyperlipidemia. Evaluation should also include the height and weight history of the parents and siblings, as well as an assessment of eating habits, appetite and hunger patterns, and physical activities of the child. A psychosocial history is also important to determine the impact that the child's weight has on his or her quality of life.

Nursing Diagnoses

After a thorough assessment of the child or adolescent, several nursing diagnoses become apparent. The prominent diagnoses are outlined in Box 40-3.

Plan of Care and Implementation

The goals of a weight loss program include the following:

1. Child will follow a diet that provides loss of body fat without interfering with growth, normal activity, and psychologic well-being.
2. Child will engage in a regular exercise program.
3. Child will modify eating behavior.
4. Child and family will receive psychologic support.

Motivation to lose weight is the key to success. Success is rarely achieved unless youngsters are motivated to lose weight and take some personal responsibility for their dietary habits and exercise program. Children who are forced by parents to seek help are seldom motivated and often become rebellious and unwilling to control dietary intake. An approach that focuses on healthy eating habits and enjoyable exercise for all members of the family is more likely to be successful.

Diet

The ideal diet for children and adolescents should meet the criteria outlined in Box 40-4. Because obesity is often a lifelong problem, it is important to provide children, adolescents, and their families with a diet that fosters healthier eating habits. Increasing dietary fiber and complex carbohydrates, modifying fat intake, and encouraging eating only in response to physical hunger cues are essential components of any diet. Recently, low-carbohydrate diets such as the Atkins Diet have been promoted for weight loss in adults and adolescents (Sondike et al, 2003). However, low-carbohydrate diets can result in ketosis, insulin resistance, and glucose intolerance. More research is needed to evaluate the long-term safety and efficacy of these diets for children and adolescents (Daniels, 2003).

A healthy diet should include high-nutrient foods such as fruits, vegetables, whole grains, and low-fat dairy and protein products. Calories and fats should be kept to a healthy level, and extremes should be avoided. The child or adolescent should not become so food conscious that they believe fats and calories are bad and that they must avoid both high-calorie and high-fat foods. Diets that contain ordinary foods in controlled portions (not adult-sized portions) rather than those that avoid specific foods are most successful. Children and adolescents need advice on how to include their favorite foods in small amounts and how to select satisfying substitutes for favorite foods. Knowing the caloric values for a wide variety of foods and snacks and how to read food labels is helpful to children, adolescents, and family members.

Snacking is an important part of the daily routine for children and adolescents. Vending machines at schools are often stocked with high-calorie, low-nutrient snacks that are easily accessible to children who have pocket money. Parents, nutritionists, and school nurses need to lobby for "treats," such as fruits, juices, and raw vegetables in school cafeterias and vending machines. Fast-food establishments, which are often located near schools, continue to present problems for children and adolescents who are attempting to lose weight.*

Children and adolescents should not initiate a reduction diet without health assessment and counseling. Significant caloric restriction for children and adolescents who are still growing is usually not recommended. Restriction diets can cause delayed or stunted growth and are often ineffective for long periods of time. The potential dangers of exotic fad diets and crash dietary programs for growing children and adolescents should be emphasized. Successful dietary programs are those that are nutritionally sound, have sufficient satiety value, produce the desired weight loss, and involve nutrition education and social support.

BOX 40-3

Nursing Diagnoses: The Child Who Is Obese

Activity intolerance
Activity intolerance, risk for
Coping, ineffective
Family processes, interrupted
Nutrition: more than body requirements, imbalanced
Nutrition: more than body requirements, risk for imbalanced
Self-esteem, chronic low
Self-esteem, situational low
Self-esteem, situational low, risk for

BOX 40-4

Essentials of an Ideal Weight Management Program

Weight maintenance or steady, slow weight loss
Nutrient, energy, and growth needs met
Feelings of hunger avoided
Preservation of lean body mass
Increased physical activity
Absence of metabolic complications
Absence of psychiatric reactions

*Information on the nutrient value of name-brand foods, including menu items from fast-food restaurants, is available from the Nutrition Coordinating Center, 1300 S. Second St., Suite 300, Minneapolis, MN 55414; phone: 612-626-9450; e-mail: nccservicecenter@epi.umn.edu; Web site: www.ncc.umn.edu.

Exercise

Physical activity is necessary to bring about weight loss, to maintain weight loss, and to redistribute body fat into muscle. Regular physical activity or exercise progressively increased over the child or adolescent's usual activity, is an integral part of a weight-reduction program. Initial goals for activity should be small and reasonable so the child does not fell overwhelmed. Physical activities should be those that stress self-improvement rather than competition. All children and teens need continued psychologic support and encouragement to participate in physical activities and exercise.

Behavioral Therapy

The most successful method for treating obesity is diet and exercise combined with behavior modification, which emphasizes identification and elimination of inappropriate eating habits and problem-solving strategies to use in situations that encourage overeating. Self-monitoring is used to increase awareness of eating behavior, and attention is focused on the social and behavioral aspects surrounding food consumption. Children are encouraged to maintain an activity log, and parents are encouraged to prohibit eating in front of the television, to limit trips to fast-food restaurants, and to omit using food for comfort or as rewards.

Group Involvement

Commercial groups or diet workshops composed primarily of adults may be helpful to some teenagers; however, a group composed of individuals their own age is more effective for children and adolescents. Groups for youngsters who are obese include summer camps designed and conducted by health professionals, school groups organized and led by the school nurse, and groups associated with special clinics. These groups should focus on weight loss as well as the development of positive self-image. Nutrition education, diet planning, and discussions centered on improvement of social skills are essential components of these groups.

Medical Therapies

No weight-loss medications are currently approved by the Food and Drug Administration (FDA) for use in the pediatric population (Moran, 2003). Appetite-suppressant drugs are no more effective than diet and exercise in maintaining weight loss, and the use of these drugs may become habit forming. Surgical techniques that bypass a substantial portion of the intestine or occlude a large segment of the stomach to produce diet restriction and weight loss are not well studied and should only be considered in extreme circumstances when medical complications have developed.

Prevention

Weight loss programs do not enjoy the success of therapeutic interventions for other disorders. Prevention of obesity should begin in early childhood with the development of healthy eating habits, regular exercise patterns, and a positive relationship between parents and children. Health care professionals should encourage frequent health visits for children who are overweight or obese and incorporate a dietary history and counseling into each health encounter.

Evaluation

The effectiveness of nursing interventions is determined by continual reassessment based on the following observational guidelines and expected outcomes:

1. Assess weight at regular intervals (usually weekly); discuss the child or adolescent's feelings, reactions, and concerns; analyze daily logs of activities (eating, behavior, exercise).
2. Review exercise program with child or teenager.
3. Interview child or adolescent about the plan of care and progress toward short- and long-term goals.

Expected Outcomes

1. Eating patterns lead to weight loss; child or adolescent expresses feelings and concerns regarding problems.
2. Child or adolescent engages in preferred exercise and activities regularly.
3. Child or adolescent demonstrates an understanding of eating patterns.
4. Child or adolescent demonstrates steady weight loss (or weight maintenance in a growing child).

Anorexia Nervosa (AN)

AN is an eating disorder characterized by a refusal to maintain a minimally normal body weight and by severe weight loss in the absence of obvious physical causes. Approximately 5% of adolescent females in the United States have AN, and 5% to 10% of all cases occur in males (Committee on Adolescence, 2003). The average age of onset is 13 years, but the disorder can occur as early as 10 years of age and as late as 25 years of age. Individuals with AN are described as perfectionists, academically high achievers, conforming, and conscientious. Typically, they have high energy levels, even with marked emaciation.

Etiology/Pathophysiology

The etiology of the disorder remains unclear. There is a distinct psychologic component, and the diagnosis is based primarily on psychologic and behavioral criteria. The dominant aspects of AN are a relentless pursuit of thinness and a fear of fatness, usually preceded by a period of mood disturbances and behavior changes. Weight loss may be triggered by a typical adolescent crisis such as the onset of menstruation or a traumatic interpersonal incident that precipitates serious out-of-control dieting. Situations of severe family stress (such as parental separation or divorce) or circumstances in which the youngster perceives a lack of personal control (such as teasing at school, changing schools, or going to college) may precipitate a desire for control and the decision not to eat. An exaggerated misinterpretation of the normal fat deposition characteristic of early adolescence or anxiety because of comments that the adolescent is putting on weight is common. Society's emphasis and the media's focus on tall, thin individuals may also play a role. Another factor in some cases is childhood sexual abuse.

Diagnostic Evaluation

Diagnosis is made on the basis of clinical manifestations (Box 40-5) and conformity to the criteria established by the American Psychiatric Association (2000) (Box 40-6).

BOX 40-5

Clinical Manifestations of Anorexia Nervosa

Severe and profound weight loss
Signs of altered metabolic activity:
- Secondary amenorrhea (if menarche attained)
- Primary amenorrhea (if menarche not attained)
- Bradycardia
- Lowered body temperature
- Decreased blood pressure
- Cold intolerance
- Dry skin and brittle nails
- Appearance of lanugo hair

BOX 40-6

Diagnostic Criteria for Anorexia Nervosa

1. Refusal to maintain body weight over a minimal normal weight for age and height (e.g., weight loss leading to maintenance of body weight less than 85% of that expected; or failure to make expected weight gain during period of growth, leading to body weight less than 85% of that expected)
2. Intense fear of gaining weight or becoming fat, even though underweight
3. Disturbance of body image, undue influence of shape or weight on evaluation, or denial of the seriousness of the current low body weight
4. In postmenarcheal females, amenorrhea (i.e., the absence of at least three consecutive menstrual cycles); a woman is considered to have amenorrhea if her periods occur only following hormone (i.e., estrogen) administration

   Specify type:

   Restricting type–no regular bingeing or purging behavior (i.e., self-induced vomiting or the misuse of laxatives, diuretics, or enemas)

   Binge eating/purging type–during the current episode of AN, the person has regularly engaged in binge eating or purging behavior (i.e., self-induced vomiting or the misuse of laxatives, diuretics, or enemas)

From American Psychiatric Association: *Diagnostic and statistical manual of mental disorders,* ed 4 (DSM-IV), Washington, DC, 1994, The Association.

Therapeutic Management

Treatment involves three major thrusts: (1) reinstitution of normal nutrition or reversal of malnutrition, (2) resolution of disturbed patterns of family interaction, and (3) individual psychotherapy to correct deficits and distortions in psychologic functioning. Most adolescents are treated on an outpatient basis, but those with severe malnutrition or electrolyte or psychiatric disturbances (severe depression or suicidal ideation) require hospitalization. An interdisciplinary team of dietitians, physicians, nurses, and counselors deliver the interventions.

Nutrition

The most important goal is to treat any life-threatening malnutrition and to restore dietary stability and weight gain. This may require the administration of tube feedings or intravenous fluids if the malnutrition is severe. In most cases, it is best to reintroduce food and snacks slowly in a stepwise manner. A reasonable goal is to reach an eventual intake of 2000 to 3000 kcal per day and a weight gain of 0.5 to 2 pounds per week (Committee on Adolescence, 2003). When restoring nutrition, health professionals must avoid the refeeding syndrome, which consists of cardiovascular, neurologic, and hematologic complications that occur when nutritional replacement is given too rapidly. This syndrome can be avoided with slow refeeding and the addition of phosphorus when total body phosphorus is depleted. Treatment goal weights are individualized and based on age, height, and stage of puberty, premorbid weight and previous growth charts. In girls who have reached menarche, resumption of menses is an objective measure of return to biologic health.

Dietary interventions are combined with psychotherapy to improve the underlying psychologic misconceptions about weight loss. Another aspect of treatment is to relieve the anxiety related to eating and the depression that accompanies the disorder. The administration of antianxiety or antidepressant medications is beneficial. However, when these drugs are used, patients should be carefully monitored for cardiovascular side effects.

Psychotherapy

Behavioral interventions are often necessary to encourage patients to accomplish the desired caloric intake and weight gain. Mental health interventions are essential. The ultimate goal is to have the child or adolescent become more realistic in their self-appraisal and capable of living as a competent individual without manipulating their body and its functions. Individual psychotherapy is aimed at helping the young person resolve the adolescent identity crisis, particularly as it relates to a distorted body image. If the disorder is related to a dysfunctional family situation, therapy is most successful when it is started soon after the onset of illness, and directed toward disengagement and redirection of malfunctioning processes in the family.

Nursing Care Management

The psychogenic nature of AN makes treatment difficult and lengthy. Only about 25% of affected individuals attain full recovery; 50% improve, but may relapse during times of stress; and 25% do poorly despite adequate treatment (Schneider & Fisher, 2001).

Nurses who care for children or teens with AN should maintain a kind, supportive, yet firm manner. The child or adolescent requires sustained support and reassurance to cope with ambivalent feelings related to the body concept. Assistance is also needed to help teens view themselves as cooperative and reliable individuals worthy of receiving kindness. Encouraging education and activities that foster self-esteem facilitates the resocialization process and promotes social acceptance among peers.

It is important for nurses to be aware of the physical side effects of AN. Patients frequently limit their fluid intake. Urinary tract problems are common, and ketones and protein may be detected in the urine as a result of breakdown of fat and protein. Vital sign instability can be severe and can include orthostatic hypotension; the pulse becomes irregular, and the heart rate decreases markedly. Bradycardia and hypothermia can result in cardiac arrest (Critical Thinking Exercise).

Health professionals, patients, and families can find assistance and information from several organizations. The Na-

Critical Thinking Exercise

ANOREXIA NERVOSA (AN)

Jane is a 13-year-old whose grades have been excellent and whom the teachers describe as a "model student." Recently, Jane's teacher told the nurse practitioner that Jane's parents were in the middle of a "messy divorce." In addition, several of Jane's friends told the nurse practitioner that they are concerned about Jane because she "jogs" every day at lunchtime and seldom eats lunch with them. Jane told her friends that she gained weight over the winter months and that she is "jogging" because she wants to qualify for the track team this spring. At the time of her routine health interview and sports physical, the nurse practitioner notes that Jane's oral temperature is 96.8° F and she weighs 34 kg. Jane has lost 9 kg since her last sports physical. When discussing her menstrual periods with the nurse practitioner, Jane states that she has not had her period for 3 months.

1. Evidence—Is there sufficient evidence to draw any conclusions about Jane's behavior?
2. Assumptions—Describe some underlying assumptions about the following:
   a. Personality characteristics of individuals with AN
   b. Factors influencing the development of AN
   c. Clinical manifestations of AN
   d. Treatment of AN
3. What implications for nursing care should be established for Jane at this time?
4. Does the evidence support your conclusion?
5. Are there alternative perspectives that you should consider?

tional Eating Disorders Organization* provides information and support services for patients and families. The National Association of Anorexia Nervosa and Associated Disorders, Inc. (ANAD),† and the American Anorexia/Bulimia Association, Inc. (AABA)‡ provide counseling, referrals, and self-help programs.

Bulimia

Bulimia is an eating disorder characterized by repeated episodes of binge eating. The binge behavior consists of secretive, frenzied consumption of large amounts of high-calorie (or "forbidden") foods during a brief period of time (usually less than 2 hours). The binge is counteracted by a variety of weight control methods (purging), including self-induced vomiting, diuretic and laxative abuse, and rigorous exercise. The frequency of bingeing can be anywhere from once a week to seven or eight times a day. Self-deprecating thoughts, a depressed mood, and awareness that the eating pattern is abnormal follow these binge-purge cycles.

The disorder is observed more frequently in older adolescent girls and young women. Affected individuals have been unsuccessful dieters, have low impulse control, and may have been self-conscious about being overweight in childhood. They fall into two categories: (1) those who purge and (2) those who do not purge. Some women are of normal weight or (more often) slightly above normal weight. Other individuals with bulimia restrict their intake and become severely underweight. This type of bulimia is called *bulimarexia.*

Diagnostic Evaluation

The diagnosis may be first suspected from the presence of complications, including fluid and electrolyte disturbances from gastrointestinal losses, abdominal complaints from laxative abuse, erosion of tooth enamel and increased dental caries from vomited gastric acid, and throat complaints. The diagnosis is established on the basis of criteria established by the American Psychiatric Association (2000) (Box 40-7).

Therapeutic Management

Therapy is similar to management of AN. Hospitalization may be required for complications such as potassium depletion and esophageal damage. Intravenous fluids, potassium replacement, and cardiac monitoring are essential elements of care. Nutrition consultation and follow-up are essential. Behavior therapy may also be used.

Nursing Care Management

Nursing care is similar to the care of the patient with AN; acute care involves careful monitoring of fluid and electrolyte alterations and observation for signs of cardiac complications. The nurse may need to help the adolescent and

BOX 40-7

Diagnostic Criteria for Bulimia

1. Recurrent episodes of binge eating. An episode of binge eating is characterized by both of the following:
   a. Eating, in a discrete period of time (e.g., within any 2-hour period), an amount of food that is definitely larger than most people would eat during a similar period of time and under similar circumstances
   b. A sense of lack of control over eating during the episode (e.g., a feeling that one cannot stop eating or control what or how much one is eating)
2. Recurrent inappropriate compensatory behavior in order to prevent weight gain, such as self-induced vomiting; misuse of laxatives, diuretics, enemas, or other medications; fasting; or excessive exercise
3. The binge eating and inappropriate compensatory behaviors both occur, on average, at least twice a week for 3 months
4. Self-evaluation is unduly influenced by body shape and weight
5. The disturbance does not occur exclusively during episodes of AN

   Specify type:

   Purging type—during the current episode of bulimia nervosa, the person has regularly engaged in self-induced vomiting or the misuse of laxatives, diuretics, or enemas

   Nonpurging type—during the current episode of bulimia nervosa, the person has used other inappropriate compensatory behaviors, such as fasting or excessive exercise, but has not regularly engaged in self-induced vomiting or the misuse of laxatives, diuretics, or enemas

From American Psychiatric Association: *Diagnostic and statistical manual of mental disorders,* ed 4 (DSM-IV), Washington, DC, 1994, The Association.

*603 Stewart St., Suite 803, Seattle, WA 98101; Web site: www.nationaleatingdisorders.org.

†PO Box 7, Highland Park, IL 60035; phone: 847-831-3438; e-mail: anad20.aol.com; Web site: www.anad.org.

‡410 East 76th St., New York, NY 10021; phone: 212-734-1114; Web site: www.aabainc.org.

family structure the environment to reduce the bingeing behavior. Relaxation techniques and telephone support networks are also helpful interventions for bingeing behavior.

SERIOUS HEALTH PROBLEMS WITH A BEHAVIORAL COMPONENT

Smoking

From 1997 until 2001, the percentage of young people who reported current cigarette use and frequent cigarette use decreased significantly (Grunbaum et al, 2002). Despite this decrease, however, a significant number of children and teenagers initiate or continue to smoke. The 2001 Youth Risk Behavior Survey indicated that 28.5% of senior high school students in the United States currently smoked cigarettes. Nationwide, 22% of young people initiate smoking by 13 years of age.

evolve CASE STUDY: TEEN SMOKING

The hazards of smoking at any age are well known, and prevention of smoking is essential in childhood and adolescence. The age at which most children initiate or experiment with smoking is approximately 11 years, and most adults who are currently addicted to tobacco developed the habit in adolescence (Moolchan, Ernst, & Henningfield, 2000). In children and adolescents, smoking produces almost immediate effects of reduced lung function, "smoker's cough," and respiratory difficulties. In addition, 24% to 50% of teens who start to smoke become nicotine-dependent (Rojas et al, 1998). Research also indicates an association between current use of tobacco and the development of depression (Goodman & Capitman, 2000) and sleep problems (Patten et al, 2000) in adolescence. Cigarettes are considered to be a gateway drug, and teenagers who smoke are 11.4 times more likely to use illicit drugs (Gordon, 2000).

Etiology

Teenagers begin smoking for various reasons, including imitation of adult behavior; peer pressure; a desire to imitate behaviors portrayed in the movies and advertisements; and a desire to control weight, especially among females (Strauss, 2000). Teenagers who do not smoke usually have family members and friends who do not smoke or who oppose smoking. Most teens who refrain from smoking have a desire to succeed in academics or athletics, particularly, high-performance sports, such as basketball, swimming, and track, and plans to go to college (Community Focus box). Although smoking among college students has increased in recent years (Rigotti, Lee, & Wechsler, 2000), rates of smoking are highest among adolescents who do not complete high school.

Smokeless Tobacco

The term smokeless tobacco refers to tobacco products that are placed in the mouth but not ignited (e.g., snuff and chewing tobacco). This popular substitute for cigarettes poses a serious hazard to children and adolescents. These products have been proven to be carcinogenic, and regular use causes foul-smelling breath and dental problems such as periodontal degeneration and oral soft tissue lesions. Use of smokeless tobacco can also lead to cigarette smoking.

Nursing Care Management

Prevention of regular smoking in teenagers is the most effective way to reduce the overall incidence of smoking. A variety of strategies have been used to prevent smoking. Because smoking is a social symbol, antismoking campaigns that address the norms of potential smokers without ridiculing or threatening their social group norms are more successful than programs that focus on the negative long-term effects of smoking. Youth-to-youth programs that emphasize the immediate personal and social consequences of smoking (e.g., unattractive stains on teeth and hands, unpleasant breath, and clothing or hair that smells of smoke) are effective in changing teenagers' attitudes toward smoking. When a significant number of influential peers "sell" their classmates on the idea that smoking is not popular, teens imitate their behavior. Teaching resistance to peer pressure to smoke is another effective strategy to prevent initiation of smoking in early adolescence. Enforcing smoking bans in schools discourages smoking and promotes a smoke-free environment as the norm. Expanding these programs to include parents, mass media, youth groups, and community organizations strengthens the impact of school-based programs (Community Focus box).

> **Community Focus**
>
> **EARLY SEXUAL MATURATION, ALCOHOL, AND CIGARETTES**
>
> Cigarette smoking and the drinking of alcohol among adolescents are complex behaviors that are not explained by any one cause or factor. Some theorists and investigators believe there is a relationship between biologic maturation and these risk-taking behaviors. For example, young girls who are sexually mature at an earlier age than their peers are often attracted to older girls and boys who may engage in risk-taking behaviors. If older teens smoke, drink, and drive while under the influence of alcohol with no adverse consequences (i.e., no motor vehicle accidents), young girls may believe that they, too, will be safe while smoking, drinking, or riding in an automobile with friends who are drinking.
>
> Although parents and nurses cannot influence the time of biologic maturation, they can identify young girls who are at risk for the initiation of risk-taking behaviors because of early puberty. Parents need to understand that an early-maturing daughter might be uncomfortable with her body, and they should take advantage of opportunities to build her self-esteem. Parental sensitivity to the importance of peer-group acceptance and parental support of a teenage daughter who feels left out or different are crucial. School nurses can provide anticipatory guidance to these girls and help them role-play coping strategies for situations that involve offers to smoke and drink. In addition, school nurses can provide information about physical development during puberty and emphasize the fact that not all teenagers mature at the same time or rate.
>
> Teachers, coaches, and church leaders can provide opportunities for these girls to "fit in" with their same-age peers through activities that stress mutual goals. For example, an early-maturing girl is typically taller than her age-mates and can be an asset in sports such as basketball and track-and-field events.

Substance Abuse

Although experimentation with drugs during childhood and adolescence is widespread, most children and teens do not become high-risk users. Experimentation is limited to 1 adolescent in 5 for stimulants and inhalants, and less than 1 in

Community Focus

NONSMOKING STRATEGIES

Nurses who work in schools, hospitals, and community agencies can take advantage of all opportunities to provide education about the dangers of smoking, to discourage smoking initiation by children and adolescents, to encourage smoking cessation, and to promote smoke-free environments. In particular, school nurses must be alert to the vulnerability of young preteens when they enter junior high school. These nurses are in an ideal position to assess stress, personal conflict, weight concerns, peer pressures, and other factors that place preteens at risk for smoking initiation. Nurses should serve as counselors to student, teacher, and parent groups and as advocates for antismoking legislative efforts. The following additional strategies are recommended*:

- Provide only brief information about long-term health consequences (e.g., cardiovascular and cancer risks).
- Discuss immediate physiologic consequences (e.g., changes in heart rate, blood pressure, respiratory symptoms, and blood carbon monoxide concentrations).
- Mention alternatives to smoking that also establish a self-image that appears independent, mature, or sophisticated (e.g., establishing a weight-lifting regimen; jogging; dancing; joining a boys' or girls' club; engaging in volunteer work for a hospital, political, religious or community group).
- Mention the negative effects in detail (e.g., earlier wrinkling of skin; yellow stains on teeth and fingers; tobacco odor on breath, hair, and clothing).
- Mention the increasing ostracism of smokers by nonsmokers, both legal and informal, in the workplace and in public places.
- Mention the increasing evidence that secondhand smoke is injurious to the health of nonsmokers who are regularly exposed, especially small children.
- Acknowledge that many adults, who were enticed to start smoking as teenagers because of its social benefits, now wish they could stop smoking.
- Give cooperative adolescents effective arguments to deal with peer pressure (e.g., by not smoking, a teenager demonstrates independence and nonconformity, traits normally prized by youth).
- Request posters or pamphlets from local agencies (e.g., American Cancer Society, American Heart Association, and American Lung Association) to display in prominent places at school.

*For information on smoking cessation, nurses can contact the Nursing Center for Tobacco Intervention, 1585 Neil Ave., Columbus, Ohio 43210-1216; phone: 614-292-0653; fax: 614-292-7976; Web site: www. con.ohio-state.edu/tobacco/. Information can also be obtained from Stop Teenage Addiction to Tobacco (STAT), a national organization devoted to educating the public and professionals, at Northeastern University, 360 Huntington Ave., 241 Cushing Hall, Boston, MA 02115; phone: 617-373-7828; e-mail: info@stat.org.

10 for hallucinogens, sedatives, and "crack" cocaine. Adolescents are the group at greatest risk for regular use of drugs; approximately 1% to 2% of teens use hard drugs regularly (US Department of Health and Human Services, 1999).

Drug abuse, misuse, and *addiction* are culturally defined and are voluntary behaviors. *Drug tolerance* and *physical dependence* are involuntary physiologic responses to the pharmacologic characteristics of the drugs, such as opioids and alcohol. Consequently, an individual can be addicted to a narcotic with or without being physically dependent. A person can also be physically dependent on a narcotic without being addicted (e.g., patients who use opioids to control pain).

Motivation

Most drug use begins with experimentation. The drug may be used only once, occasionally, or become part of a drug-centered lifestyle. Children and adolescents initiate drug use out of curiosity. For many youths, drugs produce a dreamy state of altered consciousness or a feeling of power, excitement, heightened acuity, or confidence. Others seek the visual hallucinatory experiences and sexual sensation that result from drug use. Many youngsters use drugs because their peers use them or because they want to belong to a group. Some youths also turn to drugs because they are looking for a way to cope with stress, the social and technologic changes of the world, and their feelings of powerlessness.

Types of Drugs Abused

Any drug can be abused, and most are potentially harmful to youngsters still going through formative life experiences. Although rarely considered drugs by society, the chemically active substances most frequently abused are the xanthines and theobromines contained in chocolate, tea, coffee, and colas. Ethyl alcohol and nicotine are other drugs that are legal and socially sanctioned. Any of these substances can produce mild to moderate euphoric and/or stimulant effects and can lead to physical and psychologic dependence.

Drugs with mind-altering abilities that are available on the "street" and are of medical and legal concern are the hallucinogenic, narcotic, hypnotic, and stimulant drugs. In addition, health professionals are concerned about the use of alcohol and volatile substances that are inhaled to achieve altered sensation (such as gasoline, antifreeze, plastic model airplane cement, typewriter correction fluid, and organic solvents). Recently, abuse of prescription and synthetic drugs have become a concern for professionals who work with children and adolescents. Internet Web sites have also promoted the "safe use" of some psychoactive drugs and have supplied information on new "designer" drugs that are not detectable on a standard urine drug screening test (Wax, 2002).

Alcohol

Acute or chronic abuse of alcohol (ethanol) is responsible for many acts of violence, suicide, accidental injury, and death. Alcohol drinking is likely to begin in the middle school years, and increases with age. By 18 years of age, 80% to 90% of adolescents have tried alcohol. Ethanol is a depressant that reduces inhibitions against aggressive and sexual acting out. Severe physical and psychologic symptoms accompany abrupt withdrawal, and long-term use leads to slow tissue destruction, especially of the brain and liver cells. The most noticeable effects of alcohol occur within the central nervous system, and include changes in cognitive and autonomic functions such as judgment, memory, learning ability, and other intellectual capacities. Young alcoholics often drink alone and cannot control their use of alcohol. They often rely on the substance as a defense against depression, anxiety, fear, or anger. Not all of these characteristics are observed in a youngster who is abusing alcohol, but if several signs are evident, the child or adolescent should be considered at risk. Referral to a health care professional and detoxification therapy may be necessary. Information about alcohol and answers to questions are available at the Alcohol Hotline.* Other groups that provide support and counseling for families are Al-Anon, Ala-Teen, and Ala-Tot, and Alcoholics Anonymous (an organization that has listings in all local telephone directories.

Cocaine

Although cocaine is not pharmacologically considered a narcotic, it is legally categorized as such. Cocaine is available in two forms: water-soluble cocaine hydrochloride, which is administered by "snorting" or intravenous injection; and nonsoluble alkaloid (freebase) cocaine, which is used primarily for smoking. Crack or "rock" is a purer, more menacing form of the drug. It can be produced cheaply and smoked in either water pipes or mentholated cigarettes. The use of cocaine has increased in recent years because of its availability, affordability, and its association with persons in glamorous occupations; peer pressure; and its reputation as a sexually enhancing drug.

Cocaine creates a sense of euphoria, or an indefinable high. Withdrawal does not produce the dramatic symptoms observed in withdrawal from other substances. The effects are those commonly seen in depression, including lack of energy and motivation, irritability, appetite changes, psychomotor retardation, and irregular sleep patterns. More serious symptoms include cardiovascular manifestations and seizures. Physical withdrawal should not be confused with the so-called crash after a cocaine high, which consists of a long period of sleep. Answers to questions about the risks of using cocaine are available at the National Cocaine Hotline,† which also provides referrals to support groups and treatment centers.

Narcotics

Narcotic drugs include opiates such as heroin and morphine, and opioids (opiate-like drugs) such as hydromorphone (Dilaudid), fentanyl, meperidine (Demerol), and codeine. These drugs produce a state of euphoria by removing painful feelings and creating a pleasurable experience and a sense of success accompanied by clouding of the consciousness and a dreamlike state. Physical signs of narcotic abuse include constricted pupils; respiratory depression; and, often, cyanosis. Needle marks may be visible on the arms or legs in chronic users. Physical withdrawal from opiates is extremely unpleasant unless controlled with supervised tapering doses of the opioid or substitution of methadone.

Equally as important as the physical effects are the indirect consequences related to the illegal status of narcotic use and the problems associated with securing the drug (e.g., the time-consuming searches to obtain the drug and the often illegal methods used to meet the high cost of purchasing it). Health problems also result from self-neglect of physical needs (nutrition, cleanliness, dental care), overdose, contamination, and infection, including HIV infection and hepatitis B.

Central nervous system stimulants include a variety of hypnotic drugs that produce physical dependence and withdrawal symptoms on abrupt discontinuation. They create a feeling of relaxation and sleepiness but impair general functioning. Drugs in this category include barbiturates and nonbarbiturates (e.g., methaqualone [Quaalude]), and alcohol. Barbiturates combined with alcohol produce a profound depressant effect.

Central Nervous System Stimulants

Amphetamines and cocaine do not produce strong physical dependence and can be withdrawn without much danger. However, psychologic dependence is strong, and acute intoxication can lead to violent aggressive behavior or psychotic episodes characterized by paranoia, uncontrollable agitation, and restlessness. When combined with barbiturates, the euphoric effects are particularly addictive.

Methamphetamine can be snorted, injected, swallowed, or smoked and produces a burst of energy in its users, along with intense, alternating attacks of boldness and paranoia. It provokes excitement far more intense than that caused by crack and cocaine. The drug, with the street names *crank*, *meth*, and *crystal*, is inexpensive and has a longer period of action than cocaine. Instead of a short (few minutes) high, as achieved with crack, a user can remain "up" for hours on a similar dose of crank.

Inhalants include glue "sniffing" and the inhalation of plastic cement, spray paint, and other volatile substances (e.g., gasoline, nitrous oxide, and air dusters used to remove dust from computers and camera lenses). Youngsters breathe or place these substances into paper or plastic bags or soda cans from which they rebreathe the fumes to produce a feeling of euphoria and altered consciousness. These substances contain chemical solvents and are extremely hazardous. Dusters contain freon, a substance that can cause fatal cardiac arrhythmias. The use of inhalants is increasing, and inhalants are becoming a gateway drug for young children and preteens who often progress to other harder drugs such as marijuana, heroin, and cocaine. Many young children are unaware of the dangers of "sniffing" or "huffing." In addition to rapid loss of consciousness and respiratory arrest, these substances may cause visual scanning problems, language deficiencies, motor instability, memory deficits, and attention and concentration problems.

Mind-Altering Drugs

Hallucinogens (psychedelic, psychotomimetic, psychotropic, or illusionogenic) are drugs that produce vivid hallucinations and euphoria. These drugs do not produce physical dependence, and they can be abruptly withdrawn without ill effect. However, the acute and long-term effects are variable, and in some individuals the dissociative behavior may be prolonged. Cannabis (marijuana, hashish) and lysergic acid diethylamide (LSD) are also included in this category of drugs.

Nursing Care Management Related to Therapeutic Management

Nurses who have contact with children and adolescents are in an excellent position to provide information about substance abuse and to serve as a patient advocate. The nurse

*1-800-ALCOHOL
†1-800-COCAINE

most often encounters young drug abusers when they are (1) experiencing overdose or withdrawal symptoms, (2) manifesting bizarre behavior or confusion secondary to drug ingestion, (3) worried that they are becoming or will become addicted, or (4) worried about a friend or family member who is addicted.

In particular, nurses who care for hospitalized adolescents need to know if these youths use drugs compulsively. Drug withdrawal can seriously complicate other illnesses. Nurses should be alert for any physical or behavioral clues that indicate the onset of withdrawal or the effects of drugs. Obstetric and nursery nurses may encounter drug dependence and withdrawal in newborn infants or compulsive drug-using mothers. School nurses and nurses who work in the community also play an essential role in identifying children, adolescents, and families with substance abuse problems. Early identification of children, adolescents, and families at risk for substance abuse problems is an essential aspect of prevention. Pediatric health care professionals also prevent substance abuse by creating trusting relationships so that children and adolescents feel comfortable asking questions about drugs, and health professionals can alert preadolescents and adolescents to Web sites and other aspects of society that encourage experimentation with drugs.

Acute Care

Adolescents experiencing toxic drug effects or withdrawal symptoms are usually seen initially in the emergency department. Experienced emergency department personnel are familiar with the management of acute drug toxicity, and the signs, symptoms, and behavioral characteristics of a variety of substances. When the drug is questionable or unknown, knowledge of these factors facilitates management and treatment. Often observation of or description of the child or adolescent's behavior is more valuable than reports by patients or their friends

The treatment for drug toxicity or withdrawal varies according to the drug and the method used. Every effort is made to determine the type, the time of ingestion, the amount of drug taken, the mode of administration, and the factors related to the onset of presenting symptoms. It is helpful to know the individual's pattern of use. For example, if two types of drugs are involved, they may require different treatments. Gastric lavage may be employed when the drug has been ingested recently and the cough reflex is intact, but it is of little value when the drug has been administered intravenously ("mainlined") or intranasally ("sniffed"). Because the actual content of most street drugs is highly questionable, other pharmaceutical agents are administered with caution, except perhaps the narcotic antagonists in cases of suspected opiate overdoses. It is also necessary to assess for possible trauma sustained while the patient was under the influence of the drug.

Long-term Management

A major factor in the treatment and rehabilitation of young drug users is careful assessment in the nonacute stage to determine the function that the drug plays in the youngster's life. The motivation phase is directed toward exploring the factors that influence drug use. It also involves establishing a feeling of self-worth and a commitment to self-help in the teen.

Rehabilitation begins when youngsters decide that they can and are willing to change. Rehabilitation involves fostering healthy interdependent relationships with caring and supportive adults and exploring alternate mechanisms for problem solving while simultaneously reducing or eliminating drug use. Persons working with troubled youth must be prepared for recidivism, or the tendency to relapse, and maintain a plan for reentry into the treatment process.

Family Support

Most treatment programs for substance abusers are based on adult 12-step models such as Alcoholics Anonymous. Research is needed to determine whether these adult models are effective for adolescents. Tough Love* is one such program that is based on the conviction that parents have the right and responsibility to be the policymakers in the family, to set limits on the behavior of their children, and to take control of the household from out-of-control youngsters. The premise is that allowing teenagers to experience the negative consequences of their behavior will bring them closer to accepting help and/or changing their behavior. Another group that provides support and counseling for families experiencing substance abuse and seeking strategies to copy with their children is Parents Anonymous.†

Prevention

Nurses play an important role in education efforts, as well as in individual observation, assessment, and therapy related to substance abuse. In recent years, a variety of educational programs have been applied with promising results. The most effective prevention strategies are those that are part of a broader, more general effort to promote overall health and success. Health-compromising behaviors are often interconnected and have common antecedents. Prevention efforts that focus on changing only one behavior (e.g., alcohol and other drug use) are less likely to be successful. Successful programs are those that have promoted parenting skills, social skills among distractible children, academic achievement, and skills to resist peer pressure.

Peer pressure is a powerful tool and can be used effectively in substance abuse prevention. A group that has had some success in reducing injury from drunk driving is Students Against Driving Drunk (SADD).‡ Techniques used by this group include peer counseling, parental guidelines for teenage parties, and community awareness. Nurses should encourage the formation of SADD chapters in the high schools in their communities.

---

*PO Box 1069, Doylestown, PA 18901; phone: 215-348-7090; Web site: www.toughlove.org.

†675 W. Foothill Blvd, Suite 220, Claremont, CA 91711; phone: 909-621-6184. Another source of information is the National Clearinghouse for Alcohol and Drug Information, PO Box 2345, Rockville, MD 20852; phone: 800-729-6686; email: info@health.org; Web site: www.health.org.

‡PO Box 800, Marlboro, MA 01752; phone: 508-481-3568 or 800-886-2972; Web site: www.saddonline.com

Suicide

Suicide is defined as the deliberate act of self-injury with the intent that the injury results in death. Most experts distinguish between suicidal ideation, suicide attempt (or parasuicide), and suicide.

Suicidal ideation involves a preoccupation with thoughts about committing suicide and may be a precursor to suicide. Although it is not uncommon for adolescents to experience occasional suicidal thoughts, expressions of preoccupation with suicide should be taken seriously, and an assessment should be conducted for appropriate referral. A *suicide attempt* is intended to cause injury or death. The term *parasuicide* is used to refer to behaviors ranging from gestures to serious attempts to kill oneself. Parasuicide is a preferred term because it makes no reference to intent and because a person's motive may be too difficult or complex to determine. However, all parasuicidal activity should be taken seriously.

NURSE ALERT A history of a previous suicide attempt is a serious indicator for possible suicide completion in the future. Studies of adolescent suicides have found that as many as half of the adolescents had made previous attempts. ■

Recent results from the Youth Risk Behavior Survey, 2001, indicated that 8.8% of students nationwide had attempted suicide at least once during the 12 months preceding the survey (Grunbaum et al, 2002). This number represented a significant increase from 7.8% who reported attempts in 1999 (Division of Adolescent and School Health, 2000). Approximately 15% of the students in this survey reported that they had made a specific plan to attempt suicide in the 12 months preceding the survey. In the United States, the suicide rate for adolescents has increased dramatically in the last few decades. Suicide is currently the third leading cause of death during the teenage years, surpassed only by death from injury and homicide (see Chapter 29).

Etiology

Individual, family, and social-environmental factors have all been implicated in suicide. The single most important individual factor is the presence of an active psychiatric disorder (depression, bipolar disorder, psychosis, substance abuse, or conduct disorder). Comorbidity of an affective disorder and substance abuse also increases the risk for suicide. Alcohol use has been associated with more than 50% of suicides (AAP, Committee on Adolescence, 2000). Gay and lesbian adolescents are at particularly high risk for suicide completion, especially if raised in an environment in which they are denied support systems (Community Focus box). Family factors influencing suicide include parental loss; family disruption; a family history of suicide, depression, substance abuse, or emotional disturbance; child abuse or neglect; unavailable parents; poor communication and isolation within the family; family conflict; and unrealistically high parental expectations or parental indifference with low expectations. Social/environmental factors include incarceration, isolation, acute loss of a boyfriend or girlfriend, lack of future options, and availability of firearms in the home.

Community Focus

SUICIDE, SEXUAL IDENTITY, AND SEXUAL ORIENTATION

A significant number of teenage suicides occur among homosexual youths. Gay or lesbian adolescents who live in families or communities that do not accept homosexuality are likely to suffer low self-esteem, self-loathing, depression, and hopelessness as a result of lack of acceptance from their family or community. Such internalization, without treatment and support, can lead to substance abuse and, eventually, suicide. Youths most at risk are those who struggle with gender identity issues such as gay identity formation at a young age, intrapersonal conflict regarding sexuality, and nondisclosure of orientation to others.

Supportive parents, friends, or relationships serve as protective factors against suicide. However, many gay, lesbian, and bisexual adolescents do not feel supported, understood, or accepted by their friends, parents, and families. Nurses who interact with adolescents must be aware of the association between suicide and adolescent homosexuality and gender nonconformity. School nurses may be the first individuals to discuss issues of sexual identity and orientation with adolescents and/or their families. In their professional capacity, nurses can also serve as support persons for these adolescents. Nurses can also provide guidance and resources to families so that they know and understand how best to nurture and support their child.

Nurses must also capitalize on opportunities or experiences that promote the healthy development of self-esteem in youths who choose nontraditional sexual orientation. Educational programs to raise the level of consciousness about the risk factors for and warning signs of suicide are one example. Another possibility could be programs conducted in or outside of school that are designed to foster peer relationships and competency in social skills among high-risk adolescents and young adults, such as support groups and social organizations for these young people.

Methods

Firearms are by far the most commonly used instruments in completed suicides among males and females (AAP, Committee on Adolescence, 2000). For adolescent males, the second and third most common means of suicide are hanging and overdose, respectively; for females, the second and third most common means are overdose and strangulation.

The most common method of suicide attempt is overdose or ingestion of a potentially toxic substance, such as drugs. The second most common method of suicide attempt is self-inflicted laceration.

NURSE ALERT Given what is known about youth suicide, nurses should ask parents, especially those with at-risk teenagers, if firearms are available in the house and, if so, recommend their removal. Parents must ensure that their children, especially those who are depressed, have poor problem-solving skills, or use drugs or alcohol, do not have access to firearms. Parents must also be educated on the warning signs of suicide (Box 40-8). ■

BOX 40-8

Warning Signs of Suicide

- Preoccupation with themes of death—focuses on morbid thoughts
- Wants to give away cherished possessions
- Talks of own death, desire to die
- Loss of energy, loss of interest, listlessness
- Exhaustion without obvious cause
- Changes in sleep patterns—too much or too little
- Increased irritability, argumentativeness, or stubbornness
- Physical complaints—recurrent stomachaches, headaches
- Repeated visits to physician, nurse practitioner, or emergency department for treatment of injuries
- Reckless behavior
- Antisocial behavior—engages in drinking, uses drugs, fights, commits acts of vandalism, runs away from home, becomes sexually promiscuous
- Sudden change in school performance—lowered grades, cutting classes, dropping out of activities
- Resists or refuses to go to school
- Remains distant, sad, remote—flat affect, frozen facial expression
- Describes self as worthless
- Sudden cheerfulness following deep depression
- Social withdrawal from friends, activities, interests that were previously enjoyed
- Impaired concentration
- Dramatic change in appetite

Motivation

Suicidal ideation is not uncommon in adolescents. It represents numerous fantasies, such as relief from suffering, a means of gaining comfort and sympathy, or a means of revenge against those who have hurt them. Adolescents have the erroneous perception that the act of suicide will evoke remorse and pity and that they will be able to return and witness the grief. Angry children who are unable to punish directly those who have injured or insulted them may take revenge on those who love them through self-destruction ("They'll be sorry when they find me dead." "They'll be sorry they were mean to me.").

For adolescents who are severely depressed, suicide seems to be the only release from their despair. These youngsters rarely provide evidence of their intent, and frequently conceal their suicidal thoughts. Many adolescents, however, tell their peers of their suicidal thoughts or plans but avoid telling adults. Social isolation is a significant factor in distinguishing adolescents who will kill themselves from those who will not. It is also more characteristic of those who complete suicide than of those who make attempts or threats.

The frequency of *contagion*, or *copycat suicides* (i.e., an increase in youth suicide that occurs after the suicide of one teenager is publicized) is disturbing and may indicate that teenagers perceive suicide as "glamorous." In addition, young people may not realize the finality of suicide because they have become desensitized from constantly viewing violence and death on television.

Diagnostic Evaluation

Depression is common among adolescents who attempt suicide. Depression is characterized by both subjective symptoms and objective signs that reflect the adolescent's sadness and despair. Adolescents describe feelings of sadness, despair, helplessness, hopelessness, boredom, loss of interest, and isolation. They may also feel self-reproach, self-deprecation, and guilt. Subjective symptoms of depression or specific changes in behavior place an adolescent at risk for suicide.

Therapeutic Management

Threats of suicide should always be taken seriously. There has been a tendency to dismiss a suicide attempt as an impulsive act resulting from a temporary crisis or depression. If a suicide attempt fails to draw attention to his or her problems or makes them worse, the child or adolescent may conclude that suicide is the only answer. Children need to know that someone cares and must be provided with swift and efficient crisis intervention. Although ordinary practitioners can manage an acute depressive reaction without difficulty, the youngster who has made a serious attempt or has a specific plan for suicide should receive immediate attention and competent psychiatric care.

NURSE ALERT Adolescents who express suicidal feelings and have a specific plan should be monitored at all times. They should not have access to firearms, prescription or over-the-counter drugs, belts, scarves, shoestrings, sharp objects, matches, or lighters. If they are intoxicated, they must be restrained or placed in a protective environment until a psychiatrist or psychologist can assess them. ■

Nursing Care Management

Care of the suicidal youngster includes early recognition, management, and prevention. The most important aspect of management is the recognition of warning signs that indicate a youngster is troubled and might attempt suicide. Health professionals must be alert to the signs of depression, and anyone who exhibits such behavior should be referred for thorough psychologic assessment. Depression is manifested differently in children and adolescents from that in adults. In teens it may be masked by impulsive aggressive behaviors. Defiance, disobedience, behavior problems, and psychosomatic disturbances can indicate underlying depression, suicidal ideation, and impending suicide attempts.

NURSE ALERT No threat of suicide should be ignored or challenged. Threats are a symptom that must be taken seriously. Too often, suicidal threats or minor attempts are confused with bids for attention. It is also a mistake to be lulled into a false sense of security when the adolescent's depression is apparently relieved. The improvement in attitude may mean that the youngster has made the decision and found the means to carry out the threat. ■

Peers or other confidants are valuable observers and excellent sources of information about potential suicide attempts. They may not be able to diagnose depression, but they are able to sense when a friend has undergone a marked personality change. It is important to emphasize that the peer who detects any changes in a friend is a potential rescuer and should not remain silent about the observations. Friendship does not imply collusion. A peer who believes that a friend may be suicidal should alert someone who can help (e.g., a parent, teacher, guidance counselor, school nurse, or other person).

Routine health assessments of adolescents should include questions that assess the presence of suicidal ideation or intent. The following questions can be asked (Greydanus & Pratt, 1995):

- Do you consider yourself more a happy person, an unhappy person, or somewhere in the middle?
- Have you ever been so unhappy or upset that you felt like being dead?
- Have you ever thought about hurting yourself?
- Have you ever developed a plan to hurt yourself or kill yourself?
- Have you ever attempted to kill yourself?

If a child or adolescent expresses suicidal intent, nurses make a contract, asking them to sign an agreement that they will not attempt suicide during an agreed-upon period of time and that they will call the 24-hour crisis line immediately if they feel they cannot keep their contract. The amount of time a youngster feels comfortable contracting is usually an indication of his or her risk and stability.

Because a suicide attempt is frequently an outgrowth of family distress, it is essential to intervene with the family. It is important to assess family interactions and to recognize disturbed relationships. The most effective approach is recognition of susceptible youngsters during the early stages of family distress so that family counseling can be started. Prevention must be directed toward improving childrearing practices through support and education of parents and changing societal conditions that generate defeat, despair, and maladaptive behavior.

Although confidentiality is an essential part of adolescent counseling, in the case of self-destructive behaviors, confidentiality cannot be honored. Suicidal behavior is reported to the family and other professionals, and youngsters are informed that this will be done. Such action conveys an important message to the youth—that the professionals understand and care.

Many schools have instituted suicide prevention programs. These programs include services such as drop-in counseling and a peer-counseling telephone line. Information can also be obtained from the American Association of Suicidology.*

*Suite 408, 4201 Connecticut Ave. NW, Suite 408, Washington, DC 20008; phone: 202-237-2280; Web site: www.suicidology.org.

Key Points

- The pubescent growth spurt that begins around age 10 in girls and age 12 in boys signals the beginning of adolescence.
- Biologic development during puberty is characterized by increased activity of the pituitary gland, which results in sexual maturity and the appearance of secondary sex characteristics.
- According to Erikson, the major developmental crisis of adolescence is establishing a sense of identity.
- Spiritual development is characterized by the questioning of family values and ideals, a move to more philosophic thinking, and emphasis on personal religion.
- Adolescent relationships with parents may be strained, and the influence of the peer group increases and intimate relationships assume importance.
- Teenagers demonstrate a wide variety of interests, and their increased physical and cognitive skills allow them to engage in increasingly difficult and complex activities.
- Adolescents' emotions fluctuate.
- Nutritional needs, especially for calcium, zinc, and iron, may not be met by teenagers' eating habits, such as snacking and irregular mealtimes.
- Motor vehicle injuries are the primary cause of death from injury in the adolescent years.
- The rapid changes, growth, and stress accompanying the transition to adulthood may predispose youngsters to faulty problem solving.
- Cognitive development in adolescence includes abstract thought, thinking beyond the present, logical reasoning, and a sense of idealism.
- Development of body image is closely tied to body changes and social interactions.
- According to Kohlberg's theory of moral development, adolescents begin to question existing moral values and learn to make choices.
- The most common health problems related to the female reproductive system involve menstrual dysfunction.
- Eating disorders observed in middle and late childhood are obesity, anorexia nervosa, and bulimia.
- Smoking is a widespread problem among teenagers. Reasons for smoking include social pressure, mass media influence, and a need to develop a self-concept.
- The substances abused by children and adolescents are alcohol, marijuana, narcotics, central nervous system depressants, central nervous system stimulants, hydrocarbons and fluorocarbons, and mind-altering drugs.
- Suicide, the deliberate act of self-injury with the intent to kill, may occur because of difficulties coping with stress, disturbed family environment, chemical dependency, or psychoses.
- No threat of suicide by an adolescent should be ignored or challenged.

Answer Guidelines to Critical Thinking Exercises

Discussing the Future

1. Yes, there is sufficient information to arrive at a conclusion about what advice to give Jeremy's mother.
2. (a) During adolescence, teens consider all their past relationships as they attempt to form their own personal identity. They attempt to formulate a satisfactory identity from a multiplicity of roles, aspirations, and identifications. The process of developing this identity is time-consuming and can be associated with confusion and discouragement. (b) If significant others are too persistent and demand that adolescents make specific decisions or behave in definite ways, adolescents often make prema-

ture decisions and accept roles that do not incorporate their own personal goals or aspirations. (c) Parents who communicate well with their teens have an open, nonjudgmental, nondictatorial manner. They demonstrate that they are available and willing to listen to their teenagers. However, they also wait until the teenager opens the discussion, and then they listen attentively and allow the teen to explore their issues.

3. The nursing priority in this situation is to have the mother become more aware that Jeremy is not likely to discuss his concerns on a timetable, and that it is important for her to respect his point of view. Although Jeremy wants his mother's guidance and support, he does not want to be told what to do, and he needs an opportunity to express his own feelings and views. An example of appropriate advice to give Jeremy's mother might be: "Be open and available to Jeremy. Tell him what you think, but *not what to do*."
4. Yes, the information about how teens formulate a personal identity and the principles of effective parent communication allow the nurse to formulate this response.
5. If Jeremy's mother changes her behavior and Jeremy still does not want to communicate and continues to withdraw from conversation, after a significant period of time, the nurse might explore the possibility of counseling for Jeremy and his mother. Jeremy could be suffering from depression or some other condition that causes him to withdraw from conversation and interaction with his mother.

Discussing Sexual Orientation

1. Yes, there is sufficient data to arrive at a conclusion about how to respond to John.
2. (a) Studies of gay men and lesbians indicate that adolescence is the time when individuals become aware of same-sex attraction. Homosexual and bisexual youths are at risk for health damaging behaviors such as early initiation of sexual behavior, substance abuse, suicide, and running away from home. (b) Homosexual and bisexual youths are often confronted with the antihomosexual attitudes and values of society. It is this reaction of society that makes it difficult for homosexual and bisexual youths to grow up and become healthy physically and mentally. (c) Health professionals who work with adolescents should consider the adolescent's increasing independence and responsibility while ensuring confidentiality.
3. The nurse's first priority in this situation is to give John permission to discuss his feelings about this topic. He has come to the nurse practitioner to discuss this matter, and he probably feels comfortable sharing this information with her. The nurse practitioner needs to be open and nonjudgmental in her interactions with John. He needs to know that the nurse practitioner will maintain confidentiality, appreciate his feelings, and remain sensitive to his need to talk about this topic. An example of an appropriate response for the nurse practitioner might be: "John, tell me more about how you came to this conclusion?"
4. Yes, the information about sexual orientation in adolescence and the role of the health care professional support this conclusion.
5. It might be appropriate for the nurse to gather information about John's support system and to determine the attitudes and values of John's family and peer group toward homosexuality. In addition to establishing a trusting relationship and effective communications with John, the nurse practitioner should make sure that John has a safe environment.

Respecting Privacy

1. Yes, there is sufficient evidence for the nurse to formulate a response to Jamie's mother.
2. (a) As teenagers progress through adolescence, they are able to assume more responsibility for their own health. They can take prescribed medications, keep health care appointments, and discuss their care with health care professionals. (b) Parents of adolescents should respect their teenager's independence while maintaining some level of parental involvement with their child. However, in matters of health care, they should gradually assume the role of a consultant and allow their child to take an increasingly active role in relating to health professionals. (c) Health professionals who work with adolescents must consider the adolescent's increasing independence and responsibility while also maintaining privacy and ensuring confidentiality. In most adolescent clinics, health care professionals meet with the adolescent and the parent together, followed by individual time with both the adolescent and the parent.
3. The first priority for nursing care at this point is to reassure both Jamie and her mother that they each will have an opportunity to express their concerns to the nurse practitioner. Because Jamie is the nurse practitioner's patient and the setting is an adolescent clinic, the nurse practitioner should speak with Jamie first after she has met briefly with Jamie and her mother together. An appropriate response by the nurse practitioner might be: "I would like to begin by speaking with both of you together, then spend some time just with you, Jamie, then just with you, Mrs. S." Knowing that her mother will also have an opportunity to express concerns, Jamie will likely be more open and may even say, "I know what my mother will tell you," and address the issue herself. This response will also demonstrate to Jamie that the nurse practitioner respects her privacy and will maintain confidentiality. If the nurse spoke with Mrs. S first, Jamie might feel that her privacy is being violated, and become distrustful of both the nurse practitioner and her mother. In addition, if the nurse practitioner speaks with Mrs. S first, Jamie is likely to become defensive and spend her time trying to draw from the nurse practitioner what her mother said.
4. Yes, the information about adolescent growth and development and the roles of the adolescent, their parents, and the health care professional support this conclusion.
5. The nurse practitioner should remember the circumstances under which she or he would not be able to maintain confidentiality. For example, if either Jamie or her mother share information that indicates that Jamie is at risk for either a self-destructive behavior (e.g., a suicide attempt) or maltreatment by others (child abuse), the

nurse practitioner would not be able to maintain confidentiality. However, this does not seem to be the case, based on the evidence presented at this point.

Testicular Self-Examination

1. Yes. Although testicular cancer is not common in adolescence, when it does occur it is generally malignant. Testicular cancer is very curable if detected early.
2. (a) The best way to detect testicular tumors is by performing TSE every month. (b) The usual presenting symptom for testicular cancer is a heavy, hard painless mass (either smooth or nodular) that is palpated on the testis. (c) Adolescent boys are very self-conscious about their genital anatomy. However, as a pediatric nurse practitioner at the school-based clinic, Paul is in an excellent position to teach young men how to perform this exam. It is highly probable that he has already won their trust and confidence through his routine daily nursing activities, such as providing sports physicals and treating their episodic illnesses. Paul will be able to present the class in a manner that is respectful of the young boys, while also allaying their anxieties and providing them with an important health skill. (d) The class should be presented in a matter-of-fact way, with an explanation of both the characteristics of the normal testicle as well as a description of abnormal findings.
3. The first priority is to make sure that all adolescents boys with health problems feel comfortable visiting the health suite and sharing their concerns with the nurse practitioner. The ultimate goal is to be sure that no adolescent boy with a potential testicular tumor fails to get an immediate assessment and referral for treatment.
4. Yes, the information about testicular cancer and the importance of detecting it early provide a definite rationale for the class.
5. If it is difficult to find the time for the class in the regular school health curriculum, Paul should suggest other options. Perhaps Paul could provide the information on TSE as part of an extra class that students volunteer to attend, or he could develop a self-learning packet that male students could complete when they visit the health suite.

Anorexia Nervosa

1. Using the clinical manifestations of AN (see Box 40-5) and the diagnostic criteria for AN (see Box 40-6), there is sufficient evidence to support the conclusion that Jane has AN.
2. (a) Young adolescent females with AN are often high achievers or excellent students. They have an abundance of energy, a distorted body image, and a fear of gaining weight. (b) A family crisis can influence AN. Jane's parents are currently in the middle of a divorce, and in this type of situation, some teens feel they have no control over events in their life. Consequently, some adolescents take control by refusing to eat and developing AN. (c) Jane is engaging in increased physical activity and is skipping lunch several days each week. On physical examination, she has a decreased body temperature (96.8° F), and she has lost 9 kg or 18 pounds in the past year (she is at <85% of her expected weight). She also told the nurse practitioner the she has not had her menstrual period for 3 months. These manifestations are all congruent with AN. (d) AN is treated by a team of health professionals who address the abnormal eating patterns as well as the altered body image of the individual with AN and the dysfunctional family dynamics that accompany this disorder.
3. Jane should be referred to a specialist who deals with adolescents with AN
4. Yes, the evidence supports the conclusion.
5. Because Jane has not had her menstrual period for 3 months, there is a possibility that Jane is pregnant. The nurse practitioner should obtain a pregnancy test to rule out the possibility of pregnancy.

References

Alan Guttmacher Institute: *Facts in brief, teen sex, and pregnancy,* New York, 1998, The Institute.

American Academy of Pediatrics, Committee on Adolescence: Suicide and suicide attempts in adolescents, *Pediatrics* 105(4):871-874, 2000.

American Academy of Pediatrics, Committee on Infectious Diseases, Pickering L (ed): *2003 Red Book: Report of the Committee on Infectious Diseases,* ed 26, Elk Grove Village, IL, 2003, The Academy.

American Psychiatric Association: *Diagnostic and statistical manual of mental disorders,* ed 4 (DSM-IV TR), Washington, DC, 2000, The Association.

Baker JG et al: Relationship between perceived parental monitoring and young adolescent girls' sexual and substance use behaviors, *J Pediatr Adolesc Gynecol* 12(2):17-22, 1999.

Baughcum AE et al: Maternal perceptions of overweight preschool children, *Pediatrics* 106(6):1380-1386, 2000.

Biro FM et al: Impact of timing of pubertal maturation on growth in black and white female adolescents: the National Heart Lung and Blood Institute growth and health study, *J Pediatr* 138(5):636-643, 2001.

Briggs M, Safaii S, Beall DL: Nutrition services an essential component of comprehensive school health programs, *J Am Diet Assoc* 103(4):505-514, 2003.

Brown J: Body and spirit: religion, spirituality and health among adolescents, *Adolesc Med* 12(3):509-523, 2001.

Carroll ST et al: Tattoos and body piercings as indicators of adolescent risk-taking behaviors, *Pediatr* 109(6):1021-1027, 2002.

Centers for Disease Control and Prevention: *Defining overweight and obesity,* Atlanta, 2002.

Centers for Disease Control and Prevention. Division of Adolescent and School Health, National Center for Chronic Disease Prevention and Health Promotion: Youth risk behavior surveillance—United States, 1999, *MMWR* 49(SS05):1-96, 2000.

Committee on Adolescence: Identifying and treating eating disorders, *Pediatrics* 111(1):204-211, 2003.

Daniels SR: Abnormal weight gain and weight management: are carbohydrates the enemy, *J Pediatr* 142(3):225-227, 2003.

Erikson EH: *Childhood and society,* ed 2, New York, 1963, WW Norton.

Garofalo R, Katz E: Healthcare issues of gay and lesbian youth, *Curr Opin Pediatr* 13(4):298-302, 2001.

Geller AC et al: Use of sunscreen, sunburning rates and tanning bed use among more than 10,000 U.S. children and adolescents, *Pediatrics* 109(6):1009-1014, 2002.

Goodman E, Capitman J: Depressive symptoms and cigarette smoking among teens, *Pediatrics* 106(4):748-755, 2000.

Gordon SM: *Adolescent drug use: trends in abuse, treatment and prevention,* Wernersville, 2000, Caron Foundation.

Graber JA et al: Is psychopathology associated with the timing of pubertal development? *J Am Acad Child Adolesc Psychiatry* 36(12):1768-1775, 1997.

Greydanus DE, Pratt HD: Emotional and behavioral disorders of adolescence, part 2, *Adolesc Health Update* 8(1):1-8, 1995.

Grunbaum JA et al: Youth risk behavior surveillance—United States, 2001, *MMWR* Surveillance Summaries, 51(SS04):1-64, 2002.

Hamburg DA: Toward a strategy for healthy adolescent development, *Am J Psychiatry* 154(6):7-12, 1997.

Harries M et al: Changes in the male voice at puberty: vocal fold length and its relationship to the fundamental frequency of the voice, *J Laryngol Otol* 112(5):451-454, 1998.

Hayward C et al: Psychiatric risk associated with early puberty in adolescent girls, *J Am Acad Child Psychiatry* 36(12):255-262, 1997.

Hillard PA, Nelson LM: Adolescent girls, the menstrual cycle and bone health, *J Pediatr Endoc Metab* 16(suppl 3):673-681, 2003.

Hoff T, Greene L, Davis J: *National survey of adolescent and young adult sexual health knowledge, attitudes and experiences,* California, 2003, Henry J Kaiser Family Foundation.

Hoffman RG, Rodrique JR, Johnson JH: Effectiveness of a school-based program to enhance knowledge of sun exposure: attitudes toward sun exposure and sunscreen use among children, *Child Health Care* 28(1): 69-86, 1999.

Lindeke LL, Rogers S, Finley L: An update on growth charts, old and new, *Pediatric Nursing* 28(2):138-141, 2002.

Maes L, Lievens J: Can the school make a difference? A multilevel analysis of adolescent risk and health behaviour, *Social Science & Med* 56(3): 517-529, 2003.

McArdle WD, Katch FI, Katch VL: *Essentials of exercise physiology*, ed 2, Philadelphia, 2000 Lippincott, Williams & Wilkins.

McWhorter JW, Wallmann HW, Alpert PT: The obese child: Motivation as a tool for exercise, *J Pediatr Health Care* 17(1):11-17, 2003.

Miller M, Azrael D, Hemenway D: Firearm availability and unintentional firearm deaths, suicide and homicide among 5-14 year olds, *J Trauma* 52(2):267-275, 2002.

Moolchan ET, Ernst M, Henningfield JE: A review of tobacco smoking in adolescents: treatment implications, *J Am Acad Child Adolesc Psychiatry* 39(6):682-693, 2000.

Moran R: Evaluation and treatment of childhood obesity, *Am Fam Physician* 59(4):861-868, 1999.

Moran R: Breaking the cycle of childhood obesity, *The Clinical Advisor* 6(2):62-67, 2003.

National Task Force on the Prevention and Treatment of Obesity: Overweight, obesity and health risk, *Arch Intern Med* 160(7):898, 2000.

Neinstein LS: *Adolescent health care: a practical guide,* ed 4, Baltimore, 2002, Williams & Wilkins.

Nielsen SJ, Popkin BM: Patterns and trends in food portion sizes, 1977-1998, *JAMA*, 289(4):450-453, 2003.

Ogden CL et al: Prevalence and trends in overweight among US children and adolescents, 1999-2000, *JAMA* 288(14):1728-1732, 2002.

Omar H, McElderry D, Zakharia R: Educating adolescents about puberty: what are we missing? *Int J Adolesc Med Health* 15(1):79-83, 2003.

Patten LH et al: Depressive symptoms and cigarette smoking predict development and persistence of sleep problems in US adolescents, *Pediatrics*, 106(2):E23, 2000.

Ralston SH: What determines peak bone mass and bone loss, *Baillieres Clin Rheumatol* 11(3):479-494, 1997.

Resnick MD et al: Protecting adolescents from harm: findings from the National Longitudinal Study on Adolescent Health, *JAMA* 278:823-832, 1997.

Rigotti NA, Lee JE, Wechsler H: US college student's use of tobacco products: results of a national survey, *JAMA* 284(6):699-705, 2000.

Rojas NL et al: Nicotine dependence among adolescent smokers, *Arch Pediatr Adolesc Med* 152(2):151-156, 1998.

Rosenstein NE, Fischer M, Tappero JW: Vaccine recommendations: challenges and controversies, *Infect Dis Clin N Am* 15(1):155-169, 2001.

Saewyc EM et al: Gender differences in health and risk behaviors among bisexual and homosexual adolescents, *J Adolesc Health Care* 23(3):181-188, 1998.

Schneider MB, Fisher MM: Anorexia and bulimia nervosa. In Hoeckelman RA (ed): *Primary pediatric care*, ed 4, St Louis, 2001, Mosby.

Seidell JC: Obesity: a growing problem, *Acta Paediatr* 88(suppl 428):46-50, 1999.

Simonsen RJ: Pit and fissure sealant: review of the literature, *Pediatr Dent* 24(5):393-414, 2002.

Sondike S et al: Effects of a low-carbohydrate diet on weight loss and cardiovascular risk factors in overweight adolescents, *J Pediatr* 142(3): 253-258, 2003.

Starr NB: Sun smarts: the essentials of sun protection, *J Pediatr Health Care* 13(3, part 1):136-138, 1999.

Strauss RS: Childhood obesity and self-esteem, *Pediatrics* 105(1):e15, 2000.

Timmreck LS, Reindollar RH. Contemporary issues in primary amenorrhea, *Obstet Gynecol Clin North Am* 30(2):287-302, 2003.

US Department of Health and Human Services: *National household survey on drug abuse, 1999*, Washington, DC, 1999, Substance Abuse and Mental Health Services Administration.

Wax PM: Just a click away: recreational drug web sites on the internet, *Pediatrics* 109(6):e96, 2002.

Williams AF, Ferguson SA: Rationale for graduated licensing and the risks it should address, *Injury Preven* 8(2):ii9-14, 2002.

Williams AF, McCartt AF, Geary L: Seatbelt use by high school students, *Injury Preven* 9(1):25-28, 2003.

Wilson ML, Murphy PA: Herbal and dietary therapies for primary and secondary dysmenorrhea, *Cochrane Database Syst Rev* (3):CD002124, 2001.

41 Chronic Illness, Disability, and End-of-Life Care

LEARNING OBJECTIVES

On completion of this chapter the reader will be able to:

- Identify the scope of and changing trends in care of children with special needs.
- Identify the major reactions of and effects on the family with a child with a special need.
- Define the stages of adjustment to the diagnosis of a chronic condition.
- Recognize the impact of the illness or disability on the developmental stages of childhood.
- Outline nursing interventions that promote the family's optimum adjustment to the child's chronic disorder.
- Outline nursing interventions that support the family at the time of death.
- Define the usual symptoms of normal grief.

ELECTRONIC RESOURCES

Additional information related to the content in Chapter 41 can be found on

the companion website at evolve
http://evolve.elsevier.com/Wong/maternal/

- NCLEX Review Questions
- WebLinks

or the interactive student CD-ROM
Activities for Chapter 41 include the following:

- NCLEX Review Questions
- Case Study—The Dying Child
- Critical Thinking Exercise—Neonatal Loss
- Nursing Care Plan—The Child Who is Terminally Ill or Dying

PERSPECTIVES ON THE CARE OF CHILDREN WITH SPECIAL NEEDS

Scope of the Problem

A number of terms and defining characteristics have been used to describe chronic illness and disability in children (Box 41-1). In recent years there have been continuing efforts to develop a definition that better identifies the numbers of children living with chronic conditions, as well as the impact on health and social services (Jackson, 2000). Currently, children with special health care needs are defined as those who have or are at increased risk for a chronic physical, developmental, behavioral, or emotional condition requiring health and related services of a type or amount beyond what are required by healthy children (Msall et al, 2003; Newacheck & Halfon, 1998).

Ongoing progress in medical and technologic disease management has contributed to the growing number of children with special health care needs. The number of U.S. children diagnosed with acquired immunodeficiency syndrome (AIDS) declined by 75% from 1992 to 2000 (Yogev & Chadwick, 2004). Technologic advances have substantially increased the survival of extremely-low-birth-weight and very-low-birth-weight infants (Jackson, 2000). Children with disabilities are more likely to be in poor health than children without disabilities (Newacheck & Halfon, 1998). The result of such progress is an estimated 15% to 18% of the children in the United States living with a chronic illness or disability and requiring specialized health care of a type or amount beyond that generally required by children (Perrin, 2004).

The most commonly occurring conditions causing disability are diseases of the respiratory tract and impairments of speech, special senses, and intelligence. Mental and nervous system disorders account for about one sixth of all childhood disability (Newacheck & Halfon, 1998).

The impact of chronic illness and disability in children is wide ranging. Chronic conditions in children present most families with additional tasks, responsibilities, and concerns (Ray, 2002). A child's activity level and developmental opportunities can be affected. Days can be lost from school. Children with chronic illness or disability may be at increased risk for behavior or emotional problems. Parents may lose days from work, experience financial strain, and be challenged both emotionally and physically as they cope with care of the child.

BOX 41-1

Common Terms Regarding Children with Special Needs

Chronic illness–A condition that interferes with daily functioning for more than 3 months in a year, causes hospitalization of more than 1 month in a year, or (at time of diagnosis) is likely to do either of these
Congenital disability–A disability that has existed since birth but is not necessarily hereditary
Developmental delay–A maturational lag; an abnormal, slower rate of development in which a child demonstrates a functioning level below that observed in normal children of the same age
Developmental disability–Any mental or physical disability that is manifested before age 22 years and is likely to continue indefinitely
Disability–A functional limitation that interferes with a person's ability, for example, to walk, lift, hear, or learn
Handicap–A condition or barrier imposed by society, the environment, or one's own self; not a synonym for disability
Impairment–A loss or abnormality of structure or function
Technology-dependent child–A child (from birth to age 21 years) with a chronic disability that requires the routine use of a medical device to compensate for the loss of a life-sustaining body function; daily ongoing care or monitoring is required by trained personnel

Adapted from Westbrook LE, Silver EJ, Stein RE: Implications for estimates of disability in children: a comparison of definitional components, *Pediatrics* 101(6):1025-1030, 1998; and Newacheck PW, Halfon N: Prevalence and impact of disabling chronic conditions in childhood, *Am J Public Health* 88(4):610-617, 1998.

Siblings are also affected by having a "different" brother or sister, and may simultaneously feel guilt and anger/jealousy toward their ill sibling. Additionally, secondary losses such as the ability to participate in extracurricular activities or social events occur because of routines imposed by the affected child's chronic condition.

Trends in Care

Developmental Focus

Focusing on the child's *developmental level* rather than chronologic age or diagnosis emphasizes the child's abilities and strengths rather than disabilities. Attention focuses on normalizing experiences, adapting the environment, and promoting coping skills. Nurses often are in vital positions to redirect attention from the pathologic model, with its focus on weaknesses and problems, to the developmental model to meet the unique needs of the child and family.

A developmental focus also considers family development. The life cycle of the family unit reflects changing ages and needs of family members, as well as changing external demands. A family member's serious illness or disability can cause significant stress or crisis at any stage of the family life cycle. Just as with individual development, family development may be interrupted or may even regress to an earlier level of functioning. Nurses can use the concept of family development to plan meaningful interventions and evaluate care (see Developmental Theory, Chapter 31).

Family-Centered Care

Children's physical and emotional health, as well as cognitive and social functioning, are strongly influenced by how well their families function (Schor, 2003). The importance of *family-centered care*—a philosophy that considers the family as the constant in the child's life—is especially evident in the care of children with special needs. As parents learn about the youngster's health care needs, they often become experts in delivering care. Health care providers, including nurses, are adjuncts to the child's care and need to form partnerships with parents. Collaboration is essential to forming trusting and effective partnerships and has the goal of finding the best ways to meet the needs of the child and family. Collaborative relationships are characterized by communication, dialog, active listening, awareness, and acceptance of differences (Schor, 2003).

Family–Health Care Provider Communication

The disclosure of a serious acute or chronic illness of a child is one of the most stressful aspects of communication between families and health care professionals. Often, parents have suspected for some time that there is something wrong with their child and feel that their concerns were minimized or ignored by health care professionals (Cohen, 1995; Thomlinson, 2002; Whitehead & Gosling, 2003). After a diagnosis is made, numerous studies have shown that parents are not always satisfied with the way in which information is given. Factors that influence parent dissatisfaction with communication include unsympathetic and brief diagnostic interviews, lack of privacy during diagnostic discussions, and not being provided the opportunity to ask questions. Conversely, parents report satisfaction when they perceive the health care workers providing information in an open and honest manner with respect for the parents' need for privacy and time to express emotions and ask questions (Davies, Davis, & Sibert, 2003). Similarly, these factors are important in communication of changes in the child's condition throughout the course of his or her illness.

Providing information to families with a chronically ill child should be a process of repeated discussions to allow the family to process the information, to process their reactions to that information, and to allow them to ask for clarification and further information. Nurses play an important role in ensuring that families' needs are met during discussions related to the child's diagnosis, condition, and treatment. This requires assessment regarding how much information the family is comfortable with, what they understand of the information already given to them, and how they are coping with the information both cognitively and emotionally. Nurses should ensure that the appropriate health care professionals address any concerns or further questions that families may have.

Establishing Therapeutic Relationships

Another important aspect of family-centered care of chronically ill children is establishing a therapeutic relationship with the child and family. Families, most often the mother, take on enormous responsibility in providing technical care and symptom management of their child's condition outside the health care institution (O'Brien & Wegner, 2002; Swallow & Jacoby, 2001). To build successful therapeutic relationships with families, it is necessary for nurses to recognize parents' expertise with regard to their child's condition and needs. Care conferences, especially multidisciplinary meetings that include the family and key health professionals, provide an opportunity for joint sharing of ideas and expression of feelings or concerns.

The Role of Culture in Family-Centered Care

Issues of culture, ethnicity, and race affect access to services, utilization, and follow-through with referrals and recommendations (Wise et al, 2002; Wood et al, 2002; Zuvekas & Taliaferro, 2003). For some ethnic and minority populations, cultural understandings of illness and disability, the structure of family life, social roles for individuals who are disabled, and other factors related to the perception of children may differ from those of "mainstream" American culture. These factors may affect family needs and family choices regarding the care of their child with special needs.

Although culture cannot completely explain how an individual will think and act, understanding cultural perspectives can help the nurse anticipate and understand why families may make certain decisions. Cultural attributes such as values and beliefs regarding illness or disability and its causation, social roles for the ill or disabled, family structure, the role of children, childrearing practices, self versus group orientation, spirituality, and time orientation also affect a family's response to illness or disability in a child (Carter, 2002; Marshall et al, 2003; Rehm, 1999; Sterling & Peterson, 2003).

When parents are informed of their child's chronic illness, interpreters familiar with both culture and language should be used. Children, family members, and friends of the family should not be used as translators because their presence may prevent parents from an open discussion of the issues. When working with people of different cultural backgrounds, nurses must listen carefully with an initial goal of understanding and articulating the family's perspective. The ability to interpret the mainstream medical culture to the family is also important. Furthermore, every effort is made to incorporate traditional cultural beliefs of a family into treatment plans. Developing a plan of care in conjunction with the family, considering their preferences and priorities, is an important first step in formulating a plan of care that best meets the family's needs, no matter what their cultural background (Ahmann, 1994).

Shared Decision Making

Shared decision making among the child, family, and health care team is the desired result of open, honest, culturally sensitive communication and the establishment of a therapeutic relationship between the family and health care providers. In a shared decision-making model the health care professionals provide honest, clear information regarding diagnosis, prognosis, treatment options, and risk/benefit assessment. The patient and family then share information with the health care team regarding important family values, acceptable levels of discomfort or inconvenience, and the ability to comply with treatments being recommended (Charles, Gafni, & Whelan, 1997). This process allows for all options to be discussed with regard to their consequences, risks and benefits to the child and family, the prognosis or expected course of the illness, and the impact on the family's resources (Box 41-2).

BOX 41-2

Facilitating Shared Decision Making

Continually assess the impact of the child's illness and treatment on the family.
Provide honest, accurate information regarding the trajectory of the disease, anticipated complications, and prognostic information.
Discuss what the family desires for the child's quality of life.
Avoid personal opinion or judgment of the family's questions and decisions.

Normalization

Normalization refers to behaviors and intentions of the disabled to integrate into society by living life as persons without a disability would (Morse, Wilson, & Penrod, 2000). For the chronically ill or disabled child, such behaviors could include attending school, pursuing hobbies and recreational interests, and achieving employment and a level of independence in his or her life. For the family, it may entail adapting the ill or disabled child's health and physical needs into the family routine (McDougal, 2002).

Children with chronic illness and disability and their families face numerous challenges in achieving "normalization." Families move between living with the experience of chronic childhood illness and the outside world, and often redefine "normal" based on their particular experiences, needs, and circumstances (Deatrick, Knafl, & Murphy-Moore, 1999; Nelson, 2002).

Nurses can assist families with normalizing their lives by assessing social support systems, coping strategies, family cohesiveness, and family/community resources. Interventions should focus on encouraging families to reduce stress through delegation of caregiving and family tasks, identifying ways to incorporate care into current routines, structuring the home environment to encourage the child's engagement in age-appropriate activities, and ensuring that families have access to appropriate community support services. Being supportive of the child's illness and treatment and actively including the family in all aspects of care will improve their self-esteem and promote further development (Shepard & Mahon, 2000).

Home care represents the return to a system and set of priorities in which family values are as important in the care of a child with a chronic health problem as they are in the care of other children. Home care seeks to achieve goals that are consistent with the developmental model (Stein, 1985):

- Normalize the life of a child with special needs, including those with technologically complex care, in a family and community context and setting.
- Minimize the disruptive impact of the child's condition on the family.
- Foster the child's maximum growth and development.

With appropriate training and support, families provide complex procedures and treatments in the home. Parents are challenged to retain a homelike setting among monitors, ventilators, and other sophisticated equipment. Throughout the text, home care is discussed as appropriate for specific conditions.

Paralleling normalization and home care is the process of *mainstreaming,* or integrating children with special needs into regular classrooms. Just as the home is the natural environment for children, so school must also be included as an essential component of the children's overall physical, intellectual, and social development. Children who attend school have the advantages of learning and socializing with a wide group of peers. There is an increased focus on individualization as the academic needs of these children are planned along with those of the rest of the students.

A variety of supplemental programs have been designed in the school system to accommodate special needs, both at school age and younger, through early intervention, which consists of any sustained and systematic effort to assist children from birth to age 3 years who are young, disabled, and developmentally vulnerable. This change and increasing opportunities for normalization for children with special needs in large part have resulted from the passage of Public Law 94-142 (the Education of All Handicapped Children Act of 1975) and its 1990 amendments (Public Law 101-47b), which changed the name of the act to the Individuals with Disabilities Education Act (IDEA); Public Law 99-457 (the Education of the Handicapped Act Amendments of 1986, which directs states to develop and implement statewide comprehensive, coordinated, multidisciplinary interagency programs of early intervention services for infants and toddlers with disabilities, as well as support services for their families); and the Americans with Disabilities Act (ADA) of 1990. Nurses can provide parents with information about these laws and in some cases may participate in the development of individualized educational programs (IEPs) or individualized family service plans (IFSPs) for children with special needs.

Managed Care

Managed care programs have become the major form of health care provision in the United States (Jackson, 2000). The transition to this model of care both offers opportunities and presents challenges with respect to the care of children with special health care needs. Managed care may benefit continuity and coordination of care. At the same time, some research has shown decreased access to pediatric specialists and health-related services in managed care environments.

Managing care for chronically ill children differs greatly from managing care for chronically ill adults in three major ways. First, the large number of rare disorders and low prevalence of children with such disorders makes it difficult to monitor the overall quality of care for the total population of chronically ill children. Second, the influence of the child's growth and development on aspects of onset, impact, treatment, and outcomes of chronic conditions varies with the different developmental stages. Third, children rely on adults for access to health care and follow-up with treatment regimens, making it necessary to manage the child's care in the context of the family (American Academy of Pediatrics, Committee on Children with Disabilities, 1998; Kuhlthau et al, 1998).

THE FAMILY OF THE CHILD WITH SPECIAL NEEDS

A major goal in working with the family of a child with special needs is to support the family's coping and promote their optimum functioning throughout the child's life. Long-term, comprehensive, family-centered approaches extend beyond supporting the child and family during the critical periods of diagnosis and hospitalization. Rather, comprehensive care involves forming parent-professional partnerships that can support a family's adaptation to the many changes that may be necessary in day-to-day life, determine expectations of and for the child, and provide a long-term perspective (Box 41-3).

The impact of a child's medical or developmental condition is often experienced as a crisis at the time of diagnosis, which may be at the time of birth, following a long period of physical or psychologic testing, or immediately after a tragic injury. It may also begin before the diagnosis is made, when parents are aware that something is wrong with their child but before medical confirmation (Cohen, 1995; Thomlinson, 2002; Whitehead & Gosling, 2003).

The time of diagnosis is a critical time for parents. Several factors can make it particularly difficult, including a long duration of uncertainty in the diagnostic process and negative perceptions of chronic illness or disability (Cohen, 1995; Garwick et al, 1995). Planning the setting for informing parents, assessing the family's background knowledge and experience, choosing strategies that fit the family's situation, and evaluating the family's understanding of the information will encourage optimum support at the time of diagnosis.

Impact of the Child's Chronic Illness or Disability

Each family of a child with special needs is affected by the experience. The effects on the parents and their responses are so critical that they directly influence the other members' reactions and the child's own coping.

Parents

Besides grieving for the loss of a perfect child, parents may or may not receive positive feedback from transactions with their child. Many parents feel satisfaction and fulfill-

BOX 41-3

Adaptive Tasks of Parents Having Children with Chronic Conditions

1. Accept the child's condition.
2. Manage the child's condition on a day-to-day basis.
3. Meet the child's normal developmental needs.
4. Meet the developmental needs of other family members.
5. Cope with ongoing stress and periodic crises.
6. Assist family members to manage their feelings.
7. Educate others about the child's condition.
8. Establish a support system.

From Canam C: Common adaptive tasks facing parents of children with chronic conditions, *J Adv Nurs* 18:46-53, 1993.

ment from the parenting role. For others, parenting may be a series of unrewarding experiences that contribute to parental feelings of inadequacy and failure (Box 41-4). These responses may be most evident in parents who are responsible for the child's care. For example, parents may become preoccupied with their ability to carry out certain procedures, overlooking the child's personal comfort and satisfaction or failing to offer praise for anything less than perfect cooperation or performance. They may pursue a frustrating activity until they achieve "success"—long after the child has become irritable and uncooperative. As a result, parents can become caught in a pattern of interaction that is mutually unrewarding and minimally productive. For these parents, several strategies may be helpful: education regarding what can reasonably be expected of their child, assistance in identifying the child's strengths, praise for a parental job well done, and finding respite care so that parents can renew their energies.

Parental Roles

Parenting a child with a chronic illness or disability is above and beyond that of raising a typical child. In addition to attending to the routine aspects of parenting, parents of chronically ill children take on the added responsibility of complex technical care and symptom management, advocacy, and seeking and coordinating health and social services for their ill/disabled child. These added responsibilities must then be balanced with the needs of other family members, extended family and friends, and personal health and obligations to minimize consequences to the overall functioning of the family (Ray, 2002).

Enormous demands may be placed on parental time, energy, and financial resources. Depending on the roles assumed by each partner, these responsibilities may be shared or shifted more heavily to one member. In a shared approach, parents often divide tasks in a very specific way, according to their skills or level of comfort. For example, the parent with patience for waiting may be the logical person to take the child for tests, examinations, and procedures. The parent who deals best with the sickness and side effects of treatment can ready the environment for the child's return home. It is important for nurses to realize that the absence of one parent from the hospital or clinic does not necessarily indicate that the shared parent pattern is not in effect. On the other hand, making efforts to involve both parents in decision making and in learning how to care for the child's special needs can reduce some of the burden of care often placed on mothers.

The nurse can assist parents in avoiding role conflicts by providing anticipatory guidance early on. Teaching should address stressors often identified as having an impact on the marriage: (1) the burden of care at home assumed by primarily one parent, (2) the financial burden, (3) the fear of the child dying, (4) pressure from relatives, (5) the hereditary nature of the disease (if applicable), and (6) fear of pregnancy. Other causes of tension may center on the inconveniences associated with care, such as long waits for an appointment, lack of parking near care facilities, or lack of overnight accommodations. Certainly, these last stressors are within health professionals' domain to minimize, if not eliminate.

Mother/Father Differences

Mothers and fathers in the same family often adjust and cope differently as parents of a child with special needs. Some mothers experience a peaks-and-valleys periodic crisis pattern, whereas most fathers tend to experience a steady, gradual recovery. Some research suggests that mothers of children with certain conditions may be more susceptible to psychologic distress and feeling worn out than fathers (Tong et al, 2002). Mothers are more likely to have to deal with forfeiting or delaying personal goals. Mothers often have greater needs for social support and positive reappraisal of the situation, whereas fathers are more likely to use self-controlling behaviors to cope (Goldbeck, 2001; Mastroyannopoulou et al, 1997).

The father of a child with special needs struggles with issues that may be quite distinct from those of the mother. He may feel that his role of protector is challenged because he does not know how to help and cannot protect the family from the seemingly overwhelming recurring problems. Dreams of lineage, ego fulfillment, and athletic and vocational achievement are threatened and in turn may threaten the father's self-esteem.

Single-Parent Families

Single-parent families are of special concern. The absence of a parent may result from divorce or death, or the parents may never have married. As the only parent of a child who may require extensive, sophisticated, and lifelong care, the single parent may feel an enormous burden. Available financial and emotional resources may already be stretched to the limit. A special effort should be made to assist the single parent in finding financial and support services that can ease the burden of care. Nurses can also assist the single parent in identifying helping roles that may be acceptable to relatives and friends.

Siblings

Results of studies on how siblings are affected by having a brother or sister with special needs are inconsistent. Generally, there is evidence that there is a negative effect on siblings of children with a chronic illness when compared with

BOX 41-4

Anticipated Parental Stress Points

Diagnosis of the condition—Requires considerable learning, as well as dealing with emotional response

Developmental milestones—Times that children normally achieve walking, talking, and self-care are delayed or impossible for the child

Start of schooling—Particularly stressful are situations in which appropriate schooling will not be in a regular class placement

Reaching the ultimate attainment—Situations, such as realizing that ambulation will be impossible or that the child will not learn to read, must be handled

Adolescence—Issues such as sexuality and independence become prominent

Future placement—Decisions about placement must be made when the child becomes an adult or when the parents can no longer care for the child

Death of the child

siblings of healthy children. This effect appears, however, to be decreasing in significance in recent years—most likely because of changes in public attitudes toward the ill and disabled (Sharpe & Rossiter, 2002). However, most investigators do agree that brothers and sisters of children with special needs are no more at risk for *severe* psychiatric problems than are siblings of children without chronic or disabling conditions.

A number of factors increase the risk of negative effects for siblings of ill children. Responsibility for caregiving, differential treatment by parents, and limitations in family resources and recreational time are often the experience of siblings of ill/disabled children (Lobato & Kao, 2002). Some difficulties for siblings arise from the demands of the child's condition. For example, at diagnosis the child with special needs by necessity becomes the focus of parental attention and concern. Frequent hospitalizations or trips to the physician or clinic disrupt the family routine. Siblings are pushed to the background, often staying at the homes of family and friends. The child's condition may interfere with holiday celebrations, vacations, and other special events. Siblings may resent these intrusions, which frequently demand self-sacrifice. Their parents may be unable to attend their school functions, ball games, or other activities and at times may be physically and emotionally unavailable for them. The family's financial and emotional resources may be directed toward the child with special needs. When this occurs, there is often not only a decrease in normal family activities, but a decrease in personal items for the other children as well. Not surprisingly, children with siblings who have chronic illnesses that affect day-to-day functioning appear to be more negatively affected than children of siblings with less intense daily assistance needs (Sharpe & Rossiter, 2002).

Because identification is another characteristic of sibling relationships, some siblings believe that they, too, will "catch" the condition, a reasonable assumption in light of experiences with contagious diseases, such as chickenpox. Identification, combined with a young child's egocentric thinking, may lead a sibling to feel responsible for a brother's or sister's condition. For example, siblings may believe that playing rough with their brother or sister or even thinking bad thoughts about the sibling caused the condition.

Most brothers and sisters experience mixed and sometimes contradictory feelings (Box 41-5). They may feel left out of new family developments and changing roles, guilty that they escaped getting the condition, or sad when their brother or sister is unable to participate in a particular activity or event. Some siblings feel embarrassed and ashamed; having a child in the family who is ill, disfigured, or disabled marks the family as "different" (Family Focus box). Some siblings worry about the health of the affected child (Faulkner, 1996). However, many sibling relationships show a common pattern, consisting of both conflict and companionship. This suggests that although having an ill sibling can present challenges, the relationship may be important and possibly even enhanced between the ill child and his or her sibling (Sharpe & Rossiter, 2002)

An important factor in sibling adjustment and coping is information and knowledge regarding the illness/disability. What siblings piece together or overhear is often much

BOX 41-5

Supporting Siblings of Children with Special Needs

Promote Healthy Sibling Relationships

Value each child individually and avoid comparisons. Remind each child of his or her positive qualities and contribution to other family members.

Help siblings see the differences and similarities between themselves and a child with special needs. Create a climate in which children can achieve successes without feeling guilty.

Teach siblings ways to interact with the child.

Seek to be fair in terms of discipline, attention, and resources; require the affected child to do as much for himself or herself as possible.

Let siblings settle their own differences; intervene only to prevent siblings from hurting one another.

Legitimize reasonable anger. Even children with special needs behave badly sometimes.

Respect a sibling's reluctance to be with or to include the child with special needs in activities.

Help Siblings Cope

Listen to siblings to let them know that their thoughts and suggestions are valued.

Praise siblings when they have been patient, have sacrificed, or have been particularly helpful. Do not expect siblings to always act in this manner.

Acknowledge the personal strengths siblings have and their ability to cope with stress successfully.

Provide age-appropriate information about the child's condition, and update when appropriate.

Let teachers know what is happening so they can be understanding and helpful.

Recognize special stress times for siblings and plan to minimize negative effects.

Schedule special time with siblings; have a friend or family member substitute when parent is unavailable.

Encourage siblings to join or help establish a sibling support group.

Use the services of professionals when needed. If parent feels that such a service is necessary, it should be provided in as vigorous a manner as a service for the child with special needs.

Involve Siblings

Seek out ways to realistically include siblings in the care and treatment of the child with special needs.

Limit caregiving responsibilities and give recognition when siblings perform them.

Develop a library of children's books on special needs.

Invite siblings to attend meetings to develop plans for the child with special needs (e.g., individualized educational program, individualized family service plan).

Discuss future plans with them.

Solicit their ideas on treatment and service needs.

Have them visit professionals who work with the child.

Help them develop competencies to teach the child new skills.

Provide opportunities for siblings to advocate for the child.

Allow siblings to set their own pace for learning and involvement.

Modified from Powell T, Ogle P: *Brothers and sisters—a special part of exceptional families,* Baltimore, 1985, Paul H Brooks; Spokane Washington Deaconess Medical Center, Pediatric Oncology Unit: Tips for dealing with siblings, *Candlelighters Childhood Cancer Found Q Newslett* 11(3,4):7, 1987; and Carlson J, Leviton A, Mueller M: Services to siblings: an important component of family-centered practice, *ACCH Advocate* 1(1):53-56, 1993.

Family Focus

REFLECTION OF AN OLDER BROTHER

My youngest sister, Kerry, was on an apnea monitor 3 years ago, when I was 15. I was never embarrassed about Kerry being on the monitor, except for the time it went off in church and everyone turned around to look at us.

Joey Bellino
Oldest sibling of an infant on an apnea monitor
Washington, DC

worse than the truth. Oftentimes they imagine gruesome things regarding the experiences related to the illness, treatment, and hospitalization (Shepard & Mahon, 2000). Parents are usually in the best position to impart information, although they are often overwhelmed with the medical crisis at hand (Fleitas, 2000). Nurses can encourage parents to talk with the siblings about how they perceive their sick brother or sister and to be accepting of the siblings' feelings. Nurses can be ideal educators and counselors of siblings during the course of their brother's or sister's illness (Shepard & Mahon, 2000).

Extended Family Members and Society

In addition to parents and siblings, significant nonnuclear family members or friends may experience the effects of a child's chronic illness or disability. Although extended family relationships are often helpful to parents in rearing a child with special needs, they may also be sources of stress. For example, grandparents or other well-meaning relatives may attempt to reassure the parents that the child "will grow out of" his or her slowness at a time when parents are struggling to accept reality.

Most grandparents experience some ambivalence: they love their grandchild and yet feel personal disappointment. They often experience a double grief, both for their grandchild and for their child, the parent. The future is now unpredictable not only for the grandchild, but for the child's parents as well. Grandparents do not often acknowledge these emotions and are left to adapt on their own. Support groups for grandparents, although uncommon, can be beneficial.

Considerable stress can also arise from nonfamilial sources, such as friends, neighbors, or strangers. Inability to cope with comments about the disorder or curious stares by others may foster the tendency to isolate and protect the child within the home. The family needs guidance in preparing for these inevitable experiences. Encouraging parents to dress the child as much as possible like other children is one approach. Good grooming is very important in minimizing differences in appearance.

Coping with Ongoing Stress and Periodic Crises

Professionals can help families cope with stress by providing anticipatory guidance, providing emotional support, assisting the family in assessing and identifying specific stressors, aiding the family in developing coping mechanisms and problem-solving strategies, and working collaboratively with parents so that they become empowered in the process.

Concurrent Stresses within the Family

The ability to deal with the overwhelming stresses of a lifelong disability or illness is challenged further when additional stresses are present. Stressors may be situational or developmental. They may be related to marital difficulties, sibling needs, homelessness, or social isolation. Some families may simultaneously be struggling with a family member's alcohol or other drug problem. Even the more minor stresses, such as arranging care for siblings, managing the home, and traveling to distant treatment centers, can challenge a family's ability to cope successfully.

For most families, regardless of their income or insurance coverage, financial concerns exist. The costs of caring for a child with special needs can be overwhelming. Nurses and social workers can help a family review various options for financial assistance, including insurance, managed care, or health maintenance organization (HMO) policies; Medicaid; Supplemental Security Income (SSI); Woman, Infants, and Children program (WIC); state programs for children with special health needs; disease-related associations; and local philanthropic organizations.

Coping Mechanisms

Coping mechanisms are behaviors aimed at reducing the tension caused by a crisis. *Approach behaviors* are coping mechanisms that result in movement toward adjustment and resolution of the crisis. *Avoidance behaviors* result in movement away from adjustment or maladaptation to the crisis. Several approach and avoidance behaviors used in coping with a chronic illness or disability are listed in the Guidelines box on p. 1225. None of the indexes can be used singly to assess the possible success or failure in resolving the crisis. Each behavior must be viewed in the context of all of the variables affecting the family. For example, the observation of several avoidance behaviors in an emotionally healthy family may denote significantly less risk to the successful resolution of the crisis than an equal number of avoidance behaviors in an individual who has few available supports.

Parental Empowerment

Empowerment can be seen as a process of recognizing, promoting, and enhancing competence. For parents of children with chronic conditions, empowerment may occur gradually as strength and capabilities are drawn on to master the child's care, manage family life, and plan for the future. Advocating for the child and developing parent-professional partnerships are part of taking charge (Ray, 2002).

Assisting Family Members in Managing Their Feelings

Although some previous research has postulated stages of adaptation to a chronic illness or disability, there is a great deal of individual variation in responses to the diagnosis, adjustments made, and time frames for coming to terms with a diagnosis. It is important that professionals recognize and respect a wide range of reactions and coping mechanisms. In fact, members of the family of a child with a chronic illness or disability may experience a number of difficult emotions, including fear, guilt, anger, resentment, and anxiety. Learning to manage these emotions promotes adaptive coping.

Guidelines

ASSESSING COPING BEHAVIORS

Approach Behaviors

Asks for information regarding diagnosis and child's present condition
Seeks help and support from others
Anticipates future problems; actively seeks guidance and answers
Endows the illness or disability with meaning
Shares burden of disorder with others
Plans realistically for the future
Acknowledges and accepts child's awareness of diagnosis and prognosis
Expresses feelings such as sorrow, depression, and anger and realizes reason for the emotional reaction
Realistically perceives child's condition; adjusts to changes
Recognizes own growth through passage of time, such as earlier denial and nonacceptance of diagnosis
Verbalizes possible loss of child

Avoidance Behaviors

Fails to recognize seriousness of child's condition despite physical evidence
Refuses to agree to treatment
Intellectualizes about the illness, but in areas unrelated to child's condition
Is angry and hostile to members of the staff, regardless of their attitude or behavior
Avoids staff, family members, or child
Entertains unrealistic future plans for child, with little emphasis on the present
Is unable to adjust to or accept a change in progression of disease
Continually looks for new cures with no perspective toward possible benefit
Refuses to acknowledge child's understanding of disease and prognosis
Uses magical thinking and fantasy; may seek "occult" help
Places complete faith in religion to point of relinquishing own responsibility
Withdraws from outside world; refuses help
Punishes self because of guilt and blame
Makes no change in lifestyle to meet needs of other family members
Resorts to excessive use of alcohol or drugs to avoid problems
Verbalizes suicidal intents
Is unable to discuss possible loss of child or previous experiences with death

Support from professionals, other family members, and friends can assist family members in managing their feelings. The following discussion examines some common phases of adjustment and emotional reactions.

Shock and Denial

The initial diagnosis of a chronic illness or disability is often met with intense emotion and is characterized by shock, disbelief, and sometimes denial, especially if the disorder is not obvious, such as in chronic illness. Denial as a defense mechanism is a necessary cushion to prevent disintegration and is a normal response to grieving for any type of loss. Probably all family members experience various degrees of adaptive denial as they learn of the impact that the diagnosis has on their lives.

Shock and denial can last from days to months, to even years. Examples of denial that may be exhibited at the time of diagnosis include the following:

1. "Physician shopping"
2. Attributing the symptoms of the actual illness to a minor condition
3. Refusing to believe the diagnostic tests
4. Delaying consent for treatment
5. Acting very happy and optimistic despite the revealed diagnosis
6. Refusing to tell or talk to anyone about the condition
7. Insisting that no one is telling the truth, regardless of others' attempts to do so
8. Denying the reason for admission
9. Asking no questions about the diagnosis, treatment, or prognosis

Generally, these mechanisms should be respected as short-term responses that allow individuals to distance themselves from the onslaught of a tremendous emotional impact and to collect and mobilize their energies toward goal-directed, problem-solving behaviors.

In some instances, various indicators of denial can actually be adaptive behaviors. Searching for another professional opinion may mean that parents cannot obtain answers to their questions or that they are looking for a different approach to treatment that better meets the needs of their child and family. Sometimes a delay in making decisions or a failure to ask questions simply reflects a lack of information.

In children, the importance of denial has repeatedly been demonstrated as a factor in their positive coping with the diagnosis. Denial allows the child to maintain hope in the face of overwhelming odds and to function adaptively and productively. Like hope, denial may be an adaptive mechanism for dealing with loss that persists until a family or patient is ready or needs other responses.

Denial is probably the least understood and most poorly dealt with reaction. Health professionals typically label denial as "maladaptive" and act inappropriately by attempting to strip it away by repeated and sometimes blunt explanations of the prognosis. However, denial becomes maladaptive only when it prevents recognition of treatment or rehabilitative goals necessary for the child's optimum survival or development.

Adjustment

For most families, adjustment gradually follows shock and is usually characterized by an open admission that the condition exists. This stage may be accompanied by several responses, which are quite normal parts of the adaptation process. Probably the most universal of these feelings are *guilt* and *self-accusation.* Guilt is often greatest when the cause of the disorder is directly traceable to the parent, such as in genetic diseases or from accidental injury. However, it can occur even without any scientific or realistic basis for parental responsibility. Frequently the guilt stems from a false assumption that the disability is a result of personal failing or wrongdoing, such as not doing something correctly during pregnancy or the birth. Guilt may also be associated with cultural or religious beliefs. Some parents are convinced that they are being punished for some previous misdeed. Others may see the disorder as a sacrifice sent by God to test their religious strength and faith. With correct information, support, and time, most parents master guilt and self-accusation. The ability to master resentful and self-accusatory feelings of having "caused" the child's disorder is a crucial factor in determining the parents' acceptance of their child.

Children, too, may interpret their serious illness as retribution for past misbehavior. The nurse should be particularly sensitive to the child who passively accepts all painful procedures. This child may believe that such acts are inflicted as deserved punishment. It is vital that parents and health care professionals reassure children that their illness is not their fault.

Other common and normal reactions to a diagnosis are *bitterness* and *anger.* Anger directed inward may be evident as self-reproaching or punitive behavior, such as neglecting one's health and verbally degrading oneself. Anger directed outward may be manifested in either open arguments or withdrawal from communication and may be evident in the person's relationship with any number of individuals, such as the spouse, the child, and siblings. Passive anger toward the ill child may be evident in decreased visiting, refusal to believe how sick the child is, or inability to provide comfort. Among the most common targets for parental anger are members of the staff. Parents may complain about the nursing care, the insufficient time physicians spend with them, or the lack of skill of those who draw blood or start intravenous infusions.

Children are apt to respond with anger as well, and this includes both the affected child and the well siblings. Children are aware of the loss engendered by their illness or disability and may react angrily to the restrictions imposed or the feelings of being different. Siblings may also feel anger and resentment toward the ill child and parents for the loss of routine and parental attention. It is difficult for older children and almost impossible for younger children to comprehend the plight of the affected child. Their perception is of a brother or sister who has the undivided attention of their parents, is showered with cards and gifts, and is the focus of everyone's concern.

During the period of adjustment, four types of parental reactions to the child influence the child's eventual response to the disorder: *overprotection,* in which the parents fear letting the child achieve any new skill, avoid all discipline, and cater to every desire to prevent frustration; *rejection,* in which the parents detach themselves emotionally from the child but usually provide adequate physical care or constantly nag and scold the child; *denial,* in which parents act is if the disorder does not exist or attempt to have the child overcompensate for it; and *gradual acceptance,* in which parents place necessary and realistic restrictions on the child, encourage self-care activities, and promote reasonable physical and social abilities.

Reintegration and Acknowledgment

For many families the adjustment process culminates in the development of realistic expectations for the child and reintegration of family life with the illness or disability in a manageable perspective. Because a large portion of this phase is one of grief for a loss, total resolution is not possible until the child dies or leaves home as an independent adult. Therefore one can regard adjustment as "increased comfort" with everyday living rather than a complete resolution.

This adjustment phase also involves social reintegration in which the family broadens its activities to include relationships outside of the home, with the child as an acceptable and participating member of the group. This last criterion often differentiates the reaction of gradual acceptance during the adjustment period from total acceptance, or perhaps is more descriptive of the acknowledgment process.

Many parents of children with chronic illnesses experience *chronic sorrow,* feelings of sorrow and loss that recur in waves over time. As the child's condition progresses, parents experience repeated losses that present further decline and new caregiving demands. Consequently, families must be assessed on an ongoing basis and offered appropriate support and resources as the needs of the family change over time (Gravelle, 1997).

Establishing a Support System

The diagnosis of a child with a serious health problem or disability is a major situational crisis that affects the entire family system. However, families can experience positive outcomes as they successfully deal with the many challenges that accompany a child with chronic illness or disability.

One nursing goal is to assess which families are at greater or lesser risk for succumbing to the effects of the crisis. Several variables—available support system, perception of the event, coping mechanisms, reactions to the child, available resources, and concurrent stresses within the family—influence the resolution of a crisis. Although most families cope well, the needs of families at risk are great. If they receive emotional support and guidance early, there is an increased likelihood that they will also cope successfully. Intrafamilial resources, social support from friends and relatives, parent-to-parent support, parent-professional partnerships, and community resources interweave to provide a flexible web of support for the family of a child with a chronic condition.

THE CHILD WITH SPECIAL NEEDS

Impact of Chronic Illness or Disability on the Child

The child's reaction to chronic illness or disability depends to a great extent on his or her developmental level, temperament, and available coping mechanisms; on the reactions of family members or significant others; and, to a lesser extent, on the condition itself. A child's conceptual understanding of his or her own illness is based not only on age and developmental level, but also on the duration and type of experience accumulated with the disease. Knowledge of these variables is essential in providing the kind of information and support needed by these children to cope with a sometimes overwhelming situation.

Developmental Aspects

The impact of a chronic illness or disability is influenced by the age at onset. Chronic illness affects children of all ages, but the developmental aspects of each age group dictate particular stresses and risks for the child. The nurse must also recognize that children need to redefine their condition and its implications as they develop and grow. An understanding of these developmental factors facilitates planning care to support the child and minimize the risks.

Infant

During infancy the child is engaged in the task of developing trust through an intimate, satisfying, consistent relationship with his or her parents. When illness or disability occurs, this relationship is potentially affected. For example, a visible defect can delay parent bonding as the parent mourns the loss of the perfect child. In addition, prolonged illness may impose separations that prevent the child and parent from normal attachment and deprive the infant of the nurturing relationship.

The illness itself affects the infant, especially because sensorimotor experiences are critical at this age. Illness or disability often impairs the child's motor abilities by confining the child to a crib and lessening contact with the environment. The messages transmitted to infants about their bodies are influenced by the amount of pain and discomfort they experience. Associating touch with pain can compromise the infant's ability to give and receive affection. Lack of pleasurable sensations can lead to an irritable and unhappy child. Consequently, parents may interpret the behaviors as evidence that they are not adequately meeting the child's physical and emotional needs, which further affects the parent-child relationship and the acquisition of trust. Nursing intervention can be important in helping parents work with the irritable child in a way that encourages understanding and caring.

Nurses should advocate for policies and practices that will best meet the needs of the infant and family. Twenty-four–hour visitation in the neonatal intensive care unit and other infant units is of primary importance. Showing parents how to touch and hold the infant will promote their confidence and competence. "Kangaroo care" has been shown to be both safe and beneficial to the infant. Mothers who choose to breastfeed can be encouraged, with a private space provided for them to nurse or pump and storage facilities made available for breast milk. Sibling visitation can be facilitated.

Toddler

The toddler is in the stage of autonomy; the need for mastery of locomotor and language skills is paramount. The child learning to walk and talk progresses toward becoming a separate person, both physically and psychologically. However, illness or disability can hinder mobility and deprive the child of mastery. In addition, overprotective parents can magnify the problem by setting limits on the child's exploration and experimentation for fear of injury or exertion. Even the most basic self-help skills, such as feeding and dressing, may be done for the child. Age-appropriate tasks such as toilet training may be delayed. Within the constraints of illness or disability, maximum opportunities should be provided for independence in these and other areas.

Illness can impose separations that are detrimental to the toddler. As with the infant, separation is the most anxiety-producing event. A chronic illness or disability can necessitate repeated hospitalizations and painful procedures. If the need to preserve the parent-child relationship is not appreciated, the child may become depressed and eventually detach from the parent. Children seem to have a tremendous capacity to withstand stress, provided that their attachment to the parent is maintained. Parents of toddlers may begin to look for respite care or day care, which is often difficult to find for the child with special needs.* The Americans with Disabilities Act (ADA) requires day care providers to make "reasonable modifications" for equal access to program participation (Siegel, 1995). Special medical day care centers are being developed in certain areas (Ahmann & Scher, 1996; Monical, 1995).

Preschooler

The preschooler is in the stage of initiative; numerous tasks are achieved during this age that can be hampered by chronic illness and disability. Impairment can limit the preschooler's learning about the environment, especially in terms of social development. The chronically ill preschooler confined to the home may be slow to develop social skills useful in group or school settings.

One of the major tasks of this period is establishing sexual identity, and one of the principal methods is through imitation of gender-related activities. However, the child with special needs may have fewer opportunities to engage in such activity and may view the parent predominantly in the caregiving role, because this may be the focus of their relationship. Some families expect the mother to assume the care of the child while the father provides the financial base by working outside the home. This can limit the child's identification with the male role.

In addition to sexual identity, the child's body image is forming. Children's knowledge of their bodies is limited to what they see, feel, and use. If the child is chronically ill, body awareness is focused on the personal pain and anxiety it causes. The young child may lose control over newly acquired bowel and bladder function and feel embarrassed and inferior. The child with a disability may have difficulty forming a mental image of impaired body parts, such as paralyzed extremities. This poorly developed sense of body integrity makes children especially fearful of intrusive or mutilating experiences, which can be frequent during prolonged illness.

One of the more critical influences of chronic illness or disability on preschoolers is the feeling of guilt that they "caused" the condition by a real or imagined misdeed. This is probably less a factor if the child is born with the disorder than if it occurs during the preschool years. Such guilt can greatly affect the child's developing but fragile self-esteem. Unlike the child with a temporary physical impairment who has additional opportunities for achieving mastery and thus overcoming feelings of guilt and inferiority, the child with a

---

*Access to Respite Care and Help (ARCH) is a national information center on respite programs: ARCH, c/o Chapel Hill Training Outreach Project, 800 Eastowne Dr., Chapel Hill, NC 27514; phone: 919-490-5577 or 800-473-1727 ext. 243; fax: 919-490-4905; Web site: www.chtop.com (look for ARCH icon).

chronic illness or disability experiences continual insults. Unless situations are structured for success, life can become a series of failures—of never being strong enough or good enough to compete with peers.

School-Age Child

The child of school age is striving to achieve a sense of accomplishment while overcoming a sense of inferiority. Successful mastery of this task depends on the child's ability to cooperate and compete with others. Consequently, physical impairments can greatly affect the ability to achieve and compete. For example, physical disability may hinder participation in sports, and repeated absences from school caused by illness can place the child at an academic disadvantage. To repeat a grade can saddle the child with feelings of shame, inadequacy, and inferiority. However, the decision to remain in the same grade can also enhance feelings of success because the work requirements may be easier and new classmates provide a second chance for forming friendships.

During this age there is a transition from relationships with family members to strong identification with peers. Peers increasingly influence school-age children's views of themselves and their self-esteem. Anything that labels children as "different" can affect their sense of belonging to the group (Vessey & Mebane, 2000). Nurses can help families to promote social competence in their children. For example, if children are helped to deal with their feelings of not being "normal and perfect" and to recognize their unique abilities, these children can cope very well. It is to be expected that not all children are able to master every task and that they will feel some degree of disappointment. If this is stressed to children with physical impairment, the burden to achieve is lessened.

Peer interaction is especially important in relation to cognitive development, social development, and maturation. Cognitive development is facilitated by interaction—by exploration of personal, social, and ethical values with peers, parents, and teachers. As school-age children identify more with the peer group and authority figures outside the home, there is a concurrent striving for independence from the family. However, the ill child may be forced into an extended period of dependency either from the disorder or from parental overprotectiveness. Attempts to demonstrate independence may be manifested as resentment toward the parents, refusal to comply with treatment, or risk-taking behavior such as cheating on the special diet. If parents can understand that these behaviors represent a normal phase of development, they may be more tolerant and able to find appropriate outlets for independence (e.g., increasing the child's responsibility for home care or increasing the child's control in non–disease-related activities).

Adolescent

The impact of illness or disability can be most difficult during adolescence. The major task of the adolescent is to establish a personal identity. Pubertal changes must be integrated into the self-image while the teenager is gaining control and mastery over increased physical capabilities and sexuality. During early adolescence this takes place primarily within the peer group. Illness or injury at this time interferes with teenagers' sense of mastery and control over a changing body. They are different at a stage of development when being different is unacceptable to the peer group, which may view a disability in one member as a threat to the established uniformity by which all are measured. At no other time of life is an individual so vulnerable to the emotional stress of biologic impairment. In fact, adolescents with physical differences tend to blame most of their problems on the fact that they have something wrong with them. Appearance, skills, and abilities are highly valued by peers (Fig. 41-1); a teenager who is limited in any of these qualities is subject to rejection. This is especially marked when a physical disability interferes with sexual attractiveness.

The subject of sexuality related to the effects of the disorder is a prominent concern of adolescents, but they rarely initiate a discussion of this sensitive topic. Any probable interference in sexual function because of the disability should be discussed openly and candidly with the teenager (Lock, 1998).

Teenagers with special needs are faced with the task of incorporating their disabilities into the changing self-concept. The youngster who develops the illness or acquires the disability during the crucial adolescent years has more difficulty accomplishing this task than has the teenager who has been affected since childhood. It appears that the earlier the onset of a limiting condition, the better the individual is able to adapt to it. The youngster with a newly acquired disorder will have the additional task of grieving for a lost "perfection" while adjusting to the changes taking place as a natural course of events. He or she often feels rejected because of personal appearance or an inability to engage in activities expected of a healthy adolescent. The threat is greatest during middle adolescence, when the teenager has less available energy to cope with illness because emotional resources are being used to meet the normal demands of this developmental phase.

Adolescence is a time for achieving independence from the family and planning for future goals and responsibilities. Adolescents with long-term chronic illness may be less future directed and less independent than well peers (Perrin, 2004). Enforced dependency caused by physical impairment can exacerbate the parent-child conflicts surrounding independence. Lack of understanding from both parties can re-

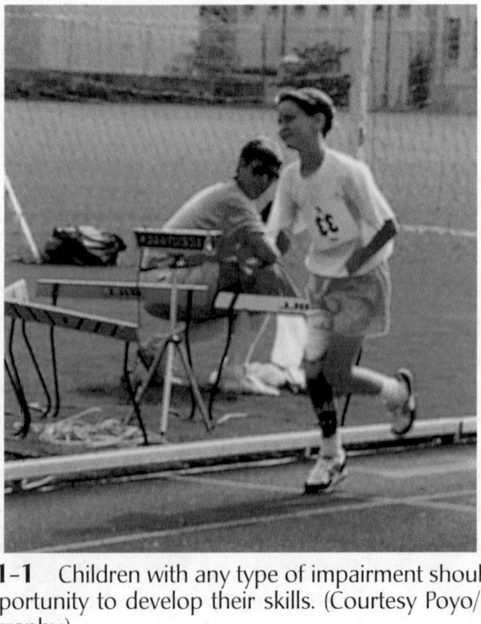

Fig. 41-1 Children with any type of impairment should have the opportunity to develop their skills. (Courtesy Poyo/Hinton Photography.)

sult in bitter feelings and intrafamilial turmoil. The tendency toward rebellion may be directed at the disorder and reflected in decreased compliance with treatment; denial of the disorder to preserve a sense of normalcy with peers; and risk-taking behavior that can place the teenager in jeopardy, such as driving a car despite a disorder that increases the chance of an injury. Such behaviors can further strain an already tense parent-child relationship. On the other hand, parents can promote independence by giving the adolescent a greater role in his or her own treatment regimen, encouraging the adolescent to develop a relationship with the health care team that is not mediated by parents, and promoting normalization principles.

Coping Mechanisms

Children's innate and learned coping mechanisms are very important in terms of their ability to deal with their disorder. Individual characteristics and the social support afforded the child are critically important influences on the child's ability to cope with stress. The better the family copes, the better the child is able to deal with the stressors imposed by the illness or disability. Individual characteristics associated with positive coping are female sex, early infancy or age older than 4 years, active or easy temperament, high self-esteem, above-average intelligence, and strong social skills.

Children with chronic conditions tend to use five distinct patterns of coping (Box 41-6). Children with more positive and accepting attitudes about their chronic illness use a more adaptive coping style characterized by optimism, competence, and compliance. They show fewer behavior problems at home and at school. The two maladaptive coping patterns—"Feels different and withdraws" and "Is irritable, moody and acts out"—are associated with poorer adaptation; children using these strategies have poorer self-concepts, more negative attitudes about their conditions, and more behavior problems at home and at school.

Well-adapted children gradually learn to accept their physical limitations but find achievement in a variety of compensatory motor and intellectual pursuits. They function well at home, at school, and with peers. They have an understanding of their disorder that allows them to accept their limitations, assume responsibility for care, and assist in treatment and rehabilitation regimens. They express appropriate emotions, such as sadness, anxiety, and anger, at times of exacerbations but confidence and guarded optimism during periods of clinical stability. They are able to identify with other similarly affected individuals, promoting positive self-images and displaying pride and self-confidence in their ability to master a productive, successful life despite the disability.

Hopefulness

Children, particularly adolescents, are sensitive to the presence or absence of hope. Hopefulness is an internal quality that mobilizes humans into goal-directed action that may be satisfying and life sustaining. A sense of hopefulness can produce increased participation in health-seeking behaviors and an improved sense of well-being (Ritchie, 2001).

Health Education and Self-Care

Health education is an intervention that promotes coping. Children need information about their condition, the therapeutic plan, and how the disease or the therapy might affect their particular situation. Children nearing puberty also need to understand the maturation process and how their disability may alter this event. For example, the youngster with Crohn's disease should understand that this disorder is associated with growth failure and delayed puberty; the child with diabetes needs to know that hormonal changes and increased growth needs will alter food and insulin requirements at this time; and the sexually active girl with sickle cell anemia or systemic lupus erythematosus needs to be aware of the risks of pregnancy. The information should not be given all at once but should be timed appropriately to meet the changing needs of the youngsters, and it should be described and repeated as often as the situation demands it.

Developing the skills and judgment needed for participation in self-care of a chronic illness or disability is a process that occurs over time. Self-care requires negotiation between parent and child. Nurses can assist families by offering information on methods for instructing children of various ages in self-care (Faulkner, 1996). Answering each child's questions as they arise in an honest and age-appropriate manner and having family discussions about the illness or disability can foster a positive family environment for health education of the child.

Responses to Parental Behavior

The parents' behavior toward the child, especially in terms of childrearing, is one of the most important influencing factors in the child's adjustment. For example, children whose parents are overprotective tend to have marked dependency (especially on the mother), fearfulness, inactivity, and lack of outside interests. Children who are raised by overly solicitous and guilt-ridden parents are often overly independent, defiant, and risk takers. Children who are reared by parents who emphasize their deficits and tend to "hide" or

BOX 41-6

Coping Patterns Used by Children with Special Needs

Develops competence and optimism. Accentuates the positive aspects of the situation and concentrates more on what he or she has or can do than on what is missing or on what he or she cannot do; is as independent as possible.

Feels different and withdraws. Sees self as being different from other children because of the chronic health condition; views being different as negative; sees self as less worthy than others; focuses on things he or she cannot do and sometimes overrestricts activities needlessly.

Is irritable, moody, and acts out. Uses proactive and self-initiated coping behaviors, although usually counterproductive in that the behaviors are not ego enhancing or socially responsible and do not result in desired outcomes; acts out irritability, which may or may not be associated with condition's symptoms.

Complies with treatment. Takes necessary medications, treatments; adheres to activity restrictions; also uses behaviors that indicate developing independence (e.g., assumes responsibility for taking medication).

Seeks support. Talks with adults, children, physicians, and nurses; develops plans to handle problems as they occur; uses downward comparison (i.e., realizes that others have it worse).

Modified from Austin J, Patterson J, Huberty T: Development of the Coping Health Inventory for children, *J Pediatr Nurs* 6(3):166-174, 1991.

isolate them appear as shy and lonely individuals who harbor resentful and hostile attitudes toward unaffected persons. In contrast, children who are reared by parents who establish reasonable limits tend to develop age-appropriate independence and achievement commensurate with their limitations. In addition, family organization and illness-related support and involvement of parents influence the child's adjustment to chronic illness (Schor, 2003). They often display pride and confidence in their ability to cope successfully with the challenges imposed by their disorder. Anticipatory guidance by the nurse and encouragement of normalizing practices may assist parents in facilitating positive adjustment in their children.

Type of Illness or Disability

The type of illness or disability also influences the child's emotional response. Interestingly, children with *more* severe disorders often cope better than those with milder conditions. However, the presence of multiple conditions may place a child at risk for more behavioral problems (Newacheck & Halfon, 1998). Considering children's cognitive ability and their delay in achieving abstract thinking until adolescence, it is likely that an obvious condition is easier to accept because its limitations are concrete. For example, children who are blind or physically disabled are constantly reminded of their inability to run. However, children with cardiac defects not only live by rules they do not understand, but also only vaguely and occasionally sense their illness, such as when they try to run and experience dyspnea and fatigue. Therefore some chronic illnesses pose special threats to children.

NURSING CARE OF THE FAMILY AND CHILD WITH SPECIAL NEEDS

Assessment

Because the nurse may meet a family during any phase of the adjustment process, several assessment areas are important. Knowledge of the family's available support system is essential and may include the marital relationship, nonmarital partners, extended family, colleagues and co-workers, friends, and professionals. The family's perception of the illness or disability is also an area that influences family adjustment. Assessment questions should focus on members' general knowledge of the condition even before the child's diagnosis was made, the influence of culture and religion on their thinking, imagined causes of the condition, and the effects of the child's disorder on the family.

Because the family's ability to cope with previous stresses influences the current situation, answers to questions about their usual coping skills are enlightening. Knowledge of concurrent stresses, such as financial, marital or nonmarital, career, or unemployment, helps identify families who may have fewer resources to cope with the child's needs.

Finally, awareness of the family members' reactions to the child and the illness or disability is important. Sample questions that the nurse and family can use to evaluate the support system, perception of the illness, coping mechanisms, resources, and concurrent stresses are listed in Table 41-1. Because factors affecting the family's response may change at any point during the illness, assessment must be a continuous process.

Special challenges exist in assessing the child's feelings about having a disability. The nurse should use a variety of communication techniques, such as drawing and play, as assessment tools rather than relying solely on parental reports. Often, children are neglected partners in their care, and their unique needs are not identified (Dixon-Woods, Young, & Henry, 1999; Young et al, 2003).

The needs of working parents and siblings also should be assessed, a goal that requires flexibility in scheduling appointments to include these important family members. When working parents know that their input is valuable, they will often change their work schedule to meet with a health professional. Because siblings can be of any age, the use of appropriate communication strategies for assessment must be considered.

Nursing Diagnoses

A number of nursing diagnoses are prominent in the nursing care of the family and child with special needs. Others specific to individual cases become evident, especially when the child's actual disorder is considered.

Plan of Care and Implementation

The nursing plan depends to a large extent on the child's actual illness or disability. However, the following are basic goals for all families of children with special needs:

1. Child and family will receive support at the time of diagnosis.
2. Family's emotional reactions will be accepted.
3. Child and family will cope with stresses of the situation.
4. Child and family will receive appropriate information about the condition.
5. Family will establish an environment of normalization for the child.
6. Family will establish realistic future goals.

The main objective in working with the family is to help them to cope effectively with those stresses imposed by the child's special needs. To achieve this goal, the entire family should be considered in every aspect of the implementation process (Family Focus box).

Provide Support at the Time of Diagnosis

Parents should be encouraged to be together when they are informed of their child's condition, thus avoiding the problem of one parent having to interpret complex findings and deal with the initial emotional reaction of the other. The informing session should take place in a private, comfortable setting free of distractions and interruptions, in an atmosphere in which the parents feel free to express their emotions (Fig. 41-2). If their feelings can be expressed and acknowledged, the

> **Family Focus**
>
> **IDENTIFYING FAMILY NEEDS**
>
> To ensure an effective plan of care, attention to family-identified needs and priorities is essential. For example, a family may have difficulty focusing on treatment issues if their current priority is obtaining enough food to feed their children.

Table 41-1

Assessment of Factors Affecting Family Adjustment

FACTORS AFFECTING ADJUSTMENT	ASSESSMENT QUESTIONS
Available support system	
Status of marital relationship Alternative support systems Ability to communicate	Whom do you talk to when you have something on your mind? (If answer is not the spouse, ask for the reason.) When something is worrying you, what do you do? What helps you most when you are upset? Does talking seem to help when you feel upset?
Perception of the illness/disability	
Previous knowledge of disorder Influence of religion Imagined cause of disorder Effects of illness or disability on family	Have you ever heard the word (name of diagnosis) before? Tell me about it (if answer is yes). Has your religion or faith been of help to you? Tell me how (if answer is yes). What are your thoughts about the causes of the disorder? How has your child's illness or disability affected you and your family? How has your lifestyle changed?
Coping mechanisms	
Reactions to previous crises Reactions to the child Childrearing practices Attitudes	Tell me one time you've had another crisis (problem, bad time) in your family. How did you solve that problem? Do you find yourself being a little more cautious with this child than with your other children? Do you feel as comfortable disciplining this child compared with your other children? How is this child different from the siblings or other children of similar age? Describe your child's personality. Is it easy, difficult, or in between? When you think of your child's future, what thoughts come to mind?
Available resources	What parts of your child's care are causing the most difficulty for you or your family? What services are available to help? What services do you need that presently are not available?
Concurrent stresses	What other problems are you facing now? (Be specific; ask about financial, marital, sibling, and extended family/friends concerns.)

parents can be helped to deal openly with them. Their emotional needs are acknowledged by showing acceptance of such expressions as crying, sadness, anger, and disappointment. Emotional support is offered by having tissues available if a family member cries and demonstrating through facial and body language that indeed this is a difficult and painful period. Although touching is a powerful expression of empathy, it must be used wisely. For example, it can prematurely terminate free expression of feelings, especially when combined with statements such as "Everything will be all right." Nurses should also be aware of cultural issues regarding touching.

Parents should receive the kind of information they desire. This can be assessed by asking the parent questions such as, "Do you prefer to hear detailed information?" Parents or other family members may have different preferences regarding the amount of information they wish to hear. Most parents want a clear, simple explanation of the diagnosis; a prediction of possible futures for the child; advice on what to do next; an opportunity to ask questions; a warm and sympathetic listener; and, most important, time. Clarification of explanations is elicited with such questions as "Do you understand what I mean?" or "Is this clear to you?" Technical terms are used with simple definitions. If the parents are unaware of the term, they are given written literature or at least a written summary of the diagnosis.

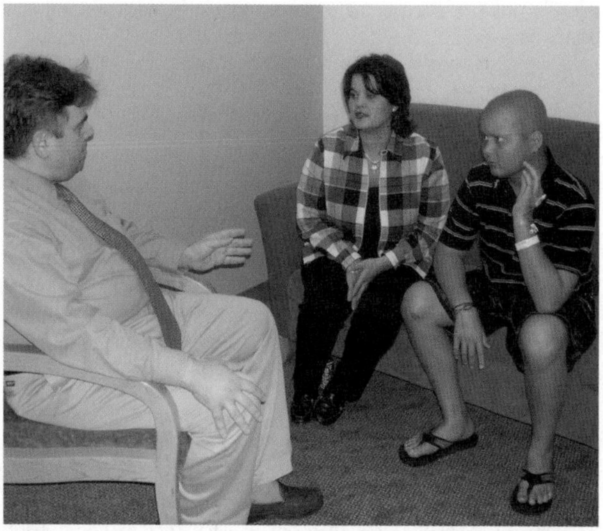

Fig. 41-2 Informing session should take place in a private, comfortable setting free of distractions and interruptions.

NURSE ALERT Develop a glossary of commonly used terms, acronyms, and "initials" to distribute to parents. The list can stand alone or become a part of patient or parent handbooks. ■

Finally, the informing conference should not end with the presentation of devastating news. Instead, the child's strengths, appealing behaviors, and potential for development are stressed, as are available rehabilitation efforts or treatment. Parents can be encouraged to view their experiences as a series of challenges that they are capable of handling, particularly with available professional feedback. The parents are assured that the nurse will be available to answer questions and to provide further assistance as needed.

The preceding discussion relates primarily to the initial informing interview. However, because of the need for long-term follow-up, it is only one in a series of continuing discussions. In all interactions, the family's input is solicited and incorporated into the plan of care. Some situations require consideration of special problems (Guidelines box).

Guidelines

SITUATIONS REQUIRING SPECIAL CONSIDERATION

Congenital Anomaly

Tension in the delivery room conveys the sense that something is seriously wrong. Communication is often delayed while the physician is involved with the mother's care. The manner in which the infant is presented may set the tone for the early parent-child relationship.

- Clarify role with physician in regard to revealing information, to enable immediate parental support.
- Explain to parents briefly in simple language what the defect is and something concerning the immediate prognosis before showing them the infant, when they are more apt to "hear" what is said.
- Be aware of nonverbal communication. Parents watch facial expressions of others for signs of revulsion or rejection.
- Present infant as something precious.
- Emphasize well-formed aspects of infant's body.
- Allow time and opportunity for parents to express their initial response.
- Encourage parents to ask questions, and provide honest, straightforward answers without undue optimism or pessimism.

Cognitive Impairment

Unless cognitive impairment (mental retardation) is associated with other physical problems, it is often easy for parents to miss clues to its presence or to make defensive excuses regarding the diagnosis.

- Plan situations that help parents become aware of the problem.
- Encourage parents to discuss their observations of child, but withhold diagnostic opinions.
- Focus on what child can do and appropriate interventions to promote progress (e.g., infant stimulation programs) to involve parents in their child's care while helping them gain an awareness of child's disability.

Physical Disability

If loss of motor or sensory ability occurs during childhood, the diagnosis is readily apparent. The challenge lies in helping the child and parents over the period of shock and grief and toward the phase of acceptance and reintegration.

- Institute early rehabilitation (e.g., using a prosthetic limb, learning to read braille, learning to read lips).
- Be aware that physical rehabilitation usually precedes psychologic adjustment.
- When the cause of the disability is accidental, avoid implying that parents or child was responsible for the injury, yet allow them the opportunity to discuss feelings of blame.
- Encourage expression of feelings (see Communication Techniques, Chapter 32).

Chronic Illness

Realization of the true impact may take months or years. Conflict over parent's versus child's concerns may result in serious problems. When condition is inherited, parents may blame themselves or child may blame parents.

- Help each family member gain an appreciation of the other's concerns.
- Discuss hereditary aspect of condition with parents at time of diagnosis to lessen guilt and accusatory feelings.
- Encourage child to express feelings by using third-person technique (e.g., "Sometimes when a person has an illness that was passed on by the parents, that person feels angry or bitter toward them").

Multiple Disabilities

The child or parent may require additional time for the shock phase and may be able to attend to only one diagnosis before hearing significant information regarding other disorders.

- Acknowledge parents' understanding and acceptance of all diagnoses, especially when an obvious and more hidden disability coexists.
- Appreciate the devastating consequences of more than one disability for a child, especially if they interfere with expressive-receptive abilities.

Terminal Illness

Parents require much support to deal with their own feelings and guidance in how to tell the child the diagnosis. They may want to conceal the diagnosis from the child. They may believe that the child is too young to know, will not be able to cope with the information, or will lose hope and the will to live.

- Approach the subject of disclosure in a positive way by asking, "How will you tell your child about the diagnosis?"
- Help parents understand the disadvantages of not telling children (e.g., deprives them of the opportunity to discuss their feelings openly and ask questions; incurs the risk of them learning the truth from outside and sometimes less tactful sources; may lessen children's trust and confidence in their parents after they learn the truth).
- Guide parents to see the potential problems involved in fostering a conspiracy.
- Offer parents guidelines for how and what to tell children about their disease or the possibility of death. Explanations should be tailored to child's cognitive ability, be based on knowledge child already has, and be honest. Honesty must be tempered with concern for child's feelings.
- Assure parents that telling a child the name of the illness and the reason for treatment instills hope, provides support from others, and serves as a foundation for explaining and understanding subsequent events.
- Acknowledge that being honest is not always easy because the truth may prompt children to ask other distressing questions, such as "Am I going to die?" However, even this difficult question must be answered.

Accept Family's Emotional Reactions

One of the most supportive interventions is to accept the family's emotional reactions to the child's condition in as nonjudgmental a manner as possible. Although all families respond differently and in varying degrees of intensity, three responses are so common and often so poorly handled that they deserve special consideration.

Denial

The nurse's response to denial is a critical component of the individual's continuing need for this defense mechanism. The most effective method of support is active listening. Silence neither reinforces nor rejects denial (or any other emotional reaction) but implies a willingness and acceptance of the person's need for this behavior. However, silence alone can be misinterpreted. For example, if the person demonstrates denial, such as by saying, "I am sure the doctors made a mistake," and the nurse responds silently and leaves, the person may infer disapproval, agreement, avoidance, or rejection from this behavior.

To be effective, silence and listening must be accompanied by physical and mental concentration and use of body language to communicate interest and concern. Direct eye contact, touch, physical closeness, and body posture, such as sitting and leaning slightly forward, demonstrate silent but effective communication.

Guilt

Because guilt is such a common response and can cause family members tremendous anxiety, they should be told directly that there is no known cause of the disorder (when appropriate) and that they are not to be blamed. Using the third-person technique is valuable in eliciting thoughts of guilt. For example, with children, an appropriate statement may be, "When people get sick, they often wonder if they did anything to make themselves sick." This allows children an opportunity to explore any feelings of responsibility they harbor.

If family members are expressing feelings of guilt, it is important to allow them to talk about their feelings rather than quickly trying to dispel them with long "scientific" explanations. Statements such as "If you believe you are responsible for Johnny's condition, then no wonder you feel so bad" acknowledge the family member's feelings. This step is frequently appreciated and necessary before the facts can be presented and absorbed.

Anger

Anger is one of the more difficult reactions to accept and deal with therapeutically. The responses to anger may be reciprocal anger, fear, acceptance, or encouragement. The first two reactions impede communication and express disapproval and rejection of the person. They most frequently occur when the listener views the anger as a personal assault. The last two responses allow the individual to express his or her feelings in an atmosphere of nonjudgmental acceptance. Two basic rules for dealing with the angry person are to avoid losing one's temper and to encourage the person to talk (Guidelines box). One essential element in the successful implementation of this process is to wait for the person to respond to a statement before proceeding to the next step. Because the objective of each statement is for the person to speak freely, the responses should avoid "yes" or "no" types of answers.

Guidelines

ENCOURAGING EXPRESSION OF EMOTION

Describe the behavior: "You seem angry at everyone."
Give evidence of understanding: "Being angry is only natural."
Give evidence of caring: "It must be difficult to endure so many painful procedures."
Help focus on feelings: "Maybe you wonder why this happened to your child."

Support Family's Coping Methods

For the family to meet the stresses of optimally adjusting to the child's condition, each member must be individually supported so that the family system is strong. Although the family can indefinitely support a member who is in need of assistance, its greatest strength lies in every member supporting each other. The nurse should bear in mind that the family member in greatest need is not necessarily the affected child but may be a parent or sibling who is dealing with stresses that require intervention.

Parents

The nurse can provide support by being attentive to families' responses to their children. Mothers and fathers need to experience success, joy, and pride in their children to give the support they need. Children, too, require support for their interactions, adjustments, and efforts. They must be reinforced for attempts to get to know their care providers and to communicate their needs to them.

Nurses must examine their attitudes to determine their ability to engage in parent-professional partnerships. An essential characteristic is the belief that parents are equal to professionals and that parents are experts regarding their child (Guidelines box).

Because most mothers and fathers of children with special needs have little or no experience with children who have chronic or disabling conditions, the nurse can serve as a role model for appropriate interactions with the child. Above all, the nurse should ensure that the parents and siblings learn to perceive the child as a child first, with unique and individual needs. The nurse needs to convey a humanistic, accepting approach to the child to enable the parents to observe this acceptance.

Guidelines

DEVELOPING SUCCESSFUL PARENT-PROFESSIONAL PARTNERSHIPS

Promote primary nursing; in nonhospital settings, designate a case manager.
Acknowledge parents' overall competence and their unique expertise with their child.
Respect parents' time as having value equal to that of other members of child's health care team.
Explain or define any medical, technical, or discipline-specific terms.
Tell families, "I am not sure" or "I don't know," when appropriate.
Facilitate family's effectiveness in team meetings (e.g., provide parents with same information as other participants).

Communication among all family members is encouraged. Parent group sessions can help parents to verbalize thoughts and feelings to each other but often do not take into account siblings' or the child's viewpoint. Therefore the nurse may need to set up a family session, such as during a home or clinic visit. Although the ideal situation is to have all of the members present at one time, this is often not possible. However, inviting members to participate at various visits is an appropriate alternative.

Parents can be encouraged to discuss their feelings toward the child, the impact of this event on their marriage, and associated stresses such as financial burdens. For most families, regardless of their income or insurance coverage, financial concerns exist. The costs of caring for a child with special needs can be overwhelming. In addition, the family wage earner may have to sacrifice job opportunities to remain close to a medical facility or to avoid losing insurance benefits.*

The nurse should regard fathers as able, effective parents, competent and capable of coping with the challenges they face. Every effort is made to include the father in visits, such as to the nursery, clinic, special school, and stimulation programs. The father should be included in the assessment process, with specific emphasis on having him describe the child's strengths and difficulties. It is not unusual to find two parents who have differing views of the child's abilities, especially in the area of developmental disabilities.

Numerous volunteer and community resources are available that provide assistance, rehabilitation, equipment, and funding for a variety of health problems.† National and local disease-oriented organizations may provide needed assistance and support to families that qualify. Many of these are discussed elsewhere in the text under the specific diagnosis. State and federal departments of health, mental health, social service, and labor may be able to help locate appropriate regional resources. For example, state programs for children with special health needs (formerly called *crippled children's services*) provide financial assistance for children with many disabling conditions. Local and national sources of respite care and medical day care may be useful to families. Nurses should become acquainted with those in their communities and with vocational programs for special groups.

*Information regarding financial issues is available from the Federation for Children with Special Needs, 95 Berkeley St., Suite 104, Boston, MA 02116; phone: 617-482-2915.

†General sources of information are the Clearinghouse for Disability Information, Room 3132, Switzer Building, C St. SW, Washington, DC 20202-2524. National Information Center for Children and Youth with Disabilities, PO Box 1492, Washington, DC 20013; phone: 202-884-8200 or 800-695-0285; Web site: www.nichcy.org. National Center for Children with Chronic Illness and Disability, Box 721-UMHC, Harvard St. at E. River Rd., Minneapolis, MN 55455; phone: 612-626-2820. A comprehensive list of books and pamphlets for parents and teachers is available from the Easter Seals National Headquarters, 230 W. Monroe St., Suite 1800, Chicago, IL 60606; phone: 312-726-6200; Web site: www.easter-seals.org. In Canada: Council of Canadians with Disabilities, Suite 926, 294 Portage Ave., Winnipeg, Manitoba R3C 0B9; phone: 204-947-0303; Web site: www.ccdonline.ca.

Parent-to-Parent Support

The support a parent receives from another parent is unique and unobtainable from any other source. A growing number of hospitals and clinics now have a parent on staff. The services these parents provide are particularly valuable for parents of children with special needs who are likely to experience frequent and lengthy hospitalizations, as well as numerous routine clinic visits.

Just being with another parent who has shared similar experiences is helpful. A parent of a child with the same diagnosis is not always necessary, because parents in the process of adjusting to a child with special needs—or finding respite services, educational or rehabilitative services, special equipment vendors, and financial counseling—tread a common path. If the agency does not have a parent staff position, the nurse can contact parent groups that will often send a representative. Another strategy is to ask another parent to talk to the parents. The nurse should seek out a parent who is a good listener, has a nonjudgmental approach to differences in families, and possesses good advocacy and problem-solving skills.

The parent self-help group is another way to promote parent-to-parent support.* Group members feel less alone and have the opportunity to observe both coping and mastery role modeling from other members. Parents' groups are rich resources for information. The nurse can foster parent participation in self-help groups by serving as a referral agent, a group advisory board member, a resource person, a group member, or an assistant in founding a group. Sometimes all that is required in starting a group is identifying one or two parents as leaders; sharing with them the names, telephone numbers, and addresses of other families who have expressed both an interest and a willingness to release their phone number and address; and guiding them in how to initiate a first meeting.†

Advocate for Empowerment

Nurses can advocate for methods that foster opportunities for parent empowerment. For example, nurses can suggest reimbursement for travel and child care, plus stipends to enable parents' voices to be heard at meetings and conferences. They can encourage parent membership on staff, committees, and boards. They can keep parents informed of pending legislation on child health issues or take action when parents inform them.

The Child

Through ongoing contacts with the child, the nurse (1) observes the child's responses to the disorder, ability to function, and adaptive behaviors within the environment and with significant others; (2) explores the child's own understanding of the nature of his or her illness or condition; and (3) provides support while the child learns to cope with his or her feelings. Children are encouraged to express their

*Information about self-help groups and books and pamphlets are available from the National Self-Help Clearinghouse, 365 5th Ave., Suite 3300, New York, NY 10016; Web site: www.selfhelpweb.org.

†New Jersey Self-Help Clearinghouse, phone: 973-326-6789; Web site: www.groups.org.

concerns rather than allowing others to express them for them, because open discussions may reduce anxiety.

One of the most important interventions is alleviating the child's feeling of being different and normalizing his or her life as much as possible (Guidelines box). Whenever possible, the nurse should assist the family in assessing the child's daily routine for indications of normalizing practices. For example, the child who remains in a bedroom all day is in need of a restructured daily routine to provide activities in different parts of the house, such as eating in the kitchen or dining room with the family. Such children may also be deprived of social, recreational, and academic activities that can be recognized by applying normalization practices. For example, home and out-of-home health-related treatments should be planned at times that least interfere with normal daily activities.

Children who are concerned that their condition detracts from their physical attractiveness need attention focused on the normal aspects of appearance and capabilities. Health professionals must help strengthen and consolidate the self-image by emphasizing the normal, while at the same time allowing children to express anger, isolation, fear of rejection, feelings of sadness, and loneliness. They need positive reinforcement for compliance and any evidence of improvement. Anything that might improve attractiveness and contribute to a positive self-image is employed, such as makeup for a teenager with a scar, clothing that disguises a prosthesis, or a hair style or wig to cover a deformity or lost hair.

Siblings

The presence of a child with special needs in a family may result in parents paying less attention to the other children. Siblings may respond by developing negative attitudes toward the child or by expressing anger in different forms. The nurse can help by using "anticipatory guidance," questioning the parents about what they believe is the best way to have siblings respond to the child and guiding them through ways to meet their other children's needs for attention. This questioning should take place before serious negative effects occur.

Siblings may also experience embarrassment associated with having a brother or sister with an illness or disability. Parents are then faced with the difficulty of responding to this embarrassment in an understanding and appropriate manner without punishing the siblings for how they feel. Parents should talk with the siblings about how they view their affected sibling. Many siblings benefit from sharing their concerns with other young people who are experiencing a similar situation.* Support groups for siblings can help decrease isolation, promote expression of feelings, and provide examples of effective coping skills.

Many parents express concern about when and how to inform the other children in the family about a sibling's disability. The answer depends on each child's level of sophistication and understanding. However, it is usually best to inform the siblings before a neighbor or other non–family member does so. Uninformed siblings may fantasize or develop apprehensions that are out of proportion to the child's actual condition. Furthermore, if parents choose to be silent or deceptive about the issue, they are setting a negative precedent for the siblings to follow, rather than encouraging the siblings to cope with the experience in a healthy and nurturing way.

The nurse must be sensitive to the reactions of siblings and whenever possible intervene to promote more positive adjustment. For example, siblings often mention that they are expected to take on additional responsibilities to help the parents care for the child. It is not unusual for them to express a positive reaction to assuming the extra duties but a negative response to feeling unappreciated for doing so. Such feelings can often be minimized by encouraging siblings to discuss this with the parents and by suggesting to parents ways of showing gratitude, such as an increase in allowance, special privileges, and, most important, verbal praise (see Box 41-5).

Extended Family Members and Community

The nurse must also be sensitive to the family's cues regarding sources of stress from extended members, such as grandparents. For example, the nurse may encourage the parents to invite the grandparents to be present during one of the child's visits to a clinic, during the diagnostic workup, or during a parent conference or to provide appropriate literature. Including grandparents in a discussion in which they can share their concerns may help them deal with their feelings, thus reducing stress on the entire family. Grandparents' feelings of blame and anger, as well as any "cure fantasies" they harbor, can be brought out in the open and dis-

Guidelines

PROMOTING NORMALIZATION

Preparation. Prepare child in advance for changes that may occur from the illness or disability; for example, the child is told in advance of the possible side effects of drug therapy.

Participation. Include child in as many decisions as possible, especially those relating to his or her care regimen; for example, the child is responsible for taking medications or scheduling home treatments.

Sharing. Allow both family members and child's peers to be a part of the care regimen whenever possible; for example, the child is given his or her medication when the other siblings receive their vitamins; the parent cooks the same menu for the whole family; and if the child is invited to another's home, the parent advises the family of the child's dietary restrictions.

Control. Identify areas where child can be in control so that feelings of uncertainty, passivity, and helplessness are decreased; for example, the child identifies activities that are appropriate to his or her energy level and chooses to rest when fatigued.

Expectation. Apply the same family rules to the child with a chronic illness or disability as to the well siblings or peers; for example, the child is disciplined, expected to fulfill household responsibilities, and attends school in accordance with abilities.

*For information on the Sibling Information Network, contact the Information Network, CUAP, 991 Main St., Suite 3A, East Hartford, CT 06108.

cussed if necessary. Grandparents can be helped to understand the effects of their behavior on the family with an appropriate statement such as "Your daughter is currently experiencing a great deal of pain and anguish. We realize that this is difficult for you, as well as your daughter; however, you can be of tremendous help by being supportive toward her."

Considerable stress can also arise from nonfamilial sources, such as friends, neighbors, or strangers. Inability to cope with comments about the disorder or curious stares by others may foster the tendency to isolate and protect the child within the home. The family needs guidance in preparing for these inevitable experiences. Encouraging parents to dress the child as much as possible like other children is one approach. Good grooming is very important in minimizing differences in appearance. Through role playing, parents can practice responses to comments such as "Is your child retarded?" or "Has he always been crippled?" Through parent groups, family members can share experiences and learn from each other how they successfully deal with probing questions or unkind remarks. Interventions should include the siblings and the affected child, who also must face and deal with these events. Nurses can teach young children about disabilities to familiarize them with the special needs and abilities of these individuals. For example, school nurses can simulate experiences such as having only one leg through role playing, can use books or films, or can invite community guests with physical limitations to visit the class.

Educate about the Disorder and General Health Care

Educating the family about the disorder is actually an extension of revealing the diagnosis. Education involves not only supplying technical information, but also discussing how the condition will affect the child. Parents may be able to digest only so much information at a time. It may be helpful to provide essential information and then follow by asking, "What else would you like to know about your child's condition?" Responding to parents' questions and concerns ensures that their information needs are met.

Activities of Daily Living

Parents also need guidance in how the condition may interfere with or alter activities of daily living, such as eating, dressing, sleeping, and toileting. One area frequently affected is nutrition. Common problems are undernutrition resulting from food being inappropriately restricted; loss of appetite, vomiting, or motor deficits that interfere with feeding; and overnutrition, usually caused by a caloric intake in excess of energy expenditure or boredom and lack of stimulation in other areas. Although the child requires the same basic nutrients as other children, the daily requirements may differ. Special nutritional considerations are discussed as appropriate throughout the text.

Safe Transportation

Modifications may also be needed regarding car safety. Children with conditions such as low birth weight or orthopedic, neuromuscular, or respiratory problems often cannot safely use conventional car restraints. For example, children with hip spica casts cannot sit properly in child safety seats. Modifications can be made to some commercial models, and for older children a special vest is available that secures the child to the back seat in a lying-down position.*

If a child requires a wheelchair, the family should consult the wheelchair manufacturer for specific instructions regarding safe car transportation. Considerations for wheelchairs used with vehicle transportation must address securing both the wheelchair and the occupant in the wheelchair. Wheelchairs should be secured facing forward with tie-downs at four points. With children who must travel with additional medical equipment, this equipment (e.g., oxygen, monitors, or ventilators) should be anchored to the floor or underneath the vehicle seat or wheelchair. Soft padding should be added around the equipment to reduce movement. A second adult should be present to monitor the condition of a medically fragile child while traveling.

Primary Health Care

Children with special needs require all the usual health care recommended for any child. Attention to injury prevention, immunizations, dental health, and regular physical examinations is essential. Nurses can play an important role in reminding parents of these aspects of care that are so often neglected when the concern is focused on the child's specific illness or disability. Specific discussions of nutrition, sleep and activity, dental health, and injury prevention are presented in the chapters on health promotion for specific age groups.

Parents also need to be aware of the importance of communicating the child's condition in the event of a medical emergency. Young children are unable to give information about their disorder, and although older children may be reliable sources, after an accident they may be physically unable to speak. Therefore all children with any type of chronic condition that may affect medical care should wear some type of identification, such as a MedicAlert bracelet,† or carry a card in their wallet that lists the medical condition and a phone number for emergency medical records and other personal information.

Children need information about their condition, the therapeutic plan, and how the disease or the therapy might affect their particular situation. Children nearing puberty also need to understand the maturation process and how their disability may alter this event. Information should not be given all at once but be timed appropriately to meet the changing needs of the youngsters, and it should be described and repeated as often as the situation demands. The subject of sexuality related to the effects of the disorder is a prominent concern of adolescents, but they rarely initiate a discussion of this sensitive topic. Any probable interference in sexual function because of the disability should be discussed openly and candidly with the teenager.

---

*Information on car safety restraints for children with special needs is available from the Automotive Safety for Children Program, Riley Hospital for Children, 575 West Dr., Room 004, Indianapolis, IN 46202; phone: 800-543-6227 or fax: 317-278-0399; Web site: www.preventinjury.org.

†PO Box 1009, Turlock, CA 95381-1009; phone: 800-ID-ALERT; Web site: www.medicalert.org.

Promote Normal Development

Aside from knowledge of the condition and its effect on the child's abilities, the family must be guided toward fostering appropriate development in their child. Although each stage may take longer to achieve, parents are guided toward helping the child to fully realize his or her potential in preparation for the next developmental stage. Table 41-2 outlines developmental aspects of chronic illness or disability and supportive interventions. With appropriate planning and knowledge of strategies to improve the child's functional abilities, most children can live fulfilling and productive lives.

Table 41-2

Developmental Aspects of Chronic Illness or Disability on Children

DEVELOPMENTAL TASKS	POTENTIAL EFFECTS OF CHRONIC ILLNESS OR DISABILITY	SUPPORTIVE INTERVENTIONS
INFANCY		
Develop a sense of trust	Multiple caregivers and frequent separations, especially if hospitalized Deprived of consistent nurturing	Encourage consistent caregivers in hospital or other care settings. Encourage parental presence, rooming-in during hospitalization, and participation in care.
Bond/attach to parent	Delayed because of separation, parental grief for loss of "dream" child, parental inability to accept the condition, especially a visible defect	Emphasize healthy, perfect qualities of infant. Help parents learn special care needs of infant for them to feel competent.
Learn through sensorimotor experiences	Increased exposure to painful experiences over pleasurable ones Limited contact with environment from restricted movement or confinement	Expose infant to pleasurable experiences through all senses (touch, hearing, sight, taste, movement). Encourage age-appropriate developmental skills (e.g., holding bottle, finger feeding, crawling).
Begin to develop a sense of separateness from parent	Increased dependency on parent for care Overinvolvement of parent in care	Encourage all family members to participate in care to prevent overinvolvement of one member. Encourage periodic respite from demands of care responsibilities.
TODDLERHOOD		
Develop autonomy Master locomotor and language skills Learn through sensorimotor experience; beginning preoperational thought	Increased dependency on parent Limited opportunity to test own abilities and limits Increased exposure to painful experiences	Encourage independence in as many areas as possible (e.g., toileting, dressing, feeding). Provide gross motor skill activity and modification of toys or equipment, such as modified swing or rocking horse. Give choices to allow simple feeling of control (e.g., choice of what book to look at, what kind of sandwich to eat). Institute age-appropriate discipline and limit setting. Recognize that negative and ritualistic behaviors are normal. Provide sensory experiences (e.g., water play, sandbox play, finger painting).
PRESCHOOL		
Develop initiative and purpose	Limited opportunities for success in accomplishing simple tasks or mastering self-care skills	Encourage mastery of self-help skills. Provide devices that make task easier (e.g., self-dressing).
Master self-care skills	Limited opportunities for socialization with peers; may appear "like a baby" to agemates	Encourage socialization (e.g., inviting friends to play, day care experience, trips to park). Provide age-appropriate play, especially associative play opportunities.
Begin to develop peer relationships	Protection within tolerant and secure family may cause child to fear criticism and withdraw	Emphasize child's abilities; dress appropriately to enhance desirable appearance.
Develop sense of body image and sexual identification	Awareness of body may center on pain, anxiety, and failure Sex-role identification focused primarily on mothering skills	Encourage relationships with same-sex and opposite-sex peers and adults. Help child deal with criticisms; realize that too much protection prevents child from realities of world.
Learn through preoperational thought (magical thinking)	Guilt (thinking he or she caused the illness/disability or is being punished for wrongdoing)	Clarify that cause of child's illness or disability is not his or her fault or a punishment.

Continued

Table 41-2

Developmental Aspects of Chronic Illness or Disability on Children—cont'd

DEVELOPMENTAL TASKS	POTENTIAL EFFECTS OF CHRONIC ILLNESS OR DISABILITY	SUPPORTIVE INTERVENTIONS
SCHOOL AGE		
Develop a sense of accomplishment	Limited opportunities to achieve and compete (e.g., many school absences, inability to join regular athletic activities)	Encourage school attendance; schedule medical visits at times other than school; encourage child to make up missed work
Form peer relationships	Limited opportunities for socialization	Educate teachers and classmates about child's condition, abilities, and special needs
Learn through concrete operations	Incomplete comprehension of the imposed physical limitations or treatment of the disorder	Encourage sports activities (e.g., Special Olympics)
		Encourage socialization (e.g., Girl Scouts, Campfire, Boy Scouts, 4-H Club; having a best friend or club membership)
		Provide child with knowledge about his or her condition
		Encourage creative activities (e.g., Very Special Arts)
ADOLESCENCE		
Develop personal and sexual identity	Increased sense of feeling different from peers and less able to compete with peers in appearance, abilities, special skills	Realize that many of the difficulties the teenager is experiencing are part of normal adolescence (rebelliousness, risk taking, lack of cooperation, hostility toward authority)
Achieve independence from family	Increased dependency on family; limited job/career opportunities	Provide instruction on interpersonal and coping skills
Form heterosexual relationships	Limited opportunities for heterosexual friendships; less opportunity to discuss sexual concerns with peers	Encourage socialization with peers, including peers with special needs and those without special needs
Learn through abstract thinking	Increased concern with issues such as why did he or she get the disorder, can he or she marry and have a family	Provide instruction on decision making, assertiveness, and other skills necessary to manage personal plans
	Decreased opportunity for earlier stages of cognition may impede achieving level of abstract thinking	Encourage increased responsibility for care and management of the disease or condition (e.g., assuming responsibility for making and keeping appointment [ideally alone], sharing assessment and planning stages of health care delivery, contacting resources)
		Encourage activities appropriate for age (e.g., attending mixed-sex parties, sports activities, driving a car)
		Be alert to cues that signal readiness for information regarding implications of condition on sexuality and reproduction
		Emphasize good appearance and wearing stylish clothes, use of makeup
		Understand that adolescent has same sexual needs and concerns as any other teenager
		Discuss planning for future and how condition can affect choices

One important aspect of promoting normal development is to encourage the child's self-care abilities in both activities of daily living and the medical regimen. An assessment of the child's age and physical, emotional, and mental capacities, as well as the support and structure provided by the family, should be considered in determining the appropriate level of self-care in the medical regimen. Even toddlers can be involved in their own care by holding supplies for the parent during a procedure. Over time, children should be encouraged toward greater autonomy in the self-care arena.

Early Childhood

During infancy the child is achieving basic *trust* through a satisfying, intimate, consistent relationship with his or her parents. However, the affected child's early existence may be stressful, chaotic, and unsatisfying. Consequently, he or she may need more parental support and expressions of affection to achieve trust. Likewise, the parents require assistance in finding ways to meet the infant's needs, such as how to hold a rigid or flaccid infant, how to feed a child with tongue thrust or episodes of dyspnea, and how to stimulate a child who seems incapable of achieving any skills. If hospitalizations are frequent or prolonged, every effort is made to preserve the parent-child relationship. Hospital policies should promote visitation by and involvement of families.

During early childhood the goal is to achieve separation from parents, autonomy, and initiative. However, the natural parental response to having a sick child is overprotection. Parents need help in realizing the importance of brief separations of the child from them and from others involved in the child's care and of providing social experiences outside the home whenever possible. Respite care, which provides temporary relief for family members, can be essential in allowing caregivers time away from the daily burdens.

When the young child has a disability that interferes with motor development, intervention must be based on providing activities that allow maximum motor development. Also, the activity must take into account the child's need for social interaction, sense of control over the body, feeling of competence and achievement, and an outlet for aggression.

When a child is unable to perform a skill independently, functional aids should be used. With innovation, many adaptations can be implemented in children's environments to increase their mobility and independence and allow them to play like other children their age. For example, with slight modifications, a child with physical limitations may be able to ride a tricycle (Fig. 41-3).

Another critical component for normal child development is discipline. Discipline and guidance serve several purposes, such as providing children with boundaries on which to test out their behavior and teaching them socially acceptable behavior. Resentment and hostility can arise among siblings if different standards are applied to each child. The nurse's responsibility is to help parents learn successful methods of managing a child's behaviors before they become problems (see Chapter 31).

School Age

For school-age children, the major tasks are entry into school and achieving a sense of *industry.* Although the importance of school in the life of all children is well known, school absences are significantly higher among children with chronic illness than among their healthy peers. The more school absences the child experiences, the more difficult it is to resume attendance, and "school phobia" may result. The child should return to school as soon as possible after diagnosis or treatments.

Preparation for entry into or resumption of school is best accomplished through a team approach with the parents, child, schoolteacher, school nurse, and primary nurse in the hospital. Ideally, this planning should begin before hospital discharge, provided that the child is well enough to resume usual activities. A structured plan should be developed, with attention to those aspects of care that must be continued during school hours, such as administration of medication or other treatments.

Children also need preparation before entering or resuming school. Having a tutor in the hospital or home as soon as children are physically able helps them realize that school will continue and gives them time to consider this prospect (Fig. 41-4). They need to investigate possible answers to the many questions others will ask. One method of anticipatory preparation is to role-play, with the child as the "returned pupil" and the nurse or parent as "other schoolmates." If the child returns to school with some obvious physical change, such as hair loss, amputation, or visible scar, the nurse might also ask questions about these alterations to prompt preparatory responses from the child.

Classroom peers also need preparation, and a joint plan of the schoolteacher, nurse, and child is best. At a minimum,

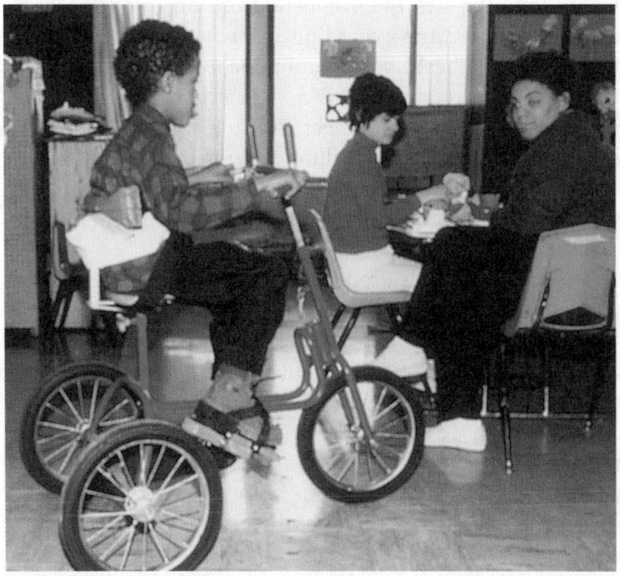

Fig. 41-3 A modified tricycle with block pedals, self-adhesive straps for support, and modified seat and handlebars can help a child with disabilities gain mobility.

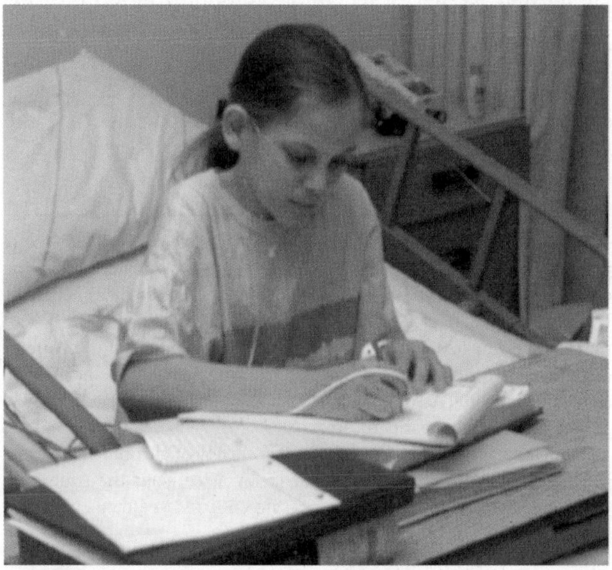

Fig. 41-4 Children with special needs should continue their schooling as soon as their condition permits.

the classmates should be given a description of the child's condition, prepared for any visible changes in the child, and allowed an opportunity to ask questions. The child should have the option of attending this session. As the child's condition changes, particularly if the illness is potentially fatal, school personnel, including the students, need periodic appraisal of the child's status and preparation for what to expect.

Children with special needs are encouraged to maintain or reestablish relationships with peers and to participate according to their capabilities in any age-appropriate activities. Alternative activities may be substituted for those that are impossible or that place a strain on the child's condition. Programs such as the Special Olympics* offer children an opportunity to compete with their peers and to achieve athletic skill. Summer camps† allow children to associate with peers and develop a wide variety of skills. Children with special needs can derive enormous benefits from expressive activities, such as art, music, poetry, dance, and drama. With adaptive equipment and imagination, children can participate in a variety of activities. Organizations such as VSA Arts (Very Special Arts) offer children an opportunity to celebrate and share their accomplishments.‡ Children need the opportunity to interact with healthy peers, as well as to engage in activities with groups or clubs composed of similarly affected age-mates. Such organizations as ostomy clubs, diabetes clubs, and cerebral palsy groups share information and provide support related to the special problems the members face.

Adolescence

Adolescence can be a particularly difficult period for the teenager and family. All of the needs discussed previously apply to this age group as well. Developing *independence* or *autonomy,* however, is a major task for the adolescent as planning for the future becomes a prominent concern. Although the emphasis in the past has been on achieving independence from physical assistance, recent developments in the fields of special education, adolescent development, and family systems suggest redefining autonomy in terms of individuals' capacities to take responsibility for their own behavior, to make decisions regarding their own lives, and to maintain supportive social relationships. Given this understanding, even individuals with severe impairment can be viewed as autonomous if they perceive their own needs and take responsibility for meeting them, either directly or by engaging the assistance of others.

Physical symptoms are high on the teenager's list of health-related concerns. Because adolescence is a time of enormous physical and emotional changes, it is important for the nurse to make a distinction between body changes that are related to disability and those that are a result of normal body development. It can be a great comfort for teenagers with disabling conditions to know that many of the changes they experience are normal developmental outcomes.

A sense of feeling different from peers can lead to loneliness, isolation, and depression. Participation in groups of teenagers with chronic conditions or disabilities can alleviate feelings of isolation and smooth the transition to a meaningful relationship with one person in adulthood.

Establish Realistic Future Goals

One of the most difficult adjustments is setting realistic future goals for the child and for those involved in his or her continued care. Sometimes the impact of this decision does not surface until the child finishes school or the parents approach retirement, when a crisis can arise because all of the family roles and relationships that maintained stability are now disrupted.

Planning for the future should be a gradual process. All along, the parents should cultivate realistic vocations for the child. For example, if children have physical disabilities, they are directed to intellectual, artistic, or musical pursuits. Children with developmental disabilities are taught manual skills. In this way, the child's development proceeds in the direction of self-support through gainful employment.

With prolonged survival, young people with chronic illnesses must deal with new decisions and problems, such as marriage, employment, and insurance coverage. With appropriate guidance, gainful employment, marriage, and a family are attainable goals. For those whose conditions are genetic, counseling is needed regarding future offspring. Prospective spouses often benefit from an opportunity to discuss their feelings regarding marriage to an individual with continued health needs and possibly a limited life span. Health insurance coverage is a critical issue because some private carriers may no longer insure a young person who leaves home or may be unwilling to reinsure the person who is independent. Life insurance is another dilemma, especially when children have serious defects, such as congenital heart anomalies.

Unfortunately, vocational pursuits and completely independent living are not realistic goals for all persons. Persons with multiple or severe disabilities may require lifelong care and assistance. In these situations parents must look to the time when they will no longer be able to care for their child. Residential placement may be very difficult unless the family mutually participates in the decision-making and planning processes. Placement outside the home should not be viewed as abandonment. Not infrequently it is the only way to preserve the family unit. The nurse should help the family investigate suitable placements, discuss their feelings regarding this decision, and explore measures to maintain meaningful communication between family members.

---

*1350 New York Ave. NW, Suite 500, Washington, DC 20005-1581; phone: 202-628-3630. Several pamphlets on sports and recreation for children with disabilities are available from the Easter Seals National Headquarters, 230 W. Monroe St., Suite 1800, Chicago, IL 60606; phone: 312-726-6200; Web site: www.easter-seals.org; and the American Alliance for Health, Physical Education, Recreation and Dance (AAHPERD), 1900 Association Dr., Reston, VA 22091; phone: 703-476-3400; Web site: www.aahperd.org.

†A directory of camps for children with a variety of chronic illnesses or general physical disabilities is available for a fee from the American Camping Association, Publications Service, 5000 State Rd., 67 N., Martinsville, IN 46151; phone: 800-428-CAMP.

‡VSA Arts has affiliate chapters in all 50 states and in selected sites internationally; yearly festivals are held throughout the world. Information is available from VSA Arts, 1300 Connecticut Ave. NW, Suite 700, Washington, DC 20036; phone: 202-737-0645; Web site: www.vsarts.org.

Evaluation

The effectiveness of nursing interventions is determined by continual reassessment and evaluation of care based on the following observational guidelines:

1. Observe family members' responses to the diagnosis and the types of questions or concerns they have.
2. Interview family members regarding their knowledge and understanding of the child's condition; observe if they have instituted suggestions, such as use of identification devices for children with certain conditions.
3. Observe responses of professionals to reactions such as denial, guilt, and anger and whether supportive interventions are used with the family.
4. Observe family members' communication patterns with each other and their ability to discuss feelings about issues such as the impact of the child's condition on the marriage or additional care responsibilities; investigate family members' use of services, such as self-help groups or other community resources.
5. Perform a developmental screening test on young children and compare results with expected milestones for the child's abilities; investigate use of functional aids to assist children in developing to their potential; question family about the child's attendance at school and interaction with peers.
6. Interview family members to determine whether their self-identified needs and concerns have been adequately addressed.

Expected Outcomes

1. Parents verbalize feelings and concerns regarding the disease or disability.
2. Parents demonstrate an attitude of acceptance and adjustment.
3. Family demonstrates an understanding of the disease and treatment options.
4. Family members set realistic goals for themselves and the child.
5. Family demonstrates positive, growth-promoting behaviors for the child and other family members.

PERSPECTIVES ON CARE OF CHILDREN AT THE END OF LIFE

Although most childhood illnesses and many injuries and other trauma respond favorably to treatment, some do not. When a child and family face a prolonged and possibly terminal illness, health professionals are faced with the challenge of providing the best possible care to meet the physical, psychologic, spiritual, and emotional needs of the child and family during the uncertain course of the illness and at the time of death. When death is sudden and unexpected, nurses are challenged to respond to grief and shock in families and provide comfort and support in the absence of a prior relationship.

Many factors affect the causes of death that nurses are likely to encounter in children: developmental factors, medical advances and technology, and changing social patterns. In infants the leading causes of death are congenital anomalies, respiratory distress syndrome, disorders related to short gestation and low birth weight, and sudden infant death syndrome (Murphy, 2000). The leading causes of death in children 5 to 9 years of age include injuries (accidents), malignant neoplasms, congenital anomalies, homicide (and legal intervention), and heart disease. In children 10 to 14 years of age, suicide is the third leading cause of death after injuries (accidents) and malignant neoplasms. In youths 15 to 19 years of age, homicide (and legal intervention), suicide, malignant neoplasms, and heart disease follow accidents as the most prevalent causes of death (Minino & Smith, 2001).

A child who is diagnosed with a life-threatening illness or who is suffering serious, life-threatening trauma needs medical diagnosis and intervention, as well as nursing assessment and care—sometimes for a short time and sometimes over a lengthy period. When cure is no longer possible and life-prolonging measures are resulting in pain and distress to the child, parents need information about care options that are available to assist them in deciding how they want the remaining time with their child to be managed by the health care team. It is important that families be reassured that although their child cannot be cured, active care will continue to be provided to maintain the child's comfort. Support must be provided to assist the child and family during the dying process. As a result, nurses may care for children and families who are making the difficult transition from curative or restorative treatments to palliative care.

Principles of Palliative Care

Palliative care involves a multidisciplinary approach to the management of a terminal illness or the dying process that focuses on symptom control and support rather than on cure or life prolongation in the absence of the possibility of a cure (Billings, 1998). The World Health Organization (1996) defines *palliative care* as the "active total care of patients whose disease is not responsive to curative treatment. Control of pain, of other symptoms, and of psychological, social and spiritual problems is paramount. The goal of palliative care is the achievement of the best possible quality of life for patients and their families." Palliative care interventions do not serve to hasten death; rather, they provide pain and symptom management, attention to issues faced by the child and family with regard to death and dying, and promotion of optimal functioning and quality of life during the time the child has remaining.

Several principles are hallmarks of palliative care. Palliative care seeks to create a therapeutic environment, as homelike as possible, if not in the child's own home. Through education and support of family members, an atmosphere of open communication is provided regarding the child's dying process and its impact on all members of the family.

Decision Making at the End of Life

Discussions concerning the possibility that a child's illness or condition is not curable and that death is an inevitable outcome causes everyone involved a great deal of stress. Physicians, other members of the health care team, and families must consider all information regarding the child's situation and make decisions that all parties agree to and that will have a profound impact on the child and family.

Ethical Considerations in End-of-Life Decision Making

A number of ethical concerns arise when parents and health care professionals are deciding on the best course of care for the dying child. Many parents and health care providers are concerned that not offering treatment that would cause potential pain and suffering, but might extend life, would be considered euthanasia or assisted suicide. To eliminate such concerns, it is necessary to understand the various terms. *Euthanasia* involves an action carried out by a person other than the patient to end the life of the patient suffering from a terminal condition. The intent of this action is based on the belief that the act is "putting the person out of his or her misery," and this action has also been called *mercy killing. Assisted suicide* occurs when someone provides the patient with the means to end his or her life and the patient uses that means to do so. The important distinction between these two actions involves who is actually acting to end the person's life.

The American Nurses Association (ANA) Code for Nurses (2001) does not support the active intent on the part of a nurse to end a person's life. However, it does permit the nurse to provide interventions to relieve symptoms in the dying patient even when the interventions involve substantial risks of hastening death. When the prognosis for a patient is poor and death is the expected outcome, it is ethically acceptable to withhold or withdraw treatments that may cause pain and suffering and provide interventions that promote comfort and quality of life. Therefore providing palliative care for patients is the ethically correct choice in such a circumstance.

Physician/Health Care Team Decision Making

Decisions by physicians regarding care are often made on the basis of the progression of the disease or amount of trauma, the availability of treatment options that would provide cure from disease or restoration of health, the impact of such treatments on the child, and the child's overall prognosis (Davis & Eng, 1998). When the physician discusses this information openly with families, a shared decision-making process can occur and decisions can be made regarding *"do not resuscitate" (DNR) orders* and care that is focused on the comfort of the child and family during the dying process. Unfortunately, many families are not given the option of terminating treatment and pursuing care that is focused on comfort and quality of life when cure is unlikely, and staff may be reluctant to raise the question of DNR orders. This occurs for a number of reasons, including the belief that not being able to "save" a child is a "failure." Also, the physician and other members of the health care team may lack knowledge of and experience with the principles of palliative care (Field & Behrman, 2003; Sahler et al, 2000; Sumner, 2003).

Parental Decision Making

Rarely are families prepared to cope with the numerous decisions that must be made when a child is dying. When the death is unexpected, as in the case of an accident or trauma, the confusion of emergency services and possibly an intensive care setting presents challenges to parents as they are asked to make very difficult choices. If the child has experienced either a life-threatening illness such as cancer or lived with a chronic illness that has now reached its terminal phase, parents are often unprepared for the reality of their child's impending death (Family Focus box). Numerous studies have found that families facing the impending death of a child depend on information provided to them by the health care team, particularly an honest appraisal of the child's prognosis, to make difficult decisions regarding care options for their child (Hinds et al, 2001; James & Johnson, 1997; Wolfe, Friebert, & Hilden, 2002).

As the group of health professionals who are most involved with families, nurses are in an excellent position to ensure that families are presented with the options available to them. The nurse's first responsibility is to explore the family's wishes. This is best done in concert with the physician, but at times may need to be initiated by the nurse. Statements such as "Tell me about your thoughts for the type of care you want your child to receive when he is dying" or "Have you considered the types of interventions you would like us to use when your child is near death?" can begin discussion of this sensitive but critical aspect of terminal care.

Family Focus

FAMILY OF THE DYING CHILD

No matter whether you have a PhD or many children, when your child dies, it is a new experience and nothing can prepare you for it. Like so many things in life, experience is the best teacher.

Three of our children have died, and by the time the third was dying, we handled many things differently. We learned a lot about dignity and the rights of the child and family. For example, at first, we didn't know that we had a right to have our child die at home. We also didn't understand pain medications and that if children are taking these medicines and are still in agony, they have not overdosed on the medication.

We learned a lot about case management. With our first two children, lots of different people were making decisions and disagreeing about what was best and what should be done. No one had primary authority. With our third child, one doctor took a primary role. Any questions and problems were handled by one person. I could call him 24 hours a day. It made a lot of difference, and I felt our concerns and needs were better heard and respected.

The nurses caring for our third child at home enabled me to step back and just be his mommy. When I could do this, I realized that we were fighting so hard for his life that we weren't really letting him die. His nurses had worked with him for a long time and really loved him. It was hard for them when we decided to let him die. In his last several days we wanted a lot of family time with our son, and I think the nurses felt left out. Something about their reaction to our increased time with him in the last few days made us feel guilty. If we had all been able to communicate a little more openly, I would have understood that they needed more time with him at the end, too. Everyone's needs could have been met.

Jeni Stepanek
Mother
Upper Marlboro, MD

The Dying Child

Children need honest and accurate information about their illness, treatments, and prognosis; this information needs to be given in clear, simple language. In most situations this best occurs as a gradual process over time, characterized by increasingly open dialogue between parents, professionals, and the child (Young et al, 2003). Providing an atmosphere of open communication early in the course of an illness facilitates answering difficult questions as the child's condition worsens. Providing appropriate literature about the disease, as well as the experience of illness and possible death, is also helpful. Exactly how and when to involve children in decisions regarding care during their dying process and death is a highly individual matter. The age or developmental level of the child is an important consideration in the process (Table 41-3). In general, parents should

Table 41-3

Children's Understanding of and Reactions to Death

CONCEPTS OF DEATH	REACTIONS TO DEATH	INTERVENTIONS
INFANTS AND TODDLERS		
Death has least significance to children younger than 6 months of age. After parent-child attachment and the development of trust is established, the loss, even if temporary, of the significant person is profound. Prolonged separation during the first several years is thought to be more significant in terms of future physical, social, and emotional growth than at any subsequent age. Toddlers are egocentric and can only think about events in terms of their own frame of reference—living. Their egocentricity and vague separation of fact and fantasy make it impossible for them to comprehend absence of life. Instead of understanding death, this age group is affected more by any change in lifestyle.	With the death of someone else, they may continue to act as though the person is alive. As children grow older, they will be increasingly able and willing to let go of the dead person. Ritualism is important; a change in lifestyle could be anxiety producing. This age group reacts more to the pain and discomfort of a serious illness than to the probable fatal prognosis. This age group also reacts to parental anxiety and sadness.	Help parents deal with their feelings, allowing them more emotional reserve to meet the needs of their children. Encourage parents to remain as near to child as possible, yet be sensitive to parents' needs. Maintain as normal an environment as possible to retain ritualism. If a parent has died, encourage having consistent caregiver for child. Promote primary nursing.
PRESCHOOL CHILDREN		
Believe their thoughts are sufficient to cause death; the consequence is the burden of guilt, shame, and punishment. Their egocentricity implies a tremendous sense of self-power and omnipotence. Usually have some connotation of its meaning. Death is seen as a departure, a kind of sleep. May recognize the fact of physical death but do not separate it from living abilities. Death is seen as temporary and gradual; life and death can change places with one another. No understanding of the universality and inevitability of death.	If they become seriously ill, they conceive of the illness as a punishment for their thoughts or actions. May feel guilty and responsible for the death of a sibling. Greatest fear concerning death is separation from parents. May engage in activities that seem strange or abnormal to adults. Because of their fewer defense mechanisms to deal with loss, young children may react to a less significant loss with more outward grief than to the loss of a very significant person. The loss is so deep, painful, and threatening that the child must deny it for the time being to survive its overwhelming impact. Behavior reactions such as giggling, joking, attracting attention, or regressing to earlier developmental skills indicate children's need to distance themselves from tremendous loss.	Help parents deal with their feelings, allowing them more emotional reserve to meet the needs of their children. Help parents to understand behavioral reactions of their children. Encourage parents to remain near the child as much as possible, to minimize the child's great fear of separation from parents. If a parent has died, encourage having a consistent caregiver for child Promote primary nursing.

Continued

Table 41-3

Children's Understanding of and Reactions to Death—cont'd

CONCEPTS OF DEATH	REACTIONS TO DEATH	INTERVENTIONS
SCHOOL-AGE CHILDREN		
Still associate misdeeds or bad thoughts with causing death and feel intense guilt and responsibility for the event Because of their higher cognitive abilities, they respond well to logical explanations and comprehend the figurative meaning of words Have a deeper understanding of death in a concrete sense Particularly fear the mutilation and punishment they associate with death Personify death as the devil, a monster, or the bogeyman May have naturalistic/physiologic explanations of death By age 9 or 10, children have an adult concept of death, realizing that it is inevitable, universal, and irreversible	Because of their increased ability to comprehend, they may have more fears, for example: • The reason for the illness • Communicability of the disease to themselves or others • Consequences of the disease • The process of dying and death itself Their fear of the unknown is greater than their fear of the known The realization of impending death is a tremendous threat to their sense of security and ego strength Likely to exhibit fear through verbal uncooperativeness rather than actual physical aggression Very interested in postdeath services May be inquisitive about what happens to the body	Help parents deal with their feelings, allowing them more emotional reserve to meet the needs of their children Encourage parents to remain near child as much as possible, yet be sensitive to parents' needs Because of children's fear of the unknown, anticipatory preparation is very important Because the developmental task of this age is industry, interventions of helping children maintain control over their bodies and increasing their understanding allow them to achieve independence, self-worth, and self-esteem and avoid a sense of inferiority Encourage children to talk about their feelings and provide aggressive outlets Encourage parents to answer questions about dying honestly rather than avoiding or fabricating euphemisms Encourage parents to share their moments of sorrow with their children Provide preparation for postdeath services
ADOLESCENTS		
Have a mature understanding of death Still very much influenced by "remnants" of magical thinking and are subject to guilt and shame Likely to see deviations from accepted behavior as reasons for their illness	Straddle transition from childhood to adulthood Have the most difficulty in coping with death Least likely to accept cessation of life, particularly if it is their own Concern is for the present much more than for the past or the future May consider themselves alienated from their peers and unable to communicate with their parents for emotional support, feeling alone in their struggle Adolescents' orientation to the present compels them to worry about physical changes even more than the prognosis Because of their idealistic view of the world, they may criticize funeral rites as barbaric, money making, and unnecessary	Help parents deal with their feelings, allowing them more emotional reserve to meet the needs of their children Avoid alliances with either parent or child Structure hospital admission to allow for maximum self-control and independence Answer adolescents' questions honestly, treating them as mature individuals and respecting their needs for privacy, solitude, and personal expressions of emotions Help parents understand their child's reactions to death/dying, especially that concern for present crises, such as loss of hair, may be much greater than for future ones, including possible death

be asked how they would like their child to be told of the prognosis, and they should be included in their child's care. Some parents may request that their child not be told that he or she is dying, even if the child asks. This often places health care providers in a difficult situation. Children, even at a young age, are very perceptive. Despite not being "told" outright that they are dying, they realize that there is something seriously wrong and that it involves them. Often, helping parents understand that honesty and shared decision making between them and their child at this time is very important to the child's emotional health, as well as the emotional health of the family, will encourage parents to allow discussion of dying with their child. Parents may require professional support and guidance in this process from a nurse, social worker, or child life specialist who has a good relationship with the child and family.

If given the opportunity, children will tell others how much they want to know. Asking questions such as "If the disease came back, would you want to know?" "Do you want others to tell you everything, even if the news isn't good?" or "If someone were not getting better (or more directly, "were dying"), do you think they would want to know?" helps children set the limits of how much truth they can accept and cope with. Children need time to process many feelings and much information so that they can assimilate and, it is hoped, accept the inevitable fact of mortality.

Care of the dying adolescent requires the nurse to become knowledgeable about any possible delays or alterations in normal growth and development. Legal and ethical issues also come to the forefront with respect to the age at which an adolescent should have autonomy in decision making with regard to care and treatment. Effective communication between the patient, family, and health care team is an important part of optimum care for the dying adolescent (Freyer, 2004).

Treatment Options for Terminally Ill Children

Based on the outcome of the decision by the child and family regarding their wishes for care, the family may choose one of several options for care.

Hospital

Families may choose to remain in the hospital to receive care if the child's illness or condition is unstable and home care is not an option or the family is uncomfortable with providing care at home. If a family chooses to remain at the hospital for terminal care, the setting should be made as homelike as possible. Families should be encouraged to bring familiar items from the child's room at home. In addition, there should be a consistent and coordinated plan of care for both the child's and the family's comfort.

Home Care

Some families may prefer to take their child home and receive services from a home care agency. Generally, these services entail periodic nursing visits to administer a treatment or provide medications, equipment, or supplies. The child's care continues to be directed by the primary physician. Home care is often the option chosen by physicians and families because of the traditional view that a child must be considered to have a life expectancy of less than 6 months to be referred to hospice care. Fortunately, a number of hospice organizations are expanding their services to children based on the presence of a life-limiting disease process for which cure is not possible, rather than on the sole criteria of a limited 6-month prognosis.

Hospice Care

Parents should be offered the option of caring for their child at home during the final phases of an illness with the assistance of a hospice organization. *Hospice* is a community health care organization that specializes in the care of dying patients by combining the hospice philosophy with the principles of palliative care. Hospice philosophy regards dying as a natural process and care of dying patients as including management of the physical, psychologic, social, and spiritual needs of the patient and family. Care is provided by a multidisciplinary group of professionals in the patient's home or an inpatient facility that employs the hospice philosophy. Hospice care for children was introduced in the 1970s, and a number of community hospice organizations now accept children into their care* (Davies et al, 2003; Faulkner & Armstrong-Dailey, 1997; Forrester, 2003; Winkler & Mardegian, 2001). Collaboration between the child's primary treatment team and the hospice care team is essential to the success of hospice care. Families may continue to see their primary care physicians as they choose.

Hospice care is based on a number of important concepts that significantly set it apart from hospital care. First, family members are the principal caregivers and are supported by a team of professional and volunteer staff. Second, the priority of care is comfort. The child's physical, psychologic, social, and spiritual needs are considered. Pain and symptom control are primary concerns, and no extraordinary efforts are used to attempt a cure or prolong life. Third, the needs of the family are considered to be as important as those of the patient. Fourth, hospice is concerned with the family's postdeath adjustment, and care may continue for a year or more.

The goal of hospice care is for children to live life to the fullest without pain, with choices and dignity, in the familiar environment of their home, and with the support of their family. Hospice care is covered under state Medicaid programs, as well as by most insurance plans. The service provides home nursing visits, as well as visits from social workers, chaplains, and, in some cases, physicians. Medications, medical equipment, and any necessary medical supplies are all provided by the hospice organization providing care.

With children, the home has been the more common environment for implementing the hospice concept; it benefits the family in a variety of ways. Children who are dying are allowed the opportunity to remain with those they love and with whom they feel secure. Many children who were thought to be in imminent danger of death have gone home and lived longer than expected. Siblings can feel more involved in the care and often have more positive perceptions of the death. Parental adaptation is often more favorable, as is shown by their perceptions of how the experience at home affected their marriage, social reorientation, religious beliefs, and views on the meaning of life and death.

If the home is chosen for hospice care, the child may or may not die in the home. Reasons for final admission to a hospital vary but may be related to the parents' or siblings' wish to have the child die outside the home; exhaustion on the part of the caregivers; and physical problems such as sudden, acute pain or respiratory distress.

*National Hospice and Palliative Care Organization, 1700 Diagonal Rd., Suite 625, Alexandria, VA 22314; phone: 703-837-1500; fax: 703-837-1233; Web site: www.nho.org. Children's Hospice International, 901 North Pitt St., Suite 230, Alexandria, VA 22314; phone: 703-684-0330 or 800-24-CHILD; Web site: www.chionline.org.

NURSING CARE OF THE CHILD AND FAMILY AT THE END OF LIFE

Regardless of where the child is cared for during the terminal stage of illness, both the child and the family usually experience the following fears: (1) fear of pain and suffering, (2) fear of dying alone (child) or of not being present when the child dies (parent), and (3) fear of actual death. Nurses can assist families by lessening their fears through attention to the care needs of the child and family (Nursing Care Plan).

Fear of Pain and Suffering

The presence of unrelieved pain in a terminally ill child can have very detrimental effects on the quality of life experienced by the child and family. Parents have reported that having their child in pain was unendurable and resulted in feelings of helplessness and a sense that they must be present and vigilant to get the necessary pain medications. Persistent pain also has an impact on the family as a whole. Nurses can alleviate the fear of pain and suffering by providing interventions aimed at treating the pain and symptoms associated with the terminal process in children.

Nursing Care Plan

THE CHILD WHO IS TERMINALLY ILL OR DYING

NURSING DIAGNOSIS: Anticipatory grieving related to terminal illness/impending death

EXPECTED OUTCOME

Child will participate in age-appropriate constructive anticipatory grief work and will exhibit free expression of feelings.

NURSING INTERVENTIONS/*RATIONALES*

Encourage children to express feelings in own way through play, drawing, or verbalization *to promote free expression in accordance with their specific cognitive and emotional abilities.*

Provide a safe, acceptable outlet for expressions of feelings (e.g., crying, sadness, anger, aggression) *because this is a needed part of the grieving process.*

Structure the care experience to allow child choices and participation in process within constraints of physical condition *to help child maintain a sense of control and self-esteem.*

Encourage family to remain near child and to stay engaged with child *to provide support and to allay child's fear of being abandoned or no longer being loved.*

NURSING DIAGNOSIS: Pain related to terminal stage of illness

EXPECTED OUTCOME

Child will exhibit minimal signs of physical discomfort.

NURSING INTERVENTIONS/*RATIONALES*

Provide and encourage family to provide the child's favorite comfort measures (e.g., rocking, stroking, storytelling, singing); move and turn carefully; avoid excessive noise or light; use noninvasive care monitoring when possible; and limit care to essentials *to minimize discomfort and promote comfort.*

Administer treatments as prescribed (e.g., oxygen *for respiratory distress,* anticonvulsants *for seizures,* analgesics *for pain,* anticholinergics *to decrease secretions*).

Talk with child in clear, distinct voice *to offer calm reassurance;* avoid whispering or talking about child *to reduce anxiety;* phrase questions to require "yes" or "no" responses *to conserve energy.*

NURSING DIAGNOSIS: Anticipatory grieving related to impending loss of a child

EXPECTED OUTCOME

Family will exhibit evidence of constructive grief process (verbalization/expression of feelings, maintenance of interpersonal relationships, use of support systems and coping mechanisms).

NURSING INTERVENTIONS/*RATIONALES*

Spend time with family to listen, answer questions, and provide information *as a way to establish trust and demonstrate support and caring.*

Provide opportunities for family to express their emotions and deal with their feelings *as a part of the grieving process.*

Help family to understand the grief process and to accept feelings being experienced (denial, sadness, guilt, anger, relief) as a normal part of the process *to enhance understanding and ability to cope.*

Encourage expression and discussion of perceptions of loss and the impact on life of the family *to provide ventilation and reinforcement of reality.*

Keep family informed of child's status, help them interpret child's responses, and encourage their participation in child's care *to allay fears and anxiety and promote involvement.*

Encourage parents to face child's fears and questions about death openly and honestly *to facilitate grief work by child and parents.*

Explore family religious and cultural beliefs related to death (e.g., prayers, rites, rituals) and arrange for appropriate spiritual care if appropriate.

Emphasize family's identified strengths and provide encouragement for decisions that demonstrate effective coping skills *to help reinforce ability to cope.*

When death is imminent, allow the family privacy and time to be with and hold, touch, and talk to the child *to facilitate saying good-bye.*

At death, allow family to remain with the child's body for as long as they wish, and to rock, hold, bathe, and talk to the child, *to facilitate grieving.*

Be physically present with the family; offer nonverbal comfort, touch if appropriate; help them move through the process of leaving the facility (e.g., gathering belongings, checking out) *to provide supportive presence and guidance in next steps.*

Determine support sources (e.g., relatives, friends, church, community) and how they can help with disruptions that occur in lifestyle (e.g., arrangements, activities of daily living, finances, transportation) *to bolster coping and provide needed support during crisis.*

Refer family to grief counseling if indicated *to aid in coping and to prevent dysfunctional grieving.*

Initiate and maintain contact; attend the funeral, visitation, or memorial service if there was a special closeness with family *to facilitate grief process and termination of therapeutic relationship with caregiver.*

Pain/Symptom Management

Pain control for children in the terminal stages of illness or injury must be given the highest priority. Despite ongoing efforts to educate physicians and nurses on pain management strategies in children, studies have reported that children continue to be undermedicated for their pain (Wolfe et al, 2000). Nearly all children experience some amount of pain in the terminal phase of their illness. The current standard for treating children's pain is according to the World Health Organization's analgesic stepladder (1996). This approach promotes tailoring the pain interventions to the child's level of reported pain. Children's pain should be assessed frequently, and medications adjusted as necessary. Pain medications should be given on a regular schedule, and extra doses for "breakthrough pain" should be available to maintain comfort. Opioid drugs such as morphine should be given for severe pain, and the dose should be increased as necessary to maintain optimum pain relief. Techniques such as distraction, relaxation techniques, and guided imagery (Lambert, 1999) should be combined with drug therapy to provide the child and family with strategies to control pain (see Chapter 44 for further discussion of pain management strategies).

In addition to pain, children experience a variety of additional symptoms during their terminal course as a result of their disease process or as a side effect of medicines used to manage pain or other symptoms. These symptoms include fatigue, nausea and vomiting, constipation, anorexia, dyspnea, congestion, seizures, anxiety, depression, restlessness, agitation, and confusion (Hellsten et al, 2000; Wolfe et al, 2002). Each of these symptoms should be aggressively managed with appropriate medications or treatments, as well as interventions such as repositioning, relaxation, massage, and other measures to maintain the child's comfort and quality of life.

Occasionally, children require very high doses of opioids to control pain. There are several reasons why this occurs. The child on long-term opioid pain management can become *tolerant* of the drug, meaning that it is necessary to give more drug to maintain the same level of pain relief. This should not be confused with *addiction,* which is a psychologic dependence on the side effects of opioids. Addiction is not a factor in managing terminal pain in children. Other obvious reasons for requiring increased doses of opioids include progression of disease and other physiologic experiences of pain. It is important to understand that there is no maximum dose that can be given to control pain. However, nurses often express concern that administering doses of opioids that exceed what they are familiar with will hasten the child's death. The principle of double effect (Box 41-7) addresses such concerns. It provides an ethical standard that supports the use of interventions that have the intention of relieving pain and suffering even though there is a foreseeable possibility that death may be hastened (Rousseau, 2001). However, in cases in which the child is terminally ill and in severe pain, using large doses of opioids and sedatives to manage pain is justified when there are no other treatment options available that would relieve the pain but make the risk of death less likely (Hawryluck & Harvey, 2000). See Chapter 44 for an extensive discussion of pain assessment and management.

BOX 41-7

Ethical Principle of Double Effect

An action that has one good (intended) and one bad (unintended but foreseeable) effect is permissible if the following conditions are met:

- The action itself must be good or indifferent. Only the good consequences of the action must be sincerely intended.
- The good effect must not be produced by the bad effect.
- There must be a compelling or proportionate reason for permitting the foreseeable bad effect to occur.

Parents' and Siblings' Need for Education and Support

Parents are the primary caregivers when the child is at home, and nurses providing care to the child and family need to teach the family about the medications being given to the child, as well as how to administer medications and use nonpharmacologic techniques. Parents should also be kept informed of all medications and treatments given to a child in the hospital, and they should be allowed to participate in the child's care to the extent that they desire.

Siblings may feel isolated and displaced during the time that their brother or sister is dying. Parents devote the majority of their time to the care and comfort of the dying child, causing siblings to feel left out of the parent–sick child relationship. Siblings may become resentful of their sick sibling and begin to feel guilty or shameful about such feelings. Nurses can assist the family by helping the parents identify ways to involve siblings in the caring process, perhaps by bringing some supply or favorite toy, game, or food item. Parents should also be encouraged to schedule some time to spend with the other children where their focus is on them. Helping parents identify a trusted friend or family member who can sit with the ill child for a short period will allow them to attend to their own needs or those of their other children.

Fear of Dying Alone or of Not Being Present When the Child Dies

When a child is being cared for at home, the burden of care experienced by parents and family members can be great. Often, as the child's condition declines, family members begin the "death vigil." Rarely is a child left alone for any length of time. This can be exhausting for family members, and nurses can assist the family by helping them arrange "shifts" so that friends or family members can be present with the child and allow others to rest. If the family has limited resources, community organizations such as hospice or churches often have volunteers who are willing to visit and sit with children. It is important that whoever is sitting with the child be aware of when the parent(s) would like to be notified to return to the child's bedside.

When a child is dying in the hospital, parents should be given full access to the child at all times. If parents need to leave for a period, they should be provided with a pager or other means of immediate communication and alerted if staff members note any change in the child that may indicate imminent death. Nurses should advocate for parents' presence in intensive care and emergency departments and attend to the parents' needs for food, drinks, comfortable chairs, blankets, and pillows.

Fear of Actual Death

Home Deaths

The majority of children receiving hospice care die at home, often in their own room with family, pets, and other loved possessions around them. The physical process of dying can be very distressing to parents, because often the child has slowly become less alert in the days before the actual death. The nurse can assist the family by providing them with information about what changes will occur as the child progresses through the dying process (Box 41-8). During this time, nursing visits often become more frequent and longer in duration to provide the family with additional support as the death nears. The most distressing change for parents to observe is the change in the respiratory pattern. In the final hours of life, the dying patient's respiration may become labored, with deep breaths and long periods of apnea, referred to as *Cheyne-Stokes respirations.* Families should be reassured that this is not distressing to the child and that it is a normal part of the dying process. However, the use of opioids can slow the respirations to make the child breathe more easily, and scopolamine, usually applied as a topical patch, can help reduce noisy respirations known as the "death rattle." Noisy respirations are more likely to occur if the child is overhydrated.

All families have the option of admitting their child to the hospital if they feel unable to deal with the death. The child who dies at home must be pronounced dead; hospice programs typically have provisions so that this may proceed smoothly. In some circumstances the police may be notified, with an explanation of the circumstances to prevent unnecessary concern regarding abuse. Providing the police with the number of the responsible practitioner is usually all that is necessary to confirm the cause of death.

Hospital Deaths

Children dying in the hospital of terminal illnesses who are receiving supportive care interventions will experience a similar process. Again, increased nursing presence and attendance to the child and family's needs provide comfort and support for many families.

Death resulting from accident or trauma or acute illness in settings such as the emergency department or intensive care unit often requires the active withdrawal of some form of life-supporting intervention, such as a ventilator or bypass machine. These situations often raise difficult ethical issues (Sine et al, 2001), and parents are often less prepared for the actual moment of death. Nurses can assist these parents by providing detailed information about what will happen as supportive equipment is withdrawn, ensuring that appropriate pain medications are administered to prevent pain during the dying process, and allowing the parents time before the start of the withdrawal to be with and speak to their child. It is important that the nurse attempt to control the environment around the family at this time by providing privacy, asking if they would like to play music, softening lights and monitor noises, and arranging for any religious or cultural rituals that the family may want performed.

After the child's death, the family should be allowed to remain with the body and hold or rock the child if they desire. After the nurse has removed all tubes and equipment from the body, parents should be given the option of assisting with the preparation of the body, such as bathing and dressing. It is important for the nurse to determine if the family has any specific needs because many cultures have adapted specific methods for coping with and mourning death, and impeding these practices may interfere with the grieving process (Clements et al, 2003).

At some point the nurse should discuss if the family has made preparations for the burial service and if the staff can help in any way. Parents often have concerns about the funeral, such as siblings' involvement in the death rituals. Although no absolute answers exist regarding the question of siblings attending the funeral or burial services, the general consensus is that the surviving children benefit from being involved in these events. However, children need preparation for postdeath services. They should be told what to expect, particularly how the deceased person will look if the coffin is open; allowed their private time to say good-bye; and permitted to stay as long as they wish. Ideally, the parents should prepare the siblings. If the parents' grief prevents this communication, a significant family member or friend should substitute (Family Focus Box).

In cases of unexplained death, violent death, or suspected suicide, autopsy is required by law. In other instances it may be optional, and parents should be informed of this choice. The procedure, as well as forms that require signing, should be explained. The family should know that the child can be in an open casket following an autopsy.

BOX 41-8

Physical Signs of Approaching Death

- Loss of sensation and movement in the lower extremities, progressing toward the upper body
- Sensation of heat, although body feels cool
- Loss of senses:
  - Tactile sensation decreases
  - Sensitive to light
  - Hearing is last sense to fail
- Confusion, loss of consciousness, slurred speech
- Muscle weakness
- Loss of bowel and bladder control
- Decreased appetite/thirst
- Difficulty swallowing
- Change in respiratory pattern:
  - Cheyne-Stokes respirations (waxing and waning of depth of breathing with regular periods of apnea)
  - "Death rattle" (noisy chest sounds from accumulation of pulmonary and pharyngeal secretions)
- Weak, slow pulse; decreased blood pressure

Family Focus

CHILDREN NEED TO SAY GOOD-BYE

As a nurse/grief counselor, I conduct grief workshops with children who have experienced the death of someone special. Children often communicate their feelings of being excluded through drawings. They may draw a picture of the dying person in a hospital bed that is raised too high for them to see the person's face clearly. Sometimes children reveal that they did not get to say good-bye because a family member told them, for example, "You don't want to see your grandma this way. She is too sick for you to visit." If the special person died at home, the children had to stay in their room when the funeral home staff took away the body.

I have learned never to underestimate the importance of allowing children to be involved with the dying person and the significance of a child's loss. Once, when I asked a 6-year-old girl to draw a picture with the theme "This is what I was doing when my ______ died," she drew a picture and completed the sentence with "when my home died." Her grandmother had been like her mother; to the child, her home was gone. We need to give children the choice of being included in the family's activities of saying good-bye.

Barbara Bilderback, MS, MA, RN
Bereavement Supervisor, Saint Francis Hospice
Tulsa, OK

Grief and Mourning

The crisis of loss does not end with the child's death. In many ways it only begins. Unfortunately, the child's death often marks the close of the family's contacts with health professionals involved in the care. Consequently, many of these families never receive the support and guidance that could assist them in resolving the loss. Fortunately, hospice programs recognize this need and provide regular follow-up after the death.

When death is the expected or possible outcome of a disorder, the child and family members experience the behavioral reactions of anticipatory grief. Anticipatory grief may be manifested in varying behaviors and intensities and may include denial, anger, depression, and other psychologic and somatic symptoms.

When death occurs—whether expected or unexpected—acute grief develops within hours to days. Acute grief is a definite syndrome with psychologic and somatic symptoms that cause intense distress (Box 41-9). Anticipatory guidance may assist grieving family members. Health professionals should emphasize that grief reactions such as hearing the dead person's voice, feeling distant from others, or seeking reassurance that they did everything possible for the lost person are normal, necessary, and expected. They in no way signify poor coping, insanity, or an approaching mental breakdown. On the contrary, such behaviors signify that the survivor is working through the acute grief. They are a necessary part of satisfactory resolution of the loss. These reactions are part of the process of resuming or restructuring a meaningful role in the social environment.

Critical Thinking Exercise: Neonatal Loss

After the death, the lengthy process of grief work or mourning begins and extends into a period of adjustment to the loss, with eventual attachment to new people and the development of new interests. Contrary to the common belief that mourning is completed in a year, research indicates that resolution of grief may take years and that there may be an *intensification* of grief during the early years. The time since a child's death is not necessarily a factor in reducing the intensity of grief for families (Davis & Eng, 1998; Murphy et al, 2003). Anticipatory guidance regarding the mourning process may be helpful to families so that they can recognize the normalcy of their experiences.

BOX 41-9

Symptomatology of Normal Grief

Sensations of Somatic Distress
Feeling of tightness in the throat
Choking, with shortness of breath
Marked tendency toward sighing
Empty feeling in the abdomen
Lack of muscular power
Intense subjective distress described as tension or mental pain

Preoccupation with Image of the Deceased
Hears, sees, or imagines that the dead person is present
Slight sense of unreality
Feeling of emotional distance from others
May believe that he or she is approaching insanity

Feelings of Guilt
Searches for evidence of failure in preventing the death
Accuses self of negligence or exaggerates minor omissions

Feelings of Hostility
Loss of warmth toward others
Tendency toward irritability and anger
Wishes to not be bothered by friends or relatives

Loss of Usual Patterns of Conduct
Restlessness, inability to sit still, aimless moving about
Continual searching for something to do or what he or she thinks should be done
Lack of capacity to initiate and maintain organized patterns of activity

Modified from Lindermann E: Symptomatology and management of acute grief, *Am J Psychiatry* 101:141-143, 1944.

A child's death can also challenge the marital relationship in several ways. Maternal and paternal reactions often differ (Birenbaum et al, 1996; Moriarty et al, 1996; Vance et al, 1995). Different grieving styles between the couple may hinder communication and support for each other. Differing needs and expectations can place a strain on the marriage.

At times family members may need assistance in their grieving (Guidelines Box: Supporting Grieving Families). Mothers, in particular, often feel a great sense of loneliness and emptiness, and part of their resolving the grief is finding a substitute role that is fulfilling and rewarding. Nurses can be instrumental in this process by (1) preparing the mother for anticipating the *normal* feelings of emptiness, loneliness, and sometimes even failure; (2) helping her reevaluate her role as parent and spouse, stressing that giving up the lost child must occur before she can reestablish emotional relationships; (3) encouraging her to explore fulfilling activities that use her special interests, talents, and qualifications; and (4) supporting her as her role changes, particularly assisting with communication between affected family members.

Guidelines

SUPPORTING GRIEVING FAMILIES*

General

Stay with the family; sit quietly if they prefer not to talk; cry with them if desired.
Accept the family's grief reactions; avoid judgmental statements (e.g., "You should be feeling better by now").
Avoid offering rationalizations for the child's death (e.g., "You should be glad your child isn't suffering anymore").
Avoid artificial consolation (e.g., "I know how you feel," or "You are still young enough to have another baby").
Deal openly with feelings such as guilt, anger, and loss of self-esteem.
Focus on feelings by using a feeling word in the statement (e.g., "You're still feeling all the pain of losing a child").
Refer the family to an appropriate self-help group or for professional help if needed.

At the Time of Death

Reassure the family that everything possible is being done for the child, if they want lifesaving interventions.
Do everything possible to ensure the child's comfort, especially relieving pain.
Provide the child and family with the opportunity to review special experiences or memories in their lives.
Express personal feelings of loss or frustrations (e.g., "We will miss him so much," "We tried everything; we feel so sorry that we couldn't save her").
Provide information that the family requests and be honest.
Respect the emotional needs of family members, such as siblings, who may need brief respites from the dying child.
Make every effort to arrange for family members, especially parents, to be with the child at the moment of death, if they want to be present.
Allow the family to stay with the dead child for as long as they wish and to rock, hold, or bathe the child.
Provide practical help when possible, such as collecting the child's belongings.
Arrange for spiritual support, based on the family's religious beliefs; pray with the family if no one else can stay with them.

Postdeath

Attend the funeral or visitation if there was a special closeness with the family.
Initiate and maintain contact (e.g., sending cards, telephoning, inviting them back to the unit, making a home visit).
Refer to the dead child by name; discuss shared memories with the family.
Discourage the use of drugs or alcohol as a method of escaping grief.
Encourage all family members to communicate their feelings rather than remaining silent to avoid upsetting another member.
Emphasize that grieving is a painful process that often takes years to resolve.

*"Family" refers to all significant persons involved in the child's life, such as the parents, siblings, grandparents, or other close relatives or friends.

Communication with the bereaved family is essential, but often there is a feeling of not knowing what to say and of helplessness in offering words of comfort (Family Focus Box: A dying child: A nurse's persspective). The most supportive approach is to avoid judging the family's reactions or offering advice or rationalizations and to focus on feelings. Perhaps the most valuable supportive measure the nurse can perform for families is to listen. Families understand that no words will relieve their pain; all they want is acceptance, understanding, and respect for their grief. A plan for regular follow-up with bereaved families can be beneficial.

Family Focus

A DYING CHILD: A NURSE'S PERSPECTIVE

Claire was unresponsive with slow, gasping breathing. Her mother asked me what I thought was happening. I replied honestly, "Your baby is dying because of her brain tumor." The mother put her arms around me and cried. We arranged for Claire to be baptized.

Honesty. As painful as the loss of a child is, my job is to assist the family through this experience. Although I usually wait until a private moment, such as driving home, I found tears streaming down my face as family and friends gathered for Claire's baptism. I went into the kitchen to compose myself, only to find several of my colleagues crying as well. Saying good-bye to a dying child will always be a difficult but shared experience.

Jeanne O'Connor Egan, RN, MSN
Pediatric Clinical Specialist, Children's Hospital
Washington, DC

It is important for families to understand that mourning takes a long time. Whereas acute grief may last only weeks or months, resolving the loss is measured in years. Holidays and anniversaries can be particularly difficult, and people who previously had been supportive may now expect the family to have "adjusted." Consequently, prolonged mourning is often silent and lonely.

For more information on end-of-life care,* visit these Web sites:

Americans for Better Care of the Dying
www.abcd-caring.com
City of Hope Pain/Palliative Care Resources Center
www.mayday.coh.org
End-of-Life Physician Education Resource Center
www.eperc.mcw.edm
Growth House
www.growthhouse.org
Last Acts
www.lastacts.org

*Other sources of publications on life-threatening illness and death are The Compassionate Friends, PO Box 3696, Oak Brook, IL 60522-3696; phone: 630-990-0010; e-mail: TCF_National@progidy.com. Centering Corporation, 1531 N. Saddle Creek Rd., Omaha, NE 68104; phone: 402-553-1200; Web site: www.centering.org. Children's Hospice International, 2202 Mt. Vernon Ave., Suite 3-C, Alexandria, VA 22314; phone: 800-24-CHILD; e-mail: chiorg@aol.com; Web site: www.chionline.org. National Cancer Institute, Cancer Information Service, Building 21, Room 10A29, Bethesda, MD 20892-2580; phone: 800-422-6237.

Key Points

- Trends in the treatment of children with chronic illness or disability have focused on developmental age, the child's strengths and uniqueness, family-centered care, establishment of normalization, early discharge, home care, mainstreaming, and early intervention.
- In response to the child with chronic illness or disability, parents may be affected by feelings of inadequacy and failure; excessive demands on time, energy, and financial resources; and strain on the marital relationship.
- Families' reactions to disability or chronic illness are manifested in the following stages: shock and denial, adjustment, reintegration, and acknowledgment.
- The child's reaction to illness or disability depends on the child's developmental level and coping mechanisms, others' reactions, and the illness itself.
- Assessment of family members' adjustment to a child's chronic illness, disability, or death includes the availability of a support system, their perception of the event, their coping mechanisms, concurrent stressors, and their response to the child.
- To help parents cope with their child's chronic illness or disability, nurses must offer attentiveness, humanistic support, solicitation of suggestions for care, facilitation of communication, verbalization of feelings, and referral to volunteer and community agencies.
- Supporting the child involves encouraging self-expression, alleviating feelings of being different, and strengthening the child's self-image.
- Children's concept of death is determined by their cognitive ability and their experience with life-threatening illness.
- Young children see death as temporary and reversible and mainly fear separation.
- School-age children view death as irreversible but not necessarily inevitable and may fear mutilation.
- Children beyond 9 to 10 years of age realize that death is irreversible, universal, and inevitable but may resist the thought of their own death.
- Siblings have special needs, including the need for information, reassurance about their own health status, assurance that they are not responsible for the illness or death, and support for their own grieving process.
- Special needs of the family facing the unexpected death of a child include support while awaiting news of the child's status; a sensitive pronouncement of death; acknowledgment of feelings of denial, guilt, and anger; an opportunity to view the body; closure; and referrals for support.
- Special decisions at the time of dying and death may involve hospital or hospice care, the child's right to die, visualization of the body, tissue donation and autopsy, and siblings' attendance at the funeral.
- Acute grief is a syndrome with intense and distressing psychologic and somatic symptoms that appear at the time of death.
- Mourning is a prolonged, painful process that consists of four phases: shock and disbelief, expression of grief, disorganization and despair, and reorganization.
- In dealing with stress related to the dying patient, the nurse can cope successfully through self-awareness, consciousness raising, knowledge and practice, an available support system, and maintenance of general good health, and by focusing on the positive rewards of involvement with dying children and their families.

References

Ahmann E: "Chunky stew": appreciating cultural diversity while providing health care for children, *Pediatr Nurs* 20(3):320-324, 1994.

Ahmann E, Scher A: Alternatives to home care for medically fragile children. In Ahmann E (editor): *Home care for the high risk infant: a family centered approach,* Gaithersburg, MD, 1996, Aspen.

American Academy of Pediatrics, Committee on Children with Disabilities: Managed care and children with special health care needs: a subject review, *Pediatrics* 102(3):657-660, 1998.

American Nurses Association: *Code of ethics for nurses with interpretive statements,* Washington, DC, 2001, ANA Publishing.

Billings JA: What is palliative care? *J Palliat Med* 1(1):73-81, 1998.

Birenbaum LK et al: Health status of bereaved parents, *Nurs Res* 45(2): 105-109, 1996.

Carter B: Chronic pain in childhood and the medical encounter: professional ventriloquism and hidden voices, *Qual Health Res* 12:28-41, 2002.

Charles C, Gafni A, Whelan T: Shared decision making in the medical encounter: what does it mean? *Soc Sci Med* 44:681-692, 1997.

Clements PT et al: Cultural perspectives of death, grief, and bereavement, *J Psychosoc Nurs Ment Health Serv* 41(7):18-26, 2003.

Cohen MH: The stages of the prediagnostic period in chronic life-threatening childhood illness: a process analysis, *Res Nurs Health* 18(1):39-48, 1995.

Davies R, Davis B, Sibert J: Parents' stories of sensitive and insensitive care by paediatricians in the time leading up to and including diagnostic disclosure of a life-limiting condition in their child, *Child Care Health Dev* 29(1):77-82, 2003.

Davis B, Eng B: Special issues in bereavement and staff support. In Doyle D, Hanks GWC, MacDonald N (editors): *Oxford textbook of palliative medicine,* ed 2, Oxford, 1998, Oxford.

Deatrick JA, Knafl KA, Murphy-Moore C: Clarifying the concept of normalization, *Image J Nurs Sch* 31:209-214, 1999.

Dixon-Woods M, Young B, Henry D: Partnerships with children, *BMJ* 319:778-780, 1999.

Faulkner KW, Armstrong-Dailey A: Care of the dying child. In Pizzo PA, Poplack DG (editors): *Principles and practice of pediatric oncology,* Philadelphia, 1997, Lippincott-Raven.

Faulkner MS: Family responses to children with diabetes and their influence on self-care, *J Pediatr Nurs* 11(2):82-93, 1996.

Field MJ, Behrman RE: Educating health care professionals. In Field MJ, Behrman RE (editors): *When children die: improving palliative and end-of-life care for children and their families,* Washington, DC, 2003, National Academies Press.

Fleitas J: When Jack fell down . . . Jill came tumbling after: siblings in the web of illness and disability, *MCN* 25:267-273, 2000.

Forrester L: One to one care in children's hospice, *Nurs Times* 99(16):44-45, 2003.

Freyer DR: Care of the dying adolescent: special considerations, *Pediatrics* 113(2):381-388, 2004.

Garwick AW et al: Breaking the news: how families first learn about their child's chronic condition, *Arch Pediatr Adolesc Med* 149(9):991-997, 1995.

Goldbeck L: Parental coping with the diagnosis of childhood cancer: gender effects, dissimilarity within couples, and quality of life, *Psychooncology* 10:325-335, 2001.

Gravelle AM: Caring for a child with a progressive illness during the complex chronic phase: parents' experience of facing adversity, *J Adv Nurs* 25:738-745, 1997.

Hawryluck LA, Harvey WR: Analgesia, virtue, and the principle of double effect, *J Palliat Care* 16(suppl):S24-S30, 2000.

Hellsten MB et al: *End-of-life care for children,* Austin, TX, 2000, Texas Cancer Council.

Hinds PS et al: End-of-life decision making by adolescents, parents, and healthcare providers in pediatric oncology: research to evidence-based practice guidelines, *Cancer Nurs* 24:122-134, 2001.

Jackson PL: The primary care provider and children with chronic conditions. In Jackson PL, Vessey PA: *Primary care of the child with a chronic condition,* ed 3, St Louis, 2000, Mosby.

James L, Johnson B: The needs of parents of pediatric oncology patients during the palliative care phase, *J Pediatr Oncol Nurs* 14(2):83-95, 1997.

Kuhlthau K et al: Assessing managed care for children with chronic conditions, *Health Affairs* 17(4):42-52, 1998.

Lambert S: Distraction, imagery, and hypnosis techniques for management of children's pain, *J Child Fam Nurs* 2(1):5-15, 1999.

Lobato DJ, Kao BT: Integrated sibling-parent group intervention to improve sibling knowledge and adjustment to chronic illness and disability, *J Pediatr Psychol* 27:711-716, 2002.

Lock J: Psychosexual development in adolescents with chronic medical illness, *Psychosomatics* 39:340-349, 1998.

Marshall ES et al: "This is a spiritual experience": perspectives of Latter-Day Saint families living with a child with disabilities, *Qual Health Res* 13: 57-76, 2003.

Mastroyannopoulou K et al: The impact of childhood non-malignant life threatening illness on parents: gender differences and predictors of parental adjustment, *J Child Psychol Psychiatry* 38(7):823-829, 1997.

McDougal J: Promoting normalization in families with preschool children with type 1 diabetes, *J Specialty Pediatr Nurs* 7(3):113-120, 2002.

Minino AM, Smith BL: Deaths: preliminary data for 2000, *Natl Vital Stat Rep* 49:1-40, 2001.

Monical W: Daycare for children who are medically fragile, *Except Parent* 25(2):27-31, 1995.

Moriarty H et al: Differences in bereavement reactions within couples following the death of a child, *Res Nurs Health* 19:461-469, 1996.

Morse JM, Wilson S, Penrod J: Mothers and their disabled children: refining the concept of normalization, *Health Care Woman Int* 21(8):659-676, 2000.

Msall ME et al: Functional disability and school activity limitations in 41,300 school-age children: relationship to medical impairments, *Pediatrics* 111:548-553, 2003.

Murphy SA et al: Bereaved parents outcomes 4 to 60 months after their child's death by accident, suicide, or homicide: a comparative study demonstrating differences, *Death Studies* 27(1):39-61, 2003.

Murphy SL: Deaths: final data for 1998, *Natl Vital Stat Rep* 48:1-105, 2000.

Nelson AM: A metasynthesis: mothering other-than-normal children, *Qual Health Res* 12:515-530, 2002.

Newacheck PW, Halfon N: Prevalence and impact of disabling chronic conditions in childhood, *Am J Public Health* 88(4):610-617, 1998.

O'Brien ME, Wegner CB: Rearing the child who is technology dependent: perceptions of parents and home care nurses, *J Spec Pediatr Nurs* 7:7-15, 2002.

Perrin JM: Chronic illness in childhood. In Behrman RE, Kleigman RM, Jensen HB (editors): *Nelson textbook of pediatrics,* ed 17, Philadelphia, 2004, WB Saunders.

Ray LD: Parenting and childhood chronicity: making visible the invisible work, *J Pediatr Nurs* 17(6):424-438, 2002.

Rehm RS: Religious faith in Mexican-American families dealing with chronic childhood illness, *Image J Nurs Sch* 31:33-38, 1999.

Ritchie MA: Self-esteem and hopefulness in adolescents with cancer, *J Pediatr Nurs* 16:35-42, 2001.

Rousseau P: Ethical and legal issues in palliative care, *Prim Care* 28:391-400, 2001.

Sahler O et al: Medical education about end-of-life care in the pediatric setting: principles, challenges, and opportunities, *Pediatrics* 105:575-584, 2000.

Schor EL: Family pediatrics: report of the Task Force on the Family, *Pediatrics* 111:1541-1571, 2003.

Sharpe D, Rossiter L: Siblings of children with a chronic illness: a meta-analysis, *J Pediatr Psychol* 27:699-710, 2002.

Shepard MP, Mahon MM: Chronic conditions and the family. In Jackson PL, Vessey JA: *Primary care of the child with a chronic condition,* ed 3, St Louis, 2000, Mosby.

Siegel RD: Child care and the ADA, *Except Parent* 25(2):34, 1995.

Sine D et al: Pediatric extubation: "pulling the tube," *J Palliat Med* 4: 519-524, 2001.

Stein REK: Home care: a challenging opportunity, *Child Health Care* 14(2):90-95, 1985.

Sterling YM, Peterson JW: Characteristics of African American women caregivers of children with asthma, *MCN* 28:32-38, 2003.

Sumner LH: Lighting the way: improving the way children die in America, *Caring* 22:14-18, 2003.

Swallow VM, Jacoby A: Mothers' evolving relationships with doctors and nurses during the chronic childhood illness trajectory, *J Adv Nurs* 36: 755-764, 2001.

Thomlinson EH: The lived experience of families of children who are failing to thrive, *J Adv Nurs* 39:537-545, 2002.

Tong H et al: Physical functioning in female caregivers of children with physical disabilities compared with female caregivers of children with a chronic medical condition, *Arch Pediatr Adolesc Med* 156:1138-1142, 2002.

Vance JC et al: Psychological changes in parents eight months after the loss of an infant from stillbirth, neonatal death, or sudden infant death syndrome—a longitudinal study, *Pediatrics* 96(5):933-938, 1995.

Vessey JA, Mebane DJ: Chronic conditions and child development. In Jackson PL, Vessey JA: *Primary care of the child with a chronic condition,* ed 3, St Louis, 2000, Mosby.

Whitehead LC, Gosling V: Parent's perceptions of interactions with health professionals in the pathway to gaining a diagnosis of tuberous sclerosis (TS) and beyond, *Res Dev Disabil* 24:109-119, 2003.

Winkler WD, Mardegian CA: Completing the continuum of care: the growth of a pediatric hospice program, *Caring* 20:22-25, 2001.

Wise PH et al: Chronic illness among poor children enrolled in the temporary assistance for needy families program, *Am J Public Health* 92: 1458-1461, 2002.

Wolfe J, Friebert S, Hilden J: Caring for children with advanced cancer: integrating palliative care, *Pediatr Clin North Am* 49:5, 2002.

Wolfe J et al: Symptoms and suffering at the end of life in children with cancer, *N Engl J Med* 342(5):326-333, 2000.

Wood PR et al: Relationships between welfare status, health insurance status, and health and medical care among children with asthma, *Am J Public Health* 92:1446-1452, 2002.

World Health Organization: *Cancer pain relief and palliative care,* Geneva, Switzerland, 1996, The Organization.

Yogev R, Chadwick EG: Acquired immunodeficiency syndrome. In Behrman RE, Kleigman RM, Jensen HB (editors): *Nelson textbook of pediatrics,* ed 17, Philadelphia, 2004, WB Saunders.

Young B et al: Managing communication with young people who have a potentially life threatening chronic illness: qualitative study of patients and parents, *BMJ* 326:1-5, 2003.

Zuvekas SH, Taliaferro GS: Pathways to access: health, insurance, the health care delivery system and racial/ethnic disparities, 1996-1999, *Health Affairs* 22(2):139-153, 2003.

Cognitive and Sensory Impairment 42

LEARNING OBJECTIVES

On completion of this chapter the reader will be able to:

- Define the classifications of mental retardation.
- Outline nursing interventions for the child with cognitive impairment that promote optimum development, including during hospitalization.
- Identify the major biologic and cognitive characteristics of the child with Down syndrome.
- Outline nursing interventions for the child with Down syndrome.
- Identify the major characteristics associated with fragile X syndrome.
- List the general classifications of hearing impairment and the effect on speech.
- Outline nursing interventions for the child with hearing impairment, including during hospitalization.
- List the common types of visual disorders in children.
- Outline nursing interventions for the child with visual impairment, including during hospitalization.
- Outline nursing interventions for the child with retinoblastoma.
- Outline nursing interventions for the child with autism.

ELECTRONIC RESOURCES

Additional information related to the content in Chapter 42 can be found on

the companion website at evolve
http://evolve.elsevier.com/Wong/maternal/

- NCLEX Review Questions
- Case Study–Down Syndrome
- WebLinks

or the interactive student CD-ROM
Activities for Chapter 42 include the following:

- NCLEX Review Questions
- Critical Thinking Exercise–Down Syndrome
- Nursing Care Plan–The Child with Mental Retardation
- Nursing Care Plan–The Child with Hearing Impairment

COGNITIVE IMPAIRMENT

General Concepts

Cognitive impairment is a general term that encompasses any type of mental difficulty or deficiency. In this chapter the term is used synonymously with *mental retardation (MR)*. The definition of MR in children comprises three components: intellectual functioning, functional strengths and weaknesses, and age younger than 18 years at time of diagnosis. Intellectual functioning is measured by an intelligence quotient (IQ) of 70 to 75 or below. In addition, the child must demonstrate functional impairment in at least 2 of 10 different adaptive skill areas: communication, self-care, home living, social skills, leisure, health and safety, self-direction, functional academics, community use, and work (Daily, 2000; Fredericks & Williams, 1998). The development of an MR classification system by the American Association of Mental Retardation (AAMR) allows for identification of the individual's specific needs in four established dimensions of care (Box 42-1). Careful evaluation to identify the needs of individuals with MR is focused on promoting habilitation for each person. It is anticipated that the functional capabilities of children with MR will improve over time when support is provided.

Diagnosis and Classification

The diagnosis of MR is usually made after a period of suspicion, by professionals or the family (or both), that the child's developmental progress is delayed. In some cases it is confirmed at birth because of recognition of distinct syndromes, such as Down syndrome. At the other extreme, the diagnosis is made when problems such as speech delays arouse concern. In all cases, a high index of suspicion for developmental delay and behavioral signs is necessary for early diagnosis (Box 42-2); routine developmental screening can assist in early identification (see Chapter 35). Delays are typically seen in gross and fine motor and speech development, although the latter is most predictive.

BOX 42-1

Dimensions of Care for Mental Retardation

Dimension I: Intellectual functioning and adaptive skills
Dimension II: Psychologic/emotional considerations
Dimension III: Physical/health/etiology considerations
Dimension IV: Environmental considerations

BOX 42-2

Early Behavioral Signs Suggestive of Cognitive Impairment

Nonresponsiveness to contact
Poor eye contact during feeding
Diminished spontaneous activity
Decreased alertness to voice or movement
Irritability
Slow feeding

From Crocker A, Nelson R: Mental retardation. In Levine M, Carey WB, Crocker AC (eds): *Developmental-behavioral pediatrics,* ed 3, Philadelphia, 1999, WB Saunders.

Results of standardized tests are used in making the diagnosis of MR. Tests for assessing adaptive behaviors include the Vineland Social Maturity Scale and the AAMR Adaptive Behavior Scale. Informal appraisal of adaptive behavior may be made by those fully acquainted with the child (e.g., teachers, parents, other care providers). Frequently these observations lead parents to seek evaluation of the child's development.

A more useful approach for clinical application is classification based on educational potential or symptom severity. For educational purposes the term *educable mentally retarded (EMR)* corresponds to the mildly retarded group, which constitutes about 85% of all people with MR. *Trainable mentally retarded (TMR)* generally applies to children with moderate levels of cognitive impairment and accounts for about 10% of the MR population (First, McQueen, & Pincus, 1996) (Table 42-1). Although nurses may be familiar with the approximate range of IQ for classifying severity, they should refrain from using numbers as the criterion for assessing or evaluating the child's abilities, because numbers are of little value in counseling parents or training these children.

Etiology

The causes of severe MR are primarily genetic, biochemical, and infectious. Although the etiology is unknown in the majority of cases, familial, social, environmental, and organic causes may predominate. General categories of events that may lead to retardation include the following (Gurrieri et al, 1999; Kabra & Gulati, 2003):

- Infection and intoxication, such as congenital rubella, syphilis, maternal drug consumption (e.g., excessive alcohol), chronic lead ingestion, or kernicterus
- Trauma or physical agent (i.e., injury to the brain suffered during the prenatal, perinatal, or postnatal period)
- Inadequate nutrition and metabolic disorders, such as phenylketonuria
- Gross postnatal brain disease, such as neurofibromatosis and tuberous sclerosis
- Unknown prenatal influence, including cerebral and cranial malformations, such as microcephaly and hydrocephalus
- Chromosomal abnormalities resulting from radiation, viruses, chemicals, parental age, and genetic mutations
- Gestational disorders, including prematurity, low birth weight, and postmaturity
- Psychiatric disorders that have their onset during the child's developmental period up to age 18 years, such as autism
- Environmental influences, including evidence of a deprived environment associated with a history of MR among parents and siblings
- Chromosomal abnormalities, such as Down syndrome and fragile X syndrome

NURSING CARE OF CHILDREN WITH COGNITIVE IMPAIRMENT

Assessment

Nurses play a major role in identifying children with cognitive impairment. In the newborn and early infancy periods, few signs are present, with the exception of Down syndrome (see p. 1259). After this age, however, delayed developmental milestones are the major clues to MR. In addition, nurses must have a high index of suspicion for early behavior patterns that may suggest cognitive impairment (see Box 42-2) and be aware of stereotypes that may delay diagnosis, such as "retarded children have to look dumb." Parental concerns, such as delayed development compared with siblings, need to be taken seriously. All children should receive regular developmental assessment, and the nurse is often the person responsible for performing such assessments (see Chapter 35). When delays are found, the nurse must use sensitivity and discretion in revealing this finding to parents.

Nursing Diagnoses

A number of nursing diagnoses are prominent in the nursing care of the child with cognitive impairment and the child's family; other diagnoses specific to individual cases become evident. The most common nursing diagnoses are outlined in the Nursing Care Plan on p 1260.

Plan of Care and Implementation

The goals of nursing care for the child with MR and family are as follows:

1. Child will be educated using effective teaching strategies.
2. Child's optimum development will be promoted.
3. Child will learn self-care skills.
4. Family will plan for future care.
5. Child will be cared for appropriately during hospitalization.

Educate Child and Family

To teach children with cognitive impairment, it is necessary to investigate their learning abilities and deficits. This is important for the nurse who may be involved in a home care type of program or who may be caring for the child in a health care setting. The nurse who understands how these

Table 42-1

Classification of Mental Retardation

LEVEL (IQ)*	PRESCHOOL (BIRTH-5 YEARS)—MATURATION AND DEVELOPMENT	SCHOOL AGE (6-21 YEARS)—TRAINING AND EDUCATION	ADULT (21 YEARS AND OLDER)—SOCIAL AND VOCATIONAL ADEQUACY
Mild: 50-55 to approximately 70-75	Often not noticed as retarded by casual observer but is slower to walk, feed self, and talk than most children; follows same sequence in development as normal children	Can acquire practical skills and useful reading and arithmetic to a third- to sixth-grade level with special education; can be guided toward social conformity; achieves mental age of 8-12 years	Can usually achieve social and vocational skills adequate to self-maintenance; may need occasional guidance and support when under unusual social or economic stress; can adjust to marriage but not childrearing
Moderate: 35-40 to 50-55	Noticeable delays in motor development, especially in speech; responds to training in various self-help activities	Can learn simple communication, elementary health and safety habits, and simple manual skills; does not progress in functional reading or arithmetic; achieves mental age of 3-7 years	Can perform simple tasks under sheltered conditions; participates in simple recreation; travels alone in familiar places; usually incapable of self-maintenance
Severe: 20-25 to 35-40	Marked delay in motor development; little or no communication skills; may respond to training in elementary self-care (e.g., self-feeding)	Usually walks, barring specific disability; has some understanding of speech and some response; can profit from systematic habit training; achieves mental age of toddler	Can conform to daily routines and repetitive activities; needs continuing direction and supervision in protective environment
Profound: below 20-25	Gross retardation; minimum capacity for functioning in sensorimotor areas; needs total care	Obvious delays in all areas of development; shows basic emotional responses; may respond to skillful training in use of legs, hands, and jaws; needs close supervision; achieves mental age of young infant	May walk; needs complete custodial care; has primitive speech; usually benefits from regular physical activity

*Data from American Psychiatric Association: *Diagnostic and statistical manual of mental disorders,* ed 5, Washington, DC, 2000, The Association.

children learn can effectively teach them basic skills or prepare them for various health-related procedures.

Children with cognitive impairment have a marked deficit in their ability to discriminate between two or more stimuli because of difficulty in recognizing the relevance of specific cues. However, these children can learn to discriminate if the cues are presented in an exaggerated, concrete form and if all extraneous stimuli are eliminated. For example, the use of colors to emphasize visual cues or the use of singing or rhymes to stress auditory cues can help them learn. Their deficit in discrimination also implies that concrete ideas are learned much more effectively than abstract ideas. Therefore demonstration is preferable to verbal explanation, and learning should be directed toward mastering a skill rather than understanding the scientific principles underlying a procedure.

Another cognitive deficit is in short-term memory. Whereas children of average intelligence can remember several words, numbers, or directions at one time, children with MR are less able to do so. Therefore they need simple, one-step directions. Learning through a step-by-step process requires a *task analysis,* in which each task is separated into its necessary components and each step is taught completely before proceeding to the next activity.

One critical area of learning that has had a tremendous impact on education for cognitively impaired individuals is *motivation.* Programs based on the motivational principles of behavior modification, employing positive reinforcement for specific tasks or behaviors, have demonstrated marked improvement in children's ability to learn. Advances in technology have greatly aided in providing reinforcement, especially in children who are severely retarded and who may have physical disabilities that limit their range of capabilities. For example, with the use of specially designed switches, children are given control of some event in the environment, such as turning on the computer or television (Fig. 42-1). The television picture becomes reinforcement for activating the switch. Repetitive use of these switches provides an early, simplistic association with a technical device that may progress to increasingly more complex aids.

Early intervention programs have been widely promoted for children with developmental disabilities, and there is considerable evidence that these programs are valuable for cognitively impaired children. Nurses working with these fami-

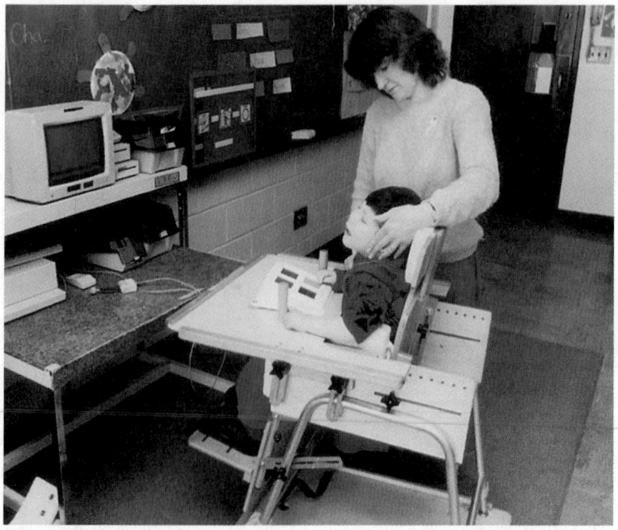

Fig. 42-1 A push panel allows a child with cognitive impairment to turn a computer on and off.

lies need to be aware of the types of programs in their community. Under Public Law 101-476, the Individuals with Disabilities Education Act of 1990, states are encouraged to provide full early intervention services and are required to provide educational opportunities for all children with disabilities from birth to 21 years of age. Services may be provided under state programs for children with special health needs (formerly Crippled Children's Program) or Head Start, or by private organizations such as the National Down Syndrome Society,* National Easter Seals,† or the Arc of the United States.‡ Parents should inquire about these programs by contacting the appropriate agencies. The child's education should begin as soon as possible, not at 5 or 6 years of age. As children grow older, their education should be directed toward vocational training that prepares them for as independent a lifestyle as possible within their scope of abilities.

Teach Child Self-Care Skills

When a child with cognitive impairment is born, parents need assistance in promoting normal developmental skills that are almost automatically learned by other children. These include self-care skills such as feeding, toileting, dressing, and grooming. Teaching these skills requires a basic knowledge of the developmental sequence in learning the skills demonstrated by children of average intelligence. For example, children with subaverage intelligence would not be expected to dress themselves as early as unaffected youngsters.

Teaching self-care skills also necessitates a working knowledge of the individual steps needed to master a skill. For example, before beginning a self-feeding program, a task analysis is performed. After a task analysis, the child is observed in a particular situation, such as eating, to determine what skills are possessed and the child's developmental readiness to learn the task. Family members are included in this process because their "readiness" is as important as the child's. Numerous self-help aids are available to facilitate independence and can be most helpful in eliminating some of the difficulties of learning, such as using a plate with suction cups to prevent accidental spills.*

Promote Child's Optimum Development

Optimum development involves more than achieving independence. It requires appropriate guidance for establishing acceptable social behavior and personal feelings of self-esteem, worth, and security. These attributes are not simply learned through a stimulation program. Rather, they must arise from the genuine love and caring that exist among family members. However, families need guidance in providing an environment that fosters optimum development. Often it is the nurse who can provide assistance in these areas of childrearing.

Another important area for promoting optimum development and self-esteem is ensuring the child's physical well-being. Any congenital defects should be repaired, such as cardiac, gastrointestinal, or orthopedic anomalies. Plastic surgery may be considered when the child's appearance may be substantially improved. Dental health is important, and orthodontic and restorative procedures can improve facial appearance immensely.

Play/Exercise

Children who are cognitively impaired have the same needs for recreation and exercise as other children. However, because of the child's slower development, parents may be less aware of the need to provide such activities. Therefore the nurse guides parents toward selection of suitable play and exercise activities (Fig. 42-2). Because play has been discussed for children in each age group in earlier chapters, only the exceptions are presented here.

The type of play is based on the child's developmental age, although the need for sensorimotor play may be prolonged for several years. Parents should use every opportunity to expose the child to as many different sounds, sights, and sensations as possible. Appropriate play includes musical mobiles, stuffed toys, water play, floating toys, a rocking chair or horse, a swing, bells, and rattles. The child should be taken on outings, such as trips to the grocery store or shopping center; other people should be encouraged to visit in the home; and the child should be related to directly, such as by cuddling, holding, rocking, talking to the child in the *en face* (face-to-face) position, and giving "rides" on the parents' shoulders.

Toys are selected for their recreational and educational value. For example, a large inflatable beach ball is a good water toy; it encourages interactive play and can be used to

---

*Information on early intervention programs in each state is available from the National Down Syndrome Society, 666 Broadway, 8th Floor, New York, NY 10012-2317; phone: 800-221-4602; fax: 212-979-2873; e-mail: info@ndss.org; Web site: www.ndss.org.

†230 W. Monroe, Suite 1800, Chicago, IL 60606-4802; phone: 800-221-6827; TTY: 312-726-4258; fax: 312-726-1494; e-mail: info@easterseals.org; Web site: www.easter-seals.com.

‡1010 Wayne Ave., Suite 650, Silver Spring, MD 20910; phone: 301-565-3842; fax: 301-565-5342; e-mail: Info@thearc.org; Web site: www.thearc.org.

*A resource for a variety of types of self-help equipment is Sammons/Preston/Rolyan, An AbilityOne Corporation, 4 Sammons Court, Bolingbrook, IL 60440; phone: 800-323-5547 (United States), 800-665-9200 (Canada); fax: 800-547-4333; Web site: www.sammonspreston.com.

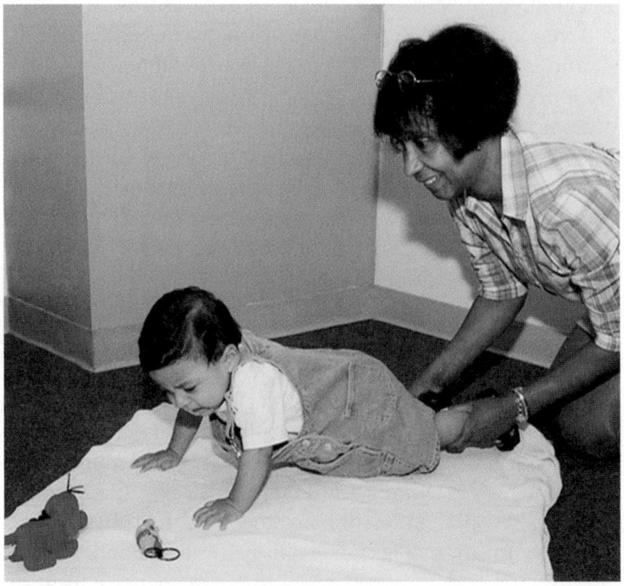

Fig. 42-2 Placing an attractive object outside of the child's reach encourages crawling movements. (Courtesy James DeLeon, Texas Children's Hospital.)

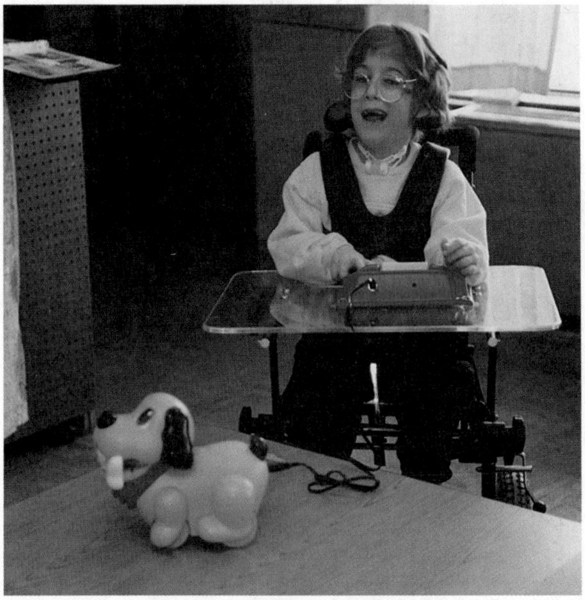

Fig. 42-3 A manual switch allows a child with cognitive impairment to play with a battery-operated toy.

learn motor skills, such as balance, rocking, kicking, and throwing. A doll with removable clothes and different types of closures can help the child learn dressing skills. Musical toys that mimic animal sounds or respond with social phrases are excellent ways of encouraging speech. Toys should be simple in design so that the child can learn to manipulate them without help. For children with severe cognitive and physical impairment, electronic switches can be used to allow them to operate toys (Fig. 42-3).

Suitable activities for physical activity are based on the child's size, coordination, physical fitness and maturity, motivation, and health (Fig. 42-4). Some children may have physical problems that prevent them from participating in certain sports, such as atlantoaxial instability in children with Down syndrome (see p. 1259). These children often have greater success in individual and dual sports than in team sports and enjoy themselves most with children of the same developmental level. The Special Olympics, Inc.,* provides these children with a unique competitive opportunity.

Safety is a major consideration in selecting recreational and exercise activities. For example, toys that may be appropriate developmentally may present dangers to a child who is strong enough to break them or use them incorrectly.

Communication

Verbal skills are typically delayed more than other physical skills. Speech requires hearing and interpretation *(receptive skills)* and facial muscle coordination *(expressive skills)*. Because both types of skills may be impaired, these children

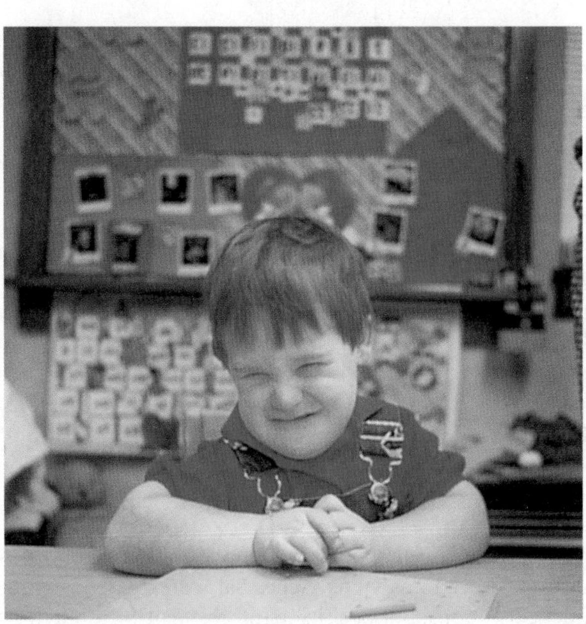

Fig. 42-4 Play activities for children with cognitive impairments need to be appropriate for their abilities.

need frequent audiometric testing and should be fitted with hearing aids if this is indicated. In addition, they may need help in learning to control their facial muscles. For example, some children may need tongue exercises to correct the tongue thrust or gentle reminders to keep the lips closed.

Nonverbal communication may be appropriate for some of these children, and various devices are available. For the child without associated physical disabilities, a talking picture board is helpful. For children with physical limitations, several adaptations or types of communication devices are available to facilitate selection of the appropriate picture or word (Fig. 42-5). Some children may be taught sign language or *Blissymbols*—a highly stylized system of graphic symbols that represent words, ideas, and concepts. Although the sym-

*1325 G Street NW, Suite 500, Washington, DC 20005; phone: 800-700-8585 or 202-628-3630; fax: 202-824-0200; Web site: www.specialolympics.org. (Website includes listing of state offices.) In Canada: Canadian Special Olympics, 60 St. Clair Ave. E., Suite 700, Toronto, Ontario M4T 2N5; phone: 416-927-9050; fax: 416-927-8475; e-mail: info@specialolympics.ca; Web site: www.cso.on.ca.

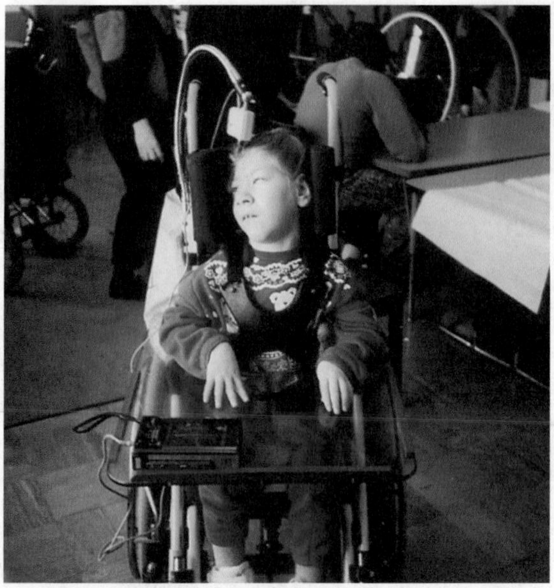

Fig. 42-5 A child with cognitive and physical impairments can play a tape recorder by moving a device near her head.

bols require education to learn their meaning, no reading skill is needed. The symbols are usually arranged on a board, and the person points or uses some type of selector to convey a message.

Discipline

Discipline must begin early. Limit-setting measures need to be simple, consistently applied, and appropriate for the child's mental age. Control measures are based primarily on teaching a specific behavior rather than on understanding the reasons behind it. Stressing moral lessons is of little value to a child who lacks the cognitive skills to learn from self-criticism or from a lesson based on previous wrongdoing. Behavior modification, especially reinforcement of desired actions, and time-out are appropriate forms of behavior control.

Socialization

Acquiring social skills is a complex task, as is learning self-care procedures. Active rehearsal with role-playing and practice sessions and positive reinforcement for desired behavior have been the most successful approaches. Parents should be encouraged early to teach their child socially acceptable behavior: waving goodbye, saying "hello" and "thank you," responding to his or her name, greeting visitors but not being overly affectionate, and sitting modestly. The teaching of socially acceptable sexual behavior is especially important to minimize sexual exploitation. Parents also need to expose the child to strangers so that he or she can practice manners, because there is no automatic transfer of learning from one situation to another.

Dressing and grooming are also important aspects of socialization. A child who is dressed in age-appropriate clothing and is well groomed is much more likely to be accepted and to develop good self-esteem. Clothes should be clean, up-to-date, and well fitted. Many attractive outfits can be adapted with self-adhering fasteners and elastic openings to facilitate self-dressing.

Children of all ages need peer relationships, and these children are no exception. As soon as possible, parents should enroll the child in appropriate preschool programs. Not only do these programs provide education and training, but they also offer an opportunity for social experiences among the children. As children grow older, they should have peer experiences similar to those of other children, including group outings, sports, and organized activities, such as Boy Scouts, Girl Scouts, or Special Olympics. They are encouraged to form a close relationship with a best friend of the same developmental age (American Academy of Pediatrics, Committee on Children and Disabilities, 2000).

Sexuality

Adolescence may be a particularly difficult time for the family, especially in terms of the child's sexual behavior, possibility of pregnancy, future plans to marry, and ability to be independent. Frequently, little anticipatory guidance has been offered parents to prepare the child for physical and sexual maturation. The nurse can help in this area by providing parents with information about sexuality education that is geared to the child's developmental level. For example, the adolescent female needs a *simple* explanation of menstruation and instructions on personal hygiene during the menstrual cycle.

These adolescents also need practical sexual information regarding anatomy, physical development, and conception.* Because of their easy persuasion and lack of judgment, they need a well-defined, concrete code of conduct. The subtleties of social sexual behavior are less beneficial than specific instructions for handling certain situations. For example, a girl should be firmly told never to go alone anywhere with any person she does not know well. A boy should be warned about intimate advances from other males. To protect him or her from abusive sexual activities, parents must closely observe their teenager's activities and associates.

The question of contraceptive protection for these adolescents is often a parental concern. Permanent contraception through sterilization is a special dilemma because of moral and ethical questions, as well as psychologic effects on the adolescent. State laws vary; some allow no sterilization, and others permit review of sterilization requests.

Parents of these adolescents are often very concerned about the advisability of marriage between two individuals with significant cognitive impairment. There is no conclusive answer; each situation must be judged individually. In some instances marriage is possible, but parenthood is usually not desirable because of the complexity of childrearing and the potential problem of perpetuating mental deficiency. The nurse should discuss this topic with parents and with the prospective couple, stressing suitable living accommodations and contraceptive methods to prevent pregnancy. If children are conceived, these parents require specialized assistance in learning to meet the needs of their offspring.

---

*Sources of information on sexuality and conception are the Arcwww.thearc.org and the Planned Parenthood Federation of America, 434 West 33rd St., New York, NY 10001; phone: 212-541-7800 or 800-829-7732; fax: 212-245-1845; e-mail: communications@ppfa.org; Web site: www.plannedparenthood.org.

Help Family Adjust to Future Care

Not all families are able to cope with home care of their affected child, especially one who is severely or profoundly retarded or with multiple disabilities. Older parents may not be able to assume care responsibilities after they reach retirement or older age. For these parents, the decision regarding residential placement is a difficult one, and the availability of such facilities varies widely. The nurse working with a family should help them investigate and evaluate various programs, in addition to assisting them in their adjustment to the decision for placement.

Care for Child during Hospitalization

Caring for the child during hospitalization can be a special challenge. Frequently, nurses are unfamiliar with children who are cognitively impaired, and they may cope with their feelings of insecurity and fear by ignoring or isolating the child. Not only is this approach nonsupportive, but it may also be destructive for the child's sense of self-esteem and optimum development, and it may hamper the parents' ability to cope with the stress of the experience. One method that successfully avoids this nontherapeutic approach is the use of the mutual participation model in planning the child's care. Parents are encouraged to stay with their child but should not be made to feel as if the responsibility is totally theirs.

When the child is admitted, a detailed history is taken (see Chapter 44), especially in terms of all self-care activity. During the interview the child's developmental age is assessed. It is best to avoid directly asking about IQ levels, because this may make the parents uncomfortable and often tells little about the child's actual abilities. Questions are approached positively. For example, rather than asking, "Is your child toilet trained yet?" the nurse may state, "Tell me about your child's toileting habits." The assessment should also focus on any special devices the child uses, effective measures of limit setting, unusual or favorite routines, and any behaviors that may require intervention. For example, if the parent states that the child engages in self-stimulatory or self-injurious activities, the nurse inquires about events that precipitate them and techniques that the parents use to manage them (Bosch & Ringdahl, 2001).

The child's functional level of eating and playing, ability to express needs verbally, progress in toilet training, and relationship with objects, toys, and other children are also assessed. The child is encouraged to be as independent as possible in the hospital.

Procedures are explained to the child through methods of communication that are at the appropriate cognitive level. Generally, explanations should be simple, short, and concrete, emphasizing what the child will experience *physically.* Demonstration, either through actual practice or with visual aids, is always preferable to verbal explanation. The nurse repeats instructions often and evaluates the child's understanding by asking questions such as "What will it feel like?" "What will the doctor look like?" "Show me how you must lie," or "Where will the dressing be?" Parents are included in preprocedural teaching for their own learning and to help the nurse learn effective methods of communicating with the child.

Assist in Measures to Prevent Retardation

Besides having a responsibility to families with a child with MR, nurses also need to be involved in programs aimed at preventing MR. Many of the familial, social, and environmental factors known to cause mild retardation are preventable. Counseling and education can reduce or eliminate such factors (e.g., poor nutrition, cigarette smoking, and chemical abuse, which increase the risk of prematurity and intrauterine growth retardation). Consequently, the major interventions are directed at improving maternal health and educating women regarding the dangers of chemicals, including alcohol during pregnancy and lead during childhood. Other preventive strategies that play an important role include adequate prenatal care; optimum medical care of high risk newborns; rubella immunization; genetic counseling and prenatal screening, especially in terms of Down syndrome or fragile X syndrome; use of folic acid supplements during the childbearing years and during pregnancy to prevent neural tube defects; newborn screening for treatable inborn errors of metabolism, such as congenital hypothyroidism, phenylketonuria, and galactosemia; and early appropriate therapies and rehabilitation services for children with developmental disabilities.

Evaluation

The effectiveness of nursing interventions is determined by continual reassessment and evaluation of care based on the following observational guidelines:

1. Observe techniques used to teach child and child's success in ability to learn; inquire if child is enrolled in early stimulation program.
2. Interview family regarding provision of appropriate socialization, discipline, and play for child; observe child's ability to communicate with others; if possible, interview child regarding feelings of self-worth.
3. Observe those activities of daily living that child can completely or partially perform.
4. Interview family members regarding any plans for future care and their awareness of community services.
5. Check patient record for evidence of nursing admission history, especially for self-help activities; observe parents' involvement in child's care; observe social interaction of child and family with other patients.
6. Investigate community programs aimed at preventing retardation and inquire as to nursing involvement in these efforts.

The *expected outcomes* are described in the Nursing Care Plan.

Nursing Care Plan: Child with Mental Retardation

Down Syndrome

Down syndrome is the most common chromosomal abnormality of a generalized syndrome, occurring in 1 in every 800 to 1000 live births (Grech, 2001; National Down Syndrome Society, 2003c). It occurs slightly more often in whites than in blacks, although the incidence is unchanged in various socioeconomic classes.

Etiology

The cause of Down syndrome is not known, but evidence from cytogenetic and epidemiologic studies supports the concept of multiple causality. Approximately 95%

Nursing Care Plan

THE CHILD WITH MENTAL RETARDATION

NURSING DIAGNOSIS: Altered growth and development related to impaired cognitive functioning

EXPECTED OUTCOME

Child exhibits evidence of appropriate growth and developmental behaviors for age and abilities.

NURSING INTERVENTIONS/RATIONALES

Involve child and family in early developmental stimulation and intervention (refer to available programs) *to maximize developmental potential.*

Assess child's developmental progress at regular intervals and note changes in functional abilities *to revise intervention as needed.*

Help family to set realistic goals and determine child's readiness for specific developmental tasks; encourage and reinforce learning of self-care skills *to facilitate development.*

Emphasize to family that this child has needs that are the same as those of other children (e.g., play, discipline, interaction, approval), and encourage interventions that help child to meet these needs at appropriate times and in appropriate ways (e.g., teaching socially acceptable behavior; encouraging appropriate grooming, hygiene, and dress; providing opportunities for peer interactions such as school, after-school activities, special events; reinforcing positive behaviors and setting limits) *to optimize development and socialization.*

As child matures, counsel child and parents on issues such as sexuality, sexual behavior, birth control, marriage and family, and vocational interests and opportunities *to assist in management of ongoing developmental issues.*

NURSING DIAGNOSIS: Altered family processes related to having a child with mental retardation

EXPECTED OUTCOME

Family members demonstrate acceptance of child.

NURSING INTERVENTIONS/*RATIONALES*

Inform family of infant problem as soon as possible after birth *to decrease anxiety of unknown.*

Provide opportunity for family to absorb and adjust to diagnosis (e.g., repeat information *to allow time for family to hear and understand;* encourage expression of concerns, fears, and feelings about diagnosis and potential impact *to facilitate adjustment;* identify support systems *to provide resources for coping*).

Provide family with written materials about child's condition *for long-term reference;* introduce family to other families with similarly affected children *to enhance support mechanisms.*

Demonstrate acceptance of child through own behavior *to serve as role model for family;* encourage family to participate in care *to form emotional attachments.*

Explore family members' reaction to the child; assist them to achieve a realistic view of child's abilities and limitations; encourage family in attempts to promote child growth and development; have family emphasize what child can do; explore ways for family to include child in family activities *to help family increase abilities to cope with and incorporate child into family structure.*

Arrange for and participate in family conferences *to provide forum for communication, mutual goal setting, and effective strategizing.*

Assess family resources and coping abilities when discussing care options on discharge *so that family can make realistic choices on the basis of their specific circumstances.*

If family opts for home care, assist them in developing a plan of care for the child and teach them the skills needed in carrying out that plan *to provide optimum care in which the entire family is involved.*

Identify additional resource systems (e.g., relatives, friends, church, health care services, community programs) and strategize with family about making good use of these systems *to develop broad base of support.*

Provide a system of ongoing follow-up and evaluation *to ensure long-term adaptation to challenges presented to family functioning by a child with mental retardation.*

As child ages, help parents explore decisions about future care options that assist in dealing with behavioral management problems, parent debility, or retirement issues *to facilitate long-term care.*

Make referrals to appropriate social agencies *for needed assistance, support, and continuity of care.*

of all cases of Down syndrome are attributable to an extra chromosome 21 (group G), thus the name *nonfamilial trisomy 21* (Grech, 2001; National Down Syndrome Society, 2003d). Although children with trisomy 21 are born to parents of all ages, there is a statistically greater risk in older women, particularly those older than 35 years of age. For example, in women 35 years of age the chance of conceiving a child with Down syndrome is about 1 in 400 live births, but in women age 40 it is about 1 in 110. However, the majority (about 80%) of infants with Down syndrome are born to women younger than age 35. In less than 5% of cases, paternal age is a factor, especially in men 55 years of age or older (Hixon et al, 1998; National Down Syndrome Society, 2003c).

About 3% to 4% of the cases may be caused by *translocation* of chromosomes 15 and 21 or 22. This type of genetic aberration is usually hereditary and is not associated with advanced parental age. From 1% to 2% of affected persons demonstrate *mosaicism,* which refers to cells with both normal and abnormal chromosomes. The degree of physical and cognitive impairment is related to the percentage of cells with the abnormal chromosome makeup.

Diagnostic Evaluation

Down syndrome can usually be diagnosed by the clinical manifestations alone (Box 42-3 and Fig. 42-6), but a chromosome analysis should be done to confirm the genetic abnormality.

Several physical problems are associated with Down syndrome. Many of these children have congenital heart malformations, the most common being septal defects. Respiratory tract infections are very prevalent and, when combined with cardiac anomalies, are the chief cause of death, partic-

BOX 42-3

Clinical Manifestations of Down Syndrome

Head
*Separated sagittal suture
Brachycephaly
Skull rounded and small
Flat occiput
Enlarged anterior fontanel
Sparse hair (variable)

Face
Flat profile

Eyes
*Oblique palpebral fissures (upward, outward slant)
Inner epicanthal folds
Speckling of iris (Brushfield spots)
Short, sparse eyelashes
Blepharitis

Nose
*Small
*Depressed nasal bridge (saddle nose)

Ears
Small
Short pinna (vertical ear length)
Overlapping upper helices
Narrow canals

Mouth
*High, arched, narrow palate
Small osseous orbit
Protruding tongue; may be fissured at lip and furrowed on surface
Hypoplastic mandible
Downward curve (especially noted when crying)
Mouth kept open

Teeth
Delayed eruption
Alignment abnormalities common
Microdontia
Periodontal disease

Chest
Shortened rib cage
Twelfth rib anomalies
Pectus excavatum/carinatum

Neck
*Skin excess; lax skin
Short and broad

Abdomen
Protruding
Muscles lax and flabby
Diastasis recti
Umbilical hernia

Genitalia
Small penis
Cryptorchidism
Bulbous vulva

Hands
Broad, short
Stubby fingers
Incurved little finger (clinodactyly)
Transverse palmar crease
Characteristic dermal ridge patterns
Distally located axial triradius
Increased ulnar loops on fingers

Feet
*Wide space between big and second toes
*Plantar crease between big and second toes
Broad, stubby, short

Musculoskeletal System
Short stature
*Hyperflexibility
*Muscle weakness
Hypotonia
Atlantoaxial instability

Skin
Dry, cracked, and frequent fissuring
Cutis marmorata (mottling)

Other
Reduced birth weight

*Most common findings in modified chart (Pueschel, 1999).

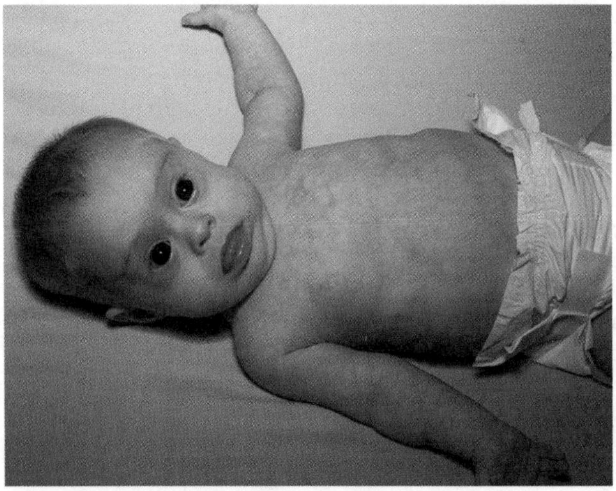

Fig. 42-6 Down syndrome in infant. Note small, square head with upward slant to the eyes, flat nasal bridge, protruding tongue, mottled skin, and hypotonia.

ularly during the first year of life. Hypotonicity of chest and abdominal muscles and dysfunction of the immune system probably predispose to the development of respiratory tract infection. Other physical problems include thyroid dysfunction, especially congenital hypothyroidism, and an increased incidence of leukemia.

Therapeutic Management

Although no cure exists for Down syndrome, a number of therapies are advocated, such as surgery to correct serious congenital anomalies and possibly the physical stigmata, although the latter is controversial. These children also benefit from regular medical care. Evaluation of sight and hearing is essential, and treatment of otitis media is required to prevent auditory loss, which can influence cognitive function. Periodic testing of thyroid function is recommended, especially if growth is severely delayed. Children participating in sports that may involve stress on the head and neck, such as gymnastics, diving, butterfly stroke in swimming, high jump, and soccer, should be evaluated radiologically for *atlantoaxial instability.* Symptoms of the disorder include neck pain, weakness, and torticollis. Affected children are at risk for spinal cord compression.

NURSE ALERT Report immediately any child with the following signs of spinal cord compression:
- Persistent neck pain
- Loss of established motor skills and bladder or bowel control
- Changes in sensation ■

Prognosis

Life expectancy for those with Down syndrome has improved in recent years but remains lower than for the general population. More than 80% survive to age 55 years and be-

Critical Thinking Exercise: Down Syndrome

yond. As the prognosis continues to improve for these individuals, it will be important to provide for their long-term health care, social, and leisure needs (National Down Syndrome Society, 2003b; Van Riper, 2003).

Nursing Care Management

Support Family at Time of Diagnosis

Because of the unique physical characteristics, the infant with Down syndrome is usually diagnosed at birth, and parents should be informed of the diagnosis at this time. Parents usually prefer that both of them be present during the informing interview so that they can support one another emotionally. They appreciate receiving reading material about the syndrome* and being referred to others for help or advice, such as parent groups or professional counseling.

After parents are aware of the diagnosis, they are confronted with the crisis of losing their perfect or dream child and grieving for and accepting their reality child. Consequently, the parents' responses to the child may greatly influence decisions regarding future care. Whereas some families willingly want to take the child home, others consider immediate residential placement. The nurse must carefully answer questions regarding developmental potential. Institutionalization is no longer an option. For families unable or unready to choose taking the newborn home, specialized foster care and adoption are other options (Critical Thinking Exercise).

Assist Family in Preventing Physical Problems

Many of the physical characteristics of Down syndrome present nursing problems. The hypotonicity of muscles and hyperextensibility of joints complicate positioning. The limp, flaccid extremities resemble the posture of a rag doll; as a result, holding the infant is difficult and cumbersome. Sometimes parents perceive this lack of molding to their bodies as evidence of inadequate parenting. The extended body position promotes heat loss because more surface area is exposed to the environment. Parents are encouraged to swaddle or wrap the infant tightly in a blanket before picking up the child to provide security and warmth. The nurse also discusses with parents their feelings concerning attachment to the child, emphasizing that the child's lack of clinging or molding is a physical characteristic, not a sign of detachment or rejection.

Decreased muscle tone compromises respiratory expansion. In addition, the underdeveloped nasal bone causes a chronic problem of inadequate drainage of mucus. The constant stuffy nose forces the child to breathe by mouth, which dries the oropharyngeal membranes, increasing the susceptibility to upper respiratory tract infections. Measures to lessen these problems include clearing the nose with a bulb-type syringe, rinsing the mouth with water after feedings, increasing fluid intake, and using a cool-mist vaporizer to keep the mucous membranes moist and the secretions liquefied. Other helpful measures include changing the child's position frequently; performing postural drainage with percussion, if necessary; practicing good handwashing; and properly disposing of soiled articles such as tissues. If antibiotics are ordered, the importance of completing the full course of therapy for successful eradication of the infection and prevention of growth of resistant organisms is stressed.

Inadequate drainage resulting in pooling of mucus in the nose also interferes with feeding. Because the child breathes by mouth, sucking for any length of time is difficult. When eating solids, the child may gag on the food because of mucus in the oropharynx. Parents are advised to clear the nose before each feeding; give small, frequent feedings; and allow opportunities for rest during mealtime.

The protruding tongue also interferes with feeding, especially of solid foods. Parents need to know that the tongue thrust is not an indication of refusal to feed, but a physiologic response. Parents are advised to use a small but long, straight-handled spoon to push the food toward the back and side of the mouth. If food is thrust out, it is refed.

Dietary intake needs supervision. Decreased muscle tone affects gastric motility, predisposing the child to constipation. Dietary measures such as increased fiber and fluid promote evacuation. The child's eating habits may need careful scrutiny to prevent obesity. Height and weight measurements should be obtained on a serial basis, especially during infancy. Because these children's growth is slower than that of the general pediatric population's trends, special growth charts developed for these children should be used (American Academy of Pediatrics, Committee on Genetics, 2001; Cohen, 1999).

Assist in Prenatal Diagnosis and Genetic Counseling

Prenatal diagnosis of Down syndrome is possible through chorionic villi sampling and amniocentesis, because chromosome analysis of fetal cells can detect the presence of trisomy or translocation. However, analysis will not identify sporadic cases in young women when there is no indication for prenatal testing. Testing for low maternal serum alpha-

??? Critical Thinking Exercise

DIAGNOSIS OF DOWN SYNDROME

The parents of Melissa, a newborn diagnosed as having Down syndrome, ask the nurse, "What are we supposed to do with her?" They further state that they already have three other children at home.

1. Evidence—Is there sufficient evidence to draw conclusions about the parents' concerns regarding their newborn daughter?
2. Assumptions—Describe an underlying assumption about each of the following:
   a. Newborn diagnosed with Down syndrome
   b. Parental care of a newborn with Down syndrome
   c. Newborn with Down syndrome and older siblings
3. What priorities for the nursing response should be established?
4. Does the evidence support your nursing intervention?
5. What alternative perspectives might you have?

*Sources of information include the Arc (see footnote, p. 1258); the American Association on Mental Retardation, 444 N. Capitol St. NW, Suite 846, Washington, DC 20001-1512; phone: 800-424-3688 or 202-387-1968; fax: 202-387-2193; Web site: www.aamr.org; the National Down Syndrome Society, 666 Broadway, 8th Floor, New York, NY 10012-2317; phone: 800-221-4602; fax: 212-979-2873; e-mail: info@ndss.org; Web site: www.ndss.org; and the National Down Syndrome Congress, 1370 Center Drive, Suite 102, Atlanta, GA 30338; phone: 800-232-6372 or 770-604-9500; Web site: www.ndsccenter.org.

evolve CASE STUDY: DOWN SYNDROME

fetoprotein, high chorionic gonadotropin, low unconjugated estriol levels, and maternal serum fetal cells marker may identify an affected fetus in women, who can then undergo amniocentesis (National Down Syndrome Society, 2003a; Yang et al, 2003).

Prenatal testing and genetic counseling should be offered to women of advanced maternal age or who have a family history of the disorder. If prenatal testing indicates that the fetus is affected, the nurse must allow the parents to express their feelings concerning elective abortion and support their decision to terminate or proceed with the pregnancy.

Fragile X Syndrome

Fragile X syndrome is the most common inherited cause of MR and the second most common genetic cause of MR after Down syndrome. It has been described in all ethnic groups and races; the incidence of affected males is 1 in 3600; the incidence of affected females is 1 in 4000 to 1 in 6000; and the incidence of carrier females is 1 in 246 to 1 in 468 (Crawford, 2001; National Fragile X Foundation, 2002).

The syndrome is caused by an abnormal gene on the lower end of the long arm of the X chromosome. Chromosome analysis may demonstrate a *fragile site* (a region that fails to condense during mitosis and is characterized by a nonstaining gap or narrowing) in the cells of affected males and females and in carrier females. This fragile site has been determined to be caused by a gene mutation that results in excessive repeats of nucleotide in a specific deoxyribonucleic acid (DNA) segment of the X chromosome. The number of repeats in a normal individual is between 6 and 50. An individual with 50 to 200 base-pair repeats is said to have a *premutation* and is therefore a carrier. When passed from a parent to a child, these base-pair repeats can expand from 200 or more, which is termed a *full mutation.* This expansion occurs only when a carrier mother passes the mutation to her offspring; it does not occur when a carrier father passes the mutation to his daughters.

The inheritance pattern has been termed *X-linked dominant with reduced penetrance.* It is in distinct contrast to the classic X-linked recessive pattern in which all carrier females are normal, all affected males have symptoms of the disorder, and no males are carriers. Consequently, genetic counseling of affected families is more complex than that for families with a classic X-linked disorder, such as hemophilia. Prenatal diagnosis of the fragile X gene mutation is now possible with direct DNA testing in a family with an established history, using amniocentesis or chorionic villi sampling (Centers for Disease Control and Prevention, 2002; Welch & Williams, 1999). Both affected sexes are fertile and therefore capable of transmitting the fragile X disorder.

Clinical Manifestations

The classic trend of physical findings in adult men with fragile X syndrome consists of a long face with a prominent jaw (prognathism); large, protruding ears; and large testes (macro-orchidism). In prepubertal children, however, these features may be less obvious, and behavioral manifestations may initially suggest the diagnosis (Box 42-4). In carrier females the clinical manifestations are extremely varied.

BOX 42-4

Clinical Manifestations of Fragile X Syndrome

Physical Features

Long, wide, and/or protruding ears
Long, narrow face with prominent jaw
In postpubertal males, enlarged testicles
Long palpebral fissures
High, arched palate
Strabismus
Increased head circumference
Mitral valve prolapse/aortic root dilation
Hypotonia
Hyperextensible finger joints
Transpalmar crease
Pes planus (flat feet)

Behavioral Features

Mild to severe cognitive impairment (occasionally, normal intelligence with learning disabilities)
Speech delay; speech may be rapid, with stuttering and repetition of words
Short attention span, hyperactivity
Mouthing beyond expected age for behavior
Hypersensitivity to taste, sounds, touch
Intolerance to change in routine
Autistic-like behaviors
May exhibit aggressive behavior

Therapeutic Management

No cure exists for fragile X syndrome. Medical treatment may include the use of serotonin agents such as carbamazepine (Tegretol) or fluoxetine (Prozac) to control violent temper outbursts and the use of central nervous system (CNS) stimulants or clonidine (Catapres) to improve attention span and decrease hyperactivity. The use of folic acid, which affects the metabolism of CNS transmitters, is controversial.

All affected children require early speech and language therapy, occupational therapy, and special education assistance. Without appropriate intervention, a progressive decline in IQ can occur.

Prognosis

Individuals with fragile X syndrome are expected to live a normal life span. Their cognitive impairment may be improved by behavioral and educational interventions.

Nursing Considerations

Because cognitive impairment is a fairly consistent finding in individuals with fragile X syndrome, the care given to these families is the same as that for any child with MR. Because the disorder is hereditary, genetic counseling is necessary to inform parents and siblings of the risks of transmission. In addition, any male or female with unexplained or nonspecific mental impairment should be referred for genetic testing and, if needed, counseling. Families with a member affected by the disorder should be referred to the National Fragile X Foundation.*

*PO Box 190488-0488, San Francisco, CA 94119; phone: 800-688-8765 or 925-938-9300; fax: 925-938-9315; e-mail: natlfx@fragilex.org; Web site: www.fragilex.org.

SENSORY IMPAIRMENT

Hearing Impairment

Hearing impairment is one of the most common disabilities in the United States. An estimated 2 in 1000 infants are born with permanent hearing loss (Applebaum, 1999). For infants admitted to the neonatal intensive care unit, the incidence rises sharply to approximately 2 to 4 per 100 neonates (American Academy of Pediatrics, Task Force on Newborn and Infant Hearing, 1999; Cunningham & Cox, 2003). There are about 1 million children with hearing impairment ranging in age from birth to 21 years in the United States, and almost one third of these children have other disabilities, such as visual or cognitive deficits.

Definition and Classification

Hearing impairment is a general term indicating disability that may range in severity from mild to profound and includes the subsets of deaf and hard-of-hearing. *Deaf* refers to a person whose hearing disability precludes successful processing of linguistic information through audition, with or without a hearing aid. *Hard-of-hearing* refers to a person who, generally with the use of a hearing aid, has residual hearing sufficient to enable successful processing of linguistic information through audition. Other terms, such as *deaf and dumb, mute,* or *deaf-mute,* are unacceptable. Hearing-impaired persons are not dumb and, if mute, have no physical speech defect other than that caused by the inability to hear.

Hearing defects may be classified according to etiology, pathology, or symptom severity. Each is important in terms of treatment, possible prevention, and rehabilitation.

Etiology

Hearing loss may be caused by a number of prenatal and postnatal conditions. These include a family history of childhood hearing impairment, anatomic malformations of the head or neck, low birth weight, severe perinatal asphyxia, perinatal infection (cytomegalovirus, rubella, herpes, syphilis, toxoplasmosis, bacterial meningitis), chronic ear infection, cerebral palsy, Down syndrome, or administration of ototoxic drugs (Berrettini et al, 1999; Holte, 2003).

In addition, high risk neonates who are surviving formerly fatal prenatal or perinatal conditions may be susceptible to hearing loss from the disorder or its treatment. For example, sensorineural hearing loss may be a result of continuous humming noises or high noise levels associated with incubators, oxygen hoods, or intensive care units, especially when combined with the use of potentially ototoxic antibiotics.

Environmental noise is a special concern. Sounds loud enough to damage sensitive hair cells of the inner ear can produce irreversible hearing loss. Very loud, brief noise, such as gunfire, can cause immediate, severe, and permanent loss of hearing. Longer exposure to less intense but still hazardous sounds, such as music, can also produce hearing loss (Roizen, 1999; Segal et al, 2003). The exact sound level that produces hearing loss is unknown.

Pathology

Disorders of hearing are divided according to the location of the defect. *Conductive* or *middle-ear hearing loss* results from interference of transmission of sound to the middle ear. It is the most common of all types of hearing loss and most frequently is a result of recurrent serous otitis media. Conductive hearing impairment involves mainly interference with loudness of sound.

Sensorineural hearing loss, also called *perceptive* or *nerve deafness,* involves damage to the inner ear structures or the auditory nerve (or both). The most common causes are congenital defects of inner ear structures or consequences of acquired conditions, such as kernicterus, infection, administration of ototoxic drugs, or exposure to excessive noise. Sensorineural hearing loss results in distortion of sound and problems in discrimination. Although the child hears some of everything going on around him or her, the sounds are distorted, severely affecting discrimination and comprehension.

Mixed conductive-sensorineural hearing loss results from interference with transmission of sound in the middle ear and along neural pathways. It frequently results from recurrent otitis media and its complications.

Central auditory imperception includes all hearing losses that do not demonstrate defects in the conductive or sensorineural structures. They are usually divided into organic or functional losses. In the *organic type* of central auditory imperception, the defect involves the reception of auditory stimuli along the central pathways and the expression of the message into meaningful communication. Examples are *aphasia,* the inability to express ideas in any form, either written or verbally; *agnosia,* the inability to interpret sound correctly; and *dysacusis,* difficulty in processing details or discrimination among sounds.

In the *functional type* of hearing loss, no organic lesion exists to explain a central auditory loss. Examples of functional hearing loss are conversion hysteria (an unconscious withdrawal from hearing to block remembrance of a traumatic event), infantile autism, and childhood schizophrenia.

Symptom Severity

Hearing impairment is expressed in terms of a *decibel (dB),* a unit of loudness (Table 42-2); it is measured at various frequencies, such as 500, 1000, and 2000 cycles/second,

Table 42-2

Intensity of Sounds Expressed in Decibels

DECIBELS	REPRESENTATIVE SOUND
0	Softest sound normal ear can hear
10	Heartbeat, rustling of leaves
20	Whisper at 1.8 meter (5 feet)
30-45	Normal conversation
60	Noise in average restaurant
70-80	Street noises
80	Loud radio in home
90-100	Train
120	Thunder, rock music
140	Thunder, rock music
>140	Pain threshold

Table 42-3

Classification of Hearing Loss Based on Symptom Severity

HEARING LEVEL (DB)	EFFECT
Slight: 16-25	Has difficulty hearing faint or (hard-of-hearing) distant speech Usually is unaware of hearing difficulty Likely to achieve in school but may have problems No speech defects
Mild to moderate: 26-55	May have speech difficulties Understands face-to-face conversational speech at 3-5 feet
Moderately severe: 56-70 (hard-of-hearing)	Unable to understand conversational speech unless loud Considerable difficulty with group or classroom discussion Requires special speech training
Severe: 71-90 (deaf)	May hear a loud voice if nearby May be able to identify loud environmental noises Can distinguish vowels but not most consonants Requires speech training
Profound: 91 (deaf)	May hear only loud sounds Requires extensive speech training

the critical listening speech range. Hearing impairment can be classified according to *hearing threshold level* (the measurement of an individual's hearing threshold by means of an audiometer) and the degree of symptom severity as it affects speech (Table 42-3). These classifications offer only general guidelines regarding the effect of the impairment on any individual child, because children differ greatly in their ability to use residual hearing.

Therapeutic Management

Conductive Hearing Loss

Treatment of hearing loss depends on the cause and type of hearing impairment. Many conductive hearing defects respond to medical or surgical treatment, such as antibiotic therapy for acute otitis media or insertion of tympanostomy tubes for chronic otitis media. When the conductive loss is permanent, hearing can be improved with the use of a hearing aid to amplify sound.

The nurse should be familiar with the types, basic care, and handling of hearing aids, especially when the child is hospitalized.* Types of aids include those worn in or behind the ear, models incorporated into an eyeglass frame, and types worn on the body with a wire connection to the ear (Fig. 42-7). One of the most common problems with a hearing aid is *acoustic feedback,* an annoying whistling sound usually caused by improper fit of the ear mold. Sometimes the whistling may be at a frequency that the child cannot hear but that is annoying to others. In this case, if children are old enough, they are told of the noise and asked to readjust the aid.

NURSE ALERT To reduce or eliminate whistling from a hearing aid, try reinserting the aid, making certain that no hair is caught between the ear mold and the canal; cleaning the ear mold or ear; or lowering the volume of the aid. ■

As children grow older, they may be self-conscious about the device. Every effort is made to make the aid inconspicuous, such as an appropriate hairstyle to cover behind-the-ear or in-the-ear models, attractive frames for glasses, and placement of the on-the-body type where it is not seen, such as under a blouse or sweater. Children are given responsibility for the care of the device as soon as they are able, because fostering independence is a primary goal of rehabilitation.

NURSE ALERT When parents express concern about their child's hearing and speech development, refer the child for a hearing evaluation. Absence of well-formed syllables ("da," "na," "yaya") by 11 months of age should result in immediate referral. ■

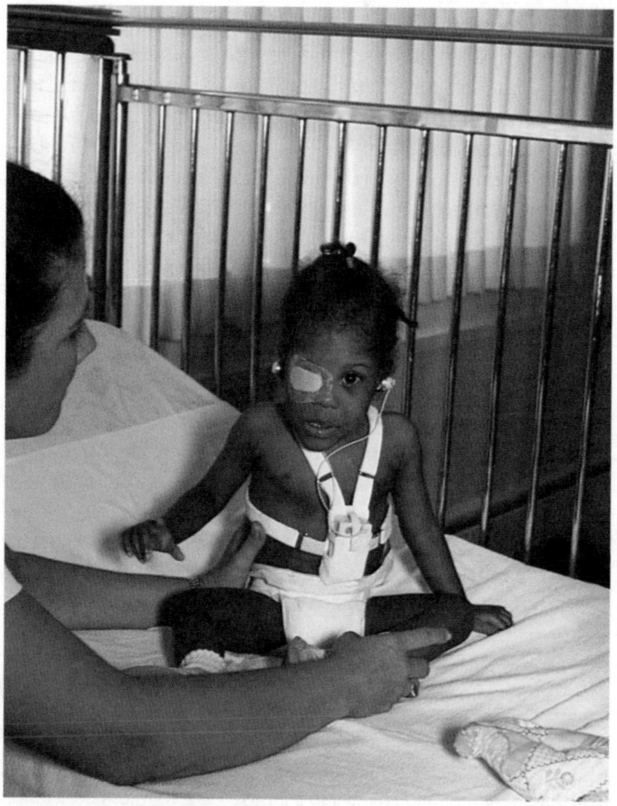

Fig. 42-7 On-the-body hearing aids are convenient for young children, such as this child with severe bilateral hearing loss. Note eye patching for strabismus.

*Information about hearing aids is available from the International Hearing Society, 16880 Middlebelt Rd., Suite 4, Livonia, MI 48154; phone: 800-521-5247; fax: 734-522-0200.

Sensorineural Hearing Loss

Treatment for sensorineural hearing loss is much less satisfactory. Because the defect is not one of intensity of sound, hearing aids are of less value in this type of defect. The use of *cochlear implants** (a surgically implanted prosthetic device) provides a sensation of hearing for individuals who have severe or profound hearing loss (Slattery & Fayad, 1999; Waltzman, Roland Jr., & Cohen, 2002). Children with sensorineural hearing loss have lost or damaged some or all of their hair cells or auditory nerve fibers. Often these children cannot benefit from conventional hearing aids because they only amplify sound that cannot be processed by a damaged inner ear. A cochlear implant bypasses the hair cells to directly stimulate surviving auditory nerve fibers so that they can send signals to the brain. These signals can be interpreted by the brain to produce sound and sensations (Allegretti, 2002).

Multichanneled implants are now available. This more sophisticated device stimulates the auditory nerve at a number of locations with differently processed signals. This type of stimulation gives a person the opportunity to use the pitch information present in speech signals, allowing the person to better understand speech.

The trend is toward early use of cochlear implants, usually by 18 months of age, to give the child maximum opportunity to develop listening, language, and speaking skills.

Nursing Care Management

Assessment

Assessment of children for hearing impairment is a critical nursing responsibility. Early detection of hearing loss, preferably within the first 3 to 6 months of life, is essential to improve the language and educational outcomes of those with hearing impairments (Holte, 2003; Yoshinaga-Itano et al, 1998). To accomplish this goal, the current recommendation is universal newborn hearing screening before discharge from the newborn nursery (American Academy of Pediatrics, Task Force on Newborn and Infant Hearing, 1999; Cunningham & Cox, 2003). This discussion focuses on developmental and behavioral indexes associated with hearing impairment. Auditory testing is presented in Chapter 35.

Infancy

At birth the nurse can observe the neonate's response to auditory stimuli, as evidenced by the startle reflex, head turning, eye blinking, and cessation of body movement. The infant may vary in the intensity of the response, depending on the state of alertness. However, a consistent absence of a reaction should lead to suspicion of hearing loss. Box 42-5 summarizes other clinical manifestations of hearing impairment in the infant.

*Cochlear Implant Association, Inc., 5335 Wisconsin Ave. NW, Suite 440, Washington, DC 20015; phone: 202-895-2781; fax: 202-895-2782; e-mail: info@cici.org; Web site: www.cici.org. Hearing Enrichment Language Program of the Hough Ear Institute, 3434 N.W. 56th St., Oklahoma City, OK 73112; phone: 405-945-7186; fax: 405-945-7188; e-mail: joanna.smith@integris-health.com; Web site: www.oraldeafed.org. Auditory-Verbal International, Inc. (AVI), 2121 Eisenhower Ave., Ste. 402, Alexandria, VA 22314; phone: 703-739-1049; TDD: 703-739-0874; fax: 703-739-0395.

BOX 42-5

Clinical Manifestations of Hearing Impairment

Infants

Lack of startle or blink reflex to a loud sound
Failure to be awakened by loud environmental noises
Failure to localize a source of sound by 6 months of age
Absence of babble or inflections in voice by age 7 months
General indifference to sound
Lack of response to the spoken word; failure to follow verbal directions
Response to loud noises as opposed to the voice

Children

Use of gestures rather than verbalization to express desires, especially after age 15 months
Failure to develop intelligible speech by age 24 months
Monotone quality, unintelligible speech, lessened laughter
Vocal play, head banging, or foot stamping for vibratory sensation
Yelling or screeching to express pleasure, annoyance (tantrums), or need
Asking to have statements repeated or answering them incorrectly
Responding more to facial expression and gestures than verbal explanation
Avoidance of social interaction; often puzzled and unhappy in such situations; prefer to play alone
Inquiring, sometimes confused facial expression
Suspicious alertness, sometimes interpreted as paranoia, alternating with cooperation
Frequently stubborn because of lack of comprehension
Irritable at not making themselves understood
Shy, timid, and withdrawn
Often appear "dreamy," "in a world of their own," or exhibit inattentiveness

Childhood

The child who is profoundly deaf is much more likely to be diagnosed during infancy than the less severely affected one. If the defect is not detected during early childhood, it likely will become evident during entry into school, when the child has difficulty in learning. Unfortunately, some of these children are mistakenly placed in special classes for students with learning disabilities or MR. Therefore it is essential that the nurse suspect a hearing impairment in any child who demonstrates the behaviors listed in Box 42-5.

Of primary importance is the effect of hearing impairment on speech development. A child with a mild conductive hearing loss may speak fairly clearly but in a loud, monotone voice. A child with a sensorineural defect usually has difficulty in articulation. For example, inability to hear higher frequencies may result in the word *spoon* being pronounced "poon." Children with articulation problems need to have their hearing tested.

NURSE ALERT Stress to parents the importance of storing batteries for hearing aids in a safe location and teaching children not to remove the battery from the hearing aid (or supervising young children to prevent them from doing so). Ingestion of batteries is most often of those from hearing aids, including the child's own aid. ■

Nursing Diagnoses

A number of nursing diagnoses are prominent in the nursing care of the child with hearing impairment and the child's family; other diagnoses specific to individual cases become evident. The most common nursing diagnoses are outlined in the Nursing Care Plan on p. 1270.

Plan of Care and Implementation

The goals of nursing care for the child with hearing impairment and the child's family are as follows:

1. Child will achieve optimum development through enhancement of the communication process and socialization.
2. Child and family will receive support.
3. Child will receive appropriate care during hospitalization.

Promote the Communication Process

The nurse's initial role in rehabilitation is to encourage the family to participate in an auditory training program.* Rehabilitation training consists of learning appropriate methods to improve communication, such as lipreading, sign language, speech language, and therapy.

Lipreading

Even though the child may become an expert at lipreading, only about 40% of the spoken word is understood, and less if the speaker has an accent, a mustache, or a beard. Exaggerating pronunciation or speaking in an altered rhythm further lessens comprehension. Parents can help the child understand the spoken word by using the suggestions in the Guidelines box. The child learns to supplement the spoken word with sensitivity to visual cues, primarily body language and facial expression (e.g., tightening the lips, muscle tension, eye contact).

Cued Speech

This method of communication is an adjunct to straight lipreading. It uses hand signals to help the child with a hearing impairment distinguish between words that look alike when formed by the lips (e.g., "mat," "bat"). It is most often used by children with hearing impairments who are using speech rather than those who are nonverbal.

Sign Language

Sign language, such as *American Sign Language (ASL)* or *British Sign Language (BSL),* is a visual gestural language that uses hand signals that roughly correspond to specific words and concepts in the English language. Family members are encouraged to learn signing because using or watching hands requires much less concentration than lipreading or talking. Also, a symbol method enables some children to learn more and to learn faster.

*Home training correspondence programs are sponsored by the John T. Tracy Clinic, 806 W. Adams Blvd., Los Angeles, CA 90007; phone: 800-522-4582; TTY: 213-747-2924; fax: 213-749-1651; Web site: www.johntracyclinic.org. Other sources of information on several aspects of hearing loss and on the International Parents' Organization are the Alexander Graham Bell Association for the Deaf, 3417 Volta Place NW, Washington, DC 20007; phone: 202-337-5220, TTY: 202-337-5221; fax: 202-337-8314; e-mail: agbell@aol.com; Web site: www.agbell.org; and Canadian Hearing Society, 271 Spadina Rd., Toronto, Ontario M5R 2V3; phone: 416-964-9595; TTY: 416-964-9595; fax: 416-928-2525; e-mail: info@chs.ca; Web site: www.chs.ca.

Guidelines

FACILITATING LIPREADING

- Attract child's attention before speaking; use light touch to signal speaker's presence.
- Stand close to child.
- Face child directly or move to a 45-degree angle.
- Stand still; do not walk back and forth or turn away to point or look elsewhere.
- Establish eye contact and show interest.
- Speak at eye level and with good lighting on speaker's face.
- Be certain nothing interferes with speech patterns, such as chewing food or gum.
- Speak clearly and at a slow and even rate.
- Use facial expression to assist in conveying messages.
- Keep sentences short.
- Rephrase message if child does not understand the words.

Speech Language Therapy

The most formidable task in the education of a child who is profoundly hearing impaired is learning to speak. Speech is learned through a multisensory approach, using visual, tactile, kinesthetic, and auditory stimulation. Parents are encouraged to participate fully in the learning process.

Additional Aids

Everyday activities present problems for older children with hearing impairment. For example, they may not be able to hear the telephone, doorbell, or alarm clock. Several commercial devices are available to help them adjust to these dilemmas. Flashing lights can be attached to a telephone or doorbell to signal its ringing. Trained hearing ear dogs can provide great assistance because they alert the person to sounds, such as someone approaching, a moving car, a signal to wake up, or a child's cry. Special *teletypewriters (TTY)* or *telecommunications devices for the deaf (TDD)* help people with impaired hearing communicate with each other over the telephone; the typed message is conveyed via the telephone lines and displayed on a small screen.*

Any audiovisual medium presents dilemmas for these children, who can see the picture but cannot hear the message. However, with *closed captioning* a special decoding device is attached to the television, and the audio portion of a program is translated into subtitles that appear on the screen.†

As children learn to compensate for their lack of hearing, they become extremely perceptive to visual and vibratory changes. Children often know when another person wants to talk to them because the person will walk close by but not pass. They learn to be alert to other people approaching them by seeing their shadows or feeling the vibrations of their footsteps. They are acutely aware of facial expressions and may comprehend the unspoken word more quickly than the spoken word.

*Directory listings stating "TDD or TTY only" before a phone number indicate that regular telephone use is not possible; "TDD or TTY and voice" indicates that both TDD/TTY users and speaking/hearing people can use the telephone number.

†Additional information is available from the National Captioning Institute, Inc., 1900 Gallows Rd., Suite 3000, Vienna, VA 22182; phone: 703-917-7600; fax: 703-917-9878; Web site: www.ncicap.org.

Socialization

Because socialization is extremely important to the child's development, the nurse discusses with the family methods of fostering social contact. If children attend a special school for the deaf, they are able to socialize with peers in that setting. Classmates become a potential source of close friendships because they communicate more easily among themselves. Parents are encouraged to promote these relationships whenever possible.

Children with a hearing impairment may need special help with school or social activities. For those children wearing hearing aids, background noise should be kept to a minimum. Because many of these children are able to attend regular classes, the teacher may need assistance in adapting methods of teaching for the child's benefit. The school nurse is often in an optimum position to emphasize methods of facilitated communication, such as lipreading (see Guidelines box). Because group projects and audiovisual teaching aids may hinder the child's learning, these educational methods should be carefully evaluated.

Support Child and Family

After the diagnosis of hearing impairment is made, parents need extensive support to adjust to the shock of learning about their child's disability and an opportunity to realize the extent of the hearing loss. If the hearing loss occurs during childhood, the child also requires sensitive, supportive care during the long and often difficult adjustment to this sensory loss. Early rehabilitation is one of the best strategies for fostering adjustment. However, progress in learning communication may not always coincide with emotional adjustment. Depression or anger is common, and such feelings are a normal part of the grieving process.

Care for Child during Hospitalization

The needs of the hospitalized child with impaired hearing are the same as those of any other child, but the disability presents special challenges to the nurse (Critical Thinking Exercise). For example, verbal explanations must be supplemented with tactile and visual aids, such as books or actual demonstration and practice. Children's understanding of the explanation needs to be constantly reassessed. If their verbal skills are poorly developed, they can answer questions through drawing, writing, or gesturing. For example, if the nurse is attempting to clarify where a spinal tap is done, the child is asked to point to where the procedure will be done on the body. Because these children often need more time to grasp the full meaning of an explanation, the nurse needs to be patient, allowing ample time for understanding.

When communicating with the child, the nurse should use the same principles as those outlined for facilitating lipreading. Ideally, nurses without foreign accents should be assigned to the child. The child's hearing aid is checked to ensure that it is working properly. If it is necessary to awaken the child at night, the nurse gently shakes the child or turns on the hearing aid before arousing the child. The nurse always makes sure that the child can see him or her before any procedures, even routine ones such as changing a diaper or regulating an infusion, are performed. It is important to remember that the child may not be aware of one's presence until alerted through visual or tactile cues.

Ideally, parents are encouraged to room with the child. However, it must be conveyed to them that this is not to serve as a convenience to the nurse but as a benefit to the child. Although the parents' aid can be enlisted in familiarizing the child with the hospital and explaining procedures, the nurse also talks directly to the youngster, encouraging expression of feelings about the experience. If there is difficulty in understanding the child's speech, an effort is made to become familiar with his or her pronunciation of words. Parents often can be helpful by explaining the child's usual speech habits. Nonverbal communication devices that employ pictures or words that the child can point to are also available (see p. 1267). Such boards can also be made by drawing pictures or writing the words of common needs on cardboard, such as *parent, food, water,* or *toilet.*

The nurse has a special role as child advocate with the child and is in a strategic position to alert other health team members and other patients to the child's special needs regarding communication. For example, the nurse should accompany other practitioners on visits to the child's room to ensure that they speak to the child and that the child understands what is said. Caregivers sometimes forget that the child has the abilities to perceive and learn despite a hearing loss, and consequently they communicate only with the parents. As a result, the child's needs and feelings remain unrecognized and unmet.

Because children with impaired hearing may have difficulty in forming social relationships with other children, the child is introduced to roommates and encouraged to engage in play activities. The hospital setting can provide growth-promoting opportunities for social relationships. With the assistance of a child-life specialist, the child can learn new recreational activities, experiment with group games, and engage in therapeutic play. The use of puppets, dollhouses, role-playing with dress-up clothes, building with a hammer and nails, finger painting, playing with syringes, and water

??? Critical Thinking Exercise

HEARING IMPAIRMENT

Four-year-old Jason has a severe congenital hearing impairment. Jason has been admitted to the outpatient surgery postanesthesia care unit (PACU) after a herniorrhaphy and after regional block. As he emerges from anesthesia, he becomes more and more agitated.

1. Evidence—Is there sufficient evidence to draw conclusions about Jason's postsurgical increasing agitation?
2. Assumptions—Describe an underlying assumption about each of the following:
   a. Severe congenital hearing impairment in a preschool child
   b. Preschooler with severe congenital hearing impairment and awakening in the PACU after surgery
   c. Preschooler with severe congenital hearing impairment and awakening from herniorrhaphy and postregional block
3. What priorities for nursing care should be established for Jason?
4. Does the evidence support your nursing intervention?
5. What alternative perspectives might you have?

play can help the child express feelings that previously were suppressed.

Assist in Measures to Prevent Hearing Impairment

A primary nursing role is prevention of hearing loss. Because the most common cause of impaired hearing is chronic otitis media, it is essential that appropriate measures be instituted to prevent infections or treat existing infections. Children with histories of ear or respiratory infections or any other condition known to increase the risk of hearing impairment should receive periodic auditory testing.

To prevent the causes of hearing loss that begin prenatally and perinatally, pregnant women need counseling regarding the necessity of early prenatal care, including genetic counseling for known familial disorders; avoidance of all ototoxic drugs, especially during the first trimester; tests to rule out syphilis, rubella, or blood incompatibility; medical management of maternal diabetes; strict control of alcohol intake; and adequate dietary intake. The necessity of routine immunization during childhood to eliminate the possibility of acquired sensorineural loss from rubella, mumps, or measles (encephalitis) is stressed.

Exposure to excessive noise pollution is a well-established cause of sensorineural hearing loss. The nurse should routinely assess the possibility of environmental noise pollution and advise children and parents of the potential danger. When individuals engage in activities associated with high-intensity noise, such as flying model airplanes, target shooting, or snowmobiling, they should wear ear protection such as earmuffs or earplugs (not ordinary dry cotton). However, any protection is better than none. Even common household equipment, such as lawn mowers, power vacuum cleaners, and cordless telephones, can be hazardous.

NURSE ALERT Suspect hazardous noise if the listener experiences (1) difficulty in communication while hearing the sound, (2) ringing in the ears (tinnitus) after exposure to the sound, or (3) muffled hearing after leaving the sound. ■

EVALUATION

The effectiveness of nursing interventions is determined by continual reassessment and evaluation of care based on the following observational guidelines:

1. Observe techniques used to communicate with child; inquire if child is enrolled in an auditory training program; inquire about socialization opportunities for child (i.e., who are child's friends, what are his or her extracurricular activities).
2. Interview family members regarding their adjustment to the sensory impairment; observe family members' relationship with child; interview child regarding feelings about the sensory impairment and its effect on activities of daily living (especially important if impairment is recent).
3. Observe types of preparation and communication used to prepare child for hospitalization or procedures; observe parents' involvement in child's care; observe interaction of child and family with other patients.
4. Investigate community programs aimed at preventing or detecting hearing loss and inquire as to nursing involvement in these efforts.

The *expected outcomes* are described in the Nursing Care Plan on p. 1270.

NURSING CARE PLAN: CHILD WITH HEARING IMPAIRMENT

Visual Impairment

Visual impairment is a common problem during childhood. In the United States the prevalence of blindness and serious visual impairment in the pediatric population is estimated at 30 to 64 children per 100,000 population. Another 100 children per 100,000 have less serious impairment (Davidson, 1999). The nurse's role is clearly one of assessment, prevention, referral, and, in some instances, rehabilitation.

Definition and Classification

Visual impairment is a general term that refers to visual loss that cannot be corrected with regular prescription lenses. However, more useful definitions for classifying visual impairments include the following. *School vision* (also known as *partially sighted*) refers to visual acuity between 20/70 and 20/200. The child should be able to obtain an education in the usual public school system with the use of normal-sized print. Near vision is almost always better than distance vision. *Legal blindness,* visual acuity of 20/200 or less and/or a visual field of 20 degrees or less in the better eye, is useful only as a legal definition, not as a medical diagnosis. It allows special considerations with regard to taxes, entrance into special schools, eligibility for aid, and other benefits.

Etiology

Visual impairment can be caused by a number of genetic and prenatal or postnatal conditions. These include perinatal infections (herpes, chlamydia, gonococci, rubella, syphilis, toxoplasmosis), retinopathy of prematurity, trauma, postnatal infections (meningitis), and disorders such as sickle cell disease, juvenile rheumatoid arthritis, Tay-Sachs disease, albinism, and retinoblastoma. In many instances, such as with refractive errors, the cause of the defect is unknown.

Refractive errors are the most common types of visual disorders in children. The term *refraction* means bending and refers to the bending of light rays as they pass through the lens of the eye. Normally, light rays enter the lens and fall directly on the retina. However, in refractive disorders the light rays either fall in front of the retina *(myopia)* or beyond it *(hyperopia)*. Other eye problems, such as strabismus, may or may not include refractive errors, but they are very important because, if untreated, they result in blindness from amblyopia. These, along with other, less common visual disorders, are summarized in Box 42-6. In addition to these disorders, other visual problems can be a result of infection or trauma.

Trauma

Trauma is a common cause of blindness in children. Injuries to the eyeball and adnexa (supporting or accessory structures, such as eyelids, conjunctiva, or lacrimal glands) can be classified as penetrating or nonpenetrating. *Penetrating wounds* are most often a result of sharp instruments, such as sticks, knives, or scissors; propulsive objects, such as

Nursing Care Plan

THE CHILD WITH HEARING IMPAIRMENT

NURSING DIAGNOSIS: Impaired verbal communication related to conductive and/or sensorineural hearing loss

EXPECTED OUTCOME

Child is able to communicate with others in the environment.

NURSING INTERVENTIONS/RATIONALES

Explore family's knowledge of hearing loss and of the speech development process *to assess baseline for interventions.*

Explain the relationship between the loss of hearing and speech; discuss how speech develops; discuss alternative methods of communication (gestures, drawing, play, sign language, lipreading) *to increase family's understanding of child's speech impairment and how to cope with the loss.*

Encourage family to pursue appropriate communication interventions (e.g., oral speech classes, signing classes) for their child and family members as dictated by the child's degree of hearing loss and the child's developmental level *to promote successful communication.*

Refer family to appropriate community resources such as American Organization for the Education of the Hearing Impaired and family support groups *to aid in coping and adaptation.*

NURSING DIAGNOSIS: Sensory/perceptual alterations (auditory) related to conductive and/or sensorineural hearing loss

EXPECTED OUTCOMES

Child exhibits uses of appropriate mechanisms to compensate for hearing loss (e.g., hearing aid, cochlear implants); child is oriented to and displays interest in external environment.

NURSING INTERVENTIONS/*RATIONALES*

If appropriate, explore mechanisms *that may enhance hearing abilities* (e.g., hearing aids, visual cues in environment, amplifier devices on telephone, doorbells, cochlear implant surgery).

If hearing aid is used, teach child and family how to use the aid, how to replace batteries, and how to prevent young children from ingesting/aspirating batteries *to promote optimum benefit and safety.*

Use tactile and visual stimuli with child *to enhance sensory stimulation through other modalities.*

Observe child's interaction with and interest in external environment *to assess orientation and function.*

Provide reality orientation *to counteract confusion and disorientation.*

NURSING DIAGNOSIS: Risk for altered growth and development related to hearing loss and impaired communication

EXPECTED OUTCOME

Child exhibits evidence of appropriate growth and development behaviors for age and abilities.

NURSING INTERVENTIONS/*RATIONALES*

If appropriate, explore mechanisms *that may enhance hearing abilities* (e.g., hearing aids, visual cues in environment, amplifier devices on telephone, doorbells, cochlear implant surgery).

Involve child and family in early stimulation and intervention exercises (refer to available programs) *to enhance development of remaining senses and maximize overall development.*

Assess child's developmental progress at regular intervals and note changes in functional abilities *to revise interventions as needed.*

Help family to set realistic goals and determine child's readiness for specific developmental tasks; encourage and reinforce learning of self-care skills *to facilitate development.*

Emphasize to family that this child has needs that are the same as those of other children (e.g., play, discipline, interaction, approval), and encourage interventions that help child to meet these needs (e.g., selecting toys that maximize visual and tactile resources, using close-captioned television, reinforcing positive behaviors and setting limits, participating in group and peer activities, giving positive feedback for successes and good efforts) *to optimize development and socialization.*

Work with school (teachers, nurse, classmates) *to enhance understanding and ensure meeting of educational needs.*

NURSING DIAGNOSIS: Altered family processes related to a diagnosis of deafness of a child

EXPECTED OUTCOME

Family members demonstrate acceptance of child.

NURSING INTERVENTIONS/*RATIONALES*

Provide opportunity for family to absorb and adjust to diagnosis (e.g., repeat information *to allow time for family to hear and understand;* encourage expression of concerns, fears, and feelings about diagnosis and potential impact *to facilitate adjustment;* identify support systems *to provide resources for coping).*

Provide family written materials about child's condition *for long-term reference;* introduce family to other families with similarly affected children *to enhance support mechanisms.*

Explore family members' reaction to the child; assist them to achieve a realistic view of child's abilities and limitations; encourage family in attempts to promote child growth and development; have family emphasize what child can do; explore ways for family to include child in family activities; encourage all family members to learn alternative communication measures *to help family increase abilities to cope with and incorporate child into family structure.*

Arrange for and participate in family conferences *to provide forum for communication, mutual goal setting, and effective strategizing.*

firecrackers, guns, bows and arrows, or slingshots; or a powerful contusion by a blunt object, which may occur during a fight or from a serious car accident. *Nonpenetrating injuries* may be a result of foreign objects in the eyes, lacerations, a blow from a blunt object such as a ball (baseball, softball, basketball, racquet sports) or fist, or thermal or chemical burns.

Treatment is aimed at preventing further ocular damage and is primarily the responsibility of the ophthalmologist. It involves adequate examination of the injured eye (with the child sedated or anesthetized in severe injuries); appropriate immediate intervention, such as removal of the foreign body or suturing of the laceration; and prevention of complications, such as administration of antibiotics or steroids and

BOX 42-6

Types of Visual Impairment

Refractive Errors

Myopia

Nearsightedness—Ability to see objects clearly at close range but not at a distance

Pathophysiology

Results from eyeball that is too long, causing image to fall in front of retina

Clinical Manifestations

Rubs eyes excessively
Tilts head or thrusts head forward
Has difficulty in reading or doing other close work
Holds books close to eyes
Writes or colors with head close to table
Clumsy; walks into objects
Blinks more than usual or is irritable when doing close work
Is unable to see objects clearly
Does poorly in school, especially in subjects that require demonstration, such as arithmetic
Dizziness
Headache
Nausea after close work

Treatment

Corrected with biconcave lenses that focus rays on retina
May be corrected with laser surgery

Hyperopia

Farsightedness—Ability to see objects at a distance

Pathophysiology

Results from eyeball that is too short, causing image to focus beyond retina

Clinical Manifestations

Because of accommodative ability, child can usually see objects at all ranges
Most children are normally hyperopic until about 7 years of age

Treatment

If correction is required, use convex lenses to focus rays on retina
May be corrected with laser surgery

Astigmatism

Unequal curvatures in refractive apparatus

Pathophysiology

Results from unequal curvatures in cornea or lens that cause light rays to bend in different directions

Clinical Manifestations

Depends on severity of refractive error in each eye
May have clinical manifestations of myopia

Treatment

Corrected with special lenses that compensate for refractive errors
May be corrected with laser surgery

Anisometropia

Different refractive strength in each eye

Pathophysiology

May develop amblyopia as weaker eye is used less

Clinical Manifestations

Depends on severity of refractive error in each eye
May have clinical manifestations of myopia

Treatment

Treated with corrective lenses, preferably contact lenses, to improve vision in each eye so they work as a unit
May be corrected with laser surgery

Amblyopia

Lazy eye—Reduced visual acuity in one eye

Pathophysiology

Results when one eye does not receive sufficient stimulation
Each retina receives different images, resulting in diplopia (double vision)
Brain accommodates by suppressing less intense image
Visual cortex eventually does not respond to visual stimulation, with resultant loss of vision in that eye

Clinical Manifestations

Poor vision in affected eye

Treatment

Preventable if treatment of primary visual defect, such as anisometropia or strabismus, begins before 6 years of age

Strabismus

"Squint" or cross-eye—Malalignment of eyes
Esotropia—Inward deviation of eye
Exotropia—Outward deviation of eye

Pathophysiology

May result from muscle imbalance or paralysis, poor vision, or congenital defect
Because visual axes are not parallel, brain receives two images, and amblyopia can result

Clinical Manifestations

Squints eyelids together or frowns
Has difficulty in focusing from one distance to another
Inaccurate judgment in picking up objects
Unable to see print or moving objects clearly
Closes one eye to see
Tilts head to one side
If combined with refractive errors, may see any of the manifestations listed for refractive errors
Diplopia
Photophobia
Dizziness
Headache
Cross-eye

Treatment

Treatment depends on cause of strabismus
May involve occlusion therapy (patching stronger eye) or surgery to increase visual stimulation to weaker eye
Early diagnosis is essential to prevent vision loss

Cataracts

Opacity of crystalline lens

Pathophysiology

Prevents light rays from entering eye and refracting on retina

Clinical Manifestations

Gradually less able to see objects clearly
May lose peripheral vision
Nystagmus (with complete blindness)
Gray opacities of lens
Strabismus
Absence of red reflex

Continued

BOX 42-6

Types of Visual Impairment—cont'd

Cataracts—cont'd

Treatment

Requires surgery to remove cloudy lens and replace lens (intraocular lens implant, removable contact lens, prescription glasses)
Must be treated early to prevent blindness from amblyopia

Glaucoma

Increased intraocular pressure

Pathophysiology

Congenital type results from defective development of some component related to flow of aqueous humor
Increased pressure on optic nerve causes eventual atrophy and blindness

Clinical Manifestations

Mostly seen in acquired types—loses peripheral vision
May bump into objects not directly in front
Sees halos around objects
May complain of mild pain or discomfort (severe pain, nausea, or vomiting if sudden rise in pressure)
Redness
Excessive tearing (epiphora)
Photophobia
Spasmodic winking (blepharospasm)
Corneal haziness
Enlargement of eyeball (buphthalmos)

Treatment

Requires surgical treatment (goniotomy) to open outflow tracts
May require more than one procedure

complete bed rest to allow the eye to heal and blood to reabsorb (Emergency box). The prognosis varies according to the type of injury. It is usually guarded in all cases of penetrating wounds because of the high risk of serious complications.

Infections

Infections of the adnexa and structures of the eyeball or globe may occur in children. The most common eye infection is *conjunctivitis*. Treatment is usually with ophthalmic antibiotics. Severe infections may require systemic antibiotic therapy. Steroids are used cautiously because they exacerbate viral infections such as herpes simplex, increasing the risk of damage to the involved structures.

Nursing Care Management

Assessment

Assessment of children for visual impairment is a critical nursing responsibility. Discovery of a visual impairment as early as possible is essential to prevent social, physical, and psychologic damage to the child. Assessment involves (1) identifying those children who by virtue of their history are at risk, (2) observing for behaviors that indicate a vision loss, and (3) screening all children for visual acuity and signs of other ocular disorders such as strabismus. This discussion focuses on clinical manifestations of various types of visual

Emergency

EYE INJURIES

Foreign Object

Examine eye for presence of a foreign body (evert upper lid to examine upper eye).
Remove a freely movable object with pointed corner of gauze pad lightly moistened with water.
Do not irrigate eye or attempt to remove a penetrating object (see following section).
Caution child against rubbing eye.

Chemical Burns

Irrigate eye copiously with tap water for 20 minutes.
Evert upper lid to flush thoroughly.
Hold child's head with eye under tap of running lukewarm water.
Take to emergency department.
Have child rest with eyes closed.
Keep room darkened.

Ultraviolet Burns

If skin is burned, patch both eyes (make sure lids are completely closed); secure dressing with Kling bandages wrapped around head rather than tape.
Have child rest with eyes closed.
Refer to an ophthalmologist.

Hematoma ("Black Eye")

Use a flashlight to check for gross *hyphema* (hemorrhage into anterior chamber; visible fluid meniscus across iris; more easily seen in light-colored than in brown eyes).
Apply ice for first 24 hours to reduce swelling if no hyphema is present.
Refer to an ophthalmologist immediately if hyphema is present.
Have child rest with eyes closed.

Penetrating Injuries

Take child to emergency department.
Never remove an object that has penetrated eye.
Follow strict aseptic technique in examining eye.
Observe for the following:
- Aqueous or vitreous leaks (fluid leaking from point of penetration)
- Hyphema
- Shape and equality of pupils, reaction to light
- Prolapsed iris (not perfectly circular)

Apply a Fox shield if available (not a regular eye patch) and apply patch over unaffected eye to prevent bilateral movement.
Maintain bed rest with child in 30-degree semi-Fowler position.
Caution child against rubbing eye.

problems (see Box 42-6). Vision testing is discussed in Chapter 35.

Infancy

At birth the nurse should observe the neonate's response to visual stimuli, such as following a light or object and cessation of body movement. The infant may vary in the intensity of the response, depending on the state of alertness.

Of special importance in detecting visual impairment during infancy are the parents' concerns regarding visual responsiveness in their child. Their concerns, such as lack of eye contact from the infant, must be taken seriously. During infancy the child should be tested for strabismus. Lack of binocularity after 4 months of age is considered abnormal and must be treated to prevent amblyopia.

NURSE ALERT Suspect blindness if the infant does not react to light and in children of any age if the parents express concern. ■

Childhood

Because the most common visual impairment during childhood is refractive errors, testing for visual acuity is essential. The school nurse usually assumes major responsibility for vision testing in schoolchildren. Besides refractive errors, the nurse should be aware of signs and symptoms that indicate other ocular problems. If a referral is made to the family requesting further eye testing, the nurse is responsible for follow-up concerning the recommendation.

Nursing Diagnoses

A number of nursing diagnoses are prominent in the nursing care of the child with visual impairment and the child's family (Box 42-7); other diagnoses specific to individual cases become evident.

Plan of Care and Implementation

The goals of care for the child with visual impairment and the child's family are as follows:

1. Child and family will receive support and education.
2. Parent-child attachment will develop.
3. Child will achieve optimum development.
4. Child will receive appropriate care during hospitalization.

Support Child and Family

The shock of learning that their child is blind or partially sighted is an immense crisis for families. Of all types of disabilities, many people fear loss of sight the most. Vision is involved in almost every activity of daily living. Parents need support during the initial phase of learning about the diagnosis and help to gain a realistic understanding of their child's abilities. The family is encouraged to investigate appropriate stimulation and educational programs for their child as soon as possible. Sources of information include state commissions for the blind, local schools for the blind, the American Foundation for the Blind,* National Federation of the Blind,† National Association for Parents of the Visually Impaired, Inc.,‡ National Association for Visually Handicapped,§ and American Council of the Blind.||

When blindness is not congenital but acquired, newly blind children need much support to help them adjust to the disability. They are usually frightened and confused by the sudden or progressive loss of sight and benefit from an environment that provides security and familiarity.

Promote Parent-Child Attachment

A crucial time in the life of blind infants is when they and their parents are getting acquainted with each other. Pleasurable patterns of interaction between the infant and parents may be lacking if there is not enough reciprocity. For example, if the parent gazes fondly at the infant's face and seeks eye contact but the infant fails to respond because he or she cannot see the parent, a troubled cycle of responses may occur. The nurse can help parents learn to look for other cues that indicate the infant is responding to them, such as whether the eyelids blink; whether the activity level accelerates or slows; whether respiratory patterns change, such as faster or slower breathing, when the parents come near; and whether the infant makes throaty sounds when they speak to the infant. In time parents learn that the infant has unique ways of relating to them. They are encouraged to show affection using nonvisual methods, such as talking or reading, cuddling, and walking the child.

Promote Child's Optimum Development

Promoting the child's optimum development requires rehabilitation in a number of important areas. These include learning self-help skills and appropriate communication techniques to become independent. Although nurses may not be directly involved in such programs, they can provide direction and guidance to families regarding the availability of programs and the need to promote these activities in their child.

BOX 42-7

Nursing Diagnoses: The Child with Vision Impairment

Altered family processes related to diagnosis of vision impairment in child

Altered growth and development related to sensory/perceptual alterations (visual)

Risk for injury related to environmental hazards, noncompliance with therapeutic plan

*11 Pennsylvania Plaza, Suite 300, New York, NY 10001; phone: 800-232-5463, 212-502-7600; TTY: 212-502-7662; fax: 212-502-7777; e-mail: afbinfo@afb.net; Web site: www.afb.org.

†1800 Johnson St., Baltimore, MD 21230; phone: 410-659-9314; fax: 410-685-5653; e-mail: nfb@nfb.org; Web site: www.nfb.org.

‡PO Box 317, Watertown, MA 02472-0317; phone: 800-562-6265; fax: 617-972-74444; Web site: www.napvi.org.

§22 W. 21st St., 6th Floor, New York, NY 10010; phone: 212-889-3141; fax: 212-727-2931; e-mail: staff@navh.org; Web site: www.NAVH.org.

||1155 15th St. NW, Suite 1004, Washington, DC 20005; phone: 800-424-8666; fax: 202-467-5085; Web site: www.acb.org. A source of information in Canada is the Canadian National Institute for the Blind, 1929 Bayview Ave., Toronto, Ontario M4G 3E8; phone: 416-480-7580; fax: 416-480-7677; Web site: www.cnib.ca.

Development and Independence

Motor development depends on sight almost as much as verbal communication depends on hearing. From earliest infancy, parents are encouraged to expose the infant to as many visual-motor experiences as possible, such as sitting supported in an infant seat or swing and being given opportunities for holding up the head, sitting unsupported, reaching for objects, and crawling.

Despite visual impairment, the child can become independent in all aspects of self-care. The same principles used for promoting independence in sighted children apply, with additional emphasis on nonvisual cues. For example, the child may need help in dressing, such as special arrangement of clothing for style coordination and braille tags to distinguish colors and prints.

The blind child also must learn to become independent in navigational skills. The two main techniques are the *tapping method* (use of a cane to survey the environment for direction and to avoid obstacles) and *guides,* such as a sighted human guide or a dog guide, such as a Seeing Eye dog. Children who are partially sighted may benefit from ocular aids, such as a monocular telescope.

Play and Socialization

Blind children do not learn to play automatically. Because they cannot imitate others or actively explore the environment as sighted children do, they depend much more on others to stimulate and teach them how to play. Parents need help in selecting appropriate play material, especially those that encourage fine and gross motor development and stimulate the senses of hearing, touch, and smell. Toys with educational value are especially useful, such as dolls with various clothing closures.

Blind children have the same needs for socialization as sighted children. Because they have little difficulty in learning verbal skills, they are able to communicate with agemates and participate in suitable activities. The nurse discusses with parents opportunities for socialization outside the home, especially regular preschools. The trend is to include these children with sighted children to help them adjust to the outside world for eventual independence.

To compensate for inadequate stimulation, these children may develop *blindisms* (self-stimulatory activities, such as body rocking, finger flicking, or arm twirling). Such habits restrict the child's social acceptance and are discouraged. Behavior modification is often successful in reducing or eliminating blindisms.

Education

The main obstacle to learning is the child's total dependence on nonvisual cues. Although the child can learn via verbal lecturing, he or she is unable to read the written word or to write without special education. Therefore the child must rely on *braille,* a system that uses raised dots to represent letters and numbers. The child can then read the braille with the fingers and can write a message using a braille writer. However, unless others read braille, this type of communication is not useful for communicating with others. A more portable system for written communication is the use of a braille slate and stylus or a microcassette tape recorder. A recorder is especially helpful for leaving messages for others and for note taking during classroom lecturing. For mathematic calculations, portable calculators with voice synthesizers are available.*

Records and tapes are significant sources of reading material other than braille books, which are large and cumbersome. The Library of Congress† has talking books, braille books, and a special records program, which are available at many local and state libraries and directly from the Library of Congress. The talking book machine and tape player are provided at no cost to families, and there is no postage fee for returning the materials. Recording for the Blind and Dyslexic‡ also provides texts and tapes of books, which are very helpful for secondary and college students who are blind.

Learning to use a regular typewriter is another form of writing but has the disadvantage of the blind person's being unable to check the accuracy of the typing. Computers eliminate this drawback; a home computer with a voice synthesizer can be adapted to speak each letter or word that has been typed.

The child with partial sight benefits from specialized visual aids, which produce a magnified retinal image. The basic devices are accommodation (e.g., bringing the object closer), special plus lenses, handheld and stand magnifiers, telescopes, video projection systems, and large print. Special equipment is available to enlarge print. Information about services for the partially sighted is available from the National Association for Visually Handicapped and American Foundation for the Blind (see previous footnote). Children with diminished vision often prefer to do close work without their glasses and compensate by bringing the object very near to their eyes. This should be allowed. The exception is the child with vision in only one eye, who should always wear glasses for protection.

Care for the Child during Hospitalization

Because nurses are more likely to care for children who are hospitalized for procedures that involve temporary loss of vision than for children who are blind, the following discussion concentrates primarily on the needs of such children. The nursing care objectives in either situation are to (1) reassure the child and family throughout every phase of treatment, (2) orient the child to the surroundings, (3) provide a safe environment, and (4) encourage independence. Whenever possible, the same nurse should care for the child to ensure consistency in the approach. These same principles also apply to a blind child who requires hospitalization.

When sighted children temporarily lose their vision, almost every aspect of the environment becomes bewildering

---

*A catalog of numerous products for people with vision problems is available from the American Foundation for the Blind (see previous footnote) and from Lighthouse International, 111 East 59th St., New York, NY 10022-1202; phone: 212-821-9200 or 800-829-0500; Web site: www.lighthouse.org.

†The National Library Service for the Blind and Visually Handicapped, 1291 Taylor St. NW, Washington, DC 20542; phone: 800-424-8567; TTY: 202-707-0744; fax: 202-707-0712; Web site: www.loc.gov/nls. (A state-by-state listing of libraries for blind and physically handicapped readers, as well as other reference circulars, is available from this office.)

‡20 Roszel Rd., Princeton, NJ 08540; phone: 800-221-4792 or 866-RFBD-585; fax: 609-987-8116; Web site: www.rfbd.org.

and frightening. They are forced to rely on nonvisual senses for help in adjusting to the blindness without the benefit of any special training. Nurses have a major role in minimizing the effects of temporary loss of vision. They need to talk to the child about everything that is occurring, emphasizing aspects of procedures that are felt or heard. They should approach the child by always identifying themselves as soon as they enter the room. Because unfamiliar sounds are especially frightening, these are explained. Parents are encouraged to room with their child and participate in the care. Familiar objects, such as a teddy bear or doll, should be brought from home to help lessen the strangeness of the hospital. As soon as the child is able to be out of bed, he or she is oriented to the immediate surroundings. If the child is able to see on admission, this opportunity is taken to point out significant aspects of the room. The child is encouraged to practice ambulating with the eyes closed to become accustomed to this experience.

The room is arranged with safety in mind. For example, a stool or chair is placed next to the bed to help the child climb in and out of bed. The furniture is always placed in the same position to prevent collisions. Cleaning personnel are reminded of the need to keep the room in order. If the child has difficulty navigating by feeling the walls, a rope can be attached from the bed to the point of destination, such as the bathroom. Attention to details such as well-fitting slippers or robes that do not hang on the floor is important in preventing tripping. Unlike the child who is blind, these children are not familiar with navigating with a cane.

The child is encouraged to be independent in self-care activities, especially if the visual loss may be prolonged or potentially permanent. For example, during bathing the nurse sets up all the equipment and encourages the child to participate. At mealtime the nurse explains where each food item is on the tray, opens any special containers, prepares cereal or toast, and encourages the child in self-feeding. Favorite finger foods, such as sandwiches, hamburgers, hot dogs, or pizza, may be good selections. The child is praised for efforts at being cooperative and independent. Any improvements made in self-care, no matter how small, are stressed.

Appropriate recreational activities are provided, and if a child-life specialist is available, such planning is done jointly. Because children with temporary blindness have a wide variety of play experiences to draw on, they are encouraged to select activities. For example, if they like to read, they may enjoy being read to. If they prefer manual activity, they may appreciate playing with clay or building blocks or feeling different textures and naming them. If they need an outlet for aggression, activities such as pounding or banging on a drum can be helpful. Simple board and card games can be played with a "seeing partner" or if the opponent helps with the game. They should have familiar toys from home to play with, because familiar items are more easily manipulated than new ones. If parents want to bring presents, they should be objects that stimulate hearing and touch, such as a radio, music box, or stuffed animal.

Assist in Measures to Prevent Visual Impairment

An essential nursing goal is to prevent visual impairment. This involves many of the same interventions discussed under hearing impairments: (1) prenatal screening for pregnant women at risk, such as those with rubella or syphilis infection and family histories of genetic disorders associated with visual loss; (2) adequate prenatal and perinatal care to prevent prematurity; (3) periodic screening of all children, especially newborns through preschoolers, for congenital blindness and visual impairments caused by refractive errors, strabismus, and other disorders; (4) rubella immunization of all children; and (5) safety counseling regarding the common causes of ocular trauma.

Safety counseling should include safe practices when working with, playing with, or carrying objects such as scissors, knives, and balls.

NURSE ALERT A helmet with a face mask should be required for children playing football, hockey, or baseball. ■

After detection of eye problems, the nurse has a responsibility to prevent further ocular damage by ensuring that corrective treatment is used. For the child with strabismus, this often necessitates occlusion patching of the stronger eye. Compliance with the procedure is greatest during the early preschool years. It is more difficult to encourage school-age children to wear the occlusive patch because the poor visual acuity of the uncovered weaker eye interferes with school work and the patch sets them apart from their peers. In school they benefit from being positioned favorably (closer to the chalkboard or other visual media) and allowed extra time to read or complete an assignment. If treatment of the eye disorder requires instillation of ophthalmic medication, the family is taught the correct procedure.

For the child with refractive errors, the nurse helps the child adjust to wearing *glasses.* Young children who often pull glasses off benefit from temporal pieces that wrap around the ears or an elastic strap attached to the frames and around the back of the head to hold the glasses on securely. After children appreciate the value of clear vision, they are more likely to wear the corrective lenses.

Glasses should not interfere with any activity. Special protective guards are available during contact sports to prevent accidental injury, and all corrective lenses should be made from safety glass, which is shatterproof. Often, corrective lenses improve visual acuity so dramatically that children are able to compete more effectively in sports. This in itself is a tremendous inducement to continue wearing glasses.

Contact lenses are a popular alternative, especially for adolescents. Several types are available, such as hard lenses, including gas-permeable ones, and soft lenses, which may be designed for daily or extended wear. Contact lenses offer several advantages over glasses, such as greater visual acuity, total corrected field of vision, convenience (especially with the extended-wear type), and optimum cosmetic benefit. Unfortunately, they are usually more expensive and require much more care than glasses, including considerable practice to learn techniques for insertion and removal. If they are prescribed, the nurse can be very helpful in teaching parents or older children how to care for the lenses.

Because trauma is the leading cause of blindness, the nurse has the major responsibility of preventing further eye injury until the specific treatment is instituted. The major principles to follow when caring for an eye injury are outlined in the Emergency box on p. 1272. Because patients with a serious eye injury fear blindness, the nurse should stay with the child and family to provide support and reassurance.

Evaluation

The effectiveness of nursing interventions is determined by continual reassessment and evaluation of care based on the following observational guidelines and expected outcomes:

1. Interview family members regarding their adjustment to the sensory impairment; observe family members' relationship with child; interview child regarding feelings about the sensory impairment and its effect on activities of daily living (especially important if a visual loss).
2. Have parents identify those cues that indicate infant is responding to them; observe nonvisual behaviors of parents as they respond to infant.
3. Observe techniques child uses to read and navigate; inquire if child is enrolled in a visual training program; inquire about socialization opportunities for child (i.e., who are child's friends, what are child's extracurricular activities).
4. Observe preparation of the room and self-care activities that provide for safety and independence during hospitalization.

Expected outcomes:

1. Parents express their feelings and concerns regarding loss of sight and demonstrate an understanding of child's disability and its implications.
2. Parents demonstrate attachment behaviors.
3. Infant or child engages in appropriate activities for level of development (specify); child demonstrates an attitude of security in the environment.
4. Child and family receive safe and supportive care during hospitalization.

Deaf-Blind Children

The most traumatic sensory impairment is loss of sight and hearing. Obviously, auditory and visual disabilities have profound effects on the child's development. They interfere with the normal sequence of physical, intellectual, and psychosocial growth. Although such children often achieve the usual motor milestones, their rate of development is slower. These children learn communication only with specialized training. *Finger spelling* is one desirable method often taught to these children. Some deaf-blind children, especially those with residual hearing or sight, can learn to speak. Whenever possible, speech is encouraged, because it allows communication with other individuals.

The future prospects for deaf-blind children are, at best, unpredictable. Congenital blindness or deafness may be accompanied by other physical or neurologic problems, which further lessen the child's learning potential. The most favorable prognosis is for children who have acquired deafness and blindness and have few, if any, associated disabilities. Their learning capacity is greatly potentiated by their developmental progress before the sensory impairments. Although total independence, including gainful vocational training, is the goal, some deaf-blind children are unable to develop to this level. They may require lifelong parental or residential care. The nurse working with such families helps them deal with future goals for the child, including possible alternatives to home care during the parents' advancing years.

Retinoblastoma

Retinoblastoma, which arises from the retina, is the most common congenital malignant intraocular tumor of childhood. Approximately 11 cases per million occur annually, primarily in children younger than 5 years of age. Retinoblastoma is caused by a mutation in a gene and may occur sporadically or be inherited (Hurwitz et al, 2002). Retinoblastoma develops when the mutated gene is unable to produce the natural signals to stop the growth of retinal cells. Of all cases, the majority are nonhereditary and unilateral, with the remainder divided between hereditary and unilateral, and hereditary and bilateral. Hereditary retinoblastomas are transmitted as an autosomal dominant trait with a 90% penetrance (Hurwitz et al, 2002; Lanzkowsky, 2000).

Diagnostic Evaluation

Retinoblastoma has few grossly obvious signs (Box 42-8). Typically it is the parent who first observes a whitish "glow" in the pupil, known as the *cat's eye reflex* (white reflex) or leukokoria. Leukokoria represents visualization of the tumor as the light momentarily falls on the mass.

The first step in diagnosis is carefully listening to and recognizing the significance of reports from family members regarding suspected abnormalities within the eye. Eye abnormalities, including cat's eye reflex, strabismus, decreased vision, and persistent painful erythematous eyes, are referred to an ophthalmologist. Definitive diagnosis is usually based on ophthalmoscopic examination under general anesthesia. Imaging studies, including ultrasonography and computed tomography of the orbit, are done to determine the extent of the disease.

Therapeutic Management

The aim of therapy is to preserve useful vision and eradicate the tumor. Treatment of retinoblastoma depends chiefly on the stage of the tumor at the time of diagnosis. *Reese-Ellsworth classification (RE)* is the commonly used standard for intraocular disease. Other staging systems such as Grabrowski and Abramson and American Joint Committee on Cancer Systems classify both intraocular and extraocular disease but are not universally used (Hurwitz et al, 2002; Schouten–van Meeteren et al, 2002).

Recently there has been a shift away from the use of external beam radiation (whole-eye irradiation that damages the cell's DNA) in the treatment of RE groups I, II, and III

BOX 42-8

Clinical Manifestations of Retinoblastoma

Cat's eye reflex (most common sign)
Strabismus (second most common sign)
Red, painful eye, often with glaucoma
Blindness (late sign)

retinoblastoma toward the use of focal intraocular therapy with or without chemotherapy (De Potter, 2002; Schouten–van Meeteren et al, 2002). Some of the common focal therapies are (1) plaque brachytherapy (surgical radioactive implant on the sclera until maximum dose has been delivered to the tumor), (2) laser photocoagulation (laser beam to coagulate blood supply to the tumor), (3) cryotherapy (freezing the tumor by destroying the microcirculation to the tumor through microcrystal formation), and (4) thermotherapy (uses microwaves or infrared radiation to deliver heat to the tumor).

Chemotherapy is being used in the early RE groups in an attempt to reduce tumor size to facilitate focal intraocular treatment (chemoreduction). Chemotherapy has been used for several years to prevent metastatic disease in RE groups IV and V and relapsed patients (chemoprevention or chemoprophylaxis). Chemoreduction and chemoprevention include two to six courses of vincristine, etoposide, and carboplatin with or without cyclophosphamide. Retinoblastoma is chemosensitive but is not yet a chemocurable disease (Schouten–van Meeteren et al, 2002). Chemoreduction and chemoprevention minimize the use of external beam radiation treatment and therefore reduce the risk of radiation-induced malignancies and facial disfigurement.

With advanced tumor growth into the optic nerve, choroid, orbit, and anterior chamber or no hope for useful vision, *enucleation* (removal) of the affected eye is the treatment of choice. After enucleation, the orbital implant is placed to provide a more natural cosmetic appearance, minimize sinking of the prosthesis, and enable motility of the prosthesis.

With bilateral disease, every attempt is made to preserve useful vision in both eyes. Chemotherapy, external beam therapy, radiotherapy, and other treatments (e.g., cryotherapy, laser therapy, plaque brachytherapy, thermotherapy) to both eyes may prevent the need for enucleation.

Trilateral retinoblastoma is a rare, usually fatal syndrome present in 1% to 8% of patients with bilateral retinoblastoma. Trilateral retinoblastoma is bilateral retinoblastoma with the involvement of pineal gland tumor or other midline structure (Hurwitz et al, 2002). Trilateral retinoblastoma is treated aggressively with chemotherapy, radiation therapy, adjuvant treatments, and gamma knife therapy with little success. However, a longer survival has been correlated with early tumor diagnosis in the asymptomatic patient and the use of initial chemoreduction at diagnosis (Hurwitz et al, 2002).

Prognosis

The overall prognosis for retinoblastoma is very favorable, with a survival rate of nearly 90% for both unilateral and bilateral tumors. Retinoblastoma is one of the tumors that may spontaneously regress.

Of major concern in long-term survivors is the development of decreased visual acuity, facial disfiguration, secondary tumors (especially osteogenic sarcoma), other sarcomas, and melanoma. Children with bilateral disease (hereditary form) are more likely to develop secondary cancers than are children with unilateral disease. It is thought that these individuals are predisposed to developing cancer and that radiation increases their risk.

Chemoprevention and high-dose chemotherapy with autologous stem cell rescue appears to be beneficial for patients with metastatic retinoblastoma (De Potter, 2002). Research studies focused on the use of monoclonal antibodies and gene therapy are being investigated to eradicate metastatic retinoblastoma.

Nursing Considerations

One of the most important nursing goals is to have a high index of suspicion for this rare malignancy. If parents report noticing a strange light in the eye, these concerns must be taken seriously. Families with a history of retinoblastoma require follow-up, and the nurse can be instrumental in reminding parents of appointments.

Because the tumor is usually diagnosed in infants or very young children, most of the preparation for diagnostic tests and treatment involves parents. After indirect ophthalmoscopy, the child may not see very clearly, or the eyes may be sensitive to light because of pupillary dilation. Parents are made aware of these normal reactions before the procedure. Screening tests, such as bone surveys and bone marrow aspiration, are rarely performed unless metastatic disease is suspected.

After the disease is staged, the practitioner confers with the parents regarding treatment. Based on the extent of the disease and the goal of eradicating the tumor and preserving useful vision, an individualized treatment plan is formulated and explained to the parents.

The treatment plan may include focal intraocular therapy with or without chemotherapy, external beam radiation, and, if necessary, enucleation. Enucleation is the treatment of choice if there is extensive disease threatening metastasis or no chance for useful vision. The enucleation procedure and the positive benefits of a prosthesis are explained to the parents. Showing them pictures of another child with an artificial eye may be helpful in their adjusting to the thought of disfigurement.

After surgery the parents are prepared for the child's facial appearance. An eye patch is in place, and the child's face may be edematous or ecchymotic. Parents often fear seeing the surgical site because they imagine a cavity in the skull. A surgically implanted sphere maintains the shape of the eyeball, and the implant is covered with conjunctiva. When the lids are open, the exposed area resembles the mucosal lining of the mouth. After the child is fitted for a prosthesis, usually within 3 weeks, the facial appearance returns to normal. Initial instructions for care of the prosthesis are given by the ocularist, who fits and manufactures the device.

Care of the socket is minimal and easily accomplished. The wound itself is clean and has little or no drainage. If an antibiotic ointment is prescribed, it is applied in a thin line on the surface of the tissues of the socket. To cleanse the site, an irrigating solution may be ordered and is instilled daily or more frequently, *before* application of the antibiotic ointment. The dressing consists of an eye pad taped over the surgical site and is changed daily. After the socket has healed completely, a dressing is no longer necessary, although it is a preventive measure against infection.

Support Family

Families with a history of the disorder may feel great guilt for transmitting the defect to their offspring. In families with no history of retinoblastoma, the discovery of the diagnosis is a shock, frequently complicated by guilt and anger for not having found it sooner. The nurse, along with the team (including a pediatric oncologic medical provider, an ophthalmologist, a radiologist, a child psychologist, social workers, a genetic counselor, and a child-life specialist), supports the family in dealing with emotional reactions, adjustment, and treatment modalities (see Chapter 44).

Autism

Autism is a complex developmental disorder of brain function accompanied by a broad range and severity of intellectual and behavioral deficits. It is manifested during early childhood primarily from 24 to 48 months of age. It occurs in 1 in 500 children; is about four times more common in males than in females (although females are more severely affected); and is not related to socioeconomic level, race, or parenting style.

Etiology

The etiology of autism is unknown. However, considerable evidence supports multiple biologic causes. Individuals with autism may have abnormal electroencephalograms, epileptic seizures, delayed development of hand dominance, persistence of primitive reflexes, metabolic abnormalities (elevated blood serotonin), and cerebellar vermal hypoplasia (the part of the brain involved in regulating motion and some aspects of memory). Brain overgrowth manifesting as a sudden increase in head size between 1 to 2 months and 6 to 14 months of age has been observed in children with autism (Courchesne, Carper, & Akshoomoff, 2003; Lainhart, 2003).

There is also strong evidence for a genetic basis that in twins is consistent with an autosomal recessive pattern of inheritance. Twin studies demonstrate a very high concordance (96%) for monozygotic (identical) twins and a 24% concordance for dizygotic (nonidentical) twins. In addition, between 5% and 16% of males with autism are positive for the fragile X chromosome.

There is a 10% to 20% risk of recurrence of autism in families with one affected child (Filipek et al, 2000). Although several genes have been suggested as possible causative factors in autism, no specific gene for the disorder has been identified (Shao et al, 2003; Tager-Flusberg & Joseph, 2003).

Contrary to previous reports, autism does not appear to be caused by the measles-mumps-rubella (MMR) vaccine (Dales, Hammer, & Smith, 2001; DeStefano et al, 2004). Autism has been reported in association with a number of conditions, such as fragile X syndrome, tuberous sclerosis, metabolic disorders, fetal rubella syndrome, *Haemophilus influenzae* meningitis, and structural brain anomalies (Williams, Dalrymple, & Neal, 2000). Recent reports have retrospectively tied autism to perinatal events such as a high incidence of uterine bleeding during pregnancy, a lower incidence of vaginal infections during pregnancy, a decreased maternal use of contraceptives, and a higher incidence of neonatal hyperbilirubinemia (Juul-Dam, Townsend, & Courchesne, 2001). These same researchers, however, urge caution in interpreting these findings.

Clinical Manifestations and Diagnostic Evaluation

Children with autism demonstrate several peculiar and often seemingly bizarre characteristics, primarily in social interactions, communication, and behavior. One hallmark characteristic is the inability to maintain eye contact with another person. Parents of autistic children have noted that their infants had difficulties with eye contact and avoidance of body contact at a very early age (Sivberg, 2003). Children with autism also display limited functional play and may interact with toys in an unusual manner (Williams et al, 2000). Autistic children may have significant gastrointestinal symptoms. Constipation is a common symptom and can be associated with acquired megarectum in children with autism (Afzal et al, 2003). Other clinical manifestations typically seen in children with autism are described in Box 42-9. Studies of these children at play suggest that deficits in social development are a primary feature of the illness. Children with autism do not always have the same manifestations; autism ranges from mild forms, requiring minimal supervision, to severe forms, in which self-abusive behavior is common. The majority (50% to 70%) of children with autism have some degree of mental retardation, with scores typically in the moderate to severe range. More females than males tend to have very low intelligence scores. Despite their relatively moderate to severe disability, some children with autism (known as *savants*) excel in particular areas, such as art, music, memory, mathematics, or perceptual skills such as puzzle building.

NURSE ALERT The therapeutic management of autism with the hormone secretin is controversial. One study failed to demonstrate significant improvement when autistic children were given one dose of synthetic human secretin (Sandler et al, 1999).* ■

Speech and language delays are also common in autistic children. The new Practice Parameter Report of the American Academy of Neurology (Filipek et al, 2000) recommends immediate evaluation of any child who does not display such language skills as babbling or gesturing by 12 months, no single word by 16 months, and lack of two-word phrases by 24 months. A sudden deterioration in extant expressive speech is also a red-flag event for further evaluation.

This report emphasizes early recognition, referral, diagnosis, and intensive early intervention to improve outcomes for children with autism. Unfortunately, diagnosis often is not made until 2 to 3 years after symptoms are first recognized. The Academy of Neurology report has a comprehensive set of suggested diagnostic criteria to be used to either rule out or establish the diagnosis of childhood autism (Filipek et al, 2000) (see Box 42-9).

*Additional information on secretin may be found at www.autism.org/secretin.html. See also Autism Society of America, 7910 Woodmont Ave, Suite 300, Bethesda, MD 20814; phone: 800-3AUTISM or 301-657-0881; Web site: www.autism-society.org.

BOX 42-9

Diagnostic Criteria for Autistic Disorder

A. A total of six (or more) items from (1), (2), and (3), with at least two from (1), and one each from (2) and (3):
  (1) Qualitative impairment in social interaction, as manifested by at least two of the following:
    (a) Marked impairment in the use of multiple nonverbal behaviors such as eye-to-eye gaze, facial expression, body postures, and gestures to regulate social interaction.
    (b) Failure to develop peer relationships appropriate to developmental level
    (c) A lack of spontaneous seeking to share enjoyment, interests, or achievements with other people (e.g., by a lack of showing, bringing, pointing out objects of interest)
    (d) Lack of social or emotional reciprocity
  (2) Qualitative impairments in communication as manifested by at least one of the following:
    (a) Delay in, or total lack of, the development of spoken language (not accompanied by an attempt to compensate through alternative modes of communication such as gestures or mime)
    (b) In individuals with adequate speech, marked impairment in the ability to initiate or sustain a conversation with others
    (c) Stereotyped and repetitive use of language or idiosyncratic language
    (d) Lack of varied, spontaneous make-believe play or social imitative play appropriate to developmental level
  (3) Restricted repetitive and stereotyped patterns of behavior, interests, and activities, as manifested by at least one of the following:
    (a) Encompassing preoccupation with one or more stereotyped and restricted patterns of interest that is abnormal either in intensity or focus
    (b) Apparently inflexible adherence to specific, nonfunctional routines or rituals
    (c) Stereotyped and repetitive motor mannerisms (e.g., hand or finger flapping or twisting, complex whole-body movements)

B. Delays or abnormal functioning in at least one of the following areas, with onset before age 3 years: (1) social interaction, (2) language as used in social communication, or (3) symbolic or imaginative play.

C. The disturbance is not better accounted for by Rett's Disorder or Childhood Disintegrative Disorder.

From American Psychiatric Association: *Diagnostic and statistical manual of mental disorders,* ed 4, (DSM-IV), Washington, DC, 1994, The Association.

Prognosis

Autism is usually a severely disabling condition. However, some children improve with acquisition of language skills and communication with others (Rapin, 1997). Some ultimately achieve independence, but most require lifelong adult supervision. Aggravation of psychiatric symptoms occurs in about half of the children during adolescence, with girls having a tendency for continued deterioration.

Early recognition of behaviors associated with autism is critical to implement appropriate interventions and family involvement. The prognosis is most favorable for children with communicative speech development by age 6 years and an IQ above 50 at the time of diagnosis.

Nursing Care Management

Therapeutic intervention for the child with autism is a specialized area involving professionals with advanced training. Although there is no cure for autism, numerous therapies have been used. The most promising results have been through highly structured and intensive behavior modification programs. In general the objective in treatment is to promote positive reinforcement, increase social awareness of others, teach verbal communication skills, and decrease unacceptable behavior. Providing a structured routine for the child to follow is a key in the management of autism.

When these children are hospitalized, the parents are essential to planning care and ideally should stay with the child as much as possible. Nurses should recognize that not all children with autism are the same, and each child will require individual assessment and treatment. Decreasing stimulation by using a private room, avoiding extraneous auditory and visual distractions, and encouraging the parents to bring in possessions the child is attached to may lessen the disruptiveness of hospitalization. Because physical contact often upsets these children, minimum holding and eye contact may be necessary to avoid behavioral outbursts. Care must be taken when performing procedures on, administering medicine to, or feeding these children, because they are either fussy eaters, who may willfully starve themselves or gag to prevent eating, or indiscriminate hoarders, swallowing any available edible or inedible items, such as a thermometer. Eating habits of autistic children may be particularly problematic for families and may involve food refusal, mouthing objects, eating nonedibles, and smelling and throwing food (Williams et al, 2000).

Children with autism need to be introduced slowly to new situations. Visits with staff caregivers are kept short whenever possible. Because these children have difficulty organizing their behavior and redirecting their energy, they need to be told directly what to do. Communication should be at the child's developmental level, brief, and concrete.

Family Support

Autism, as with so may other chronic conditions, involves the entire family and often becomes "a family disease." Nurses can help alleviate the guilt and shame often associated with this disorder by stressing what is known from a biologic standpoint, as well as how little is known about the cause of autism. It is imperative to help parents understand that they are not the cause of the child's condition.

Parents need expert counseling early in the course of the disorder and should be referred to the Autism Society of America (ASA).* ASA provides information about education, treatment programs and techniques, and facilities such as camps and group homes. There is also a siblings group called SHARE (Siblings Helping persons with Autism through Resources and Energy). Other helpful resources for parents of children with autism are the local and state de-

*7910 Woodmont Ave, Suite 300, Bethesda, MD 20814-3067; phone: 800-3AUTISM or 301-657-0881; Web site: www.autism-society.org.

partments of mental health and developmental disabilities; these organizations provide important programs for autistic children and in-school programs throughout the United States.

As much as possible, the family is encouraged to care for the child in the home. With the help of family support programs in many states, families are often able to provide home care and assist with the educational services the child needs. As the child approaches adulthood and the parents become older, the family may require assistance in locating a long-term placement facility.

Key Points

- The American Association of Mental Retardation defines *mental retardation (MR)* as significantly subaverage general intellectual functioning existing concurrently with deficits in adaptive behavior and manifested during the developmental period.
- Causes of severe MR are primarily genetic, biochemical, and infectious. Mild MR is associated primarily with familial, social, and environmental causes, whereas severe MR is more likely to be associated with specific syndromes.
- Education of children with cognitive impairment emphasizes sensory and verbal discrimination, improvement of short-term memory, motivation, and technologic support.
- Promoting optimum development may be achieved through family guidance regarding play, communication, discipline, socialization, and sexuality.
- Prevention of MR focuses on support for the premature neonate and other high risk newborns, rubella immunization, genetic counseling, and maternal education regarding the risks of chemical use and the importance of adequate nutrition.
- Down syndrome, a chromosomal abnormality, is characterized by a mild to moderate range of retardation, physical characteristics (see Box 42-3), slowed language development, congenital anomalies, sensory problems, and diminished growth and sexual development.
- Fragile X syndrome is characterized by MR and phenotypic findings in affected males. It is considered the most common hereditary cause and the second leading chromosomal cause of MR after Down syndrome.
- Hearing disorders may be classified according to the location of the defect: conductive, sensorineural, mixed conductive-sensorineural, and central auditory imperception.
- Rehabilitation for hearing loss involves parent education and support, hearing aids, lipreading, sign language, speech therapy, and promotion of socialization.
- Prevention of hearing loss includes treatment of infection, universal newborn screening and child auditory testing, immunization, pregnancy and genetic counseling, and reduction of noise pollution.
- Common visual impairments in childhood include refractive errors, amblyopia, strabismus, cataracts, glaucoma, trauma, and infections.
- Prevention of visual impairment focuses on prenatal screening, prenatal and perinatal care, periodic vision screening, immunization, and safety counseling.
- Nursing goals in visual rehabilitation include helping the family and child adjust to the child's visual impairment, promoting parent-child attachment, fostering optimum development and independence, providing for play and socialization, and being aware of educational facilities.
- For the child undergoing ocular surgery, nursing care is aimed at reassuring the child and family throughout treatment, orienting the child to the surroundings, providing a safe environment, and encouraging independence.
- Retinoblastoma is a rare congenital malignant tumor; its most common clinical manifestations are cat's eye reflex (white pupil) and strabismus.
- Autism is a complex developmental disorder of brain function accompanied by a broad range and severity of intellectual and behavioral deficits.

Answer Guidelines to Critical Thinking Exercises

Diagnosis of Down Syndrome

1. Yes. Shocked parents with three children are notified that their newborn has Down syndrome.
2. (a) Melissa is a developmentally delayed newborn who requires time-consuming care. (b) Melissa will develop a variety of medical problems causing a huge economic expense. (c) Melissa will always require parent/sibling supervision and care.
3. The first priority is to allow the parents to express their feelings of grief, anger, sadness, and guilt regarding the birth of a mentally retarded child. The nurse should not take anything for granted or give definite suggestions regarding retarded children. The nurse should demonstrate acceptance of the child because parents are sensitive to the professional's attitude.
4. Yes. The parents' response suggests unexpressed feelings of anger, loss, sadness, and confusion.
5. The nurse should guide the parents toward appropriate resources when asked, such as written information and organizations. The nurse may ask the pediatrician and the social worker to talk with the parents. Emphasize normal characteristics of the child to help the parents see the child as an individual. Encourage parents to meet other families with a similarly affected child for additional support.

Hearing Impairment

1. Yes. Jason is severely hearing impaired and awakening in an unfamiliar environment after a surgical procedure. Jason awakens in an unfamiliar environment with monitors, intravenous lines, and other equipment that may create fear, anxiety, and agitation.
2. (a) Jason's inability to hear and communicate promotes frustration and fear. (b) Jason's increasing agitation may be due to not having his hearing aid. (c) Jason, who is status postregional block for herniorrhaphy, is unable to clearly verbalize or use sign language to express needs.

3. The first priority is to establish communication with Jason by directly facing him to facilitate lipreading, touching him to get his attention, and correctly placing his hearing aids if available. Determine his usual means of communicating, and encourage expression of feelings/questions regarding environment, equipment, and procedures. Explain procedures before performing using gestures, objects, or pictures, and speak slowly and clearly. Allow ample time for Jason to show understanding of explanations. Decrease environmental noise. Listen closely as Jason speaks and focus on his pronunciation of words.
4. Yes. Jason's behavior does not suggest the transitory confusion associated with the initial emergence from anesthesia. Rather, it suggests that he became increasingly frustrated as he became aware of his environment with the inability to communicate his desires and feelings. Although pain is a possibility and needs to be evaluated, regional blocks are typically given during surgery to keep children comfortable until after they are discharged.
5. It would be appropriate to make a referral to the child-life therapist (CLT) during the hospitalization. The CLT would encourage Jason to express his feelings, fears, and anxieties regarding surgery, the hospital environment, equipment, and procedures through therapeutic play.

References

Afzal N et al: Constipation with acquired megarectum in children with autism, *Pediatrics* 112(4):939-942, 2003.

Allegretti CM: The effects of a cochlear implant on the family of a hearing-impaired child, *Pediatr Nurs* 28(6):614-620, 2002.

American Academy of Pediatrics, Committee on Children and Disabilities: Provision of educationally-related services for children and adolescents with chronic diseases and disabling conditions, *Pediatrics* 105(2):448-451, 2000.

American Academy of Pediatrics, Committee on Genetics: Health supervision for children with Down syndrome, *Pediatrics* 107(2):442-449, 2001.

American Academy of Pediatrics, Task Force on Newborn and Infant Hearing: Newborn and infant hearing loss: detection and intervention, *Pediatrics* 103(2):527-530, 1999.

Applebaum E: Detection of hearing loss in children, *Peditar Ann* 28(6):351-356, 1999.

Berrettini S et al: Progressive sensorineural hearing loss in childhood, *Pediatr Neurol* 20(2):130-136, 1999.

Bosch JJ, Ringdahl J: Functional analysis of problem behavior in children with mental retardation: what is it, and why should pediatric nurses care? *MCN* 26(6):307-311, 2001.

Centers for Disease Control and Prevention: Delayed diagnosis of fragile X syndrome–United States, 1990-1999, *MMWR* 51(33):740-742, 2002.

Cohen W (ed): Health care guidelines for individuals with Down syndrome: 1999 revisions, *Down Syndrome Q,* August 1999. Internet document available at www.denison.edu/dsq/ (accessed April 22, 2005).

Courchesne E, Carper R, Akshoomoff N: Evidence of brain overgrowth in the first year of life in autism, *JAMA* 290(3):337-344, 2003.

Crawford DC: FMR1 and the fragile X syndrome, *CDC Fact Sheet,* 2001. Internet document available at www.cdc.gov/genomics/hugenet/factsheets/FS_FragileX.htm (accessed April 22, 2005).

Cunningham M, Cox EO: Committee on Practice and Ambulatory Medicine and the Section on Otolaryngology and Bronchoesophagology: hearing assessment in infants and children: recommendations beyond neonatal screening, *Pediatrics* 111(2):436-440, 2003.

Daily DK: Identification and evaluation of mental retardation, *Am Fam Physician* 61:1059-1067, 2000.

Dales L, Hammer SJ, Smith NJ: Time trends in autism and in MMR immunization coverage in California, *JAMA* 285(9):1183-1185, 2001.

Davidson PW: Visual impairment and blindness. In Levine MD, Carey WTS, Crocker AC (editors): *Developmental-behavior pediatrics,* ed 3, Philadelphia, 1999, WB Saunders.

De Potter P: Current treatment of retinoblastoma, *Curr Opin Ophthalmol* 13(5):331-336, 2002.

DeStefano F et al: Age at first measles-mumps-rubella vaccination in children with autism and school-matched control subjects: a population-based study in metropolitan Atlanta, *Pediatrics* 113(2):259-266, 2004.

Filipek P et al: Practice parameter: screening and diagnosis of autism: report of the Quality Standards Subcommittee of the American Academy of Neurology and the Child Neurology Society, *Neurology* 55(4):468-479, 2000.

First MB, McQueen LE, Pincus HA: *DSM-IV coding update,* Washington, DC, 1996, American Psychiatric Association.

Fredericks DW, Williams WL: New definition of mental retardation for the American Association of Mental Retardation, *Image J Nurs Sch* 30(1):53-56, 1998.

Grech V: An overview and update regarding medical problems in Down syndrome, *Indian J Pediatr* 68:863-866, 2001.

Gurrieri F et al: Pervasive developmental disorder and epilepsy due to maternally derived duplication of 15q11-q13, *Neurology* 52(8):1694-1697, 1999.

Hixon M et al: FISH studies of the sperm of fathers of paternally derived cases of trisomy 21: no evidence for an increase in aneuploidy, *Hum Genet* 103(6):654-657, 1998.

Holte L: Early childhood hearing loss: a frequently overlooked cause of speech and language delay, *Pediatr Ann* 32(7):461-465, 2003.

Hurwitz R et al: Retinoblastoma. In Pizzo PA, Poplack DG (eds): *Principle and practice of pediatric oncology,* ed 4, Philadelphia, 2002, JB Lippincott.

Juul-Dam N, Townsend J, Courchesne E: Prenatal, perinatal, and neonatal factors in autism, pervasive developmental disorder not otherwise specified, and the general population, *Pediatrics* 107(4):e63, 2001.

Kabra M, Gulati S: Mental retardation, *Indian J Pediatr* 70(2):153-158, 2003.

Lainhart JE: Increased rate of head growth during infancy in autism, *JAMA* 290(3):393-394, 2003.

Lanzkowsky P: *Manual of pediatric hematology and oncology,* San Diego, 2000, Academic Press.

National Down Syndrome Society: Are any prenatal tests available to detect Down syndrome? 2003a. Internet document available at www.ndss.org (accessed April 22, 2005).

National Down Syndrome Society: Down syndrome: myths and truths, 2003b. Internet document available at www.ndss.org (accessed April 22, 2005).

National Down Syndrome Society: Questions and answers about Down syndrome, 2003c. Internet document available at www.ndss.org (accessed April 22, 2005).

National Down Syndrome Society: What causes Down syndrome? 2003d. Internet document available at www.ndss.org (accessed April 22, 2005).

National Fragile X Foundation: Prevalence of fragile X syndrome, 2002. Internet document available at www.fragilex.org/html/prevalence.htm (accessed April 22, 2005).

Pueschel SM: The child with Down syndrome. In Levine MD et al (eds): *Developmental-behavioral pediatrics,* ed 3, Philadelphia, 1999, WB Saunders.

Rapin I: Autism, *N Engl J Med* 337(2):97-103, 1997.

Roizen NJ: Etiology of hearing loss in children: nongenetic causes, *Pediatr Clin North Am* 46(1):49-64, 1999.

Sandler AD et al: Lack of benefit of a single dose of synthetic human secretin in the treatment of autism and pervasive developmental disorder, *N Engl J Med* 341(24):1801-1806, 1999.

Schouten–van Meeteren AYN et al: Overview: chemotherapy for retinoblastoma: an expanding area of clinical research, *Med Pediatr Oncol* 38:428-438, 2002.

Segal S et al: Inner ear damage in children due to noise exposure from toy cap pistols and firecrackers: a retrospective review of 53 cases, *Noise Health* 5(18):13-18, 2003.

Shao Y et al: Fine mapping of autistic disorder to chromosome 15q11-q13 by phenotypic subtypes, *Am J Hum Genet* 72(3):539-548, 2003.

Sivberg B: Parents' detection of early signs in their children having an autism spectrum disorder, *J Pediatr Nurs* 18(6):433-440, 2003.

Slattery WH, Fayad JN: Cochlear implants in children with sensorineural inner ear hearing loss, *Pediatr Ann* 28(6):359-363, 1999.

Tager-Flusberg H, Joseph RM: Identifying neurocognitive phenotypes in autism, *Philos Trans R Soc Lond B Biol Sci* 358(1430):303-314, 2003.

Van Riper M: A change of plans: the birth of a child with Down syndrome doesn't have to be a negative experience, *Am J Nurs* 103(6):71-74, 2003.

Waltzman SB, Roland JT Jr, Cohen NL: Delayed implantation in congenitally deaf children and adults, *Otol Neurotol* 23(3):333-340, 2002.

Welch JL, Williams JK: Fragile X syndrome, *Neonat Netw* 18(6):15-22, 1999.

Williams PG, Dalrymple N, Neal J: Eating habits of children with autism, *Pediatr Nurs* 26(3):259-264, 2000.

Yang YH et al: Prenatal diagnosis of fetal trisomy 21 from maternal peripheral blood, *Yonsei Med J* 44(2):181-186, 2003.

Yoshinaga-Itano C et al: Language of early- and later-identified children with hearing loss, *Pediatrics* 102(5):1161-1171, 1998.

Family-Centered Home Care 43

LEARNING OBJECTIVES

On completion of this chapter the reader will be able to:

- Differentiate home care from hospice care.
- List at least three factors contributing to the increasing emphasis on home care services.
- Describe case management/care coordination and its importance in home care.
- List general principles of a family-centered assessment and planning process.
- Identify five key characteristics of collaborative relationships.
- Describe approaches to promoting optimal development, self-care, and education in home care.
- Outline six areas in need of attention for promoting safety in home care.

ELECTRONIC RESOURCES

Additional information related to the content in Chapter 43 can be found on

the companion website at evolve
http://evolve.elsevier.com/Wong/maternal/
- NCLEX Review Questions
- WebLinks

or the interactive student CD-ROM
Activities for Chapter 43 include the following:
- NCLEX Review Questions
- Case Study—Home Care

GENERAL CONCEPTS OF HOME CARE

Definition

Home care is not a new concept in pediatrics. Over time the term has referred to parents caring for mildly ill children at home; to nursing home visits after children are discharged from the hospital; to hospice care; and, more recently, to care at home for children with more serious chronic illness and dependence on medical technology. Home care is one of the fastest growing components of the health care industry.

As discussed in this chapter, *home care* refers to care provided in the family's residence for children with complex health care needs and their families. The purpose of home care services is to promote, maintain, or restore health or to maximize the level of independence while minimizing the effects of disability and illness, including terminal illness. Home care differs from *hospice care,* which is a program of palliative and supportive care services providing physical, psychologic, social, and spiritual care for dying persons, their families, and other loved ones. Hospice services are available in both the home and inpatient settings. *End-of-life care* and planning should be considered for any child with a terminal diagnosis. Some patients may be admitted for end-of-life home care services before being ready for admission to hospice services. Many hospice programs have admission criteria that do not permit therapies such as intravenous antibiotics, total parenteral nutrition, or enteral feedings that the family may wish to continue. It is therefore important to discuss the type of care the family wishes for the child early in discharge planning to clarify expectations for home care.

Home Care Trends

The shift toward home-based health care is propelled by numerous factors. Providing quality home health care for children generally requires parental desire and ability, professional assistance, and community preparedness. A natural family environment optimizes growth and development when stress is minimal and support is optimal.

Advances in medical technology have resulted in increased survival for children with congenital and acquired illnesses. Preterm infants or children who are ventilator dependent were once cared for indefinitely in an intensive care unit or long-term care facility. These children are now able to live with their families in their own home.

Children with cancer, kidney disorders, cystic fibrosis, spina bifida, cardiac and respiratory disorders, gastrointestinal disorders, neurodegenerative diseases, and human immunodeficiency virus (HIV) infection may have ongoing health care needs as a result of the disease, its treatment, or side effects of treatment. Parents frequently have ongoing stressors after a child's hospitalization for diagnosis and treatment. Subsequent needs may include reinforcement about the disease process, addressing the physical care needs of the child, emotional support during this change in parental role, and learning in a low-stress environment. Improving the quality of life for both the child and the family is one of the driving forces in the efforts to move technology-dependent children from the hospital to the home setting. The concept of *normalization* describes the process whereby families of children with chronic illness over a period of time begin to perceive the child and their family life as normal (Knafl & Deatrick, 2002). This has important implications for pediatric home care nurses in relation to the assessment of family function and to help home care nurses gain a better understanding of family dynamics. The normalized family tends to be more flexible with treatments and incorporates the child with a disability or illness into the usual routines of daily living (Knafl & Deatrick, 2002).

The *cost of care* is another important factor in the health care delivery system today. Shorter inpatient stays are due in part to the overwhelming cost of hospitalization. Children are either not admitted to the hospital at all or are returned home as soon as possible after their acute illness. Shifting the financial burden of health care to home care agencies is an attractive alternative to third-party reimbursers. Likewise, a portion of the financial burden is shifted to the family. The family may be forced to absorb the costs of certain medications, supplies, transportation, shelter, utilities, food, laundry, housekeeping, and a portion of nursing care. Over time, chronically ill children can cause a financial burden on the family. Lifetime insurance benefits may be used up quickly, the primary caregiver may be unable to work, and many costs of health care are simply not covered by other means.

Home health care of children is not restricted to children with chronic health care needs. Several short-term, intermittent therapies such as phototherapy, apnea monitoring, and intravenous antibiotic administration may be successfully treated in a home setting, where the child may remain with the family, rather than in an acute care setting.

With the increased demand for nurses in home health and continued pervasive short supply there has been an increased focus on the role of the *family caregiver* in providing home care. A survey by the National Alliance for Caregiving (1997) revealed that 25% of U.S. households have a person being cared for by another family member; this represents care above and beyond the daily routine care of the family household. Legislation for improving resources for family caregivers, including training resources and governmental funding for such training, is currently in progress.

Effectiveness of Home Care

Providing home-based care for children gives the nurse an opportunity to assess and interact with the family in their environment. This assessment can provide the health care team with valuable information about safety, support systems, nutrition, parenting ability, and actual health care practices. This valuable information will determine future decisions for individualized care and realistic outcomes (Thompson, 2000).

There are two distinct areas of implementation of care for the pediatric home care nurse. Nurses who perform *intermittent skilled nursing visits* may see different types and numbers of patients each day. These nurses typically have an assigned patient caseload and accept responsibility for implementing the plan of care. This mode of nursing care is the one most often used today as a result of shortage of personnel and decreased reimbursements. Most home visits are now focused on helping the patient/caregiver achieve independence with care in the home to include home care by therapists, home infusion teaching by nurses, and care management, rather than direct provision of physical care. Nurses who perform *private-duty nursing*, or block nursing, are usually assigned individual patients, and they remain in the home for a predetermined amount of time (e.g., 8- or 12-hour block of time) providing patient care. The latter model is much less common. The plan of care is implemented over the course of time in the home, and short-term intermittent plans of care are more common in today's home care. An increasing trend resulting from the nursing shortage and limitations in reimbursement is to have patients receive short-term treatments in nonhospital ambulatory settings (such as ambulatory infusion centers).

A major issue in providing home care in this era is the *nursing shortage.* Agencies and families are facing much more difficulty in staffing required home care services; thus more and more of the home care provided must be carried out by family members or other caregivers. The lack of pediatric training in some nursing programs, increased acuity of home care patients, and increased pay for nurses working in acute care settings have exacerbated the nursing shortage in pediatric home health care (Page, 2001). Consideration of the caregiver's willingness, ability, and limitations is of utmost importance when assessing the appropriateness of the plan of care. It is vital to ensure that patients and families have adequate backup support and access to resources such as social services (Box 43-1). An increasing concern in pedi-

BOX 43-1

Services That Support Effective Home Care

- Adequate family training and preparation
- Primary care physician willing to oversee medical aspects of home care
- Professional caregivers trained in relevant nursing and communication skills
- Developmental intervention (e.g., physical, occupational, and speech therapy; early intervention)
- Appropriately designed and well-maintained equipment
- Supportive therapies (e.g., respiratory therapy, pharmacy, rehabilitation services, parenteral therapy, physical therapy, durable medical/infusion supplies, nutritional support)
- Adequate social and psychologic support services
- High-quality respite care
- Appropriate home renovation
- Telephone service in the home
- Appropriate transportation
- Appropriate locally available emergency facilities
- Competent case management services
- Safe environment (electricity, refrigeration)

Modified from Office of Technology Assessment (OTA), Congress of the United States: *Technology dependent children: hospital v. home care—a technical memorandum* (OTA-TM-H-38), Washington, DC, 1987, US Government Printing Office; and Bakewell-Sachs S, Porth S: Discharge planning and home care of the technology-dependent infant, *JOGNN* 24(1):77-83, 1995.

atric home health care is obtaining a managing practitioner for patients in home health. Declining reimbursements and short hospital stays have increased patients moving rapidly through the continuum of care; a patient may be seen in the emergency department or neonatal intensive care unit, then discharged to home health without ever seeing a primary care physician. It is therefore imperative that the provision of care for home patients involve multidisciplinary cooperation and communication among health care workers.

Required nursing skills are determined by patient need, parental ability, complexity of family, and the home environment. In both types of home care, the pediatric nurse is responsible for patient and family assessment and evaluating the appropriateness of the plan of care.

From technology dependence to pain management or failure to thrive, pediatric nurses are appropriate professionals to affect a child's health care needs at home. Quality interdisciplinary care can create a significant, positive impact on family coping and child outcomes (Betz, 2000; Mahony & Murphy, 1999).

Discharge Planning

Identifying appropriate local community resources is critical to a successful transfer to home care. The ultimate goal of discharge planning is for the family to become familiar with the child's needs and to be competent in providing that care. A discharge plan should include emergency management and provision of social and emotional support. General guidelines for discharge that allow for family individuality provide for ideal outcomes. The desired attributes of an appropriate home care agency are outlined in Box 43-2.

Much of the success of home care, particularly for the child who is dependent on medical technology or has complex medical problems, depends on careful planning and preparation. Discharge planning must begin early and should be based on child and family readiness, must be a multidisciplinary process that includes representatives from inpatient and home care/community settings, and must involve the family. Predischarge assessment and planning should include the following areas:

- The child's medical, nursing, educational, and other therapeutic needs
- Family members' (including siblings') education and training, coping skills, and adjustment needs
- Community readiness in areas such as availability of equipment, appropriate nursing and other personnel, educational and developmental services, respite care, and emergency plans
- Financial arrangements

Creative financial planning, including negotiating arrangements with the insurance company, health maintenance or managed care organization, and public programs, may be required.

NURSE ALERT If home care equipment is different than hospital equipment, have portable equipment to be used in the home delivered to the hospital (rather than the home), to allow family use before discharge. ■

Early involvement of the home care agency in the discharge planning process promotes continuity of care and a smooth transition from hospital to home. Before discharge, a general plan of care should be developed with multidisciplinary input. This plan should address the range of needs identified as part of the comprehensive predischarge assessment.

NURSE ALERT An excellent method of providing home care instructions is with video recordings. After the family masters the procedures, consider video recording their performance. Visual learning may be most helpful for people who cannot read or who are not fluent in English. ■

The plans for transition from hospital to home should include at least two family members learning and demonstrating all aspects of the child's care in the hospital. An in-hospital trial period during which parents provide total care for the child (such as rooming-in) is generally beneficial as well. After a successful trial, the family may benefit from taking the child home on a brief pass before making final discharge plans. (This arrangement may need to be negotiated with the insurance company before implementation.) The home care nurse plays an important role in assessing this experience with the family. A predischarge home visit allows the home care nurse to meet the family, help them assess their preparedness and the preparedness of the home environment, discuss plans for arranging the child's equipment at home (Fig. 43-1), reinforce prior discharge teaching, and implement any additional teaching that may be necessary (Bakewell-Sachs et al, 2000). Additional factors that should be considered in discharge planning include working parents, extended family, and child care arrangements.

A comprehensive discharge plan includes the plan of care or care map, specific written instructions to facilitate continuity, and detailed information about home care expectations of the family and client outcomes (Box 43-3).

BOX 43-2

Quality Pediatric Home Care Agency

Fully trained pediatric staff to provide for all aspects of care (nursing, rehabilitation therapies, pharmacy, dietitian, social worker, home medical equipment)
Prompt responsive staff with 24-hour availability
Family-centered care
Comprehensive continuing education programs
Certification of local, state, and federal regulatory agencies
Accreditation by Joint Commission on Accreditation of Healthcare Organizations (JCAHO) or Community Health Accreditation Program (CHAP)

Data from Dittbrenner H: Pediatric home care as a viable new service, *Caring* 18(2):12-15, 1999; and Lovejoy D: *Making the transition to home health nursing: a practical guide,* New York, 1997, Springer.

Case Management

Traditional definitions of *case management* generally focus on cost control, attainment of desired clinical outcomes, and monitoring and evaluation of care provided. However, for

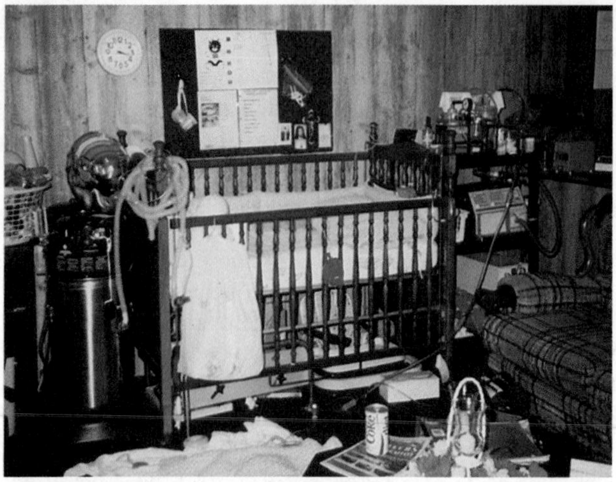

Fig. 43-1 An essential aspect of preparation for home care is arranging equipment and supplies.

BOX 43-3

Critical Home Care Referral Information

Scheduled medications
Durable medical equipment (DME)
Medical supplies
Transportation needs
Adaptive equipment
Rehabilitation therapies (e.g., occupational, physical, or speech therapy)
Psychologic counseling
Social work referral
Nursing care
Respite plans
Key family members
Demographic information
Reimbursement information

Modified from Townsend JL: Assessment of the child and family. In Votroubek WL, Townsend JL (eds): *Pediatric home care,* ed 2, Gaithersburg, MD, 1997, Aspen.

optimal home care of the child who is technology dependent, case management—or *care coordination*—should be viewed more broadly (see also Chapter 29).

Care coordination has several purposes. Its primary goal is ensuring continuity for the child and family across hospital, home, educational, therapeutic, and other settings. Other goals involve facilitating timely access to services and enhancing child and family well-being (Lindeke et al, 2002). Care should be coordinated among multiple providers to reduce the complexity of care for the child, reduce fragmentation, reduce duplication of services, and decrease the burden of care for the family. Case managers from a number of agencies may be involved in the patient's care, which may add to the parents' confusion; efforts should be made to coordinate all case managers for meetings with the family and a nurse care coordinator to minimize confusion and prevent duplication. Lindeke and colleagues (2002) propose that the ideal situation occurs when the family serves as lead care coordinator within the context of family-centered care. Care coordination should ensure that the medical, nursing, and health maintenance needs of the child, as well as financial issues, psychosocial concerns, and educational needs of the child and family, are addressed (American Academy of Pediatrics, 1999; Dittbrenner, 1999). Care coordination is most effective if a single person works with the family to accomplish the many tasks and responsibilities involved (Box 43-4).

The *nurse case manager* should have a minimum of a baccalaureate degree in nursing and 3 years' experience (American Nurses Association [ANA], 1998). The nurse case manager should be knowledgeable about community resources, including the following: primary, secondary, and tertiary health care services; speech, language, hearing, and vision resources; respite care services; financial assistance programs; parent groups; advocacy groups; local, state, and federal public officials; transportation services; and private sector individuals with an interest in children with disabilities (Thompson, 2000). With a greater focus on *outcomes of care* in home health care, the nurse case manager is challenged to be resourceful and highly skilled in communication at a number of levels (Rice, 2001). A valuable tool for nurse case managers is the *care path,* which is a multidisciplinary plan of care aimed at measuring quality patient care outcomes derived from standardized patient outcomes; the purpose of a care path is to evaluate the quality of patient care with respect to cost-effectiveness and timeliness (for samples of home care clinical care paths, see Rice, 2001). Care paths may also be used to help nurses and other health care workers learn home care and should be shared with the family members involved in patient care to provide direction and help the family see the eventual goals of care (Rice, 2001).

Care coordination should promote the family's role as primary decision maker and enhance the family's capability to meet the special needs of the child and the family as a whole. In 1999 the American Nurses Credentialing Center (ANCC), a subsidiary of the ANA, began offering specialty certification in case management.

Role of the Nurse, Training, and Standards of Care

The home care nurse must share a level of technical expertise with the acute care nurse while being able to adapt equipment, procedures, and the nursing process to the home setting. (See Chapter 45 for specific technical skills that may be required in home care practice.) The need for

BOX 43-4

Care Coordination for Children with Special Health Care Needs

Facilitate timely access to services and resources
Promote continuity of care
Provide family support and enhance family well-being
Improve health, developmental, educational, vocational, psychosocial, and functional outcomes
Maximize efficient, effective use of resources

Modified from Presler B: Care coordination for children with special health care needs, *Orthop Nurs* 17(25 suppl):45-51, 1998.

technical expertise must be matched by a knowledge of child development and the ability to work creatively with the child challenged by chronic illness and technology dependence. When caring for patients in the home setting, the nurse must be comfortable making independent nursing judgments and problem solving with no immediate assistance. At the same time, the nurse must have excellent interpersonal skills; an ability to work with other professionals and the family; and, most important, an ability to respect family autonomy (Box 43-5). Patient outcomes are more readily achievable with a balance of nursing skills that demonstrate clinical excellence, adaptability, accountability, and the ability to develop positive relationships with physicians, patients, and families.

When working with a home care agency, nurses should expect to receive patient placements appropriate to their expertise. They should also expect to receive orientation to the skills and knowledge base of the home health care nursing specialty and subsequent education to develop as expert practitioners. The minimum initial orientation should include the following areas: the individual patient's care plan and equipment needs; the agency's policies and procedures, including procedures for addressing any problems that may occur when care is provided in the home; documentation procedures; legal liability issues; and emergency procedures.

Reimbursement-driven documentation in home care differs from documentation practices in the hospital setting; increasingly, documentation must be written in specific ways to qualify for reimbursement of services and supplies. Mentoring is an ideal method of orienting a new nurse to home health care.

Nurses in pediatric home health face increasing demands for providing high-quality care with fewer resources to achieve positive patient outcomes. In doing so, the nurse often must rely on *delegation* skills to ensure that the patient and family receive the necessary care. Delegation often involves assigning nursing tasks to other health care workers; therefore the nurse must have good delegation skills as well (Timm, 2003).

Public or private home care agencies that participate in the Medicare or Medicaid programs must be certified by a federally designated, state-certification body and abide by federal and state regulations. In addition, the ANA has developed standards of nursing practice for both community health and home care nurses (ANA, 1986a, 1986b). Generalist and clinical specialist certification in both home health and community health is offered by the ANCC,* a subsidiary of the ANA. The Hospice Nurses Association offers certification in hospice nursing. Despite some important differences between pediatric and adult care in the home, as of this writing, no national standards specific to pediatric home care nursing practice have been developed. Nursing practice in pediatric home care should be guided by published guidelines, textbooks, peer-reviewed articles related to pediatric home care, and written standards of care for pediatric patients (Box 43-6). In addition, professional nursing organizations such as the Infusion Nurses Society (INS), the National Association of Neonatal Nurses (NANN), the Society of Pediatric Nurses (SPN), the Association of Pediatric Oncology Nurses (APON), the National Association of Pediatric Nurse Practitioners (NAPNAP), and others have published standards of care that apply to pediatric home health nursing practice.

The Outcome and Assessment Information Set (OASIS), as part of Medicare, has been established for adults in home health care; however, as of this writing there are no such data for children younger than age 18. As a part of OASIS, home health care quality measures have been established to measure patient care outcomes for Medicare reimbursement purposes. Other certification/licensing organizations that may oversee and regulate practice in home health include the Joint Commission on Accreditation of Healthcare Organizations (JCAHO), the Centers for Medicare/Medicaid Services (CMS) (formerly HCFA), the Occupational Safety and Health Administration (OSHA), and the Community Health Accreditation Program (CHAP). The new Health Insurance Portability and Accountability Act (HIPAA) guidelines affect the way patient records are handled in home health care to ensure patient confidentiality.

BOX 43-5

Qualities of a Pediatric Home Care Nurse

Demonstrates flexibility in skills and case management
Recognizes that the nurse is a guest in the home
Respects family culture and adapts appropriately
Works as an interdisciplinary team member
Demonstrates expertise in pediatric care (assessment and technical skills)

FAMILY-CENTERED HOME CARE

Technology dependence, chronic illness, and complex care requirements cross social, cultural, spiritual, and economic boundaries. Regardless of a family's background, family values must be respected in the provision of home care services. *The home is the family's domain,* and the child is at home because the family's central role is to nurture and raise their child. The ultimate responsibility for managing the child's health, developmental, and emotional needs lies with the family. Roush and Cox (2000) developed a framework for helping the home health care nurse understand the significance of the home to the family. The three central concepts of the model are as follows (Roush & Cox, 2000):

1. Home as familiar—the environment where one is comfortable and at ease because of the familiarity with living arrangements and routines of home
2. Home as center—the location of everyday experiences related to time, space, and one's social life

*ANCC, c/o ANA, 600 Maryland Ave. SW, Suite 100-W, Washington, DC 20024-2571; phone: 202-651-7000, 800-284-2378; Web site: www.nursingworld.org/ancc.

3. Home as protector—privacy, safety, and identity may be preserved in the environment of the home

The nurse must respect and encourage the family's central role in the care of the child and must work in collaboration with the family in efforts to care for the child. Family-centered nursing practice is essential in the home setting. Family-centered care has become acknowledged as the standard of care for children with special health care needs (Johnson, 2000).

The philosophic basis for family-centered practice is the recognition that the family is the constant in the child's life, whereas the service systems and personnel within those systems fluctuate. Professionals working with the families of children with complex chronic problems must respect the family's central, caring role; their knowledge; and their particular and unique expertise. Families have the most intimate knowledge of the child's strengths and abilities, the challenges of providing care, and the abilities and needs of other family members. Believing that no one knows the child better than the family is critical to the success of any health care plan.

BOX 43-6

Selected Resources for Home Care

American Academy of Pediatrics
141 Northwest Point Blvd.
Elk Grove Village, IL 60007-1098
Phone: 847-434-4000
Fax: 847-434-8000
Web site: www.aap.org

Association of Maternal and Child Health Programs
1220 19th St. NW
Suite 801
Washington, DC 20036
Phone: 202-775-0436
Fax: 202-775-0061
Web site: www.amchp.org

Children's Hospice International
901 N. Pitt St., Suite 230
Alexandria, VA 22314
Phone: 800-24-CHILD
Fax: 703-684-0226
Web site: www.chionline.org

National Association for Home Care
228 Seventh St. SE
Washington, DC 20003
Phone: 202-547-7424
Fax: 202-547-3540
Web site: www.nahc.org
(A special feature on the Web site is peds@home, an electronic newsletter.)

National Father's Network
16120 NE 8th St.
Bellevue, WA 98008-3937
Phone: 206-747-4404, ext. 218
Web site: www.fathersnetwork.org

National Information Center for Children and Youth with Disabilities
PO Box 1492
Washington, DC 20013-1492
Phone: 202-884-8200 (voice/TTY) or 800-695-0285 (voice/TTY)
Fax: 202-884-8441
Web site: www.nichcy.org

Pediatric Home Care Association of America
Division of National Association for Home Care
228 Seventh St., SE
Washington, DC 20003
Phone: 202-547-7424
Fax: 202-547-3540
Web site: www.nahc.org

Pediatric Nursing.com
Health Resources for Parents
Web site: www.pediatricnursing.com/parents/

Sibling Support Project
The Arc of the United States
6512 23rd Ave. NW, Suite 213
Seattle, WA 98117
Phone: 206-297-6368
Web site: www.thearc.org/siblingsupport/

Respect for Diversity

Respect for varied family structures and for racial, ethnic, cultural, spiritual, and socioeconomic diversity among families is essential in home care (see also Chapters 31 and 32). Home care nurses work in close relationship with family members and in the family's own domain. The nurse shares in these relationships, participating in care throughout the course of illness (Family Focus box). The family's background and their lifestyle choices are respected. Particular attention is given to

Family Focus

DEVELOPING RELATIONSHIPS WITH CULTURALLY DIVERSE FAMILIES

I work in the inner city, and my home care patients come from a variety of racial and ethnic backgrounds. I am Caucasian, from Australia. Often, when I first visit a family, there is an initial coolness or apprehension toward me. This is understandable because I am a stranger, and perhaps families think I'll judge them in one way or another. By the end of the first visit, however, there is usually a smile as I leave; by the second visit they often greet me with a smile at the door; and by the third visit we usually have a friendship, a trust, and an ease of communication.

If I'm working on a case for an extended time, I use a holistic nursing approach. This involves being aware of how the illness of the child affects the entire family. As I listen over many weeks to their fears and questions, and often as I share faith perspectives, a bond begins to form. I find it a privilege to share in their joys and their pain, and I feel rewarded by the trust that they invest in me.

Julie Edgerton, RN
Home Care Nurse
Children's National Medical Center
Washington, DC

Modified from Ahmann E: Thinking critically about family-centered home care nursing, *Pediatr Nurs* 20(6):588-590, 1994.

communication. The meaning of words used and the way they are said may affect various cultural groups in different ways. Families may also differ in their cultural views of children; health care; childrearing practices; and illness, its causes, and its meaning. The family's health care practices and beliefs may influence the level of investment a family will make in the child's care. The family's *religion* or spirituality is another factor that can have a major influence on a family's response to the child's special health care needs. The family will often look for spiritual meaning and purpose for the illness. Other families may choose to reject past religious ties. In some cultures, religion and beliefs about health care and illness are closely intertwined (McEvoy, 2003); thus it is important that home care nurses assess the relationships among culture, religion, and the family's beliefs about the child's illness.

A variety of cultural assessment tools are available (Giger & Davidhizar, 2002; Spruhan, 1996). The home care nurse, aware that *personal values* drive behavior, must learn about the family's culture, ask questions without implying judgment, interpret the mainstream medical culture, and help families design interventions that meet their preferences. When possible, culture-specific teaching materials should be used. Increased emphasis in health care in the United States has been placed on health care workers becoming culturally competent to effectively deliver holistic care to their patients. Home care nurses are challenged to become culturally competent to better understand the patient populations they serve (National Center for Cultural Competence, 2002).

NURSE ALERT Color-coded medication bottles, written schedules, and pillboxes or oral syringes may aid compliance with prescription administration. One should not assume that everyone who speaks English, as a primary or secondary language, is able to adequately read the language. Pictures or special symbols may be helpful when providing instructions for procedures and medication administration. ■

Respect for family diversity and awareness of both family developmental stages (see Chapter 31) and the stages of a family's adjustment to illness in a child (see Chapter 41) will assist the home care nurse in recognizing and promoting family strengths and in respecting varied coping mechanisms. Labels such as "dysfunctional," "difficult," and "noncompliant" can reinforce negative expectations and shape behaviors of both parents and professionals. On the other hand, emphasizing, identifying, and building on family strengths and coping mechanisms are strategies that promote a central goal in nursing care of the child and family: *family empowerment* (see Chapter 29). The nurse working with families should remain flexible and open-minded because new family strengths may emerge over time and coping mechanisms may wax and wane with the stresses of caring for a child with serious or multiple problems.

Parent-Professional Collaboration

Family-centered nursing practice is built on a foundation of parent-professional collaboration, which represents a shift from the traditional unidirectional relationships between health care providers and families. The *Collaborative Family Health Care Coalition* has developed core competencies for professionals collaborating with families (McDaniel & Campbell, 1996). *Collaborative caring* allows the nurse and family to work together and share outcomes in a deep and meaningful way. This approach, essential in the home care setting, is characterized by the following (Gaudet, 1997; Kellett & Mannion, 1999):

- Encouraging activities to develop self-confidence and self-esteem
- Displaying increased awareness of and respect for family caregivers
- Recognizing that families vary in defining their role
- Demonstrating an ability to understand the family's approach to caregiving
- Sharing perspectives, not just tasks and functions
- Supporting family members in their primary, irreplaceable role as caregivers
- Exchanging expertise in providing care to the child
- Assisting families in recognizing their contributions as worthwhile
- Identifying strengths and resources of child and family
- Negotiating options, priorities, and preferences
- Assisting with coping by allowing families to find meaning in caring for patient at home

Communication with the family should not be intrusive. There is no need to collect information from the family that can be obtained from the child's records. The nurse should explain to the family the reason for questions, particularly those that the family may perceive as intrusive, and should inform families of who will have access to the information. The nurse must also assure families that they have a right to expect confidentiality in regard to the data collected. When working in the home, the nurse must respect the privacy of family members' communications with each other that may be overheard.

NURSE ALERT Home care nurses should restrict their communications with other professionals to clinically relevant information about the family. ■

Home care nurses should respect the family's control of their own environment. The Guidelines box addresses "house rules" that can be negotiated.

Communication with family members should also include sharing with the family, in a supportive manner, complete and unbiased information about all aspects of the child's condition and care. Repeated explanations in simple language may be necessary. Information should be shared with families in a way that will have meaning in their cultural context. Many parents report a preference for interactions with professionals who communicate empathy and concern.

On occasion, disagreements may arise between parents and nurses over proper procedures for care of the child. Nurses should respect parental preferences in any situation that will not pose danger or risk for the child (Family Focus box). If parents wish to alter a plan of treatment that is part of medical orders, the nurse should ask that they negotiate

Guidelines

NEGOTIATING "HOUSE RULES" FOR HOME CARE

House Rules

Parking: Where to park and community regulations.
Access: Where to enter the home. Is knocking preferred or ringing the bell?
Personal belongings: Where does the nurse store own coat, boots, etc.? Does the family prefer slippers to shoes in the home?
Meals: Where may the nurse store own food? NOTE: This is very important given cultural diversity of clients.
Radio and television: Identify preferences regarding usage. Remember, this may help nurses to remain awake at night.
Patient room: The nurse is responsible for the child's immediate environment. Maintaining a clean working area and cleaning up the room at the end of the shift is the nurse's responsibility.
Telephone: Agency policy may dictate that all personal calls be limited to very brief periods and charged to the nurse making them. NOTE: Many nurses do need to check in with home at some interval during the evening.
Visitors: Identify who may enter the home when the parents are away (that is, child's friends or grandparents). A list of names should be available.
Privacy: Describe what parts of the home are off-limits to the nurse and at what times.

Child

Routine: Specify times for playtime, bathtime, and bedtime. What does the parent want to participate in regarding these routines?
Mealtime: Specify where the family wants the child fed; if tube fed, specify a preference as to how and where it is done.
Clothing: Identify who picks out the child's clothes. Identify where the laundry is and who is responsible for washing the sick child's clothing.
Discipline: Discuss specific guidelines for discipline.
Homework: Discuss when it should be done and who is responsible for it being completed.

Siblings

Discipline: Establish guidelines regarding how parents should be informed of siblings' conflicts and how discipline should be handled. NOTE: Parents or another caregiver must be in the home when siblings are home.
Patient care: Be specific regarding how children have helped with the child's care. Discuss any concerns regarding behavior that may compromise the child's or siblings' safety.

Nursing

Parental notification: Specify what information the family wishes to be aware of immediately and what can wait until they are home.
Limits of responsibility: Specify duties the nurse may not perform, such as transportation of the child to care facilities, or babysitting the siblings.
Environment: Discuss the need to have adequate lighting and a comfortable working area.

Modified from Klug R: Clarifying roles and expectations in home care, *Pediatr Nurs* 19(4):375, 1993.

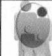

Family Focus

KNOWLEDGEABLE PARENTS

It is not unusual for parents, particularly those whose children have chronic illnesses or complex care regimens, to be more knowledgeable about their child's condition than a nurse who is assigned to the child's care. This can be disconcerting for both the parent(s) and the nurse. It is important to remember and reinforce that, regardless of the condition, parents will always know more about their child than the professional caring for the child. The nurse and parents can set goals for care in an atmosphere of mutual respect. If the parents' goal is respite from prolonged caregiving, they are less likely to want to give long explanations about their child's care, and assistance from an experienced peer may be more appropriate for the nurse to seek. If the parents wish to maintain maximum participation in care delivery, the nurse and the parents can negotiate the collaboration.

When teaching parents to perform complex chronic care regimens at home, include teaching them to expect to know more about their child's care than professionals who may come to assist them, whether that be home health, hospital, or outpatient personnel. At the same time, assure them that what various professionals who work with them will have from working with a multitude of families is a scientific knowledge base and a wealth of options for addressing and solving care problems.

Teresa L. Hall, MS, RN
Hathaway Children's Services
Sylmar, CA

the change with the physician or practitioner, because the nurse must follow the written medical orders. If disagreements cannot be resolved, a home care supervisor or case manager should be contacted to assist with problem solving.

Increasingly, home care agencies are developing ethics committees and policies for managing difficult situations such as treatment refusal (Critical Thinking Exercise).

The Nursing Process

In the home the family is a partner in each step of the nursing process. Assessment should address family strengths and resources (see Family Assessment, Chapter 34). The principles of communication discussed previously guide data collection. The nurse's observations are shared neutrally, without value judgment, and in a way that preserves the family's own role in decision making.

All the information gathered as part of the assessment process is shared with the family. The nurse should recognize that the family's perception of their most important need will generally guide their behavior and consume their attention and energy. Family priorities should guide the planning process.

Both short-term and long-term goals should be outlined and agreed on by the child, family, and professionals involved. The plan of care should integrate various disciplines that may be involved with the child in order to eliminate duplication, coordinate and consolidate care requirements. Cross-training of professionals and a transdisciplinary mode of treatment can also be useful when a child has multiple and complex care requirements. Physical or occupational therapy routines may be incorporated into the child's morning nursing procedures, or speech therapy interventions may be conducted by the parent or nurse around eating times so that the entire day is not occupied by procedures. A written schedule of daily routines should be developed and followed by all caregivers.

Critical Thinking Exercise

FAMILY-CENTERED HOME CARE AND CONFLICTS

A family wants to begin oral feeding of their 3-year-old daughter, Sarah, who is ventilator dependent, with a tracheostomy, and is being tube fed through a skin-level gastrostomy feeding tube (Mic-Key). The mother, who has assumed the role of being Sarah's primary caretaker, is adamant about starting oral feedings so that Sarah can be more like other children her age. One day the mother asks you, the nurse case manager overseeing the child's home care, to feed Sarah baby food by mouth to see how she tolerates the feeding. The child is alert and sociable yet cannot communicate her wishes except through crying and whining. She has a seizure disorder and has had several episodes of aspiration pneumonia since birth. Sarah appears to have a considerable amount of tongue thrusting and copious amounts of oral mucus that must be suctioned frequently to prevent aspiration; her cough reflex is compromised and usually only elicited with tracheal suctioning.

1. Evidence—Is there sufficient evidence to draw any conclusions about the issue of feeding Sarah at this time?
2. Assumptions—Describe some underlying assumptions about the following:
   a. Sarah's readiness for oral feedings
   b. Sarah's ability to tolerate oral feedings
   c. The mother's request for Sarah to start oral feedings
3. What implications and priorities for nursing care may be drawn at this time?
4. Does the evidence objectively support your argument (conclusion)?
5. Are there alternative perspectives to your arguments? What are they?

NURSE ALERT At each home visit, physically handle and look at all medications. Check them against the medical orders and read the labels. There may be discrepancies, duplications, or changes between hospitalizations. Clarify medication purpose, effect, and dosages with the family and physician (as necessary). ■

Goals of care are supported by intervention strategies that reflect normalization (see Chapter 41) and the interests and abilities of the child and family. Nurses can help families explore a range of alternative strategies, services, and resources so that the family can choose the best match for their situation.

Family participation in evaluating a home care plan can occur on several levels. Families and care providers should regularly review the goals of care and then update the care plan as required. The nurse can also ask the family open-ended questions at regular intervals to assess their opinions on the effectiveness of care. As part of the evaluation process, families should be acknowledged for their successes and accomplishments. Finally, families should be given an opportunity to evaluate individual home care nurses, the home care agency, and other service providers on a periodic basis. The evaluation should address the nurse's knowledge, skills, and respect for the family's choices. It also should address the agency's handling of the schedule, provision of qualified nurses, and problem-solving abilities. The evaluations should be used by the agency to improve quality of care (Family Focus box).

Home care nursing encourages a close and rewarding relationship with the family. One of the most important aspects of this relationship is maintaining professional boundaries and a therapeutic role that is supportive but not intrusive. In addition to maintaining control over their child's care, families need to control their homes and personal lives. Nurses should discuss "house rules" with the family and address issues such as physical environment, private areas in the home, responsibility for maintaining the child's environment, and interactions with siblings and extended family members (Critical Thinking Exercise).

Technologic trends that influence the nursing process in home care include the use of *laptop computers (notebooks)* to document the home visit; *personal data assistants (PDAs),* or small handheld computers that store large amounts of data, including addresses, appointments, patient tracking systems, textbooks, and important data such as pharmacologic databases (Lewis & Sommers, 2003); *Internet and e-mail* services, which increase patient-practitioner accessibility and communication; and *telemedicine or telehealth,* which has various features, including electronic systems that can transmit physiologic data directly to the practitioner via the telephone. The American Nurses Association (1999) has established a list of competencies for nurses involved in telehealth technology. *Telephone triage* has become standard in many health care institutions, and standards for triage have been published elsewhere (Schmitt, 2004).

Promotion of Optimal Development, Self-Care, and Education

There is little question that living at home offers most children with complex medical problems great social and emotional advantages over living in the hospital or another insti-

Family Focus

WHAT I LEARNED ABOUT HOME CARE

I learned many things as a result of having home care for four children over a period of 8 years. Two of the major areas I learned about were communication and families' rights. It took a long time to learn some of these things.

Initially I tried very hard to be sensitive to the professionals and often put my own feelings and needs aside. It took a while to learn that I could stand up for myself and my family and that my child could continue to receive good care. One area that was important to me was to have nurses withhold judgment on our parenting style, even if they might have parented differently.

Communication needs to be open and two-way. Families and nurses ought to tell each other what is going well. For example, "Thanks for keeping the room so neat while you're here" can help a nurse see a family's appreciation. There was so little I could do as just "Mommy" that it really meant a lot to me when nurses would say, "That's such a cute outfit you picked out for him today." Communicating about little things, even inconsequential topics such as favorite TV shows, makes it easier to communicate about more important things and about problems. Communication has to be open about problems, too.

Jeni Stepanek
Mother
Upper Marlboro, MD

Critical Thinking Exercise

MAINTAINING THERAPEUTIC BOUNDARIES

As the home care nurse who has been working with a 4-year-old ventilator-dependent child, Derek, weekly for about 5 months, you are aware that the parents have become increasingly argumentative with each other. Most of the arguments are about whether Mr. Jones helps enough with the child's care and the housecleaning. Mr. Jones works full time at one job and supplements the family income by working at a part-time job every weekend. Ms. Jones approaches you to complain about her husband's lack of involvement with the child and his care. Derek requires constant care, and the family has many expenses related to his physical care; the child is severely developmentally impaired and is not expected to improve significantly despite numerous medical interventions. He is the only child, although Ms. Jones stated that at one time they wanted to have many children.

1. Evidence–Is there sufficient evidence to draw any conclusions about the family situation at this time?
2. Assumptions–Describe some underlying assumptions about the following:
   a. Home care of the child with a chronic, terminal condition (see Ch. 41)
   b. Impact of the child's chronic condition, prognosis, and required care on the parents
   c. Status of the marriage relationship between Mr. and Ms. Jones
3. What implications and priorities for nursing care may be drawn at this time?
4. Does the evidence objectively support your argument (conclusion)?
5. Are there alternative perspectives to your arguments? What are they?

tutional setting. However, in infancy and throughout the developmental stages, a child's medical condition(s) and the dependence on medical technology can place constraints on and pose challenges to *normal development.* For example, the child may have lengthy and repeated hospitalizations; developmental regression can occur in response to stress; fatigue may be due to underlying pathology, the recurrence of an illness, or medication side effects; and equipment requirements may impede mobility, exploration, and independence. The challenge of providing support for normal development in a child who is chronically ill and technology dependent is to optimize opportunities for developmentally appropriate experiences within the constraints posed by the medical condition and the equipment requirements.

Home care plans are designed to promote optimal child development through initial and periodic assessment, planning, and referrals for further assessment or therapeutic services, and by interventions that address normalization issues and self-care. (See Chapter 41 for a discussion of normalization.) General principles for a family-centered assessment and planning process have been addressed earlier in this chapter and are applied in developmental assessment and planning as well.

Some parents may not pursue early developmental intervention because they do not view their child as needing the services. In this case professionals need to explain the child's developmental needs to parents in ways that are meaningful from the parents' own cultural and socioeconomic perspectives. Only then can parents make truly informed decisions. After parents have been fully informed of the child's condition, likely developmental sequelae, and the expected benefits of intervention, developmental goals outlined by the child and family should guide planning and intervention.

Several principles underlie appropriate developmental intervention plans for children with complex medical problems. First, understanding a child's medical condition ensures that the nurse and family can plan to maximize developmental opportunities at times when the child has the most energy and endurance and when stress signals that determine the child's tolerance for type, intensity, and duration of activity will be noted. Second, plans for developmental support should be flexible and tailored to the individual child's abilities, interests, and needs. Third, familiarity with the child's medical equipment facilitates the planning of creative ways to meet the child's developmental needs. For example, the use of lengthy oxygen tubing allows the active toddler freedom of movement during the day (Fig. 43-2); portable equipment of any type facilitates family outings; and mounting a ventilator to a wheelchair allows the adolescent greater independence.

Promoting coping and capability can buffer stress and contribute to mental health and self-esteem in a child with chronic illness. The extent to which a child is involved in his or her own care depends on many factors, including the child's developmental age, level of interest, and physical ability, as well as parental comfort and support. *Self-care,* both in activities of daily living and in regard to the medical condition, is important. The frame of reference for self-care in activities of daily living should be the goal of attaining age-appropriate competence. Some modifications in the environment, the medical equipment, or the techniques for daily

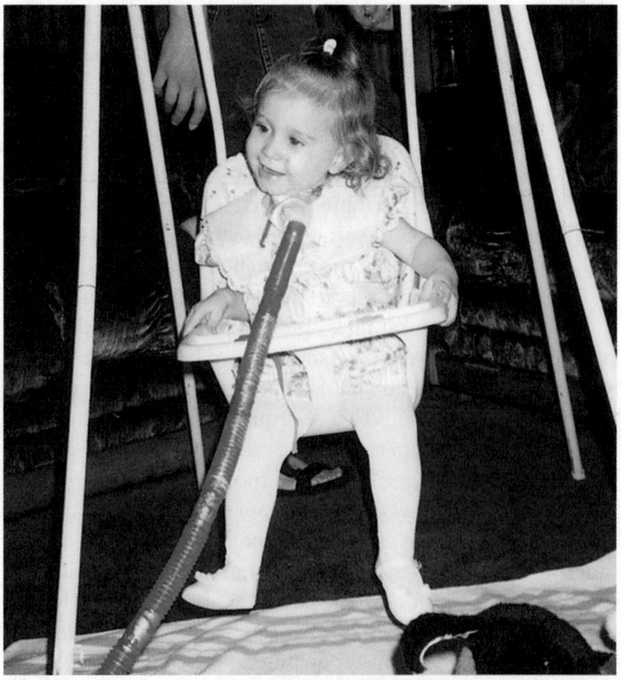

Fig. 43-2 Use of lengthy tubing facilitates a child's freedom of movement.

activities may be required to promote and support self-care. Effective teaching for self-care is focused at the child's own level of conceptual understanding and may be augmented by the use of dolls, other models and diagrams, simple explanations, and repetition.

Educational planning is important for the child who has a chronic medical condition. Federal laws ensure that all children receive a public education. Before age 3, children with developmental delays are eligible for an *early-intervention program.* The child can receive rehabilitation therapies as appropriate (e.g., physical, occupational, or speech therapy; speech pathology). After age 3, the local school system is responsible for providing this education. Some children may be eligible for special education preschools. The home care nurse should refer the family to local county programs.

Each family is entitled to an *individual family service plan (IFSP)* to help ensure early intervention. All states in the United States provide agencies that develop IFSPs; each state's plan can easily be accessed via the Internet by entering the term *individual family service plan* in an Internet search engine such as Yahoo or Google. The IFSP provides the child with disability from birth to age 3 years with a plan for integrating early intervention and rehabilitation, based on the child's and the family's needs.

When a child requiring special medical care is to be placed in an educational setting, the parents, child, school health coordinator, educational evaluation team, and education and administrative staff should meet to determine safe and appropriate placement and necessary services and personnel to enable the child to attend school in the least restrictive environment. Training of educational staff and caregivers is essential to ensuring the child's safety in the educational setting.* Special assistance can also be beneficial in reintegrating previously schooled children, such as those with cancer, into the school setting. The home care nurse may need to assist parents in developing the skills necessary to advocate effectively for their child in the educational system.

Consultation with a child-life specialist may also be arranged and can be of great assistance to the nurse and family.

Safety Issues in the Home

Safety is an important consideration in pediatric home care and should be addressed in the home care plan. First, before hospital discharge, emergency preparations must be made.

NURSE ALERT If the family does not have a telephone, arrangements may be made with the telephone company to supply service. Alternatively, one or two nearby neighbors may agree to let the family use their services. In rural areas, a local pharmacy or police or ranger station may be willing to receive messages and relay them to the family. A cell phone may be used in place of a local telephone, but it is advisable to check with the local emergency facilities regarding policies for cell phone use and emergency 911 calls. ■

The telephone and electric companies (if use of medical equipment requires electricity) are notified that the family needs to be placed on a priority service list so that the family will learn of any anticipated interruptions in service and receive priority in reinstatement of interrupted services. Prior contact with rescue squad and local emergency facility personnel can help ensure prompt and appropriate interventions if required.

Before hospital discharge, emergency protocols are developed and reviewed with both the parents and the professional caregivers. Cardiopulmonary resuscitation (CPR) guidelines, if appropriate, should be posted near the child's bedside or in another accessible location. A list of emergency telephone numbers can be placed near each home phone and should include those of the rescue squad, emergency department, managing physician(s), nursing agency, and equipment vendor(s). Additional issues to consider are *advance directives* and *out-of-hospital do not resuscitate (OHDNR)* orders (may vary by state), as indicated. If the patient and family desire advance directives to be enforced, specific guidelines must be followed that could potentially prevent undesired lifesaving measures for children with a terminal illness.

Another aspect of safety relates to the provision of care by appropriately trained individuals. Family members should receive thorough training in the child's care requirements and have the opportunity to demonstrate knowledge and confidence before hospital discharge. Professional staff caring for the child should have the appropriate background and training for the child's particular care needs. Because of the child's body size, special skill and caution are required both in performing procedures (e.g., gastrostomy feedings and suctioning) and in monitoring the use of equipment (e.g., ventilator settings, intravenous flow rates, total fluid volumes) (see Chapter 45).

The activity level and curiosity of young children raise additional safety considerations in the provision of home care. All medications, needles, and syringes, and any contaminated materials, are securely stored well out of the reach of curious hands. Special attention is paid to childproofing the control panels for ventilators, pumps, monitors, and other equipment. Use of clear plastic tape, covers, or panels to cover control knobs or buttons reduces the risk of accidental changes in settings. Much of the medical equipment now in use has special lockout capabilities that may be used to prevent accidentally altering settings. Care must be taken to prevent accidental strangulation on apnea, oximeter, or cardiac monitor wires or lengthy intravenous tubing during sleep. Electrical cords are kept short and out of reach, and safety covers are used on any open outlets. When not in use, equipment is unplugged, and any wires (e.g., lead wires for an apnea monitor) are stored out of reach.

NURSE ALERT Coiling extra tubing and taping it at the exit site, as well as running wires or tubes out of the bottoms of pajamas, is a precaution against strangulation. ■

*A thorough discussion of training issues, content, and guidelines for care in the school is provided in Porter S et al (editors): *Children and youth assisted by medical technology in educational settings: guidelines for care,* ed 2, Baltimore, 1997, Paul H. Brookes; Web site: www.pbrookes.com.

Care at night poses other safety concerns. Parents and other caregivers need to be able to clearly hear monitor, ventilator, or pump alarms at night; an inexpensive intercom system or a baby monitor can be used.

Safe transportation is a vitally important concern. Wheelchairs and other medical equipment must be properly secured to the vehicle, including vans and buses. Appropriate child restraints must be used at all times. If necessary, an extra adult should be present to monitor the child while in transit. Additional information on car safety and general health supervision is provided in Chapter 41 (see Educate about the Disorder and General Health Care).

Family-to-Family Support

Family-to-family support networks can be an important source of emotional and instrumental support and empowerment for families of children with chronic health problems. Family-to-family support does not replace professional sources of support but rather is a unique resource promoting family strengths through shared experience. Families will most likely experience increased emotional stress as a result of living with and caring for a child with special needs. Identifying meaningful sources of support can make a difference in coping abilities. The home health nurse can assist the family in increasing their involvement in community social networks. Informal support networks can be extremely beneficial. A link to a family in the same or similar situation allows the sharing of common experiences. Positive outcomes may include understanding, empathy, problem solving, or just talking to someone who will listen. The nurse should remember that the needs of each family member differ. The care plan should acknowledge each family member's needs. Peer support for school-age children and adolescents with complex care needs may be beneficial. These connections can be expanded to include letter writing, e-mails, phone calls, or specialty camping programs (Johnson, Ravert, & Everton, 2001).

Key Points

- Effective home care depends on many factors, including the child's relative medical stability; the family's willingness, training, and ability to accommodate the child's care requirements; and professional, financial, and community support.
- Comprehensive, multidisciplinary discharge planning should begin early and should include the family and a home care representative in addition to hospital personnel.
- Thorough training of the family, including a trial of care, a predischarge pass to home, and a predischarge home visit, can ease the transition to home.
- Care coordination ensures continuity of care and reduces duplication and fragmentation of services. The family may assume varying degrees of care coordination over time.
- The home care nurse must share a level of technical expertise with the critical care nurse while being able to adapt equipment, procedures, and the nursing process to the home setting. Education and training are increasingly important.
- Federal standards apply to agencies that participate in Medicare or Medicaid; standards of practice by the American Nurses Association can guide nurses in the home setting.
- Specialist and generalist credentialing is available for home care nurses.
- Family-centered nursing practice is applied in the home setting; diversity in family structures, cultural backgrounds, strengths, and coping mechanisms is respected.
- Collaborative relationships are characterized by communication, dialogue, active listening, awareness and acceptance of difference, and negotiation.
- The nursing process is adapted to involve the family in each step and to preserve the family's central role in decision making.
- "House rules" agreed on by the nurse and family allow a family to maintain a feeling of control over the home environment when professionals are present.
- Home care plans are designed to promote optimal development of the child and focus on normalization; on the impact of the child's medical condition and technologic requirements on development; on self-care; and on educational needs.
- Safety in the provision of home care services involves emergency preparations and protocols, appropriate training of family and home care personnel, and safe use and child-proofing of medical equipment.
- Family-to-family support networks can provide emotional and instrumental support and encourage family empowerment.

Answer Guidelines to Critical Thinking Exercises

Family-Centered Home Care and Conflicts

1. Yes, there is sufficient evidence to arrive at some possible conclusions (see Ch. 45, Feeding the sick child, and Box 47-5, Clinical Manifestation of Gastrointestinal Dysfunction in Children.) Sarah demonstrates tongue thrusting, which is common in healthy children from 0 to 4 or 5 months. The extrusion reflex is common in children who have little experience with oral feedings and oral stimulation.
2. (a) Given Sarah's history and assessment data, there are risks involved in starting oral feedings with Sarah, primarily choking and aspiration. (b) The mother's request is not unusual. Parents want the best for their children despite handicaps that often set them apart from other children. Although it may seem complicated to engage in communication, negotiation, and consultation over the seemingly simple issue of giving baby food to a 3-year-old, many issues must be considered. (c) The family appears to have legitimate reasons for wanting their daughter started on baby foods. The nurse should further explore reasons for wanting the child to be fed orally. They may feel that health care providers have overlooked

this aspect of normal development. The implications may be that the family is attempting to assist their daughter in achieving age-appropriate skills and may also want their daughter to participate in family mealtimes. These are legitimate, commendable goals, and the family should be supported in making such choices for their child.

3. A child who is 3 years old and has not been fed orally will benefit from an oral-motor assessment by an occupational therapist/speech therapist (OT/ST) to explore the possibility of starting minimal oral feedings. Specific plans with incremental steps to reduce oral-motor defensiveness and improve the ability to accept foods orally should precede feeding. Nutritional consultation may also be important as feeding plans shift from gastrostomy to oral feedings. The nurse and the family should continue to discuss the issue, plan for consultations and evaluations related to the child's oral-motor progress, and thereby arrange to meet the family's goals of oral feeding in safer incremental steps. Communication between the nurse and the family may also lead to other approaches to normalizing mealtimes for Sarah and her family. After the assessment has been completed by the OT/ST, specific short- and long-term goals for modified oral feedings may be developed, involving the family in such discussions. In addition, the family should be made aware of potential problems with oral feedings, including aspiration pneumonia or airway obstruction with further respiratory compromise.
4. Yes, the evidence supports implementing this plan of care. The nurse should not dismiss the parents' request for oral feedings, yet should not acquiesce to their request without assessing the situation, developing conclusions based on the assessment, and implementing an appropriate plan of care that may be evaluated by the outcomes. It would not be appropriate to begin oral feedings without first consulting an OT/ST regarding Sarah's oral-motor abilities.
5. Assessment of the child's status may reveal deficiencies that could preclude attempts at oral feedings altogether. In this case it would be important to involve other health care workers in a discussion with the parents regarding the issue of oral feedings. The home health care nurse must remember, however, that the child is the parent's responsibility and the ultimate decision about oral feedings rests with them. Home care issues that produce conflict about what constitutes the best care for the child between the primary caretaker or parents and the health care team must be handled with utmost care because the parents are ultimately responsible for the child. Such conflicts may lead to mistrust and further alienation if not handled properly. Each case should be handled on an individual basis and all available resources used to make the best care possible available to the child.

Maintaining Therapeutic Boundaries

1. Yes—there is sufficient evidence to arrive at some conclusions regarding the situation.
2. (a) Home care of any person, especially a child with a chronic debilitating condition, is stressful on any family regardless of their stability and resources. The seeming lack of coping skills and decreased financial resources make the stress worse. It is not unusual for there to be stress and conflict regarding the child's care, especially if one parent seems to be less involved in the daily care. The needs of the primary caretaker, Ms. Jones, in this instance, are not being met, and she is expressing that frustration to the nurse, who perhaps is perceived as an ally in the situation. (b) The impact of a chronic condition on parents can be devastating and can lead to misunderstandings, competition over the care of the child, and neglect of the feelings of the persons involved (in this case, Mr. and Ms. Jones). Because the child's prognosis is poor, this can further exacerbate feelings of frustration, anger, helplessness, fatigue, and conflict between parents. Parents may feel guilty about their feelings toward the child. On one hand there may be feelings of caring and loving toward the child; on the other hand, the presence of a child with a chronic condition with poor prognosis who requires constant physical care may engender feelings of wanting to see an end to the situation with the child's death. These ambivalent feelings are not unusual in parents, yet it is well known that there is gender difference in how feelings over such conditions are expressed. Unmet expectations are a source of conflict among parents with a child who is sick; expectations of each other's role in the family setting may have suffered with the loss of the "perfect" child. These feelings may last for months or even years without an appropriate resolution if adequate resources for resolution are not provided. (c) The status of the marriage appears to be strained at this time; however, there is not sufficient evidence to draw a simple conclusion without further exploration (assessment). This may be the way each parent deals with crisis situations—the mother fusses and complains and the father withdraws by going to work and being less involved. There may be some anticipatory grieving occurring, but this needs to be explored by health care persons who can be objective and properly evaluate the marriage status.
3. The concept of therapeutic boundaries supports the idea that they are not rigid and fixed. The home care nurse must be responsive to the relationship preferred by the family and the style with which the family operates. Individual roles change according to the expectations that person has about her or his role and the context within which that person is living the role. In this situation it would be appropriate for the nurse to mention that home care can be stressful for a family, indicate that referrals for counseling may be provided if desired by the parents, and listen to and reflect with Ms. Jones about her feelings. Exploring issues such as an additional home care aid to help take care of Derek might be appropriate; this would enable Ms. Jones to take a break from Derek's care and have time to herself. Additional financial aid may be explored by a qualified case manager or social worker so that Mr. Jones would not have to work as much away from home. It is important to explore the couple's feelings regarding Derek's condition and care and their role in providing for him, as well as their relationship with each other. It is not

unusual for families in crisis to become so involved in the care of the child that they forget what their marriage and relationship is about within the context of the crisis. If counseling by another professional is not desired by one or both parties, perhaps other avenues such as family support groups could be explored as an option. For any conclusion you may reach, it would be inappropriate to agree with Ms. Jones that her husband is not helping enough with the child's care. Such an action implies a judgment that is not within the nurse's role to make and undermines rather than supports the family system. Families in crisis often require professional assistance in the form of counseling to explore coping skills and help involve appropriate community resources.

4. There is some preliminary evidence to support the argument that professional help is warranted in this situation. In addition, as the feelings of Mr. and Ms. Jones are explored, additional evidence may be presented that may alter the course of action proposed.
5. Alternative perspectives may arise as more data are obtained during a family interview. It would not be appropriate for the home health care nurse to take sides with Ms. Jones or with Mr. Jones to avoid the main issues, which involve Ms. Jones' sense of isolation in the care of her child.

References

American Academy of Pediatrics: *Care coordination: integrating health and related systems of care for children with special health care needs,* Elk Grove Village, IL, 1999, The Academy.

American Nurses Association: *Standards of community health nursing practice,* Washington, DC, 1986a, The Association.

American Nurses Association: *Standards of home health nursing practice,* Washington, DC, 1986b, The Association.

American Nurses Association: *Nursing case management,* Washington, DC, 1998, The Association.

American Nurses Association: *Competencies for telehealth technologies in nursing,* Washington, DC, 1999, American Nurses Association.

Bakewell-Sachs S et al: Home care considerations for chronic and vulnerable populations, *Nurse Pract Forum* 11(1):65-72, 2000.

Betz CL: Children and youth in out-of-home placements: nursing care opportunities for pediatric nurses, *J Pediatr Nurs* 15(1):1-2, 2000.

Dittbrenner H: Pediatric home care as a viable new service, *Caring* 18(2):12-15, 1999.

Gaudet L: Stress tolerance. In Votroubek WL, Townsend JL (eds): *Pediatric home care,* ed 2, Gaithersburg, MD, 1997, Aspen.

Giger JN, Davidhizar R: The Giger and Davidhizar Transcultural Assessment Model, *J Transcult Nurs* 13(3):185-188, 2002.

Johnson BH: Family-centered care: facing the new millennium: interview by Elizabeth Ahmann, *Pediatr Nurs* 26(1):87-90, 2000.

Johnson KB, Ravert RD, Everton A: Hopkins Teen Central: assessment of an Internet-based support system for children with cystic fibrosis, *Pediatrics* 107(2):e24, 2001.

Kellett UM, Mannion J: Meaning in caring: reconceptualizing the nurse-family carer relationship in community practice, *J Adv Nurs* 29(3):697-703, 1999.

Knafl KA, Deatrick JA: The challenges of normalization for families of children with chronic conditions, *Pediatr Nurs* 28(1):49-53, 56, 2002.

Lewis JA, Sommers CO: Personal data assistants: using new technology to enhance nursing practice, *MCN* 28(2):66-71, 2003.

Lindeke LL et al: Family-centered care coordination for children with special needs across multiple settings, *J Pediatr Health Care* 16(6):290-297, 2002.

Mahony DL, Murphy JM: Neonatal drug exposure: assessing a specific population and services provided by visiting nurses, *Pediatr Nurs* 25(1): 27-34, 108, 1999.

McDaniel SH, Campbell TL: Training for collaborative family healthcare, *Fam Systems Health* 14(2):147-150, 1996.

McEvoy M: Culture and spirituality as an integrated concept in pediatric care, *MCN* 28(1):39-43, 2003.

National Alliance for Caregiving: Family caregiving in the U.S.: findings from a national survey, 1997, The Alliance. Internet document available at www.caregiving.org (accessed April 8, 2005).

National Center for Cultural Competence: Developing cultural competence in health care settings, *Pediatr Nurs* 28(2):133-137, 2002.

Page DR: Pediatric home care: nursing the shortage, *Caring* 20(6):46-47, 2001.

Rice R: Case management and leadership strategies for home care nurses. In Rice R (ed): *Home care nursing practice: concepts and application,* ed 3, St Louis, 2001, Mosby.

Roush CV, Cox JE: The meaning of home: how it shapes the practice of home and hospice care, *Home Healthc Nurse* 18(6):388-394, 2000.

Schmitt BD: *Pediatric telephone protocols: Office version,* ed 10, Elk Grove Village, IL, 2004, American Academy of Pediatrics.

Spruhan JB: Beyond traditional nursing care: cultural awareness and successful home healthcare nursing, *Home Healthc Nurse* 14(6):445-449, 1996.

Thompson J: Pediatric assessment in the home, *Home Healthc Nurse* 18(10):639-646, 2000.

Timm S: Effectively delegating nursing activities in home care, *Home Healthc Nurse* 21(4):260-265, 2003.

Reaction to Illness and Hospitalization

44

LEARNING OBJECTIVES

On completion of this chapter the reader will be able to:

- Identify the stressors of illness and hospitalization for children during each developmental stage.
- List essential priorities of nursing care for a child on admission to the hospital.
- Outline nursing interventions that prevent or minimize the stress of separation during hospitalization.
- Outline nursing interventions that minimize the stress of loss of control during hospitalization.
- Outline nursing interventions that minimize the fear of bodily injury during hospitalization.
- Describe methods of assessing and managing pain in children.
- Outline nursing interventions that support parents, siblings, and family during a child's illness and hospitalization.
- Describe nursing interventions needed when children are admitted to special units such as the emergency department.

ELECTRONIC RESOURCES

Additional information related to the content in Chapter 44 can be found on

the companion website at evolve
http://evolve.elsevier.com/Wong/maternal/
- NCLEX Review Questions
- WebLinks

or the interactive student CD-ROM
Activities for Chapter 44 include the following:
- NCLEX Review Questions
- Critical Thinking Exercise–Discharge Planning
- Nursing Care Plan–The Child in the Hospital
- Nursing Care Plan–The Family of the Ill or Hospitalized Child
- Skill–Admitting a Child to the Health Care System
- Skill–Therapeutic Play

STRESSORS OF HOSPITALIZATION AND CHILDREN'S REACTIONS

Often illness and hospitalization are the first crises children must face. Especially during the early years, children are particularly vulnerable to the crises of illness and hospitalization because (1) stress represents a change from the usual state of health and environmental routine, and (2) children have a limited number of coping mechanisms to resolve stressors (those events that produce stress). Major stressors of hospitalization include separation, loss of control, bodily injury, and pain. Children's reactions to these crises are influenced by their developmental age; their previous experience with illness, separation, or hospitalization; their innate and acquired coping skills; the seriousness of the diagnosis; and the support system available.

Separation Anxiety

The major stress from middle infancy throughout the preschool years, especially for children ages 6 to 30 months, is separation anxiety, also called *anaclitic depression*. The principal behavioral responses to this stressor during early childhood are summarized in Box 44-1.

During the phase of protest, children react aggressively to the separation from the parent. They cry and scream for their parents, refuse the attention of anyone else, and are inconsolable in their grief (Fig. 44-1). During the phase of despair, the crying stops, and depression is evident. The child is much less active, is uninterested in play or food, and withdraws from others (Fig. 44-2).

The third stage is detachment, also called denial. Superficially it appears that the child has finally adjusted to the loss. The child becomes more interested in the surroundings, plays

BOX 44-1

Manifestations of Separation Anxiety in Young Children

Phase of Protest

Observed behaviors during later infancy:
- Cries
- Screams
- Searches for parent with eyes
- Clings to parent
- Avoids and rejects contact with strangers

Additional behaviors observed during toddlerhood:
- Verbally attacks strangers (e.g., "Go away")
- Physically attacks strangers (e.g., kicks, bites, hits, pinches)
- Attempts to escape to find parent
- Attempts to physically force parent to stay

Behaviors may last from hours to days

Protest, such as crying, may be continuous, ceasing only with physical exhaustion

Approach of stranger may precipitate increased protest

Phase of Despair

Observed behaviors:
- Inactive
- Withdraws from others
- Depressed, sad
- Uninterested in environment
- Uncommunicative
- Regresses to earlier behavior (e.g., thumb-sucking, bed-wetting, use of pacifier, use of bottle)

Behaviors may last for variable length of time

Child's physical condition may deteriorate from refusal to eat, drink, or move

Phase of Detachment

Observed behaviors:
- Shows increased interest in surroundings
- Interacts with strangers or familiar caregivers
- Forms new but superficial relationships
- Appears happy

Detachment usually occurs after prolonged separation from parent; rarely seen in hospitalized children

Behaviors represent a superficial adjustment to loss

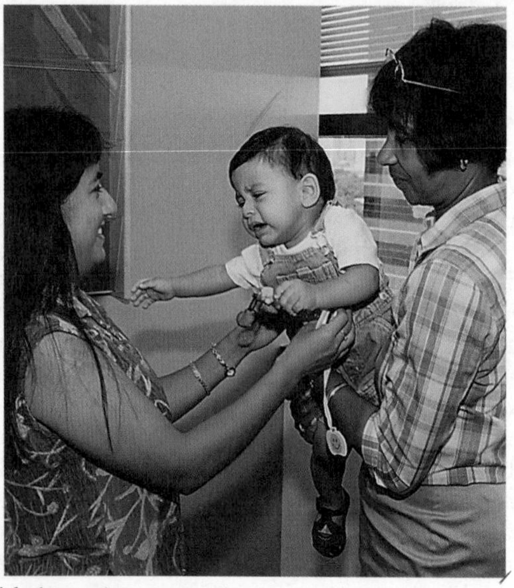

Fig. 44-1 In the protest phase of separation anxiety children cry loudly and are inconsolable.

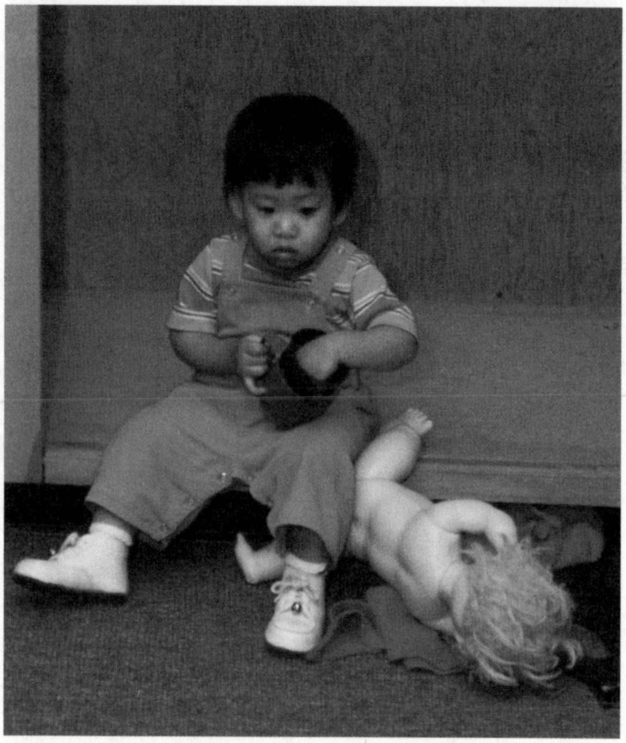

Fig. 44-2 During the despair phase of separation anxiety, children are sad, lonely, and uninterested in food and play.

with others, and seems to form new relationships. However, this behavior is the result of resignation and is not a sign of contentment. The child detaches from the parent in an effort to escape the emotional pain of desiring the parent's presence and copes by forming shallow relationships with others, becoming increasingly self-centered, and attaching primary importance to material objects. This is the most serious stage, in that reversal of the potential adverse effects is less likely to occur once detachment is established. However, in most situations the temporary separations imposed by hospitalization do not cause such prolonged parental absences that the child enters into detachment. In addition, considerable evidence suggests that even with stressors such as separation, children are remarkably adaptable and permanent ill effects are rare.

Although progression to the stage of detachment is uncommon, the initial stages are frequently observed even with very brief separations from either parent. Unless health team members understand the meaning of each stage of behavior, they may erroneously label the behaviors as positive or negative. For example, they may see the loud crying of the protest phase as "bad" behavior. Since the protesting increases when a stranger approaches the child, they may interpret that reaction as meaning they should stay away. During the quiet, withdrawn phase of despair, health team members may think that the child is finally "settling in" to the new surroundings, and they may see the detachment behaviors as proof of a "good adjustment." The faster this stage is reached, the more likely it is that the child will be regarded as the "ideal patient."

Because children seem to react "negatively" to visits by their parents, uninformed observers feel justified in restricting parental visiting privileges. For example, during the protest stage, children outwardly do not appear happy to see their parents. In fact, they may even cry louder. If they are depressed, they may reject their parents or begin to protest once more. Often they cling to their parents in an effort to ensure their continued presence. Consequently, such reactions may be regarded as "disturbing" the child's adjustment to the new surroundings. If the separation has progressed to the phase of detachment, children will respond no differently to their parents than they would to any other person.

Such reactions are distressing to parents, who are unaware of their meaning. If parents are regarded as intruders, they will see their absence as "beneficial" to the child's adjustment and recovery. They may respond to the child's behavior by staying for only short periods, visiting less frequently, or deceiving the child when it is time to leave. The result is a destructive cycle of misunderstanding and unmet needs.

Early Childhood

Separation anxiety is the greatest stress imposed by hospitalization during early childhood. If separation is avoided, young children have a tremendous capacity to withstand any other stress. During this age period, the typical reactions just described are seen. However, children in the toddler stage demonstrate more goal-directed behaviors. For example, they may plead with the parents to stay and physically try to keep the parents with them or try to find parents who have left. They may demonstrate displeasure on the parents' return or departure by having temper tantrums; refusing to comply with the usual routines of mealtime, bedtime, or toileting; or regressing to more primitive levels of development. However, temper tantrums, bed-wetting, or other behaviors may also be expressions of anger or even a physiologic response to stress.

Since preschoolers are more secure interpersonally than toddlers, they can tolerate brief periods of separation from their parents and are more inclined to develop substitute trust in other significant adults. However, the stress of illness usually renders preschoolers less able to cope with separation; as a result, they manifest many of the stage behaviors of separation anxiety, although in general the protest behaviors are more subtle and passive than those seen in younger children. Preschoolers may demonstrate separation anxiety by refusing to eat, experiencing difficulty in sleeping, crying quietly for their parents, continually asking when the parents will visit, or withdrawing from others. They may express anger indirectly by breaking their toys, hitting other children, or refusing to cooperate during usual self-care activities. Nurses need to be sensitive to these less obvious signs of separation anxiety in order to intervene appropriately.

Later Childhood and Adolescence

Previous research, usually based on adult recollections, indicated that the family does not play as important a role for school-age children as it does during the toddler and preschool years. However, in a recent study that asked children about their fears when hospitalized, children ranked "being away from my family" higher than any other fear associated with hospitalization (Wilson & Yorker, 1997). Although school-age children are better able to cope with separation in general, the stress and often accompanying regression imposed by illness or hospitalization may increase their need for parental security and guidance. This is particularly true for young school-age children who have only recently left the safety of the home and are struggling with the crisis of school adjustment. Middle and late school-age children may react more to the separation from their usual activities and peers than to the absence of their parents. These children have a high level of physical and mental activity that frequently finds no suitable outlets in the hospital environment, and even when they dislike school, they admit to missing its routine and worry that they will not be able to compete or "fit in" with their classmates when they return. Feelings of loneliness, boredom, isolation, and depression are common. Such reactions may occur more as a result of separation than from concern over the illness, treatment, or hospital setting.

School-age children may need and desire parental guidance or support from other adult figures but be unable or unwilling to ask for it. Because the goal of attaining independence is so important to them, they are reluctant to seek help directly for fear that they will appear weak, childish, or dependent. Cultural expectations to "act like a man" or to "be brave and strong" bear heavily on these children, especially boys, who tend to react to stress with stoicism, withdrawal, or passive acceptance. Often the need to express hostile, angry, or other negative feelings finds outlets in alternate ways, such as irritability and aggression toward parents, withdrawal from hospital personnel, inability to relate to peers, rejection of siblings, or subsequent behavioral problems in school.

For adolescents, separation from home and parents may be a welcomed and appreciated event. However, loss of peer-group contact may pose a severe emotional threat because of loss of group status, inability to exert group control or leadership, and loss of group acceptance. Deviations within peer groups are poorly tolerated, and although group members may express concern for the adolescent's illness or need for hospitalization, they continue their group activities, quickly filling the gap of the absent member. During the temporary separation from their usual group, ill adolescents may benefit from group associations with other hospitalized age-mates.

Loss of Control

One of the factors influencing the amount of stress imposed by hospitalization is the amount of control that persons perceive themselves as having. Lack of control increases the perception of threat and can affect children's coping skills. Many hospital situations decrease the amount of control a child feels. Although the usual sensory stimulations are lacking, the additional hospital stimuli of sight, sound, and smell may be overwhelming. Without an insight into the type of environment conducive to children's optimum growth, the hospital experience can, at best, temporarily slow development and, at worst, permanently restrict it. Because children's needs vary greatly depending on their age, the major areas of loss of control in terms of physical restriction, altered routine or rituals, and dependency are discussed for each age group.

Infants

Infants are developing the most important attribute of a healthy personality—trust. Trust is established through consistent, loving care by a nurturing person. Infants attempt to control their environment through emotional expressions, such as crying or smiling. In the hospital setting, cues may be missed or misinterpreted, and routines may be established to meet the hospital staff's needs instead of the infant's needs. Inconsistent care and deviations from the infant's daily routine may lead to mistrust and a decreased sense of control.

Toddlers

Toddlers are striving for autonomy, and this goal is evident in most of their behaviors—motor skills, play, interpersonal relationships, activities of daily living, and communication. When their egocentric pleasures meet with obstacles, toddlers react with negativism, especially temper tantrums. Any restriction or limitation of movement, such as the simple act of making toddlers lie down, can cause forceful resistance and noncompliance.

Loss of control also results from altered routines and rituals. Toddlers rely on the consistency and familiarity of daily rituals to provide a measure of stability and control in their complex world of growing and developing. The experience of hospitalization or illness severely limits their sense of expectation and predictability, since practically every detail of the hospital environment differs from that of the home.

Toddlers' main areas for rituals include eating, sleeping, bathing, toileting, and play. When the routines are disrupted, difficulties can occur in any or all of these areas. The principal reaction to such change is regression. For example, when mealtime and food choices differ from those at home, toddlers often refuse to eat, demand a bottle, or ask others to feed them. Although regression to earlier forms of behavior may seem to increase toddlers' security and comfort, in reality it is very threatening for them to relinquish their most recently acquired achievements.

Enforced dependency is a chief characteristic of the sick role and accounts for the numerous instances of toddler negativism. For example, rigid schedules, different clothes, altered caregiving activities, unfamiliar surroundings, separation from parents, and medical procedures usurp toddlers' control over their world. Although most toddlers initially react negatively and aggressively to such dependency, prolonged loss of autonomy may result in passive withdrawal from interpersonal relationships and regression in all areas of development. Therefore the effects of the sick role are most severe in instances of chronic, long-term illnesses or in those families who foster the sick role despite the child's improved state of health.

Preschoolers

Preschoolers also suffer from loss of control caused by physical restriction, altered routines, and enforced dependency. However, their specific cognitive abilities, which make them feel omnipotent and all-powerful, also make them feel out of control. This loss of control in the context of their sense of self-power is a critical influencing factor in their perception of and reaction to separation, pain, illness, and hospitalization.

Preschoolers' egocentric and magical thinking limits their ability to understand events because they view all experiences from their own self-referenced (egocentric) perspective. Without adequate preparation for unfamiliar settings or experiences, preschoolers' fantasy explanations for such events are usually more exaggerated, bizarre, and frightening than the actual facts. One typical fantasy to explain the reason for illness or hospitalization is that it represents punishment for real or imagined misdeeds. In response to such thinking the child usually feels shame, guilt, and fear.

Preschoolers' preoperational thinking means that explanations are understood only in terms of real events. Purely verbal instructions are often inadequate for them because they are unable to abstract and synthesize beyond what their senses tell them. When combined with their egocentric and magical thinking, this characteristic may lead them to interpret messages according to their particular past experiences. Even with the best preparation for a procedure, they may misconstrue the details.

School-Age Children

Because of their striving for independence and productivity, school-age children are particularly vulnerable to events that may lessen their feeling of control and power. In particular, altered family roles; physical disability; fears of death, abandonment, or permanent injury; loss of peer acceptance; lack of productivity; and inability to cope with stress according to perceived cultural expectation may result in loss of control.

Because of the nature of the patient role, many routine hospital activities usurp individual power and identity. For school-age children, dependent activities such as enforced bed rest, use of a bedpan, inability to choose a menu, lack of privacy, help with a bed bath, or transport by a wheelchair or stretcher can be a direct threat to their security. Although all of these procedures seem routine and inconsequential, they allow no freedom of choice to children who want to "act grown-up." However, when children are allowed to exert a measure of control, regardless of how limited it may be, they generally respond very well to any procedure. For example, some of the most cooperative, satisfied, and contented patients are school-age children who help make their beds, choose their schedule of activities, assist in procedures, and help the nurses care for younger children. An increased sense of control usually results from a feeling of usefulness and productivity.

In addition to the hospital environment, illness may also cause a feeling of loss of control. One of the most significant problems of children in this age group centers on boredom. When physical or enforced limitations curtail their usual abilities to care for themselves or to engage in favorite activities, school-age children generally respond with depression, hostility, or frustration. Keeping a normally active child on bed rest is difficult. However, emphasizing areas of control and capitalizing on quiet activities, particularly hobbies such as building models, promote their adjustment to physical restriction.

Adolescents

Adolescents' struggle for independence, self-assertion, and liberation centers on the quest for personal identity. Anything that interferes with this poses a threat to their sense of identity and results in a loss of control. Illness, which limits one's physical abilities, and hospitalization, which separates one from one's usual support systems, constitute major situational crises.

The patient role fosters dependency and depersonalization. Adolescents may react to dependency with rejection, uncooperativeness, or withdrawal. They may respond to depersonalization with self-assertion, anger, or frustration. Regardless of response, hospital personnel often regard them as difficult, unmanageable patients. Parents may not be a source of help, because these behaviors serve to isolate them further from understanding the adolescent. Although peers may visit, they may not be able to offer the kind of support and guidance needed. Sick adolescents often voluntarily isolate themselves from age-mates until they feel they can compete on an equal basis and meet group expectations. As a result, ill adolescents may be left with virtually no support system.

Loss of control also occurs for many of the reasons discussed for school-age children. However, adolescents are more sensitive to potential instances of loss of control and dependency than are younger children. For example, both groups seek information about their physical status and rely heavily on anticipatory preparation to decrease fear and anxiety. However, adolescents react not only to the kinds of information supplied them, but also to the means by which it is conveyed. They may feel very threatened by others who relate facts in a condescending manner. Adolescents want to know that others can relate to them on their own level. This necessitates a careful assessment of their intellectual abilities, previous knowledge, and present needs. It may also require the nurse's willingness to learn the adolescent's language.

Bodily Injury and Pain

Fears of bodily injury and pain are prevalent among children. The consequences of these fears can be far-reaching; adults who experience more medical fear and pain in childhood are more fearful of pain as adults and tend to avoid medical care (Pate et al, 1996).

In caring for children, nurses must have an appreciation of a child's concerns about bodily harm and the reactions to pain at different developmental periods. Table 44-1 summarizes developmental considerations related to children's understanding of illness and pain. Box 44-2 outlines developmental characteristics of children's reactions to pain.

Infants

Infants' responses to pain after the neonatal period are quite similar to earlier reactions, although there is marked variability in measures of distress, especially the initial cry and heart rate, which may decrease in some infants. The most consistent indicator of distress is a facial expression of discomfort (see Fig. 44-3). Infants may express pain by squirming, writhing, jerking, and flailing (Franck, Greenberg, & Stevens, 2000). Some infants may cry loudly after the procedure, whereas others are easily calmed by a gentle hug. It is important to recognize and respect such early signs of individuality and to realize that children who react less intensely may still be experiencing significant discomfort.

Infants less than 6 months of age seem to have no obvious memory of previous painful experiences and react to a potentially stressful situation with less apprehension and fear than older children. After this time, however, children's response to pain is increasingly influenced by their recall of prior painful experiences and the emotional reaction of parents during the procedure. Older infants react intensely, with physical resistance and uncooperativeness. They may refuse to lie still, attempt to push the person away, or try to escape with whatever motor activity they have achieved. Distraction does little to lessen their immediate reaction to pain, and anticipatory preparation, such as showing them the equipment, can increase their fear and resistance (see Neonatal Pain, Chapter 25).

Table 44-1

Children's Developmental Concepts of Illness and Pain

CONCEPT OF ILLNESS*	CONCEPT OF PAIN†
PREOPERATIONAL THOUGHT (2-7 YEARS)	
Phenomenism: Perceives an external, unrelated, concrete phenomenon as cause of illness (e.g., "being sick because you don't feel well") **Contagion:** Perceives cause of illness as proximity between two events that occurs by "magic" (e.g., "getting a cold because you are near someone who has a cold")	Relates to pain primarily as physical, concrete experience Thinks in terms of magical disappearance of pain May view pain as punishment for wrongdoing Tends to hold someone accountable for own pain and may strike out at person
CONCRETE OPERATIONAL THOUGHT (7-10 YEARS†)	
Contamination: Perceives cause as a person, object, or action external to the child that is "bad" or "harmful" to the body (e.g., "getting a cold because you didn't wear a hat") **Internalization:** Perceives illness as having an external cause but as being located inside the body (e.g., "getting a cold by breathing in air and bacteria")	Relates to pain physically (e.g., headache, stomachache) Is able to perceive of psychologic pain (e.g., someone dying) Fears bodily harm and annihilation (body destruction and death) May view pain as punishment for wrongdoing
FORMAL OPERATIONAL THOUGHT (13 YEARS AND OLDER)	
Physiologic: Perceives cause as malfunctioning or nonfunctioning organ or process; can explain illness in sequence of events **Psychophysiologic:** Realizes that psychologic actions and attitudes affect health and illness	Is able to give reason for pain (e.g., fell and hit nerve) Perceives several types of psychologic pain Has limited life experiences to cope with pain as adult might cope despite mature understanding of pain Fears losing control during painful experience

*From Bibace R, Walsh ME: Development of children's concepts of illness, *Pediatrics* 66(6):912-917, 1980.
†From Hurley A, Whelan EG: Cognitive development and children's perception of pain, *Pediatr Nurs* 14(1):21-24, 1988.

BOX 44-2

Developmental Characteristics of Children's Responses to Pain

Young Infant
Generalized body response of rigidity or thrashing, possibly with local reflex withdrawal of stimulated area
Loud crying
Facial expression of pain (brows lowered and drawn together, eyes tightly closed, and mouth open and squarish) (Fig. 44-3)
Demonstrates no association between approaching stimulus and subsequent pain

Older Infant
Localized body response with deliberate withdrawal of stimulated area
Loud crying
Facial expression of pain and/or anger (same facial characteristics as pain but eyes are open)
Physical resistance, especially pushing the stimulus away after it is applied

Young Child
Loud crying, screaming
Verbal expressions of "Ow," "Ouch," "It hurts"
Thrashing of arms and legs
Attempts to push stimulus away before it is applied
Uncooperative; needs physical restraint
Requests termination of procedure
Clings to parent, nurse, or other significant person
Requests emotional support, such as hugs or other forms of physical comfort
May become restless and irritable with continuing pain
All of these behaviors may be seen in anticipation of actual painful procedure

School-Age Child
May see all behaviors of young child, especially during actual painful procedure but less in anticipatory period
Stalling behavior, such as "Wait a minute" or "I'm not ready"
Muscular rigidity, such as clenched fists, white knuckles, gritted teeth, contracted limbs, body stiffness, closed eyes, wrinkled forehead

Adolescent
Less vocal protest
Less motor activity
More verbal expressions, such as "It hurts" or "You're hurting me"
Increased muscle tension and body control

Data from Craig KD et al: Developmental changes in infant pain expression during immunization injections, *Soc Sci Med* 19(12):1331-1337, 1984; and Katz ER, Kellerman J, Siegel SE: Behavioral distress in children with cancer undergoing medical procedures: developmental considerations, *J Consult Clin Psychol* 48(3):356-365, 1980.

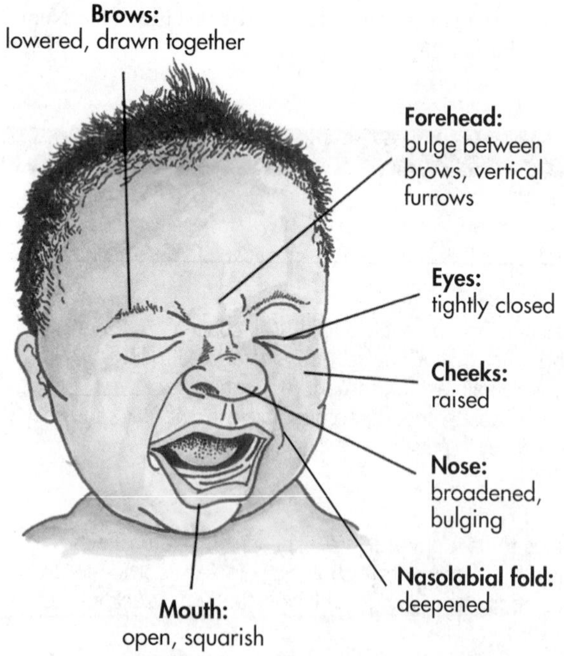

Fig. 44-3 Facial expression of physical distress is the most consistent behavioral indicator of pain in infants.

Toddlers

Toddlers' concept of body image, particularly the definition of body boundaries, is very poorly developed. Intrusive experiences, such as examining the ears or mouth or checking a rectal temperature, produce great anxiety. Toddlers may react to such painless procedures as intensely as they do to painful ones.

Toddlers' reactions to pain are similar to those seen during infancy, except that the number of variables influencing the individual response is highly complex and varied. Memory, physical restraint, separation from parents, emotional reactions of others, and lack of preparation partially determine the intensity of the behavioral response. In general, children in this age group continue to react with intense emotional upset and physical resistance to any actual or perceived painful experience. Behaviors indicating pain include grimacing; clenching their teeth and/or lips; opening their eyes wide; rocking; rubbing; and acting aggressively such as biting, kicking, hitting, or running away. Unlike adults, who usually decrease their activity when in pain, young children typically become restless and overly active; frequently this response is not recognized as a consequence of pain.

By the end of this age period, toddlers usually are able to communicate about their pain. Although they have not developed the ability to describe the type or intensity of the pain, they usually are able to localize it by pointing to a specific area.

Preschoolers

Concepts of illness begin during the preschool period and are influenced by the cognitive abilities of the preoperational stage. Preschoolers differentiate poorly between themselves and the external world. Their thinking is focused on externally perceived events, and causality is based on the proximity of two events. Consequently, children define illness according to what they are told or are given external evidence of, such as "You are sick because you have a fever." The cause of illness is seen as a concrete action the child does or fails to do, such as being told that catching a cold is the result of going out into cold weather; such statements imply a degree of responsibility and self-blame. Another explanation may base the illness on contagion, that is, the proximity of two objects or persons causes the illness (e.g., "A person gets a cold when someone else with a cold gets near him.").

The psychosexual conflicts of children in this age group make them very vulnerable to threats of bodily injury. Intrusive procedures, whether painful or painless, are threatening to preschoolers, whose concept of body integrity is still poorly developed. Preschoolers may react to an injection with as much concern for withdrawal of the needle as for the actual pain. They fear that the intrusion or puncture will not reclose and that their "insides" will leak out.

Concerns of mutilation are paramount during this age period. Loss of any body part is threatening, but preschool boys' fears of castration complicate their understanding of surgical or medical procedures associated with the genital area, such as circumcision, repair of hypospadias or epispadias, cystoscopy, or catheterization. Their limited comprehension of body functioning also increases their difficulty in understanding how or why body parts are "fixed." For example, telling preschoolers that their tonsils are to be removed may be interpreted as "taking out their voice," or having the penis "fixed" may be understood as cutting it off. Words such as "dye," "cut off," "take out," or "draw" (e.g., "draw some blood") are understood literally and can lead to confusion and fear (see Communicating with Children, Chapter 34).

Reactions to pain tend to be similar to those seen during toddlerhood, although some differences become apparent. For example, preschoolers respond more favorably than younger children to preparatory interventions, such as explanation and distraction. Physical and verbal aggression are more specific and goal directed. Instead of showing total body resistance, preschoolers may push the offending person away, try to secure the equipment, or attempt to lock themselves in a safe place. Much more thought is evident in their plan of attack or escape.

Verbal expression in particular demonstrates their advanced development in response to stress. They may verbally abuse the nurse by stating, "Get out of here," or "I hate you." They may also use the more cunning approach of trying to persuade the person to give up the intended activity. A common plea is, "Please don't give me a shot; I'll be good." Some statements are not only attempts to avoid the event but also evidence of children's perceptions about the experience.

Preschoolers can locate their pain and can use appropriate pain scales. Children as young as 3 years can use assessment tools that employ facial expressions of pain (see Table 44-2).

School-Age Children

Fears of the physical nature of the illness surface at this time. School-age children may be less concerned with pain than with disability, uncertain recovery, or possible death. Children with chronic illness are more likely to identify intrusive procedures as stressful, whereas children who are acutely ill are more likely to indicate physical symptoms (Boyd & Hunsberger, 1998). Girls tend to express more and stronger fears than boys, and previous hospitalizations may have no effect on the frequency or intensity of these fears. Because of their developing cognitive abilities, school-age children are aware of the significance of different illnesses, the indispensability of certain body parts, potential hazards of treatments, lifelong consequences of permanent injury or loss of function, and the meaning of death. A major concern of school-age children when hospitalized is their fear of being told that something is "wrong" with them. They generally take a very active interest in their health or illness. Even those children who rarely ask questions usually reveal detailed knowledge of their condition by attentively listening to all that is said around them. They request factual information and quickly perceive lies or half-truths. Seeking information tends to be one way of coping or maintaining a sense of control despite the stress and uncertainty of the illness.

School-age children define illness by a set of multiple concrete symptoms, such as signs of a cold, and view the cause as primarily germs or bacteria. The germs have a powerful, almost magical quality, so that in the child's mind, illness can be prevented by avoiding people with the germs. There is also the notion of contamination, which is similar to that seen in the younger age group; for example, the illness occurs because of physical contact or because the child engaged in a harmful action and became contaminated. Consequently, feelings of self-blame and guilt may be associated with the reason for becoming ill.

School-age children begin to show concern for the potential beneficial and hazardous effects of procedures. Besides wanting to know if a procedure will hurt, they want to know what it is for, how it will make them better, and what injury or harm could result. For example, these children may fear the actual procedure of anesthesia. Unlike preschoolers, who fear the mask and the strange surroundings, school-age children fear what may happen while they are asleep, whether they will wake up, and that they may die. Preadolescents also worry about the procedure itself, particularly if it is one that will result in visible changes in body appearance.

Intrusive procedures of a nonsexual nature, such as routine physical examination of the ears, nose, mouth, and throat, are generally well tolerated. However, concerns for privacy become evident and increasingly significant. Although school-age children may cooperate during examination of, or procedures performed on, the genital area, it is usually very stressful for them, especially in the case of preadolescents who are beginning pubertal changes. Nurses who respect children's need for privacy can provide them with much assurance and support.

By age 9 or 10, most school-age children show less fright or overt resistance to pain than younger children. They generally have learned coping methods of dealing with discomfort, such as holding rigidly still, clenching their fists or teeth, or trying to act brave through the "grin-and-bear-it" routine. If they do display signs of overt resistance, such as biting, kicking, pulling away, trying to escape, crying, or plea bargaining, they may deny such reactions later, especially to their peers for fear of embarrassment.

School-age children verbally communicate about their pain in respect to its location, intensity, and description. Unlike younger children, who may have difficulty choosing words to describe pain, children 8 years and older use a wide variety of words and phrases, such as *hurting, sore, burning, stinging, aching,* and *like a sharp knife* (Franck et al, 2000).

School-age children also use words as a means of controlling their reactions to pain. For example, these children may ask the nurse to talk to them during a procedure. Some prefer to participate in a procedure, whereas others choose to distance themselves by not looking at what is happening. Most appreciate an explanation of the procedure and seem less fearful when they know what to expect. Others try to gain control by attempting to postpone the event or bargain their way out of it. A typical request is, "Start the IV when I am finished with this." Although the ability to make decisions does increase their sense of control, unlimited procrastination results in heightened anxiety. When choices are allowed, such as selection of the intravenous (IV) site, it is best to structure the number of possible sites and to limit the number of procrastination techniques.

Similar to their more passive acceptance of pain is their nondirective request for support or help. School-age children will rarely initiate a conversation about their feelings or request someone to stay with them during a lonely or stressful period. Their visible composure, calmness, and acceptance often mask their inner longing for support. It is especially important to be aware of nonverbal clues, such as a serious facial expression, a half-hearted reply of "I'm fine," silence, lack of activity, or social isolation, as signs of the need for help. Usually when someone identifies the unspoken messages and offers support, they readily accept it.

NURSE ALERT If children's behaviors appear to differ from their rating of pain, believe their pain rating. ■

Adolescents

Although the development of body image begins at birth, its relevance is paramount during adolescence. Injury, pain, disability, and death are viewed primarily in terms of how each affects adolescents' views of themselves in the present. Any change that differentiates the adolescent from peers is regarded as a major tragedy. For example, diseases such as diabetes mellitus often present a more difficult adjustment period for children in this age group than for younger children because of the necessary changes in the adolescent's lifestyle. Conversely, serious, even life-threatening illnesses that entail no visible body changes or physical restrictions may have less immediate significance for the adolescent. Therefore the nature of bodily injury may be more important in terms of adolescents' perception of the illness than its actual degree of severity.

Adolescents' rapidly changing body image during pubertal development often makes them feel insecure about their bodies. Illness, medical or surgical intervention, and hospitalization increase their existing concerns for normalcy. They may respond to such events by asking numerous questions, withdrawing, rejecting others, or questioning the adequacy of care. Frequently their fear of loss of control and body-image change is demonstrated as overconfidence.

Because of the development of secondary sex characteristics, adolescents are very concerned about privacy. Lack of respect for this need can cause greater stress than physical pain. In addition, adolescents look for signs that indicate they are developing normally and according to acceptable standards. When illness occurs, they fear that growth may be retarded, leaving them behind their peers. Although they may not voice this concern, they may demonstrate it by carefully observing others' reactions to them.

Adolescents typically react to pain with much self-control. Physical resistance and aggression are less likely at this age unless the adolescent is totally unprepared for a procedure. As with older school-age children, adolescents are very concerned with remaining composed and feel embarrassed and ashamed of losing control. They are able to describe their pain experience and to use any of the pain assessment tools developed for adults. However, they may be reluctant to disclose their pain, requiring the nurse to listen closely and observe physical indications, such as limited movement, excessive quietness, or irritability. Adolescents may also believe that the nurse knows how they feel; thus they may see no need to ask for analgesia.

Effects of Hospitalization on the Child

Children may react to the stresses of hospitalization before admission, during hospitalization, and after discharge. A child's conception of illness is even more important than age and intellectual maturity in predicting the level of anxiety before hospitalization (Clatworthy, Simon, & Tiedeman, 1999). This may or may not be affected by the duration of the condition and/or prior hospitalizations. Therefore nurses should avoid overestimating the illness concepts of children with prior medical experience (Box 44-3).

Individual Risk Factors

A number of risk factors make certain children more vulnerable than others to the stresses of hospitalization (Box 44-4). It has also been noted that rural children exhibit significantly greater degrees of psychologic upset than urban children, possibly because urban children have opportunities to become familiar with a local hospital. Because separation is such an important issue surrounding hospitalization for young children, children who are active and strong willed tend to fare better when hospitalized than youngsters who

BOX 44-3

Posthospital Behaviors in Children

Young Children

- Initial aloofness toward parents; may last from a few minutes (most common) to a few days
- Tendency to cling to parents
- Demand parents' attention
- Vigorously oppose any separation (e.g., staying at preschool or with a babysitter)
- New fears (e.g., nightmares)
- Resistance to going to bed, night waking
- Withdrawal and shyness
- Hyperactivity
- Temper tantrums
- Food finickiness
- Attachment to blanket or toy
- Regression in newly learned skills (e.g., self-toileting)

Older Children

- Emotional coldness, followed by intense, demanding dependence on parents
- Anger toward parents
- Jealousy toward others (e.g., siblings)

BOX 44-4

Risk Factors That Increase Children's Vulnerability to the Stresses of Hospitalization

Young Children
"Difficult" temperament
Lack of fit between child and parent
Age (especially between 6 months and 5 years)
Male gender
Below-average intelligence
Multiple and continuing stresses (e.g., frequent hospitalizations)

are passive. Consequently, nurses should be alert to children who passively accept all changes and requests; these children may need more support than the "oppositional" child.

The stressors of hospitalization may cause young children to experience short- and long-term negative outcomes. Adverse outcomes may be related to the length and number of admissions, multiple invasive procedures, and the anxiety of parents. Common responses include regression, separation anxiety, apathy, fears, and sleeping disturbances, especially for children younger than 7 years of age (Melnyk, 2000). Supportive practices such as family-centered care and frequent family visiting, may lessen the detrimental effects of such admissions. Research also indicates that a child's pain experience determines how the overall hospitalization is experienced (Woodgate & Kristjanson, 1996).

Changes in the Pediatric Population

The pediatric population in hospitals today has changed dramatically over the last two decades. Although there is a growing trend toward shortened hospital stays and outpatient surgery, a greater percentage of the children hospitalized today have more serious and complex problems than those hospitalized in the past. Many of these children are fragile newborns and children with severe injuries or disabilities who have survived because of major technologic advances, yet have been left with chronic or disabling conditions that often require frequent and lengthy hospital stays. The nature of their conditions increases the likelihood that they will experience more invasive and traumatic procedures while they are hospitalized. These factors make them more vulnerable to the emotional consequences of hospitalization and result in their needs being significantly different from those of the short-term patients of the past (see Chapter 42 for further discussion on children with special needs). The majority of these children are infants and toddlers, the age group most vulnerable to the effects of hospitalization.

Concern in recent years has focused on the increasing length of hospitalization because of complex medical and nursing care, elusive diagnoses, and complicated psychosocial issues. Without special attention devoted to meeting the child's psychosocial and developmental needs in the "artificial" hospital environment, the detrimental consequences of prolonged hospitalization may be severe.

Beneficial Effects of Hospitalization

Although hospitalization can be and usually is stressful for children, it can also be beneficial. The most obvious benefit is the recovery from illness, but hospitalization also can present an opportunity for children to master stress and feel competent in their coping abilities. The hospital environment can provide children with new socialization experiences that can broaden their interpersonal relationships. The psychologic benefits need to be considered and maximized during hospitalization. Appropriate nursing strategies to achieve this goal are presented on p. 1341.

STRESSORS AND REACTIONS OF THE FAMILY OF THE CHILD WHO IS HOSPITALIZED

Parental Reactions

The crisis of childhood illness and hospitalization affects every member of the nuclear family. Parents' reactions to illness in their child depend on a variety of influencing factors. Although one cannot predict which factors are most likely to influence their response, a number of variables have been identified (Box 44-5).

Almost all parents respond to their child's illness and hospitalization with remarkably consistent reactions. Initially parents may react with disbelief, especially if the illness is sudden and serious. Following the realization of illness, parents react with anger or guilt or both. They may blame themselves for the child's illness or become angry at others for some wrongdoing. Even in the mildest of illnesses, parents question their adequacy as caregivers and review any actions or omissions that could have prevented or caused the illness. When hospitalization is indicated, parental guilt is intensified because the parents feel helpless in alleviating the child's physical and emotional pain.

Fear, anxiety, and frustration are common feelings expressed by parents. Fear and anxiety may be related to the seriousness of the illness and the type of medical procedures involved. Often great anxiety is related to the trauma and pain inflicted on the child. Feelings of frustration are often related to lack of information about procedures and treatments, unfamiliarity with hospital rules and regulations, unfriendly staff, or fear of asking questions. Much frustration can be alleviated in a pediatric unit when parents are aware of what to expect and what is expected of them, are encour-

BOX 44-5

Factors Affecting Parents' Reactions to Their Child's Illness

Seriousness of the threat to the child
Previous experience with illness or hospitalization
Medical procedures involved in diagnosis and treatment
Available support systems
Personal ego strengths
Previous coping abilities
Additional stresses on the family system
Cultural and religious beliefs
Communication patterns among family members

aged to participate in their child's care, and are regarded as the most significant contributors to the child's total health.

Parents eventually may react with some degree of depression. Mothers often comment on their feeling of physical and mental exhaustion after all of the other family members have adapted to the crisis. Parents may also worry about and miss their other children, who may be left in the care of family, friends, or neighbors. Other reasons for anxiety and depression are related to concerns for the child's future well-being, including negative effects produced by the hospitalization and any financial burden incurred from the hospitalization.

Sibling Reactions

Siblings' reactions to a sister's or brother's illness or hospitalization are discussed in Chapter 41 and differ little when a child becomes temporarily ill. Siblings experience loneliness, fear, and worry, as well as anger, resentment, jealousy, and guilt. Various factors have been identified that influence the effects of the child's hospitalization on siblings. Although these factors are similar to those seen when a child has a chronic illness, Craft (1993) reported that the following factors regarding siblings are related specifically to the hospital experience and have been found to increase the effects on the sibling:

- Younger and experiencing many changes
- Cared for outside the home by care providers who are not relatives
- Received little information about their ill brother or sister
- Perceived their parents to be treating them differently compared with before their sibling's hospitalization

Simon (1993) interviewed 45 siblings of children who were hospitalized and asked about their perceptions of the stress of the hospitalization of a brother or sister. The siblings' perceptions of the stress they experienced were equal to the level of stress of hospitalized children.

Parents are often unaware of the number of effects that siblings experience during the sick child's hospitalization and the benefit of simple interventions to minimize such effects, such as explicit explanations about the illness and provisions for the siblings to remain at home. Sibling visitation is usually beneficial to the patient, sibling, and parent but should be evaluated on an individual basis.

Altered Family Roles

In addition to the effects of separation on family roles, loss of parenting, sibling, and offspring roles may affect each family member differently. One of the most common reactions of parents is specialized and intensified attention toward the sick child. The other siblings may regard this as unfair and interpret the parents' attitude toward them as rejection. Although such responses are usually unconscious and unintended, they place unique burdens on ill children. For example, the ill child may feel obligated to play the sick role in order to meet parents' expectations, especially children who have had limited physical ability and regain normal health status, such as after corrective heart surgery. Parents may be unable to perceive the child's recovery and therefore continue the pattern of overprotection and indulgent attention.

Ill children may also feel jealousy and resentment from other siblings. Because of their singular position in the family, they may be denied the companionship of their brothers and sisters. Rivalry between siblings tends to be greatest in the sibling who is nearest in age to the ill child. Without an understanding of the interpersonal dynamics between siblings, parents are likely to blame the well children for antisocial behavior. Illness may also result in children's loss of status within either their family or social group. For example, illness in the oldest child may temporarily terminate special privileges as "big" brother or sister.

NURSING CARE OF THE CHILD WHO IS HOSPITALIZED

Preparation for Hospitalization

The rationale for preparing children for the hospital experience and related procedures is based on the principle that fear of the unknown (fantasy) exceeds fear of the known. Therefore decreasing the elements of the unknown results in less fear. When children do not have paralyzing fear to cope with, they are able to direct their energies toward dealing with the other, unavoidable stresses of hospitalization and to benefit optimally from the growth potential of the experience.

Although preparation for hospitalization is a common practice, no universal standard or program is advocated for all settings. The preparation process may be elaborate, with tours, puppet shows, and playtime with miniature hospital equipment; it may involve the use of books, videos, or films; or it may be limited to a brief description of the major aspects of any hospital stay. No firm consensus exists on the timing of the event. Some authorities recommend preparing children 4 to 7 years of age about 1 week in advance so that they can assimilate the information and ask questions. For older children the time may be longer. However, for young children, who may begin to fantasize about what they observed, 1 or 2 days before admission is sufficient time for anticipatory preparation. The length of the session should be suited to the children's attention span—the younger the child, the shorter the program. The optimum approach is one that is individualized for each child and family. Regardless of the specific type of program, all children, even those who have been hospitalized before, benefit from an introduction to the environment and routine of the unit.

NURSE ALERT In many hospitals, child-life specialists, health care professionals with extensive knowledge of child growth and development and of the special psychosocial needs of children who are hospitalized and their families, help prepare children for hospitalization, surgery, and procedures. A collaborative effort between the nurse, child-life specialist, and other members of the child's health care team helps ensure the best possible hospital experience for the child and family. ■

Assessment

Assessment is the first step in identifying nursing diagnoses and planning care for an individual child. In some instances, such as with elective admission, assessment begins even before the child is hospitalized so that appropriate preadmission preparation can be instituted. At other times, assessment occurs at the time of admission and should be integrated into other admission procedures so that the child's specific needs are recognized *early* in the hospitalization. One critical area is assessment of pain for implementing appropriate relief of discomfort (p. 1314). Although assessment is discussed under nursing care of the child who is hospitalized, a comprehensive approach must involve the child's parents or other caregivers.

The nurse's primary intent is to provide atraumatic care (see Chapter 45). Therefore patient assessment should be individualized and include an evaluation of the child's growth and development, psychosocial needs, educational needs, cultural background, and the effects of the illness on the child's family or guardian.

Admission Assessment

The nursing admission history refers to a systematic collection of data about the child and family that allows the nurse to plan individualized care. The nursing admission history presented in Box 44-6 is organized according to the Functional Health Patterns outlined by Gordon (1994, 2002) (see Nursing Diagnosis, Chapter 29). This assessment framework is a guideline for formulating nursing diagnoses. One of the main pur-

BOX 44-6

Nursing Admission History According to Functional Health Patterns*

Health Perception–Health Management Pattern

Why has your child been admitted?
How has your child's general health been?
What does your child know about this hospitalization?
  Ask the child why he or she came to the hospital.
  If the answer is "For an operation or for tests," ask the child to tell you about what will happen before, during, and after the operation or tests.
Has your child ever been in the hospital before?
  How was that hospital experience?
  What things were important to you and your child during that hospitalization? How can we be most helpful now?
What medications does your child take at home?
  Why are they given?
  When are they given?
  How are they given (if a liquid, with a spoon; if a tablet, swallowed with water; or other)?
  Does your child have any trouble taking medication? If so, what helps?
  Is your child allergic to any medications?
What, if any, forms of complementary medicine practices are being used?

Nutrition-Metabolic Pattern

What are the family's usual mealtimes?
Do family members eat together or at separate times?
What are your child's favorite foods, beverages, and snacks?
  Average amounts consumed or usual size of portions
  Special cultural practices, such as family eats only ethnic food
What foods and beverages does your child dislike?
What are your child's feeding habits (bottle, cup, spoon, eats by self, needs assistance, any special devices)?
How does your child like the food served (warmed, cold, one item at a time)?
How would you describe your child's usual appetite (hearty eater, picky eater)?
  Has being sick affected your child's appetite? In what ways?
Are there any known or suspected food allergies?
Is your child on a special diet?
Are there any feeding problems (excessive fussiness, spitting up, colic); any dental or gum problems that affect feeding?
What do you do for these problems?

Elimination Pattern

What are your child's toilet habits (diaper, toilet trained–day only or day and night, use of words to communicate urination or defecation, potty chair, regular toilet, other routines)?
What is your child's usual pattern of elimination (bowel movements)?
Do you have any concerns about elimination (bed-wetting, constipation, diarrhea)?
What do you do for these problems?
Have you ever noticed that your child sweats a lot?

Sleep-Rest Pattern

What is your child's usual hour of sleep and awakening?
What is your child's schedule for naps; length of naps?
Is there a special routine before sleeping (bottle, drink of water, bedtime story, nightlight, favorite blanket or toy, prayers)?
Is there a special routine during sleep time, such as waking to go to the bathroom?
What type of bed does your child sleep in?
Does your child have a separate room or share a room; if shares, with whom?
What are the home sleeping arrangements (alone or with others, e.g., sibling, parent, other person)?
What is your child's favorite sleeping position?
Are there any sleeping problems (falling asleep, waking during night, nightmares, sleep walking)?
Are there any problems in awakening and getting ready in the morning?
What do you do for these problems?

Activity-Exercise Pattern

What is your child's schedule during the day (preschool, day care center, regular school, extracurricular activities)?
What are your child's favorite activities or toys (both active and quiet interests)?
What is your child's usual television-viewing schedule at home?
  What are your child's favorite programs?
  Are there any TV restrictions?
Does your child have any illness or disabilities that limit activity? If so, how?
What are your child's usual habits and schedule for bathing (bath in tub or shower, sponge bath, shampoo)?
What are your child's dental habits (brushing, flossing, fluoride supplements or rinses, favorite toothpaste); schedule of daily dental care?
Does your child need help with dressing or grooming, such as hair combing?
Are there any problems with the above (dislike of or refusal to bathe, shampoo hair, or brush teeth)?
What do you do for these problems?

Continued

BOX 44-6

Nursing Admission History According to Functional Health Patterns*—cont'd

Are there special devices that your child requires help in managing (eyeglasses, contact lenses, hearing aid, orthodontic appliances, artificial elimination appliances, orthopedic devices)?

NOTE: Use the following code to assess functional self-care level for feeding, bathing/hygiene, dressing/grooming, toileting:

- O: Full self-care
- I: Requires use of equipment or device
- II: Requires assistance or supervision from another person
- III: Requires assistance or supervision from another person and equipment or device
- IV: Is dependent and does not participate

Cognitive-Perceptual Pattern

Does your child have any hearing difficulty?
- Does the child use a hearing aid?
- Have "tubes" been placed in your child's ears?

Does your child have any vision problems?
- Does the child wear glasses or contact lenses?

Does your child have any learning difficulties?
- What is the child's grade in school?

Self-Perception–Self-Concept Pattern

How would you describe your child (e.g., takes time to adjust, settles in easily, shy, friendly, quiet, talkative, serious, playful, stubborn, easygoing)?

What makes your child angry, annoyed, anxious, or sad? What helps?

How does your child act when annoyed or upset?

What have been your child's experiences with and reactions to temporary separation from you (parent)?

Does your child have any fears (places, objects, animals, people, situations)? How do you handle them?

Do you think your child's illness has changed the way he or she thinks about self (e.g., more shy, embarrassed about appearance, less competitive with friends, stays at home more)?

Role-Relationship Pattern

Does your child have a favorite nickname?

What are the names of other family members or others who live in the home (relatives, friends, pets)?

Who usually takes care of your child during the day/night (especially if other than parent, such as baby-sitter, relative)?

What are the parents' occupations and work schedules?

Are there any special family considerations (adoption, foster child, stepparent, divorce, single parent)?

Have any major changes in the family occurred lately (death, divorce, separation, birth of a sibling, loss of a job, financial strain, mother beginning a career, other)? Describe child's reaction.

Who are your child's play companions or social groups (peers, younger or older children, adults, prefers to be alone)?

Do things generally go well for your child in school or with friends?

Does your child have "security" objects at home (pacifier, bottle, blanket, stuffed animal, or doll)? Did you bring any of these to the hospital?

How do you handle discipline problems at home? Are these methods always effective?

Does your child have any condition that interferes with communication? If so, what are your suggestions for communicating with your child?

Will your child's hospitalization affect the family's financial support or care of other family members (e.g., other children)?

What concerns do you have about your child's illness and hospitalization?

Who will be staying with your child while hospitalized?

How can we contact you or another close family member outside of the hospital?

Sexuality-Reproductive Pattern

(Answer questions that apply to your child's age group.)

Has your child begun puberty (developing physical sexual characteristics, menstruation)? Have you or your child had any concerns?

Does your daughter know how to do breast self-examination?

Does your son know how to do testicular self-examination?

How have you approached topics of sexuality with your child?

Do you feel you might need some help with some topics?

Has your child's illness affected the way he or she feels about being a boy or a girl? If so, how?

Do you have any concerns with behaviors in your child, such as masturbation, asking many questions or talking about sex, not respecting others' privacy, or wanting too much privacy?

Initiate a conversation about an adolescent's sexual concerns with open-ended to more direct questions and using the terms "friends" or "partners" rather than "girlfriend" or "boyfriend":
- Tell me about your social life.
- Who are your closest friends? (If one friend is identified, could ask more about that relationship, such as how much time they spend together, how serious they are about each other, if the relationship is going the way the teenager hoped.)
- Might ask about dating and sexual issues, such as the teenager's views on sexuality education, "going steady," "living together," or premarital sex.
- Which friends would you like to have visit in the hospital?

Coping–Stress Tolerance Pattern

(Answer questions that apply to your child's age group.)

What does your child do when tired or upset?
- If upset, does your child want a special person or object? If so, explain.

If your child has temper tantrums, what causes them and how do you handle them?

Whom does your child talk to when worried about something?

How does your child usually handle problems or disappointments?

Have there been any big changes or problems in your family recently? If so, how have you handled them?

Has your child ever had a problem with drugs or alcohol or tried to commit suicide?

Do you think your child is "accident prone"? If so, explain.

Value-Belief Pattern

What is your religion?

How is religion or faith important in your child's life?

What religious practices would you like continued in the hospital (e.g., prayers before meals/bedtime; visit by minister, priest, or rabbi; prayer group)?

*The focus of the admission history is the child's psychosocial environment. Most of the questions are worded in terms of parental responses. Depending on the child's age, they should be addressed directly to the child when appropriate.

poses of the history is to assess the child's usual health habits at home to promote a more normal environment in the hospital. Therefore questions related to activities of daily living in the nutritional-metabolic, elimination, sleep-rest, and activity-exercise patterns are a major part of the assessment. The questions found under the health perception–health management pattern are directed toward evaluation of the child's preparation for hospitalization and are key factors in determining if additional preparation is needed. The questions included in the self-perception–self-concept and role-relationship patterns offer insight into the child's potential reaction to hospitalization, especially in terms of separation.

The nurse should also inquire about the use of any complementary medicine practices (Box 44-7). In a study of children with cancer, 42% had used alternative or complementary therapies, simultaneously with or following conventional treatments (Fernandez, Pyesmany, & Stutzer, 1999). Widespread use of complementary medicine is often explored, however, without discussion with the primary care physician or nurse (Moenkhoff et al, 1999; Spiegel, Stroud, & Fyfe, 1998). It is important that the use of any herbal or complementary therapy be noted in a preoperative assessment because of possible anesthesia and/or surgical complications related to herbal products (Flanagan, 2001) (Critical Thinking Exercise).

Once the data are collected, the information must be applied to the nursing process and communicated to other staff. It makes little sense to assess a child's home routine if none of this knowledge is integrated into the plan of care. Most nursing units have provisions for care plans in which specific information about the child's habits and needs are recorded.

As with any history form, the questions are only guidelines; for maximum communication, nurses should ask these questions as a part of conversation, not as a direct questionnaire. Answers to questions that are broad and nonspecific, such as "What does your child know about this hospitalization?" need to be followed by more specific questions such as "Tell me what you told him." Children may respond to questions regarding their knowledge of hospitalization with statements such as "I don't know why I am here." Although this may be correct, they have often been given some explanation concerning the reason for hospitalization. Such an answer may mean that the explanation was inadequate, their anxiety blocked the recall, or they are testing the explanation by prompting the nurse to supply additional information.

Besides taking the nursing admission history, nurses should also perform a physical assessment (see Chapter 35) or obtain the information from the medical examination before planning care. At the very least, the nurse's physical assessment of the child should include observation of the body for any bruises, rashes, signs of neglect, deformities, or physical limitations. The nurse should also listen to the heart and lungs to assess overall physical status. For example, it is impossible to evaluate improvement in respiratory function in a child admitted with pulmonary disease unless baseline data are available to compare subsequent findings.

Nursing Diagnoses

A number of nursing diagnoses are prominent in the nursing care of children who are ill and/or hospitalized. Other nursing diagnoses specific to individual cases may become evident in addition to those outlined in the Nursing Care Plan on p. 1341.

Plan of Care and Implementation

An effective plan of care for the child who is hospitalized is based on patient- and family-identified needs, as well as those identified by the nurse. Family members and the child should play active roles in developing the plan whenever possible.

BOX 44-7

Complementary Medicine Practices and Examples

Nutrition, diet, and lifestyle/behavioral health changes–Macrobiotics, megavitamins, diets, lifestyle modification, health risk reduction/health education, wellness
Mind/body control therapies–Biofeedback, relaxation, prayer therapy, guided imagery, hypnotherapy, music/sound therapy, massage, aromatherapy, education therapy
Traditional and ethnomedicine therapies–Acupuncture, ayurvedic medicine, herbal medicine, homeopathic medicine, Native-American medicine, natural products, traditional Oriental medicine
Structural manipulation and energetic therapies–Acupressure, chiropractic medicine, massage, reflexology, rolfing, therapeutic touch, Qi Gong
Pharmacologic and biologic therapies–Antioxidants, cell treatment, chelation therapy, metabolic therapy, oxidizing agents
Bioelectromagnetic therapies–Diagnostic and therapeutic application of electromagnetic fields (e.g., transcranial electrostimulation, neuromagnetic stimulation, electroacupuncture)

Critical Thinking Exercise

COMPLEMENTARY/ALTERNATIVE MEDICINE

Maria, a 10-year-old Hispanic girl, has had severe nosebleeds. She is admitted to the hospital for a complete workup in an attempt to determine the cause. Her parents and grandparents have gathered around her bed. When you enter her room to begin admitting procedures, you notice an unusual scent. Maria's mother is rubbing the contents from an unfamiliar bottle of liquid on Maria. Meanwhile, the grandmother is rubbing Maria's head. She is startled at your entry and drops something on the floor near your feet. You bend over to pick it up and discover that it is a penny.

1. Evidence–Is there sufficient evidence to draw any conclusions?
2. Assumptions–What are some underlying assumptions that may be drawn from information regarding the following issues:
   a. Complementary or alternative medical remedies
   b. The role of ethnic or folk remedies in modern healthcare practice
   c. The nurse's role in cases where alternative (vs. traditional) medicine is practiced
3. What implications and priorities for nursing care can be drawn at this time?
4. Does the evidence objectively support your argument (conclusion)?
5. Are there alternative perspectives to your arguments? If so, what are they?

The main goals for the child who is ill and/or hospitalized are as follows:

1. Child will be prepared for hospitalization.
2. Child will experience little or no separation.
3. Child will maintain a sense of control.
4. Child will exhibit decreased fear of bodily injury.
5. Child will experience a reduction of pain that is acceptable to child.
6. Child will have opportunities to participate in developmentally appropriate diversional activities.
7. Child will experience maximum benefits from hospitalization.

Preparing Child for Admission

The preparation that children require on the day of admission depends on the kind of prehospital counseling they have received. If they have been prepared in a formalized program, they will usually know what to expect in terms of initial medical procedures, inpatient facilities, and nursing staff. However, prehospital counseling does not preclude the need for support during procedures such as obtaining blood specimens, x-ray tests, or physical examination. For example, undressing young children before they feel comfortable in their new surroundings can be very upsetting. Causing needless anxiety and fear during admission may adversely affect the nurse's establishment of trust with these children. Therefore nursing assistance during the admission procedure is vital, regardless of how well prepared any child is for the experience of hospitalization. In addition, spending this time with the child gives the nurse an opportunity to evaluate the child's understanding of subsequent procedures (Fig. 44-4). Ideally, a primary nurse is assigned whenever possible to allow for individualized care and to provide a substitute support person for the child.

When a child is admitted, nurses follow several fairly universal admission procedures, which are outlined in Box 44-8. One particularly important decision is room assignment. The minimum considerations for room assignment are age, sex, and nature of the illness. Ideally, however, room selection should be based on a variety of developmental and psychobiologic needs. Determining compatible roommates, both for the children and for rooming-in parents, greatly influences the growth potential from the hospital experience.

No absolute rules govern room selection, but in general, placing children of the same age group and with similar types of illness in the same room is both psychologically and medically advantageous. However, there are many exceptions. For example, a school-age child may thrive on the responsibility of caring for a younger child. A child in traction may be very therapeutic for another child confined to bed because of a serious illness. A child who is very independent despite physical disabilities may help another child with similar or different limitations, and the parents of the child with disabilities may achieve deeper insight and acceptance of their child's disorder.

Grouping by age is especially important for adolescents. Many hospitals make an effort to place teenagers on their own unit or in a separate, designated section of the pediatric or general unit whenever possible.

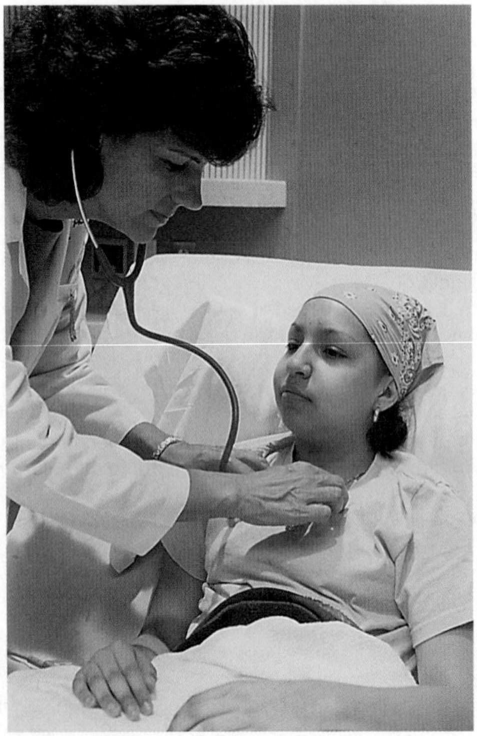

Fig. 44-4 The initial admission procedures give the nurse an opportunity to get to know the child and to assess the child's understanding of the hospital experience.

BOX 44-8

Guidelines for Admission

Preadmission

Assign a room based on developmental age, seriousness of diagnosis, communicability of illness, and projected length of stay.

Prepare roommate(s) for the arrival of a new patient; when children are too young to benefit from this consideration, prepare parents.

Prepare room for child and family, with admission forms and equipment nearby to eliminate need to leave child.

Admission

Introduce primary nurse to child and family.

Orient child and family to inpatient facilities, especially to assigned room and unit; emphasize positive areas of pediatric unit.

- Room: Explain call light, bed controls, television, bathroom, telephone, etc.
- Unit: Direct to playroom, desk, dining area, or other areas.

Introduce family to roommate and his or her parents.

Apply identification band to child's wrist, ankle, or both (if not done).

Explain hospital regulations and schedules (e.g., visiting hours, mealtimes, bedtime, limitations [give written information if available]).

Perform nursing admission history (see Box 44-6).

Take vital signs, blood pressure, height, and weight.

Obtain specimens as needed and order needed laboratory work.

Support child and assist practitioner with physical examination (for purposes of nursing assessment).

Preventing or Minimizing Separation

A primary nursing goal is to prevent separation, particularly in children under 5 years of age. Changes in hospitals' policies over recent years reflect a changed attitude toward parents; many hospitals no longer consider parents "visitors" and welcome their presence at all times throughout the child's hospitalization. Many hospitals have developed a system of family-centered care. This philosophy of care recognizes the integral role of the family in a child's life and acknowledges the family as an essential part of the child's care and illness experience. The family is considered to be partners in the care of the child (Smith & Conant Rees, 2000) (see Chapter 31).

At the least, most hospitals welcome parents at any time. Many provide facilities such as a chair or bed for at least one person per child, unit kitchen privileges, and other amenities that create a welcoming atmosphere for parents. However, not all hospitals provide such amenities, and parents' own schedules may prevent rooming-in. In such instances, strategies to minimize the effects of separation must be implemented.

A thorough, detailed nursing history specifically identifies the child's established daily routine. Usual daily activities, such as food preparation and method of feeding, help establish a complementary schedule of caregiving practices. Incorporating these normal activities also helps the parents feel that they are participating in the child's care, even if through another person. A consistent staff member can be designated to keep the family informed of the child's condition and to support the family's concerns and priorities without being judgmental (Kauffmann et al, 1998).

Nurses must have an appreciation of the child's separation behaviors. As discussed earlier, the phases of protest and despair are normal. The child is allowed to cry. Even if the child rejects strangers, the nurse provides support through physical presence. *Presence* is defined as spending time being physically close to the child while using a quiet tone of voice, appropriate choice of words, eye contact, and touch in ways that establish rapport and communicate empathy. If behaviors of detachment are evident, the nurse maintains the child's contact with the parents by frequently talking about them, encouraging the child to remember them, and stressing the significance of their visits, telephone calls, or letters.

Separation may be equally as difficult for parents, especially when they do not understand the behaviors of separation anxiety. To avoid the immediate protest, parents may sneak out or lie to the child about leaving. As a result, the child does not learn that absence is associated with a guaranteed return, but that absence means loss of parents. Helping parents recognize that separation behaviors are normal and expected can decrease the parents' anxiety and may ease their fears about leaving without telling the child. Explaining to parents how the child reacts after they leave may also be helpful. Many parents imagine that the child cries for hours after they leave, whereas in reality the child may cry for a few minutes but settle down when comforted by someone else.

Toddlers and preschoolers have a very limited concept of time. The young child's question, "Will my mommy come yesterday?" symbolizes a lack of understanding for usual measurements of time, such as days, hours, and weeks. Time is measured in associations, such as eating dinner "when Daddy comes home." Therefore, when helping parents with their fears of separation, nurses need to suggest ways of explaining leaving and returning. For example, if parents must leave to go to work or to make meals for the other family members, they should tell the child the reason for leaving. They also need to convey the expected time of return in terms of anticipated events. For example, if the parents will return in the morning, they can say to the child, "We'll see you after the sun comes up" or "We'll come back when (a favorite program) is on television."

The young child's ability to tolerate parental absence is very limited. Therefore parental visits should be frequent (e.g., visiting three times a day for short periods rather than once a day for an extended time). This may necessitate that each parent visit at different times to lessen the length of separation. When parents cannot visit, the presence of other significant people can be most comforting for the child (Fig. 44-5).

If parents leave after the child is asleep, they still need to communicate their absence. The parents of a 5-year-old boy solved this problem by devising a sign; on one side they drew a picture of a telephone, and on the other they drew a hamburger. Before they left, they turned the sign to the appropriate side to tell the child when he awoke that they were out using the telephone or eating.

Older children who know how to tell time may find it helpful to have a clock or watch. However, these children have the same need for honesty from their parents regarding visiting schedules. Because their peer groups are important, adolescents often appreciate planning visiting hours with their parents to ensure that the patient has some private time for friends.

Familiar surroundings also increase the child's adjustment to separation. If parents cannot room-in, they should leave favorite articles from home with the child, such as a blanket, toy, bottle, feeding utensil, or article of clothing. Since young

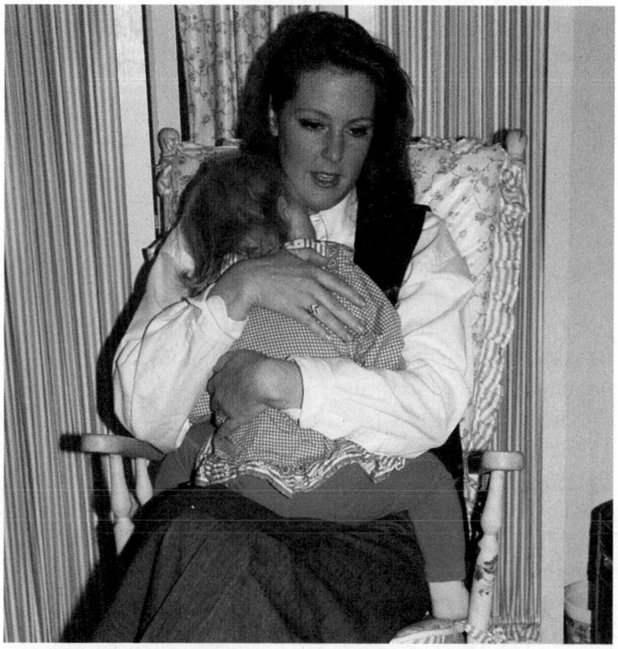

Fig. 44-5 When parents cannot visit, other significant persons can provide comfort to the hospitalized child.

children associate such inanimate objects with significant people, they gain comfort and reassurance from these possessions. They make the association that if the parents left this, the parents will surely return. Placing an identification band on the toy lessens the chances of its being misplaced and provides a symbol that the toy is experiencing the same needs as the child. Other mementos of home include photographs and audiotape or videocassette recordings of family members reading a story, singing a song, saying prayers before bedtime, relating events at home, or taking a "talking walk" through the home. The tapes can be played at lonely times, such as on awakening or before sleeping. Some units allow pets to visit, which can have therapeutic benefits for a child. Animals should be carefully screened for medical or behavioral problems, and patients should be screened for allergies.

Older children also appreciate familiar articles from home, particularly photographs, a radio, a favorite toy or game, and the usual pajamas. Often the importance of treasured objects to school-age children is overlooked or criticized. However, many school-age children have a special object to which they formed an attachment in early childhood. Therefore such treasured or transitional objects can help even older children feel more comfortable in a strange environment.

The strange sights, smells, and sounds in the hospital that are commonplace for the nurse can be frightening and confusing for children. It is important for the nurse to try to evaluate stimuli in the environment from the child's point of view (considering also what the child may see or hear happening to other patients) and to make every effort to protect the child from frightening and unfamiliar sights, sounds, and equipment. The nurse should offer explanations or prepare the child for those experiences that are unavoidable. Combining familiar or comforting sights with the unfamiliar can relieve much of the harshness of medical equipment.

NURSE ALERT "Soften" medical equipment (e.g., clip a bear or other animal to a stethoscope; use paper, fabric, or stickers to transform an IV pump into a friendly animal) to create a pleasant and more familiar environment for children. ■

Helping children maintain their usual non-home contacts also minimizes the effects of separation imposed by hospitalization. This includes continuing school lessons during the illness and confinement, visiting with friends either directly or through letter writing or telephone calls, and participating in stimulating projects whenever possible (Fig. 44-6). For extended hospitalizations, youngsters enjoy personalizing the hospital room to make it "home" by decorating the walls with posters and cards, rearranging the furniture (when possible), and displaying a collection or hobby.

Minimizing Loss of Control

Feelings of loss of control result from separation, physical restriction, changed routines, enforced dependency, and magical thinking. Although some of these cannot be prevented, most can be minimized through individualized planning of nursing care.

Promoting Freedom of Movement

Younger children react most strenuously to any type of physical restriction or immobilization. Although temporary immobilization may be necessary for some interventions such as maintaining an IV line, most physical restriction can be prevented if the nurse gains the child's cooperation.

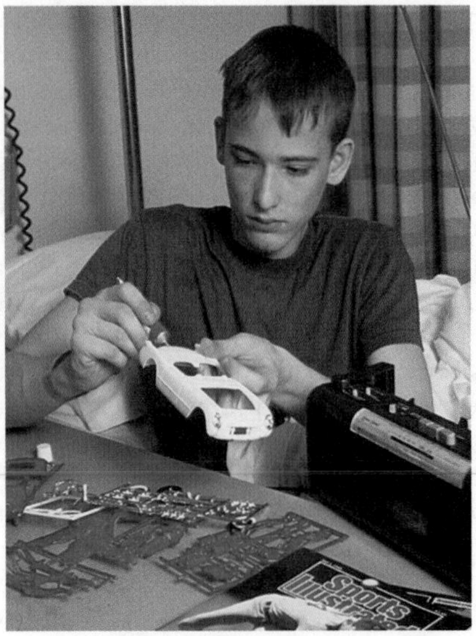

Fig. 44-6 For extended hospitalizations children enjoy having projects to occupy time. (Courtesy St. Louis Children's Hospital.)

For young children, particularly infants and toddlers, preserving parent-child contact is the best means of decreasing the need for or stress of restraint. For example, almost the entire physical examination can be done in a parent's lap, with the parent hugging the child for procedures such as otoscopy. For painful procedures the parents' preferences for assisting, observing, or waiting outside the room are evaluated.

Environmental Factors May Also Restrict Movement

Keeping children in cribs or playpens may not represent immobilization in a concrete sense, but it certainly limits sensory stimulation. Increasing mobility by transporting children in carriages, wheelchairs, carts, wagons, or on stretchers or beds provides them with mechanical freedom.

Maintaining Child's Routine

Altered daily schedules and loss of rituals are particularly stressful for toddlers and early preschoolers and may increase the stress of separation. The nursing admission history provides a baseline for planning care around the child's usual home activities.

A frequently neglected aspect of altered routines is the change in the child's daily activities. A nonhospitalized child's day, especially during the school years, is structured with specific times for eating, dressing, going to school, playing, and sleeping. However, this time structure vanishes when the child is hospitalized. Although nurses have a set schedule, the child is frequently unaware of it; new schedules are imposed that may be rigid or flexible. For example, some units have uniform nap times and bedtimes for all children, whereas others allow children to stay up late at night. Many children obtain significantly less sleep in the hospital than at home; the primary causes are delay in sleep onset and early termination of sleep because of hospital routines. Not only are hours of sleep disrupted, but waking hours are spent in passive activities. For example, few institutions impose any regulation on the amount of time the child spends watching television.

One technique that can minimize the disruption in the child's routine is *time structuring*. This approach is most suitable for the noncritically ill school-age or adolescent child who has mastered the concept of time. It involves scheduling the child's day to include all those activities that are important to the child and nurse, such as treatment procedures, schoolwork, exercise, television, playroom, and hobbies. Together, the nurse, parent, and child then plan a daily schedule with times and activities written down (Fig. 44-7). This is left in the child's room, and a clock or watch is available for the child's use. Whenever possible, a calendar is also constructed with special events marked, such as favorite television programs, visits by friends or relatives, events in the playroom, and holidays or birthdays. If specific changes in treatment are expected (e.g., beginning physical therapy in 2 days), these are added.

NURSE ALERT Ask the young child to select or draw pictures or symbols to represent daily or weekly fun activities (e.g., favorite TV programs, family visits, playroom times). Draw a clock face with the hands of the clock depicting the time each event will occur next to the child's representation. Have the child compare the clock on the schedule with a clock or watch in the room. When the two match, the child knows that it is time for a favorite activity and exactly what that activity is. ■

Encouraging Independence

The dependent role of the hospitalized patient imposes tremendous feelings of loss on older children. Principal interventions should focus on respect for individuality and the opportunity for decision making. Although these sound simple, their efficacy lies with nurses who are flexible, tolerant, and personally secure. The last is particularly important because when decision making is geared toward the patient, nurses can feel threatened by a sense of lessened control.

Promoting children's control involves maintaining independence, and the concept of self-care can be most beneficial. *Self-care* refers to the practice of activities that individuals personally initiate and perform on their own behalf in maintaining life, health, and well-being (Orem, 1995). Although self-care is limited by the child's age and physical condition, most children beyond infancy can perform some activities with little or no help. Whenever possible, these activities are encouraged in the hospital. Other approaches include jointly planning care, time structuring, wearing street clothes, making choices in food selections and bedtime, continuing school activities, and rooming with an appropriate age-mate.

ERIC'S DAILY SCHEDULE:

7:00 AM	– Breakfast, Watch TV, Brush Teeth, Wash up	3:00 PM	– Tutor (M, W, F) Study Time (T, Th)
9:00	– Tub Room, Dressing Change	4:00	– Physical Therapy
		5:00	– Dinner
10:00	– Rest, TV, Snack	6:30	– Dressing Change
11:00	– Physical Therapy	7:00 to 9:00	– TV, Reading, Snack, Friends Visit
12:00 PM	– Lunch		
1:00	– Playroom, Quiet Play, Rest, Friends Visit	9:00	– Brush Teeth, Wash up
		9:15	– Bedtime

Fig. 44-7 Time structuring is an effective strategy for normalizing the hospital environment and increasing the child's sense of control.

Promoting Understanding

Loss of control can occur from feelings of having too little influence on one's destiny, as well as from sensing overwhelming control or power over fate. Although preschoolers' cognitive abilities predispose them most to magical thinking and self-power, all children are vulnerable to misinterpreting causes for stresses such as illness and hospitalization.

Most children feel more in control when they know what to expect, because the element of fear is reduced. Anticipatory preparation and providing information help greatly to lessen stress and prevent lack of understanding (see Preparation for Procedures, Chapter 45).

Informing children of their rights while hospitalized fosters greater understanding and may relieve some of the feelings of powerlessness they typically experience. Hospitals providing services to children should have a hospital-wide policy on the rights and responsibilities of these patients and of their parents and/or guardians (Joint Commission on Accreditation of Healthcare Organizations, 1999). An increasing number of hospitals and organizations have developed a patient "Bill of Rights" that is prominently displayed throughout the hospital or is presented to children and their families on admission (Box 44-9).

Preventing or Minimizing Fear of Bodily Injury

Beyond early infancy all children fear bodily injury either from mutilation, bodily intrusion, body-image change, disability, or death. In general, preparation of children for painful procedures decreases their fears. Manipulating procedural techniques for children in each age group also minimizes fear of bodily injury. For example, since toddlers and young preschoolers are traumatized by insertion of a rectal thermometer, axillary temperatures or temperatures taken with electronic or tympanic membrane devices can effectively be substituted. Whenever procedures are performed on young children, the most supportive intervention is to do the procedure as quickly as possible while maintaining parent-child contact.

BOX 44-9

Bill of Rights for Children and Teens

In this hospital you and your family have the right to:
- Respect and personal dignity
- Care that supports you and your family
- Information you can understand
- Quality health care
- Emotional support
- Care that respects your need to grow, play, and learn
- Make choices and decisions

From Association for the Care of Children's Health: *A pediatric bill of rights*, Bethesda, MD, 1991, The Association.

Because of young children's poorly defined body boundaries, the use of bandages may be particularly helpful. For example, telling children that the bleeding will stop after the needle is removed does little to relieve their fears, whereas applying a small Band-Aid usually provides much reassurance. The size of bandages is also significant to children in this age group; the larger the bandage, the more importance is attached to the wound. Watching their surgical dressings become successively smaller is one way young children can measure healing and improvement. Prematurely removing a dressing may cause these children considerable concern for their well-being.

For children who fear mutilation of body parts, it is essential that the nurse repeatedly stress the reason for a procedure and evaluate the child's understanding. For example, explaining cast removal to preschoolers may seem simple enough, but children's comprehension of the details may vary considerably from the explanation. Asking them to draw a picture of what they think will happen presents substantial evidence of the perceived events.

Children may fear bodily injury from a great variety of sources. X-ray machines, use of strange equipment for examination, unfamiliar rooms, or awkward positions can be perceived as potentially hazardous. In addition, thoughts and actions can be imagined sources of bodily damage. For older children, masturbation or sex play may be perceived as powerful weapons of potential destruction. Therefore it is important to investigate imagined reasons, particularly of a sexual nature, for illness. Since children may fear revealing such thoughts, using projective techniques such as drawing or doll play may elicit previously undisclosed misconceptions.

Older children fear bodily injury of both internal and external origins. For example, school-age children are aware of the significance of the heart and may fear the actual operation as much as the pain, the stitches, and the possible scar. Adolescents may express concern about the actual procedure but be much more anxious over the resulting scar. An appreciation of each child's special concerns helps nurses focus on critical areas during preparation for procedures or when giving explanations of the disease processes.

Children can grasp information only if it is presented on or close to their level of cognitive development. This necessitates an awareness of the words used to describe events or processes. For example, young children told that they are going to have a CAT scan may wonder, "Will there be cats? Or something that scratches?" It is clearer to describe the procedure in simple terms and explain what the letters of the common name stand for.

When children are upset about their illness, their perception can be changed by (1) providing a somewhat different and less negative account of the disease or (2) offering an explanation that is characteristic of the next stage of cognitive development. An example of the first strategy is reassuring a preschooler who fears that after a tonsillectomy, another sore throat means a second operation. Explaining that once tonsils are "fixed" they do not need fixing again can help relieve the fear. An example of the latter strategy is to explain that germs made the tonsils sick and even though germs can cause another sore throat, they cannot cause the tonsils to ever be sick again. This higher-level explanation is based on the school-age child's concept of germs as a cause of disease.

Pain Assessment

Pain assessment is a critical component in managing pain. Pain is multifactorial and includes sensory, affective, behavioral, cognitive, sociocultural, and physiologic components. All of these require assessment (Broome & Huth, 2003; Howard, 2003). Unfortunately, health professionals, including nurses, continue to underestimate and sporadically manage pain in infants and children (Broome et al, 1996; Ellis et al, 2002;) (Evidence-Based Practice box). One of the reasons for inadequate management of pain is a lack of understanding of what pain is—a personal phenomenon that *cannot* be experienced by any other individual. Therefore defining pain in terms of another's perceptions is inappropriate and inaccurate. An operational definition that is useful in clinical practice follows: *pain is whatever the experiencing person says it is, existing whenever the person says it does* (McCaffery & Pasero, 1999). This definition implies a very important attitude toward patients—*they are believed.* It includes both verbal and nonverbal expressions of pain.

Fallacies and Facts

Children are undertreated for pain for a number of complex and interrelated reasons, including professionals' misconceptions about pain; the complexities of pain assessment, particularly in nonverbal children; and the lack of information regarding currently available pain reduction techniques. A number of fallacies continue to flourish because of incorrect knowledge about pain in infants and children, despite these fallacies having been disproved by current research on pediatric pain (Box 44-10).

Fear of Addiction

A major concern that prevents health professionals from adequately using opioids* to relieve pain is an unwarranted fear of addiction. Studies on addiction rates in patients treated with opioids have found an incidence of less than 1% (McCaffery & Pasero, 1999). One of the reasons for the unfounded and prevalent fear regarding addiction is confusion among the three terms: physical dependence, tolerance, and addiction. The American Society of Addiction Medicine (2001) has defined *physical dependence, tolerance,* and *addiction* and these definitions are found in the Community Focus box.

Fear of Respiratory Depression

Although respiratory depression is the most serious side effect of opioids, it is a rare occurrence in children. Evidence suggests that in children over 3 months of age, opioids cause no greater respiratory depression than in adults (Kart, Christrup, & Rasmussen, 1997). Respiratory depression is most likely to occur when the opioid is administered with other sedating drugs, such as hydroxyzine (Vistaril), promethazine (Phenergan), chlorpromazine (Thorazine), midazo-

*The term *opioid* refers to natural or synthetic analgesics with morphinelike actions. It is preferred to the term *narcotic,* which in a legal context refers to any substance that causes psychologic dependence, such as cocaine, which is not an opioid. The term *narcotic* also engenders unwarranted fears of addiction in older children and parents when opioids are used for pain control.

Evidence-Based Practice

UNDERMEDICATION OF PAIN IN CHILDREN

Several studies have examined the pattern of pain medication for children as compared with adults and have found remarkably consistent findings—children have been undermedicated for pain. Eland and Anderson (1977) investigated the incidence of administration of analgesics to 25 hospitalized children for postoperative pain. Twelve of the children received a total of 24 doses of analgesics; the remaining 13 children were never given any medication for pain relief. In contrast, 18 adults with identical diagnoses received 372 opioid analgesic doses and 299 nonopioid analgesic doses for a total of 671 doses. One of the saddest findings was that more than twice as many children had pain medication ordered as received it. This lack of response to the need for pain medication directly relates to the nurses who failed to administer the analgesic.

Another study investigating analgesic prescriptions given to children and adults after open heart surgery found that all of the adults received medication, for a total of 564 doses, but only three-fourths of the children were given medication, for a total of 237 doses during the first 3 postoperative days. This difference was even greater on the fifth postoperative day, when 83% of the adults continued to receive analgesics (a total of 136 doses) but only 12% of the children were medicated (a total of 10 doses) (Beyer et al, 1983).

Another study on postoperative pain found that 75% of the children reported pain on the day of surgery, and if orders for opioid or nonopioid analgesics were written, the nonopioid was given exclusively. In addition, the doses ordered were usually too small and/or too infrequent to be maximally effective. Most orders were written "PRN," which was often interpreted by nursing staff to mean "as little as possible" (Mather & Mackie, 1983).

A review of analgesic use in the emergency department reported significantly low use in children with mild-to-moderate trauma, including children with painful fractures. Head injury was associated with especially low use of analgesics (Friedland & Kulick, 1994).

Johnston and others (1992) studied 150 randomly selected hospitalized children and found that 87% reported pain, with 19% stating that their pain was severe. Of the 150 children, only 38% had received analgesics during the previous 24 hours.

An even sadder and more disappointing finding is that two decades after Eland and Anderson's (1977) seminal research, some nurses may neither have knowledge about appropriate analgesic medications for children nor appreciate the consequences of undermedication. In Boughton and others' study (1998), 25% of 36 patients were given no pain medication, and 25% of the patients stated that their pain intervention was only partially effective. All patients had PRN orders for analgesics. Clearly, the responsibility for inadequate pain control rested with the nurses.

The situation is even more serious with infants. One analysis of anesthetic practices with newborns undergoing surgical ligation of patent ductus arteriosus found that 76% of the infants received only nitrous oxide and a paralyzing agent. These infants could not move during surgery but could feel all the pain of a thoracotomy (Anand & Aynsley-Green, 1985). In a survey of nurses working in neonatal intensive care units, 79% believed that infants were undermedicated for pain. The same study found that more than half of the medications used for pain relief had no analgesic properties (Franck, 1987). A study comparing premedication for procedures such as arterial line or chest tube placement found that infants in neonatal intensive care units received no premedication much more often than children in pediatric intensive care units (Bauchner, May, & Coates, 1992). In the United States the use of analgesia and anesthesia for newborn circumcision is not routine. A survey of pediatric, obstetric, and family practice residents showed that training in the use of pain reducers during this painful procedure was inadequate (Howard et al, 1998). Unfortunately, the amount of content on pain in nursing curricula also is inadequate, and some of the textbooks contain inaccurate information (Davis, 1998; Ferrell, McCaffery, & Rhiner, 1992).

Much research has been done examining the stress response in premature infants, and the results support the belief that unrelieved pain has detrimental physiologic, anatomic, and behavioral effects (see also Neonatal Pain, Chapter 25). Much less research has been done on the long-term effects of pain on children, from both a psychologic and a physiologic point of view. Stuber and others (1997) examined the psychologic effects on survivors of childhood cancer. Many children reported long-term sequelae that resembled posttraumatic stress syndrome. Children's fears were related to their perception of the intensity of treatment, not the illness itself. Symptoms included stomachaches and bad dreams. Another study found that memory of a painful experience may cause anxiety about subsequent procedures. Weisman, Bernstein, and Schechter (1998) showed that children who had a placebo, rather than oral transmucosal fentanyl, before a painful procedure were more anxious than the medicated group for the subsequent procedure even when the analgesic was given. Based on their results, the authors argue strongly for aggressive pain control beginning with the first noxious procedure.

On a positive note, Schechter (1997) outlines the growth in research and published literature (33 articles in 1974 to 2966 articles from 1980 to 1991) in pediatric pain management that encompasses many topics such as oncology, sickle cell disease, acute pain, and chronic pain. One outcome of the large number of research studies has been the development of pain teams or pain specialists. Unfortunately, when these services exist, other health care professionals may abandon any responsibility for pain control to the pain experts or neglect to consult the pain team. Although pain teams play a very important role in treating pain adequately (Ferrell et al, 1994), in a survey of 35 pediatric pain services, only 17% had written guidelines (Tyc et al, 1998).

Guidelines are available to help practitioners assess and manage pain using methods based on the published scientific literature. In the United States the Agency for Health Care Policy and Research (AHCPR) has published guidelines developed by pain experts that focus on the issues of postoperative, procedure-related or trauma, and cancer pain. Other national and international organizations, including the Joint Commission for the Accreditation of Health Care Organizations, have also contributed research-based recommendations that nurses can use to improve pain control.

lam (Versed), or diazepam (Valium). Unlike many sedatives, opioids have the advantage of the antidote naloxone (Narcan), which rapidly reverses the respiratory depressant effect. Fortunately, the benzodiazepines, such as diazepam and midazolam, have the drug flumazenil (Romazicon) to treat respiratory depression (see Guidelines box, p. 1336).

Furthermore, as tolerance to the analgesic effect of opioids occurs, tolerance to the respiratory depressant effect also occurs. Pain acts as a natural antagonist to the respiratory depressant effect of opioids. With increased pain, a patient can receive increased doses of opioids without necessarily experiencing clinically significant respiratory depres-

BOX 44-10

Fallacies and Facts about Children and Pain

Fallacy: Infants do not feel pain.
Fact: Infants demonstrate behavioral, especially facial, and physiologic, including hormonal, indicators of pain. Neonates have the neural mechanisms to transmit noxious stimuli by 20 weeks of gestation (Anand & Hickey, 1987; Marshall, 1989; Shapiro, 1989; Stevens, Johnston, & Horton, 1993). (See also Neonatal Pain, Chapter 25.)
Fallacy: Children tolerate pain better than adults.
Fact: Children's tolerance for pain actually increases with age (Haslam, 1969; Lander & Fowler-Kerry, 1991). Younger children tend to rate procedure-related pain higher than older children (Fradet et al, 1990; Humphrey et al, 1992; Wong & Baker, 1988).
Fallacy: Children cannot tell you where they hurt.
Fact: By 4 years of age, children can accurately point to the body area or mark the painful site on a drawing (Savedra et al, 1989, 1993; Van Cleve & Savedra, 1993); children as young as 3 years old can use pain scales, such as faces (Beyer, Denyes, & Villarruel, 1992; Wong & Baker, 1988).
Fallacy: Children always tell the truth about pain.
Fact: Children may not admit having pain to avoid an injection; because of constant pain, they may not realize how much they are hurting; children may believe that others know how they are feeling and not ask for analgesia (Favaloro & Touzel, 1990; Hester, 1989).
Fallacy: Children become accustomed to pain or painful procedures.
Fact: Children often demonstrate increased behavioral signs of discomfort with repeated painful procedures (Dolgin et al, 1989; Fitzgerald, Millard, & MacIntosh, 1988; Katz, Kellerman, & Siegel, 1980; Lander & Fowler-Kerry, 1991).
Fallacy: Behavioral manifestations reflect pain intensity.
Fact: Children's developmental level, coping abilities, and temperament, such as activity level and intensity of reaction to pain, influence pain behavior (Beyer, McGrath, & Berde, 1990; Wallace, 1989; Young & Fu, 1988). Children with more active, resisting behaviors may rate pain lower than children with passive, accepting behaviors (Broome et al, 1990).
Fallacy: Narcotics are more dangerous for children than they are for adults.
Fact: Narcotics (opioids) are no more dangerous for children than they are for adults. Addiction to opioids used to treat pain is extremely rare in children (Brozovic et al, 1986; Morrison, 1991; Rodgers et al, 1988; Rogers, 1990). Reports of respiratory depression in children are also uncommon (Berde et al, 1991; Billmire, Neale, & Gregory 1985; Dilworth & MacKellar, 1987). By 3 to 6 months of age, healthy infants can metabolize opioids similarly to other children (Hertzka et al, 1989; Koren et al, 1985).

sion. Respiratory depression is rare in children receiving long-term opioid therapy because tolerance to the respiratory depression develops (Collins, 1997).

Principles of Pain Assessment in Children

The American Pain Society* (1999) created the phrase "pain: the fifth vital sign" to increase awareness of pain assessment among health care professionals. The rationale is that if pain were assessed as seriously as other vital signs, it would more likely be treated properly. Thus one principle of pain assessment is to assess patients for pain every time the nurse checks for pulse, blood pressure, temperature, and respiratory rate (Federwisch, 1999). Because pain is both a sensory and an emotional experience, several assessment strategies should be used to gather information about pain. One

Community Focus

FEAR OF OPIOID ADDICTION

One of the reasons for the unfounded but prevalent fear of addiction from opioids used to relieve pain is a misunderstanding of the differences between physical dependence, tolerance, and addiction. Health professionals and the community often confuse addiction with the physiologic effects of opioids, when in reality these three events are unrelated.

The American Society of Addiction Medicine (2001) defines these three terms as follows:

Physical dependence on an opioid is a physiologic state in which abrupt cessation of the opioid, or administration of an opioid antagonist, results in a withdrawal syndrome. Physical dependency on opioids is an expected occurrence in all individuals in the presence of continuous use of opioids for therapeutic or for nontherapeutic purposes. It does not, in and of itself, imply addiction.

Tolerance is a form of neuroadaptation to the effects of chronically administered opioids (or other medications) that is indicated by the need for increasing or more frequent doses of the medication to achieve the initial effects of the drug. Tolerance may occur both to the analgesic effects of opioids and to some of the unwanted side effects, such as respiratory depression, sedation, or nausea. The occurrence of tolerance is variable in occurrence, but it does not, in and of itself, imply addiction.

Addiction in the context of pain treatment with opioids is characterized by a persistent pattern of dysfunctional opioid use that may involve any or all of the following:

- Adverse consequences associated with the use of opioids
- Loss of control over the use of opioids
- Preoccupation with obtaining opioids, despite the presence of adequate analgesia

Unfortunately, individuals who have severe, unrelieved pain may become intensely focused on finding relief for their pain. Sometimes behaviors such as "clock watching" make patients appear to others to be preoccupied with obtaining opioids. However, this preoccupation focuses on finding relief of pain, not on using opioids for reasons other than pain control. This phenomenon has been termed *pseudoaddiction* and must not be confused with real addiction.

Nurses must educate older children, parents, and health professionals about the extremely low risk of real addiction (less than 1%) from the use of opioids to treat pain. Infants, young children, and comatose or terminally ill children simply cannot become addicted because they are incapable of a consistent pattern of drug-seeking behavior, such as stealing, drug-dealing, prostitution, and use of family income, to obtain opioids for nonanalgesic reasons.

Adapted from McCaffery M, Paseroc: Pain, ed 2, St Louis, 1999, Mosby. Data from American Society of Addiction Medicine: Public policy statement on definitions related to the use of opioids for pain treatment, February, 2001; Web site: www.asam.org.

*A number of resources on pain management are available from American Pain Society, 4700 W. Lake Ave., Glenview, IL 60025-1485; phone: 847-375-4715; Web site: www.ampainsoc.org

approach to pain assessment in children is QUEST (Baker & Wong, 1987):

Question the child.
Use a pain rating scale.
Evaluate behavioral and physiologic changes.
Secure parents' involvement.
Take the cause of pain into account.
Take action and evaluate results.

Question the Child

Children's verbal statements and descriptions of pain are the *most* important factors in assessing pain. However, young children may not know what the word *pain* means and may need help in describing it using familiar language. Using a variety of words to describe pain, such as *owie, boo-boo, feel funny,* or *hurt,* is necessary. The nurse should also use appropriate foreign language words; for example, in Spanish, *pain* may be described as *le le, duele, dolor,* or *ai ai*). Older children benefit from using simple words to describe pain. Asking children to locate the pain is also helpful, and play can provide other means for helping children reveal discomfort.

NURSE ALERT Ask child to point to where it hurts; have child mark or color the painful area on a drawing of a human figure (Fig. 44-8); ask child to tell how a puppet, doll, or stuffed animal is feeling or to point out areas on these models that "hurt" or "don't feel good." ■

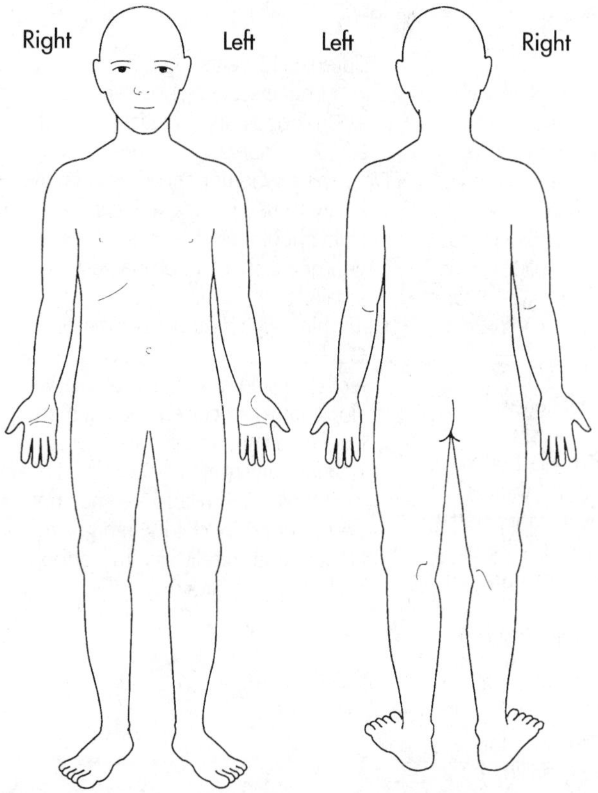

Fig. 44-8 Adolescent pediatric pain tool (APPT): body outlines for pain assessment. Instructions: "Color in the areas on these drawings to show where you have pain. Make the marks as big or as small as the place where the pain is." (From Savedra MC, Tesler MD, Holzemer WL, Ward JA, School of Nursing, University of California–San Francisco, San Francisco, CA. Copyright 1989, 1992.)

When asking children about pain, the nurse must remember that they may deny pain because they fear receiving an injectable analgesic or because they believe they deserve to suffer as punishment for some misdeed. They may also deny pain to a stranger but readily admit it to a parent. This behavior should not be interpreted as seeking attention from the parent, but as a valid indication of pain.

Use a Pain Rating Scale

Pain rating scales provide a quantitative self-reporting measure of pain. Although various pain scales exist (Table 44-2), not all of them are appropriate for young children. For the most valid and reliable pain intensity rating, a scale is selected that is suitable to the child's age, abilities, and preference. Scales using facial expressions are readily accepted by children and can be used by children as young as 3 years of age. Evidence indicates that children may prefer a faces scale to other tools (Keck et al, 1996; Luffy & Grove, 2003; Wong & Baker, 1988).

It is best to use the same scale with children to avoid confusing them with different instructions and to use the pain measurement scale for pain only. Multiple uses of the scale (e.g., as a general measure of the child's feelings) can cause the child to lose interest in the scale. Ideally, children should be taught to use the scale before pain is expected, such as preoperatively. Familiarizing children with the scale facilitates its use when children are actually in pain.

Evaluate Behavioral and Physiologic Changes

Behavioral changes are common indicators of pain and are especially valuable in assessing pain in nonverbal children. Children's behavioral responses to pain change with age and follow a developmental trend (see Box 44-2). However, children vary widely in their responses and may exhibit behaviors at one age that are more typically seen at a different age. Children with more positive moods may appear to be in less pain than they actually are. Children who use passive coping behaviors (offering no resistance, cooperating) may rate pain as more intense than children who use active coping behaviors (resisting, attacking) Recent evidence, however, indicates that temperament does not seem to be a useful predictor of response to pain (Broome, Rehwaldt, & Fogg, 1998). Cultural background may also play a role in children's pain responses (Lipson, Dibble, & Minarik, 1996). In addition, cultural and linguistic differences may hinder assessment. Unfortunately, making judgments about pain based solely on behavior may lead to underestimation of its severity and inadequate pain management (McCaffery & Pasero, 1999; Tesler, Holzemer, & Savedra, 1998).

Depending on the characteristics of pain, children may display behaviors that indicate local body pain, such as pulling the ears for ear pain, rolling the head from side to side for head and ear pain, lying on the side with legs flexed for abdominal pain, limping for leg or foot pain, and refusing to move a body part. Children who experience chronic or repeated pain often develop effective behavioral coping strategies, such as squeezing a hand, talking, counting, relaxing, or thinking about pleasant events. Once these coping skills are identified, the child is encouraged to use them in future experiences with pain.

Physiologic responses indicating pain include flushing of the skin; increases in sweating, blood pressure, pulse, and

Table 44-2

Pain Rating Scales for Children

PAIN SCALE/DESCRIPTION	INSTRUCTIONS	RECOMMENDED AGE/COMMENTS
FACES PAIN RATING SCALE* (Wong & Baker, 1988, 2000): Consists of six cartoon faces ranging from smiling face for "no pain" to tearful face for "worst pain"	**Original instructions:** Explain to child that each face is for a person who feels happy because there is no pain (hurt) or sad because there is some or a lot of pain. FACE 0 is very happy because there is no hurt. FACE 1 hurts just a little bit. FACE 2 hurts a little more. FACE 3 hurts even more. FACE 4 hurts a whole lot, but FACE 5 hurts as much as you can imagine, although you don't have to be crying to feel this bad. Ask child to choose face that best describes own pain. Record the number under chosen face on pain assessment record. Brief word instructions: Point to each face using the words to describe the pain intensity. Ask the child to choose face that best describes own pain, and record the appropriate number	Children as young as 3 years Using original instructions without affect words, such as happy or sad, or brief words resulted in same pain rating, probably reflecting child's rating of pain intensity. For coding purposes, numbers 0, 2, 4, 6, 8, 10 can be substituted for 0-5 system to accommodate 0-10 system. The FACES provides three scales in one: facial expressions, numbers, and words (Pasero, 1997). Research supports cultural sensitivity of FACES for white, black, Hispanic, Thai, Chinese, and Japanese children.

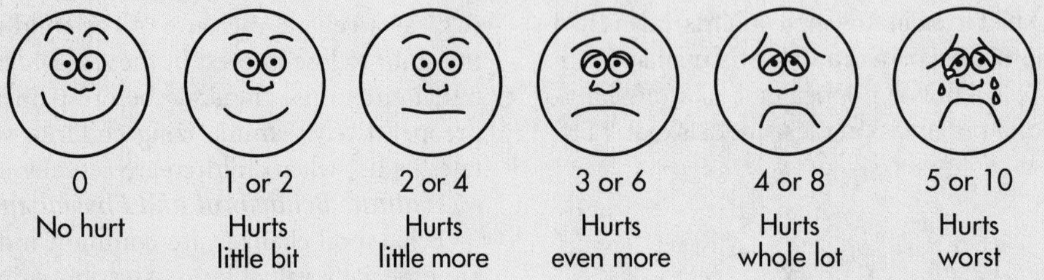

PAIN SCALE/DESCRIPTION	INSTRUCTIONS	RECOMMENDED AGE/COMMENTS
OUCHER (Beyer, Denyes, & Villarruel, 1992): Consists of six photographs of white child's face representing "no hurt" to "biggest hurt you could ever have"; also includes a vertical scale with numbers from 0 to 100; scales for black and Hispanic children have been developed (Villarruel & Denyes, 1991)	**NUMERIC SCALE** Point to each section of scale to explain variations in pain intensity: "O means no hurt." "This means little hurts" (pointing to lower part of scale, 1 to 29). "This means middle hurts" (pointing to middle part of scale, 30 to 69). "This means big hurts" (pointing to upper part of scale, 70 to 99). "100 means the biggest hurt you could ever have." Score is actual number stated by child. **PHOTOGRAPHIC SCALE** Point to each photograph on Oucher and explain variations in pain intensity using following language: first picture from the bottom is "no hurt," second is "a little hurt," third is "a little more hurt," fourth is "even more hurt than that," fifth is "pretty much or a lot of hurt," and the sixth is the "biggest hurt you could ever have." Score pictures from 0 to 5, with the bottom picture scored as 0. **GENERAL** Practice using Oucher by recalling and rating previous pain experiences (e.g., falling off a bike). Child points to number or photograph that describes pain intensity associated with experience. Obtain current pain score from child by asking, "How much hurt do you have right now?"	Children 3-13 years Use numeric scale if child can count to 100 by ones and identify larger of any 2 numbers, or by tens. Determine whether child has cognitive ability to use photographic scale; child should be able to seriate 6 geometric shapes from largest to smallest. Determine which ethnic version of Oucher to use. Allow the child to select a version of Oucher, or use version that most closely matches physical characteristics of child. (Jordan-Marsh et al, 1994). NOTE: Ethnically similar scale may not be preferred by child when given choice of ethnically neutral cartoon scale (Luffy & Grove, 2003).

*Wong-Baker FACES Pain Rating Scale reference manual describing development and research of the scale is available from the Pain/Palliative Care Resource Center, City of Hope National Medical Center, 1500 East Duarte Rd, Duarte, CA 91010; phone: 626-359-8111, ext. 3829; fax: 626-301-8941; www.elsevier-health.com/WOW/.

Table 44-2

Pain Rating Scales for Children—cont'd

PAIN SCALE/DESCRIPTION	INSTRUCTIONS	RECOMMENDED AGE/COMMENTS
POKER CHIP TOOL† (Hester et al, 1998): Uses four red poker chips placed horizontally in front of child	Say to the child: "I want to talk with you about the hurt you may be having right now." Align the chips horizontally in front of the child on the bedside table, a clipboard, or other firm surface. Tell the child, "These are pieces of hurt." Beginning at the chip nearest the child's left side and ending at the one nearest the right side, point to the chips and say, "This [first chip] is a little bit of hurt and this [fourth chip] is the most hurt you could ever have." For a young child or for any child who may not fully comprehend the instructions, clarify by saying, "That means this [one] is just a little hurt, this (two) is a little more hurt, this [three] is more yet, and this [four] is the most hurt you could ever have." Do not give children an option for zero hurt. Research with the Poker Chip Tool has verified that children without pain will so indicate by responses such as "I don't have any." Ask the child, "How many pieces of hurt do you have right now?" After initial use of the Poker Chip Tool, some children internalize the concept "pieces of hurt." If a child gives a response such as "I have one right now," before you ask or before you lay out the poker chips, record the number of chips on the Pain Flow Sheet. Clarify the child's answer by statements such as "Oh, you have a little hurt? Tell me about the hurt."	Children as young as 4 years Determine whether child has cognitive ability to use numbers by identifying larger of any two numbers.
WORD-GRAPHIC RATING SCALE‡ (Tesler et al, 1991): Uses descriptive words (may vary in other scales) to denote varying intensities of pain	Explain to child, "This is a line with words to describe how much pain you may have. This side of the line means no pain, and over here the line means worst possible pain." (Point with your finger where "no pain" is, and run your finger along the line to "worst possible pain," as you say it.) "If you have no pain, you would mark like this." (Show example.) "If you have some pain, you would mark somewhere along the line, depending on how much pain you have." (Show example.) "The more pain you have, the closer to worst pain you would mark. The worst pain possible is marked like this."(Show example.) "Show me how much pain you have right now by marking with a straight, up-and-down line anywhere along the line to show how much pain you have right now." With a millimeter rule, measure from the "no pain" end	Children 4-17 years

†Developed in 1975 by NO Hester, University of Colorado Health Sciences Center, School of Nursing, Denver, CO 80262. Also available in Spanish and French.
‡Instructions for Word-Graphic Rating Scale from Acute Pain Management Guideline Panel: *Acute pain management in infants, children, and adolescents: operative and medical procedures; quick reference guide for clinicians,* ACHPR Pub No 92-0020, Rockville, Md, 1992, Agency for Health Care Research and Quality, US Department of Health and Human Services. Word-Graphic Rating Scale is part of the Adolescent Pediatric Pain Tool and is available from Pediatric Pain Study, University of California, School of Nursing, Department of Family Health Care Nursing, San Francisco, CA 94143-0606; phone: 415-476-4040.

Continued

Table 44-2

Pain Rating Scales for Children—cont'd

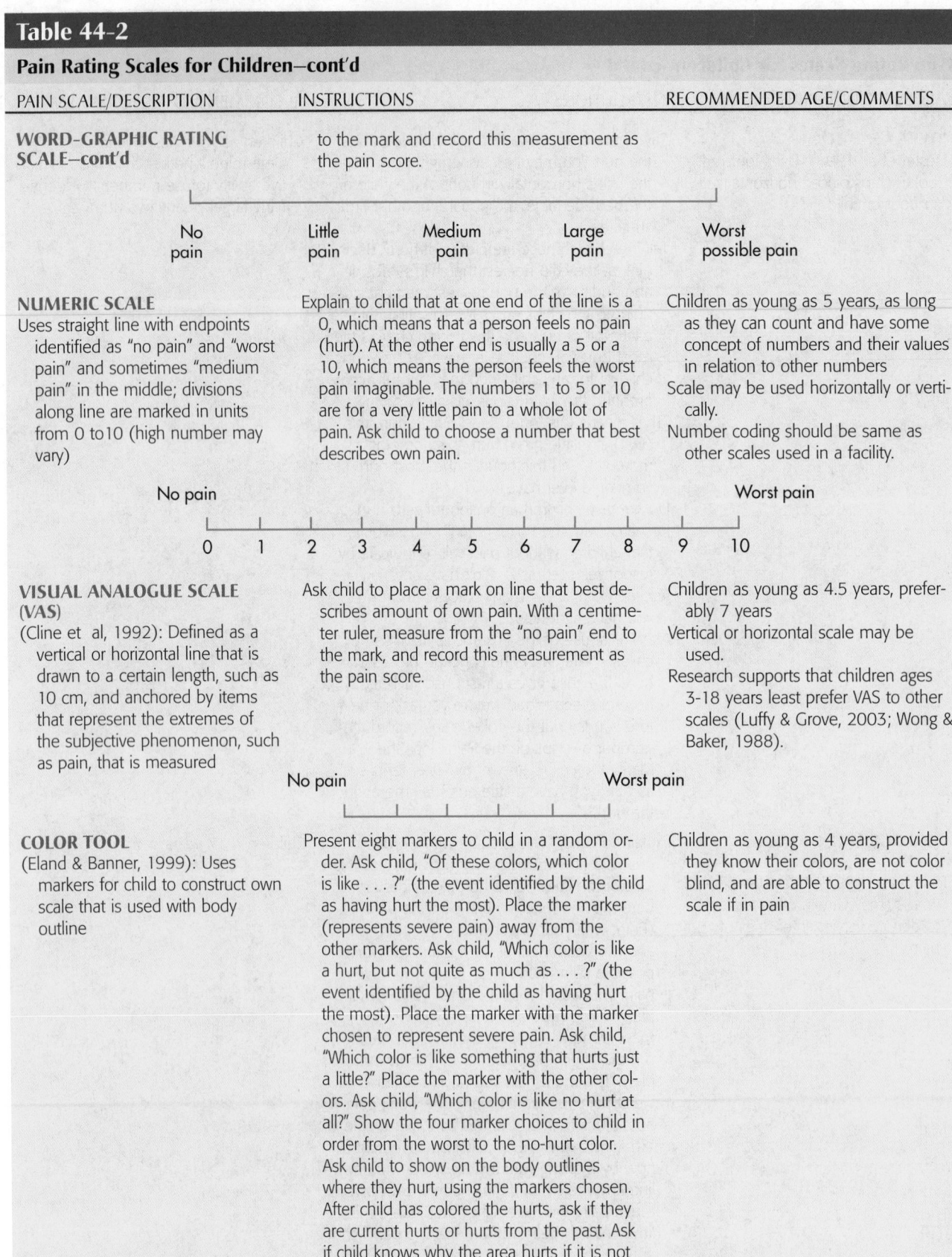

PAIN SCALE/DESCRIPTION	INSTRUCTIONS	RECOMMENDED AGE/COMMENTS
WORD-GRAPHIC RATING SCALE—cont'd	to the mark and record this measurement as the pain score.	
	No pain · Little pain · Medium pain · Large pain · Worst possible pain	
NUMERIC SCALE Uses straight line with endpoints identified as "no pain" and "worst pain" and sometimes "medium pain" in the middle; divisions along line are marked in units from 0 to10 (high number may vary)	Explain to child that at one end of the line is a 0, which means that a person feels no pain (hurt). At the other end is usually a 5 or a 10, which means the person feels the worst pain imaginable. The numbers 1 to 5 or 10 are for a very little pain to a whole lot of pain. Ask child to choose a number that best describes own pain.	Children as young as 5 years, as long as they can count and have some concept of numbers and their values in relation to other numbers Scale may be used horizontally or vertically. Number coding should be same as other scales used in a facility.
	No pain · 0 · 1 · 2 · 3 · 4 · 5 · 6 · 7 · 8 · 9 · 10 · Worst pain	
VISUAL ANALOGUE SCALE (VAS) (Cline et al, 1992): Defined as a vertical or horizontal line that is drawn to a certain length, such as 10 cm, and anchored by items that represent the extremes of the subjective phenomenon, such as pain, that is measured	Ask child to place a mark on line that best describes amount of own pain. With a centimeter ruler, measure from the "no pain" end to the mark, and record this measurement as the pain score.	Children as young as 4.5 years, preferably 7 years Vertical or horizontal scale may be used. Research supports that children ages 3-18 years least prefer VAS to other scales (Luffy & Grove, 2003; Wong & Baker, 1988).
	No pain · Worst pain	
COLOR TOOL (Eland & Banner, 1999): Uses markers for child to construct own scale that is used with body outline	Present eight markers to child in a random order. Ask child, "Of these colors, which color is like . . . ?" (the event identified by the child as having hurt the most). Place the marker (represents severe pain) away from the other markers. Ask child, "Which color is like a hurt, but not quite as much as . . . ?" (the event identified by the child as having hurt the most). Place the marker with the marker chosen to represent severe pain. Ask child, "Which color is like something that hurts just a little?" Place the marker with the other colors. Ask child, "Which color is like no hurt at all?" Show the four marker choices to child in order from the worst to the no-hurt color. Ask child to show on the body outlines where they hurt, using the markers chosen. After child has colored the hurts, ask if they are current hurts or hurts from the past. Ask if child knows why the area hurts if it is not clear to you why it does.	Children as young as 4 years, provided they know their colors, are not color blind, and are able to construct the scale if in pain

respiration; restlessness; and dilation of the pupils. However, these signs vary considerably (e.g., heart rate may actually decrease) and they may be produced by emotions such as fear, anger, or anxiety. They occur primarily in acute pain from stimulation of the sympathetic nervous system. If pain persists, the body begins to adapt and these responses decrease or stabilize. Consequently, if nurses rely primarily on observing these physiologic indications or expecting "pain" behaviors before believing that pain exists, many instances of pain will go unrecognized (Van Cleve, Johnson, & Pothier, 1996).

Several scales have been developed that use changes in behavioral and physiologic parameters to measure pain in young, nonverbal children (Table 44-3). The most common cues assessed in these instruments are facial expression, cry, activity, heart rate, and/or oxygen saturation, and body movements. One example of such a tool is the *FLACC Postoperative Pain Scale* (Merkel et al, 2002) (see Table 44-3). Unfortunately, many of these cues can be affected by events other than pain (e.g., anxiety and fear) and may be open to misinterpretation. For a discussion of pain scales for newborns, see Neonatal Pain, Chapter 25.

Table 44-3

Summary of Selected Behavioral Pain Assessment Scales for Young Children

TOOLS AND AUTHORS/ AGES OF USE	RELIABILITY AND VALIDITY	VARIABLES AND SCORING RANGE
Objective Pain Score (OPS) (Hannallah et al, 1987) Ages of use: 4 months-18 years	No testing in original publication. Later tested by original authors: 1988: concurrent validity with Linear Analogue Pain Scale, Spearman's $r = 0.721$ with scores 36 and 0.419 with scores <6 1991: interrater agreement, coefficient alpha = 0.986 for one rater and 0.983 for the other 1991: concurrent validity with CHEOPS, Pearson correlation coefficient = 0.88 and 0.94	Blood pressure (0-2) Crying (0-2) Moving (0-2) Agitation (0-2) Verbal evaluation/body language (0-2) Scoring range: 0 = no pain; 10 = worst pain
Children's Hospital of Eastern Ontario Pain Scale (CHEOPS) (McGrath et al, 1985) Ages of use: 1-5 years	Interrater reliability = 90% to 99.5% Internal correlation = significant correlations between pairs of items Concurrent validity between CHEOPS and VAS = 0.91; between individual and total scores of CHEOPS and VAS = 0.50-0.86 Construct validity with preanalgesia and postanalgesia scores = 9.9-6.3	Cry (1-3) Facial (0-2) Child verbal (0-2) Torso (1-2) Touch (1-2) Legs (1-2) Scoring range: 4 = no pain; 13 = worst pain
Nurses Assessment of Pain Inventory (NAPI) (Stevens, 1990) Ages of use: newborn-16 years	Not tested by original author. Later tested by Joyce et al (1994) Interrater agreement: weighted kappa 0.37-0.80 Discriminant validity: statistically significant differences between preanalgesia and postanalgesia scores ($p < 0.0001$) Reliability: Cronbach's alpha = 0.35-0.69	Body movement (0-2) Facial (0-3) Touching (0-2) Scoring range: 0 = no pain; 17 = worst pain
Behavioral Pain Score (BPS) (Robieux et al, 1991) Ages of use: 3-36 months	Original article stated, "reliability of the VAS and BPS scores was tested by a k test"; no further testing of reliability or validity was mentioned	Facial expression (0-2) Cry (0-3) Movements (0-3) Scoring range: 0 = no pain; 8 = worst pain
Modified Behavioral Pain Scale (MBPS) (Taddio et al, 1995) Ages of use: 4-6 months	Concurrent validity between MBPS and VAS scores = correlation coefficient 0.68 ($p < 0.001$) and 0.74 ($p < 0.001$) Construct validity using prevaccination and postvaccination scores with EMLA vs. placebo: significantly lower scores with EMLA ($p < 0.01$) Internal consistency of items = significant correlations between items Interrater agreement: ICC = 0.95, $p < 0.001$ Test-retest reliability: 0.95, $p < .001$	Facial expression (0-3) Cry (0-4) Movements (0, 2, 3) Scoring range: 0 = no pain; 10 = worst pain

Continued

Table 44-3

Summary of Selected Behavioral Pain Assessment Scales for Young Children—cont'd

TOOLS AND AUTHORS/ AGES OF USE	RELIABILITY AND VALIDITY	VARIABLES AND SCORING RANGE
Riley Infant Pain Scale (RIPS) (Schade et al, 1996) Ages of use: <36 months and children with cerebral palsy	Interrater agreement using Intraclass Correlation Coefficient = 0.53-0.83, p <0.0001 Discriminant validity using Mann-Whitney U test with preanalgesia and postanalgesia scores = statistically significant (p <0.001) Sensitivity = 0.31-0.23 Specificity = 0.86-0.90	0: Neutral face/smiling, calm, sleeping quietly, no cry, consolable, moves easily 1: Frowning/grimace, movements, restless sleep, whimpering, winces with touch 2: Clenched teeth, moderate agitation, sleeps intermittently, pain crying, difficult to console, cries with touch 3: Full cry expression, thrashing/flailing, sleeping prolonged periods interrupted by jerking or no sleep, screaming/high-pitched cry, inconsolable, screams when touched/moved Scoring range: 0 = no pain; 3 = worst pain
FLACC Postoperative Pain Tool (Merkel et al, 1997)* Ages of use: 2 months-7 years	Interrater reliability using two-way cross tabulations and kappa statistics (r[87] = 0.94; p <0.001) and kappa values above 0.50 for each category Validity using ANOVA for repeated measures to compare FLACC scores before and after analgesia; preanalgesia FLACC scores were significantly higher than postanalgesia scores at 10, 30, and 60 minutes (p <0.001 for each time) Correlation coefficients used to compare FLACC pain scores and OPS pain scores; significant positive correlation between FLACC and OPS scores (r = 0.80; p <0.001); positive correlation also found between FLACC scores and nurses' global ratings of pain (r[47] = 0.41; p <0.005)	Face (0-2) Legs (0-2) Activity (0-2) Cry (0-2) Consolability (0-2) Scoring range: 0 = no pain; 10 = worst pain

FLACC SCALE*

	0	1	2
Face	No particular expression or smile	Occasional grimace or frown, withdrawn, disinterested	Frequent to constant frown, clenched jaw, quivering chin
Legs	Normal position or relaxed	Uneasy, restless, tense	Kicking, or legs drawn up
Activity	Lying quietly, normal position, moves easily	Squirming, shifting back and forth, tense	Arched, rigid, or jerking
Cry	No cry (awake or asleep)	Moans or whimpers, occasional complaint	Crying steadily, screams or sobs, frequent complaints
Consolability	Content, relaxed	Reassurred by occasional touching, hugging, or talking to; distractable	Difficult to console or comfort

*From Merkel S et al: The FLACC: a behavioral scale for scoring postoperative pain in young children, *Pediatr Nurs* 23(3):293-297, 1997. Used with permission of Jannetti Publications, Inc and the University of Michigan Health System. Can be reproduced for clinical and research use.
NOTE: Based on accumulating clinical experience, scale can be used with full-term newborns to 2 months of age.

Assessing pain in children with developmental and/or physical disabilities or children who are in a coma, on a ventilator, or pharmacologically paralyzed is challenging and, for the most part, remains unexplored. Researchers are investigating parents' descriptions of recognizing pain in the child with serious cognitive and physical impairment (Fanurik et al, 1999; Oberlander, O'Donnell, & Montgomery, 1999).

One of the most valuable clues to pain is a change in behavior and vital signs after administration of an analgesic. Behaviors such as less irritability or cessation of crying and decreased pulse, respirations, and blood pressure provide important evidence for pain existing before treatment. Often the change in vital signs is attributed to the depressant effect of opioids, when in reality the return to more normal physiologic functioning is due to pain relief.

Encourage Parents' Involvement

Parents are often the primary source of information about how their child exhibits pain and should play a key role in the assessment of their child's pain. They are sensitive to changes in their child's behavior and typically want to be involved in their child's pain relief. Parents' ability to recognize pain in their children varies. Some parents may never have seen their child in severe pain and may not equate certain responses, such as irritability or withdrawal, with discomfort. Others are aware that certain behaviors signal pain because the child has acted similarly during previous painful events. Parents usually know what comforts their child, such as rocking, stroking, or talking. They are the persons most consistently caring for the child. Encouraging their participation gives them control and a sense of helping.

To better assess the child's pain, the nurse can interview the parents about their child's previous pain experiences. Ideally, this questioning should occur before the child is in pain, such as on admission to the hospital. Parents need to realize that their knowledge of their child is important in providing care. Parents sometimes leave the assessment of pain up to the nurse because "nurses are more experienced," and they expect the nurse to know when their child is in pain (Woodgate & Kristjanson, 1996). Consequently, parents do not report pain. Parents need to be taught nonverbal pain behaviors in children and encouraged to inform the staff when they think their child is in pain.

Take the Cause of Pain into Account

When children exhibit behaviors or other clues that suggest pain, reasons for discomfort should be investigated. The pathologic condition may give clues to the expected intensity and type of pain. For example, pain associated with vaso-occlusive crises in sickle cell disease is severe. Pain caused by bone marrow puncture is typically greater than the discomfort associated with a venipuncture. However, it is a mistake to assume that certain conditions or procedures always produce a standard amount of pain. For example, sore throat pain may be mild or severe—only the child knows the intensity.

NURSE ALERT A golden rule to follow in pain assessment is this: Whatever is painful to an adult is painful to an infant or child, until proved otherwise. Be aware that temperament affects coping style, and children with more positive moods may appear to be in less pain than they actually are. Children who use passive coping behaviors (offering no resistance, cooperating) may rate pain as more intense than children who use active coping behaviors (resisting, attacking). If children's behaviors appear to differ from their rating of pain, believe their pain rating, unless they appear to be in pain. In this case, inquire about possible reasons for denying pain (i.e., children with burns may deny pain because they believe they should suffer for setting the fire). ■

Take Action and Evaluate Results

The reason for assessing pain is to relieve it. Complete pain relief, with the combined use of pharmacologic and nonpharmacologic interventions, should be the goal. However, complete relief may not be possible.

Regardless of the type of pain intervention, *evaluation of the results is essential.* No one pain reduction technique is effective for all children. Therefore a pain assessment record is used to monitor the effectiveness of the interventions (Fig. 44-9). With nonverbal children, behavioral and physiologic signs are evaluated for evidence of pain relief. With verbal children, their statements about pain relief and pain ratings are also recorded. Changes in the medication regimen are made as needed to provide maximal pain relief with minimal side effects. Family members are often excellent partners for keeping a pain assessment record for the nurse.

NURSE ALERT Presenting practitioners with objective documentation of pain, rather than opinion, is more likely to lead to a favorable change in analgesic disorders (Walker & Wong, 1991). ■

Pain Management

Relief of pain is a basic need and right of all children. Effective pain management requires that health professionals be willing to try a number of interventions to achieve optimum results. Basically, pain-reducing methods can be grouped into two categories: nonpharmacologic and pharmacologic. Whenever possible, both should be used; however, nonpharmacologic measures are not substitutes for analgesics.

Nonpharmacologic Management

Pain is often associated with fears, anxiety, and stress. A number of nonpharmacologic techniques, such as distraction, relaxation, guided imagery, and cutaneous stimulation (Guidelines box), provide coping strategies that may help reduce pain perception, make pain more tolerable, decrease anxiety, and enhance the effectiveness of analgesics (Kachoyeanos & Friedhoff, 1993). Although research on the effectiveness of many of these interventions is inconclusive, the strategies are safe, noninvasive, and inexpensive, and most are independent nursing functions. Experimentation with several strategies that are appropriate for the child's age, pain intensity, interest, and abilities is often necessary to determine the most effective approach.

NURSE ALERT Most specific nonpharmacologic strategies require children's understanding and cooperation. Therefore try to match the strategy with the pain severity. Children in severe pain may not be able to expend the effort necessary to learn the technique, and those with very mild symptoms may not be motivated to learn. Therefore these strategies may be most useful with midrange pain. ■

In the selection of a nonpharmacologic intervention, it is best to use a technique familiar to the child or to describe several strategies and let the child select the most appealing one. Parents should be involved in the selection process; they may be familiar with the child's usual coping skills and can help identify potentially successful strategies. Involving parents also encourages their participation in learning the skill with the child and acting as coach. If the parent cannot assist the child, other appropriate persons may include a grandparent, older sibling, nurse, or child-life specialist.

Children should learn a specific strategy *before* pain occurs or before it becomes severe. To reduce the child's effort, instructions for a strategy, such as distraction or relaxation, can be audiotaped and played during a period of discomfort.

Guidelines

NONPHARMACOLOGIC STRATEGIES FOR PAIN MANAGEMENT

General Strategies

Use nonpharmacologic interventions to supplement, not replace, pharmacologic interventions and for mild pain and pain that is reasonably well controlled with analgesics.

Form a trusting relationship with child and family.
- Express concern regarding their reports of pain and intervene appropriately.
- Take an active role in seeking effective pain management strategies.

Use general guidelines to prepare child for procedure (see Chapter 45).

Prepare child before potentially painful procedures but avoid "planting" the idea of pain. For example, instead of saying, "This is going to (or may) hurt," say, "Sometimes this feels like pushing, sticking, or pinching, and sometimes it doesn't bother people. Tell me what it feels like to you."

Use "nonpain" descriptors when possible (e.g., "It feels like heat," rather than "It's a burning pain."). This allows for variation in sensory perception, avoids suggesting pain, and gives child control in describing reactions.

Avoid evaluative statements or descriptions (e.g., "This is a terrible procedure," or "It really will hurt a lot.").

Stay with child during a painful procedure.
- Allow parents to stay with child if child and parent desire; encourage parent to talk softly to child and to remain near child's head.
- Involve parents in learning specific nonpharmacologic strategies and in assisting child with their use.

Educate child about the pain, especially when explanation may lessen anxiety (e.g., that pain may occur after surgery and does not indicate something is wrong); reassure that child is not responsible for the pain.

For long-term pain control, give child a doll, which represents "the patient," and allow child to do everything to the doll that is done to the child; pain control can be emphasized through the doll by stating, "Dolly feels better after the medicine."
- Teach procedures to child and family for later use.

Specific Strategies

Distraction

Involve parent and child in identifying strong distractors.

Involve child in play; use radio, tape recorder, CD player, or computer game; have child sing or use rhythmic breathing.

Have child take a deep breath and blow it out until told to stop (French, Painter, & Coury, 1994).

Have child blow bubbles to "blow the hurt away."

Have child concentrate on yelling or saying "ouch" by focusing on "yelling as loud or soft as you feel it hurt: that way I know what's happening."

Have child look through kaleidoscope (type with glitter suspended in fluid-filled tube) and encourage to concentrate by asking, "Do you see the different designs?" (Vessey, Carlson, & McGill, 1994).

Use humor, such as watching cartoons, telling jokes or funny stories, or acting silly with child.

Have child read, play games, or visit with friends.

Relaxation

With an infant or young child:
- Hold in a comfortable, well-supported position, such as vertically against the chest and shoulder.
- Rock in a wide, rhythmic arc in a rocking chair or sway back and forth, rather than bouncing child.
- Repeat one or two words softly, such as "Mommy's here."

With a slightly older child:
- Ask child to take a deep breath and "go limp as a rag doll" while exhaling slowly; then ask child to yawn (demonstrate if needed).
- Help child assume a comfortable position (e.g., pillow under neck and knees).
- Begin progressive relaxation: starting with the toes, systematically instruct child to let each body part "go limp" or "feel heavy"; if child has difficulty with relaxing, instruct child to tense or tighten each body part and then relax it.

Allow child to keep eyes open, since children may respond better if eyes are open rather than closed during relaxation.

Guided Imagery

Have child identify some highly pleasurable real or imaginary experience.

Have child describe details of the event, including as many senses as possible (e.g., "feel the cool breezes," "see the beautiful colors," "hear the pleasant music").
- Have child write down or tape record script.

Encourage child to concentrate only on the pleasurable event during the painful time; enhance the image by recalling specific details through reading the script or playing the tape.

Combine with relaxation and rhythmic breathing.

Positive Self-Talk

Teach child positive statements to say when in pain (e.g., "I will be feeling better soon," "When I go home, I will feel better, and we will eat ice cream.").

Thought Stopping

Identify positive facts about the painful event (e.g., "It does not last long.").

Identify reassuring information (e.g., "If I think about something else, it does not hurt as much.").

Condense positive and reassuring facts into a set of brief statements and have child memorize them (e.g., "Short procedure, good veins, little hurt, nice nurse, go home.").

Have child repeat the memorized statements whenever thinking about or experiencing the painful event.

Cutaneous Stimulation

Includes simple rhythmic rubbing; use of pressure or electric vibrator; massage with hand lotion, powder, or menthol cream; application of heat or cold, such as vapocoolant spray on the site before giving injection or application of ice to the site opposite the painful area (e.g., if right knee hurts, place ice on left knee).

A more sophisticated method is *transcutaneous electrical nerve stimulation (TENS)* (use of controlled low-voltage electricity to the body via electrodes placed on the skin).

Another method is the use of *Pain Relief Therapeutic Electro-Membrane (P.R.E.M.)*, a high-technology membrane electron reservoir fabricated from a nonwoven, nonallergenic dressing that when placed in contact with the skin, releases the stored electrons in the form of microcurrent impulses.*

Behavioral Contracting

***Informal*—May be used with children as young as 4 or 5 years of age:**
- Use stars or tokens as rewards.
- Give uncooperative or procrastinating children (during a procedure) a limited time (measured by a visible timer) to complete the procedure.

*For more information contact Helio Medical Supplies, Inc., 606 Charcot Ave., San Jose, CA 95131; phone: 888-PAINTEM (724-6836); e-mail: eileen@heliomed.com.

Guidelines

NONPHARMACOLOGIC STRATEGIES FOR PAIN MANAGEMENT—cont'd

Proceed as needed if child is unable to comply.
Reinforce cooperation with a reward if the procedure is accomplished within specified time.

Formal—Use written contract that includes:
- Realistic (seems possible) goal or desired behavior
- Measurable behavior (e.g., agrees not to hit anyone during procedures)
- Contract written, dated, and signed by all persons involved in any of the agreements
- Identified rewards or consequences that are reinforcing
- Goals that can be evaluated
- Commitment and compromise requirements for both parties (e.g., while timer is used, nurse will not nag or prod child to complete procedure)

Pain Assessment Record

Directions for each column:
1. Record date and time of assessment and analgesic administration; assess analgesic effect ______________ minutes later and then ______________
2. Use a pain rating scale if child understands its use.
   Name of scale: ____________________
   Ratings: No pain = _____ Worst pain = _____ Comfort/function goals* _____
3. Record analgesic, dose, and route
4. Record possible indications or effects of pain, such as shallow breathing due to incisional pain, parental request for pain relief; record indications or effects of pain relief, such as "moves easily, playing"
5. Record any other side effects (e.g., nausea, itching)
6. Record LOS (see inset) R (respiratory function); record breaths per minute and/or other observations of respiratory status (e.g., depth of respiration, change in color of skin)
7. Signature or initials of person recording information

Level of Sedation (LOS) Scale†

S = Sleeping, easily aroused
Requires no action
1 = Awake and alert
Requires no action
2 = Occasionally drowsy, easy to arouse
Requires no action
3 = Frequently drowsy, arousable, drifts off to sleep during conversation
Notify practitioner and decrease dose
4 = Somnolent, minimal or no response to stimuli
Notify practitioner and stop opioid

1 Date/time	2 Pain rating	3 Analgesic	4 Possible effects/indications of pain or relief of pain	5 Side effects	6 LOS/R	7 Signature

*Ask the child what pain rating would be acceptable in terms of usual function (e.g., activities of daily living, playing, and attending school). From McCaffery M, Pasero C, editors: *Pain: a clinical manual,* ed 2, St Louis, 1999, Mosby.
†From Pasero C, McCaffery M: Providing epidural analgesia: how to maintain a delicate balance, *Nurs 99* 29(8):34-39, 1999.

Fig. 44-9 Pain assessment record.

Pharmacologic Management

Using pharmacologic methods to control pain requires attention to four "rights": right drug, right dose, right route, and right time. In addition, observing for side effects is an essential nursing intervention. Although nurses may not prescribe the medication, knowledge of these essential principles assists in optimally implementing analgesic orders and discussing with other practitioners possible strategies to improve pain control. In addition, observing for side effects of the drug and using supportive approaches with children when administering the drug are important nursing interventions.

Right Drug

Nonopioids, including acetaminophen (Tylenol, paracetamol) and nonsteroidal antiinflammatory drugs (NSAIDs), are suitable for mild-to-moderate pain; opioids are needed for moderate-to-severe pain. A combination of the two analgesics attacks pain on two levels: nonopioids primarily at the peripheral nervous system (PNS) and opioids primarily at

BOX 44-11

Selected Combination Opioid and Nonopioid Oral Analgesics–Nonaspirin Products*

Fioricet with Codeine	30 mg codeine 325 mg acetaminophen 50 mg butalbital 40 mg caffeine
Hydrocet	5 mg hydrocodone 500 mg acetaminophen
Lorcet-HD	5 mg hydrocodone 500 mg acetaminophen
Lorcet Plus	7.5 mg hydrocodone 650 mg acetaminophen
Lorcet 10/650	10 mg hydrocodone 650 mg acetaminophen
Lortab 2.5/500	2.5 mg hydrocodone 500 mg acetaminophen
Lortab 5/500	5 mg hydrocodone 500 mg acetaminophen
Lortab 10/500	10 mg hydrocodone 500 mg acetaminophen
Lortab Elixir (each 15 ml)	7.5 mg hydrocodone 500 mg acetaminophen
Percocet 2.5/325†	2.5 mg oxycodone 325 mg acetaminophen
Percocet-5/325	5 mg oxycodone HCl 325 mg acetaminophen
Percocet 7.5/500	7.5 mg oxycodone 500 mg acetaminophen
Percocet 10/650	10 mg oxycodone 650 mg acetaminophen
Tylenol with Codeine No. 1	7.5 mg codeine 300 mg acetaminophen
Tylenol with Codeine No. 2	15 mg codeine 300 mg acetaminophen
Tylenol with Codeine No. 3	30 mg codeine 300 mg acetaminophen
Tylenol with Codeine No. 4	60 mg codeine 300 mg acetaminophen
Tylenol and Codeine Elixir (each 5 ml)	12 mg codeine 120 mg acetaminophen 7% alcohol
Tylox†	5 mg oxycodone HCl 500 mg acetaminophen
Vicodin	5 mg hydrocodone 500 mg acetaminophen
Vicodin ES	7.5 mg hydrocodone 750 mg acetaminophen
Vicodin HP	10 mg hydrocodone 650 mg acetaminophen
Vicoprofen	7.5 mg hydrocodone 200 mg ibuprofen

*Aspirin is not recommended for children because of its possible association with Reye's syndrome. Analgesic compounds with aspirin include Darvon Compound, Darvon with A.S.A., Percodan, and Percodan-Demi. Darvon or Darvocet (propoxyphene) is not recommended; its analgesic effect is no greater than that from aspirin, acetaminophen, or other NSAIDs. Propoxyphene, an opioid, can depress respirations, and its major metabolite is cardiotoxic and is a central nervous system (CNS) stimulant that can produce seizures (Dahl, 1998).

†All medications require a prescription, but these are classified as schedule II drugs (like morphine), and each filling requires a written prescription that includes the patient's name and address, the practitioner's Drug Enforcement Agency (DEA) number, and the date. In case of emergency, verbal prescriptions for schedule II substances may be filled; however, the practitioner must provide a signed prescription within 72 hours. Schedule II prescriptions cannot be refilled but require a new prescription.

the central nervous system (CNS). This approach provides increased analgesia without increased side effects. Several commercially available combinations, such as Tylenol with Codeine, may have increasing doses of the opioid but a constant dose of the nonopioid (Box 44-11). Therefore, before increasing the opioid, it may be preferable to increase the nonopioid component (e.g., adding 300 mg of plain Tylenol to Tylenol with Codeine No. 3 before advancing to Tylenol with Codeine No. 4). However, if this approach is not successful, the pain most likely requires a stronger opioid.

Actions of various opioids differ. Morphine is considered the gold standard for the management of severe pain. When morphine is not a suitable opioid, drugs such as oxycodone, hydromorphone (Dilaudid), and fentanyl (Sublimaze) are effective substitutes. Although fentanyl is used as an anesthetic in the operating room, it is classified as an analgesic. It can be safely administered by nurses as a continuous infusion (Algren & Algren, 1998). Although methadone is usually thought of as a drug used to treat opioid-dependent patients, it is increasingly being used for postoperative analgesia or intractable pain. When administered orally or intravenously, a single dose of methadone may provide up to 36 hours of pain relief (Yaster, Kost-Byerly, & Maxwell, 2003).

Meperidine (Demerol, pethidine) is not recommended as a first-line opioid analgesic for the management of any kind of pain (American Pain Society, 1999; McCaffery & Pasero, 1999). A major drawback in the use of meperidine is its metabolite, normeperidine. Normeperidine is a CNS stimulant that can produce restlessness, irritability, twitching, jerking, agitation, tremors, and seizures. The CNS side effects caused by normeperidine are not reversed with naloxone. Another disadvantage of meperidine is the long half-life of its metabolite. Normeperidine has a half life of 15 to 20 hours, compared with meperidine's half-life of 3 hours (Tobias, 2003).

NURSE ALERT By any route of administration, the use of meperidine for any type of pain management in children should be questioned because other less toxic, more effective opioid drugs are available. Meperidine should be used only for short-term (48 hours) pain management in healthy patients who have demonstrated an unusual reaction or allergic response during treatment with other opioids. When meperidine is administered, assess the child frequently for signs of toxicity such as tremors of the outstretched hands, twitching or jerking, or increased agitation. If toxicity is suspected, discontinue the meperidine, maintain the IV infusion, and notify the practitioner immediately. An adverse drug reaction should also be reported.* ■

Opioids are frequently combined with other drugs that are considered "potentiators." However, little evidence indicates that any drug potentiates the analgesic effect of opioids; rather, drugs that produce sedation are erroneously equated with producing analgesia. One common drug combination—meperidine (pethidine [Demerol]), promethazine (Phenergan), and chlorpromazine (Thorazine), known as

*The FDA Medical Products Reporting Program, Food and Drug Administration, 5600 Fishers Lane, Rockville, MD 20852-9787; phone: 800-FDA-1088; fax: 800-FDA-0178; Web site: www.fda.gov/medwatch.

Table 44-4

Suggested Medications for Sedation

DRUG	DOSING	SIDE EFFECTS	REVERSAL AGENTS
CONSCIOUS SEDATION			
Midazolam A benzodiazepine (short acting), CNS depressant Onset: 1-5 min Peak effect: 3-5 min (IV) Half-life: 1.5-2 hr	Oral: 0.2-1 mg/kg; 30-45 min before procedure; maximum: 20 mg IV: 0.05 mg/kg 3 min before procedure (may repeat dose ×2); maximum: 2 mg/dose	Respiratory distress, depression, apnea, PVCs, amnesia, blurred vision, or hyperexcitability	Flumazenil: 0.2 mg/dose every 1 min; maximum cumulative = 1 mg
Fentanyl A narcotic analgesic Onset: 1-5 min Peak effect: no data available Half-life: 1.5-6 hr	IV: 0.5-3 mcg/kg/dose; may repeat after 30-60 min; maximum: 50 mcg/dose Use lower doses (0.5-1 mcg/kg/dose) when used in combination with other agents, such as midazolam.	Respiratory distress or depression, apnea, seizures, shock, chest wall rigidity (most rapid infusion or high doses)	Naloxone: 5-1 mcg/kg/dose; single dose should not exceed maximum likely to occur with recommended adult dose of 0.2 mg
Morphine A narcotic analgesic Onset: 15-60 min Peak effect: 30-40 min Half life: 1.5-2 hr	IV: 0.05-0.1 mg/kg 5 min before procedure; maximum: 15 mg/dose	Sedation, somnolence, respiratory distress, depression, or pruritus	Naloxone: 5-10 mcg/kg/dose; single dose should not exceed maximum recommended adult dose of 0.2 mg
UNCONSCIOUS SEDATION			
Propofol A general anesthetic Onset: within 30 sec Peak effect: 3-10 min Half life: three-compartment model Initial; 2-8 min second distribution: 40 min Terminal: 200 min	IV: 1-2 mg/kg followed by 75-100 mcg/kg/min (only with qualified anesthesia personnel available)	Pain on injection, involuntary movements, hypotension, apnea	None
Ketamine A general anesthetic Onset: 30 sec with IV administration; PO 20-45 min Peak effect: 5 min Half-life: unknown	Oral: 6-10 mg/kg given 30 min before procedure IV: 0.25-0.75 mg/kg (only with qualified anesthesia personnel available)	Laryngospasm, severe hypotension/hypertension, respiratory depression, apnea, excessive salivation	None

PO, Per os (by mouth, orally); *PVCs,* premature ventricular contractions.

DPT or lytic cocktail—has commonly been used to sedate children for procedures (see Preoperative Care, Chapter 45). Meperidine, a short-acting analgesic, provides pain relief for 2 to 3 hours but is irritating to the tissues when given intramuscularly. Promethazine has antianalgesic properties, produces excessive sedation, and can cause extrapyramidal reactions (spasms of neck, face, tongue, and back; fixed eyeballs). Besides producing prolonged deep sedation, all of these drugs can cause respiratory depression and lower the seizure threshold, a particular risk to those with a seizure disorder. In addition, the "cocktail" is usually administered intramuscularly, causing additional pain. *For these reasons, DPT is not recommended for general use* (Yaster et al, 2003). Appropriate drugs for sedation are listed in Table 44-4.

Several drugs, known as *adjuvant analgesics* or *coanalgesics,* may be used alone or with opioids to control pain symptoms. Commonly used drugs to relieve anxiety, cause sedation, and provide amnesia are diazepam (Valium) and midazolam (Versed); however, they are not analgesics. Other adjuvants include tricyclic antidepressants (i.e., amitriptyline, imipramine) and antiepileptics for neuropathic pain (brief, lancinating pain); steroids for inflammation and bone pain; and dex-

Table 44-5

Nonsteroidal Antiinflammatory Drugs (NSAIDs) Approved for Children*

DRUG (TRADE NAME)	DOSE	COMMENTS
Acetaminophen (Tylenol and other brands)	10-15 mg/kg/dose every 4-6 hr not to exceed 5 doses in 24 hr or 75 mg/kg/day, orally	Available in numerous preparations Nonprescription Higher dosage range may provide increased analgesia
Choline magnesium trisalicylate (Trilisate)	Children <37 kg: 50 mg/kg/day divided into 2 doses Children >37 kg: 2250 mg/day divided into 2 doses	Available in suspension, 500 mg/5 ml Prescription
Ibuprofen† Children's Motrin Children's Advil	Children <6 mo: 5-10 mg/kg/dose every 6-8 hr not to exceed 40 mg/kg/day	Available in numerous preparations Available in suspension, 100 mg/5 ml, and drops, 100 mg/2.5 ml Nonprescription
Naproxen (Naprosyn)	Children >2 years: 10 mg/kg/day divided into 2 doses	Available in suspension, 125 mg/5 ml, and several different dosages for tablets Prescription
Tolmetin (Tolectin)	Children >2 years: 20 mg/kg/day divided into 3 or 4 doses	Available in 200 mg, 400 mg, and 600 mg tablets Prescription

Data from Olin BR et al: *Drug facts and comparisons,* St Louis, 2002, Facts and Comparisons.

NOTE: Newer formulations of NSAIDs, such as celecoxib, (Celebrex) rofecoxib (Vioxx), or valdecoxib (Bextra), selectively inhibit one of the enzymes of cyclooxygenase (COX-2, which is responsible for pain transmission) but do not inhibit the other (COX-1). Inhibition of COX-1 decreases prostaglandin production, which is necessary for normal organ function. For example, prostaglandins help maintain gastric mucosal blood flow and barrier protection, regulate blood flow to the liver and kidneys, and facilitate platelet aggregation and clot formation. Theoretically, the COX-2 NSAIDs provide similar analgesic and antiinflammatory benefits with fewer gastric and platelet side effects than the nonselective agents. COX-2 NSAIDs are approved for use in patients over 18 years of age.

*All NSAIDs in the table (except acetaminophen) have significant antiinflammatory, antipyretic, and analgesic actions. Acetaminophen has a weak antiinflammatory action, and its classification as an NSAID is controversial. Patients respond differently to various NSAIDs; therefore, changing from one drug to another may be necessary for maximum benefit.

Acetylsalicylic acid (aspirin) is also an NSAID but is not recommended for children because of its possible association with Reye's syndrome. The NSAIDs in the table have no known association with Reye's syndrome. However, caution should be exercised in prescribing any salicylate-containing drug (e.g., Trilisate) for children with known or suspected viral infection.

†Side effects of ibuprofen, naproxen, and tolmetin include nausea, vomiting, diarrhea, constipation, gastric ulceration, bleeding nephritis, and fluid retention. Acetaminophen and choline magnesium trisalicylate are well tolerated in the gastrointestinal tract and do not interfere with platelet function. NSAIDs (except acetaminophen) should not be given to patients with allergic reactions to salicylates. All the NSAIDs should be used cautiously in patients with renal impairment.

troamphetamine and caffeine for increased analgesia and decreased sedation (McCaffery & Pasero, 1999).

At times, health professionals question whether pain really exists and administer *placebos* to "see if the pain is real." This practice is unjustified and unethical; a positive response to a placebo, such as a saline injection, is common in patients who have a documented organic basis for pain. Therefore the deceptive use of placebos does not provide useful information about the presence or severity of pain. In addition, the use of placebos can cause side effects similar to those of opioids in addition to destroying the client's trust in the health care staff, and raising serious ethical and legal questions (Pasero, 1995). The position of the American Society of Pain Management Nurses (1998) is that placebos should not be used by any route in the assessment or management of pain in any patient regardless of age or diagnosis.

Right Dosage

The optimum dosage is one that controls pain without causing severe side effects. This usually requires *titration,* the gradual adjustment of drug dosage (usually by increasing or decreasing the dose) until optimum pain relief without excessive sedation is achieved. Dosage recommendations, such as those in Tables 44-5 and 44-6, are only safe initial dosages, not optimum dosages. Children (except infants younger than about 3 to 6 months of age) metabolize drugs more rapidly than adults; younger children may require higher doses of opioids to achieve the same analgesic effect. Therefore the therapeutic effect and duration of analgesia vary. Children's dosages are usually calculated according to body weight, except in children who weigh 50 kg (110 pounds) or more, when the weight formula may exceed the average adult dose. In this case the adult dose is used.

A reasonable starting dose of opioid for infants under 6 months of age who are not mechanically ventilated is one-fourth to one-third of the recommended starting dose for older children. The infant is monitored very closely for signs of pain relief and respiratory depression. The dose is titrated to effect. Because tolerance can develop rapidly, very large opioid doses may be needed for continued severe pain (American Pain Society, 1999).

Table 44-6

Dosage of Selected Opioids for Children

DRUG	APPROXIMATE EQUI-ANALGESIC ORAL DOSE	APPROXIMATE EQUIANAL-GESIC PAREN-TERAL DOSE	Recommended Starting Dose (Children <50 kg Body Weight)[a] ORAL	PARENTERAL[b]
Morphine[c]	30 mg every 3-4 hr	10 mg every 3-4 hr	0.2-0.4 mg/kg every 3-4 hr 0.3-0.6 mg/kg time released every 12 hr	0.1-0.2 mg/kg IM every 3-4 hr (ATC dosing) 0.02-0.1 mg/kg IV bolus every 2 hr 0.015 mg/kg every 8 min PCA 0.01-0.02 mg/kg/hr IV infusion (neonates) 0.01-0.06 mg/kg/hr IV infusion (child)
Fentanyl (Sublimaze) (oral mucosal form—Actiq)[d]	Not available	0.1 mg	IV 5-15 mcg/kg; maximum dose 400 mcg	0.5-1.5 mcg/kg IV bolus every ½ hour 1-2 mcg/hr IV infusion
Codeine[e]	200 mg every 3-4 hr	130 mg every 3-4 hr	1 mg/kg every 3-4 hr	Not recommended
Hydromorphone[c] (Dilaudid)	7.5 mg every 3-4 hr	1.5 mg every 3-4 hr	0.04-0.1 mg/kg every 4-6 hr	0.02-0.1 mg/kg IM every 3-4 hr 0.005-0.2 mg/kg IV bolus every 2 hr
Hydrocodone (in Lorcet, Lortab, Vicodin, others)	30 mg every 3-4 hr	Not available	0.2 mg/kg every 3-4 hr	Not available
Levorphanol (Levo-Dromoran)	4 mg every 6-8 hr	2 mg every 6-8 hr	0.04 mg/kg every 6-8 hr	0.02 mg/kg every 6-8 hr
Meperidine (Demerol)[f]	300 mg every 2-3 hr	100 mg every 3 hr	Not recommended	0.75 mg/kg every 2-3 hr
Methadone (Dolophine, others)[g]	20 mg every 6-8 hr	10 mg every 6-8 hr	0.2 mg/kg every 6-8 hr	0.1 mg/kg every 6-8 hr
Oxycodone (Roxicodone, Oxycontin; also in Percocet, Percodan, Tylox, others)	20 mg every 3-4 hr	Not available	0.2 mg/kg every 3-4 hr[h]	Not available

Data from Acute Pain Management Guideline Panel: *Acute pain management: operative or medical procedures and trauma: clinical practice guideline,* AHCPR Pub No 92-0032, Rockville, Md, 1992, Agency for Health Care Policy and Research, Public Health Service, US Department of Health and Human Services; Berde C et al: Report of the subcommittee on disease-related pain in childhood cancer, *Pediatrics* 86(5, pt 2):820, 1990.

ATC, Around the clock; *IM,* intramuscular; *IV,* intravenous; *PCA,* patient-controlled analgesia.

NOTE: Published tables vary in the suggested doses that are equianalgesic to morphine. Clinical response is the criterion that must be applied for each patient; titration to clinical response is necessary. Because cross tolerance among these drugs is not complete, it is usually necessary to use a lower-than-equianalgesic dose when changing drugs and to retitrate to response. CAUTION: Recommended doses do not apply to patients with renal or hepatic insufficiency or other conditions affecting drug metabolism and kinetics.

[a]CAUTION: Doses listed for patients with body weight less than 50 kg cannot be used as initial starting doses in infants less than 6 months of age. For non-ventilated infants under 6 months of age, the initial opioid dose should be about one-fourth to one-third of the dose recommended for older infants and children. For example, morphine could be used at a dose of 0.03 mg/kg instead of the traditional 0.1 mg/kg.

[b]IM injections should not be used.

[c]For morphine, hydromorphone, and oxymorphone, rectal administration is an alternate route for patients unable to take oral medications, but equianalgesic doses may differ from oral and parenteral doses because of pharmacokinetic differences.

[d]Actiq is indicated only for management of breakthrough cancer pain in patients with malignancies who are already receiving and are tolerant to opioid therapy but can be used for preoperative or preprocedural sedation/analgesia.

[e]CAUTION: Codeine doses above 65 mg often are not appropriate because of diminishing incremental analgesia with increasing doses but continually increasing constipation and other side effects. Dosages are from McCaffery M, Pasero C: *Pain: a clinical manual,* ed 2, St Louis, 1999, Mosby.

[f]Meperidine is not recommended for continuous pain control (i.e., postoperatively) because of risk of normeperidine toxicity.

[g]Initial dose is 10% to 25% of equianalgesic morphine dose. Parenteral Dolophine is no longer available in the United States.

[h]CAUTION: Doses of aspirin and acetaminophen in combination with opioid/NSAID preparations must also be adjusted to patient's body weight. Daily dose of acetaminophen should not exceed 75 mg/kg or 4000 mg.

If pain relief is inadequate, the initial dosage is increased (usually by 25% to 50% and sometimes more to provide greater analgesic effectiveness). Decreasing the interval between doses may also provide more continuous pain relief. A major difference between opioids and nonopioids is that nonopioids have a ceiling effect, which means that doses higher than the recommended dose will not produce greater pain relief. Opioids do not have a ceiling effect other than that imposed by side effects; therefore, larger dosages can be given safely for increasing severity of pain.

NURSE ALERT A frequent error in attempts to improve pain control is to change to another analgesic. If an opioid, such as morphine, hydromorphone, or fentanyl, is used, rarely is the problem one of drug choice. Rather, the problem is usually one of inadequate dosage. If changing to another analgesic is warranted because of adverse side effects, the new drug should be slightly less or equal in potency to the original analgesic. ■

Parenteral and oral dosages of opioids are not the same. Because of the *first-pass effect,* an oral opioid is rapidly absorbed from the gastrointestinal tract and enters the portal circulation, where it is partially metabolized before reaching the central circulation. Therefore oral dosages must be larger to compensate for the partial loss of analgesic potency to achieve *equianalgesia* (equal analgesic effect). Conversion factors for selected opioids, when a change is made from intramuscular (IM) or IV to oral, are listed in Tables 44-7 and 44-8. Immediate conversion from IM or IV to the suggested equianalgesic oral dose may result in a substantial error in the individual child. For example, the dose may be significantly more or less than what the child requires. Small changes ensure small errors.

Right Route

Several routes of analgesic administration exist (Box 44-12). Children should not have to endure pain, such as from IM injections, to achieve pain relief. Therefore the most effective and least traumatic route of administration should be selected.

A significant advance in the administration of IV, epidural, or subcutaneous (SC) analgesics is the use of *patient-controlled analgesia (PCA).* As the name implies, the patient controls the amount and frequency of the analgesic, which is typically delivered through a special infusion device. Successfully using a PCA pump requires a patient to have enough intelligence, manual dexterity, and strength to push the button to operate the pump. Children who are able to play a video or computer game (5 to 6 years of age) often can successfully use PCA. Contraindications to use of PCA include inability to understand how to use the button, inability to push the button because of limitations of mobility (weakness or restraints), or an unwillingness to use the pump. Although it is controversial, parents and nurses have used the PCA system for the child. When used as "nurse"- or "parent"-controlled analgesia, the concept of patient control is negated, however, and the inherent safety of PCA may be compromised. Nevertheless, recent research reported safe and effective analgesia in children when the PCA was controlled by patient, parent, or nurse (Algren et al, 1998; Yaster et al, 2003).

PCA infusion devices typically allow for the following three methods or modes of drug administration to be used alone or in combination:

1. *Patient-administered boluses* that can only be infused according to the preset amount and lockout interval (time between doses); more frequent "pushing of the button" means no drug is delivered, but the patient may need the dose and/or time adjusted for better pain control
2. *Nurse-administered boluses* that are typically used to give an initial loading dose to increase blood levels rapidly and to relieve *breakthrough pain* (pain not relieved with the usual programmed dose)
3. *Continuous basal* or *background infusion* that delivers a constant amount of analgesic and prevents pain from returning during those times, such as sleep, when the patient cannot control the infusion; may decrease safety of PCA

At present the optimum use of these three modes continues to be investigated. However, as with any type of analgesic management plan, continued assessment of the child's pain relief is essential for the greatest benefit from PCA. Typical uses of PCA are for controlling perioperative pain, sickle cell crisis, trauma, and cancer.

The most commonly prescribed opioids for intravenous PCA are morphine, hydromorphone, and fentanyl. Because PCA is typically used for continuous and extended pain control, meperidine should not be administered (p. 1326). Another risk of using meperidine is confusion between its concentration (10 mg/ml) and that of morphine when the PCA pump is programmed, which can result in undermedication or overmedication.

Epidural analgesia, primarily used postoperatively or in selected cases of terminal care, can be achieved by placing a catheter in the epidural space of the spinal column. An opioid (usually fentanyl, hydromorphone, or preservative-free morphine), often with a long-acting local anesthetic (usually bupivacaine or ropivacaine) is administered via single or intermittent bolus, continuous infusion, or patient-controlled epidural analgesia (PCEA). Analgesia results from the opioid's direct effect on receptors in the dorsal horn of the spinal cord, which block transmission of pain impulses to the brain (Rasmussen, 1996). Respiratory depression is rare, but if it occurs, it develops slowly and is evident several hours after the infusion begins. It is important to examine the epidural insertion site daily for evidence of infection and to ensure the occlusive dressing is intact. A mild erythema is not uncommon when catheters have been in place for several days. Catheters should be removed, however, if a fever of unknown origin or purulent drainage is present. Occasionally when examining the insertion site, a collection of fluid is seen between the skin and the clear occlusive dressing. Usually this edema is the result of fluid leaking through the insertion site hole and is not cerebrospinal fluid. It does not require any special treatment. The dressing should be changed or reinforced.

NURSE ALERT When the epidural route is used, check the child's level of sedation and respiratory rate and depth hourly for the first 24 hours to detect delayed-onset respiratory depression (Pasero, 1999). ■

Table 44-7

Selected Analgesics (Equianalgesia)

DRUG*	EQUAL TO ORAL MORPHINE (mg)	EQUAL TO IM/IV MORPHINE (mg)
Hydromorphone (Dilaudid), 1 mg	4	1.3
Codeine, 30 mg	4.5	1.5
Meperidine (Demerol), 50 mg	4.8	1.6
Acetaminophen, 300 mg (Tylenol No. 3) Codeine, 30 mg	7.2	2.4
Acetaminophen, 325 mg (Percocet) Oxycodone, 5 mg	7.2	2.4
Aspirin, 325 mg (Percodan) Oxycodone, 5 mg	7.2	2.4
Acetaminophen, 500 mg (Vicodin, Lortab) Hydrocodone, 5 mg	9	3
Acetaminophen, 500 mg (Tylox) Oxycodone, 5 mg	9	3
Dolophine (Methadone), 10 mg	15	7.5
Acetaminophen (Tylenol), 325 mg	2.7	0.9
Aspirin, 325 mg	2.7	0.9
Acetaminophen (Tylenol Extra Strength), 500 mg	4	1.3
Acetaminophen, 300 mg (Tylenol No. 4) Codeine, 60 mg	11.7	3.9
Transdermal fentanyl patch (Duragesic) (based on 25 mcg/hr patch applied every 3 days = 50 mg oral morphine every 24 hours or divided into 6 doses = 8.3 mg) or use:	8.3	2.77

RECOMMENDED INITIAL DURAGESIC DOSE BASED ON DAILY ORAL MORPHINE DOSE†

ORAL 24-HOUR DURAGESIC MORPHINE (mg/day)	DOSE (mg/hr)
45-134	25
135-224	50
225-314	75
315-404	100
405-494	125
495-584	150
585-674	175
675-764	200
765-854	225
855-944	250
945-1034	275
1035-1124	300

Courtesy of Betty R. Ferrell, PhD FAAN, 1999. Used with permission.

NOTE: When converting to oral oxycodone from oral morphine, an appropriate conservative estimate is 15-20 mg of oxycodone per 30 mg of morphine; however, when converting to oral morphine from oral oxycodone, an appropriate conservative estimate is 30 mg of morphine per 30 mg of oxycodone. (McCaffery M, Pasero C: *Pain: a clinical manual,* ed 2, St Louis, 1999, Mosby, p 198.)

*Oral medication with exception of fentanyl.

†Data from Duragesic package insert, Janssen, Pharmaceutical Products, Titusville, NJ, 2001.

Table 44-8

SUGGESTED INTRAVENOUS PATIENT-CONTROLLED ANALGESIA OPIOID INFUSION ORDERS

DRUG	BASAL RATE (mcg/kg/hr)	BOLUS RATE (mcg/kg/dose)	LOCKOUT PERIOD (min)	MAXIMUM DOSE/HOUR (mg/kg)
Morphine	10-30	10-30	6-10	0.1-0.15
Hydromorphone	3-5	3-5	6-10	0.015-0.02
Fentanyl	0.5-1.0	0.5-1.0	6-10	0.002-0.004

From Yaster M et al: *Pediatric pain management and sedation handbook,* St Louis, 1997, Mosby.

BOX 44-12

Routes and Methods of Analgesic Drug Administration

Oral

Preferred because of convenience, cost, and relatively steady blood levels

Higher dosages of oral form of opioids required for equivalent parenteral analgesia

Peak drug effect occurs after 1-2 hours for most analgesics

- Delay in onset is disadvantage when rapid control of severe pain or of fluctuating pain is desired

Sublingual/Buccal/Transmucosal

Tablet or liquid placed between cheek and gum (buccal) or under tongue (sublingual)

Highly desirable because more rapid onset than oral route

- Less first-pass effect through liver than oral route, which normally reduces analgesia from oral opioids (unless sublingual/buccal form swallowed, which occurs often in children)

Few drugs commercially available in this form

- Many drugs can be compounded into a sublingual troche or lozenge.*

Actiq-Oral transmucosal fentanyl citrate in hard confection base on a plastic holder; indicated only for management of breakthrough cancer pain in patients with malignancies who are already receiving and are tolerant to opioid therapy but can be used for preoperative or preprocedural sedation/analgesia

Intravenous (IV) (Bolus)

Preferred for rapid control of severe pain

Provides most rapid onset of effect, usually in about 5 minutes

- Advantage for acute pain, procedural pain, and breakthrough pain

Needs to be repeated hourly for continuous pain control

- Drugs with short half-life (morphine, fentanyl, hydromorphone) are preferred, to avoid toxic accumulation of drug.

Intravenous (Continuous)

Preferred over bolus and IM for maintaining control of pain

Provides steady blood levels

Easy to titrate dosage

Subcutaneous (SC) (Continuous)

Used when oral and IV routes not available

Provides equivalent blood levels to continuous IV infusion

Suggested initial bolus dose to equal 2-hour IV dose; total 24-hour dose usually requires concentrated opioid solution to minimize infused volume. Use smallest gauge needle that accommodates infusion rate.

Patient-Controlled Analgesia (PCA)

Generally refers to self-administration of drugs, regardless of route

Typically uses programmable infusion pump (IV, epidural, SC) that permits self-administration of boluses of medication at preset dose and time interval (lockout interval is time between doses)

PCA bolus administration may be combined with initial bolus and continuous (basal or background) infusion of opioid.

Optimum lockout interval not known but must be at least as long as time needed for onset of drug

- Should effectively control pain during movement or procedures
- Longer lockout provides larger dose

Family-Controlled Analgesia

One family member (usually a parent) or other caregiver is designated child's primary pain manager and has responsibility of pressing PCA button

Guidelines for selecting a primary pain manager for family-controlled analgesia

- Spends a significant amount of time with the patient
- Is willing to assume responsibility of being primary pain manager
- Is willing to accept and respect patient's reports of pain (if able to provide) as best indicator of how much pain the patient is experiencing; knows how to use and interpret a pain rating scale
- Understands the purpose and goals of patient's pain management plan
- Understands concept of maintaining a steady analgesic blood level
- Recognizes signs of pain and side effects and adverse reactions to opioid

Nurse-Activated Analgesia

Child's primary nurse is designated primary pain manager and is only person who presses PCA button during that nurse's shift

Guidelines for selecting primary pain manager for family-controlled analgesia apply to nurse-activated analgesia

May be used in addition to a basal rate to treat breakthrough pain with bolus doses; patients are assessed every 30 minutes for the need for a bolus dose

May be used without a basal rate as a means of maintaining analgesia with ATC bolus doses

Intramuscular (IM)

NOT RECOMMENDED FOR PAIN CONTROL; NOT CURRENT STANDARD OF CARE

Painful administration (hated by children)

Some drugs (e.g., meperidine) can cause tissue and nerve damage.

Wide fluctuation in absorption of drug from muscle

Faster absorption from deltoid than from gluteal sites

Shorter duration and more expensive than oral drugs

Time consuming for staff and unnecessary delay for child

Intranasal

Available commercially as Stadol NS (butorphanol); approved for those over 18 years of age; should not be used in patient receiving morphinelike drugs because butorphanol is partial antagonist that will reduce analgesia and may cause withdrawal

Intradermal

Used primarily for skin anesthesia (e.g., before lumbar puncture, bone marrow aspiration, arterial puncture, skin biopsy)

Local anesthetics (e.g., lidocaine) cause stinging, burning sensation

- Duration of stinging may depend on type of "caine" used

To avoid stinging sensation associated with lidocaine:

- Buffer the solution by adding 1 part sodium bicarbonate (1 mEq/ml) to 9 to 10 parts 1% or 2% lidocaine with or without epinephrine (see Guidelines box p. 1335)

Normal saline with preservative, benzyl alcohol, anesthetizes venipuncture site

Use same dose as for buffered lidocaine (see Guidelines box p. 1334).

Topical/Transdermal

EMLA (eutectic mixture of local anesthetics [lidocaine/ prilocaine]) cream and anesthetic disk or ELA-Max (4% lidocaine cream)

Eliminates or reduces pain from most procedures involving skin puncture

Data primarily from American Pain Society: *Principles of analgesic use in the treatment of acute pain and chronic cancer pain,* ed 4, Skokie, Ill, 1999, The Society; and McCaffery M, Pasero C: *Pain: a clinical manual,* ed 2, St Louis, 1999, Mosby.

*For further information about compounding drugs in troche or suppository form, contact: Professional Compounding Centers of America (PCCA), Inc, 9901 South Wilcrest Dr, Houston, TX 77009, (800) 331-2498; www.pccarx.com.

BOX 44-12

Routes and Methods of Analgesic Drug Administration—cont'd

Must be placed on intact skin over puncture site and covered by occlusive dressing or applied as anesthetic disk for 1 hour or more before procedure (see Guidelines box p. XXX)

LAT (lidocaine/adrenaline/tetracaine) or tetracaine/phenylephrine (tetraphen)

Provides skin anesthesia about 15 minutes after application on nonintact skin

Gel (preferable) or liquid placed on wounds for suturing

Adrenaline must not be used on end arterioles (fingers, toes, tip of nose, penis, earlobes) because of vasoconstriction

Numby Stuff

Uses iontophoresis to transport lidocaine 2% and epinephrine 1:100,000 (Iontocaine) into the skin

A small battery-powered device delivers current via an electrode with Iontocaine and a ground electrode.

Produces local dermal anesthesia in about 10 minutes to a depth of approximately 10 mm at maximum setting

May be frightening to young children when they see the device and feel the current

Child should be observed during iontophoresis, and all metal, such as jewelry, is removed from application site to prevent burns.

Transdermal fentanyl (Duragesic)

Available as patch for continuous pain control

Safety and efficacy not established in children under 12 years

Not appropriate for initial relief of acute pain because of long interval to peak effect (12-24 hours); for rapid onset of pain relief, an immediate release opioid must be given.

Orders for "rescue doses" of an immediate release opioid should be available for breakthrough pain, a flare of severe pain that breaks through the medication being administered at regular intervals for persistent pain.

Has duration of up to 72 hours for prolonged pain relief

If respiratory depression occurs, several doses of naloxone may be needed.

Vapocoolant

Use of prescription spray coolant, such as Fluori-Methane or ethyl chloride (Pain-Ease); applied to the skin for 10-15 seconds immediately before the needle puncture; anesthesia lasts about 15 seconds.

Some children dislike the cold; spraying the coolant on a cotton ball and then applying this to the skin may be less uncomfortable.

Application of ice to the skin for 30 seconds has been found to be ineffective.

Rectal

Alternative to oral or parenteral routes

Variable absorption rate

Generally disliked by children

Many drugs can be compounded into rectal suppositories.*

Regional Nerve Block

Use of long-acting local anesthetic (bupivacaine or ropivacaine) injected into nerves to block pain at site

Provides prolonged analgesia postoperatively, such as after inguinal herniorrhaphy

May be used to provide local anesthesia for surgery, such as dorsal penile nerve block for circumcision or for reduction of fractures

Inhalation

Use of anesthetics, such as nitrous oxide, to produce partial or complete analgesia for painful procedures

Occupational exposure to high levels of nitrous oxide may cause side effects (e.g., headache)

Epidural/Intrathecal

Involves catheter placed into epidural, caudal, or intrathecal space for continuous infusion or single or intermittent administration of opioid with or without a long-acting local anesthetic (e.g., bupivacaine, ropivacaine)

Analgesia primarily from drug's direct effect on opioid receptors in spinal cord

Respiratory depression is rare but may have slow and delayed onset; can be prevented by checking level of sedation and respiratory rate and depth hourly for initial 24 hours and decreasing dose when excessive sedation is detected.

Nausea, itching, and urinary retention are common dose-related side effects from the epidural opioid.

Mild hypotension, urinary retention, and temporary motor and/or sensory deficits are common unwanted effects of epidural local anesthetic.

Catheter for urinary retention should be inserted during surgery to decrease trauma to child; if inserted when child is awake, anesthetize urethra with lidocaine.

Although opioids are usually administered parenterally, spinally, or orally, new routes such as *oral transmucosal* and *transdermal*, have recently been developed. Fentanyl is readily absorbed through the skin. However, because of its long onset, an inability to adjust drug delivery, and a long elimination half-life, transdermal fentanyl is contraindicated for acute pain management. A transdermal patch (Duragesic), however, may be used in older children and adolescents who have chronic cancer pain.

Conversely, the transmucosal route of fentanyl (Fentanyl Oralet) provides atraumatic preoperative and procedural sedation and analgesia. It is also useful in the treatment of cancer pain. Like all opioid administration, using these routes requires vigilant patient monitoring (Yaster et al, 2003).

One of the most significant improvements in the ability to provide atraumatic care to children is the anesthetic cream *EMLA*, a eutectic mixture of local anesthetics (lidocaine 2.5% and prilocaine 2.5%). The eutectic mixture, whose melting point is lower than that of the two anesthetics alone, permits effective concentrations of the drug to penetrate *intact* skin. A thick layer of cream under an occlusive transparent dressing or a "peel-and-stick" Anesthetic Disc is applied for 1 hour or more before procedures such as lumbar, venous, arterial, finger, heel, or earlobe punctures; implanted port access; insertion of peripherally inserted central catheter (PICC) lines; superficial biopsy; skin graft; laser treatment of port-wine stains; removal of epicardial (pacing) wires, chest tubes, or hair (electrolysis); bone marrow examination; allergy testing; and IM or SC injections. For deeper pain, such as IM injections, the application time should be extended up to 3 hours (Guidelines box). The duration of anesthesia is 1 to 2 hours after removal (Wong, 2003).

EMLA is approved for children 37 weeks of gestational age and older. It should be used cautiously on infants between

Guidelines

USING EMLA (EUTECTIC MIXTURE OF LOCAL ANESTHETICS-LIDOCAINE 2.5% AND PRILOCAINE 2.5%)

Explain to child that EMLA is like a "magic cream that takes hurt away." Tap or lightly scratch site of procedure to show child that "skin is now awake."

Apply the "peel-and-stick" Anesthetic Disc or a thick layer (dollop) of EMLA cream over normal intact skin to anesthetize site (about one-half of a 5 g tube; one-third of a tube may be used if puncture site is localized and superficial (e.g., intradermal injection or heel/finger puncture).

For venous access, apply to two sites; place enough cream on antecubital fossa to cover medial and lateral veins. Do not rub the cream.

If using the cream, place transparent adhesive dressing (e.g., Tegaderm) over EMLA. Make sure cream remains in a dollop or mound. A piece of plastic film (e.g., Saran Wrap) can be used, with tape to seal the edges. Use only as much adhesive as needed to prevent leakage.

To make the dressing less accessible, cover it loosely with a self-adhering Ace-type bandage (such as Coban) or an IV protector (such as I.V. House*). Label the dressing with "EMLA applied" and the date and time to distinguish it from other types of dressings. Instruct older children not to disturb the dressing. (Covering the dressing with an opaque material may reduce the attraction and discourage "fingering.") Supervise younger or cognitively compromised children throughout the application time.

Leave EMLA on skin for at least 60 minutes for superficial puncture and 2½ hours for deep penetration (e.g., IM injection, biopsy). EMLA may be applied at home and may need to be kept on longer in persons with dark and/or thicker skin. Anesthesia may last up to 4 hours after EMLA is removed.

Remove Anesthetic Disc or dressing before procedure and wipe cream from skin. For transparent dressing, grasp opposite sides, and while holding dressing parallel to skin, pull sides away from each other to stretch and loosen. An adhesive remover may be used.

Observe skin reaction (e.g., either blanched or reddened). If there is no obvious skin reaction, EMLA may not have penetrated adequately. Test skin sensitivity and reapply if needed.

Repeat tapping or lightly scratching on skin to show child that "skin is asleep" and that it cannot feel a needle.

After procedure, assess behavioral response. If child was upset, use pain scale (e.g., FACES) to help child distinguish between pain and fear. (See FACES Pain Rating Scale in Table 44-2.)

In the United States, EMLA is approved for use in infants born at 37 weeks of gestation and older. It should not be used in those rare patients with congenital or idiopathic methemoglobinemia and in infants under the age of 12 months who are receiving treatment with methemoglobin-inducing agents such as sulfonamides, phenytoin (Dilantin), phenobarbital, and acetaminophen (Tylenol). Methemoglobin, a dysfunctional form of hemoglobin, reduces the blood's oxygen-carrying capacity, causing cyanosis and hypoxemia. The use of IV methylene blue promptly eliminates the methemoglobinemia.

NOTE: Although the package insert lists under "Warnings" that patients taking drugs associated with drug-induced methemoglobinemia, such as acetaminophen, are at greater risk for developing methemoglobinemia, there have been no reported cases of this complication occurring in children taking acetaminophen and using EMLA.

Follow the manufacturer's guidelines for **maximum recommended application area to intact skin for infants and children:**

Age and body weight requirements	Maximum total dose of EMLA	Maximum application area
1 to 3 months or <5 kg	1 g	10 cm^2 (1.25 × 1.25 in)
4 to 12 months and >5 kg	2 g	20 cm^2 (1.75 × 1.75 in)
1 to 6 years and >10 kg	10 g	100 cm^2 (4 × 4 in)
7 to 12 years and >20 kg	20 g	200 cm^2 (5.5 × 5.5 in)

NOTE: If a patient over 3 months old does not meet the minimum weight requirement, the maximum total dose of EMLA should be restricted to that which corresponds to the patient's weight.

*For more information, contact I.V. House, 7400 Foxmont Dr., Hazelwood, MO 63042-2198; phone: 800-530-0400; fax: 314-831-3683; e-mail: ivhouse@ivhouse.com; Web site: www.ivhouse.com.

ages 1 and 12 months who are receiving treatment with methemoglobin-inducing agents, such as sulfonamides, phenytoin (Dilantin), and acetaminophen (Tylenol). However, the use of these drugs is not a contraindication for applying EMLA, and there are no published reports of methemoglobinemia caused by EMLA when an infant received acetaminophen. Because of their diminished levels of erythrocyte-methemoglobin reductase, infants less than 3 months old are more susceptible to prilocaine-induced *methemoglobinemia,* a very rare and reversible side effect. *Methemoglobin* is a dysfunctional form of hemoglobin that reduces the oxygen-carrying capacity of the blood, causing cyanosis and hypoxemia. The use of IV methylene blue promptly eliminates the methemoglobinemia (McCaffery & Pasero, 1999). Other side effects are mild and include pallor, erythema, or edema at the application site.

ELA-MAX is a new over-the-counter topical anesthetic that produces dermal anesthesia in 15 to 30 minutes. Researchers concluded that a 30-minute application was as effective as a 60-minute application of EMLA in reducing pain associated with intravenous cannulation in the hands of a child. Although an occlusive dressing was used in this study, an occlusive dressing is not required when using ELA-MAX (Kleiber et al, 2002).

Another topical option is *Numby Stuff,* which uses iontophoresis (mild electrical current) to actively push the drug into the skin. This preparation of Iontocaine (lidocaine HCl 2% with epinephrine, 1:100,000 topical solution) provides dermal anesthesia to a depth of 10 mm in approximately 10 minutes without causing vasoconstriction. This painless, needle-free process is noninvasive, minimizes trauma, and reduces risk of infection. It can be used for IV placement, insertion of PICC lines, lumbar punctures, implantable port needle insertion, and pulsed dye laser therapy (IOMED, 1996). In one study of children ages 5 to 12 years, iontophoresis was more effective than EMLA at reducing the pain of intravenous cannulation (Squire, Kirchoff, & Hissong, 2000). It is important to provide explanations and let the child become familiar with the equipment. Some children may be frightened by a warm or tingling sensation under the patches. This decreases after a few minutes (McCaffery & Pasero, 1999).

In some situations in which time is inadequate for preparations like EMLA to take effect, refrigerant sprays such as ethyl chloride and fluorimethane can be used. When sprayed on the skin, these sprays vaporize, rapidly cool the area, and provide superficial anesthesia. Ethyl chloride wears off in about 2 minutes with virtually no side effects (New Products, 2002).

The *intradermal route* is often used to inject a local anesthetic, typically lidocaine (Zylocaine), into the skin to reduce the pain from a lumbar puncture, bone marrow aspiration, or venous or arterial access. One problem with the use of lidocaine is the stinging and burning that initially occur. However, the use of *buffered lidocaine* reduces the stinging sensation (Wong & Pasero, 1997) (Guidelines box). Warming the lidocaine to 37° C (98.6° F) may also accomplish the same effect (Mader, Playe, & Garb, 1994).

Right Time

The right timing for administering analgesics depends on the type of pain. For continuous pain control, such as for postoperative or cancer pain, a preventive schedule of medication *around the clock (ATC)* is effective. The ATC schedule avoids low plasma concentrations that permit breakthrough pain. If analgesics are administered only when pain returns (a typical use of the PRN, or "as needed," order), pain relief may take several hours. This may require higher doses, leading to a cycle of undermedication of pain alternating with periods of overmedication and drug toxicity. This cycle of erratic pain control also promotes "clock watching," which may be erroneously equated with "addiction." Nurses can effectively use PRN orders by giving the drug at regular intervals, since "as needed" can be interpreted to mean "as needed to prevent return of pain."

Preventive pain control is best provided through continuous IV infusion rather than intermittent boluses. If intermittent boluses are given, the intervals between doses should not exceed the drug's expected duration of effectiveness. For extended pain control with fewer administration times, drugs that provide longer duration of action (e.g., some NSAIDs, time-released morphine or oxycodone, methadone, levorphanol) can be used.

NURSE ALERT Because breakthrough pain can occur even with optimum ATC scheduling, there should be an order for PRN "rescue" doses of an analgesic. ■

Continuous analgesia is not always appropriate because not all pain is continuous. Frequently, temporary pain control is needed to provide analgesia before a scheduled procedure. When pain can be predicted, the drug's peak effect should be timed to coincide with the painful event. For example, with opioids the peak effect is only a few minutes for the IV route; with nonopioids the peak effect occurs about 2 hours after oral administration. For rapid onset and peak of action, opioids that quickly penetrate the blood-brain barrier (e.g., IV fentanyl) provide excellent pain control.

Observe for Side Effects

Both NSAIDs and opioids have side effects, although the major concern is with those from opioids (Box 44-13). Respiratory depression is the most serious complication and is most likely to occur in sedated patients. The respiratory rate may decrease gradually or may cease abruptly; lower limits

Guidelines

USING BUFFERED LIDOCAINE

Supplies: 8.4% sodium bicarbonate (1 mEq/ml), 1% to 2% lidocaine with or without epinephrine, syringe with removable needle, and a 30-gauge needle

Instructions:

Use 1 part sodium bicarbonate to 10 parts lidocaine (e.g., draw up 1 ml of lidocaine and 0.1 ml of sodium bicarbonate).

Change needle used to withdraw buffered lidocaine (BL) to 30-gauge needle for intradermal injection.

For venipuncture or port access, inject 0.1 ml or less BL intradermally directly over intended puncture site; anesthesia occurs almost immediately.

Suggested maximum dose of lidocaine for local anesthesia is 4.5 mg/kg.

If buffering lidocaine vial (e.g., 20 ml lidocaine with 2 ml sodium bicarbonate), solution may be used for 7 days if unrefrigerated or 14 days if refrigerated.

BOX 44-13

Side Effects of Opioids

General

Constipation (possibly severe)
Respiratory depression
Sedation
Nausea and vomiting
Agitation, euphoria
Mental clouding
Hallucinations
Orthostatic hypotension
Pruritus
Urticaria
Sweating
Miosis (may be sign of toxicity)
Anaphylaxis (rare)

Signs of Tolerance

Decreasing pain relief
Decreasing duration of pain relief

Signs of Withdrawal Syndrome in Patients with Physical Dependence

Initial signs of withdrawal:
- Lacrimation
- Rhinorrhea
- Yawning
- Sweating

Later signs:
- Restlessness
- Irritability
- Tremors
- Anorexia
- Dilated pupils
- Gooseflesh
- Nausea/vomiting

of normal are not established for children, but any significant change from a previous rate calls for increased vigilance. A slower respiratory rate does not necessarily reflect decreased arterial oxygenation; an increased depth of ventilation may compensate for the altered rate (McCaffery & Pasero, 1999). If respiratory depression or arrest occurs, the nurse must be prepared to intervene quickly (Guidelines box).

Although respiratory depression is the most feared side effect, constipation is a common and sometimes serious side effect of opioids, which decrease peristaltic activity and increase anal sphincter tone. Prevention with stool softeners and laxatives is more effective than treatment once constipation occurs. Dietary treatment, such as increased fiber, is usually not sufficient to promote regular bowel evacuation. However, dietary measures, such as increased fluid, fruit, and bran intake, and especially activity, are encouraged.

Pruritus from epidural or IV infusion can be treated with low doses of naloxone infused slowly or with IV nalbuphine. Pruritus from IV infusion usually responds to oral antihistamines. Nausea, vomiting, and sedation usually subside after 2 days of opioid administration, although intravenous, oral, or rectal antiemetics may be necessary.

Both tolerance and physical dependence can occur with prolonged use of opioids. Treatment of tolerance involves increasing the dose or decreasing the duration between doses. Treatment of physical dependence involves gradually reducing the dose over several days to prevent occurrence of withdrawal symptoms (similar to tapering of steroid dosages after chronic steroid therapy). The following are suggested guidelines for treating physical dependence (American Pain Society, 1999):

- Gradually reduce dose (similar to tapering of steroids): Give one-half of previous daily dose in q6hr doses for first 2 days, then reduce dose by 25% every 2 days.
- Continue this schedule until total daily dose of 0.6 mg/kg/day of morphine (or equivalent) is reached.
- After 2 days on this dose, discontinue opioid.
- May also switch to oral methadone, using one-fourth of equianalgesic dose as initial weaning dose and proceeding as described above.

Use supportive statements when administering analgesics. The effectiveness of analgesics can be enhanced by a supportive attitude toward the child. By reinforcing the cause and effect of the medication and analgesia, the nurse can condition the child to expect pain relief, provided that the regimen is likely to be effective. Although IM injections should *not* be given, when they are, children need to understand that the "little hurt from the needle will take away the bigger hurt for a long time."

Parents and older children may have concerns about the use of opioids because of fear of addiction. These concerns should be addressed with assurance that any such risk is extremely low. It may be helpful to ask the question, "If you did not have this pain, would you want to take this medicine?" The answer is invariably no, which reinforces the solely therapeutic nature of the drug. It is also important to avoid making statements to the family such as "We don't want you to get used to this medicine," or "By now you shouldn't need this medicine," which may reinforce the fear of becoming addicted.

Guidelines

MANAGING OPIOID-INDUCED RESPIRATORY DEPRESSION

If respirations are depressed:

Assess sedation level .

Reduce infusion by 25% when possible.

Stimulate patient (shake gently, call by name, ask to breathe).

If patient cannot be aroused or is apneic (American Pain Society, 1999):

Administer naloxone (Narcan):

For children less than 40 kg, dilute 0.1 mg of naloxone in 10 ml of sterile saline to make 10 mcg/ml solution and give 0.5 mcg/kg.

For children over 40 kg, dilute 0.4 mg ampule in 10 ml of sterile saline and give 0.5 ml.

Administer bolus slow IV push every 2 minutes until effect is obtained.

Closely monitor patient. Naloxone's duration of antagonist action may be shorter than that of opioid, requiring repeated doses of naloxone

NOTE: Respiratory depression caused by benzodiazepines (e.g., diazepam [Valium] or midazolam [Versed]) can be reversed with flumazenil (Romazicon). Pediatric dosing experience suggests 0.01 mg/kg (0.1 ml/kg); if no (or inadequate) response after 1 to 2 minutes, administer same dose and repeat as needed at 60-second intervals for maximum dose of 1 mg (10 ml) (American Pain Society, 1999).

Providing Developmentally Appropriate Activities

A primary goal of nursing care for the child who is hospitalized is to minimize threats to the child's development. Many strategies (e.g., minimizing separation) have been discussed and may be all that the short-term patient requires. However, children who experience prolonged or repeated hospitalization are at greater risk for developmental delays or regression. The nurse who provides opportunities for the child to participate in developmentally appropriate activities further normalizes the child's environment and helps reduce interference with the child's ongoing development.

Play is the "work" of children of all ages and assumes a critical role in their development. Because of its other important purposes in the hospital setting, play is the focus of a separate discussion.

Interference with normal development may have long-term implications for the developing infant and toddler. The nurse plays a primary role in identifying children at risk and helping to plan, implement, and evaluate developmental intervention.

School is an integral part of the school-age child's and adolescent's development. Accreditation standards for hospitals serving children consider access to appropriate educational services a key factor in the accreditation decision process when a child's treatment requires a significant absence from school (Joint Commission on Accreditation of Healthcare Organizations, 1999). The nurse can encourage children to resume schoolwork as quickly as their condition permits, help them schedule and protect a selected time for studies, and help the family coordinate hospital educational services with their children's schools. Children should have the opportunity to "keep up" with art and music classes, as well as their academic subjects.

To meet the unique developmental needs of adolescents, special units have been developed that provide privacy, increased socialization, and appropriate activities for these young people. Typically these units are set apart from the general pediatric facility so that the teenagers do not share space with younger children, who are often perceived as a threat to their maturity.

These units often provide flexible routines and activities, such as more group activity, wearing of street clothes, and access to the items so critical to adolescents—telephones, compact disc and tape players, DVD players, videocasette recorders (VCRs), computers, and televisions. Because adolescents' food habits are rarely limited to the three traditional meals a day, a ready supply of snacks should be available. However, the most important benefit of these units is increased socialization with peers. In addition, staff members usually enjoy working with this age group and are well suited to establishing the trust so essential for communication.

NURSE ALERT When adolescents must share a common activity room with younger patients, referring to the area as the "activity" room rather than the "playroom" may entice them to visit the room and participate in activities. ■

Although regression is expected and normal, nurses have the responsibility of fostering the child's growth and development. Hospitalization can become a significant opportunity for learning and advancing. Extended hospitalizations for long-term chronic illness or situations of failure to thrive, abuse, or neglect represent instances in which regression must be seen as an adjustment period, to be followed by plans for promoting appropriate developmental skills.

Providing Opportunities for Play/Expressive Activities

Play is one of the most important aspects of a child's life and one of the most effective tools for managing stress. Because illness and hospitalization constitute crises in a child's life, and often involve overwhelming stresses, children need to act out their fears and anxieties as a means of coping with these stresses. Play is essential to children's mental, emotional, and social well-being. As with their developmental needs, the need for play does not stop when children are ill or in the hospital. On the contrary, play in the hospital serves many functions (Box 44-14).

Engaging in such activities gives children a sense of control. In the hospital environment, most decisions are made for the child; play and other expressive activities offer the child much-needed opportunities to make choices. Even if a child chooses not to participate in a particular activity, the nurse has offered the child a choice, perhaps one of but a few real choices the child has had that day.

Of all hospital facilities, probably no room does more to alleviate the stressors of hospitalization than the playroom or activity room. In this nonthreatening environment children temporarily distance themselves from the fears of separation, loss of control, and bodily injury. Time spent in this area should be protected. No treatments or intrusive or painful procedures should be allowed (Critical Thinking Exercise).

Diversional Activities

Almost any form of play can be used for diversion and recreation, but the activity should be selected on the basis of the child's age, interests, and limitations (Fig. 44-10). Children do not necessarily need special direction for using play

BOX 44-14

Functions of Play in the Hospital

Provides diversion and brings about relaxation
Helps the child feel more secure in a strange environment
Helps to lessen the stress of separation and the feeling of homesickness
Provides a means for release of tension and expression of feelings
Encourages interaction and development of positive attitudes toward others
Provides an expressive outlet for creative ideas and interests
Provides a means for accomplishing therapeutic goals (see Use of Play in Procedures, Chapter 45)
Places child in active role and provides opportunity to make choices and be in control

??? Critical Thinking Exercise

PLAYROOM AND HOSPITAL PROCEDURES

Hannah, a 7-year-old with cystic fibrosis, has been hospitalized numerous times with complications from the condition. She is playing Candyland with her brother, sister, and several other children in the playroom on the pediatric unit. A pediatric phlebotomist enters the playroom and says, "Hannah, I need to take some blood. I can see that you are playing a game, so I'll just do it while you play. It will just take a minute." Hannah nods her head indicating that she agrees to let the phlebotomist draw the blood at this time. The playroom is usually off-limits for invasive procedures. As Hannah's nurse, you are aware that Dr. Lung wants the results of the laboratory studies as soon as possible in order to make a decision about her course of therapy.

1. Evidence–Is there sufficient evidence to draw any conclusions about this situation at this time?
2. Assumptions–What are some underlying assumptions about the following issues:
   a. Children and painful procedures such as venipunctures
   b. The function of play in a hospitalized child
   c. The priority in performing the procedure
   d. Implications of performing the procedure in the playroom
3. What implications and priorities for nursing care can be drawn at this time? (i.e., what will you do?)
4. Does the evidence objectively support your argument (conclusion)?
5. Are there alternative perspectives to your conclusions? If so, what are they?

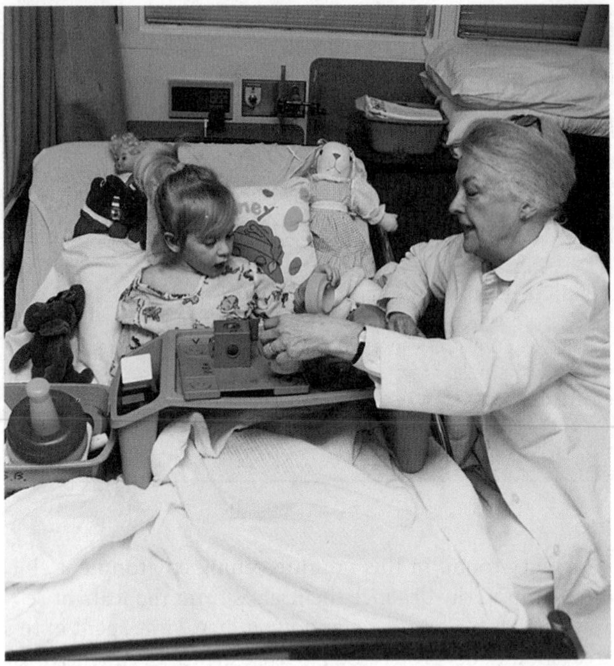

Fig. 44-10 Play materials for children in the hospital need to be appropriate for their age, interests, and limitations.

materials. All they require is the raw materials with which to work, and adult approval and supervision to help keep their natural enthusiasm or expression of feelings from getting out of control. Small children enjoy a variety of small, colorful toys that they can play with in bed or in their room, or more elaborate play equipment, such as playhouses, sandboxes, rhythm instruments, or large boxes and blocks, that may be a part of the hospital playroom.

Games that can be played alone or with another child or an adult are popular with older children, as are puzzles; reading material; quiet, individual activities, such as sewing, stringing beads, and weaving; and Lego blocks and other building materials. Assembling models is an excellent pastime, but one should make certain that all pieces and necessary materials are included in the package so that the child is not disappointed and frustrated.

Well-selected books are of infinite value to the child. Children never tire of stories; having someone read aloud gives them endless hours of pleasure and is of special value to the child who has limited energy to expend in play. A radio, VCR, electronic games, and television, included among most hospital room equipment, are useful tools for entertaining a child. Computers with access to the Internet can provide diversion, educational opportunities, and virtual support groups.

When supervising play for ill or convalescent children, it is best to select activities that are simpler than would normally be chosen according to the specific developmental level of the child. These children usually do not have the energy to cope with more challenging activities. Other limitations also influence the type of activities. Special consideration must be given to the child who is confined in terms of movement, has a restricted extremity, or is isolated. Toys for isolated children may need to be disinfected before and/or after use.

Toys

Parents of hospitalized children often ask nurses about the types of toys that would be best to bring for their child. Although parents often want to buy new toys for the hospitalized child, it is often better to wait awhile to bring new things, especially in the case of younger children. Small children need the comfort and reassurance of familiar things, such as the stuffed animal the child hugs for comfort and takes to bed at night. These familiar items are a link with home and the world outside the hospital.

Large numbers of toys often confuse and frustrate a small child. A few small, well-chosen toys are usually preferred to one large, expensive one. Children who are hospitalized for an extended time benefit from changes. Rather than a confusing accumulation of toys, older toys should be replaced periodically as interest wanes.

NURSE ALERT Have parents provide the child with a shoe box, a child's small suitcase, or a backpack to attach to the bed for an easy storage receptacle to prevent small items from becoming lost in the sheets or under the bed. ■

A highly successful diversion for a child who is hospitalized for a length of time and whose parents are unable to visit frequently is having the parents bring a box with several small, inexpensive, brightly wrapped items with a different day of the week printed on the outside of each package. The child will eagerly anticipate the time for opening each one. When the parents know when their next visit will be, they can provide the number of packages that corresponds to the days between visits. In this way the child knows that the diminishing packages also represent the anticipated visit from the parent.

Expressive Activities

Play and other expressive activities provide one of the best opportunities for encouraging emotional expression, including the safe release of anger and hostility. Nondirective play that allows children freedom for expression can be tremendously therapeutic. Therapeutic play, however, should not be confused with play therapy, a psychologic technique reserved for use by trained and qualified therapists as an interpretative method with emotionally disturbed children. *Therapeutic play,* on the other hand, is a very effective, nondirective modality for helping children deal with their concerns and fears, and at the same time it often helps the nurse to gain insights into children's needs and feelings.

Tension release can be facilitated through almost any activity, and with younger ambulatory children, large-muscle activity such as use of tricycles and wagons is especially beneficial. Much aggression can be safely directed into pounding and throwing games and activities. Beanbags are often thrown at a target or open receptacle with surprising vigor and hostility. A pounding board is employed with enthusiasm by young children; clay and play dough are marvelous media for use at any age.

Creative Expression

Although all children derive physical, social, emotional, and cognitive benefits from engaging in art or other creative activities, children's need for such activities is intensified when they are hospitalized. Children are more at ease expressing their thoughts and feelings through art, since hu-

SKILL: THERAPEUTIC PLAY

mans think first in images and later learn to translate these images into words. A child's drawing before surgery, for example, will often reveal unvoiced concerns about mutilation, body changes, and loss of self-control (Clatworthy et al, 1999). Drawing and painting are excellent media for expression. The child needs only to be supplied with the raw materials, such as crayons and paper; pots of bright poster color, large brushes, and an ample supply of newsprint supported on easels; or materials for finger painting (Fig. 44-11). Children can work individually or collaborate on a group project, such as a mural painted on a long piece of paper.

Although interpretation of children's drawing requires special training, observing changes in a series of the child's drawings over time can be helpful in assessing psychosocial adjustment and coping (Clatworthy et al, 1999). The nurse can use children's drawings, stories, poetry, and other products of creative expression as a springboard for discussion of thoughts, fears, and understanding of concepts or events (see Communication Techniques, Chapter 34).

Nurses can incorporate opportunities for musical expression into routine nursing care. For example, simple musical instruments, such as bracelets with bells, can be placed on infants' legs for them to shake to accompany mealtime music, or dressing changes. Dance and movement suggestions may encourage a child to ambulate.

Holidays provide stimulus and direction for unlimited creative projects. Children can participate in decorating the pediatric unit, and making pictures and decorations for their rooms gives the children a sense of pride and accomplishment. This is especially beneficial for children who are immobilized and isolated. Making gifts for someone at home helps maintain interpersonal ties.

Dramatic Play

Dramatic play is a well-recognized technique for emotional release, allowing children to reenact frightening or puzzling hospital experiences. Through use of puppets, replicas of hospital equipment, or some actual hospital equipment, children can play out the situations that are a part of their hospital experience. Dramatic play enables children to learn about procedures and events that will concern them and to assume the roles of the adults in the hospital environment.

Puppets are universally effective for communicating with children. Most children see them as peers and readily communicate with them. Children will relate to the puppet feelings that they hesitate to express to adults. Puppets can share children's own experiences and help them find solutions to their problems. Puppets dressed to represent figures in the child's environment—for example, a physician, nurse, child patient, therapist, and members of the child's own family—are especially useful (Fig. 44-12). Small, appropriately attired dolls are equally effective in encouraging the child to play out situations, although puppets are usually best for direct conversation.

NURSE ALERT Make a simple puppet using a large handkerchief. Place some cotton balls in the center of the cloth and wrap a rubber band over the handkerchief and cotton balls to form a "head." Place the head over the index finger so that the rubber band secures it to the finger. Let the cloth drape over the front and back of the hand. The cloth forms four parts of the puppet: the index finger is the head, the thumb and other fingers are the arms, and the draped cloth is the body. Decorate the head by drawing features on it. ■

Play must consider medical needs, but at times a procedure can be postponed for a short time to allow the child to complete a special activity (see Critical Thinking Exercise). Play must consider any limitations imposed by the child's condition. For example, small children may eat paste and other creative media; therefore, a child who is allergic to wheat should not be given finger paint made from wallpaper paste or play dough made with flour. A child on a restricted salt intake should not play with modeling dough, since salt is one of its major constituents. At home the play program can be planned around the therapy regimen. However, play can be satisfactorily incorporated into the child's care if the nurse and others involved allow some flexibility and use creativity in planning for play.

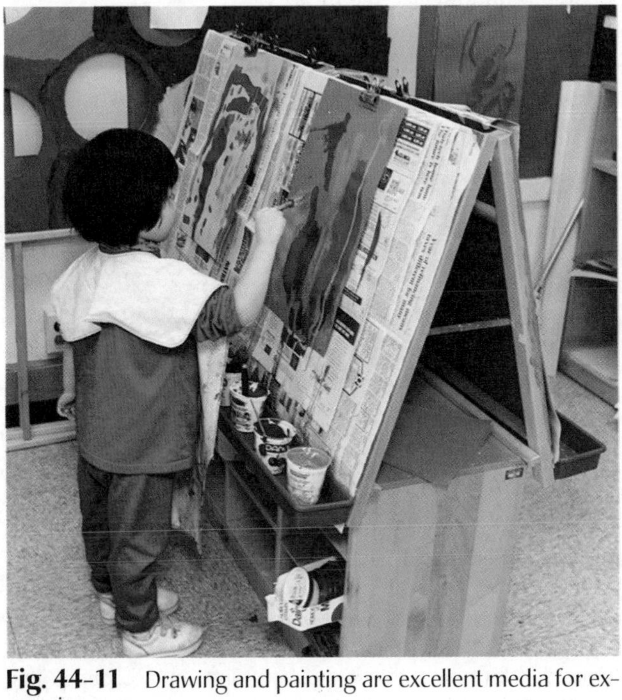

Fig. 44-11 Drawing and painting are excellent media for expression.

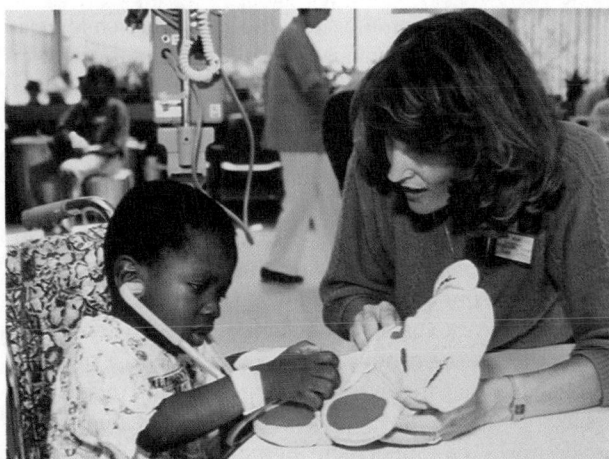

Fig. 44-12 Playing with stuffed animals allows children to safely explore feelings and concerns.

Maximizing Potential Benefits of Hospitalization

Although hospitalization generally represents a stressful time for children and families, it also represents an opportunity for facilitating positive change within the child and among family members. For some families the stress of a child's illness, hospitalization, or both can lead to strengthening of family coping behaviors and the emergence of new coping strategies (Kirby & Whelan, 1996). Therefore nursing interventions must also focus on maximizing the potential benefits of the experience.

Fostering Parent-Child Relationships

The crisis of illness and/or hospitalization can mobilize parents into more acute awareness of the needs of their children. For example, hospitalization provides opportunities for parents to learn more about their children's growth and development. When parents are helped to understand children's usual reactions to stress, such as regression or aggression, they are not only better able to support the child through the hospital experience, but also may extend their insights into childrearing practices after discharge.

Difficulties in parent-child relationships that may result in feeding problems, negative behavior, and sleep disturbances may decrease during hospitalization. The temporary cessation of such problems sometimes alerts parents to the role they may be playing in propagating the negative behavior. With assistance from health professionals, parents can restructure ways of relating to their children to foster more positive behavior.

Hospitalization may also represent a temporary reprieve or refuge from a disturbed home. Typically, abused or neglected children's dramatic physical and social improvement during hospitalization is proof of the growth potential of this experience. Hospitalized children temporarily are able to seek support, reassurance, and security from new relationships, particularly with nurses and hospitalized peers.

Providing Educational Opportunities

Illness and hospitalization represent excellent opportunities for children and other family members to learn more about their bodies, each other, and the health professions. For example, during a hospital admission for a diabetic crisis, the child may learn about the disease; the parents may learn about the child's needs for independence, normalcy, and appropriate limits; and each of them may find a new support system in the hospital staff.

Illness or hospitalization can also help older children in choosing a vocation. Frequently children have impressions of physicians or nurses that are disproportionately glorified or horrified. Actual experience with different health professionals can influence their attitude about health professionals and even a decision regarding a health career.

Promoting Self-Mastery

The experience of facing a crisis such as illness or hospitalization, coping successfully with it, and maturing as a result of it constitutes an opportunity for self-mastery. Younger children have the chance to test fantasy vs. reality fears. They realize that they were not abandoned, mutilated, castrated, or punished. In fact, they were loved, cared for, and treated with respect for their individual concerns. It is not unusual for children who have undergone hospitalization or surgery to tell others that "it was nothing" or to display proudly their scars or bandages. For older children, hospitalization may represent an opportunity for decision making, independence, and self-reliance. They are proud of having survived the experience and may feel a genuine self-respect for their achievements. Nurses can facilitate such feelings of self-mastery by emphasizing aspects of personal competence in the child and not focusing on uncooperative or negative behavior.

Providing Socialization

Hospitalization may offer children a special opportunity for social acceptance. Lonely, asocial, sometimes delinquent children find a sympathetic environment in the hospital. Children who are physically deformed or in some other way "different" from their age-mates may find an accepting social peer group (Fig. 44-13). Although this does not always spontaneously occur, nurses can structure the environment to foster a supportive child group. For example, selection of a compatible roommate can help children gain a new friend and learn more about themselves. Forming relationships with significant members of the health care team, such as the physician, nurse, child-life specialist, or minister, can greatly enhance children's adjustment in many areas of life.

Parents may also encounter a new social group in other parents who have similar problems. The waiting room or hallway "self-help" groups are inherent to every institution. Nurses can capitalize on this informal gathering by encouraging parents to discuss collectively their concerns and feelings. Nurses can also refer parents to organized parent groups or can use the help and support of recovered hospitalized patients.

Evaluation

The effectiveness of nursing interventions is determined by continual reassessment and evaluation of care based on the following observational guidelines:

1. Interview child and parents regarding the type of preparation for hospitalization the child received.
2. Review the medical record for evidence of parental visitation; interview parents and child regarding strategies used to minimize separation.
3. Observe child's hospital schedule and compare it with the schedule the child typically follows at home; interview child and family for examples of when they were allowed choices in the child's care.

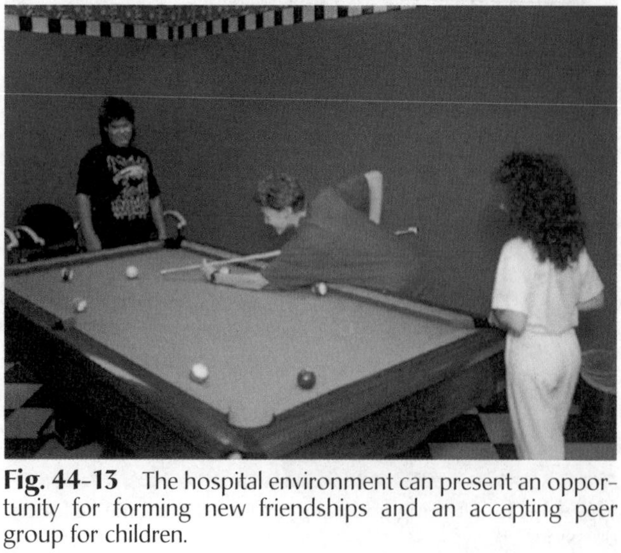

Fig. 44-13 The hospital environment can present an opportunity for forming new friendships and an accepting peer group for children.

4. Review the medical record for evidence of pain assessment and administration of analgesics or nonpharmacologic pain reducers. Compare child's behavior and pain scores before and after administration of pain reducers for evidence of pain relief.
5. Interview child regarding the types of play and other activities that were introduced by the nurses or child-life specialist and the times the child visited the playroom. For preverbal child, observe child's use of play materials.
6. Interview child and parents regarding their perception of any beneficial aspects of the hospitalization. Observe behaviors that indicate benefits, such as the formation of new friendships.

The expected outcomes are described in the Nursing Care Plan.

Nursing Care Plan

THE CHILD IN THE HOSPITAL

NURSING DIAGNOSIS: Anxiety/fear related to disruption of familiar routine, unfamiliar environment, distressing events and procedures

EXPECTED OUTCOME

Patient will exhibit minimal signs of emotional or physical distress (i.e., is calm, relaxed, cooperative; engages in nonnutritive sucking, appropriate play).

NURSING INTERVENTIONS/*RATIONALES*

Acknowledge child's fear and help child identify sources of that fear *to facilitate identification and use of coping strategies.*
Orient the child to hospital sights and sounds; provide child with accurate information about condition, procedures, and treatments; spend time with child *to promote trust and dispel fear.*
Encourage frequent family visitation with active participation in care *to prevent distress from separation.*
Use frequent touch, holding, and talking as appropriate *to provide comfort.*
Provide diversion and sensory stimulation appropriate to the child's developmental level and physical condition.
Instruct family in importance of comfort measures and in their active participation in care *to ease child's fears.*
Prepare child for procedures using developmentally appropriate approaches (therapeutic play) *to reduce fear and promote cooperation.*
Allow child choices when possible *to give some measure of control.*
Work with parents to create a routine similar to the child's usual routine at home *to increase comfort with environment.*

NURSING DIAGNOSIS: Diversional activity deficit related to illness and confinement to hospital

EXPECTED OUTCOME

Child will engage in activities that are developmentally appropriate and within physical and environmental limitations.

NURSING INTERVENTIONS/*RATIONALES*

Schedule therapies and rest periods *to allow time for play activities.*
Time play periods when child may be feeling particularly vulnerable or alone *to provide needed distraction.*
Arrange for social interactions with others *to promote socialization.*
Interview parents and child to discover the child's favorite activities and games; adapt these activities to the child's physical limitations *to provide optimum diversions.*
Have parents bring in treasured toys or objects, decorate room with familiar pictures and drawings *to familiarize an unfamiliar environment.*

NURSING DIAGNOSIS: Activity intolerance related to illness and generalized weakness

EXPECTED OUTCOME

Patient's vital signs will remain within prescribed limits during activity, and child will tolerate increasing levels of activity.

NURSING INTERVENTIONS/*RATIONALES*

Monitor child's vital signs *to assess level of physical* tolerance; monitor child's behavior and look for signs of irritability, shortened attention span, fussiness *that are indicators of a need for rest.*
Balance rest and activity, match play activities with tolerance levels *to conserve energy and prevent intolerance.*
Administer analgesics and sedatives per physician order *to decrease pain and restlessness.*
Remove stimulation and provide a quiet and calm environment during rest periods *to enhance rest and sleep.*

NURSING DIAGNOSIS: Risk for injury related to unfamiliar environment, therapies, hazardous equipment

EXPECTED OUTCOME

Patient will exhibit no evidence of injury.

NURSING INTERVENTIONS/*RATIONALES*

Employ environmental safety measures (e.g., use of side rails; bed in low position; avoidance of hazards; keeping small, sharp and breakable items out of reach) *to prevent injury.*
Transport children using age-appropriate equipment and use of locks and safety belts *to minimize risk of injury.*
Maintain vigilance during trips to bathroom, use of bathtub or shower, performance of procedures *to minimize risk of injury.*
Identify specific motor/sensory deficits and provide appropriate assistive devices *to promote function and enhance safety.*
Instruct family in standard safety practices *to promote safety.*

NURSING DIAGNOSIS: Self-care deficit; toileting, bathing/hygiene, dressing/grooming, feeding related to illness, physical restrictions, emotional regression

EXPECTED OUTCOME

Patient will exhibit self-care activities within current physical and psychologic capacities.

NURSING INTERVENTIONS/*RATIONALES*

Teach parents that some regression is expected when a child is ill so behavior can be anticipated and viewed as normal part of disease process.
Identify the level of regression and use developmental strategies appropriate to that level *to facilitate care.*
Involve child in planning and initiating daily routines as appropriate *to foster a sense of control.*
Assist child in performing activities of daily living as indicated, *allowing needed dependency and provision of support.*
Encourage child to perform activities within abilities *to promote self-confidence and independence.*

NURSING CARE OF THE FAMILY

Assessment

Assessment involves those factors that are most likely to influence the family's responses to the child's illness and/or hospitalization. Although it is not possible to predict exactly which factors are most likely to have an effect on the family's reactions, the areas discussed in Table 44-2 should be included in the assessment process. Other important variables are (1) the seriousness of the child's illness, (2) the family's previous experience with hospitalization, and (3) the medical procedures involved in the diagnosis and treatment. Important information is also obtained in the nursing admission history (see Box 44-6).

CRITICAL THINKING EXERCISE: DISCHARGE PLANNING

Discharge Assessment

Throughout the hospitalization the nurse should be aware of the need for discharge planning and those assessment factors that affect the family's ability to provide home care. Discharge planning must begin early in the hospital admission to permit sufficient time to assess the family's ability to perform care at home and to institute needed teaching. With the current concern for cost containment and recognition of children's emotional needs, home care for children with technologically complex care, such as children on ventilators, has become increasingly common. The current nursing shortage has placed more of the burden for caring for children in the home on the parents, who often become the child's *caregiver*, supervised by the nurse who acts as *case manager*.

In terms of home care for children with complex care, a thorough assessment of the family and home environment should be performed to ensure that the family's emotional and physical resources are sufficient to manage the tasks of home care. (For a discussion of family and home assessment strategies, see Chapter 43.) In addition to adequate family resources, an investigation of community services, including respite care, is needed to ensure that appropriate support agencies are available, such as emergency facilities, home health agencies, and equipment vendors. Financial resources are also a consideration. To coordinate the immense task of assessment and to plan implementation, a care coordinator or manager should be appointed early in the discharge program.

Discharge planning is also concerned with those skills that parents or children are expected to continue at home. Assessment for planning appropriate teaching includes knowledge of (1) the actual and perceived complexity of the skill, (2) the parents' or child's ability to learn the skill, and (3) the parents' or child's previous or present experience with such procedures.

Nursing Diagnoses

A number of nursing diagnoses are prominent in the nursing care of the family of the hospitalized child, and others specific to individual cases become evident. The most common nursing diagnoses are outlined in the Nursing Care Plan on p. 1341.

Plan of Care and Implementation

The main goals for the family are as follows:

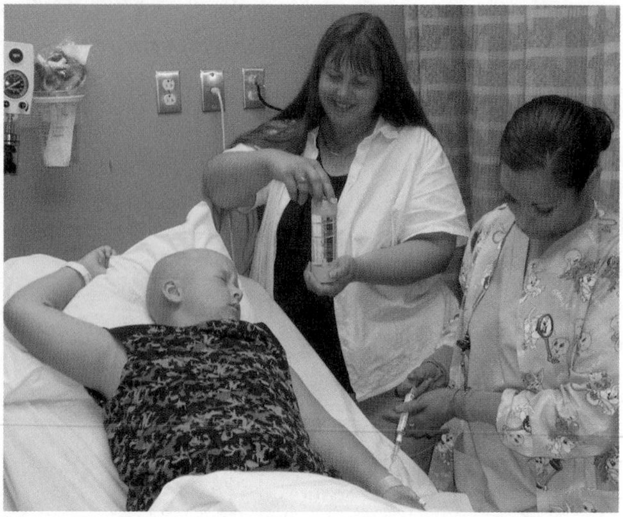

Fig. 44-14 Parental presence during hospitalization provides emotional support for the child and increases the parent's sense of empowerment in the caregiver role.

1. Family will participate in child's care to the extent they desire.
2. Family will receive support.
3. Family will be informed of child's care.
4. Family will be prepared for discharge and home care.

Encouraging Parent Participation

Preventing or minimizing separation is a key nursing goal with the child who is hospitalized, but maintaining parent-child contact is also beneficial for the family. One of the best approaches is encouraging parents to stay with their child and to participate in the care whenever possible. Although some health facilities provide special accommodations for parents, the concept of "rooming-in" can be instituted anywhere. The first requirement is the staff's positive attitude toward parents. A negative attitude toward parent participation can create barriers to collaborative working relationships (Johnson & Lindschau, 1996). Although nurses often express explicit support for the concept of family-centered care, some of their practices and beliefs suggest otherwise (Bruce & Ritchie, 1997).

When hospital staff genuinely appreciate the importance of continued parent-child attachment, they foster an environment that encourages parents to stay. When parents are included in the care planning and understand that they are a contributing factor to the child's recovery, they are more inclined to remain with their child and have more emotional reserves to support themselves and the child through the crisis. An empowerment model of helping allows the nurse to focus on parents' strengths and seek ways to promote growth and family functioning so that the parents become empowered in caring for their child (Fig. 44-14).

Because the mother tends to be the usual family caregiver, she usually spends more time in the hospital than the father. However, not all mothers (or fathers) feel equally comfortable in assuming responsibility for their child's care. Some may be under such great emotional stress that they need a temporary reprieve from total participation in caregiving activities (Remmel, 1997). Others may feel insecure in participating in specialized areas of care, such as bathing the child after surgery. On the other hand, some mothers may feel a great need to have control of their child's care. This seems particularly true of young mothers, who have more recently established their role as a parent; mothers of children too young to verbalize their needs; and ethnic minority mothers when the hospital setting is predominantly staffed by nonminority personnel. Individual assessment of each parent's preferred involvement is necessary to prevent the effects of separation while supporting parents in their needs as well.

With lifestyles and gender roles changing, fathers may assume all or some of the usual "mothering" roles in the household. In this case it may be the father-child relationship that requires preservation. Fathers need to be included in the plan of care and respected for their parental role. For some fathers the child's hospitalization may represent an opportunity to alter their usual caregiving role and increase their involvement. In single-parent families the caregiver may not be a parent but an extended family member, such as a grandparent or aunt.

One of the potential problems with continuous parent involvement is neglect of the parent's need for sleep, nutrition, and relaxation (Family Focus box). Often the sleeping accommodations are limited to a chair, and sleep is disrupted by nursing procedures. Encouraging the parents to leave for brief periods, arranging for sleeping quarters on the unit but outside the child's room, and planning a schedule of alternating visiting with another family member can minimize the stresses for the parent.

NURSE ALERT If parents are reluctant to leave the hospital (usually for fear of not being there when the child awakens or the practitioner visits), arrange for them to have a remote "beeper" that can provide immediate communication regardless of their location (Ashenberg et al, 1996). ■

All too often, nurses respond to parent participation by abandoning their patient responsibilities. Nurses need to restructure their roles to complement and augment the caregiving functions of parents. Even in units structured to provide care by parents, parents frequently feel anxiety in their caregiving responsibilities; those more involved in direct care may feel more anxiety than those less involved in direct care. Therefore 24-hour responsibility may be too much for some parents. Assistance and relief by nursing personnel should always be available to these families, and nurses must often work diligently to establish the strong bond of trust some parents need to take advantage of these opportunities.

Supporting Family Members

Support involves the willingness to stay and listen to parents' verbal and nonverbal messages. Sometimes the nurse does not give this support directly. For example, the nurse may offer to stay with the child to allow the parents time alone or may discuss with other family members the parents' need for extra relief. Often relatives and friends want to help but do not know how. Suggesting ways, such as baby-sitting, preparing meals, tending the garden or home, doing laundry, or transporting the siblings to school, can prompt others to help lessen the responsibilities that burden parents. An ongoing parent support group held on the pediatric unit during the children's traditional nap time has also proved effective in helping parents share emotions and concerns related to hospitalization (Bracht et al, 1998; Santelli, Turnbull, & Higgins, 1997).

Support may also be provided through the clergy. Parents with deep religious beliefs may appreciate the counsel of a clergy member, but because of their stress they may not have sufficient energy to initiate the contact. Nurses can be supportive by arranging for clergy to visit, upholding parents' religious beliefs, and respecting the individual meaning and significance of those beliefs.

Support involves an acceptance of cultural, socioeconomic, and ethnic values. For example, health and illness are defined differently by various ethnic groups. For some, a disorder that has few outward manifestations of illness, such as diabetes, hypertension, or cardiac problems, is not a sickness. Consequently, following a prescribed treatment may be seen as unnecessary. Nurses who appreciate the influences of culture are more likely to intervene therapeutically. (See also Chapter 32 for an extensive discussion of cultural and religious influences on health care.)

Parents need help in accepting their own feelings toward the ill child. If given the opportunity, parents often disclose their feelings of loss of control, anger, and guilt. They often resist admitting to such feelings because they expect others to disapprove of behavior that is less than perfect. Unfortunately, health personnel, including nurses, sometimes do exercise little tolerance for deviation from the expected norm. This only increases the psychologic impact of a child's illness on family members. Helping parents identify the specific reason for such feelings and emphasizing that each is a normal, expected, and healthy response to stress provides the parents with an opportunity to lessen their emotional burden.

Family Focus

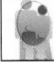

PARENTS' RELUCTANCE TO LEAVE THEIR CHILDREN UNATTENDED

Parents are often very reluctant to leave their children or to ask the nurse to watch their children while they take a break. In his research on the experiences of nurses and parents when parents room-in, Darbyshire (1994) found that many parents did not eat properly or, in some cases, at all. The following are two mothers' experiences:

I just about starved to death the first couple of days . . . just . . . I mean, it was my own fault really, 'cos I wouldn't leave the wee one. There was always going to be something else happening and I thought . . . if he gets upset I'd better be there when it finishes.

There was one day I couldn't get any of the visitors to look after the wee chap so I could go for something to eat and it was about six o'clock at night and nurse said, "You look awful, are you OK?" and I said, "No, actually I feel awful and I think I'm going to pass out," and she said, "Oh, you've just gone a funny colour," and I said, "What time is it?" and I said, "It's OK, it's just because I haven't eaten all day" because none of my family had come to take the child from me, and I didn't think to say to a nurse, "Could you watch him till I go for something to eat?"

Data from Darbyshire P: *Living with a sick child in hospital,* London, 1994, Chapman & Hall.

Family-centered care also addresses the needs of siblings. Support may involve preparing siblings for hospital visits, assessing their adjustment, and providing appropriate interventions or referrals when needed. The Home Care box suggests ways that parents can support siblings during hospitalization.

Providing Information

One of the most important nursing interventions is providing information about (1) the disease, its treatment, prognosis, and home care; (2) the child's emotional, as well as physical, reaction to illness and hospitalization; and (3) the probable emotional reactions of family members to the crisis.

For many families the child's illness is the first contact they have with the hospital experience. Often parents are not prepared for the child's behavioral reactions to hospitalization, such as separation behaviors, regression, aggression, and hostility. Providing the parents with information about these normal and expected behavioral responses can lessen the parents' anxiety during the hospital admission. The family is equally unfamiliar with hospital rules, which often adds to feelings of confusion and anxiety. Therefore the family needs clear explanations about what to expect and what is expected of them.

Parents also need to be aware of the effects of illness on the family and strategies that prevent negative changes. Specifically, parents should keep the family well informed and communicating as much as possible. They should treat all of the children as equally and as normally as before the illness occurred. Discipline, which initially may be lessened for the ill child, should be continued to provide a measure of security and predictability. When ill children know that their parents expect certain standards of conduct from them, they feel certain that they will recover. Conversely, when all limits are removed, they fear that something catastrophic will happen.

Nurses should help parents understand and accept the meaning of posthospitalization behaviors so that the parents can tolerate and support such behaviors. Consequently, parents should be forewarned of the usual continuance of such reactions after discharge (see Box 44-3). Parents who do not expect such reactions may misinterpret them as evidence of the child's "being spoiled" and demand perfect behavior at a time when the child is still reacting to the stress of illness and hospitalization. If the behaviors, especially the demand for attention, are dealt with in a supportive manner, most children are able to relinquish them and assume precrisis levels of functioning.

Nurses should also forewarn parents of siblings' reactions, particularly anger, jealousy, and resentment. Older siblings may deny such reactions because they provoke feelings of guilt. However, everyone needs outlets for emotions, and the repressed feelings may surface as problems in school, with age-mates, as psychosomatic illnesses, or in delinquent behavior.

Probably one of the most neglected areas involves giving information to siblings. Frequently age becomes the only factor that leads to an awareness of this problem, because older children may begin to ask questions or request explanations. Even in this situation, however, the information may be seriously inadequate. Children in every age group deserve some explanation of the sibling's illness or hospitalization. Although the exact wording may differ, the explanation should focus on the following concerns: (1) "Will I get sick and have to go to the hospital?" (2) "Did I cause the illness?" (for actual or imagined reasons), and (3) "Will my parents abandon me if my brother or sister doesn't recover?" If parents or nurses address the explanations to these three questions, the siblings' own fears of illness, guilt, and abandonment are minimized (Melnyk & Alpert-Gillis, 1998).

Preparing for Discharge and Home Care

Most hospitalizations necessitate some type of discharge preparation. Often this involves education of the family for continued care and follow-up in the home. Depending on the diagnosis, this may be relatively simple or highly complex. Preparing the family for home care demands a high degree of competence in planning and implementing discharge instructions. This usually is best accomplished using an *interdisciplinary team approach*, which requires a shift from the *multidisciplinary team approach* used during an acute phase of a child's illness (Hornick, 1996).

Nurses are the ones responsible for all or some of the discharge teaching, which may be further carried out by the parent as the home caregiver, with a nurse acting as resource case manager. The teaching plan incorporates levels of learning, such as observing, participating with assistance, and fi-

Home Care

SUPPORTING SIBLINGS DURING HOSPITALIZATION

Trade off staying at the hospital with spouse or have a parent surrogate who knows the siblings well stay in the home.

Offer information about the child's condition to young siblings as well as older siblings; respect the sibling who avoids information as a means of coping with the situation.

Arrange for children to visit their brother or sister in the hospital if possible.

Encourage phone visits and mail between brothers and sisters; provide children with phone numbers, writing supplies, and stamps.

Help each sibling identify an extended family member or friend to be their support person and provide extra attention during parental absence.

Make or buy inexpensive toys or trinkets for siblings, one gift for each day the child will be hospitalized.

Wrap each gift separately and place in a basket, box, or other container at each child's bedside.

Instruct siblings to open one gift each night at bedtime and to remember that he or she is in the parent's thoughts.

If the child's condition is stable and distance is not prohibitive, plan a special time at home with the siblings or have spouse or another relative or friend bring the children to meet parent(s) at a restaurant or other location near the hospital.

Have extended family members or friends schedule a visit to the child in the hospital during parental absence.

Arrange a pass for the child to leave the hospital to join the family if the child's condition permits.

Modified from Craft M, Craft J: Perceived changes in siblings of hospitalized children: a comparison of sibling and parent reports, *Child Health Care* 18(1):42-48, 1989; and Rollins J: *Brothers and sisters: a discussion guide for families*, Landover, MD, 1992, Epilepsy Foundation of America.

nally, acting without help or guidance. The skill is divided into discrete steps, and each step is taught to the family member until it is learned. Return demonstration of the skill is requested before new skills are introduced. A record of teaching and performance provides an efficient checklist for evaluation. All families need to receive detailed *written* instructions about home care, with telephone numbers for assistance, before they leave the hospital. Communication between the nurse performing discharge planning and home health care is essential for ensuring a smooth transition for the child and family.

Videocassette recordings offer another excellent vehicle for home teaching. The actual teaching session in the hospital can be recorded and played for the family as often as needed. If the family has a VCR at home, the filmed instructions serve as a refresher when parents have questions about the procedure.

Once the family is competent in performing the skill, they are given responsibility for the care. When possible, the family should have a transition or trial period to assume care with minimum health care supervision. This may be arranged on the unit, during a home pass, or in a facility, such as a motel, near the hospital. Such transitions provide a safe practice period for the family, with assistance readily available when needed, and are especially valuable when the family lives at a distance from the treating center.

In many instances parents need only simple instructions and understanding of follow-up care. However, the often overwhelming care assumed by some families, coupled with other stressors they may be experiencing, necessitates continued professional support after discharge. A follow-up home visit or telephone call gives the nurse a better opportunity to individualize care and provide information in perhaps a less stressful learning environment than the hospital (Snowdon & Kane, 1995). Appropriate referrals and resources may include visiting nurse or home health agencies, private nurse services, the school system, a physical therapist, a mental health counselor, a social worker, and any number of community agencies. Sharing the important issues surrounding the child's and family's needs is essential. Referral summaries should be concise, specific, and factual. When numerous support services are involved, periodic collaboration among the professionals involved and the family is an excellent strategy to ensure efficient usage and comprehensive delivery of services.

Evaluation

The effectiveness of nursing interventions is determined by continual reassessment and evaluation of care based on the following observational guidelines:

1. Observe schedule of parental presence and amount of participation in child's care; observe parents' willingness and ability to take care of their own needs, such as regular breaks to eat, sleep, and care for the family's needs at home.
2. Interview family regarding their concerns; observe support offered by others, such as relatives, friends, and clergy; observe if special cultural practices (if applicable) are respected in the hospital.
3. Interview family regarding their knowledge of child's illness, child's expected reactions to the hospitalization experience, and the emotional needs of the other family members, especially siblings. Observe frequency of siblings' visits and interview siblings regarding their understanding of the ill child's condition.
4. Observe family's performance of skills and determine their understanding of other aspects of home care before discharge; interview family and/or resource persons regarding the family's use of appropriate referral services.

The expected outcomes are described in the Nursing Care Plan on p. 1346.

CARE OF THE CHILD AND FAMILY IN SPECIAL HOSPITAL SITUATIONS

In addition to a general pediatric unit, children may be admitted to special facilities such as an ambulatory/outpatient setting, an isolation room, or intensive care.

Ambulatory/Outpatient Setting

The ambulatory or outpatient setting provides needed medical services for the child while eliminating the necessity of overnight admission. Among the benefits of ambulatory care are (1) minimization of the stressors of hospitalization, especially separation from the family; (2) reduced chance of infection; and (3) cost savings. Admission to the ambulatory or outpatient hospital setting usually is for surgical or diagnostic procedures, such as insertion of tympanostomy tubes, hernia repair, adenoidectomy, tonsillectomy, cystoscopy, or bronchoscopy.

In the ambulatory/outpatient setting, adequate preparation is particularly challenging Ideally, the child and parents should receive preadmission preparation, including a tour of the facility and a review of the day's events (Brewer & Lambert, 1997). Parents need information in advance to help prepare the child and themselves for surgery and enable them to care for the child at home after the procedure. Parents also appreciate suggestions for items to bring to the hospital, such as blankets or stuffed animals. When preadmission preparation is not possible, time should be allowed on the day of the procedure for children to become acquainted with their surroundings and for nurses to assess, plan, and implement appropriate teaching.

Waiting is usually inevitable in ambulatory settings. Families frequently report waiting to be the most stressful part of the experience. Providing a pager is one way to allow the family (and at times the child) to leave the area and then be paged to return when needed (Ashenberg et al, 1996).

Explicit discharge instructions are important after outpatient surgery (Home Care box, p. 1347). Parents need guidelines on when to call their practitioner regarding a change in the child's condition. A follow-up telephone call system allows for nurses to check on the child's progress within 48 to 72 hours after discharge. It also provides an opportunity for the nurse to review discharge information and answer questions.

Nursing Care Plan

THE FAMILY OF THE ILL/HOSPITALIZED CHILD

NURSING DIAGNOSIS: Altered family processes and/or ineffective family coping related to situational crisis, threat to role functioning, change in environment

EXPECTED OUTCOME
Family will exhibit use of appropriate coping mechanisms, and stress levels are reduced.

NURSING INTERVENTIONS/*RATIONALES*

Explore family background, structure, normal roles, and functions, usual coping mechanisms *to identify family strengths and weaknesses and assist in meeting needs.*

Help family arrange a schedule that balances needs of hospitalized child with functions of home and work *to help family manage stress and adapt to the situation.*

Help family prioritize needs, explore options, make decisions *to reduce stress and increase coping.*

Encourage use of available support systems (e.g., extended family, friends, church, community) and make referrals to appropriate social service agencies *to increase support and enhance available resources.*

Keep family informed about child's condition, procedures, and treatments *to reduce anxiety about the unknown.*

Give family members specific suggestions as to what each can contribute to help the child during the hospital stay and recovery *to provide for concrete family contributions and involvement.*

Provide a ready outlet for family to vent feelings, fears, and frustrations *to promote coping.*

Encourage family to take care of their own needs for rest, nutrition, relaxation, and respite *to promote coping.*

NURSING DIAGNOSIS: Powerlessness related to health care environment

EXPECTED OUTCOME
Family will exhibit a sense of control within the environment.

NURSING INTERVENTIONS/*RATIONALES*

Encourage family to identify feelings about having a child in the hospital *to enhance trust, communication, and ventilation.*

Help family identify specific modifications and adjustments that can be made within the environment (e.g., participation in child's care, decision making, scheduling; rearranging and personalizing environmental space; provision of privacy, ready access to specifically identified personnel) *to enhance feelings of control.*

Incorporate family suggestions, needs into plan of care *to enhance sense of contribution and control.*

Keep family informed about child's condition, progress; educate about treatments and procedures *to enhance knowledge.*

NURSE ALERT Help the family prepare for the transportation home by offering these suggestions:

- Have a blanket and pillow in the car. (Always use the car safety system.)
- Take a basin or plastic bag in case of vomiting.
- Use a cup with a cap and straw for the child to drink fluids.
- Give any prescribed pain medication before leaving facility. ■

Isolation

Admission to an isolation room increases all of the stressors typically associated with hospitalization. There is further separation from familiar persons, additional loss of control, and added environmental changes, such as sensory deprivation and the strange appearance of visitors. Orientation to time and place is affected. These stressors are compounded by children's limited understanding of isolation. Preschool children have difficulty understanding the rationale for isolation because they cannot comprehend the cause-and-effect relationship between germs and illness. They are likely to view isolation as punishment. Older children understand the causality better but still require information to decrease fantasizing or misinterpretation.

When a child is placed in isolation, preparation is essential for the child to feel in control. With young children the best approach is a simple explanation, such as "You need to be in this room to help you get better. This is a special place to make all the germs go away. The germs made you sick, and you could not help that."

All children, but especially younger ones, need preparation in terms of what they will see, hear, or feel in isolation. Therefore they are shown the mask, gloves, and gown and are encouraged to "dress up" in them. Playing with the strange apparel lessens the fear of seeing "ghostlike" people walk into the room. Before entering the room, nurses and other health personnel should introduce themselves and let the child see their face before donning a mask. In this way the child associates them with significant experiences and gains a sense of familiarity in an otherwise strange and lonely environment.

When the child's condition improves, appropriate play activities are provided to minimize boredom, stimulate the senses, provide a real or perceived sense of movement, orient the child to time and place, provide social interaction, and reduce depersonalization. For example, the environment can be manipulated to increase sensory freedom by moving the bed toward the door or window. Opening window shades; providing musical, visual, or tactile toys; and increasing interpersonal contact can substitute mental mobility for the limitations of physical movement. Rather than dwelling on the negative aspects of isolation, the child can be encouraged to view this experience as challenging and positive. For example, the nurse can help the child look at isolation as a method of keeping others out and letting only special people in. Children often think of intriguing signs for their doors, such as "Enter at your own risk." These signs also encourage people "on the outside" to talk with the child about the ominous greeting.

Home Care

DISCHARGE FROM AMBULATORY SETTINGS

Before beginning, explain that all instructions will also be presented in writing for the family to refer to later.

Provide an overview of the typical trajectory (expected pattern) of recovery.

Discuss expected progression of the child's activity level during the postdischarge period (e.g., "Mary will probably sleep for the rest of the day, feel kind of tired most of tomorrow, but be back to her usual activities the next day.").

Explain which activities the child is allowed and what is not permitted (e.g., bed rest, bathing).

Discuss dietary restrictions, being very specific and giving examples of "clear fluids" or what is meant by a "full liquid diet."

Discuss nausea and vomiting, if applicable, explaining how much is "normal" and what to do if more occurs (e.g., "Juan may be sick to his stomach and vomit. This is normal. However, if he vomits more than three times, please call us at this number right away.").

Discuss fever and the comfort measures to use, explaining how much fever is considered "normal," and specifically what to do if the child goes beyond the range.

Explain the amount, location, and kind of pain or discomfort the child may experience.
- Give any prescribed medication before leaving the facility.
- Send a pain scale home with the family.
- Explain how much pain and discomfort is "normal" and what to do if the child surpasses that level or if pain management interventions are unsuccessful.
- Discuss pain management, including dosage for pain medications and details on how to administer them.
- Describe appropriate nonpharmacologic comfort measures, such as holding, rocking, or swaddling.

Provide information about each medication that the child will be taking at home.
- Review the details, including dose and route.
- Demonstrate how to administer medications, if necessary (e.g., how to take wrapping off suppositories, how to insert).
- Discuss guidelines for requesting other medications.
- Request that all prescriptions be filled and with the family before discharge.

Make certain the family has all of the equipment and supplies (e.g., gauze and tape for dressing changes) they will need at home.

Discuss complications that may occur and the steps to take if they do.

Ensure that appropriate measures are in place for safe transport home.
- Remind family to use a seat belt or car seat for the child.
- Determine if there will be one person whose sole responsibility is helping ensure the child's safety and comfort during transport.
- Discuss measures the driver may need to take if this is impossible (e.g., be certain a basin is within the child's reach should vomiting occur; take a route that permits slower traffic and has places along the roadside to stop if necessary).
- Determine the availability of a blanket, pillow, and cup with a cap and straw for the child's use in the car.
- Provide a basin or plastic bag in case of vomiting.

Provide emergency phone numbers for the family to call with any concerns.

Explain that the family will be contacted (giving an approximate time) to follow-up on the child but that they should not hesitate to call if concerns arise before then.

Ask the family and child, if appropriate, if they have any questions, and problem solve with family members to meet their unique needs.

<u>NURSE ALERT</u> Have the child select a place he or she would like to visit. Help the child decorate the bed and equipment to suit the theme (e.g., truck, circus tent, spaceship, sky). At a set time each day pretend to go with the child to the special place. Consider including props such as a suitcase or picnic basket. ■

Emergency Admission

One of the most traumatic hospital experiences for the child and parents is an emergency admission. The sudden onset of an illness or the occurrence of an injury leaves little time for preparation and explanation. Sometimes the emergency admission is compounded by admission to an intensive care unit or the need for immediate surgery. However, even in those instances requiring only outpatient treatment, the child is exposed to a strange, frightening environment and to experiences that may elicit fear or cause pain. Thus every medical emergency requires psychologic intervention to reduce the fear and anxiety frequently associated with the experience. Although underutilized, child-life specialists may provide teaching and support (Krebel, Clayton, & Graham, 1996).

There is a wide discrepancy between what constitutes a medically-defined emergency and a client-defined emergency. A growing concern is the use of major emergency departments for routine primary care health visits. To offset overcrowding in emergency departments, many facilities have minor emergency units or pediatric minor emergency units for after-hour health care. Telephone triage for minor illnesses for patients is also emerging as a health care delivery mode to triage illnesses such as common cold from true life-threatening conditions that require immediate practitioner attention and intervention. Other factors contributing to the overuse of emergency departments (as opposed to the primary practitioner's office) include the increasing number of noninsured persons and households where both parents work full time and cannot afford to take off during the daytime to take the sick child to a practitioner.

In pediatric populations most visits are for respiratory infections, with skin conditions, gastrointestinal disorders, and trauma such as poisoning accounting for the remainder of cases. The most common reason parents give for bringing the child to the emergency department is concern about the illness worsening. However, practitioners may not consider the progressive symptoms as necessitating immediate or emergency care. One of the nurse's primary goals is to assess the parents' perception of the event and their reasons for considering it serious or lifethreatening.

Lengthy preparatory admission procedures are often inappropriate for emergency situations. In such instances, nurses must focus their nursing interventions on the essential components of admission counseling (Box 44-15) and complete the process as soon as the child's condition is stabilized.

Unless an emergency is life threatening, children need to participate in their care to maintain a sense of control. Because emergency departments are frequently hectic, there is a tendency to rush through procedures to save time. However, the extra few minutes needed to allow children to participate may save many more minutes of useless resistance and uncooperativeness during subsequent procedures. Other supportive measures include ensuring privacy, accepting various emotional responses to fear or pain, preserving parent-child contact, explaining all events before or as they occur, and personally remaining calm.

At times, because of the child's physical condition, little or no preparatory counseling for emergency hospitalization can be done. In such situations the implementation of *postvention,* or counseling subsequent to the event, has therapeutic value. The process of postvention involves evaluating children's thoughts regarding admission and related procedures. It is similar to precounseling techniques; however, instead of supplying information, the nurse listens to the explanations offered by the child. Projective techniques such as drawing, doll play, or storytelling are especially effective. The nurse then bases additional information on what has already been revealed.

Intensive Care Unit (ICU)

Parents who have a child in an intensive care unit are stressed (Fig. 44-15). The nature and severity of the illness and the circumstances surrounding the admission are major factors, especially for parents. Parents experience significantly more stress when the admission is unexpected rather than expected. A recent study found that parental anxiety levels reached near panic levels initially (Huckabay & Tilem-Kessler, 1999). Stressors for the child and parent are described in Box 44-16. Although several studies have described what parents perceive as most stressful, the most effective strategy may be to simply ask parents what is stressful and implement interventions that will enhance coping outcomes (Melnyk & Alpert-Gillis, 1998; Board & Ryan-Wenger, 2003). Assessment should be repeated periodically to account for changes in perceptions over time.

BOX 44-15

Guidelines for Special Hospital Admission

Emergency Admission

Lengthy preparatory admission procedures are often impossible and inappropriate for emergency situations.

Focus assessment on airway, breathing, and circulation; weigh child whenever possible for calculation of drug dosages.

Unless an emergency is life threatening, children need to participate in their care to maintain a sense of control.

Focus on essential components of admission counseling, including:
- Appropriate introduction to the family
- Use of child's name, not terms such as "honey" or "dear"
- Determination of child's age and some judgment about developmental age (if the child is of school age, asking about the grade level will offer some evidence for concurrent intellectual ability)

Information about child's general state of health, any problems that may interfere with medical treatment (e.g., allergies), and previous experience with hospital facilities

Information about the chief complaint from both the parents and the child

Admission to Intensive Care Unit (ICU)

Prepare child and parents for elective ICU admission, such as for postoperative care after cardiac surgery.

Prepare child and parents for unanticipated ICU admission by focusing primarily on the sensory aspects of the experience and on usual family concerns (e.g., persons in charge of child's care, schedule for visiting, area where family can stay).

Prepare parents regarding child's appearance and behavior when they first visit child in ICU.

Accompany family to bedside to provide emotional support and answer questions.

Prepare siblings for their visit; plan length of time for sibling visitation; monitor siblings' reactions during visit to prevent them from becoming overwhelmed.

Encourage parents to stay with their child:
- If visiting hours are limited, allow flexibility in schedule to accommodate parental needs.
- Give family members a written schedule of visiting times.
- If visiting hours are liberal, be aware of family members' needs and suggest periodic respites.
- Assure family they can call the unit at any time.

Prepare parents for expected role changes and identify ways for parents to participate in child's care without overwhelming them with responsibilities:
- Help with bath or feeding.
- Touch and talk to child.
- Help with procedures.

Provide information about child's condition in understandable language:
- Repeat information often.
- Seek clarification of understanding.
- During bedside conferences, interpret information for family members and child or, if appropriate, conduct report outside room.

Prepare child for procedures, even if this involves explanation while procedure is performed.

Assess and manage pain; recognize that a child who cannot talk, such as an infant or child in a coma or on a ventilator, can be in pain.

Establish a routine that maintains some similarity to daily events in child's life whenever possible:
- Organize care during normal waking hours.
- Keep regular bedtime schedules, including quiet times when television or radio is lowered or turned off.
- Provide uninterrupted sleep cycles (60 minutes for infant, 90 minutes for older child).
- Close and open drapes and dim lights to allow for day/night.
- Place curtain around bed for privacy.
- Orient child to day and time; have clocks or calendars in easy view for older children.

Schedule a time when child is left undisturbed (e.g., during naps, visit with family, playtime, or favorite program).

Provide opportunities for play.

Reduce stimulation in environment:

Refrain from loud talking or laughing.

Keep equipment noise to a minimum:
- Turn alarms as low as safely possible.
- Perform treatments requiring equipment at one time.
- Turn off bedside equipment that is not in use, such as suction and oxygen.

Avoid loud, abrupt noises, such as clattering bedpans or toilets flushing.

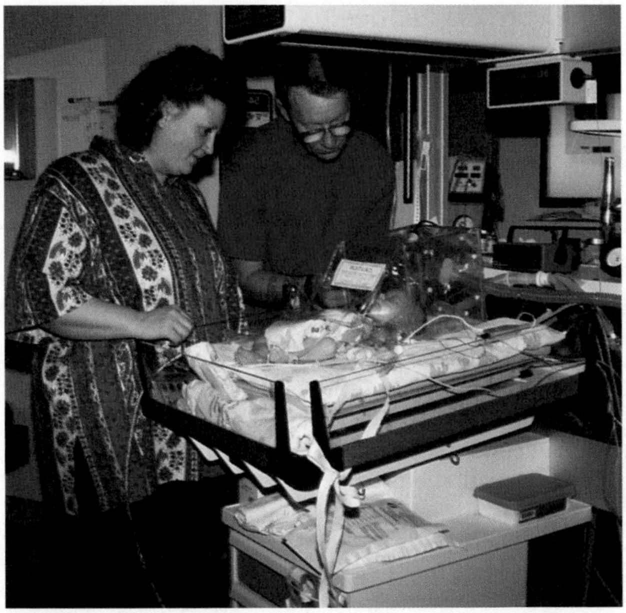

Fig. 44-15 Parents can be overwhelmed when their child is critically ill and requires care in an ICU.

BOX 44-16

Neonatal/Pediatric ICU Stressors for the Child and Family

Physical Stressors
Pain and discomfort (e.g., injections, intubation, suctioning, dressing changes, other invasive procedures)
Immobility (e.g., use of restraints, bed rest)
Sleep deprivation
Inability to eat or drink
Changes in elimination habits

Environmental Stressors
Unfamiliar surroundings (e.g., crowding)
Unfamiliar sounds
Equipment noise (e.g., monitors, telephone, suctioning, computer printout)
Human sounds (e.g., talking, laughing, crying, coughing, moaning, retching, walking)
Unfamiliar people (e.g., health care professionals, patients, visitors)
Unfamiliar and unpleasant smells (e.g., alcohol, adhesive remover, body odors)
Constant lights (disturb day/night rhythms)
Activity related to other patients
Sense of urgency among staff
Unkind or thoughtless comments from staff

Psychologic Stressors
Lack of privacy
Inability to communicate (if intubated)
Inadequate knowledge and understanding of situation
Severity of illness
Parental behavior (expression of concern)

Social Stressors
Disrupted relationships (especially with family and friends)
Concern with missing school or work
Play deprivation

Data primarily from Tichy AM et al: Stressors in pediatric intensive care units, *Pediatr Nurs* 14(1):40-42, 1988.

The emotional needs of the family are paramount when a child is admitted to an ICU. Although the same interventions discussed earlier for the stressors of separation, loss of control, and bodily injury and pain apply here, additional interventions may also benefit the family and child (see Box 44-16 and Family Focus box). Critical care must be centered on the family. Visiting hours should be liberal and flexible enough to accommodate parental needs (Hazinski, 1999).

Critically ill children become the focus of the parents' lives, and parents' most pressing need is for information (Scott, 1998). They want to know if their child will live, and if so, whether the child will be the same as before. They need to know why various interventions are being done for the child, that the child is being treated for pain and/or is comfortable, and that the child may be able to hear them even though not awake.

Despite the stresses normally associated with ICU admission, a special security develops from being carefully monitored and receiving individualized care. Therefore planning for transition to the regular unit is essential and should include (1) assignment of a primary nurse on the regular unit who visits before the transfer; (2) continued visits by the ICU staff to assess the child's and parents' adjustment and to act as a temporary liaison with the nursing staff; (3) explanation of the differences between the two units and the rationale for the change to less intense monitoring of the child's physical condition; and (4) selection of an appropriate room, such as one that is close to the nursing station, and a compatible roommate.

Family Focus

ARTISTS AS PARTNERS IN CARE

A teenaged boy with a rare genetic disorder, having made steady progress after awakening from a coma, relapsed and seemed very depressed. When told that a musician was visiting the pediatric intensive care unit (PICU), he immediately perked up and asked to have his room lights turned on. He whispered endless song requests to the musician. Family members and staff were treated to some of his first smiles in days; his biggest came when the musician held his hand and guided it across the guitar strings while they sang "Born to Be Wild" together at the boy's request. His dad was misty-eyed as he thanked the musician for the visit.

A few weeks later the boy's condition worsened and he again lapsed into a coma. There was nothing more to be done. His parents began the necessary preparations to take their son home to die.

We continued to visit our friend and his family, offering a song, a story, or just simply to say hello. I hold a vivid picture of our final visit. We stood around the boy's bed with his parents singing together songs they remembered from their youth, from more carefree times. Song and laughter filled the boy's room.

Perhaps the boy heard his parents' laughter and knew then that they would be okay. He died a few days later on the morning he was to have been discharged.

Judy Rollins, MS, RN
Washington, DC

Modified from Rollins J: *Placed in our keeping,* 1995, Unpublished.

Key Points

- Children are particularly vulnerable to the stressors of illness and hospitalization because stress represents a change from the usual state of health and routine and because they possess limited coping mechanisms.
- The three phases of separation anxiety are protest, despair, and detachment.
- Feelings of loss of control are caused by unfamiliar environmental stimuli, physical restriction, altered routine, and dependency.
- Fear of bodily pain may be manifested in the following ways: infants—facial expressions, body movements; toddlers—intense emotional upset, physical resistance; preschoolers—aggression, verbal expression, dependency; school-age children—precise verbalization of pain, passive requests for support or help, procrastination technique; adolescents—self-control, limited movement.
- Because of their separation from significant people, children who are hospitalized may lack the opportunity to form new attachments in the strange environment of the hospital and exhibit negative behaviors after discharge.
- Nursing care of the child in the hospital is aimed at preventing or minimizing separation, decreasing loss of control, minimizing fear of bodily injury, assessing and managing pain, promoting normal development, using play and/or expressive activities to lessen stress, and maximizing the potential benefits of hospitalization.
- Pain assessment includes questioning the child, using pain rating scales, evaluating behavior, securing parents' involvement, taking the cause of the pain into account, and taking action. Pain management should incorporate both pharmacologic and nonpharmacologic methods.
- The nurse can maximize potential benefits of hospitalization by fostering parent-child relations, providing educational opportunities, promoting self-mastery, and encouraging socialization.
- Family reactions are influenced by the seriousness of the illness, experience with illness or hospitalization and diagnostic or therapeutic procedures, available support systems, personal ego strengths, coping abilities, presence of additional stressors, cultural and religious beliefs, and family communication patterns.
- Fear of contracting illness, their younger age, a close relationship with the ill sibling, substitute child care, minimum explanation of the illness, and perceived changes in parenting all increase the deleterious effects of a brother's or sister's illness and hospitalization on siblings.
- Nursing care of the family involves listening to parents' verbal and nonverbal messages; providing clergy support; accepting cultural, socioeconomic, and ethnic values; giving information to families and siblings; and preparing for discharge and home care.
- Admission to an outpatient setting, emergency department, isolation room, or intensive care unit requires additional intervention strategies to meet the child's and family's needs.

Answer Guidelines to Critical Thinking Exercises

Complementary/Alternative Medicine

1. There is limited evidence to draw certain conclusions without obtaining more data from the parents. It would be appropriate to gather more information before jumping to any major conclusions at this time.
2. (a) Complementary and alternative medicine (CAM) is more common in U.S. households than previously reported. Much of the concern surrounding complementary therapies, especially in children, is the lack of sufficient data regarding their effectiveness and benefit, and the potential harm that may occur as a result of such treatments. In some cases CAM therapies may counteract certain medications or the effects of prescribed therapies. It has become more common for practitioners in emergency medicine to encounter patients who are taking CAM therapy in addition to prescription medications/treatments for conditions such as eczema, asthma, colds, and upper respiratory problems. (b) Folk remedies are quite common among certain ethnic groups and subgroups within the United States. Many are based on traditional family remedies that neither have been proved to be effective nor entirely harmful in most cases. However a few remedies remain that could be potentially harmful, especially to children if these remedies counteract the effects of prescribed treatments that are known to be effective. (c) The nurse's role in such cases is to gather sufficient data from the family about the practice, discuss the treatment (CAM) in a nonjudgmental manner, and be cognizant of the effects of the treatment on the child's current health status and potential effects on other medical treatment regimens.
3. Give the family their penny and open a dialog about the traditional practice they are using. Additional information should be gathered in a nonjudgmental manner, and the discussion should center on the family's traditional beliefs regarding the practices, the prescribed medical regimen, and whether there is conflict or potential for harm. There is no need to stop the treatment unless potential harm to the child may occur. A discussion with the primary practitioner regarding the use of CAM for Maria should ensue, followed by a discussion with the entire family if necessary.

   The contents of the bottle will more than likely be revealed during the discussion with the family. It is important to respect the family's wishes regarding traditional folk or CAM rituals, yet remain mindful of potential harmful effects on the child. It is not likely that telling the family to stop the ritual will have much success since these beliefs are deeply ingrained into cultural, religious, and medical practice; the family is more likely to continue the ritual at home on discharge and further disregard other instructions for care should a confrontational approach be adopted by the nursing and medical staff. The important concept for the staff and family to focus upon is the ultimate well-being of the child.

What you have probably observed is Santeria, the African-Caribbean religion that was brought to the New World by slaves from West Africa. It is common among immigrants from Cuba, Puerto Rico, Brazil, and Santo Domingo, and it is believed that a majority of Latin immigrants will have contact with Santeria sometime in their lives.

4. As yet, evidence to indicate that harm is being done by the CAM ritual is insufficient. Further data needs to be gathered and then a decision about further discussion of the CAM practice may occur.
5. There are no alternative views other than the notion that if the nursing and medical staff are confrontational and judgmental with the family, the family is less likely to trust the staff, thereby negating any treatments and discharge instructions for the care of the child.

Playroom and Hospital Procedures

1. There is sufficient evidence regarding this incident to draw some conclusions.
2. (a) Regardless of how minor a procedure such as a venipuncture may seem to an adult health care worker, it represents a major threat to a child. One must consider the child's age, illness, developmental level, and previous experiences with venipunctures. (b) Play is an important function of childhood whether the child is sick or well. Through play, children may act out fears, concerns, anger, and other behaviors that they may not feel comfortable expressing to adults in a confrontational manner. Play is an important part of the hospitalized child's life and it is a vehicle for promoting optimal development. (c) It is important to have the blood drawn so Dr. Lung can plan a therapeutic regimen; however, one must consider another issue and that is that there appears to have been no advanced preparation of the child's skin to minimize or prevent pain from the procedure. Regardless of the phlebotomist's skill in performing the procedure, it is also important to consider the fact that the negative repercussions for performing the procedure at this point may outweigh the positive benefits. (d) All staff on the pediatric floor must be in agreement about respecting the child's personal space in the playroom and in adhering to unit policies or rules so that respect is maintained. Failure to respect the child's space may engender further fear by other children who perceive that the playroom is not a safe place after all, when certain procedures need to be done. The fear of having other procedures performed in the playroom may prevent children from going there to participate in therapeutic and interactive play.
3. It is important to maintain a fair balance between what constitutes therapeutic management of illness and childhood recreation. It would be appropriate in this situation to intervene and ask the phlebotomist to return in 30 minutes to an hour and indicate that the child will be ready for the venipuncture in the treatment room at that time. It is important to stress that the playroom is off-limits for procedures. It would be appropriate to discuss this plan with Hannah, indicating that the procedure will be performed at the designated time. It is also important to explore pain management issues with Hannah. Does she usually use EMLA or other topical remedy to prevent pain at the site? If so, it will be necessary to make such arrangements in advance, possibly now, so her pain is managed appropriately. As the nurse, it is appropriate to discuss a delay in obtaining the lab results with Dr. Lung and the reasons for the delay. As a staff member on the pediatric floor, it is important for medical and nursing staff to communicate effectively. Should this arrangement not suite Dr. Lung's time frame for accomplishing certain tasks, one might suggest a trade-off. The nurse may draw the blood in the treatment room once preparations are made and a time is agreed upon by Hannah. Remember however that school-age children are prone to "bargain" for more time to delay or prevent the event because it is painful. One must be gently firm about the agreed-upon time of the procedure and not allow further delays to accommodate the child who simply does not want the procedure performed ever.

   Even if one accepts the conclusion that it is "okay" with Hannah, it is important to consider the possible negative implications for the other children in the room, who may be confused about even a simple procedure (e.g., checking blood pressure) or the sanctuary status of the playroom for themselves.

   To proceed with the blood draw in the playroom would violate the child's trust about what adult health care workers say regarding the purpose of the playroom as a sanctuary from painful procedures. Such action would likely result in less cooperation from the children who are present and may also make other parents present or who obtain knowledge of the incident, wonder about the sincerity of the staff. Interrupting the children's game is not necessary as this does not represent a life-threatening condition at this time.
4. Yes, there is sufficient evidence to support these decisions and the plan of action.
5. An exception is sometimes made when all of the children present are older and the procedure is a quick, painless one (e.g., checking blood pressure or giving oral medication) that all the children present have experienced. In such cases the patient and the other children are asked if it is okay and give permission before the procedure is undertaken.

References

Algren JT, Algren CL: Management of procedural and perioperative pain in children. In Weiner R (ed): *Pain management: a practical guide for clinicians,* Boca Raton, FL, 1998, St Lucie Press.

Algren JT et al: Efficacy and safety of morphine administered by patient-, parent-, or nurse-controlled analgesia in children, *Anesthesiology* 89:A1003, 1998 (abstract).

American Pain Society: *Principles of analgesic use in the treatment of acute pain and chronic cancer pain,* ed 4, Glenview, IL, 1999, The Society.
American Society of Addiction Medicine: Public policy statement on definitions related to the use of opioids for pain treatment, February, 2001.
American Society of Pain Management Nurses: ASPMN position statement: use of placebos for pain management, *Ostomy Wound Manage* 44(2): 56-57, 1998.
Anand K, Aynsley-Green A: Metabolic and endocrine effects of surgical ligation of patent ductus arteriosus in the human preterm neonate: are there implications for further improvement of postoperative outcome? *Mod Probl Paediatr* 23:143-157, 1985.
Anand KJS, Hickey P: Pain and its effects in the human neonate and fetus, *N Engl J Med* 317(21):1321-1329, 1987.
Ashenberg MD et al: Easing the wait: development of a pager program for families, *Pediatr Nurs* 22(2):103-107, 1996.
Baker C, Wong D: Q.U.E.S.T.: a process of pain assessment in children, *Orthop Nurs* 6(1):11-21, 1987.
Bauchner H, May A, Coates E: Use of analgesic agents for invasive medical procedures in pediatric and neonatal intensive care units, *J Pediatr* 121(4):647-649, 1992.
Berde C et al: Patient-controlled analgesia in children and adolescents: a randomized, prospective comparison with intramuscular administration of morphine for postoperative analgesia, *J Pediatr* 118(3):460-466, 1991.
Beyer JE, Denyes MJ, Villarruel AM: The creation, validation and continuing development of the Oucher: a measure of pain intensity in children, *J Pediatr Nurs* 7(5):335-346, 1992.
Beyer JE, McGrath PJ, Berde CB: Discordance between self-report and behavioral pain measures in children aged 3-7 years after surgery, *J Pain Symptom Manage* 5(6):350-356, 1990.
Beyer J et al: Patterns of postoperative analgesic use with adults and children following cardiac surgery, *Pain* 17(1):71-81, 1983.
Billmire DA, Neale HW, Gregory RO: Use of IV fentanyl in the outpatient treatment of pediatric facial trauma, *J Trauma* 25(11):1079-1080, 1985.
Board R, Ryan-Wenger N: Stressors and symptoms of mothers with children in the PICU, *J Pediatr Nurs* 18(3):195-201, 2003.
Boughton K et al: Impact of research on pediatric pain assessment and outcomes, *Pediatr Nurs* 24(1):31-35, 62, 1998.
Boyd, J, Hunsberger M: Chronically ill children coping with repeated hospitalizations: their perceptions and suggested interventions, *J Pediatr Nurs* 13(6):330-342, 1998.
Bracht M et al: Initiation and maintenance of a hospital-based parent group for parents of premature infants: key factors for success, *Neonatal Network* 17(3):33-37, 1998.
Brewer S, Lambert C: Preparing children for same day surgery: innovative approaches, *J Pediatr Nurs* 12(4):257-259, 1997.
Broome ME, Huth MM: Nursing management of the child in pain. In Schechter NL, Berde CB, Yaster M (eds): *Pain in infants, children, and adolescents,* ed 2, Philadelphia, 2003, Lippincott, Williams & Wilkins, pp 417-433.
Broome M, Rehwaldt M, Fogg L: Relationships between cognitive behavioral techniques, temperament, observed distress, and pain reports in children and adolescents during lumbar puncture, *J Pediatr Nurs* 13(1):48-54, 1998.
Broome M et al: Children's medical fears, coping behaviors, and pain perceptions during a lumbar puncture, *Oncol Nurs Forum* 17(3):361-367, 1990.
Broome M et al: Pediatric pain practices: a national survey of health professionals, *J Pain Symptom Manage* 11(5):312-320, 1996.
Brozovic M et al: Pain relief in sickle cell crises, *Lancet* 2(8507):624-625, 1986.
Bruce B, Ritchie J: Nurses' practices and perceptions of family centered care, *J Pediatr Nurs* 12(4):214-222, 1997.
Clatworthy S, Simon K, Tiedeman ME: Child drawing: hospital-an instrument designed to measure the emotional status of hospitalized school-aged children, *J Pediatr Nurs* 14(1):2-9, 1999.
Cline ME et al: Standardization of the visual analogue scale, *Nurs Res* 41(6):378-380, 1992.
Collins J: Intractable cancer pain in children, *Child Adolesc Psychiatr Clin* 6(4):879-888, 1997.
Craft MJ: Siblings of hospitalized children: assessment and intervention, *J Pediatr Nurs* 8(5):289-297, 1993.
Dahl JL: Darron: a drug with dubious distinction, *Cancer Pain Update* (48)3:6, Summer, 1998.
Darbyshire P: *Living with a sick child in hospital,* London, 1994, Chapman & Hall.
Davis GC: Nursing's role in pain management across the health care continuum, *Nurs Outlook* 46(1):19-23, 1998.
Dilworth NM, MacKellar A: Pain relief for the pediatric surgical patient, *J Pediatr Surg* 22(3):264-266, 1987.
Dolgin M et al: Behavioral distress in pediatric patients with cancer receiving chemotherapy, *Pediatrics* 84(1):103-110, 1989.
Eland JM, Anderson JE: The experience of pain in children. In Jacox A (ed): *Pain: a source book for nurses and other health professionals,* Boston, 1977, Little, Brown.
Eland JM, Banner W: Analgesia, sedation, and neuromuscular blockage in pediatric critical care. In Hazinski ME (ed): *Manual of pediatric critical care,* St Louis, 1999, Mosby.
Ellis JA et al: Pain in hospitalized pediatric patients: how are we doing? *Clin J Pain* 18(4):262-269, 2002.
Fanurik D et al: Children with cognitive impairment: parent report of pain and coping, *J Dev Behav Pediatr* 20(4):228-234, 1999.
Favaloro R, Touzel B: A comparison of adolescents' and nurses' postoperative pain ratings and perceptions, *Pediatr Nurs* 16(4):414-417, 424, 1990.
Federwisch A: Complete assessment: making pain the fifth vital sign, *Health Week* 4(14):18, 1999.
Fernandez C, Pyesmany A, Stutzer C: Alternative therapies in childhood cancer, *N Engl J Med* 340(7):569-570, 1999.
Ferrell BR, McCaffery M, Rhiner M: Pain and addiction: an urgent need for change in nursing education, *J Pain Symptom Manage* 7(1):48-55, 1992.
Ferrell BR et al: The experience of pediatric cancer pain. I. Impact of pain on the family, *J Pediatr Nurs* 9(6):368-379, 1994.
Fitzgerald M, Millard C, MacIntosh N: Hyperalgesia in premature infants, *Lancet* 6(8580):292, 1988.
Flanagan K: Preoperative assessment: safety considerations for patients taking herbal products, *J Perianesth Nurs* 16(1):19-26, 2001.
Fradet C et al: A prospective survey of reactions to blood tests by children and adolescents, *Pain* 40(1):53-60, 1990.
Franck L: A national survey of the assessment and treatment of pain and agitation in the neonatal intensive care unit, *J Obstet Gynecol Neonatal Nurs* 16(6):387-395, 1987.
Franck LS, Greenberg CS, Stevens B: Pain assessment in infants and children, *Pediatr Clin North Am* 47(3):487-512, 2000.
French GM, Painter EC, Coury DL: Blowing away shot pain: a technique for pain management during immunization, *Pediatrics* 93(3):384-388, 1994.
Friedland LR, Kulick RM: Emergency department analgesic use in pediatric trauma victims with fractures, *Ann Emerg Med* 23(2):203-207, 1994.
Gordon M: *Nursing diagnosis: process and application,* ed 3, St Louis, 1994, Mosby.
Gordon M: *Manual of nursing diagnosis,* ed 10, St Louis, 2002, Mosby.
Hannallah RS et al: Comparison of caudal and ilioinguinal/iliohypogastric nerve blocks for control of post-orchiopexy pain in pediatric ambulatory surgery, *Anesthesiology* 66(6):832-834, 1987.
Haslam DR: Age and the perception of pain, *Psychosom Sci* 15:86, 1969.
Hazinski MF: *Manual of pediatric critical care,* St Louis, 1999, Mosby.
Hertzka R et al: Fentanyl-induced ventilatory depression: effects of age, *Anesthesiology* 70(2):213-218, 1989.
Hester NO: Comforting the child in pain. In Funk SG et al (eds): *Key aspects of comfort,* New York, 1989, Springer.
Hester NO et al: Putting pain measurement into clinical practice. In Finley GA, McGrath PJ (eds): *Measurement of pain in infants and children,* vol 10, Seattle, 1998, International Association for the Study of Pain Press.
Hornick R: Discharge teams. In Gunter K, Manago R (eds): *Beyond discharge: interdisciplinary perspectives for transitioning children with com-*

plex medical needs from hospital to home, Bethesda, MD, 1996, Association for the Care of Children's Health.

Howard CR et al: Neonatal circumcision and pain relief: current training practices, *Pediatrics* 101(3):423-428, 1998.

Howard RF: Current status of pain management in children, *JAMA* 290(18):2464-2469, 2003.

Huckabay LMD, Tilem-Kessler D: Patterns of parental stress in PICU emergency admission, *Dimens Crit Care Nurs* 18(2):36-42, 1999.

Humphrey BG et al: The occurrence of high levels of acute behavioral distress in children and adolescents undergoing routine venipunctures, *Pediatrics* 90(1):87-91, 1992.

IOMED, Inc: Iontocaine package insert, Salt Lake City, UT, 1996, IOMED, Inc.

Johnson A, Lindschau A: Staff attitudes toward parent participation in the care of children who are hospitalized, *Pediatr Nurs* 22(2):99-102, 1996.

Johnston CC et al: A survey of pain in hospitalized patients aged 4-14 years, *Clin J Pain* 8(2):154-163, 1992.

Joint Commission on Accreditation of Healthcare Organizations: *AMH92 accreditation manual for hospitals,* Chicago, 1999, The Commission.

Jordan-Marsh M et al: Alternate Oucher form testing gender ethnicity and age variations, *Res Nurs Health* 17(2):111-118, 1994.

Joyce BA et al: Reliability and validity of preverbal pain assessment tools, *Issues Comp Pediatr Nurs* 17(3):121-135, 1994.

Kachoyeanos MK, Friedhoff M: Cognitive and behavioral strategies to reduce children's pain, *MCN Am J Matern Child Nurs* 18(1):14-19, 1993.

Kart T, Christrup LL, Rasmussen M: Recommended use of morphine in neonates, infants and children based on a literature review. I. Pharmacokinetics, *Paediatr Anaesth* 7(1):5-11, 1997.

Katz ER, Kellerman J, Siegel SE: Behavioral distress in children with cancer undergoing medical procedures: developmental considerations, *J Consult Clin Psychol* 48(3):356-365, 1980.

Kauffmann E et al: Stress-point intervention for parents of children hospitalized with chronic conditions, *Pediatr Nurs* 24(4):362-366, 1998.

Keck J et al: Reliability and validity of the FACES and Word Descriptor scales to measure procedural pain, *J Pediatr Nurs* 11(6):368-374, 1996.

Kirby R, Whelan T: The effects of hospitalization and medical procedures on children and their families, *J Fam Stud* 2(1):65-77, 1996.

Kleiber C et al: Topical anesthetics for intravenous insertion in children: a random equivalency study, *Pediatr* 110(4):758-761, 2002.

Koren G et al: Postoperative morphine infusion in newborn infants: assessment of disposition characteristics and safety, *J Pediatr* 107(6):963-967, 1985.

Krebel MS, Clayton C, Graham C: Child life programs in the pediatric emergency department, *Pediatr Emerg Care* 12(1):13-15, 1996.

Lander J, Fowler-Kerry S: Assessment of sex differences in children's and adolescents' self-reported pain from venipuncture, *J Pediatr Psychol* 16(6):783-793, 1991.

Lipson J, Dibble S, Minarik P: *Culture and nursing care: a pocket guide,* San Francisco, 1996, UCSF Nursing Press.

Luffy R, Grove SK: Examining the validity, reliability, and preference of three pediatric pain measurement tools in African-American children, *Pediatr Nurs* 29(1):54-60, 2003.

Mader TJ, Playe SJ, Garb JL: Reducing the pain of local anesthetic infiltration: warming and buffering have a synergistic effect, *Ann Emerg Med* 23(3):550-554, 1994.

Marshall RE: Neonatal pain associated with caregiving procedures, *Pediatr Clin North Am* 36(4):885-903, 1989.

Mather L, Mackie J: The incidence of postoperative pain in children, *Pain* 15(3):271-282, 1983.

McCaffery M, Pasero C: *Pain: a clinical manual,* ed 2, St Louis, 1999, Mosby.

McGrath PJ et al: The Children's Hospital of Eastern Ontario Pain Scale (CHEOPS): a behavioral scale for rating post-operative pain in children. In Fields HL, Dubner R, Cervero F (eds): *Advances in pain research and therapy,* New York, 1985, Raven Press.

Melnyk B, Alpert-Gillis L: The COPE Program: a strategy to improve outcomes of critically ill young children and their parents, *Pediatr Nurs* 24(6):521-527, 1998.

Melnyk BM: Intervention studies involving parents of hospitalized young children: an analysis of the past and future recommendations, *J Pediatr Nurs* 15(1):4-13, 2000.

Merkel S et al: The FLACC: a behavioral scale for scoring postoperative pain in young children, *Pediatr Nurs* 23(3):293-297, 1997.

Merkel S et al: Pain assessment in infants and young children: The FLACC scale, *Am J Nurs* 102 (10):55-57, 2002.

Moenkhoff M et al: Parental attitude towards alternative medicine in the paediatric intensive care unit, *Eur J Pediatr* 158(1):12-17, 1999.

Morrison R: Update on sickle cell disease: incidence of addiction and choice of opioid in pain management, *Pediatr Nurs* 17(6):503, 1991.

New Products: Gebauer's ethyl chloride topical refrigerant eases anxiety for patients and parents, *Pediatr Nurs* 28(6):636, 644, 2002.

Oberlander TF, O'Donnell ME, Montgomery CJ: Pain in children with neurological impairment, *J Dev Behav Pediatr* 20(4):234-243, 1999.

Orem D: *Nursing: concepts of practice,* ed 5, New York, 1995, Mosby.

Pasero C: Pain control: reality check on placebos, *Am J Nurs* 95(8):20, 1995.

Pasero C: Pain control, epidural analgesia in children, *Am J Nurs* 99(5):20, 1999.

Pasero CL: Using the Faces scale to assess pain, *Am J Nurs* 97(7): 19-20, 1997

Pate J et al: Childhood medical experience and temperament as predictors of adult functioning in medical situations, *Child Health Care* 25(4): 281-298, 1996.

Rasmussen G: Epidural and spinal anesthesia and analgesia. In Deshpande J, Tobias J (eds): *Pediatric pain handbook,* St Louis, 1996, Mosby.

Remmel M: Don't assume all parents want to be involved, *RN* 60(9):9, 1997 (letter).

Robieux I et al: Assessing pain and analgesia with a lidocaine-prilocaine emulsion in infants and toddlers during venipuncture, *J Pediatr* 118(6): 971-973, 1991.

Rodgers BM et al: Patient-controlled analgesia in pediatric surgery, *J Pediatr Surg* 23(3):259-262, 1988.

Rogers A: The ABC of pediatric pain, *Prim Care Cancer* 10:7-8, 1990.

Santelli B, Turnbull A, Higgins C: Parent to parent support and health care, *Pediatr Nurs* 23(3):303-306, 1997.

Savedra M et al: Pain location: validity and reliability of body outline markings by hospitalized children and adolescents, *Res Nurs Health* 12(5): 307-314, 1989.

Savedra MC et al: Assessment of postoperative pain in children and adolescents using the adolescent pediatric pain tool, *Nurs Res* 42(1):5-9, 1993.

Schade JG et al: Comparison of three preverbal scales for postoperative pain assessment in a diverse pediatric sample, *J Pain Symptom Manage* 12(6):348-359, 1996.

Schechter NL: The need for premedication for painful procedures in children, *Am J Anesthesiol* 24(suppl 1):10-12, 1997.

Scott LD: Perceived needs of parents of critically ill children, *J Soc Pediatr Nurses* 3(1):4-12, 1998.

Shapiro C: Pain in the neonate: assessment and intervention, *Neonatal Network* 8(1):7-21, 1989.

Simon K: Perceived stress of nonhospitalized children during the hospitalization of a sibling, *J Pediatr Nurs* 8(5):298-304, 1993.

Smith T, Conant Rees HL: Making family-centered care a reality, *Sem Nurs Manage* 8(3):136-142, 2000.

Snowdon A, Kane D: Parental needs following the discharge of a hospitalized child, *Pediatr Nurs* 21(5):425-428, 1995.

Spiegel D, Stroud P, Fyfe A: Complementary medicine, *West J Med* 168(4):241-247, 1998.

Squire SJ, Kirchoff KT, Hissong K: Comparing two methods of topical anesthesia used before intravenous cannulation in pediatric patients, *J Pediatr Health Care* 14(2):68-72, 2000.

Stevens B: Development and testing of a pediatric pain management sheet, *Pediatr Nurs* 16(6):543-548, 1990.

Stevens BJ, Johnston CC, Horton L: Multidimensional pain assessment in premature neonates: a pilot study, *J Obstet Gynecol Neonatal Nurs* 26(5):531-541, 1993.

Stuber M et al: Predictors of posttraumatic stress symptoms in childhood cancer survivors, *Pediatrics* 100(6):958-964, 1997.

Taddio A et al: A revised measure of acute pain in infants, *J Pain Symptom Manage* 10(6):456-463, 1995.

Tesler M, Holzemer W, Savedra M: Pain behaviors: postsurgical responses of children and adolescents, *J Pediatr Nurs* 13(1):41-47, 1998.

Tesler M et al: The word-graphic rating scale as a measure of childrens' and adolescents' pain intensity, *Res Nurs Health* 14(5):361-371, 1991.

Tobias JD: Pain management for the critically ill child in the pediatric intensive care unit. In Schechter NL, Berde CB, Yaster M (eds): *Pain in infants, children and adolescents*, ed 2, Philadelphia, 2003, Lippincott, Williams & Wilkins, pp 807-840.

Tyc V et al: A survey of pain services for pediatric oncology patients: their composition and function, *Pediatr Oncol Nurs* 15(4):207-215, 1998.

Van Cleve L, Johnson L, Pothier P: Pain responses of hospitalized infants and children to venipuncture and intravenous cannulation, *J Pediatr Nurs* 11(3):161-168, 1996.

Van Cleve L, Savedra M: Pain location: validity and reliability of body outline markings for 4- to 7-year-old children who are hospitalized, *Pediatr Nurs* 19(3):217-220, 1993.

Vessey JA, Carlson KL, McGill J: Use of distraction with children during an acute pain experience, *Nurs Res* 43(6):369-372, 1994.

Villarruel AM, Denyes MJ: Pain assessment in children: theoretical and empirical validity, *Adv Nurs Sci* 14(2):32-41, 1991.

Walker M, Wong DL: A battle plan for patients in pain, *Am J Nurs* 91(5): 32-36, 1991.

Wallace M: Temperament: a variable in children's pain management, *Pediatr Nurs* 15(2):118-121, 1989.

Weisman SJ, Bernstein B, Schechter NL: Consequences of inadequate analgesia during painful procedures in children, *Arch Pediatr Adolesc Med* 132(2):147-149, 1998.

Wilson A, Yorker B: Fears of medical events among school-age children with emotional disorders, parents and health care providers, *Issues Ment Health Nurs* 18(1):57-71, 1997.

Wong D: Topical anesthetics: two products for pain relief during minor procedures, *Am J Nurs* 103(6): 42-45, 2003.

Wong DL, Baker C: Pain in children: comparison of assessment scales, *Pediatr Nurs* 14(1):9-17, 1988.

Wong DL, Baker C: *Reference manual for the Wong-Baker FACES Pain Rating Scale,* Tulsa, OK, 2000, The Authors.

Wong DL, Baker C: *Reference manual for the Wong-Baker FACES Pain Rating Scale,* Tulsa, OK, 2004, www.us.elsevierhealth.com/wow.

Wong DL, Pasero CL: Pain control: reducing the pain of lidocaine, *Am J Nurs* 97(1):17-18, 1997.

Woodgate R, Kristjanson L: "Getting better from my hurts": toward a model of the young child's pain experience, *J Pediatr Nurs* 11(4):233-242, 1996.

Yaster M, Kost-Byerly S, Maxwell LG: Opioid agonists and antagonists. In Schechter NL, Berde CB, Yaster M (eds): *Pain in infants, children, and adolescents*, ed 2, Philadelphia, 2003, Lippincott, Williams & Wilkins, pp 181-224.

Young M, Fu V: Influence of play and temperament on the young child's response to pain, *Child Health Care* 16(3):209-215, 1988.

Pediatric Variations of Nursing Interventions

45

LEARNING OBJECTIVES

On completion of this chapter the reader will be able to:

- Identify those instances in which informed consent is required and in which minors may be considered emancipated.
- Formulate general guidelines for preparing children for procedures, including surgery.
- Implement play in therapeutic procedures.
- List general strategies for enhancing compliance in children and families.
- Outline general hygiene and care procedures for hospitalized children.
- Implement feeding techniques that encourage food and fluid intake.
- Describe methods of reducing the temperature of the child with fever or hyperthermia.
- Describe systems that can be used for infection control.
- Describe safe methods of administering oral, parenteral, rectal, optic, otic, and nasal medications to children.
- Identify nursing responsibilities in maintaining fluid balance.
- Demonstrate correct procedures for postural drainage and tracheostomy care.
- Describe the procedures involved in providing nutrition via gavage, gastrostomy, and parenteral routes.
- Describe the procedures involved in administering an enema and ostomy care to children.

ELECTRONIC RESOURCES

Additional information related to the content in Chapter 45 can be found on

the companion website at evolve
http://evolve.elsevier.com/Wong/maternal/
- NCLEX Review Questions
- Case Study–Pediatric Procedures
- WebLinks

or the interactive student CD-ROM
Activities for Chapter 45 include the following:
- NCLEX Review Questions
- Critical Thinking Exercise–Central Venous Access Device
- Nursing Care Plan–The Child Undergoing Surgery
- Skill–Administering Oral Medications

GENERAL CONCEPTS RELATED TO PEDIATRIC PROCEDURES

Informed Consent

Before undergoing any invasive procedure, including a surgical procedure, the patient or the patient's legal surrogate must receive sufficient information on which to make an informed decision. *Informed consent* refers to the legal and ethical requirement that the patient clearly, fully, and completely understand the proposed procedure or treatment to be performed. This information must include the nature of the procedure, the risks associated with the procedure, the alternatives to the procedure, and the benefits of the procedure. To obtain valid informed consent, the following three conditions must be met:

1. The person must be capable of giving consent; he or she must be over the age of majority (usually age 18) and must be considered competent (i.e., possess the mental capacity to make choices and understand their consequences).
2. The person must receive the information needed to make an intelligent decision.
3. The person must act voluntarily when exercising freedom of choice without force, fraud, deceit, duress, or other forms of constraint or coercion.

The patient has the right to accept or refuse any health care. If treated without consent, the hospital or health care provider may be charged with assault and held liable for damages.

Requirements for Obtaining Informed Consent

Written informed consent of the parent or legal guardian is usually required for medical or surgical treatment, including many diagnostic procedures. One blanket consent is not sufficient. Separate, informed permissions must be obtained for each surgical or diagnostic procedure, including the following:

- Major surgery
- Minor surgery (e.g., cutdown, biopsy, dental extraction, suturing a laceration)
- Diagnostic tests with an element of risk
- Medical treatments with an element of risk (e.g., blood transfusion, thoracentesis or paracentesis, radiation therapy, shock therapies)

Other situations that require parental consent include the following:

- Taking photographs for medical, educational, or other public use
- Removal of the child from the health care institution against medical advice
- Postmortem examinations, except in unexplained deaths, such as sudden infant death, violent death, or suspected suicide
- Release of medical information (Evidence-Based Practice box)

Decision making involving the care of older children and adolescents should include, to the extent feasible, the *assent* of the patient, as well as the parents and the physician. Assent may minimize the trauma to the child and maximize the success of the procedure. *Assent* means the child or adolescent has been informed about what will happen during the treatment or procedure and is willing to permit a health care provider to perform it. Assent should include the following elements (American Academy of Pediatrics, 1995):

- Helping the patient achieve a developmentally appropriate awareness of the nature of his or her condition
- Telling the patient what he or she can expect
- Making a clinical assessment of the patient's understanding
- Soliciting an expression of the patient's willingness to accept the proposed procedure of care

Multiple methods should be used to explain the study, including age-appropriate methods (e.g., videotapes, peer discussion, diagrams, and written materials). An assent form should be provided to each child to sign, and the child should keep a copy (Broome, 1999). By including children in the decision-making process and gaining their acceptance, children are treated with respect. Assent is not a legal requirement but an ethical one to protect the rights of children. The nurse, whether acting as a researcher, assisting in research, or caring for the child, must ultimately have the best interest of the child in mind (Algren & Schwartz, 1998).

Evidence-Based Practice

INFORMED CONSENT AND PARENTAL RIGHT TO THE CHILD'S MEDICAL CHART

Does the right to certain types of information before giving valid informed consent include the right to review medical records? Because the process of consent continues throughout the patient's treatment, is there an ongoing right of parents to see their children's medical charts?

The answer to these questions varies depending on state law. Some state statutes give parents the unrestricted right to a copy of children's medical records. Other states have no statutes that address this point. In these states, the best practice is to allow parents to review or have a copy of minors' charts under reasonable circumstances. That is, records should be available in a reasonable time. In addition, practitioners should avoid restrictive requirements such as review permitted only in the presence of a clinician. Rather, an appropriate practitioner should be available to answer any questions that parents may have during their reviews.

Eligibility for Giving Informed Consent

Informed Consent of Parents or Legal Guardians

Parents have full responsibility for the care and rearing of their minor children, including legal control over them. Therefore, as long as children are minors, their parents or legal guardians are required to give informed consent before medical treatment is rendered or any procedure is performed on them. Parents also have a right to withdraw consent later. If the parents are divorced, responsibility for informed consent rests with the parent who has legal custody.

Evidence of Consent

Obtaining informed consent varies from state to state, and policies differ at each health care facility. It is the physician's responsibility to explain the procedure, risks, benefits, and alternatives. The nurse witnesses the patient's or legal surrogate's signature on the consent form and may reinforce what the patient has been told. A signed consent form is the legal document that signifies that the process of informed consent has occurred. If parents are unavailable to sign consent forms, verbal consent may be obtained via the telephone in the presence of two witnesses. Both witnesses record that informed consent was given and by whom. Their signatures indicate that they witnessed the verbal consent.

Informed Consent of Mature and Emancipated Minors

State laws differ with regard to the so-called *age of majority,* the age at which a person is considered to have all the legal rights and responsibilities of an adult. Although some variation still exists, children become adults on their eighteenth birthday in most states. Competent adults can give informed consent on their own behalf. Nonetheless, some courts have permitted minors to consent to their treatment based on the *mature minors' doctrine,* which permits minors to give consent even though they are not technically adults as long as they demonstrate the maturity to understand the risks and benefits of the treatment or procedure (Guertler, 1997; Moskop, 1999). For example, statutes in many states permit minors to give consent on their own behalf to certain treatments, such as for sexually transmitted diseases, contraceptive services, pregnancy, or drug or alcohol abuse.

An *emancipated minor* is one who is legally under the age of majority but is recognized as having the legal capacity of an adult under circumstances prescribed by state law, such as pregnancy, marriage, high school graduation, living independently, or military service.

Treatment without Parental Consent

Exceptions to requiring parental consent before treating minor children occur in situations in which children need prompt medical or surgical treatment and a parent is not readily available to give consent or refuses to give consent. For example, a child may be brought to an emergency department accompanied by a grandparent, child care provider, teacher, older sibling, or others. In the absence of parents or legal guardians, some providers permit persons in charge of the child to give informed consent for treatment. Appropriate care for urgent or emergent problems should not be withheld or delayed because of problems obtaining consent. Efforts made to obtain consent should be documented (American Academy of Pediatrics, 2003). Emergencies include danger to life or the possibility of permanent injury.

Refusal to give consent can occur when the treatment, such as blood transfusions, conflicts with the parents' religious beliefs. All states recognize such exceptions and have statutory procedures to permit treatment if the life or health of such a minor is in jeopardy or if delayed treatment would create a risk to the minor's health. The state is also able to intervene in situations that jeopardize the health and welfare of children, as in cases in which parents neglect or impose excessive or improper punishment on a child. Most communities have procedures by which custody of the child can be transferred to a governmental or a private agency when parental neglect or abuse can be proved.

Preparation for Diagnostic and Therapeutic Procedures

Technologic advances and changes in health care have resulted in more pediatric procedures being performed in a variety of settings. Many procedures are both stressful and painful experiences for children and their parents. For most procedures, the focus of care is psychologic preparation of the child and family. Some procedures, however, require some physical preparation and the administration of sedatives or analgesics.

Psychologic Preparation

Preparing children for procedures decreases their anxiety, promotes their cooperation, supports their coping skills and may teach them new ones, and facilitates a feeling of mastery in experiencing a potentially stressful event. Many institutions have developed preadmission teaching programs designed to educate the pediatric patient and family about hospitalization and various procedures by offering hands-on experience with hospital equipment, information about the procedure to be performed, and departments they may visit (Algren, Ireland, & Stewart, 1998). Preparatory methods may be formal, such as group preparation for hospitalization. Most preparation strategies used by nurses are informal, focus on providing information about the experience, and are directed at stressful or painful procedures. Especially for painful procedures, the most effective preparation includes the provision of sensory-procedural information and helping the child develop coping skills, such as imagery, distraction, and relaxation (Broome, Rehwaldt, & Fogg, 1998).

General guidelines for preparing children for procedures are described in Box 45-1, and age-specific guidelines that consider children's developmental needs and cognitive abilities are presented in Box 45-2. In addition to these suggestions, nurses should consider the child's temperament, existing coping strategies, and previous experiences in individualizing the preparatory process. Children who are distractible and highly active, as well as those who are "slow to warm up," may need individualized sessions that are shorter for the active child but more slowly paced for the shy child. Youngsters who tend to cope well may need more emphasis on using their present skills, whereas those who appear to cope less adequately can benefit from more time de-

BOX 45-1

General Guidelines for Preparing Children for Procedures

- Determine details of exact procedure to be performed.
- Review parents' and child's present level of understanding.
- Plan actual teaching based on child's developmental age and existing level of knowledge.
- Incorporate parents in the teaching if they desire, especially if they plan to participate in care.
- Inform parents of their role during procedure, such as standing near child's head or in child's line of vision and talking softly to child.
- While preparing child and family, allow for ample discussion to prevent information overload and ensure adequate feedback.
- Use concrete, not abstract, terms and visual aids to describe procedure. For example, use a simple line drawing of a boy or girl (see Fig. 45-1), and mark the body part that will be involved in the procedure. Use nonthreatening but realistic models.*
- Emphasize that no other body part will be involved.
- If the body part is associated with a specific function, stress the change or noninvolvement of that ability (e.g., following tonsillectomy, child can still speak).
- Use words appropriate to child's level of understanding (a rule of thumb for number of words is age in years plus 1).
- Avoid words and phrases with dual meanings (see Guidelines box, p. 1360) unless child understands such words.
- Clarify all unfamiliar words (e.g., "Anesthesia is a *special* sleep").
- Emphasize sensory aspects of procedure—what child will feel, see, smell, and touch and what child can do during procedure (e.g., lie still, count out loud, squeeze a hand, hug a doll).
- Allow child to practice those procedures that will require cooperation (e.g., turning, deep breathing, using an incentive spirometer or mask).
- Introduce anxiety-laden information last (e.g., starting an intravenous line).
- Be honest with child about unpleasant aspects of a procedure, but avoid creating undue concern. When discussing that a procedure may be uncomfortable, state that it feels differently to different people and have child describe how it felt.
- Emphasize end of procedure and any pleasurable events afterward (e.g., going home, seeing parents).
- Stress positive benefits of procedure (e.g., "After your tonsils are fixed, you won't have as many sore throats").

*Soft-sculptured dolls and customized adapters and overlays for preparing children and families about procedures and as teaching models for technical care are available from Legacy Products, Inc., PO Box 267, Cambridge City, IN 47327; phone: 800-238-7951; e-mail: legacyez2b@aol.com; Web site: www.legacyproductsinc.com.

BOX 45-2

Age-Specific Guidelines for Preparing Children for Procedures Based on Developmental Characteristics

Infant: Developing a Sense of Trust and Sensorimotor Thought

Attachment to Parent

*Involve parent in procedure if desired.
Keep parent in infant's line of vision.
If parent is unable to be with infant, place familiar object with infant (e.g., stuffed toy).

Stranger Anxiety

*Have usual caregivers perform or assist with procedure.
Make advances slowly and in nonthreatening manner.
*Limit number of strangers entering room during procedure.

Sensorimotor Phase of Learning

During procedure use sensory soothing measures (e.g., stroking skin, talking softly, giving pacifier).
*Use analgesics (e.g., local anesthetic, intravenous opioid) to control discomfort.
Cuddle and hug child after stressful procedure; encourage parent to comfort child.

Increased Muscle Control

Expect older infants to resist.
Restrain adequately.
Keep harmful objects out of reach.

Memory for Past Experiences

Realize that older infants may associate objects, places, or persons with prior painful experiences and will cry and resist at the sight of them.
*Keep frightening objects out of view.
*Perform painful procedures in a separate room, not in crib (or bed).
*Use nonintrusive procedures whenever possible (e.g., axillary or tympanic temperatures, oral medications).

Imitation of Gestures

Model desired behavior (e.g., opening mouth).

Toddler: Developing a Sense of Autonomy and Sensorimotor to Preoperational Thought

Use same approaches as for infant in addition to the following:

Egocentric Thought

Explain procedure in relation to what child will see, hear, taste, smell, and feel.
Emphasize those aspects of procedure that require cooperation (e.g., lying still).
Tell child that it is okay to cry, yell, or use other means to express discomfort verbally.

Negative Behavior

Expect treatments to be resisted; child may try to run away.
Use firm, direct approach.
Ignore temper tantrums.
Use distraction techniques (e.g., singing a song *with* a child).
Restrain adequately.

Animism

Keep frightening objects out of view (young children believe objects have lifelike qualities and can harm them).

Limited Language Skills

Communicate using behaviors.
Use a few, simple terms familiar to child.
Give one direction at a time (e.g., "Lie down"; then: "Hold my hand").
Use small replicas of equipment; allow child to handle equipment.
Use play; demonstrate on doll but avoid child's favorite doll, because child may think doll is really "feeling" procedure.
Prepare parents separately to avoid child's misinterpreting words.

Limited Concept of Time

Prepare child shortly or immediately before procedure.
Keep teaching sessions short (about 5 to 10 minutes).
Have preparations completed before involving child in procedure.
Have extra equipment nearby (e.g., alcohol swabs, new needle, adhesive bandages) to avoid delays.
Tell child when procedure is completed.

Striving for Independence

Allow choices whenever possible, but realize that child may still be resistant and negative.
Allow child to participate in care and to help whenever possible (e.g., drink medicine from a cup, hold a dressing).

Preschooler: Developing a Sense of Initiative and Preoperational Thought

Egocentric

Explain procedure in simple terms and in relation to how it affects child (as with toddler, stress sensory aspects).
Demonstrate use of equipment.
Allow child to play with miniature or actual equipment.
Encourage "playing out" experience on a doll both before and after procedure to clarify misconceptions.
Use neutral words to describe the procedure (see Guidelines box, p. 1360).

Increased Language Skills

Use verbal explanation but avoid overestimating child's comprehension of words.
Encourage child to verbalize ideas and feelings.

Concept of Time and Frustration Tolerance Still Limited

Implement same approaches as for toddler but may plan longer teaching session (10 to 15 minutes); may divide information into more than one session.

Illness and Hospitalization May Be Viewed as Punishment

Clarify why each procedure is performed; a child will find it difficult to understand how medicine can make him or her feel better and can taste bad at the same time.
Ask child thoughts regarding why a procedure is performed.
State directly that procedures are never a form of punishment.

Animism

Keep equipment out of sight, except when shown to or used on child.

Fears of Bodily Harm, Intrusion, and Castration

Point out on drawing, doll, or child where procedure is performed.
Emphasize that no other body part will be involved.
Use nonintrusive procedures whenever possible (e.g., axillary temperatures, oral medication).
Apply an adhesive bandage over puncture site.
Encourage parental presence.
Realize that procedures involving genitals provoke anxiety.
Allow child to wear underpants with gown.
Explain unfamiliar situations, especially noises or lights.

*Applies to any age.

BOX 45-2—cont'd

Age-Specific Guidelines for Preparing Children for Procedures Based on Developmental Characteristics

Striving for Initiative

Involve child in care whenever possible (e.g., hold equipment, remove dressing).
Give choices whenever possible but avoid excessive delays.
Praise child for helping and attempting to cooperate; never shame child for lack of cooperation.

School-Age Child: Developing a Sense of Industry and Concrete Thought

Increased Language Skills; Interest in Acquiring Knowledge

Explain procedures using correct scientific/medical terminology.
Explain reason for procedure using simple diagrams of anatomy and physiology.
Explain function and operation of equipment in concrete terms.
Allow child to manipulate equipment; use doll or another person as model to practice using equipment whenever possible (doll play may be considered "childish" by older school-age child).
Allow time before and after procedure for questions and discussion.

Improved Concept of Time

Plan for longer teaching sessions (about 20 minutes).
Prepare in advance of procedure.

Increased Self-Control

Gain child's cooperation.
Tell child what is expected.
Suggest ways of maintaining control (e.g., deep breathing, relaxation, counting).

Striving for Industry

Allow responsibility for simple tasks (e.g., collecting specimens).
Include child in decision making (e.g., time of day to perform procedure, preferred site).
Encourage active participation (e.g., removing dressings, handling equipment, opening packages).

Developing Relationships with Peers

May prepare two or more children for same procedure or encourage one to help prepare another peer.
Provide privacy from peers during procedure to maintain self-esteem.

Adolescent: Developing a Sense of Identity and Abstract Thought

Increasingly Capable of Abstract Thought and Reasoning

Supplement explanations with reasons why procedure is necessary or beneficial.
Explain long-term consequences of procedures.
Realize that adolescent may fear death, disability, or other potential risks.
Encourage questioning regarding fears, options, and alternatives.

Conscious of Appearance

Provide privacy.
Discuss how procedure may affect appearance (e.g., scar) and what can be done to minimize it.
Emphasize any physical benefits of procedure.

Concerned More with Present Than with Future

Realize that immediate effects of procedure are more significant than future benefits.

Striving for Independence

Involve in decision making and planning (e.g., choice of time; place; individuals present during procedure, such as parents; clothing to wear).
Impose as few restrictions as possible.
Suggest methods of maintaining control.
Accept regression to more childish methods of coping.
Realize that adolescent may have difficulty in accepting new authority figures and may resist complying with procedures.

Developing Peer Relationships and Group Identity

Same as for school-age child but assumes even greater significance.
Allow adolescents to talk with other adolescents who have had the same procedure.

---

voted to simple coping strategies, such as relaxing, breathing, counting, squeezing a hand, or singing.

Children differ in their "information-seeking dimension." Some actively solicit information about the intended procedure, whereas others characteristically avoid information. Parents can often guide nurses in deciding how much information is enough for the child, because parents know whether the child is typically inquisitive or satisfied with short answers. Drawings may also be helpful in preparing children for procedures (Fig. 45-1).

The exact timing of the preparation for a procedure varies with the child's age and the type of procedure. There are no exact guidelines to govern timing, but in general the younger the child, the closer the explanation should be to the actual procedure to prevent undue fantasizing and worrying. With complex procedures, more time may be needed for assimilation of information, especially with older children. For example, the explanation for an x-ray can immediately precede the procedure for all ages, but preparation for surgery may begin the day before for young children.

Establish Trust and Provide Support

The nurse who has spent time with and who has established a positive relationship with a child will usually find it easier to gain the child's cooperation. If the relationship is based on trust, the child will associate the nurse with caregiving activities that give comfort and pleasure most of the time and not regard the nurse as someone who brings discomfort and stress. If the nurse does not know the child, it is best that the nurse be introduced by another staff person whom the child trusts. The first visit with the child should not include any painful procedure and ideally should focus on the child first, then on the explanation of the procedure. When talking with the child, the nurse uses the same guidelines for communicating with children that are discussed in Chapter 34.

Parental Presence and Support

Children need support during procedures, and for young children the greatest source of comfort is the parents. They represent security, safety, and comfort. However, controversy exists regarding the role parents should assume during

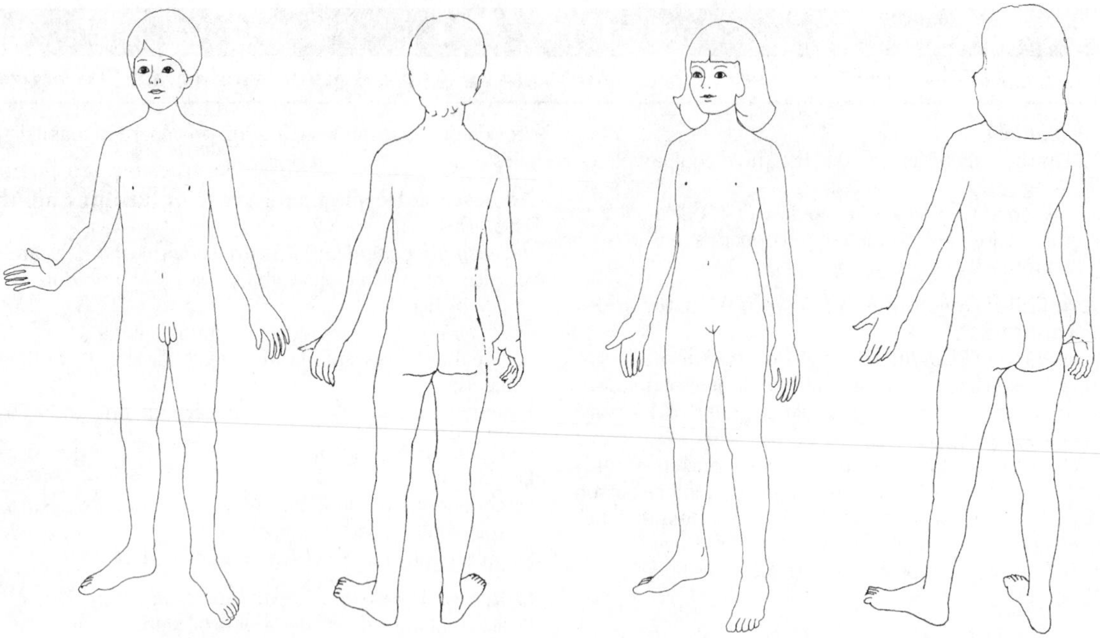

Fig. 45-1 Examples of line drawings to be used in preparing children for procedures.

the procedure, especially if discomfort is involved. Nurses need to consider the issues in deciding whether parental presence is beneficial. The parents' preferences for assisting, observing, or waiting outside the room should be assessed, as well as the child's preference for parental presence. The child's choice should be respected. Parents who want to stay should be educated, because they do not automatically know what to do, where to be, and what to say to help their child through the procedure. Simple instructions such as clarifying where parents can stand or sit in the room and positioning them where they have eye contact with the child provide support and lessen anxiety. Parents who do not want to be present or participate are supported in their decision and encouraged to remain close by so that they can be available to console the child immediately after the procedure. Parents should also know that someone will be with their child to provide support. Ideally, this person should inform the parents after the procedure about how the child did.

Provide an Explanation

Children need an explanation for anything that involves them directly. Before performing a procedure, the nurse explains to children what is to be done and what is expected of them. The explanation should be short, simple, and appropriate to the child's level of comprehension. Long explanations are not necessary and may only increase anxiety in a small child. This is especially true regarding painful procedures. When explaining the procedure to parents with the child present, the nurse uses language appropriate to the child because unfamiliar words can be misunderstood (Guidelines box). If the parents need additional preparation, this is done in an area away from the child. Teaching sessions are planned at times most conducive to the child's learning (e.g., after a rest period) and for the usual span of attention.

Special equipment is not necessary for preparing a child, but for young children who cannot yet think in concepts, using objects to supplement verbal explanation is important. Allowing children to handle actual items that will be used in their care, such as a stethoscope, a sphygmomanometer, or an oxygen mask, helps them to develop familiarity with these items and to reduce the threat often associated with their use. Miniature versions of hospital items such as gurneys and x-ray and intravenous (IV) equipment can be used to explain what the children can expect and permit them to safely experience situations that are unfamiliar and poten-

Guidelines

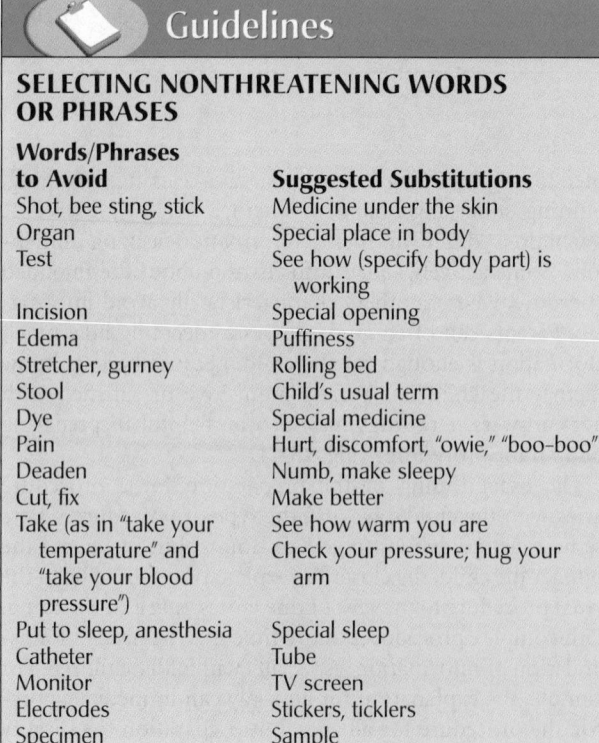

SELECTING NONTHREATENING WORDS OR PHRASES

Words/Phrases to Avoid	Suggested Substitutions
Shot, bee sting, stick	Medicine under the skin
Organ	Special place in body
Test	See how (specify body part) is working
Incision	Special opening
Edema	Puffiness
Stretcher, gurney	Rolling bed
Stool	Child's usual term
Dye	Special medicine
Pain	Hurt, discomfort, "owie," "boo-boo"
Deaden	Numb, make sleepy
Cut, fix	Make better
Take (as in "take your temperature" and "take your blood pressure")	See how warm you are Check your pressure; hug your arm
Put to sleep, anesthesia	Special sleep
Catheter	Tube
Monitor	TV screen
Electrodes	Stickers, ticklers
Specimen	Sample

tially frightening. Written and illustrated materials are also valuable aids to preparation.*

Performance of the Procedure

Supportive care continues during the procedure and can be a major factor in a child's ability to cooperate and achieve mastery. Before the procedure is begun, all equipment is assembled and the room is readied to prevent unnecessary delays and interruptions that only serve to increase the child's anxiety.

If at all possible, procedures are performed in a special treatment room rather than the child's hospital room. Traumatic procedures should never be performed in "safe" areas, such as the playroom. If the procedure is lengthy, conversation that could be misinterpreted by the child is avoided. As the procedure is nearing completion, the nurse should inform the child that it is almost over in language that the child understands.

Expect Success

Nurses who approach children with confidence and who convey the impression that they expect to be successful are less likely to encounter difficulty. It is best to approach children as though cooperation is expected. Children sense anxiety in another and may respond to a perceived threat by striking out or with active resistance. Although it is not possible to eliminate such behavior in every child, a firm approach with a positive attitude by the nurse tends to convey a feeling of security to most children.

Involve the Child

As in any other aspect of care, involving children helps to gain their cooperation. Permitting them to make choices gives them some measure of control. However, a choice is given only in situations in which one is available. Asking children, "Do you want to take your medicine now?" leads them to believe that there is an option and provides them with the opportunity to legitimately refuse or delay the medication. This places the nurse in an awkward, if not impossible, position. It is much better to state firmly, "It's time to take your medicine now." Children usually like to make choices, but the choice must be one that they may have (e.g., "It's time for your medicine. Do you want to drink it plain or with a little water?").

Many children respond to tactics that appeal to their maturity or courage. This approach also gives them a sense of participation and achievement. For example, preschool children will be proud that they can hold the dressing during the procedure or remove the tape. The same is true for the school-age child, who often cooperates with minimal resistance.

Provide Distraction

When children are occupied with an activity that interests them, they are less likely to focus on the procedure. The acute pain of procedures can be made more bearable when the patient is distracted during the process. Reading, watching television, or listening to music are a few potential activities. Other strategies for diverting attention are to have the child tightly squeeze the hands of a parent or an assistant, count aloud, sing a familiar song such as a nursery rhyme, or verbally express discomfort. For other nonpharmacologic interventions that may lessen discomfort, see Pain Management, Chapter 44.

Allow Expression of Feelings

The child should be allowed to express feelings of anger, anxiety, fear, frustration, or any other emotion. It is natural for children to strike out in frustration or to try to avoid stress-provoking situations. The child needs to know that it is all right to cry. Behavior is children's primary means of communication and coping and should be permitted unless it inflicts harm on them or those caring for them.

Postprocedural Support

After the procedure the child continues to need reassurance that he or she performed well and is accepted and loved. If the parents did not participate, the child is united with them as soon as possible so that they can provide comfort.

Encourage Expression of Feelings

Planned activity after the procedure is helpful in encouraging constructive expression of feelings. For verbal children, reviewing the details of the procedure can help clarify misconceptions and provide feedback for improving the nurse's preparatory strategies. Play is an excellent activity for all children. Infants and young children are given the opportunity for gross motor movement. Even older children can vent their anger and frustration in acceptable pounding or throwing activities. Play-Doh is a remarkably versatile medium for pounding and shaping. Dramatic play provides an outlet for anger and places the child in a position of control, in contrast to the position of helplessness in the real situation. Puppets may also be used to allow the child to communicate in a nonthreatening way. One of the most effective interventions is *therapeutic play,* which includes activities such as permitting the child to give an injection to a doll or stuffed toy to reduce the stress of injections (Fig. 45-2).

Positive Reinforcement

Children need to hear from adults that they know the youngsters did the best they could in the situation, no matter how they behaved. It is important for children to know that their worth is not being judged on the basis of their behavior in a stressful situation. Reward systems, such as earning stars, stickers, or a badge of courage, are appealing to children.

Returning to the child a short while after the procedure helps the nurse to strengthen a supportive relationship. Relating with the child during a relaxed and nonstressful period allows him or her to see the nurse not only as someone associated with stressful situations but also as someone with whom to share pleasurable experiences.

---

*Sources of preparatory materials include *Going to the Hospital* and *Going to the Doctor,* available from Family Communications, Inc., 4802 Fifth Ave., Pittsburgh, PA 15213; phone: 412-687-2990; *Hospital Friends,* available from the Centering Corporation, 1531 N. Saddle Creek Rd., Omaha, NE 68104; phone: 402-553-1200; and *Health, Illness, and Disability: A Guide to Books for Children and Young Adults,* available from Pediatric Projects, Inc., PO Box 571555, Tarzana, CA 91357-1555; phone: 800-947-0947. Other resources include *Berenstein Bears Go to the Doctor* and *Berenstein Bears Visit the Dentist* (Random House), available in most bookstores.

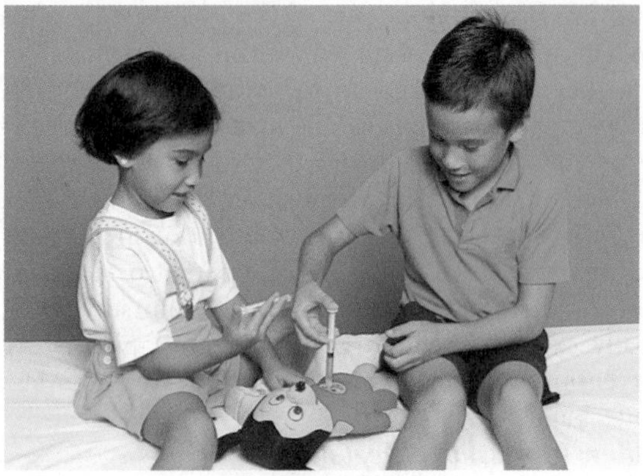

Fig. 45-2 Playing with syringes provides children with the opportunity to "play out" fears and concerns.

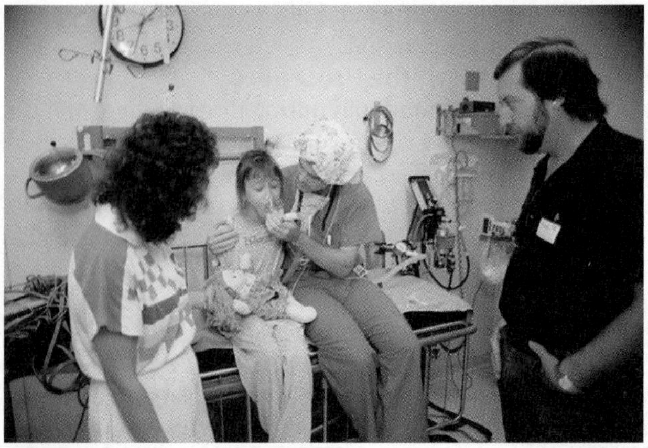

Fig. 45-3 Parental presence during induction of anesthesia can minimize child's and parents' anxiety during the preoperative period.

Use of Play in Procedures

The use of play is an integral part of relationships with children. As such, its value in specific situations is discussed throughout this book, such as in Chapter 44, in relation to hospitalization. Nurses can easily include play activities as part of nursing care. Play can be used to teach, for expression of feelings, or as a method to achieve a therapeutic goal. Consequently, it should be included in preparing children for and encouraging their cooperation during procedures. Play sessions after procedures can be structured, such as directed toward playing with syringes, or general, with a wide variety of equipment available for children to play with. Suggestions for incorporating play into nursing procedures and activities for the hospitalized child that facilitate learning and adjustment to a new situation are described in Box 45-3.

Preoperative Care

Children undergoing surgical procedures require both psychologic and physical preparation. In general, psychologic preparation is similar to that previously discussed for a procedure and employs many of the same techniques used in preparing a child for hospitalization, such as films, books, play, and tours. However, some important differences exist. Even though children are anesthetized for the actual surgical intervention, they may be subjected to numerous preoperative and postoperative procedures. Stress points before and after surgery include the admission process, blood tests, administration of preoperative medications (if prescribed), the period before and during transport to the operating room, and the return from the postanesthesia care unit (PACU).

Psychologic intervention consisting of systematic preparation, rehearsal of the forthcoming events, and supportive care during times of stress has been shown to be more effective than a single-session preparation or consistent supportive care without systematic preparation and rehearsal. Play is always an effective strategy in preparing children, and increased familiarity with medical procedures decreases anxiety.

Parental presence during induction of anesthesia is allowed in some institutions (Fig. 45-3). Potential benefits include minimizing the need for premedication and avoiding an upsetting separation of the child from the parents. Other benefits are controversial but may include decreasing the child's anxiety during induction and decreasing the long term behavioral effects of surgery (Kain, Caldwell-Andrews, & Wang, 2002). Based on the parents' favorable response to the practice and most children's desire to have parents with them during any stressful procedure, a policy of offering parents the option of attending the induction, combined with a program that prepares them for what to expect and what is expected of them, is recommended. When parents choose not to or are not allowed to attend this induction, leaving a favorite possession with the child and uniting the child and parents as soon as possible after surgery (preferably in the PACU) are important interventions. During surgery the family should have a designated place to wait and needs to be kept informed of the child's progress. Family members also should know where and when they can visit the child after surgery.

Aside from possibly being separated from the parents before and after surgery, children may be cared for by a number of unfamiliar practitioners. Although the same supportive nurse should remain with the child through as many of the procedures as possible, the child may have several nurses. Many hospitals have surgical tours for children and parents to familiarize them with the strange environment and to introduce them to other individuals who will be involved in their care.

Besides psychologic preparation, children usually require various types of physical care before surgery, such as those listed in the Nursing Care Plan on p. 1365-1366 to and in the preoperative checklist (Guidelines box). An important concern is restriction of food and fluids before surgery to avoid aspiration during anesthesia. Before fluids are restricted, children are encouraged to drink to promote hydration and minimize the dryness and thirst they experience. Infants require special attention to fluid needs. They should not be without oral fluids for an extended period preoperatively to avoid glycogen depletion and dehydration. Current preoperative fasting guidelines are found in Box 45-4.

Although most preoperative care procedures are routine, nurses should keep in mind that they can be anxiety provoking for children and parents. For example, for young children, having to wear a loose-fitting hospital gown without the security of underpants or pajama bottoms can be traumatic. Therefore these articles of clothing should be allowed to be worn to the operating room. They can be removed after induction of anesthesia.

BOX 45-3

Play Activities for Specific Procedures

Fluid Intake

Make ice pops using child's favorite juice.
Cut gelatin into fun shapes.
Make a game out of taking a sip when turning page of a book or in games such as Simon Says.
Use small medicine cups; decorate the cups.
Color water with food coloring or powdered drink mix.
Have a tea party; pour at a small table.
Let child fill a syringe and squirt it into mouth or use it to fill small, decorated cups.
Cut straws in half and place in a small container (much easier for child to suck liquid).
Decorate a straw: cut out small design with two holes and pass straw through; place small sticker on straw.
Use a "crazy" straw.
Make a "progress poster"; give rewards for drinking a predetermined quantity.

Deep Breathing

Blow bubbles with a bubble blower.
Blow bubbles with a straw (no soap).
Blow on a pinwheel, feather, whistle, harmonica, balloon, toy horn, party blower.
Practice band instruments.
Have blowing contest using balloons,* boats, cotton balls, feathers, marbles, Ping-Pong balls, pieces of paper; blow such objects on a table top over a goal line, over water, through an obstacle course, up in the air, against an opponent, or up and down a string.
Suck paper or cloth from one container to another using a straw.
Use blow bottles with colored water to transfer water from one side to the other.
Dramatize stories such as "I'll huff and puff and blow your house down" from the Three Little Pigs.
Do straw-blowing painting.
Take a deep breath and "blow out the candles" on a birthday cake.
Use a little paint brush to "paint" nails with water and blow nails dry.

Range of Motion and Use of Extremities

Throw beanbags at a fixed or movable target or throw wadded-up paper into a wastebasket.
Touch or kick Mylar balloons held or hung in different positions (if child is in traction, hang balloon from a trapeze).
Play "tickle toes"; wiggle them on request.
Play Twister game or Simon Says.
Play pretend and guess games (e.g., imitate a bird, butterfly, or horse).
Have tricycle or wheelchair races in safe area.
Play kickball or throw ball with a soft foam ball in a safe area.
Position bed so that child must turn to view television or doorway.
Climb wall like a "spider."
Pretend to teach "aerobic" dancing or exercises; encourage parents to participate.
Encourage swimming if feasible.
Play video games or pinball (fine motor movement).
Play "hide and seek": hide toy somewhere in bed (or room if ambulatory) and have child find it using specified hand or foot.
Provide clay to mold with fingers.
Paint or draw on large sheets of paper placed on floor or wall.
Encourage combing own hair; play "beauty shop" with "customer" in different positions.

Soaks

Play with small toys or objects (cups, syringes, soap dishes) in water.
Wash dolls or toys.
Bubbles may be added to bathwater if permissible; move bubbles to create shapes or "monsters."
Pick up marbles or pennies* from bottom of bath container.
Make designs with coins on bottom of container.
Pretend a boat is a submarine by keeping it immersed.
Read to child during soaks, sing with child, or play game, such as cards, checkers, or other board game (if both hands are immersed, move board pieces for child).
Sitz bath: give child something to listen to (music, stories) or look at (Viewmaster, book).
Punch holes in bottom of plastic cup, fill with water, and let it "rain" on child.

Injections

Let child handle syringe, vial, and alcohol swab, and give an injection to doll or stuffed animal.
Use syringes to decorate cookies with frosting, squirt paint, or target shoot into a container.
Draw a "magic circle" on area before injection; draw smiling face in circle after injection, but avoid drawing on puncture site.
Allow child to have a "collection" of syringes (without needles); make "wild" creative objects with syringes.
If multiple injections or venipunctures, make a "progress poster"; give rewards for predetermined number of injections.
Have child count to 10 or 15 during injection.

Ambulation

Give child something to push.
Toddler: push-pull toy
School-age child: wagon or decorated IV stand
Adolescent: a baby in a stroller or wheelchair
Have a parade; make hats, drums, etc.

Extending Environment (e.g., for Patients in Traction)

Make bed into a pirate ship or airplane with decorations.
Put up mirrors so patient can see around room.
Move patient's bed frequently, especially to playroom, hallway, or outside.

*Small objects such as marbles or coins, as well as gloves or balloons, are unsafe for young children because of possible aspiration. Latex products also carry the risk of an allergic reaction.

Historically, the most upsetting event for children has been the preoperative injection. Unfortunately, little research has been done on the value of this practice. If children have no preoperative pain, are well prepared psychologically for surgery, and have their parents nearby, preanesthetic medication may be unnecessary. When drugs are used, they should be "atraumatic" by using oral, existing IV, or rectal routes.

Numerous preanesthetic drug regimens are used with children, and no consensus exists on the optimum method. Drugs used should achieve five goals (American Academy of Pediatrics, Committee on Drugs, 1992): (1) guard the pa-

Guidelines

PREOPERATIVE PROCEDURE CHECKLIST

Vanderbilt University Medical Center

PRE-PROCEDURE CHECKLIST

Weight: ____________________

Location of Patient's Family During Procedure:

____

Date: ____________________

NPO Status Maintained Since: ____________________

PATIENT IDENTIFICATION (Indicate two identifiers):
☐ Patient Name ☐ Date of Birth ☐ Medical Record Number ☐ Social Security Number ☐ Photo ID

Source: ☐ Patient Statement ☐ Parent ☐ Guardian ☐ Spouse ☐ Domestic Partner
☐ Adult Sibling (18y or older) ☐ Adult Child ☐ Transferring Facility Representative/Documents

☐ **Identification Band On / Name, Numbers Match Patient's Statement &/or Permanent Medical Record Document**

PROCEDURE (Patient's or Other Identifying Source's Statement): ____________________

Procedure Statement Consistent With: (Check ALL that apply)
☐ **Procedure Consent** ☐ **History & Physical** ☐ Physician orders / notes ☐ Procedure Schedule ☐ Diagnostic x-rays / reports

SITE / SIDE IDENTIFICATION: ☐ Site Not Applicable (Procedure performed through a natural body orifice)

Patient's / Other Source's Statement – SITE: ____________________

SIDE: ____________________

Site / Side Statement Consistent With: (Check ALL that apply)
☐ **Procedure Consent** ☐ **History & Physical** ☐ Physician orders / notes ☐ Procedure Schedule ☐ Diagnostic x-rays / reports

Procedure / Site / Side Indentified By: ☐ Patient Statement ☐ Parent ☐ Guardian ☐ Spouse
☐ Domestic Partner ☐ Adult Sibling (18y or older) ☐ Adult Child ☐ Transferring Facility Representative/Documents

PRE-PROCEDURE PREPARATION

	Staff Initials		Staff Initials
Procedure Consent Completed	_____	Lab Work Obtained & Results Acceptable to Proceed	_____ ☐ N/A
History & Physical Completed	_____	Radiology / Cardiology / Other Studies Completed	_____ ☐ N/A
Anesthesia History & Physical Completed	_____ ☐ N/A	Pre-Procedure Scrub / Site Prep Completed	_____ ☐ N/A
Anesthesia Day of Surgery Evaluation Completed	_____ ☐ N/A	Patient Voided / Catheterized	_____ ☐ N/A
Patient ID Card in Chart (Inpatient Only)	_____ ☐ N/A	Dentures / Prostheses Removed *	_____ ☐ N/A
Current Chart(s) Available	_____ ☐ N/A	Eye Glasses / Contact Lenses Removed *	_____ ☐ N/A
"Old" Chart(s) Available	_____ ☐ N/A	Jewelry Removed *	_____ ☐ N/A
Pre-Procedure Medications Administered/Documented	_____ ☐ N/A	Other Valuables:*__________	_____ ☐ N/A
IV Patent	_____ ☐ N/A	* ☐ Given to Family ☐ Stored: __________	

SYNTHETIC / TISSUE IMPLANTS (If Applicable): ☐ Available in procedure suite ☐ Identification matches procedure request
SITE MARKING: Site Initialed By: ☐ Physician ☐ Non-Physician Proceduralist ☐ Site Marking Not Indicated ☐ See OR documentation
All Team Members Concur With Site Identification and Marking: ☐ YES ☐ Not Indicated
Site Marking Visible After Draping: ☐ YES ☐ Not Indicated ☐ See OR documentation

Comments:

Staff Confirming Patient, Procedure, Site, & Side Identification: Initials _____ **Signature/Title** ____________________

Initials _____ **Signature/Title** ____________________ **Initials** _____ **Signature/Title** ____________________

Initials _____ **Signature/Title** ____________________ **Initials** _____ **Signature/Title** ____________________

MC 0014 (04/2003)

tient's safety and welfare; (2) minimize physical discomfort or pain; (3) minimize negative psychologic responses to treatment by providing analgesia, and maximize the potential for amnesia; (4) control behavior; and (5) return the patient to a state in which safe discharge, as determined by recognized criteria, is possible.

Midazolam (Versed) provides excellent preoperative anxiety reduction, amnesia, and sedation. It is popular because of its short duration, predictable onset, and rare occurrence of respiratory depression. Oral transmucosal fentanyl (OTFC), or Fentanyl Oralet, is available as a sweetened lozenge on a plastic stick. When first approved, this appeared

BOX 45-4

Summary of Fasting Recommendations to Reduce the Risk of Pulmonary Aspiration*

Ingested Material	Minimum Fasting Period (Hours)†
Clear liquids‡	2
Breast milk	4
Infant formula	6
Nonhuman milk§	6
Light meal‖	6

From American Society of Anesthesiologists: Practice guidelines for preoperative fasting and the use of pharmacologic agents to reduce the risk of pulmonary aspiration: application to healthy patients undergoing elective procedures, *Anesthesiology* 90(3):896-905, 1999. Internet document available at www.ASAhq.org/practice/NPO/NPOguide.html (accessed April 27, 2005).

*These recommendations apply to healthy patients who are undergoing elective procedures. They are not intended for women in labor. Following the guidelines does not guarantee a complete gastric emptying has occurred.

†The fasting periods noted above apply to all ages.

‡Examples of clear liquids include water, fruit juices without pulp, carbonated beverages, clear tea, and black coffee.

§Because nonhuman milk is similar to solids in gastric emptying time, the amount ingested must be considered when determining an appropriate fasting period.

‖A light meal typically consists of toast and clear liquids. Meals that include fried or fatty foods or meat may prolong gastric emptying time. Both the amount and type of foods ingested must be considered when determining an appropriate fasting period.

to be an excellent, atraumatic route of administration. However, associated nausea and vomiting, respiratory depression, and the need for more intensive monitoring and observation than with other oral sedatives have limited its popularity to date (Cravero, Manzi, & Rice, 1998).

Children may also fear induction of anesthesia by mask. Practices that can minimize anxiety related to inhalation anesthesia include (1) disguising the unpleasant odor of anesthetic gases by applying a pleasant-smelling substance on the mask; (2) using a transparent plastic mask rather than an opaque black mask and gradually bringing it toward the face; (3) directing a stream of gas toward the child's face from the bare tube until the child becomes drowsy, and then using the mask; (4) allowing the child to sit up rather than lie down for anesthesia induction; and (5) allowing preoperative play with a mask and a doll or mannequin.

Postoperative Care

After surgical procedures, psychologic and physical observations and interventions are required to prevent or minimize possible untoward effects from anesthesia and the surgical procedure (Nursing Care Plan and Guidelines box). Although most of these interventions are prescribed by physicians, it is the nurse's responsibility to exercise judgment in their implementation. For example, vital signs are taken as frequently as necessary until they are stable. Simply recording temperature, pulse, respiration, and blood pressure without comparing the present read-

Nursing Care Plan

THE CHILD UNDERGOING SURGERY

NURSING DIAGNOSIS: Risk for injury related to surgical procedure, anesthesia

EXPECTED OUTCOME

Child shows no evidence of injury.

NURSING INTERVENTIONS/*RATIONALES*

Carry out preoperative preparations such as the following: NPO, anticholinergic medications as ordered *to prevent aspiration;* bathing, cleansing of operative site, antibiotics as ordered *to prevent infection;* emptying of bowel and bladder, insertion of catheter as ordered, cleansing enemas as ordered *to prevent distention and incontinence;* checking vital signs, laboratory values for systematic abnormality *that may complicate surgery* (e.g., elevated temperature, white blood cells [WBCs] *for signs of infection;* hemoglobin [Hb] and hematocrit [Hct] *for anemia;* platelets, clotting times *for bleeding tendencies*); clearly delineate allergies *to prevent reactions or complications;* removal of jewelry, prosthetic devices *to prevent injury;* removal of makeup, nail polish *to improve monitoring for cyanosis;* start IV per order *to provide route for fluids and medications;* dress in attire for operating room (OR) *to provide easy access to surgical site.*

Transport to surgical holding area using safety belt and side rails on stretcher *to prevent falls;* check identification and chart with surgical personnel *to ensure correct identity and completion of all preoperative preparations.*

Carry out intraoperative preparations such as the following: transfer and proper securing to surgical table *to prevent falls;* check identification *to ensure correct identity;* check chart *to ensure correct surgical procedure at correct site;* talk/play with child before anesthesia administered *to keep anxiety, fear minimal;* after child is anesthetized, careful alignment and positioning *to prevent injury to joints or pressure spots to skin;* apply restraints *to prevent falls;* place on warming blanket per order *to prevent hypothermia;* place grounding plate if electrocautery is to be used *to prevent injury;* cleanse and drape surgical site *to prevent infection;* check expiration dates on all sterile packages before use *to maintain integrity of sterile field;* monitor sterile field and institute immediate corrective measures for technique breaks *to prevent contamination of wound;* ensure correct instrument and sponge count *to prevent loss of foreign substances in wound;* dress surgical site *to prevent infection;* transfer to recovery bed, raise side rails, and transport to recovery room *for postoperative monitoring.*

Carry out recovery room procedures such as the following: monitor vital signs frequently *to assess for signs of infection, hemorrhage, aspiration;* suction as needed *to prevent aspiration, infection;* monitor neurologic status, gag and swallow reflex, cough *to assess recovery from anesthesia;* monitor intake and output, skin tone and turgor *to assess hydration status;* monitor for signs of sensory overload; orient frequently as child is waking *to prevent overload and confusion;* monitor incision site *for hemorrhage.*

Carry out postoperative procedures such as the following: employ careful wound care and good handwashing techniques *to prevent infection;* monitor vital signs *to assess for signs of infection, hemorrhage, aspiration;* turn, cough, and deep breathe *to*

See also Nursing Care Plan: The Family of the Ill/Hospitalized Child, Chapter 44.

Continued

Nursing Care Plan

THE CHILD UNDERGOING SURGERY—cont'd

prevent respiratory infection; encourage graduated nutritious oral intake after bowel sounds heard *to prevent intestinal complications and promote wound healing;* ambulate per physician order *to decrease complications of immobility;* monitor intake and output, skin turgor *to assess hydration status;* monitor and maintain bedside equipment (e.g., IV lines, IV pumps, nasogastric [NG] tubes, suction machines, wound drains, chest tubes, catheters) *to ensure function and safe operation.*

NURSING DIAGNOSIS: Anxiety/fear related to surgery, separation from support system

EXPECTED OUTCOME
Child exhibits reduced signs of fear and anxiety.

NURSING INTERVENTIONS/*RATIONALES*

Preoperatively: teach child (using developmentally appropriate approach) what to expect before, during, and after surgery; explain where parents will be during surgery *to reduce fear of unknown;* administer preoperative medications as ordered *to provide relaxation and sleep;* encourage parents to stay with child as long as possible and to touch or hold child until asleep *to reduce fear and feelings of abandonment;* allow child to take a favorite toy to the surgical holding area *to establish a sense of security.*

Postoperatively: orient child as he or she awakes, explain what is happening as it happens, be calm and reassuring *to reduce anxieties;* encourage parental presence as soon as feasible *to decrease separation anxiety.*

NURSING DIAGNOSIS: Pain related to surgical incision

EXPECTED OUTCOME
Child exhibits minimal evidence of pain.

NURSING INTERVENTIONS/*RATIONALES*

Administer postoperative pain medications as ordered before expression of pain *to prevent pain from occurring.*

Splint operative site when coughing or deep breathing: turn and position gently; avoid palpation of surgical site unless necessary *to reduce pain.*

Insert rectal tube as needed *to relieve discomfort from gas.*

Monitor bladder for fullness and encourage voiding *to prevent pain from bladder distention.*

Administer comfort measures (e.g., mouth care, lubrication of eyes if irritated, lubrication of nostril if NG tube present, massage of back) *to reduce discomfort.*

Coordinate nursing activities and procedures with administration of analgesia *to decrease pain and increase effectiveness of activity.*

Administer analgesics, antiemetics per physician order and monitor effectiveness of medications in pain and nausea relief.

NURSING DIAGNOSIS: Risk for fluid volume deficit related to NPO status, operative losses, vomiting, loss of appetite

EXPECTED OUTCOME
Child exhibits no signs of dehydration.

NURSING INTERVENTIONS/*RATIONALES*

Monitor intake and output, IV infusion rate and patency, skin turgor, mucous membranes *to evaluate hydration status.*

Offer oral fluids as ordered and tolerated; use favorite fluids *to establish oral intake after surgery.*

NURSING DIAGNOSIS: Risk for infection related to break in skin integrity, anesthesia, immobility, presence of pathogens in environment

EXPECTED OUTCOME
Lungs remain clear; surgical incision site is clean.

NURSING INTERVENTIONS/*RATIONALES*

Turn, cough, deep breathe, use incentive spirometer or blow bottle *to promote movement and clearing of lung secretions.*

Suction secretions as needed *to keep airway clear.*

Monitor respirations, auscultate breath sounds *to assess respiratory status.*

Ambulate as early as permitted *to promote increased circulation and improved gas exchange.*

Keep surgical site dressed, using careful wound care and handwashing techniques *to prevent infection.*

Monitor temperature; inspect wound for redness, swelling, pus *indicative of infection.*

NURSING DIAGNOSIS: Altered family process related to surgical procedure

EXPECTED OUTCOME
Family demonstrates understanding of surgery and related processes; family complies with directives.

NURSING INTERVENTIONS/*RATIONALES*

Teach family about surgical procedure and related tests and procedures; outline the preoperative, operative, and postoperative processes *to provide understanding of what will happen and prepare family for what is to occur;* allow time for questions; get feedback *to evaluate level of understanding.*

Be available to family *to provide support;* explore family's feelings *to offer needed emotional support.*

Let family know where to wait and whom to talk to while surgery occurring; give them an expected time frame for the procedure; let them know when they can see child after surgery *to provide support.*

Explain child's expected appearance, equipment, and attached apparatus after surgery *to prepare family and reduce fear.*

Explain care after surgery; encourage family to participate in child's care as they feel able *to facilitate a sense of control and ability to cope.*

Guidelines

POSTOPERATIVE CARE

Ensure that preparations are made to receive child.
- Bed or crib is ready.
- Intravenous equipment, such as pumps, and any other relevant equipment, such as suction apparatus, oxygen flow meter, or Gomco suction, is at bedside.

Obtain baseline information:
- Take vital signs, including blood pressure (BP); keep BP cuff in place and deflated to lessen amount of disturbance to child.
- Take and record vital signs more frequently if any value fluctuates.
- Inspect operative area.
- Check dressing if present.
- Outline any bleeding area on dressing or cast with pen.
- Reinforce, but do not remove, loose dressing.
- Observe areas below surgical site for blood that may have drained toward bed.
- Assess for bleeding and other symptoms in areas not covered with a dressing, such as throat after tonsillectomy.
- Assess skin color and characteristics.
- Assess level of consciousness and activity.

Notify physician of any irregularities in child's condition.

Assess for evidence of pain (see Pain Assessment, Chapter 44).

Review surgeon's orders after completing initial assessment, and check that any preoperative orders, such as seizure or cardiac medications, have been reordered and can be given by available routes (oral preparations may be contraindicated).

Monitor vital signs as ordered and more often if indicated.

Check dressings for bleeding or other abnormalities.

Check bowel sounds.

Observe for signs of shock, abdominal distention, and bleeding.

Assess for bladder distention.

Observe for signs of dehydration.

Detect presence of infection:
- Take vital signs every 2 to 4 hours, as ordered.
- Collect or request needed specimens.
- Inspect wound for signs of infection—redness, swelling, heat, pain, and purulent drainage.

ings with previous ones is a useless technical function. Each vital sign is evaluated in terms of side effects from anesthesia and signs of impending shock, respiratory compromise, or pain. The nurse should also be alert for the development of *malignant hyperthermia,* a potentially lethal genetic myopathy. In susceptible children, certain anesthetic agents such as succinylcholine and halothane trigger the disorder, producing elevated temperature, muscle rigidity, hypermetabolism, and muscle cell destruction. The symptoms may or may not occur during surgery; therefore alert observation in the PACU and regular care unit is essential. Early signs of the disorder include tachycardia, rising blood pressure, tachypnea, mottled skin, and muscle rigidity. An elevated temperature is considered by many to be a late sign of the disorder (Dunn, 1997).

NURSE ALERT When taking the preoperative history, ask the family if any relatives have had anesthetic difficulties suggesting malignant hyperthermia; report findings immediately. ■

Managing Pain

Comfort is a major nursing responsibility after surgery. Pain is assessed, and analgesics are administered to provide comfort and to facilitate the child's cooperation with postoperative procedures such as ambulating and deep breathing. Opioids are the most commonly used analgesics for this purpose. Routinely scheduled IV analgesics, patient-controlled analgesia (PCA), and epidural infusions, rather than as-needed (PRN) orders, provide excellent analgesia in postoperative pediatric patients.

Because respiratory infections are a potential complication, every effort is taken to aerate the lungs and remove secretions. The lungs are auscultated regularly to identify abnormal sounds or any areas of diminished or absent breath sounds. To prevent hypostatic pneumonia, respiratory movement can be encouraged with incentive spirometers or other motivating activities (see Box 45-3). If these measures are presented as games, the child is more likely to comply. The child's position is changed every 2 hours, and deep breathing is encouraged.

NURSE ALERT Early signs of respiratory involvement are abnormal rate, shallow depth, and cough. These findings are reported immediately. ■

During the recovery period, some time should be spent with children to assess their perception of surgery. Play, drawing, and storytelling are excellent methods of discovering their thoughts. With such information the nurse can support or correct their perceptions and assist children in feeling a sense of mastery for having gone through a stressful procedure.

Compliance

Compliance, also termed *adherence,* refers to the extent to which the patient's behavior in terms of taking medication, following diets, or executing other lifestyle changes coincides with the prescribed regimen. Because nurses are frequently responsible for teaching families about treatment protocols, they must have knowledge of factors that influence compliance, methods to measure compliance, and strategies to enhance adherence to prescribed treatment.

Assessment of Compliance

In developing strategies to provide compliance, the nurse must first assess factors that influence compliance in the patient. Because many children are too young to assume partial or total responsibility for their care, parents are usually the primary caregivers at home. Consequently, the nurse needs to assess their ability to carry out instructions. The first approach to assessment is knowledge of those factors that influence compliance. The second is to apply methods to objectively assess the child's and parents' levels of compliance.

Several factors influence compliance (Box 45-5), although no typical characteristics of noncompliers exist, and even education is not correlated with compliance (Rosenstock, 1988). Basically, any aspect of the health care environment that increases the family's satisfaction with the care they are receiving positively influences adherence to the treatment regimen. However, the more complex, expensive, inconvenient, and disruptive the treatment protocol, the less

BOX 45-5

Factors That Positively Influence Compliance

Individual/Family Factors
High self-esteem
Positive body image
High degree of autonomy (increased locus of control)
Supportive and well-adjusted family
Effective family communication
Family expectation for successful completion of therapy

Care-Setting Factors
Perceived satisfaction with care
Positive interactions with practitioners
Continuity of care
Individualized care
Minimum waiting time for appointments
Convenient care setting

Treatment Factors
Simple regimen
Minimum disruption in usual lifestyle
Short duration
Inexpensive
Visible benefits
Tolerable side effects

likely the family is to comply. During long-term conditions that involve multiple treatments and considerable rearrangement of lifestyle, compliance is severely affected.

Although it is helpful to know those factors that influence compliance, assessment must include more direct measurement techniques. A number of methods exist, each with advantages and disadvantages. The most successful approach includes a combination of at least two of the following methods:

Clinical judgment. The nurse judges family compliance. This is a very poor method that is subject to bias and inaccuracy unless the nurse carefully evaluates the criteria used in evaluation.

Self-reporting. The family members are asked about their ability to carry out the prescribed treatments, although most people overestimate their compliance by about 20% even when they admit to lapses in treatment.

Direct observation. The nurse directly observes the patient or family performing the treatment. This method is difficult to employ outside the health care setting, and the family's awareness of being observed frequently affects their performance.

Monitoring appointments. The family's attendance at scheduled appointments is recorded, although this method only indirectly indicates compliance with the prescribed care.

Monitoring therapeutic response. The child's response in terms of benefit from treatment is monitored and preferably recorded on a graph or chart. Unfortunately, few treatments yield directly measurable results (e.g., decreased blood pressure, weight loss).

Pill counts. The nurse counts the number of pills remaining in the original container and compares the amount missing with the number of days the medication should have been taken. Although this is a simple method, families may forget to bring the container or deliberately alter the number of pills to avoid detection. This method is also poorly suited to liquid medication, which is so often prescribed in pediatrics. Another strategy is to call the pharmacy and check on the number of refills for long-term prescriptions.

Chemical assay. For certain drugs, such as digoxin and phenytoin, measurement of plasma drug levels provides information on the amount of drug recently ingested. However, this method is expensive, indicates only short-term compliance, and requires precise timing of the assay for accurate results.

Strategies to Enhance Compliance

Strategies to improve compliance are concerned with those interventions that encourage families to follow the prescribed treatment regimen. No one approach is always successful, and the best results occur when at least two strategies are used.

Organizational strategies refer to those interventions that involve the care setting and the therapeutic plan. They include employing the factors listed in Box 45-5 that are known to positively affect compliance. Depending on the individual situation, this may involve increasing the frequency of appointments, designating a primary practitioner, reducing the cost of medication by purchasing generic brands, reducing the treatment's disruption of the family's lifestyle, and using "cues" to minimize forgetting. Numerous devices are available commercially or can be improvised for cueing, such as pill dispensers; watches with alarms; charts to record completed therapy; reminders, such as messages on the refrigerator or morning coffee pot; and treatment schedules that incorporate the treatment plan into the daily routine, such as physical therapy after the evening bath.

Educational strategies are concerned with instructing the family about the treatment plan. Although education is an important component in enhancing compliance and patients who are more knowledgeable about their condition are more likely to comply, education alone does not ensure compliant behavior. Also, for education to be effective, it must incorporate teaching principles known to enhance understanding and retention of material (Guidelines box). Written materials are essential, especially in any regimen requiring multiple or complex treatments, and need to be understandable to the average individual, who reads at about the fourth-grade level. Involvement of the immediate and extended family (e.g., grandparents) in education sessions may enhance compliance (Liptak, 1996).

Treatment strategies are related to the child's refusal or inability to take the prescribed medication. The family may also have difficulty following a prescribed treatment regimen. They may remember and understand the instructions but may not be able to give the medicine as prescribed. It is essential to assess the reason for refusal. For example, the child may not be able to swallow pills. In this case, perhaps they can be crushed or a liquid medication substituted. The opposite also may occur; the child may have difficulty drinking a liquid medication but is able to swallow pills.

Also assess the treatment and medication schedule to determine if it is reasonable for a home situation. Although an every-6-hour or every-8-hour schedule is reasonable for hospitals, a parent would have difficulty awakening one or two times at night when a medication could be given during the day at times that would be easy to remember.

Behavioral strategies encompass those interventions designed to modify behavior directly. Several strategies exist that are effective in encouraging the desired behavior and are very useful with children. Also, positive reinforcement may be employed to strengthen the behavior; this may consist of earning stars or tokens, which gains the child a special privilege or gift. At times, however, techniques such as time-out for young children or withholding privileges for older children may be needed to reduce noncompliance (see Limit Setting and Discipline, Chapter 31).

GENERAL HYGIENE AND CARE

Maintaining Healthy Skin

Skin, the largest organ of the body, is not merely a covering but also a complex structure that serves many functions, the most important of which is to protect the tissues that it encloses and to protect itself. Many routine nursing activities—maintaining an IV line, removing a dressing, positioning a child in bed, changing a diaper, using electrode patches, or maintaining restraints—have the potential to contribute to skin injury. Skin care must go beyond the daily bath and become a part of each nursing intervention. General guidelines for skin care are listed in the Guidelines box.

Assessment of the skin is most easily accomplished during the bath, but often the nurse is not the one who bathes the child. In this case the nurse needs to plan a time to observe the child's skin and to request feedback from the caregiver. The skin is examined for any early signs of injury, especially for the child who is at risk. Risk factors include impaired mobility, protein malnutrition, edema, incontinence, sensory loss, anemia, and infection. Other risk factors include not turning the patient, intubation, patients ventilated with high positive end-expiratory pressure, use of a low-air-loss bed, edema, and weight loss. Critically ill children often are at higher risk for pressure ulcers and skin breakdown because they often have several risk factors in combination. Identification of risk factors helps determine those children who

Guidelines

EFFECTIVE TEACHING OF FAMILY MEMBERS

Establish rapport; reduce anxiety and fear.
Assess what family members know and expect to learn, especially if they have concerns, and address their concerns before beginning teaching.
Assess family's learning style; ask if they prefer to have everything explained in detail or if they prefer knowing only the major facts.
Use a variety of teaching materials (lecture, demonstration, video or slide presentation, written material).
Speak family's language, avoid jargon, and clarify all terms.
Be specific when giving information.
Divide the information into small steps.
Keep information short, simple, and concrete.
Introduce most important information first.
Use "verbal" headings to organize information, such as "There are two things you need to learn: how to give the medicine and what side effects to look for. First, how to give. . . . Second, what side effects. . . ."
Stress how important the instructions are and the expected benefits; explain the detrimental effects of inadequate treatment, but avoid fear tactics.
Evaluate the teaching by eliciting feedback to ensure that family members understand the information.
Repeat information as needed.
Reward family for learning through verbal praise.
Use "teachable moments"–times when family members are most likely to accept new information (e.g., when a member asks a question or when symptoms are present).
Use "hands on" demonstration and return demonstration to encourage mastery of skills and retention of information.

Guidelines

SKIN CARE

Cleanse skin with mild nonalkaline soap or soap-free cleaning agents for routine bathing.
Provide daily cleansing of eyes, oral, and diaper or perianal areas, and any areas of skin breakdown.
Apply moisturizing agents after cleansing to retain moisture and rehydrate skin; however, cleanse skin of any old cream before adding a new layer. Commonly used agents include lactic acid, glycolic acid, mineral oil, and glycerin. Moisturizing agents are more effective when applied during or immediately after bathing.
Use minimum amounts of tape or adhesive. On very sensitive skin, use a protective, pectin-based or hydrocolloid skin barrier between skin and tape or adhesives.
Use water or possibly adhesive remover (if skin is not fragile) when removing tape or adhesives.
Place pectin-based or hydrocolloid skin barriers directly over excoriated skin. Leave barrier undisturbed until it begins to peel off, or for 5 to 7 days. With wet, oozing excoriations, place a small amount of stoma powder (as used in ostomy care) on site, remove excess powder, and apply skin barrier. Hold barrier in place for several minutes to allow barrier to soften and mold to skin surface.
Alternate electrode placement and thoroughly assess skin underneath electrodes at least every 24 to 72 hours. Alcohol-free skin sealant under leads may protect the skin from epidermal stripping with changes.
Be certain fingers or toes are visible whenever extremity is used for intravenous (IV) or arterial line.
Reduce friction by keeping skin dry (may apply absorbent powder, e.g., cornstarch) and using soft, smooth bed linen and clothes.
Use a draw sheet to move a child in bed or onto a gurney to reduce friction and shearing injuries; do not drag the child from under the arms.
Identify children who are at risk for skin breakdown before it occurs. Employ measures, such as pressure-reducing or pressure-relieving devices (e.g., mattress overlays, low-air-loss bed, gel pillows), to prevent breakdown.
Do not massage reddened bony prominences because it can cause deep tissue damage; provide pressure relief to those areas instead.
Keep skin free of excess moisture (i.e., urine or fecal incontinence, wound drainage, excessive perspiration).
Routinely assess the child's nutritional status. A child who is NPO (nothing by mouth) for several days and is only receiving IV fluid is nutritionally at risk, which can also affect the skin's ability to maintain its integrity. Parenteral nutrition should be considered for these children before they are at risk.

need a more thorough skin assessment. Assessment should occur within 24 hours of admission so that pressure ulcers and wounds that occurred before admission can be identified (Quigley & Curley, 1996; Ratcliff & Rodheaver, 1999).

When capillary blood flow is interrupted by pressure, the blood flows back into the tissue when the pressure is relieved. As the body attempts to reoxygenate the area, a bright red flush appears. This *reactive hyperemia,* or flush, is the earliest sign of tissue compromise and pressure-related ischemia. If pressure is prolonged, reactive hyperemia will not be sufficient to revitalize ischemic tissue (Calianno, 1999).

NURSE ALERT The tissue in the wound must be visible to be staged. Wounds covered with necrotic tissue or a scab should not be staged. Reverse staging should not be used to describe wounds as they heal. Accurate documentation of redness or obvious skin breakdown is essential. Color, size (height, width, and depth), location, presence of sinus tracts, odor, exudate, eschar, and response to treatment are observed and recorded at least daily. ■

The nurse must also have an understanding of the types of mechanical damage that can occur, such as pressure, friction, shearing, and epidermal stripping. When a combination of risk factors and mechanical injury is present, skin breakdown can occur (Hagelgans, 1993).

When a child is identified as being at risk for skin breakdown, nursing interventions are directed toward prevention of mechanical injury. Wounds caused by pressure can be prevented by using current technology and resources. *Pressure ulcers* can develop when the pressure on the skin and underlying tissues is greater than the capillary closing pressure, causing capillary occlusion. If the pressure remains unrelieved, vessels can collapse, resulting in tissue anoxia and cellular death. Pressure ulcers most often occur over bony prominences. These lesions are usually very deep (stage IV), extending into subcutaneous tissue or even deeper into muscle, tendon, or bone. Prevention of pressure ulcers includes measures that reduce or relieve pressure (Laurent, 1999).

A *pressure-reduction device* (e.g., gel pillows, foam mattress overlays) reduces pressure by redistributing it. These products do not prevent pressure from causing capillary closing; therefore turning and repositioning are always included when using these devices. Most of these items are overlays that are placed on top of the regular mattress. A *pressure-relief device* maintains pressure below that which would cause capillary closing. These devices are usually high-technology beds (e.g., low-air-loss beds) that are used for patients who have multiple pressure ulcer risk factors and cannot be turned effectively. Manufacturers of these beds recommend turning patients on low-air-loss beds when it can be clinically tolerated because the beds do not alleviate all interface pressure. Low-air-loss beds do not take the place of manually turning and have not been proven to relieve pressure in pediatric patients (McLane et al, 2002). Some bed manufacturers do not recommend placing patients who weigh less than 22.7 kg on a low-air-loss bed. If the bed is in the turning mode, patients may continue to pivot on one area (e.g., occiput), potentially causing friction and skin breakdown in that area.

NURSE ALERT Use of pressure-reducing devices on the bed for at-risk patients: on a bed, the device can be placed on top of a standard mattress or as a mattress replacement system; or it can be a pressure-reducing bed (Calianno, 1999). ■

Friction and shear both contribute to pressure ulcers. *Friction* occurs when the surface of the skin rubs against another surface, such as the sheets on the bed. The skin may have the appearance of an abrasion. The skin damage is usually limited to the epidermal and upper layers. It most often occurs over the elbows, heels, or occiput. Prevention of friction injury includes the use of protective sheepskin over the elbows or heels; moisturizing agents; transparent dressings over susceptible areas; and soft, smooth bed linen and clothing. Friction alone does not cause tissue necrosis, but when it acts with gravity, it results in shear injury.

Shear is the result of the force of gravity pushing down on the body and friction of the body against a surface, such as the bed or chair. For example, when a patient is in the semi-Fowler position and begins to slide to the foot of the bed, the skin over the sacral area remains in the same place because of the resistance of the bed surface. The blood vessels in the area are stretched and may cause small-vessel thrombosis and tissue death (Bryant & Doughty, 2000). The same type of damage can occur when a patient is pulled up in the bed if the skin does not move with the patient. Prevention of shear injury includes using "lift sheets" when repositioning a patient, elevating the bed no more than 30 degrees for short periods, and using the knee gatch to interrupt the pull of gravity on the body toward the foot of the bed.

Epidermal stripping results when the epidermis is unintentionally removed with tape removal. These lesions are usually shallow and irregularly shaped, and they may blister or weep after the epidermal injury. Babies are at increased risk for epidermal injury because their epidermal bond is only 40% to 60% of that of adults. Prevention of epidermal stripping includes using no tape when possible and securing dressings with laced binders (Montgomery straps) or stretchy netting (Spandage or stockinette). Use of porous or low-tack tapes (e.g., Medipore, paper, hydrogel), alcohol-free skin sealants (No Sting Barrier), and "picture framing" wounds with hydrocolloid or wafer barriers (e.g., Duoderm, Colloplast, Stomahesive) and then taping on top of the barrier also will reduce epidermal stripping.

Tape is placed so that there is no tension, traction, or wrinkles on the skin. To remove tape, the nurse slowly peels the tape away while stabilizing the underlying skin. Adhesive remover may be used to break the adhesive bond but may be drying to the skin; adhesive removers should be avoided in preterm neonates, because absorption rates vary and toxicity may occur. The adhesive is removed with water to prevent absorption and irritation. Wetting the tape with water may facilitate removal.

Chemical factors can also lead to skin damage. Fecal incontinence, especially when mixed with urine; wound drainage; or gastric drainage around gastrostomy tubes can erode epidermis. The skin can very quickly progress from redness to denudement if exposure continues. Moisture barriers, gentle cleansing as soon after exposure as possible, and skin barriers can be used to prevent damage caused by chemical factors (see also Diaper Dermatitis, Chapter 53). In addition, foam dressings that wick moisture away from the skin are helpful around gastrostomy tubes and tracheostomy sites.

Bathing

Gentle, pH-balanced soaps should be used (e.g., Dove, Nutragena, Lever 2000). Be careful of cleansers that are not pH balanced and contain artificial color, alcohol, or lanolin, because patients may have sensitivity to these cleansers. A moisturizer, if needed, is most effective when applied within minutes after the bath, after the skin has been patted dry and is still warm and moist.

Unless contraindicated, most infants and children can be bathed in a tub at the bedside, on the bed, or in a standard bathtub or shower located on the unit, which is often conveniently adapted for pediatric use. For infants and young children confined to bed, the towel method can be used. Two towels are immersed in a dilute soap solution and wrung damp. With the child lying supine on a dry towel, one damp towel is placed on top of the child and used to gently clean the body. This towel is discarded, and the child is dried and turned prone. The procedure is repeated using the second damp towel.

Infants and small children are *never* left unattended in a bathtub, and infants who are unable to sit alone are securely held with one hand during the bath. The infant's head is supported securely with one hand, or the farther arm is firmly grasped in the nurse's hand while the head rests comfortably on the nurse's wrist or arm. This hold provides secure control of the infant while the other hand is free to wash the infant's body (Fig. 45-4). Infants or children who are able to sit without assistance need only close supervision and a pad placed in the bottom of the tub to prevent slipping and loss of balance, which could result in a bumped head or submersion of the face.

In hospitalized patients, bathing regimens should be decided on an individual basis. Most children who feel well require little encouragement to participate in their daily care. Nurses need to use judgment regarding the amount of supervision the child requires. Some can be trusted to assume this responsibility unaided, whereas others will need someone in constant attendance. Children with mental or physical limitations and suicidal or psychotic children (who may commit bodily harm) require close supervision.

Areas that require special attention during bed baths and for children performing their own care are the ears, between skinfolds, the neck, the back, and the genital area. The genital area should be carefully cleansed and dried with particular care to skinfolds, and in uncircumcised boys, usually those over 3 years of age, the foreskin should be gently retracted and the exposed surfaces cleansed and then the foreskin replaced. Do not attempt to retract the foreskin in newborns. If the condition of the glans indicates inadequate cleaning, such as accumulated smegma, inflammation, phimosis, or foreskin adhesions, teaching proper hygiene is indicated. In the Vietnamese and Cambodian cultures, the foreskin is traditionally not retracted until adulthood (Krueger & Osborn, 1986). Older children have the tendency to avoid these areas; therefore they may need a gentle reminder.

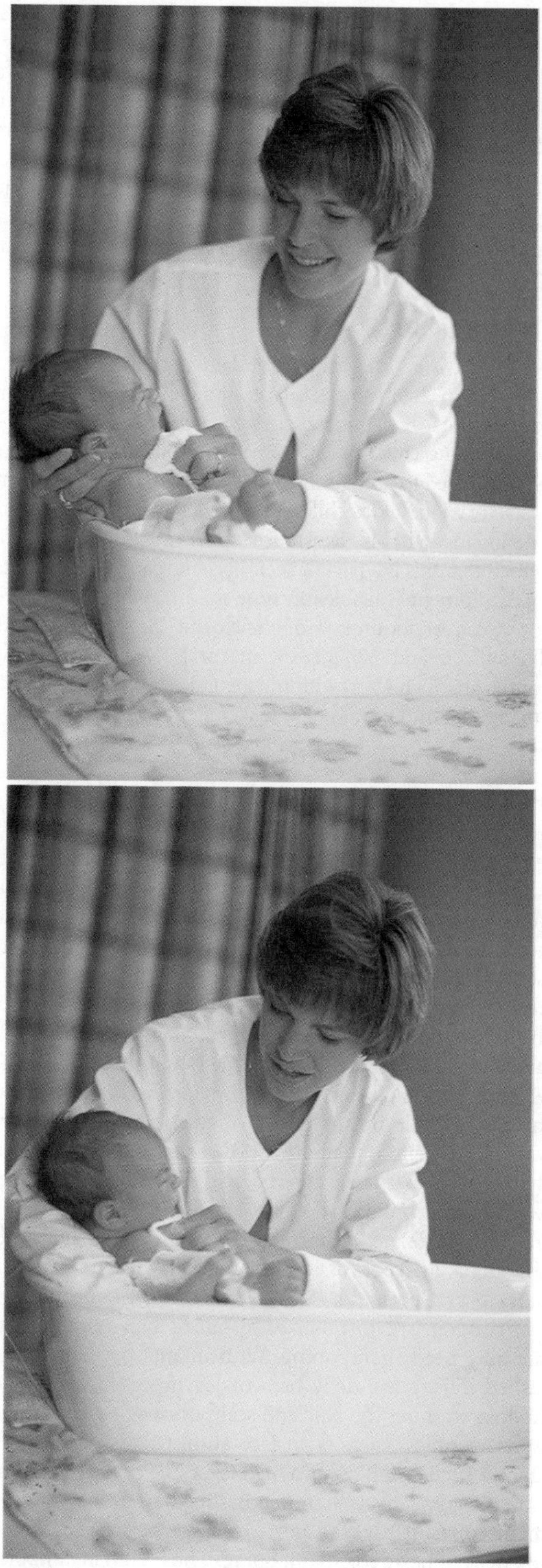

A

B

Fig. 45-4 Two methods of supporting infant during tub bath. **A**, Using hand to support neck and head. **B**, Using arm to support neck and head.

Children who are ill or debilitated need more extensive assistance with bathing and other aspects of hygienic care, but they should be encouraged to perform as much as they can without overtaxing their energies. Increasing involvement can be expected with improved strength and endurance. Children with limited capacity for self-care but no other contraindications benefit greatly from tub baths. They can be transported to the tub and, with the aid of lifting devices or an appropriate number of persons to assist, gain the advantages of a tub bath.

Oral Hygiene

Mouth care is an integral part of daily hygiene and should be continued in the hospital. Infants and debilitated children require the nurse or a family member to perform mouth care. Although young children can manage a toothbrush and should be encouraged to use it, most will need assistance to perform a satisfactory job. Older children, although capable of brushing and flossing without assistance, sometimes need to be reminded that this is a part of their hygienic care. Most hospitals have equipment available for those children who do not have a toothbrush or toothpaste of their own. (See Dental Health, Chapters 36 and 37, for specific oral hygiene techniques; mouth care of children with mucosal ulcers is discussed under nursing care of the child with leukemia in Chapter 49.)

Hair Care

Brushing and combing hair are a part of the daily care for all persons in the hospital, including infants and children. If the child does not have a brush or comb, many hospitals provide one as part of the usual admission kit. If not, the parents should be asked to bring hair care equipment for the child's use. Both boys and girls should be helped to comb or brush their hair, or it should be done for them, at least once daily. The hair is styled for comfort and in a manner pleasing to the child and parents. A satisfactory style for girls with longer hair is French braiding, which is done by starting with three equal portions of hair from the top of the scalp; as the hair is braided, segments of hair are added at successive intervals until all the hair has been incorporated into one or more neat, head-hugging braids. The ends are firmly anchored with a coated elastic band or barrette. The hair should not be cut without parental permission, although shaving hair to provide access to a scalp vein for IV needle insertion may be necessary.

If children are hospitalized for more than a few days, the hair may need shampooing. With infants the hair may be washed during the daily bath or less frequently. For most children washing the hair and scalp once or twice weekly is sufficient unless there is an indication to wash it more frequently, such as following a high fever and profuse sweating. Some hospitals have shampoo basins, but almost any child can be conveniently transported by a gurney to an accessible sink or washbasin for shampooing. Those who are unable to be transported can receive a shampoo in their beds with adequate protection or specially adapted equipment or positioning. A convenient method involves positioning the child near the edge of the bed, placing towels under the shoulders, and draping a large plastic garbage bag at the edge of the bed with one open side under the shoulders and the other side opened away from the head so that the hair is placed inside the opening. Water can be transported in a basin or placed in a clean enema bag. The nurse should fill a clean enema bag with warm water, hang the bag from an IV pole, and use the clamp on the bag's tubing to adjust the flow of water.

Teenagers, with their normally increased oily sebaceous secretions, are particularly in need of frequent hair care and usually require more frequent shampoos. Commercial no-rinse products also may prove useful on a short-term basis.

African-American children require special hair care, and this need is frequently neglected or inadequately managed. Most standard combs are inadequate and may cause hair breakage and discomfort to the child. If a special comb with widely spaced teeth is not available on the unit, the parent can be reminded to bring a comb, if possible, for the child's use. It is also much easier to comb the hair after shampooing when it is wet. This type of hair also requires a special hair dressing or pomade, which usually has a coconut oil base. The preparation is rubbed on the hands and then transferred to the hair to make it more pliable and manageable. The child's parents should be consulted regarding the preparation they want to be used on their child's hair, and they should be asked if they can provide some for use during the child's hospitalization. Petroleum jelly should *not* be used. If braiding or plaiting the hair is desired, the hair should be damp and loosely woven. The hair tightens as it dries, which could result in tension folliculitis (Jackson, 1998).

Feeding the Sick Child

Loss of appetite is a symptom common to most childhood illnesses and is frequently the initial evidence of illness, preceding fever and other overt signs of infection. In most cases children can be permitted to determine their own need for food. Because an acute illness is usually short, the nutritional state is seldom compromised. In fact, urging foods on the sick child may precipitate nausea and vomiting and in some cases even cause an aversion to the feeding situation that can extend into the convalescent period and beyond.

Refusing to eat may also be one way children can exert power and control in an otherwise helpless situation. For young children, loss of appetite may be related to the depression of separation from their parents and their natural tendency toward negativism. Parents' concern with eating can intensify the problem. Forcing a child to eat only meets with rebellion and reinforces the behavior as a control mechanism. Parents are encouraged to relax any pressure during the period of acute illness. Although it is best to encourage high-quality, nutritious foods, the child may desire foods and liquids that contain mostly empty or nonnutritional calories. Some well-tolerated foods include gelatin, clear soups, carbonated drinks, flavored ice pops, dry toast, crackers, and hard candy. Even though these substances are not nutritious, they can provide necessary fluid and calories.

Dehydration is always a hazard when children are febrile or anorexic, especially when this is accompanied by vomiting or diarrhea. An adequate fluid intake is encouraged by offering small amounts of favored fluids at frequent intervals and by offering salty foods (that increase thirst) if allowed. If diarrhea is present, high-carbohydrate liquids (e.g., carbon-

Guidelines

FEEDING THE SICK CHILD

Take a dietary history (see Chapter 34) and use information to make eating time as much like home as possible.
Encourage parents or other family members to feed child or to be present at mealtimes.
Make mealtimes pleasant; avoid any procedures immediately before or after eating; make sure child is rested and pain free.
Serve small, frequent meals rather than three large meals, or serve three meals and nutritious between-meal snacks.
Provide finger foods for young children.
Involve children in food selection and preparation whenever possible.
Serve small portions, and serve each course separately, such as soup first; followed by meat, potatoes, and vegetables; and ending with dessert. With young children, camouflage size of food by cutting meat thicker so that less appears on plate or by folding a cheese slice in half. Offer second helpings. Ensure a variety of foods, textures, and colors.
Provide food selections that are favorites of most children, such as peanut butter and jelly sandwiches, hot dogs, hamburgers, macaroni and cheese, pizza, spaghetti, tacos, fried chicken, corn on the cob, and fruit yogurt.
Avoid foods that are highly seasoned, have strong odors, are served hot, or are all mixed together, unless typical of cultural practices.
Provide fluid selections that are favorites of most children, such as fruit punch, cola, ginger ale, sweetened tea, flavored ice pops, sherbet, ice cream, milk and milkshakes, eggnog, pudding, gelatin, clear broth, or creamed soups (see also Box 45-3).
Offer nutritious snacks, such as frozen yogurt or pudding, ice cream, oatmeal or peanut butter cookies, hot cocoa, cheese slices, pieces of raw vegetable or fruit, and dried fruit or cereal.
Make food attractive and different; for example:
- Serve a "picnic lunch" in a paper bag.
- Pack food in a Chinese-food container; decorate container.
- Put a "face" or a "flower" on a hamburger or sandwich with pieces of vegetable.
- Use a cookie cutter to shape a sandwich.
- Serve pudding, yogurt, or juice frozen as an ice pop.
- Make slurpies or snow cones by pouring flavored syrup on crushed ice.
- Add food coloring to water or milk.
- Serve fluids through brightly colored or unusually shaped straws.
- Make "bowtie" sandwiches by cutting them in triangles and placing two points together.
- Slice sandwiches into "fingers."
- Grate mounds of cheese.
- Cut apples horizontally to make circles.
- Put a banana on a hot dog bun and spread with peanut butter.
- Break uncooked spaghetti into toothpick lengths and skewer cheese, cold meat, vegetables, or fruit chunks.

Praise children for what they do eat.
Do not punish children for not eating by removing their dessert or putting them to bed.

ated beverages, gelatin, flavored ice pops) are avoided because they may aggravate the diarrhea by an osmotic effect. Also, replacing abnormal losses with plain water or undiluted broth may worsen the electrolyte imbalance. Fluids should not be forced, and the child should not be wakened from rest to take fluids. Forcing fluids may create the same difficulties as urging unwanted food. Gentle persuasion with preferred beverages will usually meet with success. Using play techniques can also be very effective (Guidelines box).

When children are placed on special diets, such as clear liquids after surgery or during episodes of diarrhea, assessment of their intake and readiness to advance to more complex foods is essential.

NURSE ALERT Evidence of lack of readiness to advance the diet includes the following:
- Vomiting or diarrhea
- Decrease in appetite
- Abdominal cramping or distention
- Absence of bowel sounds
- Dehydration or weight loss ■

Once the child is feeling better, the appetite usually begins to improve. It is best to take advantage of any hungry period by serving high-quality foods and snacks. If the child still refuses to eat, nutritious fluids, such as prepared breakfast drinks, should be encouraged.

The admission nutritional assessment provides information pertinent to the patient's dietary preferences and cultural or religious preference. It is more advantageous to work with preferred food choices than with selections that children rarely eat. A number of creative approaches to food preparation can increase the child's interest in eating (see Guidelines box).

When children are placed on special diets, such as clear liquids after surgery or during episodes of diarrhea, assessment of their intake and readiness to advance to more complex foods is essential. Regardless of the type of diet, charting of the amount consumed is an important nursing responsibility. Descriptions need to be detailed and accurate, such as "4 ounces of orange juice, one pancake, no bacon, and 8 ounces of milk." Comments such as "ate well" or "ate poorly" are inadequate. Charting the percentage of the meal eaten is also inadequate unless food is measured before serving.

NURSE ALERT Ask the parent if the child ate all of the food from the tray. Occasionally a parent may eat something from the tray because the child did not want it. If a family member has eaten some of the food, this makes a marked difference in the report of how much the child ate. ■

If parents are involved in the child's care, they are encouraged to keep a list of everything eaten. Using a premeasured cup for fluids ensures a more accurate estimate of intake. A comparison of the intake at each meal can isolate food deficiencies, such as insufficient intake of meat or vegetables. Behaviors associated with mealtime also identify possible factors influencing appetite. For example, the observation that "Child eats well when with other children but plays with food if left alone in room" helps the nurse plan mealtime activities that stimulate the appetite.

Controlling Elevated Temperatures

An elevated temperature, most frequently from fever but occasionally caused by hyperthermia, is one of the most common symptoms of illness in children. This manifestation is

Table 45-1

Dosage Recommendations for Ibuprofen* (Children's Motrin)

			Oral Drops 50 mg/1.25 ml			Suspension 100 mg/5 ml		
			Rx		OTC	Rx		OTC
			Fever Under 39.2° C (102.5° F)	JRA,† Pain, and Fever ≥39.2° C (102.5° F)		Fever Under 39.2° C (102.5° F)	JRA,† Pain, and Fever ≥39.2° C (102.5° F)	
WEIGHT (lb)	WEIGHT (kg)	AGE (YEARS)	DROPPERS (5 mg/kg)	DROPPERS (10 mg/kg)	DROPPERS (7.5 mg/kg)	TEASPOONS (5 mg/kg)	TEASPOONS (10 mg/kg)	TEASPOONS (7.5 mg/kg)
12-17	5.4-7.7	6-11 mo	½	1		¼	½	
18-23	8.2-10.4	12-23 mo	1	2		½	1	
24-35	10.9-15.9	2-3	1½	3	2	¾	1½	1
36-47	16.3-21.3	4-5				1	2	1½
48-59	21.8-26.8	6-8				1¼	2½	2
60-71	27.2-32.9	9-10				1½	3	2½
72-95	32.7-43.1	11				2	4	3

Modified from McNeil Consumer Products, Fort Washington, PA, June 1997.
JRA, juvenile rheumatoid arthritis; *OTC*, over the counter; *Rx*, prescription needed.
*Doses should be administered every 6 to 8 hours. Another form of nonprescription ibuprofen is Children's Advil.
†The recommended maximum daily dose for JRA is 30 to 40 mg/kg.

frequently misunderstood and of great, but often unnecessary, concern to parents. To facilitate an understanding of fever, the following terms are defined:

Set point—The temperature around which body temperature is regulated by a thermostat-like mechanism in the hypothalamus

Fever—An elevation in set point such that body temperature is regulated at a higher level; may be arbitrarily defined as temperature above 38° C (100° F)

Hyperthermia—A situation in which body temperature exceeds the set point, which usually results from the body or external conditions creating more heat than the body can eliminate, such as in heatstroke, aspirin toxicity, seizures, or hyperthyroidism

Body temperature is regulated by a thermostat-like mechanism in the hypothalamus. This mechanism receives input from centrally and peripherally located receptors. When temperature changes occur, these receptors relay the information to the thermostat, which either increases or decreases heat production to maintain a constant set point temperature. During an infection, however, pyrogenic substances cause an increase in the body's normal set point, a process that is mediated by prostaglandins. Consequently, the hypothalamus increases heat production until the core (internal) temperature reaches the new set point (Connell, 1997).

Most fevers are of brief duration with limited consequences and are viral in nature. When fever is caused by bacteria, endotoxins are produced that activate the inflammatory process and produce fever (Rote, Huether, & McCance, 2000). In addition, fever probably plays a role in enhancing the development of both specific and nonspecific immunity and in aiding recovery and survival from infection. Contrary to popular belief, neither the rise in temperature nor its response to antipyretics indicates the severity or etiology of infection, which casts doubt on the value of using fever as a diagnostic or prognostic indicator.

Measures to Reduce Elevated Temperature

Treatment of elevated temperature depends on whether it is caused by a fever or hyperthermia. Because the set point is normal in hyperthermia but increased in fever, different approaches must be used to lower body temperature successfully.

Fever

The principal reason for treating fever is the relief of discomfort; there is no specific degree of fever that requires treatment. Relief measures include pharmacologic and environmental interventions. The most effective intervention is the use of antipyretics to lower the set point.

Antipyretic drugs include acetaminophen, aspirin, and nonsteroidal antiinflammatory drugs (NSAIDs). Acetaminophen is the preferred drug; aspirin should *not* be given to children because of the association between aspirin use in children with influenza virus or chickenpox and Reye syndrome. One nonprescription NSAID, ibuprofen, is approved for fever reduction in children as young as 6 months of age (Table 45-1). Dosage is based on the initial temperature level: 5 mg/kg of body weight for temperatures less than 39.1° C (102.5° F) or 10 mg/kg for temperatures greater than 39.1° C. The recommended dosage for pain is 10 mg/kg every 6 to 8 hours, and the recommended maximum daily dose for pain and fever is 40 mg/kg. The duration of fever reduction is generally 6 to 8 hours and is longer with the higher dose. Table 45-2 lists the recommended dosages of acetaminophen. It may be given every 4 hours but no more than five times in 24 hours. Because body temperature normally decreases at night, three to four doses in 24 hours are usually sufficient to control most fevers. The temperature is usually retaken 30

Chewable Tablets 50 mg			Chewable Tablets 100 mg			Caplets 100 mg		
Rx		OTC	Rx		OTC	Rx		OTC
Fever Under 39.2° C (102.5° F)	JRA†, Pain, and Fever ≥39.2° C (102.5° F)		Fever Under 39.2° C (102.5° F)	JRA,† Pain, and Fever ≥39.2° C (102.5° F)		Fever Under 39.2° C (102.5° F)	JRA,† Pain, and Fever ≥39.2° C (102.5° F)	
TABLETS (5 mg/kg)	TABLETS (10 mg/kg)	TABLETS (7.5 mg/kg)	TABLETS (5 mg/kg)	TABLETS (10 mg/kg)	TABLETS (7.5 mg/kg)	CAPLETS (5 mg/kg)	CAPLETS (10 mg/kg)	CAPLETS (7.5 mg/kg)
1	2		½	1				
1½	3	2	¾	1½				
2	4	3	1	2		1	2	
2½	5		1¼	2½	2	1¼	2½	2
3	6		1½	3	2½	1½	3	2½
4	8		2	4	3	2	4	3

Table 45-2

Dosage Recommendations for Acetaminophen (Tylenol)*

AGE	WEIGHT (POUNDS)	DOSE (mg)
Under 3 months	6-11	40
4-11 months	12-17	80
12-23 months	18-23	120
2-3 years	24-35	160
4-5 years	36-47	240
6-8 years	48-59	320
9-10 years	60-71	400
11 years	72-95	480
12 years and above	96+	640

*Doses should be administered four or five times daily but should not exceed five doses in 24 hours.

minutes after the antipyretic is given to assess its effect but should not be repeatedly measured; the child's level of discomfort is the best indication for continued treatment.

NURSE ALERT Acetaminophen is an effective antipyretic and analgesic when administered as recommended. However, it is important to recognize its full toxic potential in both acute overdose and excessive therapeutic administration. Several cases of acetaminophen hepatoxicity in children who received overdoses of the drug as part of therapeutic administration have been reported (Kearns, Leeder, & Wasserman, 1998). ■

Environmental measures to reduce fever may be used if tolerated by the child and if they do not induce shivering. Shivering is the body's way of maintaining the elevated set point by producing heat. Compensatory shivering greatly increases metabolic requirements above those already caused by the fever.

NURSE ALERT Treatment of shivering is directed at modifying or interfering with the rate of heat loss by warming the body, especially the extremities. ■

Traditional cooling measures, such as wearing minimum clothing, exposing the skin to the air, reducing room temperature, increasing air circulation, and applying cool, moist compresses to the skin (e.g., the forehead), are effective if employed approximately 1 hour *after* an antipyretic is given so that the set point is lowered. Cooling procedures such as sponging or tepid baths are ineffective in treating febrile children either when used alone or in combination with antipyretics, and they cause considerable discomfort (Sharber, 1997). These measures are used for hyperthermia.

Seizures associated with a fever occur in 3% to 4% of all children, usually those 3 months to 5 years of age. Although most children never have febrile seizures after the first occurrence, a younger age at onset and a family history of febrile seizures are associated with recurring episodes. For children who have febrile seizures, administration of antipyretics does not prevent recurrences (El-Radhi & Barry, 2003 ; Shinnar et al, 2001). There is little evidence to support the use of antipyretic drugs to prevent febrile seizures; nursing interventions should focus on ways in which care and comfort can be provided during a febrile illness (Purssell, 2000).

Hyperthermia

Unlike with fever, antipyretics are of no value in hyperthermia, because the set point is already normal. Consequently, cooling measures are used. Cool applications to the skin help reduce the core temperature. Cooled blood from the skin surface is conducted to inner organs and tissues, and warm blood is circulated to the surface, where it is cooled and recirculated. The surface blood vessels dilate as the body attempts to dissipate heat to the environment and facilitate this cooling process.

Commercial cooling devices, such as cooling blankets or mattresses, are available to reduce body temperature. They are placed on the bed and covered with a sheet or lightweight blanket. Frequent temperature monitoring is essential to prevent excessive cooling of the body.

Traditionally, cool compresses have been used to decrease high temperature. However, no particular temperature of water is agreed on as optimum. For tepid tub baths it is usually best to start with warm water and gradually add cool water until the desired water temperature of 37° C (98.6° F) is reached to accustom the child to the lower water temperature. Generally, the temperature of the water only has to be 1° to 2° (usually a warm temperature) less than the child's temperature to be effective (Kinmonth, Fulton, & Campbell, 1992). The child is placed directly in the tub of tepid water for 20 to 30 minutes while water is gently squeezed from a washcloth over the back and chest or gently sprayed over the body from a sprayer. In the bed or crib, cool washcloths or towels are used, exposing only one area of the body at a time. The sponging is continued for approximately 30 minutes.

After the tub or sponge bath, the child is dried and dressed in lightweight pajamas, a nightgown, or a diaper and placed in a dry bed. The temperature is retaken 30 minutes after the tub bath or sponge bath. The child is dried by gently rubbing the skin surface with a towel to stimulate circulation. The tub or sponge bath should not be continued or restarted until the skin surface is warm or if the child feels chilled. Chilling causes vasoconstriction, which defeats the purpose of the cool applications. In this condition, little blood is carried to the skin surface; the blood remains primarily in the viscera to become heated.

Whether a temperature elevation in the critically ill child is caused by fever or hyperthermia, it should be treated more aggressively. The metabolic rate increases 10% for every 1° C increase in temperature and three to five times during shivering, increasing oxygen, fluid, and caloric requirements. If the child's cardiovascular or neurologic system is already compromised, these increased needs are especially hazardous. In all children with elevated temperature, attention to adequate hydration is essential. Most children's needs can be met through additional oral fluids.

Family Teaching and Home Care

Nurses have a unique opportunity for teaching the family about health care practices while the child is hospitalized. Although most children have learned self-care and hygiene in the home or at school, many have not. For some young children, this is their first introduction to the use of a toothbrush. Much health teaching can be accomplished even when the child is hospitalized for only a short time. The daily bath, handwashing before meals and after bowel and bladder evacuation, and conscientious dental hygiene are taught by example during routine care. Clean hair, nails, and clothing, as well as good grooming, are emphasized as being essential to a pleasing appearance. Positive reinforcement of good hygiene practices helps create a positive body image, promote the development of self-esteem, and prevent health problems (e.g., teaching girls to wipe the genital area from front to back after toileting).

Although sick children's appetites may be poor and not characteristic of their home eating habits, the hospital stay provides numerous opportunities for nurses to assess the family's knowledge of good nutrition and to implement teaching as needed to improve nutritional intake.

Fever is one of the most common problems in pediatrics for which parents seek health care. Parental anxiety levels are increased with temperature elevation and its management (Liebman & Barnsteiner, 2001). Parents also need to know that sponging is indicated for elevated temperatures from hyperthermia rather than fever and that ice water and alcohol are inappropriate, potentially dangerous, solutions (Axelrod, 2000). Parents should know how to take the child's temperature and read the thermometer accurately, and should have guidelines for seeking professional care (Home Care box). Some of the newer temperature-measuring devices, such as tympanic membrane sensors, plastic strips, or digital thermometers, may be better suited for home use, because many parents are unable to read a mercury thermometer or calculate the correct decimal point (see Temperature, Chapter 35).

If the use of acetaminophen and ibuprofen is indicated, the parents need instruction in administering the drug. It is important to emphasize accuracy in both the amount of drug given and the time intervals at which the drug is administered. Because many forms of acetaminophen are available, the nurse must be certain of the type being used in the home when discussing dosage. For example, the chewable tablets come in *two* strengths (80 and 160 mg), and the specially coated, swallowable tablets for older children are 160 mg. The nurse should alert the parents to this because the tablets for older children may contain *twice* the amount of drug as the lower-dose chewable ones. If parents switch from the infant drops to the elixir, they are cautioned against using the dropper to measure the elixir, which is much less concentrated than the drops. Also, as children grow, the dosage needs to be recalculated.

Home Care

THE CHILD WITH FEVER

Call Our Office Immediately If:

Your child is less than 3 months old.
The fever is over 40.6° C (105° F).
Your child looks or acts very sick.

Call within 24 Hours If:

Your child is 3 to 6 months old (unless the fever is due to a diphtheria-pertussis-tetanus [DPT] shot).
The fever is between 40° and 40.6° C (104° and 105° F), especially if your child is less than 2 years old.
Your child has had a fever for more than 24 hours without an obvious cause or location of infection.
Your child has had a fever for more than 3 days.
The fever went away for more than 24 hours and then returned.
You have other concerns or questions.

Modified from Schmitt BD: *Instructions for pediatric patients,* ed 2, Philadelphia, 1999, WB Saunders.

SAFETY

Safety is an essential component of any patient's care, but children have special characteristics that require an even greater concern for safety. Because small children are separated from their usual environment and do not possess the capacity for abstract thinking and reasoning, it is the responsibility of everyone who comes in contact with them to maintain protective measures throughout their hospital stay. Nurses need to understand the age level at which each child is operating and plan for safety accordingly.

Name bands, a part of hospital safety practices, are particularly important for children in the pediatric age group. Infants and unconscious patients are unable to tell or respond to their names. Toddlers may answer to any name or to a nickname only. Older children may exchange places, give an erroneous name, or choose not to respond to their own names as a form of joke, unaware of the hazards of such practices.

Infection Control

The use of medical asepsis and appropriate barrier precautions to reduce the risk of *nosocomial* (hospital-acquired) infections is essential in caring for children. Children are infected frequently with organisms, such as varicella (chickenpox), that are transmissible and may be dangerous to others, especially immunocompromised patients. In addition, children may not have developed good hygiene habits, such as handwashing after toileting. Young children are especially at risk for infection because of their high oral activity. Children in diapers present infection risks if caregivers do not practice meticulous cleaning and disposal techniques.

To assist hospitals in maintaining up-to-date isolation practices, the Centers for Disease Control and Prevention (CDC) and the Hospital Infection Control Practices Advisory Committee (HICPAC) have revised the "CDC Guideline for Isolation Precautions in Hospitals," which was published in 1983. The guideline was revised to meet the following objectives: (1) to be epidemiologically sound; (2) to recognize the importance of all body fluids, secretions, and excretions in the transmission of nosocomial pathogens; (3) to contain adequate precautions for infections transmitted by the airborne, droplet, and contact routes of transmission; (4) to be as simple and user friendly as possible; and (5) to use new terms to avoid confusion with existing infection control and isolation systems.*

The revised guideline contains two levels of precautions. In the first, and most important, level are those precautions designed for the care of all patients in hospitals regardless of their diagnosis or presumed infection status. Implementation of these "standard precautions" is the primary strategy for successful nosocomial infection control. In the second level are precautions designed only for the care of specified patients. These additional "transmission-based precautions" are used for patients known or suspected to be infected or colonized with epidemiologically important pathogens that can be transmitted by airborne or droplet transmission or by contact with dry skin or contaminated surfaces.

Standard Precautions synthesize the major features of universal (blood and body fluid) precautions (UP) (designed to reduce the risk of transmission of blood-borne pathogens) and body substance isolation (BSI) (designed to reduce the risk of transmission of pathogens from moist body substances). Standard Precautions involve the use of *barrier protection,* such as gloves, goggles, gown, and/or mask, to prevent contamination from (1) blood; (2) all body fluids, secretions, and excretions *except sweat,* regardless of whether or not they contain visible blood; (3) nonintact skin; and (4) mucous membranes. Standard Precautions are designed to reduce the risk of transmission of microorganisms from both recognized and unrecognized sources of infection in hospitals.

Transmission-based precautions are designed for patients documented or suspected to be infected or colonized with highly transmissible or epidemiologically important pathogens for which additional precautions beyond Standard Precautions are needed to interrupt transmission in hospitals. There are three types of transmission-based precautions: airborne precautions, droplet precautions, and contact precautions. They may be combined for diseases that have multiple routes of transmission (Box 45-6). When used either alone or in combination, they are to be used in addition to Standard Precautions.

Airborne precautions are designed to reduce the risk of airborne transmission of infectious agents. Airborne transmission occurs by dissemination of either airborne droplet nuclei (small-particle residue [5 mcm or smaller in size] of evaporated droplets that may remain suspended in the air for long periods of time) or dust particles containing the infectious agent. Microorganisms carried in this manner can be dispersed widely by air currents and may become inhaled by or deposited on a susceptible host within the same room or over a longer distance from the source patient, depending on environmental factors; therefore *special air handling* and *ventilation* are required to prevent airborne transmission. Airborne precautions apply to patients known or suspected to be infected with epidemiologically important pathogens that can be transmitted by the airborne route. Examples of such illnesses include measles, varicella (chickenpox), and tuberculosis.

Droplet precautions are designed to reduce the risk of droplet transmission of infectious agents. Droplet transmission involves contact of the conjunctivae or the mucous membranes of the nose or mouth of a susceptible person with large-particle droplets (larger than 5 mcm in size) containing microorganisms generated from a person who has a clinical disease or who is a carrier of the microorganism. Droplets are generated from the source person primarily during coughing, sneezing, or talking and during the performance of certain procedures such as suctioning and bronchoscopy. Transmission via large-particle droplets requires close contact between source and recipient persons, because droplets do not remain suspended in the air and generally travel only short distances, usually 3 feet or less, through the air. Because droplets do not remain suspended in the air, special air handling and ventilation are not required to prevent droplet transmission. Droplet precautions

*This section is modified from Garner JS: What's in a name? The evolution of universal precautions to standard precautions: A guide to the latest recommendations in isolation practices, *Today's Surg Nurse* 19(1):14-21, 1997.

BOX 45-6

Summary of Types of Precautions and Patients Requiring Them

Standard Precautions
Use Standard Precautions for the care of all patients.

Airborne Precautions
In addition to Standard Precautions, use airborne precautions for patients known or suspected to have serious illnesses transmitted by airborne droplet nuclei. Examples of such illnesses include measles, varicella (including disseminated zoster), and tuberculosis.

Droplet Precautions
In addition to Standard Precautions, use droplet precautions for patients known or suspected to have serious illnesses transmitted by large particle droplets. Examples of such illnesses include the following:
- Invasive *Haemophilus influenzae* type b disease, including meningitis, pneumonia, epiglottitis, and sepsis
- Invasive *Neisseria meningitidis* disease, including meningitis, pneumonia, and sepsis
- Other serious bacterial respiratory infections spread by droplet transmission, including diphtheria (pharyngeal), mycoplasmal pneumonia, pertussis, pneumonic plague, streptococcal pharyngitis, pneumonia, or scarlet fever in infants and young children
- Serious viral infections spread by droplet transmission, including adenovirus, influenza, mumps, parvovirus B19, and rubella

Contact Precautions
In addition to Standard Precautions, use contact precautions for patients known or suspected to have serious illnesses easily transmitted by direct patient contact or by contact with items in the patient's environment. Examples of such illnesses include the following:
- Gastrointestinal, respiratory, skin, or wound infections or colonization with multidrug-resistant bacteria judged by the infection control program, based on current state, regional, or national recommendations, to be of special clinical and epidemiologic significance
- Enteric infections with a low infectious dose or prolonged environmental survival, including *Clostridium difficile;* for diapered or incontinent patients: enterohemorrhagic *Escherichia coli* O157:H7, *Shigella,* hepatitis A, or rotavirus
- Respiratory syncytial virus, parainfluenza virus, or enteroviral infections in infants and young children
- Skin infections that are highly contagious or that may occur on dry skin, including diphtheria (cutaneous), herpes simplex virus (neonatal or mucocutaneous), impetigo, major (noncontained) abscesses, cellulitis or decubiti, pediculosis, scabies, staphylococcal furunculosis in infants and young children, zoster (disseminated or in the immunocompromised host)
- Viral/hemorrhagic conjunctivitis
- Viral hemorrhagic infections (Ebola, Lassa, or Marburg)

From Garner JS: Guidelines for isolation precautions in hospitals, *Infect Control Hosp Epidemiol* 17(1):66, 1996.

apply to any patient known or suspected to be infected with epidemiologically important pathogens that can be transmitted by infectious droplets (see Box 45-6).

Contact precautions are designed to reduce the risk of transmission of epidemiologically important microorganisms by direct or indirect contact. *Direct-contact transmission* involves a direct body surface–to–body surface contact and physical transfer of microorganisms to a susceptible host from an infected or colonized person, such as occurs when personnel turn patients, bathe patients, or perform other patient care activities that require physical contact. Direct-contact transmission also can occur between two patients (e.g., by hand contact), with one serving as the source of infectious microorganisms and the other as a susceptible host. *Indirect-contact transmission* involves contact of a susceptible host with a contaminated intermediate object, usually inanimate, in the patient's environment (e.g., a contaminated instrument or contaminated hands that are not washed and gloves that are not changed between patients). Contact precautions apply to specified patients known or suspected to be infected or colonized (presence of microorganism in or on the patient but without clinical signs and symptoms of infection) with epidemiologically important microorganisms that can be transmitted by direct or indirect contact.

NURSE ALERT The most common piece of medical equipment, the stethoscope, can be a potent source of harmful microorganisms and nosocomial infections. One study found that 80% of 200 stethoscopes were contaminated with at least one microbe (Eckler, 1997). ■

Nurses caring for young children are frequently in contact with body substances, especially urine, feces, and vomitus. Nurses need to exercise judgment for those situations when gloves, gowns, or masks are necessary. For example, gloves and possibly gowns should be worn for changing diapers when there are loose or explosive stools. Otherwise, the plastic lining of disposable diapers provides a sufficient barrier between the hands and body substances. The type of diaper may be an important aspect of infection control. Superabsorbent disposable diapers with elastic legs contain urine and feces better than cloth diapering systems, and their use can reduce fecal contamination in the environment (Kubiak et al, 1993).

Antimicrobial-resistant organisms are causing increasing numbers of nosocomial infections. Nearly 70% of nosocomial infections can be attributed to seven pathogens: *Staphylococcus aureus,* coagulase-negative staphylococci, and enterococci; and the gram-negative organisms *Escherichia coli, Pseudomonas aeruginosa, Enterobacter,* and *Klebsiella* pneumonia. The main mode of transmission is patient to patient via the health care provider (Russell, 1999).

NURSE ALERT Handwashing is the most critical infection control practice. ■

During feedings, gowns should be worn if the child is likely to vomit or spit up, which often occurs during burping. When gloves are worn, the hands are washed thoroughly after removing the gloves, because both latex and vinyl gloves fail to provide complete protection.

Another essential practice of infection control is that all needles (uncapped and unbroken) are disposed of in a rigid, puncture-resistant container located near the site of use.

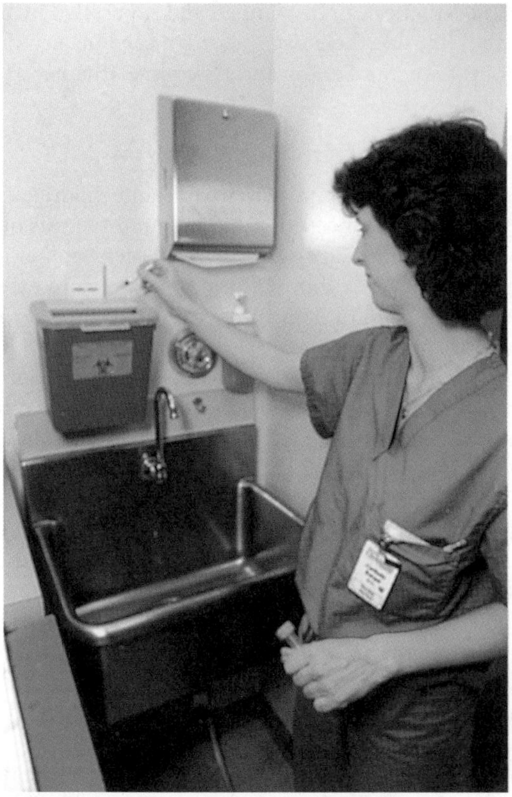

Fig. 45-5 To prevent needle-stick injuries, used needles (and other sharp instruments) are not capped or broken and are disposed of in a rigid, puncture-resistant container located near the site of use. Note placement of the container to prevent children's access to the contents.

Consequently, these containers are installed in patients' rooms. Because children are naturally curious, extra attention is needed in selecting a suitable type of container and a location that discourages access to the disposed needles (Fig. 45-5). The use of needleless systems allows secure syringe or IV tubing attachment to vascular access devices without the risk of needle-stick injury to the child or nurse.

Environmental Factors

All of the environmental safety measures in operation for the protection of adults apply to children as well and include good illumination, floors clear of fluid or objects that might contribute to falls, and nonskid surfaces in showers and tubs. Electrical equipment, which is maintained in good working order, is operated only by personnel familiar with its use and is not in contact with moisture or near tubs, where it could prove to be a shock hazard. Beds of ambulatory patients are locked in place and at a height that allows easy access to the floor. A special hazard for children is the danger of entrapment under an electronically controlled bed when it is activated to descend. Staff members should practice proper care and disposal of breakable items such as thermometers and bottles and small items such as syringe caps or needle covers. All staff members should be familiar with the area-specific fire plan.

All windows should be securely screened, and elevators and stairways made safe. Ideally, electrical outlets should be provided with covers to prevent burns in small children, whose exploratory activities may extend to inserting objects into the small openings. Bathwater is carefully checked before placing the child in it, and children must never be left alone in a bathtub. Infants are helpless in water, and small children (and some older ones) may turn on the hot water faucet and be severely burned.

Furniture is safest when it is scaled to the child's proportions, is sturdy, and is well balanced to prevent its being easily tipped over. Infants and small children must be securely strapped into infant seats, feeding chairs, and strollers. Baby walkers should be discouraged because they provide access to hazards, resulting in burns, falls, and poisonings. Infants; young children; and those who are weak, paralyzed, agitated, confused, sedated, or cognitively impaired are never left unattended on treatment tables, on scales, or in treatment areas. Even premature infants are capable of surprising mobility; therefore portholes in incubators must be securely fastened when not in use. Beds of ambulatory patients should remain locked in place and at a height that allows easy access to the floor.

Crib sides should be elevated and fastened securely unless an adult is at the bedside. It is safer to leave crib sides up, regardless of the child's ability to get out and even when the crib is unoccupied, to remove the child's temptation to climb in. Anyone attending an infant or small child in a crib with the sides down should never turn away without maintaining hand contact with the child; that is, one hand should be kept on the child's back or abdomen to prevent the child from rolling, crawling, or jumping from the open crib (Fig. 45-6). A child who is apt to or has demonstrated the inclination to climb over the sides of the crib is safest when placed in a specially constructed crib with a cover. Cribs are not placed within reach of heating units, appliances, dangling cords, or other objects that can be grabbed by curious hands, and toys are not tied to or across crib rails once children are old enough to reach them.

Toys

Toys play a vital role in the everyday life of children, and they are no less important in the hospital setting. However, nurses are responsible for assessing the safety of toys brought

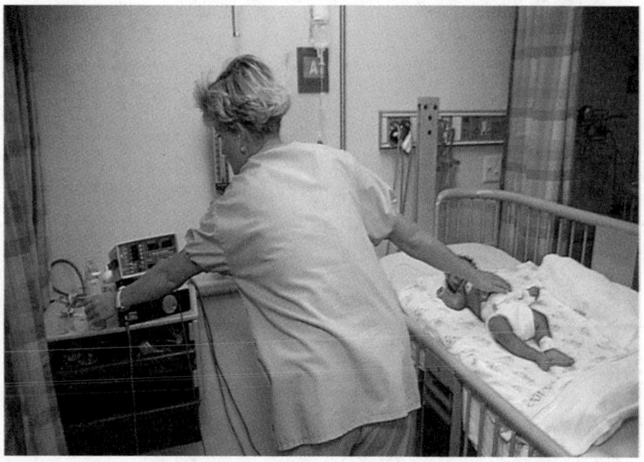

Fig. 45-6 Nurse maintains hand contact when back is turned.

to the hospital by well-meaning parents and friends. Toys and gifts should be appropriate to the child's age, condition, and treatment. For example, if the child is in an oxygen tent, electrical or friction toys cannot be placed in the tent. Toys are inspected to make certain that they are nonallergenic, washable, and unbreakable and that they have no small, removable parts that can be aspirated or swallowed or that can in other ways inflict injury to a child. Latex balloons pose a serious threat to children of all ages. If the balloon breaks, a child may put a piece of the latex in his or her mouth. If it is aspirated or swallowed, the latex piece is difficult to remove, resulting in choking. Latex balloons should *never* be permitted in the hospital setting.

NURSE ALERT Plants and flowers harbor gram-negative bacteria and molds that may be a risk to the immunocompromised child. These items may also pose the danger of poisoning to curious toddlers. ■

Limit Setting

Setting limits is essential to a child's safety. Children must understand where they are permitted to go and what they are permitted to do in the hospital. These limitations should be made clear to them, consistently enforced, and repeated as frequently as necessary to make certain that they are understood. The nurse is responsible for a child's whereabouts at all times. Children can easily wander off unnoticed, and their access to tubs, laundry chutes, medication rooms and carts, and elevators must be prevented. Normally active older children often become restless when their activity is restricted and may resort to pillow fights, water fights, and other rough play that might endanger the safety of the involved children or other children, staff, or visitors. Children in the hospital require supervision, and appropriate tension-reducing activities can be planned and supervised by nurses or by the child-life therapist. A useful discipline technique is time-out (see Limit Setting and Discipline, Chapter 31).

Transporting Infants and Children

In the course of a hospital stay, infants and children usually need to be transported within the unit and to areas outside the pediatric unit. Infants and small children can be carried for short distances within the unit, but for more extended trips the child should be securely transported in a suitable conveyance.

Small infants can be held or carried in the horizontal position with the back supported and the thigh grasped firmly by the carrying arm (Fig. 45-7, *A*). In the football hold, the infant is carried on the nurse's arm with the head supported by the hand and the body held securely between the nurse's body and elbow (Fig. 45-7, *B*). Both of these holds leave the nurse's other arm free for activity. The infant can be held in the upright position with the buttocks on the nurse's forearm and the front of the body resting against the nurse's chest. The infant's head and shoulders are supported by the nurse's other arm to allow for any sudden movement by the infant (Fig. 45-7, *C*). Older infants are able to hold their heads erect but can still make sudden movements.

Infants can be transported to other areas, such as the radiography department, in their bassinets or cribs. Baby carriages are sometimes used for infants who are not likely to stand up. Strollers and wheeled feeding chairs or tables are also convenient transporters in some situations, such as trips to the playroom or nurse's station.

The method of transporting children is determined by their age, condition, and destination. Most older children are safe in wheelchairs or on stretchers. A younger child can be transported in a crib, on a stretcher, in a wagon with raised

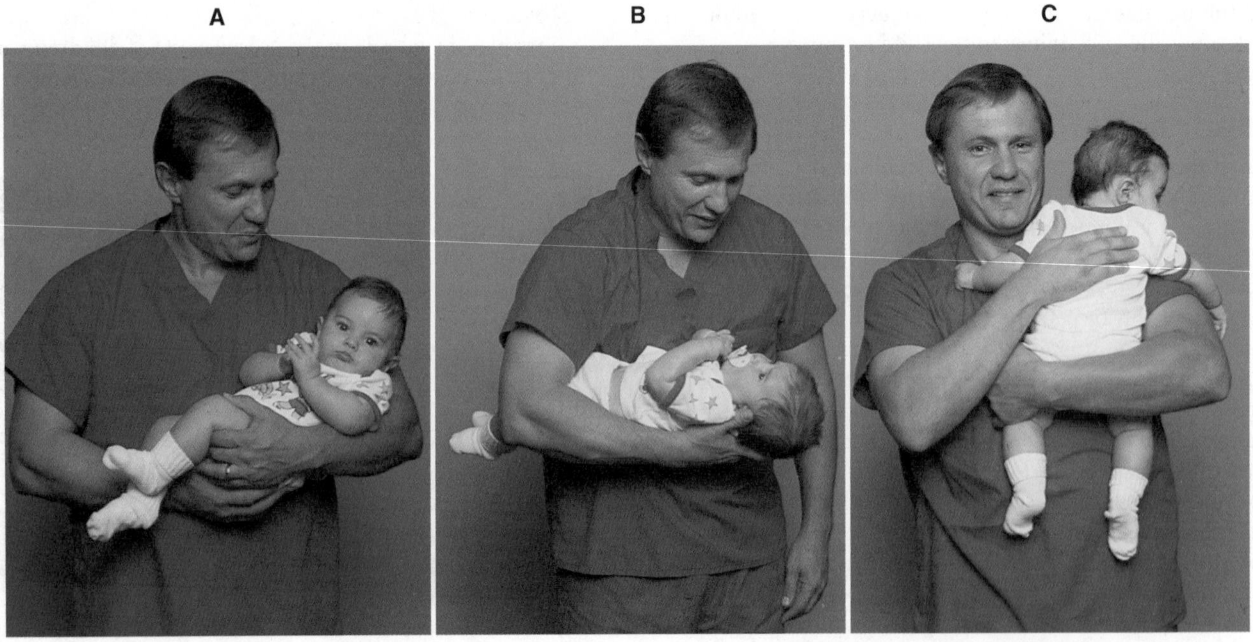

Fig. 45-7 Transporting infants. **A,** Infant's thigh firmly grasped in nurse's hand. **B,** Football hold. **C,** Back supported.

sides, or in a wheelchair with a safety belt. Stretchers should be equipped with high sides and a safety belt, both of which are secured during transport.

Restraining Methods and Therapeutic Hugging

Sometimes restraining methods and therapeutic hugging are common practices in nursing to ensure a child's safety or comfort, facilitate examination, and aid in performing diagnostic tests and therapeutic procedures. *Therapeutic hugging* is the use of a secure, comfortable, temporary holding position that provides close physical contact with the parent or caregiver (see Fig. 45-11).

Nurses need to assess whether or not restraints are needed. Restraints can often be avoided with adequate preparation of the child, parental or staff supervision of the child, and adequate protection of a vulnerable site, such as an infusion device. The nurse needs to take into account the child's development, mental status, potential threat to others or self, and safety. The Joint Commission on Accreditation of Healthcare Organizations (JCAHO) points to the need for a physician's order before application of restraint. However, alternative approaches to restraint must be attempted before seeking a physician's order for restraint (Selekman & Snyder, 1996). Therefore alternative measures to using restraints should be a careful consideration of the nurse. Creative approaches may make physical restraint unnecessary. For example, a young child might be brought to the nurses' station for observation and stimulation when parents are not present.

NURSE ALERT The Health Care Financing Administration (HCFA) and JCAHO have developed standards to guide acute care hospitals in the use of restraints. JCAHO defines restraint as "any method, physical or mechanical, which restricts a person's movement, physical activity, or normal access to his or her body" (JCAHO, 2001). JCAHO standards mandate that a policy be in effect that is clear and consistent and includes the following: the patient's need for restraint (reason for restraint) must be assessed; at least one alternative method must be attempted before restraint application; and, when restraints are applied, the least restrictive method must be used. An order must be written and an evaluation performed by a licensed independent practitioner (LIP) within 1 hour of applying the restraint. The LIP's order must include the start and stop time, date, reason for restraint, type of restraint used, and the signature of the LIP. An initial verbal order can be obtained by the registered nurse (RN) (Krozek & Scoggins, 2001). ■

When a child must be restrained, it is important to explain to the child the reason for the restraint. This information should be repeated as often as needed to gain cooperation. Have the child verbalize understanding of the need for restraint. Explain how the child can help (e.g., "Your job is to keep your arm as still as a tree".) Most important, reassure the child that the restraint is not a punishment.

Parents need to know the purpose of restraints, how to remove and reapply them, and the signs of complications from their use. Document parental consent for restraints. Sometime parents are upset when their child must be restrained and need to understand how they can help. Explain ways in which they can help to ensure maximal benefit and minimal stress (e.g., have the parent emotionally support the child by staying near the child). Position the parent at the head of the bed (provide a chair for the parent) so that the parent can soothe or calm the child by talking softly, singing, or stroking the child's skin.

After the decision is made that some restraint is necessary, it must be determined what type of restraint should be applied. For example, arm boards are less restrictive than four-point extremity restraints. Using less restrictive restraints is often possible by gaining the cooperation of the child and parents. It is the nurse's responsibility to select the most appropriate and least restrictive type of restraint.

Restraining devices are not without risk and must be checked and documented every 1 to 2 hours to ensure that they are accomplishing their purpose; that they are applied correctly; and that they do not impair circulation, sensation, or skin integrity. Restraints with ties must be secured to the bed or crib frame, not the side rails.

Selekman and Snyder (1997) recommend appropriate nursing interventions for the child who is restrained. Parental participation is always encouraged. These include, but are not limited to, the following:

- Remove and reapply restraints periodically.
- Offer comfort measures; use "therapeutic hugging" rather than mechanical restraint.
- Raise head of bed 30 degrees unless contraindicated.
- Provide range of motion as appropriate.
- Offer food, fluids, and toileting as appropriate; give pacifier.
- Discuss criteria for removal of restraint.
- Administer analgesics and sedatives if ordered or request whether needed.
- Avoid psychologic upset to other patients.
- Provide distraction (read a book) and touch.
- Maintain child's dignity.
- Provide ongoing nursing assessment.
- Document use of restraints.

Nurses play an important role in the practice of using physical restraints on children. Until more research is available, nurses need to carefully assess the children in their care and apply the nursing process in the use of restraints.

Jacket Restraint

A jacket restraint is sometimes used to keep the child safe in various chairs. The jacket is put on the child with the ties in back so that the child is unable to manipulate them. The long tapes, secured to the understructure of the crib, keep the child inside the crib. The jacket restraint is also useful as a means of maintaining the child in a desired horizontal position.

Mummy Restraint or Swaddle

When an infant or small child requires short-term restraint for examination or treatment that involves the head and neck, such as venipuncture, throat examination, and gavage feeding, the mummy device effectively controls the child's movements. A blanket or sheet is opened on the bed or crib with one corner folded to the center. The infant is placed on the blanket with shoulders at the fold and feet toward the opposite corner (Fig. 45-8, *A*). With the infant's right arm straight down against the body, the right side of the blanket is pulled firmly across the infant's right shoulder

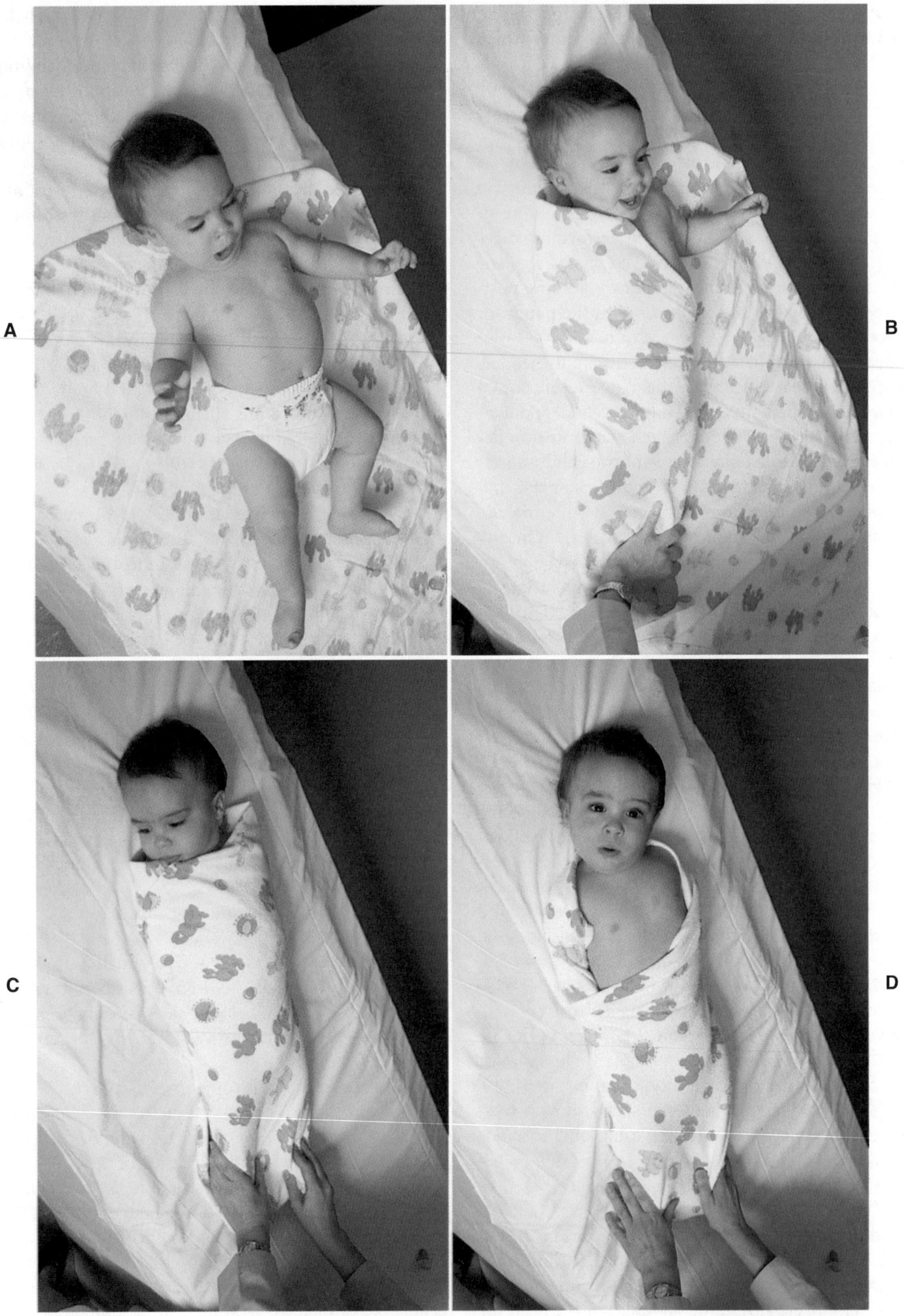

Fig. 45-8 Application of mummy restraint. **A**, Infant placed on folded corner of blanket. **B**, One corner of blanket brought across body and secured beneath body. **C**, Second corner brought across body and secured, and lower corner folded and tucked or pinned in place. **D**, Modified mummy restraint with chest uncovered.

and chest and secured beneath the left side of the body (Fig. 45-8, *B*). The left arm is placed straight against the child's side, and the left side of the blanket is brought across the shoulder and chest and locked beneath the child's body on the right side. The lower corner is folded and brought over the body and tucked or fastened securely with safety pins (Fig. 45-8, *C*). Safety pins can be used to fasten the blanket in place at any step in the process.

To modify the mummy restraint for chest examination, the folded edge of the blanket is brought over each arm and under the back, after which the loose edge is folded over and secured at a point below the chest to allow visualization of and access to the chest (Fig. 45-8, *D*).

The papoose board has the same function as the mummy restraint. It is a solid board with straps attached that secure the infant or small child to the board, similar to a mummy restraint. For maximum comfort the board should be padded. Papoose boards or mummy wraps are not substitutes for use of sedation and analgesia during painful procedures. They should be used only when no other options exist.

Arm and Leg Restraints

Arm and leg restraints are sometimes used to immobilize one or more extremities for treatment or procedures, or to facilitate healing. Several commercial restraining devices are available, including disposable wrist and ankle restraints. When this type of restraint is used, it must be appropriate to the size of the child; it must be padded to prevent undue pressure, constriction, or tissue injury; and the extremity must be observed frequently for signs of irritation or impairment of circulation. The ends of the restraints are never tied to the crib rails, because lowering the rail will disturb the extremity, frequently with a jerk that may hurt or injure the child.

Elbow Restraint

Sometimes it is important to prevent the child from bending an elbow or reaching the head or face (e.g., after lip surgery, when a scalp vein infusion is in place, or to prevent scratching in skin disorders). For this purpose, elbow restraints fashioned from a variety of materials function very well. The most common form of elbow restraint consists of a piece of muslin long enough to reach comfortably from just below the axilla to the wrist with a number of vertical pockets into which tongue depressors are inserted. The restraint is wrapped around the arm and secured with tapes or pins. It may be necessary to pin the top of the restraint to the undershirt sleeve to prevent the restraint from slipping. Similar restraints can be made from commonly available products.

Positioning for Procedures

Infants and small children are unable to cooperate for many procedures; therefore the nurse is responsible for minimizing their movement and discomfort with proper positioning. Older children usually need only minimal, if any, restraint. Careful explanation and preparation beforehand and support and simple guidance during the procedure are usually sufficient. Encourage parental participation to ease anxiety. For painful procedures, the child should receive adequate analgesia and sedation to minimize pain and the need for excessive restraint. For local anesthesia, use buffered lidocaine to reduce the stinging sensation of infiltration, or use the topical anesthetic EMLA or Numby Stuff (see Pain Management, Chapter 44).

Jugular Venipuncture

The large, superficial external jugular vein may be used to obtain blood specimens from infants and young children. For easy access to the vein, the child is first placed in a mummy restraint in which the top edge of the restraint is low enough to permit access to the vein. The child is placed so that the head and shoulders extend over the edge of a table or a small pillow, with the neck extended and the head turned sharply to the side. An alternative method (therapeutic hugging) for restraining arms and legs is with the parent holding the child's arms and legs at the same time that the child's head is restrained and positioned (Fig. 45-9). It is important for the nurse holding the child to maintain control of the child's head without interfering with the practitioner's approach to the vein. The child's crying during the procedure increases IV pressure, which facilitates visualization of the vein. After venipuncture, digital pressure is applied to the site with a dry gauze square for 3 to 5 minutes or until bleeding stops. Care must be taken not to apply excessive pressure that might compromise circulation or breathing during or after the procedure.

Femoral Venipuncture

Other frequently used sites for venipuncture are the large femoral veins. The nurse restrains the infant by placing the child supine with the legs in a frog position to provide extensive exposure of the groin area. Both the arms and the legs of the infant can be effectively controlled by the nurse's forearms and hands (Fig. 45-10). Only the side used for the venipuncture is uncovered, so the practitioner is protected should the child urinate during the procedure. Pressure is applied to the site after the withdrawal of blood to prevent oozing from the site.

Extremity Venipuncture

The most common sites of venipuncture are the veins of the extremities, especially the arm and hand. A convenient position is to place the child in the parent's (or assistant's) lap, with the child facing the parent and in the straddle po-

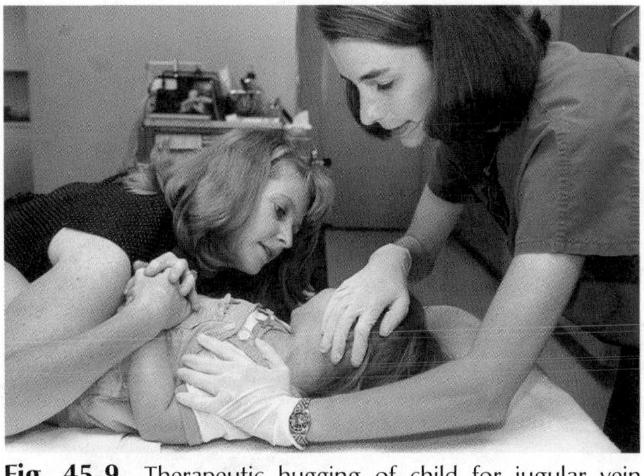

Fig. 45-9 Therapeutic hugging of child for jugular vein puncture with parental assistance.

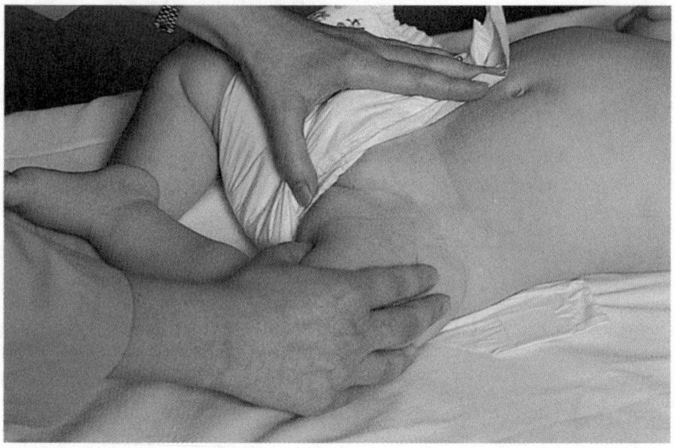

Fig. 45-10 Restraining infant for femoral vein puncture.

sition. Next, place the child's arm for venipuncture on a firm surface, such as a treatment table, for support and on top of a soft cloth or towel. Have an assistant immobilize the arm for venipuncture, or have the parent do this if an assistant is not available. Then have the parent hug the child around the body to hold the child's free arm, and place the child's legs between the parent's legs (Fig. 45-11). If the child must remain supine, have the parent (or assistant) on one side of the bed and lean over the child's upper body to apply restraint, using the hand to hold the arm for the venipuncture. Have the operator stand on the other side of the bed for access to the arm for venipuncture.

Lumbar Puncture

The technique for lumbar puncture (LP) in infants and children is similar to that in the adult, although modifications are suggested in neonates, who have less distress in a side-lying position with modified neck extension than in flexion or a sitting position (Fig. 45-12, *A*). Neonates tend to have more cardiorespiratory changes during an LP than older infants regardless of positioning; therefore oximetry and heart rate monitoring are advisable (Lehmann et al, 1990). Pediatric LP sets contain smaller spinal needles, but sometimes the practitioner will specify a particular size or type of needle that the nurse should make certain is placed on the tray.

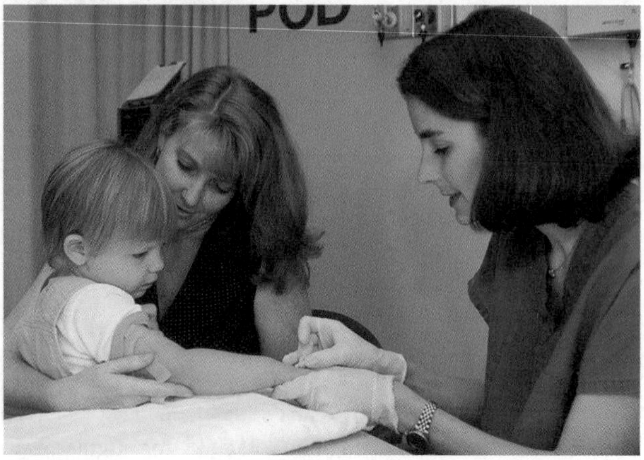

Fig. 45-11 Therapeutic hugging of child for extremity vein puncture with parental assistance.

Children should receive adequate analgesia or anesthesia to relieve pain. EMLA, a mixture of a local and topical anesthetic in a cream form, should be applied before the LP.

Children are usually controlled best in the side-lying position, with the head flexed and the knees drawn up toward the chest. Even cooperative children need to be restrained to prevent possible trauma from unexpected, involuntary movement. They can be reassured that although they are trusted, the holding will serve as a reminder to maintain the desired position. It also provides a measure of support and reassurance to them.

The child is placed on the side with the back close to the edge of the examining table on the side from which the practitioner is working. The nurse maintains the child's spine in a flexed position by holding the child with one arm behind the neck and the other behind the thighs (Fig. 45-12, *B*). The flexed position enlarges the spaces between the lumbar vertebral spines, which facilitates access to the spinal fluid space. It is helpful to wrap the legs before positioning to decrease leg movement.

An alternative position used with small infants and some older children is the sitting position. The child is placed with the buttocks at the edge of the table and with the neck flexed so that the chin rests on the chest or the nurse's arm. The infant's arms and legs are immobilized by the nurse's hands (Fig. 45-12, *C*).

NURSE ALERT The sitting position may interfere with chest expansion and diaphragm excursion, and in infants the soft, pliable trachea may collapse. Therefore observe the child for difficulty with breathing. ■

Another position that employs close and comforting contact for the child involves holding the child upright against the nurse's (or parent's) chest with the child's legs wrapped around the adult's waist. The adult's arms are used to hug and restrain the child. For ease of the examiner, the adult should be standing. A small pillow is placed between the child's abdomen and the adult to help arch the child's back. If the pillow proves unsuccessful, a third person can place an arm in this space to achieve the desired position. Care should be taken that excessive pressure does not compromise circulation or breathing and that the nose and mouth are not covered by the restrainer's body.

Specimens and spinal fluid pressure are obtained, measured, and sent for analysis in the same manner as for the adult patient. Vital signs are taken as ordered, and the child is observed for any changes in level of consciousness, motor activity, or other neurologic signs. Post-LP headache may occur and is related to postural changes; this is less severe when the child lies flat. Headache is seen much less frequently in young children than in adolescents.

Bone Marrow Aspiration or Biopsy

Positioning for a bone marrow aspiration or biopsy depends on the location of the chosen site. In children the posterior or anterior iliac crest is most frequently used, although in infants the tibia may be selected because of easy access to the site and holding of the child.

If the posterior iliac crest is used, the child is positioned prone. Sometimes a small pillow or folded blanket is placed

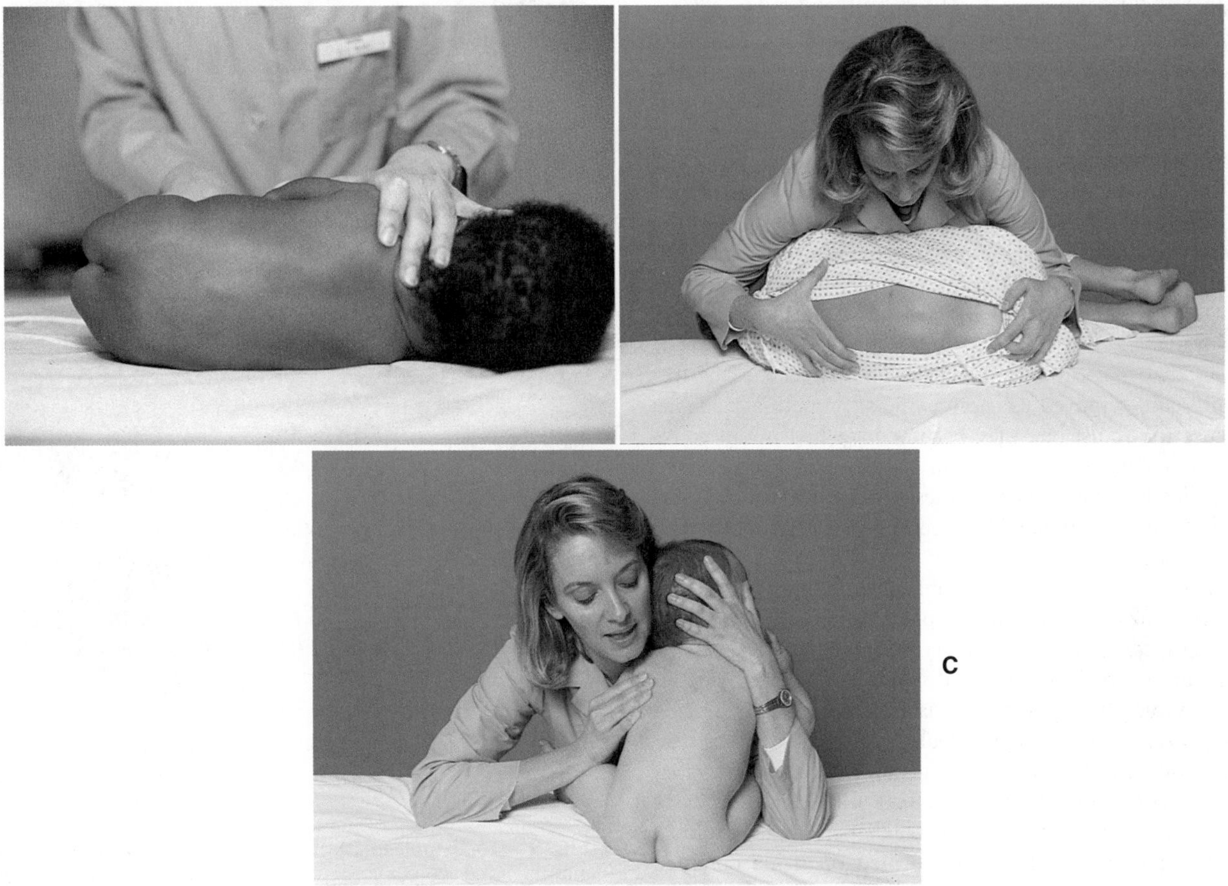

A B C

Fig. 45-12 **A**, Modified side-lying position for lumbar puncture. **B**, Older child in side-lying position. **C**, Infant sitting position allows for flexion of lumbar spine.

under the hips to facilitate obtaining the bone marrow specimen. Children should receive adequate analgesia or anesthesia to relieve pain. If the child awakens, holding may be needed, and is best done with two people—one person to immobilize the upper body and a second person to immobilize the lower extremities.

Other Procedures

For subdural puncture through a fontanel or burr hole, the infant is wrapped in a mummy restraint and placed in the supine position with the head accessible to the examiner. To control the head, the nurse uses a firm hold on each side of it. Procedures for immobilizing the head for examining the ears, nose, or throat are discussed in Chapter 35.

COLLECTION OF SPECIMENS

Urine Specimens

When children are admitted to the hospital or are seen in a clinic or office, a urine specimen may be needed. Older children and adolescents can use a bedpan or urinal or can be trusted to follow directions for collection in the bathroom. However, attention to their special needs and concerns is warranted. School-age children are cooperative but curious. They are likely to ask questions regarding the disposition of their specimen and what one expects to discover from it. Self-conscious adolescents may be reluctant to carry a specimen bottle through a hallway or waiting room and appreciate a paper bag or other means for disguising the container. The presence of menses is sometimes an embarrassment or a concern to teenage girls; therefore it is a good idea to ask if they are menstruating and to make adjustments as necessary. The specimen can be delayed, or a notation made on the laboratory slip to explain the presence of red blood cells.

Preschoolers and toddlers are usually unable to void on request. It is often best to offer them water or other liquids that they enjoy and wait about 30 minutes until they are ready to void voluntarily or to set a timer to alert them that they need to void shortly. The child will better understand what is expected if the nurse uses familiar terms, such as "pee-pee," "wee-wee," "tee-tee," or "tinkle." Some children will have difficulty voiding in an unfamiliar receptacle. Potty chairs or a potty hat placed on the toilet will usually prove satisfactory. Toddlers who have recently acquired bladder control may be especially reluctant, because they undoubtedly have been admonished for "going" in places other than those approved by parents. A useful approach is to enlist the help of parents; they are likely to be successful, and this helps them feel that they are a part of the child's care.

For infants and toddlers who are not toilet trained, special urine collection devices may be used. These devices are clear, plastic, single-use bags with self-adhering material around the opening at the point of attachment. To prepare the infant, the genitalia, perineum, and surrounding skin are washed and dried thoroughly, because the adhesive will not stick to a moist, powdered, or oily skin surface. The collection bag is easiest to apply if attached first to the perineum, progressing to the symphysis (Fig. 45-13). With little girls the perineum is stretched taut during application to that area to ensure a leakproof fit. With small boys the penis and scrotum are placed inside the bag. The adhesive portion of the bag must be firmly applied to the skin all around the genital area to avoid possible leakage. For low-birth-weight infants, small bags with adhesive that is gentle to the skin are available.* Anatomically correct urine collection bags are also available.†

The diaper is carefully replaced. The bag is checked frequently and removed as soon as the specimen is available, because the moist bag may become loosened on an active child. When urine is collected for culture, the bag is removed immediately. If the urine is not tested within 30 minutes, the specimen is refrigerated or placed in a sterile container with a preservative.

Urine obtained from disposable diapers can be tested accurately for glucose, ketones, protein, blood, bilirubin, urobilinogen, nitrates, potassium, creatinine, and urea. In one study, urine obtained from a disposable diaper provided a valid sample for diagnosing urinary tract infections (Cohen et al, 1997). Erythrocyte and leukocyte counts may be low. Superabsorbent disposable diapers may produce a false crystalluria. Specific gravity measurements are accurate for up to 4 hours provided that the disposable diapers are kept folded. The accuracy of these tests performed on urine obtained from cloth diapers is unknown. Urine samples collected by the cotton ball method were accurate for pH and specific gravity and were atraumatic to the skin of newborns (Burke, 1995). Traditionally, specific gravity refractometers have been used on nursing units to measure specific gravity. One study showed strong agreement between the use of a refractometer and regeant strip to test urine specific gravity (Barton & Holmes, 1998). However, current regulations have limited the refractometer's use to the laboratory. Urine dipsticks can be used on the nursing unit with reasonable accuracy.

At times parents may be requested to bring a urine sample to a health care facility for examination, especially when infants are unable to void during an outpatient visit. In this instance parents need instruction on applying the collection device and storage of the specimen. Ideally, the specimen should be brought to the designated place as soon as possible; if there is a delay, the sample is refrigerated and the elapsed time reported to the examiner.

Clean-Catch Specimens

The term *clean-catch specimen* traditionally refers to a urine sample obtained for culture after the urethral meatus is cleaned and the first few milliliters of urine are voided before the urine is collected *(midstream specimen)*. The procedure consists of cleaning the perineum or tip of the penis with a soap- or antiseptic-soaked sterile pad in males and of wiping from front to back only once with each pad in females. This is repeated at least two times. The area may be wiped with sterile water to prevent accidental contamination of the urine with a solution that may destroy the pathogens, although minute amounts of antiseptic such as iodine do not alter bacterial counts.

*Available from Hollister, Inc., 2000 Hollister Dr., Libertyville, IL 60048; 1-800-323-4060; Web site: www.hollister.com.

†Available from ConvaTec, CN 5254, Princeton, NJ 08543-5254; phone: 1-800-422-8811; Web site: www.convatec.com.

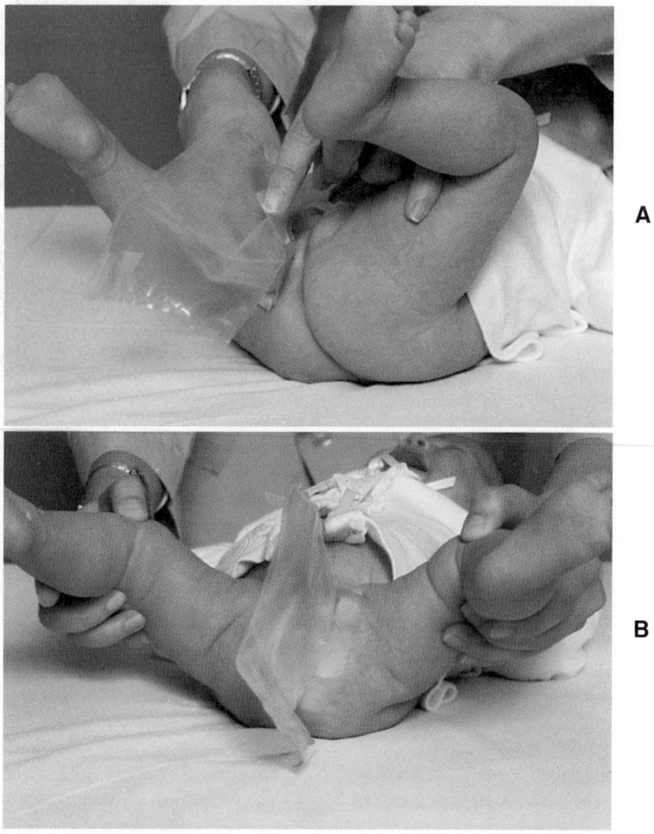

Fig. 45-13 Application of urine collection bag. **A,** On female infants, adhesive portion is applied to exposed and dried perineum first. **B,** Bag adheres firmly around perineal area to prevent urine leakage.

Although this traditional cleansing procedure is often practiced, studies have found that it does not significantly reduce contamination rates in infants, circumcised or uncircumcised males, or toilet-trained prepubertal children. Also, midstream collection does not significantly reduce contamination rates over nonmidstream specimens (Prandoni et al, 1996).

Twenty-Four–Hour Collection

Collection of urine voided over a 24-hour period creates a special challenge in infants and children. Collection bags are required to collect specimens from infants and small children. Older children require special instruction about notifying someone when they need to void or have a bowel movement so that urine can be collected separately and not discarded. Some older school-age children and adolescents can be trusted to take responsibility for collection of their own 24-hour specimens. They can keep output records and transfer each voiding to the 24-hour collection container if this is permitted.

As in any 24-hour urine collection, the collection period always starts and ends with an empty bladder. At the time the collection begins, the child is instructed to void and the specimen is discarded. All urine voided in the subsequent 24 hours is saved in a container with a preservative or is refrigerated or placed on ice. Twenty-four hours from the time the precollection specimen was discarded, the child is again instructed to void, the specimen is added to the container, and the entire collection is taken to the laboratory for examination.

Infants and small children who need a 24-hour urine collection require a special collection bag; frequent removal and replacement of adhesive collection devices can produce skin irritation. A thin coating of sealant, such as Skin-Prep, applied to the skin helps protect it and aids adhesion, unless its use is contraindicated, such as in a premature infant or a child with irritated skin. Plastic collection bags with collection tubes attached are ideal when the container must be left in place for a time. These can be connected to a collecting device or emptied periodically by aspiration with a syringe. When such devices are not available, a regular bag with a feeding tube inserted through a puncture hole at the top of the bag serves as a satisfactory substitute. However, care must be taken to empty the bag as soon as the infant urinates to prevent leakage and loss of contents. An indwelling catheter may also be placed for the collection period.

Bladder Catheterization and Other Techniques

Bladder catheterization or *suprapubic aspiration* is employed when a specimen is urgently needed or when the child is unable to void or otherwise provide an adequate specimen. Catheterization is used to obtain a sterile urine specimen and when urethral obstruction or anuria caused by renal failure is believed to be the cause of the child's failure to void. Suprapubic aspiration is useful in clarifying the diagnosis of suspected urinary tract infection in acutely ill infants.

The anxiety, fear, and discomfort experienced during catheterization can be significantly alleviated by adequate preparation of the child and parents, by selection of the correct catheter, and by the appropriate technique of insertion. Specifically, generous lubrication of the urethra before catheterization and use of a lubricant containing 2% lidocaine (Xylocaine) may significantly reduce or eliminate the burning and discomfort frequently associated with this invasive procedure.

NURSE ALERT Identify patients who have allergies to povidone-iodine or latex before using these items in catheterization. ■

Adolescent boys and children with a history of urethral surgery may be catheterized with a coudé-tipped catheter. The child with myelodysplasia or one who has been identified as being sensitive or allergic to latex is catheterized with a catheter or feeding tube manufactured of an alternative material. When an indwelling catheter is indicated for urinary drainage, a lubricious or silicone catheter is selected because these materials produce less irritation of the urethral mucosa as compared with a Silastic or latex catheter when the catheter is left in place for more than 72 hours.

A 2% lidocaine lubricant with applicator is assembled according to the manufacturer's instructions, and several drops of the lubricant are placed at the meatus. The child is advised that the lubricant is used to reduce any discomfort associated with inserting the catheter and that introduction of the lubricant into the urethra will produce a sensation of pressure and a desire to urinate (Gray, 1996).

Suprapubic aspiration, which is performed by a practitioner skilled in the procedure, involves aspirating bladder contents by inserting a 20- or 21-gauge needle in the midline approximately 1 cm above the symphysis pubis and directed vertically downward. The skin is prepared as for any needle insertion, and the bladder should contain an adequate volume of urine. This can be assumed if the infant has not voided for at least 1 hour or the bladder can be palpated above the symphysis pubis. This technique is useful for obtaining sterile specimens from young infants, because the bladder is an abdominal organ and is easily accessed. Suprapubic aspiration is painful, and therefore pain management during the procedure is important (Atraumatic Care box and Cultural Awareness box).

Stool Specimens

Stool specimens are frequently collected in children to identify parasites and other organisms that cause diarrhea, to assess gastrointestinal function, and to check for occult (hidden) blood. Ideally, stool should be collected without

Atraumatic Care

BLADDER CATHETERIZATION OR SUPRAPUBIC ASPIRATION

Use distraction to help the child relax (blowing bubbles, deep breathing, singing a song).

Use lidocaine jelly to anesthetize the area before insertion of catheter (see text). EMLA cream may lessen an infant's discomfort as the needle passes through the skin for suprapubic aspiration, but care should be taken that the site is thoroughly cleaned and prepped before the procedure.

Have the parent sit in a chair or on an examining table with a back support. Next, place the child leaning back in the parent's lap with the parent's arms hugging the child's upper body. Then place the child's legs in the frog position with the parent's legs over the child's to stabilize them. In this comfortable position, the perineum or lower abdomen is exposed for the procedure.

Children often become agitated at being restrained for either procedure. Use comfort measures through touch and voice, both during and after the procedure, to help reduce the child's distress.

Cultural Awareness

BLADDER CATHETERIZATION

Parents may be upset when their child is catheterized. Aside from the trauma the child experiences, some parents, especially those from different cultures, may fear that the procedure affects the daughter's virginity. To correct this misconception, the family may benefit from a detailed explanation of the genitourinary anatomy, preferably with a model that shows the separate vaginal and urethral openings. The nurse can also indicate that catheterization has no effect on virginity.

contamination with urine, but in children wearing diapers this is difficult unless a urine bag is applied. Children who are toilet trained should urinate first; flush the toilet; and then defecate in the toilet, a bedpan (preferably one that is placed on the toilet to avoid embarrassment), or a commercial potty hat.

Stool specimens should be large enough to obtain an ample sampling, not merely a fecal fragment. Specimens are placed in an appropriate container, which is covered and labeled. If several specimens are needed, the containers are marked with the date and time and kept in a specimen refrigerator. Special care is exercised in handling the specimen because of the risk of contamination.

Blood Specimens

Although most blood specimens are obtained by the laboratory staff, nurses are increasingly responsible for specimen collection, especially if the child has an arterial or venous device. However, whether the specimen is collected by the nurse or others, the nurse is responsible for making certain that specimens, such as serial examinations and fasting specimens, are collected on time and that the proper equipment is available, such as correct collection tubes and ice for blood gas samples. Collection, transportation, and storage of specimens can have a major impact on laboratory results (Frizzell, 1998).

Venous blood samples can be obtained by venipuncture or by aspiration from a peripheral or central access device. Withdrawing blood specimens through peripheral lock devices in small peripheral veins has met with varying degrees of success. Although it avoids an additional venipuncture for the child, attempting to aspirate blood from the peripheral lock may shorten the life of the device. When using an IV infusion site for specimen collection, it is important to consider the type of fluid being infused. For example, a specimen collected for glucose determination would be inaccurate if removed from a catheter through which glucose-containing solution were being administered.

To obtain a blood specimen from a central venous line or peripheral lock when the infusion solution may interfere with tests results, first aspirate a quantity of blood equal to the volume of fluid in the catheter and discard; then aspirate the blood sample.

For a blood culture, use the first sample of blood, because organisms are most likely to collect within the catheter itself.

NURSE ALERT On small or anemic children, keep track of the amount drawn and discarded over time. Frequent taking of blood specimens can rapidly decrease a child's blood volume. Coordinate blood samples and ask the laboratory to save blood as much as possible to reduce the frequency. ■

Arterial blood samples are sometimes needed for blood gas measurement, although noninvasive techniques, such as transcutaneous oxygen/carbon dioxide monitoring and pulse oximetry, are used frequently. Arterial samples may be obtained by arteriopuncture using the radial, brachial, or femoral arteries; by deep heel puncture; or from indwelling arterial catheters (Harrison et al, 1997). Adequate circulation should be assessed before arterial puncture by observing capillary refill or performing the *Allen test,* a procedure that assesses the circulation of the radial, ulnar, or brachial arteries. Because unclotted blood is required, only heparinized collection tubes are used. In addition, no air bubbles should enter the tube, because they can alter blood gas concentration. Crying, fear, and agitation also affect blood gas values; therefore every effort is made to comfort the child. The blood samples are packed in ice to reduce blood cell metabolism and are taken to the laboratory for immediate analysis.

Capillary blood samples are taken from children by a finger or earlobe stick, just as in the adult patient. A common method for taking peripheral blood samples from infants is by a heel stick. Before the blood sample is taken, the heel is warmed with warm, moist compresses for 5 to 10 minutes to dilate the vessels in the area. Although this is a well-accepted practice, one study questioned its effectiveness. In a study of healthy full-term infants, warming the heel with a warm gel pack (40° C [104° F]) for 10 minutes before capillary blood sampling with an automated device (Autolet) did not significantly decrease the sampling time required (Barker et al, 1996).

The area is cleansed with alcohol, and with the infant's foot firmly restrained with the free hand, the heel is punctured with a blade or an automatic lancet device. An automatic device, such as Tenderfoot* or Autolet, delivers a more precise puncture depth and is a less painful puncture than that achieved with a blade or lance (McIntosh, van Veen, & Brameyer, 1994; Vertanen et al, 2001). Although obtaining capillary blood gases is a common practice, some practitioners believe that these measures may not accurately reflect arterial values.

The most serious complication of infant heel puncture is necrotizing osteochondritis from lancet penetration of the underlying calcaneus bone. To avoid this, the puncture should be no deeper than 2.4 mm and should be made at the outer aspect of the heel. The boundaries of the calcaneus can be marked by an imaginary line extending posteriorly from a point between the fourth and fifth toes and running parallel to the lateral aspect of the heel and another line extending posteriorly from the middle of the great toe and running parallel to the medial aspect of the heel (Fig. 45-14).

The needed specimens are collected quickly, and then pressure is applied to the puncture site with a dry gauze square until bleeding stops. The arm is kept extended, not flexed, while pressure is applied for a few minutes after venipuncture in the antecubital fossa to reduce bruising. The site is then covered with an adhesive bandage. In young children, adhesive bandages pose an aspiration hazard; their use should be avoided or the adhesive bandage should be removed as soon as the bleeding stops. Applying warm compresses to ecchymotic areas increases circulation, helps remove extravasated blood, and decreases pain.

No matter how or by whom the specimen is collected, children, even some older ones, fear the loss of their blood. This is particularly true for children whose condition requires frequent blood specimens. They mistakenly believe

*Available from International Technidyne Corporation, 8 Olsen Ave., Edison, NJ 08820; phone: 732-548-5700 or 800-631-5945; Web site: www.itemed.com.

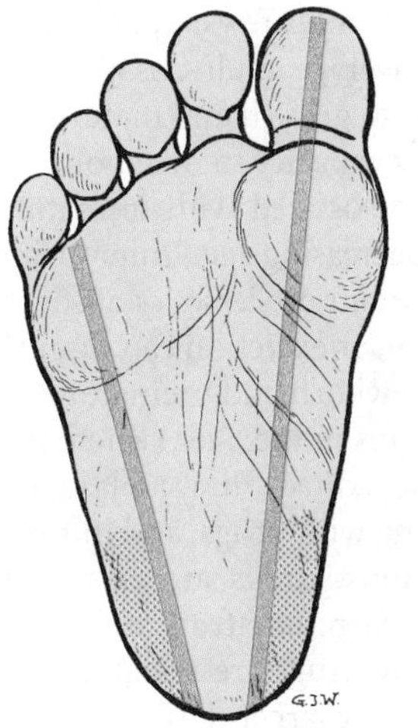

Fig. 45-14 Puncture site *(colored stippled area)* on sole of infant's foot.

that blood removed from their bodies is a threat to their lives. Explaining to them that their blood is continually being produced by their bodies provides them with a measure of reassurance regarding this aspect of the stress-provoking procedure. When the blood is drawn, a simple comment, such as "Just look how red it is. You're really making a lot of nice red blood," confirms this information and affords them an opportunity to express their concern. Covering the puncture site with an adhesive bandage strip gives them added assurance that the vital fluids will not leak out.

Children also dislike the discomfort associated with venous, arterial, or capillary punctures. In fact, children have identified these procedures as the ones most frequently causing pain during hospitalization and arterial puncture as being one of the most painful of all procedures experienced (Wong & Baker, 1988). Consequently, nurses need to institute pain reduction techniques to lessen the discomfort of these procedures (Atraumatic Care box). Younger children are more distressed by venipuncture than are older children.

Atraumatic Care

GUIDELINES FOR SKIN/VESSEL PUNCTURES

To Reduce the Pain Associated with Heel, Finger, Venous, or Arterial Punctures:

Apply EMLA topically over the site if time permits (at least 60 minutes). To remove the Tegaderm dressing atraumatically, grasp opposite sides of the film and pull the sides away from each other to stretch and loosen the film. After the film begins to loosen, grasp the other two sides of the film and pull. Use iontophoresis (Numby Stuff) over the site if time permits (8 to 20 minutes, depending on the amount of current), a vapocoolant spray, or buffered lidocaine (injected intradermally near the vein with a 30-gauge needle) to numb the skin.

Use nonpharmacologic methods of pain and anxiety control (e.g., ask child to take a deep breath when the needle is inserted and again when the needle is withdrawn; have child exhale a large breath or blow bubbles to "blow hurt away"; ask child to count slowly and then faster and louder if pain is felt).

Keep all equipment out of sight until used.

Enlist parents' presence and assistance if they wish to participate.

Restrain child *only as needed* to perform the procedure safely; use therapeutic hugging (p. 1381).

Allow the skin preparation to dry completely before penetrating the skin.

Use the smallest-gauge needle (e.g., 25 gauge) that permits free flow of blood; a 27-gauge needle can be used for obtaining 1 to 1.5 ml of blood and for prominent veins (needle length is only ½ inch).

Avoid putting an intravenous (IV) line in the dominant hand or the hand the child uses to suck the thumb.

Use an automatic lancet device for precise puncture depth of the finger or heel; press the device lightly against the skin and avoid steadying the finger against a hard surface.

Emphasize that blood entering the syringe or tube does not hurt. Reassure young children that you did not "take their blood" away and that they have a lot more inside.

Place a small bandage over the puncture site to make removal easy and less painful and to reassure young children that "their blood will not leak out."*

Have a "two try only" policy to reduce excessive insertion attempts—two operators each have two insertion attempts; if insertion is not successful after four punctures, consider alternative venous access, such as a peripherally inserted central catheter (PICC); have a policy for identifying children with difficult access and appropriate interventions (e.g., most experienced operator for the first attempt).†

For Multiple Blood Samples:

Use an intermittent infusion device (saline or heparin lock) to collect additional samples from an existing IV line; consider PICC lines early, not as a last resort. Preferably, use a saline flush for a catheter larger than 24 gauge (less painful, compatible with drugs, and less costly).

Coordinate care to allow several tests to be performed on one blood sample using micromethods of testing.

Anticipate tests (e.g., drug levels, chemistry, immunoglobulin levels) and ask the laboratory to save blood for additional testing.

For Heel Lancing in Newborns:

Heel lancing has been shown to be more painful than venipuncture (Larsson et al, 1998); consider venipuncture when the amount of blood from the heel would require much squeezing (e.g., genetic screening tests).

The effectiveness of EMLA is controversial, although application of 0.5 g for 30 minutes four times a day in preterm infants was found to be safe (Essink-Tebbes et al, 1999).

Place diapered newborn against mother's bare chest in skin-to-skin contact 10 to 15 minutes before and during heel lance (Gray, Watt, & Blass, 2000).

During the procedure, allow newborn to suck a pacifier coated with a slurry of sugar and water; to make an approximate 24% sucrose solution, add 1 teaspoon of table sugar to 4 teaspoons of sterile water. Use this solution to coat the pacifier or administer 2 ml to the tongue 2 minutes before the procedure (Blass & Watt, 1999).

*Contrary to popular belief, a study of children ages 3 to 6 years found that asking them not to look at the finger stick to avoid the sight of blood or applying a decorated bandage did not lessen their rating of pain intensity (Johnston, Stevens, & Arbess, 1993).

†For an example of one hospital's guidelines for reducing excessive IV insertion attempts, see Catudal (1999).

Respiratory Secretions and Throat Specimens

Collection of sputum or nasal discharge is sometimes required for diagnosis of respiratory infections, especially tuberculosis and respiratory syncytial virus (RSV). Older children and adolescents are able to cough as directed and supply sputum specimens when given proper directions. It must be made clear to them that a coughed specimen is needed, not mucus that is cleared from the throat. It is helpful to demonstrate a deep cough so that communication is clear. Infants and small children are unable to follow directions to cough and will swallow any sputum produced; therefore *gastric washings (lavage)* may be used to collect a sputum specimen. Sometimes it is possible to obtain a satisfactory specimen by using a suction device such as a mucous trap if the catheter is inserted into the trachea and the cough reflex is elicited. A catheter that is inserted into the back of the throat is not sufficient. For children with a tracheostomy, a specimen is easily aspirated from the trachea or major bronchi by attaching a collecting device to the suction apparatus.

Nasal washings are usually obtained to diagnose an infection of RSV. The child is placed supine, and 1 to 3 ml of sterile normal saline is instilled with a sterile syringe (without needle) into one nostril. The contents are aspirated using a small, sterile bulb syringe and are placed in a sterile container. To prevent any additional discomfort to the child, all of the equipment should be ready before the procedure is begun.

Other respiratory secretion collection methods include nasopharyngeal swabs to diagnose *Bordetella pertussis* and throat cultures. The nurse swabs both the tonsils and the posterior pharynx when obtaining a throat culture. The swab stick is inserted into the culture tube. Some culture kits require squeezing an ampule to release the culture medium.

NURSE ALERT Do not attempt to obtain a throat culture if acute epiglottitis is suspected. The trauma from the swab may increase edema, possibly occluding the airway. ■

ADMINISTRATION OF MEDICATION

Preparation for Safe Administration

The safe administration of medication to children presents a number of problems that are not encountered when giving medication to adult patients. Children vary widely in age; weight; body surface area; and the ability to absorb, metabolize, and excrete medications. Nurses must be particularly alert when computing and administering drugs to infants and children.

Determination of Drug Dosage

It is the physician's responsibility to prescribe drugs in the correct dosage to achieve the desired effect without endangering the health of the child. However, nurses must have an understanding of the safe dosage of medications they administer to children, as well as the expected action, possible side effects, and signs of toxicity (Kennedy, 1996). Unlike with adult medications, there are few standardized pediatric dosage ranges, and with a few exceptions, drugs are prepared and packaged in average adult-dosage strengths.

Factors related to growth and maturation significantly alter an individual's capacity to metabolize and excrete drugs, and deficiencies associated with immaturity become more important with decreasing age. Immaturity or defects in any or all of the important processes of absorption, distribution, biotransformation, or excretion can significantly alter the effects of a drug. Newborn and premature infants with immature enzyme systems in the liver (where most drugs are broken down and detoxified), lower plasma concentrations of protein for binding with drugs, and immaturely functioning kidneys (where most drugs are excreted) are particularly vulnerable to the harmful effects of drugs. Beyond the newborn period, many drugs are metabolized more rapidly by the liver, necessitating larger doses or more frequent administration. This is particularly important in pain control, when the dosage may need to be increased or the interval between administering analgesics may need to be decreased.

Various formulas involving age, weight, and body surface area as the basis for calculations have been devised to determine children's drug dosage from a standard adult dose. Because the administration of medication is a nursing responsibility, nurses need not only a knowledge of drug action and patient responses, but also some resources for estimating safe dosages for children. The method most often used to determine children's dosage is based on a specific dose per kilogram of body weight, such as 0.1 mg/kg.

The most reliable method for determining children's dosage is to calculate the proportional amount of *body surface area (BSA)* to body weight. The ratio of BSA to weight varies inversely with length; therefore the infant who is shorter and weighs less than an older child or adult has relatively more surface area than would be expected from the weight. The usual determination of BSA requires the use of the *West nomogram* (Fig. 45-15). The BSA is estimated from the height and weight of the child.

Checking Dosage

Administering the correct dosage of a drug is a shared responsibility between the practitioner who orders the drug and the nurse who carries out that order. Children react with unexpected severity to some drugs, and ill children are especially sensitive to drugs. Therefore checking the dose if any doubt exists about its accuracy is a professional duty. When a dose is ordered that is outside the usual range or if there is some question regarding the preparation or the route of administration, the nurse should always check with the prescribing practitioner before proceeding with the administration, because the nurse is legally liable for any drug administered.

Administering some medications requires added safeguards. Even when it has been determined that the dosage is correct for a particular child, many drugs are potentially hazardous or lethal. Most hospital units or other facilities where medications are given to children have regulations requiring that specified drugs be double-checked by another nurse before they are given to the child. Among drugs that require such safeguards are digoxin, heparin, chemotherapeutic agents, and insulin. Others frequently included are

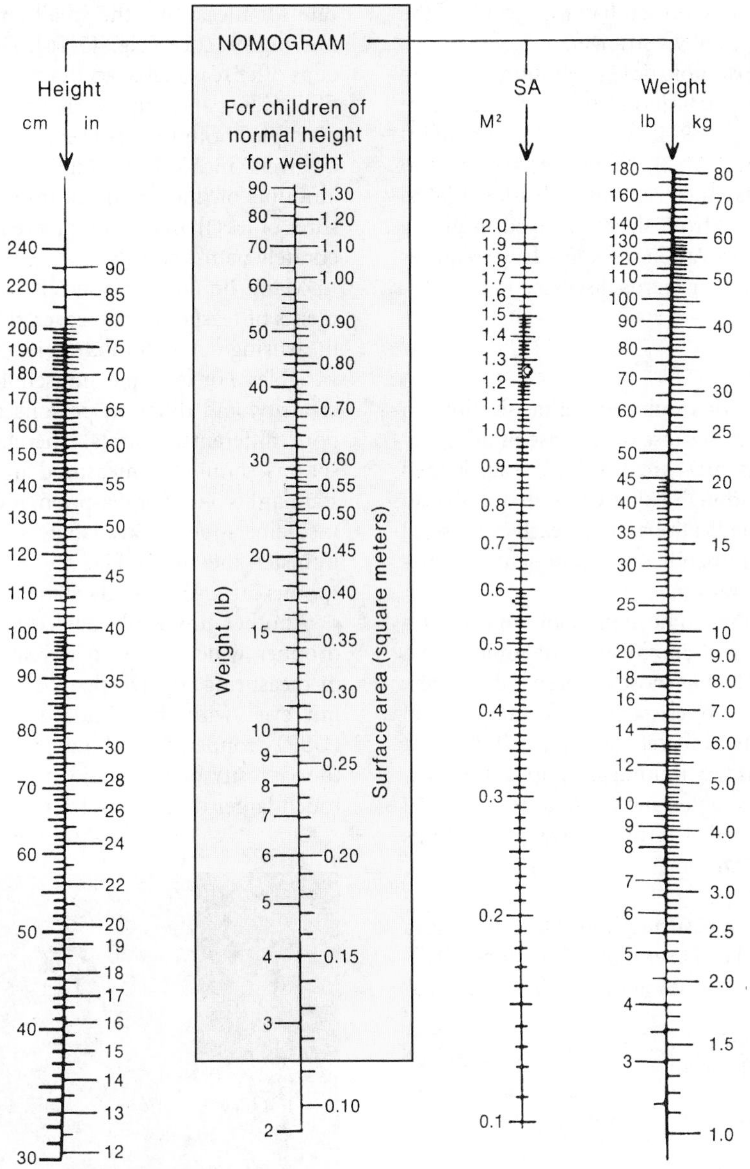

Fig. 45-15 West nomogram for estimation of surface areas. *Surface area* is indicated where a straight line connecting height and weight intersects surface area (SA) column or, if patient is approximately of normal proportion, from weight alone *(yellow area).* (Nomogram modified from data of E. Boyd by C. D. West; from Behrman RE, Kleigman RM, Jenson HB [eds]: *Nelson textbook of pediatrics,* ed 17, Philadelphia, 2000, WB Saunders.)

epinephrine, opioids, and sedatives. Even if this precaution is not mandatory, nurses are wise to take such precautions for their own sense of security. Errors in decimal point placement may easily occur and may result in a tenfold or more dosage error.

Identification

Before the administration of any medication, the child must be correctly identified, because children are not totally reliable in giving correct names on request. Infants are unable to give their name, a toddler or preschooler may admit to any name, and school-age children may deny their identity in an attempt to avoid the medication. Children sometimes exchange beds during play. Parents may be present to identify their child, but the only safe method for identifying children is to check their hospital identification band with the labeled medication or medication card. Two identifiers are required before medication administration. Identifiers include name, medical record number, and birth date.

Family Aspects

Parents can be useful sources of information regarding the child and his or her capabilities. Nearly all parents have given some kind of medication to their child and can describe approaches that they have found to be successful. In some cases it is less traumatic for the child if a parent gives the medication, provided that the nurse prepares the medication and supervises its administration and the practice is consistent with hospital or unit policy. Children being given daily medications at home are accustomed to the parent's functioning in this capacity and are less apt to object than they would if the medication were administered by a stranger.

Every child requires psychologic preparation for parenteral administration of medication and supportive care during the procedure (see p. 1397). Even if children have received several injections, they rarely become accustomed to the discomfort and have as much right as any other child to understanding and patience from those involved in giving the injection. Safe administration of any drug requires meticulous attention to the safeguards discussed here.

Oral Administration

SKILL: ADMINISTERING ORAL MEDICATIONS

The oral route is preferred for administering medications to children whenever possible. Because of the ease of administration of oral medications, most are dissolved or suspended in liquid preparations. Although some children are able to swallow or chew solid medications at an early age, solid preparations are not recommended for young children because of the danger of aspiration.

Most pediatric medications come in palatable and colorful preparations for added ease of administration. Some have a slightly unpleasant aftertaste, but most children will swallow these liquids with little if any resistance. The nurse should taste a minute amount of an oral preparation to ascertain if it is palatable or bitter. In this way legitimate complaints of dislike from the child can be accepted and the taste camouflaged whenever possible. Most pediatric units have preparations available for this purpose (Atraumatic Care box).

Preparation

Selecting a vehicle for measuring and administering a medication requires careful consideration. The devices available to measure medicines are not always sufficiently accurate for measuring the small amounts needed in pediatric nursing practice (Fig. 45-16). Disposable plastic calibrated cups offer reasonable accuracy in measuring moderate doses of liquids (paper cups are likely to have irregularly shaped or crumpled bottoms). However, the personal interpretation of a given measure is highly variable, and considerable amounts of thick medication may remain in the cup. Measures of less than a teaspoon are impossible to determine accurately with a cup.

Many liquid preparations are prescribed in measurements of teaspoons. However, the teaspoon is an inaccurate measuring device and is subject to error from a number of variables. For example, household teaspoons vary greatly in capacity, and different persons using the same spoon will pour different amounts. Therefore a drug ordered in teaspoons should be measured in milliliters; the established standard is 5 ml per teaspoon. A convenient hollow-handled medicine spoon is available to accurately measure and administer the drug (Fig. 45-16, *A*). Household *measuring* spoons can also be used when other devices are not available.

Another unreliable device for measuring liquids is the dropper, which varies to a greater extent than the teaspoon or measuring cup. Droppers are available in numerous sizes, but even with the standard United States Pharmacopeia (USP) dropper, the volume of a drop will vary according to the viscosity of the liquid measured; viscid fluids produce much larger drops than thin liquids. Many medications are

Atraumatic Care

ENCOURAGING A CHILD'S ACCEPTANCE OF ORAL MEDICATION

- Give child a flavored ice pop or small ice cube to suck to numb the tongue before giving the drug.
- Mix the drug with a small amount (about 1 teaspoon) of sweet-tasting substance, such as honey (except in infants because of the risk of botulism), flavored syrups, jam, fruit purees, sherbet, or ice cream; avoid essential food items, because the child may later refuse to eat them.
- Give a "chaser" of water, juice, soft drink, or ice pop or frozen juice bar after the drug.
- If nausea is a problem, give a carbonated beverage poured over finely crushed ice before or immediately after the medication.
- When medication has an unpleasant taste, have child pinch the nose and drink the medicine through a straw. Much of what we taste is associated with smell.
- Another alternative is to have the pharmacist prepare the drug in a flavored, chewable troche or lozenge.*
- Infants will suck medicine from a needleless syringe or dropper in small increments (0.25 to 0.50 ml) at a time. Use a nipple or special pacifier with a reservoir for the drug.

*For information about compounding drugs in troches, contact Technical Staff, Professional Compounding Centers of America (PCCA), PO Box 368, Sugarland, TX 77487; phone: 800-331-2498; Web site: www.thecompounders.com.

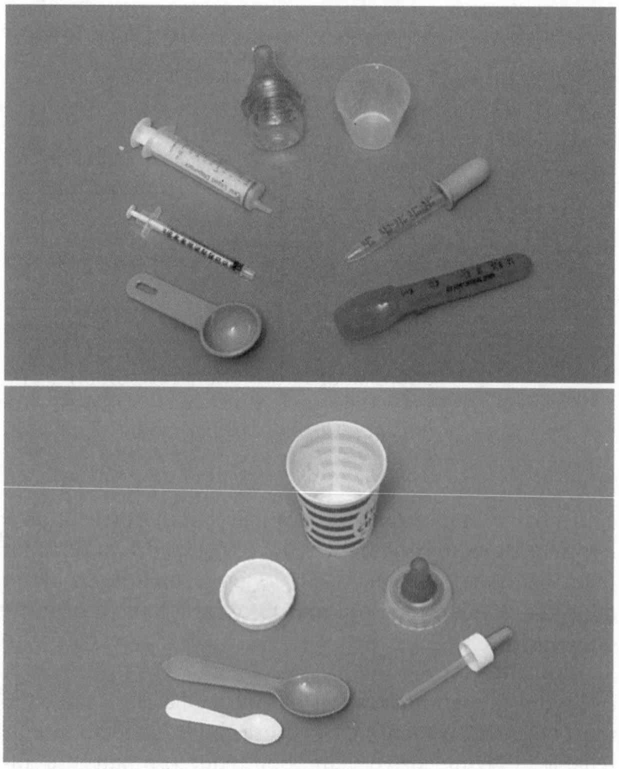

A

B

Fig. 45-16 **A,** Acceptable devices for measuring and administering oral medication to children *(clockwise):* measuring spoon, plastic syringes, calibrated nipple, plastic medicine cup, calibrated dropper, hollow-handled medicine spoon. **B,** Acceptable devices only for administering premeasured oral medication *(clockwise):* household teaspoons, paper cups, nipple, uncalibrated dropper.

supplied with caps or droppers designed for measuring each specific preparation. These are accurate when used to measure that specific medication but are not reliable for measuring other liquids. Emptying dropper contents into a medicine cup invites additional error. Because some of the liquid clings to the sides of the cup, a significant amount of the drug can be lost.

NURSE ALERT Many pediatric medications are given by drops or dropper. A misunderstanding of these terms by parents can result in a potential overdose. In addition, many droppers that come with medications are marked in tenths of cubic centimeters. If a parent were to use a syringe instead of the dropper, 0.4 cc may be thought to be the same as 4 cc. Provide education to parents on correct methods for giving medication. Demonstrate the technique. ■

The most accurate means for measuring small amounts of medication is the disposable plastic (never glass) syringe, especially the tuberculin syringe for volumes less than 1 ml. Not only does the syringe provide a reliable measure, but it also serves as a convenient means for transporting and administering the medication. The medication can be placed directly into the child's mouth from the syringe. For added safety, a short length of flexible tubing can be placed on the tip of the syringe to prevent injury to the mouth, although the tubing must be completely emptied of medication.

Young children and some older children as well have difficulty swallowing tablets or pills. Because a number of drugs are not available in pediatric preparations, the tablet needs to be crushed before it can be given to these children. Commercial devices are available,* or simple methods can be employed for crushing tablets. Not all drugs can be crushed (e.g., medication with an enteric or protective coating or formulated for slow release).

Children who must take oral medication for an extended period can be taught to swallow tablets or capsules. Training sessions include using verbal instruction, demonstration, reinforcement of progressively swallowing larger candy/capsules, no attention for inappropriate behavior, and gradual withdrawal of guidance once children can swallow their medication.

Because pediatric doses often require dividing adult preparations of medication, the nurse may be faced with the dilemma of accurate dosage. With tablets, only those that are scored can be halved or quartered accurately. If the medication is soluble, the tablet or contents of a capsule can be mixed in a small, premeasured amount of liquid and the appropriate portion given. If half a dose is required, the tablet is dissolved in 5 ml of water or flavored liquid and 2.5 ml is given.

Administration

Although administering liquids to infants is relatively easy, the nurse must be careful to prevent aspiration. With the infant held in a semireclining position, the medication is placed in the mouth from a spoon, plastic cup, plastic dropper, or plastic syringe (without needle). The dropper or syringe is best placed along the side of the infant's tongue, with the contents administered slowly in small amounts, allowing the child to swallow between deposits.

In infants up to 11 months of age and children with neurologic impairments, blowing a small puff of air in the face frequently elicits a swallow reflex.

Medicine cups can be used effectively for older infants who are able to drink from a cup. Because of the natural outward tongue thrust in infancy, medications may need to be retrieved from the lips or chin and refed. Allowing the infant to suck medication that has been placed in an empty nipple or inserting the syringe or dropper into the side of the mouth, parallel to the nipple, while the infant nurses are other convenient methods for giving liquid medications to infants. Medication is not added to the infant's formula feeding. Dispose of any plastic covers that may be on the ends of syringes. These covers are small enough to be aspirated by young children.

The young child who refuses to cooperate or resists consistently despite explanation and encouragement may require mild physical coercion. If so, it is carried out quickly and carefully. Every effort is made to determine why the child resists, and the reasons for the coercion are explained to the child in such a way that the child will know that it is being carried out for his or her well-being and is not a form of punishment. There is always a risk in using even mildly forceful techniques. A crying child can aspirate a medication, particularly when lying on the back. If the nurse holds the child in the lap with the child's right arm behind the nurse, the left hand firmly grasped by the nurse's left hand, and the head securely restrained between the nurse's arm and body, the medication can be slowly poured into the mouth (Fig. 45-17).

Intramuscular Administration

Selecting the Syringe and Needle

The volume of medication prescribed for small children and the small amount of tissue for injection require that a syringe be selected that can measure very small amounts of solution. For volumes of less than 1 ml, the tuberculin syringe, calibrated in one-hundredth increments, is appropriate. Very minute doses may require the use of a 0.5 ml, low-dose syringe. These syringes with specially constructed needles minimize the possibility of inadvertently administering incorrect amounts of a drug because of *dead space,* which allows fluid to remain in the syringe and needle after the plunger is pushed completely forward. A minimum of 0.2 ml of solution remains in a standard needle hub; therefore when very small amounts of two drugs are combined in the syringe, such as mixtures of insulin, the ratio of the two drugs can be altered significantly. Measures that minimize the effect of dead space include the following: (1) when two drugs are combined in the syringe, always draw them up in the same order to maintain a consistent ratio between the drugs; (2) use the same brand of syringe (dead space may vary between brands); and (3) use one-piece syringe units (needle permanently attached to the syringe).

*Trademark Medical manufactures a pill crusher and has compiled a list of more than 190 medications that should not be crushed or chewed. Both are available from Trademark Medical, 1053 Headquarters Park, Fenton, MO 63026-2033; phone: 800-325-9044; Web site: www.trademarkmedical.com.

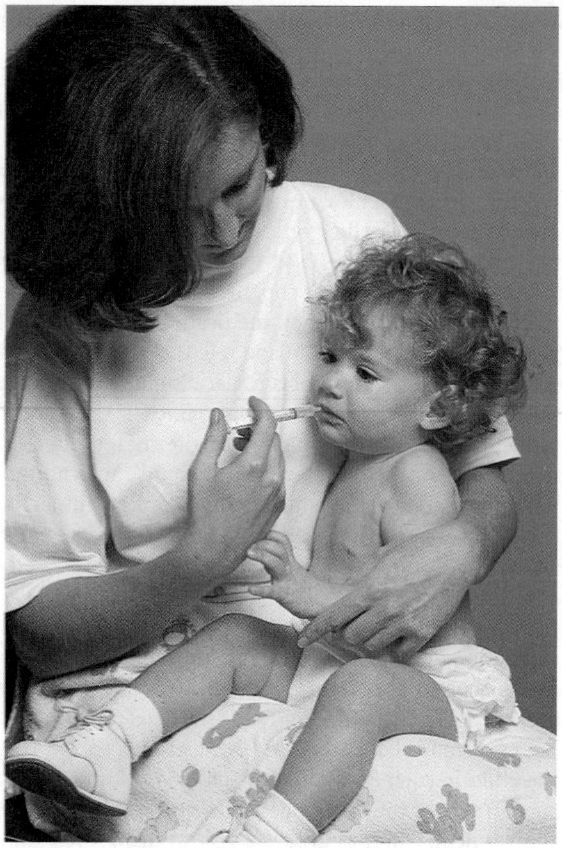

Fig. 45-17 Nurse partially restrains child for easy and comfortable administration of oral medication.

Dead space is also an important factor to consider when injecting medication, because flushing the syringe with an air bubble or parenteral fluid adds an additional amount of medication to the prescribed dose. This can be hazardous when very small amounts of a drug are given. For example, a tuberculin syringe filled to the 0.05 ml mark can deliver *more than twice* the calculated dose of medication when it is flushed with parenteral fluid from an IV line. Consequently, flushing is not advisable, especially when less than 1 ml of medication is given. Syringes are calibrated to deliver a prescribed drug dose, and the amount of medication left in the hub and needle is not part of the syringe barrel calibrations. However, the air-bubble technique (drawing up about 0.2 ml of air into the syringe after withdrawing the medication) may be beneficial with certain drugs, such as iron dextran and diphtheria and tetanus toxoid, to avoid tracking the drug through the tissue. Other techniques to minimize tracking include changing the needle after withdrawing the fluid from the vial (not always effective) and using the Z-track method.

The *needle length* must be sufficient to penetrate the subcutaneous tissue and deposit the medication in the body of the muscle. The needle gauge should be as small as possible to deliver fluid safely. Smaller-diameter (25- to 30-gauge) needles cause the least discomfort, but larger diameters are needed for viscous medication and prevention of accidental bending of longer needles (Table 45-3).

Based on ultrasonography, two injection techniques have been studied to determine the best needle length for the del-

Table 45-3

Intramuscular Injection Sites in Children

SITE	DISCUSSION
VASTUS LATERALIS 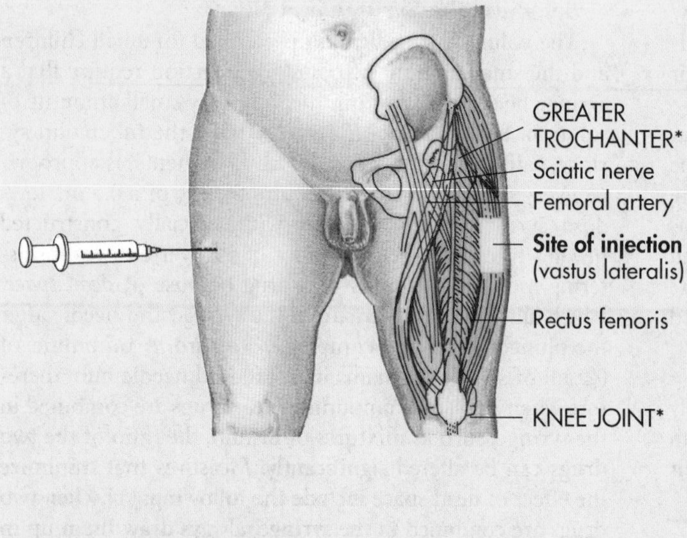 	**Location*** Palpate to find greater trochanter and knee joints; divide vertical distance between these two landmarks into thirds; inject into middle third **Needle insertion and size** Insert needle perpendicular to knee in infants and young children or perpendicular to thigh or slightly angled toward anterior thigh 22-25 gauge, 0.625-1 inch† **Advantages** Large, well-developed muscle that can tolerate larger quantities of fluid (0.5 ml [infant] to 2.0 ml [child]) Easily accessible if child is in supine, side-lying, or sitting position **Disadvantages** Thrombosis of femoral artery from injection in midthigh area Sciatic nerve damage from long needle injected posteriorly and medially into small extremity More painful than deltoid or gluteal sites

*Locations are indicated by asterisks on illustrations.

†Research has shown that a 1-inch needle is needed for adequate muscle penetration in infants 4 months old and possibly in infants as young as 2 months (Hicks et al, 1989).

Table 45-3

Intramuscular Injection Sites in Children—cont'd

SITE | DISCUSSION

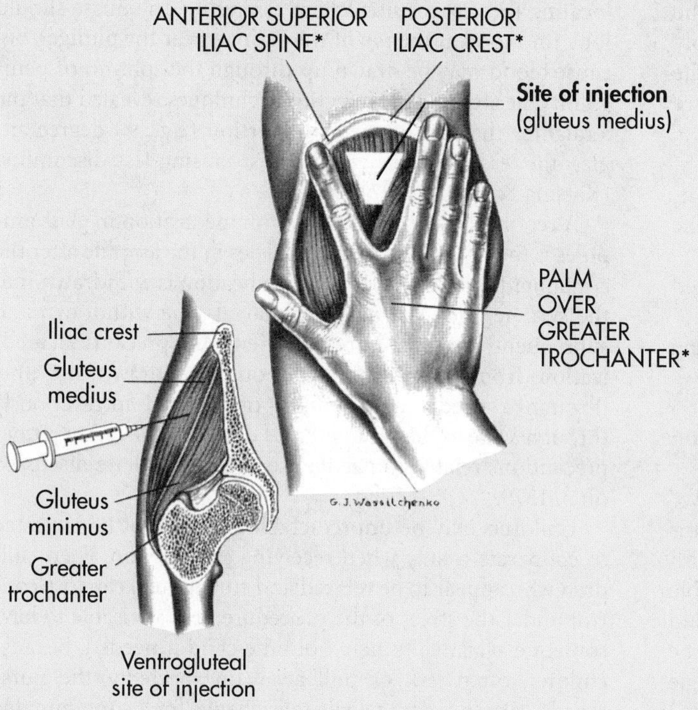

VENTROGLUTEAL

Location*

Palpate to locate greater trochanter, anterior superior iliac tubercle (found by flexing thigh at hip and measuring up to 1 to 2 cm above crease formed in groin), and posterior iliac crest; place palm of hand over greater trochanter, index finger over anterior superior iliac tubercle, and middle finger along crest of ilium posteriorly as far as possible; inject into center of V formed by fingers

Needle insertion and size

Insert needle perpendicular to site but angled slightly toward iliac crest

22-25 gauge, 0.625-1 inch‡

Advantages

Free of important nerves and vascular structures

Easily identified by prominent bony landmarks

Thinner layer of subcutaneous tissue than in dorsogluteal site, thus less chance of depositing drug subcutaneously rather than intramuscularly

Can accommodate larger quantities of fluid (0.5 ml [infant] to 2.0 ml [child])

Easily accessible if child is in supine, prone, or side-lying position

Less painful than vastus lateralis

Disadvantages

Health professionals' unfamiliarity with site

DELTOID

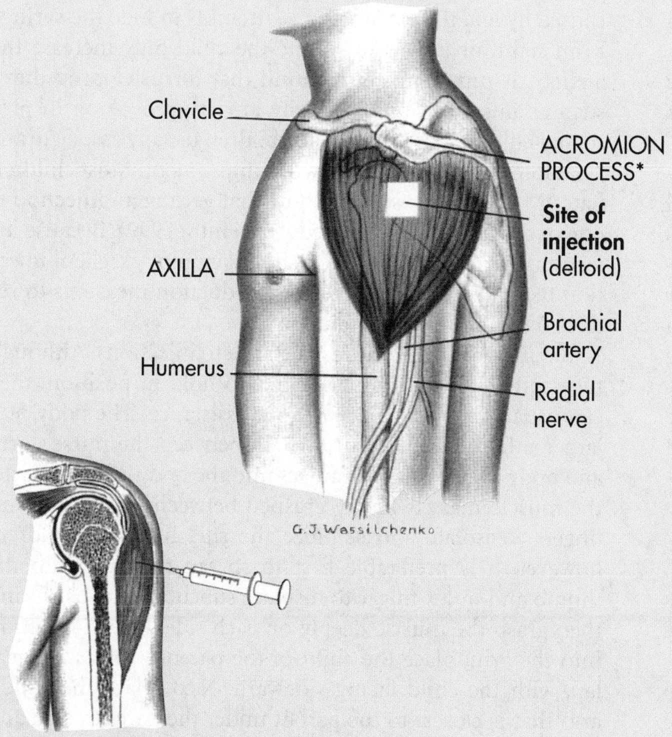

Location*

Locate acromion process; inject only into upper third of muscle that begins about 2 fingerbreadths below acromion

Needle insertion and size

Insert needle perpendicular to site but angled slightly toward shoulder

22-25 gauge, 0.625-1 inch

Advantages

Faster absorption rates than gluteal sites

Easily accessible with minimal removal of clothing

Less pain and fewer local side effects from vaccines as compared with vastus lateralis

Disadvantages

Small muscle mass; only limited amounts of drug can be injected (0.5-1.0 ml)

Small margins of safety with possible damage to radial nerve and axillary nerve (not shown, lies under deltoid at head of humerus)

‡*A Guide for Managing the Pediatric Patient, Reducing the Anxiety and Pain of Injections* (1998) is available from Becton Dickinson & Co., 1 Becton Dr., Franklin Lakes, NJ 07417; phone: 888-237-2762; fax: 201-847-4682; Web site: www.bd.com. In Canada: Becton Dickinson Canada, Inc., 2464 S. Sheridan Way, Mississauga, Ontario L5J 2M8; phone: 800-268-5430 (Ontario and Quebec) or 800-268-5450 (other areas).

toid and vastus lateralis sites. If the muscle is grasped or bunched, a needle length of 25 mm (1 inch) is recommended. If the muscle is stretched or flattened, a needle length of 16 mm ($\frac{5}{8}$ inch) is adequate (Groswasser et al, 1997). Unfortunately, the conclusions of the study fail to address whether these lengths apply to both muscles. From the data, it appears more likely that the recommendations apply to the thigh muscle only. Other recommendations for needle size and volume of fluid are based on traditional practice and have not been verified by research.

Determining the Site

Factors that are considered when selecting a site for an intramuscular (IM) injection on an infant or child include the following:

- The amount and character of the medication to be injected
- The amount and general condition of the muscle mass
- The frequency or number of injections to be given during the course of treatment
- The type of medication being given
- Factors that may impede access to or cause contamination of the site
- The child's ability to assume the required position safely

Older children and adolescents usually pose few problems in selecting a suitable site for IM injections, but infants, with their small and underdeveloped muscles, have fewer available sites. It is sometimes difficult to assess the amount of fluid that can be safely injected into a single site. Usually 1 ml is the maximum volume that should be administered in a single site to small children and older infants. The muscles of small infants may not tolerate more than 0.5 ml. As the child approaches adult size, volumes approaching those given to adults may be used. However, the larger the amount of solution, the larger the muscle must be into which it is injected.

Injections must be placed in muscles large enough to accommodate the medication; however, major nerves and blood vessels must be avoided. There is no universal agreement regarding the best IM injection site for children. The preferred site for infants is the vastus lateralis (the rectus femoris is not an acceptable site). The ventrogluteal site is relatively free of major nerves and blood vessels, is a relatively large muscle with less subcutaneous tissue than the dorsal site, has well-defined landmarks for safe site location, is less painful than the vastus lateralis, and is easily accessible in several positions. These advantages make it a preferred site over the dorsogluteal muscle and challenge the recommendation that the ventrogluteal site not be used until children have been walking. Although there are published recommendations regarding age, in clinical practice the ventrogluteal site has been used in children as young as newborns. Table 45-3 summarizes the major injection sites and illustrates the location of the preferred IM injection sites for children.

Administration

Although injections that are executed with care seldom cause trauma to the child, there have been reports of serious disability related to IM injections in children. Repeated use of a single site has been associated with fibrosis of the muscle with subsequent muscle contracture. Injections close to large nerves, such as the sciatic nerve, have been responsible for permanent disability, especially when potentially neurotoxic drugs are administered. There are several reports of tissue damage from penicillin. One of the difficulties in administering the opaque preparations, such as Bicillin, is that aspirated blood cannot be detected at the bottom of the syringe, thus increasing the risk of injecting into a blood vessel. When such drugs are injected, great care must be used in locating the correct site. When aspirating, the nurse should look for blood at the *top* of the syringe near the plunger, because blood may be drawn up through the column of penicillin. One study of IM injection techniques revealed that the straighter the path of needle insertion (e.g., 90-degree angle), the less displacement there is, causing less discomfort (Katsma & Smith, 1997).

A reported potential hazard with medication in glass ampules is the presence of glass particles in the ampule after the container is broken. When the medication is withdrawn into the syringe, the glass particles may also be withdrawn and subsequently injected into the patient. As a precaution, medication from glass ampules should be drawn up only through a needle with a filter or injected intravenously through a site in the tubing that is distal to an IV filter. Other precautions related to needle use and disposal are discussed on p. 1379.

Children may be unpredictable and cannot be expected to cooperate totally when receiving an injection. Even children who appear to be relaxed and constrained can lose control under the stress of the procedure. It is advisable to have someone available to help hold the child if needed. Because children often jerk or pull away unexpectedly, the nurse should carry an extra needle to exchange for a contaminated one so that the delay is minimal. The child, even a small one, is told that he or she is receiving an injection (preferably using a phrase such as "putting medicine under the skin"), and then the procedure is carried out as quickly and skillfully as possible to avoid prolonging the stressful experience. Delay caused by lengthy explanations, attempts to hide the syringe from sight, or efforts to soothe the child only increase the anxiety. It must be kept in mind that intrusive procedures such as injections are especially anxiety provoking in preschool children and that small children usually associate any assault to the "behind" area with punishment. Most children hate IM injections; studies show that getting an injection is one of the most feared procedures (Huth, 1999). Because injections are painful, the nurse should employ excellent injection technique and effective pain reduction measures to reduce discomfort (Guidelines box).

Small infants offer little resistance to injections. Although they squirm and may be difficult to hold in position, they can usually be restrained without assistance. The body of a larger infant can be securely held between the nurse's arm and body (Fig. 45-18). To inject into the body of the muscle, the muscle mass is firmly grasped between the thumb and fingers to isolate and stabilize the site. In obese children, however, it is preferable first to spread the skin with the thumb and index finger to displace subcutaneous tissue and then grasp the muscle deeply on each side. For an injection into the arm, place the child in the parent's (or assistant's) lap, with the child facing sideward. Next, place the child's arm that is closest to the parent under the parent's arm and wrap toward the back. Then have the parent hold the arm for the injection against the child's body.

Guidelines

INTRAMUSCULAR ADMINISTRATION OF MEDICATION

Use safety precautions in administering medication (e.g., check child's identification).
Apply EMLA topically over site if time permits (at least 60 minutes, preferably 2 to $2\frac{1}{2}$ hours for (intramuscular [IM] injection) (see Pain Management, Chapter 44).
Prepare medication.
Select needle and syringe appropriate to the following:
- Amount of fluid to be administered (syringe size)
- Viscosity of fluid to be administered (needle gauge)
- Amount of tissue to be penetrated (needle length)

Maximum volume to be administered in a single site is 1 ml for older infants and small children.
Determine site of injection (see Table 45-3); make certain that muscle is large enough to accommodate volume and type of medication.
Older children: select site as with adult patient; allow child some choice of site, if feasible.
Following are acceptable sites for infants and small or debilitated children:
- Vastus lateralis muscle
- Ventrogluteal muscle

Dorsogluteal muscle is insufficiently developed to be a safe site for infants and small children.
Administer medication.
- Provide for sufficient help in restraining child; children are often uncooperative, and their behavior is usually unpredictable.
- Explain briefly what is to be done and, if appropriate, what child can do to help.
- Expose injection area for unobstructed view of landmarks.
- Select a site where skin is free of irritation and danger of infection; palpate for and avoid sensitive or hardened areas.
- With multiple injections, rotate sites.
- Place child in a lying or sitting position; child is not allowed to stand because landmarks are more difficult to assess, restraint is more difficult, and child may faint and fall.
- Use a new, sharp needle with smallest diameter that permits free flow of the medication.
- Grasp muscle firmly between thumb and fingers to isolate and stabilize muscle for deposition of drug in its deepest part; in obese children, spread skin with thumb and index finger to displace subcutaneous tissue and grasp muscle deeply on each side.
- Allow skin preparation to dry completely before skin is penetrated.
- Have medication at room temperature.

Decrease perception of pain.
- Distract child with conversation.
- Give child something on which to concentrate (e.g., squeezing a hand or side rail, pinching own nose, humming, counting, yelling "Ouch!").
- Spray vapocoolant (e.g., ethyl chloride or fluori-methane) on site 11 to 15 seconds before injection or place a cold compress or wrapped ice cube on site about a minute before injection, or apply cold to contralateral site.
- Say to child, "If you feel this, tell me to take it out, please."
- Have child hold a small adhesive bandage and place it on puncture site after IM injection is given.

Insert needle quickly, using a dartlike motion at a 90-degree angle unless contraindicated.
Use new needle, not one that has pierced rubber stopper on vial.
Avoid tracking any medication through superficial tissues:
- Replace needle after withdrawing medication, or wipe medication from needle with sterile gauze.
- If withdrawing medication from an ampule, use a needle equipped with a filter that removes glass particles; then use a new, nonfilter needle for injection.
- Use the Z-track and/or air-bubble technique as indicated.
- Avoid any depression of the plunger during insertion of the needle.

Aspirate for blood.
- If blood is found, remove syringe from site, change needle, and reinsert into new location.
- If no blood is found, inject into a relaxed muscle:
- **Vastus Lateralis**–Place child supine or side-lying position
- **Ventrogluteal**–Place child on side with upper leg flexed and placed in front of lower leg.

Inject medication slowly.
Remove needle quickly; hold gauze sponge firmly against skin near needle when removing it to avoid pulling on tissue.
Apply firm pressure to site after injection; massage site to hasten absorption unless contraindicated, as with irritating drugs.
Place a small adhesive bandage on puncture site; with young children decorate it by drawing a smiling face or other symbol of acceptance.
Hold and cuddle young child and encourage parents to comfort child; praise older child.
Allow expression of feelings.
Discard syringe and uncapped, uncut needle in puncture-resistant container located near site of use.
Record time of injection, drug, dose, and injection site.

If the medication is given around the clock, the nurse should not try to administer an injection to a sleeping child, even though it may seem to be easier than waking the youngster. This practice can cause the child to fear going to sleep. When awakened first, the child knows that nothing will be done unless he or she is forewarned.

Subcutaneous and Intradermal Administration

Subcutaneous and intradermal injections are frequently administered to children, but the technique differs little from the method used with adults. Examples of *subcutaneous injections* include insulin, hormone replacement, allergy desensitization, and some vaccines. Tuberculin (TB) testing, local anesthesia, and allergy testing are examples of frequently administered *intradermal injections.*

Techniques to minimize the pain associated with these injections include changing the needle if it pierced a rubber stopper on a vial, using 26- to 30-gauge needles (only to inject the solution), and injecting small volumes (up to 0.5 ml). The angle of the needle for the subcutaneous injection is typically 90 degrees. In children with little subcutaneous tissue, some practitioners insert the needle at a 45-degree angle. However, the benefit of using the 45-degree angle rather than the 90-degree angle remains controversial.

Although subcutaneous injections can be given anywhere there is subcutaneous tissue, common sites include the cen-

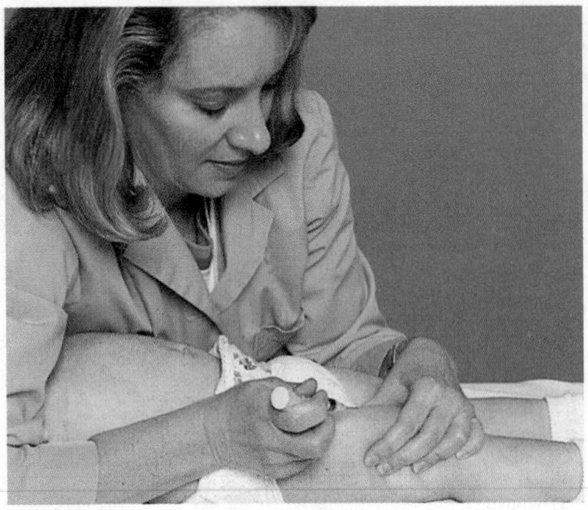

Fig. 45-18 Holding small child for intramuscular injection. Note how nurse isolates and stabilizes muscle.

ter third of the lateral aspect of the upper arm, the abdomen, and the center third of the anterior thigh. Some practitioners believe it is not necessary to aspirate before injecting subcutaneously. For example, not aspirating is an accepted practice in the administration of insulin. Automatic injector devices do not aspirate before injecting.

When giving an intradermal injection into the volar surface of the forearm, the nurse should avoid the medial side of the arm, where the skin is more sensitive.

Families often need to learn subcutaneous injection technique to administer medications, such as insulin, at home. Begin teaching as early as possible to allow the family the maximum amount of practice time possible.

Intravenous Administration

The IV route for administering medications is frequently used in pediatric therapy. For some important drugs it is the only effective route of administration. This method is used for giving drugs to children who have poor absorption as a result of diarrhea, dehydration, or peripheral vascular collapse; children who need a high serum concentration of a drug; children who have resistant infections that require parenteral medication over an extended time; children who need continuous pain relief; and children who require emergency treatment.

Insertion sites and observation of the IV infusion are discussed on p. 1404. However, several factors need to be considered in relation to IV medication. When a drug is administered intravenously, the effect is almost instantaneous and further control is limited. Most drugs for IV administration require a specified minimum dilution or rate of flow, and many are highly irritating or toxic to tissues outside the vascular system. In addition to the precautions and nursing observations related to IV therapy, factors to consider when preparing and administering drugs to infants and children by the IV route include the following:

- Amount of drug to be administered
- Minimum dilution of drug and if child is fluid restricted
- Type of solution in which drug can be diluted
- Length of time over which drug can be safely administered
- Rate of infusion that child and vessels can tolerate safely
- IV tubing volume capacity
- Time that this or another drug is to be administered
- Compatibility of all drugs that child is receiving intravenously

Before any IV infusion, the site of insertion is checked for patency. Medications are never administered with blood products. Only one antibiotic should be administered at a time.

IV infusion is suitable for children who can tolerate the necessary infusion rate and the extra fluid needed to administer the medication. For the very small infant or fluid-restricted child who is not able to tolerate the increased rate or fluids, special delivery systems, such as syringe pumps, are used. Regardless of the technique used, the nurse must know the minimum dilutions for safe administration of IV medications to infants and children. The package insert often includes this information, but if there is any doubt regarding the amount of dilution, the pharmacist should be contacted.

Peripheral Venous Access Devices

The *peripheral lock,* also known as an *intermittent infusion device* or *saline* or *heparin lock,* is used as an alternative for a keep-open infusion when extended access to a vein is required without the need for continuous fluid. It is most frequently employed for intermittent infusion of medication into a peripheral venous route. A short, flexible catheter is used as the lock device, and a site is selected where there will be minimum movement, such as the forearm. The catheter device is inserted and secured in the same manner as for any IV infusion device, but the hub is occluded with a stopper.

The type of device used may vary, and the care and use of the peripheral intermittent infusion device (PIID) are carried out according to the specific protocol of the institution or unit. However, the general concept is the same. The catheter remains in place and is flushed with saline after infusion of the medication. Many studies have shown that normal saline alone is as effective as heparin in maintaining IV patency, especially in catheters larger than 24 gauge (Beecroft et al, 1997; Heilskov et al, 1998; Kotter, 1996; Paisley et al, 1997). Two factors that may account for the difference in small-gauge catheters is frequency of flush and use of the positive-pressure technique. This technique involves instilling the final flush solution as the clamp is closed. The procedure is thought to prevent backflow of blood into the catheter, preventing a small clot from forming.

Children may be discharged with a PIID in place in order to continue receiving medications without hospitalization; this is usually reserved for children who require medications on a short-term basis and are referred to a home-based infusion company. Those with chronic illnesses who require repeated blood sampling or medications, long-term chemotherapy, or frequent hyperalimentation or antibiotic therapy are best managed with a central venous catheter or a peripherally inserted central catheter.

Central Venous Access Devices

Central venous access devices (VADs) have several different characteristics. The practitioner has to consider the best type of catheter for the individual patient's needs. Factors that can influence the decision include the reason for placement of the catheter (diagnosis), length of therapy, risk to the patient in placement of the catheter, and availability of resources to assist the family in maintaining the catheter.

Short-term or *nontunneled catheters* are used in acute care, emergency, and intensive care units. These catheters are made of polyurethane and are placed in large veins such as the subclavian, femoral, or jugular. Insertion is by surgical incision or large percutaneous threading. A chest x-ray film should be taken to verify placement of the catheter tip before administration of fluids or medications.

Peripherally inserted central catheters (PICCs) can be used for short-term to moderate-length therapy. Researchers have shown catheter longevity ranging to over 200 days (Donaldson et al, 1995; Frey, 1995). These catheters consist of silicone or polymer material and are placed by specially trained nurses, physicians, or interventional radiologists (Chung & Ziegler, 1998). The most common insertion site is above the antecubital area using the median, cephalic, or basilic vein. The catheter is threaded either with or without a guidewire into the superior vena cava. PICCs can be trimmed before insertion, and the decision can be made to insert the catheter "midline," which is considered between the insertion site and the head of the clavicle. If the catheter is threaded midline, total parenteral nutrition (TPN) and any drugs known to irritate a peripheral vein (e.g., chemotherapy drugs) should not be administered. The high concentration of glucose in TPN makes it irritating to the vessel; thus it should be infused through a central catheter.

The decision to insert a PICC needs to be made *before* there are several unsuccessful attempts at IV lines or blood sampling by phlebotomy. Once the antecubital veins have been punctured repeatedly, they are not considered to be a candidate for this type of catheter. Because this catheter is the least costly and has less chance of complications than other central VADs, it is an excellent choice for many pediatric patients. This catheter is also usually inserted either at the child's bedside or, more appropriately when available, in the unit's treatment room.

NURSE ALERT Most PICC lines are not sutured into place, so care needs to be maintained when changing the dressing. ■

Long-term central VADs include tunneled and implanted infusion ports (Table 45-4). They may have single, double, or triple lumens. Several lumens (multilumen catheters) allow more than one therapy to be administered at the same time. Reasons to use multilumen catheters include repeated blood sampling, TPN, administration of blood products or infusion of large quantities or concentrations of fluids, ability to administer incompatible drugs or fluids at the same time (through different lumens), and central venous pressure (CVP) monitoring.

With any of the central venous catheters, instilling medication through the injection cap is easily accomplished. With the implanted device the port must be palpated for placement and stabilized, the overlying skin cleansed, and only special noncoring Huber needles used to pierce the port's diaphragm on the top or side, depending on the style. To avoid repeated skin punctures, a special infusion set with a Huber needle and extension tubing with a Luer connection can be used (Fig. 45-19). With this attached, the injection procedure is the same as for an intermittent infusion device or a central venous catheter. To prevent infection, meticulous aseptic technique must be used any time the devices are entered, including instillation of heparin or saline to prevent clotting (Long et al, 1996). There should be a protocol stating that the Huber needle needs to be changed at established intervals, usually 5 to 7 days.

The children and parents are taught the procedure for care of the VAD before discharge from the hospital, including preparation and injection of the prescribed medication, the flush, and dressing changes. A protective device may be recommended for some active children to prevent their accidentally dislodging the needle. Many children take responsibility for preparing and administering medications. Both verbal and written step-by-step instructions are provided for the learners.

The use of a spandex-nylon bodysuit on active toddlers has successfully maintained central lines. One study showed that the suit could not be removed by the toddler and fit snugly over the catheter, its exit site, and its connections. The cost of two bodysuits per child, one for wearing while the other is being cleaned, is less than the costs and the risks of repeated central line insertions (Janik, Wayne, & Janik, 1995). A pocket sewn on the inside of a T-shirt provides a place in which to coil the catheter line while the child is at play if a dressing is not used. A commercial elastic vest is also available.*

Infection and an occluded catheter are two of the most common complications of central venous catheters. Although neither is an emergency, both require treatment with antibiotics for infection and a fibrinolytic agent, such as alteplase, for clots (Reed & Phillip, 1996). Uncapping can be prevented by taping the cap securely to the catheter and the clamped line to the dressing. Leaks can be prevented by using a smooth-edged clamp only. Parents are cautioned to keep scissors away from the child to prevent accidental cutting of the catheter. If the catheter leaks, they are instructed to tape it above the leak and then clamp the catheter at the taped site. The child should be taken to the practitioner as soon as possible to prevent infection or clotting after a catheter leak.

NURSE ALERT If a central venous catheter is accidentally removed, apply pressure to the entry site to the vein, not the exit site on the skin. ■

Nasogastric, Orogastric, or Gastrostomy Administration

When a child has an indwelling feeding tube or a gastrostomy, oral medications are usually given via that route. An advantage of this method is the ability to administer oral medications around the clock without disturbing the child.

*Available from Advanced Patient Devices, 3564 SabakaTrail, Verona, WI 53593; phone: 800-547-6412; fax: 608-833-6694.

Table 45-4

Comparison of Long-Term Central Venous Access Devices

DESCRIPTION	BENEFITS	CARE CONSIDERATIONS
TUNNELED CATHETER (E.G., HICKMAN/BROVIAC CATHETER)		
Silicone, radiopaque, flexible catheter with open ends One or two Dacron cuffs or Vitacuffs (biosynthetic material impregnated with silver ions) on catheter(s) enhances tissue ingrowth May have more than one lumen	Reduced risk of bacterial migration after tissue adheres to Dacron cuff or Vitacuff Easy to use for self-administered infusions Removal requires pulling catheter from site (nonsurgical procedure)	Requires daily heparin flushes Must be clamped or have clamp nearby at all times Must keep exit site dry Heavy activity restricted until tissue adheres to cuff Water sports may be restricted (risk of infection) Risk of infection still present Protrudes outside body; susceptible to damage from sharp instruments and may be pulled out; may affect body image More difficult to repair Patient/family must learn catheter care
GROSHONG CATHETER		
Clear, flexible, silicone, radiopaque catheter with closed tip and two-way valve at proximal end Dacron cuff or Vitacuff on catheter enhances tissue ingrowth May have more than one lumen	Reduced time and cost for maintenance care; no heparin flushes needed Reduced catheter damage; no clamping needed because of two-way valve Increased patient safety because of minimum potential for blood backflow or air embolism Reduced risk of bacterial migration after tissue adheres to Dacron cuff or Vitacuff Easily repaired Easy to use for self-administered IV infusions	Requires weekly irrigation with normal saline Must keep exit site dry Heavy activity restricted until tissue adheres to cuff Water sports may be restricted (risk of infection) Risk of infection still present Protrudes outside body; susceptible to damage from sharp instruments and may be pulled out; can affect body image Patient/family must learn catheter care
IMPLANTED PORTS (PORT-A-CATH, INFUS-A-PORT, MEDIPORT, NORPORT, GROSHONG PORT)		
Totally implantable metal or plastic device that consists of self-sealing injection port with top or side access with preconnected or attachable silicon catheter that is placed in large blood vessel	Reduced risk of infection Placed completely under the skin; therefore much less likely to be pulled out or damaged No maintenance care and reduced cost for family Heparinized monthly and after each infusion to maintain patency (Groshong port requires only saline) No limitations on regular physical activity, including swimming Dressing needed only when port accessed with Huber needle that is not removed No or only slight change in body appearance (slight bulge on chest)	Must pierce skin for access; pain with insertion of needle; can use local anesthetic (EMLA) or intradermal buffered lidocaine before accessing port Special noncoring needle (Huber) with straight or angled design must be used to inject into port Skin preparation needed before injection Difficult to manipulate for self-administered infusions Catheter may dislodge from port, especially if child "plays" with port site (twiddler syndrome) Vigorous contact sports generally not allowed Removal requires surgical procedure

A disadvantage is the risk of occluding or "clogging" the tube, especially when giving viscous solutions through small-bore feeding tubes. The most important preventive measure is adequate flushing after the medication is instilled. Guidelines for administration are presented in the Guidelines box on p. 1401.

NURSE ALERT Sprinkle-type medication should be avoided. However, if there is no other option and the tube is large gauge (18 Fr or greater), but usually not a Foley catheter, it may be given by mixing the sprinkles with a small amount of pureed fruit and thinning with water. The fruit keeps the sprinkles suspended so that they do not float to the top. Flush well. This

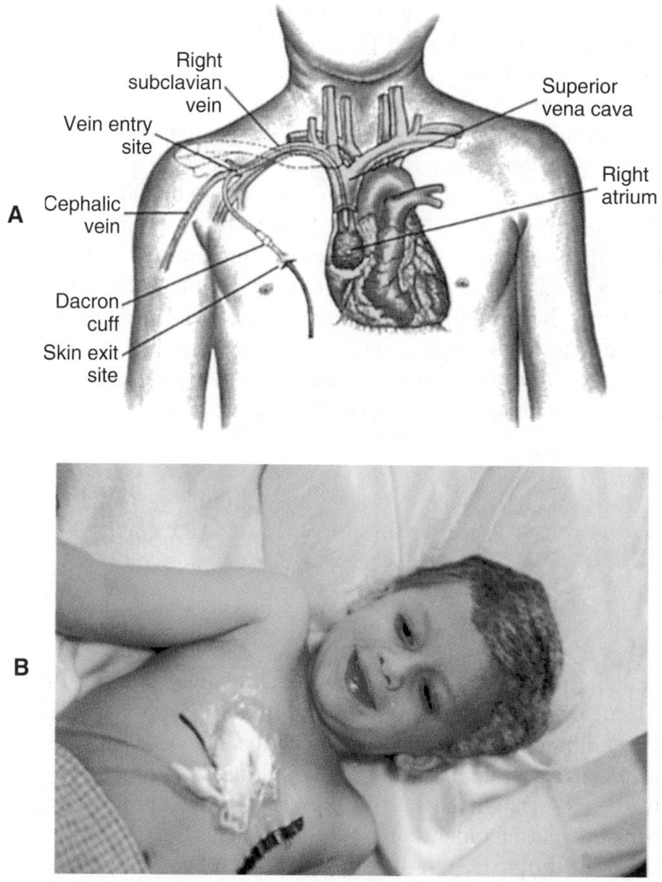

Fig. 45-19 Venous access devices. **A,** Central venous catheter insertion and exit site. **B,** Child receiving medication by way of an implantable port. Note needle and extension tubing inserted into port and secured with gauze dressings and a transparent dressing.

procedure is not recommended for skin-level gastrostomy devices. ■

Guidelines

NASOGASTRIC, OROGASTRIC, OR GASTROSTOMY MEDICATION ADMINISTRATION IN CHILDREN

Use elixir or suspension (rather than tablet) preparations of medication whenever possible.

Dilute viscous medication or syrup with a small amount of water if possible.

If administering tablets, crush tablet to a very fine powder and dissolve drug in a small amount of warm water.

Never crush enteric-coated or sustained-release tablets or capsules.

Avoid oily medications because they tend to cling to side of tube.

Do not mix medication with enteral formula unless fluid is restricted. If adding a drug:

- Check with pharmacist for compatibility.
- Shake formula well and observe for any physical reaction (e.g., separation, precipitation).
- Label formula container with name of medication, dosage, date, and time infusion started.

Have medication at room temperature.

Measure medication in a calibrated cup or syringe.

Check for correct placement of nasogastric or orogastric tube (see Guidelines box, p. 1417).

Attach syringe (with adaptable tip but without plunger) to tube.

Pour medication into syringe.

Unclamp tube and allow medication to flow by gravity.

Adjust height of container to achieve desired flow rate (e.g., increase height for faster flow).

As soon as syringe is empty, pour in water to flush tubing.

- Amount of water depends on length and gauge of tubing.
- Determine amount before administering any medication by using a syringe to fill completely an unused nasogastric or orogastric tube with water. Amount of flush solution is usually 1½ times this volume.
- With certain drug preparations (e.g., suspensions) more fluid may be needed.

If administering more than one drug at the same time, flush tube between each medication with clear water.

Clamp tube after flushing, unless tube is left open.

Rectal Administration

The rectal route for administration is less reliable but is sometimes used when the oral route is difficult or contraindicated. Some of the drugs available in suppository form are acetaminophen, sedatives, analgesics (morphine), and antiemetics. The difficulty in using the rectal route is that unless the rectum is empty at the time of insertion, the absorption of the drug may be delayed, diminished, or prevented by the presence of feces. Sometimes the drug is later evacuated, securely surrounded by stool. However, the rectal route is used most frequently in children who are unable to take anything by mouth and are unlikely to have large amounts of stool. It is also used when oral preparations are unsuitable for controlling vomiting.

To insert a suppository, the wrapper is removed and the suppository lubricated with water-soluble jelly or warm water. A gloved finger is used to quickly but gently insert the suppository into the rectum, beyond both of the rectal sphincters. The buttocks are then held or taped together firmly to relieve pressure on the anal sphincter until the urge to expel the suppository has passed—5 to 10 minutes. Sometimes the amount of drug ordered is less than the dosage available. The irregular shape of most suppositories makes the process of dividing them into a desired dose difficult if not dangerous. If the suppository must be halved, it should be cut lengthwise. However, there is no guarantee that the drug is evenly dispersed throughout the petrolatum base.

Rectal suppositories are usually inserted with the apex (pointed end) foremost. One study demonstrated easier insertion and a lower expulsion rate when the suppository was inserted with the base (blunt end) first. Reverse contractions or the pressure gradient of the anal canal may help the suppository to slip higher into the canal (Moppett & Parker, 1999).

If medication is administered via a retention enema, the same procedure is used. Drugs given by enema are diluted in the smallest amount of solution possible to minimize the likelihood of being evacuated.

Optic, Otic, and Nasal Administration

There are few differences in administering eye, ear, and nose medication to children or to adults. The major difficulty is in gaining children's cooperation. The infant's or young child's head is immobilized in the same manner as described in Fig. 35-17. Older children need only explanation and direction. Although the administration of optic, otic, and nasal medication is not painful, these drugs can cause unpleasant sensations that can be eliminated with various techniques. Parental involvement is an important component during administration. A parent's presence can decrease levels of anxiety in the child. To reduce unpleasant sensations, perform the following:

- **Eye**—Apply finger pressure to the lacrimal punctum at the inner aspect of the lid for 1 minute to prevent drainage of medication to the nasopharynx and the unpleasant "tasting" of the drug.
- **Ear**—Allow medications stored in the refrigerator to warm to room temperature before instillation.
- **Nose**—Position the child with the head hyperextended to prevent strangling sensations caused by medication trickling into the throat rather than up into the nasal passages.

To instill eye medication, the child is placed supine or sitting with the head extended, and the child is asked to look up. One hand is used to pull the lower lid downward; the hand that holds the dropper rests on the head so that it may move synchronously with the child's head, thus reducing the possibility of trauma to a struggling child or of dropping medication on the face (Fig. 45-20). As the lower lid is pulled down, a small conjunctival sac is formed; the solution or ointment is applied to this area, never directly on the eyeball. Another effective technique is to pull the lower lid down and out to form a cup, into which the medication is dropped. The lids are gently closed to prevent expression of the medication, and the child is asked to look in all directions to enhance even distribution of the preparation. Excess medication is wiped from the inner canthus outward to prevent contamination to the contralateral eye.

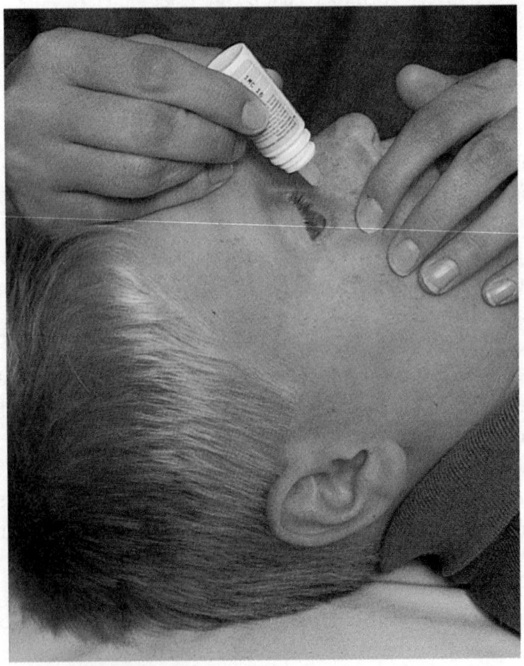

Fig. 45-20 Administering eyedrops.

Instilling eyedrops in infants can be most difficult, because they often clench the lids tightly closed. One approach is to place the drops in the nasal corner where the lids meet. The medication pools in this area, and when the child opens the lids, the medication flows onto the conjunctiva. For young children, playing a game can be helpful, such as instructing the child to keep the eyes closed until the count of 3 and then open them, at which time the drops are quickly instilled. Ointment can be applied by gently pulling down the lower lid and placing the ointment in the lower conjunctival sac.

NURSE ALERT If both eye ointment and drops are ordered, give drops first, wait 3 minutes, and then apply the ointment to allow each drug to work. When possible, administer eye ointments before bedtime or naptime, because the child's vision will be blurred temporarily. ■

Ear drops are instilled with the child in the prone or supine position and the head turned to the appropriate side. For children younger than 3 years of age, the external auditory canal is straightened by gently pulling the pinna downward and straight back. The pinna is pulled upward and back in children older than 3 years of age (see Fig. 35-20). To place the drops deep in the ear canal without contaminating the tip of the dropper, place a disposable ear speculum in the canal and administer the drops through the speculum. After instillation, the child should remain lying on the unaffected side for a few minutes. Gentle massage of the area immediately anterior to the ear facilitates the entry of drops into the ear canal. The use of cotton pledgets prevents medication from flowing out of the external canal. However, the pledgets should be loose enough to allow any discharge to exit from the ear. Premoistening the cotton with a few drops of medication prevents the wicking action from absorbing the medication instilled in the ear.

Nose drops are instilled in the same manner as in the adult patient. Unpleasant sensations associated with medicated nose drops are minimized when care is taken to position the child with the head extended well over the edge of the bed or a pillow (Fig. 45-21). Depending on size, the infant can be positioned in the football hold (see Fig. 45-7, *B*)—that is, in the nurse's arm with the head extended and stabilized between the nurse's body and elbow, and the arms and hands immobilized with the nurse's hands. After instillation of the drops, the child should remain in position for 1 minute to allow the drops to come in contact with the nasal surfaces.

Nasal spray dispensers are inserted into the naris vertically and then angled nasally to avoid trauma to the septum and to direct medication toward the inferior turbinate.

Family Teaching and Home Care

The nurse usually assumes the responsibility for preparing families to administer medications at home. The family should have an understanding of why the child is receiving

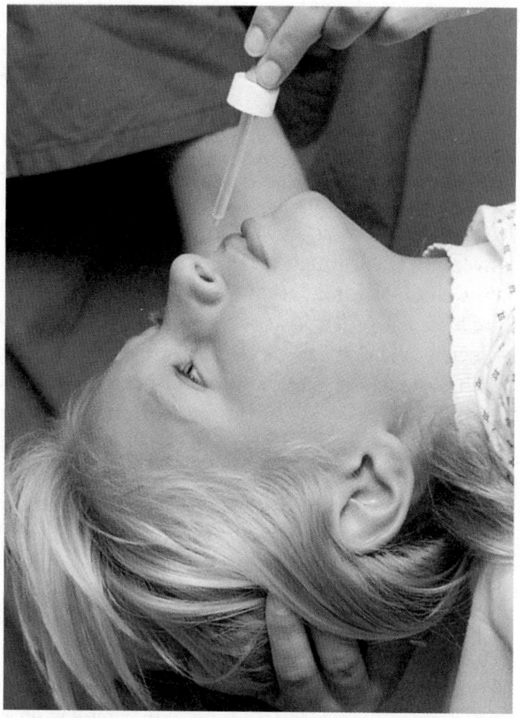

Fig. 45-21 Proper position for instilling nose drops.

the medication and the effects that might be expected, as well as the amount, frequency, and length of time the drug is to be administered. Instruction should be carried out in an unhurried, relaxed manner, preferably in an area away from busy ward or office routine, following the same guidelines for teaching as outlined in the Guidelines box on p. 1369.

The caregiver is carefully instructed regarding the correct dosage, and the nurse is responsible for preparing parents for the specifics of the task. Some persons have difficulty understanding or interpreting terminology from the pharmacy, and just because they nod or otherwise indicate an understanding, it cannot be assumed that the message is clear. It is important to ascertain their interpretation of a teaspoon, for example, and to be certain they have acceptable devices for measuring the drug. If the drug is packaged with a dropper, syringe, or plastic cup, the nurse should show and/or mark the point on the device that indicates the prescribed dose, demonstrate how the dose is drawn up into a dropper or syringe and measured, and demonstrate how any bubbles are eliminated. Also, the nurse must be certain that families understand that a prescription ordered in drops means single drops, not dropperfuls, a potential source of administration error (see Nurse Alert, p. 1393). If the nurse has any doubts about the parent's ability to administer the correct dose, the parent should be asked to give a return demonstration. This verification is especially important when the drug has potentially serious consequences from incorrect dosage, such as insulin or digoxin, or when more complex administration is required, such as parenteral injections. When teaching a parent to give an injection, adequate time for instruction and practice must be allotted.

Home modifications are often necessary because the availability of equipment or assistance can differ from that of the hospital setting. For example, the parent may need guidance in devising methods that allow for one person to hold the child and safely give the drug. One successful method is the following procedure:

- Place child supine on flat surface (bed, couch, floor).
- Sit facing child so that his or her head is between operator's thighs and his or her arms are under operator's legs.
- Place lower legs over child's legs to restrain lower body, if necessary.
- To administer oral medication, place small pillow under child's head to reduce risk of aspiration.
- To administer nasal medication, place small pillow under child's shoulders to aid flow of liquid through nasal passages.

The time that the drug is to be administered is clarified with the parent. For example, when a drug is prescribed in association with meals, the number of meals that the family is accustomed to eating influences the amount of drug the child receives. Does the child have meals twice a day or five times a day? When a drug is to be given several times during the day, together the nurse and parents can work out a schedule that accommodates the family's routine. This is particularly significant if the drug must be given at equal intervals throughout a 24-hour period. For example, telling parents that the child needs 1 teaspoon of medicine four times a day is subject to misinterpretation, because parents may routinely schedule the doses at incorrect times. Instead, a preplanned schedule based on 6-hour intervals should be set up with the number of days required for therapeutic dosage listed. Modification should also be made to accommodate sleep schedules. For example, at nighttime a 6-hour interval may be extended to 8 hours (e.g., 11 PM, 7 AM, noon, and 6 PM). Written instruction should accompany all drug prescriptions. If parents have difficulty reading or understanding English, use colors to convey instructions. For example, mark each drug with a color and place the appropriate color on a calendar chart or on a drawing of a clock to identify when the drug needs to be given. If a liquid medication and syringe are used, also mark the syringe at the place the plunger needs to be with color-coded tape.

PROCEDURES RELATED TO MAINTAINING FLUID BALANCE

Measurement of Intake and Output

One of the most important roles of the nurse in maintaining fluid balance is accurate measurement of fluid intake and output (I&O). Accurate measurements are essential to the assessment of fluid balance. Measurements from all sources—including both gastrointestinal and parenteral I&O from urine, stools, vomitus, fistulas, nasogastric suction, sweat, and drainage from wounds—must be taken and considered. Although the practitioner usually indicates when I&O measurements are to be recorded, it is a nursing responsibility to keep an accurate I&O record on patients in the following situations:

- After major surgery
- IV, diuretic, or corticosteroid therapy
- Severe thermal burns or injuries

- Renal disease or damage
- Congestive heart failure
- Dehydration (vomiting and diarrhea)
- Diabetes mellitus
- Oliguria
- Two years of age or younger
- Respiratory distress

Infants or small children who are unable to use a bedpan or those who have bowel movements with every voiding require the application of a collecting device (see p. 1386). If collecting bags are not used, wet diapers or pads are carefully weighed to ascertain the amount of fluid lost. This includes liquid stool, vomitus, and other losses. The volume of fluid in milliliters is equivalent to the weight of the fluid measured in grams. The specific gravity as a measure of osmolality is determined with a refractometer or urine dipsticks and assists in assessing the degree of hydration.

The weighed-diaper method of fluid measurement has disadvantages, including (1) inability to differentiate one type of loss from another because of admixture, (2) loss of urine or liquid stool from leakage or evaporation (especially if the infant is under a radiant warmer), and (3) additional fluid in the diaper (superabsorbent disposable type) from absorption of atmospheric moisture (from high-humidity incubators). However, when several types of diapers, including cloth, conventional disposable, and superabsorbent disposable, were compared for accuracy in terms of evaporative effects, closed superabsorbent disposable diapers followed by open superabsorbent disposable diapers were affected the least (Fox, 1992). To avoid the problem of evaporative losses and leakage of excreta, diapers should be weighed as soon as possible after becoming soiled.

Special Needs When the Child Is NPO

Infants or children who are unable or not permitted to take fluids by mouth (NPO) have special needs. To ensure that they do not receive fluids, a sign can be placed in some obvious place, such as over their beds or on their shirts, to alert others to the NPO status. To prevent the temptation to drink, fluids should not be left at the bedside.

Oral hygiene, a part of routine hygienic care, is especially important when fluids are restricted or withheld (see p. 1372). For the young child who cannot brush the teeth or rinse the mouth without swallowing fluid, the nurse can institute oral hygiene by wiping the teeth, gums, and tongue with a cloth moistened with saline. To keep the mouth feeling moist when the child is NPO, give ice chips (if this is permitted by the practitioner) or spray the mouth with a fine mist of cool water.

To keep the lips moist and prevent cracking, petrolatum (Vaseline) or some other commercial lip aid is applied. Lemon-glycerin swabs are avoided because they dry the skin, irritate open lesions, and can decay the teeth. To meet the need to suck, the infant is provided with a safe commercial pacifier.

The child who is fluid restricted presents an equal challenge. Limiting fluids is often more difficult for the child than NPO, especially when IV fluids are also eliminated. To make certain the child does not drink the entire amount allowed early in the day, the daily allotment is calculated to provide fluids at periodic intervals throughout the child's waking hours. Serving the fluids in small containers gives the illusion of larger servings. No extra liquid is left at the bedside if compliance is a problem.

Parenteral Fluid Therapy

Site and Equipment

The site selected for IV infusion depends on accessibility and convenience. Although it is possible to use any accessible vein in older children, attention must be directed toward the child's developmental, cognitive, and mobility needs when selecting a site. Ideally, in older children, the superficial veins of the forearm should be used, leaving the hands free. An older child can help select the site and thereby maintain some measure of control. For veins in the extremities it is best to start with the most distal site and avoid the child's favored hand in order to reduce the disability related to the procedure. A site is chosen that restricts the child's movements as little as possible—a site over a joint in an extremity, such as the antecubital space, is avoided. In small infants a superficial vein of the hand, wrist, forearm, foot, or ankle is usually most convenient and most easily stabilized (Fig. 45-22). Foot veins should be avoided in children learning to walk and in children already walking. Superficial veins of the scalp have no valves, insertion is easy, and they can be used

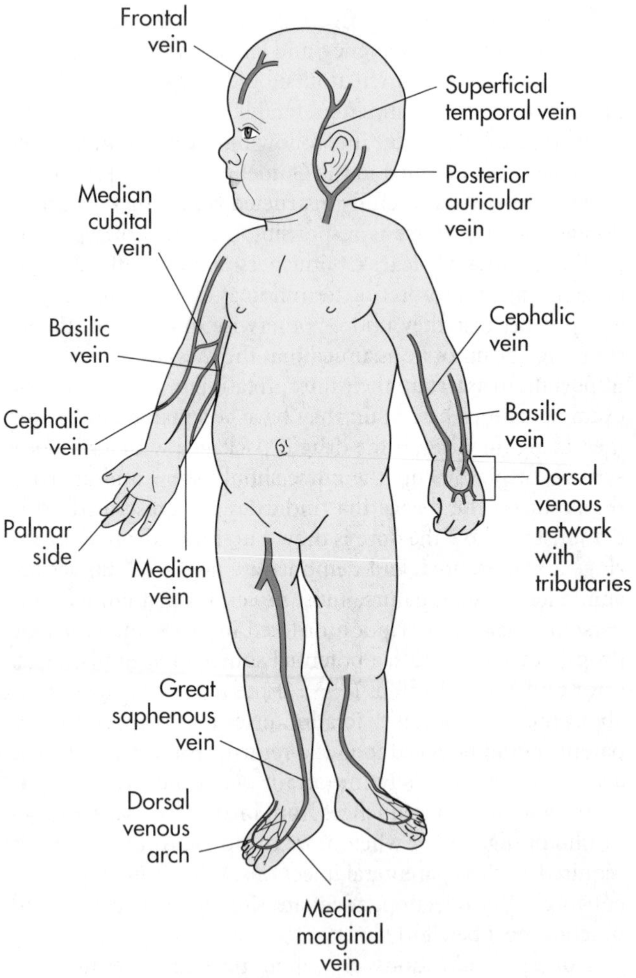

Fig. 45-22 Preferred sites for venous access in infants.

in infants up to about 9 months of age, but they should be used only when other site attempts have failed.

Selection of a scalp vein as the venipuncture site requires shaving the area around the site to visualize the vein better and to provide a smooth surface on which to tape the catheter hub and tubing. A rubber band slipped onto the head from brow to occiput will usually suffice as a tourniquet. Shaving off a portion of the infant's hair is very upsetting to parents; therefore they should be told what to expect and reassured that the hair will grow in again rapidly (save the hair because parents often wish to keep it). Remove as little as possible, directly over the insertion site and taping surface.

Situations may occur in which rapid establishment of a systemic access is vital, and venous access may be hampered by peripheral circulatory collapse, hypovolemic shock (secondary to vomiting or diarrhea, burns, or trauma), cardiopulmonary arrest, or other conditions (Banerjee et al, 1994). *Intraosseous infusion* provides a rapid, safe, and lifesaving alternate route for administration of fluids and medications until intravascular access can be attained, especially in children who are 6 years of age or younger. A large-bore needle, such as a bone marrow aspiration needle (e.g., Jamshidi) or an intraosseous needle (e.g., Cook), is inserted into the medullary cavity of a long bone, most often the proximal tibia. This procedure is usually reserved for children who are unconscious or for those who are receiving analgesia, because the procedure is painful. Local anesthesia should be used for a semiconscious patient.

For most IV infusions in children, an over-the-needle 22- to 24-gauge catheter may be used if therapy is expected to last less than 5 days. The smallest-gauge and shortest-length catheter that will accommodate the prescribed therapy should be chosen when evaluating the placement of a peripheral IV line. The length of the catheter may be directly related to infection or embolus formation—the shorter the catheter, the fewer the complications (Maki, 1994). The gauge of the catheter should maintain adequate flow of the infusate into the cannulated vein while allowing adequate blood flow around the catheter walls to promote proper hemodilution of the infusate. Because stainless steel needles tend to dislodge and infiltrate more frequently than catheters, the use of these should be limited to short-term or single-dose administration (Intravenous Nurses Society, 1998).

The goal of IV therapy is to deliver the prescribed fluids or medications without complications. Determining the best catheter for the patient early in the therapy provides the best chance of avoiding catheter-related complications (Moureau, 1999). As the length of therapy increases, decisions regarding the type of infusion device (short peripheral, midline, peripherally inserted central catheter, or central venous catheter) should be explored. Guidelines such as flow charts or algorithms are available to help in these decisions (Catudal, 1999).

Safety Catheters and Needleless Systems

One of the main causes for change in IV therapy is the concern of needle-stick injuries. To provide safer care for the patient and health care worker, manufacturers have developed safety catheters and needleless IV systems.

Over-the-needle IV catheters with hollow-bore needles carry a high risk for transmission of blood-borne pathogens from needle-stick injuries. Safety catheters prevent accidental needle sticks with the use of over-the-needle IV catheters.

Needleless IV systems, which are designed to prevent needle-stick injuries during administration of IV push medications and IV piggyback medications, may vary from manufacturer to manufacturer, but the concept is essentially the same. Some needleless systems are universal, whereas others require complete use of the entire IV delivery system for compatibility. Needleless IV systems rely on prepierced septa that are accessed by blunted plastic cannulas or systems that use valves that open and close a fluid path when activated by insertion of a syringe.

Blunt plastic cannulas and preslit injection port sites (Fig. 45-23) eliminate the need for steel needles and conventional injection port sites but remain accessible via hypodermic needles, a drawback except in emergent situations. Systems that do not permit needled access enhance safety by preventing health care workers from attempting to use needles; however, such systems are limited by the lack of needled access, especially in emergency situations (Orenstein, 1999). A syringe with a blue spike is available to access a single-dose vial (Fig. 45-23, *A*). The preslit injection port sites are identified by a white ring surrounding the port; this ring alerts users that the system is needleless (Fig. 45-23, *B*). Syringes are available with the blunt plastic cannula for accessing these sites (Fig. 45-23, *C*). A lever lock (Fig. 45-23, *D*) or threaded lock cannula (Fig. 45-23, *E*) attaches to an IV line, IV Y site, or peripheral intermittent infusion device. A preslit universal vial adapter (not pictured) provides access to standard multiple-dose vials, and syringe cannulas are then used to access the adapter.

Infusion Pumps

A variety of infusion pumps are available, refillable from the bag or bottle above or contained in a syringe pump to minimize the possibility of overloading the circulation. In-

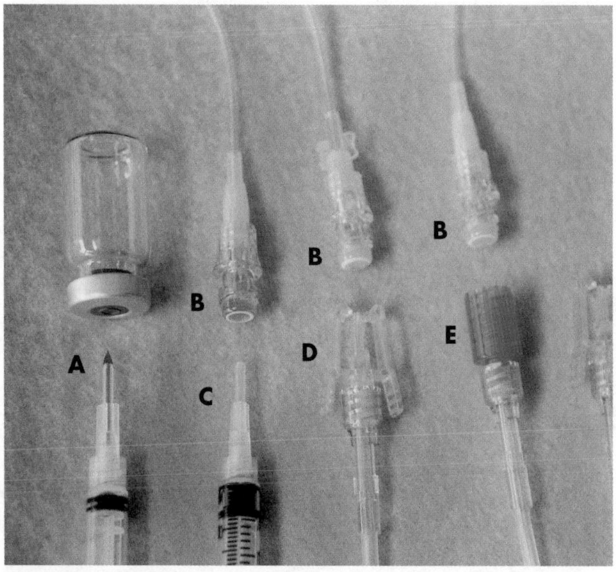

Fig. 45-23 Interlink IV access systems: **A**, blue spike syringe; **B**, preslit injection port (needleless); **C**, blunt plastic cannula syringe; **D**, lever lock cannula; **E**, threaded lock cannula.

fusion devices are almost always used in pediatrics because they can accurately infuse fluids (especially the syringe pumps, which infuse very small amounts of fluid), as well as accurately provide the prescribed amount of IV solution. It is an important nursing responsibility to calculate the amount to be infused in a given length of time, set the infusion rate, and monitor the apparatus frequently (at least every 1 to 2 hours) to make certain that the desired rate is maintained, the integrity of the system remains intact, the site remains intact (free of redness, edema, infiltration, or irritation), and the infusion does not stop.

Continuous infusion pumps, although convenient and efficient, are not without risks. Overreliance on the accuracy of the machine can cause either too much or too little fluid to be infused; therefore its use does not eliminate careful periodic assessment by the nurse. Excess pressure can build up if the machine is set at a rate faster than the vein is able to accommodate (or continues to pump when the needle is out of the lumen). This is especially true in very small infants. No matter what device is used, a thorough understanding of the apparatus is essential for safe fluid administration.

Special Care Considerations

To maintain the integrity of the IV line, adequate protection of the site is required. The catheter hub is firmly secured at the puncture site with a transparent dressing or clear, nonallergenic tape. Transparent dressings are ideal because the insertion site is easily observed. Minimal tape should be used at the puncture site and on about 1 to 2 inches of skin beyond the site to avoid obscuring the insertion site for early detection of infiltration.

A protective cover is applied directly over the catheter insertion site to protect the infusion site. Easy access to the IV site for frequent (1- to 2-hour) assessments must be considered. Improvised plastic cups that are cut in half with the ridged edges covered with tape should not be used, because they have caused injury to patients. A commercial site protector, I.V. House,* is available in different sizes (Fig. 45-24). Its ventilation holes prevent moisture from accumulating under the dome (Lee & Vallino, 1996). This device is designed to protect the IV site; allow for visibility of the site; minimize use of padded boards, splints, or other restraints and tape; and maintain skin integrity. The I.V. House may be used to protect surgical insertion sites, such as jugular, femoral, or subclavian lines; implanted ports; or peripherally inserted central catheter lines; and for the application of EMLA. The connector tubing or extension tubing can be looped to make it small enough to fit under the protective cover to prevent accidental snagging of the catheter. It is important to safely secure the IV tubing to prevent infants and children from becoming entangled in the tubing or from accidentally pulling the catheter or needle out. This securement also eliminates movement of the catheter hub at the insertion site (mechanical manipulation). A colorful and interesting sticker can be applied to the protecting device to add a positive note to the procedure.

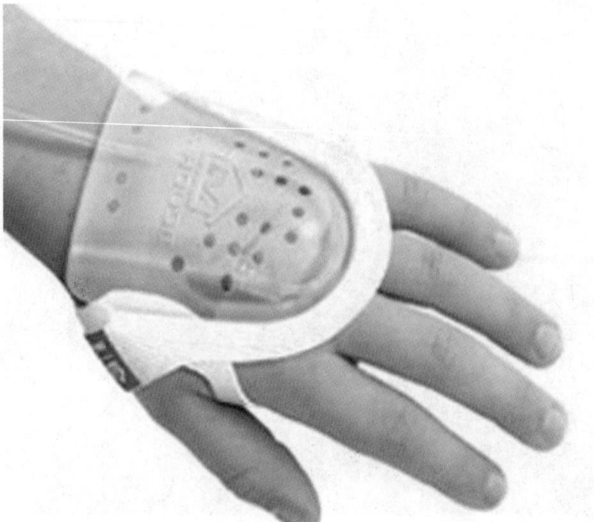

Fig. 45-24 I.V. House.

When it comes time to discontinue an IV infusion, many children are distressed by the thought of catheter removal. Therefore they need a careful explanation of the process and suggestions for helping. Encouraging children to remove or help remove the tape from the site provides them with a measure of control and often encourages their cooperation. The procedure consists of turning off any pump apparatus, occluding the IV tubing, removing the tape, pulling the catheter out of the vessel in the opposite direction of insertion, and exerting firm pressure at the site. A dry dressing (adhesive bandage strip) is placed over the puncture site. The use of adhesive-removal pads can decrease the pain of tape removal, but the skin should be washed after use because it can become irritated. To remove transparent dressings (e.g., Opsite or Tegaderm), pull the opposing edges parallel to the skin to loosen the bond. If a catheter was used for the IV infusion, the tip is inspected to make certain that the catheter is intact and that no portion remains in the vein.

Complications

The same precautions regarding maintenance of asepsis, prevention of infection, and observation for infiltration are carried out with patients of any age. However, infiltration is more difficult to detect in infants and small children than in adults. The increased amount of subcutaneous fat and the amount of tape used to secure the needle often obscure the signs of early infiltration. When the fluid appears to be infusing too slowly or ceases, the usual assessment for obstruction within the apparatus—kinks, screw clamps, shutoff valve, and positioning interference (e.g., a bent elbow)—often locates the difficulty. When these actions fail to detect the problem, it may be necessary to carefully remove some of the tape and other material that obscure a clear view of the venipuncture site. Dependent areas, such as the palm and undersides of the extremity or the occiput and behind the ears, are examined.

Whenever possible, the IV infusion should be placed in an extremity to which the identification band (or bracelet) is

*Available from I.V. House, 7400 Foxmont Dr., Hazelwood, MO 63042; phone: 800-530-0400; fax: 314-831-3863; e-mail: ivhouse@ivhouse.com; Web site: www.ivhouse.com.

not attached. Serious circulatory impairment can result from infiltrated solution distal to the band, which acts as a tourniquet, preventing adequate venous return. To check for return blood flow through the catheter, the tubing is removed from the infusion pump, and the bag is lowered below the level of the infusion site. If the tubing is connected to an infusion pump, it must be removed from the pump before lowering. A good blood return, or lack thereof, is not always an indicator of infiltration in small infants. Flushing the catheter/needle and observing for edema, redness, or streaking along the vein is an appropriate assessment of IV. Resistance during flushing or aspiration for blood return also indicates that the IV infusion may have infiltrated surrounding tissue.

NURSE ALERT Prevention of insertion site infection can be decreased by strict adherence to the following guidelines (Pearson, 1996):

- Practice good handwashing before starting an IV infusion.
- Rigorously cleanse the skin with an appropriate antiseptic, including alcohol or povidone-iodine, before catheter insertion.
- When cleansing the insertion site, use a circular motion starting from the center and working outward.
- Allow the antiseptic to dry for 30 to 60 seconds before inserting the catheter.
- Do not palpate the insertion site after the skin has been cleansed with the antiseptic. ■

Proper education of the patient and family regarding signs and symptoms of an infected site can help prevent infections from going unnoticed. When an IV infusion continues for several days, the tubing and solution are changed at regular intervals according to hospital policy, most often every 72 hours (Pearson, 1995). The dressing, whether transparent dressing or sterile gauze and tape, can be left in place for the duration of the IV infusion (Maki, 1994) unless the integrity has been compromised. To ensure that the equipment is changed regularly, it is labeled with the date and time that the new bag and tubing are attached. Any signs of inflammation, such as redness or pain, are reported immediately. This usually requires removal of the infusion and restarting it at another site or administering the medication by another route.

PROCEDURES FOR MAINTAINING RESPIRATORY FUNCTION

Inhalation Therapy

The term *inhalation therapy* is an all-inclusive term that encompasses a variety of therapies that involve changing the composition, volume, or pressure of inspired gases. These therapies include primarily increasing the oxygen concentration of inspired gas (oxygen therapy), increasing the water vapor content of inspired gas (humidification), adding airborne particles with beneficial properties (aerosol therapy), and employing various means for controlling or assisting respiration (artificial ventilation, continuous positive airway pressure).

Oxygen Therapy

Oxygen (O_2) therapy is primarily carried out in the hospital, although increasing numbers of children are receiving O_2 in the home. O_2 delivered to the infant via the incubator is satisfactory when lower levels are adequate to prevent cyanosis, but the highest concentration (almost 100%) is supplied by way of a *plastic hood* (Fig. 45-25). The humidified O_2 should not be blown directly into the infant's face, and the hood should not rub against the infant's neck, chin, or shoulder. Older, cooperative infants and children can use a *nasal cannula* or *prongs*, which can supply a concentration of O_2 of about 50%. A *mask* is not well tolerated by children.

For children beyond early infancy, the *oxygen tent* is a satisfactory means for administration of O_2 (Fig. 45-26). A tent does not require any device to come into direct contact with the face, but the concentration of O_2 within the tent is difficult to control and to maintain above 30% to 50%. A major difficulty with the use of the tent is keeping the tent closed so that the O_2 concentration is maintained.

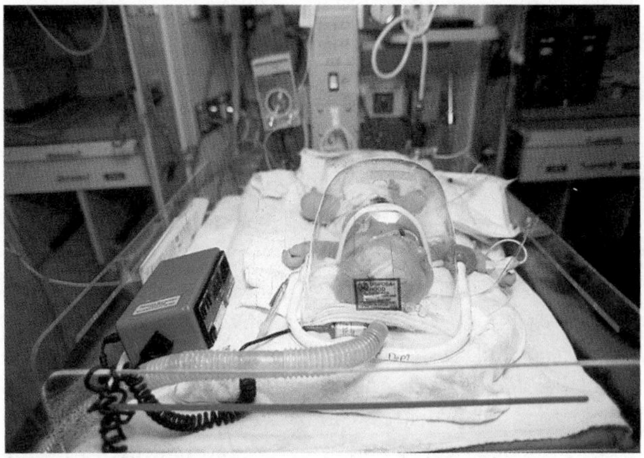

Fig. 45-25 Oxygen administered to infant by means of a plastic hood. Note oxygen analyzer (blue machine).

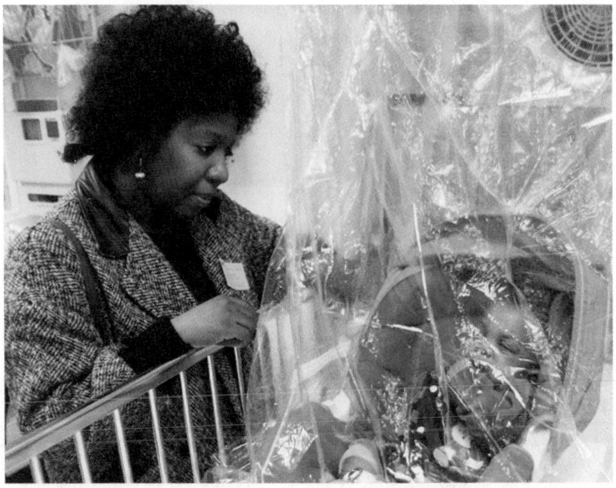

Fig. 45-26 The tent provides a comfortable method for oxygen administration. (From Wilson SF, Thompson JM: *Respiratory disorders,* St Louis, 1990, Mosby.)

To reduce O_2 loss, nursing care is planned carefully so that the tent is opened as little as possible. Because O_2 is heavier than air, loss will be greater at the bottom of the tent; therefore the tent is tucked in snugly without open edges. The bottom of the tent should be examined more often when the child is restless and fussy and liable to pull the covers loose. Some tents are even open at the top. Because of the rapid diffusing qualities of carbon dioxide (CO_2), the levels of the gas do not build up within these enclosures.

After the tent has been opened for an extended period, it is flushed with O_2 by increasing the flow meter for a few minutes to quickly raise the O_2 and mist concentration. The flow meter is then reset to the prescribed number of liters.

The enclosed tent becomes very warm; therefore some type of cooling mechanism is provided. The temperature inside the tent must be checked periodically to be certain that it is maintained at the desired level. Although the cool environment can reduce fever and airway inflammation, it can also produce hypothermia and cold stress. It is important to make certain that the child is kept warm and dry. Because O_2 is drying to the tissues, the gas is humidified, which causes moisture to condense on the tent walls.

NURSE ALERT Keep the child warm and dry by checking the temperature inside the tent and the child's bedding and clothing frequently. Adjust the temperature and change clothing as often as needed. ■

The reactions of children to the O_2 tent are variable. Some, especially older children, feel comfortable in the tent and like the cozy, close privacy it affords. Others, more often younger children, may be frightened by the forced enclosure. The plastic walls distort their view of the world and constitute a barrier between them and their source of comfort, their parent. Their distress can be minimized if they are able to see someone nearby and are reassured that they will not be left alone. A favorite toy or object can accompany the child inside the tent. However, all toys should be inspected for safety and suitability. Other familiar items can be placed at the foot of the bed or otherwise in view.

NURSE ALERT Inspect all toys for safety and suitability (e.g., vinyl or plastic, not stuffed items that absorb moisture and are difficult to keep dry). The high-level O_2 environment makes any source of sparks (e.g., mechanical or electrical toys) a potential fire hazard. ■

In most instances the child can be removed from the O_2 tent for activities such as feeding and bathing, whereas in other cases the child is placed in the tent only during periods of rest. Still other children may require O_2 continuously and can be removed from the tent or incubator only if an O_2 source is held close to the child's face. Any change in color, increased respiratory effort, or restlessness is an indication to return the child to the O_2 tent.

Oxygen Toxicity

O_2 is essential to life and a valuable therapeutic aid. However, prolonged exposure to high O_2 tensions can be damaging to some body tissues and functions. The organs most vulnerable to the adverse effects of excessive oxygenation are the retina of the premature infant and the lungs of persons at any age.

Oxygen-induced carbon dioxide narcosis is a physiologic hazard of O_2 therapy that may occur in persons with chronic pulmonary disease, such as cystic fibrosis. These children have chronic alveolar hypoventilation with a concomitant chronic CO_2 retention and hypoxemia. In these patients the respiratory center has adapted to the continuously higher arterial carbon dioxide tension ($Paco_2$) levels, and therefore hypoxia becomes the more powerful stimulus for respiration. When the arterial oxygen tension (Pao_2) level is elevated during O_2 administration, the hypoxic drive is removed, causing progressive hypoventilation and increased $Paco_2$ levels, and the child rapidly becomes unconscious. CO_2 narcosis can also be induced by the administration of sedation in these patients.

Monitoring Oxygen Therapy

Pulse oximetry is a simple, continuous, noninvasive method of determining oxygen saturation (Sao_2) to guide O_2 therapy. A sensor comprising a light-emitting diode (LED) and a photodetector is placed in opposition around a foot, hand, finger, toe, or earlobe, with the LED placed on top of the nail when digits are used (Fig. 45-27). The LED emits red and infrared lights that pass through the skin to the photodetector. The photodetector measures the amount of each type of light absorbed by functional hemoglobins. Hemoglobin saturated with O_2 (oxyhemoglobin) absorbs more infrared light than does hemoglobin not saturated with O_2 (deoxyhemoglobin). Therefore pulsatile blood flow is the primary physiologic factor that influences accuracy of the pulse oximeter.

Another noninvasive method is *transcutaneous monitoring (TCM),* which provides continual monitoring of transcutaneous partial pressure of oxygen in arterial blood ($tcPao_2$) and, with some devices, of carbon dioxide in arterial blood ($tcPaco_2$). An electrode is attached to the warmed skin to facilitate arterialization of cutaneous capillaries. The site of the electrode must be changed every 3 to 4 hours to prevent burning the skin, and the machine must be calibrated with every site change. TCM is used frequently in neonatal intensive care units, but it may not reflect Pao_2 in

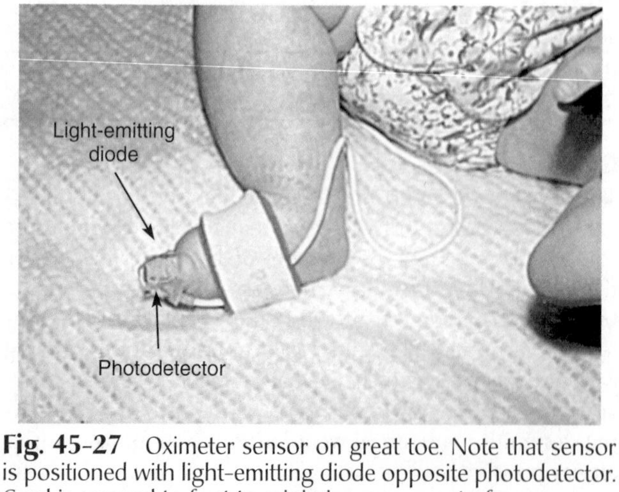

Fig. 45-27 Oximeter sensor on great toe. Note that sensor is positioned with light-emitting diode opposite photodetector. Cord is secured to foot to minimize movement of sensor.

infants with impaired local circulation or in older infants whose skin is thicker.

The PaO_2 can be correlated with the SaO_2 by means of the *oxyhemoglobin dissociation curve* (Fig. 45-28). Most important, changes in PaO_2 do not cause identical changes in SaO_2. Rather, in the steep portion of the curve, small changes in PaO_2 result in large changes in SaO_2. In the flat portion of the curve, large changes in PaO_2 result in only small changes in SaO_2. A quick formula for calculating the correlation of PaO_2 with SaO_2 is the 30-60, 60-90 rule. Assuming a normal pH, $PaCO_2$, and body temperature, this rule can apply: when $PaO_2 = 30$ mm Hg, $SaO_2 = 60\%$; when $PaO_2 = 60$ mm, $SaO_2 = 90\%$.

Also, oximetry is insensitive to hyperoxia because hemoglobin approaches 100% saturation for all PaO_2 readings greater than approximately 100 mm Hg, which is a dangerous situation for the premature infant at risk for developing retinopathy of prematurity. Therefore the premature infant being monitored with oximetry should have upper limits identified, such as 90% to 95%, and a protocol established for decreasing O_2 when saturations are high.

The degree to which O_2 combines with hemoglobin is affected by several factors. A shift of the curve to the left causes an increased affinity of hemoglobin for O_2, but the O_2 is not easily released to the tissues. This represents an increase in the SaO_2 if it is measured against the same PaO_2 of the normal oxyhemoglobin dissociation curve. This left shift can be caused by an increase in blood pH or a decrease in $PaCO_2$, body temperature, or 2,3-diphosphoglycerate (2,3-DPG), a substance in the red blood cells.

A shift of the curve to the right causes a decreased affinity of hemoglobin for O_2, but improved O_2 release to the tissues. This represents a lower SaO_2 if measured against the same PaO_2 of the normal oxyhemoglobin dissociation curve. This right shift can be caused by a decrease in blood pH or an increase in $PaCO_2$, body temperature, or 2,3-DPG.

Oximetry offers several advantages over TCM. Oximetry (1) does not require heating the skin, thus reducing the risk of burns; (2) eliminates a delay period for transducer equilibration; and (3) maintains an accurate measurement regardless of the patient's age or skin characteristics or the presence of lung disease.

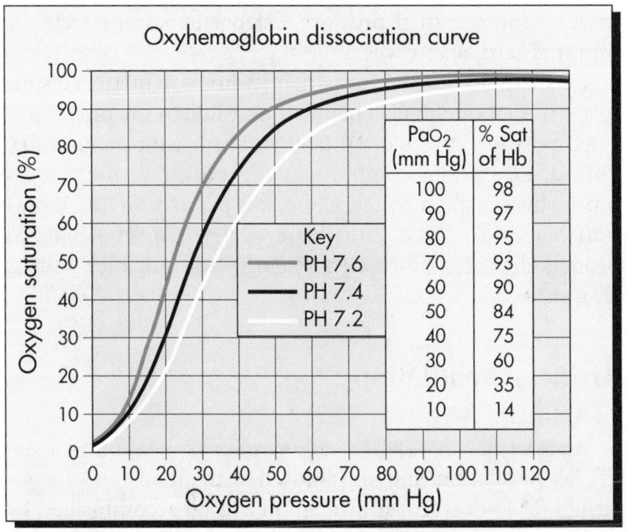

Fig. 45-28 Oxyhemoglobin dissociation curve. Changes in affinity of hemoglobin for oxygen shift position of curve. Shift to left *(colored line)* indicates increased affinity of hemoglobin for oxygen. Shift to right *(white line)* indicates decreased affinity of hemoglobin for oxygen.

NURSE ALERT It is important to make certain that sensor connectors and oximeters are compatible. Wiring that is incompatible can generate considerable heat at the tip of the sensor, causing second- and third-degree burns under the sensors. Pressure necrosis can also occur from sensors attached too tightly. Therefore inspect the skin under the sensor frequently. ■

Applying the sensor correctly is essential for accurate SaO_2 measurements. Because the sensor must identify every pulse beat to calculate the SaO_2, movement can interfere with sensing. Some devices synchronize the SaO_2 reading with the heartbeat, thereby reducing the interference caused by motion. Sensors are not placed on extremities used for blood pressure monitoring or with indwelling arterial catheters, because pulsatile blood flow can be affected. The following are general guidelines for placing sensors on infants and children:

- **Infant**—Tape the sensor securely to the great toe and tape the wire to the sole of the foot (or use a commercial holder that fastens with a self-adhering closure). Place a snugly fitting sock over the foot.
- **Child**—Tape the sensor securely to the index finger and tape the wire to the back of the hand. Use self-adhering Ace-type wrap (e.g., Coban) around the finger and/or hand to further secure the sensor and wire.

Ambient light from ceiling lights and phototherapy, as well as high-intensity heat and light from radiant warmers, can interfere with readings. Therefore the sensor should be covered to block these light sources. IV dyes; green, purple, or black nail polish; nonopaque synthetic nails; and possibly ink used for footprinting can also cause inaccurate SaO_2 measurements. The dyes should be removed or, in the case of porcelain nails, a different area used for the sensor. Skin color, thickness, and edema do not affect the readings.

Aerosol Therapy

Aerosol therapy can be effective in depositing medication directly into the airway. The value of aerosolized water, or "mist therapy," is controversial. This route of administration can be useful in avoiding the systemic side effects of certain drugs and in reducing the amount of drug necessary to achieve the desired effect. Bronchodilators, steroids, and antibiotics can be suspended in particulate form and then inhaled so that the medication reaches the small airways. The use of aerosol therapy is particularly challenging in children who are too young to cooperate with controlling the rate and depth of breathing. Administration of this therapy requires skill, patience, and creativity.

Medications can be aerosolized or nebulized with air or with O_2-enriched gas. *Handheld nebulizers* are the most frequently used equipment. The medicated "mist" is discharged into a small plastic mask, which the child holds over the nose and mouth. To avoid particle deposition in the nose and pharynx, the child is instructed to take slow, deep breaths through an open mouth during the treatment. For home use, an air compressor is necessary to force air through the liquid medication to form the aerosol. Fairly compact, portable units can be rented from health equipment companies. The *metered-dose inhaler (MDI)* is a self-contained, handheld device that allows for intermittent delivery of a specified amount of medication. Many bronchodilators are available in this form and are successfully used by children with asthma. For children under 5 or 6 years of age, a *spacer device* attached to the MDI can help with coordination of breathing and aerosol delivery. It allows the aerosolized particles to remain in suspension longer. (See also Asthma, Chapter 46.)

A major nursing responsibility during aerosol therapy is to assess the effectiveness of the treatment and the patient's tolerance of the procedure. Assessments of breath sounds and work of breathing should be done before and after treatments. Small children who become upset with having a mask held close to the face may become fatigued with fighting the procedure and may actually appear worse during and immediately after the therapy. Careful assessment is required by the nurse and practitioner to determine if the treatment is worthwhile. To accurately assess changes in breath sounds and work of breathing, it may be necessary to spend a few minutes calming the child after the procedure; this allows the vital signs to return to baseline.

Bronchial (Postural) Drainage

Bronchial drainage is indicated whenever excessive fluid or mucus in the bronchi is not being removed by normal ciliary activity and cough. Positioning the child to take maximum advantage of gravity facilitates removal of secretions. The effect is sometimes dramatic in children with chronic lung disease characterized by thick mucus, such as asthma and cystic fibrosis.

Postural drainage is carried out three to four times daily and is more effective when it follows other respiratory therapy, such as bronchodilator or nebulization medication. Bronchial drainage is generally performed before meals (or 1 to 1½ hours after meals) to minimize the chance of vomiting and is repeated at bedtime. The length and duration of treatment depend on the child's condition and tolerance level, usually 20 to 30 minutes. There are positions to facilitate drainage from all major lung segments (Fig. 45-29), but not all positions are employed at each session. Children will usually cooperate for four to six positions, but more than six tends to exceed their limits of tolerance. Older children can be expected to tolerate longer periods.

In the hospital, an older child can be positioned over an elevated knee rest. Small children and infants can be positioned with pillows or on the therapist's lap and legs (Fig. 45-30). Infants should not be placed in the Trendelenburg position because they do not have an autonomic regulation of blood flow to the head. Special modifications of the techniques are required in children whose conditions contraindicate the standard positioning, such as head injuries, some types of surgical incisions or burns, and casts or traction. At home, small children can be positioned on a padded ironing board. Children who require postural drainage over months or years may benefit from specially constructed tables padded and adjusted to their individual needs. The position used and the frequency and duration of treatment are individualized.

Chest Physiotherapy

Chest physiotherapy (CPT) usually refers to the use of postural drainage in combination with adjunctive techniques that are thought to enhance the clearance of mucus from the airway. These techniques include manual percussion, vibration, and squeezing of the chest; cough; forceful expiration; and breathing exercises. However, the efficacies of these techniques, both individually and combined, are controversial. Postural drainage in combination with forced expiration has been shown to be beneficial, but the benefit of the other techniques has yet to be demonstrated. The results of a study evaluating the effects of noninvasive inspiratory nasal pressure support ventilation (PSV) during CPT showed a significant improvement in respiratory muscle performance and a reduction in O_2 desaturation when used in combination (Fauroux et al, 1999).

The most common technique used in association with postural drainage is manual percussion of the chest wall. Nurses are often responsible for this maneuver if a respiratory therapist is not available, so they should be skilled in the technique. The patient is dressed in a lightweight shirt and placed in a postural drainage position; then the nurse gently but firmly strikes the chest wall with a cupped hand (Fig. 45-31, *A*). For infants, special devices are available for percussing small areas (Fig. 45-31, *B*). A "popping," hollow sound should be the result, not a slapping sound. The procedure should be done over the rib cage only and should be painless. Percussion can be performed with a soft circular mask (adapted to maintain air trapping) or a percussion cup marketed especially for the purpose of aiding the loosening of secretions.

CPT is contraindicated when patients have pulmonary hemorrhage, pulmonary embolism, end-stage renal disease, increased intracranial pressure, osteogenesis imperfecta, or minimal cardiac reserves.

CPT should be used for patients who have increased sputum production. It is probably of no value to the uncomplicated postoperative patient or the patient with pneumonia. Forced expiration combined with postural drainage is more effective than cough alone, but percussion and vibration have no proven value. Appropriate use of nebulized bronchodilators before CPT therapy will enhance mucus clearance.

Artificial Ventilation

Artificial Airways

An artificial airway is usually used in association with artificial ventilation and in children with upper airway obstruction. Endotracheal intubation can be accomplished by the nasal (nasotracheal), oral (orotracheal), or direct tracheal (tracheostomy) routes. Although it is more difficult to place, nasotracheal intubation is preferred to orotracheal intubation because it facilitates oral hygiene and provides more stable fixation, which reduces the complication of tra-

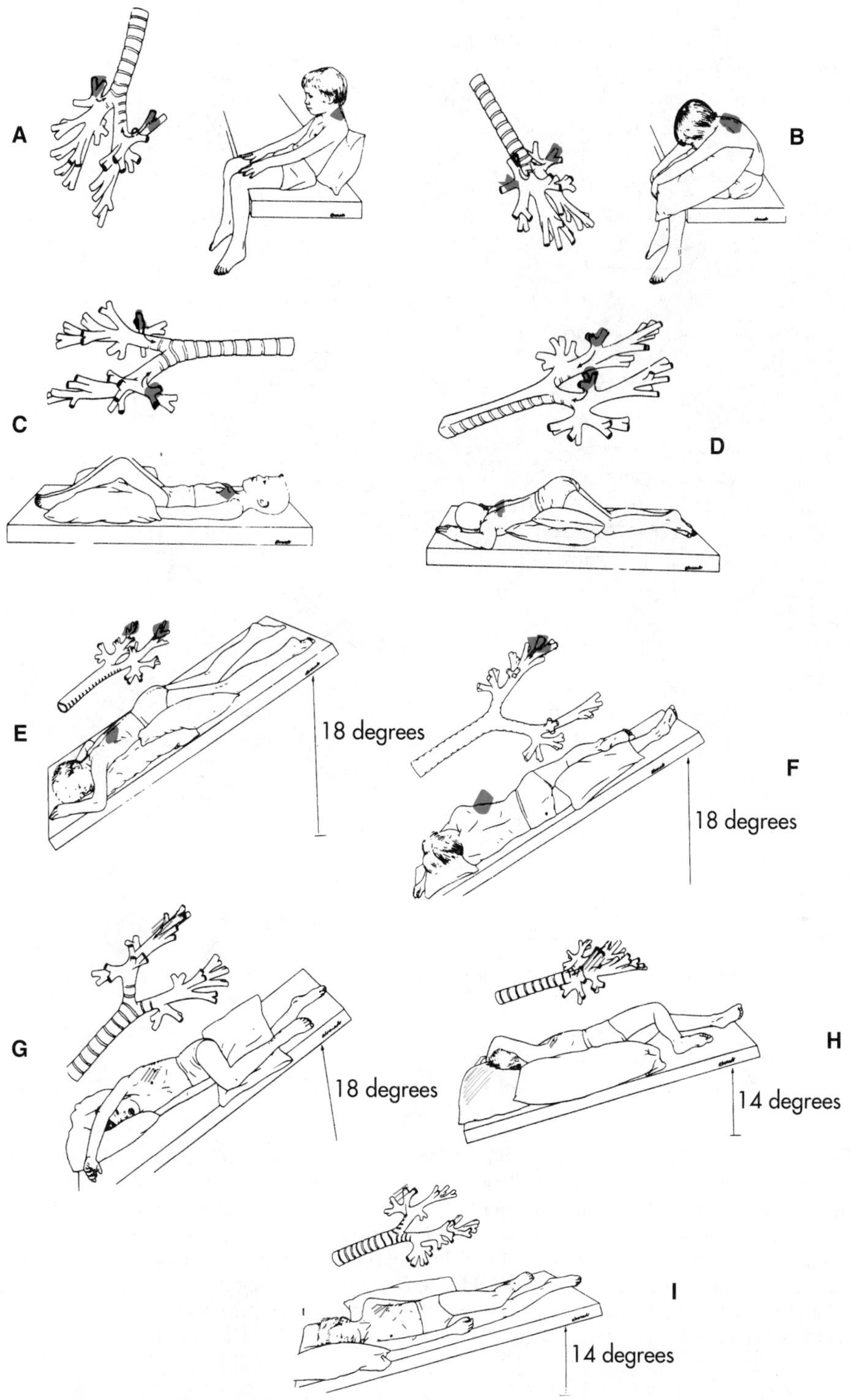

Fig. 45-29 Bronchial drainage positions for all major segments of child *(red)*. For each position, model of tracheobronchial tree is projected beside child to show segmental bronchus *(red)* being drained and pathway *(arrow)* of secretions out of bronchus. Drainage platform is horizontal unless otherwise noted. *Striped area* on child's chest indicates area to be cupped or vibrated by therapist. **A,** Apical segment of right upper lobe and apical subsegment of apical-posterior segment of left upper lobe. **B,** Posterior segment of right upper lobe and posterior subsegment of apical-posterior segment of left upper lobe. **C,** Anterior segments of both upper lobes; child should be rotated slightly away from side being drained. **D,** Superior segments of both lower lobes. **E,** Posterior basal segments of both lower lobes. **F,** Lateral basal segments of right lower lobe; left lateral basal segment would be drained by mirror image of this position (right side down). **G,** Anterior basal segment of left lower lobe; right anterior basal segment would be drained by mirror image of this position (left side down). **H,** Medial and lateral segments of right middle lobe. **I,** Lingular segments (superior and inferior) of left upper lobe (homologue of right middle lobe). (From Chernick V [ed]: *Kendig's disorders of the respiratory tract of children,* ed 6, Philadelphia, 1998, WB Saunders.)

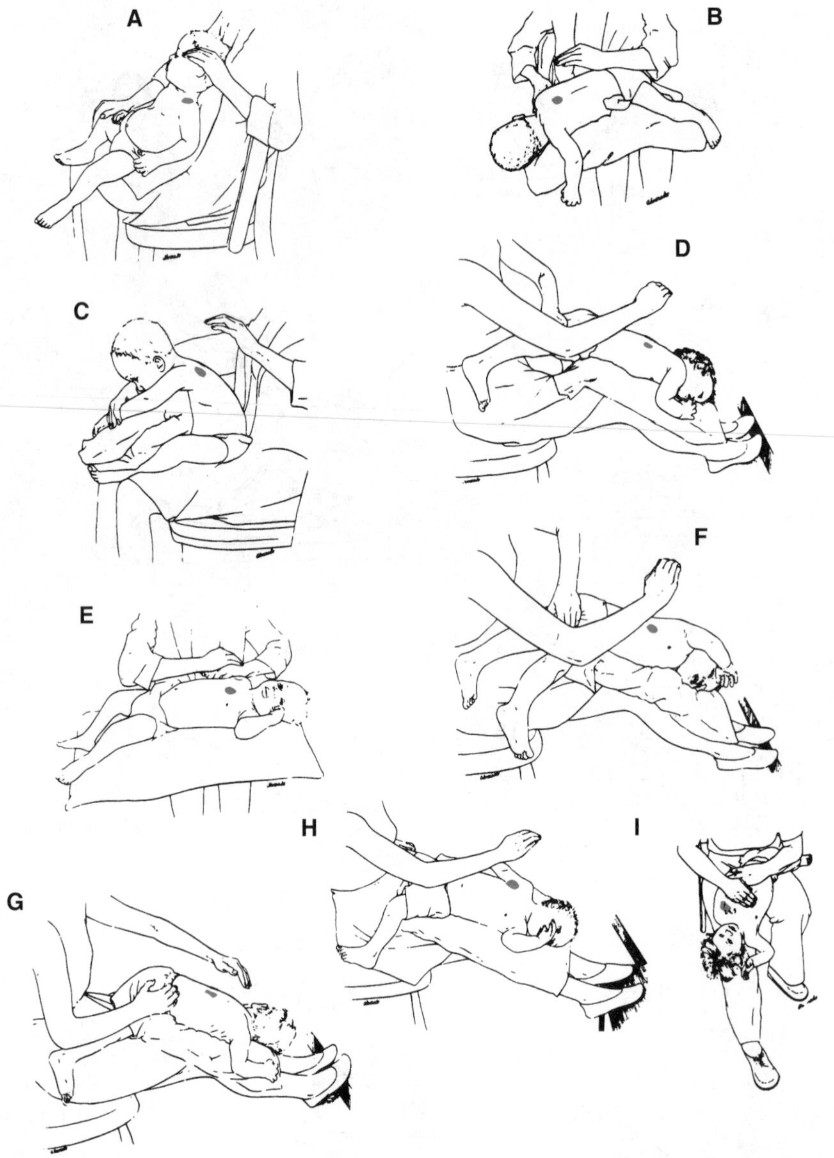

Fig. 45-30 Bronchial drainage positions for major segments of all lobes in infant *(red)*. Procedure is most easily carried out in therapist's lap. Therapist's hand on chest indicates area to be cupped or vibrated. **A**, Apical segment of left upper lobe. **B**, Posterior segment of left upper lobe. **C**, Anterior segment of left upper lobe. **D**, Superior segment of right lower lobe. **E**, Posterior basal segment of right lower lobe. **F**, Lateral basal segment of right lower lobe. **G**, Anterior basal segment of right lower lobe. **H**, Medial and lateral segments of right middle lobe. **I**, Lingular segments (superior and inferior) of left upper lobe. (Modified from Cystic Fibrosis Foundation: *Infant segmental bronchial drainage*, Rockville, MD, The Foundation.)

cheal erosion and the danger of accidental extubation. Only uncuffed endotracheal tubes should be used in children less than 8 years of age (Hazinski, 1996). Cuffed tubes may be used with adolescents to help provide an airtight seal. Air or gas delivered directly to the trachea must be humidified as in tracheostomy.

Tracheostomy

A tracheostomy is a surgical opening in the trachea; the procedure may be done on an emergency basis or may be an elective one, and it may be combined with mechanical ventilation.

Pediatric tracheostomy tubes are usually made of plastic or Silastic. The most common types are the Hollinger, Jackson, Aberdeen, and Shiley tubes. These tubes are constructed with a more acute angle than adult tubes, and they soften at body temperature, conforming to the contours of the trachea. Because these materials resist the formation of crusted respiratory secretions, they are made without an inner cannula. Some children require a metal tracheostomy tube (usually made of sterling silver or stainless steel), which contains an inner cannula. The principal advantage of metal tubes is their nonreactivity and decreased chance of causing an allergic reaction.

Children who have undergone a tracheostomy require a hospital stay. During this time the child is closely monitored for the development of complications such as hemorrhage,

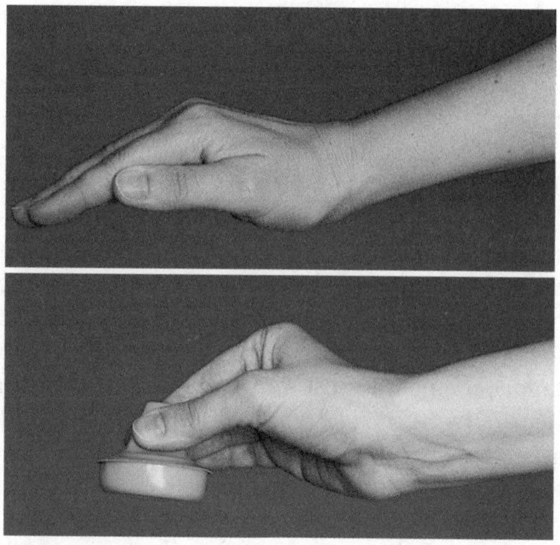

Fig. 45-31 **A,** Cupped hand position for percussion. **B,** Device for infant percussion.

edema, aspiration, accidental decannulation, tube obstruction, or the entrance of free air into the pleural cavity. The focus of postoperative nursing care is maintaining a patent airway, facilitating the removal of pulmonary secretions, providing humidified air or O_2, cleansing the stoma, monitoring the child's ability to swallow, and teaching while simultaneously preventing complications. The most dangerous complication is related to accidental decannulation and tube obstruction. Because the child may be unable to signal for help, direct observation and use of respiratory and cardiac monitors is essential. Respiratory assessments include breath sounds and work of breathing, vital signs, tightness of the tracheostomy ties, and the type and amount of secretions. Large amounts of bloody secretions are uncommon and should be considered a sign of hemorrhage. The practitioner should be notified immediately if this occurs.

The child is positioned with the head of the bed raised or in the position most comfortable to the child, with the call light easily available. Suction catheters, suction source, gloves, sterile saline, sterile gauze for wiping away secretions, scissors, an extra tracheostomy tube of the same size with ties already attached, another tracheostomy tube one size smaller, and the obturator are kept at the bedside. A source of humidification is provided, because the normal humidification and filtering functions of the airway have been bypassed. IV fluids ensure adequate hydration until the child is able to swallow sufficient amounts of fluids.

Suctioning

The airway must remain patent and requires frequent suctioning during the first few hours after a tracheostomy to remove mucous plugs and excessive secretions. Proper vacuum pressure and suction catheter size are important to prevent atelectasis and decrease hypoxia from the suctioning procedure. Vacuum pressure should range from 60 to 100 mm Hg for infants and children and from 40 to 60 mm Hg for premature infants. Unless secretions are thick and tenacious, the lower range of negative pressure is recommended. Tracheal suction catheters are available in a variety of sizes. The catheter selected should have a diameter one half the diameter of the tracheostomy tube. If the catheter is too large, it can block the airway. The catheter is constructed with a side port so that the catheter is introduced without suction and removed while simultaneous intermittent suction is applied by covering the port with the thumb (Fig. 45-32). The catheter is inserted to 0.5 cm beyond or just to the end of the tracheostomy tube. The practice of instilling sterile saline in the tracheostomy tube before suctioning is not supported by research and is no longer recommended.

NURSE ALERT Suctioning should require no more than 5 seconds. ■

Counting 1—one thousand, 2—one thousand, 3—one thousand, and so on, while suctioning is a simple means for monitoring the time. Without a safeguard, the airway may be obstructed for too long a period. Hyperventilating the child with 100% O_2 before and after suctioning (using a bag-valve-mask or increasing the fraction of inspired oxygen concentration [FiO_2] ventilator setting) is also performed to prevent hypoxia. Closed tracheal suctioning systems that allow for uninterrupted O_2 delivery may also be used.

The child is allowed to rest for 30 to 60 seconds after each aspiration to allow O_2 tension to return to normal; then the process is repeated until the trachea is clear. Suctioning should be limited to about three aspirations in one period. Oximetry is used to monitor suctioning and prevent hypoxia.

NURSE ALERT Suctioning is carried out *only as often as needed* to keep the tube patent. Signs of mucus partially occluding the airway include an increased heart rate, a rise in res-

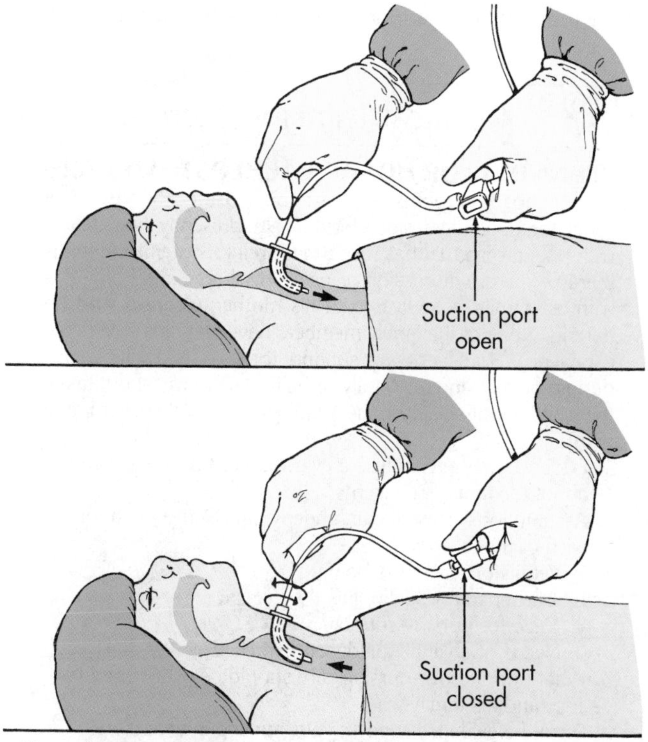

Fig. 45-32 Tracheostomy suctioning. **A,** Insertion, port open. **B,** Withdrawal, port occluded. Note that catheter is inserted just slightly beyond end of tracheostomy tube.

piratory effort, a drop in Sao_2, cyanosis, or an increase in the positive inspiratory pressure on the ventilator. ■

In the acute care setting, aseptic technique is used during care of the tracheostomy. Secondary infection is a major concern, because the air entering the lower airway bypasses the natural defenses of the upper airway. Gloves are worn during the aspiration procedure, although a sterile glove is needed only on the hand touching the catheter. A new tube, gloves, and sterile saline solution are used each time (Critical Thinking Exercise).

Routine Care

The tracheostomy stoma requires daily care. Assessments of the stoma area include observations for signs of infection and breakdown of the skin. The skin is kept clean and dry, and secretions around the stoma may be gently removed with half-strength hydrogen peroxide. Hydrogen peroxide should not be used with sterling silver tracheostomy tubes because it tends to pit and stain the silver surface. The nurse should be aware of wet tracheostomy dressings, which can predispose the peristomal area to skin breakdown. Several products are available to prevent or treat excoriation. The Allevyn tracheostomy dressing is a hydrophilic sponge with a polyurethane back that is highly absorptive. Other possible barriers to help maintain skin integrity include the use of hydrocolloid wafers (e.g., Duoderm CGF, Hollister Restore) under the tracheostomy flanges, as well as use of extra-thin hydrocolloid wafers under the chin.

The tracheostomy tube is held in place with tracheostomy ties made of a durable, nonfraying material. The ties are changed daily and when soiled. New ties are looped through the flanges and tied snugly in a triple knot at the side of the neck *before* the soiled ties are cut and removed. Some nurses have found that threading the ties through a piece of ¼-inch surgical tubing cushions the ties; others have found the tubing to be irritating to the skin. The ties should be tight enough to allow just a fingertip to be inserted between the ties and the neck (Fig. 45-33). It is easier to ensure a snug fit if the child's head is flexed rather than extended while the ties are being secured. Ties fastened with self-adhering closures are also available. These devices, such as the Dale tracheostomy tube holder, are made of a soft, cushioning, and slightly stretchy material that is very comfortable. They are becoming increasingly popular because of their ease of use and ability to maintain better skin integrity. However, nurses and family members must consider the safety factor and use them only on a child who will not pull and undo the fastener.

Routine tracheostomy tube changes are usually carried out weekly after a tract has been formed to minimize the formation of granulation tissue. The first change is usually performed by the surgeon; subsequent changes are performed by the nurse and, if the child is discharged home with the tracheostomy, by either a parent or a visiting nurse. Ideally, two caregivers participate in the procedure to assist with positioning the child.

Changing the tracheostomy tube is accomplished using sterile technique. The new, sterile tube is prepared by inserting the obturator and attaching new ties. The child is suctioned before the procedure to minimize secretions, then restrained and positioned with the neck slightly extended. One caregiver cuts the old ties and removes the tube from the stoma. The new tube is inserted gently into the stoma (using a downward and forward motion that follows the curve of the trachea), the obturator is removed, and the ties are secured. The adequacy of ventilation must be assessed after a tube change because the tube can be inserted into the soft tissue surrounding the trachea; therefore breath sounds and respiratory effort are carefully monitored.

Supplemental O_2 is always delivered with a humidification system to prevent drying of the respiratory mucosa. Humidification of room air for an established tracheostomy can be intermittent if secretions remain thin enough to be coughed or suctioned from the tracheostomy. Direct humidification via a tracheostomy mask can be provided during naps and at night so that the child is able to be up and around unencumbered during much of the day. Room humidifiers are also used successfully.

Critical Thinking Exercise

PLANNING FOR HOME TRACHEOSTOMY CARE

Jose Munoz, 18 months old, has a tracheostomy and has been ventilator dependent since birth. He is presently hospitalized with pneumonia that has responded well to systemic antibiotic therapy. You are discussing plans for discharge and home care with the family. Jose lives with his mother, Gabriela, and her parents. None of the family members have previous health care experience. Home nursing support for Jose is available only during the day, and the family verbalizes concerns about taking the child home because he requires frequent suctioning at night.

1. Evidence—Is there sufficient evidence to draw conclusions about the family's concerns?
2. Assumptions—Describe an underlying assumption about each of the following:
   a. Ventilator use in the home
   b. Tracheostomy suctioning
   c. Need for nursing support
   d. Needs of a ventilator-dependent child
3. What priorities for nursing care should be established for Jose and his family?
4. Does the evidence support your nursing intervention?
5. What alternative perspectives might you have?

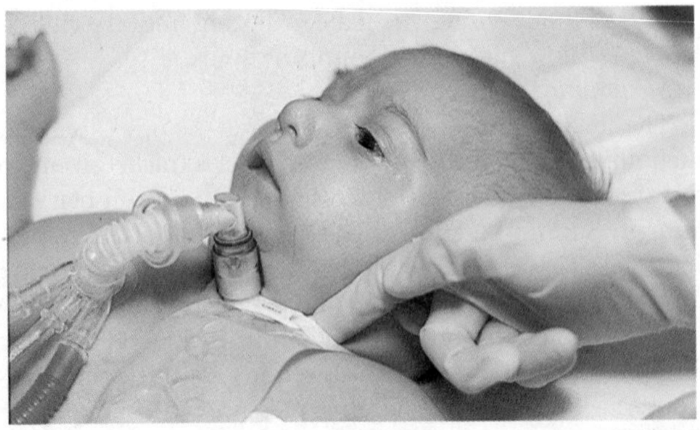

Fig. 45-33 Tracheostomy ties are snug but allow one finger to be inserted.

The inner cannula, if used, should be removed with each suctioning, cleaned with sterile saline and pipe cleaners to remove crusted material, dried thoroughly, and reinserted.

Emergency Care: Tube Occlusion and Accidental Decannulation

Occlusion of the tracheostomy tube is life threatening, and infants and children are at greater risk than adults because of the smaller diameter of the tube. Maintaining patency of the tube is accomplished with suctioning and routine tube changes to prevent the formation of crusts that can occlude the tube.

NURSE ALERT Life-threatening occlusion is apparent when the child displays signs of respiratory distress and a suction catheter cannot be passed to the end of the tube despite several attempts and instillation of saline. This situation requires an immediate tube change. ■

Accidental decannulation also requires immediate tube replacement. Some children have a fairly rigid trachea, so the airway remains partially open when the tube is removed. However, others have malformed or flexible tracheal cartilage, which causes the airway to collapse when the tube is removed or dislodged. Because many infants and children with upper airway problems have little airway reserve, if replacement of the dislodged tube is impossible, a smaller-size tube should be inserted. If the stoma cannot be cannulated with another tracheostomy tube, oral intubation should be performed.

Family Teaching and Home Care

Some of the treatments families need to continue at home are often related to respiratory procedures. Some of these treatments, such as postural drainage, require less preparation than others, such as tracheostomy care. Regardless of the home therapy, the family needs ample time to learn the skills and demonstrate them before discharge; therefore instruction should begin as soon as it is identified that the child will go home with a tracheostomy. The more comfortable they are with all the aspects of care, the more confident and less anxious the family will be when faced with total care of the child at home. For example, the family may require many practice sessions before they feel comfortable with suctioning, cleaning, and changing a tracheostomy tube and performing cardiopulmonary resuscitation (CPR) in case of an emergency. Teaching sessions should be short, and written material must accompany instructions to reinforce what is being taught. To facilitate the family's adjustment, supplies identical to the ones to which they are accustomed should be available in the home. In the event of substitution, parents need to be reassured that the unfamiliar equipment is safe to use on their child. The home should be properly equipped with all supplies and equipment needed before the child arrives.

A nurse from the public health department or other home care service should be available to the family and should periodically assess the family's ability to carry out the activities needed in the care of the child. The parents may find it helpful to talk with other parents of children with similar needs. They also need to know whom to call and where they can get help and support in times of uncertainty or in an emergency.

To prepare for any emergency, the family must be taught infant or child CPR. The local utilities company and local emergency medical services (EMS) should be notified of the child's condition and the equipment used in the home. Prior notification allows for a quicker response if help is needed.

When a child has a tracheostomy, parents are encouraged to provide as normal a life as possible for their child and other family members. Vocalization for the child with a tracheostomy has recently become a reality. Several tracheostomy speaking valves have been created to aid in the development of uninterrupted speech without the necessity of finger occlusion. One valve of several available on the market is the Passy Muir valve.* It is a one-way valve that attaches to the hub of all types and sizes of tracheostomies. It can be used in infants and in children who are ventilator assisted (Engleman & Turnage-Carrier, 1997).

The child who is physically able (e.g., a child with a tracheostomy without respiratory disability such as recurrent laryngeal polyps) can usually be allowed to engage in most activities that are appropriate for the child's age. The child may play outdoors with a scarf or other protection to loosely cover the tracheostomy stoma. Both child and parents must be cautioned regarding play near any body of water, such as a swimming pool or stream, and informed about safety precautions in the bathtub. The child should not be exposed to noxious fumes (e.g., paint, varnish, hair spray) or talc (baby powder). Young children who may spill food near the stoma should wear a fabric bib (without plastic lining) or other device to prevent dribbled food or crumbs from being aspirated. The family should have a bag with routine and emergency supplies to take with the child at all times.

PROCEDURES RELATED TO ALTERNATIVE FEEDING TECHNIQUES

Some children are unable to take nourishment by mouth because of conditions such as anomalies of the throat, esophagus, or bowel; impaired swallowing capacity; severe debilitation; respiratory distress; or unconsciousness. These children are frequently fed by way of a tube inserted orally or nasally into the stomach (*orogastric* or *nasogastric gavage*) or duodenum/jejunum (*enteral gavage*), or by a tube inserted directly into the stomach (*gastrostomy*) or jejunum (*jejunostomy*). Such feedings may be intermittent or by continuous drip. At times the entire alimentary tract must be bypassed, using IV feeding (total parenteral nutrition [TPN]). Because enteral feedings are used less often than gastric or IV feed-

*Further information can be obtained from Passy & Passy, Inc., 4521 Campus Dr., Suite 273, Irvine, CA 92612; phone: 800-634-5397; fax: 949-833-8299; e-mail: info@passy.muir.com; Web site: www.passy-muir.com.

ings, the following discussion is limited to gastric gavage, gastrostomy, and TPN.

During gavage or gastrostomy (nonoral) feedings, infants are given a pacifier. Nonnutritive sucking has several advantages, such as increased weight gain and decreased crying. However, to prevent the possibility of aspiration, only pacifiers with a safe design may be used. Using improvised pacifiers made from bottle nipples is not a safe practice. (See Injury Prevention: Aspiration in Chapter 36.)

NURSE ALERT When a child is concurrently receiving continuous-drip gastric or enteral feedings and parenteral (IV) therapy, the potential exists for inadvertent administration of the enteral formula through the circulatory system, especially when the parenteral solution is a fat emulsion, which looks milky. Safeguards to prevent this potentially serious error include the following:

- Use a separate, specifically designed enteral feeding pump mounted on a separate pole for continuous-feeding solutions.
- Label all tubing for continuous enteral feeding with brightly colored tape or labels.
- Use specifically designed continuous-feeding bags to contain the solutions instead of parenteral equipment, such as a burette. ■

Gavage Feeding

Infants and children can be fed simply and safely by a tube passed into the stomach through either the nares or the mouth. The tube can be left in place or inserted and removed with each feeding. In older children it is usually less traumatic to tape the tube securely in place between feedings. When this alternative is used, the tube should be removed and replaced with a new tube according to hospital policy, specific orders, and the type of tube used. Meticulous handwashing is practiced during the procedure to prevent bacterial contamination of the feeding, especially during continuous-drip feedings.

Preparation

The equipment needed for gavage feeding includes the following:

- A suitable tube selected according to the size of the child and the viscosity of the solution being fed. Feeding tubes are available in silicone rubber, polyurethane, polyethylene, or polyvinylchloride. Polyurethane and silicone rubber tubes are smaller in diameter and more flexible than the others and are often referred to as small-bore tubes.
- A receptacle for the fluid; for small amounts, a 10 to 30 ml syringe barrel or Asepto syringe is satisfactory; for larger amounts, a 50 ml syringe with a catheter tip is more convenient.
- A syringe to aspirate stomach contents or to inject air after the tube has been placed.
- Water or water-soluble lubricant to lubricate the tube; sterile water is used for infants.
- Paper or nonallergenic tape to mark the tube and to attach the tube to the infant's or child's cheek (and nose, if placed through the nares).
- A stethoscope to determine the correct placement in the stomach.
- The solution for feeding.

Not all feeding tubes are the same. Polyethylene and polyvinylchloride types lose their flexibility and need to be replaced frequently, usually every 3 to 4 days. The polyurethane and silicone rubber tubes are indwelling and remain flexible; thus they can remain in place longer and afford more patient comfort. Use of these small-bore tubes for continuous feeding has greatly reduced the incidence of complications such as pharyngitis, otitis media, and incompetence of the lower esophageal sphincter. Although the increased softness and flexibility of the tubes are advantages, they also result in problems such as difficult insertion (may require a stylet or metal guidewire), collapse of the tube during aspiration of gastric contents when testing for correct placement, dislodgment during forceful coughing, and unsuitability for thick feedings. Traditional methods for verifying placement are less reliable with the small-bore tubes.

Procedure

Even tiny infants with random movements can grasp and dislodge the tube. Premature infants do not ordinarily require restraint, but if they do, a small towel folded across the chest and secured beneath the shoulders is usually sufficient. Care must be taken so that breathing is not compromised.

Whenever possible, the infant should be held during the procedure to associate the comfort of physical contact with the feeding. When this is not possible, gavage feeding is carried out with the infant or child on the back or toward the right side and the head and chest elevated. Feeding the child in a sitting position helps maintain the placement of the tube in the lowest position, thus increasing the likelihood of correct placement in the stomach.

The feeding tube can be passed through either the nose (nasogastric) or the mouth (orogastric). Because most young infants are obligatory nose breathers, insertion through the mouth causes less distress and helps stimulate sucking. A tube passed through one of the nares in older infants and children is satisfactory once the tube is in place. An indwelling tube is almost always placed through the nose; the tube is alternated between nares with each insertion to minimize irritation, chance of infection, and possible breakdown of mucous membranes from pressure that occurs over time.

Two standard methods of measuring tube length for insertion are (1) measuring from the nose to the bottom of the earlobe and then to the end of the xiphoid process and (2) measuring from the nose to the earlobe and then to a point midway between the xiphoid process and the umbilicus (Fig. 45-34, *A*). Ellett (1998) found significant tube placement errors (43.5%) in a study of 39 hospitalized children. For very-low-birth-weight infants, daily weight can be used to predict insertion length.

Unfortunately, "bedside" methods used to verify the placement of the tube have serious shortcomings (Guidelines box). The most accurate method for testing tube placement is radiography, but this practice is not feasible before each feeding. One method that appears promising is the consideration of aspirate color and pH to determine placement, because respiratory, gastric, and intestinal fluids have a different pH and color. Metheny and colleagues (1998) found that acidic pH values of 4 or less were reasonable indicators of gastric tube placement, whereas respiratory fluid

A

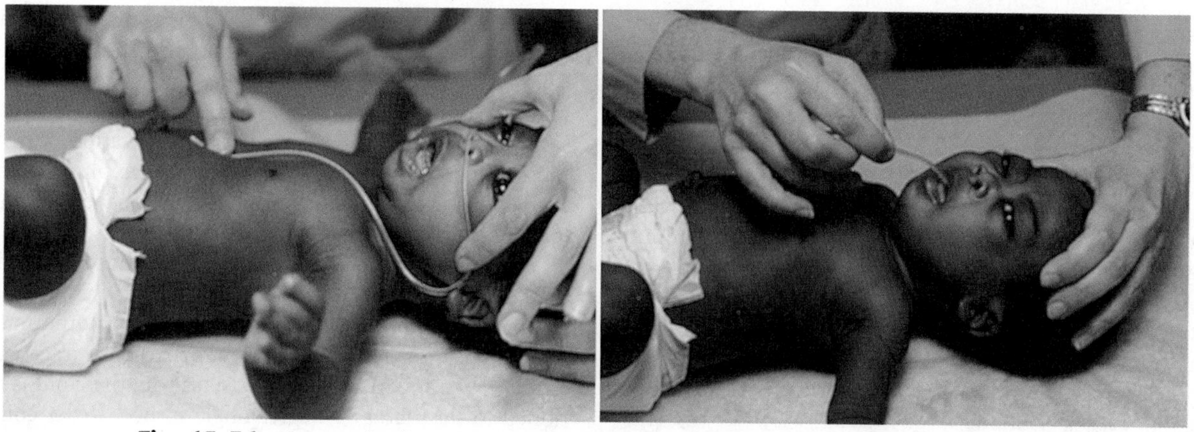

B

Fig. 45-34 Gavage feeding. **A**, Measuring tube for orogastric feeding from tip of nose to earlobe and to midpoint between end of xiphoid process and umbilicus. **B**, Inserting tube.

Guidelines

NASOGASTRIC TUBE FEEDINGS IN CHILDREN

Place child supine with head slightly hyperflexed or in a sniffing position (nose pointed toward ceiling).

Measure the tube for approximate length of insertion and mark the point with a small piece of tape.

Insert the tube, which has been lubricated with sterile water or water-soluble lubricant, through either the mouth or one of the nares to the predetermined mark. Because most young infants are obligatory nose breathers, insertion through the mouth causes less distress and helps stimulate sucking. In older infants and children, the tube is passed through the nose and alternated between nostrils. An indwelling tube is almost always placed through the nose.

When using the nose, slip the tube along the base of the nose and direct it straight back toward the occiput.

When entering through the mouth, direct the tube toward the back of the throat.

If the child is able to swallow on command, synchronize passing the tube with swallowing.

Check the position of the tube by doing *both* of the following:

Attach the syringe to the feeding tube and apply negative pressure. Aspiration of stomach contents indicates proper placement, but aspiration of respiratory secretions may be mistaken for stomach contents. However, absence of fluid is not necessarily evidence of improper placement. The stomach may be empty; the tube may not be in contact with stomach contents; or a small-bore, flexible tube may collapse. Note the amount and character of any fluid aspirated, and return the fluid to the stomach.

With the syringe, inject a small amount of air (0.5 to 1 ml in premature or very small infants to 5 ml in larger children) into the tube while simultaneously listening with a stethoscope over the stomach area. Sounds of gurgling or growling will be heard if the tube is properly situated in the stomach, although it is possible to hear the air entering the stomach even when the tube is positioned above the gastroesophageal sphincter.

Stabilize the tube by holding or taping it to the cheek, not to the forehead, because of possible damage to the nostril. To maintain correct placement, measure and record the amount of tubing extending from the nose or mouth to the distal port when the tube is first positioned. Recheck this measurement before each feeding.

Warm the formula to room temperature. Do *not* microwave! Pour formula into the barrel of the syringe attached to the feeding tube. To start the flow, give a gentle push with the plunger, but then remove the plunger and allow the fluid to flow into the stomach by gravity. The rate of flow should not exceed 5 ml every 5 to 10 minutes in premature and very small infants and 10 ml/min in older infants and children to prevent nausea and regurgitation. The rate is determined by the diameter of the tubing and the height of the reservoir containing the feeding and is regulated by adjusting the height of the syringe. A usual feeding may take from 15 to 30 minutes to complete.

Flush the tube with sterile water (1 or 2 ml for small tubes to 5 to 15 ml or more for large ones), or see discussion of flushing for administering medication through nasogastric tubes in the Guidelines box on p. 1401 to clear it of formula.

Cap or clamp indwelling tubes to prevent loss of feeding.

If the tube is to be removed, first pinch it firmly to prevent escape of fluid as the tube is withdrawn. Withdraw the tube quickly.

Position the child with the head elevated about 30 degrees and on the right side or abdomen for at least 1 hour in the same manner as following any infant feeding to minimize the possibility of regurgitation and aspiration. If the child's condition permits, bubble the youngster after the feeding.

Record the feeding, including the type and amount of residual, the type and amount of formula, and how it was tolerated. For most infant feedings, any amount of residual fluid aspirated from the stomach is refed to prevent electrolyte imbalance, and the amount is subtracted from the prescribed amount of feeding. For example, if the infant is to receive 30 ml and 10 ml is aspirated from the stomach before the feeding, the 10 ml of aspirated stomach contents is refed along with 20 ml of feeding. Another method can be used in children. If residual fluid is more than one fourth of the last feeding, return the aspirate and recheck in 30 to 60 minutes. When residual fluid is less than one fourth of the last feeding, give the scheduled feeding. If large amounts of aspirated fluid persist and the child is due for another feeding, notify the practitioner.

had pH values greater than 6. The color of the gastric fluid aspirated was found to be most often grassy green, off-white to tan, bloody, or brown, whereas the color of pleural fluid was off-white and tinged with mucus and blood. These authors suggest that an aspirate's pH and color can help determine tube placement. Until pH is studied further, especially in children, nurses need to use the traditional methods with an awareness of their limitations. If doubt exists regarding correct placement, the practitioner should be consulted.

NURSE ALERT Nurses need to take precaution when assessing tube placement. One study reported that out of 201 children, 32 had nasogastric tube placement errors as viewed by radiography (Ellett, 1998). ■

Gastrostomy Feeding

Feeding by way of a gastrostomy tube is a variation of tube feeding that is often used for children in whom passage of a tube through the mouth, pharynx, esophagus, and cardiac sphincter of the stomach is contraindicated or impossible. It is also used to avoid the constant irritation of a gastric tube in children who require tube feeding over an extended period. Placement of a gastrostomy tube may be performed with the patient under general anesthesia or percutaneously using an endoscope with the patient sedated and under local anesthesia (percutanous endoscopic gastrostomy). The tube is inserted through the abdominal wall into the stomach about midway along the greater curvature and when surgically placed is secured by a purse-string suture. The stomach is anchored to the peritoneum at the operative site. The tube used can be a Foley, wing-tip, or mushroom catheter.

Immediately after surgery the catheter is left open and attached to gravity drainage for 24 hours or more. Postoperative care of the wound site is directed toward prevention of infection and irritation. The area is cleansed with a mild, pH-balanced cleanser such as normal saline. A cotton-tipped applicator is used to remove drainage close to the tube site (O'Brien et al, 1999). After healing takes place, meticulous care is needed to keep the area surrounding the tube clean and dry to prevent excoriation and infection. Daily applications of antibiotic ointment or other preparations may be prescribed to aid in healing and prevention of irritation. Care is exercised to prevent excessive pull on the catheter that might cause widening of the opening and subsequent leakage of highly irritating gastric juices.

For children receiving long-term gastrostomy feeding, a *skin-level device* (e.g., MIC-KEY, Bard Button, Gastroport) offers several advantages. The small, flexible silicone device protrudes slightly from the abdomen, is cosmetically pleasing in appearance, affords increased comfort and mobility to the child, is easy to care for, and is fully immersible in water. The one-way valve at the proximal end minimizes reflux and eliminates the need for clamping. However, the button requires a well-established gastrostomy site and is more expensive than the conventional tube. In addition, the valve may become clogged. When functioning, the valve prevents air from escaping; therefore the child may require frequent bubbling. With some devices, during feedings the child must remain fairly still, because the tubing easily disconnects from the opening if the child moves. With other devices, extension tubing can be securely attached to the opening (Fig. 45-35). The feeding is instilled at the other end of the tubing in a manner similar to that for a regular gastrostomy. The extension tubing may also have a separate medication port. Both the feeding and the medication ports have plugs attached. Some skin-level devices require a special tube to decompress the stomach (to check residual or release air).

Feeding of water, formula, or pureed foods is carried out in the same manner and rate as in gavage feeding. A mechanical pump may be used to regulate the volume and rate of feeding. After feedings, in an effort to encourage gastric emptying and reduce potential aspiration, the child is positioned to sleep at a 30-degree angle in bed. Older children are propped up on pillows, whereas the infant can have a small wedge or pillow placed under the head end of the mattress (Holden et al, 1997). It is also recommended that the infant or child be positioned on the right side. The tube may be clamped, left open, or suspended between feedings, depending on the child's condition. A clamped tube allows more mobility but is appropriate only if the child can tolerate intermittent feedings without vomiting or prolonged backup of feeding into the tube. Sometimes a Y tube is used to allow for simultaneous decompression during feeding. If a Foley catheter is used as the gastrostomy tube, very slight tension is applied. The tube is securely taped to maintain the balloon at the gastrostomy opening to prevent leakage of gastric contents and to prevent the tube's progression toward the pyloric sphincter, where it may occlude the stomach outlet. As a precaution, the length of the tube should be measured postoperatively and then remeasured each shift to be sure it has not slipped. A mark can be made above the skin level to further ensure its placement. When the gastrostomy

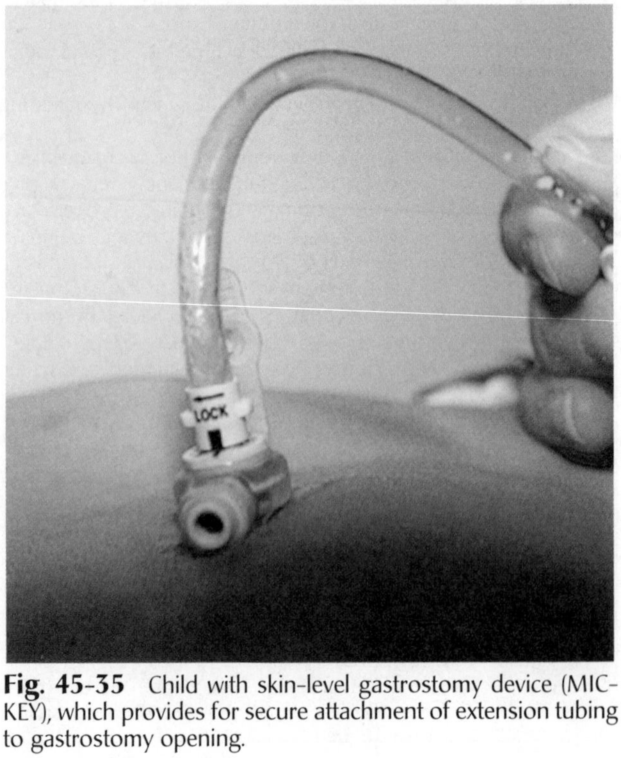

Fig. 45-35 Child with skin-level gastrostomy device (MIC-KEY), which provides for secure attachment of extension tubing to gastrostomy opening.

tube is no longer needed, it is removed; the skin opening usually closes spontaneously by contracture.

Total Parenteral Nutrition

TPN provides for the total nutritional needs of infants or children whose lives are threatened because feeding by way of the gastrointestinal tract is impossible, inadequate, or hazardous.

TPN therapy involves IV infusion of highly concentrated solutions of protein, glucose, and other nutrients. The solution is infused through conventional tubing with a special filter attached to remove particulate matter or microorganisms that may have contaminated the solution. The highly concentrated solutions require infusion into a vessel with sufficient volume and turbulence to allow for rapid dilution. The wide-diameter vessels selected are the superior vena cava and innominate or intrathoracic subclavian veins approached by way of the external or internal jugular veins. The highly irritating nature of concentrated glucose precludes the use of the small peripheral veins in most instances. However, dilute glucose-protein hydrolysates that are appropriate for infusing into peripheral veins are being used with increasing frequency. When peripheral veins are used, intralipid becomes the major calorie source. For long-term alimentation, VADs are usually used (see p. 1398).

The major nursing responsibilities are the same as for any IV therapy: control of sepsis, monitoring of the infusion rate, and assessment of the patient. The TPN solution must be prepared under rigid aseptic conditions best accomplished by specially trained technicians. The solution and tubing are changed and the infusion site redressed by specially trained nurses using meticulous aseptic precautions. In some institutions this may be a nursing responsibility. If so, the procedure is carried out according to hospital protocol.

The infusion is maintained at a constant rate by means of an infusion pump to ensure the proper concentrations of glucose and amino acids. Accurate calculation of the rate is required to deliver a measured amount in a given length of time. Because alterations in flow rate are relatively common, the drip should be checked frequently to ensure an even, continuous infusion. The TPN infusion rate should not be increased or decreased without the practitioner being informed, because alterations can cause hyperglycemia or hypoglycemia.

General assessments, such as vital signs, I&O measurements, and checking results of laboratory tests, facilitate early detection of infection or fluid and electrolyte imbalance. Additional amounts of potassium and sodium chloride are often required in hyperalimentation; therefore observation for signs of potassium or sodium deficit or excess is part of nursing care. This is rarely a problem except in children with reduced renal function or metabolic defects. Hyperglycemia may occur during the first day or two as the child adapts to the high glucose load of the hyperalimentation solution. Although occurring infrequently, insulin may be required to assist the body's adjustment to the hyperglycemia. When this occurs, nursing responsibilities include blood glucose testing. To prevent hypoglycemia at the time the hyperalimentation is disconnected, the rate of the infusion and the amount of insulin are decreased gradually.

Guidelines

ADMINISTRATION OF ENEMAS TO CHILDREN

Age	Amount	Insertion Distance
Infant	120-240 ml	2.5 cm (1 inch)
2-4 yr	240-360 ml	5.0 cm (2 inches)
4-10 yr	360-480 ml	7.5 cm (3 inches)
11 yr	480-720 ml	10.0 cm (4 inches)

In addition to children's physical needs, their developmental needs must also be considered during the often long-term use of TPN. Regular assessment of development should be performed to assess the child's progress, and appropriate interventions should be instituted to encourage expected milestones. Delays in the areas of gross motor and language skills are found most often; therefore special attention should be directed to these areas.

Family Teaching and Home Care

When alternative feedings are needed for an extended period, the family may need to learn how to feed the child with a nasogastric, gastrostomy, or TPN feeding regimen. The same principles discussed earlier in this chapter for compliance, especially in terms of education (see p. 1368), and in Chapter 44 for discharge planning and home care are applied. Because of the numerous skills the family must learn for home TPN, ample time must be planned for the family to learn and perform the procedures under supervision before assuming full responsibility for the child's care.

The family may be referred to community agencies that provide support and practical assistance. The Oley Foundation* is a nonprofit research and education organization that assists persons receiving enteral nutrition and home TPN.

PROCEDURES RELATED TO ELIMINATION

Enema

The procedure for giving an enema to an infant or child does not differ essentially from that for an adult, except for the type and amount of fluid administered and the distance for inserting the tube into the rectum. Depending on the volume, the nurse uses a syringe with rubber tubing, an enema bottle, or an enema bag (Guidelines box).

NURSE ALERT Proper insertion of the catheter tip, especially in infants, is essential to prevent rectal damage and perforation (see Fig. 35-7). If insertion of the enema tip causes discomfort, remove the tip and notify the practitioner. ■

An isotonic solution is used in children. Plain water is not used because, being hypotonic, it can cause rapid fluid shift

*214 Hun Memorial, A28, Albany Medical Center, Albany, NY 12208; phone: 800-766-OLEY; Web site: www.oley.org.

and fluid overload. The Fleet enema (pediatric or adult sized) is not advised for children because of the harsh action of its ingredients (sodium biphosphate and sodium phosphate). Commercial enemas can be dangerous to patients with megacolon and to dehydrated or azotemic children. The osmotic effect of the Fleet enema may produce diarrhea, which can lead to metabolic acidosis. Other potential complications are extreme hyperphosphatemia, hypernatremia, and hypocalcemia, which may lead to neuromuscular irritability and coma (Walton et al, 2000).

Because infants and young children are unable to retain the solution after it is administered, the buttocks must be held together for a short time to retain the fluid. The enema is administered and expelled while the child is lying with the buttocks over the bedpan and with the head and back supported by pillows. Older children are usually able to hold the solution if they understand what to do and if they are not expected to hold it for too long. The nurse should have the bedpan handy or, for the ambulatory child, ensure that the bathroom is readily available before beginning the procedure. An enema is an intrusive procedure and thus threatening to the preschool child; therefore a careful explanation is especially important to ease possible fear.

A preoperative bowel preparation solution given orally or through a nasogastric tube is increasingly being used instead of an enema. The polyethylene glycol–electrolyte lavage solution (GoLYTELY) mechanically flushes the bowel without significant absorption, thereby avoiding potential fluid and electrolyte imbalances.

Ostomies

Children may require stomas for various health problems. The most frequent causes are necrotizing enterocolitis and imperforate anus in the infant (less often, Hirschsprung disease). In the older child the most frequent causes are inflammatory bowel disease, especially Crohn's disease (regional enteritis), and ureterostomies for distal ureter or bladder defects.

Care and management of ostomies in the older child differ little from the care of ostomies in the adult patient. The major emphases in pediatric care are the preparation of the child for the procedure and teaching care of the ostomy to the child and family. The basic principles of preparation are the same as for any procedure (see p. 1357). Simple, straightforward language is most effective, together with the use of illustrations and a replica model (e.g., drawing a picture of a child with a stoma on the abdomen and explaining it as "another opening where bowel movements [or any other term the child uses] will come out"). At another time the nurse can draw a pouch over the opening to demonstrate how the contents are collected. Using a doll to demonstrate the process is an excellent teaching strategy, and special books are available.*

Children with ileostomies are fitted immediately after surgery with an appliance to protect the skin from the proteolytic enzymes in the liquid stool. Parents are usually given a choice of caring for the colostomy with or without an appliance. Pediatric appliances are available in a variety of sizes to ensure an adequate fit.†

Ostomy equipment consists of a one- or two-piece system with a hypoallergenic skin barrier to maintain peristomal skin integrity. The pouch should be large enough to contain a moderate amount of stool and flatus but not so large as to overwhelm the infant or child. A backing helps minimize the risk of skin breakdown from moisture trapped between the skin and pouch. Small clips or rubber bands should be avoided to prevent choking in the young child. Granulation tissue may grow around an ostomy site. This moist, beefy red tissue is not a sign of infection. However, if it continues to grow, the excess moisture can cause irritation of the surrounding skin.

Protection of the peristomal skin is a major aspect of stoma care. Well-fitting appliances are important to prevent leakage of contents. Before the appliance is applied, the skin is prepared with a skin sealant that is allowed to dry. Then stoma paste is applied around the base of the stoma or the back of the wafer. The sealant and paste work together to prevent peristomal breakdown.

In infants with a colostomy left unpouched, skin care is similar to that of any diapered child. However, the peristomal skin is protected with a wafer barrier, such as a hydrocolloid dressing (e.g., Duoderm) or a barrier substance (e.g., zinc oxide ointment [Desitin], karaya products, or a mixture of the zinc oxide ointment and Stoma [Stomahesive‡] powder). A gauze dressing may be applied over the stoma and water to absorb stomal drainage. If the skin becomes inflamed, denuded, or infected, the care is similar to the interventions used for diaper dermatitis (see Chapter 53). A product that helps protect healthy skin, heal excoriated skin, and minimize pain associated with skin breakdown is Preshield Plus.‡ The skin protectant adheres to denuded weeping skin. It can be applied over topical antifungal and antibacterial agents if infection is present. "No-sting" barrier film§ is a skin sealant that has no alcohol base and can be used on open skin without stinging.

With young children, protection of the pouch from being pulled off is also an important consideration. One-piece outfits keep exploring hands from reaching the pouch, and the loose waist prevents any pressure on the appliance. Keeping the child occupied with toys during the pouch change is also helpful. As children mature, their participation in ostomy care is encouraged. Even preschoolers can assist by holding supplies, pulling paper backings from the appliance, and helping clean the stoma area. Toilet training for bladder

---

**Chris Has an Ostomy* is available from United Ostomy Association, Inc., 36 Executive Park, Suite 120, Irvine, CA 92714-6744; phone: 800-826-0826.

†Little Ones Ostomy Products, ConvaTec, CN 5254, Princeton, NJ 08543-5254; phone: 800-422-8811; Web site: www.convatec.com. Parents may find the following pamphlets helpful: *A Parent's Guide to Necrotizing Enterocolitis* and *A Parent's Guide to Ostomy Care for Children*, both available from ConvaTec.

‡Healthpoint Medical, 2600 Airport Freeway, Fort Worth, TX 76111; phone: 800-441-8227; Web site: www.healthpoint.com.

§3M, St. Paul, MN; phone: 800-228-3957.

control needs to begin at the appropriate time as for any other child.

Older children and adolescents should eventually have total responsibility for ostomy care just as they would for usual bowel function. During adolescence, concerns for body image and the ostomy's impact on intimacy and sexuality emerge. The nurse should stress to teenagers that the presence of a stoma need not interfere with their activities. These youngsters can choose which ostomy equipment is best suited to their needs. Attractively designed and decorated pouch covers are well liked by teenagers.

An enterostomal therapy nurse specialist is an important member of the health care team and will have additional suggestions and assistance with skin care information and ostomy pouching options. Further information may be obtained by contacting the Wound, Ostomy, and Continence Nurses Society (WOCN).*

Family Teaching and Home Care

Because these children are almost always discharged with a functioning colostomy, preparation of the family should begin as early as possible in the hospital. The family is instructed in the application of the device (if used), care of the skin, and instructions regarding appropriate action in case skin problems develop. Early evidence of skin breakdown or stomal complications, such as ribbonlike stools, excessive diarrhea, bleeding, prolapse, or failure to pass flatus or stool, is brought to the attention of the physician, the nurse, or the stoma specialist. The same principles are applied as discussed earlier in this chapter for compliance, especially in terms of education (see p. 1367), and in Chapter 44 for discharge planning and home care.

Key Points

- Informed consent is valid when the person is capable of giving consent (is over the age of majority and is competent), is supplied with information needed to make an intelligent decision, and acts voluntarily when exercising freedom of choice.
- Informed consent is needed for major surgery, minor surgery, and diagnostic tests and medical treatments with an element of risk.
- The major tasks in psychologic preparation of the child for procedures are to establish trust, provide support, and give an explanation in easy-to-understand terms.
- Most parents and children want to be together during stressful procedures and should be offered this opportunity, along with guidance on how the parent can comfort the child.
- In the performance of a procedure the nurse should expect success, involve the child when possible in the procedure, provide distraction, and allow for expression of feelings.
- In giving postprocedural support, the nurse should encourage the child to express feelings and praise the youngster for completion of the procedure.
- Stressful times before and after surgery that produce anxiety in children include admission, blood tests, injection of preoperative medication (if used), transportation to the operating room, and return from the postanesthesia care unit.
- Assessment of compliance entails measuring factors that affect compliance through self-reporting, direct observation, monitoring of appointments and therapeutic response, pill counts, and chemical assay.
- Compliance strategies may be classified as organizational, educational, treatment, and behavioral.
- Knowledge of the sick child's eating habits and favorite foods can help in maintaining adequate nutrition.
- Control of fever may be accomplished by pharmacologic means (administration of antipyretics); hyperthermia is controlled by environmental means (minimum clothing, increased air circulation, cool compresses).
- Infection control is based on two systems. Standard Precautions provide protection when the infected person is undiagnosed. Transmission-based precautions add extra interventions for patients diagnosed with or suspected to have an infection.
- Ensuring safety in the hospital setting is a major concern and can be achieved through environmental measures, limit setting, and safe transportation.
- Restraints are used cautiously and typically require a medical order. Therapeutic hugging can avoid the use of restraints.
- Factors that affect drug dosage determination include growth and maturation, difficulty in evaluating drug response, and body surface area.
- Family teaching regarding medication administration includes telling parents why the child is receiving the drug; its possible effects; and the amount, frequency, and length of time the drug is to be administered.
- The preferred sites for intramuscular injection in children are the vastus lateralis and ventrogluteal areas.
- Intermittent venous access is accomplished by a peripheral intermittent infusion device, a peripherally inserted central catheter, a central venous catheter, or an implanted port.
- Several safety catheters and needleless device systems are available to reduce the risk of needle-stick injuries in patients and caregivers.
- Nursing assessment of fluid and electrolyte disturbances entails observation of general appearance, vital signs, and measurement of intake and output.
- Oxygen can be administered by hood, mask, nasal cannula, incubator, or oxygen tent.
- Tracheostomy suctioning involves premeasured insertion of the catheter, application of suction for 5 seconds when withdrawing the catheter, and supplemental oxygen before and after suctioning.
- Alternative forms of feeding include gavage feeding, gastrostomy feeding, and total parenteral nutrition.
- In the care of children with ostomies, nurses play an important role in family support and instruction in care of the stoma site.

*888-224-WOCN, Web site: www.wocn.org.

Answer Guidelines to Critical Thinking Exercises

Planning for Home Tracheostomy Care

1. Further evidence needs to be explored before implementing a plan for discussing home care. One item that needs clarification relates to how Jose's family managed with daytime nursing assistance before this hospitalization. Perhaps there is miscommunication between the family and nursing staff regarding the continued need for frequent nighttime suctioning. It is important to discuss with the family whether Jose's status has changed with this hospitalization. The family may need further teaching regarding home care, yet these issues must be carefully explored with the family. More information is needed regarding the family's understanding and knowledge of Jose's status.
2. (a) Because Jose has required mechanical ventilation since birth, the family is knowledgeable about his respiratory care needs and seems to be comfortable with his care. Care of a child on mechanical ventilation is a complex skill for persons without health care experience, yet in most cases families who receive adequate training, resources, and support manage the child effectively in the home environment and successfully adapt to such care. (b) Tracheal suctioning should not be performed on a set schedule, but only as needed to clear secretions that may accumulate and block the airway. Tracheal suctioning is not without inherent complications, including hypoxia and tracheal irritation. Suctioning should take place over a time frame of 10 to 25 seconds to prevent hypoxia, and the child should be adequately oxygenated before performing the procedure. Irritation of the tracheal tissues may lead to permanent damage if the suction catheter is advanced past the cannula; therefore the suction catheter is premeasured to the length of the cannula to avoid deep suctioning. Equipment needed for tracheal suctioning, such as suction catheters, manual insufflation bag, and gloves, should always be gathered before the procedure and made readily available in case of an emergency. In the event of an illness such as pneumonia, the amount of pulmonary secretions may be increased as a result of the illness; the amount usually decreases once the illness has resolved. (c) The family managed with daytime nursing assistance before this hospitalization. Once the pneumonia has resolved, frequent suctioning should not be required unless there are other intervening factors that affect his respiratory status. As noted in this case, changing the suctioning regimen decreased the frequency to a minimum of once or twice a night. (d) Jose should be discharged as soon as possible to avoid nosocomial infection, promote normalization for a toddler, and contain health care costs. The child's needs for normal growth and development are not minimized by the fact that mechanical ventilation is required. It is important that the child be involved in early developmental assessment and care in order to promote adequate growth and development.
3. Once adequate data have been gathered regarding the family's reluctance to take Jose home, a plan should be implemented to help the family cope with the care of a child on mechanical ventilation. Although the family has previously cared for Jose at home, the teaching should proceed in accordance with their level of understanding, willingness to learn, and readiness to learn. One should not assume that further teaching is not required because the family has successfully cared for him before this hospitalization. A discharge plan of care involving the family should take place to provide effective home care for Jose. While Jose was hospitalized, the nursing staff would suction him periodically when in the room, leading the family to believe that the frequency of suctioning seen in the hospital would need to be maintained at home. In this particular case, the suctioning regimen gradually decreased to a minimum of once or twice a night—a level of care the family felt they would be able to manage.
4. Yes. In talking with the night staff, you find that the nurses suction any time they walk past the room and hear Jose "gurgling." Also, if you accept the conclusion that they do not use premeasured suctioning technique, the implications are that you need to discuss with them a program of premeasured suctioning only as needed to reduce the production of secretion that may be caused from tracheal irritation.
5. Further exploration of the family's concerns and worries is warranted. A detailed assessment of the family's resources could provide insight into issues that might not be related to Jose's respiratory care.

References

Algren C, Ireland D, Stewart E: Perioperative and perianesthesia care of the child. In Albers AC et al (eds): *Comprehensive care of the pediatric patient: prehospital through rehabilitation,* Park Ridge, IL, 1998, Emergency Nurses Association.

Algren C, Schwartz P: The application of nursing research to the child. In Albers AC et al (eds): *Comprehensive care of the pediatric patient: prehospital through rehabilitation,* Park Ridge, IL, 1998, Emergency Nurses Association.

American Academy of Pediatrics: Informed consent, parental permission, and assent in pediatric practice, *Pediatrics* 95(2):314-317, 1995.

American Academy of Pediatrics: Consent for emergency medical services for children and adolescents, *Pediatrics* 111(3):703-705, 2003.

American Academy of Pediatrics, Committee on Drugs: Guidelines for monitoring and management of pediatric patients during and after sedation for diagnostic and therapeutic procedures, *Pediatrics* 86(6):1110-1115, 1992.

Axelrod P: External cooling in the management of fever, *Clin Infect Dis* 31 (5 suppl):S224-S229, 2000.

Banerjee S et al: The intraosseous route is a suitable alternative to the intravenous route for fluid resuscitation in severely dehydrated children, *Indian Pediatr* 312:1511-1520, 1994.

Barker DP et al: Capillary blood sampling: should the heel be warmed? *Arch Dis Child Fetal Neonatal Ed* 74(2):F139-F140, 1996.

Barton S, Holmes S: A comparison of regeant strips and the refractometer for measurement of urine specific gravity in hospitalized children, *Pediatr Nurs* 23(5):480-482, 1998.

Beecroft PC et al: Intravenous lock patency in children: dilute heparin versus saline, *J Pediatr Pract* 2(4):211-233, 1997.

Blass EM, Watt L: Suckling- and sucrose-induced analgesia in human newborns, *Pain* 83(3):611-623, 1999.

Broome M: Consent (assent) for research with pediatric patients, *Semin Oncol Nurs* 15(2):96-103, 1999.

Broome M, Rehwaldt M, Fogg L: Relationship between cognitive behavioral techniques, temperament, observed distress, and pain reports in children and adolescents during lumbar puncture, *J Pediatr Nurs* 13(1):48-54, 1998.

Bryant RA, Doughty D (eds): *Acute and chronic wounds: nursing management,* ed 2, St Louis, 2000, Mosby.

Burke N: Alternative methods for newborn urine sample collection, *Pediatr Nurs* 21(6):546-549, 1995.

Calianno C: Patient hygiene. II. Skin care: keeping the outside healthy, *Nursing* 29(12, suppl):1-11, 1999.

Catudal R: Pediatric IV therapy: actual practice, *J Vasc Access Devices* 4(2):27-29, 1999.

Chung DH, Ziegler NM: Central venous catheter access, *Nutrition* 14(1):119-123, 1998.

Cohen HA et al: Urine samples from disposable diapers: an accurate method for urine cultures, *J Fam Pract* 44(3):290-292, 1997.

Connell F: The causes and treatment of fever: a literature review, *Nurs Stand* 12(11):40-43, 1997.

Cravero JP, Manzi DJA, Rice LJ: The management of procedure-related pain in the child. In Ashburn MA, Rice LJ (eds): *The management of pain,* Philadelphia, 1998, Churchill- Livingstone.

Donaldson JS et al: Peripherally inserted central venous catheters: US-guided vascular access in pediatric patients, *Radiology* 197(2):542-544, 1995.

Dunn D: Malignant hypothermia, *AORN J* 65(4):728-754, 1997.

Eckler J: Combating infection, *Nursing* 27(10):20, 1997.

El-Radhi AS, Barry W: Do antipyretics prevent febrile convulsions? *Arch Dis Child* 99(7):641-642, 2003.

Ellett ML: Prevalence of feeding tube placement errors and associated risk factors in children, *MCN* 23(5):234-239, 1998.

Engleman SG, Turnage-Carrier C: Tolerance of the Passy-Muir speaking valve in infants and children less than 2 years of age, *Pediatr Nurs* 23: 571-573, 1997.

Essink-Tebbes CM et al: Safety of lidocaine-prilocaine cream application four times a day in premature neonates: a pilot study, *Eur J Pediatr* 158(5):421-423, 1999.

Fauroux B et al: Chest physiotherapy in cystic fibrosis: improved tolerance with nasal pressure support ventilation, *Pediatrics* 103(3):e32, 1999.

Fox MD: Measurement of urine output volume: accuracy of diaper weights in neonatal environments, *Neonatal Network* 11(3):11-18, 1992.

Frey AM: Pediatric peripherally inserted central catheter program report: a summary of 4,536 catheter days, *J Intravenous Nurs* 18(6):280-291, 1995.

Frizzell J: Avoiding lab test pitfalls, *Am J Nurs* 98(2):34-37, 1998.

Gray L, Watt L, Blass EM: Skin-to-skin contact is analgesic in healthy newborns, *Pediatrics* 105(1):110-111, 2000.

Gray M: Atraumatic uretheral catheterization of children, *Pediatr Nurs* 22(4):306-310, 1996.

Groswasser J et al: Needle length and injection technique for efficient intramuscular vaccine delivery in infants and children evaluated through an ultrasonographic determination of subcutaneous and muscle layer thickness, *Pediatrics* 99(3, pt 1):400-402, 1997.

Guertler AT: Pearls, pitfalls, and updates: the clinical practice of emergency medicine, *Emerg Med Clin North Am* 15(2):303-313, 1997.

Hagelgans NA: Pediatric skin care issues for the home care nurse, *Pediatr Nurs* 19(5):499-507, 1993.

Harrison A et al: Comparison of simultaneously obtained arterial and capillary blood gases in pediatric intensive care unit patients, *Crit Care Med* 25(1):1904-1908, 1997.

Hazinski MF: *Nursing care of the critically ill child,* ed 3, St Louis, 1996, Mosby.

Heilskov J et al: A randomized trial of heparin and saline for maintaining intravenous locks in neonates, *J Soc Pediatr Nurs* 3(3):111-116, 1998.

Hicks JF et al: Optimum needle length for diphtheria-inoculation of infants, *Pediatrics* 84(1):136-137, 1989.

Holden C et al: Enteral nutrition for children, *Nurs Stand* 11(32):49-54, 1997.

Huth M: Watch out: the bogeyman is in the hospital closet, *J Child Fam Nurs* 2(2):143-148, 1999.

Intravenous Nurses Society: Revised Intravenous Nursing Standards of Practice, *J Intravenous Nurs* 21(1, suppl):S35, S46-S47, S59, 1998.

Jackson F: The ABC's of black hair and skin care, *ABNFJ* 9(5):100-104, 1998.

Janik JP, Wayne ER, Janik JS: Securing central lines in rambunctious toddlers, *Pediatrics* 96(3):523-524, 1995.

Johnston CC, Stevens B, Arbess G: The effect of the sight of blood and use of decorative adhesive bandages on pain intensity ratings by preschool children, *J Pediatr Nurs* 8(3):147-151, 1993.

Joint Commission on Accreditation of Healthcare Organizations: Care of the patient: restraint and seclusion standards. In *Comprehensive accreditation manual for hospitals,* TX.7.1-TX.7.5.5, 2001.

Kain Z, Caldwell-Andrews A, Wang S: Psychological preparation of the parent and pediatric surgical patient, *Anesth Clin North Am* 20(1):29-44, 2002.

Katsma D, Smith G: Analysis of needle path during intramuscular injection, *Nurs Res* 46(5):288-292, 1997.

Kearns GL, Leeder SJ, Wasserman GS: Acetaminophen overdose with therapeutic intent, *J Pediatr* 132(1):5-8, 1998.

Kennedy D: Medication "safety checks" in pediatric acute care, *J Intravenous Nurs* 19(6):295-302, 1996.

Kinmonth AL, Fulton Y, Campbell MJ: Management of feverish children at home, *BMJ* 305(6862):1134-1136, 1992.

Kotter RW: Heparin vs saline for intermittent intravenous device maintenance in neonates, *Neonatal Network* 15(6):43-47, 1996.

Krozek J, Scoggins SA: Restraints and seclusion policy . . . amended to comply with 2001 JCAHO standards, *Cinahl Information Systems* (9p), 2001.

Krueger H, Osborn L: Effects of hygiene among the uncircumcised, *J Fam Pract* 22(4):353-355, 1986.

Kubiak M et al: Comparison of stool containment in cloth and single-use diapers using simulated infant feces, *Pediatrics* 91(3):632-636, 1993.

Larsson BA et al: Alleviation of the pain of venepuncture in neonates, *Acta Paediatr* 87(7):774-779, 1998.

Laurent C: And so to beds, *Nursing Times* 95(3):7-8, 1999.

Lee WE, Vallino LM: Intravenous insertion site protection: moisture accumulation in intravenous site protectors, *J Intravenous Nurs* 29(4): 194-197, 1996.

Lehmann M et al: Upright or lying down: is one better for doing a lumbar puncture (LP)? *Am J Dis Child* 144:427, 1990.

Liebman M, Barnsteiner J: Fever education: does it reduce parent fever anxiety? *Pediatr Emerg Care* 17(1):47-51, 2001.

Liptak GS: Enhancing compliance in pediatrics, *Pediatr Rev* 17(4):128-134, 1996.

Long CA et al: Central line associated bacteremia in the pediatric patient, *Pediatr Nurs* 22(3):247-251, 1996.

Maki DG: Infections caused by intravascular devices used for infusion therapy: pathogenesis, prevention, and management. In Bisno AL, Waldvogel FA (editors): *Infections associated with indwelling medical devices,* ed 2, Washington, DC, 1994, American Society for Microbiology.

McIntosh N, van Veen L, Brameyer H: Alleviation of the pain of heel prick in preterm infants, *Arch Dis Child Fetal Neonatal Ed* 70(3):F177-F181, 1994.

McLane KM et al: Comparison of interface pressures in the pediatric population among various support surfaces, *J Wound Ostomy Continence Nurs* 29(5):242-251, 2002.

Metheny N et al: pH, color, and feeding tubes, *RN* 61(1):25-27, 1998.

Moppett S, Parker M: Insertion of a suppository, *Nursing Times* 95(23, suppl):1-2, 1999.

Moskop JC: Ethical issues in emergency medicine: informed consent in the emergency department, *Emerg Med Clin North Am* 17(2):327-340, 1999.

Moureau N: Practical access, a back-to-basics review of intravenous therapy, *J Vasc Access Devices* 4(2, suppl):1-4, 1999.

O'Brien B et al: G-tube site care: a practical guide, *RN* 62(2):52-56, 1999.

Orenstein R: The benefits and limitations of needle protectors and needleless intravenous systems, *J Intravenous Nurs* 22(3):122-127, 1999.

Paisley MK et al: The use of heparin and normal saline flushes in neonatal intravenous catheters, *Pediatr Nurs* 23(5):521-527, 1997.

Pearson M: The Hospital Infection Control Practices Advisory Committee: guidelines for prevention of intravascular-device-related infections, *Infect Control Hosp Epidemiol* 17:438-473, 1995.

Pearson M: Special communication: guidelines for prevention of intravascular device-related infections, parts I and II, *Am J Infect Control* 24(4):262-293, 1996.

Prandoni D et al: Assessment of urine collection techniques for microbial culture, *Am J Infect Control* 24(3):219-221, 1996.

Purssell E: The use of antipyretic medications in the prevention of febrile convulsions in children, *J Pediatr Nurs* 9(4):473-480, 2000.

Quigley SM, Curley MAQ: Skin integrity in the pediatric population: preventing and managing pressure ulcers, *J Soc Pediatr Nurses* 1(1):7, 1996.

Ratcliff CR, Rodheaver GT: Pressure ulcer assessment and management, *Lippincott's Primary Care Practice* 3:242-258, 1999.

Reed T, Phillip S: Management of central venous catheter occlusion and repairs, *J Intravenous Nurs* 19(6):289-294, 1996.

Rosenstock IM: Enhancing patient compliance with health recommendations, *J Pediatr Health Care* 2(2):67-72, 1988.

Rote N, Huether S, McCance K: Hypersensitivities, infection, and immunodeficiencies. In Huether S, McCance K (eds): *Understanding pathophysiology,* ed 2, St Louis, 2000, Mosby.

Russell B: Nosocomial infections, *Am J Nurs* 99(6):24J-24P, 1999.

Selekman J, Snyder B: Uses and alternatives to restraints in pediatric settings, *AACN Clin Issues* 7(4):603-610, 1996.

Selekman J, Snyder B: Institutional policies on the use of physical restraints on children, *Pediatr Nurs* 23(5):531-537, 1997.

Sharber J: The efficacy of tepid sponge bathing to reduce fever in young children, *Am J Emerg Med* 15(2):188-192, 1997.

Shinnar S et al: Short-term outcomes of children with febrile status epilepticus, *Epilepsia* 42(1):47-53, 2001.

Vertanen H et al: An automatic incision device for obtaining blood samples from the heels of the preterm infants causes less damage than a conventional manual lancet, *Arch Dis Child Fetal Neonatal Ed* 84:F53-F55, 2001.

Walton DM et al: Morbid hypocalcaemia associated with phosphate enema in a six-week-old infant, *Pediatrics* 106:e37, 2000.

Wong DL, Baker CM: Pain in children: comparison of assessment scales, *Pediatr Nurs* 14(1):9-17, 1988.

Respiratory Dysfunction 46

LEARNING OBJECTIVES

On completion of this chapter the reader will be able to:

- Identify the factors leading to respiratory tract infection in the infant or young child.
- Contrast the effects of various respiratory infections observed in infants and children.
- Describe the postoperative nursing care of the child with a tonsillectomy.
- Outline a nursing care plan for a child with croup.
- Outline a nursing care plan for a child with acute otitis media.
- Demonstrate an understanding of the ways in which inhalation of noninfectious irritants produce pulmonary dysfunction.
- Describe the ways in which the various therapeutic measures relieve the symptoms of asthma.
- Outline a plan for teaching home care for the child with asthma.
- Describe the physiologic effects of cystic fibrosis on the gastrointestinal and pulmonary systems.
- Outline a plan of care for the child with cystic fibrosis.
- List the major signs of respiratory distress in infants and children.

ELECTRONIC RESOURCES

Additional information related to the content in Chapter 46 can be found on

the companion website at evolve
http://evolve.elsevier.com/Wong/maternal/

- NCLEX Review Questions
- Case Study–Acute Epiglottitis
- Case Study–Bronchiolitis
- Case Study–Cystic Fibrosis
- Case Study–Tonsillitis
- WebLinks

or the interactive student CD-ROM
Activities for Chapter 46 include the following:

- NCLEX Review Questions
- Anatomy Review–Location of Retractions
- Anatomy Review–Location of Tonsillar Masses
- Case Study–Cystic Fibrosis
- Case Study–Asthma
- Critical Thinking Exercise–Cystic Fibrosis Inheritance Risks
- Nursing Care Plan–The Child with Acute Respiratory Infection
- Nursing Care Plan–The Child with Asthma
- Case Study–Mononucleosis

RESPIRATORY INFECTION

General Aspects of Respiratory Infections

Infections of the respiratory tract are described according to the anatomic area of involvement. The *upper respiratory tract,* or *upper airway,* consists of the oronasopharynx, pharynx, larynx, and upper part of the trachea. The *lower respiratory tract* consists of the lower trachea, mainstem bronchi, segmental bronchi, subsegmental bronchioles, terminal bronchioles, and alveoli. In this discussion, the trachea is considered with lower tract disorders, and infections of the epiglottis and larynx are categorized as croup syndromes. However, respiratory infections seldom fall into discrete anatomic areas. Infections often spread from one structure to another because of the contiguous nature of the mucous membrane lining the entire tract. Consequently, respiratory tract infections involve several areas rather than a single structure, although the effect on one area may predominate in any given illness.

Etiology and Characteristics

Respiratory infections account for the majority of acute illnesses in children. The etiology and course of these infections are influenced by the age of the child, the season, living conditions, and preexisting medical problems.

Infectious Agents

The respiratory tract is subject to a wide variety of infective organisms. Viruses, such as the respiratory syncytial virus (RSV), cause most infections. Other agents involved in primary or secondary invasion include group A β-hemolytic streptococci, staphylococci, *Haemophilus influenzae, Chlamydia trachomatis, Mycoplasma,* and pneumococci.

Age

Infants younger than age 3 months have a lower infection rate, presumably because of the protective function of maternal antibodies. The infection rate increases from 3 to 6 months of age, the time between the disappearance of maternal antibodies and the infant's own antibody production. The viral infection rate remains high during the toddler and preschool years. By 5 years of age, viral respiratory infections are less frequent, but the incidence of *Mycoplasma pneumoniae* and group A β-hemolytic streptococcal infections increases.

Some viral agents produce a mild illness in older children but severe lower respiratory tract illness or croup in infants. For example, whooping cough is a relatively harmless tracheobronchitis in childhood but a serious disease in infancy.

Size

Anatomic differences influence the response to respiratory tract infections. The diameter of the airways is smaller in young children and subject to considerable narrowing from edematous mucous membranes and increased production of secretions. The distance between structures within the respiratory tract is also shorter in the young child, and organisms may move rapidly down the respiratory tract, causing more extensive involvement. The relatively short and open eustachian tube in infants and young children allows pathogens easy access to the middle ear.

Resistance

The ability to resist invading organisms depends on several factors. Deficiencies of the immune system place the child at risk for infection. Other conditions that decrease resistance are malnutrition, anemia, fatigue, and chilling of the body. Conditions that weaken defenses of the respiratory tract and predispose to infection also include allergies (e.g., allergic rhinitis), asthma, cardiac anomalies that cause pulmonary congestion, and cystic fibrosis. Day care attendance, especially if the caregivers smoke, increases the likelihood of infection (Blumer, 1998).

Seasonal Variations

The most common respiratory pathogens appear in epidemics during the winter and spring months. Mycoplasmal infections occur more often in autumn and early winter. Infection-related asthma (e.g., asthmatic bronchitis) occurs more frequently during cold weathers, whereas winter and spring are typically the "RSV seasons."

Clinical Manifestations

Infants and young children, especially those between 6 months and 3 years of age, react more severely to acute respiratory tract infection than older children. Young children display a number of generalized signs and symptoms, as well as local manifestations (Box 46-1).

Nursing Care Management

Assessment

Assessment of the respiratory system follows the guidelines described in Chapter 35 (for assessment of the nose, mouth and throat, chest, and lungs). Special attention should also be given to the components and observations listed in Box 46-2.

Nursing Diagnoses

After a thorough assessment, several nursing diagnoses may be identified (see Nursing Care Plan, p. 1429). Others may be apparent in individual cases.

Plan of Care and Implementation

The goals for the child with an acute respiratory infection and the child's family are as follows:

1. Child will exhibit normal respiratory efforts.
2. Child will receive adequate rest.
3. Child will remain comfortable.
4. Child will not spread primary infection to others.
5. Child's temperature will remain within normal limits.
6. Child will maintain normal hydration and adequate nutrition.
7. Child will experience no complications.
8. Child and family will receive information, especially for home care, and support.

Ease Respiratory Efforts

Many acute respiratory infections are mild and cause few symptoms. Although children may feel uncomfortable and have a "stuffy" nose and some mucosal swelling, respiratory distress occurs infrequently. Interventions delivered at home are usually sufficient to relieve minor discomfort and ease respiratory efforts. However, children with croup or epiglottitis can develop sufficient swelling to obstruct the airway and may require hospitalization and more complex therapy.

Warm or cool mist is a common therapeutic measure for symptomatic relief of respiratory discomfort. The moisture soothes inflamed membranes and is beneficial when there is hoarseness or laryngeal involvement. However, the use of steam vaporizers in the home is discouraged because of the hazards related to their use and limited evidence to support their efficacy. Shallow pans with wide surface areas for evaporation increase humidity but should be placed where they do not pose a safety hazard.

A time-honored method of producing warm mist is the shower. Running a shower of hot water into the empty bathtub or open shower stall with the bathroom door closed produces a quick source of steam. Keeping a child in this environment for 10 to 15 minutes provides the same advantages as the mist tent without the fear and restraint associated with the confines of a tent. A small child can be held on the parent's lap. Older children can sit in the bathroom under the supervision of an adult.

Promote Rest

Children who have an acute febrile illness should be placed on bed rest. This is usually not difficult while the temperature is elevated but may become a problem when children begin to feel better. Often children will comply with bed rest if they are allowed to lie quietly on a couch where they can watch television or participate in a quiet activity. If children protest, allowing them to play quietly serves the purpose of rest better than allowing them to cry excessively in bed.

Promote Comfort

Older children are usually able to manage nasal secretions with little difficulty. Parents are instructed in the correct administration of nose drops and throat irrigations, if ordered. For very young infants, who normally breathe through their

BOX 46-1

Signs and Symptoms Associated with Respiratory Infections in Infants and Small Children

Fever
May be absent in newborn infants
Greatest at ages 6 months to 3 years
Temperature may reach 39.5° to 40.5° C (103° to 105° F) even with mild infections
Often appears as first sign of infection
May be listless and irritable or somewhat euphoric and more active than normal, temporarily; some children talk with unaccustomed rapidity
Tendency to develop high temperatures with infection in certain families
May precipitate febrile seizures (see Chapter 48)
Febrile seizures uncommon after 3 or 4 years of age

Meningismus
Meningeal signs without infection of the meninges
Occurs with abrupt onset of fever
Accompanied by the following:
- Headache
- Pain and stiffness in the back and neck
- Presence of Kernig and Brudzinski signs

Subsides as the temperature decreases

Anorexia
Common with most childhood illnesses
Frequently the initial evidence of illness
Persists to a greater or lesser degree throughout febrile stage of illness; often extends into convalescence

Vomiting
Small children vomit readily with illness
Clue to onset of infection
May precede other signs by several hours
Usually short-lived but may persist during the illness

Diarrhea
Usually mild, transient diarrhea but may become severe
Often accompanies viral respiratory infections
Frequent cause of dehydration

Abdominal Pain
Common complaint
Sometimes indistinguishable from pain of appendicitis
Mesenteric lymphadenitis may be cause
Muscle spasms from vomiting may be a factor, especially in nervous, tense child

Nasal Blockage
Small nasal passages of infants easily blocked by mucosal swelling and exudation
Can interfere with respiration and feeding in infants
May contribute to the development of otitis media and sinusitis

Nasal Discharge
Frequent occurrence
May be thin and watery (rhinorrhea) or thick and purulent
Depends on the type or stage of infection
Associated with itching
May irritate upper lip and skin surrounding the nose

Cough
Common feature
May be evident only during acute phase
May persist several months after a disease

Respiratory Sounds
Sounds associated with respiratory disease:
- Cough
- Hoarseness
- Grunting
- Stridor
- Wheezing

Auscultation:
- Wheezing
- Crackles
- Absence of sound

Sore Throat
Frequent complaint of older children
Young children (unable to describe symptoms) may not complain even when highly inflamed
Child will often refuse to take oral fluids or solids

noses, an infant nasal aspirator or a rubber ear syringe is helpful in removing nasal secretions before feeding. This practice, followed by instillation of saline nose drops, may clear nasal passages and promote feeding. Saline nose drops can be prepared at home by dissolving 1 teaspoon of salt in 1 pint of warm water.

For older infants and children who can tolerate decongestants, vasoconstrictive nose drops may be administered 15 to 20 minutes before feeding and at bedtime. Two drops are instilled, and because this shrinks only the anterior mucous membranes, two more drops are instilled 5 to 10 minutes later. Phenylephrine (Neo-Synephrine) 0.25% and ephedrine 1% are frequently prescribed. Older cooperative children often prefer nasal sprays. They are taught to compress the plastic container at the moment of inspiration. Bottles of nose drops should be used only for one child and one illness because they are easily contaminated with bacteria. To avoid rebound congestion, nose drops or sprays should not be administered for more than 3 days.

Hot or cold applications sometimes provide relief for children with painful cervical adenitis. An ice bag or heating pad applied to the neck may decrease the discomfort, but safety precautions must be observed to prevent burns. The ice bag or heating device must be covered, and the heating pad should not be set at high ranges.

Prevent Spread of Infection

Careful handwashing is carried out when caring for children with respiratory infections. Children and families are taught to use a tissue or their hand to cover their nose and mouth when they cough or sneeze and to dispose of tissues properly, as well as to wash their hands. Used tissues should be immediately thrown into the wastebasket, and tissues should not be allowed to accumulate in a pile. Children with respiratory infections should not share drinking cups, washcloths, or towels.

NURSE ALERT To avoid contamination with respiratory viruses, wash hands and do not touch your eyes or nose. ■

BOX 46-2

Components for Assessing Respiratory Function

Respirations

The pattern of respirations is observed for rate, depth, ease, and rhythm of breathing:

- **Rate**–Rapid *(tachypnea)*, normal, or slow for the particular child
- **Depth**–Normal depth, too shallow *(hypopnea)*, too deep *(hyperpnea)*; usually estimated from the amplitude of thoracic and abdominal excursion
- **Ease**–Effortless; labored *(dyspnea)*; *orthopnea* (difficult breathing except in upright position); associated with intercostal or substernal retractions (inspiratory "sinking in" of soft tissues in relation to the cartilaginous and bony thorax); *pulsus paradoxus* (blood pressure falls with inspiration and rises with expiration); flaring nares; head bobbing (head of sleeping child with suboccipital area supported on caregiver's forearm bobs forward in synchrony with each inspiration); grunting; or wheezing
- **Labored breathing**–Continuous, intermittent, becoming steadily worse, sudden onset, at rest or on exertion, associated with wheezing or grunting, associated with pain
- **Rhythm**–Variation in rate and depth of respirations

Other Observations

In addition to respirations, particular attention is addressed to the following:

- **Evidence of infection**–Check for elevated temperature, enlarged cervical lymph nodes, inflamed mucous membranes, and purulent discharges from the nose, ears, or lungs (sputum)
- **Cough**–Observe the characteristics of the cough (if present); under what circumstances the cough is heard (e.g., night only, on arising), nature of the cough (paroxysmal with or without wheeze, "croupy" or "brassy"), frequency of cough, associated with swallowing or other activity, character of the cough (moist and dry), productivity
- **Wheeze**–Expiratory or inspiratory, high-pitched or musical, prolonged, slowly progressive or sudden, associated with labored breathing
- **Cyanosis**–Note distribution (peripheral, perioral, facial, trunk, and face), degree, duration, associated with activity
- **Chest pain**–May be a complaint of older children; note location and circumstances: localized or generalized, referred to base of neck or abdomen, dull or sharp, deep or superficial, associated with rapid, shallow respirations or grunting
- **Sputum**–Older children may provide sputum sample by coughing, whereas young children may need use of bulb suction to provide a sample; note volume, color, viscosity, and odor
- **Bad breath**–May be associated with some lung infections

ANATOMY REVIEW: LOCATION OF RETRACTIONS

Efforts should be made to separate affected children from contact with other children. Parents should keep affected children out of school and day care settings to prevent the spread of infection. Ideally, ill children should be isolated in a separate bedroom at the first sign of illness. However, this is a problem when living arrangements are crowded and there are several children in the family. Well children should be told to stay away from ill children.

Reduce Temperature

If the child has a significantly elevated temperature, controlling the fever is important. Parents should know how to take a child's temperature and read the thermometer accurately. Nurses should not assume that all parents can read a thermometer. Parents who cannot perform this skill should receive instruction.

If the practitioner prescribes acetaminophen or ibuprofen, parents may need help giving the drug. Most parents can read the label and calculate the desired dose, but some may require careful instruction. It is important to emphasize accuracy in determining both the amount of drug to be given and the time intervals for administration. Cool liquids are given to reduce the temperature and minimize the chances of dehydration. (See Controlling Elevated Temperatures, Chapter 45.)

Promote Hydration

Dehydration is always a hazard when children are febrile or anorexic, especially when vomiting or diarrhea is present. Offering small amounts of favorite fluids at frequent intervals encourages adequate fluid intake. High-calorie liquids, such as colas, fruit juices, water flavored and sweetened with corn syrup, or similar drinks, prevent catabolism and dehydration but should be avoided if diarrhea is present. Oral rehydration solutions, such as Infalyte or Pedialyte, should be considered for infants, and sports drinks, such as Gatorade, are recommended for older children. Fluids should not be forced, and children should not be awakened to take fluids. Forcing fluids creates the same problem as urging unwanted food. Gentle persuasion with preferred beverages is usually more successful.

To assess a child's level of hydration (see Chapter 47), parents are advised to observe the frequency of voiding and to notify the nurse or practitioner if voiding is insufficient. Counting the number of wet diapers in a 24-hour period is a satisfactory method to assess output in infants and toddlers.

Provide Nutrition

Loss of appetite is characteristic of children with acute infections. In most cases, children can be permitted to determine their own need for food. Many children show no decrease in appetite, and others respond well to foods such as gelatin, soup, and puddings (see Feeding the Sick Child, Chapter 45). Urging foods on anorexic children may precipitate nausea and vomiting and cause an aversion to feeding that may extend into the convalescent period and beyond.

Family Support and Home Care

Young children with respiratory infections are irritable and difficult to comfort; therefore the family needs support, encouragement, and practical suggestions concerning comfort measures and administration of medication. In addition to antipyretics and nose drops, the child may require antibiotic therapy. Parents of children receiving oral antibiotics must understand the importance of regular administration and of continuing the drug for the prescribed length of time, regardless of whether the child appears ill. Parents are cautioned against giving their child any medications that are not approved by the health practitioner. Adverse effects have been noted in children who have received preparations intended for adults such as long-acting nose drops (Neo-Synephrine II) and dextromethorphan cough squares that are often mistaken for candy. Parents should not give antibiotics left over from a previous illness. Self-medication with unprescribed antibiotics can produce serious adverse reactions (see Chapter 45 for administration of medications and teaching parents).

EVALUATION

Continual reassessment and evaluation determine the effectiveness of nursing interventions. The nurse should use the following guidelines:

1. Observe child's respiratory effort and movement.
2. Observe signs and symptoms for progress toward health status before illness.
3. Observe child's behavior and activity.
4. Observe other family members and contacts for evidence of infection.
5. Take temperature.
6. Observe for signs of adequate hydration.
7. Observe eating behavior.
8. Assess for complications such as dehydration, weight loss, or spread of infection to other areas of the body.
9. Observe family's behavior and interview members regarding their feelings and concerns.

The *expected outcomes* are described in the Nursing Care Plan.

Nursing Care Plan

THE CHILD WITH ACUTE RESPIRATORY INFECTION

NURSING DIAGNOSIS: Ineffective breathing pattern related to the inflammatory process

EXPECTED OUTCOME

Respiration patterns are within normal limits.

NURSING INTERVENTIONS/*RATIONALES*

Position and reposition child as needed (e.g., elevate head of bed, tripod or upright sitting position, use of support pillows and wedges) *to maintain open airway, to allow maximum use of accessory muscles,* and *to allow maximum lung and diaphragm expansion for ventilation and comfort.*

Avoid constrictive clothing or bedding *that may interfere with breathing.*

Provide increased humidity and supplemental oxygen per physician order *to aid in oxygenation and breathing.*

Suction airway as needed *to remove secretions.*

Alternate rest and activity cycles *to reduce oxygen demands.*

Administer bronchodilators and other medications as prescribed *to assist with ventilation.*

NURSING DIAGNOSIS: Ineffective airway clearance related to inflammation, increased secretions, obstruction

EXPECTED OUTCOME

Airway is patent.

NURSING INTERVENTIONS/*RATIONALES*

Position child (prone, side lying, sitting) using proper body alignment *for maximum ventilation and prevention of aspiration of secretions.*

Ensure adequate fluid intake *to keep secretions liquid* and provide humidified environment *to keep mucous membranes moist.*

Administer chest physiotherapy (percussion, vibration, postural drainage) *to promote loosening and drainage of lung secretions.*

Assist child to cough and expectorate effectively using suctioning if needed *to clear accumulated secretions.*

Administer expectorants, nebulizer treatments, and bronchodilators as prescribed *to facilitate liquefaction and clearance of secretions.*

Administer prescribed pain medications and provide splinting during coughing *to minimize discomfort and increase effectiveness of coughing.*

NURSING DIAGNOSIS: Risk for spread of infection related to presence of infective organisms

EXPECTED OUTCOME

Child shows no signs of secondary infection, and there are no signs of infection in others in environment.

NURSING INTERVENTIONS/*RATIONALES*

Maintain aseptic environment, use good handwashing techniques, and use isolation techniques and universal precautions as needed *to prevent spread of infection and avoid cross contamination and nosocomial infection.*

Administer antibiotics per physician order *to treat or prevent infection.*

Instruct child and family in appropriate precautions (e.g., handwashing, tissue disposal) *to prevent spread of infection.*

NURSING DIAGNOSIS: Activity intolerance related to inflammatory process, imbalance between oxygen supply and demand

EXPECTED OUTCOME

Child shows no signs of increased respiratory distress; child's activity tolerance is appropriate for age and abilities.

NURSING INTERVENTIONS/*RATIONALES*

Schedule activities, treatments, visits, and play around child's needs and energy levels *to maximize rest and minimize fatigue.*

Implement measures (quiet, darkened room) *to ensure sleep.*

Encourage frequent rest periods *to balance energy needs.*

Administer pain medications and sedatives per physician order *for restlessness and pain.*

Monitor vital signs *for signs of oxygen lack.*

NURSING DIAGNOSIS: Fear/anxiety related to difficulty breathing

EXPECTED OUTCOME

Child exhibits reduced signs of fear and anxiety.

NURSING INTERVENTIONS/*RATIONALES*

Acknowledge child's fear and help child identify sources of that fear *to facilitate identification and use of coping strategies.*

Explain respiratory treatments and procedures to child in developmentally appropriate terms *to allay fear of unknown.*

Show child how coughing and deep breathing help aid breathing *to allay fears and give child a measure of control.*

UPPER RESPIRATORY TRACT INFECTIONS

Nasopharyngitis

Acute nasopharyngitis (the equivalent of the "common cold") is caused by rhinovirus, RSV, adenovirus, influenza virus, and parainfluenza virus. Symptoms are more severe in infants and children than in adults. Fever is common in young children, and older children have low-grade fevers, which appear early in the course of the illness. Other clinical manifestations are listed in Box 46-3.

Therapeutic Management

Children with nasopharyngitis are managed at home. There is no specific treatment, and effective vaccines are not available. Antipyretics are prescribed for mild fever and discomfort (see Chapter 45 for management of fever). Rest is recommended until the child is free of fever for at least 1 day. Decongestants may be prescribed for children and infants older than 6 months of age to shrink swollen nasal passages. The decongestants that exert their effect by vasoconstriction are usually less effective when taken orally than when applied topically as nose drops. Because these drugs affect all vascular beds, they should be given with caution to children with diabetes.

Cough suppressants may be prescribed for a dry, hacking cough. However, some cough preparations contain up to 22% alcohol; these should not be administered to young children continuously and must be stored securely away from the reach of children.

Antihistamines are largely ineffective. These drugs have a weak atropine-like effect that dries secretions, but they can cause drowsiness or, paradoxically, have a stimulatory effect on children. There is no support for the usefulness of expectorants. Antibiotics are usually not indicated.

Prevention

Nasopharyngitis is so widespread in the general population that it is impossible to prevent. Children are more susceptible because they have not yet developed resistance to many viruses. Very young infants are subject to serious complications such as pneumonia, and attempts should be made to protect them from exposure.

Nursing Care Management

A cold is often the parents' first introduction to an illness in their infant. Most discomfort of nasopharyngitis is related to the nasal obstruction, especially in small infants. Elevating the head of the bed or crib mattress assists with drainage of secretions. Suctioning and vaporization may also provide relief. Saline nose drops and gentle suction with a bulb syringe before feeding are useful.

Maintaining adequate fluid intake is essential. Although a child's appetite for solid foods is usually diminished for several days, it is important to offer favorite fluids to prevent dehydration. Fluids can be cool or warm, depending on individual preference.

Because nasopharyngitis is spread from secretions, the best means for prevention is avoiding contact with affected persons. This goal is difficult to accomplish in family settings, classrooms, and day care centers. Family members with a cold should try to "keep it to themselves" by carefully disposing of tissues; not sharing towels, glasses, or eating utensils; covering the mouth and nose with tissues when coughing or sneezing; and washing the hands thoroughly after nose blowing or sneezing. The most frequent carriers of infection are the human hands, which deposit viruses on doorknobs, faucets, and other everyday objects. Children should be taught to wash their hands thoroughly before putting them near their eyes, nose, or mouth.

Family Support

Support and reassurance are important elements of care for families of young children with recurrent upper respiratory infections (URIs). Because URIs are common in children less than 3 years of age, families may feel as if they are on an endless roller coaster of illness. They need reassurance that frequent colds are a normal part of childhood and that by 5 years of age, their children will have developed immunity to many viruses. Parents who work outside the home should expect to take time off to care for ill children during the fall and winter months. When children spend time rou-

BOX 46-3

Clinical Manifestations of Nasopharyngitis and Pharyngitis

Nasopharyngitis

Younger Child
- Fever
- Irritability, restlessness
- Sneezing
- Vomiting or diarrhea

Older Child
- Dryness and irritation of nose and throat
- Sneezing, chilly sensation
- Muscular aches
- Cough, sometimes

Physical Signs
- Edema and vasodilation of mucosa

Pharyngitis

Younger Child
- Fever
- General malaise
- Anorexia
- Moderate sore throat
- Headache

Older Child
- Fever (may reach 40° C [104° F])
- Headache
- Anorexia
- Dysphagia
- Abdominal pain
- Vomiting

Physical Signs

Younger Child
- Mild to moderate hyperemia

Older Child
- Mild to fiery red, edematous pharynx
- Hyperemia of tonsils and pharynx; may extend to soft palate and uvula
- Often abundant follicular exudate that spreads and coalesces to form pseudomembrane on tonsils
- Cervical glands enlarged and tender

BOX 46-4

Early Evidence of Respiratory Complications

Parents are instructed to notify the health professional if any of the following are noted:
- Evidence of earache (see p. 1434)
- Respirations faster than 50 to 60 breaths/min
- Fever over 38.3° C (101° F)
- Listlessness
- Increasing irritability with or without fever
- Persistent cough for 2 days or more
- Wheezing
- Crying
- Refusal to eat
- Restlessness and poor sleep patterns

Modified from National Association of Pediatric Nurse Associates and Practitioners (NAPNAP): *Baby's first cold*, New York, 1989, Winthrop Consumer Products. Copies available from NAPNAP, 1101 Kings Hwy., N., No. 206, Cherry Hill, NJ 08034; phone: 609-667-1773; Web site: www.napnap.org.

tinely in day care centers, their infection rate is higher than if they are cared for in the home. Parents should know the signs of respiratory complications and should notify a health professional if complications occur or if the child does not improve within 2 or 3 days (Box 46-4).

Pharyngitis

Children who experience group A β-hemolytic streptococci (GABHS) infection of the upper airway *(strep throat)* are at risk for *acute rheumatic fever (ARF),* an inflammatory disease of the heart, joints, and central nervous system (see Chapter 48), and *acute glomerulonephritis,* an acute kidney infection (see Chapter 50). Permanent damage can result from these sequelae, especially ARF.

Clinical Manifestations

GABHS is generally a relatively brief illness that varies in severity from subclinical (no symptoms) to severe toxicity. The onset is often abrupt and characterized by pharyngitis, headache, fever, and abdominal pain (especially in small children). The tonsils and pharynx may be inflamed and covered with exudate (Fig. 46-1), which usually appears by the second day of illness. However, streptococcal infections should be suspected in children older than 2 years of age who have pharyngitis without exudate (Thuma, 1997). Anterior cervical lymphadenopathy (in about 30% to 50% of cases) usually occurs early, and the nodes are often tender. Pain can be relatively mild to severe enough to make swallowing difficult. Clinical manifestations usually subside in 3 to 5 days unless complicated by sinusitis or parapharyngeal, peritonsillar, or retropharyngeal abscess. Nonsuppurative complications may appear after the onset of GABHS—acute nephritis in about 10 days and ARF in an average of 18 days.

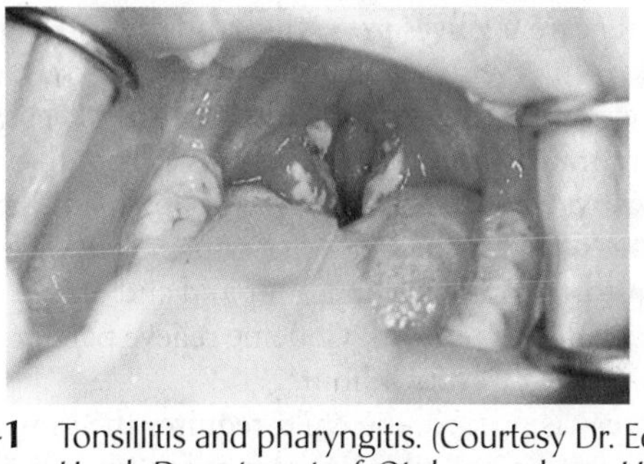

Fig. 46-1 Tonsillitis and pharyngitis. (Courtesy Dr. Edward L. Applebaum, Head, Department of Otolaryngology, University of Illinois Medical Center, Chicago.)

Diagnostic Evaluation

Although 80% to 90% of all cases of acute pharyngitis are viral, a throat culture should be performed to rule out GABHS. Because some children normally harbor streptococci in their throats, a positive culture is not always conclusive evidence of active disease. Most streptococcal infections are short-term illnesses, and antibody responses appear later than symptoms and are useful only for retrospective diagnosis.

Rapid identification of GABHS with diagnostic test kits is possible in the office or clinic setting. Because of the very high specificity of these rapid tests, a positive test result generally does not require throat culture confirmation. However, the sensitivities of these kits vary considerably, and a confirmatory throat culture is recommended in patients who have a negative test result (American Academy of Pediatrics, Committee on Infectious Diseases, 2003).

Therapeutic Management

If streptococcal sore throat infection is present, oral penicillin is prescribed in a dose sufficient to control the acute local manifestations and to maintain an adequate level for at least 10 days to eliminate any organisms that might remain to initiate ARF symptoms. Penicillin does not prevent the development of acute glomerulonephritis in susceptible children; however, it may prevent the spread of a nephrogenic strain of GABHS to others in the family. Penicillin usually produces a prompt response within 24 hours. Some patients require retreatment if the organism is not eradicated.

Intramuscular benzathine penicillin G is an appropriate therapy, but it is very painful and is not the first choice for children. Oral erythromycin is indicated for children allergic to penicillin. Other antibiotics used to treat GABHS are azithromycin, clarithromycin, oral cephalosporins, amoxicillin, and amoxicillin with clavulanic acid (McMillan & Feigin, 1999). A combination of penicillin and rifampin is more effective in eradicating GABHS than penicillin alone and is recommended for carriers.

Nursing Care Management

The nurse often obtains a throat swab for culture and instructs the parents about administering penicillin and analgesics as prescribed. Most children prefer to remain in bed during the acute phase of the illness. Cold or warm compresses to the neck may provide relief. In children who can cooperate, warm saline gargles offer relief of throat discomfort. Pain may interfere with oral intake, and children should not be forced to eat. Cool liquids or ice chips are usually more acceptable than solids.

Special emphasis is placed on correct administration of oral medication and completing the course of antibiotic therapy (see Administration of Medication: Compliance, Chapter 45). If injections are required, they must be administered deep into a large muscle mass (e.g., vastus lateralis or ventrogluteal muscle). To prevent pain, application of EMLA over the injection site for 2.5 hours before the injection is helpful (see Administration of Medication: Intramuscular Administration, Chapter 45). Parents also need to be aware of residual tenderness at the injection site, which may cause the child to limp for a day or two. Local applications of heat are helpful in relieving this discomfort.

Nurses play a key role in preventing the spread of disease. Children are considered noninfectious to others 24 hours after initiation of antibiotic therapy, but they should not return to school or day care until they have been taking antibiotics for a full 24-hour period.

NURSE ALERT When nurses become aware that children have positive throat cultures for streptococcal infection, they should remind the children to discard their toothbrush and replace it with a new one after they have been taking antibiotics for 24 hours. ■

evolve CASE STUDY: TONSILLITIS

ANATOMY REVIEW: LOCATION OF TONSILLAR MASSES

Tonsillitis

The tonsils are masses of lymphoid tissue located in the pharyngeal cavity. They filter and protect the respiratory and alimentary tracts from invasion by pathogenic organisms and play a role in antibody formation. Although their size varies, children generally have much larger tonsils than adolescents or adults. This difference is thought to be a protective mechanism because young children are especially susceptible to URIs.

Pathophysiology

Several pairs of tonsils are part of a mass of lymphoid tissue encircling the nasal and oral pharynx, known as the *Waldeyer tonsillar ring* (Fig. 46-2). The *palatine* or *faucial tonsils* are located on either side of the oropharynx, behind and below the pillars of the fauces (opening from the mouth). A surface of the palatine tonsils is usually visible during oral examination. The palatine tonsils are those removed during tonsillectomy. The *pharyngeal tonsils,* also known as the *adenoids,* are located above the palatine tonsils on the posterior wall of the nasopharynx. Their proximity to the nares and eustachian tubes causes difficulties in instances of inflammation. The *lingual tonsils* are located at the base of the tongue. The *tubal tonsils,* found near the posterior nasopharyngeal opening of the eustachian tubes, are not part of the Waldeyer tonsillar ring.

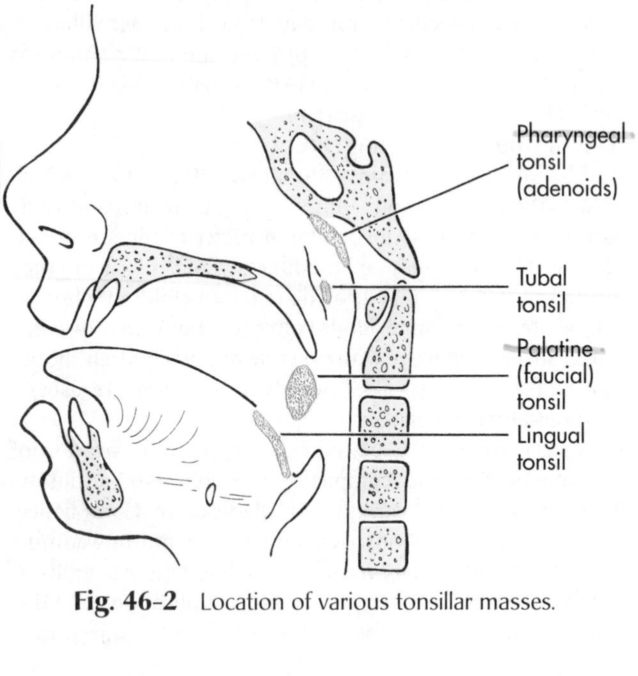

Fig. 46-2 Location of various tonsillar masses.

Etiology

Tonsillitis often occurs with pharyngitis. The causative agent may be viral or bacterial. Because of the abundant lymphoid tissue and the frequency of URIs, tonsillitis is a common cause of morbidity in young children.

Clinical Manifestations

The manifestations of tonsillitis are caused by inflammation. As the palatine tonsils enlarge from edema, they may meet in the midline (kissing tonsils), obstructing the passage of air or food. The child has difficulty swallowing and breathing. When enlargement of the adenoids occurs, the space behind the posterior nares becomes blocked, making it difficult or impossible for air to pass from the nose to the throat. As a result, the child breathes through the mouth.

Therapeutic Management

Because tonsillitis is self-limiting, treatment of viral pharyngitis is symptomatic. Throat cultures positive for GABHS infection warrant antibiotic treatment. It is important to differentiate between viral and streptococcal infection in febrile exudative tonsillitis. Because most infections are of viral origin, early rapid tests can eliminate unnecessary antibiotic administration.

Tonsillectomy is the surgical removal of the palatine tonsils. Absolute indications for a tonsillectomy are malignancy and obstruction of the airway that result in cor pulmonale. *Adenoidectomy* (the surgical removal of the adenoids) is recommended for children who have hypertrophied adenoids that obstruct nasal breathing. The American Academy of Otolaryngology—Head and Neck Surgery lists "3 or more infections of the tonsils or adenoids per year despite adequate medical therapy" as an indication for tonsillectomy or adenotonsillectomy (American Academy of Otolaryngology—Head and Neck Surgery, 2000). However, for some children the effectiveness of tonsillectomy or adenoidectomy is modest and may not justify the risk of surgery. In practice, most physicians rely on individualized decision making and do not subscribe to an absolute set of eligibility criteria for these surgical procedures (Paradise et al, 2002). Contraindications to either tonsillectomy or adenoidectomy are (1) cleft palate, because tonsils help minimize escape of air during speech; (2) acute infections at the time of surgery, because locally inflamed tissues increase the risk of bleeding; and (3) uncontrolled systemic diseases or blood dyscrasias.

Nursing Care Management

Nursing care involves providing comfort and minimizing activities or interventions that precipitate bleeding. A soft to liquid diet is preferred. A cool-mist vaporizer keeps the mucous membranes moist during periods of mouth breathing. Warm saltwater gargles, throat lozenges, and analgesic/antipyretic drugs such as acetaminophen are used to promote comfort. Combination nonopioid and opioid elixirs or tablets such as Tylenol with Codeine relieve pain and should be given routinely every 4 hours.

If surgery is needed, the child requires the same psychologic preparation and physical care as for any other surgical procedure (see Chapters 44 and 45). The following discussion focuses on postoperative nursing care for tonsillectomy and adenoidectomy (T&A), although both procedures may not be performed.

Until they are fully awake, children are placed on their abdomen or side to facilitate drainage of secretions. Suctioning is performed carefully to avoid trauma to the oropharynx. When alert, children may prefer sitting up, although they should remain in bed for the remainder of the day. They are discouraged from coughing frequently, clearing their throat, blowing their nose, or any other activity that may aggravate the operative site.

Some secretions are common, particularly dried blood from surgery. All secretions and vomitus are inspected for evidence of fresh bleeding (some blood-tinged mucus is expected). Dark brown (old) blood is usually present in the emesis, as well as in the nose and between the teeth. If parents do not expect this, they often become frightened at a time when they need to be calm and reassuring.

The throat is very sore after surgery. An ice collar provides relief, but many children find it bothersome and refuse to use it. Most children experience moderate pain after a T&A and need pain medication for at least the first 24 hours. Analgesics may be given rectally or intravenously to avoid the oral route. Because pain is continuous, analgesics should be administered at regular intervals. Local anesthetics, such as tetracaine lollipops or ice pops, and transdermal antiemetics such as promethazine (Phenergan) can be made by some pharmacists (see Pain Management, Chapter 44).

Food and fluids are restricted until children are fully alert and there are no signs of hemorrhage. Cool water, crushed ice, flavored ice pops, or diluted fruit juice is given, but fluids with a red or brown color are avoided to distinguish fresh or old blood in emesis from the ingested liquid. Citrus juice may cause discomfort and is usually poorly tolerated. Soft foods, particularly gelatin, cooked fruits, sherbet, soup, and mashed potatoes, are started on the first or second postoperative day or as the child tolerates feeding. The pain from surgery often inhibits intake, reinforcing the need for adequate pain control. Milk, ice cream, and pudding are usually not offered, because milk products coat the mouth and throat and may cause the child to clear the throat, which can initiate bleeding.

Postoperative hemorrhage is unusual but can occur. Therefore the nurse observes the throat directly for evidence of bleeding, using a good source of light and, if necessary, carefully inserting a tongue depressor. Signs of hemorrhage include increased pulse (greater than 120 beats/min), pallor, frequent clearing of the throat or swallowing by a younger child, and vomiting of bright red blood. Restlessness, an indication of hemorrhage, may be difficult to differentiate from general discomfort after surgery. Decreasing blood pressure is a late sign of shock.

NURSE ALERT The most obvious early sign of bleeding is the child's continuous swallowing of the trickling blood. While the child is sleeping, note the frequency of swallowing. If continuous bleeding is suspected, notify the surgeon immediately. ■

Family Support and Home Care

Discharge instructions include (1) avoiding irritating or highly seasoned foods, (2) avoiding gargles or vigorous toothbrushing, (3) discouraging coughing or clearing of the throat or putting objects in the mouth, (4) using analgesics or an ice collar for pain, and (5) limiting activity to decrease the potential for bleeding. Hemorrhage may occur up to 10 days after surgery as a result of tissue sloughing from the healing process. Any sign of bleeding warrants immediate medical attention.

Influenza

Influenza, or "flu," is caused by three orthomyxoviruses, which are antigenically distinct: types A and B, which cause epidemic disease, and type C, which is unimportant from an epidemiologic standpoint. Influenza is spread from one individual to another by direct contact (large-droplet infection) or by articles recently contaminated by nasopharyngeal secretions. There is no predilection for a specific age group, but attack rates are highest in young children who have had no previous contact with a strain. Influenza is frequently most severe in infants. During epidemics, infection among school-age children is believed to be a major source of transmission in a community. The disease is more common during the winter months and has a 1- to 3-day incubation period. Affected persons are most infectious for 24 hours before and after the onset of symptoms.

Clinical Manifestations

The manifestations of influenza may be subclinical, mild, moderate, or severe. Most patients have a dry throat and nasal mucosa, a dry cough, and a tendency toward hoarseness. A flushed face, photophobia, myalgia, hyperesthesia, and sometimes prostration accompany a sudden onset of fever and chills. Subglottal croup is common, especially in infants. The symptoms last for 4 to 5 days. Complications include severe viral pneumonia (often hemorrhagic), encephalitis, and secondary bacterial infections such as otitis media, sinusitis, or pneumonia.

Therapeutic Management

Uncomplicated influenza in children usually requires only symptomatic treatment: acetaminophen or ibuprofen for fever and sufficient fluids to maintain hydration. Children with influenza or other similar viruses should not receive aspirin because of its possible link with Reye syndrome. Amantadine hydrochloride is licensed for treatment of influenza in children. This medication has been effective in reducing symptoms associated with type A disease if administered within 24 to 48 hours after onset, but is ineffective against type B or C influenza or other viral diseases. It should not be given to children younger than 1 year of age but is recommended for unvaccinated high risk children. Zanamivir and rimantadine are two other drugs that have been approved for treatment of flu symptoms in children less than 18 years of age. Zanamivir is an inhaled medication that can cause bronchospasm and decreased lung function in children with asthma and chronic obstructive pulmonary disease. Zanamivir cannot be used for children less than 7 years of age, and rimantadine cannot be used for children less than 1 year of age (Palencia, 2000).

Prevention

Inactivated influenza viral vaccines are safe and effective provided the antigens in the vaccine correlate with the circulating influenza viruses (see Immunizations, Chapter 36).

In 2003, the nasal spray flu vaccine was approved by the Food and Drug Administration. However, this preparation contains a live virus and should not be used in individuals who are immunocompromised or have cancer.

Nursing Care Management

Nursing care is the same as that for any child with a URI, including implementing measures to relieve symptoms. The greatest danger to affected children is development of a secondary infection.

NURSE ALERT Prolonged fever or appearance of fever during early convalescence is a sign of secondary bacterial infection and should be reported to the practitioner for antibiotic therapy. ■

Otitis Media

Otitis media (OM) is one of the most prevalent diseases of early childhood. Its incidence is highest in the winter months. Many cases of bacterial OM are preceded by a viral respiratory infection. The two viruses most likely to precipitate OM are RSV and influenza. Most episodes of acute otitis media (AOM) occur in the first 24 months of life, but the incidence decreases with age, except for a small increase at age 5 or 6 years when children enter school. OM occurs infrequently in children older than 7 years of age. Preschool-age boys are affected more frequently than preschool-age girls. Children who have siblings or parents with a history of chronic OM have a higher incidence of OM. Children living in households with many members (especially smokers) are more likely to have OM than those living with fewer persons. Passive smoking increases the risk of persistent middle ear effusion by enhancing attachment of the pathogens that cause otitis to the respiratory epithelium in the middle ear space, by prolonging the inflammatory response, and by impeding drainage through the eustachian tube (Berman et al, 2001).

The clinical indicators used to define OM are outlined in Box 46-5.

Etiology

Streptococcus pneumoniae, H. influenzae, and *Moraxella catarrhalis* are the three most common bacteria causing AOM. The etiology of noninfectious OM is unknown, although OM may occur because of blocked eustachian tubes from the edema of URIs, allergic rhinitis, or hypertrophic adenoids. Chronic OM is frequently an extension of an acute episode.

A relationship between the incidence of OM and infant feeding methods has been noted. Breastfed infants have a lower incidence than formula-fed infants. Breastfeeding may protect infants against respiratory viruses and allergy because breast milk contains secretory immunoglobulin (Ig) A, which limits the exposure of the eustachian tube and middle ear mucosa to microbial pathogens and foreign proteins. Reflux of milk up the eustachian tubes is also less likely to occur in breastfed infants because of the semivertical positioning during breastfeeding.

BOX 46-5

What Is Acute Otitis Media?

A diagnosis of acute otitis media requires all of the following:

- Recent, usually abrupt, onset of illness
- The presence of middle ear fluid, or effusion
- Signs or symptoms of middle ear inflammation

American Academy of Pediatrics: The diagnosis and management of acute otitis media, *Pediatrics* 113(5):1451-1465, 2004.

Pathophysiology

OM is primarily the result of malfunctioning eustachian tubes. The eustachian tube, which connects the middle ear to the nasopharynx, is normally closed and flat, preventing organisms in the pharyngeal cavity from entering the middle ear. The eustachian tube opens to allow drainage of secretions produced by the middle ear mucosa and to equalize air pressure between the middle ear and the outside environment. Impaired drainage of the eustachian tube causes retention of secretions in the middle ear. Air is unable to escape through the obstructed tubes, is absorbed into the circulation, and causes negative pressure within the middle ear. If the tube opens, a difference in pressure causes bacteria to be swept into the middle ear chamber, where the organisms quickly proliferate and invade the mucosa.

Diagnostic Evaluation

Careful assessment of tympanic membrane mobility with a pneumatic otoscope is essential to differentiate AOM from otitis media with effusion (OME). If an accumulation of cerumen prevents adequate visualization of the tympanic membrane, the cerumen should be removed before inspection of the membrane (Pelton, 1998). A diagnosis of AOM is made if visual inspection of the tympanic membrane reveals a purulent discolored effusion and a bulging or full, opacified, or very reddened immobile membrane (American Academy of Pediatrics, 2004). An immobile tympanic membrane or an orange-discolored membrane indicates OME. Clinical symptoms of otitis are also helpful in making the diagnosis (Box 46-6). In AOM, symptoms such as acute ear pain, fever, and a bulging yellow or red tympanic membrane are usually present. In OME, these symptoms may be absent, and other nonspecific symptoms such as rhinitis, cough, or diarrhea are often present.

Therapeutic Management

Treatment for OM is one of the most common causes of antibiotic use in the ambulatory setting. Recently, however, concerns about drug-resistant *Streptococcus pneumoniae* and other drug resistances have caused infectious disease authorities to recommend careful and judicious use of antibiotics for treatment of this illness. Antibiotics are not required for initial treatment of OME, but may be indicated for children with persistent effusion for more than 3 months (American Academy of Pediatrics, 2004). It has been estimated that avoiding unnecessary treatment of OME with antibiotics would save up to 6 to 8 million courses of antibiotics each year (Stool et al, 1994). Recent reviews of the treatment of AOM reveal no clear evidence that antibiotics improve out-

BOX 46-6

Clinical Manifestations of Otitis Media

Acute Otitis Media
Follows an upper respiratory infection
Otalgia (earache)
Fever
Purulent discharge (otorrhea) may or may not be present

Infant or Very Young Child
Crying
Fussy, restless, irritable
Tendency to rub, hold, or pull affected ear
Rolls head from side to side
Difficulty comforting child
Loss of appetite

Older Child
Crying or verbalizes feelings of discomfort
Irritability
Lethargy
Loss of appetite

Chronic Otitis Media
Hearing loss
Difficulty communicating
Feeling of fullness, tinnitus, or vertigo may be present

comes in children younger than 2 years of age with uncomplicated AOM (O'Neill, 2001).

NURSE ALERT When should antibiotics be prescribed for AOM?

- For children age 6 months and younger—for certain or suspected AOM.
- Children age 6 months to 2 years—for certain AOM or suspected AOM with severe symptoms; observation is an option for suspected or uncertain AOM if nonsevere.
- Children age 2 to 12 years—antibiotic treatment for certain AOM with severe symptoms; observation is an option for suspected or nonsevere AOM.

The guideline provides an option to observe select children and start antibiotic treatment only if symptoms have not improved in 48 to 72 hours (American Academy of Pediatrics, 2004). ■

Current literature indicates that waiting up to 72 hours for spontaneous resolution is safe and appropriate management of AOM in healthy infants and children (American Academy of Pediatrics, 2004; Jackson, 2001). However, the watchful waiting approach is not recommended for children less than 2 years who have acute symptoms of fever and severe ear pain (Carlson & Scudder, 2004). In addition, all cases of AOM in infants younger than 6 months of age should be treated with antibiotics because of the infant's immature immune system and the potential for infection with bacteria other than the three most common organisms found in older infants and children with AOM.

When antibiotics are warranted, oral amoxicillin in high doses (80 to 90 mg/kg/day) is the treatment of choice for initial episodes of AOM in children who have not received antibiotics within the past month (Dowell et al, 1999; Jackson, 2001; Piglansky et al, 2003). The recommendation for the duration of antibiotic therapy is 10 to 14 days; in children 6 years and older, shorter courses may be sufficient (Iovino, 2003).

Second-line antibiotics used to treat OM include amoxicillin-clavulanate, azithromycin, and cephalosporins such as cefdinir, cefuroxime, and cefpodoxime. Intramuscular ceftriaxone is used when the causative organism is a highly resistant pneumococcus and when the parents are noncompliant with the therapy. The use of steroids, decongestants, and antihistamines to treat AOM is not recommended.

Myringotomy, a surgical incision of the eardrum, may be necessary to alleviate the severe pain of AOM. A myringotomy is also performed to provide drainage of infected middle ear fluid in the presence of complications (mastoiditis, labyrinthitis, or facial paralysis) or to allow purulent middle ear fluid to drain into the ear canal for culture (DeRosa & Grundfast, 2002). Recently, a minimally invasive, laser-assisted myringotomy procedure has been performed in outpatient settings (Cotter and Kosko, 2004).

Tympanostomy tube placement and adenoidectomy are surgical procedures that may be done to treat recurrent OM. Tympanostomy tubes are pressure-equalizer (PE) tubes or grommets that facilitate continued drainage of fluid and allow ventilation of the middle ear. Myringotomy with or without insertion of PE tubes should *not* be performed for initial management of OME, but may be recommended for children who have recurrent episodes of OME with a long cumulative duration (e.g., 6 months out of the previous 12) (Bluestone, 1998). Adenoidectomy is never recommended for treatment of AOM and is only performed in children with recurrent AOM or chronic OME with nasal obstruction. Tonsillectomy either alone or with adenoidectomy is not considered an effective treatment of OME (Neill, 2002).

In some children, residual middle ear effusions remain after episodes of AOM. Management options for OM with residual effusion include observation, antibiotics alone, or a combination of antibiotic and corticosteroid therapy. A hearing test should also be performed 3 months after the acute episode of AOM, and children with hearing loss should be referred to an otolaryngologist and should receive a speech and language evaluation as necessary.

Polyvalent pneumococcal polysaccharide vaccines have reduced the incidence of pneumococcal OM by 50% in children older than 2 years of age, but these vaccines are not effective in infants, who do not normally develop antibodies to polysaccharide vaccines (Andrews, 2001). For some high risk infants, an immune globulin containing antibodies against bacterial polysaccharides (BPIG) has resulted in fewer cases of AOM caused by *S. pneumoniae.*

Nursing Care Management

Nursing objectives for the child with AOM include (1) relieving pain, (2) facilitating drainage when possible, (3) preventing complications or recurrence, (4) educating the family in care of the child, and (5) providing emotional support to the child and family.

Analgesic drugs such as acetaminophen and ibuprofen are used to treat mild pain. For more severe pain, the new Centers for Disease Control and Prevention and American Academy of Pediatrics guidelines recommend a stronger analgesic such as codeine (Iovino, 2003). An ice compress placed over the affected ear may also provide comfort and reduce edema and pressure.

If the ear is draining, the external canal may be cleaned with sterile cotton swabs or pledgets coupled with topical antibiotic treatment (Ramsey, 2002). If ear wicks or lightly rolled sterile gauze packs are placed in the ear after surgical treatment, they should be loose enough to allow accumulated drainage to flow out of the ear; otherwise, infection may be transferred to the mastoid process. The wicks need to stay dry during shampoos or baths. Occasionally, drainage is so profuse that the auricle and the skin surrounding the ear become excoriated from the exudate. This is usually prevented by frequent cleansing and application of various moisture barriers (e.g., Aloe Vesta, Proshield Plus) or petrolatum jelly (e.g., Vaseline).

Parents require anticipatory guidance regarding the temporary hearing loss that accompanies OM. The nurse should caution parents that their child is not ignoring them but may be unaware of being spoken to. Parents are instructed to speak louder, at closer proximity, and facing the child. Persistent difficulty in hearing beyond the acute stage should be evaluated.

Tympanostomy tubes may allow water to enter the middle ear, but recommendations for earplugs are inconsistent. Research indicates that swimming without earplugs poses no increased risk of infection. However, lake water is contaminated, and wearing earplugs while swimming in a lake prevents total flooding of the external canal. Bathwater and shampoo water should be kept out of the ear, if possible, because soap reduces the surface tension of water and facilitates entry through the tube. Parents should be aware of the appearance of a grommet (usually a tiny, white, plastic spool-shaped tube) so that they can recognize it if it falls out. They are reassured that this is normal and requires no immediate intervention, although they should notify the practitioner.

Prevention of recurrence requires adequate education regarding antibiotic therapy. The symptoms of pain and fever usually subside within 24 to 48 hours, but nurses must emphasize that the infection is not completely eradicated until all of the prescribed medication is taken. Parents should be aware that potential complications of OM, such as hearing loss, can be prevented with adequate treatment and follow-up care.

Parents need to be taught ways to prevent OM, such as sitting or holding an infant upright during bottle-feeding and breastfeeding. Propping bottles is discouraged to avoid the supine position and to encourage human contact during feeding. Parents must recognize the initial signs of OM such as irritability and ear pulling. Eliminating tobacco smoke and known allergens from the environment is essential.

CROUP SYNDROMES

Croup is a general term applied to a symptom complex characterized by hoarseness, a resonant cough described as "barking" or "brassy" (croupy), varying degrees of inspiratory stridor, and varying degrees of respiratory distress resulting from swelling or obstruction in the region of the larynx. Acute infections of the larynx are important in infants and small children because of their increased incidence in these age groups and because the small diameter of the airway in infants and children places them at risk for significant narrowing with inflammation.

Croup syndromes can affect the larynx, trachea, and bronchi. However, laryngeal involvement often dominates the clinical picture because of the severe effects on the voice and breathing. Croup syndromes are described according to the primary anatomic area affected (i.e., epiglottitis [or supraglottitis], laryngitis, laryngotracheobronchitis [LTB], and tracheitis). In general, LTB occurs in very young children, and epiglottitis is more common in older children. A comparison of croup syndromes is provided in Table 46-1.

Acute Epiglottitis

Acute epiglottitis, or *acute supraglottitis,* is a serious obstructive inflammatory process that occurs predominantly in children 2 to 5 years of age, but can occur from infancy to adulthood. The disorder requires immediate attention. The obstruction is supraglottic as opposed to the subglottic obstruction of laryngitis. The responsible organism is usually *H. influenzae.* LTB and epiglottitis do not occur together.

evolve CASE STUDY: ACUTE EPIGLOTTITIS

Clinical Manifestations

The onset of epiglottitis is abrupt and can rapidly progress to severe respiratory distress. The child usually goes to bed asymptomatic to awaken later, complaining of sore throat and pain on swallowing. The child has a fever; appears sicker than clinical findings suggest; and insists on sitting upright and leaning forward, with the chin thrust out, mouth open, and tongue protruding *(tripod position).* Drooling of saliva is common because of the difficulty or pain on swallowing and excessive secretions.

NURSE ALERT Three clinical observations that have been found to be predictive of epiglottitis are absence of spontaneous cough, presence of drooling, and agitation. ■

The child is irritable and extremely restless and has an anxious, apprehensive, and frightened expression. The voice is thick and muffled, with a froglike croaking sound on inspiration, but the child is not hoarse. Suprasternal and substernal retractions may be visible. The child seldom struggles to breathe, and slow, quiet breathing provides better air exchange. The sallow color of mild hypoxia may progress to frank cyanosis. The throat is red and inflamed, and a distinctive large, cherry red, edematous epiglottis is visible on careful throat inspection. *Throat inspection should be attempted only when immediate intubation can be performed if needed.*

Therapeutic Management

The course of epiglottitis may be fulminant, with respiratory obstruction appearing suddenly. Progressive obstruction leads to hypoxia, hypercapnia, and acidosis followed by decreased muscular tone, reduced level of consciousness, and, when obstruction becomes more or less complete, a rather sudden death. A presumptive diagnosis of epiglottitis constitutes an emergency.

The child who is suspected of having epiglottitis should be examined in a setting where emergency equipment is readily available. Examination of the throat with a tongue depressor is contraindicated until properly experienced personnel and equipment are at hand to proceed with immediate intubation or tracheostomy in the event that the examination precipitates further or complete obstruction.

Table 46-1

Comparison of Croup Syndromes

	ACUTE EPIGLOTTITIS	ACUTE LARYNGOTRACHEO-BRONCHITIS (LTB)	ACUTE SPASMODIC LARYNGITIS	ACUTE TRACHEITIS
Age group affected	1-8 years	3 months-8 years	3 months-3 years	1 month-6 years
Etiologic agent	Bacterial, usually *Haemophilus influenzae*	Viral	Viral with allergic component	Bacterial, usually *Staphylococcus aureus*
Onset	Rapidly progressive	Slowly progressive	Sudden; at night	Moderately progressive
Major symptoms	Dysphagia Stridor aggravated when supine Drooling High fever Toxic appearance Rapid pulse and respirations	URI Stridor Brassy cough Hoarseness Dyspnea Restlessness Irritability Low-grade fever Nontoxic appearance	URI Croupy cough Stridor Hoarseness Dyspnea Restlessness Symptoms awaken child Symptoms disappear during day Tends to recur	URI Croupy cough Stridor Purulent secretions High fever No response to LTB therapy
Treatment	Antibiotics Airway protection	Humidity Racemic epinephrine	Humidity	Antibiotics

URI, upper respiratory infection.

If a lateral neck film is indicated, the same experienced personnel should accompany the child to the radiology department. Most practitioners prefer that the child not be transported but remain on the parent's lap in the examination area during portable radiology.

Endotracheal intubation or tracheostomy is usually considered for *H. influenzae* epiglottitis with severe respiratory distress. Intubation, tracheostomy, and any invasive procedure such as starting an intravenous (IV) infusion should be performed in the operating room. Whether or not there is an artificial airway, the child requires intensive observation by experienced personnel. The epiglottal swelling usually decreases after 24 hours of antibiotic therapy, and the epiglottis is near normal by the third day. Intubated children are generally extubated at this time.

Children with suspected bacterial epiglottitis are given antibiotics intravenously, followed by oral administration to complete a 7- to 10-day course. The use of corticosteroids for reducing edema may be beneficial during the early hours of treatment. Most intubated children receive a course of corticosteroids for 24 hours before extubation.

Prevention

The American Academy of Pediatrics, Committee on Infectious Diseases (2003), recommends that all children beginning at 2 months of age receive the *H. influenzae* type B conjugate vaccine (see Immunizations, Chapter 36). Since administration of the vaccine has become a routine part of the regular immunization schedule, the incidence of epiglottitis has declined.

Nursing Care Management

Epiglottitis is a serious and frightening disease for the child and family. It is important to act quickly but calmly and to provide support without increasing anxiety. The child is allowed to remain in the position that provides the most comfort and security, and parents are reassured that everything possible is being done to obtain relief for their child.

NURSE ALERT Nurses who suspect epiglottitis should not attempt to visualize the epiglottis directly with a tongue depressor or take a throat culture but should refer the child for medical evaluation immediately (Critical Thinking Exercise). ■

??? Critical Thinking Exercise

CROUP SYNDROME

Kim, a 4-year-old, is admitted to the emergency department with a sore throat, pain on swallowing, drooling, and a fever of 39° C (102.2° F). She looks ill, is agitated, and prefers to sit up and lean over. What nursing interventions should the nurse implement in this situation?

1. Evidence—Is there sufficient evidence to draw any conclusions about Kim's condition at this time?
2. Assumptions—Describe some underlying assumptions about each of the following:
   a. Epiglottitis in children
   b. Symptoms of epiglottitis
   c. Precautions to be taken when a child has suspected epiglottitis
   d. Immediate nursing interventions when caring for a child with epiglottitis
3. What priorities for nursing care can be drawn at this time?
4. Does the evidence objectively support your argument (conclusion)?
5. Are there alternative perspectives to your arguments? What are they?

Acute care of the child is the same as that described for the child with LTB. Continuous monitoring of respiratory status, including pulse oximetry and blood gases, is an important part of nursing observations, and the IV infusion is maintained as described in Chapter 45.

Acute Laryngitis

Acute infectious laryngitis is a common illness in older children and adolescents. Infants and smaller children experience more generalized involvement (see the following section on LTB). Viruses are the usual causative agents, and the principal complaint is hoarseness, which may be accompanied by other upper respiratory symptoms (e.g., coryza, sore throat, nasal congestion) and systemic manifestations (e.g., fever, headache, myalgia, malaise). Associated complaints vary with the infecting virus. Adenoviruses and influenza viruses are responsible for more systemic involvement; parainfluenza viruses, rhinoviruses, and RSV cause more mild illness.

Therapeutic Management and Nursing Care Management

The disease is usually self-limited without long-term sequelae. Treatment is symptomatic with fluids and humidified air (see Nursing Care Plan, p. 1429).

Acute Laryngotracheobronchitis

LTB is the most common croup syndrome. It primarily affects children younger than 5 years of age, and the causative organisms are the parainfluenza virus, RSV, influenza A and B, and *M. pneumoniae.* The disease is usually preceded by a URI, which gradually descends to adjacent structures. It is characterized by gradual onset of low-grade fever. Inflammation of the mucosal lining of the larynx and trachea causes a narrowing of the airway. When the airway is significantly narrowed, the child struggles to inhale air past the obstruction and into the lungs, producing the characteristic inspiratory stridor and suprasternal retractions. The typical child with LTB is a toddler who develops the classic barking or seal-like cough and acute stridor after several days of coryza. When the child is unable to inhale a sufficient volume of air, symptoms of hypoxia become evident. Obstruction that is severe enough to prevent adequate exhalation of carbon dioxide can cause respiratory acidosis and eventual respiratory failure. The progression of symptoms is outlined in Box 46-7.

Therapeutic Management

The major objective in medical management is maintaining the airway and providing adequate respiratory exchange. Children with mild croup (no stridor at rest) are managed at home. Parents are taught the signs of respiratory distress and instructed to summon professional help early if needed. Children who progress to stage II respiratory symptoms should receive medical attention.

High humidity with cool mist provides relief for most children. A cool-air vaporizer can be used at home. In the hospital setting, hoods for infants or tents for toddlers may be used to provide increased humidity and supplemental oxygen.

BOX 46-7

Progression of Symptoms in Laryngotracheobronchitis

Stage I
Fear
Hoarseness
Croupy cough
Inspiratory stridor when disturbed

Stage II
Continuous respiratory stridor
Lower rib retraction
Retraction of soft tissue of neck
Use of accessory muscles of respiration
Labored respiration

Stage III
Signs of anoxia and carbon dioxide retention
Restlessness
Anxiety
Pallor
Sweating
Rapid respirations

Stage IV
Intermittent cyanosis
Permanent cyanosis
Cessation of breathing

From Walter EB, Shurin PA: Acute respiratory infections. In Krugman S et al: *Infectious diseases of children,* ed 9, St Louis, 1992, Mosby.

NURSE ALERT Children with severe respiratory distress (traditionally, a respiratory rate greater than 60 breaths/min for infants) should not be given anything by mouth to prevent aspiration and decrease the work of breathing. ■

Nebulized epinephrine (racemic epinephrine) is often used in children with severe disease, stridor at rest, retractions, or difficulty breathing. The β-adrenergic effects cause mucosal vasoconstriction and subsequently decrease subglottic edema. The onset of action is rapid, and the peak effect is observed in 2 hours. Additional doses may be administered every 20 to 30 minutes in the intensive care unit or 3 to 4 hours in the regular hospital unit (Wald, 1999). In a significant number of children, however, improvement persists and additional treatments are not necessary.

The use of corticosteroids is beneficial because the anti-inflammatory effects decrease subglottic edema. The onset of action is clinically detectable as early as 6 hours after administration, with continued improvement over 12 to 24 hours.

It is essential to allow children with mild croup to drink beverages they like and to encourage their parents to try whatever comforting measures work best (e.g., holding their child, rocking, singing). If the child is unable to take oral fluids, IV fluid therapy may be indicated.

Nursing Care Management

The most important nursing function in the care of children with LTB is continuous, vigilant observation and accurate assessment of respiratory status. Cardiorespiratory monitoring and noninvasive pulse oximetry equipment supplement visual observations. Changes in therapy are frequently based on the nurses' observations and assessments, the child's response to therapy, and tolerance of procedures. The trend away from early intubation of children with LTB emphasizes the importance of nursing observations and the ability to recognize impending respiratory failure so that intubation can be implemented without delay. Intubation equipment must be readily accessible and taken with the child during transport to other areas (e.g., radiology, operating room).

NURSE ALERT Early signs of impending airway obstruction include increased pulse and respiratory rate; substernal, suprasternal, and intercostal retractions; flaring nares; and increased restlessness. ■

To conserve energy, children are given every opportunity to rest. Infants or small children respond to being enclosed in a tent, coughing, having laryngeal spasms, and needing IV therapy as additional sources of distress. Most infants and small children prefer to be held and to sit upright. Children also need the security of their parent's presence. Crying increases respiratory distress and hypoxia, and an extremely fussy child may tolerate procedures better when held in the parent's lap with cool mist directed toward the child's face than in a mist tent.

The rapid progression of croup, the alarming sound of the cough and stridor, and the child's apprehensive behavior and ill appearance combine to create a frightening experience for the parents. Parents need reassurance regarding their child's progress and an explanation of treatments. They may feel guilty for not having suspected the seriousness of the condition sooner. The family should be allowed to remain with their child as much as possible, especially when this decreases the child's distress.

The nurse should provide the parents with an opportunity to express their feelings, and minimize any sense of blame or guilt. Parents need frequent reassurance provided in a calm, quiet manner and education regarding what they can do to make their child more comfortable. Fortunately, as the crisis subsides and the child responds to therapy, breathing becomes easier and recovery is generally prompt. Home care includes continued humidity, adequate hydration, and nourishment.

Acute Spasmodic Laryngitis

Acute spasmodic laryngitis (*spasmodic croup,* "midnight croup," or "twilight croup") is distinct from laryngitis and LTB and is characterized by paroxysmal attacks of laryngeal obstruction that occur chiefly at night. Signs of inflammation are absent or mild, and there is often a history of previous attacks lasting 2 to 5 days, followed by uneventful recovery. This condition usually affects children ages 1 to 3 years. Some children appear to be predisposed to the condition; allergies may be implicated in some cases.

The child goes to bed feeling well or with very mild respiratory symptoms but awakens suddenly with characteristic barking, metallic cough, hoarseness, noisy inspirations, and restlessness. The child appears anxious, frightened, and prostrated. Dyspnea is aggravated by excitement; but there is no fever, the attack subsides in a few hours, and the child appears well the next day.

Therapeutic Management and Nursing Care Management

Spasmodic croup is usually self-limited, and most children are managed at home. Cool mist is recommended for the child's room. Warm mist provided by steam from hot running water in a closed bathroom is also helpful. Sometimes the spasm is relieved by sudden exposure to cold air (as when the child is taken out into the night air to see the practitioner). Parents are usually advised to have the child sleep in humidified air until the cough has subsided to prevent subsequent episodes. Children with moderately severe symptoms may be hospitalized for observation and therapy with cool mist and racemic epinephrine, as for LTB. Some patients respond to corticosteroid therapy.

Bacterial Tracheitis

Bacterial tracheitis, an infection of the mucosa of the upper trachea, is a distinct entity with features of both croup and epiglottitis. The disease occurs in children 1 month to 6 years of age, and may be a serious cause of airway obstruction that is severe enough to cause respiratory arrest. It is believed to be a complication of LTB, and although *Staphylococcus aureus* is the most frequent organism responsible, group A β-hemolytic streptococci and *H. influenzae* have also been implicated.

The manifestations of bacterial tracheitis are similar to those of LTB but are unresponsive to LTB therapy. There is a history of previous URI with croupy cough, stridor unaffected by position, toxicity, and high fever. Another prominent symptom is the production of thick, purulent tracheal secretions. Respiratory difficulties are secondary to these copious secretions.

Therapeutic Management and Nursing Care Management

Bacterial tracheitis requires vigorous management with humidified oxygen, antipyretics, and antibiotics. Most children require endotracheal intubation and frequent tracheal suctioning to prevent airway obstruction. Early recognition to prevent catastrophic airway obstruction is essential.

INFECTIONS OF THE LOWER AIRWAYS

The *reactive portion* of the lower respiratory tract includes the bronchi and bronchioles in children. Cartilaginous support of the large airways is not fully developed until adolescence. Consequently, the smooth muscle in these structures represents a major factor in the constriction of the airway, particularly in the *bronchioles,* that portion that extends from the bronchi to the alveoli. Table 46-2 compares some of the major features of bronchial and bronchiolar infections.

Bronchitis

Bronchitis (sometimes referred to as *tracheobronchitis*) is inflammation of the large airways (trachea and bronchi), which is frequently associated with a URI. Viral agents are

Table 46-2

Comparison of Conditions Affecting the Bronchi

	VIRAL-INDUCED ASTHMA*	BRONCHITIS	BRONCHIOLITIS
Description	Exaggerated response of bronchi to infection Bronchospasm, exudation, and edema of bronchi	Usually occurs in association with URI Seldom an isolated entity	More common infectious disease of lower airways Maximum obstructive impact at bronchiolar level
Age group affected	Late infancy and early childhood	Affects children in first 4 years of life	Usually children 2-12 months of age; rare after age 2 Peak incidence approximately age 6 months
Etiologic agents	Most often viruses but may be any of a variety of URI pathogens	Usually viral Other agents (e.g., bacteria, fungi, allergic disorders, airborne irritants) can trigger symptoms	Viruses, predominantly respiratory syncytial viruses; also adenoviruses, parainfluenza viruses, and *Mycoplasma pneumoniae*
Predominant characteristics	Wheezing, productive cough	Persistent dry, hacking cough (worse at night) becoming productive in 2-3 days	Dyspnea, paroxysmal nonproductive cough, tachypnea with retractions and flaring nares, emphysema; may be wheezing
Treatment	Bronchodilators, corticosteroids	Cough suppressants if needed	Oxygen mist Ribavirin may be used for high risk populations

URI, upper respiratory infection.
*See Asthma, p. 1449.

the primary cause of the disease, although *M. pneumoniae* is a common cause in children older than 6 years of age. A dry, hacking, nonproductive cough that worsens at night and becomes productive in 2 to 3 days characterizes this condition.

Bronchitis is a mild, self-limiting disease that requires only symptomatic treatment, including analgesics, antipyretics, and humidity. Cough suppressants may be useful to allow rest but can interfere with clearance of secretions. Most patients recover uneventfully in 5 to 10 days.

Respiratory Syncytial Virus/Bronchiolitis

Bronchiolitis is an acute viral infection with maximum effect at the bronchiolar level. The infection is rare in children older than 2 years of age. *Respiratory syncytial virus (RSV)* is responsible for 80% or more of the cases during epidemic periods (Long, 1999). It is considered the single most important respiratory pathogen in infancy and early childhood. Infection begins in the late fall, reaches a peak during winter, and decreases in spring. It is easily spread from hand to eye, nose, or other mucous membranes.

Pathophysiology

In RSV, the bronchiole mucosa swell, and lumina are filled with mucus and exudate. The walls of the bronchi and bronchioles are infiltrated with inflammatory cells; and peribronchiolar interstitial pneumonitis is usually present. Varying degrees of obstruction produced in the small air passages lead to hyperinflation, obstructive emphysema resulting from partial obstruction, and patchy areas of atelectasis. Dilation of bronchial passages on inspiration allows sufficient space for intake of air, but narrowing of the passages on expiration prevents air from leaving the lungs. Thus air is trapped distal to the obstruction and causes progressive overinflation *(emphysema).*

Clinical Manifestations

Bronchiolitis begins as a URI with symptoms of rhinorrhea and low-grade fever. Otitis media and conjunctivitis may also be present. In time a cough develops and, if the disease progresses, it becomes a respiratory tract infection with typical symptoms (Box 46-8). Chest radiographs show hyperaeration and areas of consolidation that are difficult to differentiate from bacterial pneumonia. Apnea may be the first recognized indicator of RSV infection in very young infants. Severe disease is followed by a rise in arterial carbon dioxide tension ($Paco_2$) (hypercapnia), leading to respiratory acidosis and hypoxemia.

evolve CASE STUDY: BRONCHIOLITIS

Diagnostic Evaluation

Positive identification of RSV is accomplished by using either enzyme-linked immunosorbent assay (ELISA) or rapid immunofluorescent antibody (IFA) from direct aspiration of nasal secretions or nasopharyngeal washings (see Respiratory Secretion and Throat Specimens, Chapter 45).

BOX 46-8

Signs and Symptoms of Respiratory Syncytial Virus

Initial
Rhinorrhea
Pharyngitis
Coughing/sneezing
Wheezing
Possible ear or eye drainage
Intermittent fever

With Progression of Illness
Increased coughing and wheezing
Air hunger
Tachypnea and retractions
Cyanosis

Severe Illness
Tachypnea, greater than 70 breaths/min
Listlessness
Apneic spells
Poor air exchange; poor breath sounds

Therapeutic Management

Bronchiolitis is treated symptomatically with high humidity, adequate fluid intake, and rest. Most children can be managed at home. Hospitalization is recommended for children with underlying lung or heart disease, associated debilitated states, or an inadequate caregiver. The child who is tachypneic, has marked retractions, seems listless, or has a history of poor fluid intake should also be admitted. Treatment involves mist therapy combined with oxygen administered by hood or tent in concentrations sufficient to alleviate dyspnea and hypoxia, after which mist alone is continued for mild dyspnea. Fluids by mouth may be contraindicated because of tachypnea, weakness, and fatigue; therefore IV fluids are preferred until the acute crisis of the disease has passed.

Clinical assessments, noninvasive oxygen monitoring, and blood gas values guide therapy. Medical therapy for bronchiolitis is controversial. Bronchodilators, corticosteroids, cough suppressants, and antibiotics are not effective in uncomplicated disease and are not recommended for routine use.

Ribavirin has in vitro antiviral activity against RSV, but ribavirin aerosol treatment for RSV infection is highly controversial. Placebo-controlled clinical trials have failed to demonstrate efficacy of this drug, and there are concerns about the drug's cost and safety. The American Academy of Pediatrics, Committee on Infectious Diseases (2003), recommends that decisions about ribavirin be made on the basis of the individual patient's clinical presentation and the physician's experience.

Prevention of RSV Infection

Two products, RSV immune globulin and palivizumab, are used to prevent RSV infection. *RSV immune globulin (RSV-IGIV)* is an IV preparation of immunoglobulin G that provides neutralizing antibodies against RSV. This drug is given in a monthly IV infusion beginning just before onset of the RSV season. The monoclonal antibody, palivizumab, is given monthly in an intramuscular (IM) injection. Both drugs have been licensed for prevention of RSV disease. The American Academy of Pediatrics, Committee on Infectious Diseases (2003), recommends that RSV-IGIV be considered for infants and children younger than 24 months of age who have chronic lung disease (CLD) and who have required medical therapy for CLD within 6 months before the anticipated start of RSV season. Palivizumab is preferred for most high risk children because of its ease of administration, safety, and effectiveness. Infants born at 32 weeks of gestation or earlier may benefit from RSV prophylaxis even if they do not have CLD. For these infants, the decision is based on their gestational age and their chronologic age at the start of RSV season. Infants born at 28 weeks of gestation or earlier may benefit by receiving the preventive drug during their first RSV season when it occurs in their first 12 months of life. Infants born at 29 to 32 weeks of gestation may benefit from prophylaxis until they are 6 months of age. Although these drugs have been shown to decrease the likelihood of hospitalization in infants born between 32 and 35 weeks of gestation, the cost of providing prophylaxis to this large group of infants should be considered carefully. The American Academy of Pediatrics, Committee on Infectious Diseases (2003), recommends prophylaxis for infants born between 32 and 35 weeks of gestation if they are younger than 6 months of age at the start of the RSV season. Prophylaxis is also recommended if infants or children have two or more of the following additional risk factors: school-age siblings, crowding in the home, day care attendance, or exposure to tobacco smoke in the home. In addition, children who are 24 months of age or younger with hemodynamically significant cyanotic and acyanotic congenital heart disease are likely to benefit from palivizumab injections. RSV-IGIV is contraindicated in children with cyanotic congenital heart disease. Neither palivizumab nor RSV-IGIV has been evaluated for immunocompromised children.

Nursing Care Management

Children admitted to the hospital with suspected RSV infection should be assigned separate rooms or grouped with other RSV-infected children. The most important infection control measures in caring for these infants and children are consistent handwashing and the use of contact precautions (gloves, gowns, masks, and goggles). Another measure is structuring patient assignments so that nurses assigned to children with RSV do not take care of other patients who are considered high risk.

If ribavirin is chosen for therapy, this drug is aerosolized and delivered via a small-particle aerosol generator through an oxygen hood, tent, mask, or ventilator. Care must be taken to minimize the escape of aerosolized ribavirin into the air.

NURSE ALERT Because of concerns about potential toxic or teratogenic effects, pregnant health care providers should not care for a child receiving ribavirin. ■

Children receiving RSV-IGIV should be monitored for symptoms of fluid volume overload during IV administration. Antibodies in RSV-IGIV may interfere with the immune response to live virus vaccines (mumps, rubella, measles, and chickenpox); therefore immunization with these vaccines should be deferred for 9 months after the last dose of RSV-IGIV infusion (American Academy of Pediatrics, Committee on Infectious Diseases, 2003). Palivizumab does not interfere with response to vaccines. However, preparations of palivizumab do not contain a preservative, so the health care professional who administers this drug must arrange to administer it within 6 hours after opening a vial. To relieve the pain of IV infusions of RSV-IGIV and the IM injections of palivizumab, EMLA cream should be applied to the IV insertion site or the IM site before the procedure.

Pneumonias

Pneumonia, inflammation of the pulmonary parenchyma, is common in childhood but occurs more frequently in infancy and early childhood. Clinically, pneumonia may occur either as a primary disease or as a complication of another illness. The various types of pneumonia include the following:

Lobar pneumonia—All or a large segment of one or more pulmonary lobes is involved. When both lungs are affected, it is known as *bilateral* or *double pneumonia.*

Bronchopneumonia—Begins in the terminal bronchioles, which become clogged with mucopurulent exudate to form consolidated patches in nearby lobules; also called *lobular pneumonia.*

Interstitial pneumonia—The inflammatory process is more or less confined within the alveolar walls (interstitium) and the peribronchial and interlobular tissues.

Although the morphologic classification is typically used, the most useful classification of pneumonia is based on the etiologic agent (i.e., viral, bacterial, mycoplasmal, or aspiration of foreign substances) (see Aspiration Pneumonia, p. 1447). Histomycosis, coccidioidomycosis, and other fungi also cause pneumonia. The causative agent is identified from the clinical history, the child's age, the general health history, the physical examination, radiography, and the laboratory examination.

Viral Pneumonia

Viral pneumonias, which occur more frequently than bacterial pneumonias, are seen in children of all ages and are often associated with viral URIs. Viruses that cause pneumonia include RSV in infants and parainfluenza, influenza, and adenovirus in older children. Few clinical symptoms are unique to a specific virus, and differentiation among viruses is usually made by laboratory examination (Box 46-9).

The prognosis is generally good, although viral infections of the respiratory tract render the affected child more susceptible to secondary bacterial invasion, especially when there is denuded bronchial mucosa. Treatment is symptomatic and includes measures to promote oxygenation and comfort, such as oxygen administration with cool mist, chest physiotherapy and postural drainage, antipyretics for fever management, fluid intake, and family support. Some authorities recommend antimicrobial therapy in the hope of reducing or preventing secondary bacterial infection, but this therapy should be reserved for children in whom a bacterial infection is demonstrated by appropriate cultures.

BOX 46-9

General Signs of Pneumonia

Fever—Usually quite high
Respiratory
  Cough—Unproductive to productive with whitish sputum
  Tachypnea
  Breath sounds—Rhonchi or fine crackles
  Dullness with percussion
  Chest pain
  Retractions
  Nasal flaring
  Pallor to cyanosis (depends on severity)
Chest x-ray film—Diffuse or patchy infiltration with peribronchial distribution
Behavior—Irritable, restless, lethargic
Gastrointestinal—Anorexia, vomiting, diarrhea, abdominal pain

Primary Atypical Pneumonia

Mycoplasma pneumoniae is the most common cause of pneumonia in children between ages 5 and 12 years. It occurs in the fall and winter months and is more prevalent in crowded living conditions. Most affected persons recover from acute illness in 7 to 10 days with symptomatic treatment followed by a week of convalescence. Hospitalization is rarely necessary.

Severe Acute Respiratory Syndrome

A severe form of atypical pneumonia identified as severe acute respiratory syndrome (SARS) was first reported in Asia in 2003. SARS is caused by a previously unrecognized coronavirus called *SARS Co-V.* Clinical manifestations of this disorder include the following: a fever greater than 100.4° F; headache; cough; shortness of breath; difficulty breathing; and, after 2 to 7 days, a dry, nonproductive cough and dyspnea. In some patients, the symptoms are severe enough to require intubation and mechanical ventilation. SARS is spread by close contact with a person who has SARS. Most cases have involved people who have cared for or lived with someone with SARS or people who have traveled to areas with reported cases of SARS (O'Connor, 2003).

In children, two distinct forms of the illness have been observed. Teenagers have malaise, myalgia, chills, and rigor, whereas young children have mainly cough and runny nose. In younger children the clinical course seems to be milder and the disease resolves more quickly than in adolescents or adults (Hon et al, 2003).

Laboratory findings include lymphopenia, leukopenia, thrombocytopenia, and elevated lactate dehydrogenase, aspartate aminotransferase, and creatinine kinase levels. The most reliable laboratory diagnostic test is positive antibodies for the SARS coronavirus 21 days after the illness. Chest radiographs in a substantial number of patients reveal focal interstitial infiltrates that progress to more generalized, patchy, interstitial infiltrates (Kuiken et al, 2003).

Treatment of SARS involves predominantly supportive care measures. Other therapies such as antibiotics, antiviral drugs, and steroids have been used with mixed results (O'Connor, 2003).

Nursing Care Management

The Centers for Disease Control and Prevention recommends that the patients with SARS receive the same treatment as any patient with serious community-acquired atypical pneumonia. This includes the use of strict handwashing, contact precautions, and airborne precautions (e.g., an isolation room with negative pressure relative to the surrounding area and the use of an N-95–filtering disposable respirator for persons entering the room). Recommendations for stopping the spread of SARS have also been developed. When triaging patients, nurses should place a surgical mask on any patient who has had close contact with SARS or who has a history of international travel to an area with cases of SARS. Health care workers who have had high risk, unprotected exposure to SARS should be excluded from duty and remain home from work to monitor their health for 10 days.

Bacterial Pneumonia

Streptococcus pneumoniae is the most common bacterial pathogen responsible for community-acquired pneumonia in both children and adults. During the last several decades, isolates of the *S. pneumoniae* organism that are resistant to penicillin and other antibiotics have become more prevalent (Tan et al, 2002). Other bacteria that cause pneumonia in children are GABHS, *S. aureus, M. catarrhalis,* and *H. influenzae.*

Beyond the neonatal period, bacterial pneumonias display distinct clinical patterns that facilitate their differentiation from other forms of pneumonia. The onset of illness is abrupt and generally follows a viral infection that disturbs the natural defense mechanisms of the upper respiratory tract.

Children with bacterial pneumonia appear ill. Symptoms include fever, malaise, rapid and shallow respirations, cough, and chest pain that is exaggerated by deep breathing. The pain of pneumonia may be referred to the abdomen and confused with appendicitis. Chills and meningeal symptoms *(meningism)* are common.

Older children with pneumococcal pneumonia can be treated at home if the condition is recognized and treatment is initiated early. Antibiotic therapy, bed rest, liberal oral intake of fluids, and administration of an antipyretic for fever are the principal therapeutic measures. Hospitalization is indicated when pleural effusion or empyema accompanies the disease. Pneumonia in the infant or young child is best treated in the hospital, because the course of illness is more variable and complications are more common in very young patients. IV fluids are frequently necessary, and oxygen is required if the child is in respiratory distress.

Complications

Some children, especially infants, with staphylococcal pneumonia can develop empyema, pyopneumothorax, or tension pneumothorax. AOM and pulmonary embolism are also common in children with pneumococcal pneumonia. A recent report indicated that the frequency of children who are hospitalized with pneumococcal pneumonia complicated by necrosis, empyema, complicated pneumonic effusion, and lung abscess may be increasing (Tan et al, 2002). Reasons for this increase in complications are unknown.

When fluid is suspected in the pleural cavity, a diagnostic needle aspiration or thoracentesis is performed. Nonpurulent effusions do not require surgical drainage. Continuous closed-chest drainage may need to be instituted when purulent fluid is aspirated.

Prognosis

The prognosis for pneumonia is generally good, with rapid recovery when symptoms are recognized and treated early. Streptococcal infections vary in duration but usually resolve spontaneously. The course of staphylococcal pneumonia is generally prolonged. The prognosis varies with the length of illness before treatment is begun, although early recognition and treatment are usually effective.

Prevention

Pneumococcal polysaccharide vaccine is recommended for use in selected individuals, such as children older than age 2 years who are at risk of acquiring pneumococcal infection or are at risk of serious disease (see Immunizations, Chapter 36).

Nursing Care Management

Nursing care of the child with pneumonia is primarily supportive and symptomatic but necessitates thorough respiratory assessment and administration of oxygen and antibiotics. The child's respiratory rate and status, as well as general disposition and level of activity, are frequently assessed. Isolation procedures are instituted according to hospital policy. Relief of physical and psychologic stress encourages rest and conservation of energy. The child is disturbed as little as possible by clustering care to encourage the child's regular sleep cycle. If the cough is disturbing, judicious use of antitussives, especially before rest times and meals, is often helpful. To prevent dehydration, fluids are frequently administered intravenously during the acute phase. Oral fluids, if allowed, are given cautiously to avoid aspiration and to decrease the possibility of aggravating a fatiguing cough.

Children may be placed in a mist tent. Cool humidification moistens the airways and provides an atmosphere that aids in temperature reduction. Children in mist tents require frequent clothing and linen changes to prevent chilling in the damp atmosphere. They are usually comfortable in a semierect position but should be allowed to determine the position of comfort. Lying on the affected side (if pneumonia is unilateral) splints the chest on that side and reduces the pleural rubbing that often causes discomfort. Fever is usually controlled by administration of antipyretic drugs as prescribed, and temperature is monitored regularly to detect a rise that might trigger a febrile seizure.

Vital signs and breath sounds are monitored to assess the progress of the disease and to detect early signs of complications. Children with ineffectual cough or those who have difficulty handling secretions require suctioning to maintain a patent airway. A simple bulb syringe is usually sufficient for infants, but mechanical suction should be readily available if needed. Older children can usually handle secretions without assistance. Postural drainage and chest physiotherapy are generally prescribed every 4 hours or more often, depending on the child's condition.

The hospitalized child is apprehensive, and treatments and tests are frightening and stress producing. Reducing anxiety and apprehension is essential. When the child is relaxed, respiratory efforts are lessened. Encouraging the presence of the caregiver provides the child with a customary source of comfort and support and often eases respiratory efforts in the child. The family needs support and reassurance. The child's dry, hacking cough can be tiring for the parents and often disturbs their sleep. Parents are kept informed of the child's progress and taught appropriate home care, such as use of a nasal aspirator and administration of antibiotics.

OTHER INFECTIONS OF THE RESPIRATORY TRACT

Pertussis (Whooping Cough)

Pertussis (whooping cough) is an acute respiratory infection caused by *Bordetella pertussis* that occurs chiefly in children younger than 4 years of age who have not been immunized. It is highly contagious and is particularly threatening in young infants, who have a high morbidity and mortality rate. (See Chapter 36 for immunization.) The incidence is highest in the spring and summer months, and a single attack confers lifetime immunity. Pertussis vaccine is effective, but the immunity diminishes with time after the initial infection or immunization.

Tuberculosis

Tuberculosis (TB) is the second leading cause of death from an infectious disease. Ten to 15 million persons in the United States are infected with TB. Case rates of TB for all ages are higher in urban, low-income areas and nonwhite racial and ethnic groups. In recent years, foreign-born children have accounted for more than one third of newly diagnosed cases of TB in children 14 years of age or younger in the United States (American Academy of Pediatrics, Committee on Infectious Diseases, 2003).

TB is caused by the *Mycobacterium tuberculosis* organism. Children are susceptible to both the human *(M. tuberculosis)* and the bovine *(Mycobacterium bovis)* organisms. Human disease caused by *M. bovis* occurs in children who ingest unpasteurized milk or milk products. Although the causative agent for TB is the tubercle bacillus, other factors influence the degree to which the organism produces an altered state in the host. These factors include heredity (resistance to the infection may be genetically transmitted), gender (higher in adolescent girls), age (lower resistance in infants, higher incidence during adolescence), stress (emotional or physical), nutritional state, and intercurrent infection (especially human immunodeficiency virus [HIV], measles, and pertussis). Children with HIV infection have an increased incidence of TB disease, and all children with TB should be tested for HIV.

The source of TB infection in children is usually an infected member of the household or a frequent visitor to the home such as a baby-sitter or domestic worker. The lung is the usual portal of entry for the organism. In the lungs a proliferation of epithelial cells surrounds and encapsulates the multiplying bacilli in an attempt to wall it off, thus forming the typical tubercle. Extension of the primary lesion at the original site causes progressive tissue destruction as it spreads within the lung, discharges material from foci to other areas of the lungs (e.g., bronchi, pleura), or produces pneumonia. Erosion of blood vessels by the primary lesion can cause widespread dissemination of the tubercle bacillus to near and distant sites *(miliary tuberculosis)*. Areas that are frequently affected include the lymph nodes, meninges, and bone.

Diagnostic Evaluation

Diagnosis is based on information derived from physical examination, history, tuberculin skin testing, radiographic examinations, and cultures of the organism. The clinical manifestations of the disease are extremely variable (Box 46-10).

The *tuberculin skin test* (TST) is the most important indicator of whether a child has been infected with the tubercle bacillus. The standard dose of purified protein derivative (PPD) is 5 tuberculin units, which is administered using a 27-gauge needle and a 1.0 ml syringe intradermally into the volar aspect of the forearm. Creation of a visible wheal is crucial to accurate testing. Recommendations for TST of children are listed in Box 46-11. Routine testing of children with no risk factors residing in communities with a low prevalence of TB is not indicated (American Academy of Pediatrics, Committee on Infectious Diseases, 2003).

A *positive reaction* indicates that the individual has been infected and has developed sensitivity to the tubercle bacillus. It does not, however, confirm the presence of active disease. After individuals react positively, they will always react positively. A previously negative reaction that becomes positive indicates that the person has been infected since the last test. Guidelines for interpreting the tuberculin skin test are listed in Box 46-12. Prompt radiographic evaluation of all children with a positive TST reaction is recommended.

NURSE ALERT The American Academy of Pediatrics, Committee on Infectious Diseases (2003), recommends that administration of the TST and interpretation of the results be performed and read by trained health care professionals. ■

The term *latent tuberculosis infection* (LTBI) is used to indicate infection in a person who has a positive TST, no physi-

BOX 46-10

Clinical Manifestations of Tuberculosis

May be asymptomatic or produce a broad range of symptoms:
- Fever
- Malaise
- Anorexia
- Weight loss
- Cough may or may not be present (progresses slowly over weeks to months)
- Aching pain and tightness in the chest
- Hemoptysis (rare)

With progression:
- Respiratory rate increases
- Poor expansion of lung on the affected side
- Diminished breath sounds and crackles
- Dullness on percussion
- Fever persists
- Generalized symptoms are manifested
- Pallor, anemia, weakness, and weight loss

BOX 46-11

Tuberculin Skin Test (TST) Recommendations for Infants, Children, and Adolescents*

Children for Whom Immediate TST Is Indicated

Contacts of persons with confirmed or suspected contagious tuberculosis (contact investigation).

Children with radiographic or clinical findings suggesting tuberculosis disease.

Children immigrating from endemic countries (e.g., Asia, Middle East, Africa, Latin America).

Children with travel histories to endemic countries or significant contact with indigenous persons from such countries.

Children Who Should Have Annual TST†

Children infected with human immunodeficiency virus (HIV).

Incarcerated adolescents.

Children Who Some Experts Recommend Should Be Tested Every 2 to 3 Years†

Children with ongoing exposure to the following people: HIV-infected people, homeless people, residents of nursing homes, institutionalized adolescents or adults, users of illicit drugs, incarcerated adolescents or adults and migrant farm workers; foster children with exposure to adults in the preceding high risk groups are included.

Children Who Some Experts Recommend Should Be Considered for TST at 4 to 6 and 11 to 16 Years

Children whose parents immigrated (with unknown TST status) from regions of the world with high prevalence of tuberculosis; continued potential exposure by travel to the endemic areas or household contact with persons from the endemic areas (with unknown TST status) should be an indication for repeat TST.

Children at Increased Risk for Progression of Infection to Disease

Children with other medical risk factors, including diabetes mellitus, chronic renal failure, malnutrition, and congenital or acquired immunodeficiencies deserve special consideration. Without recent exposure, these people are not at increased risk of acquiring tuberculosis infection. Underlying immune deficiencies associated with these conditions theoretically would enhance the possibility for progression to severe disease. Initial histories of potential exposure to tuberculosis should be included for all of these patients. If these histories or local epidemiologic factors suggest a possibility of exposure, immediate and periodic TST should be considered. An initial TST should be performed before initiation of immunosuppressive therapy, including prolonged steroid administration, for any child with an underlying condition that necessitates immunosuppressive therapy.

From American Academy of Pediatrics, Report of the Committee on Infectious Diseases: *2003 red book: report of the Committee on Infectious Diseases*, ed 26, Elk Grove Village, IL, 2003, The Academy.

*Bacille Calmette-Guérin (BCG) immunization is not a contraindication to tuberculin skin testing.

†Initial tuberculin skin testing is done at the time of diagnosis or circumstance, beginning at 3 months of age.

cal findings of disease, and normal chest radiograph findings. The term *tuberculosis disease* is used when a child has clinical symptoms or radiographic manifestations caused by the *M. tuberculosis* organism. A diagnosis of LTBI or TB disease in a child is a sentinel event usually representing recent transmission of the *M. tuberculosis* organism.

BOX 46-12

Definition of Positive TST Results in Infants, Children, and Adolescents*

Induration ≥5 mm

Children in close contact with known or suspected contagious cases of tuberculosis disease

Children suspected to have tuberculosis disease:
- Findings on chest x-ray film consistent with active or previously active tuberculosis
- Clinical evidence of tuberculosis disease†

Children receiving immunosuppressive therapy‡ or immunosuppressive conditions, including HIV infection

Induration ≥10 mm

Children at increased risk of disseminated disease:
- Those younger than 4 years of age
- Those with other medical risk conditions, including Hodgkin disease, lymphoma, diabetes mellitus, chronic renal failure, or malnutrition

Children with increased exposure to tuberculosis disease:
- Those born, or whose parents were born, in high-prevalence regions of the world
- Those frequently exposed to adults who are HIV infected, homeless, users of illicit drugs, residents of nursing homes, incarcerated or institutionalized, or migrant farm workers
- Those who travel to high-prevalence regions of the world

Induration ≥15 mm

Children 4 years of age or older without any risk factors

From American Academy of Pediatrics, Committee on Infectious Diseases: 2003 *red book: report of the Committee on Infectious Diseases*, ed 26, Elk Grove Village, IL, 2003, The Academy.

*These definitions apply regardless of previous Bacille Calmette-Guérin (BCG) immunization; erythema at TST site does not indicate a positive test result. TSTs should be read at 48 to 72 hours after placement.

†Evidence by physical examination or laboratory assessment that would include tuberculosis in the working differential diagnosis (e.g., meningitis).

‡Including immunosuppressive doses of corticosteroids.

Therapeutic Management

Medical management of TB disease in children consists of adequate nutrition, chemotherapy, general supportive measures, prevention of unnecessary exposure to other infections that further compromise the body's defenses, prevention of reinfection, and sometimes surgical procedures.

Recommended drug therapy for treating TB disease includes combinations of isoniazid (INH), rifampin, and pyrazinamide (PZA). The American Academy of Pediatrics, Committee on Infectious Diseases (2003), recommends a 6-month regimen consisting of INH, rifampin, and PZA given daily for the first 2 months, followed by INH and rifampin given two to three times a week by direct observation of therapy (DOT) for the remaining 4 months. DOT decreases the rates of relapse, treatment failures, and drug resistance, and is recommended for treatment of children and adolescents with TB in the United States.

NURSE ALERT *Direct observation of therapy* means that a health care worker or other responsible, mutually agreed-on individual is present when medications are administered to the patient. ■

When drug resistance is suspected, either ethambutol or an aminoglycoside is added to the therapeutic regimen until drug susceptibility results are available. Optimal therapy for tuberculosis in children with HIV infection has not been established, and consultation with a specialist is advised for HIV-infected children. Therapy should always include at least three drugs initially and be continued for at least 9 months. INH, rifampin, and PZA usually with ethambutol or an aminoglycoside should be given for at least the first 2 months. The three-drug regimen can be used after drug-resistant disease is excluded.

Preventive therapy is intended to keep latent infection from progressing and to prevent initial infection in persons in high risk situations. INH given daily for 9 months is recommended for latent TB infection in children (American Academy of Pediatrics, Committee on Infectious Diseases, 2003).

Surgical procedures may be required to remove the source of infection in tissues that are inaccessible to chemotherapy or that are destroyed by the disease. Orthopedic procedures may be performed for correction of bone deformities, and bronchoscopy may done for removal of a tuberculous granulomatous polyp.

Prognosis

Most children recover from primary TB infection and are often unaware of its presence. However, very young children have a higher incidence of disseminated disease. Tuberculosis is a serious disease during the first 2 years of life, during adolescence, and in children who are HIV-positive. Except in cases of tuberculous meningitis, death seldom occurs in treated children. Antibiotic therapy has decreased the death rate and the hematogenous spread from primary lesions.

Prevention

The only definite means to prevent TB is to avoid contact with the tubercle bacillus. Maintaining an optimum state of health with adequate nutrition and avoiding fatigue and debilitating infections promote natural resistance but do not prevent infection. Pasteurization and routine testing of milk and elimination of diseased cattle have reduced the incidence of bovine TB.

Bacille Calmette-Guérin (BCG) vaccine is a live virus vaccine prepared from attenuated strains of bovine bacilli. In the United States, BCG vaccine is not routinely given and should be considered only in limited circumstances such as unavoidable risk of exposure to *M. tuberculosis* and failure or unfeasibility of other methods of control of TB.

Nursing Care Management

Children with TB receive their nursing care in ambulatory settings, outpatient departments, schools, and public health settings. Most children are not contagious and require only Standard Precautions. Children with no cough and negative sputum smears can be hospitalized on an open ward. However, airborne precautions and a negative-pressure room are required for children who are contagious and hospitalized with TB disease. Infection control for hospital personnel in contagious cases should include the use of a personally fitted air-purifying respirator for all patient contacts.

Children with TB can attend school or day care facilities if they are receiving chemotherapy. They can return to regular activities as soon as effective therapy has been instituted, adherence to therapy has been documented, and clinical symptoms have diminished. Children receiving chemotherapy for TB can receive measles and other age-appropriate live virus vaccines unless they are receiving high-dose corticosteroids, are severely ill, or have specific contraindications to immunization (American Academy of Pediatrics, Committee on Infectious Diseases, 2003). Children with TB should also receive optimal nutrition and adequate rest.

Nurses assume several important roles in management of this disease, including assisting with radiographic examinations, performing skin tests, and obtaining specimens for laboratory examination. Skin tests must be performed correctly and the reaction determined in 48 to 72 hours. Sputum specimens are difficult or impossible to obtain from infants or young children, because they swallow mucus coughed from the lower respiratory tract. The best method for obtaining material for smears or culture is by *gastric washing* (i.e., aspiration of lavaged contents from the fasting stomach). The procedure is carried out and the specimen obtained early in the morning before the customary breakfast time.

Because the success of therapy depends on compliance with the drug regimen, parents are instructed about the importance of and rationale for DOT. Case finding in the community and follow-up of known contacts—individuals from whom the affected child may have acquired the disease and persons who may have been exposed to the child with the disease—are essential control measures.

PULMONARY DYSFUNCTION CAUSED BY NONINFECTIOUS IRRITANTS

Foreign Body Aspiration

Small children characteristically explore matter with their mouths and are prone to aspirate a foreign body (FB). FB aspiration can occur at any age but is most common in children 1 to 3 years of age. Severity is determined by the location, type of object aspirated, and extent of obstruction. For example, dry vegetable matter, such as a seed, nut, or piece of carrot or popcorn, that does not dissolve and that may swell when wet creates a particularly difficult problem. The high fat content of potato chips and peanuts may cause the added risk of lipoid pneumonia. "Fun foods" are the worst offenders in terms of potential for aspiration. Offending foods in the order of frequency of aspiration are hot dog, round candy, peanut or other nut, grape, cookie or biscuit, other meat, carrot, apple, and peanut butter.

A sharp or irritating object produces irritation and edema. A round, pliable object that does not break apart is more likely to occlude an airway than objects with different shapes. Latex balloons (uninflated, inflated, or in broken pieces) are especially hazardous, and a small piece of the pliable, impermeable latex can totally occlude the airway. A small object may cause little damage or pathologic changes, but objects of sufficient size to obstruct a passage can produce various changes, including atelectasis, emphysema, inflammation, and abscess.

Diagnostic Evaluation

The diagnosis of FB aspiration is suspected on the basis of the history and physical signs. Initially, an FB in the air passages produces choking, gagging, wheezing, or coughing.

Laryngotracheal obstruction most commonly causes dyspnea, cough, stridor, and hoarseness because of decreased air entry. Cyanosis may occur if the obstruction becomes worse. Bronchial obstruction usually produces cough (frequently paroxysmal), wheezing, asymmetric breath sounds, decreased airway entry, and dyspnea. When an object is lodged in the larynx, the child is unable to speak or breathe. If the obstruction progresses, the child's face may become livid, and if the obstruction is total, the child can become unconscious and die of asphyxiation. If obstruction is partial, hours, days, or even weeks may pass without symptoms after the initial period. Secondary symptoms are related to the anatomic area in which the object is lodged and are usually caused by a persistent respiratory infection distal to the obstruction. FB should also be suspected in the presence of acute or chronic pulmonary lesions. Often, by the time secondary symptoms appear, the parents have forgotten the initial episode of coughing and gagging.

Radiographic examination reveals opaque FBs but is of limited use in localizing vegetable matter. Bronchoscopy is required for definitive diagnosis of objects in the larynx and trachea. Fluoroscopic examination is valuable in detecting and localizing FBs in the bronchi.

Therapeutic Management

FB aspiration may result in life-threatening airway obstruction, especially in infants (because of the small diameter of their airways). Current recommendations for the emergency treatment of the choking child include the use of abdominal thrusts for children older than 1 year of age and back blows and chest thrusts for children younger than 1 year of age (see Airway Obstruction, p. 1470).

An FB is rarely coughed up spontaneously. Most frequently, it must be removed instrumentally by endoscopy. This procedure should be carried out as quickly as possible, because the progressive local inflammatory process triggered by the foreign material hampers removal. A chemical pneumonia soon develops, and vegetable matter begins to macerate within a few days, causing it to be even more difficult to remove. After removal of the FB, the child is placed in a high-humidity atmosphere and any secondary infection is treated with appropriate antibiotics.

Nursing Care Management

A major role of nurses caring for a child who has aspirated an FB is to recognize the signs of FB aspiration and implement immediate measures to relieve the obstruction.

All persons working with children must be prepared to deal effectively with aspiration of an FB. Choking on food or other material should not be fatal. Back blows and the Heimlich maneuver are simple procedures that can be used by both health professionals and laypersons to save lives. It is the obligation of nurses to learn these techniques and to teach them to parents and other groups (see Fig. 46-9). To aid a child who is choking, nurses must recognize the signs of distress. Not every child who gags or coughs while eating is truly choking.

NURSE ALERT The child in distress (1) *cannot speak,* (2) *becomes cyanotic,* and (3) *collapses.* These three signs indicate that the child is truly choking and requires immediate action. The child can die within 4 minutes. Follow-up care after the FB is removed includes chest physiotherapy as indicated, monitoring for respiratory distress, and education of the parents. ■

Prevention

Small children should not be allowed access to small objects that they might place in their mouth. Rubber balloons are high risk items for children; Mylar balloons are the only safe variety for children. Aluminum tabs from soft drink cans, adhesive bandages, and plastic tabs from protective coverings on containers and price tags on clothing can all become FBs. Peanut butter, a staple in the diet of children, should never be given to a child unless it is spread thinly on bread or a cracker. A spoonful of peanut butter can obstruct the airway and stick to mucous membranes, becoming difficult or impossible for the child to dislodge.

Nurses are in a position to teach prevention in a variety of settings. They can educate parents about the hazards of FB aspiration in relation to the developmental level of their children and encourage them to teach their children safety. Parents should be cautioned about behaviors that their children might imitate (e.g., holding foreign objects, such as pins, nails, and toothpicks, in their lips or mouth). Prevention based on the child's age is discussed in Chapters 36 and 38.

Aspiration Pneumonia

Aspiration pneumonia occurs when food, secretions, inert materials, volatile compounds, or liquids enter the lung and cause inflammation and a chemical pneumonitis. Aspiration of fluid or foods is a particular hazard in the child who has difficulty with swallowing or is unable to swallow because of paralysis, weakness, debility, congenital anomalies, or absent cough reflex or the child who is force-fed, especially while crying or breathing rapidly.

Nursing Care Management

Care of the child with aspiration pneumonia is the same as that described for the child with pneumonia from other causes. However, the major thrust of nursing care is aimed at prevention of aspiration. Proper feeding techniques should be carried out for weak, debilitated, and uncooperative children, and preventive measures should be used to prevent aspiration of any material that might enter the nasopharynx.

Oily nose drops and oil-based vitamin preparations are not appropriate for infants and small children. Solvents, lighter fluid, and other hydrocarbon substances should be kept away from older infants and small children, who are apt to put anything in their mouths and who may be attracted by the slightly sweet smell. Use of talcum powder should be avoided. If used, careful application (placing it on the caregiver's hand and then the child's skin) and proper storage are essential.

Infants and debilitated children should be positioned on the right side after feedings to minimize the possibility of aspirating vomitus or regurgitated feeding.

Acute (Adult) Respiratory Distress Syndrome

Acute (adult) respiratory distress syndrome (ARDS) is recognized in children, as well as adults, and has been associated with clinical conditions and injuries such as sepsis, viral pneumonia, smoke inhalation, and near-drowning. It is a syndrome characterized by respiratory distress and hypoxemia that occur within 72 hours of a serious injury or surgery in a person with previously normal lungs.

The hallmark of ARDS is increased permeability of the alveolar-capillary membrane that results in pulmonary edema. The lungs become stiff, gas diffusion is impaired, and eventually there is bronchiolar mucosal swelling and congestive atelectasis. Surfactant secretion is reduced, and the atelectasis and fluid-filled alveoli provide an excellent medium for bacterial growth. The criteria for diagnosis of ARDS in children are an acute antecedent illness or injury, acute respiratory distress or failure, no evidence of prior cardiopulmonary disease, and diffuse bilateral infiltrates evidenced on chest radiography.

Treatment involves supportive measures, such as prevention of infection; maintenance of vascular volume, hydration, and cardiac output; adequate nutrition; comfort measures; and psychologic support. Definitive therapy is directed toward improvement of oxygenation. The use of endotracheal intubation and positive end-expiratory pressure (PEEP) may be required to ensure maximum oxygen delivery. Recent advances in the treatment of ARDS include the use of lung-protective ventilator strategies, permissive hypercapnia, inhaled nitric oxide, high-frequency ventilation, and extracorporeal life support (Redding, 2001).

Prognosis

In spite of advances in treating ARDS, mortality rates in children vary greatly. The precipitating disorder influences the outcome; the worst prognosis is associated with uncontrolled sepsis, bone marrow transplantation, cancer, and multisystem involvement with hepatic failure.

Nursing care involves careful monitoring of cardiac output, heart rate, perfusion, capillary filling, and urine output, as well as assessment of respiratory status. Blood gas analysis and pulse oximetry are important evaluation tools. Respiratory distress is a frightening situation for both the child and the parents, and attention to their psychologic needs is a major element in the care of these children.

Smoke Inhalation Injury

A number of noxious substances that may be inhaled are toxic to humans. They are primarily products of incomplete combustion and cause more deaths from fires than flame injuries. The severity of the injury depends on the nature of the substances generated by the material burned, whether the victim is confined in a closed space, and the duration of contact with the smoke. Smoke inhalation results in three types of injury: heat, chemical, and systemic.

Heat injury involves thermal injury to the upper airway. Air has low specific heat; therefore the injury goes no further than the upper airway. Reflex closure of the glottis prevents injury to the lower airway.

Chemical injury involves gases that may be generated during the combustion of materials such as clothing, furniture, and floor coverings. These synthetic materials are especially toxic. Irritant gases such as nitrous oxide or carbon dioxide combine with water in the lungs to form corrosive acids; aldehydes cause denaturation of proteins, cellular damage, and edema of pulmonary tissues.

Possible inhalation injury is suspected when there is a history of flames in a closed space whether burns are present or not. Sooty material around the nose or in the sputum; singed nasal hairs; and mucosal burns of the nose, lips, mouth, or throat are all signs that the affected person requires observation for possible pulmonary injury from inhalants. A hoarse voice and cough, inspiratory and expiratory stridor, and signs of respiratory distress are further evidence of airway involvement.

Systemic injury occurs from gases that are nontoxic to the airways (e.g., carbon monoxide [CO], hydrogen cyanide). However, these gases cause injury and death by interfering with or inhibiting cellular respiration. CO is responsible for more than half of all fatal inhalation poisonings in the United States. CO is a colorless, odorless gas with an affinity for hemoglobin 230 times greater than that of oxygen. When it enters the bloodstream, CO combines readily with hemoglobin to form carboxyhemoglobin (COHb). Because it is released less readily, tissue hypoxia reaches dangerous levels before oxygen is available to meet tissue needs.

NURSE ALERT The oxygen saturation (Sa_{O_2}) obtained by pulse oximetry will be normal because the device measures only oxygenated and deoxygenated hemoglobin; it does not measure dysfunctional hemoglobin, such as COHb. ■

Accidental CO poisoning is most often a result of exposure to fumes of heaters or smoke from structural fires. Poorly ventilated recreational vehicles with improperly operated or maintained gas lamps or stoves and cooking in underventilated areas with charcoal grills or hibachis are also frequent causes. CO is produced by incomplete combustion of carbon or carbonaceous material such as wood or charcoal.

The signs and symptoms of CO poisoning are secondary to tissue hypoxia and vary with the level of COHb. Mild manifestations include headache, visual disturbances, irritability, and nausea; more severe intoxication causes confusion, hallucinations, ataxia, and coma. The bright, cherry-red lips and skin often described are less often observed; pallor and cyanosis are seen more frequently.

Therapeutic Management

Treatment of children with smoke inhalation injury is largely symptomatic. The most widely accepted treatment is placing the child on humidified 100% oxygen as quickly as possible and monitoring for signs of respiratory distress and impending failure. Baseline arterial blood gases and COHb levels are obtained. Surprisingly, arterial oxygen partial pressure (Pa_{O_2}) may be within normal limits unless there is marked respiratory depression. If CO poisoning is confirmed, 100% oxygen is continued until COHb levels fall to the nontoxic range of about 10%. The role of hyperbaric oxygen remains controversial.

Respiratory distress may occur early in the course of smoke inhalation as a result of hypoxia, or patients who are breathing well on admission may suddenly develop respiratory distress. Intubation or tracheostomy equipment should be available at the bedside. Transient edema of the airways can occur at any level in the tracheobronchial tree. Assessment and localization of the obstruction should be accomplished before severe swelling of the head, neck, or oropharynx occurs. Intubation is often necessary when (1) severe burns in the area of the nose, mouth, and face increase the likelihood of developing oropharyngeal edema and obstruction; (2) vocal cord edema causes obstruction; (3) the patient has difficulty handling secretions; and (4) progressive respiratory distress requires artificial ventilation. Controversy surrounds tracheostomy, but many prefer this procedure when the obstruction is proximal to the larynx and reserve nasotracheal intubation for lower tract involvement.

Corticosteroids have no established benefit and may increase the risk of infection. Prophylactic antibiotics offer no benefit and may lead to the development of resistant organisms (Sockrider, 1999).

Nursing Care Management

Nursing care of the child with inhalation injury is the same as that for any child with respiratory distress. Vital signs and other respiratory assessments are performed frequently, and the pulmonary status is carefully observed and maintained. Pulmonary physiotherapy is often part of the therapy, as well as mechanical ventilation if needed.

In addition to observation and management of the physical aspects of inhalation injury, the nurse also deals with the psychologic needs of a frightened child and distraught parents. As with any accidental injury, the parents feel overwhelming guilt, even when the injury occurred through no fault of their own. Parents need support, reassurance, and information regarding the child's condition, treatment, and progress.

Passive Smoking

Numerous investigations indicate that parental smoking is an important cause of morbidity in children. Children exposed to passive or environmental tobacco smoke have an increased number of respiratory illnesses, increased respiratory symptoms (i.e., cough, phlegm, and wheeze), and reduced performance on pulmonary function tests. Indoor exposure to environmental tobacco smoke has been linked to asthma in children (Morkjaroenpong et al, 2002). Among children with asthma, there is an association between parental cigarette smoking and asthma exacerbations, trips to the emergency department, medication use, and impaired recovery after hospitalization for acute asthma (Abulhosm et al, 1997). Maternal cigarette smoking is associated with increased respiratory symptoms and illnesses in children; decreased fetal growth; increased deliveries of low-birth-weight, preterm, and stillborn infants; and a greater incidence of sudden infant death syndrome (SIDS). Exposure to passive smoking during childhood may also contribute to the development of chronic lung disease in the adult.

Nursing Care Management

Nurses must provide information about the hazards of environmental smoke exposure in all their interactions with children and their family members. This information is especially important for children with respiratory and allergic illnesses.* In families where smokers refuse to quit, house rules should be established for reducing smoke in the child's environment (Home Care box). Nurses should set an example for children and families and become advocates for "no smoking" ordinances in public places and prohibition of advertising tobacco products in the media.

> **Home Care**
>
> **HOUSE RULES FOR SMOKING HOUSEHOLDS**
>
> Maintain a smoke-free home.
> Do not smoke around children.
> Restrict smoking to an isolated, outdoor area.
> Do not smoke in motor vehicles with children.
> Do not smoke in rooms children use.
> Do not allow visitors to smoke in the home.

LONG-TERM RESPIRATORY DYSFUNCTION

Asthma

Asthma is a chronic inflammatory disorder of the airways in which many cells (mast cells, eosinophils, and T lymphocytes) play a role. In susceptible children, inflammation causes recurrent episodes of wheezing, breathlessness, chest tightness, and cough, especially at night or in the early morning. These asthma episodes are associated with airflow limitation or obstruction that is reversible either spontaneously or with treatment. The inflammation also causes an increase in bronchial hyperresponsiveness to a variety of stimuli (National Asthma Education and Prevention Program, 1997).

Asthma is classified into four categories based on the symptom indicators of disease severity: mild intermittent, mild persistent, moderate persistent, and severe persistent. The mild intermittent category has the least number of symptoms; symptoms increase in frequency or intensity until the last category of severe persistent asthma (Box 46-13). These categories provide a stepwise approach to the pharmacologic management, environmental control, and educational interventions needed for each category (National Asthma Education and Prevention Program, 1997).

Asthma prevalence, morbidity, and mortality rates are increasing in the United States and other nations. These increases may result from increasing air pollution, poor access to medical care, or underdiagnosis and undertreatment. Asthma is the most common chronic disease of childhood; it is the primary cause of school absences and is responsible for a major proportion of pediatric admissions to emergency departments and hospitals.

*For a copy of the Environmental Protection Agency (EPA) report *Respiratory Health Effects of Passive Smoking,* contact CERI, U.S. EPA, 26 W. Martin Luther King Dr., Cincinnati, OH 45268; phone: 513-569-7562.

BOX 46-13

Asthma Severity Classification in Children 5 Years of Age and Older: Clinical Features before Treatment or Adequate Control*

Step 4: Severe Persistent Asthma
Continual symptoms
Frequent nighttime symptoms
Peak expiratory flow (PEF) or forced expiratory volume in 1 second (FEV_1) is ≤60% of predicted value
PEF variability >30%

Step 3: Moderate Persistent Asthma
Daily symptoms
Nighttime symptoms >1 night per week
PEF or FEV_1 is >60% to <80% of predicted value
PEF variability >30%

Step 2: Mild Persistent Asthma
Symptoms >2 times a week, but <1 time per day
Nighttime symptoms >2 times per month
PEF or FEV_1 is ≥80% of predicted value
PEF variability 20% to 30%

Step 1: Mild Intermittent Asthma
Symptoms <2 times per week
Nighttime symptoms <2 times per month
PEF or FEV_1 is ≥80% of predicted value
PEF variability <20%

From National Asthma Education and Prevention Program: Quick reference NAEPP Expert Panel report, guidelines for the diagnosis and management of asthma. Update on selected topics 2002, NIH pub no 02-5075, Bethesda, MD, 2003, National Heart, Lung, and Blood Institute.
*The presence of one clinical feature of severity is sufficient to place a patient in that category. An individual should be assigned to the most severe grade in which any feature occurs. The characteristics in this table are general and may overlap because asthma is highly variable. An individual's classification may change over time.

BOX 46-14

Triggers Tending to Precipitate or Aggravate Asthmatic Exacerbations

Allergens
Outdoor: trees, shrubs, weeds, grasses, molds, pollens, air pollution, spores
Indoor: dust or dust mites, mold, cockroach antigen
Irritants: tobacco smoke, wood smoke, odors, sprays
Exposure to occupational chemicals
Exercise
Cold air
Changes in weather or temperature
Environmental change: moving to new home, starting new school, etc.
Colds and infections
Animals: cats, dogs, rodents, horses
Medications: aspirin, nonsteroidal antiinflammatory drugs (NSAIDs), antibiotics, β-blockers
Strong emotions: fear, anger, laughing, crying
Conditions: gastroesophageal reflux, tracheoesophageal fistula
Food additives: sulfite preservatives
Foods: nuts, milk/dairy products
Endocrine factors: menses, pregnancy, thyroid disease

Etiology

Studies of children with asthma indicate that allergy influences both the persistence and severity of the disease. *Atopy,* the genetic predisposition for the development of an IgE-mediated response to common aeroallergens, is the strongest predictor for developing asthma. Although allergens play an important role in asthma, 20% to 40% of children with asthma have no evidence of allergic disease (Eggleston, 1999). In addition to allergens, other substances and conditions can serve as triggers for asthma episodes (Box 46-14). Asthma is a complex disorder involving biochemical, immunologic, infectious, endocrine, and psychologic factors.

Pathophysiology

There is general agreement that inflammation contributes to increased airway reactivity in asthma. The mechanisms contributing to airway inflammation are multiple and involve a number of different pathways. However, recognition of the importance of inflammation has made the use of antiinflammatory agents a key component of asthma therapy.

Another important component of asthma is bronchospasm and obstruction. The mechanisms responsible for the obstructive symptoms in asthma include the following (Fig. 46-3): (1) inflammation and edema of the mucous membranes; (2) accumulation of tenacious secretions from mucous glands; and (3) spasm of the smooth muscle of the bronchi and bronchioles, which decreases the caliber of the bronchioles.

NURSE ALERT Airflow is determined by the size of the airway lumen, degree of bronchial wall edema, mucous production, smooth muscle contraction, and muscle hypertrophy. ■

Bronchial constriction is a normal reaction to foreign stimuli, but in the child with asthma it is abnormally severe, producing impaired respiratory function. The smooth muscle arranged in spiral bundles around the airway causes narrowing and shortening of the airway, which significantly increases airway resistance to airflow. Because the bronchi normally dilate and elongate during inspiration and contract and shorten on expiration, the respiratory difficulty is more pronounced during the expiratory phase of respiration.

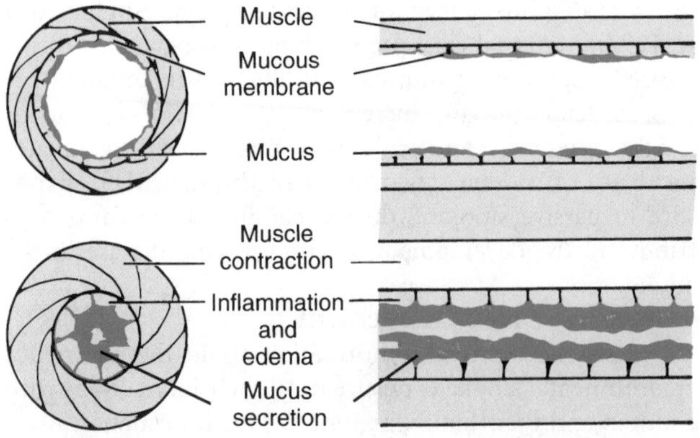

Fig. 46-3 Mechanisms of obstruction in asthma.

Increased resistance in the airway causes forced expiration through the narrowed lumen. The volume of air trapped in the lungs increases as airways are functionally closed at a point between the alveoli and the lobar bronchi. This trapping of gas forces the individual to breathe at higher and higher lung volumes. Consequently, the person with asthma fights to inspire sufficient air. This expenditure of effort for breathing causes fatigue, decreased respiratory effectiveness, and increased oxygen consumption. The inspiration occurring at higher lung volumes hyperinflates the alveoli and reduces the effectiveness of the cough. As the severity of obstruction increases, there is a reduced alveolar ventilation with carbon dioxide retention, hypoxemia, respiratory acidosis, and, eventually, respiratory failure.

Diagnostic Evaluation

The classic manifestations of asthma are dyspnea, wheezing, and coughing. However, children may experience symptoms that range from acute episodes of shortness of breath, wheezing, and cough followed by a quiet period to a relatively continuous pattern of chronic symptoms that fluctuate in severity (Box 46-15). An attack may develop gradually or appear abruptly and may be preceded by a URI. The age of the child is often a significant factor, because the first attack frequently occurs between ages 3 and 8 years. In infancy an attack usually follows a respiratory infection. Some children may experience a prodromal itching at the front of the neck or over the upper part of the back just before an attack.

NURSE ALERT Shortness of breath with air movement in the chest restricted to the point of absent breath sounds, accompanied by a sudden rise in respiratory rate, is an ominous sign indicating ventilatory failure and imminent asphyxia. ■

The diagnosis is determined primarily on the basis of clinical manifestations, history, physical examination, and, to a lesser extent, laboratory tests. Radiographic examinations are used primarily to rule out other diseases and to evaluate coexisting disease. Generally, chronic cough in the absence of infection or diffuse wheezing during the expiratory phase of respiration is sufficient to establish a diagnosis.

Pulmonary function tests (PFTs) provide an objective method of evaluating the presence and degree of lung disease, as well as the response to therapy. Spirometry can generally be performed reliably on children by age 5 or 6 years and includes either the traditional and simple mechanical spirometer often used in clinics, offices, and the home or new computerized versions. Another key measurement is the *peak expiratory flow rate (PEFR)*, which measures the maximum flow of air that can be forcefully exhaled in 1 second. PEFR is measured in liters per minute using a *peak expiratory flow meter (PEFM)*. Three zones of measurement are typically used to interpret PEFR. The zone system is patterned after a traffic light to make the categories easy to understand and remember (Guidelines box). Each child needs to establish his or her *personal best value*. A personal best value should be established during a 2- to 3-week period when the child's asthma is stable. During this period, the child records his or her PEFR at least twice a day. After the personal best value has been established, the child's current PEFR on any occasion can be compared with the personal best value.

Skin testing is useful in identifying specific allergens. Data obtained by the puncture technique correlate better than intracutaneous tests with symptoms and measurements of specific IgE antibody (Atraumatic Care box). *Provocative*

BOX 46-15

Clinical Manifestations of Asthma

Cough
- Hacking, paroxysmal, irritative, and nonproductive
- Becomes rattling and productive of frothy, clear, gelatinous sputum

Respiratory-Related Signs
- Shortness of breath
- Prolonged expiratory phase
- Audible wheeze
- May have a malar flush and red ears
- Lips deep, dark red color
- May progress to cyanosis of nail beds or circumoral cyanosis
- Restlessness
- Apprehension
- Sweating may be prominent as the attack progresses
- Older children may sit upright with shoulders in a hunched-over position, hands on the bed or chair, and arms braced
- May speak in short, panting, broken phrases

Chest
- Hyperresonance on percussion
- Coarse, loud breath sounds
- Wheezes throughout the lung fields
- Prolonged expiration
- Crackles
- Generalized inspiratory and expiratory wheezing; increasingly high pitched

With Repeated Episodes
- Barrel chest
- Elevated shoulders
- Use of accessory muscles of respiration
- Facial appearance: flattened malar bones, circles beneath the eyes, narrow nose, prominent upper teeth

Guidelines

INTERPRETING PEAK EXPIRATORY FLOW RATES*

- *Green (80% to 100% of personal best)* signals all clear. Asthma is under reasonably good control. No symptoms are present, and the routine treatment plan for maintaining control can be followed.
- *Yellow (50% to 79% of personal best)* signals caution. Asthma is not well controlled. An acute exacerbation may be present. Maintenance therapy may need to be increased. Call the practitioner if the child stays in this zone.
- *Red (below 50% of personal best)* signals a medical alert. Severe airway narrowing may be occurring. A short-acting bronchodilator should be administered. Notify the practitioner if the peak expiratory flow rate does not return immediately and stay in yellow or green zones.

*These zones are guidelines only. Specific zones and management should be individualized for each child.

> **Atraumatic Care**
>
> **SKIN TESTING**
>
> To help allay children's fears of skin tests, give them a careful and thorough explanation of what is to be done and how many "pricks" are involved (usually series of 8 on each site, for a total of 30 tests). Very young, anxious patients may benefit from one prick on the arm to demonstrate how it feels. The skin is pierced with a stylet rather than a regular needle and syringe; then a drop of allergen is placed on the site. Another helpful strategy is to have the child count off the number of pricks with the nurse as a distraction. For intradermal skin injection, EMLA, a topical anesthetic, reduces or eliminates pain without altering test results.

testing, direct exposure of the mucous membranes to a suspected antigen in increasing concentrations, helps identify inhaled allergens. The radioallergosorbent test (RAST) helps identify antigens against various foods and is often useful in determining appropriate therapy.

Therapeutic Management

The overall goals of asthma management are to prevent disability, minimize physical and psychologic morbidity, and assist the child in living as normal and happy a life as possible. This includes facilitating the child's social adjustments in the family, school, and community and normal participation in recreational activities and sports. To accomplish these goals, the child and his or her family need to recognize symptoms, learn how to manage asthma exacerbations, visit a health care provider regularly, implement appropriate therapy, and identify and eliminate environmental irritants and allergens. Adherence to the prescribed regimen is essential to successful management.

Allergen Control

Nonpharmacologic therapy is aimed at the prevention and reduction of exposure to airborne allergens and irritants. *House dust mites* and other components of house dust are one of the most frequent agents identified in children allergic to inhalants. The most important method to eliminate dust mites is to keep the humidity in the house lower than 50%, the level below which dust mites do not survive (Kaliner, Spector, & Wenzel, 1999). The *cockroach,* another common household inhabitant, is an important allergen in many locations. Exterminating live cockroaches, carefully cleaning kitchen floors and cabinets, putting food away after eating, and taking trash out in the evening are essential measures to control cockroaches. The mouse allergen is the most recent allergen to be identified in the homes of inner-city children with asthma. Researchers now recommend aggressive extermination of not only cockroaches, but also mice (Phipatanakul et al, 2000). Other recommendations for controlling allergens are found in the Home Care box.

Skin testing identifies specific allergens, and steps are taken to eliminate or avoid the offending allergens. Often, simply removing the offending environmental allergens or irritants (e.g., removal of a dog or cat from the home of a child sensitive to animal dander) will decrease the frequency of asthma episodes. Dehumidifiers or air conditioners control nonspecific factors that trigger an episode, such as extremes of temperature.

Drug Therapy

Pharmacologic therapy is used to prevent and control asthma symptoms, reduce the frequency and severity of asthma exacerbations, and reverse airflow obstruction. A stepwise approach is recommended based on the severity of the child's asthma. Because inflammation is considered an early and persistent feature of asthma, therapy is directed toward long-term suppression of inflammation.

Asthma medications are categorized into two general classes: *long-term control medications (preventer medicines)* to achieve and maintain control of inflammation and *quick-relief medications (rescue medications)* to treat symptoms and exacerbations (National Asthma Education and Prevention Program, 2002).

Many asthma medications are given by inhalation with a nebulizer or a *metered-dose inhaler (MDI).* The MDI should always be attached to a spacer when an inhaled corticosteroid is administered to prevent yeast infections in the mouth. Spacers are also important for children who have difficulty coordinating or learning proper inhalation technique (Togger & Brenner, 2001). Most pharmaceutical companies are currently striving to produce inhalers that do not contain chlorofluorocarbons (CFCs) as the propellant because CFCs have been linked to damage and depletion of the earth's ozone level. Several currently available CFC-free MDI devices, such as the Diskus inhaler and the Turbuhaler, use dry powder. These devices are breath activated, and the child needs to inhale as quickly and deeply as possible to use them effectively. Infants and very young children who have difficulty using MDIs or other inhalers can receive their asthma medications via a *nebulizer.* When this device is used, the medication is mixed with saline and nebulized with compressed air. Children are instructed to breathe normally with the mouth open to provide a direct route to the trachea.

Corticosteroids are antiinflammatory drugs used to treat reversible airflow obstruction and to control symptoms and reduce bronchial hyperreactivity in chronic asthma. Corticosteroids may be administered parenterally, orally, or by inhalation. Oral medications are metabolized slowly, with an onset of action up to 3 hours after administration and peak effectiveness occurring within 6 to 12 hours. Oral systemic steroids may be given for short periods of time (i.e., 3- or 10-day "bursts") to gain prompt control of inadequately controlled persistent asthma or to manage severe persistent asthma. These drugs should be given in the lowest effective dose. Long-term use poses the risk of adverse effects, such as osteoporosis, hypertension, Cushing syndrome, impaired immune mechanisms, and hypothalamic-pituitary-adrenal suppression (National Asthma Education and Prevention Program, 2002).

Inhaled steroids are used for long-term prevention of symptoms, as well as suppression, control, and reversal of inflammation. These medications have few side effects (cough, dysphonia, and oral thrush). There is strong evidence that these drugs improve the long-term outcomes for children of all ages with mild or moderate persistent asthma (National Asthma Education and Prevention Program, 2002). One study also indicated that regular use of low-dose inhaled corticosteroids is associated with a decreased risk of death from asthma (Suissa et al, 2000). Data from clinical trials

Home Care

"ALLERGY-PROOFING" THE HOME AND COMMUNITY

Keep humidity between 30% and 50%; use dehumidifier or air conditioner if available; keep air conditioners clean and free of mold; do not use vaporizers or humidifiers.
Encase pillows in zippered allergen-impermeable covers or wash pillows in hot water (at least 54.4° C [130° F]) every week.
Encase mattress and box springs in zippered allergen-impermeable cover.
Use foam rubber mattress and pillows or Dacron pillows and synthetic blankets.
Wash bed linens every 7 to 10 days in hot water (at least 54.4° C).
Encase polyester comforters in allergen-impermeable covers or wash in hot water (at least 54.4° C) every week; if possible, do not use comforters and use cotton blankets.
Do not use a canopy above the bed; children should not sleep on the bottom bunk of a bunk bed.
Store nothing under the bed; keep clothing in a closet with the door shut.
Use washable window shades; avoid heavy curtains; if curtains are used, launder them frequently.
Remove all carpeting if possible; if not possible, vacuum carpet once or twice a week while the child wears a mask; have child remain out of the room while vacuuming occurs and for 30 minutes after vacuuming.
If possible, use a central vacuum cleaner with a collecting bag outside of the home or use cleaner filters (e.g., high-efficiency particulate air [HEPA] filters).
Have air and heating ducts cleaned annually; change or clean filters monthly; cover heating vents with filter material (e.g., cheesecloth) to prevent circulation of dust, especially when heat is turned on after summer.
Remove unnecessary furniture, rugs, stuffed or real animals, toys, books, upholstered furniture, plants, aquariums, and wall hangings from child's room.
Use wipeable furniture (wood, plastic, vinyl, or leather) in place of upholstered furniture; avoid rattan or wicker furniture.
Cover walls with washable paint or wallpaper.
Limit child's exposure to animals (rabbits, gerbils, hamsters) at school; teach child to stay away from zoos, petting farms, and neighbor's pets.
Change child's clothes after playing outdoors; wash child's hair nightly if child is outside and pollen count is high.
Keep child indoors while lawn is being mowed, bushes/trees are being trimmed, or pollen count is high.
Keep windows and doors closed during pollen season; use air conditioner if possible or go to places that are air conditioned, such as libraries and shopping malls, when the weather is hot.
Wet-mop bare floors weekly; wet-dust and clean child's room weekly; child should not be present during cleaning activities.
Wash showers and shower curtains with bleach or Lysol at least once a month.
Limit or avoid child's exposure to tobacco and wood smoke; do not allow cigarette smoking in the house or car; select day care centers, play areas, and shopping malls that are smoke free.
Avoid odors or sprays (e.g., perfumes, talcum powder, room deodorizers, chalk dust at school, fresh paint, cleaning solutions).
Avoid cellar (basement) as a play area if it is damp, and use a dehumidifier in damp basement.
Cover all food, including pet food, and put food away in cabinets.
Store garbage in closed containers.
Use pesticide sprays, roach bait traps, and boric acid powder to kill cockroaches; if living in an apartment or adjacent housing, encourage neighbors to work together to get rid of cockroaches and mice.
Repair leaking or dripping faucets; seal cracks and crevices in cabinets and pantry areas.

that followed children for 6 years indicate that the use of inhaled corticosteroids at recommended doses does not have long-term, significant effects on growth, bone mineral density, ocular toxicity, or suppression of adrenal/pituitary axis (National Asthma Education and Prevention Program, 2002). However, primary care providers should monitor the growth of children and adolescents taking corticosteroids frequently (at least every 3 to 6 months) to assess the systemic effects of these drugs and make appropriate reductions in dosages or changes to other types of asthma therapy when necessary (Daley-Yates and Richards, 2004).

Cromolyn sodium is a nonsteroidal antiinflammatory drug (NSAID) used for asthma. It stabilizes mast cell membranes, inhibits activation and release of mediators from eosinophil and epithelial cells, and inhibits the acute airway narrowing after exposure to exercise, cold dry air, and sulfur dioxide. There is no reliable way to predict whether a child will respond to the drug. Cromolyn sodium has minimal side effects (occasional coughing on inhalation of the powder formulation) and may be given via nebulizer or MDI. *Nedocromil sodium* is another drug used for maintenance therapy in asthma. This drug has both antiallergic and antiinflammatory properties and few side effects.

β-Adrenergic agonists (primarily *albuterol*, *metaproterenol*, and *terbutaline*) are used for treatment of acute exacerbations and for the prevention of exercise-induced bronchospasm. They can be given via inhalation or as oral or parenteral preparations. The inhaled drug has a more rapid onset of action than the oral form. Inhalation also reduces troublesome systemic side effects: irritability, tremor, nervousness, and insomnia.

Inhaled β-adrenergic agents should not be taken more than three to four times daily for acute symptoms. *Salmeterol (Serevent)* is a long-acting bronchodilator that is used twice a day. This drug is added to antiinflammatory therapy and used for long-term prevention of symptoms, especially nighttime symptoms, and exercise-induced bronchospasm.

Methylxanthines, principally *theophylline*, have been used for decades to relieve symptoms and prevent asthma attacks. Theophylline, however, is now considered a third-line agent and unnecessary for treating asthma exacerbations. Theophylline may be taken intravenously, intramuscularly, orally, or rectally (seldom used). The drug is also available in sustained-release oral form. In addition to its bronchodilator effect, theophylline is a central respiratory stimulant and increases respiratory muscle contractility.

When theophylline is used, serum concentrations must be monitored. Therapeutic effects are maintained at plasma levels between 5 and 15 mcg/ml. Maximum levels of 15 mcg/ml are recommended for outpatient care (Eggleston, 1999).

NURSE ALERT Theophylline toxicity can occur with serum levels of 20 mcg/ml or greater. Side effects from theophylline include nausea, vomiting, headache, irritability, and insomnia. Early signs of toxicity are nausea, tachycardia, and irritability; seizures and dysrhythmias occur at blood theophylline levels greater than 30 mcg/ml. ■

Leukotriene Modifiers

Leukotrienes are mediators of inflammation that cause increases in airway hyperresponsiveness. Leukotriene modifiers (e.g., zafirlukast, zileuton, and montelukast sodium) block inflammatory and bronchospasm effects. These drugs are not used to treat acute episodes, but are given orally in combination with β-adrenergic agonists and steroids to provide long-term control and prevention of symptoms in mild persistent asthma (Fost & Spahn, 1998).

Recently, the Food and Drug Administration approved the drug omalizumab (Xolair) for treatment of asthma in patients older than 12 years of age. Omalizumab is a monoclonal antibody that blocks the binding of IgE to mast cells. Blocking this interaction eventually inhibits the inflammation that is associated with asthma. Because many patients with asthma are atopic and possess specific IgE antibodies to allergens responsible for airway inflammation, this drug is a promising adjunct to the treatment of asthma. The drug is administered once or twice a month via subcutaneous injection. Clinical trials of the drug indicate that it can be an effective therapy for patients with symptomatic moderate to severe allergic asthma that is poorly controlled with inhaled corticosteroids (Rosenwasser & Nash, 2003).

Exercise

Exercise-induced bronchospasm (EIB) is an acute, reversible, usually self-terminating airway obstruction that develops during or after vigorous activity, peaks 5 to 10 minutes after stopping the activity, and usually stops in another 20 to 30 minutes. Patients with EIB have cough, shortness of breath, chest pain or tightness, wheezing, and endurance problems during exercise, but an exercise challenge test in a laboratory is necessary to make the diagnosis.

The problem is rare in activities that require short bursts of energy (e.g., baseball, sprints, gymnastics, skiing) and more common in those that involve endurance exercise (e.g., soccer, basketball, distance running). Swimming is well tolerated by children with EIB, because they are breathing air fully saturated with moisture and because of the type of breathing required in swimming. Exhaling under water is beneficial because it prolongs expiration and increases the end-expiratory pressure within the respiratory tract (essentially pursed-lip breathing).

Children with asthma are often excluded from exercise by parents, teachers, and practitioners, as well as by the children themselves, because they are reluctant to provoke an attack. However, this practice can seriously hamper peer interaction and physical health. Exercise is advantageous for children with asthma, and most children can participate in activities at school and in sports with minimum difficulty, provided their asthma is under control. Participation should be evaluated on an individual basis. Appropriate prophylactic treatment with β-adrenergic agents or cromolyn sodium before exercise will usually permit full participation in strenuous exertion.

Chest Physiotherapy

Chest physiotherapy (CPT) includes breathing exercises and physical training. These therapies help produce physical and mental relaxation, improve posture, strengthen respiratory musculature, and develop more efficient patterns of breathing. For the motivated child, breathing exercises and controlled breathing are of value in preventing overinflation and improving efficiency of the cough. However, CPT is not recommended during acute, uncomplicated exacerbations of asthma.

Hyposensitization

The role of hyposensitization in childhood asthma has become controversial. In the past, immunotherapy was used for seasonal allergies and when single substances were identified as the offending allergen. It is not recommended for allergens that can be eliminated, such as foods, drugs, and animal dander.

Injection therapy is usually limited to clinically significant allergens. The initial dose of the offending allergen(s), based on the size of the skin reaction, is injected subcutaneously. The amount is increased at weekly intervals until a maximum tolerance is reached, after which a maintenance dose is given at 4-week intervals. This may be extended to 5- or 6-week intervals during the off-season for seasonal allergens. Successful treatment is continued for a minimum of 3 years and then stopped. If no symptoms appear, acquired immunity is assumed; if symptoms recur, treatment is reinstituted.

NURSE ALERT Hyposensitization injections should be administered only with emergency equipment and medications readily available in the event of an anaphylactic reaction. ■

Prognosis

The outlook for children with asthma varies widely. Some children's asthma symptoms may improve at puberty, but up to two thirds of children with asthma continue to have symptoms through puberty and into adulthood. The prognosis for control or disappearance of symptoms varies in children from those who have rare and infrequent attacks to those who are constantly wheezing or are subject to status asthmaticus. In general, when symptoms are severe and numerous, when symptoms have been present for a long time, and when there is a family history of allergy, there is a greater likelihood of a poor prognosis. Many children who outgrow their exacerbations continue to have airway hyperresponsiveness and cough as adults. Furthermore, airway hyperresponsiveness in adults appears to be associated with decreased lung function.

Although death from asthma is rare, the death rate has increased in recent years. The adolescent age group appears to be the most vulnerable, with the greatest increase occurring in ages 10 to 14 years. No reliable data exist to explain this increase. Factors that have been postulated include exposure of atopic persons to more allergens, change in severity of the disease, abuse of drug therapy (toxicity), failure of families and practitioners to recognize the severity of asthma, and psychologic factors such as denial and refusal to accept the disease. Risk factors for asthma deaths include early onset, frequent attacks, difficult-to-manage disease, adolescence, history of respiratory failure, psychologic problems (refusal to take medications), dependency on or misuse of drugs (high use), presence of physical stigmata (barrel chest, intercostal retractions), and abnormal pulmonary function tests (Capen & Sherman, 1998).

Status Asthmaticus

Children who continue to display respiratory distress despite vigorous therapeutic measures, especially use of sympathomimetics, are considered to be in *status asthmaticus*. The condition may develop gradually or rapidly, and often occurs with complicating conditions (e.g., pneumonia) that can influence the duration and treatment of the attack. A child with status asthmaticus is usually seen in the emergency department and frequently admitted to a pediatric intensive care unit for close observation and continuous cardiorespiratory monitoring.

NURSE ALERT Status asthmaticus is a medical emergency that can result in respiratory failure and death if untreated. The child who sweats profusely, remains sitting upright, and refuses to lie down is in severe respiratory distress. Also, the child who suddenly becomes agitated, or the agitated child who suddenly becomes quiet, may be seriously hypoxic and requires immediate intervention. ■

Therapy for status asthmaticus is aimed at improvement of ventilation, correction of dehydration and acidosis, and treatment of any concurrent infection. Bronchospasm is relieved by giving inhaled aerosolized short-acting β_2-adrenergic agonists (either intermittently or continuously), along with corticosteroids (either orally or intravenously). For the child not responding to either of these therapies, subcutaneous epinephrine (1:1000) at a dose of 0.01 ml/kg, with a maximum dose of 0.3 ml, or subcutaneous terbutaline is administered. The child is given IV fluids and nothing by mouth except liquids if the condition permits. IV fluids are infused at maintenance rates, and the child is monitored for pulmonary edema.

NURSE ALERT Dehydration should be corrected slowly; overhydration can increase the accumulation of interstitial pulmonary fluid, exacerbating small airway obstruction. ■

Correction of dehydration, acidosis, hypoxia, and electrolyte imbalance is guided by frequent monitoring of oxygenation (pulse oximetry), blood gases, and serum electrolytes. Nasal prongs, hood, or face mask is used to administer humidified oxygen. Because oxygen is a stimulus for respiration, high levels may significantly depress respirations.

The latest recommendations for the management of asthma state that antibiotics should not be used to treat acute asthma attacks except when a bacterial infection resulting from another condition such as pneumonia or sinusitis is present (National Asthma Education and Prevention Program, 2002). As the attack subsides, fluids and medications are given orally, adrenergic agonists are administered via an MDI, and plans for discharge and follow-up care are made.

Nursing Care Management

Assessment

Physical assessment of asthma involves the same observations and techniques described in the general discussion of assessment of respiratory infection and physical assessment of the chest (see Chapter 35). In addition, some physical characteristics of chronic respiratory involvement are noted and evaluated, including chest configuration, posturing, and type of breathing.

Nurses assist with diagnostic tests, pulmonary function tests, and skin testing, as well as a general health assessment. Nurses also assess how asthma affects the child's everyday activities and self-concept, as well as the child's and the family's adherence to prescribed therapy. The nurse should determine any cultural or ethnic beliefs or practices that influence self-management and that may necessitate modifications in educational approaches to meet the needs of the family.

Nursing Diagnoses

Based on a thorough assessment, several nursing diagnoses are identified. The more common diagnoses are included in the Nursing Care Plan on p. 1458. Others may apply in specific situations.

Plan of Care and Implementation

The goals for the child with asthma and the child's family include the following:

1. Child will not experience an asthmatic episode.
2. Child will exhibit improved ventilatory capacity.
3. Child will maintain optimum health.
4. Child will not develop complications.
5. Child will engage in normal activities for age.
6. Child and family will receive appropriate support and education regarding the disease and its management.

Avoid Allergens

One goal of asthma management is avoidance of an exacerbation. Parents need to know how to avoid allergens and relieve asthma episodes. The nurse assists the parent in modifying the environment to reduce contact with the offending allergen(s) (see Home Care box). Parents are cautioned to avoid exposing a sensitive child to excessive cold, wind, or other extremes of weather and to smoke, sprays, or other irritants. Foods known to provoke symptoms should be eliminated from the diet.

Approximately 2% to 6% of children with asthma are sensitive to aspirin; therefore nurses should caution parents to use other analgesic/antipyretic drugs for discomfort or fever and to read package labeling. Although aspirin is rarely given to children in the United States, salicylate compounds are in other common medicines such as Pepto-Bismol. Children with aspirin-induced asthma may also be sensitive to NSAIDs and tartrazine (yellow dye number 5, a common food coloring).

Relieve Bronchospasm

Parents and older children are taught to recognize early signs and symptoms of an impending attack so that it can be controlled before symptoms become distressing. Most children can recognize prodromal symptoms well before an attack (about 6 hours) and implement preventive therapy. Objective signs that parents may observe include rhinorrhea, cough, low-grade fever, irritability, itching (especially in the front of the neck and chest), apathy, anxiety, sleep disturbance, abdominal discomfort, and loss of appetite. A variety of easy-to-use, inexpensive PEFMs are available for use in the home and at school to assess changes in pulmonary function (Home Care box).

Children who use a nebulizer, MDI, Diskus, or Turbuhaler to deliver drugs need to learn how to use the device correctly. A study of school-age children with asthma indicated that only 7% of these children had effective MDI skills (Winkelstein et al, 2000). The MDI device (Fig. 46-4) delivers medication directly to the airways; therefore the child needs to learn to breathe slowly and deeply for better distribution to narrowed airways (Home Care box).

Young children and those who are unable to manipulate the MDI or coordinate breathing should use spacers. These devices allow the parent or child to deliver the medication from the MDI into the spacer, from which the child then inhales the medication. Spacers also prevent yeast infections in the mouth when inhaled corticosteroids are administered via an MDI.

The child and parents also need to be cautioned about the adverse effects of prescribed drugs and the dangers of overuse of β_2-adrenergic agonists. They should know that it is important to use these drugs when needed but not indis-

Home Care

USE OF A PEAK EXPIRATORY FLOW METER

1. Before each use, make sure the sliding marker or arrow on the peak expiratory flow meter points to zero or is at the bottom of the numbered scale.
2. Stand up straight.
3. Remove gum or any food from the mouth.
4. Close your lips tightly around the mouthpiece. Be sure to keep your tongue away from the mouthpiece.
5. Blow out as hard and as quickly as you can, a "fast hard puff."
6. Note the number by the marker on the numbered scale.
7. Repeat entire routine three times; wait 30 seconds between each routine.
8. Record the highest of the three readings, not the average.
9. Measure the peak expiratory flow rate (PEFR) close to the same time and same way each day (e.g., morning and evening; before or 15 minutes after taking medication).
10. Keep a chart of your PEFRs.

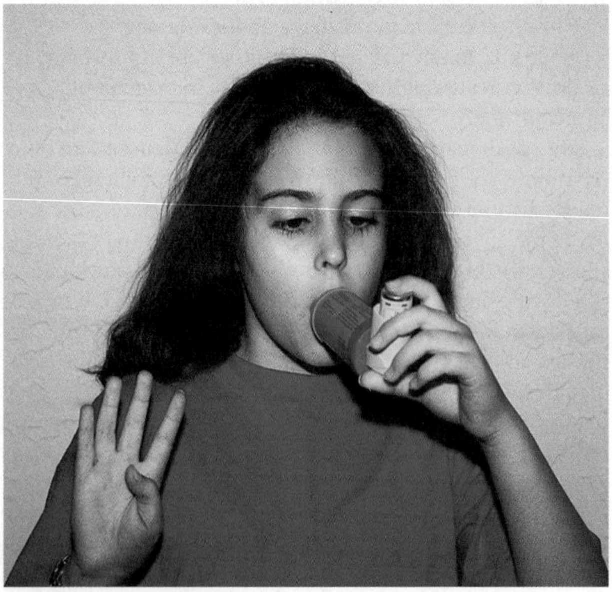

Fig. 46-4 Child using metered-dose inhaler with spacer. Fingers are used for counting to 10 seconds.

Home Care

USE OF A METERED-DOSE INHALER*

Steps for Checking How Much Medicine Is in the Canister

1. If the canister is new, it is full.
2. If the canister has been used repeatedly, it might be empty. (Check product label to see how many inhalations should be in each canister.)
3. The most accurate way to determine how many doses remain in a metered-dose inhaler (MDI) is to count and record each actuation as it is used.
4. Many dry-powder inhalers have a dose-counting device or dose indicator on the canister to let you know when the canister is empty.
5. Placing dry-powder inhalers or MDIs with hydrofluoroalkanes in water will destroy these inhalers.

Steps for Using the Inhaler

1. Remove the cap and hold inhaler upright.
2. Shake the inhaler.
3. Tilt the head back slightly and breathe out slowly.
4. With the inhaler in an upright position, position the mouthpiece:
   a. About 3 to 4 cm from the mouth *or*
   b. Insert into an AeroChamber *or* spacer (this method is recommended for young children and for people using corticosteroids)
5. At the end of a normal expiration, depress the top of the inhaler canister firmly to release the medication (into either the AeroChamber or the mouth), and breathe in slowly (about 3 to 5 seconds). Relax the pressure on the top of the canister.
6. Hold the breath for at least 5 to 10 seconds to allow the aerosol medication to reach deeply into the lungs.
7. Remove the inhaler and breathe out slowly through the nose.
8. Wait 1 minute between puffs (if additional one is needed).

Adapted from National Asthma Education and Prevention Program: *Expert panel report II: guidelines for the diagnosis and management of asthma,* pub no 97-4051, Bethesda, MD, 1997, National Heart, Lung, and Blood Institute.

*NOTE: Some dry-powder inhalers require a different inhalation technique. To use these dry-powder inhalers, it is important to close the mouth tightly around the mouthpiece of the inhaler and inhale rapidly and deeply.

criminately or as a substitute for avoiding the symptom-provoking allergen. Parents are cautioned against purchasing over-the-counter preparations because these medications can place the children at risk for increased dosage of a drug and toxicity.

NURSE ALERT Long-acting β-adrenergic inhalers (salmeterol [Serevent]) should be used only as directed (usually every 12 hours) and not more frequently. They are not intended to relieve acute asthmatic symptoms. ■

The family should obtain a PEFM and learn to use this device to monitor their child's asthma. A written asthma action plan that includes the three peak flow meter zones and the child's asthma medications should be obtained from the child's primary care provider. This action plan should be used to make decisions about asthma management at home and at school.

Parents are cautioned to avoid exposing the child with asthma to excessive cold, wind, or other extremes of weather and to smoke, sprays, or other irritants. Foods known to provoke symptoms should be eliminated from the diet, and parents are advised to read labels on prepared foods and snacks to determine the presence of allergens.

The child should be protected from a respiratory infection that can trigger an attack or aggravate the asthmatic state, especially in young children whose airways are mechanically smaller and more reactive. Annual influenza vaccinations are recommended for patients with persistent asthma (American Academy of Pediatrics, Committee on Infectious Diseases, 2003). Equipment used for the child, such as nebulizers, must be kept absolutely clean to decrease the chances of contamination with bacteria and fungi.

Breathing exercises and controlled breathing are taught and encouraged for motivated youngsters, and the nurse should provide information concerning activities that promote diaphragmatic breathing, side expansion, and improved mobility of the chest wall. Play techniques that can be used for younger children to extend their expiratory time and increase expiratory pressure include blowing cotton balls or a Ping-Pong ball on a table, blowing a pinwheel, blowing bubbles, and preventing a tissue from falling by blowing it against the wall.

Self-care and asthma self-management programs are important in helping the child and family cope with asthma. Most asthma self-management programs for children convey several principles. First, asthma is a common disease that can be controlled with appropriate drug therapy, environmental control, education, and management skills. Second, it is much easier to prevent than to treat an asthma episode; adherence to a therapeutic program is necessary to prevent exacerbations. Third, children with asthma can live full and active lives.

Asthma camps provide an opportunity for children with asthma to engage in physical activity while learning about their disease in a controlled environment with their peers and health professionals. Children who attend asthma camps often demonstrate improved asthma self-management skills.

Several organizations provide education and services for health professionals and families of children with asthma.* Asthma education and awareness are important aspects of asthma management.

Provide Acute Asthma Care

Children who are admitted to the hospital with acute asthma are ill, anxious, and uncomfortable. In many instances, they are admitted from the emergency department in status asthmaticus and in acute distress. Nebulized β-adrenergic agonists with oxygen and a systemic corticosteroid are administered to relieve bronchospasm. The child is monitored closely and continuously during therapy for relief of respiratory distress and any side effects. Vital signs are checked frequently. An IV infusion may be started to provide a means for hydration and a route for medications.

Older children usually prefer the high-Fowler position, although they may be more comfortable sitting upright or leaning slightly forward. When possible, the nurse communicates in such a way that the child can reply in a few words to avoid fatigue, because shortness of breath makes talking difficult.

Children with acute asthma are apprehensive and anxious. The calm, efficient presence of a nurse helps reassure them that they are safe and will be cared for during this stressful period. It is important to assure children that they will not be left alone and that their parents are allowed to remain with them.

Parents need reassurance and want to be informed of their child's condition and therapies. They may feel that they have in some way contributed to the child's condition or could have prevented the episode. Reassurance regarding their efforts expended on the child's behalf and their parenting capabilities can help alleviate their stress. Efforts to reduce parental apprehension will also reduce the child's distress. Anxiety is easily communicated to the child from parents and members of the staff.

Support Child and Family

The nurse working with children with asthma can provide support in a number of ways. Many children voice frustration because their exacerbations interfere with their daily activities and social lives. They need education about what to do to prevent an asthma episode. These children also need reassurance from the health team that they can learn to control and cope with their asthma and live a normal life.

NURSE ALERT Be aware of children, especially adolescents, who are depressed and may not comply with therapy as a means of passive suicide. Refer these youngsters for psychologic support. ■

*Asthma and Allergy Foundation of America (AAFA), 1125 15th St., Washington, DC 20005; phone: 202-466-7643 or 800-7-ASTHMA; Web site: www.aafa.org. American Lung Association, 1740 Broadway, New York, NY 10019; phone: 212-315-8700 or 800-LUNG-USA; Web site: www.lungusa.org. National Heart, Lung, and Blood Institute, Information Center, Code AS-ASHA, PO Box 30105, Bethesda, MD 20824-0105; fax: 301-251-1223; Web site: www.nhlbi.nih.gov/nhlbi.htm.

The short-term and long-term adaptation of children with asthma often depends on the family's acceptance of the disorder. The task of living day-to-day with affected children involves the family continually. There are periodic crises and the ever-present threat of a crisis, requiring parental vigilance; sleepless nights; frequent trips to the doctor, emergency department, or hospital; and often overwhelming medical expenses. Throughout these stresses, parents are encouraged to promote as normal a life as possible for their children.

Evaluation

Continual reassessment and evaluation determine the effectiveness of nursing interventions. The following observational guidelines and expected outcomes are important:

1. Interview family about removal or avoidance of known allergens.
2. Observe child for evidence of respiratory symptoms.
3. Assess child's general health.
4. Observe child and interview family about any infections or other complications.
5. Interview child about daily activities.
6. Determine the degree to which the family and child understand the child's condition and the extent to which the therapies are carried out.

The *expected outcomes* are described in the Nursing Care Plan.

Nursing Care Plan

THE CHILD WITH ASTHMA

NURSING DIAGNOSIS: Risk for suffocation related to interaction of child with allergens

EXPECTED OUTCOME

Asthmatic episodes are reduced or eliminated.

NURSING INTERVENTIONS/*RATIONALES*

Make an inventory of allergens that trigger reactions or asthmatic episodes *to establish a baseline for prevention.*

Teach child and family how to avoid, limit exposure to, modify, or eliminate conditions *that trigger allergy attacks and asthmatic episodes.*

Teach child and family to recognize early signs *so an impending asthmatic episode can be treated early.*

Instruct child and family in correct use of prescribed bronchodilators, antiinflammatories, and other asthma medications *to avoid underuse or overuse of the drugs.*

Instruct child and family in correct use of equipment (e.g., inhalers, nebulizers, peak flow meters) *to ensure correct use and optimum benefit.*

Encourage sound health practices (good nutrition, adequate rest, appropriate exercise, good hygiene) *to support body's natural defenses.*

Encourage child and family to prevent exposure to respiratory infections *because they can serve as triggers for asthma attacks.*

NURSING DIAGNOSIS: Ineffective airway clearance related to allergenic response and inflamed bronchial tree

EXPECTED OUTCOME

The patient will exhibit evidence of improved ventilatory capacity (i.e., absence of dyspnea, respiration rate and rhythm within normal limits).

NURSING INTERVENTIONS/*RATIONALES*

Implement breathing exercises and controlled breathing *to improve chest wall mobility and diaphragmatic expansion.*

Use developmentally appropriate play techniques *to increase expiratory pressure and extend expiratory time.*

Use coughing, percussion, and postural drainage as needed *to clear secretions.*

Supervise use of equipment (e.g., inhalers, nebulizers, peak flow meters) *to evaluate use patterns and optimum benefit.*

Administer medications as ordered *to decrease inflammatory response and improve breathing.*

NURSING DIAGNOSIS: Activity intolerance related to imbalance between oxygen supply and demand

EXPECTED OUTCOME

The patient's activity level will be within normal limits.

NURSING INTERVENTIONS/*RATIONALES*

Balance rest and physical activity, increasing activity levels as tolerated, *to regain balance between oxygen supply and demand.*

NURSING DIAGNOSIS: Altered family processes related to having a child with chronic health problem

EXPECTED OUTCOME

Family exhibits positive adaptive behaviors to child's condition.

NURSING INTERVENTIONS/*RATIONALES*

Identify and praise positive coping mechanisms of child and family members *to reinforce long-term use.*

Explore child's and family's understanding of the disease and treatment process *to evaluate family's ability to carry out preventive and emergency intervention.*

Reinforce need for consistent use of preventive measures and need for early response to signs of impending attack *to prevent severe exacerbation.*

Be alert to signs of maladaptation (e.g., parental rejection or overprotection, nonadherence to treatment regimen, lack of alterations in environment or lifestyle, sporadic health care follow-up).

Encourage family to work with school *to develop a consistent plan of care in the school setting.*

Refer family to appropriate support groups and community resources *to provide ongoing support.*

See also Nursing Care Plan: The Child with Chronic Illness or Disability, Chapter 41.

CRITICAL THINKING EXERCISE: CYSTIC FIBROSIS INHERITANCE RISKS

Cystic Fibrosis

Cystic fibrosis (CF) is inherited as an autosomal recessive trait; the affected child inherits the defective gene from both parents, with an overall incidence of 1:4 (see Appendix C). The mutated gene responsible for CF is located on the long arm of chromosome 7, along with its protein product, *cystic fibrosis transmembrane regulator (CFTR).*

Pathophysiology

CF is characterized by several clinical features: increased viscosity of mucous gland secretions, a striking elevation of sweat electrolytes, an increase in several organic and enzymatic constituents of saliva, and abnormalities in autonomic nervous system function. Although both sodium and chloride are affected, the defect appears to be primarily a result of abnormal chloride movement; the CFTR appears to function as a chloride channel. Children with CF demonstrate decreased pancreatic secretion of bicarbonate and chloride and an increase in sodium and chloride in both saliva and sweat. This characteristic is the basis for the sweat chloride diagnostic test.

The primary factor, and the one that is responsible for many of the clinical manifestations of the disease, is mechanical obstruction caused by the increased viscosity of mucous gland secretions (Fig. 46-5). Instead of forming a thin, freely flowing secretion, the mucous glands produce a thick mucoprotein that accumulates and dilates them. Small passages in organs such as the pancreas and bronchioles become obstructed as secretions precipitate or coagulate to form concretions in glands and ducts. The earliest manifestation of CF is *meconium ileus* in the newborn, in which the small intestine is blocked with thick, puttylike, tenacious, mucilaginous meconium.

In the pancreas the thick secretions block the ducts, eventually causing *pancreatic fibrosis.* This blockage prevents essential pancreatic enzymes from reaching the duodenum, which causes marked impairment in the digestion and absorption of nutrients. The disturbed function is reflected in bulky stools that are frothy from undigested fat *(steatorrhea)* and foul smelling from putrefied protein *(azotorrhea).* The islands of Langerhans may decrease in number as pancreatic fibrosis progresses, and a type of diabetes called *CF-related diabetes* is a frequent finding in adolescents and adults with CF (Balinsky & Zhu, 2004). In the liver, localized biliary obstruction and fibrosis are common and become more extensive with time.

A common gastrointestinal (GI) complication associated with CF is *prolapse of the rectum,* which occurs in infancy and childhood and is related to large, bulky stools, malnutrition, and increased intraabdominal pressure secondary to paroxysmal cough. Affected children of all ages are subject to intestinal obstruction from inspissated or impacted feces. Gumlike masses can obstruct the bowel and produce a partial or complete obstruction, a condition that is referred to as *distal intestinal obstruction syndrome.*

Pulmonary complications constitute the most serious threat to life in children with CF. Many children demonstrate respiratory symptoms before 1 year of age; others may not develop symptoms for weeks, months, or years. In the respiratory tract, bronchial and bronchiolar obstruction by the

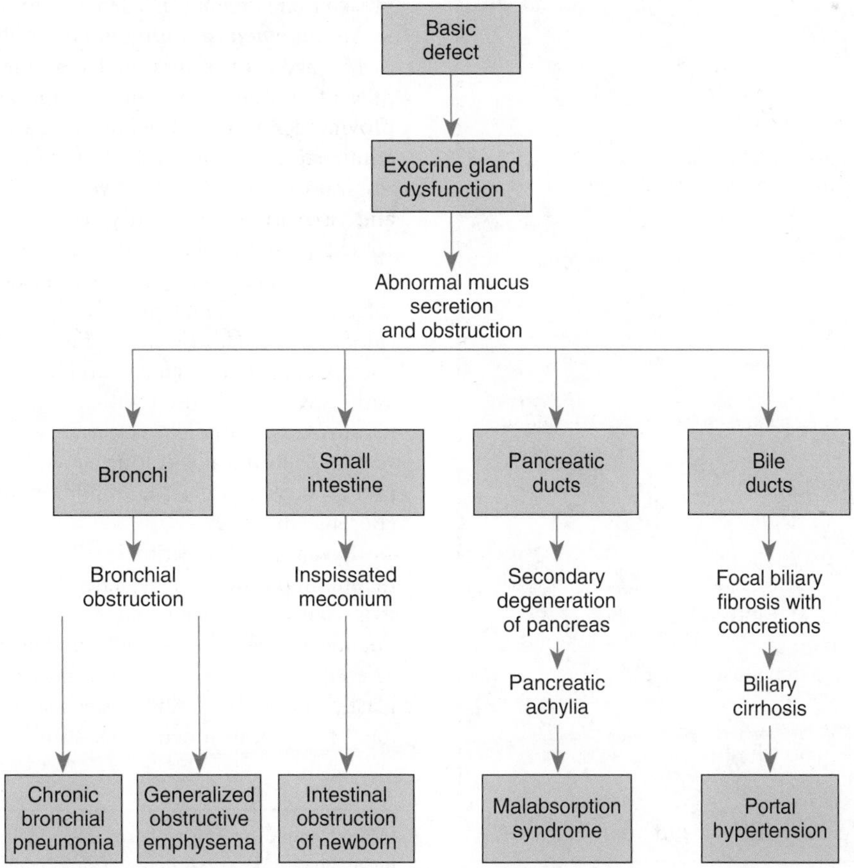

Fig. 46-5 Various effects of exocrine gland dysfunction in cystic fibrosis.

abnormally thick, tenacious mucus causes patchy atelectasis with hyperinflation. The child is unable to expectorate the mucus because of its increased viscosity. This retained mucus serves as an excellent medium for bacterial growth. Reduced oxygen–carbon dioxide exchange causes variable degrees of hypoxia, hypercapnia, and acidosis.

evolve CASE STUDY: CYSTIC FIBROSIS

Diagnostic Evaluation

An initial evaluation is conducted with overall appraisal in the areas of general activity, physical findings, nutritional status, and findings on chest radiograms (Box 46-16). The diagnosis of CF is established on the basis of (1) a history of the disease in the family, (2) absence of pancreatic enzymes, (3) increase in electrolyte concentration of sweat, and (4) chronic pulmonary involvement.

The consistent finding of abnormally high sodium and chloride concentrations in the sweat is a unique characteristic of CF. Parents frequently report that their infants taste "salty" when they kiss them. For diagnostic purposes the quantitative *sweat chloride test* is performed on sweat obtained by iontophoresis of pilocarpine. Normally the sweat chloride content is less than 40 mEq/L; a chloride concentration greater than 60 mEq/L is diagnostic of CF. In infants, a value greater than 40 mmol/L is highly suggestion of CF.

Chest radiography reveals characteristic patchy atelectasis and obstructive emphysema. PFTs are sensitive indexes of lung function, providing evidence of abnormal function of the small airways in CF. Other diagnostic tools that may aid in diagnosis include stool fat analysis and enzyme analysis. Stool analysis requires a 72-hour sample with accurate recording of food intake during that time. Radiographs, including barium enema, are used for diagnosis of meconium ileus.

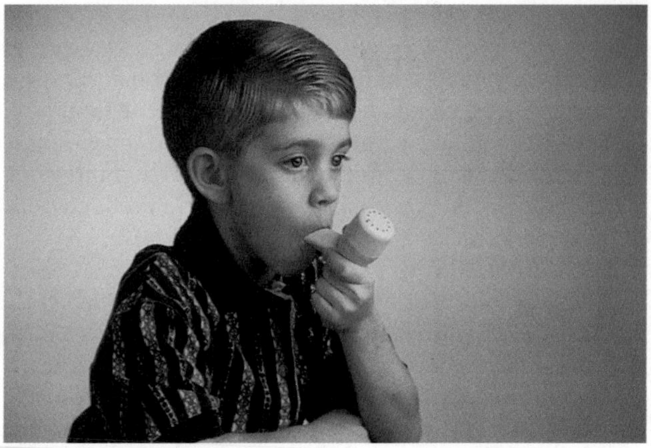

Fig. 46-6 Child using Flutter mucous clearance device. (Courtesy Scandipharm, Inc.)

BOX 46-16

Clinical Manifestations of Cystic Fibrosis

Meconium Ileus*
Abdominal distention
Vomiting
Failure to pass stools
Rapid development of dehydration

Gastrointestinal Manifestations
Large, bulky, loose, frothy, extremely foul-smelling stools
Voracious appetite (early in disease)
Loss of appetite (later in disease)
Weight loss
Marked tissue wasting
Failure to grow
Distended abdomen
Thin extremities
Sallow skin
Evidence of deficiency of fat-soluble vitamins A, D, E, and K
Anemia

Pulmonary Manifestations
Initial signs:
- Wheezy respirations
- Dry, nonproductive cough

Eventually:
- Increased dyspnea
- Paroxysmal cough
- Evidence of obstructive emphysema and patchy areas of atelectasis

Progressive involvement:
- Overinflated, barrel-shaped chest
- Cyanosis
- Clubbing of fingers and toes
- Repeated episodes of bronchitis and bronchopneumonia

*In about 10% of cases.

Therapeutic Management

The improved survival rate of patients with CF is due to antibiotic therapy and improved nutritional management. Goals of therapy are to (1) prevent or minimize pulmonary complications, (2) ensure adequate nutrition for growth, (3) encourage appropriate physical activity, and (4) promote a reasonable quality of life for the child and the family. A multisystem approach to treatment is needed to accomplish these goals.

Management of Pulmonary Problems

Management of pulmonary problems is directed toward prevention and treatment of pulmonary infection by improving aeration, removing mucopurulent secretions, and administering antimicrobial agents. Most children develop respiratory symptoms by 3 years of age. The large amounts and viscosity of respiratory secretions in children with CF contribute to the likelihood of respiratory infections.

CASE STUDY: CYSTIC FIBROSIS

The most common pathogens responsible for pulmonary infections are *Pseudomonas aeruginosa, Burkholderia cepacia, S. aureus, H. influenzae, Escherichia coli,* and *Klebsiella pneumoniae. P. aeruginosa* and *B. cepacia* are particularly pathogenic for children with CF, and infections with these organisms are difficult to clear. In addition, children with CF who are chronically colonized with these organisms have poorer survival rates than children who are not colonized (Rosenstein, 1999).

Prevention of infection involves a daily routine of CPT to maintain pulmonary hygiene. CPT is usually performed twice daily (on rising and in the evening) and more frequently if needed, especially during pulmonary infection. The Flutter mucous clearance device* is a small, handheld plastic pipe with a stainless-steel ball on the inside that facilitates removal of mucus (Fig. 46-6). It has the advantage of

*Manufactured by Scandipharm, Inc., 22 Inverness Center Parkway, Birmingham, AL 35242; phone: 205-991-8085 or 800-950-8085; Web site: www.scandipharm.com.

increasing sputum expectoration and being used without an assistant.

Bronchodilator medication delivered in an aerosol opens bronchi for easier expectoration and is administered before CPT when the patient exhibits evidence of reactive airway disease or wheezing. Another aerosolized medication is *recombinant human deoxyribonuclease (D-Nase),* known generically as *dornase alfa (Pulmozyme),* which decreases the viscosity of mucus. It is well tolerated and has no major adverse effects; minor reactions are voice alterations and laryngitis. The drug causes improvement in PFTs and perceptions of well-being, as well as a reduction in the viscosity of sputum.

Physical exercise is an important adjunct to daily CPT. Exercise stimulates mucous secretion and provides a sense of well-being and increased self-esteem. Any aerobic exercise that is enjoyed by the patient should be encouraged. The ultimate aim of exercise is to establish an adequate breathing pattern.

Pulmonary infections are treated as soon as they are recognized. Some practitioners prefer to prescribe oral antibiotics prophylactically at the time of diagnosis; others begin therapy when pulmonary symptoms occur. Sputum culture and sensitivity guide the choice of antibiotic. Aerosolized antibiotics such as tobramycin, ticarcillin, and gentamicin are beneficial for patients with frequent pulmonary exacerbations.

IV antibiotics are often administered at home as an alternative to hospitalization. Most children with CF have central venous access devices for home administration of IV medications. However, when pulmonary function does not improve with outpatient management, hospitalization may be recommended for continued antibiotic therapy and vigorous CPT. Oxygen administration is used for children with acute episodes, but must be used cautiously because many children with CF have chronic carbon dioxide retention, and the unsupervised use of oxygen can be harmful (see Oxygen Therapy: Oxygen Toxicity, Chapter 45). Pneumothorax can occur in children and adolescents with more advanced disease if there is a rupture of subpleural blebs through the visceral pleura.

NURSE ALERT Signs of a pneumothorax are usually nonspecific and include tachypnea, tachycardia, dyspnea, pallor, and cyanosis. ■

Management of Gastrointestinal Problems

The principal treatment for pancreatic insufficiency is replacement of pancreatic enzymes, which are administered with meals and snacks to ensure that digestive enzymes are mixed with food in the duodenum. Enteric-coated products prevent the neutralization of enzymes by gastric acids, thus allowing activation to occur in the alkaline environment of the small bowel. The amount of enzymes depends on the severity of the insufficiency, the response of the child to enzyme replacement, and the philosophy of the practitioner. Usually one to five capsules are administered with a meal, and a smaller amount is taken with snacks. Capsules can be swallowed whole or taken apart and the contents sprinkled on a small amount of food to be taken at the beginning of the meal. The amount of enzyme is adjusted to achieve normal growth and a decrease in the number of stools to one or two per day.

Children with CF require a well-balanced, high-protein, high-caloric diet (because of the impaired intestinal absorption). In fact, they often require up to 150% of the recommended daily allowances to meet their needs for growth. Breastfeeding with enzyme supplementation should be continued whenever possible for parents who prefer this method and, when necessary, supplemented with a higher-calorie-per-ounce formula. For formula-fed infants, commercial cow's milk formulas are usually adequate, although frequently a hydrolysate formula with medium-chain triglycerides (e.g., Pregestimil, Alimentum) may be recommended. Enzymes are mixed into cereal or fruit, such as applesauce. Because the uptake of fat-soluble vitamins is decreased, water-miscible forms of these vitamins (A, D, E, and K) are given, along with multivitamins and the enzymes. When high-fat foods are eaten, the child is encouraged to add extra enzymes. Sometimes patients will be placed on supplemental tube feedings or parenteral alimentation in an effort to build up nutritional reserves if there has been a history of inability to maintain weight.

Prognosis

Despite considerable progress and a recent surge in new treatments, CF remains a progressive and incurable disease. The pulmonary involvement ultimately determines the patient's outcome, because pancreatic enzyme deficiency is less of a problem if adequate nutrition is ensured. With advances in technology, parents and adolescents are challenged to set future goals that include college, careers, social relationships, and marriage.

Screening

In utero diagnosis of CF is possible based on detection of two CF mutations in the fetus. Newborn screening has been available since 1979. The standard method of diagnosis is detection of abnormal chloride secretions in sweat. Sometimes testing of DNA to detect the F508 gene may be substituted for the sweat test. Carrier screening is also available and reliable for siblings and family members of a child with CF (Balinsky & Zhu, 2004).

Nursing Care Management

Assessment of the child with CF involves both pulmonary and GI observations. Pulmonary assessment is the same as that described for asthma, with special attention to lung sounds, observation of cough, and evidence or degree of finger clubbing. GI assessment involves observing the frequency and nature of the stools and abdominal distention. The nurse should also be alert to evidence of failure to thrive (e.g., weight loss, wasting, pallor, fatigue). Family members are interviewed to determine the child's eating and eliminating habits, to determine salty perspiration, and to confirm a history of frequent respiratory infections or bowel obstruction in infancy.

On initial contact, which frequently occurs in the hospital setting, nurses are involved in performing or assisting with diagnostic tests, primarily sweat for laboratory analysis of chloride content and, less often, collection of stool specimens for trypsin and fat analyses.

Hospital Care

When patients with CF are hospitalized, Standard Precautions with meticulous handwashing should be implemented to decrease the nosocomial spread of organisms among CF patients and to other patients in the hospital. Sputum and soiled tissues from all CF patients should be discarded in a covered no-touch receptacle whenever possible. In some hospitals, patients with CF who are colonized or infected with organisms with antimicrobial resistance are placed in a private room. In addition, CF patients who are colonized or infected with *B. cepacia* complex may be hospitalized in a private room on a separate nursing unit, away from other CF patients, and have limitations placed on their activities while in the hospital. Such limitations include not using the playroom or hospital cafeteria when other CF patients are present.

When the child with is hospitalized for diagnosis or treatment of pulmonary complications, aerosol therapy is instituted or continued. Respiratory therapists often initiate, supervise, and provide these treatments. If the hospital or institution does not have respiratory therapists assigned to this therapy, the nurse administers the aerosol therapy, performs CPT, and teaches breathing exercises. CPT should not be performed before or immediately after meals. Planning CPT so that it does not coincide with meals is difficult in the hospital situation, but essential to the effectiveness of this treatment.

Oxygen is cautiously administered to children in respiratory distress, and the child requires frequent assessment. The hazard of *oxygen narcosis* is a constant threat in children with CF. The child requires close observation to assist with cough and expectoration.

The diet is implemented for the newly diagnosed child or continued for the child who is hospitalized for pulmonary disease. Children in the early stages of CF often have a good appetite, and some will eat excessively. With infection and increased lung involvement, their appetite diminishes, and eventually it becomes a challenge to tempt failing appetites. Some younger children may object to the extra fluids that are encouraged to prevent dehydration. Food is considered therapy for these patients. The caloric intake should be increased as necessary. Pancreatic enzymes are supplied for each meal or snack, and adequate salt is provided, especially for febrile children. (See Feeding the Sick Child, Chapter 45.)

Frequent skin care is performed to prevent irritation and skin breakdown over bony prominences. Particular attention is necessary after use of the bedpan or when the diaper is changed. Careful cleansing helps reduce irritation and odor from offensive stools, and the use of moisture barriers protects the skin. (See Maintaining Healthy Skin, Chapter 45.)

The child needs support during the many treatments and tests that are a part of the hospitalization. IV fluids and blood tests are almost always a part of the treatment, and the child soon associates hospitalization with these stress-provoking procedures. Because these children are usually quite thin with little muscle mass, careful selection of injection sites is required.

Providing support to both the child and the family is essential. The progressive nature of the disease makes each illness requiring hospitalization a potentially life-threatening event. Skilled nursing care and sympathetic attention to the emotional needs of the child and family help them cope with the stresses associated with repeated respiratory infections and hospitalization.

Home Care

After the diagnosis is confirmed and after each hospitalization, home care is implemented. The plan of care should be flexible so that family activities are disrupted as little as possible. Parents need help contacting the vendors who will provide home care equipment. They also need opportunities to learn how to use the equipment, as well as how to solve problems they may encounter while delivering therapy at home.

Patients and family members need education about the preferred diet of nutritious meals with tolerated fat, increased protein and carbohydrate, and the administration of pancreatic enzymes. For infants and young children, the enzymes can be mixed with pureed fruit, such as applesauce, and fed with a spoon. Capsules are usually suitable for older children. It is important to stress to parents that the enzymes, in the amount regulated to the child's needs, should be administered at the beginning of all meals and snacks. They are cautioned about not restricting salt, especially during hot weather, and ensuring an adequate fluid intake, because dehydration aggravates the thick mucous secretions. Oral hygiene is important because of interference with salivation and the increased susceptibility to oral infections.

One of the most important aspects of educating parents for home care is teaching CPT and breathing exercises. The success of a therapy program depends on conscientious performance of these treatments regularly as prescribed. The number of times these therapies are performed each day is determined on an individual basis, and often parents readily learn to adjust the number and intensity of the treatments to the child's needs. For the young child, postural drainage can be achieved with simple activities such as hanging by the knees from a bar or low-hanging trapeze, turning somersaults, or playing "wheelbarrow" with the child suspended head down and propelling with the hands while the adult holds on to the feet. Most children respond to a challenge, such as "How long can you stand on your head?" Small children can stand on their head with their head on the cushion of a large chair with or without an adult holding on to their feet. Parents soon learn to respond to cues from their children and incorporate spontaneous and fun activities into the treatment regimen.

Another important aspect of home care is the administration of IV antibiotics. As a result of the current use of venous access devices, such as peripherally inserted central catheter (PICC) lines, Infus-a-port, and central lines, parents and children can now assume responsibility for home administration of IV antibiotics.* When this occurs, families need detailed information about how to give the medications, their possible side effects, and how to troubleshoot any problems with the venous access device.

---

*Two excellent publications available from the Cystic Fibrosis Foundation are *What Everyone Should Know about Cystic Fibrosis* and *Cystic Fibrosis: A Summary of Symptoms, Diagnosis, and Treatment.* For information about specialized medications (e.g., Pulmozyme), equipment for CF, or home infusions, contact Home Infusion and Pharmacy Services, a subsidiary of the Cystic Fibrosis Pharmacy, Inc., H.H.C.S. Pharmacy Services, 633 E. Colonial Dr., Orlando, FL 32803; phone: 800-741-4427.

Children with CF should receive routine primary care with special attention to diet, growth and development, and immunizations. In addition to all recommended immunizations, patients with CF should receive the influenza vaccine starting at age 6 months and followed by a yearly booster (American Academy of Pediatrics, Committee on Infectious Diseases, 2003).

The nurse can assist the family in contacting resources that provide help to families. Various child health services and many local clinics, private agencies, service clubs, and other community groups offer equipment and medications either free or at reduced rates. The Cystic Fibrosis Foundation has chapters throughout the United States to provide education and services to families and professionals.*

Family Support

The most challenging aspect of providing care for the family of a child with CF is meeting the emotional needs of the child and family. The diagnosis, treatment, and prognosis of CF are often associated with many problems and frustrations. The diagnosis can evoke feelings of guilt and self-recrimination in parents. These feelings may be particularly strong if the newly diagnosed child is the second affected child in the family and the parents had been counseled about the 1:4 risk of such an event occurring.

The long-range problems for an infant, child, or adolescent with CF are those encountered in any chronic illness (see Chapter 41). Both the child and the family must make many adjustments, the success of which depends on their ability to cope and also on the quality and quantity of support they receive from outside sources. Combined efforts of a variety of health professionals are needed to provide the most comprehensive services to families. It is often the nurse who organizes and coordinates these services, assesses the home situation, and collects the data needed to evaluate the effectiveness of the services.

The persistent need for treatment several times a day places tremendous strain on the family. When the child is young, a family member must perform postural drainage and CPT. Children often balk at these treatments, and the parents are placed in the position of insisting on adherence. The stress and anxiety related to this continual routine may produce feelings of resentment in both the child and the family members. When possible, occasional trusted respite care should be available to the parents to allow them the opportunity to leave the situation for short periods without undue anxiety about the child's welfare.

The affected child may become resentful about the disease, its relentless routine of therapy, and the necessary curtailment it places on activities and relationships. The child's activities are interrupted or built around treatments, medications, and diet. This imposes hardships and influences the child's quality of life. For example, the child may need to carry medication to school and other places if he or she eats away from home. Some aspects of the disease such as growth retardation and persistent coughing may be the cause of ridicule from other children. However, the child should be encouraged to attend school and to join age-appropriate peer groups to foster a life that is as normal and productive as possible.

As the disease progresses, family stress should be expected, and the patient may become angry and noncompliant. As the disease progresses, family members may become more aware of the possibility of death. It is important for the nurse to recognize the changing needs of the family, and provide sources for counseling if necessary when stressful setbacks occur. Patients need to be guided into activities that enable them to express anger, sorrow, and fear without guilt.

Anticipatory grieving and other aspects related to care of a child with a terminal illness are another important part of nursing care. For example, it is important to prepare family members for end-of-life decisions and care. Families may need information about specific interventions such as hospice and treatments for pain and dyspnea (see Chapter 41).

As life expectancy increases for children with CF, issues related to marriage, childbearing, and career choice become relevant. Men must be informed at some point that they will be unable to produce offspring. However, a distinction should be made between sterility and impotence. Normal sexual relationships can be expected. Female patients may be able to bear children but should be informed of the possible deleterious effects on the respiratory system created by the burden of pregnancy. They also need to know that their children will be carriers of the CF gene.

Life as an independent adult, the goal that most families have for their children, should be encouraged for children with CF. From the time that children can take partial responsibility for their own care (e.g., CPT, taking enzymes), independence and accountability should be fostered. The prognosis for children with CF has improved, and many children with CF are well adjusted despite numerous hospitalizations and unpleasant complications.

RESPIRATORY EMERGENCIES

Respiratory Failure

In general, the term *respiratory insufficiency* is applied to two situations: (1) when there is increased work of breathing but gas exchange function is near normal and (2) when normal blood gas tensions cannot be maintained and hypoxemia and acidosis develop secondary to carbon dioxide retention.

Respiratory failure is defined as the inability of the respiratory apparatus to maintain adequate oxygenation of the blood, with or without carbon dioxide retention. *Respiratory arrest* is the cessation of respiration. *Apnea* is the cessation of breathing for more than 20 seconds or for a shorter period when associated with hypoxemia or bradycardia (Curley & Moloney-Harmon, 2001).

Effective pulmonary gas exchange requires clear airways, normal lungs and chest wall, and adequate pulmonary circulation. Anything that affects these functions or their relationships can compromise respiration.

Diagnostic Evaluation

Respiratory failure that occurs as a result of acute obstruction of a major airway or cardiac arrest is sudden and readily apparent. Gradual or progressive deterioration of

*6931 Arlington Rd., Bethesda, MD 20814-3205; phone: 800-FIGHT-CF or 301-951-4422; Web site: www.cff.org. In Canada: Canadian Cystic Fibrosis Foundation, 586 Eglinton Ave. E., Suite 204, Toronto, Ontario M4P 1P2.

respiratory function is less easily recognized. Nursing observation and judgment are vital to the recognition and early management of respiratory failure. Nurses must be able to assess a situation and initiate appropriate action within moments. Signs of respiratory failure are listed in Box 46-17.

Therapeutic Management

The interventions used in the management of respiratory failure are often dramatic, requiring special skills and emergency procedures. Some techniques used to assist ventilation include artificial ventilation, artificial airway, and cardiopulmonary resuscitation (CPR).

Artificial Ventilation

A variety of methods for controlling or assisting ventilation are available. Temporary assistance involves the use of a manual self-inflating ventilation bag with a mask and valve to prevent rebreathing. With the mask placed over the child's nose and mouth, an open airway is established by correct positioning with the chin forward and the neck extended to the "sniffing" position. The bag is rhythmically compressed, forcing the gas from the bag into the child's lungs.

For prolonged assistance, mechanical ventilation is used to replace the bellows function of the diaphragm and thoracic wall muscles. The lungs are inflated by the application of either positive or negative pressure. The positive-pressure machine inflates the lung by increasing airway pressure above atmospheric pressure, and a negative-pressure ventilator creates a subatmospheric pressure around the chest wall while airway pressure remains atmospheric. Application of positive pressure by mechanical means usually improves the distribution of gas within the lung and often reinflates partially collapsed lung segments. The overall effect is the improvement of gas exchange.

Nursing Care Management

For families whose child has a respiratory arrest, support is aimed at keeping the family informed of the child's status and helping them to cope with a near-death experience or an actual death (see Chapter 41). Knowing that their child requires CPR is a frightening and often overwhelming experience for parents. Uncertainty regarding the outcome—both mortality and morbidity—is a primary concern. Traditionally, family members are not allowed to be present during resuscitation efforts. However, recent studies indicate that family presence during emergencies alleviates the family's anger about being separated from the patient during a crisis, reduces their anxiety, eliminates doubts about what was done to help the patient, and facilitates the grieving process when the patients dies (Tucker, 2003). Regardless of whether an institution permits parental presence during CPR, nurses must consider the needs, fears, and concerns of family members during an arrest situation. If family presence is not permitted, nurses should arrange for someone to remain with the family during the code. After the child's recovery or death, the family will continue to need support and thorough medical information regarding lifesaving measures, the prognosis if the child survives, and the cause of death if the child dies.

BOX 46-17

Clinical Manifestations of Respiratory Failure

Cardinal Signs
- Restlessness
- Tachypnea
- Tachycardia
- Diaphoresis

Early but Less Obvious Signs
- Mood changes, such as euphoria or depression
- Headache
- Altered depth and pattern of respirations
- Hypertension
- Exertional dyspnea
- Anorexia
- Increased cardiac output and renal output
- Central nervous system symptoms (decreased efficiency, impaired judgment, anxiety, confusion, restlessness, irritability, depressed level of consciousness)
- Flaring nares
- Chest wall retractions
- Expiratory grunt
- Wheezing or prolonged expiration

Signs of More Severe Hypoxia
- Hypotension or hypertension
- Dimness of vision
- Somnolence
- Stupor
- Coma
- Dyspnea
- Depressed respirations
- Bradycardia
- Cyanosis, peripheral or central

Cardiopulmonary Resuscitation

Cardiac arrest in children is less often of cardiac origin than from prolonged hypoxemia secondary to inadequate oxygenation, ventilation, and circulation (shock). Some causes of cardiac arrest include injuries, suffocation (e.g., FB aspiration), smoke inhalation, SIDS, and infection. Respiratory arrest has been associated with a better survival rate than cardiac arrest. After cardiac arrest occurs, the outcome of resuscitative efforts is poor.

Complete apnea signals the need for rapid, vigorous action to prevent cardiac arrest. In such situations, nurses must initiate action immediately. In the hospital, emergency equipment must be available and easily accessible in all patient care areas. The status of emergency equipment must be checked at least once daily. Regardless of the cause of the arrest, basic procedures are carried out and modified somewhat according to the child's size.

NURSE ALERT Rescuers who have infections that may be transmitted by blood or saliva or who believe they have been exposed to such an infection should not perform mouth-to-mouth resuscitation if a barrier device or mask with a one-way valve is not available. If CPR efforts are anticipated in the workplace or other out-of-hospital setting, rescuers should have access to these devices (American Heart Association, 2000). ■

Outside the hospital situation, the first action in an emergency is to quickly assess the extent of any injury and determine whether the child is unconscious. A child who is struggling to breathe but conscious should be transported immediately to an *advanced life support (ALS)* facility, with the child maintaining whatever position affords the most comfort. Attempting to transport a child by automobile wastes valuable time in obtaining help. Transport by an *emergency medical service (EMS)* is recommended. Services in most large communities can institute ALS immediately or en route to a medical facility.

An unconscious child is managed with care to prevent additional trauma if a head or spinal cord injury has been sustained. The circumstances in which the child is found offer clues to a possible injury. For example, a child who has been thrown from a bicycle or fallen from a tree is more likely to have sustained trauma than a child who is discovered in bed. The child should be turned as a unit with firm support provided to the head and neck to prevent rolling, twisting, or tilting backward or forward.

Resuscitation Procedure

Current CPR guidelines incorporate the use of the automated external defibrillator (AED) in the treatment of cardiorespiratory arrest if the child has a weight greater than 25 kg (55 lb, or approximately 8 years of age) (American Heart Association, 2000) (Box 46-18 and Figures 46-7 *A-E*). In out-of-hospital situations, the use of an AED in children 1 to 8 years of age is appropriate if the defibrillating machine is approved for use in children. In a hospital situation, where weight-based defibrillation dosing is possible, manual defibrillation is the mode of choice (American Heart Association, 2003). When using an AED, health care providers are advised to give adults and children older than 8 years a defibrillatory shock within 5 minutes of collapse outside the hospital and within 3 minutes in the hospital.

For effective CPR, the victim is placed on his or her back on a firm, flat surface, employing appropriate precautions (Fig. 46-8). Unlike rescuers of adults, who initiate EMS first, pediatric rescuers provide 1 minute of basic life support (BLS) before activating EMS. Because pediatric arrest is most commonly the result of a respiratory arrest, maintaining ventilation is a primary consideration. With loss of consciousness, the tongue, which is attached to the lower jaw, relaxes and falls back, obstructing the airway. To open the airway, the head is positioned with either the head tilt/chin lift or jaw thrust. Health professionals should be able to use both maneuvers. *Head tilt* is accomplished by placing one hand on the victim's forehead and applying firm, backward pressure with the palm to tilt the head back. The fingers of the free hand are placed under the bony portion of the lower jaw near the chin to lift and bring the chin forward *(chin lift)*. This supports the jaw and helps tilt the head back (Fig. 46-9, *A*).

The *jaw thrust* is accomplished by grasping the angles of the victim's lower jaw and lifting with both hands, one on each side, displacing the mandible upward and outward (Fig. 46-9, *B*). In suspected neck injuries the jaw thrust method should be used while the cervical spine is completely immobilized. After restoration of a patent airway by removal of foreign material and secretions (if indicated), and if the child is not breathing, continuation of the airway is maintained and rescue breathing is initiated. To ventilate the lungs in the infant (birth to 1 year of age), the bag-valve-mask or operator's mouth is placed in such a way that both the mouth and the nostrils are covered (Fig. 46-9, *C*). Children (older than 1 year of age) are ventilated through the mouth while the nostrils are firmly pinched for airtight contact (Fig. 46-9, *D*).

NURSE ALERT The volume of air in an infant's lungs is small, and the air passages are considerably smaller, with resistance to flow potentially higher than in adults. Therefore small puffs of air are delivered. ■

If air enters freely and the chest rises, the airway is assumed to be clear. The correct volume for each breath must be provided without causing abdominal distention. Gastric distention, which interferes with diaphragmatic excursion, frequently occurs when more volume than necessary is delivered and the breaths are delivered too rapidly.

After the initial two breaths, the pulse is palpated to determine the presence of a heartbeat. The carotid is the most central and accessible artery in children older than 1 year of age (Fig. 46-9, *E*). However, the very short and often fat neck of the infant renders the carotid pulse difficult to palpate. Therefore, in the infant, it is preferable to use the brachial pulse, located on the inner side of the upper arm midway between the elbow and shoulder (Fig. 46-9, *F*). Absence of a carotid or brachial pulse is considered sufficient indication to begin external cardiac massage.

Chest Compression

External chest compression consists of serial, rhythmic compressions of the chest to maintain circulation to vital organs until the child achieves spontaneous vital signs or ALS can be provided. *Chest compressions are always interspersed with ventilation of the lungs.* For optimum compressions, it is essential that the child's spine is supported on a firm surface during compressions of the sternum and that sternal pressure is forceful but not traumatic. For an infant the hard surface can be the rescuer's hand or forearm, with the palm supporting the infant's back. The child's head is positioned for optimum airway opening using the head tilt/chin lift maneuver. It is essential to prevent overextension of the head of small infants, because this tends to close the flexible trachea.

The placement of the fingers for compression in infants is at a point on the lower sternum one fingerbreadth below the intersection of the sternum and an imaginary line drawn between the nipples (Fig. 46-9, *G*). Compressions on the child 1 to 8 years of age are applied to the lower half of the sternum (Fig. 46-9, *H*). Sternal compression to infants is applied with two or three fingers on the sternum exerting a firm downward thrust; for children, pressure is applied with the heel of one hand. Current guidelines include the addition of the two-thumb technique for chest compressions for infants when two health care providers are present. In the two-thumb technique, one of the two rescuers places both thumbs side by side over the lower half of the infant's sternum; the remaining fingers encircle the infant's chest and support the back. The depth of compression is adapted to the child's size. The location, rate, and depth for children older than 8 years of age are the same as for adults.

BOX 46-18

Infant Cardiopulmonary Resuscitation (CPR)*

Establish unresponsiveness by gently shaking the infant's shoulder or flicking the heel. If bystander is near, shout for help to activate the emergency response system.

Place the infant on his or her back on a firm surface.

Open the *airway* by tilting the head back into a "sniff" position (Fig. 46-7, *A*)—place one hand on infant's forehead and the fingers on the bony part of the lower jaw near the middle of the chin. Avoid hyperextending the airway, which will collapse the trachea and occlude the airway.

Check *breathing* for 3 to 5 seconds—look for chest rise; listen for air as evidence of infant breathing; feel for air coming from infant's mouth on rescuer's cheek.

Remove any mucus or emesis (if present) with fingers, bulb syringe, or catheter to clear airway.

Breaths—Give two slow breaths by covering infant's mouth with rescuer's mouth† and pinching the nose shut (depends on size) or by covering mouth and nose to maintain a good seal (Fig 46-7, *B*). Each breath should be sufficient only to make infant's chest rise. Each breath is given over 1 to 1.5 seconds each, allowing for exhalation after each breath.

Circulation—Check brachial pulse (Fig. 46-7, *C*) and other signs of circulation (breathing, coughing, or movement in response to the two breaths). If signs of circulation are present but breathing is absent or inadequate, provide rescue breathing (give one breath every 3 seconds, or about 20 breaths per minute).

If signs of circulation are present and heart rate is less than 60 beats per minute with signs of poor perfusion, begin *chest compressions* by compressing with middle and index finger of one hand on the breastbone one fingerbreadth below an imaginary line drawn across the infant's nipples (Fig. 46-7, *D*). Give five chest compressions, compressing the chest to a depth of 1 inch; after each five chest compressions, give one breath, and then resume with five chest compressions interspersed with one breath. Perform chest compressions and breathing for approximately 1 minute (Fig. 46-7, *E*).

Evaluate effectiveness of chest compressions and breathing. If alone and emergency response system has not been activated, perform 1 minute of CPR, and then carry infant to the nearest phone and activate the emergency response system. Continue chest compressions and breaths at a 5:1 ratio until the infant responds and shows signs of breathing or circulation. Continue rescue breathing—one breath every 3 seconds if signs of circulation are present but infant is not breathing on his or her own (or effectively).

Recovery position—If infant begins breathing on his or her own and there is no evidence of trauma, place on side with head resting on infant's arm and the top leg slightly bent at the knees resting on the firm surface

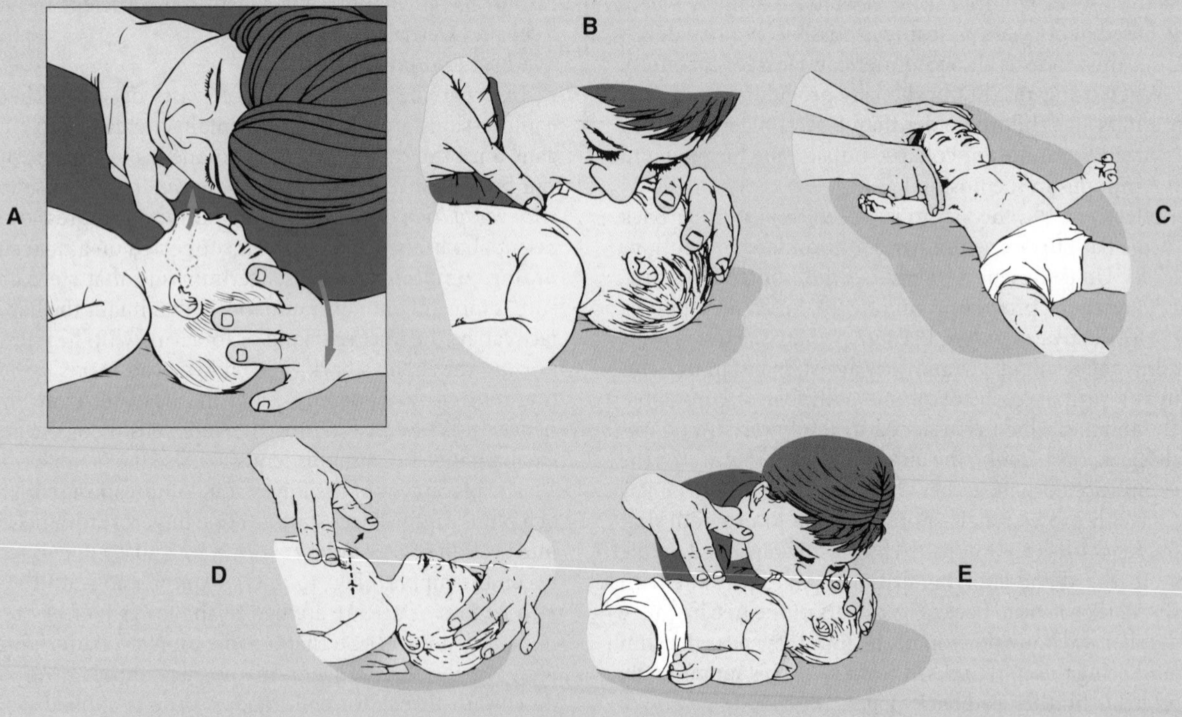

Fig. 46-7 A, Opening airway: proper positioning to open the infant's airway. **B**, Covering the nose and mouth for breathing. **C**, Checking the arm (brachial) pulse. **D**, Finding the proper location for chest compressions. **E**, Combining breathing with chest compressions.

Figures are reproduced with permission from Chandra NC, Hazinski MF: *Textbook of basic life support for healthcare providers,* Dallas, 1994, American Heart Association.

*These guidelines should not be used as substitutes for basic life support (BLS). It is important that you participate in an infant/child CPR class in your neighborhood. These guidelines do not replace the Neonatal Resuscitation Program (NRP) guidelines; special situations involving the resuscitation of newly born and preterm infants require health care providers to use appropriate clinical judgment and established, written protocols for resuscitation that fall outside the realm of infant CPR guidelines listed here.

†BLS-trained health care providers should use an appropriate-size bag and mask to deliver ventilations.

		ACTIONS		
	Objectives	**Adult (over 8 yr)**	**Child (1 to 8 yr)**	**Infant (under 1 yr)**
A. AIRWAY	1. Assessment: Determine unresponsiveness.	Tap or gently shake shoulder.		
		Say, "Are you okay?"		Speak loudly.
	2. Get help.	Activate EMS.	Shout for help. If second rescuer available, have person activate EMS.	
	3. Position the victim.	Turn on back as a unit, supporting head and neck if necessary (4-10 seconds).		
	4. Open the airway.	Head-tilt/chin-lift.		
B. BREATHING	5. Assessment: Determine breathlessness.	Maintain open airway. Place ear over mouth, observing chest. Look, listen, feel for breathing (3-5 seconds).*		
	6. Give 2 rescue breaths.	Maintain open airway.		
		Seal mouth to mouth.		Mouth to nose/mouth.
		Give 2 slow breaths. Observe chest rise. Allow lung deflation between breaths.		
		1½ to 2 seconds each	1 to 1½ seconds each	
	7. Option for obstructed airway.	a. Reposition victim's head. Try again to give rescue breaths.		
			b. Activate EMS.	
		c. Give 5 subdiaphragmatic abdominal thrusts (the Heimlich maneuver).		c. Give 5 back blows. c. Give 5 chest thrusts.
		d. Tongue-jaw lift and finger sweep.	d. Tongue-jaw lift, but finger sweep only if you see a foreign object.	
		If unsuccessful, repeat a, c, and d until successful.		
C. CIRCULATION	8. Assessment: Determine pulselessness.	Feel for carotid pulse with one hand; maintain head-tilt with the other (5-10 seconds).		Feel for brachial pulse: keep head-tilt.
CPR	Pulse absent: Begin chest compressions: 9. Landmark check.	Run middle finger along bottom edge of rib cage to notch at center (top of sternum).		Imagine a line drawn between the nipples.
	10. Hand position.	Place index finger next to finger on notch:		Place 2-3 fingers on sternum. 1 finger's width below line. Depress ½-1 in.
		Two hands next to index finger. Depress 1½-2 in.	Heel of one hand next to index finger. Depress 1-1½ in.	
	11. Compression rate.	80-100 per minute	100 per minute	At least 100 per minute
	12. Compressions to breaths.	2 breaths to every 15 compressions	1 breath to every 5 compressions	
	13. Number of cycles.	4	20 (approximately 1 minute)	
	14. Reassessment.	Feel for carotid pulse.		Feel for brachial pulse.
		If no pulse, resume CPR, starting with compressions.	If alone, activate EMS. If no pulse, resume CPR, starting with compressions.	
	Pulse present; not breathing: Begin rescue breathing.	1 breath every 5 seconds (12 per minute)	1 breath every 3 seconds (20 per minute)	

*If victim is breathing or resumes effective breathing, place in recovery position: (1) move head, shoulders, and torso simultaneously; (2) turn onto side; (3) leg not in contact with ground may be bent and knee moved forward to stabilize victim; (4) victim should not be moved in any way if trauma is suspected and should not be placed in recovery position if rescue breathing or CPR is required.

Fig. 46-8 One-rescuer CPR. (Modified from Stapleton ER et al: *BLS for healthcare providers,* Dallas, 2001, American Heart Association.)

CPR is continued at the appropriate ratio of breaths to compressions for age until signs of recovery appear. These signs include palpable peripheral pulses, return of pupils to normal size, the disappearance of mottling and cyanosis, and possibly return of spontaneous respiration.

Medications

Medications are an important adjunct to CPR, especially cardiac arrest, and are used during and after resuscitation in children. Appropriate fluid therapy is initiated immediately in the hospital or by EMS personnel during transport (see Parenteral Fluid Therapy, Chapter 45, and Shock, Chapter 48). A complete supply of emergency medications is kept and maintained in all EMS vehicles and on all hospital units. The supply is checked on a regular basis (usually once on each 8-hour shift). Resuscitation medications are listed in Table 46-3.

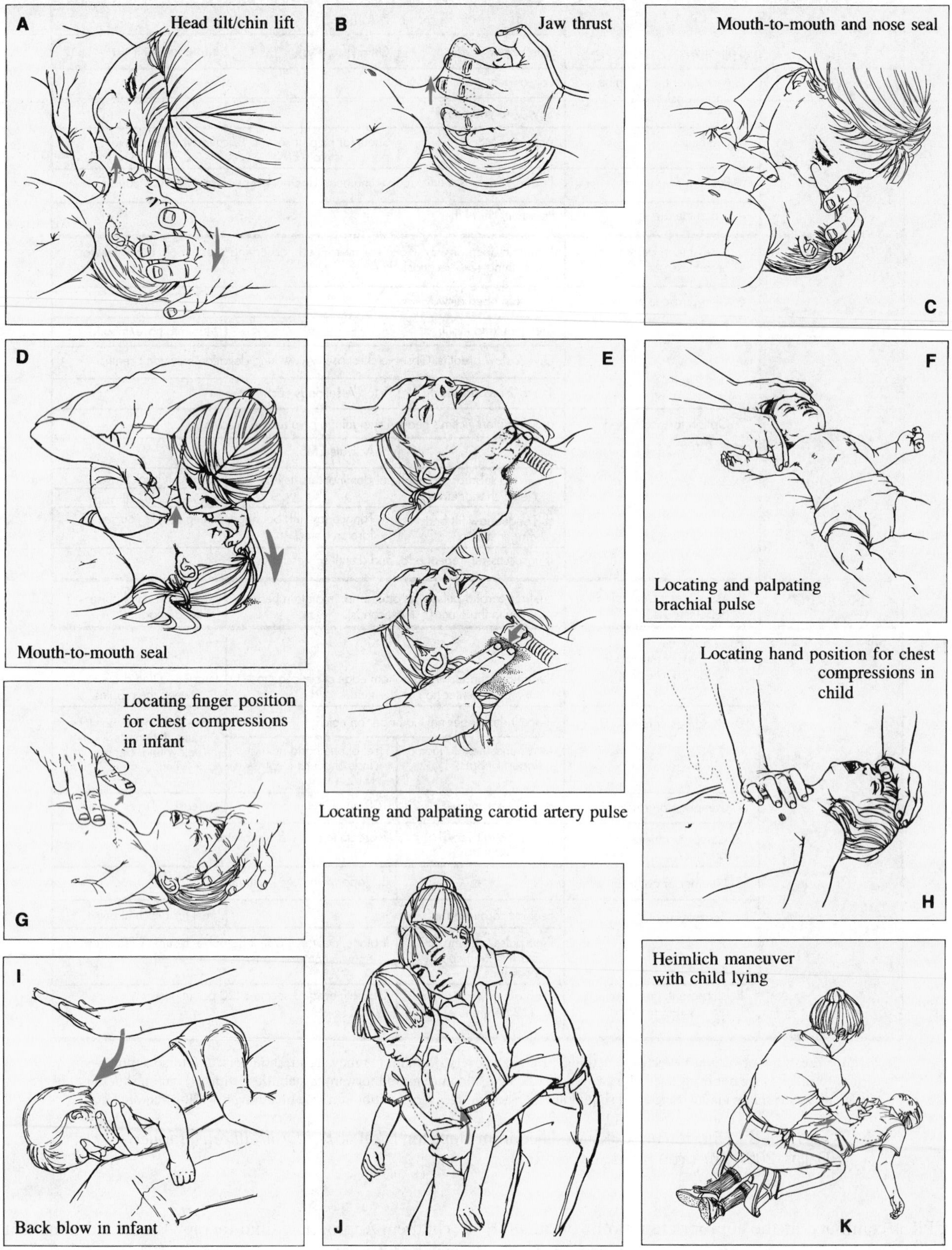

Fig. 46-9 Procedures for cardiopulmonary resuscitation, **A** to **H**, and airway obstruction, **I** to **K.** (From Chandra NC, Hazinski MF [eds]: *Textbook of basic life support for healthcare providers,* Dallas, 1997, American Heart Association.)

Table 46-3
Drugs for Pediatric Cardiopulmonary Resuscitation

DRUG/DOSE	ACTION	IMPLICATION
Epinephrine HCl* IV/IO: 0.01 mg/kg (1:10,000) Endotracheal tube (ET): 0.1 mg/kg (1:1000) Repeat doses = 0.1 ml/kg (1:1000)	Adrenergic Acts on both α- and β-receptor sites, especially heart and vascular and other smooth muscle	Most useful drug in cardiac arrest Disappears rapidly from bloodstream after injection; instill 2-3 ml saline after ET administration May produce renal vessel constriction and decreased urine formation
Sodium bicarbonate IV/IO: 1 mEq/kg Newborn: 0.5 mEq/ml 2 mg/kg	Alkalinizer Buffers pH	Infuse slowly and only when ventilation is adequate; flush with saline before and after administration
Atropine sulfate* 0.02 mg/kg/dose Minimum dose: 0.1 mg Maximum single dose: infants and children, 0.5 mg; adolescents, 1 mg	Anticholinergic-parasympatholytic Increases cardiac output, heart rate by blocking vagal stimulation in heart	Do not mix with catecholamines or calcium Used to treat bradycardia after ventilatory assessment Always provide adequate ventilation and monitor O_2 saturation Produces pupillary dilation, which constricts with light
Calcium chloride 10% 20 mg/kg IV 0.2 mg/kg/dose q10min	Electrolyte replacement Needed for maintenance of normal cardiac contractility	Used only for hypocalcemia, calcium blocker overdose, hyperkalemia, or hypermagnesemia Administer slowly; very sclerosing; administer in central vein Incompatible with phosphate solutions
Lidocaine HCl* 1 mg/kg/dose	Antidysrhythmic Inhibits nerve impulses from sensory nerves	Used for ventricular arrhythmias only
Amiodarone IV: 5 mg/kg Over 30 min followed by continuous infusion Starting at 5 mcg/kg/min May increase to maximum 10 mcg/kg/min	Antidysrhythmic agent Inhibits adrenergic stimulation; prolongs action potential and refractory period in myocardial tissues; decreased atrioventricular (AV) conduction and sinus node function	Recommended as first choice for shock-refractory ventricular tachycardia Contraindicated in severe sinus node dysfunction, marked sinus bradycardia, second- and third-degree AV block Monitor for hypotension
Adenosine 0.1 mg/kg as a rapid IV bolus Maximum initial dose: 6 mg (given over 1-2 sec) Repeat administration: double initial dose (maximum dose = 12 mg) Follow with ≥5 ml normal saline flush	Antidysrhythmic, for supraventricular tachycardia (SVT) Causes a temporary block through the atrioventricular node and interrupts reentry circuits	Administer by rapid IV push followed by saline flush May cause transient bradycardia
Naloxone (Narcan)* 0.1 mg/kg/dose† May repeat q2-3min	Reverses respiratory arrest due to excessive opiate administration	Evaluate level of pain following administration because analgesic effects of opioids are reversed with large doses of naloxone
Magnesium 25-50 mg/kg Maximum: 2 g	Inhibits calcium channels and causes smooth muscle relaxation	Given by rapid IV infusion for suspected hypomagnesemia Have calcium gluconate (IV) available as antidote
INFUSIONS		
Epinephrine HCl infusion 0.05 mcg/kg/min	Adrenergic See above	Titrated to desired hemodynamic effect

*These drugs may be administered via the endotracheal tube if an IV line is not available.
†Dose of naloxone to reverse respiratory depression without reversing analgesia from opioids is 0.5 mcg/kg in children <40 kg (American Pain Society, 1992).
IV, intravenous; *IO*, intraosseous.

Continued

Table 46-3—cont'd

Drugs for Pediatric Cardiopulmonary Resuscitation

DRUG/DOSE	ACTION	IMPLICATION
Dopamine HCl infusion 2 mcg/kg/min	Agonist Acts on alpha receptors, causing vasoconstriction	Titrated to desired hemodynamic response
Dobutamine HCl infusion 2 mcg/kg/min	Increases cardiac output Direct-acting β2-adrenergic agonist Increases contractility and heart rate	Titrated to desired hemodynamic response Little vasoconstriction, even at high rates
Lidocaine HCl infusion 10 mcg/kg/min	Antidysrhythmic Increases electrical stimulation threshold of ventricle	See above Lower infusion dose used in shock

NURSE ALERT When administering drugs during CPR (or a "code"), use a saline flush between medications to prevent drug interactions. Document all drugs, dosages, and the time and route of administration. ■

Airway Obstruction

Attempts at clearing the airway should be considered for (1) children in whom aspiration of a foreign body is witnessed or strongly suspected and (2) unconscious, nonbreathing children whose airways remain obstructed despite the usual maneuvers to open them. When aspiration is strongly suspected, the child is encouraged to continue coughing as long as the cough remains forceful. If the cough becomes ineffective, mechanical maneuvers should be used in an attempt to dislodge the object.

NURSE ALERT In a conscious choking child, attempt to relieve the obstruction only if all of the following occur:
- The child is unable to make any sounds.
- The cough becomes ineffective.
- There is increasing respiratory difficulty with stridor. ■

Blind finger sweeps are avoided in both infants and children. A combination of *back blows* (over the spine between the shoulder blades) and *chest thrusts* (on the sternum, same location as for chest compressions) is recommended to relieve the foreign body obstruction in infants (Fig. 46-10). The Heimlich maneuver or abdominal thrusts are recommended for children older than 1 year of age.

Infants

A choking infant is placed face down over the rescuer's arm with the head lower than the trunk and the head supported (Fig. 46-9, *I*). For additional support, the rescuer should support the arm firmly against the thigh. Up to five quick, sharp, back blows are delivered between the infant's shoulder blades with the heel of the rescuer's hand. Less force is required than would be applied to an adult. After delivery of the back blows, the rescuer's free hand is placed flat on the infant's back so that the infant is "sandwiched" between the two hands, making certain the neck and chin are well supported. While the rescuer maintains support with the infant's head lower than the trunk, the infant is turned and placed supine on the rescuer's thigh, where up to five quick downward chest thrusts are applied in rapid succession in the same location as external chest compressions described for CPR. Back blows and chest thrusts are continued until the object is removed or the infant becomes unconscious.

Children

The *Heimlich maneuver*, a series of *subdiaphragmatic abdominal thrusts*, is recommended for children older than 1 year of age. The maneuver creates an artificial cough that forces air, and with it the foreign body, out of the airway. The procedure is carried out with the child in a standing, sitting, or lying position (Fig. 46-9, *J* and *K*). In the conscious choking child, upward thrusts are delivered to the upper abdomen with the fisted hand at a point just below the rib cage (Fig. 46-9, *J*). To prevent damage to the internal organs, the rescuer's hands should not touch the xiphoid process of the sternum or the lower margins of the ribs. Up to five thrusts are repeated in rapid succession until the foreign body is expelled.

It is neither necessary nor desirable to squeeze or compress the arms during the procedure. It is not a punch or a bear hug. The child may vomit after relief of the obstruction and should be positioned to prevent aspiration. After breathing is restored, the child should receive medical attention and be assessed for complications.

The success of the technique is primarily a result of the obstruction occurring at the end of a maximum respiration. The victim is most likely to choke on food during inspiration; therefore the tidal volume plus expiratory reserve volume is present in the lungs. When pressure is exerted on the diaphragm by the maneuver, the food bolus is ejected with considerable force by this trapped air.

NURSE ALERT If the victim is breathing or resumes effective breathing after emergency interventions, place in the recovery position: move the head, shoulders, and torso simultaneously and turn onto the side. The leg not in contact with the ground may be bent and the knee moved forward to stabilize the victim (Fig. 46-11). The victim should not be moved in any way if trauma is suspected and should not be placed in the recovery position if rescue breathing or CPR is required. ■

Signs of life-threatening obstruction

The truly choking child *cannot speak, becomes cyanotic,* and *collapses.*

		Actions		
	Objectives	**Adult (over 8 yr)**	**Child (1 to 8 yr)**	**Infant (under 1 yr)**
CONSCIOUS VICTIM	1. Assessment: Determine airway obstruction.	Ask, "Are you choking?" Determine if victim can cough or speak.		Observe breathing difficulty, ineffective cough, no strong cry.
	2. Act to relieve obstruction.	Perform up to 5 subdiaphragmatic abdominal thrusts (Heimlich maneuver).		Give 5 back blows. Give 5 chest thrusts.
	Be persistent.	Repeat Step 2 until obstruction is relieved or victim becomes unconscious.		
VICTIM WHO BECOMES UNCONSCIOUS	3. Position the victim: call for help.	Turn on back as a unit, supporting head and neck, face up, arms by sides. Call out, "Help!" Activate EMS. If second rescuer available, have person activate EMS.		
	4. Check for foreign body.	Perform tongue-jaw lift and finger sweep.	Perform tongue-jaw lift. Remove foreign object only if you actually see it.	
	5. Give rescue breaths.	Open the airway with head-tilt/chin-lift. Try to give rescue breaths. If airway is obstructed, reposition head and try to ventilate again.		
	6. Act to relieve obstruction.	Perform up to 5 subdiaphragmatic abdominal thrusts (Heimlich maneuver).		Give 5 back blows. Give 5 chest thrusts.
	7. Be persistent.	Repeat steps 4-6 until obstruction is relieved.		
UNCONSCIOUS VICTIM	1. Assessment: Determine unresponsiveness.	Tap or gently shake shoulder. Shout, "Are you okay?"	Tap or gently shake shoulder.	
		If unresponsive, activate EMS.		
	2. Call for help: position the victim.	Turn on back as a unit, supporting head and neck, face up, arms by sides.		
			Call out for help.	
	3. Open the airway.	Head-tilt/chin-lift.		Head-tilt/chin-lift, but do not tilt too far.
	4. Assessment: Determine breathlessness.	Maintain an open airway. Ear over mouth; observe chest. Look, listen, feel for breathing (3-5 seconds).		
	5. Give rescue breaths.	Make mouth-to-mouth seal.		Make mouth-to-nose-and-mouth seal.
		Try to give rescue breaths.		
	6. If chest is not rising, try again to give rescue breaths.	Reposition head. Try rescue breaths again.		
	7. Activate the EMS system.		If airway obstruction not relieved after about 1 minute, activate EMS as rapidly as possible.	
	8. Act to relieve obstruction.	Perform up to 5 subdiaphragmatic abdominal thrusts (Heimlich maneuver).		Give 5 back blows. Give 5 chest thrusts.
	9. Check for foreign body.	Perform tongue-jaw lift and finger sweep.	Perform tongue-jaw lift. Remove foreign object only if you actually see it.	
	10. Rescue breaths.	Open the airway with head-tilt/chin-lift. Try again to give rescue breaths. If airway is obstructed, reposition head and try to ventilate again.		
	11. Be persistent.	Repeat steps 8-10 until obstruction is relieved.		

Fig. 46-10 Foreign body airway obstruction management. (Modified from Stapleton ER et al: *BLS for healthcare providers,* Dallas, 2001, American Heart Association.)

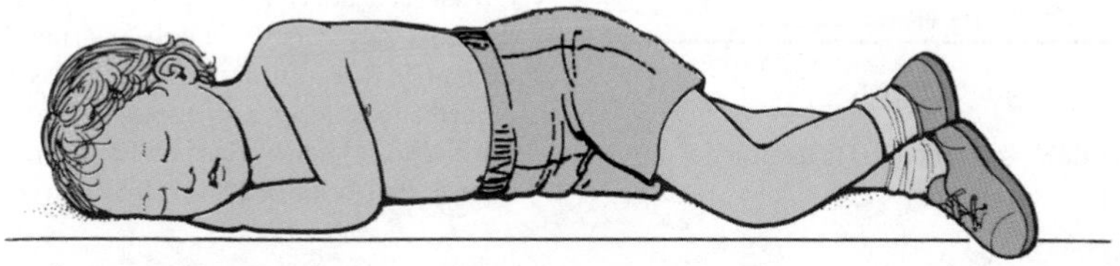

Fig. 46-11 Recovery position for child after respiratory emergency.

Key Points

- Acute infection of the respiratory tract is the most common cause of illness in infancy and childhood.
- The incidence and severity of respiratory tract infections are influenced by the infectious agents involved, the child's age, and the child's natural defenses.
- Common respiratory tract infections of childhood include nasopharyngitis, pharyngitis (including tonsillitis), influenza, and otitis media.
- Croup syndromes involve acute inflammation and variable degrees of obstruction of the epiglottis, larynx, or trachea.
- The primary goals in the care of children with croup are observation for signs of respiratory distress and relief of laryngeal obstruction.
- Common infections of the lower airways are bacterial tracheitis, bronchitis, and respiratory syncytial virus (RSV)/bronchiolitis.
- Pneumonias are classified according to site (lobar, bronchial, or interstitial) or by etiologic agent (viral, bacterial, mycoplasmal) or are associated with aspiration of foreign material.
- In tuberculosis, susceptibility to bacillus can be influenced by heredity, age, stress, poor nutrition, and intercurrent infection.
- Passive inhalation of or exposure to environmental tobacco smoke is a major environmental pollutant contributing to respiratory illness in children.
- Asthma is the leading cause of chronic illness in children.
- General therapeutic management of asthma includes allergen control, drug therapy, and sometimes hyposensitization.
- Support for the family of the child with asthma includes education about the disease and its therapy and facilitation of self-management.
- Cystic fibrosis is the most common inherited disease in children.
- The diagnosis of cystic fibrosis is based on the family history, increased sweat electrolyte content, absent pancreatic enzymes, and chronic pulmonary involvement.
- Choking and respiratory failure are respiratory emergencies that necessitate immediate intervention.
- The Heimlich maneuver is reserved for children in whom foreign body aspiration is witnessed or strongly suspected. A combination of back blows and chest thrusts is used for infants with foreign body aspiration.
- In a conscious choking child, attempts to relieve the obstruction are used only if the child is unable to make any sounds, the cough becomes ineffective, or the child has increasing respiratory difficulty with stridor.

Answer Guidelines to Critical Thinking Exercises

Croup Syndrome

1. Yes, there are sufficient data to arrive at a possible conclusion in this situation.
2. (a) Epiglottitis is a serious obstructive inflammatory process that occurs in children 2 to 5 years of age. (b) Symptoms of epiglottitis include throat pain, restlessness, drooling, and a desire to sit upright and lean forward. (c) Because epiglottitis can quickly progress to severe respiratory distress, the nurse should never examine the child's throat with a tongue depressor or take a throat culture. (d) Nursing interventions for the child with epiglottitis include monitoring the child's respiratory status, allowing the child to remain in the position that is most comfortable, having a tracheostomy tray and emergency equipment available, and assisting with insertion of an IV line and administration of antibiotics.
3. The suspicion of epiglottitis constitutes an emergency. The priority for nursing care at this time is to maintain the child's airway.
4. Yes, the evidence supports the conclusion.
5. Alternative perspectives to this situation are not apparent at this time. However, after Kim's respiratory condition stabilizes and her treatment is begun, it would be worthwhile to determine whether her immunizations are up to date. Recently, the number of cases of epiglottitis has been reduced significantly by administration of the *Haemophilus influenzae* type B conjugate vaccine.

References

Abulhosm RS et al: Passive smoke exposure impairs recovery after hospitalization for acute asthma, *Arch Pediatr Adolesc Med* 151:135-139, 1997.

American Academy of Otolaryngology—Head and Neck Surgery: Why do kids have earaches, www.entnet.org/KidsENT/earaches.cfm, 2003.

American Academy of Pediatrics: The diagnosis and management of acute otitis media, *Pediatrics* 113(5):1451-1465, 2004.

American Academy of Pediatrics, Committee on Infectious Diseases: *2003 red book: report of the Committee on Infectious Diseases,* ed 26, Elk Grove Village, IL, 2003, The Academy.

American Heart Association: Part 9: pediatric basic life support, *Resuscitation* 46:301-341, 2000.

American Heart Association, ILCOR Advisory Statement: *Use of automated external defibrillators for children: an update,* June 2003, Dallas, Texas.

American Pain Society: *Principles of analgesic use in the treatment of acute pain and chronic cancer pain,* ed 3, Glenview, IL, 1992, The Society.

Andrews JS: Otitis media and otitis externa. In Hoekelman RA et al (eds): *Primary pediatric care,* ed 4, St Louis, 2001, Mosby.

Balinsky W, Zhu CW: Pediatric cystic fibrosis: evaluating costs and genetic testing, *J Pediatr Health Care* 18:30-34, 2004.

Berman S et al: Ear, nose and throat. In Hay WW et al (eds): *Current pediatric diagnosis and treatment,* ed 15, New York, 2001, Lange Medical Books/McGraw-Hill.

Bluestone CD: Recent advances in pediatric otolaryngology: modern management of otitis media, *Pediatr Clin North Am* 36:1371-1385, 1998.

Blumer JL: Traditional management of acute otitis media. In Klein JO (ed): *Otitis media management strategies for the 21st century,* Bala Cynwyd, PA, 1998, Meniscus Educational Institute.

Capen CL, Sherman JM: Fatal asthma in children: a nurse managed model for prevention, *J Pediatr Nurs* 13(6):367-375, 1998.

Carlson L, Scudder L: Controversies in the management of pediatric otitis media, *Adv Nurse Pract,* Feb 2004, pp 73-77.

Cotter CS, Kosko JR: Effectiveness of laser-assisted myringotomy for otitis media in children, *Laryngoscope* 114(3):486-9, 2004.

Curley MA, Moloney-Harmon PA: *Critical care nursing of infants and children,* Philadelphia, 2001, WB Saunders.

Daley-Yates PT, Richards DH: Relationship between systemic corticosteroid exposure and growth velocity: development and validation of a pharmacokinetic/pharmacodynamic model, *Clin Ther* 26(11):1905-19, 2004.

DeRosa J, Grundfast KM: Surgical management of otitis media, *Pediatr Ann* 31(12):814-820, 2002.

Dowell SF et al: Acute otitis media: management and surveillance in an era of pneumococcal resistance—a report from the Drug-Resistant *Streptococcus pneumoniae* Therapeutic Working Group, *Pediatr Infect Dis J* 18: 1-9, 1999.

Eggleston PA: Asthma. In McMillan J et al (eds): *Oski's pediatrics: principles and practice,* ed 3, Philadelphia, 1999, Lippincott Williams & Wilkins.

Fost DA, Spahn JD: The leukotriene modifiers: a new class of asthma medication, *Contemp Pediatr* 15:95-107, 1998.

Hon KL et al: Clinical presentations and outcome of severe acute respiratory syndrome in children, *Lancet* 361(9370):1701-1703, 2003.

Iovino LA: New acute otitis media guidelines chart several new areas of care, *Infect Dis Child* 16(3):30-31, 2003.

Jackson PL: *Healthy people 2010* objective: reduce number and frequency of courses of antibiotics for ear infections in young children, *Pediatr Nurs* 27(6):591-593, 605, 2001.

Kaliner MA, Spector SL, Wenzel SE: Treating allergic rhinitis for better asthma control, *Patient Care N P,* May 1999, pp 2-7.

Kuiken T et al: Newly discovered coronavirus as the primary cause of severe acute respiratory syndrome, *Lancet* 362(9380):263-270, 2003.

Long SS: Respiratory syncytial virus. In McMillan J et al (eds): *Oski's pediatrics: principles and practice,* ed 3, Philadelphia, 1999, Lippincott Williams & Wilkins.

McMillan JA, Feigin RD: Group A streptococcal infections. In McMillan J et al (eds): *Oski's pediatrics: principles and practice,* ed 3, Philadelphia, 1999, Lippincott Williams & Wilkins.

Morkjaroenpong V et al: Environmental tobacco smoke exposure and nocturnal symptoms among inner-city children with asthma, *J Allergy Clin Immunol* 110(1):147-153, 2002.

National Asthma Education and Prevention Program: *Expert Panel report II: guidelines for the diagnosis and management of asthma,* pub no 97-4051, Bethesda, MD, 1997, National Heart, Lung, and Blood Institute, National Institutes of Health.

National Asthma Education and Prevention Program: Guidelines for the diagnosis and management of asthma, update on selected topics 2002, *J Allergy Clin Immunol* 110(5):S145-S219, 2002.

Neill RA: What are the indications for tonsillectomy in children? *J Fam Pract* 51:314, 2002.

O'Connor BB: SARS—The latest menacing microbe, *Nurs Spectrum* 13(12), June 16, 2003.

O'Neill P: Acute otitis media: child health. In *Clinical evidence,* London, 2001, BMJ Publishing Group, 181-188.

Palencia S: Treating the flu: available medications, *Allergy Asthma Health,* Fall 2000, pp 30-32.

Paradise JL et al: Tonsillectomy and adenotonsillectomy for recurrent throat infection in moderately affected children, *Pediatrics* 110:7-15, 2002.

Pelton SI: Otoscopy for the diagnosis of otitis media, *Pediatr Infect Dis J* 17:540-543, 1998.

Phipatanakul W et al: Mouse allergen I. The prevalence of mouse allergen in inner-city homes: the National Cooperative Inner-City Asthma Study, *J Allergy Clin Immunol* 106(6):1070-1074, 2000.

Piglansky L et al: Bacteriologic and clinical efficacy of high dose amoxicillin for therapy of acute otitis media in children, *Pediatr Infect Dis J* 22(5):405-413, 2003.

Ramsey AM: Diagnosis and treatment of the child with a draining ear, *J Pediatr Health Care* 16(4):161-169, 2002.

Redding GJ: Current concepts in adult respiratory distress syndrome in children, *Curr Opin Pediatr* 13(3):261-266, 2001.

Rosenstein BJ: Cystic fibrosis. In McMillan J et al (eds): *Oski's pediatrics: principles and practice,* ed 3, Philadelphia, 1999, Lippincott Williams & Wilkins.

Rosenwasser LJ, Nash DB: Incorporating omalizumab into asthma treatment guidelines: consensus panel recommendations, *Pharmacy Therapeutics* 28(6):400-413, 2003.

Sockrider MM: Respiratory complications of burns and smoke inhalation (respiratory burns). In McMillan J et al (eds): *Oski's pediatrics: principles and practice,* ed 3, Philadelphia, 1999, Lippincott Williams & Wilkins.

Stool SE et al: *Otitis media with effusion in young children. Clinical practice guideline,* AHCPR pub no 94-0622, 1994, Washington, DC.

Suissa S et al: Low-dose inhaled corticosteroids and the prevention of death from asthma, *N Engl J Med* 343(5):332-336, 2000.

Tan TQ et al: Clinical characteristics of children with complicated pneumonia caused by *Streptococcus pneumoniae, Pediatrics* 110(1):1-6, 2002.

Thuma PE: Pharyngitis and tonsillitis. In Hoekelman RA et al (eds): *Primary pediatric care,* ed 3, St Louis, 1997, Mosby.

Togger DA, Brenner PS: Metered dose inhalers, *Am J Nurs* 101(10):26-32, 2001.

Tucker TL: Open doors—family presence at codes, *Nurs Spectrum* 13(12DC):8-9, 2003.

Wald ER: Croup. In McMillan J et al (eds): *Oski's pediatrics: principles and practice,* ed 3, Philadelphia, 1999, Lippincott Williams & Wilkins.

Winkelstein ML et al: Factors associated with medication self-administration in children with asthma, *Clin Pediatr* 39(6):337-345, 2000.

Unit 11

47 Gastrointestinal Dysfunction

LEARNING OBJECTIVES

On completion of this chapter the reader will be able to:

- Describe the characteristics of infants that affect their ability to adapt to fluid loss or gain.
- Formulate a plan of care for the infant with acute diarrhea.
- Compare and contrast the inflammatory diseases of the gastrointestinal tract.
- Describe the nursing care of the child with hepatitis.
- Formulate a plan for teaching parents preoperative and postoperative care of the child with a cleft lip or palate.
- Formulate a plan of care for the child with an obstructive disorder.
- Identify nutritional therapies for the child with a malabsorption syndrome.

ELECTRONIC RESOURCES

Additional information related to the content in Chapter 47 can be found on

the companion website at evolve
http://evolve.elsevier.com/Wong/maternal/
- NCLEX Review Questions
- Case Study–Appendicitis
- Case Study–Acute Diarrhea (Gastroenteritis)
- WebLinks

or the interactive student CD-ROM
Activities for Chapter 47 include the following:
- NCLEX Review Questions
- Case Study–Cleft Lip and Palate
- Case Study–Dehydration and Diarrhea
- Nursing Care Plan–The Child with Diarrhea (Gastroenteritis)
- Nursing Care Plan–The Child with Cleft Lip and/or Palate

NUTRITIONAL DISTURBANCES

Vitamin Disturbances

Although true vitamin deficiencies are rare in the United States, subclinical deficiencies are commonly seen in population subgroups in which either maternal or child dietary intake of foods containing adequate amounts of vitamins is imbalanced. Vitamin D–deficiency rickets, once rarely seen because of vitamin D–fortified milk, has increased. Populations at risk include (1) children breastfed by mothers with an inadequate intake of vitamin D or breastfed longer than 6 months without adequate maternal vitamin D intake or supplementation; (2) children who are exposed to minimal sunlight because of their particular clothing, religious, or cultural beliefs, housing in areas of high pollution, or dark skin pigmentation; (3) those with diets that are low in sources of vitamin D and calcium; and (4) individuals who use milk products not supplemented with vitamin D (e.g., yogurt, raw cow's milk) as the primary source of milk. Thus the American Academy of Pediatrics (2003a) now recommends that infants who are exclusively breastfed begin to receive 200 international units of vitamin D per day by age 2 months. Furthermore, children who have minimal sun exposure, who do not consume at least 500 ml of vitamin D–fortified milk per day, or who are not taking a vitamin supplement with vitamin D should take vitamin D supplements daily to prevent rickets and vitamin D deficiency. The 200 international units of vitamin D may be obtained by taking a multivitamin supplement containing 400 international units of vitamin D per milliliter or per tablet (American Academy of Pediatrics, 2003a). Inadequate maternal ingestion of cobalamin (vitamin B_{12}) may contribute to infant neurologic impairment when exclusive breastfeeding (past 6 months) is the only source of the infant's nutrition (MMWR Weekly, 2003).

Children may also be at risk secondary to disorders or their treatment. For example, vitamin deficiencies of the fat-soluble vitamins A and D may occur in malabsorptive disorders. Preterm infants may develop rickets in the second month of life as a result of inadequate intake of vitamin D, calcium, and phosphoros. Children receiving high doses of salicylates, such as for rheumatoid arthritis, may have impaired vitamin C storage. Environmental tobacco smoke exposure has been implicated with decreased concentrations of ascorbate in children; therefore increased intake of sources of vitamin C should be encouraged even in children minimally exposed to environmental tobacco smoke (Preston et al, 2003). Children with chronic illnesses resulting in anorexia, decreased food intake, or possible nutrient malabsorption as a result of multiple medications should be carefully evaluated for adequate vitamin and mineral intake in some form (parenteral or enteral).

Vitamin A deficiency correlates with increased morbidity and mortality rates in children with measles. Complications from diarrhea and infections are often increased in infants and children with vitamin A deficiency. The American Academy of Pediatrics (2003a) recommends that vitamin A supplementation be considered in children hospitalized with measles and associated complications (diarrhea, croup, pneumonia), especially children between 6 months and 2 years of age.

Of particular concern is the overuse of vitamins as a part of complementary and alternative medicine.* One recent survey found that a relatively small group of parents routinely gave their children megavitamin therapy; however, the researcher recommends further research to ascertain a more realistic number of children using multivitamin preparations (Loman, 2003). There is concern among health care workers that terms often used to market supplements, such as *megavitamins,* may mislead parents regarding the actual benefits (or harm) of such therapies. The intention herein is not to discredit the use of complementary and alternative medicine such as vitamin supplements; rather, it is to ensure safety and efficacy in children who may experience inadvertent harm.

The use of various herbal therapies, or intake of herbs, is also becoming more popular; many of these have been a part of medicine for centuries and are beneficial in some cases. Herbs known to have adverse effects in children include ephedra, comfrey, and pennyroyal; some herbs may not be harmful taken alone but may counteract or potentiate prescription medications when taken together (Loman, 2003). Parents should be fully cognizant of the use of herbs to ensure that there is more benefit than potential harm in the ingredient being used. Health care workers also need to be knowledgeable of the benefits or potential harm in herbs to appropriately counsel parents and address their concerns. Little research has been performed in children on many over-the-counter herbal medicines yet some herbs are known to cause harm in children (Kemper & Gardiner, 2004; Lanski et al, 2003; Loman, 2003). Parents should be cautioned not to exceed the upper limits of vitamin intake according to the new Dietary Reference Intakes (see Dietary Reference Intakes, p. 1486, and recommended dietary allowances in Appendix G.

An excessive dose of a vitamin is generally defined as 10 or more times the recommended dietary allowance (RDA), although the fat-soluble vitamins, especially A and D, tend to cause toxic reactions at lower doses. With the addition of vitamins to commercially prepared foods, the potential for hypervitaminosis has increased, especially when combined with the excessive use of vitamin supplements. Hypervitaminosis of vitamins A and D presents the greatest problems, because these fat-soluble vitamins are stored in the body. Vitamin D is the most likely of all vitamins to cause toxic reactions in relatively small overdoses. The water-soluble vitamins, primarily niacin, vitamin B_6, and vitamin C, can also cause toxicity. Poor outcomes in infants have been associated with megavitamin therapy, namely a fatal hypermagnesemia, as a result of high doses of magnesium oxide (McGuire, Kulkarni, & Baden, 2000), and severe anemia and thrombocytopenia resulting from megadoses of vitamin A (Perrotta et al, 2002).

One vitamin supplement that is recommended for all women of childbearing age is a daily dose of 0.4 mg of folic acid, the usual RDA. Folic acid taken before conception and during early pregnancy can reduce the risk of neural tube defects such as spina bifida by as much as 70%. Drugs such as oral contraceptives and antidepressants may decrease folic acid absorption; thus adolescent females taking such medications should consider supplementation. Factors that may influence iron absorption are listed in Box 47-1.

Deficiencies and excesses of vitamins A, B complex, C, D, E, and K are summarized in Table 47-1, and the RDAs are listed in Appendix G .

BOX 47-1

Factors That Affect Iron Absorption

Increase

Acidity (low pH)—Administer iron between meals (gastric hydrochloric acid)
Ascorbic acid (vitamin C)—Administer iron with juice, fruit, or multivitamin preparation
Vitamin A
Calcium
Tissue need
Meat, fish, poultry
Cooking in cast iron pots

Decrease

Alkalinity (high pH)—Avoid any antacid preparation
Phosphates—Milk is unfavorable vehicle for iron administration
Phytates—Found in cereals
Oxalates—Found in many fruits and vegetables (plums, currants, green beans, spinach, sweet potatoes, tomatoes)
Tannins—Found in tea, coffee
Tissue saturation
Malabsorptive disorders
Disturbances that cause diarrhea or steatorrhea
Infection

Mineral Disturbances

A number of minerals are essential nutrients. The *macrominerals* refer to those with daily requirements greater than 100 mg and include calcium, phosphorus, magnesium,

Text continued on p. 1481.

*Helpful Web sites for health care and consumer information concerning herbs include the National Center for Complementary and Alternative Medicine: www.nccam.nih.gov; the American Botanical Council: www.herbalgram.org; and the Herb Research Foundation: www.herb.org.

Table 47-1

Vitamins and Their Nutritional Significance

PHYSIOLOGIC FUNCTIONS/SOURCES	RESULTS OF DEFICIENCY OR EXCESS	NURSING CONSIDERATIONS
VITAMIN A (RETINOL)*		
Functions Necessary component in formation of pigment rhodopsin (visual purple) Formation and maintenance of epithelial tissue Normal bone growth and tooth development Needed for growth and spermatogenesis Involved in thyroxine formation Antioxidant	**Deficiency** Night blindness Keratinization (hardening and scaling) of epithelium Xerophthalmia (hardening and scaling of cornea and conjunctiva) Phrynoderma (toad skin) Drying of respiratory, gastrointestinal, and genitourinary tracts Defective tooth enamel Retarded growth Impaired bone formation Decreased thyroxine formation Decreased resistance to infections	Encourage foods rich in vitamin A, such as whole cow's milk. As milk consumption decreases, encourage foods rich in vitamin A. Ensure adequate intake in preterm infants. Advise parents of safe use of supplements in child with measles.
Sources *Natural form*—Liver, kidney, fish oils, milk and nonskim milk products, egg yolk *Provitamin A (carotene)*—Carrots, sweet potatoes, squash, apricots, spinach, collards, broccoli, cabbage, artichokes	**Excess** Early signs—Irritability, anorexia, pruritus, fissures at corners of nose and lips *Later signs*—Hepatomegaly, jaundice, retarded growth, poor weight gain, thickening of the cortex of long bones with pain and fragility, hard tender lumps in extremities and occiput of the skull Can cause birth defects if excessive maternal intake NOTE: Overdose results from ingestion of large quantities of the vitamin only, not the provitamin; large amounts of carotene (carotenemia) cause yellow or orange discoloration of the skin (not the sclera, urine, or feces as in jaundice) but none of the above symptoms.	Emphasize correct use of vitamin supplements and potential hazards of excess. Investigate child's dietary habits to calculate approximate intake; if excessive, remove supplemental source (e.g., daily feeding of liver). Advise parents of the benign nature of carotenemia; treatment is avoidance of excess pigmented fruits or vegetables, especially carrots; skin color returns to normal in 2 to 6 weeks.
VITAMIN B_1 (THIAMIN)‡		
Functions Coenzyme (with phosphorus) in carbohydrate metabolism Needed for healthy nervous system Digestion and normal appetite	**Deficiency** *Gastrointestinal*—Anorexia, constipation, indigestion *Neurologic*—Apathy, fatigue, emotional instability, polyneuritis, tenderness of calf muscles, partial anesthesia, muscle weakness, paresthesia, hyperesthesia, decreased or absent tendon reflexes, convulsions, coma (in infants) *Cardiovascular*—Palpitations, cardiac failure, peripheral vasodilation, edema	
Sources Pork, beef, liver, legumes, nuts, whole or enriched grains and cereals, green vegetables, fruits, milk, brown rice	**Excess** Headache Irritability Insomnia Rapid pulse Weakness	**Vitamin B complex** Encourage foods rich in B vitamins. Stress proper cooking and storage techniques to preserve potency, such as minimum cooking of vegetables in small amount of liquid, storage of milk in opaque container.

*Fat soluble.
‡Water soluble

Table 47-1

Vitamins and Their Nutritional Significance—cont'd

PHYSIOLOGIC FUNCTIONS/SOURCES	RESULTS OF DEFICIENCY OR EXCESS	NURSING CONSIDERATIONS
VITAMIN B_1 (THIAMIN)—cont'd		**Vitamin B complex—cont'd** Advise against fad diets that severely restrict groups of food, such as vegetarianism (vegans or macrobiotics). Explore need for vitamin supplements when dieting, when using goat milk exclusively for infant feeding (deficient in folic acid), or when the breastfeeding mother is a strict vegetarian (vitamin B_{12}). Emphasize correct use of vitamin supplements and potential hazards of excess.
VITAMIN B_2 (RIBOFLAVIN)‡		
Functions Coenzyme (with phosphorus) in carbohydrate, protein, and fat metabolism Maintains healthy skin, especially around mouth, nose, and eyes	**Deficiency** Ariboflavinosis *Lips*—Cheilosis (fissures at corners of lips), perlèche (inflammation at corners of lips) *Tongue*—Glossitis *Nose*—Irritation and cracks at nasal angle *Eyes*—Burning, itching, tearing, photophobia, corneal vascularization, cataracts *Skin*—Seborrheic dermatitis, delayed wound healing and tissue repair	Same as vitamin B complex
Sources Milk and its products, eggs, organs (liver, kidney, heart), enriched cereals, some green leafy vegetables,† legumes	**Excess** Paresthesia, pruritus	
NIACIN (NICOTINIC ACID, NICOTINAMIDE)‡		
Functions Coenzyme (with riboflavin) in protein and fat metabolism Needed for healthy nervous system and skin and for normal digestion May lower cholesterol	**Deficiency** Pellagra *Oral*—Stomatitis, glossitis *Cutaneous*—Scaly dermatitis on exposed areas *Gastrointestinal*—Anorexia, weight loss, diarrhea, fatigue *Neurologic*—Apathy, anxiety, confusion, depression, dementia Death	Same as vitamin B complex If used as hypolipidemic agent, stress safe dosage to prevent child's accidental ingestion.
Sources Meat, poultry, fish, peanuts, beans, peas, whole or enriched grains (except corn and rice) Milk and its products are sources of tryptophan (60 mg tryptophan = 1 mg niacin)	**Excess** Release of histamine, a vasodilator (flushing, decreased blood pressure, increased cerebral blood flow; aggravates asthma) Dermatologic problems (pruritus, rash, hyperkeratosis, acanthosis nigricans) Increased gastric acidity (aggravates peptic ulcer disease) Hepatotoxicity Increased serum uric acid levels Elevated plasma glucose levels Certain cardiac arrhythmias	

†Green leafy vegetables include spinach, broccoli, kale, turnip greens, mustard greens, collards, dandelion greens, and beet greens.
‡Water soluble

Continued

Table 47-1

Vitamins and Their Nutritional Significance—cont'd

PHYSIOLOGIC FUNCTIONS/SOURCES	RESULTS OF DEFICIENCY OR EXCESS	NURSING CONSIDERATIONS
VITAMIN B_6 (PYRIDOXINE)‡		
Functions Coenzyme in protein and fat metabolism Needed for formation of antibodies and hemoglobin Needed for utilization of copper and iron Aids in conversion of tryptophan to niacin	**Deficiency** Scaly dermatitis, weight loss, anemia, retarded growth, irritability, convulsions, peripheral neuritis	Same as vitamin B complex Stress proper cooking and storing techniques to preserve potency. Cook food covered in small amount of water. Do not soak food in water. Store in light-resistant container.
Sources Meats, especially liver and kidney, cereal grains (wheat, corn), yeast, soybeans, peanuts, tuna, chicken, salmon	**Excess** Peripheral nervous system toxicity (unsteady gait, numb feet and hands, clumsiness of hands, sometimes perioral numbness) May cause peptic ulcer disease or seizures	
FOLIC ACID (FOLACIN; REDUCED FORM CALLED FOLINIC ACID OR CITROVORUM FACTOR)‡		
Functions Coenzyme for single-carbon transfer (purines, thymine, hemoglobin) Necessary for formation of red blood cells May prevent neural tube defects (i.e., myelomeningocele)	**Deficiency** Macrocytic anemia, bone marrow depression, glossitis, intestinal malabsorption	Same as vitamin B complex Stress proper cooking and storing techniques to preserve potency: Cook food covered in small amount of water. Do not soak food in water. Store in light-resistant container. Women of childbearing age should supplement to prevent neural tube defects.
Sources Green leafy vegetables,† cabbage, asparagus, liver, kidneys, nuts, eggs, whole grain cereals, legumes, bananas	**Excess** Rare because megadoses not available over the counter May cause insomnia and irritability	
VITAMIN B_{12} (COBALAMIN)‡		
Functions Coenzyme in protein synthesis; indirect effect on formation of red blood cells (particularly on formation of nucleic acids and folic acid metabolism) Needed for normal functioning of nervous tissue	**Deficiency** Pernicious anemia (one form of deficiency from absence of intrinsic factor in gastric secretions) General signs of severe anemia Lemon-yellow tinge to skin Spinal cord degeneration Delayed brain growth	Same as vitamin B complex
Sources Meat, liver, kidney, fish, shellfish, poultry, milk, eggs, cheese, nutritional yeast, sea vegetables	**Excess** Rare	
BIOTIN‡		
Functions Coenzyme in carbohydrate, protein, and fat metabolism Interrelated with functions of other B vitamins	**Deficiency** Deficiency is uncommon because synthesized by bacterial flora	Same as vitamin B complex

‡Water soluble
†Green leafy vegetables include spinach, broccoli, kale, turnip greens, mustard greens, collards, dandelion greens, and beet greens.

Table 47-1

Vitamins and Their Nutritional Significance—cont'd

PHYSIOLOGIC FUNCTIONS/SOURCES	RESULTS OF DEFICIENCY OR EXCESS	NURSING CONSIDERATIONS
BIOTIN—cont'd		
Sources Liver, kidney, egg yolk, tomatoes, legumes, nuts	**Excess** Unknown	
PANTOTHENIC ACID‡		
Functions Coenzyme in carbohydrate, protein, and fat metabolism Synthesis of amino acids, fatty acids, and steroids	**Deficiency** Deficiency is uncommon because of its multiple food sources and synthesis by bacterial flora	Same as vitamin B complex
Sources Liver, kidney, heart, salmon, eggs, vegetables, legumes, whole grains	**Excess** Minimum toxicity (occasional diarrhea and water retention)	
VITAMIN C (ASCORBIC ACID)‡		
Functions Essential for collagen formation Increases absorption of iron for hemoglobin formation Enhances conversion of folic acid to folinic acid Affects cholesterol synthesis and conversion of proline to hydroxyproline Probably a coenzyme in metabolism of tyrosine and phenylalanine May play role in hydroxylation of adrenal steroids May have stimulating effect on phagocytic activity of leukocytes and formation of antibodies Antioxidant agent (spares other vitamins from oxidation)	**Deficiency** Scurvy *Skin*—Dry, rough, petechiae, perifollicular hyperkeratotic papules (raised areas around hair follicles) *Musculoskeletal*—Bleeding muscles and joints, pseudoparalysis from pain, swelling of joints, costochondral beading (scorbutic rosary) *Gums*—Spongy, friable, swollen, bleed easily, bluish red or black, teeth loosen and fall out *General disposition*—Irritable, anorexic, apprehensive, in pain, refuses to move, assumes semi-froglike position when supine (scorbutic pose) Signs of anemia Decreased wound healing Increased susceptibility to infection	Encourage foods rich in vitamin C. Investigate infant's diet for sources of vitamin, especially when cow's milk is principal source of nutrition. Stress proper cooking and storing techniques to preserve potency: Wash vegetables quickly; do not soak in water. Cook vegetables in covered pot with minimum water and for short time; avoid copper or cast iron cookware. Do not add baking soda to cooking water. Use fresh fruits and vegetables as soon as possible; store in refrigerator. Store juice in airtight, opaque container. Wrap cut fruit or eat soon after exposing to air.
Sources Citrus fruits, strawberries, tomatoes, potatoes, cabbage, broccoli, cauliflower, spinach, papaya, mango, cantaloupe, watermelon, enriched fruit juice	**Excess** Diarrhea Increased excretion of uric acid and acidification of urine (may cause urate precipitation and formation of oxalate stones)	In caring for child with scurvy: Position for comfort and rest. Handle very gently and minimally. Administer analgesics as needed. Prevent infection. Provide good oral care. Provide soft, bland diet. Emphasize rapid recovery when vitamin is replaced. Emphasize correct use of vitamin supplement and potential hazards of excess. Identify groups at risk for vitamin C supplements (e.g., those with thalassemia or those receiving anticoagulant or aminoglycoside antibiotic therapy).

‡Water soluble

Continued

Table 47-1

Vitamins and Their Nutritional Significance—cont'd

PHYSIOLOGIC FUNCTIONS/SOURCES	RESULTS OF DEFICIENCY OR EXCESS	NURSING CONSIDERATIONS
VITAMIN C (ASCORBIC ACID)—cont'd	**Excess—cont'd** Hemolysis Impaired leukocytosis activity Damage to beta cells of pancreas and decreased insulin production Reproductive failure "Rebound scurvy" from withdrawal of large amounts	
VITAMIN D_2 (ERGOCALCIFEROL) AND VITAMIN D_3 (CHOLECALCIFEROL)*		
Functions Absorption of calcium and phosphorus and decreased renal excretion of phosphorus	**Deficiency** Rickets *Head*—Craniotabes (softening of cranial bones, prominence of frontal bones), deformed shape (skull flat and depressed toward middle), delayed closure of fontanels *Chest*—Rachitic rosary (enlargement of costochondral junction of ribs), Harrison groove (horizontal depression in lower portion of rib cage), pigeon chest (sharp protrusion of sternum) *Spine*—Kyphosis, scoliosis, lordosis *Abdomen*—Pot belly, constipation *Extremities*—Bowing of arms and legs, knock-knee, saber shins, instability of hip joints, pelvic deformity, enlargement of epiphyses at ends of long bones *Teeth*—Delayed calcification, especially of permanent teeth *Rachitic tetany*—Seizures	Encourage foods rich in vitamin D, especially fortified cow's milk. In breastfed infants, encourage use of vitamin D supplements if maternal diet is inadequate or if infant is exposed to minimal sunlight. In caring for child with rickets: Maintain good body alignment. Reposition frequently to prevent decubiti and respiratory infection. Handle very gently and minimally. Prevent infection. Institute seizure precautions. Have 10% calcium gluconate available in case of tetany. Observe for possibility of overdose from supplements. If prescribed, supervise proper use of orthopedic splints and braces. Same as vitamin A; may include low-calcium diet during initial therapy
Sources Direct sunlight Cod liver oil, herring, mackerel, salmon, tuna, sardines Enriched food sources—milk, milk products, enriched cereals, margarine, breads, many breakfast drinks	**Excess** *Acute*—Vomiting, dehydration, fever, abdominal cramps, bone pain, convulsions, coma *Chronic*—Lassitude, mental slowness, anorexia, failure to thrive, thirst, urinary urgency, polyuria, vomiting, diarrhea, abdominal cramps, bone pain, pathologic fractures *Calcification of soft tissue*—Kidneys, lungs, adrenal glands, vessels (hypertension), heart, gastric lining, tympanic membrane (deafness) Osteoporosis of long bones Elevated serum levels of calcium and phosphorus	
VITAMIN E (TOCOPHEROL)*		
Functions Production of red blood cells and protection from hemolysis Muscle and liver integrity Coenzyme factor in tissue respiration Minimizes oxidation of polyunsaturated fatty acids and vitamins A and C in intestinal tract and tissues	**Deficiency** Hemolytic anemia from hemolysis caused by shortened life of red blood cells, especially in premature infants; focal necrosis of tissues Causes infertility in rats but not in humans (does not increase human male virility or potency)	Initiate early feeding in premature infants; may need supplementation.

*Fat soluble

Table 47-1

Vitamins and Their Nutritional Significance—cont'd

PHYSIOLOGIC FUNCTIONS/SOURCES	RESULTS OF DEFICIENCY OR EXCESS	NURSING CONSIDERATIONS
VITAMIN E (TOCOPHEROL)*—cont'd		
Sources Vegetable oils, wheat germ oil, milk, egg yolk, fish, whole grains, nuts, legumes, spinach, broccoli	**Excess** Little is known; less toxic than other fat-soluble vitamins	
VITAMIN K*		
Functions Catalyst for production of prothrombin and blood-clotting factors II, VII, IX, and X by the liver	**Deficiency** Hemorrhage	Administer prophylactically to all newborns. Other indications include intestinal disease, lack of bile, prolonged antibiotic therapy; may be used in management of blood-clotting time when anticoagulants such as warfarin (Coumadin) and dicumarol (bishydroxycoumarin), which are vitamin K antagonists, are used.
Sources Pork, liver, green leafy vegetables,† cabbage, tomatoes, egg yolk, cheese	**Excess** Hemolytic anemia in individuals who are deficient in glucose-6-phosphate dehydrogenase	

*Fat soluble

†Green leafy vegetables include spinach, broccoli, kale, turnip greens, mustard greens, collards, dandelion greens, and beet greens.

sodium, potassium, chloride, and sulfur. *Microminerals,* or trace elements, have daily requirements of less than 100 mg and include several essential minerals whose exact role in nutrition is still unclear. The greatest concern with minerals is deficiency, especially iron, calcium, phosphorus, magnesium, and zinc. Low levels of zinc can cause nutritional failure to thrive.

The regulation of mineral balance in the body is a complex process. Dietary extremes of mineral intake can cause a number of mineral-mineral interactions that could result in unexpected deficiencies or excesses. For example, excessive amounts of one mineral, such as zinc, can result in a deficiency of another mineral, such as copper, even if sufficient amounts of copper are ingested. Thus megadose intake of one mineral may cause an inadvertent deficiency of another essential mineral by blocking its absorption in the blood or intestinal wall, or by competing with binding sites on protein carriers needed for metabolism.

Deficiencies can also occur when various substances in the diet interact with minerals. For example, iron, zinc, and calcium can form insoluble complexes with phytates or oxalates (substances found in plant proteins), which impair the bioavailability of the mineral. This type of interaction is important in vegetarian diets because plant foods such as soy are high in phytates. Contrary to popular opinion, spinach is not an ideal source of iron or calcium because of its high oxylate content.

Deficiencies and excesses of the essential macrominerals and microminerals are summarized in Table 47-2. General nursing considerations are discussed on p. 486, and specific interventions are discussed in Table 47-2.

Vegetarian Diets

Vegetarian diets are becoming more popular in the United States because people are concerned about hypertension, obesity, cardiovascular disease, and cancers of the stomach, intestine, and colon. A survey of adolescent vegetarians indicated that this group was more likely than nonvegetarians to meet the *Healthy People 2010* objectives for overall nutrient consumption (Perry et al, 2002). Although there are many health benefits to vegetarian diets in adults, the importance of such diets and their relationship to potential nutritional deficiencies in children cannot be overemphasized. The stricter the vegetarian diet, the more difficult it becomes to ensure adequate nutrition for infants and children.

The major types of vegetarianism are as follows:

- **Lacto-ovo vegetarians** exclude meat from their diet but consume dairy products and, rarely, fish.
- **Lacto-vegetarians** exclude meat and eggs but drink milk.
- **Pure vegetarians (vegans)** eliminate any food of animal origin, including milk and eggs.
- **Zen macrobiotics** are even more restrictive than pure vegetarians; small amounts of fruits, vegetables, and legumes are allowed.
- **Semivegetarians** consume a lacto-ovo vegetarian diet with some fish and poultry; this is an increasingly popular form

Text continued on p. 1486.

Table 47-2

Minerals and Their Nutritional Significance

PHYSIOLOGIC FUNCTIONS/SOURCES	RESULTS OF DEFICIENCY OR EXCESS	NURSING CONSIDERATIONS
CALCIUM*		
Functions Bone and tooth development and maintenance (in combination with phosphorus) Muscle contractions, especially the heart Blood clotting Absorption of vitamin B_{12} Enzyme activation Nerve conduction Integrity of intracellular cement substances and various membranes	**Deficiency** Rickets Tetany Impaired growth, especially of bones and teeth Osteoporosis	Encourage foods rich in calcium, especially dairy products. Caution that oxalates in leafy vegetables (spinach), oxalates in chocolates, and a high phosphorus intake (especially from carbonated beverages) can decrease calcium absorption. Discourage use of whole cow's milk in newborns because the phosphorus/calcium ratio favors excretion of calcium. Advise against fad diets, especially those that restrict dairy products. Emphasize correct use of calcium supplements, especially the possible interaction between megadoses of calcium and resulting deficiency states of other minerals.
Sources Dairy products, egg yolk, sardines, canned salmon with bones, green leafy vegetables† (except spinach), soybeans, dried beans, peas	**Excess** Drowsiness, extreme lethargy Impaired absorption of other minerals (iron, zinc, manganese) Calcium deposits in tissues (renal failure)	
CHLORIDE*		
Functions Acid-base and fluid balance Enzyme activation in saliva Component of hydrochloric acid in stomach	**Deficiency** Acid-base disturbances (hypochloremic alkalosis, dehydration); occurs mostly in combination with sodium loss	Deficiency and excess are unusual; most diets supply adequate chloride (usually in combination with sodium). Disease states such as excessive vomiting can necessitate chloride replacement.
Sources Salt, meat, eggs, dairy products, many prepared and preserved foods	**Excess** Acid-base disturbance	
CHROMIUM†		
Functions Involved in glucose metabolism and energy production	**Deficiency** Possible abnormal glucose metabolism	No specific recommendations are needed.
Sources Meat (liver, dark meat of chicken), cheese, whole-grain breads and cereals, legumes, peanuts, brewer's yeast, vegetable oils	**Excess** Unknown	
COPPER†		
Functions Production of hemoglobin Essential component of several enzyme systems	**Deficiency** Anemia, leukopenia, neutropenia	Deficiency from inadequate food sources is less likely than from excess intake of other minerals, especially zinc and possibly iron; therefore emphasize the correct use of any vitamin supplement. Caution against cooking acidic foods in unlined copper pots, which can lead to chronic and toxic accumulation of copper.

*Macrominerals—required intake >100 mg/day.
†Microminerals or trace elements—required intake <100 mg/day.

Table 47-2

Minerals and Their Nutritional Significance—cont'd

PHYSIOLOGIC FUNCTIONS/SOURCES	RESULTS OF DEFICIENCY OR EXCESS	NURSING CONSIDERATIONS
COPPER—cont'd		
Sources Organ meats, oysters, nuts, seeds, legumes, corn oil margarine	**Excess** Severe vomiting and diarrhea Hemolytic anemia	
FLUORIDE†		
Functions Formation of caries-resistant teeth Strong bone development	**Deficiency** Increased susceptibility to tooth decay	In areas with optimally fluoridated water, encourage sufficient intake to supply recommended amount of fluoride. In areas of unfluoridated water or when ready-to-use formula, bottled water, or breast milk is used, stress the importance of fluoride supplements. In areas with excess fluoride in the water, consider the use of bottled water in drinking and cooking to reduce the fluoride intake to safe levels. Fluoride has the narrowest range of safe and adequate intake; therefore stress the importance of storing supplements in a safe area.
Sources Fluoridated water and foods or beverages prepared with fluoridated water, fish, tea, commercially prepared chicken for infants	**Excess** Fluorosis (mottling or pitting of enamel) Severe bone deformities	
IODINE†		
Functions Production of thyroid hormone Normal reproduction	**Deficiency** Goiter (enlarged thyroid from decreased thyroxine formation)	Encourage use of iodized salt for individuals living far from the sea. If iodine preparations are in the home, stress the importance of safe storage.
Sources Seafood, kelp, iodized salt, sea salt, enriched bread, milk (from dairy processing)	**Excess** Unknown from food sources; may occur from ingestion of iodine preparations, such as saturated solutions of potassium iodide	
IRON†		
Functions Formation of hemoglobin and myoglobin Essential part of several enzymes and proteins	**Deficiency** Anemia	Discourage excessive milk consumption, especially more than 1 L per day (milk is a very poor source of iron). If iron supplements are prescribed, teach parents factors that affect absorption (see Box 47-1). Stress the importance of storing iron supplements in a safe area.
Sources Liver, especially pork, followed by calf, beef, and chicken; kidney, red meat, poultry, shellfish, whole grains, iron-enriched infant formula and cereal, enriched cereals and bread, legumes, nuts, seeds, green leafy vegetables (except spinach), dried fruits, potatoes, molasses, tofu, prune juice	**Excess** Hemosiderosis (excess iron storage in various tissues of the body, especially the spleen, liver, lymph glands, heart, and pancreas) Hemochromatosis (excess iron storage with cellular damage)	

†Microminerals or trace elements—required intake <100 mg/day.

Continued

Table 47-2

Minerals and Their Nutritional Significance—cont'd

PHYSIOLOGIC FUNCTIONS/SOURCES	RESULTS OF DEFICIENCY OR EXCESS	NURSING CONSIDERATIONS
MAGNESIUM*		
Functions Bone and tooth formation Production of proteins Nerve conduction to muscles Activation of enzymes needed for carbohydrate and protein metabolism	**Deficiency** Tremors, spasm Irregular heartbeat Muscular weakness Lower extremity cramps Convulsions, delirium	
Sources Whole grains, nuts, soybeans, meat, green leafy vegetables (uncooked), tea, cocoa, raisins	**Excess** Nervous system disturbances caused by imbalance in calcium/magnesium ratio	Deficiency and excess are unusual, except in disease states such as prolonged vomiting or diarrhea or kidney dysfunction, where replacement may be needed.
MANGANESE†		
Functions Activation of enzymes involved in reproduction, growth, and fat metabolism Normal bone structure Nervous system functioning	**Deficiency** Unknown	No specific recommendations are needed.
Sources Nuts, whole grains, legumes, green vegetables, fruit	**Excess** Unknown	
MOLYBDENUM†		
Functions Essential component of several oxidative enzymes	**Deficiency** Very rare; diagnosed in patients on complete total parenteral alimentation	No specific recommendations are needed.
Sources Legumes, whole grains, organs, some dark green vegetables	**Excess** Produces secondary copper deficiency (growth failure, anemia, disturbed bone development)	
PHOSPHORUS*		
Functions Bone and tooth development (in combination with calcium) Involved in numerous chemical reactions, including protein, carbohydrate, and fat metabolism Acid-base balance	**Deficiency** Weakness, anorexia, malaise, bone pain	Dietary deficiency is uncommon, although prolonged use of antacids can produce deficiency, in which case supplementation is recommended. To preserve calcium/phosphorus ratio in newborns, discourage use of whole cow's milk.
Sources Dairy products, eggs, meat, poultry, legumes, carbonated beverages	**Excess** Produces secondary calcium deficiency from disturbed calcium/phosphorus ratio	
POTASSIUM*		
Functions Acid-base and fluid balance (major extracellular fluid areas) Nerve conduction Muscular contraction, especially the heart Release of energy	**Deficiency** Cardiac arrhythmias Muscular weakness Lethargy Kidney and respiratory failure Heart failure	Dietary deficiency and excess are unlikely, although disease states such as prolonged nausea and vomiting or the use of diuretics can result in hypokalemia; in such instances, encourage replacement with supplements of rich food sources, such as bananas.
Sources Bananas, citrus fruit, dried fruits, meat, fish, bran, legumes, peanut butter, potatoes, coffee, tea, cocoa	**Excess** Cardiac arrhythmias Respiratory failure Mental confusion Numbness of extremities	

*Macrominerals—required intake >100 mg/day.

Table 47-2

Minerals and Their Nutritional Significance—cont'd

PHYSIOLOGIC FUNCTIONS/SOURCES	RESULTS OF DEFICIENCY OR EXCESS	NURSING CONSIDERATIONS
SELENIUM†		
Functions Antioxidant, especially protective of vitamin E Protects against toxicity of heavy metals Associated with fat metabolism	**Deficiency** Keshan disease (cardiomyopathy in children; found in China)	Deficiency and excess are uncommon in North America, although selenium deficiency can occur in patients receiving prolonged total parenteral alimentation; in these instances, supplementation is required.
Sources Seafood, organs, egg yolk, whole grains, chicken, meat, tomatoes, cabbage, garlic, mushrooms, milk	**Excess** Eye, nose, and throat irritation Increased dental caries Liver and kidney degeneration	
SODIUM*		
Functions Acid-base and fluid balance (major extracellular fluid cation) Cell permeability; absorption of glucose Muscle contraction	**Deficiency** Dehydration Hypotension Convulsions Muscle cramps	Deficient intake is very rare, although losses secondary to nausea, vomiting, excessive sweating, and use of diuretics can occur and require replacement. Encourage parents to limit excessive use of salt in preparing foods and to limit commercial foods with high sodium content, such as smoked meats.
Sources Table salt, seafood, meat, poultry, numerous prepared foods	**Excess** Edema Hypertension Intracranial hemorrhage	
SULFUR*		
Functions Essential component of cell protein, especially of hair and skin Enzyme activation Associated with energy metabolism Detoxification of certain chemical reactions	**Deficiency** Unknown	No specific recommendations are needed.
Sources Dairy products, eggs, meat, fish, nuts, legumes	**Excess** Unknown	
ZINC†		
Functions Component of about 100 enzymes Synthesis of nucleic acids and protein in immune system and coagulation Release of vitamin A from liver Improved wound healing with vitamin C Normal taste sensitivity	**Deficiency** Loss of appetite Diminished taste sensation Delayed healing *Skin lesions*—Erythematous, crusted lesions around body orifices Alopecia Diarrhea Growth failure Retarded sexual maturity	Encourage food sources rich in zinc, especially protein. Caution that fiber, phytates, oxalates, tannins (in tea or coffee), iron, and calcium adversely affect zinc absorption. Recognize groups at risk for zinc deficiency, such as vegetarians and Mexican-Americans, whose diets may have restricted or low meat content and high fiber and phytate content; and patients with malabsorption syndromes. Emphasize correct use of zinc supplements and the possible interaction with other minerals.
Sources Seafood (especially oysters), meat, poultry, eggs, wheat, legumes	**Excess** Vomiting and diarrhea Malaise, dizziness Anemia, gastric bleeding Impaired absorption of calcium and copper	

*Macrominerals—required intake >100 mg/day.
†Microminerals or trace elements—required intake <100 mg/day.

of vegetarianism and poses little or no nutritional risk to infants unless dietary fat and cholesterol intake is severely restricted.

Many individuals who are concerned about healthy diets subscribe to vegetarian diets that may not be typified by these categories. Therefore during nutritional assessment it is necessary to clearly list exactly what the diet includes and excludes.*

The major deficiencies in the stricter vegetarian diets are inadequate protein for growth; inadequate calories for energy and growth; poor digestibility of many of the bulky natural, unprocessed foods, especially for infants; and deficiencies of vitamin B_6, niacin, riboflavin, vitamin D, iron, calcium, and zinc. Strict vegetarian diets also require supplements of vitamin B_{12} and vitamin D. Vitamin D is essential if exposure to sunlight is inadequate (less than 5 to 15 minutes per day on the hands, arms, and face) or in persons who are dark skinned or who live in northern latitudes or cloudy or smoky areas.

Iron deficiency anemia and rickets may also be seen in children on strict vegetarian and macrobiotic diets as a result of consuming plant foods such as unrefined cereals, which impair the absorption of iron, calcium, and zinc.

Nursing Care Management

Identification of nutrient imbalance is the initial nursing goal and requires assessment based on a dietary history and physical examination for signs of deficiency or excess. Once assessment data are collected, this information is evaluated against standard intakes to identify areas of concern.

The Dietary Reference Intakes (DRIs)

The DRIs are quantitative estimates of nutrient requirements for planning and evaluating diets for healthy infants, and are comprised of four categories. These include Estimated Average Requirements (EARs) for age and gender categories, tolerable upper-limit (UL) nutrient intakes that are associated with a low risk of adverse effects, adequate intakes (AIs) of nutrients, and new standard RDAs. The guidelines present information about lifestyle factors that may affect nutrient function, such as caffeine intake and exercise, and about how the nutrient may be related to chronic disease. The first DRIs published included calcium, magnesium, phosphorus, vitamin D, and fluoride. Additional groups of nutrients include folate and other B vitamins, dietary antioxidants, micronutrients, macronutrients, trace elements, electrolytes, and food components such as dietary fiber. The comprehensive set of guidelines covers nutrient needs across the life span, including infancy. An important factor in the development of the DRIs that affects children, particularly infants 0 to 6 months, is that the Adequate Intakes are based on the nutrient intake of term, healthy, breastfed infants (by well-nourished mothers), which now represents the gold standard for infant nutrition in this age group. This represents a major change in infant nutrition recommendations; specific needs to meet the nutrient requirements for formula-fed infants were not included in DRI reports (Devaney & Barr, 2002; Institute of Medicine, 2000).*

The U.S. Department of Health and Human Services together with the U.S. Department of Agriculture have released the 2005 Dietary Guidelines for Americans, providing advice to promote health while reducing the risk for major chronic diseases. The primary premise is that nutritional needs should be met through eating a balanced diet from a variety of foods, not supplements; maintaining a healthy weight by balancing caloric intake with physical activity; consuming adequate amounts of fruits, vegetables, and whole grains, drinking 3 cups daily of fat-free or low-fat milk or equivalent; and limiting intake of fat, cholesterol, sugar, salt, and alcohol. The new Food Guidance System includes a revised food guide system, My Pyramid, which replaces the basic four food groups and the previous edition of the Food Guide Pyramid and is used to convey nutrition information to the public. This new Food Guide System is comprehensive and applies to children as young as 2 years of age (Fig. 47-1).

NURSE ALERT When solid foods are introduced, the safety and digestibility of the selections must be considered. Raw fruits with seeds, vegetables, and nuts are hazardous for infants and young children because of the danger of aspiration. Beans, grain cereals, and vegetables should be served well cooked and mashed during infancy. ■

The number of servings and serving sizes are important components of the new My Pyramid, Steps to a Healthier You. Guidelines for serving sizes from the five food groups are listed in Box 47-2. Young children need the same variety of foods as older children but may need less than the 1600 calories provided by the suggested minimum number of servings in each food group. To meet their caloric needs, adjustments are made by using the minimum number of servings and smaller serving sizes. However, it is important that children have the equivalent of at least 3 cups of milk per day. For children 2 to 8 years of age, 2 cups of milk per day is recommended. Adolescents, who require increased calories for growth, should have at least 3 cups of milk per day and more fruits, and may require the maximum number of suggested servings. Current recommendations for fat intake for children 2 to 3 years of age are that no more than 30% to 35% of calories should come from fat and the remainder of calories should come from carbohydrates and protein, and 25% to 35% of calories for children and adolescents 4 to 18 years of age.

Because one of the best assurances of nutritional adequacy is eating a variety of foods, families need guidelines for selecting foods that provide essential nutrients without exceeding energy requirements. With a varied diet, most children do not need vitamin or mineral supplements. Unfortunately, there are no restrictions on the availability of toxic doses of vitamins or minerals. Nurses need to inquire

*Further information regarding vegetarian diets may be found at the Vegetarian Resource Group (VRG), PO Box 1463, Baltimore, MD 21203; phone: 410-366-VEGE; Web site: www.vrg.org.

*Further information may be found regarding the nutrition guidelines at MyPyramid.gov.

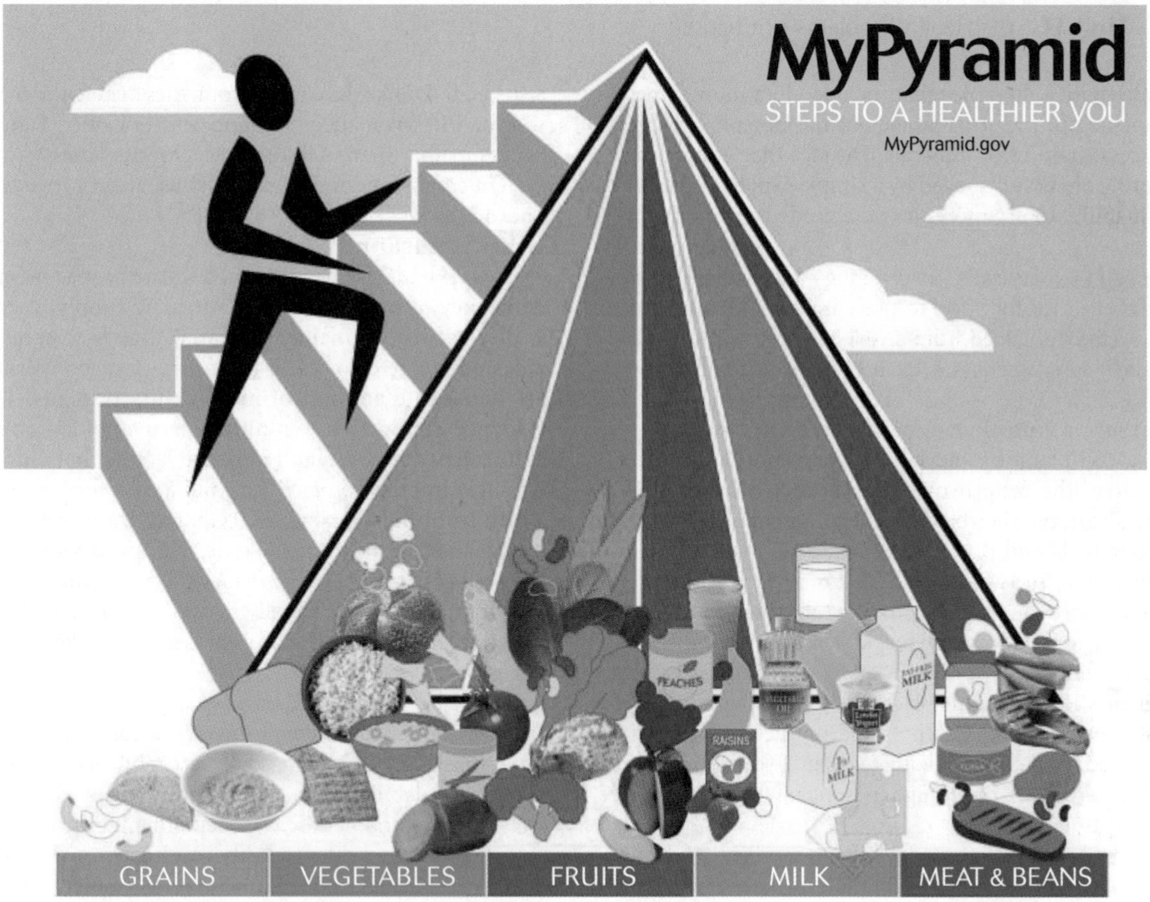

Fig. 47-1 MyPyramid Steps to a Healthier You. US Department of Agriculture Center for Policy and Promotion, 2005.

BOX 47-2

GRAINS Make half your grains whole	VEGETABLES Vary your veggies	FRUITS Focus on fruits	MILK Get your calcium-rich foods	MEAT & BEANS Go lean with protein
Eat at least 3 oz. of whole-grain cereals, breads, crackers, rice, or pasta every day 1 oz. is about 1 slice of bread, about 1 cup of breakfast cereal, or 1/2 cup of cooked rice, cereal, or pasta	Eat more dark-green veggies like broccoli, spinach, and other dark leafy greens Eat more orange vegetables like carrots and sweet potatoes Eat more dry beans and peas like pinto beans, kidney beans, and lentils	Eat a variety of fruit Choose fresh, frozen, canned, or dried fruit Go easy on fruit juices	Go low-fat or fat-free when you choose milk, yogurt, and other milk products If you don't or can't consume milk, choose lactose-free products or other calcium sources such as fortified foods and beverages	Choose low-fat or lean meats and poultry Bake it, broil it, or grill it Vary your protein routine — choose more fish, beans, peas, nuts, and seeds
For a 2,000-calorie diet, you need the amounts below from each food group. To find the amounts that are right for you, go to MyPyramid.gov.				
Eat 6 oz. every day	Eat 2 1/2 cups every day	Eat 2 cups every day	Get 3 cups every day; for kids aged 2 to 8, it's 2	Eat 5 1/2 oz. every day

Find your balance between food and physical activity

- Be sure to stay within your daily calorie needs.
- Be physically active for at least 30 minutes most days of the week.
- About 60 minutes a day of physical activity may be needed to prevent weight gain.
- For sustaining weight loss, at least 60 to 90 minutes a day of physical activity may be required.
- Children and teenagers should be physically active for 60 minutes every day, or most days.

Know the limits on fats, sugars, and salt (sodium)

- Make most of your fat sources from fish, nuts, and vegetable oils.
- Limit solid fats like butter, margarine, shortening, and lard, as well as foods that contain these.
- Check the Nutrition Facts label to keep saturated fats, *trans* fats, and sodium low.
- Choose food and beverages low in added sugars. Added sugars contribute calories with few, if any, nutrients.

MyPyramid.gov
STEPS TO A HEALTHIER YOU

U.S. Department of Agriculture
Center for Nutrition Policy and Promotion
April 2005
CNPP-15

USDA

From MyPyramid.gov, 2005.

about alternative therapies that include vitamin or mineral supplements and inform families of the potential dangers from excess vitamins or minerals. The idea that "more is better" is probably best dispelled by a simple explanation of the body's inability to use more than the needed requirement.

NURSE ALERT Educate childbearing adolescent females about the need for folic acid to prevent neural tube birth defects. It is easily obtained from a well balanced diet or a daily multivitamin supplement (see Table 47-1). ■

Achieving a nutritionally adequate vegetarian diet requires careful planning and knowledge of nutrient sources. For children, the lacto-ovo vegetarian diet is nutritionally adequate; however, the vegan diet requires supplementation with vitamins D and B_{12} for children ages 2 to 12 years. Infants should be breastfed for the first 6 months and preferably for 1 year, be fed solid foods after about 4 months, and receive iron-fortified cereal for at least 18 months. The American Dietetic Association (1997) recommends iron supplementation in infants exclusively breastfed after 4 to 6 months by vegetarian mothers and no dietary fat restrictions in vegetarian children younger than 2 years. The use of vitamin C juices with foods high in iron will further improve iron absorption.

However, breast milk from vegetarian mothers can be deficient in vitamin B_{12}; supplementation of both mother and child is advisable. If whole fortified cow's or human milk or commercial infant formula is not given, fortified soy milk is recommended. A variety of foods should be introduced during the early years to ensure a more well-balanced intake. Mothers who continue exclusive or partial breastfeeding past 6 months should have a careful evaluation of their particular vegetarian diet to ensure adequate intake of nutrients.

To ensure sufficient protein in the diet, foods with incomplete proteins (those that do not have all of the essential amino acids) should be eaten with other foods that supply the missing amino acids. The three basic combinations of foods consumed by vegetarians that generally provide the appropriate amounts of essential amino acids are as follows:

1. Grains (cereal, rice, pasta) and legumes (beans, peas, lentils, peanuts)
2. Grains and milk products (milk, cheese, yogurt)
3. Seeds (sesame, sunflower) and legumes

Protein and Energy Malnutrition

Malnutrition continues to be a major health problem in the world today, particularly in children younger than 5 years of age. Lack of food, however, is not always the primary cause for malnutrition. In many developing and underdeveloped nations, diarrhea is a major factor. Additional factors are bottle-feeding (in poor sanitary conditions), inadequate knowledge of proper child care practices, parental illiteracy, economic and political factors, and simply the lack of adequate food for children. The most extreme forms of malnutrition, or protein and energy malnutrition (PEM), are kwashiorkor and marasmus.

Milder forms of PEM are seen in the United States, although the classic cases of marasmus and kwashiorkor may also occur. Unlike developing countries, where the main reason for PEM is inadequate food, in the United States PEM occurs primarily in children with chronic illnesses or inadvertent malnourishment as a consequence of caretaker knowledge inadequacy.

Kwashiorkor

Kwashiorkor has been defined in the past as primarily a deficiency of protein with an adequate supply of calories. A diet consisting mainly of starch grains or tubers provides adequate calories in the form of carbohydrates but an inadequate amount of high-quality proteins. There is evidence supporting a multifactorial etiology, including cultural, psychologic, and infective factors that may jointly or singly interact to place the child at risk for kwashiorkor. Taken from the Ga language (Ghana), the word *kwashiorkor* means "the sickness the older child gets when the next baby is born" and aptly describes the syndrome that develops in the first child, usually between 1 and 4 years of age, when weaned from the breast after the second child is born.

The child with kwashiorkor has thin, wasted extremities and a prominent abdomen from edema (ascites). The edema often masks the severe muscular atrophy, making the child appear less debilitated than he or she actually is. The skin is scaly and dry and has areas of depigmentation. Several dermatoses may be evident, partly resulting from the vitamin deficiencies. Permanent blindness often results from the severe lack of vitamin A. Mineral deficiencies are common, especially iron, calcium, and zinc. The hair is thin, dry, coarse, and dull. Depigmentation is common, and patchy alopecia may occur.

Diarrhea commonly occurs from a lowered resistance to infection and produces electrolyte imbalance. A large number of fatalities in children with kwashiorkor occurred in those who developed human immunodeficiency virus (HIV) infection, many of whom were breastfed. Protein deficiency increases the child's susceptibility to infection, which eventually results in death. Behavioral changes are evident as the child grows progressively more irritable, lethargic, withdrawn, and apathetic. Fatal deterioration may be caused by diarrhea and infection or may occur as the result of circulatory failure.

Marasmus

Marasmus results from general malnutrition of both calories and protein. It is a common occurrence in underdeveloped countries during times of drought, especially in cultures where adults eat first; the remaining food is often insufficient in quality and quantity for the children.

Marasmus is usually a syndrome of physical and emotional deprivation and is not confined to geographic areas where food supplies are inadequate. It may be seen in children with failure to thrive in whom the cause is not solely nutritional but primarily emotional. Marasmus may be seen in infants as young as 3 months of age if breastfeeding is not successful and there are no suitable alternatives. *Marasmic kwashiorkor* is a form of PEM in which clinical findings of both kwashiorkor and marasmus are evident; the child has edema, severe wasting, and stunted growth.

Marasmus is characterized by gradual wasting and atrophy of body tissues, especially of subcutaneous fat. The child appears to be very old, with flabby and wrinkled skin, unlike the child with kwashiorkor, who appears more rounded from the edema. Fat metabolism is less impaired than in kwashiorkor, so that deficiency of fat-soluble vitamins is usually minimal or absent.

The child is fretful, apathetic, withdrawn, and so lethargic that prostration frequently occurs. Intercurrent infection with debilitating diseases such as tuberculosis, parasitosis, HIV, and dysentery is common.

Therapeutic Management

The treatment of PEM includes providing a diet with high-quality proteins, carbohydrates, vitamins, and minerals. When PEM occurs as a result of diarrhea, three management goals are identified: (1) rehydration with an oral rehydration solution that also replaces electrolytes, (2) medications such as antibiotics and antidiarrheals, and (3) provision of adequate nutrition either by breastfeeding or a proper weaning diet. When the child is too ill to tolerate oral fluids, intravenous administration of fluids, electrolytes, minerals, and vitamins is required to prevent death. Additional management of PEM is aimed at restoring or replacing essential vitamins and minerals, namely vitamin E, vitamin A, selenium, and zinc, which have been shown to have significant roles in infection and congestive heart failure related to PEM.

Nursing Care Management

Provision of essential physiologic needs, such as protection from infection, adequate hydration, skin care, and restoration of physiologic integrity, is paramount. Because children are usually weak and withdrawn, they depend on others for feeding. Poor skin integrity increases the chance of infections and further skin breakdown. Tube feedings may be required in infants too weak to breastfeed or bottle-feed. Oral rehydration with an approved oral rehydration solution is commonly used in cases of PEM where diarrhea and infection are not immediately life threatening.

A larger problem is the prevention of these conditions through education concerning the importance of proper nutrition, whether breastfeeding or bottle-feeding, when being weaned to semisolid foods. There are reported cases of kwashiorkor in children in the United States as a result of ingestion of improper types of nutrients; in both cases, toddlers were being fed a health food milk alternative and very few solids (Carvalho et al, 2001). It is imperative that nurses be at the forefront in educating and reinforcing healthy nutrition habits in parents of small children to prevent malnutrition. Because children with marasmus may suffer from emotional starvation as well, care should be consistent with care of the child with failure to thrive.

Food Sensitivity

Food sensitivity is a general term that includes any type of adverse reaction to food or food additives. Food sensitivities can be divided into two broad categories:

1. *Food allergy* or *hypersensitivity,* which refers to reactions involving immunologic mechanisms, usually immunoglobulin E (IgE); the reactions may be immediate or delayed and mild or severe, such as an anaphylactic reaction.
2. *Food intolerance,* which refers to reactions involving known or unknown nonimmunologic mechanisms; lactose intolerance is an example of a reaction that looks like allergy but is due to deficiency of the enzyme lactase.

However, this classification is not universally accepted; therefore the terms *food sensitivity, hypersensitivity, allergy,* and *intolerance* are often used interchangeably.

Food allergy is caused by exposure to allergens, usually proteins (but not the smaller amino acids) that are capable of inducing IgE antibody formation ("sensitization") when ingested. Sensitization refers to the initial exposure of an individual to an allergen, resulting in an immune response; subsequent exposure induces a much stronger response that is clinically apparent. Consequently, food hypersensitivity typically occurs after the food has been ingested one or more times. The most common food allergens are listed in Box 47-3.

Allergies in general demonstrate a genetic component: children who have one parent with allergy have a 50% or greater risk of developing allergy; children who have both parents with allergy have up to a 100% risk of developing allergy. Allergy with a hereditary tendency is referred to as *atopy.* Some infants with atopy can be identified at birth from elevated levels of IgE in cord blood.

Deaths have been reported in children who suffered an anaphylactic reaction to food. Onset of the reactions occurred shortly after ingestion, usually within seconds or minutes. In most of the children the reactions did not begin

BOX 47-3

Hyperallergenic Foods/Sources

Milk*—Ice cream, butter, margarine (if it contains dairy products), yogurt, cheese, pudding, baked goods, wieners, bologna, canned creamed soups, instant breakfast drinks, powdered milk drinks, milk chocolate
Eggs*—Mayonnaise, creamy salad dressing, baked goods, egg noodles, some cake icing, meringue, custard, pancakes, French toast, root beer
Wheat*—Almost all baked goods, wieners, bologna, pressed or chopped cold cuts, gravy, pasta, some canned soups
Legumes—Peanuts,* peanut butter or oil, beans, peas, lentils
Nuts*—Some chocolates, candy, baked goods, cherry soda (may be flavored with a nut extract), walnut oil
Fish or shellfish*—Cod liver oil, pizza with anchovies, Caesar salad dressing, any food fried in same oil as fish
Soy*—Soy sauce, teriyaki or Worcestershire sauce, tofu, baked goods using soy flour or oil, soy nuts, soy infant formulas or milk, soybean paste, tuna packed in vegetable oil, many margarines
Chocolate—Cola beverages, cocoa, chocolate-flavored drinks
Buckwheat—Some cereals, pancakes
Pork, chicken—Bacon, wieners, sausage, pork fat, chicken broth
Strawberries, melon, pineapple—Gelatin, syrups
Corn—Popcorn, cereal, muffins, cornstarch, corn meal, corn bread, corn tortilla
Citrus fruits—Orange, lemon, lime, grapefruit; any of these in drinks, gelatin, juice, or medicines
Tomatoes—Juice, some vegetable soups, spaghetti, pizza sauce, catsup
Spices—Chili, pepper, vinegar, cinnamon

*Most common allergens.

with skin signs such as hives, red rash, and flushing, but rather as an acute asthma attack. Additional clinical features that individuals with acute anaphylactic food reactions have include (1) asthma, (2) accidental ingestion of the food allergen, (3) immediate symptoms, and (4) a prior allergic reaction to the food (Burks, 2000). Other symptoms of anaphylaxis to food allergens include wheezing; cough, dyspnea, urticaria, abdominal cramps, vomiting, diarrhea, a drop in systemic blood pressure or shock, and, in small preverbal children, restlessness, urticaria, irritability, listlessness, and unresponsiveness. A grading system of clinical signs and symptoms associated with food anaphylaxis has been proposed to measure the severity of the reaction (Sampson, 2003). Children with suspected food anaphylaxis should be watched closely because a biphasic response has been recorded in a number of cases in which there is an immediate response, apparent recovery, and then acute recurrence of symptoms. The most common foods causing anaphylaxis are peanut, tree nut, fish, and shellfish (Pongracic, 2000).

The spectrum of food allergy symptoms may include clinical manifestations that involve the skin (urticaria), gastrointestinal tract, and respiratory tract. Oral allergy syndrome occurs when a food allergen is ingested (commonly fruits and vegetables) and there is subsequent edema and pruritus involving the lips, tongue, palate, and throat; recovery from symptoms is usually rapid. Immediate gastrointestinal hypersensitivity is an IgE-mediated reaction to a food allergen, and reactions include nausea, abdominal pain, cramping, diarrhea, vomiting, anaphylaxis, or all of these (Burks, 2000). Additional food hypersensitivities seen in young children include allergic eosinophilic gastritis, allergic eosinophilic gastroenterocolitis, dietary protein enterocolitis (or milk protein intolerance), and dietary protein proctitis (Burks, 2000).

Parents, teachers, and day care workers should be educated regarding signs and symptoms of food allergies. Those with food sensitivity should avoid unfamiliar foods, as well as restaurants and fast-food establishments that do not disclose food ingredients. Peanut allergy warnings are now standard on products that contain peanut fragments from the manufacturing process, but hidden ingredients remain an issue for children with food hypersensitivity.

Although the reason is unknown, many children "outgrow" their food allergies; children may outgrow milk and egg allergies, but peanut allergies may persist. Children who are allergic to more than one food may develop tolerance to each food at different times. Because of the tendency to lose the hypersensitivity, allergic foods should be reintroduced into the diet after a period of abstinence (usually a year or more) to evaluate if the food can be safely added to the diet. However, foods that are associated with severe anaphylactic reactions will continue to present a lifelong risk and must be avoided. Because children with food allergies (usually two or more) are at risk for inadequate nutrient intake and growth failure, it is recommended that they have an annual nutritional assessment to prevent such problems (Christie et al, 2002).

Breastfeeding is now considered to be a primary consideration for avoiding atopy in families with known food sensitivities; however, there is some evidence that cow's milk protein is transferred via breast milk. The breastfeeding mother is encouraged to avoid foods such as peanuts, tree nuts, fish, and shellfish during the first 6 months of breastfeeding. In addition, supplementation, if required, is best with hydrolysated or amino acid formulas, not soy formulas. The strategies listed in the Guidelines box are those recommended by most authorities for infants with a family history of atopy.*

Guidelines

PREVENTING ATOPY IN CHILDREN

Identify Children at Risk

Family history of allergy
Increased IgE in cord blood and postnatal serum
Dry, flaky skin

Prenatal Precautions (Last Trimester)

Avoid any known food allergens
Avoid milk and other dairy products, peanuts, and eggs
Minimize ingestion of other hyperallergenic foods

Postnatal Precautions

Breast milk (preferred) or casein/whey hydrolysate formula (e.g., Nutramigen, Pregestimil, Alimentum) or amino acid formula such as Neocate exclusively for at least 6 months
No solid food for first 6 months
No cow's milk or soy formula for 12 months
No eggs, fish, corn, citrus, peanuts, nuts, or chocolate for 12 months
One new food added at 5-day intervals to identify possible reaction

Environmental Control

Limited exposure to dust mites, molds, furry animals, latex products, and cigarette smoke

Data from Johnstone D: Strategy for intervention of food allergy in infants, *Int Pediatr* 4(4):319-325, 1989; Zeiger R et al: Effectiveness of dietary manipulation in the prevention of food allergy in infants, part 2, *J Allergy Clin Immunol* 78(1, pt 2):224-238, 1986; and Wood RA: Prospects for the prevention of allergy in children, *Curr Opin Pediatr* 8(6):601-605, 1995.

NURSE ALERT Children with extremely sensitive food allergies should wear medical identification such as a bracelet and have an injectable epinephrine cartridge readily available and know how to use it. It is also helpful for the child to have a copy of the individualized written treatment plan on hand for prompt diagnosis and treatment (such plans can be downloaded from www.foodallergy.org and completed by the practitioner). ■

Cow's Milk Allergy

Cow's milk allergy (also referred to as cow's milk protein allergy [CMPA]) is a multifaceted disorder representing ad-

*Further information for parents of infants with food allergies is available from the American Academy of Allergy, Asthma, and Immunology, 611 E. Wells St., Milwaukee, WI 52202; phone: 800-822-2762; Web site: www.aaaai.org. Additional helpful Web sites for information on food allergies include Medline Plus Health Information (sponsored by the National Institutes of Health): http://medlineplus.gov/; the Food Allergy and Anaphylaxis Network: www.foodallergy.org; and the National Institute of Allergy and Infectious Diseases: www.niaid.nih.org.

verse systemic and local gastrointestinal reactions to cow's milk protein. (This discussion is centered on cow's milk protein found in commercial infant formulas; whole milk is not recommended for infants younger than 1 year of age.) The hypersensitivity may be manifested within the first 4 months of life through a variety of signs and symptoms (Box 47-4) that may appear within several minutes of milk ingestion or after a period of several days. The diagnosis may initially be made from the history, although the history alone is not diagnostic; the timing and diversity of clinical manifestations vary greatly. For example, cow's milk allergy may be manifested as colic, chronic constipation, gastroesophageal reflux, or sleeplessness in an otherwise healthy infant. The incidence of CMPA is reported to range from 2% to 7.5% in developed countries, although the percentage may appear to be higher because of parental report of symptoms rather than actual confirmation of CMPA (Host, 2002; Salvatore & Vandenplas, 2002).

Diagnostic Evaluation

A number of diagnostic tests may be performed, including stool analysis for blood (both frank and occult bleeding can occur from the colitis), serum IgE levels, skin-prick or scratch testing, and radioallergosorbent test (measures IgE antibodies to specific allergens in serum by radioimmunoassay). Both skin and radioallergosorbent testing help identify the offending food, but the results are not always conclusive. The CAP system FEIA test is reported to have a 95% or greater predictive value in identifying children with allergies to egg, milk, peanut, and fish; use of this test would negate the need for the double-blind placebo-controlled food challenge in many children (Sampson, 2001).

The most definitive diagnostic strategy is elimination of milk, followed by challenge testing after improvement of symptoms. Challenge testing involves reintroducing small quantities of milk in the diet to detect resurgence of symptoms; at times challenge testing involves the use of a placebo so that the parent is unaware of or "blind" to the timing of allergen ingestion. A double-blind placebo-controlled food challenge is the gold standard for diagnosing food allergies such as CMPA, yet is not used very often for diagnosing cow's milk protein allergy (Baron, 2000).

Therapeutic Management

Treatment of cow's milk allergy is elimination of all dairy products. For infants fed cow's milk formula, this primarily involves changing the formula to a casein hydrolysate milk formula (Pregestimil, Nutramigen, or Alimentum), in which the protein has been broken down (or "predigested") into its amino acids through enzymatic hydrolysis. Another choice is the amino acid–based formula, Neocate. Soy-based formula is not recommended because of cross-reactivity to soy (American Academy of Pediatrics, Committee on Nutrition, 1998). Goat's milk is not an acceptable substitute because it cross-reacts with cow's milk protein, is deficient in folic acid, and is unsuitable as the only source of calories. Infants who are breastfed but have symptoms of cow's milk hypersensitivity are treated by eliminating all dairy products from the lactating mother's diet, although there is some evidence that restricting maternal dairy intake is not necessary. If maternal dairy intake is restricted, these women need vitamin D and calcium supplementation to prevent deficiency. Infants are maintained on the dairy-free diet for a year or more, depending on the type of reaction and severity, at which time very small quantities of milk are reintroduced.

Nursing Care Management

The principal nursing objectives are identification of potential milk allergy and appropriate counseling of parents regarding substitute formulas. The protein hydrolysate formulas tend to be less palatable than milk-based formulas. Consequently, reluctance to accept the new formula may be a problem. This can be overcome by introducing the formula gradually over a few days using 1 ounce of new formula to 7 ounces of old formula, then 2 to 6 ounces, 3 to 4, and as needed, or by adding nonnutritive flavor packets available in a number of different flavors (Ross Laboratories). Parents also need to be reassured that the infant will receive complete nutrition from the new formula and will suffer no ill effects from the absence of cow's milk. Carnation Good Start, a whey protein hydrolysate, is not appropriate for CMPA because some children may react to it (Anderson, 1997).

After solid foods are started, parents need guidance in avoiding all associated milk products, although many children reportedly outgrow cow's milk protein sensitivity by 3 to 4 years of age (Sicherer, 2001) (see Box 47-3). Carefully reading all food labels helps avoid ingesting prepared foods containing milk products.

Lactose Intolerance

Lactose intolerance refers to at least three different entities that involve a deficiency of the enzyme lactase, which is needed for the hydrolysis or digestion of lactose in the small intestine; lactose is hydrolyzed into glucose and galactose. Congenital lactase deficiency occurs soon after birth after the newborn has consumed lactose-containing milk (human milk or commercial formula). This inborn error of metabolism involves the complete absence or severely reduced pres-

BOX 47-4

Common Clinical Manifestations of Cow's Milk Sensitivity

Gastrointestinal
Diarrhea
Vomiting
Colic
Abdominal pain

Respiratory
Rhinitis
Bronchitis
Asthma
Wheezing
Sneezing
Coughing
Chronic nasal discharge

Other Signs and Symptoms
Eczema
Excessive crying
Pallor (from anemia secondary to chronic blood loss in gastrointestinal tract)

ence of lactase, is rare, and requires lifelong lactose-free or extremely reduced lactose diet.

Late-onset lactase deficiency, sometimes referred to as primary lactase deficiency, is the most common type of lactose intolerance and is manifested usually around 3 to 7 years of age, although the time of onset is variable. Ethnic groups with a high incidence of lactase deficiency include Asians, southern Europeans, Arabs, Israelis, and African-Americans.

Lactose intolerance (secondary lactase deficiency) may occur secondary to damage of the intestinal lumen, which decreases or destroys the enzyme lactase. Cystic fibrosis, sprue, kwashiorkor, and certain infections (e.g., giardiasis, HIV, or rotavirus) may cause a temporary or permanent lactose intolerance.

The primary symptoms of lactose intolerance include abdominal pain, bloating, flatulence, and diarrhea, and severity may range from mild to severe. The onset of symptoms occurs within 30 minutes to several hours of lactose consumption. Lactose intolerance is often perceived as an allergy, and, in several studies of acute gastrointestinal symptoms ascribed to lactose intolerance, measurement of lactase activity is normal (Goldberg, Folta, & Must, 2002).

Lactose intolerance may be diagnosed on the basis of the history and improvement with a lactose-reduced diet. The breath hydrogen test is used to positively diagnose the condition. Breath samples in lactose-deficient individuals will yield a higher percentage of hydrogen (20 parts per million or more above baseline).

Treatment of lactose intolerance is elimination of offending dairy products; however, some advocate decreasing the amount of dairy products rather than total elimination, especially in small children. In infants, soy-based formula can be substituted for cow's milk formula or human milk (American Academy of Pediatrics, Committee on Nutrition, 1998). Most people are able to tolerate small amounts of lactose even in the presence of deficient lactase activity and should be encouraged to continue their intake of dairy products in small amounts to obtain much-needed nutrients (Goldberg et al, 2002). Milk taken at meals may be better tolerated than when taken alone (Home Care box). Pretreated milk (with microbial-derived lactase) is reported to be effective in improving lactose absorption. Because dairy products are a major source of calcium and vitamin D, supplementation of these nutrients is needed to prevent deficiency. Yogurt contains inactive lactase enzyme, which is activated by the temperature and pH of the duodenum; this lactase activity substitutes for the lack of endogenous lactase. Fresh yogurt may be tolerated better than frozen yogurt; hard cheeses, lactase-treated dairy products, and lactase tablets taken with dairy products are also viable options. An important distinction between lactose intolerance and food hypersensitivity is that lactose intolerance will not manifest as an anaphylactic-type reaction.

Nursing Care Management

Nursing care is similar to the interventions discussed for cow's milk allergy: explaining the dietary restrictions to the family; identifying alternative sources of calcium, such as yogurt; explaining the importance of supplementation; and discussing sources of lactose, especially hidden sources such as its use as a bulk agent in certain medications, and ways of controlling the symptoms (see Home Care box). Parents are advised to check with the pharmacist regarding this possibility when obtaining medication.

> **Home Care**
>
> **CONTROLLING SYMPTOMS OF LACTOSE INTOLERANCE**
>
> In infants, substitute soy-based formula for cow's milk formula or human milk.
>
> Limit milk consumption to one glass at a time.
>
> Drink milk with other foods rather than alone.
>
> Eat hard cheese, cottage cheese, or yogurt instead of drinking milk.
>
> Use enzyme tablets (Lactaid, Lactrase, Dairy Ease) to metabolize the lactose in milk or supplement the body's own lactase (add tablets to milk or sprinkle on dairy products such as ice cream).
>
> Eat small amounts of dairy foods daily to help colonic bacteria adapt to ingested lactose.

GASTROINTESTINAL DYSFUNCTION

The extensive surface area of the gastrointestinal (GI) tract and its digestive function represent the major means of exchange between the human organism and the environment. Inflammatory and malabsorptive disorders impair the functional integrity of the GI tract. In addition, the intestine of the infant is extremely vulnerable to infection. Acute infectious diarrhea causes significant alterations in fluid and electrolyte balance in both infants and children.

Numerous observations provide clues to specific GI problems (Box 47-5). In any disorder that involves GI losses of large amounts of fluid, dehydration poses a serious threat to life and demands immediate attention.

Dehydration

Dehydration is a common body fluid disturbance in infants and children and occurs whenever the total output of fluid exceeds the total intake, regardless of the cause. Dehydration may result from a number of diseases that cause insensible losses through the skin and respiratory tract, through increased renal excretion, and through the GI tract. Although dehydration can result from lack of oral intake (especially in elevated environmental temperatures), more often it is a result of abnormal losses, such as those that occur in vomiting or diarrhea, when oral intake only partially compensates for the abnormal losses. Other significant causes of dehydration are diabetic ketoacidosis and extensive burns.

Water Balance in Infants

Infants and young children have a greater need for water and are more vulnerable to alterations in fluid and electrolyte balance. Compared with older children and adults, infants have a greater fluid intake and output relative to size. Water and electrolyte disturbances occur more frequently and more rapidly, and infants and children adjust less promptly to these alterations.

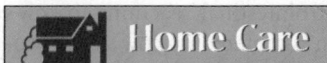

BOX 47-5

Clinical Manifestations of Gastrointestinal Dysfunction in Children

Failure to thrive–Weight consistently below the 3rd percentile or BMI (body mass index) below the 5th percentile or a decrease from established growth pattern.

Spitting up or regurgitation–Passive transfer of gastric contents into the esophagus or mouth.

Vomiting–Forceful ejection of gastric contents; involves a complex process under central nervous system control that causes salivation, pallor, sweating, and tachycardia; usually accompanied by nausea.

Projectile vomiting–Vomiting accompanied by vigorous peristaltic waves and typically associated with pyloric stenosis or pylorospasm.

Nausea–Unpleasant sensation vaguely referred to the throat or abdomen with an inclination to vomit.

Constipation–Delay or difficulty with the passage of stools that is present for 2 weeks or longer; associated with symptoms that may include blood-streaked stools and abdominal discomfort.

Encopresis–Involuntary overflow of incontinent stool causing soiling or incontinence secondary to fecal retention or impaction.

Diarrhea–Increase in the number of stools with an increased water content as a result of alterations of water and electrolyte transport by the gastrointestinal (GI) tract; may be acute or chronic.

Hypoactive, hyperactive, or absent bowel sounds–Evidence of intestinal motility problems that may be caused by inflammation or obstruction.

Abdominal distention–Protuberant contour of the abdomen that may be caused by delayed gastric emptying, accumulation of gas or stool, inflammation, or obstruction.

Abdominal pain–Pain associated with the abdomen that may be localized or diffuse, acute or chronic; often caused by inflammation, obstruction, or hemorrhage.

Gastrointestinal bleeding–May be from an upper or lower GI source and may be acute or chronic.

Hematemesis–Vomiting of bright red blood or denatured blood that results from bleeding in the upper GI tract or from swallowed blood from the nose or oropharynx.

Hematochezia–Passage of bright red blood per rectum, usually indicating lower GI tract bleeding.

Melena–Passage of dark-colored, "tarry" stools resulting from denatured blood, suggesting upper GI tract bleeding or bleeding from the right colon.

Jaundice–Yellow coloration of the skin and sclerae associated with liver dysfunction.

Dysphagia–Difficulty swallowing caused by abnormalities in the neuromuscular function of the pharynx or upper esophageal sphincter or by disorders of the esophagus.

Dysfunctional swallowing–Impaired swallowing caused by central nervous system defects or structural defects of the oral cavity, pharynx, or esophagus; can cause feeding problems or aspiration.

Fever–Common manifestation of illness in children with GI disorders; usually associated with dehydration, infection, or inflammation.

The fluid compartments in the infant vary significantly from those in the adult, primarily because of an expanded extracellular compartment. The *extracellular fluid (ECF)* compartment constitutes more than half the total body water at birth and has a greater relative content of extracellular sodium and chloride. The infant loses a large amount of fluid at birth and maintains a larger amount of ECF than the adult until about 2 years of age. This contributes to greater and more rapid water loss during this age period.

Fluid losses create compartment deficits that are reflected throughout the duration of dehydration. In general, approximately 60% of fluid is lost from the ECF, and the remaining 40% comes from the *intracellular fluid (ICF)*. The amount of fluid lost from the ECF increases with acute illness and decreases with chronic loss.

Fluid losses vary with age and are divided into insensible, urinary, and fecal losses. Approximately two thirds of *insensible losses* occur through the skin; the remaining one third is lost through the respiratory tract. Heat and humidity, body temperature, and respiratory rate influence insensible fluid loss. Infants and children have a greater tendency to become highly febrile than do adults. Fever increases insensible water loss by approximately 7 ml/kg/24 hr for each degree of rise in temperature above 37.2° C (99° F). Fever and increased surface area relative to volume are factors that contribute to greater insensible fluid losses in young patients.

Body Surface Area

The infant's relatively greater body surface area (BSA) allows larger quantities of fluid to be lost in insensible perspiration through the skin. It is estimated that the BSA of the premature neonate is five times as great, and that of the newborn is two to three times as great, as that of the older child or adult. The proportionately longer GI tract in infancy is another source of fluid loss, especially from diarrhea.

Basal Metabolic Rate

The rate of metabolism in infancy is significantly higher than in adulthood because of the larger BSA in relation to the mass of active tissue. Consequently, there is a greater production of metabolic wastes that must be excreted by the kidneys. Any condition that increases metabolism causes greater heat production, insensible fluid loss, and an increased need for water for excretion. The basal metabolic rate (BMR) in infants and children is higher to support growth.

Kidney Function

The kidneys of the infant are functionally immature at birth and are inefficient in excreting waste products of metabolism. Of particular importance for fluid balance is the inability of the infant's kidneys to concentrate or dilute urine, to conserve or excrete sodium, and to acidify urine. The infant is less able to handle large quantities of solute-free water than is the older child, and infants are more likely to become dehydrated when given concentrated formulas or overhydrated when given excessive water or dilute formula.

Fluid Requirements

Infants ingest and excrete a greater amount of fluid per kilogram of body weight than do older children. Because electrolytes are excreted with water and the infant has limited ability for conservation, maintenance requirements include both water and electrolytes. The daily exchange of ECF in the infant is greatly increased over that of older children, which leaves the infant little fluid volume reserve in dehydrated states. Fluid requirements depend on hydration status, size, environmental factors, and underlying disease (Box 47-6).

BOX 47-6

Daily Maintenance Fluid Requirements

1. Calculate weight of child in kilograms:
   Weight of child (in pounds) divided by 2.2 pounds/kg =
   Weight in kilograms.
2. Allow 100 ml/kg for first 10 kg.
3. Allow 50 ml/kg for second 10 kg.
4. Allow 20 ml/kg for remainder of weight in kilograms.
5. Divide total amount by 24 hours to obtain rate in milliliters per hour.

Types of Dehydration

The pathophysiology of dehydration is understood by recognizing that the distribution of water between the ECF and ICF spaces depends on active transport of potassium into and sodium out of cells by energy-requiring processes. Sodium is the chief solute in ECF and is the primary determinant of ECF volume. Potassium is primarily intracellular. When ECF volume is reduced in acute dehydration, the total body sodium content is almost always reduced as well, regardless of serum sodium measurements. Replacement of fluid volume should therefore be accompanied by sodium repletion. Sodium depletion in diarrhea occurs in two ways: out of the body in stool and into the ICF compartment to replace potassium to maintain electrical equilibrium.

Dehydration is classified into three categories on the basis of osmolality and depends primarily on the serum sodium concentration: (1) isotonic, (2) hypotonic, and (3) hypertonic (Fann, 1998; Ledwith, 1997).

Isotonic (*isosmotic* or *isonatremic*) *dehydration,* the primary form of dehydration in children, occurs in conditions in which electrolyte and water deficits are present in approximately balanced proportions. Water and salt are lost in approximately equal amounts. The observable fluid losses are not necessarily isotonic, because losses from other avenues make adjustments so that the sum of all losses, or the net loss, is isotonic. There is no osmotic force between the ICF and the ECF, so the major loss is sustained from the ECF compartment. This significantly reduces the plasma volume and the circulating blood volume, which affects the skin, muscles, and kidneys. Shock is the greatest threat to life, and the child with isotonic dehydration displays symptoms characteristic of hypovolemic shock. Plasma sodium remains within normal limits, between 130 and 150 mEq/L.

Hypotonic (*hyposmotic* or *hyponatremic*) *dehydration* occurs when the electrolyte deficit exceeds the water deficit, leaving the serum hypotonic. Because ICF is more concentrated than ECF in hypotonic dehydration, water moves from the ECF to the ICF to establish osmotic equilibrium. This movement further increases the ECF volume loss, and shock is a frequent finding. Because there is a greater proportional loss of ECF in hypotonic dehydration, the physical signs tend to be more severe, with smaller fluid losses than with isotonic or hypertonic dehydration. Serum sodium concentration is less than 130 mEq/L.

Hypertonic (*hyperosmotic* or *hypernatremic*) *dehydration* results from water loss in excess of electrolyte loss and is usually caused by a proportionately larger loss of water or a larger intake of electrolytes. This type of dehydration is the most dangerous, and it requires more specific fluid therapy. Hypertonic diarrhea may occur in infants who are given fluids by mouth that contain large amounts of solute, or in children who receive high-protein nasogastric tube feedings that place an excessive solute load on the kidneys. In hypertonic dehydration, fluid shifts from the lesser concentration of the ICF to the ECF. Plasma sodium concentration is greater than 150 mEq/L (Behrman, Kliegman, & Arvin, 2000).

Because the ECF volume is proportionately larger, hypertonic dehydration consists of a greater degree of water loss for the same intensity of physical signs. Shock is less apparent. However, neurologic disturbances (e.g., alterations in consciousness, poor ability to focus attention, lethargy, increased muscle tone with hyperreflexia, and hyperirritability to stimuli) are more likely to occur. Cerebral changes are serious and may result in permanent damage.

Diagnostic Evaluation

Diagnosis of the type and degree of dehydration is necessary to develop an effective plan of therapy. The degree of dehydration has been described as a percentage: 5% (mild), 10% (moderate), or 15% (severe). Water constitutes only 60% to 70% of the infant's weight. However, adipose tissue contains little water and is highly variable in individual infants and children. A more accurate means of describing dehydration is to reflect acute loss (over 48 hours or less) in milliliters per kilogram of body weight. For example, a loss of 50 ml/kg is considered to be a mild fluid loss, whereas a loss of 100 ml/kg produces severe dehydration. Weight is the most important determinant of the percent of total body fluid loss in infants and younger children. However, often the preillness weight is unknown. Other predictors of fluid loss include a changing level of consciousness (irritability to lethargy), response to stimuli, decreased skin elasticity and turgor, prolonged capillary refill, increased heart rate, and sunken eyes and fontanels. Clinical signs provide clues to the extent of dehydration (Table 47-3). Using multiple predictors increases the sensitivity of assessing the fluid deficit, and early studies have shown a reasonably high degree of agreement between experienced observers in assessment of the level of dehydration. Objective signs of dehydration are present at a fluid deficit of less than 5%. Any two of the following signs are predictors of a deficit of at least 5%: capillary refill of 2 seconds, absent tears, dry mucous membranes, and an ill general appearance. Generally, three or more clinical findings are present at a deficit of 5% to 9%, and six or more findings are found with a deficit of 10% or more (Gorelick, Shaw, & Murphy, 1997). Shock, tachycardia, and very low blood pressure are common features of severe depletion of ECF volume.

Therapeutic Management

See discussion on therapeutic management of diarrhea, p. 1500.

Nursing Care Management

Nursing observation and intervention are essential to the detection and therapeutic management of dehydration. A variety of circumstances cause fluid losses in infants, and changes can take place quickly. An important nursing responsibility is observation for signs of dehydration. Nursing assessment should begin with observation of general appearance and proceed to more specific observations. Condi-

Table 47-3

Evaluating Extent of Dehydration

LEVEL OF DEHYDRATION	MILD	MODERATE	SEVERE
Weight loss—infants	5%	10%	15%
Weight loss—children	3%-4%	6%-8%	10%
Pulse	Normal	Slightly increased	Very increased
Blood pressure	Normal	Normal to orthostatic (>10 mm Hg change)	Orthostatic to shock
Behavior	Normal	Irritable, more thirsty	Hyperirritable to lethargic
Thirst	Slight	Moderate	Intense
Mucous membranes*	Normal	Dry	Parched
Tears	Present	Decreased	Absent, sunken eyes
Anterior fontanel	Normal	Normal to sunken	Sunken
External jugular vein	Visible when supine	Not visible except with supraclavicular pressure	Not visible even with supraclavicular pressure
Skin* (less useful in children >2 years)	Capillary refill >2 seconds	Slowed capillary refill (2-4 seconds [decreased turgor])	Very delayed capillary refill (>4 seconds) and tenting; skin cool, acrocyanotic or mottled
Urine specific gravity	>1.020	>1.020; oliguria	Oliguria or anuria

Adapted from Jospe N, Forbes G: Fluids and electrolytes—clinical aspects, *Pediatr Rev* 17(11):395-403, 1996.
*These signs are less prominent in patients who have hypernatremia.

tions in which dehydration may develop quickly include diarrhea; vomiting; sweating; fever; disorders such as diabetes, renal disease, and cardiac anomalies; administration of certain drugs (such as diuretics and steroids); and trauma (major surgery, burns, and other extensive injury).

Intake and Output

Accurate measurements of fluid intake and output are vital to the assessment of dehydration. This includes oral and parenteral intake and losses from urine, stools, vomiting, fistulas, nasogastric suction, sweat, and wound drainage:

Urine—Frequency, color, consistency, and volume (when weighing diapers, approximately 1 g wet diaper weight equals 1 ml urine)
Stools—Frequency, volume, and consistency
Vomitus—Volume, frequency, and type
Sweating—Can be estimated from frequency of clothing and linen changes

In addition to fluid intake and output, the following observations assist in assessment of dehydration:

Vital signs—Temperature (normal, elevated, or lowered depending on degree of dehydration), pulse (tachycardia), respirations (tachypnea), and blood pressure (hypotension)
Skin—Color, temperature, turgor, presence or absence of edema, and capillary refill
Mucous membranes—Moisture, color, and presence and consistency of secretions
Body weight—Decreased in relation to degree of dehydration
Fontanel (infants)—Sunken, soft, or normal
Sensory alterations—Presence of thirst

For nursing interventions, see discussion under specific disorders.

DISORDERS OF MOTILITY

Diarrhea

Diarrhea is a symptom that results from disorders involving digestive, absorptive, and secretory functions. Diarrhea is caused by abnormal intestinal water and electrolyte transport. Worldwide, there are an estimated 1.3 billion episodes of diarrhea each year. Approximately 24% of all deaths in children living in developing countries are related to diarrhea and dehydration. Most children living in developed countries have mild forms of gastroenteritis. However, in the United States, approximately 220,000 children younger than age 5 are hospitalized and approximately 300 children younger than 5 years die of diarrhea and dehydration each year (Endsley & Galbraith, 1998).

Diarrheal disturbances involve the stomach and intestines (gastroenteritis), the small intestine (enteritis), the colon (colitis), or the colon and intestines (enterocolitis). Diarrhea is classified as acute or chronic.

Acute diarrhea, a leading cause of illness in children younger than 5 years of age, is defined as a sudden increase in frequency and a change in consistency of stools, often caused by an infectious agent in the GI tract. It may be associated with upper respiratory or urinary tract infections, antibiotic therapy, or laxative use. Acute diarrhea is usually self-limited (less than 14 days' duration) and subsides without specific treatment if dehydration does not occur. *Acute infectious diarrhea (infectious gastroenteritis)* is caused by a variety of viral, bacterial, and parasitic pathogens (Table 47-4).

evolve CASE STUDY: ACUTE DIARRHEA (GASTROENTERITIS)

Table 47-4

Infectious Causes of Acute Diarrhea

ORGANISM	PATHOLOGY	CHARACTERISTICS	COMMENTS
VIRAL AGENTS			
Rotavirus Incubation: 48 hours Diagnosis: enzyme immunoassay (EIA)	Fecal-oral transmission 7 groups (A-G): Most group A virus replicates in mature villus epithelial cells of small intestine; leads to (1) imbalance in ratio of intestinal fluid absorption to secretion and (2) malabsorption of complex carbohydrates	Mild to moderate fever Vomiting followed by the onset of watery stools Fever and vomiting generally abate in approximately 2 days, but diarrhea persists 5-7 days	Most common cause of diarrhea in children <5 years of age. Infants 6-12 months are most vulnerable. Peak occurrences in winter months. Important cause of nosocomial infections. Affects all ages; usually milder in children >3 years of age; immune-compromised children at greater risk for complications
Norwalk-like organisms Incubation: 12-48 hours Also called caliciviruses Diagnosis: EIA	Fecal-oral; contaminated water Pathology similar to rotavirus Affects villus epithelial cells of small intestine Leads to (1) imbalance in ratio of intestinal fluid absorption to secretion and (2) malabsorption of complex carbohydrates	Abdominal cramps; nausea, vomiting, malaise, low-grade fever, watery diarrhea without blood; duration brief, 2-3 days; tends to resemble so-called food poisoning symptoms with nausea predominating	Affects all ages Multiple strains often named for the location of outbreak (e.g., Norwalk, Sapporo, Snow Mountain, Montgomery)
BACTERIAL AGENTS			
Escherichia coli Incubation: 3-4 days Variable depending on strain Diagnosis: sorbitol MacConkey agar (SMAC agar) + for blood but fecal leukocytes are absent or rare	*E. coli* strains produce diarrhea as result of enterotoxin production, adherence, or invasion (enterotoxigenic-producing *E. coli* [ETEC]; enterohemorrhagic *E. coli* [EHEC]; enteroaggregative *E. coli*)	Watery diarrhea 1-2 days; then severe abdominal cramping and bloody diarrhea Can progress to hemolytic uremic syndrome (HUS)	Food-borne pathogen Traveler's diarrhea Highest incidence in summer Cause of nursery epidemics Symptomatic treatment Antibiotics may worsen course Antimotility agents and opioids should be avoided
***Salmonella* groups** (nontyphoidal; gram-negative rods, nonencapsulated, nonsporulating) Incubation 6-72 hours Diagnosis: gram-stained stool culture	Invasion of mucosa in the small and large intestine; edema of the lamina propria; focal acute inflammation with disruption of the mucosa and microabscesses	Nausea, vomiting, colicky abdominal pain, bloody diarrhea, fever; symptoms variable: mild to severe May have headache, cerebral manifestations (e.g., drowsiness, confusion, meningismus, seizures) Infants may be afebrile and nontoxic May result in life-threatening septicemia and meningitis Nausea/vomiting typically short duration; diarrhea may persist as long as 2-3 weeks Typically shed virus for average of 5 weeks; cases reported up to 1 year	Incidence highest in warm months: July to November Food-borne outbreaks common Usually transmitted person to person but may transmit via undercooked meats, poultry Poultry and poultry products cause about half the cases In children: pets (e.g., dogs, cats, hamsters, turtles) Communicable as long as organisms are excreted Antibiotics not recommended in uncomplicated cases Antimotility agents also not recommended—prolong transit time and carrier state Incidence decreasing over past 10 years

Table 47-4

Infectious Causes of Acute Diarrhea—cont'd

ORGANISM	PATHOLOGY	CHARACTERISTICS	COMMENTS
BACTERIAL AGENTS—cont'd			
Salmonella typhi Produces enteric fever—systemic syndrome Incubation usually 7-14 days but could be 3-30 days depending on size of inoculum Diagnosis: positive blood cultures; also sometimes positive stool and urine Late stage: positive bone marrow culture	Bloodstream invasion; after ingestion, organism attaches to microvilli of ileal brush borders and bacteria invades the intestinal epithelium via Peyer's patches; is then transported to intestinal lymph nodes and enters bloodstream via thoracic ducts, and circulating organisms reach reticuloendothelial cells causing bacteremia	Manifestations depend on age Abdominal pain; diarrhea; nausea, vomiting, high fever, lethargy Must be treated with antibiotics	Incidence is much lower in developed countries; United States has about 400 cases/year 65% of U.S. cases acquired via international cases Ingestion of foods/water contaminated with human feces is most common mode of transmission Congenital and intrapartum transmission can occur Three vaccines are available
***Shigella* groups** Gram-negative organisms Nonmotile Anaerobic bacilli Incubation: 1-7 days Diagnosis: stool culture Loaded with polymorphonuclear leukocytes	Enterotoxins: invade the epithelium with superficial mucosal ulcerations	Patients appear sick Symptoms begin with fever, fatigue, anorexia Crampy abdominal pain precedes watery or bloody diarrhea Symptoms usually subside in 5-10 days	Most cases in children younger than 9 years with about one third of cases in children ages 1-4 weeks Antibiotics shorten illness and lower mortality risk All patients are at risk for dehydration Acute symptoms may persist for 1 week or more Antidiarrheal medications not recommended; may predispose to toxic megacolon
***Yersinia* enterocolitis** Incubation period: dose dependent, 1-3 weeks Diagnosis: stool culture serology; enzyme-linked immunosorbent assay (ELISA) Patients have leukocytosis; elevated sedimentation rate	Pathology is poorly understood; believe production of enterotoxin	Mucoid diarrhea, sometimes bloody; abdominal pain suggestive of appendicitis; fever, vomiting	Seen more frequently in the winter months Transmitted by pets and food Antibiotics usually do not alter the clinical course in uncomplicated cases; antibiotics should be used in complicated infections and compromised hosts
Campylobacter jejuni Microaerophilic, motile, gram-negative bacilli Incubation period: 1-7 days Ability to cause illness appears dose related Diagnosis by stool culture, sometimes in the blood Commonly found in GI tract of wild or domestic animals	Not fully understood; possibly (1) adherence to intestinal mucosa by toxin; (2) invasion of the mucosa in the terminal ileum and colon; (3) translocation, in which the organisms penetrate the mucosa and replicate in the lamina propria	Fever, abdominal pain, diarrhea, can be bloody; vomiting Watery, profuse, foul-smelling diarrhea Clinically similar to *Salmonella* or *Shigella* Fecal-oral transmission	Most infections in humans relate to consumption of contaminated foods or water; undercooked meats, particularly chicken Also acquired from contaminated household pets (e.g., dogs, cats, hamsters) Bimodal peaks in infants <1 year and again at ages 15-29 months Antibiotics do not prolong the carriage of bacteria and may eliminate organism more quickly Erythromycin is the drug of choice Antimotility agents not recommended and tend to prolong symptoms

Continued

Table 47-4

Infectious Causes of Acute Diarrhea—cont'd

ORGANISM	PATHOLOGY	CHARACTERISTICS	COMMENTS
BACTERIAL AGENTS—cont'd			
Vibrio cholerae Gram-negative, motile, curved bacillus living in bodies of salt water Incubation period: 1-3 days Diagnosis by stool culture	Enters via oral route in contaminated food or water; if survives acid stomach environment, travels to the small intestine and adheres to the mucosa and produces toxin	Onset abrupt; vomiting, watery diarrhea without cramping or tenesmus Dehydration can occur quickly	More prevalent in developing countries Rehydration most important treatment Antibiotics can shorten diarrhea Despite continued efforts, still no vaccine
Clostridium difficile Gram-positive anaerobic bacillus Diagnosis by detecting *C. difficile* toxin in stool culture	Produces two important toxins (A and B) Toxin binds to the enterocyte surface receptor resulting in alteration of permeability, protein synthesis, and direct cytotoxicity	Most cases: mild, watery diarrhea lasting few days Some cases: prolonged diarrhea and illness May cause pseudomembranous colitis Some individuals are extremely ill with high fever, leukocytosis, hypoalbuminemia	Associated with alteration of normal intestinal flora by antibiotics Adults tend to have more severe symptoms than children Treatment with antibiotics in symptomatic patients—metronidazole Resistant strains have developed Relapse is common
Clostridium perfringens Incubation period: 8-24 hours; anaerobic, gram-positive, spore-producing bacilli	Toxins produced in the intestine after ingestion of organism	Acute onset: watery diarrhea, crampy abdominal pain Fever, nausea, and vomiting rare Duration of illness usually 24 hours	Transmitted by contaminated food products, most often meats and poultry Usually self-limiting and medical intervention not needed Oral rehydration usually sufficient Antibiotics serve no purpose and should not be used
Clostridium botulinum Incubation period: 12-26 hours (range, 6 hours to 8 days) Gram-positive, anaerobic, spore-producing bacilli Blood and stool culture should be obtained and transmitted to special laboratory (usually state health department) to detect toxin	Botulism caused by binding of toxin to the neuromuscular junction	Clinical presentation related to age and the strain of the botulism Abdominal pain, cramping, and diarrhea Other strains: respiratory compromise, central nervous system symptoms	Transmitted in contaminated food products Can be acquired via wound infection Treatment involves supportive care and neutralization of the toxin
Staphylococcus Incubation period is generally short, 1-8 hours Gram-positive, nonmotile, aerobic, or facultative anaerobic bacteria Diagnosis by identifying organism in food, blood, pus, aspirate	Direct tissue invasion and production of toxin	Clinical presentation depends on site of entry In food poisoning: profuse diarrhea, nausea, and vomiting	GI illness transmitted in inadequately cooked or refrigerated foods Self-limiting in GI illness Symptomatic treatment

Chronic diarrhea is defined as an increase in stool frequency and increased water content with a duration of more than 14 days. It is often caused by chronic conditions, such as malabsorption syndromes, inflammatory bowel disease, immune deficiency, food allergy, lactose intolerance, or chronic nonspecific diarrhea, or it may occur as a result of inadequate management of acute diarrhea.

Intractable diarrhea of infancy is a syndrome that occurs in the first few months of life, persists for longer than 2 weeks with no recognized pathogens, and is refractory to treatment. The most common cause is acute infectious diarrhea that was not managed adequately.

Chronic nonspecific diarrhea (CNSD), also known as irritable colon or childhood and toddlers' diarrhea, is a common cause of chronic diarrhea in children 6 to 54 months of age. These children have loose stools, often with undigested food particles, and diarrhea of greater than 2 weeks' duration. Children with CNSD grow normally and have no evidence of malnutrition, no blood in their stool, and no enteric infection (Huffman, 1999). Dietary indiscretions and food sensitivities have been linked to chronic diarrhea. The excessive intake of juices and artificial sweeteners such as sorbitol, a substance found in many commercially prepared beverages and foods, may be a factor.

Etiology

Most pathogens that cause diarrhea are spread by the fecal-oral route through contaminated food or water or are spread from person to person where there is close contact (e.g., day care centers). Lack of clean water, crowding, poor hygiene, nutritional deficiency, and poor sanitation are major risk factors, especially for bacterial or parasitic pathogens. The increased frequency and severity of diarrheal disease in infants is also related to age-specific alterations in susceptibility to pathogens. For example, the immune system of infants has not been exposed to many pathogens and has not acquired protective antibodies. Worldwide, infectious agents, viruses, bacteria, and parasites are the most common causes of acute gastroenteritis. In developed nations, viruses, primarily rotavirus, cause 70% to 80% of infectious diarrhea.

Rotavirus is the most important cause of serious gastroenteritis among children and a significant nosocomial (hospital-acquired) pathogen. Rotavirus disease is most severe in children 3 to 24 months of age. Children younger than 3 months of age have some protection from the disease because of maternally acquired antibodies. Approximately 25% of severe cases of rotavirus occur in older children (Coffin, 2001).

Salmonella, Shigella, and *Campylobacter* organisms are the most frequently isolated bacterial pathogens. *Salmonella* has the highest occurrence in infants; *Giardia* and *Shigella* have the highest incidence among toddlers. *Shigella* infection is uncommon in the United States, accounting for less than 5% of diarrheal illnesses in infants and toddlers. *Campylobacter* has a bimodal presentation (highest in children less than 12 months with a second rise in incidence at 15 to 19 years). *Giardia* and *Cryptosporidium* organisms are parasites. *Giardia* represents 15% of nondysenteric illness in the United States; *Cryptosporidium* is often associated with outbreaks in young children in day care centers. *Clostridium difficile, Plesiomonas,* and *Yersinia* are parasites that are frequently responsible for causing diarrhea that lasts more than 10 days in a previously healthy adolescent. Traveler's diarrhea is also more common in adolescents than in other age groups (Ramaswamy & Jacobson, 2001).

Antibiotic administration is frequently associated with diarrhea because antibiotics alter the normal intestinal flora, resulting in an overgrowth of other bacteria such as *C. difficile.* Antibiotic-associated diarrhea can also be caused by *Salmonella, Clostridium porringers* type A, and *Staphylococcus aureus* pathogens (Jabbar & Wright, 2003).

Pathophysiology

Invasion of the GI tract by pathogens results in increased intestinal secretion as a result of enterotoxins, cytotoxic mediators, or decreased intestinal absorption secondary to intestinal damage or inflammation. Enteric pathogens attach to the mucosal cells and form a cuplike pedestal on which the bacteria rests. The pathogenesis of the diarrhea depends on whether the organism remains attached to the cell surface resulting in a secretory toxin (noninvasive, toxin-producing, noninflammatory type) diarrhea, or penetrates the mucosa (systemic) diarrhea. Noninflammatory diarrhea is the most common diarrheal illness, resulting from the action of enterotoxin that is released after attachment to the mucosa (Ramaswamy & Jacobson, 2001). The most serious and immediate physiologic disturbances associated with severe diarrheal disease are (1) dehydration, (2) acid-base imbalance with acidosis, and (3) shock that occurs when dehydration progresses to the point that circulatory status is seriously impaired.

Diagnostic Evaluation

Evaluation of the child with acute gastroenteritis begins with a careful history that seeks to discover the possible cause of diarrhea, to assess the severity of symptoms and the risk of complications, and to elicit information about current symptoms indicating other treatable illnesses that could be causing the diarrhea. The history should include questions about recent travel, exposure to untreated drinking or washing water sources, contact with animals or birds, day care center attendance, recent treatment with antibiotics, or recent diet changes. History questions should also explore the presence or absence of other symptoms such as the presence of fever, vomiting, frequency, character of stools (e.g., watery, bloody), urine output, dietary habits, and recent food intake (Burkhart, 1999).

Extensive laboratory evaluation is not indicated in children who have uncomplicated diarrhea and no evidence of dehydration because most diarrheal illnesses are self-limiting. Laboratory tests are indicated for children who are severely dehydrated and receiving intravenous therapy. Watery, explosive stools suggest glucose intolerance; foul-smelling, greasy, bulky stools suggest fat malabsorption. Diarrhea that develops after the introduction of cow's milk, fruits, or cereal may be related to enzyme deficiency or protein intolerance (Savilahti, 2000). Neutrophils or red blood cells in the stool indicate bacterial gastroenteritis or inflammatory bowel disease. The presence of eosinophils suggests protein intolerance or parasitic infection. There is debate about the benefit of obtaining stool cultures in children with domestically acquired gastroenteritis. Stool cultures should be performed when blood, mucus, or polymorphonuclear leukocytes are present in the stool; when symptoms are severe; when there is a history of travel to a developing country; and when there is suspicion of a specific pathogen. Gross blood or occult blood may indicate pathogens such as *Shigella, Campylobacter,* or hemorrhagic *Escherichia coli* strains. An enzyme-linked immunosorbent assay (ELISA) may be used to confirm the presence of rotavirus or *Giardia.* If there is a history of recent antibiotic use, the stool should be tested for *C. difficile* toxin. When bacterial and viral cultures are negative and when diarrhea persists for more than a few days, stools should be examined for ova and parasites. A stool specimen with a pH of less than 6 and the presence of reducing substances may indicate carbohydrate malabsorption or secondary lactase deficiency. Stool electrolyte measurements may help identify children with secretory diarrhea.

Urine specific gravity should be determined if dehydration is suspected. A complete blood count (CBC), serum electrolytes, creatinine, and blood urea nitrogen (BUN) should be obtained in the child who requires hospitalization. The hemoglobin, hematocrit, creatinine, and BUN levels are usually elevated in acute diarrhea and should normalize with rehydration.

Therapeutic Management

CASE STUDY: DEHYDRATION AND DIARRHEA

The major goals in the management of acute diarrhea include (1) assessment of fluid and electrolyte imbalance, (2) rehydration, (3) maintenance fluid therapy, and (4) reintroduction of an adequate diet. Infants and children with acute diarrhea and dehydration should be treated first with *oral rehydration therapy (ORT).* ORT is one of the major worldwide health care advances of the past decade. It is more effective, safer, less painful, and less costly than intravenous (IV) rehydration. The American Academy of Pediatrics, World Health Organization, and Centers for Disease Control and Prevention all recommend ORT as the treatment of choice for most cases of dehydration caused by diarrhea (American Academy of Pediatrics, Provisional Committee on Quality Improvement, 1996; Gastanaduy & Begue, 1999; Nappert et al, 2000). Oral rehydration solutions (ORSs) enhance and promote the reabsorption of sodium and water, and studies indicate that these solutions greatly reduce vomiting, volume loss from diarrhea, and the duration of the illness. ORSs are available in the United States as commercially prepared solutions and are successful in treating the majority of infants with isotonic, hypotonic, or hypertonic dehydration. Guidelines for rehydration recommended by the American Academy of Pediatrics are included in Box 47-7.

After rehydration, an ORS may be used during maintenance fluid therapy by alternating the solution with a low-sodium fluid such as water, breast milk, lactose-free formula, or half-strength lactose-containing formula. In older children, an ORS can be given and a regular diet continued. Ongoing stool losses should be replaced on a 1:1 basis with an ORS. If the stool volume is not known, approximately 10 ml/kg (4 to 8 ounces) of ORS should be given for each diarrhea stool.

Solutions for oral hydration are useful in most cases of dehydration, and vomiting is not a contraindication. A child who is vomiting should be given an ORS at frequent intervals and in small amounts. In young children, the fluid may be given with a spoon or small syringe in 5 to 10 ml increments every 1 to 5 minutes by the caregiver. An ORS may also be given via nasogastric or gastrostomy tube infusion. Infants without clinical signs of dehydration do not need ORT. They should, however, receive the same fluids recommended for infants with signs of dehydration in the maintenance phase and for ongoing stool losses.

BOX 47-7

Model for Rehydration

Rehydration solution should consist of 75 to 90 mEq of sodium (Na^-) per liter.
Give 40 to 50 ml/kg of rehydration solution over 4 hours.
Replacement and maintenance solution should consist of 40 to 60 mEq of Na^- per liter.
Reevaluate the need for further rehydration; initiate maintenance therapy using maintenance formulations, with daily volumes not to exceed 150 ml/kg/day.
In children with diarrhea without significant dehydration, the maintenance phase may be initiated without the need for rehydration solution).
If additional fluids are needed, use low-salt fluids such as breast milk or water.

Modified from American Academy of Pediatrics, Provisional Committee on Quality Improvement, Subcommittee on Acute Gastroenteritis: Practice parameter: the management of acute gastroenteritis in young children, *Pediatrics* 97(3):424-435, 1996.

NURSE ALERT Diarrhea is not managed by encouraging intake of clear fluids by mouth, such as fruit juices, carbonated soft drinks, and gelatin. These fluids usually have a high carbohydrate content, a very low electrolyte content, and a high osmolality (Lasche & Duggan, 1999). Caffeinated soda is avoided, because caffeine is a mild diuretic and may lead to increased loss of water and sodium. Chicken or beef broth is not given, because it contains excessive sodium and inadequate carbohydrate. A BRAT diet (bananas, rice, applesauce, and toast or tea) is contraindicated for the child and especially for the infant with acute diarrhea, because this diet has little nutritional value (low in energy and protein), is high in carbohydrates, and is low in electrolytes. ■

Early reintroduction of nutrients is desirable and is gaining more widespread acceptance. Continued feeding or early reintroduction of a normal diet has no adverse effects and actually lessens the severity and duration of the illness and improves weight gain when compared with the gradual reintroduction of foods (Lasche & Duggan, 1999). Infants who are breastfeeding should continue to do so, and an ORS should be used to replace ongoing losses in these infants.

The use of nonhuman milk for infants and children with diarrhea remains controversial. Cow's milk and cow's milk formulas are of concern because poor digestion of lactose can occur in children with infectious diarrhea. However, some studies indicate that well-hydrated infants may resume full-strength nonhuman milk feeding immediately without adverse reactions (Hugger, Harkless, & Rentschler, 1998).

Many infants and children are safely managed with a diet containing cow's milk. Some practitioners advocate the use of a lactose-free formula only if milk or regular formula is not tolerated. In older children, a regular diet can generally be offered after rehydration has been achieved. In toddlers, there is no contraindication to continuing soft or pureed foods. A diet of easily digestible foods such as cereals, cooked vegetables, and meats is adequate for the older child.

In cases of severe dehydration and shock, IV fluids are initiated whenever the child is unable to ingest sufficient amounts of fluid and electrolytes to (1) meet ongoing daily physiologic losses, (2) replace previous deficits, and (3) replace ongoing abnormal losses. Patients who usually require IV fluids are those with severe dehydration, those with uncontrollable vomiting, those who are unable to drink for any reason (e.g., extreme fatigue, coma), and those with severe gastric distention.

The IV solution is selected on the basis of what is known regarding the probable type and cause of the dehydration—usually a saline solution containing 5% dextrose in water. Sodium bicarbonate may be added, because acidosis is usually associated with severe dehydration. Although the initial phase of fluid replacement is rapid in both isotonic and hypotonic dehydration, it is contraindicated in hypertonic dehydration because of the risk of water intoxication, especially in the brain cells.

After the severe effects of dehydration are under control, specific diagnostic and therapeutic measures are begun to detect and treat the cause of the diarrhea. Because of the self-limiting nature of vomiting and its tendency to improve when dehydration is corrected, the use of antiemetic agents is not recommended. The use of antibiotic therapy in children with acute gastroenteritis is controversial. Antibiotics may shorten the course of some diarrheal illnesses (e.g., those caused by *Shigella*). However, most bacterial diarrheas are self-limiting, and the diarrhea often resolves before the causative organism can be determined. Antibiotics may prolong the carrier period for bacteria such as *Salmonella*. Antibiotics may be considered, however, in patients with immunosuppression, patients with severe symptoms or persistent disease, or patients who have had transplantation (Burkhart, 1999; Jabbar & Wright, 2003).

Nursing Care Management

Assessment

The nursing assessment of diarrhea begins with observation of the infant or child's general appearance and behavior. Physical assessment includes all the parameters described for assessment of dehydration, such as decreased urine output; decreased weight; dry mucous membranes; poor skin turgor, sunken fontanel; and pale, cool, dry skin. With severe dehydration, increased pulse and respiration, decreased blood pressure, and a prolonged capillary refill time (longer than 2 seconds) may indicate impending shock.

A history provides information about probable etiologic agents, such as introduction of a new food, exposure to infectious agents, travel to an area of high susceptibility, contact with foods that might be contaminated, and contact with pets known to be sources of enteric infections. An allergic, drug, and dietary history may indicate food allergies, use of laxatives or antibiotics, or sources of excess sorbitol and fructose (e.g., apple juice).

Nursing Diagnoses

Several nursing diagnoses are identified following a thorough physical assessment. The major diagnoses appropriate for the infant or child are described in the Nursing Care Plan on p. 1503. Other diagnoses may be evident depending on the age, condition, and etiology of the diarrhea.

Plan of Care and Implementation

The goals for the dehydrated infant or child and for the family are as follows:

1. Infant or child will maintain adequate hydration.
2. Infant or child will maintain appropriate nutrition for age.
3. Infant or child will not spread infection (if etiologic agent) to others.
4. Family will receive appropriate support and education, especially regarding home care.

The management of most cases of acute diarrhea takes place in the home with education of the caregiver. Caregivers are taught to monitor for signs of dehydration (especially the number of wet diapers or voidings) and the amount of fluids taken by mouth, and to assess the frequency and amount of stool losses. Education relating to ORT, including the administration of maintenance fluids and replacement of ongoing losses, is important (Critical Thinking Exercise). An ORS should be administered in small quantities at frequent intervals. Vomiting is not a contraindication to ORT unless it is severe. Information concerning the introduction of a normal diet is essential. Parents need to know that a slightly higher

Critical Thinking Exercise

DIARRHEA

A mother brings her 8-month-old infant, Mary, to the primary care clinic. The mother reports that Mary has had a "cold" for about 2 days, and this morning she began to vomit and has had diarrhea for the past 8 hours. The mother states that Mary is still breastfeeding, but that she is not taking as much fluid as usual, and she is having three times as many stools as usual (the stools are watery in consistency). When the nurse practitioner examines Mary, she notes that her temperature is 100.4° F, her pulse and blood pressure are in the normal range, her mucous membranes are moist, and she has tears when she cries. The nurse practitioner also notes that Mary's weight has not changed from what it was when she was seen in the clinic 2 weeks ago for her well-child visit. What interventions should the nurse practitioner include in her initial management of Mary?

1. Evidence—Is there sufficient evidence for the nurse practitioner to draw any conclusions for the initial plan of management?
2. Assumptions—Describe some underlying assumptions about the following:
   a. Clinical manifestations of various levels of dehydration
   b. Management of acute diarrhea
   c. Breastfeeding and the management of acute diarrhea
   d. Use of antidiarrheal medications for acute diarrhea
3. What nursing interventions should the nurse practitioner implement at this time?
4. Does the evidence support the nurse practitioner's conclusion?
5. Are there any alternative perspectives that the nurse practitioner should consider?

stool output initially occurs with continuation of a normal diet and with ongoing replacement of stool losses. The benefits of a better nutritional outcome with fewer complications and a shorter duration of illness outweigh the potential increase in stool frequency. Parents' concerns should be addressed to ensure adherence to the treatment plan.

If the child with acute diarrhea and dehydration is hospitalized, an accurate weight must be obtained, as well as careful monitoring of intake and output. The child may be placed on parenteral fluid therapy with nothing by mouth (NPO) for 12 to 48 hours. Monitoring the IV infusion is an important nursing function. The nurse must ensure that the correct fluid and electrolyte concentration is infused, that the flow rate is adjusted to deliver the desired volume in a given time, and that the IV site is maintained.

Accurate measurement of output is essential to determine if renal blood flow is sufficient to permit the addition of potassium to the IV fluids. The nurse is responsible for examination of stools and collection of specimens for laboratory examination (see Collection of Specimens, Chapter 44). Care should be taken when obtaining and transporting stools to prevent possible spread of infection. A clean tongue depressor can be used to obtain specimens for laboratory examination or as an applicator for transfer to a culture medium. Stool specimens should be transported to the laboratory in appropriate containers and media according to hospital policy.

Diarrheal stools are highly irritating to the skin, and extra care is needed to protect the skin of the diaper region from excoriation (see Diaper Dermatitis, Chapter 53). Rectal temperatures are avoided because they stimulate the bowel, increasing passage of stool.

Support for the child and family involves the same care and consideration given all hospitalized children (see Chapter 43). Parents are kept informed of the child's progress and instructed in the use of frequent and proper handwashing and the disposal of soiled diapers, clothes, and bed linen. Everyone caring for the child must be aware of "clean" areas and "dirty" areas, especially in the hospital, where the sink in the child's room is used for many purposes. Soiled diapers and linen should be discarded in receptacles close to the bedside. To remind caregivers to keep diapers and other soiled articles away from clean areas, place signs identifying "clean" (e.g., bed table) and "dirty" (e.g., sink, bathroom) areas. List the articles that may be stored in each area on these signs.

Prevention

The best intervention for diarrhea is prevention. The fecal-oral route spreads most infections, and parents need information about preventive measures such as personal hygiene, protecting the water supply from contamination, and careful food preparation.

NURSE ALERT To reduce the risk of bacteria transmitted via food, encourage parents to do the following:

- Quickly freeze or refrigerate all ground meat and other perishable foods.
- Never thaw food on the counter or let it sit out of the refrigerator for more than 2 hours.
- Wash hands, utensils, and work areas with hot, soapy water after contact with raw meat to keep bacteria from spreading.
- Check ground meat with a fork to make sure no pink is showing before taking a bite.
- Cook all dishes made with ground meat until brown or gray inside or to an internal temperature of 71° C (160° F). ■

Meticulous attention to perianal hygiene, disposal of soiled diapers, proper handwashing, and isolation of infected persons also minimizes the transmission of infection (see Infection Control, Chapter 44).

Parents need information about preventing diarrhea while traveling. They are cautioned against giving their children adult medications that are used to prevent traveler's diarrhea. Until vaccines or other prophylactic measures are proved to be safe for children, the best measure during travel to areas where water may be contaminated is to allow children to drink only bottled water and carbonated beverages (from the container through a straw supplied from home). Tap water, ice, unpasteurized dairy products, raw vegetables, unpeeled fruits, meats, and seafood should also be avoided.

Evaluation

The effectiveness of nursing interventions is determined by continued reassessment according to the following observational guidelines:

1. Monitor fluid losses with careful intake and output measurements and daily weights.
2. Monitor food intake, especially calories.
3. Observe for evidence of complications from underlying disease (specify) or therapy.
4. Observe and interview family to determine extent and effectiveness of care.

The *expected outcomes* are described in the Nursing Care Plan.

NURSING CARE PLAN: CHILD WITH DIARRHEA (GASTROENTERITIS)

Constipation

Constipation is an alteration in the frequency, consistency, or ease of passing stool. Parents often define constipation as 3 or more days without the passage of stool (Castiglia, 2001). It may also be defined as painful bowel movements, which are often blood streaked, or include the retention of stool, with or without soiling, even with a stool frequency of more than three stools per week (Loening-Baucke, 1995). The frequency of bowel movements, however, is not considered a diagnostic criterion because it varies widely among children. Having extremely long intervals between defecation is termed *obstipation.* Constipation with fecal soiling is referred to as *encopresis.*

Constipation may arise secondary to a variety of organic disorders or in association with a wide range of systemic disorders. Structural disorders of the intestine, such as strictures, ectopic anus, and Hirschsprung disease, may be associated with constipation. Systemic disorders associated with constipation include hypothyroidism, hypercalcemia resulting from hyperparathyroidism or vitamin D excess, and chronic lead poisoning. Constipation may be associated with drugs such as antacids, diuretics, antiepileptics, antihistamines, opioids, and iron supplementation. Spinal cord lesions may be associated with loss of rectal tone and sensation. Affected children are prone to chronic fecal retention and overflow incontinence.

Nursing Care Plan

THE CHILD WITH DIARRHEA (GASTROENTERITIS)

NURSING DIAGNOSIS: Fluid volume deficit related to excessive GI losses from diarrhea/emesis

EXPECTED OUTCOME

Patient exhibits signs of adequate hydration (i.e., skin–normal turgor, moist mucous membranes; vital signs within normal limits [WNL]; balanced intake and output [I&O]; no thirst; blood–electrolytes, hemoglobin/hematocrit, and osmolality WNL; urine–appearance, specific gravity, and osmolality WNL; clear mental processes).

NURSING INTERVENTIONS/*RATIONALES*

Administer prescribed oral rehydration solutions (ORSs) and/or intravenous (IV) solutions alternated with small amounts of low-sodium fluids such as water, breast milk, or lactose-reduced formula *for rehydration and replacement.* (**Avoid fluids with high-carbohydrate, low-electrolyte values such as carbonated drinks, fruit juices, and gelatin.**)

Monitor thirst, skin turgor, capillary refill, mucous membranes, mental status, I&O, vital signs, and appropriate blood and urine laboratory results *to assess hydration status.*

Describe all episodes of diarrhea/emesis *to evaluate for continuing fluid loss.*

Instruct family about appropriate administration of fluids, maintenance of I&O records, and signs and symptoms of continuing dehydration *to optimize compliance.*

NURSING DIAGNOSIS: Altered nutrition: less than body requirements related to diarrheal losses, inadequate intake

EXPECTED OUTCOME

Patient exhibits adequate intake of appropriate nourishment and satisfactory regain of any lost weight.

NURSING INTERVENTIONS/*RATIONALES*

After rehydration, begin refeeding by reintroducing foods from a normal diet as tolerated *to reduce number of stools and weight loss and to shorten the duration of illness.* (**Avoid bananas, rice, apples, and toast or tea [BRAT] diet because it is low in protein, electrolytes, and energy and too high in carbohydrates.**)

Observe and record response to feedings *to assess feeding tolerance.*

Weigh *to monitor weight status.*

Instruct family about appropriate foods *to optimize compliance;* instruct breastfeeding mothers to continue breastfeeding *because it reduces duration and severity of the illness.*

NURSING DIAGNOSIS: Risk for transmitting infection related to invasion of the GI tract by microorganisms

EXPECTED OUTCOME

Patient shows no evidence of transmission of infection to patient contacts.

NURSING INTERVENTIONS/*RATIONALES*

Implement appropriate Standard Precautions, careful handwashing techniques, and use of snug-fitting and superabsorbent disposable diapers *to reduce likelihood of fecal transmission.*

Instruct all members in the environment in isolation procedures and handwashing techniques *to optimize compliance and reduce spread of organisms.*

NURSING DIAGNOSIS: Impaired skin integrity related to irritation caused by frequent, loose stools

EXPECTED OUTCOME

Patient's skin is intact.

NURSING INTERVENTIONS/*RATIONALES*

Keep skin clean and dry through frequent diaper changes, use of superabsorbent disposable diapers, and use of gentle nonalkaline soap and water solution *to protect skin from irritation.* (**Avoid commercial baby wipes that contain alcohol because they add to the irritation.**)

Inspect skin for redness and excoriation; expose reddened areas to air *to promote healing;* use a moisture barrier ointment or cream *to protect excoriated areas.*

Inspect perineum and buttocks *for signs of infection such as fungal growth or Candida* and treat with appropriate medication as prescribed.

Instruct family about skin inspection *for early detection of skin problems.*

NURSING DIAGNOSIS: Anxiety/fear related to separation from parents, unfamiliar environment, distressing procedures

EXPECTED OUTCOME

Patient exhibits minimal signs of emotional or physical distress (e.g., is calm, relaxed, cooperative; engages in nonnutritive sucking, appropriate play).

NURSING INTERVENTIONS/*RATIONALES*

Encourage frequent family visitation with active participation in care *to prevent distress from separation.*

Use frequent touch, holding, and talking *to provide comfort;* use pacifier and mouth care for infants who are on nothing-by-mouth (NPO) status.

Provide diversion and sensory stimulation appropriate to the child's developmental level and physical condition.

Instruct family in importance of comfort measures and in their active participation in care *to ease child's fears.*

The majority of children have *idiopathic* or *functional constipation,* because no underlying cause can be identified. Chronic constipation may occur as result of environmental factors, psychosocial factors, or a combination of both. Transient illness, withholding and avoidance secondary to painful or negative experiences with stooling, and dietary intake with decreased fluid and fiber all play a role in the etiology of constipation.

Newborn Period

Normally the newborn infant passes a first meconium stool within 24 to 36 hours of birth. Any infant who does not do so should be assessed for evidence of intestinal atresia or stenosis, Hirschsprung disease (congenital aganglionic megacolon), hypothyroidism, meconium plugs, or meconium ileus. *Meconium plugs* are caused by meconium that has reduced water content and are usually evacuated after digital examination but may require irrigations with a hypertonic solution or contrast medium.

Meconium ileus, the initial manifestation of cystic fibrosis, is the luminal obstruction of the distal small intestine by abnormal meconium. Treatment is the same as for a meconium plug; early surgical intervention may be needed to evacuate the small intestine.

Infancy

The onset of constipation frequently occurs during infancy and may result from organic causes such as Hirschsprung disease, hypothyroidism, and strictures. It is important to differentiate these conditions from functional constipation. Constipation in infancy is often related to dietary practices. It is less common in breastfed infants, who have softer stools than bottle-fed infants. Breastfed infants may also have decreased stools because of more complete use of breast milk with little residue. When constipation occurs with a change from human milk or modified cow's milk to whole cow's milk, simple measures such as adding or increasing the amount of cereal, vegetables, and fruit in the diet of the infant usually corrects the problem. When a bottle-fed infant passes a hard stool that results in an anal fissure, stool-withholding behaviors may develop in response to pain on defecation (Critical Thinking Exercise).

??? Critical Thinking Exercise

CONSTIPATION

Harry, an 8-month-old infant, is seen by the pediatric nurse practitioner for his well-child visit. Harry's mother states that he usually has one hard stool every 4 to 5 days, which causes discomfort when the stool is passed. He has also had one episode of diarrhea and two episodes of ribbonlike stools. Abdominal distention and vomiting have not accompanied the constipation, and Harry's growth has been normal. Currently, his diet consists of cow's milk formula only. Harry's mother reports that the infrequent passage of hard stools began approximately 6 weeks ago when she stopped breastfeeding. Which interventions should the nurse practitioner include in the initial management of Harry's problem?

1. Evidence—Is there sufficient evidence for the nurse practitioner to draw any conclusions about the management of Harry's problem?
2. Assumptions—Describe some underlying assumptions about the following:
   a. Causes of constipation in infants
   b. Factors associated with functional constipation in infants
   c. Management of functional constipation in infants
3. What interventions should the nurse practitioner implement at this time?
4. Does the evidence support these interventions?
5. Are there alternative perspectives that the nurse practitioner should consider? What are they?

Childhood

Most constipation in early childhood is due to environmental changes or normal development when a child begins to attain control over bodily functions. A child who has experienced discomfort during bowel movements may deliberately try to withhold stool. Over time, the rectum accommodates to the accumulation of stool, and the urge to defecate passes. When the bowel contents are ultimately evacuated, the accumulated feces are passed with pain, thus reinforcing the desire to withhold stool.

Constipation in school-age children may represent an ongoing problem, or it may be a first-time event. The onset of constipation at this age is often the result of environmental changes, stresses, and changes in toileting patterns. A common cause of new-onset constipation at school entry is fear of using the school bathrooms, which are noted for their lack of privacy. Early and hurried departure for school immediately after breakfast may also impede bathroom use.

The management of simple constipation consists of a plan to promote regular bowel movements. Often this is as simple as changing the diet to provide more fiber and fluids, eliminating foods known to be constipating, and establishing a bowel routine that allows for regular passage of stool. Stool-softening agents such as docusate or lactulose may also be helpful. If other symptoms such as vomiting, abdominal distention, or pain and evidence of growth failure are associated with the constipation, the condition should be investigated further.

Nursing Care Management

Constipation tends to be self-perpetuating. A child who has difficulty or discomfort when attempting to evacuate the bowels has a tendency to retain the bowel contents, and this may initiate a vicious circle. Nursing assessment begins with an accurate history of bowel habits; diet; events associated with the onset of constipation; drugs or other substances that the child may be taking; and the consistency, color, frequency, and other characteristics of the stool. If there is no evidence of a pathologic condition, the major task is to educate the parents regarding normal stool patterns and to participate in the education and treatment of the child.

Dietary modifications are essential in preventing constipation. During infancy, simply increasing the carbohydrate (sugar or corn syrup) in the infant's formula will often relieve the problem. During childhood, the diet should contain increased amounts of fiber and fluid. Parents benefit from guidance in selecting foods that facilitate bowel movements (Box 47-8). They need reassurance concerning the benign nature of the condition. It is also important to discuss their attitudes and expectations regarding toilet habits.

When constipation persists despite dietary intervention, more aggressive management may be necessary. It is important to differentiate an acute episode of constipation from chronic functional constipation, which can result from chronic stool-withholding behavior. As the rectal vault becomes distended over time, further complications such as fecal impaction and encopresis may develop.

Hirschsprung Disease

Hirschsprung disease (congenital aganglionic megacolon) is a mechanical obstruction caused by inadequate motility of

BOX 47-8

High-Fiber Foods

Bread, Grains
Whole-grain bread or rolls
Whole-grain cereals
Bran
Pancakes, waffles, and muffins with fruit or bran
Unrefined (brown) rice

Vegetables
Raw vegetables, especially broccoli, cabbage, carrots, cauliflower, celery, lettuce, and spinach
Cooked vegetables, such as those listed above, and asparagus, beans, Brussels sprouts, corn, potatoes, rhubarb, squash, string beans, and turnips

Fruits
Raw fruits, especially those with skins or seeds, other than ripe banana or avocado
Raisins, prunes, or other dried fruits

Miscellaneous
Nuts, seeds, legumes, popcorn
High-fiber snack bars

part of the intestine. It accounts for about one fourth of all cases of neonatal obstruction, although it may not be diagnosed until later in infancy or childhood. The incidence is 1 in 5000 live births. It is four times more common in males than in females, and it may follow a familial pattern in a small number of cases. Hirschsprung disease is usually an isolated birth defect, but it has been associated with other syndromes, including Down syndrome. Depending on its presentation, it may be an acute, a life-threatening, or a chronic condition (DiLorenzo, 2001).

Pathophysiology

The term *congenital aganglionic megacolon* describes the primary defect, which is the absence of ganglion cells in one or more segments of the colon. In Hirschsprung disease, there is an abnormal migration of the precursor ganglion cells that derive from the neural crest in the developing brain. The result is an impaired colonization of ganglion cells in the distal portion of the GI tract resulting in aganglionosis. In about 75% of cases, the disease is limited to the rectosigmoid area with the aganglionic segment beginning at the internal anal sphincter and extending proximally, blending into the normal colon. Lack of enervation produces the functional defect that results in absence of propulsive movements (peristalsis). Stool accumulates with distention of the bowel proximal to the defect (megacolon). The internal sphincter fails to relax because the ganglion segment is missing the inhibitory neurotransmitter, nitric oxide. The result is an obstruction because the evacuation of stool, gas, and liquids is prevented (Fig. 47-2). Intestinal distention and ischemia may also occur as a result of distention of the bowel wall, which contributes to the development of *enterocolitis* (inflammation of the small bowel and colon). Enterocolitis is the leading cause of death in children with Hirschsprung disease (DiLorenzo, 2001).

Diagnostic Evaluation

Most children with Hirschsprung disease are diagnosed in the first few months of life. Clinical manifestations vary according to the age when symptoms are recognized and the presence of complications, such as enterocolitis (Box 47-9). In infants, the findings include a distended abdomen, a contracted anal sphincter, and small-caliber empty rectum. In older children, a careful history is helpful. Radiographs, an unprepped barium enema, and anorectal manometric examinations assist in the differential diagnosis, which is confirmed by a full-thickness rectal biopsy demonstrating the absence of ganglion cells in the myenteric and submucosal plexus.

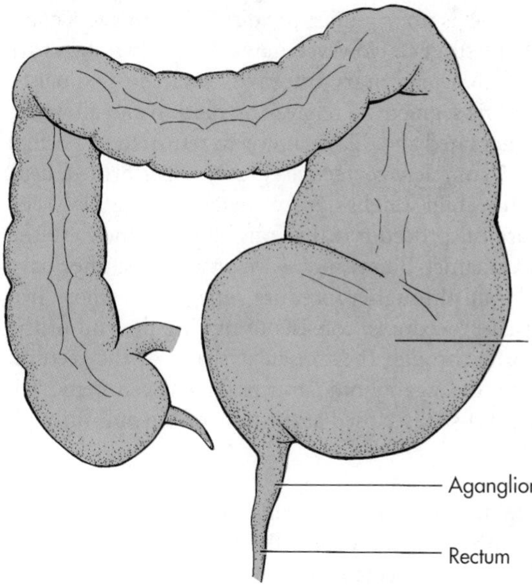

Fig. 47-2 Hirschsprung disease.

Therapeutic Management

Treatment is primarily surgical to remove the aganglionic portion of the bowel to relieve obstruction and restore normal bowel motility and function of the internal anal sphinc-

BOX 47-9

Clinical Manifestations of Hirschsprung Disease

Newborn Period
Failure to pass meconium within 24 to 48 hours after birth
Refusal to feed
Bilious vomiting
Abdominal distention

Infancy
Failure to thrive
Constipation
Abdominal distention
Episodes of diarrhea and vomiting
Signs of enterocolitis
Explosive, watery diarrhea
Fever
Appears significantly ill

Childhood (Symptoms Appear More Chronic)
Constipation
Ribbonlike, foul-smelling stools
Abdominal distention
Visible peristalsis
Easily palpable fecal mass
Undernourished, anemic appearance

ter. If the bowel is not significantly distended, this is accomplished in one surgery. However, in most cases two stages are required. First, a temporary ostomy is created proximal to the aganglionic segment to relieve obstruction and allow the normally enervated and dilated bowel to return to its normal size. Second, complete corrective surgery is performed, usually when the child weighs approximately 9 kg (20 lb). The various surgical procedures that can be performed are the Swenson, Duhamel, Boley, and Soave procedures. The Soave endorectal pull-through procedure, one of the most frequently used procedures, consists of pulling the end of the normal bowel through the muscular sleeve of the rectum, from which the aganglionic mucosa has been removed. The ostomy is usually closed at the time of the pull-through procedure.

Prognosis

Most children with Hirschsprung disease require surgery rather than medical therapy. Once the patient is stabilized with fluid and electrolyte replacement, if needed, the temporary colostomy is performed and has a high rate of success. After the later pull-through procedure, anal stricture and incontinence are potential complications that may occur, requiring further therapy, including dilation or bowel-retraining therapy.

Nursing Care Management

The nursing concerns depend on the child's age and the type of treatment. If the disorder is diagnosed during the neonatal period, the main objectives are (1) to help the parents adjust to a congenital defect in their child, (2) to foster infant-parent bonding, (3) to prepare them for the medical/surgical intervention, and (4) to assist them in colostomy care after discharge.

Preoperative Care

The child's preoperative care depends on the age and clinical condition. A child who is malnourished may not be able to withstand surgery until the physical status improves. Often this involves symptomatic treatment with enemas; a low-fiber, high-calorie, and high-protein diet; and in severe situations, the use of total parenteral nutrition (TPN).

Physical preoperative preparation includes the same measures that are common to any surgery (see Surgical Procedures, Chapter 44). In the newborn, whose bowel is sterile, no additional preparation is necessary. However, in other children, preparation for the pull-through procedure involves emptying the bowel with repeated saline enemas and decreasing bacterial flora with systemic antibiotics and colonic irrigations using antibiotic solution. Oral antibiotics may also be prescribed.

Enterocolitis is the most serious complication of Hirschsprung disease. Emergency preoperative care includes frequent monitoring of vital signs and blood pressure for signs of shock; monitoring fluid and electrolyte replacements, as well as plasma or other blood derivatives; and observing for symptoms of bowel perforation, such as fever, increasing abdominal distention, vomiting, increased tenderness, irritability, dyspnea, and cyanosis.

Because progressive distention of the abdomen is a serious sign, the nurse measures abdominal circumference with a paper tape measure, usually at the level of the umbilicus or at the widest part of the abdomen. The point of measurement is marked with a pen to ensure reliability of subsequent measurements. Abdominal measurement can be obtained with the vital sign measurements and is recorded in serial order so that any change is obvious. To reduce stress to the acutely ill child when frequent measurements of abdominal circumference are needed, the tape measure can be left in place beneath the child rather than removed each time.

The child's age dictates the type and extent of psychologic preparation. Because a colostomy is usually performed, the child who is of at least preschool age is told about the procedure in concrete terms, with the use of visual aids (see Chapter 44). It is important to time explanations appropriately to prevent the anxiety and confusion that could result from too much information. It is also important to stress to parents and older children that the colostomy for Hirschsprung disease is temporary, unless so much bowel is involved that a permanent ileostomy must be performed. In most instances the extent of bowel resection is known before surgery, although the nurse should be aware of those instances when doubt exists concerning repair. The nurse should remember that although a temporary colostomy is favorable in terms of future health and adjustment, it requires additional surgery, which may be very stressful to parents and children.

Postoperative Care

Postoperative care is the same as that for any child or infant with abdominal surgery (see Surgical Procedures, Chapter 44). When a colostomy is part of the corrective procedure, stomal care is a major nursing task (see Ostomies, Chapter 44). To prevent contamination of the abdominal wound with urine in the infant, the diaper should be pinned below the dressing. Sometimes a Foley catheter is used in the immediate postoperative period to divert the flow of urine away from the abdomen.

Discharge Care

After surgery, parents need instruction concerning colostomy care. Even a preschooler can be included in the care by handing articles to the parent, rolling up the colostomy pouch after it is emptied, or applying barrier preparations to the surrounding skin. Although the diagnosis of Hirschsprung disease is less frequent in school-age children or adolescents, children this age can often be involved in colostomy care to the point of total responsibility.

Some institutions and communities have enterostomal therapists who provide expert assistance in planning home care. If families require financial assistance and psychologic support, referral to a social worker, home health care agency, or community health nurse provides continuity of care.

Vomiting

Vomiting is the forceful ejection of gastric contents through the mouth. It is a well-defined, complex, coordinated process that is under central nervous system control and is often accompanied by nausea and retching. Vomiting may be divided into two categories: nonbilious and bilious. Some small intestinal reflux is common in all vomiting. In nonbilious vomiting, the majority of bile drains into the more distal portions of the intestine. If an obstruction is present, nonbilious vomiting suggests a more proximal obstruction. Bilious vomiting implies a disorder of motility or distal physical blockage. Causes of nonbilious vomiting include infectious, inflammatory, metabolic/endocrinologic, neurologic, and psychologic causes, as well as obstructive lesions. Causes of bilious vomiting include intestinal atresia and stenosis, malrotation with or without volvulus, ileus, intussusceptions, intestinal duplication, mass lesions, incarcerated inguinal hernia, and appendicitis. Vomiting may also be associated with other processes, including acute infectious diseases, increased intracranial pressure (ICP), toxic ingestions, food intolerances and allergies, mechanical obstruction of the GI tract, metabolic disorders, and psychogenic problems. Vomiting is common in childhood, is usually self-limited, and requires no specific treatment. However, complications may occur, including dehydration and electrolyte disturbances, malnutrition, aspiration, and Mallory-Weiss syndrome (small tears in the distal esophageal mucosa).

Therapeutic Management

Management is directed toward detection and treatment of the cause of the vomiting and prevention of complications from the loss of fluid. Fluids are administered in the same manner and in a similar electrolyte composition to those administered for diarrhea. Although most children respond to these measures, antiemetic drugs may be needed. Antiemetics such as ondansetron (Zofran) and trimethobenzamide (Tigan) block receptors in the chemoreceptor trigger zone; others enhance gastroduodenal peristalsis (e.g., metoclopramide [Reglan]) or compete for H_1-receptor sites (e.g., promethazine [Phenergan]). For children who are prone to motion sickness, it is helpful to administer an appropriate dose of dimenhydrinate (Dramamine) before a trip.

Nursing Care Management

The major focus of nursing care is observation and reporting of vomiting behavior and associated symptoms and the implementation of measures to reduce the vomiting. Accurate assessment of the type of vomiting, the appearance of the vomitus, and the child's behavior in association with the vomiting helps establish a diagnosis.

Nursing interventions are determined by the cause of the vomiting. When the vomiting is a manifestation of improper feeding methods, establishing proper techniques through teaching and example will usually correct the situation. If vomiting is believed to be an indication of obstruction, food is usually withheld or special feeding techniques are implemented. In situations in which vomiting is related to concurrent infection, dietary indiscretion, or emotional factors, efforts are directed toward maintaining hydration or preventing dehydration.

The thirst mechanism is the most sensitive guide to fluid needs, and ad libitum administration of a glucose-electrolyte solution to an alert child will restore water and electrolytes satisfactorily. It is important to include carbohydrate to spare body protein and avoid ketosis resulting from exhaustion of glycogen stores. Small, frequent feedings of fluids or foods are preferred. After vomiting has stopped, more liberal amounts of fluids are offered, followed by gradual resumption of the regular diet.

The vomiting infant or child is positioned on the side or semireclining to prevent aspiration and observed for evidence of dehydration. It is important to emphasize the need for the child to brush the teeth or rinse the mouth after vomiting to dilute hydrochloric acid that comes in contact with the teeth. A flavored mouthwash or toothbrushing will freshen the mouth. Careful monitoring of fluid and electrolyte status is necessary to prevent an electrolyte disturbance.

Gastroesophageal Reflux

Gastroesophageal reflux (GER) is defined as the transfer of gastric contents into the esophagus. Approximately 1 in 300 to 1 in 1000 children have gastroesophageal reflux. It is important to differentiate GER from *gastroesophageal reflux disease (GERD)*. GERD represents symptoms or tissue damage that result from GER. However, GER may occur without reflux disease (GERD), and conversely, GERD may occur without regurgitation (Orenstein, 1999). GER becomes a disease when complications such as failure to thrive, bleeding, or dysphagia develop. GERD is associated with respiratory symptoms, including apnea, bronchospasm, laryngospasm, and pneumonia (Zeiter & Hyams, 1999).

The causes of GER are related to dysfunction of the *lower esophageal sphincter (LES)*, delay in gastric emptying, poor clearance of esophageal acid, and the susceptibility of esophageal mucosa to acid injury (Zeiter & Hyams, 1999). In the past, GER was thought to be the result of decreased LES tone. However, it now appears that *transient relaxation of the lower esophageal sphincter (TRLES)* is the mechanism that leads to GER. Factors that cause LES pressure to vary include gastric distention, increased abdominal pressure caused by coughing, central nervous system disease, delayed gastric emptying, hiatal hernia, and gastrostomy placement.

Infants and children who are especially prone to GER include premature infants; infants with bronchopulmonary dysplasia; and children who have had tracheoesophageal or esophageal atresia repair, neurologic disorders, scoliosis, asthma, cystic fibrosis, or cerebral palsy.

Reflux of stomach contents into the esophagus predisposes the infant or child to aspiration and the development of respiratory symptoms, particularly pneumonia. Other concerns include (1) the association of life-threatening apnea with GER and (2) repeated irritation of the esophageal lining with gastric acid, which can lead to esophagitis and subsequent bleeding. Bleeding produces anemia, hematemesis, or melena (blood in stools). Heartburn is also a frequent symptom in children who are able to describe it. Box 47-10 lists the clinical manifestations and complications of GER.

Diagnostic Evaluation

The history and physical examination is usually sufficiently reliable to establish the diagnosis of GER. However, the upper GI series is helpful to evaluate the presence of anatomic abnormalities (e.g., pyloric stenosis, malrotation, annular pancreas, hiatal hernia, esophageal stricture). Esophageal pH monitoring establishes the presence of acid reflux. Endoscopy may be helpful to assess the presence and severity of esophagitis and strictures and to exclude other disorders, such as Crohn's disease. *Scintigraphy* detects radioactive substances in the esophagus after a feeding of the compound and assesses gastric emptying.

Therapeutic Management

Therapeutic management of GER depends on its severity. No therapy is needed for the infant who is thriving and has no respiratory complications. Some children require small,

BOX 47-10

Clinical Manifestations and Complications of Gastroesophageal Reflux

Symptoms in Infants
Spitting up, regurgitation, vomiting (may be forceful)
Excessive crying, irritability, arching of the back, stiffening
Weight loss, failure to thrive
Respiratory problems (cough, wheeze, stridor, gagging, choking with feedings)
Hematemesis
Apnea or apparent life-threatening event (ALTE)

Symptoms in Children
Heartburn
Abdominal pain
Noncardiac chest pain
Chronic cough
Dysphagia
Nocturnal asthma
Recurrent pneumonia

Complications
Esophagitis
Esophageal stricture
Laryngitis
Recurrent pneumonia
Anemia
Barrett's esophagus

Adapted from Rudolph CD et al: Guidelines for evaluation and treatment of gastroesophageal reflux in infants and children: recommendations of the North American Society for Pediatric Gastroenterology and Nutrition, *J Pediatr Gastroenterol Nutr* 32(suppl 2):S1-S31, 2001.

frequent feedings of thickened formula and positioning therapy, which helps minimize the symptoms until the child grows and a normal physiologic barrier to reflux develops.

Although study continues on this topic, there is evidence to support a 1- to 2-week trial of a hypoallergenic formula in formula-fed infants. Controversies surround thickened feedings. Milk-thickening agents do not improve reflux index scores, but this therapy has been shown to decrease the number of episodes of vomiting and to increase the caloric density of the formula. Feedings thickened with 1 teaspoon to 1 tablespoon of rice cereal per ounce of formula may be recommended. This may benefit infants who are underweight as a result of GER. Constant nasogastric feedings may be necessary for the infant with severe reflux and failure to thrive.

Several studies have examined the effectiveness of positioning therapy for infants. Esophageal pH monitoring has demonstrated that infants have significantly less GER in the prone position than in the supine position. Despite the potential benefit of the prone position in relationship to GERD, because of its association with sudden infant death syndrome (SIDS), the American Academy of Pediatrics recommends the nonprone positioning for sleep. The prone position should only be considered in cases where the risk of death from the complications of GER outweighs the risk of SIDS. If the prone position is used, parents need to be cautioned to avoid soft bedding, which can increase the risk of SIDS. In children older than 1 year, there is a benefit to the left-side position during sleep and the elevation of the head of the bed.

Pharmacologic therapy may be used as an adjunct therapy to treat infants and children with persistent symptoms of GER. H_2 antagonists, such as cimetidine (Tagamet), ranitidine (Zantac), and famotidine (Pepcid), have proved effective in reducing the amount of acid present in gastric contents and may prevent esophagitis. Proton pump inhibitors such as esomeprazole (Nexium), lansoprazole (Prevacid), omeprazole (Prilosec), pantoprazole (Protonix), and rabeprazole (Aciphex), are very effective in blocking acid production. Current investigations are ongoing to examine the effectiveness and potential side effects of these drugs in infants and children. Metoclopramide (Reglan) has been found to increase resting LES pressure mildly and to increase rates of gastric emptying. However, side effects, including restlessness, drowsiness, and extrapyramidal reaction, may occur, and in some patients, metoclopramide actually increases the number of reflux episodes. Bethanechol has been shown to increase LES pressure, but it has not been proved to decrease reflux by pH probe studies. Bethanechol has a side effect of respiratory symptoms such as wheezing. In practice, metoclopramide and bethanechol have not been shown to be effective in treating GERD in children (Rudolph et al, 2001).

Cisapride (Propulsid), a drug used to promote gastric emptying, was taken off the market in 2000 because of the risk of serious cardiac arrhythmias and death associated with its use. However, the drug is available through an investigational limited-access program.

Surgical management of GER is reserved for children with severe complications such as recurrent aspiration pneumonia, apnea, severe esophagitis, or failure to thrive, and for children who have failed to respond to medical therapy. The *Nissen fundoplication* (Fig. 47-3) is the most common surgical procedure. This surgery involves passage of the gastric fundus behind the esophagus to encircle the distal esophagus. The most recent surgical advance is the introduction of the laparoscopic Nissen fundoplication (Rothenberg, 1998; Trovar et al, 1998). Complications following fundoplication include breakdown of the wrap, small bowel obstruction, gas-bloat syndrome, infection, and retching and dumping syndrome (Rudolph et al, 2001).

Prognosis

The majority of infants with GER have a mild problem that generally improves by 12 to 18 months of age and requires only conservative lifestyle changes or medical therapy. If GER is severe and remains unsuccessfully treated, multiple complications can occur. Presence of esophageal strictures caused by persistent esophagitis with scarring is the most significant complication. Recurrent respiratory distress with aspiration pneumonia, another serious complication, is an indication for surgery. Failure to thrive caused by GER is generally managed with medical therapy and nutritional support.

Nursing Care Management

Nursing care is directed at (1) identifying children with symptoms; (2) educating parents regarding home care, including feeding, positioning, and medications; and (3) if appropriate, providing care for the child undergoing surgical repair (see Surgical Procedures, Chapter 44). Early in the

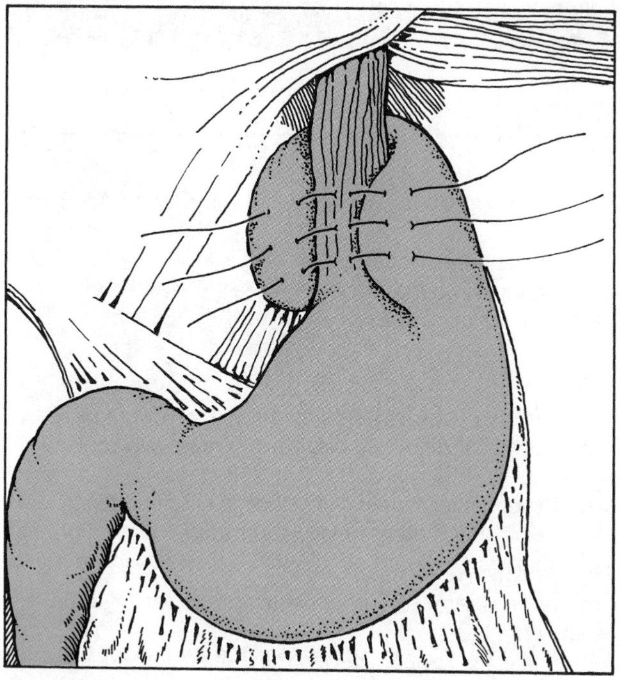

Fig. 47-3 Nissen fundoplication sutures passing through esophageal musculature. (Redrawn from Campbell A, Ferrara B: *AORN J* 57:671-679, 1993.)

treatment program, parents should be reassured that most infants and children outgrow GER, and often conservative lifestyle changes are sufficient. Parents need support and reassurance to implement lifestyle changes. Although it is not known if lifestyle changes bring additional benefit to patients receiving pharmacologic interventions, some changes may be helpful. Older children and adolescents need to know that caffeine, chocolate, and spicy foods may weaken the LES and aggravate symptoms. Tobacco and alcohol are also associated with GER. Obesity increases abdominal pressure, and weight management may reduce GER symptoms. To help parents cope with the inconvenience of dealing with a child, who spits up frequently, simple measures such as using bibs and protective cloths during and after feedings are beneficial. When medical management is necessary, parents need information about the medications and their potential side effects. Prokinetic medications must be given before feedings. Medications for acid control must be given regularly and timed to provide coverage two or three times a day as ordered.

INTESTINAL PARASITIC DISEASES

Intestinal parasitic diseases, including helminths (worms) and protozoa, constitute the most frequent infections in the world. In the United States, the incidence of intestinal parasitic disease, especially giardiasis, has increased among young children who attend day care centers. Young children are especially at risk because of typical hand-mouth activity and uncontrolled fecal activity.

Intestinal parasitic diseases in humans are caused by various infecting organisms. This discussion is limited to the two most common parasitic infections among children in the United States: giardiasis and pinworms. Table 47-5 describes the outstanding features of selected helminths that belong to the family of nematodes.

General Nursing Care Management

Nursing responsibilities related to intestinal parasitic infections involve assistance with identification of the parasite, treatment of the infection, and prevention of initial infection or reinfection. Identification of the organism is accomplished by laboratory examination of substances containing the worm, its larvae, or ova. Most are identified by examining fecal smears from the stools of persons suspected of harboring the parasite. Fresh specimens are best for revealing parasites or larvae; therefore collected specimens should be taken directly to the laboratory for examination. If this is not feasible, the specimen is placed in a container with a preservative. Parents need clear instructions on obtaining an adequate sample and the number of samples required (see Stool Specimens, Chapter 44). In most parasitic infections, examination of other family members, especially children, may be carried out to identify those who are similarly affected.

After the diagnosis is confirmed and appropriate treatment is planned, parents need further explanation and reinforcement. Compliance in terms of drug therapy and other measures, such as thorough handwashing, are essential for eradication of the parasite. The family needs to understand the nature of transmission and that in some cases the medication must be repeated in 2 weeks to 1 month to kill organisms hatched since initial treatment.

The nurse's most important function is preventive education of children and families regarding hygiene and health habits. Thorough handwashing before eating or handling food and after using the toilet is the most important precautionary method.

Giardiasis

Giardiasis is caused by the protozoan *Giardia lamblia* (also called *Giardia intestinalis, Giardia duodenalis,* and *Lamblia intestinalis*). It is the most common intestinal parasitic pathogen in the United States. Child care centers are common sites for urban giardiasis, and the children may pass cysts for months. Giardiasis should also be considered in those with a history of recent travel to an endemic area (Pickering, 2003).

The potential for transmission is great, because the cysts—the nonmotile stage of the protozoa—can survive in the environment for months. Chief modes of transmission are person to person; water, especially mountain lakes, streams, and pools frequented by diapered infants; food; and animals, especially puppies. In children, person-to-person transmission is the most likely cause. Although individuals infected with giardiasis may be asymptomatic, common symptoms include abdominal cramps and diarrhea (Box 47-11).

Diagnosis of giardiasis may be made by microscopic examination of stool specimens or duodenal fluid, or by identification of *G. lamblia* antigens in these specimens by tech-

Table 47-5

Selected Intestinal Parasites

CLINICAL MANIFESTATIONS	COMMENTS
ASCARIASIS—*ASCARIS LUMBRICOIDES* (COMMON ROUNDWORM)	
Light infections: asymptomatic Heavy infections: anorexia, irritability, nervousness, enlarged abdomen, weight loss, fever, intestinal colic Severe infections: intestinal obstruction, appendicitis, perforation of intestine with peritonitis, obstructive jaundice, lung involvement—pneumonitis	Transferred to mouth by way of contaminated food, fingers, or toys Largest of the intestinal helminths Affects principally young children 1-4 years of age Prevalent in warm climates
HOOKWORM DISEASE—*NECATOR AMERICANUS*	
Light infections in well-nourished individuals: no problems Heavier infections: mild to severe anemia, malnutrition May be itching and burning followed by erythema and a papular eruption in areas to which the organism migrates	Transmitted by discharging eggs on the soil, which are picked up, causing infection from direct skin contact with contaminated soil Wearing shoes is recommended, although children playing in contaminated soil expose many skin surfaces
STRONGYLOIDIASIS—*STRONGYLOIDES STERCORALIS* (THREADWORM)	
Light infection: asymptomatic Heavy infection: respiratory signs and symptoms; abdominal pain, distention; nausea and vomiting; diarrhea—large, pale stools, often with mucus Threat to life in children with weakened immunologic defenses	Transmission is same as for hookworm except autoinfection common Older children and adults affected more often than young children Severe infections may lead to severe nutritional deficiency
VISCERAL LARVA MIGRANS—*TOXOCARA CANIS* (DOGS); INTESTINAL TOXOCARIASIS—*TOXOCARA CATI* (CATS)	
Depends on reactivity of infected individual May be asymptomatic except for eosinophilia Specific diagnosis difficult	Transmitted by direct contamination of hands from contact with dog, cat, or objects or by ingestion of soil Dogs and cats should be kept away from areas where children play; sandboxes are especially important transmission areas Periodic deworming of diagnosed dogs and cats Control of dog and cat population Continued education and laws to prevent indiscriminate canine and feline defecation
TRICHURIASIS—*TRICHURIS TRICHIURA* (WHIPWORM)	
Light infections: asymptomatic Heavy infections: abdominal pain and distention, diarrhea	Transmitted from contaminated soil, vegetables, toys, and other objects Most frequent in warm, moist climates Occurs most often in undernourished children living in unsanitary conditions

BOX 47-11

Clinical Manifestations of Giardiasis

Infants and young children:
- Diarrhea
- Vomiting
- Anorexia
- Failure to thrive

Children older than 5 years of age:
- Abdominal cramps
- Intermittent loose stools
- Constipation
- Stools may be malodorous, watery, pale, and greasy

Most infections resolve spontaneously in 4 to 6 weeks

Rarely, chronic form occurs:
- Intermittent loose, foul-smelling stools
- Possibility of abdominal bloating, flatulence, sulfur-tasting belches, epigastric pain, vomiting, headache, and weight loss

niques such as enzyme immunoassay (EIA). Because the *Giardia* organisms live in the upper intestine and are excreted in a highly variable pattern, repeated microscopic examination of stool specimens may be required to identify trophozoites (active parasites) or cysts. Duodenal specimens are obtained by direct aspiration, biopsy, or the *string test.* In the string test, the child swallows a gelatin capsule with a nylon string attached. Several hours later, the string is withdrawn and the contents are sent for laboratory analysis. With the availability of EIA techniques to identify *Giardia* antigens in stool specimens, other tests are being used less often.

Therapeutic Management

The drugs available for treatment of giardiasis are quinacrine (Atabrine), furazolidone (Furoxone), and metronidazole (Flagyl). The drug of choice is furazolidone, unless cost is a factor, in which case quinacrine is substituted. Quinacrine is less than one tenth the cost of furazolidone, and its long-term safety is established over the use of metronidazole. Unfortunately, quinacrine has the highest frequency of side effects, especially nausea and vomiting; temporary yellow staining of the skin, sclera, and urine; and a very bitter taste.

Nursing Care Management

The most important nursing consideration is prevention of giardiasis, especially among children and staff of day care centers. Attention to meticulous sanitary practices, especially during diaper changes, is essential (Fig. 47-4). Nurses can play an important role in educating day care staff regarding appropriate sanitation practices.

After children are infected, family education regarding drug administration is essential. Parents often need suggestions for encouraging the child to take quinacrine. If other household members are infected, the nurse should inquire about their understanding and management of the disease.

To decrease the side effects of quinacrine and increase its palatability, crush tablets and mix them with a strong flavoring such as jam or syrup and administer the drug with or after meals.

Enterobiasis (Pinworms)

Enterobiasis, or pinworms, caused by the nematode *Enterobius vermicularis,* is the most common helminthic infection in the United States. It is universally present in temperate climatic zones and may infect more than 30% of all children at any one time. Crowded conditions, such as in classrooms and day care centers, favor transmission.

Infection begins when the eggs are ingested or inhaled (the eggs float in the air). The eggs hatch in the upper intestine, then mature and migrate through the intestine. After mating, adult females migrate out the anus and lay eggs (Pickering, 2003). The movement of the worms on skin and mucous membrane surfaces causes intense itching. As the child scratches, eggs are deposited on the hands and underneath the fingernails. The typical hand-to-mouth activity of youngsters makes them especially prone to reinfection. Pinworm eggs persist in the indoor environment for 2 to 3 weeks, contaminating anything they contact, such as toilet seats, doorknobs, bed linen, underwear, and food. Except for the intense rectal itching associated with pinworms, the clinical manifestations are nonspecific (Box 47-12).

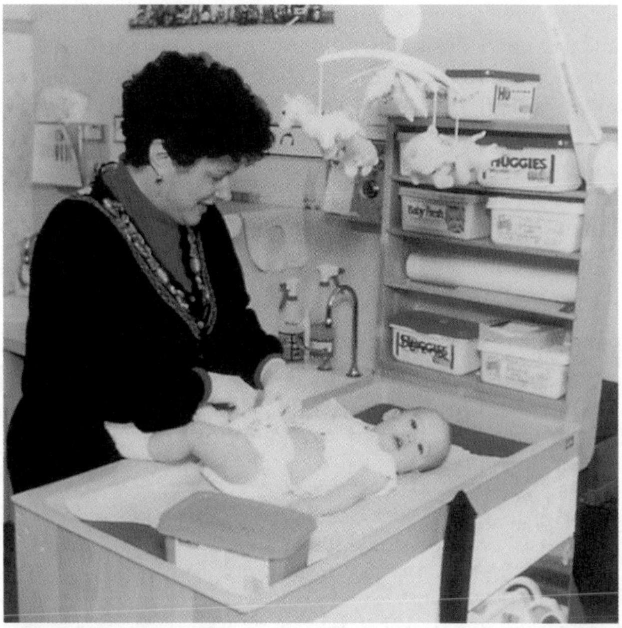

Fig. 47-4 Prevention of giardiasis, especially in day care centers, requires sanitary practices during diaper changes, such as discarding paper diapers in a covered receptacle, changing paper covers on the diaper-changing surface, and having facilities for handwashing nearby. NOTE: Soiled cloth diapers and clothing should be stored in a plastic bag for transport home.

Diagnostic Evaluation

Diagnosis is most commonly made from the tape test (see Nursing Care Management). Repeated tests to collect eggs may be necessary, and if there is a possibility that other family members may be infected, a tape test should be performed on them.

Therapeutic Management

The drugs available for treatment of pinworms include mebendazole (Vermox), pyrantel pamoate (Antiminth), piperazine phosphate, and pyrvinium pamoate (Povan). The drug of choice is mebendazole, which is safe, effective, and convenient, with few side effects. However, it is not recommended for children younger than 2 years of age. If pyrvinium pamoate is prescribed, parents are advised that the drug stains stool and vomitus bright red, as well as clothing or skin that comes in contact with the drug. Because pinworms are easily transmitted, all household members are treated. The drugs should be repeated in 2 weeks to prevent reinfection.

Nursing Care Management

Nursing care is directed at identifying the parasite, eradicating the organism, and preventing reinfection. Parents need clear, detailed instructions for the *tape test.* A loop of transparent (not "frosted" or "magic") tape, sticky side out, is placed around the end of a tongue depressor, which is then firmly pressed against the child's perianal area. A convenient, commercially prepared tape is also available for this purpose. Pinworm specimens are collected in the morning as soon as the child awakens and *before* the child has a bowel movement or bathes. The procedure may need to be performed more than once before eggs are collected. Parents are instructed to place the tongue blade in a glass jar or loosely

BOX 47-12

Clinical Manifestations of Pinworms

Intense perianal itching (principal symptom); evidence of itching in young children includes the following:
- General irritability
- Restlessness
- Poor sleep
- Bed-wetting
- Distractibility
- Short attention span

Perianal dermatitis and excoriation secondary to itching
If worms migrate, possible vaginal and urethral infection

in a plastic bag so that it can be brought in for microscopic examination. For specimens collected in the hospital, practitioner's office, or clinic, the tape is placed smoothly on a glass slide, sticky side down, for examination.

Adherence to the drug regimen is usually excellent, because the duration of treatment is typically only one dose. However, the family is reminded of the need to take a second dose in 2 weeks. Posting a reminder on the refrigerator door or bathroom mirror is helpful.

To prevent reinfection, washing all clothes and bed linens in hot water and vacuuming the house may be recommended. However, there is little documentation on the effectiveness of these measures, because pinworms survive on many surfaces. Helpful suggestions include handwashing after toileting and before eating, keeping the child's fingernails short to minimize the chance of ova collecting under the nails, dressing children in one-piece sleeping outfits, and daily showering rather than tub bathing. Families should be informed that recurrence is common. Repeated infections should be treated in the same manner as the first one.

INFLAMMATORY DISORDERS

Acute Appendicitis

Appendicitis, inflammation of the *vermiform appendix* (blind sac at the end of the cecum), is the most common cause of emergency abdominal surgery in childhood. In the Unites States, 60,000 to 80,000 cases are diagnosed each year. The average age of children with appendicitis is 10 years, with boys and girls equally affected before puberty. Despite emphasis on early surgical intervention, the mortality rate of acute appendicitis in children is high. Death rates from nonperforated and perforated appendicitis are 0.1% and 5%, respectively. Death is usually the result of complications associated with a delayed diagnosis. At the time of initial presentation, about one third of all cases involve an already perforated appendix. Abdominal pain is a common complaint in children, and perforation of the appendix can occur within approximately 48 hours of the initial complaint of pain. Early recognition is essential.

Etiology

The cause of appendicitis is obstruction of the lumen of the appendix, usually by hardened fecal material (fecalith). Swollen lymphoid tissue, frequently occurring after a viral infection, can also obstruct the appendix. A rare cause of obstruction is a parasite such as *E. vermicularis* or pinworms, which can obstruct the appendiceal lumen.

Pathophysiology

With acute obstruction, the outflow of mucous secretions is blocked and pressure builds within the lumen, resulting in compression of blood vessels. The resulting ischemia is followed by ulceration of the epithelial lining and bacterial invasion. Subsequent necrosis causes perforation or rupture, with fecal and bacterial contamination of the peritoneal cavity. The resulting inflammation spreads rapidly throughout the abdomen *(peritonitis)*, especially in young children, who are unable to localize infection. Progressive peritoneal inflammation results in functional intestinal obstruction of the small bowel *(ileus)* because intense GI reflexes severely inhibit bowel motility. Because the peritoneum represents a major portion of total body surface, the loss of ECF to the peritoneal cavity leads to electrolyte imbalance and hypovolemic shock.

Diagnostic Evaluation

Diagnosis is not always straightforward. Numerous infections and inflammatory processes have similar features to that of appendicitis. Fever, vomiting, abdominal pain, and an elevated blood count are associated with appendicitis, but are also seen in inflammatory bowel disease, pelvic inflammatory disease, gastroenteritis, urinary tract infection, right lower lobe pneumonia, constipation, mesenteric adenitis, Meckel diverticulum, and intussusception. Prolonged symptoms and delayed diagnosis often occur in preschool-age children; the risk of perforation is greatest in this age group because of their inability to verbalize their complaints.

The diagnosis is based primarily on the history and physical examination (Box 47-13). Pain, the cardinal feature, is initially generalized (usually periumbilical); however, it usually descends to the lower right quadrant. The most intense site of pain may be at *McBurney point,* located at a point midway between the anterior superior iliac crest and the umbilicus. Rebound tenderness is not a reliable sign and is extremely painful to the child. Referred pain, elicited by light percussion around the perimeter of the abdomen, indicates the presence of peritoneal irritation. Movement, such as riding over bumps in an automobile or gurney, aggravates the pain. In addition to pain, significant clinical manifestations include fever, a change in behavior, anorexia, and vomiting.

Laboratory studies usually include a complete blood count; urinalysis (to rule out a urinary tract infection); and in adolescent females, a serum human chorionic gonadotropin (to rule out an ectopic pregnancy). A white blood cell (WBC) count greater than 10,000/mm is common, but not necessarily specific for appendicitis. However, a normal WBC count and a temperature less than 100.5° F may be helpful to exclude appendicitis. An elevated percentage of bands (often referred to as "a shift to the left") may indicate an inflammatory process. Recently, some primary care providers have been adding the C-reactive protein (CRP) to the laboratory studies. CRP is an acute-phase reactant that rises within 12 hours of the onset of infection. However, the CRP test has low specificity, and any infectious process can cause an elevated CRP.

BOX 47-13

Clinical Manifestations of Appendicitis

Right lower quadrant abdominal pain
Fever
Rigid abdomen
Decreased or absent bowel sounds
Vomiting (typically follows onset of pain)
Constipation or diarrhea may be present
Anorexia
Tachycardia; rapid, shallow breathing
Pallor
Lethargy
Irritability
Stooped posture

evolve CASE STUDY: APPENDICITIS

Ultrasonography (US) and a computed topography (CT) scan are helpful in differentiating pediatric abdominal pain from other causes. Findings such as visualization of the appendix and the presence of fluid around the appendix are important sonographic signs (Irish et al, 1998).

NURSE ALERT Signs of peritonitis in addition to fever include sudden relief from pain after perforation, subsequent increase in pain (usually diffuse and accompanied by rigid guarding of the abdomen), progressive abdominal distention, tachycardia, rapid shallow breathing, pallor, chills, and irritability. ■

Therapeutic Management

Treatment of appendicitis before perforation includes rehydration, antibiotics, and surgical removal of the appendix *(appendectomy)*. The operation is usually performed through a right lower quadrant incision (open appendectomy). Laparoscopic surgery is now commonly used to treat nonperforated acute appendicitis (Holcomb, 2001). Recovery is rapid, and, if no complications occur, the hospital stay is short.

Ruptured Appendix

Management of the child diagnosed with peritonitis caused by a ruptured appendix often begins preoperatively with IV administration of fluid and electrolytes, systemic antibiotics, and nasogastric suction. Postoperative management includes IV fluids, continued administration of antibiotics, and nasogastric suction for abdominal decompression until intestinal activity returns. The child with peritonitis is given antibiotics, including ampicillin, gentamicin, and clindamycin, for 7 to 10 days.

In some instances the wound is closed following irrigation of the peritoneal cavity. Many surgeons, however, leave the wound open (delayed closure) to prevent wound infection. A Penrose drain may be used to permit transperitoneal drainage. When delayed closure is used, wound irrigations and wet-to-dry dressings are a routine part of postoperative care.

Prognosis

Complications are uncommon following a simple appendectomy. The mortality rate from perforating appendicitis has improved from nearly certain death a century ago to 1% or less at present (Strahlman, 2001). The most common complications include wound infection and intraabdominal abscess. Early recognition of the illness is essential to prevent complications.

Nursing Care Management

Because abdominal pain is the most common childhood complaint with appendicitis, it is important to assess the severity of pain (see Pain Assessment, Chapter 44). One of the most reliable estimates is the degree of change in behavior. For example, a child who stays home from school and voluntarily lies down or refuses to play is much more likely to have considerable discomfort than the child who is absent from school but plays contentedly at home. The younger, nonverbal child will assume a rigid, motionless, side-lying posture with the knees flexed on the abdomen, and there is decreased range of motion of the right hip. Older children may exhibit all of these behaviors while complaining of abdominal pain. They can always indicate a point at which the pain is worse than at any other location.

NURSE ALERT In any instance when severe abdominal pain is expected, be aware of the danger of administering laxatives or enemas or applying heat to the area. Such measures stimulate bowel motility and increase the risk of perforation. ■

Postoperative Care

Postoperative care for the nonperforated appendix is the same as that for most abdominal procedures. Care of the child with a ruptured appendix and peritonitis involves more complex care, and the course of recovery is considerably longer (usually 7 to 10 days of hospitalization). The child is maintained on IV fluids, allowed nothing by mouth, and kept on low continuous gastric decompression until there is evidence of intestinal activity. Listening for bowel sounds and observing for other signs of bowel activity (e.g., passage of stool) are part of the routine assessment. Management of IV therapy is the same as that for any child receiving fluids and parenteral antibiotics. A drain is often placed in the wound during surgery, and frequent dressing changes with meticulous skin care are essential to prevent excoriation of the area surrounding the surgical site. Wound care includes irrigation with antibacterial solution.

Management of pain from the incision and repeated dressing changes and irrigations are an essential part of the child's care. Psychologic care of the child and parents is similar to that used in other emergency situations (see Emergency Admission, Chapter 44). Parents and older children need to express their feelings and concerns regarding the events surrounding the illness and hospitalization. The nurse can provide education and psychosocial support to promote adequate coping and alleviation of anxiety for both the child and the family.

Meckel Diverticulum

Meckel diverticulum is a remnant of the fetal omphalomesenteric duct that connects the yolk sac with the primitive midgut during fetal life. Normally this structure is obliterated by the seventh to eighth week of gestation, when the placenta replaces the yolk sac as the source of nutrition for the fetus. Failure of obliteration may result in an *omphalomesenteric fistula* (a fibrous band connecting the small intestine to the umbilicus, known as Meckel diverticulum).

Meckel diverticulum is a true diverticulum because it arises from the antimesenteric border of the small intestine, and all layers of the intestinal wall are present. The diverticulum is usually found within 100 cm (40 inches) of the ileocecal valve and averages 1 to 10 cm (2.625 to 4 inches) in length (Schwartz, 1999).

Meckel diverticulum is the most common congenital malformation of the GI tract and is present in 1% to 4% of the population (Schwartz, 1999). It is twice as common in males as in females, and complications are more frequent in males. Most symptomatic cases are seen in childhood. Patients requiring surgery are generally less than 10 years of age, and about 50% are less than 2 years of age (Schwartz, 1999).

Pathophysiology

The possible symptomatic complications of this condition are bleeding, obstruction, and inflammation; bleeding is the most common problem in children. Gastric mucosa is the most common ectopic tissue found in Meckel diverticulum. Bleeding is caused by peptic ulceration or perforation because of the unbuffered acidic secretion. Several other mechanisms can cause obstruction. Obstruction may also be caused by entanglement of the small intestine around a fibrous cord, trapping of a loop of intestine under the band, incarceration within a hernia sac, or volvulus of the intestinal segment containing the diverticulum. Diverticulitis occurs when peptic ulceration or obstruction leads to inflammation.

Diagnostic Evaluation

Diagnosis is usually based on the history, physical examination, and a specialized radiographic study. The most common clinical presentation in children includes painless rectal bleeding, abdominal pain, or signs of intestinal obstruction (Box 47-14). Bleeding, which may be mild or profuse, often appears as dark red or "currant jelly" stools; bleeding may be significant enough to cause hypotension. The more common obstructive symptoms in children are volvulus and intussusception. The Meckel scan, a radionucleotide *scintigraphy,* detects the presence of gastric mucosa with an overall diagnostic accuracy of 90%. Abdominal radiographs, barium enema, and arteriography are not successful diagnostic tools. Blood studies are performed to screen for bleeding disorders and anemia (Schwartz, 1999).

Therapeutic Management

The standard treatment is surgical removal of the diverticulum. When severe hemorrhage increases the surgical risk, interventions to correct hypovolemic shock, such as blood replacement, IV fluids, and oxygen, may be necessary. Antibiotics may be used preoperatively to control infection. If intestinal obstruction has occurred, appropriate preoperative measures are used to reverse electrolyte imbalances and prevent abdominal distention.

Prognosis

If this condition is diagnosed and treated early, full recovery is likely. The mortality rate of untreated Meckel diverticulum ranges from 2.5% to 15%. Complications of untreated Meckel diverticulum include GI hemorrhage and bowel obstruction.

Nursing Care Management

Nursing objectives are similar to those for any child undergoing surgery (see Chapter 44). Because the onset of this condition is often rapid, parents require psychologic support. The massive intestinal bleeding that can accompany a Meckel diverticulum is traumatic to both the child and the parents and may significantly affect their emotional reaction to hospitalization and surgery.

Specific preoperative considerations with intestinal bleeding include (1) frequent monitoring of vital signs and blood pressure for shock, (2) keeping the child on bed rest, and (3) recording the approximate amount of blood lost in stools. In the absence of frank hemorrhage, the nurse tests the stools for occult blood. Postoperatively, the child requires IV fluids and a nasogastric tube for the decompression and evacuation of gastric contents.

BOX 47-14

Clinical Manifestations of Meckel Diverticulum

Abdominal Pain
Similar to appendicitis
May be vague and recurrent

Bloody Stools*
Painless
Bright or dark red with mucus ("currant jelly" stool)
In infants, bleeding may be accompanied by pain

Sometimes
Severe anemia
Shock

*Often an initial sign.

INFLAMMATORY BOWEL DISEASE

Inflammatory bowel disease (IBD) is a term that is used for two forms of chronic intestinal inflammation—*ulcerative colitis (UC)* and *Crohn's disease (CD).* Although UC and CD have similar epidemiologic, immunologic, and clinical features, they are two distinct conditions with very important differences (Table 47-6).

GI symptoms, extraintestinal and systemic inflammatory responses, and exacerbations and remissions without complete resolution characterize these diseases. Growth failure, particularly common in CD, is an important problem unique to the pediatric population. CD is more disabling, has more serious complications, and has less effective medical and surgical treatment than UC. Because UC is confined to the colon, theoretically it may be cured with a colectomy. Over the past 30 years, the incidence of CD has risen, whereas the incidence of UC in children has remained stable. The incidence of UC in children has been estimated as 3.5 new cases per 100,000 per year; the incidence of CD is 3.11 per 100,000 (Jackson & Grand, 1999).

Etiology

Despite decades of research, the etiology of IBD is not completely understood and there is no known cure. There is evidence to indicate a multifactorial etiology. It is proposed that IBD is the result of one or more environmental influences, such as infectious organisms, dietary habits, and environmental toxins that promote disease in genetically susceptible individuals. Research is focused on theories of defective immunoregulation of the inflammatory response to bacteria or viruses in the GI tract in individuals with a genetic predisposition. A familial tendency is apparent in approximately 20% to 25% of cases. Individuals from higher socioeconomic levels and more whites are affected, and the condition occurs more frequently among Jews living in Europe and North America and among people living in urban settings. Males and females are affected equally (Leichtner, Jackson, & Grand, 1996). A primary role for psychologic factors has not been supported, although psychologic problems may occur as a result of IBD and may intensify symptoms and influence the course of the disease.

Pathophysiology: Ulcerative Colitis

The inflammation is limited to the colon and rectum, with the distal colon and rectum the most severely affected. Inflammation affects the mucosa and submucosa and involves continuous segments along the length of the bowel

Table 47-6

Clinical Manifestations of Inflammatory Bowel Diseases

CHARACTERISTICS	ULCERATIVE COLITIS	CROHN'S DISEASE
Rectal bleeding	Common	Uncommon
Diarrhea	Often severe	Moderate to severe
Pain	Less frequent	Common
Anorexia	Mild or moderate	May be severe
Weight loss	Moderate	May be severe
Growth retardation	Usually mild	May be severe
Anal and perianal lesions	Rare	Common
Fistulas and strictures	Rare	Common
Rashes	Mild	Mild
Joint pain	Mild to moderate	Mild to moderate

with varying degrees of ulceration, bleeding, and edema. The presentation may be mild, moderate, or severe, depending on the extent of mucosal inflammation and systemic symptoms. Most cases include bloody diarrhea or occult fecal blood, abdominal pain that is most intense during defecation, and varying degrees of systemic manifestations and growth abnormalities (Leichtner et al, 1996). Thickening of the bowel wall and fibrosis are unusual, but long-standing disease can result in shortening of the colon and strictures. Extraintestinal manifestations are less common in UC than in CD.

Pathophysiology: Crohn's Disease

The chronic inflammatory process of CD involves any part of the GI tract from the mouth to the anus but most often affects the terminal ileum. The disease involves all layers of the bowel wall (transmural) in a discontinuous fashion, meaning that between areas of intact mucosa, there are areas of affected mucosa (skip lesions). The most common symptoms are abdominal pain with cramps, diarrhea, and weight loss. Other manifestations include fever; anorexia; rectal bleeding; and perineal discomfort, including anal fissures or fistulas. The presence of perianal disease is a strong indication for CD. Mild GI symptoms, poor growth, and extraintestinal manifestations may be present for several years before overt GI symptoms occur. The inflammation may result in ulcerations, fibrosis, and adhesions; stiffening of the bowel wall; stricture formation; and fistulas to other loops of bowel, bladder, vagina, or skin. Extraintestinal manifestations are common, including erythema nodosum, large joint arthritis, uveitis, mouth ulcers, liver disease, and renal calculi.

Diagnostic Evaluation

The diagnosis of UC and CD is derived from the history, physical examination, laboratory evaluation, and other diagnostic procedures. Because the diseases have similar symptoms, it is difficult to distinguish CD from UC. UC is confined to the large bowel and affects only the inner lining (the mucosa and submucosa). CD involves all layers of the bowel (transmural). Laboratory tests include a CBC to evaluate anemia and an erythrocyte sedimentation rate or CRP to assess the systemic reaction to the inflammatory process. Levels of total protein, albumin, iron, zinc, magnesium, vitamin B_{12}, and fat-soluble vitamins may be low in children with CD. Stools are examined for the presence of blood, leukocytes, and infectious organisms. A serologic panel is often used in combination with clinical findings to diagnose IBD and to differentiate between CD and UC. In IBD, autoantibodies called *antineutrophil cytoplasm antibodies (ANCAs)* may be detected in the blood. The perinuclear antineutrophil cytoplasm antibody (pANCA) is associated with UC. Approximately 60% to 70% of patients with UC and 15% of those with CD are pANCA positive. Anti-*Saccharomyces cerevisiae* antibodies (ASCAs) have been found in 67% to 92% of individuals with CD (Baron, 2002).

In patients with CD, an upper GI series with small bowel follow-through reveals images that demonstrate narrowing or modularity of the small bowel. The terminal ileum may be narrowed or rigid with partial obstruction. In about one third of the patients, lesions pierce the walls of the small intestine and colon, creating tracts called *fistulas* between the intestine and adjacent structures such as the bladder, anus, vagina, or skin. Fistulas may become infected, causing discharge of pus and mucus. A CT scan is helpful in evaluating abscesses, fistulas, and bowel wall thickening. *Endoscopy,* direct visualization of the surface of the GI tract with biopsies, is necessary to confirm the diagnosis, assess the extent of inflammation, and evaluate for strictures. Endoscopy may be both upper and lower colonoscopy depending on the clinical presentation of the child.

Therapeutic Management

The goals of therapy are to (1) control the inflammatory process to reduce or eliminate the symptoms, (2) obtain long-term remission, (3) promote normal growth and development, and (4) allow as normal a lifestyle as possible. Treatment is individualized and managed according to the type and the severity of the disease, its location, and the response to therapy.

Medical Treatment

Drugs that mediate and control inflammation (corticosteroids, aminosalicylates, sulfasalazine, immunosuppressives, and biologic therapies) are used to treat IBD. *Cortico-*

steroids, such as prednisone and prednisolone, are used in short bursts to suppress the inflammatory response in moderate to severe IBD. These drugs inhibit the production of adhesion molecules, cytokines, and leukotrienes. Although these drugs reduce the acute symptoms of IBD, they have side effects that relate to long-term use, including growth suppression (adrenal suppression), weight gain, and decreased bone density (Baron, 2002). High doses of IV corticosteroids may be administered in acute episodes and tapered according to clinical response. *Aminosalicylates* are useful in decreasing the frequency of recurrences in mild cases of IBD. *Sulfasalazine* decreases inflammation by inhibiting prostaglandin synthesis. Because it is only active in the colon, it is not effective in the treatment of small bowel disease. Sulfasalazine may decrease the absorption of folic acid; therefore daily supplements of folic acid are needed in long-term therapy. Side effects of this drug include headache, nausea, vomiting, neutropenia, and oligospermia. The side effects are caused primarily by the sulfapyridine component of the drug, so alternative nonabsorbable salicylate drugs such as olsalazine and mesalamine may be prescribed. Mesalamine comes in a variety of formulations that are active in different parts of the bowel. Asacol is active in the terminal ileum and the colon. Pentasa targets the jejunum, and Rowasa is a topical preparation administered rectally by enema to relieve inflammation of the distal colon and rectum.

Immunomodulatory medications are used when the symptoms of IBD persist despite the use of steroids or when the patient cannot be weaned from corticosteroids (e.g., when reducing the dose of steroids results in return of symptoms such as diarrhea, pain, and bleeding). *Azathioprine* and its metabolite *6-MP* block the synthesis of purine, thus inhibiting the ability of deoxyribonucleic acid (DNA) and ribonucleic acid (RNA) to hinder lymphocyte function, especially that of T cells. Side effects include infection, pancreatitis, hepatitis, bone marrow toxicity, arthralgia, and malignancy. Other immunomodulatory medications include *methotrexate, cyclosporin,* and *mycophenolate mofetil.* Patients on these medications require regular monitoring of their CBC and differential to assess for changes that reflect suppression of the immune system.

Antibiotics, such as metronidazole and ciprofloxacin, may be used as an adjunctive therapy to treat complications such as perianal disease or small bowel bacterial overgrowth. Side effects of this drug are peripheral neuropathy, nausea, and a metallic taste.

Biologic therapies act to regulate inflammatory and antiinflammatory cytokines. Tumor necrosis factor–alpha (TNF-α) is believed to influence active inflammation. Infliximab (Remicade) is an antibody to TNF-α. This drug is given via IV infusions 6 to 12 weeks apart. Approximately 5% of patients have acute allergic reactions to infliximab and require premedication with prednisone and diphenhydramine before infusion to prevent reactions. Long intervals between infusions may predispose patients to serum sickness (an immune response causing fever, muscle pain, arthritis, and hives) (Baron, 2002). Severe complications of this drug include lupus-like syndrome and lymphoma. Other biologic medications include methotrexate, interleukin-10, and thalidomide.

Nutritional Support

Nutritional support is a primary component of the treatment of IBD. Growth failure is a common serious complication, especially in CD. Growth failure is characterized by weight loss, alteration in body composition, retarded height, and delayed sexual maturation. Malnutrition causes the growth failure, and its etiology is multifactorial. Malnutrition occurs as a result of inadequate dietary intake, excessive GI losses, malabsorption, drug-nutrient interaction, and increased nutritional requirements. Inadequate dietary intake occurs with anorexia and episodes of increased disease activity. Excessive loss of nutrients (protein, blood, electrolytes, and minerals) occurs secondary to intestinal inflammation and diarrhea. Carbohydrate, lactose, fat, vitamin, and mineral malabsorption, as well as vitamin B_{12} and folic acid deficiencies, occur with disease episodes and with drug administration and when the terminal ileum is resected. Finally, nutritional requirements are increased with inflammation, fever, and fistulas and during periods of rapid growth (e.g., adolescence).

The goals of nutritional support include (1) correction of nutrient deficits and replacement of ongoing losses, (2) provision of adequate energy and protein for healing, and (3) provision of adequate nutrients to promote normal growth. Nutritional support includes both enteral and parenteral nutrition. A well-balanced, high-protein, high-calorie diet is recommended for children whose symptoms do not prohibit an adequate oral intake. There is little evidence that avoiding specific foods influences the severity of the disease. Supplementation with multivitamins, iron, and folic acid is recommended.

Special enteral formulas, given either by mouth or continuous nasogastric infusion (often at night) may be required. Elemental formulas are completely absorbed in the small intestine with almost no residue. Several studies have demonstrated that a diet consisting only of elemental formula not only improved nutritional status but also induced disease remission, either without steroids or with a diminished dosage of steroids required. An elemental diet is a safe and potentially effective primary therapy for patients with CD.

TPN has also improved nutritional status in patients with IBD. Short-term remissions have been achieved after TPN, although complete bowel rest has not reduced inflammation or added to the benefits of improved nutrition by TPN (Leichtner et al, 1996). Nutritional support is less likely to induce a remission in UC than in CD. Improvement of nutritional status is important, however, in preventing deterioration of the patient's health status and in preparing the patient for surgery.

Surgical Treatment

Surgery is indicated for UC when medical and nutritional therapies fail to prevent complications. Surgical options include a *subtotal colectomy* and *ileostomy* that leaves a rectal stump as a blind pouch. A reservoir pouch is created in the configuration of a J or an S to help improve continence postoperatively. An ileoanal pull-through preserves the normal pathway for defecation. In many cases UC can be cured with a total colectomy.

Surgery may be required in children with CD when complications cannot be controlled by medical and nutritional therapy. Segmental intestinal resections are performed for small bowel obstructions, strictures, or fistulas. Partial colonic resection is not curative, and the disease often recurs.

Prognosis

IBD is a chronic disease. Relatively long periods of quiescent disease may follow exacerbations. The outcome of the disease is influenced by the regions and severity of involvement, as well as by appropriate therapeutic management. Malnutrition, growth failure, and bleeding are serious complications. The overall prognosis for UC is good.

The development of carcinoma of the colon is a long-term complication of IBD. In UC, removal of the diseased bowel prevents development of carcinoma. In CD, however, surgical removal of the affected bowel does not prevent bowel cancer, and routine screening of stool specimens is necessary for early detection.

Nursing Care Management

The nursing considerations in the management of IBD extend beyond the immediate period of hospitalization. These interventions involve (1) continued guidance of families in terms of dietary management; (2) coping with factors that increase stress and emotional lability; (3) adjusting to a disease of remissions and exacerbations; and (4) when indicated, preparing the child and parents for the possibility of diversionary bowel surgery.

Because nutritional support is an essential part of therapy, encouraging the anorectic child to consume sufficient quantities of food is often a challenge. Successful interventions include the following: involving the child in meal planning; encouraging small, frequent meals or snacks rather than three large meals a day; serving meals around medication schedules when diarrhea, mouth pain, and intestinal spasm are controlled; and preparing high-protein, high-calorie foods such as eggnog, milkshakes, cream soups, puddings, or custard (if lactose is tolerated) (see Feeding the Sick Child, Chapter 44). Foods that are known to aggravate the condition are avoided. Using bran or a high-fiber diet for IBD is questionable. Bran, even in small amounts, has been shown to worsen the patient's condition. Occasionally the occurrence of aphthous stomatitis further complicates adherence to dietary management. Mouth care before eating and the selection of bland foods help relieve the discomfort of mouth sores.

When nasogastric feedings or TPN is indicated, nurses play an important role in explaining the purpose and the expected outcomes of this therapy. The nurse should acknowledge the anxieties of family members and give them adequate time to demonstrate the skills necessary to continue the therapy at home if needed (Critical Thinking Exercise).

The importance of continued drug therapy despite remission of symptoms must be stressed to the child and family members. Failure to adhere to the pharmacologic regimen can result in exacerbation of the disease (see Compliance, Chapter 44).

Family Support

The nurse should attend to the emotional components of the disease and assess any sources of stress. Frequently, the nurse can help children to adjust to problems of growth retardation, delayed sexual maturation, dietary restrictions, feelings of being "different" or "sickly," inability to compete with peers, and necessary absence from school during exacerbations of the illness.

If a permanent colectomy/ileostomy is required, the nurse can teach the child and family how to care for the ileostomy. The nurse can also emphasize the positive aspects of the surgery, particularly accelerated growth and sexual development, permanent recovery, and the eliminated risk of colonic cancer in UC; and the normality of life despite bowel diversion. Introducing the child and parents to other ostomy patients, especially those who are the same age, can be effective in fostering eventual acceptance. Whenever possible, the continent ostomies should be offered as options to the child, although they are not performed in all centers in the United States.

Because of the chronic and often lifelong nature of the disease, families benefit from the educational services provided by organizations such as the Crohn's and Colitis Foundation of America, Inc. (CCFA).* If diversionary bowel surgery is indicated, the United Ostomy Association† and the Wound Ostomy and Continence Nurses Society‡ are avail-

??? Critical Thinking Exercise

INFLAMMATORY BOWEL DISEASE

Susan, a 13-year-old girl, was admitted to the hospital because of bloody diarrhea, abdominal pain, and weight loss. After a thorough evaluation, including laboratory tests, radiographic studies, and gastrointestinal endoscopy procedures, the diagnosis of Crohn's disease (CD) was made. Medical treatment, including corticosteroid drugs and nutritional support, was implemented during this hospitalization.

Susan has improved considerably and is to be discharged home this week. Enteral formula administered by continuous nighttime nasogastric (NG) tube infusion will be continued at home, and both Susan and her family are eager to learn how to perform these feedings. You are the nurse who is responsible for Susan's discharge planning. Which interventions relating to these feedings should you include in Susan's preparations for discharge?

1. Evidence—Are there sufficient data to formulate any specific interventions for discharge?
2. Assumptions—Describe some underlying assumptions about the following:
   a. The goals of nutritional support for children with CD
   b. Teaching required by an adolescent or family member who is administering NG tube feedings at home
   c. Psychosocial issues related to CD
3. What are the priorities for discharge planning at this time?
4. Does the evidence support your conclusion?
5. Are there alternative perspectives to your conclusion? What are they?

---

*386 Park Ave. S., 17th Floor, New York, NY 10016; phone: 800-932-2423; Web site: www.ccfa.org.

†19772 MacArthur Blvd., Suite 200, Irvine, CA 92612-2405; phone: 714-660-8624; Web site: www.uoa.org.

‡1550 South Coast Highway, Suite 201, Laguna Beach, CA 92651; phone: 888-224-9626; Web site: www.wocn.org. In Canada: Crohn's and Colitis Foundation of Canada; Web site: www.ccfc.ca; and United Ostomy Association, Canada, PO Box 46057, College Park, PO 444, Yonge St., Toronto, Ontario M5B2L8; phone: 416-595-5452, fax: 416-595-9924.

able to assist with ileostomy care and provide important psychologic support through their self-help groups. Adolescents often benefit by participating in peer-support groups, which are sponsored by the CCFA.

Peptic Ulcer Disease

Peptic ulcers may be classified as acute or chronic, and peptic ulcer disease (PUD) is a chronic condition that affects the stomach or duodenum. Ulcers are described as gastric or duodenal and as primary or secondary. A *gastric ulcer* involves the mucosa of the stomach; a *duodenal ulcer* involves the pylorus or duodenum. Most *primary ulcers* occur in the absence of a predisposing factor and tend to be chronic, occurring more frequently in the duodenum. *Stress ulcers* result from the stress of a severe underlying disease or injury (e.g., severe burns, sepsis, intracranial disease, severe trauma, multisystem organ failure) and are more frequently acute and gastric.

About 1.7% of children in general pediatric practices have PUD, and the disease represents about 3.4 per 10,000 pediatric hospital admissions. Primary ulcers are more common in children older than 6 years, and stress ulcers are more common in infants younger than 6 months. Except for very young children, the incidence is two to three times greater in boys than in girls (Motil, 1999).

Etiology

The exact cause is unknown, although infectious, genetic, and environmental factors are important. There is an increased familial incidence, and the disease is increased in persons with blood group O.

There is a significant relationship between the bacterium *Helicobacter pylori* (previously called *Campylobacter pylori*) and ulcers. *H. pylori* is known to colonize the gastric mucosa and has been identified in 90% to 100% of adult patients with PUD. It may cause ulcers by weakening the gastric mucosal barrier and allowing acid to damage the mucosa. It is believed that *H. pylori* is acquired via the fecal-oral route, and this hypothesis is supported by finding viable *H. pylori* in feces. The exact mechanism by which it causes gastric inflammation is unclear; however, the large amount of urease present in *H. pylori* may be a factor. Urease hydrolyses urea to ammonia and bicarbonate in the gastric mucosa, and ammonia can be toxic to gastric cells (Chelimsky & Czinn, 2001).

In addition to ulcerogenic drugs, both alcohol and smoking contribute to ulcer formation. There is no conclusive evidence to implicate particular foods, such as caffeine-containing beverages or spicy foods, but polyunsaturated fats and fiber may play a role in ulcer formation.

Psychologic factors may play a role in the development of PUD, and stressful life events, dependency, passiveness, and hostility have all been implicated as contributing factors.

Pathophysiology

Most likely, the pathology is due to an imbalance between the destructive (cytotoxic) factors and defensive (cytoprotective) factors in the GI tract. The toxic mechanisms include acid, pepsin, medications such as aspirin, nonsteroidal anti-inflammatory drugs (NSAIDs), bile acids, and infection with *H. pylori.* The defensive factors include the mucous layer, local bicarbonate secretion, epithelial cell renewal, and mucosal blood flow (Motil, 1999). Prostaglandins play a role in mucosal defense because they stimulate both mucus and alkali secretion. The primary mechanism that prevents the development of peptic ulcer is the secretion of mucus by the epithelial and mucous glands throughout the stomach. The thick mucous layer acts to diffuse acid from the lumen to the gastric mucosal surface, thus protecting the gastric epithelium. The stomach and the duodenum produce bicarbonate, and production of bicarbonate decreases acidity on the epithelial cells, thereby minimizing the effects of the low pH (Chelimsky & Czinn, 2001). When abnormalities in the protective barrier exist, the mucosa is vulnerable to damage by acid and pepsin. Exogenous factors, such as aspirin and NSAIDs, cause gastric ulcers by inhibition of prostaglandin synthesis. Zollinger-Ellison syndrome may occur in children who have multiple, large, or recurrent ulcers. This syndrome is characterized by hypersecretion of gastric acid, intractable ulcer disease, and intestinal malabsorption caused by a gastrin-secreting tumor of the pancreas (Motil, 1999).

Diagnostic Evaluation

Diagnosis is based on the history of symptoms, physical examination, and diagnostic testing. The focus is on symptoms such as epigastric abdominal pain, nocturnal pain, oral regurgitation, heartburn, weight loss, hematemesis, and melena (Box 47-15). History should include questions relating to the use of potentially causative medications such as NSAIDS, corticosteroids, alcohol, and tobacco. Laboratory studies may include a CBC to detect anemia; stool analysis for occult blood, liver function tests, sedimentation rate, or CRP to evaluate inflammatory bowel disease; amylase and lipase to evaluate pancreatitis; and gastric acid measure-

BOX 47-15

Characteristics of Peptic Ulcer

Neonates
- Usually gastric and secondary
- Commonly has a history of prematurity, respiratory distress, sepsis, hypoglycemia, or an intraventricular hemorrhage
- Perforation may be first sign that massive bleeding may occur

Infants to 3-Year-Old Children
- Most likely to have a secondary ulcer located equally in the stomach or duodenum
- Primary ulcers less common and usually located in stomach
- Likely to occur in relation to illness, surgery, or trauma
- Hematemesis, melena, or perforation

2- to 6-Year-Old Children
- Primary or secondary ulcers
- Located equally in stomach and duodenum
- Perforation more likely in secondary ulcers
- Periumbilical pain, poor eating, vomiting, irritability, nighttime waking, hematemesis, melena

Children 6 Years and Older
- Usually primary and most often duodenal
- More typical of adult type
- Chance of recurrence greater
- Often associated with *H. pylori*
- Epigastric pain or vague abdominal pain
- Nighttime waking, hematemesis, melena, and anemia may occur

ments to identify hypersecretion. A lactose breath test may be performed to detect lactose intolerance.

Radiographic studies such as an upper GI series may be performed to evaluate obstruction or malrotation. An upper endoscopy is the most reliable procedure to diagnose PUD. A biopsy is taken to determine the presence of *H. pylori. H. pylori* can also be diagnosed by a blood test that identifies the presence of the antigen to this organism. The C urea breath test measures bacterial colonization in the gastric mucosa. This test is used to screen for *H. pylori* in adults and is now being evaluated for children.

Therapeutic Management

The major goals of therapy for children with PUD are to relieve discomfort, promote healing, prevent complications, and prevent recurrence. Management is primarily medical and consists of administration of medications to treat the infection and to reduce or neutralize gastric acid secretion.

Antacids are beneficial medications to neutralize gastric acid. However, in terms of healing the ulcer or eradication of *H. pylori,* antacids are not as effective as medications that inhibit acid secretion.

Histamine (H_2)–receptor antagonists (antisecretory drugs) act to suppress gastric acid production. Cimetidine (Tagamet), ranitidine (Zantac), and famotidine (Pepcid) are examples of these medications. These medications have few side effects.

Proton pump inhibitors (PPIs), such as omeprazole and lansoprazole, act to inhibit the hydrogen ion pump in the parietal cells, thus blocking the production of acid. Controlled studies of these drugs have been done in adults, and these drugs are now commonly used to treat ulcers in children. They appear to be well tolerated and to have infrequent side effects (e.g., headache, diarrhea, nausea, and vomiting).

Mucosal protective agents, such as sucralfate and bismuth-containing preparations, may be prescribed for PUD. Sucralfate is an aluminum-containing agent that forms a protective barrier over ulcerated mucosa to protect against acid and pepsin. Sucralfate is available in both pill and liquid forms. Because sucralfate blocks the absorption of other medications, it should be given separately from other medications.

Bismuth compounds are sometimes prescribed for the relief of ulcers, but they are used less frequently than PPIs. Although these compounds inhibit the growth of microorganisms, the mechanism of their activity is poorly understood. In combination with antibiotics, bismuth is effective against *H. pylori.* Although concern has been expressed about the use of bismuth salts in children because of potential side effects, none of these side effects have been reported when these compounds have been used in the treatment of *H. pylori* infection.

Triple-drug therapy is the recommended treatment regimen for *H. pylori.* Combination therapy has demonstrated 90% effectiveness in eradication of *H. pylori* when compared with antibiotic monotherapy (Motil, 1999). Examples of drug combinations used in triple-drug therapy are (1) bismuth, clarithromycin, and metronidazole; (2) lansoprazole, amoxicillin, and clarithromycin; and (3) metronidazole, clarithromycin, and omeprazole.

In addition to medications, the child with PUD should be given a nutritious diet and advised to avoid caffeine. Adolescents are warned about gastric irritation associated with alcohol use and smoking.

Children with an acute ulcer who have developed complications, such as massive hemorrhage, require emergency care. The administration of IV fluids, blood, or plasma depends on the amount of blood loss. Replacement with whole blood or packed cells may be necessary for significant loss.

Surgical intervention may be required for complications such as hemorrhage, perforation, or gastric outlet obstruction. Ligation of the source of bleeding or closure of a perforation is performed. A vagotomy and pyloroplasty may be indicated in children with recurring ulcers despite aggressive medical treatment.

Prognosis

The long-term prognosis for PUD is variable. Many ulcers are successfully treated with medical therapy; however, primary duodenal peptic ulcers often recur. Complications such as GI bleeding can occur and extend into adult life. The effect of maintenance drug therapy on long-term morbidity remains to be established with further studies.

Nursing Care Management

The primary nursing goal is to promote healing of the ulcer through compliance with the medication regimen. If an analgesic/antipyretic is needed, acetaminophen, not aspirin or NSAIDs, is used. Critically ill neonates, infants, and children in intensive care units should receive antacids and H_2 blockers to prevent stress ulcers. Critically ill children receiving IV H_2 blockers should have their gastric pH values checked at frequent intervals and buffered with antacid if necessary.

The role of stress in ulcer formation should be considered for nonhospitalized children with chronic illnesses. In children, many ulcers occur secondarily to other conditions, and the nurse should be aware of family and environmental conditions that may aggravate or precipitate ulcers. Children may benefit from psychologic counseling and from learning how to cope constructively with stress.

HEPATIC DISORDERS

Acute Hepatitis

Etiology

Hepatitis is an acute or chronic inflammation of the liver that can result from several different causes (e.g., a virus, a chemical or drug reaction, or other diseases). Nonviral causes of hepatitis include autoimmune hepatitis, Wilson's disease, α_1-antitrypsin deficiency, and steatohepatitis. The following six viruses cause most cases (90%) of viral hepatitis (Table 47-7):

- Hepatitis A virus (HAV)
- Hepatitis B virus (HBV)
- Hepatitis C virus (HCV)
- Hepatitis D virus (HDV)
- Hepatitis E virus (HEV)
- Hepatitis G virus (HGV)

Hepatitis A

HAV is the most common form of acute viral hepatitis in most parts of the world. It is a member of the picornavirus family. The virus produces a contagious disease transmitted

Table 47-7

Comparison of Types A, B, and C Hepatitis

CHARACTERISTICS	TYPE A	TYPE B	TYPE C
Incubation period	15-50 days, average 25-30 days	30-180 days, average 50 days	6-7 weeks, average 2 weeks-6 months
Period of communicability	Believed to be later half of incubation period to the first week after the onset of clinical illness	Variable Virus in blood or other body fluids during late incubation period and acute stage of disease; may persist in carrier state for years to lifetime	Begins before onset of symptoms May persist in carrier state for years
Mode of transmission	Principal route—fecal-oral Rarely—parenteral	Principal route—parenteral Less frequent route—oral, sexual, any body fluid Perinatal transfer—transplacental blood (last trimester), at delivery, or during breastfeeding, especially if mother has cracked nipples	Principal route—parenteral Nonparenteral spread possible
Clinical features			
Onset	Usually rapid, acute	More insidious	Usually insidious
Fever	Common and early	Less frequent	Less frequent
Anorexia	Common	Mild to moderate	Mild to moderate
Nausea and vomiting	Common	Sometimes present	Mild to moderate
Rash	Rare	Common	Sometimes present
Arthralgia	Rare	Common	Rare
Pruritus	Rare	Sometimes present	Sometimes present
Jaundice	Present (many cases anicteric)	Present	Present
Immunity	Present after one attack; no crossover to type B or C	Present after one attack; no crossover to type A or C	Present after one attack; no crossover to type A or B
Carrier state	No	Yes	Yes
Chronic infection	No	Yes	Yes
Prophylaxis			
Immune globulin (IG)	Passive immunity Successful, especially in early incubation period and preexposure prophylaxis	Passive immunity Inconsistent benefits; probably of no use	Not currently recommended by Centers for Disease Control and Prevention
HAV vaccine	Two inactivated vaccines are approved for children ages 2-18 years: Havrix and Vaqta; given in a two-dose schedule (6-12 months between doses)		
HBV immune globulin (HBIG)	No benefit	Postexposure protection possible if given immediately after definite exposure	No benefit
HBV vaccine		Provides active immunity Universal vaccination recommended for all newborns	
Mortality rate	0.1%-0.2%	0.5%-2.0% in uncomplicated cases; may be higher in complicated cases	1%-2.0% in uncomplicated cases; may be higher in complicated cases

primarily in contaminated stool spread via the fecal-oral route from person to person. HAV has been associated with miniepidemics in areas of poor hygiene and high population density. There is no chronic or carrier state. HAV infection affects individuals of all ages, but the highest incidence occurs among preschool- or school-age children younger than 15 years. Children may serve as the source of HAV infection in adults, such as in child care center exposures. Usually HAV disease in children is mild. It is frequently anicteric and often subclinical. Infected children who show no symptoms may still spread the virus to others. HAV can be severe in children with immunodeficiency disorders. The incubation period is approximately 3 weeks. Although some cases may be prolonged, the prognosis is excellent. A highly effective vaccine for HAV was introduced in 1997 (Balistreri et al, 2002; Regev & Schiff, 2000).

Hepatitis B

HBV infection can occur as an acute or a chronic infection and may range from being asymptomatic and limited to causing fatal fulminant (rapid and severe) hepatitis. HBV varies greatly throughout the world. High-prevalence areas have been identified in Africa and Asia; the United States is considered a low-prevalence area. Transmission is usually via the parenteral route through the exchange of blood or any bodily secretion or fluid. Infections from blood transfusion have been reduced as a result of blood product–screening procedures. Transplantation of organs, intimate physical contact, transmission from mother to infant, and the splashing of contaminated fluids into the mouth or eyes are other sources of infection. Adults whose occupations are associated with exposure to blood or blood products (such as health care workers) are at increased risk for infection and should receive HBV vaccination.

Most HBV infection in children is acquired perinatally. Newborns are at risk for hepatitis if the mother is infected with HBV or was a carrier of HBV during pregnancy. Possible routes of maternal-fetal-infant transmission include (1) leakage of virus across the placenta late in pregnancy or during labor and (2) ingestion of amniotic fluid or maternal blood.

HBV infection occurs in children and adolescents in the following high risk groups: (1) individuals with hemophilia and others who have received multiple transfusions, (2) children and adolescents involved in IV drug abuse, (3) institutionalized children and adolescents, (4) preschool-age children in endemic areas, and (5) individuals engaged in heterosexual or homosexual activity with infected partners. The incubation period of HBV infection varies from 45 to 160 days.

Hepatitis C

About 0.2% to 0.4% of children younger than 12 years of age are infected with HCV. It is estimated that 4 million people in the United States are anti-HCV positive. Approximately 7% of HCV-infected mothers transmit the HCV to their newborns (Balistreri et al, 2002). The second most common route of infection is by percutaneous exposure, which occurs through transfusion of blood or blood products, transplantation of organs or tissues, or sharing used needles. Transfusion-associated HCV infection is low, but a common cause of infection is injection drug use. The American Academy of Pediatrics, Committee on Infectious Diseases (1998), suggests screening the following groups: (1) all infants born to HCV-infected women, (2) individuals who received blood products before 1992, (3) individuals involved in injection drug use, and (4) individuals who receive hemodialysis. The length of time that maternal antibody is present in infants born to HCV-infected women must be considered, and screening should be done after the infant is 12 months old. However, a routine screening program, such as that for HBV, is not recommended.

The clinical course of HCV infection is variable. Incubation averages 6 to 7 weeks, with a range of 2 weeks to 6 months. HCV causes acute hepatitis that progresses to chronic disease in more than 70% of affected individuals and can cause end-stage liver disease in 10% of these patients. However, both acute and chronic HCV infections often produce only mild, nonspecific symptoms or no symptoms at all (Bonkovsky & Mehata, 2001).

Current recommendations are to evaluate HCV-infected children at regular intervals to monitor for chronic hepatitis. Most children will be asymptomatic with evidence of chronic hepatitis on liver biopsy. Liver enzyme levels may fluctuate between periods of normal and elevated values (Balistreri, 1999).

Hepatitis D

HDV is an important cause of acute and chronic liver disease. HDV is a defective RNA virus that requires the function of HBV. HDV infection occurs primarily in hemophiliac patients and IV drug abusers. The incubation period is 2 to 8 weeks. Both acute and chronic forms are more severe than HBV infection and can lead to cirrhosis. Testing for HDV infection is recommended in children with chronic HBV infection or severe liver disease and in children with acute exacerbation of a previously stable liver disease.

Hepatitis E

HEV infection is enterally transmitted. Transmission may occur through the fecal-oral route or from contaminated water. The incubation period is 2 to 9 weeks. This illness is uncommon in children, does not cause chronic liver disease, is not a chronic condition, and has no carrier state. The mortality rate resulting from submassive hepatic necrosis is low except in pregnant women in their third trimester, in whom mortality rates approach 20%.

Hepatitis G

HGV is a blood-borne virus that may also be transmitted by organ transplantation. High risk groups include transfusion recipients, IV drug users, and individuals infected with HCV. Individuals with the virus are often asymptomatic, and most infections are chronic. The incubation period is unknown.

Diagnostic Evaluation

Diagnosis is based on the history (especially regarding possible exposure to a hepatitis virus), physical examination, and serologic markers (antibodies or antigens) indicating the presence of active infection with hepatitis A, B, or C or previous infection. Because the liver has a large function reserve, abnormal laboratory tests may be the only indication of hepatitis. However, liver function tests (LFTs) are not specific for the diagnosis of viral hepatitis. Although serum aspartate aminotransferase (AST) and alanine aminotransferase (ALT) levels are markedly elevated in viral hepatitis, other diseases or conditions may also cause their elevation. When hepatitis is severe, albumin levels are depressed and prothrombin times are increased. Serum bilirubin levels peak 5 to 10 days after clinical jaundice appears.

Diagnosis of viral hepatitis is based on the presence of specific viral markers. Diagnosis of acute HAV infection is based on the presence of anti-HAV immunoglobulin M (IgM) antibody in the serum. HBV diagnosis depends on the presence of hepatitis B surface antigen (HBsAG) or anti-HBV core (anti-HBc) IgM antibody. Chronic HBV infection is associated with the persistence of HBsAg and HBV DNA markers. The diagnosis of HCV is based on the detection of anti-HCV antibodies and confirmation by polymerase chain reaction for hepatitis C RNA.

Other diagnostic studies include a urinalysis to evaluate the bilirubinemia and to rule out other causes of hepatitis. An abdominal ultrasound provides measurement of liver size, detection of cystic lesions and stones, and imaging of the gallbladder. Cholescintigraphy radionuclide imaging detects abnormalities in liver uptake, concentration, and excretory function. Liver biopsy aids in assessing the severity of the disease.

Pathophysiology

Pathologic changes occur primarily in the parenchymal cells of the liver and result in varying degrees of swelling, infiltration of liver cells by mononuclear cells, subsequent degeneration, necrosis, and fibrosis.

Hepatitis can be self-limited, and complete regeneration of liver cells without scarring may occur. However, some forms of hepatitis do not result in complete return of liver function. These include *fulminant hepatitis,* which is characterized by a severe, acute course and massive destruction of the liver, which results in liver failure and death in 1 to 2 weeks. *Subacute* or *chronic active hepatitis* is characterized by progressive liver destruction, uncertain regeneration, scarring, and potential cirrhosis.

The initial *anicteric* (absence of jaundice) *phase* usually lasts 5 to 7 days and is often mistaken for influenza. Symptoms include nausea, vomiting, extreme anorexia, malaise, easy fatigability, arthralgia, skin rashes, slight to moderate fever, and epigastric or upper right quadrant abdominal pain. Dark urine is a symptom of the *icteric* (jaundice) *phase.* Pruritus may accompany jaundice and can be bothersome, but many children with acute viral hepatitis do not develop jaundice.

Therapeutic Management

Treatment options for viral hepatitis are limited. The goals of management include early detection, recognition of chronic liver disease, support and monitoring, and prevention of spread of the disease.

HAV infection is an acute disease that resolves with support and management of symptoms. HBV and HCV treatment is directed at managing the viral load to prevent further destruction of the liver. Currently, interferons are used to treat HBV and HCV. Interferons are naturally occurring proteins that exert antiviral, antiproliferative, and immunomodulatory effects. A recent interferon formulation, pegylated interferon, can be administered once a week and has been found to sustain plasma levels and enhance viral suppression (Karnam & Reddy, 2003). Lamivudine and adefovir are two other interferon analogues that suppress the replication of HBV (Yuen & Lai, 2001). A combination of interferon-α and ribavirin has resulted in a sustained response in some adult patients with HBV and HCV (Regev & Schiff, 2000).

Another important aspect of the therapeutic management of hepatitis involves hospitalization. Hospitalization is necessary if coagulopathy or fulminant hepatitis is present.

Prevention

Proper handwashing and standard isolation precautions can prevent the spread of hepatitis. Prophylactic use of standard immune globulin (Ig) is effective in preventing HAV infection in situations of preexposure (e.g., anticipated travel to areas where HAV is prevalent) or in situations of postexposure during the early part of the incubation period. Hepatitis B immune globulin (HBIG) is effective in preventing HBV infection after exposure. IG must be administered less than 2 weeks after exposure.

Vaccines have been developed to prevent HAV and HBV infection. HBV vaccination is recommended for all newborns and for high risk groups. HAV is also recommended for high risk groups (see Immunizations, Chapter 36). Active immunizations are not available against HCV. It is possible to prevent HDV infection by preventing HBV infection.

Prognosis

The prognosis for children with hepatitis is variable and depends on the type of virus. HAV usually causes a mild and brief illness with no carrier state. HBV causes a wide spectrum of acute and chronic illness. Chronic HBV infection leads to cirrhosis in approximately one fourth to one third of the cases. Hepatocellular carcinoma is a potentially fatal complication of HBV infection. HCV infection frequently becomes chronic, and cirrhosis may develop in some patients. Chronic HCV infection is the leading indication for liver transplantation in adults in the United States (Regev & Schiff, 2000). Fulminant hepatic failure occurs in a small number of cases of viral hepatitis, regardless of the etiology, and is associated with a high mortality rate.

Nursing Care Management

Nursing objectives depend on the severity of the hepatitis, the medical management, and factors influencing the control and transmission of the disease. Children with benign viral hepatitis are frequently cared for at home, and the clinic or office nurse must explain the medical therapy and control measures. If further assistance is needed for parents to comply with therapy, a public health nursing referral may be necessary.

A well-balanced diet and a realistic schedule of rest and activity adjusted to the child's condition are encouraged. HAV is not infectious within a week after the onset of jaundice, and children may feel well enough to resume school. Parents are cautioned about administering any medication to the child, because normal doses of many drugs may become dangerous because of the liver's inability to detoxify and excrete them. Handwashing is the single most critical measure in reducing risk of transmission. The nurse should explain to parents and children the ways in which HAV (oral-fecal route) and HBV (parenteral route) are spread.

Children who are hospitalized are not usually isolated in a separate room unless they are fecally incontinent or their toys and other items become contaminated with feces. They are discouraged from sharing their toys. (For further discussion, see Infection Control, Chapter 45.)

Nurses who care for young people with HBV infection who have a known or suspected history of illicit drug use should help these teens to realize the dangers of drug abuse. Nurses should stress the parenteral mode of transmission of hepatitis, and encourage them to seek counseling through a drug program. HBV and HCV are chronic diseases that require frequent monitoring and management. Many communities have multidisciplinary clinics dedicated to the management of these diseases.

Cirrhosis

Cirrhosis occurs at the end stage of many chronic liver diseases, including biliary atresia and chronic hepatitis. Cirrhosis can also result from infectious, autoimmune, or toxic factors and from chronic diseases such as hemophilia and cystic fibrosis. A cirrhotic liver is irreversibly damaged.

Clinical manifestations in children are similar to those seen with all chronic liver disorders. Children exhibit jaundice, poor growth, anorexia, muscle weakness, and lethargy. Ascites, edema, GI bleeding, anemia, and abdominal pain may be present with impaired intrahepatic blood flow. Pulmonary function may be impaired because of pressure against the diaphragm from hepatosplenomegaly and ascites. Dyspnea and cyanosis may occur, especially on exertion. Intrapulmonary arteriovenous shunts may develop and cause hypoxemia. Spider angiomas and prominent blood vessels are often present on the upper torso.

Therapeutic Management

Therapy is directed toward (1) frequent assessment of liver status with physical examination and LFTs and (2) management of specific complications. The only successful treatment for end-stage liver disease and liver failure may be *liver transplantation,* which has improved the prognosis substantially for many children with cirrhosis. Currently, the 1-year survival rate for liver transplantation is 85%. Increasing numbers of recipients are reaching their second decade after transplant. The increasing life span after transplantation is due to advances in surgical techniques and improved preoperative, intraoperative, and postoperative care (Atkison et al, 2002).

Prognosis

Liver transplantation has revolutionized the approach to liver cirrhosis. Liver failure and cirrhosis are indications for transplantation. Liver transplantation reflects the failure of other medical and surgical measures to prevent or treat cirrhosis. Careful monitoring of the child's condition and quality of life are necessary to evaluate the need for and timing of transplantation (Family Focus box).

Nursing Care Management

Nursing care of the child with cirrhosis is determined by the cause of the cirrhosis, the severity of complications, and the prognosis. The prognosis for life is poor unless successful liver transplantation occurs. Nursing care of this child is similar to that for any child with a life-threatening illness (see Chapter 41). Hospitalization is usually required when complications occur.

> **Family Focus**
>
> **END-STAGE LIVER DISEASE**
>
> In many cases the child and family must cope with an uncertain progression of the disease. The only hope for long-term survival may be liver transplantation. Transplantation can be very successful, but the waiting period may be long, and there are many more children in need of organs than there are donors. The procedure is very expensive and is performed only at designated medical centers that are often far from the family's home. The nurse should recognize the unique stresses of coping with end-stage liver disease and waiting for transplantation and assist the family in coping with these stressors. The assistance of social workers and support from other parents can be very beneficial.

Biliary Atresia

Biliary atresia, or *extrahepatic biliary atresia (EHBA),* is a progressive inflammatory process that causes both intrahepatic and extrahepatic bile duct fibrosis, resulting in obstructed bile flow. EHBA has been detected in 1 in 10,000 to 1 in 15,000 live births. The disorder is more common in girls and premature infants. In the United States, the incidence is twice as high in African-American infants as in white infants, and more common in Chinese than in either Japanese or white populations. If untreated, EHBA usually leads to cirrhosis, liver failure, and death in the first 2 years of life.

Etiology/Pathophysiology

The exact cause of biliary atresia is unknown. Because EHBA has two distinct forms, postnatal and fetal/embryonic, different pathogenic mechanisms are suggested. Postnatal EHBA represents 65% to 90% of cases and is probably the result of infection or an immune-mediated mechanism. Direct hyperbilirubinemia first appears after the resolution of physiologic jaundice. Histology demonstrates bile duct remnants and a progressive inflammatory process. In the fetal embryonic form, which represents 10% to 35% of cases, there is a congenital absence of biliary ductal patency and an absence of bile duct remnants. Many infants have associated congenital anomalies. The pathology of EHBA varies. Varying degrees of cholestasis occur, resulting in retention of irritants and toxins. Cholestasis is the accumulation of compounds that cannot be excreted because of occlusion or obstruction of the biliary tree. Injury to the liver occurs as the result of the inflammation caused by homeostasis.

Diagnostic Evaluation

Early diagnosis is the key to the survival of the child with EHBA. Infants who undergo surgery in the first 60 days of life have an 80% chance of establishing bile flow. Between 60 and 90 days of life, the chance of reestablishing flow drops to 50%; after 90 days, it drops to 10% (Sinatra, 2001). Growth parameters and nutritional status should be assessed, because many infants and children have nutritional deficiencies and poor growth. Several clinical signs may indicate the presence of EHBA (Box 47-16). Blood tests should include a CBC, electrolytes, bilirubin, and liver enzymes. Additional

BOX 47-16

Clinical Manifestations of Extrahepatic Biliary Atresia

Jaundice
- Earliest manifestation and most striking feature of disorder
- First observed in sclera
- May be present at birth
- Usually not apparent until age 2 to 3 weeks

Urine dark and stains diaper
Stools lighter than expected or white or tan
Hepatomegaly and abdominal distention common
Splenomegaly occurs later
Poor fat metabolism results in:
- Poor weight gain
- General failure to thrive

Pruritus
Irritability
Difficult to comfort infant

laboratory analyses include α_1-antitrypsin level, TORCH titers (see Maternal Infections, Chapter 28), hepatitis serology, alpha-fetoprotein, urine cytomegalovirus, and a sweat test, which is indicated to rule out other conditions that cause persistent cholestasis and jaundice. Abdominal ultrasonography allows inspection of the liver and biliary system. Hepatobiliary scintigraphy demonstrates biliary patency but does not provide diagnostic certainty. Endoscopic retrograde cholangiopancreatography (ERCP) is performed in very young infants. This procedure, which is done under general anesthesia, has an 80% reported diagnostic accuracy. Percutaneous liver biopsy is highly reliable when the biopsy contains specimens from a number of portal areas. Definitive diagnosis of EHBA is obtained during surgical laparotomy and an intraoperative cholangiogram.

Therapeutic Management

The primary treatment of biliary atresia is *hepatic portoenterostomy (Kasai procedure)* in which a segment of intestine is anastomosed to the resected porta hepatis to attempt bile drainage. Bile drainage is achieved in approximately 80% to 90% of infants who undergo surgery when younger than 10 weeks of age (Halamek & Stevenson, 1997). However, progressive cirrhosis still occurs in many children, and up to 80% to 90% eventually require liver transplantation (Andres, 1996). Prophylactic antibiotics are given following the Kasai procedure to minimize the risk of ascending cholangitis.

Medical management is primarily supportive. It includes nutritional support with infant formulas that contain medium-chain triglycerides and essential fatty acids. Supplementation with fat-soluble vitamins, multivitamin, and minerals, including iron, zinc, and selenium, is usually required. Aggressive nutritional support with continuous tube feedings or TPN is indicated for moderate to severe failure to thrive. The enteral solution should be low in sodium. Ursodeoxycholic acid is used to treat pruritus and hypercholesterolemia.

Prognosis

Untreated biliary atresia results in progressive cirrhosis and death in most children by 2 years of age. The Kasai procedure improves the prognosis but is not a cure. Biliary drainage can often be achieved if the surgery is done before the intrahepatic bile ducts are destroyed. Long-term survival has been reported in children who receive the Kasai procedure; however, even with successful bile drainage, many children ultimately develop liver failure.

Advances in surgical techniques and the use of immunosuppressive and antifungal drugs have improved the success of transplantation. The major obstacle continues to be a shortage of donor livers. Reduced-size transplantation, split-liver transplantation, retransplantation, and increased public awareness may improve donor organ availability in the future.

Nursing Care Management

Nursing interventions for the child with biliary atresia include support of the family before, during, and after surgical procedures, as well as education regarding the treatment plan. In the postoperative period of a portoenterostomy, nursing care is similar to that after major abdominal surgery. Family members need education relating to the proper administration of medications and nutritional therapy, including special formulas, vitamin and mineral supplements, tube feedings, or parenteral nutrition. Pruritus can often be relieved by drug therapy or comfort measures such as baths and trimming of fingernails.

Children and their families also need psychosocial support. The uncertain prognosis, discomfort, and waiting for transplantation produce stress, and hospitalizations, pharmacologic therapy, and nutritional therapy impose financial burdens on the family. Families can receive help from the Children's Liver Disease Foundation,* an organization that provides educational materials, programs, and support systems.

STRUCTURAL DEFECTS

Cleft Lip and Cleft Palate

Clefts of the lip and palate are facial malformations that occur during embryonic development and are the most common congenital deformities of the head and neck. They may appear separately or, more often, together. Cleft lip (CL) results from failure of the maxillary and median nasal processes to fuse; cleft palate (CP) is a midline fissure of the palate that results from failure of the two sides to fuse. This discussion is concerned primarily with cleft lip and palate (CL/P).

CL may vary from a small notch to a complete cleft extending into the base of the nose (Fig. 47-5). Clefts can be unilateral or bilateral. Deformed dental structures are associated with CL. CP alone occurs in the midline and may involve the soft and hard palates. When associated with CL, the defect may involve the midline and extend into the soft palate on one or both sides.

CL/P is more common than CP and varies by ethnicity. The occurrence in whites is 1 in every 1000 births; the occurrence in Native Americans and Asians is 1 in every 500 births; and the occurrence in African-Americans is 1 in every 2000 births. CP occurs alone in only 1 in every 2500 cases and does not display variation by ethnicity (Wilkins-Haug,

*36 Great Charles St., Birmingham, B33 JY, United Kingdom; phone: 0121-212-3839; fax: 0121-212-4300; Web site: www.childliverdisease.org.

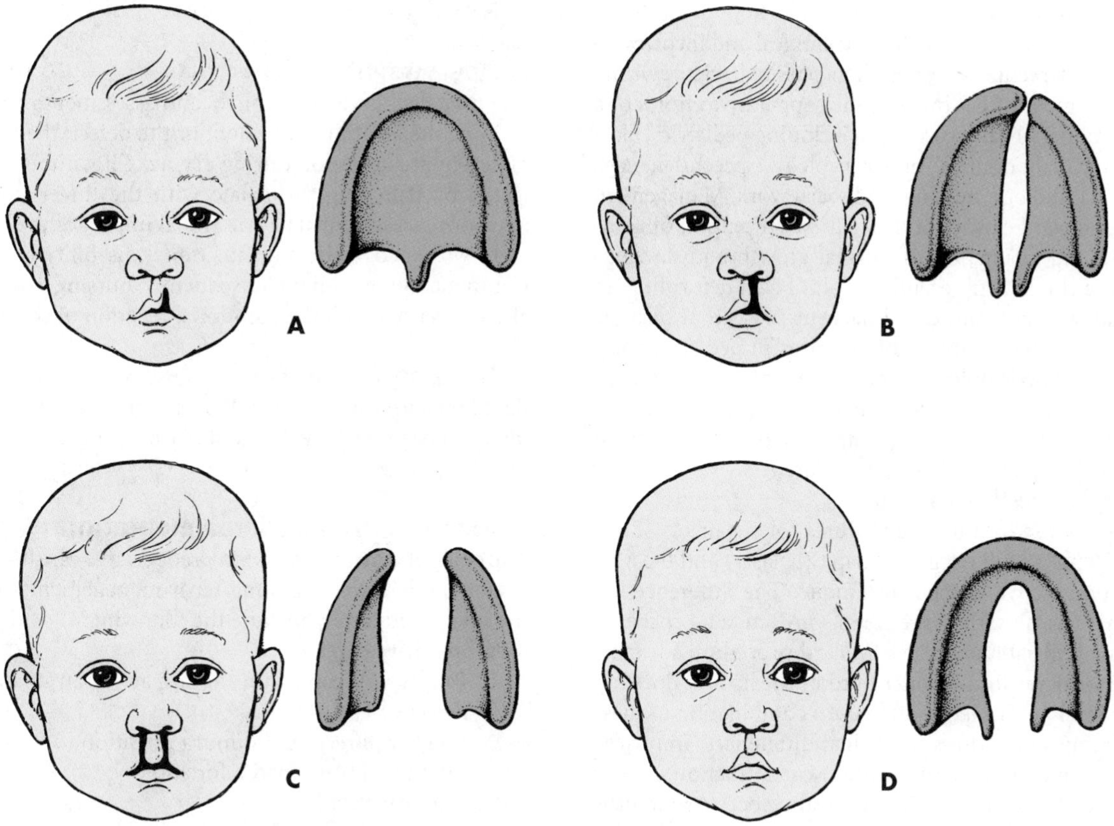

Fig. 47-5 Variations in clefts of lip and palate at birth. **A,** Notch in vermilion border. **B,** Unilateral cleft lip and palate. **C,** Bilateral cleft lip and palate. **D,** Cleft palate.

2003). Approximately 60% to 80% of children born with cleft lip and palate are male. Females have a higher frequency of isolated clefts of the secondary palate. Unilateral clefts are nine times more common than bilateral clefs and occur twice as frequently on the left side. Isolated bilateral CLs are uncommon; approximately 86% have palatal clefts. Approximately 68% of unilateral CLs have an associated palatal cleft (Kirschner & LaRossa, 2000).

Etiology

Cleft deformities may be an isolated anomaly or they may occur with a recognized syndrome. CL with or without CP is distinct from isolated CP. Clefts of the secondary palate alone are more likely to be associated with syndromes than isolated CL or CL/P.

CL/P may be caused by exposure to teratogens such as alcohol, anticonvulsants, and isotretinoin, but there is little evidence to link isolated clefts to any single teratogenic agent with the exception of phenytoin. Use of phenytoin during pregnancy is associated with a tenfold increase in the incidence of CL. The incidence of CL among mothers who smoke during pregnancy is twice as great as the incidence in mothers who do not smoke during pregnancy (Kirschner & LaRossa, 2000).

Pathophysiology

Cleft deformities represent a genetic defect in cell migration that results in a failure of the maxillary and premaxillary processes to come together between the third and twelfth week of embryonic development. Although often appearing together, CL and CP are distinct malformations embryologically, occurring at different times during the developmental process. Merging of the upper lip at the midline is completed between the seventh and eleventh weeks of gestation. Fusion of the secondary palate (hard and soft palate) takes place later, between the seventh and twelfth weeks of gestation. In the process of migrating to a horizontal position, they are separated by the tongue for a short time. If there is delay in this movement, or if the tongue fails to descend soon enough, the remainder of development proceeds but the palate never fuses.

Diagnostic Evaluation

CL with or without CP is apparent at birth. The defect elicits severe emotional reactions in parents. CP is less obvious than CL and may not be detected without a thorough assessment of the mouth. CP is identified when the examiner places a finger directly on the palate. Clefts of the hard palate form a continuous opening between the mouth and the nasal cavity. The severity of the CP has an impact on feeding; the infant is unable to generate negative pressure and create suction in the oral cavity. This impairs feeding, even though in most cases the infant's ability to swallow is normal.

Prenatal diagnosis with fetal ultrasound is not reliable until the soft tissues of the fetal face can be visualized at 13 to 14 weeks. The sensitivity of fetal ultrasound for facial clefting is almost 100% when CL/P is associated with other structural anomalies. In isolated CL/P, sensitivity may be 50% with CP; an intact lip is the most difficult to diagnose prenatally (Wilkins-Haug, 2003).

Therapeutic Management

Treatment of the child with CL is surgical and involves no long-term interventions other than possible scar revision. The management of CP involves the cooperative efforts of a multidisciplinary health care team, including pediatrics, plastic surgery, orthodontics, otolaryngology, speech/language pathology, audiology, nursing, and social work. Management is directed toward closure of the cleft(s), prevention of complications, and facilitation of normal growth and development in the child. Until recently, repair of cleft deformities in the neonate was not considered safe. Surgery is now possible in younger neonates because of advances in pediatric anesthesiology and neonatology. However, the infant must be free of any oral, respiratory, or systemic infections. In deformities of both the lip and palate, the palate is repaired first to avoid disrupting the lip after it has been repaired.

Surgical Correction: Cleft Lip

The two most common procedures for repair of CL are the Tennison-Randall triangular flap (Z-plasty) and the Millard rotational advancement technique. The difference between these two is that the Tennison-Randall procedure crosses the philtral line and the Millard procedure advances a triangle of tissue in the upper third of the lip and does not cross the midline. Surgeons often use a combination of these two techniques to address individual differences. Improved surgical techniques have minimized scar retraction, and in the absence of infection or trauma, healing occurs with little scar formation. Optimum cosmetic results, however, are difficult to obtain in severe defects. Additional revisions may be necessary at a later age.

Surgical Correction: Cleft Palate

CP repair was previously postponed until a later age than the repair of the CL to take advantage of palatal changes that take place with normal growth. With advanced surgical and anesthesia techniques, many surgeons are currently performing palatal repairs in the neonatal period (Sandberg, Magee, & Denk, 2002). The timing of repair remains controversial. Most surgeons prefer to close the cleft before the child develops faulty speech habits.

Prognosis

Even with good anatomic closure, most children with CL/P have some degree of speech impairment that requires speech therapy. Physical problems result from inefficient functioning of the muscles of the soft palate and nasopharynx, improper tooth alignment, and varying degrees of hearing loss. Improper drainage of the middle ear, as a result of inefficient function of the eustachian tube, contributes to recurrent otitis media with scarring of the tympanic membrane, which leads to hearing impairment in many children with CP. Upper respiratory infections require immediate and meticulous attention, and extensive orthodontics and prosthodontics may be needed to correct problems of malposition of teeth and maxillary arches.

Long-term problems are related to social adjustment of the child. The better the physical care, the better the chance for emotional and social adjustment, although the presence of the defect and the degree of residual disability are not always directly related to a satisfactory adjustment. Physical defects are a threat to the self-image, and abnormal speech quality is an impediment to social expression.

Nursing Care Management

Assessment

The lip defect is visible at birth, and assessment involves describing the location and extent of the defect; the CP is estimated by visualization during crying. CP without CL is detected by palpating the palate with the finger during the newborn assessment. The emotional impact of the birth of a child with a cosmetic and functional disability is especially traumatic to the family. Consequently, nursing assessment is also concerned with the emotional reaction of the family.

Nursing Diagnoses

Based on a thorough physical assessment, a number of nursing diagnoses are evident and described in the Nursing Care Plan on p. 1529.

Plan of Care and Implementation

The goals of care are related to preoperative care, short-term postoperative care, and long-term management. Goals for the infant and family include the following:

- **Preoperative care:**
  1. Family will cope with the impact of an infant with a defect.
  2. Infant will receive optimum nutrition.
  3. Infant will be prepared for surgery.
- **Postoperative care:**
  1. Infant will experience no trauma and minimal or no pain.
  2. Infant will receive optimum nutrition.
  3. Infant will experience no complications.
  4. Infant and family will receive adequate support.
  5. Family will be prepared for care at home and long-term needs of a child with CP.

The immediate nursing problems for an infant with CL/P deformities are related to feeding and dealing with the parental reaction to the defect. Facial deformities are particularly disturbing to parents. CL is a visible defect that may produce a strong negative response in parents, which could influence maternal-infant attachment. However, a study of infants with CL or CP indicated that maternal-infant attachment was not negatively affected when measured at 1 year of age (Speltz et al, 1997). During the initial phase following birth, it is important for the nurse to place emphasis not only on the infant's physical needs, but also on the parents' emotional needs (Speltz et al, 1997). The manner of handling the infant should convey to the parents that the infant is a precious human being. (See Chapter 41 for interventions in assisting parents in accepting a birth defect.) Throughout the course of therapy, parents need explanations of the immediate and long-range problems associated with CP. They may be unaware that more is involved than repairing the defect. Whenever possible, they should be referred to a comprehensive CP team.

Case Study: Cleft Lip and Palate

Feeding

Feeding the infant presents a challenge to nurses and parents. Growth failure in infants with CL or CP has been attributed to preoperative feeding difficulties. After surgical repair, most infants who have isolated CL or CP with no associated syndromes gain weight or achieve adequate weight and height for age (Lee, Nunn, & Wright, 1997).

CL or CP reduces the infant's ability to suck, making bottle-feeding and breastfeeding difficult. In breastfeeding, the CL or CP interferes with compression of the areola. Liquid taken into the mouth escapes via the cleft through the nose. Feeding is best accomplished with the infant's head in an upright position, either held in the caregiver's hand or cradled in the arm. Normal nipples are unsuitable for these infants, who are unable to generate the suction required. A variety of special "cleft palate" nipples have been devised and used with some success. However, large, soft nipples with large holes; Nursettes; or the long, soft lamb's nipples appear to offer the best means for nipple feeding. The newer "gravity flow" nipple* attached to a squeezable plastic bottle allows formula to be deposited directly into the mouth in the same manner as with a bulb syringe. Success has also been achieved by modification of a standard nipple. A single small slit or crosscut is made in the end of the nipple with a sharp surgical blade or pair of sharp thin scissors. The enlarged opening, which can be adjusted to the infant's individual needs, allows the infant to swallow the formula easily, bypassing the suction problem.

The enlarge, stimulate, swallow, and rest (ESSR) feeding technique also works well with these infants. The steps in the ESSR feeding technique are as follows: (1) *enlarge* the nipple; (2) *stimulate* the suck reflex; (3) *swallow* fluid appropriately; and (4) *rest* when the infant signals with facial expression. Infants fed with the ESSR method revealed a significantly greater increase in their mean weight before surgery than infants fed with traditional methods (Richard, 1994).

Using special or modified nipples or feeding techniques helps meet the infant's sucking needs. Muscle development is important for later development of speech. During feeding, the nipple is positioned so that it is compressed by the infant's tongue and existing palate. If a single-slit nipple is used, the slit is placed vertically so that the infant will be able to produce and stop a flow of milk by alternately opening and closing the opening. No matter which type of nipple is used, gentle, steady pressure on the base of the bottle reduces the chance of choking or coughing. The person feeding should resist the temptation to remove the nipple because of the noise the infant makes or for fear that the infant will choke. These infants swallow excessive amounts of air, and they require frequent burping.

When the infant has trouble with nipple feeding, a rubber-tipped medicine dropper, Asepto syringe, or Breck feeder (a large syringe with soft rubber tubing) provides an efficient, safe feeding device. The rubber extension should be long enough to extend back into the mouth to reduce the likelihood of regurgitation through the nose. The formula is deposited on the back of the tongue, and the flow is controlled by bulb or syringe compression that is adjusted to the infant's needs. With some infants, spoon feeding works best, especially if the formula is slightly thickened with cereal. After feeding, the infant is given water to rinse the mouth.

Breastfeeding is also an option. The nipple is positioned and stabilized well back in the oral cavity so that tongue action facilitates milk expression. The suction required to stimulate milk may be absent initially, and a breast pump may be useful before nursing to stimulate the let-down reflex.

*Ross Laboratories, Columbus, OH 43216.

Regardless of the feeding method used, the mother should begin feeding the infant as soon as possible, preferably after the initial nursery feeding. When maternal feeding is initiated early, the mother can help determine the method best suited to her and the infant and can become adept in the technique before discharge from the hospital.

Preoperative Care

In preparation for surgical repair, parents are frequently taught to accustom the infant to the needs of the early postoperative period, especially if surgery is delayed for several months. It is mandatory for the infant to be positioned on the back or side postoperatively. Most infants tolerate these positions well because they are accustomed to being supine for sleeping. It is also helpful to place the infant or child in arm restraints periodically before admission and to feed the infant with a rubber-tipped Asepto syringe or other device that will be used postoperatively.

Postoperative Care: Cleft Lip

The major efforts in the postoperative period are directed toward protecting the operative site. After CL repair *(cheiloplasty)*, a metal appliance or adhesive strips are securely taped to the cheeks to relax the surgical site and prevent tension on the suture line caused by crying or other facial movement. Elbow restraints are used to prevent the infant from rubbing or disturbing the suture line and are applied immediately after surgery. It is advisable to pin the cuff of the restraints to the infant's clothing to keep the restraints in place. Older infants who roll over will require a jacket restraint in addition to restricting arm movement to prevent rolling on the abdomen and rubbing the face on the sheet, especially if the repair involves the lip. It is important to remove the elbow restraints periodically to exercise the arms, to provide relief from restrictions, to observe the skin for signs of irritation, and to provide an opportunity for cuddling and body contact. Restraints should be released one at a time. Sitting the infant in an infant seat provides a change of position and a different view of the environment. Adequate analgesia is required to relieve postoperative pain and to provide restlessness.

Clear liquids are offered when the infant has fully recovered from the anesthesia, and feeding is resumed when tolerated. The suture site is carefully cleansed of formula or serosanguineous drainage as needed with a cotton-tipped swab dipped in saline. A thin layer of antibiotic ointment may be prescribed for application to the suture line after cleansing. Meticulous care of the suture line is essential because inflammation or infection will interfere with optimum healing and the ultimate cosmetic effect of the surgical repair. Gentle aspiration of mouth and nasopharyngeal secretions may be necessary to prevent aspiration and respiratory complications. An upright or infant seat position is helpful in the immediate postoperative period (especially for the infant who has difficulty in handling secretions).

Postoperative Care: Cleft Palate

The child with CP repair *(palatoplasty)* is allowed to lie on the abdomen immediately postoperatively. The child may resume feeding by bottle, breast, or cup shortly after surgery.

NURSE ALERT Avoid the use of suction or other objects in the mouth, such as tongue depressors, thermometers, spoons, or straws. ■

Oral packing may be secured to the palate after palatoplasty; this packing is usually removed after 2 to 3 days. Sometimes the infant will have difficulty breathing following surgery, because it is often necessary to alter an established pattern of breathing and adjust to breathing through the nose. This is frustrating but seldom requires more than positioning and support. The elbows may be restrained to keep the child's hands away from the mouth. Parents are instructed to maintain elbow restraints at home until the palate is healed, usually in 4 to 6 weeks. They are instructed to remove the restraints (one at a time) frequently to allow the child to exercise the arms.

The nurse must assess the infant's or child's level of postoperative pain. Opioids may be prescribed initially, and acetaminophen may be given as needed thereafter.

The older infant or child may be discharged on a blenderized or soft diet, and parents are instructed to continue the diet until the surgeon directs them otherwise. Parents are cautioned against allowing the child to eat hard items (such as toast, hard cookies, and potato chips) that can damage the repaired palate.

Long-Term Care

Children with CL/P often require a variety of services during recovery. Family members need support and encouragement by health professionals and guidance in activities that facilitate a normal outcome for their child. Financial stress is frequently cited as a difficult issue by parents. With the combined efforts of the family and the health team, most children achieve a satisfactory outcome. Many children with CL/P have surgical correction that creates a near-normal–appearing lip and permits good function. Parents need to understand the function of therapy and the purpose and care of all appliances, as well as the importance of establishing good mouth care and proper brushing habits.

Throughout the child's development, an important goal is the development of a healthy personality and self-esteem. Many communities have CP parents' groups that offer help and support to families. Agencies that provide services and information for children with CL/P and their families include the American Cleft Palate Association, the Cleft Palate Foundation, the Association of Birth Defect Children, the March of Dimes–Birth Defects Foundation, and the various state children's medical services.

Evaluation

To determine the effectiveness of nursing interventions, continual reassessment and evaluation of care is based on the following observational guidelines:

- **Preoperative care:**
  1. Observe and interview family members about their understanding, feelings, and concerns regarding the defect, any anticipated surgery, and their interactions with the infant.
  2. Observe infant during feeding.
  3. Complete preoperative checklist.
- **Postoperative care:**
  1. Inspect operative site, including the protective device.
  2. Observe for behavioral and physiologic indicators of pain and response to analgesics.
  3. Observe infant during feeding, measure intake and output, and weigh infant daily.
  4. Observe operative site for evidence of infection, bleeding, sloughing, or irritation.
  5. Observe and interview family members regarding their understanding and concerns about the infant, including long-term needs.

The *expected outcomes* are described in the Nursing Care Plan on p. 1529.

Esophageal Atresia with Tracheoesophageal Fistula

Congenital atresia of the esophagus and tracheoesophageal fistula (TEF) are rare malformations that are believed to result from failed separation of the esophagus and trachea by a septum that forms by the fourth week of gestation. These defects occur as separate entities or in combination (Fig. 47-6). They have a fatal outcome without early diagnosis and treatment.

Etiology

Esophageal atresia (EA) with or without an associated TEF is the most common esophageal malformation. It occurs in 1 in every 2000 to 1 in every 5000 live births. There appears to be an equal sex incidence, but the birth weight of most affected infants is significantly lower than average, and there is an unusually high incidence of prematurity in infants with EA. A history of maternal polyhydramnios is present in approximately 50% of infants with the defects. EA/TEF is often present with the VATER or VACTERL syndromes. VATER and VACTERL are acronyms that describe the associated anomalies. These syndromes involve a combination of vertebral, anorectal, cardiovascular, tracheoesophageal, renal, and limb abnormalities. The cardiac anomalies occur most frequently with EA/TEF.

Pathophysiology

The cause of EA/TEF is unknown. In the most frequently encountered form of esophageal atresia and TEF (80% to 95% of cases), the proximal esophageal segment terminates in a blind pouch, and the distal segment is connected to the trachea or primary bronchus by a short fistula at or near the bifurcation (Fig. 47-6, *C*). The second most common variety (5% to 8%) consists of a blind pouch at each end, widely separated and with no communication to the trachea (Fig. 47-6, *A*). Less frequently, an otherwise normal trachea and esophagus are connected by a common fistula (Fig. 47-6, *E*). Extremely rare anomalies involve a fistula from the trachea to the upper esophageal segment (Fig. 47-6, *B*) or to both the upper and the lower segments (Fig. 47-6, *D*).

Diagnostic Evaluation

The disorder is suspected on the basis of clinical manifestations (Box 47-17). EA should also be suspected in cases of maternal polyhydramnios. Although the diagnosis is established on the basis of clinical signs and symptoms, the exact type of anomaly is determined by radiographic studies. A radiopaque catheter is inserted into the hypopharynx and advanced until it encounters an obstruction. Chest films are taken to ascertain esophageal patency or the presence and level of a blind pouch. Sometimes fistulas are not patent, which makes their presence more difficult to diagnose. The

Nursing Care Plan

THE CHILD WITH CLEFT LIP OR CLEFT PALATE (OR BOTH)

NURSING DIAGNOSIS: Altered nutrition: less than body requirements, related to physical defect of oral cavity

EXPECTED OUTCOME

Patient exhibits signs of adequate nutritional intake (e.g., appropriate weight gain).

NURSING INTERVENTIONS/*RATIONALES*

Administer diet appropriate for age and nutritional needs *to ensure adequate nutritional content.*

If infant is breastfeeding, teach mother to stimulate let-down reflex before feeding with a breast pump or manually *because required suction from infant may be lacking.*

Have mother position and stabilize nipple well back in infant's oral cavity against existing palate *to facilitate expression of milk.*

Hold child in upright position to feed *to prevent aspiration* and burp frequently *because infant takes in excess amounts of air.*

If child is unable to maintain adequate suction on a nipple, try using alternative feeding appliances (e.g., Breck feeder, Aesepto syringe) *to facilitate feeding.*

Postoperatively, administer prescribed intravenous fluids *to ensure adequate hydration.*

Maintain feeding records and weigh regularly *to assess adequacy of intake.*

NURSING DIAGNOSIS: Potential for altered parenting related to having child with highly visible physical defect

EXPECTED OUTCOME

Parents demonstrate acceptance of the infant.

NURSING INTERVENTIONS/*RATIONALES*

Allow parents to express feelings, fears *to facilitate coping.*

Convey attitudes and behaviors of acceptance of infant *to serve as a role model for parents.*

Describe results of surgical correction of defect with photos of satisfactory results *to alleviate fears of the unknown and foster hope.*

Arrange for parents to meet with others who have experienced and successfully coped with similar situations *to provide ongoing support.*

NURSING DIAGNOSIS: Risk for trauma of surgical site related to position of site

EXPECTED OUTCOME

Operative site is undamaged.

NURSING INTERVENTIONS/*RATIONALES*

For cleft lip repair, use a lip protective device; position on back or side *to protect suture line.*

For cleft palate repair, prevent sustained crying, placement of objects in mouth *to protect suture line.*

Restrain infant at elbows *to prevent access to operative site;* use jacket restraints on older infants *to prevent rolling onto abdomen and rubbing of suture line on bedding.*

Cleanse suture line after feeding *to reduce presence of foreign materials that may irritate suture line.*

Teach restraint and cleansing techniques to parents *to minimize complications after discharge.*

NURSING DIAGNOSIS: Pain related to surgical procedure

EXPECTED OUTCOME

Infant is resting comfortably.

NURSING INTERVENTIONS/*RATIONALES*

Administer pain medications per physician order *to prevent or minimize pain.*

Remove restraints periodically under careful supervision *to exercise arms and provide relief from restrictions.*

Monitor vital signs and behavior for evidence of pain or discomfort.

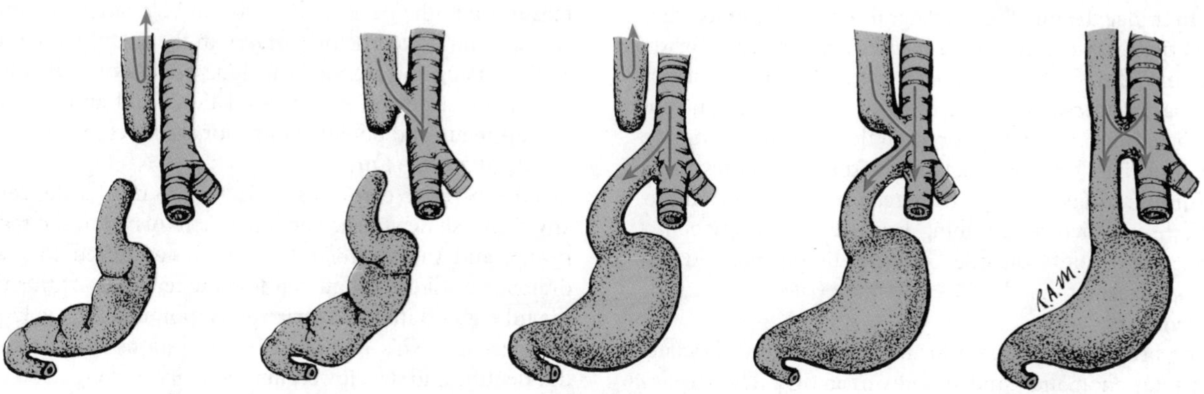

Fig. 47-6 Five most common types of esophageal atresia and tracheoesophageal fistula.

BOX 47-17

Clinical Manifestations of Tracheoesophageal Fistula

Excessive salivation and drooling
Three *C*'s of tracheoesophageal fistula:
- Coughing
- Choking
- Cyanosis

Apnea
Increased respiratory distress after feeding
Abdominal distention

presence of gas in the stomach or small bowel is indicative of a coexisting TEF.

Therapeutic Management

EA is a surgical emergency. The treatment includes maintenance of a patent airway, prevention of pneumonia, gastric or blind pouch decompression, and surgical repair of the anomaly. When EA/TEF is suspected, the infant is immediately taken off oral intake, started on IV fluids, and placed in the position least likely to cause aspiration of either mouth or stomach secretions. Removal of secretions from the mouth and upper pouch requires frequent or continuous suction. Because aspiration pneumonia is almost inevitable and appears early, broad-spectrum antibiotic therapy is often instituted.

Primary surgical correction consists of a thoracotomy with division and ligation of the TEF and an end-to-side anastomosis of the esophagus. This may consist of one operation or be staged with two or more procedures. For infants who are premature, have multiple anomalies, or are in very poor condition, a staged procedure is preferred that involves palliative measures, including gastrostomy, ligation of the TEF, and provision of constant drainage of the esophageal pouch. A delayed esophageal anastomosis is usually attempted after several weeks to months when the upper pouch elongates. Further surgical techniques may be performed later to facilitate esophageal lengthening. If an esophageal anastomosis still cannot be accomplished, a *cervical esophagostomy* (to allow drainage of saliva) and gastrostomy are performed.

A primary anastomosis may be impossible because of insufficient length of the two segments of the esophagus. In these cases, an esophageal replacement procedure using a part of the colon or gastric tube interposition may be necessary to bridge the missing esophageal segment. Endotracheal intubation may be required, because many infants (10% to 20%) also have *tracheomalacia,* a weakness in the tracheal wall that occurs when a dilated proximal pouch compresses the trachea in early fetal life or when the trachea does not develop normally because of a loss of intratracheal pressure.

Complications of a primary repair include an anastomotic leak, strictures resulting from tension or ischemia, esophageal motility disorders causing dysphagia, and gastroesophageal reflux.

Prognosis

The prognosis is related to the birth weight, associated congenital anomalies, and time of diagnosis. The survival rate is nearly 100% in full-term infants without severe respiratory distress or other anomalies. In premature low-birth-weight infants with associated anomalies, the incidence of complications is high. The overall mortality rate is 50% (Ryckman, Flake, & Balistreri, 1997).

Nursing Care Management

Nursing responsibility for detection of this malformation begins *immediately* after birth. Ideally, the diagnosis should be made before the initial feeding, but often it is not. If fed, the infant swallows normally but suddenly coughs and struggles, and the fluid is aspirated or returns through the nose and mouth. For this reason, it is customary for the nurse to give the infant the first feeding of plain water or to be present when a parent feeds the child to observe the infant's response. Early breastfeeding should not be prevented unless there is a strong suspicion of EA.

NURSE ALERT Any infant who has an excessive amount of frothy saliva in the mouth or difficulty with secretions and unexplained episodes of cyanosis should be suspected of having an EA/TEF, and referred *immediately* for medical evaluation. ■

Cyanosis is usually the result of laryngospasm caused by overflow of saliva into the larynx from the proximal esophageal pouch. It normally clears after removal of the secretions from the oropharynx by suctioning. Any suspicion of TEF is reported immediately. The infant is placed in an incubator or a radiant warmer, and oxygen is administered to help relieve respiratory distress. Intubation and assisted mechanical ventilation may be necessary if the infant is in respiratory distress. When a newborn is suspected of having a TEF, the most desirable position is supine with the head elevated on an inclined plane of at least 30 degrees. This position minimizes the reflux of gastric secretions up the distal esophagus into the trachea and bronchi.

It is imperative that the source of aspiration be removed at once. Oral fluids are withheld, and the infant's fluid needs are met parenterally or via gastrostomy. Until surgery, the blind pouch is kept empty by intermittent or continuous suction through an indwelling nasal catheter that extends to the end of the pouch. The catheter needs attention because it has a tendency to become clogged with mucus. It is usually replaced daily by the practitioner. In the event that a staged repair is performed, a gastrostomy tube is inserted and left open so that air entering the stomach through the fistula can escape, thus minimizing the danger of gastric contents being regurgitated into the trachea. The tube empties by gravity drainage. Feedings through the gastrostomy tube and irrigations with fluid are contraindicated before surgery in the infant with a distal TEF. Nursing interventions include respiratory assessment, airway management, thermoregulation, fluid and electrolyte management, and potential nutritional support.

Postoperative Care

Postoperative care is essentially the same as the care of any high risk newborn. The infant is returned to the radiant heater, and the gastrostomy tube is connected to gravity drainage until the infant can tolerate feedings. At this time, the tube is elevated and secured at a point above the level of the stomach. This allows gastric secretions to pass to the duodenum and swallowed air to escape through the open tube. Tracheal suction should only be done using a premeasured catheter and with extreme caution to avoid injury to the suture line. If tolerated, gastrostomy feedings may be started and continued until the esophageal anastomosis is healed. Before oral feedings are initiated and the chest tube is removed, a contrast study or esophagram is performed to verify the integrity of the esophageal anastomosis.

The initial attempt at oral feeding must be carefully observed to make sure that the infant can swallow without choking. Oral feedings are begun with sterile water, followed by frequent small feedings of formula. Until the infant can take a sufficient amount by mouth, gastrostomy feedings or parenteral nutrition may supplement oral intake. Infants are usually not discharged until they are taking oral fluids well and the gastrostomy tube is removed. However, the infant who has palliative surgery will be discharged with the gastrostomy tube in place. The nurse is responsible for making certain that the caregiver is educated and has practiced the care of the gastrostomy (see Chapter 44).

Special Problems

Upper respiratory complications are a threat to life in both the preoperative and the postoperative period. In addition to pneumonia, there is a constant danger of respiratory distress resulting from atelectasis, pneumothorax, and laryngeal edema. Any persistent respiratory difficulty after removal of secretions is reported to the surgeon immediately. The infant is monitored for anastomotic leaks, as evidenced by purulent chest tube drainage, increased WBC count, and temperature instability.

In the infant awaiting esophageal replacement surgery, the catheter is removed and the upper esophageal segment is drained through a cervical esophagostomy. An esophagostomy is difficult to care for because the skin becomes irritated by moisture from the continuous discharge of saliva. Frequent removal of drainage and application of a layer of protective ointment may remedy the problem. A dressing or ostomy appliance may be applied to collect the drainage, and an enterostomal therapist can provide additional guidance to prevent or treat skin breakdown.

For the infant who requires esophageal replacement, nonnutritive sucking is provided by a pacifier. Sometimes small amounts of water or formula are given orally, and although the liquid drains from the esophagostomy, this process allows the infant to develop mature sucking patterns. Other appropriate oral stimulation prevents feeding aversions. Infants who remain NPO for an extended period or who have not received oral stimulation have difficulty with eating by mouth after corrective surgery and may develop oral hypersensitivity and food aversion. They require patient, firm guidance to learn how to take food into the mouth and swallow after repair. A referral to a multidisciplinary feeding behavior program is often necessary.

As with any congenital anomaly, parents need support in adjusting to the child's condition. One difficulty is the immediate transfer of the sick newborn to the intensive care unit and the length of hospitalization. Encouraging parents to visit the infant, participate in care when appropriate, and express their feelings regarding the infant's condition facilitates the attachment process. The nurse in the intensive care unit should assume responsibility for ensuring that the parents are kept fully informed of the infant's progress.

Preparing parents for discharge involves teaching them skills that they will need at home. Parents are taught to observe for behaviors that indicate the need for suctioning, as well as signs of respiratory distress and constriction of the esophagus (e.g., poor feeding, dysphagia, drooling, regurgitation of undigested food). Discharge planning also includes obtaining the necessary equipment and home nursing services to provide home care.

Hernias

A *hernia* is a protrusion of a portion of an organ or organs through an abnormal opening. The danger from herniation arises when the organ protruding through the opening is constricted to the extent that circulation is impaired or when the protruding organs encroach on and impair the function of other structures. A hernia that cannot be reduced easily is called an *incarcerated hernia*. A *strangulated hernia* is one in which the blood supply to the herniated organ is impaired. The herniations of concern are those that protrude through the diaphragm, the abdominal wall, or the inguinal wall. The other hernias of significance to the pediatric age groups are outlined in Table 47-8.

OBSTRUCTIVE DISORDERS

Obstruction in the GI tract occurs when the passage of nutrients and secretions is impeded by a constricted or occluded lumen or when there is impaired motility *(paralytic ileus)*. Obstructions may be congenital or acquired. Many congenital obstructions, such as atresia, imperforate anus, meconium plug, and meconium ileus, usually appear in the neonatal period. Other obstructions of congenital etiology, such as malrotation, Hirschsprung disease, volvulus, incarcerated hernia, and Meckel diverticulum, appear after the first few weeks of life. Intestinal obstruction from acquired causes such as intussusception, pyloric stenosis, and tumors may occur in infancy or childhood. Intestinal obstructions from any cause are characterized by similar signs and symptoms (Box 47-18).

Hypertrophic Pyloric Stenosis

Hypertrophic pyloric stenosis (HPS) occurs when the circumferential muscle of the pyloric sphincter becomes thickened, resulting in elongation and narrowing of the pyloric channel. This produces an outlet obstruction and compensatory dilation, hypertrophy, and hyperperistalsis of the stomach. This condition usually develops in the first few weeks of life, causing projectile vomiting, dehydration, metabolic alkalosis, and failure to thrive. The precise etiology is unknown. There is a genetic predisposition, and siblings and offspring of affected persons are at increased risk of developing HPS. Firstborn children and males are affected five times more frequently than females. HPS is more common in full-term than in premature infants, and it is seen less frequently in African-American and Asian infants than in Caucasian infants.

Pathophysiology

The circular muscle of the pylorus thickens as a result of hypertrophy (increased size) and hyperplasia (increased mass). This produces severe narrowing of the pyloric canal between the stomach and the duodenum, causing partial obstruction of

Table 47-8

Summary Outline of Hernias

TYPE	MANIFESTATIONS/DIAGNOSTIC EVALUATION	MANAGEMENT
DIAPHRAGMATIC Protrusion of abdominal organs through opening in diaphragm	**Symptoms:** Mild to severe respiratory distress within a few hours after birth; tachypnea, cyanosis, dyspnea, absent breath sounds in affected area; impaired cardiac output; possible symptoms of shock, severe acidosis **Diagnosis** suspected on basis of symptoms—confirmed by radiographic study; often diagnosed prenatally as early as twenty-fifth week of gestation	**Therapeutic:** Supportive treatment of respiratory distress and correction of acidosis; possible use of endotracheal intubation, GI decompression, and extracorporeal membrane oxygenation (ECMO) Prophylactic antibiotic administration Surgical reduction of hernia and repair of defect **Nursing:** *Preoperative:* Reduce stimulation—environmental/care activities Prompt recognition; resuscitation and stabilization Maintain suction, oxygen, and IV fluids Positioning—head up Administer medications *Postoperative:* Carry out routine postoperative care and observation Relieve pain and provide comfort Support family because this is a critical illness
HIATAL **Sliding:** Protrusion of an abdominal structure (usually stomach) through esophageal hiatus	**Symptoms:** Dysphagia, failure to thrive, vomiting, neck contortions, frequent unexplained respiratory problems, bleeding; usually associated with gastroesophageal reflux (GER); may cause gastric volvulus and obstruction **Diagnosis** made by fluoroscopy	**Therapeutic:** Management of GER symptoms; positioning; pharmacologic treatment; and dietary management Surgical treatment when complications are related to GER despite medical management **Nursing:** Be alert to significant signs and carry out routine postoperative care
ABDOMINAL **Umbilical:** Weakness in abdominal wall around umbilicus; incomplete closure of abdominal wall, allowing intestinal contents to protrude through opening	**Symptoms:** Noted by inspection and palpation of the abdomen High incidence in premature and African-American infants Usually closes spontaneously by 1-2 years of age	**Therapeutic:** No treatment of small defects Operative repair if persists to age 4-6 years or if defect is >1.5-2.0 cm by age 2 years Strangulation requires immediate attention **Nursing:** Discourage use of home remedies (e.g., belly bands, coins) Reassure parents
Omphalocele: Protrusion of intraabdominal viscera into base of umbilical cord; sac is covered with peritoneum without skin **Gastroschisis:** Protrusion of intraabdominal contents through defect in abdominal wall lateral to umbilical ring; there is never a peritoneal sac	**Symptoms:** Obvious on inspection Observe for other malformations	**Therapeutic:** Surgical repair of defect *Preoperative:* Large lesions—gradual reduction of abdominal contents Prophylactic antibiotic administration **Nursing:** *Preoperative:* Keep sac or viscera moist with saline-soaked pads Use overhead warming unit Carry out routine care of IV line Nasogastric suction NPO

BOX 47-18

Clinical Manifestations of Mechanical/Paralytic Intestinal Obstruction

Colicky abdominal pain—From peristalsis attempting to overcome the obstruction
Abdominal distention—As a result of accumulation of gas and fluid above the level of the obstruction
Vomiting—Often the earliest sign of a high obstruction; a later sign of lower obstruction (may be bilious or feculent)
Constipation and obstipation—Early signs of low obstructions; later signs of higher obstructions
Dehydration—From losses of large quantities of fluid and electrolytes into the intestine
Rigid and boardlike abdomen—From increased distention
Bowel sounds—Gradually diminish and cease
Respiratory distress—Occurs as the diaphragm is pushed up into the pleural cavity
Shock—Plasma volume diminishes as fluids and electrolytes are lost from the bloodstream into the intestinal lumen
Sepsis—Caused by bacterial proliferation with invasion into the circulation

the lumen (Fig. 47-7, *A*). Over time, inflammation and edema further reduce the size of the opening, resulting in complete obstruction. The hypertrophied pylorus may be palpable as an olive-like mass in the upper abdomen. Pyloric stenosis is not a congenital disorder. Evidence suggests that local innervation is involved in the pathogenesis. In most cases this is an isolated lesion; however, it may be associated with intestinal malrotation, esophageal and duodenal atresia, and anorectal anomalies.

Diagnostic Evaluation

The diagnosis of HPS is often made after the history and physical examination. The olive-like mass is easily palpated when the stomach is empty, the infant is quiet, and the abdominal muscles are relaxed. Vomiting usually occurs 30 to 60 minutes after feeding, and becomes projectile as the obstruction progresses. Emesis is nonbilious, usually consisting of stale milk. Often these infants become dehydrated and lethargic and appear significantly malnourished.

If the diagnosis is inconclusive from the history and physical signs (Box 47-19), ultrasonography will demonstrate an elongated, sausage-shaped mass with an elongated pyloric channel. If ultrasound fails to demonstrate a hypertrophied pylorus, upper GI radiography should be done to rule out other causes of vomiting. Laboratory findings reflect the metabolic alterations created by severe depletion of both fluid and electrolytes from extensive and prolonged vomiting. There are decreased serum levels of both sodium and potassium, although these may be masked by the hemoconcentration from ECF depletion. Of greater diagnostic value is a decrease in serum chloride levels and increases in pH and bicarbonate (carbon dioxide content) characteristic of metabolic alkalosis. The BUN level will be elevated as evidence of dehydration.

Therapeutic Management

Surgical relief of the pyloric obstruction by *pyloromyotomy* (sometimes called *Fredet-Ramstedt procedure)* is the standard treatment for this disorder. The procedure is performed through a right upper quadrant incision (lapa-

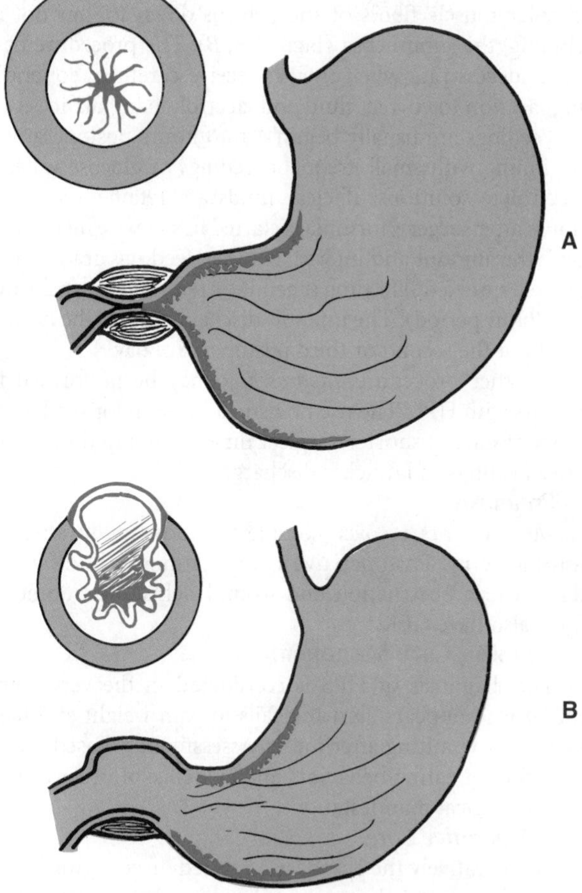

Fig. 47-7 Hypertrophic pyloric stenosis. **A,** Enlarged muscular area nearly obliterates pyloric channel. **B,** Longitudinal surgical division of muscle down to submucosa establishes adequate passageway.

BOX 47-19

Clinical Manifestations of Hypertrophic Pyloric Stenosis

Projectile vomiting
- May be ejected 3 to 4 feet from the child when in a side-lying position, 1 foot or more when in a back-lying position
- Occurs shortly after a feeding (may not occur for several hours)
- May follow each feeding or appear intermittently
- Nonbilious vomitus; may be blood tinged

Infant hungry, avid nurser; eagerly accepts a second feeding after vomiting episode
No evidence of pain or discomfort except that of chronic hunger
Weight loss
Signs of dehydration
Distended upper abdomen
Readily palpable olive-shaped tumor in the epigastrium just to the right of the umbilicus
Visible gastric peristaltic waves that move from left to right across the epigastrium

rotomy) and consists of a longitudinal incision through the circular muscle fibers of the pylorus down to, but not including, the submucosa (Fig. 47-3, *B*). The procedure has a high success rate when infants receive careful preoperative preparation to correct fluid and electrolyte imbalances.

Feedings are usually begun 4 to 6 hours postoperatively, beginning with small, frequent feedings of glucose water or electrolyte solutions. If clear fluids are retained, about 24 hours after surgery, formula is started in stepwise increments, with the amount and interval between feedings gradually increased until a full feeding schedule is reinstated (usually over a 48-hour period). The infant is discharged from the hospital by about the second or third postoperative day.

Another procedure, *laparoscopy,* may be performed for infants with HPS. The use of a small incision for the laparoscope results in shorter surgical time, more rapid postoperative feeding, and quicker discharge.

Prognosis

Most infants recover completely and rapidly after pyloromyotomy. Postoperative complications include persistent pyloric obstruction and wound dehiscence. Some infants also have GER.

Nursing Care Management

The diagnosis of HPS is considered in the very young infant who appears alert but fails to gain weight and has a history of vomiting after meals. Assessment is based on observation of eating behaviors and evidence of other characteristic clinical manifestations.

Preoperative Care

Preoperatively the emphasis is placed on restoring hydration and electrolyte balance. Infants are usually given no oral feedings and receive IV fluids with glucose and electrolyte replacement based on laboratory serum electrolyte values. Careful monitoring of the IV infusion and diligent attention to intake, output, and urine specific gravity measurements are important. Vomiting and the number and character of stools are observed and recorded accurately.

Observations also include assessment of vital signs, particularly those that might indicate fluid or electrolyte imbalances. These infants are prone to metabolic alkalosis from loss of hydrogen ions and to potassium, sodium, and chloride depletion. The skin and mucous membranes, as well as daily weight, are assessed for alterations in hydration status and water gain or loss.

If stomach decompression and gastric lavage are used preoperatively, the nurse is responsible for ensuring that the tube is patent and functioning properly and for measuring and recording the type and amount of drainage. The infant is usually positioned flat or with the head slightly elevated. Infants who are receiving IV fluids and infants who have a nasogastric tube for continuous drainage must be observed to prevent the needle or tube from becoming dislodged.

General hygienic care, with attention to the skin and mouth in dehydrated infants, is essential. Protection from infection is also important, because infants with impaired nutritional status are more susceptible than normal newborns. Parental involvement is encouraged and promoted.

Postoperative Care

Postoperative vomiting may occur, and most infants, even with successful surgery, exhibit some vomiting during the first 24 to 48 hours. IV fluids are administered until the infant can retain adequate amounts by mouth. Observation of physical signs, monitoring of IV fluids, careful observation, and recording of intake and output is maintained. The infant is also observed for evidence of pain, and appropriate analgesics are given. The nasogastric tube may be maintained after surgery for a variable time.

Feedings are usually instituted soon after surgery, beginning with clear liquids containing glucose and electrolytes. They are offered slowly, in small amounts, and at frequent intervals as ordered by the practitioner. If the infant has been breastfed, breast milk, expressed by the mother, is given by bottle when the infant is able to tolerate feedings. Breastfeeding is resumed as soon as feasible. Observation and recording of feedings and the infant's responses to feedings are a vital part of postoperative care. Positioning with the head elevated is usually continued postoperatively. Care of the operative site consists of observation for any drainage or signs of inflammation and care of the incision as directed by the surgeon.

Parents are encouraged to remain with their child and become involved in the child's care. Vomiting of a projectile nature is frightening to parents, and they often believe that they may have done something wrong or that surgery was not successful. Most parents need support and reassurance that the condition is caused by a structural problem and is in no way a reflection on their parenting skills and capacities.

Intussusception

Intussusception is one of the most frequent causes of intestinal obstruction in children between 3 months and 3 years of age. The peak occurrence is between ages 5 and 9 months (Brandt, 1999). Intussusception is more common in males than in females and in children with cystic fibrosis. Although specific intestinal lesions can be found in a small percentage of these children, the cause is usually not known. More than 90% of intussusceptions do not have a pathologic lead point, such as a polyp, lymphoma, or Meckel diverticulum. The idiopathic cases are most likely a result of hypertrophy of intestinal lymphoid tissue secondary to viral infection.

Pathophysiology

Intussusception occurs when a proximal segment of the bowel telescopes into a more distal segment, pulling the mesentery with it. The mesentery is compressed and angled, resulting in lymphatic and venous obstruction. As edema from the obstruction increases, pressure within the area of intussusception increases. When the pressure equals the arterial pressure, arterial blood flow stops, resulting in ischemia and the pouring of mucus into the intestine. Venous engorgement also leads to leaking of blood and mucus into the intestinal lumen, forming the classic currant jelly stools (Brandt, 1999). The most common site is the *ileocecal valve* (ileocolic), where the ileum invaginates into the cecum and colon (Fig. 47-8). Other forms include ileoileal (one part of the ileum invaginates into another section of the ileum) and colocolic (one part of the colon invaginates into another area of the colon), usually in the area of the hepatic or splenic flexure or at some point along the transverse colon.

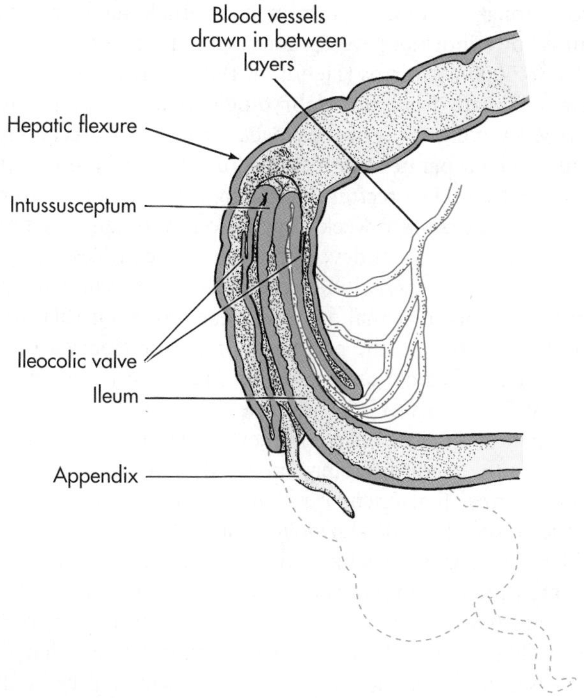

Fig. 47-8 Ileocolic intussusception.

NURSE ALERT The classic signs (e.g., severe colicky abdominal pain in a child with vomiting, currant jelly stools) may not be present. A more chronic picture, characterized by diarrhea, anorexia, weight loss, occasional vomiting, and periodic pain, may be present. Because intussusception is potentially life threatening, the nurse should be aware of alternate presentations and observe these children closely and refer them for further evaluation. ■

Diagnostic Evaluation

Frequently the diagnosis can be made on subjective findings alone (Box 47-20). However, definitive diagnosis is based on a barium enema, which clearly demonstrates the obstruction to the flow of barium. Initially, however, an abdominal radiograph is obtained to detect intraperitoneal air from a bowel perforation, which would contraindicate a barium enema. A rectal examination reveals mucus, blood, and, occasionally, a low intussusception itself.

Therapeutic Management

In most cases the initial treatment of choice is nonsurgical hydrostatic reduction traditionally by barium enema. In this procedure, correction of the invagination is carried out at the same time as the diagnostic testing. The force exerted by the flowing barium is usually sufficient to push the invaginated portion of the bowel into its original position, similar to pushing an inverted "finger" out of a glove. This procedure is not recommended if there are clinical signs of shock or perforation.

The use of barium as the contrast agent is becoming less routine, and a high percentage of radiologists use water-soluble contrast and air pressure to reduce intussusceptions. The increased use of water-soluble contrast reflects concern regarding the risk of barium peritonitis. The administration of air pressure to reduce intussusception is as successful as, and more rapid than, barium, without the risk of peritonitis and with decreased exposure to radiation. Some use carbon dioxide instead of air. It has the advantage of being absorbed by the gut and is associated with less discomfort. It also eliminates the risk of an air embolism. IV fluids, nasogastric decompression, and antibiotic therapy may be used before hydrostatic reduction is attempted. If these procedures are not successful, the child may require surgical intervention. Surgery involves manually reducing the invagination and, when indicated, resecting any nonviable intestine.

Prognosis

Nonoperative reduction is successful in approximately 75% of cases. Surgery is required for patients in whom the contrast enema is unsuccessful. With early diagnosis and treatment, serious complications and death are uncommon.

Nursing Care Management

The nurse can help establish a diagnosis by listening to the parent's description of the child's physical and behavioral symptoms. It is not unusual for parents to express that they felt something was seriously wrong before others shared their concerns. The description of the child's severe colicky abdominal pain combined with vomiting is a significant sign of intussusception.

As soon as a possible diagnosis of intussusception is made, the nurse prepares the parents for the immediate need for hospitalization, the nonsurgical technique of hydrostatic reduction, and the possibility of surgery. It is important to explain the basic defect of intussusception. A model of the defect is easily demonstrated by pushing the end of a finger on a rubber glove back into itself or using the example of a telescoping rod. The principle of reduction by hydrostatic pressure can be simulated by filling the glove with water, which pushes the "finger" into a fully extended position.

Physical care of the child does not differ from that for any child undergoing abdominal surgery. Even though nonsurgical intervention may be successful, the usual preoperative procedures, such as withholding of fluids by mouth, routine laboratory testing (CBC and urinalysis), signed parental consent, and preanesthetic sedation, are performed. For the child with signs of electrolyte imbalance, hemorrhage, or peritonitis, additional preparation, such as replacement fluids, whole blood or plasma, and nasogastric suctioning, may be needed. Before surgery the nurse monitors all stools.

BOX 47-20

Clinical Manifestations of Intussusception

- Sudden acute abdominal pain
  - Child screams and draws the knees toward the chest
  - Child appears normal and comfortable during intervals between episodes of pain
- Vomiting
- Lethargy
- Passage of red, currant jelly–like stools (stool mixed with blood and mucus)
- Tender, distended abdomen
- Palpable sausage-shaped mass in upper right quadrant
- Empty lower right quadrant (Dance sign)
- Eventual fever, prostration, and other signs of peritonitis

NURSE ALERT Passage of a normal brown stool usually indicates that the intussusception has reduced itself. This is immediately reported to the practitioner, who may choose to alter the diagnostic/therapeutic plan of care. ■

Postprocedural care includes observations of vital signs, blood pressure, intact sutures and dressing, and the return of bowel sounds. After hydrostatic reduction or autoreduction, the nurse observes for passage of barium or water-soluble contrast material and the stool patterns, because there may be recurrences of the intussusception. Children may be admitted to the hospital or monitored on an outpatient basis. A recurrence of intussusception is treated with hydrostatic reduction, but a laparotomy is considered for multiple recurrences.

Because hospitalization may be the child's first separation from the parents, it is important to preserve the parent-child relationship by encouraging rooming-in or extended visiting. It may be the parents' first experience with hospitalization, necessitating their preparation for procedures such as IV therapy, frequent vital sign and blood pressure monitoring, dressings, and special orders, such as NPO. Because of the rapidity of the onset, diagnosis, and treatment, parents may feel stunned or numb. They may ask few questions, or they may constantly make inquiries, sometimes the same ones several times. If the nurse realizes the circumstances surrounding this condition, the parents' reactions are more likely to be understood and accepted.

Malrotation and Volvulus

Malrotation of the intestine is due to the abnormal rotation of the intestine around the superior mesenteric artery during embryologic development. Malrotation may manifest in utero or may be asymptomatic throughout life. Infants with malrotation have intermittent vomiting, recurrent abdominal pain, distention, or lower GI bleeding. Malrotation is the most serious type of intestinal obstruction, because if the intestine undergoes complete volvulus (the intestine twisting around itself), compromise of the blood supply will result in intestinal necrosis, peritonitis, perforation, and death.

Diagnostic Evaluation

It is imperative that malrotation and volvulus be diagnosed promptly and surgical treatment instituted quickly. Any infant with bilious vomiting should be evaluated carefully for malrotation, volvulus, and obstruction. An upper GI series is the definitive procedure to diagnose this condition.

Therapeutic Management

Surgery is indicated to remove the affected area. Because of the extensive nature of some lesions, short-gut syndrome is a postoperative complication.

Nursing Care Management

Preoperatively, the nursing care is the same as that provided to an infant or child with intestinal obstruction. Postoperatively, the nursing care is similar to that provided to the infant or child who has undergone abdominal surgery.

Anorectal Malformations

Anorectal malformations include a number of anomalies of the genitourinary and pelvic organs. These malformations are among the more common congenital malformations caused by abnormal development, with an incidence of 1 in 2000 to 5000 live births (Hendren, 1998). The anus and rectum originate from an embryologic structure called the *cloaca.* Lateral growth of the cloaca forms the urorectal septum, which separates the rectum dorsally from the urinary tract ventrally. The rectum and urinary tract separate completely by the seventh week of gestation. Anomalies that occur reflect the stage of development of these processes.

Imperforate anus includes several forms of malformation without an obvious anal opening. Many have a fistula from the distal rectum to the perineum or genitourinary system. Anorectal malformations may occur in isolation or as part of the VACTERL or VATER syndromes.

A persistent cloaca is a complex anorectal malformation in which the rectum, vagina, and urethra drain into a common channel that opens onto the perineum via the usual urethral site. *Cloacal exstrophy* is a rare, severe defect in which there is externalization of the bladder and bowel through the abdominal wall. Often the genitalia are indefinite, and chromosome studies are necessary to determine the child's sex. Gender assignment is almost always female. The exstrophic bladder is separated into two halves by the cecum; other features may include an omphalocele, an imperforate anus, and, at times, a neural tube defect. With improved surgical techniques, survival rates for this condition are 88% to 90% in some centers (Smith et al, 1997).

Anorectal anomalies are classified according to sex and abnormal anatomic features, including genitourinary and associated pelvic anomalies. The level of rectal descent is determined by the relationship of the termination of the bowel to the puborectalis sling of the levator ani musculature. Anorectal malformations are classified according to sex and the level of the malformation (high, intermediate, and low) (Table 47-9). About 50% of children with anorectal anomalies have a urologic problem.

Table 47-9

Classification of Anorectal Malformations

LEVEL	MALE	FEMALE
High	Anorectal agenesis With rectoprostatic-urethral fistula Without fistula Rectal atresia	Anorectal agenesis With rectovaginal fistula Without fistula Rectal atresia
Intermediate	Recto-bulbar-urethral fistula Agenesis without fistula	Rectovestibular fistula Rectovaginal fistula Agenesis without fistula
Low	Anocutaneous fistula Anal stenosis Rare malformations	Anovestibular fistula Anocutaneous fistula Anal stenosis Cloaca Rare malformations

From Stephens FD et al: *Pediatr Surg Int* 1:200, 1986.

Diagnostic Evaluation

Checking for patency of the anus and rectum is a routine part of the newborn assessment and should include observations regarding the passage of meconium. Inspection of the perineal area reveals absence of the normal anal opening; however, the appearance of the perineum alone does not accurately predict the level of the lesion. Genitourinary and pelvic anomalies associated with anorectal malformations should be considered.

In the newborn, the presence of meconium on the perineum does not always indicate anal patency (particularly in girls), because a fistula may be present and allow evacuation of meconium through the vagina. Fistulas may not be apparent at birth but may become obvious as peristalsis gradually forces the meconium through the fistula. Rectourinary fistulas should be suspected if there is meconium in the urine. Anal stenosis may not be identified until the child is older and has a history of difficult defecation, abdominal distention, and ribbonlike stools.

Abdominal ultrasound is performed to determine the existence of other malformations. An intravenous pyelogram (IVP) and voiding cystourethrogram are recommended for the infant with a high malformation to identify anomalies of the urinary tract. Further examination is also indicated when there is evidence of urinary tract infection or other symptoms. If a syndrome is suspected, cardiac evaluation and spinal films should be obtained.

Therapeutic Management

Successful treatment for anal stenosis is generally accomplished by manual dilations. The procedure is initiated by a physician, and it is repeated on a regular basis by the nurses in the hospital. Parents are taught to continue the dilations at home. Perineal fistulas are treated by anoplasty during the newborn period. The opening is moved to the center of the external sphincter and dilations are begun. More extensive defects are usually managed with a colostomy and corrective surgical repair performed later in the first year (Pena, 2000).

The type of defect, the sacral anatomy, and the quality of muscles influence the long-term prognosis. In general, if the newborn has a deep midline groove, two well-formed buttocks, and an anal dimple, the prognosis for bowel control is better than if the infant has a flat or "rocker" bottom and no midline groove because of associated neurologic problems (Flake & Ryckman, 1997). A functioning interior anal sphincter is important to achieve continence. In its absence, the child may need a bowel program to achieve socially acceptable bowel continence. Other potential complications after surgical treatment include strictures, recurrent rectourinary fistula, mucosal prolapse, and constipation.

Nursing Care Management

The first nursing responsibility is identification of undetected anorectal malformations. A poorly developed anal dimple, a genitourinary fistula, or vertebral abnormalities suggest a high lesion. A newborn who does not pass a stool within 24 hours of birth requires further assessment. In addition, meconium that appears at an inappropriate orifice is reported. Preoperative care includes diagnostic evaluation, GI decompression, and IV fluids.

Nursing care after an anorectoplasty is directed toward healing the surgical site without infection or complications. Care involves keeping the anal area as clean as possible with scrupulous perineal care. A temporary dressing and drain may be placed initially to manage the continuous passage of stool. Protective ointments such as zinc oxide and occlusive dressings such as hydrocolloids decrease skin irritation from frequent loose stools. The preferred position is a side-lying prone position with the hips elevated or a supine position with the legs suspended at a 90-degree angle to the trunk to prevent pressure on perineal sutures.

There may be a nasogastric tube for abdominal decompression and IV feedings. The infant is given formula when normal peristalsis is noted. Care of the infant with a colostomy involves frequent dressing changes, meticulous skin care, and correct application of a collection device (see Chapter 44).

Family Support, Discharge Planning, and Home Care

Long-term follow-up is important for children with high malformations. After the definitive pull-through procedure, toilet training is delayed, and complete continence is seldom achieved at the usual age of 2 to 3 years. Prevention of constipation is important, and breastfeeding is encouraged postoperatively. If a cow's milk–based formula is used, a laxative may be prescribed. Bowel habit training, diet modification, and administration of stool softeners or fiber are important aspects of bowel management. Optimum bowel function may not be achieved until late childhood or adolescence. Support and reassurance are important during the slow progression to normal function.

Parents are instructed in perineal and wound care or care of the colostomy. Anal dilations may be necessary for some infants. Parents are advised to observe stooling patterns and to notify the physician if there are any signs of anal stricture or complications.

MALABSORPTION SYNDROMES

Chronic diarrhea and malabsorption of nutrients characterize malabsorption syndromes. An important complication of malabsorption syndromes in children is failure to thrive. Most cases are classified according to the location of the supposed anatomic or biochemical defect. The term *celiac disease* is often used to describe a symptom complex with four characteristics: (1) steatorrhea (fatty, foul, frothy, bulky stools), (2) general malnutrition, (3) abdominal distention, and (4) secondary vitamin deficiencies.

Digestive defects are conditions in which the enzymes necessary for digestion are diminished or absent, such as (1) cystic fibrosis, in which pancreatic enzymes are absent; (2) biliary or liver disease, in which bile flow is affected; or (3) lactase deficiency, in which there is congenital or secondary lactose intolerance.

Absorptive defects are conditions in which the intestinal mucosal transport system is impaired. This may occur because of a primary defect (e.g., celiac disease) or secondary to inflammatory disease of the bowel that results in impaired absorption because bowel motility is accelerated (e.g., ulcerative colitis). Obstructive disorders (e.g., Hirschsprung disease) also cause secondary malabsorption from enterocolitis.

Anatomic defects, such as extensive resection of the bowel or short-bowel syndrome, affect digestion by decreasing the transit time of substances and affect absorption by severely compromising the absorptive surface.

Celiac Disease

Celiac disease (CD), also known as *gluten-induced enteropathy, gluten-sensitive enteropathy (GSE),* and *celiac sprue,* is a disease of the proximal small intestine characterized by abnormal mucosa and permanent intolerance to gluten. CD is second only to cystic fibrosis as a cause of malabsorption in children. The age at which this condition first appears and its prevalence have changed over the past 30 to 40 years. Celiac sprue used to be considered a disease of childhood, but adult manifestation is becoming more common. It is seen more frequently in Europe than in America and is rarely reported in Asians or blacks. Although previous figures suggested that CD affected 1 in 6000 individuals, recent studies suggest that the prevalence is more likely to be 1 in 250 individuals (American Gastroenterological Association Medical Position Statement, 2001). The exact cause of CD is unknown, but there appears to be an inherited predisposition with an influence by environmental factors.

Pathophysiology

The disease is characterized by intolerance to the protein *gluten,* found in wheat, barley, rye, and oats. Although the pathologic process is still obscure, susceptible individuals are unable to digest the gliadin component of gluten, resulting in an accumulation of a toxic substance that is damaging to the mucosal cells.

Diagnostic Evaluation

Symptoms of CD are usually noted several months after the introduction of gluten-containing grains into the diet, typically between ages 1 and 5 years (Box 47-21). The clinical manifestations are usually insidious and chronic. The first evidence may be failure to thrive and diarrhea.

BOX 47-21

Clinical Manifestations of Celiac Disease

Impaired Fat Absorption
Steatorrhea (excessively large, pale, oily, frothy stools)
Exceedingly foul-smelling stools

Impaired Absorption of Nutrients
Malnutrition
Muscle wasting (especially prominent in legs and buttocks)
Anemia
Anorexia
Abdominal distention

Behavioral Changes
Irritability
Fretfulness
Uncooperativeness
Apathy

Celiac Crisis*
Acute, severe episodes of profuse watery diarrhea and vomiting
May be precipitated by:
- Infections (especially gastrointestinal)
- Prolonged fluid and electrolyte depletion
- Emotional disturbance

*In very young children.

The diagnosis of celiac disease is based on a biopsy of the small intestine demonstrating the characteristic changes of mucosal inflammation, crypt hyperplasia, and villous atrophy (Dieterich, Esslinger, & Schuppan, 2003). Within a day or two of instituting the diet, most children with CD demonstrate a favorable response, including weight gain and improved appetite. Within a few weeks there is resolution of the diarrhea and steatorrhea.

Serologic testing to detect antibodies to connective tissue (endomysium and reticulin) and to gliadin are available. The presence of antigliadin, antireticulin, and antiendomysial IgG and IgA antibodies (and the disappearance of these antibodies when gluten is removed from the diet) aids in diagnosis (Walker-Smith, 1999). The autoantibodies of antireticulin IgA and antiendomysial IgA are more specific markers for active celiac disease than circulating IgA antigliadin antibodies, which may be present in other diseases and conditions. A more specific test is the enzyme tissue transglutaminase (tTG), which has been found to be the autoantigen recognized by antiendomysial antibody (Walker-Smith, 1999).

Although these markers are useful in the diagnosis and screening of CD, they vary in sensitivity and specificity and are usually followed by a biopsy to confirm the diagnosis (Murray, 1999).

Therapeutic Management

Treatment of chronic CD is primarily dietary. Although the diet is called "gluten free," it is actually *low* in gluten, because it is impossible to remove every source of this protein. Studies indicate that most patients can tolerate restricted amounts of gluten. Because gluten is found primarily in the grains of wheat and rye, but also in smaller quantities in barley and oats, these four foods are eliminated. Corn and rice become substitute grain foods.

Children with untreated celiac disease may have associated lactose intolerance related to intestinal mucosal lesions, which usually improve with gluten withdrawal and intestinal healing. Specific nutritional deficiencies are treated with appropriate supplements, including vitamins, iron, and calories.

Prognosis

CD is regarded as a chronic disease. Its extent varies among children. The most severe symptoms usually occur in early childhood and again in adult life. Strict dietary avoidance of gluten prevents symptoms and may minimize the risk of developing lymphoma, the most serious complication of the disease.

Nursing Care Management

The main nursing consideration is helping the child adhere to dietary management. Considerable time is involved in explaining to the child and the parents the disease process, the specific role of gluten in aggravating the condition, and those foods that must be restricted. It is especially difficult to maintain a diet indefinitely when the child has no symptoms and temporary transgressions result in no difficulties. However, evidence indicates that most individuals who relax their diet experience a relapse of their disease and possibly exhibit growth retardation, anemia, or osteomalacia. There is also the risk of developing malignant lymphoma of the small intestine or other GI malignancies.

Although the chief source of gluten is cereal and baked goods, grains are frequently added to processed foods as thickeners or fillers. Gluten is also added to many foods as "hydrolyzed vegetable protein." The nurse must advise parents to read carefully all ingredients on labels to avoid hidden sources of gluten. Many gluten-containing products are easily eliminated from the infant's or young child's diet, but monitoring the diet of a school-age child or adolescent is more difficult. Many "favorite" foods, such as hot dogs, pizza, and spaghetti, are chief offenders. Luncheon preparation away from home is particularly difficult, because bread, luncheon meats, and instant soups are not tolerated.

In addition to restricting gluten, other dietary alterations may be necessary initially. For example, in some children who have more severe mucosal damage, disaccharide digestion is impaired, especially lactose. Therefore these children often need a temporary lactose-free diet, which necessitates eliminating all milk products.

Generally, management includes a diet high in calories and proteins, with simple carbohydrates, such as fruits and vegetables, but low in fats. Initially the bowel may be inflamed, as a result of the pathologic process, so high-fiber foods, such as nuts, raisins, raw vegetables, and raw fruits with skin, are avoided until inflammation has subsided.

Several organizations and resources are available to help families cope with this condition. The Celiac Sprue Association/United States of America* is an organization that provides support, guidance, and educational materials to families concerning a gluten-free diet, food sources, recipes, and travel information. There are also several published cookbooks that contain gluten-free recipes†.

Short-Bowel Syndrome

Short-bowel syndrome (SBS) is a malabsorptive disorder that occurs when there is decreased mucosal surface area, usually as a result of extensive resection of the small intestine. The most common causes of SBS in children include congenital anomalies (jejunal and ileal atresia, gastroschisis), ischemia (necrotizing enterocolitis), and trauma or vascular injury (volvulus [twisting of bowel on itself]). Other causes include volvulus that results in massive resection, long-segment Hirschsprung disease, and omphalocele. The prognosis for infants and children with SBS has dramatically improved in the past 25 years as a result of advances in parenteral nutrition and enteral feeding. Both the amount and the location of bowel lost are important in determining the severity of the condition. The preservation of the terminal ileum and ileocecal valve influences fluid and nutrient absorption and may avoid problems of bacterial overgrowth by preventing the entrance of bacteria from the colon into the small intestine.

*PO Box 31700, Omaha, NE, 68131-0700; phone: 402-558-0600; e-mail: celia-cusa@aol.com. In Canada: Canadian Celiac Association, Inc., 190 Britannia Rd. E., Unit 11, Mississauga, Ontario, L4Z 1W6; phone: 905-507-6208; Web site: www.celiac.ca.

†A booklet, *Pointers for Parents: Coping with Celiac Sprue,* provides information on shopping, cooking, and living with an affected child. It is available from the Clinical Dietetics Department, Children's Memorial Hospital, 2300 Children's Plaza, Chicago, IL 60614; phone: 773-880-4793.

The small intestine has significant capacity for adaptation after resection. During the *adaptation process,* the villus height increases (villus hyperplasia), and the cell number and absorptive surface area are also increased. As villus length and the number of enterocytes available for absorption per centimeter of bowel increase, nutrient absorption increases. Intraluminal enteral feedings stimulate the adaptation process and maintain the structural and functional integrity of the small intestine.

Therapeutic Management

The goals of treatment are (1) to preserve as much length of bowel as possible during surgery; (2) to maintain the child's nutritional status, growth, and development while intestinal adaptation occurs; (3) to stimulate intestinal adaptation with enteral feeding; and (4) to minimize complications related to the disease process and therapy.

Nutritional support is the long-term focus of care. The *initial phase* of therapy includes TPN as the primary source of nutrition. Complications associated with SBS and long-term TPN include central venous catheter infection or occlusion, catheter migration, thrombosis or emboli, bacterial overgrowth, metabolic complications, cholestasis, and liver dysfunction.

The *second phase* is the introduction of enteral feeding, which usually begins as soon as possible after surgery. Elemental formulas containing glucose, sucrose and glucose polymers, hydrolyzed proteins, and medium-chain triglycerides facilitate absorption. Usually these formulas are given by continuous infusion through a nasogastric or gastrostomy tube. As the enteral feedings are advanced, the TPN solution is decreased in terms of calories, amount of fluid, and total hours of infusion per day.

The *final phase* of nutritional support occurs when growth and development are sustained exclusively by enteral feedings. When TPN is discontinued, there is a risk of nutritional deficiency secondary to malabsorption of fat-soluble vitamins (A, D, E, K), and trace minerals (iron, selenium, zinc). Serum vitamin and mineral levels should be obtained, and enteral supplementation of vitamins and minerals may be required. Pharmacologic agents have been used to reduce secretory losses. H_2 blockers, proton pump inhibitors, and octreotide inhibit gastric or pancreatic secretion. Cholestyramine is often prescribed to improve diarrhea that is associated with bile salt malabsorption. Growth factors have also been used to hasten adaptation and to enhance mucosal growth, but these uses are still experimental.

Numerous complications are associated with SBS and long-term TPN (see Chapter 45). Infectious, metabolic, and technical complications can occur. Catheter sepsis can occur after improper care of the catheter. The GI tract can also be a source of microbial seeding of the catheter. Bowel atrophy may foster increased intestinal permeability of bacteria. A lack of adequate sites for central lines may become a significant problem for the child in need of long-term TPN. Hepatic dysfunction, hepatomegaly with abnormal liver function tests, and cholestasis may also occur.

Bacterial overgrowth is likely to occur when the ileocecal valve is absent or when stasis exists as a result of a partial obstruction or a dilated segment of bowel with poor motility. Alternating cycles of broad-spectrum antibiotics are used to reduce bacterial overgrowth. This treatment may also decrease the risk of bacterial translocation and subsequent central venous catheter infections. Other complications of bacterial overgrowth and malabsorption include metabolic acidosis and gastric hypersecretion.

Many surgical interventions (e.g., intestinal valves, tapering enteroplasty or stricturoplasty, intestinal lengthening, and interposed segments) have been used to slow intestinal transit, reduce bacterial overgrowth, or increase mucosal surface area. *Intestinal transplantation* has been performed successfully in children. However, the experience is limited and the long-term results are unknown. Only children with a permanent dependence on TPN or severe complications of long-term parenteral nutrition are candidates for transplantation.

Prognosis

The prognosis for infants with SBS has improved with advances in TPN and with the understanding of the importance of intraluminal nutrition. Improved surgical techniques for the management of therapy-related problems and the development of more specific immunosuppressive medications for transplantation have all contributed to improved management. The prognosis depends in part on the length of the residual small intestine. An intact ileocecal valve also improves the prognosis. Infants and children with SBS usually die of TPN-related problems, such as fulminant sepsis or severe TPN cholestasis.

Nursing Care Management

The most important components of nursing care are administration and monitoring of nutritional therapy. During TPN therapy, care must be taken to minimize the risk of complications related to the central venous access device (i.e., catheter infections, occlusions, dislodgment, or accidental removal). Care of the enteral feeding tubes and monitoring of enteral feeding tolerance are also important nursing responsibilities.

When long-term parenteral nutrition is required, preparing the family for home care is a major nursing responsibility that should be initiated early to prevent a lengthy hospitalization with subsequent problems such as family dysfunction and developmental delays. Many infants and children can be successfully cared for at home with enteral and parenteral nutrition when the family is prepared and provided with adequate support services. Follow-up by a multidisciplinary nutritional support service is essential. The nurse plays an active and important role in the success of a home nutrition program. Home infusion companies provide portable equipment, which enables the child and family to maintain a more normal lifestyle.

When hospitalization is prolonged, the child's developmental and emotional needs must be met. This often requires special planning to promote normal family adjustment and adaptation of the hospital routines. Care of the hospitalized child is discussed in Chapter 44.

INGESTION OF INJURIOUS AGENTS

Since the passage of the Poison Prevention Packaging Act of 1970, which requires that certain potentially hazardous drugs and household products be sold in child-resistant containers, the incidence of poisonings in children has decreased dramatically. However, despite these advances, poisoning remains a significant health concern, with most cases occurring in children younger than 6 years of age. Although pharmaceuticals such as analgesics, cough and cold preparations, topical preparations, antibiotics, vitamins, GI preparations, hormones, and antihistamines are frequently the agents of poisonings, children may be poisoned by a variety of substances. The most frequently ingested poisons include the following (Litovitz et al, 2000; Powers, 2000):

- Cosmetics and personal care products (perfume, cologne, aftershave)*
- Cleaning products (hypochlorite ["household"] bleach, pine oil disinfectants)
- Plants (nontoxic GI irritants, oxalates) (Box 47-22)
- Foreign bodies, toys, and miscellaneous substances (desiccants, thermometers, bubble-blowing solutions)

More than 90% of poisonings occur in the home, although a significant number take place elsewhere, such as in a grandparent's or friend's home, in a school, or in a health care facility.

NURSE ALERT The following five commonly used and easily available drugs (first four are over-the-counter products) can cause serious or fatal consequences if as little as $^1/_4$ teaspoon or $^1/_2$ tablet is ingested: methyl salicylate, camphor, topical imidazolines (sympathomimetics such as those contained in Visine, Afrin, Otrivin, and Clear Eyes), benzocaine, and diphenoxylate-atropine (Lomotil and others). Stress to parents the importance of keeping such drugs away from children. If these agents are ingested, advise parents to seek medical treatment immediately. Emesis is not induced for significant camphor, topical imidazoline, or Lomotil ingestions (Powers, 2000). ■

The developmental characteristics of young children predispose them to poisoning by ingestion. Infants and toddlers explore their environment through oral experimentation. Because the sense of taste is not discriminating at this age, many unpalatable substances are ingested. In addition, toddlers and preschoolers are developing autonomy and initiative, which increase their curiosity and noncompliant behavior. Imitation is also a powerful motivator, especially when combined with lack of awareness of danger.

This section is primarily concerned with the immediate emergency treatment of ingestion of injurious agents. Specific management of corrosive, hydrocarbon, acetaminophen, salicylate, plant, and iron poisoning is summarized in Box 47-23. Because of the importance of lead poisoning among young children, ingestion of lead is discussed separately. Appropriate suggestions for poison prevention are discussed on p. 1545.

Principles of Emergency Treatment

A poisoning may or may not require emergency intervention, but in every instance medical evaluation is necessary to initi-

*The most common substances in each category are in parentheses. Substances ingested are not necessarily most toxic but often represent ready availability.

BOX 47-22

Poisonous and Nonpoisonous Plants

Poisonous Plants: Toxic Parts

Apple: leaves, seeds
Apricot: leaves, stem, seed pits
Azalea: all parts
Buttercup: all parts
Cherry (wild or cultivated): twigs, seeds, foliage
Daffodil: bulbs
Dumb cane, Dieffenbachia: all parts
Elephant ear: all parts
English ivy: all parts
Foxglove: leaves, seeds, flowers
Holly: berries and leaves
Hyacinth: bulbs
Ivy: leaves
Mistletoe*: berries, leaves
Oak tree: acorn, foliage
Philodendron: all parts
Plum: pit
Poinsettia†: leaves, stems, sap
Poison ivy, poison oak: leaves, fruit, stems, smoke from burning plants
Pothos: all parts
Rhubarb: leaves
Tulip: bulbs
Water hemlock: all parts
Wisteria: seeds, pods
Yew: all parts

Nonpoisonous Plants

African violet
Aluminum plant
Asparagus fern
Begonia
Boston fern
Christmas cactus
Coleus
Gardenia
Grape ivy
Jade plant
Piggyback begonia
Piggyback plant
Prayer plant
Rubber tree
Snake plant
Spider plant
Swedish ivy
Wax plant
Weeping fig
Zebra plant

*Eating one or two berries or leaves is probably nontoxic.
†Mildly toxic if ingested in massive quantities.

Critical Thinking Exercise

POISONING

Mrs. Berry, a neighbor, calls you. She is very upset because her 2-year-old son has eaten several chewable multivitamins with iron. She asks you if she should give her son syrup of ipecac. What should you advise her to do?

1. Evidence—Is there sufficient evidence to formulate an answer for Mrs. Berry?
2. Assumptions—Answer the following questions and describe some underlying assumptions on which your answers are based:
   a. What is the best initial response when a child ingests a potentially poisonous substance?
   b. What is syrup of ipecac?
   c. What are the dangers involved in the use of syrup of ipecac?
3. What is the priority for nursing care at this time?
4. Does the evidence support your conclusion?
5. What alternative perspectives might you have?

Emergency

POISONING

1. Assess the victim:
   Take vital signs; reevaluate routinely.
   Initiate cardiorespiratory support if needed.
   Treat other symptoms, such as seizures.
2. Terminate exposure:
   Empty mouth of pills, plant parts, or other material.
   Flush eyes continuously with normal saline (room-temperature tap water at home) for 15 to 20 minutes.
   Flush skin and wash with soap and a soft cloth; remove contaminated clothes, especially if a pesticide, acid, alkali, or hydrocarbon is involved.
   Bring victim of an inhalation poisoning into fresh air.
   Give one sip of water to dilute ingested poison.
3. Identify the poison:
   Question the victim and witnesses.
   Look for environmental cues (empty container, nearby spill, odor on breath) and save all evidence of poison (container, vomitus, urine).
   Be alert to signs and symptoms of potential poisoning in absence of other evidence, including symptoms of ocular or dermal exposure.
   Call poison control center or other competent emergency facility for immediate advice regarding treatment.
4. Remove poison and prevent absorption:
   Place child in side-lying, sitting, or kneeling position with head below chest to prevent aspiration.
   Administer activated charcoal if ordered (unless used repeatedly, usual dose is 1 g/kg unless amount of toxin is known).

ate appropriate action. Parents are advised to call the Poison Control Center (PCC) *before* initiating any intervention. The local PCC telephone number (usually listed in the front of the telephone directory) should be posted near each phone in the house (Critical Thinking Exercise; Emergency box).*

*Also available by calling 800-222-1222 or online at American Association of Poison Control Centers: www.aapcc.org.

Based on the initial telephone assessment, the PCC counsels the parents to begin treatment at home or to take the child to an emergency facility. When a call is taken, the name and telephone number of the caller are recorded to reestablish contact if the connection is interrupted. Because most poisonings are managed in the home, expert advice is essential in minimizing adverse effects. When the exact quantity or type of ingested toxin is not known, admission to a hos-

BOX 47-23

Selected Poisonings in Children

Corrosives (Strong Acids or Alkali)

Drain, toilet, or oven cleaners
Electric dishwasher detergent (liquid, because of higher pH, is more hazardous than granular)
Mildew remover
Batteries
Clinitest tablets
Denture cleaners
Bleach

Clinical Manifestations

Severe burning pain in mouth, throat, and stomach
White, swollen mucous membranes; edema of lips, tongue, and pharynx (respiratory obstruction)
Violent vomiting (hemoptysis)
Drooling and inability to clear secretions
Signs of shock
Anxiety and agitation

Comments

Household bleach is a frequently ingested corrosive but rarely causes serious damage
Liquid corrosives cause more damage than granular preparations

Treatment

Inducing emesis is contraindicated (vomiting redamages the mucosa)
Dilute corrosive with water or milk (usually no more than 120 ml [4 ounces])
Do not neutralize—neutralization can cause an exothermic reaction (which produces heat and causes increased symptoms or produces a thermal burn in addition to a chemical burn)
Maintain patent airway if needed
Administer analgesics
Do not allow oral intake
Esophageal stricture may require repeated dilations or surgery

Hydrocarbons

Gasoline
Kerosene
Lamp oil
Mineral seal oil (found in furniture polish)
Lighter fluid
Turpentine
Paint thinner and remover (some types)

Clinical Manifestations

Gagging, choking, and coughing
Nausea
Vomiting
Alterations in sensorium, such as lethargy
Weakness
Respiratory symptoms of pulmonary involvement
Tachypnea
Cyanosis
Retractions
Grunting

Comments

Immediate danger is aspiration (even small amounts can cause bronchitis and chemical pneumonia)
Gasoline, kerosene, lighter fluid, mineral seal oil, and turpentine cause severe pneumonia

Treatment

Inducing emesis is generally contraindicated
Gastric decontamination and emptying are questionable, even when the hydrocarbon contains a heavy metal or pesticide; if gastric lavage must be performed, a cuffed endotracheal tube should be in place before lavage because of a high risk of aspiration
Symptomatic treatment of chemical pneumonia includes high humidity, oxygen, hydration, and antibiotics for secondary infection

Acetaminophen

Clinical Manifestations

Occurs in four stages:

1. Initial period (2 to 4 hours after ingestion)
   Nausea
   Vomiting
   Sweating
   Pallor
2. Latent period (24 to 36 hours)
   Patient improves
3. Hepatic involvement (may last up to 7 days and be permanent)
   Pain in right upper quadrant
   Jaundice
   Confusion
   Stupor
   Coagulation abnormalities
4. Patients who do not die in hepatic stage gradually recover

Comments

Most common drug poisoning in children
Occurs from acute ingestion
Toxic dose is 150 mg/kg or greater in children
Because of multiple formulations and concentrations, chronic acetaminophen toxicity is a significant problem
Parents should be counseled to read product packaging carefully and to consult a health care professional to avoid inappropriate dosing (Abruzzi & Stork, 2002)

Treatment

Antidote *N*-acetylcysteine (Mucomyst) can usually be given orally but is first diluted in fruit juice or soda because of the antidote's offensive odor
Given as 1 loading dose and usually 17 maintenance doses in different dosages
May be given intravenously, but use is investigational

Aspirin (Acetylsalicylic Acid [ASA])

Clinical Manifestations

Acute poisoning
Nausea
Disorientation
Vomiting
Dehydration
Diaphoresis
Hyperpnea
Hyperpyrexia
Oliguria
Tinnitus
Coma
Convulsions
Chronic poisoning

BOX 47-23

Selected Poisonings in Children—cont'd

Same as above but subtle onset (often mistaken for viral illness)
Dehydration, coma, and seizures may be more severe
Bleeding tendencies

Comments

May be caused by acute ingestion (severe toxicity occurs with 300 to 500 mg/kg)
May be caused by chronic ingestion (i.e., more than 100 mg/kg/day for 2 or more days); can be more serious than acute ingestion
Time to peak serum salicylate level can vary with enteric aspirin or the presence of concretions (bezoars)

Treatment

Hospitalization for severe toxicity
Emesis, lavage, activated charcoal, or cathartic
Lavage will not remove concretions of ASA
Activated charcoal is important early in ASA toxicity
Sodium bicarbonate transfusions to correct metabolic acidosis and urinary alkalinization may be effective in enhancing elimination; urinary alkalinization is very difficult to achieve
Be aware of the risk for fluid overload and pulmonary edema
External cooling for hyperpyrexia
Anticonvulsants
Oxygen and ventilation for respiratory depression
Vitamin K for bleeding
In severe cases, hemodialysis (not peritoneal dialysis) may be used

Iron

Mineral supplement or vitamin containing iron

Clinical Manifestations

Occurs in five stages:

1. Initial period (0.5 to 6 hours after ingestion) (if child does not develop gastrointestinal symptoms in 6 hours, toxicity is unlikely)
   Vomiting
   Hematemesis
   Diarrhea
   Hematochezia (bloody stools)
   Gastric pain
2. Latency (2 to 12 hours)
   Patient improves
3. Systemic toxicity (4 to 24 hours after ingestion)
   Metabolic acidosis
   Fever
   Hyperglycemia
   Bleeding
   Shock
   Death (may occur)
4. Hepatic injury (48 to 96 hours)
   Seizures
   Coma
5. Rarely, pyloric stenosis develops at 2 to 5 weeks

Comments

Factors related to frequency of iron poisoning:
  Widespread availability
  Packaging of large quantities in individual containers
  Lack of parental awareness of iron toxicity
  Resemblance of iron tablets to candy (e.g., M&M's)
  Toxic dose is based on the amount of elemental iron in various salts (sulfate, gluconate, fumarate), which ranges from 20% to 33%; ingestions of 60 mg/kg are considered dangerous

Treatment

Emesis or lavage
For toxic doses, lavage may be necessary for all chewable tablets or liquids if spontaneous vomiting has not occurred
Chelation therapy with deferoxamine in severe intoxication (may turn urine a red to orange color)
If intravenous deferoxamine is given too rapidly, hypotension, facial flushing, rash, urticaria, tachycardia, and shock may occur; stop the infusion, maintain the intravenous line with normal saline, and notify the practitioner immediately

Plants

See Box 47-22.

Clinical Manifestations

Depends on type of plant ingested
May cause local irritation of oropharynx and entire gastrointestinal tract
May cause respiratory, renal, and central nervous system symptoms
Topical contact with plants can cause dermatitis

Comments

Some of most frequently ingested substances
Rarely cause serious problems, although some plant ingestions can be fatal
Can also cause choking and allergic reactions

Treatment

Induce emesis
Wash from skin or eyes
Supportive care as needed

pital for laboratory evaluation and surveillance is critical during the time after ingestion.

Assessment

The first and most important principle in dealing with a poisoning is to treat the child first, not the poison. This necessitates an immediate concern for life support. Vital signs are taken and respiratory or circulatory support is instituted as needed. The victim's condition is routinely reevaluated. Because shock is a complication of several types of household poisons, particularly corrosives, measures to reduce the effects of shock, such as elevation of the legs and head to the level of the heart to promote venous drainage and provision of warmth and rest, are important. Maintenance of respiratory function may require insertion of an airway or mechanical ventilation.

The emergency department nurse's responsibility is to be prepared for immediate intervention with all of the necessary equipment. Because time and speed are critical factors in recovery from serious poisonings, anticipation of potential problems and complications means the difference between life and death.

Gastric Decontamination

In general, the immediate treatment is to remove the ingested poison by adsorbing the toxin with activated charcoal, performing gastric lavage, or increasing bowel motility (catharsis). Because of continuing controversy regarding the use of these methods, each toxic ingestion should be treated individually (Abruzzi & Stork, 2002). Specific antidotes may be administered for certain poisonings. *Syrup of ipecac,* an emetic that exerts its action through irritation of the gastric mucosa and by stimulation of the vomiting center, is no longer recommended for immediate treatment at home. The American Academy of Pediatrics, Committee on Injury, Violence, and Poison Prevention (2003b), recommends that existing ipecac in the home should be disposed of safely. The first action for a caregiver of a child who may have ingested a toxic substance is to consult the local PCC. If the PCC cannot be reached, the child should be taken to the nearest emergency department.

NURSE ALERT Syrup of ipecac is contraindicated in cases of ingestion of corrosive substances and in the child who is comatose or having seizures. In children who have ingested hydrocarbons, ipecac is contraindicated if the risk of aspiration outweighs the benefit of gastric evacuation. Ipecac may cause prolonged vomiting (enduring as long as 12 hours), which makes it relatively contraindicated in ingestions that may cause sedation, coma, or seizures (Powers, 2000). ■

No emetic or other substance should be given at home without consultation with a PCC or physician.

If the child is admitted to an emergency facility, *gastric lavage* may be performed to empty the stomach of the toxic agent. Lavage is indicated for young infants in whom ipecac is contraindicated; if the patient is comatose or convulsing or requires a protected airway; or if the ingested poison is rapidly absorbed (strychnine or cyanide). The use of lavage in petroleum distillate poisoning remains controversial because of the danger of aspiration. When lavage is performed, the largest-diameter tube that can be inserted is used to facilitate passage of gastric contents.

Another method of decontaminating the stomach is the use of *activated charcoal,* an odorless, tasteless, fine black powder that adsorbs many compounds, creating a stable complex. In the future, activated charcoal may replace syrup of ipecac as the home remedy of choice (Ford & Delaney, 2001), but the American Academy of Pediatrics, Committee on Injury, Violence, and Poison Prevention (2003b), believes it is premature to recommend the administration of activated charcoal in the home. Activated charcoal is mixed with water or a saline cathartic to form a slurry. Slurries are neither gritty nor distasteful but resemble black mud. To increase the child's acceptance of activated charcoal, the nurse should mix it with diet soda and serve it through a straw in an opaque container with a cover (such as a disposable coffee cup with lid) or an ordinary cup covered with aluminum foil or placed inside a small paper bag. Potential complications from the use of activated charcoal include aspiration (usually in patients with impaired gag reflexes), constipation, and intestinal obstruction (in multiple doses). Cathartics, such as sorbitol, sodium, or magnesium, may be administered to stimulate evacuation of the bowel, thus decreasing systemic absorption of the poison and aiding in the removal of the charcoal. Many commercial preparations of activated charcoal contain cathartics. However, the use of cathartics is controversial.

In a minority of poisonings, specific *antidotes* are available to counteract the poison. They are highly effective and should be available in all emergency facilities. The supply of antidotes should be checked routinely and replaced as used or according to expiration dates. Among the more frequently employed antidotes are *N*-acetylcysteine for acetaminophen poisoning, oxygen for carbon monoxide inhalation, naloxone for opioid overdose, flumazenil (Romazicon) for benzodiazepine (Valium, Versed) overdose, Digibind for digoxin toxicity, and antivenin for certain poisonous bites.

Prevention of Recurrence

The ultimate objective is to prevent poisonings from occurring or recurring. One effective counseling method is first to discuss the difficulties of constantly watching and safeguarding young children (Family Focus box). In this way the challenging task of raising children can lead to a discussion of injury prevention as part of the parental role. This approach also incorporates contributory causes for the incident, such as inadequate support systems, marital discord, discipline techniques (especially use of physical punishment), and maternal distress. A visit to the home, especially after a repeat poisoning situation, is recommended as part of the follow-up care to assess hazards, including family factors, and to evaluate appropriate injury-proofing measures. One method of identifying risk areas is to ask specific questions or to have the parent complete a questionnaire designed to isolate factors that predispose children to poisoning.

Another approach is to encourage parents to bend down to the child's eye level and survey the home environment for potential hazards. Have the parents try to open cabinets and reach shelves to access poisons.

Passive measures (those that do not require active participation) have been the most successful in preventing poisoning and include child-resistant closures and limiting the number of tablets in one container. However, these measures alone are not sufficient to prevent poisoning, because most toxic agents in the home do not have safety closures. Therefore *active measures* (those that require participation) are essential. Guidelines for preventing the occurrence or recurrence of a poisoning are listed in the Guidelines box.

Family Focus

POISONING

A poisoning is more than a physical emergency for the child—it usually represents an emotional crisis for the parents, particularly in terms of guilt, self-reproach, and insecurity in the parenting role. The emergency department is no place to admonish the family for negligence, lack of appropriate supervision, or failure to injury-proof the home. Rather, it is a time to calm and support the child and parents, while unaccusingly exploring the circumstances of the injury. If the nurse prematurely attempts to discuss ways of preventing such an incident from recurring, the parents' anxiety will block out any suggestions or offered guidance. Therefore it is preferable for the nurse to delay the discussion until the child's condition is stabilized or, if the child is discharged immediately after emergency treatment, to make a public health referral or send a packet of information.

Guidelines

POISON PREVENTION

Assess possible contributing factors in occurrence of injury, such as discipline, parent-child relationship, developmental ability, environmental factors, and behavior problems.
Institute anticipatory guidance for possible future injuries based on child's age and maturational level.
Refer to visiting nurse agency to evaluate home environment and need for injury-proofing measures.
Provide assistance with environmental manipulation when necessary, such as lead removal.
Educate parents regarding safe storage of toxic substances.
Advise parents to take drugs out of sight of children.
Teach children the hazards of ingesting nonfood items.
Advise parents against using plants for teas or medicine.
Discuss problems of discipline and children's noncompliance and offer strategies for effective discipline.
Instruct parents regarding correct administration of drugs for therapeutic purposes and to discontinue drug if there is evidence of mild toxicity.
Advise parents to contact the poison control center or practitioner immediately when a poisoning occurs.
Post number of regional poison control center with emergency phone list by telephone.
Include by the telephone the home address with nearest cross street in case an ambulance is needed. (In an emergency, family members may not remember the house address, and baby-sitters may not be aware of the information.)

Heavy Metal Poisoning

Heavy metal poisoning can occur from the ingestion of a variety of substances, the most common being lead. Other sources that are important in terms of children are iron and mercury. *Mercury toxicity,* a rare form of heavy metal poisoning, has occurred in children from a variety of sources, such as broken thermometers or thermostats, broken fluorescent lights, and interior latex house paint (Etzel, 2000). Elemental mercury (also called metallic mercury or quicksilver) is nontoxic if ingested and if the GI tract is healthy (e.g., has no fistulas). However, mercury is volatile at room temperature and enters the bloodstream after it is inhaled, causing toxicity (tremors, memory loss, insomnia, gingivitis, diarrhea, anorexia, weight loss). The classic form of mercury poisoning is called *acrodynia* (or "painful extremities").

NURSE ALERT Mercury thermometers are no longer recommended for use because, if broken, the inhaled vapors can cause toxicity. To prevent inhalation, spilled mercury must be cleaned up quickly, using disposable towels and rubber gloves and washing the hands well after removing the spill. ■

Heavy metals have an affinity for certain essential tissue chemicals, which must remain free for adequate cell functioning. When metals are bound to these substances, cellular enzyme systems are inactivated. Treatment involves *chelation,* use of a chemical compound that combines with the metal for rapid and safe excretion.

Lead Poisoning

Poisoning from lead has been a problem throughout history and throughout the world. In the United States the problem began in the early 1900s when white lead was added to paints and when tetraethyl lead was added to gasoline as an antiknock compound. Lead content in paint was decreased in 1950, and in 1978 the use of lead in household paint was banned. The greatest problems remaining for young children are the presence of deteriorating lead-based paint in many older homes and the the presence of soil in yards that has a high lead content. Chipping, flaking, and chalking lead-based paint contributes to the environmental dust found in households. Normal hand-to-mouth behavior, coupled with the presence of lead dust in the environment, is the most common method of poisoning (Jacob et al, 2000).

Independent risk factors for having an elevated blood lead level include poverty, age less than 6 years, African-American ethnicity, and dwelling in the city (Markowitz, 2000). Any child, however, is at risk for becoming lead poisoned if hazardous conditions for lead are present in the child's environment.

Causes of Lead Poisoning

Although there are numerous sources of lead (Box 47-24), in most instances of acute childhood lead poisoning, the source is nonintact lead-based paint in an older home or lead-contaminated bare soil in the yard. Microparticles of lead gain entrance into a child's body through ingestion or inhalation and, in the case of an exposed pregnant woman, by placental transfer. Inhalation exposure usually occurs during renovation and remodeling activities in the home; ingestion happens during normal day-to-day play and mouthing activities. Sometimes a child will actually swallow loose chips of lead-based paint, because it has a sweet taste. Water and food may also be contaminated with lead.

Nurses must be aware of their patients' cultural and ethnic practices and product use. Substances used as natural therapies have been found to contain lead (Cultural Awareness box).

Pathophysiology and Clinical Manifestations

Lead can affect any part of the body, including the renal, hematologic, and neurologic systems (Fig. 47-9). Of most concern for young children is the developing brain and nervous system, which is more vulnerable than that of an older child or adult. Lead in the body moves via an equilibration process between the blood, the soft tissues and organs, and the bones and teeth. At the cellular level it competes with molecules of calcium, interfering with the regulating action of calcium. The inorganic lead found in lead-based paint is not fat soluble and consequently should not cross the blood-brain barrier. However, it does so by impairing the endothelial cells there. Lead interferes with several neurotransmitter mechanisms in the brain. Massive body burdens of lead can lead to cerebral edema and encephalopathy.

Lead can also interfere with the binding of iron onto the heme molecule. This sometimes creates a picture of anemia, even though the child is not iron deficient. Lead toxicity to the erythrocytes leads to the release of the enzyme erythrocyte protoporphyrin (EP). Because EP is not sensitive to

BOX 47-24

Sources of Lead*

Lead-based paint in deteriorating condition
Lead solder
Lead crystal
Battery casings
Lead fishing sinkers
Lead curtain weights
Lead bullets
The following may contain lead:
- Ceramic ware
- Water
- Pottery
- Pewter
- Dyes
- Industrial factories
- Vinyl mini-blinds
- Playground equipment
- Collectible toys
- Artists' paints
- Pool cue chalk

Occupations and hobbies involving lead:
- Battery and aircraft manufacturing
- Lead smelting
- Brass foundry work
- Radiator repair
- Construction work
- Bridge repair work
- Painting contracting
- Mining
- Ceramics work
- Stained-glass making
- Jewelry making

*The U.S. Consumer Product Safety Commission issues alerts and recalls for products that contain lead and that may unexpectedly pose a hazard to young children.

blood lead levels of less than about 16 to 25 mcg/dl, it is no longer used as a screening test. However, elevation of the EP level (above 35 mcg/dl of whole blood) is a good indicator of toxicity from lead and reflects the length of exposure and body burden of lead in the individual child.

Diagnostic Evaluation

Children with lead poisoning rarely have symptoms, even at levels requiring chelation therapy. A diagnosis of lead poisoning is based only on the lead testing of a venous blood specimen from a venipuncture. The level of concern for an elevated blood lead level has dropped from 80 mcg/dl in 1950 to 10 mcg/dl today.

Anticipatory Guidance

Anticipatory guidance lends support to primary prevention efforts. The Centers for Disease Control and Prevention (CDC) (1997a) recommends that the following information be made available to families beginning during prenatal care, at 3 to 6 months, and at 1 year of age:

- Hazards of lead-based paint in older housing
- Ways to control lead hazards safely
- Hazards accompanying repainting and renovation of homes built before 1978
- Other exposure sources, such as traditional remedies, that might be relevant for a family

Cultural Awareness

SOURCES OF LEAD

In some cultures the use of traditional ethnic remedies that contain lead may increase children's risk of lead poisoning. These remedies include the following:

Azarcon (Mexico)—For digestive problems; a bright orange powder; usual dose is 0.25 to 1 teaspoon, often mixed with oil, milk, or sugar or sometimes given as a tea; sometimes a pinch is added to a baby bottle or tortilla dough for preventive purposes

Greta (Mexico)—A yellow-orange powder, used in the same way as azarcon

Paylooah (Southeast Asia)—Used for rash or fever; an orange-red powder given as 0.5 teaspoon straight or in a tea

Surma (India)—Black powder applied to the inner lower eyelid that is used as a cosmetic to improve eyesight

Unknown ayurvedic (Tibet)—Small, gray-brown balls used to improve slow development; two balls are given orally three times a day

Tamarindo jellied, fruit candy (Mexico)—Fruit candy packaged in ceramic jars (which are lead contaminated)

Lozeena (Iraq)—A bright orange powder used by Iraqis to color meat and rice

Modified from Lead poisoning associated with use of traditional ethnic remedies—California, 1991-1992, *MMWR* 42(27):521-524, 1993; and Lead poisoning associated with imported candy and powdered food coloring—California and Michigan, *MMWR* 47(48):1041-1043, 1998.

Screening for Lead Poisoning

When primary prevention fails, the secondary prevention effort of screening for elevated blood lead levels can identify children much earlier than in the past. The most recent CDC guidelines (1997a, 1997b) recommend either universal screening or targeted screening, depending on the risk factors and blood lead level surveillance information available for the area.

Universal screening should be done at ages 1 and 2 years. Any child between ages 3 and 6 years who has not been previously screened should also be tested. Any child with risk factors should be screened more often.

Targeted screening is acceptable when an area has been determined by existing data to have less risk. Children should be screened when they live in a high risk geographic area or are members of a group determined to be at risk (e.g., Medicaid recipients), or if their family cannot answer "no" to the following personal risk questions:

- Does your child live in or regularly visit a house that was built before 1950?
- Does your child live in or regularly visit a house built before 1978 with recent or ongoing renovations or remodeling within the past 6 months?
- Does your child have a sibling or playmate who has or did have lead poisoning?

Therapeutic Management

The degree of concern, urgency, and need for medical intervention changes as the lead level increases. Education is one of the most important elements of the treatment process. The CDC (1997a) has identified several areas that should be discussed with the family of every child who has an elevated blood lead level (10 mcg/dl and above):

- The child's blood lead level and what it means

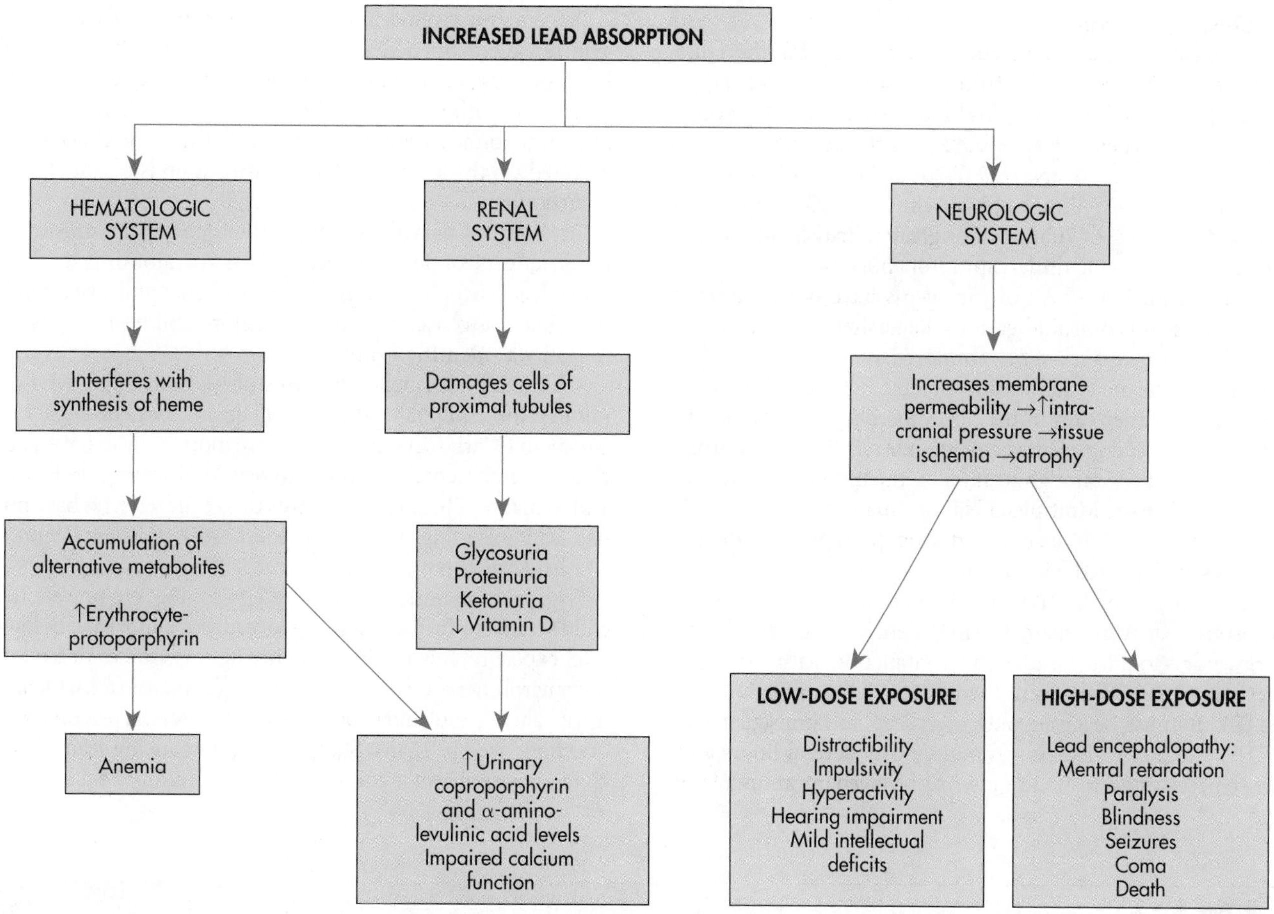

Fig. 47-9 Main effects of lead on body systems.

- Potential adverse health effects of an elevated blood lead level
- Sources of lead exposure and suggestions on how to reduce exposure
- The importance of wet cleaning to remove lead dust on floors, window sills, and other surfaces
- The importance of good nutrition, particularly adequate amounts of calcium and iron
- The need for follow-up testing to monitor the child's blood lead level
- Results of an environmental investigation when applicable
- The hazards of improper removal of lead paint (dry sanding, scraping, or open-flame burning)

Treatment actions vary depending on the child's blood lead level. Based on a diagnosis from a venous blood lead level test, the CDC (1997a) recommends the following actions:

Blood lead level (mcg/dl)	Action
<10	Reassess or rescreen in 1 year. If exposure status changes, do this sooner.
10-14	Provide family with lead poisoning education, follow-up testing, and social service referral if necessary.
15-19	Provide family with lead poisoning education, follow-up testing, and social service referral as needed; if blood lead level persists, initiate actions for blood lead level of 20 to 44 mcg/dl.
20-44	Provide coordination of care, clinical management, environmental investigation, and lead hazard control.
45-69	Within 48 hours, provide coordination of care and clinical management, including *chelation therapy* (medication that removes lead from the blood and, to some extent, from other places in the body), environmental investigation, and lead hazard control. The child must not remain in a lead hazardous environment if resolution is to occur.
≥70	*Immediately* provide medical treatment and chelation therapy, and begin coordination of care, clinical management, environmental investigation, and lead hazard control.

Chelation Therapy

Medical treatment and chelation therapy for the child with lead poisoning varies from practice to practice. However, when a child has a venous blood lead level of 45 mcg/dl or above, two chelating agents are used consistently: calcium disodium edetate (CaNa2EDTA or EDTA) and succimer (Chemet, meso-2,3 dimercaptosuccinic acid [DMSA]). With a blood lead level of 70 mcg/dl or greater, British antilewisite (BAL, dimercaprol, dimercaptopropanol) is used in conjunction with EDTA. All of the agents have potential toxic side effects and contraindications. Renal, hepatic, and hematologic parameters must be monitored.

Because of the equilibration process between blood, soft tissues, and other sites in the body, there is often a rebound of the blood lead level after chelation. After the body burden of lead is reduced enough to stabilize the blood lead level, rebound will cease. Multiple chelations may be necessary. Adequate hydration is essential during therapy because the chelates are excreted via the kidneys.

BAL must not be used in the presence of a glucose-6-phosphate dehydrogenase (G6PD) deficiency or peanut allergy, nor should it be given in conjunction with iron. It is never used as a single-agent therapy, only in conjunction with EDTA. It must be given only at a deep intramuscular site. EDTA should be given intravenously over several hours and, when necessary to restrict fluids, may be given intramuscularly.

Succimer is given orally over a 19-day course of treatment. The capsule is opened and sprinkled on a small amount of food or may be swallowed whole. Adverse effects include nausea, vomiting, diarrhea, loss of appetite, rash, elevated liver function tests, and neutropenia. Because the chelates are excreted via the kidneys, adequate hydration is essential.

Prognosis

The central nervous system is the focus of the most dramatic effects of lead exposure. Massive amounts of lead cause lead encephalopathy. Seizures, coma, and even death were known to occur in the days before children's exposure to lead was identified early.

Children with smaller amounts of lead poisoning who do not develop encephalopathy are still at risk for neurologic impairment (Markowitz, 2000). They are more likely to have a decrease in intellectual functions, to develop learning problems, and to manifest behavior problems than children who have not had lead poisoning (Finkelstein, Markowitz, & Rosen, 1998).

Nursing Care Management

The primary nursing goal in lead poisoning is to prevent the child's initial or further exposure to lead. For children with low-level exposure, this requires identifying the sources of lead in the environment. Careful history taking is the most useful and most valuable tool and should concentrate on the personal risk questions (see p. 1546). Suggestions for reducing lead in the child's environment are listed in the Community Focus box.

Community Focus

REDUCING BLOOD LEAD LEVELS

Make sure child does not have access to peeling paint or chewable surfaces painted with lead-based paint, especially window sills and wells.

If a house was built before 1960 (possibly before 1980) and has hard-surface floors, wet mop them at least once per week. Wipe other hard surfaces (e.g., window sills, baseboards). If there are loose paint chips in an area, such as a window well, use a wet disposable cloth to pick up and discard them. Do not vacuum hard-surfaced floors or window sills or wells, because this spreads dust. Use vacuum cleaners with agitators to remove dust from rugs rather than vacuum cleaners with suction only. If a rug is known to contain lead dust and cannot be washed, it should be discarded.

Wash and dry child's hands and face frequently, especially before eating.

Wash toys and pacifiers frequently.

If soil around home is or is likely to be contaminated with lead (e.g., if home was built before 1960 or is near a major highway), plant grass or other ground cover; plant bushes around outside of house so that child cannot play there.

During remodeling of older homes, be sure to follow correct procedures. Be certain children and pregnant women are not in the home, day or night, until process is completed. After deleading, thoroughly clean house using cleaning solution to damp mop and dust before inhabitants return.

In areas where lead content of water exceeds the drinking water standard and a particular faucet has not been used for 6 hours or more, "flush" the cold-water pipes by running the water until it becomes as cold as it will get (30 seconds to greater than 2 minutes). The more time water has been sitting in pipes, the more lead it may contain.*

Use only cold water for consumption (drinking, cooking, and especially for making infant formula).

Hot water dissolves lead more quickly than cold water and thus contains higher levels of lead. May use first-flush water for nonconsumption uses.

Have water tested by a competent laboratory. This action is especially important for apartment dwellers; flushing may not be effective in high-rise buildings or in other buildings with lead-soldered central piping.

Do not store food in open cans, particularly if cans are imported.

Do not use pottery or ceramic ware that was inadequately fired or is meant for decorative use for food storage or service. Do not store drinks or food in lead crystal.

Avoid folk remedies or cosmetics that contain lead.

Make sure that home exposure is not occurring from parental occupations or hobbies. Household members employed in occupations such as lead smelting should shower and change into clean clothing before leaving work. Construction and lead abatement workers may also bring home lead contaminants.

Make sure child eats regular meals, because more lead is absorbed on an empty stomach.

Make sure child's diet contains sufficient iron and calcium and not excessive fat.

Modified from Centers for Disease Control and Prevention: *Preventing lead poisoning in young children,* Atlanta, 1991, The Centers.

*For more information, contact the county or state department of health or environment for information on local water quality. For general information on lead, call the National Lead Information Center (National Safety Council), 1019 19th St. NW, Suite 401, Washington, DC 20036-5105; phone: 1-800-424-LEAD; Web site: www.nsc.org/ehc/lead.htm; or Alliance to End Childhood Lead Poisoning; phone: 202-543-1147; Web site: www.qec/p.org.

Atraumatic Care

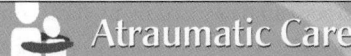

LEAD CHELATION THERAPY

To lessen the pain from intramuscular injection of $CaNa_2EDTA$, the local anesthetic procaine is injected with the drug. Apply eutectic mixture of local anesthetic (i.e., EMLA) cream over the puncture site 2.5 hours before the injection of EDTA and BAL. Administer intravenous EDTA whenever possible.

Children who must undergo chelation therapy are prepared for the injections and allowed to express their pain and anger. Playing with syringes and aggressive play (e.g., pounding clay, throwing beanbags) provides an excellent outlet for children and their frustrations. Children also deserve an explanation of the need for the treatment, particularly that it is not a punishment for eating lead or paint. During home or chelation therapy, parents need to understand the importance of giving the drug as prescribed.

Chelating agents are administered deeply into a large muscle mass (Atraumatic Care box). To lessen the pain from $CaNa_2EDTA$, the local anesthetic procaine is injected with the drug. Rotation of sites is essential to prevent the formation of painful areas of fibrotic tissue. Because $CaNa_2EDTA$ and lead are toxic to the kidneys, records are kept of intake and output, and the results of urinalysis are assessed to monitor renal functioning. Because of the risk of seizures, appropriate precautions are instituted at the bedside of children with high blood lead levels.

NURSE ALERT $CaNa_2EDTA$ is never given in the absence of an adequate urinary output. Children receiving the drug intramuscularly must be able to maintain adequate oral intake of fluids. ■

Discharge planning for children with lead poisoning must include thorough education of families regarding safety from lead hazards, clear instructions regarding medication administration and follow-up, and confirmation that the child will be discharged to a home without lead hazards. Although caution must be used to avoid alarming parents unnecessarily, it is important that they know the risk implications for their child's behavior and cognitive functions. Nurses should observe the development and behavior of children who are hospitalized. Any concerns that are identified should be thoroughly evaluated. Referral to a child development or speech and language specialist may be indicated.

As in any situational crisis, parents need support and understanding if their child is treated for lead poisoning. Many families at the highest risk for lead poisoning have the fewest resources to comply with measures such as relocation or deleading the home. Appropriate referrals are essential.

Key Points

- Infants are subject to fluid depletion because of their greater surface area relative to body mass, high rate of metabolism, and immature kidney function.
- Dehydration can be classified as isotonic, hypotonic, and hypertonic.
- Vomiting and diarrhea account for significant fluid depletion, especially in infants and small children.
- The amount, frequency, and characteristics of stool and vomitus are important nursing observations.
- Diarrhea can be caused by an inflammatory process of infectious origin, a toxic reaction to ingestion of poisonous substances, dietary indiscretions, or infections outside the alimentary tract. The primary treatment of diarrhea is the use of an oral rehydrating solution.
- Hirschsprung disease requires surgical removal of aganglionic segments of bowel.
- Postoperative care of the child with abdominal surgery involves assessing the abdomen, providing hydration and nutrition, intravenous fluids, proper positioning, wound care, and psychologic support.
- Nursing care of gastrointestinal (GI) reflux is aimed at identifying children with suggestive symptoms, helping parents with home care feeding and positioning, and caring for the child undergoing surgical intervention.
- Although the cause of appendicitis is poorly understood, it is typically a result of obstruction of the lumen, usually by a fecalith. Common signs and symptoms are right lower quadrant abdominal pain, tenderness, and fever.
- Meckel diverticulum is a congenital malformation of the GI tract characterized by bloody stools.
- Inflammatory bowel disease refers to ulcerative colitis and Crohn's disease. Chronic diarrhea is the most common feature. It is treated by dietary management and medication, although surgery is needed in some cases.
- Peptic ulcers are poorly understood, but contributing factors include interference with the normal protective mechanisms of the mucosal lining and the presence of *Helicobacter pylori*.
- Viral hepatitis is caused by six types of virus: hepatitis A virus, hepatitis B virus, hepatitis C virus, hepatitis D virus, hepatitis E virus, and hepatitis G virus.
- Hepatitis A virus is spread by the fecal-oral route, whereas hepatitis B and C viruses are transmitted primarily by the parenteral route. The most effective measure in prevention and control of hepatitis in any setting is handwashing.
- Structural disorders of the GI tract include cleft lip, cleft palate, esophageal atresia with tracheoesophageal fistula, anorectal malformations, and biliary atresia.
- Biliary atresia is a serious disorder, often causing progressive liver failure, which is an indication for liver transplantation.
- Cleft lip and palate, the most common facial malformation, may involve nutritional, dental, and speech problems.
- Hernias related to the GI tract can be minor (umbilical) or life threatening (diaphragmatic, gastroschisis, omphalocele).
- General signs of obstruction include colicky abdominal pain, nausea and vomiting, abdominal distention, and decreased stool output.
- Hypertrophic pyloric stenosis is recognized by characteristic projectile vomiting, malnutrition, dehydration, and a palpable mass in the epigastrium and is relieved by pyloromyotomy.
- Intussusception is one of the most common causes of intestinal obstruction during infancy and is characterized by abdominal pain and blood in stools. Treatment is either nonsurgical hydrostatic reduction or surgical reduction.

- Malabsorption syndromes are disorders associated with some degree of impaired digestion or absorption. They include digestive defects, absorptive defects, and anatomic defects.
- Celiac disease is characterized by an intolerance to gluten. It is thought to be either an inborn error of metabolism or an immunologic response.
- Short-bowel syndrome is characterized by a loss of intestine resulting in a diminished ability to absorb a regular diet normally. Specialized enteral and parenteral nutrition is a major element of care for these children.

Answer Guidelines to Critical Thinking Exercises

Diarrhea

1. Yes, there are sufficient data for the nurse practitioner to arrive at some conclusions.
2. (a) See Table 47-3 and note the criteria for mild dehydration. (b) Infants and children with mild dehydration are managed with oral rehydration therapy and early reintroduction of an adequate diet. In cases of severe dehydration, or when infants and children have uncontrollable vomiting, intravenous fluids are used in the management of acute diarrhea. (c) Breastfeeding generally can be continued in mild dehydration. (d) Antidiarrheal medications are not recommended for the treatment of acute infectious diarrhea. These medications have adverse effects such as slowed motility and can prolong the illness.
3. At the present time, Mary meets all the criteria for mild dehydration. It is highly probable that she has acute infectious diarrhea because her mother noted that she has had a "cold" for several days, she is vomiting, she is having diarrhea, and she has an elevated temperature. The priority for nursing care at this time is to provide rehydration via an oral rehydration solution (ORS). ORS use is an effective, safe, and cost-effective way to treat mild dehydration. The nurse practitioner should provide the mother with instructions to give Mary the ORS at frequent intervals and in small amounts. The mother should also be instructed to continue with breastfeeding and normal feedings. Early reintroduction of normal nutrients is desirable in cases of mild dehydration; delayed introduction of food may be harmful and can prolong the illness. Mary's mother should also be told to avoid the use of antidiarrheal medications.
4. Yes, the evidence supports this initial plan of management.
5. Mary's mother should be instructed to continue to monitor Mary for signs of improvement (an increase in the number of voidings or the number of wet diapers, and a decrease in vomiting). However, if Mary's condition does not improve, Mary's mother should be instructed to bring Mary back to the clinic or to the local emergency department. Mary's mother should be told to use frequent handwashing when caring for Mary to avoid transferring this infection to other members of the family.

Constipation

1. Yes, there are sufficient data to arrive at some conclusions for an initial plan of management.
2. (a) Constipation in infancy can be caused by medical conditions such as Hirschsprung disease, hypothyroidism, or strictures, or it can be simple functional constipation. (b) In infancy, changes in dietary practices such as a change from human milk to cow's milk may precipitate functional constipation. (c) Functional constipation is usually treated by dietary modifications such as increasing the amount of carbohydrate, fruit, or vegetables in the infant's diet.
3. Initially, the nurse practitioner can tell Harry's mother that functional constipation may occur with changes in the diet (e.g., the change from breastfeeding 6 weeks ago to bottle-feeding of cow's milk). The nurse practitioner can recommend that Harry's mother slowly introduce cereal and prune juice into Harry's diet. Cereal and one or two offerings of fruit juice each day may help prevent further constipation. Often, simple measures such as the introduction of solid foods or other dietary modifications help remedy functional constipation.
4. The initial data seem to point to the conclusion that Harry has functional constipation. However, the one episode of diarrhea and the two episodes of passage of ribbonlike stools do not usually occur with functional constipation
5. The nurse practitioner should remember that constipation can be caused by medical conditions such as Hirschsprung disease; therefore a referral to a gastroenterologist for further evaluation is also warranted at this time.

Inflammatory Bowel Disease

1. Yes, there is sufficient evidence to arrive at some conclusions about what to include in Susan's discharge planning.
2. (a) The goals of nutritional support for a patient with CD include (1) correction of nutrient deficits and replacement of ongoing losses, (2) provision of adequate energy and protein for healing, and (3) provision of adequate nutrients to support normal growth. (b) See Chapter 45, Gavage Feeding, pp. 1416. (c) Adolescents who are diagnosed with CD must adjust to the fact that they have a chronic illness that is characterized by remissions and exacerbations. CD may affect their activities of daily living, their social interactions with peers, and their ability to attend school. An important goal of therapy for adolescents with CD is to allow them to have as normal a lifestyle as possible.
3. The most immediate priority for discharge is to teach Susan and her family how to insert the nasogastric (NG) tube, how to administer the feedings, how to obtain the supplies needed for the tube feedings at home, and how to observe for any untoward effects of the NG feedings. As Susan's discharge nurse, you should have Susan and another family member insert the NG tube, demonstrate how to check the placement of the NG tube, and demonstrate how to start and stop the feedings while Susan is in the hospital. As Susan's nurse, you will also need to arrange for the appropriate vendors to deliver the feeding tube supplies and feeding pump to Susan's home before discharge so that the supplies will be in place when Susan is discharged. While doing all this teaching, you should also be alert to any questions, worries, or anxieties that Susan or her family members may express.
4. Yes, Susan is to receive nighttime NG tube infusions at home, and her family has expressed a desire to perform

this procedure at home. Therefore this discharge teaching is required.

5. Now that the acute disease exacerbation is under control, Susan will be able to resume school attendance and activities with her peers. However, some of her activities of daily living have been changed (e.g., the nighttime NG feedings), and she will need to adjust to remissions and exacerbations that characterize CD. To help Susan and her family cope with these changes, you should refer them to the services of the Crohn's and Colitis Foundation of America, Inc. Perhaps Susan can become involved in one of the adolescent peer-support groups that are sponsored by this group.

Poisoning

1. Yes, there is sufficient evidence to formulate an answer for Mrs. Berry.
2. (a) When a child ingests a poisonous substance, the initial goal is to remove the poison. Specific actions that are taken to remove poisons include inducing vomiting, administering activated charcoal to adsorb the toxin, and performing gastric lavage. (b) Syrup of ipecac is an emetic that induces vomiting by producing an irritant effect on the gastric mucosa. In the past, syrup of ipecac was recommended for home treatment of some cases of ingestion. However, ipecac is no longer recommended for routine home treatment of poisoning. (c) Syrup of ipecac is contraindicated when a corrosive substance or a hydrocarbon has been ingested or in cases when a child is comatose or having seizures.
3. The first priority for nursing care is to advise Mrs. Berry to call the poison control center immediately to obtain guidance. Each ingestion is treated individually, and information from the poison control center is essential to determine the most appropriate action. The most toxic ingredient in a chewable multivitamin is iron, which produces symptoms after several hours. Therefore treatment, if needed, should begin long before symptoms appear.
4. Yes, there is sufficient evidence to make sure that Mrs Berry knows syrup of ipecac should not be used in the home.
5. This situation is very straightforward, and the response is easily derived from the information. No other alternative perspectives are apparent at this time.

References

Abruzzi G, Stork CM: Pediatric toxicological concerns, *Emerg Med Clin North Am* 20(1):223-247, 2002.

American Academy of Pediatrics: Prevention of rickets and vitamin D deficiency: New guidelines for vitamin D intake, *Pediatrics* 111(4): 908-910, 2003a.

American Academy of Pediatrics, Committee on Infectious Diseases: Hepatitis C virus infection, *Pediatrics* 101(3):481-485, 1998.

American Academy of Pediatrics, Committee on injury, Violence, and Poison Prevention: Poison treatment in the house, *Pediatrics,* 112(5): 1182-1185, 2003b.

American Academy of Pediatrics, Committee on Nutrition: Soy protein-based formulas: recommendations for its use in infant feeding, *Pediatrics* 101(1):148-153, 1998.

American Academy of Pediatrics, Provisional Committee on Quality Improvement, Subcommittee on Acute Gastroenteritis: Practice parameter: the management of acute gastroenteritis in young children, *Pediatrics* 97(3):424-435, 1996.

American Dietetic Association: ADA Reports. Position of the American Dietetic Association: vegetarian diets, *J Am Dietetic Assoc* 97(11):1317-1321, 1997.

American Gastroenterological Association Medical Position Statement: Celiac sprue, *Gastroenterology* 120(6):1522-1525, 2001.

Anderson JA: Milk, eggs, and peanuts: food allergies in children, *Am Fam Physician* 56(5):1365-1375, 1997.

Andres JM: Neonatal hepatobiliary disorders, *Clin Perinatol* 23(2):321-352, 1996.

Atkison RP et al: Long-term results of pediatric liver transplantation in a combined pediatric and adult transplant program, *Can Med Assoc J* 166(13):1663-1671, 2002.

Balistreri AF: Hepatitis C—pediatric implications. Presented at the Thirty-Fourth Annual Pediatric Postgraduate Course—Perspective in Pediatrics, Bal Harbour, FL, Feb 5-11, 1999.

Balistreri WF et al: Acute and chronic hepatitis: working group report of the First World Congress of Pediatric Gastroenterology, Hepatology, and Nutrition, *J Pediatr Gastroenterol Nutr* 35(2 suppl):S62-S73, 2002.

Baron ML: Assisting families in making appropriate feeding choices: cow's milk protein allergy versus lactose intolerance, *Pediatr Nurs* 26(5): 516-520, 2000.

Baron ML: Crohn disease in children: this chronic illness can be painful and isolating, but new treatments may help, *Am J Nurs* 102(10):26-34, 2002.

Behrman RE, Kliegman RM, Arvin AM: *Nelson textbook of pediatrics,* ed 16, Philadelphia, 2000, WB Saunders.

Bonkovsky HL, Mehata S: Hepatitis C: a review and update, *J Am Acad Dermatol* 44(2):159-182, 2001.

Brandt ML: Intussusception. In McMillan JA et al (eds): *Oski's pediatrics: principles and practice,* ed 3, Philadelphia, 1999, Lippincott Williams & Wilkins.

Burkhart DM: Management of acute gastroenteritis in children, *Am Fam Physician* 60(9):2555-2563, 2565-2566, 1999.

Burks W: Diagnosis of allergic reactions to food, *Pediatr Ann* 29(12): 744-752, 2000.

Carvalho NF and others: Severe nutritional deficiencies in toddlers resulting from health food milk alternatives, *Pediatrics* 107(4):e46, 2001.

Castiglia PT: Constipation in children, *J Pediatr Health Care* 15(4):200-202, 2001.

Centers for Disease Control and Prevention: *Screening young children for lead poisoning: guidance for state and local public health officials,* Atlanta, 1997a, The Centers.

Centers for Disease Control and Prevention: Update: blood lead levels—United States, 1991-1994, *MMWR* 46(7):141-146, 1997b.

Chelimsky G, Czinn S: Peptic ulcer disease in children, *Pediatr Rev* 22(10):349-355, 2001.

Christie L et al: Food allergies in children affect nutrient intake and growth, *J Am Diet Assoc* 102(11):1648-1651, 2002.

Coffin SE: Future vaccines: recent advances and future prospects, *Primary Care* 28(4):869-887, 2001.

Devaney BL, Barr SI: DRI, EAR,RDA,AI,UL: Making sense of this alphabet soup, *Pediatr Basics* 97(Winter):2-9, 2002.

Dieterich W, Esslinger B, Schuppan D: Pathomechanisms in celiac disease, *Int Arch Allergy Immunol* 132(2):98-108, 2003.

DiLorenzo C: Disorders of the anorectum: pediatric anorectal disorders, *Gastroenterol Clin* 30(1):269-287, 2001.

Endsley S, Galbraith A: Are you overlooking oral rehydration therapy in childhood diarrhea? It's not just for use in developing countries, *Postgrad Med* 104(4):159-162, 1998.

Etzel R: The "fatal four' indoor air pollutants, *Pediatr Ann* 29(6):344-350, 2000.

Fann B: Fluid and electrolyte balance in the pediatric patient, *J Intravenous Nurs* 21(3):153-159, 1998.

Finkelstein Y, Markowitz ME, Rosen JF: Low-level lead induced neurotoxicity in children: an update on central nervous system effects, *Brain Res Rev* 27:168-176, 1998.

Flake AW, Ryckman FC: Selected anomalies and intestinal obstruction. In Fanaroff AA, Martin RJ (eds): *Neonatal-perinatal medicine: diseases of the fetus and infant,* ed 6, St Louis, 1997, Mosby.

Ford M, Delaney KA: Activated charcoal alone. In Ford MD: *Clinical toxicology,* St Louis, 2001, WB Saunders.

Gastanaduy AS, Begue RE: Acute gastroenteritis, *Clin Pediatr* 38(1):1-12, 1999.

Goldberg JP, Folta SC, Must A: Milk: Can a "good" food be so bad? *Pediatrics* 110(4):826-831, 2002.

Gorelick MH, Shaw KN, Murphy KO: Validity and reliability of clinical signs in the diagnosis of dehydration in children, *Pediatrics* 99(5):e6, 1997.

Halamek LP, Stevenson DK: Neonatal jaundice and liver disease. In Fanaroff AA, Martin RJ (eds): *Neonatal-perinatal medicine: diseases of the fetus and infant,* ed 6, St Louis, 1997, Mosby.

Hendren WH: Pediatric rectal and perineal problems, *Pediatr Clin North Am* 45(6):1353-1371, 1998.

Holcomb GW: Minimally invasive surgery. In Hoekelman RA et al (eds): *Primary pediatric care,* ed 4, St Louis, 2001, Mosby.

Host A : Frequency of cow's milk allergy in childhood, *Ann Allergy Asthma Immunol* 89(6 suppl 1):33-37, 2002.

Huffman S: Toddler's diarrhea, *J Pediatr Health Care* 13:32-33, 1999.

Hugger J, Harkless G, Rentschler D: Oral rehydration therapy for children with acute diarrhea, *Nurse Pract* 23(12):52-62, 1998.

Institute of Medicine, Food and Nutrition Board: *Dietary Reference Intakes: applications in dietary assessment,* National Academy Press, Washington D.C., 2000.

Irish MS et al: The approach to common abdominal diagnoses in infants and children, *Pediatr Clin North Am* 45(4):729-772, 1998.

Jabbar A, Wright RA: Gastroenteritis and antibiotic-associated diarrhea, *Primary Care* 30(1):63-80, 2003.

Jackson WD, Grand RJ: Crohn's disease. In McMillan JA et al (eds): *Oski's pediatrics: principles and practice,* ed 3, Philadelphia, 1999, Lippincott Williams & Wilkins.

Jacob B et al: The effect of low level blood on hematological parameters in children, *Environ Res* 82(2):150-159, 2000.

Karnam US, Reddy KR: Pegylated interferons, *Clin Liver Dis* 7(1):139-148, 2003.

Kemper KJ, Gardiner P: Herbal medicines. In Behrman RE, Kliegman RM, Jenson HB, eds, *Nelson textbook of pediatrics,* ed 17, Philadelphia, Saunders, 2004.

Kirschner RE, LaRossa D: Cleft lip and palate, *Otolaryngol Clin North Am* 33(6):1191-1215, 2000.

Lanski et al: Herbal therapy use in a pediatric emergency department population: expect the unexpected. *Pediatrics.* May;111(5 Pt 1):981-5. 2003.

Lasche J, Duggan C: Managing acute diarrhea: what every pediatrician needs to know, *Contemp Pediatr* 16(2):74-83, 1999.

Ledwith C: Fluids and electrolytes. In Merenstein G, Kaplan D, Rosenberg A (eds): *Handbook of pediatrics,* Stamford, CT, 1997, Appleton & Lange.

Lee J, Nunn J, Wright C: Height and weight achievement in cleft lip and palate, *Arch Dis Child* 76(1):70-72, 1997.

Leichtner AM, Jackson WD, Grand RJ: Ulcerative colitis. In Walker WA et al (eds): *Pediatric gastrointestinal disease: pathophysiology, diagnosis, management,* ed 2, St Louis, 1996, Mosby.

Litovitz T et al: 1999 Annual report of the American Association of Poison Control Centers Toxic Exposure Surveillance System, *Am J Emerg Med* 18(5):517-574, 2000.

Loening-Baucke V: Functional constipation, *Semin Pediatr Surg* 4(10): 26-34, 1995.

Loman: The use of complementary and alternative health care practices among children, *J Pediatr Health Care.* 17(2):58-63. 2003.

Markowitz M: Lead poisoning, *Pediatr Rev* 21(10):327-335, 2000.

McGuire JK, Kulkarni MS, and Baden HP: Fatal hypermagnesemia in a child treated with megavitamin/megamineral therapy, *Pediatrics* 105(2): 414, 2000.

MMWR Weekly: Neurologic impairment in children associated with maternal dietary deficiency of cobalamin—Georgia, 2001, *MMWR Weekly* 52(4):61-64, 2003.

Motil K: Peptic ulcer disease. In McMillan JA et al (eds): *Oski's pediatrics: principles and practice,* ed 3, Philadelphia, 1999, Lippincott Williams & Wilkins.

Murray JA: The widening spectrum of celiac disease, *Am J Clin Nutr* 69: 354-365, 1999.

Nappert G et al: Oral rehydration solutions therapy in the management of children with rotavirus diarrhea, *Nutr Rev* 58(3):80-87, 2000.

Orenstein SR: Gastroesophageal reflux, *Pediatr Rev* 20(1):24-28, 1999.

Pena A: Anorectal malformations. In Behrman RE, Kliegman RM, Jenson HB (eds): *Nelson textbook of pediatrics,* ed 16, Philadelphia, 2000, WB Saunders.

Perrotta S et al: Infant hypervitaminosis A causes severe anemia and thrombocytopenia: evidence of a retinol-dependent bone marrow cell growth inhibition, *Blood* 99(6):2017-2022, 2002.

Perry CL et al: Adolescent vegetarians: how well do their dietary patterns meet the Healthy People 2010 objectives? *Arch Pediatr Adolesc Med* 156(5):426-427, 2002.

Pickering L, Ed: *Red Book: report of the Committee on Infectious Diseases,* ed 26, Elk Grove Village, IL, 2003, American Academy of Pediatrics, The Academy.

Pongracic JA: Is it food allergy? *Contemp Pediatr* 17(12):101-122, 2000.

Powers K: Diagnosis and management of common toxic ingestions and inhalations, *Pediatr Ann* 29(6):330-342, 2000.

Preston AM et al: Influence of environmental tobacco smoke on vitamin C status in children. Am J Clin Nutr. 77(1):167-72, 2003.

Ramaswamy K, Jacobson K: Infectious diarrhea in children, *Gastroenterol Clin* 30(3):611-624, 2001.

Regev A, Schiff ER: Viral hepatitis A, B, and C, *Clin Liver Dis* 4(1):47-71, 2000.

Richard ME: Weight comparisons of infants with complete cleft lip and palate, *Pediatr Nurs* 20(20):191-196, 1994.

Rothenberg SS: Experience with 220 consecutive laparoscopic Nissen fundoplication in infants and children, *J Pediatr Surg* 33(2):274-278, 1998.

Rudolph CD et al: Guidelines for evaluation and treatment of gastroesophageal reflux in infants and children: recommendations of the North American Society for Pediatric Gastroenterology and Nutrition, *J Pediatr Gastroenterol Nutr* 32(suppl 2):S1-S31, 2001.

Ryckman F, Flake AW, Balistreri WF: Upper gastrointestinal disorders. In Fanaroff AA, Martin RJ (eds): *Neonatal-perinatal medicine: diseases of the fetus and infant,* ed 6, St Louis, 1997, Mosby.

Salvatore S, Vandenplas Y: Gastroesophageal reflux and cow milk allergy: Is there a link? *Pediatrics* 110(5):972-984, 2002.

Sampson HA: Utility of food-specific IgE concentrations in predicting symptomatic food allergy, *J Allergy Clin Immunol* 107(5):891-896, 2001.

Sampson HA: Anaphylaxis and emergency treatment, *Pediatrics* 111(6): 1601-1608, 2003.

Sandberg SJ, Magee WP, Denk MJ: Neonatal cleft lip and cleft palate repair, *AORN Online* 75(3):488, 490-499, 501, 503-504, 506-508, 2002.

Savilahti E: Food-induced malabsorption syndromes, *J Pediatr Gastroenterol Nutr* 30(S1):S61-S66, 2000.

Schwartz MZ: Meckel diverticulum. In Wyllie R, Hyams JS (Eds): *Pediatric gastrointestinal disease: physiology, diagnosis, management,* ed 2, Philadelphia, 1999, Mosby.

Sicherer SH: Diagnosis and management of childhood food allergy, *Curr Prob Pediatr* 21(2):39-57, 2001.

Sinatra FR: Liver transplantation for biliary atresia, *Pediatr Rev* 22(5): 166-180, 2001.

Smith EA et al: Current urologic management of cloacal exstrophy: experience with 11 patients, *J Pediatr Surg* 32(2):256-262, 1997.

Speltz ML et al: Early predictors of attachment in infants with cleft lip and/or palate, *Child Dev* 68(1):12-25, 1997.

Strahlman RS: Appendicitis. In Hoekelman RA et al (eds): *Primary pediatric care,* ed 4, St Louis, 2001, Mosby.

Trovar JA et al: Functional results of laparoscopic fundoplication in children, *J Pediatric Gastroenterol Nutr* 26(4):429-431, 1998.

Walker-Smith J: Celiac disease. In Wyllie R, Hyams JS (eds): *Pediatric gastrointestinal disease: pathophysiology, diagnosis, management,* ed 2, St Louis, 1999, Mosby.

Wilkins-Haug L: Prenatal diagnosis of orofacial clefts, *Up to Date,* Jan 7, 2003. Internet document available at www.uptodate.com (accessed Jan 2003).

Yuen MF, Lai CL: Treatment of chronic hepatitis B, *Lancet Infect Dis* 1(4):383-393, 2001.

Zeiter DK, Hyams JS: Gastroesophageal reflux: pathogenesis, diagnosis, and treatment, *Allergy Asthma Proc* 20(1):45-49, 1999.

Cardiovascular Dysfunction 48

LEARNING OBJECTIVES

On completion of this chapter the reader will be able to:

- Design a plan for assisting a child during a cardiac diagnostic procedure.
- Demonstrate an understanding of the hemodynamics, distinctive manifestations, and therapeutic management of congenital heart disease.
- Outline a plan of care for an infant or a child with congestive heart failure.
- Describe the care for a child who has hypoxia.
- Describe the care for an infant or a child with a congenital heart defect and its surgical repair.
- Discuss the role of the nurse in helping the child and family cope with congenital heart disease.
- Differentiate between rheumatic fever and rheumatic heart disease.
- List the criteria for selected cholesterol screening of children.
- Discuss the assessment and management of hypertension in children and adolescents.
- Outline a plan of care for a child with Kawasaki disease.
- Describe the emergency treatment for shock, including anaphylaxis.

ELECTRONIC RESOURCES

Additional information related to the content in Chapter 48 can be found on

the companion website at evolve
http://evolve.elsevier.com/Wong/maternal/
- NCLEX Review Questions
- WebLinks

or the interactive student CD-ROM
Activities for Chapter 48 include the following:
- NCLEX Review Questions
- Anatomy Review—Changes in Circulation at Birth
- Anatomy Review—Conduction System of the Heart
- Case Study—Patent Ductus Arteriosus
- Critical Thinking Exercise—Cardiac Catheterization
- Nursing Care Plan—The Child with Congestive Heart Failure

CARDIOVASCULAR DYSFUNCTION

Cardiovascular disorders in children are divided into two major groups: congenital heart disease and acquired heart disorders. *Congenital heart disease* includes primarily anatomic abnormalities present at birth that result in abnormal cardiac function. The clinical consequences of congenital heart defects fall into two broad categories: congestive heart failure and hypoxemia. *Acquired cardiac disorders* refer to disease processes or abnormalities that occur after birth and can be seen in the normal heart or in the presence of congenital heart defects. They result from various factors, including infection, autoimmune responses, environmental factors, and familial tendencies.

Assessment of Cardiac Function

History and Physical Examination

Taking an accurate health history is an important first step in assessing an infant or a child for possible heart disease. Parents may have specific concerns such as poor feeding or fast breathing in their infant or that their 7-year-old can no longer keep up with friends on the soccer field. Others may not always realize that their child has a medical problem; their child has always been pale and a fussy baby.

Asking for details about the mother's health history, pregnancy, and birth history is important in assessing infants. Mothers with chronic health conditions, such as diabetes or lupus, are more likely to have infants with heart disease. Some medications, such as phenytoin (Dilantin), are teratogenic to the fetus. Maternal alcohol use or illicit drug use increases the risk of congenital heart defects. Exposures to infections, such as rubella, early in pregnancy may result in congenital anomalies. Infants with low birth weight resulting from intrauterine growth retardation are more likely to have congenital anomalies. High-birth-weight infants have an increased incidence of heart disease.

A detailed family history is also important. There is an increased incidence of congenital cardiac defects if either parent of a sibling has a heart defect. Some diseases, such as

Marfan syndrome, and some cardiomyopathies are hereditary. A family history of frequent fetal loss, sudden infant death, and sudden death in adults may indicate heart disease. Congenital heart defects are seen in many syndromes, such as Down syndrome and Turner syndrome.

The physical assessment of suspected cardiac disease begins with observation of general appearance; it then proceeds with more specific observations. The following assessment techniques are supplementary to the general assessment techniques described for physical assessment of the chest and heart in Chapter 35.

Inspection

Nutritional state. Failure to thrive or poor weight gain is associated with heart disease.

Color. Cyanosis is a common feature of congenital heart disease, and pallor is associated with poor perfusion.

Chest deformities. An enlarged heart sometimes distorts the chest configuration.

Unusual pulsations. Visible pulsations of the neck veins are seen in some patients.

Respiratory excursion. This refers to the ease or difficulty of respiration (e.g., tachypnea, dyspnea, presence of expiratory grunt).

Clubbing of fingers. This is associated with cyanosis.

Palpation and Percussion

Chest. These maneuvers help discern heart size and other characteristics (e.g., thrills) associated with heart disease.

Abdomen. Hepatomegaly or splenomegaly may be evident.

Peripheral pulses. Rate, regularity, and amplitude (strength) may reveal discrepancies.

Auscultation

Heart rate and rhythm. Listen for fast heart rates (tachycardia), slow heart rates (bradycardia), or irregular rhythms.

Character of heart sounds. Listen for distinct or muffled sounds, murmurs, and additional heart sounds.

Diagnostic Evaluation

A variety of invasive and noninvasive tests may be used in the diagnosis of heart disease (Table 48-1). Some of the more common diagnostic tools that require nursing assessment and intervention are described here.

Table 48-1

Procedures for Cardiac Diagnosis

PROCEDURE	DESCRIPTION
Chest radiograph (x-ray)	Provides information on heart size and pulmonary blood flow patterns
Electrocardiography (ECG)	Graphic measure of electrical activity of heart
Holter monitor	24-hour continuous ECG recording used to assess dysrhythmias
Echocardiography	Use of high-frequency sound waves obtained by a transducer to produce an image of cardiac structures
Transthoracic	Done with transducer on chest
M-mode	One-dimensional graphic view used to estimate ventricular size and function
Two-dimensional (2-D)	Real-time, cross-sectional views of heart used to identify cardiac structures and cardiac anatomy
Doppler	Identifies blood flow patterns and pressure gradients across structures
Fetal	Imaging fetal heart in utero
Transesophageal (TEE)	Transducer placed in esophagus behind heart to obtain images of posterior heart structures or in patients with poor images from chest approach
Cardiac catheterization	Imaging study using radiopaque catheters placed in a peripheral blood vessel and advanced into heart to measure pressures and oxygen levels in heart chambers and visualize heart structures and blood flow patterns
Hemodynamics	Measures pressures and oxygen saturations in heart chambers
Angiography	Use of contrast material to illuminate heart structures and blood flow patterns
Biopsy	Use of special catheter to remove tiny samples of heart muscle for microscopic evaluation; used in assessing infection, inflammation, or muscle dysfunction disorders; also to evaluate for rejection after heart transplant
Electrophysiology (EPS)	Special catheters with electrodes employed to record electrical activity from within heart; used to diagnose rhythm disturbances
Exercise stress test	Monitoring of heart rate, blood pressure, electrocardiogram (ECG), and oxygen consumption at rest and during progressive exercise on a treadmill or bicycle
Cardiac magnetic resonance imaging (MRI)	Noninvasive imaging technique; used in evaluation of vascular anatomy outside of heart (i.e., coarctation of the aorta, vascular rings), estimates of ventricular mass and volume; uses for MRI are expanding

Bedside cardiac monitoring with the electrocardiogram (ECG) is commonly used in pediatrics, especially in the care of children with heart disease. The bedside monitor provides valuable information about heart rate and rhythm through a graphic display of the ECG tracing and a digital display. An alarm can be set with parameters for individual patient requirements and will sound if the heart rate is above or below the set parameters. Gelfoam electrodes are commonly used and placed on the right side of the chest (above the level of the heart) and on the left side of the chest, and a ground electrode is placed on the abdomen. Electrodes should be changed every 1 to 2 days because they are irritating to the skin. Bedside monitors are an adjunct to patient care and should never be substituted for direct assessment and auscultation of heart sounds. The nurse should assess the patient, not the monitor.

NURSE ALERT Electrodes for cardiac monitoring are often color coded: white for right, green (or red) for ground, and black for left. Always check to ensure that these colors are placed correctly. ■

Echocardiography

Echocardiography is one of the most frequently used tests for detecting cardiac dysfunction in children. Recent improvements in echocardiographic techniques have made it increasingly possible to confirm the diagnosis without resorting to cardiac catheterization. In an increasing number of instances, a prenatal diagnosis of congenital heart disease can be made by fetal echocardiography.

Echocardiography involves the use of ultrasonic waves to produce an image of the heart's structure. A transducer placed directly on the chest wall delivers repetitive pulses of ultrasound and processes the returned signals (echoes).

Although the test is noninvasive, painless, and associated with no known side effects, it can be stressful for children. The child must lie quietly in the standard echocardiographic positions; crying, nursing, or sitting up often leads to diagnostic errors or omissions. Therefore infants and young children may need a mild sedative; older children benefit from psychologic preparation for the test. The distraction of a video or movie is often helpful.

Cardiac Catheterization

Critical Thinking Exercise: Cardiac Catheterization

Cardiac catheterization is an invasive diagnostic procedure in which a radiopaque catheter is inserted through a peripheral blood vessel into the heart (Uzurk, 2001). The catheter is usually introduced through percutaneous technique, in which the catheter is threaded through a large-bore needle that is inserted into the vein. The catheter is guided through the heart with the aid of fluoroscopy. After the tip of the catheter is within a heart chamber, contrast material is injected, and films are taken of the dilution and circulation of the material *(angiography)*. Types of cardiac catheterizations include the following:

Diagnostic catheterizations. These studies are used to diagnose congenital cardiac defects, particularly in symptomatic infants and before surgical repair. They are divided into right-sided catheterizations, in which the catheter is introduced through a vein (usually the femoral vein) and threaded to the right atrium (most common), and left-sided catheterizations, in which the catheter is threaded through an artery into the aorta and into the heart.

Interventional catheterizations (therapeutic catheterizations). A balloon catheter or other device is used to alter the cardiac anatomy. Examples include dilating stenotic valves or vessels or closing abnormal connections (Table 48-2).

Table 48-2

Current Interventional Cardiac Catheterization Procedures in Children

INTERVENTION	DIAGNOSIS
Balloon atrioseptostomy (BAS) Well established in newborns May also be done under echo guidance	Transposition of great arteries Some complex single-ventricle defects
Balloon dilation Treatment of choice	Valvular pulmonic stenosis Branch pulmonary artery stenosis Congenital valvular aortic stenosis Rheumatic mitral stenosis Recurrent coarctation of aorta Further follow-up required in native coarctation of aorta in patients older than 7 months and in congenital mitral stenosis
Coil occlusion Accepted alternative to surgery	Patent ductus arteriosus (<4 mm)
Transcatheter device closure Several devices in clinical trials	Atrial septal defect
Stent placement	Pulmonary artery stenosis Other lesions investigational
Radiofrequency ablation	Some tachydysrhythmias

Data from Allen HD et al: Pediatric therapeutic cardiac catheterization: AHA Scientific Statement, *Circulation* 97:609-625, 1998.

Electrophysiology studies. Catheters with tiny electrodes that record the impulses of the heart directly from the conduction system are used to evaluate dysrhythmias and sometimes to destroy accessory pathways that cause some tachydysrhythmias.

Nursing Care Management

Cardiac catheterization has become a routine diagnostic procedure and may be done on an outpatient basis. However, it is not without risks, especially in neonates and seriously ill infants and children. Typical reactions include acute hemorrhage from the entry site (more likely with interventional procedures because larger catheters are used), low-grade fever, nausea, vomiting, loss of pulse in the catheterized extremity (usually transient, resulting from a clot, hematoma, or intimal tear), and transient dysrhythmias (generally catheter induced) (Uzurk, 2001). Rare risks include stroke, seizures, tamponade, and death.

Preprocedural Care

A complete nursing assessment is necessary to ensure a safe procedure with minimum complications. This assessment should include accurate height (essential for correct catheter selection) and weight. Obtaining a history of allergic reactions is important, because some of the contrast agents are iodine based. Specific attention to signs and symptoms of infection is crucial. Severe diaper rash may be a reason to cancel the procedure if femoral access is required. Because assessment of pedal pulses is important after catheterization, the nurse should assess and mark pulses (dorsalis pedis, posterior tibial) before the child goes to the catheterization room. The presence and quality of pulses in both feet are clearly documented. Baseline oxygen saturation using pulse oximetry in children with cyanosis is also recorded.

Preparing the child and family for the procedure is the joint responsibility of the physician, nurse, and parents. School-age children and adolescents benefit from a description of the catheterization laboratory and a chronologic explanation of the procedure, emphasizing what they will see, feel, and hear. Older children and adolescents may bring earphones and their favorite music so they can listen during the catheterization procedure.

Methods of sedation vary among institutions and may include oral or intravenous (IV) medications (see Chapter 45). The child's age, heart defect, clinical status, and type of catheterization procedure planned are considered when sedation is determined. General anesthesia may be needed for some interventional procedures. Children are allowed nothing by mouth (NPO) for 4 to 6 hours or more before the procedure, according to institutional guidelines. Infants and patients with polycythemia may need IV fluids to prevent dehydration and hypoglycemia.

Postprocedural Care

Patients may recover from the procedure in a recovery unit or their hospital room; occasionally, intensive care may be required. Patients are usually placed on a cardiac monitor and a pulse oximeter for the first few hours of recovery. The most important nursing responsibility is observation of the following for signs of complications:

- Pulses, especially below the catheterization site, for equality and symmetry (pulse distal to the site may be weaker for the first few hours after catheterization but should gradually increase in strength)
- Temperature and color of the affected extremity, because coolness or blanching may indicate arterial obstruction
- Vital signs, which are taken as frequently as every 15 minutes, with special emphasis on heart rate, which is counted for 1 full minute for evidence of dysrhythmias or bradycardia
- Blood pressure, especially for hypotension, which may indicate hemorrhage from cardiac perforation or bleeding at the site of initial catheterization
- Dressing, for evidence of bleeding or hematoma formation in the femoral or antecubital area
- Fluid intake, both IV and oral, to ensure adequate hydration (blood loss in the catheterization laboratory, the child's NPO status, and diuretic actions of dyes used during the procedure put children at risk for hypovolemia and dehydration)
- Hypoglycemia, especially in infants, who should receive dextrose-containing IV fluids; blood glucose levels should be checked

NURSE ALERT If bleeding occurs, direct continuous pressure is applied 2.5 cm (1 inch) above the percutaneous skin site to localize pressure over the vessel puncture. ■

Depending on hospital policy, the child may be kept in bed with the affected extremity maintained straight for 4 to 6 hours after venous catheterization and for 6 to 8 hours after arterial catheterization to facilitate healing of the cannulated vessel. If younger children have difficulty complying, they can be held in the parent's lap with the leg maintained in the correct position. The child's usual diet can be resumed as soon as tolerated, beginning with sips of clear liquids and advancing as the condition allows. The child is encouraged to void to clear the contrast material from the blood. Generally, there is only slight discomfort at the percutaneous site. To prevent infection, the catheterization area is protected from possible contamination. If the child wears diapers, the dressing can be kept dry by covering it with a piece of plastic film and sealing the edges of the film to the skin with tape. However, the nurse must be careful to continue to observe the site for any evidence of bleeding (Home Care box and Critical Thinking Exercise).

Home Care

AFTER CARDIAC CATHETERIZATION

Remove pressure dressing the day after catheterization. Cover site with an adhesive bandage strip for several days.
Keep site clean and dry. Avoid tub baths for several days; may shower.
Observe site for redness, swelling, drainage, and bleeding. Monitor for fever. Notify practitioner if these occur.
Avoid strenuous exercise for several days. May attend school.
Resume regular diet without restrictions.
Use acetaminophen or ibuprofen for pain.
Keep follow-up appointments per practitioner's instruction.

Modified from Children's Hospital (Boston) Cardiovascular Program, 1994.

Critical Thinking Exercise

CARDIAC CATHETERIZATION

Tommy, a 4-year-old with tetralogy of Fallot, has just returned to his hospital room from the cardiac catheterization recovery room. His mother calls you to the bedside to tell you that he is vomiting and bleeding. You arrive to find Tommy, anxious, pale, crying, and sitting in a puddle of blood.

1. Evidence—Is there sufficient evidence to draw conclusions about Tommy's situation?
2. Assumptions—Describe an underlying assumption about each of the following:
   a. Risks of cardiac catheterization
   b. Association between vomiting and bleeding following heart catheterization
   c. Concerns related to acute blood loss
3. What priorities for nursing care should be established for Tommy?
4. Does the evidence support your nursing interventions?
5. What alternative perspectives might you have?

CONGENITAL HEART DISEASE

The incidence of congenital heart disease (CHD) in children is generally believed to be 5 to 8 per 1000 live births (Behrman, Kliegman, & Jenson, 2000). About 2 to 3 in 1000 infants will be symptomatic during the first year of life. CHD is the major cause of death (other than prematurity) in the first year of life. Although there are more than 35 well-recognized defects, the most common heart anomaly is ventricular septal defect (VSD).

The exact etiology of 90% of the congenital cardiac defects is unknown. Most are thought to be a result of multifactorial inheritance: a complex interaction of genetic and environmental factors. The tremendous amount of information being discovered in molecular biology and the Human Genome Project will likely increase our understanding of the genetic etiologies of congenital heart defects.

Some risk factors are known to increase the incidence of congenital heart defects. Maternal factors include chronic illnesses such as diabetes or poorly controlled phenylketonuria (PKU), alcohol consumption, and exposure to environmental toxins and infections. Family history of a cardiac defect in a parent or sibling increases the likelihood of a cardiac anomaly. The risk of congenital heart disease increases if a first-degree relative (parent or sibling) is affected (Behrman et al, 2000). The familial risk is higher with left-sided obstructive lesions.

Congenital heart anomalies are often associated with chromosomal abnormalities, syndromes, or congenital defects in other body systems. Down syndrome (trisomy 21), trisomy 13, and trisomy 18 are highly correlated with congenital heart defects.

Circulatory Changes at Birth

During fetal life, blood carrying oxygen and nutritive materials from the placenta enters the fetal system through the umbilicus via the large umbilical vein. Oxygenated blood enters the heart by way of the inferior vena cava. Because of the higher pressure of blood entering the right atrium, it is directed posteriorly in a straight pathway across the right atrium and through the *foramen ovale* to the left atrium. In this way, the better-oxygenated blood enters the left atrium and ventricle to be pumped through the aorta to the head and upper extremities. Blood from the head and upper extremities entering the right atrium from the superior vena cava is directed downward through the tricuspid valve into the right ventricle. From here it is pumped through the pulmonary artery, where the major portion is shunted to the descending aorta via the *ductus arteriosus.* Only a small amount flows to and from the nonfunctioning fetal lungs (Fig. 48-1, *A*).

Before birth, the high pulmonary vascular resistance created by the collapsed fetal lung causes greater pressures in the right side of the heart and the pulmonary arteries. At the same time, the free-flowing placental circulation and the ductus arteriosus produce a low vascular resistance in the remainder of the fetal vascular system. With the cessation of placental blood flow from clamping of the umbilical cord and the expansion of the lungs at birth, the hemodynamics of the fetal vascular system undergo pronounced and abrupt changes (Fig. 48-1, *B*).

With the first breath, the lungs are expanded, and increased oxygen causes pulmonary vasodilation. Pulmonary pressures start to fall as systemic pressures, given the removal of the placenta, start to rise. Normally the foramen ovale closes as the pressure in the left atrium exceeds the pressure in the right atrium. The ductus arteriosus starts to close in the presence of increased oxygen concentration in the blood and other factors.

ANATOMY REVIEW: CHANGES IN CIRCULATION AT BIRTH

Altered Hemodynamics

To appreciate the physiology of heart defects, it is necessary to understand the role of pressure gradients, flow, and resistance within the circulation. As with any fluid, blood flows from an area of high pressure to one of lower pressure and toward the path of least resistance in response to the pumping action of the heart. In general, the higher the pressure gradient, the greater the rate of flow; the higher the resistance, the lesser the rate of flow.

Normally the pressure on the right side of the heart is lower than that on the left side, and the resistance in the pulmonary circulation is less than that in the systemic circulation. Vessels entering or exiting these chambers have corresponding pressures. Therefore if an abnormal connection exists between the heart chambers (such as a septal defect), blood will necessarily flow from an area of higher pressure (left side) to one of lower pressure (right side). Such a flow of blood is termed a *left-to-right shunt.* Anomalies resulting in cyanosis may result from a change in pressure so that the blood is shunted from the right to the left side of the heart *(right-to-left shunt)* because of either increased pulmonary vascular resistance or obstruction to blood flow through the pulmonic valve and artery. Cyanosis may also result from a defect that allows mixing of oxygenated and deoxygenated blood within the heart chambers or great arteries, such as occurs in truncus arteriosus.

ANATOMY REVIEW: CONDUCTION SYSTEM OF THE HEART

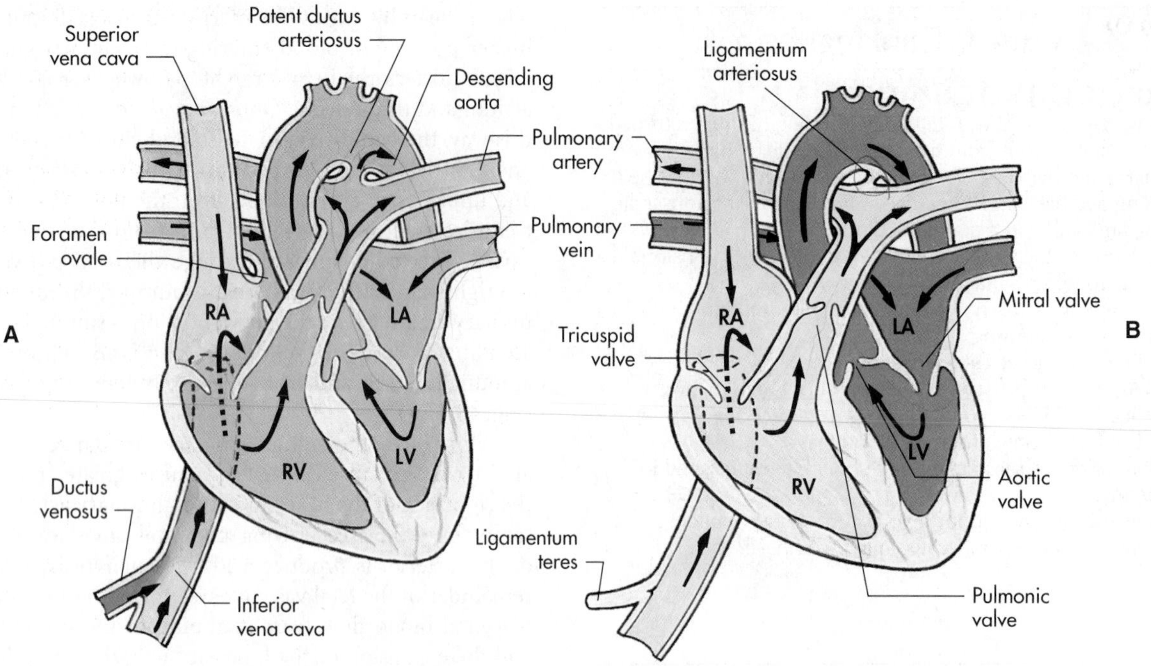

Fig. 48-1 Changes in circulation at birth. **A**, Prenatal circulation. **B**, Postnatal circulation. *Arrows* indicate direction of blood flow. Although four pulmonary veins enter the LA, for simplicity this diagram shows only two. *RA*, right atrium; *LA*, left atrium; *RV*, right ventricle; *LV*, left ventricle.

Classification of Defects

Congenital heart defects have been divided into two categories. Traditionally, cyanosis, a physical characteristic, has been used as the distinguishing feature, dividing the anomalies into *acyanotic defects* and *cyanotic defects*. In clinical practice this system is problematic because children with acyanotic defects may develop cyanosis. Also, more often, those with cyanotic defects may appear pink and have more clinical signs of congestive heart failure (CHF).

A more useful classification system is based on hemodynamic characteristics (blood flow patterns within the heart). These blood flow patterns are (1) *increased pulmonary blood flow*, (2) *decreased pulmonary blood flow*, (3) *obstruction to blood flow* out of the heart, and (4) *mixed blood flow*, in which saturated and desaturated blood mix within the heart or great arteries. As a comparison, both classification systems are outlined in Fig. 48-2.

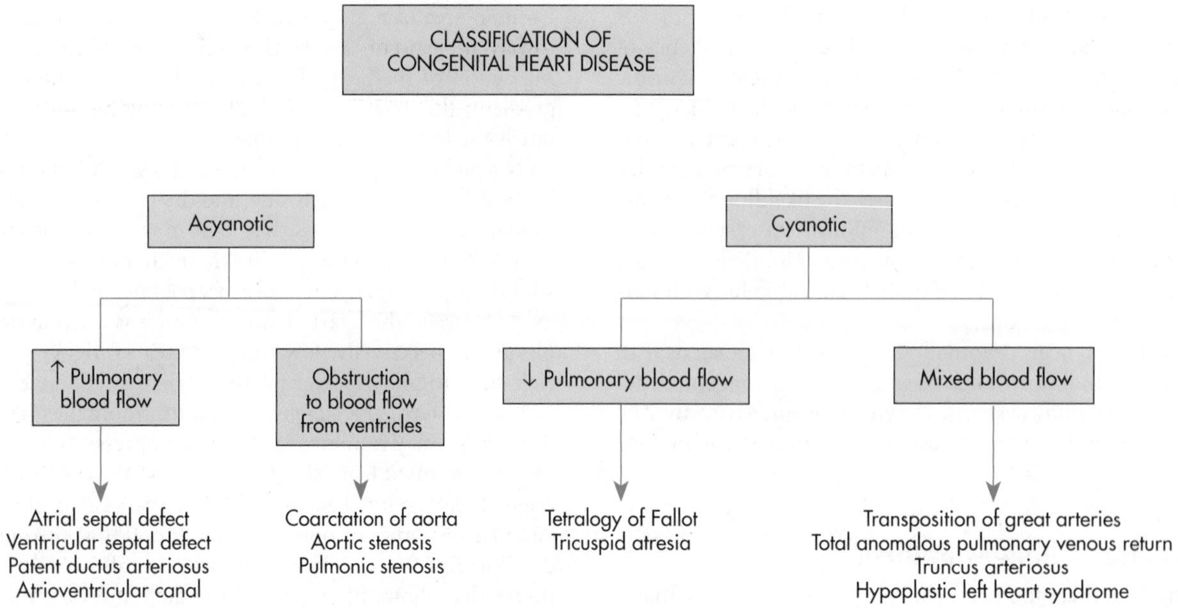

Fig. 48-2 Comparison of acyanotic-cyanotic and hemodynamic classification systems of congenital heart disease.

With the hemodynamic classification system, the clinical manifestations of each group are more uniform and predictable. Defects that allow blood flow from the higher pressure left side of the heart to the lower pressure right side (left-to-right shunt) result in increased pulmonary blood flow and cause CHF. Obstructive defects impede blood flow out of the ventricles; obstruction on the left side of the heart results in CHF, whereas severe obstruction on the right side causes cyanosis. Defects that cause decreased pulmonary blood flow result in cyanosis. Mixed lesions present a variable clinical picture based on the degree of mixing and amount of pulmonary blood flow; hypoxemia (with or without cyanosis) and CHF usually occur together. This system is used in the following discussion.

Defects with Increased Pulmonary Blood Flow

In this group of cardiac defects, intracardiac communications along the septum or an abnormal connection between the great arteries allows blood to flow from the higher pressure left side of the heart to the lower pressure right side of the heart (Fig. 48-3). Increased blood volume on the right side of the heart increases pulmonary blood flow at the expense of systemic blood flow. Clinically, patients demonstrate signs and symptoms of CHF. Atrial and ventricular septal defects and patent ductus arteriosus are typical anomalies in this group (Box 48-1).

Obstructive Defects

Obstructive defects are those in which blood exiting the heart meets an area of anatomic narrowing *(stenosis)*, causing obstruction to blood flow. The pressure in the ventricle and in the great artery before the obstruction is increased, and the pressure in the area beyond the obstruction is decreased. The location of the narrowing is usually near the valve (Fig. 48-4), as follows:

Valvular—At the site of the valve itself

Subvalvular—Narrowing in the ventricle below the valve (also referred to as the *ventricular outflow tract*)

Supravalvular—Narrowing in the great artery above the valve

Coarctation of the aorta (narrowing of the aortic arch), aortic stenosis, and pulmonic stenosis are typical defects in this group (Box 48-2). Hemodynamically, there is a pressure load on the ventricle and decreased cardiac output. Clinically, infants and children exhibit signs of CHF. Children with mild obstruction may be asymptomatic. Rarely, as in severe pulmonic stenosis, hypoxemia may be seen.

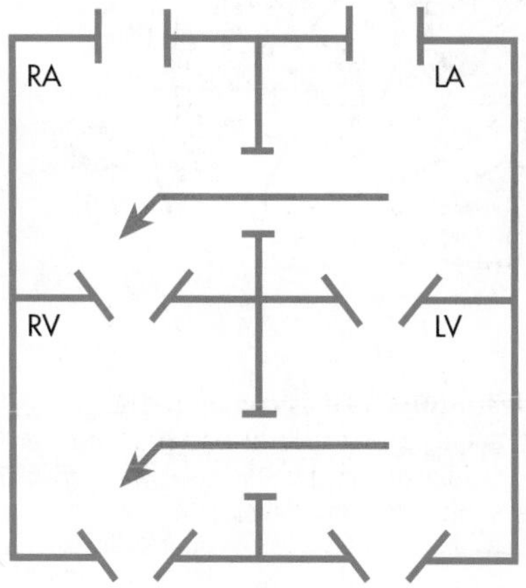

Fig. 48-3 Hemodynamics in defects with increased pulmonary blood flow.

Defects with Decreased Pulmonary Blood Flow

In this group of defects, there is obstruction of pulmonary blood flow and an anatomic defect (atrial septal defect [ASD] or VSD) between the right and left sides of the heart (Fig. 48-5). Because blood has difficulty exiting the right side of the heart via the pulmonary artery, pressure on the right side increases, exceeding left-sided pressure. This allows desaturated blood to shunt right to left, causing desaturation in the left side of the heart and in the systemic circulation. Clinically, these patients are hypoxemic and usually appear cyanotic. Tetralogy of Fallot and tricuspid atresia are the more common defects in this group (Box 48-3).

Mixed Defects

Many complex cardiac anomalies are classified together in the *mixed* category because survival in the postnatal period depends on mixing of blood from the pulmonary and systemic circulations within the heart chambers (Box 48-4). Hemodynamically, fully saturated systemic blood flow mixes with the desaturated pulmonary blood flow, causing a relative desaturation of the systemic blood flow. Pulmonary congestion occurs because the differences in pulmonary artery pressure and aortic pressure favor pulmonary blood flow. Cardiac output decreases because of a volume load on the ventricle. Clinically, these patients have a variable picture that combines some degree of desaturation (although cyanosis is not always visible) and signs of CHF. Some defects, such as transposition of the great arteries, cause severe cyanosis in the first days of life and later cause CHF. Others, such as truncus arteriosus, cause severe CHF in the first weeks of life and mild desaturation.

CLINICAL CONSEQUENCES OF CONGENITAL HEART DISEASE

Congestive Heart Failure

CHF is the inability of the heart to pump an adequate amount of blood to the systemic circulation at normal filling pressures to meet the metabolic demands of the body. In children, CFH most frequently occurs secondary to structural abnormalities (e.g., septal defects) that result in increased blood volume and pressure within the heart. It can also result from myocardial failure in which the contractility of the ventricle is impaired. This can occur with cardiomyopathy, dysrhythmias, or severe electrolyte disturbances. CHF can also occur because of excessive demands on a normal heart muscle, such as in sepsis or severe anemia.

Pathophysiology

Heart failure is often separated into two categories: right-sided and left-sided failure. In *right-sided failure*, the right ventricle is unable to pump blood effectively into the pulmonary artery, resulting in increased pressure in the right atrium and systemic venous circulation. Systemic venous hypertension causes hepatosplenomegaly and occasionally edema. In *left-sided failure*, the left ventricle is unable to pump blood into the systemic circulation, resulting in in-

BOX 48-1

Defects with Increased Pulmonary Blood Flow

Atrial Septal Defect (ASD)

Description: Abnormal opening between the atria, allowing blood from the higher pressure left atrium to flow into the lower pressure right atrium. There are three types:

Ostium primum (ASD 1)—Opening at lower end of septum; may be associated with mitral valve abnormalities

Ostium secundum (ASD 2)—Opening near center of septum

Sinus venosus defect—Opening near junction of superior vena cava and right atrium; may be associated with partial anomalous pulmonary venous connection

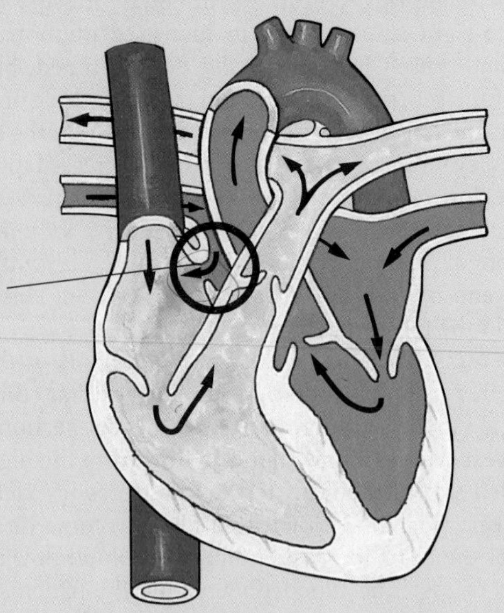

Pathophysiology: Because left atrial pressure slightly exceeds right atrial pressure, blood flows from the left to the right atrium, causing an increased flow of oxygenated blood into the right side of the heart. Despite the low pressure difference, a high rate of flow can still occur because of low pulmonary vascular resistance and the greater distensibility of the right atrium, which further reduces flow resistance. This volume is well tolerated by the right ventricle because it is delivered under much lower pressure than in a ventricular septal defect. Although there is right atrial and ventricular enlargement, cardiac failure is unusual in an uncomplicated ASD. Pulmonary vascular changes usually occur only after several decades if the defect is unrepaired.

Clinical manifestations: Patients may be asymptomatic. They may develop congestive heart failure (CHF). There is a characteristic murmur. Patients are at risk for atrial dysrhythmias (probably caused by atrial enlargement and stretching of conduction fibers) and pulmonary vascular obstructive disease and emboli formation later in life from chronic increased pulmonary blood flow.

Surgical treatment: Surgical Dacron patch closure of moderate to large defects similar to closure of ventricular septal defects. Open repair with cardiopulmonary bypass is usually performed before school age. In addition, the sinus venosus defect requires patch placement, so the anomalous right pulmonary venous return is directed to the left atrium with a baffle. The ASD 1 may require repair or, rarely, replacement of the mitral valve.

Nonsurgical treatment: ASD 2 may also be closed using devices during cardiac catheterization. This technique is in clinical trials in some centers (Uzurk, 2001).

Prognosis: Very low operative mortality rate, less than 1%.

Ventricular Septal Defect (VSD)

Description: Abnormal opening between the right and left ventricles. May be classified according to location: membranous (accounting for 80%) or muscular. May vary in size from a small pinhole to absence of the septum, resulting in a common ventricle. Frequently associated with other defects, such as pulmonary stenosis, transposition of the great vessels, patent ductus arteriosus, atrial defects, and coarctation of the aorta. Many VSDs (20% to 60%) are thought to close spontaneously. Spontaneous closure is most likely to occur during the first year of life in children having small or moderate defects. A left-to-right shunt is caused by the flow of blood from the higher pressure left ventricle to the lower pressure right ventricle.

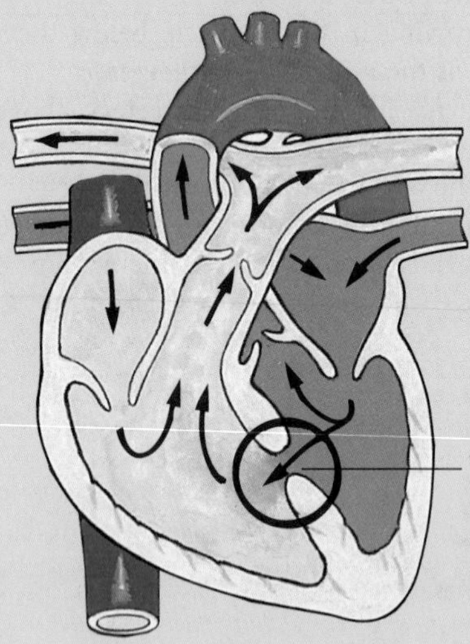

Pathophysiology: Because of the higher pressure within the left ventricle and because the systemic arterial circulation offers more resistance than the pulmonary circulation, blood flows through the defect into the pulmonary artery. The increased blood volume is pumped into the lungs, which may eventually result in increased pulmonary vascular resistance. Increased pressure in the right ventricle as a result of left-to-right shunting and pulmonary resistance causes the muscle to hypertrophy. If the right ventricle is unable to accommodate the increased workload, the right atrium may also enlarge as it attempts to overcome the resistance offered by incomplete right ventricular emptying.

Clinical manifestations: CHF is common. There is a characteristic murmur. Patients are at risk for bacterial endocarditis and pulmonary vascular obstructive disease. In severe defects, Eisenmenger syndrome may develop.

BOX 48-1

Defects with Increased Pulmonary Blood Flow—cont'd

Surgical treatment:

Palliative: Pulmonary artery banding (placing a band around the main pulmonary artery to decrease pulmonary blood flow) in infants with severe CHF was common in the past. It is unusual now because improvements in surgical techniques and postoperative care make complete repair in infancy the preferred approach.

Complete repair (procedure of choice): Small defects are repaired with a purse-string approach. Large defects usually require a knitted Dacron patch sewn over the opening. Both procedures are performed via cardiopulmonary bypass. The repair is generally approached through the right atrium and the tricuspid valve. Postoperative complications include residual VSD and conduction disturbances.

Nonsurgical treatment: Device closure during cardiac catheterization is under clinical trials in some centers for closure of muscular defects that carry a high operative risk.

Prognosis: Risks depend on the location of the defect, number of defects, and other associated cardiac defects. Single membranous defects have a low mortality rate (less than 5%); multiple muscular defects can have a risk of more than 20%.

Atrioventricular Canal (AVC) Defect

Description: Incomplete fusion of endocardial cushions. Consists of a low atrial septal defect that is continuous with a high ventricular septal defect and clefts of the mitral and tricuspid valves, creating a large central atrioventricular (AV) valve that allows blood to flow between all four chambers of the heart. The directions and pathways of flow are determined by pulmonary and systemic resistance, left and right ventricular pressures, and the compliance of each chamber, although flow is generally from left to right. It is the most common cardiac defect in children with Down syndrome.

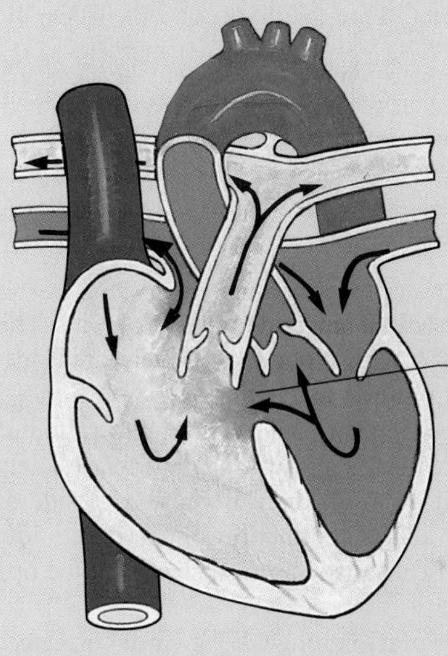

Pathophysiology: The alterations in the hemodynamics depend on the defect's severity and the child's pulmonary vascular resistance. Immediately after birth, while the newborn's pulmonary vascular resistance is high, there is minimum shunting of blood through the defect. After this resistance falls, left-to-right shunting occurs and pulmonary blood flow increases. The resultant pulmonary vascular engorgement predisposes to development of CHF.

Clinical manifestations: Patients usually have moderate to severe CHF. There is a characteristic murmur. There may be mild cyanosis that increases with crying. Patients are at high risk for developing pulmonary vascular obstructive disease.

Surgical treatment:

Palliative: Pulmonary artery banding for infants with severe symptoms that are caused by increased pulmonary blood flow in some centers. Most centers perform complete repair in infancy.

Complete repair: Surgical repair consists of patch closure of the septal defects and reconstruction of the AV valve tissue (either repair of the mitral valve cleft or fashioning two AV valves). If the mitral valve defect is severe, a valve replacement may be needed. Postoperative complications include heart block, CHF, mitral regurgitation, dysrhythmias, and pulmonary hypertension.

Prognosis: Operative mortality rate is less than 10%. A potential later problem is mitral regurgitation, which may require valve replacement.

Patent Ductus Arteriosus (PDA)

Description: Failure of the fetal ductus arteriosus (artery connecting the aorta and pulmonary artery) to close within the first weeks of life. The continued patency of this vessel allows blood to flow from the higher pressure aorta to the lower pressure pulmonary artery, causing a left-to-right shunt.

Pathophysiology: The hemodynamic consequences of PDA depend on the size of the ductus and the pulmonary vascular resistance. At birth the resistance in the pulmonary and systemic circulations is almost identical, thus equalizing the resistance in the aorta and pulmonary artery. As the systemic pressure exceeds the pulmonary pressure, blood begins to shunt from the aorta, across the duct, to the pulmonary artery (left-to-right shunt). The additional blood is recirculated through the lungs and returned to the left atrium and left ventricle. The effect of this altered circulation is increased workload on the left side of the heart, increased pulmonary vascular congestion and possibly resistance, and potentially increased right ventricular pressure and hypertrophy.

Clinical manifestations: Patients may be asymptomatic or show signs of CHF. There is a characteristic machinery-like murmur. A widened pulse pressure and bounding pulses result from runoff of blood from the aorta to the pulmonary artery. Patients are at risk for bacterial endocarditis and pulmonary vascular obstructive disease in later life from chronic excessive pulmonary blood flow.

CASE STUDY: PATENT DUCTUS ARTERIOSUS

Continued

BOX 48-1

Defects with Increased Pulmonary Blood Flow—cont'd

Patent Ductus Arteriosus (PDA)—cont'd

Medical management: Administration of indomethacin (prostaglandin inhibitor) has proved successful in closing a patent ductus in premature infants and some newborns (Pham & Carlos, 2002).

Surgical treatment: Surgical division or ligation of the patent vessel via a left thoracotomy. A newer technique, visual-assisted thoracoscopic surgery (VATS), uses a thoracoscope and instruments placed through three small incisions on the left side of the chest to place a clip on the ductus. It is used in some centers and eliminates the need for a thoracotomy, thereby speeding postoperative recovery.

Nonsurgical treatment: Use of coils to occlude the PDA in the catheterization laboratory is done in many centers. Small infants (with small-diameter femoral arteries) and those patients with large or unusual PDAs may require surgery.

Prognosis: Both procedures can be done at low risk with less than 1% mortality rate.

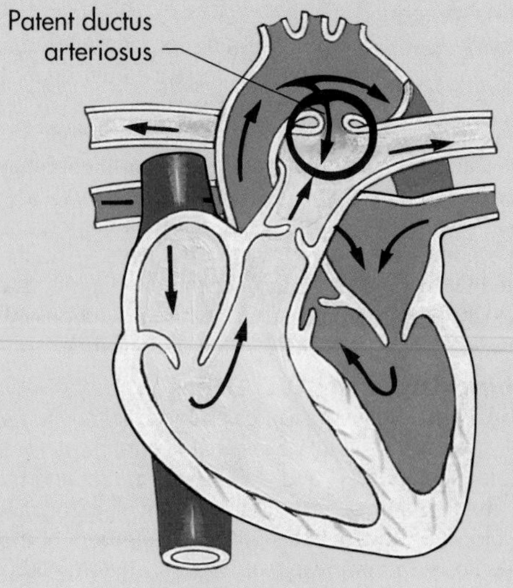

creased pressure in the left atrium and pulmonary veins. The lungs become congested with blood, causing elevated pulmonary pressures and pulmonary edema.

Although each type of heart failure produces different signs and symptoms, clinically it is unusual to observe solely right- or left-sided failure in children. Because each side of the heart depends on adequate function of the other side, failure of one chamber causes a reciprocal change in the opposite chamber.

If the abnormalities precipitating CHF are not corrected, the heart muscle becomes damaged. Despite compensatory mechanisms, the heart is unable to maintain an adequate cardiac output. Decreased blood flow to the kidneys continues to stimulate sodium and water reabsorption, leading to

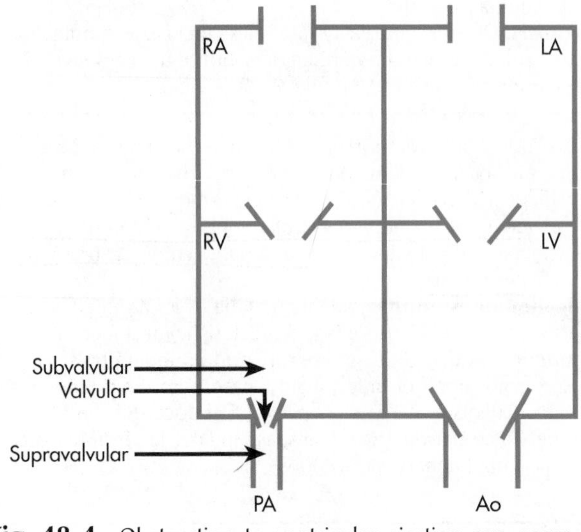

Fig. 48-4 Obstruction to ventricular ejection can occur at the valvular level (shown), below the valve (subvalvular), or above the valve (supravalvular). Pulmonary stenosis is shown here. See Fig. 48-1 for abbreviations.

fluid overload, increased workload on the heart, and congestion in the pulmonary and systemic circulations (Fig. 48-6).

The signs and symptoms of CHF can be divided into three groups: (1) impaired myocardial function, (2) pulmonary congestion, and (3) systemic venous congestion (Box 48-5). Because these hemodynamic changes occur from different causes and at differing times, the clinical presentation may vary among children.

Diagnostic Evaluation

Diagnosis is made on the basis of clinical symptoms such as tachypnea and tachycardia at rest, dyspnea, retractions, activity intolerance (especially during feeding in infants), weight gain caused by fluid retention, and hepatomegaly. A chest x-ray film demonstrates cardiomegaly and increased pulmonary blood flow. Ventricular hypertrophy appears on the ECG. An echocardiogram is done to determine the cause of CHF, such as a congenital heart defect or poor ventricular function.

Therapeutic Management

The goals of treatment are to (1) improve cardiac function (increase contractility and decrease afterload), (2) remove accumulated fluid and sodium (decrease preload), (3) decrease cardiac demands, and (4) improve tissue oxygenation and decrease oxygen consumption. For most infants diagnosed with CHF, the cause is CHD. Infants are stabilized on medical therapy and then referred for surgical repair. For children newly diagnosed with CHF, the cause may be worsening ventricular function after a previous cardiac repair, cardiomyopathy, arrhythmia, or other causes. In addition to management of CHF, the underlying cause is treated if possible.

Improve Cardiac Function

Myocardial efficiency is improved through administration of digitalis glycosides. The beneficial effects are increased cardiac output, decreased heart size, decreased venous pressure, and relief of edema. In pediatrics, digoxin

BOX 48-2

Obstructive Defects

Coarctation of the Aorta (COA)

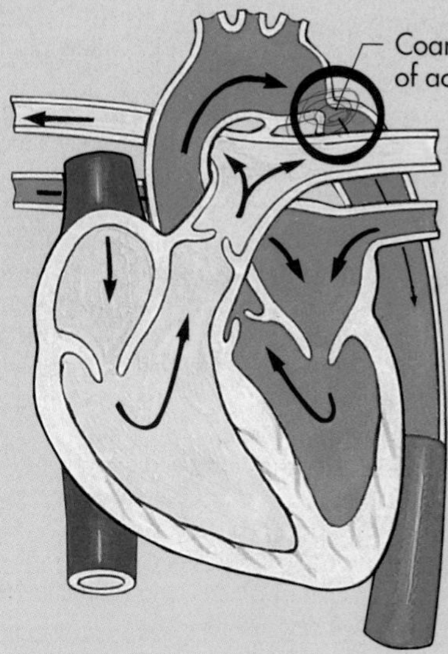

Description: Localized narrowing near the insertion of the ductus arteriosus, resulting in increased pressure proximal to the defect (head and upper extremities) and decreased pressure distal to the obstruction (body and lower extremities).

Pathophysiology: The effect of a narrowing within the aorta is increased pressure proximal to the defect and decreased pressure distal to it. In the preductal type of COA, the lower half of the body is supplied with blood by the right ventricle through the ductus arteriosus. In the postductal type, right ventricular outflow cannot maintain blood flow to the descending aorta. Therefore collateral circulation develops during fetal life to maintain flow from the ascending to the descending aorta.

Clinical manifestations: There may be high blood pressure and bounding pulses in arms, weak or absent femoral pulses, and cool lower extremities with lower blood pressure. There are signs of congestive heart failure (CHF) in infants. Often these patients' hemodynamic condition deteriorates rapidly and they are admitted to the intensive care unit near death, usually severely acidotic and hypotensive. Mechanical ventilation and inotropic support are often necessary before surgery. Older children may experience dizziness, headaches, fainting, and epistaxis resulting from hypertension. Patients are at risk for hypertension, ruptured aorta, aortic aneurysm, or stroke.

Surgical treatment: Either resection of the coarcted portion with an end-to-end anastomosis of the aorta or enlargement of the constricted section using a graft of prosthetic material or a portion of the left subclavian artery. Because this defect is outside the heart and pericardium, cardiopulmonary bypass is not required and a thoracotomy incision is used. Postoperative hypertension (greater than 160 mm Hg) is treated with intravenous sodium nitroprusside or amrinone, followed by oral medications, such as captopril, hydralazine, and/or propranolol. Residual permanent hypertension after repair of COA seems to be related to age and time of repair. To prevent both hypertension at rest and exercise-provoked systemic hypertension after repair, elective surgery for COA is advised within the first 2 years of life. There is a 5% to 10% risk of recurrent narrowing in patients who underwent surgical repair as infants (Hougen & Sell, 1995). Percutaneous balloon angioplasty techniques have proved to be highly effective in relieving residual postoperative coarctation gradients.

Nonsurgical treatment: Balloon angioplasty as a primary intervention for COA is being performed in some centers, but concerns about inadequate relief of gradients, risk of aneurysm formation, and restenosis have limited its widespread use. Studies have demonstrated that balloon angioplasty is effective in children and that aneurysm formation is rare. The high restenosis rate in infants younger than 7 months of age limits its application in this group, and further study is needed (Allen et al, 1998; Uzurk, 2001).

Prognosis: Less than 5% mortality rate in patients with isolated coarctation; increased risk in infants with other complex cardiac defects.

Aortic Stenosis (AS)

Description: Narrowing or stricture of the aortic valve, causing resistance to blood flow in the left ventricle, decreased cardiac output, left ventricular hypertrophy, and pulmonary vascular congestion. The prominent anatomic consequence of AS is the hypertrophy of the left ventricular wall, which eventually will lead to increased end-diastolic pressure, resulting in pulmonary venous and pulmonary arterial hypertension. Left ventricular hypertrophy also interferes with coronary artery perfusion and may result in myocardial infarction or scarring of the papillary muscles of the left ventricle, causing mitral insufficiency. *Valvular stenosis,* the most common type, is usually caused by malformed cusps resulting in a bicuspid rather than tricuspid valve or fusion of the cusps. *Subvalvular stenosis* is a stricture caused by a fibrous ring below a normal valve; *supravalvular stenosis* occurs infrequently. Valvular AS is a serious defect for the following reasons: (1) the obstruction tends to be progressive; (2) sudden episodes of myocardial ischemia, or low cardiac output, can result in sudden death; and (3) surgical repair rarely results in a normal valve. This is one of the rare instances in which strenuous physical activity may be curtailed because of the cardiac condition.

Pathophysiology: A stricture in the aortic outflow tract causes resistance to ejection of blood from the left ventricle. The extra workload on the left ventricle causes hypertrophy. If left ventricular failure develops, left atrial pressure will increase; this causes increased pressure in the pulmonary veins, resulting in pulmonary vascular congestion (pulmonary edema).

Clinical manifestations: Infants with severe defects demonstrate signs of decreased cardiac output with faint pulses, hypotension, tachycardia, and poor feeding. Children show signs of exercise intolerance, chest pain, and dizziness when standing for a long period. There is a characteristic murmur. Patients are at risk for bacterial endocarditis, coronary insufficiency, and ventricular dysfunction.

Continued

BOX 48-2

Obstructive Defects—cont'd

Valvular Aortic Stenosis

Surgical treatment: Aortic valvotomy under inflow occlusion (Uzurk, 2001).

Prognosis: Aortic valvotomy in critically ill neonates and infants still carries a mortality rate of 10% to 20% in major medical centers (Hawkins et al, 1998). Results of aortic valvotomy in older children are very good, with mortality rate close to 0%. However, aortic valvotomy remains a palliative procedure, and approximately 25% of patients require additional surgery within 10 years for recurrent stenosis. A valve replacement may be required at the second procedure. An aortic homograft with a valve may also be used *(extended aortic root replacement)*, or the pulmonary valve may be moved to the aortic position and replaced with a homograft valve *(Ross procedure)*.

Nonsurgical treatment: Dilating narrowed valve with balloon angioplasty in the catheterization laboratory.

Prognosis: Complications include aortic insufficiency or valvular regurgitation, tearing of the valve leaflets, and loss of pulse in the catheterized limb. Relief of obstruction is similar to that for surgical valvotomy (Allen et al, 1998).

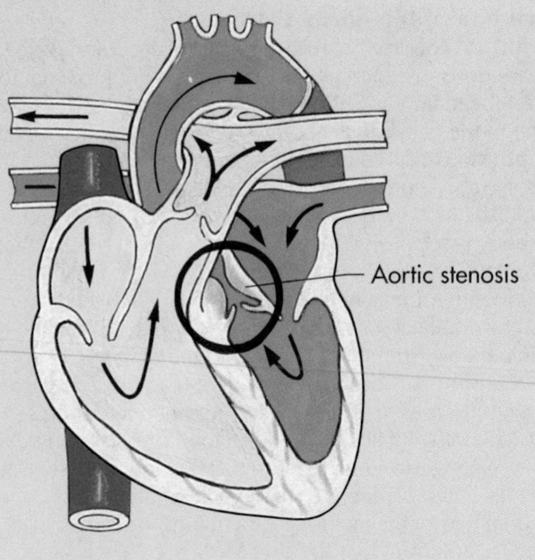

Subvalvular Aortic Stenosis

Surgical treatment: May involve incising a membrane if one exists or cutting the fibromuscular ring. If the obstruction results from narrowing of the left ventricular outflow tract and a small aortic valve annulus, a patch may be required to enlarge the entire left ventricular outflow tract and annulus and replace the aortic valve, an approach known as the *Konno* procedure.

Prognosis: Mortality rate from surgical repairs of subvalvular AS is less than 5% in major centers; however, about 20% of these patients develop recurrent subaortic stenosis and require additional surgery (Freed, 2001).

Pulmonic Stenosis (PS)

Description: Narrowing at the entrance to the pulmonary artery. Resistance to blood flow causes right ventricular hypertrophy and decreased pulmonary blood flow. *Pulmonary atresia* is the extreme form of PS in that there is total fusion of the commissures and no blood flows to the lungs. The right ventricle may be hypoplastic.

Pathophysiology: When PS is present, resistance to blood flow causes right ventricular hypertrophy. If right ventricular failure develops, right atrial pressure will increase, and this may result in reopening of the foramen ovale, shunting of unoxygenated blood into the left atrium, and systemic cyanosis. If PS is severe, congestive heart failure (CHF) occurs, and systemic venous engorgement will be noted. An associated defect such as a patent ductus arteriosus (PDA) partially compensates for the obstruction by shunting blood from the aorta to the pulmonary artery and into the lungs.

Clinical manifestations: Patients may be asymptomatic; some have mild cyanosis or CHF. Newborns with severe narrowing will be cyanotic. There is a characteristic murmur. Cardiomegaly is evident on chest x-ray film. Patients are at risk for bacterial endocarditis, with progressive narrowing causing increased symptoms.

Surgical treatment: In infants, transventricular (closed) valvotomy *(Brock)* procedure. In children, pulmonary valvotomy with cardiopulmonary bypass. Need for surgical treatment is uncommon with widespread use of balloon angioplasty techniques (Uzurk, 2001).

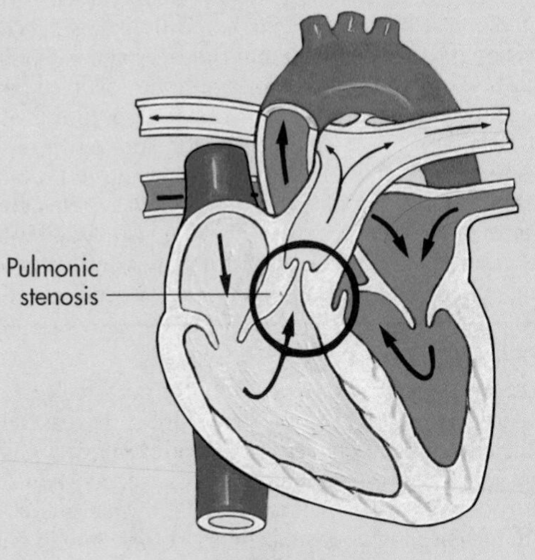

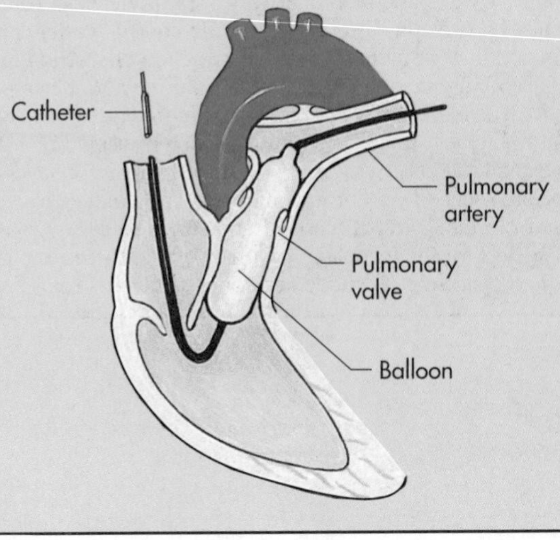

BOX 48-2

Obstructive Defects—cont'd

Pulmonic Stenosis (PS)—cont'd

Nonsurgical treatment: Balloon angioplasty in the cardiac catheterization laboratory to dilate the valve. A catheter is inserted across the stenotic pulmonic valve into the pulmonary artery, and a balloon at the end of the catheter is inflated and rapidly passed through the narrowed opening (see figure, bottom of p. 1564). The procedure is associated with few complications and has proved to be highly effective. It is the treatment of choice for discrete PS in most centers and can be done safely in neonates.

Prognosis: Low risk for both procedures; less than 2% mortality rate. Both balloon dilation and surgical valvotomy leave the pulmonic valve incompetent because they involve opening the fused valve leaflets; however, these patients are clinically asymptomatic. Long-term problems with restenosis or valve incompetence may occur.

(Lanoxin) is used almost exclusively because of its more rapid onset. It is available as an elixir (0.05 mg/ml) for oral administration. For infants the dose is calculated in micrograms (1000 mcg = 1 mg).

Treatment consists of a digitalizing dose, given orally or intravenously in divided doses over 24 hours to produce optimum cardiac effects, and a maintenance dose, given orally twice a day to maintain blood levels. During digitalization the child is monitored by means of an ECG to observe for the desired effects (prolonged P-R interval and reduced ventricular rate) and to detect side effects, especially dysrhythmias.

A newer group of drugs used in the treatment of CHF are the *angiotensin-converting enzyme (ACE) inhibitors.* As their name implies, these drugs inhibit the normal function of the renin-angiotensin system in the kidney. The ACE inhibitors block the conversion of angiotensin I to angiotensin II so that, instead of vasoconstriction, vasodilation occurs. Vasodilation results in decreased pulmonary and systemic vascular resistance, decreased blood pressure, and a reduction in afterload. Two ACE inhibitors are frequently used in pediatrics: *captopril (Capoten),* given three times a day, and *enalapril (Vasotec),* given twice a day. The principal side effects of ACE inhibitors are hypotension, cough, and renal dysfunction. Captopril is given to infants and young children because it can be given in smaller doses.

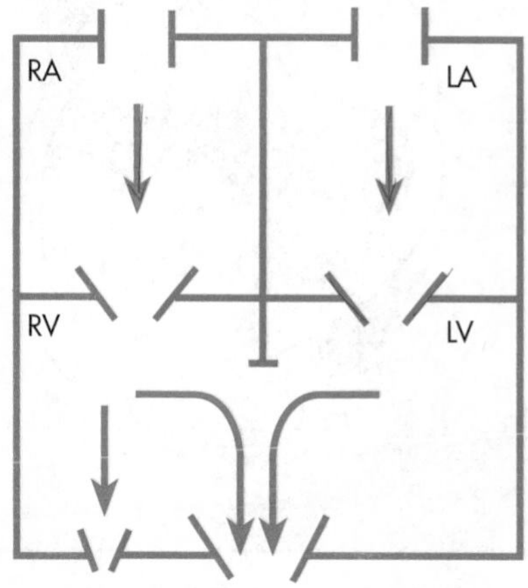

Fig. 48-5 Hemodynamic defects with decreased pulmonary blood flow. See Fig. 48-1 for abbreviations.

NURSE ALERT Because ACE inhibitors also block the action of aldosterone, the addition of potassium supplements or spironolactone (Aldactone) to the drug regimen of patients taking diuretics is usually not needed and may cause hyperkalemia. ■

Remove Accumulated Fluid and Sodium

Treatment consists of diuretics, possible fluid restriction, and possible sodium restriction. Diuretics are the mainstay of therapy to eliminate excess water and salt to prevent reaccumulation. The most frequently used agents are listed in Table 48-3. Because furosemide and the thiazides are potassium-losing diuretics, potassium supplements may be prescribed, and rich sources of the electrolyte are encouraged in the diet.

NURSE ALERT A fall in the serum potassium level enhances the effects of digitalis, increasing the risk of digoxin toxicity. Therefore serum potassium levels must be carefully monitored. ■

Fluid restriction may be required in the acute states of CHF and must be carefully calculated to avoid dehydrating the child, especially if cyanotic CHD and significant polycythemia are present. Infants rarely need fluid restrictions because CHF makes feeding so difficult that they struggle to take maintenance fluids.

Sodium-restricted diets are used less often in children than in adults to control CHF because of their potential negative effects on appetite. If salt intake is restricted, additional table salt and highly salted foods are avoided.

Decrease Cardiac Demands

The workload on the heart is reduced when metabolic needs are kept to a minimum. This is accomplished by limiting physical activity (bed rest), preserving body tempera-

BOX 48-3

Defects with Decreased Pulmonary Blood Flow

Tetralogy of Fallot (TOF)

Description: The classic form includes four defects: (1) ventricular septal defect, (2) pulmonic stenosis, (3) overriding aorta, and (4) right ventricular hypertrophy.

Pathophysiology: The altered hemodynamics vary widely, depending primarily on the degree of pulmonary stenosis, but also on the size of the ventricular septal defect (VSD) and the pulmonary and systemic resistance to flow. Because the VSD is usually large, pressures may be equal in the right and left ventricles. Therefore the shunt direction depends on the difference between pulmonary and systemic vascular resistance. If pulmonary vascular resistance is higher than systemic resistance, the shunt is from right to left. If systemic resistance is higher than pulmonary resistance, the shunt is from left to right. Pulmonic stenosis decreases blood flow to the lungs and, consequently, the amount of oxygenated blood that returns to the left side of the heart. Depending on the position of the aorta, blood from both ventricles may be distributed systemically.

Clinical manifestations:

Infants: Some infants may be acutely cyanotic at birth; others have mild cyanosis that progresses over the first year of life as the pulmonic stenosis worsens. There is a characteristic murmur. There may be acute episodes of cyanosis and hypoxia, called blue spells or tet spells (see p. 1577). Anoxic spells occur when the infant's oxygen requirements exceed the blood supply, usually during crying or after feeding.

Surgical treatment:

Palliative shunt: In infants who cannot undergo primary repair, a palliative procedure to increase pulmonary blood flow and increase oxygen saturation may be performed. The preferred procedure is the *Blalock-Taussig* or *modified Blalock-Taussig shunt,* which provides blood flow to the pulmonary arteries from the left or right subclavian artery (see Table 48-4). In general, however, shunts are avoided because they may result in pulmonary artery distortion.

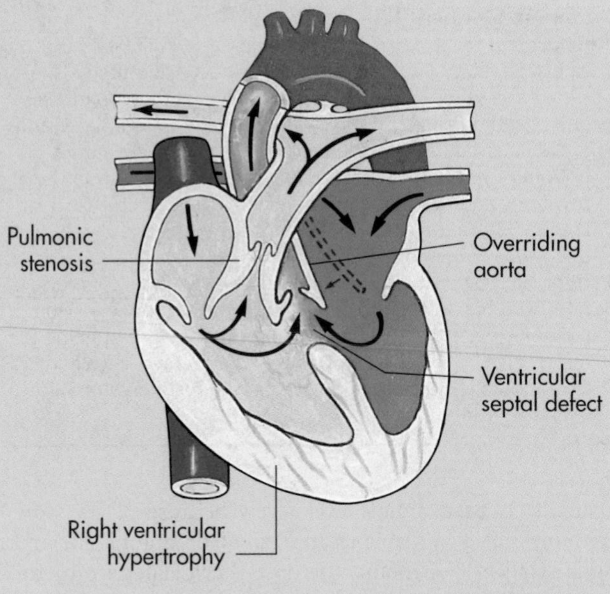

Complete repair: Elective repair is usually performed in the first year of life. Indications for repair include increasing cyanosis and the development of hypercyanotic spells. Complete repair involves closure of the VSD and resection of the infundibular stenosis, with a pericardial patch to enlarge the right ventricular outflow tract. The procedure requires a median sternotomy and the use of cardiopulmonary bypass.

Prognosis: The operative mortality rate for total correction of TOF is less than 5%. With improved surgical techniques there is a lower incidence of dysrhythmias and sudden death; surgical heart block is rare. Congestive heart failure may occur postoperatively.

Tricuspid Atresia

Description: Failure of the tricuspid valve to develop; consequently, there is no communication from the right atrium to the right ventricle. Blood flows through an atrial septal defect (ASD) or a patent foramen ovale to the left side of the heart and through a VSD to the right ventricle and out to the lungs. It is often associated with pulmonic stenosis and transposition of the great arteries. There is complete mixing of unoxygenated and oxygenated blood in the left side of the heart, resulting in systemic desaturation and varying amounts of pulmonary obstruction, causing decreased pulmonary blood flow.

Pathophysiology: At birth the presence of a patent foramen ovale (or other atrial septal opening) is required to permit blood flow across the septum into the left atrium; the patent ductus arteriosus allows blood flow to the pulmonary artery into the lungs for oxygenation. A VSD allows a modest amount of blood to enter the right ventricle and pulmonary artery for oxygenation. Pulmonary blood flow usually is diminished.

Clinical manifestations: Cyanosis is usually seen in the newborn period. There may be tachycardia and dyspnea. Older children have signs of chronic hypoxemia with clubbing. Patients are at risk for bacterial endocarditis, brain abscess, and stroke.

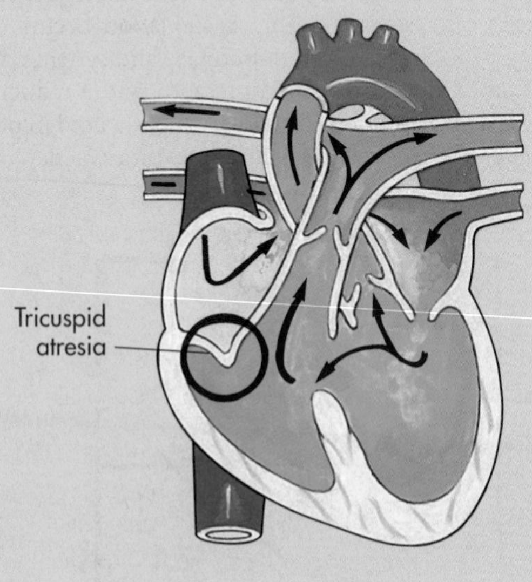

BOX 48-3

Defects with Decreased Pulmonary Blood Flow—cont'd

Tricuspid Atresia—cont'd

Therapeutic management: For the neonate whose pulmonary blood flow depends on the patency of the ductus arteriosus, a continuous infusion of prostaglandin E_1 is started until surgical intervention can be arranged.

Surgical treatment: *Palliative* treatment is the placement of a shunt *(pulmonary-to-systemic artery anastomosis)* to increase blood flow to the lungs. If the ASD is small, an atrial septostomy is done during cardiac catheterization. Some children have increased pulmonary blood flow and require *pulmonary artery banding* to lessen the volume of blood to the lungs. A *bidirectional Glenn shunt* (cavopulmonary anastomosis) may be performed at 6 to 9 months as a second stage.

Modified Fontan procedure: Systemic venous return is directed to the lungs without a ventricular pump through surgical connections between the right atrium and the pulmonary artery. A fenestration (opening) in the right atrial baffle is sometimes done to relieve pressure. The patient must have normal ventricular function and a low pulmonary vascular resistance for the procedure to be successful. The modified Fontan procedure separates oxygenated and unoxygenated blood inside the heart and eliminates the excess volume load on the ventricle but does not restore normal anatomy or hemodynamics (O'Brien & Boisvert, 2001).

Prognosis: Surgical mortality rate varies. It is less than 10% in many centers and increases with more complex anatomy and other risk factors. Postoperative complications include dysrhythmias, systemic venous hypertension, pleural and pericardial effusions, and ventricular dysfunction. Although initial results have been encouraging, long-term survival and morbidity must await future studies.

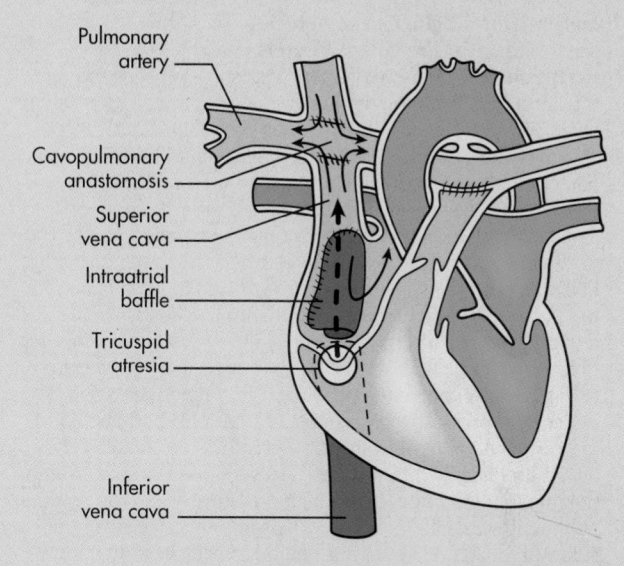

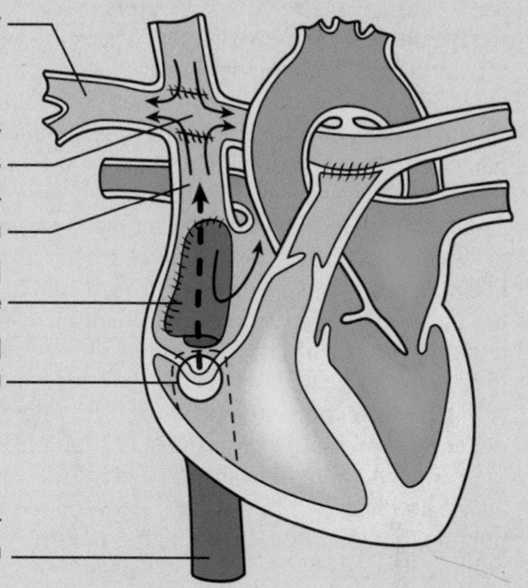

ture, treating any infections, reducing the effort of breathing (semi-Fowler position), and using medication to sedate an irritable child.

Improve Tissue Oxygenation

All of the preceding measures serve to increase tissue oxygenation, either by improving myocardial function or by lessening tissue oxygen demands. In addition, supplemental cool, humidified oxygen may be administered to increase the amount of available oxygen during inspiration. Oxygen administration is especially helpful in patients with pulmonary edema, intercurrent respiratory infections, and increased pulmonary vascular resistance (oxygen is a vasodilator that decreases pulmonary vascular resistance).

NURSE ALERT Oxygen is a drug and is administered only with an appropriate order. There are some uncommon circumstances in patients with complex hemodynamics in which oxygen can be detrimental. ■

An oxygen hood is preferred with young infants to provide increased concentration of the gas. A nasal cannula or face tent may be useful with older infants and children. Nasal cannulas are ideal for long-term oxygen administration because the child can be ambulatory and can easily eat and drink. Cool humidification is necessary to counteract the drying effect of oxygen. The amount of cool humidity is carefully regulated to prevent chilling.

Nursing Care Management

The infant or child with CHF is usually admitted to the hospital, where intensive nursing care is available. The child is positioned for optimum ventilation and administered oxygen by the most effective means, IV access is established, and cardiac and respiratory function is monitored continuously using a cardiac monitor and pulse oximeter to monitor oxygen saturation. Urine output and serum electrolytes are evaluated frequently.

Assessment

Nurses need to be alert to signs of CHF in infants and children with suspected or known congenital defects. Signs of CHF indicate a worsening clinical condition; the earlier they are detected, the sooner treatment can be begun.

Text continued on p. 1571.

BOX 48-4

Mixed Defects

Transposition of the Great Arteries (TGA) or Transposition of the Great Vessels (TGV)

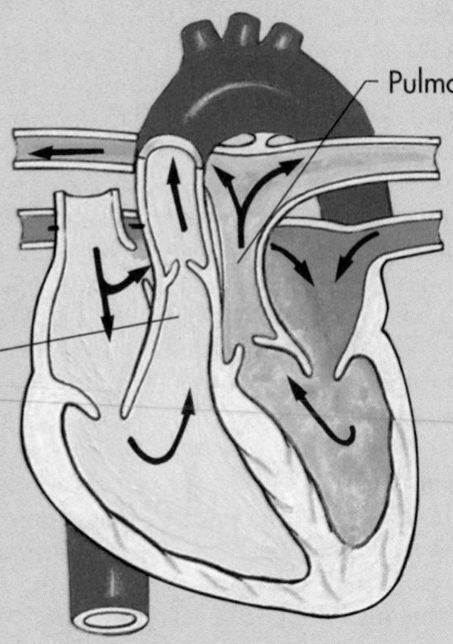

Description: The pulmonary artery leaves the left ventricle, and the aorta exits from the right ventricle, with no communication between the systemic and pulmonary circulations.

Pathophysiology: Associated defects such as septal defects or patent ductus arteriosus (PDA) must be present to permit blood to enter the systemic circulation and/or the pulmonary circulation for mixing of saturated and desaturated blood. The most common defect associated with TGA is a patent foramen ovale. At birth there is also a PDA, although in most instances this closes after the neonatal period. Another associated anomaly may be a ventricular septal defect (VSD). The presence of these defects increases the risk of congestive heart failure (CHF), because they often produce high pulmonary blood flow under high pressure. For example, a large VSD permits blood to flow from the right to the left ventricle, into the pulmonary artery, and finally to the lungs. However, it also produces high pulmonary blood flow under high pressure, which can result in pulmonary vascular resistance. The same series of events occurs with a large PDA, because blood directly from the aorta flows under high pressure into the pulmonary artery and lungs.

Clinical manifestations: Depend on the type and size of the associated defects. Children with minimum communication are severely cyanotic and depressed at birth. Those with large septal defects or a PDA may be less severely cyanotic but may have symptoms of CHF. Heart sounds vary according to the type of defect present. Cardiomegaly is usually evident a few weeks after birth.

Therapeutic management:

To provide intracardiac mixing: The administration of intravenous prostaglandin E_1 may be initiated to temporarily increase blood mixing if systemic and pulmonary mixing is inadequate to provide an oxygen saturation of 75% or to maintain cardiac output. During cardiac catheterization a balloon atrial septostomy *(Rashkind procedure)* may also be performed to increase mixing and maintain cardiac output over a longer period.

Surgical treatment:

Arterial switch procedure: Procedure of choice performed in first weeks of life. Involves transecting the great arteries and anastomosing the main pulmonary artery to the proximal aorta (just above the aortic valve) and anastomosing the ascending aorta to the proximal pulmonary artery. The coronary arteries are switched from the proximal aorta to the proximal pulmonary artery, creating a new aorta. Reimplantation of the coronary arteries is critical to the infant's survival, and they must be reattached without torsion or kinking to provide the heart with its supply of oxygen. The advantage of the arterial switch procedure is the reestablishment of normal circulation, with the left ventricle acting as the systemic pump. Potential complications of the arterial switch include narrowing at the great artery anastomoses or coronary artery insufficiency.

Intraatrial baffle repairs: Intraatrial baffle repairs are rarely performed, although many adolescents and adults survive today with repairs that were done 10 to 25 years ago. An intraatrial baffle is created to divert venous blood to the mitral valve and pulmonary venous blood to the tricuspid valve using the patient's atrial septum *(Senning procedure)* or a prosthetic material *(Mustard procedure)*. They are performed in the first year of life. A disadvantage is the continuing role of the right ventricle as the systemic pump and the late development of right ventricular failure and rhythm disturbances. Other potential postoperative complications include loss of normal sinus rhythm, baffle leaks, and ventricular dysfunction.

Rastelli procedure: Operative choice in infants with TGA, VSD, and severe pulmonic stenosis (PS). It involves closure of the VSD with a baffle, directing left ventricular blood through the VSD into the aorta. The pulmonic valve is then closed, and a conduit is placed from the right ventricle to the pulmonary artery, creating a physiologically normal circulation. Unfortunately, this procedure requires multiple conduit replacements as the child grows.

Prognosis: Operative mortality rate is about 5% to 10% with all procedures; with atrial level repairs, there is a later risk of dysrhythmias and ventricular dysfunction.

BOX 48-4

Mixed Defects—cont'd

Total Anomalous Pulmonary Venous Connection (TAPVC)

Description: Rare defect characterized by failure of the pulmonary veins to join the left atrium. Instead, the pulmonary veins are abnormally connected to the systemic venous circuit via the right atrium or various veins draining toward the right atrium, such as the superior vena cava. The abnormal attachment results in mixed blood being returned to the right atrium and shunted from the right to the left through an atrial septal defect (ASD). The type of TAPVC is classified according to the pulmonary venous point of attachment as follows:

Supracardiac—Attachment above the diaphragm, such as to the superior vena cava (most common form)

Cardiac—Direct attachment to the heart, such as to the right atrium or coronary sinus

Infracardiac—Attachment below the diaphragm, such as to the inferior vena cava (most severe form)

TAPVC is also called *total anomalous pulmonary venous return (TAPVR)* or *total anomalous pulmonary venous drainage (TAPVD)*.

Pathophysiology: The right atrium receives all the blood that normally would flow into the left atrium. As a result, the right side of the heart hypertrophies, whereas the left side, especially the left atrium, may remain small. An associated ASD or patent foramen ovale allows systemic venous blood to shunt from the higher pressure right atrium to the left atrium and into the left side of the heart. As a result, the oxygen saturation of the blood in both sides of the heart (and ultimately, in the systemic arterial circulation) is the same. If the pulmonary blood flow is large, pulmonary venous return is also large and the amount of saturated blood is relatively high. However, if there is obstruction to pulmonary venous drainage, pulmonary venous return is impeded, pulmonary venous pressure rises, and pulmonary interstitial edema develops and eventually contributes to CHF. Infracardiac TAPVC is often associated with obstruction to pulmonary venous drainage and is a surgical emergency.

Clinical manifestations: Most infants develop cyanosis early in life. The degree of cyanosis is inversely related to the amount of pulmonary blood flow—the more pulmonary blood, the less cyanosis. Children with unobstructed TAPVC may be asymptomatic until pulmonary vascular resistance decreases during infancy, increasing pulmonary blood flow, with resulting signs of CHF. Cyanosis becomes worse with pulmonary vein obstruction; after obstruction occurs, the infant's condition usually deteriorates rapidly. Without intervention, cardiac failure will progress to death.

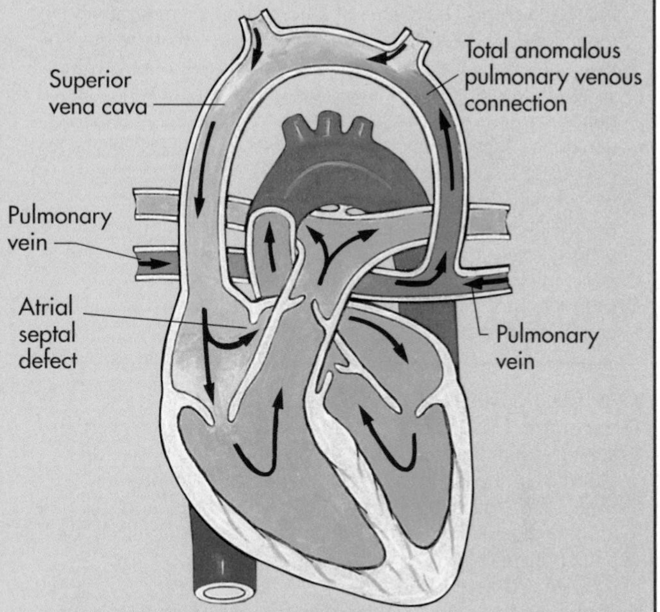

Surgical treatment: Corrective repair in early infancy. The surgical approach varies with the anatomic defect. In general, however, the common pulmonary vein is anastomosed to the left atrium, the ASD is closed, and the anomalous pulmonary venous connection is ligated. The cardiac type is most easily repaired; the infracardiac type has the highest morbidity and mortality rates because of the higher incidence of pulmonary vein obstruction. Potential postoperative complications include reobstruction; bleeding; dysrhythmias, particularly heart block; pulmonary artery hypertension; and persistent heart failure.

Prognosis: The cardiac type has a surgical mortality rate of less than 5%; morbidity and mortality rates are greater with the other types and increase with the presence of pulmonary vein obstruction.

Truncus Arteriosus (TA)

Description: Failure of normal septation and division of the embryonic bulbar trunk into the pulmonary artery and the aorta, resulting in a single vessel that overrides both ventricles. Blood from both ventricles mixes in the common great artery, causing desaturation and hypoxemia. Blood ejected from the heart flows preferentially to the lower pressure pulmonary arteries, causing increased pulmonary blood flow and reduced systemic blood flow. There are three types:

Type I—A single pulmonary trunk arises near the base of the truncus and divides into the left and right pulmonary arteries.

Type II—The left and right pulmonary arteries arise separately but in close proximity and at the same level from the back of the truncus.

Type III—The pulmonary arteries arise independently from the sides of the truncus.

Pathophysiology: Blood ejected from the left and right ventricles enters the common trunk, mixing pulmonary and systemic circulations. Blood flow is distributed to the pulmonary and systemic circulations according to the relative resistances of each system. The amount of pulmonary blood flow depends on the size of the pulmonary arteries and the pulmonary vascular resistance. Generally, resistance to pulmonary blood flow is less than systemic vascular resistance, resulting in preferential blood flow to the lungs. Pulmonary vascular disease develops at an early age in patients with truncus arteriosus.

Clinical manifestations: Most infants are symptomatic with moderate to severe CHF and variable cyanosis, poor growth, and activity intolerance. There is a characteristic murmur.

Surgical treatment: Early repair in the first few months of life. Corrective repair involves closing the VSD so that the truncus arteriosus receives the outflow from the left ventricle, excising the pulmonary arteries from the aorta, and attaching them to

Continued

BOX 48-4

Mixed Defects—cont'd

the right ventricle by means of a homograft. Homografts (segments of cadaver aorta and pulmonary artery that are treated with antibiotics and cryopreserved) are preferred over synthetic conduits to establish continuity between the right ventricle and pulmonary artery. Homografts are more flexible and easier to use during the procedure and are thought to be less prone to obstruction. Postoperative complications include persistent heart failure, bleeding, pulmonary artery hypertension, dysrhythmias, and residual VSD. These children require additional procedures to replace the conduit as its size becomes inadequate in relation to the children's growth.

Prognosis: Mortality rate is greater than 10%; future operations are required to replace the conduits.

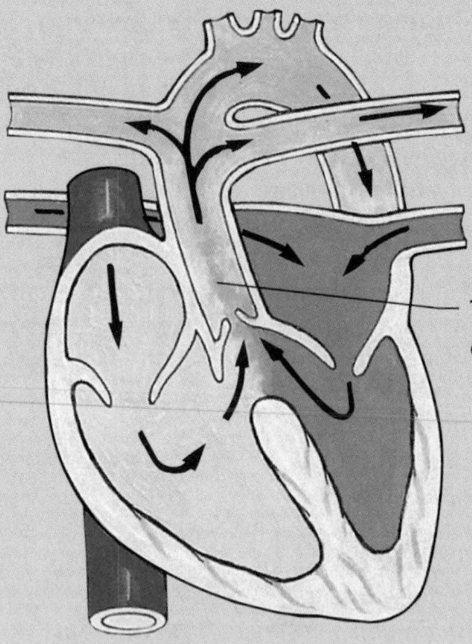

Hypoplastic Left Heart Syndrome (HLHS)

Description: Underdevelopment of the left side of the heart, resulting in a hypoplastic left ventricle and aortic atresia. Most blood from the left atrium flows across the patent foramen ovale to the right atrium, to the right ventricle, and out the pulmonary artery. The descending aorta receives blood from the patent ductus arteriosus supplying systemic blood flow (O'Brien & Boisvert, 2001).

Pathophysiology: An ASD or patent foramen ovale allows saturated blood from the left atrium to mix with desaturated blood from the right atrium, and to flow through the right ventricle and out into the pulmonary artery. From the pulmonary artery the blood flows to the lungs, then through the ductus arteriosus into the aorta and out to the body. The amount of blood flow to the pulmonary and systemic circulations depends on the relationship between the pulmonary and systemic vascular resistances. The coronary and cerebral vessels receive blood by retrograde flow through the hypoplastic ascending aorta.

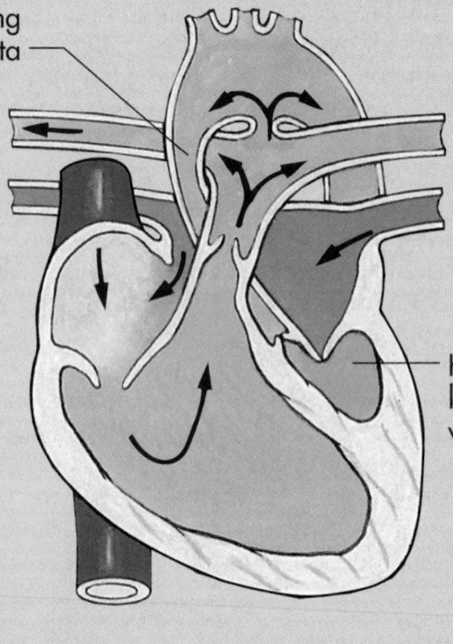

Clinical manifestations: Patients are usually symptomatic in the first week of life with cyanosis and CHF when the PDA starts to close with progressive deterioration and decreased cardiac output, leading to cardiovascular collapse. It is usually fatal in the first months of life without intervention.

Therapeutic management: Neonates require stabilization with mechanical ventilation and inotropic support preoperatively. A prostaglandin E_1 infusion is needed to maintain ductal patency, ensuring adequate systemic blood flow.

Surgical treatment: Several-staged approach. First stage is *Norwood procedure:* anastomosis of the main pulmonary artery to the aorta to create a new aorta, placement of a shunt or inserting a conduit from the right ventricle to pulmonary artery to provide pulmonary blood flow, and creation of a large ASD. Postoperative complications include imbalance of systemic and pulmonary blood flow, bleeding, low cardiac output, and persistent heart failure. The second stage is often a *bidirectional Glenn shunt* done at 6 to 9 months of age to relieve cyanosis and reduce the volume load on the right ventricle. The final repair is a *modified Fontan procedure* (see Tricuspid Atresia in Box 48-3).

Transplantation: Some programs believe that heart transplantation in the newborn period is the best option for these infants. Problems include the shortage of newborn organ donors, risk of rejection, long-term problems with chronic immunosuppression, and infection (see Heart Transplantation, p. 1591).

Prognosis: Mortality risks of more than 25% with both surgery and transplantation. Results vary widely in different centers. This may improve in the future. Because of the high risk nature of both surgical palliation and neonatal heart transplantation, some cardiologists continue to recommend no treatment for this defect.

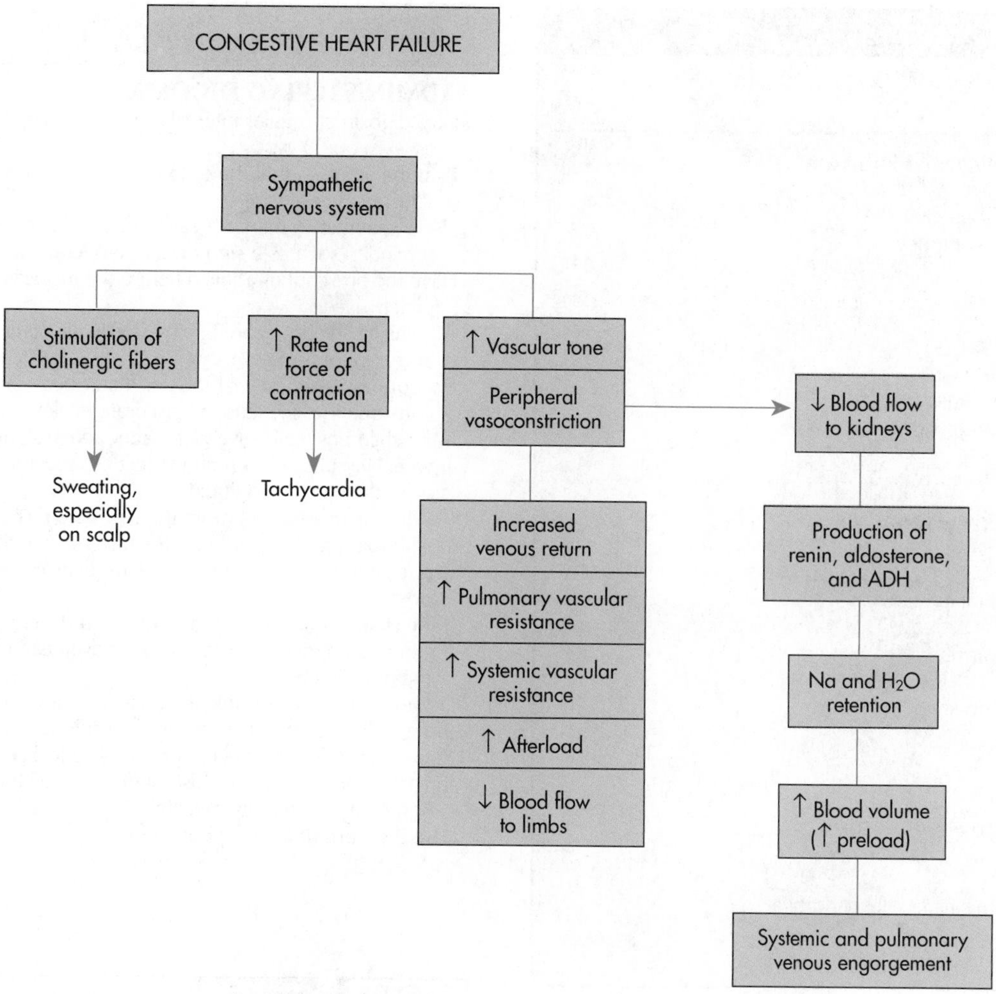

Fig. 48-6 Pathophysiology of congestive heart failure.

Nursing Diagnoses

Several nursing diagnoses are identified after a thorough assessment. Some of these are included in the Nursing Care Plan on p. 1576. Others may become apparent in special circumstances and with children in different age groups.

Plan of Care and Implementation

The goals for the infant or child with CHF and the infant's or child's family are as follows:

1. Infant or child will exhibit improved cardiac output.
2. Infant or child will experience decreased cardiac demands.
3. Infant or child will exhibit improved respiratory function.
4. Infant or child will maintain adequate nutritional status.
5. Infant or child will exhibit no evidence of fluid excess.
6. Infant or child and family will receive adequate support and education.

Although the objectives of nursing care are the same, interventions for infants differ from those for older children.

Assist in Measures to Improve Cardiac Function

The nurse's responsibility in administering digoxin includes observing for signs of toxicity, calculating and administering the correct dosage, and instituting parental teaching regarding drug administration at home. The child's apical pulse is always checked before administering digoxin. As a general rule, the drug is not given if the pulse is below 90 to 110 beats/min in infants and young children or below 70 beats/min in older children (the cutoff point for adults is 60 beats/min). However, because the pulse rate varies in children in different age groups, the written drug order should specify at what heart rate the drug is withheld. The nurse should also use judgment in evaluating the pulse rate. If it is significantly lower than the previous recording, the dose should be withheld until the practitioner is notified.

The apical rate is taken because a pulse deficit (radial pulse rate lower than apical) may be present with decreased cardiac output. It is auscultated for 1 full minute to evaluate alterations in rhythm. If the child is monitored by means of an ECG, a rhythm strip is obtained and attached to the chart for rate and rhythm analysis, such as abnormal lengthening of the P-R interval (more than a 50% increase over predigitalization interval) and dysrhythmias.

Digoxin is a potentially dangerous drug because the margin of safety of therapeutic, toxic, and lethal doses is very narrow. Many toxic responses are extensions of its therapeu-

BOX 48-5

Clinical Manifestations of Congestive Heart Failure

Impaired Myocardial Function
Tachycardia
Sweating (inappropriate)
Decreased urine output
Fatigue
Weakness
Restlessness
Anorexia
Pale, cool extremities
Weak peripheral pulses
Decreased blood pressure
Gallop rhythm
Cardiomegaly

Pulmonary Congestion
Tachypnea
Dyspnea
Retractions (infants)
Flaring nares
Exercise intolerance
Orthopnea
Cough, hoarseness
Cyanosis
Wheezing
Grunting

Systemic Venous Congestion
Weight gain
Hepatomegaly
Peripheral edema, especially periorbital
Ascites
Neck vein distention (children)

tic effects. Therefore the nurse must maintain a high index of suspicion for signs of toxicity when administering digoxin (Box 48-6).

Because digoxin toxicity can occur from accidental overdose, great care must be taken in properly calculating and measuring the dosage. When converting milligrams to micrograms to milliliters, the nurse carefully checks the placement of the decimal point, because an error causes a significant change in dosage. For example, 0.1 mg is 10 times the dosage of 0.01 mg.

NURSE ALERT Infants rarely receive more than 1 ml (50 mcg or 0.05 mg) in one dose; a higher dose is an immediate warning of a dosage error. To ensure safety, compare the calculation with another staff member's calculation before giving the drug. ■

These same principles are taught to parents in preparation for discharge, although the correct dose in milliliters is usually specified on the container, thus reducing potential errors in calculation. The nurse watches the parent measure the elixir in the dropper and stresses the level mark as the meniscus of the fluid that is observed at eye level. Other instructions for administering digoxin are listed in the Home Care box and the Critical Thinking Exercise.

Home Care

ADMINISTERING DIGOXIN

Give digoxin at regular intervals, usually every 12 hours, such as 8 AM and 8 PM.
Plan the times so that the drug is given 1 hour before or 2 hours after feedings.
Use a calendar to mark off each dose that is given, or post a reminder, such as a sign on the refrigerator.
Have the prescription refilled before the medication is completely used.
Administer the drug carefully by slowly directing it on the side and back of the mouth.
Do not mix it with other foods or fluids, because refusal to consume these results in inaccurate intake of the drug.
If the child has teeth, give water after administering the drug; whenever possible, brush the teeth to prevent tooth decay from the sweetened liquid.
If a dose is missed and more than 4 hours has elapsed, withhold the dose and give the next dose at the regular time; if less than 4 hours has elapsed, give the missed dose.
If the child vomits, do not give a second dose.
If more than two consecutive doses have been missed, notify the practitioner.
Do not increase or double the dose for missed doses.
If the child becomes ill, notify the practitioner immediately.
Keep digoxin in a safe place, preferably a locked cabinet.
In case of accidental overdose of digoxin, call the nearest poison control center immediately; the number is usually listed in the front of the telephone directory.

Critical Thinking Exercise

DIGOXIN TOXICITY

You are visiting a 3-month-old infant at home who began receiving digoxin and furosemide (Lasix) 5 days ago for management of CHF. A brief assessment indicates that the infant appears well but is not very active, has a weak suck reflex, and does not exhibit much spontaneous movement during interaction with the mother. The mother mentions that the infant is a good baby and does not cry much except when he is very hungry. She also mentions that he vomited several times yesterday and vomited twice this morning; this was not perceived as unusual because her 3-year-old did the same thing and was diagnosed with gastroesophageal reflux. Further assessment of the infant reveals an irregular heartbeat of 86 to 104 beats/min at rest, and the heart rhythm is also noted to be irregular. No murmur or other significant sounds are auscultated.

1. Evidence—Is there sufficient evidence to draw conclusions about this infant?
2. Assumptions—Describe an underlying assumption about each of the following:
   a. Side effects of furosemide (Lasix)
   b. Side effects of digoxin
   c. Infants with CHF
3. What priorities for nursing care should be established for this infant?
4. Does the evidence support your nursing interventions?
5. What alternative perspectives might you have?

Table 48-3

Diuretics Used in Congestive Heart Failure

ACTIONS	COMMENTS	NURSING CONSIDERATIONS
FUROSEMIDE (LASIX)		
Blocks reabsorption of sodium and water in proximal renal tubule and interferes with reabsorption of sodium	Drug of choice in severe congestive heart failure (CHF) Causes excretion of chloride and potassium (hypokalemia may precipitate digitalis toxicity)	Begin to record output as soon as drug is given Observe for dehydration caused by profound diuresis Observe for side effects (nausea and vomiting, diarrhea, ototoxicity, hypokalemia, dermatitis, postural hypotension) Encourage foods high in potassium and/or give potassium supplements Monitor chloride and acid-base balance with long-term therapy Observe for signs of digoxin toxicity
CHLOROTHIAZIDE (DIURIL)		
Acts directly on distal tubules to decrease sodium, water, potassium, chloride, and bicarbonate absorption	Less frequently used drug Causes hypokalemia, acidosis from large doses	Observe for side effects (nausea, weakness, dizziness, paresthesia, muscle cramps, skin eruptions, hypokalemia, acidosis) Encourage foods high in potassium and/or give potassium supplements
SPIRONOLACTONE (ALDACTONE)		
Blocks action of aldosterone, which promotes retention of sodium and excretion of potassium	Weak diuretic Has potassium-sparing effect; frequently used with thiazides, furosemide Poorly absorbed from gastrointestinal tract Takes several days to achieve maximum actions	Observe for side effects (skin rash, drowsiness, ataxia, hyperkalemia) Do not administer potassium supplements

BOX 48-6

Common Signs of Digoxin Toxicity in Children

Gastrointestinal	Cardiac
Nausea	Bradycardia
Vomiting	Dysrhythmias
Anorexia	

Parents are also advised of the signs of toxicity. According to the practitioner's preference, they may be taught to take the pulse before giving the drug. A return demonstration of the procedure from both parents and any other principal caregivers is included as part of the teaching plan. Their level of anxiety in counting the pulse is assessed, because overconcern about the heart rate may result in excessive withholding of the drug.

Afterload Reduction

For patients receiving ACE inhibitors for afterload reduction, the nurse should carefully monitor blood pressure before and after dose administration, observe for symptoms of hypotension, and notify the practitioner if blood pressure is low. Numerous medications affecting the kidney can potentiate renal dysfunction, so children taking multiple diuretics and an ACE inhibitor require careful assessment of serum electrolytes and renal function.

Decrease Cardiac Demands

The infant requires rest and conservation of energy for feeding. Every effort is made to organize nursing activities to allow for uninterrupted periods of sleep. Whenever possible, parents are encouraged to stay with their infant to provide the holding, rocking, and cuddling that help children sleep more soundly. To minimize disturbing the infant, changing bed linen and complete bathing are done only when necessary. Feeding is planned to accommodate the infant's sleep and wake patterns. The child is fed when hungry, such as when sucking on fists rather than when crying for a bottle, because the stress of crying exhausts the limited energy supply. Because infants with CHF tire easily and may sleep through feedings, smaller feedings every 3 hours may be helpful. Gavage feedings may be instituted to provide adequate nutrition and allow the infant to rest.

Every effort is made to minimize unnecessary stress. Older children need an explanation of what is happening to them to decrease anxiety about their illness and necessary treatments such as cardiac monitoring, oxygen administration, and medications. Outlining a plan for the day, preparing the child for tests and procedures, providing quiet activities, and providing adequate rest periods are all helpful interventions with older children. Some infants and children require sedation during the acute phase of illness to allow them to rest (Smith, 2001).

Temperature is carefully monitored because hyperthermia or hypothermia increases the need for oxygen. Febrile states are reported to the physician, because infection must be promptly treated. Maintaining body temperature is of special importance in children who are receiving cool, humidified oxygen and in infants, who tend to be diaphoretic and lose heat by way of evaporation.

Skin breakdown from edema is prevented with a change of position every 2 hours (from side to side while in semi-Fowler position) and use of a pressure-relieving mattress or bed. The skin, especially over the sacrum, is checked for evidence of redness from pressure.

Reduce Respiratory Distress

Careful assessment, positioning, and oxygen administration can reduce respiratory distress. Respirations are counted for 1 full minute during a resting state. Any evidence of increased respiratory distress is reported, because this may indicate worsening CHF.

Infants are positioned to encourage maximum chest expansion, with the head of the bed elevated; they should sit up in an infant seat or be held at a 45-degree angle. Children prefer to sleep on several pillows and remain in a semi-Fowler or high-Fowler position during waking hours. Shirts and diapers are pinned loosely to allow maximum chest expansion. Safety restraints, such as those used with infant seats, are applied low on the abdomen and loosely enough to provide both safety and maximum expansion.

The infant or child is often given humidified supplemental oxygen via oxygen hood or tent, nasal cannula, or mask. The child's response to oxygen therapy is carefully evaluated by noting respiratory rate, ease of respiration, color, and especially oxygen saturations, as measured by oximetry.

Respiratory infections can exacerbate CHF and should be appropriately treated and prevented if possible. The child should be protected from persons with respiratory infections and have a noninfectious roommate. With an older child, it is advantageous to choose a roommate who is also confined to bed and relatively quiet to promote a restful environment. Good handwashing is practiced before and after caring for any hospitalized child. Antibiotics may be given to combat respiratory infection. The nurse ensures that the drug is given at equally divided times over a 24-hour schedule to maintain high blood levels of the antibiotic.

Maintain Nutritional Status

Meeting the nutritional needs of infants with CHF or serious cardiac defects is a nursing challenge. The metabolic rate of these infants is greater because of poor cardiac function and increased heart and respiratory rates. Their caloric needs are greater than those of the average infant because of their increased metabolic rate, yet their ability to take in adequate calories is hampered by their fatigue (Smith, 2001). Feeding for a fragile infant with serious CHD is similar to exercise in an adult, and the infant often does not have the energy or cardiac reserve to do extra work. The nurse seeks measures to enable the infant to feed easily without excess fatigue and to increase the caloric density of the formula.

The infant should be well rested before feeding and fed soon after awakening so as not to expend energy on crying. A 3-hour feeding schedule works well for many infants. (Feeding every 2 hours does not provide enough rest between feedings, and a 4-hour schedule requires an increased volume of feeding, which many infants are unable to take.) The feeding schedule should be individualized to the infant's needs. A soft preemie nipple or a slit in a regular nipple to enlarge the opening decreases the energy expenditure of the infant while sucking. Infants should be well supported and fed in a semiupright position. The infant may need to rest frequently and may need to have the jaw and cheeks stroked to encourage sucking. Generally, giving an infant about a half hour to complete a feeding is reasonable. Prolonging the feeding time can exhaust the infant and decrease the rest period between feedings.

Infants with feeding difficulties are often gavage fed using a nasogastric tube to supplement their oral intake and ensure adequate calories. If they are very stressed and fatigued, in respiratory distress, or tachypneic to 80 to 100 breaths/min, oral feedings may be withheld and all nutrition given by gavage feedings. Gavage feedings are usually a temporary measure until the infant's medical status improves and nutritional needs can be met through oral feedings. Some infants with severe CHF, neurologic deficits, or significant gastroesophageal reflux may need placement of a gastrostomy tube to allow adequate nutrition.

Increasing the caloric density of formulas by concentration and then adding corn oil, medium-chain triglycerides (MCT oil), or Polycose is frequently done. Infant formulas provide 20 calories per ounce, and the use of additives can increase the calories to 30 calories or more per ounce. This allows the infant to obtain more calories despite a smaller volume intake of formula. The caloric density of the formula needs to be increased slowly (by two calories per ounce per day) to prevent diarrhea or formula intolerance. Breastfeeding mothers are encouraged to provide the infant with alternating feedings of breast milk and high-calorie formulas. Some lactating mothers will prefer to feed the child expressed breast milk that has been fortified with Similac or Enfamil powder, Polycose, or corn oil to increase caloric intake. A supplemental nurser may also be helpful. A diet plan specific to the individual infant's needs is calculated and prescribed by the nutritionist in collaboration with the other health personnel. The nurse needs to reinforce this information with the parents as necessary.

Assist in Measures to Promote Fluid Loss

When diuretics are given, the nurse records fluid intake and output and monitors body weight at the same time each day to evaluate benefit from the drug. Because profound diuresis may cause dehydration and electrolyte imbalance (loss of sodium, potassium, chloride, and bicarbonate), the nurse observes for signs indicating either complication, as well as signs and symptoms suggesting reactions to the drugs. Diuretics should be given early in the day to children who are toilet trained to avoid the need to urinate at night. If potassium-losing diuretics are given, the nurse encourages foods high in potassium, such as bananas, oranges, whole grains, legumes, and leafy vegetables, and administers prescribed supplements. Serum potassium levels are checked frequently.

NURSE ALERT Mix the elixir with fruit juice (red punch or grape juice works well) to disguise the bitter taste and to prevent intestinal irritation from a concentrated solution. ■

Fluid restriction is rarely necessary in infants because of their difficulty in feeding. However, if fluids are restricted, the nurse plans fluid intake schedules for a 24-hour period, allowing for most fluids during waking hours. Toddlers and preschoolers should be given small amounts of liquid in small cups so that the containers appear full. It is also important to avoid leaving extra fluids at the bedside, because older children may help themselves to additional servings. Older children's cooperation is gained by placing them in charge of recording fluid intake.

If salt is limited, the nurse discusses food sources of sodium with the family and discourages their bringing salt-containing treats to the child. At mealtime the child's tray is checked to make sure the appropriate diet is given.

Support Child and Family

CHF is a serious complication of heart disease. Parents and older children are usually acutely aware of the critical nature of the condition. Because stress places additional demands on cardiac function, the nurse should focus on reducing anxiety through anticipatory preparation, frequent communication with the parent regarding the child's progress, and constant reassurance that everything possible is being done.

Home care involves many of the same interventions discussed under Plan for Discharge and Home Care (see p. 1583). The nurse teaches the family about the medications that need to be administered and alerts them to the signs of worsening CHF that require medical attention, such as increased sweating, decreased urine output (noted in fewer wet diapers or infrequent use of the toilet), or poor feeding. Compliance is a major issue, and every effort is extended to improve the family's adherence to the medication schedule (see Chapter 45). Written instructions regarding correct administration of digoxin are essential (see Home Care box, p. 1572), including an explanation regarding signs of toxicity.

If CHF is the end stage of a severe heart defect, the nurse cares for this child as for any child who is terminally ill, using the principles discussed in Chapter 41 .

Evaluation

The effectiveness of nursing interventions for the child with CHF and the child's family is determined by continual reassessment and evaluation of care based on the following observational guidelines:

1. Monitor heart rate and quality, respiratory rate and effort, and color, and observe behaviors that provide clues to expended effort.
2. Observe nutritional intake, feeding behaviors, and weight.
3. Monitor intake, output, and weight.
4. Interview and observe behaviors of family.

The *expected outcomes* are described in the Nursing Care Plan on p. 1576.

Hypoxemia

Hypoxemia refers to an arterial oxygen tension (or pressure, PaO_2) that is less than normal and can be identified by a decreased arterial saturation or a decreased PaO_2. *Hypoxia* is a reduction in tissue oxygenation that results from low oxygen saturations and PaO_2 and results in impaired cellular processes. *Cyanosis* is a blue discoloration in the mucous membranes, skin, and nail beds of the child with reduced oxygen saturation. It results from the presence of deoxygenated hemoglobin (hemoglobin not bound to oxygen) in a concentration of 5 g/dl of blood. Cyanosis is usually apparent when arterial oxygen saturations are 80% to 85%. Determination of cyanosis is subjective. It can vary depending on skin pigment, quality of light, color of the room, or clothing worn by the child. The presence of cyanosis may not accurately reflect arterial hypoxemia, because both oxygen saturation and the amount of circulating hemoglobin are involved. Children with severe anemia may not be cyanotic despite severe hypoxemia, because the hemoglobin level may be too low to produce the characteristic blue color. Conversely, patients with polycythemia may appear cyanotic despite a near-normal PaO_2. Heart defects that cause hypoxemia and cyanosis result from desaturated venous blood (blue blood) entering the systemic circulation without passing through the lungs.

Adolescents and young adults may become cyanotic because of unrepaired septal defects in which the increased pulmonary blood flow over many years results in pulmonary vascular changes. *Eisenmenger complex (syndrome)* refers to the clinical situation in which a left-to-right shunt becomes a right-to-left shunt because of a progressive increase in pulmonary vascular resistance. With increasing pulmonary vascular thickening, the resistance in the pulmonary circulation can exceed or equal that in the systemic circulation, causing a reversal of blood flow from the right to the left ventricle.

Clinical Manifestations

Over time, two physiologic changes occur in the body in response to chronic hypoxemia: polycythemia and clubbing. *Polycythemia*, an increased number of red blood cells, increases the oxygen-carrying capacity of the blood. However, anemia may result if iron is not readily available for the formation of hemoglobin. Polycythemia increases the viscosity of the blood and crowds out clotting factors. *Clubbing*, a thickening and flattening of the tips of the fingers and toes, is thought to occur because of chronic tissue hypoxemia and polycythemia (Fig. 48-7). Infants with mild hypoxemia may

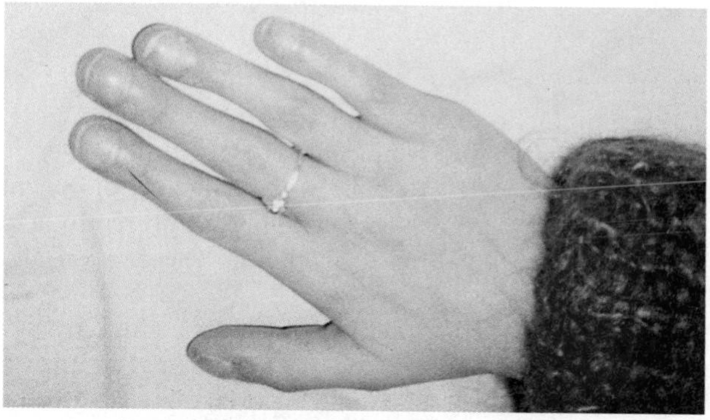

Fig. 48-7 Clubbing of the fingers.

Nursing Care Plan

THE CHILD WITH CONGESTIVE HEART FAILURE

NURSING DIAGNOSIS: Decreased cardiac output related to structural defect, myocardial dysfunction

EXPECTED OUTCOME

Patient exhibits signs of improved cardiac output (i.e., strong, regular pulse with rates within normal limits [WNL]; blood pressure WNL; absence of pallor; adequate capillary refill).

NURSING INTERVENTIONS/*RATIONALES*

Administer digoxin (Lanoxin) per physician order *to improve myocardial efficiency:* make certain dosage is within safe limits; count pulse for 1 minute before giving drug and withhold if too slow; monitor for adverse or toxic effects. Ensure adequate intake of potassium and monitor potassium levels, *because decreased levels enhance toxicity of digoxin.*

Administer medications *to decrease afterload as ordered;* monitor for hypotension and electrolyte levels.

Administer oxygen per physician order *to increase supply to myocardium.*

Monitor apical and radial pulses frequently for rate and rhythm *to detect presence of dysrythmias;* monitor skin color, temperature, capillary refill, and vital signs *to assess for status of cardiac output.*

Plan child's care and activities to prevent overexertion, *which increases myocardial oxygen demand.*

Administer stool softeners as ordered *to prevent straining at stool and resultant bradycardia.*

NURSING DIAGNOSIS: Ineffective breathing pattern related to pulmonary congestion

EXPECTED OUTCOME

Patient exhibits signs of improved respiratory function (i.e., regular, even respirations with rates WNL; good color; adequate oxygen saturations; decreased restlessness).

NURSING INTERVENTIONS/*RATIONALES*

Place in inclined posture of 30 to 45 degrees and avoid constrictive clothing or restraints around abdomen or chest *to encourage maximum chest expansion.*

Administer humidified oxygen as ordered *to reduce hypoxia.*

Monitor respiratory rate, rhythm, ease of breathing, skin color, oxygen saturations by oximetry, breath sounds, and restlessness *to assess pulmonary status.*

Suction airway as needed *to remove secretions.*

Plan child's care and activities with adequate rest *to prevent fatigue and reduce oxygen demand.*

NURSING DIAGNOSIS: Fluid volume excess related to pulmonary congestion and fluid accumulation

EXPECTED OUTCOME

Patient exhibits evidence of fluid loss (i.e., increased urine output, weight loss, reduction of edema).

NURSING INTERVENTIONS/*RATIONALES*

Administer diuretics as prescribed *to induce diuresis.*

Monitor weight, intake and output, level of edema, urine specific gravity, and electrolytes *to assess fluid status;* monitor blood urea nitrogen and creatinine levels *to assess renal function.*

Monitor intravenous and oral intake carefully *to prevent further fluid overload.*

Provide skin care and reposition frequently when edematous *to prevent skin breakdown;* provide oral care *to prevent drying of mucous membranes.*

Monitor skin turgor *to assess for dehydration.*

NURSING DIAGNOSIS: Activity intolerance related to oxygen imbalance

EXPECTED OUTCOME

Patient's activity level is within normal limits.

NURSING INTERVENTIONS/*RATIONALES*

Maintain neutral thermal environment *to decrease oxygen demands.*

Feed small volumes at frequent intervals using soft nipple with moderately large opening *to decrease fatigue;* implement gavage feeding if necessary *to prevent fatigue and ensure adequate intake.*

Implement measures to reduce anxiety, crying, and signs of distress, *which increase demand for oxygen.*

Perform only necessary functions *to reduce fatigue and energy expenditure.*

Balance rest and physical activity, increasing activity levels as tolerated, *to regain balance between oxygen supply and demand.*

See also Nursing Care Plan: The Family of the Ill/Hospitalized Child, Chapter 44 .

be asymptomatic except for cyanosis and exhibit near-normal growth and development. Those with more severe hypoxemia may exhibit fatigue with feeding, poor weight gain, tachypnea, and dyspnea. Severe hypoxemia resulting in tissue hypoxia is manifested by clinical deterioration and signs of poor perfusion.

Squatting, most characteristic of children with tetralogy of Fallot, is seen in toddlers and older children as an unconscious attempt to relieve chronic hypoxia, especially during exercise. Because of early surgical intervention during infancy, squatting is rarely seen.

Hypercyanotic spells, also referred to as *blue spells* or *tet spells* because they are often seen in infants with tetralogy of Fallot, may occur in any child whose heart defect includes obstruction to pulmonary blood flow and communication between the ventricles. The infant becomes acutely cyanotic and hyperpneic because sudden infundibular spasm decreases pulmonary blood flow and increases right-to-left shunting (the proposed mechanism in tetralogy of Fallot). Spells, rarely seen before 2 months of age, occur most frequently in the first year of life. They occur more often in the morning and may be preceded by feeding, crying, defecation, or stressful procedures (Critical Thinking Exercise). Because profound hypoxemia causes cerebral hypoxia, hypercyanotic spells require prompt assessment and treatment to prevent brain damage or possibly death.

Persistent cyanosis as a result of cyanotic cardiac defects places the child at risk for significant *neurologic complications.* Cerebrovascular accident (CVA, or stroke), brain abscess, and developmental delays (especially in motor and cognitive development) may result from chronic hypoxia.

Therapeutic Management

Hypercyanotic spells occur suddenly, and prompt recognition and treatment are essential. In the hospital setting, spells are often seen during blood drawing or IV insertion, when the child is highly agitated, or after cardiac catheterization. Treatment of a hypercyanotic spell is outlined in the Guidelines box. Morphine, administered subcutaneously or through an existing IV line, helps reduce infundibular spasm. A spell indicates the need for prompt surgical treatment if possible. In infants with defects not amenable to surgical repair, a shunt may be created surgically to increase blood flow to the lungs. Several commonly used shunt procedures are described in Table 48-4 and Fig. 48-9.

The cyanotic infant and child are well hydrated to keep the hematocrit and blood viscosity within acceptable limits to reduce the risk of CVAs. Fevers are carefully evaluated because bacteremia can result in bacterial endocarditis. The in-

Critical Thinking Exercise

HYPERCYANOTIC SPELL

A 4-month-old infant known to have tetralogy of Fallot is seen in the emergency department because of a 2-day history of diarrhea, low-grade fever, and poor oral intake. When blood tests are obtained, he becomes acutely cyanotic with rapid, shallow respirations.

1. Evidence—Is there sufficient evidence to draw conclusions about this infant's condition?
2. Assumptions—Describe an underlying assumption about each of the following:
   a. Symptoms associated with tetralogy of Fallot
   b. Diarrhea, low-grade fever, and poor oral intake in a 4-month-old infant
   c. Acute cyanotic episodes in a 4-month-old infant
3. What priorities for nursing care should be established for this infant?
4. Does the evidence support your nursing interventions?
5. What alternative perspectives might you have?

Guidelines

TREATING HYPERCYANOTIC SPELLS

Place infant in knee-chest position (Fig. 48-8).
Employ calm, comforting approach.
Administer 100% oxygen by face mask.
Give morphine subcutaneously or through existing intravenous (IV) line.
Begin IV fluid replacement and volume expansion if needed.
Repeat morphine administration.

Table 48-4

Selected Shunt Procedures for Children with Cardiac Defects

SHUNT LOCATION	COMMENTS
MODIFIED BLALOCK-TAUSSIG (BT) SHUNT	
Subclavian artery to pulmonary artery using Gore-Tex or Impra tube graft	Shunt flow sometimes excessive, requiring use of diuretics Possibility of thrombosis; antiplatelet therapy may be used postoperatively Easy to ligate at time of definitive correction Shunt size fixed and may become too small as child grows
CENTRAL SHUNT	
Ascending aorta to main pulmonary aorta using Gore-Tex graft	Length of shunt acts to restrict blood flow, limiting symptoms of congestive heart failure; may require diuretics Uncommon; used when modified BT shunt cannot be done Easy to perform and remove at time of repair
GLENN SHUNT	
Superior vena cava to side of right pulmonary artery, which is ligated from main pulmonary artery Blood flow to right lung only	Used as a second shunt procedure if complete repair is not possible High mortality rate in infants younger than age 6 months Superior vena cava syndrome may occur Pulmonary arteriovenous fistulas may occur many years later Difficult to take down at time of definitive repair
BIDIRECTIONAL GLENN (CAVOPULMONARY ANASTOMOSIS) SHUNT	
Superior vena cava to side of right pulmonary artery Blood flow to both lungs	Done as a second shunt; often as a staging step to a Fontan procedure Can be incorporated into eventual modified Fontan procedure Relieves cyanosis and decreases volume overload on ventricle

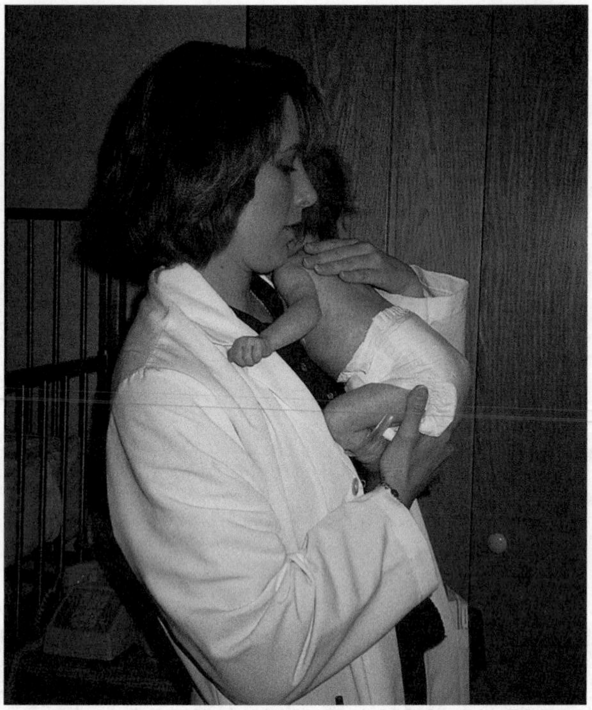

Fig. 48-8 Infant held in knee-chest position.

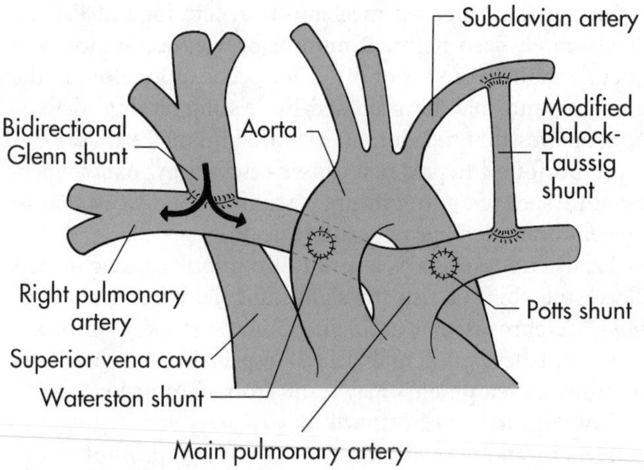

Fig. 48-9 Schematic diagram of cardiac shunts. NOTE: Two early shunt procedures–Waterston shunt (ascending aorta to right pulmonary artery) and Potts shunt (descending aorta to left pulmonary artery)–are no longer performed because of problems with excessive pulmonary blood flow and distortion of the pulmonary arteries. Adult patients may have had these shunts done as their initial repair.

fant is monitored closely for anemia because of the risk of CVAs and the reduced arterial oxygen-carrying capacity that occurs. Iron supplementation and possibly blood transfusion are used as needed.

Respiratory infections or reduced pulmonary function from any cause can worsen hypoxemia in the cyanotic child. Aggressive pulmonary hygiene, chest physiotherapy, administration of antibiotics, and use of oxygen to improve arterial saturations are important interventions.

Nursing Care Management

The general appearance of infants and children with significant cyanosis poses unique concerns. Blue lips and fingernails are obvious signs of their hidden cardiac defect. Clubbing and small, thin stature in older children further indicate severe heart disease. Adolescents are especially concerned about their body image; children with cyanosis are often teased about their appearance and singled out as different. Many children, when asked what surgery will do, reply, "Make me pink." Their joy and excitement after surgery are evident when they see their pink fingers. Accentuating the normal and positive and being careful not to call attention to their cyanosis are helpful interventions. Meeting other children in the clinic or hospital who are cyanotic reassures them that they are not the only ones who are blue.

Parents are often fearful of their child's bluish color, because cyanosis is usually associated with lack of oxygen and severe illness. They also must deal with comments from relatives, friends, and strangers about their child's abnormal color. They need a simple explanation of hypoxemia and cyanosis and reassurance that cyanosis does not imply a lack of oxygen to the brain. Their questions and fears need to be addressed in a calm, supportive manner, and positive aspects of their child's growth and development are emphasized. They are taught the treatment for hypercyanotic spells (see Guidelines box, p. 1577).

Dehydration must be prevented in hypoxemic children because it potentiates the risk of CVAs. Fluid status is carefully monitored, with accurate intake and output and daily weight measurements. Maintenance fluid therapy is the minimum requirement, supplemental fluids should be readily available, and gavage feeding or IV hydration is given to children unable to take adequate oral fluids. Fever, vomiting, and diarrhea can cause dehydration and require prompt treatment. Parents are instructed in the importance of adequate fluid intake and measures to prevent dehydration. An oral electrolyte solution should be available at home in the event that the infant is unable to tolerate the usual formula. The practitioner should be notified of fever, vomiting, diarrhea, or other problems.

Preventive measures and accurate assessment of respiratory infection are important nursing considerations. Any compromise in pulmonary function will increase the infant's hypoxemia. Good handwashing and protection from individuals with an obvious respiratory infection are important. Aggressive pulmonary hygiene, treatment with antibiotics or antiviral agents as indicated, and supplemental oxygen to decrease hypoxemia are necessary measures. Infants may need to be gavage fed or given parenteral hydration if respiratory distress prevents oral feeding.

NURSE ALERT Intracardiac shunting of blood from the right side (desaturated) to the left side of the heart allows air in the venous system to go directly to the brain, resulting in an air embolism. Therefore all IV lines should have filters in place to prevent air from entering the system; the entire tubing should be checked for air; all connections should be taped securely; and any air should be removed. ■

NURSING CARE OF THE FAMILY AND CHILD WITH CONGENITAL HEART DISEASE

When a child is born with a severe cardiac anomaly, the parents are faced with the immense psychologic and physical tasks of adjusting to the birth of a child with special needs. The reactions and nursing interventions required to support the family are similar to those of other parents whose children have serious chronic conditions and are discussed in Chapter 41.

The following discussion is primarily directed (1) toward the family of an infant who has a serious heart defect and requires home care before definitive repair and (2) toward preparation and care of the child and family when heart surgery is performed. For nursing care related to the child with hypoxemia and CHF, the reader should refer to earlier discussions of these topics.

Nursing care of the child with a congenital heart defect begins as soon as the diagnosis is suspected. Prenatal diagnosis of congenital heart defects is becoming increasingly frequent. Those with severe congenital cardiac defects are usually diagnosed in infancy.

Help Family Adjust to the Disorder

After parents learn of the heart defect, whether it is soon after the child's birth or at a later period, they are initially in a period of shock, followed by high anxiety and fear that the child will die. The family needs time to grieve before they can assimilate the meaning of the defect. Unfortunately, the demands for medical treatment may not allow this, instead necessitating that the parents immediately give informed consent for diagnostic or therapeutic procedures. The nurse can be instrumental in supporting parents in their loss, assessing their level of understanding, supplying information as needed, and helping other members of the health care team to understand the parents' reactions (Family Focus box).

Severely distressed newborns usually remain in the hospital. This can seriously affect parent-infant attachment unless parents are encouraged to hold, touch, and look at their child. Every effort must be made by health personnel to foster attachment.

The effect of a child with a serious heart defect on the family is complex. No member, regardless of the degree of positive adjustment, is unaffected. Mothers frequently feel inadequate in their mothering ability because they gave birth to a child with a defect and are unable to keep the child well. They often feel constantly exhausted from the pressures of caring for these children and the other family members. Fathers and siblings may feel neglected and resentful, a reaction similar to the feelings of family members toward other chronic conditions (see Chapter 41). Often, parents do not feel confident leaving the child in another's care. This often sets up a trap for parents, especially mothers, who become locked into the child's care with no relief. Although the fears are justified, they can be minimized by gradually teaching someone (a reliable relative or neighbor) how to care for the child.

> **Family Focus**
>
> **THE DIAGNOSIS OF HEART DISEASE**
>
> Remember, we don't have your experience. We don't see children every day who have heart disease. We would have been upset finding out our child had to have his tonsils out. How could we ever be prepared for this? Please remember, we only know people who have trivial heart murmurs. How could we ever expect this to happen? And to us, this is the worst problem we've ever heard of.
>
> We still fear most what we don't know and understand. Be honest with us. If you don't know either, tell us. But at least don't leave us wondering about what you know and we don't. Not knowing anything really can be worse than knowing something bad. Be honest, but don't strip us of hope. . . .
>
> Please, remember we are trying to learn complex information in a moment of time. And trying to learn it in a context of great pain and emotional investment. This is our lives you're talking about. Please be thorough, but keep it simple. Tell us again, maybe even again and again, when we can hear better.

From Schrey C, Schrey M: A parent's perspective: our needs and our message, *Crit Care Nurs Clin North Am* 6(1):113-119, 1994.

The need to maintain discipline and set consistent limits cannot be overemphasized. Using behavior modification techniques, either in the form of concrete rewards (e.g., a favorite activity) or social reinforcement (e.g., approval), can be effective. However, it is most beneficial if employed *before* the child learns to control the family. Therefore it is necessary to guide parents toward the need for discipline while the child is in infancy to prevent later problems.

Another issue that may develop within family relationships is the child's overdependency. This is often the result of parental fear that the child may die. The best approach to dealing with this dilemma is prevention. Parents need guidance to recognize the eventual hazards of continuing dependency and protectiveness as the child grows older, and the nurse can assist parents in learning ways to foster optimum development. Unless parents are shown what activities the child can do, they may focus on physical limitations and encourage dependency.

A child with CHD may constitute a long-term family crisis. Frequently the continuing unremitting stresses of care—physical exhaustion, financial costs, emotional upset, fear of death, and concern for the child's future—are not fully appreciated by those caring for the family. Even when the child's condition is stabilized or corrected, the family may need to make new adjustments in their lifestyle. Introducing them to other families with similarly affected children can help them adjust to the daily stresses. (Some local chapters of the American Heart Association have organized parent groups.)

Educate Family about the Disorder

When parents are ready to hear about the heart condition, they require a clear explanation based on their level of understanding. A review of the basic structure and function of the heart is helpful before describing the defect. A simple diagram, pictures, or a model of the heart can help parents visualize the heart and the congenital defect.* Parents appreciate receiving written information about the specific condition. A glossary of frequently used terms is also helpful. Parents also require information about prognosis and treatment options.

Increasingly, families are using the Internet as a source of information about heart disease in children.† They are also finding support through contacts with other parents and parent groups. Several Internet sites with pertinent information are listed in the footnote on this page. It is important for parents to realize that not all Web sites offer medically accurate information, and information from other parents might not be applicable to their own situation. Some children with rare, complex heart defects require individualized treatment plans, and general information on the Internet or in books may not apply to their child. Parents should use their health care team, in particular their cardiologist, to discuss information they have received from other sources.

Infants and children with CHD require good nutrition. Providing infants with adequate nutrition is especially difficult because of their high caloric requirements and inability to suck effectively because of fatigue and tachypnea. Instructing parents in feeding methods that decrease the work of the infant and giving high-calorie formula are important interventions. (See p. 1574 for a discussion on feeding the infant with CHF.)

Children with severe cardiac defects are often anorexic. Encouraging them to eat can be a tremendous challenge. Because of the parents' concern over eating, children learn early to manipulate parents through eating, such as making unrealistic demands for foods that are not available. The nurse advises parents of the potential problem, because prevention yields greater success than intervention. For example, the child should be given a choice of available high-quality foods. Suggestions for feeding sick children are discussed in Chapter 45.

The family also needs to be knowledgeable regarding the therapeutic management of the disorder, especially in terms of the medications the child is receiving. Parents are taught the correct procedure for giving drugs and cautioned to keep them in a safe area to prevent accidental ingestion.

Children of various ages have different ideas about their heart. Children between ages 4 and 6 years have heard about the heart, know its approximate anatomic location in the chest or back, illustrate it as valentine shaped, and characterize it by sounds such as *tick-tock* and *thump.* Children ages 7 to 10 have a clearer concept of the heart, realizing that it is not shaped like a valentine and that it has vital functions, such as "It makes you live." However, their knowledge of its integrated functions to pump blood through a system of vessels to all parts of the body is still hazy. By age 10 or 11, children have a much more involved concept of the heart, with knowledge of veins, valves, pumping action, and circulation. They are beginning to appreciate why death occurs when the heart stops.

Information given to the child must be tailored to the child's developmental age. As the child matures, the level of information is revised to meet the child's new cognitive level. Preschoolers need basic information about what they will experience more than what is actually occurring physiologically. School-age children benefit from a concrete explanation of the defect. Preadolescents and adolescents often appreciate a more detailed description of how the defect affects their heart. Children of all ages need to express their feelings concerning the diagnosis.

Help Family Cope with Effects of the Disorder

Parents should be aware of the symptoms of their child's cardiac condition (if the child is symptomatic). Parents of children who may develop CHF should be familiar with these symptoms and know when to contact the practitioner. Parents of children with cyanosis should be informed about fluid management and hypercyanotic spells. Parents should know how to contact their child's cardiologist at all times and know what to do in an emergency.

Another area of parental concern is the child's level of physical activity. Children do not need to restrict activity, and the best approach is to treat the child normally and allow self-limited activity. Exceptions to self-determined activity primarily involve strenuous recreational and competitive sports in children with specific cardiac problems. Activities and exercise restrictions should be discussed with the child's cardiologist. Deliberately attempting to prevent crying should be avoided because it can establish a maladaptive parental pattern of relating to the infant.

NURSE ALERT Although decisions regarding activity restrictions are made on an individual basis on the cardiologist's advice, children with moderate to severe aortic stenosis or insufficiency are usually not permitted to engage in strenuous activity (Koster, 1994). ■

Prepare Child and Family for Surgery

Few surgical procedures demand as much planning for preoperative preparation and postoperative care as heart surgery. The reader is urged to review the general principles for preparing children for procedures, such as surgery, discussed in Chapter 45. This discussion focuses on those measures specific to cardiovascular procedures. Preoperative preparation is often done in the outpatient setting, and children are admitted the day of surgery. Some infants and patients with other medical needs may be admitted the day before surgery.

No well-documented research exists on how extensive the preoperative preparation should be, and the nurse must use considerable judgment in planning the aspects of teaching. Preparation can be divided into three categories: environment, equipment, and procedures.

*The booklet *If Your Child Has a Congenital Heart Defect: A Guide for Parents,* as well as other information, is available from the American Heart Association, 7272 Greenville Avenue, Dallas, TX 75231; phone: 214-373-6300 or 800-AHA-USA1; Web site: www.americanheart.org.

†The Children's Health Information Network; Web site: www.tchin.org; PediHeart; Web site: www.pediheart.org/parents/index.html; NASPE (information on arrhythmias); Web site: www.naspe.org; Kids with Heart National Association for Children's Heart Disorders, 1578 Careful Drive, Green Bay, WI 54304; Web site: www.kidswithheart.org.

Introduce Child and Family to the Environment

If a visit to the recovery room or intensive care unit (ICU) is planned, it should take place when there is least activity in the area, the parents can accompany the child, and the child is well rested. Usually a day before surgery is ample time to allow the child to ask questions and to prevent undue fantasizing about the experience. If a visit is included in the teaching plan, the nurse can use a book, preferably with pictures or photographs of the actual rooms, to explain the environment to the child.

During the visit to the ICU, the child and parents should experience everything that directly affects the child's care, such as the sounds of ECG monitors, oxygen tents, and placement of the bed. All positive, nonfrightening aspects of the environment are emphasized, such as the play area, visitors' section, pictures or mobiles in the room, or television. If it is a pediatric ICU, the nurse can introduce the family to other children who may be recovering from surgery. The child should be protected from the frightening sights in the unit, and equipment not in view postoperatively, such as equipment located behind or below the bed, needs less attention. The child and parents are encouraged to ask questions or to explore further any equipment in the room, but they should not be pushed to assimilate more information than they appear to be tolerating.

Familiarize Child and Family with Equipment and Procedures

Some of the equipment, such as the stethoscope, blood pressure apparatus, and thermometer, will already be familiar to the child and parents. However, the nurse emphasizes that procedures involving such equipment will be done more frequently. If monitoring devices, such as blood pressure or oximetry, are used, the child is told about the placement of the sensor on the skin.

Types of equipment new to many families are the oxygen mask, suction, chest tubes, endotracheal tubes, incentive spirometers, nasogastric tube, and IV tubing. Each of these is shown and demonstrated either on the child or on a doll, if he or she appears ready. With a younger child, miniaturized equipment suitable for use with a doll or puppet is often less anxiety producing than the actual samples. If other children in the unit have an IV infusion or are in oxygen tents, the older child may benefit from seeing them, but this must be planned carefully to avoid frightening the child.

Several IV lines are inserted perioperatively: (1) an ordinary line for infusion of fluids, inserted in a peripheral vein; (2) a venous pressure line, inserted into the right subclavian or jugular vein; and (3) an arterial line for direct measurement of arterial pressure. Younger children need only know the location of each line. Older children may appreciate knowing the reason for each infusion. Because the lines are inserted during surgery, they are not painful; they only cause discomfort because movement is restricted.

The type and size of incision the child will have after surgery are discussed and can be shown on a doll. Usually one of two types of incisions is made: a *median sternotomy,* which splits the sternum, or a *lateral thoracotomy,* which extends from the midaxillary line to the scapula. Minimally invasive surgical techniques using a *ministernotomy* (opening the lower half of the sternum) are becoming more widely used to decrease postoperative pain and speed postoperative recovery. Frequently, no sutures are visible, because subcuticular, absorbable sutures may be used. If this is done, it should be pointed out to the child and parents, who may fear the incision will open.

An endotracheal (ET) tube is inserted during surgery and may be left in place for ventilatory assistance and tracheobronchial suctioning. However, it may be best to prepare older children for the ET tube only if *prolonged* ventilatory support is planned. The ET tube can be presented as a "breathing tube" that is placed in the nose or mouth. The nurse explains that while the tube is in, the child will feel it in the throat and will not be able to talk, but nothing is wrong. The child can express desires by pointing or using a picture communication board. At this point, communicating the amount of discomfort from the surgery can also be discussed, especially using measurement tools such as numbers or faces (see Pain Assessment, Chapter 44). The nurse stresses that the tube will be removed as soon as possible, often during the first postoperative day. The child may be told about chest tubes and their purpose in draining fluid from around the heart and lungs.

Preoperative physical care differs little, if any, from that for any other surgery and is discussed in Chapter 45. The child should be assured that the parents will be there when he or she wakes up; parents should be allowed to accompany their child as far as possible to the operating suite. After all the equipment and procedures have been explained, it is important to talk about "getting well" and going home. If a doll was used during the preparatory session, the tubes can be removed, and the doll can be dressed in regular clothes in anticipation of discharge.

Provide Postoperative Care

Immediate postoperative care is usually provided by specially trained nurses in ICUs. Many of the procedures, such as arterial pressure and central venous pressure (CVP) monitoring, and the observations related to vital functions require advanced educational training (the reader should refer to critical care texts for further information). However, nurses caring for the child before surgery and during the convalescent period need to be familiar with the major principles of care. Selected complications that may occur postoperatively are described in Box 48-7.

Observe Vital Signs

Vital signs and blood pressure are recorded frequently until stable. Heart rate and respirations are counted for 1 full minute, compared with the ECG monitor, and recorded with activity. The heart rate is normally increased after surgery. The nurse observes cardiac rhythm and notifies the practitioner of any changes in regularity. Dysrhythmias may occur postoperatively secondary to anesthetics, acid-base and electrolyte imbalance, hypoxia, surgical intervention, or trauma to conduction pathways (see p. 1588).

At least hourly, the lungs are auscultated for breath sounds. Diminished or absent sounds most likely indicate an area of atelectasis, which necessitates further medical assessment.

Temperature changes are typical during the early postoperative period. Hypothermia is expected immediately after

BOX 48-7

Selected Complications after Cardiac Surgery and Treatment Approaches

Cardiac

- **Congestive heart failure:** Digoxin, diuretics (see p. 1572)
- Low cardiac output: Intravenous inotropes (see Shock, p. 1596)
- **Dysrhythmias:** Identification, drug treatment, possible pacing, cardioversion (see p. 1588)
- **Tamponade** (blood or fluid in the pericardial space constricting the heart): Prompt removal of fluid by pericardiocentesis

Respiratory

- **Atelectasis:** Chest physiotherapy, coughing, deep breathing, ambulation
- **Pulmonary edema:** Diuretics
- **Pleural effusions:** Diuretics, possible chest tube drainage
- **Pneumothorax:** Possible chest tube drainage

Neurologic

- **Seizures:** Assessment, antiepileptic drugs
- **Cerebrovascular accident (stroke), cerebral edema, neurologic deficits:** Assessment and treatment

Infectious Disease

- **Infections** (especially wound, pneumonia, otitis media, and sepsis): Antibiotics

Hematologic

- **Anemia:** Iron supplementation, possible transfusion
- **Postoperative bleeding:** Initially, clotting factors, blood products; may need repeat surgery to locate and ligate source of bleeding

Other

- **Postpericardiotomy syndrome** (syndrome of fever, leukocytosis, friction rub, pericardial and pleural effusions, lethargy seen about 7 to 21 days after cardiac surgery; possible viral or autoimmune etiologies): Antipyretics, diuretics, antiinflammatory medications

surgery from hypothermia procedures, effects of anesthesia, and loss of body heat to the cool environment. During this period the child is kept warm to prevent additional heat loss. Infants may be placed under radiant heat warmers. During the next 24 to 48 hours the body temperature may rise to 37.7° C (100° F) or slightly higher as part of the inflammatory response to tissue trauma. After this period, an elevated temperature is most likely a sign of infection and warrants immediate investigation for probable cause.

Maintain Respiratory Status

Infants usually require mechanical ventilation in the immediate postoperative period. Early extubation in the operating room or early postoperative period is becoming more common. Children may be extubated in the operating room or in the first few postoperative hours, especially children who did not require cardiopulmonary bypass. Suctioning is performed only as needed and performed carefully to avoid vagal stimulation (which can trigger cardiac dysrhythmias) and laryngospasm, especially in infants. Suctioning is intermittent and maintained for no more than 5 seconds at a time to prevent depleting the oxygen supply. Supplemental oxygen is administered with a manual resuscitation bag before and after the procedure to prevent hypoxia. The heart rate is monitored after suctioning to detect changes in rhythm or rate, especially bradycardia. The child should always be positioned facing the nurse to permit assessment of the child's color and tolerance of the procedure.

<u>NURSE ALERT</u> During suctioning, observe for signs and symptoms of respiratory distress, such as tachypnea, use of accessory muscles for breathing, and restlessness. ■

When weaning and extubation are completed, humidified oxygen is delivered by mask, hood, or nasal cannula to prevent drying of mucosa. The child is encouraged to turn and deep breathe at least hourly. Every measure is employed to enhance ventilation and decrease pain, such as splinting of the operative site and use of analgesics. Chest tubes are inserted into the pleural or mediastinal space during surgery or in the immediate postoperative period to remove secretions and air to allow reexpansion of the lung. Drainage is checked hourly for color and quantity. Immediately after surgery the drainage may be bright red, but afterward it should be serous. The largest volume of drainage occurs in the first 12 to 24 hours and is greater in extensive heart surgery.

<u>NURSE ALERT</u> Chest tube drainage greater than 3 ml/kg/hr for more than 3 consecutive hours or 5 to 10 ml/kg in any 1 hour is excessive and may indicate postoperative hemorrhage. The surgeon is notified immediately because cardiac tamponade can develop rapidly and is life threatening. ■

Chest tubes are usually removed on the first to third postoperative day. Removal of chest tubes is a painful, frightening experience. Analgesics such as morphine sulfate, often combined with midazolam (Versed), should be given before the procedure. Older children are forewarned that they will feel a sharp, momentary pain. After the suture is cut, the tubes are quickly pulled out at the end of full inspiration to prevent intake of air into the pleural cavity. A purse-string suture (placed when the tubes were inserted) is pulled tight to close the opening. A petrolatum-covered gauze dressing is immediately applied over the wound and securely taped on all four sides to the skin so that an airtight seal is formed. The dressing is checked for signs of drainage and any evidence of infection.

Monitor Fluids

Intake and output of all fluids must be accurately calculated. Intake is primarily IV fluids; however, a record of fluid used to flush the arterial and CVP lines or to dilute medications is also kept. Output includes hourly recordings of urine (usually a Foley catheter is inserted and attached to a closed collecting device), drainage from chest and nasogastric tubes, and blood drawn for analysis. Urine is analyzed for specific gravity to assess the concentrating ability of the kidneys and to assess the body's approximate degree of hydration. Renal failure is a potential risk from a transient period of low cardiac output.

NURSE ALERT The signs of renal failure are decreased urine output (less than 1 ml/kg/hr) and elevated levels of blood urea nitrogen and serum creatinine. ■

Fluids are restricted during the immediate postoperative period to prevent hypervolemia, which places additional demands on the myocardium, predisposing to cardiac failure. To monitor fluid retention, the child is weighed daily, and the same scale is used at approximately the same time each day to avoid errors in measurement. The child is usually given nothing by mouth for the first 24 hours. If an ET tube is inserted, oral fluids are usually withheld until the child is extubated. Fluid restriction may be imposed even when oral fluids are given. The nurse calculates the distribution over a 24-hour period based on the child's preoperative weight and drinking habits. The distribution should allow for most fluid to be given during the child's most wakeful and active periods.

Provide Rest and Progressive Activity

After heart surgery, rest should be provided to decrease the workload of the heart and promote healing. The simplest way to ensure individualized, efficient, high-quality care is to plan at the beginning of the shift the nursing procedures to be done, with periods of rest identified. The schedule should be shared with parents to allow them to visit at the most advantageous times, such as after a rest period when no special treatments are anticipated.

A progressive schedule of ambulation and activity is planned, based on the child's preoperative activity patterns and postoperative cardiovascular and pulmonary function. Ambulation is initiated early, usually by the second postoperative day, when chest tubes, arterial lines, and assisted ventilatory equipment may be removed. Activity progresses from sitting on the edge of the bed and dangling the legs to standing up and to sitting in a chair. Heart rate and respirations are carefully monitored to assess the degree of cardiac demand imposed by each activity. Tachycardia, dyspnea, cyanosis, desaturation, progressive fatigue, or dysrhythmias indicate the need to limit further energy expenditure.

Provide Comfort and Emotional Support

Heart surgery is both painful and frightening for children, and comfort is a primary nursing concern. Continuous IV opioid infusions, particularly morphine and fentanyl, are safe and effective analgesics. Patient-controlled analgesia may be used with children old enough to understand the concept. Nonsteroidal antiinflammatory drugs (NSAIDs) such as ketorolac (Toradol) may be used intravenously. Epidural morphine may be another option, because it affords very good pain control when a thoracotomy is performed. Paralyzing agents such as pancuronium (Pavulon) or metocurine (Metubine) may also be used with the analgesics for children who are very agitated or hemodynamically unstable.

Most patients need IV analgesics for pain control during the immediate postoperative period. After extubation and removal of lines and tubes, pain can be satisfactorily controlled with oral medications such as ibuprofen, codeine with acetaminophen (Tylenol), or oxycodone and acetaminophen (Tylox). Acetaminophen alone provides adequate pain relief for most children at discharge. Sternotomy incisions are usually well tolerated, with some discomfort when walking and coughing. Thoracotomy incisions are usually more painful because the incision is through muscle; a more aggressive pain management plan with around-the-clock medications for several days is often necessary to allow for adequate rest, ambulation, and pulmonary hygiene.

In addition to pharmacologic pain control, every effort is made to minimize the discomfort of procedures, such as using a firm pillow or favorite stuffed animal placed against the chest incision during movement and performing treatments *after* pain medication is given, preferably at a time that coincides with the drug's peak effect. Nonpharmacologic measures are used to lessen the perception of pain, and parents are encouraged to comfort their child as much as possible. (See also Pain Assessment: Pain Management, Chapter 44.)

The first few postoperative days are particularly difficult because parents see their child in pain and realize the potential risks from surgery. They often are overwhelmed by the physical environment of the ICU and feel useless because they can do so little for their child. The importance of their presence in making the child feel more secure is stressed, even if they do not provide physical care.

Plan for Discharge and Home Care

Ideally, discharge planning begins on admission for cardiac surgery and includes an assessment of the parents' adjustment to the child's altered state of health. The family will need both verbal and written instructions on medication, nutrition, activity restrictions, subacute bacterial endocarditis, return to school, wound care, and signs and symptoms of infection or complications (Home Care box). Referrals to community agencies may be warranted to assist parents in the transition from hospital to home and to reinforce the teaching.

The parents will also need clear instructions on when to seek medical care, such as for a change in the child's behavior or an unexplained fever. Follow-up with the cardiologist is also arranged before discharge. Appropriate identification, such as a MedicAlert device, is indicated for children with a pacemaker or a heart transplant and for those receiving anticoagulation therapy or antidysrhythmic medication.

Home Care

TOPICS TO INCLUDE IN DISCHARGE TEACHING AFTER CARDIAC SURGERY

Medication teaching (for digoxin, see Home Care box, p. 1572)
Activity restrictions
Diet and nutrition
Wound care (include dressings if any, suture removal, bathing)
Bacterial endocarditis prophylaxis (see Box 48-9)
Follow-up appointments (cardiologist, primary care provider)
Community agencies as needed (visiting nurse service, early developmental intervention)
When to call practitioner; signs and symptoms of postoperative problems
Review of cardiac defect and surgical repair

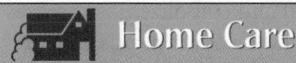

The nurse also discusses common behavior disturbances that may occur after discharge, such as nightmares, sleep disturbances, separation anxiety, and overdependence. A supportive, consistent response is essential to allow the child to overcome the surgical experience. The child should be encouraged to work out feelings and fears through therapeutic play.

Although surgical correction of heart defects has improved dramatically, it is still not possible to completely repair many of the complex anomalies. For many children, repeat procedures are required to replace conduits or grafts or to manage complications such as restenosis. Consequently, the long-term prognosis is uncertain, and full recovery is not always possible. For these families, medical follow-up and continued emotional support are essential. The nurse can often serve as an important primary health professional and as a resource for referrals when needed.

BOX 48-8

Clinical Manifestations of Infective Endocarditis

Onset usually insidious
Unexplained fever (low grade and intermittent)
Anorexia
Malaise
Weight loss
Characteristic findings caused by extracardiac emboli formation:
- Splinter hemorrhages (thin black lines) under the nails
- Osler nodes (red, painful intradermal nodes found on pads of phalanges)
- Janeway lesions (painless hemorrhagic areas on palms and soles)
- Petechiae on oral mucous membranes

May be present:
- Congestive heart failure
- Cardiac dysrhythmias
- New murmur or change in previously existing one

ACQUIRED CARDIOVASCULAR DISORDERS

Bacterial (Infective) Endocarditis

Bacterial endocarditis (BE), or *infective endocarditis (IE),* also referred to as *subacute bacterial endocarditis (SBE),* is an infection of the valves and inner lining of the heart. Although it can occur without underlying heart disease, it is most often a sequela of bacteremia in the child with acquired or congenital anomalies of the heart or great vessels. It especially affects children with valvular abnormalities, prosthetic valves, recent cardiac surgery with invasive lines, and rheumatic heart disease with valve involvement. The most common causative agent is *Streptococcus viridans;* other causative agents are *Staphylococcus aureus,* gram-negative bacteria, and fungi such as *Candida albicans.*

Pathophysiology

Organisms may enter the bloodstream from any site of localized infection. The most common portals of entry are oral from dental work *(S. viridans);* the urinary tract, such as from urinary tract infection after catheterization (gram-negative bacilli); the heart, from cardiac surgery, especially if synthetic material is used (valves, patches, conduits); and the bloodstream from long-term indwelling catheters. The microorganisms grow on the endocardium, forming vegetations (verrucae), deposits of fibrin, and platelet thrombi. The lesion may invade adjacent tissues, such as aortic and mitral valves, and may break off and embolize elsewhere, especially in the spleen, kidney, and central nervous system.

Diagnostic Evaluation

The diagnosis of IE is suspected on the basis of clinical manifestations (Box 48-8). Several laboratory findings may suggest IE (e.g., ECG changes [prolonged P-R interval], radiographic evidence of cardiomegaly, anemia, elevated erythrocyte sedimentation rate, leukocytosis, microscopic hematuria). Vegetations on the valve and abnormal valve function can often be visualized by echocardiography. Definitive diagnosis rests on growth and identification of the causative agent in the blood.

Therapeutic Management

Treatment should be instituted immediately and consists of administration of high doses of appropriate antibiotics intravenously for 2 to 8 weeks. Blood cultures are taken periodically to evaluate response to antibiotic therapy.

Prevention involves administration of prophylactic antibiotic therapy 1 hour before procedures known to increase the risk of entry of organisms. Drugs of choice include amoxicillin, ampicillin, clindamycin, cephalexin, cefadroxil, azithromycin, and clarithromycin (Box 48-9).

Nursing Care Management

Ideally, the objective of nursing care is to counsel parents of high risk children concerning the need for prophylactic antibiotic therapy before procedures such as dental work. The family's regular dentist should be advised of existing cardiac problems in the child as an added precaution to ensure preventive treatment. These children should also maintain the highest level of oral health to reduce the chance of bacteremia from oral infections.

Parents should also have a high index of suspicion regarding potential infections. Without unduly alarming them, the nurse stresses that any unexplained fever, weight loss, or change in behavior (lethargy, malaise, anorexia) must be brought to the practitioner's attention. Such symptoms should not be self-diagnosed as a cold or flu. Early treatment is important in preventing further cardiac damage, embolic complications, and growth of resistant organisms.

Treatment of endocarditis requires long-term parenteral drug therapy. In many cases, IV antibiotics may be administered at home with nursing supervision for part of the treatment course. Nursing goals during this period are (1) preparation of the child for IV infusion, usually with an intermittent-infusion device, and several venipunctures for blood cultures; (2) observation for side effects of antibiotics, especially inflammation along venipuncture sites; (3) observation for complications, including embolism and CHF; and (4) education regarding the importance of follow-up visits for cardiac evaluation, echocardiographic monitoring, and blood cultures.

BOX 48-9

Endocarditis Prophylaxis Recommendations

Dental Procedures
Dental extractions
Periodontal procedures, including surgery, scaling and root planing, probing, and recall maintenance
Dental implant placement and reimplantation of avulsed teeth
Endodontic (root canal) instrumentation or surgery only beyond the apex
Subgingival placement of antibiotic fibers/strips
Initial placement of orthodontic bands but not brackets
Intraligamentary local anesthetic injections
Prophylactic cleaning of teeth or implants where bleeding is anticipated

Other Procedures
Respiratory Tract
Surgeries that involve respiratory mucosa
Bronchoscopy with a rigid bronchoscope
Tonsillectomy and/or adenoidectomy

Gastrointestinal Tract
Sclerotherapy for esophageal varices
Esophageal stricture dilation
Endoscopic retrograde cholangiography with biliary obstruction
Biliary tract surgery
Surgical operations that involve intestinal mucosa

Genitourinary Tract
Prostatic surgery
Cystoscopy
Urethral dilation

From Dajani AS et al: Prevention of bacterial endocarditis: recommendations by the American Heart Association, *JAMA* 277:1794-1801, 1997.

Rheumatic Fever

Rheumatic fever (RF) is a poorly understood inflammatory disease that occurs after infection with group A β-hemolytic streptococcal pharyngitis. It is a self-limited illness that involves the joints, skin, brain, serous surfaces, and heart. Cardiac valve damage (referred to as *rheumatic heart disease*) is the most significant complication of RF. In developed countries, RF and rheumatic heart disease have become uncommon. However, RF remains a devastating problem in developing countries and has reappeared in some parts of the United States (Gentles et al, 2001).

Etiology

Strong evidence supports a relationship between upper respiratory infection with group A streptococci and subsequent development of RF (usually within 2 to 6 weeks). In almost all cases of RF, a previous infection with group A streptococci can be documented by laboratory evidence of rising antibody titers. Prevention or treatment of group A streptococcal infection prevents RF.

Diagnostic Evaluation

Diagnosis is based on a set of guidelines recommended by the American Heart Association. These guidelines, known as *modifications of the Jones criteria,* suggest that the presence of two major manifestations or one major and two minor manifestations, such as fever and arthralgia, with supportive evidence of recent streptococcal infection, indicates a high probability of RF (Guidelines box).

Guidelines

DIAGNOSIS OF INITIAL ATTACK OF RHEUMATIC FEVER (JONES CRITERIA, 1992 UPDATE)*

Major Manifestations
Carditis
Tachycardia out of proportion to degree of fever
Cardiomegaly
New murmurs or change in preexisting murmurs
Muffled heart sounds
Pericardial friction rub
Chest pain
Changes in ECG (especially prolonged P-R interval)

Polyarthritis
Swollen, hot, red, painful joint(s)
After 1 to 2 days affects different joint(s)
Favors large joints—knees, elbows, hips, shoulders, wrists

Erythema Marginatum
Erythematous macules with clear center and wavy, well-demarcated border
Transitory
Nonpruritic
Primarily affects trunk and extremities (inner surfaces)

Chorea (St. Vitus Dance, Sydenham chorea)
Sudden aimless, irregular movements of extremities
Involuntary facial grimaces
Speech disturbances
Emotional lability
Muscle weakness (can be profound)
Muscle movements exaggerated by anxiety and attempts at fine motor activity; relieved by rest

Subcutaneous Nodes
Nontender swelling
Located over bony prominences
May persist for some time, then gradually resolve

Minor Manifestations
Clinical findings
  Arthralgia
  Fever

Laboratory Findings
Elevated acute-phase reactants
  Erythrocyte sedimentation rate
  C-reactive protein

Supporting Evidence of Antecedent Group A Streptococcal Infection
Positive throat culture or rapid streptococcal antigen test
  Elevated or rising streptococcal antibody titer

From Special Writing Group of the Committee on Rheumatic Fever, Endocarditis, and Kawasaki Disease of the Council on Cardiovascular Disease in the Young of the American Heart Association: Guidelines for the diagnosis of rheumatic fever: Jones criteria, 1992 (update), *JAMA* 268:2069-2073, 1992.
*If supported by evidence of preceding group A streptococcal infection, the presence of two major manifestations or of one major and two minor manifestations indicates a high probability of acute rheumatic fever.

Children suspected of having RF are tested for streptococcal antibodies. The most reliable and best standardized test is an elevated or rising *antistreptolysin-O (ASO* or *ASLO) titer,* which occurs in 80% of children with RF.

Therapeutic Management

The goals of medical management are (1) eradication of hemolytic streptococci, (2) prevention of permanent cardiac damage, (3) palliation of the other symptoms, and (4) prevention of recurrences of RF. Penicillin is the drug of choice, with erythromycin as a substitute in penicillin-sensitive children. Salicylates are used to control the inflammatory process, especially in the joints, and reduce the fever and discomfort. Bed rest is recommended during the acute febrile phase but need not be strict.

Prophylactic treatment against recurrence of RF is started after the acute therapy and involves monthly intramuscular injections of benzathine penicillin G (1.2 million units), two daily oral doses of penicillin (200,000 units), or one daily dose of sulfadiazine (1 g). The duration of long-term prophylaxis is uncertain.

Children who have had acute RF are susceptible to recurrent RF for the rest of their lives and should be followed medically for at least 5 years. Children and families must be aware of the need for continuing antibiotic prophylaxis for dental work, infection, and invasive procedures.

Nursing Care Management

The objectives of nursing care for the child with RF are to (1) encourage compliance with drug regimens, (2) facilitate recovery from the illness, (3) provide emotional support, and (4) prevent the disease. Because compliance is a major concern in long-term drug therapy, every effort is made to encourage adherence to the therapeutic plan (see Compliance, Chapter 45). When compliance is poor, monthly injections may be substituted for daily oral administration of antibiotics, and children need preparation for this often-dreaded procedure.

Interventions during home care are primarily concerned with providing rest and adequate nutrition. Usually, after the febrile stage is over, children can resume moderate activity, and their appetite improves. If carditis is present, the family must be aware of any activity restrictions and may need help in choosing less strenuous activities for the child.

One of the most disturbing and frustrating manifestations of the disease is *chorea.* The onset is gradual and may occur weeks to months after the illness; it sometimes even occurs in children who have not been diagnosed with RF. It may be mistaken for nervousness, clumsiness, behavioral changes, inattentiveness, and learning disability. It is usually a source of great frustration to the child because the movements, incoordination, and weakness severely limit physical ability. The child needs an opportunity to verbalize feelings. Of utmost importance is stressing to parents and schoolteachers the involuntary, sudden nature of the movements, that the chorea is transitory, and that all manifestations eventually disappear.

Nurses also have a role in prevention, primarily in screening school-age children for sore throats caused by group A streptococci. This may involve actively participating in throat culture screening programs or in referring children with a possible streptococcal infection for testing.

Hyperlipidemia (Hypercholesterolemia)

Hyperlipidemia is a general term for excessive lipids (fat and fatlike substances); *hypercholesterolemia* refers to excessive cholesterol in the blood. High lipid or cholesterol levels are believed to play an important role in producing atherosclerosis (fatty plaques on the arteries), which eventually can lead to coronary artery disease, a primary cause of morbidity and mortality in the adult population. Research indicates that a presymptomatic phase of atherosclerosis begins in childhood. Preventive cardiology is focusing on the screening and management of lipid levels in childhood. The goal is to identify those children at high risk and intervene early.

Cholesterol is part of the lipoprotein complex in plasma that is essential for cellular metabolism. Triglycerides, natural fats synthesized from carbohydrates, are used for energy. Both are major lipids transported on *lipoproteins,* a combination of lipids and proteins, which include the following:

Low-density lipoproteins (LDLs)—Contain low concentrations of triglycerides, high levels of cholesterol, and moderate levels of protein. LDL is the major carrier of cholesterol to the cells. Cells use cholesterol for synthesis of membranes and steroid production. Elevated circulating LDL is a strong risk factor in cardiovascular disease.

High-density lipoproteins (HDLs)—Contain very low concentrations of triglycerides, relatively little cholesterol, and high levels of protein. They transport free cholesterol to the liver for excretion in the bile. High levels of HDL are thought to protect against cardiovascular disease.

Diagnostic Evaluation

Hyperlipidemia is diagnosed on the basis of analysis of blood for a full lipid profile. Two samples drawn in the fasting state (12 hours) should be analyzed, and the average of the values used for diagnosis. Blood samples should be collected after having the child sit for 5 minutes. The tourniquet should be applied immediately before the needle puncture, because posture and vascular stasis may affect results. Diagnostic values for acceptable, borderline, and high total cholesterol and LDL cholesterol levels are listed in Table 48-5.

Screening children for hypercholesterolemia is a controversial issue, with some authorities advocating universal screening and others proposing selective screening. Guidelines recommended by the American Academy of Pediatrics (1998) recommend a strategy that combines two comple-

Table 48-5

Classification of Cholesterol Levels in Children from Families with a History of Heart Disease

CATEGORY	TOTAL CHOLESTEROL (mg/dl)	LDL CHOLESTEROL (mg/dl)
Acceptable	<170	<110
Borderline	170-199	110-129
High	≥200	≥130

From National Cholesterol Education Program: Report of the Expert Panel on Blood Cholesterol Levels in Children and Adolescents, *Pediatrics* 89(3 pt 2):527, 1992.

mentary approaches: (1) a *population approach* that aims to lower the average levels of blood cholesterol among all American children through population-wide changes in nutrient intake and eating patterns, and (2) an *individualized approach* based on selective screening (Evidence-Based Practice).

Therapeutic Management

Treatment of high cholesterol is primarily dietary. The American Academy of Pediatrics guidelines recommend a two-step dietary approach that restricts the intake of cholesterol and fat. Children with borderline LDL cholesterol are advised to follow the *step-one diet.* It recommends the same nutrient intake as for the general population (i.e., less than 10% of total calories from saturated fatty acids, no more than 30% of calories from total fat, less than 300 mg/day of cholesterol, and adequate calories to support growth and development and to reach or maintain desirable body weight). Children with high LDL cholesterol levels initially are also placed on this diet. If these dietary modifications fail to achieve satisfactory levels of LDL after 3 months of therapy, the *step-two diet* is initiated. These dietary restrictions include a further reduction of saturated fatty acid intake to 7% of calories and of cholesterol intake to less than 200 mg/day.

New research continues to support the benefit of diets low in saturated fats. Current thinking favors a "Mediterranean"-type diet. Whole grains, fruits, and vegetables form the foundation of this diet. In addition, this diet allows the use of monounsaturated fats, such as olive oil and canola oil, which have beneficial effects on HDL-cholesterol values. The use of these fats also makes the diet more realistic.

NURSE ALERT The Report of the Expert Panel on Blood Cholesterol Levels in Children and Adolescents regarding recommendations for fat intake are not intended for infants from birth to 2 years of age, whose fast growth requires a higher percentage of calories from fat. Toddlers 2 to 3 years of age may safely make the transition to the recommended eating pattern as they begin to eat with the family. No treatment recommendations are made for any child younger than 2 years of age. ■

For children with severe hypercholesterolemia who fail to respond to dietary modifications, drug therapy may be necessary. Two drugs recommended for treatment are the bile acid–binding resins or sequestrants *cholestyramine* and *colestipol.* These two drugs act by binding bile acids in the intestinal lumen. Because they are not absorbed by the intestine, they do not produce systemic toxicity and are safe for children. Cholestyramine (Questran) and colestipol (Colestid) are both powders that are mixed with water or juice just before ingestion. Some patients cannot tolerate the medication because of the taste and the side effects, the most significant being constipation, abdominal pain, gastrointestinal bloating, flatulence, and nausea.

Patients should be instructed to take one multivitamin supplement with iron daily, because cholestyramine may interfere with the absorption of fat-soluble vitamins. It may also interfere with the absorption of other medications, which should be given at least 1 hour before or 6 hours after the resin-binding agent is ingested.

Nursing Care Management

Nurses play an important role in the screening, education, and support of children with hyperlipidemia and their families. When a child is referred to a lipid clinic, it is essential that the family be adequately prepared for the first visit. Generally, the parents will be asked to keep a dietary history of the child before this visit. Sometimes they will need to complete a questionnaire regarding the child's normal dietary habits during the preceding year. Families should be instructed to keep their child fasting for at least 12 hours before screening. It is important to schedule the blood test early in the morning and to arrange for nourishment immediately thereafter. At the visit, a full family history should be taken, including the health of both parents and all first-degree relatives. Specific questions should be asked regard-

Evidence-Based Practice

CHOLESTEROL SCREENING FOR CHILDREN

Practitioners' opinions differ regarding lipid screening in childhood. In 1992 the National Cholesterol Education Program (NCEP) issued a consensus statement that provides guidelines for cholesterol screening in the pediatric population. Currently, selective screening is recommended for children who have a family history of premature cardiovascular disease (younger than 55 years old) or children who have at least one parent with a high blood cholesterol level (greater than 240 mg/dl). In addition, if a child's complete family history is not available, practitioners may consider screening. Finally, cholesterol values should be obtained in children who have any individual risk factors, such as a history of diabetes, Kawasaki disease, hypertension, or obesity.

Selective screening is favored by many experts because high blood cholesterol levels aggregate in families as a result of shared genetic and environmental factors (American Academy of Pediatrics, 1998). In addition, the most severely affected children generally come from families in which there is a high incidence of early heart disease.

Advocates of selective screening oppose universal screening for various reasons. Screening is costly, and the laboratory data may vary significantly from center to center, resulting in inappropriate diagnosis.

Those favoring universal screening believe that selective screening is too limited and overlooks many children with hyperlipidemia. With varying family constellations a common situation today, family history may be incomplete. In addition, a negative history from a parent may be inaccurate, because approximately half of well-educated adults do not know their own cholesterol levels.

In your practice, how many adult family members know their "numbers"? Also, observe how often pediatric practitioners ask about parents' cholesterol levels and heart disease as part of the child's health assessment. From your observations, do you believe that selective screening is being implemented?

ing early heart disease, hypertension, strokes (CVAs), sudden death, hyperlipidemia, diabetes, and endocrine abnormalities. Nurses may also uncover risk factors when obtaining a health history for other purposes. It is therefore important that nurses be familiar with current screening practices and the availability of resources for children with positive family histories.

Parents and extended families should be informed about cholesterol and hyperlipidemia. This education should include a brief introduction to the different lipoprotein categories, including cholesterol, HDL, LDL, and triglycerides. Also, behavioral risk factors for heart disease, such as smoking and exercise, should be reviewed. For management to be effective, parents need to understand the rationale for dietary or pharmacologic intervention. The key is prevention of future cardiovascular disease.

Stringent dietary guidelines may become an issue of control and a source of great stress for many families. Children should not be viewed as having a disease. Rather, the positive aspects of healthy eating, regular exercise, and avoiding smoking should be emphasized. Basic dietary changes should be encouraged for the whole family so that the affected child is not singled out. Cultural differences must be considered and recommendations individualized. Substitution rather than elimination needs to be emphasized. Visual aids are often helpful, especially for the children (e.g., test tubes depicting the amount of fat in a hot dog). Diets should be flexible and individually tailored by a nutritionist experienced in combining recommendations that meet both the nutritional demands of the growing child and the lipid modifications. Parents are encouraged to participate in dietary and educational sessions, ask questions, and share ideas and experiences.

Parents often feel guilty about the hereditary component of hyperlipidemia. Many also believe they have failed if the diet alone is not making a significant difference in their child's lipid profile. They need to be reassured that a dietary approach alone is often not sufficient, especially for children with values greater than the 95th percentile.

Parents of children who require pharmacologic therapy need to understand the purpose, dosage, and possible side effects of the various drugs. Medication schedules should remain flexible and should not interfere with the child's daily activities. For example, children of elementary school age may have better compliance if they take a resin-binding agent (e.g., cholestyramine, colestipol) twice a day (i.e., before school and at night) rather than the standard three times a day.

Cardiac Dysrhythmias

Dysrhythmias, or *abnormal heart rhythms,* can occur in children with structurally normal hearts, as features of some congenital heart defects, and in patients after surgical repair of congenital heart defects. They are also seen in patients with cardiomyopathy and with cardiac tumors. They can occur secondary to metabolic and electrolyte imbalances. They can be classified in several ways, including by heart rate characteristics (bradycardia and tachycardia) or by the origin of the dysrhythmia in the atria or ventricles (Hanisch, 2001). Some dysrhythmias are well tolerated and self-limiting. Others may cause decreased cardiac output with associated symptoms. Some dysrhythmias can cause sudden death. Treatment depends on the cause of the dysrhythmia and its severity. Many advances have been made in the diagnosis and treatment of pediatric dysrhythmias in the past decade. Improvements in technology have allowed better diagnosis, the development of ablation techniques, and the expansion of pacemaker capabilities. New anti-arrhythmic medications have proven safe and effective in children. Radiofrequency ablation has offered a cure for some dysrhythmias. Pediatric electrophysiology has become a highly specialized field, and the student is referred to more detailed sources for an in-depth discussion. The following sections address diagnostic studies and the most common forms of tachycardia (supraventricular tachycardia [SVT]) and bradycardia (complete heart block) that require treatment in the pediatric population.

Diagnostic Evaluation

Nurses must be familiar with the standards of normal heart rate for the particular age group (see Appendix J). An initial nursing responsibility is recognition of an abnormal heartbeat, either in rate or rhythm. When a dysrhythmia is suspected, the apical rate is counted for a full minute and compared with the radial rate, which may be lower because not all of the apical beats are felt. Consistently high or low heart rates should be regarded as suspicious. The patient should be placed on a cardiac monitor with recording capabilities. A 12-lead ECG yields more information than the monitor recording and should be done as soon as possible.

The basic diagnostic procedure is the ECG, including 24-hour Holter monitoring. *Electrophysiologic cardiac catheterization* allows for identification of the conduction disturbance and immediate investigation of drugs that may control the dysrhythmia. Another procedure that may be employed is *transesophageal recording.* An electrode catheter is passed to the lower esophagus and, when in position at a point proximal to the heart, is used to stimulate and record dysrhythmias.

Classification

Dysrhythmias can be classified according to various criteria, such as effect on heart rate and rhythm, as follows:

Bradydysrhythmias—abnormally slow rate
Tachydysrhythmias—abnormally rapid rate
Conduction disturbances—irregular heart rate

Bradydysrhythmias

Sinus bradycardia (slower than normal rate) in children can be due to the influence of the autonomic nervous system, as with hypervagal tone, or can occur in response to hypoxia and hypotension (Hanisch, 2001). Sinus bradycardias are also known to develop after some complex cardiac surgical repairs involving extensive atrial suture lines such as atrial baffle repairs (Mustard and Senning repairs) and the Fontan procedure.

Complete atrioventricular block (AV block) is also referred to as *complete heart block.* This can be either congenital (occurring in children with structurally normal hearts) or acquired after surgery to repair cardiac defects. AV blocks are most often related to edema around the conduction system and resolve without treatment. Temporary epicardial wires are placed in most patients at surgery; if a rhythm disturbance occurs, temporary pacing can be employed. Several days after surgery, the health practitioner removes the wires by pulling slowly and deliberately down on them from the site of insertion.

A permanent pacemaker may be needed in some children. The pacemaker takes over or assists in the conduction function of the heart. The surgical implantation of a pacemaker is usually a low risk procedure. After the wire has been introduced, a small incision is made and a pocket is formed under the muscle to house and protect the generator. Continuous ECG monitoring is necessary during the recovery phase to assess pacemaker function. The nurse should be aware of the programmed rate and expected individual generator variations. The pacemaker insertion site is monitored for signs of infection. Analgesics are given for pain.

Pacemaker functions have become more sophisticated, and some models can adjust heart rate to activity demands or be programmed for overdrive pacing or cardioversion.

When a pacemaker is implanted, the education of the parents and child includes an explanation of the device, a description of the component parts and the surgical procedure, and discharge teaching. For example, discharge teaching includes information about the signs and symptoms of infection, general wound care, and any specific limitations to activity. Instructions for telephone transmission of ECG readings are also given. Children with pacemakers should wear a medical alert device, and their parents should have a pacer identification card with specific pacer data in case of an emergency.

Discharge teaching includes information about the signs and symptoms of infection, general wound care, and activity restrictions. Parents and older children and adolescents should be taught to take a pulse and know the settings of the pacemaker. If the patient's low rate is set at 80 and the heart rate is only 68, there is a problem with the pacemaker that needs to be investigated. Instructions for telephone transmission of ECG readings are also given. Telephone transmission can be used to transmit ECG strips and also to monitor battery life and pacemaker function. The pacemaker generator will have to be replaced periodically because of battery depletion. Children with pacemakers should wear a medical-alert device, and their parents should have a pacemaker identification card with specific pacer data in case of emergency. Cardiopulmonary resuscitation (CPR) instruction is suggested for parents.

Tachydysrhythmias

Sinus tachycardia (abnormally fast heart rate) secondary to fever, anxiety, pain, anemia, dehydration, or any other etiologic factor requiring increased cardiac output should be ruled out first before diagnosing an increased heart rate as pathologic. SVT is the most common tachydysrhythmia found in children and refers to a rapid, regular heart rate of 200 to 300 beats per minute (Hanisch, 2001). The onset of SVT is often sudden, the duration is variable, and the rhythm may end abruptly and convert back to a normal sinus rhythm. Clinical signs in infants and young children are poor feeding, extreme irritability, and pallor. Children may experience palpitations, dizziness, chest pain, and diaphoresis. If SVT is sustained, signs of CHF may be seen.

The treatment of SVT depends on the degree of compromise imposed by the dysrhythmia. In some cases, vagal maneuvers, such as applying ice to the face, massaging the carotid artery (on one side of the neck only), or having an older child perform a Valsalva maneuver (e.g., exhaling against a closed glottis, blowing on a thumb as if it were a trumpet for 30 to 60 seconds), have terminated SVT. If vagal maneuvers fail or the child is hemodynamically unstable, adenosine (a drug that impairs AV conduction) may be used. Adenosine is given by rapid IV push with a saline bolus immediately after the drug because of its very short half-life. If this is unsuccessful or cardiac output is compromised, esophageal overdrive pacing or synchronized cardioversion (delivering an electrical shock to the heart) can be employed in the intensive care setting (Hanisch, 2001). Sedation is needed for both procedures. Cardioversion should never be done in a conscious patient. More long-term pharmacologic treatment includes digoxin or possibly Inderal or amiodarone for severe or recurrent SVT.

A primary focus of nursing care is education of the family regarding the symptoms of SVT and its treatment. SVT may occur again despite therapy. Parents should be taught to take a radial pulse for a full minute. If medication is prescribed, instructions regarding accurate dosage and the importance of administering the correct dose at specified intervals are stressed.

Radiofrequency ablation has become first-line therapy for some types of SVT. The procedure is done in the cardiac catheterization laboratory and begins with mapping of the conduction system to identify the dysrhythmia focus. A catheter delivering radiofrequency current is directed at the site, and the area is heated to destroy the tissue in the area. These are lengthy procedures, often 6 to 8 hours, and sedation or general anesthesia is required. Preparation is similar to that for cardiac catheterization.

Conduction Disturbances

Most rhythm disturbances are seen postoperatively in the child undergoing cardiac surgery and are of little significance. AV blocks are most often related to treatment. Temporary epicardial wires are placed in most patients at surgery; if a rhythm disturbance occurs, temporary pacing can be used.

Pulmonary Artery Hypertension

Pulmonary artery hypertension (PAH) describes a group of rare disorders that result in an elevation of pulmonary artery pressure above 25 mm Hg at rest after the neonatal period (Barst, 1999). These disorders are poorly understood, and until recently there was no treatment beyond supportive care. PAH is a progressive, eventually fatal disease for which there is no known cure. It can be difficult to diagnose in the early stages. Often when patients become symptomatic and a diagnosis is made, their disease is rapidly progressing, treatment is unsuccessful, and death occurs within several years.

PAH can be caused by increased pulmonary blood flow or increased pulmonary vascular resistance. Why some children develop the disease and others do not is unclear. There are many possible causes of PAH. Cardiac causes occur primarily in patients with a large left-to-right shunt producing increased pulmonary blood flow. If these defects are not repaired early, the high pulmonary flow will cause changes in the pulmonary artery vessels and the vessels will lose their elasticity. Other causes of PAH include hypoxic lung diseases, thromboembolic diseases causing pulmonary vascular obstruction, collagen vascular diseases, and exposure to toxic substances. Many of the patients have no identifiable cause for PAH and have primary or idiopathic PAH.

Clinical Manifestations

The clinical manifestations include dyspnea with exercise, chest pain, and syncope. Dyspnea is the most common symptom and is caused by impaired oxygen delivery. Chest pain is the result of coronary ischemia in the right ventricle from severe hypertrophy. Syncope reflects a limited cardiac output leading to decreased cerebral blood flow. Right-sided heart dysfunction is steadily progressive, and when symptoms of venous congestion and edema are present, prognosis is poor.

Therapeutic Management

Although no cure is known, several therapies have shown promise in slowing the progression of the disease and improving quality of life. In general, situations that may exacerbate the disease and cause hypoxia, such as exercise and high altitudes, are avoided. Supplemental oxygen, especially at night while sleeping, is commonly used to relieve hypoxia. Patients are at risk for thromboembolic events leading to pulmonary emboli, so anticoagulation with Coumadin is often prescribed.

Vasodilator therapy (which relaxes vascular smooth muscle and reduces pulmonary artery pressure) has improved the survival of patients with PAH. Oral calcium-channel blockers have been successful in some children. Continuous IV prostacyclin and chronic inhaled nitric oxide have been used with some success in children who did not respond to oral therapy. Both of these therapies, although promising, have only been used in small numbers of patients and are very expensive. Lung transplantation may be another treatment option.

Cardiomyopathy

Cardiomyopathy refers to abnormalities of the myocardium in which the cardiac muscles' ability to contract is impaired. Cardiomyopathies are relatively rare in children. Possible etiologic factors include familial or genetic causes, infection, deficiency states, metabolic abnormalities, and collagen vascular diseases. Most cardiomyopathies in children are considered primary or idiopathic, in which the cause is unknown and the cardiac dysfunction is not associated with systemic disease. Some of the known causes of *secondary* cardiomyopathy are anthracycline toxicity (the antineoplastic agents doxorubicin [Adriamycin] and daunomycin), hemochromatosis (from excessive iron storage), Duchenne muscular dystrophy, Kawasaki disease, collagen diseases, and thyroid dysfunction.

Cardiomyopathies can be divided into three broad clinical categories according to the type of abnormal structure and dysfunction present: dilated cardiomyopathy, hypertrophic cardiomyopathy, and restrictive cardiomyopathy. *Dilated cardiomyopathy* is characterized by ventricular dilation and greatly decreased contractility resulting in symptoms of CHF. This is the most common type of cardiomyopathy in children. Its cause is often unknown. Clinical findings include CHF with tachycardia, dyspnea, hepatosplenomegaly, fatigue, and poor growth. Dysrhythmias may be present and may be more difficult to control with worsening heart failure.

Hypertrophic cardiomyopathy is characterized by an increase in heart muscle mass without an increase in cavity size, usually occurring in the left ventricle and associated with abnormal diastolic filling. Half of these patients have a familial autosomal dominant genetic abnormality (Burch & Blair, 1999). Clinical symptoms usually occur during the school-age period or adolescence and may include anginal chest pain, dysrhythmias, and syncope. Sudden death is possible. Manifestation in infancy includes signs of CHF and has a poor prognosis. Chest radiography shows a mildly enlarged heart; the ECG demonstrates left ventricular (LV) hypertrophy, often with ST-T changes. The ECG is most helpful and demonstrates asymmetric septal hypertrophy and an increase in LV wall thickness, with a small LV cavity.

Restrictive cardiomyopathy, rare in children, describes a restriction to ventricular filling caused by endocardial or myocardial disease or both. It is characterized by diastolic dysfunction and absence of ventricular dilation or hypertrophy. Symptoms are similar to those of CHF (see p. 1572).

Therapeutic Management

Treatment is directed toward correcting the underlying cause whenever feasible. However, in most affected children this is not possible, and treatment is aimed at managing CHF and dysrhythmias. Digoxin, diuretics, and aggressive use of afterload reduction agents have been found to be helpful in managing symptoms in those with dilated cardiomyopathy. Digoxin and inotropic agents are usually not helpful in the other forms of cardiomyopathy, because increasing the force of contraction may exacerbate the muscular obstruction and actually impair ventricular ejection. Beta blockers such as propranolol (Inderal) or calcium-channel blockers such as verapamil (Calan) have been used to reduce left ventricular outflow obstruction and improve diastolic filling in those with hypertrophic cardiomyopathy.

Careful monitoring and treatment of dysrhythmias is essential. Anticoagulants may be given to reduce the risk of thromboemboli, a complication of the sluggish circulation through the heart. For worsening heart failure and signs of poor perfusion, IV inotropic or vasodilating drugs may be needed. Severely ill children may require mechanical ventilation, oxygen administration, and IV medications. Heart transplantation may be a treatment option for patients who have worsening symptoms despite maximum medical therapy.

Nursing Care Management

Because of the poor prognosis in many children with cardiomyopathy, nursing care is consistent with that for any child with a life-threatening disorder (see Chapter 41). One of the most difficult adjustments for the child (especially the normally active youngster with hypertrophic cardiomyopathy) may be the realization of failing health and the need for restricted activity. The child should be included in decisions regarding activity and allowed to discuss feelings, particularly if the disease follows a progressively fatal course. After symptoms of CHF or dysrhythmias develop, the same nursing interventions are implemented as discussed on pp. 1571-1575. If cardiac transplantation is considered, the needs of the child and family are great in terms of psychologic preparation and postoperative care. The nurse plays an important role in assessing the family's understanding of the procedure and long-term consequences. Children of school age and older should be fully informed to give their assent to the procedure (see Informed Consent, Chapter 45).

Heart Transplantation

Heart transplantation has become a treatment option for infants and children with worsening heart failure and a limited life expectancy despite maximum medical and surgical management. Indications for cardiac transplantation in children are cardiomyopathy and end-stage congenital heart disease. It is also an option for patients with some forms of complex congenital cardiac defects, such as hypoplastic left heart syndrome, for whom conventional surgical approaches have a high mortality rate (Luikart, 2001).

The heart transplant procedure may be orthotopic or heterotopic. *Orthotopic heart transplantation* refers to removing the recipient's own heart and implanting a new heart from a donor who has had brain death but a healthy heart. The donor and recipient are matched by weight and blood type. *Heterotopic heart transplantation* refers to leaving the recipient's own heart in place and implanting a new heart to act as an additional pump or "piggyback" heart; this type of transplant is rarely done in children.

Before transplantation, potential recipients undergo a careful cardiac evaluation to determine if there are any other medical or surgical options to improve the patient's cardiac status. Other organ systems are assessed to identify problems that might preclude or increase the risk of transplantation. A psychosocial evaluation of the patient and family is done to assess family function, support systems, and the family's ability to comply with the complex medical regimen after the transplant. Support services to help the family successfully care for their child are provided when possible. Parents and older adolescents need extensive education about the risks and benefits of transplantation so that they can make an informed decision (Higgins, 2001). Patients are listed on a national computer network organized by the United Network for Organ Sharing (UNOS) to match donors and recipients.

The number of heart transplants in pediatric patients has been constant for the last decade, between 340 and 400 transplants per year (Boucek et al, 2001). This probably reflects a limit in the number of available donors. Infants are the largest group of pediatric transplant recipients. Data from the International Society for Heart and Lung Transplantation Registry for pediatric heart transplants between 1996 and 1999 showed a 1-year actuarial survival rate of 86% and a 4-year actuarial survival rate of 79% (Boucek et al, 2001). The posttransplant course is complex. Although heart function is greatly improved or normal after transplantation, the risk of rejection is serious. The leading cause of death after heart transplantation is rejection (Fortuna, Chinnock, & Bailey, 1999). Rejection of the heart is diagnosed primarily by endomyocardial biopsy in older children. Serial echocardiograms are often used in infants and young children to reduce the need for invasive biopsies. Immunosuppressants must be taken for life and have many systemic side effects (Luikart, 2001). Infection is always a risk. Potential long-term problems that may limit survival include chronic rejection, causing coronary artery disease; renal dysfunction and hypertension resulting from cyclosporine administration; lymphoma; and infection. In the short term, after successful transplantation, children are able to return to full participation in age-appropriate activities and appear to adapt well to their new lifestyle. Transplantation is not a cure, because patients must live with the lifetime consequences of chronic immunosuppression. The long-term prognosis is unknown because heart transplantation is a relatively new therapy in the pediatric population, begun in 1985.

Nursing Care Management

Nursing care after transplantation is demanding and complex, with careful attention to both the physical needs of the child and the emotional needs of the child and family. Successfully caring for a child after a heart transplant requires the expertise and dedication of many members of the health care team. Nurses play vital roles in assessment, coordination of care, psychosocial support, and patient and family education. The heart transplant recipient must be carefully monitored for signs of rejection, infection, and the side effects of the immunosuppressant medications. The patient's and the family's psychosocial well-being also needs to be assessed to identify issues such as increased family stress, depression, substance abuse, and school problems. Noncompliance with an intense medication regimen, especially during adolescence, can lead to serious medical problems and can be fatal. Psychosocial concerns and appropriate interventions for the child with a life-threatening disorder are presented in Chapter 44.

The first 6 months to 1 year after the transplant are most intense, because the risk of complications is greatest and the patient and family are adjusting to a new lifestyle. Patients are monitored closely by the health care team, with frequent visits and laboratory tests. Care is usually shared between local health care providers and the transplant center. Many patients are able to return to school and other age-appropriate activities within 2 to 3 months after the transplant.

VASCULAR DYSFUNCTION

Systemic Hypertension

Hypertension is defined as the consistent elevation of blood pressure (BP) beyond values considered to be the upper limits of normal. The two major categories are *essential hypertension* (no identifiable cause) and *secondary hypertension* (subsequent to an identifiable cause). Hypertension is the most common cause of CVAs and a major risk factor for myocardial infarction in adults. In recent years there has been increasing interest in this disorder in adolescents and children, particularly in terms of prevention of later morbidity and mortality. Routine BP measurements have detected hypertension with surprising frequency in asymptomatic children, especially teenagers. Although the prevalence of the condition in adolescents is difficult to evaluate, evidence is accumulating to indicate that the essential hypertension of adulthood may have its origin in childhood; thus its early detection has significance for prevention and treatment.

Etiology

Most instances of hypertension observed in young children occur secondary to a structural abnormality or an underlying pathologic process, although this is being challenged by screening programs of relatively healthy children. The most common cause of secondary hypertension is renal disease, followed by cardiovascular, endocrine, and some neurologic disorders. As a rule, the younger the child and the more severe the hypertension, the more likely it is to be secondary.

The causes of essential hypertension are undetermined, but evidence indicates that both genetic and environmental factors play a role. The incidence of hypertension has been shown to be higher in children whose parents are hypertensive. American blacks have a higher incidence of hypertension than whites, and in these persons it develops earlier, is frequently more severe, and results in death at an earlier age. Environmental factors that contribute to the risk of developing hypertension include obesity, salt ingestion, smoking, and stress.

Diagnostic Evaluation

From the increasing numbers of hypertensive or potentially hypertensive children and adolescents being identified, a BP determination should be a routine part of annual assessment in children. Although clinical manifestations associated with hypertension depend largely on the underlying cause, some observations can provide clues to the examiner that an elevated BP may be a factor (Box 48-10). In infants and very young children who cannot communicate symptoms, observation of behavior provides clues, although gross behavioral changes may not be apparent until complications are present.

No definitive cutoff values are used in the diagnosis of hypertension in the pediatric patient. The National Institutes of Health (1996) has suggested the classification found in Appendix J. *Significant hypertension* is a BP persistently between the 95th and 99th percentiles for age, sex, and height. *Severe hypertension* is a BP persistently at or above the 99th percentile for age, sex, and height. These newer guidelines take into account the differences in body size. It is important to note that a child who is large for his or her age may normally have a higher BP than a child of average size. Before a diagnosis is made, BP should be measured on at least three separate occasions.

A careful family history should be obtained to screen for other relatives with hypertension or other cardiovascular risk factors. In children with suspected primary hypertension, initial laboratory data are also obtained. This generally includes a urinalysis, renal function studies such as creatinine and blood urea nitrogen, a lipid profile, complete blood count, and electrolytes.

Therapeutic Management

Therapy for secondary hypertension involves diagnosis and treatment of the underlying cause. In cases amenable to surgical repair, the nature of the condition, the type of surgery, and the age of the child are all important considerations. Children or adolescents with consistently elevated BP readings from no known cause or those with secondary hypertension not amenable to surgical correction may be treated with a combination of nonpharmacologic and pharmacologic interventions. Dietary practices and lifestyle changes are important in the control of hypertension both for children and for adults. Nonpharmacologic measures, such as limitation of dietary salt, weight control, increased exercise, and avoidance of stress and smoking, carry no risk and should be instituted first, except in severe cases. Because the long-term effects of antihypertensive agents on children are not known, drug treatment of asymptomatic children with mild or borderline hypertension is not recommended.

Drug therapy is instituted with caution in children with significant elevations of BP resistant to nonpharmacologic intervention. The treatment should begin with one drug and should add other drugs only if control is not obtained. Compliance with antihypertensive drug regimens is extremely difficult. The oral antihypertensive drugs used most often in children include the beta blockers (propranolol), ACE inhibitors, diuretics, and occasionally a vasodilator (hydralazine). The goal is to achieve a normotensive state throughout the day without accompanying drug side effects.

Nursing Care Management

The nurse is active in detection, diagnosis, and therapy in many settings. Nurses are frequently the persons who operate well-child care and follow-up units and are usually the primary contact between health services and the child and family.

BP measurement should always be a part of the routine assessment of infants and children. To obtain an accurate reading, care is taken to quiet the child or relax the adolescent while the measurement is recorded to avoid false readings caused by excitement. The chief cause of falsely elevated BP readings is the use of improperly fitting, narrow cuffs. Therefore attention to correct measurement technique is essential (see Blood Pressure, Chapter 35).

Nursing counseling and guidance of affected children are challenges. Education aimed at understanding hypertension and its implication over the life span is essential in promoting patient and family compliance with both nonpharmacologic and pharmacologic therapies (see Compliance, Chapter 45).

Home BP measurements can facilitate surveillance in youngsters with chronic hypertension and can document effectiveness of therapy. A family member can be instructed in how to take and record accurate BP measurements, thus de-

BOX 48-10

Clinical Manifestations of Hypertension

Adolescents and Older Children
Frequent headaches
Dizziness
Changes in vision

Infants and Young Children
Irritability
Head banging or head rubbing
May wake up screaming in the night

creasing the number of trips to a health care facility. This individual needs to understand when to contact the practitioner regarding elevated values. The school nurse can often be a valuable resource in monitoring BP.

The nurse plays an important role in assessing individual families and providing targeted information regarding nonpharmacologic modes of intervention, such as diet, weight loss, smoking, and exercise programs. If extensive dietary counseling is required, the child should be referred to a nutritionist with expertise in working with children and adolescents. Exercise regimens should be individualized. School-age children and young adolescents generally prefer team sports rather than individual training, which they may view as a burden rather than an enjoyable activity. If peers and family members can be encouraged to participate in any of the management strategies, the child's compliance is likely to be greater.

Young hypertensive women should avoid oral contraceptives because of their pressor effects. Other options need to be presented before this form of birth control is discontinued (see Contraception, Chapter 40).

If drug therapy is prescribed, the nurse needs to provide information to the family regarding the reasons for it, how the drug works, and possible side effects. General instructions for antihypertensive drugs include the following:

- Rise slowly from a horizontal position and avoid sudden position changes.
- Take drug as prescribed.
- Notify practitioner if unpleasant side effects occur, but do not discontinue drug.
- Avoid alcohol and stay on prescribed diet.

The need for follow-up is stressed, especially because antihypertensive therapy can sometimes be safely discontinued if BP remains under control over time.

Kawasaki Disease (Mucocutaneous Lymph Node Syndrome)

Kawasaki disease (KD) is an acute systemic vasculitis of unknown cause. It is seen in every racial group, and about 80% of the cases occur in children younger than 5 years of age, with peak incidence in the toddler age group. The acute disease is self-limited. Without treatment, however, approximately 20% of children with KD develop cardiac sequelae. Infants younger than 1 year of age are most seriously affected by KD and are at the greatest risk for heart involvement.

The etiology of KD remains a mystery. Although it is not spread by person-to-person contact, several factors support infectious etiologic factors. It is often seen in geographic and seasonal outbreaks, with most cases reported in the late winter and early spring.

Pathophysiology

The principal area of involvement is the cardiovascular system. During the initial stage of the illness, extensive inflammation of the arterioles, venules, and capillaries occurs, which later progresses to the formation of coronary artery aneurysms in some children. When death occurs, it is usually the result of coronary thrombosis or severe scar formation and stenosis of the main coronary artery.

Clinical Manifestations

Because no specific diagnostic test exists for KD, the diagnosis is established on the basis of clinical findings and associated laboratory results (Box 48-11). These criteria should be used as guidelines. Many children with KD do not fulfill standard diagnosis criteria, and infants often have an atypical presentation. It is therefore important to consider KD as a possible diagnosis in any infant or child with prolonged elevated temperature that is unresponsive to antibiotics and is not attributable to another cause.

KD manifests in three phases: acute, subacute, and convalescent. The *acute phase* begins with the abrupt onset of high fever that is unresponsive to antibiotics and antipyretics. The child then develops the remaining diagnostic symptoms. During this stage the child is typically *very* irritable. The *subacute phase* begins with resolution of the fever and lasts until all clinical signs of KD have disappeared. During this phase the child is at greatest risk for the development of coronary artery aneurysms. Echocardiograms are used to monitor myocardial and coronary artery status. A baseline echocardiogram should be obtained at the time of diagnosis for comparison with future studies. Irritability persists during this phase. In the *convalescent phase,* all the clinical signs of KD have resolved, but the laboratory values have not returned to normal. This phase is complete when all blood values are normal (6 to 8 weeks after onset). At the end of this stage the child has regained his or her usual temperament, energy, and appetite.

Cardiac Involvement

The most serious complication of KD is the potential for myocardial infarction, which generally results from thrombotic occlusion of a coronary aneurysm. The main symptoms of acute myocardial infarction in children are abdominal pain, vomiting, restlessness, inconsolable crying, pallor, and shock.

Therapeutic Management

The current treatment of KD includes high-dose IV gamma globulin along with salicylate therapy. Gamma globulin has been demonstrated to be effective at reducing the incidence of coronary artery abnormalities when given within the first 10 days of the illness. A single, large infusion of 2 g/kg

BOX 48-11

Diagnostic Criteria for Kawasaki Disease

The child must exhibit five of the following six criteria, including fever:

1. Fever for 5 or more days (often diagnosed with shorter duration of fever if other symptoms are present)
2. Bilateral conjunctival injection (inflammation) without exudation
3. Changes in the oral mucous membranes, such as erythema, dryness, and fissuring of the lips; oropharyngeal reddening; or "strawberry tongue" (large papillae are exposed)
4. Changes in the extremities, such as peripheral edema, erythema of the palms and soles, and periungual desquamation (peeling) of the hands and feet
5. Polymorphous rash
6. Cervical lymphadenopathy (one lymph node larger than 1.5 cm)

over 10 to 12 hours is recommended (American Academy of Pediatrics, Committee on Infectious Diseases, 2000).

Aspirin is given initially in an antiinflammatory dose (80 to 100 mg/kg/day in divided doses every 6 hours) to control fever and symptoms of inflammation. After fever has subsided, aspirin is continued at an antiplatelet dose (3 to 5 mg/kg/day). Low-dose aspirin is continued in patients without echocardiographic evidence of coronary abnormalities until the platelet count has returned to normal (6 to 8 weeks). If the child develops coronary abnormalities, salicylate therapy is continued indefinitely. Additional anticoagulation with Coumadin may be indicated in children with giant aneurysms.

Prognosis

Most children with KD recover fully after treatment. However, when cardiovascular complications occur, serious morbidity may result. Death occurs rarely but almost always results from coronary thrombosis.

Nursing Care Management

In the initial phase the nurse must monitor the child's cardiac status carefully. Intake and output and daily weight measurements are recorded. Although the child may be reluctant to eat and therefore may be partially dehydrated, fluids need to be administered with care because of the usual finding of myocarditis. The child should be assessed frequently for signs of CHF, including decreased urine output, gallop rhythm (an additional heart sound), tachycardia, and respiratory distress.

Administration of gamma globulin should follow the same guidelines as for any blood product, with frequent monitoring of vital signs. Patients must be watched for allergic reactions. Cardiac status must be monitored because of the large volume being administered to patients with myocarditis and diminished left ventricular function.

Most nursing care focuses on symptomatic relief. To minimize skin discomfort, cool cloths, unscented lotions, and soft, loose clothing are helpful. During the acute phase, mouth care, including lubricating ointment to the lips, is important for the mucosal inflammation. Clear liquids and soft foods can be offered.

Patient irritability is perhaps the most challenging problem. These children need a quiet environment that promotes adequate rest. Their parents need to be supported in their efforts to comfort an often inconsolable child. They may need time away from their child, and nurses can often provide respite care for the family. Parents need to understand that irritability is a hallmark of KD and that they need not feel guilty or embarrassed about their child's behavior.

Discharge Teaching

Parents need accurate information about the progression of KD, including the importance of follow-up monitoring and when they should contact their practitioner. Irritability is likely to persist for up to 2 months after the onset of symptoms. Peeling of the hands and feet is painless and occurs primarily in the second and third weeks. Arthritis, especially of the larger weight-bearing joints, may persist for several weeks. Children are typically most stiff in the mornings, during cold weather, and after naps. Passive range of motion in the bathtub is often helpful in increasing flexibility. Any live immunizations (e.g., measles-mumps-rubella, varicella) should be deferred for 11 months after the administration of gamma globulin because the body might not produce the appropriate amount of antibodies (American Academy of Pediatrics, Committee on Infectious Diseases, 2000). The decision to give the varicella (chickenpox) vaccine while the child is receiving aspirin therapy is made individually by the practitioner. Temperature should be recorded after discharge until the child has been afebrile for several days.

All parents should understand the unlikely but real possibility of myocardial infarction, as well as the signs and symptoms of cardiac ischemia, in a child. At discharge the ultimate cardiac sequela is generally not known, because changes occur up to a month after the onset of KD. In addition, the parents of children with known severe coronary artery sequelae may be taught CPR.

Shock

Shock, or *circulatory failure,* is a complex clinical syndrome characterized by inadequate tissue perfusion to meet the metabolic demands of the body, resulting in cellular dysfunction and eventual organ failure. Although the causes are different, the physiologic consequences are the same: hypotension, tissue hypoxia, and metabolic acidosis.

Circulatory failure in children is a result of hypovolemia, altered peripheral vascular resistance, or pump failure. Types of shock are listed in Box 48-12.

Pathophysiology

A healthy child's circulatory system is able to transport oxygen and metabolic substrates to body tissues, which require a constant source for these essential needs. The cardiac output and distribution to the various body tissues can change very rapidly in response to intrinsic (myocardial and intravascular) or extrinsic (neuronal) control mechanisms. In shock states these mechanisms are altered or challenged.

Reduced blood flow, as in hypovolemic shock, causes diminished venous return to the heart, low CVP, low cardiac output, and hypotension. Vasomotor centers in the medulla are signaled, causing a compensatory increase in the force and rate of cardiac contraction and constriction of arterioles and veins, thereby increasing peripheral vascular resistance. Simultaneously the lowered blood volume leads to the release of large amounts of catecholamines, antidiuretic hormone, adrenocorticosteroids, and aldosterone in an effort to conserve body fluids. This causes reduced blood flow to the skin, kidneys, muscles, and viscera to shunt the available blood to the brain and heart. Consequently, the skin feels cold and clammy, there is poor capillary filling, and glomerular filtration and urine output are significantly reduced.

As a result of impaired perfusion, oxygen is depleted in the tissue cells, causing them to revert to anaerobic metabolism, producing lactic acidosis. The acidosis places an extra burden on the lungs as they attempt to compensate for the metabolic acidosis by increased respiratory rate to remove excess carbon dioxide. Prolonged vasoconstriction results in fatigue and atony of the peripheral arterioles, which leads to vessel dilation. Venules, less sensitive to vasodilator substances, remain constricted for a time, causing massive pooling in the capillary and venular beds, which further depletes blood volume.

Complications of shock create further hazards. Central nervous system hypoperfusion may eventually lead to cerebral edema, cortical infarction, or intraventricular hemorrhage. Renal hypoperfusion causes renal ischemia with possible tubular or glomerular necrosis and renal vein thrombosis. Reduced blood flow to the lungs can interfere with surfactant secretion and result in adult respiratory distress syndrome (ARDS), characterized by sudden pulmonary congestion and atelectasis with formation of a hyaline membrane. Gastrointestinal tract bleeding and perforation are always a possibility after splanchnic ischemia and necrosis of intestinal mucosa. Metabolic complications of shock may include hypoglycemia, hypocalcemia, and other electrolyte disturbances.

BOX 48-12

Types of Shock

Hypovolemic

Characteristics

Reduction in size of vascular compartment
Falling blood pressure
Poor capillary filling
Low central venous pressure

Most Frequent Causes

Blood loss (hemorrhagic shock)—trauma, gastrointestinal bleeding, intracranial hemorrhage
Plasma loss—increased capillary permeability associated with sepsis and acidosis, hypoproteinemia, burns, peritonitis
Extracellular fluid loss—vomiting, diarrhea, glycosuric diuresis, sunstroke

Distributive

Characteristics

Reduction in peripheral vascular resistance
Profound inadequacies in tissue perfusion
Increased venous capacity and pooling
Acute reduction in return blood flow to the heart
Diminished cardiac output

Most Frequent Causes

Anaphylaxis (anaphylactic shock)—extreme allergy or hypersensitivity to a foreign substance
Sepsis (septic shock, bacteremic shock, endotoxic shock)—overwhelming sepsis and circulating bacterial toxins
Loss of neuronal control (neurogenic shock)—interruption of neuronal transmission (spinal cord injury)
Myocardial depression and peripheral dilation—exposure to anesthesia or ingestion of barbiturates, tranquilizers, opioids, antihypertensive agents, or ganglionic blocking agents

Cardiogenic

Characteristic

Decreased cardiac output

Most Frequent Causes

After surgery for congenital heart disease
Primary pump failure—myocarditis, myocardial trauma, biochemical derangements, congestive heart failure
Dysrhythmias—supraventricular tachycardia, atrioventricular block, and ventricular dysrhythmias; secondary to myocarditis or biochemical abnormalities (occasionally)

Diagnostic Evaluation

The etiology of shock can be discerned from the history and the physical examination. The severity of the shock is determined by measurements of vital signs, including CVP and capillary filling (Box 48-13). Shock can be regarded as a form of compensation for circulatory failure. Because of the progressive nature of shock, it can be divided into the following three stages or phases:

1. *Compensated shock.* Vital organ function is maintained by intrinsic compensatory mechanisms; blood flow is usually normal or increased but generally uneven or maldistributed in the microcirculation.
2. *Uncompensated shock.* Efficiency of the cardiovascular system gradually diminishes, until perfusion in the microcirculation becomes marginal despite compensatory adjustments. The outcomes of circulatory failure that progress beyond the limits of compensation are tissue hypoxia, metabolic acidosis, and eventual dysfunction of all organ systems.
3. *Irreversible, or terminal, shock.* Damage to vital organs, such as the heart or brain, is of such magnitude that the entire organism will be disrupted regardless of therapeutic intervention. Death occurs even if cardiovascular measurements return to normal levels with therapy.

At all stages, the principal differentiating signs are observed in (1) the degree of tachycardia and perfusion to extremities, (2) the level of consciousness, and (3) the BP. Additional signs or modifications of these more universal signs may be present depending on the type and cause of the shock. Initially the child's ability to compensate is effective;

BOX 48-13

Clinical Manifestations of Shock

Compensated

Apprehensiveness
Irritability
Unexplained tachycardia
Normal blood pressure
Narrowing pulse pressure
Thirst
Pallor
Diminished urine output
Reduced perfusion of extremities

Uncompensated

Confusion and somnolence
Tachypnea
Moderate metabolic acidosis
Oliguria
Cool, pale extremities
Decreased skin turgor
Poor capillary filling

Irreversible

Thready, weak pulse
Hypotension
Periodic breathing or apnea
Anuria
Stupor or coma

therefore early signs are subtle. As the shock state advances, signs are more obvious and indicate early decompensation.

Additional signs may be present, depending on the type and etiology of the shock. In early septic shock there are chills, fever, and vasodilation, with increased cardiac output that results in warm, flushed skin (hyperdynamic or "hot" shock). A later and ominous development is disseminated intravascular coagulation (see Chapter 49), the major hematologic complication of septic shock. Anaphylactic shock is frequently accompanied by urticaria and angioneurotic edema, which is life threatening when it involves the respiratory passages (see Anaphylaxis, this page).

Laboratory tests that assist in assessment include blood gas measurements, pH, and sometimes liver function tests. Coagulation tests are evaluated when there is evidence of bleeding, such as oozing from a venipuncture site, bleeding from any orifice, or petechiae. Cultures of blood and other sites are indicated when there is a high suspicion of sepsis. Renal function tests are performed when impaired renal function is evident.

Therapeutic Management

Treatment of shock consists of three major thrusts: (1) ventilation, (2) fluid administration, and (3) improvement of the pumping action of the heart (vasopressor support). The first priority is to establish an airway and administer oxygen. After the airway is ensured, circulatory stabilization is the major concern.

Ventilatory Support

The lung is the organ most sensitive to shock. Decreased or redistribution of blood flow to respiratory muscles plus the increased work of breathing can rapidly lead to respiratory failure. Critically ill patients are unable to maintain an adequate airway. To place the lung at rest and improve ventilation, tracheal intubation is initiated early with positive-pressure ventilation. Supplemental oxygen is always given as soon as possible. Blood gases and pH are monitored frequently.

Increased extravascular lung water caused by edema contributes to the development of respiratory complications. Therapy is directed toward maintaining normal arterial blood gas measurements, normal acid-base balance, and circulation. Efforts are made to remove fluid and prevent its accumulation with the use of diuretics.

Cardiovascular Support

In most cases, rapid restoration of blood volume is all that is needed for resuscitation of the child in shock. An isotonic crystalloid solution (normal saline or Ringer's lactate) is the fluid of choice; colloids such as albumin are also used. Successful resuscitation is reflected by an increase in BP and a reduction in heart rate; increased cardiac output will result in improved capillary circulation and skin color. CVP measurements of right atrial pressure help guide fluid therapy, and urine output measurement is an important indicator of adequacy of circulation. Correction of acidosis, hypoxemia, hypoglycemia, hypothermia, and any metabolic derangements is mandatory.

Temporary pharmacologic support may be required to enhance myocardial contractility, reverse metabolic or respiratory acidosis, or maintain arterial pressure. The principal agents used to improve cardiac output and circulation are the catecholamines, such as dopamine (Intropin) and epinephrine (Adrenalin). Vasodilators that are sometimes used include nitroprusside (Nipride) and milrinone.

Nursing Care Management

When shock is a likely complication, the child is observed carefully for any early signs, which are reported immediately for further medical evaluation.

NURSE ALERT Early clinical signs include apprehension, irritability, normal BP, narrowing pulse pressure (difference between diastolic and systolic BP), thirst, pallor, diminished urine output, unexplained mild tachycardia, and a decrease in perfusion of the hands and feet. ■

The child who is in shock requires intensive observation and care. *The initial action is to ensure adequate tissue oxygenation.* The nurse should be prepared to administer oxygen by the appropriate route and to assist with any intubation and ventilatory procedures indicated. Other procedures and activities that require immediate attention are establishing an IV line, weighing the child, obtaining baseline vital signs, placing an indwelling catheter, obtaining blood gases and other measurements, and administering medications as indicated. The child is best positioned flat with the legs elevated.

The nurse's responsibilities are to monitor the IV infusion, intake and output, vital signs (including CVP), and general systems assessments on a routine basis. IV medications are titrated according to patient responses, and vital signs are taken every 15 minutes during the critical periods and thereafter as needed. Urine output is measured hourly; blood gases, hematocrit, pH, and electrolytes are monitored frequently to assess the status of the child and the efficacy of therapy. An apnea and cardiac monitor is attached and monitored continuously. In the initial stages of acute shock, the care of the child often requires the attendance of more than one nurse to manage all the necessary activities that must be carried out simultaneously (Emergency box).

Anaphylaxis

Anaphylaxis is the acute clinical syndrome resulting from the interaction of an allergen and a patient who is hypersensitive to that allergen. When the antigen enters the circulatory system, a generalized reaction rapidly takes place. Vasoactive amines (principally histamine or a histamine-like substance) are released and cause vasodilation, bronchoconstriction, and increased capillary permeability.

Severe reactions are immediate in onset, are often life threatening, and frequently involve multiple systems, primarily the cardiovascular, respiratory, gastrointestinal, and integumentary systems. Exposure to the antigen can be by ingestion, inhalation, skin contact, or injection. Examples of common allergens associated with anaphylaxis include drugs (e.g., antibiotics, chemotherapeutic agents, radiologic contrast media), latex, foods, venoms from bees or snakes, and biologic agents (antisera, enzymes, hormones, blood products).

Emergency

SHOCK

Ventilation

Establish airway—be prepared for intubation
Administer oxygen, usually 100% by mask

Fluid Administration

Obtain vascular access (preferably IV, intraosseous in emergency)
Restore fluid volume as ordered (initial volume resuscitation is 20 ml/kg of isotonic crystalloid [normal saline or Ringer's lactate] over 5 to 20 minutes)

Cardiovascular Support

Administer vasopressors; especially epinephrine IV (dose: 0.01 mg/kg = 0.1 ml/kg of 1:10,000 solution)
May repeat every 3 to 5 minutes in cardiac arrest

General Support

Continuous ECG monitoring
Monitor pulse oximetry
Keep child warm and calm

In Addition

Septic Shock
Administer broad-spectrum antibiotics intravenously

Anaphylaxis
Remove allergen if possible, intramuscular epinephrine, corticosteroids as ordered

Data from American Heart Association: Pediatric advanced life support provider manual, Dallas, 2002, The Association.

NURSE ALERT Penicillin allergy is associated with immediate onset (within an hour of administration) or accelerated onset (1 to 72 hours after administration) of skin eruption, especially a urticarial rash, or more serious symptoms such as laryngeal edema or anaphylactic shock. ■

Clinical Manifestations

The onset of clinical symptoms usually occurs within seconds or minutes of exposure to the antigen, and the rapidity of the reaction is directly related to its intensity: the sooner the onset, the more severe the reaction. The reaction may be preceded by symptoms of uneasiness, restlessness, irritability, severe anxiety, headache, dizziness, paresthesia, and disorientation. The patient may lose consciousness. Cutaneous signs of flushing and urticaria are common early signs, followed by angioedema, most notable in the eyelids, lips, tongue, hands, feet, and genitalia.

Bronchiolar constriction may follow, causing narrowing of the airway; pulmonary edema and hemorrhage also may occur. Laryngeal edema with severe acute upper airway obstruction may be life threatening and requires rapid intervention. Shock occurs as a result of mediator-induced vasodilation, which causes capillary permeability and loss of intravascular fluid into the interstitial space. Sudden hypotension and impaired cardiac output with poor perfusion are seen.

Therapeutic Management

Successful outcome of anaphylactic reactions depends on rapid recognition and institution of treatment. The goals of treatment are to provide ventilation, restore adequate circulation, and prevent further exposure by identifying and removing the cause when possible.

A mild reaction with no evidence of respiratory distress or cardiovascular compromise can be managed with subcutaneous administration of antihistamines, such as diphenhydramine (Benadryl) and epinephrine.

Moderate or severe distress presents a potentially life-threatening emergency. Establishing an airway is the first concern, as with all shock states. Epinephrine is given subcutaneously or intravenously as an antihistamine and to support the cardiovascular system and increase blood pressure. Other routes for giving epinephrine are intramuscular and via the airway, either nebulized or injected through an ET tube. In severe anaphylaxis, epinephrine by any route is better than none. Fluids are given to restore blood volume. Additional vasopressors may be given to improve cardiac output.

Prevention of a reaction is preferable. Preventing exposure is more easily accomplished in children known to be at risk, including those with (1) a history of previous allergic reaction to a specific antigen, (2) a history of atopy, (3) a history of severe reactions in immediate family members, and (4) a reaction to a skin test, although skin tests are not available for all allergens. Desensitization may be recommended in certain cases.

Nursing Care Management

The major nursing responsibility in anaphylaxis is anticipating which children are likely to develop a reaction, recognizing the early signs, and intervening appropriately. When an anaphylactic reaction is suspected, both immediate intervention and preparation for medical therapy are nursing responsibilities. Ventilation is ensured by placing the child in a head-elevated position, unless contraindicated by hypotension, to facilitate breathing and administer oxygen. If the child is not breathing, CPR is initiated, and emergency medical services are summoned.

If the cause can be determined, measures are implemented to slow the spread of the offending substance. An IV infusion is established immediately. Emergency medications are given intravenously whenever possible; however, epinephrine may be given subcutaneously (see Emergency box). Vital signs and urine output are monitored frequently. Medications are administered as prescribed, with regular assessment to monitor effectiveness and to detect signs of side effects of medication and fluid overload.

To prevent an anaphylactic reaction, parents are always asked about possible allergic responses to foods, latex, medications, and environmental conditions (see Guidelines box, Taking an Allergy History, p. 971). These are displayed prominently on the patient's chart. The specific allergen is noted, as is the type and severity of the reaction. Parents are excellent historians, especially when the child has displayed a pronounced reaction to a substance. Drugs, including related drugs (e.g., penicillin, nafcillin), and other items, such as latex, that have produced a reaction previously are *never* used. If the child is allergic to insect venom, the family is instructed to purchase an emergency kit to be kept with the child at all times. Both the family and the child, if the child is old enough, are taught how to use the equipment. Medical identification should be carried by the patient at all times.

Toxic Shock Syndrome

Toxic shock syndrome (TSS) is a relatively rare condition caused by the toxins produced by the *Staphylococcus* bacteria. First described in 1978, TSS can cause acute multisystem organ failure and a clinical picture that resembles septic shock. TSS became well known in 1980 because of the striking relationship between the disease and tampon use (Nakase, 2000). An aggressive health education campaign about the dangers of prolonged tampon use and a change in the chemical composition of tampons has markedly reduced the incidence of TSS in menstruating women. Cases of TSS have also been reported in men, older women, and children.

Diagnostic Evaluation

Diagnosis is established on the basis of the criteria established by the Centers for Disease Control and Prevention's toxic case definition (Box 48-14). A history of tampon use contributes to the diagnosis. Additional laboratory tests include cultures from blood, the vagina, the cervix, and any discharge. Other laboratory tests are those that facilitate the management of shock.

Therapeutic Management

The management of TSS is the same as management of shock of any etiology and may range from supportive care in mild cases to hospitalization and intensive care in severe cases. Appropriate parenteral antibiotics are usually administered after cultures are obtained.

Nursing Care Management

Nursing care and observation of the acutely ill patient are the same as those described for shock of any etiology. Because the disease is relatively rare, the major efforts of nursing are directed toward prevention. The association between the disease and the use of tampons provides some direction for education. Avoiding the use of tampons offers the most certain preventive measure, although this approach is probably unacceptable to most adolescent girls, who prefer the freedom, comfort, and inconspicuousness that tampons afford.

Adolescent girls who use tampons can be taught general hygiene measures, such as handwashing before insertion of the tampon and not to use a tampon that has been dropped or otherwise soiled. Tampons should be inserted carefully to avoid vaginal abrasion. Also, it is wise to modify their use. For example, tampons may be used intermittently during the menstrual cycle, alternating with sanitary napkins—perhaps using the napkins during the night, when at home during the day, and when flow is slight. Young girls are advised not to use superabsorbent tampons and not to leave any tampon in the body for more than 4 to 6 hours.

Patients who use tampons need to understand that they should remove the tampon and consult their health professional if they develop a sudden high fever, vomiting, diarrhea, muscle pain, dizziness, fainting or near fainting when standing up, or rash that resembles a sunburn.

BOX 48-14

Criteria for Definition of Toxic Shock Syndrome

1. Fever of 38.9° C (102° F) or higher
2. Presence of diffuse macular erythroderma
3. Desquamation, particularly of palms and soles, 1 to 2 weeks after onset of illness
4. Hypotension, defined as a systolic blood pressure of 90 mm Hg or less for adults and below the 5th percentile for children younger than 16 years of age; or an orthostatic drop in diastolic blood pressure of 15 mm Hg or more with a change from lying to sitting; or orthostatic syncope; or orthostatic dizziness
5. Involvement of three or more of the following organ systems: gastrointestinal, muscular, mucous membrane, renal, hepatic, hematologic, or central nervous system

Toxic shock syndrome is probable when four of the five major criteria are fulfilled. In addition, if blood and cerebrospinal fluid cultures are obtained, they must be negative for any organisms other than *Staphylococcus aureus.* Serologic tests for Rocky Mountain spotted fever, leptospirosis, and measles also must be negative.

Modified from American Academy of Pediatrics, Committee on Infectious Diseases, Pickering L, ed: *2003 red book: report of the Committee on Infectious Diseases,* ed 26, Elk Grove Village, IL, 2003, The Academy.

Key Points

- Congenital heart disease (CHD) is the most common form of cardiac disease in children.
- Major categories to investigate in the cardiac history are poor weight gain, poor feeding habits, and fatigue during feeding; frequent respiratory infections and difficulties; and evidence of exercise intolerance.
- The most common tests used in assessing cardiac function are radiography, electrocardiography, echocardiography, and cardiac catheterization.
- Cardiac catheterization procedures can be divided into three groups: (1) diagnostic procedures, including angiography, that measure pressures and saturations to establish cardiac diagnosis; (2) interventional procedures, in which catheters or balloon devices are used to correct cardiac defects; and (3) electrophysiology studies, in which catheters with electrodes are used to evaluate dysrhythmias.
- Diagnostic cardiac catheterization provides important information about oxygen saturation of blood within the chambers and great vessels, pressure changes, changes in cardiac output or stroke volume, and anatomic abnormalities.
- Several prenatal factors may predispose children to CHD: maternal rubella during pregnancy, maternal alcoholism, maternal age older than 40 years, and maternal type 1 diabetes.
- Congenital heart defects can be divided into four main groups, as determined by hemodynamic patterns: (1) defects that result in increased pulmonary blood flow, (2) obstructive defects, (3) defects that result in decreased pulmonary blood flow, and (4) mixed defects.
- Clinical consequences of congenital heart defects include congestive heart failure (CHF) and hypoxemia. A child can have both hypoxemia and CHF, although usually they occur independently.
- Clinical manifestations of CHF are impaired myocardial function (tachycardia, cardiomegaly), pulmonary congestion (dyspnea, tachypnea, orthopnea, cyanosis), and sys-

temic congestion (hepatosplenomegaly, edema, distended veins).

- Nursing measures in the care of a child with CHF are to assist in improving cardiac function, decrease cardiac demands, reduce respiratory distress, maintain nutritional status, promote fluid loss, and provide family support.
- Clinical manifestations of hypoxemia are cyanosis, polycythemia, clubbing, and delayed growth and development. The child is at increased risk for hypercyanotic spells, cerebrovascular accidents, brain abscess, and bacterial endocarditis.
- Caring for the child with CHD and the family requires helping them to adjust to the disorder and to cope with the effects of the defect, and fostering growth-promoting family relationships.
- Preoperative care of the child with a congenital heart defect involves introducing the child and family to the hospital and preparing them for preoperative and postoperative procedures.
- Providing postoperative care includes observing vital signs and arterial/venous pressures, maintaining respiratory status, allowing maximum rest, providing comfort, monitoring fluids, planning for progressive activities, giving emotional support, observing for complications of surgery, and planning for discharge and home care.
- Acquired cardiovascular disorders include bacterial endocarditis, rheumatic fever, hyperlipidemia (hypercholesterolemia), and cardiac dysrhythmias.
- Prevention of bacterial endocarditis in certain children with CHD involves administration of prophylactic antibiotics when specific procedures are performed.
- Acute rheumatic fever is a systemic inflammatory disease that can damage the cardiac valves and is associated with previous group A streptococcal infection. Its incidence has increased in some areas of the United States.
- Cholesterol screening in children is controversial; currently, children with known risk factors for hyperlipidemia are screened and treated as needed. The influence of childhood cholesterol levels on later development of coronary artery disease is under investigation.
- Common dysrhythmias in children include slow rhythms (bradycardias, heart block) and fast rhythms (sinus tachycardia, supraventricular tachycardia).
- Heart transplantation has been extended to infants and children with cardiomyopathy and complex congenital heart defects involving ventricular dysfunction, such as hypoplastic left heart syndrome.
- Education of the child with hypertension and the family focuses on drug therapy, diet control, and appropriate exercise.
- Kawasaki disease is an extensive inflammation of small vessels and capillaries that may progress to involve the coronary arteries, causing aneurysm formation. The administration of gamma globulin is an important aspect of treatment.
- Emergency treatment for shock includes ensuring ventilation; administering vasopressors, fluids or blood, and antibiotics as needed; and providing supportive measures such as correct positioning, warmth, and psychologic reassurance to the child and family.
- Persons at risk for anaphylaxis may be identified by a history of previous allergic reaction, history of atopy, history of severe reactions in family, and positive skin test to the allergen.
- Nursing management of the patient with toxic shock syndrome focuses on prevention primarily through education concerning safe tampon use.

Answer Guidelines to Critical Thinking Exercises

Cardiac Catheterization

1. Yes. This patient has just undergone an invasive surgical procedure. Bleeding is a potential risk after cardiac catheterization.
2. (a) Complications after cardiac catheterization can include acute hemorrhage from the catheterization entry site, low-grade fever, nausea and vomiting, loss of pulses in the catheterized extremity, and transient dysrhythmias. (b) Nausea and vomiting can occur after heart catheterization, but are not directly related to acute blood loss. However, if the child had significant vomiting occurring immediately after the procedure and was not able to keep his leg straight, the vomiting might have increased the chance of bleeding at the catheterization entry site. (c) Significant blood loss can occur in a short time after the use of an artery for cardiac catheterization.
3. The first priority is to prevent bleeding. Pressure is applied above the visible catheterization site where the vessel was accessed. Place the child flat in bed to decrease the effect of gravity on the rate of bleeding. Notify the practitioner immediately. Replacement fluids may need to be administered, and pharmacologic control of emesis is important.
4. This may be an arterial bleed, and Tommy is at risk for losing a large amount of blood in a short time. Your first priority should be to control the bleeding. Appropriate measures are to treat the patient like a shock patient by immediately lying the child flat to help with the control of bleeding.
5. In this case it is essential for the nurse to understand the complications associated with heart catheterization. Observation of acute blood loss at the site of catheter entry does not provide other alternative perspectives but supports an immediate need to control bleeding.

Digoxin Toxicity

1. Yes. The infant has been vomiting since yesterday and has an irregular heartbeat.
2. (a) Lasix is a diuretic that is a mainstay of therapy to eliminate excess water and salt to prevent reaccumulation of fluid. Side effects can include nausea and vomiting, diarrhea, ototoxicity, hypokalemia, and postural hypotension. (b) Digoxin is a potentially dangerous drug because the margin of safety of therapeutic, toxic, and lethal doses is very narrow. Common signs of digoxin toxicity are bradycardia, anorexia, nausea, and vomiting. Dysrhythmias can occur with digoxin toxicity. The dose of digoxin must be calculated exactly. (c) The goals of treatment for CHF are to improve cardiac output, remove excess fluid

and stabilize the sodium level, decrease cardiac demands and improve tissue oxygenation, and decrease oxygen consumption. Digoxin is used because of its rapid onset and decreased risk of toxicity as a result of a relatively short half-life compared with other digitalis preparations.

3. The home health nurse should notify the health care provider of the findings before giving digoxin. The assessment reveals a slow, irregular heartbeat and intermittent vomiting. These are common signs of digoxin toxicity in infants. Because the medication was started only 5 days ago, digoxin toxicity should be a major concern. Because furosemide (Lasix) is a non–potassium-sparing diuretic, a concomitant problem with the vomiting is hypokalemia, which is a common finding in children with CHF, Lasix administration, and vomiting. This should also be further evaluated at this visit.
4. Yes. The implications of the assessment are essential because the margin of safety for digoxin blood levels is narrow. Continuing to give the digoxin can cause a toxic reaction. Further evaluation is important.
5. Vomiting in a young child is a concern, but with a history of CHD and digoxin therapy, the first priority is to evaluate for digoxin toxicity. As noted previously, hypokalemia is also a concern. The vomiting may cause fluid loss above that for which the infant is able to compensate, and the possibility of mild dehydration should be evaluated.

Hypercyanotic Spell

1. Yes. The patient has a history of tetralogy of Fallot, which is associated with acute episodes of cyanosis and hypoxia. Hypercyanotic episodes occur suddenly and are common with crying.
2. (a) Infants with tetralogy of Fallot may be acutely cyanotic at birth; others have mild cyanosis that progresses over the first year of life as pulmonic stenosis worsens. (b) Symptoms of diarrhea, low-grade fever, and poor oral intake can be indicative of an acute infection in a young child. However, the hypercyanotic spell requires immediate attention. (c) Acute cyanotic spells, called blue spells or "tet" spells, can occur suddenly when the infant's oxygen requirements exceed oxygen availability. This may occur during crying or after feeding.
3. The priorities are to immediately calm the infant, place in the knee-chest position, administer blow-by oxygen, and call for assistance.
4. Yes. The infant is having a hypercyanotic, or tet, spell, and the first actions should be to calm the infant, place in the knee-chest position, and give supplemental oxygen. A hypercyanotic spell will likely worsen without immediate intervention, so prompt action is needed. If the nurse fails to accept the conclusions, negative implications may result, because a severe hypercyanotic spell may require intravenous medications, hydration, and resuscitative measures to stabilize the infant. To decrease the pain at the phlebotomy site and possibly decrease the hypercyanotic spell, place EMLA or Elamax on the site 1 hour before the procedure to decrease pain.
5. An alternative perspective is the concern for an infection because of a history of diarrhea and low-grade fever for the past 2 days. However, in the presence of a diagnosis of tetralogy of Fallot, the immediate presentation of a hypercyanotic episode needs immediate attention. There should be a record or notation on the plan of care of calming measures that have been effective in calming the child in the past—this information is crucial in the care of such children.

References

Allen HD et al: Pediatric therapeutic cardiac catheterization, AHA Scientific Statement, *Circulation* 97:609-625, 1998.

American Academy of Pediatrics: Cholesterol in childhood, *Pediatrics* 101 (1 pt 1):141-147, 1998.

American Academy of Pediatrics, Committee on Infectious Diseases, Pickering L, ed: *2000 red book: report of the Committee on Infectious Diseases,* ed 25, Elk Grove Village, IL, 2000, The Academy.

Barst RJ: Recent advances in the treatment of pediatric pulmonary artery hypertension, *Pediatr Clin North Am* 46(2):333-345, 1999.

Beekman RH: Coarctation of the aorta. In Allen HD et al, eds: *Moss and Adams' heart disease in infants, children, and adolescents,* ed 6, Philadelphia, 2001, Lippincott Williams & Wilkins.

Behrman RE, Kliegman RM, Jenson HA: *Nelson textbook of pediatrics,* ed 16, Philadelphia, 2000, WB Saunders.

Boucek MM et al: The registry of the International Society of Heart and Lung Transplantation: fourth official pediatric report 2000, *J Heart Lung Transplant* 20:39-52, 2001.

Burch M, Blair E: The inheritance of hypertrophic cardiomyopathy, *Pediatr Cardiol* 20(5):313-316, 1999.

Fortuna RS, Chinnock RE, Bailey LL: Heart transplantation among 233 infants during the first six months of life: the Loma Linda experience, *Clin Transpl* 263-272, 1999.

Freed MD: Aortic stenosis. In Allen HD et al, eds: *Moss and Adams' heart disease in infants, children, and adolescents,* ed 6, Philadelphia, 2001, Lippincott Williams & Wilkins.

Gentles T et al: Left ventricular mechanics during and after acute rheumatic fever: contractile dysfunction is closely related to valve regurgitation, *J Am Coll Cardiol* 37(1):201-207, 2001.

Hanisch D: Pediatric arrhythmias, *J Pediatr Nurs* 16(5):351-362, 2001.

Hawkins JA et al: Late results and reintervention after aortic valvotomy for critical aortic stenosis, *Ann Thorac Surg* 65:1758-1762, 1998.

Higgins SS: Parental role in decision making about pediatric cardiac transplantation: familial and ethical considerations, *J Pediatr Nurs* 16(5): 332-337, 2001.

Hougen TJ, Sell J: Recent advances in the diagnosis and treatment of coarctation of the aorta, *Curr Opin Cardiol* 10(5):524-529, 1995.

Koster NK: Physical activity and congenital heart disease, *Nurs Clin North Am* 29(2):345-356, 1994.

Luikart H: Pediatric cardiac transplantation management issues, *J Pediatr Nurs* 16(5):320-331, 2001.

Nakase J: Update on emerging infections from the Center for Disease Control and Prevention, *Ann Emerg Med* 36(3):268-270, 2000.

National Institutes of Health, National Heart, Lung, and Blood Institute: *Update on the Task Force Report (1987) on High Blood Pressure in Children and Adolescents,* Bethesda, MD, 1996, The Institutes.

O'Brien P, Boisvert JT: Current management of infants and children with single ventricle anatomy, *J Pediatr Nurs* 16(5):338-350, 2001.

Pham JT, Carlos MA: Current treatment strategies of symptomatic patent ductus arteriosus, *J Pediatr Health Care* 16(6):306-310, 2002.

Smith P: Primary care in children with congenital hearth disease, *J Pediatr Nurs* 16(5):308-319, 2001.

Uzurk K: Therapeutic cardiac catheterization for congenital heart disease: a new era in pediatric care, *J Pediatr Nurs* 16(5):300-307, 2001.

Hematologic and Immunologic Dysfunction

49

LEARNING OBJECTIVES

On completion of this chapter the reader will be able to:

- Distinguish between the various categories of anemia.
- Describe the prevention of iron deficiency anemia and the care of the child with iron deficiency anemia.
- Compare sickle cell anemia and β-thalassemia major in relation to pathophysiology and nursing care.
- Describe the mechanisms of inheritance and nursing care of the child with hemophilia.
- Relate the pathophysiology and clinical manifestations of leukemia.
- Demonstrate an understanding of the rationale of therapies for neoplastic disease.
- Outline a plan of care for the child with neoplastic disease and the family.
- Contrast the pathophysiology and management of the immunodeficiency disorders.
- List nursing precautions and responsibilities during blood transfusion.
- Describe the types of hematopoietic stem cell transplants.

ELECTRONIC RESOURCES

Additional information related to the content in Chapter 49 can be found on

the companion website at evolve
http://evolve.elsevier.com/Wong/maternal/

- NCLEX Review Questions
- Case Study—Sickle Cell Anemia
- WebLinks

or the interactive student CD-ROM
Activities for Chapter 49 include the following:

- NCLEX Review Questions
- Case Study—Acute Lymphoid Leukemia
- Critical Thinking Exercise—Bone Marrow Test
- Nursing Care Plan—The Child with Cancer
- Nursing Care Plan—The Child with HIV Infection

HEMATOLOGIC/IMMUNOLOGIC DYSFUNCTION

Assessment of Hematologic Function

Several tests can be performed to assess hematologic function, including additional procedures to identify the cause of the dysfunction. The following discussion is limited to a description of the most common and one of the most valuable tests, the *complete blood cell count (CBC)*. Other procedures, such as those related to iron, coagulation, and immune status, are discussed throughout the chapter as appropriate. The nurse should be familiar with the significance of the findings from the CBC (Table 49-1) and aware of normal values for age, which are listed in Appendix F.

As with any disorder, the history and physical examination are essential to identification of hematologic dysfunction, and the nurse is often the first person to suspect a problem based on information from these sources. Comments by the parent regarding the child's lack of energy, food diary of poor sources of iron, frequent infections, and bleeding that is difficult to control offer clues to the more common disorders affecting the blood. A careful physical appraisal, especially of the skin, can reveal findings (e.g., pallor, petechiae, bruising) that may indicate minor or serious hematologic conditions. Nurses need to be aware of the clinical manifestations of blood diseases to assist in recognizing symptoms and establishing a diagnosis.

NURSE ALERT A common term used in describing an abnormal CBC is *shift to the left,* which refers to the presence of immature neutrophils in the peripheral blood from hyperfunction of the bone marrow, as seen during a bacterial infection. ■

RED BLOOD CELL DISORDERS

Anemia

The term *anemia* describes a condition in which the number of red blood cells (RBCs) or the hemoglobin (Hgb or Hb) concentration is reduced below normal values for age. As a result of this decrease, the oxygen-carrying capacity of the

Table 49-1

Tests Performed as Part of the Complete Blood Cell Count

TEST (AVERAGE VALUE)*	DESCRIPTION/COMMENTS
Red blood cell (RBC) count (4.5-5.5 million/mm³)	Number of RBCs/mm³ of blood Indirectly estimates Hgb content of blood Reflects function of bone marrow
Hemoglobin (Hgb) determination (11.5-15.5 g/dl)	Amount of Hgb/g/dl of whole blood Total blood Hgb primarily depends on number of circulating RBCs, but also on amount of Hgb in each cell
Hematocrit (Hct) (35%-45%)	Percentage or volume of packed RBCs to whole blood Indirectly measures Hgb content Is approximately three times Hgb content
RBC indexes	
Mean corpuscular volume (MCV) (77-95 mcm³)	Average of mean volume (size) of a single RBC MCV values expressed as cubic microns (mcm³) or femtoliters (fl)
Mean corpuscular hemoglobin (MCH) (25-33 pg/cell)	Average or mean quantity (weight) of Hgb in a single RBC MCH values expressed as picograms (pg) or micromicrograms (μμg) MCV and MCH depend on accurate counts of RBCs, whereas MCHC does not; therefore MCHC is often more reliable All indexes depend on average cell measurements and do not show individual RBC variations (anisocytosis)
Mean corpuscular hemoglobin concentration (MCHC) (31%-37% Hgb [g]/dl RBC)	Average concentration of Hgb in a single RBC MCHC values expressed as % Hgb (g)/cell or Hgb (g)/dl RBC
RBC volume distribution width (RDW) (13.4% ± 1.2%)	Average size of RBCs Differentiates some types of anemia
Reticulocyte count (0.5%-1.5% erythrocytes)	% Reticulocytes to RBCs Index of production of mature RBCs by bone marrow Decreased count indicates depressed bone marrow function Increased count indicates erythrogenesis in response to some stimulus When reticulocyte count is extremely high, other forms of immature RBCs (normoblasts, even erythroblasts) may be present Indirectly estimates hypochromic anemia Usually elevated in patients with chronic hemolytic anemia
White blood cell (WBC) count (4.5-13.5 × 10³ cells/mm³)	Number of WBCs/mm³ of blood Total number of WBCs less important than differential count
Differential WBC count	Inspection and quantification of WBC types present in peripheral blood Values are expressed as percentages; to obtain absolute number of any type of WBCs, multiply its respective percentage by total number of WBCs
Neutrophils (polys) (54%-62%) (3-5.8 × 10³ cells/mm³)	Primary defense in bacterial infection; capable of phagocytizing and killing bacteria
Bands (3%-5%) (0.15-0.4 × 10³ cells/mm³)	Immature neutrophil Increased numbers in bacterial infection Also capable of phagocytosis and killing
Eosinophils (1%-3%) (0.05-0.25 × 10³ cells/mm³)	Named for their staining characteristics with eosin dye Increased in allergic disorders, parasitic diseases, certain neoplasms, and other diseases
Basophils (0.075%) (0.015-0.030 cells/mm³)	Named for their characteristic basophilic stippling Contain histamine, heparin, and serotonin; believed to cause increased blood flow to injured tissues while preventing excessive clotting

*See Appendix F for normal values according to ages.

Table 49-1

Tests Performed as Part of the Complete Blood Cell Count—cont'd

TEST (AVERAGE VALUE)*	DESCRIPTION/COMMENTS
Lymphocytes (25%-33%) (1.5-3.0 × 10^3 cells/mm^3)	Involved in development of antibody and delayed hypersensitivity
Monocytes (3%-7%)	Large phagocytic cells that are involved in early stage of inflammatory reaction
Absolute neutrophil count (ANC) (>1000)	% Neutrophils WBC count Indicates body's capability to handle bacterial infections
Platelet count (150-400 10^3/mm^3)	Number of platelets/mm^3 of blood Cellular fragments that are necessary for clotting to occur
Stained peripheral blood smear	Visual estimation of amount of Hgb in RBCs and overall size, shape, and structure of RBCs Various staining properties of RBC structures may be evidence of immature forms of erythrocytes Shows variation in size and shape of RBCs: microcytic, macrocytic, poikilocytic (variable shapes)

blood is diminished, causing a reduction in the oxygen available to the tissues. Anemia is the most common hematologic disorder of infancy and childhood and is not a disease itself but an indication or manifestation of an underlying pathologic process.

Classification

Anemias are classified in relation to (1) *etiology* or *physiology,* manifested by erythrocyte and/or Hgb depletion, and (2) *morphology,* the characteristic changes in RBC size, shape, and color (Box 49-1). Although the morphologic classification is more useful in terms of laboratory evaluation of anemia, the etiologic approach provides direction for planning nursing care. For example, anemia with reduced Hgb concentration may be caused by a dietary depletion of iron, and the principal intervention is replenishing iron stores (Fig 49-1).

Consequences of Anemia

The basic physiologic defect caused by anemia is a decrease in the oxygen-carrying capacity of blood and consequently a reduction in the amount of oxygen available to the cells. When the anemia has developed slowly, the child usually adapts to the declining Hgb level.

The effects of anemia on the circulatory system can be profound. Because the viscosity of blood depends almost entirely on the concentration of RBCs, the resulting hemodilution of severe anemia decreases peripheral resistance, causing greater quantities of blood to return to the heart. The increased circulation and turbulence within the heart may produce a murmur. Because the cardiac workload is greatly increased, especially during exercise, infection, or emotional stress, cardiac failure may ensue.

Children seem to have a remarkable ability to function well despite low levels of Hgb. *Cyanosis* (the result of the quantity of deoxygenated Hgb in arterial blood) is typically not evident. Growth retardation, resulting from decreased cellular metabolism and coexisting anorexia, is a common finding in chronic severe anemia and is frequently accompanied by delayed sexual maturation in the older child.

Diagnostic Evaluation

In general, anemia may be suspected from findings on the history and physical examination, such as lack of energy, easy fatigability, and pallor; however, unless the anemia is severe, the first clue to the disorder may be alterations in the CBC, such as decreased RBCs, and decreased Hgb and hematocrit (Hct) levels. Although anemia is sometimes defined as an Hgb level below 10 or 11 g/dl, this arbitrary cutoff is inappropriate for all children, because Hgb levels normally vary with age (see Table 49-1 and Appendix F).

Other tests specific to a particular type of anemia are employed to determine the underlying cause of anemia. These are discussed in relation to the particular disorder.

BOX 49-1

Red Blood Cell Morphology

Characteristics of Red Blood Cells (RBCs)

Size (Cell Size)

Variation in RBC sizes (anisocytocytes)
- Normocytes (normal cell size)
- Microcytes (smaller than normal cell size)
- Macrocytes (larger than normal cell size)

Shape (Irregular Shape)

Variation in RBC shapes (poikilocytes)
- Spherocytes (globular cells)
- Drepanocytes (sickle-shaped cells)
- Numerous other irregular-shaped cells

Color (Staining Characteristics)

Variation in hemoglobin concentration in the RBC
- Normochromic (sufficient or normal amount of hemoglobin per RBC)
- Hypochromic (reduced amount of hemoglobin per RBC)
- Hyperchromic (increased amount of hemoglobin per RBC)

Therapeutic Management

The objective of medical management is to reverse the anemia by treating the underlying cause and to make up for any deficiency of blood, blood component, or substance the blood needs for normal functioning. For example, blood or blood cells are replaced after hemorrhage; in nutritional anemias, the specific deficiency is replaced.

In patients with severe anemia, supportive medical care may include oxygen therapy, bed rest, and replacement of intravascular volume with intravenous (IV) fluids. The prognosis for anemia depends on the correction of the cause.

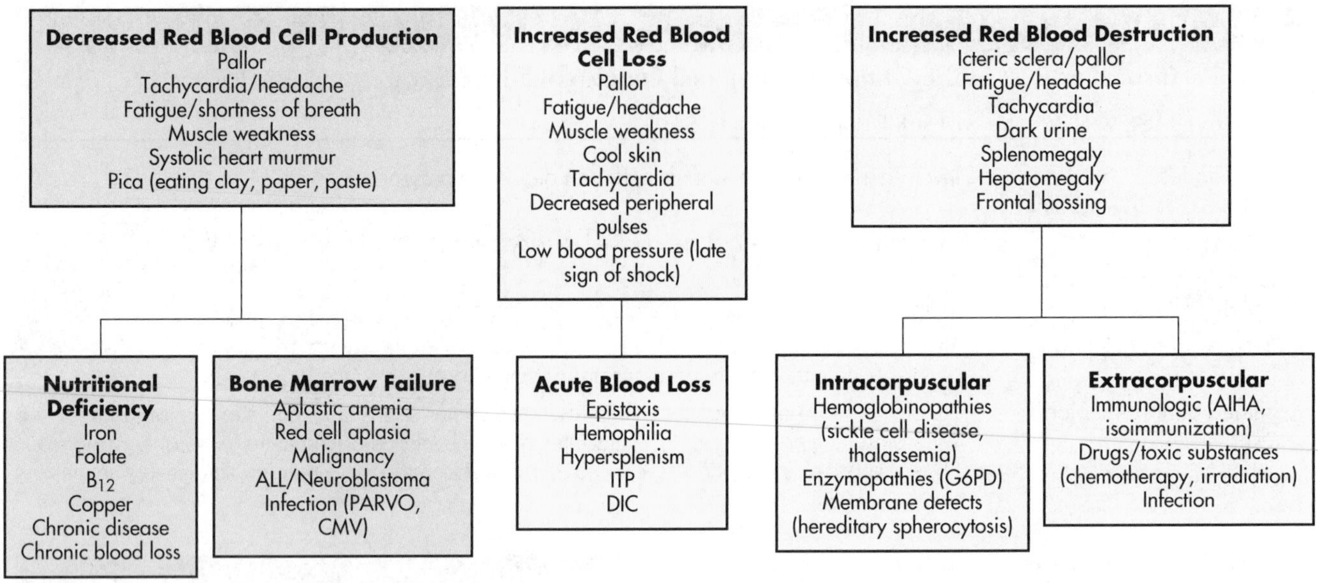

Fig. 49-1 Classification of anemias.

Nursing Care Management

The assessment of anemia includes the basic techniques that are applicable to any condition. The age of the infant or child provides some clues regarding the possible etiology of the anemia. For example, iron deficiency anemia occurs more frequently in the toddler between 12 and 36 months of age and during the growth spurt of adolescence.

Racial or ethnic background is significant. For example, the anemias related to abnormal Hgb levels are found in Southeast Asians and persons of African or Mediterranean ancestry. These same groups may be genetically deficient in the enzyme lactase after the period of infancy. Affected individuals are unable to tolerate lactose in the diet, with consequent intestinal irritation and chronic blood loss.

Special emphasis is placed on a careful history to elicit any information that might help identify the cause of the anemia. For example, a statement such as "My child drinks lots of milk" is a frequent finding in toddlers with iron deficiency anemia. An episode of diarrhea may have precipitated a temporary lactose intolerance in a young child.

Stool examination for occult (microscopic) blood (Hemoccult test) can identify chronic intestinal bleeding that results from a primary or secondary lactase deficiency. It is also important to understand the significance of various blood tests (see Table 49-1).

Prepare Child and Family for Laboratory Tests

Usually, several blood tests are ordered, but because they are generally done sequentially rather than at one time, the child is subjected to multiple finger or heel punctures or venipunctures. Laboratory technicians frequently are not aware of the trauma that repeated punctures represent to a child. However, these invasive procedures need not be painful (see Blood Specimens, Chapter 45). For example, the topical application of EMLA or Elamax before needle punctures can eliminate any pain (see Pain Management, Chapter 44). Therefore the nurse is responsible for preparing the child and family for the tests by (1) explaining the significance of each test, particularly why the tests are not done at one time; (2) encouraging parents or another supportive person to be with the child during the procedure; and (3) allowing the child to play with the equipment on a doll or participate in the actual procedure (e.g., by cleansing the finger with an alcohol swab). Older children may appreciate the opportunity to observe the blood cells under a microscope or in photographs. This experience is an especially important consideration if a serious blood disorder, such as leukemia, is suspected, because it serves as a foundation for explaining the pathophysiology of the disorder.

Bone marrow aspiration is not a routine hematologic test but is essential for definitive diagnosis of the leukemias, lymphomas, and certain anemias.

NURSE ALERT The following are suggested explanations for teaching children about blood components:

- *Red blood cells*—Carry the oxygen you breathe from your lungs to all parts of your body
- *White blood cells*—Help keep germs from causing infection
- *Platelets*—Small parts of cells that help make bleeding stop; platelets help your body stop bleeding by forming a clot (scab) over the hurt area
- *Plasma*—The liquid portion of blood; has clotting factors that help make bleeding stop ■

Decrease Tissue Oxygen Needs

Because the basic pathology in anemia is a decrease in oxygen-carrying capacity, an important nursing responsibility is to assess the child's energy level and minimize excess demands. The child's level of tolerance for activities of daily living and play is assessed, and adjustments are made to allow as much self-care as possible without undue exertion. During periods of rest, the nurse takes vital signs and observes behavior to establish a baseline of nonexertion energy expenditure. During periods of activity, the nurse repeats these measurements and observations to compare them with resting values.

NURSE ALERT Signs of exertion include tachycardia, palpitations, tachypnea, dyspnea, shortness of breath, hyperpnea, breathlessness, dizziness, light-headedness, diaphoresis, and change in skin color. The child looks fatigued (sagging, limp posture; slow, strained movements; inability to tolerate additional activity; difficulty sucking in infants). ■

Diversional activities are planned that promote rest but prevent boredom and withdrawal. Because short attention span, irritability, and restlessness are common in anemia and increase stress demands on the body, appropriate activities are planned, such as listening to music; using a tape recorder; watching television; reading or listening to stories or comics; continuing a favorite hobby, such as stamp collecting, coloring, or drawing; playing board and card games; or being wheeled in a carriage or chair. Choosing the appropriate roommate, such as a child of similar age with a diagnosis that also requires restricted activity, is a helpful intervention.

If infants or young children are hospitalized, the importance of preventing separation from parents must be considered. Crying and fretfulness place increased stress demands on the body, which increases oxygen needs. Parents need help in understanding the importance of their presence, even though the child may be less responsive than usual. The nurse also explains the reason for mood changes and the necessity of allowing the child's dependency.

Prevent Complications

Children who are so severely anemic that they are hospitalized may require oxygen to prevent or reduce tissue hypoxia. Because these children are susceptible to infection, every effort is expended to prevent exposure to infectious agents. All the usual precautions are taken to prevent infection, such as practicing thorough handwashing, selecting an appropriate room in a noninfectious area, restricting visitors or hospital personnel with active infection, and maintaining adequate nutrition. The nurse also observes for signs of infection, particularly temperature elevation and leukocytosis.

Iron Deficiency Anemia

Anemia caused by an inadequate supply of dietary iron is the most prevalent nutritional disorder in the United States and the most common mineral disturbance. Children 12 to 36 months of age are at risk for anemia as a result of cow's milk being a major staple of the child's diet (Segel, Hirsch, & Feig, 2002a). The prevalence of iron deficiency anemia has decreased, probably in part because of families' participation in the Women, Infants, and Children (WIC) program, which provides iron-fortified formula for the first year of life and routine screening of Hgb levels during early childhood (Bogen, Krause, & Serwint, 2001). Premature infants are especially at risk because of their reduced fetal iron supply. Adolescents are also at risk because of their rapid growth rate combined with poor eating habits.

Pathophysiology

Iron deficiency anemia can be caused by any number of factors that decrease the supply of iron, impair its absorption, increase the body's need for iron, or affect the synthesis of Hgb. Although the clinical manifestations and diagnostic evaluation are similar regardless of the cause, the therapeutic and nursing considerations depend on the specific reason for the iron deficiency. The following discussion is limited to iron deficiency anemia resulting from inadequate iron in the diet.

During the last trimester of pregnancy, iron is transferred from mother to fetus. Most of the iron is stored in the circulating erythrocytes of the fetus, with the remainder stored in the fetal liver, spleen, and bone marrow. These iron stores are usually adequate for the first 5 to 6 months in a full-term infant but for only 2 to 3 months in premature infants or multiple births. If dietary iron is not supplied to meet the infant's growth demands after the fetal iron stores are depleted, iron deficiency anemia results. Physiologic anemia should not be confused with iron deficiency anemia resulting from nutritional causes.

Although most toddlers with iron deficiency anemia are underweight, many infants are overweight because of excessive milk ingestion (known as *milk babies*). These children become anemic for two reasons: milk, a poor source of iron, is given almost to the exclusion of solid foods, and 50% of iron-deficient infants fed cow's milk have an increased fecal loss of blood.

Therapeutic Management

After the diagnosis of iron deficiency anemia is made, therapeutic management focuses on increasing the amount of supplemental iron the child receives. This is usually done through dietary counseling and the administration of oral iron supplements.

In formula-fed infants, the most convenient and best sources of supplemental iron are iron-fortified commercial formula and iron-fortified infant cereal. Iron-fortified formula provides a relatively constant and predictable amount of iron and is not associated with an increased incidence of gastrointestinal (GI) symptoms, such as colic, diarrhea, or constipation. Infants younger than 12 months of age should *not* be given fresh cow's milk because it may increase the risk of GI blood loss occurring from allergy to the milk protein or from GI mucosal damage resulting from a lack of cytochrome iron (heme protein) (Segel, Hirsch, & Feig, 2002b). If GI bleeding is suspected, the child's stool should be guaiac tested on at least four or five occasions to identify any intermittent blood loss.

Dietary addition of iron-rich foods is usually inadequate as the sole treatment of iron deficiency anemia, because the iron is poorly absorbed and provides insufficient supplemental quantities of iron. If dietary sources of iron cannot replace body stores, oral iron supplements are prescribed for approximately 3 months. Ferrous iron, more readily absorbed than ferric iron, results in higher Hgb levels. Ascorbic acid (vitamin C) appears to facilitate absorption of iron and may be given as vitamin C–enriched foods and juices with the iron preparation.

If the Hgb level fails to rise after 1 month of oral therapy, it is important to assess for persistent bleeding, iron malabsorption, noncompliance, improper iron administration, or other causes of the anemia. Parenteral (IV or intramuscular [IM]) iron administration is safe and effective, but it is painful, expensive, and occasionally associated with regional lymphadenopathy or allergic reaction (Andrews, 2003). Therefore parenteral iron is reserved for children who have iron malabsorption or chronic hemoglobinuria. Transfusions are indicated for the most severe anemia and in cases of serious infection, cardiac dysfunction, or surgical emergency when anesthesia is required. Packed RBCs (2 to 3 ml/kg), not whole blood, are used to minimize the chance of circulatory overload. Supplemental oxygen is administered when tissue hypoxia is severe.

Prognosis

The prognosis for a child with this condition is very good. However, there is some evidence that if the iron deficiency anemia is severe and long-standing, cognitive, behavioral, and motor impairment may result (Andrews, 2003; Halterman et al, 2001).

Nursing Care Management

An essential nursing responsibility is instructing parents in the administration of iron. Oral iron should be given as prescribed in two divided doses between meals, when the presence of free hydrochloric acid is greatest, because more iron is absorbed in the acidic environment of the upper GI tract. A citrus fruit or juice taken with the medication aids in absorption.

NURSE ALERT Cow's milk contains substances that bind the iron and interfere with absorption. Iron supplements should not be administered with milk or milk products (Carley, 2003). ■

An adequate dosage of oral iron turns the stools a tarry green color. The nurse advises parents of this normally expected change and inquires about its occurrence on follow-up visits. Absence of the greenish black stool may be a clue to poor administration of iron, either in schedule or in dosage. Vomiting and diarrhea can occur with iron therapy. If the parents report these symptoms, the iron can be given with meals and the dosage reduced and then gradually increased until tolerated.

Liquid preparations of iron may temporarily stain the teeth. If possible, the medication should be taken through a straw or given through a syringe or medicine dropper placed toward the back of the mouth. Brushing the teeth after administration of the drug lessens the discoloration.

If parenteral iron preparations are prescribed, iron dextran must be injected deeply into a large muscle mass using the Z-tract method. The injection site is *not* massaged after injection to minimize skin staining and irritation. Because no more than 1 ml should be given in one site, the IV route should be considered to avoid multiple injections. Careful observation is required because of the risk of adverse reactions, such as anaphylaxis, with IV administration. A test dose is recommended before routine use.

Diet

A primary nursing objective is to prevent nutritional anemia through family education. Because breast milk is a poor iron source after 5 months of lactation, the nurse must reinforce the importance of administering iron supplementation in the exclusively breastfed infant by 4 to 6 months of age (Andrews, 2003; Griffins & Abrams, 2001).

In the formula-fed infant, the nurse discusses with parents the importance of using iron-fortified formula and the introduction of solid foods at the appropriate age during the first year of life. Traditionally, cereals are one of the first semisolid foods to be introduced into the infant's diet at approximately 4 months of age (Davidsson, 2003). The best solid-food source of iron is commercial iron-fortified cereals. It may be difficult at first to teach the infant to accept foods other than milk. The same principles are applied as those for introducing new foods (see Nutrition, Chapter 36), especially feeding the solid food before the milk. Predominantly milk-fed infants rebel against solid foods, and parents are cautioned about this and the need to be firm in not relinquishing control to the child. It may require intense problem solving on the part of both the family and the nurse to overcome the child's resistance.

A difficulty encountered in discouraging the parents from feeding milk to the exclusion of other foods is dispelling the popular myth that milk is a "perfect food." Many parents believe that milk is best for the infant and equate the weight gain with a "healthy child" and "good mothering." The nurse can also stress that overweight is not synonymous with good health.

Diet education of teenagers is especially difficult, especially because teenage girls are particularly prone to following weight-reduction diets. Emphasizing the effect of anemia on appearance (pallor) and energy level (difficulty maintaining popular activities) may be useful.

Sickle Cell Anemia

evolve CASE STUDY: SICKLE CELL ANEMIA

Sickle cell anemia (SCA) is one of a group of diseases collectively termed *hemoglobinopathies,* in which normal adult hemoglobin (hemoglobin A [HbA]) is partly or completely replaced by abnormal sickle hemoglobin (HbS). *Sickle cell disease (SCD)* includes all those hereditary disorders whose clinical, hematologic, and pathologic features are related to the presence of HbS. Even though SCD is sometimes used to refer to SCA, this use is incorrect. Other correct terms for SCA are *SS* and *homozygous sickle cell disease.*

The following are the most common forms of SCD in the United States:

- *Sickle cell anemia* is the homozygous form of the disease (HbSS or SS).
- *Sickle cell–C disease* is a heterozygous variant of SCD, including both HbS and HbC (SC).
- *Sickle cell–hemoglobin E disease* is a variant of SCD in which glutamic acid has been substituted for lysine in the number-26 position of the β-chain (SE).
- *Sickle thalassemia disease* is a combination of sickle cell trait and β-thalassemia trait (Sβthal). β^1 refers to the ability to still produce some normal HbA. β^0 indicates that there is no ability to produce HbA.

Of the SCDs, SCA is the most common form in African-Americans, followed by sickle cell–C disease and sickle β-thalassemia.

SCA is found primarily in African-Americans, Hispanics, and other ethnic groups. SCA occurs infrequently in Caucasians (especially those of Mediterranean descent). The incidence of the disease varies in different geographic locations. Among African-Americans, the incidence of sickle cell trait is about 8%. In West Africa, the incidence is reported to be as high as 40% among native Africans. The high incidence of sickle cell trait in West Africans is believed by some to be the result of selective protection afforded trait carriers against one type of malaria.

The gene that determines the production of HbS is situated on an autosome and, when present, is always detectable and therefore dominant. Heterozygous persons who have both normal HbA and abnormal HbS are said to have *sickle cell trait.* Persons who are homozygous have predominantly HbS and have *sickle cell anemia.* The inheritance pattern is essentially that of an autosomal recessive disorder (see Appendix C). Therefore when both parents have sickle cell trait, there is a 25% chance with each pregnancy of producing an offspring with SCA.

Although the defect is inherited, the sickling phenomenon is usually not apparent until later in infancy because of the presence of fetal hemoglobin (HbF). As long as the child has predominantly HbF, sickling does not occur because there is less HbS. The newborn with SCA is generally asymptomatic because of the protective effect of Hgb F (60% to 80% HbF), but this rapidly decreases during the first year, so the child is at risk for sickle cell–related complications (Dover & Platt, 2003).

Pathophysiology

The clinical features of SCA are primarily the result of (1) *obstruction* caused by the sickled RBCs and (2) increased RBC *destruction* (Fig. 49-2). The entanglement and enmeshing of rigid sickle-shaped cells with one another intermittently block the microcirculation, causing vaso-occlusion. The resultant absence of blood flow to adjacent tissues causes local hypoxia, leading to tissue ischemia and infarction (cellular death). Most of the complications seen in SCA can be traced to this process and its impact on various organs of the body. The effect of sickling and infarction on organ structures occurs in the following sequence (see also consequences in Box 49-2):

1. Stasis with enlargement
2. Infarction with ischemia and destruction
3. Replacement with fibrous tissue (scarring)

Clinical Manifestations

The clinical manifestations of SCA vary greatly in severity and frequency. The most acute symptoms of the disease occur during periods of exacerbation called *crises.* There are several types of episodic crises: vaso-occlusive, acute splenic sequestration, aplastic, hyperhemolytic, cerebrovascular accident (stroke), chest syndrome, and infection. The crises may occur individually or concomitantly with one or more other crises. The episode may be a *vaso-occlusive crisis,* preferably called a "painful episode," characterized by distal

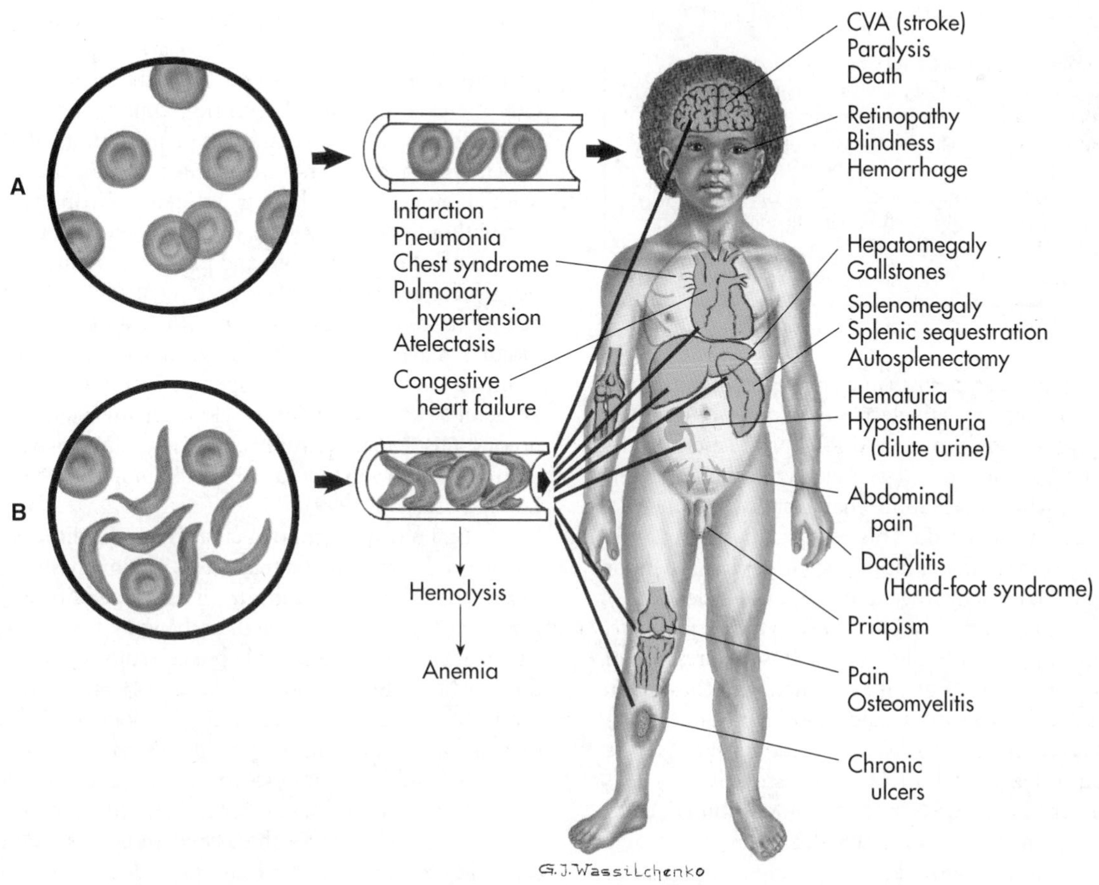

Fig. 49-2 Differences between effects of **A**, normal and **B**, sickled red blood cells on circulation with related complications.

BOX 49-2

Clinical Manifestations of Sickle Cell Anemia

General
Possible growth retardation
Chronic anemia (Hgb 6 to 9 g/dl)
Possible delayed sexual maturation
Marked susceptibility to sepsis

Vaso-Occlusive Crisis
Pain in area(s) of involvement
Manifestations related to ischemia of involved areas:
- Extremities—painful swelling of hands and feet (sickle cell dactylitis, or "hand-foot syndrome"), painful joints
- Abdomen—severe pain resembling acute surgical condition
- Cerebrum—stroke, visual disturbances
- Chest—symptoms resembling pneumonia, protracted episodes of pulmonary disease
- Liver—obstructive jaundice, hepatic coma
- Kidney—hematuria
- Genital—priapism (painful penile erection)

Sequestration Crisis
Pooling of large amounts of blood:
- Hepatomegaly
- Splenomegaly
- Circulatory collapse

Effects of Chronic Vaso-Occlusive Phenomena
Heart—cardiomegaly, systolic murmurs
Lungs—altered pulmonary function, susceptibility to infections, pulmonary insufficiency
Kidneys—inability to concentrate urine, progressive renal failure, enuresis
Liver—hepatomegaly, cirrhosis, intrahepatic cholestasis
Spleen—splenomegaly, susceptibility to infection, functional reduction in splenic activity progressing to autosplenectomy
Eyes—intraocular abnormalities with visual disturbances, sometimes progressive retinal detachment and blindness
Extremities—skeletal deformities such as lordosis and kyphosis, avascular necrosis of hip/shoulder, chronic leg ulcers, susceptibility to osteomyelitis
Central nervous system—hemiparesis, seizures

ischemia and pain; a *sequestration crisis,* a pooling of blood in the liver and spleen with decreased blood volume and shock; an *aplastic crisis,* diminished RBC production resulting in profound anemia; or a *hyperhemolytic crisis,* an accelerated rate of RBC destruction characterized by anemia, jaundice, and reticulocytosis. This complication frequently suggests other coexisting conditions, such as viral illness or glucose-6-phosphate dehydrogenase (G6PD) deficiency.

Another serious complication is *acute chest syndrome,* which is clinically similar to pneumonia. It is the presence of a new pulmonary infiltrate and is associated with chest pain, fever, cough, tachypnea, wheezing, and hypoxia. A *cerebrovascular accident (CVA, stroke)* is a sudden and severe complication, often with no related illnesses. Sickled cells block the major blood vessels in the brain, resulting in cerebral infarction, which causes variable degrees of neurologic impairment. Repeat CVAs causing progressively greater brain damage occur in approximately 70% of untreated children who have already experienced one stroke (Dover & Platt, 2003).

Diagnostic Evaluation

Newborn screening for SCA is mandatory in most of the United States so that infants can be identified before symptoms occur. At birth the infant has up to 80% of HbF, which does not carry the defect. Because levels of HbS are low at birth, Hgb electrophoresis or other tests that measure Hgb concentrations are indicated. Early diagnosis (before 3 months of age) enables initiation of appropriate interventions to minimize complications. The family is taught to administer prophylactic antibiotics, to identify early signs of infection, and to seek medical therapy as soon as possible.

If SCA is not diagnosed in early infancy, it is likely to manifest symptoms during the toddler and preschool years. SCA is occasionally first diagnosed during a crisis that follows an acute respiratory or GI infection. Routine hematologic tests are done to evaluate the anemia. Several specific tests detect the presence of the abnormal Hbg in the heterozygote and/or the homozygote. For *screening* purposes the *sickle-turbidity test (Sickledex)* is frequently used, because it can be performed on blood from a finger stick and yields accurate results in 3 minutes. However, if the test is positive, Hgb electrophoresis is necessary to distinguish between those children with the trait and those with the disease. *Hemoglobin electrophoresis* ("fingerprinting" of the protein) is an accurate, rapid, and specific test for detecting the homozygous and heterozygous forms of the disease, as well as the percentages of the various types of Hgb.

Therapeutic Management

The aims of therapy are (1) to prevent conditions that enhance sickling phenomena, which are responsible for the pathologic sequelae; and (2) to treat the medical emergencies of sickle cell crisis. Prevention consists of maintaining hemodilution. The successful implementation of this goal depends more often on nursing interventions than on medical therapies. Research is investigating hydroxyurea with and without erythropoietin, which may increase the concentration of fetal hemoglobin and ultimately reduce complications (Charache et al, 1996; Ferster et al, 2001). Hematopoietic stem cell transplantation with stabilization of prior organ damage is a possible cure for SCD (Karayalcin, 2000). Limiting factors include proper patient selection and the availability of suitable donors (Karayalcin, 2000). This technology raises many ethical issues regarding patient access and availability of therapy (Platt & Guinan, 1996; Simon, Lobo, & Jackson, 1999).

Medical management of a crisis is usually directed at supportive and symptomatic treatment. The main objectives are to provide (1) rest to minimize energy expenditure and oxygen use; (2) hydration through oral and IV therapy; (3) electrolyte replacement, because hypoxia results in metabolic acidosis, which also promotes sickling; (4) analgesics for the severe pain from vaso-occlusion; (5) blood replacement to treat anemia and hydration to reduce the viscosity of the sickled blood; and (6) antibiotics to treat any existing infection.

Administration of pneumococcal and meningococcal vaccines is recommended for these children because of their susceptibility to infection as a result of a functional asplenia. In addition to routine immunizations, the child with SCD should receive a yearly influenza vaccination. (See Immunizations, Chapter 36.) Oral penicillin prophylaxis is also recommended by 2 months of age (American Academy of Pediatrics, Section on Hematology/Oncology, Committee on Genetics, 2002; National Institutes of Health, National Heart, Lung, and Blood Institute [NIH/NHLBI], 2002; Segel et al, 2002b).

Short-term oxygen therapy may be helpful if a child has symptoms of respiratory difficulty. Severe hypoxia must be prevented because this causes massive systemic sickling that can be fatal. Although oxygen may prevent more sickling, it usually is not effective in reversing sickling, because the oxygen is unable to reach the enmeshed sickled erythrocytes in clogged vessels (Chiocca, 1996; Perkins, 2001). In addition, prolonged administration can depress bone marrow, further aggravating the anemia (Khoury & Grimsley, 1995).

Exchange transfusion, which reduces the number of circulating sickle cells and slows down the vicious circle of hypoxia, thrombosis, tissue ischemia, and injury, has been successful. The procedure is sometimes advocated as a possible preventive technique. A transcranial Doppler (TCD) test identifies the child with SCD who is at high risk for developing a CVA by monitoring the intracranial vascular flow (American Academy of Pediatrics, Section on Hematology/Oncology, Committee on Genetics, 2002; Segel et al, 2002b). The TCD is performed yearly on children from 2 to 16 years of age. If the TCD is abnormal, magnetic resonance imaging of the brain is done to detect cerebral arterial stenosis or ischemia. The recommended treatment for a confirmed abnormal TCD is chronic transfusion therapy (Segel et al, 2002b). However, multiple transfusions carry the risk of transmission of viral infection, hyperviscosity, transfusion reactions, alloimmunization, and hemosiderosis (Karayalcin, 2000; Orkin & Nathan, 2003). After a CVA has occurred, blood transfusions are usually given every 3 to 4 weeks to help prevent a repeat stroke. To reduce iron overload, home subcutaneous chelation therapy may be started (see p. 1612).

In children with recurrent life-threatening splenic sequestration, splenectomy may be a lifesaving measure. However, because the spleen usually atrophies on its own through progressive fibrotic changes *(functional asplenia)*, routine splenectomy is not recommended because of the risk of overwhelming infection. Any procedure that requires anesthesia has increased risk for these children. *Painful priapism (continual or intermittent erection)* may be treated by aspiration of the corpora cavernosum. This complication is particularly frequent in vaso-occlusive crises.

The most frequent problem for patients with SCA is *vaso-occlusive pain* (Fig. 49-3). The chronic nature of this pain can greatly affect the child's development. A multidisciplinary approach is best for its management. When mild to moderate pain is reported, ibuprofen or acetaminophen is used initially. If these drugs are not effective alone, codeine can be added. The dosages of both drugs are titrated (adjusted) to a therapeutic level. Opioids such as immediate- and sustained-release morphine, oxycodone, hydromorphone (Dilaudid), and methadone are administered intravenously or orally for severe pain and are given around the clock. Patient-controlled analgesia (PCA) has been used successfully for sickle cell–related pain. PCA reinforces the patient's role and responsibility in managing the pain and provides flexibility in dealing with pain, which may vary in severity over time. The use of high-dose IV methylprednisolone has decreased the duration of severe pain in children (Dover & Platt, 2003; Griffin, McIntire, & Buchanan, 1994). (See Pain Management, Chapter 44.)

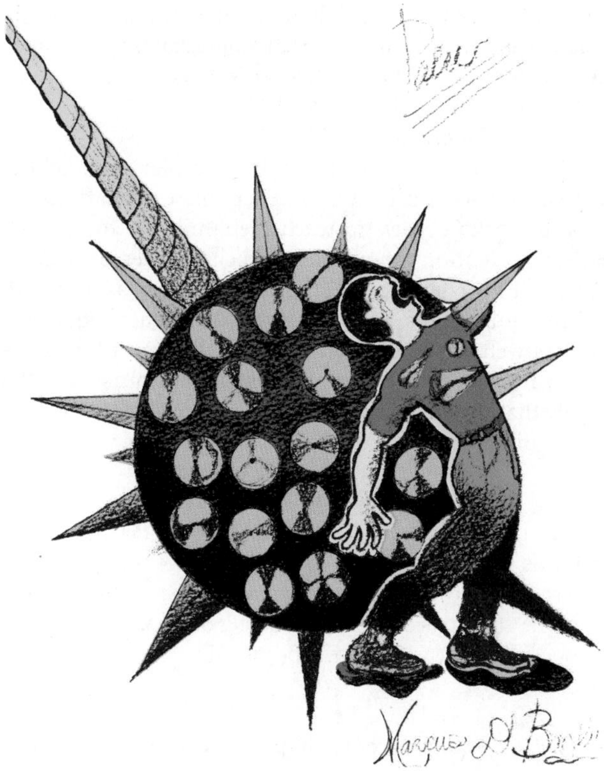

Fig. 49-3 Drawing of sickle cell pain by a 17-year-old boy. When asked what message he would like to give health professionals about treating pain, he stated, "Tell them to listen to the patient and family. They know about the pain."

NURSE ALERT Meperidine (pethidine [Demerol]) is not recommended. Normeperidine, a metabolite of meperidine, is a central nervous system stimulant that produces anxiety, tremors, myoclonus, and generalized seizures when it accumulates with repetitive dosing. Patients with SCD are particularly at risk for normeperidine-induced seizures (NIH/NHLBI, 2002; American Pain Society, 1999). ■

Prognosis

The prognosis varies. Most of the time, children are without symptoms and participate in normal activities without restrictions. The greatest risk is usually in children younger than 5 years of age, and the majority of deaths in these children are caused by overwhelming infection. Consequently, SCA is a chronic illness with a potentially terminal outcome.

Individuals with higher levels of HbF are more likely to have fewer complications than those with lower levels (Segel et al, 2002b; Steinberg et al, 2003). Long-term follow up of patients taking hydroxyurea alone revealed a 40% reduction in mortality rate (Steinberg et al, 2003).

Physical and sexual maturation are delayed in adolescents with SCA. Although adults achieve normal height, weight, and sexual function, the delay may present problems to the adolescent (Dover & Platt, 2003; Gribbons, Zahr, & Opas, 1995). Hematopoietic stem cell transplantation offers the hope of a cure for some children, although the mortality rate is approximately 8% and the graft failures after transplantation range from 9% to 14% (Dover & Platt, 2003).

Nursing Care Management

Educate Family and Child

Family education begins with an explanation of the disease and its consequences. After this explanation, the most important issues to teach the family are to (1) seek early intervention for problems, such as fever of 38.5° C (101.5° F) or greater; (2) give penicillin as ordered; (3) recognize signs and symptoms of splenic sequestration, as well as respiratory problems that can lead to hypoxia; and (4) treat the child normally. The nurse tells the family that the child is normal but can get sick in ways that other children cannot.

NURSE ALERT One simple yet graphic way to demonstrate the effect of sickling is to roll rounded objects, such as marbles or beads, through a tube to simulate normal circulation and then roll pointed objects, such as screws or jacks, through the tube. The effect of sickling and clumping of the pointed objects is especially noticeable at a bend or slight narrowing of the tube. ■

The nurse emphasizes the importance of adequate hydration to prevent sickling and to delay the stasis-thrombosis-ischemia cycle in a crisis. It is not sufficient to advise parents to "force fluids" or "encourage drinking." They need specific instructions on how many daily glasses or bottles of fluid are required. Many foods are also a source of fluid, particularly soups, flavored ice pops, ice cream, sherbet, gelatin, and puddings.

Increased amounts of fluids combined with impaired kidney function result in the problem of *enuresis.* Parents who are unaware of this fact frequently employ the usual measures to discourage bed-wetting, such as limiting fluids at night, and may resort to punishment and shame to force bladder control. Enuresis is treated as a complication of the disease, such as joint pain or some other symptom, to alleviate parental pressure on the child.

Promote Supportive Therapies during Crises

The success of many of the medical therapies relies heavily on nursing implementation. Management of pain is an especially difficult problem and often involves experimenting with various analgesics, including opioids, and schedules before relief is achieved. Unfortunately, these children tend to be undermedicated, resulting in their "clock watching" and demands for additional doses sooner than might be expected. Often this incorrectly raises suspicions of drug addiction, when in fact the problem is one of improper dosage (Family Focus box). In choosing and scheduling analgesics, the goal should be *prevention* of pain.

NURSE ALERT Advise parents to be particularly alert to situations in which dehydration may be a possibility, such as hot weather, and to recognize early signs of reduced intake, such as decreased urine output (e.g., fewer wet diapers) and increased thirst. ■

Any pain program should be combined with psychologic support to help the child deal with the depression, anxiety, and fear that may accompany the disease. This includes regular visits with the child to discuss any concerns during the hospitalization and positive reinforcement of coping skills, such as successful methods of dealing with the pain and compliance with treatment prescriptions. To reduce the negative connotation associated with the term "crisis," it is best to say "pain episode."

> **Family Focus**
>
> **FEAR OF ADDICTION**
>
> Although pain is usually severe and opioids are warranted, many families fear that their child will become addicted to the narcotic. Unfortunately, misinformed health professionals may foster this unfounded fear, resulting in needless suffering. Few, if any, children who receive opioids for severe pain become behaviorally addicted to the drug (NIH/NHLBI, 2002). Families and older children, especially adolescents, need to be reassured that opioids are medically indicated, high doses may be needed, and addiction is rare.

Frequently, heat to the affected area is soothing. Cold compresses are not applied to the area because this enhances sickling and vasoconstriction. Bed rest is usually well tolerated during a crisis, although actual rest depends greatly on pain alleviation and organized schedules of nursing care. Some activity, particularly passive range-of-motion exercises, is beneficial to promote circulation. Usually the best course of action is to let children dictate their activity tolerance.

If blood transfusions or exchange transfusions are given, the nurse has the responsibility of observing for signs of transfusion reaction . Because hypervolemia from too-rapid transfusion can increase the workload of the heart, the nurse also is alert to signs of cardiac failure.

In splenic sequestration, the size of the spleen is gently measured by abdominal palpation (see Abdomen, Chapter 35). The nurse should be aware of spleen size because an increasing splenomegaly is an ominous sign. A decreasing spleen size denotes response to therapy. Vital signs and blood pressure are also closely monitored for impending shock. Anemia is typically not a complication in vaso-occlusive crises but is a critical problem in other types of crises. The nurse monitors for evidence of increasing anemia and institutes appropriate nursing interventions (see p. 1604). Oxygen is not beneficial in vaso-occlusive episodes unless hypoxemia is present (Chiocca, 1996; Karayalcin, 2000). It does not reverse sickled RBCs, and if used in the nonhypoxic patient, it will decrease erythropoiesis (Khoury & Grimsley, 1995). Because prolonged use of oxygen can aggravate the anemia, signs of lack of therapeutic benefit, such as restlessness, increased pallor, and continued pain, are reported.

Intake, especially of IV fluids, and output are recorded. The child's weight should be taken on admission, because it serves as a baseline for evaluating hydration. Because diuresis can result in electrolyte loss, the nurse also observes for signs of hypokalemia and should be familiar with normal serum electrolyte values to report changes.

Recognize Other Complications

Nurses also need to be aware of the signs of chest syndrome and CVA, both potentially fatal complications.

NURSE ALERT Report signs of the following immediately:

Chest syndrome:

- Severe chest, back, or abdominal pain
- Fever of 38.5° C (101.5° F) or higher
- Very congested cough
- Dyspnea, tachypnea
- Retractions
- Declining oxygen saturation (oximetry)

Cerebrovascular accident (CVA, stroke):

- Severe, unrelieved headaches
- Severe vomiting
- Jerking or twitching of the face, legs, or arms
- Seizures
- Strange, abnormal behavior
- Inability to move an arm and/or a leg
- Stagger or an unsteady walk
- Stutter or slurred speech
- Weakness in the hands, feet, or legs
- Changes in vision

Support Family

Families need the opportunity to discuss their feelings regarding transmitting a potentially fatal, chronic illness to their child. Because of the widely publicized prognosis for children with SCA, many parents express their prevalent fear of the child's death. Three manifestations of SCD that may appear in the first 2 years of life (dactylitis, severe anemia, and leukocytosis) can be predictors of disease severity (Miller et al, 2000). However, nursing care for the family should be the same as that for any family with a child with a life-threatening illness. Particular emphasis is placed on the siblings' reactions, the stress on the marital relationship, and the childrearing attitudes displayed toward the child (see Chapter 31). Several resources are available to the family with a sickling disorder.*

*National Association for Sickle Cell Disease, Inc., 3345 Wilshire Boulevard, Suite 1106, Los Angeles, CA 90010-1880; phone: 800-421-8453; Web site: www.sicklecelldisease.org. Center for Sickle Cell Disease, Howard University, 2121 Georgia Avenue NW, Washington, DC 20059; phone: 202-806-7930. National Heart, Lung, and Blood Institute, 9000 Rockville Pike, Building 31, Room 4A-21, Bethesda, MD 20892; phone: 301-496-4236; Web site: www.nhlbi.nih.gov/nhlbi/nhlbi.htm. The Agency for Healthcare Research Quality (AHRQ) (formerly AHCPR) has published three booklets on sickle cell disease: *Sickle Cell Disease: Comprehensive Screening, Diagnosis, Management, and Counseling in Newborns and Infants,* Clinical Practice Guideline no. 6, pub. no. AHCPR-0562; *Sickle Cell Disease: Comprehensive Screening and Management in Newborns and Infants,* Quick Reference Guide for Clinicians no. 6, pub. no. AHCPR-0563; and *Sickle Cell Disease in Newborns and Infants: A Guide for Parents,* pub. no. AHCPR 93-0564. They are available from the AHCPR Publications Clearinghouse, PO Box 8547, Silver Spring, MD 20907; phone: 800-358-9295; Web site: www.ahcpr.gov. *Guideline for the Management of Acute and Chronic Pain in Sickle-Cell Disease,* from American Pain Society, 4700 W. Lake Avenue, Glenview, IL 60025-1485; phone: 847-375-4715; fax: 847-375-6315; email: info@ampainsoc.org; Web site: www.ampainsoc.org. *Clinical Reference Guide for Health Care Providers; Sickle Cell Related Pain: Assessment and Management—A Guide for Patients and Parents,* from the New England Regional Genetics Groups (NERGG), No. 28 Clarendon Street, Newton, MA 02460; phone: 617-243-3033, email: maryaten @mediaone.net; Web site: www.acadia.net/NERGG. A video, *Sickle Cell Disease Is More Than Pain Management,* is available from Maxishare, PO Box 2041, Milwaukee, WI 53201; phone: 800-444-7747. Information is also available from the Sickle Cell Disease Association of America, Inc., 200 Cooperate Pointe, Suite 495, Culver City, CA 90230-7633.

The nurse advises parents to inform all treating personnel of the child's condition. The use of medical identification, such as a bracelet, is another way of ensuring awareness of the disease.

If family members have the SCD trait or SCA, genetic counseling is necessary. A primary goal is informing parents who carry the trait, in language they can understand, of the 25% chance with each pregnancy of having a child with the disease.

β-Thalassemia (Cooley Anemia)

The term *thalassemia,* which is derived from the Greek word *thalassa,* meaning "sea," is applied to a variety of inherited blood disorders characterized by deficiencies in the rate of production of specific globin chains in Hgb. The name appropriately refers to those people living near the Mediterranean Sea, as well as their descendants, who have the highest incidence of the disease, namely Italians, Greeks, and Syrians. Evidence suggests that the high incidence of the disorders among these groups is a result of selective advantage of the trait to malaria, as is postulated in sickle cell disease. However, the disorder has a wide geographic distribution, probably as a result of genetic migration through intermarriage or possibly as a result of spontaneous mutation.

β-Thalassemia is the most common of the thalassemias and occurs in four forms: two heterozygous forms—*thalassemia minor,* an asymptomatic silent carrier, and *thalassemia trait,* which produces a mild microcytic anemia; *thalassemia intermedia,* which is manifested as splenomegaly and moderate to severe anemia; and a homozygous form, *thalassemia major* (also known as *Cooley anemia*), which results in a severe anemia that would lead to cardiac failure and death in early childhood without transfusion support.

Pathophysiology

Normal postnatal Hgb is composed of two β-chains and two β-polypeptide chains. In β-thalassemia there is a partial or complete deficiency in the synthesis of the β-chain of the Hgb molecule. Consequently, there is a compensatory increase in the synthesis of β-chains, and β-chain production remains activated, resulting in defective Hgb formation. This unbalanced polypeptide unit is very unstable; when it disintegrates, it damages RBCs, causing severe anemia.

To compensate for the hemolytic process, an overabundance of erythrocytes is formed unless the bone marrow is suppressed by transfusion therapy. Excess iron from hemolysis of supplemental RBCs in transfusions and from the rapid destruction of defective cells is stored in various organs *(hemosiderosis).*

Diagnostic Evaluation

The onset of thalassemia major may be insidious and not recognized until the latter half of infancy. The clinical effects of thalassemia major are primarily attributable to (1) defective synthesis of HbA, (2) structurally impaired RBCs, and (3) shortened life span of erythrocytes (Box 49-3).

Hematologic studies reveal the characteristic changes in RBCs (i.e., microcytosis, hypochromia, anisocytosis, poikilocytosis, target cells, and basophilic stippling of various stages). Low Hgb and Hct levels are seen in severe anemia, although they are typically lower than the reduction in RBC count because of the proliferation of immature erythrocytes.

BOX 49-3

Clinical Manifestations of β-Thalassemia

Anemia (Before Diagnosis)
Pallor
Unexplained fever
Poor feeding
Enlarged spleen/liver

With Progressive Anemia
Signs of chronic hypoxia:
- Headache
- Precordial and bone pain
- Decreased exercise tolerance
- Listlessness
- Anorexia

Other Features
Small stature
Delayed sexual maturation
Bronzed, freckled complexion (if not chelated)

Bone Changes (Older Children If Untreated)
Enlarged head
Prominent frontal and parietal bosses
Prominent malar eminences
Flat or depressed bridge of the nose
Enlarged maxilla
Protrusion of the lip and upper central incisors and eventual malocclusion
Generalized skeletal osteoporosis

Hgb electrophoresis confirms the diagnosis, and radiographs of involved bones reveal characteristic findings.

Therapeutic Management

The objective of supportive therapy is to maintain sufficient Hgb levels to prevent bone marrow expansion and the resulting bony deformities, and to provide sufficient RBCs to support normal growth and normal physical activity. Transfusions are the foundation of medical management. Recent studies have evaluated the benefits of maintaining the child's Hgb level above 9.5 g/dl, a goal that may require transfusions as often as every 3 to 5 weeks. The advantages of this therapy include (1) improved physical and psychologic well-being because of the ability to participate in normal activities, (2) decreased cardiomegaly and hepatosplenomegaly, (3) fewer bone changes, (4) normal or near-normal growth and development until puberty, and (5) fewer infections.

One of the potential complications of frequent blood transfusions is iron overload. Because the body has no effective means of eliminating the excess iron, the mineral is deposited in body tissues. To minimize the development of hemosiderosis, *deferoxamine (Desferal),* an iron-chelating agent, is given with oral supplements of vitamin C. Vitamin C should be used only in patients who are ascorbate depleted and only while deferoxamine is being administered. As ferritin levels decrease toward normal, the role of vitamin C in increasing iron excretion disappears (Orkin & Nathan, 2003). Deferoxamine is given intravenously or subcutaneously, often at home using a portable infusion pump, over 8 to 24 hours (usually during sleep) for 5 to 7 days a week. It is also given intravenously over 4 hours at the time of blood transfusion in many centers. Creative strategies such as behavioral contracting have been used to assist the child in complying with the deferoxamine regimen.

In some children with severe splenomegaly who demonstrate increased transfusion requirements, a splenectomy may be necessary to decrease the disabling effects of abdominal pressure and to increase the life span of supplemental RBCs. Over time, the spleen may accelerate the rate of RBC destruction and thus increase transfusion requirements. After a splenectomy, children generally require fewer transfusions, although the basic defect in Hgb synthesis remains unaffected. A major postsplenectomy complication is severe and overwhelming infection. Therefore these children continue to receive prophylactic antibiotics with close medical supervision for many years and should receive the pneumococcal and meningococcal vaccines in addition to the regularly scheduled immunizations (see Immunizations, Chapter 36).

NURSE ALERT Ensure that the patient (if old enough) and the patient's family understand the need to notify the health professional of all fevers of 38.5° C (101.5° F) or greater because of the risk of sepsis in a child with asplenia. ■

Prognosis

Most children treated with blood transfusion and early chelation therapy survive well into adulthood. The most common cause of death is iron-induced heart disease, multiple organ failure, postsplenectomy sepsis, liver disease, and malignancy (Paley, 2000). Hematopoietic stem cell transplantation has the best results in the least symptomatic patients with a 75% rate of complication-free survival (Orkin & Nathan, 2003; Paley, 2000).

Nursing Care Management

The objectives of nursing care are to (1) promote compliance with transfusion and chelation therapy, (2) assist the child in coping with the anxiety-provoking treatments and the effects of the illness, (3) foster the child's and family's adjustment to a chronic illness, and (4) observe for complications of multiple blood transfusions. Basic to each of these goals is explaining to parents and older children the defect responsible for the disorder, its effect on RBCs, and the potential effects of untreated iron overload (such as diabetes and heart disease). Because the prevalence of this condition is high among families of Mediterranean descent, the nurse also inquires about the family's previous knowledge about thalassemia. All families with a child with thalassemia should be tested for the trait and referred for genetic counseling.

As with any chronic illness, the needs of the family must be met for optimum adjustment to the stresses imposed by the disorder (see Chapter 41). Sources of information for the family include the Cooley's Anemia Foundation* and the Thalassemia Action Group.† Genetic counseling for the par-

*129-09 26th Avenue, Suite 203, Flushing, NY 11354; phone: 718-321-2873 or 800-522-7222; fax: 718-321-3340; Web site: www.thalassemia.org.

†129-09 26th Avenue, Suite 203, Flushing, NY 11354; phone: 718-321-2873 or 800-522-7222; fax: 718-321-3340; Web site: www.geocities.com/hotsprings/8730/.

ents and fertile offspring is mandatory, and both prenatal diagnosis using amniocentesis at 20 weeks of gestation or fetal blood sampling at 10 weeks and screening for thalassemia trait are available.

Aplastic Anemia

Aplastic anemia (AA) refers to a condition in which the formed elements of the blood are simultaneously depressed as a result of bone marrow failure. The peripheral blood smear demonstrates pancytopenia or the triad of profound anemia, leukopenia, and thrombocytopenia. *Hypoplastic anemia* is characterized by a profound depression of RBCs, but normal or slightly decreased white blood cells (WBCs) and platelets.

Etiology

AA can be *primary* (*congenital,* or present at birth) or *secondary (acquired).* The best-known congenital disorder of which AA is an outstanding feature is *Fanconi syndrome,* a rare hereditary disorder characterized by pancytopenia, hypoplasia of the bone marrow, and patchy brown discoloration of the skin resulting from the deposit of melanin and associated with multiple congenital anomalies of the musculoskeletal and genitourinary systems. The syndrome appears to be inherited as an autosomal recessive trait with varying penetrance; therefore affected siblings may demonstrate several different combinations of defects.

Several etiologic factors contribute to the development of acquired hypoplastic anemia; however, about 70% of all cases are considered idiopathic (Box 49-4). Acquired AA is classified as either severe acquired AA or moderate acquired AA. The following discussion focuses on severe acquired AA, which carries a poorer prognosis and follows a more rapidly fatal course than the primary types.

Diagnostic Evaluation

The onset of clinical manifestations, which include anemia, leukopenia, and decreased platelet count, is usually insidious. Definitive diagnosis is determined from bone marrow aspiration, which demonstrates the conversion of red bone marrow to yellow, fatty bone marrow. *Severe AA* is defined as less than 25% bone marrow cellularity with at least two of the following findings: granulocyte count less than 500/mm^3; platelet count less than 20,000/mm^3; and reticulocyte count less than 40,000/mm^3 (Shende, 2000; Shimamura & Guinan, 2003). *Moderate AA* is defined as more than 25% bone marrow cellularity with at least two of the following findings: granulocyte count greater than 500/mm^3; platelet count greater than 20,000/mm^3; and reticulocyte count greater than 40,000/mm^3 (Shende, 2000; Shimamura & Guinan, 2003).

BOX 49-4

Common Causes of Acquired Aplastic Anemia

- Infection with the human parvovirus, hepatitis, or overwhelming infection
- Irradiation
- Drugs such as the chemotherapeutic agents and several antibiotics, one of the most notable being chloramphenicol
- Industrial and household chemicals, including benzene and its derivatives, which are found in petroleum products, dyes, paint remover, shellac, and lacquers
- Infiltration and replacement of myeloid elements, such as in leukemia or the lymphomas
- Idiopathic, in which no identifiable precipitating cause can be found

Therapeutic Management

The objectives of treatment are based on the recognition that the underlying disease process is failure of the bone marrow to carry out its hematopoietic functions. Therefore therapy is directed at restoring function to the marrow and involves two main approaches: (1) immunosuppressive therapy to remove the presumed immunologic functions that prolong aplasia or (2) replacement of the bone marrow through transplantation. Bone marrow transplantation is the treatment of choice for severe AA when a suitable donor exists (see p. 1639).

Antilymphocyte globulin (ALG) or *antithymocyte globulin (ATG)* is the principal drug treatment used for AA. The rationale for using ATG is based on the theory that AA may be a result of autoimmunity. ATG and cyclosporine suppress T-cell–dependent autoimmune responses but do not cause bone marrow suppression. Cyclosporine is administered orally for several weeks to months. The optimum schedule for ATG administration is still under investigation. It is usually given intravenously over 12 to 16 hours for 4 days, after a test dose to check for hypersensitivity. A course may be repeated, depending on the reduction in circulating lymphocytes and the patient's response. Because of the hypersensitivity response associated with ATG (i.e., fever, chills, myalgias), methylprednisolone is given intravenously to prevent these side effects. Colony-stimulating factor (CSF) and granulocyte-macrophage colony-stimulating factor (GM-CSF), given parenterally, may be used to enhance bone marrow production. Androgens may be used with ATG to stimulate erythropoiesis if the AA is nonresponsive to initial therapies. Cyclosporine may be administered in children who fail to respond to ATG, and success has also been achieved using high-dose methylprednisolone.

Hematopoietic stem cell transplantation should be considered *early* in the course of the disease if a compatible donor can be found. Transplantation is more successful when performed before multiple transfusions have sensitized the child to leukocyte and *human leukocyte antigens (HLAs).* Hematopoietic stem cell transplantation is associated with an 85% survival rate in untransfused patients compared with a 70% survival rate in transfused patients (Shende, 2000).

Nursing Care Management

The care of the child with AA is similar to that of the child with leukemia (see p. 1621)—specifically, preparing the child and family for the diagnostic and therapeutic procedures, preventing complications from the severe pancytopenia, and emotionally supporting them in terms of a potentially fatal outcome. Information and support are available from the Aplastic Anemia and MDS International Foundation, Inc.*

*PO Box 613, Annapolis, MD 21404-0613; phone: 800-747-2828; fax: 410-867-0240; Web site: www.aamds.org.

Because each of these nursing considerations is discussed in the section on leukemia, only the exceptions are presented here. The drug ATG is usually administered by way of a central vein. If not, vigilant care must be directed to the IV infusion to prevent extravasation. Meticulous care of the venous access is essential because of the child's susceptibility to infection. CSFs are usually given by subcutaneous injection over several days. Chemotherapeutic agents have been reported in the treatment of the relapsed patient with AA after ATG/CSF therapy. Many of the side effects associated with chemotherapy such as nausea and vomiting, alopecia, and mucositis are experienced by children receiving treatment for AA. Specialized care is required for children who have hematopoietic stem cell transplantation (see p. 1639).

DEFECTS IN HEMOSTASIS

Hemostasis is the process that stops bleeding when a blood vessel is injured. Vascular and plasma clotting factors, as well as platelets, are required. A complex system of clotting, anticlotting, and clot breakdown *(fibrinolysis)* mechanisms exists in equilibrium to ensure clot formation only in the presence of blood vessel injury and to limit the clotting process to the site of vessel wall injury. Dysfunction in these systems will lead to bleeding or abnormal clotting. Although the coagulation process is complex, clotting depends on three factors: (1) vascular influence, (2) platelet role, and (3) clotting factors.

Hemophilia

The term *hemophilia* refers to a group of bleeding disorders in which there is a deficiency of one of the factors necessary for coagulation of the blood. Although the symptomatology is similar regardless of which clotting factor is deficient, the identification of specific factor deficiencies allows definitive treatment with replacement agents.

In about 80% of all cases of hemophilia, the inheritance pattern is demonstrated as X-linked recessive (see Appendix C). The two most common forms of the disorder are *factor VIII deficiency* (*hemophilia A,* or *classic hemophilia*) and *factor IX deficiency* (*hemophilia B,* or *Christmas disease*). *von Willebrand disease* (*vWD*) is another hereditary bleeding disorder characterized by a deficiency, an abnormality, or an absence of the protein called *von Willebrand factor* (*vWF*) and a deficiency of factor VIII. Unlike hemophilia, vWD affects both males and females. The following discussion is primarily concerned with factor VIII deficiency, which accounts for 80% to 85% of all hemophilia cases.

Pathophysiology

The basic defect of hemophilia A is a deficiency of *factor VIII (antihemophilic factor [AHF])*. AHF is produced by the liver and is necessary for the formation of thromboplastin in phase I of blood coagulation. The less AHF found in the blood, the more severe the disease. Individuals with hemophilia have two of the three factors required for coagulation: vascular influence and platelets. Therefore they may bleed for longer periods, but not at a faster rate.

Bleeding into subcutaneous and intramuscular tissue is common. Hemarthrosis, which is bleeding into a joint space, is the most frequent type of internal bleeding. Bony changes and crippling deformities occur after repeated bleeding episodes over several years. Signs of hemarthrosis are swelling, warmth, redness, pain, and loss of movement. Bleeding in the neck, mouth, or thorax is serious, because the airway can become obstructed. Intracranial hemorrhage can have fatal consequences and is one of the major causes of death. Hemorrhage anywhere along the GI tract can lead to anemia, and bleeding into the retroperitoneal cavity is especially hazardous because of the large space for blood to accumulate. Hematomas in the spinal cord can cause paralysis.

Diagnostic Evaluation

Overt, prolonged hemorrhage is readily apparent; bleeding into tissues is less apparent (Box 49-5). The diagnosis is usually made from a history of bleeding episodes, evidence of X-linked inheritance (only one third of the cases are new mutations), and laboratory findings. The tests specific for hemophilia plasma depend on specific factors for a reaction to occur, such as the partial thromboplastin time (PTT). Specific determination of factor deficiencies requires assay procedures normally performed in specialized laboratories. Carrier detection is possible in classic hemophilia using deoxyribonucleic acid (DNA) testing and is an important consideration in families in which female offspring may have inherited the trait.

Therapeutic Management

The primary therapy for hemophilia is replacement of the missing clotting factor. The products available are *factor VIII concentrate* from pooled plasma or a genetically engineered recombinant, to be reconstituted with sterile water immediately before use, and *DDAVP (1-deamino-8-d-arginine vasopressin),* a synthetic form of vasopressin that increases plasma factor VIII and vWF levels. DDAVP is the treatment of choice in mild hemophilia and vWD if the child shows an appropriate response. DDAVP is not effective in the treatment of severe hemophilia A, severe vWD, or any form of hemophilia B. Vigorous therapy is instituted to prevent chronic crippling effects from joint bleeding.

Other drugs may be included in the therapy plan, depending on the source of the hemorrhage. Corticosteroids are given for hematuria, acute hemarthrosis, and chronic synovitis. Nonsteroidal antiinflammatory drugs (NSAIDs), such as ibuprofen, are effective in relieving pain caused by

BOX 49-5

Clinical Manifestations of Hemophilia

Prolonged bleeding anywhere from or in the body
Hemorrhage from any trauma—loss of deciduous teeth, circumcision, cuts, epistaxis, injections
Excessive bruising—even from a slight injury, such as a fall
Subcutaneous and intramuscular hemorrhages
Hemarthrosis (bleeding into the joint cavities), especially the knees, ankles, and elbows
Hematomas—pain, swelling, and limited motion
Spontaneous hematuria

synovitis; however, they must be used with caution because they inhibit platelet function (Dragone & Karp, 1996; National Hemophilia Foundation, 2003). Oral administration or local application of epsilon-aminocaproic acid (Amicar) prevents clot destruction; however, its use is limited to mouth or trauma surgery, and a dose of factor concentrate must be given first.

A regular program of exercise and physical therapy is an important aspect of management. Physical activity within reasonable limits strengthens muscles around joints and may decrease the number of spontaneous bleeding episodes.

Treatment without delay results in more rapid recovery and a decreased likelihood of complications; therefore most children are treated at home. The family is taught the technique of venipuncture and to administer the AHF to children older than 2 to 3 years of age. The child learns the procedure for self-administration at 8 to 12 years of age. Home treatment is highly successful, and the rewards, in addition to the immediacy, are less disruption of family life, fewer school or work days missed, and enhancement of the child's self-esteem and independence.

Primary prophylaxis in hemophilia patients has been practiced for many years in European countries (Fischer et al, 2001) and has proved to be effective in preventing arthropathy. Primary prophylaxis involves the infusion of factor VIII concentrate on a regular basis before the onset of joint damage. Secondary prophylaxis involves the infusion of factor VIII concentrate on a regular basis after the child experiences his first joint bleed. The infusions are given three times a week. Aggressive factor replacement may be a cost-effective alternative to primary prophylaxis. This involves the infusion of a high dose of factor VIII concentrate when a joint bleed occurs, followed by 2 days of more standard doses of factor VIII concentrate with consideration of additional treatment every other day for one week (Montgomery, Gill, & Scott, 2003; Nolan et al, 2003).

Prognosis

Although there is no cure for hemophilia, its symptoms can be controlled and its potentially crippling deformities greatly reduced or even avoided. Today many children with hemophilia function with minimal or no joint damage. They are normal children with an average life expectancy in every respect but one: they have a tendency to bleed, which is a significant inconvenience but not necessarily a life-threatening event.

Unfortunately, those individuals with hemophilia who were treated before current purification techniques for factor VIII concentrate (between 1979 and 1985) may have been exposed to the human immunodeficiency virus (HIV). It is estimated that more than 50% of these patients have seroconverted to HIV-positive status (Butler et al, 2003). As these individuals become sexually active, the issue of sexual transmission of HIV becomes increasingly important. The adolescent must be knowledgeable regarding safe sexual behavior. Individuals with hemophilia diagnosed and treated with factor concentrates since 1985 are at virtually no risk for developing HIV infection from treatment. Current manufacturing techniques have also greatly reduced the risk of hepatitis transmission.

Gene therapy may prove to be a treatment option in the future. This therapy involves introducing a working copy of the factor VIII gene into a patient who has a flawed copy of the gene. Problems exist with appropriate selection of the vector, identification of the cell for gene expression, and control of side effects (Montgomery et al, 2003).

Nursing Care Management

The earlier a bleeding episode is recognized, the more effectively it can be treated. Signs that indicate internal bleeding are especially important to recognize. Children are aware of internal bleeding and are very reliable in telling the examiner where an internal bleed is. In addition to the manifestations described (see Box 49-5), the nurse maintains a high level of suspicion when a child with hemophilia demonstrates signs such as headache, slurred speech, loss of consciousness (from cerebral bleeding), and black tarry stools (from GI bleeding).

Prevent Bleeding

The goal of prevention of bleeding episodes is directed toward decreasing the risk of injury. Prevention of bleeding episodes is geared mostly toward appropriate exercises to strengthen muscles and joints and to allow age-appropriate activity. During infancy and toddlerhood, the normal acquisition of motor skills creates innumerable opportunities for falls, bruises, and minor wounds. Restraining the child from mastering motor development can herald more serious long-term problems than allowing the behavior. However, the environment should be made as safe as possible, with close supervision maintained during playtime, to minimize incidental injuries.

For older children, the family usually needs assistance in preparing for school. A nurse who knows the family can be instrumental in discussing the situation with the school nurse and in jointly planning an appropriate schedule of activity. Because almost all persons with hemophilia are boys, the physical limitations in regard to active sports may be a difficult adjustment, and activity restrictions must be tempered with sensitivity to the child's emotional, as well as physical, needs. Use of protective equipment, such as padding and helmets, is particularly important, and noncontact sports, especially swimming, walking, jogging, tennis, golf, fishing, and bowling, are encouraged (National Hemophilia Foundation, 2003).

To prevent oral bleeding, some readjustment in terms of dental hygiene may be needed to minimize trauma to the gums, such as use of a water irrigating device, softening the toothbrush in warm water before brushing, or using a sponge-tipped disposable toothbrush. A regular toothbrush should be soft bristled and small in size.

Because any trauma can lead to a bleeding episode, all persons caring for these children must be aware of their disorder. These children should wear medical identification, and older children should be encouraged to recognize situations in which disclosing their condition is important, such as during dental extraction or injections. Health personnel need to take special precautions to prevent the use of procedures that may cause bleeding, such as IM injections. The subcutaneous route is substituted for IM injections whenever possible. Venipunctures for blood samples are usually preferred for these children. There is usually less bleeding after the venipuncture than after finger or heel punctures. Neither aspirin nor any aspirin-containing compound should be used. Acetaminophen (Tylenol) is a suitable aspirin substitute, especially for use during control of pain at home.

Recognize and Control Bleeding

As noted, the earlier a bleeding episode is recognized, the more effectively it can be treated. Factor replacement therapy should be instituted according to established medical protocol, and supportive measures may be implemented, such as *RICE,* which is (1) *rest,* (2) *ice,* (3) *compression,* and (4) *elevation.* When parents and older children are taught such measures beforehand, they can be prepared to initiate immediate treatment. Plastic bags of ice or cold packs should be kept in the freezer for such emergencies. However, such measures do not take the place of factor replacement.

Prevent Crippling Effects of Bleeding

As a result of repeated episodes of hemarthrosis, incompletely absorbed blood in the joints, and limitation of motion, bone and muscle changes occur that result in flexion contractures and joint fixation. During bleeding episodes the joint is elevated and immobilized. Active range-of-motion exercises are usually instituted after the acute episode. This allows the child to control the degree of exercise and discomfort. If an exercise program is instituted in the home, a physical therapist or public health nurse may need to supervise compliance with the regimen. Rarely, orthopedic intervention, such as casting, application of traction, or aspiration of blood, may be necessary to preserve joint function. Diet is also an important consideration, because excessive body weight can increase the strain on affected joints, especially the knees, and predispose to hemarthrosis. Consequently, calories need to be supplied in accordance with energy requirements.

Support Family and Prepare for Home Care

Genetic counseling is essential as soon as possible after diagnosis. Unlike many other disorders in which both parents carry the trait, the feeling of responsibility for this condition usually rests with the mother. Without an opportunity to discuss her feelings, the marital relationship can suffer. Technology is now available to identify carriers in approximately 80% of cases and may reduce the anxiety regarding childbearing in females who may be at risk of carrying the defective gene, such as sisters or maternal aunts of an affected male. The discovery of factor concentrates has greatly changed the outlook for these children. Bleeding can be minimized, and the child can live a much more normal, unrestricted life. Children are taught to take responsibility for their disease at an early age. They learn their limitations and other preventive measures, as well as self-administration of the prophylactic AHF.

The needs of families who have children with hemophilia are best met through a comprehensive team approach of physicians (pediatrician, hematologist, orthopedist), nurse practitioner, nurse, social worker, and physical therapist. Parent-group discussions are beneficial in meeting those needs often best met by similarly affected families. For example, with the improved prognosis for these children, parents and adolescents with hemophilia are faced with vocational and financial problems, in addition to concern over future childbearing. After children reach 21 years of age, many insurance companies will no longer carry them. This can be disastrous in terms of the cost of treatment. The National Hemophilia Foundation* and the Canadian Hemophilia Society† provide numerous services and publications for both health providers and families. Financial support is particularly important. A person with severe hemophilia may require factor replacement therapy and other medical treatments that cost in excess of $70,000 to $90,000 a year.

Children who have become infected with HIV through transfusions and factor replacement products are faced with the consequences of this dreaded disease. Consequently, they need the support of health professionals, especially in the areas of safe sexual practices to avoid disease transmission, public education regarding acquired immunodeficiency syndrome (AIDS), and ways to deal with public reactions to persons who have AIDS (see p. 1632).

Idiopathic Thrombocytopenic Purpura

Idiopathic thrombocytopenic purpura (ITP) is an acquired hemorrhagic disorder characterized by (1) *thrombocytopenia,* excessive destruction of platelets; (2) *purpura,* a discoloration caused by petechiae beneath the skin; and (3) a *normal bone marrow with normal or increased number of immature platelets (megakaryocytes) and eosinophils.* Although the cause is unknown, it is believed to be an autoimmune response to disease-related antigens. It is the most frequently occurring thrombocytopenia of childhood. The greatest frequency of occurrence is between 2 and 10 years of age.

The disease occurs in one of two forms: an acute, self-limiting course or a chronic condition (greater than 6 months' duration). The acute form is most often seen after upper respiratory infections; after the childhood diseases measles, rubella, mumps, and chickenpox; or after infection with parvovirus B19.

Diagnostic Evaluation

The diagnosis is suspected on the basis of clinical manifestations (Box 49-6). In ITP the platelet count is reduced to below 20,000/mm^3; therefore tests that depend on platelet function, such as the tourniquet test, bleeding time, and clot retraction, are abnormal. Although there is no definitive test on which to establish a diagnosis of ITP, several are usually performed to rule out other disorders in which thrombocytopenia is a manifestation, such as systemic lupus erythematosus, lymphoma, or leukemia.

Therapeutic Management

Management of ITP is primarily supportive, because the course of the disease is self-limited in the majority of cases. Activity is restricted at the onset while the platelet count is low and while active bleeding or progression of lesions is occurring. Treatment for acute illness is symptomatic and has included prednisone, IV immune globulin (IVIG), and anti-

*National Hemophilia Foundation, 116 West 43rd Street, 11th Floor, New York, NY 10001; phone: 800-42HANDI or 212-328-3700; fax: 212-328-3777; e-mail: info@hemophilia.org; Web site: www.hemophilia.org.

†Canadian Hemophilia Society, 625 President Kennedy, Suite 1210, Montreal, Quebec H3A 1K2; phone: 514-848-0503; e-mail: chs@odysee.net.

BOX 49-6

Clinical Manifestations of Idiopathic Thrombocytopenic Purpura

- Easy bruising
  - Petechiae
  - Ecchymoses
  - Most often over bony prominences
- Bleeding from mucous membranes
  - Epistaxis
  - Bleeding gums
- Internal hemorrhage evidenced by
  - Hematuria
  - Hematemesis
  - Melena
  - Hemarthrosis
  - Menorrhagia
- Hematomas over lower extremities

D antibody. These are not curative therapies. Some experts suggest that no therapy is necessary for the asymptomatic patient, with no difference in the recovery of platelet counts over time. *Anti-D antibody* is a relatively new therapy for ITP. Infusion of anti-D antibody causes a transient hemolytic anemia in the patient. Along with the clearance of antibody-coated RBCs, there is prolonged survival of platelets resulting from the blockade of the Fc receptors of the reticuloendothelial cells. The platelet count does not increase until 48 hours after an infusion of anti-D antibody; therefore it is not appropriate therapy for patients who are actively bleeding. The benefits of choosing anti-D antibody therapy over prednisone or IVIG is that anti-D antibody can be given in one dose over 5 to 10 minutes and is significantly less expensive than IVIG. Historically, patients who are treated with prednisone must first undergo a bone marrow examination to rule out leukemia. Therefore the use of anti-D antibody alleviates the need for a bone marrow examination. Patients must meet certain criteria before the administration of anti-D antibody (Box 49-7). Premedication with acetaminophen (such as Tylenol) 5 to 10 minutes before infusion is recommended.

BOX 49-7

Criteria for Anti-D Antibody Therapy

- Children between age 1 year and 19 years
- Rh(D)-positive blood type
- Normal white blood cell count and hemoglobin for age: platelets less than 30,000/mm^3
- No active mucosal bleeding
- No prior history of reaction to plasma products
- No patient known to be immunoglobulin A deficient
- No concurrent infection
- No patient with Evans syndrome (characterized by the combination of idiopathic thrombocytopenic purpura and autoimmune hemolytic anemia)
- No patient with suspected lupus or other collagen/vascular disorder

NURSE ALERT After administration of anti-D antibody, observe the child for a minimum of 1 hour and maintain a patent IV line. Obtain baseline vital signs before the infusion and again 5, 20, and 60 minutes after beginning the infusion. Fever, chills, and headache may occur during or shortly after the infusion. If fever, chills, or headache occurs, diphenhydramine (Benadryl) and Solu-Cortef should be given and the patient should be observed for an additional hour. ■

Splenectomy is reserved for those patients in whom ITP has persisted for 1 year or longer. It is the only treatment associated with long-term remission for 60% to 90% of children. Splenectomy removes the risk of hemorrhage, but increases the risk of septicemia (Bell, 2002; Chu, Korb, & Sakamoto, 2000; Wilson, 2003). Before considering splenectomy, it is generally recommended to wait until the child is older than 5 years of age because of the increased risk of bacterial infection. Pneumococcal and meningococcal vaccines are recommended before splenectomy. The child also receives penicillin prophylaxis after splenectomy. The length of prophylactic therapy is controversial, but in general, a minimum of 3 years is recommended.

Prognosis

The majority of children have a self-limited course without major complications. Some children will develop chronic ITP and require ongoing therapy. A splenectomy may modify the disease process, and the child will be asymptomatic.

Nursing Care Management

Nursing care is largely supportive and should include teaching regarding possible side effects of therapy and limitation in activities while the child's platelet count is 50,000 to 100,000/mm^3. Children with ITP should not participate in *any* contact sports, bike riding, skateboarding, in-line skating, gymnastics, climbing, or running. Parents are encouraged to engage their children in quiet activities and to prevent any injuries to the child's head. The harmful effects of using aspirin and NSAIDs to control pain are critical for these children; therefore salicylate substitutes (such as acetaminophen) are always used. As in any condition with an uncertain outcome, the family needs emotional support.

Disseminated Intravascular Coagulation

Disseminated intravascular coagulation (DIC), also known as *consumption coagulopathy,* is characterized by diffuse fibrin deposition in the microvasculature, consumption of coagulation factors, and endogenous generation of thrombin and plasmin. DIC is a secondary disorder of coagulation that occurs as a complication of a number of pathologic processes, such as hypoxia, acidosis, shock, and endothelial damage. It can result from many severe systemic diseases, such as congenital heart disease, necrotizing enterocolitis, gram-negative bacterial sepsis, rickettsial infections, and some severe viral infections.

Pathophysiology

DIC occurs when the first stage of the coagulation process is abnormally stimulated. Although no well-defined sequence of events occurs, two distinct phases can be identified. First, when the clotting mechanism is triggered in the circulation, thrombin is generated in greater amounts than can be neutralized by the body. Consequently, there is rapid conversion of fibrinogen to fibrin, with aggregation and destruction of platelets. If local and widespread fibrin deposition in blood vessels takes place, obstruction and eventual necrosis of tissues occur. Second, the fibrinolytic mechanism is activated, causing extensive destruction of clotting factors. With a deficiency of clotting factors, the child is vulnerable to uncontrollable hemorrhage into vital organs. An additional complication is damage and hemolysis of RBCs (Fig. 49-4).

Diagnostic Evaluation

DIC is suspected when the patient has an increased tendency to bleed (Box 49-8). Hematologic findings include prolonged prothrombin time (PT), PTT, and thrombin time (TT). There is a profoundly depressed platelet count, fragmented RBCs, and depleted fibrinogen.

Therapeutic Management

Treatment of DIC is directed toward control of the underlying or initiating cause, which in most instances stops the coagulation problem spontaneously. Platelets and fresh-frozen plasma may be needed to replace lost plasma components, especially in the child whose underlying disease remains uncontrolled. The extremely ill newborn infant may require exchange transfusion with fresh blood. The IV administration of heparin to inhibit thrombin formation is most often restricted to patients who have not responded to treatment of the underlying disease or replacement of coagulation factors and platelets.

Nursing Care Management

The goals of nursing care are to be aware of the possibility of DIC in the severely ill child and to recognize signs that might indicate its presence. The skills needed to monitor IV infusion and blood transfusions and to administer heparin are the same as those for any child receiving these therapies (see p. 1636). (See Chapter 44 for care of the child with a life-threatening illness.)

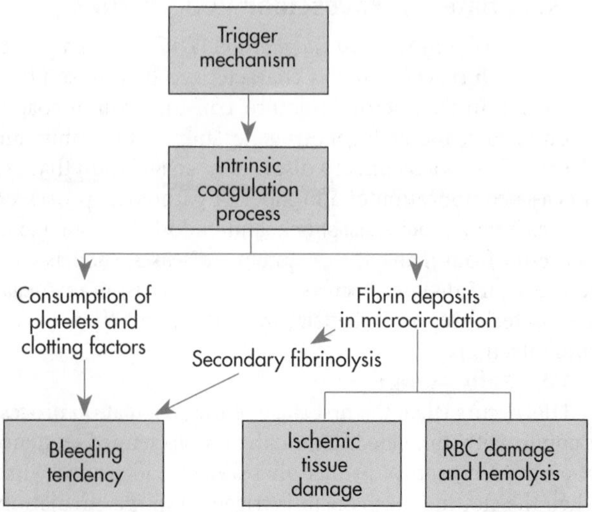

Fig. 49-4 Effects of disseminated intravascular coagulation.

BOX 49-8

Clinical Manifestations of Disseminated Intravascular Coagulation

Petechiae
Purpura
Bleeding from openings in the skin
Venipuncture site
Surgical incision
Bleeding from umbilicus, trachea (newborn)
Evidence of gastrointestinal bleeding
Hypotension
Organ dysfunction from infarction and ischemia

Epistaxis (Nosebleeding)

Isolated and transient episodes of epistaxis, or nosebleeding, are common in childhood. The nose, especially the septum, is a highly vascular structure, and bleeding usually results from direct trauma, including blows to the nose, foreign bodies, and nose picking, or from mucosal inflammation associated with allergic rhinitis and upper respiratory infections. The bleeding ordinarily stops spontaneously or with minimum pressure and requires no medical evaluation or therapy.

Recurrent epistaxis and severe bleeding may indicate an underlying disease, particularly vascular abnormalities, leukemia, thrombocytopenia, and clotting factor deficiency diseases (e.g., hemophilia, von Willebrand disease). Nosebleeds are sometimes associated with administration of aspirin, even in normal amounts. Persistent episodes of epistaxis require medical evaluation.

Nursing Care Management

In the event of a nosebleed, an essential intervention is to remain calm. Otherwise, the child will become more agitated, the blood pressure will increase, and the child will not cooperate. Although in most instances a nosebleed is not serious, it can be very upsetting to family members as well. They need reassurance that the loss of blood is not serious and that the bleeding usually stops within 10 to 15 minutes.

To control the bleeding, the child is instructed to sit up and lean forward (not to lie down) to avoid aspiration of blood. Most of the nosebleeding originates in the anterior part of the nasal septum and can be controlled by applying pressure to the soft lower portion of the nose with the thumb and forefinger (Emergency box). During this time the child breathes through the mouth.

If hemorrhage continues, the child should be evaluated by a practitioner, who may pack the nose with epinephrine-soaked gauze. After a nosebleed, petroleum or water-soluble jelly can be inserted into each nostril to prevent crusting of old blood and to lessen the likelihood of the child's picking

Emergency

EPISTAXIS

Have child sit up and lean forward (not lying down).
Apply continuous pressure to nose with thumb and forefinger for at least 10 minutes.
Insert cotton or wadded tissue into each nostril, and apply ice or cold cloth to bridge of nose if bleeding persists.
Keep child calm and quiet.

at the nose and restarting the hemorrhage. If a child has numerous nosebleeds, factors believed to increase the likelihood of bleeds are eliminated, such as discouraging nose picking or altering the household humidity by placing a cool-mist humidifier in the child's room. Repeated bleeding episodes lasting longer than 30 minutes may be an indication to refer the child for evaluation for the possibility of a bleeding disorder.

NEOPLASTIC DISORDERS

Neoplastic disorders are the leading cause of death from disease in children past infancy, and almost half of all childhood cancers involve the blood or blood-forming organs. Leukemias and lymphomas are discussed here. Malignant solid tumors of childhood are discussed elsewhere in relation to the tissues or organs involved.

Leukemias

CASE STUDY: ACUTE LYMPHOID LEUKEMIA

Leukemia, cancer of the blood-forming tissues, is the most common form of childhood cancer. The annual incidence is 3 to 4 cases per 100,000 white children younger than 15 years of age (Margolin, Steuber, & Poplack, 2002). It occurs more frequently in males than in females after age 1 year, and the peak onset is between 2 and 6 years of age. It is one of the forms of cancer that has demonstrated dramatic improvements in survival rates. Current long-term disease-free survival for children with acute lymphoid leukemia approaches 80%, whereas acute nonlymphoid leukemia has a 45% to 50% survival rate (Redner, 2000). (See also Prognosis, p. 1621.)

Classification

Leukemia is a broad term given to a group of malignant diseases of the bone marrow and lymphatic system. Research has revealed that it is a complex disease of varying heterogeneity. Consequently, classification has become increasingly complex, sophisticated, and essential, because identification of the subtype of leukemia has therapeutic and prognostic implications. The following is a brief overview of the major classification systems currently being used.

Morphology

Two forms are generally recognized in children: *acute lymphoid leukemia (ALL)* and *acute nonlymphoid (myelogenous) leukemia (ANLL* or *AML).* Synonyms for ALL include *lymphatic, lymphocytic, lymphoblastic,* and *lymphoblastoid leukemia.* Usually the terms *stem cell* or *blast cell leukemia* also refer to the lymphoid type of leukemia. Synonyms for the AML type include *granulocytic, myelocytic, monocytic, myelogenous, monoblastic,* and *monomyeloblastic leukemia.*

Cytochemical Markers

Several chemical stains aid in differentiation between ALL and ANLL. For instance, terminal deoxynucleotidyl transferase (TdT) is able to differentiate between ALL and non-ALL (Margolin et al, 2002).

Chromosome Studies

Chromosome analysis has become an important tool in the diagnosis of ALL. For example, children with trisomy 21 have 20 times the risk of other children for developing ALL. Children with more than 50 chromosomes on the leukemic cells (hyperdiploid) have the best prognosis (Margolin et al, 2002). Translocations of chromosomes also found on the leukemic cells can denote good prognosis, as in the trisomies 4 and 10, or a poor prognosis, as in the t(9:22) or Philadelphia chromosome.

Cell-Surface Immunologic Markers

Cell-surface antigens have permitted differentiation of ALL into three broad classes: non-T, non-B ALL; B-cell ALL; and T-cell ALL. Children with non-T, non-B ALL have the best prognosis, especially if they have the common acute lymphocytic leukemia antigen, known as CALLA positive, on their cell surfaces (Margolin et al, 2002).

Pathophysiology

Leukemia is an unrestricted proliferation of immature WBCs in the blood-forming tissues of the body. Although not a "tumor" as such, the leukemic cells demonstrate the same neoplastic properties as solid cancers. Therefore the resulting pathologic condition and clinical manifestations are caused by infiltration and replacement of any tissue of the body with nonfunctional leukemic cells. Highly vascular organs, such as the spleen and liver, are the most severely affected.

To understand the pathophysiology of the leukemic process, it is important to clarify two common misconceptions. First, although leukemia is an overproduction of WBCs, most often in the acute form the leukocyte count is low (thus the term *leukemia*). Second, these immature cells do not deliberately attack and destroy the normal blood cells or vascular tissues. Cellular destruction takes place by infiltration and subsequent competition for metabolic elements (Table 49-2).

In all types of leukemia, the proliferating cells depress the production of formed elements of the blood in bone marrow by competing for and depriving the normal cells of the essential nutrients for metabolism. The most common signs and symptoms of leukemia are a result of infiltration of the bone marrow. The three main consequences are (1) *anemia* from decreased RBCs, (2) *infection* from neutropenia, and (3) *bleeding* from decreased platelet production. The invasion of the bone marrow with leukemic cells gradually causes a weakening of the bone and a tendency toward fractures. As leukemic cells invade the periosteum, increasing pressure causes severe pain.

The spleen, liver, and lymph glands demonstrate marked infiltration, enlargement, and eventually fibrosis. Hepatosplenomegaly is typically more common than lymphadenopathy. The next most important site of involvement is the central nervous system (CNS) secondary to leukemic infiltration, which may cause increased intracranial pressure.

Leukemic cells may also invade the testes, kidneys, prostate, ovaries, GI tract, and lungs. With long-term survivors becoming more common, such sites of leukemia invasion, especially the testes, are becoming more important clinically.

Diagnostic Evaluation

Leukemia is usually suspected by the history, physical manifestations (see Table 49-2), and a peripheral blood smear that contains immature forms of leukocytes, frequently combined with low blood counts. Definitive diagnosis is based on flow cytometry of the cells obtained in the

Table 49-2

Pathology and Related Clinical Manifestations of Leukemia

ORGAN OR TISSUE	CONSEQUENCES	MANIFESTATIONS
Bone marrow dysfunction	Decreased RBCs—anemia	Pallor, fatigue
	Neutropenia—infection	Fever
	Decreased platelets—bleeding tendencies	Hemorrhage (petechiae)
	Invasion of bone marrow—bone weakness; invasion of periosteum	Tendency toward fractures Pain
Liver	Infiltration, enlargement, eventual fibrosis	Hepatomegaly
Spleen	Infiltration, enlargement	Splenomegaly
Lymph glands	Infiltration, enlargement	Lymphadenopathy
Central nervous system: meninges	Increased intracranial pressure, ventricular enlargement	Severe headache Vomiting Irritability, lethargy Papilledema
	Meningeal irritation	Eventual coma Pain Stiff neck and back
Hypermetabolism	Cell deprivation of nutrients by invading cells	Muscle wasting Weight loss Anorexia Fatigue

bone marrow aspiration or biopsy. Flow cytometry identifies the specific type of blast cell. Typically, the bone marrow is hypercellular, with primarily blast cells. After the diagnosis is confirmed, a lumbar puncture is performed to determine if there is any CNS involvement. A few of the children will have CNS involvement at diagnosis, although most are asymptomatic.

Therapeutic Management

Treatment of leukemia involves the use of chemotherapeutic agents, with or without cranial irradiation, in four phases: (1) *induction therapy,* which achieves a complete remission or less than 5% leukemic cells in the bone marrow; (2) *CNS prophylactic therapy,* which prevents leukemic cells from invading the CNS; (3) *intensification therapy* (consolidation), which eradicates residual leukemia cells, followed by delayed intensification, which prevents emergence of resistant leukemic clones; and (4) *maintenance therapy,* which serves to maintain the remission phase. Although the combination of drugs and radiation may vary according to institutions, the prognostic or risk characteristics of the patient, and the type of leukemia being treated, the following general principles for each phase are consistently employed.

Remission Induction

Almost immediately after confirmation of the diagnosis, induction therapy is begun and lasts for 4 to 6 weeks. The principal drugs used for induction in ALL are corticosteroids, vincristine, and L-asparaginase, with or without doxorubicin. Recent clinical trials have substituted dexamethasone for prednisone because of its effectiveness in crossing the blood-brain barrier and reducing CSF relapse (Colby-Graham & Chordas, 2003). However, the toxicities of dexamethasone continue to be evaluated. Drug therapy for AML includes doxorubicin or daunorubicin (daunomycin) and cytosine arabinoside; various other drugs such as etoposide or thioguanine may be used.

Because many of the drugs also cause myelosuppression of normal blood elements, the period immediately after a remission can be critical. The body is defenseless against and highly susceptible to infection and spontaneous hemorrhage. Consequently, supportive therapy during this time is essential.

CNS Prophylactic Therapy

Treatment of the CNS consists of prophylactic therapy using intrathecal chemotherapy with methotrexate, cytarabine, and hydrocortisone. Sometimes methotrexate, as well as cytarabine, may be given as single agents intrathecally. Because of the concern regarding late effects of cranial irradiation, this treatment is reserved for high risk patients and those with CNS disease.

Intensification or Consolidation Therapy

After complete remission is obtained, a period of intensified treatment is administered to eradicate residual leukemic cells; this is followed by delayed intensification to prevent emergence of resistant leukemic clones. Intrathecal along with systemic chemotherapy, including L-asparaginase, high-dose or intermediate-dose methotrexate, cytarabine, vincristine, and mercaptopurine, is administered over a period of several months.

Maintenance Therapy

Maintenance therapy is begun after completion of successful induction and consolidation therapy to preserve the remission and further lessen the number of leukemic cells.

Combined drug regimens, including daily mercaptopurine, weekly methotrexate, and periodic intrathecal therapy, are administered over the remaining 2-year period. Also, during maintenance therapy, periodic CBCs are taken to evaluate the marrow's response to the drugs.

Reinduction after Relapse

The presence of leukemic cells in the bone marrow, CNS, or testes constitutes a relapse. Therapy for the child who has relapsed includes reinduction with prednisone and vincristine, along with a combination of other drugs not previously used. CNS preventive therapy and maintenance therapy follow as outlined previously, after remission occurs.

Hematopoietic Stem Cell Transplantation

Hematopoietic stem cell transplantation (HSCT) has been used successfully for treating children who have ALL and AML. HSCT is *not* recommended for children with ALL during the first remission because of the excellent results possible with chemotherapy. Because of the poorer prognosis in children with AML, recent studies support HSCT during first remission. From 60% to 70% of children with AML who undergo HSCT experience long-term remission (Colby-Graham & Chordas, 2003).

Bone marrow used for HSCT may not only be from antigen-matched related donors, but also from matched unrelated donors or mismatched donors. Peripheral blood stem cell transplants are capable of differentiating into specialized cells of the hematologic system and can be obtained from related or unrelated donors or from umbilical cord blood (see p. 1640). Regardless of the type of transplant, it is accompanied by significant risk of morbidity and mortality, including graft-versus-host disease (GVHD), overwhelming infection, and severe organ damage.

Prognosis

The most important prognostic factors for determining long-term survival for children with ALL (in addition to treatment) are (1) the initial WBC count, (2) the child's age at the time of diagnosis, (3) the type of cell involved, (4) the sex of the child, and (5) karyotype analysis. Children with a normal or low WBC count and who have non-T, non-B ALL and are CALLA positive have a much better prognosis than those with a high count or other cell types. Children diagnosed between 2 and 9 years of age have consistently demonstrated a better outlook than those diagnosed before 2 or after 10 years of age, and girls appear to have a more favorable prognosis than boys. Children with a DNA index greater than 1.16 (hyperdiploid) and translocation of chromosomes 4 and 10 have a better prognosis (Margolin et al, 2002).

Late Effects of Treatment

Although vigorous treatment of childhood cancers has resulted in dramatically improved survival rates, increasing concern surrounds late effects—adverse changes related to treatment modalities—and recurrence of the disease process. Almost no organ is exempt, and almost every antineoplastic agent, including and especially irradiation, is responsible for some adverse effect.

The most devastating late effect is development of a second malignancy. Children who received cranial irradiation at age 5 years or younger are most susceptible to developing brain tumors (Silverman & Sallan, 2003). Treatment with anthracycline is associated with cardiomyopathy; cranial irradiation and intrathecal chemotherapy are associated with cognitive and neuropsychologic deficits, which are just a few of the long-term sequelae. Consequently, close monitoring for late effects is essential, especially with the advent of additional clinical trials.

Nursing Care Management

Nursing care of the child with leukemia is directly related to the regimen of therapy. General psychologic interventions are necessary during each phase of therapy.

Assessment

The history and physical examination often yield the first clues to the presence of neoplastic disease. Vague complaints such as fatigue, pain in a limb, night sweating, lack of appetite, headache, and general malaise may be the earliest clues of leukemia.

Nursing Diagnoses

Many nursing diagnoses become apparent after an assessment of the child with leukemia and the child's family. Some are considered in the Nursing Care Plan on p. 1628. Others are identified in specific situations.

Plan of Care and Implementation

The goals of nursing care of the child with leukemia and the child's family include the following:

1. Child will receive appropriate primary health care.
2. Child and family will be prepared for diagnostic and therapeutic procedures.
3. Child will experience minimal complications of myelosuppression.
4. Problems of irradiation and drug toxicity will be managed.
5. Child and family will receive adequate support and education.

Nursing care of the child with leukemia is directly related to the regimen of therapy. Nurses working with families of children with cancer have a significant supportive role in helping them understand the various therapies, preventing or managing expected side effects or toxicities, observing for late effects of treatment, and helping the child and family live as normal a life as possible and cope with the emotional aspects of the disease. Education is a constant feature of the nursing role, especially in terms of clinical trials and home care. Diagnosis of leukemia tends to generate anxiety in families and patients. The nurse is instrumental in providing support and reassurance, as well as accurate explanation regarding diagnostic tests, procedures, and treatment plans.

Prepare Child and Family for Diagnostic and Therapeutic Procedures

From the time before diagnosis to cessation of therapy, children must undergo several tests; the most traumatic are bone marrow aspiration or biopsy and lumbar punctures. Multiple finger sticks and venipunctures for blood analysis and drug infusion are common occurrences. Therefore the child needs an explanation of each procedure and what can be expected. In addition, effective pharmacologic measures, including conscious and unconscious sedation, and non-

CRITICAL THINKING EXERCISE: BONE MARROW TEST

pharmacologic strategies are used to reduce discomfort associated with these painful procedures.

Relieve Pain

The effective use of analgesia is especially important when the malignant process is uncontrolled and causes acute pain. Dosages of opioids (narcotics) are adjusted or *titrated to the child's needs* and administered *around the clock* for optimum pain control. Nonpharmacologic strategies should be implemented as needed but are not substitutes for pharmacologic management. The reader is encouraged to review the principles of pain assessment and management presented in Chapter 44 and Preparation for Procedures in Chapter 45 when caring for a child with leukemia.

Prevent Complications of Myelosuppression

The leukemic process and most of the chemotherapeutic agents cause myelosuppression. The reduced numbers of blood cells result in secondary problems of infection, bleeding tendencies, and anemia. Supportive care involves both medical and nursing management. Because these are so closely linked, they are discussed together rather than separately.

Infection

A frequent complication of treatment for childhood cancer is overwhelming infection secondary to neutropenia. The child is most susceptible to overwhelming infection during three phases of the disease: (1) at the time of diagnosis and relapse when the leukemic process has replaced normal leukocytes, (2) during immunosuppressive therapy, and (3) after prolonged antibiotic therapy that predisposes to the growth of resistant organisms. However, the use of granulocyte colony–stimulating factor (G-CSF) has reduced the incidence and duration of infection in children receiving treatment for cancer.

The first defense against infection is prevention. When the child is hospitalized, the nurse employs all measures to control transfer of infection. These typically include the use of a private room, restriction of all visitors and health personnel with active infection, and strict handwashing technique with an antiseptic solution. In some research centers, special germ-free environments are available during complete myelosuppression from intensive chemotherapy or for bone marrow transplant.

NURSE ALERT Because the usual viral infections of childhood are particularly dangerous, the child is not immunized against these diseases (measles, rubella, mumps, and polio) until the immune system is capable of responding appropriately to the vaccine. If given when the immune system is depressed, the attenuated virus can result in an overwhelming infection. The child can receive the Salk (inactivated) vaccine for poliomyelitis. Children with cancer should not routinely receive the varicella vaccine. Siblings and other family members can receive the varicella vaccine without risk to the child with cancer (American Academy of Pediatrics, Committee on Infectious Diseases, 2003). ■

The child is evaluated for potential sites of infection (e.g., mucosal ulceration; skin abrasion; skin tear, such as a hangnail) and observed for any elevation in temperature. To identify the source of infection, chest radiographs and blood, stool, urine, and nasopharyngeal cultures are taken. IV antibiotics are administered; if this therapy is prolonged, a venous access device, such as a peripherally inserted central catheter (PICC), an intermittent infusion device (saline lock or PRN adaptor), a catheter, or an implanted infusion port, is used to maintain IV access.

Prevention of infection continues to be a priority after discharge from the hospital. Ordinarily, the child is allowed to return to school when the WBC count is at a satisfactory level, usually an absolute neutrophil count (ANC) greater than 500/mm^3 (Guidelines box). At all times, family members are encouraged to practice good handwashing to prevent introducing pathogens into the home. The child may need to be isolated from school contacts in the event of an outbreak of a childhood disease, especially chickenpox.

Nutrition is another important component of infection prevention. An adequate protein-caloric intake provides the child with better host defenses against infection and increased tolerance to chemotherapy and irradiation. However, providing optimum nutrition during periods of anorexia and vomiting from chemotherapy is a tremendous challenge (see Feeding the Sick Child, Chapter 45).

Hemorrhage

Before the use of transfused platelets, hemorrhage was a leading cause of death in patients with leukemia. Now most bleeding episodes can be prevented or controlled with the administration of platelet concentrates or platelet-rich plasma.

Because infection increases the tendency toward hemorrhage, and because bleeding sites become more easily infected, skin punctures are avoided whenever possible. When finger sticks, venipunctures, IM injections, and bone marrow aspirations are performed, aseptic technique must be employed, as well as continued observation for bleeding. Meticulous mouth care is essential, because gingival bleeding with resultant mucositis is a frequent problem. Because the rectal area is prone to ulceration from various drugs, feces and urine are removed immediately, and the perianal area is washed. Taking rectal temperatures is avoided to prevent trauma. Children are advised to avoid activities that might cause injury or bleeding, such as riding bicycles or skateboards, climbing trees or playground equipment, and playing contact sports.

Platelet transfusions are generally reserved for active bleeding episodes that do not respond to local treatment and

Guidelines

CALCULATING THE ABSOLUTE NEUTROPHIL COUNT

Determine the total percent of neutrophils ("polys" or "segs" and "bands").

Multiply white blood cell (WBC) count by percent of neutrophils.

Example:

WBC = 1000, neutrophils = 7%, nonsegmented neutrophils (bands) = 7%

Step 1: 7% + 7% = 14%

Step 2: 0.14 × 1000 = 140 absolute neutrophil count (ANC)

that may occur during induction or relapse therapy. Epistaxis and gingival bleeding are the most common. The nurse teaches parents and older children measures to control nosebleeding (see p. 1628). Pressure at the site without disturbing clot formation is the general rule.

During bleeding episodes the parents and child need much emotional support. Often parents will request a platelet transfusion, unaware of the need for trying local measures first. The nurse can be instrumental in allaying anxiety by acknowledging the feelings of the child and family and explaining the reason for delaying a platelet transfusion until absolutely necessary.

Anemia

Initially, anemia may be profound from complete replacement of the bone marrow by leukemic cells. During induction therapy, blood transfusions may be necessary. The usual precautions in caring for the child with anemia are instituted (see p. 1604).

Use Precautions in Administering and Handling Chemotherapeutic Agents

Many chemotherapeutic agents are vesicants (sclerosing agents) that can cause severe cellular damage if even minute amounts of the drug infiltrate surrounding tissue. Only nurses experienced with chemotherapeutic agents should administer vesicants. Guidelines are available* and must be followed exactly to prevent tissue damage to patients. Interventions for extravasation vary, but each nurse should be aware of the institution's policies and implement them at once.

In addition to extravasation, a potentially fatal complication is anaphylaxis, especially from L-asparaginase, teniposide (VM-26), etoposide (VP-16), bleomycin, and cisplatin. Nursing responsibilities include prevention of, recognition of, and preparation for serious reactions. Prevention begins with a careful history for known allergy.

In addition to the many responsibilities nurses must have in regard to the child and family, they must also use safeguards to protect themselves. Handling chemotherapeutic agents may present risks to handlers and to their offspring, although the exact degree of risk is not known.

Some children have a venous access device, which facilitates administration of IV drugs. During treatment and remission, many drugs are taken orally at home. Compliance with the medication schedule is essential, and nurses play an important role in educating the family about the drugs and encouraging adherence to the plan.

NURSE ALERT Chemotherapeutic drugs must be given through a free-flowing IV line. The infusion is stopped *immediately* if any sign of infiltration (pain, stinging, swelling, or redness at the cannulation site) occurs. ■

NURSE ALERT When chemotherapeutic and immunologic agents are given, the child must be observed for 20 minutes after the infusion for signs of anaphylaxis (cyanosis, hypotension, wheezing, severe urticaria). Emergency equipment (especially blood pressure monitor and bag-valve-mask) and emergency drugs (especially oxygen, epinephrine, antihistamine, aminophylline, corticosteroids, and vasopressors) must be available. If a reaction is suspected, the drug is discontinued, the IV line is flushed with saline, and the child's vital signs and subsequent responses are monitored. ■

Manage Problems of Drug Toxicity

Chemotherapy presents several nursing challenges. The complexity of the treatment protocols is often overwhelming to families. In addition, each therapy is associated with a number of predictable side effects. Nurses must be aware of these side effects and use judgment in recognizing actions, as well as toxicities (Box 49-9).

Nausea and Vomiting

The nausea and vomiting that occur shortly after administration of several of the drugs and from cranial or abdominal radiation can be profound. The serotonin-receptor antagonists (e.g., ondansetron [Zofran]) are effective in the control of nausea and vomiting occurring after emetogenic chemotherapy and radiation therapy. When combined with dexamethasone, these agents are the treatment of choice in the prevention of cisplatin-induced delayed emesis (Bryant, 2003).

The most beneficial regimen for antiemetic control has been the administration of the antiemetic *before* the chemotherapy begins. The goal is to prevent the child from ever experiencing nausea or vomiting, thus preventing development of anticipatory symptoms (the conditioned response of developing nausea and vomiting before receiving the drug).

Anorexia

Loss of appetite is a direct consequence of the chemotherapy or irradiation. It is a major problem for parents because it is the one area they feel responsible for, particularly when so many other facets of care are outside their control. There are no universally successful techniques for encouraging a sick child to eat. However, the guidelines in Chapter 45 can be helpful during the anorexic period and can prevent additional problems during the remission.

Some children still do not eat despite these approaches. When loss of appetite and weight persist, the nurse should investigate the family situation to determine if any factors (e.g., conditioned aversion to food, environmental stress related to eating, controlling behavior, anger) might be contributing to the problem. Nasogastric tube feedings or total parenteral nutrition may be implemented for children with significant nutritional problems.

Mucosal Ulceration

One of the most distressing side effects of several drugs is GI mucosal cell damage, which can produce ulcers anywhere along the alimentary tract. Oral ulcers greatly compound anorexia because eating is extremely uncomfortable, but the following interventions may be helpful: (1) provide a bland, moist, soft diet appropriate for the child's age and preferences; (2) use a soft sponge toothbrush (Toothettes)* or cotton-tipped applicator; (3) provide frequent mouthwashes with normal saline (using a solution of 1 teaspoon of table salt and 1 pint of water) or sodium bicarbonate mouth rinses (using a solution of 1 teaspoon of baking soda in

---

**Cancer Chemotherapy Guidelines* can be obtained from the Oncology Nursing Society, 501 Holiday Drive, Pittsburgh, PA 15220-2749; phone: 412-921-7373; Web site: www.ons.org.

*Manufactured by Halbrand, Inc., Willoughby, Ohio.

BOX 49-9

Summary of Selected Chemotherapeutic Agents Used in the Treatment of Childhood Leukemias and Lymphomas*

Bleomycin (Blenoxane)
Administration
IV, IM, SC

Side Effects and Toxicity
Allergic reaction—fever, chills, hypotension, anaphylaxis
Fever (nonallergic)
N/V (mild)†
Stomatitis
Cumulative dose effects include the following:
Skin—rash, hyperpigmentation, thickening, ulceration, peeling, nail changes, alopecia
Lungs—pneumonitis with infiltrate that can progress to fatal fibrosis

Comments and Specific Nursing Considerations
Should give test dose (SC) before therapeutic dose is administered
Have emergency drugs at bedside
Hypersensitivity occurs with first one to two doses
May give acetaminophen before drug to reduce likelihood of fever
Concentration of drug in skin and lungs accounts for toxic effects
Perform pulmonary function tests at baseline, during and following therapy

Corticosteroids (Hormones)
Administration
PO, IT; IM or IV rarely used

Side Effects and Toxicity, Short-Term Use
For short-term use, no acute toxicity
Usual side effects are mild: moon face, fluid retention, weight gain, mood changes, increased appetite, gastric irritation, insomnia, susceptibility to infection

Comments and Specific Nursing Considerations
Explain expected effects, especially in terms of body image, increased appetite, and personality changes
Monitor weight gain
Recommend moderate salt restriction
Administer with antacid and early in morning (sometimes given every other day to minimize side effects)
May need to disguise bitter taste (crush tablet and mix with syrup, jam, ice cream, or other highly flavored substance; use ice to numb tongue before administration; place tablet in gelatin capsule if child can swallow it)
Observe for potential infection sites; usual inflammatory response and fever are absent

Side Effects and Toxicity, Long-Term Use
Long-term effects of chronic steroid administration are mood changes, hirsutism, trunk obesity (buffalo hump), thin extremities, muscle wasting and weakness, osteoporosis, poor wound healing, bruising, potassium loss, gastric bleeding, hypertension, diabetes mellitus, growth retardation

Comments and Specific Nursing Considerations
Same as for short-term use; in addition, encourage foods high in potassium (bananas, raisins, prunes, coffee, chocolate)
Test stools for occult blood
Monitor blood pressure
Test blood for sugar and urine for acetone
Observe for signs of abrupt steroid withdrawal: flulike symptoms, hypotension, hypoglycemia, shock

Daunorubicin (Daunomycin, Rubidomycin) and Doxorubicin (Adriamycin, Doxorubicin)
Administration
IV

Side Effects and Toxicity
N/V (moderate)
Stomatitis
BMD (7 to 14 days later)
Fever, chills
Local phlebitis
Alopecia
Cumulative-dose toxicity includes the following:
Cardiac abnormalities
Electrocardiographic changes
Heart failure

Comments and Specific Nursing Considerations
Vesicant‡ (extravasation may not cause pain)
Use only sterile distilled water as a diluent
Observe for any changes in heart rate or rhythm and signs of failure
Cumulative dose must not exceed 375 mg/m^2 (less with radiation)
Warn parents that drug causes urine to turn red (for up to 12 days after administration); this is normal, not hematuria

L-Asparaginase (Elspar)
Administration
SC, IV

Side Effects and Toxicity
Allergic reactions (including anaphylactic shock)
Fever
N/V (mild)
Anorexia
Weight loss
Arthralgia
Toxicity:
Liver dysfunction
Hyperglycemia
Renal failure
Pancreatitis
Coagulation abnormalities

Comments and Specific Nursing Considerations
Have emergency drugs at bedside
Record signs of allergic reaction, such as urticaria, facial edema, hypotension, or abdominal cramps
Check weight daily
Normally, blood urea nitrogen and ammonia levels rise as a result of drug; not evidence of liver damage
Check urine for sugar and blood amylase
Observe for thrombotic events

*Includes principal drugs used in the treatment of childhood leukemias and lymphomas. Several other conventional and investigational chemotherapeutic agents may be employed in the treatment regimen.
†*N/V,* nausea and vomiting. Mild, 20% incidence; moderate, 20% to 70% incidence; severe, 75% incidence.
‡Vesicants (sclerosing agents) can cause severe cellular damage if even minute amounts of the drug infiltrate surrounding tissue.
BMD, bone marrow depression; *IM,* intramuscular; *IT,* intrathecal; *IV,* intravenous; *PO,* by mouth; *SC,* subcutaneous.

BOX 49-9

Summary of Selected Chemotherapeutic Agents Used in the Treatment of Childhood Leukemias and Lymphomas—cont'd

Mechlorethamine (Nitrogen Mustard, Mustargen)

Administration

IV

Side Effects and Toxicity

N/V (30 minutes to 8 hours later) (severe)
BMD (2 to 3 weeks later)
Alopecia
Local phlebitis

Comments and Specific Nursing Considerations

Vesicant

Mercaptopurine (6-MP, Purinethol)

Administration

PO, IV

Side Effects and Toxicity

N/V (mild)
Diarrhea
Anorexia
Stomatitis
BMD (4 to 6 weeks later)
Immunosuppression
Dermatitis
Less often may be hepatic dysfunction

Comments and Specific Nursing Considerations

6-MP is an analog of xanthine; therefore allopurinol (Zyloprim) delays its metabolism and increases its potency, necessitating a lower dose (one third to one quarter) of 6-MP

Methotrexate (MTX, Amethopterin)

Administration

PO, IV, IM, IT
May be given in conventional doses (mg/m^2) or high doses (g/m^2)

Side Effects and Toxicity

N/V (severe at high doses)
Diarrhea
Mucosal ulceration (2 to 5 days later)
BMD (10 days later)
Immunosuppression
Dermatitis
Photosensitivity
Alopecia (uncommon)
Toxic effects include the following:
- Hepatitis (fibrosis)
- Osteoporosis
- Nephropathy
- Pneumonitis (fibrosis)

Neurologic toxicity with IT use—pain at injection site, meningismus (signs of meningitis without actual inflammation), especially fever and headache; potential sequelae—transient or permanent hemiparesis, seizures, dementia, death

Comments and Specific Nursing Considerations

Side effects and toxicity are dose related
Potency and toxicity are increased by reduced renal function, salicylates, sulfonamides, and aminobenzoic acid; avoid use of these substances, such as aspirin
Avoid exposure to sun and use sun block
High-dose therapy:
- Citrovorum factor (folinic acid or leucovorin) decreases cytotoxic action of MTX; used as an antidote for overdose and to enhance normal cell recovery after high-dose therapy; avoid use of vitamins containing folic acid during MTX therapy unless prescribed by physician

IT therapy:
- Drug must be mixed with preservative-free diluent
- Report signs of neurotoxicity immediately

Procarbazine (Matulane)

Administration

PO

Side Effects and Toxicity

N/V (moderate)
BMD (3 to 4 weeks later)
Lethargy
Dermatitis
Myalgia
Arthralgia
Less often:
- Stomatitis
- Neuropathy
- Alopecia
- Diarrhea
- Amenorrhea

Comments and Specific Nursing Considerations

Central nervous system (CNS) depressants (phenothiazines, barbiturates) enhance CNS symptoms
Monoamine oxidase inhibition sometimes occurs; therefore all other drugs are avoided unless medically approved; red wine, fava beans, and broad bean pods are avoided

Vincristine (Oncovin) and Vinblastine (Velban)

Administration

IV

Side Effects and Toxicity

Neurotoxicity (less severe with vinblastine)—paresthesia (numbness); ataxia; weakness; footdrop; hyporeflexia; constipation (dynamic ileus); hoarseness (vocal cord paralysis); abdominal, chest, and jaw pain; mental depression
Fever
N/V (mild)
BMD (minimal; 7 to 14 days later)
Alopecia
Syndrome of inappropriate antidiuretic hormone excretion (SIADH)

Comments and Specific Nursing Considerations

Vesicant
Report signs of neurotoxicity because may necessitate cessation of drug
Individuals with underlying neurologic problems may be more prone to neurotoxicity
Monitor stool patterns closely; administer stool softener
Excreted primarily by liver into biliary system; administer cautiously to anyone with biliary disease
Maximum vincristine dose is 2 mg

Continued

BOX 49-9

Summary of Selected Chemotherapeutic Agents Used in the Treatment of Childhood Leukemias and Lymphomas*—cont'd

Cytosine Arabinoside (Ara-C, Cytosar, Cytarabine, Arabinosyl Cytosine)

Administration

IV, IM, SC, IT

Side Effects and Toxicity

Alopecia
N/V (mild)
BMD (7 to 14 days later)
Mucosal ulceration
Immunosuppression
Hepatitis (usually subclinical)
Fever, conjunctivitis, and maculopapular rash with high doses

Comments and Specific Nursing Considerations

Crosses blood-brain barrier
Use with caution in patients with hepatic dysfunction
Administer steroid eyedrops to prevent conjunctivitis with high doses

Cyclophosphamide (Cytoxan, CTX, Neosar)

Administration

PO, IV, IM

Side Effects and Toxicity

N/V (3 to 4 hours later) (severe at high doses)
BMD (10 to 14 days later)
Alopecia
Hemorrhagic cystitis
Severe immunosuppression
Stomatitis (rare)
Hyperpigmentation
Transverse ridging of nails
Infertility
Cardiac toxicity
SIADH

Comments and Specific Nursing Considerations

BMD has platelet-sparing effect
Give dose early in day to allow adequate fluids afterward
Force fluids before administering drug and for 2 days after to prevent chemical cystitis; encourage frequent voiding even during night
Warn parents to report signs of burning on urination or hematuria to practitioner
Mesna is given to prevent hemorrhagic cystitis

Dacarbazine (DTIC-Dome)

Administration

IV

Side Effects and Toxicity

N/V (especially after first dose) (severe)
BMD (7 to 14 days later)
Alopecia
Flulike syndrome
Burning sensation in vein during infusion (not extravasation)

Comments and Specific Nursing Considerations

Vesicant (less sclerosive)
Must be given cautiously in patients with renal dysfunction
Decrease IV rate or use warm, moist towels on IV site to decrease burning

*Includes principal drugs used in the treatment of childhood leukemias and lymphomas. Several other conventional and investigational chemotherapeutic agents may be employed in the treatment regimen.

1 quart of water); and (4) use local anesthetics (e.g., Chloraseptic lozenges) or nonprescription preparations without alcohol (e.g., Orabase, Ulcerase, Benadryl/Maalox solution). Although local anesthetics are effective in temporarily relieving the pain, many children dislike the taste and the numb feeling they produce.

NURSE ALERT Viscous lidocaine is not recommended for young children; if applied to the pharynx, it may depress the gag reflex, increasing the risk of aspiration. Seizures have been rarely associated with the use of oral viscous lidocaine (Cho, Cheng, & Cheng, 2000). ■

Other preparations that may be used to prevent or treat mucositis include chlorhexidine gluconate (Peridex) because of its dual effectiveness against candidal and bacterial infections, antifungal troches (lozenges) or mouthwash, and lip balm (e.g., Aquaphor) to keep the lips moist. Agents that should not be used include lemon glycerin swabs (irritate eroded tissue and can decay teeth), hydrogen peroxide (delays healing by breaking down protein), and milk of magnesia (dries mucosa).

Stomatitis may cause such difficulty with eating that the child may require hospitalization for hydration, parenteral nutrition, and pain control (often with IV morphine). The child will usually choose the foods that are best tolerated, and the nurse should encourage parents to relax any eating pressures. Because the stomatitis is a temporary condition, the child can resume good food habits after the ulcers heal. Dental hygiene can become a serious problem for children with orthodontic appliances. Sometimes it may be necessary to remove the braces to allow chemotherapy to continue.

Rectal ulcers are managed by meticulous toilet hygiene, warm sitz baths after each bowel movement, and use of an occlusive ointment or dressing applied to the ulcerated area to promote epithelialization. Stool softeners are necessary to prevent further discomfort. Parents are advised to record bowel movements, because the child may voluntarily avoid defecation to prevent discomfort. Rectal thermometers and suppositories are contraindicated because insertion may further traumatize the area.

Neuropathy

Vincristine and, to a lesser extent, vinblastine can cause various neurotoxic effects. Nursing interventions for management of these effects include (1) administering stool softeners or laxatives for severe constipation caused by decreased bowel innervation; (2) maintaining good body alignment and, if on bed rest, using a footboard or high-top shoes to minimize or prevent footdrop; (3) carrying out safety measures during ambulation because of weakness and numbing of the extremities, which may cause difficulty in walking or fine hand movement; and (4) providing a soft or liquid diet for severe jaw pain.

Hemorrhagic Cystitis

Sterile hemorrhagic cystitis, a side effect of chemical irritation to the bladder from cyclophosphamide, can be decreased and often prevented by (1) a liberal fluid intake (at least one and a half times the recommended daily fluid requirement); (2) frequent voiding immediately after feeling the urge, before bed, and after arising; (3) administering the drug early in the day to allow for sufficient oral intake and voiding; and (4) administering mesna (an agent that provides protection to the bladder) as ordered. If oral home administration is prescribed, the family needs *specific* instructions regarding exactly how much fluid the child must have.

NURSE ALERT If signs of cystitis occur, such as burning or bleeding on urination, prompt medical evaluation is needed. ■

Alopecia

Hair loss is a common side effect of several chemotherapeutic drugs and cranial irradiation, although not all children lose their hair during drug therapy. It is better to warn children and parents of this side effect than to allow them to think that it is only a remote possibility. A soft cotton cap is the most comfortable head wear for children. Polyester increases perspiration and causes itching. Other options include scarves, hats, or a wig.

NURSE ALERT If the child chooses to wear a wig, encouraging the child to select one similar to the child's own hairstyle and color before the hair falls out is helpful in fostering later adjustment to hair loss. ■

The nurse should also inform the family that hair regrows in 3 to 6 months and may be of a different color and texture. Frequently the hair is darker, thicker, and curlier than before. If the child chooses not to wear a wig, attention to some type of head covering, especially in cold climates and during exposure to sun, and scalp hygiene are important. The scalp should be washed like any other body part.

Moon Face

Short-term steroid therapy produces no acute toxicities and produces two beneficial reactions: increased appetite and a sense of well-being. However, it does produce alterations in body image, which, although not clinically significant, can be extremely distressing to older children. One of these is moon face, in which the child's face becomes rounded and puffy. It is not unusual for other children to make fun of the child with such remarks as "Miss Piggy," "Porky Pig," or "fat face." It is helpful to reassure children who experience such name-calling that after cessation of the drug the facial changes will return to normal. Unlike hair loss, little can be done to camouflage this obvious change. If the child resumes activity early in the course of treatment, the change may be less noticeable to peers than after a long absence.

Mood Changes

Shortly after beginning steroid therapy, children experience a number of mood changes that range from feelings of well-being and euphoria to depression and irritability. If parents are unaware of these drug-induced changes, they may become unduly concerned. Therefore the nurse should warn them of the reactions and encourage them to discuss the behavioral changes with each other and the child.

Provide Continued Physical Care and Emotional Support

Because of the improved survival of these children, continued monitoring of physical and intellectual growth and development is essential. Nurses should stress the importance of regular follow-up care.

An important aspect of continued emotional support involves the prognosis. Although leukemia is no longer invariably fatal, it must be remembered that survival statistics are only average estimates and apply to those children treated with the latest protocols since diagnosis. For the low risk child the chances may be better, but for the high risk child they may be significantly poorer. Of those who do survive after discontinuing therapy, some will relapse. At present, only the passage of time is positive confirmation of the child's being ultimately "cured" of the disease. Remission, even in excess of 5 years, cannot be equated with a cure. With increasing concern regarding late effects of treatment, continued surveillance of the child's health status is needed. The nurse who is working with family members must individualize information regarding the "numbers" and the potential risks. An understanding of each member's emotional needs, as well as competent care of physical ones, is essential to the positive, growth-promoting support of the family. Comprehensive emotional support for the family of the child with a potentially fatal illness is discussed in Chapter 41.

Evaluation

The effectiveness of nursing interventions is determined by continual reassessment and evaluation of care based on the following observational guidelines:

1. Compare number of visits for primary health with recommended schedule of health supervision.
2. Monitor growth, development, and other aspects of regular health assessment; check mouth for adequacy of dental hygiene; review immunization record for age-appropriate vaccines and use of nonliving virus preparations.
3. Interview child and family regarding their understanding of treatments and diagnostic tests.
4. Employ pain assessment techniques for procedural pain.
5. Make careful observations of physical status.
   a. Take vital signs regularly.
   b. Observe for evidence of bleeding, infection, neuropathy, cystitis, and mucosal ulceration.
   c. Observe and record intake and output.
6. Interview child and family and observe behaviors as a result of complications of therapies.
7. Interview child and family and observe behaviors that provide clues to their response to the disease, its therapy, and nursing interventions.

The *expected outcomes* are described in the Nursing Care Plan on pp. 1628-1630.

Nursing Care Plan

THE CHILD WITH CANCER

NURSING DIAGNOSIS: Risk for injury related to malignant process and treatment

EXPECTED OUTCOME

Complications from chemotherapy are minimized, and the child exhibits signs of complete or partial remission.

NURSING INTERVENTIONS/*RATIONALES*

Administer chemotherapeutic agents per physician order and monitor IV site closely for signs of infiltration *to prevent severe tissue damage.*

Obtain allergy history *to prevent anaphylaxis.*

Observe child for at least 20 minutes after chemotherapy infusion *for signs of anaphylaxis* (cyanosis, wheezing, hypotension, urticaria); stop infusion and flush IV line *to minimize reaction;* have emergency equipment and drugs readily available *to prevent delay in treatment of anaphylactic reaction.*

NURSING DIAGNOSIS: Risk for injury (hemorrhage, hemorrhagic cystitis) related to interference with cell proliferation

EXPECTED OUTCOME

The child exhibits no evidence of bleeding or hematuria.

NURSING INTERVENTIONS/*RATIONALES*

Monitor platelet counts and administer platelets per physician order *to raise platelet count and minimize bleeding tendencies.*

Do not administer aspirin products *because they interfere with platelet function.*

Teach child and family to limit activity when platelet count drops *to minimize chances of accidental injury.*

Use care in the administration of therapy (e.g., avoid grabbing with fingers and friction with clothing and bedclothes when turning; keep skin clean and dry and sheets clean and wrinkle free; use soft sponge for oral care) *to reduce bruising and injury.*

Turn and reposition frequently, use pressure-relieving mattresses *to prevent pressure ulcers.*

Implement only essential skin puncturing procedures; monitor puncture site carefully; apply gentle pressure, ice to bleeding sites *to minimize bleeding.*

Teach child and parents how to manage nosebleeds *to reduce blood loss.*

Administer ordered drugs that are irritating to the bladder mucosa early in day *to allow sufficient fluid intake and voiding for flushing of irritants.*

Ensure increased oral intake as ordered and encourage frequent voiding *to flush metabolites from system and prevent irritation.*

Observe for and report signs of cystitis (burning and pain on urination) *to ensure prompt medical treatment.*

NURSING DIAGNOSIS: Risk for infection related to depressed body defenses

EXPECTED OUTCOME

The child exhibits no evidence of infection.

NURSING INTERVENTIONS/*RATIONALES*

Place child in private room and screen all visitors and staff for signs of infection *to minimize exposure to infective organisms.*

Teach child and family about good hygiene and careful handwashing techniques *to prevent spread of infection.*

Use good handwashing for all contacts with child and scrupulous aseptic technique for all invasive procedures *to minimize exposure to infection.*

Encourage a nutritionally complete diet *to support body's natural defenses.*

Administer antibiotics and GCSF per physician order *to prevent infection.*

Monitor vital signs and observe skin and mucosa *to detect signs of infection.*

Do not administer live attenuated virus vaccines (i.e., measles-mumps-rubella, oral polio, varicella zoster) to child with depressed immune system *to prevent overwhelming the system and introducing an infectious disease;* use inactivated virus vaccines as prescribed (i.e., chickenpox, Salk polio, influenza) *to prevent common childhood illnesses.*

NURSING DIAGNOSIS: Risk for fluid volume deficit related to chemotherapy-induced nausea and vomiting

EXPECTED OUTCOME

The child is adequately hydrated.

NURSING INTERVENTIONS/*RATIONALES*

Administer initial dose of antiemetic before starting chemotherapy *to reduce incidence of nausea and vomiting.*

Administer regular doses of antiemetic as ordered for the duration of expected cycle of nausea and vomiting *to decrease or prevent nausea and vomiting episodes.*

Administer IV fluids as ordered *to maintain hydration;* encourage oral fluids and foods in small amounts *to increase tolerance.*

Monitor child's response to antiemetic *because reactions are idiosyncratic and adjustments in drugs or dose may be needed.*

Monitor intake and output *to ensure adequate hydration.*

Avoid foods with strong odors *because they may induce nausea and vomiting.*

Encourage frequent intake of fluids in small amounts *because small portions are usually better tolerated.*

NURSING DIAGNOSIS: Altered mucous membranes related to administration of chemotherapeutic agents

EXPECTED OUTCOME

The child exhibits no evidence of oral mucositis or rectal ulceration.

NURSING INTERVENTIONS/*RATIONALES*

Institute meticulous oral hygiene (e.g., soft-sponge toothbrush *to avoid trauma;* frequent mouthwashes *to promote healing;* lip balm *to keep lips moist*). Do not use lemon glycerin swabs, *which irritate eroded tissue and induce tooth decay;* hydrogen peroxide, *which delays healing of ulcers;* and milk of magnesia, *which dries oral mucosa.*

Inspect oral mucosa daily for ulcers and report immediately *to ensure early treatment.*

Nursing Care Plan

THE CHILD WITH CANCER—cont'd

Apply local anesthetics as ordered to ulcerated areas before meals *to relieve pain and increase food intake.* Do not use viscous lidocaine in young children *because it may depress gag reflex.*
Serve a bland, moist, soft diet; avoid juices with ascorbic acid; use a straw for fluids; avoid oral and rectal temperature-taking *to decrease pain and injury to ulcerated areas.*
Administer prescribed antiinfective agents *to prevent or treat mucositis,* analgesics *to control pain.*
Wash perianal area after stools *to lessen irritation.*
Use warm sitz baths *to ease pain and promote healing.*
Expose reddened mucosal areas to air; apply protective skin barriers to perianal area *to protect mucosa and promote healing.*
Use stool softeners, bulk laxatives *to prevent constipation.*
Track frequency and description of bowel movements *to assess for constipation.*

NURSING DIAGNOSIS: Altered nutrition: less than body requirements related to chemotherapeutically induced loss of appetite

EXPECTED OUTCOME
Nutritional intake is adequate.

NURSING INTERVENTIONS/*RATIONALES*
Allow child any food tolerated, fortify foods with supplements, use small frequent feedings, make food appealing, and involve child in selection and preparation *to increase intake and tolerance.*
Take family history *to assess any food issues that may require intervention* (e.g., use of food as control mechanism or reward and punishment).

NURSING DIAGNOSIS: Impaired skin integrity related to administration of chemotherapy, radiotherapy, immobility

EXPECTED OUTCOME
Skin is clean and intact.

NURSING INTERVENTIONS/*RATIONALES*
Provide meticulous skin care, turn and reposition frequently *to prevent skin breakdown.*
Inspect skin frequently *to assess for areas of impending breakdown.*
Encourage adequate caloric-protein intake *to prevent negative nitrogen balance.*

NURSING DIAGNOSIS: Impaired physical mobility related to neuromuscular impairment (neuropathy)

EXPECTED OUTCOME
The child is as mobile as condition permits, and signs of neuropathy are minimal.

NURSING INTERVENTIONS/*RATIONALES*
Match activity level to physical condition and abilities *to prevent overexertion and injury.*
If bedridden, have patient perform passive range of motion *to retain full range of motion;* use a footboard or high-top shoes *to prevent footdrop;* position body in correct alignment with adequate support *to prevent pain and contractures.*

NURSING DIAGNOSIS: Pain related to cancer and treatments

EXPECTED OUTCOME
The child exhibits no signs of discomfort.

NURSING INTERVENTIONS/*RATIONALES*
Be judicious in caregiving and handling *to minimize pain.*
Administer analgesics as prescribed on a regular schedule *to prevent start or recurrence of pain.*
Implement appropriate nonpharmacologic pain reduction techniques *as an adjunct to analgesics.*
Monitor child for vital signs, signs of irritability, restlessness *to assess need for and effectiveness of pain management techniques.*

NURSING DIAGNOSIS: Fear related to diagnosis, prognosis, treatment procedure

EXPECTED OUTCOME
The child exhibits signs of reduced fear.

NURSING INTERVENTIONS/*RATIONALES*
Acknowledge child's fear and help child to identify sources of that fear *to facilitate identification and use of coping strategies.*
Orient child to hospital sights and sounds; provide child with accurate information about condition, procedures, and treatments; and spend time with child *to promote trust and dispel fear.*
Encourage frequent family visitation with active participation in care *to prevent distress from separation.*
Use frequent touch, holding, and talking as appropriate *to provide comfort.*
Provide diversion and sensory stimulation appropriate to the child's developmental level and physical condition.
Instruct family in importance of comfort measures and in their active participation in care *to ease child's fears.*
Prepare child for procedures using developmentally appropriate approaches (therapeutic play) *to reduce fear and promote cooperation.*
Allow child choices when possible *to give child some measure of control.*
Work with parents to create a routine that is similar to the child's usual routine at home *to increase comfort with environment.*

NURSING DIAGNOSIS: Altered family processes related to situational crises (child with life-threatening disease), treatment approaches

EXPECTED OUTCOME
The family members exhibit adaptation of their usual roles and functions to accommodate the child's special needs, and they exhibit growth-promoting behaviors.

Continued

Nursing Care Plan

THE CHILD WITH CANCER—cont'd

NURSING INTERVENTIONS/*RATIONALES*

Provide opportunity for family to absorb and adjust to diagnosis (e.g., repeat information *to allow time for family to hear and understand;* encourage expression of concerns, fears, and feelings about diagnosis and potential impact *to facilitate adjustment;* identify support systems *to provide resources for coping.*

Assist family to understand expected treatment, rationale, and implications *to provide a sound basis for decision making.*

Teach family about expected side effects and toxicities of treatment *to prevent surprises and prepare them for what will happen.*

Explore family members' reaction to child; assist them to achieve a realistic view of child's condition; have family emphasize what child can do; explore ways for family to include child in family activities *to help family increase abilities to cope with child's illness and to help child remain a part of the family structure.*

Arrange for and participate in family conferences *to provide a forum for communication, mutual goal setting, and effective strategizing.*

Have parents spend special time with siblings *so that they do not feel neglected or left out.*

Identify additional resource systems (e.g., relatives, friends, church, health care services, community programs) and strategize with family about making good use of these systems *to develop broad base of support.*

NURSING DIAGNOSIS: Anticipatory grieving related to impending loss of a child

See Nursing Care Plan: The Child Who Is Terminally Ill or Dying, Chapter 41.

Lymphomas

Pediatric lymphomas are the third most common group of malignancies in children and adolescents. The lymphomas, a group of neoplastic diseases that arise from the lymphoid and hemopoietic systems, are divided into Hodgkin disease and non-Hodgkin lymphoma (NHL). These diseases are further subdivided according to tissue type and extent of disease. NHL is more prevalent in children younger than 14 years of age, whereas Hodgkin disease is prevalent in adolescence and the young adult period, with a striking increase between ages 15 and 19 years.

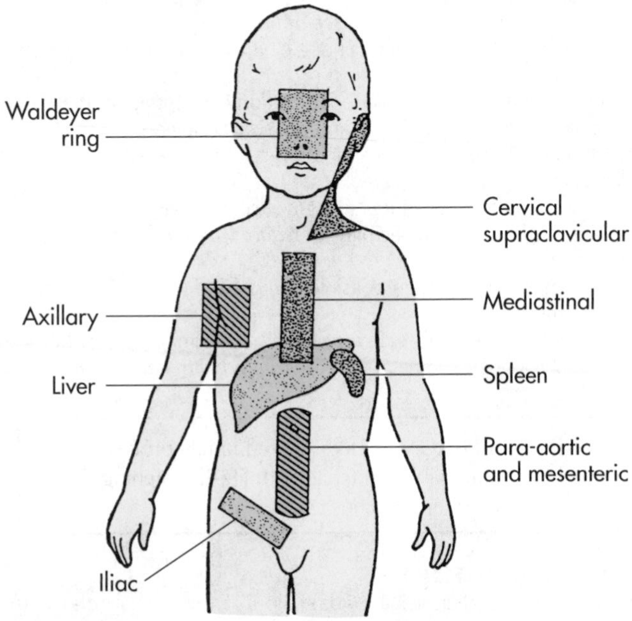

Fig. 49-5 Main areas of lymphadenopathy and organ involvement in Hodgkin disease.

Hodgkin Disease

Hodgkin disease is a neoplastic disease that originates in the lymphoid system and primarily involves the lymph nodes. It predictably metastasizes to nonnodal or extralymphatic sites, especially the spleen, liver, bone marrow, and lungs, although no tissue is exempt from involvement (Fig. 49-5). It is classified according to four histologic types: (1) lymphocytic predominance, (2) nodular sclerosis, (3) mixed cellularity, and (4) lymphocytic depletion. Accurate staging of the extent of disease is the basis for treatment protocols and expected prognoses.

The Ann Arbor staging system (Box 49-10) assigns stage based on the number of sites of lymph node involvement, presence of extranodal disease, and history of any symptoms. Patients are classified as A if asymptomatic and as B if they have the following symptoms: temperature of 38° C (100.4° F) or higher for 3 consecutive days, drenching night sweats, or unexplained loss of body weight (10% or more) over the preceding 6 months (Hudson & Donaldson, 2002).

BOX 49-10

Stages of Hodgkin Disease

Stage I: Lesions are limited to one lymph node area or only one additional extralymphatic site (IE), such as the liver, lungs, kidney, or intestines.

Stage II: Two or more lymph node regions on the same side of the diaphragm or one additional extralymphatic site or organ (IIE) on the same side of the diaphragm is involved.

Stage III: Lymph node regions on both sides of the diaphragm are involved, or one extralymphatic site (IIIE), spleen (IIIS), or both (IIISE).

Stage IV: Cancer has metastasized diffusely throughout the body to one or more extralymphatic sites with or without involvement of associated lymph nodes.

Asymptomatic enlarged cervical or supraclavicular lymphadenopathy is the most common manifestation of Hodgkin disease (Box 49-11). Other systemic symptoms, including fever, weight loss, and night sweats, as well as cough, abdominal discomfort, anorexia, nausea, and pruritus, may occur. Because multiple organs may be involved, diagnosis is based on several tests and the extent of metastatic disease. Tests include a CBC, erythrocyte sedimentation rate, serum copper, ferritin level, fibrinogen, immunoglobulins, uric acid level, liver function tests, T-cell function studies, and urinalysis. Radiographic tests include computed tomography (CT) scans of the neck, chest, abdomen, and pelvis; a gallium scan (identifies metastatic/recurrent disease); a chest x-ray film; and, if clinically indicated, a bone scan to identify metastatic disease. With the advent of CT and gallium scans, a lymphangiogram may not be needed, although elimination is controversial.

Although used rarely, *lymphangiography* may be performed. This is visualization of the lymphatic circulation of the lower extremities, groin, ileopelvic and abdominal-aortic regions, and thoracic duct by way of a radiopaque medium injected in the feet or hands.

A lymph node biopsy is essential to establish histiologic diagnosis and staging. The presence of Reed-Sternberg cells is characteristic of Hodgkin disease. These large cells, which are multilobed and nucleated with abundant cytoplasm and a typically halolike clear zone around the nucleolus, are often described as having an "owl's eyes" appearance (Hudson & Donaldson, 2002). A bone marrow aspiration or biopsy is usually performed. With the advent of CT and gallium scans to identify metastatic disease and multiagent chemotherapy to eradicate metastatic disease, a laparotomy without splenectomy is avoided except in a few selected cases.

Therapeutic Management

The primary modalities of therapy are radiation and chemotherapy. Each may be used alone or in combination based on the clinical staging. Radiation may involve only the involved field (IF), an extended field (EF) (involved areas plus adjacent nodes), or total nodal irradiation (TNI), depending on the extent of involvement.

Two effective, widely used combinations of chemotherapy are mechlorethamine, vincristine (Oncovin), procarbazine, and prednisone (MOPP) or doxorubicin (Adriamycin), bleomycin, vinblastine, and dacarbazine (ABVD). However, the MOPP therapy combination caused severe late effects, especially secondary malignancies. At present, use of ABVD with cyclophosphamide, vincristine, prednisone, and procarbazine (COPP) as a substitute for MOPP has minimized late effects.

Follow-up care of children no longer receiving therapy is essential to identify relapse and secondary cancers. In children with splenectomy resulting from laparotomy or splenic irradiation, prophylactic antibiotics are administered for an indefinite period. Also, immunizations against pneumococci and meningococci are recommended before the splenectomy.

Prognosis

Long-term survival for all stages of Hodgkin disease is excellent. Early-stage disease can have survival rates greater than 90%, with advanced stages having rates between 65% and 75%.

Nursing Care Management

Nursing care involves the same objectives as for patients with other types of cancer—specifically, (1) preparation for diagnostic and operative procedures, (2) explanation of treatment side effects (see Box 49-9), and (3) child and family support (see Chapter 41). Because this is most often a disease of adolescents and young adults, the nurse must have an appreciation of their psychologic needs and reactions during the diagnostic and treatment phases (see Nursing Care Plan, pp. 1628-1630).

After the child is hospitalized for suspected Hodgkin disease, a battery of diagnostic tests is ordered. The family needs an explanation of why each test is performed, because many of them, such as bone marrow aspiration and lymph node biopsy, are invasive procedures.

The most common side effect of irradiation is fatigue. This is particularly difficult for active, outgoing school-age children and adolescents, because it prevents them from keeping up with their peers. Sometimes adolescents will push themselves to the point of physical exhaustion rather than admit and succumb to the decreased activity tolerance. The nurse cautions parents to observe for behavior such as extreme fatigue at the end of the day, falling asleep at the dinner table, inability to concentrate on homework, or an increased susceptibility to infection. A regular bedtime and scheduled rest periods are important for these children, especially during chemotherapy, when myelosuppression increases the risk of infection and debilitation. Before discharge, the nurse should discuss a feasible school schedule with the parents and child.

An area of concern for adolescents is the high risk of sterility from irradiation and chemotherapy. Both drugs, particularly procarbazine and alkylating agents, and irradiation to the gonads can lead to infertility. Adolescents should be informed of these side effects early in the course of the diagnosis and treatment. Sperm banking is now offered at

BOX 49-11

Clinical Manifestations of Hodgkin Disease

- Painless enlargement of the lymph nodes:
  - Enlarged, firm, nontender, movable nodes in the cervical area are most common
  - "Sentinel" node located near the left clavicle may be first enlarged node
  - Axillary and inguinal lymph nodes less frequently
- Other signs and symptoms of lymphadenopathy:
  - Enlarged mediastinal nodes cause persistent nonproductive cough
  - Enlarged retroperitoneal nodes produce unexplained abdominal pain
- Systemic symptoms (usually indicate advanced involvement):
  - Low-grade or intermittent fever
  - Anorexia
  - Nausea
  - Weight loss
  - Night sweats
  - Pruritus

many cancer centers before the initiation of treatment in adolescent boys. Sexual function is not altered, although the appearance of secondary sexual characteristics and menstruation may be delayed in the pubescent child. Delayed sexual maturation may be an extremely sensitive and stressful issue for children (see Chapter 52).

Non-Hodgkin Lymphoma

Non-Hodgkin lymphoma (NHL) occurs more frequently in children than Hodgkin disease. NHL is diagnosed in approximately 750 to 800 children each year in the United States (Link & Donaldson, 2003). Histologic classification of childhood NHL is strikingly different from that of Hodgkin disease, as demonstrated in the following statements:

- The disease is usually diffuse rather than nodular.
- The cell type is either undifferentiated or poorly differentiated.
- Dissemination occurs early, more often, and rapidly.
- Mediastinal involvement and invasion of meninges are common.

NHL exhibits a variety of morphologic, cytochemical, and immunologic features, not unlike the diversity seen in leukemia. Classification is based on the histologic pattern: (1) lymphoblastic, (2) Burkitt or non-Burkitt, or (3) large cell. Immunologically these cells are also classified as T-cells; B-cells; or non-T, non-B cells (lacking immunologic properties).

The clinical staging system used in Hodgkin disease is of little value in NHL, although it has been modified and other systems have been developed.

Diagnostic Evaluation

Because the clinical presentation of most children with NHL is widespread disseminated disease, thorough pathologic staging is unnecessary. Clinical manifestations depend on the anatomic site and extent of involvement. These manifestations include many of those seen in Hodgkin disease and leukemia, as well as organ symptoms related to pressure from enlargement of adjacent lymph nodes, such as intestinal or airway obstruction, cranial nerve palsies, and spinal paralysis.

Recommendations for staging include a surgical biopsy of an enlarged node, histopathologic confirmation of disease with cytochemical and immunologic evaluation, bone marrow examination, radiographic studies (especially tomograms of the lungs and GI organs), and lumbar puncture.

Therapeutic Management

The treatment protocols for NHL include aggressive use of irradiation and chemotherapy. Similar to leukemia therapy, the protocols include induction, consolidation, and maintenance phases, some with intrathecal chemotherapy. Antineoplastic agents used in the treatment of NHL include vincristine, prednisone, L-asparaginase, methotrexate, 6-mercaptopurine, cytarabine, cyclophosphamide, anthracyclines, and teniposide or etoposide (Link & Donaldson, 2003).

Prognosis

The prognosis is excellent for children with localized disease, and long-term remissions are possible in many patients, even in those with disseminated disease. Because relapse after 2 years is rare, survival after 24 months is considered a cure.

Nursing Care Management

Nursing care of the child with NHL is similar to that required for children with leukemia. Many of the same drugs are employed, although the schedules differ. Because of the intense chemotherapy, nursing care is primarily directed toward managing the side effects of these agents and providing supportive care to the child and family (see Nursing Care Plan, pp. 1628-1630).

IMMUNOLOGIC DEFICIENCY DISORDERS

A number of disorders can cause profound, often life-threatening alterations within the body's immune system. The most serious are those conditions that completely depress immunity, such as severe combined immunodeficiency disease. However, the one disorder that generates the most anxiety, within both the family and the community at large, is HIV infection/AIDS.

Several classifications of immune dysfunction exist. *AIDS, severe combined immunodeficiency syndrome (SCID),* and *Wiskott-Aldrich syndrome* are syndromes wherein the body is unable to mount an immune response. The immune response can also be misdirected. In *autoimmune disorders,* antibodies, macrophages, and lymphocytes attack healthy cells.

Human Immunodeficiency Virus Infection and Acquired Immunodeficiency Syndrome

Since the first cases of AIDS were identified in the early 1980s, HIV infection has generated intense medical investigation. Research has led to early diagnosis of and improved medical treatments for HIV infection, changing this disease from a rapidly fatal one to a chronic, but terminal, disease of childhood.

Epidemiology

The first AIDS cases in the pediatric population in the United States were identified in children born to HIV-infected mothers and in children who received blood products. More than 90% of these children acquired the disease perinatally from their mothers. Smaller numbers of children were infected through the transfusion of contaminated blood or blood products before 1985 or were infected through sexual abuse. In contrast, sexual activity and IV drug use are major sources of HIV infection in adolescents.

The estimated number of children with perinatally acquired AIDS peaked during 1992; subsequent years have seen significant declines. This trend is a result of implementation of recommended HIV counseling and voluntary testing practices and the use of zidovudine therapy to prevent perinatal transmission. Zidovudine therapy in HIV-infected pregnant women, and subsequently in their infants, has significantly reduced the transmission of HIV (Ioannidis et al, 2001; Lyall, 2002). The effectiveness of other HIV drugs such as Nevirapine to prevent perinatal transmission is being studied (Meldrum, 2003; Merchant & Keshavarz, 2001). Routine HIV counseling and voluntary testing for pregnant

BOX 49-12

Common Clinical Manifestations of HIV Infection in Children

Lymphadenopathy
Hepatosplenomegaly
Oral candidiasis
Chronic or recurrent diarrhea
Failure to thrive
Developmental delay
Parotitis

women are recommended (American Academy of Pediatrics, Committee on Pediatric AIDS, 2000b), and guidelines for the use of antiretroviral drugs in HIV-infected pregnant women to reduce perinatal transmission are available (Lyall, 2002).

Etiology

HIV is a retrovirus that is transmitted by lymphocytes and monocytes. It is found in the blood, semen, vaginal secretions, and breast milk. It has an incubation period of months to years (Ezekowitz & Stockman, 2003). There are different strains of HIV. HIV-2 is prevalent in Africa, whereas HIV-1 is the dominant strain in the United States and elsewhere. *Horizontal transmission* of HIV occurs through intimate sexual contact or parenteral exposure to blood or body fluids containing visible blood. *Perinatal (vertical) transmission* occurs when an HIV-infected pregnant woman passes the infection to her infant. There is no evidence that *casual* contact between infected and uninfected individuals can spread the virus.

Pathophysiology

HIV primarily infects a specific subset of T-lymphocytes, the CD_4+ T-cells. The virus takes over the machinery of the CD_4+ lymphocyte, using it to replicate itself, rendering the CD_4+ cell dysfunctional. The CD_4+ lymphocyte count gradually decreases over time, leading to progressive immune deficiency. The count eventually reaches a critical level below which there is substantial risk of opportunistic illnesses followed by death.

BOX 49-13

Common AIDS-Defining Conditions in Children

Pneumocystis carinii pneumonia
Lymphoid interstitial pneumonitis
Recurrent bacterial infections
Wasting syndrome
HIV encephalopathy
Candidal esophagitis
  Cytomegalovirus disease
  Mycobacterium avium-intracellulare complex infection
  Severe herpes simplex infection
  Pulmonary candidiasis
Cryptosporidiosis

Clinical Manifestations

Common clinical manifestations of HIV infection in children are varied (Box 49-12). The diagnosis of AIDS is associated with certain illnesses or conditions. The most common AIDS-defining conditions observed among American children are listed in Box 49-13. Other problems in these children may include short stature, malnutrition, and cardiomyopathy. CNS abnormalities resulting from HIV infection may include neuropsychologic deficits; developmental disabilities; and deficits in motor skills, communication, and behavioral functioning.

Diagnostic Evaluation

For children 18 months of age and older, the HIV enzyme-linked immunosorbent assay (ELISA) and Western blot immunoassay are performed to determine HIV infection. In infants born to HIV-infected mothers, these assays will be positive because of the presence of maternal antibodies derived transplacentally. Maternal antibodies may persist in the infant up to 18 months of age. Therefore other diagnostic tests are employed, most commonly the HIV polymerase chain reaction (PCR) for detection of proviral DNA. With this technique, more than 95% of infected infants can be diagnosed by 1 month of age (Ezekowitz & Stockman, 2003).

The Centers for Disease Control and Prevention (CDC) (1994) has developed a classification system to describe the spectrum of HIV disease in children (Table 49-3). The sys-

Table 49-3

Pediatric HIV Classification*

IMMUNOLOGIC CATEGORIES	N: NO SIGNS/ SYMPTOMS	A: MILD SIGNS/ SYMPTOMS	B: MODERATE SIGNS/ SYMPTOMS†	C: SEVERE SIGNS/ SYMPTOMS†
No evidence of suppression	N1	A1	B1	C1
Evidence of moderate suppression	N2	A2	B2	C2
Severe suppression	N3	A3	B3	C3

From Centers for Disease Control and Prevention: 1994 revised classification system for human immunodeficiency virus infection in children less than 13 years of age, *MMWR* 43(RR-12):1-10, 1994.

*Children whose HIV infection status is not confirmed are classified by using the above table with the letter *E* (for perinatally exposed) placed before the appropriate classification code (e.g., EN2).

†Both category C and lymphoid interstitial pneumonitis in category B are reportable to state and local health departments as AIDS.

tem indicates the severity of clinical signs and symptoms and the degree of immunosuppression. Mild signs and symptoms include lymphadenopathy, parotitis, hepatosplenomegaly, and recurrent or persistent sinusitis or otitis media. Moderate signs and symptoms include lymphoid interstitial pneumonitis (LIP) and a variety of organ-specific dysfunctions or infections. Severe signs and symptoms include AIDS-defining illnesses with the exception of LIP. Children with LIP have a better prognosis than those with other AIDS-defining illnesses. In children whose HIV infection is not yet confirmed, the letter *E* (vertically exposed) is placed in front of the classification. The immune categories are based on CD_4+ lymphocyte counts and percentages. Age adjustment of these numbers is necessary because normal counts, which are relatively high in infants, decline steadily until 6 years of age, when they reach adult norms (Table 49-4).

Therapeutic Management

The goals of therapy for HIV infection include slowing the growth of the virus, preventing and treating opportunistic infections, and providing nutritional support and symptomatic treatment. *Antiretroviral drugs* work at various stages of the HIV life cycle to prevent reproduction of functional new virus particles. Although not a cure, these drugs can suppress viral replication, preventing further deterioration of the immune system, and thus delay disease progression. Classes of antiretroviral agents include nucleoside reverse transcriptase inhibitors (e.g., zidovudine, didanosine, stavudine, lamivudine, abacavir), nonnucleoside reverse transcriptase inhibitors (e.g., nevirapine, delavirdine, efavirenz), nucleotide reverse transcriptase inhibitors (e.g., adefovir), protease inhibitors (e.g., indinavir, saquinavir, ritonavir, nelfinavir, amprenavir), and adjunctive antiretrovirals (e.g., hydroxyurea). Combinations of these drugs are used to forestall the emergence of drug resistance. Antiretroviral therapy regimens and guidelines are continually evolving. Therapy is lifelong, making adherence difficult. Laboratory markers (CD_4+ lymphocyte count, viral load) assist in monitoring both disease progression and response to therapy.

Pneumocystis carinii pneumonia (PCP) is the most common opportunistic infection of children infected with HIV. It occurs most frequently between 3 and 6 months of age. All infants born to HIV-infected women should receive prophylaxis during the first year of life according to guidelines set by the CDC (1995) and American Academy of Pediatrics, Committee on Pediatric AIDS (2000b). After 1 year of age, the need for prophylaxis is determined by the presence of severe immunosuppression or a history of PCP (CDC, 1995; National Institute of Allergy and Infectious Diseases, National Institutes of Health, 2003). Trimethoprim-sulfamethoxazole (TMP-SMZ) is the agent of choice. If adverse effects are experienced with TMP-SMZ, dapsone or pentamidine can be used.

Prophylaxis is often employed for other opportunistic infections, such as disseminated *Mycobacterium avium-intracellulare* complex (MAC), candidiasis, and herpes simplex. IV immunoglobulin has been helpful in preventing recurrent or serious bacterial infections in some HIV-infected children.

Immunization against common childhood illnesses is recommended for all children exposed to and infected with HIV (American Academy of Pediatrics, Committee on Pediatric AIDS, 2000a). Varicella (chickenpox) vaccine and measles-mumps-rubella (MMR) vaccine can be administered if there is no evidence of severe immunocompromise. The pneumococcal and influenza vaccines are recommended. Because antibody production to vaccines may be poor or decrease over time, immediate prophylaxis after exposure to several vaccine-preventable diseases (e.g., measles, varicella) is warranted. It should be recognized that children receiving IV gamma globulin prophylaxis may not respond to the MMR vaccine (Morbidity and Mortality Weekly Report [MMWR], 2003).

HIV infection often leads to marked failure to thrive and multiple nutritional deficiencies. Nutritional management may be difficult because of recurrent illness, diarrhea, and other physical problems. Intensive nutritional interventions should be instituted when the child's growth begins to slow or weight begins to decrease.

Prognosis

Early recognition and improved medical care have changed HIV disease from a rapidly fatal illness to a chronic disease. After the introduction of combination antiretroviral therapy, the numbers of new AIDS cases and deaths declined

Table 49-4

Immunologic Categories Based on Age-Specific CD_4^+ T-Lymphocyte Counts and Percent of Total Lymphocytes

	Age of Child					
	<12 Months		1-5 Years		6-12 Years	
	MCL	(%)	MCL	(%)	MCL	(%)
IMMUNOLOGIC CATEGORY						
No evidence of suppression	≥1500	(≥25)	≥1000	(≥25)	≥500	(≥25)
Evidence of moderate suppression	750-1499	(15-24)	500-999	(15-24)	200-499	(15-24)
Severe suppression	<750	(<15)	<500	(<15)	<200	(<15)

From Centers for Disease Control and Prevention: 1994 revised classification system for human immunodeficiency virus infection in children less than 13 years of age, *MMWR* 43(RR-12):1-10, 1994.

substantially. Between 1995 and 1998, the annual number of AIDS cases declined by 38% and deaths declined by 63% (MMWR, 2003). The annual numbers of AIDS cases and deaths have remained stable since 1998 (CDC, 2001). The number of children with AIDS, attributed to perinatal HIV transmission, peaked in 1992 at 954 cases and declined by 89% to 101 cases in 2001 (CDC, 2001).

Nursing Care Management

Education concerning transmission and control of infectious diseases, including HIV infection, is essential for children with HIV infection and anyone involved in their care. The basic tenets of Standard Precautions should be presented in an age-appropriate manner, with careful consideration of the educational levels of the individuals (see Infection Control, Chapter 45). Safety issues, including appropriate storage of special medications and equipment (e.g., needles and syringes), are emphasized. Unfortunately, relatives, friends, and others in the general public may be fearful of contracting HIV infection, and criticism and ostracism of the child and family may occur. In an effort to protect the child, the family may limit the child's activities outside the home. Although certain precautions are justified in limiting exposure to sources of infections, they must be tempered with concern for the child's normal developmental needs. Both the family and the community need ongoing education about HIV to dispel many of the myths that have been perpetuated by uninformed persons.*

Prevention is a key component of HIV education. Educating adolescents about HIV is essential in preventing HIV infection in this age group. Education should include the routes of transmission, the hazards of IV and other recreational drug use, and the value of sexual abstinence and safe sex practices. Such education should be a part of anticipatory guidance provided to all adolescent patients. Nurses can also encourage adolescents at risk to undergo HIV counseling and testing. In addition to identifying infected teenagers and getting them into care, such counseling affords adolescents an opportunity to learn about, and possibly change, their risk behaviors.

The nurse's role in the care of the child with HIV is multifaceted (see Nursing Care Plan, p. 1637). The nurse serves as educator, direct care provider, case manager, and advocate. As with all chronic illnesses, these children will have much involvement with the health care system. The need for HIV medications is lifelong. Nurses are instrumental in encouraging and empowering these children (and their caretakers) to adhere to their medication regimens. Clinic visits and hospitalizations may become frequent as the disease progresses. The physiologic care of the child is directed at minimum exposure to infections; nutritional support; comfort measures, including pain management; and assessment and recognition of changes in status that may indicate new complications. The scope of nursing care will change with new symptoms, changes in treatment, and disease progression. The unpredictability of the course of pediatric HIV infection is a continual source of stress to these children and their caretakers. Psychologic interventions will vary with the unique circumstances of each child and family.

The multiple complications associated with HIV disease are potentially painful (Ezekowitz & Stockman, 2003; Sullivan & Woda, 2003). Aggressive pain management is essential for these children to have an acceptable quality of life. Their pain may be due to infections (e.g., otitis media, dental abscess), encephalopathy (e.g., spasticity), adverse effects of medications (e.g., peripheral neuropathy), or an unknown source (e.g., deep musculoskeletal pain). Sources of pain are related not only to disease processes, but also to various treatments these children often undergo, including venipunctures, lumbar punctures, biopsies, and endoscopies. Ongoing assessment of pain is crucial and is most easily accomplished in older children who are able to communicate. Nonverbal and developmentally delayed children are more difficult to assess. Be alert for other signs of pain: emotional detachment, lack of interactive play, irritability, and depression. Effective pain management depends on the appropriate use of pharmacologic agents, including EMLA cream, acetaminophen, NSAIDs, muscle relaxants, and opioids. Tolerance to opioids may indicate increased dosing; monitored use ensures safety. Nonpharmacologic interventions (guided imagery, hypnosis, and relaxation and distraction techniques) are useful adjuncts.

Common psychosocial concerns include disclosure of the diagnosis to the child, making custody plans when the parent is infected, and anticipating the loss of a family member. Other stressors may include financial difficulties, HIV-associated stigma, striving to keep the diagnosis secret, other infected family members, and the multiple losses associated with HIV. Most mothers of these children are single mothers who are also HIV infected. As primary caretakers, they often attend to the needs of their child first, neglecting their own health in the process (Family Focus box). The nurse can encourage the mother to receive regular health care. Family members are often involved in the care of the child, particu-

Family Focus

CAREGIVERS AND THE INFANT WITH HIV INFECTION

Unlike other fatal pediatric diseases, HIV infection is associated with special family alterations. The infant infected in utero faces multiple physical and parental problems. Because the mother is infected, she may be ill or dying and therefore unable to care for the child. If possible, grandparents or other relatives may assume care. Foster care is often difficult to arrange because of the nature of the disease, especially in relation to the social stigma and the child's multiple medical needs. These children may require frequent hospitalizations with progression of their HIV disease. When children remain in the hospital, the importance of consistent caregivers, especially primary nurses, who attend to the youngsters' physical, developmental, and emotional needs cannot be overemphasized. However, primary nurses may face the risk of overinvolvement and must be aware of the boundaries of a therapeutic relationship.

*Additional information is available from the AIDS Hotline: 800-342-2437 (AIDS); and from the National Pediatric and Family HIV Resource Center, 30 Bergen Street, ADMC 4, Newark, NJ 07103; phone: 973-972-0410 or 800-362-0071; Web site: www.pedhivaids.org.

larly if the mother has symptomatic illness. After the death of the mother, a grandparent or other relative typically assumes responsibility for the care of the child. Nursing can provide support and encouragement for the new surrogate parent, particularly during the transition phase. If no family member is available, the child may be placed in a foster or group home. Nursing is an integral part of the multidisciplinary team necessary for the successful management of the complex medical and social problems of these families.

Children with HIV infection attend day care centers and schools. It is well established that the risk of HIV transmission in these settings is minimal. These institutions are required to follow CDC and Occupational Safety and Health Administration (OSHA) guidelines for infection control measures. Standard Precautions describing proper management of blood and body fluids should also be followed. It is recommended that school personnel receive current HIV information and include it in the health education curriculum for kindergarten through twelfth grade (American Academy of Pediatrics, Committee on Pediatric AIDS, 2000a; American Academy of Pediatrics, Committee on Pediatric AIDS and Committee on Infectious Diseases, 1999). School nurses play a vital role in educating the school staff, students, and parents. They are also invaluable in monitoring the needs of known affected children.

Confidentiality is a major issue in day care or school attendance. Parents and legal guardians have the right to decide whether to inform these agencies of their child's HIV diagnosis. Unfortunately, myths about HIV infection continue to exist, and the family often wishes to avoid any potential criticism or ostracism of the child.

Nursing care of the child with HIV infection is summarized in the Nursing Care Plan on p. 1637.

Severe Combined Immunodeficiency Disease

SCID is a defect characterized by absence of both humoral and cell-mediated immunity. The terms *Swiss-type lymphopenic agammaglobulinemia* (an autosomal recessive form of the disease) and *X-linked lymphopenic agammaglobulinemia* have been used to describe this disorder, which, as the names imply, can follow either mode of inheritance.

Susceptibility to infection occurs early in life, most often in the first month of life. The child suffers from chronic infection, fails to completely recover from an infection, is frequently reinfected, and is infected with unusual agents. Failure to thrive is a consequence of the persistent illnesses.

Diagnosis is usually based on a history of recurrent, severe infections from early infancy; a familial history of the disorder; and specific laboratory findings, which include lymphopenia, lack of lymphocyte response to antigens, and absence of plasma cells in the bone marrow. Documentation of immunoglobulin (Ig) deficiency is difficult during infancy because of the normally delayed response of infants in producing their own immunoglobulins and material transfer of IgG.

Therapeutic Management

The only definitive treatment for SCID is HSCT from a histocompatible donor (usually a sibling), a haplo-identical donor (usually a parent), or a match-unrelated donor. IVIG infusions and PCP prophylaxis are used to augment the humoral immunity until the transplant is performed. Several investigators are attempting gene therapy with some success, but there is a potential complication of insertional mutagenesis (Buckley, 2002).

Nursing Care Management

Nursing care focuses on the prevention of infection and supporting the child and family. The care is consistent with that needed for HSCT for any condition (see p. 1638). Because the prognosis for SCID is very poor if a compatible bone marrow donor is not available, nursing care is directed at supporting the family in caring for a child with a life-threatening illness (see Chapter 41). Genetic counseling is essential because of the modes of transmission in either form of the disorder.

Wiskott-Aldrich Syndrome

The Wiskott-Aldrich syndrome (WAS) is an X-linked recessive disorder characterized by a triad of abnormalities: (1) thrombocytopenia, (2) eczema, and (3) immunodeficiency of selective functions of B-lymphocytes and T-lymphocytes. A defective gene has been identified and designated the WAS protein (Bonilla & Geha, 2003). At birth, the symptoms may be bloody diarrhea as a result of thrombocytopenia. As the child grows older, recurrent infection and eczema become more severe, and the bleeding becomes less frequent.

Eczema is typical of the allergic type and easily becomes superinfected. Chronic infection with herpes simplex is a frequent problem and may lead to chronic keratitis of the eye with loss of vision. Chronic pulmonary disease, sinusitis, and otitis media result from repeated infections. In those children who survive the bleeding episodes and overwhelming infections, malignancy presents an additional risk to survival.

Medical treatment involves (1) counteracting the bleeding tendencies with platelet transfusions, (2) using IV gamma globulin to provide passive immunity, and (3) administering prophylactic antibiotics to prevent and control infection. Splenectomy alone or with HSCT may extend the survival to adulthood (Bonilla & Geha, 2003; Champi, 2002).

Nursing Care Management

Because of the poor prognosis for these children, the main nursing consideration is supporting the family in the care of a fatally ill child. Physical care is directed at controlling the problems imposed by the disorder. The measures used to control bleeding are similar to those for hemophilia and vWD (see previous discussions). Another major goal is prevention or control of infection. Because eczema is a troublesome problem, nursing measures specific to this condition are especially important. The genetic implications of this X-linked recessive disorder differ little from those of any other X-linked disorder.

TECHNOLOGIC MANAGEMENT OF HEMATOLOGIC/IMMUNOLOGIC DISORDERS

Blood Transfusion Therapy

Technologic advances in blood banking and transfusion medicine enable the administration of only the blood component needed by the child, such as packed RBCs in anemia or platelets for bleeding disorders. However, regardless

Nursing Care Plan

THE CHILD WITH HIV INFECTION

NURSING DIAGNOSIS: Risk for infection related to impaired body defenses

EXPECTED OUTCOME

The child exhibits no evidence of infection and no evidence of spread of the virus.

NURSING INTERVENTIONS/*RATIONALES*

Place child in private room and screen all visitors and staff for signs of infection *to minimize exposure to infective organisms.*

Teach child and family about good hygiene and careful hand-washing techniques *to prevent spread of infection.*

Use good handwashing for all contacts with child and scrupulous aseptic technique for all invasive procedures *to minimize exposure to infection.*

Encourage a nutritionally complete diet *to support body's natural defenses.*

Administer prescribed antibiotics *to prevent infection,* antiretroviral drugs *to increase lymphocyte production,* trimethoprim-sulfamethoxazole tablets *to prevent pneumocystis pneumonia,* and rifabutin *to prevent* Mycobacterium avium.

Monitor vital signs and observe skin and mucosa, auscultate lungs *to detect signs of infection.*

Do not administer live attenuated virus vaccines (i.e., MMR, oral polio, varicella zoster) to child with depressed immune system *to prevent overwhelming the system and introducing an infectious disease;* use inactivated virus vaccines as prescribed (i.e., Salk polio, influenza) *to prevent common childhood illnesses.*

Instruct child and family about protective methods (e.g., hand-washing after using bathroom; avoidance of blood and body fluids by others; avoidance of biting, scratching behaviors) *to prevent spread of virus.*

Use appropriate universal precautions when administering care and performing invasive procedures *to prevent spread of HIV.*

NURSING DIAGNOSIS: Altered nutrition: less than body requirements related to recurrent illness, diarrhea, loss of appetite, oral thrush

EXPECTED OUTCOME

The child's nutritional intake is adequate.

NURSING INTERVENTIONS/*RATIONALES*

Provide high-calorie, high-protein diet *to meet body requirements for metabolism and growth;* fortify foods with nutritional supplements *to maximize quality of intake.*

Involve child in selection and preparation *to increase intake and tolerance.*

Use creativity to encourage child to eat (see Feeding the Sick Child, Chapter 45).

Monitor height and weight *to assess for slowed growth or weight loss.*

Administer antifungal medications as ordered *to prevent or treat thrush.*

NURSING DIAGNOSIS: Impaired social interaction related to recurrent illness, social stigma of HIV

EXPECTED OUTCOME

The child is involved in age-appropriate peer-group and family activities.

NURSING INTERVENTIONS/*RATIONALES*

Assist child to identify personal strengths *to facilitate coping.*

Educate school personnel and classmates about HIV *so child is not unnecessarily isolated.*

Encourage family to plan activities that include child as a participating member *to increase family interaction.*

Encourage child to maintain phone contact with friends during hospitalization *to reduce feelings of isolation.*

Introduce child to other children with HIV *to provide mutual support system.*

NURSING DIAGNOSIS: Altered sexuality pattern related to risk of disease transmission

EXPECTED OUTCOME

The adolescent displays appropriate sexual behavior and exhibits positive sexual identity.

NURSING INTERVENTIONS/*RATIONALES*

Educate adolescent about sexual transmission risks, perinatal infection risks, avoidance of high risk behavior, abstinence/use of condoms *so adolescent can make informed decisions about safe and healthy expressions of sexuality.*

Encourage adolescent to talk about feelings and concerns related to sexuality *to facilitate coping.*

NURSING DIAGNOSIS: Altered family processes related to situational crises (child with life-threatening disease) and treatment approaches

See Nursing Care Plan: The Child with Cancer, p. 1628, and Nursing Care Plan: The Child Who Is Terminally Ill or Dying, p. 1246.

of the blood component infused, all transfusions have some risks. Therefore nurses need to be aware of the possible complications and the appropriate interventions. Table 49-5 summarizes the major hazards of transfusions, the signs and symptoms typically associated with each, and nursing responsibilities. The following general guidelines apply to all transfusions:

- Take vital signs, including blood pressure, *before* administering blood to establish baseline data for intratransfusion and posttransfusion comparison, and then every 15 minutes for 1 hour while blood is infusing.
- Check the identification of the recipient with the donor's blood group and type, regardless of the blood product used.
- Administer the first 50 ml of blood or 20% of the volume (whichever is smaller) *slowly* and stay with the child.
- Administer with normal saline on a piggyback setup or have normal saline available.

Table 49-5

Nursing Care of the Child Receiving Blood Transfusions

COMPLICATION	SIGNS/SYMPTOMS	PRECAUTIONS/NURSING RESPONSIBILITIES
IMMEDIATE REACTIONS		
Hemolytic Reactions		
Most severe type, but rare Incompatible blood Incompatibility in multiple transfusions	Chills Shaking Fever Pain at needle site and along venous tract Nausea/vomiting Sensation of tightness in chest Red or black urine Headache Flank pain Progressive signs of shock or renal failure Sudden severe headache	Identify donor and recipient blood types and groups before transfusion is begun; verify with another nurse or practitioner Transfuse blood slowly for first 15-20 minutes and/or initial 20% of blood volume; remain with patient Stop transfusion immediately in event of signs or symptoms, maintain patent intravenous line, and notify practitioner Save donor blood to re-crossmatch with patient's blood Monitor for evidence of shock Insert urinary catheter and monitor hourly outputs Send sample of patient's blood and urine to laboratory for presence of hemoglobin (indicates intravascular hemolysis) Observe for signs of hemorrhage resulting from disseminated intravascular coagulation (DIC) Support medical therapies to reverse shock
Febrile Reactions		
Leukocyte or platelet antibodies Plasma protein antibodies	Fever Chills	May give acetaminophen for prophylaxis Leukocyte-poor red blood cells (RBCs) are less likely to cause reaction Stop transfusion immediately; report to practitioner for evaluation
Allergic Reactions		
Recipient reacts to allergens in donor's blood	Urticaria Pruritus Flushing Asthmatic wheezing Laryngeal edema	Give antihistamines for prophylaxis to children with tendency toward allergic reactions Stop transfusions immediately Administer epinephrine for wheezing or anaphylactic reaction
Circulatory Overload		
Too rapid transfusion (even a small quantity) Excessive quantity of blood transfused (even slowly)	Precordial pain Dyspnea Rales Cyanosis Dry cough Distended neck veins Hypertension	Transfuse blood slowly Prevent overload by using packed RBCs or administering divided amounts of blood Use infusion pump to regulate and maintain flow rate Stop transfusion immediately if signs of overload Place child upright with feet in dependent position to increase venous resistance
Air Emboli		
May occur when blood is transfused under pressure	Sudden difficulty in breathing Sharp pain in chest Apprehension	Normalize pressure before container is empty when infusing blood under pressure Clear tubing of air by aspirating air with syringe at nearest Y connector if air is observed in tubing; disconnect tubing and allow blood to flow until air has escaped only if a Y connector is not available
Hypothermia		
	Chills Low temperature Irregular heart rate Possible cardiac arrest	Allow blood to warm at room temperature (less than 1 hour) Use approved mechanical blood warmer or electric warming coil to warm blood rapidly; never use microwave oven Take temperature if patient complains of chills; if subnormal, stop transfusion

Table 49-5

Nursing Care of the Child Receiving Blood Transfusions—cont'd

COMPLICATION	SIGNS/SYMPTOMS	PRECAUTIONS/NURSING RESPONSIBILITIES
IMMEDIATE REACTIONS—cont'd		
Electrolyte Disturbances		
Hyperkalemia (in massive transfusions or in patients with renal problems)	Nausea, diarrhea Muscular weakness Flaccid paralysis Paresthesia of extremities Bradycardia Apprehension Cardiac arrest	Use washed RBCs or fresh blood if patient is at risk
DELAYED REACTIONS		
Transmission of Infection		
Hepatitis Human immunodeficiency virus (HIV) Malaria Syphilis Bacteria or viruses	Signs of infection (e.g., jaundice) Toxic reaction: high fever, severe headache or substernal pain, hypotension, intense flushing, vomiting/diarrhea	Blood is tested for antibodies to HIV, hepatitis C virus (HCV), and hepatitis B core antigen (HBcAg); in addition, blood is tested for hepatitis B surface antigen (HBsAg) and alanine aminotransferase (ALT), and a serology test is performed for syphilis; positive units are destroyed; individuals at risk for carrying certain viruses are deferred from donation Report any sign of infection and, if occurring during transfusion, stop transfusion immediately, send sample for culture and sensitivity tests, and notify practitioner
Other alloimmunization Antibody formation Occurs in patients receiving multiple transfusions	Increased risk of hemolytic, febrile, and allergic reactions	Use limited number of donors Observe carefully for signs of reactions
Delayed Hemolytic Reaction	Destruction of RBCs and fever 5-10 days after transfusion	Observe for posttransfusion anemia and decreasing benefit from successive transfusion

- Administer blood through an appropriate filter to eliminate particles in the blood and prevent the precipitation of formed elements; gently shake the container frequently.
- Use blood within 30 minutes of its arrival from the blood bank; if it is not used, return to the blood bank—do not store in the regular unit refrigerator.
- Infuse a unit of blood (or the specified amount) within 4 hours. If the infusion will exceed this time, the blood should be divided into appropriately sized quantities by the blood bank and the unused portion refrigerated under controlled conditions.
- If a reaction of any type is suspected, take vital signs, stop the transfusion, maintain a patent IV line with normal saline and new tubing, and notify the practitioner. Do *not* restart the transfusion until the child's condition has been medically evaluated.

Although hemolytic reactions are rare, ABO incompatibility remains the most common cause of death from blood transfusion, and human error is usually responsible (administration of the wrong type to the patient or mislabeling of the blood product) (Norville & Bryant, 2002). Hemolysis can also cause the release of large quantities of phospholipids, which are capable of stimulating disseminated intravascular coagulation (see p. 1617). Acute kidney shutdown and eventual renal failure are a result of renal vasoconstriction from antigen-antibody complexes derived from the RBC surface.

Blood is usually administered to children by infusion pump; therefore the usual precautions and management related to pumps apply. When the blood is started with a standard transfusion set, the filter chamber is filled to allow the total filter to be used. The drip chamber is partially filled with blood to permit counting of the drops. In adjusting the flow rate, it is important to remember that blood administration sets do not use microdrops (60 drops/ml) but regular drops (usually 10 or 15 drops/ml). Therefore this must be considered when calculating the flow rate.

Hematopoietic Stem Cell Transplantation

HSCT is used to establish healthy hematopoiesis in both malignant and nonmalignant disease. Candidates for transplantation are children who have disorders that are unlikely to be cured by other means. Most HSCT patients undergo ablative therapy that is intensive, using high-dose combination chemotherapy with or without total body irradiation (Ryan et al, 2002). After the body is free of cells and the immune system is suppressed to prevent rejection of the transplanted marrow, the stem cells harvested from the bone marrow, peripheral blood, or the umbilical vein of the placenta are given to the patient by IV transfusion. The newly transfused stem cells will begin to repopulate the ablative bone marrow. In essence, a new blood-forming organ will be accepted by the recipient.

The selection process of a suitable donor and the potential complications in transplantation are related to the *HLA system complex.* Some of the major HLA antigens are A, B, C, D, and DR. There is a wide diversity for each of these HLA loci. There are more than 20 different HLA-A antigens that can be inherited and more than 40 different HLA-B antigens.

The genes are inherited as a single unit or *haplotype.* A child inherits one unit from each parent; thus a child and each parent have one identical and one nonidentical haplotype. Because the possible haplotype combinations among siblings follow the laws of mendelian genetics, there is a 1-in-4 chance that two siblings have two identical haplotypes and are perfectly matched at the HLA loci.

The importance of HLA matching is to prevent the serious complication known as *graft-versus-host disease (GVHD).* Because the child's immune system is essentially rendered nonfunctional, there is little difficulty with bone marrow rejection by the recipient. However, the donor's marrow may contain antigens not matched to the recipient's antigens, which begin attacking body cells. The more closely the HLA systems match, the less likely GVHD is to develop. However, it can occur even with a perfect HLA match, because there are as yet unidentified and thus unmatched histocompatibility antigens (Guinan, Krance, and Lehmann, 2002).

Different types of bone marrow transplantation (BMT) are now performed in children with cancer. *Allogeneic* BMT involves the matching of a histocompatible donor with the recipient. However, allogeneic BMT is limited by the presence of a suitable marrow donor.

Because of the limited numbers of patients having HLA-identical siblings, other types of allogeneic transplants have evolved. *Umbilical cord blood stem cell transplantation* is an established, rich source of hematopoietic stem cells for use in children with cancer (Ryan et al, 2002). Because stem cells can be found with high frequency in the circulation of newborns, cord blood transplantation has become an alternative for some children (Ryan et al, 2002). The benefit of using umbilical cord blood is the blood's relative immunodeficiency at birth, allowing for partially matched unrelated cord blood transplants to be successful, with a lower risk of GVHD-related problems (Ryan et al, 2002).

Autologous BMTs use the patient's own marrow that was collected from disease-free tissue, frozen, and sometimes treated to remove malignant cells. Children with solid tumors such as neuroblastoma, Hodgkin disease, NHL, rhabdomyosarcoma, Ewing's sarcoma, and Wilms' tumor have been treated with autologous BMTs.

Peripheral stem cell transplants (PSCTs) are also used in children with cancer. PSCT, a type of autologous transplant, differs in the way stem cells are collected from the patient. CSF is first given to stimulate the production of many stem cells (Ryan et al, 2002). After the WBC count is high enough, the stem cells are collected by an "apheresis" machine. This machine filters out peripheral stem cells from whole blood, returning the remainder of the blood cells and plasma to the child. Stem cells have been collected in very small children without problems (Guinan et al, 2002). The peripheral stem cells are then frozen until the patient is ready for the PSCT.

Nursing Care Management

The care of children undergoing BMT is similar to that of any child receiving chemotherapy and radiotherapy. The hospitalization is typically 3 to 6 weeks in an isolated environment, during which time the child is subjected to numerous procedures and side effects of therapy. Throughout this long ordeal, there is the family's concern for successful engraftment and fear of fatal complications (Family Focus box). Consequently, nurses involved with the child and family need to provide sensitive care and maintain a supportive attitude during the many crises that may arise. If the procedure is not successful, the care needed by these families is consistent with that required by the family of any child with a life-threatening disorder (see Chapter 41).

Apheresis

Apheresis is the removal of blood from an individual, separation of the blood into its components, retention of one or more of these components, and reinfusion of the remainder of the blood into the individual. Apheresis is most often used to remove large quantities of platelets from healthy adult donors. These transfusion products have greatly prolonged the survival of patients with hematologic and oncologic diseases.

This technique is used to remove peripheral blood stem cells (PBSCs) from children before they receive HSCT or high-dose chemotherapy and/or radiation therapy, which is severely toxic to the bone marrow. These PBSCs can then be used to restore the child's bone marrow. Apheresis is also used as a therapeutic modality. The blood component that is diseased or toxic is separated from the blood, and the remainder is returned to the individual. Therapeutic apheresis is considered part of standard therapy for many diseases. Plasma is selectively removed from individuals with hyperviscosity, life-threatening complications of myasthenia gravis, Guillain-Barré syndrome, thrombotic thrombocytopenic purpura, and certain drug overdoses. WBCs are removed from individuals with high-WBC-count leukemia.

Family Focus

THE DECISION FOR A HEMATOPOIETIC STEM CELL TRANSPLANT

A family's decision for a child to undergo hematopoietic stem cell transplantation (HSCT) may be fraught with challenges. Often the child is facing certain death from the malignancy. The preparation of the child for the transplant also places the patient at great medical risk.

After the preparatory regimen is begun and the child's immune system is destroyed, there is no turning back. Unlike kidney transplantation, HSCT does not have a "rescue" procedure, such as dialysis, for supportive therapy. If the donor is a sibling, the issue of his or her marrow "saving" the brother or sister can be a concern, especially if the transplant fails. Parents often must leave the home to stay at the transplant center and encounter additional stressors such as arranging child care, taking a leave from work, and managing finances. The patient faces the greatest stress—fear of HSCT failure or life-threatening complications.

Nursing Care Management

Difficult venous access and small blood volume can limit the ability to use this therapy in the infant and young child. Education of the family and child focuses on the purposes of the therapy, as well as the technology.

Specially trained individuals perform the apheresis procedure. Attention focuses on rate of removal, blood component separation, and reinfusion of blood into the child. Vital signs are monitored, and the child is continuously observed for any adverse reactions secondary to the circulatory volume changes and the anticoagulant used.

When apheresis components are infused, nursing measures will differ if the product is autologous (blood component from the child) or allogeneic (blood component from another individual). Autologous components are the child's own blood; therefore a major precaution is proper identification to ensure the correct component. The rate of infusion should be adjusted to the child's tolerance. If the product is allogeneic, all precautions for blood transfusions apply.

Key Points

- *Anemia* is defined as reduction of red blood cells or hemoglobin concentration to levels below normal for age; disorders are classified either by etiology/physiology or by morphology.
- The role of the nurse in treatment of anemia is to assist in establishing a diagnosis, prepare the child for laboratory tests, administer prescribed medications, decrease tissue oxygen needs, implement safety precautions, and observe for complications.
- The main nursing goal in prevention of nutritional anemia is parent education regarding correct feeding practices.
- Sickle cell anemia is a hereditary hemoglobinopathy caused by adult hemoglobin (Hgb A) being partly or completely replaced by sickle hemoglobin (Hgb S).
- Nursing care of the child with sickle cell anemia is focused on teaching the family how to prevent and recognize sickle cell problems, manage pain during crises, and help the child and parents adjust to a lifelong, chronic disease.
- Nursing care of the child with thalassemia includes observing for complications of multiple blood transfusions, assisting the child in coping with the effects of illness, and fostering parent-child adjustment to long-term illness.
- Causes of acquired aplastic anemia include irradiation, drugs, industrial and household chemicals, infections, and infiltration and replacement of myeloid elements; however, the majority of the causes are idiopathic.
- Clotting depends on three processes: vascular spasm, platelet aggregation, and coagulation and clot formation.
- Nursing care of the child with hemophilia involves preventing bleeding by decreasing the risk of injury, recognizing and managing bleeding with factor replacement, preventing the crippling effects of joint degeneration, and preparing and supporting the child and family for home care.
- Goals in the care of the child with leukemia are to prepare the family for diagnostic and therapeutic procedures, prevent complications of myelosuppression, manage problems of irradiation and drug toxicity, and provide continued emotional support.
- The lymphomas include Hodgkin and non-Hodgkin lymphoma and are disorders involving the lymphoid system.
- Immunodeficiency disorders render the affected individual unable to fight infectious organisms.
- HIV infection is primarily acquired in infants from a parent with HIV infection and in adolescents from engaging in high risk behaviors.
- Blood transfusions supply needed blood components.
- Hematopoietic stem cell transplantation replaces the diseased or malfunctioning bone marrow with viable blood stem cells.
- Apheresis is the selective removal of a blood component. It can be used to supply cellular elements needed for therapy (i.e., platelets or stem cells) or to remove diseased components.

References

American Academy of Pediatrics, Committee on Infectious Diseases, Pickering L (ed): *2003 red book: report of the Committee on Infectious Diseases,* ed 26, Elk Grove Village, IL, 2003, The Academy.

American Academy of Pediatrics, Committee on Pediatric AIDS: Identification and care of HIV-exposed and HIV-infected infants, children, and adolescents in foster care, *Pediatrics* 106(1):149-153, 2000a.

American Academy of Pediatrics, Committee on Pediatric AIDS: Technical report: perinatal human immunodeficiency virus testing and prevention of transmission, *Pediatrics* 106(6):1-12, 2000b.

American Academy of Pediatrics, Committee on Pediatric AIDS and Committee on Infectious Diseases: Issues related to human immunodeficiency virus transmission in schools, child care, medical settings, the home, and community, *Pediatrics* 104(2):318-324, 1999.

American Academy of Pediatrics, Section on Hematology/Oncology, Committee on Genetics: Health supervision for children with sickle cell disease, *Pediatrics* 109(3):526-536, 2002.

American Pain Society: *Guidelines for the management of acute and chronic pain in sickle-cell disease,* Glenview, IL, 1999, American Pain Society.

Andrews NC: Disorders of iron metabolism and sideroblastic anemia. In Nathan D et al (eds): *Nathan and Oski's hematology of infancy and childhood,* ed 6, Philadelphia, 2003, WB Saunders.

Bell WR: Role of splenectomy in immune (idiopathic) thrombocytopenic purpura, *Blood Rev* 16:39-41, 2002.

Bogen DL, Krause JP, Serwint JR: Outcome of children identified as anemic by routine screening in an inner-city clinic, *Arch Pediatr Adolesc Med* 155:366-371, 2001.

Bonilla FA, Geha RS: Primary immunodeficiency diseases. In Nathan D et al (eds): *Nathan and Oski's hematology of infancy and childhood,* ed 6, Philadelphia, 2003, WB Saunders.

Bryant R: Managing side effects of childhood cancer treatment, *J Pediatr Nurs* 18(2):113-125, 2003.

Buckley RH: Gene therapy for SCID—a complication after remarkable progress, *Lancet* 360:1185-1186, 2002.

Butler RB et al: Promoting safer sex among HIV-positive youth with haemophilia: theory, intervention, and outcome, *Haemophilia* 9(2): 214-222, 2003.

Carley A: Anemia: when is it iron deficiency? *Pediatr Nurs* 29(2):127-133, 2003.

Centers for Disease Control and Prevention: 1994 revised classified system for human immunodeficiency virus infection in children less than 13 years of age, *MMWR* 43(RR-12):1-10, 1994.

Centers for Disease Control and Prevention: 1995 revised guidelines for prophylaxis against *Pneumocystis carinii* pneumonia for children infected with or perinatally exposed to human immunodeficiency virus, *MMWR* 44(RR-4):1-11, 1995.

Centers for Disease Control and Prevention: *HIV/AIDS surveillance report,* 2001, 13:2, 2001.

Champi C: Primary immunodeficiency disorders in children: prompt diagnosis can lead to lifesaving treatment, *J Pediatr Health Care* 16:16-21, 2002.

Charache S et al: Hydroxyurea and sickle cell anemia: clinical utility of a myelosuppressive switching agent, *Medicine* 75(6):300-326, 1996.

Chiocca EM: Sickle cell crisis: severe pain and potential tissue necrosis are the major concerns, *Am J Nurs* 96(9):49, 1996.

Cho S, Cheng AC, Cheng MCK: Oral care for children with leukemia, *Hong Kong Med J* 6(2):203-208, 2000.

Chu YW, Korb J, Sakamoto KM: Idiopathic thrombocytopenia purpura, *Pediatr Rev* 21(3):95-104, 2000.

Colby-Graham MF, Chordas C: The childhood leukemias, *J Pediatr Nurs* 18(2):87-95, 2003.

Davidsson L: Approaches to improve iron bioavailability from complementary foods, *J Nutr* 133(5 suppl 1):1560S-1562S, 2003.

Dover GJ, Platt OS: Sickle cell disease. In Nathan D et al (eds): *Nathan and Oski's hematology of infancy and childhood,* ed 6, Philadelphia, 2003, WB Saunders.

Dragone MA, Karp S: Bleeding disorders. In Jackson PL, Vessey JA (eds): *Primary care of the child with a chronic condition,* ed 2, St Louis, 1996, Mosby.

Ezekowitz RAB, Stockman III JA: Hematologic manifestations of systemic diseases. In Nathan D et al (eds): *Nathan and Oski's hematology of infancy and childhood,* ed 6, Philadelphia, 2003, WB Saunders.

Ferster A et al: Five years of experience with hydroxyurea in children and young adults with sickle cell disease, *Blood* 97(11):3628-3632, 2001.

Fischer K et al: Changes in treatment strategies for severe haemophilia over the last 3 decades: effects of clotting factor consumption and arthropathy, *Haemophilia* 7:446-452, 2001.

Gribbons D, Zahr LK, Opas SR: Nursing management of children with sickle cell disease: an update, *J Pediatr Nurs* 10(4):232-242, 1995.

Griffin TC, McIntire D, Buchanan GR: High-dose intravenous methylprednisolone therapy for pain in children and adolescents with sickle cell disease, *N Engl J Med* 330(11):733-737, 1994.

Griffins IJ, Abrams SA: Iron and breastfeeding, *Pediatr Clin North Am* 48:401, 2001.

Guinan ED, Krance RA, Lehmann LE: Stem cell transplantation in pediatric oncology. In Pizzo PA, Poplack DG (eds): *Principles and practice of pediatric oncology,* ed 4, Philadelphia, 2002, JB Lippincott.

Halterman JS et al: Iron deficiency and cognitive achievement among school-aged children and adolescents in the United States, *Pediatrics* 107(6):1381-1386, 2001.

Hudson MM, Donaldson SS: Hodgkins disease. In Pizzo PA, Poplack DG (eds): *Principles and practice of pediatric oncology,* ed 4, Philadelphia, 2002, JB Lippincott.

Ioannidis JP et al: Perinatal transmission of human immunodeficiency virus type I by pregnant women with RNA virus loads <1000 copies 1 ml, *J Infect Dis* 183:539-545, 2001.

Karayalcin G: Hemolytic anemia (sickle cell anemia). In Lanzkowsky P (ed): *Manual of pediatric hematology and oncology,* ed 3, San Diego, 2000, Academic Press.

Khoury H, Grimsley E: Oxygen inhalation in nonhypoxic sickle cell patients during vaso-occlusive crisis, *Blood* 86(10):3998, 1995.

Link MP, Donaldson SS: The lymphomas and lymphadenopathy. In Nathan D et al (eds): *Nathan and Oski's hematology of infancy and childhood,* ed 6, Philadelphia, 2003, WB Saunders.

Lyall EGH: Paediatric HIV in 2002—a treatable and preventable infection, *J Clin Virol* 25:107-119, 2002.

Margolin JF, Steuber CP, Poplack DG: Acute lymphoblastic leukemia. In Pizzo PA, Poplack DG (eds): *Principles and practice of pediatric oncology,* ed 4, Philadelphia, 2002, JB Lippincott.

Meldrum J: Nevirapine efficacy underestimated for protecting babies from HIV? *AIDSmap.* Internet document available at www.aidsmap.com (accessed August 18, 2003).

Merchant RC, Keshavarz R: Human immunodeficiency virus postexposure prophylaxis for adolescents and children, *Pediatrics* 108(2):1-13, 2001.

Miller ST et al: Prediction of adverse outcomes in children with sickle cell disease, *N Engl J Med* 342(2):83-89, 2000.

Montgomery RR, Gill JC, Scott JP: Hemophilia and von Willebrand disease. In Nathan D et al (eds): *Nathan and Oski's hematology of infancy and childhood,* ed 6, Philadelphia, 2003, WB Saunders.

Morbidity and Mortality Weekly Report: Advancing HIV prevention: new strategies for a changing epidemic—United States, *MMWR* 52(15): 329-332, 2003.

National Hemophilia Foundation, Bleeding Disorders Information Center: Newly diagnosed: parents FAQ 2003. Internet document available at www.hemophilia.org/bdi/bdi_newly7c.htm (accessed August 23, 2003).

National Institute of Allergy and Infectious Diseases, National Institutes of Health: HIV infection and AIDS: an overview. Anthrax, NIAID fact sheet, 2003. Internet document available at www.niaid.nih.gov/factsheets/hivinf.htm (accessed August 18, 2003).

National Institutes of Health, National Heart, Lung, and Blood Institute, Division of Blood Disease and Resources: *The management of sickle cell disease,* NIH pub no 02-2117, Bethesda, MD, 2002, NHLBI Health Information Network.

Nolan B et al: Unsuspected haemophilia in children with a single swollen joint, *Br Med J* 326:151-152, 2003.

Norville R, Bryant R: Blood component deficiencies. In Baggott C et al (eds): *APON nursing care of children and adolescents with cancer,* ed 3, Philadelphia, 2002, WB Saunders.

Orkin SH, Nathan DG: The thalassemias. In Nathan D et al (eds): *Nathan and Oski's hematology of infancy and childhood,* ed 6, Philadelphia, 2003, WB Saunders.

Paley C: Hemolytic anemia (thalassemias). In Lanzkowsky P (ed): *Manual of pediatric hematology and oncology,* ed 3, San Diego, 2000, Academic Press.

Perkins S: Disorders of hematopoiesis. In Collins RD, Swerdlow SH (eds): *Pediatric hematopathology,* Philadelphia, 2001, Churchill Livingstone.

Platt OS, Guinan EC: Bone marrow transplantations in sickle cell anemia: the dilemma of choice, *N Engl J Med* 335(6):426-427, 1996.

Redner A: Leukemias. In Lanzkowsky P (ed): *Manual of pediatric hematology and oncology,* ed 3, San Diego, 2000, Academic Press.

Ryan LG et al: Hematopoietic stem cell transplantation. In Baggott CR et al (eds): *Nursing care of children and adolescents with cancer,* ed 3, Philadelphia, 2002, WB Saunders.

Segel GB, Hirsch MG, Feig SA: Managing anemia in a pediatric office practice: part 1, *Pediatr Rev* 23(3):75-83, 2002a.

Segel GB, Hirsch MG, Feig SA: Managing anemia in a pediatric office practice: part 2, *Pediatr Rev* 23(4):111-121, 2002b.

Shende A: Bone marrow failure. In Lanzkowsky P (ed): *Manual of pediatric hematology and oncology,* ed 3, San Diego, 2000, Academic Press.

Shimamura A, Guinan EC: Acquired aplastic anemia. In Nathan D et al (eds): *Nathan and Oski's hematology of infancy and childhood,* ed 6, Philadelphia, 2003, WB Saunders.

Silverman LB, Sallan SE: Acute lymphoblastic leukemia. In Nathan D et al (eds): *Nathan and Oski's hematology of infancy and childhood,* ed 6, Philadelphia, 2003, WB Saunders.

Simon K, Lobo ML, Jackson S: Current knowledge in the management of children and adolescents with sickle cell disease: part 1, physiological issues, *J Pediatr Nurs* 14(5):281-295, 1999.

Steinberg MH et al: Effect of hydroxyurea on mortality and morbidity in adult sickle cell anemia: risks and benefits up to 9 years of treatment, *JAMA* 289(13):1645-1651, 2003.

Sullivan JL, Woda BA: Lymphohistiocytic disorders. In Nathan D et al (eds): *Nathan and Oski's hematology of infancy and childhood,* ed 6, Philadelphia, 2003, WB Saunders.

Wilson DB: Acquired platelet defects. In Nathan D et al (eds): *Nathan and Oski's hematology of infancy and childhood,* ed 6, Philadelphia, 2003, WB Saunders.

Genitourinary Dysfunction 50

LEARNING OBJECTIVES

On completion of this chapter the reader will be able to:

- Describe the various factors that contribute to urinary tract infections in infants and children.
- Discuss the preoperative preparation of the child and parents when the child has a structural defect of the genitourinary tract.
- Demonstrate an understanding of the causes and mechanisms of edema formation in nephrotic syndrome.
- Outline a nursing care plan for a child with nephrotic syndrome.
- Compare the child with minimal-change nephrotic syndrome and the child with acute glomerulonephritis in terms of clinical manifestations and nursing care.
- Contrast the causes, complications, and management of acute and chronic renal failure.
- List the types of renal dialysis.
- Recognize signs of kidney transplant rejection.

ELECTRONIC RESOURCES

Additional information related to the content in Chapter 50 can be found on

the companion website at evolve
http://evolve.elsevier.com/Wong/maternal/
- NCLEX Review Questions
- WebLinks

or the interactive student CD-ROM
Activities for Chapter 50 include the following:
- NCLEX Review Questions
- Nursing Care Plan—The Child with Chronic Renal Failure

GENITOURINARY DYSFUNCTION

Assessment of Renal Function

Assessment of kidney and urinary tract integrity and diagnosis of renal or urinary tract disease are based on several evaluative tools. Physical examination, history taking, and observation of symptoms are the initial procedures. In suspected urinary tract diseases or disorders, further assessment by laboratory, radiologic, and other evaluative methods is carried out.

Clinical Manifestations

As in most disorders of childhood, the incidence and type of kidney or urinary tract dysfunction change with the age and maturation of the child. In addition, the presenting complaints and the significance of these complaints vary with maturation. For example, a complaint of enuresis has greater significance at age 8 years than at age 4. In the newborn, urinary tract disorders are associated with a number of obvious malformations of other body systems, including the curious and unexplained but frequent association between malformed or low-set ears and urinary tract anomalies.

Many of the clinical manifestations of renal disease are common to a variety of childhood disorders, but their presence is an indication to obtain further information from the child's history, family history, and laboratory studies as part of a complete physical examination. Suspected renal disease can be further evaluated by means of radiographic studies and renal biopsy (Table 50-1).

Laboratory Tests

Both urine and blood studies contribute vital information for detection of renal problems. The single most important test is probably routine urinalysis. Specific urine and blood tests provide additional information. Because nurses are usually the persons who collect the specimens for examination and who often perform many of the screening tests, they should be familiar with the test, its function, and factors that can alter or distort the results of the test. The major urine and blood tests are outlined in Tables 50-2 and 50-3.

Nursing Care Management

Nursing responsibilities in assessment of genitourinary disorders or diseases begin with observation of the child for any manifestations that might indicate dysfunction. Many conditions have specific characteristics that distinguish them

Table 50-1

Radiologic and Other Tests of Urinary System Function

TEST	PROCEDURE	PURPOSE	COMMENTS AND NURSING RESPONSIBILITIES
Urine culture and sensitivity	Collection of sterile specimen	Determines presence of pathogens and the drugs to which they are sensitive	Does not require specific parental permission Send specimen to laboratory immediately after collection Catheterization, clean-catch, or suprapubic specimen
Renal/bladder ultrasound	Transmission of ultrasonic waves through renal parenchyma, along ureteral course, and over bladder	Allows visualization of renal parenchyma, renal pelvis without exposure to external beam radiation or radioactive isotopes Visualization of dilated ureters and bladder wall also possible	Noninvasive procedure
Testicular (scrotal) ultrasound	Transmission of ultrasonic waves through scrotal contents and testis	Allows visualization of scrotal contents, including testis Testicular ultrasound is used to identify masses, and Doppler-enhanced ultrasound is used to differentiate hyperemia of epididymo-orchitis from ischemia of torsion	Noninvasive procedure
Scout film	Flat plate roentgenogram of abdomen and pelvis for kidney, ureters, bladder (KUB)	Detects and establishes renal outlines, presence of calculi, or opaque foreign bodies in bladder	Prepare as for routine x-ray film
Voiding cystourethrography	Contrast medium injected into bladder through urethral catheter until bladder is full; films taken before, during, and after voiding	Visualizes bladder outline and urethra, reveals reflux of urine into ureters, and shows complications of bladder emptying	Prepare child for catheterization
Radionuclide (nuclear) cystogram	Radionuclide-containing fluid injected through urethral catheter until bladder is full; images generated before, during, and after voiding	Alternative to voiding cystourethrography in children with allergy to intravesical contrast material Allows evaluation of reflux, although visualization of anatomic details is relatively poor	Prepare child for catheterization Reassure patient and parents that allergic response to contrast materials is avoided by use of radionuclide
Radioisotope imaging studies	Contrast medium injected intravenously; computer analysis to measure uptake or washout (excretion) for analysis of organ function	DTPA is a radioisotope used to measure glomerular filtration rate; estimate of differential renal function and renal washout to determine presence and location of upper urinary tract obstruction DMSA is a radioisotope that allows visualization of renal scars and differential renal function; ureters and bladder are not visualized MAG 3 radioisotope combines features of DTPA (evaluation of upper urinary tract obstruction) with features of DMSA radioisotope (differential renal function)	Insert or assist with insertion of intravenous infusion Monitor intravenous infusion Urethral catheterization may accompany DTPA radioisotope scan; prepare child for catheterization when indicated

Table 50-1

Radiologic and Other Tests of Urinary System Function—cont'd

TEST	PROCEDURE	PURPOSE	COMMENTS AND NURSING RESPONSIBILITIES
Intravenous pyelography (IVP) (intravenous urogram; excretory urogram)	Intravenous injection of a contrast medium Medium secreted and concentrated by tubules X-ray films made 5, 10, and 15 minutes after injection; delayed films (30, 60 minutes, etc.), are obtained if obstruction suspected	Defines urinary tract Provides information about integrity of kidneys, ureters, and bladder Retroperitoneal masses visualized when they shift position of ureters	Preparation for test: Infants less than 2 years of age—no solid food, omit one bottle on morning of examination; studies should be performed early to avoid withholding of fluids Children 2-14 years of age—give cathartic evening before examination, nothing orally after midnight, enema (Fleet [see Nurse Alert, p. 1419] or soapsuds) morning of examination
Computed tomography (CT)	Narrow-beam x-rays and computer analysis provide precise reconstruction of area	Visualizes vertical or horizontal cross section of kidney Especially valuable to distinguish tumors and cysts	Noncontrast scan is noninvasive Contrast-enhanced CT scan preparation is similar to IVP
Cystoscopy	Direct visualization of bladder and lower urinary tract through small scope inserted via urethra	Investigation of bladder and lower tract lesions; visualizes ureteral openings, bladder wall, trigone, and urethra	Give nothing orally after midnight Carry out preoperative preparations
Retrograde pyelography	Contrast medium injected through ureteral catheter	Visualizes pelvic calyces, ureters, and bladder	Prepare the child for cystoscopy
Renal angiography	Contrast medium injected directly into renal artery via catheter placed in femoral artery (or umbilical artery in newborn) and advanced to renal artery	Visualizes renal vascular system, especially for renal arterial stenosis	Give cathartic if ordered Give preoperative medication if ordered Observe for reaction to contrast medium Monitor vital signs after procedure
Whitaker perfusion test	Injection of contrast material through renal pelvis and ureters Pressures are measured in renal pelvis and urinary bladder	Determine presence of obstruction causing upper urinary tract dilation	Prepare child for insertion of a spinal needle or perfusion catheter in renal pelvis (anesthetic often required)
Renal biopsy	Removal of kidney tissue by open or percutaneous technique for study by light, electron, or immunofluorescent microscopy	Yields histologic and microscopic information about glomeruli and tubules; helps to distinguish between types of nephritic syndromes Distinguishes other renal disorders	Give nothing orally 4-6 hours before test Premedicate as ordered Prepare setup for procedure Assist with procedure Take vital signs Apply pressure to area with pressure dressing and, if feasible, a sandbag Bed rest for 24 hours Observe for abdominal pain, tenderness Monitor input and output; surgical incision may be required in infants
Urodynamics	Set of tests designed to measure bladder filling, storage, and evacuation functions Uroflowmetry is a test to determine efficiency of urination Cystometrogram is a graphic comparison of bladder pressure as a function of volume Voiding pressure study is a comparison of detrusor contraction pressure, sphincter electromyelogram, and urinary flow	Determine characteristic of voiding dysfunction Used to identify type (cause) of incontinence or urinary retention Especially valuable for voiding dysfunction complicated by urinary infection, urinary retention, or neurogenic bladder dysfunction	Prepare child for catheterization Insertion of a rectal tube will produce feelings of rectal fullness or pressure Insertion of needles may be required for sphincter electromyography

Table 50-2

Urine Tests of Renal Function

TEST	NORMAL RANGE	DEVIATIONS	SIGNIFICANCE OF DEVIATIONS
PHYSICAL TESTS			
Volume	Age related: Newborn: 30-60 ml Children: bladder capacity (oz) = age (years) + 2	Polyuria Oliguria	Osmotic factors (urinary glucose level in diabetes mellitus) Retention caused by obstructive disease Inadequate bladder emptying caused by neurogenic bladder or obstructive disorder
		Anuria	Obstruction of urinary tract; acute renal failure
Specific gravity	With normal fluid intake: 1.016-1.022 Newborn: 1.001-1.020	High	Dehydration Presence of protein or glucose Presence of radiopaque contrast medium after radiologic examinations
	Others: 1.001-1.030	Low	Excessive fluid intake Distal tubular dysfunction Insufficient antidiuretic hormone Diuresis
		Fixed at 1.010	Chronic glomerular disease
Osmolality	Newborn: 50-600 mOsm/L Thereafter: 50-1400 mOsm/L	High or low	Same as for specific gravity More sensitive index than specific gravity
Appearance	Clear pale yellow to deep gold	Cloudy Cloudy reddish pink to reddish brown	Contains sediment Blood from trauma or disease Myoglobin after severe muscle destruction
		Light Dark Red	Dilute Concentrated Trauma
CHEMICAL TESTS			
pH	Newborn: 5-7	Weak acid or neutral	If associated with metabolic acidosis, suggests tubular acidosis
	Thereafter: 4.8-7.8 Average: 6		If associated with metabolic alkalosis, suggests potassium deficiency Urinary infection
		Alkaline	Metabolic alkalosis
Protein level	Absent	Present	Abnormal glomerular permeability (e.g., glomerular disease, changes in blood pressure) Most kidney disease Orthostatic in some individuals
Glucose level	Absent	Present	Diabetes mellitus Infusion of concentrated glucose-containing fluids Glomerulonephritis Impaired tubular reabsorption
Ketone levels	Absent	Present	Conditions of acute metabolic demand (stress) Diabetic ketoacidosis
Leukocyte esterase	Absent	Present	Can identify both lysed and intact white blood cells via enzyme detection
Nitrites	Absent	Present	Most species of bacteria convert nitrates to nitrites in the urine

Table 50-2

Urine Tests of Renal Function—cont'd

TEST	NORMAL RANGE	DEVIATIONS	SIGNIFICANCE OF DEVIATIONS
MICROSCOPIC TESTS			
White blood cell count	Less than 1 or 2	More than 5 polymorphonuclear leukocytes/field	Urinary tract inflammatory process
		Lymphocytes	Allograft rejection Malignancy
Red blood cell count	Less than 1 or 2	4-6/field in centrifuged specimen	Trauma Stones Glomerular injury Infection Neoplasms
Presence of bacteria	Absent to a few	More than 100,000 organisms/ml in centrifuged specimen	Urinary tract infection
Presence of casts	Occasional	Granular casts	Tubular or glomerular disorders Degenerative process in advanced renal disease
		Cellular casts	Pyelonephritis
		White blood cell	Glomerulonephritis
		Red blood cell	Proteinuria; usually transient
		Hyaline casts	

Table 50-3

Blood Tests of Renal Function

TEST	NORMAL RANGE (MG/DL)	DEVIATIONS	SIGNIFICANCE OF DEVIATIONS
Blood urea nitrogen (BUN)	Newborn: 4-18 Infant, child: 5-18	Elevated	Renal disease—acute or chronic (the higher the BUN, the more severe the disease) Increased protein catabolism Dehydration Hemorrhage High protein intake Corticosteroid therapy
Uric acid	Child: 2.0-5.5	Increased	Severe renal disease
Creatinine	Infant: 0.2-0.4 Child: 0.3-0.7 Adolescent: 0.5-1.0	Increased	Severe renal impairment

from other disorders. These are discussed as appropriate throughout the chapter.

The nurse is generally the one who is responsible for preparing infants, children, and parents for tests and for collection of urine and (sometimes) blood specimens (see Preparation for Procedures, Chapter 44, and Collection of Specimens, Chapter 45) for observation and laboratory analysis. An important nursing responsibility is to maintain careful *intake and output* and *blood pressure* measurements on most children with genitourinary dysfunction and those who might be at risk for developing renal complications (e.g., children in shock, postoperative patients). For example, any significant degree of renal disease can diminish the glomerular filtration rate, a measure of the amount of plasma from which a given substance is totally cleared in 1 minute. A number of substances can be used, but the most useful clinical estimation of glomerular filtration is the clearance of *creatinine,* an end product of protein metabolism in muscle and a substance that is freely filtered by the glomerulus and secreted by renal tubular cells. The nurse's responsibility in this test is collection of urine, usually a 12- or 24-hour specimen.

GENITOURINARY TRACT DISORDERS/DEFECTS

Urinary Tract Infection

Infection of the genitourinary tract is one of the most common conditions of childhood. Up to 10% of children will have a febrile urinary tract infection (UTI) during the first 2 years of life (Rosenthal, 2004). UTIs may involve the urethra and bladder (lower urinary tract) or the ureters, renal pelvis, calyces, and renal parenchyma (upper urinary tract). Because it is often impossible to localize the infection, the broad designation UTI is applied to the presence of significant numbers of microorganisms anywhere within the urinary tract, except the distal third of the urethra, which is usually colonized with bacteria. The peak incidence of UTI not caused by structural anomalies occurs between 2 and 6 years of age, and except for the neonatal period, females have a higher risk for developing UTI. This coincides with toilet training and establishing voiding habits.

Classification

Infection of the urinary tract may be present with or without clinical symptoms. As a result, the site of infection is often difficult to pinpoint with any degree of accuracy. Terms used to describe urinary tract disorders include the following:

Bacteriuria—Presence of bacteria in the urine

Asymptomatic bacteriuria—Significant bacteriuria with no evidence of clinical infection (usually defined as greater than 100,000 colony-forming units [CFUs])

Symptomatic bacteriuria—Bacteriuria accompanied by physical signs of urinary infection (dysuria, suprapubic discomfort, hematuria, fever)

Recurrent UTI—Repeated episode of bacteriuria or symptomatic UTI

Persistent UTI—Persistence of bacteriuria despite antibiotic treatment

Febrile UTI—Bacteriuria accompanied by fever and other physical signs of urinary infection; presence of a fever typically implies a pyelonephritis

Cystitis—Inflammation of the bladder

Urethritis—Inflammation of the urethra

Pyelonephritis—Inflammation of the upper urinary tract and kidneys

Urosepsis—Febrile urinary tract infection coexisting with systemic signs of bacterial illness; blood culture reveals presence of urinary pathogen

Etiology

A variety of organisms can be responsible for UTI. *Escherichia coli* (80% of cases) and other gram-negative enteric organisms are most frequently implicated; these organisms are usually found in the anal and perineal region. Other organisms associated with UTI include *Proteus, Pseudomonas, Klebsiella, Staphylococcus aureus, Haemophilus,* and coagulase-negative *Staphylococcus.* Several factors contribute to the development of UTI in childhood.

Anatomic and Physical Factors

The structure of the lower urinary tract is believed to account for the increased incidence of bacteriuria in females (Rosenthal, 2004). The short urethra, which measures about 2 cm (0.75 inch) in young girls and 4 cm (1.5 inches) in mature women, provides a ready pathway for invasion of organisms. In addition, the closure of the urethra at the end of micturition may return contaminated bacteria to the bladder. The longer male urethra (as long as 20 cm [8 inches] in an adult) and the antibacterial properties of prostatic secretions inhibit the entry and growth of pathogens.

NURSE ALERT Considerable evidence suggests there are fewer UTIs among circumcised male infants than among uncircumcised male infants, but the difference is not significant enough to recommend routine circumcision in newborns (American Academy of Pediatrics, 1999). ■

The single most important host factor influencing the occurrence of UTI is *urinary stasis.* Ordinarily, urine is sterile, but at 37° C (98.6° F) it provides an excellent culture medium. Under normal conditions the act of completely and repeatedly emptying the bladder flushes away any organisms before they have an opportunity to multiply and invade surrounding tissue. However, urine that remains in the bladder allows bacteria from the urethra to rapidly become established in the rich medium. Incomplete bladder emptying (stasis) may result from *reflux* (see Vesicoureteral Reflux later in this chapter), anatomic abnormalities (especially those involving the ureters), dysfunction of the voiding mechanism, or extrinsic ureteral or bladder compression that may be caused by constipation. The key to preventing UTI is to maintain adequate blood supply to the bladder wall by avoidance of overdistention and high bladder pressure.

Altered Urine and Bladder Chemistry

Several mechanical and chemical characteristics of the urine and bladder mucosa help maintain urinary sterility. An increased fluid intake promotes flushing of the normal bladder and lowers the concentration of organisms in the infected bladder. Diuresis also seems to enhance the antibacterial properties of the renal medulla.

Most pathogens favor an alkaline medium. Normally, urine is slightly acidic. A urine pH of about 5 hampers bacterial multiplication, although the acidification rarely eliminates the bacteriuria. Much has been reported about the use of cranberry juice for the prevention of UTI. This mechanism was initially thought to result from increased urine acidity. However, a study of children with neurogenic bladder shows that ingestion of cranberry juice results in a median pH of only 6.0. Urine is bacteriostatic to *E. coli* at a pH of 5.0 (attainable only by injection of pure hippuric acid). Further findings from this study suggest the antiadherence properties of cranberries are most often observed in UTI caused by fimbriated *E. coli* strains, which are more common in healthy patients with UTI and less common in patients with chronic medical illnesses or urinary tract anomalies (Schlager et al, 1999). Further research is needed to determine the efficacy of cranberry products in children with UTI.

Diagnostic Evaluation

The clinical manifestations of UTI depend on the age of the child (Box 50-1). Diagnosis of UTI is confirmed by detection of bacteriuria in urine culture, but urine collection is often difficult, especially in infants and very small children. Several factors may alter a urine specimen, and contamina-

BOX 50-1

Signs and Symptoms of Urinary Tract Disorders or Disease at Different Ages

Neonatal Period (Birth to 1 Month)
Poor feeding
Vomiting
Failure to gain weight
Rapid respiration (acidosis)
Respiratory distress
Spontaneous pneumothorax or pneumomediastinum
Frequent urination
Screaming on urination
Poor urine stream
Jaundice
Seizures
Dehydration
Other anomalies or stigmata
Enlarged kidneys or bladder

Infancy (1 to 24 Months)
Poor feeding
Vomiting
Failure to gain weight
Excessive thirst
Frequent urination
Straining or screaming on urination
Foul-smelling urine
Pallor
Fever
Persistent diaper rash
Seizures (with or without fever)
Dehydration
Enlarged kidneys or bladder

Childhood (2 to 14 Years)
Poor appetite
Vomiting
Growth failure
Excessive thirst
Enuresis, incontinence, frequent urination
Painful urination
Swelling of face
Seizures
Pallor
Fatigue
Blood in urine
Abdominal or back pain
Edema
Hypertension
Tetany

tion of a specimen by organisms from sources other than the urine, such as perineal and perianal flora in bag specimens, is the most frequent cause of false-positive results. Unless the specimen is a first morning sample, a recent high fluid intake may indicate a falsely low organism count. Therefore children should not be encouraged to drink large volumes of water in an attempt to obtain a specimen quickly.

NURSE ALERT A child who exhibits the following should be evaluated for UTI:
- Incontinence in a toilet-trained child
- Strong-smelling urine
- Frequency or urgency ■

More accurate estimates of bacterial content are obtained from *suprapubic aspiration* (in children younger than 2 years of age) and properly performed bladder catheterization (as long as the first few milliliters are excluded from collection). The specimen should be taken directly to the laboratory for culture immediately.

Tests to detect bacteriuria are being used with increased frequency in screening for UTI. The dipstick tests that test for leukocyte esterase or nitrite are quick and inexpensive methods for detecting infection before obtaining final culture results.

Localization of the infection site may involve more specific tests, including percutaneous kidney taps and bladder washout procedures. Other tests such as ultrasonography, voiding cystourethrogram (VCUG), intravenous pyelogram (IVP), and dimercaptosuccinic acid (DMSA) scan may be performed after the infection subsides to identify anatomic abnormalities contributing to the development of infection and existing kidney changes from recurrent infection.

Therapeutic Management

The objectives of treatment of children with UTI are (1) to eliminate current infection, (2) to identify contributing factors to reduce the risk of recurrence, (3) to prevent systemic spread of the infection, and (4) to preserve renal function. Antibiotic therapy should be initiated on the basis of identification of the pathogen, the child's history of antibiotic use, and the location of the infection. Several antimicrobial drugs are available for treating UTI, but all of them can occasionally be ineffective because of resistance of organisms. Common antiinfective agents used for UTI include the penicillins, sulfonamide (including trimethoprim and sulfisoxazole in combination), the cephalosporins, and nitrofurantoin.

If anatomic defects such as primary reflux or bladder neck obstruction are present, surgical correction of these abnormalities may be necessary to prevent recurrent infection. Follow-up study is an important component of medical management, because the relapse rate is high and recurrent infection tends to occur 1 to 2 months after termination of treatment. The aim of therapy and careful follow-up is to reduce the chance of renal scarring. However, recurrent infection of the urinary bladder predisposes the individual to transient episodes of vesicoureteral reflux.

Vesicoureteral Reflux

Vesicoureteral reflux (VUR) refers to the abnormal retrograde flow of bladder urine into the ureters. During voiding, urine is swept up the ureters and then flows back into the empty bladder, where it acts as a reservoir for bacterial growth until the next void. *Primary reflux* results from congenitally abnormal insertion of ureters into the bladder; *secondary reflux* occurs as a result of an acquired condition.

It is not clear that reflux necessarily causes infections. What is clear is that reflux is more likely to be associated with recurring kidney infections rather than simple bladder infections (cystitis). In the presence of reflux, infected urine (bacteria) from the bladder has access to the kidney, resulting in kidney infections (pyelonephritis). These children are usually very symptomatic with high fevers, vomiting, and chills. Reflux when associated with UTI is the most common cause of renal scarring in children. Renal scarring may occur with the first episode of febrile UTI. Reflux in the presence of sterile urine does not cause renal damage. Therefore the most important concept in managing VUR is preventing bacteria from reaching the kidneys. VUR is managed conservatively with daily low-dose antibiotic therapy. A urine culture should be done every 2 to 3 months and any time the child has a fever. This method of management requires a motivated, reliable, and cooperative family. Many children will outgrow the reflux over a period of years. An annual voiding cystourethrogram is done to assess the status of the reflux.

Indications for surgical intervention include significant anatomic abnormality at the ureterovesical junction, recurrent UTIs, severe forms of VUR, noncompliance with medical therapy, intolerance to antibiotics, and VUR after puberty in females.

Prognosis

With prompt and adequate treatment at the time of diagnosis, the long-term prognosis for UTI is usually excellent. However, the hazard of progressive renal injury is greatest when infection occurs in young children (especially those younger than 2 years of age) and is associated with congenital renal malformations and reflux. Therefore early diagnosis of children at risk is particularly important during infancy and toddlerhood.

Nursing Care Management

Nurses should instruct parents to observe regularly for clues suggesting UTI. Unfortunately, the signs of UTI are not as evident as those of upper respiratory tract infection. Therefore many cases go undetected because no one thought to investigate this common problem.

Because infants and young children often are unable to express their feelings and sensations verbally, it is difficult to detect discomfort they may be experiencing from dysuria. A careful history regarding voiding habits, stooling pattern, and episodes of unexplained irritability may assist in detecting less obvious cases of UTI. Consequently, parents should be cautioned to observe for specific clues of UTI in suspected cases.

NURSE ALERT Check the diaper every half hour. This increases the opportunity for observing the stream for such findings as straining or fretting before voiding begins, signs of discomfort before and during urinating, starting and stopping the stream intermittently, and frequent dripping of small amounts of urine. ■

When infection is suspected, collecting an appropriate specimen is essential. It is the nurse's responsibility to take every precaution to obtain acceptable clean-voided specimens to avoid the use of other collecting procedures except when absolutely indicated. Because of the unreliability of a specimen obtained via a urine collection bag, suprapubic aspiration of urine or sterile catheterization should be done in the infant or young child who has a fever.

Frequently, additional tests are performed to detect anatomic defects. Children are prepared for these tests as appropriate for their age. This includes an explanation of the procedure, its purpose, and what the children will experience (see Preparation for Procedures, Chapter 44). Sometimes a simple description of the urinary system is helpful. Especially for preschool children, the nurse must clarify that the urinary tract is separate from any sexual function and that the test is for a problem that they did not cause. Children may associate blame for perceived wrongdoing (e.g., masturbation) or unacceptable thoughts with the reason for the illness or the tests. For children younger than 3 to 4 years of age, the procedure can be explained on a doll. For those who are older, a simple drawing of the bladder, urethra, ureters, and kidneys makes the procedure more understandable.

Handling actual equipment when feasible can be helpful in allaying anxiety in children of all ages. Anticipatory instruction on distraction techniques such as deep breathing, storytelling, and imagery may help the child relax and be more cooperative during the actual procedures. If surgery is indicated, the child will be able to encounter the impending procedure with facts and understanding of the procedure that will help to decrease his or her fear and anxiety concerning more extensive medical-surgical intervention.

Because antibacterial drugs are indicated in UTI, the nurse advises parents of proper dosage and administration. When antiseptics such as nitrofurantoin are used for prolonged therapy to maintain urine sterility, parents need an explanation of the drug's continued necessity when no signs of infection are present. For all children, an adequate or increased fluid intake is encouraged.

Prevention

Prevention is the most important goal in both primary and recurrent infection, and most preventive measures are simple hygienic habits that should be a routine part of daily care (Guidelines box). For example, parents are taught to cleanse their infant's genital areas from front to back to avoid contaminating the urethral area with fecal organisms. Female children are taught to wipe from front to back after voiding or defecating. Children should void as soon as they feel the urge (Critical Thinking Exercise).

Sexually active adolescent females are advised to urinate as soon as possible after they have intercourse to flush out bacteria introduced during the activity. Children who have recurrent UTIs or neurogenic bladder are frequently maintained on daily low-dose antibiotics. Giving the dose at bedtime allows the drug to remain in the bladder overnight. The nurse should reinforce the importance of compliance to parents and older children.

Obstructive Uropathy

Structural or functional abnormalities of the urinary system that obstruct the normal flow of urine can produce renal disorders. When there is interference with urine flow, the backup of urine above the obstruction causes *hydronephrosis* (dilation of the renal pelvis from distention) with even-

Guidelines

PREVENTION OF URINARY TRACT INFECTION

Factors Predisposing to Development	Measures of Prevention
Short female urethra close to vagina and anus	Perineal hygiene: wipe from front to back. Avoid tight clothing or diapers; wear cotton panties rather than nylon. Check for vaginitis or pinworms, especially if child scratches between legs.
Incomplete emptying (reflux) and overdistention of bladder	Avoid "holding" urine; encourage child to void frequently, especially before long trip or other circumstances in which toilet facilities are not available. Empty bladder completely with each void. Have the child "double void" (void, wait a few minutes, and void again). Severe cases may require clean, intermittent catheterization or biofeedback instruction. Avoid straining during defecation and avoid constipation.
Concentrated urine	Encourage generous fluid intake.

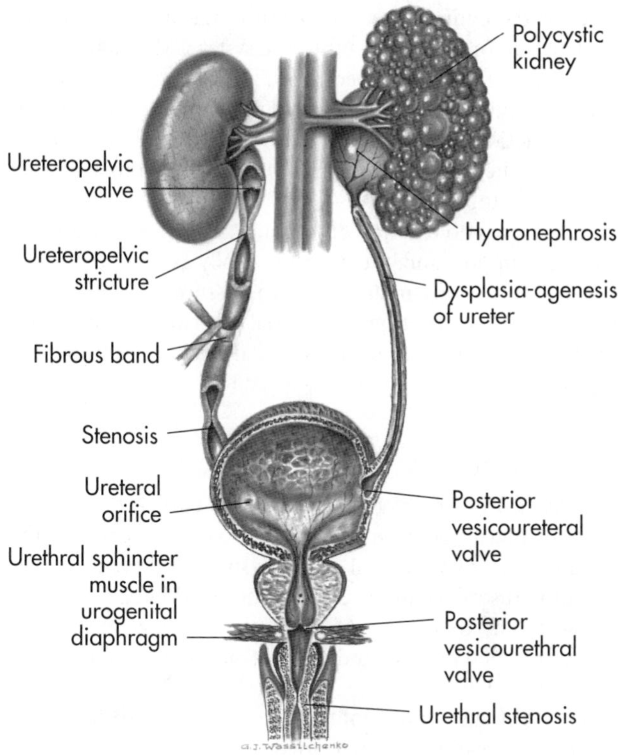

Fig. 50-1 Major sites of urinary tract obstruction.

Critical Thinking Exercise

URINARY TRACT INFECTION AND CONSTIPATION

During your assessment of Ginger, a 4-year-old admitted to the hospital for a severe urinary tract infection (UTI), her mother tells you that Ginger has bowel movements every third to fourth day. They are usually large, hard-formed stools, and Ginger sometimes has trouble evacuating the stool.

1. Evidence—Is there sufficient evidence to draw a conclusion about Ginger's UTI and constipation?
2. Assumptions—Describe an underlying assumption about each of the following:
   a. Urinary tract infections and females
   b. Normal bowel patterns for 4-year-old children
   c. Association between UTIs and constipation
3. What priorities for nursing care should be established for Ginger?
4. Does the evidence support your nursing intervention?
5. What alternative perspectives might you have?

tual pressure destruction to renal parenchyma, although the dilating ureters form a reservoir that reduces the effect on the kidneys for a long time.

Obstruction may be congenital or acquired, unilateral or bilateral, and complete or incomplete, and the manifestations may be acute or chronic. The obstruction can occur at any level of the upper or lower urinary tract (Fig. 50-1). Partial obstruction may not be symptomatic unless there is a water or solute diuresis. Boys are affected more frequently than girls, and malformations should be suspected when patients have some other congenital defects (e.g., prune belly syndrome, chromosomal anomalies, anorectal malformations, defects of the pinna of the ear).

Damage to distal nephrons in chronic uropathy alters the ability to concentrate urine, contributing to increased urine flow and metabolic acidosis occurring from decreased excretion of acid secondary to impaired ability of the distal nephron to secrete hydrogen ions. Partial obstruction results in progressive loss of renal function as a result of irreversible damage to the nephrons. Pooled urine serves as a medium for bacterial growth; therefore UTIs further increase the extent of renal damage.

Early diagnosis and surgical correction or procedures that divert the flow of urine to bypass the obstruction, such as placement of a temporary percutaneous nephrostomy tube or cutaneous ureterostomy, are essential to prevent progressive renal damage. Medical complications of acute or chronic renal failure or infection are managed as described for those disorders.

Nursing Care Management

Nursing goals in urinary tract obstruction include helping to identify cases, assisting with diagnostic procedures, and caring for children with complications (described elsewhere). Preparing parents and children for procedures is a major nursing responsibility. Preparation for urinary diversion procedures is of special importance (see Preparation for Procedures, Chapter 44).

Parents and children need emotional support and counseling during the lengthy management of these disorders. Many children are discharged with ureteral drainage systems in place that must be protected from damage, and the danger of infection is a constant concern. Parents are taught to care for the equipment and recognize the signs of possible obstruction or infection within the system. Maintaining adequate urine flow is imperative. Fluids should be encouraged. The tube should be observed frequently for indications of obstruction resulting from sediment, small blood clots, or kinking. The physician should inspect any drainage from around the tube.

Children with external diversional systems will need psychologic support and guidance, especially as they reach adolescence and body-image concerns assume more prominence. Those with progressive renal deterioration may face the prospect of dialysis or transplantation and the emotional aspects that accompany these procedures.

External Defects

Defects of the external genitourinary tract are serious conditions primarily because of the psychologic impact on the child. Satisfactory surgical repair is successful for the more common disorders and is carried out or initiated as early as possible. The major anomalies of the lower genitourinary tract, their description, and their management are outlined in Table 50-4.

Psychologic Problems Related to Genital Surgery

Surgery involving sexual organs can be particularly disruptive to children, especially preschoolers fearing punishment, retaliation, body mutilation, or castration. Some of the problems of hospitalization, separation, and anxiety can be eased by hospital practices that are sensitive to the needs of the child (see Chapter 44).

The body image of a child is largely derived as a result of feedback from the primary caregivers, and parental anxiety regarding an acceptable physical appearance and adequate future sexual competency is readily communicated to an affected child. Therefore children with birth defects are at risk for developing a distorted body image that reflects the caregiver's subtly communicated evaluation of their bodies. The trend toward repair of visible genital defects is based in large part on these psychologic variables. The earlier a repair can be achieved, the more likely the possibility that the child will develop a normal body image.

During the years from 3 to 6, the phallic-oedipal period, children show a strong interest in and concern about the genital area, sex differences, and genital normality or its lack. It is also a time when children are frightened of what they perceive to be threats to their body and bodily function. They also view any untoward happening as a punishment for real or imagined wrongdoing or unacceptable sexual feelings, such as masturbation, sex play, or erotic feelings. Surgical repair is recommended before these fears and anxieties develop.

After extensive review of the emotional, cognitive, and body-image problems that may occur in children undergoing surgical reconstruction of a genital deformity, it was recommended that surgery be accomplished between ages 6 and 15 months to minimize the psychologic effects of surgery and anesthesia (Kass, 1996).

Nursing Care Management

Preparing children and their families for diagnostic and surgical procedures (see Preparation for Procedures, Chapter 44) and for home care are major nursing functions. Most postoperative care involves care of the surgical site. Tub baths are discouraged for 1 week after simple surgeries. The surgical site is kept clean and otherwise protected from infection and is inspected for signs of infection. Dressings, if any, are inspected regularly. More complex surgeries require additional care and observation (e.g., catheter care for urethral reconstruction and care of urinary diversion stomas and collection devices).

Some older children's activities, such as pushing, lifting, playing with straddle toys or in sandboxes, swimming, and rough activities, may be restricted for some types of surgical repairs. Precise restrictions depend on the specific type of surgery. Activities of infants and toddlers are not limited.

In most cases the results of surgery are quite satisfactory. However, in some of the more severe defects, such as exstrophy and those that require stomas, additional emotional interventions may be needed. A major concern of parents and children is related to surgery affecting the genitalia directly. Concerns about penile size, appearance of the genitalia, potential ability to procreate, and rejection by peers (especially the opposite sex) are potential fears that require psychologic adjustment, particularly during adolescence.

GLOMERULAR DISEASE

Nephrotic Syndrome

Nephrotic syndrome is a clinical state that includes massive proteinuria, hypoalbuminemia, hyperlipemia, and edema. The disorder can occur as (1) a primary disease known as *idiopathic nephrosis, childhood nephrosis,* or *minimal-change nephrotic syndrome (MCNS);* (2) a secondary disorder that occurs as a clinical manifestation after or in association with glomerular damage of known or presumed etiology; or (3) a congenital form inherited as an autosomal recessive disorder. The disorder is characterized by increased glomerular permeability to plasma protein, which results in massive urinary protein loss. The glomerulus is responsible for the initial step in the formation of urine, and the filtration rate depends on an intact glomerular membrane. This discussion is devoted to MCNS because it constitutes 80% of nephrotic syndrome cases.

Pathophysiology

The onset of MCNS can occur at any age but predominantly occurs in children between 2 and 7 years of age. It is rare in children younger than 6 months of age, uncommon in infants younger than 1 year of age, and unusual after age 8 years. Patients with MCNS are twice as likely to be male.

The pathogenesis of MCNS is not understood. There may be a metabolic, biochemical, physiochemical, or immune-mediated disturbance that causes the basement membrane of the glomeruli to become increasingly permeable to protein, but the cause and mechanisms are only speculative.

The glomerular membrane, normally impermeable to albumin and other proteins, becomes permeable to proteins, especially albumin, which leak through the membrane and are lost in urine *(hyperalbuminuria).* This reduces the serum albumin level *(hypoalbuminemia),* decreasing the colloidal osmotic pressure in the capillaries. As a result, the vascular hydrostatic pressure exceeds the pull of the colloidal osmotic

Table 50-4

Defects of the Genitourinary Tract

DEFECT	THERAPEUTIC MANAGEMENT
INGUINAL HERNIA	
Protrusion of abdominal contents through inguinal canal into scrotum	Detected as painless inguinal swelling of variable size Surgical closure of inguinal defect
HYDROCELE	
Fluid in scrotum	Surgical repair indicated if spontaneous resolution not accomplished in 1 year
PHIMOSIS	
Narrowing or stenosis of preputial opening of foreskin	Mild cases: manual retraction of foreskin and proper cleansing of area Severe cases: circumcision or vertical division and transverse suturing of foreskin
HYPOSPADIAS	
Urethral opening located behind glans penis or anywhere along ventral surface of penile shaft	Objectives of surgical correction: To enable child to void in standing position and direct stream voluntarily in usual manner Improve physical appearance of genitalia Produce a sexually adequate organ
CHORDEE	
Ventral curvature of penis, often associated with hypospadias	Surgical release of fibrous band causing the deformity
EPISPADIAS	
Meatal opening located on dorsal surface of penis	Surgical correction, usually including penile and urethral lengthening and bladder neck reconstruction (if necessary)
CRYPTORCHIDISM	
Failure of one or both testes to descend normally through inguinal canal	Detected by inability to palpate testes within scrotum Medical: administration of human chorionic gonadotropin (older child) Surgical: orchiopexy Objectives of therapy: Prevent damage to undescended testicle Decrease incidence of malignant tumor formation Avoid trauma and torsion Close inguinal canal Prevent cosmetic and psychologic disability from empty scrotum
EXSTROPHY OF BLADDER	
Eversion of posterior bladder through anterior bladder wall and lower abdominal wall; associated with open pubic arch (a severe defect)	Potential objectives of surgical correction: Preserve renal function Attain urinary control Adequate reconstructive repair Improve sexual function (especially in males)
AMBIGUOUS GENITALIA	
Types	**Therapeutic Management**
Masculinized female (female pseudohermaphrodite)	Gender assignment—female; assign gender, but do *not* perform irreversible surgery, because some children may change gender later in life; family participation essential
Incompletely masculinized male (male pseudohermaphrodite)	Assign gender, but do *not* perform irreversible surgery, because some children may change gender later in life; family participation essential
True hermaphrodite (both ovaries and testes)	Assign gender, but do *not* perform irreversible surgery, because some children may change gender later in life; gender assignment depends on predominant characteristics; family participation essential
Mixed gonadal dysgenesis	Assign gender, but do *not* perform irreversible surgery, because some children may change gender later in life; gender assignment depends on predominant characteristics; family participation essential

pressure, causing fluid to accumulate in the interstitial spaces *(edema)* and body cavities, particularly in the abdominal cavity *(ascites)*. The shift of fluid from the plasma to the interstitial spaces reduces the vascular fluid volume *(hypovolemia)*, which in turn stimulates the renin-angiotensin system and the secretion of antidiuretic hormone and aldosterone. Tubular reabsorption of sodium and water is increased in an attempt to increase intravascular volume. The elevation of serum lipids is unexplained. The sequence of events in nephrotic syndrome is diagrammed in Fig. 50-2.

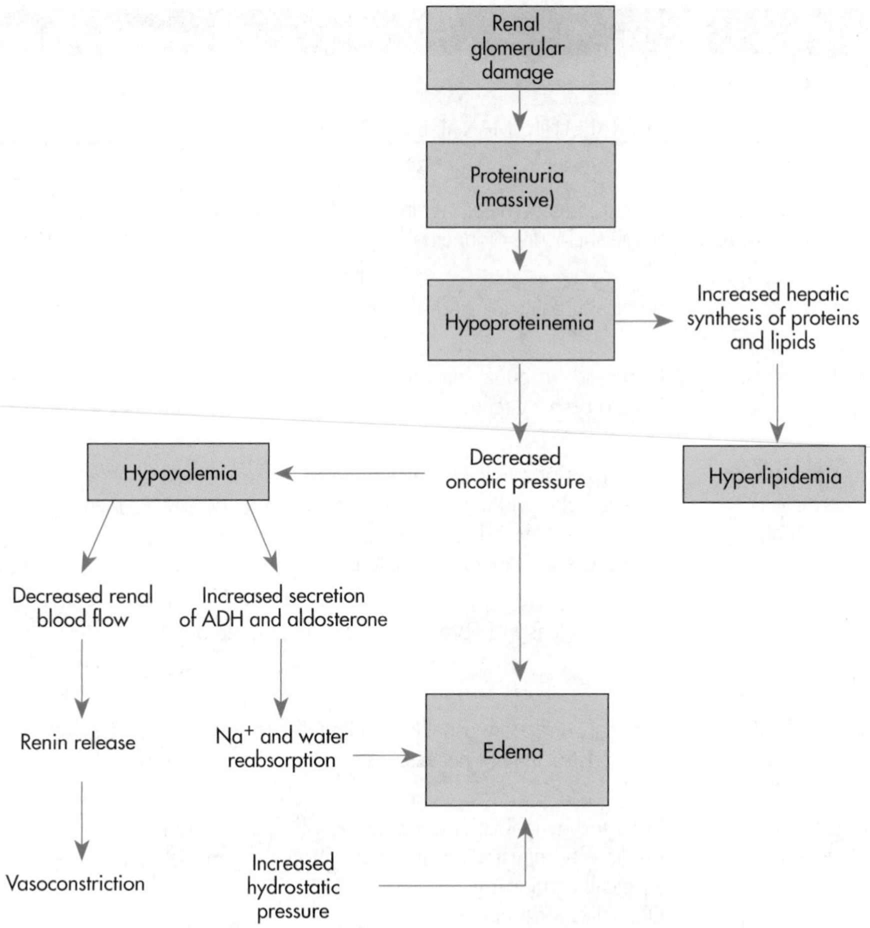

Fig. 50-2 Sequence of events in nephrotic syndrome.

NURSE ALERT A child who exhibits the following should be evaluated for the possibility of nephrotic syndrome:
- Weight gain over that expected based on previous pattern
- Parent observation that the child's clothes fit tightly
- Decreased urine output
- Pallor, fatigue ■

Diagnostic Evaluation

The disease is suspected on the basis of clinical manifestations (Box 50-2), especially when weight gain in a previously well child increases slowly over days or weeks. The generalized edema may develop rapidly or gradually but eventually prompts the family to seek medical attention. Parents usually give a history of the child being well but steadily gaining weight and then becoming anorexic, irritable, and less active.

The diagnosis of MCNS is suspected on the basis of the history and clinical manifestations (edema, proteinuria, hypoalbuminemia, and hypercholesterolemia in the absence of hematuria and hypertension) in children between 2 and 8 years of age. The hallmark of MCNS is massive proteinuria (higher than 3+ on urine dipstick). Hyaline casts, oval fat bodies, and a few red blood cells can be found in the urine of some affected children, although there is seldom gross hematuria. The glomerular filtration rate is usually normal or high.

Total serum protein concentration is low, with the serum albumin significantly reduced and plasma lipids elevated. Hemoglobin and hematocrit are usually normal or elevated as a result of hemoconcentration. The platelet count may be elevated. Serum sodium concentration may be low. If the patient does not respond to a 4- to 8-week course of steroids, a renal biopsy may be needed to distinguish between other types of nephrotic syndrome. The biopsy results of children with MCNS is remarkable for effacement of the foot processes of the epithelial cells lining the basement membrane, but otherwise the kidney tissue is normal.

Therapeutic Management

Objectives of therapeutic management include (1) reducing excretion of urinary protein, (2) reducing fluid retention in the tissues, (3) preventing infection, and (4) minimizing complications related to therapies. Dietary restrictions include a low-salt diet and fluid restriction. If complications of edema develop, diuretic therapy may be initiated to provide temporary relief from edema. Sometimes infusions of 25% albumin are used. Acute infections are treated with appropriate antibiotics.

Corticosteroids are the first line of therapy for MCNS. The starting dose for prednisone is usually 2 mg/kg body weight per day, in one or more divided doses. In most children this response occurs within 7 to 21 days. The medication is then tapered over a period of several weeks and eventually stopped

BOX 50-2

Clinical Manifestations of Nephrotic Syndrome

Weight gain
Puffiness of face (facial edema):
- Especially around the eyes
- Apparent on arising in the morning
- Subsides during the day

Abdominal swelling (ascites)
Pleural effusion
Labial or scrotal swelling
Edema of intestinal mucosal may cause the following:
- Diarrhea
- Anorexia
- Poor intestinal absorption

Ankle/leg swelling
Irritability
Easily fatigued
Lethargic
Blood pressure normal or slightly decreased
Susceptibility to infection
Urine alterations:
- Decreased volume
- Frothy

if the child remains asymptomatic. About two thirds of children with MCNS have a relapse, heralded first by increased urine protein. Relapses can be diagnosed early if parents are taught routine home monitoring of urine protein by dipstick. Relapses are treated with a repeated course of high-dose steroid therapy. Side effects of the steroids include weight gain, rounding of the face, and increased appetite. Long-term therapy may result in hirsutism, growth retardation, cataracts, hypertension, gastrointestinal bleeding, bone demineralization, infection, and hyperglycemia. Children who do not respond to steroid therapy, those who have frequent relapses, and those in whom the side effects threaten their growth and general health may be considered for a course of therapy using other immunosuppressant medications (cyclophosphamide, chlorambucil, or cyclosporine).

MCNS episodes, both the first episode and relapse, often happen in conjunction with a viral or bacterial infection. Relapses can also be triggered by allergies and immunizations. Relapses in children with MCNS may continue over many years.

Complications of nephrotic syndrome include infection, circulatory insufficiency secondary to hypovolemia, and thromboembolism. Infections that may be seen in children with nephrotic syndrome include peritonitis, cellulitis, and pneumonia and require prompt recognition and vigorous treatment with appropriate antibiotic therapy.

Prognosis

The prognosis for ultimate recovery in most cases is good. It is a self-limiting disease, and in children who respond to steroid therapy the tendency to relapse decreases with time. With early detection and prompt implementation of therapy to eradicate proteinuria, progressive basement membrane damage is minimized, so that when the tendency to exacerbations is past, renal function is usually normal or near normal. It is estimated that approximately 80% of affected children have this favorable prognosis.

Nursing Care Management

Continuous monitoring of fluid retention or excretion is an important nursing function. Strict intake and output records are essential but may be difficult to obtain from very young children. Application of collection bags is highly irritating to edematous skin that is readily subject to breakdown. Application of diapers or weighing wet pads may be necessary.

<u>NURSE ALERT</u> Another strategy for obtaining a daily urine protein is to place cotton balls in the diaper at night before bedtime and then squeeze them out in the morning. ■

Other methods of monitoring progress include urine examination for albumin, daily weight, and measurement of abdominal girth. Assessment of edema (e.g., increased or decreased swelling around the eyes and dependent areas), the degree of pitting, and the color and texture of skin are part of nursing care. Vital signs are monitored to detect any early signs of complications such as shock or an infective process.

Infection is a constant source of danger to edematous children and those receiving corticosteroid therapy. These children are particularly vulnerable to upper respiratory infection; therefore they must be kept warm and dry, active, and protected from contact with infected individuals (i.e., roommates, visitors, and personnel). Vital signs are monitored to detect any early signs of an infective process.

Loss of appetite accompanying active nephrosis creates a perplexing problem for nurses. During this time the combined efforts of nurse, dietitian, parents, and the child are needed to formulate a nutritionally adequate and attractive diet. Salt is usually restricted (but not eliminated) during the edema phase, and fluid restriction (if prescribed) is limited to short-term use during massive edema. Every effort should be made to serve attractive meals with preferred foods and a minimum of fuss, but it usually requires a considerable amount of ingenuity and enticement to get the child to eat (see Feeding the Sick Child, Chapter 44).

Children usually adjust activities according to their tolerance level. However, they may require guidance in selecting play activities. Suitable recreational and diversional activities are an important part of their care. Irritability and mood swings that accompany steroid therapy are not unusual in these children and may create an additional challenge to the nurse and the family.

Family Support and Home Care

Continuous support of the child and family is one of the major nursing considerations. Many children are treated at home during exacerbations. Parents are taught to detect signs of relapse and to call for changes in treatment at the earliest indications. Unless the edema and proteinuria are severe or the parents, for some reason, are unable to care for the ill child, *home care is preferred.* Parents are instructed in testing urine for albumin, administration of medications, and general care. Parents are also instructed regarding avoiding contact with infected playmates, but the child should attend school.

The prolonged course of the relapsing form of nephrotic syndrome is taxing to both the child and the family. The up-and-down course of remissions and exacerbations with periodic disruption of family life by hospitalization places a severe strain on the child and the family, both psychologically and financially. Reassurance regarding this characteristic of the course of the disease, with emphasis on the importance of long-term care, needs to be provided to parents and children to gain their cooperation. A satisfactory response is more likely when relapses are detected and therapy is instituted early, and remissions are prolonged when instructions are carried out faithfully. Continuous support of the child and family is one of the major nursing considerations (see Chapter 41).

Acute Glomerulonephritis

Acute glomerulonephritis (AGN) may be a primary event or a manifestation of a systemic disorder that can range from minimal to severe. Common features include oliguria, edema, hypertension and circulatory congestion, hematuria, and proteinuria. Most cases are postinfectious and have been associated with pneumococcal, streptococcal, and viral infections. *Acute poststreptococcal glomerulonephritis (APSGN)* is the most common of the postinfectious renal diseases in childhood and the one for which a cause can be established in the majority of cases. APSGN can occur at any age but affects primarily early school-age children, with a peak age of onset of 6 to 7 years. It is uncommon in children younger than 2 years of age, and males outnumber females 2:1.

Etiology

APSGN is an immune-complex disease that occurs after an antecedent streptococcal infection with certain strains of the group A β-hemolytic streptococcus. Most streptococcal infections do *not* cause APSGN. A latent period of 10 to 21 days occurs between the streptococcal infection and the onset of clinical manifestations. Disease secondary to streptococcal pharyngitis is more common in the winter or spring, but when APSGN is associated with pyoderma (principally *impetigo*), it may be more prevalent in later summer or early fall, especially in warmer climates. Second episodes of AGN are rare.

Pathophysiology

The pathophysiology of APSGN is still uncertain. Immune complexes are deposited in the glomerular basement membrane. The glomeruli become edematous and infiltrated with polymorphonuclear leukocytes, which occlude the capillary lumen. The resulting decrease in plasma filtration results in an excessive accumulation of water and retention of sodium that expands plasma and interstitial fluid volumes, leading to circulatory congestion and edema. The cause of the hypertension associated with AGN cannot be completely explained by fluid retention. Excess renin may also be produced.

Diagnostic Evaluation

Typically, affected children are in good health until they experience the streptococcal infection. In some instances there is a history of only a mild cold or no previous infection at all. The onset of nephritis appears after an average latent period of about 10 days (Box 50-3). Because the child appears to be well during the latest period, the association is not recognized by the parents. The edema is relatively moderate and may not be appreciated by someone unfamiliar with the child's normal appearance.

BOX 50-3

Clinical Manifestations of Acute Poststreptococcal Glomerulonephritis

Edema:
- Especially periorbital
- Facial edema more prominent in the morning
- Spreads during the day to involve extremities and abdomen

Anorexia

Urine:
- Cloudy, smoky brown (resembles tea or cola)
- Severely reduced volume

Pallor

Irritability

Lethargy

Child appears ill

Child seldom expresses specific complaints

Older children may complain of the following:
- Headaches
- Abdominal discomfort
- Dysuria

Vomiting possible

Mild to moderately elevated blood pressure

Urinalysis during the acute phase characteristically shows hematuria and proteinuria. Proteinuria generally parallels the hematuria and may be 3+ or 4+ in the presence of gross hematuria. Gross discoloration of the urine reflects red blood cell and hemoglobin content. Microscopic examination of the sediment shows many red blood cells, leukocytes, epithelial cells, and granular and red blood cell casts. Bacteria are not seen.

Azotemia that results from impaired glomerular filtration is reflected in elevated blood urea nitrogen and creatinine levels in at least 50% of cases. Occasionally proteinuria is excessive and the patient may have nephrotic syndrome (i.e., hypoproteinemia and hyperlipidemia).

Cultures of the pharynx are rarely positive for streptococci, because the renal disease occurs weeks after the infection.

NURSE ALERT A child who exhibits the following should be evaluated for possible AGN:
- Orbital edema, which parents report is worse in the morning
- Loss of appetite
- Decreased output
- Dark-colored urine
- Antecedent streptococcal infection ■

Some serologic tests are necessary to make the diagnosis of AGN. Circulating serum antibodies to streptococcus indicate the presence of a previous infection. The antistreptolysin O (ASO) titer is the most familiar and readily available test for streptococcal infection. Other antibodies that may aid in diagnosis are elevated antihyaluronidase (AHase), antideoxyribonuclease B (ADNase-B), and streptozyme.

All patients with APSGN have reduced serum complement (C3) activity in the early stages of the disease. Rising

C3 levels are used as a guide to indicate improvement of the disease and should be normal in almost all patients 8 weeks after the disease onset.

Studies that may be useful include chest x-ray examination, which generally shows cardiac enlargement, pulmonary congestion, or pleural effusion during the edematous phase of acute disease. Renal biopsy for diagnostic purposes is seldom required but may be useful in the diagnosis of atypical cases.

Therapeutic Management

Management consists of general supportive measures and early recognition and treatment of complications. Children who have normal blood pressure and a satisfactory urine output can generally be treated at home. Those with substantial edema, hypertension, gross hematuria, or significant oliguria should be hospitalized because of the unpredictability of complications.

Dietary restrictions depend on the stage and severity of the disease, especially the extent of edema. Moderate sodium restriction and even fluid restriction may be instituted for children with hypertension and edema. Foods with substantial amounts of potassium are generally restricted during the period of oliguria.

Regular measurement of vital signs, body weight, and intake and output is essential to monitor the progress of the disease and to detect complications that may appear at any time during the course of the disease. *A record of daily weight is the most useful means for assessing fluid balance.* Rarely, children with AGN will develop acute renal failure with oliguria that significantly alters the fluid and electrolyte balance (resulting in hyperkalemia, acidosis, hypocalcemia, or hyperphosphatemia). These children require careful management. Peritoneal dialysis or hemodialysis is seldom needed.

Acute hypertension must be anticipated and identified early. Blood pressure measurements are taken every 4 to 6 hours. A variety of antihypertensive medications, as well as diuretics, are used to control hypertension. Antibiotic therapy is indicated only for those children with evidence of persistent streptococcal infections. It is used to prevent transmission of nephritogenic streptococci to other family members.

Prognosis

Almost all children correctly diagnosed as having APSGN recover completely, and specific immunity is conferred, so that subsequent recurrences are uncommon. Some of these children have been reported to develop chronic disease, but most of these cases are now believed to be different glomerular diseases misdiagnosed as poststreptococcal disease.

Nursing Care Management

Nursing care of the child with glomerulonephritis involves careful assessment of the disease status, with regular monitoring of vital signs (including frequent measurement of blood pressure), fluid balance, and behavior.

Vital signs provide clues to the severity of the disease and early signs of complications. They are carefully measured, and any deviations are reported and recorded. The volume and character of urine are noted, and the child is weighed daily. Children with restricted fluid intake, especially those who are not severely edematous or those who have lost weight, are observed for signs of dehydration.

Assessment of the child's appearance for signs of cerebral complications is an important nursing function, because the severity of the acute phase is variable and unpredictable. The child with edema, hypertension, and gross hematuria may be subject to complications, and anticipatory preparations such as seizure precautions and intravenous equipment are included in the nursing care plan.

For most children a regular diet is allowed, but it should contain no added salt. Foods high in sodium and salted treats are eliminated, and parents and friends are advised not to bring snacks such as potato chips or pretzels. However, the total amount of salt ingested is usually less than prescribed because of the child's poor appetite. Fluid restriction, if prescribed, is more difficult, and the amount permitted should be evenly divided throughout the waking hours. Meal preparation and service require special attention, because the child is indifferent to meals during the acute phase. Again, collaboration with parents and the dietitian and special consideration for food preferences facilitate meal planning.

During the acute phase, children are generally content to lie in bed. As they begin to feel better and their symptoms subside, they will want to be up and about. Activities should be planned to allow for frequent rest periods and avoidance of fatigue. Children who have mild edema and no hypertension, as well as convalescent children who are being treated at home, need follow-up care. Parents are instructed regarding general measures, including diet, and prevention of infection.

Health supervision is continued with weekly, followed by monthly, visits for evaluation and urinalysis. Parent education and support in preparation for discharge and home care include education in home management and the need for follow-up care and health supervision.

MISCELLANEOUS RENAL DISORDERS

Hemolytic-Uremic Syndrome

Hemolytic-uremic syndrome (HUS) is an uncommon, acute renal disease that occurs primarily in infants and small children between 6 months and 5 years of age. HUS is the most common cause of acquired acute renal failure in children (Brandt et al, 1994). The clinical features of the disease include acquired hemolytic anemia, thrombocytopenia, renal injury, and central nervous system symptoms. The etiology of HUS is thought to be associated with bacterial toxins, chemicals, and viruses. The appearance of the disease has been associated with *Rickettsia,* viruses (especially coxsackievirus, echovirus, and adenovirus), *Escherichia coli,* pneumococci, *Shigella,* and *Salmonella* and may represent an unusual response to these infections. Multiple cases of HUS caused by enteric infection of the *E. coli* 0157:H7 serotype have been traced to undercooked meat, especially ground beef. Often sources are unpasteurized milk or fruit juice, especially apple, alfalfa sprouts, lettuce, and salami, and drinking or swimming in sewage-contaminated water. The clinical presentation is usually a history of a prodromal illness (most often gastroenteritis or an upper respiratory infection) followed by the sudden onset of hemolysis and renal failure.

Pathophysiology

The primary site of injury appears to be the endothelial lining of the small glomerular arterioles, which become swollen and occluded with deposits of platelets and fibrin clots (intravascular coagulation). Red blood cells are damaged as they attempt to move through the partially occluded blood vessels. These damaged cells are removed by the spleen, causing acute hemolytic anemia. The platelet aggregation within the damaged blood vessels or the damage and removal of platelets produce the characteristic thrombocytopenia.

Diagnostic Evaluation

The triad of anemia, thrombocytopenia, and renal failure is sufficient for diagnosis (Box 50-4). Renal involvement is evidenced by proteinuria, hematuria, and the presence of urinary casts; blood urea nitrogen and serum creatinine levels are elevated. A low hemoglobin and hematocrit and a high reticulocyte count confirm the hemolytic nature of the anemia.

Therapeutic Management

The goals of therapy are early diagnosis and aggressive, supportive care of the acute renal failure and hemolytic anemia. The most consistently effective treatment of HUS is hemodialysis or peritoneal dialysis, which is instituted in any child who has been anuric for 24 hours or who demonstrates oliguria with uremia or hypertension and seizures. Other treatments include use of pharmacologic agents, fresh-frozen plasma, and plasma pheresis. Blood transfusions with fresh, washed packed cells are administered for severe anemia but are used with caution to prevent circulatory overload from added volume.

Prognosis

With prompt treatment the recovery rate is about 95%, but residual renal impairment ranges from 10% to 50% in various areas. Long-term complications include chronic renal failure, hypertension, and central nervous system disorders. Death is usually caused by residual renal impairment or central nervous system injury.

Nursing Care Management

Nursing care is the same as that provided in acute renal failure and, for children with continued impairment, includes management of chronic disease. Because of the sudden and life-threatening nature of the disorder in a previously well child, parents are often not prepared for the impact of hospitalization and treatment. Therefore support and understanding are especially important aspects of care.

BOX 50-4

Clinical Manifestations of Hemolytic Uremic Syndrome

- Vomiting
- Irritability
- Lethargy
- Marked pallor
- Hemorrhagic manifestations:
  - Bruising
  - Petechiae
  - Jaundice
  - Bloody diarrhea
- Oliguria or anuria
- Central nervous system involvement:
  - Seizures
  - Stupor/coma
- Signs of acute heart failure (sometimes)

Wilms' Tumor

Wilms' tumor, or *nephroblastoma,* is the most common malignant renal and intraabdominal tumor of childhood. Its frequency is estimated to be 7.6 cases per 1 million white children less than 15 years of age (Gundy et al, 2002). Wilms' tumor occurs about three times more often in blacks than in East Asians in the United States. The peak age at diagnosis is approximately 3 years, and occurrence is slightly more frequent in boys than in girls. The majority of patients with Wilms' tumor are diagnosed at younger than 5 years of age, with 1% to 2.5% having a familial origin. Unfortunately, there is no method of identifying gene carriers at this time.

Etiology

Wilms' tumor probably arises from a malignant, undifferentiated cluster of primordial cells capable of initiating the regeneration of an abnormal structure. Its occurrence slightly favors the left kidney, which is advantageous because surgically this kidney is easier to manipulate and remove. In about 10% of cases both kidneys are involved. Studies have shown that development of Wilms' tumor is frequently associated with aniridia, hemihypertrophy, Beckwith-Wiedemann syndrome, and genitourinary anomalies (Gundy et al, 2002; Kline & Sevier, 2003).

Diagnostic Evaluation

In a child suspected of having Wilms' tumor, special emphasis is placed on the history and physical examination for the presence of congenital anomalies, a family history of cancer, and signs of malignancy (e.g., weight loss, size of liver and spleen, indications of anemia, or lymphadenopathy). Most children with Wilms' tumor are brought to the practitioner because of abdominal swelling or an abdominal mass (Box 50-5). Specific tests include radiographic studies, including abdominal ultrasound, abdominal and chest computed tomography scan, hematologic studies, biochemical studies, and urinalysis. Studies to demonstrate the relationship of the tumor to the ipsilateral kidney and the presence of a normally functioning kidney on the contralateral side are essential. If a large tumor is present, an inferior ve-

BOX 50-5

Clinical Manifestations of Wilms' Tumor

- Abdominal swelling or mass:
  - Firm
  - Nontender
  - Confined to one side
- Hematuria (less than one fourth of cases)
- Fatigue/malaise
- Hypertension (occasionally)
- Weight loss
- Fever
- Manifestations resulting from compression of tumor mass
- Secondary metabolic alterations from tumor or metastasis
- If metastasis, symptoms of lung involvement:
  - Dyspnea
  - Cough
  - Shortness of breath
  - Chest pain (sometimes)

nacavogram is necessary to demonstrate possible tumor involvement adjacent to the vena cava. A bone marrow aspiration may be performed to rule out metastasis, which is rare in children with Wilms' tumor.

NURSE ALERT To reinforce the need for caution, it may be necessary to post a sign on the bed that reads "DO NOT PALPATE ABDOMEN." Careful bathing and handling are also important in preventing trauma to the tumor site. ■

Therapeutic Management

Combined treatment of surgery and chemotherapy with or without radiation is based on the histologic pattern and clinical stage.

Surgery is scheduled as soon as possible after confirmation of a renal mass, usually within 24 to 48 hours of admission. A large transabdominal incision is performed for optimum visualization of the abdominal cavity. The tumor-affected kidney and adjacent adrenal gland are removed. Great care is taken to keep the encapsulated tumor intact, because rupture can seed cancer cells throughout the abdomen, lymph channel, and bloodstream. The contralateral kidney is carefully inspected for evidence of disease or dysfunction. Regional lymph nodes are inspected, and a biopsy is performed when indicated. Any involved structures, such as part of the colon, diaphragm, or vena cava, are removed. Metal clips are placed around the tumor site for exact marking during radiotherapy.

If both kidneys are involved, the child may be treated with radiotherapy or chemotherapy before surgery to decrease the size of the tumor, allowing more conservative surgery. It may be possible to perform a partial nephrectomy on the less affected kidney, with a total nephrectomy on the opposite side. When a transplant is feasible, such as from a twin, sibling, or parent, bilateral nephrectomy is considered as a last resort.

Postoperative radiation therapy is indicated for children with large tumors, metastasis, residual postoperative disease, unfavorable histology, or recurrence. Chemotherapy is indicated for all stages. The most effective agents for treating Wilms' tumor are actinomycin D (dactinomycin), vincristine, and doxorubicin (Adriamycin) with the addition of cyclophosphamide for unfavorable histology or advanced disease (Gundy et al, 2002). The duration of therapy varies, ranging from 6 to 15 months.

Prognosis

Survival rates for Wilms' tumor are the highest among all childhood cancers. Children with localized tumor (stages I and II) have a 90% chance of cure with multimodal therapy. Factors that favorably affect the success of further therapy include initial treatment with only vincristine and dactinomycin, relapse to the lungs only, relapse in the abdomen of a patient who received no prior abdominal irradiation, and relapse more than 12 months after diagnosis. Wilms' tumor may recur, especially in the lungs. Both chemotherapy and radiation therapy can induce second tumors, usually in areas that have been irradiated (Gundy et al, 2002).

Nursing Care Management

Nursing care of the child with Wilms' tumor is similar to that of children with other cancers treated with surgery, irradiation, and chemotherapy. However, there are some significant differences; these are discussed for each phase of nursing intervention.

Preoperative Care

The preoperative period is one of swift diagnosis. The nurse is faced with the challenge of preparing the child and parents for all laboratory and operative procedures within 24 to 48 hours of admission. Because of the minimal amount of available preparatory time, explanations should be simple, repetitive, and focused on the child's actual experiences. In addition to the usual preoperative observations, blood pressure is monitored, because hypertension from excess renin production is a possibility.

There are several special preoperative concerns, the most important of which is that the *tumor is not palpated* unless absolutely necessary, because manipulation of the mass may cause dissemination of cancer cells to adjacent and distant sites.

Because radiotherapy and chemotherapy are usually begun immediately after surgery, parents need an explanation of what to expect, such as major benefits and side effects. The timing of the information should be considered to avoid overwhelming the family. Ideally, the nurse should be present during physician-parent conferences to answer questions as they arise. It is usually better to postpone telling the child about these side effects until after surgery. Alopecia, usually of most concern to older children, does not occur until approximately 2 weeks after the initial treatment regimen. Therefore the child can be prepared for the hair loss postoperatively.

Postoperative Care

Despite the extensive surgical intervention necessary in many children with Wilms' tumor, the recovery is usually rapid. The major nursing responsibilities are the same as those after any abdominal surgery (see Surgical Procedures, Chapter 44). Because these children are at risk for intestinal obstruction from vincristine-induced ileus, radiation-induced edema, and postsurgical adhesion formation, gastrointestinal activity, such as bowel movements, bowel sounds, distention, vomiting, and pain, are carefully monitored.

The nurse also monitors blood pressure, urine output, and signs of infection, as well as instituting pulmonary hygiene to prevent postoperative pulmonary complications.

Family Support

The postoperative period is frequently difficult for parents. The shock of seeing their child immediately after surgery may be the first realization of the seriousness of the diagnosis. It also marks the confirmation of the stage of the tumor. During this period, the nurse should be with the parents to assure them of the child's recovery after surgery and to assess the parent's understanding of the total experience. They need an opportunity to express their feelings and need to be provided the same emotional care discussed in Chapter 41 for families who have a child with a life-threatening disorder.

Older children need an opportunity to deal with their feelings concerning the many procedures to which they have been subjected in rapid succession. Play therapy with dolls or puppets or through drawing can be extremely beneficial in helping them adjust. It is not unusual for children to feel angry because of the extent of surgery, the need for additional therapy, or the seriousness of the disorder.

NURSE ALERT Because the child is left with one kidney, certain precautions, such as avoiding contact sports, are recommended to prevent injury to the remaining organ. Prompt detection and treatment of any genitourinary signs or symptoms are mandatory. ■

RENAL FAILURE

Renal failure is the inability of the kidneys to excrete waste material, concentrate urine, and conserve electrolytes. It can occur suddenly *(acute renal failure [ARF])* in response to inadequate perfusion, kidney disease, or urinary tract obstruction, or it can develop slowly *(chronic renal failure)* as a result of long-standing kidney disease or an anomaly.

Azotemia and *uremia* are terms often used in relation to renal failure. *Azotemia* is the accumulation of nitrogenous waste within the blood. *Uremia* is a more advanced condition in which retention of nitrogenous products produces toxic symptoms. Azotemia is not life threatening, whereas uremia is a serious condition that often involves other body systems.

Acute Renal Failure

ARF is said to exist when the kidneys suddenly are unable to regulate the volume and composition of urine appropriately in response to food and fluid intake and the needs of the organism. The principal feature of ARF is oliguria* associated with azotemia, metabolic acidosis, and diverse electrolyte disturbances. ARF is not common in childhood, but the outcome depends on the cause, associated findings, and prompt recognition and treatment.

The pathologic conditions that produce ARF caused by glomerulonephritis and HUS have been discussed in relation to those disorders. ARF can also develop as a result of a large number of related or unrelated clinical conditions: poor renal perfusion, urinary tract obstruction, acute renal injury, or the final expression of chronic, irreversible renal disease. The most common cause in children is transient renal failure resulting from severe dehydration or other causes of poor perfusion that may respond to restoration of fluid volume.

Pathophysiology

ARF is usually reversible, but the deviations of physiologic function can be extreme, and the mortality rate in the pediatric age group remains high. There is severe reduction in the glomerular filtration rate, an elevated blood urea nitrogen level, and a significant reduction in renal blood flow.

The clinical course is variable and depends on the cause. In reversible ARF there is a period of severe oliguria, or a low-output phase, followed by an abrupt onset of diuresis, or a high-output phase, and then a gradual return to, or toward, normal urine volumes.

Diagnostic Evaluation

In many instances of ARF the infant or child is already critically ill with the precipitating disorder, and the explanation for development of oliguria may or may not be readily apparent (Box 50-6). When a previously well child develops ARF without obvious cause, a careful history is taken to reveal symptoms that may be related to glomerulonephritis, obstructive uropathy, or exposure to nephrotoxic chemicals (e.g., ingestion of heavy metals, inhalation of carbon tetrachloride or other organic solvents or drugs known to be toxic to the kidneys). Significant laboratory measurements during renal shutdown that serve as a guide for therapy are blood urea nitrogen, serum creatinine, pH, sodium, potassium, and calcium.

NURSE ALERT Diminished urine output and lethargy in a child who is dehydrated, in shock, or recently postoperative should be evaluated for possible acute kidney failure. ■

NURSE ALERT Any of the following signs of hyperkalemia constitute an emergency and are reported immediately:

- Serum potassium concentrations in excess of 7 mEq/L
- Presence of electrocardiographic abnormalities, such as prolonged QRS complex, depressed ST segment, high-peaked T waves, bradycardia, or heart block ■

Therapeutic Management

Treatment of ARF is directed toward (1) treatment of the underlying cause, (2) management of the complications of renal failure, and (3) provision of supportive therapy within the constraints imposed by the renal failure.

Treatment of poor perfusion resulting from dehydration consists of volume restoration, as described in Chapter 47 in treatment of dehydration. If oliguria persists after restoration of fluid volume or if the renal failure is caused by intrinsic renal damage, the physiologic and biochemical abnormalities that have resulted from kidney dysfunction must be corrected or controlled. Initially a Foley catheter is inserted to rule out urine retention, to collect available urine for analysis, and to monitor results of diuretic administration. The catheter may or may not be removed during the oliguric phase.

BOX 50-6

Clinical Manifestations of Acute Renal Failure

Specific:
- Oliguria
- Anuria uncommon (except in obstructive disorders)

Nonspecific (may develop):
- Nausea
- Vomiting
- Drowsiness
- Edema
- Hypertension

Manifestations of underlying disorder or pathologic condition

*The definition of oliguria varies extensively in the literature, from 1.8 to 4 dl/m²/24 hr.

The amount of exogenous water provided should not exceed the amount needed to maintain zero water balance. It is calculated on the basis of estimated endogenous water formation and losses from sensible (primarily gastrointestinal) and insensible sources. No allotment is calculated for urine as long as oliguria persists.

When the output begins to increase, either spontaneously or in response to diuretic therapy, the intake of fluid, potassium, and sodium must be monitored and adequate replacement provided to prevent depletion and its consequences. Some patients pass enormous amounts of electrolyte-rich urine.

Complications

The child with ARF has a tendency to develop water intoxication and hyponatremia, which makes it difficult to provide calories in sufficient amounts to meet the needs of the child and reduce the tissue catabolism, metabolic acidosis, hyperkalemia, and uremia. If the child is able to tolerate oral foods, food sources high in concentrated carbohydrate and fat but low in protein, potassium, and sodium may be provided. However, many children have functional disturbances of the gastrointestinal tract, such as nausea and vomiting; therefore the intravenous (IV) route is generally preferred and usually consists of essential amino acids or a combination of essential and nonessential amino acids administered by the central venous route.

Control of water balance in these patients requires careful monitoring of feedback information, such as accurate intake and output, body weight, and electrolyte measurements. In general, during the oliguric phase, no sodium, chloride, or potassium is given unless there are other large, ongoing losses. Regular measurement of plasma electrolyte, pH, blood urea nitrogen, and creatinine levels is required to assess the adequacy of fluid therapy and to anticipate complications that require specific treatment.

Hyperkalemia is the most immediate threat to the life of the child with ARF. Hyperkalemia can be minimized and sometimes avoided by eliminating potassium from all food and fluid, by reducing tissue catabolism, and by correcting acidosis. Measures employed for the reduction of serum potassium levels are oral or rectal administration of an ion-exchange resin such as sodium polystyrene sulfonate (Kayexalate) and peritoneal dialysis or hemodialysis (see p. 1665). The resin produces its effect by exchange of its sodium for the potassium, thus binding potassium for removal from the body. This increased sodium concentration may contribute to fluid overload, hypertension, and cardiac failure. Dialysis removes potassium and other waste products from the serum by diffusion through a semipermeable membrane.

Hypertension is a frequent and serious complication of ARF, and to detect it early, blood pressure measurements are made every 4 to 6 hours. The most common cause of hypertension in ARF is overexpansion of extracellular fluid and plasma volume together with activation of the renin-angiotensin system. Hypertension is controlled with antihypertensive drugs. Other measures that may be used include limiting fluids and salt.

Anemia is frequently associated with ARF, but transfusion is not recommended unless the hemoglobin drops below 6 g/dl. Transfusions, if used, consist of fresh, packed red blood cells given slowly to reduce the likelihood of increasing blood volume, hypertension, and hyperkalemia.

Seizures occur often when renal failure progresses to uremia and are also related to hypertension, hyponatremia, and hypocalcemia. Treatment is directed to the specific cause when known. More obscure causes are managed with antiepileptic drugs.

Cardiac failure with pulmonary edema is almost always associated with hypervolemia. Treatment is directed toward reduction of fluid volume, with water and sodium restriction and administration of diuretics.

Prognosis

The prognosis of ARF depends largely on the nature and severity of the causative factor or precipitating event and the promptness and competence of management. The outcome is least favorable in children with rapidly progressive nephritis and cortical necrosis. Children in whom ARF is a result of HUS or acute glomerulitis may recover completely, but residual renal impairment or hypertension is more often the rule. Complete recovery is usually expected in children whose renal failure is a result of dehydration, nephrotoxins, or ischemia. ARF following cardiac surgery is less favorable. It is often impossible to assess the extent of recovery for several months.

Nursing Care Management

Meticulous attention to fluid intake and output is mandatory and includes all of the physical measurements discussed previously in relation to problems of fluid balance. Monitoring fluid balance and vital signs is a continuous process, and observers are constantly on the alert for signs of complications so that appropriate interventions can be implemented. Because these children require intensive observation and, often, specialized treatment, such as dialysis, they are usually admitted to an intensive care unit in which needed equipment and trained personnel are available.

Limiting fluid intake requires ingenuity on the part of caregivers to cope with the child who is thirsty. Rationing the daily intake in small amounts of fluid served in containers that give the impression of larger volumes is one strategy. Older children who understand the rationale of fluid limits can help determine how their daily ration should be distributed.

Meeting nutritional needs is sometimes a problem; the child may be nauseated, and encouraging concentrated foods without fluids may be difficult. When nourishment is provided by the IV route, careful monitoring is essential to prevent fluid overload. In addition, nursing measures such as maintaining an optimum thermal environment, reducing any elevation of body temperature, and reducing restlessness and anxiety are employed to decrease the rate of tissue catabolism.

The nurse must be continually alert for changes in behavior that indicate the onset of complications. Infection from reduced resistance, anemia, and general morbidity is a constant threat. Fluid overload and electrolyte disturbances can precipitate cardiovascular complications such as hypertension and cardiac failure. Fluid and electrolyte imbalances, acidosis, and accumulation of nitrogenous waste products can produce neurologic involvement manifested by coma, seizures, or alterations in sensorium.

Although children with ARF are usually quite ill and voluntarily diminish their activity, infants may become restless and irritable, and children are often anxious and frightened. There are frequent, painful, and stress-producing treatments and tests that must be performed. The presence of a supportive, empathetic nurse can provide comfort and stability in a threatening and unnatural environment.

Family Support

Providing support and reassurance to parents is among the major nursing responsibilities. The seriousness of ARF and its emergency nature are stressful to parents, and most feel some degree of guilt regarding the child's condition, especially when the illness is a result of ingestion of a toxic substance, dehydration, or a genetic disease. They need reassurance and a sympathetic listener. They also need to be kept informed of the child's progress and provided explanations regarding the therapeutic regimen. The equipment and the child's behavior are sometimes frightening and anxiety provoking. Nurses can do much to help parents comprehend and deal with the stresses of the situation.

Chronic Renal Failure

The kidneys are able to maintain the chemical composition of fluids within normal limits until more than 50% of functional renal capacity is destroyed by disease or injury. Chronic renal insufficiency, or *chronic renal failure (CRF),* begins when the diseased kidneys can no longer maintain the normal chemical structure of body fluids under normal conditions. Progressive deterioration over months or years produces a variety of clinical and biochemical disturbances that eventually culminate in the clinical syndrome known as *uremia.*

A variety of diseases and disorders can result in CRF. The most frequent causes are congenital renal and urinary tract malformations, vesicoureteral reflux associated with recurrent urinary tract infection, chronic pyelonephritis, hereditary disorders, chronic glomerulonephritis, and glomerulonephropathy associated with systemic diseases such as anaphylactoid purpura and lupus erythematosus.

Pathophysiology

Early in the course of progressive nephrotic destruction, the child remains asymptomatic with only minimal biochemical abnormalities. Unless the presence of CRF is detected during the process of routine assessment, signs and symptoms that indicate advanced renal damage frequently emerge only late in the course of the disease. Midway in the disease process, as increasing numbers of nephrons are totally destroyed and most others are damaged to varying degrees, the few that remain intact are hypertrophied but functional. These few normal nephrons are able to make sufficient adjustments to stresses to maintain reasonable degrees of fluid and electrolyte balance. Definitive biochemical examination at this time will reveal restricted tolerance to excesses or restrictions. As the disease progresses to the end stage, because of a severe reduction in the number of functioning nephrons, the kidneys are no longer able to maintain fluid and electrolyte balance, and the features of uremic syndrome appear.

The accumulation of various biochemical substances in the blood, those that result from diminished renal function, produces complications such as the following:

- Retention of waste products, especially the blood urea nitrogen and creatinine
- Water and sodium retention, which contributes to edema and vascular congestion
- Hyperkalemia of dangerous levels
- Metabolic acidosis of a sustained nature because of continual hydrogen ion retention and bicarbonate loss
- Calcium and phosphorus disturbances, resulting in altered bone metabolism, which in turn causes growth arrest or retardation, bone pain, and deformities known as *renal osteodystrophy*
- Anemia caused by hematologic dysfunction, including shortened life span of red blood cells, impaired red blood cell production related to decreased production of erythropoietin, prolonged bleeding time, and nutritional anemia
- Growth disturbance, probably caused by such factors as renal osteodystrophy, poor nutrition associated with dietary restrictions and loss of appetite, and biochemical abnormalities

Children with CRF seem to be more susceptible to infection, especially pneumonia, urinary tract infection, and septicemia, although the reason for this is unclear. These children become extraordinarily sensitive to changes in vascular volume that may cause pulmonary overload, central nervous system symptoms, hypertension, and cardiac failure.

Diagnostic Evaluation

The diagnosis of CRF is usually suspected on the basis of any number of clinical manifestations, a history of prior renal disease, or biochemical findings. The onset is usually gradual, and the initial signs and symptoms are vague and nonspecific (Box 50-7).

Laboratory and other diagnostic tools and tests are of value in assessing the extent of renal damage, biochemical disturbances, and related physical dysfunction (see Tables 50-1 to 50-3). Often they can help establish the nature of the underlying disease and differentiate between other disease processes and the pathologic consequences of renal dysfunction.

Therapeutic Management

In irreversible renal failure the goals of medical management are to (1) promote maximal renal function, (2) maintain body fluid and electrolyte balance within safe biochemical limits, (3) treat systemic complications, and (4) promote as active and normal a life as possible for the child for as long as possible. The child is allowed unrestricted activity and is allowed to set his or her own limits regarding rest and extent of exertion. School attendance is encouraged as long as the child is able. When the effort is too great, home tutoring is arranged.

Diet regulation is the most effective means, short of dialysis, for reducing the quantity of materials that require renal excretion. The goals of the diet in renal failure are to provide sufficient calories and protein for growth while limiting the excretory demands made on the kidney, to minimize metabolic bone disease *(osteodystrophy),* and to minimize fluid and electrolyte disturbances. Dietary protein intake is limited only to the recommended daily allowance (RDA) for the child's age. Restriction of protein intake below the RDA is

BOX 50-7

Clinical Manifestations of Chronic Renal Failure

Early signs:
- Loss of normal energy
- Increased fatigue on exertion
- Pallor, subtle (may not be noticed)
- Elevated blood pressure (sometimes)

As the disease progresses:
- Decreased appetite (especially at breakfast)
- Less interest in normal activities
- Increased or decreased urine output with compensatory intake of fluid
- Pallor more evident
- Sallow, muddy appearance of skin

Child may complain of the following:
- Headache
- Muscle cramps
- Nausea

Other signs and symptoms:
- Weight loss
- Facial edema
- Malaise
- Bone or joint pain
- Growth retardation
- Dryness or itching of the skin
- Bruised skin
- Sensory or motor loss (sometimes)
- Amenorrhea (common in adolescent girls)

Uremic syndrome (untreated):
- Gastrointestinal symptoms
  - Anorexia
  - Nausea and vomiting
- Bleeding tendencies
  - Bruises
  - Bloody diarrheal stools
  - Stomatitis
  - Bleeding from lips and mouth
  - Intractable itching
- Uremic frost (deposits of urea crystals on skin)
- Unpleasant "uremic" breath odor
- Deep respirations
- Hypertension
- Congestive heart failure
- Pulmonary edema
- Neurologic involvement
  - Progressive confusion
  - Dulled sensorium
  - Coma (ultimately)
  - Tremors
  - Muscular twitching
  - Seizures

believed to negatively affect growth and neurodevelopment. Malnutrition may develop in patients with CRF even before they need dialysis (Steiber, 1999).

Sodium and water are not usually limited unless there is evidence of edema or hypertension, and potassium is not usually restricted. However, restrictions of any or all three may be imposed in later stages or at any time that abnormal serum concentrations are evident.

Dietary phosphorus is controlled to prevent or correct the calcium/phosphorus imbalance by the reduction of protein and milk intake. Phosphorus levels can be further reduced by oral administration of calcium carbonate preparations that combine with the phosphorus to decrease gastrointestinal absorption and thus the serum levels of phosphate. At the same time that serum calcium levels are increased from the calcium carbonate, vitamin D therapy is begun to increase calcium absorption.

Metabolic acidosis is alleviated through administration of alkalizing agents such as sodium bicarbonate or a combination of sodium and potassium citrate.

Growth failure is one major consequence of CRF, especially in the preadolescent. These children grow poorly both before and after the initiation of hemodialysis. The use of recombinant human growth hormone to accelerate growth in children with growth retardation secondary to CRF has been successful (Mehls et al, 2002; Schaefer et al, 1999). *Osseous deformities* that result from renal osteodystrophy, especially those related to ambulation, are troublesome and require correction if they occur. *Dental defects* are common in children with CRF, and the earlier the onset of the disease, the more severe the dental manifestations (including hypoplasia, hypomineralization, tooth discolorization, alteration in size and shape of teeth, malocclusion, and ulcerative stomatitis). Therefore regular dental care is especially important in these children.

Anemia in children with CRF is related to decreased production of erythropoietin. Recombinant human erythropoietin (rHuEPO) is being offered to these children as thrice-weekly or weekly subcutaneous injections and is replacing the need for frequent blood transfusions. The drug corrects the anemia and in turn increases appetite, activity, and general well-being in the children who receive it.

Hypertension of advanced renal disease may be managed initially by cautious use of a low-sodium diet, fluid restriction, and perhaps diuretics such as hydrochlorothiazide or furosemide. Severe hypertension requires the use of antihypertensive agents, singly or in combinations.

Intercurrent infections are treated with appropriate antimicrobials at the first sign of infection; however, any drug eliminated through the kidneys is administered with caution. Other complications are treated symptomatically (e.g., central-acting antiemetics for *nausea*, antiepileptics for *seizures*, and diphenhydramine [Benadryl] for *pruritus*).

Once evidence of *end-stage renal disease (ESRD)* appears in a child, the disease runs its relentless course and results in death in a few weeks, unless waste products and toxins are removed from body fluids by dialysis or kidney transplantation. Because these techniques have been adapted for infants and small children, these alternatives have been implemented in most cases of renal failure after conservative management is no longer effective (see Technologic Management of Renal Failure, p. 1665).

Prognosis

Dialysis and transplantation are the only treatments currently available for children with ESRD. Although children may survive on dialysis, it is not an ideal long-term modality. Complications include infection of access sites, growth failure, and disruption of normal socialization. Many pediatric centers encourage families of children with ESRD to consider renal transplantation. The North American Renal Transplantation in Children Report of the Pediatric Renal Transplant Cooperative Study reports a graft survival rate of 90% at 1 year and 74% at 6 years for living donor kidneys, and 80% at 1 year and 58% at 6 years for cadaver kidneys (Benfield et al, 2003).

Posttransplant complications include infection, hypertension, steroid toxicity, hyperlipidemia, aseptic necrosis, malignancy, and growth retardation (Suthanthiran & Strom, 1994). Long-term graft survival is not guaranteed, and many children require a second or third transplant. Successful renal transplantation does improve rehabilitation of children with CRF, both educationally and psychologically. Increasing use of primary or preemptive renal transplants is becoming the optimum form of renal replacement therapy, leading to substantial improvement in quality of life (Laine et al, 1998).

Nursing Care Management

Assessment

Assessment of the child with CRF is primarily one of observation for signs of complications and evidence of improvement through therapy. Some of the first changes observed are growth failure, developmental delay, bone disease, and hypertension.

Nursing Diagnoses

A number of nursing diagnoses become evident on assessment of the child. The most relevant in the majority of cases are outlined in the Nursing Care Plan on pp. 1666-1667. Others will be appropriate for individual children and their families.

Plan of Care and Implementation

The goals of care for the child with CRF, especially one in ESRD, and the child's family are as follows:

1. Child will receive encouragement in his or her normal growth and development, minimizing the impact of the disease process.
2. Child will remain free of complications.
3. Child and family will receive appropriate support, guidance, and education.

The multiple complications of ESRD are managed according to medical protocols prescribed for the care of those specific problems. However, progressive disease places a number of stresses on the child and family, including those of a potentially fatal illness (see Chapter 41). There is a continuing need for repeated examinations that often entail painful procedures, side effects, and frequent hospitalizations. Diet therapy becomes progressively more restricted and intense, and the child is required to take a variety of medications. Ever present in all aspects of the treatment regimen is the agonizing realization that without treatment, death is inevitable.

Some specific stresses related to ESRD and its treatment are predictable. When it first becomes apparent that ESRD is inevitable, both parents and child experience depression and anxiety. Acceptance is particularly difficult if renal failure progresses rapidly after diagnosis. Denial and disbelief are usually pronounced, especially among the parents. After kidney failure is established and symptoms become progressively more distressing, the initiation of dialysis is usually perceived as a positive experience, and after experiencing initial concerns regarding the treatment, the child begins to feel better and parental anxiety is relieved for a time.

Initiating a dialysis regimen is a traumatic and anxiety-provoking experience for most children, because it involves surgery for implantation of a graft, fistula, or peritoneal catheter. The initial experience with the dialysis procedure is frightening to most children. They need reassurance about the nature of the preparations for dialysis and the conduct of the treatment.

Both the graft and the fistula require needle insertions at each dialysis. The goal is to perform pain-free venipuncture. Using buffered lidocaine with a small-gauge needle (30 gauge) to anesthetize the area before venipuncture of the graft/fistula is one method. Using an anesthetizing topical preparation such as EMLA (eutectic mixture of local anesthetics [lidocaine and prilocaine]) 1 hour before venipuncture is another approach (see Pain Management, Chapter 44).

External dual-lumen venous access devices eliminate the need for needles but are more prone to infection and other central line complications.

Adolescents, with their increased need for independence and their urge for rebellion, usually adapt less well. They resent the control and enforced dependence imposed by the rigorous and unrelenting therapy program. They resent being dependent on hemodialysis technology, their parents, and the professional staff. Depression and hostility are common in adolescents undergoing hemodialysis.

The availability of home peritoneal dialysis has offered a greater degree of freedom for persons undergoing long-term dialysis. The nurse is responsible for teaching the family about (1) the disease, its implications, and the therapeutic plan; (2) the possible psychologic effects of the disease and the treatment; and (3) the technical aspects of the procedure. The family learns to manage the various aspects of the dialysis procedure, how to maintain accurate records, and how to observe for signs of complications that need to be reported to the proper persons.

Body changes related to the disease process, such as skin color, growth retardation, and lack of sexual maturation, are stress provoking. Dietary restrictions are particularly burdensome for both children and parents. Children feel deprived when they are unable to eat foods previously enjoyed and that are unrestricted for other family members. Consequently, failure to cooperate may occur. Diet restrictions may be interpreted as punishment. Some children, unable to understand fully the purpose of restrictions, will sneak forbidden food items at every opportunity. Allowing children, especially adolescents, maximum participation in and responsibility for their own treatment program is helpful.

Family Focus

FAMILY PRIORITIES

Families who have children with long-term chronic illnesses, such as end-stage renal disease, spend much time in hospitals, outpatient clinics, and primary health care facilities. When they miss appointments or respond less quickly than anticipated, sometimes they are quickly labeled "noncompliant." It is important to remember that families have to develop priorities for the unit as a whole. Sometimes the family may decide that it is more important for the parent to go to work or to attend a sibling's school performance than to attend an appointment scheduled for them by health care personnel. The chronically ill child cannot and should not always be the number one priority for the family. The professional staff who works with the family can help the parents prioritize the needs of the ill child within the needs of the family constellation.

Teresa Hall, MS, RN
Hathaway Children's Services
Sylmar, CA

After months or years of dialysis, the parents and child feel anxiety associated with the prognosis and continued pressures of the treatment. The relentless need for treatment interferes with family plans. The time spent in transportation to and from the dialysis unit and the time spent undergoing dialysis treatments cut into time for outside activities, including school. Graft and fistula problems, as well as peritoneal catheter exit site infections, may develop and are a common source of aggravation (Family Focus box).

The possibility of renal transplantation often provides hope for relief from the rigors of hemodialysis and peritoneal dialysis. Most children and families respond well to a kidney transplant, and most children can be successfully rehabilitated.

The National Kidney Foundation* and other agencies provide a number of services and information for families of children with renal disease.

Evaluation

The effectiveness of nursing interventions is determined by continual reassessment and evaluation of care based on the following observational guidelines:

1. Observe and interview family members regarding their compliance with the medical and dietary regimen.
2. Monitor vital signs, growth measurements, laboratory reports, behavior, and appearance.
3. Observe and interview child and family regarding their feelings, concerns, and fears; observe reactions to therapies and prognosis.

The *expected outcomes* are described in the Nursing Care Plan on pp. 1666-1667.

*30 East 33rd Street, New York, NY 10016; phone: 212-889-2210 or 800-622-9010; Web site: www.kidney.org. In Canada: Kidney Foundation of Canada, 300-5165, Sherbrooke Street West, Montreal, QC H4A 1T6; phone: 514-369-4806 or 800-361-7494; Web site: www.kidney.ca.

TECHNOLOGIC MANAGEMENT OF RENAL FAILURE

Dialysis

Dialysis is the process of separating colloids and crystalline substances in solution by the difference in their rate of diffusion through a semipermeable membrane. Methods of dialysis currently available for clinical management of renal failure are *peritoneal dialysis,* wherein the abdominal cavity acts as a semipermeable membrane through which water and solutes of small molecular size move by osmosis and diffusion according to their respective concentrations on either side of the membrane, and *hemodialysis,* in which blood is circulated outside the body through artificial membranes that permit a similar passage of water and solutes. A third type of dialysis is *hemofiltration,* in which blood filtrate is circulated outside the body by hydrostatic pressure exerted across a semipermeable membrane with simultaneous infusion of a replacement solution. Types of hemofiltration include *continuous venovenous hemofiltration (CVVH), continuous venovenous hemodialysis (CVVHD),* and *continuous venovenous hemodiafiltration (CVVHDF).* These continuous renal replacement therapies are used in cases of ARF, severe fluid overload, and inborn errors of metabolism, as well as after bone marrow transplantation (Goldstein, 2003).

Peritoneal dialysis is the preferred form of dialysis for infants, children and parents who wish to remain independent, families who live a long distance from the medical center, and children who prefer fewer dietary restrictions and a gentler form of dialysis. Chronic peritoneal dialysis is most often performed at home. The two types of peritoneal dialysis are *continuous ambulatory peritoneal dialysis (CAPD)* and *continuous cycling peritoneal dialysis (CCPD).* In both methods, commercially available sterile dialysis solution is instilled into the peritoneal cavity through a surgically implanted indwelling catheter tunneled subcutaneously and sutured into place. The warmed solution is allowed to enter the peritoneal cavity by gravity and remains a variable length of time according to the rate of solute removal and glucose absorption in individual patients. The care and management of the procedure are the responsibility of the parents of young children. Use of home health nurses to give parents respite from care has been initiated in some centers (Cascio et al, 1994). Older children and adolescents can carry out the procedure themselves, which provides them with some control and less dependency. This is especially important for adolescents.

NURSE ALERT Observe for changes in the color of the dialysate draining from the child. The spent solution should be clear. If the color is cloudy, notify the practitioner immediately (Schaefer, 2003). ■

Hemodialysis requires the creation of a vascular access and the use of special dialysis equipment—the hemodialyzer, or so-called artificial kidney. Vascular access may be one of three types: fistulas, grafts, or external vascular access devices. An *arteriovenous fistula* is an access in which a vein

Nursing Care Plan

THE CHILD WITH CHRONIC RENAL FAILURE

NURSING DIAGNOSIS: Risk for injury related to accumulated electrolytes and waste products

EXPECTED OUTCOME
Child exhibits no evidence of accumulation of waste products and no evidence of injury.

NURSING INTERVENTIONS/*RATIONALES*

Provide diet low in protein, potassium, sodium, and phosphorus; high in calories and calcium; and supplemented with essential amino acids as ordered *to reduce excretory demand on kidneys.*

Assist and monitor renal or peritoneal dialysis as prescribed *to maintain excretory function.*

Administer potassium-removing resins as prescribed *to reduce potassium levels;* antihypertensives *for hypertension;* diuretics *for edema;* phosphate binders *for hyperphosphatemia;* antiinfectives *for infection;* and antipruritics *for itching.*

Monitor for signs of accumulating waste products (e.g., elevated blood urea nitrogen, creatinine; hyperkalemia, hyperphosphatemia; muscle twitching; muscle cramps; anorexia, nausea, vomiting; hypertension; pruritis; yellowing skin; confusion, lethargy) *to ensure prompt treatment.*

Balance activity and rest and plan appropriate activities *to reduce fatigue and chances of injury.*

Provide meticulous skin care and avoid shearing and frictional forces *to reduce injury to skin.*

NURSING DIAGNOSIS: Fluid volume excess related to failure of renal regulatory mechanisms

EXPECTED OUTCOME
Child exhibits no evidence of increase in fluid accumulation.

NURSING INTERVENTIONS/*RATIONALES*

Instruct child and family about fluid restrictions and strategize ways to maintain those restrictions (e.g., keep mouth moist with hard candies, gum, ice chips; keep lips lubricated; divide fluids into small, even quantities throughout day) *to decrease chances of fluid overload.*

Monitor intake and output, weight changes, and girth measurements *to track fluid accumulation.*

NURSING DIAGNOSIS: Altered nutrition: less than body requirements related to restricted diet and loss of appetite

EXPECTED OUTCOME
Child exhibits adequate and appropriate food intake.

NURSING INTERVENTIONS/*RATIONALES*

Provide dietary instructions for child and family, including allowed foods, recipes, and menus, *to increase successful use of restrictive diet and to reduce excretory demand on kidneys.*

NURSING DIAGNOSIS: Body-image/self-esteem disturbance related to altered appearance, chronic illness, frequent treatments, feelings of being different

EXPECTED OUTCOME
Child exhibits signs of acceptance of self and of alteration in appearance; child exhibits signs of coping with disease process.

NURSING INTERVENTIONS/*RATIONALES*

Relate to child on appropriate cognitive level, conveying an attitude of caring and acceptance, *to encourage positive feelings about self;* serve as role model for others *to foster positive attitudes of acceptance toward child.*

Encourage child to verbalize feelings and perceptions about CRF (e.g., repeated treatments and hospitalizations, feelings of differentness, implications of functional limits, difficulty in making friends, views of self) *to facilitate coping and open expression of problems, fears, wants, wishes, and needs.*

Have child identify strengths, assets, and things he or she likes about self *to increase positive feelings about self and abilities.*

Support positive coping behaviors.

Involve child in care and management of disease *to promote a sense of control, independence, and self-esteem.*

Introduce child to other children who have similar disabilities; arrange for support groups for child and parents *to increase coping skills.*

Refer child for counseling if needed *to enhance adaptation.*

Encourage use of regular hygiene and grooming practices *to promote positive appearance.*

NURSING DIAGNOSIS: Impaired social interaction related to repeated hospitalizations, confinement, activity intolerance

EXPECTED OUTCOME
Child engages in appropriate family and peer interactions.

NURSING INTERVENTIONS/*RATIONALES*

Encourage regular school attendance and promote peer contacts *to provide opportunity to develop and maintain peer relationships.*

Encourage selection of play activities and recreational outlets *that encourage interaction;* restrict time spent in solo activities *that promote social isolation.*

Encourage contact with peers and siblings by telephone or visit when hospitalized or confined *to maintain social interaction and reduce sense of isolation.*

Plan specific periods of developmentally appropriate diversional activity suited to child's physical condition and energy level *to decrease feelings of boredom and negative self-absorption.*

Nursing Care Plan

THE CHILD WITH CHRONIC RENAL FAILURE—cont'd

NURSING DIAGNOSIS: Altered family processes related to child with chronic illness

EXPECTED OUTCOME

Family exhibits adaptation of usual roles and functions to accommodate special needs of child; family exhibits growth-promoting behaviors.

NURSING INTERVENTIONS/*RATIONALES*

Provide opportunity for family to absorb and adjust to diagnosis (e.g., repeat information *to allow time for family to hear and understand;* encourage expression of concerns, fears, and feelings about diagnosis and potential impact *to facilitate adjustment;* identify support systems *to provide resources for coping*).

Assist family to understand expected treatment, rationales, and implications *to provide a sound basis for decision making.*

Explore family members' reaction to child, assist them to achieve a realistic view of child's abilities and limitations, encourage family in attempts to promote child growth and development, have family emphasize what child can do, and explore ways for family to include child in family activities *to help family increase abilities to cope with and incorporate child into family structure.*

Arrange for and participate in family conferences *to provide forum for communication, mutual goal setting, and effective strategizing.*

Have parents spend special time with siblings *so that they do not feel neglected or left out.*

Identify additional resource systems (e.g., relatives, friends, church, health care services, community programs) and strategize with family about making good use of these systems *to develop broad base of support.*

Provide a system of ongoing follow-up and evaluation *to ensure long-term adaptation to challenges presented to family functioning by a child with chronic disease.*

and an artery are connected surgically. The preferred site is the radial artery and a forearm vein, which produces dilation and thickening of the superficial vessels of the forearm to provide easy access for repeated venipuncture. An alternative is the creation of a subcutaneous (internal) *arteriovenous graft* by anastomosing artery and vein, with a synthetic prosthetic graft for circulatory access. The most commonly used material is expanded polytetrafluoroethylene (ePTFE). Both the graft and the fistula require needle insertions with each dialysis treatment.

For external vascular access devices, percutaneous catheters are inserted in the femoral, subclavian, or internal jugular veins, even in very small children. A more permanent form of external access is available via a central catheter inserted surgically into the internal jugular vein. This catheter has a dual lumen, which allows a larger volume of blood flow with minimum recirculation. Catheters eliminate the need for skin punctures but may require some home care.

Hemodialysis is best suited to children who do not have someone in the family who is able to perform home peritoneal dialysis and to those who live close to a dialysis center. The procedure is usually performed three times per week for 4 to 6 hours, depending on the size of the child. Hemodialysis achieves rapid correction of fluid and electrolyte abnormalities but can cause problems in association with this rapid change, such as muscle cramping and hypotension. Disadvantages include school absence during dialysis and strict fluid and dietary restrictions between dialysis sessions. Boredom for the child and family is often a problem during dialysis, and planned activities should be introduced (Fig. 50-3) (Currier & Brewer, 1999).

Most children show rapid clinical improvement with the implementation of dialysis, although it is directly related to the duration of uremia before dialysis and good nutrition. Growth rate and skeletal maturation improve, but recovery of normal growth occurs infrequently. In many cases, sexual development, although delayed, progresses to completion.

Transplantation

Renal transplantation is now an acceptable and effective means of therapy in the pediatric age group. Although peritoneal dialysis and hemodialysis are life preserving, both require major alterations in lifestyle. Transplantation offers the opportunity for a relatively normal life and is the preferred form of treatment for children with ESRD. Primary or preemptive transplants maintain the greatest amount of normalcy in the family's life.

Kidneys for transplant are available from two sources: a *living related donor (LRD),* usually a parent or a sibling, or a *cadaver donor (CAD),* wherein the family of a dead or brain-dead patient consents to donation of a healthy kidney. Retransplantation occurs frequently.

The primary goal in transplantation is the long-term survival of grafted tissue by securing tissue that is antigenically similar to that of the recipient and by suppressing the recipient's immune mechanism. The immunosuppressant therapy of choice has been corticosteroids (prednisone) in conjunction with cyclosporine and azathioprine. Other ther-

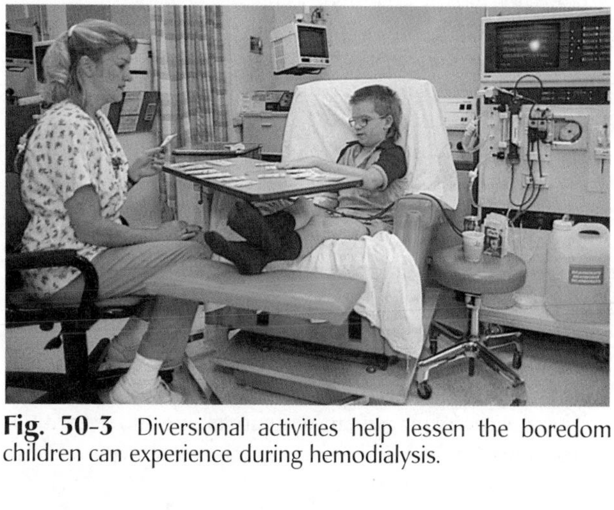

Fig. 50-3 Diversional activities help lessen the boredom children can experience during hemodialysis.

apies include antilymphoblast globulin and monoclonal antibodies. New immunosuppressant medications are rapidly coming into clinical trials and into use in large transplant centers. It is important for the nurse to learn about the medications and their side effects used in the antirejection protocols. Because the immunosuppressant medications are taken indefinitely, transplant patients experience many side effects of the drugs, including hypertension, growth retardation, cataracts, risk of infection, obesity, characteristics of Cushing syndrome, and hirsutism (Currier, McCarley, & Brewer, 2001).

NURSE ALERT The child with a recent kidney transplant (a few days) or one who was grafted approximately 6 months previously who exhibits any of the following should be evaluated immediately for possible rejection:

- Fever
- Swelling and tenderness over graft area
- Diminished urine output
- Elevated blood pressure ■

Rejection of the transplanted kidney is the most common cause of transplant failure. Rejection is treated aggressively with immunosuppressant medications and can often be reversed. Some patients do not respond to treatment of acute rejection or develop chronic rejection and must eventually return to dialysis or undergo another kidney transplant.

Key Points

- Common inflammatory disorders of the genitourinary tract include urinary tract infection, nephrotic syndrome, and acute glomerulonephritis.
- Management of urinary tract infections is directed at eliminating infection, detecting and correcting functional or anatomic abnormalities, preventing recurrences, and preserving renal function.
- Vesicoureteral reflux is the retrograde flow of bladder urine into the ureters.
- Obstructive uropathy is a result of structural or functional abnormalities of the urinary system that obstruct the normal flow of urine.
- The more common defects of the genitourinary tract include phimosis, cryptorchidism, inguinal hernia, hydrocele, and hypospadias.
- Body-image concerns and castration anxiety are particularly intense in children with defects in the genital area.
- Nephrotic syndrome is characterized by increased glomerular permeability to protein, with massive urinary loss of protein resulting in hypoproteinemia and edema.
- Management of nephrotic syndrome is aimed at reducing excretion of protein, reducing or preventing fluid retention by tissues, and preventing infection and other complications.
- Common features of acute glomerulonephritis are oliguria, edema, hypertension, circulatory congestion, hematuria, and proteinuria.
- Therapeutic management of acute glomerulonephritis is maintenance of fluid balance, treatment of hypertension, and antibiotic therapy.
- Management of hemolytic-uremic syndrome is aimed at control of complications and hematologic manifestations of renal failure.
- Wilms' tumor is the most common malignant neoplasm of the kidney in infants and children.
- In acute renal failure, management is directed at determining treatment of the underlying cause, management of complications of renal failure, and supportive therapy.
- Abnormalities in chronic renal failure are waste product retention, water and sodium retention, hyperkalemia, acidosis, calcium and phosphorus disturbance, anemia, and growth disturbances.
- The types of dialysis used in end-stage renal disease are peritoneal dialysis and hemodialysis.
- When the child will need home dialysis, the nurse educates the family about the disease, its implications, the therapeutic plan, possible psychologic effects of the disease, and the treatment and technical aspects of the procedure.
- The major concerns in renal transplantation are tissue matching and prevention of rejection; psychologic concerns involve self-image as related to possible body changes as a result of the effects of corticosteroid therapy.

Answer Guidelines to Critical Thinking Exercise

Urinary Tract Infection and Constipation

1. Yes. Ginger's mother reports a history of constipation with large, hard-formed stools occurring only every 3 to 4 days. She was diagnosed with a UTI severe enough to be admitted to the hospital.
2. (a) The structure of the lower urinary tract is believed to account for the increased incidence of bacteriuria in females. (b) A history of hard, large stools occurring every 3 to 4 days is not a normal elimination pattern for 4-year-old children. (c) The presence of a large stool mass within the colon is likely to cause pressure on the bladder and urethra and not allow the bladder to empty completely. Stasis of the urine can lead to infection.
3. The first priority at this time is to begin treatment for the UTI. Ginger's diet and fluid intake should be evaluated, and a plan to prevent constipation in the future should be developed.
4. Yes. Ginger's history reflects chronic problems with constipation that must be addressed.
5. Ginger might have other risk factors associated with UTIs in children, and this should be explored further. The single most important host factor influencing the occurrence of UTI is urinary stasis. Other possible causes of urinary stasis may need to be considered.

References

American Academy of Pediatrics: Task Force on Circumcision, *Pediatrics* 103(3):686-693, 1999.

Benfield MR et al: Changing trends in pediatric transplantation: 2001 annual report of the North American Pediatric Renal Transplant Cooperative Study, *Pediatr Transplant* 7(4):321-335, 2003.

Brandt JR et al: More on *E. coli*–induced hemolytic-uremic syndrome, *J Pediatr* 125(4):519-526, 1994.

Cascio C et al: Use of private duty nurses for daily CCPD and family relief in pediatric PD patients, *Adv Perit Dial* 10:304-306, 1994.
Currier H, Brewer ED: Pediatric hemodialysis. In Gutch CF, Stoner MH, Corea AL (eds): *Review of hemodialysis for nurses and dialysis personnel,* ed 6, St Louis, 1999, Mosby.
Currier H, McCarley PB, Brewer ED: The pediatric renal failure-dialysis-transplant patient. In Lancaster L (ed): *ANNA core curriculum,* ed 4, Pitman, NJ, 2001, American Nephrology Nurses' Association.
Goldstein SL: Overview of pediatric renal replacement therapy in AFT, *Artificial Organs* 27(9):770-783, 2003.
Gundy PE et al: Wilms tumor. In Pizzo PA, Poplack DP (eds): *Principles and practices of pediatric oncology,* ed 4, Philadelphia, 2002, JB Lippincott.
Kass E: Timing of elective surgery on the genitalia of male children with particular reference to the risks, benefits, and psychological effects of surgery and anesthesia, *Pediatrics* 97(4):590-594, 1996.
Kline NE, Sevier N: Solid tumors in children, *J Pediatr Nurs* 18(2):96-102, 2003.
Laine J et al: Pediatric kidney transplantation, *Ann Med* 30(1):45-57, 1998.
Mehls O et al: Effectiveness of growth hormone treatment in short children with chronic renal failure, *J Pediatr* 141(1):147-148, 2002.
Rosenthal M: Current concept in managing UTIs in children, *Infect Dis Child* 17(3):30-31, 2004.
Schaefer F: Management of peritonitis in children receiving chronic peritoneal dialysis, *Paediatr Drugs* 5(5):315-325, 2003.
Schaefer F et al: Long-term experience with growth hormone treatment in children with chronic renal failure, *Perit Dial Int* 19(suppl 2):S467-S472, 1999.
Schlager TA et al: Effect of cranberry juice on bacteriuria in children with neurogenic bladder receiving intermittent catheterization, *J Pediatr* 135(6):698-702, 1999.
Steiber AL: Clinical indicators associated with poor oral intake of patients with chronic renal failure, *J Ren Nutr* 9(2):84-88, 1999.
Suthanthiran M, Strom TB: Renal transplantation, *N Engl J Med* 331(6):365-375, 1994.

Unit 11

51 Cerebral Dysfunction

LEARNING OBJECTIVES

On completion of this chapter the reader will be able to:

- Describe the various modalities for assessment of cerebral function.
- Differentiate between the stages of consciousness.
- Formulate a plan of care for the unconscious child.
- Distinguish between the types of head injuries and the serious complications.
- Describe the nursing care of a child with a tumor of the central nervous system.
- Outline a plan of care for the child with bacterial meningitis.
- Differentiate between the various types of seizure disorders.
- Demonstrate an understanding of the manifestations of a seizure disorder and the management of a child with such a disorder.
- Describe the preoperative and postoperative care of a child with hydrocephalus.

ELECTRONIC RESOURCES

Additional information related to the content in Chapter 51 can be found on

the companion website at evolve
http://evolve.elsevier.com/Wong/maternal/
- NCLEX Review Questions
- Case Study–Meningitis
- WebLinks

or the interactive student CD-ROM
Activities for Chapter 51 include the following:
- NCLEX Review Questions
- Case Study–Hydrocephalus with Myelomeningocele
- Critical Thinking Exercise–Seizures
- Nursing Care Plan–The Unconscious Child

CEREBRAL DYSFUNCTION

Assessment of Cerebral Function

Most of the information about the status of the brain is obtained by indirect measurements. Some of these measurements are discussed elsewhere in relation to numerous aspects of child care (e.g., as part of assessments of health [Chapter 35], newborn status [Chapter 25], mental retardation [Chapter 42], hypoxic injury [cerebral palsy, Chapter 55], and attainment of developmental milestones at each stage of development). Since increased intracranial pressure and altered states of consciousness have such prominent places in neurologic dysfunction, they are described here, followed by techniques for neurologic assessment and diagnostic tests.

General Aspects

Children younger than 2 years of age require special evaluation because they are unable to respond to directions designed to elicit specific neurologic responses in infants. Early neurologic responses in infants are primarily reflexive; these responses are gradually replaced by meaningful movement in the characteristic cephalocaudal direction of development. This evidence of progressive maturation reflects more extensive myelinization and changes in neurochemical and electrophysiologic properties.

Most information about infants and small children is gained by observing their spontaneous and elicited reflex responses as they develop increasingly complex locomotor and fine motor skills and by eliciting progressively sophisticated communicative and adaptive behaviors. Delay or deviation from expected milestones helps identify high risk children. Persistence or reappearance of reflexes that normally disappear indicates a pathologic condition. In evaluating the infant or young child, it is also important to obtain the pregnancy and delivery history to determine the possible effect of intrauterine environmental influences known to affect the orderly maturation of the central nervous system (CNS). These influences include maternal infections, chemicals, trauma, and metabolic insults.

General aspects of assessment that provide clues to the etiology of dysfunction include the following:

Family history—Sometimes offers clues regarding possible genetic disorders with neurologic manifestations

Health history—May provide valuable clues regarding the cause of dysfunction (e.g., an injury, short febrile illness, encounter with an animal or insect, ingestion of neurotoxic substances, inhalation of chemicals, a past illness, or known diabetes mellitus)

Physical evaluation of infants—Includes observation of the following:
- Size and shape of the head
- Spontaneous activity and postural reflex activity
- Sensory responses
- Attitude—normal flexed posture, extreme extension, opisthotonos, hypotonia
- Symmetry in movement of extremities
- Excessive tremulousness or frequent twitching movements
- Altered expiratory cycle:
  - Prolonged apnea
  - Ataxic breathing
  - Paradoxical chest movement
  - Hyperventilation
- Skin and hair texture
- Distinctive facial features
- Presence of a high-pitched, piercing cry
- Abnormal eye movements
- Inability to suck or swallow
- Lip smacking
- Asymmetric contraction of facial muscles
- Yawning (may indicate cranial nerve involvement)
- Muscular activity and coordination
- Level of development

Increased Intracranial Pressure

The brain, tightly enclosed in the solid bony cranium, is well protected but highly vulnerable to pressure that may accumulate within the enclosure. The cranium's total volume—brain (80%), cerebrospinal fluid (CSF) (10%), and blood (10%)—must remain approximately the same at all times. A change in the proportional volume of one of these components (e.g., increase or decrease in intracranial blood) must be accompanied by a compensatory change in another. In this way the volume and pressure normally remain constant. Examples of compensatory changes are reduction in blood volume, decrease in CSF production, increase in CSF absorption, or shrinkage of brain mass by displacement of intracellular and extracellular fluid. Children with open fontanels compensate by skull expansion and widened sutures. However, at any age the capacity for spatial compensation is limited. An increase in intracranial pressure (ICP) may be caused by tumors or other space-occupying lesions, accumulation of fluid within the ventricular system, bleeding, or edema of cerebral tissues. Once compensation is exhausted, any further increase in volume will result in a rapid rise in ICP.

Early signs and symptoms of increased ICP are often subtle and assume many patterns (Box 51-1). As pressure increases, signs and symptoms become more pronounced and the level of consciousness deteriorates.

BOX 51-1

Clinical Manifestations of Increased Intracranial Pressure in Infants and Children

Infants
- Tense, and/or bulging fontanel
- Separated cranial sutures
- Macewen sign (cracked-pot sound on percussion)
- Irritability
- High-pitched cry
- Increased occipitofrontal circumference
- Distended scalp veins
- Changes in feeding
- Crying when disturbed
- Setting-sun sign

Children
- Headache
- Nausea
- Vomiting
- Diplopia, blurred vision
- Seizures

Personality and Behavior Signs
- Irritability, restlessness
- Indifference, drowsiness
- Decline in school performance
- Diminished physical activity and motor performance
- Increased sleeping
- Memory loss
- Inability to follow simple commands
- Lethargy and drowsiness

Late Signs
- Bradycardia
- Lowered level of consciousness
- Decreased motor response to command
- Decreased sensory response to painful stimuli
- Alterations in pupil size and reactivity
- Decerebrate or decorticate posturing
- Cheyne-Stokes respirations
- Papilledema
- Coma

Altered States of Consciousness

Consciousness implies awareness—the ability to respond to sensory stimuli and have subjective experiences. There are two components of consciousness: *alertness,* an arousal-waking state, including the ability to respond to stimuli; and *cognitive power,* including the ability to process stimuli and produce verbal and motor responses.

An altered state of consciousness usually refers to varying states of unconsciousness that may be momentary or may extend for hours, days, or indefinitely. *Unconsciousness* is depressed cerebral function—the inability to respond to sensory stimuli and have subjective experiences. *Coma* is defined as a state of unconsciousness from which the patient cannot be aroused even with powerful stimuli.

Levels of Consciousness

Assessment of level of consciousness (LOC) remains the earliest indicator of improvement or deterioration in neurologic status. LOC is determined by observations of the child's responses to the environment. Other diagnostic tests, such as motor activity, reflexes, and vital signs, are more variable and do not necessarily directly parallel the depth of the comatose state. The most consistently used terms are described in Box 51-2.

BOX 51-2

Levels of Consciousness

Full consciousness—Awake and alert; oriented to time, place, and person; behavior appropriate for age
Confusion—Impaired decision making
Disorientation—Disorientation to time and place, decreased level of consciousness
Lethargy—Limited spontaneous movement, sluggish speech, drowsy
Obtundation—Arousable with stimulation
Stupor—Remains in a deep sleep, responsive only to vigorous and repeated stimulation
Coma—No motor or verbal response to noxious (painful) stimuli
Persistent vegetative state (PVS)—The permanently lost function of the cerebral cortex—eyes follow objects only by reflex or when attracted to the direction of loud sounds; all four limbs are spastic but can withdraw from painful stimuli; hands show reflexive grasping and groping; the face can grimace, some food may be swallowed, and the child may groan or cry but utters no words.

Modified from Seidel HM et al (eds): *Mosby's guide to physical examination,* ed 5, St Louis, 1999, Mosby.

Coma Assessment

Several scales have been devised in an attempt to standardize the description and interpretation of the degree of depressed consciousness. The most popular of these is the *Glasgow Coma Scale (GCS),* which consists of a three-part assessment: eye opening, verbal response, and motor response (Fig. 51-1). When LOC is being assessed in young children, it is often useful to have a parent present to help elicit a desired response. An infant or child may not respond in an unfamiliar environment or to unfamiliar voices. Children older than 3 years of age should be able to give their name, although they may not be cognizant of place or time.

Numeric values of 1 through 5 are assigned to the levels of response in each category. The sum of these numeric values provides an objective measure of the patient's LOC. The lower the score, the deeper the coma. A person with an unaltered LOC would score the highest, 15; a score of 8 or below is generally accepted as a definition of coma; the lowest score, 3, indicates deep coma. The Task Force for the Determination of Brain Death in Children has established physical examination criteria for cases of irreversible coma.

NURSE ALERT Lack of response to painful stimuli is abnormal and should be reported immediately. ■

Neurologic Examination

The purpose of the neurologic examination is to establish an accurate, objective baseline of neurologic information. It is essential that the neurologic examination be documented in a fashion that is able to be reproduced by others. This allows for a comparison of the findings that allows the observer to detect subtle changes in the neurologic status that might not otherwise be evident. Descriptions of behaviors should be simple, objective, and easily interpreted: "Drowsy but awake and conversationally rational/oriented"; "Sleepy but arousable with vigorous physical stimuli. Pressure to nail

NEUROLOGIC ASSESSMENT

Pupils	Right	Size	
		Reaction	
	Left	Size	
		Reaction	

++ = Brisk
\+ = Sluggish
− = No reaction
C = Eye closed by swelling

GLASGOW COMA SCALE

Eyes open	Spontaneously	4	
	To speech	3	
	To pain	2	
	None	1	
Best motor response	Obeys commands	6	
	Localizes pain	5	
	Flexion withdrawal	4	
	Flexion abnormal	3	
	Extension	2	
	None	1	

Usually record best arm or age-appropriate response

	>2 years		<2 years
Best response to auditory and/or visual stimulus	Orientation	5	5 Smiles, listens, follows
	Confused	4	4 Cries, consolable
	Inappropriate words	3	3 Inappropriate persistent cry
	Incomprehensible words	2	2 Agitated, restless
	None	1	1 No response
	Endotracheal tube or trach	T	
COMA SCALE TOTAL			

Pupil scale (mm): 1, 2, 3, 4, 5, 6, 7, 8

HAND GRIP:
Equal
Unequal
R____L
Weakness

LOC:
Alert/oriented x4
Sleepy
Irritable
Comatose
Disoriented
Combative
Lethargic
Awake
Sleeping
Drowsy
Agitated

MUSCLE TONE:
Normal
Arching
Spastic
Flaccid
Weak
Decorticate
Decerebrate
Other ________

EYE MOVEMENT:
Normal
Nystagmus
Strabismus
Other ________

FONTANEL/WINDOW:
Soft
Flat
Sunken
Tense
Bulging
Closed
Other ________

MOOD/AFFECT:
Happy
Content
Quiet
Withdrawn
Sad
Flat
Hostile

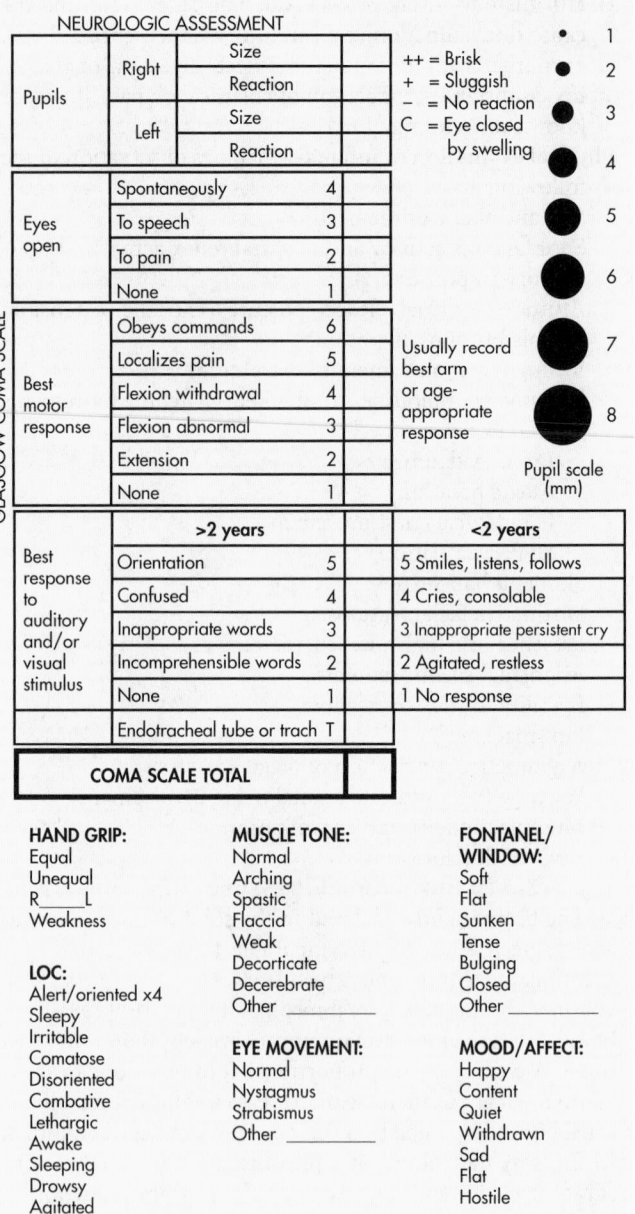

Fig. 51-1 Pediatric coma scale.

base of right hand results in upper extremity flexion/lower extremity extension."

Vital Signs

Pulse, respiration, and blood pressure provide information regarding the adequacy of circulation and the possible underlying cause of altered consciousness. Autonomic activity is most intensively disturbed in cases of deep coma or brainstem lesions.

Body temperature is often elevated, and sometimes the elevation may be extreme. Coma of a toxic origin may produce hypothermia. High temperature is most frequently a sign of an acute infectious process or heat stroke but may be caused by ingestion of some drugs (especially salicylates, alcohol, and barbiturates) or by intracranial bleeding, especially subarachnoid hemorrhage. Hypothalamic involvement may cause elevated or decreased temperature.

The *pulse* is variable and may be rapid, slow and bounding, or feeble. *Blood pressure* may be normal, elevated, or at shock levels. The Cushing reflex, or pressor response, which causes a slowing of the pulse and an increase in blood pressure, is uncommon in children; when it occurs, it is a very late sign. Vital signs are also affected by medications. For assessment purposes, actual *changes* in pulse and blood pressure are more important than the direction of the change.

Respirations are often slow, deep, and irregular. Slow, deep breathing is often seen in the heavy sleep caused by sedatives, after seizures, or in cerebral infections. Slow, shallow breathing may result from sedatives or opioids (narcotics). Hyperventilation (deep and rapid respirations) is usually a result of metabolic acidosis or abnormal stimulation of the respiratory center in the medulla caused by salicylate poisoning, hepatic coma, or Reye's syndrome.

Breathing patterns have been described with a number of terms (e.g., apneustic, cluster, ataxic, Cheyne-Stokes). However, it is better to describe what is being observed rather than placing a label on it because the traditional terms are often used and interpreted incorrectly. Periodic or irregular breathing is an ominous sign of brainstem (especially medullary) dysfunction that often precedes complete apnea. The *odor* of the breath may provide additional clues (e.g., the fruity, acetone odor of ketosis; the foul odor of uremia; the fetid odor of hepatic failure; or the odor of alcohol).

Skin

The skin may offer clues to the cause of unconsciousness. The body surface should be examined for the presence of injury, needle marks, petechiae, bites, and ticks. Evidence of toxic substances may be found on the hands, face, mouth, and clothing, especially in small children.

Eyes

Pupil size and reactivity are assessed (Fig. 51-2; see also Fig. 51-1). Pinpoint pupils are commonly observed in poisoning, such as opiate or barbiturate poisoning, or in brainstem dysfunction. Widely dilated and reactive pupils are often seen after seizures and may involve only one side. Dilated pupils may also be caused by eye trauma. Widely dilated and fixed pupils suggest paralysis of cranial nerve III secondary to pressure from herniation of the brain through the tentorium. A unilateral fixed pupil usually suggests a lesion on the same side. If pupils are fixed bilaterally for more than 5 minutes, brainstem damage is usually implied. Dilated and nonreactive pupils are also seen in hypothermia, anoxia, ischemia, poisoning with atropine-like substances, or prior instillation of mydriatic drugs.

NURSE ALERT The sudden appearance of a fixed and dilated pupil(s) is a neurosurgical emergency. ■

The description of eye movements should indicate whether one or both eyes are involved and how the reaction was elicited. The parents should be asked about preexisting strabismus, which will cause the eyes to appear normal under compromise. A posttraumatic strabismus indicates cranial nerve VI damage.

Special tests, usually performed by qualified persons, include the following:

Doll's head maneuver—Elicited by rotating the child's head quickly to one side and then to the other. Conjugate (paired or working together) movement of the eyes in the direction opposite to the head rotation is normal. Absence of this response suggests dysfunction of the brainstem or oculomotor nerve (cranial nerve III).

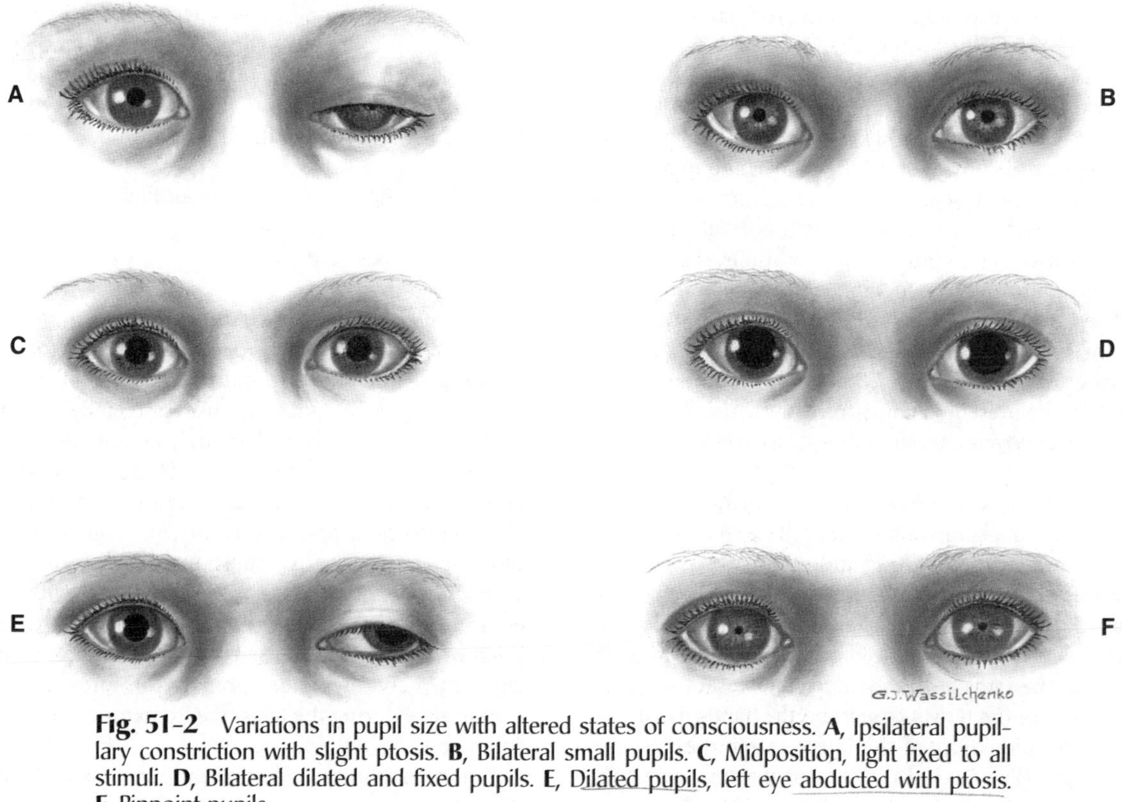

Fig. 51-2 Variations in pupil size with altered states of consciousness. **A**, Ipsilateral pupillary constriction with slight ptosis. **B**, Bilateral small pupils. **C**, Midposition, light fixed to all stimuli. **D**, Bilateral dilated and fixed pupils. **E**, Dilated pupils, left eye abducted with ptosis. **F**, Pinpoint pupils.

NURSE ALERT Any tests that require head movement are not attempted until after cervical spine injury has been ruled out. ■

Caloric test, or oculovestibular response—Elicited with the child's head up (head of bed is elevated 30 degrees) by irrigating the external auditory canal with 10 ml of ice water for 20 seconds, which normally causes conjugate movement of the eyes toward the side of stimulation. This movement is lost when the pontine centers are impaired, thus providing important information in assessment of the comatose patient.

NURSE ALERT The caloric test is painful and is never performed on a child who is awake or on an individual with a ruptured tympanic membrane. ■

Funduscopic examination—Reveals additional clues. Papilledema will not be evident early in the course of unconsciousness because it takes 24 to 48 hours to develop, if it develops at all. Papilledema is characterized by optic disc swelling, indistinct optic disc margins, hemorrhage, tortuosity of vessels, and absence of venous pulsations. The presence of preretinal (subhyaloid) hemorrhages in children is almost invariably a result of acute trauma with intracranial bleeding, usually subarachnoid or subdural hemorrhage.

Motor Function

Observing spontaneous activity, posture, and response to painful stimuli provides clues to the location and extent of cerebral dysfunction. Even subtle movements (e.g., the outward rotation of a hip) should be noted and the child observed for other signs. Asymmetric movements of the limbs or absence of movement suggests paralysis. In hemiplegia the affected limb lies in external rotation and will fall uncontrollably when lifted and allowed to drop. These observations should be described rather than labeled.

In the deeper comatose states, little or no spontaneous movement is present, and the musculature tends to be flaccid. There is considerable variability in the motor behavior in lesser degrees of coma. For example, the child may be relatively immobile or restless and hyperkinetic; muscle tone may be increased or decreased. Tremors, twitching, and spasms of muscles are common observations. The patient may display purposeless plucking or tossing movements. Combative or negativistic behavior is not uncommon. Hyperactivity is more common in acute febrile and toxic states than in cases of increased ICP. Seizures are common in children and may be present in coma from any cause. Any repetitive or seizure movements should be described.

Posturing

Because cortical control over motor function is lost in brain dysfunction, primitive postural reflexes emerge. These reflexes are evident in posturing and motor movements directly related to the area of the brain involved. *Decorticate posturing* (Fig. 51-3, *A*) is seen when dysfunction of the cerebral cortex is severe. Typical decorticate posturing includes adduction of the arms at the shoulders, flexion of the arms on the chest with the wrists flexed and the hands fisted, and extension and adduction of the lower extremities. *Decerebrate posturing* (Fig. 51-3, *B*), a sign of dysfunction at the level of the midbrain, is characterized by rigid extension and pronation of the arms and legs. The posturing may not be evident when the child is quiet but can usually be elicited by applying painful stimuli, such as a blunt object pressed on the base of the nail.

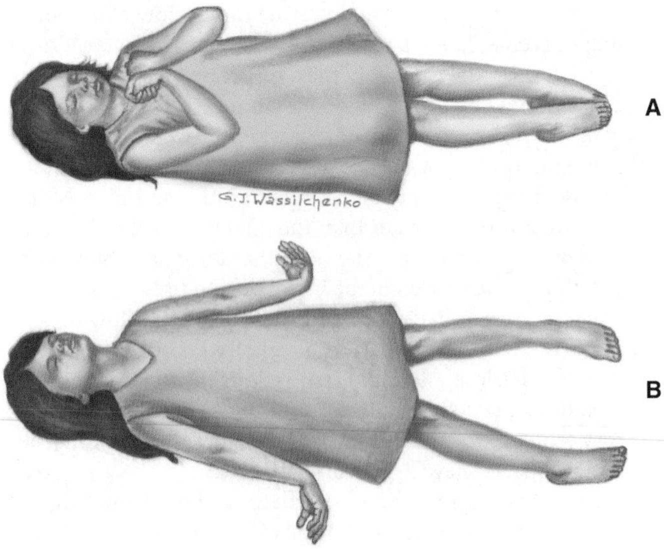

Fig. 51-3 **A**, Decorticate posturing. **B**, Decerebrate posturing.

Reflexes

Testing of some reflexes may be of limited value. In general, the corneal, pupillary, muscle-stretch, superficial, and plantar reflexes tend to be absent in deep coma. The state of reflexes is variable in lighter grades of unconsciousness and depends on the underlying pathologic process and the location of the lesion. Absence of corneal reflexes and presence of a tonic neck reflex are associated with severe brain damage. The Babinski reflex (see Extremities, Chapter 35) may be of value if it is found to be present consistently in children older than 18 months. A positive Babinski reflex is significant in assessment of pyramidal tract lesions when it is unilateral and associated with other pyramidal signs.

NURSE ALERT Three key reflexes that demonstrate neurologic health in young infants are the Moro, tonic neck, and withdrawal reflexes. ■

Special Diagnostic Procedures

Numerous diagnostic procedures are used for assessment of cerebral function. Laboratory tests that may help determine the cause of unconsciousness include blood glucose, urea nitrogen, and electrolyte (pH, sodium, potassium, chloride, calcium, and bicarbonate) tests; clotting studies, hematocrit, and a complete blood cell count; liver function tests; blood cultures (if fever is present); and sometimes studies to detect lead or other toxic substances, such as drugs.

Highly sophisticated tests are carried out with specialized equipment by skilled personnel. Most of these tests are outlined in Box 51-3. Because such tests can be threatening to children, a child will need preparation for and support and reassurance during the tests (see Preparation for Procedures, Chapter 45).

Children who are old enough to understand will require careful explanation of the procedure, why it is being done,

BOX 51-3

Procedures Used in Cerebral Assessment

Lumbar Puncture (LP)
Diagnostic: measures spinal fluid pressure, obtains cerebrospinal fluid (CSF) for visualization and laboratory analysis

Subdural Tap
Helps rule out subdural effusions
Relieves intracranial pressure

Electroencephalography (EEG)
Measures electric activity of cerebral cortex
Detects electric abnormalities
Used to determine brain death

Video EEG
Split-screen simultaneous visualization of whole-body, facial, and EEG recording

Computed Tomography (CT) Scan
Visualizes horizontal and vertical cross section of brain at any axis
Distinguishes density of various intracranial tissues and structures—congenital abnormalities, hemorrhage, tumors, and demyelinating and inflammatory processes

Nuclear Brain Scan
Test material accumulates in areas where blood-brain barrier is defective
Identifies focal brain lesions (e.g., tumors, abscesses)
Positive uptake of material with encephalitis and subdural hematoma
Visualizes CSF pathways

Transillumination
Varying degrees of localized glowing may be seen in abnormal fluid accumulation in various areas of head

Echoencephalography
Identifies shifts in midline structures from their normal positions as a result of intracranial lesions
May show ventricular dilation

Radiography
Shows fractures, dislocations, spreading suture lines, and craniostenosis
Shows degenerative changes, bone erosion, and calcifications

Magnetic Resonance Imaging (MRI)
Permits visualization of morphologic features of target structures
Permits tissue discrimination unavailable with many other techniques

Positron Emission Transaxial Tomography (PETT) or Positron Emission Tomography (PET)
Detects and measures such functions as blood volume and flow in brain, metabolic activity, and biochemical changes within tissues

Real-Time Ultrasonography (RTUS)
Allows high-resolution anatomic visualization in a variety of imaging planes

Digital Subtraction Angiography (DSA)
Visualizes vasculature of target tissue
Visualizes finite vascular abnormalities

what they will experience, and how they can help. School-age children usually appreciate a more detailed description of why contrast material is injected. The importance of lying still for tests must be stressed. Children unfamiliar with the machines can be shown a picture beforehand. Although radiographic examinations are not painful, the machinery is often so frightening in appearance that the child protests because of anxiety.

Tests such as computed tomography (CT) and magnetic resonance imaging (MRI) require that children be immobilized. Chin and cheek pads are sometimes used to prevent the slightest head movement, and straps are applied to the body to prevent any change in body position. The nurse can explain these events to a frightened child by comparing them to an astronaut's preparation for a space flight. It is very important to emphasize to the child that at no time is the procedure painful.

Usually young children are developmentally unable to cooperate, and sedation will be required. Numerous agents are used for sedation during diagnostic procedures; chloral hydrate remains a safe and frequently used medication before diagnostic imaging tests. The suggested oral chloral hydrate dose is as follows (Lee, Nechyba, & Gunn, 2002):

- 75 to 100 mg/kg (to a maximum dose of 1 g for infants and 2 g for children).
- If child is still awake after 20 minutes, supplementary doses of 100 mg/kg may be given up to a total dose of 1 g for infants and 2 g for children.
- The drug should be given 35 to 45 minutes before the anticipated imaging time.

It is helpful for nurses to become acquainted with the equipment and the general environment in which the test will take place so that they can better explain the procedure to children at their level of understanding. Equipment is often strange and ominous to children and may be perceived as a frightening monster. They need constant reassurance from a trusted companion. Because children are particularly frightened of needles, they need to be informed of any medication or contrast media to be administered intravenously.

Physical preparation may involve administering a sedative or providing intravenous (IV) access for infusion of contrast material. If so, children should be given a local topical anesthetic such as EMLA (eutectic mixture of local anesthetic) before the IV is placed and helped through the preparation and administration and assured that someone will remain with them (if possible). Children will need continual support and reinforcement during procedures for which they remain conscious. Vital signs and physiologic response to the procedure are monitored throughout. Conscious sedation records become part of the child's chart. Many diagnostic procedures performed on an outpatient basis require sedation, and children need recovery time and observation. Written instructions should be reviewed with parents if the child is discharged to home following a procedure.

Children who have undergone a procedure while under general anesthesia require postanesthesia care, including positioning to prevent aspiration of secretions and frequent assessment of vital signs and LOC. In addition, other neurologic functions, such as pupillary responses, motor strength, and movement, are tested at regular intervals. Any surgical wound resulting from the test is checked for bleeding, CSF leakage, and other complications. Children who undergo repeated subdural taps should have their hematocrit measured daily to detect any blood loss from the procedure.

Children's emotional reactions to procedures are also considered. They should be allowed to express their feelings about their experiences verbally and through the use of therapeutic play. Parents also seek—and are entitled to—an explanation of results of tests and procedures performed on their children. Nurses are in a unique position to provide support and education to parents regarding procedures.

NURSING CARE OF THE UNCONSCIOUS CHILD

The unconscious child requires continuous nursing attendance, with observation, recording, and evaluation of changes in objective signs. These observations provide valuable information regarding the patient's progress. Often they serve as a guide to diagnosis and treatment. Therefore careful and detailed observations are essential for the patient's welfare. In addition, vital functions must be maintained and complications prevented through conscientious and meticulous nursing care. The outcome of unconsciousness may be early with complete recovery, death within a few hours or days, persistent and permanent unconsciousness, or recovery with varying degrees of residual mental and/or physical disability. The outcome and recovery of the unconscious child may depend on the level of nursing care and observational skills.

Emergency measures are directed toward ensuring a patent airway, treatment of shock, and reduction of ICP (if present). Delayed treatment often leads to increased damage. As soon as emergency measures have been implemented—and in many cases concurrently—therapies for specific causes are begun. Because nursing care is closely related to medical management, both are considered here.

Assessment

Continual observation of LOC, pupillary reaction, and vital signs is essential to management of CNS disorders. Regular assessment of neurologic signs is a vital part of nursing comatose children. Vital signs are measured and recorded regularly. The frequency depends on the cause of coma, the status, and the progression of cerebral involvement. Intervals may be as short as every 15 minutes or as long as every 2 hours. Significant alterations are reported immediately. Temperature is taken every 2 to 4 hours, depending on the patient's condition.

An elevated temperature may occur in children with CNS dysfunction; therefore, a light covering is sufficient. Vigorous efforts, such as tepid sponge baths or application of a hypothermia blanket, are needed to prevent brain damage if temperature exceeds 40° C (104° F) rectally.

The LOC is assessed periodically, including size, equality, and reaction of pupils to light; as well as signs of meningeal irritation such as nuchal rigidity. Other aspects of LOC assessment include response to vocal commands, spontaneous behavior, resistance to care, and response to painful stimuli. Motions of any type, changes in muscle tone or strength, and body position are noted. Seizure activity is described according to the type and length of seizure and body areas involved (see Box 51-13). An antiepileptic drug such as phenytoin (Dilantin) or phenobarbital is ordered for control of seizure activity.

Pain management for the comatose child requires astute nursing observation and management. Signs of pain include changes in behavior (e.g., increased agitation and rigidity, alterations in physiologic parameters); increased heart rate, respiratory rate, and blood pressure; and decreased oxygen saturation. Since these findings are not specific for pain, the nurse should observe for their appearance during times of induced or suspected pain and their disappearance after the inciting procedure or the administration of analgesia. A pain assessment record should be used to document indications of pain and the effectiveness of interventions (see Pain Assessment, Chapter 44).

The use of opioids, such as morphine, to relieve pain is controversial because they may mask signs of altered consciousness or depress respirations. However, unrelieved pain activates the stress response, which can elevate ICP. In order to block the stress response, some authorities advocate the use of analgesics, sedatives, and, in some cases such as head injury, paralyzing agents via continuous IV infusion. A frequently used combination is fentanyl (Sublimaze), midazolam (Versed), and vecuronium (Norcuron). If there are concerns about assessing the LOC or respiratory depression, naloxone can be used to reverse the opioid effects. Acetaminophen and codeine may also be effective analgesics for mild to moderate pain. Regardless of which drugs are used, adequate dosage and regular administration are essential in order to provide optimal pain relief (see Pain Management, Chapter 44).

Other measures to relieve discomfort include providing a quiet, dimly lit environment; limiting visitors to a minimum; preventing any sudden, jarring movement, such as banging into the bed; and preventing an increase in ICP. The last is most effectively achieved by proper positioning and prevention of straining, such as during coughing, vomiting, or defecating.

NURSE ALERT When opioids are used, bowel elimination must be closely monitored because of the potential constipating effect. Stool softeners should be given with laxatives as needed to prevent constipation. ■

Nursing Diagnoses

Based on a thorough assessment, several nursing diagnoses are identified. The more common diagnoses for the unconscious child are included in the Nursing Care Plan on pp. 1682-1683. Others may apply in specific situations.

Plan of Care and Implementation

The goals for the unconscious child and the family include the following:

1. Child will maintain respiratory integrity.
2. Child will not experience increasing ICP.

3. Child will have basic needs (hygiene, nutrition, hydration, elimination) met.
4. Child will not experience complications of immobility.
5. Family will receive adequate support and education.

Respiratory Management

Respiratory effectiveness is the primary concern in the care of the unconscious child, and establishment of an adequate airway is *always* the first priority. Carbon dioxide has a potent vasodilating effect and will increase cerebral blood flow (CBF) and ICP. Cerebral hypoxia that lasts longer than 4 minutes nearly always causes irreversible brain damage.

NURSE ALERT Respiratory obstruction and subsequent compromise leads to cardiac arrest. Maintaining an adequate, patent airway is of the utmost importance. ■

Children in lighter states of coma may be able to cough and swallow, but those in deeper states are unable to handle secretions, which tend to pool in the throat and pharynx. Dysfunction of cranial nerves IX and X places the child at risk for aspiration and cardiac arrest; therefore, the child is positioned to prevent aspiration of secretions, and the stomach is emptied to reduce the likelihood of vomiting. In infants, blockage of air passages from secretions can happen in seconds. In addition, upper airway obstruction from laryngospasm is a frequent complication in comatose children.

An oral airway can be used for the child who is suffering a temporary loss of consciousness, such as after a contusion, seizure, or anesthesia. For children who remain unconscious for a longer time, a nasotracheal or orotracheal tube is inserted to maintain the open airway and facilitate removal of secretions. A tracheostomy is performed in cases in which laryngoscopy for introduction of an endotracheal tube would be difficult or dangerous. Suctioning is used only as needed to clear the airway, exerting care to prevent increasing ICP. Respiratory status is observed and evaluated regularly. Signs of respiratory embarrassment may be an indication for ventilatory assistance.

When the respiratory center is involved, mechanical ventilation is usually indicated (see Chapter 46). Blood gas analysis is performed regularly, and oxygen is administered when indicated. Moderately severe hypoxia and respiratory acidosis are often present but are not always evident from clinical manifestations. Hyperventilation frequently accompanies unconsciousness and may lead to respiratory alkalosis, or it may represent the body's attempt to compensate for metabolic acidosis. Therefore blood gas and pH determinations are essential guides for electrolyte therapy. Chest physiotherapy is carried out on a regular basis, and the child's position is changed at least every 2 hours to prevent pulmonary complications.

Intracranial Pressure Monitoring

Management of the child with increased ICP is possibly the most formidable task and the most controversial subject in pediatric critical care. It appears that the outcome in pediatric neurologic injury may reflect the initial cerebral damage more than the subsequent intracranial hypertension. Of note, ICP gives little indication of the severity of the initial insult (Bayir, Kochanek, & Clark 2003).

When increased ICP is a result of accumulation of CSF from obstruction of CSF flow, a ventricular tap will provide relief quickly and effectively. Evacuation of a hematoma reduces pressure from this source. Indications for inserting an ICP monitor are as follows:

1. Glasgow Coma Scale evaluation of 8
2. Glasgow Coma Scale evaluation of less than 8 with respiratory assistance
3. Deterioration of condition
4. Subjective judgment regarding clinical appearance and response.

Four major types of ICP monitors are

1. Intraventricular catheter with fibroscopic sensors attached to a monitoring system
2. Subarachnoid bolt (Richmond screw)
3. Epidural sensor
4. Anterior fontanel pressure monitor.

Transducers for both ventricular and subarachnoid monitoring should be set up without the use of a flush device. Direct ventricular pressure measurement remains the gold standard of ICP monitoring.

The catheter method involves introduction of a catheter into the lateral ventricle on the nondominant side, if known, or placement in the subdural space. The catheter has the advantage of providing a means of extraventricular (or continuous) drainage to reduce pressure. A drainage bag attached to the system is kept at the level of the ventricles and can be lowered to decrease ICP (Critical Thinking Exercise).

NURSE ALERT If the external ventricular drain (EVD) is unclamped for CSF drainage, carefully monitor the level of the collection container. If the container is too low, improper CSF decompression could lower ICP too rapidly, causing bleeding and pain. ■

Critical Thinking Exercise

HYDROCEPHALUS

Three-year-old Emma is 5 days postoperative for removal of a posterior fossa tumor. Although an external ventricular drain (EVD) was placed to treat her hydrocephalus, she continues to demonstrate signs of increased ICP, including holding the back of her head, anorexia, crying when moved or when strangers enter the room, and intermittent lethargy. On examination, fluid drainage is noted on the mother's clothes, and Emma is experiencing repetitive, rapid eyelid blinking.

1. Evidence—Is there sufficient evidence to draw conclusions about Emma's behavior, physical assessment findings, and ICP?
2. Assumptions—Describe any underlying assumption about each of the following:
   a. A preschool-age child who had a posterior fossa tumor removed 5 days ago.
   b. A preschool-age child who has an EVD placed to treat the hydrocephalus.
   c. A preschool-age child with an EVD who continues to demonstrate physical signs associated with increased ICP after recent surgery.
3. What priorities for nursing care should be established?
4. Does the evidence support your nursing intervention?
5. What alternative perspectives might you have?

With the bolt method the end of the bolt is placed into the subarachnoid space. The bolt cannot be adequately secured in a small child's pliant skull, although special modifications have been developed for children younger than 6 years of age.

NURSE ALERT The bolt is stabilized with dressings, but these are not changed or disturbed, even to check the site. ■

The placement of the bolt is not adjusted by anyone except the neurosurgeon who placed the device. The neurosurgeon is notified if a satisfactory waveform is not observed.

An epidural sensor can be placed between the dura and the skull through a burr hole and connected to a stopcock assembly and a transducer, which provides a readout of the pressure. Correlation of pressure readings is less invasive but may be inconsistent. In infants a fontanel transducer can be used to detect impulses from a pressure sensor and convert them to electrical energy. The electrical energy is then converted to visible waves or numeric readings on an oscilloscope. ICP measurement from the anterior fontanel is noninvasive but may prove to be inaccurate if the equipment is poorly placed or inconsistently recalibrated. The intraparenchymal pressure monitoring device (e.g., Camino) is a result of fiberoptic technology and performs reliably.

ICP can be increased by instillation of solutions; therefore, antibiotics are administered systemically if a positive CSF culture is obtained. However, IV ICP monitoring rarely causes infection. Because CSF is a body fluid, standard precautions are implemented according to hospital policy (see Infection Control, Chapter 45).

Nurses caring for patients with intracranial monitoring devices must be acquainted with the system, assist with insertion, interpret the monitor readings, and be able to distinguish between danger signals and mechanical dysfunction.

For increased ICP resulting from cerebral edema, several medical measures are available. Osmotic diuretics may provide rapid relief in emergency situations. Although their effect is transient, lasting only about 6 hours, they can be lifesaving in emergencies. These substances are rapidly excreted by the kidneys and carry with them large quantities of sodium and water. Mannitol (or sometimes urea) administered intravenously is the drug most frequently used for rapid reduction. The infusion is generally given slowly but may be pushed rapidly in cases of herniation or impending herniation. Because of the profound diuretic effect of the drug, an indwelling catheter is inserted to ensure bladder emptying. Adrenocorticosteroids are not recommended for cerebral edema secondary to head trauma. $PaCO_2$ should be maintained at 25 to 30 mm Hg to produce vasoconstriction, which reduces CBF, thereby decreasing ICP.

Nursing Activities

In cases of high levels of increased ICP, nursing procedures tend to trigger reactive pressure waves in many patients. For example, increased intrathoracic or abdominal pressure will be transmitted to the cranium. Particular care should be taken in positioning these patients to avoid neck vein compression, which may further increase ICP by interfering with venous return.

The child can be propped to one side or the other, and the use of an alternating-pressure mattress reduces the chance of prolonged pressure to vulnerable areas. Frequent clinical assessment of the child cannot be replaced by an ICP monitoring device.

NURSE ALERT The head of the bed is elevated 15 to 30 degrees, and the child is positioned so that the head is maintained in midline to facilitate venous drainage and avoid jugular compression. Turning side to side is contraindicated because of the risk of jugular compression. ■

It is important to avoid activities that may increase ICP by causing pain or emotional stress. Gentle range-of-motion exercises can be carried out but should not be performed vigorously. Nontherapeutic touch can cause an increase in ICP. Any disturbing procedures to be performed should be scheduled to take advantage of therapies that reduce ICP, such as osmotherapy and sedation. Efforts are taken to minimize or eliminate environmental noise. Assessment and intervention to relieve pain are important nursing functions to decrease ICP. Individualizing nursing activities and minimizing environmental stimuli by decreasing noxious procedures help to control ICP (El Bashir, Laundy, & Booy, 2003; Vernon-Levett, 1998).

Suctioning

Suctioning and percussion are poorly tolerated and are therefore contraindicated unless concurrent respiratory problems exist. Hypoxia and the Valsalva maneuver associated with cough both acutely elevate ICP. Vibration, which does not increase ICP, accomplishes excellent results and should be tried first if treatment is needed. If suctioning is necessary, it should be brief and preceded by hyperventilation with 100% oxygen, which can be monitored during suctioning with a pulse oxygen sensor reading to determine oxygen saturation.

Nutrition and Hydration

Fluids and calories are supplied initially by the IV route (see Chapter 45). An IV infusion is started early, and the type of fluid administered is determined by the general condition of the patient. Fluid therapy requires careful monitoring and adjustment based on neurologic signs and electrolyte determinations. Often, comatose children are unable to cope with the same amounts of fluid they could tolerate at other times, and overhydration must be avoided to prevent fatal cerebral edema.

Later, nutrition is provided in a balanced formula given by nasogastric or gastrostomy tube. The nasogastric tube is usually taped in place with care to prevent pressure on the nares. Most children have continuous feedings, but if bolus feedings are used, the tube is rinsed with water after each feeding. Tubes are replaced according to unit policy. Nostrils are alternated with each replacement to prevent nasal irritation and pressure. Overfeeding should be avoided to prevent vomiting with its attendant danger of aspiration. Stomach contents are aspirated and measured before feeding to ascertain the amount remaining in the stomach. If the residual volume is excessive (depending on the size of the child), the dietitian and physician should be consulted about altering the formula's composition so as to provide the needed calo-

Table 51-1

Effects of Altered Pituitary Secretion

MEASUREMENT	DIABETES INSIPIDUS	SYNDROME OF INAPPROPRIATE ANTIDIURETIC HORMONE SECRETION
Urine output	Increased	Decreased
Specific gravity	Decreased	Increased
Serum sodium	Increased (hypernatremia)	Decreased (hyponatremia)

ries and nutrients in a smaller volume. The aspirated contents should always be refed.

Hydration is maintained in the same manner (initially by IV and later by feeding tube). When cerebral edema is a threat, fluids may be restricted to reduce the chance of fluid overload. Skin and mucous membranes are examined for signs of dehydration. Observation for signs of altered fluid balance related to abnormal pituitary secretions is a part of nursing care.

Altered Pituitary Secretion

An altered ability to handle fluid loads is attributed in part to the syndrome of inappropriate antidiuretic hormone (SIADH) and diabetes insipidus (DI) resulting from hypothalamic dysfunction (see Chapter 52). SIADH frequently accompanies CNS diseases such as head injury, meningitis, encephalitis, brain abscess, brain tumor, and subarachnoid hemorrhage. In the patient with SIADH, scant quantities of urine are excreted, electrolyte analysis reveals hyponatremia and hyposmolality, and manifestations of overhydration are evident. It is important to evaluate all parameters because the reduced urine output might be erroneously interpreted as a sign of dehydration.

The treatment of SIADH consists of restriction of fluids until serum electrolytes and osmolality return to normal levels. Since SIADH frequently occurs with meningitis in children, fluid restriction is often prescribed. Likewise, DI may occur following intracranial trauma. There is increased urine volume and the accompanying danger of dehydration (see Table 51-1 for comparison of fluid changes in SIADH and DI). Adequate replacement of fluids is essential, and observation of electrolyte balance is necessary to detect signs of hypernatremia and hyperosmolality. Exogenous vasopressin may be administered.

Medications

The cause of unconsciousness determines specific drug therapies. Children with infectious processes are given antibiotics appropriate to the disease and the infecting organism, and corticosteroids are prescribed for inflammatory conditions and edema. Cerebral edema is an indication for osmotherapy with osmotic diuretics. Sedatives or antiepileptics are prescribed for seizure activity (see p. 1706). Sedation in the combative child provides amnesic and anxiolytic properties in conjunction with a paralytic agent. The combination decreases ICP and allows treatment of cerebral edema. Usual drugs include morphine, midazolam (Versed), and pancuronium (Pavulon). Midazolam is attractive because of its short half-life.

Deep coma, induced by administration of barbiturates, is controversial in the management of ICP. Barbiturates are currently reserved for the reduction of increased ICP when all else has failed. Barbiturates decrease the cerebral metabolic rate for oxygen and protect the brain during times of reduced cerebral perfusion pressure (CPP). Barbiturate coma requires extensive monitoring, cardiovascular and respiratory support, and ICP monitoring to assess response to therapy. Paralyzing agents such as pancuronium also may be needed to aid in performing diagnostic tests, improving effectiveness of therapy, and reducing risks of secondary complications. Elevation of ICP and/or heart rate of patients who are being given paralyzing agents or are under sedation may indicate the need for another dose of either or both medications.

Thermoregulation

Hyperthermia often accompanies cerebral dysfunction; if it is present, measures are implemented to reduce the temperature to prevent brain damage and to reduce metabolic demands generated by the increased body temperature. Antipyretics are the method of choice for fever reduction; cooling devices are used for hyperthermia. Laboratory tests and other methods are used in an attempt to determine the cause, if any, of the hyperthermia.

Elimination

A retention catheter is usually inserted in the acute phase, although diapers may be used and weighed to record urine output. The child who formerly had bowel and bladder control is generally incontinent. If the child remains comatose for a long period, the indwelling catheter may be removed and periodic bladder emptying accomplished by intermittent catheterization. Stool softeners are usually sufficient to maintain bowel function, but suppositories or enemas may be needed occasionally for adequate elimination and to prevent an impaction. The passage of liquid stool after a period of no bowel activity is usually a sign of an impaction. To avoid this preventable problem, daily recording of bowel activity is essential.

Hygienic Care

Routine measures for cleansing and maintaining skin integrity are an integral part of nursing care of the unconscious child. Skinfolds require special attention to prevent excoriation. The child who is unable to move is prone to develop tissue breakdown and pressure necrosis; therefore, the child may be placed on a pressure-reducing or pressure-relieving device to prevent pressure on prominent areas of the body. The goal is prevention by regular change of position and inspection of vulnerable areas, such as the ankle, trochanter, and shoulder. Since unconscious children undergo numerous invasive procedures, these skin sites require special assessment and intervention to promote healing and to prevent infection. Bed linen and any clothing are kept dry and free of wrinkles. If the child requires surgery or radiography, the nurse checks all dressings, bony sites, catheters, and IV access lines.

Mouth care is performed at least twice daily, since the mouth tends to become dry or coated with mucus. The teeth are carefully brushed with a soft toothbrush or cleaned with gauze saturated with saline. Commercially prepared cleansing devices, such as Toothettes, are convenient for cleansing the mouth and teeth. Lips are coated with ointment or other preparations to protect them from drying, cracking, or blistering.

The deeply comatose child is also prone to eye irritation. The corneal reflexes are absent; therefore, the eyes are easily irritated or damaged by linen, dust, or other substances that may come in contact with them. Excessive dryness results from incomplete closure of the eyes and/or decreased secretions, especially if the child is undergoing osmotherapy to reduce or prevent brain edema.

NURSE ALERT The eyes should be examined regularly and carefully for early signs of irritation or inflammation. Artificial tears (methylcellulose) are placed in the eyes every 1 to 2 hours. Eye dressings may sometimes be needed to protect the eyes from possible damage. ■

The hair is combed and styled neatly. Long hair is usually braided and secured with ponytail bands. The scalp should be kept clean with dry or wet shampoos as needed. The child's head may be shaved for tests or surgical procedures. If so, the hair is saved, if possible, and given to the family.

Positioning and Exercise

The unconscious child is positioned to prevent aspiration of saliva, nasogastric secretions, and vomitus, and to minimize ICP. The head of the bed is elevated, and the child is placed in a side-lying or semiprone position. A small, firm pillow is placed under the head, and the uppermost limbs are flexed and supported with pillows. The weight of the body should not rest on the dependent arm. In the semiprone position the child lies with the dependent arm at the side behind the body, the opposite side supported on pillows, and the uppermost arm and leg flexed and resting on the pillows. This position prevents undue pressure on the dependent extremities. The dependent position of the face encourages drainage of secretions and prevents the flaccid tongue from obstructing the airway.

Normal range-of-motion exercises help maintain function and prevent contractures of joints. Exercises should be done gently and with full range of motion. A small rolled pad can be placed in the palms to help maintain proper position of fingers; footboards or boots can be used to help prevent footdrop; splinting may be needed to prevent severe contractures of the wrist, knee, or ankle in decerebrate children.

Stimulation

Sensory stimulation is important in the care of the unconscious child, just as it is in the care of the alert child. For the temporarily unconscious or semiconscious child, sensory stimulation helps arouse the child to the conscious state and orient the child in terms of time and place. Auditory and tactile stimulation are especially valuable. Tactile stimulation is not appropriate for the child in whom it may elicit an undesirable response. However, for other children, tactile contact often has a relaxing and calming effect. When the child's condition permits, holding or rocking has a soothing effect and provides the body contact needed by young children.

The auditory sense is often present in a state of coma. Hearing is the last sense to be lost and the first one to be regained; therefore, the child should be spoken to as any other child. Conversation around the child should not include thoughtless or derogatory remarks. A radio playing soft music or a music box or CD player is frequently used to provide auditory stimulation. Singing the child's favorite songs or reading a favorite story is a tactic used to maintain the child's contact with a familiar world. Playing songs or stories recorded in the parents' voices can provide a continuous source of familiar stimulation.

Regaining Consciousness

Awakening from a coma is a gradual process; however, sometimes children regain consciousness within a short time. Regaining orientation involves knowing person, place, and time, in that order.

Certain behaviors have been observed when children awaken from the unconscious state. The stress and anxiety they appear to feel in a strange and unfamiliar environment are consistently expressed in silent and withdrawn behavior. Children respond to basic questioning but usually do not display their prehospitalization personality and social behavior until they are transferred from the critical care area.

Family Support

Helping parents of an unconscious child cope with the situation is especially difficult. They may demonstrate all the guilt, fear, hostility, and anxiety of any parent of a seriously ill child (see Chapter 44). In addition, these parents are faced with the uncertain outcome of the cerebral dysfunction. The fear of death, mental retardation, or other permanent disability is present. Nursing intervention with parents depends on the nature of the pathologic condition, the personality of the parents, and the parent-child relationship before the injury or illness.

If there is little or no residual effect, the child will be dismissed to home care fairly soon. The parents need the most intensive nursing intervention during the period of crisis and uncertainty. During the recovery phase they are given information, information is clarified, and they are encouraged to become involved in the child's care. Often the child's hospitalization is brief; however, some children require extended hospitalization for intensive therapy and rehabilitation.

The parents of children who die within hours or days require the support and guidance that the parents of any dying child would need in coping with the reality of the death and resolving their grief (see Chapter 41).

Probably the most difficult situations are those that involve children who are unconscious permanently or for an indefinite period. Unlike parents who lose a child through death, the finality is lacking for these parents, often leaving them in a state of suspended grief. The presence of the child renders the parents unable to resolve the loss. Like parents of dying children, parents of the comatose child search for any signs of hope. Well-meaning friends and relatives relate instances of miraculous recoveries. The parents seek confirmation and support for such possibilities and assign erroneous meanings to any sign in the child, such as reflexive muscle contractions, that might be interpreted as evidence of recovery.

At these times nurses need to respond with compassion and gentle honesty. They can acknowledge that miraculous recoveries do occur, but they are rare. The important message is to maintain open communication with the family.

Like parents who lose a child through death, the parents of the child lost to their world attempt to reconstitute a representation of the child. They bring items that belong to the child, such as favorite toys, music, and other objects cherished by the child. This is interpreted as an attempt to provide stimulation for the child in the hope of eliciting a response, to let the hospital staff know the child as the unique individual he or she was so that the parents' distress can be better appreciated, and to reconstitute an image of the child "lost" to them and for whom they mourn. An awareness of these behaviors and coping mechanisms provides nurses with the understanding that helps them support the parents in their grief process.

Superimposed on the process of grieving for the "lost" child, parents may be faced with difficult decisions. When the child's brain is so severely damaged that vital functions must be maintained by artificial means, the parents must make the final decision to remove life-support systems. Because the decision is so difficult for parents, the practitioner is frequently placed in a position of making the decision indirectly. After providing the parents with all of the information, the practitioner will suggest that the child be removed from the life support to "see if the child can make it without help." The approach relieves the parents of the decision and can be effective, but it is based on an evaluation of the parents' intellectual level and emotional state. Sometimes parents may even choose to refuse treatment if they believe it to be best for the child and the family (informed dissent). At other times parents request that "everything possible" be done for the child.

The nurses can be instrumental in providing guidance and clarifying information—a valued but demanding undertaking. It is not unusual for the family to ask the same questions and to compare responses elicited from different staff members. A child's death is an intensely personal issue that deserves direct involvement by the nurse and auxiliary support systems.

When the child has survived the illness or injury that produced the brain damage but is left unconscious permanently, the parents must decide whether to place the child in a chronic care facility or arrange to care for the child at home. The nurse can listen to the parents' discussions regarding alternatives, provide information when appropriate, and support the family in their decision. The nurse can help the family prepare for the transfer of the child and make referrals to persons or agencies that can provide additional assistance.

When the child has survived the cerebral insult and is not comatose, but physical and/or mental capacity is limited, either minimally or severely, families must cope with the long and tedious rehabilitation process and the uncertain outcome. The drain on financial, emotional, and social resources can be enormous.

For parents who choose to care for their child at home, planning for home care begins early in the process of recovery. The family should become involved with the care of the child as soon as they indicate an interest and ability to do so. They need education and support in learning to care for the child, regular follow-up observation and assessment of the home management, and planning for some respite care of the child. Parents need to understand that it is important to plan for periodic relief from the continual care of the child (see Preparing for Discharge and Home Care, Chapter 44; and Family-Centered Home Care, Chapter 43).

Evaluation

The effectiveness of nursing interventions for the unconscious child is determined by continual reassessment and evaluation of care based on the following observational guidelines:

1. Monitor child's neurologic signs, vital signs, and behavior.
2. Observe child's response to nursing activities, therapies, and diagnostic procedures; monitor ICP.
3. Observe child's color, position, and motor activity; measure fluid and nutritional intake and output.
4. Monitor status of child's respiratory, renal, and gastrointestinal systems and skin.
5. Observe family behaviors and interview members regarding their understandings and their feelings and concerns.

The expected outcomes are described in the Nursing Care Plan on pp. 1682-1683.

CEREBRAL TRAUMA

Head Injury

Head injury is a pathologic process involving the scalp, skull, meninges, or brain as a result of mechanical force. According to national statistics and the Safe Kids Campaign,* injuries are the number-one health risk for children and the leading cause of death in children older than 1 year of age. Yearly, 1 in 4 children in the United States will suffer an injury serious enough to require medical attention. Tragically, 8000 children are killed every year by injuries. It has been estimated that 300 per 100,000 children per year have a traumatic brain injury and that 10 per 100,000 children per year die as a result of the brain injury. Studies indicate that as many as three-fourths of the childhood deaths caused by mechanical trauma are the direct result of a brain injury.

Etiology

The three major causes of brain damage in childhood in order of importance are falls, motor vehicle injuries, and bicycle injuries. Neurologic injury accounts for the highest mortality, with boys affected twice as often as girls. In motor

*SAFE KIDS, 1301 Pennsylvania Avenue NW, Suite 1000, Washington, DC 20004-1707; phone: 202-662-0600; fax: 202-393-2072; Web site: www.safekids.org.

Nursing Care Plan

THE UNCONSCIOUS CHILD

NURSING DIAGNOSIS: Risk for suffocation (aspiration) related to ineffective airway clearance secondary to depressed sensorium, impaired motor function

EXPECTED OUTCOME
Patent airway is maintained; no signs of cerebral hypoxia are present.

NURSING INTERVENTIONS/*RATIONALES*
Position semiprone or side-lying with neck slightly extended, nose in "sniffing" position *to provide optimal ventilation and prevent aspiration.* **Avoid neck hyperextension, which can block airway.**
Insert oral airway if indicated *to promote ventilation.*
Remove pooled secretions promptly *to prevent aspiration.*
Have emergency equipment available for insertion of endotracheal tube or tracheostomy *to prevent delay in treatment response to blocked airway.*
Administer oxygen, hyperventilate as ordered *to increase oxygenation to tissues.*
Monitor vital signs, blood gases, and pH *for evidence of hypoxia.*

NURSING DIAGNOSIS: Risk for infection (respiratory) related to coma, immobility, pooling or respiratory secretions

EXPECTED OUTCOME
Patient exhibits no evidence of infection; lungs are clear.

NURSING INTERVENTIONS/*RATIONALES*
Place child in private room and screen all visitors and staff for signs of infection *to minimize exposure to infective organisms.*
Teach family about good hygiene and careful handwashing techniques *to prevent spread of infection.*
Observe careful asepsis in all procedures *to prevent spread of infection.*
Remove nasal and oral secretions as they form and provide good oral hygiene *to remove medium for growth of microorganisms.*
Monitor vital signs, auscultate lungs *to detect signs of infection.*

NURSING DIAGNOSIS: Risk for injury related to depressed sensorium, intracranial abnormality

EXPECTED OUTCOME
Child exhibits no evidence of injury (i.e., no increased ICP, cerebral edema, seizure activity).

NURSING INTERVENTIONS/*RATIONALES*
Elevate head of bed 15 to 30 degrees with child's head in midline position *to facilitate venous drainage and prevent jugular compression.*
Prevent constipation, excessive stimuli in environment, painful stimuli, vigorous suctioning, or percussing *because these activities can lead to increased ICP and seizure activity.*
Use stool softeners as ordered; monitor bowel movements *to prevent constipation and Valsalva maneuver.*
Keep room darkened, quiet; play soothing background music: place earphones over child's ears; use touching and calm, soothing voice to talk with child when performing care *to reduce environmental stimuli.*
Use sedation as ordered *for episodes of agitation or restlessness.*
Observe child for signs of pain (e.g., agitation, increases in pulse, blood pressure), and medicate with analgesic or paralyzing agents as ordered *to reduce pain.*
Arrange painful procedures to occur after sedation or analgesic administration *to decrease chances of increasing ICP.*
Administer antiseizure medication as ordered *to prevent seizure activity.*
Monitor neurologic vital signs *to assess neurosensory status.*

NURSING DIAGNOSIS: Ineffective thermoregulation related to intracranial abnormality; CNS dysfunction

EXPECTED OUTCOME
Child maintains body temperature at normothermic levels.

NURSING INTERVENTIONS/*RATIONALES*
Monitor and record body temperature frequently *to assess status of thermoregulatory system and effectiveness of interventions.*
Administer antipyretics as ordered *for fever.*
Remove blankets, administer tepid sponge bath, use hypothermia blankets *to reduce hyperthermia.*
Maintain adequate hydration *to reduce or prevent fever.*
Use blankets, bed warmers *to reduce hypothermia.*
Prevent shivering, which can increase ICP and metabolic rate.
Monitor blood urea nitrogen (BUN), pH, electrolyte, glucose levels *because they may be affected by thermal instability.*

NURSING DIAGNOSIS: Risk for disuse syndrome related to coma, prolonged immobility

EXPECTED OUTCOME
Child maintains full range of motion; muscle tone (no contractures, footdrop); skin integrity (no skin redness, irritation, breakdown, decubiti); normal patterns of elimination (no constipation, renal retention, renal calculi); normal circulatory function (no thrombus formation, venous stasis); adequate dietary intake (no weight loss, muscle wasting).

NURSING INTERVENTIONS/*RATIONALES*
Turn and reposition every 2 hours *to promote circulation and prevent skin breakdown* (align properly, provide positional supports, use handrolls or splints *to position hands in functional position;* use footboard or hightop tennis shoes *to prevent footdrop*); perform passive range of motion frequently *to maintain full range in all joints and prevent contracture formation:* seat in chair *to improve circulation;* place on tilt table *to prevent loss of bone density to long bones.*
Use pressure reduction mattress overlay *to prevent pressure necrosis;* use foam pads on ankles, heels, elbows *to protect bony prominences;* massage skin with lotion regularly *to stimulate circulation and prevent friction and shearing effects;* keep bedclothes clean, dry, and wrinkle-free *to prevent skin irritation;* lubricate lips *to prevent drying and cracking;* lubricate eyes and keep them closed *to prevent drying and corneal irritation;* cleanse skin, mucous membranes of mouth and perianal area regularly *to prevent irritation and breakdown;* keep skin folds clean and dry *to prevent*

Nursing Care Plan

THE UNCONSCIOUS CHILD—cont'd

excoriation; inspect skin, mucous membranes, corneas regularly *to assess for early signs of irritation or breakdown.*

Ensure adequate fluid intake, administer stool softeners *to maintain urinary output, prevent calculi, and aid bowel elimination;* monitor intake and output (I & O), hydration status, electrolytes, BUN, creatinine, urine characteristics *to assess for adequate hydration.*

Apply elastic stockings as indicated to promote venous return, prevent stasis.

Provide tube feedings that are adequate to support the nutritional and metabolic needs of child (e.g., increased fiber, protein, vitamin C; decreased calcium); monitor weight daily to assess nutritional adequacy.

NURSING DIAGNOSIS: Altered family processes related to situational crises (child in coma)

EXPECTED OUTCOME

Family exhibits adaptation of usual roles and functions to accommodate special needs of child; family exhibits growth-promoting behaviors.

NURSING INTERVENTIONS/*RATIONALES*

Provide opportunity for family to absorb and adjust to diagnosis (e.g., repeat information *to allow time for family to hear and understand;* encourage expression of concerns, fears, and feelings about diagnosis and potential impact *to facilitate adjustment;* identify support systems *to provide resources for coping*).

Keep family informed of child's status, assist family to understand expected treatment *to promote trust and provide a sound basis for decision making.*

Explore parents' reaction to the child, involve them in child's daily care routines, have them touch and hold child *to provide some measure of control.*

Have parents spend special time with siblings *so they don't feel neglected or left out.*

Identify additional resource systems (e.g., relatives, friends, church, health care services, community programs) and strategize with family about making good use of these systems *to develop broad base of support.*

Provide a system of ongoing follow-up observation and evaluation *to ensure long-term adaptation to challenges presented to family functioning by a child who is in a long-term comatose state.*

vehicle accidents children younger than 2 years of age are almost exclusively injured as passengers, whereas older children may also be injured as pedestrians or cyclists. The majority of deaths from brain trauma caused by bicycle injuries occur between the ages of 5 and 19 years. Bicycle helmet laws have been effective in reducing the risk of head injury by 85% and brain injury by 88% (Rivara & Grossman, 2004).

The exposed nature of the head renders it particularly vulnerable to external violence, and many of the physical characteristics of children predispose them to craniocerebral trauma. For example, infants are frequently left unattended on beds, in high chairs, and in other places from which they can fall. Because the head of an infant or toddler is proportionately larger and heavier in relation to other body parts, it is the most likely to be injured. Incomplete motor development contributes to falls at young ages, and the natural curiosity and exuberance of children also increase their risk of injury.

Pathophysiology

The pathology of brain injury is directly related to the force of impact. Intracranial contents (brain, blood, CSF) are damaged because the force is too great to be absorbed by the skull and musculoligamentous support of the head. The elastic, pliable skull of the infant and young child absorbs much of the direct energy of physical impact to the head and affords some protection to intracranial structures. Although nervous tissue is delicate, it usually requires a severe blow to cause significant damage.

A child's response to head injury is different from that of an adult. The larger head size and insufficient musculoskeletal support render the very young child particularly vulnerable to acceleration-deceleration injuries.

Primary head injuries are those that occur at a time of trauma and include skull fracture, contusions, intracranial hematoma, and diffuse injury. Subsequent complications include hypoxic brain damage, increased ICP, infection, and cerebral edema. The predominant feature of a child's brain injury is the amount of diffuse swelling that occurs. Hypoxia and hypercapnia threaten the energy requirements of the brain and increase cerebral blood flow. The added volume across the blood-brain barrier, along with the loss of autoregulation, exacerbates cerebral edema. Pressure inside the skull that is greater than arterial pressure results in inadequate perfusion.

Cerebral hyperemia occurs more often in children, and this volume expansion may account for their tendency to develop intracranial hypertension. However, because the cranium of very young children has the ability to expand and the thin skull is more compliant, they may tolerate increases in ICP better than older children and adults do. Children have a significantly higher percentage of good outcomes and a lower mortality rate, as well as a lower incidence of surgical mass lesions after severe head trauma. However, their thinner, softer skull may sustain greater long-term damage than previously suggested.

Physical forces act on the head through *acceleration, deceleration,* or *deformation.* Acceleration or deceleration is more descriptive of the circumstances responsible for most head injuries. When the stationary head receives a blow, the sudden acceleration causes deformation of the skull and mass movement of the brain. Continued movement of the intracranial contents allows the brain to strike parts of the skull (e.g., the sharp edges of the sphenoid or the irregular surface of the anterior fossa) or the edges of the tentorium.

Although the brain volume remains unchanged, significant distortion takes place as the brain changes shape in response to the force of impact to the skull. This movement can cause bruising at the point of impact *(coup)* and/or at a distance as the brain collides with the unyielding surfaces far removed from the point of impact *(contrecoup)* (Fig. 51-4). Thus a blow to the occipital region can cause severe injury to the frontal and temporal areas of the brain. Sudden deceleration, such as takes place during a fall, causes the greatest cerebral injury at the point of impact. Children with an acceleration/deceleration injury demonstrate diffuse generalized cerebral swelling produced by increased blood volume or a redistribution of cerebral blood volume (cerebral hyperemia) rather than by increased water content (edema), as seen in adults.

Another effect of brain movement is shearing stresses, which may tear small arteries and cause subdural hemorrhages. Damage can also occur when severe compression of the skull causes the brain to be forced through the tentorial opening. This can produce irreparable damage to the brainstem (Fig. 51-5).

Concussion

The most common head injury is *concussion,* a transient and reversible neuronal dysfunction, with instantaneous loss of awareness and responsiveness, that results from trauma to the head and persists for a relatively short time, usually minutes or hours. It is generally followed by amnesia for the moment of the injury and a variable period after the injury. The common misconception that loss of consciousness is the hallmark of concussion is not true, especially for children. Concussion is correctly defined as "a traumatically induced alteration in mental status." Confusion and amnesia following head injury are the hallmarks of concussion.

The pathogenesis of concussion is still unclear but may be a result of shearing forces that cause stretching, compression, and tearing of nerve fibers, particularly in the area of the central brainstem, the seat of the reticular activating system. It has also been suggested that the anatomic alterations of nerve fibers cause the release of large quantities of acetylcholine into the CSF and a reduction in oxygen consumption with increased lactate production.

Contusion and Laceration

The terms *contusion* and *laceration* are used to describe visible bruising and tearing of cerebral tissue. Contusions represent petechial hemorrhages along the superficial aspects of the brain at the site of impact (coup injury) and/or a lesion remote from the site of direct trauma (contrecoup injury). In serious accidents there may be multiple sites of injury.

The major areas of the brain susceptible to contusion or laceration are the occipital, frontal, and temporal lobes. Also, the irregular surfaces of the anterior and middle fossae at the base of the skull are capable of producing bruises or lacerations on forceful impact. Contusions may cause focal disturbances in strength, sensation, or visual awareness. The degree of brain damage in the contused areas varies according to the extent of vascular injury. Signs will vary from mild, transient weakness of a limb to prolonged unconsciousness

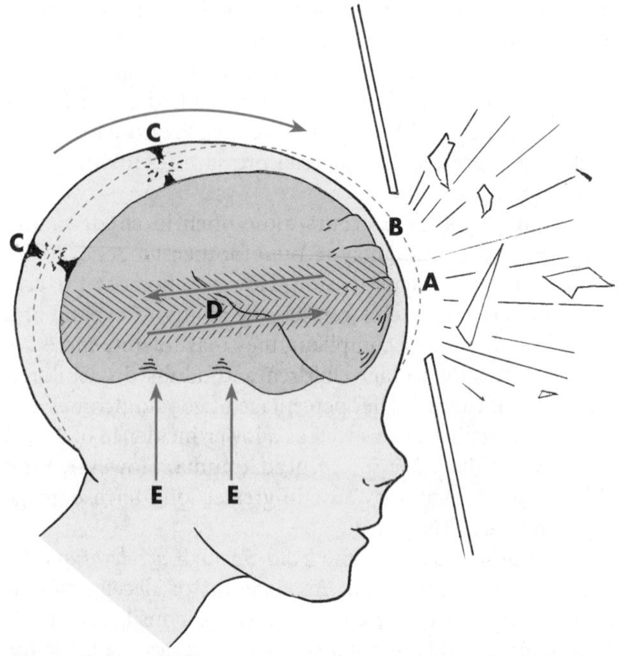

Fig. 51-4 Mechanical distortion of cranium during closed head injury. **A,** Preinjury contour of skull. **B,** Immediate postinjury contour of skull. **C,** Torn subdural vessels. **D,** Shearing forces. **E,** Trauma from contact with floor of cranium. (Redrawn from Grubb RL, Coxe WS: Central nervous system trauma: cranial. In Eliasson SG, Presky AL, Hardin WB Jr [eds]: *Neurological pathophysiology,* New York, 1974, Oxford University Press.)

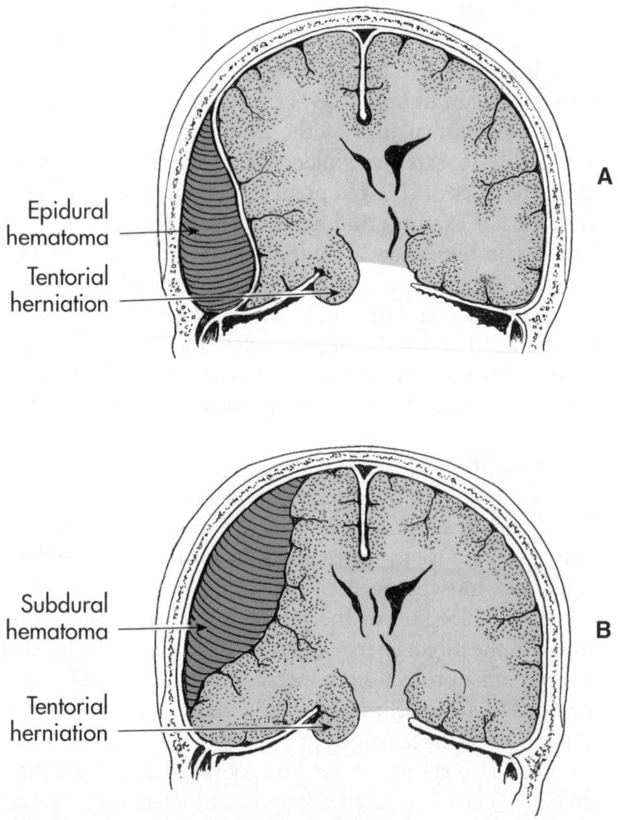

Fig. 51-5 **A,** Epidural (extradural) hematoma and compression of temporal lobe through tentorial hiatus. **B,** Subdural hematoma.

and paralysis. However, the signs and symptoms may be clinically indistinguishable from those of concussion.

The lower incidence of cerebral contusion in infancy has been attributed to the infant's pliable skull with less convolutional markings of the inner space between brain tissue and bone. In addition, the infant's brain tissue has a softer consistency, which also reduces surface injury. However, infants who are roughly shaken (shaken baby syndrome) can sustain profound neurologic impairment, seizures, retinal hemorrhages, and intracranial subarachnoid or subdural hemorrhages. In addition to these classic injuries, high cervical spinal cord hemorrhages and contusions can occur.

Cerebral lacerations are generally associated with penetrating or depressed skull fractures. However, they may occur without fracture in small children. When brain tissue is actually torn, with bleeding into and around the tear, usually more severe and prolonged unconsciousness and paralysis occur, leaving permanent scarring and some degree of disability.

Fractures

Because of its flexibility, the immature skull is able to sustain a greater degree of deformation than the adult skull before it incurs a fracture. A great deal of force is required to produce a fracture in the skull of an infant. However, the undersurface of the skull contains grooves in which the meningeal arteries lie. A fracture that runs through one of these grooves may tear the artery and produce severe and damaging hemorrhage. Hypovolemic hypotension can occur in infants with skull fractures.

The types of fractures that occur are as follows:

Linear fractures are those in which the lines of the fracture are predetermined by the site and velocity of the impact, as well as by the strength of the bone. These are uncommon before 2 to 3 years of age but constitute the majority of childhood skull fractures. Most linear skull fractures are associated with an overlying hematoma or soft-tissue swelling (Schutzman & Greenes, 2001).

Depressed fractures are those in which the bone is locally broken, usually into several irregular fragments that are pushed inward, causing pressure on the brain. The inner portion of the bone is more extensively fragmented than the outer portion, which almost invariably produces tears in the dura. These are uncommon before 2 to 3 years of age. In infants and very young children, the soft, malleable bone may become dented in a peculiar rounded or "Ping-Pong ball" depression, without laceration of either skin or dura.

Comminuted fractures consist of multiple associated linear fractures. They usually result from intense impact. These types of fractures often result from repeated blows against an object and may suggest child abuse.

Basilar fractures involve the basilar portion of the frontal, ethmoid, sphenoid, temporal, or occipital bones. Because of the proximity of the fracture line to structures surrounding the brainstem, this is a serious head injury. Approximately 80% of the cases may include clinical features such as subcutaneous bleeding in the posterior neck area and over the mastoid process (Battle's sign). Bleeding around the eyes (raccoon eyes) or bleeding behind the tympanic membrane may occur (hemotympanum).

Open fractures cause communication between the skull and the scalp or the surfaces of the upper respiratory tract. Open fractures increase the risk of central nervous system infection. They may have an overlying laceration called a *compound fracture.* Open fractures can also create an opening in the paranasal sinuses or middle ear that can lead to CSF rhinorrhea or otorrhea. Facial paralysis, vertigo, tinnitus, or hearing loss may develop.

Diastatic fractures are traumatic separations of the cranial sutures. These most frequently affect the lambdoid suture and are rarely seen beyond the first 3 years of life. They require no specific treatment but should be observed for "growing fractures." Growing fractures are skull fractures associated with an underlying dural tear that may be caused by a leptomeningeal cyst, dilated ventricles, or a herniated brain. Neurologic symptoms include headache, seizures, and asymmetric cranial growth (Schutzman & Greenes, 2001). Infants and young children who have isolated skull fractures should be evaluated for growing skull fractures from 1 to 2 months after the injury (Schutzman & Greenes, 2001.)

Complications

The major complications of trauma to the head are hemorrhage, infection, edema, and herniation through the tentorium. Infection is always a hazard in open injuries, and edema is related to tissue trauma. Vascular rupture may occur even in minor head injuries, causing hemorrhage between the skull and cerebral surfaces. Compression of the underlying brain produces effects that can be rapidly fatal or insidiously progressive.

NURSE ALERT Posttraumatic meningitis should be suspected in children with increasing drowsiness and fever who also have basilar skull fractures. ■

Epidural Hemorrhage

The blood accumulates between the dura and the skull to form a hematoma, which, because of the difficulty with which dura is stripped from bone, forces the underlying brain contents downward and inward as the brain expands (see Fig. 51-5, *A*). Since bleeding is generally arterial, brain compression occurs rapidly. Most often the expanding hematoma is located in the parietotemporal region, forcing the medial portion of the temporal lobe under the edge of the tentorium, where it causes pressure on nerves and blood vessels. The lower incidence of epidural hematoma in childhood has been attributed to the fact that the middle meningeal artery is not embedded in the bone surface of the skull until approximately 2 years of age. Therefore a fracture of the temporal bone is less likely to lacerate the artery. Second, the dura closely adheres to the inner table of the skull, especially at the level of the sutures, making separation from bleeding less likely. However, a child's skull can be indented with sufficient force to tear the middle meningeal artery and rebound intact without causing a fracture. Hemorrhage can also derive from dural veins or the dural sinuses, especially in infants and small children, in whom fracture is less likely to occur. In 20% to 40% of children a skull fracture is not detectable. The classic clinical picture of epidural hemorrhage (momentary unconsciousness followed by a normal period, then lethargy or coma) is seldom evident in children (see Box 51-4 for clinical manifestations). The period of impaired consciousness is frequently lacking, and the symptom-free period is atypical because of nonspecific complaints such as irritability, headache, and vomiting. When it does occur, the symptom-free period frequently lasts longer than 48 hours. Clinically significant epidural hematomas are uncommon in children younger than 4 years of age. These differences may be caused by the decreased tendency of the resilient skull to fracture; the ability of blood to escape through widened sutures, an open fontanel, or a fracture; bleeding from smaller vessels with less rapid and massive bleeding; lower systolic blood pressure in children; and possibly the decreased susceptibility of the child's brain to pressure changes.

Subdural Hemorrhage

A subdural hemorrhage is bleeding between the dura and the cerebrum, usually as a result of rupture of cortical veins that bridge the subdural space (see Fig. 51-5, *B*). Subdural hematomas are 10 times more frequent than epidural hematomas, occurring most often in infancy, with a peak incidence at 6 months.

Unlike epidural hemorrhage, which develops inwardly against the less resistant brain tissue, subdural hemorrhage tends to develop more slowly and spreads thinly and widely until it is limited by the dural barriers—the falx and tentorium. Subdural hematoma is fairly common in infants, frequently as a result of birth trauma, falls, assaults, or violent shaking. The small subdural space and dura firmly attached to the skull in this area are highly vulnerable to increased ICP.

NURSE ALERT Children with a subdural hematoma and retinal hemorrhages should be evaluated for the possibility of child abuse, especially shaken baby syndrome (SBS). ■

Repeated subdural taps often provide relief in the infant, as revealed by follow-up CT scans, improved neurologic status, and a flat anterior fontanel. Surgical evacuation of the hematoma is the treatment of choice in the older child and is frequently required in infants.

Cerebral Edema

Some degree of brain edema is expected, especially 24 to 72 hours after craniocerebral trauma. Cerebral edema caused by direct cellular injury or vascular injury induces vascular stasis, anoxia, and further vasodilation. If the progression continues unchecked, ICP exceeds arterial pressure and fatal anoxia ensues, and/or the pressure causes herniation of a portion of the brain over the edge of the tentorium, compressing the brainstem and occluding the posterior cerebral arteries. Diffuse cerebral swelling and changes in CBF are common patterns following head injury in children.

NURSE ALERT If a child loses consciousness or vomits more than three times, medical attention should be sought. ■

BOX 51-4

Clinical Manifestations of Acute Head Injury

Minor Injury

May or may not lose consciousness
Transient period of confusion
Somnolence
Listlessness
Irritability
Pallor
Vomiting (one or more episodes)

Signs of Progression

Altered mental status (e.g., difficulty rousing child)
Mounting agitation
Development of focal lateral neurologic signs
Marked changes in vital signs

Severe Injury

Signs of increased intracranial pressure (see Box 51-1)
Increased head size (infant)
Bulging or full fontanel (infant)
Retinal hemorrhage
Extraocular palsies (especially cranial nerve VI)
Hemiparesis
Quadriplegia
Elevated temperature
Unsteady gait (older child)
Papilledema (older child)
Retinal hemorrhages

Associated Signs

Scalp trauma
Other injuries (e.g., to extremities)

Diagnostic Evaluation

A detailed history, especially a health history, both past and present, is essential in evaluating the child with a craniocerebral trauma. Certain disorders, such as drug allergies, hemophilia, diabetes mellitus, or epilepsy, may produce similar symptoms. Furthermore, even minor traumatic injury can aggravate a preexisting disease process. Events surrounding the injury often supply significant data. It must be determined whether the infant or child exhibited alterations in consciousness, and any other signs and behaviors exhibited by the child must be noted. Since head injuries are frequently accompanied by injuries in other areas, the examination is performed with care to avoid further damage.

NURSE ALERT Stabilize a child's spine after head injury until a spinal cord injury is ruled out.

Initial Assessment

Priorities in the initial stabilization phase of a child with a head injury include assessment of the ABCs (airway, breathing, circulation); evaluation for shock; a neurologic examination, especially LOC; pupillary symmetry and response to light; and seizures (Bayir et al, 2003). The assessment is carried out quickly in relation to vital signs (Emergency box). Excited and irritable children may have a rapid pulse, hyperventilate, appear pale, and feel clammy shortly after an injury.

NURSE ALERT Deep, rapid, periodic, or intermittent and gasping respirations; wide fluctuations or noticeable slowing of the pulse; and widening pulse pressure or extreme fluctuations in blood pressure are signs of brainstem involvement. It is important to note that marked hypotension may represent internal injuries. ■

Ocular signs such as fixed and dilated pupils, fixed and constricted pupils, and pupils that are poorly reactive or nonreactive to light and accommodation indicate increased ICP or brainstem involvement. It is important to remain with the child who demonstrates fixed and dilated pupils, since these are ominous signs, with the probability of respiratory arrest. Dilated, nonpulsating blood vessels indicate increased ICP before the appearance of papilledema. Retinal hemorrhages are seen in acute head injuries.

NURSE ALERT Observation of asymmetric pupils or one dilated, nonreactive pupil in a comatose child is a neurosurgical emergency. ■

Less urgent but important additional assessments include examination of the scalp for lacerations and palpation for other abnormalities. A significant amount of blood loss can occur from scalp lacerations.

NURSE ALERT Bleeding from the nose or ears needs further evaluation, and a watery discharge from the nose (rhinorrhea) that is positive for glucose (as tested with Dextrostix) suggests leaking of CSF from a skull fracture. ■

An accurate assessment of clinical signs provides baseline information. Serial evaluations, preferably by a single observer, help detect changes in the neurologic status. Alterations in mental status, evidenced by increased difficulty in rousing the child, mounting agitation, development of focal lateral neurologic signs, or marked changes in vital signs, usually indicate extension or progression of the basic pathologic process.

Special Tests

After a thorough clinical examination, a variety of diagnostic tests are helpful in providing a more definitive diagnosis of the type and extent of the trauma. The severity of a head injury may not be apparent on clinical examination of a child, but it will be detectable on a CT scan. Whenever the child has a history consistent with a serious head injury (unrestrained occupant in a severe motor vehicle accident or a fall from a significant height), it is important that a scan be performed even if the child initially appears alert and oriented. All children with head injuries who have any alteration of consciousness, headache, vomiting, skull fracture, seizure, or a predisposing medical condition should also undergo CT scanning.

MRI and neurobehavioral assessment following early head injury may be useful in documenting cognitive impairment in relation to structural alterations in the young brain. MRI provides details of soft tissues better than any other noninvasive device. Electroencephalography is not particularly helpful for early diagnosis but is useful for defining seizure activity or focal destructive lesions after the acute phase of illness. Lumbar puncture is rarely used in craniocerebral trauma and is contraindicated in the presence of increased ICP because of the possibility of herniation. In some centers monitoring ICP is part of the assessment.

Posttraumatic Syndromes

Posttraumatic syndromes can be clinically manifested because of structural complications resulting from a head injury and through the signs and symptoms demonstrated by the child. Structural complications can include hydrocephalus and focal deficits such as optic atrophy, cranial nerve palsies, motor deficits, diabetes insipidus, aphasia, and seizures. Behavioral disturbances include sleep disturbances, phobias, emotional lability, altered school performance, and changes related to aggressiveness or withdrawal. *Postconcussion syndrome* is a common sequela to brain injury and can occur within minutes to an hour after a head injury. The manifestations vary with the age of the child. The syndrome occurs very frequently in children younger than 1 year of age. The syndrome in adolescents is similar to that in adults. The duration of manifestations can vary from several days to several months. Death from concussion is preventable unless overwhelming secondary brain injury has occurred (Durkin et al, 1998; Gennarelli, 1999).

Posttraumatic seizures occur in a number of children who survive a head injury and are more common in children than in adults. Seizures are more likely to occur within the first few days of the head injury (Chiaretti et al, 2000). *Structural complications* (e.g., hydrocephalus) may occur follow-

Emergency

HEAD INJURY

Assess child:
- **A**—Airway (with cervical-spine immobilization); use jaw thrust to open airway
- **B**—Bleeding
- **C**—Circulation

Clean any abrasions with soap and water.
Apply clean dressing.
If bleeding, apply ice to relieve pain and swelling.
Keep NPO until instructed otherwise.
Assess pain, but do not give analgesics or sedatives.
Check pupil reaction every 4 hours (including twice during night) for 48 hours.
Awaken twice during the night to check level of consciousness.
Seek medical attention if any of the following apply:
- Injury sustained:
  - At high speed (e.g., automobile)
  - Fall from a significant distance (e.g., roof, tree, or height greater than that of the child)
  - From great force (e.g., baseball bat)
  - Under suspicious circumstances
- Loss of consciousness
- Amnesia
- Discomfort (crying) more than 10 minutes after injury
- Headache that is severe, worsening, interferes with sleep
- Fluid leak from ears or nose
- Vomiting three or more times
- Swelling in front of or above earlobe or increased swelling
- Confused or not behaving normally
- Difficult to rouse from sleep
- Difficulty speaking
- Blurred vision or seeing double
- Unsteady gait
- Difficulty using extremities
- Neck pain
- Pupils dilated, unequal, or fixed
- Infant with full or bulging fontanel
- Bruising below the eyes

Family Focus

MAINTAINING CONTACT

Maintaining contact with parents for continued observation and reevaluation of the child, when indicated, facilitates early diagnosis and treatment of possible complications from head injury, such as hematoma, hydrocephalus, cysts, and posttraumatic seizures. Children are generally hospitalized for 24 to 48 hours of observation if their family lives far from medical facilities or lacks transportation or a telephone that would provide access to immediate help. Other circumstances such as language or other communication barriers, or even emotional trauma, may hinder learning and make it difficult for families to feel confident in caring for their child at home.

Atraumatic Care

NONINVASIVE LOCAL ANESTHESIA

The use of topical lidocaine, epinephrine, and tetracaine (LET) solution (Pasero & McCaffery, 1999) or lidocaine, adrenaline, and tetracaine (LAT) gel provides noninvasive anesthesia for suturing (Ernst et al, 1997). Both of these preparations provide an acceptable alternative to tetracaine, adrenaline, and cocaine (TAC), which is more expensive, is a restricted narcotic, and carries a higher potential for toxicity (Pasero & McCaffery, 1999).

ing a head injury. The type of residual effect depends on the location and nature of the disorder. True mental retardation occurs only after severe injuries.

Therapeutic Management

The majority of children with mild-to-moderate concussion who have not lost consciousness can be cared for and observed at home after careful examination reveals no serious intracranial injury. Nurses should provide parents with clear explanations and instructions and should encourage them to ask questions both before and after leaving the medical facility if clarification is needed (Family Focus box).

The parents are instructed to check the child every 2 hours to determine any changes in responsiveness. The sleeping child should be wakened to see if he or she can be roused normally. Parents are advised to maintain contact with the health professional, who usually wishes to examine the child again in 1 or 2 days. The manifestations of epidural hematoma in children do not generally appear until 24 hours or more after injury.

Children with severe injuries, those who have lost consciousness for more than a few minutes, and those with prolonged and continued seizures or other focal or diffuse neurologic signs must be hospitalized until their condition is stable and their neurologic signs have diminished.

The child is maintained on nothing by mouth or restricted to clear liquids, if able to take fluids by mouth, until it is determined that vomiting will not occur. IV fluids are indicated in the child who is comatose or displays dulled sensorium and/or in the child with persistent vomiting. Fluid balance is closely monitored by daily weights; accurate intake and output measurements; and serum osmolality to detect early signs of water retention, excessive dehydration, and states of hypertonicity or hypotonicity.

The volume of IV fluid is carefully monitored to avoid aggravating any cerebral edema and to minimize the possibility of overhydration in case of SIADH. However, damage to the hypothalamus or pituitary gland may produce diabetes insipidus with its accompanying hypertonicity and dehydration.

Restlessness can be satisfactorily managed, if necessary, with mild sedation, and headache is usually controlled with acetaminophen (Tylenol). Antiepileptics are used for seizure control and frequently in cases of suspected contusion or laceration. Antibiotics may be administered if lacerations, CSF leakage, or excessive cerebral tissue damage are present. Prophylactic tetanus toxoid is given as appropriate. Cerebral edema is managed as described for the unconscious child. Hyperthermia is controlled with tepid sponges or a hypothermia blanket.

Surgical Therapy

Scalp lacerations are sutured after the underlying bone is carefully examined (Atraumatic Care box). Depressed fractures require surgical reduction and removal of bone fragments. Torn dura is sutured. "Ping-Pong ball" skull fractures in very young infants ordinarily correct themselves within a few weeks and do not require specific treatment, although they can be reduced by pressure against the bone.

Prognosis

The outcome of craniocerebral trauma depends on the extent of injury and complications. However, the outlook is generally more favorable for children than for adults (Faillace, 2002; Masson et al, 2003). More than 90% of children with concussions or simple linear fractures recover without symptoms after the initial period. The incidence of fatalities and neurologic sequelae is lower in children than in adults, even in those with severe head injuries. The prognosis for recovery is primarily related to the duration of coma and the degree of injury. The combination of impaired consciousness and skull fracture carries the highest risk of complication.

The concern regarding outcome is increasingly focused on cognitive, emotional, and/or mental problems. Recent studies indicate that children experience a higher frequency of psychologic disturbances following head injury, whereas adults are more prone to complaints of a physical nature.

Children may be more vulnerable than adults to long-term cognitive and behavioral dysfunction after diffuse brain injury. Even with recovery, the effects of brain injury on a child's potential can never be known.

True coma (not obeying commands, eyes closed, and not speaking) usually does not last more than 2 weeks. A child's eventual outcome can range from brain death to a persistent vegetative state to complete recovery. However, even the best recovery may be associated with personality changes, including mood lability and loss of confidence, impaired short-term memory, headaches, and subtle cognitive impairments. Many children are left with significant disabilities after head injury that appear months later as learning difficulties, behavioral changes, or emotional disturbances (Faillace, 2002). Generally, within 6 months to 1 year after the injury, 90% of the long-term neurologic outcome has been achieved.

Nursing Care Management

The hospitalized child requires careful neurologic assessment and evaluation (including vital signs) repeated at frequent intervals to provide information needed to establish a correct diagnosis, reveal signs and symptoms of increased ICP, determine clinical management, prevent many complications, and provide support to the child and family during the recovery phases.

The child is placed on bed rest, usually with the head of the bed elevated slightly, and appropriate safety measures, such as side rails kept up for older children and seizure precautions for children of all ages, are implemented. For the extremely restless child, hard surfaces may have to be padded and restraint used to prevent the possibility of further injury. Care is individualized according to the specific needs of the child. The unconscious child is managed as described in the previous section, but most childhood head injuries are those causing momentary stunning or temporary unconsciousness. Children may be restless and irritable, but more often their reaction is to fall asleep when left undisturbed. A quiet environment helps reduce the restlessness and irritability. Shining bright lights directly into the child's face is irritating and often aggravates the child, making assessment of ocular responses difficult.

Frequent examinations of vital signs, neurologic signs, and LOC are extremely important nursing observations. When possible, they should be performed by a single observer to better detect subtle changes that may indicate worsening of neurologic status. Pupils are checked for size, equality, reaction to light, and accommodation. After the initial elevations usually seen following injury, the vital signs generally return to normal unless there is brainstem involvement. An axillary measurement of temperature is the safest method, since seizures are not uncommon and vomiting is a frequent response in children, especially when the child is disturbed.

The most important nursing observation is assessment of the child's LOC. Alterations in consciousness appear earlier in the progression of an injury than alterations of vital signs or focal neurologic signs. Some expected responses may be misinterpreted as deviations from the normal. Frequent examinations of alertness are fatiguing to the child; therefore, the child often desires to fall asleep, which may be confused with depressed consciousness. When left alone, the child promptly dozes. It is not uncommon to observe ocular divergence through the partially closed eyelids.

A key nursing role is to provide sedation and analgesia for the child. The conflict between the need to promote comfort and relieve anxiety in the child versus the need to be able to assess for neurologic changes presents a dilemma. However, both goals can be achieved with close observation of the child's LOC and response to analgesics, use of a pain assessment record, and effective communication with the practitioner. To differentiate between sedation from an opioid or the injury, naloxone (Narcan) can be given *slowly* to reverse the opioid's sedative effect. Decreasing restlessness after administration of an analgesic most likely reflects pain control rather than a decreasing LOC.

Observations of position and movement provide additional information. Any abnormal posturing is noted, as well as whether it occurs continuously or intermittently. Are the child's handgrips strong and equal in strength? Are there any signs of decerebrate or decorticate posturing? What is the child's response to stimulation? Is movement purposeful, random, or absent? Are movement and/or sensation equal on both sides or restricted to one side only?

The child may complain of headache or other discomfort. The child who is too young to describe a headache will be fussy and resist being handled. The child who suffers from vertigo will often assume a position of comfort and vigorously resist efforts to be moved. Forcible movement causes the child to vomit and display spontaneous nystagmus. Seizures, relatively common in children with craniocerebral trauma, may be of any type but are more often generalized, regardless of the type of injury. Any seizure activity should be carefully observed and described in detail. Children in postictal (postseizure) states are lethargic, with sluggish pupils.

Drainage from any orifice is noted. Bleeding from the ear suggests the possibility of a basal skull fracture. The amount and characteristics of the drainage are observed, and since the auditory canal may be a source of infection, dry, sterile cotton can be placed loosely at the orifice and changed when soiled.

NURSE ALERT Suctioning through the nares is contraindicated because there is a risk of the catheter entering the brain parenchyma through a fracture in the skull. ■

Head trauma is frequently accompanied by other undetected injuries; therefore, any bruises, lacerations, or evidence of internal injuries or fractures of the extremities are noted and reported. Associated injuries are evaluated and treated appropriately.

The child with normal LOC is usually allowed clear liquids unless fluid is restricted. If the child has an IV infusion, it is maintained as prescribed. The diet is advanced to that appropriate for the child's age as soon as the condition permits. Intake and output are measured and recorded, and any incontinence of bowel or bladder is noted in the child who has been toilet trained.

The child should be observed for any unusual behavior, but behavior should be interpreted in relation to the child's normal behavior. For example, urinary incontinence during sleep would be of no consequence in a child who routinely wets the bed but would be highly significant for one who is always dry. In addition, a child who is subject to nightmares might cry out and demonstrate agitated behavior at night. Parents are valuable resources. Information obtained from parents at or shortly after admission is helpful in evaluating the child's behavior (e.g., the case with which the child is roused normally, the usual sleeping position, how much the child sleeps during the day, motor activity the child is capable of [rolling over, sitting up, climbing], hearing and visual acuity, appetite, and manner of eating [spoon, bottle, cup]). There would be less concern about a child who falls asleep several times during the day if this is consistent with the child's usual behavior.

Family Support

The emotional and educational support of the family of children who have suffered head injury presents a formidable, challenging aspect to nursing care. Witnessing the parents' ordeal of grief and helplessness on seeing their child in an intensive care unit connected to monitoring equipment in an altered state evokes empathy. The nurse can encourage the family to be involved in the child's care, to bring in familiar belongings, or to make a tape recording of familiar voices and sounds. Parents may need a demonstration on how to touch or cuddle their child and may want to talk about their grief. The nurse can listen attentively, reinforce what is being done to assist the child, and direct parents toward signs and symptoms of recovery to instill hope without promises. A common phenomenon is for families to seek information from all health care providers, asking, "What will she be like? What do you know?" as they search for some clue that the child is recovering. Honesty and kindness, along with competent care, distinguish excellent nursing abilities.

When the child is discharged, the parents are advised of probable posttraumatic symptoms that may be expected, such as behavioral changes, sleep disturbances, phobias, and seizures. They should understand observations that should be made and how to contact the physician, nurse, or health facility in case the child develops any unusual signs or symptoms. The importance of follow-up evaluation should be emphasized. It is often advisable to refer the family to a public health agency for home follow-through to be certain that the child receives posthospital evaluation.

Rehabilitation

The rehabilitation and management of the child with permanent brain injury are essential aspects of care. Rehabilitation of brain-injured children is begun as soon as feasible and usually involves the family and a rehabilitation team. Careful assessment of the child's capabilities, limitations, and probable potential is made as early as possible, and appropriate interventions are implemented to maximize the residual capacities. The Brain Injury Association of America* "arose from the mutual frustration and sense of hopelessness experienced by families in their search for appropriate facilities and support to return head-injured loved ones to their maximum functioning potential." It provides information and listings of rehabilitation services and support groups throughout the country.

Pediatric trauma rehabilitation is a national concern. Coordinating care and services for early rehabilitation involves identifying the child and family's response to the traumatic injury and disability, securing available resources, and recognizing the parental role in the process.

The child with a disability resulting from head trauma requires assessment on a physical, cognitive, emotional, and social level. The child has experienced separation, pain, sensory deprivation and overload, changes in circadian cycle, and fear of the unknown. Recovery and transition require new coping strategies at the same time that regressive and acting-out behavior may start. Parents and children need honest communication for decision making. A rehabilitation facility or home rehabilitation is advocated when the child has progressed beyond what can be provided in a hospital setting. The Rancho Los Amigos Scale provides a systematic assessment of the possible progress a child may achieve following a severe head injury.

*105 North Alfred Street, Alexandria, VA 22314; phone: 703-236-6000; fax: 703-236-6001; Web site: www.biausa.org.

Prevention

Tremendous strides have been taken in the prevention of cerebral damage after head injury in children. New developments requiring research point to the prevention of cellular injury or the primary insult. However, the greatest benefit lies in prevention of head injuries. Nurses can exert a valuable influence on behalf of children through education. The reason injuries remain preventable is that unnecessary risks go unchecked. Inadequate supervision combined with a child's natural sense of indestructibility and exploration can lead to lethal results. Nurses are in the unique position of influencing caregivers in terms of growth and development. Banning the use of infant walkers is an example. This equipment does not help develop motor skills but places infants at risk for head and neck injuries from falls, especially down steps. Public education, coupled with legislative support, can prevent childhood injuries. (For extensive discussions of childhood injuries, see the discussions on injury prevention in Chapters 36, 37, 38, 39, 40. See also Childhood Mortality, Chapter 29).

Near-Drowning

Drowning ranks second as a cause of accidental death in children. Most cases of drowning are accidental, usually involving the following individuals:

1. Children who are helpless in water, such as inadequately attended children in or near swimming pools or infants in bathtubs
2. Small children who fall into ponds, streams, and flooded excavations, usually near home
3. Occupants of pleasure boats who fail to wear life preservers
4. Children who have diving accidents
5. Children who are able to swim but overestimate their endurance.

Accidental drowning occurs five times more often in boys than in girls; almost 40% of children are younger than age 5, and 90% of cases occur in private swimming pools (Kallas, 2004).

Drowning can take place in any body of water, including such unlikely ones as a pail of water. Top-heavy toddlers fall head first into a pail of water, their arms become trapped, and they are unable to free themselves. Hot tubs and whirlpool spas have been implicated in childhood drowning injury. The suction created at the outlet is strong enough to trap even larger children underwater. Drowning as a form of fatal child abuse has also been recognized as a problem. Homicidal drownings are unwitnessed, they usually occur in the home, and the victims are either infants or toddlers. With expeditious treatment many children are being saved. For purposes of this discussion, two terms need clarification:

Drowning—Death from asphyxia while submerged, regardless of whether fluid has entered the lungs

Near-drowning—Survival at least 24 hours after submersion in a fluid medium

Pathophysiology

The major pulmonary changes that occur in drowning are directly related to the length of submersion (regardless of the type and amount of fluid aspirated), the physiologic response of the victim, and the development and degree of immersion hypothermia. In addition, cerebral recovery depends on the effectiveness of initial resuscitation and subsequent critical care measures to support cerebral salvage.

Physiologic factors that influence the extent of damage from immersion include resistance to asphyxia and anoxia, which shows some individual variation. There is greater resistance with diminishing age; young children can withstand longer periods of submersion. More important is the drowning, or diving, reflex. This neurologic response is triggered by immersion of the face in cold water. Blood is shunted away from the periphery, and the flow is concentrated to the brain and heart predominantly.

The problems created by near-drowning are (1) hypoxia and asphyxiation, (2) aspiration, and (3) hypothermia (except near-drowning in hot tubs). Cardiopulmonary arrest is secondary to asphyxiation.

Hypoxia is the primary problem because it results in global cell damage, and different cells tolerate variable lengths of anoxia. Neurons, especially cerebral cells, sustain irreversible damage after 4 to 6 minutes of submersion. The heart and lungs can survive up to 30 minutes. Regardless of the amount of water aspirated, there is arterial hypoxemia (resulting from atelectasis with shunting of blood through the nonventilated alveoli) and a combined respiratory acidosis (resulting from retained carbon dioxide) and metabolic acidosis (caused by buildup of acid metabolites from anaerobic metabolism). The pathologic events are directly related to the duration of submersion. The major difficulty is acute ventilatory insufficiency. Approximately 10% of drowning victims die without aspirating fluid but succumb from acute asphyxia as a result of prolonged reflex laryngospasm.

Aspiration of fluid occurs in the majority of drownings. The aspirated fluid results in pulmonary edema, atelectasis, airway spasm, and pneumonitis, which aggravates the hypoxia. It was previously thought that submersion in saltwater versus fresh water altered the physiologic response to near-drowning. However, there is no clinically significant difference in the response of human survivors, and the type of water does not alter the therapy or outcome.

Hypothermia occurs rapidly in infants and children, partly because of their large surface area relative to body mass and partly as a result of the cold water itself. Water is an excellent heat conductor, and the contact with the skin is increased by struggling. Hypothermia may make resumption or maintenance of cardiac function possible if body temperature is less than 30° C (86° F). Profound hypothermia is usually evidence of lengthy submersion.

Therapeutic Management

Resuscitative measures should begin at the scene of a drowning, and the victim should be transported to the hospital with maximal ventilatory and circulatory support. Many victims need care for some time after aspiration of fluid. In the hospital, intensive pulmonary care is implemented and continued according to the needs of the patient.

In general, the management of the near-drowning victim is based on the degree of cerebral insult (Box 51-5). The first priority is to restore oxygen delivery to the cells and prevent further hypoxic damage. A spontaneously breathing child will do well in an oxygen-enriched atmosphere; the more severely affected child will require endotracheal intubation and mechanical ventilation. Blood gases and pH are monitored frequently as a guide to oxygen, fluid, and electrolyte therapies.

NURSE ALERT All children who have a near-drowning experience should be admitted to the hospital for observation. Although many patients do not appear to have suffered adverse effects from the event, complications (e.g., respiratory compromise, cerebral edema) may occur 24 hours after the incident. ■

Aspiration pneumonia is a frequent complication that occurs about 48 to 72 hours after the episode. Bronchospasm, alveolocapillary membrane damage, atelectasis, abscess formation, and acute respiratory distress syndrome are other complications that occur after aspiration of fluid.

Prognosis

Studies report that the best predictors of a good outcome were length of submersion in non-icy water (<5° C [41° F]) for less than 5 minutes and the presence of sinus rhythm, reactive pupils, and neurologic responsiveness at the scene. The worst prognoses—for death or severe neurologic impairment—were in children submerged for more than 10 minutes and not responding to advanced life support within 25 minutes. All children without spontaneous, purposeful movement and normal brainstem function 24 hours after near-drowning suffered severe neurologic deficits or death (Kallas, 2004; Zuckerman, Gregory, & Santos-Damiani, 1998).

Nursing Care Management

Nursing care depends on the condition of the child. A child who survives may need intensive respiratory nursing care with attention to vital signs, mechanical ventilation and/or tracheostomy, blood gas determination, chest therapy,

BOX 51-5

Clinical Manifestations of Near-Drowning

CATEGORY	CHARACTERISTICS
A	Awake, minimal injury Fully conscious; may have mild hypothermia, mild chest radiograph changes, mild arterial blood gas abnormalities
B	Blunted sensorium, moderate injury Obtund, stuporous, purposeful response to painful stimuli, mild-to-moderate hypothermia, frequent respiratory distress, abnormal chest radiographs, arterial blood gas abnormalities
C	Comatose, severe anoxia Unarousable, abnormal response to pain, ab normal respiratory pattern, seizures, shock, marked arterial blood gas abnormalities, abnormal chest radiographs, arrhythmias, metabolic acidosis, hyperkalemia, hyperglycemia, disseminated intravascular coagulation **C1:** Decorticate, Cheyne-Stokes respirations **C2:** Decerebrate, central hyperventilation **C3:** Flaccid, apneic or cluster breathing **C4:** Flaccid, apneic, no detectable circulation

and IV infusion. Frequently the child is comatose for an indefinite period and requires the same care as an unconscious child. A difficult aspect in the care of the child victim of near-drowning is helping the parents cope with severe guilt reactions. The magnitude of the event is so great that efforts to provide comfort and support are of only limited success. Parents need to hear that everything possible is being done to treat the child, and this message needs to be repeated often.

The parents of the child who is saved from death are also faced with the anxiety of not knowing what the outcome will be, and sometimes they wish for the death of the child. Because their situation generates such intense feelings of loneliness, it is important for families to know that they are not alone. They need to be reminded frequently that there are caring people to assist them both during the crisis and later. Additional sources of support that can be recommended are psychiatric and social work consultants, community services, and religious support. Self-help groups are excellent if these are available in the community.

Nurses often have difficulty relating to the parents if obvious neglect has precipitated the accident and subsequent problems; therefore, it is important for those who care for these children and their families to assess their own feelings about the situation, as well as the coping abilities and resources of the family. Caring for near-drowning victims and their families requires nurses to be sensitive to the needs of the child and the family and to recognize their own reactions and emotions.

Prevention

Most drownings, particularly of infants or small children, can be prevented with adequate supervision. Water safety and survival training should be required for all school-age children, and nurses can be active advocates in their communities. Nurses are also in a position to emphasize the importance of adequate adult supervision when children are in the water. Aquatic programs for infants and toddlers do not decrease the risk of drowning; young children should never be left unattended when in or near the water (American Academy of Pediatrics [AAP], Committee on Sports Medicine and Fitness and Committee on Injury and Poison Prevention, 2000; Kallas, 2004). Parents with pools should know cardiopulmonary resuscitation (CPR) techniques. See also Injury Prevention in Chapters 36, 37, 38, 39, 40.

NERVOUS SYSTEM TUMORS

Brain tumor and neuroblastoma are two major forms of childhood cancer derived from neural tissue. CNS tumors account for approximately 20% of all childhood cancers, and approximately 65 cases per million occur in children under 15 years of age (Redner, 2000). Both of these tumors are difficult to treat and have not demonstrated the dramatic improvements in survival seen in other forms of childhood cancer.

Brain Tumors

Brain tumors are the most common solid tumors in children and are the second most common childhood cancer. The majority of tumors (about 60%) are *infratentorial* (below the tentorium cerebelli), which means that they occur in the posterior third of the brain, primarily in the cerebellum or brainstem. This anatomic distribution accounts for the frequency of symptoms resulting from increased ICP. The other tumors are *supratentorial,* or within the anterior two thirds of the brain, mainly the cerebrum.

Brain tumors, whether benign or malignant, can arise from any cell within the cranium. Consequently, the cranial cells' origin provides a histologic classification for major tumors. For instance, astrocytes (cells that form the supportive tissue for neurons) may form a common glial tumor called an astrocytoma. The major infratentorial tumors are medulloblastomas, cerebellar astrocytomas, brainstem gliomas, and ependymomas, and the major supratentorial tumors are astrocytomas, hypothalamic tumors, optic pathway tumors, and craniopharyngiomas.

Diagnostic Evaluation

The signs and symptoms of brain tumors are directly related to their anatomic location and size and, to some extent, the age of the child. In infants, whose cranial sutures are still open, virtually no early detectable symptoms develop. It is not until spinal fluid obstruction causes markedly increased head size that a lesion may be suspected. Even in older children, clinical manifestations are nonspecific. However, the most common symptoms are headache, especially on awakening, and vomiting that is not related to feeding. The common clinical manifestations and assessment of brain tumors are presented in Table 51-2.

Diagnosis of a brain tumor is based subjectively on presenting clinical signs and objectively on neurologic tests and histologic diagnosis via surgery. Because the signs and symptoms are vague and easily overlooked, early diagnosis necessitates a high index of suspicion during history taking. A number of tests may be used in the neurologic evaluation, but the most common diagnostic procedure is MRI, which determines the location and extent of the tumor. Other tests that may be used include CT, angiography, electroencephalography, and lumbar puncture. Lumbar puncture is dangerous in the presence of increased ICP because of the possibility of brainstem herniation following a sudden release of pressure. The definitive diagnosis is based on brain tissue specimens obtained during surgery.

Therapeutic Management

Treatment may involve the use of surgery, radiation therapy, and chemotherapy. All three may or may not be used, depending on the type of tumor. The treatment of choice is total removal of the tumor without residual neurologic damage. Patients with the most complete tumor removal have the greatest chance of survival. Radiation therapy is used to treat most tumors and to shrink the size of the tumor before attempting surgical removal. Chemotherapy has emerged in the past decade to delay radiation in children younger than 3 years of age because of the rapid brain development occurring in the first 3 years of life (Murray-Ryan & Petriccione, 2002; Strother et al, 2002). Chemotherapy is also used as adjunct therapy for residual tumor, nonresectable tumor, or recurrent tumor. Water-soluble agents are able to penetrate the disrupted blood-brain barrier and attack brain tumor cells (Murray-Ryan & Petriccione, 2002; Strother et al, 2002). Typically, the most commonly used chemotherapy is cisplatin, carboplatin, vincristine, cyclophosphamide, lomustine, carmustine, etoposide,

Table 51-2

Clinical Manifestations and Assessment of Brain Tumors

SIGNS AND SYMPTOMS	ASSESSMENT
HEADACHE	
Recurrent and progressive In frontal or occipital areas Usually dull and throbbing Worse on arising, less during day Intensified by lowering head and straining, such as during bowel movement, coughing, sneezing	Record description of pain, location, severity, and duration Use pain rating scale to assess severity of pain (see Chapter 44) Note changes in relation to time of day and activity Observe changes in behavior in infants (persistent irritability, crying, head rolling)
VOMITING	
With or without nausea or feeding Progressively more projectile More severe in morning Relieved by moving about and changing position	Record time, amount, and relationship to feeding, nausea, and activity
NEUROMUSCULAR CHANGES	
Incoordination or clumsiness Loss of balance (use of wide-based stance, falling, tripping, banging into objects) Poor fine motor control Weakness Hyporeflexia or hyperreflexia Positive Babinski sign Spasticity Paralysis	Test muscle strength, gait, coordination, and reflexes (see Chapter 35)
BEHAVIORAL CHANGES	
Irritability Decreased appetite Failure to thrive Fatigue (frequent naps) Lethargy Coma Bizarre behavior (staring, automatic movements)	Observe behavior regularly Compare observations with parental reports of normal behavioral patterns Monitor growth and food intake Monitor activity and sleep
CRANIAL NERVE NEUROPATHY	
Cranial nerve involvement varies according to tumor location Most common signs: Head tilt	Assess cranial nerves, especially VII (facial), IX (glossopharyngeal), X (vagus), V (trigeminal, sensory roots), and VI (abducens) (see Chapter 35)
Visual defects (nystagmus, diplopia, strabismus, episodic "graying out" of vision, visual field defects)	Assess visual acuity, binocularity, and peripheral vision (see Chapter 35)
VITAL SIGN DISTURBANCES	
Decreased pulse and respiration Increased blood pressure Decreased pulse pressure Hypothermia or hyperthermia	Measure vital signs frequently Monitor pulse and respirations for 1 full minute Record pulse pressure (difference between systolic and diastolic blood pressure)
OTHER SIGNS	
Seizures Cranial enlargement* Tense, bulging fontanel at rest* Nuchal rigidity Papilledema (edema of optic nerve)	Record seizure activity Measure head circumference daily (infant and young child) Perform funduscopic examination if skilled in procedure

*Present only in infants and young children.

ifosfamide, and topotecan. Surgery (biopsy, resection, laser, or stereotactic), radiation therapy (hyperfractionated, fractionated, or stereotactic), and/or multiagent chemotherapy are all instrumental in the treatment of brain tumors.

Prognosis

The prognosis for the child with a brain tumor depends on the type of brain tumor, the size of the tumor, the extent of the disease, and the age of the child. Problems associated with treatment and a relatively poor prognosis, primarily in infants and young children, are compounded by serious late effects of therapy. A decline in incidence of children with medulloblastoma has been significantly linked with a protective effect of maternal folate, iron, and multivitamin supplementation. Along with the recent advances of surgical instrumentation allowing aggressive surgical intervention (e.g., stereotactic surgery, radiosurgery), modifications in radiation (e.g., hyperfractionation, brain mapping) and use of chemotherapy (e.g., intrathecal, intratumoral) have increased the long-term survival rates for many children with brain tumors (Alston et al, 2003; Gupta & Berger, 2003; Murray-Ryan & Petriccione, 2002; Strother et al, 2002).

Nursing Care Management

A brain tumor is often suspected in a child admitted to the hospital with neurologic dysfunction, although the actual diagnosis may not as yet be confirmed. Establishing a baseline of data with which to compare preoperative and postoperative changes is an essential step toward planning physical care and preventing complications. It also allows the nurse to assess the degree of physical incapacity and the family's emotional reaction to the diagnosis.

Vital signs, including blood pressure and pulse pressure (the difference between systolic and diastolic pressures), are taken routinely and more often when any change is noted. Any sudden variations are reported immediately. It is especially important to note a change in vital signs during or after diagnostic procedures. A routine neurologic assessment is also performed at the same time as vital signs, and head circumference is measured on infants and very young children.

The child is observed for evidence of headache, vomiting, and any seizure activity. The location, severity, and duration of the headache are noted, as well as its relationship to activity and time of day. Behaviors such as lying flat and facing away from light or refusing to engage in play are clues to discomfort in the nonverbal child. The child's gait is observed at least once daily. Head tilt and other changes in posturing are always noted.

Prepare Child and Family for Diagnostic/Operative Procedures

The child's preparation for the diagnostic tests depends on his or her age and previous experience. Since most of the tests involve x-ray equipment, the child may be familiar with the procedure. By the time most children are late preschoolers, they know that the head and brain are important parts of their bodies. It may be helpful to have them draw their concept of the brain in order to clarify misconceptions and base the explanation on their level of understanding.

Although the temptation is to justify the need for surgery by stating that removing the tumor will take away various symptoms, the nurse should refrain from emphasizing this point too strenuously. Postsurgery headaches and cerebellar symptoms, such as ataxia, may be aggravated rather than improved. Surgery may not improve vision. With optic gliomas the child will be blind in one eye. Finally, surgical removal of the mass may be impossible, and after surgery there may be temporary deterioration of functioning. Being honest before surgery most often makes honesty after the operation easier because no false hopes were created.

However, honesty does not negate instilling hope. A truthful explanation regarding the operation is: "The surgeon will see exactly where the tumor is. If it is small and in one place, it will be removed. If it is large, as much of it as possible will be removed so that some of your symptoms will go away." It is best to deliver information in small amounts and let the child pursue additional answers. For example, some children will ask about what happens when part of the tumor is left in. An honest reply is that after surgery the practitioner will attempt to destroy the remaining tumor with radiation and/or chemotherapy. A further explanation of radiation or chemotherapy should be delayed until a decision regarding these treatments is made.

The hair may be shaved in the operating room just before surgery or in the child's room, usually the night before surgery. When shaving is done with the child awake, the procedure is approached in a sensitive, positive way. If the child's hair is long, it should be braided so that the long swatch can be saved. Showing children how they look at different stages of the process helps them prepare for the final appearance.

Once the hair is clipped very short or shaved, the child can be given a cap or scarf to wear to camouflage the baldness. Every precaution is taken to provide privacy during the procedure and to protect the child from teasing or ridicule by other children before surgery. It is also emphasized that the hair will regrow shortly after surgery. Depending on the child's immediate adjustment to the hair loss, the nurse may introduce the idea of wearing a wig until the hair is grown in, particularly if additional irradiation or chemotherapy is anticipated.

The child is also told about the size of the dressing. Usually the entire scalp is covered to maintain a tight wound closure, even if only a small incision is made. Infratentorial head dressings may be attached to the upper back and extend forward on the neck to maintain slight extension and alignment as a precaution against wound rupture. Applying a similar dressing or "special hat" to a doll is often a less traumatic way of demonstrating the physical appearance.

The child also needs a brief explanation of how he or she will feel after surgery and where he or she will be. Ordinarily children will return to a special intensive care unit, which they should visit beforehand. The child should be aware that he or she may be sleepy for some time after surgery and that a headache is likely, although it should last only a few days.

Parents need similar explanations before surgery, especially in terms of special equipment used in the intensive care unit, dressings, and their child's behavior. For example, they should know that it is not unusual for the child to be comatose or lethargic for a few days after surgery. The nurse may wish to encourage less frequent visiting during this period so that parents can rest and be able to provide support when the child awakens.

The nurse should participate in preoperative conferences with the physician and parents. The nurse needs to know what information the parents have been given in order to be able to give further explanations or emotional support when necessary.

Prevent Postoperative Complications

Usually the surgeon prescribes specific orders for vital signs, neurologic checks, positioning, fluid regulation, and medication. These vary somewhat, depending on the location of the craniotomy. The following are general principles of care for infratentorial or supratentorial surgery. Additional aspects of care that are discussed elsewhere may include care of the child with seizures and care of the unconscious child in terms of neurologic assessment.

Vital signs are taken as frequently as every 15 to 30 minutes until stable. Temperature measurement is particularly important because of hyperthermia resulting from surgical intervention in the hypothalamus or brainstem and from some types of general anesthesia. To prepare for this reaction, a cooling blanket should be placed on the bed *before* the child returns to the unit so that it is ready for use when needed. The temperature is monitored carefully when any cooling measures are taken because hypothermia can occur suddenly. Recognizing signs of other complications such as increased ICP, meningitis, and respiratory tract infection is imperative.

NURSE ALERT When temperature is elevated, an infectious process must always be suspected, particularly if the febrile state occurs 1 to 2 days after surgery. ■

Neurologic checks are an essential aspect of care and include pupillary reaction to light, LOC, sleep patterns, and response to stimuli. Although children may be comatose for a few days, once they regain consciousness, there should be a steady increase in alertness. Regression to a lethargic, irritable state indicates increasing pressure, possibly caused by meningitis or cerebral edema.

NURSE ALERT Sluggish, dilated, or unequal pupils are reported immediately because they may indicate increased ICP and potential brainstem herniation, a medical emergency. ■

Observations for function are not instituted until the child regains consciousness. However, as soon as possible the nurse should begin testing reflexes, handgrip, and functioning of the cranial nerves. Muscle strength is usually diminished as a result of general weakness after surgery but should improve daily. Ataxia may be significantly worse with cerebellar intervention, but it will slowly improve. Edema near the cranial nerves may depress important functions such as the gag, blink, or swallowing reflex.

Dressings are observed for evidence of drainage. If soiled, the dressing is not removed but is reinforced with dry sterile gauze. The approximate amount of drainage is estimated and recorded. A drain may be placed in the operative site.

NURSE ALERT To keep an accurate account of drainage, the soiled area is circled with a pen every hour or so. In this way, continuous bleeding is easily recognized. The presence of colorless drainage is reported immediately, since it most likely is CSF from the incisional area. A foul odor from the dressing may indicate an infection. Such a finding is reported, and a culture is taken. ■

Once the younger child is alert, the arms may need to be restrained to preserve the dressing. Even a child who has been cooperative before surgery must be closely supervised during the initial stages of regaining consciousness, when disorientation and restlessness are common. Correct positioning after surgery is critical to prevent pressure against the operative site, reduce ICP, and avoid the danger of aspiration. If a large tumor was removed, the child is not placed on the operated side, since the brain may suddenly shift to that cavity, causing trauma to the blood vessels, linings, and the brain itself. The nurse confers with the surgeon to be certain of the correct position, including degree of neck flexion. The first 24 to 48 hours after brain surgery are critical. If the child's position is restricted, notice of this is posted above the head of the bed. When the child is turned, every precaution is used to prevent jarring or malalignment in order to prevent undue strain on the sutures. Two nurses are needed—one supporting the head and the other supporting the body. The use of a turning sheet may facilitate turning a heavy child.

The child with an infratentorial procedure is usually positioned flat and on either side. Pillows should be placed against the child's back, not head, to maintain the desired position. Ordinarily the head and neck are kept in midline with the body and slightly extended. In a supratentorial craniotomy the head is usually elevated above the heart to facilitate CSF drainage and decrease excessive blood flow to the brain to prevent hemorrhage.

NURSE ALERT The Trendelenburg position is contraindicated in both infratentorial and supratentorial surgeries because it increases ICP and the risk of hemorrhage. If shock is impending, the practitioner is notified immediately, before the head is lowered. ■

With an infratentorial craniotomy the child is allowed nothing by mouth for at least 24 hours, or longer if the gag and swallowing reflexes are depressed or the child is comatose. With a supratentorial operation, clear fluids may be resumed soon after the child is alert, sometimes within 24 hours. If the child vomits, oral liquids are stopped. Vomiting not only predisposes to aspiration, but also increases ICP and the potential for incisional rupture.

The child should be fed to conserve energy and minimize movement. If there is any sign of facial paralysis, the child is fed slowly to prevent choking or aspiration. Sometimes gavage feeding is necessary when body functions are too depressed to permit safe oral feedings or when the child refuses to eat or drink. IV fluids are continued until oral fluids are well tolerated. Because of the postoperative cerebral edema and danger of increased ICP, fluids are carefully monitored.

Headache may be severe and is largely a result of cerebral edema. Measures to relieve some of the discomfort include providing a quiet, dimly lit environment; restricting visitors to a minimum; preventing any sudden jarring movement, such as banging into the bed; and preventing an increase in ICP. Avoiding increased ICP is most effectively achieved by proper positioning and prevention of straining, such as during coughing, vomiting, or defecating. The use of opioids, such as morphine, to relieve pain is controversial because it is thought that they may mask signs of altered consciousness or depress respirations. However, they can be given safely, since naloxone can be used to reverse opioid effects, such as sedation or respiratory depression. Acetaminophen and codeine are also effective analgesics for mild-to-moderate pain. Regardless of the drugs used, adequate dosage and regular administration are essential to providing optimal pain relief. (See also Pain Assessment and Pain Management, Chapter 44.) Placing an ice bag on the forehead may also provide some headache relief, especially if facial edema is severe.

Bowel movements are monitored to prevent constipation. Stool softeners may be given as soon as liquids are tolerated to facilitate easy passage of stool. Saline drops, or artificial tears, may be needed to prevent corneal ulceration if the eyelids do not close completely.

Support Child and Family

The emotional needs of the family are immense when the diagnosis is a brain tumor, and feelings are influenced by the extent of surgery, any neurologic deficits, the expected prognosis, and additional therapy. Since few definitive answers can be given before surgery, the surgeon's report is a significant finding that can vary from a completely benign, resected neoplasm to a highly malignant, invasive, and only partially removed tumor. Although parents try to prepare themselves for a potentially fatal diagnosis, it is a shock for them.

Ideally, a nurse should be with the parents when the physician visits with them to discuss the expected prognosis and plan of therapy. Although parents may hear only a fraction of what they are told, they can begin to put the future into perspective. While some children will be cured, those with residual tumor may live for several years or die within a relatively short period of time. Regardless of the future prospects, the parents' thinking must be directed toward helping the child recover and resume a normal life to his or her maximal potential.

It is also a time to encourage parents to verbalize their feelings about the diagnosis. Often they express tremendous guilt for attributing the insidious onset of symptoms, such as ataxia, visual difficulty, or headache, to "minor complaints" by the child. Any comments that insinuate that the parents should have sought medical advice sooner are avoided, since such remarks only add to the parents' guilt feelings.

During this period the nurse should also discuss with parents what they plan to tell the child. If the child was prepared honestly, as described previously, the diagnosis can be expressed in a similar manner. During recovery the child will need additional explanation about the treatment, as well as the reason for any residual neurologic effects, such as ataxia or blindness.

Promote Return to Optimal Functioning

The ultimate goal is a cured child who has maximal functioning. As soon as possible, the child should resume usual activities within tolerable limits, especially returning to school.* Until the skull is completely healed, the child may need to wear a helmet when engaging in any active sport. The school nurse and teacher should confer with the parents to discuss activity restrictions, such as physical education, and the reactions of schoolmates to the child's appearance. Since children often equate brain surgery with "going crazy," it is important to prepare the child for possible remarks to this effect. As one child told a classmate, "It's *your* head they should have fixed, because you're crazy. Can't you see that I'm all better?"

After discharge, the family needs continuing medical and emotional support from health care personnel. Children who are long-term survivors after treatment for a brain tumor may have residual disabilities, such as growth retardation, cranial nerve palsies, sensory defects, motor abnormalities (especially ataxia), intellectual deficits, memory loss, dysphagia, dysgraphia, and behavioral problems. The high frequency of late effects attests to the tremendous need for follow-up care despite successful treatment of the tumor. See Nursing Care Plan: The Child With Cancer, Chapter 49.

Neuroblastoma

Neuroblastomas are the most common malignant extracranial solid tumors in children, accounting for 8% to 10% of all childhood cancers (Brodeur & Maris, 2002). They occur in about 1 per 10,000 live births, with a slightly higher incidence in males. The majority of children with neuroblastoma present before 10 years of age, with the median age of occurrence at 22 months (Brodeur & Maris, 2002). These tumors originate from embryonic neural crest cells that normally give rise to the adrenal medulla and the sympathetic ganglia. Consequently, the majority of tumors develop in the adrenal gland or the retroperitoneal sympathetic chain. Other sites may be in the head, neck, chest, or pelvis.

Neuroblastoma is a "silent" tumor. In more than 70% of cases, diagnosis is made after metastasis occurs, with the first signs caused by involvement in the nonprimary site, usually the lymph nodes, bone marrow, skeletal system, skin, or liver.

Diagnostic Evaluation

The objective of diagnosis is to locate the primary site and areas of metastasis. The signs and symptoms of neuroblastoma depend on the location and stage of the disease. Most presenting signs are caused by compression of adjacent structures (Box 51-6). Skeletal survey; skull, neck, chest, abdominal, and bone CT scans; and bilateral bone marrow aspirations and biopsies are used to locate a tumor mass and/or metastasis. A metaiodobenzylguanidine (MIBG) scan is used to determine involvement of bone and/or tissue; however, it is only available at certain centers.

Urinary excretion of catecholamines is detected in approximately 95% of children with adrenal or sympathetic tumors. Analyzing the breakdown products excreted in the urine, namely vanillylmandelic acid (VMA), homovanillic acid (HVA), dopamine, and norepinephrine permits detection of suspected tumor before and after medical/surgical intervention (Brodeur & Maris, 2002; Kline & Sevier, 2003). Amplification of proto-oncogene, known as the *N-myc* gene, and chromosomal abnormalities correlates strongly with

*Excellent publications are available from the National Brain Tumor Foundation, 414 13th Street, Suite 700, Oakland, CA 94712; phone: 800-934-CURE; fax: 510-839-9779; e-mail: *mdts@braintumor.org*; Web site: www.braintumor.org. The pamphlet *When Your Child Is Ready to Return to School* is available from the American Brain Tumor Association, 2720 River Road, Des Plaines, IL 60018; phone: 847-827-9910; fax: 847-827-9918; e-mail: info@abta.org; Web site: www.abta.org.

BOX 51-6

Clinical Manifestations of Neuroblastoma

Abdominal Tumors
Firm, nontender, irregular mass
Crosses the midline
Compression of kidney, ureter, or bladder may cause urinary frequency or retention

Distant Metastasis
Ocular:
- Supraorbital ecchymosis
- Periorbital edema
- Proptosis (exophthalmos) from invasion of retrobulbar soft tissue
- Lymphadenopathy, especially cervical and supraclavicular

Skeletal: bone pain may or may not be present
Intracranial: neurologic impairment
Thoracic: respiratory obstruction
Spinal cord: varying degrees of paralysis
Adrenal:
- Increased catecholamine excretion
- Flushing
- Hypertension
- Tachycardia
- Diaphoresis

Widespread Metastasis
Pallor
Weakness
Irritability
Anorexia
Weight loss

advanced-stage disease, rapid tumor progression, and a poor prognosis (Brodeur & Maris, 2002).

Therapeutic Management

Accurate clinical staging is important for establishing initial treatment. Therefore surgery is used both to remove as much of the tumor as possible and to obtain biopsies. In early stages, complete surgical removal of the tumor is the treatment of choice. If the tumor is large, partial resection is attempted, with a course of irradiation postoperatively to shrink the tumor in the hope of complete removal at a later date. Surgery is usually limited to biopsy in stages III and IV because of the extensive metastasis, although the use of additional surgery to assess tumor regression or remove a regressed tumor is not unlikely.

The precise role of radiation therapy is unclear. It does not appear to be of any benefit in children with stage I and II disease. It is commonly used with stage III disease; although it may not improve survival expectancy, it may make a large tumor operable. Radiation therapy provides emergency management of a massive neuroblastoma that is causing spinal cord compression (Kline & Sevier, 2003; Nguyen et al, 2000). Radiation therapy also offers palliation for metastatic lesions in the bones, lung, liver, or brain.

Chemotherapy is the mainstay of therapy for extensive local or disseminated disease. Agents used in various combinations include cyclophosphamide, doxorubicin, cisplatin, etoposide, vincristine, ifosfamide, carboplatin, topotecan, and teniposide. In children with high risk disease or recurrent disease, retinoic acid, radiation therapy, and myeloablative chemotherapy with peripheral stem cell rescue may be used to obtain a longer remission, even though a poor overall survival rate is seen (Brodeur & Maris, 2002; Kline & Sevier, 2003).

Prognosis

If all stages are grouped together, the 5-year disease-free survival rates range from 88% to 90% for children in the low risk stage, and from 22% to 30% in children in the high risk stage (Brodeur & Maris, 2002). Generally, the younger the child at diagnosis (especially younger than 1 year of age), the better the survival rate. Neuroblastoma is one of the few tumors that demonstrate spontaneous regression (especially stage IV-S), possibly as a result of maturity of the embryonic cell or the development of an active immune system.

Nursing Care Management

Nursing considerations are similar to those discussed for leukemia and brain tumors, including psychologic and physical preparation for diagnostic and operative procedures; prevention of postoperative complications for abdominal, thoracic, or cranial surgery; and explanation of chemotherapy and radiation therapy and their side effects.

Since this tumor carries a poor prognosis for many children, every consideration must be given the family in terms of coping with a life-threatening illness (see Chapter 41). Because of the high degree of metastasis at the time of diagnosis, many parents suffer substantial guilt for not having recognized signs earlier. Parents need much support in dealing with these feelings and expressing them to the appropriate people.

INTRACRANIAL INFECTIONS

The nervous system and its coverings are subject to infection by the same organisms that affect other organs of the body. However, the nervous system is limited in the ways in which it responds to injury. Infectious processes share virtually the same clinical and pathologic features. They differ primarily in the growth and virulence of the specific organism. It is generally difficult to distinguish between the various etiologic agents by looking at clinical manifestations. Laboratory studies are needed to identify the causative agent. The inflammatory process can affect the meninges *(meningitis)*, the brain *(encephalitis)*, or the spinal cord *(myelitis)*.

Meningitis is the most common infection of the CNS. It can be caused by a variety of organisms, but the three main types are the following:

1. *Bacterial*, or pyogenic, caused by pus-forming bacteria, especially the meningococcus, pneumococcus, and *Haemophilus* organisms
2. *Tuberculous*, caused by the tubercle bacillus
3. *Viral*, or aseptic, caused by a wide variety of viral agents

evolve CASE STUDY: MENINGITIS

Bacterial Meningitis

Bacterial meningitis is an acute inflammation of the meninges and the CNS. The advent of antimicrobial therapy has had a marked effect on the course and prognosis of the illness, although the use of conjugate vaccines against *Haemophilus influenzae* type B (Hib vaccine) in 1990 has led to the most dramatic change in the epidemiology of bacterial meningitis (Bonthius & Karacay, 2002; Centers for Disease Control and Prevention [CDC], 2002). In the early 1990s, the incidence of *H. influenzae* decreased from 41 cases per 100,000 children to 3 cases per 100,000 children younger than 5 years of age (CDC, 2002). Today *H. influenzae* type B infection has virtually been eradicated in areas of the world where the vaccine is administered routinely (Bonthius & Karacay, 2002; CDC, 2002). However, bacterial meningitis caused by other organisms remains a serious illness in children. It is significant because of the residual damage caused by undiagnosed and untreated or inadequately treated cases. The majority of reported cases occur in children between 1 month and 5 years of age (Bonthius & Karacay, 2002; Saez-Llorens & McCracken, 2003).

Bacterial meningitis can be caused by any of a variety of bacterial agents. *Streptococcus pneumoniae* (pneumococcal) and *Neisseria meningitidis* (meningococcal) organisms are responsible for bacterial meningitis in 95% of children older than 2 months of age. The leading causes of neonatal meningitis are the group B streptococci and *Escherichia coli* organisms. *E. coli* infection is seldom seen beyond infancy. Meningococcal (epidemic cerebrospinal) meningitis occurs in epidemic form and is the only form readily transmitted to others. It is transmitted by droplet infection from nasopharyngeal secretions. Although it may develop at any age, the risk of meningococcal infection increases with the number of contacts; therefore, it occurs predominantly in school-age children and adolescents.

Pathophysiology

Meningitis appears to occur as an extension of a variety of bacterial infections, probably as a result of the lack of acquired resistance to the various causative organisms. The most common route of infection is by vascular dissemination from a focus of infection elsewhere. Organisms also gain entry by direct implantation after penetrating wounds, skull fractures that provide an opening into the skin or sinuses, lumbar puncture or surgical procedures, anatomic abnormalities such as spina bifida, or foreign bodies such as a ventricular shunt. Once implanted, the organisms spread into the CSF, which serves as a conduit for spread of infection throughout the subarachnoid space.

The infective process is that seen in any bacterial infection—inflammation, exudation, white blood cell accumulation, and varying degrees of tissue damage. The brain becomes hyperemic and edematous, and the entire surface of the brain is covered with a layer of purulent exudate. As infection extends to the ventricles, thick pus, fibrin, or adhesions may occlude the narrow passages, obstructing the flow of CSF.

NURSE ALERT Any child who is ill and develops a purpuric or petechial rash may have overwhelming meningococcemia and must receive medical attention immediately (Box 51-7). ■

Diagnostic Evaluation

A lumbar puncture (LP) is the definitive diagnostic test. The fluid pressure is measured, and samples are obtained for culture, Gram stain, blood cell count, and determination of glucose and protein content. The findings are usually diagnostic. Culture and stain are needed to identify the causative organism. Spinal fluid pressure is usually elevated, but interpretation is often difficult when the child is crying. Sedation with meperidine (Demerol) or fentanyl (Sublimaze) and midazolam (Versed) can alleviate the child's pain and fear associated with this procedure. EMLA, a topical anesthetic cream applied to the skin overlying L3 to L5 an hour before LP, reduces pain for children undergoing this procedure.

There is generally an elevated white blood cell count, predominantly polymorphonuclear leukocytes, but it may be extremely variable. The glucose level is reduced, generally in proportion to the duration and severity of the infection. The protein concentration is usually increased. A blood culture is advisable for all children with suspected meningitis and occasionally proves positive when results of CSF culture are negative. Nose and throat cultures may provide helpful information in some cases.

Therapeutic Management

Acute bacterial meningitis is a medical emergency that requires early recognition and immediate institution of therapy to prevent death and avoid residual disabilities. The initial therapeutic management includes the following:

- Isolation precautions
- Initiation of antimicrobial therapy
- Maintenance of optimal hydration
- Maintenance of ventilation
- Reduction of increased ICP
- Management of bacterial shock
- Control of seizures
- Control of extremes of temperature
- Correction of anemia
- Treatment of complications

The child is isolated from other children, usually in an intensive care unit for close observation. An IV infusion is started to facilitate the administration of antimicrobial agents, fluids, antiepileptic drugs, and blood if needed. The child is placed on a cardiac monitor.

The choice of antibiotic is based on the known sensitivity of the organism. Except under special circumstances, the drugs are administered intravenously throughout the course of treatment. They are given in large doses, and the period of therapy is determined by CSF findings (normal glucose level and negative culture) and the child's clinical condition. Dexamethasone is currently recommended for the treatment of *H. influenzae* type b meningitis to decrease the risk of neurologic sequelae, and it should be considered for use in other types of bacterial meningitis (AAP, Committee on Infectious Diseases, 2003; Bonthius & Karacay, 2002; El Bashir et al, 2003). It should not be used if aseptic or nonbacterial meningitis is suspected (Bonthius & Karacay, 2002).

Maintaining hydration is a prime concern, and the decision to administer IV fluids and the type and amount of fluid are determined by the patient's condition. Optimal hydration involves correction of any fluid deficits followed by maintenance hydration at minimal levels to prevent cerebral edema. Electrolyte disturbances and cerebral edema are complications associated with poor neurologic outcomes

BOX 51-7

Clinical Manifestations of Bacterial Meningitis

Children and Adolescents

Usually abrupt onset
Fever
Chills
Headache
Vomiting
Alterations in sensorium
Seizures (often the initial sign)
Irritability
Agitation
May develop:
- Photophobia
- Delirium
- Hallucinations
- Aggressive behavior
- Drowsiness
- Stupor
- Coma

Nuchal rigidity
- May progress to opisthotonos

Positive Kernig and Brudzinski signs
Hyperactive but variable reflex responses
Signs and symptoms peculiar to individual organisms:
- Petechial or purpuric rashes (meningococcal infection), especially when associated with a shocklike state
- Joint involvement (meningococcal and *H. influenzae* infection)
- Chronically draining ear (pneumococcal meningitis)

Infants and Young Children

Classic picture (above) rarely seen in children between 3 months and 2 years of age
Fever
Poor feeding
Vomiting
Marked irritability
Frequent seizures (often accompanied by a high pitched cry)
Bulging fontanel
Nuchal rigidity may or may not be present
Brudzinski and Kernig signs are not helpful in diagnosis
- Difficult to elicit and evaluate in this age group

Subdural empyema (*H. influenzae* infection)

Neonates: Specific Signs

Extremely difficult to diagnose
Manifestations vague and nonspecific
Well at birth but within a few days begins to look and behave poorly
Refuses feedings
Poor sucking ability
Vomiting or diarrhea
Poor tone
Lack of movement
Weak cry
Full, tense, and bulging fontanel may appear late in course of illness
Neck usually supple

Neonates: Nonspecific Signs That May Be Present

Hypothermia or fever (depending on the maturity of the infant)
Jaundice
Irritability
Drowsiness
Seizures
Respiratory irregularities or apnea
Cyanosis
Weight loss

(Bonthius & Karacay, 2002). If indicated, measures are taken to reduce ICP as described previously (p. 1678).

Complications are treated appropriately, such as aspiration of subdural effusion in infants and heparin therapy for children who develop disseminated intravascular coagulation syndrome. If shock occurs, it is managed by restoration of blood volume and maintenance of electrolyte balance. Seizures, which occur in a large number of children, are controlled with anticonvulsants.

Lumbar puncture is carried out as needed to determine the effectiveness of therapy. The patient is evaluated neurologically during the convalescent period and at regular intervals during the succeeding year.

Prognosis

The age of the child, the type of organism, the severity of the infection, the duration of the illness before the onset of therapy, and the sensitivity of the organism to antimicrobial drugs are important factors in determining the prognosis. Sequelae are most commonly seen when the disease occurs in the first 2 months of life and least often in children with meningococcal meningitis. The residual deficits in infants are primarily a result of communicating hydrocephalus and the greater effects of cerebritis on the immature brain. In older children the residual effects are related to the inflammatory process itself or result from vasculitis associated with the disease. The mortality rate and incidence of poor neurologic outcome are highest in patients with pneumococcal meningitis (Prober, 2004; Saez-Llorens & McCracken, 2003). Evaluation of cranial nerve VIII is needed for at least a 6-month follow-up period to assess for possible hearing loss.

Prevention

Vaccines are available for types A, C, Y, and W-135 meningococci and *H. influenzae* type b. Routine meningococcal vaccination of children is not recommended. However, routine vaccinations for *H. influenzae* type b are recommended for all children beginning at 2 months of age (see Immunizations, Chapter 36). Pneumococcal conjugate vaccine is recommended for all children beginning at 2 months of age (AAP, Committee on Infectious Diseases, 2003; Kaplan, 2002).

Nursing Care Management

Nurses should take necessary precautions to protect themselves and others from possible infection. Parents are taught the proper procedures and supervised in their application.

NURSE ALERT A major priority of nursing care of a child with suspected meningitis is to administer the antibiotic as soon as it is ordered. The child is also placed on respiratory isolation for at least 24 hours after implementation of antimicrobial therapy. ■

The room should be kept as quiet as possible, and environmental stimuli kept at a minimum, because most affected children are sensitive to noise, bright lights, and other external stimuli. Most children are more comfortable without a pillow and with the head of the bed slightly elevated. A side-lying position is more often assumed because of nuchal rigidity. The nurse should avoid actions, such as lifting the child's head, that cause pain or increase discomfort. Measures are taken to ensure safety because children with meningitis are often restless and subject to seizures.

The nursing care of the child with meningitis is determined by the child's symptoms and treatment. Observation of vital signs, neurologic signs, LOC, urine output, and other pertinent data is carried out at frequent intervals. The child who is unconscious is managed as described previously (see p. 1676), and all children are observed carefully for signs of complications just described, especially signs of increased ICP, shock, or respiratory distress. Head circumference is measured on the infant because subdural effusions and obstructive hydrocephalus can develop as a complication of meningitis.

Fluids and nourishment are determined by the child's status. The child with dulled sensorium is usually given nothing by mouth. Other children are allowed clear liquids initially and progressed to a diet suitable for their age. Careful monitoring and recording of intake and output are needed to determine deviations that might indicate impending shock or increasing fluid accumulation, such as cerebral edema or subdural effusion.

One of the problems in nursing care of children with meningitis is maintaining the IV infusion for the length of time needed to provide adequate antimicrobial therapy (usually 10 days). Since continuous IV fluids are usually not necessary, an intermittent infusion device is used. In some cases children who are recovering uneventfully are sent home with the device, and parents are taught IV drug administration.

Family Support

The sudden onset of the illness makes emotional support of the child and parents extremely important. Parents are very upset and concerned about their child's condition and frequently feel guilty for not having suspected the seriousness of the illness sooner. They need much reassurance that the natural onset of meningitis is sudden and that they acted responsibly in seeking medical assistance when they did. The nurse encourages them to openly discuss their feelings to minimize blame and guilt. They also are kept informed of the child's progress and of all procedures and treatments. In the event that the child's condition worsens, they need the same psychologic care as parents facing the possible death of their child (Family Focus box; see also Chapter 41).

Family Focus

PREVENTING BACTERIAL MENINGITIS

With immunization schedules calling for administration of Hib vaccine and pneumococcal conjugate vaccine to infants at 2 months of age, parents should be encouraged to bring their child to a health facility so that the full series of inoculations is completed. With the 10% to 15% mortality rate associated with bacterial meningitis, early immunization can prevent families from experiencing the tragic death of a child. Nurses play a significant role in educating families regarding preventive measures, such as early vaccination.

Nonbacterial (Aseptic) Meningitis

Aseptic meningitis is caused by a number of agents, principally viruses, and is frequently associated with other diseases, such as measles, mumps, herpes, and leukemia. Enteroviruses and mumps viruses account for a large number of cases.

The onset may be abrupt or gradual. The initial manifestations are headache, fever, malaise, gastrointestinal symptoms, and signs of meningeal irritation that develop a day or two after the onset of illness. Abdominal pain and nausea and vomiting are common; back and leg pain, sore throat, chest pain, photophobia, and generalized muscular aches or pains are found occasionally. A maculopapular rash may be present. These symptoms usually subside spontaneously and rapidly, and the child is well in 3 to 10 days, with no residual effects.

Diagnosis is based on clinical features and CSF findings, which include increased lymphocytes, predominantly mononuclear cells. It is important to differentiate this self-limited disorder from the more serious form of meningitis and to diagnose and treat any disease of which it is a manifestation.

Treatment is primarily symptomatic, such as acetaminophen for headache and muscle pain and positioning for comfort. Antimicrobial agents may be administered and isolation enforced until a definitive diagnosis is made as a precaution against the possibility that the disease might be of bacterial origin.

Nursing care is similar to nursing care of the child with bacterial meningitis.

Encephalitis

Encephalitis is an inflammatory process of the CNS that produces altered function of various portions of the brain and spinal cord. Encephalitis can be caused by a variety of organisms, including bacteria, spirochetes, fungi, protozoa, helminths, and viruses. Most infections are associated with viruses, and this discussion is limited to these etiologic agents.

Etiology

Encephalitis can occur as a result of either direct invasion of the CNS by a virus or postinfectious involvement of the CNS after a viral disease. Often the specific type of encephalitis in a particular child may not be identified for some time or at all. The majority of cases of known etiology are associated with childhood viral diseases. Most other viral infections are those involved with arthropod vectors and those associated with hemorrhagic fevers. The vector reservoir for most agents pathogenic for humans and detected in the United States are mosquitoes and ticks; therefore, most cases of encephalitis appear during the hot summer months.

Herpes simplex encephalitis is an uncommon disease, but 30% of cases involve children. The initial clinical findings are nonspecific (fever, altered mental status), but most cases evolve to demonstrate focal neurologic signs and symptoms. Children may experience focal seizures. The CSF is abnormal in most cases. Because of a rise in the number of children with herpes simplex virus encephalitis, suspected cases require prompt attention, especially since the diagnosis can be difficult. The clinical diagnosis can be confirmed by the rapid appearance of IgM antibody to herpes simplex virus type 1 in CSF and serum. The early use of IV acyclovir reduces mortality and morbidity.

Diagnostic Evaluation

The clinical features are similar, regardless of the agent involved. Manifestations can range from a mild, benign form that resembles aseptic meningitis, lasts a few days, and is followed by rapid and complete recovery, to a fulminating encephalitis with severe CNS involvement (Box 51-8).

The diagnosis is made on the basis of clinical findings, circumstances associated with the disease, and (when possible) identification of the specific virus. Arboviruses are rarely detected in the blood or spinal fluid, but viruses of herpes, mumps, measles, and enteroviruses may be found in CSF. Serologic diagnosis may be reached by means of a variety of antibody tests. The first blood for testing should be drawn as soon after onset as possible, with the second 2 or 3 weeks later. Laboratory detection of herpes simplex virus DNA in CSF may be used to expedite diagnosis of herpes simplex encephalitis.

Therapeutic Management

Patients with suspected encephalitis are hospitalized promptly for skilled nursing care and observation. Treatment is primarily supportive, including conscientious nursing care, control of cerebral manifestations, and adequate nutrition and hydration, with observations and management as for other disorders involving cerebral injury. Follow-up care with periodic reevaluation and rehabilitation are important requisites to survivors with residual effects of the disease.

Prognosis

The prognosis for the child afflicted with encephalitis depends on the child's age, the type of organism, and residual neurologic damage. Very young children (younger than 2 years of age) may exhibit increased neurologic disability, including learning difficulties and seizure disorders.

Nursing Care Management

Nursing care of the child with encephalitis is the same as for any unconscious child and the child with meningitis. Neurologic monitoring, administration of medications, and support of the child and parents are the major aspects of care.

BOX 51-8

Clinical Manifestations of Encephalitis

Onset: Sudden or Gradual
Malaise
Fever
Headache
Dizziness
Apathy
Lethargy
Neck stiffness
Nausea and vomiting
Ataxia
Tremors
Hyperactivity
Speech difficulties: mutism
Altered mental status

Severe Cases
High fever
Stupor
Seizures
Disorientation
Spasticity
Coma (may proceed to death)
Ocular palsies
Paralysis

Reye's Syndrome

Reye's syndrome (RS) is a disorder defined as toxic encephalopathy associated with other characteristic organ involvement. It is characterized by fever, profoundly impaired consciousness, and disordered hepatic function.

The etiology of the disorder is obscure, but most cases of RS follow a common viral illness, most frequently influenza or varicella. The potential association between aspirin therapy for the treatment of fever in children with varicella or influenza and the development of RS precludes its use in these patients (Bhutta, Van Savell, & Schexnayder, 2003; McGovern, Glasgow, & Stewart, 2001).

Pathophysiology

RS has been defined by the CDC as an acute noninflammatory encephalopathy and hepatopathy, with no reasonable explanation for the cerebral and hepatic abnormalities. The pathology of RS is a mitochondrial insult induced by different viruses, drugs, exogenous toxins, and genetic factors.

Diagnostic Evaluation

Elevated ammonia levels tend to correlate with the clinical manifestations and prognosis. Definitive diagnosis is established by liver biopsy (Box 51-9). Children who in the past would have been diagnosed with RS are now given other diagnoses, such as metabolic disorders, as a result of improved diagnostic techniques.

Therapeutic Management

The most important aspect of successful management of the child with RS is early diagnosis and aggressive therapy. Rapid progression through coma stages and high peak ammonia concentrations are associated with a more serious

BOX 51-9

Staging Criteria for Reye's Syndrome

Stage I: Vomiting, lethargy, and drowsiness; liver dysfunction; type I electroencephalogram (EEG); follows commands; pupillary reaction brisk
Stage II: Disorientation, combativeness, delirium, hyperventilation, hyperactive reflexes, appropriate responses to painful stimuli; evidence of liver dysfunction; type I EEG; pupillary reaction sluggish
Stage III: Obtunded, coma, hyperventilation, decorticate rigidity, preservation of pupillary light reaction and oculovestibular reflexes (although sluggish); type II EEG
Stage IV: Deepening coma, decerebrate rigidity, loss of oculocephalic reflexes, large and fixed pupils, loss of doll's eye reflex, loss of corneal reflexes; minimal liver dysfunction; type III or IV EEG; evidence of brainstem dysfunction
Stage V: Seizures, loss of deep tendon reflexes, respiratory arrest, flaccidity; type IV EEG; usually no evidence of liver dysfunction

prognosis. Cerebral edema with increased ICP represents the most immediate threat to life. Recovery from RS is rapid and usually without sequelae if diagnosis is determined early and implementation of therapy is prompt.

Prognosis

Although the incidence of Reye's syndrome has markedly decreased, health professionals must remind parents and caregivers to avoid using both aspirin and non-aspirin-containing salicylates during febrile illnesses in children (Bhutta et al, 2003; Kamienski, 2003). Survivors may have subtle neuropsychologic deficits. Generally, recovery is good given the gravity of the disease (Bhutta et al, 2003; Kamienski, 2003).

Nursing Care Management

The child who is acutely ill with RS requires continuous and intensive nursing care. In addition to appraising vital functions and neurologic status, the nurse assists with a lumbar puncture, obtains blood for laboratory examination, and inserts various IV lines such as peripheral, arterial, and central venous pressure. A retention catheter and a nasogastric tube are inserted, and when respirations are compromised, an endotracheal tube is inserted and attached to a ventilator for controlled respirations.

Care and observations are implemented as for any child with an altered state of consciousness (p. 1671) and increasing ICP. Accurate and frequent monitoring of intake and output is essential for adjusting fluid volumes to prevent both dehydration and cerebral edema. The child who is paralyzed and in a drug-induced coma is totally dependent on the caregivers, and meticulous vigilance and attention to all biologic needs are mandatory. Since hypovolemic shock is a constant danger in children with controlled fluid intake and osmotic diuresis, vital signs, including central venous pressure and/or cardiac output (Swan-Ganz catheter), are monitored frequently. Because of related liver dysfunction, the nurse must observe for signs of impaired coagulation such as prolonged bleeding time.

Family Support

Parents of children with RS need a great deal of emotional support. They are usually frightened by the child's appearance, the treatment, and the life-threatening severity and suddenness of the illness. Their distress is increased if they believe that their actions may have contributed to a delay in diagnosis. They need to be kept informed regarding the child's progress, to have diagnostic procedures and therapeutic management explained, and to be given concerned and sympathetic support.

The National Reye's Syndrome Foundation* was established by the parents of a child who died of this disease in hope of encouraging research on the disease and of educating parents and health professionals.

Human Immunodeficiency Virus Encephalopathy

Children with human immunodeficiency virus (HIV) encephalopathy, a complication of acquired immunodeficiency syndrome (AIDS), present a nursing challenge. Progressive encephalopathy has been greatly reduced in infants and children as a result of a dramatic decrease in perinatal HIV transmission and the availability of combination antiretroviral therapy (AAP, Committee on Infectious Diseases, 2003).

Neurologic manifestations in children suggest that the progressive encephalopathy is a result of primary and persistent infection of the brain with the virus. Unexplained neurodevelopmental regression and focal seizures are the dominant clinical features of the disorder. Others include progressive motor dysfunction and atypical CNS infections. These manifestations indicate a poor prognosis and, almost invariably, a fatal outcome. However, earlier implementation of therapies for AIDS may allow for slower progression of these neurologic complications.

Appropriate precautions are practiced by nurses when caring for these children. Careful handling of the child is a hallmark of excellent nursing, since these children may experience pain, isolation, social stigma, susceptibility to infection, and abandonment resulting in less than minimum sensorimotor stimulation. Nursing assessment and intervention warrant planning time to meet developmental needs, especially if it means holding, rocking, and comforting the child. Pain management is essential and may require use of several drugs to effectively treat the neuropathic pain (see Pain Assessment and Pain Management, Chapter 44). (See also Chapter 49 for a more extensive discussion of AIDS.)

Rabies

Rabies is an acute infection of the nervous system caused by a virus that is almost invariably fatal if left untreated. It is transmitted to humans by the saliva of an infected mammal introduced through a bite or skin abrasion. After entry into a new host, the virus multiplies in muscle cells and is spread through neural pathways without stimulating a protective host immune response.

Approximately 88% of rabies cases come from wild animals, and 12% from domestic animals. Emergency depart-

*National Reye's Syndrome Foundation, Inc.; phone: 800-233-7397; fax: 419-636-9897; Web site: www.reyessyndrome.org.

ments across the country have observed that the majority of dog bites occurring in children were found to be provoked (Brady, 2000). The risk of infection from a dog bite is 5%, compared to a 20% to 50% risk of infection from a cat bite (Avner, 1999). Cats are now the most common domestic animals and should be the target of rabies vaccination programs. Carnivorous wild animals (especially raccoons, skunks, and foxes) and bats are the animals most often infected with rabies and the cause of most indigenous cases of human rabies in the United States (CDC, 2001). The likelihood of human exposure to a rabid domestic animal has decreased greatly. The circumstances of a biting incident are important. An unprovoked attack is more likely to indicate a rabid animal than a provoked attack. Bites inflicted on a child attempting to feed or handle an apparently healthy animal can generally be regarded as provoked. Any child bitten by a wild animal is assumed to be exposed to rabies.

NURSE ALERT Unusual behavior in an animal is cause for suspicion; children should be warned to beware of wild animals that appear friendly. ■

The disease is uncommon in humans, but the highest incidence occurs in children younger than 15 years of age. The incubation period usually ranges from 1 to 3 months but may be as short as 10 days or as long as 8 months. Only 10% to 15% of persons bitten develop the disease, but once symptoms are present, rabies progresses inexorably to a fatal outcome. Diagnosis is made on the basis of the history and clinical features (Box 51-10). Although treatment is of little avail once symptoms appear, the long incubation period allows time for induction of active and passive immunity before the onset of illness.

Therapeutic Management

Two types of immunizing products are available for use in humans: the *inactivated rabies vaccines,* which induce an active immune response; and the *globulins,* which contain preformed antibodies. The two types of products should be used concurrently for postexposure rabies treatment when prophylaxis is indicated.

The current therapy for a rabid animal bite consists of thorough cleansing of the wound and passive immunization with *human rabies immune globulin (HRIG)* as soon as possible after exposure. A tetanus shot should be administered and antibiotics given if indicated (CDC, 1999; Molf, 2002).

Postexposure active immunity is conferred by administration of the *human diploid cell rabies vaccine (HDCV).* The first dose of the vaccine is given at the same time as the immune globulin and followed by intramuscular injections on days 3, 7, 14, and 28 after the first dose (Molf, 2002). An additional dose in 90 days is recommended by the World Health Organization. Before antirabies prophylaxis is initiated, the local or state health department is consulted.

Nursing Care Management

Both parents and children are frightened by the urgency and seriousness of the situation. They need anticipatory guidance for the therapy and support and reassurance regarding the efficacy of the preventive measures for this dreaded disease. Animal bites require treatment in an emergency department to allow for wound care and rabies prophylaxis. Prevention strategies for young children include close supervision of interactions between children and animals (Bernardo et al, 2002). Certain circumstances may warrant vaccination, such as when a child is being taken to an area of the world where rabies in stray dogs is still a problem.

BOX 51-10

Clinical Manifestations of Rabies

Initial Signs
General malaise
Fever
Sore throat

Excitement Phase
Hypersensitivity
Increased reaction to external stimuli
Seizures
Maniacal behavior
Choking

Severe Spasm of Respiratory Muscles*
Apnea
Cyanosis
Anoxia

*From attempts at swallowing (characteristics from which the term *hydrophobia* was derived).

SEIZURE DISORDERS

Seizures are caused by malfunctions of the brain's electrical system that result from cortical neuronal discharge. The manifestations of seizures are determined by the site of origin and may include unconsciousness or altered consciousness; involuntary movements; and changes in perception, behaviors, sensations, and posture. Seizures are the most commonly observed neurologic dysfunction in children and can occur with a wide variety of conditions involving the CNS.

Epilepsy

Seizures result from paroxysmal discharges in cortical neurons and are symptoms of abnormal brain function. They are considered to be a symptom of an underlying disease process. Once it is determined that the child has had a seizure, it is important to distinguish whether the episode was an epileptic or a non-epileptic seizure. Although seizures are indispensably characteristic of epilepsy, not every seizure is epileptic. Epilepsy is a chronic seizure disorder with recurrent and unprovoked seizures.

Etiology

Seizure disorders have numerous and varied causes (e.g., tumors, infections, neoplasms). Most seizures are *idiopathic.* Although the cause of idiopathic epilepsy is unknown, genetic factors may in some way alter the seizure threshold to influence neuronal discharge. A seizure disorder also can be *acquired* as a result of brain injury during prenatal, perinatal, or postnatal periods. This injury may be caused by trauma, hypoxia, infections, exogenous or endogenous toxins, and a variety of other factors. Biochemical events (e.g., hypoglycemia, hypocalcemia, and certain nutritional deficiencies) produce seizure activity.

The incidence of causative factors associated with childhood seizures is frequently related to the age of the child. Seizures are more common during the first 2 years of life than during any other period of childhood. In very young infants the most frequent causes are birth injuries (e.g., intracranial trauma, hemorrhage, or anoxia) and congenital defects of the brain. Acute infections commonly cause seizures in late infancy and early childhood but become an infrequent cause in middle childhood. In children older than 3 years of age, the most common factor is idiopathic epilepsy.

Seizure activity is believed to be caused by spontaneous electric discharge initiated by a group of hyperexcitable cells referred to as the *epileptogenic focus.* These cells display increased electric excitability in response to any of a variety of physiologic stimuli, such as cellular dehydration, abnormal blood glucose levels, electrolyte imbalance, fatigue, emotional stress, and endocrine changes. When neuronal excitation from the epileptogenic focus spreads to the brainstem, a generalized seizure develops. Seizures are designated as *focal (localized), focal with rapid generalization,* and *generalized,* on the basis of the characteristic neuronal discharges. In a large proportion of children focal seizures spread to other areas, ultimately becoming generalized with loss of consciousness.

Classification

There are many different types of epileptic seizures, and each has unique characteristics. The onset of a seizure is abrupt, paroxysmal, and transitory, and signs are highly variable. The current classification system divides seizures into two major categories: partial and generalized (Box 51-11). Some of these are described in the following section.

Partial seizures are caused by abnormal electric discharges from epileptogenic foci limited to a more-or-less circumscribed region of the cerebral cortex. Focal seizures may arise from any area of the cerebral cortex, but the frontal, temporal, and parietal lobes are the ones that are most often affected. The area of cerebral involvement is reflected by clinical manifestations. Partial seizures are subdivided into three types. *Simple partial seizures* have elementary or simple symptoms and are accompanied by no alteration of consciousness (also called an *aura*). *Complex partial seizures* involve complex symptoms and impairment of consciousness. These seizures may begin with an *aura,* a simple partial seizure that is usually a sensation or sensory phenomenon that reflects the complicated connections and integrative functions of that area of the brain. The aura is part of the seizure event and is associated with electroencephalogram (EEG) changes (Johnston, 2004; Shafer, 1999). *Simple* or *complex seizures secondarily generalized* develop into generalized seizures, usually a tonic-clonic event.

Generalized seizures without a focal onset appear to arise in the reticular formation, and the clinical observations indicate that the initial involvement is from both hemispheres. Frequently loss of consciousness occurs and is the initial clinical manifestation. Unlike partial seizures that become generalized, there is no aura. Episodes occur at any time, day or night, and the interval between episodes may be minutes, hours, weeks, or even years. Most affected persons first experience seizures in childhood, and children whose seizures begin before age 4 years have mental retardation and behavioral and learning problems more frequently than those whose seizures begin after age 4.

Diagnostic Evaluation

Establishing a diagnosis is critical. The process of diagnosis in a child with a seizure disorder has two major foci: (1) to ascertain the type of seizure the child has experienced and (2) to attempt to understand the cause of the events. The assessment and diagnosis rely heavily on a thorough history, skilled observation, and use of several diagnostic tests.

During the assessment process it is unusual to observe the child having a seizure; therefore, a complete, accurate, and detailed history should be obtained from a reliable and knowledgeable informant. This history involves prenatal, perinatal, and neonatal periods, including any instances of infection, apnea, colic, or poor feeding, and information regarding any previous accidents or serious illnesses.

Another treatment for refractory seizures is the use of the *ketogenic diet,* which severely restricts carbohydrate and protein intake and uses fat as the primary fuel to produce ketosis. A recent review of the effects of the diet supports that some children have reduced seizures during treatment, but the long-term effects, such as increased blood lipid levels, are not known (Lefevre & Aronson, 2000).

History of the seizure(s) should be equally detailed, including the type of seizure or description of the child's behavior during the event(s), the age at onset, and the time at which the seizure occurs (e.g., early morning, before meals, while awake, or during sleep). Any factors that may have precipitated the seizure are important, including fever, infection, falls that may have caused trauma to the head, anxiety, fatigue, activity (e.g., hyperventilation), and environmental events (exposure to strong stimuli such as bright, flashing lights or loud noises). If the child can describe any sensory phenomena, these are recorded. The duration and progression of the seizure (if any) and the *postictal* (period after the seizure) feelings and behavior, such as confusion, inability to speak, amnesia, headache, and sleep, are recorded. The ability to identify seizure types accurately has resulted from the technologic advances in video recording and long-term EEG monitoring.

A complete physical and neurologic examination, including developmental assessment of language, learning, behavior, and motor abilities, often provides clues to neurologic disturbances. A family history can offer clues to paroxysmal disorders such as migraine, breath-holding spells, febrile seizures, or neurologic diseases that may be related to the seizure disorder.

Laboratory studies that may prove to be of value include a complete blood cell count and white blood cell count (for signs of infection). Blood and CSF glucose may give evidence of hypoglycemic episodes or infection, and serum electrolytes, blood urea nitrogen, calcium, and other blood studies might indicate metabolic disturbances. Lumbar puncture can confirm a suspected diagnosis of cerebrospinal infection.

BOX 51-11

Classification and Clinical Manifestations of Seizures

Partial Seizures

Simple Partial Seizures with Motor Signs

Characterized by:
- Localized motor symptoms
- Somatosensory, psychic, autonomic symptoms
- Combination of these
- Abnormal discharges remain unilateral

Manifestations:
- Aversive seizure (most common motor seizure in children)
  - Eye or eyes and head turn away from the side of the focus
  - Awareness of movement or loss of consciousness
- Rolandic (Sylvan) seizure
  - Tonic-clonic movements involving the face
  - Salivation
  - Arrested speech
  - Most common during sleep
- Jacksonian march (rare in children)
  - Orderly, sequential progression of clonic movements beginning in a foot, hand, or face and moving or "marching" to adjacent body parts

Simple Partial Seizures with Sensory Signs

Characterized by various sensations, including:
- Numbness, tingling, prickling, paresthesia, or pain originating in one area (e.g., face or extremities) and spreading to other parts of the body
- Visual sensations or formed images
- Motor phenomena such as posturing or hypertonia
- Uncommon in children younger than 8 years of age

Complex Partial Seizures (Psychomotor Seizures)

Observed more often in children from 3 years through adolescence

Characterized by:
- Period of altered behavior
- Amnesia for event (no recollection of behavior)
- Inability to respond to environment
- Impaired consciousness during event
- Drowsiness or sleep usually follows seizure
- Confusion and amnesia may be prolonged
- Complex sensory phenomena (aura)
  - Most frequent sensation—strange feeling in the pit of the stomach that rises toward the throat
- Often accompanied by:
  - Odd or unpleasant odors or tastes
  - Complex auditory or visual hallucinations
  - Ill-defined feelings of elation or strangeness (e.g., déjà vu, a feeling of familiarity in a strange environment)
- May be strong feelings of fear and anxiety, distorted sense of time and self
- Small children may emit a cry or attempt to run for help

Patterns of motor behavior:
- Stereotypic
- Similar with each subsequent seizure
- May suddenly cease activity, appear dazed, stare into space, become confused and apathetic, and become limp or stiff or display some form of posturing
- May be confused
- May perform purposeless, complicated activities in a repetitive manner (automatisms), such as walking, running, kicking, laughing, or speaking incoherently, most often followed by postictal confusion or sleep; may be oropharyngeal activities, such as smacking, chewing, drooling, swallowing, and nausea or abdominal pain followed by stiffness, a fall, and postictal sleep; rarely manifests such as rage or temper tantrums; aggressive acts uncommon during seizure

Generalized Seizures

Tonic-Clonic Seizures (Formerly Known as Grand Mal)

Most common and most dramatic of all seizure manifestations

Occur without warning

Tonic phase: lasts approximately 10 to 20 seconds

Manifestations:
- Eyes roll upward
- Immediate loss of consciousness
- If standing, falls to floor or ground
- Stiffens in generalized, symmetric tonic contraction of entire body musculature
- Arms usually flexed
- Legs, head, and neck extended
- May utter a peculiar piercing cry
- Apneic, may become cyanotic
- Increased salivation and loss of swallowing reflex

Clonic phase: lasts about 30 seconds but can vary from only a few seconds to a half hour or longer

Manifestations:
- Violent jerking movements as the trunk and extremities undergo rhythmic contraction and relaxation
- May foam at the mouth
- May be incontinent of urine and feces
- As event ends, movements become less intense, occur at longer intervals, then cease entirely
- Status epilepticus: series of seizures at intervals too brief to allow the child to regain consciousness between the time one event ends and the next begins
- Requires emergency intervention
- Can lead to exhaustion, respiratory failure, and death

Postictal state:
- Appears to relax
- May remain semiconscious and difficult to arouse
- May awaken in a few minutes
- Remains confused for several hours
- Poor coordination
- Mild impairment of fine motor movements
- May have visual and speech difficulties
- May vomit or complain of severe headache
- When left alone, usually sleeps for several hours
- On awakening is fully conscious
- Usually feels tired and complains of sore muscles and headache
- No recollection of entire event

Absence Seizures (Formerly Called Petit Mal or Lapses)

Characterized by:
- Onset usually between 4 and 12 years of age
- More common in girls than in boys
- Usually cease at puberty
- Brief loss of consciousness
- Minimal or no alteration in muscle tone
- May go unrecognized because of little change in child's behavior
- Abrupt onset; suddenly develops 20 or more attacks daily
- Event often mistaken for inattentiveness or daydreaming
- Events can be precipitated by hyperventilation, hypoglycemia, stresses (emotional and physiologic), fatigue, or sleeplessness

Continued

BOX 51-11

Classification and Clinical Manifestations of Seizures—cont'd

Manifestations:
- Brief loss of consciousness
- Appear without warning or aura
- Usually last about 5 to 10 seconds
- Slight loss of muscle tone may cause child to drop objects
- Able to maintain postural control; seldom falls
- Minor movements such as lip smacking, twitching of eyelids or face, or slight hand movements
- Not accompanied by incontinence
- Amnesia for episode
- May need to reorient self to previous activity

***Atonic and Akinetic Seizures (Also Known as* Drop Attacks)**

Characterized by:
- Onset usually between 2 and 5 years of age
- Sudden, momentary loss of muscle tone and postural control
- Events recur frequently during the day, particularly in the morning hours and shortly after awakening

Manifestations:
- Loss of tone causes child to fall to the floor violently
  - Unable to break fall by putting out hand
  - May incur a serious injury to the face, head, or shoulder
- Loss of consciousness only momentary

Myoclonic Seizures

A variety of seizure episodes
May be isolated as benign essential myoclonus
May occur in association with other seizure forms
Characterized by:
- Sudden, brief contractures of a muscle or group of muscles
- Occur singly or repetitively
- No postictal state
- May or may not be symmetric
- May or may not include loss of consciousness

Infantile Spasms

Also called infantile myoclonus, massive spasms, hypsarrhythmia, salaam episodes, or infantile myoclonic spasms
Most commonly occur during the first 6 to 8 months of life
Twice as common in males as in females
Child may have numerous seizures during the day without postictal drowsiness or sleep
Outlook for normal intelligence is poor
Manifestations:
- Possible series of sudden, brief, symmetric, muscular contractions
- Head flexed, arms extended, and legs drawn up
- Eyes may roll upward or inward
- May be preceded or followed by a cry or giggling
- May or may not include loss of consciousness
- Sometimes flushing, pallor, or cyanosis

Infants who are able to sit but not stand:
- Sudden dropping forward of the head and neck with trunk flexed forward and knees drawn up-the "salaam" or "jackknife" seizure
- Less often: alternate clinical forms observed
  - Extensor spasms rather than flexion of arms, legs, and trunk, and head nodding
  - Lightning events involving a single, momentary, shocklike contraction of the entire body

Skull radiographs, CT scans, and other studies help to identify skull abnormalities, separation of sutures, and intracranial calcifications. Focal seizures in children younger than 1 year of age are indications for MRI to rule out a supratentorial tumor. An EEG is obtained for all children with seizure activity and is the most useful tool for evaluating seizure disorders. The EEG is carried out under varying conditions, including with the child asleep, awake, awake with provocative stimulation (flashing lights, noise), and hyperventilating. Stimulation elicits abnormal electrical activity, which is recorded on the EEG.

Variations of the EEG are video recordings and simultaneous polygraphs of the patient during waking and/or sleeping. These techniques can be used concurrently and are especially valuable in differentiating epileptic activity from paroxysmal behavior or non-epileptic motor events.

Therapeutic Management

The objectives of treatment of seizure disorders are to (1) control the seizures or reduce their frequency, (2) discover and correct the cause when possible, and (3) help the child who has recurrent seizures to live as normal a life as possible. Seizures of a recurrent nature are treated as soon as the diagnosis is established. If the seizure activity is a manifestation of an infectious, traumatic, or metabolic process, the seizure therapy is instituted as a part of the general therapeutic regimen. Seizure control is considered to prevent secondary brain cell injury from the neuronal discharge and hypoxia.

It is known that persons predisposed to epilepsy have seizures when their basal level of neuronal excitability exceeds a critical point or threshold; no event occurs if the excitability is maintained below this threshold. The administration of antiepileptic drugs serves to raise this threshold and prevent seizures. Consequently, the primary therapy for seizure disorders is the administration of the appropriate antiepileptic drug or combination of drugs in a dosage that provides the desired effect without causing undesirable side effects or toxic reactions.

Numerous drugs are available for control of seizures. The primary drugs prescribed for partial seizures and/or generalized tonic-clonic seizures are carbamazepine (Tegretol), phenytoin (Dilantin), fosphenytoin (Cerebyx), and valproic acid (Depakote or Depakene). The drug of choice for absence seizures is ethosuximide (Zarontin) and valproic acid. The dosage is determined by monitoring serum drug levels. Complete control can be achieved in only 50% to 75% of affected children, however, even with careful attention to details of therapy.

There is increasing evidence that diminishing polypharmacy can bring about a better quality of life; therefore, single-drug therapy is recommended. Several new drugs have also increased seizure control for many children. These include gabapentin (Neurontin), lamotrigine (Lamictal), and Felbamate (Felbatol). The use of Felbamate is controversial because of the side effects of aplastic anemia or hepatic failure.

Once seizures are controlled, the drug or drugs are continued for a prolonged time. However, periodic reevaluation of the drug is important to assess the continued effectiveness and to alter the dosage if indicated. The dosage will need to be increased as the child grows.

Withdrawal of antiepileptic therapy follows a predesigned protocol, usually begun when the child has been seizure free for at least 2 years with a normal EEG. Recurrence is most likely within the first year after discontinuance of the medication. When a medication is discontinued, the dosage should be reduced gradually over 1 to 2 weeks. Sudden withdrawal of a drug can cause an increase in the number and severity of seizures, often precipitating status epilepticus. If the time for reducing the medication coincides with puberty or, in younger children, occurs during periods when the child is subject to frequent infections, the drug is continued for a longer period. Repeat EEGs are generally obtained every 6 months to 2 years.

When seizure activity is determined to be caused by a hematoma, tumor, or other progressive cerebral lesion, surgical removal is the treatment. Surgery also may be indicated for those who suffer from repetitive, incapacitating seizures that are caused by a focal brain abnormality, if removal of the lesion does not result in significant loss of vital functions, such as speech and movement. The risks of brain surgery cannot be underestimated. Also, the costs of surgical interventions must be taken into consideration, as well as the numerous tests necessary to assess the child before surgery.

Status Epilepticus

Status epilepticus is a continuous seizure that lasts more than 30 minutes or a series of seizures from which the child does not regain a premorbid level of consciousness. The initial treatment is directed toward support and maintenance of vital functions, including maintaining an adequate airway, administration of oxygen, and hydration, and followed by IV administration of either diazepam (Valium) or phenobarbital. Rectal diazepam is a simple, effective, and safe treatment for prehospital management (Lee et al, 2002; Mitchell et al, 1999). Lorazepam (Ativan) may be replacing IV diazepam as the drug of choice. It has a longer duration of action and causes less respiratory distress in children older than 2 years of age.

NURSE ALERT Fosphenytoin (Cerebyx) is often used to treat seizures instead of IV phenytoin because of possible complications and drug interactions associated with IV phenytoin. If IV phenytoin is used, it should be administered via slow IV push and at a rate that does not exceed 50 mg/min. Because phenytoin precipitates when mixed with glucose, only normal saline is used to flush the tubing or catheter. Fosphenytoin may be given in saline or glucose solutions at a rate of up to 150 mg PE (phenytoin equivalent)/min, and it may be given intramuscularly if necessary. ■

The child must be closely monitored during administration to detect early alterations in vital signs that may indicate impending cardiac arrest or respiratory depression. When diazepam is ineffective, phenobarbital, often in extremely high levels that may require respiratory support, is given intravenously as the initial medication. Patients who do not respond to drug therapy may require the use of IV lidocaine, general anesthesia, or a potent skeletal muscle relaxant such as curare. This should be administered by an anesthesiologist.

NURSE ALERT Status epilepticus is a medical emergency requiring immediate intervention to prevent permanent injury to the brain, respiratory failure, and death. ■

Prognosis

The course and prognosis for children with seizures depend on the etiology, type of seizure, age at onset, and family and medical histories. At diagnosis the best predictors of long-term remission were children with idiopathic syndromes, younger than 9 years of age at onset, and no prior neonatal seizures before treatment (Berg et al, 2001).

Risk factors associated with recurrence of epilepsy include the following:

1. Adolescent age and older
2. Family history of epilepsy
3. Frequent seizures on antiepileptic medication
4. Multiple antiepileptic therapy (polytherapy)
5. Abnormal EEG
6. Seizures that result from past injury or insult (Berg et al, 2001).

The prognosis following treatment for status epilepticus is more favorable than previously reported. The majority of children will probably have no intellectual impairment. The highest morbidity is found in patients with a nonidiopathic, nonfebrile cause, compared to children with idiopathic or febrile status epilepticus who have a more favorable outcome (Barnard & Wirrell, 1999; Johnston, 2004).

Nursing Care Management

An important nursing function during a seizure is observing the seizure and describing its pertinent features. Any alterations in behavior and characteristics of the seizure, such as sensory-hallucinatory phenomena (e.g., an aura), motor effects (e.g., eye movements, muscular contractions, laterality, and complex activities), alterations in consciousness, and postictal state, are noted and recorded (Box 51-12).

Generalized seizures and others with dramatic manifestations are easily detected, but absence seizures may be more difficult to detect. They are easily misinterpreted as inattention. Any unusual behavior, even seemingly inconsequential behavior such as a momentary interruption of activity, staring, or mental blankness, should be described. The more detailed these descriptions, the more valuable they are for assessment. The nurse notes the time that the seizure began and the duration of the seizure.

History taking is a vital tool for helping identify factors that are significant in establishing a cause of the seizures. Interviewing the child and family helps elicit problems related to the psychologic impact of the disorder on their lives.

The child must be protected from injury during the seizure (Emergency box). It is impossible to halt a seizure once it has begun, and no attempt should be made to do so. The nurse must remain calm, stay with the child, and prevent the child from sustaining any harm during the seizure. If possible, the child should be isolated from the view of others by closing a door or pulling screens. A seizure can be very upsetting to the child, other visitors, and their families.

BOX 51-12

General Observations of the Child During a Seizure

Observe Seizure

Describe

Order of events (before, during, and after)
Duration of seizure
Tonic-clonic—from first signs of event until jerking stops
Absence—from loss of consciousness until consciousness regained
Complex partial—from first sign of unresponsiveness, motor activity, automatisms until signs of responsiveness to environment return

Onset

Time of onset
Significant preseizure precipitating events—bright lights, noise, excitement, stress
Behavior
Change in facial expression
Cry or other sound
Stereotyped or automatous movements
Random activity (wandering)
Position of eyes, head, body, extremities
Unilateral or bilateral posturing of one or more extremities

Movement

Change of position, if any
Site of commencement—hand, thumb, mouth, generalized
Tonic phase—length, parts of body involved
Clonic phase—twitching or jerking movements, parts of body involved, sequence of parts involved, generalized, change in character of movements
Lack of movement or muscle tone of body part or entire body

Face

Color change—pallor, cyanosis, flushing
Perspiration
Mouth—position, deviating to one side, teeth clenched, tongue bitten, frothing at mouth, flecks of blood or bleeding
Lack of expression
Asymmetric expression

Eyes

Position—straight ahead, deviation upward or outward, conjugate or divergent gaze
Pupils—change in size, equality, reaction to light and accommodation

Respiratory Effort

Presence and length of apnea

Other

Incontinence of urine or stool

Observe Postictally

Duration of postictal period
State of consciousness
Orientation
Arousable
Motor ability
Any change in motor function
Ability to move all extremities
Paresis or weakness
Speech
Sensations
Complaint of discomfort or pain
Any sensory impairment
Recollection of preseizure sensations, aura

If other persons are present, they should be assured that everything is being done for the child. After the seizure, they can be given a simple explanation about the event as needed.

NURSE ALERT Do not move or forcefully restrain the child during a tonic-clonic seizure and do not place a solid object between the teeth. ■

If the nurse is able to reach the child in time, a child who is standing or is seated in a chair (including a wheelchair) is eased to the floor immediately. During and sometimes after the tonic-clonic seizure, the swallowing reflex is lost, salivation increases, and the tongue is hypotonic. Therefore the child is at risk for aspiration and airway obstruction. Placing the child on the side facilitates drainage and helps maintain a patent airway. If the child becomes cyanotic, oxygen is administered. After the seizure the child is kept on the side in bed to allow the youngster to sleep. When feasible, the child is reintegrated into the environment as soon as possible. Sending a child with a chronic seizure disorder home from school is not necessary, unless the parents request this.

Children who are known to have seizures or who are under observation for seizures will require some precautions. The extent of these measures depends on the type and frequency of the seizure (Box 51-13).

Long-Term Care

Care of the child with a recurrent seizure disorder involves physical care and instruction regarding the importance of the drug therapy and, probably more significant, the problems related to the emotional aspects of the disorder. Few diseases generate as much anxiety among relatives as epilepsy. Fears and misconceptions about the disease and its treatment abound in the layperson's mind. For many it represents the archetype of severe hereditary affliction. Therefore the foci of nursing care are directed toward helping the child and the family deal with the psychologic and sociologic problems related to the disorder and educating the child, the family, peers, and the public toward a more realistic and liberal view of the disease.

Children subject to seizures are placed on some type of drug therapy. The nurse can help the parents plan the administration of the medication at convenient times to minimize disruption to the family routine. The most convenient times for administration seem to be with meals or at bedtime. Although antiepileptic drugs are available in liquid extracts or emulsions, the tablet form is preferred by neurologists. The unequal distribution of the drug in the solute and

Emergency

SEIZURES

Tonic-Clonic Seizure

During the Seizure

Remain calm.
Time the seizure episode.
If child is standing or seated, ease child down to the floor.
Place pillow or folded blanket under child's head.
Loosen restrictive clothing.
Remove eyeglasses.
Clear area of any hazards or hard objects.
Allow seizure to end without interference.
If vomiting occurs, turn child to one side.
Do not:
- Attempt to restrain child or use force
- Put anything in child's mouth
- Give any food or liquids

After the Seizure

Time the postictal period.
Check for breathing. Check position of head and tongue. Reposition if head is hyperextended. If child is not breathing, give rescue breathing and call emergency medical service (EMS).
Keep child on side.
Remain with child.
Do not give food or liquids until fully alert and swallowing reflex has returned.
Call EMS when necessary.
Look for medical identification and determine what factors occurred before onset of seizure that may have been triggering factors.
Check head and body for possible injuries.
Check inside of mouth to see if tongue or lips have been bitten.

Complex Partial Seizure

During the Seizure

Do not restrain.
Remove harmful objects from area.
Redirect to safe area.
Do not agitate; instead, talk in calm, reassuring manner.
Do not expect child to follow instructions.
Watch to see if seizure generalizes.

After the Seizure

Stay with child and reassure until fully conscious.

Call Emergency Medical Services If:

Child stops breathing
There is evidence of injury or child is diabetic or pregnant
Seizure lasts for more than 5 minutes (unless duration of that child's seizures is typically longer than 5 minutes) and written medical order is present
Status epilepticus occurs
Pupils are not equal in size after seizure
Child vomits continuously 30 minutes after seizure has ended (sign of possible acute problem)
Child cannot be awakened and is unresponsive to painful stimuli after seizure has ended
Seizure occurs in water
This is child's first seizure

Modified from *Seizure recognition and first aid*, 2001, Epilepsy Foundation; www.efa.org.

the increased likelihood of inaccurate measurements make liquid medication less desirable. For small children the tablet of the proper dosage can be crushed and administered in syrup, jelly, or other palatable substances.

NURSE ALERT Children taking phenobarbital and/or phenytoin should receive adequate vitamin D and folic acid, since deficiencies of both have been associated with these antiepileptics. Phenytoin should not be taken with milk. ■

It is important to impress on the family the need to continue the medication regularly without interruption for as long as required. The parents and the child will need to know the common side effects of the drug prescribed and observe for signs that might indicate unfavorable reactions.

Parents need to be warned of possible behavioral changes as the seizures are controlled in children taking primidone, phenobarbital, or phenytoin. Changes in personality, indifference to school activities and family, hyperactivity, or even psychotic behavior may sometimes be observed. The potential effects of antiepileptics on learning and behavior should be considered. Progressive intellectual deterioration in a child with epilepsy requires investigation of present medication plus the role of the underlying cerebral pathology. Parents should notify the health professional if the child has an illness, including vomiting or fever. Vomiting can interfere with drug absorption; fever may increase metabolic requirements; both can precipitate seizure activity.

BOX 51-13

Seizure Precautions

Extent of precautions depends on type, severity, and frequency of seizures
May include the following:
- Side rails raised when child is sleeping or resting
- Side rails and other hard objects padded
- Waterproof mattress/pad on bed/crib
- Appropriate precautions during potentially hazardous activities:
  - Swimming with a companion
  - Use of protective helmet and padding during bicycle riding, skateboarding, in-line skating
  - Supervision during use of hazardous machinery/equipment
- Have child carry or wear medical identification
- Alert other caregivers to need for any special precautions
- Identify and avoid triggering factors whenever possible

Rectal preparations of some medications are highly useful and effective when a child is unable to take oral medications because of repeated vomiting, gastrointestinal surgery, or status epilepticus. Administration of rectal drugs can be learned by parents for home treatment during a seizure. Rectal Ativan is useful as an adjunctive home treatment for children at risk for prolonged seizures.

The degree to which activities are restricted is individualized for each child and depends on the following factors:

1. Type, frequency, and severity of the seizures
2. The child's response to therapy
3. The length of time the seizures have been controlled

Normal healthy activities are encouraged for children, and participation in competitive sports is determined on an individual basis. With encouragement, most older children can accept the restrictions placed on activities. Only essential restrictions should be placed on children regarding sports and peer activity to reduce the likelihood of needlessly accentuating differences.

Because the child is encouraged to attend school, camp, and other normal activities, the school nurse and the teacher should be made aware of the child's condition and therapy. They can help ensure regularity of medication and any special care the child might need. Teachers, child care providers, camp counselors, youth organization leaders, coaches, and other adults who assume responsibility for children should be instructed regarding care of the child during a seizure so that they can act in a calm manner to promote the welfare of the child and to positively influence the attitude of the child's peers.*

Triggering Factors

Careful and detailed documentation of seizures over a period of time may reveal a pattern. When this occurs, the nurse or responsible adult may intervene to identify the triggering factors and make changes in the environment that may prevent the seizures or decrease their frequency. The necessary changes are often very simple and cost free but can make an enormous difference in the child's and family's lives (Critical Thinking Exercise).

CRITICAL THINKING EXERCISE: SEIZURES

Factors that may trigger seizures in children include the following:

Changes in dark-light patterns, such as those that occur with a flash on a camera, automobile headlights, passing a picket fence, reflections of light on snow or water, or rotating blades on a fan
Sudden loud noises, specific voices, songs, or nursery rhymes
Startling or sudden movements
Extreme or drastic changes in temperature
Dehydration
Fatigue
Hyperventilation
Hypoglycemia
Ingestion of caffeine
Insufficient protein in the diet (protein is needed to metabolize some antiepileptic drugs).

Although there have been reports of seizures triggered by flashing video games, this relationship has not been confirmed by controlled studies. Seizures may be caused by the length of playing time, which may cause sleep deprivation, fatigue, excitement, or photosensitivity (Johnston, 2004). On the basis of current knowledge, the overwhelming majority of children with seizures can play video games without the risk of seizures.†

??? Critical Thinking Exercise

SEIZURES

Since age 2 years, Jane Little has had epilepsy that is well controlled with medication. However, now that she has begun elementary school, her seizures have returned. On the way home Jane usually has a seizure on the bus; however, on weekends and holidays she is seizure free. Jane's parents are concerned that a triggering factor at school may bring on the seizures and are considering taking her out of school. As the school nurse, what should you advise Jane's parents to do?

1. Evidence—Is there sufficient evidence to draw conclusions about the reoccurrence of Jane's seizures when riding on the school bus?
2. Assumptions—Describe an underlying assumption about each of the following:
   a. A 6-year-old school-age girl diagnosed with epilepsy and seizures at 2 years of age.
   b. A school-age child whose seizures are no longer totally controlled, despite adequate pharmacologic management.
   c. A school-age child with epilepsy who is exposed to a seizure trigger when she rides the school bus and attends school.
3. What priorities for nursing care should be established?
4. Does the evidence support your nursing intervention?
5. What alternative perspectives might you have?

If a child is photosensitive, avoiding such things as wallpaper with stripes, ceiling fans, and blinking lights may be necessary; viewing the TV screen from a distance of at least 2 yards and covering one eye may be beneficial.

Family Support

Parental attitudes and management of a child with a seizure disorder are as varied as those of other parents of children with a chronic disorder, and they are subject to the same long-term problems (see Chapter 41). Whether the seizures result from illness, injury, or unknown etiology, the parents may feel guilt, anxiety, and often humiliation. They want to know if the condition will affect the child's mental capacities. To many persons, epilepsy is erroneously associated with mental deficiency. Seizures do frequently accompany other manifestations of severe brain damage from disease or injury, but the majority of children with seizures, like any population of healthy children, display a wide range of intelligence.

Parents also wonder how the illness will affect the child's future and need reassurance that it will not shorten the life of the child and that the child can attend school, marry, and elect to have children. The child will need vocational guidance, and the parents should become familiar with the laws in their state regarding any limitations that might be imposed on the child because of the disorder. It should be emphasized that seizures can be controlled or greatly reduced in the majority of children and that new studies hold the promise of progress in future treatment. Parents also need reas-

*An excellent resource is Santilli N, Dodson WE, Walton AV: *Students with seizures: a manual for school nurses*, ed 2, Landover, Md, 2001, Epilepsy Foundation of America.

†For more information on video games and epilepsy, contact the Epilepsy Foundation National Office, 4351 Garden City Drive, Landover, MD 20785; phone: 301-459-3700 or 800-EFA-1000; Web site: www.efa.org.

surance that less stigma is attached to the disease than has been in the past.

It is important to encourage a healthy attitude toward the child and the disease and to help the parents feel competent in their ability to meet their responsibilities. The child should be reared as any normal child, with natural concern tempered by the understanding of the need of the child not to be overprotected. Many parents refrain from correcting or punishing the child, especially if they have had the experience of such an emotional stress precipitating a seizure. The child must not be made to feel different in any way. Parents should be encouraged to be honest and open about the disorder with the child and with others. Some parents are tempted to try to conceal the nature of the child's illness because of their belief that the disorder is shameful or a disgrace to the family.

Restrictions on the child's activities is necessary for safety, but this area can be approached in a positive way in terms of what the child *can* do rather than what the child cannot do. Sometimes parents curtail the child's activities more than necessary. The child needs to experience the maturing influences of play and work. The Epilepsy Foundation* is a national organization that works toward and for the welfare of persons with epilepsy and their families; helps with employment and legal problems; and provides education to patients, families, and communities.

The Child with Epilepsy

The child who is provided the security of a loving family, rewards and punishments no different from those of other children, and support in acquiring self-esteem is more apt to have a positive attitude toward the disease. Children derive their self-concept and self-esteem from observations of others' reactions to them and their own perception of their capabilities. The suddenness and unpredictability of seizures and the reactions of others further influence their feelings. When others consider children to be different, inferior, or objects of ridicule, they come to view themselves as different, inferior, and incapable.

Children with epilepsy need to learn about their disease and the role that the medication plays in contributing to their prolonged well-being. As soon as they are old enough, children should assume responsibility for taking their own medication and be advised to carry medical identification with pertinent information about their condition. Planning activities with children and emphasizing the activities in which they can engage rather than those in which they cannot will help them succeed and gain satisfaction in their achievements. They should be offered opportunities and encouraged to exercise judgment in their daily lives.

The adolescent period may be a trying time for the child with epilepsy. Limits imposed on the young person's activities at a time when freedom and independence are desired may bring the disability into sharp focus. For example, some states do not allow persons with epilepsy to obtain a driver's license, even when the disease is controlled; in others there are restrictions on employment insurance.

Epilepsy should not be a severe impairment to most youngsters, and the nurse, by assuming the role of patient advocate, helping to educate the public regarding the disease, working toward making opportunities available to persons with the disorder, and lobbying for legislation that recognizes the needs of the individual with a seizure disorder, can help erase the stigma that still remains regarding the disease.

Febrile Seizures

Febrile seizures are transient disorders of children that occur in association with a fever. They are one of the most common neurologic disorders of childhood, affecting about 4% of children. Most febrile seizures occur after 6 months of age and usually before age 3 years, with increased frequency in children younger than 18 months. They are unusual after 5 years of age. Boys are affected about twice as often as girls, and there appears to be an increased susceptibility in families. Most febrile seizures are generalized and last less than 5 minutes (Fishman, 1999; Johnston, 2004).

The cause of febrile seizures is still uncertain. In most children the severity but not the rapidity of the temperature elevation seems to be a factor. The fever usually exceeds 38.8° C (101.8° F) and occurs during the temperature rise rather than after a prolonged elevation. Sometimes it constitutes the dramatic beginning of an illness. Febrile seizures usually accompany an upper respiratory or gastrointestinal infection. Although the pertussis and MMR (measles-mumps-rubella) vaccine do not cause febrile seizures, these immunizations can be precipitating factors in initial episodes of febrile seizures in children prone to having seizures (Barlow et al, 2001).

Most febrile seizures have stopped by the time the child is taken to a medical facility. However, if the seizure continues, treatment consists of controlling the seizure with diazepam (Valium) and reducing the temperature by administration of acetaminophen. In children with simple febrile seizures, prophylactic antiepileptic therapy is not recommended. The most important interventions are parental education and emotional support (AAP, Committee on Quality Improvement, Subcommittee on Febrile Seizures, 1999; Johnston, 2004). Little risk of neurologic deficit, epilepsy, mental retardation, or altered behavior has been observed as sequelae of febrile seizures.

Parents need reassurance of the *benign* nature of febrile seizures (almost 95% of children with febrile seizures will not develop epilepsy or any neurologic damage). They should be told that their child is in no danger of dying during a febrile seizure. They also need education regarding protecting the child from harm and observing exactly what happens to the child during the event. Attempts to lower the temperature with acetaminophen or to use diazepam to prevent a seizure are of no benefit in most children (Uhari et al, 1995). Tepid sponge baths are ineffective in significantly lowering the temperature; the shivering effect further increases metabolic output, and cooling causes discomfort in the child.

NURSE ALERT If a febrile seizure lasts more than 5 minutes, parents should seek medical attention immediately. Parents should call for emergency assistance (911) and not try to take a child in a car if he/she is actively seizing. ■

---

*Epilepsy Foundation National Office, 4351 Garden City Drive, Landover, MD 20785; phone: 301-459-3700 or 800-EFA-1000; Web site: www.efa.org.

CEREBRAL MALFORMATIONS

Cranial Deformities

In the normal newborn the cranial sutures are separated by membranous seams several millimeters wide. For the first few hours to 1 to 2 days after birth, the cranial bones are highly mobile, which allows them to mold and slide over one another, adjusting the circumference of the head to accommodate to the changing shape and character of the birth canal. The principal sutures in the infant's skull are the sagittal, coronal, and lambdoidal sutures, and the major soft areas at the juncture of these sutures are the anterior and posterior fontanels.

Following birth, growth of the skull bones occurs in a direction *perpendicular* to the line of the suture, and normal closure occurs in a regular and predictable order. Although there are wide variations in the age at which closure takes place in individual children, normally all sutures and fontanels are ossified by the following ages:

8 weeks: Posterior fontanel closed
6 months: Fibrous union of suture lines and interlocking of serrated edges
18 months: Anterior fontanel closed
12 years: Sutures unable to be separated by increased ICP

Solid union of all sutures is not completed until very late childhood. Closure of a suture before the expected time inhibits the perpendicular growth. Since normal increase in brain volume requires expansion, the skull is forced to grow in a direction *parallel* to the fused suture. This alteration in skull growth always produces a distortion of the head shape when the underlying brain growth is normal. The small head with closed and normal shape is a result of deficient brain growth; the suture closure is secondary to this brain growth failure. Failure of brain growth is not secondary to suture closure.

Various types of cranial deformities are encountered in early infancy. These include the enlarged head with frontal protrusion (bossing; characteristic of hydrocephalus), the parietal bossing that is seen in chronic subdural hematoma, the small head, and a variety of skull deformities (Box 51-14). Some occur during prenatal development; in others, head circumference is usually within normal limits at birth, and the deviation from normal development becomes apparent with advancing age.

Prognosis

The majority of infants presenting with craniosynostosis have normal brain development. The exceptions are those genetic disorders that involve brain pathology.

Nursing Care Management

Nursing care of families in which there is a child with a cranial defect involves identifying children with deformities and referring them for evaluation. Because no therapy is available for children with microcephaly, nursing care is directed toward helping parents adjust to rearing a child with brain damage (see Chapter 42).

Caring for infants who benefit from surgery requires special emphasis on observation for signs of decreased hematocrit and hemoglobin because of the large blood loss during surgery (Family Focus box). A cardiac monitor may demonstrate a resting heart rate of 200. Nursing care includes observation for signs of hemorrhage, infection, pain, and swelling, as well as parental education for suture care and safety. Surgical sutures should remain dry and intact. Parents need to observe for any signs of redness, drainage, or swelling and report any temperature greater than 38.4° C (101° F).

Early surgical management of craniosynostosis allows proper expansion of the brain and the creation of an acceptable appearance. Parents require special support and education during this time, especially from the health care team (Stal, Chebret, & McElroy, 1998).

BOX 51-14

Cranial Deformities

Microcephaly—Head circumference more than 2 standard deviations below average for age, sex, and gestation; caused by failure of brain development
Management—No treatment available
Craniosynostosis—Premature closure of single or multiple sutures of cranial vault, face, and base of skull
- **Scaphocephaly**—Premature closure of sagittal suture causes skull to become elongated in an anteroposterior direction, with a high cranial vault and a subnormal transverse diameter
- **Brachycephaly**—Premature closure of coronal sutures causes skull to become shortened in an anteroposterior direction, with flattening of occiput and forehead
- **Oxycephaly**—Premature closure of both coronal and sagittal sutures causes an excessively high and narrow skull that tapers upward on all sides
- **Plagiocephaly**—Unilateral closure of one coronal or lambdoidal suture causes skull to become asymmetric
- **Craniofacial dysostosis (Crouzon disease)**—Premature closure of any or all cranial sutures, most frequently the coronal, and a typical facial deformity (widely spaced eyes, hypoplastic maxilla, and beaklike nose; tongue appears large and protruding; frequently with exophthalmos)

Management—Surgical release of closed sutures; Crouzon disease—surgical correction of major facial deformities

Hydrocephalus

Hydrocephalus is a condition caused by an imbalance in the production and absorption of CSF in the ventricular system. When production is greater than absorption, CSF accumulates within the ventricular system, usually under increased pressure, producing passive dilation of the ventricles.

CASE STUDY: HYDROCEPHALUS WITH MYELOMENINGOCELE

Family Focus

BLOOD DONATION

Parents may wish to provide a compatible blood donor for their infant undergoing a planned surgical correction for craniosynostosis. Nurses need to inform and guide parents through this blood bank procedure.

Pathophysiology

The two mechanisms by which CSF is formed include secretion by the choroid plexuses and lymphatic-like drainage by the extracellular fluid of the brain. CSF circulates throughout the ventricular system and then is absorbed within the subarachnoid spaces by a mechanism that is not entirely clear. Prenatal diagnosis is undoubtedly having an impact on the current prevalence at birth of hydrocephalus. The advent of MRI and CT scanning has provided valuable information about the pathophysiology of various diseases. The causes are diverse; they are either congenital (maldevelopment or intrauterine infection) or acquired (neoplasm, hemorrhage, or infection).

Hydrocephalus is a symptom of an underlying brain disorder resulting in either (1) impaired absorption of CSF within the subarachnoid space (ventricles communicate; *communicating hydrocephalus*) or (2) obstruction to the flow of CSF within the ventricles (ventricles do not communicate; *noncommunicating hydrocephalus*). Any imbalance of secretion and absorption causes an increased accumulation of CSF in the ventricles, which become dilated and compress the brain substance against the surrounding rigid bony cranium. When this occurs before fusion of the cranial sutures, it produces enlargement of the skull, as well as dilation of the ventricles (Fig. 51-6). In children younger than 10 to 12 years of age, previously closed suture lines, especially the sagittal suture, may become diastatic or opened.

Most cases of noncommunicating hydrocephalus are a result of developmental malformations. Although the defect usually is apparent in early infancy, it may become evident at any time from the prenatal period to late childhood or early adulthood. Other causes include neoplasms, infections, and trauma. An obstruction to the normal flow can occur at any point in the CSF pathway to produce increased pressure and dilation of the pathways proximal to the site of obstruction.

Developmental defects (e.g., Arnold-Chiari malformations [ACMs], aqueduct stenosis, aqueduct gliosis, and atresia of the foramina of Luschka and Magendie [Dandy-Walker syndrome]) account for most cases of hydrocephalus from birth to 2 years of age. Hydrocephalus is so often associated with myelomeningocele that all such infants should be observed for its development. In the remainder of cases there is a history of intrauterine infection, perinatal hemorrhage, and neonatal meningoencephalitis. In older children hydrocephalus is most often a result of space-occupying lesions, intracranial infections, hemorrhage, or preexisting developmental defects, such as aqueduct stenosis or the *Arnold-Chiari malformation* (a congenital anomaly in which the cerebellum and medulla oblongata extend down through the foramen magnum).

Diagnostic Evaluation

The two factors that influence the clinical picture in hydrocephalus are the time of onset and the presence of preexisting structural lesions. In infancy, before closure of the cranial sutures, head enlargement is the predominant sign, whereas in older infants and children the lesions responsible for hydrocephalus produce other neurologic signs through pressure on adjacent structures before causing CSF obstruction (Box 51-15).

In infancy the diagnosis of hydrocephalus is based on head circumference that crosses one or more grid lines on the measurement chart within a period of 2 to 4 weeks and on associated neurologic signs that are present and progressive. However, other diagnostic studies are needed to localize the site of CSF obstruction. Routine daily head circumference measurements are carried out in infants with myelomeningocele and intracranial infections. In evaluation of a premature infant, specially adapted head circumference charts are consulted to distinguish abnormal head growth from rapid head growth that takes place normally.

The signs and symptoms in early to late childhood are caused by increased ICP, and specific manifestations are related to the focal lesion. Most commonly resulting from posterior fossa neoplasms and aqueduct stenosis, the clinical

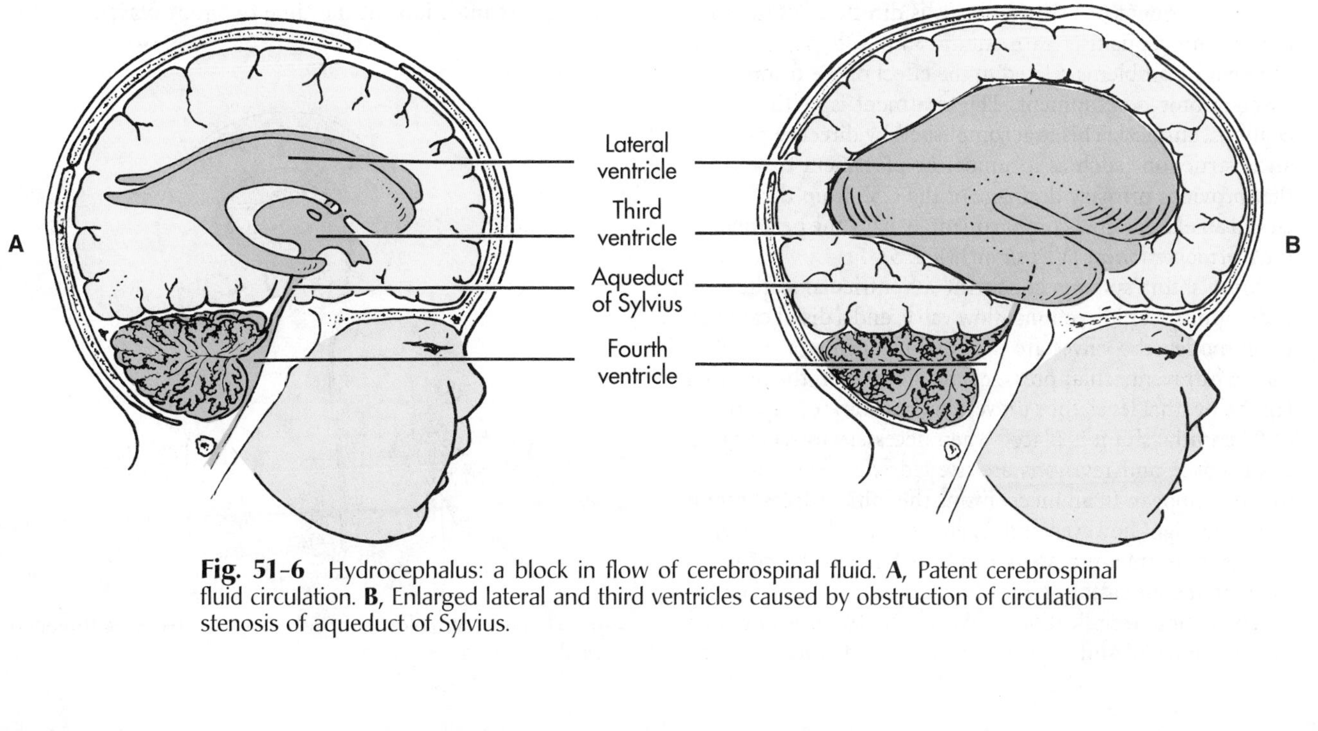

Fig. 51-6 Hydrocephalus: a block in flow of cerebrospinal fluid. **A**, Patent cerebrospinal fluid circulation. **B**, Enlarged lateral and third ventricles caused by obstruction of circulation—stenosis of aqueduct of Sylvius.

BOX 51-15

Clinical Manifestations of Hydrocephalus

Infancy (Early)
Abnormally rapid head growth
Bulging fontanels (especially anterior) sometimes without head enlargement:
- Tense
- Nonpulsatile

Dilated scalp veins
Separated sutures
Macewen sign (cracked-pot sound on percussion)
Thinning of skull bones

Infancy (Later)
Frontal enlargement, or bossing
Depressed eyes
Setting sun sign (sclera visible above the iris)
Pupils sluggish, with unequal response to light

Infancy (General)
Irritability
Lethargy
Infant cries when picked up or rocked and quiets when allowed to lie still
Early infantile reflex acts may persist
Normally expected responses fail to appear

May display:
- Change in level of consciousness
- Opisthotonos (often extreme)
- Lower extremity spasticity
- Vomiting

Advanced cases:
- Difficulty in sucking and feeding
- Shrill, brief, high-pitched cry
- Cardiopulmonary embarrassment

Childhood
Headache on awakening; improvement following emesis or upright posture
Papilledema
Strabismus
Extrapyramidal tract signs (e.g., ataxia)
Irritability
Lethargy
Apathy
Confusion
Incoherence
Vomiting

manifestations are primarily those associated with space-occupying lesions.

The primary diagnostic tools for detecting hydrocephalus are CT and MRI. Sedation is required, since the child must remain absolutely still for an accurate picture to be produced. Diagnostic evaluation of children who have symptoms of hydrocephalus after infancy is similar to that used in those with suspected intracranial tumor. In the neonate, echoencephalography is useful in comparing the ratio of lateral ventricle to cortex.

Therapeutic Management

The treatment of hydrocephalus is directed toward relief of the hydrocephalus, treatment of complications, and management of problems related to the effect of the disorder on psychomotor development. The treatment is, with few exceptions, surgical. This is accomplished by direct removal of an obstruction (such as a tumor) or placement of a shunt that provides primary drainage of the CSF from the ventricles to an extracranial compartment, usually the peritoneum *(ventriculoperitoneal [VP] shunt)* (Fig. 51-7).

Most shunt systems consist of a ventricular catheter, a flush pump, a unidirectional flow valve, and a distal catheter. In all models the valves are designed to open at a predetermined intraventricular pressure and close when the pressure falls below that level, thus preventing backflow of secretions.

The initial shunt is placed when necessary to relieve CSF obstruction, and revisions are needed when signs of malfunction appear. In all mechanisms the initial success rate is relatively high; however, shunts are associated with complications that interfere with continued shunt function or threaten the life of the child.

The major complications of VP shunts are infection and malfunction. All shunts are subject to mechanical difficulties, such as kinking, plugging, or separation or migration of the tubing. Malfunction is most often caused by mechanical obstruction either within the ventricles from particulate matter (tissue or exudate) or at the distal end from thrombosis or displacement as a result of growth. The child with a shunt obstruction is often first seen in an emergency department with clinical manifestations of increased ICP, frequently accompanied by worsening neurologic status.

The most serious complication, shunt infection, can occur at any time, but the period of greatest risk is 1 to 2 months after placement. The infection is generally a result of intercurrent infections at the time of shunt placement. In-

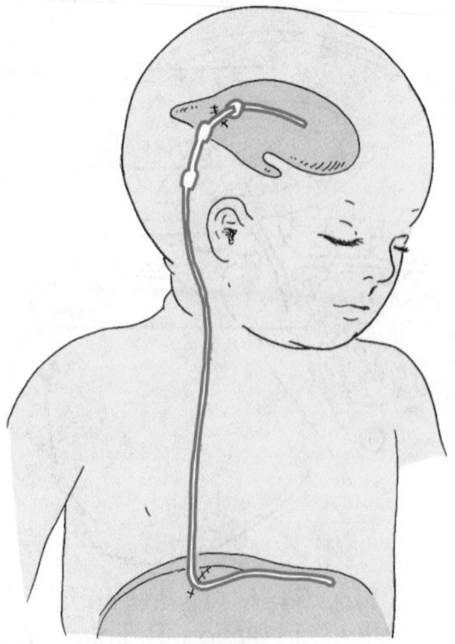

Fig. 51-7 Ventriculoperitoneal shunt. Catheter is threaded beneath the skin.

fections include septicemia, bacterial endocarditis, wound infection, shunt nephritis, meningitis, and ventriculitis. Meningitis and ventriculitis are of greatest concern, since any complicating CNS infection is a significant predictor of intellectual outcome. Infection is treated with massive doses of antibiotics administered by the IV route. A persistent infection requires removal of the shunt until the infection is controlled. External ventricular drainage (EVD) is used until CSF is sterile. The EVD allows for removal of CSF through a tube placed in the child's ventricle that flows by gravity into a collection device.

An alternative procedure to shunt placement is the endoscopic third ventriculostomy in children with noncommunicating hydrocephalus. In this procedure, an endoscope is used to make a small opening in the floor of the third ventricle that allows the CSF to flow freely through the previously blocked ventricle. Aldana and others (2003) have shown that endoscopic septal fenestration has an overall patency rate of 81%, which may eliminate the need for a CSF shunt. The complication rate of the endoscopic septal fenestration procedure was 9.3% and included intraventricular hemorrhage, sterile meningitis, and septostomy failure (Aldana et al, 2003).

Prognosis

The prognosis of children with treated hydrocephalus depends largely on the rate at which hydrocephalus develops, the duration of increased ICP, the frequency of complications, and the cause of the hydrocephalus. For example, malignant tumors may have a high mortality regardless of other complicating factors.

Surgically treated hydrocephalus with continued neurosurgical and medical management has a survival rate of about 80%, with the highest incidence of mortality occurring within the first year of treatment. Of the surviving children, approximately one-third are both intellectually and neurologically normal, and one-half have neurologic disabilities.

Nursing Care Management

Preoperatively the infant with diagnosed or suspected hydrocephalus is observed carefully for signs of increasing ICP. In infants the head is measured daily at the point of largest measurement—the occipitofrontal circumference (OFC) (see Head Circumference, Chapter 35, for technique). Fontanels and suture lines are gently palpated for size, signs of bulging, tenseness, and separation. An infant with normal ICP will display bulging under certain circumstances such as straining or crying; therefore, such accompanying behavior should be noted. Irritability, lethargy, or seizure activity, as well as altered vital signs and feeding behavior, may indicate an advancing pathologic condition.

In older children, who are usually admitted to the hospital for elective or emergency shunt revision, the most valuable indicator of increasing ICP is an alteration in the child's LOC and the way in which the child interacts with the environment. Changes are identified by observation and by comparison of present behavior with customary behavior, sleep patterns, developmental capabilities, and habits, all obtained through a detailed history and a baseline assessment. This baseline information serves as a guide for postoperative assessment and evaluation of shunt function.

General nursing care of the infant with hydrocephalus may present special problems. Maintaining adequate nutrition often requires flexible feeding schedules to accommodate diagnostic procedures, since feeding before or after handling can precipitate an episode of vomiting. Small feedings at more frequent intervals are often better tolerated than larger ones spaced farther apart. These infants are often difficult to feed and require extra time and innovation.

The nurse is responsible for preparing the child for diagnostic tests such as tomography and for assisting the practitioner with procedures such as a ventricular tap, which is often performed to relieve excessive pressure during the preoperative period and for CSF examination. Sedation is required, since the child must remain absolutely still during diagnostic testing. IV pentobarbital or oral chloral hydrate is commonly used for these procedures. (See Chapter 45 for information about preparing children for procedures.)

NURSE ALERT If surgery is anticipated, IV lines should not be placed in a scalp vein on a child with hydrocephalus. ■

Fortunately, almost all affected children are recognized, and treatment is begun early. For those children with significant head enlargement, care must be exercised to see that the head is well supported when the infant is fed or moved to prevent extra strain on the infant's neck, and measures must be taken to prevent development of pressure areas. As the hydrocephalus progresses, untreated children become increasingly helpless and prone to the multiple problems of immobility (e.g., pressure sores and contracture deformities). Not infrequently, infants with irreversible brain damage or with severe developmental defects such as hydranencephaly, in which both cerebral hemispheres fail to develop and are replaced with a membranous sac filled with CSF, are placed in long-term care facilities.

Postoperative Care

Routine postoperative care and observation are instituted. In addition, the infant or child is positioned carefully on the unoperated side to prevent pressure on the shunt valve and pressure areas. The child is kept flat to help avert complications resulting from too-rapid reduction of intracranial fluid. When the ventricular size is reduced too rapidly, the cerebral cortex may pull away from the dura and tear the small interlacing veins, producing a subdural hematoma. This is not a problem in children with elective shunt revision, since their intraventricular size and pressure have been normal. The surgeon indicates the position to be maintained and the extent of activity allowed. If there is increased ICP, the surgeon will prescribe elevation of the head of the bed and/or that the child be allowed to sit up to enhance gravity flow through the shunt. Pain management can usually be achieved with acetaminophen with or without codeine for mild-to-moderate pain and opioids for severe pain (see Pain Management, Chapter 44).

Observation is continued for signs of increased ICP, which indicates obstruction of the shunt. Neurologic assessment includes evaluation of pupillary dilation (pressure causes compression or stretching of the oculomotor nerve, producing dilation on the same side as the pressure) and blood pressure (hypoxia to the brainstem causes variability in these vital signs).

NURSE ALERT Arbitrary pumping of the shunt may cause obstruction or other problems and should not be performed unless indicated by the neurosurgeon. ■

The child is also observed for abdominal distention, because CSF may cause peritonitis or a postoperative ileus as a complication of distal catheter placement. In addition, intake and output are carefully monitored. Children may be placed on fluid restriction with nothing by mouth for 24 hours. The IV infusion is closely monitored to prevent fluid overload. Routine feeding is resumed after the prescribed NPO period, but the presence of bowel sounds is determined before feeding a child with a VP shunt.

Since infection is the greatest hazard of the postoperative period, nurses are continually on the alert for the usual manifestations of CSF infection, which may include elevated vital signs, poor feeding, vomiting, decreased responsiveness, and seizure activity. There may be signs of local inflammation at the operative sites and along the shunt tract. The child's diaper should be kept off the peritoneal dressing site or suture line. Antibiotics are administered by the IV route as ordered, and the nurse may also need to assist the practitioner with intraventricular instillation. The incision site is inspected for leakage, and any suspected drainage is tested for glucose, an indication of CSF.

Meticulous skin care is continued postoperatively, with extra care taken to prevent tissue damage from pressure. A pressure-reducing mattress or overlay pad underneath the child helps prevent pressure on prominent areas. Skin is inspected regularly for any signs of pressure, irritation, or infection.

Family Support

Specific needs and concerns of parents during periods of hospitalization are related to the reason for the child's hospitalization (shunt revision, infection, diagnosis) and the diagnostic and/or surgical procedures to which the child must be subjected. Often parents have very little understanding of anatomy; therefore, they need further exploration and reinforcement of information that was given to them by the physician and neurosurgeon, as well as information about what they can expect. They are especially frightened of any procedure that involves the brain, and the fear of retardation or brain damage is very real and pervasive. Nurses can do much to allay their anxiety by explaining the rationale underlying the various nursing and medical activities, such as positioning or testing, and by simply being available and willing to listen to their concerns.

To prepare for the child's discharge and home care, the parents are instructed on how to recognize signs that indicate shunt malfunction or infection and how to pump the shunt, if necessary. Active children may have accidents, such as a fall, that can damage the shunt, and the tubing may pull out of the distal insertion site or become disconnected during normal growth.

Safe transportation is an essential issue to discuss with parents. The tendency for the enlarged head to fall forward and to turn to the side, combined with poor head control, influences the type of child restraint system needed. Small infants can be restrained reclining in an approved car-restraint bed.

The management of hydrocephalus in a child is a demanding task for both family and health professionals, and helping a family cope with the child is an important nursing responsibility. It is important to emphasize that hydrocephalus is a lifelong problem and that the child will require evaluation on a regular basis. The overall aim is to establish realistic goals and an appropriate educational program that will help the child achieve his or her optimum potential.

Anticipatory guidance prepares parents for possible problems and helps them avoid being overprotective of the child. Few restrictions (mainly contact sports) need be placed on the child's activities, and the child should be encouraged to live as would any other child of the same age and abilities. Parents need support and encouragement in coping with the child and with problems the child may encounter in relationships with peers and others. Reactions of other children when the child has a noticeably enlarged head or requires shaving at the times of revision are stressful situations for both child and parents. (See Chapter 41 for a discussion on problems and coping with the child with a disability.)

Families can be referred to community agencies for support and guidance. The National Hydrocephalus Foundation (NHF)* and the Hydrocephalus Association† provide information on the condition for families and assist interested groups in establishing local organizations. Helpful booklets are available from these and other sources.

Key Points

- Level of consciousness (LOC) is the most important indicator of neurologic health; altered levels include full consciousness, confusion, disorientation, lethargy, obtundation, stupor, coma, and persistent vegetative state.
- Complete neurologic examination includes LOC; posture; motor, sensory, cranial nerve, and reflex testing; and vital signs.
- Nursing care of the unconscious child focuses on ensuring respiratory management; performing neurologic assessment; monitoring intracranial pressure (ICP); supplying adequate nutrition and hydration; providing drug therapy; promoting elimination, hygienic care, proper positioning, exercise, and stimulation and providing family support.
- Fractures resulting from head injuries may be classified as depressed, compound, basilar, and diastatic.
- Primary head injury involves features that occur at the time of trauma, including fractured skull, contusions, intracranial hematoma, and diffuse injury. Secondary complications include hypoxic brain damage, increased ICP, infection, cerebral edema, and posttraumatic syndromes.

---

*12413 Centralia Road, Lakewood, CA 90715-1623; phone: 562-402-3523 or 888-857-3434; fax: 562-924-6666; Web site: www.nhfonline.org.
†870 Market Street, Suite 955, San Francisco, CA 94102; phone: 415-732-7040; Web site: www.hydroassoc.org. A booklet entitled, *About hydrocephalus: a book for parents,* is available in English or Spanish.

- The young child's response to head injury is different because of the following features: larger head size, expandable skull, larger blood volume to the brain, small subdural spaces, and thinner, softer brain tissue.
- Problems resulting from near-drowning include hypoxia and asphyxiation, aspiration, and hypothermia.
- Nursing care of the child with a brain tumor includes observing for signs and symptoms related to the tumor, preparing the child and family for diagnostic tests and operative procedures, preventing postoperative complications, planning for discharge, and promoting a return to optimal health.
- Nursing care of the child with meningitis includes administering antibiotics, taking isolation precautions, removing environmental stimuli, ensuring correct positioning, monitoring vital signs, administering intravenous therapy, promoting adequate fluid and nutritional status, and providing supportive care to the family.
- Routine immunization of infants against *Haemophilus influenzae* type B infection has reduced the incidence of bacterial meningitis.
- Encephalitis may result from direct invasion of the central nervous system by a virus or from involvement of the central nervous system after viral disease.
- A seizure is a symptom of an underlying pathologic condition and may be manifested by sensory-hallucinatory phenomena, motor effects, sensorimotor effects, or loss of consciousness.
- Partial seizures are categorized as simple (without associated impairment of consciousness) or complex (with impaired consciousness); both types may become generalized.
- Generalized seizures are categorized as tonic-clonic convulsive absence, atonic and akinetic, myoclonic, and infantile spasms.
- Long-term care of the child with recurrent seizure disorders includes physical care as well as education regarding the importance of drug therapy and problems related to emotional aspects of the disorder.
- Febrile seizures are the most common type of childhood seizure.
- Many cranial deformities are amenable to surgical correction.
- Hydrocephalus is a symptom of underlying brain pathology demonstrated by impaired absorption of cerebrospinal fluid (CSF) or obstruction to the flow of CSF within the ventricles.
- Therapy for hydrocephalus involves relief of the hydrocephalus, treatment of the underlying brain disorder if possible, prevention and/or treatment of complications, and management of problems related to psychomotor development.

Answer Guidelines to Critical Thinking Exercises

Hydrocephalus

1. Yes. Emma's fussiness; holding the back of her head; intermittent periods of lethargy; and repetitive, rapid eye blinking are signs of increased ICP.
2. (a) Emma's posterior fossa tumor removal places her at risk for cerebral edema with associated increased ICP. (b) Emma's EVD may be occluded and should be assessed. Positioning of the EVD is important to evaluate since the CSF drains by gravity; repositioning may be necessary to promote adequate drainage and decrease ICP. (c) The physical signs and behavior are indicative of increased ICP, which may occur if Emma's EVD is obstructed or is draining improperly. There is evidence that CSF is draining on the mother's clothing, which is an abnormal finding with an EVD; the EVD is a closed system, and breakage or malfunction may cause the child further harm if bacteria colonize the reservoir.
3. The nurse should inspect the EVD site, assess Emma's neurologic status, and notify the medical provider of the findings. A transparent dressing should be placed over the EVD site to observe for CSF drainage, an abnormal finding. The EVD should remain positioned so that gravity drainage of CSF is enhanced (at the level of the external auditory meatus with the head at a 20- to 30-degree elevation); rapid CSF drainage is undesirable since this may result in subdural complications. A CT scan may be useful in determining the status of the drainage device.
4. Yes. Emma's signs of increased ICP and CSF drainage on her mother's clothes support the nurse's actions.
5. Another consideration for some of Emma's fussiness in the postoperative period is discomfort and pain. However, pain management should be monitored closely to avoid masking the signs of increased ICP. Once it is evident that the ICP is elevated, pain management measures should be performed, including an assessment of what Emma has taken previously to relieve pain. In addition, the nurse should explain the signs of elevated ICP to the mother and convey that obstruction of CSF flow from the EVD can cause these clinical signs and behaviors. Reassurance that the increased ICP will subside with removal of the EVD obstruction is important.

Seizures

1. Yes. Jane is a school-age child with previously controlled seizures who is now having seizures while riding on the school bus. Although there appears to be a pattern to the seizure activity, until further assessment is performed, the exact reason for the seizure activity may not be found.
2. (a) Jane's seizures have been controlled in the past with anticonvulsant medication. (b) This abrupt onset of seizures after having control for years needs further evaluation. With the consistent pattern and abrupt onset of the seizures, seeking medical reevaluation should be advised if no triggering event is identified. (c) Many environmental factors may trigger seizures in children who have had adequate pharmacologic management of seizures. These include but are not necessarily limited to the following: changes in dark-light patterns such as a camera flash, automobile lights, reflections on light surfaces such as snow or water, or rotating fan blades; sudden noises or startling movements; drastic changes in temperature; dehydration; fatigue; hypoglycemia; caffeine; and inadequate amounts of protein in the diet. Since the seizures appear to have a pattern, that is, when

Jane rides the bus home from school, further investigation and assessment are required.

3. Your first priority is to help the family identify triggering events that would yield pertinent and necessary information. Because the bus ride appears to be a focal event surrounding the recurrence of seizures, this must be assessed for potential triggers. At your suggestion, Mrs. Little rode the school bus home with Jane. As on previous rides Jane began to seize as a long white picket fence was passed; her mother noted that the child stared intently at the fence and that is when the seizure activity started. Because the fence was perceived as a potential triggering factor, actions were taken to minimize exposure to the repetitive motion of observing the white picket fence as the bus passed. Once Jane was seated on the other side of the bus, the seizure episodes stopped. As the school nurse, it would be appropriate for you to continue discussing Jane's progress with her parents and explore their feelings about taking her out of school. With a thorough assessment of their feelings about the matter and reassurance that the trigger for the recurrence of seizure activity is removed, the parents may be more amenable to leaving Jane in school. Parents of children with chronic illness such as epilepsy are encouraged to make the child's life as normal as possible, and taking her out of school would not promote that goal.
4. An accurate interpretation of the information is that it is not within the scope of nursing practice for the school nurse to change the dosage of the antiepileptic medication. As Jane grows, adjustments in medication will be necessary when she visits her primary care practitioner. An option that was explored was having the parents take Jane to school in their car; however, the seizures may still occur if Jane sits in the same position as on the school bus and is exposed to the fence that was the triggering mechanism in this case.
5. One alternate perspective that may need to be explored is whether the antiepileptic medication is within the therapeutic range for the size of the child. If recent antiepileptic drug levels have not been obtained, this may be something to consider. A visit to the primary care practitioner is encouraged.

References

Aldana PR et al: Results of endoscopic septal fenestration in the treatment of isolated ventricular hydrocephalus, *Pediatr Neurosurg* 38(6):286-294, 2003.

Alston RD et al: Childhood medulloblastoma in northwest England, 1954 to 1977: incidence and survival, *Dev Med Child Neurol* 45(5):308-314, 2003.

American Academy of Pediatrics, Committee on Infectious Diseases In Pickering L (ed): *2003 red book: report of the Committee on Infectious Diseases,* ed 26, Elk Grove Village, IL, 2003, The Academy.

American Academy of Pediatrics, Committee on Quality Improvement, Subcommittee on Febrile Seizures: Practice parameter: long-term treatment of the child with simple febrile seizures, *Pediatrics* 103(6): 1307-1309, 1999.

American Academy of Pediatrics, Committee on Sports Medicine and Fitness and Committee on Injury and Poison Prevention: Swimming programs for infants and toddlers, *Pediatrics* 105(4):868-870, 2000.

Avner JR: Animal and human bites and bite-related infections. In Burg FD, Ingelfinger JR, Wald WR (eds): *Gellis and Kagan's current pediatric therapy,* ed 16, Philadelphia, 1999, WB Saunders.

Barlow WE et al: The risks of seizures after receipt of whole-cell pertussis or measles, mumps and rubella vaccine, *N Engl J Med* 345(9):656-661, 2001.

Barnard C, Wirrell E: Does status epilepticus cause developmental deterioration and development of epilepsy? *J Child Neurol* 14(12):787-794, 1999.

Bayir H, Kochanek PM, Clark RS: Traumatic brain injury in infants and children: mechanisms of secondary damage and treatment in the intensive care unit, *Crit Care Clin* 19(3):529-549, 2003.

Berg AT et al: Two-year remission and subsequent relapse in children with newly diagnosed epilepsy, *Epilepsia* 42(12):1553-1562, 2001.

Bernardo LM et al: A comparison of dog bite injuries in younger and older children treated in a pediatric emergency department, *Pediatr Emerg Care* 18(3):247-249, 2002.

Bhutta AT, Van Savell H, Schexnayder SM: Reye's syndrome: down but not out, *South Med J* 96(1):43-45, 2003.

Bonthius DJ, Karacay B: Meningitis and encephalitis in children: an update, *Neurol Clin* 20(4):1013-1038, 2002.

Brady M: Common injuries. In Burns CE et al (eds): *Pediatric primary care, a handbook for nurse practitioners,* ed 2, Philadelphia, 2000, WB Saunders.

Brodeur GM, Maris JM: *Neuroblastoma.* In Pizzo PA, Poplack DG (eds): *Principles and practice of pediatric oncology,* ed 4, Philadelphia, 2002, Lippincott-Raven.

Centers for Disease Control and Prevention: Human rabies prevention—United States, 1999, *MMWR* 48(RR-1):1-21, 1999a.

Centers for Disease Control and Prevention: Progress toward elimination of *Haemophilus influenza* type b invasive disease among infants and children—United States, 1998-2000, *MMWR* 51:234-239, 2002.

Centers for Disease Control and Prevention: Compendium of animal rabies prevention and control, 2001, National Association of State Public Health Veterinarians, Inc, *MMWR* 50(RR-8):1-9, 2001.

Chiaretti A et al: Early post-traumatic seizures in children with head injury, *Childs Nerv Syst* 16(12):862-866, 2000.

Durkin MS et al: The epidemiology of urban pediatric neurological trauma: evaluation of, and implications for, injury prevention programs, *Neurosurgery* 42(2):300-310, 1998.

El Bashir H, Laundy M, Booy R: Diagnosis and treatment of bacterial meningitis, *Arch Dis Child* 88(7):814-819, 2003.

Ernst AA et al: Topical lidocaine adrenaline tetracaine (LAT gel) versus injectable buffered lidocaine for local anesthesia in laceration repair, *West J Med* 167(2): 79-81, 1997.

Faillace WJ: Management of childhood neurotrauma, *Surg Clin North Am* 82(2):349-363, 2002.

Fishman MA: Febrile seizures. In McMillan JA and others (eds): *Principles and practice of pediatrics,* ed 3, Philadelphia, 1999, JB Lippincott.

Gennarelli TA: Trauma to the head: general considerations. In Schwartz GR, editor: *Principles and practices of emergency medicine,* ed 4, Philadelphia, 1999, Lippincott Williams & Wilkins.

Gupta N, Berger MS: Brain mapping for hemispheric tumors in children, *Pediatr Neurosurg* 38(6):302-306, 2003.

Johnston MV: Seizures in childhood. In Behrman RE, Kliegman RM, Jenson HTS (eds): *Nelson textbook of pediatrics,* ed 17, Philadelphia, 2004, WB Saunders.

Kallas HJ: Drowning and near-drowning. In Behrman RE, Kliegman RM, Jenson HTS (eds): *Nelson textbook of pediatrics,* ed 17, Philadelphia, 2004, WB Saunders.

Kamienski MC: Reye syndrome, *Am J Nurs* 103(7):54-57, 2003.

Kaplan SL: Management of pneumococcal meningitis, *Pediatr Infect Dis J* 21(6):589-591, 2002.

Kline NE, Sevier N: Solid tumors in children, *J Pediatr Nurs* 18(2):96-102, 2003.

Lee C, Nechyba C, Gunn V: Drug doses. In The John Hopkins Hospital, Gunn V, Nechyba C (eds): *The Harriet Lane handbook,* ed 16, Philadelphia, 2002, Mosby.

Lefevre F, Aronson N: Ketogenic diet for the treatment of refractory epilepsy in children: a systematic review of efficacy, *Pediatrics* 105(4):e46, 2000. Internet document available at www.pediatrics.org/cgi/content/full/105/4/e46 (accessed June 6, 2005).

Masson F et al: Epidemiology of traumatic comas: a prospective population-based study, *Brain Inj* 17(4):279-293, 2003.

McGovern MC, Glasgow JFT, Stewart MC: Lesson of the week: Reye's syndrome and aspirin: lest we forget, *BMJ* 322(7302):1591-1592, 2001.

Mitchell WG et al: An open-label study of repeated use of diazepam rectal gel (Diastat) for episodes of acute breakthrough seizures and clusters: safety, efficacy, and tolerance, *North Am Diastat Group*, *Epilepsia* 40(11):1610-1617, 1999.

Molf I: Immunoprophylaxis. In The John Hopkins Hospital, Gunn V, Nechyba C (eds): *The Harriet Lane handbook,* ed 16, Philadelphia, 2002, Mosby.

Murray-Ryan J, Petriccione MM: Central nervous system tumors. In Baggott CR et al (eds): *Nursing care of children and adolescents with cancer*, ed 3, Philadelphia, 2002, WB Saunders.

Nguyen NP et al: Neuroblastoma producing spinal cord compression: rapid relief with low dose of radiation, *Anticancer Res* 20(6c):4687-4690, 2000.

Pasero C, McCaffery M: Procedural pain management. In McCaffery M, Pasero C (eds): *Pain: clinical manual,* ed 2, St Louis, 1999, Mosby.

Prober CG: Central nervous system infections. In Behrman RE, Kliegman RM, Jenson HTS (eds): *Nelson textbook of pediatrics,* ed 17, Philadelphia, 2004, WB Saunders.

Redner A: Central nervous system malignancies. In Lanzkowsky P (ed): *Manual of pediatric hematology and oncology*, ed 3, San Diego, 2000, Academic Press.

Rivara FP, Grossman D: Injury control. In Behrman RE, Kliegman RM, Jenson HTS (eds): *Nelson textbook of pediatrics,* ed 17, Philadelphia, 2004, WB Saunders.

Saez-Llorens X, McCracken GH Jr: Bacterial meningitis in children, *Lancet* 361(9375):2139-2148, 2003.

Schutzman SA, Greenes DS: Pediatric minor head trauma, *Ann Emerg Med* 37(1):65-74, 2001.

Shafer PO: Epilepsy and seizures: advances in seizure assessment, treatment, and self-management, *Nurs Clin North Am* 34(3):743-759, 1999.

Stal S, Chebret L, McElroy C: The team approach in the management of congenital and acquired deformities, *Clin Plast Surg* 25(4):485-491, 1998.

Strother DR et al: Tumors of the central nervous system. In Pizzo PA, Poplack DG (eds): *Principles and practice of pediatric oncology*, ed 4, Philadelphia, 2002, Lippincott-Raven.

Uhari M et al: Effect of acetaminophen and of low intermittent doses of diazepam on prevention of recurrences of febrile seizures, *J Pediatr* 126(6):991-995, 1995.

Vernon-Levett P: Neurologic system. In Slota MC (ed): *Core curriculum for pediatric critical care nursing,* Philadelphia, 1998, WB Saunders.

Zuckerman GB, Gregory PM, Santos-Damiani SM: Predictors of death and neurologic impairment in pediatric submersion injuries: the pediatric risk of mortality score, *Arch Pediatr Adolesc Med* 152:134-140, 1998.

52 Endocrine Dysfunction

LEARNING OBJECTIVES

On completion of this chapter the reader will be able to:

- Differentiate between the disorders caused by hypopituitary and hyperpituitary dysfunction.
- Describe the manifestations of thyroid hypofunction and hyperfunction and the management of children with the disorders.
- Distinguish between the manifestations of adrenal hypofunction and hyperfunction.
- Differentiate among the various categories of diabetes mellitus.
- Discuss the management and nursing care of the child with diabetes mellitus in the acute care setting.
- Distinguish between a hypoglycemic and a hyperglycemic reaction.
- Design a teaching plan for a child with diabetes mellitus.
- Formulate a teaching plan for instructing the parents of a child with diabetes mellitus.

ELECTRONIC RESOURCES

Additional information related to the content in Chapter 52 can be found on

the companion website at evolve
http://evolve.elsevier.com/Wong/maternal/
- NCLEX Review Questions
- WebLinks

or the interactive student CD-ROM
Activities for Chapter 52 include the following:
- NCLEX Review Questions
- Case Study–Diabetes Mellitus
- Critical Thinking Exercise–Hypothyroidism
- Nursing Care Plan–The Child with Diabetes Mellitus

DISORDERS OF PITUITARY FUNCTION

The *pituitary gland*, or *hypophysis*, is often referred to as the *master gland* because of its role in regulating other endocrine glands. Under the influence of secretions from the hypothalamus, the anterior lobe of the pituitary (adenohypophysis) releases or withholds seven hormones (Table 52-1). These hormones control the secretion of hormones from other endocrine glands and influence somatic and sexual development. Because of this relationship, a dysfunction observed in target tissues can be a result of malfunction of the hypothalamus, the pituitary gland, or the target gland. If the tropic hormones are involved, the resulting disorder reflects the altered stimulus to the target gland. For example, if thyroid-stimulating hormone is deficient, thyroid hormone is also deficient, and the child displays the manifestations of hypothyroidism. Overproduction of pituitary hormone is thought to be caused by hyperplasia of the pituitary cells or by a primary hypothalamic defect that results in excess production of the hormone's releasing factor.

Deficiencies of the anterior pituitary hormones may be a result of organic defects or of idiopathic etiology and may occur as a single hormonal problem or in combination with other hormonal deficiencies. The clinical manifestations depend on the hormones involved and the age of onset. This discussion is limited to dysfunction related primarily to the secretion of growth hormone.

Hypopituitarism: Growth Hormone Deficiency

Hypopituitarism is primarily a disorder associated with deficient secretion of *growth hormone (GH) (somatotropin)*. It may be caused by a variety of conditions: development defects; destructive lesions such as tumors, trauma, vascular abnormalities, or surgery; certain hereditary disorders; or functional disorders such as anorexia nervosa or psychosocial dwarfism. In more than half of children with hypopituitarism, no lesion is evident and the cause is unknown—*idiopathic hypopituitarism* or *idiopathic pituitary growth failure.*

GH deficiency inhibits somatic growth in all body cells (Fig. 52-1). The primary site of dysfunction in the syndrome appears to be in the hypothalamus. The extent of idiopathic GH deficiency may be complete or partial, but the cause is

Table 52-1

Endocrine Glands and Their Function

HORMONE	PRIMARY EFFECT
ADENOHYPOPHYSIS (ANTERIOR PITUITARY GLAND)	
Growth hormone (GH)	Promotes growth of bone and soft tissues
Thyroid-stimulating hormone (TSH)	Stimulates thyroid hormone secretion
Adrenocorticotropic hormone (ACTH)	Stimulates adrenal cortex to secrete glucocorticoids and androgens
Gonadotropins • Follicle-stimulating hormone (FSH) • Luteinizing hormone (LH)	Stimulate gonads to mature and produce sex hormones and germ cells
Prolactin	Stimulates milk secretion
Melanocyte-stimulating hormone (MSH)	Promotes pigmentation of skin
NEUROHYPOPHYSIS (POSTERIOR PITUITARY GLAND)	
Antidiuretic hormone (ADH)	Acts on kidney tubules to reabsorb water
Oxytocin	Stimulates uterine contractions Causes milk ejection reflex
THYROID GLAND	
Thyroid hormones	Regulate metabolic rate Control rate of body cell growth
Thyrocalcitonin	Influences ossification and development of bone
PARATHYROID GLANDS	
Parathyroid hormone (PTH)	Regulates calcium metabolism
ADRENAL CORTEX	
Aldosterone	Regulates sodium retention and excretion
Sex hormones	Influence development of bones, reproductive organs, and secondary sex characteristics
Glucocorticoids	Promote metabolism Mobilize body defenses during stress Suppress inflammatory reaction
ADRENAL MEDULLA	
Catecholamines	Produce a sympathetic response Increase blood pressure and blood glucose levels
ISLETS OF LANGERHANS OF PANCREAS	
Insulin	Promotes utilization of glucose by cells; decreases blood glucose levels
Glucagon	Increases blood glucose levels Accelerates glyconeogenesis
Somatostatin	Inhibits secretion of insulin and glucagon
OVARIES	
Estrogen	Stimulates ripening of ova Produces female secondary sex characteristics Promotes epiphyseal closure of bones
Progesterone	Prepares uterus for fertilization
TESTES	
Testosterone	Stimulates spermatogenesis Produces male secondary sex characteristics Promotes epiphyseal closure of bones

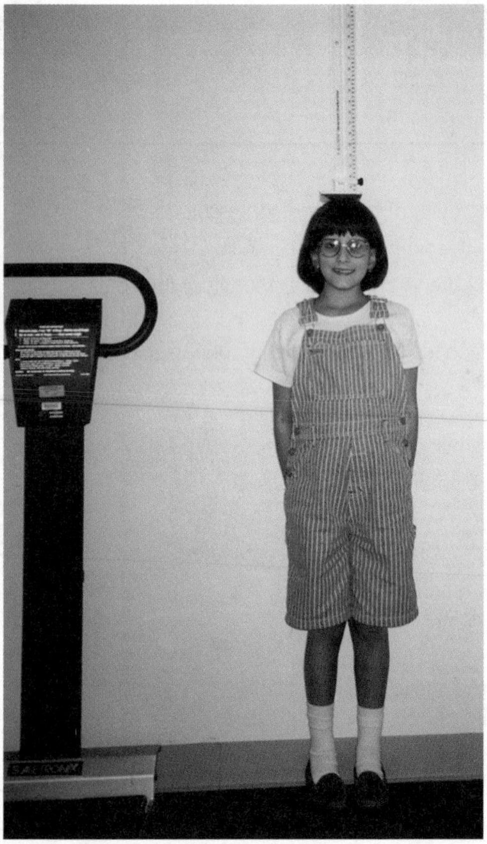

Fig. 52-1 Thirteen-year-old girl with short stature. Height is 133 cm. Normal height for age is 145 to 168 cm.

BOX 52-1

Clinical Manifestations of Hypopituitarism

Reason for seeking treatment–Presenting complaint–short stature
- Usually normal growth first year
- Growth during second year drops below established percentile
- Growth measurements below 5th percentile

Premature aging common in later life
Height may be retarded more than weight
Appear well nourished
Skeletal proportions normal
Tend to be relatively inactive
Less apt to participate in aggressive, sporting-type activities
Bone age nearly always retarded but closely related to height age
Usually primary teeth appear at expected age; eruption of permanent teeth delayed
Teeth are overcrowded and malpositioned (because of underdeveloped jaw)
Sexual development usually delayed but normal

unknown. It is frequently associated with other pituitary hormone deficiencies and is treated more frequently in boys than in girls.

Diagnostic Evaluation

Only a small number of children with delayed growth or short stature have hypopituitary dwarfism. In the majority of instances the cause is constitutional delay. Although children with hypopituitarism are normal at birth, they show growth patterns that progressively deviate from the normal growth rate, often beginning in infancy. The chief complaint in most instances is short stature (Box 52-1).

A complete diagnostic evaluation should include a family history, a history of the child's growth patterns and previous health status, physical examination, psychosocial evaluation, drug intake, parental heights, birth size, nutritional state, review of systems, radiographic surveys, and endocrine studies. Many endocrinologists recommend magnetic resonance imaging of the brain before starting GH therapy to rule out a pituitary abnormality or lesion (Arends et al, 2002). The diagnosis is based on radioimmunoassay of plasma GH levels stimulated pharmacologically with two different stimulation tests. GH levels below 10 ng/ml after two provocative tests establish the diagnosis (Guyda, 2000; Shulman & Bercu, 1998). Serum levels of the hormones directly responsible for skeletal growth (insulin-like growth factor 1, insulin-like growth factor–binding protein 3) are now used to evaluate GH deficiency error (Durham, 2003).

Radiographic examination of the hand and wrist for centers of ossification is an important procedure in evaluating growth. Endocrine studies to detect tropic hormone deficiencies are also performed if there is evidence of hypothyroidism, hypersecretion of cortisol, or gonadal aplasia.

Therapeutic Management

Treatment of GH deficiency caused by organic lesions is directed toward correction of the underlying disease process (e.g., surgical removal or irradiation of a tumor). The definitive treatment of GH deficiency is replacement of GH. *Biosynthetic GH* prepared by recombinant deoxyribonucleic acid (DNA) technology is the therapy of choice. Children with other hormone deficiencies require replacement therapy to correct the specific disorders. This may involve administration of thyroid extract, cortisone, testosterone, or estrogens and progesterone. The sex hormones are usually begun during adolescence to promote normal sexual maturation. Currently, much controversy exists over the use of GH in children who are short but not GH deficient.

Prognosis

GH replacement is successful in 80% of affected children. Children who respond to therapy typically increase their growth rate from 3.5 to 4 cm/year before treatment to 8.7 ± 1.5 cm/year. Young children, obese children, and severely GH-deficient children respond best. Growth responses to GH will vary depending on age, length of treatment, frequency of administration, dosage, weight, and GH receptor amount (Blethen et al, 1996). Overall, studies have noted improved actual or near-final adult height. Early diagnosis and initiation of therapy is important to successful therapy (August, Julius, & Blethen, 1998). A recent investigation revealed that patients diagnosed with GH deficiency in childhood are no longer GH deficient at the end of therapy after attainment of final height (Thomas et al, 2003).

Nursing Care Management

Nursing care is primarily directed toward assisting in establishing the diagnosis and providing emotional support to the child and family (see Chapter 41). Because these children appear younger than their chronologic age, others frequently relate to them in childish ways. Parents and teachers benefit from guidance directed toward realistic expectations of the child based on age and abilities (Zimet et al, 1997).

Children undergoing hormone replacement require additional support, such as preparation for daily subcutaneous injections and education for self-management during the school-age years.

NURSE ALERT Injections are given at bedtime to most closely approximate physiologic release of GH. ■

Even when hormone replacement is successful, these children attain their eventual adult height at a slower rate than their peers; thus they need assistance in setting realistic expectations regarding the expected outcome. Professionals and families may find education and support from the Human Growth Foundation.* The treatment is expensive—up to $20,000 to $30,000 per year depending on dosage.

Pituitary Hyperfunction

Excess GH before closure of the epiphyseal shafts results in proportional overgrowth of long bones until the individual reaches a height of 8 feet or more. Vertical growth is accompanied by rapid and increased development of muscles and viscera. Weight is increased but is usually in proportion to height. Proportional enlargement of head circumference also occurs and may result in delayed closure of the fontanels. Children with a pituitary-secreting tumor may also demonstrate signs of increasing intracranial pressure, especially headache.

If hypersecretion of GH occurs after epiphyseal closure, growth is in the transverse direction, producing a condition known as *acromegaly.* Typical facial features include overgrowth of the head, lips, nose, tongue, jaw, and paranasal and mastoid sinuses; separation and malocclusion of the teeth in the enlarged jaw; disproportion of the face to the cerebral division of the skull; increased facial hair; and thickened, deeply creased skin.

Diagnostic Evaluation

Diagnosis is based on a history of excessive growth during childhood and evidence of increased levels of GH. Radiologic studies may reveal a tumor in an enlarged sella turcica; normal bone age; enlargement of bones, such as the paranasal sinuses; and evidence of joint changes. Endocrine studies to confirm excess of other hormones, such as cortisol and sex hormones, are also included in the differential diagnosis.

Therapeutic Management

If a lesion is present, surgical treatment, including cryosurgery or hypophysectomy, may be warranted to remove the tumor whenever feasible. Other therapies that destroy pituitary tissue include external irradiation and radioactive implants. Depending on the extent of surgical extirpation and the degree of pituitary insufficiency, hormone replacement with thyroid extract, cortisone, and sex hormones may be necessary.

Nursing Care Management

The primary nursing consideration is early identification of children with excessive growth rates. Although medical management does not diminish the height already attained, it can retard further growth. The earlier the treatment is begun, the better the chance to attain a normal adult height.

Children with excessive growth rates require as much emotional support as those with short stature. However, girls may suffer from the effects of excessive height much more than boys, who may find their height an asset when pursuing sports such as basketball. A compassionate nurse can be very supportive to these children, especially before adolescence, when they are larger than their peers. The nurse can emphasize to a tall girl that as boys grow older, they become taller, and she will not always be looking down at them. Because early adolescence is a time of idol worship, the nurse can point out marriages of celebrities in which the woman is taller than the man to help the girl gain a perspective that not all heterosexual relationships must follow stereotypic models.

Precocious Puberty

Manifestations of sexual development before age 9 years in boys or age 8 years in girls are considered precocious and should be investigated (Kempers & Otten, 2002; Midyett et al, 2003). Girls with a higher percentage of body fat at 5 years of age are more likely to exhibit earlier pubertal development (Davison, Susman, & Birch, 2003). African-American girls usually enter puberty first, followed by Mexican-Americans, and then white girls (Anderson, Dallal, & Must, 2003; Chumlea et al, 2003; Wu, Mendola, & Buck, 2002). Early sexual development can have a number of causes and may result from a disorder of the gonad, the adrenal gland, or the hypothalamic-pituitary gonadal axis. The disorder occurs far more frequently in girls than in boys. No causative factor can be found in 80% to 90% of girls. A central nervous system insult or structural injury in boys is more common (Root, 2000).

True, or *complete, precocious puberty* is always isosexual and results from premature activation of the hypothalamic-pituitary-gonadal axis, which produces early maturation and development of the gonads with secretion of sex hormones, development of secondary sex characteristics, and sometimes production of mature sperm or ova. Precocious puberty is explained only as an unusually early activation of the maturation process that is regarded as a normal course of events at a later age. There is early acceleration of linear growth with early epiphyseal fusion and ultimate height less than what would have been anticipated with later pubertal onset. *Precocious pseudopuberty,* or *incomplete puberty,* differs from true sexual precocity in that there is no early secretion of gonadotropin. Most cases result from early overproduction of sex hormone, usually caused by a tumor of the

*997 Glen Cove Ave., Glen Head, NY 11545; phone: 800-451-6434; e-mail: hgf1@hgfound.org; Web site: www.hgfound.org.

ovary or testis, a tumor or hyperplasia of the adrenal gland, or exogenous sources of androgens or estrogens.

Therapeutic Management

Treatment of precocious pseudopuberty is directed toward the specific cause when known. Precocious puberty of central origin is managed with monthly subcutaneous injections of a synthetic analog of luteinizing hormone–releasing hormone (LHRH, Lupron), which regulates pituitary secretions. This therapy slows the prepubertal growth to normal rates in affected children. Treatment is discontinued at a chronologically appropriate time, allowing pubertal changes to resume.

Nursing Care Management

Psychologic support and guidance of the child and family are the most important aspects of management. Parents need a detailed explanation and reassurance of the benign nature of the condition. Dress and activities for the physically precocious child should be appropriate to the chronologic age.

Despite the early sexual development, maturation of the gonads and the appearance of secondary sexual characteristics proceed in the usual order. After puberty, physical differences from peers are no longer present. Heterosexual interest is not usually advanced beyond the child's chronologic age; however, the nurse should emphasize to parents that the child is fertile. No form of contraception is necessary unless the child is sexually active.

Diabetes Insipidus

The principal disorder of posterior pituitary hypofunction is *diabetes insipidus (DI),* also known as *neurogenic DI.* The disease is a result of hyposecretion of *antidiuretic hormone (ADH),* or *vasopressin,* which produces a state of uncontrolled diuresis. Primary causes are familial or idiopathic; secondary causes include trauma (accidental or surgical), tumors, granulomatous disease, infections (meningitis or encephalitis), or vascular anomalies (aneurysm). The disorder is not to be confused with nephrogenic DI, a rare hereditary disorder caused by unresponsiveness of the renal tubules to the hormone.

Clinical Manifestations

The cardinal signs of DI are polyuria and polydipsia. In the older child, excessive urination accompanied by a compensatory insatiable thirst may be so intense that the child does little other than drink fluids and void (Cheetham & Baylis, 2002). Not infrequently, the first sign is enuresis. In the infant the initial symptom is irritability that is relieved with feedings of water but not milk. The infant is also prone to dehydration, electrolyte imbalance, hyperthermia, azotemia, and potential circulatory collapse.

NURSE ALERT The child with DI complicated by congenital absence of the thirst center must be encouraged to drink sufficient quantities of liquid to prevent electrolyte imbalance. ■

Diagnostic Evaluation

The simplest test used to diagnose this condition is restriction of oral fluids and observation of consequent changes in urine volume and concentration. In DI, fluid restriction has little or no effect on urine formation but causes weight loss from dehydration. If this test is positive, the child should be given a test dose of injected *aqueous vasopressin (Pitressin),* which should alleviate the polyuria and polydipsia. Unresponsiveness to exogenous vasopressin usually indicates nephrogenic DI.

NURSE ALERT Small children require close supervision during fluid restriction to prevent them from drinking, even from toilet bowls, plants, or other unlikely sources of fluid. ■

Therapeutic Management

The usual treatment requires daily hormone replacement of vasopressin. The drug of choice is *desmopressin acetate (DDAVP),* a synthetic analog of vasopressin. DDAVP may also be given orally. Recent studies have found this to be an effective alternative (Boulgourdjian et al, 1997). Nasal DDAVP has widely replaced the use of vasopressin tannate in peanut oil. The injectable form has the advantage of lasting 48 to 72 hours, which affords the child a full night's sleep. However, it has the disadvantages of requiring frequent injections and proper preparation of the drug.

NURSE ALERT To be effective, vasopressin must be thoroughly resuspended in the oil by being held under warm running water for 10 to 15 minutes and shaken vigorously before being drawn into the syringe. If this is not done, the oil may be injected without ADH. Small brown particles, which indicate drug dispersion, must be seen in the suspension. ■

DDAVP is available and administered intranasally by way of a flexible tube to achieve adequate control. It is usually administered twice daily. The response pattern of the child is variable, with duration ranging from 8 to 20 hours. Children receiving DDAVP need to be observed for a possible overdose of the drug. The signs of overdosage are those of water intoxication and are similar to manifestations of inappropriate antidiuretic hormone secretion.

Nursing Care Management

The initial objective of care is identification of the disorder. After confirmation of the diagnosis, parents need a thorough explanation of the condition, with special emphasis on distinguishing the difference between diabetes insipidus and diabetes mellitus. The parents must realize that treatment is lifelong. If the child is to receive the injectable vasopressin, ideally both parents, as well as children who are over 7 years of age, should be taught the correct procedure for preparation and administration of the drug. Once children are old enough, they should be encouraged to assume full responsibility for care.

For emergency purposes these children should wear medical-alert identification. Older children are advised to carry the nasal vasopressin spray with them for temporary relief of symptoms. School personnel should be made aware of the problem so that the child is granted unrestricted use of the lavatory and drinking water. Failure to permit this may result in embarrassing accidents that often result in the child's unwillingness to attend school.

Syndrome of Inappropriate Antidiuretic Hormone Secretion

Hypersecretion of the posterior pituitary ADH (vasopressin) produces the disorder known as *syndrome of inappropriate antidiuretic hormone (SIADH).* SIADH is observed with increased frequency in a variety of conditions, especially those involving infections, tumors, and trauma of the central nervous system.

The manifestations observed are directly related to fluid retention and hypotonicity. Increased secretion of ADH causes the kidneys to reabsorb water, which increases the fluid volume and decreases serum osmolality. When serum sodium levels are lowered to 120 mEq/L, the child displays anorexia, nausea (sometimes vomiting), stomach cramps, irritability, and personality changes. With progressive reduction in sodium, other neurologic signs, stupor, and seizures may be evident. The symptoms disappear when the underlying disorder is corrected. Immediate management consists of restricting fluids.

NURSE ALERT Children with SIADH develop an expanded circulatory volume but do not form edema, which is an excess of both water and sodium. ■

Nursing Care Management

The first goal of nursing management is recognizing the presence of SIADH from symptoms described in patients at risk. Accurately measuring intake, output, and daily weight and observing for signs of fluid overload are primary nursing functions, especially in the child receiving intravenous (IV) fluids.

Seizure precautions are implemented, and the child and family need education regarding the rationale for fluid restriction. The rare child with chronic SIADH will be placed on a long-term regimen of ADH-antagonizing medication and will require instructions for its administration.

DISORDERS OF THYROID FUNCTION

The thyroid gland secretes two types of hormones: *thyroid hormone (TH),* which consists of the hormones *thyroxine* (T_4) and *triiodothyronine* (T_3), and *thyrocalcitonin.* The secretion of thyroid hormones is controlled by *thyroid-stimulating hormone (TSH)* from the anterior pituitary. Hypothyroidism or hyperthyroidism may result from a defect in the target gland or from a disturbance in secretion of TSH or its releasing factor in the hypothalamus.

Because the functions of T_3 and T_4 are qualitatively the same, the term *thyroid hormone (TH)* is used throughout this discussion.

The synthesis of TH depends on available sources of dietary iodine and tyrosine. The thyroid is the only endocrine gland capable of storing excess amounts of hormones for release as needed. The main physiologic action of TH is to regulate the basal metabolic rate and thereby control the processes of growth and tissue differentiation.

Thyrocalcitonin helps maintain blood calcium levels by decreasing the calcium concentration. Its effect is the opposite of that of parathyroid hormone; it inhibits skeletal demineralization and promotes calcium deposition in the bone.

Juvenile Hypothyroidism

CRITICAL THINKING EXERCISE: HYPOTHYROIDISM

Hypothyroidism is one of the most common endocrine problems of childhood. It may be either congenital or acquired and represents a deficiency in secretion of TH. Hypothyroidism from dietary insufficiency of iodine is rare in the United States because iodized salt is a readily available source of the nutrient. This discussion is limited to the juvenile form of hypothyroidism.

Beyond infancy, primary hypothyroidism may be caused by a number of defects. For example, a congenital hypoplastic thyroid gland may provide sufficient amounts of TH during the first year or two but be inadequate when rapid body growth increases demands on the gland. A partial or complete thyroidectomy for cancer or thyrotoxicosis can leave insufficient thyroid tissue to furnish hormones for body requirements. Irradiation for Hodgkin disease or other malignancies or infectious processes may be a cause of hypothyroidism (Pizzo & Poplack, 2001).

Clinical manifestations depend on the extent of dysfunction and the age of the child at the onset (Box 52-2). Because brain growth is nearly complete by 2 to 3 years of age, mental retardation and neurologic sequelae are not associated with juvenile hypothyroidism.

Therapy is oral TH replacement, the same as for hypothyroidism in the infant, although the prompt treatment needed for brain growth in the infant is not required in the child. In children with severe symptoms, the restoration of euthyroidism is achieved more gradually, with administration of increasing amounts of L-thyroxine over 4 to 8 weeks to avoid symptoms of hyperthyroidism that can occur with treatment of chronic hypothyroidism.

Nursing Care Management

Cessation or retardation of growth in a child whose growth has previously been normal should alert the observer to the possibility of hypothyroidism. Following diagnosis and implementation of thyroxine therapy, the importance of compliance and periodic monitoring of the response to therapy should be stressed to the parents. Children should

BOX 52-2

Clinical Manifestations of Juvenile Hypothyroidism

- Decelerated growth
  - Less when acquired at later age
- Myxedematous skin changes
  - Dry skin
  - Puffiness around eyes
  - Sparse hair
  - Constipation
  - Sleepiness
  - Mental decline

learn to take responsibility for their health as soon as they are old enough, at about 9 to 10 years of age.

Goiter

A goiter is an enlargement or hypertrophy of the thyroid gland. It can be congenital or acquired. Congenital disease usually occurs as a result of antithyroid drugs or iodides administered to the mother during pregnancy. The acquired disease can result from increased secretion of pituitary thyrotropic hormone in response to decreased circulating levels of TH, neoplastic or inflammatory processes, or dietary iodine deficiency.

Enlargement of the thyroid gland may be mild and noticeable only when there is an increased demand for TH (e.g., during periods of rapid growth). Enlargement of the thyroid at birth can be sufficient to cause severe respiratory distress. TH replacement is necessary to treat the hypothyroidism and reverse the TSH effect on the gland.

Nursing Care Management

Large goiters are identified by their obvious appearance. Smaller nodules may be evident only on palpation. Nurses in ambulatory settings need to be aware of the possibility of neck enlargement from goiters and report such findings.

NURSE ALERT If an infant is born with a goiter, immediate precautions are instituted for emergency ventilation, such as supplemental oxygen and a tracheostomy set. Positioning the child with the neck hyperextended often facilitates breathing. ■

Immediate surgery to remove part of the gland may be lifesaving. When thyroid replacement is necessary, parents have the same needs regarding its administration as discussed for the parents of children who have hypothyroidism.

Lymphocytic Thyroiditis

Lymphocytic thyroiditis *(Hashimoto disease, juvenile autoimmune thyroiditis)* is the most common cause of thyroid disease in children and adolescents, and it accounts for the largest percentage of juvenile hypothyroidism. It also accounts for many of the enlarged thyroid glands formerly designated as thyroid hyperplasia of adolescence, or "adolescent goiter." The disease is more common in girls than in boys and in white persons than in black persons. It occurs more frequently after age 6, reaching a peak incidence in adolescence; there is evidence that the disease is self-limited.

Pathophysiology

There is a strong genetic predisposition to the development of autoimmune thyroiditis, although no mode of inheritance has been delineated and the basic stimulus or autoimmune defect is unknown. The disease is characterized by lymphocytic infiltration of the gland, inflammation, and, in many patients, replacement with fibrous tissue. In the early stages there may be only hyperplasia.

Diagnostic Evaluation

The enlarged thyroid gland may be detected by the practitioner during a routine examination, although it may be noted by parents when the youngster swallows. Most children are euthyroid, but some display symptoms of hypothyroidism. Others have signs that suggest hyperthyroidism (Box 52-3).

BOX 52-3

Clinical Manifestations of Lymphocytic Thyroiditis

Enlarged Thyroid Gland
Usually symmetric
Firm
Freely movable
Nontender

Tracheal Compression
Sense of fullness
Hoarseness
Dysphagia

Hyperthyroidism (Possible)
Nervousness
Irritability
Increased sweating
Hyperactivity

Thyroid function tests are usually normal, although TSH levels may be slightly or moderately elevated. With progressive disease the T_4 decreases, followed by a decrease in T_3 levels and an increase in TSH. A variety of abnormalities in radioactive iodine uptake may be noted. The majority of children have serum antibody titers to thyroid antigens, but fewer children have a positive red blood cell hemagglutination test. When both tests are used, almost all children with thyroid autoimmunity are detected.

Therapeutic Management

In many cases the goiter is transient and asymptomatic and regresses spontaneously within a year or two. Therapy of a nontoxic diffuse goiter is usually simple, uncomplicated, and effective. Oral administration of TH depresses TSH, thus decreasing the size of the gland significantly. Surgery is contraindicated in this disorder.

Nursing Care Management

Nursing care consists of identifying the youngster with thyroid enlargement, reassuring the child that the condition is probably only temporary, and reinforcing instructions for thyroid therapy.

Hyperthyroidism (Graves Disease)

The largest percentage of hyperthyroidism in childhood is caused by Graves disease, which is usually associated with an enlarged thyroid gland and exophthalmos (Thompson, 2002). The peak incidence of the disease occurs between 12 and 14 years of age, but it may be present at birth in children of thyrotoxic mothers. The incidence is five times higher in girls than in boys. The disease is apparently caused by a serum thyroid-stimulating immunoglobulin, but no specific etiology has been identified. There is definitive evidence for familial association; a large number of persons with the disease possess the histocompatibility antigen HLA-B8.

Diagnostic Evaluation

The development of manifestations is highly variable (Box 52-4). Manifestations develop gradually, with an interval between onset and diagnosis of approximately 6 to 12 months. Diagnosis is established on the basis of increased levels of T_4 and T_3. Thyrotropin (TSH) is suppressed to unmeasurable levels. Other tests are rarely indicated.

Therapeutic Management

Therapy for hyperthyroidism is controversial, but all methods are directed toward retarding the rate of hormone secretion. The three acceptable modes available are (1) the antithyroid drugs, which interfere with the biosynthesis of TH, including propylthiouracil (PTU) and methimazole (MTZ, Tapazole); (2) subtotal thyroidectomy; and (3) ablation with radioiodine (^{131}I-iodide) (Rivkees & Cornelius, 2003). When affected children exhibit signs and symptoms of hyperthyroidism, their activity should be limited. Vigorous exercise is restricted until thyroid levels are decreased to normal or near-normal values.

Thyrotoxicosis (thyroid "crisis" or thyroid "storm") may occur from sudden release of the hormone. Although it is unusual in children, a crisis can be life threatening. A crisis may be precipitated by acute infection, surgical emergencies, or discontinuation of antithyroid therapy. Treatment, in addition to antithyroid drugs, is administration of β-adrenergic blocking agents (propranolol), which provide relief from the disturbing side effects of the reaction.

BOX 52-4

Clinical Manifestations of Hyperthyroidism (Graves Disease)

Cardinal Signs
Emotional lability
Physical restlessness, characteristically at rest
Decelerated school performance
Voracious appetite with weight loss in 50% of cases
Fatigue

Physical Signs
Tachycardia
Widened pulse pressure
Dyspnea on exertion
Exophthalmos (protruding eyeballs)
Wide-eyed, staring expression with lid lag
Tremor
Goiter (hypertrophy and hyperplasia)
Warm, moist skin
Accelerated linear growth
Heat intolerance (may be severe)
Hair fine and unable to hold a curl
Systolic murmurs

Thyroid Storm
Acute onset:
- Severe irritability and restlessness
- Vomiting
- Diarrhea
- Hyperthermia
- Hypertension
- Severe tachycardia
- Prostration

May progress rapidly to:
- Delirium
- Coma
- Death

Nursing Care Management

The initial nursing objective is identification of children with hyperthyroidism. Because the clinical manifestations often appear gradually, the goiter and ophthalmic changes may not be noticed, and the excessive activity may be attributed to behavioral problems. Nurses in ambulatory settings, particularly those caring for children in school, need to be alert to signs that suggest this disorder, especially weight loss despite an excellent appetite, academic difficulties resulting from a short attention span and inability to sit still, unexplained fatigue and sleeplessness, and difficulty with fine motor skills (such as writing). Exophthalmos may develop long before the onset of signs and symptoms of hyperthyroidism and may be the only initial sign (Thompson, 2002).

Much of the care during diagnosis and initial medical therapy is related to the physical symptoms. The child needs a quiet, unstimulating environment that is conducive to rest, and sometimes hospitalization is necessary during the immediate treatment phase. A regular routine is beneficial, with frequent rest periods, minimizing the stress of coping with unexpected demands and meeting the child's needs promptly. Physical activity is restricted. For example, school physical education classes are discontinued. Despite the excessive activity of these children, they tire easily, experience muscle weakness, and are unable to relax to recoup their strength.

Once therapy is instituted, the nurse explains the drug regimen, emphasizing the importance of observing for side effects of antithyroid drugs. Untoward effects of PTU and related compounds include skin rash, drug fever, enlargement of the salivary and cervical lymph glands, diminished sense of taste, hepatitis, and edema of the lower extremities.

NURSE ALERT Children being treated with PTU must be carefully monitored for side effects of the drug. Because sore throat and fever accompany the grave complication of leukopenia, these children should be seen by a practitioner if such symptoms occur. Parents and children should be taught to recognize and report symptoms immediately. ■

Parents should also be aware of the signs of hypothyroidism, which can occur from overdose of the drugs. The most common indications are lethargy and somnolence.

Surgical Care

If surgery is anticipated, iodine is usually administered for a few weeks before the procedure. Because oral iodine preparations are unpalatable, they should be mixed with a strong-tasting fruit juice, such as grape or punch flavors, and be given through a straw. Compliance with iodine therapy is essential to avoid the danger of thyroid crisis after sudden discontinuation.

Psychologic preparation of children for thyroidectomy is similar to that for any other surgical procedure (see Chapter 45). However, of special consideration is the site of the incision. The fear of having the throat cut is very real and in older children is associated with death. The nurse should explain that the throat is not cut, only the skin, to allow for removal of the gland. Showing children a picture of the anatomic location of the thyroid around the trachea is often helpful. Children should be prepared for the dressing around the neck and the possibility of an endotracheal or "breathing" tube after surgery.

Postoperative care involves positioning with the neck slightly flexed to avoid strain on the sutures and observation for bleeding and complications. The children are taught to support the neck in this position when they sit up. Damage to the recurrent laryngeal nerve is evidenced by severe stridor or hoarseness (or both), although some hoarseness is expected. Observation for signs of hypoparathyroidism, which causes hypocalcemia, should be implemented in the immediate postoperative period.

NURSE ALERT The earliest indication of hypoparathyroidism may be anxiety and mental depression, followed by paresthesia and evidence of heightened neuromuscular excitability, such as the following:

Chvostek sign–Facial muscle spasm elicited by tapping the facial nerve in the region of the parotid gland

Trousseau sign–Carpal spasm elicited by pressure applied to nerves of the upper arm

Tetany–Carpopedal spasm (sharp flexion of wrist and ankle joints), muscle twitching, cramps, seizures, and sometimes stridor ■

DISORDERS OF PARATHYROID FUNCTION

The parathyroid glands secrete *parathyroid hormone (PTH)*, whose main function, along with vitamin D, is to maintain homeostasis of blood calcium concentration. PTH exerts its effect by (1) increasing the release of calcium and phosphate from the bone (bone demineralization), (2) increasing the absorption of calcium and the excretion of phosphate by the kidneys, and (3) promoting calcium absorption in the gastrointestinal tract. The net result of these actions is to increase the plasma calcium concentration while lowering the plasma phosphate concentration.

Hypoparathyroidism

Two classic forms of hypoparathyroidism are observed during childhood. *Autoimmune hypoparathyroidism,* in which there is deficient production of PTH, may occur as a component of multiglandular failure, usually in relation to autoimmune phenomena. Familial hypoparathyroidism is inherited as an autosomal recessive trait, with early onset, usually in the first month of life. In *pseudohypoparathyroidism,* production of PTH is increased but end-organ responsiveness to the hormone is deficient. Pseudohypoparathyroidism is also thought to be inherited as an X-linked dominant trait with variable expressivity. Transient hypoparathyroidism may also be observed in infants born to mothers with the disease or in infants fed a milk formula with a high phosphate-to-calcium ratio.

Diagnostic Evaluation

The diagnosis of hypoparathyroidism is made on the basis of clinical manifestations associated with *decreased serum calcium* and *increased serum phosphorus levels* (Box 52-5). Levels of plasma PTH are low in idiopathic hypoparathyroidism but high in pseudohypoparathyroidism. End-organ responsiveness is tested by the administration of PTH with measurement of urinary cyclic adenosine monophosphate (cAMP). Kidney function tests are included in the differential diagnosis to rule out renal insufficiency. Although bone radiographs are usually normal, they may demonstrate increased bone density and suppressed growth.

Therapeutic Management

The objective of treatment is to maintain normal serum calcium and phosphate levels with a minimum of complications. Acute or severe tetany is corrected immediately by IV and oral administration of calcium gluconate and follow-up daily doses to achieve normal levels. When the diagnosis is confirmed, *vitamin D therapy* is begun. Long-term management consists of administration of massive doses of vitamin D; oral

BOX 52-5

Clinical Manifestations of Hypoparathyroidism

Pseudohypoparathyroidism
Short stature
Round face
Short, thick neck
Short, stubby fingers and toes
Dimpling of skin over knuckles
Subcutaneous soft tissue calcifications
Mental retardation a prominent feature

Idiopathic Hypoparathyroidism
None of the above physical characteristics observed
Papilledema may be seen
May be mental retardation

Both Types
Dry, scaly, coarse skin with eruptions
Hair often brittle
Nails thin and brittle with characteristic transverse grooves
Dental and enamel hypoplasia
Muscle contractions:
- Tetany
- Carpopedal spasm
- Laryngospasm (laryngeal stridor)
- Muscle cramps and twitching
- Positive Chvostek sign or Trousseau sign (or both) (see Nurse Alert, above left)

Paresthesias, tingling
Neurologic:
- Headache
- Seizures (generalized, absence, or focal)
- Swings of emotion
- Loss of memory
- Depression
- Confusion can occur

Gastrointestinal:
- Muscle cramps
- Diarrhea
- Vomiting

Retarded skeletal growth

calcium supplementation may be useful, although it is not essential.

Nursing Care Management

The initial objective is recognition of hypocalcemia. Unexplained seizures, irritability (especially to external stimuli), gastrointestinal symptoms (e.g., diarrhea, vomiting, abdominal cramps), and positive signs of tetany should lead the nurse to suspect this disorder. Much of the initial nursing care is related to the physical manifestations and includes institution of seizure and safety precautions, reduction of environmental stimuli (e.g., sudden noises or movements, bright lights), and observation for signs of laryngospasm.

NURSE ALERT Signs of *laryngospasm* are stridor, hoarseness, and a feeling of tightness in the throat. A tracheostomy set and injectable calcium gluconate should be placed near the bedside for emergency use. The IV administration of calcium gluconate requires precautions against extravasation of the drug and tissue destruction. ■

After initiation of treatment, the nurse discusses with the parents the need for continuous daily administration of calcium salts and vitamin D. Because vitamin D toxicity can be a serious consequence of therapy, parents are advised to watch for signs, which include weakness, fatigue, lassitude, headache, nausea, vomiting, and diarrhea. Early renal impairment is manifested by polyuria, polydipsia, and nocturia.

Hyperparathyroidism

Hyperparathyroidism is rare in childhood but can be primary or secondary. The most common cause of primary hyperparathyroidism is adenoma of the gland. The most common causes of secondary hyperparathyroidism are chronic renal disease, renal osteodystrophy, and congenital anomalies of the urinary tract. The common factor is hypercalcemia. The manifestations of hyperparathyroidism are listed in Box 52-6.

Diagnostic Evaluation

Blood studies to confirm the presence of *elevated calcium* and *lowered phosphorus levels* are routinely performed. Measurement of PTH, as well as several tests to isolate the cause of the hypercalcemia, such as renal function studies, should be included. Other procedures employed to substantiate the physiologic consequences of the disorder include electrocardiography and radiographic bone surveys.

Therapeutic Management

Treatment depends on the cause. The treatment of primary hyperparathyroidism is surgical removal of the tumor or hyperplastic tissue. Treatment of secondary hyperparathyroidism is directed at the underlying contributing cause, thus subsequently restoring the serum calcium balance. However, in some instances the underlying disorder is irreversible, such as in chronic renal failure (see Chapter 50). In this instance treatment is the same as the treatment for renal osteodystrophy.

Nursing Care Management

Surgical removal is the major treatment modality, and nursing care is similar to that discussed for the child with hyperthyroidism (see p. 1727). Because hypocalcemia is a potential complication, observation for signs of tetany, institution of seizure precautions, and having calcium gluconate available for emergency use are part of the nursing care.

BOX 52-6

Clinical Manifestations of Hyperparathyroidism

Gastrointestinal
Nausea
Vomiting
Abdominal discomfort
Constipation

Central Nervous System
Delusions
Confusion
Hallucinations
Impaired memory
Lack of interest and initiative
Depression
Varying levels of consciousness

Neuromuscular
Weakness
Easy fatigability
Muscle atrophy (especially proximal muscles of lower limbs)
Tongue twitching
Paresthesias in extremities

Skeletal
Vague bone pain
Subperiosteal resorption of phalanges
Spontaneous fractures
Absence of lamina dura around teeth

Renal
Polyuria
Polydipsia
Renal colic
Hypertension

DISORDERS OF ADRENAL FUNCTION

The *adrenal cortex* secretes three main groups of hormones collectively called *steroids* and classified according to their biologic activity: (1) *glucocorticoids* (cortisol, corticosterone), (2) *mineralocorticoids* (aldosterone), and (3) *sex steroids* (androgens, estrogens, and progestins). Alterations in the levels of these hormones produce significant dysfunction in a variety of body tissues and organs. Because the adrenocortical cells are capable of producing any of the steroids, pathologic conditions may result in a deficiency or an excess of more than one type of hormone. However, most are rare in children.

The *adrenal medulla* secretes the *catecholamines epinephrine* and *norepinephrine.* Both hormones have essentially the same effects on various organs as those caused by direct sympathetic stimulation, except that the hormonal effects last several times longer. Catecholamine-secreting tumors are the primary cause of adrenal medullary hyperfunction.

Acute Adrenocortical Insufficiency

The acute form of adrenocortical insufficiency *(adrenal crisis)* may result from a number of causes during childhood. Although a rare disorder, some of the more common etiologic factors include hemorrhage into the gland from trauma, which may be caused by a prolonged, difficult labor; fulminating infections, such as meningococcemia, that result in hemorrhage and necrosis (Waterhouse-Friderichsen syndrome); abrupt withdrawal of exogenous sources of cortisone or failure to increase exogenous supplies during stress; or congenital adrenogenital hyperplasia of the salt-losing type.

Diagnostic Evaluation

There is no rapid, definitive test for confirmation of acute adrenocortical insufficiency. Routine procedures such as measurement of plasma cortisol levels are too time consuming to be practical. Therefore diagnosis is usually based on clinical symptoms (Box 52-7). Improvement with cortisol therapy confirms the diagnosis.

Therapeutic Management

Treatment involves replacement of cortisol, replacement of body fluids to correct dehydration and hypovolemia, administration of glucose solutions to correct hypoglycemia, and specific antibiotic therapy in the presence of infection. If hemorrhage has been severe, whole blood may be replaced. In the event that these measures do not reverse the circulatory collapse, vasopressors are used for immediate vasoconstriction and elevation of blood pressure. Once the child's condition is stabilized, oral doses of cortisone, fluids, and salt are given, similar to the regimen used for chronic adrenal insufficiency.

BOX 52-7

Clinical Manifestations of Acute Adrenocortical Insufficiency

Early Symptoms
Increased irritability
Headache
Diffuse abdominal pain
Weakness
Nausea and vomiting
Diarrhea

Generalized Hemorrhagic Manifestations (Waterhouse-Friderichsen Syndrome)
Fever—increases as condition worsens
Central nervous system signs
- Nuchal rigidity
- Seizures
- Stupor
- Coma

Shocklike State
Weak, rapid pulse
Decreased blood pressure
Shallow respirations
Cold, clammy skin
Cyanosis
Circulatory collapse (terminal event)

Newborn
Hyperpyrexia
Tachypnea
Cyanosis
Seizures
Gland may be evident as palpable retroperitoneal mass (hemorrhagic)

Nursing Care Management

Because of the abrupt onset and potentially fatal outcome of this condition, prompt recognition is essential. Vital signs and blood pressure are measured often to monitor the hyperpyrexia and shocklike state. Seizure precautions are instituted, because seizures from the elevated temperature are not uncommon. As soon as therapy is instituted, the nurse monitors the child's response to fluid and cortisol replacement, being alert to too rapid administration of fluids and drugs. Overtreatment with cortisol and sodium chloride can precipitate complications such as an ascending flaccid paralysis. The nurse should observe for signs of hypokalemia and should evaluate serum electrolyte levels. The condition is rapidly corrected with IV and oral potassium replacement. Intake and urine output are measured and recorded.

NURSE ALERT Monitor serum electrolyte levels and observe for signs of hypokalemia or hyperkalemia, (e.g., weakness, poor muscle control, paralysis, cardiac dysrhythmias, and apnea). ■

NURSE ALERT When the oral preparation is given, the potassium supplement should be mixed with a small amount of strongly flavored fruit juice to disguise its bitter taste. ■

The sudden, severe nature of this disorder requires considerable emotional support for the child and family. The child is usually in an intensive care unit, where the surroundings are strange and frightening. Because recovery within 24 hours is often dramatic, the nurse should keep the parents apprised of the child's condition, emphasizing signs of improvement, such as a lowered temperature and elevated blood pressure. If paralysis occurs, the nurse should assure them that this condition is temporary and quickly reversed.

Chronic Adrenocortical Insufficiency (Addison Disease)

Chronic adrenocortical insufficiency is rare in children. When it does occur, it is usually caused by a destructive lesion of the adrenal glands or a neoplasm, or it has an idiopathic cause.

Evidence of this disorder is usually gradual in onset, because 90% of adrenal tissue must be nonfunctional before signs of insufficiency are manifested (Box 52-8). However, during periods of stress, when demands for additional cortisol are increased, symptoms of acute insufficiency may appear in a previously well child.

Definitive diagnosis is based on measurements of functional cortisol reserve. The cortisol and urinary 17-hydroxycorticosteroid levels are low and fail to rise, whereas plasma adrenocorticotropic hormone (ACTH) levels are elevated with corticotropin stimulation, the definitive test for the disease.

Therapeutic Management

Treatment involves replacement of *glucocorticoids (cortisol)* and *mineralocorticoids (aldosterone)*. Some children are able to be maintained solely on oral supplements of cortisol

BOX 52-8

Clinical Manifestations of Chronic Adrenocortical Insufficiency

Neurologic Symptoms
Muscular weakness
Mental fatigue
Irritability, apathy, and negativism
Increased sleeping, listlessness

Pigmentary Changes
Previous scars
Palmar creases
Mucous membranes
Hair
Hyperpigmentation over pressure points (elbows, knees, or waist)
Less frequently, vitiligo (loss of pigmentation)

Gastrointestinal Symptoms
Dehydration
Anorexia
Weight loss

Circulatory Symptoms
Hypotension
Small heart size
Dizziness
Syncopal (fainting) attacks

Hypoglycemia
Headache
Hunger
Weakness
Trembling
Sweating

Other Signs (Seen in Some Children)
Recurrent, unexplained seizures
Intense craving for salt
Acute abdominal pain
Electrolyte imbalances

(cortisone or hydrocortisone preparations) with a liberal intake of salt. Other forms of therapy include monthly injections of desoxycorticosterone acetate or implantation of desoxycorticosterone acetate pellets subcutaneously every 9 to 12 months. During stressful situations, such as infection, emotional upset, or surgery, the dosage must be tripled to accommodate the body's increased need for glucocorticoids. Failure to meet this requirement will precipitate an acute crisis. Overdosage produces cushingoid signs (Fig. 52-2).

Nursing Care Management

Once the disorder is diagnosed, parents need guidance concerning drug therapy. They must be aware of the continuous need for cortisol replacement. Sudden termination of the drug because of inadequate supplies or inability to ingest the oral form because of vomiting places the child in danger of an acute adrenal crisis. Ideally, the parents should have a prefilled syringe of hydrocortisone in the home and should be taught the proper technique for intramuscular administration of the drug in case of a crisis. Unnecessary administration of cortisone will not harm the child but, if needed, may be lifesaving. Any evidence of acute insufficiency is reported to the practitioner immediately.

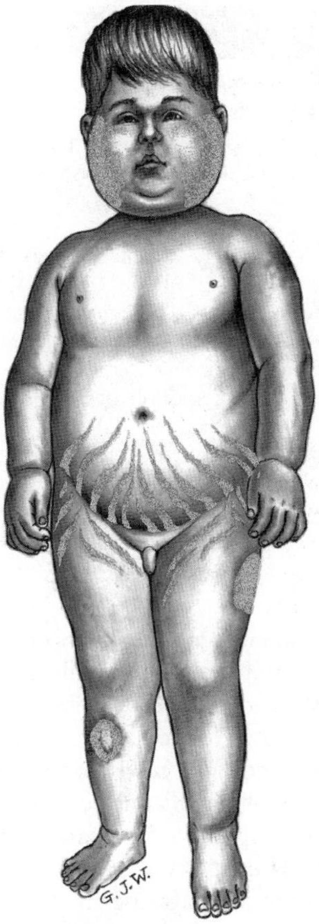

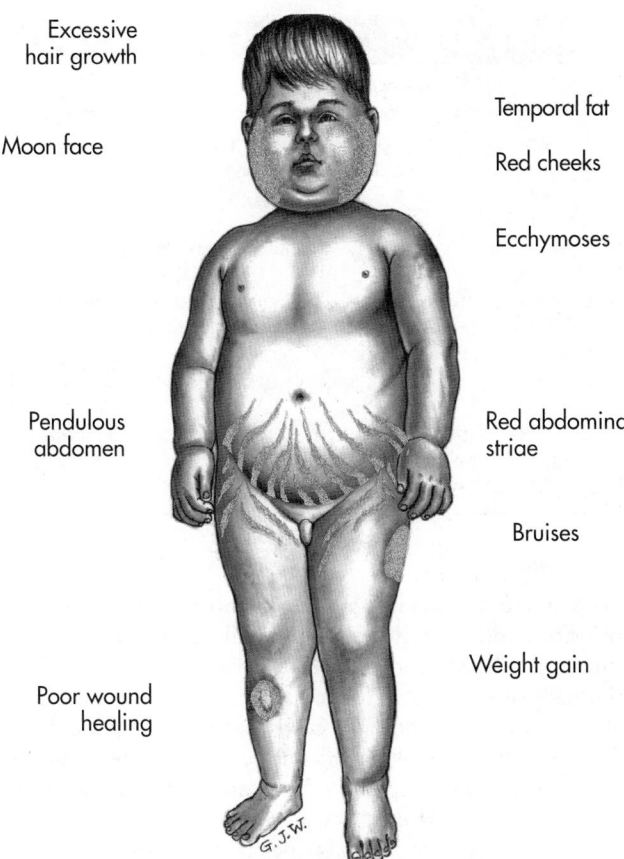

Fig. 52-2 Characteristics of Cushing syndrome.

Because the body cannot supply endogenous sources of cortical hormones during times of stress, the home environment should be stable and relatively unstressful. Parents need to be aware that during periods of emotional or physical crisis the child requires additional hormone replacement. The child should wear medical identification to permit medical personnel to adjust the requirements during emergency care.

Cushing Syndrome

Cushing syndrome is a characteristic group of manifestations caused by excessive circulating free cortisol. It can result from a variety of etiologies, which generally fall into one of five categories (Box 52-9). Cushing syndrome in young children may be due to an adrenal tumor (Moshang, 2003).

Cushing syndrome is uncommon in children. When seen, it is often caused by excessive or prolonged steroid therapy, which produces a cushingoid appearance (Box 52-10). This condition is reversible once steroids are discontinued. Abrupt withdrawal may precipitate acute adrenal insufficiency; gradual withdrawal of exogenous supplies is necessary to allow the anterior pituitary an opportunity to secrete increasing amounts of ACTH to stimulate the adrenals to produce cortisol.

Diagnostic Evaluation

Several tests are helpful in confirming excess cortisol levels. These include fasting blood glucose levels for hyperglycemia, serum electrolyte levels for hypokalemia and alkalosis, 24-hour urinary levels of elevated 17-hydroxycorticoids and

BOX 52-9

Etiology of Cushing Syndrome

Pituitary—Cushing syndrome with adrenal hyperplasia, usually attributed to an excess of adrenocorticotropic hormone (ACTH)
Adrenal—Cushing syndrome with hypersecretion of glucocorticoids, generally a result of adrenocortical neoplasms
Ectopic—Cushing syndrome with autonomous secretion of ACTH, most often caused by extrapituitary neoplasms
Iatrogenic—Cushing syndrome, frequently a result of administration of large amounts of exogenous corticosteroids
Food dependent—Inappropriate sensitivity of adrenal glands to normal postprandial increases in secretion of gastric inhibitory polypeptide (Magiakou et al, 1994)

17-ketosteroids, and radiographic studies of bone for evidence of osteoporosis and of the skull for enlargement of the sella turcica. Administration of an exogenous supply of cortisone normally suppresses ACTH production. However, in individuals with Cushing syndrome, cortisol levels remain elevated. This test is helpful in differentiating between children who are obese and those who appear to have cushingoid features.

Therapeutic Management

Treatment depends on the cause. In most cases surgical intervention involves bilateral adrenalectomy and postoperative replacement of the cortical hormones (the therapy for this is the same as that outlined for chronic adrenal insufficiency). If a pituitary tumor is found, surgical extirpation or irradiation may be chosen. In either of these instances, treatment of panhypopituitarism with replacement of growth hormone, thyroid extract, antidiuretic hormone, gonadotropins, and steroids may be necessary for an indefinite period.

Nursing Care Management

Nursing care also depends on the cause. When cushingoid features are caused by steroid therapy, the effects may be lessened with administration of the drug early in the morning and on an alternate-day basis. Giving the drug early in the day maintains the normal diurnal pattern of cortisol secretion. If given during the evening, the drug is more likely to produce symptoms, because endogenous cortisol levels are already low and the additional supply exerts more pronounced effects. An alternate-day schedule allows the anterior pituitary an opportunity to maintain more normal hypothalamic-pituitary-adrenal control mechanisms.

If an organic cause is found, nursing care is related to the treatment regimen. Although a bilateral adrenalectomy permanently solves one condition, it also produces another syndrome. Before surgery, parents need to be adequately informed of the operative benefits and disadvantages. Postoperative teaching regarding drug replacement is a nursing function.

NURSE ALERT Postoperative complications of adrenalectomy are related to the sudden withdrawal of cortisol. Observe for signs of a shocklike state, especially hypotension and hyperpyrexia. ■

BOX 52-10

Clinical Manifestations of Cushing Syndrome

- Centripetal fat distribution
  - Truncal obesity
  - Supraclavicular fat pads
  - Fat pads on neck and back ("buffalo hump")
- Rounded or "moon" face
- Muscular wasting
  - Thin extremities
  - Pendulous abdomen
  - Muscle weakness
- Thin skin and subcutaneous tissue
- Poor wound healing
- Increased susceptibility to infection
- Decreased inflammatory response
- Excessive bruising
- Petechial hemorrhages
- Facial plethora ("red cheeks")
- Reddish purple abdominal striae
- Hypertension
- Hypokalemia
- Alkalosis
- Osteoporosis
  - Compression fractures of vertebrae
  - Kyphosis
  - Backache
  - Retarded linear growth
- Hypercalciuria—renal calculi
- Psychoses
  - Irritability
  - Insomnia
  - Euphoria
  - Depression
  - Frank psychoses
- Peptic ulcer
- Hyperglycemia
  - Glycosuria
  - Latent or overt diabetes
- Virilization
  - Hirsutism (excessive body hair)
  - Acne
  - Deepening of voice
  - Clitoral enlargement
  - Tendency toward male physique in female
- Amenorrhea
- Impotence

Congenital Adrenal Hyperplasia

Congenital adrenal hyperplasia (CAH) is a family of disorders caused by decreased enzyme activity required for cortisol production in the adrenal cortex. The most common defect is 21-hydroxylase deficiency, which constitutes more than 90% of all cases of CAH (Levine, 2000). This deficiency occurs in approximately 1 per 12,000 to 1 per 15,000 births and causes overproduction of the adrenal androgens, resulting in virilization of the female fetus.

Pathophysiology

Interference in the biosynthesis of cortisol during fetal life results in an increased production of ACTH, which stimulates hyperplasia of the adrenal gland. Depending on the enzymatic defect, increased quantities of cortisol precursors and androgens are secreted. There are six major types of biochemical defects. In each there is excess production of androgens, which causes ambiguous genitalia in females and precocious genital development in males. In both sexes, linear growth is accelerated and epiphyseal closure is premature, ultimately resulting in short stature. Other forms of CAH do not result in excess production of androgens but cause various degrees of hypoaldosteronism or hyperaldosteronism.

The most common biochemical defect is partial or complete *21-hydroxylase deficiency.* With partial deficiency, enough aldosterone is produced to preserve sodium and adequate cortisol is produced to prevent signs of adrenocortical insufficiency. In the complete or salt-losing form, insufficient amounts of aldosterone and cortisol are produced, so that circulatory collapse occurs without immediate replacement of the mineralocorticoids and glucocorticoids.

Diagnostic Evaluation

Clinical diagnosis is initially based on congenital abnormalities that lead to difficulty in assigning sex to the newborn (Box 52-11) and on signs and symptoms of adrenal insufficiency or hypertension. Definitive diagnosis is confirmed by evidence of increased 17-ketosteroid levels in most types of CAH (Levine, 2000). Blood electrolytes demonstrate loss of sodium and chloride and elevation of potassium. A karyotype for positive sex determination should always be done in any case of ambiguous genitalia.

Ultrasonography can also be used to visualize the presence of pelvic structures. It is especially useful in CAH to identify the absence or presence of female reproductive organs in a newborn or child with ambiguous genitalia. Because it yields immediate results, it has the advantage of determining the child's gender long before the more complex laboratory results for chromosome analysis or steroid levels are available.

Therapeutic Management

The initial medical objective is to confirm the diagnosis and assign a sex to the child, usually according to the genotype. In both sexes cortisone is administered to suppress the abnormally high secretions of ACTH. Cortisone depresses the secretion of ACTH by the adenohypophysis, which in turn inhibits the secretion of adrenocorticosteroids, which stems the progressive virilization. If cortisol is given early enough, the signs and symptoms of masculinization in the female gradually disappear, and excessive early linear growth is slowed. Puberty occurs normally at the appropriate age.

Because these children are unable to produce cortisol in response to stress, the dosage is increased during episodes of infection, fever, or other stresses. Acute emergencies require immediate IV or intramuscular administration. Children with the salt-losing type of CAH require aldosterone replacement and supplementary dietary salt.

Depending on the degree of masculinization in the female, reconstructive surgery may be required to reduce the size of the clitoris, separate the labia, and create a vaginal orifice. This should be done after the infant is physically able to tolerate the procedure and before she is old enough to be aware of the abnormal genitalia. Plastic surgery is generally done in stages and yields excellent cosmetic results. The capacity for orgasm is not necessarily impaired, and fertility is preserved.

Unfortunately, not all children with CAH are diagnosed at birth and raised in accordance with their genetic sex. Particularly in the case of affected females, masculinization of the external genitalia may have led to sex assignment as a male. In these situations, it is advisable to continue rearing the child as a male in accordance with the assigned sex and phenotype. Hormone replacement may be required to permit linear growth and to initiate male pubertal changes. Surgery is usually indicated to remove the female organs and reconstruct the phallus for satisfactory sexual relations. These individuals are not fertile. Males with the non–salt-losing variant of CAH may go undiagnosed until early childhood when premature virilism occurs.

Nursing Care Management

The nursing care of the child with CAH and the child's family is concerned primarily with identifying the condition and providing support and assistance. Of major importance is recognition of ambiguous genitalia in newborns. If there is any question regarding assignment of sex, the parents need to be told immediately in order to prevent the embarrassing situation of informing family members of the child's sex and then having to change the announcement. As with any congenital defect, the parents require an adequate explanation of the condition and a period of time to grieve for the loss of perfection. Parents need an explanation regarding this disorder that facilitates their explaining it to others. The external genitalia are referred to as sex organs, and the similarity between the penis/clitoris and scrotum/labia during fetal development is emphasized to help parents understand

BOX 52-11

Clinical Manifestations of Adrenogenital Hyperplasia

Female
- Masculinization
- Enlarged clitoris (appears as small phallus)
- Fusion of labia (saclike structure resembling a scrotum)
- Vaginal orifice usually closed by fused labia

Male
- Precocious genital development
- Genital enlargement (macrogenitosomia precox)
- Frequent erections

Untreated
- Early sexual maturation
- Enlargement of external sexual organs
- Development of axillary, pubic, and facial hair
- Deepening of voice
- Acne
- Marked increase in musculature (changes toward an adult male physique)
- Accelerated linear growth
- Premature epiphyseal closure (short stature by end of puberty)

Female
- No breast development
- Females remain amenorrheic and infertile

Male
- Testes remain small

that too much male hormone secretion caused some organs to overdevelop. Using a correct vocabulary allows parents to explain the abnormalities to others in a straightforward manner, just as if the defect involved the heart or an extremity. As soon as the sex is determined, parents are informed of the findings and encouraged to choose an appropriate name, and the child is identified as a male or female, with no reference to ambiguous sex. If the appearance of the enlarged genitalia in a female child concerns the parents, they are encouraged to discuss their feelings.

Nursing considerations regarding cortisol and aldosterone replacement are the same as those for chronic adrenocortical insufficiency. A follow-up visit by a home health nurse may be desirable to ensure that parents understand and comply with the treatment regimen. Likewise, nurses in well-child facilities should assume responsibility for guidance and supervision regarding this aspect of care during each visit.

Because these infants are especially prone to dehydration and salt-losing crises, parents need to be aware of signs of dehydration and the urgency of immediate medical intervention to stabilize the child's condition. Parents, and later the child, need to understand that the medical regimen must be a lifelong commitment; therefore they should be provided with the education and counseling that is most likely to ensure informed and willing compliance. They also need to know that growth retardation that may have occurred before therapy cannot be overcome and that normal stature is not a realistic expectation, even though growth velocity may improve with medication. The parents are also taught to give necessary injections using the guidelines discussed in Chapter 45.

In the unfortunate situation in which the sex is erroneously assigned and the correct sex determined later, parents need a great deal of help in understanding the reason for the incorrect sex identification and the options for sex reassignment and/or medical/surgical intervention.

NURSE ALERT The parents should be advised that there is no physical harm in treating for suspected adrenal insufficiency that is not present, whereas the consequence of not treating acute adrenal insufficiency can be fatal (Ruble, 1996).

Because the hereditary form of adrenogenital hyperplasia is an autosomal-recessive disorder, parents should be referred to genetic counseling before conceiving another child. Prenatal treatment with glucocorticoid (dexamethasone) can be offered to the mother during subsequent pregnancies to prevent the occurrence of sex ambiguity. Likewise, affected offspring also require genetic counseling, because both sexes are generally able to reproduce. (See genetic counseling in Appendix C.)

Hyperaldosteronism

Excessive secretion of aldosterone may be caused by an adrenal tumor; also, in some types of adrenogenital syndromes, symptoms are caused by increased sodium levels, water retention, and potassium loss. The clinical diagnosis is suspected when there are findings of hypertension, hypokalemia, and polyuria that fail to respond to ADH administration.

Therapeutic Management

Temporary treatment of the disorder involves replacement of potassium and administration of *spironolactone (Aldactone),* a diuretic that blocks the effects of aldosterone. Definitive treatment is similar to that for chronic adrenocortical insufficiency.

Nursing Care Management

An important nursing consideration is recognition of the syndrome, particularly in children who demonstrate high blood pressure. After the diagnosis, nursing care is related to the treatment regimen, such as education about the diuretic and potassium supplements (see Nurse Alert, p. 1730). Parents need to be aware of the signs of hypokalemia and hyperkalemia (see Nurse Alert, p. 1730).

Pheochromocytoma

Pheochromocytoma is an adrenal tumor characterized by secretion of catecholamines. The tumor most commonly arises from the chromaffin cells of the adrenal medulla but may occur wherever these cells are found, such as along the paraganglia of the aorta or thoracolumbar sympathetic chain. In children this type of tumor is most frequently bilateral or multiple and is generally benign. Often there is a familial transmission of the condition as an autosomal dominant trait that tends to favor males. The clinical manifestations of pheochromocytoma are caused by an increased production of catecholamines, and they mimic those of other disorders, such as hyperthyroidism, diabetes mellitus, or functional hyperventilation (Box 52-12).

Therapeutic Management

Definitive treatment consists of surgical removal of the tumor. In children the tumors may be bilateral, requiring a bilateral adrenalectomy and lifelong glucocorticoid and mineralocorticoid therapy.

Nursing Care Management

An initial nursing objective is identification of children with this disorder. Outstanding clues are hypertension and hypertensive attacks. Preoperative nursing care involves

BOX 52-12

Clinical Manifestations of Pheochromocytoma

Hypertension
Tachycardia
Headache
Decreased gastrointestinal activity; resultant constipation
Anorexia
Weight loss
Hyperglycemia
Polyuria
Polydipsia
Hyperventilation
Nervousness
Heat intolerance
Diaphoresis
Signs of congestive heart failure in severe cases

frequent monitoring of vital signs and observing for evidence of hypertensive attacks and congestive heart failure. Urine should be tested at least daily for glucose and ketones. Any signs of hyperglycemia are noted and reported immediately.

NURSE ALERT DO *NOT* PALPATE MASS. Preoperative palpation may facilitate release of catecholamines, which can stimulate severe hypertension and tachyarrythmias. ■

The environment should be conducive to rest and free of emotional stress. This requires adequate preparation during hospital admission and before surgery. Parents are encouraged to room-in with their child and to participate in the care. Play activities need to be tailored to the child's energy level but should not be overly strenuous or challenging, because these can increase the metabolic rate and promote frustration and anxiety.

After surgery the child is observed for signs of shock from removal of excess catecholamines. If a bilateral adrenalectomy was performed, the nursing interventions are those discussed for chronic adrenocortical insufficiency.

DISORDERS OF PANCREATIC HORMONE FUNCTION

The islets of Langerhans of the pancreas have three major functioning cells:

1. The *alpha cells* produce *glucagon,* which increases the blood glucose levels by stimulating the liver and other cells to release stored glucose (glycogenolysis).
2. The *beta cells* produce *insulin,* which lowers blood glucose levels by facilitating the entrance of glucose into the cells for metabolism.
3. The *delta cells* produce *somatostatin,* which is believed to regulate the release of insulin and glucagon.

The discussion of disorders of pancreatic hormone secretion is limited to diabetes mellitus.

CASE STUDY: DIABETES MELLITUS

Diabetes Mellitus

Diabetes mellitus (DM) is a disease of metabolism characterized by a total or partial deficiency of the hormone *insulin,* resulting in a metabolic adjustment or physiologic change in almost all areas of the body. It is the most common endocrine disorder of childhood, with the peak incidence reached during early adolescence (Ross, 2003).

Classification

Traditionally DM had been classified according to the type of treatment needed. The old categories were insulin-dependent diabetes mellitus (IDDM), or type I, and non–insulin-dependent diabetes mellitus (NIDDM), or type II. In 1997 these terms were eliminated because treatment can vary (some people with NIDDM require insulin) and because the terms do not indicate the underlying problem. The new terms are type 1 and type 2, using Arabic symbols to avoid confusion (e.g., type II could be read as type eleven) (American Diabetes Association, 2001).

Type 1 diabetes is characterized by destruction of the pancreatic beta cells, which produce insulin; this usually leads to absolute insulin deficiency. Type 1 diabetes has two forms. *Immune-mediated diabetes mellitus* results from an autoimmune destruction of the beta cells. It typically starts in children or young adults who are slim, but it can arise in adults of any age. *Idiopathic type 1 diabetes* refers to rare forms of the disease that have no known cause.

Type 2 diabetes usually arises because of insulin resistance, in which the body fails to use insulin properly, combined with relative (rather then absolute) insulin deficiency. People with type 2 can range from predominantly insulin resistant with relative insulin deficiency to predominantly deficient in insulin secretion with some insulin resistance. In the past, type 2 diabetes occured in those who are over 45, are overweight and sedentary, and have a family history of diabetes.

Changes in food consumption and exercise patterns have increased the rate of type 2 diabetes mellitus in children and adolescents in the United States (Kiess et al, 2003; Steinberger & Daniels, 2003; Stephenson, 2003).

Etiology

The clinical syndrome of DM results from a large variety of etiologic and pathogenic mechanisms. Type 1 DM is now believed to be an autoimmune disease that arises when a person with a genetic predisposition is exposed to a precipitating event, such as a viral infection.

Genetic Factors

Type 1 DM is not inherited, but heredity is a prominent factor in the etiology. A variety of genetic mechanisms have been proposed, but most authorities favor a multifactorial inheritance or a recessive gene somehow linked to the human lymphocyte antigen (HLA). However, the genetic influence in type 1 DM and type 2 DM appears to differ in several ways. Studies of type 2 DM in identical twins demonstrate a 90% to 100% concordance throughout the life span, whereas studies of type 1 DM in identical twins demonstrate a 30% to 50% concordance rate (Redondo, Fain, & Eisenbarth, 2001; Stephenson, 2003). Children diagnosed with type 1 diabetes before 5 years of age may have different autoimmune and genetic characteristics related to their diabetes than older children (Hathout et al, 2003).

Autoimmune Mechanisms

An autoimmune process is involved in persons who develop type 1 DM. The current theory is that the presence of the HLA genes causes a defect in the immune system that renders the possessor susceptible to a trigger event, which can be a dietary source (Kimpimaki et al, 2001), virus, bacterium, or chemical irritant. The predisposing event initiates an autoimmune process that gradually destroys beta cells. Without beta cells no insulin can be produced. There is also a strong association between type 1 DM and other autoimmune endocrine disorders, such as thyroiditis and Addison disease.

Pathophysiology

Insulin is needed to support the metabolism of carbohydrates, fats, and proteins, primarily by facilitating the entry of these substances into the cell, with the exception of nerve cells and vascular tissue. With a deficiency of insulin, glucose is unable to enter the cell, and its concentration in the blood-

Table 52-2

Comparison of Manifestations of Hypoglycemia and Hyperglycemia

VARIABLE	HYPOGLYCEMIA	HYPERGLYCEMIA
Onset	Rapid (minutes)	Gradual (days)
Mood	Labile, irritable, nervous, weepy	Lethargic
Mental status	Difficulty concentrating, speaking, focusing, coordinating Nightmares	Dulled sensorium Confused
Inward feeling	Shaky feeling, hunger Headache Dizziness	Thirst Weakness Nausea/vomiting Abdominal pain
Skin	Pallor Sweating	Flushed Signs of dehydration
Mucous membranes	Normal	Dry, crusty
Respirations	Shallow, normal	Deep, rapid (Kussmaul)
Pulse	Tachycardia, palpitations	Less rapid, weak
Breath odor	Normal	Fruity, acetone
Neurologic	Tremors Late: hyperflexia, dilated pupils, seizure	Diminished reflexes Paresthesia
Ominous signs	Shock, coma	Acidosis, coma
Blood:		
• Glucose	Low: below 60 mg/dl	High: 250 mg/dl or more
• Ketones	Negative	High/large
• Osmolarity	Normal	High
• pH	Normal	Low (7.25 or less)
• Hematocrit	Normal	High
• HCO_3	Normal	Less than 20 mEq/L
Urine:		
• Output	Normal	Polyuria (early) to oliguria (late) Enuresis, nocturia
• Glucose	Negative	High
• Ketones	Negative/trace	High
Visual	Diplopia	Blurred vision

stream *(hyperglycemia)* increases (Table 52-2). The increased concentration of glucose produces an osmotic gradient that causes the movement of body fluid from the intracellular space to the extracellular space; from there the body fluid is excreted by the kidneys. When the serum glucose level exceeds the renal threshold (±180 mg/dl), glucose "spills" into the urine *(glycosuria)*, along with an osmotic diversion of water *(polyuria)*, a cardinal sign of diabetes. The urinary fluid losses cause the excessive thirst *(polydipsia)* observed in diabetes. As might be expected, this water washout results in a depletion of other essential chemicals.

Protein is also wasted during insulin deficiency. Because glucose is unable to enter the cells, protein is broken down and converted to glucose by the liver *(glucogenesis)*; this glucose then contributes to the hyperglycemia. Without the use of carbohydrates for energy, fat and protein stores are depleted as the body attempts to meet its energy needs. The hunger mechanism is triggered, but the increased food intake *(polyphagia)* enhances the problem by further elevating the blood glucose.

Ketoacidosis

When insulin is absent, glucose is unavailable for cellular metabolism and the body chooses alternative sources of energy, principally fat. Consequently, fats break down into fatty acids, and glycerol in the fat cells and liver is converted to ketone bodies (β-hydroxybutyric acid, acetoacetic acid, acetone). The ketone bodies can be used as an alternative source of fuel for glucose, but they are used in the cells at a limited rate. Any excess is eliminated in the urine *(ketonuria)* or the lungs (acetone breath). The ketone bodies in the blood *(ketonemia)* are strong acids that lower serum pH, producing *ketoacidosis.* The respiratory system attempts to eliminate the excess carbon dioxide by increased depth and rate—*Kussmaul respirations,* the hyperventilation characteristic of metabolic acidosis.

With cellular death, potassium is released from the cell into the interstitial spaces and then into the bloodstream. It is then excreted by the kidney, where the loss is accelerated by osmotic diuresis. The total-body potassium is then decreased, even though the serum potassium level may be elevated as a result of the decreased fluid volume in which it circulates. Alteration in serum and tissue potassium can make cardiac arrest a potential problem.

If these conditions are not reversed by insulin therapy in combination with correction of the fluid deficiency and electrolyte imbalance, progressive deterioration occurs, with dehydration, electrolyte imbalance, acidosis, coma, and death. *Diabetic ketoacidosis (DKA)* is a pediatric emergency and should be diagnosed promptly, with therapy instituted.

Long-Term Complications

Long-term complications of diabetes involve the small, as well as larger, blood vessels. The principal microvascular complications are *nephropathy* and *retinopathy.* The process appears to be one of *glycosylation,* wherein proteins from the blood become deposited in the basement membrane of small vessels (e.g., glomeruli, retina), where they become trapped by "sticky" glucose compounds (glycosyl radicals). The buildup of these substances over time causes narrowing of the vessels with subsequent interference with microcirculation to the affected areas. With poor control, vascular changes appear as early as 2.5 to 3 years after diagnosis; with good control, changes have been postponed for 20 or more years.

Neuropathy appears to be an identical process, but glycosylation occurs on the sheath of nerves, interrupting neurotransmission of stimuli. Macrovascular disease may develop after 25 years of diabetes and creates the predominant complications in patients with type 2 DM. Intensive insulin therapy appears to delay the onset and slow the progression of clinically important retinopathy, including vision loss, nephropathy, and neuropathy, by 35% to more than 70% (Wunderlich et al, 1998).

NURSE ALERT Recurrent urinary tract and vaginal infections, especially with *Candida albicans,* are often an early sign of type 1 DM, especially in adolescents. ■

Diagnostic Evaluation

Three groups of children who should be considered at risk for diabetes are (1) those who have glycosuria, polyuria, and a history of weight loss or failure to gain despite a hearty appetite; (2) those with transient or persistent glycosuria; and (3) those who display manifestations of metabolic acidosis, with or without stupor or coma. Clinical manifestations of type 1 DM are outlined in Box 52-13. Diabetes is a great imitator; influenza, gastroenteritis, and appendicitis are the conditions most often diagnosed.

An 8-hour fasting blood glucose level $\geq$126 mg/dl, a random blood glucose value of $\geq$200 accompanied by classic signs of diabetes, or an oral glucose tolerance test (OGTT) finding $\geq$200 mg/dl in the 2-hour sample is almost certain to indicate diabetes (American Diabetes Association, 2001; Hoffman, 2003). Postprandial blood glucose determinations and the traditional OGTTs have yielded low detection rates in children and are not usually necessary for establishing a diagnosis. Serum insulin levels may be normal or moderately elevated at the onset of diabetes; delayed insulin response to glucose indicates the presence of impaired glucose tolerance.

Ketoacidosis must be differentiated from other causes of acidosis or coma, including hypoglycemia, uremia, gastroenteritis with metabolic acidosis, salicylate intoxication encephalitis, and other intracranial lesions. DKA is a state of relative insulin insufficiency and may include the presence of hyperglycemia (blood glucose level $\geq$330 mg/dl), ketonemia (strongly positive), acidosis (pH <7.30 and bicarbonate <15 mmol/L), glycosuria, and ketonuria (Magee & Bhatt, 2001). Tests used to determine glycosuria and ketonuria are the glucose oxidase tapes (Keto-Diastix).

BOX 52-13

Clinical Manifestations of Type 1 Diabetes Mellitus

Polyphagia
Polyuria
Polydipsia
Weight loss
Enuresis or nocturia
Irritability; "not himself" or "not herself"
Shortened attention span
Lowered frustration tolerance
Fatigue
Dry skin
Blurred vision
Poor wound healing
Flushed skin
Headache
Frequent infections
Hyperglycemia:
- Elevated blood glucose levels
- Glucosuria

Diabetic ketosis:
- Ketones, as well as glucose, in urine
- Dehydration may or may not be present

Diabetic ketoacidosis:
- Dehydration
- Electrolyte imbalance
- Acidosis
- Deep, rapid breathing (Kussmaul)

Therapeutic Management

The definitive treatment is replacement of insulin. However, insulin needs are affected by nutritional intake, activity, emotions, and other life events, such as illnesses and puberty. Medical and nutritional guidance are primary, but management also includes continuing diabetes education, family guidance, and emotional support.

Insulin Therapy

Insulin is available in highly purified pork preparations and in human insulin manufactured by biosynthesis. Most clinicians suggest human insulin as the treatment of choice. It is available in rapid-, short-, intermediate-, and long-acting preparations, and all are packaged in the strength of 100 units/ml (Box 52-14). (Other dosages are available for situations where extraordinarily large or small dosages are required.)

NURSE ALERT Insulin comes dissolved in liquids at different strengths. Most people use U-100 insulin. This means it has 100 units of insulin per milliliter (ml) of fluid. Be sure that the syringe you use matches the insulin strength. U-100 insulin needs a U-100 syringe. ■

BOX 52-14

Types of Insulin

There are four types of insulin, based on the following:
- How soon the insulin starts working (onset)
- When the insulin works the hardest (peak time)
- How long the insulin lasts in your body (duration)

However, each person responds to insulin in his or her own way. That is why onset, peak time, and duration are given as ranges.

Rapid-acting (lispro) insulin reaches the blood within 15 minutes after injection. The insulin peaks 30 to 90 minutes later and may last for as long as 5 hours.

Short-acting (regular) insulin usually reaches the blood within 30 minutes after injection. The insulin peaks 2 to 4 hours later and stays in the blood for about 4 to 8 hours.

Intermediate-acting (NPH and Lente) insulins reach the blood 2 to 6 hours after injection. The insulins peak 4 to 14 hours later and stay in the blood for about 14 to 20 hours.

Long-acting (Ultralente) insulin takes 6 to 14 hours to start working. It has no peak or a very small peak 10 to 16 hours after injection. The insulin stays in the blood for 20 to 24 hours.

Some insulins come mixed together. For example, you can buy regular insulin and NPH insulins already mixed in one bottle. This makes it easier to inject two kinds of insulin at the same time. However, you cannot adjust the amount of one insulin without also changing the amount of the other insulin.

Daily insulin is administered subcutaneously by twice-daily injections, by multiple-dose injections, or by means of a portable pump. Diabetes can be controlled satisfactorily in most children with a *twice-daily insulin* regimen consisting of a combination of *rapid-acting (lispro)* or *short-acting (regular)* and *intermediate-acting (NPH or Lente)* insulin given in the same syringe before breakfast and before the evening meal. The amount of insulin is determined by measurements of the blood glucose level after the peak effect of the insulin has occurred. For example, the amount of regular insulin at breakfast is determined by a pattern of the previous lunchtime blood glucose values. Regular insulin is best given at least 30 minutes before meals to allow sufficient time for absorption. On the other hand, lispro insulin is best given no more than 10 to 15 minutes before the meal. Some children require more frequent administration of insulin. This includes children with difficult-to-control diabetes and children during the adolescent growth spurt. An intensive insulin management program has been shown to reduce microvascular complications in young, healthy patients who have type 1 DM.

NURSE ALERT Never store insulin at very cold (under 36° F) or very hot (over 86° F) temperatures. Extreme temperatures destroy insulin. ■

Insulin may lose some potency if the bottle has been open for more than 30 days. Examine the bottle of insulin closely to make sure the insulin looks normal. Regular insulin should be perfectly clear—there should be no floating pieces or color. NPH or Lente insulin should be cloudy, with no floating pieces or crystals on the bottle.

The *insulin pump* is designed to deliver fixed amounts of regular or lispro insulin continuously, thereby more closely imitating the release of the hormone by the islet cells (Olohan & Zappitelli, 2003). The system consists of a syringe to hold the insulin, a plunger, and a computerized mechanism to drive the plunger. The insulin flows from the syringe through a catheter to a needle inserted into subcutaneous tissue (the abdomen or thigh), and the lightweight device is worn on a belt or a shoulder holster. The tubing and catheter are changed every 48 hours by the child or parent, using aseptic technique, and taped in place.

Although the pump provides more even insulin release, it has disadvantages. It should not be removed for more than 1 to 2 hours, which may limit some activities (e.g., bathing and swimming, although some water-safe models are now available); skin infections are common; and, like any other mechanical device, it is subject to malfunction. However, the pumps are equipped with alarms that signal problems that may arise, such as depleted batteries, an occluded needle or tubing, or a microprocessor malfunction.

Researchers are experimenting with *intranasal* and *inhaled insulin administration* (Skyler et al, 2001). Given nasally or deep into the lungs, the insulin is able to cross the mucosa to increase serum levels. The duration of action is not long enough to be a total replacement for injections but may be of value as insulin supplementation at mealtime.

Islet cell or *whole pancreas transplantation* may offer hope to patients in the future. Viable insulin-producing cells have been injected into the portal vein, where they take root in the liver and eventually produce up to two thirds of the needed insulin. The major use of transplants has been in persons who have serious complications, particularly those whose deteriorating kidneys have required renal transplants and who are receiving immunosuppression therapy. However, islet cell and pancreatic transplants tend not to be sustainable over time despite continuation of therapy. The use of nonhuman islets encapsulated in immunoprotective, semipermeable membranes may have a future in the treatment of type 1 DM (Lanza et al, 1999; Robertson et al, 2000).

Monitoring

Self-monitoring of blood glucose (SMBG) has improved diabetes management and is used successfully by children from the onset of their diabetes. By testing their own blood, children and parents are able to change their insulin regimen to maintain their glucose level in the euglycemic (normal) range of 80 to 120 mg/dl. Diabetes management depends to a great extent on SMBG. New devices that measure and record blood glucose levels automatically have been approved by the Food and Drug Administration (FDA) for use in children (Chase et al, 2003; Cox, 2002; Olohan & Zappitelli, 2003). The Glucowatch Biographer uses reverse iontophoresis to draw interstial fluid through the skin to measure the glucose level with an electrochemical sensor (Chase et al, 2003; Olohan & Zappitelli, 2003; Plotnick, 2003).

Laboratory measurement of *glycosylated hemoglobin (hemoglobin A_{1c})* levels reflects the average blood glucose levels during the previous 2 to 3 months and is of value in assessing glucose control in any person with diabetes. As red blood cells circulate in the bloodstream, glucose molecules gradually attach to the hemoglobin A molecules and remain there for the lifetime of the red blood cell, approximately 120 days. Nondiabetic hemoglobin A_{1c} values are generally between 4% and 6% but can vary by laboratory. Acceptable diabetes control for children is typically a hemoglobin A_{1c} value of 7.5%.

Urine testing for glucose is no longer used for diabetes management; there is poor correlation between simultaneous glycosuria and blood glucose concentrations. However, urine testing can be carried out to detect evidence of ketonuria.

Nutrition

Essentially, the nutritional needs of children with diabetes are no different from those of unaffected children. Children with diabetes require no special foods or supplements. They need sufficient calories to balance daily expenditure for energy and to satisfy the requirement for growth and development. They also need consistent intake and timing of food, especially carbohydrates.

Normally, insulin is secreted in response to food intake. However, insulin injected subcutaneously has a relatively predictable time of onset, peak effect, duration of action, and absorption rate, depending on the type of insulin used. Consequently, the timing of food consumption is regulated to correspond to the time and action of the insulin prescribed. Meals and snacks must be eaten at the same times each day, and the total number of calories and proportions of basic nutrients must be consistent from day to day. The distribution of calories, especially carbohydrates, is determined to fit the activity pattern of each child. Alterations in food intake are made so that food, insulin, and exercise are balanced. Extra food is needed for extra activity.

There is no one diet for diabetes. General guidelines exist, such as "eat less fat and less saturated fat" and "eat more whole grains, fruits, and vegetables." Sugars and sweets, or "simple sugars," do not raise blood glucose any quicker than starches, or "complex carbohydrates." Provide healthy nutrition advice—eat sugars and sweets in moderation. The diabetes meal plan must be based on individual needs and developed with expert assistance from a registered dietitian.

Exercise

Exercise is encouraged and never restricted unless indicated by other health conditions, because it lowers blood glucose levels. It is included as part of diabetes management and is planned around the child's interests and capabilities. However, in most instances children's activities are unplanned, and the resulting decrease in the blood glucose level can be compensated for by providing extra snacks before (and, if prolonged, during) the activity. Besides providing a feeling of well-being, regular exercise aids in the body's use of food and often decreases insulin requirements.

Hypoglycemia

Even a child with well-controlled diabetes may often experience mild symptoms of hypoglycemia, but if the signs and symptoms are recognized early (see Table 52-2) and relieved promptly by appropriate therapy, the child's activity should not be interrupted for more than a few minutes.

NURSE ALERT Hypoglycemic episodes most commonly occur before meals, or when the insulin effect is peaking. ■

The most common causes of hypoglycemia, *insulin reaction,* are bursts of physical activity without additional food, or delayed, omitted, or incompletely consumed meals or snacks. Reglycosalation of muscles and replenishment of liver glycogen may occur over the ensuing 24 hours. Therefore particular vigilance related to hypoglycemia may be necessary during the night after vigorous exertion.

In the majority of cases, simple concentrated sugar, such as honey, that can be held in the mouth for a short time will elevate the blood glucose level and alleviate the symptoms. The simpler the carbohydrate, the more rapidly it will be absorbed. For a mild reaction, low-fat milk is a good food to use in children. It supplies them with lactose or milk sugar, as well as providing a more prolonged action from the protein and fat (aids in decreased absorption). All children with diabetes should carry with them a source of glucose, such as glucose tablets, Insta-glucose, hard candy, or sugar cubes. The rapid-releasing sugar is followed by a complex carbohydrate and protein, such as a slice of bread or a cracker spread with peanut butter.

Glucagon is sometimes prescribed for home treatment of severe hypoglycemia. It is available by prescription as a prefilled syringe and is administered intramuscularly or subcutaneously. Glucagon functions by releasing stored glycogen from the liver and requires about 10 minutes to elevate the blood glucose level. Once the child is responsive, the lost glycogen stores are replaced by small amounts of sugar-containing fluid administered frequently until the child feels comfortable about trying solid foods.

NURSE ALERT Vomiting may occur after administration of glucagon; therefore precautions against aspiration must be taken (e.g., placing the child on the side), because the child will be unconscious. ■

The *Somogyi phenomenon,* or *Somogyi effect,* should be recognized as a separate response from hypoglycemia. This phenomenon occurs when the blood glucose level decreases to the point where stress hormones (epinephrine, growth hormone, and corticosteroids) are released, causing a rebound hyperglycemia. Prevention consists of increasing the amount of food eaten, decreasing the insulin, or both.

Illness Management

Illness alters diabetes management. Maintaining blood glucose control is usually related to the seriousness of the illness. As the illness runs its course, the goal of diabetes management is to maintain some euglycemia while recognizing and treating urinary ketones and preventing dehydration. Some hyperglycemia and ketonuria are expected in most illnesses, even with diminished food intake, and indicate the need for increased insulin. Insulin should never be omitted during an illness, although dosage requirements may increase, decrease, or remain unchanged, depending on the severity of the illness and the child's appetite. In addition, supplemental doses of lispro or regular insulin are often used to manage the hyperglycemia associated with illness. Illness management must always include careful attention to fluid balance. Hyperglycemia contributes to dehydration, and the child will require extra oral fluids while ill.

Management of Diabetic Ketoacidosis

DKA, the most complete state of insulin deficiency, is a life-threatening situation. The child is admitted to an intensive care facility for management, which consists of rapid assessment, adequate insulin to reduce the elevated blood glucose level, fluids to overcome dehydration, and electrolyte replacement (especially potassium). The preferred method for administering insulin to the child with ketoacidosis is a continuous IV infusion of low-dose regular insulin.

Current trends suggest cautious fluid resuscitation and blood glucose management to reduce risk of cerebral edema. The fluid deficit is replaced evenly over 24 to 48 hours. Serum potassium levels may be normal on admission, but rapid return of potassium to cells following initiation of fluid and insulin can seriously deplete serum levels, with the attendant risk of cardiac arrhythmias. A cardiac monitor is employed as a guide to therapy and to determine changes that might indicate alterations in potassium concentration.

NURSE ALERT Potassium must never be given until the serum potassium level is known to be normal or low and voiding of urine is observed. All maintenance IV fluids should include 20 to 40 mEq/L of potassium. Never give potassium as a rapid IV bolus, or cardiac arrest may result. ■

When the critical period is over, the task of regulating insulin dosage to diet and activity is begun. Children should be actively involved in their own care and are given responsibility according to their ability and guidance of the nurse.

NURSE ALERT Because insulin can chemically bind to plastic tubing and in-line filters, thereby reducing the amount of the medication reaching the bloodstream, an insulin mixture is run through the tubing to saturate the insulin binding sites before the infusion is begun. ■

Nursing Care Management

Assessment

Daily monitoring of blood glucose levels; periodic urine analysis for ketones; and observation for signs of hypoglycemia, hyperglycemia, or other complications is part of the daily life of the child with diabetes and the child's family. Diabetes should be suspected in any child who exhibits the manifestations outlined in Box 52-13, and the child should be referred for further assessment and appropriate testing.

The signs and symptoms of hypoglycemia are caused by both increased adrenergic activity and impaired brain function, and it is often difficult to distinguish between hyperglycemia and a hypoglycemic reaction (see Table 52-2). Because the symptoms are similar and usually begin with changes in behavior, the simplest way to differentiate between the two is to test the blood glucose level (low in hypoglycemia; elevated in hyperglycemia).

Education is the cornerstone of diabetes management and the major responsibility in diabetes nursing care. Whether teaching is conducted on an outpatient basis or in a preparatory, in-depth manner on an inpatient basis, the ability and readiness of the individual learner must be accurately assessed. This includes assessment of the educational background and emotional stability of the individual(s) involved and the use of appropriate measurement tools, such as a pretest or an objective assessment of the learner's educational level and literacy.

Nursing Diagnoses

A number of nursing diagnoses are prominent in the nursing management of type 1 DM, and others specific to individual cases become evident. The most common are outlined in the Nursing Care Plan on p. 1746.

Plan of Care and Implementation

The goals of care for the child with DM and the child's family are as follows:

1. Child and family will be educated about the disease, assessment techniques, and therapy.
2. Child will experience a minimum of complications of diabetes.
3. Child will develop a positive self-image.
4. Child and family will receive adequate support.

Once the child with diabetes is diagnosed and insulin therapy initiated, the major nursing responsibility is the education of the family and reinforcement of information. The parents must supervise and manage the child's therapeutic program, but the child should assume responsibility for self-management as soon as he or she is capable. Children can assist with blood glucose testing at a relatively young age (4 to 5 years), and most should be able to administer their own insulin with supervision at about 9 years of age. In situations in which the parents are inconsistent or unreliable, the child is taught self-care at an earlier age and additional adult support is sought.

Several organizations are prepared to assist with education and dissemination of knowledge about diabetes. The American Diabetes Association, Inc.,* Canadian Diabetes Association,† Juvenile Diabetes Foundation International,‡ Juvenile Diabetes Research Foundation—Canada,§ and American Association of Diabetes Educators|| are valuable resources for a wide variety of educational materials. The National Diabetes Information Clearinghouse¶ publishes a number of comprehensive annotated bibliographies, including *Educational Materials for and about Young People with Diabetes* (a compilation of resource materials for children, siblings, parents, teachers, and health professionals) and *Sports and Exercise for People with Diabetes.*

Self-management, the ultimate goal for the child with diabetes, is more likely to occur when the child understands

---

*1660 Duke St., Alexandria, VA 22314; phone: 800-232-3472; Web site: www.diabetes.org.

†15 Toronto St., Suite 800, Toronto, Ontario M5C 2E3; phone: 416-363-3373 or 800-BANTING; Web site: www.diabetes.ca.

‡120 Wall St., New York, NY 10005; phone: 800-223-1138; Web site: www.jdf.org.

§89 Granton Dr., Richmond Hill, Ontario L4B 2N5; phone: 800-668-0274; Web site: www.jdfc.ca.

||100 W. Monroe, Suite 400, Chicago, IL 60603; phone: 800-338-3633; Web site: www.aadenet.org.

¶1 Information Way, Bethesda, MD 20892-3560; phone: 301-654-3327; fax: 301-907-8906; e-mail: ndic@info.niddk.gov; Web site: www.niddk.nih.gov/health/diabetes/ndic.htm.

the disorder and the care it requires. Properly educated and with adequate resources, any family should be able to follow a program of regulated control satisfactorily. The following information will allow the family to manage the daily aspects of care.

Identification

One of the first issues to raise with parents is the need for the child to wear medical identification. This essential and immediate information could save the child's life. Identification tags come in a variety of forms, including neck chains, bracelets, and tags for shoes.

Nature of Diabetes

The better the parents understand the pathophysiology of diabetes and the function and action of insulin and glucagon in relation to caloric intake and exercise, the better their understanding of the disease and its effect on the child. Parents need answers to a number of questions (voiced or unvoiced), because those answers will provide them with an increased feeling of security in coping with the disease. Parents initially may worry about what diabetes is, how their child developed diabetes, and if their other children are at risk of developing diabetes. In addition, they will worry about what to tell family, friends, and school personnel. They may have fears about complications and about how they will afford the cost of diabetes care.

Meal Planning

Normal nutrition is a major aspect of the family education program. Diet instruction is usually conducted by the nutritionist, with reinforcement and guidance from the nurse. Learning about foods within specific food groups helps in making choices. Weights and measures of foods, used as eye-training devices in defining portion sizes, should be practiced repeatedly, with gradual conversion to estimating foods. Members of the family are also guided in reading labels for the nutritional value of foods and food contents. Meals and snacks are modified to suit the child and the present food menu, preserving cultural patterns and preferences as much as possible.

Lists of popular fast-food items and items served at the major fast-food chains can be obtained from the American Diabetes Association to help guide food selections. Children are advised to use sugar substitutes with moderation in items such as soft drinks. "Sugar-free" chewing gum and candy made with sorbitol may be used in moderation. However, sorbitol is metabolized to fructose and then to glucose, and large amounts of sorbitol can cause an osmotic diarrhea. Dietetic foods that contain sorbitol are more expensive than regular foods, and often the total carbohydrate content of the food is the same or even greater.

Insulin

Families need to understand the treatment method and the insulin prescribed, including the effective duration, onset, and peak action. They also need to know the characteristics of the various types of insulins, and the proper mixing and dilution of insulins. Insulin, once opened, should be discarded in 1 month (even if refrigerated). Unopened insulin is good until the expiration date on the bottle.

Injection Procedure

Learning to give the insulin injections is a source of anxiety for the family and the child. It is helpful for the learner to know that this important aspect of care will become as routine as brushing the teeth. First, the basic injection technique is taught, using an orange or similar item and normal saline for practice. To gain the confidence of the child, the nurse demonstrates the technique by giving a skillful injection to the parent, who then returns the demonstration by giving the nurse an injection. With practice, family members soon are able to give the insulin injection to the child. Both parents should participate, and as little time as possible should elapse between instruction and the actual injection, especially with parents and the teenage learner.

Insulin is injected at a 90-degree angle into subcutaneous tissue, where it is slowly absorbed (Fig. 52-3). Newly diagnosed children may have lost adipose tissue, and care should be exercised not to inject into the muscle. The pinch technique is the most effective method for obtaining skin tightness to allow easy entrance of the needle into subcutaneous tissues in children. The site selected will sometimes depend on whether the child or parent administers the insulin. The upper arms, thighs, hips, and abdomen are usual injection sites for insulin. The child can reach the thighs, abdomen, and part of the hip and arm easily but may require help to inject other sites. For example, a parent can pinch a loose fold of skin on the arm while the child injects the insulin.

Injections are rotated to various areas of the body to enhance absorption, because insulin absorption is slowed by the fat pads that develop in overused areas of injection. The parents and child are helped to work out a rotation pattern, which involves giving about four to six injections in one area (each injection about 1 inch, or the diameter of the insulin vial, from the previous injection) and then moving to another area. In this way injection sites for an entire month can

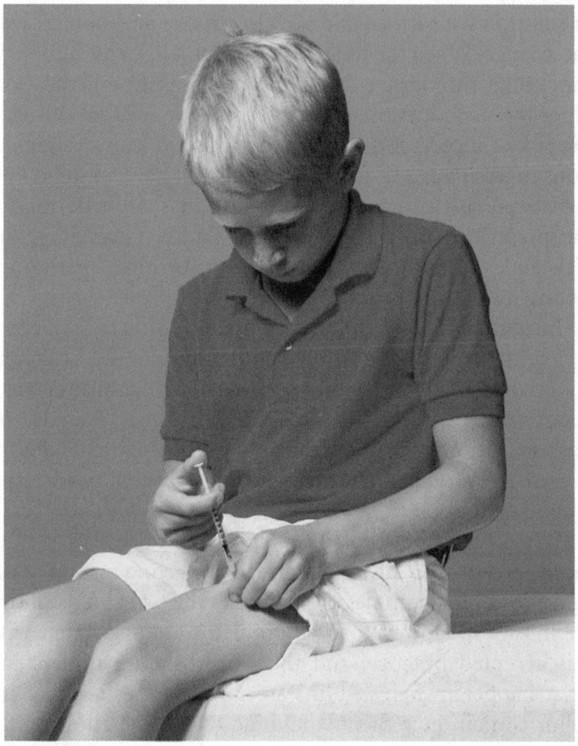

Fig. 52-3 School-age children are able to administer their own insulin.

Table 52-3

Onset and Duration of Action Related to Injection Site

	Site of Injection			
	ABDOMEN	ARM	LEG	BUTTOCK
Rate	Very fast	Fast	Slow	Very slow
Duration	Very short	Short	Long	Very long

From Albisser AM, Sperlich M: Adjusting insulins, *Diabetes Educ* 18(3): 211-218, 1992.

be planned in advance on a simple chart or illustration, such as an outline of a body or a teddy bear. It is a good idea for the parents each to give one or two injections a week in the areas that are difficult to reach in order to keep in practice.

It is important to remember that the absorption rate varies in different parts of the body (Table 52-3). Methodically using one anatomic area and then moving to another minimizes variation in absorption rates. Recommendations suggest rotating injections within an anatomic area (Fleming, 1999). An example of this would be using the abdomen for morning injections and the thighs for evening injections. This may assist with obtaining more consistent blood glucose levels. Injecting *small* doses of insulin also minimizes changes in plasma glucose levels. Absorption is also altered by vigorous exercise, which enhances absorption from exercised muscles. Therefore it is recommended that excess exercise be avoided during the time the insulin is expected to peak or that other sites be used.

Teaching includes the proper way to equalize pressure in the bottle by injecting an amount of air equal to the amount of solution withdrawn and how to remove air bubbles from the syringe. When insulin dosages are small, an air bubble in the syringe can displace a significant amount of medication. Since the introduction of the 5/10 ml and 3/10 ml syringes, the risk of incorrect dosage has diminished. However, injections of less than 2 units of U-100 insulin have an unacceptably large risk of error. Diluted insulin should be used if the prescribed dose is less than 2 units (Gnanalingham, Newland, & Smith, 1998). Aspiration for blood before injecting the insulin is not routinely done.

Insulin syringes should be compared for accuracy, comfort, and strength. The family and/or child should be able to choose both "their" insulin and "their" syringe from a variety of samples. Use of the same type of syringe (even during hospitalization) is recommended to prevent errors in dosage caused by varying markings and amounts of dead space among syringes.

When the child's dosage requires the injection of both rapid- or short-acting and intermediate-acting insulin at the same time, most families prefer to mix the two and use a single injection. However, some problems are associated with this accepted practice, and the family should understand what happens when insulins are mixed. Longer-acting insulins contain ingredients that bind to insulin, allowing for gradual release after injection. Some brands contain extra binding compounds that can bind with rapid- or short-acting insulin, blunting the action of the quicker insulin and altering the effect on blood glucose. The degree of alteration depends on the type of longer-acting insulin, the ratio of rapid- or short-acting insulin to long-acting insulin, and how long the mixture is allowed to stand before injection. The mixture should be injected less than 5 minutes after mixing (before the zinc content of the long-acting insulin affects the action time of the rapid- or short-acting insulin) or longer than 15 minutes after mixing (to allow the insulins to resume long-acting and short-acting properties).

To obtain the maximum benefit from mixing insulins, the following procedure is recommended:

1. Inject the measured amount of air (equivalent to the dosage) into the longer-acting insulin (cloudy).
2. Inject the measured amount of air into the rapid- or short-acting (clear) insulin and, without removing the needle, withdraw the clear insulin.
3. Insert the needle (already containing the clear insulin) into the longer-acting insulin and withdraw the desired amount.

NURSE ALERT When mixing types of insulin, always withdraw the clear insulin first, and then the longer-acting insulin next to avoid contaminating the clear insulin with the longer-acting insulin. ■

It has become acceptable practice (though not recommended by all professionals) to reuse disposable needles and syringes. Bacteria counts are unaffected, and there is a considerable cost saving. It is important to stress the importance of vigorous handwashing before handling any equipment, as well as capping the syringe immediately after use. Syringes may be stored at room temperature. Nurses should also teach proper disposal of equipment after use in the home. Although it is not standard practice in the hospital, the use of a needle clipper is recommended to safely remove and house the used needle. In addition, the syringe plunger can be broken before disposal. An excellent means for syringe disposal is use of an opaque, puncture-resistant container, such as an empty coffee can, bleach bottle, or milk carton that is labeled "biohazardous waste" and is discarded with similar material only, not with household refuse. Many pharmacies now carry commercially produced sharps containers.

Other devices are available for insulin injection and may offer advantages to some children. Children who do not wish to give themselves injections can be taught to use a syringe-loaded injector (Injectease). With the device, puncture is always automatic. Adolescents respond well to a self-contained and compact device resembling a fountain pen (e.g., NovoPen), which eliminates conventional vials and syringes. Preloaded pens may also cause less pain, because the needle is not blunted by piercing the rubber top of the insulin vial (Lteif & Schwenk, 1999).

Some children are considered candidates for continuous subcutaneous insulin infusion with a portable insulin pump. The child and the parents are taught to operate the device, including the mechanics of the pump, battery changes, and alarm systems. They learn how to load the syringe, insert the catheter, adjust the insulin flow for routine needs and for illnesses, and connect and disconnect the catheter. Nurses who work where the pumps are part of the therapeutic regimen should become familiar with the operation of the specific device being used and the protocol of the regimen.

Glucose Monitoring

Nurses should also be prepared to teach and supervise blood glucose monitoring. Blood for testing can be obtained by two different methods: manually or with a spring-loaded puncturing device. The automatic lancet device is recommended because its precise puncture depth produces better blood flow and less pain. However, the child and family should learn to use both methods in the event of mechanical failure. Several lancet devices are available from which to choose, and each provides a means for obtaining enough blood for testing (Fig. 52-4). Many lancet devices may be adjusted for depth of puncture.

NURSE ALERT Caution children not to allow anyone else to use their lancet or lancet device because of the risk of contracting hepatitis B virus or human immunodeficiency virus (HIV) infection. ■

Repeated finger punctures can be painful, but most children become accustomed to the procedure (Atraumatic Care box). However, persistent signs of redness and soreness at the puncture site should be investigated. It may be evidence of poor technique or poor skin healing relative to poor control. Alternative site testing (AST) meters were approved by the FDA in 1999; however, results of AST in comparison with fingertip measures have not been consistent (Lock et al, 2002; Seley, 2003). Further studies on AST meters need to be conducted to determine the effectiveness of the meters.

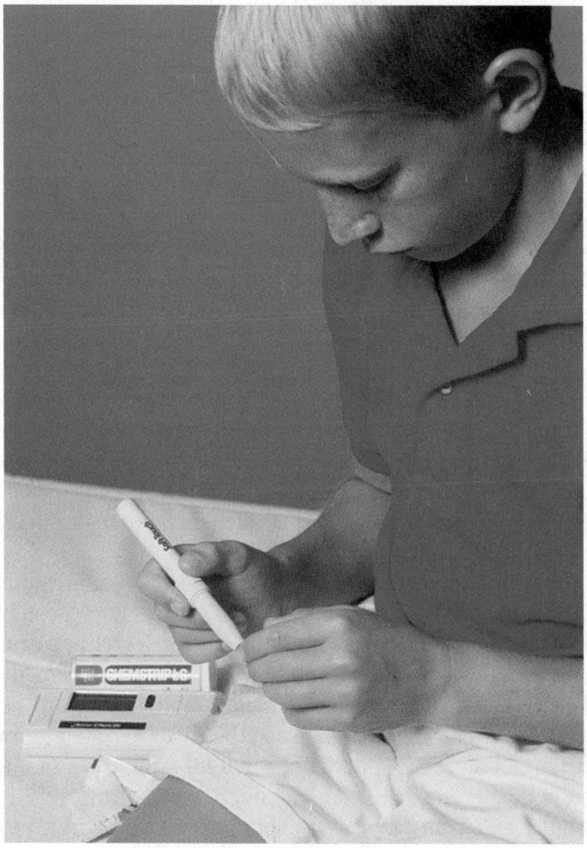

Fig. 52-4 Child using finger-stick device to obtain blood sample. Blood glucose monitor and reagent strips are nearby.

The least expensive testing method uses a visually read reagent strip to which blood is applied. After blotting, the color change is compared with a color scale for an estimation of the blood glucose level. The strips can be cut in half (although this is not recommended by all professionals) to obtain two readings per strip. This method might be ideal for use at school, where expensive equipment can be lost or broken.

Many types of glucose monitors are available for home use. The family should be shown features of several meters, including advantages and disadvantages, and allowed to choose equipment that best meets their needs. One important consideration is the amount of blood needed. Choosing devices that require small amounts may prevent repunctures.

Urine Testing

Urine ketone testing is easily taught but requires careful attention to technique. The test strip must be used accurately and the test timed precisely. Because the test strip is visually read, adequate lighting must be available. Testing for ketones is recommended during times of illness or when glucose readings are high. Moisture will cause changes to take place in both glucose and ketone strips; therefore families are instructed to discard strips that are discolored, that have been open for a specified time, or after an expiration date. Test strips are available for testing both glucose and ketones.

Hyperglycemia and Hypoglycemia

Severe hyperglycemia is most often caused by illness, growth, emotional upset, or inaccurate or missed insulin doses. With careful glucose monitoring, most elevations can be managed by adjustment of insulin or food intake. Parents should understand how to adjust food, activity, and insulin at the time of illness or when the child is treated for an illness with a medication known to raise the blood glucose level, such as cough syrup or steroids. The hyperglycemia is managed by increasing insulin soon after the increased glucose is noted.

Hypoglycemia is caused by imbalances of food intake, insulin, and activity. Ideally, hypoglycemia should be pre-

Atraumatic Care

MINIMIZING PAIN OF BLOOD GLUCOSE MONITORING

To enhance blood flow to the finger, hold it under warm water for a few seconds before the puncture.

When obtaining blood samples, use the ring finger or thumb (blood flows more easily to these areas), and puncture the finger just to the side of the finger pad (more blood vessels and fewer nerve endings).

To prevent a deep puncture, press the platform of the lancet device lightly against the skin and do not steady the finger against a hard surface.

Use glucose monitors that require very small blood samples to avoid repunctures (e.g., Glucometer Elite).

Apply EMLA to the puncture site, especially when the child is newly diagnosed and the skin is still very sensitive (see Pain Management, Chapter 44).

vented, and parents need to be prepared to prevent, recognize, and treat the problem. They should be familiar with the signs of hypoglycemia and instructed in treatment, including care of the child with seizures (see Chapter 51). Hypoglycemia can be managed effectively as outlined in the Emergency box.

Exercise

Exercise should be planned (as may be necessary for the sedentary teenager) or observed (as in most active children). If the child is more active at one time of the day than at another, food and/or insulin can be altered to meet the activity pattern of the individual. Food should be increased in the summer, when children tend to be more active. Decreased activity on return to school may require a decrease in food intake. The child who is active in team sports will need additional food intake on the days of activity in the form of a carbohydrate snack about 30 minutes before the anticipated activity. Races or other competition may call for a slightly higher food intake than practice times.

Food will usually need to be repeated for prolonged activity periods, often as frequently as every 45 minutes to 1 hour. Families should be informed that if increased food is not tolerated, decreased insulin is the next course of action. If the blood glucose level is elevated (240 mg/dl or greater) and ketone values are positive before planned exercise, the activity should be postponed until the blood glucose is controlled. Moderate to large ketone values should be reported to the practitioner.

Record Keeping

Recording information about food, insulin, blood glucose measurements, and ketonuria is useful to the practitioner, as well as to the family. Insulin reactions are noted, including the time, severity, treatment, and response to treatment. Dietary variations are noted so that an increased blood glucose level can be analyzed in relation to the insulin dose, food intake, and activity level. Record keeping should also include identified stresses, such as school exams, birthday parties, and injuries.

Self-Management

Self-management is the key to close control. Being able to make changes when they are needed rather than waiting until the next contact with health professionals is important for self-management and gives the child and parents the feeling that they have control over the disease. As children grow and assume more and more responsibility for self-management, they develop confidence in their ability to manage their disease and in themselves as persons. Self-management techniques to be mastered are the testing of blood and urine, administration of insulin, and adjustment of insulin and diet with alterations in day-to-day activities and unusual occurrences.

Hygiene

All aspects of personal hygiene are emphasized for the child with diabetes. The child should be cautioned against wearing shoes without socks, wearing sandals, or walking barefoot. The correct method of nail and extremity care instituted for each particular child (with the guidance of a podiatrist) can begin health practices that last a lifetime. Eyes should be checked once a year, unless the child wears glasses, and then as directed by the ophthalmologist. Regular dental care is emphasized, and cuts and scratches should be treated with plain soap and water unless otherwise indicated.

Acute Care

Children with diabetes may be admitted to the hospital at the time of their initial diagnosis, during illness or surgery, or during episodes of DKA—especially in the small number who exhibit a degree of metabolic lability or who have repeated episodes of DKA. Most children with diabetes are able to keep the disease under control with periodic assessment and adjustment of insulin, diet, and activity as needed under health supervision.

The child with DKA requires intensive nursing care. On admission to the hospital, usually an intensive care unit, an IV infusion is started immediately to hydrate the child and to administer insulin, usually as a continuous infusion (see Management of Diabetic Ketoacidosis, p. 1740). The blood glucose level is monitored at regular intervals, and the insulin is administered as ordered.

Sodium, potassium, and bicarbonate levels are monitored and replaced as indicated. Because potassium and sodium reenter the cells rapidly after administration of insulin, depletion of these electrolytes can be a serious consequence. The child is attached to a cardiac monitor for continual assessment of cardiac status, especially when potassium levels are markedly altered.

Careful and accurate records are maintained, including vital signs, blood pressure, IV fluids, electrolytes, insulin, blood glucose level, intake and output, and weight. A urine collection device is used to obtain the urine measurements, which include volume, specific gravity, and glucose and ketone values. The volume relative to the glucose content is important, because 5% glucose in a 300 ml sample is a significantly greater amount than a similar reading from a 75 ml sample. A diabetic flow sheet maintained at the bedside provides an ongoing record of the vital signs, urine and blood

Emergency

HYPOGLYCEMIA

Mild Reaction: Adrenergic Symptoms

Give child 10 to 15 g of simple carbohydrate (preferably liquid; e.g., 3 to 6 ounces of orange juice).
Follow with starch-protein snack.

Moderate Reaction: Neuroglycopenic Symptoms

Give child 10 to 15 g of simple carbohydrate as above.
Repeat in 10 to 15 minutes if symptoms persist.
Follow with larger snack.
Watch child closely.

Severe Reaction: Unresponsive, Unconscious, or Seizures

Administer glucagon as prescribed.
Follow with planned meal or snack when child is able to eat, or add a snack.

Nocturnal Reaction

Give child 10 to 15 g of simple carbohydrate.
Follow with a snack.

tests, amount of insulin given, and intake and output of the patient. The level of consciousness is assessed and recorded at frequent intervals. Any change or deterioration in the level of consciousness must be reported to the health care provider. Such changes may indicate an increase in intracranial pressure and must be managed aggressively. The comatose child generally regains consciousness fairly soon after initiation of therapy but is managed as is any unconscious child during that time.

Family Support

In any educational program, the psychologic needs of the child are just as important as the physical needs. Adjustment to a chronic illness is difficult and follows the grief process (see Chapter 41). A noticeable adjustment cycle occurs during the week-long education course. First, there is interest and perhaps some anger and doubt, followed by denial and accompanied by the overwhelming feeling of "Why me?" There are doubts regarding the ability to absorb so much essential information. Then there are the acceptance and synthesis of material, as the learners realize that they are able to state and demonstrate their understanding of the material.

Young children usually adjust well to problems related to the disease. However, challenges exist, such as providing regular feedings to the sick infant or to the negative toddler. With toddlers and preschoolers, insulin injections and glucose testing may be difficult at first. However, they usually accept the procedures when the parents use a matter-of-fact approach without calling attention to a "hurt" and treat the procedure like any other routine part of a child's life. Following the injection, time with some special and positive attention, such as reading, talking, or some other pleasant activity, is one way to convert children who initially refuse injections to those who accept them.

School-age children tend to accept their condition more easily than adolescents. School-age children can understand the basic concepts related to their disease and its treatment. They are able to test blood glucose and urine; recognize food groups; give injections; keep records; and distinguish between feelings of fear, excitement, and hypoglycemia. They understand how to recognize, prevent, and treat hypoglycemia. However, they still need considerable parental involvement.

Adolescents appear to have the most difficulty in adjusting. Adolescence is a time when there is much stress to be "perfect" and to be like peers; however, no matter what others say, having diabetes is being different. Some youngsters are more upset about not being able to have a candy bar than about injections, diet, and other aspects of management. If children can accept the difference as a part of life—in other words, if they can accept that each person is different in some way—then, with adequate family support, they should be able to adjust well (Family Focus box and Critical Thinking Exercise).

For all families, daily compliance with numerous procedures and structured living schedules is difficult. Maintaining good blood glucose control requires ongoing motivation. Nurses can encourage families to adhere to treatment regimens and lifestyle adjustments by emphasizing the benefits of preventing complications such as hypoglycemia. In some families, complications can have a favorable impact.

Family Focus

THE ADOLESCENT WITH TYPE 1 DIABETES MELLITUS

As a nurse caring for adolescents with type 1 diabetes mellitus (DM), I am constantly aware of the wide range of adolescent behaviors that affect the course of this disease. Education of the child and the parents can often make the difference between a disease in control of the teenager and a teenager in control of the disease.

I have cared for many adolescent girls who have episodes of hyperglycemia at the time of menstruation that can result in diabetic ketoacidosis (DKA). I have found that education regarding sick-day protocol with sliding-scale rapid-acting insulin instituted at the first sign of hyperglycemia, which may occur 1 to 2 days before onset of menses, can keep the adolescent girl out of the intensive care unit and in control of her diabetes.

Eating disorders, such as bulimia or anorexia nervosa, in the teenager with type 1 DM pose a serious health hazard. Also, insulin manipulation or omission has been identified as a weight-loss method used by some adolescents (Barber & Lowes, 1998). Poor disease control may also be used by depressed teens as a method of suicide. Nurses working with these adolescents must be aware of the hazards and openly discuss the risks with the young person. A referral for specialized intervention may be needed.

Another group of adolescents with diabetes who are at risk are those who drink alcohol. I have found that confusion about the effects of alcohol on blood glucose is common. Teenagers may believe that alcohol will increase blood glucose levels, when in fact the opposite occurs. Ingestion of alcohol inhibits the release of glycogen from the liver, therefore resulting in hypoglycemia. Teenagers with diabetes who drink alcohol may become hypoglycemic but be treated as if they were inebriated (drunk). Behaviors may be similar, such as shakiness, combativeness, slurred speech, and loss of consciousness.

Education regarding the effects of alcohol is important and must be included in a teaching plan. If teenagers insist on drinking alcohol, they can be cautioned to use sweetened mixers or eat snacks when consuming alcoholic beverages.

Episodes of hyperglycemia or hypoglycemia may become a serious issue for adolescents who are leaving home for the first time. One teenager confided that her mother always recognized her combative, antisocial behavior as impending hypoglycemia and treated her with the appropriate intervention. The teenager feared that a college roommate might be offended by the behavior and leave her alone with impending hypoglycemia.

One young man realized he could not live alone when he "took a nap because of feeling tired" and woke up 4 days later in the hospital. Fortunately, his family realized he was in a coma and summoned emergency medical services. The fatigue signaled the beginning of a viral infection, which led to a blood glucose level of 410 mg/dl. Nurses need to address these fears openly and facilitate ways in which the teenager can enlist the aid of significant peers who may be available during hyperglycemic or hypoglycemic episodes.

Susan Zekauskas, MSN, RN, PNP

Nursing Care Plan

THE CHILD WITH DIABETES MELLITUS

NURSING DIAGNOSIS: Risk for injury related to hypoglycemia or hyperglycemia

EXPECTED OUTCOME
Child demonstrates normal blood glucose levels.

NURSING INTERVENTIONS/*RATIONALES*
Obtain blood glucose level *to determine appropriate insulin dose and monitor glucose level.*
Administer insulin as ordered *to maintain normal glucose level.*
Make sure nutritional intake is appropriate, timely, and adequate *to maintain blood glucose level.*
Monitor for signs of hypoglycemia (e.g., sweating, shaky, nervousness, faintness, fatigue, palpitations, confusion) and hyperglycemia (nausea, urinary frequency, thirst, hunger, tiredness, fruity breath) and correct appropriately (e.g., readily absorbed carbohydrates followed by complex carbohydrate and protein for hypoglycemia; insulin for hyperglycemia) *to maintain glucose balance and prevent long-term complications.*

NURSING DIAGNOSIS: Knowledge deficit related to new health condition (diabetes mellitus)

EXPECTED OUTCOME
Child and family delineate plan of care for management of diabetes; child and family exhibit evidence of incorporation of care behaviors into daily routine.

NURSING INTERVENTIONS/*RATIONALES*
Ascertain family's general knowledge of diabetes *to assess baseline knowledge.* Set up an environment conducive to learning (e.g., teaching methods appropriate to age of child and family; use of written materials, pictures, and audiovisuals; use of short, repetitive teaching sessions with ongoing reinforcement of information and feedback; encouragement of questions; clarification of misconceptions) *to maximize learning.*
Discuss the pathology and potential sequelae of diabetes, the function and actions of insulin in relation to eating and exercise, the need for careful adherence to the plan of care, and the importance of regular health care *to ensure adequate understanding and promote compliance.*
Help family understand diabetic diet and dietary exchanges and to plan any needed dietary changes within family cultural and food preferences; help with menus, recipes, shopping strategies (refer to dietitian if available) *to promote successful adaptation of dietary practices.*
Teach family the importance of careful blood glucose monitoring *to maintain consistent blood glucose levels and prevent ketoacidosis.*
Teach family about importance of judicious exercise and the need for glucose monitoring after vigorous exercise *to prevent hypoglycemia.*
Teach family about need for careful oral and body hygiene; prompt treatment of cuts and scrapes; careful foot care; and regular visits to the dentist, ophthalmologist, and endocrinologist *to prevent or detect early signs of complications.*
Teach family how to use and interpret glucose monitoring equipment; how to store, draw up, and administer insulin; how to rotate injection sites; and use of any needed supplies or equipment by using a demonstration–return demonstration technique *to ensure comfort and ability to perform needed procedures and handle equipment.*
Have child wear a medical-identification device (bracelet, necklace) at all times *to ensure prompt and proper emergency care if needed.*
Increase child's role in self-management of disease by using age-appropriate guidelines *to move child into a long-term role as independent manager of the disease process and associated treatments.*

NURSING DIAGNOSIS: Altered family processes related to situational crises (child with chronic disease/disability)

Once parents experience the child's having a severe insulin reaction with a seizure, or once the adolescent has one in a public place, the desire to maintain better control is reinforced. They must understand how to prevent problems and how to handle problems calmly if they occur. (See Compliance, Chapter 45.)

NURSE ALERT Ongoing motivation to adhere to a regimen is difficult. An older child and parent (or another caregiver) may enjoy negotiating a "day off," when the responsibility for testing and recording blood glucose is delegated from the child to the caregiver (or vice versa). ■

Camps for children with diabetes and other special groups are very useful. In the special camp these children learn that they are not alone. As a result, most children become more independent and resourceful outside the camp setting. Camp time also provides parents a respite from the child's daily regimen. Information about such camps and organizations can be obtained from the American Diabetes Association. A free list of accredited camps specifically for children and teenagers with diabetes is also available.*

Evaluation

The effectiveness of nursing interventions is determined by continual reassessment and evaluation of care based on the following observational guidelines:

1. Interview family to determine their understanding of the disease; have child and family demonstrate and discuss the needed assessment and therapeutic techniques.
2. Interview family regarding their understanding of tight control; analyze and evaluate management records.

*Camp Directory, 1660 Duke St., Alexandria, VA 22314; phone: 800-232-3472.

Critical Thinking Exercise

TYPE 1 DIABETES MELLITUS

Rebecca is a 15-year-old with a 3-year history of type 1 diabetes mellitus who has been admitted to the pediatric intensive care unit for treatment of diabetic ketoacidosis (DKA). This is her fifth hospital admission for DKA in the past year. Rebecca's parents are divorced and she has four younger siblings, none of whom have diabetes. Rebecca's mother has maintained two jobs for the past 5 years and frequently leaves Rebecca in charge of the household. In anticipation of her discharge, you are to plan a patient education program for Rebecca and her mother. What important issues regarding Rebecca's unstable diabetic management must you consider in order to plan the education program?

1. Evidence—Is there sufficient evidence to draw conclusions about Rebecca's recurrent episodes of DKA?
2. Assumptions—Describe an underlying assumption about each of the following:
   a. Type 1 DM in adolescence
   b. Type 1 DM and menses
   c. Emotional stress and elevated blood glucose levels
   d. Blood glucose monitoring for insulin management
3. What priorities for nursing care should be established for Rebecca?
4. Does the evidence support your nursing intervention?
5. What alternative perspectives might you have?

3. Discuss child's disease with him or her.
4. Interview family and child regarding their feelings and concerns about the disease.

The *expected outcomes* are described in the Nursing Care Plan on p. 1746.

Key Points

- The endocrine system has three components: the cell, which sends a chemical message via a hormone; target cells, which receive the message; and the environment through which the chemical is transported from the site of synthesis to the sites of cellular action.
- Pituitary dysfunction is manifested primarily by growth disturbance.
- The main physiologic action of thyroid hormone is to regulate the basal metabolic rate and control the processes of growth and tissue differentiation.
- Disorders of thyroid function include hypothyroidism, autoimmune thyroiditis, goiter, and hyperthyroidism.
- Therapy for hyperthyroidism is directed at retarding the rate of hormone secretion and may include drug therapy, thyroidectomy, or radioiodine therapy.
- Classic forms of hypoparathyroidism in childhood are idiopathic—deficient production of parathyroid hormone (PTH)—and pseudohypoparathyroidism—increased PTH production with end-organ unresponsiveness to PTH.
- The adrenal cortex secretes three important groups of hormones: glucocorticoids, mineralocorticoids, and sex steroids.
- Disorders of adrenal function include acute adrenocortical insufficiency, chronic adrenocortical insufficiency, Cushing syndrome, congenital adrenogenital hyperplasia, and hyperaldosteronism.
- Four categories of Cushing syndrome are pituitary, adrenal, ectopic, and iatrogenic.
- Management of congenital adrenogenital hyperplasia includes assignment of a sex according to genotype, administration of cortisone, and, possibly, reconstructive surgery.
- Diabetes mellitus is categorized as type 1 diabetes, type 2 diabetes, and maturity-onset diabetes of the young.
- The focus of type 1 diabetes management is insulin replacement, diet, and exercise.
- Education of families includes explanation of diabetes, meal planning, administering insulin injection, monitoring, general hygienic practices, promoting exercise, record keeping, and observing for complications.

Answer Guidelines to Critical Thinking Exercise

Type 1 Diabetes Mellitus

1. Yes. Rebecca has had five hospital admissions for DKA in the past year. Numerous factors must be involved with her unstable disease.
2. (a) The normal tasks of adolescence can play a significant role in blood glucose instability. (b) Adolescent girls with diabetes have frequent fluctuations of blood glucose levels immediately before, during, or after their menses. (c) Rebecca's personal loss from the divorce, her mother's absence due to a heavy work schedule, and the added responsibilities of the household may cause significant stress, resulting in elevated blood glucose levels. (d) Careful, frequent, consistent monitoring of blood glucose levels is essential for effective insulin management during adolescence.
3. The first priority would be to focus directly on the issue of hyperglycemia. Determination of Rebecca's practice of monitoring and management of her diabetes at home is essential. Areas of diabetic management that should be emphasized include careful dietary management, an appropriate exercise program, conscientious self-testing of blood glucose, appropriate administration of daily insulin, and adherence to sliding-scale insulin therapy. Discussion of the emotional stressors she identifies at this time is appropriate.
4. Yes, Rebecca's history of DKA over the past year supports her inability to monitor and manage her diabetes.
5. It would be appropriate to make a referral for special support services for counseling and possible home care follow-up to assess her diabetic management skills at home.

References

American Diabetes Association: Report of the Expert Committee on the Diagnosis and Classification of Diabetes Mellitus, *Diabetes Care* 24(suppl 1):S5-S20, 2001.

Anderson SE, Dallal GE, Must A: Relative weight and race influence average age at menarche: results from two nationally representative surveys of US girls studied 25 years apart, *Pediatrics* 111(4):844-850, 2003.

Arends NJT et al: MRI findings of the pituitary gland in short children born small for gestational age (SGA) in comparison with growth hormone–

deficient (GHD) children and children with normal stature, *Clin Endocrinol* 57:719-724, 2002.

August GP, Julius JR, Blethen SL: Adult height in children with growth hormone deficiency who are treated with biosynthetic growth hormone: the National Cooperative Growth Study Experience, *Pediatrics* 102(2):512-516, 1998.

Barber CJ, Lowes L: Eating disorders and adolescent diabetes: is there a link? *Br J Nurs* 7(7):398-402, 1998.

Bercu B: The growing conundrum: growth hormone treatment of the non–growth hormone deficient child, *JAMA* 276(7):567-568, 1996.

Blethen SL et al: Safety of recombinant deoxyribonucleic acid–derived growth hormone, *J Clin Endocrinol Metab* 81(5):1704-1710, 1996.

Boulgourdjian EM et al: Oral desmopressin treatment of central diabetes insipidus in children, *Acta Pediatr* 86:1261-1262, 1997.

Chase HP et al: Use of the GlucoWatch Biographer in children with type 1 diabetes, *Pediatrics* 111(4):790-794, 2003.

Cheetham T, Baylis PH: Diabetes insipidus in children: pathophysiology, diagnosis and management, *Paediatr Drugs* 4(12):785-796, 2002.

Chumlea WC et al: Age at menarche and racial comparisons in US girls, *Pediatrics* 111(1):110-113, 2003.

Cox M: A better mousetrap: what's new in blood glucose monitoring? *J Pediatr Health Care* 16(3):314-316, 2002.

Davison KK, Susman EJ, Birch LL: Percent body fat at age 5 predicts earlier pubertal development among girls at age 9, *Pediatrics* 111(4):815-821, 2003.

Durham E: Growth hormone deficiency in children, a change in diagnostic approach, *Adv Nurse Pract* 11(1):41-67, 2003.

Fleming DF: Challenging traditional insulin injection practices, *Am J Nurs* 99(2):72-74, 1999.

Gnanalingham MG, Newland P, Smith CP: Accuracy and reproducibility of low dose insulin administration using pen-injectors and syringes, *Arch Dis Child* 79(1):59-62, 1998.

Guyda HJ: Growth hormone testing and the short child, *Pediatr Res* 48(5):579-580, 2000.

Hathout EH et al: Clinical, autoimmune, and HLA characteristics of children diagnosed with type 1 diabetes before 5 years of age, *Pediatrics* 111(4):860-863, 2003.

Hoffman RP: Juvenile diabetes: avoiding problems during therapy, *Clinical Advisor,* May 2003, pp 70-75.

Kempers MJE, Otten BJ: Idiopathic precocious puberty versus puberty in adopted children; auxological response to gonadotrophin-releasing hormone agonist treatment and final height, *Eur J Endocrinol* 147:609-616, 2002.

Kiess W et al: Type 2 diabetes mellitus in children and adolescents: a review from a European perspective, *Horm Res* 59(suppl 1):77-84, 2003.

Kimpimaki T et al: Short term exclusive breastfeeding predisposes young children to increased genetic risk of type 1 diabetes to progressive beta-cell autoimmunity, *Diabetolgia* 44(1):63-69, 2001.

Lanza RP et al: Xenotransplantation of cells using biodegradable microcapsules, *Transplant* 67(8):1105-1111, 1999.

Levine LS: Congenital adrenal hyperplasia, *Pediatr Rev* 21(5):159-170, 2000.

Lock JP et al: Whole-blood glucose testing at alternative sites: glucose values and hematocrit of capillary blood drawn from fingertip and forearm, *Diabetes Care* 25(6):961-964, 2002.

Lteif AN, Schwenk WF: Accuracy of pen injectors versus insulin syringes in children with type 1 diabetes, *Diabetes Care* 22(10):137-140, 1999.

Magee MF, Bhatt BA: Management of decompensated diabetes: diabetic ketoacidosis and hyperglycemic hyperosmolar syndrome, *Crit Care Clin* 17(1):75-106, 2001.

Magiakou MA et al: Cushing's syndrome in children and adolescents: presentation, diagnosis, and therapy, *N Engl J Med* 331(10):629-636, 1994.

Midyett LK et al: Are pubertal changes in girls before age 8 benign? *Pediatrics* 111(1):47-51, 2003.

Moshang T: Editorial: Cushing's disease, 70 years later…and the beat goes on, *J Clin Endocrinol Metab* 88(1):31-33, 2003.

Olohan K, Zappitelli D: The insulin pump: making life with diabetes easier, *Am J Nurs* 103(4):48-56, 2003.

Pizzo PA, Poplack DG: *Principles and theories of pediatric oncology,* Philadelphia, 2001, Lippincott Williams & Wilkins.

Plotnick LP: The next step in blood glucose monitoring? *Pediatrics* 111(4):885, 2003.

Redondo M, Fain P, Eisenbarth G: Genetics of type 1A diabetes, *Recent Prog Horm Res* 56:69-89, 2001.

Rivkees SA, Cornelius EA: Influence of iodine-131 dose on the outcome of hyperthyroidism in children, *Pediatrics* 111(4):745-748, 2003.

Robertson RP et al: Pancreas and islet transplantation for patients with diabetes (technical review), *Diabetes Care* 23:112-116, 2000.

Root AW: Precocious puberty, *Pediatr Rev* 21(1):10-19, 2000.

Ross LF: Minimizing risks: the ethics of predictive diabetes mellitus screening research in newborns, *Arch Pediatr Adolesc Med* 157:89-95, 2003.

Ruble JA: Congenital adrenal hyperplasia. In Jackson PL, Vessey JA (eds): *Primary care of the child with a chronic condition,* ed 2, St Louis, 1996, Mosby.

Seley J: Giving the fingers a rest: alternative site testing eases blood glucose monitoring, *Am J Nurs* 103(3):73-77, 2003.

Shulman DI, Bercu BB: Growth hormone therapy: an update, *Contemp Pediatr* 15(8):95-108, 1998.

Skyler J et al: Efficacy of inhaled human insulin in type 1 diabetes mellitus: a randomized proof-of-concept study, *Lancet* 357(9253):324-325, 2001.

Steinberger J, Daniels SR: Obesity, insulin resistance, diabetes, and cardiovascular risk in children, *Circulation* 107:1448-1453, 2003.

Stephenson M: Type 2 diabetes: a growing epidemic in children, *Infect Dis Child* 16(4):34, 36-37, 2003.

Thomas M et al: Growth hormone (GH) secretion in patients with childhood-onset GH deficiency: retesting after one year of therapy and at final height, *Horm Res* 59:7-15, 2003.

Thompson GB: Surgical management in Graves' disease, *Panminerva Med* 44(4):287-293, 2002.

Wu T, Mendola P, Buck GM: Ethnic differences in the presence of secondary sex characteristics and menarche among US girls: the third national health and nutrition examination survey, 1988-1994, *Pediatrics* 110(4):752-756, 2002.

Wunderlich RP et al: Pathophysiology and treatment of painful diabetic neuropathy of the lower extremity, *South Med J* 91(10):894-898, 1998.

Zimet GD et al: Psychosocial outcome of children evaluated for short stature, *Arch Pediatr Adolesc Med* 151(10):1017-1023, 1997.

Integumentary Dysfunction 53

LEARNING OBJECTIVES

On completion of this chapter the reader will be able to:

- Describe the distribution and configuration of the various skin lesions.
- List the benefits of a moist environment for wound healing.
- Discuss the nursing care related to therapies for skin disorders.
- Contrast the manifestations of and therapies for bacterial, viral, and fungal infections of the skin.
- Compare the skin manifestations related to age in children.
- Outline a plan of care to prevent and treat diaper dermatitis.
- Outline a plan of care for a child with atopic dermatitis.
- Formulate a teaching plan for an adolescent with acne.
- Describe the methods for assessing a burn wound.
- Discuss the physical and emotional care of a child with a severe burn wound.

ELECTRONIC RESOURCES

Additional information related to the content in Chapter 53 can be found on

the companion website at evolve
http://evolve.elsevier.com/Wong/maternal/

- NCLEX Review Questions
- Case Study–Poison Ivy
- Case Study–Impetigo
- WebLinks

or the interactive student CD-ROM
Activities for Chapter 53 include the following:

- NCLEX Review Questions
- Case Study–Acne Vulgaris
- Case Study–Burns
- Critical Thinking Exercise–Drug Reactions
- Nursing Care Plan–The Child with a Full-Thickness Burn

INTEGUMENTARY DYSFUNCTION

Skin Lesions

Lesions of the skin result from a variety of etiologic factors. Skin lesions originate from (1) contact with injurious agents (infective organisms, toxic chemicals, and physical trauma); (2) hereditary factors; (3) external factors (e.g., allergens); or (4) systemic diseases (e.g., measles, lupus erythematosus, nutritional deficiency diseases). Responses to these agents or factors are highly individualized. An agent that may be harmless to one individual may be damaging to another, and a single agent may produce different responses in different individuals.

An important factor in the etiology of skin manifestations is the age of the child. Infants are subject to "birthmark" malformations and atopic dermatitis that appear early in life; the school-age child is susceptible to ringworm of the scalp; and acne is a characteristic skin disorder of puberty. Contact dermatitis, such as poison ivy, is seen only when the noxious agent is found in the environment. Tension and anxiety may produce, modify, or prolong skin conditions.

Skin of Younger Children

The major skin layers arise from different embryologic origins. Early in the embryonic period, a single layer of epithelium forms from the ectoderm, while simultaneously the corium develops from the mesenchyme. In the infant and small child, the epidermis is loosely bound to the dermis.

This poor adherence causes the layers to separate easily during an inflammatory process to form blisters. This is especially true in preterm infants, who have a propensity to blister formation and separation of the skin during careless handling (such as removal of adhesive tape). In contrast, the skin of the older child is thinner, and the cells of all the strata are more compressed.

Pathophysiology of Dermatitis

Over half of the dermatologic problems in children are forms of dermatitis. This implies a sequence of inflammatory changes in the skin that is grossly and microscopically similar but diverse in course and causation. Acute responses produce intercellular and intracellular edema, the formation of intradermal vesicles, and an initial infiltration of inflammatory cells into the epidermis. In the dermis there is edema, vascular dilation, and early perivascular cellular infiltration. The location and manner of these reactions produce the lesions characteristic of each disorder. The changes are usually reversible, and the skin ordinarily recovers without blemish unless complicating factors such as ulceration from the primary irritant, scratching, and infection are introduced or underlying vascular disease develops. In chronic conditions, permanent effects are seen that vary according to the disorder, the general condition of the affected individual, and the available therapy.

Diagnostic Evaluation

The history and subjective symptoms of skin lesions are explored first, and the objective characteristics of the lesions are noted simultaneously. Many skin lesions are easily diagnosed after careful inspection.

History and Subjective Symptoms

Many cutaneous lesions are associated with local symptoms. The most common local symptom is itching *(pruritus)*, which varies in intensity. Pain or tenderness often accompanies some skin lesions. Other skin sensations such as burning, prickling, stinging, or crawling are also described. Alterations in local feeling include absence of sensation *(anesthesia)*, excessive sensitiveness *(hyperesthesia)*, diminished sensation (*hypesthesia* or *hypoesthesia*), or abnormal sensation, such as burning or prickling *(paresthesia)*. These symptoms may remain localized or migrate, may be constant or intermittent, and may be aggravated by a specific activity, such as exposure to sunlight.

It is important to determine whether the child has an allergic condition such as asthma or hay fever or history of a previous skin disease. Atopic dermatitis, often associated with allergies, frequently begins in infancy. Important questions for the parent include when the lesion or symptom first appeared; whether it occurred with ingestion of a food or other substance, including any medication; and whether the condition was related to activity such as contact with plants, insects, or chemicals.

CRITICAL THINKING EXERCISE: DRUG REACTIONS

Objective Findings

The distribution, size, morphology, and arrangement of skin lesions provide significant information. Extrinsic causes usually result from physical, chemical, or allergic irritants or from an infectious agent such as bacteria, fungi, viruses, or animal parasites. Skin manifestations are also produced by intrinsic causes such as an infection (measles or chickenpox), drug sensitization, or other allergic phenomena.

Lesion

Skin lesions assume distinct characteristics that are related to the pathologic process. Nurses should become familiar with the common terms that are applied to skin lesions because these terms are used in the processes of record keeping and communication. These terms include the following:

Erythema—A reddened area caused by increased amounts of oxygenated blood in the dermal vasculature

Macule—flat; nonpalpable; circumscribed; less than 1 cm in diameter; brown, red, purple, white, or tan in color
Examples: Freckles; flat moles; rubella; rubeola

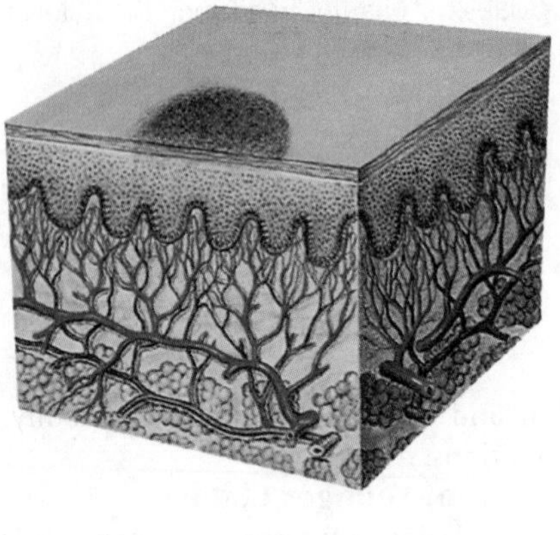

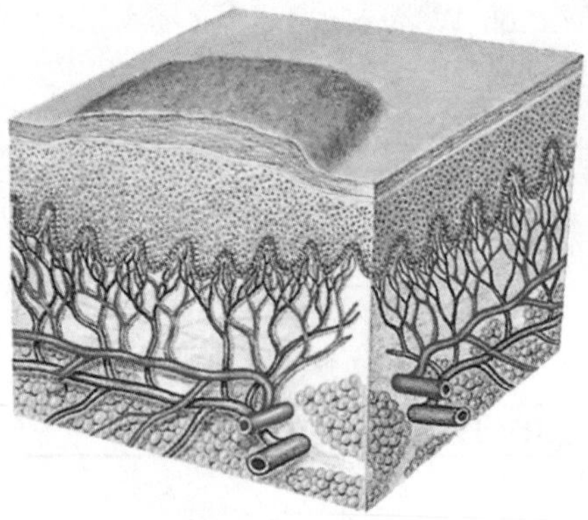

Plaque—elevated; flat topped; firm; rough; superficial papule greater than 1 cm in diameter; may be coalesced papules
Examples: Psoriasis; seborrheic and actinic keratoses

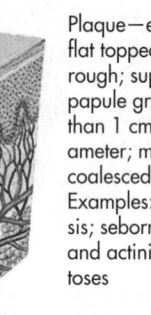

Patch—flat; nonpalpable; irregular in shape; macule that is greater than 1 cm in diameter
Examples: Vitiligo; port-wine marks

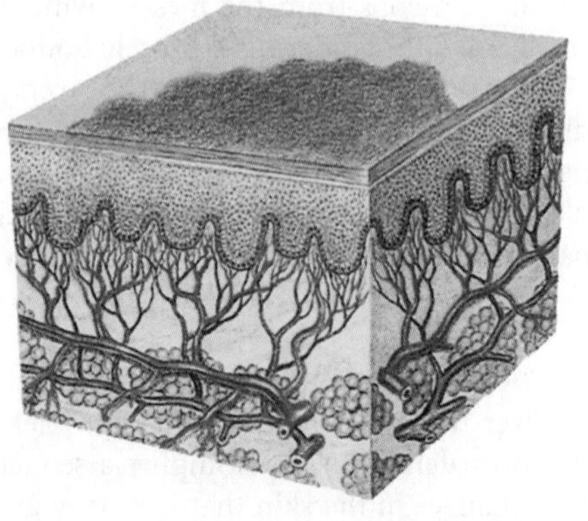

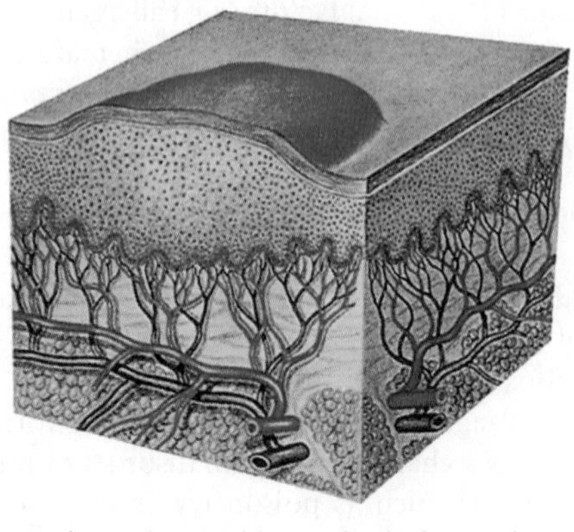

Wheal—elevated, irregularly shaped area of cutaneous edema; solid, transient, changing, variable diameter; pale pink with lighter center
Examples: Urticaria; insect bites

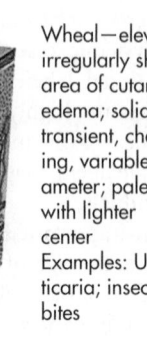

Fig. 53-1 Primary skin lesions. (From Seidel HM et al: *Mosby's guide to physical examination*, ed 5, St Louis, 2003, Mosby.)

Ecchymoses (bruises)—Localized red or purple discolorations caused by extravasation of blood into dermis and subcutaneous tissues

Petechiae—Pinpoint, tiny, and sharp circumscribed spots in the superficial layers of the epidermis

Primary lesions—Skin changes produced by a causative factor; common primary lesions in pediatric skin disorders are macules, papules, and vesicles (Fig. 53-1)

Secondary lesions—Changes that result from alteration in the primary lesions, such as those caused by rubbing,

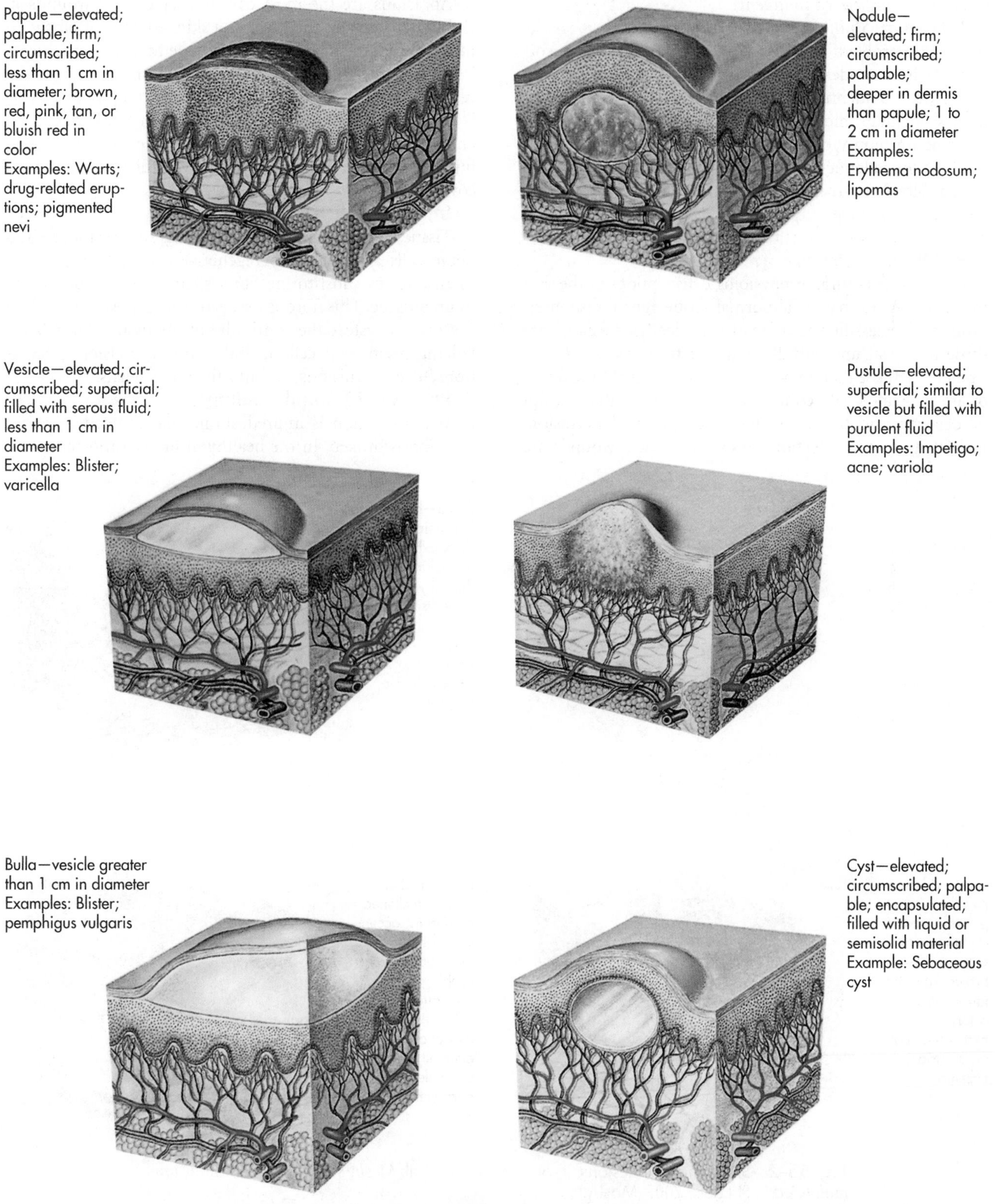
Papule—elevated; palpable; firm; circumscribed; less than 1 cm in diameter; brown, red, pink, tan, or bluish red in color
Examples: Warts; drug-related eruptions; pigmented nevi
Nodule—elevated; firm; circumscribed; palpable; deeper in dermis than papule; 1 to 2 cm in diameter
Examples: Erythema nodosum; lipomas
Vesicle—elevated; circumscribed; superficial; filled with serous fluid; less than 1 cm in diameter
Examples: Blister; varicella
Pustule—elevated; superficial; similar to vesicle but filled with purulent fluid
Examples: Impetigo; acne; variola
Bulla—vesicle greater than 1 cm in diameter
Examples: Blister; pemphigus vulgaris
Cyst—elevated; circumscribed; palpable; encapsulated; filled with liquid or semisolid material
Example: Sebaceous cyst

Fig. 53-1, cont'd Primary skin lesions.

scratching, medication, or involution and healing (Fig. 53-2)

Distribution pattern—The pattern in which lesions are distributed over the body, whether local or generalized, and the specific areas associated with the lesions

Configuration and arrangement—The size, shape, and arrangement of a lesion or groups of lesions (e.g., *discrete, clustered, diffuse,* or *confluent*)

Laboratory Studies

If a skin problem is related to a systemic disease (e.g., collagen or immunodeficiency disease), laboratory studies are performed to identify these conditions. Diagnostic techniques include microscopic examination, cultures, skin scrapings or biopsy, cytodiagnosis, patch testing, Wood light examination, allergic skin testing, and other laboratory tests such as blood count and sedimentation rate.

Wounds

Wounds are structural or physiologic disruptions of the skin that activate normal or abnormal tissue repair responses. Wounds are classified as acute or chronic. *Acute wounds* are those that heal uneventfully within 2 to 3 weeks. *Chronic wounds* are those that do not heal in the expected time frame or are associated with complications. Cofactors that disrupt or delay wound healing include compromised perfusion, malnutrition, and infection. In children, most wounds are acute and can be prevented from becoming chronic wounds through appropriate nursing care. Wounds are also classified as surgical and nonsurgical and then further classified in the same manner as burns: superficial wounds, partial-thickness wounds, and full-thickness wounds (complex wounds that include muscle, bone, or both).

Epidermal Injuries

Abrasions are the most common epidermal wounds in children, usually in the form of a skinned knee or elbow. In most injuries the margins of the abraded area are superficial, involving only the outer layers of epidermis, although the central portion may extend into the dermis. Epithelial tissue is composed of labile cells, which are constantly destroyed and replaced throughout the life span. Therefore epidermal injuries usually result in rapid, uneventful healing and recovery.

Injury to Deeper Tissues

Tissues composed of permanent cells such as muscle and nerve cells are unable to regenerate. These tissues repair themselves by substituting fibrous connective tissue for the injured tissue. This fibrous tissue, or *scar,* serves as a patch to preserve or restore the continuity of the tissue. Wounds involving permanent cells include surgical incisions, lacerations, ulcers, evulsions, and full-thickness burns.

Process of Wound Healing

When the skin is injured, its normal protective barrier function is broken. In the healthy immunocompetent indi-

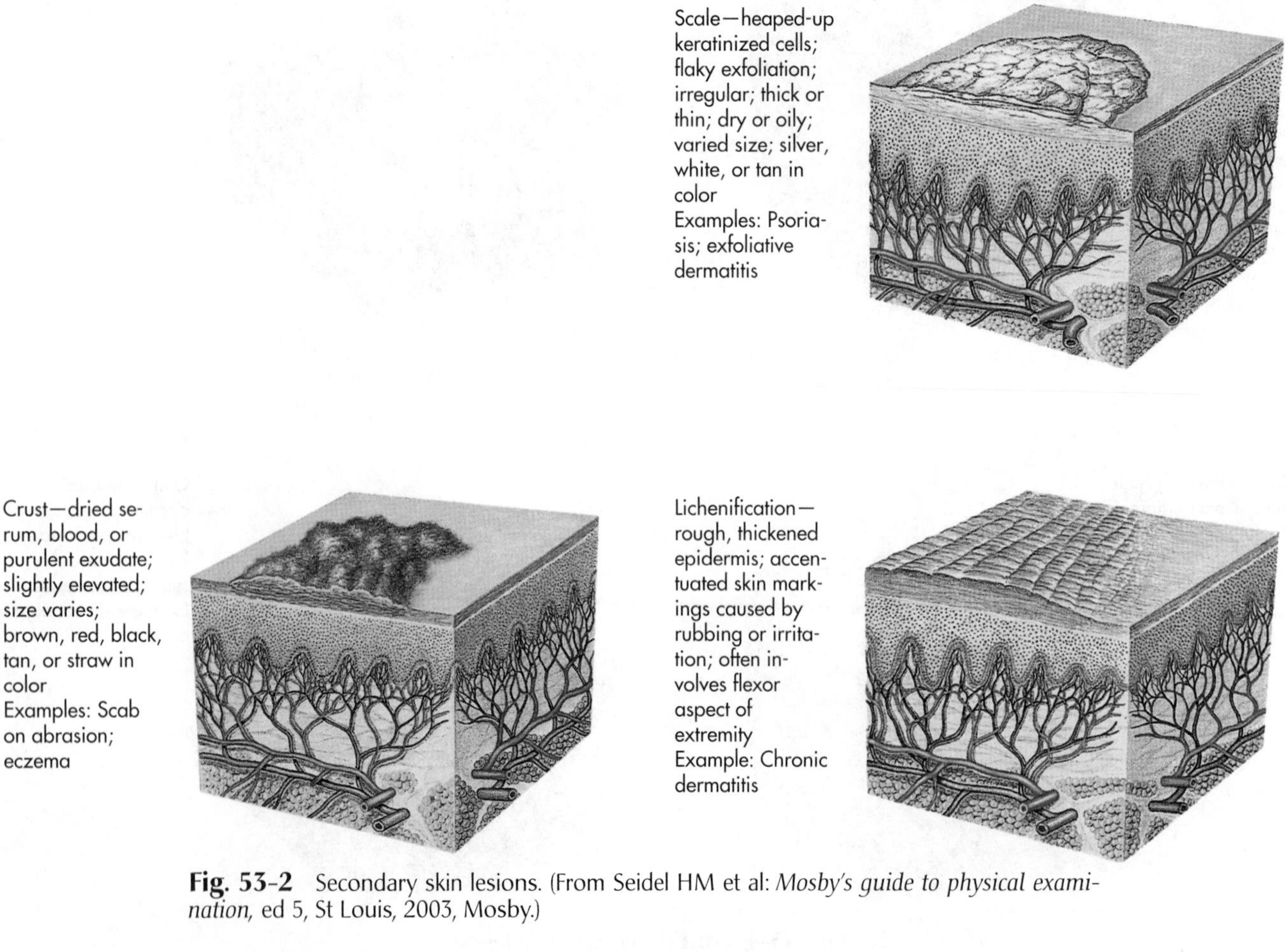
Scale—heaped-up keratinized cells; flaky exfoliation; irregular; thick or thin; dry or oily; varied size; silver, white, or tan in color
Examples: Psoriasis; exfoliative dermatitis
Crust—dried serum, blood, or purulent exudate; slightly elevated; size varies; brown, red, black, tan, or straw in color
Examples: Scab on abrasion; eczema
Lichenification—rough, thickened epidermis; accentuated skin markings caused by rubbing or irritation; often involves flexor aspect of extremity
Example: Chronic dermatitis

Fig. 53-2 Secondary skin lesions. (From Seidel HM et al: *Mosby's guide to physical examination,* ed 5, St Louis, 2003, Mosby.)

Scar—thin to thick fibrous tissue replacing injured dermis; irregular; pink, red, or white in color; may be atrophic or hypertrophic
Example: Healed wound or surgical incision

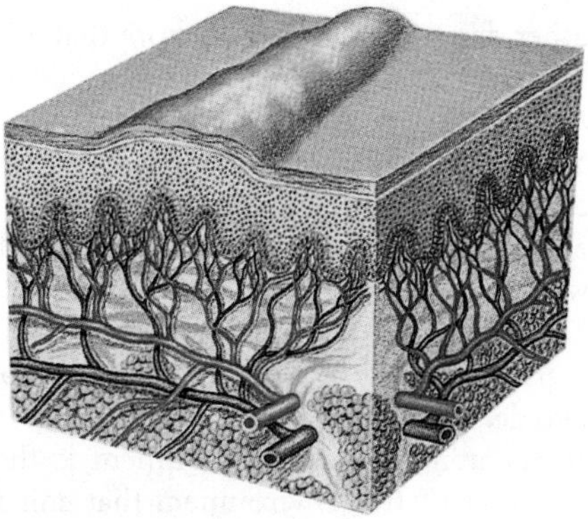

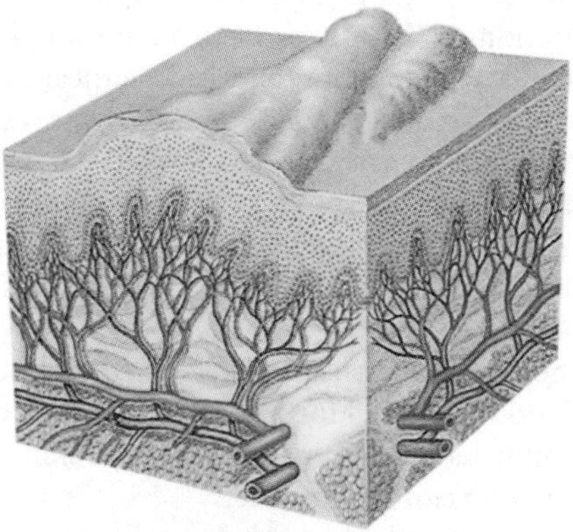

Keloid— irregularly shaped, elevated, progressively enlarging scar; grows beyond boundaries of wound; caused by excessive collagen formation during healing
Example: Keloid from ear piercing or burn scar

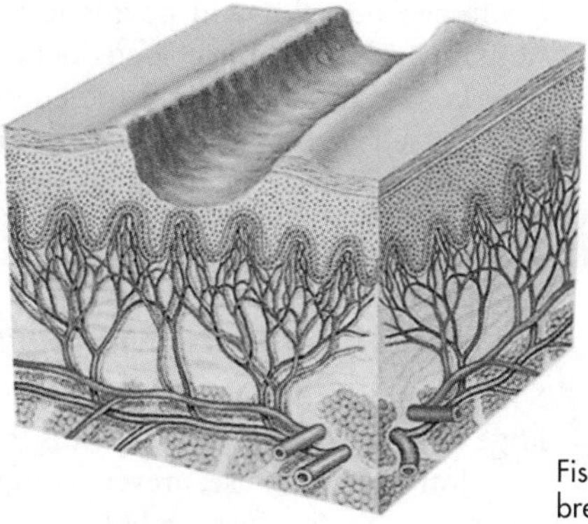

Excoriation—loss of epidermis; linear or hollowed-out crusted area; dermis exposed
Examples: Abrasion; scratch

Fissure—linear crack or break from epidermis to dermis; small; deep; red
Examples: Athlete's foot; cheilosis

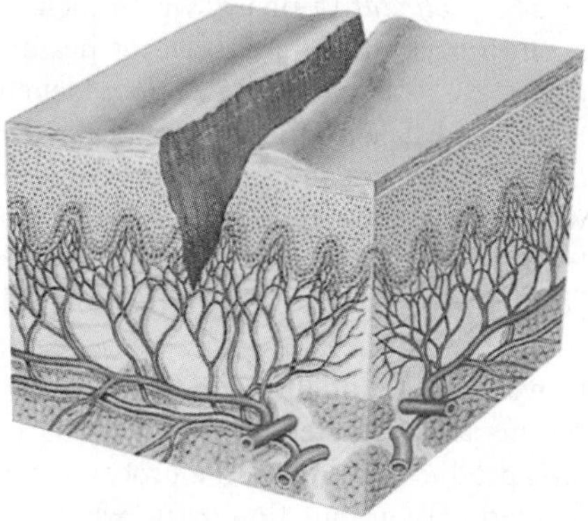

Erosion—loss of all or part of epidermis; depressed; moist; glistening; follows rupture of vesicle or bulla; larger than fissure
Examples: Varicella; variola following rupture

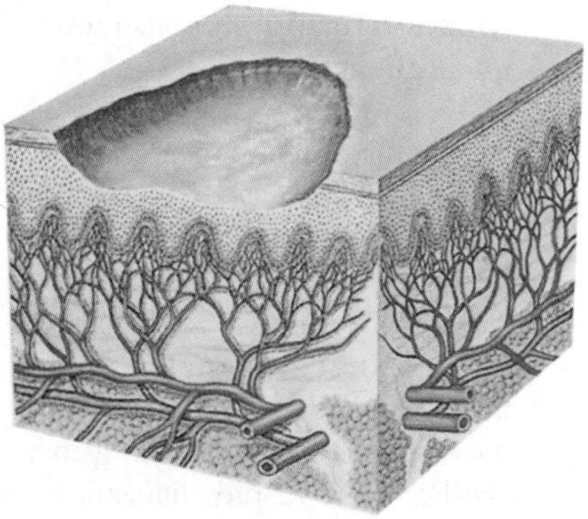

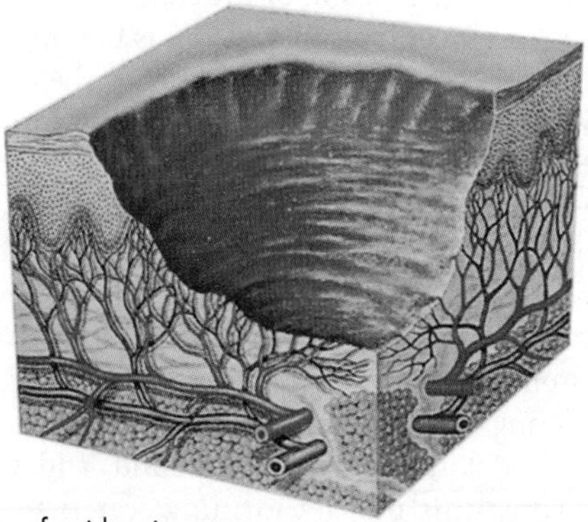

Ulcer—loss of epidermis and dermis; concave; varies in size; exudative; red or reddish blue
Examples: Decubiti; stasis ulcers

Fig. 53-2, cont'd Secondary skin lesions.

vidual, acute traumatic abrasions, lacerations, and superficial skin and soft tissue injuries heal spontaneously without complications. The process of tissue healing involves complex cellular interactions and biochemical reactions. The healing process is segregated into four phases that are characterized by the particular cells involved and the chemicals produced. The four stages of wound healing are hemostasis, inflammation, proliferation, and remodeling (Krasner, Rodeheaver, & Sibbald, 2001). Some authorities combine the first two phases.

In the *hemostasis* phase, platelets act to seal off the damaged blood vessels and form a stable clot. Hemostasis occurs within minutes of the initial injury to the skin unless there is an underlying clotting disorder.

Inflammation, the second stage of wound healing, presents a clinical picture that involves erythema, swelling, and warmth often associated with pain at the wound site. This stage usually lasts up to 4 days after the injury. The inflammation phase involves white blood cells such as the neutrophils, monocytes, and macrophages. These cells mount an initial defense against microbial invasion and secrete proteolytic enzymes that destroy nonviable tissue and microorganisms in the wound area.

The proliferative phase, which includes *granulation* and *contracture*, is the third stage of healing. This phase lasts from 4 to 21 days in acute wounds, depending on the size of the wound. The proliferative phase involves the replacement of dermal tissues and subdermal tissues in deep wounds, as well as the contraction of the wound. This phase is characterized clinically by the presence of granulation tissue, the "beefy," pebbled red tissue in the wound base. *Fibroblasts*, or immature connective tissue cells, secrete collagen, which provides the foundation for dermal regeneration. Angiocytes regenerate the outer layers of capillaries, and endothelial cells produce the lining in a process called *angiogenesis*. The formation of granulation tissue, which provides the foundation for the wound, is dependent on angiogenesis. The keratinocytes are responsible for epithelialization. In the final stage of epithelialization, contracture occurs as the keratinocytes differentiate and form the protective outer layer, or *stratum corneum*, of the skin.

Remodeling or *maturation* is the final phase of the healing process. This phase occurs in the dermis as fibroblasts increase the tissue tensile strength and gradually replace type 3 collagen in the scar tissue with type 1 collagen, thicken the collagen fibers, and reorient the collagen fibers along the lines of tissue tension. Fibroblasts disappear as the wound becomes stronger. The wound edges are brought closer together and a mature scar is formed. Children heal aggressively with abundant scar tissue, especially during growth spurts. The highly elastic quality of children's skin pulls on the wound, and the wound defends against this pull by forming scar tissue. Remodeling and maturation occur over several months and can take up to 2 years. Thus some wounds that appear to be completely healed can break down suddenly if attention is not paid to the initial causative factors.

The phases of wound healing are complex, and healing may be interrupted by disease conditions, medications, and other systemic and local factors that influence the healing process. When a wound does not follow the *normal wound healing trajectory*, it may become stuck in one of the stages and become a chronic wound. It is important that health care providers understand and address the factors that influence wound healing and prevent the development of chronic wounds.

Factors That Influence Healing

A revolution in wound healing has occurred in the last two decades. Emphasis has shifted from interventions aimed at maintaining a dry environment to those that promote a moist, crust-free environment that enhances the migration of epithelial cells across the wound and facilitates remodeling. An acute full-thickness wound kept in a moist environment usually reepithelializes in 12 to 15 days, whereas the same wound when kept open to the air heals in about 25 to 30 days.

Numerous factors can delay healing (Table 53-1). For example, traditional practices, such as the use of antiseptics (hydrogen peroxide and povidone-iodine [Betadine] solutions), which were once thought to prevent infection, are now known to have a cytotoxic effect on healthy cells and minimal effect on controlling infections. Povidone-iodine may also be absorbed through the skin in neonates and young children.

General Therapeutic Management

Some skin disorders demand aggressive therapy, but by and large the major aim of treatment is to prevent further damage, eliminate the cause, prevent complications, and provide relief from discomfort while tissues undergo healing. Factors that contribute to the development of dermatitis and that prolong the course of the disease should be eliminated when possible. The most common causative agents of dermatitis in infants, children, and adolescents are environmental factors (soaps, bubble baths, shampoos, rough or tight clothing, wet diapers, blankets, and toys) and the natural elements (such as dirt, sand, heat, cold, moisture, and wind). Dermatitis may also result from home remedies and medications.

Dressings

No one dressing meets the needs of all wounds. The traditional *dry* gauze dressing should not be used on open wounds, because it allows the wound surface to dry, does little to prevent bacterial invasion, and adheres to the dried scab so that removal disturbs the newly regenerating epithelial cells. In most instances, traditional gauze dressings have been replaced with moist wound healing dressings (Table 53-2). Moist wound healing increases the rate of collagen synthesis and reepithelialization and decreases pain and inflammation. It also creates an environment for autolytic debridement of necrotic tissue, which creates a clean wound bed and enhances granulation. However, a balance must be achieved between creating a moist wound bed and maintaining a dry periwound area that protects the skin and wound from maceration. The dressing type and frequency of dressing changes help to achieve this balance. The frequency of dressing changes is based on the presence of infection, the

Table 53-1

Factors That Delay Wound Healing

FACTOR	EFFECT ON HEALING
Dry wound environment	Allows epithelial cells to dry out and die; impairs migration of epithelial cells across wound surface
Nutritional deficiencies	
Vitamin A	Results in inadequate inflammatory response
Vitamin B_1	Results in decreased collagen formation
Vitamin C	Inhibits formation of collagen fibers and capillary development
Protein	Reduces supply of amino acids for tissue repair
Zinc	Impairs epithelialization
Immunocompromise	Results in inadequate or delayed inflammatory response
Impaired circulation	Reduces supply of nutrients to wound area Inhibits inflammatory response and removal of debris from wound area
Stress (pain, poor sleep)	Releases catecholamines that cause vasoconstriction
Antiseptics	
Hydrogen peroxide	Toxic to fibroblasts; can cause subcutaneous gas formation (mimics gas-forming infection)
Povidone-iodine	Toxic to white and red blood cells and fibroblasts
Chlorhexidine	Toxic to white blood cells
Medications	
Corticosteroids	Impair phagocytosis Inhibit fibroblast proliferation Depress formation of granulation tissue Inhibit wound contraction
Chemotherapy	Interrupts the cell cycle, damages DNA or prevents DNA repair
Antiinflammatory drugs	Decrease the inflammatory phase
Foreign bodies	Inhibit wound closure Increase inflammatory response
Infection	Increases inflammatory response Increases tissue destruction
Mechanical friction	Damages or destroys granulation tissue
Fluid accumulation	Accumulation in area inhibits tissues from approximating
Radiation	Inhibits fibroblastic activity and capillary formation May cause tissue necrosis
Diseases	
Diabetes mellitus	Inhibits collagen synthesis Impairs circulation and capillary growth Hyperglycemia impairs phagocytosis
Anemia	Reduces oxygen supply to tissues
Peripheral vascular disease	Reduces oxygen supply to wounds
Uremia	Decreases collagen and granulation tissue

type of dressing, the location of the wound, and the amount of drainage. Dressings should always be changed when they are loose or soiled. They should be changed more frequently in areas where contamination is likely (e.g., the sacral area, the buttocks, the tracheal area) or when wound infection is suspected or present.

Topical Therapy

A variety of agents and methods are available for treatment. In selecting a therapeutic regimen, the practitioner considers (1) the choice of active ingredient, (2) the proper vehicle or base, (3) the cosmetic effect, (4) the cost, and (5) instructions for use. Several basic concepts must also be considered. Overtreatment is avoided. For example, when the dermatitis is acute, topical applications should be mild and bland to avoid further irritation. Broken or inflamed skin, especially in children, is more absorbent than intact skin, and chemicals that are nonirritating to intact skin may be highly irritating to inflamed skin.

Topical applications may be applied to treat the disorder, reduce itching, decrease external stimuli, or apply external heat or cold. The emollient action of soaks, baths, and lotions provides a soothing film over the skin surface that reduces external stimuli. Ordinarily lukewarm, tepid, or cool applications offer the greatest relief.

Table 53-2

Commonly Used Occlusive Dressings and Other Products*

EXAMPLES	INDICATIONS	ADVANTAGES	DISADVANTAGES	CONSIDERATIONS
Polyurethane films Op-Site, Tegaderm, Bioclusive, Blisterfilm, Acu-derm, Polyskin II, Transorb, EpiView	Protection of partial-thickness red wounds Cover dressing for hydrophilic preparations and hydrogels Autolytic debridement of wounds with dry eschar	Transparent; good adhesion; reduces pain, minimizes friction forces to wound; time saving; easy to store; cost effective Moisture, vapor, and oxygen transmission Impermeable to water and bacteria	Adhesive injury to intact and new skin; nonabsorbent; some products difficult to apply; variable barrier function; can promote wound infection Unsuitable for electrical stimulation wound healing	Protect wound margins; avoid in wounds with infection, copious drainage, tracts or fragile skin surrounding lesion Change only if dressing leaks Contraindicated in third-degree burns
Polymeric forms Allevyn, Allevyn Adhesive, Allevyn Cavity, Nu-Derm, Lyofoam, PolyMem	Used when a nonadherent dressing is needed Used for wounds with moderate to heavy exudates	Moisture is absorbed into foam; maceration is decreased Removal does not cause reinjury to wound Comfortable, easy to apply; cushions and protects wound	Requires an additional dressing to secure if the foam does not have an adhesive surface	Do not use on infected wounds Contraindicated for third-degree burns
Hydrocolloids Duoderm CGF, Duoderm Extra Thin, Comfeel, Restore, Tegasorb, SignaDress, Cutinova Hydro, Ultec, Actiderm, Replicare	Protection of superficial and small, deep red wounds Autolytic debridement of small, noninfected yellow wounds* Partial thickness, stages 2 and 3; shallow full thickness, granulating with minimal to moderate exudates, stage 4	Absorbent; nonadhesive to healing tissue; waterproof; reduces pain; easy to apply; time saving; easy to store Moldable to area; occlusive; provides insulation; maintains moist wound surface; wet-to-dry adherence	Nontransparent; may soften and lose shape with heat or friction; odor and brown drainage on removal (melted dressing material)	Frequency of changes depends on amount of exudates (change as needed for leakage). DO *NOT* USE for heavily exudative wounds, sinus tracts, or infected wounds; shape dressing to wound area Contraindicated in third-degree burns
Hydrogels/sheets Vigilon, Elastogel, Aquasorb, Nu-Gel, Duoderm Gel, Second Skin, Hypergel, IntraSite Gel, Carrasyn	Protection of superficial and moderately deep red wounds Autolytic debridement of small, noninfected yellow or black wounds* Delivery system for topical antimicrobial creams (increases penetration) Partial and full thickness	Absorbent; nonadhesive; reduces pain; compatible with topicals; good conformity; easy to store Maintains a moist wound surface, has a "cooling" effect	Poor barrier; semitransparent; requires cover dressing to secure; can promote growth of *Pseudomonas* and other gram-negative bacteria and yeast Unused portion will dessicate Not for weight-bearing ulcers Expensive; nonadhesive High water content can macerate surrounding skin	Do not use in infected wounds; change every 8 hours or as needed for leakage Cut and shape to wound DO *NOT* REMOVE poly backing Monitor wound for overhydration and skin maceration around wound edges

Modified from Bryant RA: *Acute and chronic wounds, nursing management,* St Louis, 2000, Mosby; and McCulloch JM, Cloth LC, Feedar JA: *Wound healing alternatives in management,* Philadelphia, 1995, FA Davis.

*NOTE: Users should read package inserts for any contraindications to use of these products. Some dressings, such as Duoderm CGF, have been approved for application to infected wounds if wound is cultured and treated for infection. Many products should not be used on third-degree burns.

Table 53-2

Commonly Used Occlusive Dressings and Other Products—cont'd

EXAMPLES	INDICATIONS	ADVANTAGES	DISADVANTAGES	CONSIDERATIONS
Hydrocolloid absorption powders, pastes, beads, and granules Bard absorption dressing, Comfeel Ulcus paste, Comfeel Ulcus powder, Multidex powder and gel, Debrisan	Used on uneven and exudating ulcers	Controls bacteria Cleanses wound Reduces odor Cost effective		Cleans with lukewarm water or saline to remove Contraindicated in third-degree burns
Alginates Sorbsan, Kaltostat, Curasorb, Algi Site, restore, CalciCare	Used for leg ulcers, donor sites, infected traumatic or exudating wounds	Nonallergenic; biodegradable; little to no local tissue reaction Decreases pain at wound site	Expensive; easily displaced by mechanical forces Permeable to bacteria, urine	Change daily after proper cleansing if used on infected wounds Requires a secondary cover dressing Contraindicated in third-degree burns

NURSE ALERT Application of heat tends to aggravate most conditions, and its use is usually reserved for reducing specific inflammatory processes, such as folliculitis and cellulitis.

Ointments in a petrolatum base provide protection from moisture. Therefore this type of ointment is indicated around gastrostomy tubes, in skinfolds, and on the diaper area. Creams are absorbed by the skin and are used for areas where a nongreasy "feel" is desired (e.g., face or hands). ■

Topical Corticosteroid Therapy

Glucocorticoids are the therapeutic agents used most frequently for skin disorders. Their local antiinflammatory effects are merely palliative, so the medication must be applied until the condition undergoes a remission or the causative agent is eliminated. Corticosteroids are applied directly to the affected area, are essentially nonsensitizing, and have only minor side effects. As with the use of any steroids, their use in large amounts may mask signs of infection, and symptoms may be exacerbated following termination of the drug. Families are cautioned that the medication cannot be used for all skin disorders. The concentrations available without prescription are not adequate for stubborn skin conditions (e.g., psoriasis) and may cause worsening of inflammation caused by fungus or bacteria. Most parents and children apply too much topical hydrocortisone; therefore they should be counseled that it is both effective and economical to apply only a thin film and to massage it into the skin. Parents and children should also be advised to use the application for no more than 5 to 7 days because these agents may cause depigmentation and other changes in the skin.

Other Topical Therapies

Other topical treatments include chemical cautery (especially useful for warts), cryosurgery, electrodesiccation (chiefly used for warts, granulomas, and nevi), ultraviolet therapy (primarily used in psoriasis and acne), laser therapy (especially for birthmarks), and acne therapies such as dermabrasion and chemical peels. New drugs called *topical immunomodulators* are very effective in reducing the itching of atopic dermatitis (eczema) and preventing the recurrence of "flares."

Systemic Therapy

Systemic drugs may be used as an adjunct to topical therapy in some dermatologic disorders. The drugs most frequently used are corticosteroids, antibiotics, and antifungal agents. Corticosteroids are valuable because of their capacity to inhibit inflammatory and allergic reactions. Dosage is carefully adjusted and gradually tapered to the minimum dose that is effective and tolerated. In infants and children, dosage is larger than is usually calculated from body weight ratios. However, prolonged use may temporarily suppress growth.

Antibiotics are used in severe or widespread skin infections. However, because these drugs tend to produce hypersensitivity in some patients, they are used with caution. Antifungal agents are the only means for treating systemic fungal infections.

Nursing Care of the Child with a Skin Disorder

The child's subjective symptoms and the parent's history provide valuable information to help establish a diagnosis. Older children often describe the condition as painful, itching, or tingling or in other descriptive terms. However, much can be determined by also observing the younger child's behavior. Does the child scratch? Is the child restless or irritable? Does the child favor or avoid using a body part? A careful history provides important clues. Has the child had access to chemicals or been in the woods or around a woodpile? Has the child eaten a new food? Is the child taking medication? Has the child any known allergy? Do siblings or playmates have similar lesions? What soap or bubble bath is used for bathing?

It is important for nurses to not only describe but also to assess skin lesions and wounds. The color, shape, and distribution of lesions and wounds are important. Individual lesions are described according to standard terminology. Sometimes two descriptors are used to describe a particular characteristic (e.g., *maculopapular rash*). To confirm or amplify the findings made by inspection, the skin may be gently palpated to detect characteristics such as temperature, moisture, texture, elasticity, and the presence of edema. Wounds are assessed for depth of tissue damage, evidence of healing, and signs of infection.

NURSE ALERT Signs of wound infection include the following:
- Increased erythema, especially beyond the wound margin
- Edema
- Purulent exudate
- Pain
- Increased temperature ■

The frequency of wound assessment depends on the severity and complexity of the wound. For example, simple or chronic wounds are assessed weekly; infected or complex wounds are assessed daily. Wounds are measured at least weekly (height, width, and depth). The wound bed is assessed for color, drainage, odor, necrosis, granulation tissue, fibrin slough, undermining and condition of the wound edges, and the color and condition of the surrounding skin.

Therapeutic programs are designed to include general measures such as rest, protection, and relief of discomfort and specific treatments such as medication and physical techniques. Only a few skin diseases are contagious; therefore it is usually not necessary to isolate the affected child unless there is a danger of acquiring a secondary infection (e.g., the child receiving large doses of corticosteroids or other immunosuppressant drugs or the child with an immunologic deficiency disorder). However, if the skin manifestation is caused by a viral exanthema, such as measles or chickenpox, the child is prevented from exposing other susceptible children.

Wound Care

Parents can generally manage small skin lesions or wounds at home. The parents are instructed to wash their hands and then wash the wound gently with mild soap and water or normal saline. They are cautioned to avoid betadine, alcohol, and hydrogen peroxide because these products are toxic to wounds.

NURSE ALERT Do not put anything in a wound that you would not put in the eye. The safest solution is normal saline. ■

Open wounds are covered with a dressing, such as a commercial adhesive bandage, although larger wounds may benefit from the use of occlusive dressings (see Table 53-2). If occlusive dressings are applied, parents should learn how to apply and remove the dressings correctly. For example, hydrocolloid dressings adhere best if a wide margin is left around the wound and the dressing is pressed against intact skin until it adheres.* If a dressing needs to be secured, a nonalcohol skin barrier can be applied to protect the skin, or the wound can be "picture framed" with a hydrocolloid and dressing tape can be secured to the hydrocolloid. This method of securing the dressing protects the skin when the tape is removed. Montgomery straps or stretch netting can also be used to secure dressings and to avoid the use of tape.

NURSE ALERT Advise parents that the yellow gel forming under hydrocolloid dressings may look like pus and has a distinct odor (somewhat fruity) but is normal leakage. ■

Dressings are removed carefully to protect intact skin and the epithelial surface of the wound. When removing transparent or hydrocolloid dressings, the nurse or parent should raise one edge of the dressing and pull *parallel* to the skin to loosen the adhesive. The longer the dressings are left on, the easier they are to remove. Less frequent dressing changes decrease wound contamination.

Lacerations present a special challenge. The injured child and family are usually very distressed by the bleeding. In particular, scalp lacerations tend to bleed profusely. Parental feelings of guilt and shock usually accompany the injury. The initial nursing intervention is to apply pressure to the area and to attempt to calm the child before further examination. Unless there is bleeding from a severed artery, the wound is cleansed with a forced jet of sterile tepid water or saline (via syringe) and examined for extent, depth, and presence of foreign material such as dirt, glass, or fabric fragments.

The location of the wound facilitates assessment. Wounds over bony areas may contain bone chips, and clear fluid seeping from severe head wounds may indicate cerebrospinal fluid. A pressure dressing is applied for transfer to medical care. Once the child is in a medical facility, he or she is prepared for suturing (Atraumatic Care box).

Puncture wounds that do not require a tetanus booster are soaked in warm water and soap for several minutes. Causing the wound to rebleed may be helpful. An adhesive bandage can be applied if desired. Puncture wounds of the head, chest, or abdomen or those that could still contain a portion of the puncturing object must be evaluated carefully.

Parents are cautioned against opening blisters or kissing a wound "to make it better." The wound can easily become contaminated from germs in the human mouth. If scabs form, they are allowed to slough off without assistance; picking or early removal may cause scarring and secondary infection. Parents are advised to seek medical help if there is evidence of infection.

Relief of Symptoms

Most therapeutic regimens for skin lesions are directed toward relief of pruritus, the most common subjective complaint. Cooling the affected area and increasing the skin pH

---

*Information on the use of the hydrocolloid dressing Duoderm is available from ConvaTec Professional Services, PO Box 5254, Princeton, NJ 08543; phone: 800-422-8811; fax: 908-281-2405; Web site: www.convatec.com.

Atraumatic Care

PAINLESS SUTURING AND WOUND CLEANSING

A variety of topical anesthetic solutions, such as lidocaine, adrenaline, and tetracaine (LAT) combined and tetracaine-phenylephrine (tetraphen), applied to wounds, especially on the head, scalp, and face, provide anesthesia in 10 to 15 minutes (Smith et al, 1996). Tetracaine, adrenaline, and cocaine (TAC) combined or AC (without tetracaine) should not be used because of the potential for lethal cocaine intoxication. LAT is as effective as, is safer than, and is much less expensive than TAC. If further anesthesia is required or if the topical preparations are not available, using buffered lidocaine administered with a 30-gauge needle reduces the stinging and burning of the injection (see Pain Management, Chapter 44). The use of a noninvasive tissue adhesive (e.g., Derma Bond*) provides a faster and less painful method of facial laceration repair with cosmetic results comparable to those obtained with suturing (Osmond, Klassen, & Quinn, 1995).

*Manufactured by Closure Medical Corporation, Raleigh, NC.

with cool baths or compresses and alkaline applications (e.g., baking soda baths) are helpful in cooling the affected area and reducing the itching. Clothing and bed linen should be soft and lightweight to decrease the irritation from friction and stimulation.

During treatment, both the affected and unaffected skin is protected from damage and secondary infection. Preventing scratching is very important. Older children can cooperate, although they may need to be reminded to stop scratching or rubbing. However, small or uncooperative children may require the use of devices such as mittens (especially during sleep) or special coverings. Keeping fingernails clean, short, and trimmed reduces the risk of secondary infection.

Antipruritic medications, such as diphenhydramine (Benadryl) or hydroxyzine (Atarax), may be prescribed for severe itching, especially if it disturbs the child's rest. Pain and discomfort are usually managed with nonpharmacologic measures and mild analgesia. Severe pain requires more potent medication. Occlusive dressings over wounds reduce pain. For suturing wounds, a topical anesthetic or intradermal buffered lidocaine should be used. (See Pain Management, Chapter 44.)

Topical Therapy

The specific type of topical therapy and the mode of application depend on the nature and location of the lesion. It is especially important to wash the hands before and after application of any topical therapy. The skin is assessed before the application and reassessed after treatment. Any observed changes are noted and described.

Wet compresses or *dressings* cool the skin by evaporation, relieve itching and inflammation, and cleanse the area by loosening and removing crusts and debris. A variety of ingredients, such as plain water or Burow solution (available without a prescription), can be applied on Kerlix gauze, plain gauze, or (preferably) soft cotton cloths such as freshly laundered handkerchiefs or strips from diaper, sheeting, or pillowcase material.

Dressings immersed in the desired solution are wrung out slightly and applied to the affected area wet but not dripping. They are applied flat and smooth in such a way that motion is not totally restricted—fingers are wrapped separately, and arms and legs are wrapped so that elbows and knees can bend. Dressings are held in place by Kerlix or other cotton wrap, tubular stockinette, mittens, and socks (two pairs—one to hold the dressings in place, the other to take up movement). When evaporation begins to dry them, the dressings are removed, rewet in the solution, and reapplied using aseptic technique. The solution is *not* poured or applied with a syringe directly over the dressings. As fluid evaporates, the solution becomes more concentrated, and this occurrence could damage sensitive lesions.

Fresh solution at room temperature is applied at 2-, 3-, or 4-hour intervals and allowed to remain on the lesion for 30 minutes to 1.5 hours. Wet dressings are seldom continued after about 48 hours. The child is protected against chilling during treatment, and no more than 20% of the body is covered at one time to avoid the risk of hypothermia. After treatment, the skin is dried thoroughly by patting with a towel. Lotion or other medication (if prescribed) is applied at this time.

When children are uncooperative in the use of wet dressings, *soaks* are often used for removal of crusts and for their mild astringent action. The same solutions are used as for wet compresses. Gaining young children's cooperation for hand or foot soaks is difficult unless the procedure is accompanied by play. Older infants and toddlers delight in playing with brightly colored objects or poker chips scattered over the bottom of the receptacle, and preschoolers can be challenged to hold a floating item beneath the water's surface. However, these activities require supervision; infants and small children place items in their mouths, and children easily lose control with water play. Washing dishes, cars, dolls, or doll clothes will also occupy time during soaks.

Although older children can cooperate, they, too, need something to do during the procedure, such as listening to music or a story, or watching television. Placing the solution and the extremity in a plastic sealable bag is an effective method to soak a hand or foot.

Baths are useful in the treatment of widespread dermatitis by evenly distributing the soothing antipruritic and anti-inflammatory effects of the solution, usually oatmeal or mineral oil preparations. The solution is added to a tub of lukewarm water. The temperature of the bath is tepid, and the treatment usually lasts 15 to 30 minutes. Therapeutic baths are more interesting when toy boats or other items for water play accompany the procedure.

Topical applications are applied to skin lesions to ease discomfort, prevent further injury, and facilitate healing. A thin application of the ointment or cream may be covered with a plastic film and anchored with adhesive, covered with a commercial transparent dressing or wrapped in Kerlix gauze and held in place by a stretchy net dressing. Topical preparations are applied systematically with the contour of the body surface (not simply up and down). Children love to be "painted," and lotion applications can be fun when an ordinary paintbrush is used. Regardless of the type of preparation used, parents need detailed information on how to apply it and how long the preparation should remain on the skin.

NURSE ALERT Provide written instructions and demonstrate to parents the correct amount of topical medication to apply (e.g., size of a pea; thin film to cover). If more than one preparation is applied, mark the containers with numbers so the parents remember the correct order of application. Stress that more is not necessarily better with some medications, such as steroids. ■

Home Care and Family Support

Dermatologic conditions always involve the family, but few situations require hospitalization and most care is delivered at home. Because the family must carry out the treatment plan, their cooperation is essential. Regimens that are simple to accomplish in the clinic, hospital, or primary care provider's office may be frustrating and baffling at home. The family may also need assistance in adapting equipment available for home therapy.

It is important that the child and family be given as detailed an explanation as possible about both the expected and unexpected results of treatment, including any ill effects that might occur. If unexplained reactions develop, the family is directed to discontinue treatment and report the reactions to the appropriate person. The use of over-the-counter medicines is discouraged unless the preparations have been discussed with the health care provider and have received approval.

Because the skin is the most visible portion of the body, defects in its surface alter its appearance and cause distress for the child. Skin problems may also result in rejection by others. Parents of other children may fear that their children will "catch" the disorder. Occasionally the affected child's own family members reduce their interaction or physical contact with the child. This is seldom a problem with dermatitis of short duration, but chronic conditions can frequently create problems and affect the child's self-esteem (Family Focus box).

> **Family Focus**
>
> **SKIN LESIONS AND SELF-ESTEEM IN THE SCHOOL-AGE CHILD**
>
> When I was 8 years old, a lot of small, oval, tannish brown spots developed, especially around my neck and waist. The dermatologist said it was a rare condition and it should disappear by the time I was 11 or 12. They actually disappeared when I was 10. Because the spots were kind of unusual, the dermatologist invited me to attend a dermatology meeting where people with strange skin problems were placed in private clinic rooms and doctors came in and looked at each person's skin. They were all nice, but I felt a little like an animal in the zoo. The thing I mostly remember about the spots was that I always tried to keep them covered. People stared, and kids made fun of me. The spots didn't hurt or itch, but I always knew they were there. I would not wear a two-piece swimsuit, even though my friends wore them. My mom and I tried to think of anything that might have caused the spots, but I never knew why they developed on me. I remember thinking it wasn't fair that it happened to me. I learned that many times, people cannot prevent the bad things that happen to them.
>
> Marissa White, age 16
> Tulsa, OK

INFECTIONS OF THE SKIN

evolve CASE STUDY: IMPETIGO

Bacterial Infections

Normally, the skin harbors a variety of bacterial flora, including the major pathogenic varieties of staphylococci and streptococci. The degree of pathogenicity of the organism depends on its invasiveness and toxicity, the integrity of the skin, and the immune and cellular defenses of the host. Children with congenital or acquired immunodeficiency disorders (e.g., acquired immunodeficiency syndrome), those in a debilitated condition, those receiving immunosuppressant therapy, and those with a generalized malignancy such as leukemia or lymphoma are at risk for developing bacterial infections.

Because of the characteristic "walling-off" process of the inflammatory reaction (abscess formation), staphylococci are more difficult to treat, and the local infected area is associated with an increase in bacteria all over the skin surface that serves as a source of continuing infection. Staphylococcal infections occur most often in younger children, and the incidence decreases with advancing age. Common bacterial skin disorders are outlined in Table 53-3 (Figs. 53-3 and 53-4).

Nursing Care Management

The major nursing interventions related to bacterial skin infections are to prevent the spread of infection and to prevent complications. Handwashing is mandatory before and after contact with an affected child, and this practice is emphasized to all those who care for the child. The child should be provided with towels separate from those of other family members. Impetigo contagiosa is easily spread by self-inoculation; therefore children with this condition must be cautioned against touching the involved area. This is difficult to accomplish. Although distraction and reminders are useful, these measures do not work when children are unsupervised or sleeping.

Children and parents are often tempted to squeeze follicular lesions. They must be warned that squeezing will not hasten the resolution of the infection and that there is a risk of making the lesion worse or spreading the infection. No attempt should be made to puncture the surface of the pustule with a needle or sharp instrument. A child with a sty may waken with the eyelids of the affected eye sealed shut with exudate. The child or the parents are instructed to gently wipe the lid from the inner to the outer edge with warm water and a clean washcloth until the exudate is removed.

The child with limited cellulitis of an extremity is usually managed at home on a regimen of oral antibiotics and warm compresses. The parents are taught the procedures and instructed in administration of the medication. Children with more extensive cellulitis, especially around a joint with lymphadenitis or on the face, are usually admitted to the hospital for parenteral antibiotics with continued treatment at home. Nurses are responsible for teaching the family to administer the medication and apply compresses.

Table 53-3

Bacterial Infections

DISORDER/ORGANISM	MANIFESTATIONS	MANAGEMENT	COMMENTS
Impetigo contagiosa (see Fig. 53-3)—*Staphylococcus*	Begins as a reddish macule Becomes vesicular Ruptures easily, leaving superficial, moist erosion Tends to spread peripherally in sharply marginated irregular outlines Exudate dries to form heavy, honey-colored crusts Pruritus common Systemic effects: minimal or asymptomatic	Careful removal of undermined skin, crusts, and debris by softening with 1:20 Burow solution compresses Topical application of bactericidal ointment Systemic administration of oral or parenteral antibiotics (penicillin) in severe or extensive lesions	Tends to heal without scarring unless secondary infection Autoinoculable and contagious Very common in toddler, preschooler May be superimposed on eczema
Pyoderma—*Staphylococcus, Streptococcus*	Deeper extension of infection into dermis Tissue reaction more severe Systemic effects: fever, lymphangitis	Soap and water cleansing Wet compresses Bathing with antibacterial soap as prescribed	Autoinoculable and contagious May heal with or without scarring
Folliculitis (pimple), **furuncle** (boil), **carbuncle** (multiple boils)—*Staphylococcus aureus*	Folliculitis: infection of hair follicle Furuncle: larger lesion with more redness and swelling at a single follicle Carbuncle: more extensive lesion with widespread inflammation and "pointing" at several follicular orifices Systemic effects: malaise, if severe	Skin cleanliness Local warm, moist compresses Topical application of antibiotic agents Systemic antibiotics in severe cases Incision and drainage of severe lesions, followed by wound irrigations with antibiotics or suitable drain implantation	Autoinoculable and contagious Furuncle and carbuncle tend to heal with scar formation A lesion should never be squeezed
Cellulitis—*Streptococcus, Staphylococcus, Haemophilus influenzae* (see Fig. 53-4)	Inflammation of skin and subcutaneous tissues with intense redness, swelling, and firm infiltration Lymphangitis "streaking" frequently seen Involvement of regional lymph nodes common May progress to abscess formation Systemic effects: fever, malaise	Oral or parenteral antibiotics Rest and immobilization of both affected area and child Hot moist compresses to area	Hospitalization may be necessary for child with systemic symptoms Otitis media may be associated with facial cellulitis
Staphylococcal scalded skin syndrome—*S. aureus*	Macular erythema with "sandpaper" texture of involved skin Epidermis becomes wrinkled (in 2 days or less), and large bullae appear	Systemic administration of antibiotics Gentle cleansing with saline, Burow solution, or 0.25% silver nitrate compresses	Infant subject to fluid loss, impaired body temperature regulation, and secondary infection, such as pneumonia, cellulitis, and septicemia Heals without scarring

Viral Infections

Viruses are intracellular parasites that produce their effect by using the intracellular substances of the host cells. Composed of only a deoxyribonucleic acid (DNA) or ribonucleic acid (RNA) core enclosed in an antigenic protein shell, viruses are unable to provide for their own metabolic needs or to reproduce themselves. After a virus penetrates a cell of the host organism, it sheds the outer shell and disappears within the cell, where the nucleic acid core stimulates the host cell to form more virus material from its intracellular substance. In a viral infection, the epidermal cells react with inflammation and vesiculation (as in herpes simplex) or by proliferating to form growths (warts).

Many of the communicable viral diseases of childhood are associated with rashes, and each rash is characteristic. Common viral disorders of the skin are outlined in Table 53-4.

Table 53-4

Viral Infections

INFECTION	MANIFESTATIONS	MANAGEMENT	COMMENTS
Verruca (warts) Cause: human papillomavirus (various types)	Small, benign tumors Usually well-circumscribed, gray or brown, elevated, firm papules with a roughened, finely papillomatous texture Occur anywhere, but usually appear on exposed areas such as fingers, hands, face, and soles May be single or multiple Asymptomatic	Not uniformly successful Local destructive therapy, individualized according to location, type, and number—surgical removal, electrocautery, curettage, cryotherapy (liquid nitrogen), caustic solutions (lactic acid and salicylic acid in flexible collodion, retinoic acid, salicylic acid plasters), x-ray treatment, laser Hypnotherapy may be effective	Common in children Tend to disappear spontaneously Course unpredictable Most destructive techniques tend to leave scars Autoinoculable Repeated irritation will cause to enlarge Apply topical anesthetic (EMLA)
Verruca plantaris (plantar wart)	Located on plantar surface of feet and, because of pressure, are practically flat; may be surrounded by a collar of hyperkeratosis	Apply caustic solution to wart, wear foam insole with hole cut to relieve pressure on wart; soak 20 minutes after 2-3 days; repeat until wart comes out	Destructive techniques tend to leave scars, which may cause problems with walking Apply topical anesthetic (EMLA)
Herpes simplex virus • Type I (cold sore, fever blister) • Type II (genital)	Grouped, burning, and itching vesicles on inflammatory base, usually on or near mucocutaneous junctions (lips, nose, genitals, buttocks) Vesicles dry, forming a crust, followed by exfoliation and spontaneous healing in 8-10 days May be accompanied by regional lymphadenopathy	Avoidance of secondary infection Burow solution compresses during weeping stages Topical therapy (penciclovir) can shorten duration of cold sores Oral antiviral (acyclovir) for initial infection or to reduce severity in recurrence Valacyclovir (Valtrex), an oral antiviral used for episodic treatment of recurrent genital herpes, reduces pain, stops viral shedding, and has a more convenient administration schedule than acyclovir	Heal without scarring unless secondary infection Type I cold sores can be prevented by using sunscreens protecting against ultraviolet A (UVA) and ultraviolet B (UVB) light to prevent lip blisters Aggravated by corticosteroids Positive psychologic effect from treatment May be fatal in children with depressed immunity
Varicella zoster virus (herpes zoster; shingles)	Caused by same virus that causes varicella (chickenpox) Virus has affinity for posterior root ganglia, posterior horn of spinal cord, and skin; crops of vesicles usually confined to dermatome following along course of affected nerve Usually preceded by neuralgic pain, hyperesthesias, or itching May be accompanied by constitutional symptoms	Symptomatic Analgesics for pain Mild sedation sometimes helpful Local moist compresses Drying lotions may be helpful Ophthalmic variety: systemic corticotropin (adrenocorticotropic hormone [ACTH]) and/or corticosteroids Acyclovir Lidoderm topical anesthetic	Pain in children usually minimal Postherpetic pain does not occur in children Chickenpox may follow exposure; isolate affected child from other children in a hospital or school May occur in children with depressed immunity; can be fatal
Molluscum contagiosum Cause: pox virus	Flesh-colored papules with a central caseous plug (umbilicated) Usually asymptomatic	Cases in well children resolve spontaneously in about 18 months Treatment reserved for troublesome cases Apply topical anesthetic (EMLA) and remove with curette Use tretinoin gel 0.01% or cantharidin (Cantharone) liquid Curettage or cryotherapy	Common in school-age children Spread by skin-to-skin contact, including autoinoculation and fomite-to-skin contact

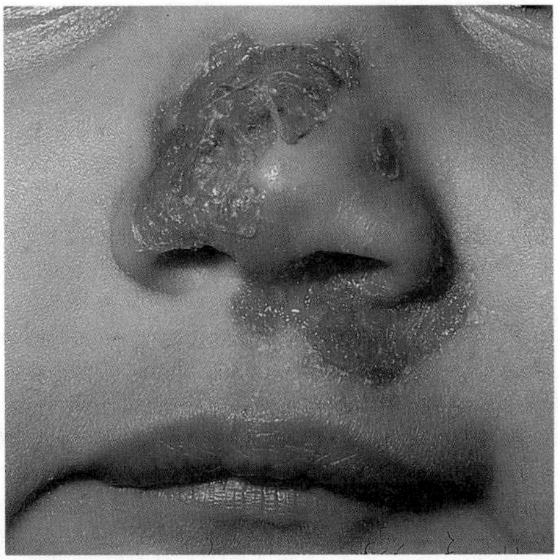

Fig. 53-3 Impetigo contagiosa. (From Weston WL, Lane AT: *Color textbook of pediatric dermatology,* ed 3, St Louis, 2002, Mosby.)

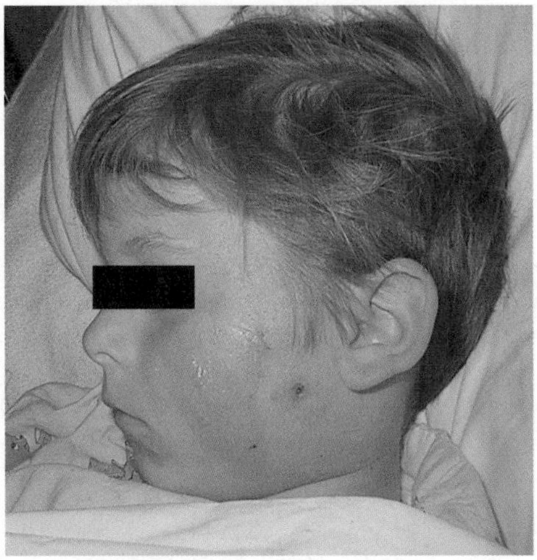

Fig. 53-4 Cellulitis of cheek from puncture wound. (From Weston WL, Lane AT: *Color textbook of pediatric dermatology,* ed 3, St Louis, 2002, Mosby.)

Dermatophytoses (Fungal Infections)

The *dermatophytoses* (collectively termed *ringworm*) are infections caused by a group of closely related filamentous fungi that invade primarily the stratum corneum, hair, and nails. These are superficial infections that live on, not in, the skin. They are confined to the dead keratin layers and are unable to survive in the deeper layers. Because the keratin is desquamated constantly, the fungus must multiply at a rate that equals the rate of keratin production to maintain itself; otherwise, the infection would be shed with the discarded skin cells. Common dermatophytoses are outlined in Table 53-5 (Fig. 53-5).

Dermatophytoses are designated by the Latin word *tinea,* with further designation related to the area of the body where they are found (e.g., tinea capitis [ringworm of the scalp]). Dermatophyte infections are most often transmitted from one person to another or from infected animals to humans. Diagnosis is made from microscopic examination of scrapings taken from the advancing periphery of the lesion, which almost always produces a scale.

Nursing Care Management

When teaching families how to care for ringworm, the nurse should emphasize good health and hygiene. Because of the infectious nature of the disease, affected children should not exchange grooming items, headgear, scarves, or other articles of apparel that have been in proximity to the infected area with other children. Affected children are provided with their own towels and directed to wear a protective cap at night to avoid transmitting the fungus to bedding, especially if they sleep with another person. Because the infection can be acquired by animal-to-human transmission, all household pets should be examined for the presence of the disorder. Other sources of infection are seats with headrests (theater seats), seats in public transportation vehicles, helmets, and gymnasium mats.

Treatment with the drug griseofulvin frequently continues for weeks or months, and because subjective symptoms subside, children or parents may be tempted to decrease or discontinue the drug. The nurse should emphasize to family members the importance of maintaining the prescribed dosage schedule and of taking the medication with high-fat foods for best absorption. They are also instructed regarding possible drug side effects, such as headache, gastrointestinal upset, fatigue, insomnia, and photosensitivity. For children who take the drug over many months, periodic testing is required to monitor leukopenia and assess liver and renal function.

A

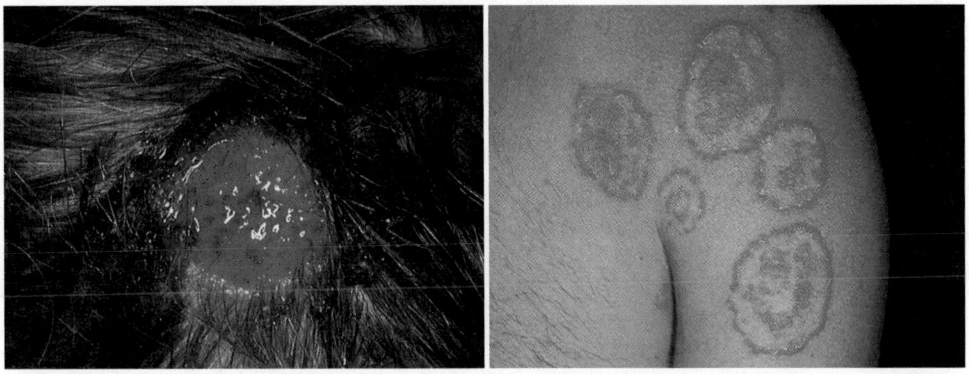

B

Fig. 53-5 **A,** Tinea capitis. **B,** Tinea corporis. Both infections are caused by *Microsporum canis,* the "kitten" or "puppy" fungus. (From Habif TP: *Clinical dermatology: a color guide to diagnosis and therapy,* ed 4, St Louis, 2004, Mosby.)

Table 53-5

Dermatophytoses (Fungal Infections)

DISEASE/ORGANISM	MANIFESTATIONS	MANAGEMENT	COMMENTS
Tinea capitis—*Trichophyton tonsurans, Microsporum audouini, Microsporum canis* (see Fig. 53-5, *A*)	Lesions in scalp but may extend to hairline or neck Characteristic configuration of scaly, circumscribed patches and/or patchy, scaling areas of alopecia Generally asymptomatic, but severe, deep inflammatory reaction may occur that manifests as boggy, encrusted lesions (kerions) Pruritic Microscopic examination of scales is diagnostic	Oral griseofulvin Oral ketoconazole for difficult cases Selenium sulfide shampoos Topical antifungal agents (e.g., clotrimazole, haloprogin, miconazole)	Person-to-person transmission Animal-to-person transmission Rarely, permanent loss of hair *M. audouini* transmitted from one human being to another directly or from personal items; *M. canis* usually contracted from household pets, especially cats Atopic individuals more susceptible
Tinea corporis—*Trichophyton rubrum, Trichophyton mentagrophytes, M. canis, Epidermophyton* (see Fig. 53-5, *B*)	Generally round or oval, erythematous scaling patch that spreads peripherally and clears centrally; may involve nails (tinea unguium) Diagnosis: direct microscopic examination of scales Usually unilateral	Oral griseofulvin Local application of antifungal preparation such as tolnaftate, haloprogin, miconazole, clotrimazole; apply 1 inch beyond periphery of lesion; continual application 1 to 2 weeks after no sign of lesion	Usually of animal origin from infected pets Majority of infections in children caused by *M. canis* and *M. audouini*
Tinea cruris ("jock itch")—*Epidermophyton floccosum, T. rubrum, T. mentagrophytes*	Skin response similar to tinea corporis Localized to medial proximal aspect of thigh and crural fold; may involve scrotum in males Pruritic Diagnosis: same as for tinea	Local application of tolnaftate liquid Wet compresses or sitz baths may be soothing	Rare in preadolescent children Health education regarding personal hygiene
Tinea pedis ("athlete's foot")—*T. rubrum, Trichophyton interdigitale, E. floccosum*	On intertriginous areas between toes or on plantar surface of feet Lesions vary: • Maceration and fissuring between toes • Patches with pinhead-sized vesicles on plantar surface • Pruritic • Diagnosis: direct microscopic examination of scrapings	Oral griseofulvin Local applications of tolnaftate liquid and antifungal powder containing tolnaftate Acute infections: compresses or soaks followed by application of glucocorticoid cream Elimination of conditions of heat and perspiration by clean, light socks and well-ventilated shoes; avoidance of occlusive shoes	Most common in adolescents and adults; rare in children, but occurrence increases with wearing of plastic shoes Transmission to other individuals rare despite general opinion to contrary Ointments not successful
Candidiasis (moniliasis)—*Candida albicans corporis*	Grows in chronically moist areas Inflamed areas with white exudate, peeling, and easy bleeding Pruritic Diagnosis: characteristic appearance	Amphotericin B, nystatin ointment, or other antifungal preparations to affected areas	Common form of diaper dermatitis (see Fig. 53-11) Oral form common in infants Vaginal form in older females May be disseminated in immunosuppressed children

Systemic Mycotic (Fungal) Infections

Mycotic (systemic or deep fungal) infections have the capacity to invade the viscera, as well as the skin. The most common infections are the lung diseases, which are usually acquired by inhalation of fungal spores. These fungi produce a variable spectrum of disease, and some are common in certain geographic areas. They are not transmitted from person to person but appear to reside in the soil, from which their spores are airborne. The cutaneous lesions caused by deep fungal infections are granulomatous and appear as ulcers, plaques, nodules, fungating masses, and abscesses. The course of deep fungal diseases is chronic with slow progression that favors sensitization (Table 53-6).

SKIN DISORDERS RELATED TO CHEMICAL OR PHYSICAL CONTACTS

Contact Dermatitis

Contact dermatitis is an inflammatory reaction of the skin to chemical substances, natural or synthetic, that evokes a hypersensitivity response or direct irritation. The initial reaction occurs in an exposed region, most commonly the face and neck, backs of the hands, forearms, male genitalia, and lower legs. Early in the reaction, there is usually a sharp delineation between inflamed and normal skin that ranges from a faint, transient erythema to massive bullae on an erythematous, swollen base. Itching is a constant symptom.

Table 53-6

Systemic Mycoses

DISORDER/ ORGANISM	SKIN MANIFESTATIONS	SYSTEMIC MANIFESTATIONS	TREATMENT	COMMENTS
North American blastomycosis—*Blastomyces dermatitidis*	Chronic granulomatous lesions and microabscesses in any part of body Initial lesion is a papule; undergoes ulceration and peripheral spread	Pulmonary symptoms, such as cough, chest pain, weakness, and weight loss May have skeletal involvement, with bone destruction and formation of cutaneous abscesses	Intravenous (IV) administration of amphotericin B	Usual portal of entry is lungs Source of infection unknown Noninfectious Pulmonary infections may be mild and self-limiting and require no treatment Progressive disease often fatal
Cryptococcosis—*Cryptococcus neoformans (Torula histolytica)*	Usually on face; acneiform, firm, nodular, painless eruption	Central nervous system (CNS) manifestations: headache, dizziness, stiff neck, and signs of increased intracranial pressure Low-grade fever, mild cough, lung infiltration	IV amphotericin B; may be administered intrathecally for CNS involvement 5-Flurocytosine for meningitis Excision and drainage of local lesions	Acquired by inhalation of dust but may enter through skin Prognosis serious Noninfectious Increased incidence in persons receiving corticosteroids with lymphoreticular malignancies, or type 2 diabetes
Histoplasmosis—*Histoplasma capsulatum*	Not distinctive or uniform but most appear as punched-out or granulomatous ulcers	General systemic symptoms may include pallor, diarrhea, vomiting, irregular spiking temperature, hepatosplenomegaly, and pulmonary symptoms Any tissue of body may be involved with related symptoms	IV amphotericin B for severe cases Oral ketoconazole	Organism cultured from soil, especially where contaminated with fowl droppings Fungus enters through skin or mucous membranes of mouth and respiratory tract Endemic in Mississippi and Ohio River valleys Disseminated diseases most common in infants and children
Coccidioidomycosis (valley fever)—*Coccidioides immitis*	Erythema nodosum Erythema multiforme Erythematous maculopapular rash	Primary lung disease usually asymptomatic May be sign of acute febrile illness Disseminated disease is very serious	IV amphotericin B IV miconazole (synthetic imidazole) Intraventricular miconazole plus oral ketoconazole for CNS involvement Surgical resection of persistent pulmonary cavities	Inhalation of aerospores from soil Endemic in southwestern United States Usually resolves spontaneously Increased incidence in dark-skinned races (Filipino, black, Mexican, Asian)

The cause may be a primary irritant or a sensitizing agent. A *primary irritant* is one that irritates any skin. A *sensitizing agent* produces an irritation on those individuals who have met the irritant or something chemically related to it, have undergone an immunologic change, and have become sensitized. Prior exposure is not necessarily a factor in the reaction. In relatively low concentrations, a sensitizer irritates only persons who are allergic to it.

In infants, contact dermatitis occurs on the convex surfaces of the diaper area (see Diaper Dermatitis, p. 1775). Other agents that produce contact dermatitis include plants (poison ivy, oak, or sumac); animal irritants (wool, feathers, and furs); metal (nickle found in jewelry, sleeper snaps and snaps on denim); vegetable irritants (oleoresins, oils, and turpentine); and synthetic fabrics (e.g., shoe components), dyes, cosmetics, perfumes, and soaps (including bubble baths). The list is endless.

The major goal in treatment is to prevent further exposure of the skin to the offending substance. Provided there is no further irritation, the normal recuperative powers of the skin will often produce healing without treatment. Otherwise, treatment of contact dermatitis is based on severity. Mild cases are treated with topical steroids. Mild to moderately severe cases may require a 2-week course of strong topical corticosteroids. Very severe cases require systemic corticosteroids (Kronemyer, 2003).

Nursing Care Management

Nurses frequently detect evidence of contact dermatitis during routine physical assessments. Skin manifestations in specific areas suggest limited contact, such as around the eyes (mascara), areas of the body covered by clothing but not protected by undergarments (wool), or areas of the body not covered by clothing (ultraviolet injury). Generalized involvement is more likely to be caused by bubble bath or soap. Often nurses can determine the offending agent and counsel families regarding management. However, if the lesions persist, are extensive, or show evidence of infection, medical evaluation is indicated.

Poison Ivy, Oak, and Sumac

evolve CASE STUDY: POISON IVY

Contact with the dry or succulent portions of any of three poisonous plants (ivy, oak, and sumac) produces localized, streaked or spotty, oozing, and painful impetiginous lesions. The offending substance in these plants is *urushiol*, an extremely potent oil. Sensitivity to urushiol is not inborn but is developed after one or two exposures and may change over a lifetime. All parts of the plants contain the oil, including dried leaves and stems (Fig. 53-6). Even smoke from burning brush piles can produce a reaction.

Animals do not seem to be affected by the oil; however, dogs or other animals that have run or played in the plants may carry the sap on their fur, and animals that eat the plants can transfer the oil in their saliva. Shoes, tools, and toys can transfer the oil. Golf balls that have been in the rough are another source of contact.

Urushiol takes effect as soon as it touches the skin. It penetrates through the epidermis and bonds with the dermal layer, where it initiates an immune response. The full-blown reaction is evident after about 2 days, with redness, swelling, and itching at the site of contact. Several days later, streaked or spotty blisters oozing serum from damaged cells produce the characteristic impetiginous lesions (Fig. 53-7). The lesions dry and heal spontaneously, and itching stops by 10 to 14 days.

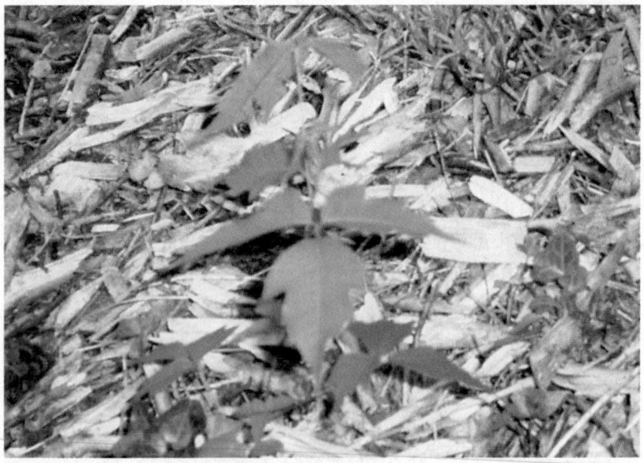

Fig. 53-6 Poison ivy plants.

Therapeutic Management

Treatment of the lesions includes calamine lotion, soothing Burow solution compresses, and/or Aveeno baths to relieve discomfort. Topical corticosteroid gel is very effective for prevention or relief of inflammation, especially when applied before blisters form. Oral corticosteroids may be needed for severe reactions, and a sedative such as diphenhydramine (Benadryl) may be ordered.

Nursing Care Management

When it is known that the child has made contact with the plant, the area is immediately flushed (preferably within 15 minutes) with *cold* running water to neutralize the urushiol not yet bonded to the skin. If there is a stream nearby, an effective method is to have the child enter the water (clothes and all) and allow the water to rinse the oil from both skin and clothing. Harsh soap is contraindicated because it removes protective skin oils and dilutes the urushiol, allowing it to spread; hard scrubbing irritates the skin. All clothing

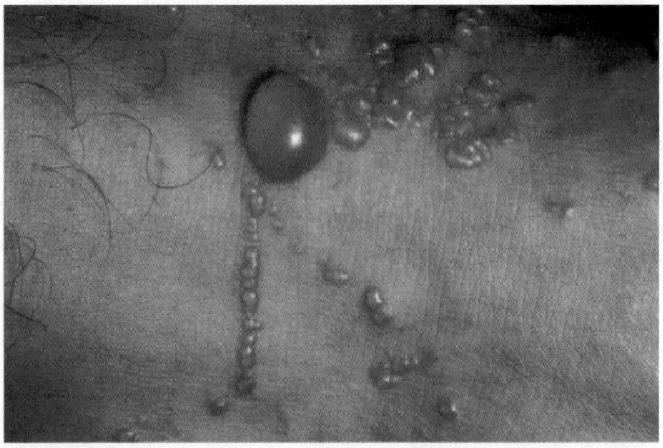

Fig. 53-7 Poison ivy; note "streaked" blisters surrounding one large blister. (From Habif TP: *Clinical dermatology: a color guide to diagnosis and therapy,* ed 4, St Louis, 2004, Mosby.)

Critical Thinking Exercise

POISON IVY

While at an overnight camp near a stream, Billy, age 9, runs up to the campfire and shows the nurse some leaves he has picked in the woods. The nurse recognizes the leaves as poison ivy. One of the adolescent assistants wants to throw the leaves on the campfire, and scrub Billy's hands vigorously with soap. Billy's cabin mates ask the nurse: "Is poison ivy catching? Are we going to get it too?" What nursing actions should the camp nurse implement?

1. Evidence—Is there sufficient evidence to draw any conclusions at this time?
2. Assumptions—Describe some underlying assumptions about the following:
   a. The agent that causes poison ivy
   b. Effects of poison ivy on the skin
   c. Immediate treatment for poison ivy
   d. Contraindicated treatments for poison ivy
3. What implications and priorities for nursing care can be drawn at his time?
4. Does the evidence support your conclusion?
5. Are there alternative perspectives to your arguments?

that has come in contact with the plant is removed with care and thoroughly laundered in hot water and detergent. Every effort is made to prevent the child from scratching the lesions. Although the lesions do not spread by contact with the blister serum or from scratching, they can become secondarily infected (Critical Thinking Exercise).

Prevention

Prevention is best accomplished by avoiding contact and removing the plant from the environment. All children, especially those known to be sensitive, should be taught to recognize the plant. Information regarding means for destroying plants can be obtained from the U.S. Department of Agriculture or Forestry Service. A cream that protects exposed skin from poison oak and ivy is Stokogard.*

Drug Reactions

Adverse reactions to drugs are seen more often in the skin than in any other organ, although any organ of the body can be affected. The reaction may be a result of toxicity related to drug concentration, individual intolerance to the average dosage of the drug, or an allergic or idiosyncratic response. The manifestations may be associated with side effects or secondary effects of a drug, either of which are unrelated to its primary pharmacologic actions.

Although any drug is capable of producing a reaction in the susceptible individual, some drugs have a tendency to produce a particular reaction consistently, and others are more likely to produce an untoward effect. Many are allergenic responses that occur following a previous administration of the drug, even a topical application. Other factors influence a drug response in a particular individual. For example, the incidence increases with the amount and number of drugs given.

NURSE ALERT Intravenous (IV) drugs are more likely to cause a reaction than oral drugs. Stop the drug, but maintain the infusion with normal saline. ■

Manifestations of drug reactions may be delayed or immediate. A period of 7 days is usually required for a child to develop sensitivity to a drug that has never been administered previously. With prior sensitivity the manifestations appear almost immediately. Rashes are the most common manifestation of adverse drug reactions in children. However, individual drug reactions may vary from a single lesion to extensive, generalized epidermal necrosis such as that seen in Stevens-Johnson syndrome (see Table 53-9). Cutaneous manifestations can resemble almost any skin disease and can be seen in almost any degree of severity. With few exceptions, the distribution of a drug eruption is widespread, because it results from a circulating agent, appears as an inflammatory response with itching, is sudden in onset, and may be associated with constitutional symptoms such as fever, malaise, gastrointestinal upsets, anemia, or liver and kidney damage.

In most cases treatment for simple cutaneous reactions consists of discontinuing the drug. Sometimes a decision is made to continue the drug (such as an antibiotic in an infant or small child) until the cause of the rash is clearly indicated. In urticarial-type eruptions antihistamines may be ordered, and for widespread and severe lesions corticosteroids are beneficial. Severe anaphylactic reactions are a medical emergency (see Anaphylaxis, Chapter 45).

Nursing Care Management

The most effective means of management is prevention. Parents always remember a severe reaction. A careful history will elicit evidence of a previous drug reaction. The history should include the name of the drug, nature of the reaction, drug dose, and how soon after administration the reaction occurred.

Nurses who suspect that a rash is caused by a medication should withhold any further dose and report the eruption to the practitioner. Frequent offenders in drug reactions are penicillin and sulfonamides, and nurses must be alert to this possibility. However, even commonplace drugs, including aspirin, barbiturates, chemical agents in some foods, flavoring agents, and preservatives, are capable of producing an undesired response. Persons who have severe reactions should wear an identification bracelet or chain in case of emergency or inadvertent administration of the offending drug.

Foreign Bodies

Parents can remove small wooden splinters with a needle and tweezers that have been sterilized with alcohol or a flame. The area around the sliver is washed with soap and water before removal is attempted. The sliver is exposed with the needle, then grasped firmly by the tweezers and pulled out. Some foreign bodies, such as a fishhook, pieces of glass, a difficult-

*Distributed in the United States by Stockhausen, Inc., Greensboro, NC 27406; phone: 800-334-0242.

to-see object, or a deeply embedded object (such as a needle in a foot or near a joint), require medical evaluation.

Small cactus prickles or spines are troublesome to remove, but the following methods may prove helpful:

- Apply a thin layer of water-soluble household glue and cover with gauze; when the glue dries, peel off the gauze.
- Apply hair removal wax or body sugar (Aplon*), let dry, and remove.
- Place cellophane tape, sticky side down, over the spines and lift off.

SKIN DISORDERS RELATED TO INSECT AND ANIMAL CONTACTS

Scabies

Scabies is an endemic infestation caused by the scabies mite, *Sarcoptes scabiei.* Lesions are created as the impregnated female burrows into the stratum corneum of the epidermis (never into living tissue) to deposit her eggs and feces. The inflammatory response and intense itching occur after the host becomes sensitized to the mite, approximately 30 to 60 days following initial contact. If the person has been previously sensitized to the mite, the response occurs within 48 hours after exposure. After this time, the areas over which the mite has traveled will begin to itch and develop the characteristic eruption (Box 53-1). Consequently, mites will not necessarily be located at all sites of eruption.

There is great variability in the type of lesions. Infants often develop an eczematous eruption; therefore the observer must look for discrete papules, burrows, or vesicles.

BOX 53-1

Clinical Manifestations of Scabies

Lesion

Children—minute grayish-brown, threadlike (mite burrows), pruritic
Black dot at end of burrow (mite)
Infants—eczematous eruption, pruritic

Distribution

Generally in intertriginous areas—interdigital, axillary-cubital, popliteal, inguinal
Children over 2 years of age—primarily hands and wrists
Children younger than 2 years of age—primarily feet and ankles

Nursing Care Management

The treatment of scabies consists of the application of a scabicide such as permethrin 5% cream (Elimite). Alternative drugs are 1% lindane cream or lotion and 10% crotamiton. Permethrin is preferred because it is safer, avoids the risk of neurotoxicity, and is more effective than lindane. Nurses instructing families in the use of scabicides should emphasize the importance of following directions carefully. Permethrin is applied to all skin surfaces (not just areas with rash, but also areas between the fingers and toes, the umbilicus, and the cleft of the buttocks). The cream should remain on the skin for 8 to 14 hours, and then be removed by bathing. Lindane is removed by bathing after 8 to 12 hours. One application of premethrin and lindane is sufficient. Lindane should not be used for patients with crusted scabies, premature infants, young infants, people with known seizure disorders, people with hypersensitivity to the product, or patients with extensive dermatitis. Lindane should not be used immediately after a bath or shower. Crotamiton is applied once a day for 2 days followed by a cleansing bath 48 hours after the last application. Families need to know that although the mite that causes scabies will be killed with these treatments, the rash and the itch will not be eliminated until the stratum corneum is replaced in approximately 2 to 3 weeks. Soothing ointments or lotions can be applied for itching. Antibiotics may be given for secondary infection.

Another prescription drug used to treat scabies is ivermectin (Frankowski & Weiner, 2002). Ivermectin is administered orally in a single dose for treatment of severe or crusted scabies. It should be considered for patients whose infestation is refractory or those who cannot tolerate topical scabicides (Offidani et al, 1999). However, the safety and efficacy of ivermectin for pediatric patients less than 5 years of age or children weighing less than 15 kg (33 pounds) is not established. This drug is not currently licensed for treatment of scabies by the U.S. Food and Drug Administration (American Academy of Pediatrics, Committee on Infectious Diseases, 2003).

Pediculosis Capitis

Pediculosis capitis (head lice) is an infestation of the scalp by *Pediculus humanus capitis,* a common parasite in school-age children. The adult louse lives only about 48 hours when away from a human host, and the life span of the average female is 1 month. The female lays her eggs at night at the junction of a hair shaft and close to the skin because the eggs need a warm environment. The *nits,* or eggs, hatch in approximately 7 to 10 days. Itching is usually the only symptom. Common areas involved are the occipital area, behind the ears, and the nape of the neck (Box 53-2).

Diagnostic Evaluation

Diagnosis is made by observation of the white eggs (nits) firmly attached to the hair shafts (Fig. 53-8). Because of their brief life span and mobility, adult lice are more difficult to

BOX 53-2

Clinical Manifestations of Pediculosis

Pruritus (caused by crawling insect and insect saliva on skin)
Nits observable on hair shaft (see Fig. 53-8)

Distribution

Occipital area
Behind ears
Nape of neck
Eyebrows and eyelashes (occasionally) (caused by pubic lice)

*Distributed by Corsa, Ltd., 555 N. Lane, Suite 5025, Conshohocker, PA 19428; phone: 610-834-1555; Web site: www.corsa.com.

A 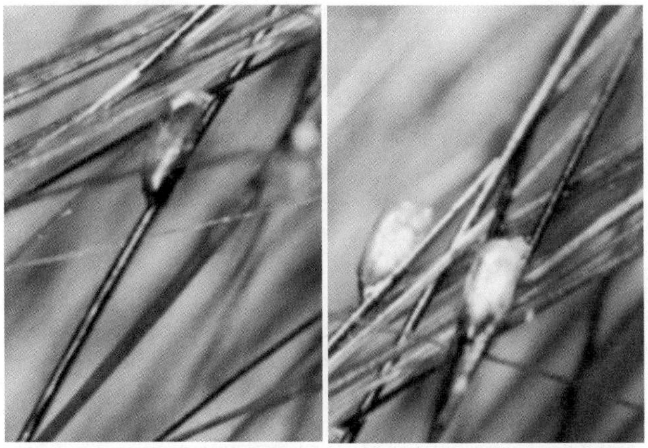 B

Fig. 53-8 **A**, Empty nit case. **B**, Viable nits. (From *The contemporary approach to the control of head lice in schools and communities,* Pittsburgh, 1991, SmithKline Beecham.)

locate. Nits must be differentiated from dandruff, lint, hair spray, and other items of similar size and shape. Scratch marks or inflammatory papules, caused by secondary infection, may also be found on the scalp in the vulnerable areas.

Therapeutic Management

Treatment consists of the application of pediculicides and manual removal of nit cases. The drug of choice for infants and children is permethrin 1% cream rinse (Nix), which kills adult lice and nits. This product and preparations of pyrethrin with piperonyl butoxide (RID or A-200 pyrinate) can be obtained without a prescription and are more effective and safer than lindane. The Food and Drug Administration (FDA) has issued a warning regarding the use of lindane because of the potential for neurotoxicity (FDA, 2003). Although the FDA believes that the benefits of lindane outweigh the risks when used as directed, patients should be treated with lindane only when other treatments are not tolerable or have failed. Another product approved for treatment of head lice, malathion 0.5% (Ovide), is available only by prescription. However, malathion contains flammable alcohol, must remain on the hair for 8 to 12 hours, and is not recommended for children less than 2 years of age.

Nursing Care Management

An important nursing role is providing the parents with education about pediculosis. Nurses should emphasize that *anyone* can get pediculosis; it has no respect for age, socioeconomic level, or cleanliness. The louse does not jump or fly, but it can be transmitted from one person to another on personal items. Lice are more apt to infest white children, those with straight hair, and girls. Children are cautioned against sharing combs, hair ornaments, hats, caps, scarves, coats, and other items used on or near the hair. Children who share lockers are more likely to become infested, and slumber parties place children at risk. Lice are not carried or transmitted by pets.

Nurses or parents should carefully inspect a child who scratches his or her head more than usual for bite marks, redness, and nits. The hair is systematically spread with two flat-sided sticks or tongue depressors, and the scalp is observed for any movement that indicates a louse. Nurses should wear gloves when examining the hair. Lice are small and grayish tan, have no wings, and are visible to the naked eye. The nits, or eggs, appear as tiny whitish oval specks adhering to the hair shaft about ¼ inch from the scalp. The adherent nature of the nits distinguishes them from dandruff, which falls off readily. *Empty nit cases,* indicating hatched lice, are translucent rather than white and are located more than ¼ inch from the scalp (see Fig. 53-8).

If evidence of infestation is found, it is important to treat the child according to the directions on the label of the pediculicide. Parents are advised to read the directions carefully before beginning treatment. The child is made as comfortable as possible during the application process, because the pediculicide must remain on the scalp and hair for several minutes. Playing "beauty parlor" during the shampoo is a useful strategy. The child lies supine, with the head over a sink or basin, and covers the eyes with a dry towel or washcloth. This prevents medication, which can cause chemical conjunctivitis, from splashing into the eyes. If eye irritation occurs, the eyes must be flushed well with tepid water. It is not necessary to remove the nits after treatment because only live lice cause infestation. However, because none of the pediculicides are 100% effective in killing all the eggs, the makers of some pediculocides recommend manual removal of the nits following treatment. An extra-fine-tooth comb that is included in many commercial pediculocides or available at community pharmacies facilitates manual removal. If the comb is ineffective in removing the nit cases, they should be removed by scraping them off the strands of hair with the examiner's fingernails.

Live lice survive for up to 48 hours away from the host, but nits are shed into the environment and are capable of hatching in 7 to 10 days. Therefore measures must be taken to prevent further infestation (Community Focus box). Spraying with insecticide is not recommended because of the danger to children and animals. Families should also be advised that

Community Focus

PREVENTING THE SPREAD AND RECURRENCE OF PEDICULOSIS

- Machine wash all washable clothing, towels, and bed linens in hot water, and dry in a hot dryer for at least 20 minutes. Dry-clean nonwashable items.
- Thoroughly vacuum carpets, car seats, pillows, stuffed animals, rugs, mattresses, and upholstered furniture.
- Seal nonwashable items in plastic bags for 14 days if unable to dry-clean or vacuum.
- Soak combs, brushes, and hair accessories in lice-killing products for 1 hour or in boiling water for 10 minutes.
- In day care centers, store children's clothing items such as hats and scarves and other headgear in separate cubicles.
- Discourage the sharing of items such as hats, scarves, hair accessories, combs, and brushes among children in group settings such as day care centers.
- Avoid physical contact with infested individuals and their belongings, especially clothing and bedding.
- Inspect children in a group setting regularly for head lice.
- Provide educational programs on the transmission of pediculosis, its detection, and its treatment.

Modified from Chin J (ed): *Control of communicable diseases manual,* Washington, DC, 2000, American Public Health Association.

the pediculicide is relatively expensive, especially when several members of the household require treatment.

The psychologic effects of lice infestations are stressful to children. They are influenced by the reactions of others, including their parents, school nurses, and officials. Some children feel ashamed or guilty. Parents are strongly cautioned against cutting a child's hair or, worse, shaving a child's head. Lice infest short hair as readily as long hair, and these actions only compound the child's distress and serve as a continual reminder to peers, who are prone to taunt children who have a different appearance.

Prevention

The increasing incidence of pediculosis in schoolchildren is a serious concern for school nurses, parents, and community health agencies. However, school head lice screening programs have not proven to have a significant effect on the incidence of head lice in the school setting; parent education programs may be more helpful in the management of head lice. Children with head lice should be allowed to return to school after proper treatment. Both the American Academy of Pediatrics and the National Association of School Nurses discourage a "no nit" policy for schools (Frankowski & Weiner, 2002).

Arthropod Bites and Stings

Bites and stings account for a significant amount of mild to moderate discomfort in children. Most bites and stings are managed by simple symptomatic measures, such as compresses, calamine lotion, and prevention of secondary infection. *Arthropods* include insects and arachnids, such as mites, ticks, spiders, and scorpions. Most arthropods in the United States are relatively harmless, including tarantulas. Although all spiders produce venom that is injected via fangs, some are unable to pierce the skin and others produce venom that is insufficiently toxic to be harmful. Only scorpions and two spiders—the brown recluse (Fig. 53-9) and the black widow—inject venom deadly enough to require immediate attention. Children bitten by these arachnids must receive medical attention as soon as possible. Major offending creatures, their manifestations, and management are outlined in Table 53-7.

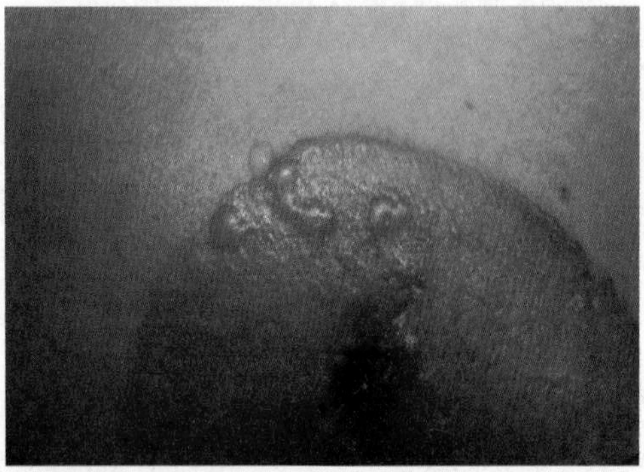

Fig. 53-9 Brown recluse spider bite; note central necrosis surrounded by purplish area and blisters. (From Weston WL, Lane AT: *Color textbook of pediatric dermatology,* St Louis, 1991, Mosby.)

When a hymenopteran (bees in particular) stings, its barbed stinger penetrates into the skin. As long as the stinger remains in the skin, the muscles push the stinger deeper and the venom is pumped into the wound. The best approach is to remove the stinger as quickly as possible and to get away from the vicinity of other insects to prevent further injury. Children who have become sensitized to hymenopteran bites may demonstrate a severe systemic response that can be life threatening. One sting can produce generalized urticaria, respiratory difficulty (from laryngeal edema), hypotension, and death. Intramuscular administration of epinephrine provides immediate relief and must be available for emergency use.

Hypersensitive children should wear a medical identification bracelet. They should also have a kit that contains epinephrine and a hypodermic syringe. Families are reminded to check the expiration date on the kit and to replace an outdated one. They should determine if a nurse is available at the school and the school policy regarding administration of drugs. If a school nurse is not present, someone at the school should be designated to inject the epinephrine in case of an emergency.

Infections Transmitted by Arthropods

The organisms responsible for a number of disorders are transmitted to human beings via arthropods (Table 53-8). Mammals become infected only through the bites of infected lice, fleas, ticks, and mites, all of which serve as both infectors and reservoirs. *Rickettsiae* are intracellular parasites, similar in size to bacteria, that inhabit the alimentary tract of a wide range of natural hosts. Rickettsial diseases are more common in temperate and tropical climates where humans live in association with arthropods. Infection in humans is incidental (except epidemic typhus) and not necessary for the survival of the rickettsial species. However, once the organism invades a human, it causes a disease that varies in intensity from a benign, self-limiting illness to a disease that is fulminating and fatal.

Lyme Disease

Lyme disease is the most common tick-borne disorder in the United States. It is caused by the spirochete, *Borrelia burgdorferi,* which enters the skin and bloodstream through the saliva and feces of ticks, especially the deer tick. Most cases of Lyme disease are reported in the northeastern United States from southern Maine to northern Virginia. Lyme disease may present in any of three stages. *Stage 1* consists of the tick bite at the time of inoculation, followed in 3 to 31 days by the development of *erythema migrans* at the site of the bite (Fig. 53-10). *Stage 2,* the most serious stage of the disease, is characterized by systemic involvement of neurologic, cardiac, and musculoskeletal systems that appears several weeks after the cutaneous phase is completed. *Stage 3,* or the late stage, includes musculoskeletal pain that involves the tendons, bursae, muscles, and synovia. Arthritis may occur, and late neurologic problems include deafness and chronic encephalopathy.

Table 53-7

Skin Lesions Caused by Arthropods

MECHANISM/CHARACTERISTICS	MANIFESTATIONS	MANAGEMENT
INSECT BITES—FLIES, GNATS, MOSQUITOES, FLEAS		
Mechanism: Foreign protein in insects' saliva introduced when skin is penetrated for a blood-sucking meal Distribution: Almost everywhere—fleas, mosquitoes, ants Suburbs and rural areas—bees Urban areas—hornets, wasps, yellow jackets	Hypersensitivity reaction Papular urticaria Firm papules; may be capped by vesicles or excoriated Little or no reaction in nonsensitized person	Treatment: Use antipruritic agents and baths Administer antihistamines Prevent secondary infection Prevention: Avoid contact Remove focus, such as treating furniture, mattresses, carpets, and pets, where insects may live Apply insect repellent when exposure is anticipated
CHIGGERS—HARVEST MITE		
Mechanism: Attach with claws and secrete a digestive substance that liquefies the host's epidermis Manifestations: Erythematous papules Intense itching	Same as insect bites Favor warm areas of body, especially intertriginous areas and areas covered with clothing	Avoid contact, especially in areas of tall grass and underbrush Apply insect repellant when exposure is anticipated; insecticides such as diazinon can also be sprayed in yards May require systemic steroids for extensive bites
HYMENOPTERANS—BEES, WASPS, HORNETS, YELLOW JACKETS, FIRE ANTS		
Mechanism: Injection of venom through stinging apparatus Venom contains histamine, allergenic proteins, and often a spreading factor, hyaluronidase Severe reactions caused by hypersensitivity and/or multiple stings	Local reaction: small red area, wheal, itching, and heat Systemic reactions: may be mild to severe, including generalized edema, pain, nausea and vomiting, confusion, respiratory embarrassment, and shock	Treatment: Carefully scrape off stinger or pull out stinger as quickly as possible Cleanse with soap and water Apply cool compresses Apply common household product (e.g., lemon juice, paste made with aspirin or baking soda) Administer antihistamines Severe reactions: administer epinephrine, corticosteroids; treat for shock Prevention: Teach child to wear shoes; to avoid wearing bright clothing, flowery prints, shiny jewelry, or perfumed grooming products (cologne, scented hairspray), which might attract the insect; and to avoid places where the insect may be contacted Hypersensitive children should wear medical identification to indicate allergy and therapy needed; family should keep emergency medication and be taught its administration
BLACK WIDOW SPIDER		
Mechanism: Venom injected through a clawlike appendage; has neurotoxic action Characteristics: Spider is shiny black, with a body about 1.25 cm (0.5 inches) long and a red or orange hourglass-shaped marking on underside Avoids light and bites in self-defense	Mild sting at time of bite Area becomes swollen, painful, and erythematous Dizziness, weakness, and abdominal pain May produce delirium, paralysis, seizures, and (if large amount of venom absorbed) death	Treatment: Cleanse wound with antiseptic Apply cool compresses Administer antivenin Administer muscle relaxant, such as calcium gluconate; analgesics and/or sedatives; hydrocortisone or diazepam intravenously Prevention: Teach children to avoid places that harbor the spider (e.g., woodpiles)

Continued

Table 53-7
Skin Lesions Caused by Arthropods—cont'd

MECHANISM/CHARACTERISTICS	MANIFESTATIONS	MANAGEMENT
BROWN RECLUSE SPIDER		
Mechanism: Venom injected via fangs Venom contains powerful necrotoxin Characteristics: Spider is slender, with long legs and body length of 1 to 2 cm; color is fawn to dark brown; recognized by fiddle-shaped mark on head Shy; bites only when annoyed or surprised Prefers dark areas where seldom disturbed	Mild sting at time of bite Transient erythema followed by bleb or blister; mild to severe pain in 2-8 hours; purple, star-shaped area in 3-4 days; necrotic ulceration in 7-14 days (see Fig. 53-9) Systemic reactions may include fever, malaise, restlessness, nausea, vomiting, and joint pain Generalized petechial eruption Wounds heal with scar formation	Treatment: Apply cool compresses locally Administer antibiotics, corticosteroids Relieve pain Wound may require skin graft Prevention: Teach children to avoid possible nesting sites
SCORPIONS		
Mechanism: Sting by means of a hooked caudal stinger that discharges venom Venom of more venomous species contains hemolysins, endotheliolysins, and neurotoxins Characteristics: Usual habitat is southwestern United States	Intense local pain, erythema, numbness, burning, restlessness, vomiting Ascending motor paralysis with seizures, weakness, rapid pulse, excessive salivation, thirst, dysuria, pulmonary edema, coma, and death Some species produce only local tissue reaction with swelling at puncture site (distinctive) Symptoms subside in a few hours Deaths occur among children under 4 years of age, usually in first 24 hours	Treatment: Delay absorption of venom by keeping child quiet; place involved area in dependent position Administer antivenin Relieve pain Admit to pediatric intensive care unit for surveillance Prevention: Teach children to avoid possible nesting sites
TICKS		
Mechanism: In process of sucking blood, head and mouth parts are buried in skin Characteristics: Feed on blood of mammals Significant in humans because of pathologic organism carried May be vectors of various infectious diseases, such as Rocky Mountain spotted fever, Q fever, tularemia, relapsing fever, Lyme disease, tick paralysis Must attach and feed for 1-2 hours to transmit disease Usual habitat is very wooded area	Tick usually attached to skin, head embedded Produce firm, discrete, intensely pruritic nodules at site of attachment May cause urticaria or persistent localized edema	Treatment: Grasp tick with tweezers (forceps) as close as possible to point of attachment Pull straight up with steady, even pressure; if bare hands, use a tissue to touch tick during removal; wash hands thoroughly with soap and water Remove any remaining part (e.g., head) with sterile needle Cleanse wounds with soap and disinfectant Prevention: Teach children to avoid areas where prevalent Inspect skin (especially scalp) after being in wooded areas

Diagnostic Evaluation
Diagnosis is best made clinically during the early stages by recognizing the characteristic rash, erythema migrans. Serologic testing may be used to establish the diagnosis in later stages of the disease.

Therapeutic Management
Early and appropriate treatment is essential to prevent complications. Children over 8 years of age are treated with oral doxycycline; amoxicillin is recommended for children under 8 years of age (American Academy of Pediatrics,

Table 53-8

Eruptions Caused by Rickettsiae

DISORDER/ORGANISM/HOST	MANIFESTATIONS	MANAGEMENT	COMMENTS
Rocky Mountain spotted fever—*R. rickettsii* Arthropod: tick Transmission: tick Mammal source: wild rodents; dogs	Gradual onset: fever, malaise, anorexia, myalgia Abrupt onset: rapid temperature elevation, chills, vomiting, myalgia, severe headache Maculopapular or petechial rash primarily on extremities (ankles and wrists) but may spread to other areas, characteristically on palms and soles	Control: protection from tick bite by wearing proper apparel, tick repellent Tetracycline or chloramphenicol Vigorous supportive therapy	Usually self-limited in children Onset in children may resemble any infectious disease Severe disease rare in children Children and dogs should be inspected regularly if they play in wooded areas See Table 53-7 for management of ticks
Epidemic typhus—*R. prowazekii* Arthropod: body louse Transmission: infected feces into broken skin Mammal source: humans	Abrupt onset of chills, fever, diffuse myalgia, headache, malaise Maculopapular rash becomes petechial 4 to 7 days later, spreading from trunk outward	Control: immediate destruction of vectors Tetracycline or chloramphenicol Supportive treatment	Patient should be isolated until deloused See discussion on p. 1768 for management of pediculosis Excreta from infected lice also in dust—disinfect patient's clothing, bedding, and possessions and wash in hot water
Endemic typhus—*R. typhi* Arthropod: rat fleas or lice Transmission: flea bite; inhaling or ingesting flea excreta Mammal source: rats	Headache, arthralgia, backache followed by fever; may last 9-14 days Maculopapular rash after 1-8 days of fever; begins in trunk and spreads to periphery; rarely involves face, palms, soles	Control: eliminate rat reservoir, insect vectors, or both Tetracycline or chloramphenicol Supportive treatment	Fairly common in United States Shorter duration than epidemic typhus Mild, seldom fatal illness Difficult to distinguish from epidemic typhus
Rickettsialpox—*R. akari* Arthropod: mouse mite Transmission: mite Mammal source: house mouse	Maculopapular rash following primary lesion; eschar at site of bite; fever, chills, headache	Control: eradication of rodent reservoir and mite vector Tetracycline or chloramphenicol Supportive treatment	Self-limited nonfatal disease Endemic in New York City Found in many cities in United States

Committee on Infectious Diseases, 2003). For patients allergic to penicillin, alternative drugs include cefuroxime and erythromycin (Wade, 2000). Most experts treat individuals with early Lyme disease for 14 to 21 days. Treatment of erythema migrans almost always prevents development of later stages of Lyme disease.

In 1998 the FDA licensed a Lyme disease vaccine for people 15 to 70 years of age. However, the vaccine was withdrawn in 2002 because of low market demand, and it is no longer available.

Nursing Care Management

The major thrust of nursing care should be educating parents to protect their children from exposure to ticks. Children should avoid tick-infested areas or wear light-colored clothing so that ticks can be spotted easily, tuck pant legs into socks, and wear a long-sleeved shirt tucked into

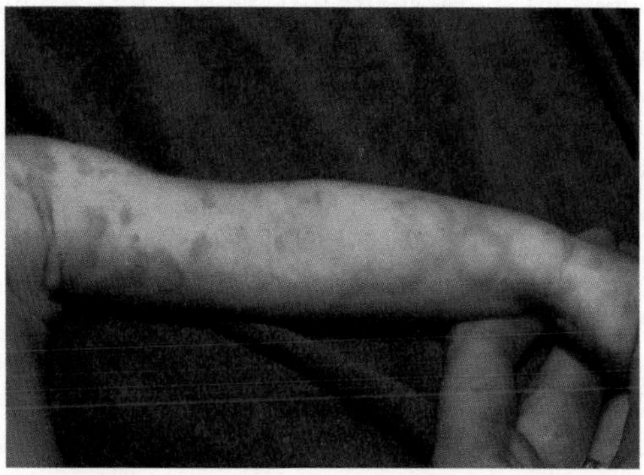

Fig. 53-10 Lyme disease. Note annular red rings in erythema migrans. (From Weston WL, Lane AT: *Color textbook of pediatric dermatology,* St Louis, 1991, Mosby.)

pants when in wooded areas. Grass and shrubbery where ticks may be lurking should be avoided, and children and adults should walk in the center of trails. Parents and children need to perform regular tick checks when they are in infested areas. After a hike, a bare skin check (with special attention to the scalp, neck, armpits, and groin areas) is important to spot any ticks and remove them. Parents should also be alert for signs of the skin lesion, especially if their children have been in tick-infested areas. Insect repellents containing diethyltoluamide (DEET) and permethrin can protect against ticks, but parents should use these chemicals cautiously. Although there have been reports of serious neurologic complications in children resulting from frequent and excessive application of DEET repellants, the risk is low when they are used properly. Products with DEET should be applied sparingly according to label instructions and not applied to a child's face, hands, or any areas of irritated skin. After the child returns indoors, treated skin should be washed with soap and water. Information about Lyme disease can be obtained from the American Lyme Disease Foundation, Inc.*

Animal Bites

Animal bites are common in childhood. However, children are bitten more often by animals belonging to the family or to neighbors than by stray animals. More than half the victims of dog bites are less than 5 years of age; boys are bitten more frequently than girls (Bernardo et al, 2000). Most dog or cat injuries are to the upper extremities. Small children are likely to be bitten or scratched on the head, face, and neck because they tend to put their heads near the animal's head and flail their arms rather than protecting their heads. Animal bites are potentially serious because of the likelihood of significant infection. Injuries vary in intensity from small puncture wounds to complete evulsion of tissue that is associated with significant crush injury.

Therapeutic Management

General wound care consists of rinsing the wound with copious amounts of saline or Ringer's lactate under pressure via a large syringe and washing the surrounding skin with mild soap. A clean pressure dressing is applied, and the extremity is elevated if the wound is bleeding. Medical evaluation is advised, because there is danger of tetanus and rabies, although dogs in most urban areas must be immunized against rabies. Bites from wild animals, such as squirrels, bats, raccoons, foxes, and skunks, are also dangerous.

Prophylactic antibiotics are indicated for puncture wounds and wounds in areas that may prove to be cosmetically or functionally impaired if infected. Extensive lacerations are debrided and loosely sutured to allow for drainage in the event of infection. Tetanus toxoid is administered according to standard guidelines (see Immunizations, Chapter 36), and rabies protocol is followed (see Rabies, Chapter 51). Injuries to poorly vascularized areas, such as the hands, are more likely to become infected than those in more vascularized areas, such as the face; puncture wounds are more apt to become infected than lacerations.

Nursing Care Management

The most important aspect related to animal bites is prevention. Children should understand animal behavior and develop respect for animals (Community Focus box). Parents should monitor their children's behavior with a dog and instruct them not to tease or surprise a dog, invade its territory, interfere with its feeding or sleeping, take its toy, or interact with a sick or injured dog or a dog with pups. Parents who are considering getting a pet, especially a dog, for themselves or their children should select a dog that has a high level of sociability with children and that is unlikely to be a danger to their children.

Human Bites

Children often acquire lacerations from the teeth of other humans in rough play, during fights, or as victims of child abuse. Many preschool children bite others out of frustration or anger. Because human dental plaque and gingiva harbor pathogenic organisms, all human bites should receive attention. Delayed treatment increases the risk of infection.

If the laceration is less than one-quarter inch in length, the wound can be treated at home. The wound is washed vigorously with soap and water, and a pressure dressing is

Community Focus

ANIMAL SAFETY

- Teach children to avoid strange animals, especially animals who are wild or appear to be sick, frightened, or injured. It is very important that children do not approach dogs who are chained up or behind a fence, as they can be particularly aggressive.
- If a child would like to pet a friend's or neighbor's animal, they should always ask permission first and let the dog see and sniff them before proceeding.
- If two animals are fighting, children should never try to break up the fight. They should call an adult that they know for help.
- Teach children that it is not OK to mistreat pets. They should never hit, kick, or pull on an animal's tail. They should also never disturb an animal who is eating, sleeping, has a special toy, or caring for puppies or kittens.
- If confronted with a threatening dog, avoid eye contact and remain motionless with your hands at your sides until the dog leaves the area. Visit www.NoDogBites.org for more suggestions.
- Do not let children walk dogs they cannot control should the animal try to run.
- Do not adopt animals whose care will be the responsibility of one or more children. All animals are ultimately the responsibility of the adults in the home.
- Make sure that your pets are up to date on all of their required vaccinations.
- Spay or neuter your pets; it keeps them healthier and makes them less likely to bite.
- Train and socialize your dog for appropriate behavior using humane, reward-based training methods.

From The Humane Society of the United States, 2005.

*Mill Pond Offices 293, Route 100, Suite 204, Somers, NY 10589; phone: 914-277-6970 or 800-876-LYME, fax: 914-277-6974; Web site: www.aldf.com.

applied to stop bleeding. Ice applications minimize discomfort and swelling. Increased pain or redness at the wound site is an indication that the child should receive medical attention for antibiotic therapy. Tetanus toxoid is needed if the child is insufficiently immunized. Wounds greater than one-quarter inch should receive medical attention.

Cat Scratch Disease

Cat scratch disease is the most common cause of regional lymphadenitis in children and adolescents. It usually follows the scratch or bite of an animal (a cat or kitten in 99% of cases). The disease is usually a benign, self-limiting illness that resolves spontaneously in about 2 to 4 months. Diagnosis is made on the basis of (1) history of contact with a cat or kitten, (2) the presence of regional lymphadenopathy for several days, and (3) serologic identification of the causative organism by indirect fluorescent antibody assay or polymerase chain reaction test. The disease may persist for several months before gradual resolution. In some children, especially those who are immunocompromised, the adenitis may progress to suppuration and serious complications. Treatment is primarily supportive, but antibiotic therapy may hasten the resolution of adenopathy in the disease (Centers for Disease Control and Prevention, 2002).

MISCELLANEOUS SKIN DISORDERS

A number of miscellaneous skin lesions occur in children. Some occur as a result of congenital disorders and are inherited as an autosomal dominant trait (Table 53-9). *Ichthyoses* are a heterogeneous group of disorders characterized by scaling that create challenging problems in treatment. These disorders are not discussed in detail here because of their wide variability.

SKIN DISORDERS ASSOCIATED WITH SPECIFIC AGE GROUPS

Several common dermatologic conditions are confined to children in specific age groups. These conditions include diaper dermatitis, atopic dermatitis, and seborrheic dermatitis, which occur predominantly in infants, and acne, which is most common in adolescence.

Diaper Dermatitis

Diaper dermatitis is common in infants and is one of several acute inflammatory skin disorders caused either directly or indirectly by the wearing of diapers. The peak age of occurrence is 9 to 12 months of age, and the incidence is greater in bottle-fed infants than in breastfed infants.

Pathophysiology and Clinical Manifestations

Diaper dermatitis is caused by prolonged and repetitive contact with an irritant (e.g., urine, feces, soaps, detergents, ointments, and friction). Although the irritant in the majority of cases is urine and feces, the specific components that contribute to irritation include a combination of factors.

Prolonged contact of the skin with diaper wetness produces higher friction, greater abrasion damage, increased transepidermal permeability, and increased microbial counts. Healthy skin is less resistant to potential irritants.

Although ammonia was once thought to cause diaper rash because of the association between the strong odor on diapers and dermatitis, ammonia alone is not sufficient. The irritant quality of urine is related to an increase in pH from the breakdown of urea in the presence of fecal urease. The increased pH promotes the activity of fecal enzymes, principally the proteases and lipases, which act as irritants. Fecal enzymes also increase the permeability of skin to bile salts, another potential irritant in feces.

The eruption of diaper dermatitis is manifested primarily on convex surfaces or in folds. The lesions represent a variety of types and configurations. Eruptions involving the skin in most intimate contact with the diaper (e.g., the convex surfaces of buttocks, inner thighs, mons pubis, and scrotum) but sparing the folds are likely to be caused by chemical irritants, especially from urine and feces (Fig. 53-11). Other causes are detergents or soaps from inadequately rinsed cloth diapers or the chemicals in disposable wipes. Perianal involvement is usually the result of chemical irritation from feces, especially diarrheal stools. *Candida albicans* infection produces perianal inflammation and a maculopapular rash with satellite lesions that may cross the inguinal fold (Fig. 53-12). It is seen in up to 90% of infants with chronic diaper

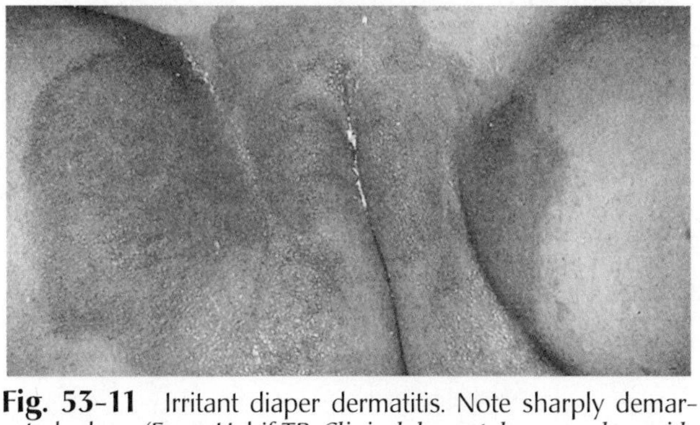

Fig. 53-11 Irritant diaper dermatitis. Note sharply demarcated edges. (From Habif TP: *Clinical dermatology: a color guide to diagnosis and therapy*, ed 3, St Louis, 1996, Mosby.)

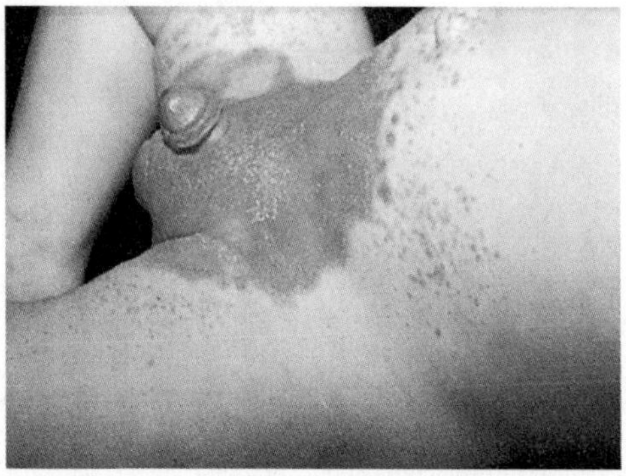

Fig. 53-12 Candidiasis of diaper area. Note beefy red central erythema with satellite pustules. (From Weston WL, Lane AT, Morelli JG: *Color textbook of pediatric dermatology*, ed 2, St Louis, 1996, Mosby.)

Table 53-9

Miscellaneous Skin Disorders

DISEASE/CAUSATIVE AGENT	LOCAL MANIFESTATIONS	MANAGEMENT	COMMENTS
Urticaria—usually allergic response to drugs or infection	Development of wheals Vary in size and configuration and tend to appear quickly, spread irregularly, and fade within a few hours May be constant or intermittent, sparse or profuse, small or large, discrete or confluent May be acute, chronic, or recurrent in acute attacks	Local soothing and antipruritic applications Antihistamines Epinephrine or ephedrine Cortisone in severe cases Severe upper respiratory involvement may require tracheostomy	Known etiologic agents should be avoided May be accompanied by malaise, fever, lymphadenopathy Severe cases may involve mucous membranes, internal organs, and joints Obstruction to air passages is a medical emergency
Intertrigo—mechanical trauma and aggravating factors of excessive heat, moisture, and sweat retention	Red, inflamed, moist, partially denuded, marginated areas, the shapes of which are determined by location Appears where opposing skin surfaces rub together, such as intergluteal folds, groin, neck, and axilla Excessive moisture and obesity are often factors	Affected areas kept clean and dry Skinfolds kept separated with a generous supply of nonmedicated powder Expose to air and light Remove excess clothing	A form of diaper irritation Prevent recurrence by keeping susceptible areas clean and dry Frequently associated with overheating from too much clothing; common in trached patients with short necks and copious secretions
Psoriasis—unknown; hereditary predisposition; may be triggered by stress	Round, thick, dry, reddish patches covered with coarse, silvery scales over trunk and extremities; first lesions commonly appear in scalp; facial lesions more common in children than in adults Affected cells proliferate at a much more rapid rate than normal cells	Tar preparations in combination with ultraviolet (UV) B light or natural sunlight Topical corticosteroids Topical vitamin D analog calcipotriene Phenol and saline solutions followed by a tar shampoo to remove scales Keratolytic agents (salicylic acid) Acitretin Emollients may provide relief	Uncommon in children under age 6 years Persons are otherwise healthy individuals Coal tar acts synergistically with ultraviolet light Keratolytic agents enhance absorption of corticosteroids Humidifiers may help in winter
Alopecia* Alopecia areata	Sudden onset of asymptomatic, noninflammatory, round, bald patches in hairy parts of body	Psychologic support Inducement of allergic contact dermatitis to stimulate growth of hair Minoxidil (peripheral vasodilator)	Family history in 10%-26% of cases Some concern regarding drug therapy safety Refer to support groups*
Traumatic alopecia	Traction alopecia around scalp margins from tight hair styles (e.g., braids, pony tails, corn rows)	Counseling regarding hair styling, use of hair cosmetics, hot combs, rollers	More prevalent in black children and adolescents Prolonged traction can produce fibrosis of hair root and permanent loss
Trichotillomania	Compulsive hair pulling	Determine and treat cause	Chronic hair pulling may require psychologic therapy
Tinea capitis	See Table 53-5	See Table 53-5	See Table 53-5

*National Alopecia Areata Foundation, 710 C St., Suite 11, San Rafael, CA 94901; phone: 415-456-4644; fax: 415-456-4274; e-mail: 74301.1642@compuserve.com.

Table 53-9

Miscellaneous Skin Disorders—cont'd

DISEASE/CAUSATIVE AGENT	LOCAL MANIFESTATIONS	MANAGEMENT	COMMENTS
Erythema multiforme (Stevens-Johnson syndrome)—unknown; associated with ingestion of some drugs; often follows upper respiratory infection	Erythematous papular rash Lesions enlarge by peripheral expansion; develop central vesicle Involves most skin surfaces except scalp May extend to mucous membranes, especially oral, ocular, and urethral	Symptomatic and supportive Maintain adequate intake of fluids (oral or intravenous), calories, and protein Moist wound care, hydrogels such as Carragauze, Vaseline, or Aquaphor Appropriate treatment of complications Diligent monitoring of urine volume and specific gravity, hemoglobin and hematocrit, serum electrolyte levels, total body weight	Rash often preceded by fever and malaise Complications include renal failure and severe eye disease Respiratory involvement in a number of cases Self-limiting, but recovery may extend for weeks; skin lesions may subside without scarring; mucous membrane lesions may persist for months Recurrence rate 20%; mortality rate as high as 10%
Neurofibromatosis—inherited disorder; autosomal dominant inheritance pattern	Café-au-lait spots, pigmented nevi, axillary freckling Slow-growing cutaneous and subcutaneous neurofibromas	Symptomatic treatment of associated manifestations (e.g., speech defects, seizures, skeletal defects [scoliosis, kyphosis], learning disabilities) Surgical removal of troublesome tumors	High mutation rate Refer to support groups† Family needs to know about genetic implications

†National Neurofibromatosis Foundation, Inc., 95 Pine St., 16th Floor, New York, NY 10005; phone: 800-323-7938 or 212-344-6633; fax: 212-747-0004; e-mail: nnff@nf.org; website: www.nf.org.

dermatitis and should be considered in diaper rashes that are recalcitrant to treatment.

Nursing Care Management

Nursing interventions are aimed at altering the three factors that produce dermatitis—wetness, pH, and fecal irritants. The most significant factor amenable to intervention is the moist environment created in the diaper area. Changing the diaper as soon as it becomes wet eliminates a large part of the problem, and removing the diaper to expose healthy skin to air facilitates drying. The use of a hair dryer or heat lamp is not recommended because these devices can cause burns.

Diaper construction has a significant impact on the incidence and severity of diaper dermatitis. Superabsorbent disposable paper diapers reduce diaper dermatitis. They contain an absorbent gelling material that binds water tightly to decrease skin wetness, maintains pH control by providing a buffering capacity, and decreases skin irritation by preventing mixing of urine and feces in the diaper. Another advance in diapers is the addition of an inner layer or top sheet that is impregnated with petrolatum (as in Ultra Pampers with Tender Touch Liner*).

Guidelines for controlling diaper rash are presented in the Home Care box. A common misconception about using cornstarch on skin is that it promotes the growth of *Candida albicans.* Neither cornstarch nor talc promotes the growth of fungi under conditions normally found in the diaper area. Cornstarch is more effective in reducing friction and tends to cake less than talc when the skin is wet. On the basis of these properties and its safety in terms of inhalation injury, cornstarch is the preferred product. Talc should not be used.

*Manufactured by Procter & Gamble Company, Cincinnati, OH 45224; phone: 800-285-6064; Web site: www.pampers.com.

Atopic Dermatitis (Eczema)

Eczema or *eczematous inflammation of the skin* refers to a descriptive category of dermatologic diseases and not to a specific etiology. *Atopic dermatitis (AD)* is a type of pruritic eczema that usually begins during infancy and is associated with allergy with a hereditary tendency *(atopy).* AD occurs in three forms based on the age of the child and the distribution of lesions:

1. **Infantile (infantile eczema)**—Usually begins at 2 to 6 months of age; generally undergoes spontaneous remission by 3 years of age.
2. **Childhood**—May follow the infantile form; occurs at 2 to 3 years of age; 90% of children have manifestations by age 5 years.
3. **Preadolescent and adolescent**—Begins at about 12 years of age; may continue into the early adult years or indefinitely.

Home Care

CONTROLLING DIAPER RASH

Keep skin dry.*

Use superabsorbent disposable diapers to reduce skin wetness.

If using cloth diapers, use only overwraps that allow air to circulate; avoid rubber pants.

Change diapers as soon as soiled, especially with stool, whenever possible, preferably once during the night.

Expose healthy or only slightly irritated skin to air, not heat, to dry completely.

Apply ointment, such as zinc oxide or petrolatum, to protect skin, especially if skin is very red or has moist, open areas.

Do not remove skin barrier cream with each diaper change; remove waste material and reapply skin barrier cream.

To completely remove ointment, especially zinc oxide, use mineral oil; do not wash vigorously.

Do not overwash the skin, especially with perfumed soaps or commercial wipes, which may be irritating.

May use a moisturizer or nonsoap cleanser, such as cold cream or Cetaphil, to wipe urine from skin.

Gently wipe stool from skin using water and mild soap, such as Dove.

When traveling, fill an old baby wipe container with soft paper towels and warm water.

*Powder helps keep the skin dry, but talc is very dangerous if breathed into the lungs. Plain cornstarch or cornstarch-based powder is safer. When using any powder product, shake it first into your hand, and then apply it to the diaper area. Store the container away from the infant's reach; keep the container closed when not in use.

The diagnosis of AD is based on a combination of history and morphologic findings (Box 53-3 and Fig. 53-13). Children with AD have a lower threshold for cutaneous itching, and many authorities believe the dermatologic manifestations appear subsequent to scratching from the intense pruritus. For example, infants rub their faces against bed linen, and their crawling (a form of scratching) results in irritation of knees and elbows. Lesions disappear if the scratching is stopped.

The majority of children with infantile AD have a family history of eczema, asthma, food allergies, or allergic rhinitis, which strongly supports a genetic predisposition. The cause is unknown but appears to be related to abnormal function of the skin, including alterations in perspiration, peripheral vascular function, and heat tolerance. Manifestations of the chronic disease improve in humid climates and get worse in the fall and winter, when homes are heated and environmental humidity is lower. The disorder can be controlled but not cured.

Therapeutic Management

The major goals of management are to (1) hydrate the skin, (2) relieve pruritus, (3) reduce flare-ups or inflammation, and (4) prevent and control secondary infection. The general measures for managing AD focus on reducing pruritus, as well as other aspects of the disease. Management strategies include avoiding exposure to skin irritants or allergens, avoiding overheating, avoiding skin hydration, and administrating medications such as antihistamines, topical steroids, and (sometimes) mild sedatives as indicated.

Enhancing skin hydration and preventing dry, flaky skin is accomplished in a number of ways, depending on the child's skin characteristics and individual needs. A tepid bath with a mild soap (Dove or Neutrogena), no soap, or an emulsifying oil, followed immediately by application of an emollient (within 3 minutes), assists in trapping moisture and preventing moisture loss. Bubble baths and harsh soaps should be avoided. The bath may need to be repeated once or twice daily, depending on the child's status; excessive bathing without emollient application only dries out the skin. Some lotions are not effective, and emollients should be chosen carefully to prevent excessive skin drying. Aquaphor, Cetaphil, and Eucerin are acceptable lotions for skin hydration. A nighttime bath, followed by emollient application and dressing in soft cotton pajamas, may help alleviate most nighttime pruritus.

BOX 53-3

Clinical Manifestations of Atopic Dermatitis

Distribution of Lesions

Infantile form—generalized, especially cheeks, scalp, trunk, and extensor surfaces of extremities (see Fig. 53-13)

Childhood form—flexural areas (antecubital and popliteal fossae, neck), wrists, ankles, and feet

Preadolescent and adolescent form—face, sides of neck, hands, feet, face, and antecubital and popliteal fossae (to a lesser extent)

Appearance of Lesions

Infantile form:
- Erythema
- Vesicles
- Papules
- Weeping
- Oozing
- Crusting
- Scaling
- Often symmetric

Childhood form:
- Symmetric involvement
- Clusters of small erythematous or flesh-colored papules or minimally scaling patches
- Dry and may be hyperpigmented
- Lichenification (thickened skin with accentuation of creases)
- Keratosis pilaris (follicular hyperkeratosis) common

Adolescent/adult form:
- Same as childhood manifestations
- Dry, thick lesions (lichenified plaques) common
- Confluent papules

Other Physical Manifestations

Intense itching

Unaffected skin dry and rough

African-American children likely to exhibit more papular and/or follicular lesions than Caucasian children

May exhibit one or more of the following:
- Lymphadenopathy, especially near affected sites
- Increased palmar creases (many cases)
- Atopic pleats (extra line or groove of lower eyelid)
- Prone to cold hands
- Pityriasis alba (small, poorly defined areas of hypopigmentation)
- Facial pallor (especially around nose, mouth, and ears)
- Bluish discoloration beneath eyes ("allergic shiners")
- Increased susceptibility to unusual cutaneous infections (especially viral)

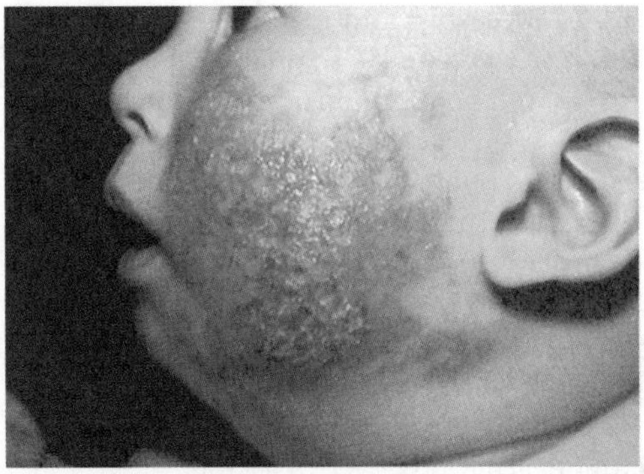

Fig. 53-13 Infantile atopic dermatitis with oozing and crusting of lesions. (From Weston WL, Lane AT, Morelli JG: *Color textbook of pediatric dermatology,* ed 3, St Louis, 2002, Mosby.)

Sometimes colloid baths, such as the addition of 2 cups of cornstarch to a tub of warm water, provide temporary relief of itching and may help the child sleep if given before bedtime. Cool wet compresses are soothing to the skin and provide antiseptic protection.

Oral antihistamine drugs (hydroxyzine [Atarax] or diphenhydramine [Benadryl]) usually relieve moderate or severe pruritus. Nonsedating antihistamines such as loratadine (Claritin) or fexofenadine (Allegra) may be preferred for daytime pruritis relief. Because pruritus increases at night, a mildly sedating antihistamine may be needed.

Occasional flare-ups require the use of topical steroids to diminish inflammation. Low-, moderate-, or high-potency topical corticosteroids are prescribed, depending on the degree of involvement, the area of the body to be treated, the age of the child, the potential for local side effects (striae, skin atrophy, and pigment changes), and the type of vehicle to be used (e.g., cream, lotion, or ointment). Topical immunomodulators, a new nonsteroidal treatment for atopic dermatitis, are best used at the beginning of a flare-up just as the skin becomes read and itches. Two new immunomodulator medications used in children with AD are tacrolimus and pimecrolimus (Kronemyer, 2003). Tacrolimus is available in two ointment strengths (0.03% and 0.1%); the 0.03% concentration has been approved for use in children 2 years of age and older. Tacrolimus is recommended for intermittent therapy in patients who are not adequately responsive to, or are intolerant of, conventional therapy (Yetman & Parks, 2002). Pimecrolimus is available in a 1% cream that has no systemic accumulation or effects. This drug is approved for use in children with mild to moderate AD. Both drugs can be used freely on the face without worrying about steroid side effects

If secondary skin infections occur in children with AD, these infections are managed with appropriate systemic antibiotics.

Nursing Care Management

Assessment

Assessment of the child with AD includes a family history for evidence of atopy, a history of previous involvement, and any environmental or dietary factors associated with the present and previous exacerbations. The skin lesions are examined for type, distribution, and evidence of secondary infection. Parents are interviewed regarding the child's behavior, especially in relation to scratching, irritability, and sleeping patterns. Exploration of the family's feelings and methods of coping is also important.

Nursing Diagnoses

Nursing diagnoses identified for the child with AD include the following:

- Impaired skin integrity related to eczematous lesions
- Risk for infection related to risk of secondary infection of primary lesions
- Interrupted family processes related to the child's discomfort and lengthy therapy

Others diagnoses will be apparent in individual cases.

Plan of Care and Implementation

The objectives for nursing care of the child with AD and the child's family are as follows:

1. Child will experience no or minimal pruritus.
2. Child will receive appropriate treatment for skin hydration.
3. Child will experience no complications.
4. Child and family will receive adequate support.

The nursing care of the child with AD is challenging. Controlling the intense pruritus is imperative if the disorder is to be successfully managed, because scratching leads to new lesions and may cause secondary infection. In addition to the medical regimen, other measures can be taken to prevent or minimize the scratching. Fingernails and toenails are cut short, kept clean, and filed frequently to prevent sharp edges. Gloves or cotton stockings can be placed over the hands and pinned to shirtsleeves. One-piece outfits with long sleeves and long pants also decrease direct contact with the skin. If gloves or socks are used, the child needs time to be free from such restrictions. An excellent time to remove gloves, socks, or other protective devices is during the bath or after receiving sedative or antipruritic medication.

Conditions that increase itching are eliminated when possible. Woolen clothes or blankets, rough fabrics, and furry stuffed animals are removed from the child's environment. Because heat and humidity cause perspiration (which intensifies itching), proper dress for climatic conditions is essential. Pruritus is often precipitated by exposure to the irritant effects of certain components of common products such as soaps, detergents, fabric softeners, perfumes, and powders. Most children experience less itching when soft cotton fabrics are worn next to the skin. During cold months, synthetic fabrics (not wool) should be used for overcoats, hats, gloves, and snowsuits. Exposure to latex products, such as gloves and balloons, should also be avoided.

Clothes and sheets are laundered in a mild detergent and rinsed thoroughly in clear water (without fabric softeners or antistatic chemicals). Putting the clothes through a second complete wash cycle without using detergent reduces the amount of residue remaining in the fabric.

Preventing infection is usually accomplished by preventing scratching. Baths are given as prescribed, the water is kept tepid, and soaps (except as indicated) and bubble baths are avoided, as well as oils or powders. Skinfolds and diaper areas need frequent cleansing with plain water. A room humidifier or vaporizer may benefit children with extremely dry skin. The skin lesions are examined for signs of infection, usually the presence of honey-colored crusts with surrounding erythema. Any signs of infection are reported to the practitioner.

NURSE ALERT If the child is being treated with baths for hydration, it is imperative that the emollient preparation be applied immediately following bathing (while the skin is still slightly moist) to prevent drying. ■

Wet soaks and compresses are applied and medications for pruritus or infection are administered as directed. The family is given explicit instructions on the preparation and use of soaks, special baths, and topical medications, including the order of application if more than one is prescribed. It is important to emphasize that one thick application of topical medication is *not* equivalent to several thin applications, and that excessive use of an agent (particularly steroids) can be hazardous. If children have difficulty remaining still for a 10- or 15-minute soak, bath, or dressing application, these can be carried out at naptime or when the child is engrossed in watching television, listening to a story, or playing with tub toys.

Because adequate rest is important for these children, who are usually fretful and irritable, planning meals, baths, medications, and treatments during periods when they are awake is essential. Sleepy, tired children are normally cranky, and such behavior only intensifies the urge to scratch. During periods of irritability, these children tend to have a poor appetite, which is worsened by restriction of their usual foods.

Diet modification is another source of frustration to parents. When a hypoallergenic diet is prescribed, parents need help to understand the reason for the diet and the guidelines for avoiding hyperallergic foods (Guidelines box). Because hypoallergenic diets take time before visible effects are apparent, parents need reassurance that results may not be seen immediately. If airborne allergens make eczema worse, the family is counseled about "allergy proofing" the home.

Family Support

Parents are assured that the lesions will not produce scarring (unless secondarily infected) and that the disease is not contagious. However, the child may have repeated exacerbations and remissions. Spontaneous and permanent remission takes place at approximately 2 to 3 years of age in most children with the infantile disorder.

During acute phases, emotional stress can become intense for the family. They need time to discuss negative feelings and to be reassured that these feelings are normal. Stress tends to aggravate the severity of the condition. Therefore efforts to relieve as much anxiety as possible in both the parents and the child have beneficial emotional and physical effects.

Evaluation

The effectiveness of nursing interventions is determined by continual reassessment and evaluation of care based on the following observational guidelines:

1. Observe child's behavior, clothing, and activities.
2. Examine skin for evidence of dryness.
3. Examine skin lesions for evidence of secondary infection.
4. Interview family members and encourage dialogue regarding the child and aspects of care.

Expected outcomes include the following:

1. Child does not scratch and rests or plays quietly.
2. Skin appears well hydrated.
3. There is no evidence of secondary infection.
4. Family members comply with the therapeutic regimen, freely discuss their feelings and concerns, and appear to be coping with the inconveniences imposed by the disorder (specify).

Guidelines

PREVENTING ATOPY IN CHILDREN

Identify Children at Risk

Family history of allergy
Increased IgE in cord blood and postnatal serum
Dry, flaky skin

Prenatal Precautions (Last Trimester)

Avoid any known food allergens
Avoid milk and other dairy products, peanuts, and eggs
Minimize ingestion of other hyperallergenic foods

Postnatal Precautions

Breast milk or casein/whey hydrolysate formula (e.g., Nutramigen, Pregestimil, Alimentum) exclusively for at least 6 months
No solid food for first 6 months
No cow's milk or soy formula for 12 months
No egg, fish, corn, citrus, peanuts, nuts, or chocolate for 12 to 18 months
One new food added at 5- to 7-day intervals to identify possible reaction

Environmental Control

Limited exposure to dust, molds, furry animals, and cigarette smoke

Data from Johnstone D: Strategy for intervention of food allergy in infants, *Int Pediatr* 4(4):319-325, 1989; Zeiger R et al: Effectiveness of dietary manipulation in the prevention of food allergy in infants, part II, *J Allergy Clin Immunol* 78(1, pt 2):224-238, 1986; and Wood RA: Prospects for the prevention of allergy in children, *Curr Opin Pediatr* 8(6):601-605, 1995.

Seborrheic Dermatitis

Seborrheic dermatitis is a chronic, recurrent, inflammatory reaction of the skin. It occurs most commonly on the scalp (cradle cap) but may involve the eyelids (blepharitis), external ear canal (otitis externa), nasolabial folds, and inguinal region. The cause is unknown, although it is more common in early infancy, when sebum production is increased. The lesions are characteristically thick, adherent, yellowish, scaly, oily patches that may or may not be mildly pruritic. Unlike atopic dermatitis, seborrheic dermatitis is not associated with a positive family history for allergy and is common in infants shortly after birth and in adolescents after puberty. Diagnosis is made primarily on the basis of the appearance and the location of the crusts or scales.

Nursing Care Management

Cradle cap may be prevented with adequate scalp hygiene. Not infrequently, parents omit shampooing the infant's hair for fear of damaging the "soft spots," or fontanels. The nurse should discuss how to shampoo the infant's hair and emphasize that the fontanel is like skin anywhere else on the body—it does not puncture or tear with mild pressure.

When seborrheic lesions are present, the treatment is directed at removing the crusts. Parents are taught the appropriate procedure to clean the scalp. Education may need to include a demonstration. Shampooing should be done daily with a mild soap or commercial baby shampoo; medicated shampoos are not necessary, but an antiseborrheic shampoo containing sulfur and salicylic acid may be used. Shampoo is applied to the scalp and allowed to remain on the scalp until the crusts are softened. Then the scalp is thoroughly rinsed. A fine-tooth comb or a soft facial brush after shampooing helps remove the loosened crusts from the strands of hair after shampooing.

Acne

Case Study: Acne Vulgaris

Acne vulgaris is the most common skin problem treated by physicians during adolescence. Acne involves anatomic, physiologic, biochemical, genetic, immunologic, and psychologic factors.

One half of the adolescent population experiences acne by the end of the teenage years. Although the disorder can appear before age 10 years, the peak incidence occurs in middle to late adolescence (at age 16 to 17 years in girls and 17 to 18 years in boys). It is more common in boys than in girls. The degree to which an individual is affected may range from nothing more than a few isolated comedones to a severe inflammatory reaction. Although the disease is self-limited and not life threatening, it has great significance to the adolescent. Health professionals should not underestimate the impact that acne has on teens.

Numerous factors affect the development and course of acne. Its distribution in families and a high degree of concordance in identical twins suggest hereditary factors. Premenstrual flares of acne occur in nearly 70% of adolescent girls, suggesting a hormonal cause. Studies do not indicate a clear association between stress and acne, but adolescents commonly cite stress as a cause for acne outbreaks. Cosmetics containing lanolin, petrolatum, vegetable oils, lauryl alcohol, butylstearate, and oleic acid can increase comedome production. Exposure to oils in cooking grease can be a precursor in adolescents who work over fast-food restaurant hot oils. There is no known link between dietary intake and the development or worsening of acne.

Pathophysiology

Acne is a disease that involves the *pilosebaceous follicles* (the hair follicle and sebaceous gland complex) of the face, neck, chest, and upper back. Three pathophysiologic factors are involved in the development of acne: excessive sebum production, comedogenesis, and the overgrowth of *Propionibacterium acnes* (Mancini, 2000).

Comedogenesis (formation of comedones) results in a noninflammatory lesion that may be either an open comedone ("blackhead") or a closed comedone ("whitehead"). Inflammation occurs with the proliferation of *P. acnes,* which draws in neutrophils causing inflammatory papules, pustules, nodules, and cysts (Fig. 53-14).

A

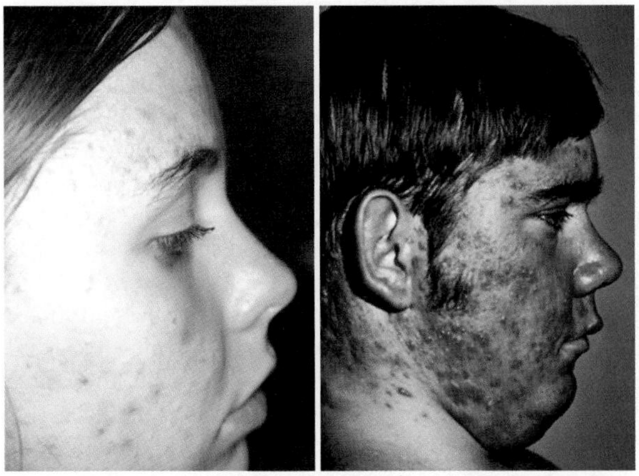

B

Fig. 53-14 Acne vulgaris. **A,** Comedones with a few inflammatory pustules. **B,** Papulopustular acne. (From Weston WL, Lane AT: *Color textbook of pediatric dermatology,* St Louis, 1991, Mosby.)

Therapeutic Management

Successful management of acne depends on a cooperative effort between the health care provider, the adolescent, and the parents. Unlike many other dermatologic conditions, acne lesions resolve slowly, and improvement may not be apparent for at least 6 weeks. Individual comedones can take several weeks to months to resolve, and papules and pustules usually resolve in about 1 week. The multifactorial causes of acne necessitate a combined approach for successful treatment. Treatment consists of general measures of care and specific treatments determined by the type of lesions involved.

General Measures

Improvement of the adolescent's overall health status is part of the general management. Adequate rest, moderate exercise, a well-balanced diet, reduction of emotional stress, and elimination of any foci of infection are all part of general health promotion.

Cleansing

Dirt or oil on the surface of the skin does not cause acne. Gentle cleansing with a mild cleanser once or twice daily is usually sufficient. Antibacterial soaps are ineffective and may be too drying when used in combination with topical acne medications. For some adolescents, hygiene of the hair and scalp appears to be related to the clinical activity of the acne. Acne on the forehead may improve with brushing the hair away from the forehead and more frequent shampooing.

Medications

Treatment success depends on commitment from the adolescent. Before prescribing treatment, the adolescent's level of comfort and readiness to begin treatment should be determined.

Tretinoin (Retin-A) is the only drug that effectively interrupts the abnormal follicular keratinization that produces microcomedones, the invisible precursors of the visible comedones. Tretinoin alone is usually sufficient for management of comedonal acne (Russell, 2000). Tretinoin is available as a cream, gel, or liquid. This drug can be extremely irritating to the skin and requires careful patient education for optimum usage. The patient should be instructed to begin with a pea-sized dot of medication, which is divided into the three main areas of the face and then gently rubbed into each area. The medication should not be applied for at least 20 to 30 minutes after washing to decrease the burning sensation. The avoidance of sun and the daily use of sunscreen must be emphasized, because sun exposure can result in severe sunburn. Adolescents should be advised to apply the medication at night and to use a sunscreen with a sun protection factor (SPF) of at least 15 in the daytime.

Topical *benzoyl peroxide* is an antibacterial agent that inhibits the growth of *P. acnes* organisms. It is effective against both inflammatory and noninflammatory acne, and is an effective first-line agent. This medication is available as a cream, lotion, gel, or wash. The patient should be informed that the medication may have a bleaching effect on sheets, bedclothes, and towels. The adolescent can be reassured that skin bleaching will not occur. Accommodation to the medication can be gained with a gradual increase in the strength and frequency of application.

When inflammatory lesions accompany the comedones, a *topical antibacterial agent* may be prescribed. These agents are used to prevent new lesions, as well as to treat preexisting acne. Clindamycin, erythromycin, metronidazole, azelaic acid, and the combination of either benzoyl peroxide and erythromycin (Benzamycin) or benzoyl peroxide and glycolic acid are all choices for topical antibacterial therapy (Leyden, 1997). The combination of 5% benzoyl peroxide and 3% erthromycin is especially beneficial although the exact mechanism of action is not understood (Burkhart, Specht, & Neckers, 2000). Tretinoin improves the penetration of other topical agents, and combination therapy with tretinoin and an antibacterial treatment is the only way to address three of the pathogenic causes of acne: keratinization, *P. acnes,* and inflammation (Laude, 2000).

Systemic antibiotic therapy is used when moderate to severe acne does not respond to topical treatments. Oral antibiotics are considered safe to use to treat acne. These antibiotics include tetracycline, erythromycin, minocycline, doxycycline, clindamycin, and trimethoprim-sulfamethoxazole (Leyden, 1997).

Girls with mild to moderate acne may respond well to topical treatment and the addition of an *oral contraceptive pill (OCP).* OCPs reduce the endogenous androgen production and decrease the bioavailability of the woman's circulating androgens. Both of these actions result in decreased acne.

Isotretinoin, 13-cis retinoic acid (Accutane), is a potent and effective oral agent that is reserved for severe cystic acne that has not responded to other treatments. Isotretinoin is the only agent available that affects factors involved in the development of acne. However, treatment with isotretinoin should be managed *only* by a dermatologist. Adolescents with multiple, active, deep dermal or subcutaneous cystic and nodular acne lesions are treated for 20 weeks. Multiple side effects can occur, including dry skin and mucous membranes, nasal irritation, dry eyes, decreased night vision, photosensitivity, arthralgia, headaches, mood changes, aggressive or violent behaviors, depression, and suicidal ideation. Adolescents on this drug should be monitored for depression, depressive symptoms, and suicidal ideation (Jacobs, Deutsch, & Brewer, 2001). The drug should be given only at the recommended doses for no longer than the recommended duration of time. The most significant side effects of this drug are the teratogenic effects. Isotretinoin is absolutely contraindicated in pregnant women. Sexually active young women must use an effective contraceptive method during treatment and for 1 month after treatment. Patients receiving isotretinoin should also be monitored for elevated cholesterol and triglyceride levels. Significant elevation may require discontinuation of the medication.

Nursing Care Management

Because acne is so common and its appearance may seem so mild, the health care provider may underestimate the relative importance of the disease to the adolescent. The nurse should assess the individual adolescent's level of distress, current management, and perceived success of any regimen before initiating a referral. If adolescents do not perceive the acne to be a problem, motivation to follow the treatment plan may be absent.

The nurse can provide ongoing support for the adolescent when a treatment plan is initiated. The family is also encouraged to support the adolescent in his or her efforts. Use of medications and basic skin care information should be discussed in detail with the adolescent. Written instructions should accompany the verbal discussion. Information to dispel myths regarding the use of abrasive cleansing products can prevent unnecessary costs and trauma to the skin.

Teenagers need education about the factors that aggravate and damage the skin, such as too vigorous scrubbing. In addition, picking, squeezing, and manual expression with fingernails breaks down the ductal walls of lesions and causes the acne to worsen. Mechanical irritation, such as vinyl helmet straps that rub areas predisposed to acne, can also cause the development of lesions.

THERMAL INJURY

Burns

CASE STUDY: BURNS

Burn injuries are usually attributed to extreme heat sources but may also result from exposure to cold, chemicals, electricity, or radiation. Most burns are relatively minor and do not require definitive medical treatment. However, burns involving a large body surface area, critical body parts, or the geriatric or pediatric population often benefit from treatment in specialized burn centers. The American Burn Association has established criteria to guide decisions regarding the severity of injury and the need for transfer for specialized care.

When burns are characterized by patients' age and type of injury, the following patterns become apparent: (1) hot-water scalds are most frequent in toddlers; (2) flame-related burns are more common in older children; (3) 10% to 20% of documented cases of child abuse include burn injuries (Herndon et al, 2002); and (4) children playing with matches or lighters account for 1 in 10 house fires.

The extent of tissue destruction is determined by the intensity of the heat source, the duration of contact or exposure, the conductivity of the tissue involved, and the rate at which the heat energy is dissipated by the skin. A brief exposure to high-intensity heat from a flame can produce burn injuries similar to those induced by long exposure to less intense heat in hot water.

Characteristics of Burn Injury

The physiologic responses, therapy, prognosis, and disposition of the injured child are all directly related to the *amount of tissue destroyed.* Therefore the severity of the burn injury is assessed on the basis of the percentage of surface burned and the depth of the burn. Among children in the school-age group or younger age groups, a burn that is 10% of the *total body surface area (TBSA)* can be life threatening if not treated correctly. Other important factors in determining the seriousness of the injury are the location of the wounds, the age of the child, the causative agent, the presence of respiratory involvement, the general health of the child, and the presence of any associated injury or condition.

Type of Injury

The majority of burns result from contact with thermal agents such as a flame, hot surfaces, or hot liquids. Electrical injuries caused by household current have the greatest incidence in young children, who insert conductive objects into electrical outlets and bite or suck on connected electrical cords (Herndon et al, 2002). These burns occur most commonly during the spring and summer months and are also associated with risk-taking behaviors in boys. Direct contact with high- or low-voltage current, as well as lightning strikes, is the most frequent mechanism of injury. The resistance of the tissue and the path of the electric current are responsible for the damage incurred. Electric current travels through the body following the path of least resistance, which involves the tissues, fluid, blood vessels, and nerves. A more localized burn is produced if skin resistance is high at the area of contact, and a more systemic pattern of injury is produced if skin resistance is low. Often compared with a crush injury, serious electrical trauma results from current passing through vital organs, muscle compartments, and nerve or vascular pathways. Loss of limbs, cardiac fibrillation, respiratory collapse, and burns are common occurrences following exposure to electrical energy.

Chemical burns are seen in the pediatric population and can cause extensive injury. The severity of injury is related to the chemical agent (acid, alkali, or organic compound) and the duration of contact. The mechanism of injury differs from other burns in that there is a chemical disruption and alteration of the physical properties of the exposed body area. Noxious agents exist in many cleaning products commonly found in the home. In addition to concern for localized damage, the potential for systemic toxicity must be addressed. Of particular concern is the exposure of the eyes to chemical agents, the ingestion of caustic substances, and inhalation of toxic gases produced from chemicals.

Extent of Injury

The extent of a burn is expressed as a percentage of the TBSA. This is most accurately estimated by using specially designed age-related charts (Fig. 53-15). It is more efficient to use a chart designed to assign body proportions to children of different ages.

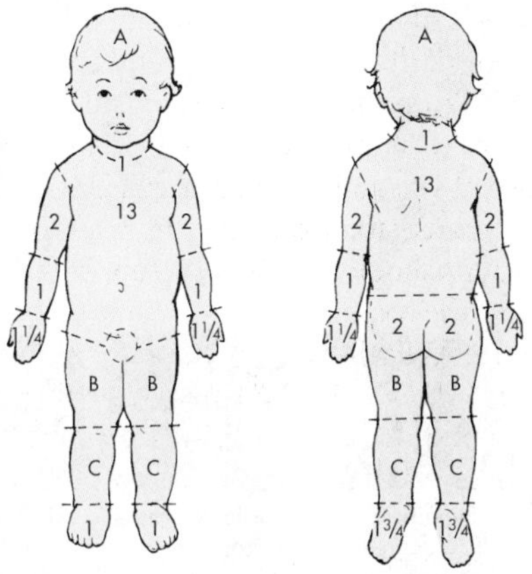

A

RELATIVE PERCENTAGES OF AREAS AFFECTED BY GROWTH

AREA	BIRTH	AGE 1 YR	AGE 5 YR
A = ½ of head	9½	8½	6½
B = ½ of one thigh	2¾	3¼	4
C = ½ of one leg	2½	2½	2¾

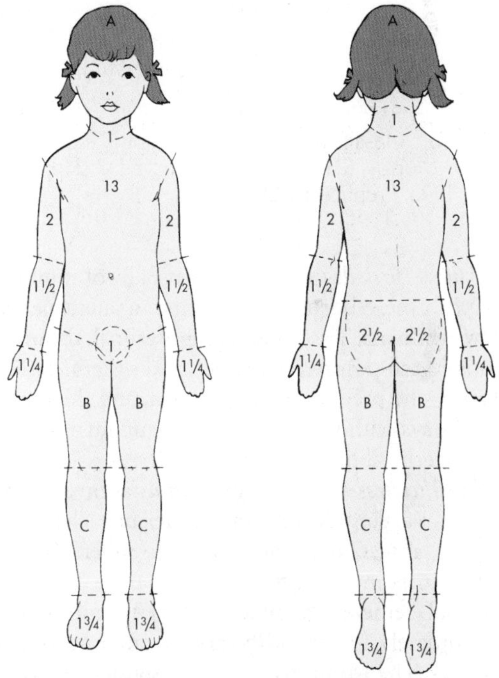

B

RELATIVE PERCENTAGES OF AREAS AFFECTED BY GROWTH

AREA	AGE 10 YR	AGE 15 YR	ADULT
A = ½ of head	5½	4½	3½
B = ½ of one thigh	4½	4½	4¾
C = ½ of one leg	3	3¼	3½

Fig. 53-15 Estimation of distribution of burns in children. **A**, Children from birth to age 5 years. **B**, Older children.

Depth of Injury

A thermal injury is a three-dimensional wound that is also assessed in relation to depth of injury. Traditionally the terms *first-, second,-* and *third-degree burn* have been used to describe the depth of tissue injury. However, with the current emphasis on wound healing, these have been replaced by more descriptive terms based on the extent of destruction to the epithelializing elements of the skin (Fig. 53-16).

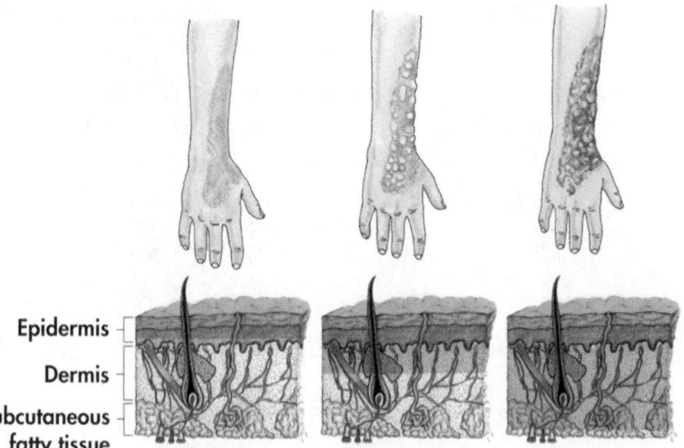

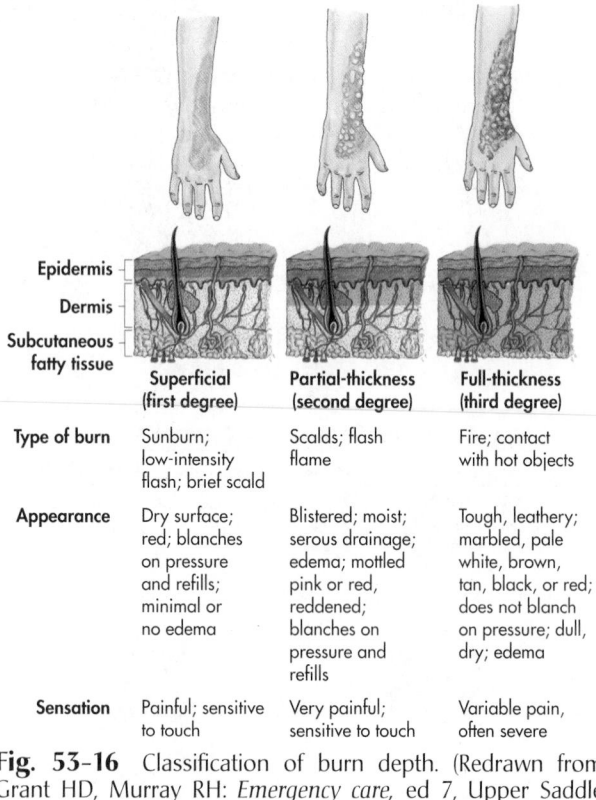

	Superficial (first degree)	Partial-thickness (second degree)	Full-thickness (third degree)
Type of burn	Sunburn; low-intensity flash; brief scald	Scalds; flash flame	Fire; contact with hot objects
Appearance	Dry surface; red; blanches on pressure and refills; minimal or no edema	Blistered; moist; serous drainage; edema; mottled pink or red, reddened; blanches on pressure and refills	Tough, leathery; marbled, pale white, brown, tan, black, or red; does not blanch on pressure; dull, dry; edema
Sensation	Painful; sensitive to touch	Very painful; sensitive to touch	Variable pain, often severe

Fig. 53-16 Classification of burn depth. (Redrawn from Grant HD, Murray RH: *Emergency care,* ed 7, Upper Saddle River, NJ, 1995, Prentice-Hall.)

A

B

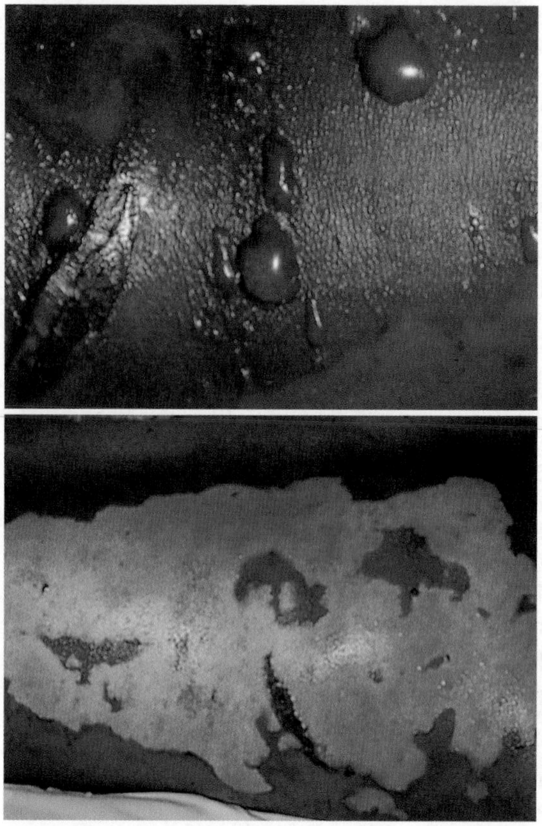

Fig. 53-17 Superficial partial-thickness burns on a black child. **A,** Blisters intact. **B,** Blisters removed. (Courtesy Hillcrest Medical Center, Tulsa, OK.)

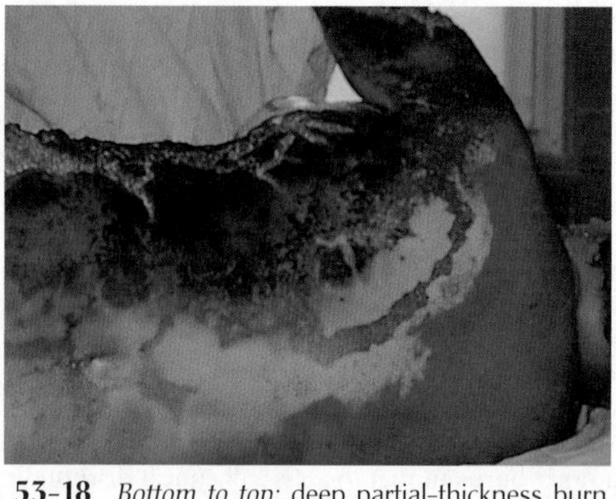

Fig. 53-18 *Bottom to top:* deep partial-thickness burn (red area); full-thickness burn (white area); full-thickness burn with eschar (brown area). (Courtesy Hillcrest Medical Center, Tulsa, OK.)

Superficial (first-degree) burns are usually of minor significance. With these burns, there is often a latent period followed by erythema. Tissue damage is minimal, the protective functions of the skin remain intact, and systemic effects are rare. Pain is the predominant symptom, and the burn heals in 5 to 10 days without scarring. Mild sunburn is an example of a superficial first-degree burn.

Partial-thickness (second-degree) injuries involve the epidermis and varying degrees of the dermis. These wounds are painful, moist, red, and blistered. Superficial partial-thickness burns involve the epidermis and part of the dermis. Dermal elements are intact, and the wound should heal in approximately 14 days with variable amounts of scarring (Fig. 53-17). The wound is extremely sensitive to temperature changes, exposure to air, and light touch. Although classified as second-degree or partial-thickness burns, deep dermal burns resemble full-thickness injuries in many respects. Sweat glands and hair follicles remain intact. The burn may appear mottled, with pink, red, or waxy white areas exhibiting blisters and edema formation. Systemic effects are similar to those encountered with full-thickness burns. Although many of these wounds heal spontaneously, they often heal with extensive scarring.

Full-thickness (third-degree) burns are serious injuries that involve the entire epidermis and dermis and extend into subcutaneous tissue (see Fig. 53-16). Nerve endings, sweat glands, and hair follicles are destroyed. The burn varies in color from red to tan, waxy white, brown, or black and is distinguished by a dry, leathery appearance (Fig. 53-18). Normally, full-thickness burns lack sensation in the area of injury because of the destruction of nerve endings. However, most full-thickness burns have superficial and partial-thickness burned areas at the periphery of the burn, where nerve endings are intact and exposed. Excised eschar and donor sites also cause exposed nerve fibers. As the peripheral fibers regenerate, painful sensations return. Consequently, children often experience severe pain related to the size and depth of the burn. Full-thickness wounds are not capable of reepithelialization and require surgical excision and grafting to close the wound.

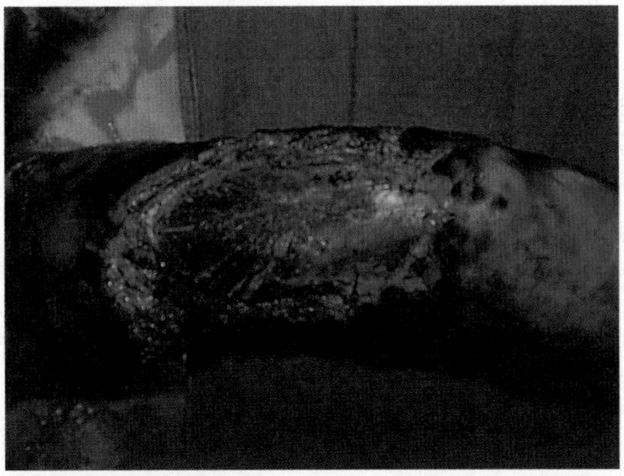

Fig. 53-19 Full-thickness burn with muscle and fascia involved. (Courtesy Hillcrest Medical Center, Tulsa, OK.)

Fourth-degree burns are full-thickness injuries that involve underlying structures such as muscle, fascia, and bone. The wound appears dull and dry, and ligaments, tendons, and bone may be exposed (Fig. 53-19).

Severity of Injury

Burns are classified as minor, moderate, or major, which is useful in determining the disposition of the patient for treatment. Burn patients are categorized as (1) those with a *major burn injury,* who require the services and facilities of a specialized burn center; (2) those with a *moderate burn,* who may be treated in a hospital with expertise in burn care; and (3) those with *minor injuries,* who may be treated on an outpatient basis. The extent and depth of the burn (Table 53-10), the causative agent, the body area involved, the patient's age, and concomitant injuries and illnesses determine the severity of the injury.

Because the skin of infants is so thin, it is likely to sustain deeper injuries. Children younger than 2 years of age, especially 6 months or younger, have a significantly higher mortality rate than older children with burns of similar magnitude. Acute or chronic illnesses or superimposed injuries also complicate burn care and response to treatment.

Inhalation Injury

Trauma to the tracheobronchial tree often follows inhalation of the heated gases and toxic chemicals produced during combustion. Although direct thermal injury to the upper airway may occur, heat damage below the vocal cords is rare. Inspired heated air is cooled in the upper airway before reaching the trachea. Reflex closure of the cords and laryngeal spasm also prevents full inhalation. However, evidence of direct thermal injury to the upper airway includes burns of the face and lips, singed nasal hairs, and laryngeal edema. Clinical manifestations may be delayed as long as 24 to 48 hours. Wheezing, increasing secretions, hoarseness, wet rales, and carbonaceous secretions are signs of respiratory tract involvement. Upper airway obstruction is often associated with burn shock and fluid resuscitation. In such situations, endotracheal intubation may also be necessary to preserve a patent airway.

Inhalation of carbon monoxide is suspected when the injury has occurred in an enclosed space. Mucosal erythema and edema followed by sloughing of the mucosa are manifestations of respiratory injury. A mucopurulent membrane replaces the mucosal lining and seriously compromises respiration and ventilation.

Early in the postburn period, most pulmonary infections result from nosocomial exposure, immobility, and abdominal distention. The hematogenous variety occurs later and is related to the septic burn wound or other foci, such as phlebitis at the site of an invasive IV line. A significant increase in mortality rate has been observed when inhalation injury and pneumonia are both present.

Deep burns, especially those circling the thorax, may cause restriction of chest excursion as a result of edema and inelastic eschar formation. Young children are particularly at risk because of the pliability of the skeletal structure. Hypoxia is relieved by an escharotomy incision, which allows expansion of the chest wall to facilitate ventilation.

Pathophysiology

Thermal injuries produce both local and systemic effects that are related to the extent of tissue destruction. In superficial burns the tissue damage is minimal. In partial-thickness burns there is considerable edema and more severe capillary damage. With a major burn greater than 30% of the TBSA, there is a systemic response involving an increase in capillary permeability, allowing plasma proteins, fluids, and electrolytes to be lost. Maximum edema formation in a small wound occurs about 8 to 12 hours after injury. After a larger injury, hypovolemia, associated with this phenomenon, will slow the rate of edema formation, with maximum effect at 18 to 24 hours.

Table 53-10

Severity Grading System Adopted by the American Burn Association

	MINOR*	MODERATE	MAJOR
Partial-thickness burns	<10% of total body surface area (TBSA)	10%-20% of TBSA	>20% of TBSA
Full-thickness burns			All
Treatment	Usually outpatient; may require 1- to 2-day admission	Admission to hospital, preferably one with expertise in burn care	Admission to a burn center

From Vaccaro P, Trofino RB: Care of the patient with minor to moderate burns. In Trofino RB (ed): *Nursing care of the burn-injured patient,* Philadelphia, 1991, FA Davis.

*Minor burns exclude any burn involving the face, hands, feet, perineum, or crossing joints; electrical burns; any injury complicated by the presence of inhalation injury or concomitant trauma; and children with psychosocial factors affecting the injury.

Another systemic response is anemia, caused by direct heat destruction of red blood cells, hemolysis of injured red blood cells, and trapping of red blood cells in the microvascular thrombi of damaged cells. A long-term decrease in the number of red blood cells may result in diminished red blood cell life span. Initially there is an increased blood flow to the heart, brain, and kidneys, with decreased blood flow to the gastrointestinal tract. There is an increase in metabolism to maintain body heat, providing for the increased energy needs of the body.

Complications

Thermally injured children are subject to a number of serious complications, both from the wound and from systemic alterations resulting from the injury. The immediate threat to life is related to airway compromise and profound shock. During healing, infection—both local and systemic sepsis—is the primary complication. Mortality rates associated with thermal trauma in children increase with the severity of injury and decrease as age advances. In children older than 3 years, the mortality rate is similar to that of adults. Below this age, the survival rate with burns and their associated complications lessens considerably.

A less apparent respiratory injury is inhalation of carbon monoxide. Carbon monoxide has a greater affinity for hemoglobin than does oxygen, thereby depriving peripheral tissues and oxygen-dependent organs (such as the heart and brain) of the oxygen needed for survival. Treatment for either of these two problems is 100% oxygen, which reverses the situation rapidly.

Pulmonary problems are a major cause of death in children with either thermal burns or complications in the respiratory tract. Respiratory problems include inhalation injuries, aspiration in unconscious patients, bacterial pneumonia, pulmonary edema, pulmonary embolus, posttraumatic pulmonary insufficiency, and atelectasis. The most common cause of respiratory failure in the pediatric age group is bacterial pneumonia, which requires prolonged intubation and sometimes necessitates a tracheostomy. Tracheostomies increase the incidence of serious complications and are performed only in extreme cases.

A less common complication is pulmonary edema resulting from fluid overload or acute respiratory distress syndrome (ARDS) in association with gram-negative sepsis. This syndrome results from pulmonary capillary damage and leakage of fluid into the interstitial spaces of the lung. A loss of compliance and interference with oxygenation are the consequences of pulmonary insufficiency in conjunction with systemic sepsis.

Wound Sepsis

Sepsis is a critical problem in the treatment of burns and an ever-present threat following the shock phase. Initially, burn wounds are relatively pathogen free unless they are contaminated with potentially infectious material, such as dirt or polluted water. However, dead tissue and exudate provide a fertile field for bacterial growth. On approximately the third postburn day, early colonization of the wound surface by a preponderance of gram-positive organisms (primarily staphylococci) changes to predominantly gram-negative opportunistic organisms, particularly *Pseudomonas aeruginosa*. By the fifth postburn day, bacterial invasion is well underway beneath the surface of the burn wound. Early surgical excision of eschar together with placement of autograft reduces the incidence of sepsis.

Therapeutic Management

Emergency Care

The initial management of the burn patient begins at the scene of injury. The first priority is to stop the burning process (Emergency box). The child should then be transported immediately to the nearest medical facility for treatment and evaluation. The child and the family are usually extremely frightened and anxious; sensitivity to their emotional state and reassurance should be provided during the transport process.

Stop the Burning Process

The chief aim of rescue in flame burns is to smother the fire, not fan it. Children tend to panic and run, which spreads the flames and makes assistance more difficult. The injured child should be placed in a horizontal position and rolled in a blanket, rug, or similar article, with care taken not to cover the head and face because of the danger of inhalation of toxic fumes. If nothing is available, the victim should lie down and roll over slowly to extinguish the flames. Remaining in the vertical position may cause the hair to ignite or the inhalation of flames, heat, or smoke.

Major burns with large amounts of denuded skin should not be cooled. Heat is rapidly lost from burned areas, and additional cooling leads to a drop in core body temperature and potential circulatory collapse. Wet dressings also promote vasoconstriction because of cooling, resulting in impaired circulation to the burned area and increased tissue damage. Chemical burns require continuous flushing with large amounts of water before transport to a medical facility.

Emergency

BURNS

Minor Burns

Stop the burning process:
- Apply cool water to the burn or hold the burned area under cool running water. Do not use ice.

Do not disturb any blisters that form, unless the injury is from a chemical substance.
Do not apply anything to the wound.
Cover with a clean cloth if risk of damage or contamination.
Remove burned clothing and jewelry.

Major Burns

Stop the burning process:
- Flame burns—smother the fire.
- Place victim in the horizontal position.
- Roll victim in a blanket or similar object; do not cover the head.

Assess for an adequate airway and breathing.
If not breathing, begin mouth-to-mouth resuscitation.
Remove burned clothing and jewelry.
Cover wound with a clean cloth.
Keep victim warm.
Transport to medical aid.
Begin intravenous and oxygen therapy as prescribed.

The use of neutralizing agents on the skin is contraindicated, because a chemical reaction is initiated and further injury may result. If the chemical is in powder form, the addition of water may spread the caustic agent. The powder should be brushed off if possible.

Burned clothing is removed to prevent further damage from smoldering fabric and hot beads of melted synthetic materials. Jewelry is removed to eliminate the transfer of heat from the metal and constriction resulting from edema formation. This also provides access to the wound and prevents painful removal later.

Assess the Victim's Condition

As soon as the flames are extinguished, the child is assessed. Airway, breathing, and circulation are the primary concerns. Cardiopulmonary complications may result from exposure to electric current, inhalation of toxic fumes and smoke, hypovolemia, and shock. Emergency measures are instituted as appropriate.

Cover the Burn

The burn wound should be covered with a clean cloth to prevent contamination, decrease pain by eliminating air contact, and prevent hypothermia. No attempt should be made to treat the burn. Application of topical ointments, oils, or other home remedies is contraindicated.

Transport the Child to Medical Aid

The child with an extensive burn is not given anything by mouth to avoid aspiration in the presence of paralytic ileus and upper airway edema and to prevent water intoxication. The child is transported to the nearest medical facility. If this cannot be accomplished within a relatively short period of time, IV access should be established, if possible, with a large-bore catheter. Oxygen is administered, if available, at 100%. A report of the initial assessment and any interventions implemented is given to the medical facility assuming care of the child.

Provide Reassurance

Providing reassurance and psychologic support to both the family and the child helps immeasurably during the period of postinjury crisis. Reducing anxiety conserves energy the family and child will need to cope with the physiologic and emotional stress of injury.

Minor Burns

Treatment of burns classified as minor can usually be managed adequately on an outpatient basis when it is determined that the parent can be relied on to carry out instructions for care and observation. Patients with less than optimum circumstances may require close follow-up to ensure adherence with treatment.

The wound is cleansed with a mild soap and tepid water. Debridement of the wound includes removal of any embedded debris, chemicals, and devitalized tissue. Removal of intact blisters remains controversial. Some authorities argue that blisters provide a barrier against infection; others maintain that blister fluid is an effective medium for the growth of microorganisms. However, blisters should be broken if the injury is due to a chemical agent to control absorption. Most practitioners favor covering the wound with an antimicrobial ointment to reduce the risk of infection and to provide some form of pain relief. The dressing consists of nonadherent fine mesh gauze placed over the ointment and a light wrap of gauze dressing that does not interfere with movement. This helps keep the wound clean and protect it from trauma. The caregiver is instructed to wash the wound, reapply the dressing, and return the child to the office or clinic as directed for wound observation. The frequency of dressing changes may vary from every other day to once a day.

Some practitioners prefer an occlusive dressing, such as a hydrocolloid, which is placed over the wound after cleansing. Hydrogel dressings, which are soothing and nonadherent, may also be used. The dressing is changed when leakage occurs, at regular intervals, or at least weekly. This method eliminates the discomfort associated with frequent dressing changes but impairs visualization of the wound surface.

If there is a high probability of infection or other complications or if there is doubt about the ability to carry out instructions, the caregiver may be directed to bring the patient in daily for dressing changes and inspection. Another option is have a nurse make a home visit to inspect the wound and perform the dressing change. Frequent removal of the dressing is an effective mode of debridement. Soaking the dressing in tepid water or normal saline before removal helps loosen the dressing and debris and reduce discomfort. Burns of the face are usually treated by an open method. The wound is washed and debrided in the same manner, and a thin film of antimicrobial ointment is applied.

A tetanus history is obtained on admission. If there is no history of immunization, or if more than 5 years have passed since the last immunization, tetanus prophylaxis is administered. There is no evidence that systemic antibiotic prophylaxis decreases the incidence of infection in small burn wounds (Herndon et al, 2002). Therefore antibiotics should be used only when there is evidence of infection. A mild analgesic such as acetaminophen is usually sufficient to relieve discomfort; the antipyretic effect of the drug also alleviates the sensation of heat.

Most minor burns heal without difficulty, but hospitalization is indicated if the wound margin becomes erythematous, gross purulence is noted, or the child develops evidence of systemic reaction (e.g., fever or tachycardia). The child should also be evaluated for functional impairment, and the caregiver should be instructed in the exercise and ambulation program. Following wound healing, an evaluation of scar maturation and range of motion will indicate any need for further therapy.

Major Burns

The first priority is airway maintenance. The inhalation of noxious agents or respiratory burns is suggested when there is a history of injury in an enclosed space; edema of the oral and nasal membranes; thermal injury to the face, nares, and upper torso; hyperemia; and blisters or evidence of trauma to the upper respiratory passages. When respiratory involvement is suspected or evident, 100% oxygen is administered and blood gas values, including carbon monoxide levels, are determined.

If the child exhibits changes in sensorium, air hunger, or other signs of respiratory distress, an endotracheal tube is inserted to maintain the airway. When severe edema of the face and neck is anticipated, intubation is performed before swelling makes intubation difficult or impossible. Controlled intubation is preferred to an emergency procedure. Intubation allows for the delivery of humidified oxygen, the removal of secretions from respiratory passages, and the provision of ventilatory support.

When full-thickness burns encircle the chest, constricting eschar may limit chest wall excursion, and ventilation of the child becomes more difficult. Escharotomy of the chest relieves this constriction and improves ventilation.

Fluid Replacement Therapy

The objectives of fluid therapy are to (1) compensate for water and sodium lost to traumatized areas and interstitial spaces, (2) reestablish sodium balance, (3) restore circulating volume, (4) provide adequate perfusion, (5) correct acidosis, and (6) improve renal function.

Fluid replacement is required during the first 24 hours because of fluid shifts that occur following the injury. Various formulas are used to calculate fluid needs, and the one adopted depends on practitioner preference. Crystalloid solutions are used during this initial phase of therapy. Parameters such as vital signs (especially heart rate), urine output volume, adequacy of capillary filling, and state of sensorium determine adequacy of fluid resuscitation.

After the initial 24-hour period, theoretically there is a capillary seal, and capillary permeability is restored. Colloid solutions such as albumin, plasmalyte, or fresh frozen plasma are useful in maintaining plasma volume. However, children with burn injuries usually require fluids in excess of their calculated maintenance and replacement volume. Reasons for this may include underestimation of burn size (particularly in pediatric patients), pulmonary injury that sequesters resuscitation fluid in the lung, electrical injury with greater tissue destruction than that which is visible, and a delay in the initiation of fluid resuscitation. Irreversible burn shock that persists despite aggressive fluid resuscitation remains a significant cause of death in the immediate postburn period. Fluid balance may continue to be a problem throughout the course of treatment, especially during periods in which there may be considerable evaporative loss from the wound.

Nutrition

The enhanced metabolic requirements and catabolism in severe burns make nutritional needs of paramount importance and often difficult to satisfy. The diet must provide sufficient calories to meet the increased metabolic needs and enough protein to avoid protein breakdown. Hypoglycemia can result from the stress of the burn injury as the liver glycogen stores are rapidly depleted.

A high-protein, high-calorie diet is encouraged after resolution of paralytic ileus. However, many children have poor appetites and are unable to meet energy requirements solely by oral feeding. Most children with burns in excess of 25% of the TBSA require supplementation with tube feeding. Early and continued nutritional support is an important part of therapy for seriously burned patients. Enteral feeding provides direct nourishment to the gastrointestinal tract and helps reverse the defective gut barrier that accompanies burn shock (Hansbrough, 1998).

If nutritional requirements cannot be met entirely by the enteral route, parenteral hyperalimentation is used to supplement intake. However, enteral feeding increases blood flow in the intestinal tract, preserves gastrointestinal function, and minimizes bacterial translocation by decreasing mucosal atrophy of the intestines. These factors make enteral feeding the preferred route of nutritional support (Herndon et al, 2002).

To facilitate growth and proliferation of epithelial cells, administration of vitamins A and C is begun early in the postburn period. Zinc is also supplemented because of its important role in wound healing and epithelialization.

Medication

Antibiotics are usually not administered prophylactically. The administration of systemic antibiotics to control wound colonization is not indicated, because decreased circulation to the injured area prevents delivery of the medication to areas of deepest injury. Surveillance cultures and monitoring of the clinical course provide the most reliable indicators of developing infection. Appropriate antibiotics are instituted to treat the specific identified organism. Otitis media should not be overlooked as a source of fever in the pediatric population.

Some form of sedation and analgesia is required in the care of burned children. Morphine sulfate is the drug of choice for severe burn injuries. Morphine has extensive distribution but is metabolized rapidly; continuous infusion or frequent administration is needed for pain management in burns. Morphine is administered intravenously and titrated to individual need. The unstable circulatory status and edema formation preclude intramuscular or subcutaneous administration. When combined, midazolam (Versed) and fentanyl (Sublimaze) also provide excellent IV sedation and analgesia to control procedural pain in children with burns (Herndon et al, 2002). The oral form of fentanyl, Fentanyl Oralet, provides effective analgesia in a convenient form that the child can suck. Dosage monitoring is important because tolerance to opioids may develop. IV analgesics are most effective when they are administered just before the onset of procedural pain.

The use of short-acting anesthetic agents, such as propofol and nitrous oxide, has proved beneficial in eliminating procedural pain. Pharyngeal reflexes remain intact, thus ensuring a patent airway. Propofol (Deprivan) is an IV sedative-hypnotic agent that produces sedation in less than 1 minute and lasts only a few minutes.

Nitrous oxide is a useful short-term analgesic when given in a mixture of gases on a fixed ratio of 50% nitrous oxide and 50% oxygen (Annequin et al, 2000). Initiation of action is approximately 1 minute, with peak effect reached in 3 to 5 minutes. Nitrous oxide is useful to alleviate anxiety and raise the threshold of pain during procedures. The child may self-administer the nitrous oxide mixture with assistance. For any conscious or unconscious sedation, the child must be monitored continuously during the procedure. (See Preoperative Care, Chapter 45, and Pain Assessment and Pain Management, Chapter 44.)

Management of the Burn Wound

After the initial period of shock and the restoration of fluid balance, the primary concern is the burn wound. The objectives of wound management include prevention of infection, removal of devitalized tissue, and closure of the wound. The application of dressings and topical antimicrobial therapy reduce pain by minimizing the exposure to air.

Primary Excision

In children with large, full-thickness burn wounds, excision is performed as soon as the patient is hemodynamically stable after initial resuscitation. Because the burn wound precipitates an exaggerated physiologic response, many complications do not resolve until the eschar is excised and the wound is closed. Early excision of deep partial-thickness and full-thickness burns reduces the incidence of infection and the threat of sepsis.

Debridement

Partial-thickness wounds require debridement of devitalized tissue to promote healing. Debridement is very painful and requires analgesia and a sedative before the procedure. Medications given for pain need to be readily available during this procedure and may need to titrated up during the procedure. Hydroxyzine (Atarax) and diphenhydramine (Benadryl) are often needed for itching, which occurs after whirlpool and debridement. The itching becomes particularly bothersome as the burns heal.

Hydrotherapy is employed to cleanse the wound and involves soaking in a tub or showering once or twice a day for no more than 20 minutes. The water acts to loosen and remove sloughing tissue, exudate, and topical medications. Hydrotherapy helps to cleanse not only the wound but the entire body and aids in maintenance of range of motion. Mesh gauze serves to entrap the exudative slough and is readily removed during hydrotherapy. Any loose tissue is carefully trimmed away before the wound is redressed.

Topical Antimicrobial Agents

Methods used for managing the burn wound include the following:

Exposure—Wounds are left open to air; crust forms on partial-thickness wounds, and eschar forms on full-thickness burns.

Open—Topical antimicrobial agent is applied directly to the wound surface, and the wound is left uncovered.

Modified—Antimicrobial agent is applied directly or impregnated into thin gauze and applied to the wound; gauze or net secures the area.

Occlusive—Antimicrobial agent is impregnated in gauze or applied directly to the wound; multiple layers of bulky gauze are placed over the primary layer and secured with gauze or net.

All of these methods provide wound coverage and employ some type of topical agent. Topical agents do not eliminate organisms from the wound but can effectively inhibit bacterial growth. To be effective, a topical application must be nontoxic, capable of diffusing through eschar, harmless to viable tissue, inexpensive, and easy to apply. A topical ointment should not encourage the development of resistant strains of bacteria and should produce minimum electrolyte derangement. A comparison of commonly used agents is summarized in Table 53-11.

Biologic Skin Coverings

Permanent coverage of extensive burns is a prolonged process that requires repeated operations for debridement and grafting. Early closure shortens the period of metabolic stress and decreases the likelihood of burn wound sepsis. In the acute phase, biologic dressings cover and protect the wound from contamination, reduce fluid and protein loss, increase the rate of epithelialization, reduce pain, and facilitate movement of joints to retain range of motion.

Allograft (homograft) skin is obtained from human cadavers that are screened for communicable diseases. Homograft is particularly useful in the coverage of surgically excised deep partial-thickness and full-thickness wounds in extensive burns when available donor sites are limited. Severe immunosuppression occurs in massively burned children and the allograft becomes adherent. The homograft can remain in place until suitable donor sites become available. Typically, rejection is seen approximately 14 days after application. The availability of tissue banks and a supply of suitable donors limit the use of homografts.

Xenograft from a variety of species, most notably pigs, is commercially available. In large burns, the porcine xenograft is commonly applied when extensive early debridement is indicated to cover a partial-thickness burn; this provides a temporary covering for the wound until an available autograft can be applied to the full-thickness areas (Herndon et al, 2002). Pigskin dressings are replaced daily or every 2 to 3 days. They are particularly effective in children with partial-thickness scald burns of the hands and face, because they allow relatively pain-free movement, which reduces contracture formation and has the added benefit of improving appetite and morale.

When applied early to a superficial partial-thickness injury, biologic dressings stimulate epithelial growth and faster wound healing. However, biologic dressings must be applied to clean wounds. If the dressing covers areas of heavy microbial contamination, infection occurs beneath the dressing. In the case of partial-thickness burns, such infection may convert the wound to a full-thickness injury.

Synthetic skin coverings are available for the management of partial-thickness burn wounds. Ideally, the dressing should provide the properties of human skin: adherence, elasticity, durability, and hemostasis. Synthetic skin substitutes are readily available, have an indefinite shelf life, and are relatively inexpensive.

Synthetic dressings are composed of a variety of materials and can be used successfully in the management of superficial partial-thickness burns and donor sites. Examples include adherent elastic films, hydroactive materials, or colloidal suspensions that are usually permeable to air, vapor, and fluids. BCG Matrix* consists of a film-backed mesh-reinforced hydrocolloid dressing.

Biobrane† is a flexible silicone-nylon membrane bonded to collagenous peptides of porcine skin. Calcium alginate is another treatment for donor sites. As with biologic dressings, it is important that the wound be free of debris before the dressing is applied. Body temperature elevation or evidence of purulence, erythema, or cellulitis around the wound edges may indicate that the wound has become infected beneath the dressing. If this occurs, prompt discontinuance of the synthetic dressing is indicated. All synthetic

---

*Brennan Medical, Inc., St. Paul, MN.

†Dow Hickman Pharmaceuticals, Inc., Sugar Land, TX.

Table 53-11

Comparison of Common Topical Preparations

AGENT	DRESSINGS	ADVANTAGES	DISADVANTAGES
Silver nitrate 0.5% ($AgNO_3$)	Open, modified, or occlusive; impedes joint movement; dressings changed twice daily; keep dressing moist, rewet at least every 2 hours	Greatly reduces evaporative losses; does not interfere with wound healing; bacteriostatic action against major burn flora, including *Pseudomonas* and *Staphylococcus;* inexpensive	Does not penetrate eschar; ineffective on established burn wound infections; little effect on *Klebsiella* and *Aerobacter* groups; stains skin, clothing, linens; makes assessment of the wound difficult because of staining; hypotonicity pulls electrolytes from the wound, depleting sodium, potassium, chloride, and magnesium; stings on application
Silver sulfadiazine 1% (AgSD)	Occlusive; motion of joints maintained; applied twice daily; do not use with a history of allergy to sulfa	Little pain on application; bactericidal by altering DNA and cell metabolism; effective against gram-positive and gram-negative bacteria; easy to apply; nontoxic	Transient neutropenia; does not penetrate eschar; forms proteinaceous gel on wound surface that is painful to remove; occasional rashes and pruritus; decreases granulocyte formation
Mafenide acetate 10% (Sulfamylon)	*Cream:* Usually open; do not apply to face; apply twice daily *Solution:* Occlusive; keep dressing moist (rewet at least every 2 hours); protect solution from light	Penetrates eschar and diffuses rapidly into burn wound and underlying tissues; effective in deep flame, electrical, and infected wounds; bacteriostatic against many gram-positive and gram-negative organisms, including *Pseudomonas* and *Clostridium*	Difficult and painful to remove cream; pain on application; metabolic acidosis, hypercapnia, and carbonic anhydrase inhibition; inhibits wound healing; hypersensitivity in some patients
Bacitracin	Open, modified; motion of joints maintained; change dressing twice daily	Bactericidal and bacteriostatic against gram-positive organisms; low toxicity; painless application; ease of application	Limited activity against gram-negative organisms; allergic reaction in sensitive individuals

dressings are reputed to hasten wound healing and reduce discomfort.

PERMANENT SKIN COVERINGS

Permanent coverage of deep partial-thickness and full-thickness burns is usually accomplished with a split-thickness skin graft. This graft consists of the epidermis and a portion of the dermis removed from an intact area of skin by a special instrument, the *dermatome* (Fig. 53-20). *The removal of skin with a dermatome is a very painful procedure; this procedure should always be done in an atraumatic fashion with the help of conscious sedation.*

With extensive burns, it is often difficult to find enough viable skin to cover the wounds; therefore available donor sites and special techniques are used. Split-thickness skin grafts may be sheet graft or mesh graft:

Sheet graft. A sheet of skin, removed from the donor site, is placed intact over the recipient site and sutured in place; it is used in areas where cosmetic results are most visible (Fig. 53-21).

Mesh graft. A sheet of skin is removed from the donor site and passed through a mesher, which produces tiny slits in the skin that allow the skin to cover 1.5 to 9 times the area of the sheet graft; this results in a less desirable cosmetic and functional outcome (Fig. 53-22).

The donor site is dressed with synthetic wound coverings or fine-mesh gauze until the dressing separates at 10 to 14 days when the wound is healed. Dressings are not changed on donor sites to avoid damage to newly healed, delicate epithelium. Healed donor sites are available for reharvesting in patients with extensive burns and limited undamaged skin, but the quality of skin is decreased when multiple grafts are taken.

ARTIFICIAL SKIN

The development of Integra,* a product that allows the dermis to regenerate, has produced significant improvement in burn wound healing and decreased scar formation. It is applied

*Integra Life Sciences Corporation, Plainsboro, NJ.

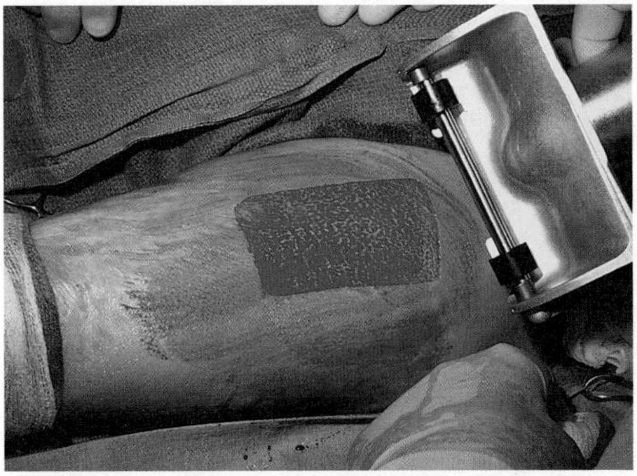

Fig. 53-20 Removal of split-thickness skin graft with a dermatome.

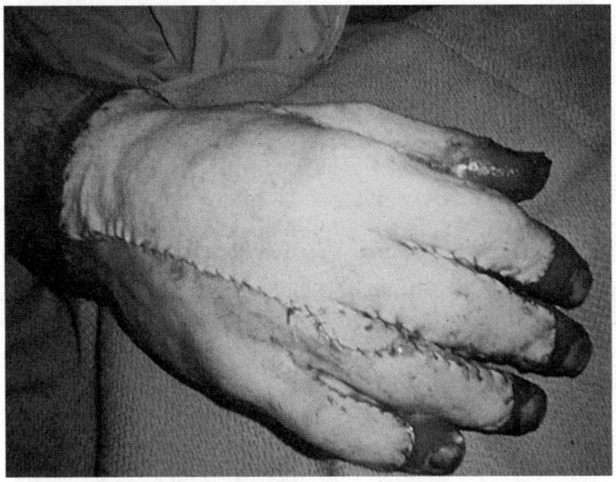

Fig. 53-21 Sheet graft.

to partial-thickness and full-thickness burns. The two-layer membrane is made of collagen (a fibrous protein from animal tendons and cartilage) and silicone rubber (i.e., Silastic). The Silastic layer is peeled off after the dermis is formed. The application of artificial skin does not replace the grafting procedure, but it prepares the burn wound to accept an ultrathin autograft. Advantages include faster healing of the burn wound when integrity of the dermis is restored, faster healing of donor sites with the use of ultrathin grafts, and restoration of sweat glands and hair follicles. A disadvantage is its high cost.

CULTURED EPITHELIUM

When burns are extensive and donor sites for split-thickness skin grafting are limited, it is possible to culture cells from a full-thickness skin biopsy and produce coherent sheets that can be applied to clean, excised full-thickness wounds. Epithelial cell culture grafts offer the possibility of an unlimited source of autografts in patients with extensive burns. Cultured epithelial autografts are effective in early wound closure. The child's own skin is fractionated and cultured in a porcine medium to form a thin epithelial layer that is applied to the burn wound. This technique offers an improved rate of survival in patients with extensive burns and limited donor sites.

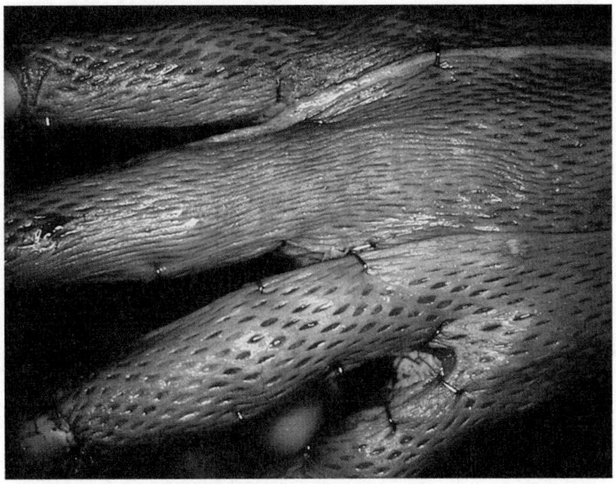

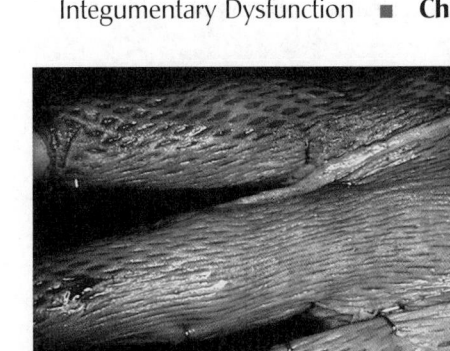

Fig. 53-22 Mesh graft.

Prognosis

Children differ from adults in their responses to thermal injury, and the mortality rates in young children are significantly higher than those in older children and adults. Mortality rate is greatest for children younger than 48 months of age. Many children who do survive have long-term functional and cosmetic impairments.

Nursing Care Management

Because the care of burned children encompasses a broad range of skills, nursing care has been divided into segments that correspond with the major phases of burn treatment. The *acute phase,* also referred to as the *emergent* or *resuscitative phase,* involves the first 24 to 48 hours. The *management phase* extends from the completion of adequate resuscitation through wound coverage. The *rehabilitative phase* begins once the majority of the wounds have healed and rehabilitation has become the predominant focus of the plan of care. This phase continues until all reconstructive procedures and corrective measures are accomplished (often a period of months or years).

Acute Phase

The primary emphasis during the emergent phase is the treatment of burn shock and the management of pulmonary status. Monitoring vital signs, output, fluid infusion, and respiratory parameters are ongoing activities in the hours immediately following injury. IV infusion is begun immediately and is regulated to maintain a urine output of at least 1 to 2 ml/kg in children weighing less than 30 kg; an output of 30 to 50 ml/hr is expected in children weighing more than 30 kg. Urine output and specific gravity, vital signs, laboratory data, and objective signs of adequate hydration guide the rate of fluid administration.

Children who are hospitalized with burns require constant observation and assessment for complications. Alterations in electrolyte balance produce clinical symptoms of confusion, weakness, cardiac irregularities, and seizures. Changes in respiratory function and gas exchange are reflected clinically by restlessness, irritability, increased work of breathing, and alterations in blood gas values. The loss of protective function of the skin exposes burned children to increased risk of hypothermia. Edema formation and circulatory impairment result in the loss of sensation and in deep, throbbing pain.

NURSE ALERT Evaluate the extremity and check the pulse every hour. If unable to palpate, use Doppler to ascertain loss of circulation and pulse. If the pulse is lost, escharotomy may be necessary to relieve the edema causing pressure on blood vessels, to restore adequate circulation. ■

Burn units maintain a pictorial record of the wound to record progress and for legal purposes (if child abuse is suspected). The burn wound is treated according to the protocol of the specific burn facility. The burn team monitors infection control procedures and ensures that staff and visitors comply with established protocols to prevent cross-contamination in the burn unit.

Throughout the acute phase of care, the psychosocial needs of the children and their families should not be overlooked. The child is frightened, uncomfortable, and often confused. Children may be isolated from familiar persons and surroundings; the overwhelming physical needs at this time are the primary focus of the staff and parents. In addition to feeling concern for their child, the family experiences guilt, which may be related to the fact that the parents did not or could not protect their child from injury. Consistency in the information presented and in the attitude of the staff creates a sense of familiarity and stability during the acute phase of care. Consistent caregivers can also help decrease the patient's and the family's anxiety and provide coordination of care. For example, when many teams of consultants and specialists are involved in the care of the child, appointing one "spokesperson" decreases the confusion and enhances communication regarding the child's care.

Management and Rehabilitative Phases

After the patient's condition is stabilized, the management phase begins. The multidisciplinary team concentrates on preventing wound infections, closing the wound as quickly as possible, and managing the numerous complications. Although the rehabilitative phase begins when permanent wound closure has been achieved, rehabilitation issues are identified on admission and are included in the plan of care throughout the hospital course.

Assessment

Wound assessment and comprehensive assessment of the child's general condition and behaviors are of major importance. The nurse must assess signs of complications, infection, and the need for and effectiveness of pain management.

NURSE ALERT Disorientation in the burned patient is one of the first signs of overwhelming sepsis and may indicate inadequate hydration. Assessment of the sensorium is another important indicator of the adequacy of hydration. A spiking fever and diminished bowel sounds accompanied by paralytic ileus are noted and progressively increase over 48 to 72 hours, after which the temperature falls to subnormal limits. At this time the wound deteriorates, the white blood cell count is depressed, and septic shock becomes manifest. ■

Nursing Diagnoses

Nursing diagnoses identified for the child with severe or extensive burns are included in the Nursing Care Plan on pp. 1797-1798. Additional diagnoses may be ascertained for individual children.

Plan of Care and Implementation

The goals for the child with a burn injury and the child's family are as follows:

1. Child will experience reduction of pain.
2. Child will exhibit evidence of wound healing.
3. Child will receive adequate nutrition and will achieve reduction in metabolic losses.
4. Child will not experience complications during acute care.
5. Child will not experience complications during long-term care.
6. Child and family will receive emotional support.

Comfort Management

The severe pain of the wound and resultant therapies, the anxiety generated by these experiences, sleep deprivation, itching related to wound healing, and the conscious and unconscious interpretations of traumatic events contribute to the psychologic behaviors commonly observed in children with burns. It is always difficult to deal with a child in pain, and inflicting pain on a helpless child is contrary to the empathic nature of nursing. Interventions to promote comfort may include medications (including IV morphine or midazolam and short-term anesthetics such as propofol), relaxation techniques, distraction therapy, behavioral techniques, operant conditioning (tokens, star chart, etc.), and family participation.

Children need age-appropriate explanations before all procedures. When children appear to accept pain with little or no response, psychologic consultation may be needed. Consistency in caregivers is important. If this is not possible, a carefully developed, multidisciplinary plan of care is necessary to provide consistency.

Care of the Burn Wound

The nurse has a major responsibility for cleansing, debriding, and applying topical medications and dressings to the burn wound. Pain medication should be administered so that the peak effect of the drug coincides with the procedure. Children who have an understanding of the procedure to be performed and some perceived control demonstrate less maladaptive behavior. Children also respond well to participating in decisions (Guidelines box).

Outer dressings are removed. Any dressings that have adhered to the wound can be more easily removed by applying tepid water or normal saline. Loose or easily detached tissue is debrided during the cleansing process. In dressing the wound, it is important that all areas be clean, that medication be amply applied, and that no two burned surfaces touch each other (e.g., fingers or toes, or ears touching the side of the head). If they are touching, the burned surfaces will heal together, causing deformity and/or dysfunction.

Topical medications may be applied directly to the wound with a tongue blade or gloved hand or impregnated into fine-mesh gauze before application. Dressings are then applied to assist in exudate absorption, wound debridement, and increased patient comfort. All dressings applied circumferentially should be wrapped in a distal-to-proximal man-

Guidelines

REDUCING THE STRESS OF BURN CARE PROCEDURES

Have all materials ready before beginning.
Administer appropriate analgesics and anxiolytics.
Remind the child of the impending procedure to allow sufficient time to prepare.
Allow the child to test and approve the temperature of the water.
Allow the child to select the area of the body on which to begin.
Allow the child to request a short rest period during the procedure.
Allow the child to remove the dressings if desired.
Provide something constructive for the child to do during the procedure (e.g., holding a package of dressings or a roll of gauze).
Inform the child when the procedure is near completion.
Praise the child for cooperation.

ner. The dressing is applied with sufficient tension to remain in place but not so tightly as to impair circulation or limit motion. Elastic bandages are applied over dressings to prevent epithelial breakdown, decrease edema formation, stimulate circulation, and improve mobility. A stable dressing is especially important when the child is ambulatory.

Standard Precautions, including the use of protective garb and barrier techniques, should be followed when caring for patients with thermal injuries. Frequent handwashing and forearm washing is the single most important element of the infection control program. Strict policies for cleaning the environment and patient care equipment should be implemented to minimize the risk of cross-contamination. All visitors and members of other departments should be oriented to the infection control policies, including the importance of handwashing and forearm washing and use of protective garb. Visitors should be screened for infection and contagious diseases before patient contact.

Nutrition

Oral feedings are encouraged unless the child is intubated or paralytic ileus persists. Because children often lack an appetite, the child needs encouragement, help, and patience. Consultation between the caregiver and the dietitian helps determine food preferences. Children who are old enough to participate should be included in meal planning. In addition, many children prefer an atmosphere more nearly like that provided at home. Therefore, when possible, many children enjoy sitting at a table and interacting with other children at mealtimes. Painful procedures should not be scheduled near mealtimes, because most children will be too physically exhausted and emotionally upset to eat.

Children who require enteral supplementation must be monitored for feeding intolerance and tube malposition. The nurse should also monitor and report any abdominal distention, diarrhea, or electrolyte and metabolic deviations.

Prevention of Complications

Acute Care

The maintenance of body temperature is important to the child with burns. Core body temperature is supported when energy is conserved with an environmental temperature of 28° to 33° C (82° to 91° F). Large areas of the body should not be exposed simultaneously during dressing changes. Warmed solutions, linens, occlusive dressings, heat shields, a radiant warmer, and warming blankets assist in preventing hypothermia.

The chief danger during acute care is infection—wound infection, generalized sepsis, or bacterial pneumonia. Accurate and ongoing assessments of all parameters that provide clues to the early diagnosis and treatment of infection are essential. Symptoms of sepsis include a change in the level of consciousness, a rising or falling white blood cell count, hypothermia or hyperthermia, a loss of the progression of wound healing, increasing fluid requirements, hypoactive or absent bowel sounds, a rising or falling blood glucose level, tachycardia, tachypnea, and thrombocytopenia.

Children are reluctant to move if movement causes pain, and they are likely to assume a position of comfort. Unfortunately, the most comfortable position often encourages the formation of contractures and loss of function. Ongoing efforts to prevent contractures include maintaining proper body alignment, positioning and splinting involved extremities in extension, active and passive physical therapy, and encouragement of spontaneous movement when feasible. Frequent position changes are important to promote adequate bronchopulmonary hygiene and capillary perfusion to common pressure areas. Low-air-loss beds are beneficial for the morbidly obese or children with posterior grafts. Special attention should be given to areas at risk for increased pressure, such as the posterior scalp, heels, sacrum, and areas exposed to mechanical irritation from splints and dressings.

Long-Term Care

The rehabilitative phase of care begins once wound coverage is achieved. Scar formation becomes a major problem as burn wounds heal (Fig. 53-23). Contractile properties of the scar tissue can result in disabling contractures, deformity, and disfigurement.

Uniform pressure applied to the scar decreases the blood supply. When pressure is removed, blood supply to the scar is immediately increased; therefore periods without pressure should be brief to avoid nourishment of the hypertrophic tissue. Continuous pressure to areas of scarring can be achieved by elastic bandages or commercially available pressure garments. Because these custom-made garments are often worn for months, revisions may be required as the child grows. It is much easier to prevent scarring and contracture of the wound than to resolve an existing problem. Splints and appliances may also be needed until wound maturation is achieved (Fig. 53-24).

Scar tissue has certain significant properties, particularly for growing children. Intense itching occurs in healing burn wounds and scar tissue until the scar is no longer active. Itching is usually treated with a combination of H1 and H2 antagonists such as cetirizine (Zytrec) and cimetidine (Tagamet) (Baker et al, 2001); an H1 antagonist alone; and frequent applications of a moisturizer, such as Vaseline, Cetaphil, Aquaphor, Eucerin, cocoa butter, or Nivea. Petrolatum-based ointments (Vaseline, Aquaphor) seem to spread more easily on friable skin than thick creams. Massage therapy during the application of moisturizers is also beneficial to stretch scar tissue and aid in contracture prevention. Scar

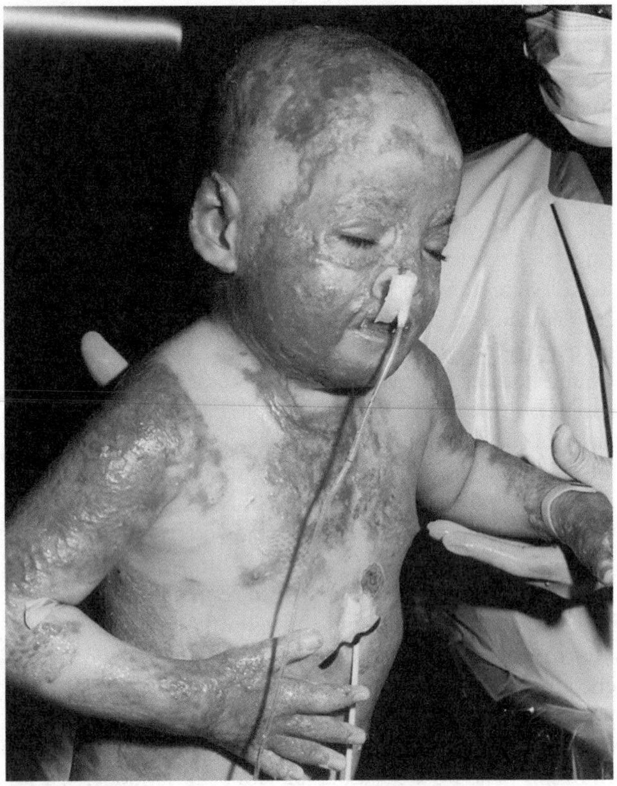

Fig. 53-23 Extensive scars from flame burn. (Courtesy C.R. Boeckman, MD, Regional Burn Center, Akron, OH.)

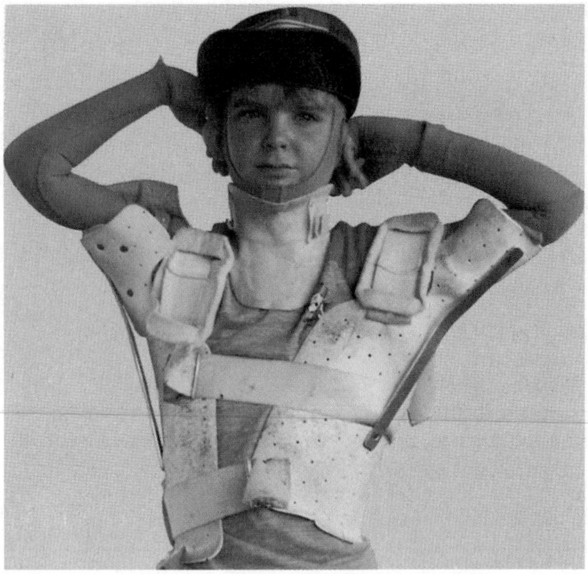

Fig. 53-24 Child in elasticized (Jobst) garment and "airplane" splints.

tissue has no sweat glands, and children with extensive scarring may experience difficulty during hot weather. Caregivers should be alerted to this possibility and be prepared to institute alternative methods of cooling when necessary.

Scar tissue does not grow and expand, as does normal tissue, which may create difficulties, especially in functional areas such as the hands and over joints. Additional surgery is sometimes required to allow independent functioning in daily activities, to improve cosmetic appearance, or to restore anatomic integrity.

The nursing activities in the rehabilitative phase of treatment focus on the child's and the family's adaptation to the burn injury and their ability to reintegrate into the community. The psychologic pain and sequelae of severe burn injury are as intensive as the physical trauma. The impact of severe burns taxes the coping mechanisms at all ages. Very young children, who suffer acutely from separation anxiety, and adolescents, who are developing an identity, are probably the most affected psychologically. Toddlers cannot understand why the parents they love and who have protected them can leave them in such a frightening and unfamiliar place. Adolescents, in the process of achieving independence from the family, find themselves in a dependent role with a damaged body. Being different from others at a time when conformity with peers is so important is difficult to accept.

Anticipation of the return to school can be overwhelming and frightening. It is essential that health care professionals recognize the importance of preparing teachers and classmates for the child's return. Teachers need to be provided with information to assist the child and family and to promote the child's optimum adjustment. Hospital-sponsored school reentry programs use a variety of methods to provide education and information about the implications of the injury, the garments and appliances, and the need for support and acceptance. Telephone calls, videotapes, information packets, and visits by members of the health care team offer opportunities to help with reintegration into the school environment—a focal point of the child's life.

Psychosocial Support of the Child

Children should begin early to do as much for themselves as possible and to be active participants in their care. Loss of control and perceived helplessness may result in acting-out behaviors. During illness, children regress to a previous developmental level that allows them to deal with stress. As children begin to participate in their care, they gain confidence and self-esteem. Fears and anxieties diminish with accomplishment and self-confidence. If the child demonstrates nonadherence in the rehabilitative phase, a behavior modification program can be initiated to promote or reward the child's accomplishments in care.

Children need to know that their injury and the treatments are not punishment for real or imagined transgressions and that the nurse understands their fear, anger, and discomfort. They also need body contact. This is often difficult to arrange for the child with massive burns. Stroking areas of unburned skin is comforting. Even older children enjoy sitting on the parent's lap and being cuddled and hugged. This can be a reward or a comfort in times of stress, but most of all it should be kept in mind that it is a natural part of childhood.

Psychosocial Support of the Family

Recognizing and respecting each family's strengths, differences, and methods of coping allows the nurse to respond to their unique needs by implementing a family-centered approach to care. In the acute phase, all attention is focused on the child, and the parents feel powerless and ineffectual. Most parents feel overwhelming guilt, regardless of whether the guilt is justified. They feel responsible for the injury.

These feelings may impede the child's rehabilitation. Parents may indulge the child and allow nonadherent behaviors that affect physical and emotional recovery. Parents need to be informed of the child's progress and helped to cope with their feelings while providing support to their child. The nurse can help them understand that it is not selfish to look after themselves and their own needs in order to meet the needs of their child. It is important to recognize the parents' need to grieve the change in the normal appearance of their child as a part of the grieving process. Definitive professional help may be needed for parents whose response to the injury is severe or whose response to stress is manifested in destructive behavior.

The parents are members of the multidisciplinary team and participate in the development of the plan of care. It is important to facilitate their input; to consider all aspects of the physical, emotional, social, and cultural factors affecting the child and family; and to establish a realistic home therapy program. The family's willingness to assume responsibility for care and their ability to implement the therapeutic regimen are assessed. Home, school, and other environmental factors are explored; financial concerns and available community resources are discussed; and a specific plan of care for the child, with an anticipated follow-up program, is developed.

Prevention of Burn Injury

The best intervention is to prevent burns from occurring. Hot liquids in the kitchen and bathroom most commonly injure infants and toddlers. Hot liquids should be kept out of reach; tablecloths and dangling appliance cords are often pulled by toddlers, who spill hot grease and liquids on themselves. Electrical cords and outlets represent a potential risk to small children, who may chew on accessible cords and insert objects into outlets.

The Consumer Product Safety Commission recommends a reduction of water heater thermostats to a maximum of 48.9° C (120° F). The "dial-down" recommendation has been suggested by utility companies, burn treatment centers, medical personnel, and others interested in public safety. However, many water heaters continue to remain set at levels well above the safe level. Small children are especially at risk for scald injuries from hot tap water because of their decreased reaction time and agility, their curiosity, and the thermal sensitivity of their skin. Caregivers should never leave a child unattended in a bath and without adult supervision. Water should always be tested before a child is placed in the tub or shower.

The increased use of microwave ovens has resulted in burn injuries from the extremely hot internal temperatures generated in heated items. Baby formula, jelly-filled pastries, and hot liquids and dishes may result in cutaneous scalds or the ingestion of overheated liquids. Parents should use caution when removing items from the microwave oven and should always test the food before giving it to children.

As children mature, risk-taking behaviors increase. Matches and lighters are very dangerous in the hands of the young. Adults must remember to keep potentially hazardous items out of the reach of children; a lighter, like a match, is a tool for adult use.

Education related to fire safety and survival should begin with the very young. "Stop, drop, and roll" to extinguish a fire can be practiced. The fire escape route, including a safe meeting place away from the home in case of fire, also should be practiced.

Community activities are also very helpful in supporting burn survivors and preventing burns. The Aluminum Cans for Burned Children (ACBC) is an exemplary effort based in the Clifford R. Boeckman, MD, Regional Burn Center, Akron, Ohio.* Activities funded by ACBC include Burn Survivors Support Group, Burn Camp, and meetings of Juvenile Firestoppers (for children with fire-setting behavior). Adult weekend retreats and school and family education sessions are a part of this program. Burn center staff and fire department staff provide the personnel to present programs.

Additional information on burn care and prevention can be obtained from the American Burn Association† and the National Safety Council.‡ The Alisa Ann Ruch Burn Foundation§ provides assistance to burn victims and burn centers. The Shriners Burn Institutes are staffed to treat pediatric patients following acute burn injuries and those requiring rehabilitative and reconstructive services as a result of scarring and functional impairment. Information can be obtained from local Shrine Temples and Shrine Clubs, from Shriners Hospitals, or by contacting the International Shrine Headquarters.|| The Alisa Ann Ruch Foundation and Shriners Hospitals for Crippled Children support research to improve burn care and treatment and promote public education in burn prevention.

Evaluation

The effectiveness of nursing interventions is determined by continual reassessment and evaluation of care based on the following observational guidelines:

1. Observe the child's behavior during all aspects of care; listen to verbal cues; use a pain assessment record to evaluate the effectiveness of analgesia.
2. Observe the burn wound and the child's general condition.
3. Observe the child's eating behavior and the amount of food consumed; weigh daily or as indicated.
4. Inspect the burn wound for signs of infection; measure vital signs; and observe for evidence of respiratory complications, gastric bleeding, altered hemoglobin level, and neurologic signs.
5. Observe for evidence of healing, scar formation, and contracture; assess effectiveness of physical therapy and appliances (splints, pressure garments).

---

*Children's Hospital Medical Center of Akron, 1 Perkins Square, Akron, OH 44308-1062; phone: 330-543-8224; fax: 330-379-8152; Web site: www.akronchildrens.org.

†625 North Michigan Ave., Suite 1530, Chicago, IL 60611; phone: 312-642-9260 or 800-548-2876; fax: 312-642-9130; e-mail: aba@ameriburn.org.

‡1121 Spring Lake Dr., Itasca, IL 60143-3201; phone: 800-621-7615; Web site: www.nsc.org.

§20944 Sherman Way, Suite 115, Canoga Park, CA 91303; phone: 818-883-7700; Web site: www.aarbf.org.

||*2900 Rocky Point Dr., Tampa, FL 33607; phone: 800-237-5055 (in Florida: 800-282-9161); International Shrine Headquarters Web site: www.shrinershq.org; Shriners Burn Institutes Web site: www.shrinershq.org/Hospitals/BurnInst/.

6. Observe the child's and the family's behaviors; interview the child and family regarding their feelings and concerns.

The *expected outcomes* are described in the Nursing Care Plan on pp. 1797-1798.

Sunburn

Sunburn is a common skin injury caused by overexposure to ultraviolet (UV) light waves. The sun emits a continuous spectrum of visible and nonvisible light rays that range in length from very short to very long. The shorter, higher-frequency waves are more damaging than longer wavelengths, but much of the light is filtered out as it travels through the atmosphere. Of the light that does filter through, *ultraviolet A (UVA) waves* are the longest and cause only minimum burning, but play a significant role in photosensitive and photoallergic reactions. They are also responsible for premature aging of the skin and potentiate the effects of *ultraviolet B (UVB) waves.* UVB waves are shorter and are responsible for tanning, burning, and most of the harmful effects attributed to sunlight, especially skin cancer.

Numerous factors influence the amount of UVB exposure. Maximum exposure occurs at midday (10 AM to 3 PM), when the distance from the sun to a given spot on the earth is shortest. There is more exposure at higher altitudes and near the equator, and less when the sky is hazy (although the amount of UV radiation that does penetrate is easily underestimated). Window glass effectively screens out UVB but not UVA rays. Fresh snow, water, and sand reflect UV rays, especially when the sun is directly overhead.

Sunburn is usually an epidermal burn, although severe sunburn can be a partial-thickness burn with blister formation. Treatment of sunburn involves stopping the burning process, decreasing the inflammatory response, and rehydrating the skin. Local application of cool tap water soaks, or immersion in a tepid-water bath (temperature slightly below 36.7° C [98° F]) for 20 minutes or until the skin is cool limits tissue destruction and relieves the discomfort. After the cool applications, a bland oil-in-water moisturizing lotion can be applied. Partial-thickness burns are treated the same as those from any heat source (see earlier discussion on burns).

Nursing Care Management

Protection from sunburn is the major goal of management, and the harmful effects of the sun on the delicate skin of infants and children are currently receiving increased attention. To protect skin exposed to the sun for extended periods, skin should be covered with clothing, and FDA-approved sun protection agents should be applied.

Two types of products are available for sun protection: *topical sunscreens,* which partially absorb UV light, and *sun blockers,* which block out UV rays by reflecting sunlight. The most frequently recommended sun blockers are zinc oxide and titanium dioxide ointments. Sunscreens are products containing a *sun protection factor (SPF)* based on evaluation of effectiveness against UV rays. The SPF is a number, such as 15, which indicates that if individuals normally burn in 10 minutes without a sunscreen, use of a sunscreen with SPF 15 allows them to remain in the sun 15 times 10, or 150 minutes (2.5 hours) before acquiring the same degree of burns. The most effective sunscreens against UVB are *p-aminobenzoic acid (PABA)* and *PABA-esters.*

Sunscreens are applied evenly to all exposed areas, with special attention to skinfolds and areas that might become exposed as clothing shifts. Parents are directed to read labels of sunscreen products carefully for the SPF and follow the manufacturer's directions for application.

NURSE ALERT Sunscreens are not recommended for infants under 6 months of age. However, infants under 6 months of age may have sunscreen applied over small areas of skin such as the back of hands that may not be adequately covered by clothing when they are in the sun (American Academy of Pediatrics, Committee on Environmental Health, 1999). Infants should be kept out of the sun or physically shaded from it. Fabric with a tight weave, such as cotton, offers good protection. ■

Individuals who work in the community, such as teachers, day care workers, coaches, and youth-group leaders, and relatives, should all be made aware of sun safety for children. Sunscreens must be applied *liberally.*

Cold Injury

Cold injuries are most commonly seen in very cold regions. The nature of the heat-regulating mechanisms of the body are such that the inner portion of the body, or core, produces heat and the periphery, or outer area, conserves or dissipates heat. When the body attempts to conserve heat, the outer tissues are subjected to low temperatures, and local trauma may result.

Chilblain, redness and swelling of the skin, occurs when extremities, usually the hands, are exposed intermittently to temperatures of −1.1° to 15.5° C (30° to 60° F). The response may vary but is characterized by intense vasodilation that increases the temperature of involved tissues above that of unaffected tissue and produces edematous, reddish blue patches that itch and burn. As warming takes place, the sensations become more intense, but ordinarily they subside in a few days.

Frostbite is the term used to describe tissue damage caused when excessive heat loss to local tissues allows ice crystals to form in tissues. The frostbitten part appears white or blanched, feels solid, and is without sensation. Rapid rewarming is associated with less tissue necrosis than slow thawing. It restores blood flow and shortens the period of cellular damage. Rewarming produces a flush (sometimes deep purple) and a return of sensation, which is extremely painful. Large blisters may appear in 24 to 48 hours after rewarming, and begin to reabsorb within 5 to 10 days, followed by the formation of a hard black eschar. Superficial injury often heals without incident. Rewarming is accomplished by immersing the part in well-agitated water at 37.8° to 42.2° C (100° to 108° F). Discomfort is managed with analgesics and sedatives. Care of blistered skin is similar to that described for burns. It is seldom possible to estimate the extent of tissue loss until new skin layers are revealed after the eschar layer separates.

Nursing Care Plan

THE CHILD WITH A FULL-THICKNESS BURN MORE THAN 25% TBSA

NURSING DIAGNOSIS: Impaired skin integrity related to thermal injury

EXPECTED OUTCOME

The child exhibits signs of wound healing, and skin grafts remain intact.

NURSING INTERVENTIONS/*RATIONALES*

Thoroughly cleanse wound and debride devitalized skin *to decrease infection and promote healing.*

Apply topical and systemic bacterial agents to wounds as ordered *to decrease chances of infection.*

Dress wounds as ordered *to protect against infection and fluid loss.*

Monitor serum electrolytes and blood gases *for potential adverse effects of topical agents.*

Monitor wound appearance for signs of infection or healing *to guide ongoing treatment.*

Monitor grafts for evidence of hematoma/fluid collection; aspirate or express fluids *to maintain graft contact with base of site.*

Use appropriate measures (e.g., splints, dressings, restraints) *to prevent child from touching or picking at wound and graft sites.*

Offer high-calorie, high-protein meals and snacks *to meet nutritional requirements caused by increased metabolism and catabolism.*

Administer supplemental vitamins A, B, and C; iron; and zinc *to facilitate wound healing and epithelialization.*

NURSING DIAGNOSIS: Fluid volume deficit related to active loss of body fluids secondary to thermal injury

EXPECTED OUTCOME

The child exhibits signs of adequate fluid volume and electrolyte balance.

NURSING INTERVENTIONS/*RATIONALES*

Administer intravenous fluids with sodium as ordered *to prevent burn shock and maintain perfusion.*

Monitor vital signs, skin turgor, and mucous membranes *for signs of fluid volume/electrolyte balance.*

Monitor intake and output (including wound drainage and urinary output) *to assess fluid balance and circulatory status.*

Monitor electrolytes, blood gases, and specific gravity *to assess hydration and electrolyte balance.*

NURSING DIAGNOSIS: Risk for fluid volume excess related to retention of fluids and sodium secondary to intravenous therapy, edema formation

EXPECTED OUTCOME

The child exhibits signs of adequate fluid volume and electrolyte balance.

NURSING INTERVENTIONS/*RATIONALES*

Discontinue intravenous fluids as ordered when an established rate of urinary output is reached and adequate circulatory volume is restored *to prevent fluid overload.*

Monitor respiratory status *for signs of fluid accumulation in lungs;* tissue pressures *for signs of edema that may cause permanent injury to underlying nerves and muscles.*

NURSING DIAGNOSIS: Risk for infection related to denuded or absence of skin, presence of pathogenic organisms, and altered immune response

EXPECTED OUTCOME

The child exhibits no evidence of infection.

NURSING INTERVENTIONS/*RATIONALES*

Place child in appropriate protective environment (e.g., laminar air flow, isolation, private room) and screen all visitors and staff for signs of infection *to minimize exposure to infective organisms.*

Teach child and family about good hygiene and careful handwashing techniques *to prevent spread of infection.*

Use good handwashing for all contacts with child and scrupulous aseptic technique with gown, cap, mask, and gloves for all wound care procedures *to minimize exposure to infection.*

Cleanse and debride eschar, crust, and blisters *to remove infection reservoir.*

Administer prescribed topical antimicrobials and cover wound with dry dressings per protocol *to provide a barrier to organisms.*

Encourage a nutritionally complete diet (high-calorie, high-protein diet) *to support body's natural defenses.*

Monitor vital signs, observe wounds, and obtain wound cultures *to detect signs of infection.*

NURSING DIAGNOSIS: Anxiety/pain related to trauma from burns and debridement therapy and other treatments

EXPECTED OUTCOME

The child exhibits a reduced level of pain and/or anxiety.

NURSING INTERVENTIONS/*RATIONALES*

Monitor closely for pain relief needs and administer medications as ordered *to decrease pain;* anticipate need and administer medication before onset of severe pain and at regular intervals *to better manage pain levels;* medicate before procedures such as debridement, hydrotherapy, and dressing changes *to better manage pain levels.*

Administer medications as prescribed, apply lotions *for the relief of itching of scar tissue.*

Prepare child and family for procedures and allow the child to make active choices during procedures (e.g., testing temperature of water for hydrotherapy, selecting which site to start debridement, saying when to stop procedure for a rest, helping with the procedure) *to promote sense of control and cooperation.*

Implement nonpharmacologic pain reduction techniques as appropriate (e.g., distraction, relaxation, guided imagery, positive self-talk, cutaneous stimulation) *to relieve pain.*

NURSING DIAGNOSIS: Impaired physical mobility related to pain, scar formation, joint contracture

EXPECTED OUTCOME

The child maintains physical mobility, minimal scar formation, and joint contractures.

Continued

Nursing Care Plan

THE CHILD WITH A FULL-THICKNESS BURN MORE THAN 25% TBSA—cont'd

NURSING INTERVENTIONS/*RATIONALES*

Implement active/passive range of motion *to prevent contractures, keep joints mobile, and minimize pain.*

Use positioning techniques, splinting, conformers, and pressure garments *to prevent flexion and scar contractures.*

Ambulate as soon as possible, promote self-help activities, and encourage play *to maintain mobility.*

Use lotion and massage healed areas *to soften scars and promote relaxation.*

Administer analgesic before painful activity (e.g., physical therapy) *so that child is more likely to cooperate and be mobile.*

NURSING DIAGNOSIS: Ineffective thermoregulation related to loss of skin surface, sweat glands

EXPECTED OUTCOME

The child exhibits tolerance to the environment.

NURSING INTERVENTIONS/*RATIONALES*

Carefully control and monitor temperature in environment, limit exposure to temperature extremes *to prevent hypothermia or hyperthermia.*

Avoid vigorous physical activity *that may lead to heat prostration.*

Monitor temperature *to assess for hypothermia or hyperthermia.*

NURSING DIAGNOSIS: Body-image/self-esteem disturbance related to scar formation, alterations in appearance and function

EXPECTED OUTCOME

The child demonstrates an acceptance of self, his or her own physical appearance, and physical abilities.

NURSING INTERVENTIONS/*RATIONALES*

Relate to child, conveying an attitude of caring and acceptance, *to encourage positive feelings about self;* serve as role model for others *to foster positive attitudes of acceptance toward child.*

Encourage child to verbalize feelings and perceptions about the burn incident, wounds, and scarring (e.g., nightmares, fears of fire, pain of therapy, multiple treatments and prolonged and multiple hospitalizations, feelings of differentness, implications of functional limits, difficulty in making friends, views of self) *to facilitate coping and open expression of problems, fears, wants, wishes, and needs.*

Have child identify strengths, assets, and things he or she likes about self *to increase positive feelings about self and abilities.*

Support positive coping behaviors.

Introduce child to other children who have had similar experiences; arrange for support groups for child and parents *to increase coping skills.*

Refer child and family for counseling as needed *to enhance adaptation.*

Encourage use of regular hygiene and grooming practices, use of accessories (e.g., wigs, concealing makeup, concealing clothing) *to promote positive appearance.*

Prepare peers for child's appearance *to encourage acceptance and support.*

NURSING DIAGNOSIS: Altered family processes related to situational crises (child with scarring, altered appearance and function)

EXPECTED OUTCOME

Family members exhibit adaptation of usual roles and functions to accommodate special needs of the child and exhibit growth-promoting behaviors.

NURSING INTERVENTIONS/*RATIONALES*

Provide opportunity for family to absorb and adjust to diagnosis (e.g., repeat information *to allow time for family to hear and understand;* encourage expression of concerns, fears, and feelings about diagnosis and potential impact *to facilitate adjustment;* identify support systems *to provide resources for coping*).

Assist family to understand expected treatment, rationale, and implications *to provide a sound basis for decision making.*

Explore family's reaction to the child; assist them to achieve a realistic view of child's abilities and limitations; encourage family in attempts to promote child's growth and development; have family emphasize what child can do; explore ways for family to include child in family activities *to help family increase abilities to cope with and incorporate child into family structure.*

Arrange for and participate in family conferences *to provide forum for communication, mutual goal setting, and effective strategizing.*

Have parents spend special time with siblings *so they do not feel neglected or left out.*

Identify additional resource systems (e.g., relatives, friends, church, health care services, community programs) and strategize with family about making good use of these systems *to develop broad base of support.*

Provide a system of ongoing follow-up and evaluation *to ensure long-term adaptation to challenges presented in family functioning by a child with severely altered appearance and scarring.*

Key Points

- A variety of factors can produce lesions of the skin.
- It is important for nurses to be able to describe skin lesions accurately.
- The process of wound healing consists of hemostasis, inflammation, proliferation, and remodeling.
- A moist environment promotes wound healing.
- Bacterial, viral, and fungal infections are common in childhood.
- Some skin diseases are transmitted by arthropod vectors, especially ticks.
- The most common skin infestations of childhood—scabies and pediculosis capitis—affect children of any age and from any social class.
- Contact dermatitis may involve a primary irritant or a sensitizing agent.
- Adverse reactions to drugs are manifested more often in the skin than in any other body organ.

- The most common skin disorders of infancy are diaper dermatitis, seborrheic dermatitis, and atopic dermatitis.
- Acne, a disorder affecting many adolescents, is related to excessive sebum production, the formation of comedones, and the overgrowth of the *Propionibacterium acnes* organism.
- Medication and gentle facial cleansing are the treatments of choice for acne.
- Burns are caused by thermal, chemical, electric, or radioactive agents.
- Burns are assessed on the extent, depth, and severity of the wound.
- Essentials of emergency care of burn injury include stopping the burning process, covering the burn, transporting the injured child to medical aid, and providing reassurance to the child and family.
- Management of minor burns consists of facilitating wound healing, relieving discomfort, and preventing complications.
- Management of major burns consists of facilitating wound healing, relieving discomfort, replacing destroyed skin, preventing and/or treating complications, and providing rehabilitation.
- Sunscreen is recommended for use when the skin is exposed to the damaging effects of the sun's rays.
- Thermal injuries to the skin can result from exposure to extreme cold.

Answer Guidelines to Critical Thinking Exercise

Poison Ivy

1. Yes, there are sufficient data to determine an effective intervention.
2. (a) The leaves and stems of the poison ivy plant contain urushiol, an oil that produces an immune reaction in the skin. (b) When urushiol comes in contact with the skin, it penetrates the epidermis and bonds with the dermal layer. After about 2 days, localized, oozing, and painful impetiginous lesions are produced in the skin. (c) When a child has contact with any part of the poison ivy plant, the skin areas should be immediately flushed with cold running water to neutralize the urushiol, and calamine lotion should be applied. Clothing that has come in contact with the plant should be removed and thoroughly laundered in hot water and detergent. (d) Harsh soap is contraindicated because it removes the protective skin oils and dilutes the urushiol, allowing it to spread; hard scrubbing irritates the skin.
3. The most important immediate intervention is to rinse Billy's hands in cool water and apply calamine lotion. Billy's camp is near a stream, so he can enter the water where it is shallow and allow the water to rinse the oil of the poison ivy from his hands and clothes. The leaves should not be burned because contact with the smoke can cause a skin reaction and is also dangerous to the lungs if it is inhaled. Billy's clothes should be washed in hot water with detergent. Poison ivy lesions are not contagious, so the camp nurse should tell Billy's cabin mates that they will not "catch" his poison ivy.
4. Yes, the evidence supports these interventions.
5. The camp nurse should use this experience as an opportunity to provide the young campers and the adolescent assistants with education about common hazardous plants, insects, and ticks found in the outdoor environment; strategies to prevent contact with these agents; and first aid measures to implement if contact does occur.

References

American Academy of Pediatrics, Committee on Environmental Health: Ultraviolet light: a hazard to children, *Pediatrics* 104(2):328-333, 1999.

American Academy of Pediatrics, Committee on Infectious Diseases: *2003 red book: report of the Committee on Infectious Diseases,* ed 26, Elk Grove Village, IL, 2003, The Academy.

Annequin D et al: Fixed 50% nitrous oxide oxygen mixture for painful procedures: a French survey, *Pediatrics* 105(4):e47, 2000. Internet document available at www.pediatrics.org/cgi/content/full/105/4/e47 (accessed May 31, 2005).

Baker RAU et al: Burn wound itch control using H1 and H2 antagonists, *J Burn Care Rehabil* 22(4):263-268, 2001.

Bernardo LM et al: Dog bites in children treated in a pediatric emergency department, *JSPN* 5(2):87-95, 2000.

Burkhart CN, Specht K, Neckers D: Synergistic activity of benzoyl peroxide and erythromycin, *Skin Pharmacol Appl Skin Physiol* 13(5):292-296, 2000.

Centers for Disease Control and Prevention: Cat-scratch disease in children—Texas, September 2000–August 2001, *MMWR* 51(10):212-214, 2002.

Food and Drug Administration: FDA issues health advisory regarding labeling changes for lindane products, *HealthInfo Tx Report,* April 2003. Internet document available at www.fda.gov/bbs/topics/ANSWERS/2003/ANS01205.html (accessed May 31, 2005).

Frankowski BL, Weiner LB: Head lice, *Pediatrics* 110(3):638-643, 2002.

Hansbrough JF: Enteral nutritional support in burn patients, *Gastrointest Endosc Clin North Am* 8(3):645-647, 1998.

Herndon DN et al: *Total burn care,* ed 2, London, 2002, WB Saunders.

Jacobs DG, Deutsch NL, Brewer M: Suicide, depression, and isotretinoin: is there a causal link? *J Am Acad Dermatol* 45(5):S168-S175, 2001.

Krasner DL, Rodeheaver GT, Sibbald RG: *Chronic wound care: a clinical source book for healthcare professionals,* ed 3, Wayne, PA, 2001, HMP Communications.

Kronemyer B: Scratching the surface of atopic and contact dermatitis, *Infect Dis Child* 16(3):40, 2003.

Laude TA: Acne in childhood and adolescence: update on treatment choices, *Consultant* 3:457-465, 2000.

Leyden JJ: Therapy for acne vulgaris, *N Engl J Med* 336:1156-1162, 1997.

Mancini AJ: Acne vulgaris: a treatment update, *Contemp Pediatr* 17(12):122-133, 2000.

Offidani A et al: Treatment of scabies with ivermectin, *Eur J Dermatol* 9(2):100-101, 1999.

Osmond MH, Klassen TP, Quinn JV: Economic comparison of a tissue adhesive and suturing in the repair of pediatric facial lacerations, *J Pediatr* 126(6):892-895, 1995.

Russell JJ: Topical therapy for acne, *Am Fam Physician* 61(2):357-366, 2000.

Smith GA et al: Comparison of topical anesthetics without cocaine to tetracaine-adrenaline-cocaine and lidocaine infiltration during repair of lacerations: bupivacaine-norepinephrine is an effective new topical anesthetic agent, *Pediatrics* 97(3):301-307, 1996.

Wade CF: Keeping Lyme disease at bay, an integrated approach to prevention, *Am J Nurs* 100(7):26-31, 2000.

Yetman RJ, Parks D: Diagnosis and management of atopic dermatitis, *J Pediatr Health Care* 16(3):143-145, 2002.

Unit 11

54 Musculoskeletal or Articular Dysfunction

LEARNING OBJECTIVES

On completion of this chapter the reader will be able to:

- Outline a plan for the care of a child immobilized with an injury or a degenerative disease.
- Formulate a teaching plan for the parents of a child in a cast.
- Explain the functions of the various types of traction.
- Devise a nursing care plan for a child in traction.
- Differentiate among the various congenital skeletal defects.
- Design a teaching plan for the parents of a child with a congenital skeletal deformity.
- Describe the therapies and nursing care of a child with scoliosis.
- Outline a plan of care for a child with osteomyelitis.
- Differentiate between osteosarcoma and Ewing sarcoma.
- Describe the nursing care of a child with juvenile rheumatoid arthritis.
- Demonstrate an understanding of the management of systemic lupus erythematosus.

ELECTRONIC RESOURCES

Additional information related to the content in Chapter 54 can be found on

the companion website at evolve
http://evolve.elsevier.com/Wong/maternal/

- NCLEX Review Questions
- Case Study—Osteomyelitis
- WebLinks

or the interactive student CD-ROM
Activities for Chapter 54 include the following:

- NCLEX Review Questions
- Case Study—Fractures
- Case Study—Developmental Dysplasia of the Hip
- Critical Thinking Exercise—Osteogenic Sarcoma
- Nursing Care Plan—The Child Who is Immobilized
- Skill—Monitoring Neurovascular Status

THE IMMOBILIZED CHILD

Immobilization

One of the most difficult aspects of illness in children is the immobility it imposes. Children by nature are usually quite active, and immobility, however temporary, may have lasting consequences on the child's developmental progress. The most frequent reasons for immobility are congenital defects (e.g., spina bifida, arthrogryposis), degenerative disorders (e.g., muscular dystrophy), and infections or injuries that impair the integumentary system (severe burns), the musculoskeletal system (e.g., multiple fractures, osteomyelitis), or the neurologic system (e.g., spinal cord injury, polyneuritis, head injury). At times therapies such as traction and spinal fusion are responsible for prolonged immobilization, although the increasing trends in health care are early mobilization and discharge and outpatient treatment.

Physiologic Effects of Immobilization

Many clinical studies, including space program research, have documented predictable consequences that occur after immobilization and the absence of gravitational force. Functional and metabolic responses to restricted movement can be noted in most of the body systems. Each has a direct influence on the child's growth and development because homeostatic mechanisms thrive on normal use and need feedback to maintain dynamic equilibrium. Inactivity leads to a decrease in the functional capabilities of the whole body as dramatically as the lack of physical exercise leads to muscle weakness.

Disuse from illness, injury, or a sedentary lifestyle can limit function and potentially delay age-appropriate milestones. Most of the pathologic changes that occur during immobilization arise from decreased muscle strength and mass, decreased metabolism, and bone demineralization, which are closely interrelated, with one change leading to or affecting the other. Some results of immobilization are primary and produce a direct effect; other pathophysiologic consequences occur frequently but seem to be more indirect and are therefore secondary effects. Many pathophysiologic changes affect more than one body system, with the primary or secondary effect being demonstrated in both systems.

The major effects of immobilization are outlined briefly in Table 54-1 and are related directly or indirectly to decreased muscle activity, which produces numerous primary changes in the musculoskeletal system with secondary alterations in the cardiovascular, respiratory, metabolic, and renal systems. The musculoskeletal changes that occur during disuse are a result of alterations in gravity and stress on the muscles, joints, and bones. Muscle disuse leads to tissue breakdown and loss of muscle mass *(atrophy)*. Muscle atrophy causes decreased strength and endurance, which may take weeks or months to restore.

During immobilization a joint contracture begins when the arrangement of collagen, the main structural protein of connective tissues, is altered, resulting in a denser tissue that does not glide as easily. Eventually muscles, tendons, and ligaments can shorten and reduce joint movement, ultimately producing contractures that restrict function. The daily stresses on bone created by motion and weight bearing maintain the balance between bone formation (osteoblastic activity) and bone reabsorption (osteoclastic activity). During immobilization, increased calcium leaves the bone, causing osteopenia (demineralization of the bones), which may predispose bone to pathologic fractures. The major musculoskeletal consequences of immobilization are (1) significant decrease in muscle size, strength, and endurance; (2) bone demineralization leading to osteoporosis; and (3) contractures and decreased joint mobility. The larger the portion of the body immobilized and the longer the immobilization, the greater the hazards of immobility.

Psychologic Effects of Immobilization

For children, one of the most difficult aspects of illness is immobilization. Throughout childhood, physical activity is an integral part of daily life and is essential for physical growth and development. The activity helps children deal with a variety of feelings and impulses and provides a mechanism by which they can exert control over inner tensions. Children respond to anxiety with increased activity. Removal of this power deprives them of necessary input and a natural outlet for their feelings and fantasies.

When children are immobilized by disease or as part of a treatment regimen, they experience diminished environmental stimuli with a loss of tactile input and an altered perception of themselves and their environment. Sudden or gradual immobilization narrows the amount and variety of environmental stimuli children receive by means of all of their senses: touch; sight; hearing; taste; smell; and proprioception, or the feeling of where they are in their environment. This sensory deprivation commonly leads to feelings of isolation and boredom, and of being forgotten, especially by peers.

Physical interference with the activity of infants and young children gives them a feeling of helplessness. Even speech and language skills require sensorimotor activity and experience. Children who are restrained by casts, splints, or straps during the first 3 years of life may have more difficulty with language than children whose activities are unrestricted.

For the toddler, exploration and imitative behaviors are essential to developing a sense of autonomy; the preschooler's expression of initiative is evidenced by the need for vigorous physical activity; the school-age child's development is strongly influenced by physical achievement and competition; and the adolescent relies on mobility to achieve independence. The quest for mastery at every stage of development is related to mobility.

The monotony of immobilization can lead to sluggish intellectual and psychomotor responses, decreased communication skills, increased fantasizing, and even hallucinations and disorientation. Children are likely to become depressed over their loss of ability to function or any marked changes in body image. They may seek the attention of others by reverting to earlier developmental behaviors, such as wanting to be fed, bed-wetting, and baby talk.

Limbs in casts or traction transmit less than normal sensory data. Children who have limited ability to feel others touching them not only experience less tactile stimuli in a physical sense, but are also deprived of warm, loving feelings that arise from being touched. The loss of feeling derived from touch can further add to their sense of being isolated and unwanted.

Children may react to immobility by active protest, anger, and aggressive behavior; or they may become quiet, passive, and submissive. Children should be allowed to discharge their anger, but it should be within the limits of safety to their self-esteem and not damaging to the integrity of others. For example, providing an object to attack rather than a person or a valued possession is safe and therapeutic. When children are unable to express anger, aggression is often displayed inappropriately through regressive behavior and outbursts of crying or temper tantrums.

Effect on Families

Even brief periods of immobilization may disrupt family function, and catastrophic illness or disability may severely tax their resources and coping abilities.

The family's needs often must be met by the services of a multidisciplinary team, and nurses play a key role in anticipating the services they will need and in coordinating conferences to plan care. In preparation for discharge, home visits are advisable, and home management is commonly planned weeks in advance of the actual discharge. Such planning includes special considerations for cultural, economic, physical, and psychologic needs. A child with a severe disability is very dependent, and caregivers need rest periods to revitalize themselves. Individual and group counseling is beneficial for preproblem-solving situations and provides an emotional support system. Parent groups are also helpful and often allow nonthreatening social contact. The families of children with permanent disabilities need long-term resources because some of the most difficult problems arise as they try to sustain high-quality care for many years (see Chapter 41).

Table 54-1

Summary of Physical Effects of Immobilization*

PRIMARY EFFECTS	SECONDARY EFFECTS
MUSCULAR SYSTEM	
Decreased muscle strength, tone, and endurance	Decreased venous return and decreased cardiac output Decreased metabolism and need for oxygen Decreased exercise tolerance Bone demineralization
Disuse atrophy and loss of muscle mass	Catabolism Loss of strength
Loss of joint mobility	Contractures, ankylosis of joints
Weak back muscles	Secondary spinal deformities
Weak abdominal muscles	Impaired respiration
SKELETAL SYSTEM	
Bone demineralization—osteoporosis, hypercalcemia	Negative calcium balance Pathologic fractures Calcium deposits Extraosseous bone formation, especially at hip, knee, elbow, and shoulder Renal calculi
Negative calcium balance	Life-threatening electrolyte imbalance
METABOLISM	
Decreased metabolic rate	Slowing of all systems Decreased food intake
Negative nitrogen balance	Decline in nutritional state Impaired healing
Hypercalcemia	Electrolyte imbalance
Decreased production of stress hormones	Decreased physical and emotional coping capacity
CARDIOVASCULAR SYSTEM	
Decreased efficiency of orthostatic neurovascular reflexes	Inability to adapt readily to upright position Pooling of blood in extremities in upright posture
Diminished vasopressor mechanism	Orthostatic hypotension (intolerance) with syncope—hypotension, decreased cerebral blood flow, tachycardia
Altered distribution of blood volume	Decreased cardiac workload
Venous stasis	Decreased exercise tolerance
Dependent edema	Pulmonary emboli and/or thrombi Tissue breakdown and susceptibility to infection
RESPIRATORY SYSTEM	
Decreased need for oxygen	Altered oxygen—carbon dioxide exchange and metabolism
Decreased chest expansion and diminished vital capacity	Diminished oxygen intake Dyspnea and inadequate arterial oxygen saturation; acidosis
Poor abdominal tone and distention	Interference with diaphragmatic excursion
Mechanical or biochemical secretion retention	Hypostatic pneumonia
Loss of respiratory muscle strength	Bacterial and viral pneumonia Atelectasis Poor cough Upper respiratory infection
GASTROINTESTINAL SYSTEM	
Distention caused by poor abdominal muscle tone	Interference with respiratory movements
No specific primary effect	Difficulty in feeding in prone position; gravitation effect on feces through ascending colon, or weakened smooth muscle tone may cause constipation Anorexia
URINARY SYSTEM	
Alteration of gravitational force	Difficulty in voiding in prone position
Impaired ureteral peristalsis	Urinary retention in calyces and bladder Infection Renal calculi
INTEGUMENTARY SYSTEM	
No specific primary effect	Decreased circulation and pressure leading to tissue injury and decreased healing capacity Difficulty with personal hygiene

*Not all problems will apply in every situation.

Nursing Care Management

Assessment

Physical assessment of the child who is immobilized as a result of an injury or a degenerative disease focuses not only on the injured part (e.g., fracture or damaged joint) but also on the functioning of other systems that may be affected secondarily (e.g., the circulatory, renal, respiratory, muscular, and gastrointestinal systems). With long-term immobilization there may also be neurologic impairment and changes in electrolytes (especially calcium), nitrogen balance, and the general metabolic rate. The psychologic impact of immobilization should also be assessed.

Nursing Diagnoses

Nursing diagnoses for the immobilized child are outlined in the Nursing Care Plan on p. 1805. Others are identified in specific cases.

Plan of Care and Implementation

The general goals of care for the immobilized child and family include the following:

1. Child will experience no physical injury.
2. Child will experience no psychologic complications.
3. Child will engage in appropriate diversional activities.
4. Child and family will receive adequate support.

Children who require prolonged total immobility and are unable to move themselves in bed should be placed on a special mattress to prevent skin breakdown. Frequent position changes also help prevent dependent edema and stimulate circulation, respiratory function, gastrointestinal motility, and neurologic sensation. Children at greater risk for skin breakdown include those with prolonged immobilization, orthotic and prosthetic devices including wheelchairs, and plaster casts (Samaniego, 2003). Additional risk factors include poor nutrition, friction (from bed linen with traction) and moist skin (from urine or perspiration). Nursing care of children at risk includes proactive strategies for preventing skin breakdown when such conditions are present. The Modified Braden Q Scale is a reliable, objective tool that may be used in the assessment for pressure ulcer development in children who are acutely ill or who are at risk for skin breakdown from neurologic conditions and immobilization (Curley et al, 2003). Frequent position changes help prevent dependent edema and stimulate circulation, respiratory function, gastrointestinal motility, and neurologic sensations.

NURSE ALERT On admission each child should have a skin assessment and a skin score documented in the medical record. ■

Children are encouraged to be as active as their condition and restrictive devices allow. This poses few problems for children, whose innate ingenuity and natural inclination toward mobility provide them with the impetus for physical activity. They need the opportunity, the materials or objects to stimulate activity, and the encouragement and participation of others. Those who are unable to move need passive exercise and movement, perhaps in consultation with a physical therapist (PT).

When possible, transporting the child by stretcher, stroller, or wagon outside the confines of the room increases environmental stimuli and provides social contact with others. While hospitalized, children benefit from same-age visitors, computers, books, video games, and other items brought from their own room at home, all of which help them function in a more normal way. An activity center or tray that slants can be particularly helpful for the child with limited mobility to use for drawing, coloring, writing, and playing with small toys such as trucks and cars. A play therapist or child-life specialist should be consulted for recreational planning. As soon as possible, hospitalized children should be allowed to wear their own clothes (street clothes, especially in preadolescent and adolescent girls) and resume school and previous activities. A parent or siblings should be allowed to stay overnight and room in with the hospitalized child to prevent the effects of family disruption from hospitalization. All efforts should be made to minimize family disruption resulting from the hospitalization. Although most of the suggestions discussed relate to hospital care, the same consultations (PT/occupational therapist/child-life/speech therapy) and environment may be considered in the home as well to help assist the child and family achieve independence and normalization. The use of play (see Chapter 44) and any activity that is tolerated (e.g., turning in bed or changing the location of the bed within the room) help alter the monotony of immobilization and decrease tension and frustration.

Using dolls, stuffed animals, or puppets to illustrate and explain the immobilization is a valuable tool for small children. Placing a cast, tubing, or other restraining equipment on the doll offers the child a nonthreatening opportunity to express, through the doll, feelings concerning the restrictions and feelings toward the nurse and other health care providers. Children typically dislike hospital food, which is usually not tailored to their age. Parents and friends should be allowed to bring in meals from home or other sources, provided they meet necessary requirements for the illness; this enables children to have more control of their environment and will decrease resistance to treatments and schedules, which is usually common behavior evidenced when adults and children are not given any choices in an acute care setting.

One of the most useful interventions to help children cope with immobility is participation in their own care. Self-care is usually well received by children. They can help plan their daily routine; select their diet (when possible); and choose "street clothes," including innovative adornments such as baseball caps or brightly colored stockings, to express their autonomy and individuality. They are encouraged to do as much as they are able to for themselves in order to keep muscles active and their interest alive. It is important for children to understand behavioral limitations or rules, and their questions should be answered. In some situations they have a choice; in others they do not. They may or may not be permitted to sleep late, but they can choose their own clothing. Most of children's activity of daily living is play; therefore, therapies that incorporate this concept are more apt to gain their cooperation.

Visits from significant persons, such as family members and friends, offer occasions for emotional support and also provide opportunities for learning how to care for the child.

Some privacy is needed, particularly by the teenager, and most long-term health care facilities recognize that rooms shared by two to four children, rather than large wards, are better environments for habilitation or rehabilitation. If a traumatic incident caused the child's disability, guilt feelings may be displayed overtly or masked behind regressive or aggressive behavior. The feeling that "I must have been bad for this to happen" is common, and honest feedback stating, "It just happened—it was an accident," needs to be repeated many times.

With the increased trend in early mobilization, early discharge and home health care, many children are discharged home within a few days of hospitalization. Follow-up treatment may take place in the home setting or an outpatient ambulatory facility.

Family Support and Home Care

The needs of a child with severe disabilities can be very complex, and family members require time to assimilate the teachings and demonstrations needed to understand the child's situation and care. Even the child who is confined on a short-term basis can be a challenge for the family, which is usually unprepared for the problems imposed by the child's special needs. Home modification is usually needed for facilitating care, especially when it involves traction, large casts, or extended confinement. Suitable child care may be needed for times when all family members work.

Just as in the hospital, the child at home is encouraged to be as independent as possible and to follow a schedule that approximates his or her normal lifestyle as nearly as possible, such as continuing school lessons, regular bedtime, and suitable recreational activities.

Evaluation

The effectiveness of nursing interventions is determined by continual reassessment and evaluation of care based on the following observational guidelines and expected outcomes:

1. Observe vital signs, neurologic signs, and respiratory, gastrointestinal, and renal functioning; inspect skin; observe effects of correct functioning of equipment and appliances (e.g., traction, cast, and braces).
2. Observe child's behavior; engage in dialogue to elicit feelings, concerns, and interests.
3. Observe child's activities and interests.
4. Interview child and family regarding their feelings and concerns; observe family interaction at home, if possible.

Expected outcomes are contained in the Nursing Care Plan.

TRAUMATIC INJURY

Soft Tissue Injury

Injuries to the muscles, ligaments, and tendons are common in children (Fig. 54-1). In young children, soft tissue injury usually results from mishaps during play. In older children and adolescents, participation in sports is the more common cause.

Contusions

A contusion is damage to the soft tissue, subcutaneous structures, and muscle. The tearing of these tissues and small blood vessels and the inflammatory response lead to hemorrhage, edema, and associated pain when the child attempts to move the injured part. The escape of blood into the tissues is observed as *ecchymosis,* a black-and-blue discoloration.

Large contusions cause gross swelling, pain, and disability, and those sustained while the child is participating in sports usually receive immediate attention from health personnel. The less spectacular, smaller injuries may go unnoticed, allowing continued participation; however, they can become disabling after rest because of pain and muscle spasm. The young athlete is commonly instructed to "work it out" or disregard the pain. Instead of this approach, an assessment of the affected area should be first carried out by a qualified health care worker or certified athletic trainer because further damage to the site may result if the area is severely traumatized. Immediate treatment consists of cold application, as in the treatment of sprains described in the following section. Return to participation is allowed when the strength and range of motion of the affected extremity are equal to those of the opposite extremity or is demonstrated under conditions such as sport-specific tests. *Myositis ossificans* may occur from deep contusions to the biceps or quadriceps muscles; this condition may result in a restriction of flexibility of the affected limb.

Related to contusions are crush injuries that occur in children when they slam their fingers (in doors, folding chairs, or equipment) or hit their fingers (as when hammer-

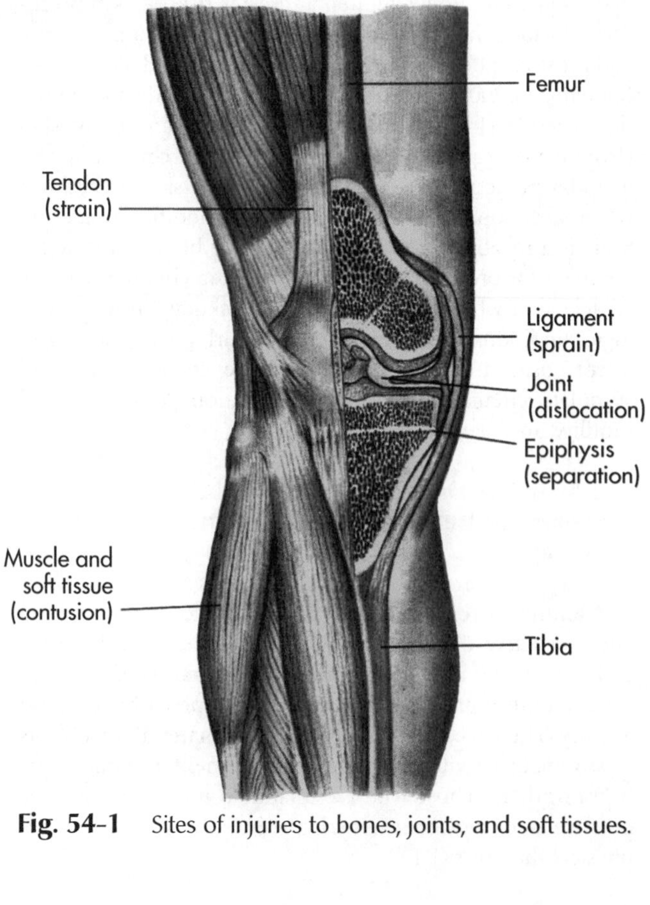

Fig. 54-1 Sites of injuries to bones, joints, and soft tissues.

Nursing Care Plan

THE CHILD WHO IS IMMOBILIZED

NURSING DIAGNOSIS: Impaired physical mobility related to mechanical restrictions, physical disability

EXPECTED OUTCOME
Child engages in activities appropriate to physical limitations.

NURSING INTERVENTIONS/*RATIONALES*
Arrange for appropriate transport (e.g., wheelchair, stretcher, crutches, stroller) *to maintain mobility;* plan trips outside confines of room *to prevent isolation.*
Rearrange furniture in room when child is confined for long term *to break monotony and provide variety.*
Encourage mobility freedom of movement, independence in activities of daily living, and play within physical limits *to maintain sense of autonomy and control.*
Encourage child to make choices about daily routine, food, clothing, play within physical limits *to maintain sense of control.*

NURSING DIAGNOSIS: Risk for impaired skin integrity related to immobility, therapeutic devices

EXPECTED OUTCOME
Skin is clean, dry, and intact.

NURSING INTERVENTIONS/*RATIONALES*
Turn and reposition every 2 hours *to promote circulation and prevent skin breakdown* (align properly, provide positional supports; use handrolls or splints *to position hands in functional position;* use footboard, high top tennis shoes or splints *to prevent footdrop*); perform passive range of motion frequently *to maintain full range in all joints and prevent contracture formation;* seat child in chair *to improve circulation;* place on tilt table *to prevent loss of bone density to long bones.*
Use pressure reduction mattress overlay *to prevent pressure necrosis;* use foam pads on ankles, heels, elbows *to protect bony prominences;* massage skin with lotion regularly *to stimulate circulation and prevent friction and shearing effects;* keep bedclothes clean, dry, and wrinkle-free *to prevent skin irritation;* cleanse skin, mucous membranes of mouth, and perianal area regularly *to prevent irritation and breakdown;* keep skinfolds clean and dry *to prevent excoriation;* inspect skin and mucous membranes regularly *to assess for early signs of irritation or breakdown.*

NURSING DIAGNOSIS: Risk for injury related to impaired mobility

EXPECTED OUTCOME
Child exhibits no evidence of injury.

NURSING INTERVENTIONS/*RATIONALES*
Promote and teach child and family proper transfer techniques, use of mobilizing devices (e.g., wheelchairs, crutches, walkers, braces) *to enhance safety.*
Modify environment as appropriate (e.g., place call bell in easy reach, remove hazards and barriers, clear traffic areas) *to enhance safety.*

NURSING DIAGNOSIS: Diversional activity deficit related to mobility impairment and confinement

EXPECTED OUTCOME
Child engages in activities that are developmentally appropriate and within physical and environmental limitations.

NURSING INTERVENTIONS/*RATIONALES*
Schedule therapies and rest periods *to allow time for play activities.* Time play periods when child may be feeling particularly vulnerable or alone *to provide needed distraction.*
Arrange for social interactions with others *to promote socialization.*
Interview parents and child *to discover the child's favorite activities and games;* adapt activities to the child's physical limitations *to provide optimal diversions.*
Have parents bring in treasured toys or objects; decorate room with familiar pictures and drawings *to familiarize child with an unfamiliar environment.*

ing a nail). A severe crush injury involves the bone, with swelling and bleeding beneath the nail (subungual) and sometimes laceration of the pulp of the distal phalanx. The *subungual hematoma* can be released by creating a hole at the proximal end of the nail with a battery-operated microcautery device or a heated 18-gauge needle.

Dislocations

Long bones are held in approximation to one another at the joint by ligaments. A dislocation occurs when the force of stress on the ligament is so great as to displace the normal position of the opposing bone ends or to displace the bone end from its socket. The predominant symptom is pain that increases with attempted passive or active movement of the extremity. In dislocations there may be an obvious deformity and inability to move the joint. Dislocation of the phalanges is the most common type seen in children, followed by elbow dislocation. The most common injury in young children is subluxation or partial dislocation of the radial head, also called "pulled elbow" or *"nursemaids' elbow."* In the majority of cases the injury occurs in a child younger than 5 years who receives a sudden longitudinal pull or traction at the wrist while the arm is fully extended and the forearm pronated. It usually occurs when an adult or older sibling who is holding the child by the hand or wrist gives a sudden pull or jerk to prevent a fall, attempts to lift the child by pulling the wrist, or when the child pulls away by dropping to the floor or ground. The child often cries, appears anxious, and refuses to use the affected limb. The practitioner manipulates the arm by applying firm finger pressure to the head of the radius, then supinates and flexes the forearm to return the bone structure to normal alignment. A click may be heard or felt, and functional use of the arm returns within minutes (Greene, 2001). However, the longer the subluxation is present, the longer it takes for the child to recover mobility after treatment. No anesthetic is usually required but a mild pain reliever such as acetaminophen may be given. In an older child, severe elbow injury or dislocation should be carefully evaluated by a practitioner immediately; likewise, a traumatic elbow injury in the younger child that is not a subluxation should be carefully evaluated.

In children younger than 5 years of age, the hip can be dislocated by a fall. The greatest risk after this injury is the potential loss of blood supply to the head of the femur. Relocation of the hip within 60 minutes after the injury provides the best chance for prevention of damage to the femoral head.

Shoulder dislocations occur most often in older adolescents and are often sports related. Temporary restriction of the joint, with a sling or bandage that secures the arm to the chest, in a shoulder dislocation, can provide sufficient comfort and immobilization until medical attention is received.

Simple dislocations should be reduced as soon as possible with the child under mild sedation and often local anesthesia. Anesthetics such as intravenous ketamine (Ketalar) and midazolam (Versed), IV propofol (Diprivan), or fentanyl (Sublimaze) can be used to produce partial or complete analgesia. An unreduced dislocation will be complicated by increased swelling, making reduction difficult and increasing the risk of neurovascular problems. Treatment depends on the severity of the injury.

Sprains

A sprain occurs when trauma to a joint is so severe that a ligament is partially or completely torn or stretched by the force created as a joint is twisted or wrenched, often accompanied by damage to associated blood vessels, muscles, tendons, and nerves.

The presence of joint laxity is the most valid indicator of the severity of a sprain. In a severe injury the child complains of the joint "feeling loose" or as if "something is coming apart," and may describe hearing a "snap," "pop," or "tearing." Pain is seldom the principal subjective symptom. There is a rapid onset with swelling (often diffuse), accompanied by immediate disability and appreciable reluctance to use the injured joint.

Strains

A strain is a microscopic tear to the musculotendinous unit and has features in common with sprains. The area is painful to touch and swollen. Most strains are incurred over time rather than suddenly, and the rapidity of the appearance provides clues regarding severity. In general, the more rapidly the strain occurs, the more severe the injury. When the strain involves the muscular portion, there is more bleeding, often palpable soon after injury and before edema obscures the hematoma.

Therapeutic Management

The first minutes to 12 hours is the most critical period for virtually all soft tissue injuries. Basic principles of managing sprains and other soft tissue injuries are summarized in the acronyms *RICE* and *ICES:*

R–Rest	**I**–Ice
I–Ice	**C**–Compression
C–Compression	**E**–Elevation
E–Elevation	**S**–Support

Soft tissue injuries should be iced immediately. This is best accomplished with crushed ice wrapped in a towel or encased in a screw-top ice bag or resealable storage bag. A wet elastic wrap, which transfers cold better than dry wrap, is applied to provide compression and to keep the ice pack in place. Chemical-activated ice packs are also effective for immediate treatment but are not reusable and must be closely monitored for leakage. A cloth barrier should be used between the ice container and the skin to prevent trauma to the tissues. Ice has a rapid cooling effect on tissues and reduces the pain threshold. However, ice should never be applied for more than 30 minutes at a time because of the body's homeostatic response to cold, which may trigger a decrease in vascularization at the injury site.

Elevating the extremity uses gravity to facilitate venous return and to reduce edema formation in the damaged area. The point of injury should be kept several inches above the level of the heart for therapy to be effective. Several pillows can be used effectively for elevation. Allowing the extremity to be dependent causes excessive fluid accumulation in the area of injury, delaying healing and causing painful swelling.

NURSE ALERT A plastic bag of frozen vegetables, such as peas, serves as a convenient ice pack for soft tissue injuries. It is clean, watertight, and easily molded to the injured part. When available, snow placed in a plastic bag may serve as an ice bag. ■

Torn ligaments, especially those in the knee, are usually treated by immobilization with a knee immobilizer or range-of-motion brace until the child is able to walk without a limp. Crutches are used for mobility to rest the affected extremity. Passive leg exercises, gradually increased to active ones, are begun as soon as sufficient healing has taken place. Parents and children are cautioned against using any form of liniment or other heat-producing preparation before examination. If the injury requires casting or splinting, the heat generated in the enclosed space can cause extreme discomfort and may even cause tissue damage. In some cases torn knee ligaments are managed with arthroscopy and ligament repair or reconstruction as necessary, depending on the extent of the tear, ligaments involved, and age of the child. Surgical reconstruction of the anterior cruciate ligament (ACL) may be performed in young athletes who wish to continue in active sports (Greene, 2001).

Fractures

Case Study: Fractures

Bone fractures occur when the resistance of bone against the stress being exerted yields to the stress force. Fractures are a common injury at any age but are more likely to occur in children and older adults. Because childhood is a time of rapid bone growth, the pattern of fractures, problems of diagnosis, and methods of treatment differ in the child and the adult. In children fractures heal much faster than in adults. Consequently, children may not require as long a period of immobilization of the affected extremity as an adult with a fracture.

Fracture injuries in children are most often a result of traumatic incidents at home, at school, in a motor vehicle, or in association with recreational activities. Children's everyday activities include vigorous play that predisposes them to injury—climbing, falling down, running into immovable objects, skateboarding, and receiving blows to any part of their bodies.

Aside from automobile accidents or falls from heights, true injuries that cause fractures rarely occur in infancy; therefore, bone injury in children of that age group warrants further investigation. In any small child, radiographic evidence of fractures at various stages of healing are, with few exceptions, a result of physical abuse. Any investigation of fractures in infants, particularly multiple fractures, should include consideration of *osteogenesis imperfecta.*

The clavicle is probably the bone most commonly broken in childhood, with approximately half of clavicle fractures occurring in children under 10 years of age. Common mechanisms of injury include a fall with an outstretched hand or direct trauma to the bone.

Fractures in school-age children are often a result of bicycle, automobile, or skateboard injuries. Adolescents are vulnerable to multiple and severe trauma because they are mobile on bicycles, all-terrain vehicles, skateboards, skis, snowboards, bicycles, and motorcycles and are active in sports.

Epiphyseal (or Physeal) Injuries

The weakest point of long bones is the cartilage growth plate or epiphyseal plate. Consequently, this is a common site of damage during trauma. Detection of epiphyseal injuries is sometimes difficult, but critical. Fractures involving the epiphysis or epiphyseal plate present special problems in determining whether or not bone growth will be affected. Treatment of these fractures may include open reduction and internal fixation to prevent or reduce growth disturbances.

BOX 54-1

Types of Fractures in Children

Bend–Occurs when the bone is bent but not broken. A child's flexible bone can be bent 45 degrees or more before breaking. However, if bent, the bone will straighten slowly, but not completely, to produce some deformity but without the angulation seen when the bone breaks. Bends occur most commonly in the ulna and fibula, often in association with fractures of the radius and tibia.

Buckle, or torus, fracture–Produced by compression of the porous bone; appears as a raised or bulging projection at the fracture site. These fractures occur in the most porous portion of the bone near the metaphysis (the portion of the bone shaft adjacent to the epiphysis) and are more common in young children.

Greenstick fracture–Occurs when a bone is angulated beyond the limits of bending. The compressed side bends, and the tension side fails, causing an incomplete fracture similar to the break observed when a green stick is broken.

Complete fracture–Divides the bone fragments. These fragments often remain attached by a periosteal hinge, which can aid or hinder reduction.

Types of Fractures

A fractured bone consists of fragments—the fragment closer to the midline, or the proximal fragment; and the fragment farther from the midline, or the distal fragment. When fracture fragments are separated, the fracture is *complete;* when fragments remain attached, the fracture is *incomplete.* The fracture line can be any of the following:

Transverse—Crosswise, at right angles to the long axis of the bone

Oblique—Slanting but straight, between a horizontal and a perpendicular direction

Spiral—Slanting and circular, twisting around the bone shaft

The twisting of an extremity while the bone is breaking results in a spiral break. If the fracture does not produce a break in the skin, it is a *simple,* or *closed fracture. Open,* or *compound fractures* are those with an open wound through which the bone is or has protruded. If the bone fragments cause damage to other organs or tissues (such as the lung or bladder), the injury is said to be a *complicated fracture.* When small fragments of bone are broken from the fractured shaft and lie in the surrounding tissue, the injury is a *comminuted fracture.* This type of fracture is rare in children. The types of fractures seen most often in children are described in Box 54-1 and in Fig. 54-2.

NURSE ALERT A spiral fracture in children may indicate child abuse. Further assessment and immediate involvement of interdisciplinary team members, such as a social worker, are necessary. ■

Immediately after a fracture occurs, the muscles contract and physiologically splint the injured area. This phenome-

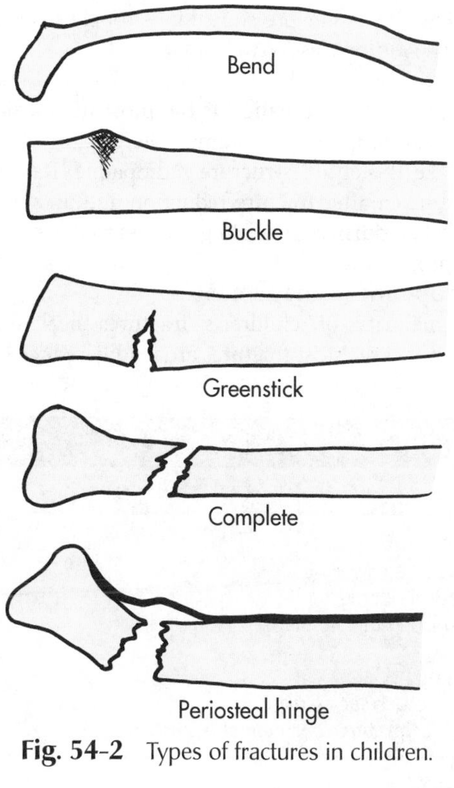

Fig. 54-2 Types of fractures in children.

non accounts for the muscle tightness observed over a fracture site and the deformity that is produced as the muscles pull the bone ends out of alignment. This muscle response must be overcome by traction or complete muscle relaxation (e.g., with anesthesia) in order to realign the distal bone fragment to the proximal bone fragment.

Bone Healing and Remodeling

Bone healing is characteristically rapid in children because of the thickened periosteum and generous blood supply. When there is a break in the continuity of bone, the osteoblasts are stimulated to maximum activity. New bone cells are formed in immense numbers almost immediately after the injury and, in time, are evidenced by a bulging growth of new bone tissue between the fractured bone fragments. This is followed by deposition of calcium salts to form a *callus.*

Fractures heal in less time in children than in adults. The approximate healing times for a femoral shaft are as follows:

- Neonatal period—2 to 3 weeks
- Early childhood—4 weeks
- Later childhood—6 to 8 weeks
- Adolescence—8 to 12 weeks

Diagnostic Evaluation

A history is often lacking in childhood injuries. Infants are unable to communicate, and older children seldom volunteer information (even under direct questioning) when the injury occurred during suspicious activities. Unless they are witnesses to the injury, parents may misinterpret what the child is trying to say. In cases of child abuse, parents may give false information to protect themselves.

The child may exhibit the same manifestations seen in adults (Box 54-2). However, often a fracture is remarkably stable because of intact periosteum. The child may even be able to use an affected arm or walk on a fractured leg.

NURSE ALERT A fracture should be strongly suspected in a small child who refuses to walk or crawl. ■

Radiographic examination is the most useful diagnostic tool for assessing skeletal trauma. The calcium deposits in bone make the entire structure radiopaque. Radiographic films are taken after fracture reduction and, in some cases, may be taken during the healing process to determine satisfactory progress.

Therapeutic Management

The majority of children's fractures heal well, and nonunion is rare. Most fractures are readily reduced by simple traction and immobilization until healing takes place. However, the position of the bone fragments in relation to one another influences the rapidity of healing and the residual deformity. Healing is prompt and complete with end-to-end apposition, but a gap between fragments delays (or prevents) healing. The goals of fracture management are the following:

1. To regain alignment and length of the bony fragments (reduction)
2. To retain alignment and length (immobilization)
3. To restore function to the injured parts
4. To prevent further injury

In children the bone fragments are usually realigned and immobilized by traction or by closed manipulation and casting until an adequate callus is formed. Weight bearing on lower extremity fractures and active movement for the purpose of regaining function can begin after the fracture site is stable. The child's natural tendency to be active is usually sufficient to restore normal mobility, and physical therapy is rarely needed. In most cases children's fractures can be managed by closed reduction and cast immobilization, which is most often provided on an outpatient basis with reevaluation in 7 to 10 days.

Children are most frequently hospitalized for fractures of the femur and the supracondylar area of the distal humerus, which may require internal fixation and pinning; displaced supracondylar fractures in children should be treated surgically (Do & Herrera-Soto, 2003). If simple reductions cannot be achieved or if a neurovascular problem is detected after injury, observation in a hospital is indicated. Severe contusions with profound swelling cannot be treated with a cast, which would act as a tourniquet on the extremity. A badly malaligned fracture requires traction for a period before a cast is applied.

The major methods for immobilizing a fracture—casting and traction—are described in the following sections on casting and traction.

Nursing Care Management

Nurses are frequently the persons who make the initial assessment of a child with a suspected fracture (Emergency box). The child and parents may be frightened and upset, and the child is often in pain. Therefore, if the child is alert and there is no evidence of hemorrhage, the initial nursing interventions are directed toward calming and reassuring the child and parents so that a more extensive assessment can be more easily accomplished.

While remaining calm and speaking in a quiet voice, the nurse can ask the parents and older child to describe what happened and how they feel about it. Because the child usually arrives with the limb supported in some manner, this time does not delay or endanger the treatment. Initially it is best not to touch the child but to ask him or her to point to the painful area and to wiggle the fingers or toes. By this time the child usually feels relatively safe and will allow someone to gently touch the area just enough to feel the pulse and test for sensation. A child's anxiety is greatly influenced by previous experiences with injury and with health personnel; however, he or she needs to be told what will happen and what to do to help. The affected limb need not be palpated, and it should not be

BOX 54-2

Clinical Manifestations of a Fracture

Signs of injury:
- Generalized swelling
- Pain or tenderness
- Diminished functional use of affected part

May be:
- Bruising
- Severe muscular rigidity
- Crepitus (grating sensation at fracture site)

Emergency

FRACTURE

Assess the extent of injury—5 *Ps*;
- Pain and point of tenderness
- Pulses—distal to the fracture site
- Pallor
- Paresthesia—sensation distal to the fracture site
- Paralysis—movement distal to the fracture site

Determine the mechanism of injury.
Move the injured part as little as possible.
Cover open wounds with a sterile or clean dressing.
- Immobilize the limb, including joints above and below the fracture site; do not attempt to reduce the fracture or push protruding bone under the skin.
- Soft splint (pillow or folded towel)
- Rigid splint (rolled newspaper or magazine)
- Uninjured leg can serve as a splint for a leg fracture if no splint available

Reassess neurovascular status.
Apply traction if circulatory compromise is present.
Elevate the injured limb if possible.
Apply cold to the injured area.
Call emergency medical service or transport to medical facility.

moved unless properly splinted. If the child is at home or if the practitioner is not present to examine the child, some type of splint is applied carefully for transport to the medical facility. Parental anxiety may be heightened by the child's pain reaction and fear, and possibly other events surrounding the accident, thus it is important to communicate to the parent that the child will receive the necessary care, including pain management.

NURSE ALERT The five "Ps" of ischemia from a vascular injury should be included in an assessment of the injury:

1. Pain
2. Pallor
3. Pulselessness
4. Paresthesia
5. Paralysis ■

The Child in a Cast

The completeness of the fracture, the type of bone involved, and the amount of weight bearing influence how much of the extremity must be included in the cast to immobilize the fracture site completely. In most cases the joints above and below the fracture are immobilized to eliminate the possibility of movement that might cause displacement at the fracture site. Four major categories of casts are used for fractures: *upper extremity* to immobilize the wrist or elbow, *lower extremity* to immobilize the ankle or knee, *spinal* and *cervical* for immobilization of the spine, and *spica casts* to immobilize the hip and knee.

The Cast

Casts are constructed from gauze strips and bandages impregnated with plaster of paris or, more commonly, from synthetic lighter weight and water-resistant materials (e.g., fiberglass and polyurethane resin).

Both types of casting produce heat from chemical reaction activated by water immediately after application. Plaster casts mold closely to the body part, take 10 to 72 hours to dry, have a smooth exterior, and are inexpensive. The newer synthetic casting material is lighter, dries in 5 to 30 minutes, permits earlier weight bearing, and is water-resistant. The disadvantage of synthetic casting is its inability to mold closely to body parts; its rough exterior, which may scratch surfaces; and increased cost.

NURSE ALERT Synthetic casts have special advantages for children. They come in different colors and with designs (e.g., cartoons, stripes); they are lightweight, durable, easy to clean, and relatively water-resistant, depending on the type of inner lining used; only those with a Gore-Tex inner lining may be immersed in water without affecting the cast integrity. Bathing with a synthetic cast may be accomplished by covering the cast with a plastic bag; if the synthetic cast gets wet, it should be dried thoroughly. One drawback to immersion is the time necessary to completely dry the cast. The synthetic casts are difficult to write on. A waterproof marker or color markers may be used for writing on the cast. ■

Cast Application

The developmental age of the child should be considered before the cast is applied. For preschoolers who fear bodily harm and fantasize loss of an extremity, instead of immobilization, it may be helpful to use a plastic doll or stuffed animal to explain the procedure beforehand. It is also helpful to explain that the synthetic cast material will become warm but will not burn. During the application of the cast, various distraction methods may be used including a discussion of favorite pets, activities at school, blowing bubbles, and so forth. In this age group explanations such as "This will help your arm get better" are futile because the child has no concept of causality.

Before the cast is applied, the extremities are checked for any abrasions, cuts, or other alterations in the skin surface and for the presence of rings or other items that might cause constriction from swelling; such objects are removed. A tube of cloth stockinette is stretched over the area to be casted, and bony prominences are padded with soft cotton sheeting. Some practitioners use a Gore-Tex liner under a hip spica cast to prevent continuous exposure to moisture and possible skin breakdown. Dry rolls of casting material are immersed in a pail of water. The (plaster) wet rolls are put on in a bandage fashion and molded to the extremity. During application of the plaster cast, the underlying stockinette is pulled over the rough edges of the cast and secured with a layer of wet plaster 0.5 to 1 inch below the rim to form a smooth, padded edge to protect the skin.

If the practitioner does not form such a protective edge with stockinette, the rough edges of the plaster cast can be protected by a "petaled" edge. Small pieces approximately 2 to 3 inches long are cut from 1- or 1.5-inch-wide adhesive tape or moleskin. The edges are rounded with scissors, and these "petals" are placed over the edge of the cast, with each petal slightly overlapping the previous petal to form a smooth, neat edge. It is easier to apply the petal to the underside of the cast first and then bring the loose edge to the front, pressing firmly so that the edges remain securely attached. Synthetic casts usually do not require additional padding on the edges because they do not crack like plaster material.

Nursing Care Management

The complete evaporation of the water from a hip spica cast can take 24 to 48 hours when older types of plaster materials are used. Drying occurs within minutes with fiberglass cast material. The cast must remain uncovered to allow it to dry from the inside out. Turning the child in a plaster cast at least every 2 hours will help dry a body cast evenly and prevent complications related to immobility. A regular fan or cool-air hair dryer to circulate air may be helpful when the humidity is high.

NURSE ALERT Heated fans or dryers are not used, because they cause the cast to dry on the outside and remain wet beneath or cause burns from heat conduction by way of the cast to the underlying tissue. ■

A wet plaster cast should be supported by a pillow that is covered with plastic and handled by the palms of the hands to prevent indenting the cast, which can create pressure areas. A dry plaster-of-paris cast produces a hollow sound when it is tapped with the finger. If "hot spots" are felt on the cast surface (usually indicating infection beneath the area), this should be reported so that a window can be made in the cast to observe the site.

SKILL: MONITORING NEUROVASCULAR STATUS

During the first few hours after a cast is applied, the chief concern is that the extremity may continue to swell to the extent that the cast becomes a tourniquet, shutting off circulation and producing neurovascular complications. To reduce the likelihood of this potential problem, the body part can be elevated, thereby increasing venous return. If edema is excessive, casts are bivalved (i.e., cut to make anterior and posterior halves that are held together with an elastic bandage). The cast and the involved extremity are observed frequently for neurovascular integrity and any signs of compromise. Permanent muscle and tissue damage can occur within 6 to 8 hours.

NURSE ALERT Observations such as pain (unrelieved by pain medication 1 hour after administration), swelling, discoloration (pallor or cyanosis) of the exposed portions, decreased pulses, decreased temperature, or the inability to move the distal exposed part(s) should be reported immediately. ■

When an extremity that has sustained an open fracture is casted, a window is often left over the wound area to allow for observation and for dressing of the wound. In some cases a cast may not be applied for days in order to permit access to the wound for observation; instead, a temporary immobilization device such as a splint may be applied. For the first few hours after surgery, there may be substantial bleeding that will soak through the cast. Periodically the circumscribed blood-stained area should be outlined with a ballpoint pen or pencil, and the time indicated to provide a guide for assessing the amount of bleeding.

Usually the child is discharged to home care after a cast is applied in the emergency department or clinic. Parents need instructions on drying and caring for the cast and on checking for signs and symptoms that indicate the cast is too tight (Home Care box). They should also be told to take the child to the health professional for attention if the cast becomes too loose, because a loose cast no longer serves its purpose. A cast is a badge of honor for the child and serves as visible evidence of an otherwise invisible injury.

Nurses can help families adapt the child's home environment to meet the temporary encumbrance of a cast. Home care creates problems of various magnitudes, especially for children in large casts (e.g., a hip spica). Commonplace situations become problematic (e.g., transporting a child safely and comfortably in a car). Standard seat belts and car seats may not be readily adapted for use by children in some casts. Specially designed car seats and restraints that meet safety requirements are available.* Alterations to standard car seats to accommodate the cast are not recommended because the structure may be adversely altered.

Parents are taught the proper care of the cast (or orthotic device) and are helped to devise means for maintaining cleanliness. A superabsorbent disposable diaper (newborn size) is tucked beneath the entire perineal opening of the cast. A larger (toddler size) diaper can be applied and fastened over the small diaper and cast.

For tightly fitting casts, transparent film dressings can be cut into strips as for petaling, and one edge applied to the cast edge and the other directly to the perineum; this forms a continuous, waterproof bridge between the perineum and the cast to prevent leakage. An additional advantage to the use of this transparent dressing is that it keeps both the skin and the cast dry while allowing for observation of skin beneath the dressing.

Older infants and small children may stuff bits of food, small toys, or other items under the cast; parents should be alerted to this possibility so that suitable preventive measures can be initiated.

Feeding the infant in a hip spica cast offers problems in positioning. Very young infants can be fed in the supine position with the head elevated; with the infant's hips and legs supported on a pillow at the side, the parent can cuddle the infant in his or her arms during feeding. A somewhat similar position can be used for breastfeeding (i.e., with the infant supported on pillows or held in a "football" hold facing the mother with the legs behind her). An alternate position is to hold the infant upright on the caregiver's lap with the legs of the infant astride the adult's leg.

Children in spica casts usually find the prone position easier for self-feeding from a small table placed next to the dining table. The use of a conventional toilet is almost impossible. Small bedpans or other containers offer alternatives for elimination. The nurse may suggest waterproofing methods, using plastic wraps that can help with elimination and showers. Baths are possible only if the plaster cast is kept out of the water and covered to prevent it from becoming wet

---

*For additional information contact the Automotive Safety for Children Program, James Whitcomb Riley Hospital for Children, Indiana University School of Medicine, 575 West Drive, Room 004, Indianapolis, IN 46202; phone: 317-274-2977 (in Indianapolis 800-543-6227); Web site: www.preventinjury.org.

Home Care

CAST CARE

Keep the casted extremity elevated on pillows or similar support for the first day, or as directed by the health professional.

Avoid indenting the cast (use palms of hand to handle) while still wet to avoid creating pressure points.

Observe the extremities (fingers or toes) for any evidence of swelling or discoloration (darker or lighter than a comparable extremity), and contact the health professional if noted.

Check movement and sensation of the visible extremities frequently.

Follow health professional's orders regarding any restriction of activities.

Restrict strenuous activities for the first few days.
- Engage in quiet activities but encourage use of muscles.
- Move the joints above and below the cast on the affected extremity.

Encourage frequent rest for a few days, keeping the injured extremity elevated while resting.

Avoid allowing the affected limb to hang down for any length of time.
- Keep an injured upper extremity elevated (e.g., on a pillow) while upright.
- Elevate a lower limb when sitting and avoid standing for too long.

Do not allow the child to put anything inside the cast.
- Keep small items that might be placed inside the cast away from small children.

Keep a clear path for ambulation.
- Remove toys, hazardous floor rugs, pets, or other items over which the child might stumble.

Use crutches appropriately if lower limb fracture.
- The crutches should fit properly, have a soft rubber tip to prevent slipping, and be well padded at the axilla.

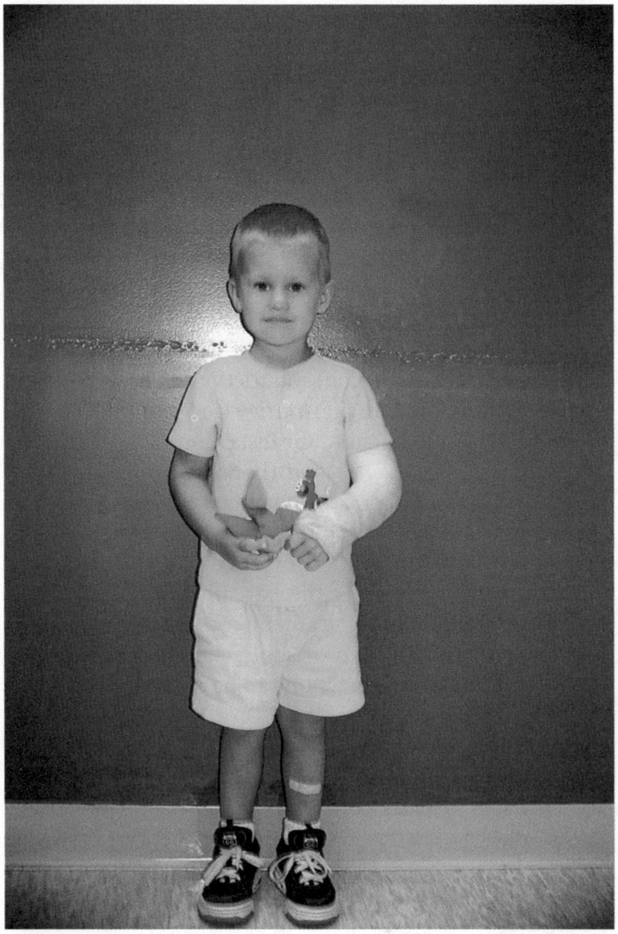

Fig. 54-3 Young children usually adapt well to a cast but often fear the removal.

from splashes. Synthetic casts can be immersed in water if a special type of cast liner is used.

Cast Removal

Cutting the cast to remove it or to relieve tightness is frequently a frightening experience for children. They fear the sound of the cast cutter and are terrified that their flesh, as well as the cast, will be cut. The oscillating blade vibrates very rapidly back and forth and will not cut when placed *lightly* on the skin. Children have described it as producing a "tickly" sensation. The vibration also generates heat that may be felt by the child. Both of these feelings should be explained. Preparation for the procedure will help reduce anxiety, especially if a trusting relationship has been established between the child and the nurse. Many young children come to regard the cast as part of themselves, which intensifies their fear of removal (Fig. 54-3). Using the analogy of having fingernails trimmed or a haircut sometimes helps reduce their anxiety. They need continual reassurance that all is going well and that their behavior is accepted. One concern with fiberglass casts during removal is the potential for inhalation of fiberglass particles; this may be avoided by only using a cast saw with a built in vacuum or placing a mask on the child as age permits (Adkins, 1997).

After the cast is removed, the skin surface will be caked with desquamated skin and sebaceous secretions. Simple soaking in a bathtub is usually sufficient for their removal, but several days may be required to eliminate the accumulation completely. Application of oil or skin lotion may provide comfort. The parents and child should be instructed not to pull or forcibly remove this material with vigorous scrubbing because it may cause excoriation and bleeding.

The Child in Traction

The ever-changing health care arena has witnessed the demise of many long-term treatments involving lengthy hospitalization; one such change is in the area of traction. Most balanced skeletal traction is applied in children after a severe or complex injury to allow physiologic stability, align bone fragments, and permit closer evaluation of the injured site. Newer technology has produced orthopedic fixation devices that allow partial or full mobility, thus preventing long-term immobilization and its consequences. In many situations, surgical intervention may be carried out within a matter of days; therefore, skeletal traction devices described herein may be used infrequently in many cases.

Bone fragments that cannot be aligned initially by simple traction and stabilization with a cast require the extended pulling force supplied by continuous traction.

Traction may be used for other purposes, including the following:

- To provide rest for an extremity
- To help prevent or improve contracture deformity
- To correct a deformity
- To treat a dislocation
- To allow preoperative or postoperative positioning and alignment
- To provide immobilization of specific areas of the body
- To reduce muscle spasms (rare in children)

Purposes of Traction

The three essential components of traction management are traction, countertraction, and friction (Fig. 54-4). To reduce or realign a fracture site, *traction* (forward force) is produced by attaching weight to the distal bone fragment; body weight provides *countertraction* (backward force); and the patient's contact with the bed constitutes the *frictional* force. These forces are used to align the distal and proximal bone fragments by adjusting the line of pull upward or downward and adducting or abducting the extremity.

To attain equilibrium, the amount of forward force is adjusted by adding weight to or subtracting weight from the traction, and/or countertraction can be increased by elevating the foot of the bed to create a greater gravitational pull to the backward force. A bed board placed under the mattress of heavy children prevents sagging, which might otherwise change the direction of the forces applied to the fracture.

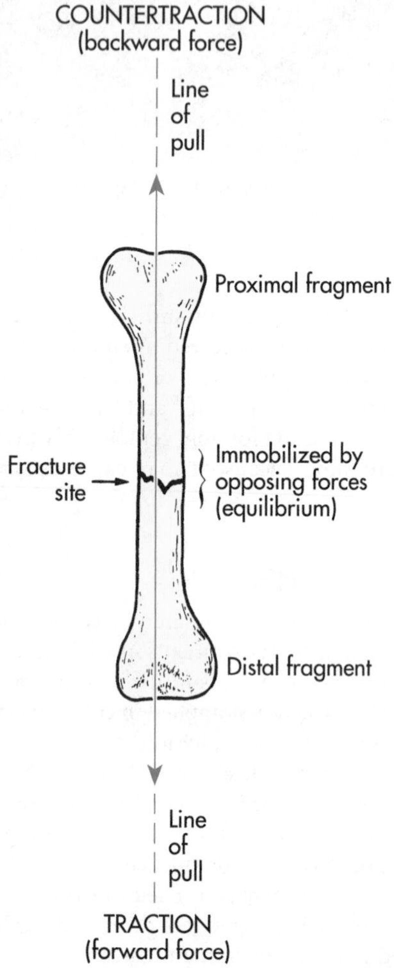

Fig. 54-4 Application of traction for maintaining equilibrium.

The three primary purposes of traction for reduction of fractures are:

1. To fatigue the involved muscle and reduce muscle spasm so that bones can be realigned
2. To position the distal and proximal bone ends in desired realignment to promote satisfactory bone healing
3. To immobilize the fracture site until realignment has been achieved and sufficient healing has taken place to permit casting or splinting

The *all-or-none law,* characteristic of muscle contractibility, influences the complete relaxation. When muscle is stretched, muscle spasm ceases and permits the realignment of the bone ends. The continuous maintenance of traction is important during this phase because releasing the traction allows the normal contracting ability of the muscle to again cause a malpositioning of the bone ends.

The realignment of the fragments is a gradual process that is achieved more rapidly in infants, who have limited muscle tone, than in muscular teenagers. The desired line of pull and callus formation are checked periodically by radiographic examination. The traction pull to some degree immobilizes the fracture site; however, adjunctive immobilizing devices such as splints or casts are sometimes used with skeletal traction. In injuries in which there is severe soft tissue swelling or vascular and nerve damage, it is customary to use traction until these complications have been resolved and it is safe to apply a cast. Immobilization with traction will be maintained until the bone ends are in satisfactory realignment, after which a less-confining type of immobilization—a cast, pins, or external stabilization device—will be applied.

Types of Traction (General)

The pull needed for traction can be applied to the distal bone fragment in several ways (Box 54-3). The type of traction applied is determined primarily by the age of the child, the condition of the soft tissues, and the type and degree of displacement of the fracture. Fractures most commonly treated by application of traction are those involving the

BOX 54-3

Types of Traction

Manual traction–Applied to the body part by the hands placed distally to the fracture site. Nurses frequently provide manual traction during cast application.

Skin traction–Applied directly to the skin surface and indirectly to the skeletal structures. The pulling mechanism is attached to the skin with adhesive material or an elastic bandage. Both types are applied over soft, foam-backed traction straps to distribute the traction pull.

Skeletal traction–Applied directly to the skeletal structure by a pin, wire, or tongs inserted into or through the diameter of the bone distal to the fracture.

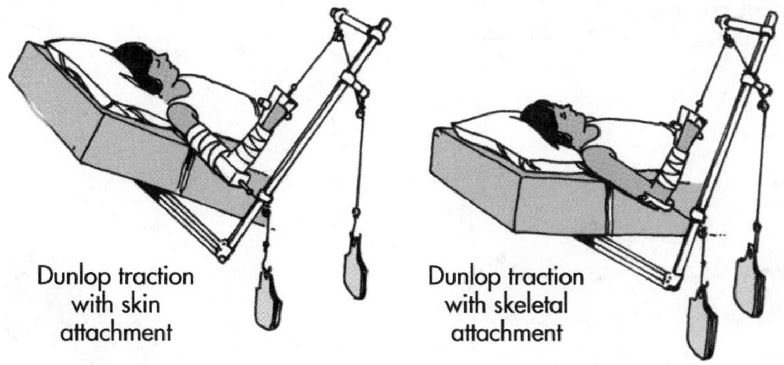

Fig. 54-5 Dunlop traction. (Figs. 54-5 to 54-9, *A* redrawn from Hilt NE, Schmitt EW: *Pediatric orthopedic nursing,* St Louis, 1975, Mosby.)

humerus, femur, and vertebrae. The major types of traction for specific fractures are discussed in the following sections.

Upper Extremity Traction

Treatment of fractures of the humerus by traction is accomplished by (1) *overhead suspension,* in which the arm, bent at the elbow, is suspended vertically by skin or skeletal attachment and traction is applied to the distal end of the humerus; or (2) *Dunlop traction.* With Dunlop traction (Fig. 54-5), the arm is suspended horizontally, using either skin or skeletal attachment. A skeletal wire placed in the upper arm to allow additional weight may be applied in certain instances, such as a supracondylar fracture. When skin traction is used, straps are placed on the lower and upper arm with the arm flexed to accomplish pull in two directions, one along the longitudinal direction of the upper arm and one to maintain vertical alignment of the lower arm.

Fractures of the humerus, which usually result from a fall with the arm in extension, frequently involve the supracondylar portion. These fractures especially place the patient at risk for nerve damage and angulation deformities; therefore, the fractures must be reduced carefully, sometimes with the patient under anesthesia. Because of the danger of complications, children with closed reduction of supracondylar fractures require close observation for neurovascular status and may need hospitalization. In severely malaligned fractures, closed reduction and pinning with the patient under anesthesia is followed by application of skeletal traction for a given period, then casting.

Lower Extremity Traction

The severity of the fracturing force and the ability of the muscles to hold the fracture out of alignment will determine the fracture type and the amount of overriding of the fragments. The periosteum may remain intact, which helps maintain alignment. A fracture in the middle third of the shaft of the femur results in significant overriding but minimal displacement. In a fracture in the lower one third of the shaft, the pull of the gastrocnemius muscle causes the distal fragment to become downwardly displaced.

Fractures of the femur can often be reduced with immediate application of a hip spica cast in young children. When traction is required, several types may be used, based on the initial assessment.

Bryant traction is a type of running traction in which the pull is only in one direction. Skin traction is applied to the legs, which are flexed at a 90-degree angle at the hips. The child's trunk (buttocks are raised slightly off the bed) provides countertraction.

Buck extension is a type of skin traction with the legs in an extended position. Except for fracture cases, turning from side to side with care is permitted, to maintain the involved leg alignment. Buck extension is used primarily for short-term immobilization, preoperatively with dislocated hips, for correcting contractures, or for bone deformities such as Legg-Calvé-Perthes disease.

Russell traction (Fig. 54-6) uses skin traction on the lower leg and a padded sling under the knee. Two lines of pull, one along the longitudinal line of the lower leg and one perpendicular to the leg, are produced. This combination of pulls allows realignment of the lower extremity and immobilizes the hip and knee in a flexed position. The hip flexion must be kept at the prescribed angle to prevent fracture malalignment, because there is no direct support under the fracture and the skin traction may slip. Special nursing measures include carefully checking the position of the traction so that the amount of desired hip flexion is maintained and damage to the common peroneal nerve under the knee does not produce footdrop.

One of the most common types of skeletal traction is *90-degree–90-degree* traction (Fig. 54-7). The lower leg is supported by a boot cast or a calf sling, and a skeletal Steinmann pin or Kirschner wire is placed in the distal fragment of the femur, resulting in a 90-degree angle at both the hip and the knee. From a nursing standpoint, this traction facilitates position changes, toileting, and prevention of complications related to traction.

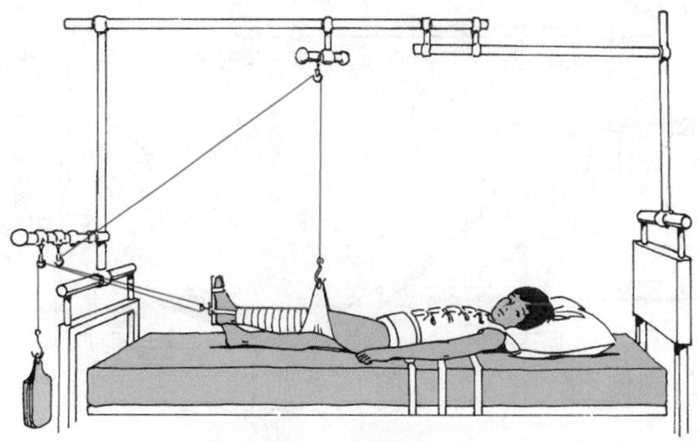

Fig. 54-6 Russell traction.

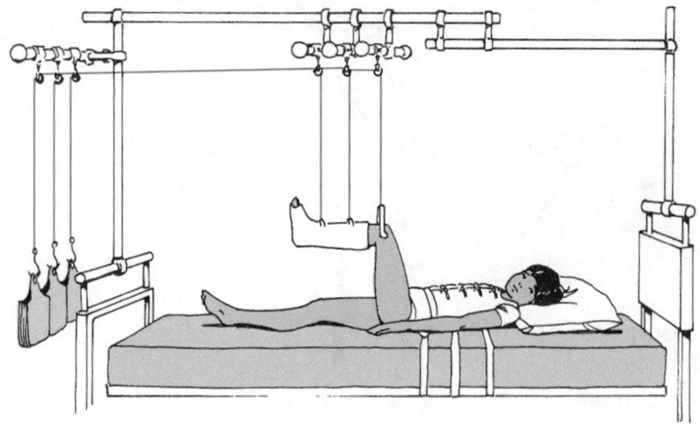

Fig. 54-7 "Ninety-ninety" traction.

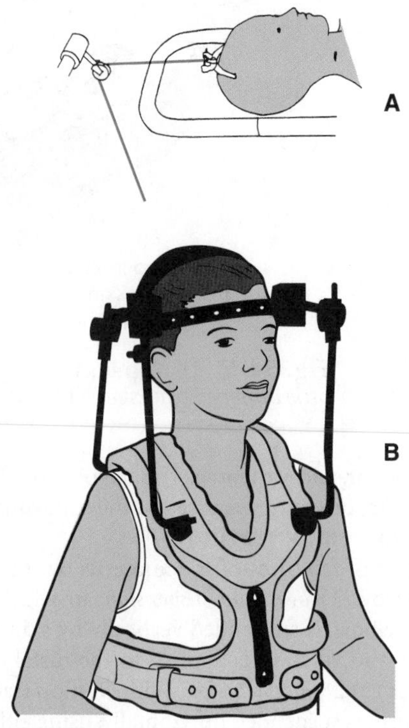

Fig. 54-9 **A**, Crutchfield tong traction. **B**, Halo vest.

Balance suspension traction (Fig. 54-8) may be used with or without skin or skeletal traction. Unless used with another traction, the balanced suspension merely suspends the leg in a desired flexed position to relax the hip and hamstring muscles and does not exert any traction directly on a body part. A *Thomas ring splint* extends from the groin to midair above the foot, and a *Pearson attachment* supports the lower leg. Towels or pieces of felt covered with stockinette are clipped or pinned to the splints for leg support. When the child is lifted off the bed, the traction lifts with the child without loss of alignment. This traction requires very careful checking of splints and ropes to make certain that no slippage or fraying has occurred. The traction is of great value in an older and heavier child when it is essential to lift the patient for care.

Cervical Traction

The cervical area is a vulnerable site for flexion or extension injuries to muscle, vertebrae, or the spinal cord. Cervical muscle trauma without other complications is treated with a cervical hard collar to relieve the weight of the head from the fracture site. When a child displaces or fractures a cervical vertebra, it may be necessary to reduce and immobilize the site with cervical skeletal traction. The spinal cord runs through the intravertebral canal, and dislocation or fracture of the vertebrae can also cause spinal cord injury. Nursing assessment of neurologic function is essential to prevent further injury during the application and use of cervical skeletal traction.

Most cervical traction is accomplished with the use of a *halo brace* or *halo vest* (Fig. 54-9, *B*). This device consists of a steel halo attached to the head by four screws inserted into the outer skull; several rigid bars connect the halo to a vest that is worn around the chest, thus providing greater mobility of the rest of the body while avoiding cervical spinal motion altogether. If the injury has been limited to a vertebral fracture without neurologic deficit, a halo brace can be applied to permit earlier ambulation.

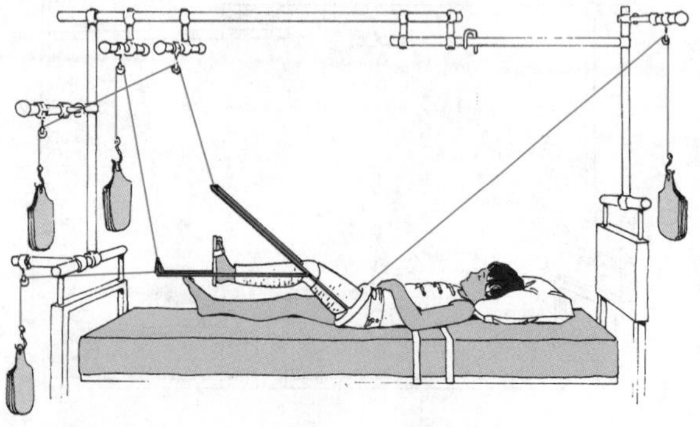

Fig. 54-8 Balance suspension with Thomas ring splint and Pearson attachment.

Cervical traction may also be accomplished by the insertion of *Crutchfield, Barton,* or *Gardner-Wells tongs* through burr holes in the skull and weights attached to the hyperextended head (Fig. 54-9, *A*). As the neck muscles fatigue with constant traction pull, the vertebral bodies gradually separate so that the cord is no longer pinched between the vertebrae. Immobilization until fracture healing or surgical fixation can occur is an essential goal of cervical traction.

Nursing Care Management

To assess the child in traction, it is essential to know the purpose for which the traction is applied and to understand the basic principles of traction. Regular assessment of both the child and the traction apparatus is required (Guidelines box). Many of the nursing problems associated with a child in traction are related to immobility or improper maintenance and care of the traction device, which may lead to complications.

<u>NURSE ALERT</u> Skeletal traction should be maintained as originally set by the practitioner. When the child needs to be moved in the bed or if the traction needs to be adjusted or released for any other reason, an orthopedist is consulted. ■

Complications that may occur with skin traction include skin breakdown and ischemia to the lower extremities; thus it is important to observe the 5 *Ps*. A pressure reducing air mattress may be required to prevent skin breakdown. In ad-

Guidelines

TRACTION CARE

Understand Therapy

Understand purpose of traction.
Understand function of traction in each specific situation.

Maintain Traction

Check desired line of pull and relationship of distal fragment to proximal fragment.
Check whether fragment is being directed upward, adducted, or abducted.
Check function of each component.
- Position of bandages, frames, splints
- Ropes: In center tract of pulley, taut, no fraying, knots tied securely
- Pulleys:
- In original position on attachment bar; have not been displaced from original site
- Wheels freely moveable
- Weights:
- Correct amount of weight
- Hanging freely
- In safe location

Check bed position—head or foot elevated as directed for desired amount of pull and countertraction.
Do not remove skeletal traction or adhesive traction straps on skin traction.

Maintain Alignment

Observe for correct body alignment with emphasis on alignment of shoulder, hip, and leg.
- Check after child has moved.
- Maintain correct angles at joints.

Skin Traction

Replace nonadhesive straps and/or elastic bandage on skin traction *when permitted* and/or absolutely necessary, but make certain that traction on limb is maintained by someone during procedure.
Assess bandages to ascertain if they are correctly applied (diagonal or spiral), not too loose or too tight, which could cause slippage and malalignment of traction.

Skeletal Traction

Check pin sites frequently for signs of bleeding, inflammation, or infection.
Cleanse pin sites per institution protocol or as ordered.
Apply topical antiseptic or antibiotic daily as ordered.
Cover ends of pins with protective rubber or padding to prevent child's being scratched by pin.
Note pull of traction on pin; pull should be even.
Check pin screws to be certain that screws are tight in metal clamp that attaches traction apparatus to pin.

Prevent Skin Breakdown

Provide foam overlay or alternating-pressure mattress underneath hips and back.
Make total-body skin checks for redness or breakdown, especially over areas that receive greatest pressure.
Wash and dry skin at least daily.
Inspect pressure points daily or more often if risk of breakdown is observed.
Use a skin breakdown assessment scale such as Modified Braden Q.
Stimulate circulation with gentle massage over pressure areas.
Change position at least every 2 hours to relieve pressure.

Prevent Complications

Check pulses in affected area and compare with pulses in contralateral site.
Assess circular dressings for excessive tightness.
Assess restrictive bandages or devises used to maintain traction on affected limb. Make certain that they are not too loose or too tight.
Remove periodically and check for pressure areas.
Encourage deep breathing frequently with maximum inspiratory chest expansion.
Note any neurovascular changes, such as:
- Color in skin and nail beds
- Alterations in sensation, increased pain
- Alterations in motor ability

Take immediate action to correct problem or report to practitioner if neurovascular changes are found.
Record findings of neurovascular changes.
Carry out passive, active, or active-with-resistance exercises of uninvolved joints.
Note if any tightness, weakness, or contractures are developing in uninvolved joints and muscles.
Take measures to correct or prevent further development of weakness, such as applying foot plate to prevent footdrop.

dition to routine skin observation and care, the child in skeletal traction will need special skin care at the pin site according to hospital policy or practitioner preference. Frequent pin care and assessment of the insertion and exit sites are important to prevent infection. In an extensive study of pin site care Holmes and colleagues (2005) concluded that there is insufficient evidence on which to recommend any single method of pin care as being beneficial over another. The authors did however make several recommendations which have research-based support. The recommendations for pin site care are as follows:

1. Pins located in areas with a considerable amount of soft tissue (femur, tibia, across the knee) should be considered as being at higher risk for infection.
2. After the first 48 to 72 hours (once drainage has diminished) pin site care should be performed daily or weekly for sites with mechanically stable bone-pin interfaces.
3. A chlorhexidine 2 mg/ml solution may be the most effective cleanser for pin site care (Holmes et al, 2005).

The authors did not specifically address the pediatric population and issues such as the management of crusts, skin adherence to the pin, and the use of dressings are discussed in the Holmes and colleagues (2005) article.

When the child is first placed in traction, an increase in discomfort is common as a result of the traction pull fatiguing the muscle. It has been determined that orthopedic conditions are associated with a higher-than-average number of painful events and a higher percentage of bodily symptoms than other common conditions. Intravenous opioids, including analgesics and muscle relaxants, help during this phase of care and should be administered liberally.

NURSE ALERT For skeletal traction to be effective ensure that the weights are hanging freely at all times. ■

The specific nursing responsibilities for the patient in traction are outlined in the Guidelines box.

Distraction

Unlike traction, which helps bones realign and fuse properly, distraction is the process of separating opposing bone to encourage regeneration of new bone in the created space. Distraction can also be used when limbs are of unequal lengths and new bone is needed to elongate the shorter limb.

External Fixation

The *Ilizarov external fixator (IEF)* is a common external fixation device. The IEF uses a system of wires, rings, and telescoping rods that permits limb lengthening to occur by manual distraction. In addition to lengthening bones, the device can be used to correct angular or rotational defects or to immobilize fractures (Gugenheim, 2000). The device is attached surgically by securing a series of external full or half rings to the bone with wires. External telescoping rods connect the rings to each other. Manual distraction is accomplished by manipulating the rods to increase the distance between the rings. A percutaneous osteotomy is performed when the device is applied to create a "false" growth plate. A special osteotomy or corticotomy involves cutting only the cortex of the bone while preserving its blood supply, bone marrow, endosteum, and periosteum. Capillary blood flow to the transected area is essential for proper bone growth. Cut bone ends typically grow at a rate of 1 cm/month. The IEF can result in up to a 15-cm gain in length.

Nursing Care Management

Success of the IEF depends on the child's and family's cooperation; therefore, before surgery they must be fully informed of the appearance of the device, how it accomplishes bone growth, needed alterations in activities, and home and follow-up care. Children are involved in learning to adjust the device to accomplish distraction. Children, as well as parents, should be instructed in pin care, including observation for infection and loosening of the pins. Cleaning routines for the pin sites vary among practitioners but should not traumatize the skin.

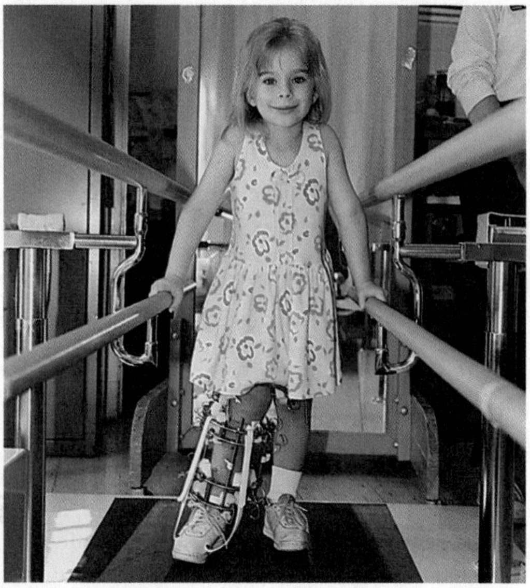

Fig. 54-10 Child with Ilizarov external fixator (right leg) during physical therapy on parallel bars.

Children who participate actively in their care report less discomfort. Because the device is external and quite bulky, the child and family may need to modify clothing for increased comfort and accessibility (Fig. 54-10). Partial weight bearing is allowed, and the child needs to learn to walk with crutches. Alterations in activity include modifications at school and in physical education. Full weight bearing is not allowed until the distraction is completed and bone consolidation has occurred. Follow-up care is essential to maintaining appropriate distraction until the desired leg length is achieved. The device is removed surgically after the bone has consolidated, and the child may need to use crutches or have a cast for 4 to 6 weeks following removal.

Amputation

A child may be born with the congenital absence of a body part, have a traumatic loss of an extremity, or need a surgical amputation for a pathologic condition such as *osteosarcoma* (see p. 1831). With today's surgical technology and the quick thinking of bystanders who save a traumatically amputated body part, some children have had fingers and arms sewn back on with variable degrees of functional use regained.

NURSE ALERT For an amputated limb or body part that may be reattached, do the following:
- Rinse limb gently with normal saline
- Loosely wrap limb in sterile gauze
- Place wrapped limb in a watertight bag
- Cool (without freezing) bag in ice water (do not pack in ice because this may harm tissue)
- Label with child's name, date, time, and transport with the child to the hospital ■

Surgical amputation or the surgical repair of a permanently severed limb focuses on constructing an adequately nourished stump. A smooth, healthy, padded stump, free of nerve endings, is important in prosthesis fitting and subsequent ambulation. In some situations in which there is no vascular or neurologic deficit, a cast is applied to the stump immediately after the procedure, and a pylon, metal extension, and artificial foot are attached so that the patient can walk on the temporary prosthesis within a few hours.

Nursing Care Management

Stump shaping is done postoperatively with special elastic bandaging using a figure-8 bandage, which applies pressure in a cone-shaped fashion. This technique decreases stump edema, controls hemorrhage, and aids in developing desired contours so that the child will bear weight on the posterior aspect of the skin flap rather than on the end of the stump. Stump elevation may be used during the first 24 hours, but after this time the extremity should not be left in this position because contractures will develop in the proximal joint and seriously hamper ambulation. Monitoring proper body alignment will further decrease the risk of flexion contractures.

For older children and adolescents, arm exercises (as well as parallel bars, which are used in prosthesis-training programs) help build up the arm muscles necessary for walking with crutches. Full range-of-motion exercises of joints above the amputation must be performed several times daily using active and isotonic exercises.

Depending on the age of the child, children or their parents will need to learn stump hygiene, including careful soap and water washing every day and checking for skin irritation, breakdown, or infection. A tube of stockinette or powder is used to slide the prosthesis on more easily. Skin must be checked carefully every time the prosthesis is removed, and prosthesis tolerance time must be adjusted to prevent skin breakdown.

For children who have had an amputation, *phantom limb sensation* is an expected experience because the nerve-brain connections are still present. Gradually these sensations fade, although in many amputees they persist for years. Preoperative discussion of this phenomenon will aid a child in understanding these "unusual feelings" and in not hiding the experiences from others. Limb pain, especially pain that increases with ambulation, should be evaluated for the possibility of a neuroma at the free nerve endings in the stump, or other problems such as a poorly fitting prosthesis or joint instability.

Developmental Dysplasia of the Hip (DDH)

The broad term *developmental dysplasia of the hip* (DDH) describes a spectrum of disorders related to abnormal development of the hip that may develop at any time during fetal life, infancy, or childhood. A change in terminology from congenital hip dysplasia (CHD) and congenital dislocation of the hip (CDH) to DDH more properly reflects a variety of hip abnormalities in which there is a shallow acetabulum, subluxation, or dislocation.

The incidence of hip instability of some kind is approximately 10 per 1000 live births. The incidence of frank dislocation or a dislocatable hip is 1 per 1000 live births (Wall, 2000), and approximately 30% to 50% of infants with DDH were born breech (Thompson, 2004a). The left hip is involved in 60% of cases, the right hip in 20%, and both hips in 20%. Sixty percent of the patients are girls. Caucasian children have a higher incidence of developmental dysplasia than other groups (Maher, Salmond, & Pellino, 2002).

Cultural Awareness ▶▶

DEVELOPMENTAL DYSPLASIA OF THE HIP

A striking relationship exists between the development of the dislocation and methods of handling infants. Among the cultures with the highest incidence of dislocation, newly born infants are tightly wrapped in blankets or other swaddling material or are strapped to cradle boards. In cultures such as the Far East, where mothers traditionally carry infants on their backs or hips in the widely abducted straddle position, the disorder is virtually unknown.

Pathophysiology

The cause of DDH is unknown but certain factors such as gender, birth order, family history, intrauterine position, delivery type, joint laxity, and postnatal positioning are believed to affect the risk of DDH. Predisposing factors associated with DDH may be divided into three broad categories: (1) physiologic factors, which include maternal hormone secretion and intrauterine positioning; (2) mechanical factors, which involves breech presentation, multiple fetus, oligohydramnios, and large infant size; other mechanical factors may include continued maintenance of the hips in adduction and extension that will in time cause a dislocation (Cultural Awareness box); and (3) genetic factors, which entail a higher incidence (6%) of DDH in siblings of affected infants, and an even greater incidence (36%) of recurrence if sibling and one parent were affected.

Three degrees of DDH are illustrated in Fig. 54-11:

Acetabular dysplasia (or preluxation)—mildest form of DDH in which there is neither subluxation nor dislocation. There is a delay in acetabular development evidenced by osseous hypoplasia of the acetabular roof that is oblique and shallow, although the cartilaginous roof is comparatively intact. The femoral head remains in the acetabulum.

Subluxation—The largest percentage of DDH, subluxation, implies incomplete dislocation of the hip and is sometimes regarded as an intermediate state in the development from primary dysplasia to complete dislocation. The femoral head remains in contact with the acetabu-

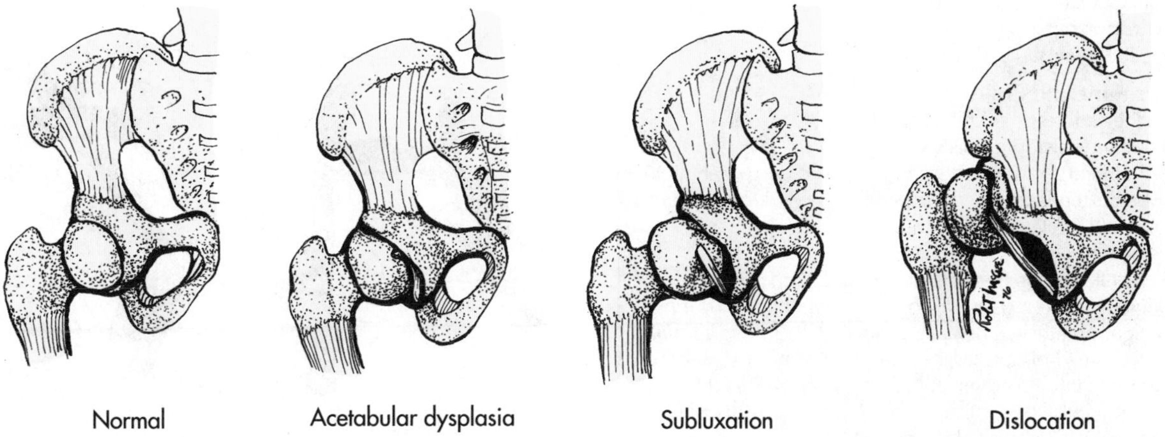

Fig. 54-11 Configuration and relationship of structures in developmental dysplasia of the hip.

lum, but a stretched capsule and ligamentum teres cause the head of the femur to be partially displaced. Pressure on the cartilaginous roof inhibits ossification and produces a flattening of the socket.

Dislocation—The femoral head loses contact with the acetabulum and is displaced posteriorly and superiorly over the fibrocartilaginous rim. The ligamentum teres is elongated and taut.

Diagnostic Evaluation

DDH is often not detected at the initial examination after birth; thus, all infants should be carefully monitored for hip dysplasia at follow-up visits throughout the first year of life. In the newborn period dysplasia usually appears as hip joint laxity rather than as outright dislocation (Box 54-4).

NURSE ALERT The Ortolani and Barlow tests must be performed by an experienced clinician to prevent further damage to the hip. If these tests are performed too vigorously in the first 2 days of life, when the hip subluxates freely, persistent dislocation may occur. (See Fig. 24-8, p. 702.) ■

Universal newborn screening by serial hip examinations, performed by properly trained health care providers, is now recommended for early detection and treatment of DDH (American Academy of Pediatrics [AAP], Committee on Quality Improvement and Subcommittee on Developmental Dysplasia of the Hip, 2000; Witt, 2003).

Radiographic examination in early infancy is not reliable, because ossification of the femoral head does not normally take place until the third to sixth month of life. However, the cartilaginous head can be visualized directly by ultrasonography. Experts suggest that ultrasound be used to screen hips at 2 weeks after birth in infants with clinical signs of DDH, infants with a higher risk of DDH (according to the predisposing factors listed above), and to monitor the efficacy of treatment in infants with DDH (Roberts et al, 2002). In infants older than age 4 months and in children, radiographic examination is useful in confirming the diagnosis. An upward slope in the roof of the acetabulum (the acetabular angle) greater than 40 degrees with upward and outward displacement of the femoral head is a frequent finding in older children. Computed tomography (CT) scan may be useful to assess the position of the femoral head relative to the acetabulum after closed reduction and casting.

BOX 54-4

Clinical Manifestations of Developmental Dysplasia of the Hip

Infant

Shortening of limb on affected side (Galleazzi sign, Allis sign)
Restricted abduction of hip on affected side
Unequal gluteal folds (infant prone)
Positive Ortolani test
Positive Barlow test

Older Infant and Child

Affected leg shorter than the other
Telescoping or piston mobility of joint
  Head of femur can be felt to move up and down in buttock when extended thigh is pushed first toward child's head and then pulled distally
Trendelenburg sign
  When child stands first on one foot and then on the other (holding onto a chair, rail, or someone's hands) bearing weight on affected hip, pelvis tilts downward on normal side instead of upward, as it would with normal stability
Greater trochanter is prominent and appears above a line from anterior superior iliac spine to tuberosity of ischium
Marked lordosis (bilateral dislocations)
Waddling gait (bilateral dislocations)

Therapeutic Management

Treatment is begun as soon as the condition is recognized because early intervention is more favorable to the restoration of normal bony architecture and function. The longer treatment is delayed, the more severe the deformity, the more difficult the treatment, and the less favorable the prognosis. The treatment varies with the age of the child and the extent of the dysplasia. The goal of treatment is to obtain and maintain a safe, congruent position of the hip joint to promote normal hip joint development.

Newborn to Age 6 Months

The hip joint is maintained by splinting with the proximal femur centered in the acetabulum in an attitude of flexion. Of the numerous devices available, the *Pavlik harness* is the most widely used, and with time, motion, and gravity, the hip works into a more abducted, reduced position (Fig. 54-12). The harness is worn continuously until the hip is clinically and radiographically stable, usually in about 3 to 6 months.

When adduction contracture is present, other devices such as skin traction are used to slowly and gently stretch the hip to full abduction, after which wide abduction is maintained until stability is attained. When maintaining stable reduction is difficult, a hip spica cast is applied and changed periodically to accommodate the child's growth. After 3 to 6 months, sufficient stability is acquired to allow transfer to a removable protective abduction brace. The duration of treatment depends on development of the acetabulum but is usually accomplished within the first year.

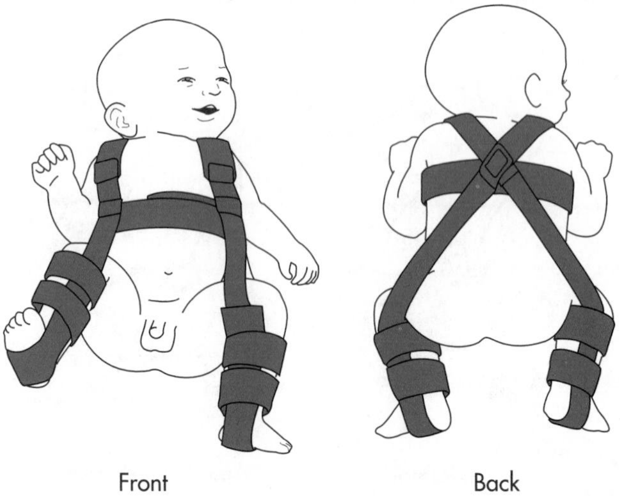

Fig. 54-12 Child in Pavlik harness. (From Ball JW: *Mosby's pediatric patient teaching guides,* St Louis, 1998, Mosby.)

Ages 6 to 18 Months

In this age group the dislocation is not recognized until the child begins to stand and walk, when attendant shortening of the limb and contractures of hip adductor and flexor muscles become apparent (see Fig. 24-8). Gradual reduction by traction is used for approximately 3 weeks. An individualized home traction program may be developed for the child preoperatively to decrease the length of hospitalization and maintain the home environment. The child then undergoes an attempted closed reduction of the hip under general anesthesia if the hip is not reducible and open reduction is performed. After reduction, the child is placed in a hip spica cast for 2 to 4 months until the hip is stable, at which time a flexion-abduction brace is applied.

Older Child

Correction of the hip deformity in older children is inherently more difficult than in the preceding age groups, because secondary adaptive changes and other etiologic factors (such as juvenile rheumatoid arthritis or nonambulatory cerebral palsy) complicate the condition. Operative reduction, which may involve preoperative traction, tenotomy of contracted muscles, and any one of several innominate osteotomy procedures designed to construct an acetabular roof, is usually required. After cast removal and before weight bearing is permitted, range-of-motion exercises help restore movement. Successful reduction and reconstruction become increasingly difficult after the age of 4 years and are usually impossible or inadvisable in children older than 6 years of age because of severe shortening and contracture of muscles and deformity of the femoral and acetabular structures.

Nursing Care Management

Assessment

Nurses are in a unique position to detect DDH in early infancy. During the infant assessment process and routine nurturing activities, the hips and extremities are inspected for any deviations from normal. These observations are reported to the attending practitioner, and the ambulatory child who displays a limp or an unusual gait should be referred for evaluation. This may indicate an orthopedic or neurologic problem. Nonambulatory children with cerebral palsy should also be assessed for evidence of dislocation.

The major nursing problems in the care of an infant or child in a cast or other device are related to maintenance of the device and adaptation of nurturing activities to meet the needs of the infant or child. Generally, treatment and follow-up care of these children are carried out in a clinic, practitioner's office, or outpatient unit. Hospitalization may be necessary for cast application or brace fitting but seldom exceeds 24 to 48 hours. Longer hospitalization is required for open reduction.

Nursing Diagnoses

Nursing diagnoses identified for the child with developmental dysplasia of the hip are:

Impaired physical mobility related to correction device

Risk for impaired skin integrity related to presence of correction device

Altered family processes related to care of a child in a corrective device

Plan of Care and Implementation

The goals of care for the child in a mechanical device for correction of DDH are as follows:

1. Child will maintain correct position of hip in acetabulum.
2. Child will experience no complications related to wearing corrective device.
3. Family will adapt routine nurturing activities to accommodate corrective device.

NURSE ALERT The former practice of double- or triple-diapering for DDH is not recommended because it promotes hip extension, thus worsening proper hip development. ■

The primary nursing goal is teaching parents to apply and maintain the reduction device. The Pavlik harness allows for easy handling of the infant and usually produces less apprehension in the parent than heavy braces and casts. Because of the infant's rapid growth, the straps should be checked every 1 to 2 weeks for possible adjustments. It is important that parents understand the correct use of the appliance, which may or may not allow for its removal during bathing. Unbuckling or removal of the harness is determined individually on the basis of the family's level of understanding and the degree of deformity in the hip. In general, parents should not adjust the harness without supervision. The child should be examined by the practitioner before any adjustment is attempted to make certain the hips are in correct placement before the harness is resecured.

Casts and orthotics devices (braces) offer more challenging nursing problems because they cannot be removed for routine care, although sometimes a brace may be removed for bathing. Care of an infant or small child with a cast requires nursing innovation to reduce skin pressure or friction and to maintain cleanliness of both the child and the cast, particularly in the diaper area. (See p. 1809 for care of the child in a cast.)

It is important for nurses, parents, and other caregivers to understand that children in corrective devices need to be involved in all the activities of any child in the same age group. Toys are chosen that can be used in a prone position on the floor or in the seats devised for feeding and other activities. Confinement in a cast or appliance should not exclude children from family (or unit) activities. They can be held astride the lap for comfort and transported to areas of activity. An adapted wheelchair, stroller, or scooter can offer mobility to the older infant or child.

Evaluation

The effectiveness of nursing interventions is determined by continual assessment and evaluation of care based on the following observational guidelines and expected outcomes:

1. Inspect corrective device regularly.
2. Inspect child's skin and circulation regularly.
3. Observe family's behavior with child and interview them regarding identified problems and solutions.

Expected outcomes include the following:

1. Hip remains in desired abducted position; corrective device is positioned properly.

2. Skin remains free of irritation; circulation is unimpaired.
3. Family adjusts nurturing activities to accommodate corrective device.

CONGENITAL DEFECTS

Some skeletal defects may be diagnosed at birth or within days, weeks, or months after birth. In other cases the deviation may be difficult to detect without careful inspection. Therefore it is imperative that nurses become acquainted with signs of these defects and understand the principles of therapy in order to direct others in the care and management of these children.

Congenital Clubfoot

Congenital *clubfoot* is a complex deformity of the ankle and foot that includes forefoot adduction, midfoot supination, hindfoot varus, and ankle equinus. Deformities of the foot and ankle are described according to the position of the ankle and foot. The more common positions involve the following variations:

Talipes varus—An inversion or a bending inward

Talipes valgus—An eversion or bending outward

Talipes equinus—Plantar flexion in which the toes are lower than the heel

Talipes calcaneus—Dorsiflexion, in which the toes are higher than the heel

Most cases of clubfoot are a combination of these positions, and the most commonly occurring type of clubfoot (approximately 95%) is the composite deformity *talipes equinovarus (TEV),* in which the foot is pointed downward and inward in varying degrees of severity (Fig. 54-13). Unilateral clubfoot is somewhat more common than bilateral clubfoot and may occur as an isolated defect or in association with other disorders or syndromes, such as chromosomal defects, arthrogryposis (a generalized immobility of the joints), cerebral palsy, or spina bifida.

The incidence of clubfoot in the general population is 1 to 2 per 1000 live births, with boys affected twice as often as girls. Bilateral clubfeet occur in 50% of the cases (Gilmore & Thompson, 2003). The precise cause of clubfoot is unknown. Some authorities attribute the defect to abnormal positioning and restricted movement in utero, although the evidence is not conclusive. Other experts implicate arrested or abnormal embryonic development. Arrested development during this early stage tends to result in a rigid deformity, whereas mechanical pressures from intrauterine positioning are likely causes of more flexible deformities.

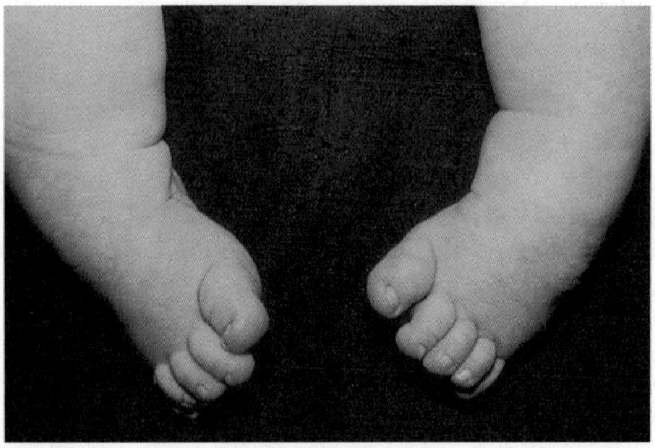

Fig. 54-13 Bilateral congenital talipes equinovarus (congenital clubfoot) in 2-month-old infant. (From Zitelli BJ, Davis HW: *Atlas of pediatric physical diagnosis,* ed 4, St Louis, 2002, Mosby.)

Classification

The literature describes three major categories of clubfoot: (1) positional clubfoot (also called transitional, mild, or postural clubfoot), which is believed to occur primarily from intrauterine crowding and responds to simple stretching and casting; (2) syndromic (or teratologic) clubfoot, which is associated with other congenital anomalies such as myelomeningocele or arthrogryposis and is a more severe form of clubfoot that is often resistant to treatment; (3) congenital clubfoot, also referred to as idiopathic, which may occur in an otherwise normal child and has a wide range of rigidity and prognosis. The third category may be detected in utero by ultrasonography and is the most common type of TEV seen.

The mild, or postural, clubfoot may correct spontaneously or may require passive exercise or serial casting. There is no bony abnormality, but there may be tightness and shortening of the soft tissues medially and posteriorly. The teratologic clubfoot is associated with other congenital anomalies such as myelodysplasia or arthrogryposis. These feet usually require surgical correction and have a high incidence of recurrence. The congenital idiopathic clubfoot, or "true clubfoot," almost always requires surgical intervention because there is bony abnormality.

Diagnostic Evaluation

The deformity is readily apparent and easily detected prenatally through ultrasonography or at birth. However, it must be differentiated from some positional deformities that can be passively corrected or overcorrected. Paralytic changes in the lower extremity of children with neuromuscular involvement often produce equinovarus deformity. An increased risk of hip dysplasia is associated with clubfoot deformities.

Therapeutic Management

The goal of treatment for clubfoot is to achieve a painless, plantigrade, and stable foot. Treatment of clubfoot involves three stages: (1) correction of the deformity, (2) maintenance of the correction until normal muscle balance is regained, and (3) follow-up observation to avert possible recurrence of the deformity. Some feet respond to treatment readily; some respond only to prolonged, vigorous, and sustained efforts; and the improvement in others remains disappointing even with maximum effort on the part of all concerned.

Serial casting is begun shortly after birth, before discharge from the nursery. Successive casts allow for gradual stretching of skin and tight structures on the medial side of the foot (Fig. 54-14). Manipulation and casting are repeated frequently (every few days for 1 to 2 weeks, then at 1- to 2-week intervals) to accommodate the rapid growth of early infancy. The extremity or extremities are casted until maximum cor-

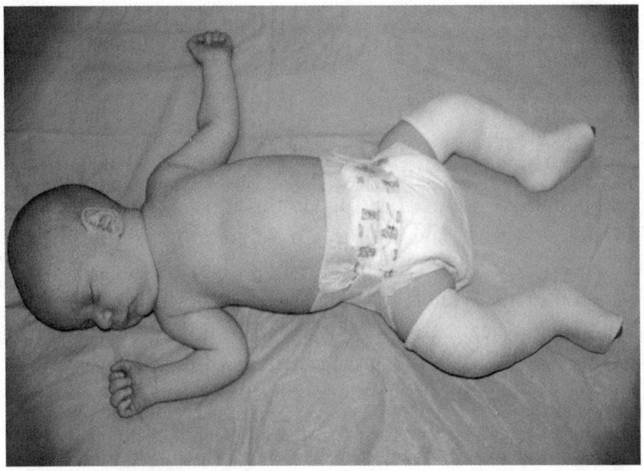

Fig. 54-14 Feet casted for correction of bilateral congenital talipes equinovarus.

rection is achieved, usually within 8 to 12 weeks. A Denis Browne splint may be used to manage feet that correct with casting and manipulation. A radiograph or ultrasound is then evaluated to see the relationship of the bones to each other. Failure to achieve normal alignment by 3 months indicates the need for surgical intervention, which may take place between 6 and 12 months of age. The foot (or feet) is immobilized postoperatively for approximately 6 to 12 weeks and the child is allowed to walk after the cast is removed (Gilmore & Thompson, 2003).

Surgical intervention for clubfoot involves pin fixation and the releasing of tight joints and tendons. Casting of the affected foot and leg is performed, and after 2 or 3 months, a varus-prevention brace is used to maintain correction. With severe deformities, repeated surgical tendon or joint releases may be necessary.

In recent years several nonsurgical approaches to clubfoot have been reintroduced. These methods (Ponseti manipulation and French physical therapy) involve daily or weekly manipulation and stretching of tissues with either casting (Ponseti) or taping and splinting of the affected extremity (French). A percutaneous tendoachilles lengthening may be performed prior to the final casting at 6 to 7 weeks to correct the equines deformity. A continuous passive motion (CPM) machine may be used several hours daily to stretch and strengthen muscle groups involved with the French physical therapy treatment (Faulks & Luther, 2005).

Nursing Care Management

Nursing care of the child with clubfoot is the same as for any child who has a cast (see p. 1809). Because the child will spend considerable time in a corrective device, nursing care plans include both long-term and short-term goals. Conscientious observation of the skin and circulation is particularly important in young infants because of their normally rapid growth rate. Because treatment and follow-up care are handled in the orthopedist's office, clinic, or outpatient department, parent education and support are important in nursing care of these children.

Parents need to understand the overall treatment program, the importance of regular cast changes, and the role they play in the long-term effectiveness of the therapy. Reinforcing and clarifying the orthopedist's explanations and instructions, teaching parents about care of the cast or appliance (including vigilant observation for potential problems), and encouraging parents to facilitate normal development within the limitations imposed by the deformity or therapy are all part of nursing responsibilities.

Metatarsus Adductus (Varus)

Metatarsus adductus, or metatarsus varus, is probably the most common congenital foot deformity. In most instances it is a result of abnormal intrauterine positioning, particularly in the firstborn child, and is usually detected at birth. The deformity is characterized by medial adduction of the toes and forefoot, frequently in association with inversion, and by convexity of the lateral border of the foot. Metatarsus adductus may be divided into three categories: type I, in which the forefoot is flexible and corrects easily with manipulation; type II, in which there is only partial flexibility in the forefoot, and it corrects passively past neutral position but only to neutral position with active manipulation; and type III, in which the forefoot is rigid and will not stretch to neutral position with manipulation (Gilmore & Thompson, 2003). Unlike TEV, with which it is often confused, the angulation occurs at the tarsometatarsal joint, whereas the heel and ankle remain in a neutral position. Ankle range of motion is normal. This deformity often causes a pigeon-toed gait in the child.

Management depends on the rigidity and type of the deformity. Correction can usually be accomplished by gentle manipulation and passive stretching of the foot with types I and II, which the parent is taught to perform. Repeated and consistent stretching is continued for the first 6 weeks, after which the treatment is based on the flexibility of the foot. With type III, the child will usually require serial manipulation and casting to correct the defect. Casting is performed every 1 to 2 weeks for 6 to 8 weeks after which a corrective shoe or orthosis may be used. Surgical correction is rarely required for the condition unless there is residual deformity at 4 years of age at which time soft tissue release and serial casting is performed; older children with deformity may require more extensive surgery (Thompson, 2004b).

Nursing Care Management

The nursing role primarily involves identifying the defect, so that early therapy and instruction of the parents can be initiated. The nurse teaches the parents how to hold the heel firmly and to stretch only the forefoot; otherwise, undue force on the heel may produce a valgus deformity. If casting or orthosis is required, the nurse instructs the parents in cast care and observation of the corrective device (see p. 1809).

Skeletal Limb Deficiency

Congenital limb deficiencies, or reduction malformations, are manifested by a variety of degrees of loss of functional capacity. They are characterized by underdevelopment of skeletal elements of the extremities. The range of malformation can extend from minor defects of the digits to serious abnormalities such as *amelia,* absence of an entire extremity; or *meromelia,* partial absence of an extremity that includes *phocomelia* (seal limbs), interposed deficiency of long bones with relatively good development of hands and feet attached at or near the shoulder or the hips. Most reduction defects are primary defects of development of the limb, but prenatal destruction of the limb can occur, such as the amputation of a limb in utero from constriction of an amniotic band (amniotic band syndrome).

Pathophysiology

Limb deficiencies can be attributed to both heredity and environment and can originate at any stage of limb development. Formation of limbs may be suppressed at the time of limb bud formation, or there may be interference in later stages of differentiation and growth. Heredity appears to play a prominent role, and prenatal environmental insults have been implicated in a number of cases. The latter includes the well-publicized thalidomide tragedy of the 1950s and early 1960s, which demonstrated a clear relationship between the time of exposure of the pregnant woman to the antiemetic drug and the presence and type of limb deformity in the newborn. Many drugs may still have similar *teratogenic* effects in the first trimester of pregnancy; therefore, medication administration during this period should be carefully evaluated by the practitioner. Unfortunately, during this period, the woman may not realize her pregnant condition unless the event is highly anticipated, and inadvertent consumption of harmful medications may occur. Deletion or shortening of digits or limbs may also be associated with *chorionic villus sampling,* especially before 10 to 12 weeks of gestation; however, the incidence and relationship remain uncertain.

Therapeutic Management

Children with congenital limb deficiencies should be fitted with prosthetic devices whenever possible, and the devices should be applied at the earliest possible stage of development in an attempt to match the motor readiness of the infant. This favors natural progression of prosthetic use. For example, a young infant with an upper extremity deficiency is fitted with a simple passive device, such as a mitten prosthesis, to encourage limb exploration, sitting (with the extremities needed for support), and bilateral hand activities.

Lower limb prostheses are applied when the infant begins sitting up and can maintain balance. In preparation for prosthetic devices, surgical modification may be necessary to ensure the most favorable use of the device, because severe deformity can interfere with its effective use. Phocomelic digits are preserved for controlling switches of externally powered appliances in upper extremities. Digits (in both upper and lower extremities) provide the child with surfaces for tactile exploration and stimulation. Prostheses are replaced to accommodate growth and increasing capabilities of the child.

Nursing Care Management

Prosthetic application training and habilitation are most successfully carried out in a center that specializes in meeting the special needs of these children, especially very young children and those with amputations or missing limbs. It involves a ***prosthetist,*** who specializes in the development, fitting, and maintenance of prosthetic limbs, and other health care workers such as PTs and occupational therapists. Parents need special attention and support and are encouraged to assist the child in making age-commensurate adjustments to the environment.

Osteogenesis Imperfecta (OI)

Osteogenesis imperfecta (OI) is the most common osteoporosis syndrome in children. OI is a heterogeneous, group-inherited syndrome characterized by excessive fractures and bone deformity. There are at least five types of OI, accounting for significant disease variability. Clinical features may include the following: varying degrees of bone fragility, deformity, and fracture; blue sclerae; hearing loss; and dentinogenesis imperfecta (hypoplastic discolored teeth). The inheritance pattern is autosomal dominant in the majority of cases, although the most severe form demonstrates autosomal-recessive inheritance (Box 54-5).

Most types of OI have defects in the COL1A1 or COL1A2 genes, which code for polypeptide chains in type 1 procollagen, a precursor of type 1 collagen, a major structural component of bone. The error results in faulty bone mineralization, abnormal bone architecture, and increased susceptibility to fracture.

Classifications for OI are based on clinical features and patterns of inheritance (see Box 54-5). Clinically, type I is the most common, with wide variability of bone fragility; some affected family members have significant deformity and disability, whereas others lead agile active lives. Type II variants are the most severe and are considered lethal in infancy. Type III OI is characterized by multiple fractures, bone deformity, and severe disability; affected individuals rarely live to 30 years of age. Type IV is similar to type I with blue or white sclerae. A new variant, or type V, has been described in which

BOX 54-5

Classification of Osteogenesis Imperfecta

Type		Characteristics
I*	A	Mild bone fragility; blue sclerae; normal teeth; hearing loss (occurs between ages 20 and 30 years); autosomal-dominant inheritance
	B	Same as A except dentinogenesis imperfecta instead of normal teeth
	C	Same as B; no bone fragility
II		Lethal; stillborn or die in early infancy; severe bone fragility, multiple fractures at birth; 10% of cases of osteogenesis imperfecta (OI); autosomal recessive inheritance
III		Severe bone fragility leads to severe progressive deformities; normal sclerae; marked growth failure; most autosomal-recessive inheritance; few autosomal-dominant inheritance
IV	A	Mild to moderate bone fragility; normal sclerae; short stature; variable deformity; autosomal-dominant inheritance
	B	Same as A except dentinogenesis imperfecta instead of normal teeth; approximately 6% of cases of OI
V		Clinically similar to Type IV; hyperplastic callus; collagen mutation is negative

*Two thirds of cases are type I.

those affected have a hyperplastic callus; no collagen mutations are noted in this group (Marini, 2004).

Therapeutic Management

The treatment for OI is primarily supportive, although patients and families are optimistic about new research advances. Bone marrow transplant for severe OI was first reported in 1999 with positive results; however, this is still considered an experimental treatment (Horwitz et al, 2001). The use of bisphosphonate therapy to promote increased bone density and prevent fractures is also being evaluated. Several studies report increased bone density; decreased bone pain; and decreased fractures with intravenous pamidronate, a potent inhibitor of bone resorption (Falk et al, 2003; Zeitlin, Fassier, & Glorieux, 2003).

The goals of a rehabilitative approach to management are directed at preventing (1) positional contractures and deformities, (2) muscle weakness and osteoporosis, and (3) malalignment of lower extremity joints prohibiting weight bearing.

Lightweight braces and splints help support limbs, prevent fractures, and aid in ambulation. Physical therapy helps prevent disuse osteoporosis and strengthens muscles, which in turn improves bone.

Surgery is sometimes used to help treat the manifestations of the disease. Surgical techniques are used to correct deformities that interfere with bracing, standing, or walking. For the child with recurrent fractures, inserting an intramedullary rod provides stability to bones.

Nursing Care Management

Infants and children with this disorder require careful handling to prevent fractures. They must be supported when they are being turned, positioned, moved, and held. Even changing a diaper may cause a fracture in severely affected infants. These children should never be held by the ankles when being diapered but should be gently lifted by the buttocks or supported with pillows.

Both parents and the affected child need education regarding the child's limitations and guidelines in planning suitable activities that promote optimum development and protect the child from harm. Realistic occupational planning and genetic counseling are part of the long-term goals of care. Educational materials and information can be obtained from the Osteogenesis Imperfecta Foundation, Inc.,* which also has a network that can put a family in contact with other families with a similar problem.

OI is a differential diagnosis that must be ruled out in the event of multiple fractures that may be attributed to nonaccidental injury. A detailed history, no evidence of associated soft-tissue injury, and the presence of other symptoms related to OI help determine the diagnosis.

NURSE ALERT Children with current fractures or healing fractures should be screened for osteogenesis imperfecta—the assumption that abuse or neglect is the cause of fractures in children must be carefully evaluated by a multidisciplinary team. ■

*804 West Diamond Avenue, Suite 210, Gaithersburg, MD 20878; phone: 800-981-2663; Web site: www.oif.org.

ACQUIRED DEFECTS

Legg-Calvé-Perthes Disease

Legg-Calvé-Perthes disease (LCPD) is a self-limited juvenile idiopathic avascular necrosis of the femoral head. The disease affects children ages 2 to 12 but most commonly boys between 4 and 8 years of age. Unilateral hip involvement is present in 90% of cases, it rarely occurs in African Americans, and has a worse prognosis when detected in older children and those with severe involvement (Greene, 2001).

Pathophysiology

The cause of the disease is unknown, but there is a disturbance of circulation to the femoral capital epiphysis that produces an ischemic aseptic necrosis of the femoral head. During middle childhood, circulation to the femoral epiphysis is more tenuous than at other ages and can become obstructed by trauma, inflammation, coagulation defects, and a variety of other causes. The pathologic events seem to take place in four stages (Box 54-6). The entire process may encompass as little as 18 months or continue for several years. The reformed femoral head may be severely altered or appear entirely normal.

Clinical Manifestations and Diagnostic Evaluation

The onset of LCPD is usually insidious, and the history may reveal only intermittent appearance of a limp on the affected side or a symptom complex including hip soreness, ache, or stiffness that can be constant or intermittent. The parents may report seeing the child limping, and the limp becomes more pronounced with increased activity. The pain may be experienced in the hip, along the entire thigh, or in the vicinity of the knee joint. The pain and limp are usually most evident on arising and at the end of a long day of activities. The pain is usually accompanied by joint dysfunction and limited range of motion. There may be a vague history of trauma. The diagnosis is established by radiographic examination, with the definitive diagnosis being

BOX 54-6

Stages of Legg-Calvé-Perthes Disease

Stage I: Aseptic necrosis or infarction of the femoral capital epiphysis with degenerative changes producing flattening of the upper surface of the femoral head—the **avascular stage**

Stage II: Capital bone absorption and revascularization with fragmentation (vascular resorption of the epiphysis) that gives a mottled appearance on radiographs—the **fragmentation**, or **revascularization stage**

Stage III: New bone formation, which is represented on radiographs as calcification and ossification or increased density in the areas of radiolucency; this filling-in process appears to take place from the periphery of the head centrally—the **reparative stage**

Stage IV: Gradual reformation of the head of the femur without radiolucency and, it is hoped, to a spherical form—the **regenerative stage**

magnetic resonance imaging (MRI), which demonstrates osteonecrosis.

Therapeutic Management

Because deformity occurs early in the disease process, the aim of treatment is to keep the head of the femur contained in the acetabulum, which serves as a mold to preserve the spherical shape of the head and to maintain a full range of motion. Because LCPD is a biologic process involving revascularization of the femoral head, removal of necrotic bone, and replacement with viable bone (Greene, 2001), or mechanical intervention may not produce optimal results (Roy, 1999). However, there is no agreement regarding the best treatment in terms of conservative versus surgical approaches. There has reportedly been no particular treatment that has yielded good outcomes on a consistent basis (Greene, 2001). Often, treatment approaches vary with the severity of presentation. Activity causes microfractures of the soft, ischemic epiphysis, which tend to induce synovitis, stiffness, and adductor contractures. The initial therapy is rest and non–weight bearing, which helps reduce inflammation and restore motion. Later, active motion is encouraged. In some cases traction is applied to stretch tight adductor muscles.

Containment can be accomplished in several ways. One is the use of non–weight-bearing devices, such as an abduction brace, leg casts, or a leather harness sling, which prevent weight bearing on the affected limb. Another includes the use of various weight-bearing appliances, such as abduction-ambulation braces or casts after a period of bed rest and traction. A third consists of surgical reconstruction and containment procedures. Conservative therapy must be continued for 2 to 4 years, although braces constructed from lightweight materials allow the child to maintain a nearly normal activity level. Surgical correction, although subjecting the child to additional risks (e.g., from anesthesia, infection, blood transfusion), returns the child to normal activities in 3 to 4 months. The use of home traction has also been explored.

Prognosis

The disease is self-limited, but the ultimate outcome of therapy depends on early and efficient treatment and the age of the child at onset of the disorder. Younger children, whose epiphyses are more cartilaginous, have the best prognosis for complete recovery; however, a recent report suggests that patients younger than 5 years of age do not always have the optimal outcomes previously predicted (Fabry, Fabry, & Moens, 2003). The later the diagnosis is made, the more femoral damage has occurred before treatment is implemented. In many cases, with good patient compliance, the prognosis is excellent.

Nursing Care Management

Nurses may be the first health professionals to identify affected children and to refer them for medical evaluation. They are also persons on whom the child and the family can rely to help them understand and adjust to the therapeutic measures. Because most of the child's care is conducted on an outpatient basis, the major emphasis of nursing care is teaching the family the care and management of the corrective appliance selected for therapy. The family needs to learn the purpose, function, application, and care of the corrective device and the importance of compliance to achieve the desired outcome (Family Focus box).

One of the most difficult aspects associated with the disorder is coping with a normally active child who feels well but must remain relatively inactive. Suitable activities must be devised to meet the needs of the child in the process of developing a sense of initiative or industry. Activities that meet the creative urges are well received.

> **Family Focus**
>
> **LEGG-CALVÉ-PERTHES DISEASE**
>
> A family with five healthy children was one day startled to learn that their 2-year-old son could no longer walk. He was diagnosed with Legg-Calvé-Perthes disease. Through several years of prosthetic devices and numerous physician visits, hospitalizations, and surgeries, this family turned a potentially devastating experience into one with cherished memories.
>
> Today, the parents reflect upon how their family coped with the reality of a debilitating disease. It was difficult for the parents to observe an eager, energetic child watch other children riding bicycles, running, or playing outdoor games. Also, they are warmed by memories of watching their other children make the difference for their sibling. They all developed a strong bond through caring and sharing with one another. Coping as a family was an easy adjustment and, most of all, therapeutic. Today, over 20 years later, the parents feel that each family member has grown with feelings of faith and trust. The experience proved to them that life will go on, and that life is what you make it!
>
> Shona Swenson Lenss, MS, RN, FNP
> Cheyenne, Wyoming

Slipped Femoral Capital Epiphysis (SFCE)

Slipped femoral capital epiphysis (SFCE), or coxa vara, refers to the spontaneous displacement of the proximal femoral epiphysis in a posterior and inferior direction. It develops most frequently shortly before or during accelerated growth and the onset of puberty (children between the ages of 10 and 16 years: median age, 13 for boys, 12 for girls) and is most frequently observed in males and obese children. Bilateral involvement occurs in up to 40% to 50% of cases (Greene, 2001).

Pathophysiology

Most cases of SFCE are idiopathic, although it can be associated with endocrine disorders, renal osteodystrophy, and radiation therapy. The cause of idiopathic SFCE is multifactorial and includes obesity, physeal architecture and orientation, and pubertal hormone changes that affect physeal strength. Although obesity stresses the physeal plate, SFCE can also occur in children who are not obese. Radiographs show medial displacement of the epiphysis and uncovered upper portion of the femoral neck adjacent to the physis. There is a widened growth plate and irregular metaphysis. The capital femoral epiphysis remains in the acetabulum, but the femoral neck slips, deforming the femoral head and stretching blood vessels to the epiphysis.

Diagnostic Evaluation

The disorder is suspected when an adolescent or preadolescent youngster displays clinical signs or complains of

BOX 54-7

Clinical Manifestations of Slipped Femoral Capital Epiphysis

May be obese
Limp on affected side
Pain in hip
Continuous or intermittent
Frequently referred to groin, anteromedial aspect of thigh, or knee
Restricted internal rotation on adduction with external rotation deformity
Loss of abduction and internal rotation as severity increases
Shortening of lower extremity

thigh pain (Box 54-7). The diagnosis is confirmed by radiographic examination.

Therapeutic Management

Treatment goals include avoiding further slipping of the femoral head, avoiding chondrolysis and osteonecrosis, and correcting the deformity. Surgical treatment varies with the degree of displacement; methods include presurgery bed rest/traction followed by a single pin, multiple pins and screws, or osteotomy for deformity correction if needed. Postsurgery care includes non-weight bearing with crutch ambulation until acceptable, painless range of motion is achieved. SFCE with severe displacement is an emergency and requires surgical reduction and stabilization.

Nursing Care Management

Nursing care is the same as that for a child in a cast or a child in traction, as discussed earlier in this chapter. Postoperative care involves hemodynamic stabilization and assessment for complications.

Kyphosis and Lordosis

The spine, consisting of numerous segments, can acquire deformity curves of three types: kyphosis, lordosis, and scoliosis (Fig. 54-15). *Kyphosis* is an abnormally increased convex angulation in the curvature of the thoracic spine (Fig. 54-15, *B*). It can occur secondary to disease processes such as tuberculosis, chronic arthritis, osteodystrophy, or compression fractures of the thoracic spine. The most common form of kyphosis is "postural." Children, especially during the time when skeletal growth outpaces growth of muscle, are prone to exaggeration of a normal kyphosis. They assume abnormal sitting and standing positions. This is particularly common in self-conscious adolescent girls who assume a round-shouldered slouching posture in an attempt to hide their

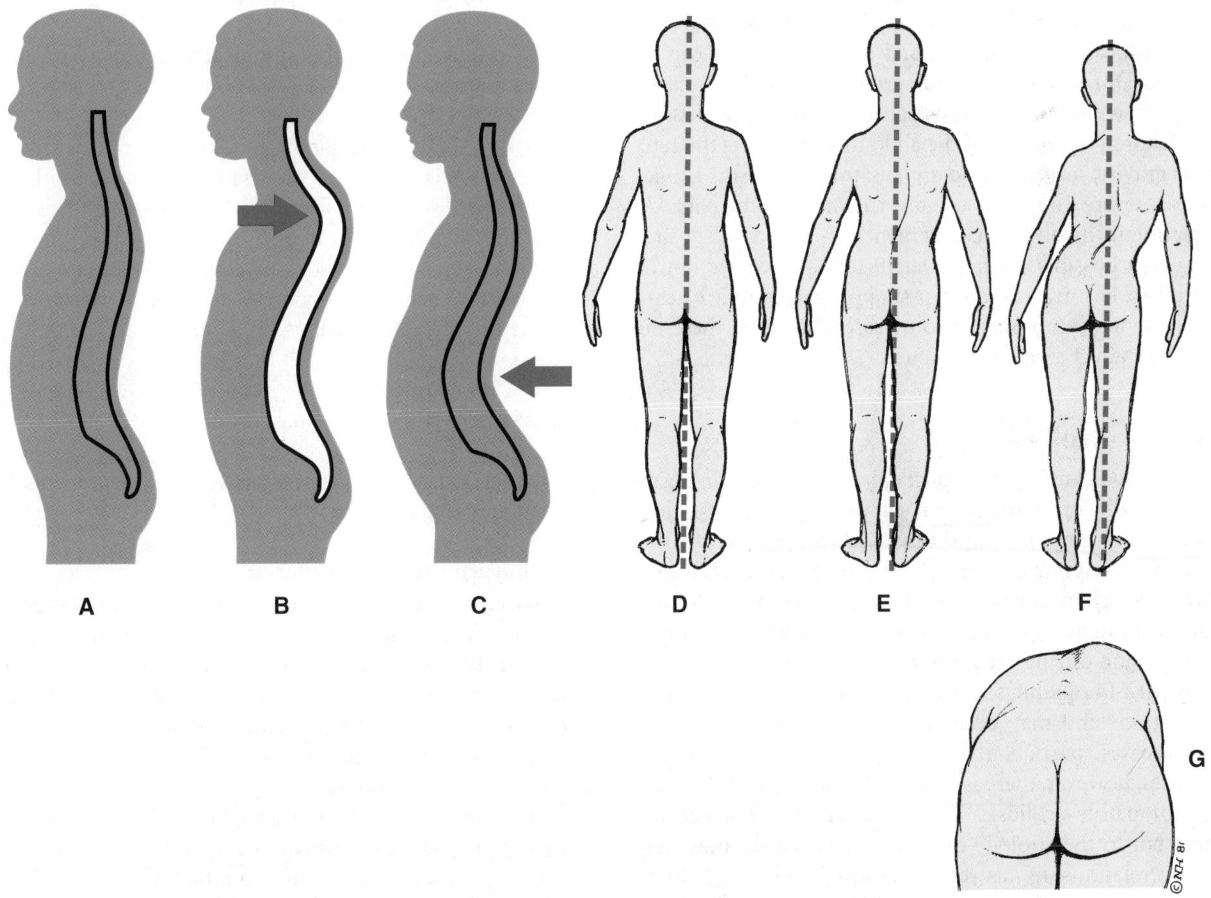

Fig. 54-15 Spinal column curvatures. **A**, Normal spine. **B**, Kyphosis. **C**, Lordosis. **D**, Normal spine in balance. **E**, Mild scoliosis in balance. **F**, Severe scoliosis not in balance. **G**, Rib hump and flank asymmetry seen in flexion caused by rotary component. (Redrawn from Hilt NE, Schmitt EW: *Pediatric orthopedic nursing*, St Louis, 1975, Mosby.)

developing breasts. *Scheuermann kyphosis* is a thoracic curve greater than 45 degrees with wedging greater than 5 degrees of at least three adjacent vertebral bodies and vertebral irregularity.

Postural kyphosis is almost always accompanied by a compensatory postural lordosis, an abnormally exaggerated concave lumbar curvature. Treatment of kyphosis consists of exercises to strengthen shoulder and abdominal muscles and bracing for more marked deformity. With adolescents who are significantly self-conscious in relation to their appearance, the best approach is to emphasize the cosmetic value of corrective therapy and to place the responsibility on the adolescent for carrying out an exercise program at home with regular visits to and assessments by a therapist. Most adolescents respond well to selected sports as a supplement to regular exercise. Boys prefer weight lifting and other upper body strength-building sports. Girls may prefer swimming, ballet, or dancing. Swimming is excellent and has the added advantages of exercising all muscles, eliminating gravity, and teaching breath control. Treatment with a brace may be indicated until skeletal maturity, and surgical fusion may be considered for severe, painful, or progressive thoracic curves such as Scheuermann kyphosis.

Lordosis is an accentuation of the cervical or lumbar curvature beyond physiologic limits (Fig. 54-15, *C*). It may be a secondary complication of a disease process, a result of trauma, or idiopathic. It is often seen in association with flexion contractures of the hip, scoliosis, obesity, developmental dislocation of the hip, and slipped femoral capital epiphysis. During the pubertal growth spurt, lordosis of varying degrees is observed in teenagers, especially girls. In obese children the weight of the abdominal fat alters the center of gravity, causing a compensatory lordosis. Unlike kyphosis, severe lordosis is usually accompanied by pain.

Treatment involves management of the predisposing cause when possible, such as weight loss and correction of deformities. Postural exercises or support garments are helpful in relieving symptoms in some cases; however, these do not usually effect a permanent cure.

Idiopathic Scoliosis

Idiopathic scoliosis is a complex spinal deformity in three planes, usually involving lateral curvature, spinal rotation causing rib asymmetry, and thoracic hypokyphosis. It is the most common spinal deformity and can be further classified according to age of onset: *infantile,* at birth or up to 3 years of age, or it can develop during childhood *(juvenile),* but it is most common during the growth spurt of early adolescence *(adolescent).* Idiopathic scoliosis can be caused by a number of conditions and may occur alone or in association with other diseases, particularly neuromuscular conditions. In most cases, however, there is no apparent cause, and thus the name idiopathic scoliosis. There appears to be a genetic component to the etiology of idiopathic scoliosis; however, the exact relationship has yet to be established. The following section is limited to a discussion of adolescent idiopathic scoliosis.

Idiopathic scoliosis is most noticeable during the preadolescent growth spurt. Parents frequently bring a child for follow-up on an abnormal school scoliosis screening or because of "ill-fitting" clothes, such as poorly fitting slacks. School screening is somewhat controversial, because there are no controlled studies to demonstrate improved outcomes; however, many experts suggest that school screening has increased public and professional awareness of scoliosis and has decreased the number of significant cases of serious deformity (Newton & Wenger, 2001). The AAP recommends scoliosis screening at the time of primary practitioner visits in all preadolescent and adolescent children.

Diagnostic Evaluation

Observation is performed behind an undressed (in underpants and bra, if female) standing child, noting asymmetry of shoulder height, scapular or flank shape, or hip height and alignment. When the child bends forward at the waist (the Adams test) with hanging arms, asymmetry of the ribs and flanks may be noted. A scoliometer is also used in the initial screening to measure truncal rotation (as does the Adams test). Often a primary curve and a compensatory curve will place the head in alignment with the gluteal cleft. However, in the uncompensated curve, the head and hips are not aligned (Fig. 54-15 *E* and *F*). (See Spine, Chapter 35, for additional information.) Definitive diagnosis is made by radiographs of the child in the standing position and use of the Cobb technique (standard measurement of angle curvature), which establishes the degree of curvature. The Risser scale is used to evaluate skeletal maturity on the radiographs; the scale assists in making a determination of the likely progression of the spinal angulature as the child's bones mature.

NURSE ALERT Intraspinal conditions or other disease processes that can cause scoliosis must be ruled out. The presence of pain, sacral dimpling or hairy patches, cutaneous vascular changes, absent or abnormal reflexes, bowel or bladder incontinence, or left thoracic curve may indicate an intraspinal abnormality such as syringomyelia, diastematomyelia, or tethered cord syndrome. A MRI scan should be obtained for evaluation. ■

NURSE ALERT Not all spinal curvatures are scoliosis. A curve of less than 10 degrees is considered a postural variation. Curves of under 20 degrees are mild and, if nonprogressive, do not require treatment. ■

Therapeutic Management

Current management options include observation with regular clinical and radiographic evaluation, orthotic intervention (bracing), and surgical spinal fusion. Treatment decisions are based on the magnitude, location, and type of curve; the age and skeletal maturity of the child; and any underlying or contributing disease process.

Bracing and Exercise

For many curves in the growing child and adolescent, bracing may be the treatment of choice. It is important to realize that *bracing is not curative,* but that it may slow the progression of the curvature to allow skeletal growth and maturity. The two most common types of bracing are (1) the *Boston* and *Wilmington braces,* which are underarm orthoses customized from prefabricated plastic shells, with corrective forces for each patient using lateral pads and decreasing lumbar lordosis, and (2) a *TLSO (thoracolumbosacral orthotic),* which is an underarm orthosis made of plastic that is custom molded to the body and then shaped to correct or hold the deformity (Fig. 54-16). The *Milwaukee brace,* which is an individually adapted brace that includes a neck ring, is rarely used in scoliosis but is sometimes used in the treatment of kyphosis. The *Charleston nighttime bending brace* is worn only when the child is in bed because it prevents walking because of the severity of the trunk bend (Newton & Wenger, 2001). Bracing, although used as the gold standard treatment for mild to moderate curvatures, has not proved to be entirely effective in the treatment of scoliosis (Newton & Wenger, 2001), and retrospective studies show only slight variation in outcomes in regard to type of brace used (Thompson, 2004c). Compliance in wearing the brace is difficult because of the age of the child and preoccupation with body image and appearance.

Exercises alone and chiropractic treatment are rarely of value to manage scoliosis (Thompson, 2004c); transcutaneous electrical stimulation has also proved to be an ineffective treatment for this condition. Exercises are of benefit when used in conjunction with bracing to maintain and strengthen spinal and abdominal muscles during treatment.

Surgical Management

Surgical intervention may be required for correction of severe curves (usually 40 degrees or more). The degree of curvature and the cause determine the decision for surgery. Bracing and exercise have been universally disappointing in curves greater than 40 degrees, and paralytic and congenital curves, which will eventually progress, are best treated with early surgical stabilization if the health status of the child will allow major surgery. The age of the child and location of the curvature influence the decision for surgery, and any progressive or severe curve that does not respond to more conservative orthotic measures requires surgical correction. Difficulties with balance or seating, respiratory excursion, or pain are also considered.

The surgical technique consists of realignment and straightening with internal fixation and instrumentation combined with bony fusion *(arthrodesis)* of the realigned spine. The goals of surgical intervention are to correct the curvatures on the sagittal and coronal planes and to have a solid, pain-free fusion in a well-balanced torso, with maximum mobility of the remaining spinal segments.

Many instrumentation systems, including Harrington, Dwyer, Zielke, Luque, Cotrel-Dubousset, Isola, TSRH (Texas Scottish Rite Hospital), and Moss-Miami, are available. Se-

A B C

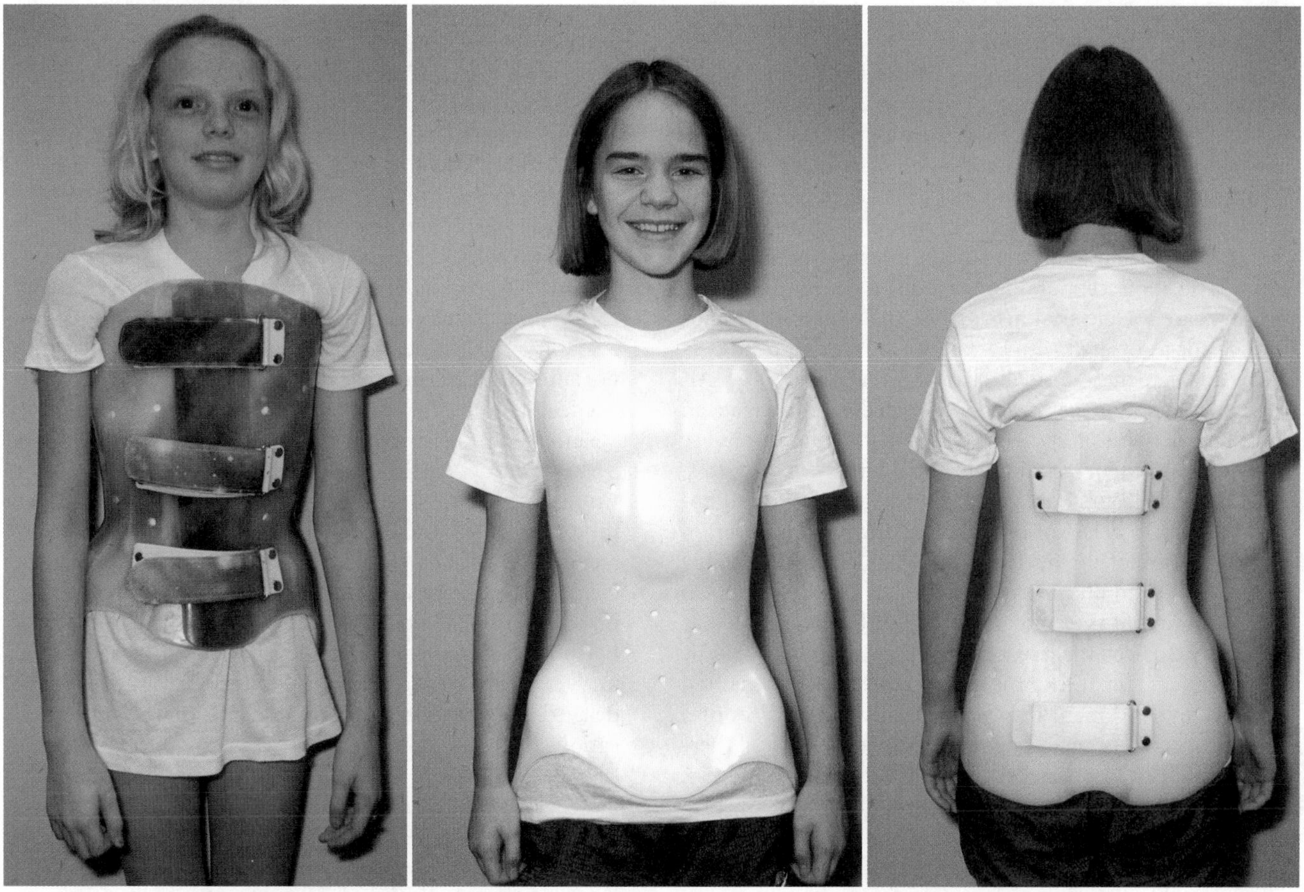

Fig. 54-16 **A,** Standard TLSO brace for idiopathic scoliosis. Note the color and design incorporated into the brace to make it more acceptable to children and adolescents. **B,** Variation of a standard TLSO that fastens in the back, **C,** to provide needed support for the spine curvature.

lection of the system is individualized according to the needs of the patient and the preference of the surgeon. Posterior or anterior surgical approaches can be used.

The Harrington system, the first internal spinal instrumentation device, consists of distraction and compression rods, hooks, and nuts. The posterior elements are decorticated, and bone from the iliac crest or donor bone is placed across the vertebrae to provide fusion. Postoperatively the child is log-rolled to prevent spinal motion and a molded plastic jacket is used to stabilize the spine until the fusion is solid.

The Luque-rod segmental spinal instrumentation provides segmental stability by the use of wires and L-shaped rods. By way of a posterior approach, the wires are threaded beneath the lamina of each vertebra and tightened around the rods resting along the transverse processes to stabilize the spine. Bone from the iliac crest or donor bone is used to fuse the spine. The advantage of this method is that the patient can be mobile within a few days and no postoperative immobilization is required. The disadvantage is the risk of nerve damage.

The Cotrel-Dubousset (CD) instrumentation combines the Harrington and L-rod approaches by using bilateral rods and hooks at many sites. Anterior approaches using the Dwyer or Zielke instrumentation involve screws into the vertebral bodies connected by a cable or rod. These systems require postoperative immobilization with a custom-fitted plastic jacket.

Nursing Care Management

Treatment for scoliosis extends over a significant portion of the affected child's period of growth. In adolescents this period is the one in which their identity, physical and psychologic, is formed. The identification of scoliosis as a "deformity," in combination with unattractive appliances and a significant surgical procedure, can have a negative effect on the already fragile adolescent body image (Noonan et al, 1997). The adolescent and family require not only excellent nursing care for physical needs to be met, but also psychologic needs associated with the diagnosis, surgery, postoperative recovery, and eventual rehabilitation (Slote, 2002). Although these adolescents are encouraged to participate in most peer activities, necessary therapeutic modifications are likely to make them feel different and apart.

When a child first faces the prospect of a prolonged period in a brace, jacket, or other device, the therapy program and the nature of the device must be explained thoroughly to both the child and the parents so that they will have an understanding of the anticipated results, how the appliance corrects the defect, the freedoms and constraints imposed by the device, and what they can do to help achieve the desired goal. The management involves the skills and services of a team of specialists, including the orthopedist, physical therapist, orthotist (a specialist in fitting orthopedic braces), nurse, social worker, and sometimes a thoracic or pulmonary specialist.

It is difficult for a child to be restricted at any phase of development, but the adolescent needs continual positive reinforcement, encouragement, and as much independence as can be safely assumed during this time. Guidance and assistance regarding anticipated problems, such as selection of clothing and participation in social activities, are appreciated by adolescents. Socialization with peers is strongly encouraged, and every effort is expanded to help the adolescent feel attractive and worthwhile.

Preoperative Care

The preoperative workup usually involves a radiographic series, including bending and traction films, pulmonary function studies, and a number of routine laboratory studies. Because spinal surgery usually involves considerable blood loss, several options are considered preoperatively to maintain or replace blood volume. Autologous blood donations may be obtained from the patient before the surgery to replace blood loss during the operation. Other options include intraoperative blood salvage, intraoperative hemodilution, erythropoietin administration, or controlled induced hypotension, which must be carefully monitored at all times to prevent physiologic instability (Newton & Wenger, 2001).

Surgery for spinal fusion is quite complex, and often adolescents who require the procedure because of idiopathic scoliosis are not familiar with medical terms, procedures, or experiences. Preoperative teaching is critical for the adolescent to be able to cooperate and participate in his or her treatment and recovery. Extensive preoperative teaching is essential to prepare the adolescent for the postoperative and recovery course; because the surgery is quite extensive, the patient is taught how to manage his or her own patient-controlled analgesia (PCA) pump, how to log roll, the use and function of other equipment that will be used such as a chest tube (for anterior repair), Foley catheter, and so on. It is recommended that the child or adolescent bring a favorite toy (age-dependent), or personal items such as a favorite stuffed animal, laptop computer or portable compact disc player for postoperative use. Meeting with a peer who has undergone a similar surgery is also valuable (Slote, 2002).

Postoperative Care

After surgery, patients are monitored in an acute care setting and log rolled when changing position to prevent damage to the fusion and instrumentation. Skin care is very important, and pressure-relieving mattresses or beds may be needed to prevent pressure wounds (see Maintaining Healthy Skin, Chapter 45).

In addition to the usual postoperative assessments of wound, circulation, and vital signs, the neurologic status of the patient's extremities requires special attention. Prompt recognition of any neurologic impairment is imperative because delayed paralysis may develop that requires surgical intervention. The most common postoperative problems after spinal fusion include neurologic injury or spinal cord injury, hypotension from acute blood loss, wound infection, delayed neurologic injury, and implanted hardware complications (Newton & Wenger, 2001).

The child usually has considerable pain for the first few days after surgery and requires frequent administration of pain medication, preferably the use of opioids administered intravenously on a regular schedule. For children able to understand the concept, PCA is recommended (see Pain Assessment; Pain Management, Chapter 44). In most cases the patient begins walking as soon as possible. Depending on the instrumentation used, most patients are walking by the second or third postoperative day and are discharged by 1 week, depending on the surgical approach. In addition to pain management, the patient is evaluated for skin integrity, adequate urinary output, fluid and electrolyte balance, and ileus (Slote, 2002). The latter may be particularly distressful for the adolescent who is self-conscious. Discharge planning should include a timetable for follow-up with the practitioner and resumption of regular activities.

All patients are started on physical therapy as soon as they are able, beginning with range-of-motion exercises on the first postoperative day, and many of the activities of daily living in the following days. Self-care, such as washing and eating, is always encouraged. Throughout the hospitalization, age-appropriate activities and contact with family and friends are important parts of nursing care and planning (see Immobilization, p. 1800).

The family is encouraged to become involved with the patient's care to facilitate the transition from hospital to home management. An organization that provides education and services to both families and professionals is the National Scoliosis Foundation, Inc.* The American Academy of Orthopaedic Surgeons† and Scoliosis Research Society (SRS),‡ an organization of physicians and scientists, have published an excellent book, *Scoliosis,* and the SRS has educational information available on its Web site.

INFECTIONS OF BONES AND JOINTS

evolve CASE STUDY: OSTEOMYELITIS

Osteomyelitis

Osteomyelitis is an infection in the bone. *Acute osteomyelitis* is a bone infection present less than 2 weeks, *subacute osteomyelitis* is a bone infection lasting 2 to 6 weeks, and in *chronic osteomyelitis* the infection lasts more than 6 weeks. Osteomyelitis can occur at any age but is more common in young children and older adults. It occurs more often in boys than girls with a 2 to 3:1 ratio. Other than sickle cell anemia, most children with osteomyelitis do not have significant risk factors.

Pathophysiology

Osteomyelitis can be acquired exogenously by direct inoculation of bone during trauma, puncture, or surgery; the hand and foot are common sites. Hematogenous osteomyelitis is seeded by organisms from a preexisting infection such as tonsillitis or impetigo or by seeding from a contiguous source such as an adjacent infected bone or joint. Hematogenous osteomyelitis usually occurs in the metaphyses of long bones, the femur or tibia. The infecting organism travels from the site of infection to the small end-artery capillary loops in the bone metaphyses causing obstruction and initiating infection, with complications of bone destruction and abscess formation. Any bacteria can cause osteomyelitis, but *Staphylococcus aureus* is the most common pathogen. *Haemophilus influenzae* used to be a common pathogen in the younger child; however, the incidence has decreased since the advent of *H. influenzae* vaccine. Children with sickle cell anemia are at increased risk for *Salmonella* as a causative organism.

Most cases involve the femur or tibia. In infants the diagnosis is challenging because of difficulty localizing symptoms and the increased likelihood of multiple bone involvement.

Diagnostic Evaluation

Typically children with acute hematogenous osteomyelitis present with a 2- to 7-day history of pain, warmth, tenderness, and decreased range of motion in the affected limb, and systemic symptoms of fever, irritability, and lethargy (Box 54-8). Symptoms often resemble those observed in other diseases involving bones such as arthritis or leukemia. There may be nonspecific elevation of the white blood cell count, erythrocyte sedimentation rate, and C-reactive protein. Blood cultures may be positive but can be negative in children already receiving antibiotics. Direct bone aspirates are more likely to yield a causative organism. Early plain radiographs are often normal but help rule out other diseases. Technetium-labeled bone scans are more sensitive in early disease (Karwowska et al, 1998). Ultrasound, CT, and MRI can also be useful to help make the diagnosis of osteomyelitis.

Therapeutic Management

As soon as blood and bone aspirate cultures are obtained, empiric parenteral antibiotics are administered pending culture results. Because *S. aureus* is the most prevalent causative organism the empiric antibiotics are typically penicillinase-resistant penicillin and a third-generation cephalosporin. When cultures are received the appropriate antibiotic is continued for 4 to 6 weeks. In select cases oral antibiotics may follow a shorter, intensive IV course with good results (Karwowska et al, 1998). Because of prolonged high-dose therapy, it is important to monitor hematologic, renal, he-

BOX 54-8

Clinical Manifestations of Acute Osteomyelitis

General Manifestations
History of trauma to affected bone (frequent)
Child appears very ill
Irritability
Restlessness
Elevated temperature
Rapid pulse
Dehydration

Local Manifestations
Tenderness
Increased warmth
Diffuse swelling over involved bone
Involved extremity painful, especially on movement
Involved extremity held in semiflexion
Surrounding muscles tense and resist passive movement

*5 Cabot Place, Stoughton, MA 02072; phone: 781-341-6333 or 800-673-6922; Web site: www.scoliosis.org.

†6300 North River Road, Rosemont, IL 60018-4262; phone: 847-698-1627.

‡611 East Wells Street, Milwaukee, WI 53202; phone: 414-289-9107; Web site: www.srs.org.

patic, and other organ systems that might be adversely affected by the drugs (e.g., ototoxic).

Opinions differ regarding surgical intervention, but typically chronic osteomyelitis will not respond without débridement and the removal of dead bone. Débridement and amputation are frequently required in osteomyelitis in the diabetic foot and in other conditions with impaired blood flow. Antibiotic-impregnated seed implants and direct antibiotic solution instillation and drainage may be used to improve local antibiotic delivery.

Nursing Care Management

During the acute phase of illness any movement of the affected limb will cause discomfort; therefore, the child is positioned comfortably with the affected limb supported. Moving and turning are carried out carefully and gently to minimize pain. Pain medication is administered to provide comfort. Vital signs are taken and recorded frequently, and measures are implemented to reduce a significant temperature elevation.

Antibiotic therapy requires careful observation and monitoring of the IV equipment and site. Because more than one antibiotic is usually administered, the compatibility of the drugs is determined and care is taken to avoid mixing noncompatible drugs. For long-term antibiotic therapy, an intermittent infusion device or peripherally inserted central catheter (PICC) is used (see Peripheral Venous Access Devices, Chapter 45). Antibiotic therapy is often continued at home.

The child with an open wound may be placed on contact isolation. The wound is managed as prescribed. Antibiotic solution administered directly into the wound is most efficiently accomplished with a regular IV infusion setup that is prepared and regulated in the same manner as any other. If used, drainage tubes are connected to low Gomco or wall suction devices for continuous removal. Intake and output are measured and recorded, and the character of the wound drainage is noted. The amount and character of drainage on the wound dressing are also noted.

Casts are sometimes used for immobilization, and if so, routine cast care is carried out. The extremity is examined for sensation, circulation, and pain, and the area over the inflammation is usually left open for observation. The affected area, casted or uncasted, is assessed for color, swelling, heat, and tenderness.

The child usually has a poor appetite at first. Nourishment in the form of high-calorie liquids, such as 100% fruit juices, gelatin, and flavored ice pops, is encouraged until the child begins to feel better. The appetite returns as the acute symptoms subside. During convalescence adequate nutrition must be maintained to aid healing and formation of new bone.

When the acute stage subsides, the child begins to feel better, the appetite improves, and the child becomes interested in the surroundings and relationships and may move about in bed. However, weight bearing on the affected limb is not permitted until healing is well under way to avoid pathologic fractures. Diversional and constructive activities become important nursing interventions. The child is usually confined to bed for some time after the acute phase but may be allowed to move about in a wheelchair when isolation and bed rest are no longer necessary. As the infection subsides, physical therapy is instituted to ensure restoration of optimum function. If amputation is required, evaluation of emotional and social support is essential for successful adaptation.

Septic (Suppurative, Pyogenic, Purulent) Arthritis

Infections of the joints, like those of bone, usually develop through hematogenous dissemination from another focus; occasionally they result from direct extension of a soft tissue infection. Joint infections occur predominantly in males, especially in the adolescent age group. In infancy, however, the incidence in boys and girls is nearly equal. Any joint may be involved, but the hip, knee, shoulder, and other large joints are most commonly affected. Usually only one joint is involved.

Therapeutic Management and Nursing Care Management

The affected joint is aspirated and evaluated for type of organism and subsequent fluid accumulation. An infection involving the hip, however, is considered a surgical emergency to prevent compromised blood supply to the head of the femur (Lampe, 2004). Antibiotic therapy is initiated after cultures and fluid aspirate occur. Follow-up serial aspirations may be necessary, and antibiotic regimen is maintained according to the isolated organism and the response to antibiotic therapy. Surgical intervention may also be required if there was a penetrating wound or possibly a foreign object involved. Physical therapy may be used for the child who is immobilized in a cast or traction to prevent flexion contractures. Pain management is an important aspect of nursing care, particularly for large joint involvement such as the hip. Additional nursing care is the same as for osteomyelitis.

Skeletal Tuberculosis

In children infection of bones and joints is acquired by lymphohematogenous spread at the time of primary infection. Occasionally, infection is from chronic pulmonary tuberculosis. Skeletal tubercular infection is not common in the United States but must be considered in communities with high tuberculosis case rates. The infection most likely involves the vertebrae, causing a tubercular spondylitis. If the infection is progressive, it causes Pott's disease with destruction of the vertebral bodies and resultant kyphosis.

Symptoms and onset are usually insidious; the child may report persistent or intermittent pain. Other findings include joint swelling and stiffness; fever and weight loss are not common. Tubercular arthritis can also affect single joints such as a knee or hip and tends to cause severe destruction of adjacent bone. Diagnosis requires isolation of *Mycobacterium tuberculosis* from the site (bone biopsy) and patients with positive cultures are started on treatment of combined antituberculosis chemotherapy, isoniazid, rifampin, and pyrazinamide; streptomycin or other antituberculosis drugs may be required if drug-resistance is encountered. Reliance on a positive PPD (purified protein derivative) skin test alone is not considered diagnostic for tuberculous arthritis. Supervised drug therapy is recommended to ensure treatment compliance. In some cases surgical débridement may be required. Tuberculous spondylitis and hip infection may involve immobilization, casting, and spinal fusion.

Nursing Care Management

The nursing responsibilities are similar to those for other types of osteomyelitis and septic arthritis, but include monitoring tuberculosis drug therapy and identifying positive family or environmental active disease contacts.

BONE AND SOFT TISSUE TUMORS

General Concepts: Bone Tumors

Neoplastic disease can arise from any tissues involved in bone growth. In children the two types that account for 85% of all primary malignant bone tumors are osteogenic sarcoma (osteosarcoma) and Ewing sarcoma.

The peak ages for occurrence during childhood are 15 to 19 years. The sexes are affected equally until puberty, at which time the ratio approaches 2:1 in favor of males. This propensity for males, with a peak incidence during adolescence, is thought to be related to the accelerated growth rate of osseous tissue. These two bone tumors have several characteristics in common, which are discussed. Specific information related to each tumor is also presented.

Diagnostic Evaluation

A primary objective in diagnosis of bone neoplasm is to rule out causes such as trauma or infection. A history and careful questioning regarding pain help determine the duration and rate of tumor growth (Box 54-9). Physical assessment focuses on the functional status of the affected area, signs of inflammation, size of the mass, involvement of regional lymph nodes, and any systemic indication of generalized malignancy.

Definitive diagnosis is based on radiologic studies such as chest radiograph, MRI, CT scans, and radioisotope bone scans that determine the extent of the disease. A needle or surgical bone biopsy is performed to determine the histologic type. Radiologic findings are characteristic for each type of tumor. In osteogenic sarcoma, the needlelike bone projections present a "sunburst" appearance, whereas the layers of new bone in Ewing sarcoma will have an "onion-skin" or "hair-on-end" appearance (Ginsberg et al, 2002; Link, Gebhardt, & Meyers, 2002). MRI provides information regarding neurovascular structures, intramedullary bone involvement, and soft-tissue extension (Rednek, 2000).

There is no reliable biochemical test for bone cancers, although elevated alkaline phosphatase levels may occur in osteoid tumors. Several tests may be performed to rule out metastatic disease from other neoplasms. Chest CT is usually a standard procedure, because pulmonary metastasis is the most common complication of primary bone tumors. Bone marrow aspiration is helpful in diagnosing Ewing sarcoma in the rare event that the child has bone marrow metastasis.

BOX 54-9

Clinical Manifestations of Bone Tumors

- Pain localized at affected site
  - May be severe or dull
  - Often relieved by position of flexion
  - Frequently brought to attention when child:
    - Limps
    - Curtails own physical activity
    - Is unable to hold heavy objects

Osteogenic Sarcoma

Osteogenic sarcoma is the most commonly encountered malignant bone cancer in children, with a peak incidence between 10 and 25 years of age. Most primary tumor sites are in the metaphysis of long bones (i.e., the wider part of the shaft, next to epiphyseal growth plate), especially in the lower extremities. More than half occur in the femur, particularly the distal portion, with the rest involving the humerus, tibia, pelvis, jaw, and phalanges.

CRITICAL THINKING EXERCISE: OSTEOGENIC SARCOMA

Therapeutic Management

Optimum treatment of osteosarcoma is surgery and chemotherapy. The surgical approach consists of radical surgical resection or amputation. Depending on the tumor site, preoperative response to chemotherapy, and location of the tumor, the goal of surgery is to remove the diseased bone surrounded by a large margin of healthy bone. With tumors of the distal femur, preservation of the hip joint may be possible. Other surgical procedures include an above-the-knee amputation for tumors of the tibia or fibula, a hemipelvectomy for tumors of the innominate (hip) bone, and a forequarter amputation (removal of the arm, the scapula, and a portion of the clavicle on the affected side) for tumors of the upper humerus. *Limb-salvage procedures* entail en bloc resection of tumor-bearing bone with prosthetic replacement of the involved bone. Partial limb salvage by a *rotationplasty procedure* involves resection of the tumor, including the knee joint, with the lower part of the leg rotated 180 degrees and retransplanted to the thigh, creating a shortened leg with the ankle joint at the position of the former knee joint (Link et al, 2002).

All children with osteosarcoma receive chemotherapy to treat microscopic disease (Kline & Sevier, 2003). Antineoplastic drugs, such as high-dose methotrexate with citrovorum rescue, Adriamycin, actinomycin D, cyclophosphamide, ifosfamide, etoposide, and cisplatin may be administered in combination or singly, both before and after surgery.

Prognosis

Surgical procedures (limb-salvage procedures, amputation, thoracotomy) accompanied by multiagent chemotherapy have significantly improved survival rates in patients with osteosarcoma. Approximately 65% to 85% of patients with nonmetastatic osteosarcoma can expect long-term survival (Rednek, 2000). The patient with metastatic osteosarcoma has a survival prognosis rate of less than 50%. To improve long-term survival, a compound known as muramyl tripeptide phosphatidylethanolamine (MTP-PE) is being studied. MTP-PE is designed to stimulate macrophages to kill tumor cells, consequently reducing the risk of recurrence in patients with osteosarcoma (Dzierzbicka et al, 2003; Link et al, 2002).

Nursing Care Management

Nursing care depends on the type of surgical approach, and in either instance preparation of the child and family is crucial. Obviously, the family may have more difficulty adjusting to an amputation than a limb-salvage procedure.

Honesty is essential to gain the cooperation and trust of the child. The diagnosis of cancer should not be disguised with falsehoods such as "infection." To accept the need for radical surgery, the child must be aware of the lack of alternatives for treatment. Although the task of informing the child is the responsibility of the physician, the nurse should be present for the discussion or be aware of exactly what is said to the child. The child should be told a few days before surgery, so that he or she has time to think about the diagnosis and consequent treatment and to ask questions.

Sometimes children have many questions about the prosthesis, limitations on physical ability, and prognosis in terms of cure. At other times they react with silence or with a calm manner that masks their concern and fear. Either response is part of the grieving process that accompanies a loss and must be accepted. Children should not be overwhelmed with information. A supportive approach is to answer their questions without offering additional information and to express a willingness to talk.

The child is also informed of the need for chemotherapy and its side effects before surgery. Caution must be exercised in offering too much information at one time. It is wise to discuss hair loss with emphasis on positive aspects, such as wearing a wig or baseball cap. Because bone tumors affect adolescents and young adults, it is not unusual for them to become angry about the radical body alterations.

If an amputation is performed, the child may be fitted with a temporary prosthesis immediately after surgery, which permits early functioning and fosters psychologic adjustment. If this is not done, the child requires stump care, which is the same as for any amputee. A permanent prosthesis is usually fitted within 6 to 8 weeks. During hospitalization the child begins physical therapy to become proficient in the use and care of the device.

In rotationplasty, a prosthesis is fitted over the newly created knee joint. However, the appearance of a foot placed backward on the leg to create a substitute knee is a major change in body image. Children often need help in dealing with their own feelings and other people's reactions to the leg.

Phantom limb pain may develop after amputation. This symptom is characterized by pain, tingling, itching, burning, or cramping in the area of the amputated leg (Olsson, 1999). The child and family need to know that the sensations are real, not imagined. Amitriptyline (Elavil) has been used successfully in children to decrease the pain (Berde, Billett, & Collins 2002).

Discharge planning must begin early during the postoperative period. Every effort is made to promote normality and gradual resumption of realistic preamputation activities.* Role-playing in anticipation of such experiences is very beneficial in preparing the child for the inevitable confrontation by others. Environmental barriers, such as stairs, are assessed in terms of the accessibility of the school or home, especially because the child may need to use crutches or a wheelchair before complete healing and prosthetic competency are achieved.

The family and child need a great deal of support in adjusting not only to a life-threatening diagnosis, but also to alteration in body image and function. Because loss of a limb involves a grieving process, those caring for the child need to recognize that anger and depression are normal and necessary reactions. Often parents view the anger as a direct affront to them for allowing the amputation, or they view the depression as rejection. These are not personal attacks but the child's attempts to cope with the loss.

Ewing Sarcoma (Primitive Neuroectodermal Tumor)

Ewing sarcoma, a primitive neuroectodermal tumor, is the second most common malignant bone tumor (after osteogenic sarcoma) in children and adolescents (Ginsberg et al, 2002). It arises in the marrow spaces of the bones such as the femur, tibia, fibula, ulna, humerus, vertebrae, pelvis, scapula, ribs, and skull. The disease occurs almost exclusively in individuals younger than age 30, with most occurrences in individuals between 4 and 20 years of age (Grier, 1997).

Therapeutic Management

Surgical amputation is not routinely recommended but may be considered when the results of radiotherapy render the extremity useless or deformed (such as from retarded growth in young children) or when the tumor appears resectable. The treatment of choice is intensive radiation therapy of the involved bone combined with chemotherapy. A widely used drug regimen includes vincristine, actinomycin D, and cyclophosphamide; or ifosfamide, VP-16, and Adriamycin.

Prognosis

The prognosis is best for children who do not have metastasis at the time of diagnosis. Children with massive tumors or lung and bone marrow metastasis have a much poorer prognosis. Children with distal lesions have the best chance for cure.

Nursing Care Management

The psychologic adjustment to Ewing sarcoma is typically less traumatic than to osteogenic sarcoma because of the preservation of the affected limb. Many families accept the diagnosis with a sense of relief in knowing that this type of bone cancer does not necessitate amputation, and initially they may not be aware of the deleterious effects on the irradiated site, especially severely affected growth, function, and appearance. Consequently, they need preparation for the various diagnostic tests, including bone marrow aspiration and surgical biopsy, and adequate explanation of the treatment regimen.

High-dose radiation therapy often causes a skin reaction of dry or moist desquamation followed by hyperpigmentation. The nurse advises the child to wear loose-fitting clothes over the radiated area to minimize additional skin irritation. Because of increased sensitivity, the radiated skin is protected

*Information about special programs for children with amputations is available from the Candlelighters Childhood Cancer Foundation, PO Box 498, Kensington, MD 20895; phone: 800-366-2223; Web site: www.candlelighters.org. Information about prostheses can be obtained from the National Amputation Foundation, Inc., 40 Church Street, Malverne, NY 11565; phone: 516-887-3600; Web site: http://www.nationalamputation.org/. In Canada: War Amputations of Canada, 1 Maybrook Drive, Scarborough, ON M1V 5K9; phone: 800-250-3030 (United States and Canada); phone: 416-297-2660; Web site: www.waramps.ca.

from sunlight and from sudden changes in temperature, such as those caused by the use of heating pads or ice packs. The child is encouraged to use the extremity as tolerated. Occasionally an active exercise program may be planned by the physical therapist to preserve maximum function.

The child needs the same considerations as any other patient with cancer in adjusting to the effects of chemotherapy, such as hair loss, severe nausea and vomiting, peripheral neuropathy, and possibly cardiotoxicity. Every effort should be made to outline a treatment plan that allows the child maximum resumption of a normal lifestyle and activities. (See also Nursing Care Plan: The Child with Cancer in Chapter 49.)

Rhabdomyosarcoma

The most common soft-tissue sarcoma in children is rhabdomyosarcoma. These malignant neoplasms originate from undifferentiated mesenchymal cells in muscles, tendons, bursae, and fascia or from such cells in fibrous, connective, lymphatic, or vascular tissue. These disorders derive their name from the specific tissue(s) of origin, such as *myosarcoma* (*myo,* muscle) or *rhabdomyosarcoma* (*rhabdo,* striated). Because striated (skeletal) muscle is found almost anywhere in the body, these tumors occur in many sites, the most common of which are the head and neck, especially the orbit. Sixty-five percent of the tumors occur in children younger than age 6 years, with most of the remaining cases between 10 to 18 years of age.

Diagnostic Evaluation

The initial signs and symptoms are related to the site of the tumor and compression of adjacent organs (Box 54-10). Some tumor locations, particularly the orbit, produce symptoms early in the course of the illness and contribute to rapid diagnosis and improved prognosis. Other tumors, such as those of the retroperitoneal area, produce no symptoms until they are large, invasive, and widely metastasized. Unfortunately, many of the signs and symptoms attributable to rhabdomyosarcoma are vague and commonly suggest a common childhood illness, such as "earache" or "runny nose." In some instances a primary tumor site is never identified.

Diagnosis begins with a careful examination of the head and neck area, particularly palpation of a nontender, firm, hard mass. The nasopharynx and oropharynx are inspected for any evidence of a visible mass. Radiographic studies are performed to isolate a tumor site; accompanied by chest radiographic examinations, chest CT scans, bone surveys, and bone marrow aspiration to rule out metastasis. A lumbar puncture is indicated for head and neck tumors. An excisional biopsy is performed to confirm the histologic type.

Therapeutic Management

Because this tumor is highly malignant, with metastasis frequently occurring at the time of diagnosis, aggressive multimodal therapy (i.e., surgery, chemotherapy, and radiation) is recommended. Complete removal of the primary tumor is advocated whenever possible. The intergroup rhabdomyosarcoma staging system incorporates the size, invasiveness, lymph node involvement, and primary tumor site in the determination of treatment and prognosis (Shamberger, Jaksic, & Ziegler, 2002).

High-dose irradiation to the primary tumor is recommended for most tumors. Radiation usually begins after several chemotherapy courses have been given to shrink the tumor. Drugs that are cytotoxic for rhabdomyosarcoma are vincristine, actinomycin D, and cyclophosphamide, with or without Adriamycin; as well as ifosfamide, cisplatin, etoposide, and carboplatin. These may be given for 1 to 2 years.

Prognosis

With current treatment protocols, survival rates for children with tumors detected at all clinical stages have increased considerably. Tumors of the orbit, superficial head, neck, testes, vagina, and uterus all have a 4-year survival rate

BOX 54-10

Clinical Manifestations of Rhabdomyosarcoma According to Tumor Site

Orbit
Rapidly developing unilateral proptosis
Ecchymosis of conjunctiva
Loss of extraocular movements (strabismus)
Orbital cellulitis

Nasopharynx
Stuffy nose (earliest sign)
Nasal obstruction-dysphagia, nasal voice (obstruction of posterior nasal conchae)
Pain (sore throat and ear)
Epistaxis
Palpable neck nodes
Visible mass in oropharynx (late sign)

Paranasal Sinuses
Nasal obstruction
Local pain/swelling
Discharge (may be unilateral)
Sinusitis
Swelling

Middle Ear
Signs of chronic serous otitis media
Pain/swelling
Mass in external canal
Sanguinopurulent drainage
Facial nerve palsy

Retroperitoneal Area
(Usually a "silent" tumor)
Abdominal mass
Pain
Signs of intestinal or genitourinary obstruction

Perineum
Visible superficial mass (scrotum, vaginal, or cervical areas)
Bowel or bladder dysfunction (from tumor compression)
Vaginal bleeding or mucosanguineous discharge

Extremity
Pain
Palpable fixed mass
Regional lymph enlargement

of 90%. Tumors of the parameningeal area, bladder, prostate, and limbs have an approximately 65% survival rate (Shamberger et al, 2002).

Nursing Care Management

The nursing responsibilities are similar to those for other types of cancer, especially the solid tumors when surgery is used. Specific objectives include (1) careful assessment for signs of the tumor, especially during well-child examinations; (2) preparation of the child and family for the multiple diagnostic tests; and (3) supportive care during each stage of multimodal therapy. The reader is urged to review nursing care management under Leukemias in Chapter 49 for physical care of the child, and Chapter 41 for emotional support of the family in the event of a poor prognosis.

DISORDERS OF JOINTS

Juvenile Rheumatoid Arthritis (Juvenile Idiopathic Arthritis)

Juvenile idiopathic arthritis (JIA) is a new name replacing juvenile rheumatoid arthritis (JRA) in the research literature and more slowly in clinical practice. JIA is an autoimmune inflammatory disease causing inflammation of joints and other tissue with an unknown cause. JIA has two peak ages of onset: between 1 and 3 years of age and between 8 and 10 years of age. Twice as many girls as boys are affected. The exact incidence is unknown but studies suggest a minimum incidence of 4.08 per 100,000 children (Malleson, Fung, & Rosenberg, 1996). A popular theory is an infectious (virus) or environmental agent triggers an abnormal inflammatory response in a genetically predisposed child resulting in chronic arthritis, but there is no substantiating evidence.

Pathophysiology

The disease process is characterized by chronic inflammation of the synovium with joint effusion and eventual erosion, destruction, and fibrosis of the articular cartilage. Adhesions between joint surfaces and ankylosis of joints occur if the inflammatory process persists.

Clinical Manifestations

The outcome of JIA is variable and unpredictable. The disease, even in severe forms, is rarely life-threatening but can cause significant disability. The arthritis tends to wax and wane and eventually becomes inactive in approximately 70% of the cases; however, these children may have severe or minimal joint damage remaining when active arthritis abates. Approximately 30% of the children will have progressive arthritis into adulthood. Their arthritis can cause significant joint deformity and functional disability requiring medication, physical therapy, and perhaps future joint replacement. Chronic and acute uveitis can cause permanent vision loss if undiagnosed and not aggressively treated.

Classification of Juvenile Idiopathic Arthritis

JIA is not a single disease, but a heterogenous group of diseases. The three subtypes include pauciarticular onset, polyarticular onset, and systemic onset. Pauciarticular (oligoarthritis) onset, which involves arthritis in four or less joints, accounts for 50% of all cases. Polyarticular onset, which involves more than four joints, accounts for 40% of all cases. Systemic onset has variable arthritis with systemic features of high fevers with late-evening spikes, transient maculopapular rash, hepatosplenomegaly, pericarditis, pleuritis, and lymphadenopathy. Systemic onset represents 10% to 15% of all cases. Although JIA and adult disease both involve arthritis, the diseases are distinct. In contrast to adult disease, JIA occurs in children younger than 16 years of age, children have negative rheumatoid factor in 90% of the cases, systemic features in 10% of the cases, and the associated complication of uveitis (inflammation of the iris and ciliary body) in 8% to 20% of the cases. A large portion of JIA cases—60% to 70%—tends to "burn out" and become inactive.

The universal Durban classification of JIA revised and published in 1998 lists seven disease categories, each with its own set of criteria end exclusions: systemic arthritis, oligoarthritis, rheumatoid factor–negative polyarthritis, rheumatoid factor–positive arthritis, psoriatic arthritis, enthesitis-related arthritis, and other arthritis (Petty et al, 1998). Recently the International League of Associations for Rheumatology further refined the definitions for JIA to provide improved categorization and treatment of the disease (Petty et al, 2004).

Diagnostic Evaluation

JIA is a diagnosis of exclusion; there are no definitive tests. The diagnosis is based in part on the classification criteria of the American College of Rheumatology, which includes clinical criteria of age of onset before 16 years, arthritis in one or more joints for 6 weeks or longer, onset defined by type of disease in first 6 months (systemic, polyarthritis, or pauciarticular), and exclusion of other etiologies (Brewer et al, 1997; Miller & Cassidy, 2004; Petty et al, 1998). Laboratory tests may provide supporting evidence of disease. An elevated erythrocyte sedimentation rate (ESR) may or may not be present. Leukocytosis is frequently present during exacerbations of systemic JIA. Antinuclear antibodies (ANA) are common in JIA but are not specific for arthritis; however, they help identify children with pauciarticular disease who are at greater risk for uveitis. The rheumatoid factor (RF) may be positive in older children with polyarticular involvement but both ANA and RF may also be present with certain viral infections such as Epstein-Barr virus (Miller & Cassidy, 2004). Plain radiographs are the best initial imaging studies and may show soft-tissue swelling and joint space widening from increased synovial fluid in the joint. Later films can reveal osteoporosis, narrow joint space, erosions, subluxation, and ankylosis.

Therapeutic Management

There is no cure for JIA. The major goals of therapy are to control pain, preserve joint range of motion and function, minimize effects of inflammation such as joint deformity, and promote normal growth and development. Outpatient care is the mainstay of therapy; lengthy hospitalizations are infrequent in this era of managed care. The treatment plan can be exhaustive and intrusive for the child and family, including medications, physical and occupational therapy, ophthalmologic slit lamp examinations, splints, comfort measures, dietary management, school modifications, and psychosocial support.

Medications

Many arthritis medications are available and most are effective in suppressing the inflammatory process and relieving pain. These drugs may be given alone or in combination and are prescribed in a stepwise manner dependent on disease response to each level.

Nonsteroidal anti-inflammatory drugs (NSAIDs) are the first drugs used. Naproxen, ibuprofen, and tolmetin are approved for use in children. They are effective with few common side effects other than gastrointestinal irritation and bruising; with naproxen, skin fragility is a possible side effect. NSAIDs must be taken with food. There is unofficial use of other NSAIDs approved for arthritis in adults but not yet children. Aspirin, once the drug of choice, has been replaced by NSAIDs because they have fewer side effects and easier administration schedules.

Methotrexate is the second-line medication used in children who have failed with NSAIDS alone. It is started in combination with an NSAID. It is effective, with acceptable toxicity, which requires monitoring of complete blood cell counts and liver functions. Patient education about possible side effects, including discussions with teens about birth defects and avoiding alcohol is essential.

Corticosteroids are potent immunosuppressives used for life-threatening complications, incapacitating arthritis, and uveitis. They are administered at the lowest effective dose for the briefest period and discontinued on a tapering schedule. They may be administered orally, as intraarticular joint injections, as intravenous pushes, or in eye drop form for uveitis. A single intraarticular injection may provide effective relief for children with pauciarticular disease unresponsive to NSAIDS (Padeh & Passwell, 1998). Prolonged use of systemic steroids is associated with significant side effects, including Cushing syndrome, osteoporosis, increased infection risk, glucose intolerance, cataracts, and growth suppression.

Etanercept is a tumor necrosis factor (inhibitor) alpha receptor blocker and an effective drug for children with JIA who are nonresponsive to methotrexate (Lovell et al, 2003). It is given as twice per week via subcutaneous injections. Possible side effects include transient allergic reaction at injection site, increased infection risk, and rare reports of demyelinating disease and pancytopenia. Another TNF inhibitor, Infliximab, will soon be available for patients with JIA.

Slow-acting antirheumatic drugs (SAARDs) may require months to be effective and typically work in combination with NSAIDs. SAARDs include sulfasalazine, hydroxychloroquine, gold, and D-penicillamine. SAARDs are used less often because methotrexate has been recognized as second-line therapy.

Physical Management

Programs of physical management are individualized for each child and designed to reach the ultimate goal-preserving function or preventing deformity. Physical therapy is directed toward specific joints, focusing on strengthening muscles, mobilizing restricted joint motion, and preventing or correcting deformities. Occupational therapy assumes responsibility for generalized mobility and performance of activities of daily living.

General treatment or maintenance programs vary; physiotherapists may be involved several times weekly to monthly in management of a home program, or their visits may be limited to infrequent review of the home program for compliance, effectiveness, and need. Normal activities of daily living and the child's natural tendency to be active are usually sufficient to maintain muscle strength and joint mobility.

Exercising in a pool is excellent therapy, because it allows freedom of movement with support. If there is pain on motion, a hot pack or warm bath before therapy may help.

Practitioners may recommend nighttime splinting to help minimize pain and reduce flexion deformity. Joints most frequently splinted are the knees, wrists, and hands. Positioning during rest is also important. The child rests on a firm mattress with no pillow or a very low one. Loss of extension in the knee, hip, and wrist causes special problems and requires vigilance to detect the earliest signs of involvement and vigorous attention to prevent deformity with specialized passive stretching, positioning, and resting splints.

Prognosis

The course of JIA is highly variable and depends on onset type. As many as 45% of JIA patients will have active disease lasting into early adulthood with often severe physical limitations. The prognosis is best for children with pauciarticular JIA and worst for children with chronic, polyarticular disease, especially those positive for RF. Chronic uveitis is a common occurrence and may develop in females with onset before age 6 with pauciarticular (oligoarthritis) disease (Miller & Cassidy, 2004).

Nursing Care Management

Assessment

Nursing the child with JIA involves assessment of the child's general health, the status of involved joints, and the child's emotional response to all ramifications of the disease (e.g., discomfort, physical restrictions, therapies, and self-concept).

Nursing Diagnoses

Nursing diagnoses and management identified for the child with *JIA* include the following:

- Chronic pain related to joint inflammation
- Impaired physical mobility related to joint discomfort and stiffness
- Bathing/hygiene, dressing/grooming, feeding, or toileting self-care deficit related to impaired joint mobility
- Altered family processes related to a situational crisis (child with a chronic illness)

Plan of Care and Implementation

Goals for the child with JIA and family include the following:

1. Child will experience reduction of pain to level acceptable to child.
2. Child will remain healthy.
3. Child will exhibit signs of adequate joint function.
4. Child will perform activities of daily living.
5. Child and family will receive adequate support.

The effects of JIA are manifest in every aspect of the child's life, physical activities, social experiences, and personality development. Although children with severe disease may have more physical barriers to overcome, studies show that emotional and behavioral functioning is most closely linked with maternal depression and parental distress, not with physical disability (Frank et al, 1998). Nursing interventions to support the parents may foster a successful adaptation for the entire family. Parental concerns about the disease prognosis, financial and insurance issues, spouse/sibling relationships, and job and schedule conflicts must all be addressed. Referral to social workers, counselors, or support groups may be needed.

Relieve Pain

In one recent study, children with polyarticular arthritis reported having pain an average of 73% of days; a majority reported having mild to moderate pain with 31% reporting severe pain (Schanberg et al, 2003).The pain of JIA is multifactorial—disease severity, functional status, individual pain threshold, family variables, and psychologic adjustment. The aim is to provide as much relief as possible with medication and other therapies to help children tolerate the pain and complete activities of daily living. Opioid administration is not a routine therapy for the chronic pain of JIA. Nonpharmacologic modalities have proved effective in modifying pain perception (see Pain Management, Chapter 44) and activities that aggravate pain. Behavioral and cognitive therapy, such as relaxation techniques, and anxiety reduction may be useful tools in treating arthritis pain in children (Schanberg et al, 1997; 2003).

Promote General Health

The general health of the child must be considered. A well-balanced diet with sufficient calories to maintain growth is essential. If the child is relatively inactive, caloric intake needs to match energy needs to avoid excessive weight gain, which places additional stress on affected joints. Sleep and rest are essential for children with JIA. Children with JIA report frequent disrupted nighttime sleep, daytime sleepiness, fatigue, anxiety, and altered mood (Labyak, Bourguignon, & Docherty, 2003). Some children will require rest during the day; however, daytime napping that interferes with nighttime sleepiness should be avoided. A bedtime routine that involves comfort measures can help induce sleep. A firm mattress, heated water bed, electric blanket, or sleeping bag help provide warmth, comfort, and rest. Children with joint contractures may wear nighttime splints and this might initially be a source of bedtime conflict. The family needs instruction on how to use the splint appropriately so that it does not cause pain or impede sleep. Behavior modification programs that reward splint and exercise compliance may be helpful in reducing compliance barriers. Well-child care to assess growth and development as well as immunization requirements needs to be coordinated between the primary care provider and the rheumatologist. Common childhood illnesses such as upper respiratory infections may cause arthritis to worsen; consequently, medical attention must be sought quickly for relatively minor illness to prevent flares. Effective communication between the family, the primary care provider, and the rheumatology team is essential for care coordination.

Children are encouraged to attend school, even on days when there may be some pain or discomfort. The aid of the school nurse is enlisted so that a child is permitted to take the prescribed medication at school and to arrange for rest in the nurse's office during the day. Split days or half days may help a child remain involved in school. Permitting the child to come to school late allows time to gain joint movement and reduces the time at school to avoid exhaustion. It is important that the child attend school to learn skills and engage in social interaction, especially if the JIA continues to limit physical skills. Arranging for two sets of textbooks eliminates the need to carry heavy or numerous books to and from school, thus reducing discomfort and difficulty ambulating. A formal school hearing may be necessary to obtain an individualized education plan, ensured by public law, which includes intensive school modifications.

Facilitate Compliance

The child and family are involved in the therapeutic plan. They need to know the purpose and correct use of any splints and appliances and the medication regimen. The family is instructed regarding administration of medications, as well as the value of a regular schedule of administration to maintain a satisfactory drug level in the body. They need to know that NSAIDs should not be given on an empty stomach and to be alert for signs of medication toxicity. If evidence of drug toxicity is noted, the family is instructed to notify the health professional and follow that person's instructions.

Encourage Heat and Exercise

Heat has been shown to be beneficial to children with arthritis. Moist heat is best for relieving pain and stiffness, and the most efficient and practical method is in the bathtub with warm water. Sometimes a daily whirlpool bath, paraffin bath, or hot packs may be used as needed for temporary relief of acute swelling and pain. Hot packs are easily applied using a bath towel wrung out after being immersed in hot water or heated in a microwave oven; covered with plastic, it is applied to the area for 20 minutes. Commercial pads that warm in only a few minutes in the microwave are also available. Painful hands or feet can be immersed in a pan of warm water for 10 minutes two or three times daily in addition to tub baths.

Pool therapy is the easiest method for exercising a large number of joints. Swimming activities strengthen muscles and maintain mobility in larger joints. Very small children who are frightened of the water can carry out their exercises in the bathtub. Small children love to splash, kick, and throw things in the water. A weekly aquatic program of 1 hour per week for 20 sessions was perceived as being beneficial to children with JIA even though results were not statistically significant (Takken et al, 2003). Activities of daily living provide satisfactory exercise for older children to maintain maximum mobility with minimum pain. These children are encouraged in their efforts to be independent and patiently allowed to dress and groom themselves, to assume daily tasks, and to care for their belongings. It is often difficult for children to manipulate buttons, to comb or brush hair, and to operate faucets; but unless there is an acute flare-up, parents and other caregivers should not offer assistance. In addition, children should learn and understand why others do not help them. A child's natural affinity for play offers many opportunities for incorporating therapeutic exercises. Throwing or kicking a ball and riding a tricycle (with the seat raised to achieve maximum leg extension) are excellent moving and stretching exercises for a very young child whose daily living activities are physically limited.

NURSE ALERT Another method of supplying warmth before the child arises is to plug an electric blanket into an appliance timer. Set the blanket to medium or high and adjust the timer to turn on the blanket 1 hour before the child awakens (McIlvain-Simpson & Singsen, 1997). ■

An effective approach to beginning the day's activities is to awaken children early to give them their medication and then to allow them to sleep for an hour. On arising, children take a hot bath (or shower) and perform a simple ritual of limbering-up exercises, after which they commence the activities of the day, such as going to school. Exercise, heat, and rest are spaced throughout the remainder of the day according to the child's individual needs and schedules. Parents are instructed in exercises that meet the needs of the child.

The Arthritis Foundation* and its council, the American Juvenile Arthritis Organization, provide services for both parents and professionals, and nurses should refer families to this agency as an added resource.

Support Child and Family

JIA affects every aspect of life for the child and family. Physical limitations may interfere with self-care, school participation, and recreational activities. The intensive treatment plan, including multiple medications, physical therapy, comfort measures, and medical appointments, is intrusive and very disruptive to the parents' work schedule and the family's routine. To prevent isolation and encourage independence, the family is encouraged to pursue their normal activities. Unfortunately, the adaptations necessary to make that happen take resourcefulness and commitment from all family members. At diagnosis and throughout the span of JIA, it is essential to recognize signs of stress and counterproductive coping and provide the necessary support to maximize adaptation. The problems and needs of the family with a chronic illness like JIA are discussed in Chapter 41, and the reader is directed to that chapter for guidance in planning care.

Evaluation

The effectiveness of nursing interventions is determined by continual reassessment and evaluation of care based on the following observational guidelines:

1. Observe child's behavior and use pain assessment techniques.
2. Conduct routine assessment of child's general health.
3. Observe child during planned and unplanned activities, assess mobility of joints, and observe the use of prescribed appliances.
4. Observe child's ability to perform activities of daily living.
5. Observe and interview child and family regarding feelings and concerns.

Expected outcomes include the following:

1. Child is able to complete activities of daily living with minimum or no discomfort.
2. Child attains and maintains optimal health status (specify).
3. Child engages in activities suitable to interests, capabilities, and developmental level; joints are mobile, flexible, and free of deformity.
4. Child is involved in self-care activities to maximum capabilities.
5. Child and family demonstrate an understanding of the child's disease and therapies; they verbalize their feelings and concerns.

*PO Box 7669, Atlanta, GA 30357-0669; phone: 800-283-7800; Web site: www.arthritis.org. In Canada, **The Arthritis Society** may be accessed for location of all local Canadian province offices; Web site: www.arthritis.ca. Another resource is the **American College of Rheumatology;** Web site: www.rheumatology.org.

Systemic Lupus Erythematosus (SLE)

Systemic lupus erythematosus (SLE) is a chronic, multisystem, autoimmune disease of the connective tissues and blood vessels characterized by inflammation in potentially any body tissue. Its course and symptoms are variable and unpredictable, with mild to life-threatening complications. SLE in children tends to be more severe at onset and has a more aggressive clinical course than adult-onset disease. In addition to SLE, there are other forms of lupus, such as neonatal lupus, which occurs when maternal autoantibodies cross the placenta and cause transient lupus-like symptoms in the newborn with the potential serious complication of heart block. The remaining discussion focuses on SLE.

The estimated minimum incidence of SLE is 0.28 per 100,000 children younger than 16 years of age (Malleson, Fung, & Rosenberg, 1996). SLE is more common in girls, with an approximate 5:1 female-to-male ratio, and typically occurs between the ages of 10 and 19 years. There is a familial tendency, although many newly diagnosed patients are unaware of other affected family members. SLE has been reported in all cultures, but within the United States there has been a disproportionately higher report in African-American, Asian, and Hispanic children.

The cause of SLE is unknown. Potential triggers include hormonal imbalance, immune abnormalities, and environmental exposures, including drugs, infection, sun exposure, stress, and chemical agents.

Clinical Manifestations and Diagnostic Evaluation

The child with SLE may have any clinical manifestation (Box 54-11) with mild to life-threatening severity. The diagnosis is established when 4 of the 11 diagnostic criteria are met (Box 54-12). Renal involvement is common in children and adolescents with SLE; approximately 40% to 50% will develop diffuse profilerative glomerulonephritis (Klein-Gitelman, Reiff, & Silverman, 2002).

Therapeutic Management

The goal of treatment is to ensure the health of the child by balancing the medications necessary to avoid exacerbation and complications while preventing or minimizing treatment-associated morbidity. Therapy involves the use of specific medications and general supportive care. The drugs

BOX 54-11

Clinical Manifestations of Systemic Lupus Erythematosus Related to Tissues Involved

Cutaneous lesions include the classic photosensitive erythematous malar butterfly rash extending across the nose and cheeks and sparing the nasolabial folds. Other skin findings include maculopapular rashes on any surface, discoid lesions, periungual erythema, livedo reticularis, infarcts, and alopecia.

Musculoskeletal findings include arthritis, arthralgia, myositis, and myalgia.

Central nervous system symptoms vary from headache, memory loss, and depression to seizures, psychosis, and paralysis.

Heart and lung findings may include pericarditis, myocarditis, myocardial infarction, and valvulitis. Pleural effusions, pleuritis, and pneumonitis are possible pulmonary complications.

Renal involvement, glomerulonephritis, is a serious and common complication in childhood systemic lupus erythematosus.

Lymphatic tissue involvement may include splenomegaly and generalized lymphadenopathy.

Blood abnormalities may include anemia, leukopenia, and thrombocytopenia.

Gastrointestinal symptoms include abdominal pain, nausea, vomiting, elevated lipase and amylase, and hepatomegaly.

Constitutional symptoms include weight loss, overwhelming fatigue, and low-grade fever.

used to control inflammation are corticosteroids administered in doses sufficient to control inflammation, then tapered to the lowest suppressive dose. Many (77%) children with SLE require moderate-to-high dose corticosteroid therapy, which will affect growth and development in the affected child. Other drugs include antimalarial preparations (hydroxychloroquine), which are useful for rash and arthritis; NSAIDs, which relieve muscle and joint inflammation; and immunosuppressive agents, such as cyclophosphamide or azathioprine, for renal and central nervous system involvement. General supportive care includes sufficient nutrition, sleep and rest, and exercise. Exposure to the sun and ultraviolet B (UVB) light is limited because of its association with SLE exacerbation.

Nursing Care Management

The principal nursing goal is to help the child and family positively adjust to the disease and therapy. High-dose corticosteroids may cause growth retardation and infection; therefore, plans for interventions to meet the child's growth needs should be implemented; the child's family is educated regarding signs and symptoms of opportunistic infections as well as the regular administration of childhood immunizations. Referral to a social worker, psychologist, or support group may help the child and family make a successful adjustment. Support groups include the Lupus Foundation of America, Inc.,* and the Arthritis Foundation (p. 1837).

*2000 L Street, NW, Suite 710, Washington, DC 20036; phone: 202-349-1155 or 800-558-0121; Web site: www.lupus.org.

BOX 54-12

Classification Criteria of Systemic Lupus Erythematosus

(Requires four criteria for classification.)

1. Malar rash: fixed malar erythema
2. Discoid rash: patchy erythematous lesions
3. Photosensitivity: rash with sun exposure
4. Oral ulcers: painless ulcers in mouth/nose
5. Arthritis: swelling, tenderness or effusion in two or more peripheral joints (nonerosive)
6. Serositis: pleuritis/pericarditis
7. Renal disorder: proteinuria/casts
8. Neurologic disorder: psychosis/seizures
9. Hematologic disorder: hemolytic anemia, thrombocytopenia, leukopenia, lymphopenia
10. Immunologic disorder; anti-dsDNA, anti-SM, antiphospholipid antibodies, lupus anticoagulant, false-positive syphilis test (RPR)
11. Antinuclear antibody

Key issues include therapy compliance; body-image problems associated with rash, hair loss, and steroid therapy; school attendance; vocational activities; social relationships; sexual activity; and pregnancy.* (See Chapter 41 for a discussion on adjusting to a chronic illness.) Specific instructions for avoiding exposure to the sun and UVB light, such as sunscreens, sun-resistant clothing, and altering outdoor activities, must be provided with great sensitivity to ensure compliance while minimizing the associated feeling of being different from peers (see Sunburn, Chapter 53). Patients need to be instructed to maintain regular medical supervision and seek attention quickly during illness or before elective surgical procedures, such as dental extraction, because of potential needs for increased steroids or prophylactic antibiotics. People with SLE should carry medical identification for their disease and steroid dependence.

Key Points

- Immobility has a profound effect on all aspects of growth and development.
- The major physical consequences of immobilization are loss of muscle strength, endurance, and muscle mass; bone demineralization; loss of joint mobility; and contractures.
- Features of children's fractures not observed in the adult include presence of growth plate, thicker and stronger periosteum, bone porosity, more rapid healing, and less joint stiffness.
- The goals of fracture management are to regain alignment and length of bony fragments, retain alignment and length, and restore function to injured parts.
- The method of fracture reduction is determined by the age of the child, degree of displacement, amount of overriding, amount of edema, condition of the skin and soft tissues, sensation, and circulation distal to the fracture.

*A recommended booklet available from the Arthritis Foundation is *Meeting the Challenge: A Young Person's Guide to Living with Lupus.*

- The primary purposes of traction are to fatigue involved muscles and reduce muscle spasm, position bone ends in desired realignment, and immobilize the fracture site until realignment has been achieved to permit casting or splinting.
- The etiology of developmental dysplasia of the hip appears to be related to intrauterine, genetic, and cultural factors.
- Treatment of clubfoot consists of manipulation and casting to correct the deformity, maintenance of the correction, and prevention of possible recurrence of the deformity.
- Acquired hip deformities are managed with non–weight-bearing devices (Legg-Calvé-Perthes disease) or surgical stabilization (slipped femoral capital epiphysis).
- Observation for scoliosis is an important part of a routine physical assessment.
- Scoliosis is managed by bracing and exercise or surgical correction.
- Bone infections are managed with vigorous antibiotic therapy, immobilization of the affected part, and (sometimes) surgical drainage.
- Osteosarcoma is a neoplasm of bone-forming tissues; Ewing sarcoma is a neoplasm that arises from bone marrow spaces.
- Rhabdomyosarcoma may occur almost anywhere in the body, but the most common sites are the head and neck.
- Nursing care of the child with juvenile arthritis consists of promoting general health, relieving discomfort, preventing deformity, and preserving function.
- Systemic lupus erythematosus is a chronic autoimmune disorder that affects the collagen tissues of the body.

References

Akins LM: Cast changes: synthetic versus plaster, *Pediatr Nurs* 23(4): 422-426,1997.

American Academy of Pediatrics, Committee on Quality Improvement and Subcommittee on Developmental Dysplasia of the Hip: Clinical practice guideline: early detection of developmental dysplasia of the hip, *Pediatrics* 105(4):896-905, 2000.

Berde CB, Billett AL, Collins JJ: Symptom management in supportive care. In Pizzo PA, Poplack DG (eds): *Principles and practice of pediatric oncology*, ed 4, Philadelphia, 2002, JB Lippincott.

Brewer EJ et al: Current proposed revision of JRA criteria, *Arthritis Rheum* 29(suppl 2):195-199, 1997.

Cryer B, Feldman M: Cyclooxygenase-1 and cyclooxygenase-2 selectivity of widely used nonsteroidal anti-inflammatory drugs, *Am J Med* 104: 413-421, 1998.

Curley MA et al: Predicting pressure ulcer risk in pediatric patients: the Braden Q Scale, *Nurs Research* 52(1):22-33, 2003.

Do T, Herrera-Soto J: Elbow injuries in children, *Curr Opin Pediatr* 15(1):68-73, 2003.

Dzierzbicka K et al: Synthesis and cytotoxic activity of conjugates of muramyl and normuramyl dipeptides with batracylin derivatives, *J Med Chem* 46(6):978-986, 2003.

Fabry K, Fabry G, Moens P: Legg-Calvé-Perthes disease in patients under 5 years of age does not always result in a good outcome; personal experience and meta-analysis of the literature, *J Pediatr Orthop B* 12(3): 222-227, 2003.

Falk MJ et al: Intravenous biphosphonate therapy in children with osteogenesis imperfecta, *Pediatrics* 111(3):573-578, 2003.

Faulks S, Luther B: Changing paradigm for the treatment of clubfeet, *Orthop Nurs* 24(1):25-30, 2005.

Frank RG et al: Disease and family contributors to adaptation in juvenile rheumatoid arthritis and juvenile diabetes, *Arthritis Care Res* 11(3): 166-176, 1998.

Gilmore A, Thompson GH: Common childhood foot deformities, *Consult Pediatricians* 2(2):63-71, 2003.

Ginsberg JP et al: Ewing's sarcoma family of tumors: Ewing's sarcoma of bone and soft tissue and the peripheral primitive neuroectodermal tumors. In Pizzo PA, Poplack DG (eds): *Principles and practice of pediatric oncology*, ed 4, Philadelphia, 2002, JB Lippincott.

Greene WB (ed): *Essentials of musculoskeletal care*, ed 2, Rosemont, IL, 2001, American Academy of Orthopaedic Surgeons.

Grier H: The Ewing family of tumors: Ewing's tumors, *Pediatr Clin North Am* 44(4):991-1004, 1997.

Gugenheim JJ Jr.: The Ilizarov fixator for pediatric and adolescent supracondylar fracture variants, *J Pediatr Orthop* 20(2):177-182, 2000.

Holmes SB et al: Skeletal pin site care: National Association of Orthopaedic Nurses guidelines for orthopaedic nurses, *Orthop Nurs* 24(2): 99-107, 2005.

Horwitz EM et al: Clinical responses to bone marrow transplantation in children with severe osteogenesis imperfecta, *Blood* 97(5):1227-1331, 2001.

Karwowska A et al: Epidemiology and outcomes of osteomyelitis in the era of sequential intravenous-oral therapy, *Pediatr Infect Dis J* 17:1021-1026, 1998.

Klein-Gitelman M, Reiff A, Silverman ED: Systemic lupus erythematosus in childhood, *Rheum Dis Clin North Am* 28(3):561-577, 2002.

Kline NE, Sevier N: Solid tumors in children, *J Pediatr Nurs* 18(2):96-102, 2003.

Labyak SR, Bourguignon C, Docherty S: Sleep quality in children with juvenile rheumatoid arthritis, *Holistic Nurs Prac* 17(4):193-200, 2003.

Lampe RM: Osteomyelitis and suppurative arthritis. In Behrman RE, Kliegman RM, Jenson HB (eds): *Nelson textbook of pediatrics*, ed 17, Philadelphia, 2004, WB Saunders.

Link M, Gebhardt MC, Meyers PA: Osteosarcoma. In Pizzo PA, Poplack DG (eds): *Principles and practice of pediatric oncology*, ed 4, Philadelphia, 2002, JB Lippincott.

Loder RT: Slipped capital femoral epiphysis, *Am Fam Physician* 59(9): 2135-2142, 1998.

Lovell DJ et al: Long-term efficacy and safety of etanercept in children with polyarticular-course juvenile rheumatoid arthritis: interim results from an ongoing multicenter, open-label, extended-treatment trial, *Arthritis Rheum* 48(1):218-226, 2003.

Maher AB, Salmond SW, Pellino TA: *Orthopaedic nursing*, ed 3, Philadelphia, 2002, WB Saunders.

Malleson P, Fung M, Rosenberg A: The incidence of pediatric rheumatic diseases: results from the Canadian Ped Rheumatology Association Disease Registry, *J Rheumatol* 23(11):1981-1987, 1996.

Marini JC: Osteogenesis imperfecta. In Behrman RE, Kliegman RM, Jenson HB (eds): *Nelson textbook of pediatrics*, ed 17, Philadelphia, 2004, WB Saunders.

McIlvain-Simpson G, Singsen B: Decreasing morning stiffness, *Small Talk* 3(6):8, 1997.

Meyers PA, Gorlick R: Osteosarcoma, *Pediatr Clin North Am* 44(4):973-989, 1997.

Miller ML, Cassidy JT: Juvenile rheumatoid arthritis, In Behrman RE, Kliegman RM, Jenson HB (eds): *Nelson textbook of pediatrics*, ed 17, Philadelphia, 2004, WB Saunders.

Newton PO, Wenger DR: Idiopathic and congenital scoliosis. In Morrissy RT, Weinstein SL (eds): *Lovell and Winter's pediatric orthopaedics*, Philadelphia, 2001, Williams & Wilkins.

Noonan KJ et al: Long term psychosocial characteristics of patients treated for idiopathic scoliosis, *J Pediatr Orthop* 17:712-717, 1997.

Olsson GL: Neuropathic pain in children. In McGrath PJ, Finley GA (eds): *Chronic and recurrent pain in children and adolescents*, Seattle, 1999, IASP Press.

Padeh S, Passwell P: Intraarticular corticosteroid injection in the management of children with chronic arthritis, *Arthritis Rheum* 41(7): 1210-1214, 1998.

Pearson M: Historical perspective of the treatment of osteosarcoma: an interview with Dr. Norman Jaffe, *J Pediatr Oncol Nurs* 15(2):90-94, 1998.

Petty RE et al: Revision of the proposed classification criteria for juvenile idiopathic arthritis: Durban, 1997, *J Rheumatol* 25(10):1991-1994, 1998.

Petty RE et al: International League of Associations for Rheumatology classification of juvenile idiopathic arthritis: second revision, Edmonton, 2001, *J Rheumatol* 31(2):390-392, 2004.

Rednek A: Malignant bone tumors. In Lanzkowsky P (ed): *Pediatric hematology and oncology*, ed 3, New York, 2000, Academic Press.

Roberts CS et al: Review article: diagnostic ultrasonography: applications in orthopaedic surgery, *Clin Orthop Rel Res* 401:248-264, 2002.

Roy D: Current concepts in Legg-Calvé-Perthes disease, *Pediatr Ann* 28(12):748-751, 1999.

Samaniego IA: A sore spot in pediatrics: risk factors for pressure ulcers, *Pediatr Nurs* 29(4):278-283,2003.

Schanberg LE et al: Pain coping and the pain experience in children with juvenile chronic arthritis, *Pain* 73(2):181-189, 1997.

Schanberg LE et al: Daily pain and symptoms in children with polyarticular arthritis, *Arthritis Rheum* 48(5):1390-1397, 2003.

Shamberger RC, Jaksic T, Ziegler MM: General principles of surgery. In Pizzo PA, Poplack DG (eds): *Principles and practice of pediatric oncology*, ed 4, Philadelphia, 2002, JB Lippincott.

Slote RJ: Psychological effects of caring for the adolescent undergoing spinal fusion for scoliosis, *Orthop Nurs* 21(6):19-28, 2002.

Takken T et al: Aquatic fitness training for children with juvenile idiopathic arthritis, *Rheumatology* (Oxford) 42(11):1408-1414, 2003.

Thompson GH: The hip. In Behrman RE, Kliegman RM, Jenson HB (eds): *Nelson textbook of pediatrics*, ed 17, Philadelphia, 2004a, WB Saunders.

Thompson GH: The foot and toes. In Behrman RE, Kliegman RM, Jenson HB (eds): *Nelson textbook of pediatrics*, ed 17, Philadelphia, 2004b, WB Saunders.

Thompson GH: The spine. In Behrman RE, Kliegman RM, Jenson HB (eds): *Nelson textbook of pediatrics*, ed 17, Philadelphia, 2004c, WB Saunders.

Wall EJ: Practical primary pediatric orthopaedics, *Nurs Clin North Am* 35(1):95-113, 2000.

Wexler LH, Helman LJ: Rhabdomyosarcoma and the undifferentiated sarcoma. In Pizzo PA, Poplack DG (eds): *Principles and practice of pediatric oncology*, ed 3, Philadelphia, 1997, JB Lippincott.

Witt C: Detecting developmental dysplasia of the hip, *Adv Neonatal Care* 13(2):65-75, 2003.

Zeitlin L, Fassier F, Glorieux FH: Modern approach to children with osteogenesis imperfecta, *J Pediatr Orthop B* 12(2):77-87, 2003.

Neuromuscular or Muscular Dysfunction

55

LEARNING OBJECTIVES

On completion of this chapter the reader will be able to:

- Discuss the nursing role in helping parents cope with a child with cerebral palsy.
- Formulate a nursing care plan for the preoperative and postoperative care of a child with myelomeningocele.
- Outline a plan of care for a child with Duchenne muscular dystrophy.
- Discuss the prevention and treatment of tetanus.
- Identify the causes of botulism in infants and children.
- List three causes of spinal cord injury in children.

ELECTRONIC RESOURCES

Additional information related to the content in Chapter 55 can be found on

the companion website at evolve
http://evolve.elsevier.com/Wong/maternal/
- NCLEX Review Questions
- WebLinks

or the interactive student CD-ROM
Activities for Chapter 55 include the following:
- NCLEX Review Questions
- Critical Thinking Exercise–Guillain-Barré Syndrome
- Nursing Care Plan–The Child with Cerebral Palsy

CONGENITAL NEUROMUSCULAR OR MUSCULAR DISORDERS

Cerebral Palsy

Cerebral palsy (CP) is a nonspecific term applied to disorders characterized by early onset of impaired movement and posture. It is nonprogressive and may be accompanied by perceptual problems, language deficits, and intellectual impairment. The etiology, clinical features, and course are variable and are characterized by abnormal muscle tone and coordination as the primary disturbances. CP is the most common permanent physical disability of childhood, and the incidence is reported to be between 1.5 and 3 in every 1000 live births in the United States (Dabney, Lipton, & Miller, 1997; Winter et al, 2002). In population-based surveys the incidence of CP has risen slightly in term infants (Winter et al, 2002).

A variety of prenatal, perinatal, and postnatal factors contribute to the etiology of CP singly or multifactorially. Although the prevalent hypothesis has been that CP results from perinatal problems, especially birth asphyxia, it is now believed that CP results more often from existing *prenatal* brain abnormalities; however, the exact cause of these abnormalities remains elusive. Intrauterine exposure to maternal infection is associated with an increased risk of CP in infants of normal birth weight and preterm infants (Gibson et al, 2003; Volpe, 2001); however, not all term infants exposed to chorioamnionitis develop CP (Grether et al, 2003). The prevalence of CP in infants born before 36 weeks of gestation and weighing less than 2000 g has been reported to be 12%; the strongest independent risk factor for development of CP was periventricular leukomalacia (Han et al, 2002). Preterm birth of extremely-low-birth-weight and very-low-birth-weight infants continues to be the single most important risk factor for CP, yet, in many cases, no identifiable cause is determined. Kernicterus, caused by high levels of unbound bilirubin in the neonatal period in full-term infants, has also been implicated as a causative factor of CP (Centers for Disease Control and Prevention [CDC], 2001a). Damage occurring as a result of shaken baby syndrome may also result in CP in survivors (Smith, 2003).

Pathophysiology

It is difficult to establish a precise location of neurologic lesions based on etiology or clinical signs because no characteristic pathologic pattern exists. Some patients have gross malformations of the brain; others may have evidence of vascular occlusion, atrophy, loss of neurons, and degeneration. *Anoxia* plays the most significant role in the pathologic state of brain damage, which is often secondary to other causative mechanisms. A few exceptions occur and are related to anatomic areas such as spastic diplegia (associated with prematurity), caused by hypoxic infarction or hemorrhage in the area adjacent to the lateral ventricles. Ataxic CP may occur in relation to cerebral hypoplasia and, in some cases, severe hypoglycemia (Volpe, 2001). The American College of Obstetricians and Gynecologists, in conjunction with the American Academy of Pediatrics, has recently published a report in which neonatal encephalopathy is defined (American Academy of Pediatrics & American College of Obstetricians and Gynecologists, 2003). The report affirms that approximately 70% of cases of neonatal encephalopathy occur as a result of events occurring *before* the onset of labor; criteria are established to define events sufficiently capable of causing intrapartum asphyxia and CP. Evidence indicates that events that cause the majority of CP cases occur not as a result of intrapartum asphyxia, but other causes that have been discussed previously (American Academy of Pediatrics & American College of Obstetricians and Gynecologists, 2003).

CP has been classified in several ways, but the most useful classification is based on the nature and distribution of neuromuscular dysfunction (Box 55-1).

Diagnostic Evaluation

The neurologic examination and history are the primary modalities for diagnosis of CP. A thorough knowledge of normal variations of motor development is required for detecting abnormal progress, and a careful history is elicited to detect possible etiologic factors. Early recognition is made more difficult by the lack of reliable neonatal neurologic signs; however, infants with known etiologic risk factors should be followed and evaluated closely in the first several months of life. The alert observer may be suspicious when a child demonstrates some of the manifestations outlined in Box 55-2. The child's spontaneous movements (particularly gait analysis in ambulatory children) and behavior are observed, including posture; attitude; and muscle size, function, and tone. The persistence of primitive reflexes may be of value, and two of these aid in the diagnosis: the asymmetric tonic neck reflex, or persistent Moro reflex (beyond 4 months of age), and the crossed extensor reflex (Nehring & Steele, 1996). Magnetic resonance imaging (MRI) is useful in identifying the location and extent of structural lesions and any associated pathology or anomaly; an MRI of the spine is also helpful in excluding spinal cord pathology (Johnston, 2004). Supplemental diagnostic tests may be employed, such as hearing and vision function, electroencephalography, and a genetic evaluation.

Therapeutic Management

The goals of therapy for children with CP are early recognition and promotion of optimum development to enable affected children to attain normalization and their potential

BOX 55-1

Clinical Classification of Cerebral Palsy

Spastic—May involve one or both sides
- Hypertonicity with poor control of posture, balance, and coordinated motion
- Impairment of fine and gross motor skills
- Active attempts at motion increase abnormal postures and overflow of movement to other parts of the body

Dyskinetic/athetoid—Abnormal involuntary movement
- Athetosis, characterized by slow, wormlike, writhing movements that usually involve the extremities, trunk, neck, facial muscles, and tongue
- Involvement of the pharyngeal, laryngeal, and oral muscles causes drooling and dysarthria (imperfect speech articulation)
- Involuntary movements may take on choreoid (involuntary, irregular, jerking movements) and dystonic (disordered muscle tone) manifestations that increase in intensity with emotional stress and around adolescence

Ataxic
- Wide-based gait
- Rapid, repetitive movements performed poorly
- Disintegration of movements of the upper extremities when the child reaches for objects

Mixed type/dystonic—Combination of spasticity and athetosis

BOX 55-2

Clinical Signs and Symptoms of Cerebral Palsy

Spastic Type
- Increased muscle tone
- Increased deep tendon reflexes and clonus (sudden dorsiflexion of the ankle or rapid distal movement of the patella results in alternating spasm and relaxation of the muscles being stretched)
- Flexor, adductor, and internal rotator muscles more involved than extensor, abductor, and external rotator muscles
- Difficulty with fine and gross motor skills
- Most common contracture is that of the heel cord
- Hip adductor contractures lead to progressive subluxation and dislocation
- Knee contractures
- Scoliosis common
- Typical gait is crouched, intoeing, scissoring
- Elbow, wrist, and fingers in flexed position with thumb adducted
- Motor weakness of antagonist muscle groups

Athetoid Type
- Purposeless, involuntary, uncontrollable movements of face and extremities
- Increased movements with stress and voluntary movements, absent during sleep
- Contractures rare
- Normal deep tendon reflexes

Ataxic Type
- Disturbed coordination
- Lack of equilibrium
- Unsteady gait
- Few orthopedic problems
- Hyporeflexia
- Loss of ability to gauge distance, speed, power of movement
- Muscles hypotonic
- Speech slurred, jerky, explosive
- Nystagmus common

Other Manifestations
- Visual deficits (most common in spastic type)
- Hearing impairment (most common in athetoid type)
- Oral motor involvement resulting in drooling and feeding problems
- Developmental delay (40% to 60%; most common in atonic and rigid types and spastic quadriparesis)
- Sensory impairment
- Seizures (approximately 40% of those with spastic hemiplegia affected)

From Maher AB, Salmond SW, Pellino TA: *Orthopaedic nursing,* ed 3, Philadelphia, 2002, WB Saunders.

within the limits of their existing health problems. The disorder is permanent, and therapy is primarily preventive and symptomatic.

The broad aims of therapy are (1) to establish locomotion, communication, and self-help; (2) to gain optimum appearance and integration of motor functions; (3) to correct associated defects as effectively as possible; (4) to provide educational opportunities adapted to the individual child's needs and capabilities; and (5) to promote socialization experiences with other affected and unaffected children. Each child is evaluated and managed on an individual basis. The plan of therapy may involve a variety of settings, facilities, and specially trained persons, including the parents.

Ankle-foot orthoses (AFOs; braces) are worn by many of these children and are used to help prevent or reduce deformity, increase the energy efficiency of gait, and control alignment. Other mobilization devices include wheeled scooter boards that allow children to propel themselves while on the abdomen, wheeled go-carts that provide sitting balance and serve as early "wheelchair" experience for young children, and special devices that leave the upper extremities free (Figs. 55-1 and 55-2).

Orthopedic surgery may be required to correct contracture or spastic deformities, to provide stability for an uncontrollable joint, and to provide balanced muscle power. This includes tendon-lengthening procedures (especially heel cord lengthening), release of spastic wrist flexor muscles, and correction of hip and adductor muscle spasticity or contracture to improve locomotion. A neurosurgical intervention, *selective dorsal rhizotomy,* is used selectively in some children with CP. The procedure involves selectively cutting dorsal column sensory rootlets that have an abnormal response to electrical stimulation. Achieving the benefits from the surgery requires intensive physical therapy and family commitment. Because the procedure results in flaccid muscles, the child must be retaught to sit, stand, and walk.

Surgical intervention is usually reserved for the child who does not respond to the more conservative measures, but it is also indicated for the child whose spasticity causes progressive deformities. Surgery is primarily used to improve function rather than for cosmetic purposes and is followed by physical therapy.

Intense pain may occur with muscle spasms in patients with CP. Pharmacologic agents given orally (dantrolene sodium, baclofen, and diazepam) have had little effectiveness in improving muscle coordination in children with CP; however, they are effective in decreasing overall spasticity (Jacobs, 2001). The most common side effects of these agents include hepatotoxicity (dantrolene [Dantrium]), drowsiness, fatigue, and muscle weakness. Less commonly, diaphoresis and constipation may be seen with baclofen (Lioresal). Diazepam (Valium) is used frequently but should be restricted to older children and adolescents. Botulinum toxin (Botox) has become an important drug in the treatment of spasticity for CP (Jacobs, 2001). Botox is injected into the muscle, where it acts to inhibit the release of acetylcholine into a specific muscle group, thereby preventing muscle movement. When administered early in the course of the illness, affected muscle contractures may be prevented, particularly in lower extremities, and surgical procedures with possible adverse effects may be avoided. The goal is to allow stretching of the muscle as it relaxes and permit ambulation with an AFO (Jacobs, 2001). The major reported adverse effect of Botox injection is pain at the injection site (Roscigno, 2002). Currently there is reportedly no strong evidence to support or refute the use of Botulinum toxin A to reduce muscle tone and spasticity and improve function in

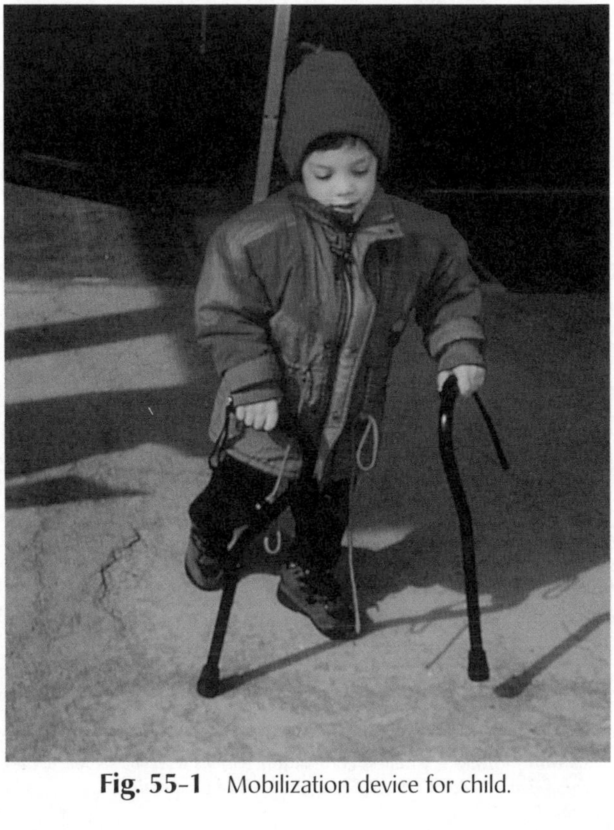

Fig. 55-1 Mobilization device for child.

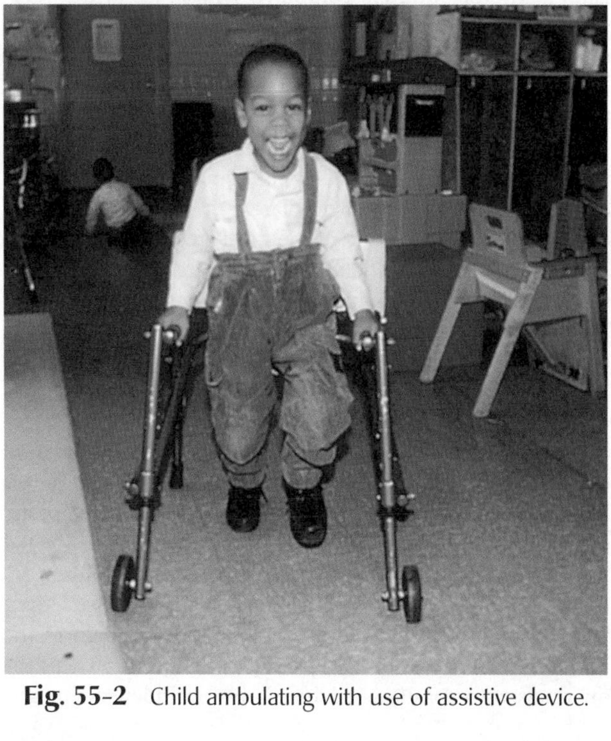

Fig. 55-2 Child ambulating with use of assistive device.

children with CP; individual results varied in the studies reviewed (Wasiak, Hoare, & Wallen, 2004).

The neurosurgical and pharmacologic approach to managing the spasticity associated with CP involves the implantation of a pump to infuse baclofen directly into the intrathecal space surrounding the spinal cord to provide relief of spasticity. Intrathecal baclofen therapy is best suited for children with severe spasticity that interferes with activities of daily living and ambulation (Jacobs, 2001). Patients are screened before pump placement by the infusion of a "test dose" of intrathecal baclofen delivered via a lumbar puncture. Close monitoring for side effects (hypotonia, somnolence, seizures, nausea, vomiting, headache, and catheter- or pump-related problems) (Albright et al, 2003) and relief of spasticity occurs for several hours after the infusion. If a positive effect is noted, the patient is considered a candidate for pump placement. Benefits of intrathecal baclofen include fewer systemic side effects, dosage titration for maximizing effects, and reversibility of therapy with removal of the pump if so desired (Jacobs, 2001).

Antiepileptic drugs (AEDs), such as carbamazepine (Tegretol) and valproic acid (Depakote), are prescribed routinely for children who have seizures. Care of visual and auditory deficits requires the attention of appropriate specialists, and speech therapy involves the services of a speech therapist. Regular visits to the dentist and prophylaxis, including brushing, fluoride, and flossing, should be instituted as soon as the teeth erupt. Dental care is especially important for children being given phenytoin, because they often develop gum hyperplasia.

A wide variety of technical aids are available to improve the functioning of children with CP. These include electromechanical toys that employ the concept of biofeedback and operate from a head unit. The toy is manipulated only when the head and trunk are in correct alignment. Eye-hand coordination can also be enhanced by computerized toys and games. Microcomputers combined with voice synthesizers aid children with speech difficulties to "speak." These and others print messages onto screen monitors and paper. These devices have made it apparent that some children have been erroneously considered to be mentally retarded. The application of this technology makes it possible for persons with CP to function eventually in their own residences and can be extended into the workplace.

Physical therapy is one of the most frequently used conservative treatment modalities. It requires the specialized skills of a qualified therapist with an extensive repertoire of exercise methods who can design a program to stimulate each child to achieve his or her functional goals.

Prognosis

Approximately 30% to 50% of individuals with CP are mentally retarded, and an even higher percentage have mild cognitive and learning deficits (Green, Greenberg, & Hurwitz, 2003); however, many children with severe spastic quadriplegic CP have normal intelligence. Growth is affected in children with spastic quadriplegia, and many children remain below the 5th percentile for age and sex. As children with CP transition to adulthood, about 30% remain in the home and are cared for by a parent or caregiver; 50% of individuals with spastic quadriplegia live in independent settings and function at appropriate social levels considering their disability (Green et al, 2003).

Nursing Care Management

Assessment

Early recognition of CP is often a result of alert observation by the nurse. Although the diagnosis may not be established until later in infancy, the nurse should be especially observant for signs in an infant who has a history that includes any of the prenatal or perinatal conditions that predispose to neonatal encephalopathy. Children who have one or more risk factors for CP should be carefully evaluated and followed from birth to identify abnormal signs of development. In addition, factors in the postnatal period that may contribute to hypoxic events should be monitored and prevented. Delayed attainment of developmental milestones is one of the most valuable clues to recognizing CP; therefore developmental delays in a child offer one of the earliest indications of neurologic impairment (Box 55-3).

Nursing Diagnoses

Based on a thorough assessment, several nursing diagnoses identified for the child with CP are primarily related to self-help and to facilitating mobility (see Nursing Care Plan, p. 1847). Other diagnoses may apply in specific cases.

Plan of Care and Implementation

The goals of nursing care for the child with CP and the child's family are as follows:

1. Child will acquire mobility within personal capabilities.
2. Child will acquire communication skills or use appropriate assistive devices.
3. Child will engage in self-help activities.
4. Child will receive appropriate education.
5. Child will develop a positive self-image.
6. Family members will receive appropriate education and support in their efforts to meet the child's needs.
7. Child will receive appropriate care if hospitalized.

BOX 55-3

Potential Warning Signs of Cerebral Palsy

Physical Signs

Poor head control after 3 months of age
Stiff or rigid arms or legs
Pushing away or arching back
Floppy or limp body posture
Cannot sit up without support by 8 months
Uses only one side of the body, or only the arms to crawl

Behavioral Signs

Extreme irritability or crying
Failure to smile by 3 months
Feeding difficulties
- Persistent gagging or choking when fed
- After 6 months of age, tongue pushes soft food out of the mouth

Data from Pathways Awareness Foundation: *Parents . . . if you see any of these warning signs . . . don't delay,* Chicago, 1991, The Foundation.

Because children are being treated at an earlier age, parents are participating earlier in treatment programs for their disabled child. Parents are taught the proper handling and home care of young children with CP and need a carefully planned program so that their change of role from parent to therapist can be melded into the already-established relationship. Nurses reinforce the plan of care and assist the family in devising and modifying equipment and activities to continue the therapy program in the home (see also Home Care, Chapter 43).

Passive range-of-motion exercises, stretching, and elongation exercises are valuable at any age, even at early ages when the child is unable to cooperate. They are of particular value for postural abnormalities around various joints.

Training in manual skills and activities of daily living proceeds along developmental lines and according to the child's functional level. Sitting, balancing, crawling, and walking are encouraged at appropriate ages, accompanied by stimulation of protective extension and equilibrium reactions. Hand activities are begun early to improve motor function and provide the child with sensory experiences and information about the environment. As the child progresses from simple feeding and self-care activities, training is extended to include other tasks, such as cooking or typing, that are within the child's developmental and functional capabilities.

Incorporating play into the therapeutic program often requires great ingenuity and inventiveness from those involved in the child's care. Objects and toys are chosen to provide needed sensory input, using a variety of shapes, forms, and textures.

The child may need considerable help (and patience) in learning to feed, dress, and care for personal hygiene needs. Children should be fed in the normal eating position. When they have difficulty with sucking and swallowing, it is tempting to hold them in a semireclining posture to make use of gravity flow. This method does not promote active swallowing, however, and the neck hyperextension may even interfere with swallowing. A more flexed sitting position with arms brought forward to decrease the tendency toward back and neck extension is more natural during bottle- or spoon-feeding and encourages active swallowing (Suresh-Babu et al, 1998).

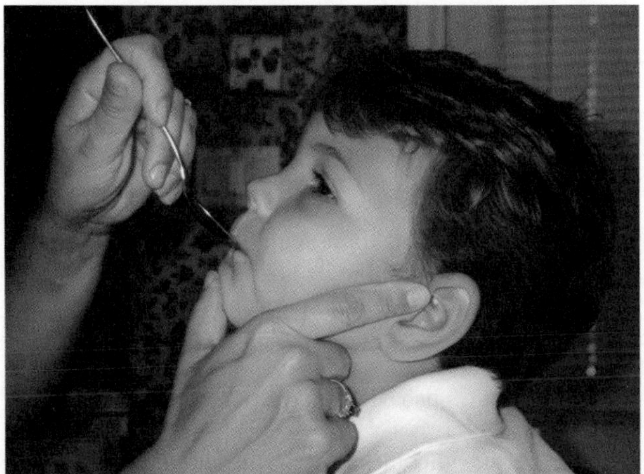

Fig. 55-3 Manual jaw control provided anteriorly.

Because jaw control is compromised, more normal control can be achieved if the feeder provides stability of the oral mechanism from the side or front of the face. When directed from the front, the middle finger of the nonfeeding hand is placed posterior to the body portion of the chin, the thumb is placed below the bottom lip, and the index finger is placed parallel to the child's mandible (Fig. 55-3). Manual jaw control from the side assists with head control, correction of neck and trunk hyperextension, and jaw stabilization. The middle finger of the nonfeeding hand is placed posterior to the bony portion of the chin, the index finger is placed on the chin below the lower lip, and the thumb is placed obliquely across the cheek to provide lateral jaw stability (Fig. 55-4).

Speech training under the supervision of a speech therapist is begun early, before the child learns poor habits of communication. Feeding techniques that force the child to use the lips and tongue in eating help facilitate speech (e.g., placing food at the side of the tongue, first one side and then the other; making the child use the lips to take food from a spoon rather than placing it directly on the tongue; and avoiding using the teeth to remove the food from the utensil). If severe dysarthria prevents articulate speech and the child has reasonable intelligence, nonverbal communication, such as sign language, is taught. Children may also communicate through specially adapted computers with artificial intelligence to augment motor and language function and talking typewriters (Johnston, 2004).

Educational requirements are determined by the child's needs and potential. Children with mild to moderate involvement are generally able to participate in regular classes. Resource rooms are available in most schools to provide more individualized attention to a child's particular needs. Integration of these children into regular classrooms should be the initial goal. For those who are unable to benefit from formal education, a training program may be appropriate.

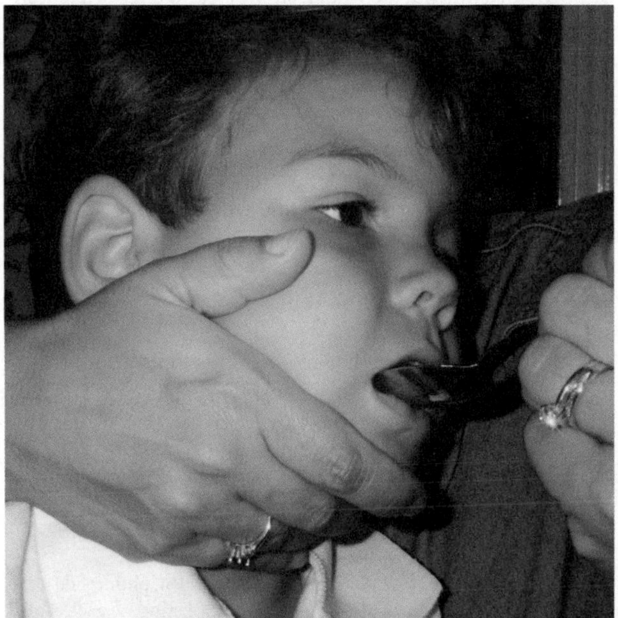

Fig. 55-4 Manual jaw control provided from the side.

At adolescence, prevocational and vocational counseling and guidance are arranged.

Recreational outlets and after-school activities should be considered for the child who is unable to participate in the regular athletic programs and other peer activities. Some children can compete in athletic and artistic endeavors, and many games and pastimes are suited to their capabilities. Competitive sports are also becoming increasingly available to children with disabilities and offer an added dimension to physical activities. Information on training programs and competition on local, state, regional, and national levels can be obtained from the National Disability Sports Alliance.*

Recreational activities serve to stimulate children's interest and curiosity, help them adjust to their disability, improve their functional abilities, and build self-esteem. Any accomplishment that helps children approach a "normal" way of life enhances their self-concept.

Family Support

Probably the nursing interventions most valuable to the family are support and help in coping with the emotional aspects of the disorder, many of which are discussed in relation to the child with a disability (see Chapter 41). Initially, the parents need supportive counseling directed toward understanding the implications of the diagnosis and all of the feelings that it engenders. Later they need clarification regarding what they can expect from the child and from health professionals. Having a child with CP creates numerous challenges of daily management and changes in family life.

The nurse needs to support the parents in their frustration, their problem solving, their concerns, their approaches to helping the child, and their lack of gratification, as well as the positive approaches they use. All of these aspects must be explored and discussed. Parents, as well as other members of the family, require support and counseling. Siblings of a child with a disability are affected and may respond to the presence of the child with overt or less evident behavioral problems. The family needs a relationship with nurses who can provide continued contact, support, and encouragement through the long process of habilitation.

Parents can also find help and solace from parent support groups. They can share problems and concerns with, and derive comfort and practical information from, others. Parent groups are most helpful through sharing experiences and accomplishments. For example, parents can understand from others what it is like to have a child with CP, which is generally not possible from professionals (Family Focus box). The national organization, United Cerebral Palsy Association,† has branches in most communities.

The Hospitalized Child

CP is not a disorder that requires hospitalization; therefore when children with CP are hospitalized, they are usually admitted for another reason or for corrective surgery. Children with CP should be approached and treated the same as any children in the hospital. To facilitate the care and management of children with CP, the therapy program should be continued, insofar as their condition allows, during the time they are hospitalized. This should be incorporated into the nursing care plan, and every effort should be made to ensure that the ground that has been so laboriously gained is not lost. Encouraging the parent to room-in and actively participate in the child's care facilitates a continuation of the home therapy program and helps the child adjust to an unfamiliar environment.

It is equally important to remember that a hospitalization may be the first time a parent can defer care to a nurse and not be the primary caregiver. This respite may be crucial to the parent's well-being.

Family Focus

THE REALITY OF ACCEPTANCE OF CEREBRAL PALSY

Acceptance is rarely achieved in the length of time implied in the literature.

In the first place, what is it? To me, it is the end of comparing my son with every other child I see. I focus on *his* gains, not society's expectations.

It is also being able to laugh periodically *at* his "clumsiness." It is "gallows humor" as he achieves adulthood; jokes about CP can be funny now.

The bitterness is gone; I am now happy for people who have children without CP.

I no longer feel sorry for my son, but rather for the people who cannot see him for the great person he is; the CP does *not* come first.

He is now a young man of 25 years and I am learning to accept his independence.

It is a "never-ending story."

Elaine A. Dunham, RN
Shriner's Hospital
Springfield, MA

Evaluation

The effectiveness of nursing interventions is determined by continual reassessment and evaluation of care based on the following observational guidelines:

1. Observe child's movements and use of mobilization devices.
2. Observe child's speech and ability to use communication devices.
3. Observe child's activities, especially those related to self-care.
4. Interview family regarding child's activities and school attendance.
5. Observe child's interactions with others and choice of activities; interview child regarding feelings and concerns.
6. Interview family members regarding their feelings and concerns and observe family members' interaction with the child.
7. Observe child's behavior and responses during hospitalization.

The expected outcomes are described in the Nursing Care Plan.

*25 West Independence Way, Kingston, RI 02881; phone: 401-792-7130; Web site: www.ndsaonline.org.

†1660 L Street NW, Suite 700, Washington, DC 20036; phone: 800-872-5827; Web site: www.ucpa.org (also provides a listing of each state's United Cerebral Palsy organization).

NURSING CARE PLAN: CHILD WITH CEREBRAL PALSY

Nursing Care Plan

THE CHILD WITH CEREBRAL PALSY

NURSING DIAGNOSIS: Impaired physical mobility related to neuromuscular impairment

EXPECTED OUTCOME

Child acquires locomotion within capabilities (specify).

NURSING INTERVENTIONS/*RATIONALES*

Encourage gross and fine motor activities (e.g., sitting, crawling, walking, grasping, throwing) at appropriate ages *to facilitate optimum motor development.*

Refer to therapeutic modalities (physical therapy) that strengthen muscles, relax increased muscle tone, and improve control and balance *to facilitate optimum motor development.*

Balance rest and activity *to provide optimum energy for motor trials.*

Use aids such as parallel bars, crutches, and orthoses (braces) *to facilitate locomotion.*

Use passive and active range-of-motion and stretching exercises *to facilitate muscle development, prevent flexion contractures, and maintain joint flexibility.*

NURSING DIAGNOSIS: Bathing/hygiene, dressing/grooming, feeding, toileting self-care deficits related to physical disability

EXPECTED OUTCOME

Child engages in self-care activities commensurate with capabilities.

NURSING INTERVENTIONS/*RATIONALES*

Encourage child to assist in self-care activities as age and capabilities permit, discourage parents from doing them for the child *to foster independence and confidence in abilities.*

Modify environment, introduce use of assistive devices and specialized equipment, and devise alternative methods of completing tasks as needed *to facilitate maximum functioning.*

Use therapeutic play and adapted toys *to increase developmental and functional abilities and encourage cooperation of child.*

Emphasize child's abilities, praise effort and accomplishments, and promote and reinforce successful endeavors *to foster a sense of self-esteem and competence.*

Refer to therapeutic modalities (e.g., physical therapy [PT], speech therapy, and occupational therapy [OT]) for strengthening of oral motor muscles, development of swallowing control, and evaluation and work with adaptive devices *to enhance functional ADLs.*

NURSING DIAGNOSIS: Risk for injury related to physical disability, neuromuscular, perceptual and cognitive impairment

EXPECTED OUTCOME

Child will experience no injury.

NURSING INTERVENTIONS/*RATIONALES*

Promote and teach child and family proper use of adaptive and protective devices (e.g., crutches, walkers, braces, helmets, large-handled utensils) *to enhance safety.*

Modify environment as appropriate (e.g., pad furniture; avoid throw rugs, polished floors, deep carpets; put side rails on bed; remove hazards and barriers, clear traffic areas) *to enhance safety.*

Provide adequate rest *to prevent fatigue, which increases injury risk.*

Use feeding techniques and assistive devices (feed in upright position, stroke throat to aid swallowing), which encourage intake and proper swallowing *to minimize choking and aspiration.*

Use restraints in car and when seated *to enhance safety.*

Institute seizure precautions if appropriate and administer seizure medications as ordered *to prevent seizure activity and possible injury.*

NURSING DIAGNOSIS: Impaired verbal communication related to hearing loss, neuromuscular impairment, cognitive impairment

EXPECTED OUTCOME

Child will engage in communication process within limits of impairment.

NURSING INTERVENTIONS/*RATIONALES*

Refer to therapeutic modalities (OT, speech therapy) for strengthening of oral motor muscles, evaluation of oral motor abilities, exercises that promote vocalizations/verbalizations, development of verbal and nonverbal communication modalities *to enhance communication.*

Teach caregivers (family, schoolteachers, therapists, nurses) how to use various verbal and nonverbal communication methods and adaptive communications equipment (e.g., communication boards, sign language, computer aids, voice synthesizers) *to enhance communication with others in environment.*

NURSING DIAGNOSIS: Fatigue related to increased energy expenditure

EXPECTED OUTCOME

Child exhibits signs of adequate rest and optimum nutritional intake.

NURSING INTERVENTIONS/*RATIONALES*

Balance activity with frequent rest periods; monitor for any signs of tiredness *to reduce fatigue.*

Provide high-calorie, high-protein diet *to meet increased energy expenditure needs.*

Monitor weight *to evaluate adequacy of intake.*

Carry out a regular schedule of health promotion and maintenance (regular checkups with physician, dentist; immunizations; avoidance of people with infections) *to enhance general state of health.*

NURSING DIAGNOSIS: Disturbed body image related to perception of disability

EXPECTED OUTCOME

Child demonstrates acceptance of self, physical appearance, and physical and developmental abilities.

NURSING INTERVENTIONS/*RATIONALES*

Relate to child on appropriate cognitive level, conveying an attitude of caring and acceptance, *to encourage positive feelings about self;* serve as role model for others *to foster positive attitudes of acceptance toward child.*

Continued

Nursing Care Plan

THE CHILD WITH CEREBRAL PALSY—cont'd

Encourage child to communicate feelings about the disability (e.g., feelings of differentness, implications of functional limit, difficulty in making friends, views of self) *to facilitate coping.*
Have child identify strengths, assets, and things he or she likes about self *to increase positive feelings about self.*
Support positive coping behaviors.
Introduce child to other children who have similar disabilities, arrange for support groups for child and parents *to increase coping skills.*
Refer child for counseling if needed *to enhance adaptation.*
Encourage use of good grooming and age-appropriate dress *to enhance appearance.*

NURSING DIAGNOSIS: Interrupted family processes related to a child with a lifelong disability

EXPECTED OUTCOME

Family members will exhibit adaptation of usual roles and functions to accommodate special needs of child, and they will exhibit growth-promoting behaviors.

NURSING INTERVENTIONS/*RATIONALES*

Provide opportunity for family to absorb and adjust to diagnosis (e.g., repeat information *to allow time for family to hear and understand;* encourage expression of concerns, fears, and feelings about diagnosis and potential impact *to facilitate adjustment;* identify support systems *to provide resources for coping*).
Assist family to understand expected treatment, rationale, and implications *to provide a sound basis for decision making.*
Explore family reaction to the child; assist them to achieve a realistic view of child's abilities and limitations; encourage family in attempts to promote child growth and development; have family emphasize what child can do; explore ways for family to include child in family activities *to help family increase abilities to cope with and incorporate child into family structure.*
Identify additional resource systems (e.g., relatives, friends, church, health care services, community programs) and strategize with family about making good use of these systems *to develop broad base of support.*
Provide a system of ongoing follow-up and evaluation *to ensure long-term adaptation to challenges presented to family functioning by a child with a chronic disability.*

Spina Bifida (Myelomeningocele)

Abnormalities that are derived from the embryonic neural tube *(neural tube defects [NTDs])* constitute the largest group of congenital anomalies that is consistent with multifactorial inheritance. Normally the spinal cord and cauda equina are encased in a protective sheath of bone and meninges (Fig. 55-5, *A*). Failure of neural tube closure produces defects of varying degrees (Box 55-4). They may involve the entire length of the neural tube or may be restricted to a small area.

In the United States, rates of NTDs have declined from 1.3 per 1000 births (1970) to 0.3 per 1000 births after the introduction of mandatory food fortification with folic acid in 1998 (Honein, 2001). Increased use of prenatal diagnostic techniques and termination of pregnancies have also affected the overall incidence of NTDs. (See also Prevention, p. 1852.) *Myelodysplasia* refers broadly to any malformation of the spinal canal and cord. Midline defects involving failure of the osseous (bony) spine to close are called *spina bifida (SB),* the most common defect of the central nervous system. SB is categorized into two types: spina bifida occulta and spina bifida cystica.

Spina bifida occulta refers to a defect that is not visible externally. It occurs most commonly in the lumbosacral area (L5 and S1) (Fig. 55-5, *B*). SB occulta may not be apparent unless there are associated cutaneous manifestations or neuromuscular disturbances.

Spina bifida cystica refers to a visible defect with an external saclike protrusion. The two major forms of SB cystica are *meningocele,* which encases meninges and spinal fluid but no neural elements (Fig. 55-5, *C*), and *myelomeningocele* (or *meningomyelocele*), which contains meninges, spinal fluid, and nerves (Fig. 55-5, *D*). Meningocele is not associated with neurologic deficit, which occurs in varying, often serious, degrees in myelomeningocele. Clinically the term *spina bifida* is used to refer to myelomeningocele.

Pathophysiology

Most authorities believe that the primary defect in NTDs is a failure of neural tube closure during early development (the first 3 to 5 weeks) of the embryo. However, there is also evidence implicating a multifactorial etiology, including drugs, radiation, maternal malnutrition, chemicals, and possibly a genetic mutation in folate pathways in some cases, which may result in abnormal development (Johnston & Kinsman, 2004). Additional factors predisposing to an increased risk of NTDs include prepregnancy maternal obesity, previous NTD pregnancy, and the use of antiepilectic drugs (AEDs) in pregnancy (Finnell, Gould, & Spiegelstein, 2003; Frey and Hauser, 2003; Watkins et al, 2003). The degree of neurologic dysfunction depends on where the sac protrudes through the vertebrae, the anatomic level of the defect, and the amount of nerve tissue involved (Rintoul et al, 2002). Most myelomeningoceles involve the lumbar or lumbosacral area. Hydrocephalus is a frequently associated anomaly in 80% to 90% of the children.

Diagnostic Evaluation

The diagnosis of SB is made on the basis of clinical manifestations (Box 55-5) and examination of the meningeal sac (Fig. 55-6, *A*). Diagnostic measures used to evaluate the brain and spinal cord include MRI, ultrasound, computed tomography, and myelography.

Laboratory examinations are used primarily to determine causative organisms for the major complications of myelomeningocele—meningitis and urinary tract infections.

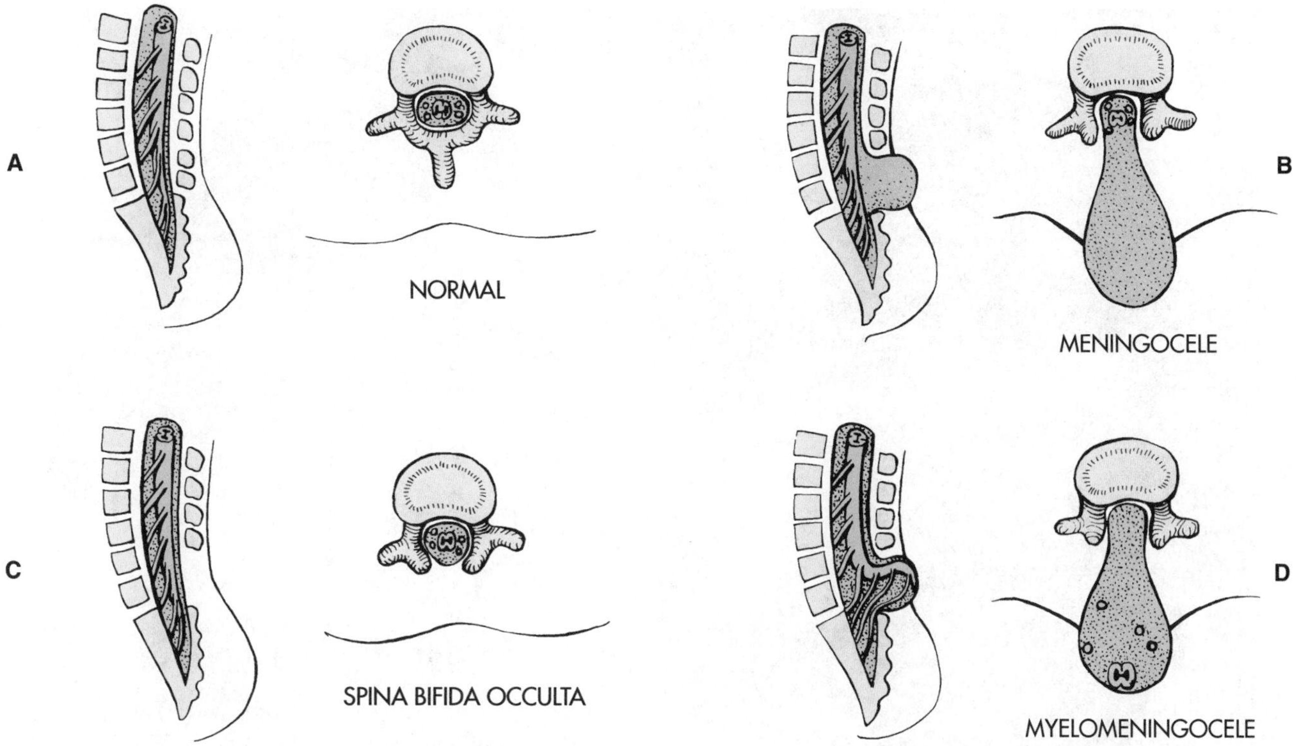

Fig. 55-5 Midline defects of osseous spine with varying degrees of neural herniations.

BOX 55-4

Neural Tube Defects

Cranioschisis—A skull defect through which various tissues protrude

Exencephaly—Brain totally exposed or extruded through an associated skull defect; fetus usually aborted

Anencephaly—If fetus with exencephaly survives, degeneration of the brain to a spongiform mass with no bony covering; incompatible with life usually beyond a few days

Encephalocele—Herniation of brain and meninges through a defect in the skull producing a fluid-filled sac

Rachischisis or **spina bifida**—Fissure in the spinal column that leaves the meninges and spinal cord exposed

Meningocele—Hernial protrusion of a saclike cyst of meninges filled with spinal fluid (see Fig. 55-5, *C*)

Myelomeningocele (meningomyelocele)—Hernial protrusion of a saclike cyst containing meninges, spinal fluid, and a portion of the spinal cord with its nerves (see Fig. 55-5, *D*)

Prenatal Detection

It is possible to determine the presence of some major open NTDs prenatally. Fetal ultrasound and elevated concentrations of alpha-fetoprotein (AFP), a fetal-specific gamma$_1$-globulin, in amniotic fluid may indicate the presence of anencephaly or myelomeningocele. The optimum time for performing these diagnostic tests is between 16 and 18 weeks of gestation, before AFP concentrations normally diminish and in sufficient time to permit a therapeutic

BOX 55-5

Characteristics of Spina Bifida

Spina Bifida Cystica

Sensory disturbances usually parallel motor dysfunction
- *Below second lumbar vertebra:*
  - Flaccid, partial paralysis of lower extremities
  - Varying degrees of sensory deficit
  - Overflow incontinence with constant dribbling of urine
  - Lack of bowel control
  - Rectal prolapse (sometimes)
- *Below third sacral vertebra:*
  - No motor impairment
  - May be saddle anesthesia with bladder and anal sphincter paralysis

Joint deformities (sometimes produced in utero):
- Talipes valgus or varus contractures
- Kyphosis
- Lumbosacral scoliosis
- Hip dislocations

Spina Bifida Occulta

Often no observable manifestations

May be associated with one or more cutaneous manifestations:
- Skin depression or dimple
- Port-wine angiomatous nevi
- Dark tufts of hair
- Soft, subcutaneous lipomas

May be neuromuscular disturbances:
- Progressive disturbance of gait with foot weakness
- Bowel and bladder sphincter disturbances

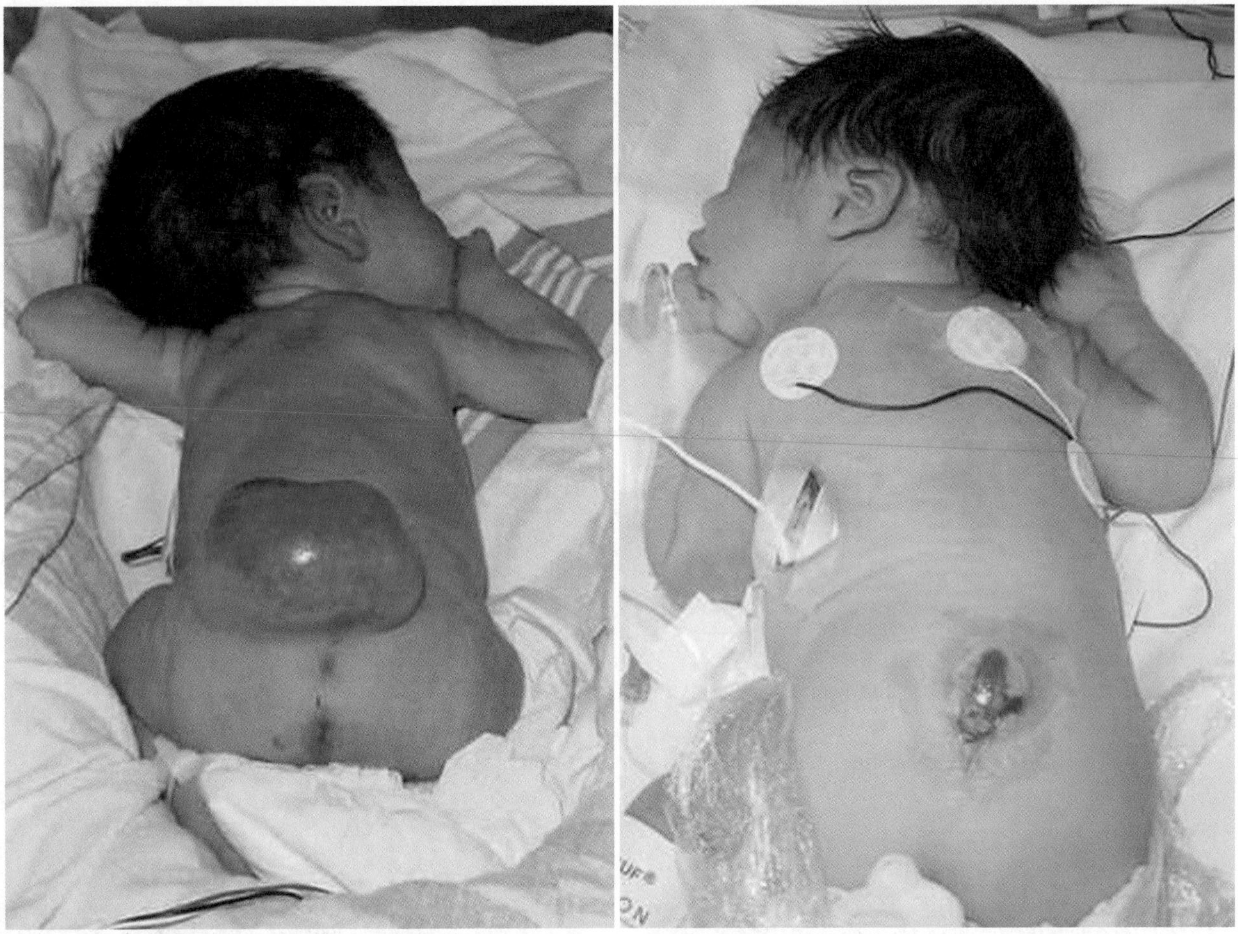

Fig. 55-6 **A,** Meningomyelocele with intact sac. **B,** Myelomeningocele with ruptured sac. (Photo courtesy of Dr. Robert C. Dauser, Neurosurgery, Baylor College of Medicine, Houston, Texas.)

abortion (should this option be desired). Chorionic villus sampling (CVS) is also a measure for prenatal diagnosis of NTDs; however, it carries certain risks (skeletal limb depletion) and is not recommended before 10 weeks of gestation. It is recommended that such diagnostic procedures be considered for all mothers who have borne an affected child, and testing is offered to all pregnant women. In addition, elective prelabor cesarean birth may result in less motor dysfunction.

Therapeutic Management

Early surgical closure of the myelomeningocele sac through fetal surgery is being evaluated in relation to prevention of injury to the exposed spinal cord tissue and the improvement of neurologic and urologic outcomes in the affected child (Hirose, Farmer, & Albanese, 2001; Holmes et al, 2001; Olutoye & Adzick, 1999; Tulipan & Bruner, 1998). Initial fetal surgical success and survival rates appear to be positive; however, reports vary in relation to the success of fetal surgery in the actual reduction of urologic problems, improvement of lower leg function, and prevention of hydrocephalus in the postnatal period (Holmes et al, 2001; Tubbs et al, 2003). Some have suggested that the ethical issues surrounding fetal surgery, outcomes, and the risks involved have yet to be satisfactorily discussed and settled (Lyerly & Mahowald, 2003). Management of the child who has a myelomeningocele requires a multidisciplinary approach involving the specialties of neurology, neurosurgery, pediatrics, urology, orthopedics, rehabilitation, physical therapy, and social services, as well as intensive nursing care in a variety of specialty areas. The collaborative efforts of these specialists are focused on (1) the myelomeningocele and the problems associated with the defect—hydrocephalus, paralysis, orthopedic deformities, and genitourinary abnormalities; (2) possible acquired problems that may or may not be associated, such as meningitis, hypoxia, and hemorrhage; and (3) other abnormalities, such as cardiac or gastrointestinal malformations.

Infancy

Initial care of the newborn involves prevention of infection; preservation of neurologic function; neurologic assessment, including observation for associated anomalies; and dealing with the impact of the anomaly on the family. Although meningoceles are repaired early, especially if there is danger of rupture of the sac, the philosophy regarding skin closure of myelomeningocele varies. Most authorities believe that early closure, within the first 24 to 72 hours, offers the most favorable outcome. Surgical closure within the first 24 hours is recommended if the sac is leaking (Kaufman, 2004). Early closure, preferably in the first 12 to 18 hours, not only prevents local infection and trauma to the exposed tissues but also avoids stretching of other nerve roots, which may occur as the meningeal sac expands during the first hours after birth, thus preventing further motor impairment.

Associated problems are assessed and managed by appropriate surgical and supportive measures. Shunt procedures provide relief from imminent or progressive hydrocephalus (see Chapter 51). Meningitis, urinary tract infection, and pneumonia are treated with vigorous antibiotic therapy and supportive measures. Surgical intervention for Arnold-Chiari malformation (a downward herniation of the brain into the brainstem) or for tethered cord (scar tissue binding the spinal cord) is indicated only when the child is symptomatic.

Improved surgical techniques do not alter the major physical disability, spinal defect, or chronic urinary tract infections that affect the quality of life for these children. Superimposed on the physical problems are the effects that the disorder has on family life and finances, including the need for specialized school and hospital services.

Orthopedic Considerations

According to most orthopedists, musculoskeletal problems that will affect later locomotion should be evaluated early, and treatment, where indicated, should be instituted without delay. Neurologic assessment will determine the neurosegmental level of the lesion, recognition of spasticity and progressive paralysis, potential for deformity, and functional expectations. Orthopedic management includes preventing joint contractures, correcting the existing deformity, preventing or minimizing the effects of motor and sensory deficits, preventing skin breakdown, and obtaining the best possible function of affected lower extremities. Common orthopedic problems requiring attention in SB include deformities of the knees, hips, feet, and spine; fractures and insensate skin further complicate orthopedic care (Brown, 2001). Other problems that may occur later include kyphosis and scoliosis (Brown, 2001). Because children with this condition often have decreased sensitivity in lower extremities, preventive skin care is very important. A high percentage (60%) of children seen in a wound clinic for skin breakdown had myelomeningocele (Samaniego, 2003). The status of the neurologic deficit remains the most important factor in determining the child's ultimate functional abilities.

With technologic advances, a variety of lightweight orthoses are available to provide mobility to children with spinal cord lesions, including braces, special "walking" devices, and custom-built wheelchairs (see also Chapter 42). Early in infancy, intervention with passive range-of-motion exercises, positioning, and stretching exercises may help decrease the incidence of muscle contractures (Brown, 2001). Corrective surgical procedures, when indicated, are best initiated at an early age so that the child will not lag significantly behind age-mates in developmental progress. Where there is little hope for lower extremity functioning, surgery is seldom recommended unless it will improve sitting position in a wheelchair and function for activities of daily living (ADLs) and mobility.

Management of Genitourinary Function

Myelomeningocele is one of the most common causes of *neuropathic (neurogenic) bladder dysfunction* among children. In infants the goal of treatment is to preserve renal function. In older children the goal is to preserve renal function and achieve optimum urinary continence. Urinary incontinence is a chronic, often debilitating problem for the child. In addition, the neuropathic bladder may produce *urinary system distress,* characterized by symptomatic urinary tract infections, ureterohydronephrosis, and vesicoureteral reflux or renal insufficiency. The characteristics of bladder dysfunction in children vary according to the level of the neurologic lesion and the influence of bony growth and development on the spine. Therefore ongoing urologic monitoring is essential. There is growing evidence that early intervention, based on evaluation during the neonatal period and before complications occur, serves to improve bladder function, reduce the risk of subsequent urinary system distress, and decrease the need for reconstructive surgery of the lower urinary tract (Holzbeierlein et al, 2000; Kaefer et al, 1999).

Treatment of renal problems includes (1) regular urologic care with prompt and vigorous treatment of infections; (2) some type of regular emptying of the bladder, such as *clean intermittent catheterization (CIC)* taught to and performed by parents and self-catheterization taught to children; (3) medications to improve bladder storage and continence, such as oxybutynin chloride (Ditropan) and tolterodine (Detrol); and (4) surgical procedures such as *vesicostomy* (stoma created on the abdominal wall for urinary drainage) and *augmentation enterocystoplasty* (or gastrocystoplasty) (increases bladder capacity, reverses or halts the deleterious effects of the poorly compliant bladder wall, and reduces harmfully high bladder pressures caused by detrusor hyperreflexia with vesicosphincter dyssynergia).

Infrequently, children with myelodysplasia may develop severe dysfunction of the bladder that compromises renal function or produces debilitating urinary incontinence that is intractable to other treatments. *Urinary diversion,* typically using a continent neobladder constructed from bowel or stomach, may be required. Whenever feasible, the neobladder is constructed in a way that allows continence, and CIC is used to regularly evacuate urine. The appendix may also be used to create a stoma from the bladder to the abdominal wall or, in older children, the umbilicus, whereby intermittent catheterization may be done on a less conspicuous basis for normalization of daily activities (also referred to as the Mitrofanoff route). The ureter may be used as an alternative to the appendix for some children. If the appendix is insufficient a segment of tapered intestine, ileum, or colon may be used to create a conduit (Monti tube) (Mitrofanoff & Liard, 2001).

Bowel Control

Some degree of fecal continence can usually be achieved in most children with myelomeningocele with diet modification, regular toilet habits, and prevention of constipation and impaction. It is frequently a lengthy process. Fiber supplements, laxatives, suppositories, or enemas aid in producing regular evacuation. Older children and adolescents seeking more independence may attain bowel continence and higher quality of life after undergoing the Malone antegrade continence enema (MACE) procedure (Yerkes et al, 2003). In this procedure, the appendix or ileum is used to create a catheterizable channel with attachment of the proximal end to the colon. The distal end of the channel exits through a small abdominal stoma. Every 1 to 2 days, a catheter is passed through the stoma allowing enema solution to be instilled directly into the colon. After administration of the enema solution, the child sits on the toilet for 30 to 60 minutes as stool is flushed out through the rectum. Frequency of enemas and volume of solution used to completely evacuate the bowel vary among individuals.

Prognosis

The early prognosis for the child with myelomeningocele depends on the neurologic deficit present at birth, including motor ability and bladder innervation and the presence of associated anomalies. Early surgical repair of the spinal defect, antibiotic therapy to reduce the incidence of meningitis and ventriculitis, prevention of urinary system dysfunction, a program of bowel management, and early detection and correction of hydrocephalus have significantly increased the survival rate and quality of life in such children. Based on current medical knowledge and ethical considerations, aggressive management is favored for the child with myelomeningocele.

Prevention

The widespread use of folic acid among women of childbearing age is expected to significantly decrease the incidence of SB. It has been estimated that a daily intake of 0.4 mg of folic acid in women of childbearing age will prevent 50% to 70% of all cases of NTDs (CDC, 2001b). Preliminary data show a 24% decrease in cases of SB between 1996 and 2001 (Matthews, Honein, & Erickson, 2002). For women who have had a previous pregnancy affected by NTDs, folic acid intake is increased to 4 mg under supervision of a practitioner beginning 1 month before a planned pregnancy and continuing during the first trimester. Supplementation of 4 mg of folate should not be given in multivitamin preparations because of the risk of overdose of other vitamins. However, despite the recommendations of several health care and public agencies for the daily intake of 0.4 mg of folic acid in the periconceptual period, one survey revealed that only a small percentage (42%) of women of childbearing age actually follow these guidelines (CDC, 2001b). Awareness of the benefits of folic acid for the prevention of birth defects was highest in women who were 25 to 29 years of age, college educated, married, Caucasian, and not considered overweight. These results indicate that nurses and other health care workers have an important task in disseminating information that may decrease the incidence of birth defects in children by promoting maternal consumption of folic acid.*

To ensure adequate daily intake of the recommended amount of folic acid, women must take a folic acid supplement, eat a fortified breakfast cereal containing 100% of the recommended dietary allowance (RDA) of folic acid (e.g., Kellogg's Product 19, General Mills Total, Multigrain Cheerios Plus), or increase their consumption of fortified foods (cereal, bread, rice, grits, pasta) and foods naturally rich in folate (green leafy vegetables and citrus fruits). The only population in which folic acid has not proved to be effective in decreasing the incidence of NTDs is epileptic women taking antiepileptic medications during pregnancy (Finnell et al, 2003).

NURSE ALERT Because approximately one half of all pregnancies in the United States are unplanned (Henshaw, 1998), adolescent girls and women of childbearing age need to be educated about the necessity of folic acid to prevent neural tube defects. The daily dose of 0.4 mg (400 mcg) is most easily obtained from a multivitamin supplement. ■

Nursing Care Management

At birth, an examination is performed to assess the intactness of the membranous cyst. During transport to the nursery, every effort is made to prevent trauma to this protective covering (see Fig. 55-6, *A*). In addition to the routine assessment of the newborn (see Chapter 24), the infant is assessed for the level of neurologic involvement. Movement of extremities or skin response, especially an anal reflex, that might provide clues to the degree of motor or sensory impairment is noted. It is important to observe the infant's behavior in conjunction with the stimulus, because limb movements can be induced in response to spinal cord reflex activity that has no connection with the higher centers. Observation of urine output, especially if a diaper remains dry, may indicate urinary retention. Abdominal assessment revealing bladder distention, even with a wet diaper, may indicate urinary overflow in a retentive bladder.

NURSE ALERT Do not take rectal temperatures in infants with SB. Because bowel sphincter function is commonly affected, the thermometer can cause irritation and rectal prolapse. ■

Care of the Myelomeningocele Sac

The infant is usually placed in an incubator or warmer so that temperature can be maintained without clothing or covers that might irritate the delicate lesion. When an overhead warmer is used, the dressings over the defect require more frequent moistening because of the dehydrating effect of the radiant heat.

Before surgical closure, the myelomeningocele is prevented from drying by the application of a sterile, moist, nonadherent dressing over the defect. The moistening solution is usually sterile normal saline solution. Dressings are changed frequently (every 2 to 4 hours), and the sac is closely inspected for leaks, abrasions, irritation, or any signs of infection. The sac must be carefully cleansed if it becomes soiled or contaminated. Sometimes the sac ruptures during delivery or transport, and any opening in the sac greatly increases the risk of infection to the central nervous system (Fig. 55-6, *B*).

NURSE ALERT Observe for early signs of infection, such as elevated temperature (axillary), irritability, and lethargy. ■

One of the most difficult, important, and challenging aspects in the early care of the infant with myelomeningocele

*Information is available from the Centers for Disease Control and Prevention, Division of Birth Defects and Pediatric Genetics, NCBDDD, CDC, 4770 Buford Highway NE, MS F-45, Atlanta, GA 30341; phone: 888-232-6789, e-mail: flo@cdc.gov; Web site: www.cdc.gov/ncbddd/folicacid; and the **March of Dimes** Resource Center, 1275 Mamaroneck Avenue, White Plains, NY 10605; phone: 888-MODIMES; Web site: www.modimes.org.

is positioning. Before surgery the infant is kept in the prone position to minimize tension on the sac and the risk of trauma. The prone position allows for optimum positioning of the legs, especially in cases of associated hip dysplasia. The infant is placed flat with the hips only slightly flexed to reduce tension on the defect. The legs are maintained in abduction with a pad between the knees to counteract hip subluxation, and a small roll is placed under the ankles to maintain a neutral foot position. A variety of aids, including diaper rolls, rolled blankets, or specially designed frames and appliances, can be used to maintain the desired position.

Prevent Complications

The prone position affects other aspects of the infant's care. For example, in this position the infant is more difficult to keep clean, pressure areas are a constant threat, and feeding becomes a problem. The infant's head is turned to one side for feeding. Fortunately, most defects are repaired early, and the infant can be held for feeding soon after surgery. Special care must be taken to avoid pressure on the operative site.

Diapering the infant may be contraindicated until the defect has been repaired and healing is well advanced or epithelialization has taken place. The padding beneath the diaper area is changed as needed to keep the skin dry and free of irritation. If urinary retention is detected, CIC may be used. Because the bowel sphincter is commonly affected, there is continual passage of stool, often misinterpreted as diarrhea, which is a constant irritant to the skin and a source of infection to the spinal lesion.

Areas of sensory and motor impairment are subject to skin breakdown and therefore require meticulous care. Placing the infant on a special mattress or mattress overlay reduces pressure on the knees and ankles. Periodic cleansing, application of lotion, and gentle massage aid circulation.

Range-of-motion exercises are sometimes carried out to prevent contractures, and stretching of contractures is performed when indicated. However, these exercises may be restricted to the foot, ankle, and knee joint. Where the hip joints are unstable, stretching against tight hip flexors or adductor muscles, which act much like bowstrings, may aggravate a tendency toward subluxation. Consultation with a physical therapist is an important aspect of the short- and long-term management of infants with myelomeningocele.

Provide Postoperative Care

Postoperative care of the infant with myelomeningocele involves the same basic care as that of any postsurgical infant: monitoring vital signs, monitoring intake and output, providing nourishment, observing for signs of infection, and managing pain as needed. Care of the operative site includes close observation for signs of leakage of cerebrospinal fluid. General care is continued as preoperatively.

The prone position is maintained after surgical closure, although a side-lying or partial side-lying position is usually acceptable unless it aggravates a coexisting hip dysplasia or permits undesirable hip flexion. This offers an opportunity for position changes, which reduce the risk of pressure sores and facilitate feeding. Ankle splints may be used to prevent muscle contractures. The infant can often be held by the parents shortly after surgery, with care taken to avoid pressure on the operative site. Once the effects of anesthesia have subsided and the infant is alert, feedings may be resumed unless there are other anomalies or associated complications. Head circumference is monitored frequently and the infant is evaluated for any signs of increased intracranial pressure (bulging or taut anterior fontanel, poor feeding, irritability, fussiness, setting sun sign).

Because children who have SB are prone to develop an allergy to latex, reducing exposure to latex from birth on is hoped to decrease the chance of allergy development. Parent education must emphasize preventive measures to avoid latex sensitization. The establishment of a latex-safe environment is being accomplished in many health care facilities where patients (and health care workers) are at high risk (see Latex Allergy, later in this chapter).

Support Family and Educate about Home Care

Parents are encouraged to become involved in the child's care as soon as possible. They need to learn how to continue at home the care that has been initiated in the hospital—positioning, feeding, skin care, and range-of-motion exercises when appropriate. Parents are taught CIC technique when it is prescribed. They need to know the signs of complications and how to obtain assistance when needed. The long-range planning with and support of the parents and child begin in the hospital and extend throughout childhood and even beyond. Nurses assume an important role as a central member of the health team. Children with SB are usually followed on an outpatient basis for ongoing screening of health problems and early detection and management of such problems; a multidisciplinary outpatient clinic allows the child and parents to see a variety of specialists in one location for ongoing care and support. (See Chapter 41 for a discussion of care of the child with a disability.)

Habilitation and normalization involve not only solving problems of self-help and locomotion but also solving problems related to genitourinary dysfunction and bowel incontinence which may affect the child's socialization. The child's acceptance by family members is extremely important to the success of normalization and socialization to school and other children's activities. The Spina Bifida Association of America* is organized to provide services and support for families of children with spinal lesions.

Latex Allergy

Latex allergy was identified as being a serious health hazard when a report linked intraoperative anaphylaxis with latex in children with SB. The high prevalence of latex allergy (up to 80%) in children with SB has been attributed to the repeated exposure to latex products during surgery and from numerous bladder catheterizations, as well as possible disease-associated factors (Mazon et al, 2000; Szepfalusi et al, 1999). Allergic reactions range from mild (urticaria, wheezing, watery eyes, and rashes) to severe (anaphylactic shock). More severe reactions tend to occur when latex comes in contact with mucous membranes, wet skin, the bloodstream, or an airway. There also can be cross-reactions to a number of foods (e.g., banana, avocado, kiwi, chestnut). In

*4590 MacArthur Boulevard, NW, Suite 250, Washington, DC 20007-4226; phone: 202-944-3285 or 800-621-3141; Web site: www.sbaa.org.

Guidelines

IDENTIFYING LATEX ALLERGY

Does your child have any symptoms, such as sneezing, coughing, rashes, or wheezing, when handling rubber products (e.g., balloons, tennis or Koosh balls, adhesive bandage strips), or when in contact with rubber hospital products (e.g., gloves, catheters)?
Has your child ever had an allergic reaction during surgery?
Does your child have a history of rashes, asthma, or allergic reactions to medication or foods, especially milk, kiwi, bananas, or chestnuts?
How would you identify or recognize an allergic reaction in your child?
What would you do if an allergic reaction occurred?
Has anyone ever discussed latex or rubber allergy or sensitivity with you?
Has your child had any allergy testing?
When did your child last come in contact with any type of rubber product? Were you present?

Modified from Romanczuk A: Latex use with infants and children: it can cause problems, *MCN* 18(4):208-212, 1993.

addition to patients with SB, high risk populations include patients with urogenital anomalies or multiple surgeries, as well as health care workers. (See Box 55-6 for medical conditions associated with SB.)

The most important goals are prevention of latex allergy and identification of children with a known hypersensitivity (Guidelines box). High risk and latex-allergic individuals must be managed in a *latex-safe environment.* Care must be taken so that they do not come in direct or secondary contact with products or equipment containing latex at any time during medical treatment. Allergy testing has been used with varying success to identify latex allergy. Skin prick testing and provocation testing carry the risk of allergic reaction or anaphylaxis. The radioallergosorbent test (RAST) has been used to measure the serum level of latex-specific immunoglobulin E (IgE). The RAST has been shown to be 90% to 95% sensitive (Kellett, 1997). Pretreatment with antihistamines and steroids (dexamethasone) before and after surgery to reduce the possibility of a serious reaction remains controversial because it may interfere with healing.

Latex, a natural product derived from the rubber tree, is used in combination with other chemicals to give elasticity, strength, and durability to many products.

Avoiding contact with latex is the most important intervention. The establishment of a latex-safe environment is being accomplished in many health care facilities where patients and health care workers are at high risk. In addition, lists of products (e.g., vinyl gloves) that may be substituted for latex have been published.* Allergic reactions to latex protein can also occur when the substance is transferred to food by food handlers wearing latex gloves, prompting several states to pass legislation that prohibits the use of latex gloves in food service

*For an updated list of latex-free items (medical and community) and alternative products, contact the Spina Bifida Association of America, 4590 MacArthur Boulevard. NW, Suite 250, Washington, DC 20007-4226; phone: 202-944-3285 or 1-800-621-3141; Web site: www.sbaa.org.

BOX 55-6

Medical Conditions Associated with Risk of Latex Allergy

Spina bifida
Urogenital anomalies
Imperforate anus
Tracheoesophageal fistula
VATER association (*v*ertebral defects, imperforate *a*nus, *t*racheo*e*sophageal fistula, and *r*adial and renal dysplasia)
Preterm infants
Ventriculoperitoneal shunt
Mental retardation
Cerebral palsy
Quadriplegia
Multiple surgeries
Atopy

(Beezhold et al, 2000; Liddle, 2001). In the health care arena, it is important to use products with the lowest potential risk of sensitizing patients and staff members. User labeling for latex-containing devices that come into contact directly or indirectly with live human tissue was proposed by the Food and Drug Administration (FDA) in 1996.

The American Nurses Association (ANA) (1997), National Institute for Occupational Safety and Health (NIOSH) (1997), Occupational Safety and Health Administration (OSHA) (1999), National Association of Neonatal Nurses (NANN) (2000), and other state, school, and health care organizations have issued statements on latex allergies directing all health care institutions to abandon the unnecessary use of powdered latex gloves and provide latex-free equipment and latex-safe environments for patients and staff known to have, or who are at high risk for developing, an allergy to latex. Procedures for the identification and treatment of latex-sensitive patients, provision of latex-free medical products, and reporting of allergic events related to latex medical devices to the FDA MedWatch Program are also strongly advocated by the ANA.* In addition, the ANA recommends that each health care facility have a multidisciplinary task force to develop occupational health guidelines to ensure a safe environment for health care workers to minimize latex exposure, identify those at risk for reaction to latex, and accommodate the needs of latex-sensitive employees.

NURSE ALERT Ask *all* patients about allergic reactions to latex, not only those at risk, during the health interview with the parent or child. Be sure that this is a routine part of all preoperative and preprocedural histories. Stress the importance of the allergy history to *all* personnel (e.g., phlebotomists). ■

*The FDA Medical Products Reporting Program, Food and Drug Administration, 5600 Fishers Lane, Rockville, MD 20852-9787; phone: 800-FDA-1088; fax: 800-FDA-0178; Web site: www.fda.gov/medwatch. Additional information regarding latex allergy may be found at the following Web sites: www.latexallergyhelp.com; www.latexallergyresources.org (American Latex Allergy Association); http://latexallergylinks.tripod.com; www.sbaa.org.

The identification of those sensitive to latex is best accomplished through careful screening of *all* patients. (See Guidelines box for questions related to latex allergy.)

Children with latex allergy should carry or wear some form of medical identification. Education programs regarding latex hypersensitivity are aimed at those who care for high risk groups, such as children with SB, and may include relatives, school nurses, teachers, child care workers, and baby-sitters. In addition to educating caregivers about the child's exposure to medical products that contain latex, nurses need to inform them of common nonmedical latex objects. Items brought to the hospital, such as floral bouquets, are also screened for latex balloons, which have been banned in many hospitals, and latex toys. Parents should also be given literature explaining signs and symptoms of latex hypersensitivity and appropriate emergency treatment (see Anaphylaxis, Chapter 48).

Progressive Infantile Spinal Muscular Atrophy (Werdnig-Hoffmann Disease)

Progressive infantile spinal muscular atrophy (SMA) (Werdnig-Hoffmann disease), or *SMA type 1,* is a disorder characterized by progressive weakness and wasting of skeletal muscles caused by degeneration of anterior horn cells. It is inherited as an autosomal recessive trait and is the most common paralytic form of the *floppy infant syndrome (congenital hypotonia).* The sites of the pathologic condition are the anterior horn cells of the spinal cord and the motor nuclei of the brainstem, but the primary effect is atrophy of skeletal muscles. The age of onset is variable, but the earlier the onset, the more disseminated and severe the motor weakness. The disorder may be manifested early—often at birth—and almost always before 2 years of age. The manifestations (Box 55-7) and prognosis are categorized according to the age of onset, severity of weakness, and clinical course; some children may fluctuate between exhibiting symptoms of types 1 and 2, or between types 2 and 3 in regard to clinical function (Sarnat, 2004).

Diagnosis and Therapeutic Management

The diagnosis is the molecular genetic marker for the survival motor neuron (SMN) gene, which is located on chromosome 5q13. Prenatal diagnosis may be made by genetic analysis of circulating fetal cells in maternal blood (Beroud et al, 2003) or circulating fetal cells in amniotic fluid. The risk of subsequent affected offspring in carriers of the mutant gene or in families with known cases of SMA may also be evaluated genetically. Further diagnostic studies include muscle electromyography (EMG), which demonstrates a denervation pattern, and muscle biopsy; however, the genetic analysis has become the gold standard for diagnosis of the condition. There is no cure for the disease, and treatment is symptomatic and preventive, primarily preventing joint contractures and treating orthopedic problems, the most serious of which is scoliosis; hip subluxation and dislocation may also occur. Many children benefit from powered chairs, lifts, special pressure-adjustable mattresses, and accessible environmental controls. Muscle and joint contractures require careful attention and care to prevent further complications. The use of lower extremity orthoses may assist with ambulation, but eventually the child may be confined to a

BOX 55-7

Clinical Manifestations of Spinal Muscular Atrophy

Type 1 (Werdnig-Hoffmann Disease)

- Disease acquired in utero or during first 2 months of life
- Hypotonia and inactivity are most prominent features
- Infant lies in the frog position with legs externally rotated, abducted, and flexed at knees
- Weakness
- Absent deep tendon reflexes
- Limited movements of shoulder and arm muscles
- Active movement is usually limited to fingers and toes
- Diaphragmatic breathing with intercostal retractions (diaphragmatic paralysis may occur)
- Abnormal tongue movements
- Weak cry and cough
- Secretions tend to pool in oropharynx
- Alert facies
- Normal sensation and intellect
- Tire quickly during feedings (if breastfed, may lose weight before noticeable)
- Affected infants do not progress to sit alone, roll over, or walk
- Early death (usually by 2 years of age) from respiratory failure or infection

Type 2 (Intermediate SMA)

- Symptoms manifest between 2 and 12 months of age
- Early–weakness confined to arms and legs
- Later–becomes generalized
- Legs usually involved to greater extent than arms
- Prominent pectus excavatum
- Movements absent during complete relaxation or sleep
- Some infants able to sit if placed in position
- Failure to walk is common
- Life span varies from 7 months to 7 years or even longer in some cases

Type 3 (Kugelberg-Welander Disease)

- Onset of symptoms in late childhood or adolescence (may be initially misdiagnosed as muscular dystrophy [limb girdle])
- Normal head control and can sit unassisted by 6 to 8 months of age
- Thigh and hip muscles weak
- In those who manage to walk:
  - Lumbar lordosis
  - Waddling gait
  - Genu recurvatum
  - Protuberant abdomen
  - Ambulation becomes increasingly difficult
  - Age of onset influences ambulatory difficulty–the later (after 2 years) the onset, the better the prognosis
  - Confined to a wheelchair by second decade (may vary)
- Deep tendon reflexes may be present early but disappear
- Scoliosis is common

NOTE: These classifications are general, and experts suggest there may be variations in life span and other characteristics (Iannaccone & Burghes, 2002; Russman, 1996; Russman et al, 1992).

wheelchair as muscle atrophy progresses. Upper respiratory infections may occur and are treated with antibiotic therapy.

Prognosis

Prognosis varies according to age of onset or group as described in Box 55-7. Individuals with SMA type 1 commonly succumb to respiratory infections or failure between 1 and 24 months of age (Iannaccone & Burghes, 2002; Thompson & Berenson, 2001); however, some may live into their third or fourth decade of life. Some affected persons do not demonstrate progressive loss of strength and function (Russman, 1996).

Nursing Care Management

The infant or small child with progressive muscle weakness requires nursing care similar to that of the immobilized patient. However, the underlying goal of treatment should be to assist the child and family in dealing with the illness while progressing toward a life of normalization within the child's capabilities. Special attention to preventing muscle and joint contractures, promoting independence in performance of ADLs, and becoming incorporated into the mainstream of school when possible should be the focal point of care. In addition, parents need support and resources to be able to provide for the child and remain an intact family. Because children with neuromuscular disease have abnormal breathing patterns that often contribute to early death, it is important to assess adequate oxygenation, especially during the sleep phase when shallow breathing occurs and hypoxemia may develop. Home pulse oximetry may be used to assess the child during sleep and provide supplemental oxygenation treatment as necessary (Birnkrant, 2002) (see section on Duchenne muscular dystrophy, later in this chapter, for respiratory management). Supportive care also includes management of orthoses and other orthopedic equipment as required. Because children with SMA are intellectually normal, verbal, tactile, and auditory stimulation are important aspects of developmental care. Supporting them so that they can see the activities around them and transporting them in appropriate conveyances (e.g., wagon, power wheelchair) for a change of environment provide stimulation and a broader scope of contacts.

Children who are able to sit require proper support and attention to alignment to prevent deformities and other complications. Children who survive beyond infancy will need attention to educational needs and opportunities for social interaction with other children. The parents of a child who is chronically ill require much support and encouragement (see Chapter 41). Parents who have not sought genetic counseling should be encouraged to do so to evaluate further risk potential.

Juvenile Spinal Muscular Atrophy (Kugelberg-Welander Disease)

Juvenile spinal muscular atrophy (Kugelberg-Welander disease, juvenile proximal hereditary muscular atrophy) is also a result of anterior horn cell and motor nerve degeneration. The disease is characterized by a pattern of muscular weakness similar to that of infantile spinal muscular atrophy (see Box 55-7). Several modes of inheritance have been reported for the disease: autosomal recessive, autosomal dominant, and X-linked recessive.

The onset occurs from younger than 1 year of age into adulthood, with symptoms resembling type 3 infantile spinal muscular atrophy; proximal muscle weakness (especially of the lower limbs) and muscular atrophy are the predominant features. The disease runs a slowly progressive course. Some children lose the ability to walk 8 to 9 years after the onset of symptoms, but many can still walk after 30 years or more. Many affected persons have a normal life expectancy (Iannaccone, 1998).

Therapeutic Management and Nursing Care Management

The management is primarily symptomatic and supportive and is related to maintaining mobility as long as possible, preventing complications, and providing support to the child and family.

Muscular Dystrophies

Muscular dystrophies (MDs) constitute the largest and most important single group of muscle diseases of childhood. The MDs have a genetic origin in which there is gradual degeneration of muscle fibers, and they are characterized by progressive weakness and wasting of symmetric groups of skeletal muscles, with increasing disability and deformity. In all forms of MD there is insidious loss of strength, but each type differs in regard to muscle groups affected (Fig. 55-7), age of onset, rate of progression, and inheritance pattern. The most common form, *Duchenne muscular dystrophy,* is considered separately in the next section.

Facioscapulohumeral (Landouzy-Déjérine) muscular dystrophy is inherited as an autosomal dominant disorder with onset in early adolescence. It is characterized by difficulty in raising the arms over the head, lack of facial mobility, and a forward slope of the shoulders. The progression is slow, and the life span is usually unaffected.

Limb-girdle muscular dystrophy is an autosomal recessive disease of later childhood or adolescence with variable but usually slow progression; it is characterized by weakness of proximal muscles of the pelvic and shoulder girdles.

Treatment of the MDs consists mainly of supportive measures, including physical therapy, orthopedic procedures to minimize deformity, and assistance for the affected child in meeting the demands of daily living.

Pseudohypertrophic (Duchenne) Muscular Dystrophy

Duchenne muscular dystrophy (DMD) is the most severe and the most common muscular dystrophy of childhood. It is inherited as an X-linked recessive trait, and the single gene defect is located on the short arm of the X chromosome. DMD has a reportedly high mutation rate, with a positive family history in 65% of all cases (Thompson & Berenson, 2001); therefore genetic counseling is an important aspect of the care of the family. As in all X-linked disorders, males are affected almost exclusively. At the genetic level, DMD results from mutation of the gene that encodes *dystrophin,* a protein found in skeletal muscle. The incidence is approximately 1 per 3600 male births (Sarnat, 2004). Box 55-8 describes the characteristics of DMD.

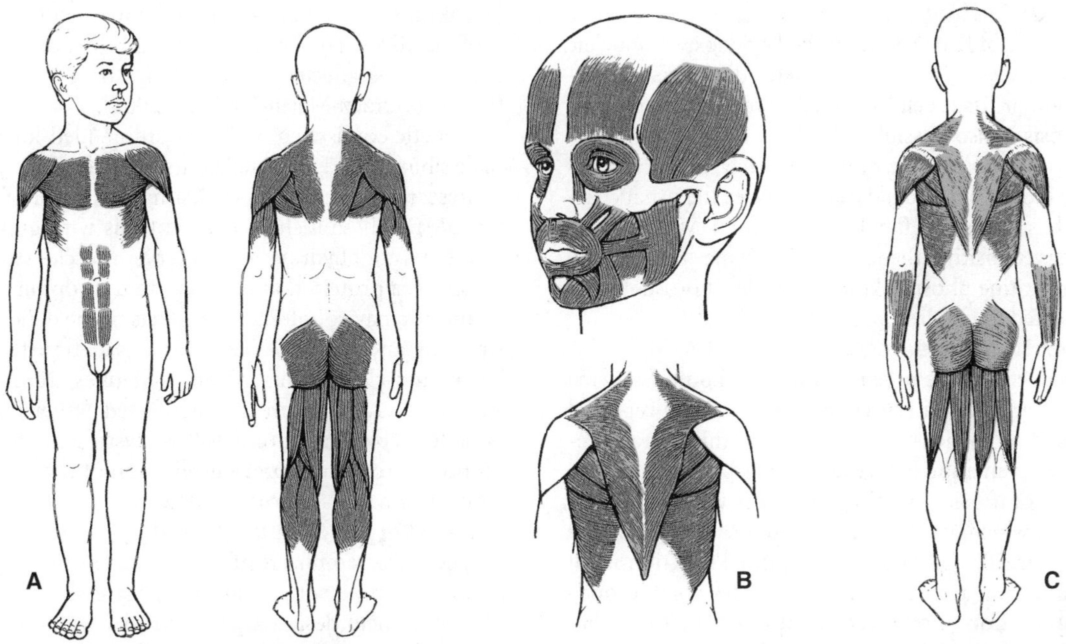

Fig. 55-7 Initial muscle groups involved in muscular dystrophies. **A**, Pseudohypertrophic. **B**, Facioscapulohumeral. **C**, Limb-girdle.

Most children with DMD reach the appropriate developmental milestones early in life, although there may be mild, subtle delays. Evidence of muscle weakness usually appears during the third year, although there may have been a history of delay in motor development, particularly walking. Difficulties in running, riding a bicycle, and climbing stairs are usually the first symptoms noted. Later, abnormal gait on a level surface becomes apparent. In the early years, rapid developmental gains may mask the progression of the disease. Questioning the parents may reveal that the child has difficulty in rising from a sitting or supine position. Parents may also notice that the child has enlarged calves (Box 55-9).

The term *pseudohypertrophy* is derived from muscular enlargement caused by fatty infiltration. Profound muscular atrophy occurs in later stages, and as the disease progresses, contractures and deformities involving large and small joints are common complications. Ambulation usually becomes impossible by 12 years of age. Facial, oropharyngeal, and respiratory muscles are often spared until the terminal stages of the disease. Ultimately the disease process involves the diaphragm and auxiliary muscles of respiration, and cardiovascular involvement (cardiomyopathy, dysrhythmias, and heart failure) is common. Mild mental delay is common in roughly 30% of all individuals with MD, and many have permanent learning disabilities; however, children with DMD should be transitioned into early learning programs and eventually into regular classrooms as much as possible. The eventual cause of death is usually respiratory tract infection or cardiac failure; however, much progress has been made in providing ventilatory methods to prolong and maintain quality of life.

BOX 55-8

Characteristics of Duchenne Muscular Dystrophy

- Early onset, usually between 3 and 5 years of age
- Progressive muscular weakness, wasting, and contractures
- Calf muscle hypertrophy in most patients
- Loss of independent ambulation by 9 to 11 years of age
- Slowly progressive, generalized weakness during teenage years
- Relentless progression until death from respiratory or cardiac failure

BOX 55-9

Clinical Manifestations of Duchenne Muscular Dystrophy

- Relentless progression until death from respiratory or cardiac failure
- Waddling gait
- Lordosis
- Frequent falls
- Gower sign (child turns onto side or abdomen, flexes knees to assume a kneeling position, then with knees extended gradually pushes torso to an upright position by "walking" the hands up the legs)
- Enlarged muscles (especially thighs and upper arms)
  - Feel unusually firm or woody on palpation
- Later stages: profound muscular atrophy
- Mental deficiency (common)
  - Mild (about 20 IQ points below normal)
  - Mental deficit present in 25% to 30% of patients
- Complications:
  - Contracture deformities of hips, knees, and ankles
  - Disuse atrophy
  - Obesity

Diagnostic Evaluation

The diagnosis of DMD is established by deoxyribonucleic acid (DNA) analysis (molecular genetic diagnosis) of peripheral blood or tissue cells obtained by muscle biopsy. Prenatal diagnosis is also possible as early as 12 weeks of gestation. Additional diagnostic evaluation may include EMG and muscle biopsy. If the child demonstrates the usual characteristics, has a positive family history for DMD, and the DNA analysis is positive, the muscle biopsy may be deferred. The serum creatine phosphokinase (CK) level is usually extremely elevated in children with DMD.

Therapeutic Management

No effective treatment exists for childhood MD. Increased muscle bulk and muscle power have been reported after a course of corticosteroids; however, this therapy requires further evaluation before it becomes routine management because of the side effects, particularly weight gain and osteoporosis, which may further complicate the disease process (Sarnat, 2004). Maintaining optimal function in all muscles for as long as possible is the primary goal; secondary is the prevention of contractures. It has been found that children who remain as active as possible are able to avoid wheelchair confinement for a longer time. Maintenance of function often includes stretching exercises, strength and muscle training, breathing exercises and use of incentive spirometry to increase and maintain vital lung capacity, range-of-motion exercises, surgery to release contracture deformities, bracing, and performance of ADLs. Parents should always be involved in making decisions about the child's care, and teaching regarding home safety and prevention of falls is important as well (Metules, 2002). Parents should also be encouraged to have the child keep follow-up appointments for medical care and physical and occupational therapy. Because respiratory infections are most troublesome in these children, influenza and pneumococcal vaccines are encouraged and contact with persons with respiratory infections should be avoided. Baseline pulmonary function testing, electrocardiograms, and echocardiograms are recommended (Metules, 2002).

Eventually, respiratory and cardiac problems become the central focus of the debilitating illness. Children with neuromuscular disease have abnormal breathing patterns, particularly during rapid-eye-movement sleep, and hypoxia may occur as a result of inadequate oxygenation (Birnkrant, 2002). The child and parents should be involved in a discussion of long-term ventilation options. Cardiac and respiratory assessment during wake-sleep cycles is imperative. The use of incentive spirometry helps maintain vital capacity, and breathing exercises should be taught early. Respiratory care later in life may involve the use of noninvasive intermittent positive pressure ventilation (IPPV) on a temporary or full-time basis, mechanically assisted coughing (MAC), or tracheotomy and relieving airway obstruction with coughing and suctioning devices; the tracheotomy, however, is associated with more complications. Home pulse oximetry may be used to monitor oxygenation during sleep or as an adjunct to decision making regarding the use of MAC to clear the airways. Several devices are available to children with neuromuscular disease to assist in clearing the airway when the cough reflex is ineffective or diminished (Birnkrant, 2002). Survival in individuals with DMD may be prolonged several years with the use of noninvasive IPPV and MAC as alternatives to tracheotomy and airway suctioning (Gomez-Merino & Bach, 2002).

Genetic counseling is also recommended for parents, female siblings, and maternal aunts and their female offspring.

Research is in progress evaluating a number of treatments for DMD. These include clinical trials with glutamine and creatine monohydrate to preserve muscle strength; and utrophin, a protein that is similar to dystrophin and in large quantities may counteract the effects of the deficiency of dystrophin and the enzyme CT GalNac transferase, which blocks muscle wasting in mice (Metules, 2002). Myoblast transfer therapy (from the unaffected father) offers some hope for replacement of defective dystrophin; however, immunosuppression to prevent rejection of the foreign cells is a major drawback (Sarnat, 2004).

Nursing Care Management

The major emphasis of nursing care is to help the child and family cope with a chronic, progressive, incapacitating disease; to help design a program that will afford maximal independence and reduce the predictable and preventable disabilities associated with the disorder; and to help the child and family deal constructively with the limitations the disease imposes on their daily lives. Because of newer advances in technology, children with MD may live into early adulthood; therefore the goals of care should also involve decisions regarding quality of life, achieving independence, and transition to adulthood.

Working closely with other health care team members, nurses assist the family in developing the child's self-help skills to give the child the satisfaction of being as independent as possible for as long as possible. This requires continual evaluation of the child's capabilities, which are often difficult to assess.

Practical difficulties faced by families are physical limitations of housing and mobility. Parents also need assistance in buying and modifying clothing for their child. It is difficult to find clothing and footwear to wear comfortably in a wheelchair and to fit hypertrophied muscles. The parent's social activities are also restricted, and the family's activities must be continually modified to the needs of the affected child.

When the child becomes increasingly incapacitated, the family may consider home-based care, a skilled nursing facility, or respite care to provide the care needed. Unless the child is severely incapacitated, he should also be involved in the decisions regarding such care. Nurses can assist with decision making by exploring all available options and resources and support the child and family in the decision. Older boys with MD may also need psychiatric or psychologic counseling to deal with issues such as depression, anger, and quality of life (Bothwell et al, 2002). Parents also need to be encouraged to become involved in support groups because there is evidence that adequate social support from family, community, and other parents is crucial to appropriate coping in families with children with chronic illness (Bothwell et al, 2002).

Regardless of how successful the program is or how well the family adapts to the disorder, superimposed on the physical and emotional problems associated with a child with a long-term disability is the constant presence of the ultimate outcome of the disease. All of the manifestations seen in the child with a chronic fatal illness are encountered in these families (see Chapter 41). The guilt feelings of the mother may be particularly pronounced in this disorder because of the mother-to-son transmission of the defective gene.

The Muscular Dystrophy Association of America, Inc.,* has branches in most communities to provide assistance to families in which there is a member with muscular dystrophy.

ACQUIRED NEUROMUSCULAR DISORDERS

Guillain-Barré Syndrome

CRITICAL THINKING EXERCISE: GUILLAIN-BARRÉ SYNDROME

Guillain-Barré syndrome (GBS), also known as *postinfectious polyneuritis,* is an uncommon acute demyelinating polyneuropathy with a progressive, usually ascending flaccid paralysis. Children are less often affected than adults, with children between ages 4 and 10 years having higher susceptibility. *Congenital GBS* is rare yet may be seen in the neonatal period and consists of hypotonia, weakness, and decreased or absent reflexes; maternal neuromuscular disease may or may not be present. Diagnosis is established by the same criteria as in older children, but the symptoms gradually subside over the first few months of life and there is no presence of disease by 12 months (Sarnat, 2004).

Pathophysiology

GBS is an immune-mediated disease often associated with a number of viral or bacterial infections or the administration of certain vaccines. It has been associated with infectious mononucleosis, measles, mumps, *Campylobacter jejuni* (gastroenteritis), *Borrelia burgdorferi* (Lyme disease), *Helicobacter pylori,* and *Mycoplasma* and *Pneumocystis* infections. Onset of GBS symptoms usually occurs within 10 days of the primary infection. Pathologic changes in spinal and cranial nerves consist of inflammation and edema with rapid, segmented demyelination and compression of nerve roots within the dural sheath. Nerve conduction is impaired, producing ascending partial or complete paralysis of muscles innervated by the involved nerves. GBS has three phases (Sulton, 2002):

1. *Acute*—begins with onset of symptoms and continues until new symptoms stop appearing or deterioration ceases; may last as long as 4 weeks
2. *Plateau*—symptoms remain constant without further deterioration; may last from days to weeks
3. *Recovery*—patient begins to improve and progress to complete recovery; usually lasts a few days to a few weeks

Diagnostic Evaluation

Diagnosis of GBS is based on clinical manifestations (Box 55-10), cerebrospinal fluid (CSF) analysis, and EMG findings. CSF analysis reveals an increased protein concentration, and EMG shows evidence of acute muscle denervation; other laboratory studies are usually noncontributory. The symmetric nature of the paralysis helps differentiate this disorder from spinal paralytic poliomyelitis, which usually affects sporadic muscles.

BOX 55-10

Clinical Manifestations of Guillain-Barré Syndrome

Initial Symptoms
Muscle tenderness
Paresthesia and cramps (sometimes)
Proximal symmetric muscle weakness

Paralysis
Ascending paralysis from lower extremities
Frequently involves muscles of trunk, upper extremities, and those supplied by cranial nerves (especially facial)
Flaccid paralysis with loss of reflexes
May involve facial, extraocular, labial, lingual, pharyngeal, and laryngeal muscles
Intercostal and phrenic nerves:
Breathlessness in vocalizations
Shallow, irregular respirations

Other Manifestations
Tendon reflexes depressed or absent
Variable degrees of sensory impairment
Muscle tenderness or sensitivity to slight pressure
Urinary incontinence or retention and constipation

Therapeutic Management

Treatment of GBS is primarily supportive. In the acute phase, patients are hospitalized because respiratory and pharyngeal involvement may require assisted ventilation, sometimes with a temporary tracheotomy. Treatment modalities include aggressive ventilatory support, intravenous administration of immunoglobulin, and steroids; plasmapheresis and immunosuppressive drugs may also be used. Plasmapheresis has been shown to decrease the length of recovery in patients with severe GBS; however, it is expensive and side effects include hypotension, fever, chills, urticaria, and bradycardia (Sulton, 2002). Further evidence reports equal benefits to treatment of GBS with intravenous immunoglobulin administration or plasmapheresis; both sped up recovery time in studies reviewed (Hughes et al, 2003).

Course and Prognosis

Better outcomes are associated with younger age, no requirement for mechanical ventilatory assistance, slower progression of disease, normal peripheral nerve function on EMG, and treatment by plasmapheresis (Graf et al, 1999). Recovery usually begins within 2 to 3 weeks, and most patients regain full muscle strength; the recovery of muscle strength progresses in the reverse order of onset of paralysis, with lower extremity strength being the last to recover. Poor prognosis with subsequent residual effects in children is reportedly associated with the following: cranial nerve involvement, extensive disability at time of presentation, and intubation (Sarnat, 2004).

Almost all deaths are caused by respiratory failure; therefore early diagnosis and access to respiratory support are especially important. The rate of recovery is usually related to the degree of involvement, which may extend from a few

*3300 East Sunrise Drive, Tucson, AZ 85718; phone: 800-572-1717; Web site: www.mdausa.org. In Canada: 2345 Yonge Street, Suite 900, Toronto, Ontario M4P 2E5; phone: 416-488-0030, 800-567-2873; Web site: www.mdac.ca.

weeks to months. The greater the degree of paralysis, the longer the recovery phase.

Nursing Care Management

Nursing care is essentially supportive and is the same as that required for the child with immobilization and respiratory depression. The emphasis of care is on close observation to assess the extent of paralysis and on prevention of complications, including autonomic dysfunction (hypertension, orthostatic hypotension, syndrome of inappropriate antidiuretic hormone secretion, life-threatening dysrhythmias), respiratory dysfunction, fear and anxiety, and pain management (Sulton, 2002).

During the acute phase of GBS the child's condition should be carefully observed for possible difficulty in swallowing and respiratory involvement. The child's respiratory function is closely monitored, and oxygen source, appropriate-sized insufflation bag and mask, endotracheal intubation and suctioning equipment, tracheotomy tray, and vasoconstrictor drugs are kept available. Vital signs, including neurologic signs and level of consciousness, are monitored frequently. For the child who develops respiratory impairment, the care is the same as that for any child with respiratory distress requiring mechanical ventilation.

Respiratory care, should intubation be required, requires close monitoring of oxygenation status (usually by pulse oximetry and sometimes arterial blood gases), maintenance of an open airway with suctioning, and postural changes to prevent pneumonia. Children with oral and pharyngeal involvement may be fed via a nasogastric tube to ensure adequate feeding. Immobilization, which occurs with GBS, decreases gastrointestinal function; therefore attention to problems such as decreased gastric emptying, constipation, and feeding residuals require nursing assessment and appropriate collaborative interventions. Temporary urinary catheterization may be required; urinary retention is not uncommon, and appropriate assessment of urinary output is vital. Sensory impairment and paralysis in the lower extremities makes the child susceptible to skin breakdown; therefore attention should be given to meticulous skin care. A key to recovery in the child with GBS is the prevention of muscle and joint contractures, so passive range-of-motion exercises must be carried out routinely to maintain vital function. Although the child may have a generalized paralysis, cognitive function remains intact; therefore it is important for nursing care to involve communication with the child regarding procedures and treatments that may be frightening, especially if mechanical ventilation is required. Parents are encouraged to talk to the child and make eye and physical contact as much a possible to reassure the child during the illness.

Physical therapy is limited to passive range-of-motion exercises during the evolving phase of the disease. Later, as the disease stabilizes and recovery begins, an active physical therapy program is implemented to prevent contracture deformities and facilitate muscle recovery. This may include active exercise, gait training, and bracing.

Throughout the course of the illness, support of the child and parents is paramount. The usual rapidity of the paralysis and the long period of recovery greatly tax the emotional reserves of all family members. The parents and child benefit from repeated reassurance that recovery is occurring and from realistic information regarding the possibility of permanent disability. In the event of a residual disability, the family needs assistance in accepting and adjusting to the loss of function (see Chapter 41). The Guillain-Barré Syndrome Foundation International* is a nonprofit organization devoted to support, education, and research. It provides support to families of recovered persons, publishes informational literature and a newsletter, and maintains a list of practitioners experienced with the disease.

Tetanus

Tetanus, or *lockjaw,* is an acute, preventable, and often fatal disease caused by an exotoxin produced by the anaerobic, spore-forming, gram-positive bacillus *Clostridium tetani.* The disorder is characterized by painful muscular rigidity primarily involving the masseter and neck muscles. There are four requirements for the development of tetanus: (1) presence of tetanus spores or vegetative forms of the bacillus, (2) injury to the tissues, (3) wound conditions that encourage multiplication of the organism, and (4) a susceptible host.

Tetanus spores are found in soil, dust, and the intestinal tracts of human beings and animals, especially herbivorous animals. The organisms are more prevalent in rural areas but are readily carried to urban areas by the wind. The organisms are not invasive but enter the body by way of wounds, particularly a puncture wound, burn, or crushed area. They may enter through a very minor, unnoticed break in the skin, such as a thorn or needle prick, bee sting, or scratch. In the newborn, infection may occur through the umbilical cord, usually in situations in which infants are delivered in severely contaminated surroundings. The disease has the greatest incidence in months when persons are more involved in outdoor activities. Substance abusers are especially susceptible from poor injection technique and the use of street heroin, which is often mixed with quinine, a protoplasmic poison that favors the growth of the organism (American Academy of Pediatrics, Committee on Infectious Diseases, 2003).

Pathophysiology

When prevention efforts are not effective and conditions are favorable, the organisms proliferate and form potent exotoxins, one of which is tetanospasmin. Tetanospasmin affects the central nervous system to produce the clinical manifestations of the disease. The ideal conditions for growth of the organisms are devitalized tissues without access to air, such as wounds that have not been washed or kept clean and those that have crusted over, trapping pus beneath. The exotoxin appears to reach the central nervous system by way of either the neuron axons or the vascular system. The toxin becomes fixed on nerve cells of the anterior horn of the spinal cord and the brainstem. The toxin acts at the myoneural junction to produce muscular stiffness and lower the threshold for reflex excitability.

---

*PO Box 262, Wynnewood, PA 19096; phone: 610-667-0131; Web site: www.guillain-barre.com.

The incubation period for tetanus varies from 3 days to 3 weeks and averages 8 days; most cases occur within 14 days. In neonates it is usually 3 to 14 days. Shorter incubation periods have been associated with more heavily contaminated wounds, more severe disease, and a worse prognosis (American Academy of Pediatrics, Committee on Infectious Diseases, 2003).

The manner of onset varies, but the initial symptoms are usually a progressive stiffness and tenderness of the muscles in the neck and jaw. Eventually all voluntary muscles are affected (Box 55-11). As the child recovers from the disease, the paroxysms become less frequent and gradually subside. Survival beyond 4 days usually indicates recovery, but complete recovery may require weeks. The mortality rate is about 30%, but the disease is almost invariably fatal in the newborn. The incubation period is short, with the appearance of symptoms 3 to 10 days after exposure. The first symptom in the neonate is difficulty sucking, which progresses to total inability to suck, excessive crying, irritability, and nuchal rigidity (American Academy of Pediatrics, Committee on Infectious Diseases, 2003).

Therapeutic Management

Preventive measures are based on the immune status of the affected child and the nature of the injury. Specific prophylactic therapy after trauma is administration of *tetanus toxoid* (tetanus antitoxin [TAT] is no longer available in the United States) (see Immunizations, Chapter 36, for age-specific recommendations).

BOX 55-11

Clinical Manifestations of Tetanus

Initial Symptoms

Progressive stiffness and tenderness of muscles in neck and jaw
Characteristic difficulty in opening the mouth (trismus)
Risus sardonicus (sardonic smile) caused by facial muscle spasm

Progressive Involvement

Opisthotonic positioning
Boardlike rigidity of abdominal and limb muscles
Difficulty swallowing
High sensitivity to external stimuli (slight noise, gentle touch, or bright light):
- Trigger paroxysmal muscular contractions that last seconds to minutes
- Contractions recur with increased frequency until almost continuous (sustained tetanic)

Laryngospasm and tetany of respiratory muscles:
- Accumulated secretions
- Respiratory arrest
- Atelectasis
- Pneumonia

Other Aspects

Mentation unaffected; patient alert
Pain and distress are reflected in:
- Rapid pulse
- Sweating
- Anxious expression

Fever usually absent or only mild

The unprotected or inadequately immunized child who sustains a "tetanus-prone" wound (such as, but not limited to, wounds contaminated with dirt, feces, soil, and saliva; puncture wounds; avulsions; and wounds resulting from missiles, crushing, burns, and frostbite) should receive *tetanus immune globulin (TIG)*. Concurrent administration of both TIG and tetanus toxoid at separate sites is recommended both to provide protection and to initiate the active immune process. Completion of active immunization is carried out according to the usual pattern (American Academy of Pediatrics, Committee on Infectious Diseases, 2003). Antibiotic treatment with penicillin G (alternatively erythromycin or tetracycline in older children with allergy to penicillin) is important in the management of tetanus as an adjunct against *Clostridia* (Arnon, 2004).

Aggressive supportive care is necessary to treat tetanus in the acute phase. The acutely ill child is best treated in an intensive care facility, where close and constant observation and equipment for monitoring and respiratory support are readily available. A quiet environment is preferred to reduce external stimuli.

General supportive care, including maintenance of adequate fluid and electrolyte balance and caloric intake, is indicated. Indwelling oral or nasogastric feedings are used when necessary, but severe laryngospasm may require intravenous (IV) parenteral nutrition or gastrostomy feeding. Recurrent laryngospasm or excessive accumulation of secretions may require endotracheal intubation. TIG therapy to neutralize toxins is the most specific therapy for tetanus. Antibiotics are administered to control the proliferation of the vegetative forms of the organism at the site of infection. Local care of the wound by surgical débridement and cleansing helps reduce the numbers of proliferating organisms at the site of injury. The cleansing should be repeated several times during the first 48 hours, and deep, infected lacerations are usually exposed and débrided.

Diazepam (Valium) is the drug of choice for seizure control and muscle relaxation (Arnon, 2004), but lorazepam (Ativan) may be used in some cases. Other AEDs may be administered as well. Intrathecal baclofen, magnesium sulfate, dantrolene sodium, and midazolam may also be used in the management of tetanus (Arnon, 2004). Patients with severe tetanus and those who do not respond to other muscle relaxants may require the administration of a neuromuscular blocking agent, such as rocuronium or vecuronium. Because of their paralytic effect on respiratory muscles, use of these drugs requires mechanical ventilation with endotracheal intubation or tracheotomy and constant cardiopulmonary monitoring. Endotracheal tube insertion or tracheostomy is often indicated and should be performed before severe respiratory distress develops.

Nursing Care Management

In caring for the child with tetanus during the acute phase, every effort is made to control or eliminate stimulation from sound, light, and touch. Although a darkened room is ideal, sufficient light is essential so that the child can be carefully observed; light appears to be less irritating than vibratory or auditory stimuli. The infant or child is handled as little as possible, and extra effort is expended to avoid any sudden or loud noise to prevent seizures.

Medications are administered, and vital signs, including neurologic signs, are observed and recorded at frequent intervals. The location and extent of muscle spasms and assessment of their severity are important nursing observations. Respiratory status is carefully evaluated for any signs of distress, and appropriate emergency equipment is kept available at all times. Muscle relaxants, opioids, and sedatives that may be prescribed can also cause respiratory depression; therefore the child must be assessed for excessive central nervous system depression. Oxygen saturation is monitored, and when needed, blood gases are obtained to evaluate respiratory status. Attention to hydration and nutrition may involve monitoring an IV infusion, monitoring nasogastric or gastrostomy feedings, and suctioning oropharyngeal secretions when indicated.

If a muscle paralyzing agent such as vecuronium is used, the total paralysis (including respirations) makes oral communication impossible. The drug is not a sedative, however, and anxiety should be considered in children who are intubated. Therefore all of the child's needs must be anticipated and procedures carefully explained beforehand.

Because their mental status is clear, children with tetanus are aware of what is happening to them and are often in a state of terror. They should not be left alone, and all efforts should be made to reduce anxiety, which can contribute to muscular spasms. A calm and reassuring manner and sympathetic understanding can assist immeasurably in helping a child through this crisis. Parents are encouraged to stay with the child to offer security and support.

Botulism

Botulism is an acute flaccid paralysis caused by the preformed toxin produced by the anaerobic bacillus *Clostridium botulinum.* In classic or food-borne botulism, the most common source of the toxin is a contaminated food source. It was previously believed that home-canned foods were the most common source; however, this has been disproved in outbreaks associated with restaurant food. Other forms of botulism include wound botulism, infant botulism, and human-made botulism, usually a result of bioterrorism (Schechter & Arnon, 2004). In food-borne illness, central nervous system symptoms appear abruptly within a few hours or gradually over several days after ingestion of contaminated food and may not be preceded by acute digestive disturbance (Box 55-12).

Treatment consists of IV administration of botulism antitoxin and general supportive measures, primarily respiratory and nutritional. Toxins vary in protein-binding capacity. Some have a relatively short half-life and do not bind to tissues firmly; therefore therapy is continued until paralysis abates. Other toxins appear to bind irreversibly to nerve endings and are therefore not amenable to neutralization.

Infant Botulism

Infant botulism, unlike the disease in older persons, is caused by ingestion of spores or vegetative cells of *C. botulinum* and the subsequent release of the toxin from organisms colonizing the gastrointestinal tract. *C. botulinum* types A and B are the most common causative strains of infant botulism. These forms of botulism have become more prevalent than any other forms. There appears to be no common food or drug source of the organisms; however, the *C. botulinum* organisms have been found in honey and light or dark corn syrup fed to affected infants (American Academy of Pediatrics, Committee on Infectious Diseases, 2003). Botulism may occur in infants as young as 3 weeks of age or up to 6 months of age, with peak incidence between 2 and 4 months of age (Aneja, Thomas, & Elberger, 2000).

There is wide variation in the severity of the disease, from mild constipation to progressive sequential loss of neurologic function and respiratory failure (see Box 55-12). The affected infant is usually well before the onset of symptoms. Constipation is a common initial symptom, and almost all infants exhibit generalized weakness and a decrease in spontaneous movements. Deep tendon reflexes are usually diminished or absent; cranial nerve deficits are common, as evidenced by loss of head control, difficulty in feeding, weak cry, and reduced gag reflex. The most frequently recognized form of the disease is consistent with the hypotonic infant. Clinical signs often mimic those of sepsis in young infants. Botulism toxin exerts its effect by inhibiting the release of acetylcholine at the myoneural junction, thereby impairing motor activity of muscles innervated by affected nerves.

Diagnosis is made on the basis of the clinical history, physical examination, and laboratory detection of the organism in the patient's blood or stool. However, isolation of the organism may take several days; therefore suspicion of botulism by clinical presentation should involve emergent treatment (Schechter & Arnon, 2004). EMG may be helpful in establishing the diagnosis; however, results may be normal early in the course of the illness. Treatment consists of immediate administration of botulism immune globulin intravenous (BIGIV) (American Academy of Pediatrics, Committee on Infectious Diseases, 2003) after the diagnosis is

BOX 55-12

Clinical Manifestations of Botulism

General Signs
Weakness
Dizziness
Headache
Difficulty talking and speaking
Diplopia
Vomiting
Progressive, life-threatening respiratory paralysis

Infant Botulism*
Constipation (a common symptom)
Generalized weakness
Decrease in spontaneous movements
Diminished or absent deep tendon reflexes
Loss of head control
Difficulty feeding
Weak cry
Reduced gag reflex
Progressive respiratory paralysis

*Most commonly diagnosed as a "rule out sepsis" in the acute phase because of clinical presentation.

confirmed and supportive measures, primarily respiratory and nutritional management. Approximately 50% of affected infants will require intubation and mechanical ventilation. Trivalent equine botulinum antitoxin and bivalent antitoxin, used in adults and older children, is not administered to infants. A human-derived botulism antitoxin (BIGIV) has been recently evaluated and is now available for use in infants by the California Department of Health Services*; initial clinical trials are promising, and there was a decreased need for mechanical ventilation, decreased length of stay, and decreased requirement for tube feeding (Schechter & Arnon, 2004). Antibiotic therapy is not part of the management because the botulinum toxin is an intracellular molecule and antibiotics would not be effective; aminoglycosides in particular should not be administered because they may potentiate the blocking effects of the neurotoxin (Schechter & Arnon, 2004).

The prognosis is generally good if the patient is adequately treated, although recovery may be very slow, requiring a few weeks after severe illness; the average length of stay for infant botulism is 44 days, and the fatality rate is reported to be less than 2% (Cox & Hinkle, 2002). Untreated patients may require a longer hospitalization.

NURSE ALERT Honey should not be given to infants younger than 12 months old because *C. botulinum* spores, which cause infant botulism, have been isolated in the natural sweetener (Centers for Disease Control and Prevention, 2002). ■

Nursing Care Management

Nursing responsibilities include observing for and reporting signs of neuromuscular weakness or impairment and providing intensive nursing care when the infant is hospitalized. Parental support and reassurance are important (Community Focus box). Most infants recover when the disorder is recognized and therapy is implemented. Parents should be aware that during recovery, patients tire easily when muscular action is sustained. This has important implications for timing the resumption of feedings, because of the risk of aspiration. Parents should also be advised that normal bowel action may not return for several weeks; therefore a stool softener can be beneficial. Cathartics and enemas are not advised.

Community Focus

PREVENTING BOTULISM

Home supervision and education regarding possible modes of infection (such as the use of honey as formula sweetener or to coat a pacifier nipple) are nursing responsibilities. Because the prime sources of botulism toxin are usually inadequately cooked or improperly canned foods, families are advised about the danger of home-canned foods, especially vegetables, fruits, fish, and condiments. Improperly cooked seafood is a common source of botulism as well. Boiling is not always adequate, particularly at high altitudes, where water boils at a lower temperature, which does not destroy the organisms.

Spinal Cord Injuries

Spinal cord injuries (SCIs) with major neurologic involvement are not a common cause of physical disability in children. However, a significant number of children with these injuries are admitted to major medical centers, and because of the increased survival rate as a result of improved management, nurses are more likely to be involved in the care of children with SCIs.

Mechanisms of Injury

The most common cause of serious spinal cord damage in children is trauma involving motor vehicle crashes (MVCs) (including automobile-bicycle, all-terrain vehicles, and snowmobiles), sports injuries (especially from diving, trampoline activities, gymnastics, and football), birth trauma, and child abuse. The increased use of recreational activities involving motorized vehicles such as jet water skis, all-terrain vehicles, and motorcycles has also increased the incidence of SCIs in young children. Congenital defects of the spine such as myelomeningocele may, in some cases, produce the effects of SCI.

Transverse myelitis (inflammation of the spinal cord) has also been reported to develop from inadvertent intraarterial administration of long-acting penicillin injected into the buttocks. Damage can be extensive enough to result in paraplegia or even lower limb amputation.

In MVCs, most SCIs in children are a result of indirect trauma caused by sudden hyperflexion or hyperextension of the neck, often combined with a rotational force. Trauma to the spinal cord without evidence of vertebral fracture or dislocation (SCIWORA) is particularly likely to occur in an MVC when proper safety restraints are not used. An unrestrained child becomes a projectile during sudden deceleration and is subject to injury from contact with a variety of objects inside and outside the vehicle. Individuals who use only a lap seat belt restraint are at greater risk of spinal cord injury than those who use a combination lap and shoulder restraint. High cervical spine injuries have been reported in children younger than 2 years of age who are restrained in forward-facing car seats. Infants who are improperly restrained in an infant car seat may experience cervical trauma in an MVC. Small children may also be severely injured by deploying front seat air bags.

Falling from heights occurs less often in children than in adults, but vertebral compression from blows to the head or buttocks can occur in water sports (diving and surfing), falls from horses, or other athletic activities. Birth injuries may occur in breech deliveries from traction force on the spinal cord during delivery of the head and shoulders. An increasing number of adolescents receive SCIs secondary to gunshot wounds, stabbings, or other violently inflicted injury.

The injury sustained can affect any of the spinal nerves, and the higher the injury, the more extensive the damage. The child can be left with complete or partial paralysis of the lower extremities *(paraplegia)* or with damage at a higher level and without functional use of any of the four extremities *(quadriplegia)*. A high cervical cord injury that affects

*Phone: 510-540-2646 (24-hour telephone availability).

the phrenic nerve paralyzes the diaphragm and leaves the child dependent on mechanical ventilation.

A mild but equally frightening form of cord trauma is *spinal cord compression,* a temporary neural dysfunction without visible damage to the cord. Complete quadriplegia can result but initially may not be differentiated from serious cord injury.

Therapeutic Management

The management of the child with SCI has changed dramatically in the last two decades as a result of improved technology, surgical procedures, and research into the complexity of the spinal cord and its neurologic components. Initial care begins at the scene of the accident; therefore education and training of first responder personnel in spinal immobilization, stabilization, and transfer techniques to prevent or reduce the severity of injury is critically important. Evidence indicates that as many as one fourth of SCIs occur *after* the initial traumatic injury during transit or as a result of management during the early stages of the injury. Because of the complexity of these injuries, it is usually recommended that these persons be transported to a spinal injury center for care by specially trained health care personnel as soon as possible after the injury for appropriate diagnostic evaluation and intervention.

SCI management guidelines and standards of care have recently been published for adult and pediatric patients with spinal injuries by the American Association of Neurological Surgeons and the Congress of Neurological Surgeons. For information regarding these guidelines and a more in-depth review of SCI care, see Barker and Saulino (2002).

Nursing Care Management

The nursing care of the paraplegic or quadriplegic child is complex and challenging. A multidisciplinary SCI team is equipped to manage the acute phase of the injury, and some members, including the nurse, may follow the patient to eventual recovery. Nursing management is concerned with ensuring adequate initial stabilization of the entire spinal column with a rigid cervical collar with supportive blocks on a rigid backboard (Barker & Saulino, 2002). During the acute phase of the injury, it is imperative that airway patency be maintained and respiratory function monitored. It is important to evaluate the extent of the neurologic damage early to establish a baseline for neurologic functioning; continual assessment of function should occur to prevent further deterioration of neurologic status as a result of spinal cord edema. The American Spinal Injury Association (ASIA) Impairment Scale may be used to assess neurologic function on a routine basis during the patient's recovery (Barker & Saulino, 2002).

NURSE ALERT In any situation in which spinal cord injury is suspected or a possibility, the child should be calmed, reassured, and told not to move; no one should be allowed to move the child unless he or she is able to stabilize the entire spine. A rigid cervical collar is used to immobilize the cervical spine, and the child is placed supine on a rigid immobilization board. Infants and small children are removed in their car seats with cervical stabilization with towels if the proper rigid collar size is unavailable; no attempt should be made to take them out of the seat. ■

Additional nursing care is aimed at monitoring and maintenance of adequate systemic blood pressure, administration of pharmacologic agents such as methylprednisolone, and assessment for concomitant injuries or complications such as hemorrhage, which might hinder adequate recovery. Because SCI patients are particularly labile during the first few weeks after the injury, it is also important to monitor for cardiovascular complications and respiratory failure. When surgery is required, the nursing care for the child is the same as that with any other major surgery involving prolonged anesthesia and major organ or skeletal trauma; preoperative teaching using age-appropriate props is essential to helping the child understand postoperative equipment, monitoring procedures, and pain management. Patients with SCI and subsequent immobilization have the same needs as those mentioned in Chapter 54. During the recovery and rehabilitation phase, patients with SCI must be carefully monitored for complications of immobility such as deep vein thrombosis and pulmonary embolus.

The goals of rehabilitation include preparing the child and family to live at home and function as independently as possible. Treatment with *functional electrical stimulation (FES)* (an implantable electrical stimulator with leads attached to the paralyzed muscles or nerves) has allowed children with certain SCIs greater mobility and functional use of paralyzed muscles; FES enables these children to sit, stand, and walk with the aid of crutches, a walker, or other orthoses. Administration of pharmacologic agents such as clonidine hydrochloride may improve ambulation in patients with partial SCI, and exercise therapy through interactive locomotor training has been beneficial in helping some individuals with SCI regain ambulatory function (Kalb, 2003).

Key Points

- Clinical manifestations of cerebral palsy include delayed gross motor development; abnormal motor performance; alterations of muscle tone; abnormal postures; reflex abnormalities; and associated disabilities such as mental retardation, seizures, and sensory impairment.
- Therapy for cerebral palsy takes into account the nature of the physical disability, defects associated with the disorder, and interpersonal and social influences encountered by the affected child.
- Care of the infant and child with myelomeningocele is directed toward protecting the meningeal sac, preventing infection and skin breakdown, observing for signs of urologic and bowel complications, and planning appropriate interventions to optimize the child's development.
- Spinal muscular atrophy type 1 disease (Werdnig-Hoffmann disease) is characterized by progressive weakness and wasting of skeletal muscles caused by degeneration of anterior horn cells of the spinal cord.
- Muscular dystrophies are the greatest and most important cause of muscular dysfunction of childhood.
- Major complications of Duchenne muscular dystrophy include joint contractures, disuse atrophy, obesity, and respiratory and cardiac problems.

- Nursing care of the child with Guillain-Barré syndrome consists of monitoring vital signs, providing respiratory support and physical therapy, providing reassurance, and providing support to the child and family.
- Tetanus occurs when tetanus spores or vegetative bacilli enter a wound and multiply in a susceptible host.
- Infant botulism results from the release of toxins from *Clostridium botulinum* colonizing the gastrointestinal tract.
- Therapeutic management of spinal cord injury is directed toward immobilizing the entire spinal column at the scene of the traumatic event, safe transportation by health care personnel trained to transport possible spinal trauma victims, evaluating neurologic damage, preventing further neurologic damage, and implementing an aggressive rehabilitation program designed to help achieve independence and movement.

References

Albright AL et al: Long-term intrathecal baclofen therapy for severe spasticity of cerebral origin, *J Neurosurg* 98(2):291-295, 2003.

American Academy of Pediatrics, American College of Obstetricians and Gynecologists: *Neonatal encephalopathy and cerebral palsy: defining the pathogenesis and pathophysiology,* Washington, DC, 2003, American College of Obstetricians and Gynecologists.

American Academy of Pediatrics, Committee on Infectious Diseases, Pickering L (ed): *2003 red book: report of the Committee on Infectious Diseases,* ed 26, Elk Grove Village, IL, 2003, The Academy.

American Nurses Association: Position statement on latex allergy, *Okla Nurse* 42(4):32-33, 1997.

Aneja R, Thomas C, Elberger S: Early infantile botulism, *Emerg Med* 32(6):36-41, 2000.

Arnon SS: Tetanus *(Clostridium tetani).* In Behrman RE, Kliegman RM, Jenson HB (eds): *Nelson textbook of pediatrics,* ed 17, Philadelphia, 2004, WB Saunders.

Barker E, Saulino MF: Special report: first-ever guidelines for spinal cord injuries, *RN* 65(10):32-37, 2002.

Beezhold DH et al: Latex protein: a hidden "food" allergen? *Allergy Asthma Proc* 21(5):301-306, 2000.

Beroud C et al: Prenatal diagnosis of spinal muscular atrophy by genetic analysis of circulating fetal cells, *Lancet* 361(9362):1013-1014, 2003.

Birnkrant DJ: The assessment and management of the respiratory complications of pediatric neuromuscular diseases, *Clin Pediatr* 41(5):301-308, 2002.

Bothwell JE et al: Duchenne muscular dystrophy—parental perceptions, *Clin Pediatr* 41(2):105-109, 2002.

Brown JP: Orthopaedic care of children with spina bifida: you've come a long way, baby! *Orthop Nurs* 20(4):51-58, 2001.

Centers for Disease Control and Prevention: Kernicterus in full term infants—United States, 1994-1998, *MMWR* 50(23):491-494, 2001a.

Centers for Disease Control and Prevention: Knowledge and use of folic acid among women of reproductive age—Michigan, 1998, *MMWR* 50(10):185-189, 2001b.

Centers for Disease Control and Prevention: Botulism in the United States, 1899-1996. 2002. Internet document available at www.cdc.gov/ncidod/dbmd/diseaseinfo/botulism.pdf (accessed July 1, 2003).

Cox N, Hinkle R: Radiologic decision-making: infant botulism, *Am Fam Physician* 65(7):1388-1392, 2002.

Dabney KW, Lipton GE, Miller F: Cerebral palsy, *Curr Opin Pediatr* 9(1): 81-88, 1997.

Finnell RH, Gould A, Spiegelstein O: Pathobiology and genetics of neural tube defects, *Epilepsia* 44(suppl 3):14-23, 2003.

Frey L, Hauser WA: Epidemiology of neural tube defects, *Epilepsia* 44(suppl 3):4-13, 2003.

Gibson CS et al: Antenatal causes of cerebral palsy: associations between inherited thrombophilias, viral and bacterial infection, and inherited susceptibility to infection, *Obstet Gynecol Surv* 58(3):209-220, 2003.

Gomez-Merino E, Bach JR: Duchenne muscular dystrophy: prolongation of life by noninvasive ventilation and mechanically assisted coughing, *Am J Phys Med Rehabil* 81(6):411-415, 2002.

Graf WD et al: Outcome in severe pediatric Guillain-Barré syndrome after immunotherapy or supportive care, *Neurology* 52(7):1494-1497, 1999.

Green L, Greenberg GM, Hurwitz E: Primary care of children with cerebral palsy, *Clin Fam Pract* 5(2):1-21, 2003.

Grether JK et al: Intrauterine exposure to infection and risk of cerebral palsy in very preterm infants, *Arch Pediatr Adolesc Med* 157(1):26-32, 2003.

Han TR et al: Risk factors of cerebral palsy in preterm infants, *Am J Phys Med Rehabil* 81(4):297-303, 2002.

Henshaw SK: Unintended pregnancy in the United States, *Fam Plan Perspect* 30:24-29, 1998.

Hirose F, Farmer DL, Albanese CT: Fetal surgery for myelomeningocele, *Curr Opin Obstet Gynecol* 13(2):215-222, 2001.

Holmes NM et al: Fetal intervention for myelomeningocele: effect on postnatal bladder function, *J Urol* 166(6):2383-2386, 2001.

Holzbeierlein J et al: The urodynamic profile of myelodysplasia in childhood with spinal closure during gestation, *J Urol* 164(4):1336-1339, 2000.

Honein MA: Impact of folic acid fortification of the US food supply and occurrence of neural tube defects, *JAMA* 285(23):2981-2986, 2001.

Hughes RAC et al: Intravenous immunoglobulin for Guillain-Barré syndrome, *Cochrane Library* (2):CD002063, 2003.

Iannaccone ST: Spinal muscular atrophy, *Semin Neurol* 18(1):19-26, 1998.

Iannaccone ST, Burghes A: Spinal muscular atrophies, *Adv Neurol* 88:83-98, 2002.

Jacobs JM: Management options for the child with spastic cerebral palsy, *Orthop Nurs* 20(3):53-59, 2001.

Johnston MV: Cerebral palsy. In Behrman RE, Kliegman RM, Jenson HB (eds): *Nelson textbook of pediatrics,* ed 17, Philadelphia, 2004, WB Saunders.

Johnston MV: Encephalopathies. In Behrman RE, Kliegman RM, Jenson HB (eds): *Nelson textbook of pediatrics,* ed 17, Philadelphia, 2004, WB Saunders.

Johnston MV, Kinsman S: Congenital anomalies of the central nervous system. In Behrman RE, Kliegman RM, Jenson HB (eds): *Nelson textbook of pediatrics,* ed 17, Philadelphia, 2004, WB Saunders.

Kaefer M et al: Improved bladder function after prophylactic treatment of the high risk neurogenic bladder in newborns with myelomeningocele, *J Urol* 162(3 pt 2):1068-1071, 1999.

Kalb RG: Getting the spinal cord to think for itself, *Arch Neurol* 60(6): 805-808, 2003.

Kaufman BA: Neural tube defects, *Pediatr Clin North Am* 51(2):389-419, 2004.

Kellett PB: Latex allergy: a review, *J Emerg Nurs* 23(1):27-36, 1997.

Liddle A: Arizona announces updates to state food-safety health codes, *Nation's Restaurant News ,p.4,* Oct 8, 2001.

Lyerly AD, Mahowald MB: Maternal-fetal surgery for treatment of myelomeningocele, *Clin Perinatol* 30(1):155-165, 2003.

Matthews TJ, Honein MA, Erickson JD: Spina bifida and anencephaly prevalence—United States, 1991-2001, *MMWR Recomm Rep* 51(RR-13):9-11, 2002.

Mazon A et al: Latex sensitization in children with spina bifida: follow-up comparative study after two years, *Ann Allergy Asthma Immunol* 84: 207-210, 2000.

Metules T: Duchenne muscular dystrophy, *RN* 65(10):39-47, 2002.

Mitrofanoff P, Liard A: Bladder reconstruction and substitution. In Gearhart JP, Rink RC, Mouriquand PDE (eds), *Pediatric urology,* Philadelphia, 2001, Saunders.

National Association of Neonatal Nurses: Position statement on latex allergy, Central Lines, Jan 2000. Internet document available at www.nann.org (accessed May 26, 2005).

National Institute for Occupational Safety and Health: *NIOSH alert: preventing allergic reactions to natural rubber latex in the workplace,* 1997, DHHS pub no 97-135.

Nehring WM, Steele S: Cerebral palsy. In Jackson PL, Vessey JA (eds): *Primary care of the child with a chronic illness,* ed 2, St Louis, 1996, Mosby.

Occupational Safety and Health Administration: *Technical information bulletin—potential for allergy to natural rubber latex gloves and other natural rubber products,* April 12, 1999, US Department of Labor.

Olutoye OO, Adzick NS: Fetal surgery for myelomeningocele, *Semin Perinatol* 23(6):462-473, 1999.

Rintoul NE et al: A new look at myelomeningoceles: functional level, vertebral level, shunting, and the implications for fetal intervention, *Pediatrics* 109(3):409-413, 2002.

Roscigno CI: Addressing spasticity-related pain in children with spastic cerebral palsy, *J Neurosci Nurs* 34(3):123-131, 2002.

Russman BS: Function changes in spinal muscular atrophy II and III: the DCN/SMA group, *Neurology* 47(4):973-976, 1996.

Russman BS et al: Spinal muscular atrophy: new thoughts on the pathogenesis and classification schema, *J Child Neurol* 7(4):347-353, 1992.

Samaniego IA: A sore spot in pediatrics: risk factors for pressure ulcers, *Pediatr Nurs* 29(4):278-232, 2003.

Sarnat HB: Neuromuscular disorders. In Behrman RE, Kliegman RM, Jenson HB (eds): *Nelson textbook of pediatrics,* ed 17, Philadelphia, 2004, WB Saunders.

Schechter R, Arnon SS: Anaerobic bacterial infections: botulism *(Clostridium botulinum).* In Behrman RE, Kliegman RM, Jenson HB (eds): *Nelson textbook of pediatrics,* ed 17, Philadelphia, 2004, WB Saunders.

Smith J: Shaken baby syndrome, *Orthop Nurs* 22(3):196-203, 2003.

Sulton LL: Meeting the challenge of Guillain-Barré syndrome, *Nurs Manage* 33(7):25-30, 2002.

Suresh-Babu MV et al: Nutrition in children with cerebral palsy, *J Pediatr Gastroenterol Nutr* 26(4):484-485, 1998.

Szepfalusi Z et al: Latex sensitization in spina bifida appears disease-associated, *J Pediatr* 134(3):344-348, 1999.

Thompson GH, Berenson FR: Other neuromuscular disorders. In Morrissy RT, Weinstein SL (eds): *Lovell and Winter's pediatric orthopaedics,* ed 5, Philadelphia, 2001, Lippincott Williams & Wilkins.

Tubbs RS et al: Late gestational intrauterine myelomeningocele repair does not improve lower extremity function, *Pediatr Neurosurg* 38(3):128-132, 2003.

Tulipan N, Bruner JP: Myelomeningocele repair in utero: a report of three cases, *Pediatr Neurosurg* 28(4):177-180, 1998.

Volpe JJ: *Neurology of the newborn,* ed 4, Philadelphia, 2001, WB Saunders.

Wasiak J, Hoare B, Wallen M: Botulinum toxin A as an adjunct to treatment in the management of the upper limb in children with spastic cerebral palsy, *Cochrane Database Syst Rev* 2004(3):CD003469, 2004.

Watkins ML et al: Maternal obesity and risk for birth defects, *Pediatrics* 111(5 pt 2):1152-1158, 2003.

Winter S et al: Trends in the prevalence of cerebral palsy in a population-based study, *Pediatrics* 110(6):1220-1225, 2002.

Yerkes EB et al: The Malone antegrade continence enema procedure: quality of life and family perspective, *J Urol* 169(1):320-323, 2003.

Appendix

Relationship of Drugs to Breast Milk and Effect on Infant

A

The drugs listed in this appendix have been categorized by their major use. The ratings given are those published by the American Academy of Pediatrics (AAP) Committee on Drugs. These ratings label drugs that transfer into human milk. Drugs without a rating were not included in the AAP list. The ratings are described as follows:

1. Drugs that are contraindicated during breastfeeding
2. Drugs of abuse that are contraindicated during breastfeeding
3. Radioactive compounds that require temporary cessation of breastfeeding
4. Drugs with unknown effects on breastfeeding but may be of concern
5. Drugs that have been associated with significant effects on some breastfeeding infants and should be given to breastfeeding mothers with caution
6. Maternal medication usually compatible with breastfeeding
7. Food and environmental agents that have an effect on breastfeeding

DRUG	EXCRETED IN MILK	% ADULT DOSE IN MILK	AAP RATING	COMMENTS
ANALGESICS AND ANTIINFLAMMATORY DRUGS (Nonnarcotic)				
Acetaminophen (Datril, Tylenol, Darvocet, Comtrex, Excedrin)	Yes	0.04 to 1.85	6	Drug found in milk; drug and metabolite found in infant's urine
Aspirin (Bayer, Anacin, Bufferin, Excedrin, Fiorinal, Empirin, etc.)	Yes	0.5 to 21	5	Metabolized in liver.
Ibuprofen (Advil, Nuprin, Motrin, etc.)	Yes	<0.8	6	Metabolites are inert. Food slows absorption.
Indomethacin (Indocin)	Yes	0.07 to 0.98	6	Food delays absorption.
Ketorolac tromethamine (Toradal)	Yes	0.16 to 0.4	6	Food decreases rate but not amount of absorption
Mefenamic acid (Ponstel)	Yes	0.036 to 0.8	6	Infant able to excrete via urine.
Nalbuphine (Nubain)	Yes	<1	NR	Has active metabolites.
Naproxen (Naproxyn, Anaprox, Naprosyn, Aleve)	Yes	0.26 to 1.1	6	Food delays absorption.
Propoxyphene (Darvon, Wygesic)	Yes	Unknown	6	Metabolized in liver.

Compiled from Lawrence RA & Lawrence RM: *Breastfeeding: a guide for the medical profession*, ed 6, St Louis, 2005, Mosby.
NR = not rated.

Continued

DRUG	EXCRETED IN MILK	% ADULT DOSE IN MILK	AAP RATING	COMMENTS
ANTIINFECTIVES (may change intestinal flora of infant and sensitize for later allergic reaction)				
Acyclovir (Zovirax)	Yes	5.6 ± 4.4	6	Minimal absorption through skin.
Amoxicillin (Amoxil, Augmentin)	Yes	0.7	6	Dose-dependent oral availability.
Ampicillin (Polycillin, Amcill, Omnipen, Penbritin, Unasyn)	Yes	0.05 to 0.4	NR	In neonates, up to 12% plasma protein bound, oral availability increases.
Carbenicillin (Pyopen, Geopen, Geocillin)	Yes	0.001	NR	Drug is given to neonate. Not well absorbed from gastrointestinal (GI) tract.
Cefazolin (Ancef, Kefzol)	Yes	0.075	6	Detected in milk if given intravenously (IV).
Cephalexin (Keflex)	Yes	0.85 ± 0.35	NR	Completely gone by 8 hours; absorption less in first few months.
Cephalothin (Keflin)	Yes	0.4	NR	Higher volume of distribution in infant.
Chloramphenicol (Chloromycetin)	Yes	1.3 to 7.4	4	Possible idiosyncratic bone marrow depression.
Colistin (Coly-Mycin)	Yes	0.07	NR	Not absorbed orally.
Demeclocycline (Declomycin)	Yes		NR	Drug remains in milk 3 days after dose.
Erythromycin (Ilosone, E-Mycin, Erythrocin, Benzamycin)	Yes	0.1 to 2.1	6	Should not be given under 1 month of age because of risk of jaundice.
Gentamicin (Garamycin, G-Myticin)	Yes	Unknown	NR	Appreciable absorption in neonate.
Isoniazid (Nydrazid, INH, Rifamate)	Yes	2.3	6	Not detected in infant's blood but in urine.
Kanamycin (Kantrex)	Yes	0.95	6	Serum half-life in infant is inversely related to age.
Metronidazole (Flagyl, MetroGel, Protostat)	Yes	0.13 to 36	4	AAP says to discard milk for 12 hours if mother takes 2 g dose.
Nitrofurantoin (Furadantin, Macrodantin)	Yes	0.6	6	Caution needed in infants with glucose-6-phosphate dehydrogenase (G6PD) deficiency.
Novobiocin (Albamycin, Cathomycin)	Yes	0.15	NR	Infant can be given drug directly.
Nystatin (Mycostatin)	No	Not absorbed orally	NR	Can be given to infant directly.
Oxacillin (Prostaphlin, Bactocill)	Yes	Trace	NR	Displaces bilirubin from albumin in infants.
Penicillin G, benzathine (Bicillin)	Yes	0.8	NR	Best on empty stomach, increased in neonate.
Streptomycin	Yes	0.5	6	Is given to infants directly.
Sulfisoxazole (Gantrisin, Pediazole)	Yes	0.45	6	Jaundice may develop, avoid in infants with G6PD.
Tetracycline HCl (Achromycin, Panmycin, Sumycin)	Yes	0.03 to 4.8	6	Probably chelated by calcium in milk.
ANTICOAGULANTS				
Dicumarol (bishydroxy-coumarin), warfarin (Panwarfin)	Yes	0.5	NR	Not measureable in all milk samples. Has been associated with bleeding in breastfed infants.
Heparin	No	None	NR	Heparin ineffective orally.

Compiled from Lawrence RA & Lawrence RM: *Breastfeeding: a guide for the medical profession,* ed 6, St Louis, 2005, Mosby.

DRUG	EXCRETED IN MILK	% ADULT DOSE IN MILK	AAP RATING	COMMENTS
ANTICONVULSANTS AND SEDATIVES (barbiturates may pass into milk but do not sedate infant)				
Magnesium sulfate (Eldertonic, Vicon Forte)	Yes	0.5	6	May produce sedation in infant.
Pentobarbital (Nembutal)	Yes	Traces	NR	Depends on liver for detoxification so may accumulate in newborn.
Phenobarbital (Luminal, Donnatal, Tedral)	Yes	1.5	5	Sleepiness and decreased sucking possible.
Phenytoin (Dilantin)	Yes	1.4 to 7.2	6	No problem if mother's plasma concentration is in therapeutic range.
ANTIHISTAMINES (may suppress lactation; administer after breastfeeding; all pass into breast milk)				
Brompheniramine maleate (Dimetane, Dristan)	Yes	Unknown	NR	Well absorbed from GI tract.
Diphenhydramine (Benadryl)	Yes	Unknown	NR	Metabolism shows ethnic variation. Volume of distribution is greater in Asians than Caucasians.
Promethazine (Phenergan, Mepergan)	Yes	Unknown	NR	Passage into human milk is expected; increases serum prolactin level.
AUTONOMIC DRUGS				
Amphetamine (Adderall)	Yes	6.1 ± 0.1	2	Jitteriness, irritability, and sleepiness may be seen in nursing infants.
Atropine sulfate* (Donnatol, Lomotil, Urised)	Yes	Unknown	6	May inhibit lactation.
Ergotamine (Cafergot)	Yes	Unknown	5	May inhibit lactation. Vomiting, diarrhea, convulsions in infant.
Neostigmine (Prostigmin)	No	None	NR	Poorly absorbed from GI tract.
Propranolol (Inderal)	Yes	0.05 to 1	6	Risk of effect almost nonexistent; some Caucasians poor absorbers.
Propantheline bromide (Pro-Banthine)	No	Uncontrolled data indicate no measurable levels	NR	Activity of long-acting dose not studied.
CARDIOVASCULAR DRUGS				
Diazoxide (Hyperstat)	Unknown	Unknown	NR	Antihypertensive.
Digoxin (Lanoxin)	Yes	0.07 to 14	6	Not detected in infant's plasma.
Hydralazine (Apresoline)	Yes	0.8	6	Antihypertensive.
Methyldopa (Aldomet, Aldoril, Aldoclor)	Yes	0.02 to 0.09	6	Antihypertensive.
Nifedipine (Procardia)	Yes	0.00163 ± 0.00125	6	Calcium channel blocker. Minimal amount in milk.
Quinidine (Quinaglute)	Yes	4.1	6	May suppress prolactin secretion.
DIURETICS				
Chlorothiazide (Aldochlor, Diupres, Diuril)	Yes	Minimal	6	Absorption from GI tract is incomplete and dose dependent.
Furosemide (sulfamoylanthranilic acid) (Lasix)	Possible	Not found in all samples	NR	Drug is given to neonates under medical management.
Spironolactone (Aldactazide, Aldactone)	Yes	Unknown	6	80% of drug converted to canrenone.
GASTROINTESTINAL AGENTS				
Casanthranal (Peri-Colace)	Yes	Low	NR	Can cause diarrhea and colic in infant.
Cascara sagrada (Milk of Magnesia)	Yes	Low	6	May increase bowel activity in infant.
Senna (Senakot)	No	None	6	None.

*Atropine sulfate is an ingredient in many prescription and nonprescription drugs.

Continued

DRUG	EXCRETED IN MILK	% ADULT DOSE IN MILK	AAP RATING	COMMENTS
HORMONES AND CONTRACEPTIVES				
Cortisone (Cortone)	Yes	Significant amounts	NR	Probably OK to use as replacement therapy in Addison's disease.
Epinephrine (Adrenalin, EpiPen)	Yes	Unknown	NR	Destroyed in GI tract of infant.
Estradiol (Emcyt, Estrace)	Yes	0.004 to <10	6	
Estrogen	Yes	0.1	6	May alter quality and quantity of milk.
Insulin	No	None	NR	Not excreted in human milk.
Levonorgestrel (Norplant, Levlen, Triphasil)	Yes	1.1	6	Does not affect milk production.
Medroxyprogesterone acetate (Amen, Cycrin, Depo-Provera)	Yes	0.86 to 5	6	Increased prolactin level before and after sucking. 6-month injection may affect milk supply; 3-month injection should not decrease supply.
Prednisone (Deltasone)	Yes	0.15 ± 0.11	6	
Progesterone (Crinone, Prometrium, Cyclogest, Gesterol, Gestone)	Unknown	Unknown	6	In low doses, progesterone-only oral contraceptives are OK.
Propylthiouracil	Yes	0.03 to 2.6	6	Get baseline levels of T_3, T_4, TSH in infant before and 6 weeks after mother starts taking medication.
Thyroid and thyroxine (T_4)	Yes	0.3 to 2.0	6	Appears to protect infants of hypothyroid mothers who are breastfed.
Tolbutamide (Orinase)	Yes	18	6	Watch for jaundice.
NARCOTICS				
Cocaine	Yes	Significant levels in milk	2	No metabolites or drug found in milk after 36 hours or in infant's urine after 60 hours.
Codeine	Yes	5 ± 2	6	Chinese metabolize or less drug than Caucasians do.
Heroin	Yes	Significant	2	Level in milk enough to cause addiction in infant.
Marijuana (*Cannabis sativa* L.)	Yes	Unknown	2	Shown in laboratory animals to produce structural changes in nursling's brain cells. Infant at risk of inhaling smoke during feeding or when held by person who is smoking.
Meperidine (Demerol, Mepergan)	Yes	Unknown	6	Renal excretion of drug and metabolite is pH dependent.
Methadone	Yes	2.2	6	No signs in infant if mother getting less than 20 mg/24 hr. If more than that, withdrawal may be a problem. Suggest that mother take daily dose after evening feeding and supplement with formula at next feeding.
Morphine	Yes	0.8 to 1.2	6	Amounts in breast milk too variable to consider breastfeeding as means of treating withdrawal symptoms. May cause galactorrhea and prolactin increase.
Oxycodone	Yes	Unknown	NR	
PSYCHOTROPIC AND MOOD-CHANGING DRUGS				
Alcohol (Ethanol)	Yes	1 to 19.5	6	Milk may smell like alcohol. High amounts cause depression of milk-ejection reflex (dose dependent). Infant cannot metabolize ethanol.

Compiled from Lawrence RA & Lawrence RM: *Breastfeeding: a guide for the medical profession*, ed 6, St Louis, 2005, Mosby.

DRUG	EXCRETED IN MILK	% ADULT DOSE IN MILK	AAP RATING	COMMENTS
PSYCHOTROPIC AND MOOD-CHANGING DRUGS—cont'd				
Amitriptyline (Elavil, Etrafon, Triavil)	Yes	0.8 ± 0.2	4	Galactorrhea or prolactin increase.
Caffeine	Yes	0.66 to 2.3	6	Caffeine present in many hot and cold drinks. Consider if infant very wakeful.
Chlordiazepoxide (Librium)	Yes	Unknown	NR	May contribute to jaundice. May cause drowsiness.
Chlorpromazine (Thorazine)	Yes	0.07 to 0.2	4	Drowsiness and lethargy in infants.
Desipramine (Norpramin, Pertofrane)	Yes	1	4	Neither drug nor metabolite recovered from nursing infant's serum or urine. Some Caucasians are poor metabolizers.
Diazepam (Valium)	Yes	2 to 12	4	Sedation if fed 4 hr but not 8 hr after dose. More in evening milk.
Haloperidol (Haldol)	Yes	0.15 to 2	4	Causes prolactin increase. In animals, nurslings have behaviorial abnormalities. These effects not seen in humans.
Imipramine (Tofranil)	Yes	0.1	4	Causes galactorrhea and prolactin increase.
Lithium carbonate (Eskalith, Lithane, Lithonate)	Yes	1.8	5	Measurable lithium in infant's serum. Inhibits cAMP, which is significant for brain growth. Cyanosis, poor muscle tone, and ECG changes seen in breastfeeding infant.
Meprobamate (Miltown, Equanil)	Yes	Unknown	NR	Galactorrhea seen in some women.
Phencyclidine (PCP)	Yes	Unknown	2	Animal studies show PCP in milk even after drug has been discontinued for 40 days.
Theobromine	Yes	20	NR	Chocolate the most common cause of exposure. If mother consumes more than a pound a day, may see irritability or increased bowel activity.
Thioridazine (Mellaril)	Yes	Unknown	NR	Galactorrhea reported in some women.
Trifluoperazine (Stelazine)	Yes	Unknown	4	Excretion into milk not significant after therapeutic doses. Galactorrhea reported in some women. Increase in serum prolactin levels.
MISCELLANEOUS				
DPT	Yes	Minimum	NR	Does not interfere with immunization schedule.
Methotrexate (Folex, Rheumatrex)	Yes	0.93	1	Food delays absorption. Peaks at 19 hours in milk.
Nicotine	Yes	Unknown	NR	May suppress lactation. Decreased response of prolactin and oxytocin to suckling. Smoke exposure may be a concern.
Poliovirus vaccine	No	None	NR	Live vaccine taken orally. Not necessary to withhold breastfeeding.
Rh antibodies	Yes	Unknown	NR	Inactivated by gastric juices. Not a contraindication for breastfeeding.
Rubella virus vaccine	Yes	Minimum		Will not confer passive immunity.
Theophylline (Marax, Quibron, Theolair)	Yes	<1 to 15	6	Extremely low clearance in infants less than 6 months old.
Tuberculin test	Yes	Unknown	NR	Tuberculin-sensitive mothers can immunize their infants through breast milk. Immunity may last several years.

DPT, diphtheria, pertussis, tetanus

B Family Assessment

Family APGAR Questionnaire

PART I

The following questions have been designed to help us better understand you and your family. You should feel free to ask questions about any item in the questionnaire.

The space for comments should be used when you wish to give additional information or if you wish to discuss the way the question is applied to your family. Please try to answer all questions.

Family is defined as the individual(s) with whom you usually live. If you live alone, your "family" consists of persons with whom you now have the strongest emotional ties.*

For each question, check only one box

	Almost always	**Some of the time**	**Hardly ever**
I am satisfied that I can turn to my family for help when something is troubling me.	☐	☐	☐
I am satisfied with the way my family talks over things with me and shares problems with me.	☐	☐	☐
I am satisfied that my family accepts and supports my wishes to take on new activities or directions.	☐	☐	☐
I am satisfied with the way my family expresses affection and responds to my emotions, such as anger, sorrow, and love.	☐	☐	☐
I am satisfied with the way my family and I share time together.	☐	☐	☐

A

Comments (after each question): ____________________

*According to which member of the family is being interviewed the interviewer may substitute for the word "family" either spouse, significant other, parents, or children.

Fig. B-1 Family APGAR questionnaire; may be photocopied for clinical use. **A**, Part I. (Modified from Smilkstein G, Ashworth C, Montano D: Validity and reliability of the family APGAR as a test of family function, *J Fam Pract* 15(2):303-311, 1982.)

Family APGAR Questionnaire

PART II

Who lives in your home?* List by relationship (e.g., spouse, significant other,†child, or friend).

Please check below the column that best describes how you now get along with each member of the family listed.

Relationship	Age	Sex	Well	Fairly	Poorly
____________	__	__	☐	☐	☐
____________	__	__	☐	☐	☐
____________	__	__	☐	☐	☐
____________	__	__	☐	☐	☐
____________	__	__	☐	☐	☐
____________	__	__	☐	☐	☐

If you don't live with your own family, please list below the individuals to whom you turn for help most frequently. List by relationship, (e.g., family member, friend, associate at work, or neighbor).

Please check below the column that best describes how you now get along with each person listed.

Relationship	Age	Sex	Well	Fairly	Poorly
____________	__	__	☐	☐	☐
____________	__	__	☐	☐	☐
____________	__	__	☐	☐	☐
____________	__	__	☐	☐	☐
____________	__	__	☐	☐	☐
____________	__	__	☐	☐	☐

*If you have established your own family, consider home to be the place where you live with your spouse, children, or significant other; otherwise, consider home as your place of origin, e.g., the place where your parents or those who raised you live.

†"Significant other" is the partner you live with in a physically and emotionally nurturing relationship, but to whom you are not married.

Fig. B-1, cont'd **B**, Part II.

C Patterns of Inheritance

GLOSSARY

congenital The condition is present at birth. The disorder may be brought about by genetic causes, nongenetic causes, or a combination of these.

familial A disorder that "runs in families" or is present in more members of a family than would be expected by chance.

genetic The disorder is caused by a single harmful gene, by several genes, or by a deviation in chromosome number or structure. It may or may not be apparent at birth.

genotype The genetic constitution that determines the physical and chemical characteristics of an individual.

heterozygous Having dissimilar genes at a given position (locus) on a pair of chromosomes.

homozygous Having the same genes at a given position (locus) on a pair of chromosomes.

inherited (heritable, hereditary) Synonymous with *genetic,* although in the past often used to describe a disorder that appeared in parent and offspring over several generations.

mutation Structural or chemical alteration in genetic material that, when changed, remains changed and is transmitted to future generations. Mutations usually occur naturally *(spontaneous)*, or they can be *induced* by a variety of external agents, or *mutagens,* including temperature, certain chemicals, and radiation.

phenotype The physical or chemical characteristics of an individual, produced by the interaction of the environment with the genotype.

Modifications of Basic Inheritance Patterns

heterogeneity The same or similar manifestations that result from (1) different mutant genes at the same location on a chromosome or (2) mutant genes at different locations on a chromosome (such as the hemophilias, which produce defects in coagulation, and the muscular dystrophies, which produce muscular weakness) that exhibit different inheritance patterns.

linkage Some genes are located too close together on a chromosome, so they segregate and migrate together during cell division; therefore the characteristics they produce always appear together in the phenotype.

penetrance The regularity with which an inherited trait is manifested in the person who carries the gene. When a gene produces its effect on the phenotype each time it is present in the genotype, it is said to be *fully penetrant* or to exhibit *complete penetrance.* For example, achondroplasia (a form of dwarfism) is always evident whenever the gene is present. If a trait is not recognized in a person who carries the responsible gene, it is said to be *nonpenetrant* in that individual. This phenomenon accounts for what appears to be skipped generations.

pleiotropy The multiple, different, and seemingly unrelated effects associated with a particular disorder; the varied clinical features that constitute a syndrome. For example, Marfan syndrome, a disorder of the elastic fibers of connective tissue, may be manifested in an individual by any or all of the symptoms associated with it—aortic aneurysm, dislocation of the optic lens, or any of a number of skeletal deformities.

variable expressivity The degree of severity of, or the variability in, the manifestations seen in persons of a particular genotype. For instance, polydactyly can be expressed as any number of extra digits, or the extra digits may be fingers in one generation and toes in another. The severity of a disorder may be so mild as to be almost undetected or so severe that the affected individual is totally incapacitated.

Autosomal Dominant Inheritance

Characteristics of a condition caused by a dominant gene on an autosome include the following (Fig. C-1):

1. Males and females are affected with equal frequency.
2. Affected individuals have an affected parent (unless the condition is caused by a fresh mutation).
3. Half the children of a heterozygous affected parent will possess the defective gene, although it may be nonpenetrant.
4. Unaffected children of affected parents will have unaffected children (unless the gene is nonpenetrant).

		Affected parent	
	Gametes	A	a
Normal parent	a	A a Affected	a a Normal
	a	A a Affected	a a Normal

Fig. C-1 Possible offspring of mating between normal parent, aa, and parent with an autosomal dominant trait, Aa.

		Heterozygous parent A/a	
	Gametes	A	a
Heterozygous parent A/a	A	AA Normal	Aa Carrier
	a	Aa Carrier	aa Affected

Fig. C-2 Possible offspring of mating between two parents with a recessive gene, a, on an autosome.

Autosomal Recessive Inheritance

Characteristics of a condition caused by a recessive gene on an autosome include the following (Fig. C-2):

1. Males and females are affected with equal frequency.
2. Affected individuals have unaffected parents who are heterozygous for the trait.
3. There is a one in four chance that any child of two unaffected heterozygous parents will be affected.
4. Two affected parents will have affected children exclusively.
5. Affected individuals married to unaffected individuals will have normal children, all of whom will be carriers.
6. There is usually no evidence of the trait in previous generations—a negative family history.

X-Linked Dominant Inheritance

Characteristics of a condition caused by a dominant gene on an X chromosome include the following (Fig. C-3):

1. Affected individuals have an affected parent.
2. All the daughters but none of the sons of an affected male will be affected.
3. Half the sons and half the daughters of an affected female will be affected.
4. Normal children of an affected parent will have normal offspring.
5. There are no carriers.
6. The inheritance pattern shows a positive family history.

X-Linked Recessive Inheritance

Characteristics of a disorder caused by a recessive gene on the X chromosome include the following (Fig. C-4):

1. Affected individuals are principally males.
2. Affected individuals have unaffected parents (except in the rare possibility that the father is affected and the mother is a carrier).
3. Half of the female siblings of an affected male will be carriers of the trait.
4. Unaffected male siblings of an affected male cannot transmit the disorder.
5. Sons of an affected male are unaffected.
6. Daughters of an affected male are carriers.
7. The unaffected male children of a carrier female do not transmit the disorder.

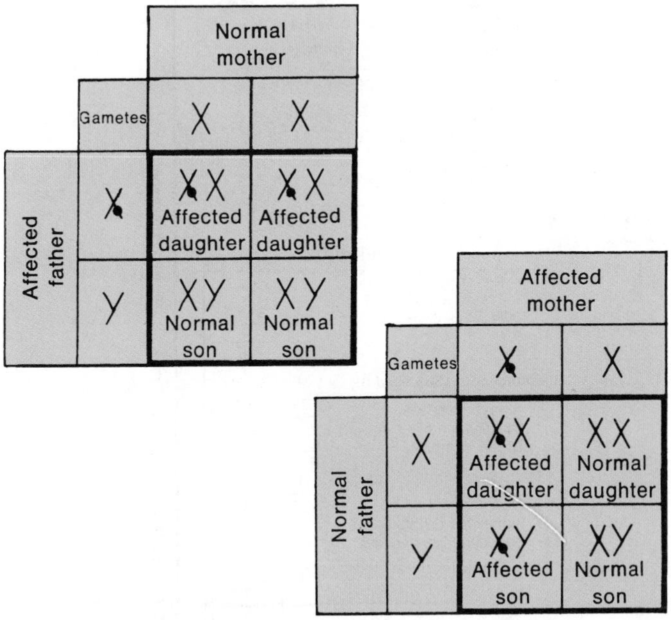

Fig. C-3 Sex differences in offspring ratios in X-linked dominant inheritance. ●, Dominant allele on X chromosome.

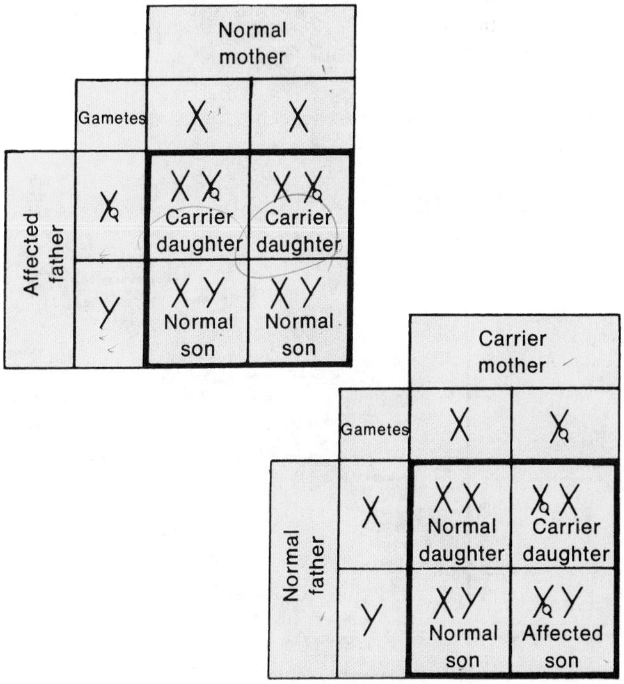

Fig. C-4 Differences in offspring ratios in X-linked recessive inheritance. ○, Recessive allele on X chromosome.

D Developmental/Sensory Assessment

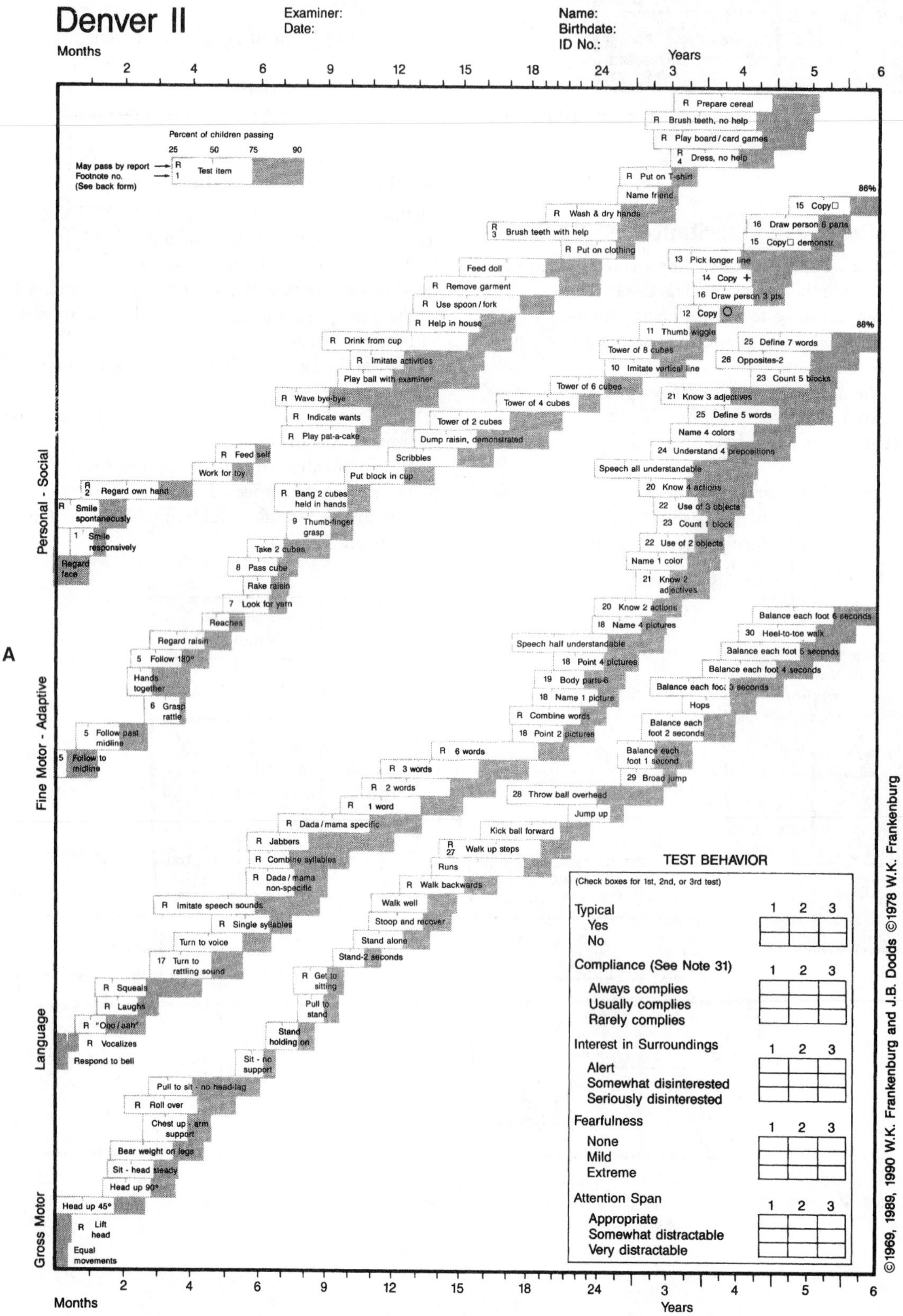
Denver II
Examiner:
Date:
Name:
Birthdate:
ID No.:
Months
Years
2
4
6
9
12
15
18
24
3
4
5
6
Percent of children passing
25
50
75
90
May pass by report
Footnote no.
(See back form)
R
1
Test item
R Prepare cereal
R Brush teeth, no help
R Play board/card games
R 4 Dress, no help
R Put on T-shirt
Name friend
R Wash & dry hands
R 3 Brush teeth with help
R Put on clothing
Feed doll
R Remove garment
R Use spoon/fork
R Help in house
R Drink from cup
R Imitate activities
Play ball with examiner
R Wave bye-bye
R Indicate wants
R Play pat-a-cake
R Feed self
Work for toy
R 2 Regard own hand
R Smile spontaneously
1 Smile responsively
Regard face
86%
15 Copy □
16 Draw person 6 parts
15 Copy □ demonstr.
13 Pick longer line
14 Copy +
16 Draw person 3 pts.
12 Copy ○
11 Thumb wiggle
Tower of 8 cubes
10 Imitate vertical line
Tower of 6 cubes
Tower of 4 cubes
Tower of 2 cubes
Dump raisin, demonstrated
Scribbles
Put block in cup
R Bang 2 cubes held in hands
9 Thumb-finger grasp
Take 2 cubes
8 Pass cube
Rake raisin
7 Look for yarn
Reaches
Regard raisin
5 Follow 180°
Hands together
6 Grasp rattle
5 Follow past midline
5 Follow to midline
88%
25 Define 7 words
26 Opposites-2
23 Count 5 blocks
21 Know 3 adjectives
25 Define 5 words
Name 4 colors
24 Understand 4 prepositions
Speech all understandable
20 Know 4 actions
22 Use of 3 objects
23 Count 1 block
22 Use of 2 objects
Name 1 color
21 Know 2 adjectives
20 Know 2 actions
18 Name 4 pictures
Speech half understandable
18 Point 4 pictures
19 Body parts-6
18 Name 1 picture
R Combine words
18 Point 2 pictures
R 6 words
R 3 words
R 2 words
R 1 word
R Dada/mama specific
R Jabbers
R Combine syllables
R Dada/mama non-specific
R Imitate speech sounds
R Single syllables
Turn to voice
17 Turn to rattling sound
R Squeals
R Laughs
R "Ooo/aah"
R Vocalizes
Respond to bell
Balance each foot 6 seconds
30 Heel-to-toe walk
Balance each foot 5 seconds
Balance each foot 4 seconds
Balance each foot 3 seconds
Hops
Balance each foot 2 seconds
Balance each foot 1 second
29 Broad jump
28 Throw ball overhead
Jump up
Kick ball forward
R 27 Walk up steps
Runs
R Walk backwards
Walk well
Stoop and recover
Stand alone
Stand-2 seconds
R Get to sitting
Pull to stand
Stand holding on
Sit - no support
Pull to sit - no head-lag
R Roll over
Chest up - arm support
Bear weight on legs
Sit - head steady
Head up 90°
Head up 45°
R Lift head
Equal movements
A
Personal - Social
Fine Motor - Adaptive
Language
Gross Motor
TEST BEHAVIOR
(Check boxes for 1st, 2nd, or 3rd test)
Typical
Yes
No
Compliance (See Note 31)
Always complies
Usually complies
Rarely complies
Interest in Surroundings
Alert
Somewhat disinterested
Seriously disinterested
Fearfulness
None
Mild
Extreme
Attention Span
Appropriate
Somewhat distractable
Very distractable
1 2 3
©1969, 1989, 1990 W.K. Frankenburg and J.B. Dodds ©1978 W.K. Frankenburg

Fig. D-1 **A**, Denver II. (From W. K. Frankenburg and J. B. Dodds, 1990.)

DIRECTIONS FOR ADMINISTRATION

1. Try to get child to smile by smiling, talking or waving. Do not touch him/her.
2. Child must stare at hand several seconds.
3. Parent may help guide toothbrush and put toothpaste on brush.
4. Child does not have to be able to tie shoes or button/zip in the back.
5. Move yarn slowly in an arc from one side to the other, about 8" above child's face.
6. Pass if child grasps rattle when it is touched to the backs or tips of fingers.
7. Pass if child tries to see where yarn went. Yarn should be dropped quickly from sight from tester's hand without arm movement.
8. Child must transfer cube from hand to hand without help of body, mouth, or table.
9. Pass if child picks up raisin with any part of thumb and finger.
10. Line can vary only 30 degrees or less from tester's line.
11. Make a fist with thumb pointing upward and wiggle only the thumb. Pass if child imitates and does not move any fingers other than the thumb.

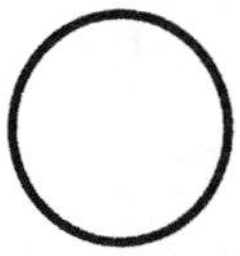

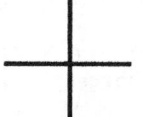

12. Pass any enclosed form. Fail continuous round motions.

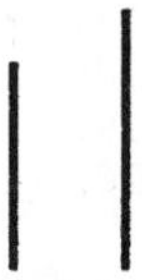

13. Which line is longer? (Not bigger.) Turn paper upside down and repeat. (pass 3 of 3 or 5 of 6)

14. Pass any lines crossing near midpoint.

15. Have child copy first. If failed, demonstrate.

When giving items 12, 14, and 15, do not name the forms. Do not demonstrate 12 and 14.

16. When scoring, each pair (2 arms, 2 legs, etc.) counts as one part.
17. Place one cube in cup and shake gently near child's ear, but out of sight. Repeat for other ear.
18. Point to picture and have child name it. (No credit is given for sounds only.)
    If less than 4 pictures are named correctly, have child point to picture as each is named by tester.

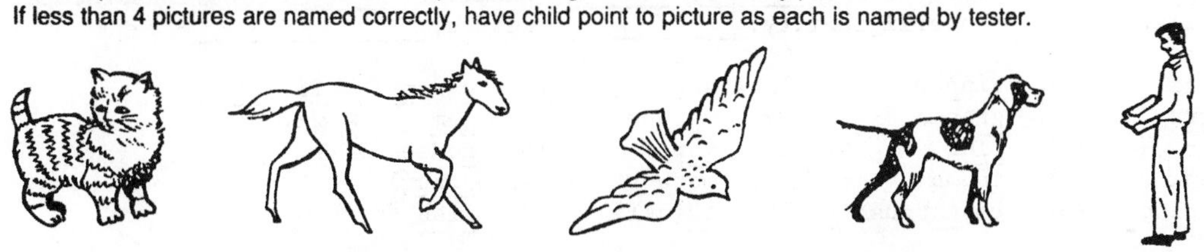

19. Using doll, tell child: Show me the nose, eyes, ears, mouth, hands, feet, tummy, hair. Pass 6 of 8.
20. Using pictures, ask child: Which one flies?... says meow?... talks?... barks?... gallops? Pass 2 of 5, 4 of 5.
21. Ask child: What do you do when you are cold?... tired?... hungry? Pass 2 of 3, 3 of 3.
22. Ask child: What do you do with a cup? What is a chair used for? What is a pencil used for?
    Action words must be included in answers.
23. Pass if child correctly places <u>and</u> says how many blocks are on paper. (1, 5).
24. Tell child: Put block **on** table; **under** table; **in front of** me, **behind** me. Pass 4 of 4.
    (Do not help child by pointing, moving head or eyes.)
25. Ask child: What is a ball?... lake?... desk?... house?... banana?... curtain?... fence?... ceiling? Pass if defined in terms of use, shape, what it is made of, or general category (such as banana is fruit, not just yellow). Pass 5 of 8, 7 of 8.
26. Ask child: If a horse is big, a mouse is __? If fire is hot, ice is __? If the sun shines during the day, the moon shines during the __? Pass 2 of 3.
27. Child may use wall or rail only, not person. May not crawl.
28. Child must throw ball overhand 3 feet to within arm's reach of tester.
29. Child must perform standing broad jump over width of test sheet (8 1/2 inches).
30. Tell child to walk forward, ∞∞∞∞→ heel within 1 inch of toe. Tester may demonstrate.
    Child must walk 4 consecutive steps.
31. In the second year, half of normal children are non-compliant.

OBSERVATIONS:

B

Fig. D-1, cont'd **B,** Directions for administration of numbered items on Denver II. (From W. K. Frankenburg and J. B. Dodds, 1990.)

DENVER ARTICULATION SCREENING EXAM
for children 2½ to 6 years of age

Instructions: Have child repeat each word after you. Circle the underlined sounds that he pronounces correctly. Total correct sounds is the Raw Score. Use charts on reverse side to score results.

Name:

Hosp. No.:

Address: ______________________
____

Date: __________ Child's age: __________ Examiner: __________ Raw score: ____
Percentile: ______ Intelligibility: __________ Result: __________

1. table	6. zipper	11. sock	16. wagon	21. leaf
2. shirt	7. grapes	12. vacuum	17. gum	22. carrot
3. door	8. flag	13. yarn	18. house	
4. trunk	9. thumb	14. mother	19. pencil	
5. jumping	10. toothbrush	15. twinkle	20. fish	

Intelligibility: (circle one)
1. Easy to understand
2. Understandable ½ the time
3. Not understandable
4. Can't evaluate

Comments:

A

Date: __________ Child's age: __________ Examiner: __________ Raw score: ____
Percentile: ______ Intelligibility: __________ Result: __________

1. table	6. zipper	11. sock	16. wagon	21. leaf
2. shirt	7. grapes	12. vacuum	17. gum	22. carrot
3. door	8. flag	13. yarn	18. house	
4. trunk	9. thumb	14. mother	19. pencil	
5. jumping	10. toothbrush	15. twinkle	20. fish	

Intelligibility: (circle one)
1. Easy to understand
2. Understandable ½ the time
3. Not understandable
4. Can't evaluate

Comments:

Date: __________ Child's age: __________ Examiner: __________ Raw score ____
Percentile: ______ Intelligibility: __________ Result: __________

1. table	6. zipper	11. sock	16. wagon	21. leaf
2. shirt	7. grapes	12. vacuum	17. gum	22. carrot
3. door	8. flag	13. yarn	18. house	
4. trunk	9. thumb	14. mother	19. pencil	
5. jumping	10. toothbrush	15. twinkle	20. fish	

Intelligibility: (circle one)
1. Easy tc understand
2. Understandable ½ the time
3. Not understandable
4. Can't evaluate

Fig. D-2 **A**, Denver Articulation Screening Examination (DASE) for children 2½ to 6 years of age. (From A. F. Drumwright, University of Colorado Medical Center, 1971.)

To score DASE words: Note raw score for child's performance. Match raw score line (extreme left of chart) with column representing child's age (to the closest previous age group). Where raw score line and age column meet number in that square denotes percentile rank of child's performance when compared to other children that age. Percentiles above heavy line are ABNORMAL percentiles, below heavy line are NORMAL.

PERCENTILE RANK

Raw Score	2.5 yr.	3.0	3.5	4.0	4.5	5.0	5.5	6 years
2	1							
3	2							
4	5							
5	9							
6	16							
7	23							
8	31	2						
9	37	4	1					
10	42	6	2					
11	48	7	4					
12	54	9	6	1	1			
13	58	12	9	2	3	1	1	
14	62	17	11	5	4	2	2	
15	68	23	15	9	5	3	2	
16	75	31	19	12	5	4	3	
17	79	38	25	15	6	6	4	
18	83	46	31	19	8	7	4	
19	86	51	38	24	10	9	5	1
20	89	58	45	30	12	11	7	3
21	92	65	52	36	15	15	9	4
22	94	72	58	43	18	19	12	5
23	96	77	63	50	22	24	15	7
24	97	82	70	58	29	29	20	15
25	99	87	78	66	36	34	26	17
26	99	91	84	75	46	43	34	24
27		94	89	82	57	54	44	34
28		96	94	88	70	68	59	47
29		98	98	94	84	84	77	68
30		100	100	100	100	100	100	100

B

To score intelligibility:

	NORMAL	ABNORMAL
2½ years	Understandable ½ the time, or, "easy"	Not understandable
3 years and older	Easy to understand	Understandable ½ time Not understandable

Test result: 1. NORMAL on DASE and Intelligibility = NORMAL

2. ABNORMAL on DASE and/or Intelligibility = ABNORMAL

*If abnormal on initial screening, rescreen within 2 weeks.
If abnormal again, child should be referred for complete speech evaluation.

Fig. D-2, cont'd **B**, Percentile rank. (From A. F. Drumwright, University of Colorado Medical Center, 1971.)

DENVER EYE SCREENING TEST

Name:
Hospital No.:
Ward:
Address:

	1ST SCREENING: DATE:						RESCREENING: DATE:					
	Right Eye			Left Eye			Right Eye			Left Eye		
Vision Tests	Normal	Abnormal	Untestable	Normal	Abnormal	Untestable	Normal	Abnormal	Untestable	Normal	Abnormal	Untestable
1. "E" (3 years and above—3 to 5 trials)	3P	3F	U	3P	3F	U	3P	3F	U	3P	3F	U
2. Picture card (2 1/2 - 2 11/12 yrs.—3 to 5 trials)	3P	3F	U	3P	3F	U	3P	3F	U	3P	3F	U
3. Fixation (6 months - 2 5/12 years)	P	F	U	P	F	U	P	F	U	P	F	U
4. Squinting		yes			yes			yes			yes	

Tests for Non-Straight Eyes	Normal	Abnormal	Untestable	Normal	Abnormal	Untestable
1. Do your child's eyes turn in or out, or are they ever not straight?	NO	YES	U	NO	YES	U
2. Cover Test	P	F	U	P	F	U
3. Pupillary Light Reflex	P	F	U	P	F	U

Total Test Rating (Both Eyes)		
Normal (passed vision test plus no squint, plus passed 2/3 tests for non-straight eyes)	Normal	Normal
Abnormal (abnormal on any vision test, squinting or 2 of 3 procedures for non-straight eyes)	Abnormal	Abnormal
Untestable (untestable on any vision test or untestable on 2/3 tests for non-straight eyes)	Untestable	Untestable
Future Rescreening Appointment for Total Test Rating (Abnormal or Untestable)	Date:	Date:

Fig. D-3 Denver Eye Screening Test. (From W. K. Frankenburg and J. B. Dodds, University of Colorado Medical Center, 1969.)

SNELLEN SCREENING*

Preparation

1. Hang the Snellen chart on a light-colored wall so that the 20- to 30-foot lines are at eye level when children 6 to 12 years old are tested in the standing position (Fig. D-4).
2. Secure the chart to the wall with double-stick tape on the back side of all four corners. If the chart must be reversed for use of letter or E chart, secure it at the top and bottom with tacks. Make sure that the chart does not swing when in place.
3. The illumination intensity on the chart should be 10 to 30 foot candles, without any glare from windows or light fixtures. The illumination should be checked with a light meter.
4. Mark an exact 20-foot distance from the chart. Mark the floor with a piece of tape or "footprints" positioned so that the heels touch the 20-foot line.

Procedure

1. Place the child at the 20-foot mark, with the heel edging the line if the child is standing or with the back of the chair placed at the marker if the child is seated.
2. If the E chart is used, accustom the child to identifying which direction the "legs of the E" are pointing. Use a demonstration E card for this purpose.
3. Teach the child to use the occluder to cover one eye. Instruct the child to keep both eyes open during the test. Provide a clean cover card for each child and then discard after use.
4. If the child wears glasses, test only with glasses on.
5. Test both eyes together, then the right eye, then the left eye.
6. Begin with the 40- or 30-foot line and proceed with the test to include the 20-foot line.
7. With a child suspected of low vision, begin with the 200-foot line, and proceed until child can no longer correctly read three out of four or four out of six symbols on a line.
8. Use covers on the Snellen chart to expose only one symbol or one line at a time. When screening kindergarten or older children, expose one line but use a pointer to point to one symbol at a time.

*Modified from recommendations of the National Society to Prevent Blindness: *Guide to testing distance visual acuity,* Schaumburg, IL, 1988, The Society.

Recording and Referral

1. Record the last line the child read correctly (three out of four or four out of six symbols).
2. Record visual acuity as a fraction. The numerator represents the distance from the chart, and the denominator represents the last line read correctly. For example, 20/30 means that the child read the 30-foot line at a 20-foot distance.
3. Observe the child's eyes during testing and record any evidence of squinting, head tilting, thrusting the head forward, excessive blinking, tearing, or redness.
4. Only make referrals after a second screening has been made on children who are potential candidates for referral.
5. The following children should be referred for a complete eye examination:
   a. Three-year-old children with vision in either eye of 20/50 or less (inability to correctly identify one more than half the symbols on the 40-foot line) *or* a two-line difference in visual acuity between the eyes in the passing range (e.g., 20/20 in one eye and 20/40 in the other)
   b. All other ages and grades with vision in either eye of 20/40 or less (inability to correctly identify one or more than half the symbols on the 30-foot line)
   c. All children who consistently show any of the signs of possible visual disturbances, regardless of visual acuity

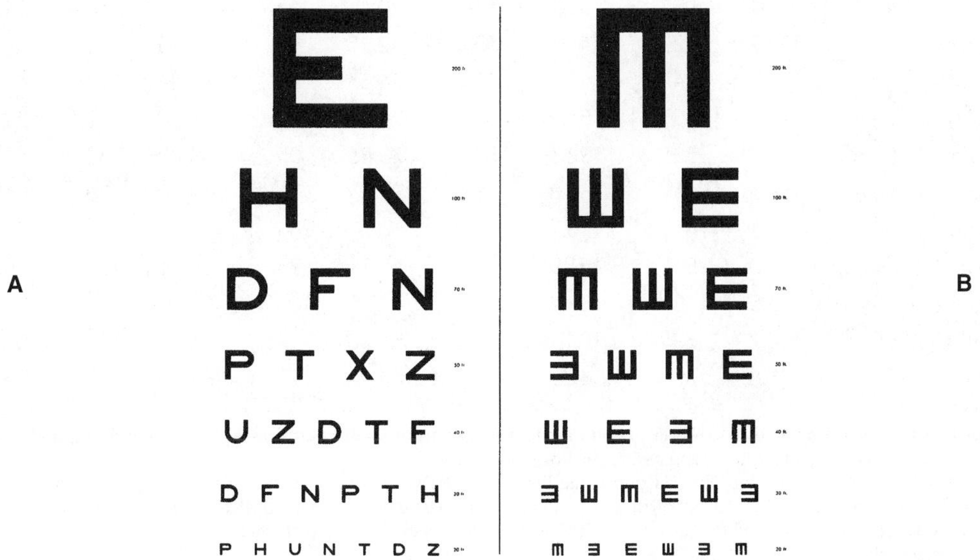

Fig. D-4 Snellen chart. **A**, Letter (alphabet) chart. **B**, Symbol E chart. (From National Society to Prevent Blindness, Inc., Schaumburg, IL.)

Appendix

E Growth Measurements

HEIGHT AND WEIGHT MEASUREMENTS FOR BOYS

	Height by Percentiles						Weight by Percentiles					
	5		50		95		5		50		95	
AGE*	cm	INCHES	cm	INCHES	cm	INCHES	kg	lb	kg	lb	kg	lb
Birth	46.4	18¼	50.5	20	54.4	21½	2.54	5½	3.27	7¼	4.15	9¼
3 months	56.7	22¼	61.1	24	65.4	25¾	4.43	9¾	5.98	13¼	7.37	16¼
6 months	63.4	25	67.8	26¾	72.3	28½	6.20	13¾	7.85	17¼	9.46	20¾
9 months	68.0	26¾	72.3	28½	77.1	30¼	7.52	16½	9.18	20¼	10.93	24
1	71.7	28¼	76.1	30	81.2	32	8.43	18½	10.15	22½	11.99	26½
1½	77.5	30½	82.4	32½	88.1	34¾	9.59	21¼	11.47	25¼	13.44	29½
2†	82.5	32½	86.8	34¼	94.4	37¼	10.49	23¼	12.34	27¼	15.50	34¼
2½†	85.4	33½	90.4	35½	97.8	38½	11.27	24¾	13.52	29¾	16.61	36½
3	89.0	35	94.9	37¼	102.0	40¼	12.05	26½	14.62	32¼	7.77	39¼
3½	92.5	36½	99.1	39	106.1	41¾	12.84	28¼	15.68	34½	18.98	41¾
4	95.8	37¾	102.9	40½	109.9	43¼	13.64	30	16.69	36¾	20.27	44¾
4½	98.9	39	106.6	42	113.5	44¾	14.45	31¾	17.69	39	21.63	47¾
5	102.0	40¼	109.9	43¼	117.0	46	15.27	33¾	18.67	41¼	23.09	51
6	107.7	42½	116.1	45¾	123.5	48½	16.93	37¼	20.69	45½	26.34	58
7	113.0	44½	121.7	48	129.7	51	18.64	41	22.85	50¼	30.12	66½
8	118.1	46½	127.0	50	135.7	53½	20.40	45	25.30	55¾	34.51	76
9	122.9	48½	132.2	52	141.8	55¾	22.25	49	28.13	62	39.58	87¼
10	127.7	50¼	137.5	54¼	148.1	58¼	24.33	53¾	31.44	69¼	45.27	99¾
11	132.6	52¼	143.3	56½	154.9	61	26.80	59	35.30	77¾	51.47	113½
12	137.6	54¼	149.7	59	162.3	64	29.85	65¾	39.78	87¾	58.09	128
13	142.9	56¼	156.5	61½	169.8	66¾	33.64	74¼	44.95	99	65.02	143¼
14	148.8	58½	163.1	64¼	176.7	69½	38.22	84¼	50.77	112	72.13	159
15	155.2	61	169.0	66½	181.9	71½	43.11	95	56.71	125	79.12	174½
16	161.1	63½	173.5	68¼	185.4	73	47.74	105¼	62.10	137	85.62	188¾
17	164.9	65	176.2	69¼	187.3	73¾	51.50	113½	66.31	146¼	91.31	201¼
18	165.7	65¼	176.8	69½	187.6	73¾	53.97	119	68.88	151¾	95.76	211

Modified from National Center for Health Statistics (NCHS), Health Resources Administration, Department of Health, Education, and Welfare, Hyattsville, MD. Conversion of metric data to approximate inches and pounds by Ross Laboratories.

AUTHOR'S NOTE: As of this writing, the Centers for Disease Control and Prevention (CDC), National Center for Health Statistics (NCHS), has published revised growth charts for the United States. The 14 NCHS growth charts and new body mass index–for–age (BMI-for-age) charts are available for boys and girls from birth to age 20 years. The growth charts can be printed from the CDC Web site: www.cdc.gov/growthcharts.

*Years unless otherwise indicated.

†Height data include some recumbent length measurements, which make values slightly higher than if all measurements had been of stature (standing height).

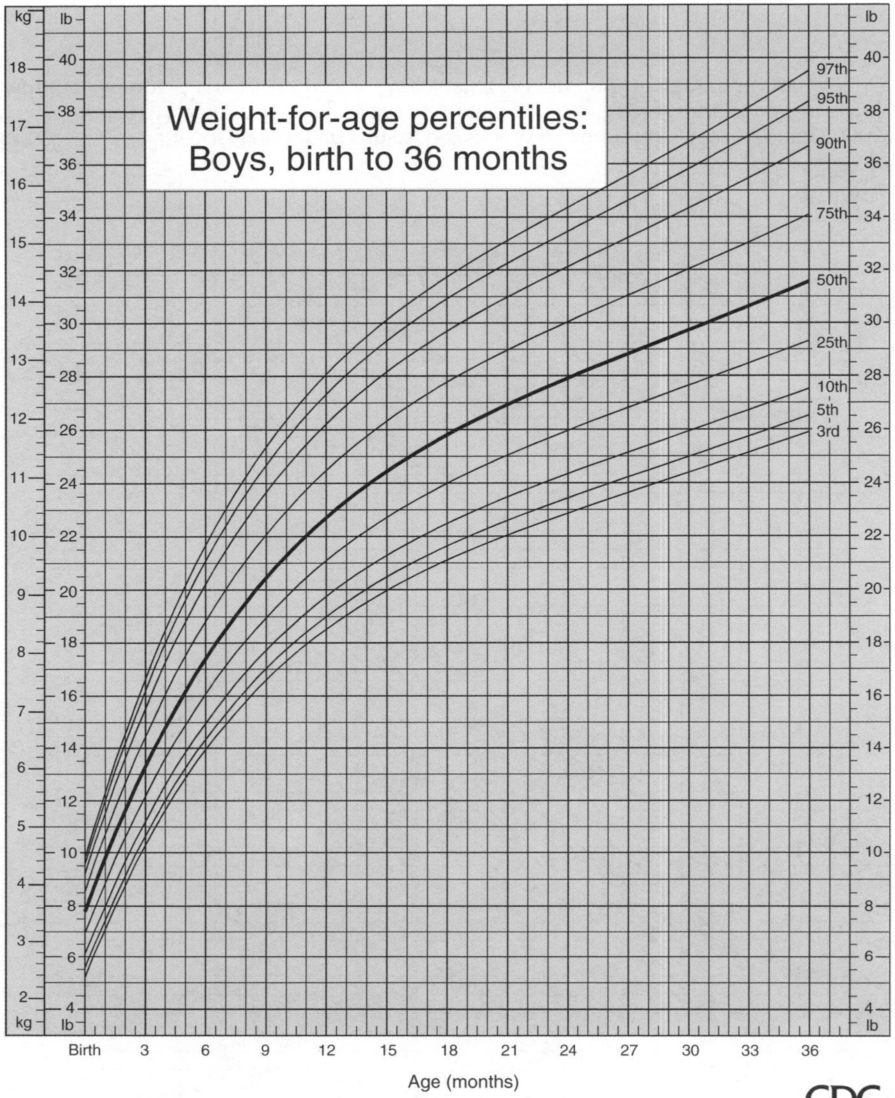

Fig. E-1 Weight-for-age percentiles, boys, birth to 36 months, CDC growth charts: United States. (Developed by the National Center for Health Statistics in collaboration with the National Center for Chronic Disease Prevention and Health Promotion [2000].)

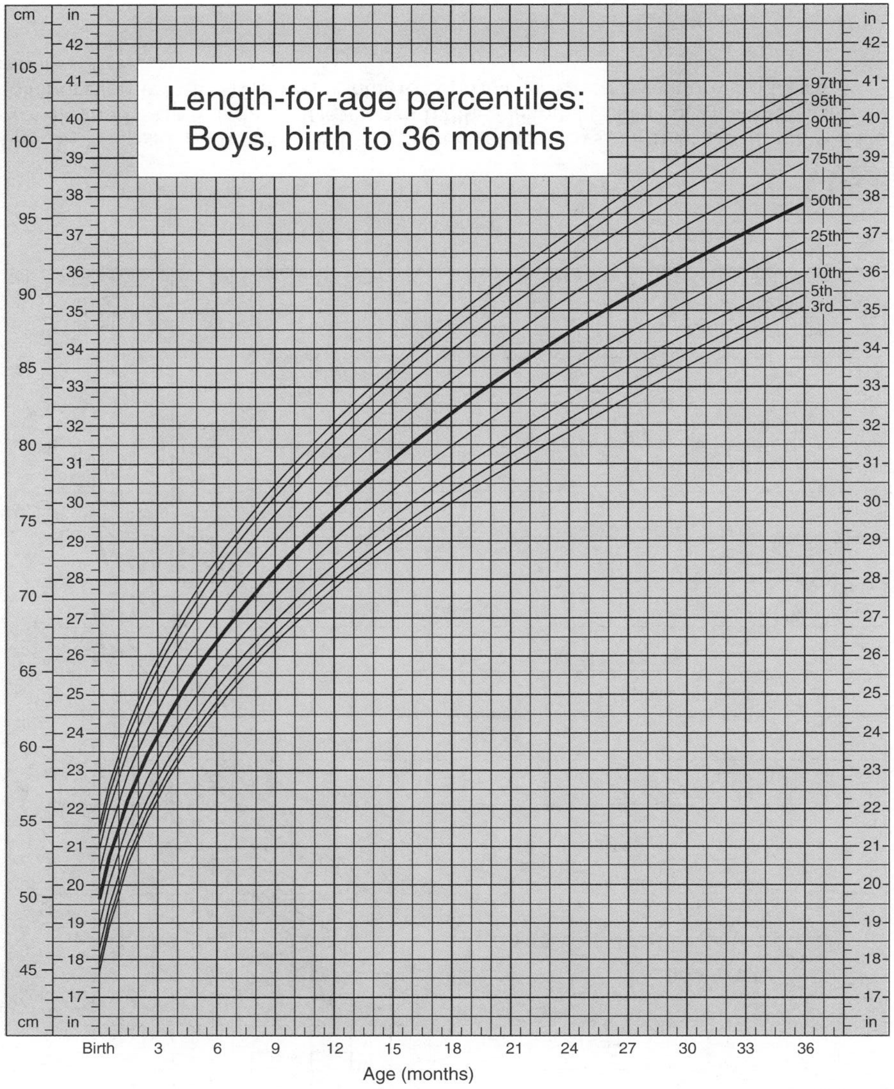

Fig. E-2 Length-for-age percentiles, boys, birth to 36 months, CDC growth charts: United States. (Developed by the National Center for Health Statistics in collaboration with the National Center for Chronic Disease Prevention and Health Promotion [2000].)

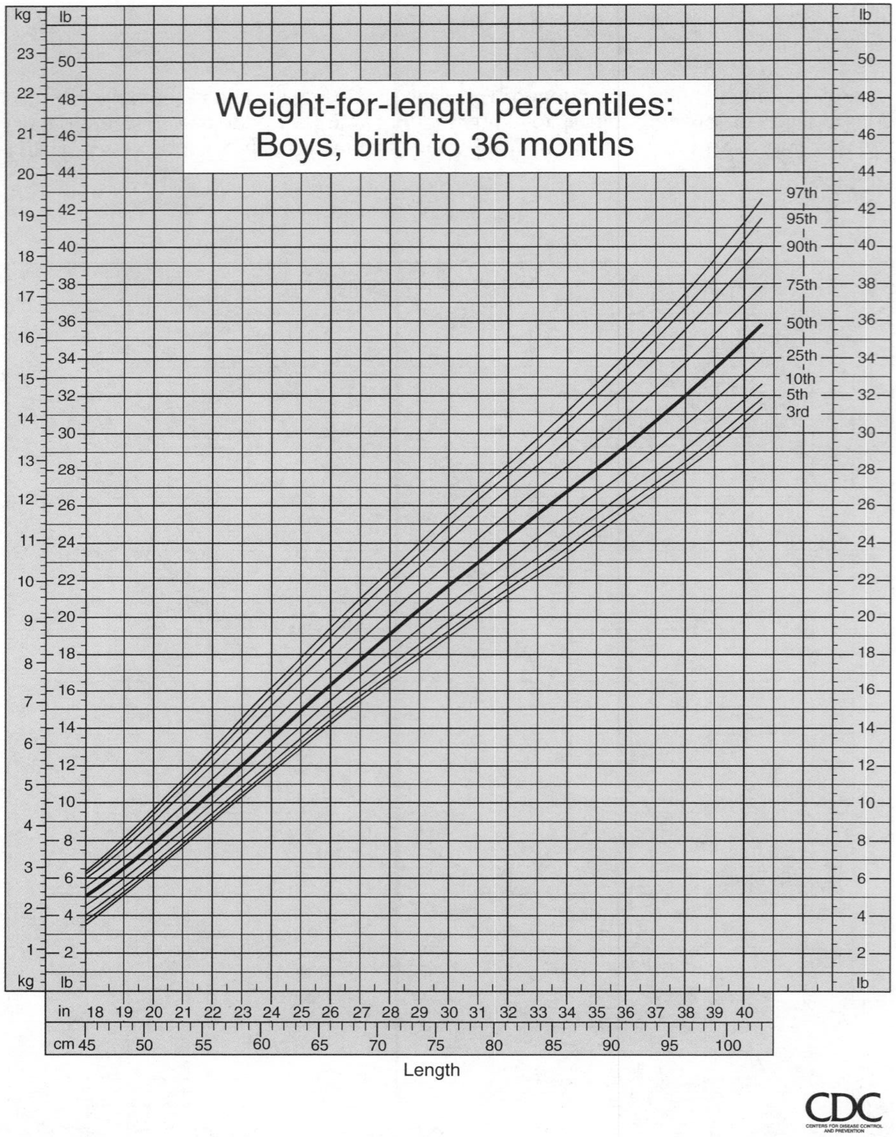

Fig. E-3 Weight-for-length percentiles, boys, birth to 36 months, CDC growth charts: United States. (Developed by the National Center for Health Statistics in collaboration with the National Center for Chronic Disease Prevention and Health Promotion [2000].)

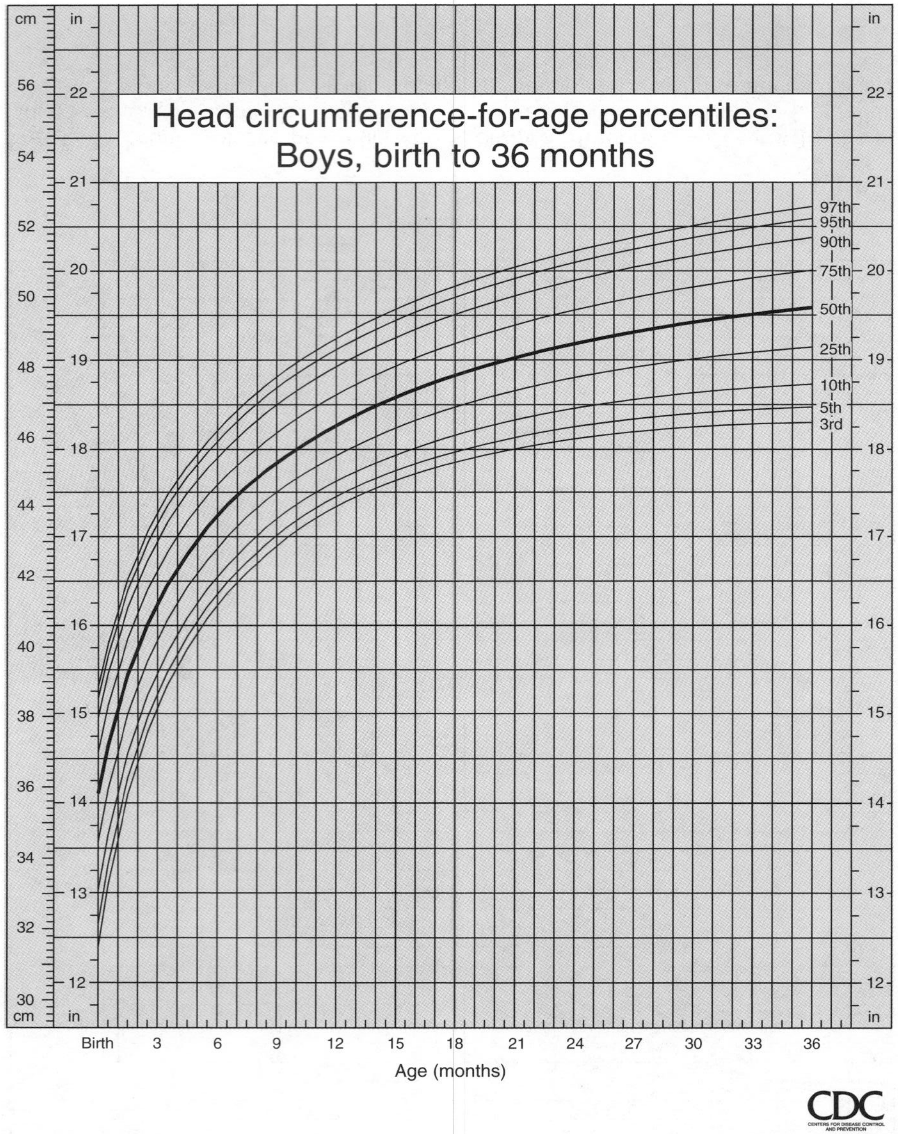

Fig. E-4 Head circumference–for–age percentiles, boys, birth to 36 months, CDC growth charts: United States. (Developed by the National Center for Health Statistics in collaboration with the National Center for Chronic Disease Prevention and Health Promotion [2000].)

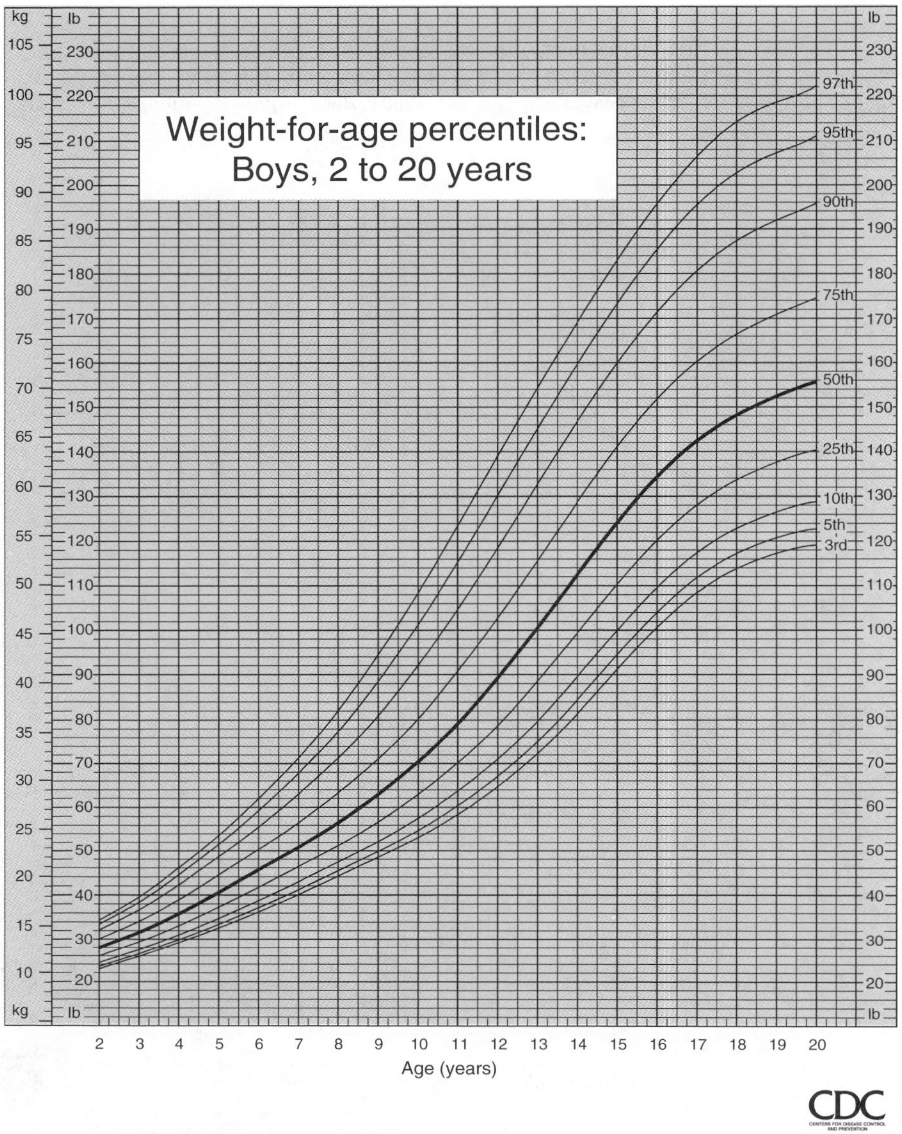

Fig. E-5 Weight-for-age percentiles, boys, 2 to 20 years, CDC growth charts: United States. (Developed by the National Center for Health Statistics in collaboration with the National Center for Chronic Disease Prevention and Health Promotion [2000].)

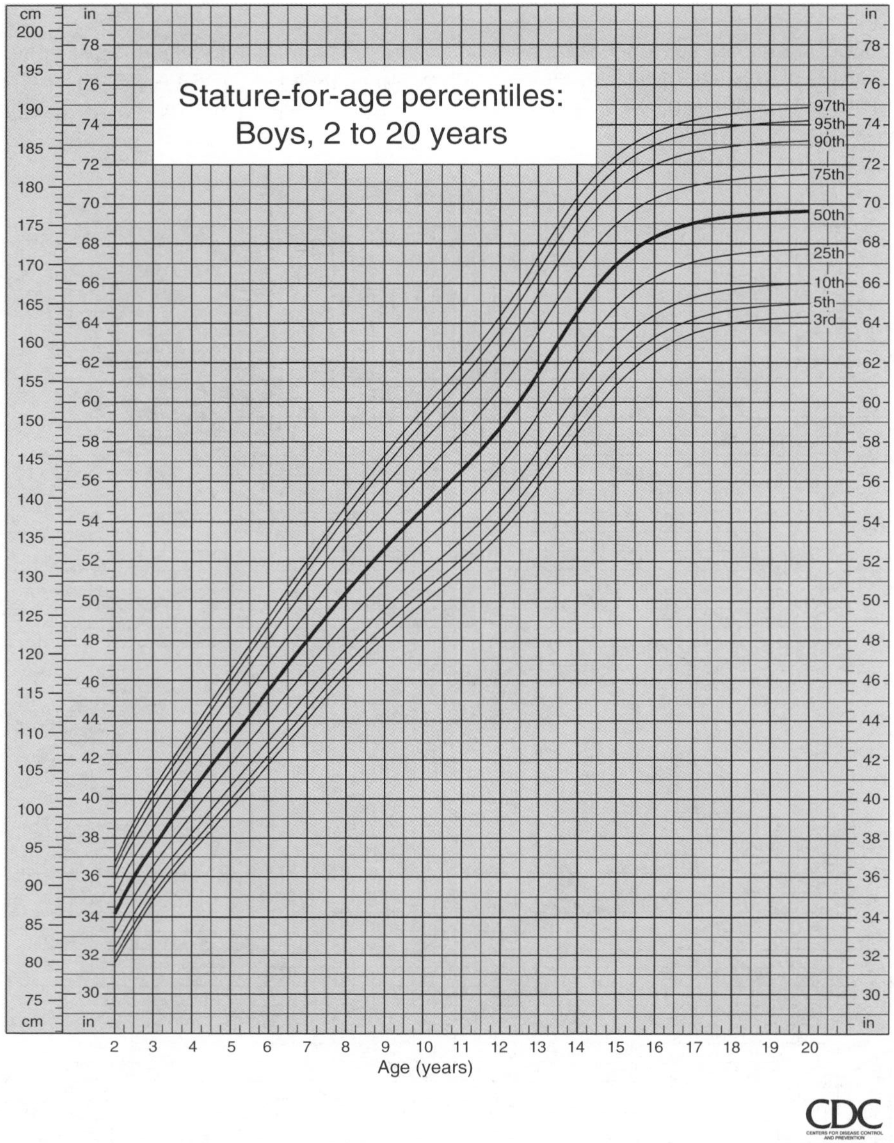

Fig. E-6 Stature-for-age percentiles, boys, 2 to 20 years, CDC growth charts: United States. (Developed by the National Center for Health Statistics in collaboration with the National Center for Chronic Disease Prevention and Health Promotion [2000].)

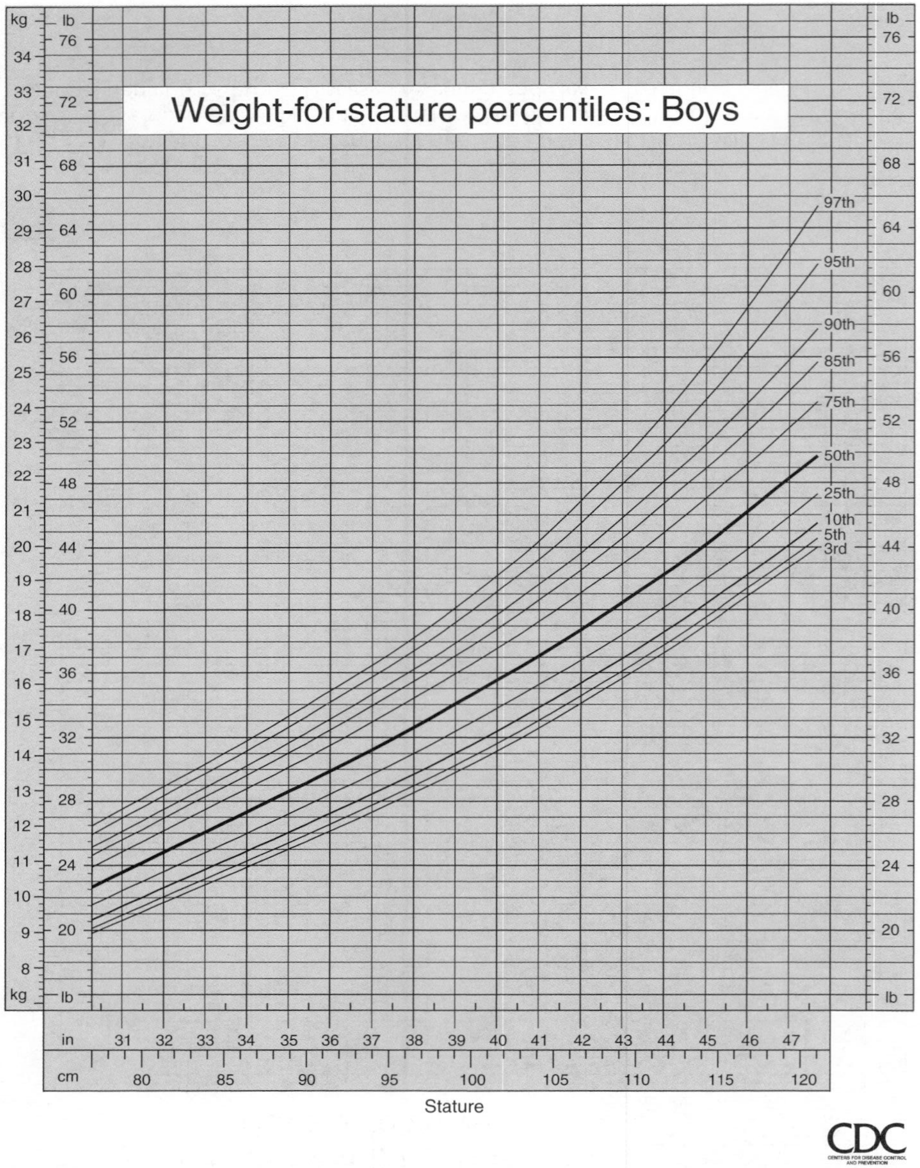

Fig. E-7 Weight-for-stature percentiles, boys, CDC growth charts: United States. (Developed by the National Center for Health Statistics in collaboration with the National Center for Chronic Disease Prevention and Health Promotion [2000].)

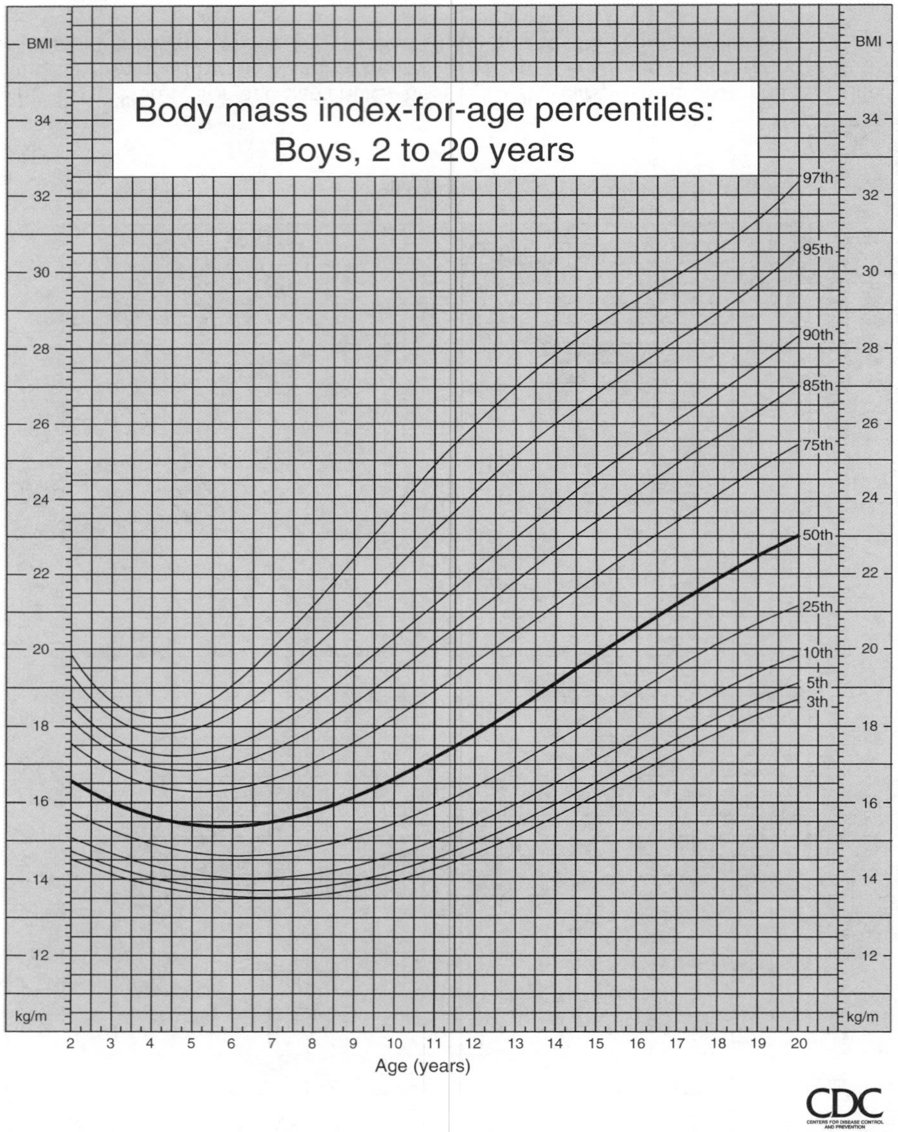

Fig. E-8 Body mass index-for-age percentiles, boys, 2 to 20 years, CDC growth charts: United States. (Developed by the National Center for Health Statistics in collaboration with the National Center for Chronic Disease Prevention and Health Promotion [2000].)

HEIGHT AND WEIGHT MEASUREMENTS FOR GIRLS

	Height by Percentiles						Weight by Percentiles					
	5		50		95		5		50		95	
AGE*	cm	INCHES	cm	INCHES	cm	INCHES	kg	lb	kg	lb	kg	lb
Birth	45.4	17¾	49.9	19¾	52.9	20¾	2.36	5¼	3.23	7	3.81	8½
3 months	55.4	21¾	59.5	23½	63.4	25	4.18	9¼	5.4	12	6.74	14¾
6 months	61.8	24¼	65.9	26	70.2	27¾	5.79	12¾	7.21	16	8.73	19¼
9 months	66.1	26	70.4	27¾	75.0	29½	7.0	15½	8.56	18¾	10.17	22½
1	69.8	27½	74.3	29¼	79.1	31¼	7.84	17¼	9.53	21	11.24	24¾
1½	76.0	30	80.9	31¾	86.1	34	8.92	19¾	10.82	23¾	12.76	28¼
2†	81.6	32¼	86.8	34¼	93.6	36¾	9.95	22	11.8	26	14.15	31¼
2½†	84.6	33¼	90.0	35½	96.6	38	10.8	23¾	13.03	28¾	15.76	34¾
3	88.3	34¾	94.1	37	100.6	39½	11.61	25½	14.1	31	17.22	38
3½	91.7	36	97.9	38½	104.5	41¼	12.37	27¼	15.07	33¼	18.59	41
4	95.0	37½	101.6	40	108.3	42¾	13.11	29	15.96	35¼	19.91	44
4½	98.1	38½	105.0	41¼	112.0	44	13.83	30½	16.81	37	21.24	46¾
5	101.1	39¾	108.4	42¾	115.6	45½	14.55	32	17.66	39	22.62	49¾
6	106.6	42	114.6	45	122.7	48¼	16.05	35½	19.52	43	25.75	56¾
7	111.8	44	120.6	47½	129.5	51	17.71	39	21.84	48¼	29.68	65½
8	116.9	46	126.4	49¾	136.2	53½	19.62	43¼	24.84	54¾	34.71	76½
9	122.1	48	132.2	52	142.9	56¼	21.82	48	28.46	62¾	40.64	89½
10	127.5	50¼	138.3	54½	149.5	58¾	24.36	53¾	32.55	71¾	47.17	104
11	133.5	52½	144.8	57	156.2	61½	27.24	60	36.95	81½	54.0	119
12	139.8	55	151.5	59¾	162.7	64	30.52	67¼	41.53	91½	60.81	134
13	145.2	57¼	157.1	61¾	168.1	66¼	34.14	75¼	46.1	101¾	67.3	48¼
14	148.7	58½	160.4	63¼	171.3	67½	37.76	83¼	50.28	110¾	73.08	161
15	150.5	59¼	161.8	63¾	172.8	68	40.99	90¼	53.68	118¼	77.78	171½
16	151.6	59¾	162.4	64	173.3	68¼	43.41	95¾	55.89	123¼	80.99	178½
17	152.7	60	163.1	64¼	173.5	68¼	44.74	98¾	56.69	125	82.46	181¾
18	153.6	60½	163.7	64½	173.6	68¼	45.26	99¾	56.62	124¾	82.47	181¾

Modified from National Center for Health Statistics (NCHS), Health Resources Administration, Department of Health, Education, and Welfare, Hyattsville, MD. Conversion of metric data to approximate inches and pounds by Ross Laboratories.

*Years unless otherwise indicated.

†Height data include some recumbent length measurements, which make values slightly higher than if all measurements had been of stature.

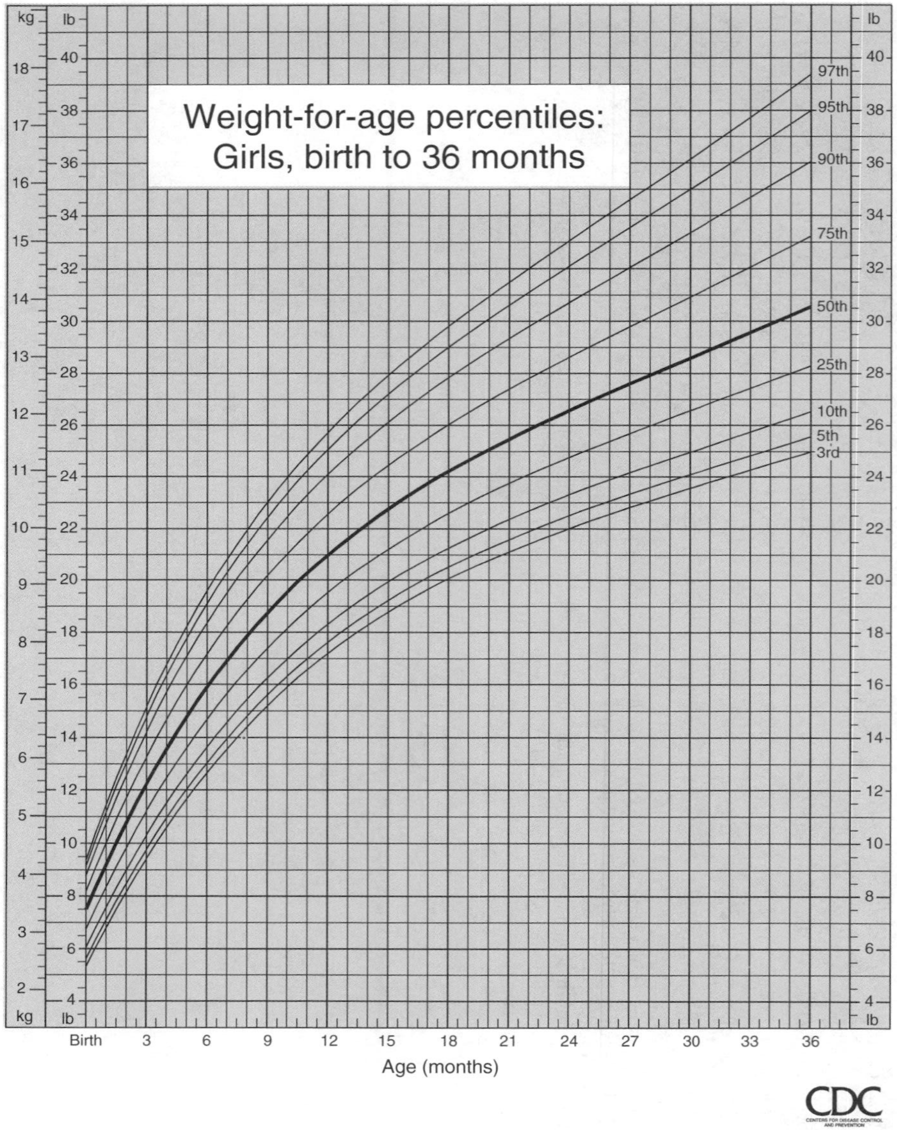

Fig. E-9 Weight-for-age percentiles, girls, birth to 36 months, CDC growth charts: United States. (Developed by the National Center for Health Statistics in collaboration with the National Center for Chronic Disease Prevention and Health Promotion [2000].)

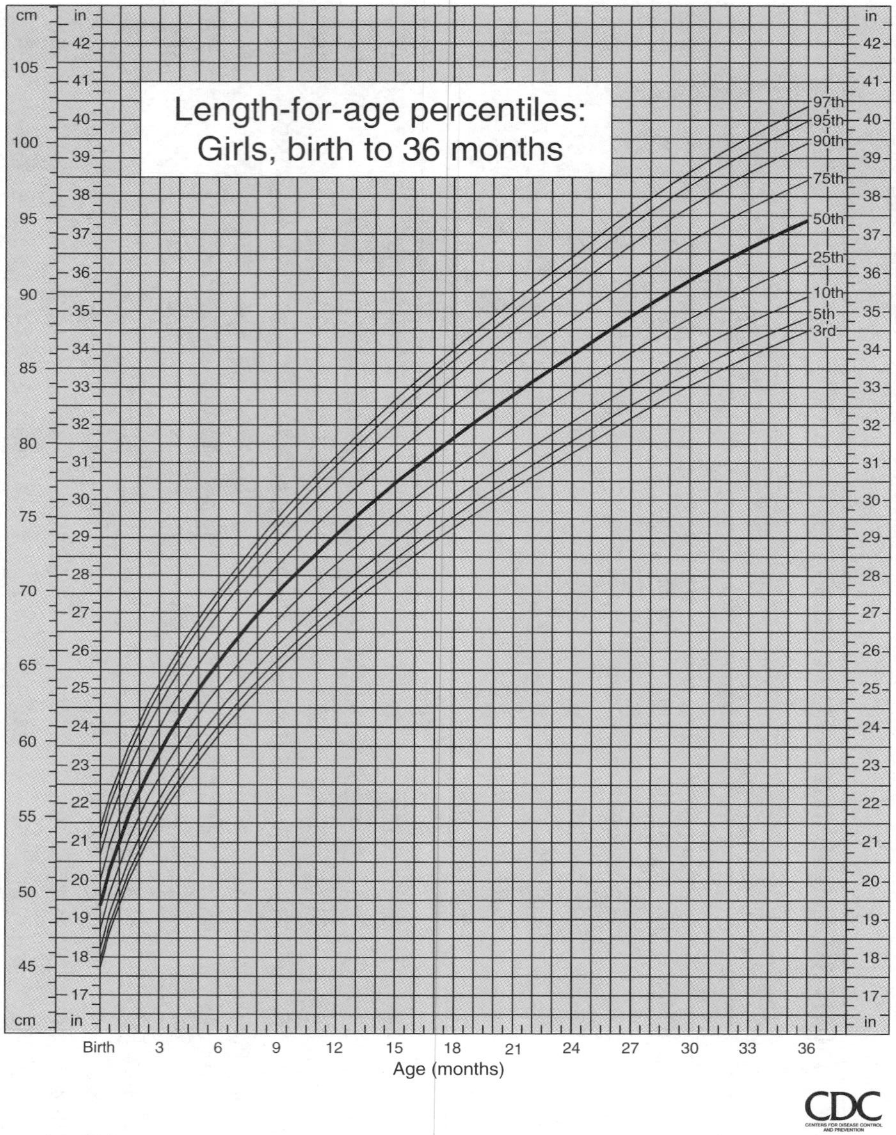

Fig. E-10 Length-for-age percentiles, girls, birth to 36 months, CDC growth charts: United States. (Developed by the National Center for Health Statistics in collaboration with the National Center for Chronic Disease Prevention and Health Promotion [2000].)

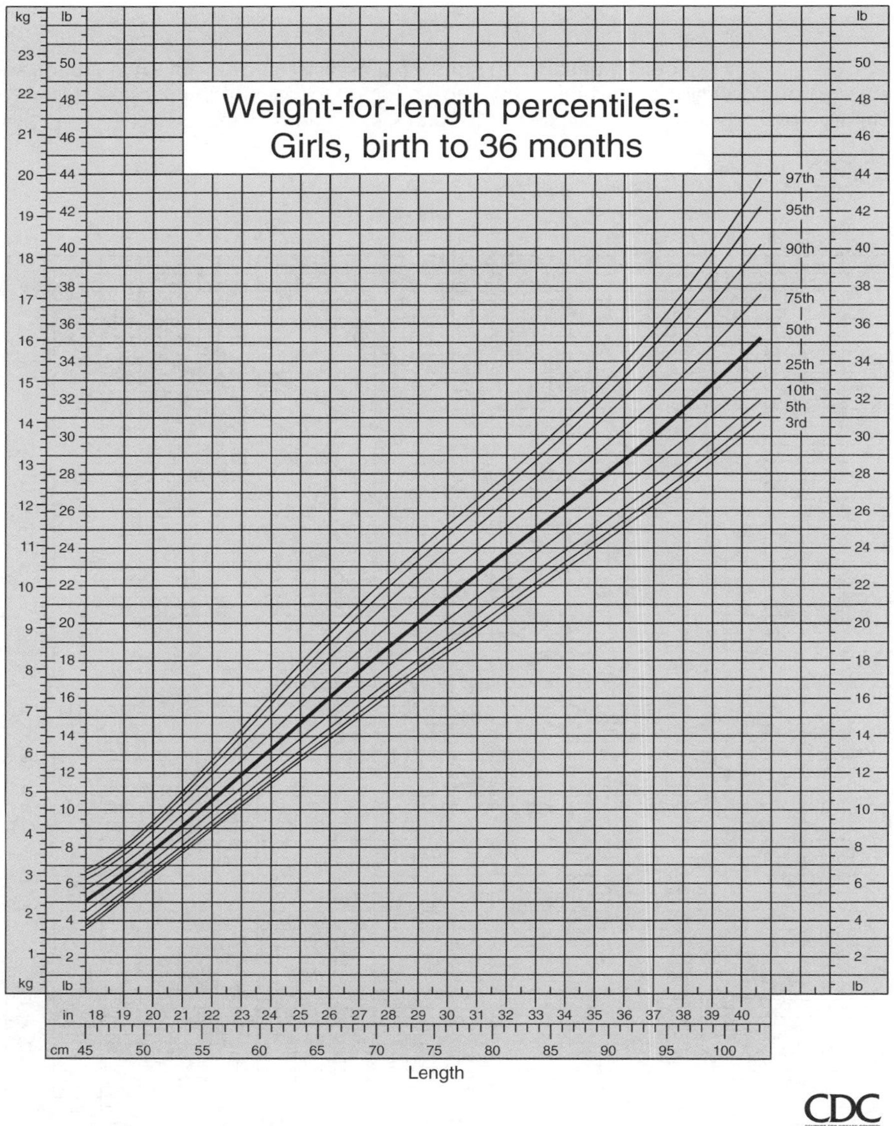

Fig. E-11 Weight-for-length percentiles, girls, birth to 36 months, CDC growth charts: United States. (Developed by the National Center for Health Statistics in collaboration with the National Center for Chronic Disease Prevention and Health Promotion [2000].)

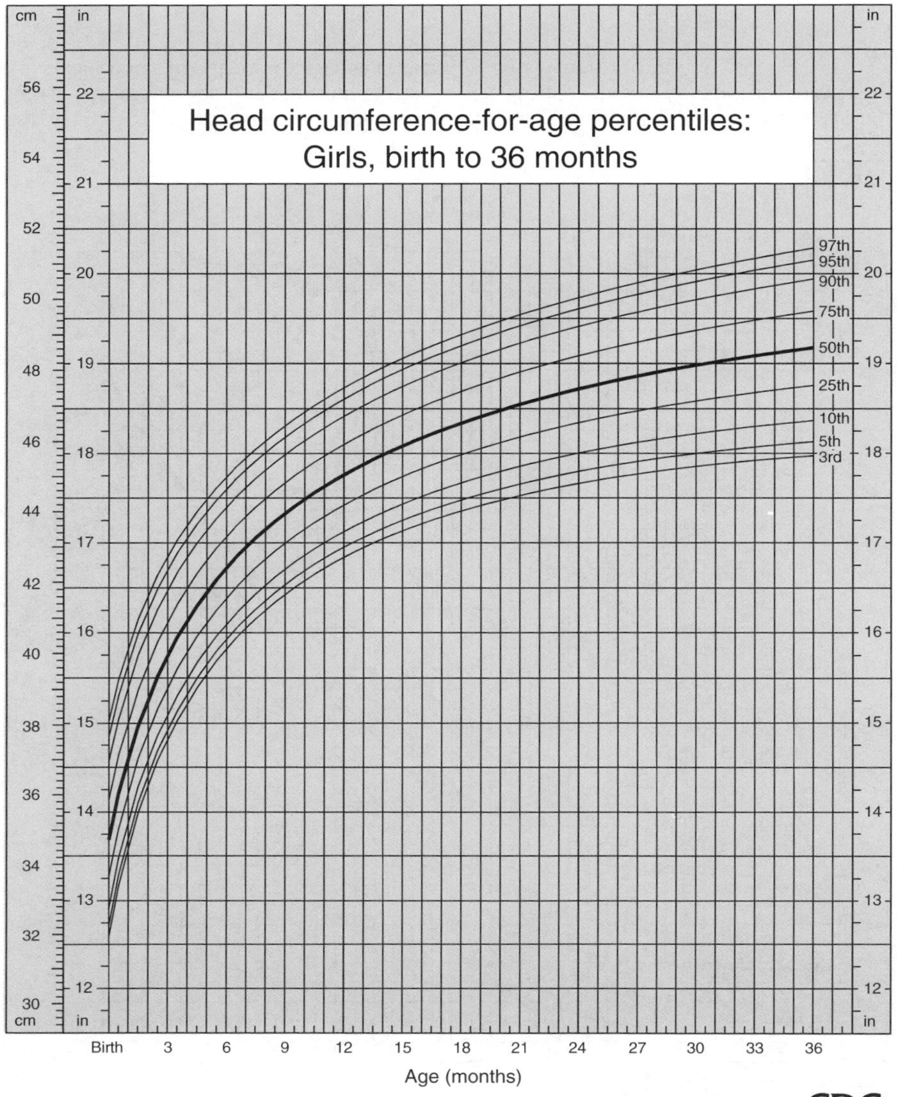

Fig. E-12 Head circumference–for–age percentiles, girls, birth to 36 months, CDC growth charts: United States. (Developed by the National Center for Health Statistics in collaboration with the National Center for Chronic Disease Prevention and Health Promotion [2000].)

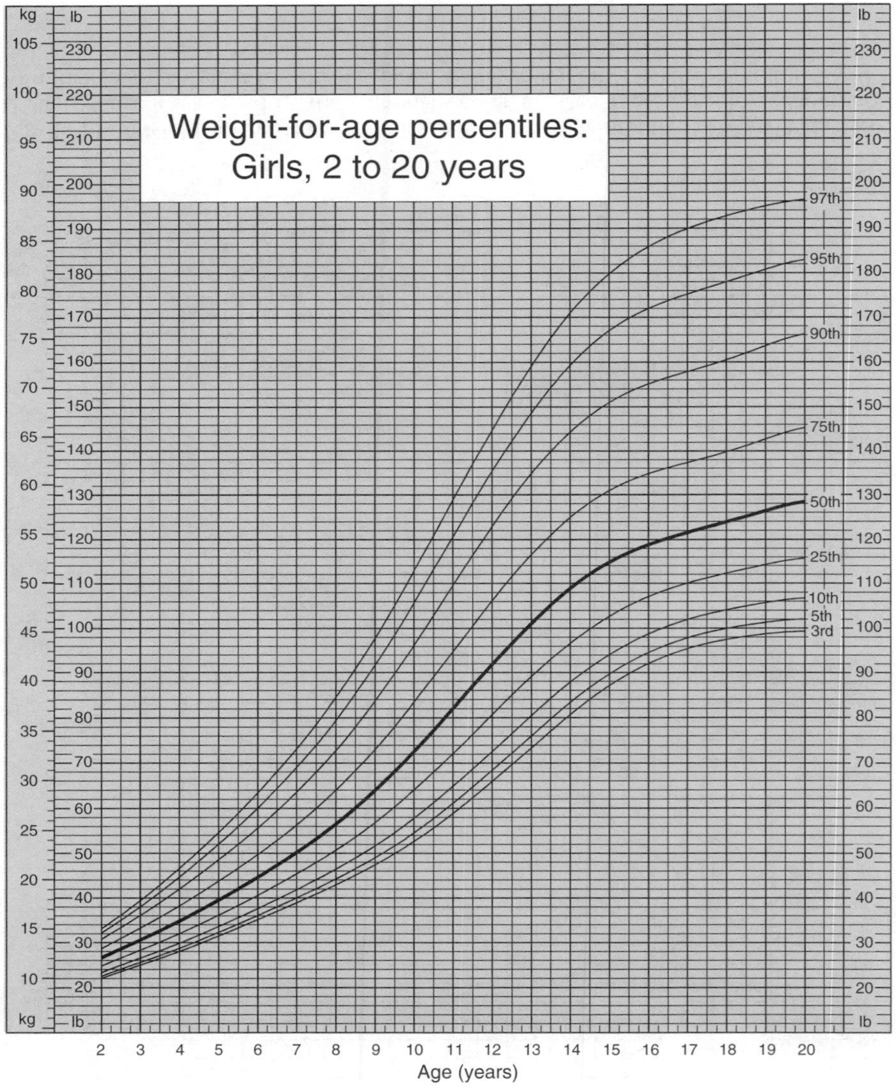

Fig. E-13 Weight-for-age percentiles, girls, 2 to 20 years, CDC growth charts: United States. (Developed by the National Center for Health Statistics in collaboration with the National Center for Chronic Disease Prevention and Health Promotion [2000].)

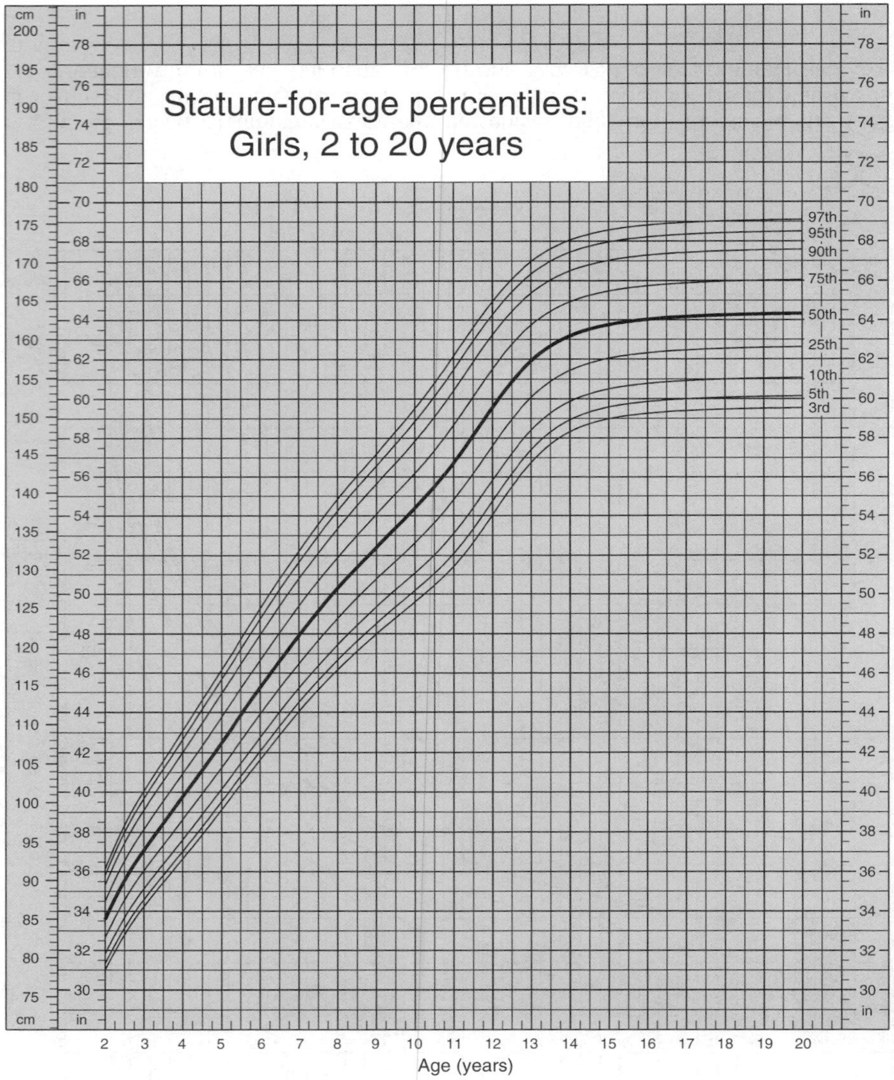

Fig. E-14 Stature-for-age percentiles, girls, 2 to 20 years, CDC growth charts: United States. (Developed by the National Center for Health Statistics in collaboration with the National Center for Chronic Disease Prevention and Health Promotion [2000].)

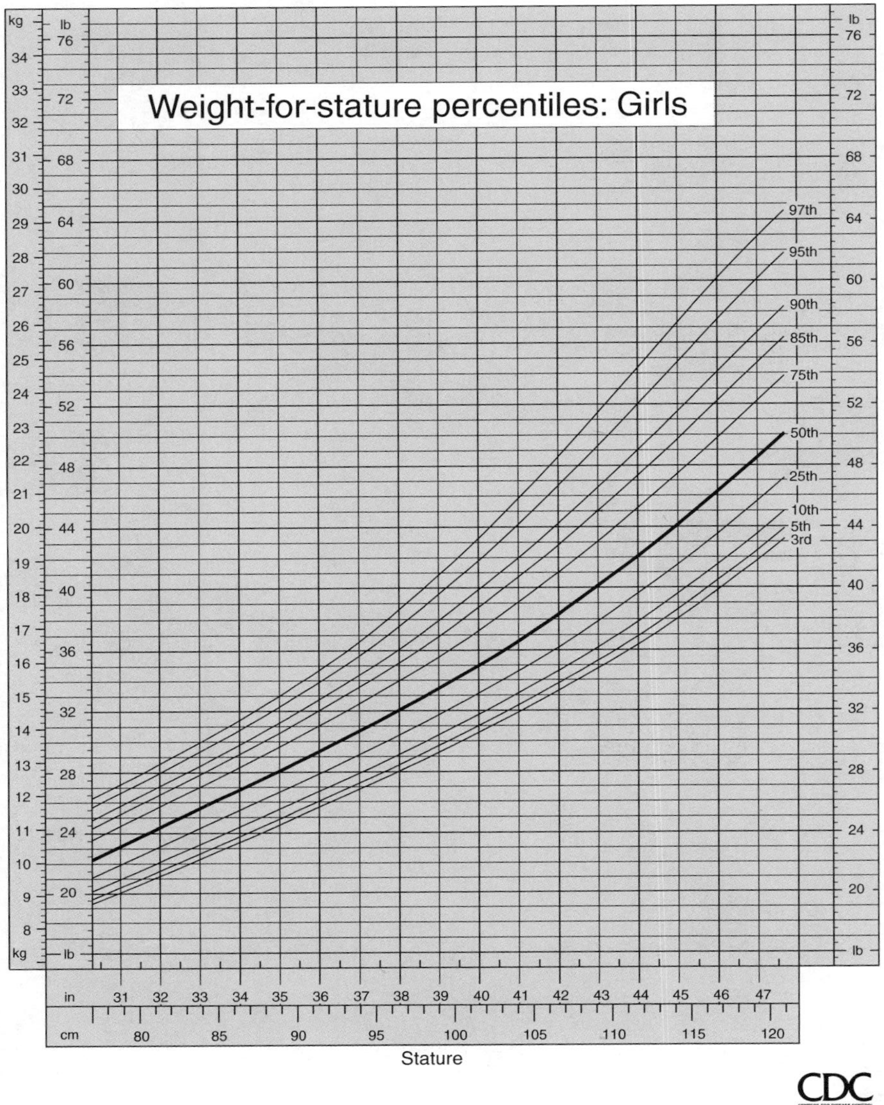

Fig. E-15 Weight-for-stature percentiles, girls, CDC growth charts: United States. (Developed by the National Center for Health Statistics in collaboration with the National Center for Chronic Disease Prevention and Health Promotion [2000].)

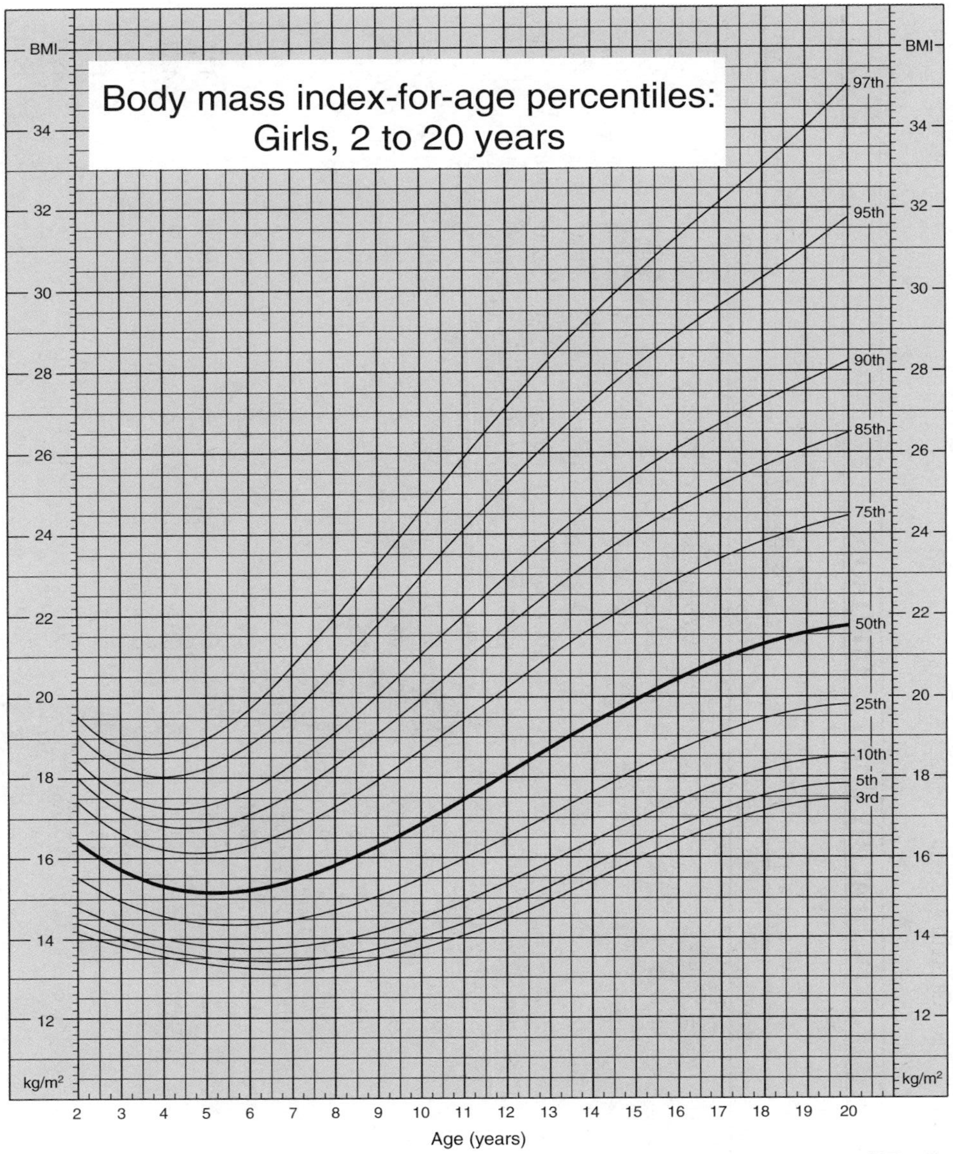

Fig. E-16 Body mass index-for-age percentiles, girls, 2 to 20 years, CDC growth charts: United States. (Developed by the National Center for Health Statistics in collaboration with the National Center for Chronic Disease Prevention and Health Promotion [2000].)

GROWTH STANDARDS OF HEALTHY CHINESE CHILDREN

	Weight (kg)		Height (cm)		Head Circumference (cm)	
AGE	BOYS	GIRLS	BOYS	GIRLS	BOYS	GIRLS
Birth	3.27	3.17	50.6	50.0	34.3	33.7
1 month	4.97	4.64	56.5	55.5	38.1	37.3
2 months	5.95	5.49	59.6	58.4	39.7	38.7
3 months	6.73	6.23	62.3	60.9	41.0	40.0
4 months	7.32	6.69	64.4	62.9	42.0	41.0
5 months	7.70	7.19	65.9	64.5	42.9	41.9
6 months	8.22	7.62	68.1	66.7	43.9	42.8
8 months	8.71	8.14	70.6	69.0	44.9	43.7
10 months	9.14	8.57	72.9	71.4	45.7	44.5
12 months	9.56	9.04	75.6	74.1	46.3	45.2
15 months	10.15	9.54	78.3	76.9	46.8	45.6
18 months	10.67	10.08	80.7	79.4	47.3	46.2
21 months	11.18	10.56	83.0	81.7	47.8	46.7
24 months	11.95	11.37	86.5	85.3	48.2	47.1
12.5 years	12.84	12.28	90.4	89.3	48.8	47.7
3 years	13.63	13.16	93.8	92.8	49.1	48.1
3.5 years	14.45	14.00	97.2	96.3	49.4	48.5
4 years	15.26	14.89	100.8	100.1	49.7	48.9
4.5 years	16.07	15.63	103.9	103.1	50.0	49.1
5 years	16.88	16.46	107.2	106.5	50.2	49.4
5.5 years	17.65	17.18	110.1	109.2	50.5	49.6
6 years	19.25	18.67	114.7	113.9	50.8	50.0
7 years	21.01	20.35	120.6	119.3	51.1	50.2
8 years	23.08	22.43	125.3	124.6	51.4	50.6
9 years	25.33	24.57	130.6	129.5	51.7	50.9
10 years	27.15	27.05	134.4	134.8	51.9	51.3
11 years	30.13	30.51	139.2	140.6	52.3	51.7
12 years	33.05	34.74	144.2	146.6	52.7	52.3
13 years	36.90	38.52	149.8	150.7	53.0	52.8

Data from Bejing Children's Hospital, 1987, China.

PERCENTILES FOR TRICEPS SKINFOLD

	Triceps Skinfold Percentiles (mm)									
	Males					Females				
AGE GROUP (YEARS)	5	25	50	75	95	5	25	50	75	95
1-1.9	6	8	10	12	16	6	8	10	12	16
2-2.9	6	8	10	12	15	6	9	10	12	16
3-3.9	6	8	10	11	15	7	9	11	12	15
4-4.9	6	8	9	11	14	7	8	10	12	16
5-5.9	6	8	9	11	15	6	8	10	12	18
6-6.9	5	7	8	10	16	6	8	10	12	16
7-7.9	5	7	9	12	17	6	9	11	13	18
8-8.9	5	7	8	10	16	6	9	12	15	24
9-9.9	6	7	10	13	18	8	10	13	16	22
10-10.9	6	8	10	14	21	7	10	12	17	27
11-11.9	6	8	11	16	24	7	10	13	18	28
12-12.9	6	8	11	14	28	8	11	14	18	27
13-13.9	5	7	10	14	26	8	12	15	21	30
14-14.9	4	7	9	14	24	9	13	16	21	28
15-15.9	4	6	8	11	24	8	12	17	21	32
16-16.9	4	6	8	12	22	10	15	18	22	31
17-17.9	5	6	8	12	19	10	13	19	24	37
18-18.9	4	6	9	13	24	10	15	18	22	30
19-24.9	4	7	10	15	22	10	14	18	24	34

From Frisancho A: New norms of upper limb fat and muscle areas for assessment of nutritional status, *Am J Clin Nutr* 34:2540-2545, 1981.

PERCENTILES OF UPPER ARM CIRCUMFERENCE

	Arm Circumference Percentiles (mm)									
	Males					Females				
AGE GROUP (YEARS)	5	25	50	75	95	5	25	50	75	95
1-1.9	142	150	159	170	183	138	148	156	164	177
2-2.9	141	153	162	170	185	142	152	160	167	184
3-3.9	150	160	167	175	190	143	158	167	175	189
4-4.9	149	162	171	180	192	149	160	169	177	191
5-5.9	153	167	175	185	204	153	165	175	185	211
6-6.9	155	167	179	188	228	156	170	176	187	211
7-7.9	162	177	187	201	230	164	174	183	199	231
8-8.9	162	177	190	202	245	168	183	195	214	261
9-9.9	175	187	200	217	257	178	194	211	224	260
10-10.9	181	196	210	231	274	174	193	210	228	265
11-11.9	186	202	223	244	280	185	208	224	248	303
12-12.9	193	214	232	254	303	194	216	237	256	294
13-13.9	194	228	247	263	301	202	223	243	271	338
14-14.9	220	237	253	283	322	214	237	252	272	322
15-15.9	222	244	264	284	320	208	239	254	279	322
16-16.9	244	262	278	303	343	218	241	258	283	334
17-17.9	246	267	285	308	347	220	241	264	295	350
18-18.9	245	276	297	321	379	222	241	258	281	325
19-24.9	262	288	308	331	372	221	247	265	290	345

From Frisancho A: New norms of upper limb fat and muscle areas for assessment of nutritional status, *Am J Clin Nutr* 34:2540-2545, 1981.

F Common Laboratory Tests

TEST/SPECIMEN (SI)	AGE/GENDER/REFERENCE	Normal Ranges: CONVENTIONAL UNITS		INTERNATIONAL UNITS (SI)	
Acetaminophen					
Serum or plasma	Therap. conc.	10-30 mcg/ml		66-200 mcmol/L	
	Toxic conc.	>200 mcg/ml		>1300 mcmol/L	
Ammonia nitrogen					
Plasma or serum	Newborn	90-150 mcg/dl		64-107 mcmol/L	
	0-2 wk	79-129 mcg/dl		56-92 mcmol/L	
	>1 mo	29-70 mcg/dl		21-50 mcmol/L	
	Thereafter	0-50 mcg/dl		0-35.7 mcmol/L	
Antistreptolysin O titer (ASO)					
Serum	2-4 yr	<160 Todd units			
	School-age children	170-330 Todd units			
Base excess					
Whole blood	Newborn	(−10)-(−2) mEq/L		(−10)-(−2) mmol/L	
	Infant	(−7)-(−1) mEq/L		(−7)-(−1) mmol/L	
	Child	(−4)-(+2) mEq/L		(−4)-(+2) mmol/L	
	Thereafter	(−3)-(+3) mEq/L		(−3)-(+3) mmol/L	
Bicarbonate (HCO_3)	Arterial	21-28 mEq/L		21-28 mmol/L	
Serum					
	Venous	22-29 mEq/L		22-29 mmol/L	
		Premature (mg/dl)	**Full term (mg/dl)**	**Premature (mcmol/L)**	**Full term (mcmol/L)**
Bilirubin, total					
Serum	Cord	<2.0	<2.0	<34	<34
	0-1 d	<8.0	<6.0	<137	<103
	1-2 d	<12.0	<8.0	<205	<137
	2-5 d	<16.0	<12.0	<274	<205
	Thereafter	<20.0	<10.0	<340	<171
Bilirubin, direct (conjugated)					
Serum		0.0-0.2 mg/dl		0-3.4 mcmol/L	
Bleeding time					
Blood from skin puncture					
Ivy	Normal	2-7 min		2-7 min	
	Borderline	7-11 min		7-11 min	
Simplate (G-D)		2.75-8 min		2.75-8 min	
Blood volume					
Whole blood	Male	52-83 ml/kg		0.052-0.083 L/kg	
	Female	50-75 ml/kg		0.050-0.075 L/kg	
C-reactive protein (CRP)					
Serum	Cord	52-1330 ng/ml		52-1330 mcg/L	
	2-12 yr	67-1800 ng/ml		67-1800 mcg /L	
Calcium, ionized					
Serum, plasma, or whole blood	Cord	5.0-6.0 mg/dl		1.25-1.50 mmol/L	
	Newborn, 3-24 hr	4.3-5.1 mg/dl		1.07-1.27 mmol/L	
	24-48 hr	4.0-4.7 mg/dl		1.00-1.17 mmol/L	

Modified from Behrman RE et al (eds): *Nelson textbook of pediatrics*, ed 17, Philadelphia, 2004, WB Saunders; and McMillan A et al (eds): *Oski's pediatrics—principles and practice*, ed 3, Philadelphia, 1999, Lippincott Williams & Wilkins.

Continued

	Normal Ranges		
TEST/SPECIMEN	AGE/GENDER/REFERENCE	CONVENTIONAL UNITS	INTERNATIONAL UNITS (SI)
Calcium, ionized—cont'd			
Serum, plasma, or whole blood—cont'd	Thereafter	4.8-4.92 mg/dl or 2.24-2.46 mEq/L	1.12-1.23 mmol/L
Calcium, total			
Serum	Cord	9.0-11.5 mg/dl	2.25-2.88 mmol/L
	Newborn, 3-24 hr	9.0-10.6 mg/dl	2.3-2.65 mmol/L
	24-48 hr	7.0-12.0 mg/dl	1.75-3.0 mmol/L
	4-7 d	9.0-10.9 mg/dl	2.25-2.73 mmol/L
	Child	8.8-10.8 mg/dl	2.2-2.70 mmol/L
	Thereafter	8.4-10.2 mg/dl	2.1-2.55 mmol/L
Carbon dioxide, partial pressure (Pco_2)			
Whole blood, arterial	Newborn	27-40 mm Hg	3.6-5.3 kPa
	Infant	27-41 mm Hg	3.6-5.5 kPa
	Thereafter: Male	35-48 mm Hg	4.7-6.4 kPa
	Female	32-45 mm Hg	4.3-6.0 kPa
Carbon dioxide, total (tCO_2)			
Serum or plasma	Cord	14-22 mEq/L	14-22 mmol/L
	Premature (1 wk)	14-27 mEq/L	14-27 mmol/L
	Newborn	13-22 mEq/L	13-22 mmol/L
	Infant, child	20-28 mEq/L	20-28 mmol/L
	Thereafter	23-30 mEq/L	23-30 mmol/L
Cerebrospinal fluid (CSF)			
Pressure		70-180 mm water	70-180 mm water
Volume	Child	60-100 ml	0.06-0.10 L
	Adult	100-160 ml	0.10-0.16 L
Chloride			
Serum or plasma	Cord	96-104 mEq/L	96-104 mmol/L
	Newborn	97-110 mEq/L	97-110 mmol/L
	Thereafter	98-106 mEq/L	98-106 mmol/L
Sweat	Normal (homozygote)	<40 mEq/L	<40 mmol/L
	Marginal (e.g., asthma, Addison disease, malnutrition)	45-60 mEq/L	45-60 mmol/L
	Cystic fibrosis	<60 mmol/L	<60 mmol/L
Cholesterol, total			
Serum or plasma	Acceptable	<170 mg/dl	<4.4 mmol/L
	Borderline	170-199 mg/dl	4.4-5.1 mmol/L
	High	≥200 mg/dl	≥5.2 mmol/L
Clotting time (Lee-White)			
White blood		5-8 min (glass tubes)	5-8 min
		5-15 min (room temp)	5-15 min
		30 min (silicone tube)	30 min
Creatine kinase (CK, CPK)			
Serum	Cord blood	70-380 units/L	70-380 units/L
	5-8 hr	214-1175 units/L	214-1175 units/L
	24-33 hr	130-1200 units/L	130-1200 units/L
	72-100 hr	87-725 units/L	87-725 units/L
	Adult	5-130 units/L	5-130 units/L
Creatinine			
Serum	Cord	0.6-1.2 mg/dl	53-106 mcmol/L
	Newborn	0.3-1.0 mg/dl	27-88 mcmol/L
	Infant	0.2-0.4 mg/dl	18-35 mcmol/L
	Child	0.3-0.7 mg/dl	27-62 mcmol/L
	Adolescent	0.5-1.0 mg/dl	44-88 mcmol/L
	Adult: Male	0.6-1.2 mg/dl	53-106 mcmol/L
	Female	0.5-1.1 mg/dl	44-97 mcmol/L

Continued

TEST/SPECIMEN	AGE/GENDER/REFERENCE	Normal Ranges: CONVENTIONAL UNITS	Normal Ranges: INTERNATIONAL UNITS (SI)
Creatinine—cont'd			
Urine, 24 hr	Premature	8.1-15.0 mg/kg/24 hr	72-133 mcmol/kg/24 hr
	Full term	10.4-19.7 mg/kg/24 hr	92-174 mcmol/kg/24 hr
	1.5-7 yr	10-15 mg/kg/24 hr	88-133 mcmol/kg/24 hr
	7-15 yr	5.2-41 mg/kg/24 hr	46-362 mcmol/kg/24 hr
Creatinine clearance (endogenous)			
Serum or plasma and urine	Newborn	40-65 ml/min/1.73 m²	
	<40 yr: Male	97-137 ml/min/1.73 m²	
	Female	88-128 ml/min/1.73 m²	
Digoxin			
Serum, plasma; collect at least 12 hr after dose	Therap. conc.		
	CHF	0.8-1.5 ng/ml	1.0-1.9 nmol/L
	Arrhythmias	1.5-2.0 ng/ml	1.9-2.6 nmol/L
	Toxic conc.		
	Child	>2.5 ng/ml	>3.2 nmol/L
	Adult	>3.0 ng/ml	>3.8 nmol/L
Eosinophil count			
Whole blood, capillary blood		50-250 cells/mm³ (mcl)	50-250 × 10⁶ cells/L
Erythrocyte (RBC) count			
Whole blood	Cord	3.9-5.5 million/mm³	3.9-5.5 × 10¹² cells/L
	1-3 d	4.0-6.6 million/mm³	4.0-6.6 × 10¹² cells/L
	1 wk	3.9-6.3 million/mm³	3.9-6.3 × 10¹² cells/L
	2 wk	3.6-6.2 million/mm³	3.6-6.2 × 10¹² cells/L
	1 mo	3.0-5.4 million/mm³	3.0-5.4 × 10¹² cells/L
	2 mo	2.7-4.9 million/mm³	2.7-4.9 × 10¹² cells/L
	3-6 mo	3.1-4.5 million/mm³	3.1-4.5 × 10¹² cells/L
	0.5-2 yr	3.7-5.3 million/mm³	3.7-5.3 × 10¹² cells/L
	2-6 yr	3.9-5.3 million/mm³	3.9-5.3 × 10¹² cells/L
	6-12 yr	4.0-5.2 million/mm³	4.0-5.2 × 10¹² cells/L
	12-18 yr: Male	4.5-5.3 million/mm³	4.5-5.3 × 10¹² cells/L
	Female	4.1-5.1 million/mm³	4.1-5.1 × 10¹² cells/L
Erythrocyte sedimentation rate (ESR)			
Whole blood			
Westergren (modified)	Child	0-10 mm/hr	0-10 mm/hr
	<50 yr: Male	0-15 mm/hr	0-15 mm/hr
	Female	0-20 mm/hr	0-20 mm/hr
Wintrobe	Child	0-13 mm/hr	0-13 mm/hr
	Adult: Male	0-9 mm/hr	0-9 mm/hr
	Female	0-20 mm/hr	0-20 mm/hr
Fibrinogen			
Plasma	Newborn	125-300 mg/dl	1.25-3.00 g/L
	Thereafter	200-400 mg/dl	2.00-4.00 g/L
Galactose			
Serum	Newborn	0-20 mg/dl	0-1.11 mmol/L
	Thereafter	<5 mg/dl	<0.28 mmol/L
Urine	Newborn	≤60 mg/dl	≤3.33 mmol/L
	Thereafter	≤14 mg/24 hr	<0.08 mmol/d
Glucose			
Serum	Cord	45-96 mg/dl	2.5-5.3 mmol/L
	Newborn, 1 d	40-60 mg/dl	2.2-3.3 mmol/L
	Newborn, >1 d	50-90 mg/dl	2.8-5.0 mmol/L
	Child	60-100 mg/dl	3.3-5.5 mmol/L
	Thereafter	70-105 mg/dl	3.9-5.8 mmol/L

TEST/SPECIMEN	AGE/GENDER/REFERENCE	Normal Ranges CONVENTIONAL UNITS		INTERNATIONAL UNITS (SI)	
Glucose–cont'd					
Whole blood					
CSF	Adult	65-95 mg/dl		3.6-5.3 mmol/L	
Urine (quantitative)	Adult	40-70 mg/dl		2.2-3.9 mmol/L	
(qualitative)					
Glucose tolerance test					
(GTT), oral		<0.5 g/d		<2.8 mmol/d	
Serum		Negative		Negative	
Dosages		**Normal**	**Diabetic**	**Normal**	**Diabetic**
Adult: 75 g	Fasting	70-105 mg/dl	≥126 mg/dl	3.9-5.8 mmol/L	≥7.0 mmol/L
Child: 1.75 g/kg of ideal	60 min	120-170 mg/dl	≥200 mg/dL	6.7-9.4 mmol/L	≥11 mmol/L
weight up to maximum of	90 min	100-140 mg/dl	≥200 mg/dl	5.6-7.8 mmol/L	≥11 mmol/L
75 g	120 min	70-120 mg/dl	≥200 mg/dl	3.9-6.7 mmol/L	≥11 mmol/L
Growth hormone (hGH, somatotropin)					
Plasma	1 d	5-53 ng/mL		5-53 mcg /L	
	1 wk	5-27 ng/mL		5-27 mcg/L	
	1-12 mo	2-10 ng/mL		2-10 mcg/L	
	Fasting child/adult	<0.7-6.0 ng/mL		<0.7-6.0 mcg/L	
Hematocrit (HCT, Hct)					
Whole blood	1 d (cap)	48%-69%		0.48-0.69 vol. fraction	
	2 d	48%-75%		0.48-0.75 vol. fraction	
	3 d	44%-72%		0.44-0.72 vol. fraction	
	2 mo	28%-42%		0.28-0.42 vol. fraction	
	6-12 yr	35%-45%		0.35-0.45 vol. fraction	
	12-18 yr: Male	37%-49%		0.37-0.49 vol. fraction	
	Female	36%-46%		0.36-0.46 vol. fraction	
Hemoglobin (Hb)					
Whole blood	1-3 d (cap)	14.5-22.5 g/dl		2.25-3.49 mmol/L	
	2 mo	9.0-14.0 g/dl		1.40-2.17 mmol/L	
	6-12 yr	11.5-15.5 g/dl		1.78-2.40 mmol/L	
	12-18 yr: Male	13.0-16.0 g/dl		2.02-2.48 mmol/L	
	Female	12.0-16.0 g/dl		1.86-2.48 mmol/L	
Hemoglobin A					
Whole blood		>95% of total		>0.95 fraction of Hb	
Hemoglobin F					
Whole blood	1 d	63%-92% HbF		0.63-0.92 mass fraction HbF	
	5 d	65%-88% HbF		0.65-0.88 mass fraction HbF	
	3 wk	55%-85% HbF		0.55-0.85 mass fraction HbF	
	6-9 wk	31%-75% HbF		0.31-0.75 mass fraction HbF	
	3-4 mo	<2%-59% HbF		<0.02-0.59 mass fraction HbF	
	6 mo	<2%-9% HbF		<0.02-0.09 mass fraction HbF	
	Adult	<2.0% HbF		<0.02 mass fraction HbF	
Immunoglobulin A (IgA)					
Serum	Cord blood	1.4-3.6 mg/dl		14-36 mg/L	
	1-3 mo	1.3-53 mg/dl		13-530 mg/L	
	4-6 mo	4.4-84 mg/dl		44-840 mg/L	
	7 mo-1 yr	11-106 mg/dl		110-1060 mg/L	
	2-5 yr	14-159 mg/dl		140-1590 mg/L	
	6-10 yr	33-236 mg/dl		330-2360 mg/L	
	Adult	70-312 mg/dl		700-3120 mg/L	
Immunoglobulin D (IgD)					
Serum	Newborn	None detected		None detected	
	Thereafter	0-8 mg/dl		0-80 mg/L	

Continued

TEST/SPECIMEN	AGE/GENDER/REFERENCE	Normal Ranges CONVENTIONAL UNITS	 INTERNATIONAL UNITS (SI)
Immunoglobulin E (IgE)			
Serum	Male	0-230 international units/ml	0-230 kinternational units/L
	Female	0-170 international units/ml	0-170 kinternational units/L
Immunoglobulin G (IgG)			
Serum	Cord blood	636-1606 mg/dl	6.36-16.06 g/L
	1 mo	251-906 mg/dl	2.51-9.06 g/L
	2-4 mo	176-601 mg/dl	1.76-6.01 g/L
	5-12 mo	172-1069 mg/dl	1.72-10.69 g/L
	1-5 yr	345-1236 mg/dl	3.45-12.36 g/L
	6-10 yr	608-1572 mg/dl	6.08-15.72 g/L
	Adult	639-1349 mg/dl	6.39-13.49 g/L
Immunoglobulin M (IgM)			
Serum	Cord blood	6.3-25 mg/dl	63-250 mg/L
	1-4 mo	17-105 mg/dl	170-1050 mg/L
	5-9 mo	33-126 mg/dl	330-1260 mg/L
	10 mo-1 yr	41-173 mg/dl	410-1730 mg/L
	2-8 yr	43-207 mg/dl	430-2070 mg/L
	9-10 yr	52-242 mg/dl	520-2420 mg/L
	Adult	56-352 mg/dl	560-3520 mg/L
Iron			
Serum	Newborn	100-250 mcg/dl	18-45 mcmol/L
	Infant	40-100 mcg/dl	7-18 mcmol/L
	Child	50-120 mcg/dl	9-22 mcmol/L
	Thereafter: Male	65-170 mcg/dl	12-30 mcmol/L
	Female	50-170 mcg/dl	9-30 mcmol/L
	Intoxicated child	280-2550 mcg/dl	50.12-456.5mcmol/L
	Fatally poisoned child	>1800 mcg/dl	>322.2 mcmol/L
Iron-binding capacity, total (TIBC)			
Serum	Infant	100-400 mcg/dl	17.90-71.60 mcmol/L
	Thereafter	250-400 mcg/dl	44.75-71.60 mcmol/L
Lead			
Whole blood	Child	<10 mcg/L	<0.48 mcmol/L
Urine, 24 hr		<80 mcg/L	<0.39 mcmol/L
Leukocyte count (WBC count)		**× 1000 cells/mm³ (mcl)**	**× 10⁹ cells/L**
Whole blood	Birth	9.0-30.0	9.0-30.0
	24 hr	9.4-34.0	9.4-34.0
	1 mo	5.0-19.5	5.0-19.5
	1-3 yr	6.0-17.5	6.0-17.5
	4-7 yr	5.5-15.5	5.5-15.5
	8-13 yr	4.5-13.5	4.5-13.5
	Adult	4.5-11.0	4.5-11.0
		× 1000 cells/mm³ (mcl)	**× 10⁶ cells/L**
CSF	Premature	0-25 mononuclear	0-25
		0-10 polymorphonuclear	0-10
		0-1000 RBC	0-1000
	Newborn	0-20 mononuclear	0-20
		0-10 polymorphonuclear	0-10
		0-800 RBC	0-800
	Neonate	0-5 mononuclear	0-5
		0-10 polymorphonuclear	0-10
		0-50 RBC	0-50
	Thereafter	0-5 mononuclear	0-5

TEST/SPECIMEN	AGE/GENDER/REFERENCE	Normal Ranges: CONVENTIONAL UNITS		INTERNATIONAL UNITS (SI)
Leukocyte differential count				
Whole blood	Myelocytes	0%	0 cells/mm^3 (mcl)	Number fraction 0
	Neutrophils ("bands")	3%-5%	150-400 cells/mm^3 (mcl)	Number fraction 0.03-0.05
	Neutrophils ("segs")	54%-62%	3000-5800 cells/mm^3 (mcl)	Number fraction 0.54-0.62
	Lymphocytes	25%-33%	1500-3000 cells/mm^3 (mcl)	Number fraction 0.25-0.33
	Monocytes	3%-7%	285-500 cells/mm^3 (mcl)	Number fraction 0.03-0.07
	Eosinophils	1%-3%	50-250 cells/mm^3 (mcl)	Number fraction 0.01-0.03
	Basophils	0%-0.75%	15-50 cells/mm^3 (mcl)	Number fraction 0-0.0075
Mean corpuscular hemoglobin (MCH)	Birth	31-37 pg/cell		0.48-0.57 fmol/cell
Whole blood	1-3 d (cap)	31-37 pg/cell		0.48-0.57 fmol/cell
	1 wk-1 mo	28-40 pg/cell		0.43-0.62 fmol/cell
	2 mo	26-34 pg/cell		0.40-0.53 fmol/cell
	3-6 mo	25-35 pg/cell		0.39-0.54 fmol/cell
	0.5-2 yr	23-31 pg/cell		0.36-0.48 fmol/cell
	2-6 yr	24-30 pg/cell		0.37-0.47 fmol/cell
	6-12 yr	25-33 pg/cell		0.39-0.51 fmol/cell
	12-18 yr	25-35 pg/cell		0.39-0.54 fmol/cell
	18-49 yr	26-34 pg/cell		0.40-0.53 fmol/cell
Mean corpuscular hemoglobin concentration (MCHC)				
Whole blood	Birth	30%-36% Hb/cell or g Hb/dl RBC		4.65-5.58 mmol Hb/L RBC
	1-3 d (cap)	29%-37% Hb/cell or g Hb/dl RBC		4.50-5.74 mmol Hb/L RBC
	1-2 wk	28%-38% Hb/cell or g Hb/dl RBC		4.34-5.89 mmol Hb/L RBC
	1-2 mo	29%-37% Hb/cell or g Hb/dl RBC		4.50-5.74 mmol Hb/L RBC
	3 mo-2 yr	30%-36% Hb/cell or g Hb/dl RBC		4.65-5.58 mmol Hb/L RBC
	2-18 yr	31%-37% Hb/cell or g Hb/dl RBC		4.81-5.74 mmol Hb/L RBC
	>18 yr	31%-37% Hb/cell or g Hb/dl RBC		4.81-5.74 mmol Hb/L RBC
Mean corpuscular volume (MCV)				
Whole blood	1-3 d (cap)	95-121 mcm^3		95-121 fl
	0.5-2 yr	70-86 mcm^3		70-86 fl
	6-12 yr	77-95 mcm^3		77-95 fl
	12-18 yr: Male	78-98 mcm^3		78-98 fl
	Female	78-102 mcm^3		78-102 fl
Osmolality				
Serum	Child, adult	275-295 mOsmol/kg H_2O		
Urine, random		50-1400 mOsm/kg H_2O, depending on fluid intake; after 12-hr fluid restriction: >850 mOsm/kg H_2O		
Urine, 24 hr		≃300-900 mOsmol/kg H_2O		

Continued

TEST/SPECIMEN	AGE/GENDER/REFERENCE	Normal Ranges CONVENTIONAL UNITS	 INTERNATIONAL UNITS (SI)
Oxygen, partial pressure (Po_2)			
Whole blood, arterial	Birth	8-24 mm Hg	1.1-3.2 kPa
	5-10 min	33-75 mm Hg	4.4-10.0 kPa
	30 min	31-85 mm Hg	4.1-11.3 kPa
	>1 hr	55-80 mm Hg	7.3-10.6 kPa
	1 d	54-95 mm Hg	7.2-12.6 kPa
	Thereafter (decreased with age)	83-108 mm Hg	11-14.4 kPa
Oxygen saturation (Sao_2)			
Whole blood, arterial	Newborn	85%-90%	Fraction saturated 0.85-0.90
	Thereafter	95%-99%	Fraction saturated 0.95-0.99
Partial thromboplastin time (PTT)			
Whole blood (Na citrate)			
Nonactivated		60-85 sec (Platelin)	60-85 sec
Activated		25-35 sec (differs with method)	25-35 sec
pH			**H^+ concentration**
Whole blood, arterial	Premature (48 hr)	7.35-7.50	31-44 nmol/L
	Birth, full term	7.11-7.36	43-77 nmol/L
	5-10 min	7.09-7.30	50-81 nmol/L
	30 min	7.21-7.38	41-61 nmol/L
	>1 hr	7.26-7.49	32-54 nmol/L
	1 d	7.29-7.45	35-51 nmol/L
	Thereafter	7.35-7.45	35-44 nmol/L
	Must be corrected for body temperature		
Urine, random	Newborn/neonate	5-7	0.1-10 mcmol/L
	Thereafter	4.5-8	0.01-32 mcmol/L (average ≃1.0 mcmol/L)
Stool		7.0-7.5	31-100 nmol/L
Phenylalanine			
Serum	Premature	2.0-7.5 mg/dl	120-450 mcmol/L
	Newborn	1.2-3.4 mg/dl	70-210 mcmol/L
	Thereafter	0.8-1.8 mg/dl	50-110 mcol/L
Urine, 24 hr	10 d-2 wk	1-2 mg/day	6-12 mcmol/day
	3-12 yr	4-18 mg/d	24-110 mcmol/day
	Thereafter	Trace-17 mg/day	Trace-103 mcmol/day
Plasma volume	Male	25-43 ml/kg	0.025-0.043 L/kg
Plasma	Female	28-45 ml/kg	0.028-0.045 L/kg
Platelet count (thrombocyte count)			
Whole blood (EDTA)	Newborn (After 1 wk, same as adult)	84-478 × 10^3/mm^3 (mcl)	84-478 × 10^9/L
Potassium	Adult	150-400 × 10^3/mm^3 (mcl)	150-400 × 10^9/L
Serum	Newborn	3.0-6.0 mEq/L	3.0-6.0 mmol/L
Plasma (heparin)	Thereafter	3.5-5.0 mEq/L	3.5-5.0 mmol/L
Urine, 24 hr		3.4-4.5 mEq/L	3.4-4.5 mmol/L
Protein		2.5-125 mEq/d varies with diet	2.5-125 mmol/L
Serum, total	Premature	4.3-7.6 g/dl	43-76 g/L
	Newborn	4.6-7.4 g/dl	46-74 g/L
	1-7 yr	6.1-7.9 g/dl	61-79 g/L
	8-12 yr	6.4-8.1 g/dl	64-81 g/L
	13-19 yr	6.6-8.2 g/dl	66-82 g/L

	Normal Ranges		
TEST/SPECIMEN	AGE/GENDER/REFERENCE	CONVENTIONAL UNITS	INTERNATIONAL UNITS (SI)
Protein—cont'd			
Total			
Urine, 24 hr		1-14 mg/dl 50-80 mg/day (at rest) <250 mg/day after intense-exercise	10-140 mg/L 50-80 mg/day <250 mg/d after intense exercise
CSF		Lumbar: 8-32 mg/dl	80-320 mg/L
Prothrombin time (PT)			
One-stage (Quick)			
Whole blood (Na citrate)	In general	11-15 sec (varies with type of thromboplastin)	11-15 sec
	Newborn	Prolonged by 2-3 sec	Prolonged by 2-3 sec
Two-stage modified (Ware and Seegers)			
Whole blood (Na citrate)		18-22 sec	18-22 sec
RBC count: see Erythrocyte count			
Red blood cell volume			
Whole blood	Male	20-36 ml/kg	0.020-0.036 L/kg
Reticulocyte count	Female	19-31 ml/kg	0.019-0.031 L/kg
Whole blood	Adults	0.5%-1.5% of erythrocytes or 25,000-75,000/mm³ (mcl)	0.005-0.015 (number fraction) or 25,000-75,000 × 10^6/L
Capillary	1 d	0.4%-6.0%	0.004-0.060 (number fraction)
	7 d	<0.1%-1.3%	<0.001-0.013 (number fraction)
	1-4 wk	<0.1%-1.2%	<0.001-0.012 (number fraction)
	5-6 wk	<0.1%-2.4%	<0.001-0.024 (number fraction)
	7-8 wk	0.1%-2.9%	0.001-0.029 (number fraction)
	9-10 wk	<0.1%-2.6%	<0.001-0.026 (number fraction)
	11-12 wk	0.1%-1.3%	0.001-0.013 (number fraction)
Salicylates			
Serum, plasma	Therap. conc.	15-30 mg/dl	1.1-2.2 mmol/L
	Toxic conc.	>30 mg/dl	>18.5 mmol/L
Sedimentation rate: see Erythrocyte sedimentation rate			
Sodium			
Serum or plasma	Newborn	134-146 mEq/L	134-146 mmol/L
	Infant	139-146 mEq/L	139-146 mmol/L
	Child	138-145 mEq/L	138-145 mmol/L
	Thereafter	136-146 mEq/L	136-146 mmol/L
Urine, 24 hr		40-220 mEq/L (diet dependent)	40-220 mmol/L
Sweat	Normal	<40 mEq/L	<40 mmol/L
	Indeterminate	45-60 mEq/L	45-60 mmol/L
	Cystic fibrosis	>60 mEq/L	>60 mmol/L
Specific gravity			
Urine, random	Adult	1.002-1.030	1.002-1.030
	After 12 hr fluid restriction	>1.025	>1.025

Continued

TEST/SPECIMEN	AGE/GENDER/REFERENCE	Normal Ranges: CONVENTIONAL UNITS		INTERNATIONAL UNITS (SI)	
Theophylline					
Serum, plasma	Therap. conc.				
	Bronchodilator	10-20 mcg/ml		56-110 mcmol/L	
	Premature apnea	5-10 mcg/ml		28-56 mcmol/L	
	Toxic conc.	>20 mcg/ml		>110 mcmol/L	
Thrombin time					
Whole blood (Na citrate)		Control time ± 2 sec when control is 9-13 sec		Control time ± 2 sec when control is 9-13 sec	
Thyroxine, total (T_3)					
Serum	Cord	8-13 mcg/dl		103-168 nmol/L	
	Newborn	11.5-24 (lower in low-birth-weight infants)		148-310 nmol/L	
	Neonate	9-18 mcg/dl		116-232 nmol/L	
	Infant	7-15 mcg/dl		90-194 nmol/L	
	1-5 yr	7.3-15 mcg/dl		94-194 nmol/L	
	5-10 yr	6.4-13.3 mcg/dl		83-172 nmol/L	
	Thereafter	5-12 mcg/dl		65-155 nmol/L	
	Newborn screen (filter paper)	6.2-22 mcg/dl		80-284 nmol/L	
Triglycerides (TG)					
Serum, after ≥12 hr fast		**mg/dl**		**g/L**	
		Male	**Female**	**Male**	**Female**
	Cord blood	10-98	10-98	0.10-0.98	0.10-0.98
	0-5 yr	30-86	32-99	0.30-0.86	0.32-0.99
	6-11 yr	31-108	35-114	0.31-1.08	0.35-1.14
	12-15 yr	36-138	41-138	0.36-1.38	0.41-1.38
	16-19 yr	40-163	40-128	0.40-1.63	0.40-1.28
Triiodothyronine, free					
Serum	Cord	20-240 pg/dl		0.3-3.7 pmol/L	
	1-3 d	200-610 pg/dl		3.1-9.4 pmol/L	
	6 wk	240-560 pg/dl		3.7-8.6 pmol/L	
	Adults (20-50 yr)	230-660 pg/dl		3.5-10.0 pmol/L	
Triiodothyronine, total (T_3-RIA)					
Serum	Cord	30-70 ng/dl		0.46-1.08 nmol/L	
	Newborn	72-260 ng/dl		1.16-4 nmol/L	
	1-5 yr	100-260 ng/dl		1.54-4 nmol/L	
	5-10 yr	90-240 ng/dl		1.39-3.70 nmol/L	
	10-15 yr	80-210 ng/dl		1.23-3.23 nmol/L	
	Thereafter	115-190 ng/dl		1.77-2.93 nmol/L	
Urea nitrogen					
Serum or plasma	Cord	21-40 mg/dl		7.5-14.3 mmol/L	
	Premature (1 wk)	3-25 mg/dl		1.1-9 mmol/L	
	Newborn	3-12 mg/dl		1.1-4.3 mmol/L	
	Infant/child	5-18 mg/dl		1.8-6.4 mmol/L	
	Thereafter	7-18 mg/dl		2.5-6.4 mmol/L	
Urine volume					
Urine, 24 hr	Newborn	50-300 ml/d		0.050-0.3 L/day	
	Infant	350-550 ml/d		0.350-0.5 L/day	
	Child	500-1000 ml/d		0.500-1 L/d	
	Adolescent	700-1400 ml/d		0.700-1.4 L/d	
	Thereafter: Male	800-1800 ml/d		0.800-1.8 L/d	
	Female	600-1600 ml/d (varies with intake and other factors)		0.600-1.6 L/d	
WBC: see Leukocyte count					

ABBREVIATIONS USED IN LABORATORY TESTS

Abbreviation	Term
cap	capillary
CHF	congestive heart failure
conc.	concentration
CSF	cerebrospinal fluid
d	day; diem
EDTA	ethylenediaminetetraacetate
g	gram
m	meter
hr	hour
L, l	liter
mEq	milliequivalent
min	minute
mm	millimeter
mm^3	cubic millimeter
mo	month
mol	mole
mOsmol	milliosmole
s	second
SI	International system of units
Therap.	therapeutic
U, unit	International unit of enzyme activity
vol	volume
wk	week
yr	year
>	greater than
≥	greater than or equal to
<	less than
≤	less than or equal to
±	plus or minus
≈	approximately equal to

PREFIXES DENOTING DECIMAL FACTORS

Prefix	Symbol	Amount
deci	d	one tenth (10^{-1})
centi	c	one hundredth (10^{-2})
milli	m	one thousandth (10^{-3})
micro	μ, mc	one millionth (10^{-6})
nano	n	one billionth (10^{-9})
pico	p	one trillionth (10^{-12})
femto	f	one quadrillionth (10^{-15})

Appendix

G Dietary Reference Intakes

DIETARY REFERENCE INTAKES: RECOMMENDED DIETARY ALLOWANCES (RDA) AND ADEQUATE INTAKE (AI)*

CATEGORY	AGE (YEARS) OR CONDITION	Weight (kg)	Weight (lb)	Height (cm)	Height (in)	PROTEIN RDA (g/kg)	Fat-Soluble Vitamins: VITAMIN A RDA (mcg/d)[a]	VITAMIN D AI (mcg/d)[b]	VITAMIN E RDA (mg/d)[c]	VITAMIN K AI (mcg/d)
Infants	0.0-0.5	6	13	62	24		400	5	4	2
	0.5-1.0	9	20	71	28		500	5	5	2.5
Children	1-3	12	27	86	34	1.10	300	5	6	30
	4-8	20	44	115	45	0.95	400	5	7	55
Males	9-13	36	79	144	57	0.95	600	5	11	60
	14-18	61	134	174	68	0.85	900	5	15	75
	19-30	70	154	177	70	0.80	900	5	15	120
Females	9-13	37	81	144	57	0.95	600	5	11	60
	14-18	54	119	163	64	0.85	700	5	15	75
	19-30	57	126	163	64	0.80	700	5	15	90
Pregnant	≤18					+25 g/d	750	5	15	75
Lactating	≤18					+25 g/d	1200	5	19	75

*NOTE: For all nutrients, values for infants are AI.

Modified from the *Dietary Reference Intake* series, National Academy of Sciences, National Academies Press, 1997, 1998, 2000, 2001; and American Academy of Pediatrics: *Pediatric nutrition handbook*, ed 5, Washington, DC, 2004, National Academies Press.

[a]Retinol equivalent (RAE). 1 RAE = 1 mcg retinol.

[b]Cholecalciferol, 1 mcg cholecalciferol = 40 international units vitamin D. Assumes an absence of adequate exposure to sunlight.

[c]Expressed as α-tocopherol.

[d]Expressed as niacin equivalents (NE); except for infants < 6 months of age, expressed as preformed niacin. 1 mg niacin = 60 mg tryptophan.

[e]Expressed as dietary folate equivalents (DFE); 1 DFE − 1 mcg food folate = 0.6 mcg folic acid from fortified food or as a supplement consumed with food = 5 mcg of a supplement taken on an empty stomach.

[f]In view of evidence linking folate intake with neural tube defects in the fetus, it is recommended that all women capable of becoming pregnant consume 400 mcg from supplements or fortified foods in addition to intake of food folate from the diet.

[g]It is assumed all women will continue consuming 400 mcg from supplements or fortified food until their pregnancy is confirmed and they enter prenatal care, which ordinarily occurs after the end of the preconceptional period—the critical time for formation of the neural tube.

Water-Soluble Vitamins							Minerals						
VITAMIN C RDA (mg/d)	THIAMIN RDA (mg/d)	RIBOFLAVIN RDA (mg/d)	NIACIN RDA (mg/d)[d]	VITAMIN B_6 RDA (mg/d)	FOLATE RDA (mcg/d)[e]	VITAMIN B_{12} RDA (mcg/d)	CALCIUM AI (mg/d)	PHOSPHORUS RDA (mg/d)	MAGNESIUM RDA (mg/d)	IRON RDA (mg/d)	ZINC RDA (mg/d)	IODINE RDA (mcg/d)	SELENIUM RDA (mcg/d)
40	0.2	0.3	2	0.1	65	0.4	210	100	30	0.27	2	110	15
50	0.3	0.4	4	3	80	0.5	270	275	75	11	3	130	20
15	0.5	0.5	6	0.5	150	0.9	500	460	80	7	3	90	20
25	0.6	0.6	8	0.6	200	1.2	800	500	130	10	5	90	30
45	0.9	0.9	12	1	300	1.8	1300	1250	240	8	8	120	40
75	1.2	1.3	16	1.3	400	2.4	1300	1250	410	11	11	150	55
90	1.2	1.3	16	1.3	400	2.4	1000	700	400	8	11	150	55
45	0.9	0.9	12	1	300	1.8	1300	1250	240	8	8	120	40
65	1	1	14	1.2	400	2.4	1300	1250	360	15	9	150	55
75	1.1	1.1	14	1.3	400[f]	2.4	1000	700	310	18	8	150	55
80	1.4	1.4	18	1.9	600[g]	2.6	1300	1250	400	27	13	220	60
115	1.4	1.6	17	2	500	2.8	1300	1250	360	10	14	290	70

ESTIMATED SAFE AND ADEQUATE DAILY DIETARY INTAKES OF SELECTED VITAMINS AND MINERALS[a]

		Vitamins		Trace Elements[b]				
CATEGORY	AGE (YEARS)	BIOTIN (mcg)	PANTOTHENIC ACID (mg)	COPPER (mg)	MANGANESE (mg)	FLUORIDE (mg)	CHROMIUM (mcg)	MOLYBDENUM (mcg)
Infants	0-0.5	10	2	0.4-0.6	0.3-0.6	0.1-0.5	10-40	15-30
	0.5-1	15	3	0.6-0.7	0.6-1.0	0.2-1.0	20-60	20-40
Children and adolescents	1-3	20	3	0.7-1.0	1.0-1.5	0.5-1.5	20-80	25-50
	4-6	25	3-4	1.0-1.5	1.5-2.0	1.0-2.5	30-120	30-75
	7-10	30	4-5	1.0-2.0	2.0-3.0	1.5-2.5	50-200	50-150
	11+	30-100	4-7	1.5-2.5	2.0-5.0	1.5-2.5	50-200	75-250
Adults		30-100	4-7	1.5-3.0	2.0-5.0	1.5-4.0	50-200	75-250

From Food and Nutrition Board, National Research Council: *Recommended dietary allowances,* ed 10, Washington, DC, 1989, National Academy of Sciences.
[a]Because there is less information on which to base allowances, these figures are not given in the main table of RDAs and are provided here in the form of ranges of recommended intakes.
[b]Because the toxic levels for many trace elements may be only several times usual intakes, the upper levels for the trace elements given in this table should not be habitually exceeded.

ESTIMATED SODIUM, CHLORIDE, AND POTASSIUM MINIMUM REQUIREMENTS OF HEALTHY PERSONS[a]

AGE	WEIGHT (kg)[a]	SODIUM (mg)[a,b]	CHLORIDE (mg)[a,b]	POTASSIUM (mg)[c]
Months				
0-5	4.5	120	180	500
6-11	8.9	200	300	700
Years				
1	11.0	225	350	1000
2-5	16.0	300	500	1400
6-9	25.0	400	600	1600
10-18	50.0	500	750	2000
>18[d]	70.0	500	750	2000

From Food and Nutrition Board, National Research Council: *Recommended dietary allowances,* ed 10, Washington, DC, 1989, National Academy of Sciences.
[a]No allowance has been included for large, prolonged losses from the skin through sweat.
[b]There is no evidence that higher intakes confer any health benefit.
[c]Desirable intakes of potassium may considerably exceed these values (~3500 mg for adults).
[d]No allowance included for growth. Values for those younger than 18 years of age assume a growth rate at the 50th percentile reported by the National Center for Health Statistics and averaged for males and females.

MEDIAN HEIGHTS AND WEIGHTS AND RECOMMENDED ENERGY INTAKE

CATEGORY	AGE (YEAR) OR CONDITION	Weight (kg)	Weight (lb)	Height (cm)	Height (in)	Ree[A] (kcal/day)	Average Energy Allowance (kcal)[b] MULTIPLES OF Ree	PER kg	PER DAY[C]
Infants	0.0-0.5	6	13	60	24	320		108	650
	0.5-1.0	9	20	71	28	500		98	850
Children	1-3	13	29	90	35	740		102	1300
	4-6	20	44	112	44	950		90	1800
	7-10	28	62	132	52	1130		70	2000
Males	11-14	45	99	157	62	1440	1.70	55	2500
	15-18	66	145	176	69	1760	1.67	45	3000
	19-24	72	160	177	70	1780	1.67	40	2900
	25-50	79	174	176	70	1800	1.60	37	2900
	51+	77	170	173	68	1530	1.50	30	2300
Females	11-14	46	101	157	62	1310	1.67	47	2200
	15-18	55	120	163	64	1370	1.60	40	2200
	19-24	58	128	164	65	1350	1.60	38	2200
	25-50	63	138	163	64	1380	1.55	36	2200
	51+	65	143	160	63	1280	1.50	30	1900
Pregnant	1st trimester								+0
	2nd trimester								+300
	3rd trimester								+300
Lactating	1st 6 months								+500
	2nd 6 months								+500

From Food and Nutrition Board, National Research Council: *Recommended dietary allowances,* ed 10, Washington, DC, 1989, National Academy of Sciences.

[a]Resting energy expenditure (Ree).

[b]In the range of light to moderate activity, the coefficient of variation is ±20%.

[c]Figure is rounded.

The data in this table have been assembled from the observed median heights and weights of children together with desirable weights for adults for the mean heights of men (70 inches) and women (64 inches) between ages 18 and 34 years as surveyed in the U.S. population (HEW/NCHS data). The energy allowances for the young adults are for men and women doing light work. The allowances for the two older age groups represent mean energy needs over these age spans, allowing for a 2% decrease in basal (resting) metabolic rate per decade and a reduction in activity of 200 kcal/day for men and women between 51 and 75 years of age, 500 kcal for men over 75, and 400 kcal for women over 75. The customary range of daily energy output is shown for adults in parentheses and is based on a variation in energy needs of ±400 kcal at any one age, emphasizing the wide range of energy intakes appropriate for any age group of people. Energy allowances for children through age 18 are based on medium energy intakes of children these ages followed in longitudinal growth studies.

Appendix

H NANDA-Approved Nursing Diagnoses 2005-2006

Activity intolerance
Activity intolerance, risk for
Adjustment, impaired
Airway clearance, ineffective
Allergy response, latex
Allergy response, latex, risk for
Anxiety
Anxiety, death
Aspiration, risk for
Attachment, impaired parent/infant/child, risk for
Autonomic dysreflexia
Autonomic dysreflexia, risk for
Body image, disturbed
Body temperature, imbalanced, risk for
Bowel incontinence
Breastfeeding, effective
Breastfeeding, ineffective
Breastfeeding, interrupted
Breathing pattern, ineffective
Cardiac output, decreased
Caregiver role strain
Caregiver role strain, risk for
Comfort, impaired
Communication, verbal, impaired
Communication, readiness for enhanced
Conflict, decisional (specify)
Conflict, parental role
Confusion, acute
Confusion, chronic
Constipation
Constipation, perceived
Constipation, risk for
Coping, ineffective
Coping, readiness for enhanced
Coping, community, ineffective
Coping, community, readiness for enhanced
Coping, defensive
Coping, family, compromised
Coping, family, disabled
Coping, family, readiness for enhanced
Death syndrome, sudden infant, risk for
Denial, ineffective
Dentition, impaired
Development, delayed, risk for
Diarrhea
Disuse syndrome, risk for
Diversional activity, deficient
Energy field, disturbed
Environmental interpretation syndrome, impaired
Failure to thrive, adult
Falls, risk for
Family processes: alcoholism, dysfunctional
Family processes, interrupted
Family processes, readiness for enhanced
Fatigue
Fear
Fluid balance, readiness for enhanced
Fluid volume, deficient
Fluid volume, excess
Fluid volume, deficient, risk for
Fluid volume, imbalanced, risk for
Gas exchange, impaired
Grieving
Grieving, anticipatory
Grieving, dysfunctional
Grieving, risk for dysfunctional
Growth and development, delayed
Growth disproportionate, risk for
Health maintenance, ineffective
Health-seeking behaviors
Home maintenance, impaired
Hopelessness
Hyperthermia
Hypothermia
Identity, personal, disturbed
Incontinence, urinary, functional
Incontinence, urinary, reflex
Incontinence, urinary, stress
Incontinence, urinary, total
Incontinence, urinary, urge
Incontinence, urinary, urge, risk for
Infant behavior, disorganized
Infant behavior, disorganized, risk for
Infant behavior, organized, readiness for enhanced
Feeding pattern, infant, ineffective
Infection, risk for
Injury, risk for
Injury, perioperative positioning, risk for
Intracranial adaptive capacity, decreased
Knowledge, deficient
Knowledge of (Specify), readiness for enhanced
Lifestyle, sedentary
Loneliness, risk for
Memory, impaired
Mobility, bed, impaired
Mobility, physical, impaired
Mobility, wheelchair, impaired
Nausea
Neglect, unilateral
Noncompliance
Nutrition, readiness for enhanced
Nutrition: less than body requirements, imbalanced
Nutrition: more than body requirements, imbalanced
Nutrition: more than body requirements, risk for imbalanced
Oral mucous membrane, impaired
Pain, acute
Pain, chronic
Parenting, readiness for enhanced
Parenting, impaired
Parenting, impaired, risk for
Peripheral neurovascular dysfunction, risk for
Poisoning, risk for
Post-trauma syndrome
Post-trauma syndrome, risk for

North American Nursing Diagnosis Association International: *Nursing diagnoses: definitions and classification 2005-2006.* Philadelphia, 2005, NANDA.

Powerlessness
Powerlessness, risk for
Protection, ineffective
Rape-trauma syndrome
Rape-trauma syndrome: compound reaction
Rape-trauma syndrome: silent reaction
Religiosity, impaired
Religiosity, readiness for enhanced
Religiosity, risk for impaired
Relocation stress syndrome
Relocation stress syndrome, risk for
Role performance, ineffective
Self-care deficit, bathing/hygiene
Self-care deficit, dressing/grooming
Self-care deficit, feeding
Self-care deficit, toileting
Self-concept, readiness for enhanced
Self-esteem, chronic low
Self-esteem, situational low
Self-esteem, situational low, risk for
Self-mutilation
Self-mutilation, risk for
Sensory perception, disturbed
Sexual dysfunction
Sexuality patterns, ineffective
Skin integrity, impaired
Skin integrity, impaired, risk for
Sleep deprivation
Sleep patterns, disturbed
Sleep, readiness for enhanced
Social interaction, impaired
Social isolation
Sorrow, chronic
Spiritual distress
Spiritual distress, risk for
Spiritual well-being, readiness for enhanced
Suffocation, risk for
Suicide, risk for
Surgical recovery, delayed
Swallowing, impaired
Therapeutic regimen management, effective
Therapeutic regimen management, ineffective
Therapeutic regimen management, readiness for enhanced
Therapeutic regimen management, community, ineffective
Therapeutic regimen management, family, ineffective
Thermoregulation, ineffective
Thought processes, disturbed
Tissue integrity, impaired
Tissue perfusion, ineffective
Transfer ability, impaired
Trauma, risk for
Urinary elimination, readiness for enhanced
Urinary elimination, impaired
Urinary retention
Ventilation, spontaneous, impaired
Ventilatory weaning response, dysfunctional
Violence, other-directed, risk for
Violence, self-directed, risk for
Walking, impaired
Wandering

Appendix

I Translations of FACES Pain Rating Scale*

TRANSLATIONS OF WONG-BAKER FACES PAIN RATING SCALE*

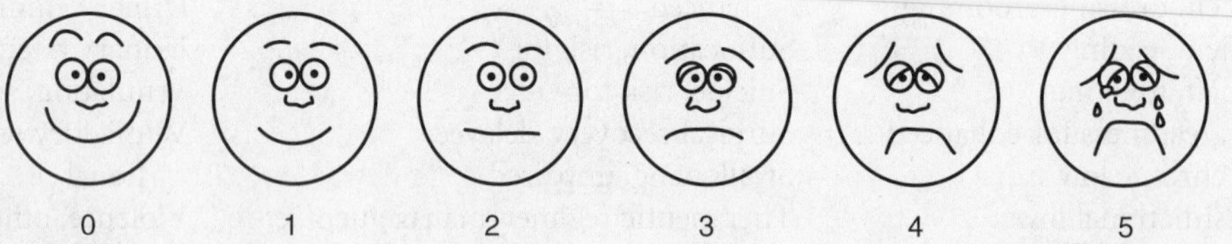

0–5 coding	0	1	2	3	4	5
0-10 coding	0	2	4	6	8	10
ENGLISH	No hurt	Hurts little bit	Hurts little more	Hurts even more	Hurts whole lot	Hurts worst
SPANISH	No duele	Duele un poco	Duele un poco más	Duele mucho	Duele mucho más	Duele el máximo
FRENCH	Pas mal	Un petit peu mal	Un peu plus mal	Encore plus mal	Très mal	Très très mal
ITALIAN	Non fa male	Fa male un poco	Fa male un po di piu	Fa male ancora di piu	Fa molto male	Fa maggior-mente male
PORTUGUESE	Não doi	Doi um pouco	Doi um pouco mais	Doi muito	Doi muito mais	Doi o máximo
BOSNIAN	Ne boli	Boli samo malo	Boli malo više	Boli još više	Boli puno	Boli najviše
VIETNAMESE	Không dau	Hỏi dau	Dau hỏn chút	Dau nhiêu hỏn	Dau thât nhiêu	Dau qúa dô
CHINESE	無痛	微痛	較痛	更痛	很痛	劇痛
GREEK	Δεν Πovaï	Πovaï Λιγo	Πovaï Λιγo Πιo Πoλν	Πovaï Πoλν	Πovaï Πιo Πoλν	Πovaï Παρa Πoλν
ROMANIAN	No doare	Doare puţin	Doare un pic mai mult	Doare şi mai mult	Doare foarte tare	Doare cel mai mult

Brief word instructions (above): Point to each face using the words to describe the pain intensity. Ask the child to choose face that best describes own pain and record the appropriate number. *Note:* In a study of 148 children ages 4 to 5 years, there were no differences in pain scores when children used the original or brief word instructions. (In Wong D, Baker C: *Reference manual for the Wong-Baker FACES Pain Rating Scale,* Duarte, CA, 1998, City of Hope Mayday Pain Resource Center; also available on the following Web site: http://www.mosby.com/MERLIN/Wong/Essentials/).

*__Wong-Baker FACES Pain Rating Scale:__ Available at no charge from The Purdue Frederick Company, 100 Connecticut Ave., Norwalk, CT 06850-3590; phone: 203-853-0123, ext. 7378 or 7314. Spanish and Portuguese translations by Ellen Johnsen; French translation by Thomas Angelo; Italian translation by Madeline Mitchko; Romanian translation by Florin Nicolae; Vietnamese translation by Yen B. Isle; Chinese translation by Hung-Shen Lin; Japanese translation from *After the announcement of cancer,* Tokyo, 1993, Iwanami Shoten, Pub; German translation from Wong DL: *Pediatric quick reference,* Berlin, Wiesbaden, 1997, Ullstein Mosby.

ORIGINAL INSTRUCTIONS:

English

Explain to the person that each face is for a person who feels happy because he has no pain (hurt) or sad because he has some or a lot of pain. Face 0 is very happy because he doesn't hurt at all. Face 1 hurts just a little bit. Face 2 hurts a little more. Face 3 hurts even more. Face 4 hurts a whole lot. Face 5 hurts as much as you can imagine, although you don't have to be crying to feel this bad. Ask the person to choose the face that best describes how he is feeling.

Rating scale is recommended for persons age 3 years and older.

Spanish

Explíquele a la persona que cada cara representa una persona que se siente feliz porque no tiene dolor o triste porque siente un poco o mucho dolor. **Cara 0** se siente muy feliz porque no tiene dolor. **Cara 1** tiene un poco de dolor. **Cara 2** tiene un poquito más de dolor. **Cara 3** tiene más dolor. **Cara 4** tiene mucho dolor. **Cara 5** tiene el dolor más fuerte que usted pueda imaginar, aunque usted no tiene que estar llorando para sentirse así de mal. Pídale a la persona que escoja la cara que mejor describe su propio dolor.

Esta escala se puede usar con personas de tres años de edad o más.

French

Expliquez à la personne que chaque visage représent un personne qui est heureux parce qu'elle n'a pas point du mal ou triste parce qu'il a un peu ou beaucoup du mal. **Visage 0** est trés heureux parce qu'elle n'a pas point du mal. **Visage 1** a un petit peu de mal. **Visage 2** a plus du mal. **Visage 3** a encore plus du mal. **Visage 4** a beaucoup du mal. **Visage 5** a autant mal que vous pouvez imaginer, bien que ces mauvais sentiments ne finissent pas nécessairement a vous faire pleurer. Demandez à la personne de choisir le visage qui convient le mieux avec ses sentiments.

Ces evaluations sont recommendés pour des personnes de trois ans et davantage.

Italian

Spiegare a la persona che ogni facien è per una persona che si sente felice perchè non tiene dolore oppure triste perchè ha poco o molto dolore. **Faccia O** è molto felice perchè non tiene dolore. **Faccia 1** tiene poco dolore. **Faccia 2** tiene un po più di dolore. **Faccia 3** tiene più dolore. **Faccia 4** tiene molto dolore. **Faccia 5** tiene molto dolore che non puoi immaginare però non devi piangere per tenere dolore. Domandi ala persona di scegliere quale faccia meglio descrive come si sente.

Grado scale è raccomandata a la persona di tre anni in sù.

Portuguese

Explique a pessoa que cada face representa uma pessoa que está feliz porque não têm dor, ou triste por ter um pouco ou muita dor. **Face 0** está muito feliz porque não têm nenhuma dor. **Face 1** tem apenas um pouco de dor. **Face 2** têm um pouco mais de dor. **Face 3** têm ainda mais dor. **Face 4** têm muita dor. **Face 5** têm uma dor máxima, apesar de que nem sempre provoca o choro. Peça a pessoa que escolhe a face que melhor descreve como ele se sente.

Esta escala é aplicável a pessoas de tres anos de idade ou mais.

Romanian

Explicati copilului că fiecare desen (figură) corespunde unei persoane care este veselă, pentru ca nu are nici o durere, sau unei persoane care este tristă, pentru că are dureri. **Figura 0** este foarte fericită pentru că nu are nici o durere. **Figura 1** arată că doare doar un pic. **Figura 2** arată că doare ceva mai mult. **Figura 3** arată că doare şi mai mult. **Figura 4** arată că doare foarte tare. **Figura 5** arată că doare atât de tare cât se poate imagina, chiar dacă nu este însoţita neapărat de lacrimi. Cereţi copilului (persoanei) să indice figura care exprimă cel mai bine cum se simte el.

Scala de evaluare a durerii este recomandată pentru copiii în vârstă de 3 ani şi peste.

Bosnian

Objasnite osobi da je svako lice namjenjeno za osobu koja se osjeća sretnom jer ne osjeća bol ili tužnom jer osjeća malo ili puno boli. **Lice 0** je sretno jer ne osjeća nikakvu bol. **Lice 1** osjeća samo malu bol. **Lice 2** osjeća malo više boli. **Lice 3** osjeća još veću bol. **Lice 4** osjeća puno boli. **Lice 5** osjeća onoliku bol koju je moguće zamisliti, što ne znači da osoba koja osjeća tu bol mora plakati. Upitajte osobu da izabere lice koje najbolje opisuju kako se osjeća. Skala procijene bola se preporućuje za osobe starosti 3 godine ili više.

Upirati prstom na svako lice objašnjavajući riječima intensitet boli. Pitajte dijete da izabere lice koje najbolje opisuje njihovu bol i zabilježite odgovarajući broj.

German

Erläutern Sie dem Kind, daβ jedes Gesicht zu einer Person gehört, die froh darüber ist, keine Schmerzen zu haben, oder die sehr traurig ist, weil sie mäβige bis starke Schmerzen hat. **Gesicht 0** ist sehr froh, weil es keine Schmerzen hat. **Gesicht 1** sagt, es tut ein biβchen weh. **Gesicht 2** hat ein biβchen mehr Schmerzen. **Gesicht 3** sagt, es tut noch mehr weh, und **Gesicht 4,** es tut ziemlich weh. **Gesicht 5** leidet unter so starken Schmerzen, wie Du Dir nur vorstellen kannst, auch wenn dabei nicht unbedingt Tränen flieβen müssen. Bitten Sie das Kind, das Gesicht auszuwählen, das seinem Empfinden am besten entspricht. Empfohlen für Kinder ab 3 Jahren.

Vietnamese

Xin cắt nghĩa cho mổi người, từng khuôn mặt của một người cãm thấy vui vẽ tại vì không có sự đau đớn hoặc, buồn vì có chút ít hay rất nhiều sự đau đớn.

Cái **mặt** với **số 0** thì rất là vui tại vì mặt ấy không có sự đau đớn. **Mặt số 1** chỉ đau một chút thôi. **Mặt số 2** hơi đau hơn một chút nữa. **Mặt số 3** đau hơn chút nữa. **Mặt số 4** đau thật nhiều. **Mặt số 5** đau không thể tưởng tượng, mặc dù người ta không cần phải khóc mới cảm thấy được sự buồn khổ như thế.

Bạn hỏi từng người tự chọn khuôn mặt nào diển tả được sự đau đớn của chính mình.

Japanese

３歳以上の患者に望ましい。それぞれの顔は、患者の痛み (pain, hurt) がないのでご機嫌な感じ、または、ある程度の痛み・沢山の痛みがあるので悲しい感じを表現していることを説明して下さい。0＝痛みがまったくないから、とても幸せな顔をしている、1＝ほんの少し痛い、2＝もう少し痛い、3＝もっと痛い、4＝とっても痛い、5＝痛くて涙を流す必要はないけれども、これ以上の痛みは考えられないほど痛い。今、どのように感じているか最もよく表わしている顔を選ぶよう、患者に求めて下さい。

Chinese

解釋給人聽用每張臉譜來代表著一個人的感覺是因爲沒有疼痛〔傷痛〕而感快樂或是因爲些許疼痛或者是許多疼痛而感傷心。第零張臉是很快樂的因爲他一點也不覺得疼痛。第一張臉只痛一丁點兒。第二張臉又痛多了一些。第三張臉痛得更多了。第四張臉是非常痛了。第五張臉是爲人們所能想像到的劇痛既使感到這樣難過，卻不一定哭出來。請這人選擇出最能代表他現在感覺的一張臉譜。此量表適用於三歲以上的人。

Pediatric Vital Signs and Parameters

CENTIGRADE TO FAHRENHEIT TEMPERATURE CONVERSIONS

°C	°F	°C	°F	°C	°F
35.0	95.0	37.0	98.6	39.0	102.2
35.2	95.4	37.2	99.0	39.2	102.6
35.4	95.7	37.4	99.3	39.4	102.9
35.6	96.1	37.6	99.7	39.6	103.3
35.8	96.4	37.8	100.0	39.8	103.6
36.0	96.8	38.0	100.4	40.0	104.0
36.2	97.2	38.2	100.8	40.2	104.4
36.4	97.5	38.4	101.1	40.4	104.7
36.6	97.9	38.6	101.5	40.6	105.1
36.8	98.2	38.8	101.8	40.8	105.4
				41.0	105.8

Conversion Formulas

$°F = (°C \times 9/5) + 32$ or $(°C \times 1.8) + 32$

$°C = (°F - 32) + 5/9$ or $(°F - 32) + 0.55$

NORMAL HEART RATES FOR INFANTS AND CHILDREN

	Rate (Beats/Min)		
AGE	RESTING (AWAKE)	RESTING (SLEEPING)	EXERCISE (FEVER)
Newborn	100-180	80-160	Up to 220
1 week to 3 months	100-220	80-200	Up to 220
3 months to 2 years	80-150	70-120	Up to 200
2 years to 10 years	70-110	60-90	Up to 200
10 years to adult	55-90	50-90	Up to 200

From Gillette PC: Dysrhythmias. In Adams FH, Emmanoulides GC, Riemenschneider TA (eds): *Moss, heart disease in infants, children, and adolescents,* ed 4, Baltimore, 1989, Williams & Wilkins.

NORMAL TEMPERATURES IN CHILDREN

	Temperature	
AGE	°F	°C
3 months	99.4	37.5
6 months	99.5	37.5
1 year	99.7	37.7
3 years	99.0	37.2
5 years	98.6	37.0
7 years	98.3	36.8
9 years	98.1	36.7
11 years	98.0	36.7
13 years	97.8	36.6

Modified from Lowrey GH: *Growth and development of children,* ed 8, St Louis, 1986, Mosby.

NORMAL RESPIRATORY RATES FOR CHILDREN

AGE	RATE (BREATHS/MIN)
Newborn	35
1 to 11 months	30
2 years	25
4 years	23
6 years	21
8 years	20
10 years	19
12 years	19
14 years	18
16 years	17
18 years	16-18

BP LEVELS FOR BOYS BY AGE AND HEIGHT PERCENTILE

AGE, y	BP PERCENTILE	SBP, mm Hg Percentile of Height							DBP, mm Hg Percentile of Height						
		5th	10th	25th	50th	75th	90th	95th	5th	10th	25th	50th	75th	90th	95th
1	50th	80	81	83	85	87	88	89	34	35	36	37	38	39	39
	90th	94	95	97	99	100	102	103	49	50	51	52	53	53	54
	95th	98	99	101	103	104	106	106	54	54	55	56	57	58	58
	99th	105	106	108	110	112	113	114	61	62	63	64	65	66	66
2	50th	84	85	87	88	90	92	92	39	40	41	42	43	44	44
	90th	97	99	100	102	104	105	106	54	55	56	57	58	58	59
	95th	101	102	104	106	108	109	110	59	59	60	61	62	63	63
	99th	109	110	111	113	115	117	117	66	67	68	69	70	71	71
3	50th	86	87	89	91	93	94	95	44	44	45	46	47	48	48
	90th	100	101	103	105	107	108	109	59	59	60	61	62	63	63
	95th	104	105	107	109	110	112	113	63	63	64	65	66	67	67
	99th	111	112	114	116	118	119	120	71	71	72	73	74	75	75
4	50th	88	89	91	93	95	96	97	47	48	49	50	51	51	52
	90th	102	103	105	107	109	110	111	62	63	64	65	66	66	67
	95th	106	107	109	111	112	114	115	66	67	68	69	70	71	71
	99th	113	114	116	118	120	121	122	74	75	76	77	78	78	79
5	50th	90	91	93	95	96	98	98	50	51	52	53	54	55	55
	90th	104	105	106	108	110	111	112	65	66	67	68	69	69	70
	95th	108	109	110	112	114	115	116	69	70	71	72	73	74	74
	99th	115	116	118	120	121	123	123	77	78	79	80	81	81	82
6	50th	91	92	94	96	98	99	100	53	53	54	55	56	57	57
	90th	105	106	108	110	111	113	113	68	68	69	70	71	72	72
	95th	109	110	112	114	115	117	117	72	72	73	74	75	76	76
	99th	116	117	119	121	123	124	125	80	80	81	82	83	84	84
7	50th	92	94	95	97	99	100	101	55	55	56	57	58	59	59
	90th	106	107	109	111	113	114	115	70	70	71	72	73	74	74
	95th	110	111	113	115	117	118	119	74	74	75	76	77	78	78
	99th	117	118	120	122	124	125	126	82	82	83	84	85	86	86
8	50th	94	95	97	99	100	102	102	56	57	58	59	60	60	61
	90th	107	109	110	112	114	115	116	71	72	72	73	74	75	76
	95th	111	112	114	116	118	119	120	75	76	77	78	79	79	80
	99th	119	120	122	123	125	127	127	83	84	85	86	87	87	88
9	50th	95	96	98	100	102	103	104	57	58	59	60	61	61	62
	90th	109	110	112	114	115	117	118	72	73	74	75	76	76	77
	95th	113	114	116	118	119	121	121	76	77	78	79	80	81	81
	99th	120	121	123	125	127	128	129	84	85	86	87	88	88	89
10	50th	97	98	100	102	103	105	106	58	59	60	61	61	62	63
	90th	111	112	114	115	117	119	119	73	73	74	75	76	77	78
	95th	115	116	117	119	121	122	123	77	78	79	80	81	81	82
	99th	122	123	125	127	128	130	130	85	86	86	88	88	89	90
11	50th	99	100	102	104	105	107	107	59	59	60	61	62	63	63
	90th	113	114	115	117	119	120	121	74	74	75	76	77	78	78
	95th	117	118	119	121	123	124	125	78	78	79	80	81	82	82
	99th	124	125	127	129	130	132	132	86	86	87	88	89	90	90
12	50th	101	102	104	106	108	109	110	59	60	61	62	63	63	64
	90th	115	116	118	120	121	123	123	74	75	75	76	77	78	79
	95th	119	120	122	123	125	127	127	78	79	80	81	82	82	83
	99th	126	127	129	131	133	134	135	86	87	88	89	90	90	91
13	50th	104	105	106	108	110	111	112	60	60	61	62	63	64	64
	90th	117	118	120	122	124	125	126	75	75	76	77	78	79	79
	95th	121	122	124	126	128	129	130	79	79	80	81	82	83	83
	99th	128	130	131	133	135	136	137	87	87	88	89	90	91	91
14	50th	106	107	109	111	113	114	115	60	61	62	63	64	65	65
	90th	120	121	123	125	126	128	128	75	76	77	78	79	79	80
	95th	124	125	127	128	130	132	132	80	80	81	82	83	84	84
	99th	131	132	134	136	138	139	140	87	88	89	90	91	92	92
15	50th	109	110	112	113	115	117	117	61	62	63	64	65	66	66
	90th	122	124	125	127	129	130	131	76	77	78	79	80	80	81
	95th	126	127	129	131	133	134	135	81	81	82	83	84	85	85
	99th	134	135	136	138	140	142	142	88	89	90	91	92	93	93
16	50th	111	112	114	116	118	119	120	63	63	64	65	66	67	67
	90th	125	126	128	130	131	133	134	78	78	79	80	81	82	82
	95th	129	130	132	134	135	137	137	82	83	83	84	85	86	87
	99th	136	137	139	141	143	144	145	90	90	91	92	93	94	94
17	50th	114	115	116	118	120	121	122	65	66	66	67	68	69	70
	90th	127	128	130	132	134	135	136	80	80	81	82	83	84	84
	95th	131	132	134	136	138	139	140	84	85	86	87	87	88	89
	99th	139	140	141	143	145	146	147	92	93	93	94	95	96	97

The 90th percentile is 1.28 SD, the 95th percentile is 1.645 SD, and the 99th percentile is 2.326 SD over the mean.

BP LEVELS FOR GIRLS BY AGE AND HEIGHT PERCENTILE

AGE, y	BP PERCENTILE	SBP, mm Hg Percentile of Height 5th	10th	25th	50th	75th	90th	95th	DBP, mm Hg Percentile of Height 5th	10th	25th	50th	75th	90th	95th
1	50th	83	84	85	86	88	89	90	38	39	39	40	41	41	42
	90th	97	97	98	100	101	102	103	52	53	53	54	55	55	56
	95th	100	101	102	104	105	106	107	56	57	57	58	59	59	60
	99th	108	108	109	111	112	113	114	64	64	65	65	66	67	67
2	50th	85	85	87	88	89	91	91	43	44	44	45	46	46	47
	90th	98	99	100	101	103	104	105	57	58	58	59	60	61	61
	95th	102	103	104	105	107	108	109	61	62	62	63	64	65	65
	99th	109	110	111	112	114	115	116	69	69	70	70	71	72	72
3	50th	86	87	88	89	91	92	93	47	48	48	49	50	50	51
	90th	100	100	102	103	104	106	106	61	62	62	63	64	64	65
	95th	104	104	105	107	108	109	110	65	66	66	67	68	68	69
	99th	111	111	113	114	115	116	117	73	73	74	74	75	76	76
4	50th	88	88	90	91	92	94	94	50	50	51	52	52	53	54
	90th	101	102	103	104	106	107	108	64	64	65	66	67	67	68
	95th	105	106	107	108	110	111	112	68	68	69	70	71	71	72
	99th	112	113	114	115	117	118	119	76	76	76	77	78	79	79
5	50th	89	90	91	93	94	95	96	52	53	53	54	55	55	56
	90th	103	103	105	106	107	109	109	66	67	67	68	69	69	70
	95th	107	107	108	110	111	112	113	70	71	71	72	73	73	74
	99th	114	114	116	117	118	120	120	78	78	79	79	80	81	81
6	50th	91	92	93	94	96	97	98	54	54	55	56	56	57	58
	90th	104	105	106	108	109	110	111	68	68	69	70	70	71	72
	95th	108	109	110	111	113	114	115	72	72	73	74	74	75	76
	99th	115	116	117	119	120	121	122	80	80	80	81	82	83	83
7	50th	93	93	95	96	97	99	99	55	56	56	57	58	58	59
	90th	106	107	108	109	111	112	113	69	70	70	71	72	72	73
	95th	110	111	112	113	115	116	116	73	74	74	75	76	76	77
	99th	117	118	119	120	122	123	124	81	81	82	82	83	84	84
8	50th	95	95	96	98	99	100	101	57	57	57	58	59	60	60
	90th	108	109	110	111	113	114	114	71	71	71	72	73	74	74
	95th	112	112	114	115	116	118	118	75	75	75	76	77	78	78
	99th	119	120	121	122	123	125	125	82	82	83	83	84	85	86
9	50th	96	97	98	100	101	102	103	58	58	58	59	60	61	61
	90th	110	110	112	113	114	116	116	72	72	72	73	74	75	75
	95th	114	114	115	117	118	119	120	76	76	76	77	78	79	79
	99th	121	121	123	124	125	127	127	83	83	84	84	85	86	87
10	50th	98	99	100	102	103	104	105	59	59	59	60	61	62	62
	90th	112	112	114	115	116	118	118	73	73	73	74	75	76	76
	95th	116	116	117	119	120	121	122	77	77	77	78	79	80	80
	99th	123	123	125	126	127	129	129	84	84	85	86	86	87	88
11	50th	100	101	102	103	105	106	107	60	60	60	61	62	63	63
	90th	114	114	116	117	118	119	120	74	74	74	75	76	77	77
	95th	118	118	119	121	122	123	124	78	78	78	79	80	81	81
	99th	125	125	126	128	129	130	131	85	85	86	87	87	88	89
12	50th	102	103	104	105	107	108	109	61	61	61	62	63	64	64
	90th	116	116	117	119	120	121	122	75	75	75	76	77	78	78
	95th	119	120	121	123	124	125	126	79	79	79	80	81	82	82
	99th	127	127	128	130	131	132	133	86	86	87	88	88	89	90
13	50th	104	105	106	107	109	110	110	62	62	62	63	64	65	65
	90th	117	118	119	121	122	123	124	76	76	76	77	78	79	79
	95th	121	122	123	124	126	127	128	80	80	80	81	82	83	83
	99th	128	129	130	132	133	134	135	87	87	88	89	89	90	91
14	50th	106	106	107	109	110	111	112	63	63	63	64	65	66	66
	90th	119	120	121	122	124	125	125	77	77	77	78	79	80	80
	95th	123	123	125	126	127	129	129	81	81	81	82	83	84	84
	99th	130	131	132	133	135	136	136	88	88	89	90	90	91	92
15	50th	107	108	109	110	111	113	113	64	64	64	65	66	67	67
	90th	120	121	122	123	125	126	127	78	78	78	79	80	81	81
	95th	124	125	126	127	129	130	131	82	82	82	83	84	85	85
	99th	131	132	133	134	136	137	138	89	89	90	91	91	92	93
16	50th	108	108	110	111	112	114	114	64	64	65	66	66	67	68
	90th	121	122	123	124	126	127	128	78	78	79	80	81	81	82
	95th	125	126	127	128	130	131	132	82	82	83	84	85	85	86
	99th	132	133	134	135	137	138	139	90	90	90	91	92	93	93
17	50th	108	109	110	111	113	114	115	64	65	65	66	67	67	68
	90th	122	122	123	125	126	127	128	78	79	79	80	81	81	82
	95th	125	126	127	129	130	131	132	82	83	83	84	85	85	86
	99th	133	133	134	136	137	138	139	90	90	91	91	92	93	93

The 90th percentile is 1.28 SD, the 95th percentile is 1.645 SD, and the 99th percentile is 2.326 SD over the mean.

Appendix

K Spanish-English Translations

PHYSICAL EXAMINATION

Open your mouth	abre la boca
Breathe deeply	respira profundo
Turn over	cambio
Hoarse	ronco
Rash or skin lesion produced by insect bite	rosadura o una lesión en la piel producida por una picadura de insecto
Rash	roncha, salpullido, rosadura
Ringworm	tiña
To tighten (grip)	apretar
To loosen	relajar, aflojar
Bruise	moretón
Skin "spot"—like a blanching	mancha
Snore, stertor	roncar
Snoring sound	ronquido
Swollen	hinchado

SYMPTOMS

I would like to know if you have . . .	- Quisiera saber si tienes
. . . . or have had	...o has tenido
cough	tos
runny nose	catarro
fever	fiebre o calentura
vomiting or nausea	vómito o náusea
diarrhea	diarrhea
constipation	estreñimiento
pain	dolor
Allergic reaction	- reacción alérgica
Seizure	convulsion
Sore throat	dolor de garganta
Diaper dermatitis	dermatitis del pañal
Dizzy	mareado(a)

HISTORY

Are you sleeping well?	¿Estás durmiendo bien?
Have you had any trauma?	¿Has tenido algún trastorno o algún trauma?
Have you had any hemorrhage or loss of blood?	¿Has tenido una hemorragia o pérdida de sangre?
Problems during pregnancy or delivery?	¿Problemas en el embarazo o parto?
Born at term or premature?	¿Nació a tiempo o fue prematuro?
Did he or she get better after the treatment or the medicine given?	¿Mejoró después del tratamiento o después de haberle dado la medicina?
How many times did (he, she) urinate today?	¿Cuántas veces orinó hoy?
How many wet diapers has (he, she) had?	¿Cuántos pañales ha mojado?
How many dirty diapers?	¿Cuántos pañales sucios?
Where does it hurt?	¿Dónde te duele?
When did it start?	¿Cuándo empezó?
Does (he, she) have any allergies to medicine or food?	¿Tiene alergia a alguna medicina o comida?
Up-to-date	al corriente
Contagious	contagioso
Stool	escremento, heces, popo
Has (she, he) had any chronic illnesses?	¿Ha tenido enfermedades crónicas?
How many times did he, she vomit today?	¿Cuántas veces vomitó hoy?
Wheezing or adventitious sounds (in lungs)	pillido o ruidos en los pulmones
Nasal secretions	secreción nasal
Stuffy nose	bloqueo nasal
Breathing problems	dificultad para respirar
Thick discharge	flujo grueso
Wound	herida
Blood pressure	presión arterial
Temperature	temperatura
Fever	calentura, fiebre
Pulse	pulso
Heartbeat	latido del corazón
Airway	vía respiratoria
Vital signs	signos vitales

SPECIFIC CONDITIONS

Flu	gripa
Croup	crup
Bronchitis	bronquitis
Burn	quemadura
Rash or dermatitis	erupción o rosadura
Pneumonía	neumonía

Pertussis	tos ferina
Measles	sarampión
Mumps	paperas
Chicken pox	varicela
Rubella	rubeola
Polio	polio
Tetanus	tétano
Vomiting	vómito
Diarrhea	diarrhea
Asthma	asma
Mucous	moco
Seizures	convulsions
Drainage	drenaje
Immunization	vacuna
Poison ivy	hiedra venenosa
Bacterial infection	infección bacterial
Viral infection	infección viral
Diaper dermatitis	rosadura del pañal
Rash or skin lesion produced by insect bite	rosadura o lesión de la piel hecha por una picadura de insecto
Ulcer (as in mouth ulcers or chancre sores)	úlceras o llagas en la boca
Gastritis	gastritis, agruras
Constipation	estreñimiento
Home remedies	tratamientos caseros
Fracture	fractura
Intensive care	cuidado intensivo
Immunizations	vacunas
Animal bite	mordida de animal
Menstrual period	menstruación
Birth control	anticonceptivo

EQUIPMENT

Can also mean NG tube or urinary catheter, can be any tube that has to be inserted into body (MicKey button; gastrostomy)	sonda, catéter urinario, tubo que se introduce al cuerpo
Gown	bata
Suction	succión
Sheet	sábana
Diaper	pañal
Bulb syringe	bombilla
Clothes, clothing	ropa
Splint or cast	férula o yeso
Dressing, bandage	bendaje, gaza
Infusion pump	máquina para infusion
Tape	cinta
Teaspoon	cucharadita
Cup (as in small medicine cup or drinking cup)	taza
Syringe	jeringa
Pill	pastille
Needle	aguja
Antibiotic	antibiótico
Cotton swab	algodón
Pacifier	chupón
Bottle, as in baby bottle or medicine bottle	botella
Juice	jugo
Milk	leche

BODY PARTS

Bone	hueso
Blood	sangre
Tongue	lengua
Head	cabeza
Arm	brazo
Finger	dedo
Leg	pierna
Neck	cuello
Elbow	codo
Foot	pie
Ear	oreja, oido
Nose	nariz
Mouth	boca
Bladder	vejiga
Back	espalda
Chest	pecho
Spleen	bazo
Gallbladder	vesícula biliar

PAIN MANAGEMENT

Do you have any pain in the . . . ?	¿Tienes dolor….?
headache	de cabeza
stomachache	del estómago
backache	de la espalda
chest pain	en el pecho
in the arm	en el brazo
in the legs	en las piernas
in the mouth	en la boca
in the eyes	en los ojos
in the bladder	en la vejiga
How many hours, days, months, years have you had pain in the. . . .	¿Por cuántos (as) horas, días, meses, años has tenido dolor en…?
Please show me where it hurts	Muéstreme dónde te duele, por favor.
What medicine are you taking for pain? What medicine have you taken for pain?	¿Qué medicina estás tomando para el dolor? ¿Qué medicina has tomado para el dolor?
Calm down	cálmate
This won't hurt	esto no te va a doler

PROCEDURES

Injection	inyección
Lumbar puncture	punción lumbar
"Oral hydration solution" such as Pedialyte usually means	suero por boca
IV fluids	suero en la vena o intravenoso
Start an IV	ponerle suero por vena
Normal saline drops	gotas de solución salina
Humidity	humedad
Vaporizer	vaporizador de aire
Breathing treatment	tratamiento pulmonary
Humidity in the bathroom with a hot shower running	vapor de la regadera
Stool sample	muestra de heces (popo) escremento
We need to take some blood to see what exactly (illness) (he, she) has . . .	le tenemos que hacer una prueba de sangre para averiguar la enfermedad…
"The results of your blood test show . . ."	"los resultados de la sangre muestran"
The most important thing is to decrease the fever with Tylenol or Motrin	lo más importante es reducír la fiebre con Tylenol o Motrin
We will have to catheterize (him, her)	tendremos que ponerle una sonda en la vejiga
Topical treatment	tratamiento tópico
To suture	suturar
A suture	sutura
To swab (as in "swab the mouth" or "to place a cream on . . .")	untar
He, she should take lots of clear liquids	debe tomar bastantes líquidos claros
To nurse, breastfeed	amamantar
To burp	eructar
X-ray	radiografía
CT scan	tomografía
Nasal drops	gotas nasales
Put ice on it	aplicarle hielo

MISCELLANEOUS PHRASES

He, she will need to be hospitalized for treatment . . . observation	Tendrá que ser hospitalizado para dar….tratamiento… o ser observado…
We need a urine specimen in this cup	necesitamos una muestra de orina en esta taza
Take him, her to the primary doctor tomorrow	llévelo al doctor o a la clínica mañana
He, she is very sick	está muy enfermo

Index

A

Page numbers followed by *b* indicate boxes; *f* indicates figures; *t* indicates tables.

C

F

I

S

V